TEXTBOOK OF
GASTROENTEROLOGY

TEXTBOOK OF
GASTROENTEROLOGY

Ian A.D. Bouchier
MD, FRCP, FRCP(Ed)
Professor of Medicine, University of Dundee;
Honorary Consultant Physician,
Ninewells Hospital and Medical School, Dundee, Scotland

Robert N. Allan
MD, PhD, FRCP
Senior Clinical Lecturer,
University of Birmingham;
Consultant Physician,
The General Hospital,
Birmingham, England

Humphrey J.F. Hodgson
DM, FRCP
Senior Lecturer in Medicine,
Royal Postgraduate Medical School;
Honorary Consultant Physician,
Hammersmith Hospital,
London, England

Michael R.B. Keighley
MS, FRCS
Reader in Surgery, University of Birmingham;
Consultant Surgeon, The General Hospital,
Birmingham, England

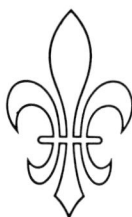

Baillière Tindall
LONDON PHILADELPHIA TORONTO
MEXICO CITY RIO DE JANEIRO SYDNEY TOKYO HONG KONG

Baillière Tindall   1 St Anne's Road
W.B. Saunders   Eastbourne, East Sussex BN21 3UN, England

West Washington Square
Philadelphia, PA 19105, USA

1 Goldthorne Avenue
Toronto, Ontario M8Z 5T9, Canada

Apartado 26370 – Cedro 512
Mexico 4, DF Mexico

Rua Evaristo da Veiga 55, 20° andar
Rio de Janeiro – RJ, Brazil

ABP Australia Ltd, 44–50 Waterloo Road
North Ryde, NSW 2113, Australia

Ichibancho Central Building, 22–1 Ichibancho
Chiyoda-ku, Tokyo 102, Japan

10/FL, Inter-Continental Plaza, 94 Granville Road
Tsim Sha Tsui East, Kowloon, Hong Kong

© 1984 Baillière Tindall

First published 1984

Typeset by Santype International Ltd., Salisbury, Wilts.
Printed and bound in Great Britain by
William Clowes Ltd., Beccles and London

British Library Cataloguing in Publication Data

Textbook of gastroenterology.
  1. Digestive organs—Diseases
  I. Bouchier, Ian A. D.
  616.3   RC801

ISBN 0 7020 1027 8

Preface

As the practice of medicine changes so must the textbooks which form such an important basis for the transmission of knowledge. Gastroenterology is a dynamic discipline which is developing rapidly because of the impact of new concepts and technology involving endoscopy, radioimmunoassay, ultrasonography, computerized tomography as well as biochemistry and molecular biology. But the focus of this change must remain with the clinician and the way in which he practises the art and science of medicine. We have attempted to bring together these developments in a completely new authoritative text, which retains the traditional format of specific diseases and avoids divisions into structure, function and clinical syndromes. Good gastroenterological practice combines sound clinical ability and judgement with an understanding of the scientific basis of the specialty. Thus while emphasizing the clinical practice of gastroenterology we have neither ignored relevant aspects of the basic sciences nor eschewed controversy.

The book is intended for specialist gastroenterologists and all other clinicians with an interest in gastroenterology. The content has been determined to some extent by the physical problem of producing a single volume which is neither too large to handle nor too indigestible to absorb. We therefore have been deliberately selective but, because we believe that reference books are as often used to obtain information about rare disorders as for the common stuff of everyday practice, we have discussed many uncommon conditions at length. Our self-imposed restrictions on size and the availability of a comprehensive companion book on the liver (*Liver and Biliary Disease*, edited by R. Wright *et al.*) from our publisher led us to exclude consideration of liver disease.

We have taken the decision that the *Textbook of Gastroenterology* should reflect to a large extent the practice of British Gastroenterology, which has such a strong tradition of sound clinical practice. However, there are many aspects which are best covered by experts in other centres around the world and we have been fortunate to have contributions from distinguished clinicians in Europe, the Americas, Africa, India, the Far East and Australasia. It has been our purpose to involve as many gastroenterologists as necessary to cover all the topics; this presents problems in style and balance but has the overriding advantage of ensuring that each topic is dealt with by an expert. We are extremely grateful to all our contributors; the work stands as a testimony to their professional ability and skills in communication.

We have been fortunate in the friendly and highly competent support which we have enjoyed from our publisher and in particular we would like to express our thanks to Joyce Brown, David Cross, William Wolvey and David Inglis.

We also wish to record our appreciation of our secretaries, who so willingly and ably typed the manuscripts. Finally we thank our wives and families for their whimsical tolerance during the book's gestation.

Ian A. D. Bouchier
Robert N. Allan

Humphrey J. F. Hodgson
Michael R. B. Keighley

Contents

Contributors

J. Alexander-Williams, MD, ChM, FRCS, FACS
Honorary Clinical Senior Lecturer, University of Birmingham; Consultant Surgeon, The General Hospital, Steelhouse Lane, Birmingham B4 6NH, UK.
Complications of Gastric Surgery

Robert N. Allan, MD, PhD, FRCP
Senior Clinical Lecturer, University of Birmingham; Consultant Physician, The General Hospital, Steelhouse Lane, Birmingham B4 6NH, UK.
Endometriosis; Crohn's Disease: Clinical Presentation and Diagnosis

Michael Atkinson, MD, FRCP
Consultant Physician, University Hospital, Queen's Medical Centre, Nottingham NG7 2UH, UK.
The Oesophagus: Cricopharyngeal Disorders, Diverticula of the Pharynx and Oesophagus, Oesophageal Webs, Oesophageal Rings, Infections, Foreign Bodies, Perforation, Chemical and Physical Damage, Oesophageal Involvement by Systemic Disease

A. T. R. Axon, MD, FRCP
Consultant Physician, The General Infirmary, Great George Street, Leeds LS1 3EX, UK.
Evaluation of Pancreatic Disease

V. Balakrishnan, MD, DM
Professor of Gastroenterology, Medical College, Trivandrum; Professor and Head, Department of Gastroenterology, Medical College Hospital, Trivandrum, Kerala 695011, India.
Calcific Pancreatitis; Shwachman Syndrome

J. E. Banatvala, MA, MD, FRCPath
Professor of Clinical Virology, St Thomas' Hospital Medical School, London SE1 7EH, UK.
Virus Infections of the Gastrointestinal Tract

John G. Banwell, DM, FRCP
Professor, Division of Medicine, Case Western Reserve University School of Medicine, Lakeside Hospital, Cleveland, Ohio 44106; Director, Division of Gastroenterology and Clinical Nutrition, University Hospital of Cleveland, Ohio, USA.
Worm Infections of the Gastrointestinal Tract

D. N. Baron, MD, DSc, FRCP, FRCPath
Professor, Department of Chemical Pathology, Royal Free Hospital School of Medicine, Rowland Hill Street, London NW3 2PF; Honorary Consultant Chemical Pathologist, Royal Free Hospital, London, UK.
Reference Ranges in Theory and Practice

J. H. Baron, DM, FRCP
Senior Lecturer and Consultant, Departments of Surgery and Medicine, Royal Postgraduate Medical School and Hammersmith Hospital, Ducane Road, London W12 0HS; Consultant Physician, St Charles's Hospital; Sub-Dean, St Mary's Hospital Medical School, London, UK.
Gastric Secretion

R. E. Barry, BSc, MD, FRCP
Consultant Senior Lecturer, Department of Medicine, Bristol University; Honorary Consultant in Medicine, Bristol Royal Infirmary, Marlborough Street, Bristol BS2 8HW, UK.
Surgical Causes of Malabsorption: Jejuno-ileal Bypass

John G. Bartlett, MD
Professor of Medicine, Johns Hopkins University School of Medicine; Chief, Division of Infectious Diseases, Johns Hopkins Hospital, Blalock 1111, Baltimore, Maryland 21205, USA.
Pseudomembranous Colitis and Antibiotic-Associated Colitis

M. K. Basu, BDS, FDS, RCS(Ed), DDS
Senior Lecturer, Department of Oral Pathology, University of Birmingham Dental School, St Chad's Queensway, Birmingham B4 6NN, UK.
Oral Manifestations of Gastrointestinal Disease

Robert W. Beart Jr, MD
Section of Colon and Rectal Surgery, Mayo Clinic, Rochester, Minnesota 55905, USA.
Anal Tumours

G. D. Bell, MD, MRCP, MRCS
Consultant Gastroenterologist, Ipswich Hospital, Heath Road Wing, Ipswich, Suffolk, UK.
Clinical Features and Medical Treatment of Gallstones

J. R. Bennett, MD, FRCP
Consultant Physician, Gastrointestinal Unit, Hull Royal Infirmary, Anlaby Road, Kingston-upon-Hull HU3 2JZ, UK.
Oesophagitis

Agostinho Bettarello, MD
Professor of Medicine; Chief, Division of Clinical Gastroenterology, Hospital das Clínicas de Faculdade de Medicina da Universidade de São Paulo, Caixa Postal 8091, São Paulo, Brazil.
Chagas' Disease

P. G. Bevan, ChM, FRCS, LRCP
Professor of Surgery, University of Birmingham; Consultant Surgeon, Dudley Road Hospital, Birmingham B18 7QH, UK.
Late Problems after Cholecystectomy

Richard L. Blackett, ChM, FRCS
Senior Registrar in General Surgery, Cardiff Royal Infirmary, Newport Road, Cardiff CF2 1SZ, UK.
Chronic Duodenal Ulcer: Surgical Treatment

S. R. Bloom, MA, DSc, MD, FRCP
Professor of Endocrinology, Royal Postgraduate Medical School; Consultant Physician, Hammersmith Hospital, Ducane Road, London W12 0HS, UK.
VIPomas and Other Pancreatic Tumours

L. H. Blumgart, MD, FRCS
Director and Professor, Royal Postgraduate Medical School; Professor of Surgery, Hammersmith Hospital, Ducane Road, London W12 0HS, UK.
Tumours of the Gallbladder and Biliary Tract

C. C. Booth, MD, FRCP
Director, Clinical Research Centre, Northwick Park Hospital, Harrow, Middlesex, UK.
Malignant Complications of Coeliac Disease

Ian A. D. Bouchier, MD, FRCP, FRCP(Ed)
Professor of Medicine, University of Dundee; Honorary Consultant Physician, Ninewells Hospital and Medical School, Dundee DD1 9SY, UK.
Gallbladder Disease in Children; Hyperplastic Cholecystoses; Vasculitis of the Gallbladder and Biliary Tract; Emphysematous Cholecystitis; Haemobilia; Intrahepatic Lithiasis; Ascites

Contributors

Martin J. Brodie, MD, MRCP
Honorary Clinical Lecturer, University of Glasgow; Consultant Clinical Pharmacologist, Western Infirmary, Glasgow G11 6NT, and Garnaval Hospital, Glasgow, UK.
Drugs and the Small Intestine

Keith D. Buchanan, MD, PhD, FRCP
Professor of Metabolic Medicine, Queen's University of Belfast, Institute of Clinical Science, Grosvenor Road, Belfast BT12 6BJ; Consultant Physician, Royal Victoria Hospital, Belfast, UK.
Zollinger–Ellison Syndrome

Michael Camilleri, MD, MPhil, MRCP
Mayo Clinic, Gastroenterology Unit, Saint Mary's Hospital, Rochester, Minnesota 55901, USA.
Genetic and Congenital Vascular Disorders of the Intestine; Internal Paraneoplastic Syndromes Associated with Cancer

David C. A. Candy, MSc, MB BS, MRCP
Clinical Lecturer in Paediatrics and Child Health, University of Birmingham, Institute of Child Health, Francis Road, Birmingham B16 8ET, UK.
Paediatric Gastroenteritis

Martin C. Carey, MD
Associate Professor of Medicine and Lawrence J. Henderson Associate Professor of Health Sciences and Technology, Harvard Medical School, Boston; Associate in Medicine, Division of Gastroenterology, Department of Medicine, Brigham and Women's Hospital, 75 Francis Street, Boston, Massachusetts 02115, USA.
Formation of Cholesterol Gallstones

D. L. Carr-Locke, MA, MB BChir, MRCP
Consultant Physician and Lecturer in Gastroenterology, Department of Medicine, Clinical Sciences Building, Leicester Royal Infirmary, Leicester LE1 5WW, UK.
Gallbladder Dyskinesia and Biliary Stenosis

L. R. Celestin, MB BS, FRCS
Consultant Surgeon, 8 Church Avenue, Stoke Bishop, Bristol BS9 1LD, UK.
Tumours of the Oesophagus

V. S. Chadwick, MD, FRCP
Professor of Experimental Medicine, The Wellcome Research Institute, University of Otago Medical School, Dunedin, New Zealand.
Mechanisms of Malabsorption and Diarrhoea; Clinical Investigation of Patients with Malabsorption and Diarrhoea

I. Chanarin, MD, FRCPath
Head, Section of Haematology, Clinical Research Centre; Consultant Haematologist, Northwick Park Hospital, Harrow, Middlesex, UK.
Pernicious Anaemia and the Gut

Derrick M. Chisholm, BDs, PhD, FDS, RCPS
Professor and Consultant, Dental Hospital and School, Department of Dental Surgery, Park Place, Dundee DD1 4HN, UK.
Oral Manifestations of Gastrointestinal Disease

J. Cinqualbre, MD
Associate Professor of Surgery, Pavillon Chirurgical A, Hospices Civils, Strasbourg, 67005 Cedex, France.
Chronic Ischaemia of the Gut

John Clark, ChM, FRCS
Clinical Teacher, Welsh National School of Medicine; Consultant Surgeon, Glan Clwyd Hospital, Bodelwyddan, Rhyl, Clwyd LL18 5UJ, UK.
Congenital Abnormalities of the Oesophagus

M. L. Clark, MD, FRCP
Senior Lecturer, St Bartholomew's Hospital Medical College; Consultant Physician, St Bartholomew's Hospital, London EC1A 7BE, and St Leonard's and Hackney Hospitals, London, UK.
Coeliac Disease

Jennifer C. Clay, MB BS, MRCOG
Senior Clinical Lecturer in Venereology, University of Birmingham Medical School; Consultant, The General Hospital, Steelhouse Lane, Birmingham B4 6NH, UK.
Sexually Transmitted Diseases and the Gastrointestinal Tract

Roy Cockel, MA, MB, FRCP
Senior Clinical Lecturer in Medicine, University of Birmingham Medical School; Consultant Physician, Selly Oak Hospital, Birmingham B29 6JD, UK.
Late Problems after Cholecystectomy

G. C. Cook, MD, DSc, FRCP, FRACP
Senior Lecturer, London School of Hygiene and Tropical Medicine, Keppel Street, London, WC1E 7HT; Honorary Consultant Physician, University College Hospital and Hospital for Tropical Diseases, London, UK.
Post-infective Malabsorption

B. T. Cooper, MD, MRCP
Lecturer in Medicine, University of Bristol, Bristol Royal Infirmary, Bristol BS2 8HW, UK.
Diabetes Mellitus and the Gut; Ménétrier's Disease

Timothy M. Cox, MSc, MD, MRCP
Wellcome Senior Clinical Fellow, Department of Medicine, Royal Postgraduate Medical School, Ducane Road, London W12 0HS; Honorary Consultant Physician, Hammersmith Hospital, London, UK.
Haemochromatosis and the Gut

Brian Creamer, MD, FRCP
Senior Lecturer in Medicine, St Thomas' Hospital Medical School; Consultant Physician, St Thomas' Hospital, London SE1 7EH, UK.
Immunoproliferative Small Intestinal Disease

A. Cuschieri, MD, ChM, FRCS(Eng), FRCS(Ed)
Professor and Head, University Department of Surgery, Ninewells Hospital and Medical School, Dundee DD1 9SY; Honorary Senior Consultant, Tayside Health Board, UK.
Cancer of the Exocrine Pancreas

Sidney Cywes, MMed(Surg), FACS(Ped), FRCS(Eng)
Professor and Head, Department of Paediatric Surgery, University of Cape Town Medical School; Chief of Paediatric Surgery, Red Cross War Memorial Children's Hospital, Rondebosch, Cape Town 7700, Republic of South Africa.
Congenital Abnormalities of the Gallbladder and Biliary Tract

R. J. Davies, MA, MD, MRCP
Senior Lecturer, St Bartholomew's Hospital Medical College; Consultant Chest Physician, St Bartholomew's Hospital, London EC1A 7BE, UK.
Respiratory Disease and the Gut

Joseph S. Davison, PhD
Professor and Senior Alberta Heritage Research Scholar, Department of Medical Physiology, Faculty of Medicine, University of Calgary Health Sciences Centre, 3330 Hospital Drive NW, Calgary, Alberta, Canada T2N 4N1.
Physiology of Extrahepatic Bile Transport

Stephen A. Deane, MB BS, FRACS, FRCS(C)
Senior Lecturer in Surgery, University of Sydney; Visiting Medical Officer (General Surgery), Westmead Centre, Westmead, New South Wales 2145, Australia.
Embryology and Anatomy of the Stomach and Duodenum

H. Brendan Devlin, MA, MD, MCh, FRCS
Consultant Surgeon, North Tees General Hospital, Hardwick, Stockton-on-Tees, Cleveland TS19 8PE, UK.
Stomas and Stoma Care

Ian A. Donovan, MD, FRCS
Senior Lecturer in Surgery, University of Birmingham Medical School; Consultant Surgeon, Dudley Road Hospital, Birmingham B18 7QH, UK.
Gastroduodenal Motility

P. W. Dykes, MB ChB(NZ), FRACP, FRCP
Senior Lecturer in Immunology, University of Birmingham; Consultant Physician, The General Hospital, Birmingham B4 6NH, UK.
Acute Upper Gastrointestinal Haemorrhage

Martin A. Eastwood, MB ChB, MSc, FRCP(Ed)
Senior Lecturer, University of Edinburgh; Consultant Physician, Western General Hospital, Edinburgh EH4 2XU, UK.
Diverticular Disease

D. A. W. Edwards, MD, MB BChir, FRCP
Surgical Unit, University College Hospital Medical School, The Rayne Institute, 5 University Street, London WC1E 6JJ, UK.
Physiology of the Oesophagus

Serge Erlinger, MD
Associate Professor of Medicine, Faculty of Medicine Xavier-Bichat, University of Paris 7; Hôpital Beaujon, 100 Boulevard Avenue General Leclerc, Clichy, France.
Physiology of Bile Secretion

Peter D. Fairclough, MD, MRCP
Senior Lecturer, Gastroenterology Department, St Bartholomew's Hospital Medical College, London EC1 7BE; Consultant Physician, Hackney and St Bartholomew's Hospitals, London, UK.
Digestion and Malabsorption of Carbohydrate; Absorption and Malabsorption of Vitamins

Michael J. G. Farthing, MD
Division of Geographic Medicine, Tufts–New England Medical Center, 136 Harrison Avenue, Boston, Massachusetts 02111, USA.
Shigellosis

J. W. L. Fielding, MD, FRCS
Senior Lecturer in Surgery, University of Birmingham; Honorary Consultant Surgeon, Department of Surgery, Queen Elizabeth Hospital, Edgbaston, Birmingham B15 2TH, UK.
Gastric Carcinoma: Clinical Features, Diagnosis and Treatment

J. M. Findlay, MB ChB, MRCP, DMRD

Consultant Physician and Gastroenterologist, Bradford Royal Infirmary, Duckworth Lane, Bradford, Yorkshire BD9 6RJ, UK.

Gastrointestinal Tuberculosis

Robert S. Fisher, MD

Professor of Medicine, Temple University School of Medicine, Philadelphia, Pennsylvania 19140; Co-Chief, Gastroenterology Section, Temple University Hospital, Philadelphia, PA, USA.

Progressive Systemic Sclerosis (Scleroderma) and the Gut; Systemic Lupus Erythematosus and the Gut; Polymyositis/Dermatomyositis and the Gut; Rheumatoid Arthritis and the Gut

Gordon G. Forstner, MD, FRCP(C)

Professor, Department of Pediatrics, University of Toronto; Director, Kinsmen Cystic Fibrosis Research Centre, Hospital for Sick Children, 555 University Avenue, Toronto, Ontario, Canada M5G 1X8.

Cystic Fibrosis

Stanley M. Goldberg, MD, FACS

Clinical Professor and Director, Division of Colon and Rectal Surgery, Department of Surgery, 1731 Medical Arts Building, University of Minnesota, Minneapolis, Minnesota 55402, USA.

Anal Fissure

Stephen E. Goldfinger, MD

Associate Professor of Medicine and Associate Dean for Continuing Education, Harvard Medical School; Physician, Massachusetts General Hospital, Gastrointestinal Unit, Boston, Massachusetts 02114, USA.

Familial Mediterranean Fever (Recurrent Polyserositis)

Roger H. Grace, MB, FRCS

Consultant Surgeon, Royal Hospital, Wolverhampton WV2 1BT, and New Cross Hospital, Wolverhampton, UK.

Anorectal Sepsis

S. N. Gyde, MA, BM BCh

Research Associate, Gastroenterology Unit, The General Hospital, Steelhouse Lane, Birmingham B4 6NH, UK.

Cancer in Ulcerative Colitis; Cancer in Crohn's Disease

David R. W. Haddock, MD, FRCP

Senior Lecturer in Tropical Medicine, Liverpool School of Tropical Medicine, Pembroke Place, Liverpool L3 5QA; Honorary Consultant Physician, Merseyside Regional Health Authority, UK.

Cholera

J. Hardcastle, MA, MChir, FRCS, MRCP

Professor, University of Nottingham; Professor of Surgery, University Hospital, Nottingham NG7 2UH, UK.

Tumours of the Small Intestine

Anita E. Harding, MD, MRCP

Lecturer in Neurology, Institute of Neurology, Queen Square, London, and Royal Postgraduate Medical School, Ducane Road, London W12 0HS, UK.

Neurological Disorders and the Gut

Philip S. E. G. Harland, MB BCh, MRCP

Senior Physician and Head, Department of Paediatrics, Riyadh Armed Forces Hospital, P.O. Box 7897, Riyadh 11472, Kingdom of Saudi Arabia.

Deficiency Diseases

John T. Harries, MD, MSc, FRCP (Deceased)
Professor of Paediatric Gastroenterology, Department of Child Health, University of London, Institute of Child Health, London; Honorary Consultant Physician, The Hospital for Sick Children, Great Ormond Street, London, UK.
Familial Pancreatitis

P. C. Hawker, MD, MRCP
Senior Medical Registrar, The General Hospital, Steelhouse Lane, Birmingham B4 6NH, UK.
Acute Upper Gastrointestinal Haemorrhage

Clifford Hawkins, MD, FRCP
Consultant Physician, Queen Elizabeth Hospital, Birmingham B15 2TH, UK.
An Approach to the Patient with Chronic Abdominal Pain

K. W. Heaton, MA, MD, FRCP
Reader in Medicine, University of Bristol, Department of Medicine, Bristol Royal Infirmary, Bristol BS2 8HW; Honorary Consultant Physician, Bristol and Weston Health Authority, UK.
Irritable Bowel Syndrome

Mike M. Henry, MB, FRCS
Consultant Surgeon, Department of General Surgery, Central Middlesex Hospital, Acton Lane, London NW10 7NS, UK.
Conditions of the Pelvic Floor

Graham L. Hill, MD, ChM, FRCS, FRACS
Professor and Chairman, Department of Surgery, University of Auckland School of Medicine, Auckland Hospital, Park Road, Auckland 3, New Zealand.
Therapeutic Nutrition

Oscar Hill, MB BChir, FRCP, FRCPsych
Consultant Psychiatrist, St Luke's–Woodside Hospital, Woodside Avenue, Muswell Hill, London N10 3HU, UK.
Anorexia Nervosa and Related Disturbances

Takeshi Hirayama, MD
Professor and Chief, Epidemiology Division, National Cancer Centre Research Institute, Tsukiji 5-Chome, Chuo-ku, Tokyo, Japan.
Gastric Carcinoma: Epidemiology and Screening

Humphrey J. F. Hodgson, DM, FRCP
Senior Lecturer in Medicine, Royal Postgraduate Medical School; Honorary Consultant Physician, Hammersmith Hospital, Ducane Road, London W12 0HS, UK.
Whipple's Disease; Immunodeficiency and the Gut; Lymphomas of the Small Intestine; Immunological Aspects of the Aetiology and Pathogenesis of Inflammatory Bowel Disease; Polyarteritis and the Gut; Henoch–Schönlein Purpura and the Gut; Other Vasculitic Disorders and the Gut; Carcinoid Tumours and the Carcinoid Syndrome

Allan Victor Hoffbrand, MA, DM, FRCP, FRCPath
Professor of Haematology, Royal Free Hospital Medical School; Honorary Consultant, Royal Free Hospital, Pond Street, London NW3 2QG, UK.
Absorption and Malabsorption of Haematinics

Vendie H. Hooks III, MD
Assistant Professor of Surgery, Medical College of Georgia, Augusta, Georgia 30912, USA.
Anal Fissure

David Hopwood, BSc, MD, PhD, MRCPath
Reader, Department of Pathology, Ninewells Hospital and Medical School, Dundee DD1 9SY, UK.
Embryology and Anatomy of the Oesophagus; Anatomy and Embryology of the Gallbladder and Biliary Tract

L. E. Hughes, DS, FRCS, FRACS
Professor of Surgery, Welsh National School of Medicine, Heath Park, Cardiff CF4 4XN; Consultant Surgeon, University Hospital of Wales, Cardiff, UK.
Perianal Crohn's Disease

R. H. Hunt, FRCP, FRCP(C)
Professor, McMaster University; Professor and Head, Division of Gastroenterology, McMaster University Medical Centre, 1200 Main Street, West Hamilton, Ontario, Canada L8N 3Z5.
Angiodysplasia of the Gut; Acute Colonic Haemorrhage

Clement W. Imrie, BSc, ChB, FRCS
Honorary Lecturer in Surgery, University of Glasgow; Consultant Surgeon, General Surgery, Royal Infirmary, Glasgow G4 0SF, UK.
Acute Pancreatitis

O. F. W. James, MA, FRCP
Reader in Medicine (Geriatrics), University of Newcastle upon Tyne; Consultant Physician, Freeman Hospital, Freeman Road, High Heaton, Newcastle upon Tyne NE7 7DN, UK.
The Aged Gut

Jozef Janssens, MD, AggHO
Associate Professor, Department of Medicine, Division of Gastroenterology and Gastroenterology Research Centre, University of Leuven, 3000 Leuven, Belgium.
Motor Disorders of the Oesophagus

D. P. Jewell, MA, DPhil, FRCP
Consultant Physician, Gastroenterology Unit, John Radcliffe Hospital, Oxford, UK.
Ulcerative Colitis: Pathology, Symptoms and Signs, Complications, Diagnosis and Medical Treatment

Stephen N. Joffe, MD, FRCS
Professor of Surgery, University of Cincinnati Medical Center, Medical Sciences Building, 231 Bethesda Avenue, Cincinnati, Ohio 45267; Consultant Surgeon, University Hospital, Cincinnati, OH, USA.
Duodenitis

Alan G. Johnson, MChir, FRCS
Professor of Surgery, University of Sheffield, Royal Hallamshire Hospital, Sheffield S10 2SJ; Honorary Consultant Surgeon, Royal Hallamshire Hospital, Sheffield, UK.
Complications of Chronic Peptic Ulcer

David Johnston, MD, ChM, FRCS
Professor and Head of University Department of Surgery, The General Infirmary, Leeds LS1 3EX; Honorary Consultant Surgeon, The General Infirmary, Leeds, UK.
Chronic Duodenal Ulcer: Surgical Treatment

Roland T. Jung, MA, MD, MRCP
Honorary Senior Lecturer, University of Dundee; Consultant Physician, Department of Medicine, Ninewells Hospital and Medical School, Dundee DD1 9SY, UK.
Obesity; Appetite and Satiety

Michael R. B. Keighley, MS, FRCS
Reader in Surgery and Consultant Surgeon, The General Hospital, Steelhouse Lane, Birmingham B4 6NH, and The University of Birmingham, UK.
Physiology and Sphincter Control in the Large Intestine; Surgical Treatment of Crohn's Disease

T. L. Kennedy, MB BS, FRCS, FRC(I)
Surgeon, Department of Surgery, Royal Victoria Hospital, Belfast, UK.
Zollinger–Ellison Syndrome

M. G. W. Kettlewell, MA, MChir, FRCS
Lecturer in Surgery, University of Oxford; Fellow of Green College, Oxford; Consultant Surgeon, John Radcliffe Hospital, Headington, Oxford OX3 9DU, UK.
Intestinal Obstruction and Ileus

C. T. Keusch, MD
Professor of Medicine and Chief, Division of Geographic Medicine, Tufts–New England Medical Center, 136 Harrison Avenue, Boston, Massachusetts 02111, USA.
Shigellosis

W. Milo Keynes, MD, MChir, FRCS
Department of Anatomy, University of Cambridge, Cambridge CB2 1TN, UK.
Clinical Anatomy and Congenital Abnormalities of the Pancreas

R. Kieny, MD
Professor and Head, Department of Cardiovascular Surgery, Pavillon Chirurgical A, Hospices Civils, Strasbourg 67005 Cedex, France.
Chronic Ischaemia of the Gut

Barbara S. Kirschner, MD
Assistant Professor of Pediatrics, University of Chicago; Head, Section of Pediatric Gastroenterology, Wyler Children's Hospital, Department of Pediatrics, 950 East 59th Street, Chicago, Illinois 60637, USA.
Inflammatory Bowel Disease in Childhood

Steve Kohl, MD
Associate of Infectious Diseases, Program of Infectious Diseases, University of Texas Health Science Center at Houston, Medical School, 6431 Fannin, P.O. Box 20708, Houston, Texas 77025; Attending Pediatrician, Hermann Hospital, Houston, and Infectious Diseases Consultant, Anderson Hospital and Tumor Research Institute, Houston, TX, USA.
Yersinia Infections

Guenter J. Krejs, MD
Associate Professor of Internal Medicine, Department of Internal Medicine, University of Texas Health Science Center, Southwestern Medical School, 5323 Harry Hines Boulevard, Dallas, Texas 75235, USA.
Short Gut Syndrome

Parveen J. Kumar, MB, MRCP
Senior Lecturer, Department of Gastroenterology, St Bartholomew's Hospital, West Smithfield, London EC1A 7BE, UK.
Food Allergy

M. J. S. Langman, MD, FRCP
Professor of Therapeutics, University of Nottingham Medical School, Nottingham NG7 2UH; Honorary Consultant Physician, Nottingham Group Hospitals, UK.
Incidence, Epidemiology and Genetics of Inflammatory Bowel Disease

Jeremy O. N. Lawson, MB BS, FRCS
Consultant Paediatric Surgeon, St Thomas' Hospital, London SE1 7EH, and Westminster Children's Hospital, London, UK.
Hirschsprung's Disease; Anorectal Malformation

E. C. G. Lee, MB BCh, FRCS
Consultant Surgeon, Gastroenterology Unit, John Radcliffe Hospital, Headington, Oxford OX3 9DU, UK.
Surgical Treatment of Ulcerative Colitis

John R. Lee, FRCS, FRCR
Senior Clinical Lecturer, University of Birmingham; Radiologist, The General Hospital, Steelhouse Lane, Birmingham B4 6NH, UK.
Radiology and Endoscopy of Crohn's Disease

Leslie S. Leighton, MD
Post-Doctoral Research Fellow, Gastroenterology Division, Department of Medicine, Brigham and Women's Hospital, 75 Francis Street, Boston, Massachusetts 02115, USA.
Formation of Cholesterol Gallstones

Richard Lendrum, MA, MB BChir, FRCP
Senior Lecturer in Medicine, University of Newcastle upon Tyne; Consultant Physician, Freeman Hospital, High Heaton, Newcastle upon Tyne NE7 7DN, and the General Hospital, Newcastle upon Tyne, UK.
Aetiology and Epidemiology of Chronic Gastric Ulcer

J. E. Lennard-Jones, MD, FRCP
Professor of Gastroenterology, London Hospital Medical College; Consultant Gastroenterologist, St Mark's Hospital for Diseases of the Colon and Rectum, City Road, London EC1V 2PS, UK.
Constipation, Faecal Impaction and Laxative Abuse; Drug Treatment of Crohn's Disease

A. J. Levi, MD, FRCP
Consultant Gastroenterologist, Northwick Park Hospital and Clinical Research Centre, Watford Road, Harrow, Middlesex HA1 3UJ, UK.
Extraintestinal Manifestations of Inflammatory Bowel Disease

M. D. Levitt, MD
VA Hospital, Research Office, 54th Street and 48th Avenue S., Minneapolis, Minnesota 55417, USA.
Macroamylasaemia

Paul D. Lewis, BSc, MD, MRCP, FRCPath
Reader in Histopathology, Royal Postgraduate Medical School; Consultant Pathologist and Neurologist, Hammersmith Hospital, Ducane Road, London W12 0HS, UK.
Neurological Disorders and the Gut

C. Martin Lockwood, MB BCh, MRCP
Senior Lecturer, Royal Postgraduate Medical School; Honorary Consultant Physician, Hammersmith Hospital, Ducane Road, London W12 0HS, UK.
Polyarteritis and the Gut; Henoch–Schönlein Purpura and the Gut

Richard G. Long, MD, MRCP
Clinical Teacher, Nottingham University Medical School; Consultant Physician and Gastroenterologist, City Hospital, Hucknall Road, Nottingham NG5 1PB, and University Hospital, Nottingham, UK.
Systemic Endocrine Disorders and the Gut: Parathyroid Diseases, Thyroid Diseases, Pituitary Diseases, Adrenal Disorders, Multiple Endocrine Adenomatosis

M. S. Losowsky, MD, FRCP
Professor, Department of Medicine, St James's Hospital, Leeds LS9 7TF, UK.
The Consequences of Malabsorption

M. H. Lyall, ChM, FRCS(Ed)
Honorary Senior Lecturer, University of Dundee; Consultant Surgeon, Ninewells Hospital and Medical School, Dundee DD1 9SY, UK.
Embryology and Anatomy of the Large Intestine; Congenital Abnormalities of the Anterior Abdominal Wall, Peritoneum and Mesentery

Juan-Ramón Malagelada, MD
Professor of Medicine, Mayo Medical School; Consultant in Gastroenterology, Mayo Clinic and Mayo Foundation, Gastroenterology Unit, Saint Mary's Hospital, Rochester, Minnesota 55905, USA.
The Gut Response to a Meal and its Hormonal Control

Christopher Niels Mallinson, MB, FRCP
Consultant Physician, Lewisham Hospital, London SE13 6LH, UK.
Insulinoma including Nesidioblastosis; Glucagonoma

Bibhat K. Mandal, FRCP(Ed)
Lecturer in Communicable Diseases, University of Manchester; Consultant Physician, Regional Department of Infectious Diseases, Monsall Hospital, Newton Heath, Manchester M10 8WR, UK.
Salmonella Infections

Janet M. Marks, DM, FRCP
Senior Lecturer in Dermatology, University of Newcastle upon Tyne, University Department of Dermatology, Royal Victoria Infirmary, Newcastle upon Tyne NE1 4LP; Honorary Consultant Dermatologist, Newcastle upon Tyne Health Authority, UK.
Skin Disease and the Gut

V. I. Mathan, MD, PhD, MRCP, FAMS
Professor of Medicine and Gastroenterology, and Director, Wellcome Research Unit and Department of Gastroenterology, Christian Medical College Hospital, Vellore 632 004, Tamil Nadu, India.
Tropical Sprue

P. N. Maton, MSc, MB BS, MRCP
Digestive Diseases Branch, National Institutes of Health, Bethesda, Maryland 20205, USA.
Carcinoid Tumours and the Carcinoid Syndrome; Internal Paraneoplastic Syndromes Associated with Cancer

H. B. McMichael, MD, FRCP
Honorary Senior Lecturer in Medicine, Royal Postgraduate Medical School; Consultant Physician, General Wing, Ealing Hospital, Uxbridge Road, Southall, Middlesex UB1 3HW, and Hammersmith Hospital, London, UK.
Digestion and Malabsorption of Fat

A. S. McNeish, MSc, MB ChB(Glas), FRCP
Professor of Paediatrics and Child Health and Director of the University of Birmingham Institute of Child Health, Francis Road, Birmingham B16 8ET; Honorary Consultant Paediatrician, Children's Hospital, Ladywood, Birmingham, UK.
Paediatric Gastroenteritis

Laurence J. Miller, MD, MS
Assistant Professor of Internal Medicine, Mayo Medical School; Consultant in Gastroenterology, Mayo Clinic and Mayo Foundation, Gastroenterology Unit, Saint Mary's Hospital, Rochester, Minnesota 55905, USA.
The Gut Response to a Meal and its Hormonal Control

C. J. Mitchell, BSc, MB, MRCP
Consultant Physician, Scarborough Hospital, Scalby Road, Scarborough, North Yorkshire, UK.
Evaluation of Pancreatic Disease

Robert Modigliani, MD
Professor, CHU Lariboisiere-Saint-Louis; Gastroenterology Clinic, Hospital Saint-Lazare, 75010
Paris, France.
Chronic Non-specific Ulcerative Enteritis

A. G. Morgan, MD, FRCP
Consultant Physician, Airedale General Hospital, Steeton, Keighley, Yorkshire BD20 6TD, UK.
Chronic Gastric Ulcer: Clinical Features, Investigation and Diagnosis and Medical Treatment

Leon Morgenstern, MD, FACS
Clinical Professor of Surgery, UCLA School of Medicine, Los Angeles, California; Director of
Surgery, Department of Surgery, Cedars–Sinai Medical Center, 8700 Beverly Boulevard, Los
Angeles, California 90048, USA.
Radiation Enteropathy

David L. Morris, MB ChB, FRCS
Lecturer, Department of Surgery, University of Nottingham, University Hospital, Queens Medical
Centre, Nottingham NG7 2UH; Honorary Senior Registrar, Trent Region, UK.
Congenital Abnormalities of the Stomach and Duodenum; Benign Gastric Tumours

T. J. Muscroft, MSc, FRCS
Senior Surgical Registrar, Queen Elizabeth Hospital, Birmingham B15 2TH, UK.
**Gastric Bezoar; Phlegmonous Gastritis; Carcinoma of the Duodenum; Acute Dilatation of the
Stomach**

Allen R. Myers, MD
Professor of Medicine, Temple University School of Medicine, Philadelphia, Pennsylvania 19140;
Deputy Chairman, Department of Medicine, Temple University Hospital, Philadelphia, PA, USA.
**Progressive Systemic Sclerosis (Scleroderma) and the Gut; Systemic Lupus Erythematosus and the
Gut; Polymyositis/Dermatomyositis and the Gut; Rheumatoid Arthritis and the Gut**

Graham Neale, MA, BSc, MB, FRCP
Consultant Physician, Addenbrooke's Hospital, Cambridge; Clinical Scientist, MRC Dunn Clini-
cal Nutrition Centre, Addenbrooke's Hospital, Trumpington Street, Cambridge CB2 1QE, UK.
Bacteriology of the Small Gut and Bacterial Overgrowth

R. J. Nicholls, MChir, FRCS
Consultant Surgeon, St Mark's Hospital for Diseases of the Colon and Rectum, City Road,
London EC1V 2PS, and St Thomas' Hospital, London, UK.
**Skin Tags; Thrombosed Perianal Varix; Hypertrophied Papilla; Condylomata Acuminata; Anal
Stenosis; Hidranenitis Suppurativa; Pilonidal Sinus**

Santhat Nivatvongs, MD, FACS
Associate Professor of Surgery, Division of Colon and Rectal Surgery, Department of Surgery,
1731 Medical Arts Building, University of Minnesota, Minneapolis, Minnesota 55402, USA.
Anal Fissure

M. M. T. O'Hare, BSc, PhD
Department of Medicine, Queen's University of Belfast, Institute of Clinical Science, Grosvenor
Road, Belfast BT12 6BJ, UK.
Zollinger–Ellison Syndrome

Colm A. Ó Morain, MD, MSc, MRCP(I)
Consultant Gastroenterologist, Meath and Adelaide Hospitals, Dublin, Irish Republic.
Extraintestinal Manifestations of Inflammatory Bowel Disease

J. Osman, MB, MRCP
Senior Registrar, St Bartholomew's Hospital, London EC1A 7BE, UK.
Respiratory Disease and the Gut

Leslie W. Ottinger, MD
Associate Professor of Surgery, Harvard Medical School; Visiting Surgeon, Massachusetts
General Hospital, Ambulatory Care Center, 15 Parkman Street, Boston, Massachusetts 02114,
USA.
Acute Ischaemia of the Gut

C. R. Pennington, BSc, MB ChB, MRCP
Honorary Senior Lecturer, Dundee University; Consultant Physician, King's Cross Hospital,
Clepington Road, Dundee DD3 8EA, UK.
Campylobacter Enterocolitis; Ascites

B. Pentecost, MD, MB BS, FRCP
Senior Clinical Lecturer, University of Birmingham; Consultant Physician, The General Hospital,
Steelhouse Lane, Birmingham B4 6NH, UK.
Cardiac Disease and the Gut

O. H. Petersen, PhD
Professor, The Physiological Laboratory, University of Liverpool, Liverpool L69 3BX, UK.
Physiology of the Pancreas

Ross A. Pettigrew, FRACS
Research Fellow, Department of Surgery, University of Auckland School of Medicine, Auckland
Hospital, Park Road, Auckland 3, New Zealand.
Therapeutic Nutrition

Henrique Watter Pinotti, MD
Associate Professor of Surgery; Chief, Division of Surgery of the Digestive Tract, Hospital das
Clínicas da Faculdade de Medicina da Universidade de São Paulo, Caixa Postal 8091, São Paulo,
Brazil.
Chagas' Disease

D. W. Piper, MD, FRCP, FRACP
Professor, Department of Medicine, Royal North Shore Hospital, Saint Leonards, New South
Wales 2065, Australia.
Acute Gastritis and Acute Peptic Ulcer

J. M. Polak, MD, DSc, MRCPath
Reader in Histochemistry, Department of Pathology, Royal Postgraduate Medical School; Con-
sultant Histopathologist, Hammersmith Hospital, Ducane Road, London W12 0HS, UK.
VIPomas and Other Pancreatic Tumours

A. V. Pollock, MB ChB, FRCS
Consultant Surgeon, Scarborough Hospital, Scalby Road, Scarborough, Yorkshire, UK.
Acute Appendicitis

R. E. Pounder, MA, MD, FRCP
Senior Lecturer in Medicine, Royal Free Hospital School of Medicine; Honorary Consultant
Physician and Gastroenterologist, Royal Free Hospital, Pond Street, London NW3 2QG, UK.
Chronic Duodenal Ulcer: Clinical Features, Investigation and Diagnosis and Medical Treatment

D. M. Preston, MB, MRCP
Senior Medical Registrar, John Radcliffe Hospital, Headington, Oxford OX3 9DU, UK.
Constipation, Faecal Impaction and Laxative Abuse

Ashley B. Price, BM, FRCPath
Consultant Histopathologist, Northwick Park Hospital, Watford Road, Harrow, Middlesex, UK.
Benign Tumours of the Large Intestine – Polyps and Polyposis

T. Richard Price, PhD, MRCP
Senior Registrar, Guy's Hospital, St Thomas Street, London SE1 9RT, UK.
Calcium, Vitamin D and Metabolic Bone Disease

Alan E. Read, MD, FRCP
Professor of Medicine and Head, University Department of Medicine, Bristol Royal Infirmary, Bristol BS2 8HW, UK.
Retroperitoneal Fibrosis (Ormond's Disease)

N. W. Read, MD, MRCP
Senior Lecturer in Physiology, University of Sheffield; Honorary Consultant Gastroenterologist, Royal Hallamshire Hospital, Glossop Road, Sheffield S10 2JF, UK.
Intestinal Transport of Fluid and Electrolytes

Jonathan Reeve, DM, FRCP
MRC Clinical Scientific Staff, Division of Radioisotopes, MRC Clinical Research Centre, Watford Road, Harrow, Middlesex HA1 3UJ; Honorary Consultant Physician, Northwick Park Hospital, Harrow, UK.
Calcium, Vitamin D and Metabolic Bone Disease

James M. Richter, MD
Instructor In Medicine, Harvard Medical School; Assistant in Medicine, Massachusetts General Hospital, Boston, Massachusetts 02114, USA.
Chronic Pancreatitis

David A. Rothenberger, MD
Clinical Assistant Professor of Surgery, Division of Colon and Rectal Surgery, Department of Surgery, 1731 Medical Arts Building, University of Minnesota, Minneapolis, Minnesota 55402, USA.
Anal Fissure

R. C. G. Russell, MS, FRCS
Consultant Surgeon, The Middlesex Hospital, Mortimer Street, London W1N 8AA, UK.
Peritonitis

R. I. Russell, MD, PhD, FRCP(Ed), FRCP(Glas)
Honorary Lecturer, University of Glasgow; Consultant in Charge, Gastroenterology Unit, The Royal Infirmary, Glasgow G4 0SF, UK.
Chronic Gastrointestinal Haemorrhage

Thomas R. Russell, MD, FACS
Assistant Clinical Professor of Surgery, University of California School of Medicine, San Francisco, California 94143; Chief of Surgery, Presbyterian Hospital, San Francisco, California, USA.
Pruritus Ani and Proctalgia Fugax

M. Y. Sankar, FRCS
Visiting Professor of Surgery; Consultant Gastroenterologist Surgeon, Endoscopy Diagnostic and Research Centre, Bangalore, India.
Duodenitis

C. O. S. Savage, BSc, MRCP
MRC Research Fellow, Royal Postgraduate Medical School; Honorary Registrar, Hammersmith Hospital, Ducane Road, London W12 0HS, UK.
Polyarteritis and the Gut; Henoch–Schönlein Purpura and the Gut

S. H. Saverymuttu, BSc, MRCP
Research Fellow, Royal Postgraduate Medical School; Honorary Registrar, Hammersmith Hospital, Ducane Road, London W12 0HS, UK.
Graft-versus-Host Disease and the Gut

Philip J. Shorvon, MA(Cantab), MB BS, MRCP
Department of Gastroenterology, The Middlesex Hospital, Mortimer Street, London W1N 8AA, UK.
Amyloidosis and the Gut

D. B. A. Silk, MD, FRCP
Consultant Physician, Department of Gastroenterology and Nutrition, Central Middlesex Hospital, Acton Lane, London NW10 7NS, UK.
Digestion and Malabsorption of Protein; Absorption and Malabsorption of Minerals

J. M. Sloan, MD, MB BCh, MRCPath, DObst RCOG
Senior Lecturer, Department of Pathology, Queen's University of Belfast, Institute of Clinical Science, Grosvenor Road, Belfast BT12 6BJ, UK.
Zollinger–Ellison Syndrome

Adam N. Smith, MD, FRCS(Ed), FRS(Ed)
Reader in Surgery, University of Edinburgh; Consultant Surgeon, Western General Hospital, Edinburgh EH4 2XU, UK.
Diverticular Disease

Sat Somers, MB ChB, FRCP(C), DABR
Associate Professor, McMaster University; Consultant Radiologist, McMaster University Medical Centre, 1200 Main Street West, Hamilton, Ontario, Canada L8N 3Z5.
Acute Colonic Haemorrhage

John Spencer, MS, FRCS
Senior Lecturer in Surgery, Royal Postgraduate Medical School; Consultant Surgeon, Hammersmith Hospital, Ducane Road, London W12 0HS, UK.
Diaphragmatic Hernia

R. C. Spiller, MSc, MRCP
Research Fellow and Honorary Registrar, Department of Gastroenterology and Nutrition, Central Middlesex Hospital, Acton Lane, London NW10 7NS, UK.
Absorption and Malabsorption of Minerals

Christopher J. F. Spry, MRCP, DPhil, MRCPath
Senior Lecturer, Department of Immunology, Royal Postgraduate Medical School; Honorary Consultant in Medicine, Hammersmith Hospital, Ducane Road, London W12 0HS, UK.
Eosinophilic Gastroenteritis

William Kinear Stewart, MD, PhD, FRCP, FRCP(Ed)
Senior Lecturer, University of Dundee; Honorary Consultant in Medicine, Tayside Health Board at Royal Infirmary and Ninewells Hospital, Dundee DD1 9SY, UK.
Chronic Renal Failure and the Gut

R. G. Strickland, MD

Professor of Medicine, University of New Mexico School of Medicine, Albuquerque, New Mexico 87131; Chief, Division of Gastroenterology, University of New Mexico Hospital, Albuquerque, NM, USA.
Chronic Gastritis

Warren Strober, MD

Chief, Mucosal Immunity Section, Laboratory of Clinical Investigation, National Institute of Allergy and Infectious Diseases, National Institutes of Health, Bethesda, Maryland 20205, USA.
Protein-losing Enteropathy

Christine M. Swinson, BM BCh, MRCP

Formerly Member of the Scientific Staff (Clinical) and Honorary Senior Registrar, Northwick Park Hospital and Clinical Research Centre, Harrow, Middlesex; Currently Locum at the Royal National Orthopaedic Hospital, London, UK.
Malignant Complications of Coeliac Disease

B. N. Tandon, MD, FAMS

Professor of Medicine and Head, Department of Gastroenterology and Human Nutrition, All-India Institute of Medical Sciences, Ansari Nagar, New Delhi 110029, India.
Giardiasis

J. Temple, MB(Hons), ChM, FRCS(Ed), FRCS(Eng)

Honorary Senior Clinical Lecturer, University of Birmingham; Consultant Surgeon, Queen Elizabeth Hospital, Birmingham B15 2TH, UK.
Abscess; Abdominal Tuberculosis; Foreign Bodies; Blunt Trauma

John Terblanche, ChM, FRCS, FCS(SA)

Professor and Head, Department of Surgery, University of Cape Town Medical School, Observatory 7925, Cape Town; Co-Director, Medical Research Council Liver Research Group, University of Cape Town, Republic of South Africa.
Congenital Abnormalities of the Gallbladder and Biliary Tract

G. R. Thompson, MD, FRCP

Honorary Senior Lecturer in Medicine, Royal Postgraduate Medical School; Honorary Consultant Physician, Hammersmith Hospital, Ducane Road, London W12 0HS, UK.
Lipid Abnormalities and the Gut

Henry Thompson, MD, FRCPath

Reader in Pathology, University of Birmingham; Honorary Consultant in Pathology, The General Hospital, Steelhouse Lane, Birmingham B4 6NH, UK.
Histopathology of Crohn's Disease

James P. S. Thomson, MS, FRCS

Consultant Surgeon and Dean of Postgraduate Studies, St Mark's Hospital for Diseases of the Rectum and Colon, City Road, London EC1V 2PS; Consultant Surgeon, Hackney Hospital; Honorary Consultant Surgeon, St Mary's Hospital; Honorary Lecturer in Surgery, St Bartholomew's Hospital Medical College, London, UK.
Haemorrhoids

Andrew M. Tomkins, MB, FRCP

Senior Lecturer and Consultant Physician, Department of Human Nutrition, London School of Hygiene and Tropical Medicine, Keppel Street (Gower Street), London WC1E 7HT, UK.
Traveller's Diarrhoea

James Toouli, B(Med)Sci, MB BS, PhD, FRACS
Lecturer, Department of Surgery, Flinders University of South Australia; Staff Specialist, Department of Surgery, Flinders Medical Centre, Bedford Park, South Australia 5042; Visiting Specialist, Repatriation General Hospital, Adelaide, Australia.
Cholecystitis and Cholelithiasis

Bruce W. Trotman, MD
Associate Professor of Medicine, University of Pennsylvania School of Medicine, Philadelphia, Pennsylvania 19104; Hospital of the University of Pennsylvania and Philadelphia Veterans Administration Medical Center, Philadelphia, PA, USA.
Formation of Pigment Gallstones

J. N. Udall, MD, PhD
Assistant Professor of Pediatrics, Harvard Medical School; Assistant in Pediatrics, Pediatric Gastrointestinal and Nutrition Unit, Massachusetts General Hospital, Boston, Massachusetts 02114, USA.
Basic Gastrointestinal Immunology

Gaston N. Vantrappen, MD, AggHO
Professor of Medicine, University of Leuven; Head, Department of Medicine, Division of Gastroenterology and Gastroenterology Research Centre, University of Leuven, 3000 Leuven, Belgium.
Motor Disorders of the Oesophagus

Easwaran P. Variyam, MD
Assistant Professor of Medicine, Case Western Reserve University School of Medicine, Cleveland, Ohio; Head, Endoscopy Unit, Gastroenterology Section, Veterans Administration Medical Center, 10701 East Boulevard, Cleveland, Ohio 44106, USA.
Worm Infections of the Gastrointestinal Tract

C. W. Venables, MS, MB BS, FRCS
Lecturer in Surgery, University of Newcastle upon Tyne; Consultant Surgeon in Gastroenterology, Freeman Hospital, High Heaton, Newcastle upon Tyne NE7 7DN, UK.
Surgical Treatment of Chronic Gastric Ulcer

Gary C. Vitale, MD
Visiting Lecturer and Research Fellow, Department of Surgery, Ninewells Hospital and Medical School, Dundee DD1 9SY, UK; Department of Surgery, University of Louisville School of Medicine, Louisville, Kentucky, USA.
Cancer of the Exocrine Pancreas

W. Allan Walker, MD
Professor of Pediatrics, Harvard Medical School; Chief, Pediatric Gastrointestinal and Nutritional Unit, Department of Pediatrics, Massachusetts General Hospital, Boston, Massachusetts 02114, USA.
Basic Gastrointestinal Immunology

J. A. Walker-Smith, MD(Sydney), FRACP, FRCP(Edin), FRCP(Lond)
Reader in Paediatric Gastroenterology, Academic Department of Child Health, Queen Elizabeth Hospital for Children, Hackney Road, London E2 8PS, UK.
Chronic Diseases of the Small Intestine in Childhood

M. Walport, MB BChir, MRCP
MRC Unit on Mechanisms in Tumour Immunity, MRC Centre, University Medical School, Hills Road, Cambridge CB2 2QH, UK.
Behçet's Syndrome and the Gut

Alexander J. Walt, MS(Minn), MB ChB, FRCS(Can). FRCS(Eng), FACS
Penberthy Professor of Surgery and Chairman of the Department of Surgery, Wayne State University School of Medicine, 6-C University Health Center, 4201 St Antoine, Detroit, Michigan 48201; Chief of Surgery, Harper–Grace Hospitals, Detroit, MI, USA.
Injuries to the Pancreas

Andrew L. Warshaw, MD
Associate Professor of Surgery, Harvard Medical School; Associate Visiting Surgeon, Massachusetts General Hospital, Ambulatory Care Center, 15 Parkman Street, Boston, Massachusetts 02114, USA.
Chronic Pancreatitis

W. C. Watson, MD
Department of Gastroenterology, University of Western Ontario, London, Ontario, Canada N6A 5C1.
Coeliac Axis Compression Syndrome

James McK. Watts, MB BS, FRACS
Professor of Surgery, Flinders University of South Australia; Chairman, Department of Surgery, Flinders Medical Centre, Bedford Park, South Australia 5042; Repatriation General Hospital, Adelaide, Australia.
Cholecystitis and Choledocholithiasis

Gerald Webbe, DSc, MSc, FIBiol
Head, Department of Medical Helminthology and Professor of Applied Parasitology, London School of Hygiene and Tropical Medicine, Keppel Street, London WC1E 7HT, UK.
Schistosomiasis

P. J. Whorwell, MD, BSc, MRCP
Senior Lecturer in Medicine, University of Manchester; Consultant Physician, University Hospital of South Manchester, Manchester M20 8DB, UK.
Aetiology and Pathogenesis of Inflammatory Bowel Disease

Christopher B. Williams, BM, FRCP
Consultant Physician, St Mark's Hospital for Diseases of the Rectum and Colon, City Road, London EC1V 2PS, and St Bartholomew's Hospital, London, UK.
Benign Tumours of the Large Intestine – Polyps and Polyposis

Norman S. Williams, MS, FRCS
Senior Lecturer, University Department of Surgery; Honorary Consultant Surgeon, The General Infirmary, Leeds LS1 3EX, UK.
Malignant Tumours of the Large Intestine

C. P. Willoughby, MA, DM, MRCP
Consultant Physician and Gastroenterologist, Basildon and Thurrock Health District, Basildon Hospital, Nether Mayne, Basildon, Essex, UK.
Inflammatory Bowel Disease and Pregnancy

D. L. Wingate, MA, MSc, DM, FRCP
Senior Lecturer in Gastroenterology, The London Hospital Medical College; Honorary Consultant Gastroenterologist, The London Hospital, Whitechapel, London E1 1BB, UK.
Motility Disorders of the Small Intestine

Bruce G. Wolff, MD
Instructor in Surgery, Mayo Medical School, Rochester, Minnesota 55901; Consultant in Colon and Rectal and General Surgery, Rochester Methodist Hospital and St Mary's Hospital, Rochester, MN, USA.
Anal Tumours

R. A. B. Wood, MB ChB, FRCS

Senior Lecturer in Surgery, Ninewells Hospital and Medical School, Dundee, DD1 9SY, UK.
Sclerosing Cholangitis

Nicholas A. Wright, MA, MD, PhD, MRCPath

Professor of Histopathology, Royal Postgraduate Medical School; Director of Histopathology, Hammersmith Hospital, Ducane Road, London W12 0HS, UK.
Anatomy and Congenital Abnormalities of the Small Intestine

A. P. Wyatt, FRCS

Honorary Tutor in Surgery, King's College Hospital and St Thomas' Hospital, London; Consultant General Surgeon, Brook General Hospital, London SE18 4LW, UK.
Pneumatosis Coli (Pneumatosis Cystoides Intestinalis)

Isidoro Zaidman, MD

Director, Residency Training Program, School of Medicine, Universidad Central de Venezuela; Head, Department of Gastroenterology, Hospital Padre Machado, Unidad Clinica Esmeralda, 1B. Av. Los Proceres, San Bernardino, Caracas, Venezuela.
Intestinal Amoebiasis

Chapter 1
Oral Manifestations of Gastrointestinal Disease

M. K. Basu and D. M. Chisholm

Although there are obvious differences between the mouth and the rest of the gastrointestinal tract, there are similarities in terms of exocrine secretion, constituents and the species of bacteria and food products present. For example, secretions from both the mouth and the gastrointestinal tract contain mucin, electrolytes, secretory IgA and lactoferrin,[19] gastrointestinal commensals, such as lactobacilli, enterococci, bacteroides, and some members of the Enterobacteriaceae can also be isolated from human mouths.[45]

Furthermore, basic research has indicated a primary immunological association between the mouth and the remainder of the gastrointestinal tract in terms of recirculation and homing of lymphoid cells.[29, 52] The pharynx and oesophagus are also lined by the same type of epithelium as the mouth, namely stratified squamous epithelium. It is not surprising, in view of these similarities, to find that some gastrointestinal diseases have oral manifestations. Changes that may occur include ulceration, nodularity, inflammation, ulceration oedema, fibrosis and mobility of the teeth (Table 1.1).[9]

RECURRENT ORAL ULCERATION

The presence of oral ulcers is frequently observed in many gastrointestinal, dermatological and other disorders. Ulceration is the most common lesion of the oral mucosa (Table 1.1).

Recurrent oral ulceration (aphthous ulcers) can be grouped into three varieties: minor aphthous ulcers, major aphthous ulcers and herpetiform ulcers (Table 1.2).[36]

Aetiology

Whilst in some patients a cause cannot be determined, in others predisposing factors such as trauma, stress, nutritional deficiency and/or hormonal imbalance can be identified. A family history is found in 25–50% of patients. It is possible that the oral mucosa in patients prone to aphthous ulcers might be more than usually susceptible to mechanical injury, thereby precipitating ulceration. There is no convincing evidence to implicate any particular virus. Despite the existence of a substantial literature on the immunological and cellular responses of patients with recurrent aphthous ulcers a consistent pattern fails to be revealed. A slight increase in serum IgM and IgG is found and autoantibodies to saline homogenates of oral mucosa have been reported. Although it has been suggested that there is an increased frequency of HLA-A1, -B12 and -Aw29 in patients with recurrent oral ulceration, further confirmatory

Table 1.1　Oral changes associated with gastrointestinal disease.

Glossitis	*Ulceration*	*Cheilitis*	*Gingivitis*
Crohn's disease	Recurrent aphthous ulcers	Crohn's disease	Crohn's disease
Alcohol abuse	Crohn's disease	Acrodermatitis enteropathica	Coeliac disease
Coeliac disease	Ulcerative colitis	Alcohol abuse	Scurvy
Kwashiorkor	Behçet's syndrome	Coeliac disease	Kwashiorkor
Pernicious anaemia	Corticosteroid therapy	Kwashiorkor	
Folic acid deficiency	Coeliac disease	Iron deficiency anaemia	
Niacin deficiency	Acrodermatitis enteropathica	Vitamin B deficiencies	
Riboflavin deficiency	Anorexia nervosa	Paterson–Kelly syndrome	
Pyridoxine deficiency	Iron deficiency anaemia		
Paterson–Kelly syndrome	Pernicious anaemia	*Bullous lesions*	
Carcinoid syndrome	Riboflavin deficiency	Virus infections – herpes simplex, Coxsackie	
	Pyridoxine deficiency	Bullous lichen planus	
Pigmentation	Pemphigus	Bullous pemphigoid	
Peutz–Jeghers syndrome	Tuberculosis	Erythema bullosa	
Addison's disease		Benign mucosa pemphigoid	
Haemochromatosis	*Vascular*	Pemphigus vulgaris	
Acanthosis nigricans	Hereditary haemorrhagic		
Pseudoxanthoma elasticum	telangiectasia		
	Scleroderma		
	Blue rubber bleb naevus		
	Kaposi's sarcoma		

evidence is required. A very small number of female patients develop the ulcers regularly before the onset of the menstrual period.

Clinical features

During a prodromal phase of 1–2 days the patient may experience a burning or mildly painful sensation in particular areas of the buccal mucosa or tongue. This is followed by the appearance of ulcers at various sites in the lips, cheek and tongue. Aphthous stomatitis appears primarily as an erosive phenomenon and lacks a vesiculobullous stage. Once the ulcers have appeared the pain increases in severity, lasting for a few days. Thereafter the pain subsides even though a prominent ulcer may be present. There is no constitutional reaction and local lymphadenopathy occurs uncommonly.

The distinction between the three types of recurrent aphthous ulcers is shown in Table 1.2. Minor oral ulcers occur as small, single oral ulcers on the mucosa of the lips, cheeks and side of tongue and account for 80% of all recurrent aphthous ulcers. The ulcers are shallow with a yellow/white base and surrounding rim of erythema. Ulcers of the major aphthous type are larger and involve additionally the oropharynx and dorsum of the tongue (Figure 1.1). Severe pain and difficulty in eating and swallowing is experienced by most patients. Healing is associated with fibrosis and scar formation so that in chronic sufferers there is thickening and nodularity of the lips and cheeks which can be unsightly.

Table 1.2　The distinction between the different varieties of recurrent oral ulcers.

	Minor aphthous ulcers	Major aphthous ulcers	Herpetiform ulcers
Male : female	1.3 : 1	0.8 : 1	2.6 : 1
Peak age of onset (year)	10–20	10–20	20–30
Number of ulcers	1–5	1–10	10–100
Size (mm)	<10	>10	1–2
Duration (days)	4–14	10–30	7–10
Healing with scars (%)	<10	>60	±30
Recurrence (month)	1–4	<monthly	<monthly
Site	Lips, cheek, tongue	Lips, cheek, tongue, pharynx, palate	Lips, cheek, tongue, pharynx, palate, gums
Duration (year)	<5	>15	>5
Local treatment	Corticosteroids	Corticosteroids	Tetracycline

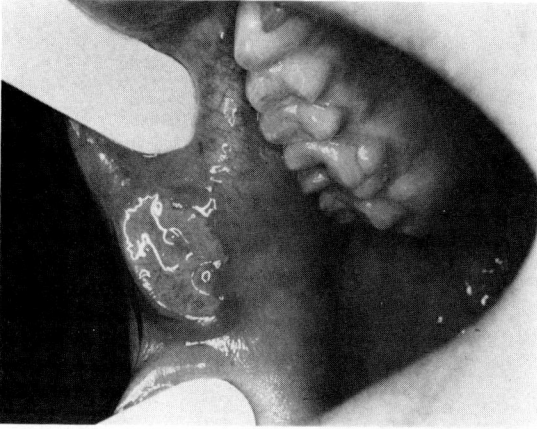

Fig. 1.1 Major aphthous ulcer of several days' duration affecting the angle of the mouth and the right buccal mucosa.

Differential diagnosis

Oral ulceration of a local nature requires to be differentiated from that associated with a systemic disease, namely: Behçet's syndrome, Crohn's disease, ulcerative colitis, *Yersinia* infection, coeliac disease and vasculitis. The ulceration is neither specific nor pathognomonic in any of these conditions. Consequently, the diagnosis of idiopathic recurrent oral ulceration can only be made after a careful clinical examination, supported by appropriate laboratory investigation, to exclude disease in other parts of the gastrointestinal tract. Behçet's syndrome includes genital ulcers, a variety of cutaneous lesions (erythema nodosum, erythema multiforme), ocular, neurological, joint and intestinal manifestations.

Common viral diseases of the oral mucosa, including herpes zoster and the Coxsackie viruses, cause a vesiculoerosive lesion, frequently associated with malaise and fever. Bullous lichen planus, bullous pemphigoid, pemphigus vulgaris and erythema bullosa all demonstrate the presence of bullae. The erosive lesions of tuberculosis are secondary to severe pulmonary disease. Candidiasis has a prominent creamy/white exudate in association with the ulcers. Bacterial infections, such as Vincent's stomatitis, secondary syphilis or gonorrhoea, should not cause confusion. Appropriate microbiological investigations will be of diagnostic value and should be undertaken.

Iron, vitamin B_{12} and folate deficiency states may be accompanied by recurrent oral ulceration. The lesions are commoner in males and tend to be more chronic. The diagnosis is readily made on appropriate haematological investigation.

Treatment

Predisposing factors should be removed and management is based upon local therapy using a combination of corticosteroids, analgesics and antibiotics.

Topical steroids

These are of most benefit if used during the prodromal stage and the most useful preparations are 0.1% triamcinolone in Orabase, 2.5 mg tablets of hydrocortisone sodium succinate and 0.1 mg tablets of betamethasone valerate. These drugs are used 3–4 times daily, the latter being dissolved in water and used as a mouthwash.

Topical antibiotics

Tetracycline is the antibiotic of choice and in order to prevent acute candidiasis it is best given in combination with nystatin in the form of Mysteclin capsules (250 mg tetracycline hydrochloride plus 250 000 units nystatin). The capsules should be used four times daily and dissolved in 5 ml water which is kept in the mouth for two minutes.

Others

Local anaesthetic lozenges or viscous solutions give symptomatic relief. The immunostimulant drug levamisole has been tried but remains to be fully evaluated. Attempts to prevent ovulation in women have not met with success. Idiopathic recurrent aphthous ulceration does not respond to prolonged treatment with iron, vitamin B_{12} or other members of the vitamin B group and this therapy is best given when there is clear evidence of a nutritional deficiency.

PATERSON–KELLY (PLUMMER–VINSON) SYNDROME

The triad of dysphagia, glossitis and anaemia constitutes the Paterson–Kelly syndrome. Almost all patients are postmenopausal women, although occasionally the syndrome may occur in men. Pale dry skin, spoonshaped nails (koilonychia) and splenomegaly are frequently present. Patients may complain of dryness of the eyes with a burning sensation, burning and itchiness of the vulva, and atrophy of the vaginal and anal mucosa. However, dysphagia is the outstanding symptom in all patients and has been attributed to the formation of webs in the oesophagus at the level of fifth or sixth cervical vertebra.

There is a 10–30% incidence of cancer of the upper alimentary tract in these patients, thus highlighting the precancerous nature of the syndrome.[54, 69]

Aetiology

It is generally accepted that the majority of the symptoms of the disease (dysphagia, glossitis, anaemia and koilonychia) are due to iron deficiency.[44, 62]

Clinical features

As mentioned above, dysphagia is the main symptom. The oesophageal web consists of a thin, crescentic membrane arising usually from the anterior wall, and can be visualized directly by oesophagoscopy or radiographically after a barium swallow. The pharyngeal mucosa appears dry, shiny and atrophic, whilst webs, fissures and superficial ulcerations may be present.[44] The majority of the patients with Paterson–Kelly syndrome have hypochromic, microcytic anaemia and this may be associated with a low serum iron concentration. The patients often suffer from achlorhydria. The epithelium of the hypopharynx and oesophagus shows hyperkeratosis and atrophy when submitted for histopathological examination, whilst the underlying tissues of the lamina propria and muscle show atrophic changes.[49, 57] Evidence of increased mitotic activity may be found in the basal layers of the affected epithelium.[62]

Oral manifestations

Careful examination of patients with Paterson–Kelly syndrome often reveals the presence of a thin vermilion border of the lips, angular cheilitis and reduced width of the mouth. The oral mucosa appears thin and atrophic whilst the tongue may be smooth and devoid of papillae (Figure 1.2). The latter may be red in colour, painful and enlarged. Fissuring of the tongue surface has been described[11] and there is leucoplakia of the oral mucosa, especially on the dorsum of the tongue.[13, 49, 54] Histological changes in the affected oral mucosa are essentially similar to those found in the pharyngeal and oesophageal mucosa.

Treatment

The Paterson–Kelly syndrome is treated by correcting the iron deficiency and dilating the oesophagus with the oesophagoscope or by bou-

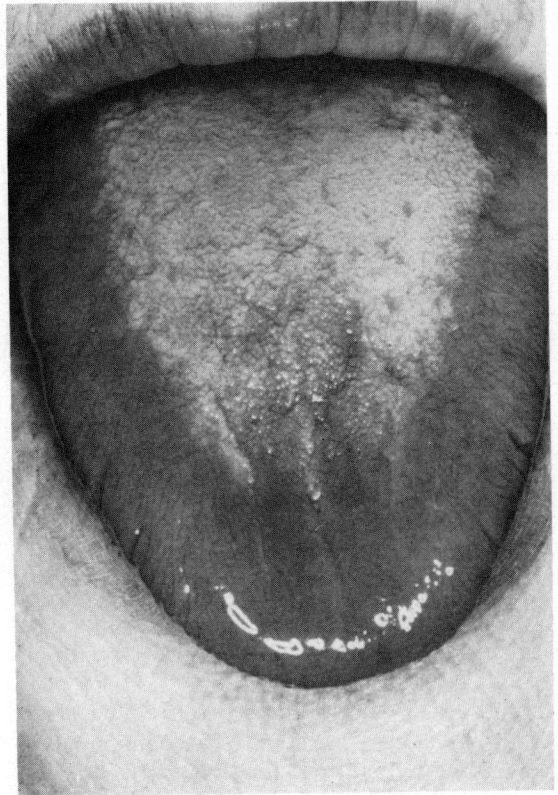

Fig. 1.2 Atrophic glossitis in a middle-aged female with iron-deficiency anaemia. Note the smooth tip and lateral borders.

gienage. Treatment of the mouth symptoms should include the use of 2% lignocaine viscous to reduce painful and burning sensations. Leucoplakic lesions should be excised and submitted for histological examination, to exclude cellular atypia or malignant transformation.

CANDIDAL OROPHARYNGO-OESOPHAGITIS

Candidal infection of the mucous membranes of the mouth, pharynx and oesophagus is an increasingly recognized disease entity.[22, 33] It has been defined as a disease in which hyphal forms of *Candida albicans* have invaded the mucosa of the upper alimentary tract with resulting destructive changes.[46] Most patients complain of persistent dysphagia and oropharyngeal discomfort of varying intensity, or a burning retrosternal pain or both. In the majority of patients there is underlying malignant disease, or endocrine or immunological disorders.[31, 46] A history of prior treatment with antibiotics is obtainable in a minority of other patients. Prolonged treatment with cortico-steroids and other immunosuppressive agents predisposes to this condition.[26] The mucosal involvement may be acute or chronic and it may be associated with a disseminated and life-threatening candidal infection.[32, 46] Evidence of skin, nail or hair involvement may be lacking.[20]

Aetiology

Candida albicans invades the upper alimentary tract mucosa and fungal mycelia can be demonstrated in the superficial layers of the epithelium.[60] Evidence of impaired cell-mediated immunity specifically to *Candida* may be found.[20, 60] It remains to be determined whether this immune defect is primary and causative, in the sense of allowing *C. albicans* to invade the tissue.

Clinical features

Oesophagoscopy reveals severe inflammation of the pharyngeal and oesophageal mucous membrane with ulceration and frequently pseudo-membrane formation. An associated stricture of the upper oesophagus is usually present. The radiological features include an irregular, ragged mucosal pattern with numerous small indentations and protrusions. Smears made from pharyngeal and oesophageal swabs show numerous yeast and mycelial forms of the fungus and luxurious growth of *C. albicans* can be obtained with culture. The patients usually have elevated *Candida* agglutinating antibody titres, suggesting intact humoral immunological responses, but in vivo and in vitro allergy to *Candida* antigen is usually present. However, cell-mediated immune responses to dinitro-chlorobenzene, *Trichophyton*, mumps and PPD remain normal.[20, 60]

Oral manifestations

In the mouth, typical white lesions of 'candidal leucoplakia' are found (Figure 1.3). Some of these may show evidence of erosion. The white lesions may form a reticulate pattern, mimicking oral lichen planus. Angular cheilitis may also be present.[60] Candidal organisms are found in smears made from oral swabs and microscopic examination shows the presence of fungal mycelia within the affected oral epithelium.

Treatment

Treatment should be directed first to supportive measures and correction of the underlying pre-

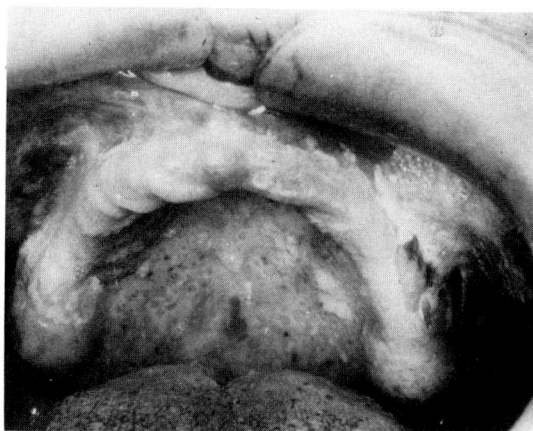

Fig. 1.3 Plaque-like lesions of *Candida albicans* in a middle-aged, edentulous female.

disposing factors. The *Candida* infection may subside spontaneously if immunosuppression, steroids or antibiotics can be discontinued. Hourly ingestion of nystatin in a viscous suspension with methylcellulose, or of miconazole viscous suspension, has been reported to be successful.[60] In some cases, also, the use of intravenous amphotericin B has been judged successful.[20] Oesophageal bougienage may be necessary to dilate strictures when they are present.

CYSTIC FIBROSIS

This disease entity, first recognized in 1938, was considered to be a pancreatic disease resulting in maldigestion and loss of fat and nitrogen in the stool. It is now recognized to be a generalized abnormality of exocrine glands. The disease occurs in approximately one per 2000 live births in Caucasians,[50] and follows an autosomal recessive pattern of inheritance (Chapter 18).

Oral manifestations

The major salivary glands appear to be affected differently according to the glycoprotein content of their secretions. The submandibular glands may enlarge and there may be a reduction in saliva volume, while the parotid glands are less affected.[6] The values of total protein, many of the enzymes, calcium and phosphorus are elevated in submandibular saliva, while sodium, chloride and potassium concentrations are within normal limits.[14, 39] Eosinophilic plugs are frequently found in the ducts of the labial salivary glands.[58] There is a paucity of dental studies but it would appear that treated cystic fibrosis patients have no evidence of increased dental caries or periodontal disease.[70] Meticulous oral hygiene measures are necessary in view of the tendency to calculus formation and *Pseudomonas aeruginosa* colonization of the mouth in cystic fibrosis patients.[34, 38, 66]

FOOD ALLERGY

Food constituents can act as allergens, and allergic responses to many different foods are known to occur (e.g. allergy to cow's milk protein). Although in allergies of this kind the alimentary tract acts as the portal of entry for the allergen and also possibly as the route of immunization,[30] the site of reaction can be extra-intestinal and take the form of skin rash, asthma, migraine, etc. The terms 'alimentary allergy' or 'gastrointestinal allergy' have been used to describe the condition.[59] Alternatively, gastrointestinal symptoms may predominate and give rise to the descriptive term 'gastrointestinal allergy' (see Chapter 8).

Oral manifestations include cheilitis and aphthous stomatitis.[25, 61] Recent in vitro studies have indicated that food sensitivity may play a minor role in the development of recurrent aphthous stomatitis.[68]

Treatment consists of removing the offending foodstuffs from the diet, and although corticosteroids may relieve symptoms they should be used only as a temporary or emergency measure.

CROHN'S DISEASE

Crohn's disease (CD) is a granulomatous inflammatory disease of the bowel of unknown aetiology. It almost invariably runs a chronic course, periods of quiescence being interrupted by exacerbation of varying acuteness, severity and duration. It usually affects young adults and most commonly involves the ileocaecal region, but it may involve, either concurrently or consecutively, any part of the alimentary tract from the mouth to the anus (Chapter 12).

Oral manifestations

The occurrence of oral lesions in patients with CD is not uncommon and incidence figures of 6–20% have been reported.[8, 18, 28, 35] They occur more commonly in patients with colonic disease (granulomatous colitis) or ileocolitis as opposed to disease confined to the small bowel[8, 28] and occur most frequently when

patients have other extra-intestinal manifestations such as skin and joint lesions.[28] The oral lesions can precede the onset of intestinal disease, and in one instance histologically typical oral lesions occurred some time before bowel lesions could be demonstrated.[12] The oral lesions have the following appearances: aphthous ulcers, diffuse swelling of the lips and cheek, well-defined areas on the oral mucosa showing inflammatory hyperplasia and fissuring (cobblestone – Figure 1.4), indurated polypoid

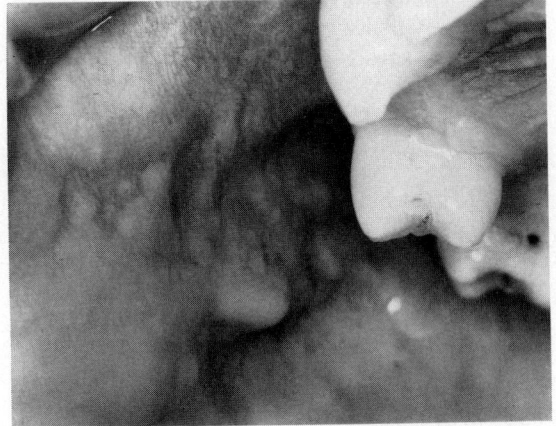

Fig. 1.4 Multiple, discrete swellings of right buccal mucosa giving rise to 'cobblestone' appearance in a 12-year-old boy with Crohn's disease.

tag-like lesions on vestibular and retromolar mucosa and persistent deep linear ulcers with hyperplastic margins and indurated fissures on the mid-line of the lower lip.[51] The lesions can be either painful and tender or asymptomatic, and they vary in duration, sometimes lasting for months. As with the bowel disease, the oral lesions run a chronic course with periods of quiescence interrupted by exacerbations of varying severity. In about 10% of patients histological examination of the oral lesions shows the presence of characteristic non-caseating granulomas and diffusely distributed lymphocytes, plasma cells and histiocytes in the lamina propria and submucosa. The overlying oral epithelium is infiltrated by lymphocytes and a few neutrophils, but it may be ulcerated. A dense and conspicuous perivascular infiltrate is frequently present in the submucosa and focal collections of lymphocytes may be found within the fibrous tissue stroma of the minor salivary glands.[8] In the other 90% of patients the surface epithelium may be ulcerated and there is frequently evidence of fissuring on the surface. Focal collections of lymphocytes are found in the lamina propria and submucosa, which may also contain secondary lymphoid follicles. Perivascular mononuclear cell infiltration is prominent, and there are other non-specific signs of chronic inflammation such as neuronal hyperplasia and intimal thickening.

In the unaffected oral mucosa and minor salivary glands of CD patients, abnormalities such as focal lymphocytic infiltrates are found in 67% at routine histological screening.[10] Immunohistochemical studies show an increase in the number of IgA-containing plasma cells but this is not correlated with disease activity.[17] In contrast a significant correlation between disease activity and the number of IgM-containing cells is found.

Immunofluorescence studies in which normal mucosa of CD patients is incubated with CD serum show the presence of circulating antibodies against buccal epithelium in some.[63] Although this procedure was suggested as a diagnostic test, its value has not been confirmed.[10, 45]

Treatment

The oral lesions should be treated with local application of 2% lignocaine viscous to reduce pain. Corsodyl (0.2% w/v chlorhexidine gluconate) mouth washes three or four times a day may be used to reduce the risk of secondary infection of the mouth ulcers. Local application of steroids in the form of Corlan (hydrocortisone sodium succinate) or mouth washes containing prednisolone sodium phosphate will reduce inflammation. Mouth washing with Predsol enema solution (Glaxo) or a solution containing one 5 mg tablet of Prednesol (Glaxo) in 100 ml of water has been used with success. Infiltration of the oral lesion with slow-release steroids has also been tried with variable success. Longstanding single ulcers, tags and other localized lesions can be treated by surgical excision. The oral lesions usually show signs of regression when the bowel symptoms are brought under control.

ULCERATIVE COLITIS

Ulcerative colitis is an inflammatory disease of unknown aetiology which involves the colonic and rectal mucosa in a diffuse pattern (Chapter 12).

Oral manifestations

In patients with ulcerative colitis, the following oral lesions may be found: recurrent aphthous ulceration; ulcers analogous to pyoderma gangrenosum of the skin; pyostomatitis vegetans; and haemorrhagic ulcers of the oral mucosa and skin.

RECURRENT APHTHOUS ULCERATION

Recurrent aphthous ulcers develop fairly commonly in patients with ulcerative colitis – incidence figures from 4–20% have been reported.[9, 28, 48] Clinically the ulcers resemble either major or minor aphthae. Their onset is usually sudden and coincides with recurrence of diarrhoea and other symptoms. Frequently the serum albumin levels of these patients are low and the serum seromucoid concentration elevated.

Histological examination of the oral epithelium reveals infiltration of the lamina propria and submucosa by lymphocytes and histiocytes. A few plasma cells, eosinophils and neutrophils are also present. Frequently there is evidence of angiitis with leucocytoclasia (nuclear fragmentation) in the submucosa and the involved blood vessels stain for complement C3.

PYODERMA GANGRENOSUM

Lesions analogous to pyoderma gangrenosum were found in two out of 100 patients in one study[9] and two other cases have also been reported.[41] Macroscopically the lesions appear as irregular shaped ulcers of 15–20 mm diameter, with rolled out margins and a greyish coloured base. Over a period of four to eight weeks the painful lesions develop during a stage when bowel symptoms are present, serum albumin levels are low and serum seromucoid levels high. There may be associated skin lesions. The oral lesions can develop in patients who have symptoms attributable to complications with their ileostomy stoma. Microscopic examination of oral biopsy specimens shows evidence of ulceration, the ulcer being covered by a fibrinopurulent membrane. The lamina propria is heavily infiltrated by chronic inflammatory cells among which numerous histiocytes and a few multinucleate 'foreign body'-type giant cells are present. There is evidence of perivascular hyalinization and fibrin deposition.

PYOSTOMATITIS VEGETANS

McCarthy and Shklar in 1963 first described the syndrome of pyostomatitis vegetans and ulcerative colitis.[43] They coined the term 'pyostomatitis vegetans' since the oral lesions resembled, both macroscopically and microscopically, the skin lesions of pyoderma vegetans of Hallopeau, a variant of pemphigus vegetans.[37]

In pyostomatitis vegetans the lip and cheek mucosae are diffusely swollen and inflamed, with deep fissure-like ulcerations separating papillary projections of mucous membrane. The gingivae and the palatal mucosa may also be involved, whilst the submandibular lymph nodes are swollen and tender and the patient may be febrile. The lesions develop over a period of 6–8 weeks.

Suprabasal separation of the oral epithelium together with intraepithelial abscesses filled with eosinophils and a few acantholytic cells characterize the histopathological picture. In addition, the lamina propria is heavily infiltrated by inflammatory cells consisting mainly of eosinophils, histiocytes and lymphocytes, but a few plasma cells and neutrophils are also present. A perivascular infiltrate composed almost exclusively of eosinophils may affect the lamina propria and submucosa.

HAEMORRHAGIC ULCERS OF THE SKIN AND ORAL MUCOSA

These appear on the oral mucosa as discrete irregular-shaped haemorrhagic ulcers of varying size. Similar ulcers occur on the skin of the cheeks, inner aspects of the thighs, buttocks and lower abdomen. The lesions, starting as haemorrhagic bullae which subsequently burst to become ulcers, develop within 1–3 days. Microscopic examination reveals evidence of cutaneous necrotizing vasculitis in the affected lamina propria and submucosa. Thus there is fibrinoid necrosis of the venules and an infiltrate rich in neutrophils; extravasation of erythrocytes and leucocytoclasia are associated findings.

Treatment

The oral lesions in patients with ulcerative colitis should be treated by 2% lignocaine viscous to relieve pain; Corsodyl (chlorhexidine gluconate) mouth washes should be prescribed to reduce risk of secondary infection of the mouth ulcers and topical steroids can be used to reduce the severity of mucosal inflammation. When the symptoms of colitis are controlled by medical or surgical therapy, the oral lesions usually resolve.

COELIAC DISEASE

Coeliac disease is a malabsorptive disorder of the small intestinal mucosa associated with the ingestion of the cereal-protein gluten by susceptible individuals (see Chapter 8).

Oral manifestations

Patients with malabsorption commonly complain of oral ulceration of the recurrent aphthous type. A study of patients with idiopathic steatorrhoea showed that 59% had aphthous ulceration as one of their presenting symptoms.[16] In patients with adult coeliac disease 12% have aphthous ulceration at presentation.[7] It is of interest that the incidence of coeliac disease in individuals suffering from recurrent aphthous ulceration appears to be much higher than the incidence of coeliac disease in the population, and incidence figures range from 2%[36] to 25%.[4, 24] In patients with coeliac disease the aphthous ulcers are usually of the minor type. The patients may or may not have other signs and symptoms relating to their bowel disease. Eczematous skin lesions may be present and childhood coeliacs may show evidence of dental hypoplasia.

Microscopic examination of the aphthous ulcers reveals profound lymphocyte–monocyte infiltration of the lamina propria and submucosa with variable numbers of neutrophils. There are collections of plasma cells beneath the intact epithelium. A perivascular infiltrate of neutrophils is frequently present and some of these show evidence of nuclear fragmentation (leucocytoclasia). The presence of IgM and IgG plasma cells within the lamina propria is demonstrated by direct immunofluorescence in biopsy material of the ulcers.

Treatment

The aphthous ulcers in patients with coeliac disease should be treated on a symptomatic basis with 2% lignocaine viscous, Corsodyl mouth washes and topical steroids. The ulcers do not respond to treatment with haematinics and permanent cure is obtained when gluten is withdrawn from the patients' diets.[24, 67]

CIRRHOSIS OF THE LIVER

Oral manifestations

Painless, bilateral enlargement of parotid glands (sialosis) occurs in patients with alcoholic cirrhosis.[47] In a prospective study of 70 consecutive patients with cirrhosis of the liver, Summerskill *et al.*[56] found sialosis of the parotid glands in 9 out of 35 alcoholic subjects.

Histological examination of enlarged glands demonstrates hypertrophy of the glandular acini and fatty infiltration[39] without any obvious inflammatory change. Parotid saliva flow rate is increased in patients with alcoholic cirrhosis and the saliva contains elevated levels of potassium, calcium, total protein and amylase.[1] The immunoglobulin levels remain unaffected.[39]

The cause of parotid gland enlargement in alcoholic cirrhosis is not clear and both alcohol- and cirrhosis-associated nutritional deficiency have been suggested as possible factors.[65] The parotid gland enlargement in alcoholic cirrhosis is reversible and often disappears if the patient abstains from alcohol and the nutritional status improves.[56]

Components of Sjögren's disease are frequently present in patients with autoimmune liver disease, and symptoms suggestive of sicca syndrome occur in a high proportion of patients with chronic active hepatitis, primary biliary cirrhosis or cryptogenic cirrhosis.[2, 27, 55] It has been suggested that the development of sicca symptoms in autoimmune liver disease is a consequence of sensitization to cross-reacting antigens shared by the biliary tree and the salivary and lachrymal glands.[55]

REFERENCES

1 Abelson, D. C., Mandel, I. D. & Karmiol, M. (1976) Salivary studies in alcoholic cirrhosis. *Oral Surgery*, **11**, 188–192.

2 Alarcon-Segovia, D., Diaz-Jouanen, E. & Fishbein, E. (1973) Features of Sjögren's syndrome in primary biliary cirrhosis. *Annals of Internal Medicine*, **79**, 31–36.

3 Aronson, M. D., Phillips, C. A. & Beeken, W. L. (1974) Isolation of a viral agent from intestinal tissue of patients with Crohn's disease and other intestinal disorders. *Gastroenterology*, **66**, 661.

4 Asquith, P. & Basu, M. K. (1978) Aphthous ulceration. The incidence of coeliac disease and gluten sensitivity. In *Perspective in Coeliac Disease* (Ed.) McNicholl, B., McCarthy, C. F. & Fottrell, P. F. Lancaster: MTP.

5 Asquith, P., Kraft, S. C. & Rothberg, R. M. (1973) Lymphocyte responses to non-specific mitogens in inflammatory bowel disease. *Gastroenterology*, **65**, 1–7.

6 Barbero, G. J. & Sibinga, M. S. (1962) Enlargement of the submaxillary glands in cystic fibrosis. *Pediatrics*, **29**, 788–793.

7 Barry, R. E., Baker, P. & Read, A. E. (1974) The clinical presentation. *Clinics in Gastroenterology*, **3**(1), 55–69.

8 Basu, M. K., Asquith, P., Thompson, R. A. & Cooke, W. T. (1975) Oral manifestations of Crohn's disease. *Gut*, **16**, 249–254.

9 Basu, M. K., Asquith, P., Cooke, W. T. & Thompson, H. (1979) Oral mucosal lesions in ulcerative colitis. (Personal communication.)

10 Basu, M. K., Chesner, I. M., Thompson, R. A. &

11 Beitman, R. G., Frost, S. S. & Roth, J. L. A. (1981) Oral manifestations of gastrointestinal disease. *Digestive Diseases and Sciences*, **26**, 741–747.

12 Bishop, R. P., Brewster, A. C. & Antonioli, D. A. (1972) Crohn's disease of the mouth. *Gastroenterology*, **62**, 302–306.

13 Cahn, L. R. (1952) A case of Plummer–Vinson syndrome. *Oral Surgery*, **5**, 325–329.

14 Chernick, W. S., Barbero, G. J. & Parkins, F. M. (1961) Studies on submaxillary saliva in cystic fibrosis. *Journal of Pediatrics*, **59**, 890–898.

15 Cook, M. G. & Dixon, M. F. (1973) An analysis of the reliability of detection and diagnostic value of various pathological features of Crohn's disease and ulcerative colitis. *Gut*, **14**, 255–262.

16 Cooke, W. T., Peerey, A. L. P. & Hawkins, C. F. (1953) Symptoms, signs and diagnostic features of steatorrhoea. *Quarterly Journal of Medicine*, **22**, 59–77.

17 Crama-Bohbouth, G., Bosman, F. T., Vermeer, B. J., van der Wal, A. M., Biemond, I., Weterman, I. T. & Pena, A. S. (1983) Immunohistological findings in lip biopsy specimens from patients with Crohn's disease and healthy subjects. *Gut*, **24**, 202–205.

18 Croft, C. B. & Wilkinson, A. R. (1972) Ulceration of the mouth, pharynx and larynx in Crohn's disease of the intestine. *British Journal of Surgery*, **59**, 249–252.

19 Drasar, B. S. & Hill, M. J. (1974) *Human Intestinal Flora*. London: Academic Press.

20 Dutta, S. K. & Al-Ibrahim, M. S. (1978) Immunological studies in acute pseudo-membranous esophageal candidiasis. *Gastroenterology*, **75**, 292–296.

21 Dyer, N. H., Child, J. A., Mollin, D. L. & Dawson, A. M. (1972) Anaemia in Crohn's disease. *Quarterly Journal of Medicine*, new series **41**(164) 419–436.

22 Eras, P., Goldstein, M. J. & Sherlock, P. (1972) Candida infection of the gastrointestinal tract. *Medicine* (Baltimore), **51**, 367–379.

23 Ferguson, M. M. (1975) Oral mucous membrane markers of internal disease. Part II. In *Oral Mucosa in Health and Disease* (Ed.) Dolby, A. E. pp. 233–299. Oxford: Blackwell.

24 Ferguson, R., Basu, M. K., Asquith, P. & Cooke, W. T. (1976) Jejunal mucosal abnormalities in patients with recurrent aphthous ulceration. *British Medical Journal*, **i**, 11–13.

25 Finn, R. & Cohen, N. H. (1978) 'Food allergy', fact or fiction. *Lancet*, **i**, 426–428.

26 Frenkel, J. K. (1962) Role of corticosteroids as predisposing factors in fungal diseases. *Laboratory Investigation*, **11**, 1192–1208.

27 Golding, P. L., Brown, R., Mason, A. M. & Taylor, E. (1970) 'Sicca complex' in liver disease. *British Medical Journal*, **iv**, 340–342.

28 Greenstein, A. J., Janowitz, H. D. & Sachar, D. B. (1976) The extra-intestinal complications of Crohn's disease and ulcerative colitis. *Medicine*, **55**, 401–402.

29 Hall, J. G. & Smith, M. E. (1970) Homing of lymph-borne immunoblasts to the gut. *Nature*, **226**, 262–263.

30 Hemmings, W. A. (1978) Food allergy, *Lancet*, **i**, 608.

31 Jensen, K. B., Stenderup, A., Thomson, J. B. & Bichel, J. (1964) Esophageal moniliasis in malignant neoplastic disease. *Acta Medica Scandinavica*, **175**, 455–459.

32 Kirkpatrick, C. H., Rich, R. R. & Bennett, J. E. (1971) Chronic mucocutaneous candidiasis: model building in

cellular immunity. *Annals of Internal Medicine,* **74,** 955–978.

33 Kodsi, B. E., Wickremsinghe, P. C., Kozinn, P. J. *et al.* (1976) Candida esophagitis: a prospective study of 27 cases. *Gastroenterology,* **71,** 715–719.

34 Komiyama, K. & Gibbons, R. J. (1984) Co-aggregation between indigenous oral bacteria and Ps. aeruginosa strains isolated from cystic fibrosis patients. *Journal of Dental Research,* **63** (special issue), 186.

35 Kyle, J. (1972) *Crohn's Disease.* London: Heinemann.

36 Lehner, T. (1977) Oral ulceration and Behçet's syndrome. *Gut,* **18,** 491–511.

37 Lever, W. F. & Schaumberg-Lever, G. (1975) *Histopathology of the Skin.* Philadelphia: Lippincott.

38 Lindemann, R. A., Newman, M. G., Kaufman, A. K. & Stiehm, E. R. (1984) Pseudomonas aeruginosa from cystic fibrosis patients: oral colonization. *Journal of Dental Research,* **63** (special issue), 186.

39 Mandel, I. D. & Baurmash, H. (1978) Salivary immunoglobulins in diseases affecting the salivary glands. In *Secretory Immunity and Infection* (Ed.) McGhee, J. R., Mestecky, J. & Babb, J. L. pp. 839–847. New York: Plenum.

40 Mandel, I. D., Kutscher, A., Denning, C. R. *et al.* (1967) Salivary studies in cystic fibrosis. *American Journal of Diseases of Children,* **113,** 431–438.

41 Margoles, J. S. & Wenger, J. (1961) Stomal ulceration association with pyoderma gangrenosum and ulcerative colitis: report of two cases. *Gastroenterology,* **41,** 594–598.

42 Matthews, N., Tapper-Jones, L., Mayberry, F. & Rhodes, J. (1979) Buccal biopsies in diagnosis of Crohn's disease. *Lancet,* **i,** 500–501.

43 McCarthy, P. & Shklar, G. (1963) A syndrome of pyostomatitis vegetans and ulcerative colitis. *Archives of Dermatology,* **88,** 913–919.

44 McNab Jones, R. F. (1961) The Paterson–Brown Kelly syndrome: its relationship to iron deficiency and postcricoid carcinoma. *Journal of Laryngology and Otology,* **75,** 529–561.

45 Nolte, W. A. (1977) *Oral Microbiology,* 3rd edn. St Louis: C. V. Mosby.

46 Quie, P. G. & Chilgren, R. A. (1971) Acute disseminated and chronic mucocutaneous candidiasis. *Seminars in Hematology,* **8,** 227–242.

47 Rothbell, E. N. & Duggan, J. J. (1957) Enlargement of parotid gland in disease of liver. *American Journal of Medicine,* **22,** 367–372.

48 Samitz, M. H. & Greenberg, M. S. (1951) Skin lesions in association with ulcerative colitis. *Gastroenterology,* **19,** 476–479.

49 Savilahti, R. R. (1946) On the pathologic anatomy of Plummer–Vinson syndrome. *Acta Medica Scandinavica,* **125,** 40–54.

50 Schaap, T. & Cohen, M. M. (1976) A proposed model for the inheritance of cystic fibrosis. In *Cystic Fibrosis, Projections into the Future* (Ed.) Mangos, J. A. & Talamo, R. C. pp. 291–303. Florida: Symposia Specialists.

51 Schiller, K. F. R., Golding, P. L., Peebles, R. A. & Whitehead, R. (1971). Crohn's disease of the mouth and lips. *Gut,* **12,** 864–865.

52 Sewell, H. F., Gell, P. G. H. & Basu, M. K. (1979) Immune responsiveness and oral immunization. *International Archives of Allergy and Applied Immunology,* **58,** 414–425.

53 Sherlock, P., Goldstein, M. J. & Eras, P. (1970) Oesophageal moniliasis. *Modern Treatment,* **7,** 1250–1260.

54 Simpson, R. R. (1939) Anaemia with dysphagia: a precancerous condition. *Journal of Laryngology and Otology,* **54,** 738–746.

55 Sullivan, S., MacFarlane, I. G., Wojcicka, B. M., Eddleston, A. L. W. F. & Williams, R. (1978) Sicca syndrome and immune responses to bile and salivary antigens. In *Immune Reactions in Liver Diseases* (Ed.) Eddleston, A. L. W. F., Weber, J. C. P. & Williams, R. pp. 144–148. Tunbridge Wells: Pitman Medical.

56 Summerskill, W. H. J., Davidson, C. S., Dible, J. H. *et al.* (1960) Cirrhosis of the liver. A study of alcoholic and non-alcoholic patients in Boston and London. *New England Journal of Medicine,* **262,** 1–9.

57 Suzman, N. M. (1933) Syndrome of anaemia, glossitis and dysphagia. Report of eight cases with special reference to observations at autopsy in one instance. *AMA Archives of Internal Medicine,* **51,** 1–21.

58 Sweeney, L. R., Hedrick, M. C., Meskin, L. H. & Warwick, W. J. (1967) The involvement of the labial mucous salivary gland in patients with cystic fibrosis. II. The heterozygote state. *Pediatrics,* **40,** 421–424.

59 Truelove, S. C. & Jewell, D. P. (1975) The intestine in allergic diseases. In *Clinical Aspects of Immunology* (Ed.) Gell, P. G. H., Coombs, R. R. A. & Lachmann, P. J. Oxford: Blackwell.

60 Tytgal, G. N. (1977) A case of oropharyngooesophageal candidiasis. *Gastroenterology,* **72,** 536–540.

61 Vaughan, V. C. (1969) *Textbook of Pediatrics* (Ed.) Nelson, W. E., Vaughan, V. C. & McKay, R. J. p. 509. Philadelphia: Saunders.

62 Waldenström, J. (1938) Iron and epithelium. Some clinical observations. *Acta Medica Scandinavica* (supplement), **90,** 380–397.

63 Walker, J. E. G. (1978) Possible diagnostic test for Crohn's disease by the use of buccal mucosa. *Lancet,* **ii,** 759–760.

64 Watts, J. McK. (1961) The importance of the Plummer–Vinson syndrome in the aetiology of carcinoma of the upper gastro-intestinal tract. *Postgraduate Medical Journal,* **37,** 523–533.

65 Wolfe, S. J., Summerskill, W. H. J. & Davidson, C. S. (1957) Parotid swelling, alcoholism and cirrhosis. *New England Journal of Medicine,* **256,** 491–495.

66 Wotman, S., Mercadente, J., Mandel, I. D. *et al.* (1973) The occurrence of calculus in normal children, children with cystic fibrosis and children with asthma. *Journal of Periodontology,* **44,** 278–280.

67 Wray, D., Ferguson, M. M., Mason, D. K., Hutcheon, A. W. & Dagg, J. H. (1975) Recurrent aphthae: treatment with vitamin B_{12}, folic acid and iron. *British Medical Journal,* **ii,** 490–493.

68 Wray, D., Vlagopoulos, T. P. & Siraganian, R. P. (1982) Food allergens and basophil histamine release in recurrent aphthous stomatitis. *Oral Surgery,* **54,** 388–395.

69 Wynder, E. L., Hultberg, S., Jacobsson, F. & Bross, I. J. (1957) Environmental factors in cancer of the upper alimentary tract. A Swedish study with special reference to Plummer–Vinson (Patterson–Kelly) syndrome. *Cancer,* **10,** 470–487.

70 Yule, A. J. (1970) Fibro-cystic disease of the pancreas (mucoviscidosis). Case Report. *Australian Dental Journal,* **15,** 519–520.

Chapter 2
The Oesophagus

EMBRYOLOGY AND ANATOMY

EMBRYOLOGY

Initially the oesophagus is a short tube stretching from the respiratory diverticulum to the fusiform dilatation, which becomes the stomach in the developing part of the foregut. The endodermal lining is at first columnar. With the growth of the embryo and descent of the heart and lungs the oesophagus lengthens rapidly, with a temporary obliteration of the lumen. When this reappears it is lined by stratified squamous epithelium. The visceral mesoderm which surrounds the oesophagus develops into connective and muscular tissue. The upper two-thirds of the muscular tissue becomes mainly striated, while the lower one-third, like the rest of the gut, is mainly non-striated.

ANATOMY

The oesophagus is a muscular tube 25 cm long connecting the pharynx, opposite the sixth vertebra, to the cardia, slightly to the left of the eleventh thoracic vertebra and some 40 cm from the incisor teeth. It has three parts – cervical, thoracic and abdominal – each segment has important relations.

The outermost layer of the oesophagus is a condensation of fascia of the posterior mediastinum. The lower end is fixed by the phreno-oesophageal ligament and posteriorly to the preaortic fascia. The muscular coat has two layers: the outer longitudinal layer and the inner circular layer. In the upper portion both layers are striated; in the lower third both are smooth and continuous with the muscle layers of the stomach. Recently, a muscular lower oesophageal sphincter has been documented in detail

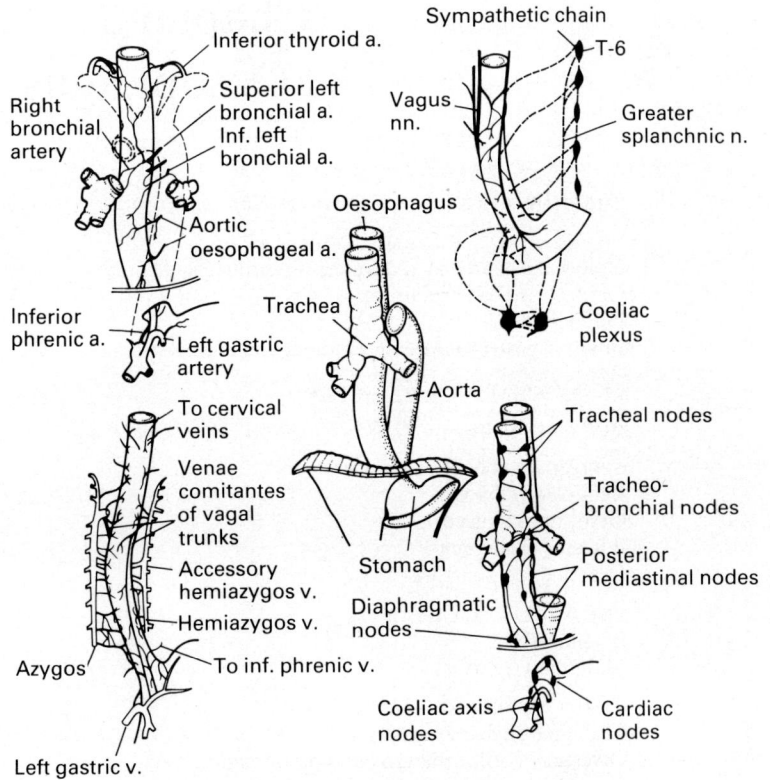

Fig. 2.1 Anatomy of the human oesophagus: arterial supply (upper left), venous drainage (lower left), innervation (upper right) and lymphatic system (lower right). From Ellis, F. H. (1981) The oesophagus. In *Davis-Christopher Textbook of Surgery* (Ed.) Sabiston, D. C. p. 794, with kind permission of the author, the editor and the publisher, W. B. Saunders.

by Liebermann-Meffert *et al*:[8] previously none was thought to be present.[7] Between the muscle layers is the myenteric plexus, but there is no submucosal plexus.[10] Most neurones of the myenteric plexus are cholinesterase-positive and probably motor in function; the others (20–40%) are argyrophil and thought to be concerned with the coordination of swallowing. The vagi and glossopharyngeal nerves carry motor fibres to the striped muscle (Figure 2.1). The vagi supply parasympathetic fibres. The sympathetic innervation is derived from several sources – the fourth to sixth thoracic segments and the greater splanchnic nerves. There are more autonomic nerves reaching the lower oesophagus than any other segment of the alimentary tract.

The submucosa contains nerve fibres, large blood vessels, lymphatics and oesophageal mucous glands, which have a longitudinal linear arrangement. The mucosa is formed by a stratified, squamous, non-keratinized epithelium, through which the mucous glands open, and is arranged in a series of longitudinal folds. The epithelium changes abruptly to cardiac mucosa[7] 1–2 cm superior to the lower end of the anatomical oesophagus, but merges with that of the mouth proximally. The muscularis mucosae, which is split in the upper part of the oesophagus, fuses in the middle and lower parts and is

continuous with the equivalent smooth muscle of the stomach.

The arterial supply is segmental and derived from the inferior thyroid, bronchial, left phrenic and left gastric arteries and from a series of small twigs from the aorta (Figure 2.1). There is a well-developed submucous venous plexus which drains into the thyroid azygos and hemiazygos veins and the left gastric vein. This constitutes an important anastomosis between the systemic and portal venous systems.

The lymphatic drainage from the upper third of the oesophagus is to the deep cervical, retropharyngeal and paratracheal nodes. In the middle third the drainage is to the paraoesophageal and tracheobronchial nodes and directly into the thoracic duct. The lower third drains towards the abdomen into the left gastric and pericardial nodes.

HISTOLOGY AND CELL BIOLOGY

The oesophagus is lined by stratified, squamous, non-keratinized epithelium. There is a basal cell compartment which forms up to 15% of the normal epithelial thickness.[6] Papillae (dermal pegs) with capillaries project from the lamina propria up to 33% of the distance towards the luminal surface.

Electron microscopy has delineated three layers of epithelial cells: basal, prickle and functional.[5] The deepest is the basal cell compartment, which is normally one or two cells deep and is the site of mitosis. In oesophagitis there is an increase in the volume density of the basal cell compartment and in the more severe forms a significant increase in tritiated thymidine labelling of epithelial cells in this compartment in response to cells shed. Increased papillary length helps increase the volume of this compartment by increasing the surface area of the basement membrane and the increased capillary length will increase metabolic exchange with the epithelium.

Above the basal cell layer, the cells differentiate in the prickle cell layer. Numerous desmosomes on cell processes give the layer its name and, together with abundant tonofilaments, its

mechanical strength. These suprabasal cells contain glycogen and small, round bodies, the membrane coating granules (Figure 2.2). Membrane coating granules also occur in the skin and in vaginal and buccal mucosa.[9] In the oral mucosa, their volume density rises to about 0.25%. They contain lysosomal enzymes, mucosubstances and a small amount of lipid. These are secreted into the intercellular space, where the mucosubstances form a partial intercellular barrier. A stimulus for their secretion is low pH. The process of exocytosis inserts new undamaged membrane into the cell surface; this can replace damaged plasmalemma, which may subsequently be retrieved.

Finally, there is the functional layer abutting onto the lumen and capable of withstanding mechanical, chemical and physical trauma from the passing boli of food and regurgitated gastric

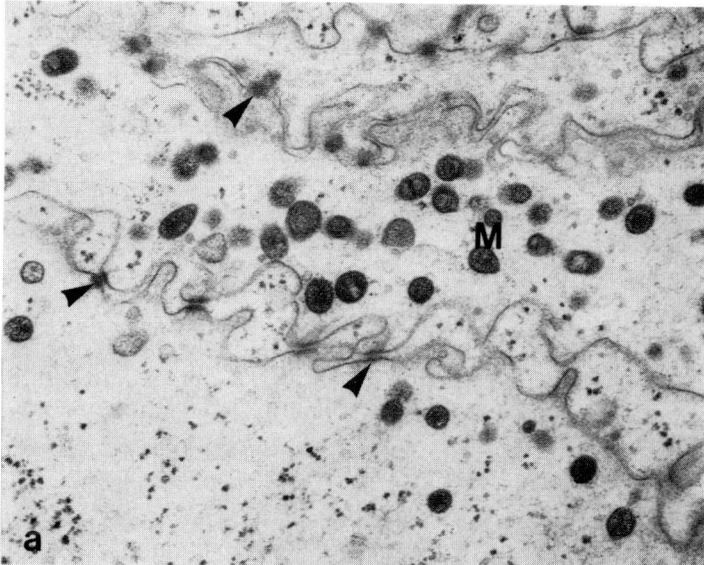

Fig. 2.2 (a) Several oesophageal epithelial cells from the functional layer from a patient with a mild oesophagitis. There are moderate numbers of membrane coating granules (M), showing variation in form but mostly with granular cores. In the intercellular spaces there are glycogen rosettes. The cells are held together by desmosomes (arrowheads). × 30 000. (b) Membrane coating granule (arrowheads) fusing with cell membrane in exocytosis. The intercellular space is marked ICS. There are abundant tonofilaments (T) in the cytoplasm. × 110 000. From Hopwood, Logan and Bouchier (1978),[5] with kind permission of the authors and the editor of *Virchows Archiv.*

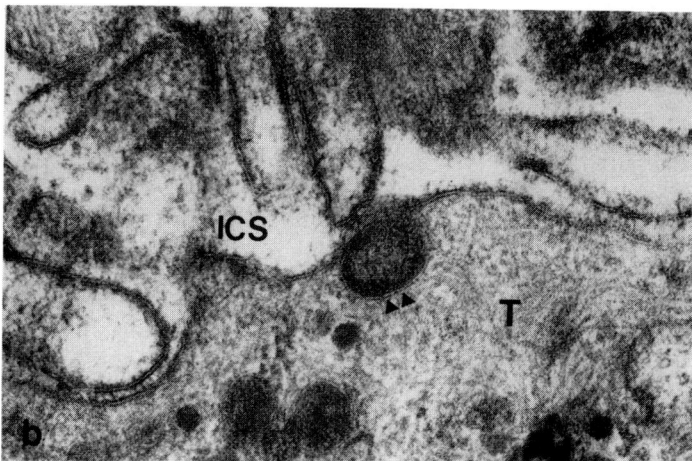

contents. The lowest 5 cm of the oesophagus is frequently subject to peptic reflux even in normal individuals and as a consequence shows evidence of damage. This may be produced by various proteases, lipases and the detergent bile acids.[2, 4]

Langerhans' cells may be seen not infrequently, and melanocytes are reported among the epithelial cells.

Histochemical techniques at light and electron microscopic levels have shown the presence of glycogen in the suprabasal epithelial cells. Neutral mucosubstances, including glycosyl and mannosyl residues, are also present in the glycocalyx. Neuraminidase-sensitive sialyl groups are also present. Incubation of biopsies with cationized ferritin, which labels the plasmalemma, demonstrates fluidity of the cell membranes and their retrieval.[5] Acid phosphatase and β-glucuronidase activity has been demonstrated in membrane coating granules. Amounts of triglyceride have been shown as fine droplets in the functional and upper prickle cell layers, although their role remains obscure.[5] By light microscopy, sugar residues in the glycocalyx can be seen to increase in amount as the cells differentiate towards the luminal surface.

Submucosal glands
The submucosal glands are similar to the mucus-secreting inner salivary glands, with myoepithelial cells and occasional oncocytes as well as the principal and subsidiary mucus cells of the acini.[1] No APUD cells are present.

Function

These morphological features may reflect defence mechanisms against refluxed gastric and duodenal juices, which rapidly produce marked damage to the oesophageal epithelium. An excessive loss of cells from the functional layer induces mitosis and extension of the basal compartment. Refluxing of hydrogen ions induces the exocytosis of membrane coating granules with the insertion of new membrane and membrane retrieval from the plasmalemma. The mucosubstances of the membrane coating granules also act as a partial barrier to the refluxing materials. Parakeratinization may be induced. Acid in the oesophagus also induces peristalsis, with subsequent clearance of the refluxed material.

REFERENCES

1   Al Yassin, T. M. & Toner, P. G. (1977) Fine structure of squamous epithelium and submucosal glands of human oesophagus. *Journal of Anatomy*, **123**, 703–721.

2   Bateson, M. C., Hopwood, D., Milne, G. & Bouchier, I. A. D. (1981) Oesophageal epithelial ultrastructure after incubation with gastrointestinal fluids and their components. *Journal of Pathology*, **133**, 33–51.

3   Hopwood, D, Ross, P. E. & Bouchier, I. A. D. (1981) Reflux oesophagitis. *Clinics in Gastroenterology*, **10**, 505–520.

4   Hopwood, D., Bateson, M. C., Milne, G. & Bouchier, I. A. D. (1981) The effects of bile acids and hydrogen ion on the fine structure of oesophageal epithelium. *Gut*, **22**, 306–311.

5   Hopwood, D., Logan, Kathleen R. & Bouchier, I. A. D. (1978) The electron microscopy of normal human oesophageal epithelium. *Virchows Archiv B*, **26**, 345–358.

6   Hopwood, D., Ross, P. E., Logan, Kathleen R. *et al.* (1979) Changes in enzyme activity in normal and histologically inflamed oesophageal epithelium. *Gut*, **20**, 769–774.

7   Lendrum, F. C. (1937) Anatomic features of the cardiac orifice of the stomach. *Archives of Internal Medicine*, **59**, 474.

8   Liebermann-Meffert, D., Allgöwer, M., Schmid, P. & Blum, A. L. (1979) Muscular equivalent of the lower oesophageal sphincter. *Gastroenterology*, **76**, 31–38.

9   Odland, G. F. & Holbrook, K. (1981) The lamellar granules of epidermis. *Current Problems in Dermatology*, **9**, 29–49.

10 Smith, B. (1972) *The Neuropathology of The Alimentary Tract*. London: Arnold.

CONGENITAL ABNORMALITIES

Congenital oesophageal disorders usually present in the neonatal period and the majority relate to the common embryological origin of the respiratory tract and oesophagus, to failure of recanalization or innervation or to reduplication.

OESOPHAGEAL ATRESIA AND TRACHEO-OESOPHAGEAL FISTULA

Oesophageal atresia occurs in approximately one in 3000 live births. Prematurity is common. Various lengths of oesophagus may be completely atretic and strictures in the distal third represent partial failure of recanalization. In 90% of cases of atresia there is a fistulous communication between a patent segment of oesophagus and the trachea or right main bronchus. Half of these infants have a congenital abnormality, frequently life-threatening, in another system. One-fifth of the other abnormalities are gastrointestinal and half of these are anorectal. One fifth have heart and major vascular anomalies, one-tenth genitourinary problems and the remainder have central nervous or skeletal anomalies, Down's syndrome or facial clefts. The VATER association describes the coincidence of vertebral, anal and radial anomalies with tracheo-oesophageal fistula. The abnormalities develop in the fourth to sixth week of intrauterine life, possibly as a result of external influences on the embryo. Familial associations are rare.

Clinical features and investigation

The relative incidences of the various anatomical arrangements of the oesophageal atresia and tracheo-oesophageal fistula are illustrated in Figure 2.3. The consequences of an obstructed upper segment of oesophagus are maternal polyhydramnios, dilatation of the segment with tracheal compression and overflow of frothy saliva, which drools from the mouth. Initially, the infant feeds eagerly, but regurgitates almost immediately through the nose and mouth and chokes. Pulmonary aspiration is a serious problem, particularly in the premature infant whose cough and swallowing reflexes are immature.

A 10 French gauge radiopaque infant nasogastric tube is passed into the oesophagus. The catheter normally arrests at 9–13 cm or it may curl. It is aspirated by syringe as soon as it is passed and every 15 minutes thereafter. A plain radiograph demonstrates the blind pouch. The safest contrast medium is air, 10 ml being injected down the catheter for the second radiograph, which is alateral. It is important to distinguish atresia from a long stenosis which can be treated by dilatation, and the air contrast film must be taken during head-down tilting. Pneumonitis is inevitable if an upper pouch fistula exists, but a fistula may be very difficult to detect because it is not constantly patent and visualization is not guaranteed even by opaque contrast radiography. Opaque contrast should not be used because of the risk of pulmonary aspiration. Inhalation from the nasopharynx will obscure evidence of a tracheo-oesophageal fistula.

The lower segment of the oesophagus is narrow, underdeveloped and usually in communication with the airway at the tracheal bifurcation or right main bronchus. The result is that the high airway pressure during crying inflates the stomach and intestines. Diaphragmatic splinting adds rapidly and dangerously to respiratory embarrassment. A thin column of air between the tracheal bifurcation and cardia may indicate the lower oesophageal pouch. Gastrooesophageal reflux is usual in neonates and in the presence of a lower segment fistula is highly dangerous because of the volume and high acidity of fluid which can enter the respiratory tract. Duodenal and small-intestinal atresia can coexist; in that event bile is aspirated from the trachea. Infrequently, the lower segment fistula is absent and consequently no intestinal gas is seen on the plain radiograph. If there is associated duodenal atresia the stomach is hugely distended with fluid.

Immediate management

Oesophageal atresia is an emergency which requires prompt recognition and efficient treatment. The upper oesophageal pouch must be emptied immediately and kept empty; in particular, the pouch is aspirated before any change in the baby's position and during transit. Body temperature is maintained in an incubator with a high humidity to facilitate clearance of airway secretions. The requirement to nurse head-down to drain the bronchial tree conflicts with the need to nurse head-up to reduce gastrooesophago-tracheal reflux through a lower pouch fistula. As a compromise, the baby should be nursed horizontally on its side, turning hourly. Gastric decompression is achieved at the earliest opportunity by a distally placed gastrostomy, with the tube left open to drain and with frequent aspiration by hand. Sump suction drainage of the upper oesophageal pouch is ideal,[10] but a sufficiently small catheter may not be available for nasal passage, in which case a lateral pharyngostomy may be used.

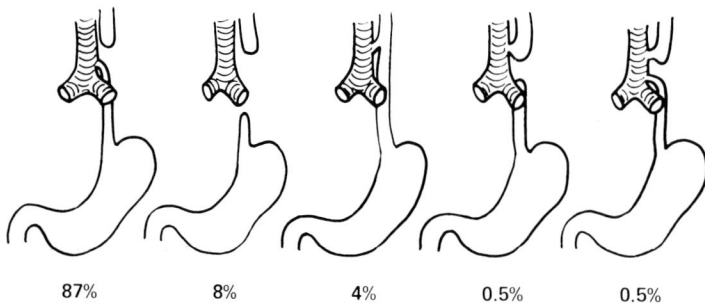

87%   8%   4%   0.5%   0.5%

Fig. 2.3   The various forms of oesophageal atresia and tracheo-oesophageal fistula and their relative incidence.

Respiratory distress requires oxygen, physiotherapy, intubation and endotracheal toilet. The bacteriology of the tracheal and upper oesophageal pouch aspirates is monitored and appropriate antibiotic therapy given. Fluid therapy is administered through a reliable intravenous cannula and intravenous feeding maintained until it is certain that there is no risk of gastrostomy feeds refluxing into the trachea and the oesophageal anastomosis is safe.

Specialist treatment

Babies must be presented to a specialist unit very quickly, and they should have as good pulmonary function as possible. The electrolyte, nutritional, blood volume and passive immune status is not as important as small size, prematurity, pneumonia, hyperbilirubinaemia and other congenital malformations, which militate against a successful result from surgical intervention. In a fit baby weighing over 2.5 kg a virtually 100% survival rate can be achieved after primary repair, but in smaller babies the success rate drops to 45%. The outlook is extremely poor for any baby with severe pneumonitis or serious congenital anomaly.[6, 13]

Surgical procedures

Freeman[5] has described the surgical techniques and their development. A gastrostomy is performed as an isolated procedure for the lower-end fistula. Most of the fistulas require thoracotomy for transfixion or suture and division and this is undertaken when the baby's condition is optimal. Primary anastomosis is performed in the fit infant in whom there is little separation of the ends of the oesophagus. Widely separated ends require a colonic interposition graft when the baby is bigger (10–15 kg); until that time the proximal pouch may be elongated by the regular passage of bougies. The distal pouch becomes dilated by repeated gastro-oesophageal reflux but it may be elongated by the passage of bougies through the gastrostomy. Further elongation may be obtained at operation by circular oesophageal myotomy. In this way it is often possible to avoid an interposition. Booss, Höllwarth and Sauer described the passage of a nylon 6 (Perlon) thread under endoscopic control through the gastrostomy, lower pouch, intervening connective tissue, upper pouch and pharynx.[1] Bougies were passed over this thread until the two ends were approximated and continuity of the lumen established by pressure necrosis. It may be necessary to control aspiration pneumonitis by cervical oesophagostomy, and a balloon catheter in the lower oesophageal segment can be used to control a fistula from the point of view of reflux and the lower-pressure leak in the respiratory system.[4] The postoperative problems which may occur are anastomotic leak and stricture, tracheomalacia, recurrent tracheo-oesophageal fistula, recurrent laryngeal palsy, incoordinated peristalsis or aperistalsis in the distal oesophageal segment, iatrogenic hiatal hernia, and reflux oesophagitis with a subsequent late stricture.

Isolated tracheo-oesophageal fistula

Isolated tracheo-oesophageal fistulas are commonly called H fistulas, but the letter N more accurately depicts the direction of the fistula, which passes downwards towards the oesophagus. The condition presents after the neonatal period and must be suspected in any infant who suffers recurrent bronchopneumonia and yet feeds normally. Respiratory distress occurs when the abdomen is distended. About 60% of these fistulas occur between the level of the seventh cervical and second thoracic vertebrae. It is therefore possible to repair them through a cervical incision. The greatest difficulty is in confirming the diagnosis: several techniques may be necessary. Bubbles can be observed oesophagoscopically during endotracheal ventilation, and cine-oesophagography and direct catheterization under vision may be successful.[3]

Laryngo-tracheo-bronchial clefts and 'oesophageal lung' are rare major anomalies. In the latter case the right main bronchus arises from the oesophagus and a pneumonectomy is required.

OESOPHAGEAL OBSTRUCTION

Congenital stenosis at the junction of the distal and middle thirds is relatively common and is diagnosed by an oesophagogram. It is suggested by dysphagia, regurgitation and aspiration when weaning commences. Food impaction occurs. There may be a web or a 2–3 mm long stricture and there is frequently an associated oesophageal motor disorder. Rarely, an intramural bronchial hamartoma is present. Spontaneous oesophageal rupture is uncommon but may be associated with distal atresia. Herpes simplex infection acquired during delivery or in the neonatal period can cause oesophageal stenosis at a later stage. Rare causes of obstruction are distal muscular hypertrophy, which requires the same treatment as hypertrophic pyloric stenosis, oesophageal varices, foreign body impaction and pharyngo-oesophageal diverticulum, which presents with a neck lump and dysphagia in the early months of life and is presumed to be congenital.

DUPLICATIONS

Spherical duplication cysts, called neuroenteric cysts, occur separately from the oesophagus in the posterior mediastinum or neck and are often an incidental finding. They do not erode vertebrae as do neuroblastomas, but vertebral malformations often coexist. Gastric cysts secrete and may perforate or fistulate into the oesophagus, skin or pulmonary system.

INFANTILE GASTRO-OESOPHAGEAL REFLUX AND HIATAL HERNIA

Gastro-oesophageal reflux is a common condition in normal infants but is a particular hazard in recumbent, retarded children and in cerebellar disease. Sandifer's syndrome describes reflux associated with involuntary torsion spasms of the neck and abnormal posture. A degree of cardio-oesophageal incompetence is normal but abnormal reflux is signified by postprandial vomiting, especially when lying flat. This vomiting starts soon after birth. Copious vomiting leads to failure to thrive and fluid and electrolyte depletion. Oesophagitis can be severe enough to cause haematemesis, but blood transfusion is rarely required. Severe oesophagitis with eventual formation of a stricture can cause dysphagia. Cot deaths could follow from reflex cardiac arrythmia caused by gastric content refluxing into the oesophagus.[11,12]

Pathological reflux can be confirmed by 24-hour pH monitoring[8] and this technique identifies those children in whom pneumonitis and bronchospasm is a result of aspiration of refluxed material.[8] Reflux should not be neglected: thickened feeds are given for mild cases, but if this is unsuccessful the infant is nursed day and night in a semi-sitting position. Suitable chairs are readily available commercially. A Nissen fundoplication is rarely required.

Hiatal hernia is not a prerequisite for gastro-oesophageal reflux. The oesophagus never appears tortuous when an axial (sliding) hiatal hernia is present and so it is commonly and incorrectly assumed that the oesophagus is congenitally short. Only rarely can the gastro-oesophageal junction not be delivered into the abdomen and then it is more likely that oesophageal immobility is due to postinflammatory mural fibrosis than to a congenitally short organ. Severe gastro-oesophageal reflux in young adults is frequently traced back to early life and 50% of infants with proven hiatal hernia still have the hernia or reflux many years later.[2,9]

REFERENCES

1 Booss, D., Höllwarth, M. & Sauer, H. (1982) Endoscopic oesophageal anastomosis. *Journal of Pediatric Surgery*, **17**, 138–143.

2 Carré, I. J. & Astley, R. (1960) The fate of the partial thoracic stomach (hiatus hernia) in children. *Archives of Diseases in Childhood*, **35**, 484–486.

3 Filston, H. C., Rankin, J. S. & Kirks, D. R. (1982) The diagnosis of primary and recurrent tracheoesophageal fistulas: value of selective catheterisation. *Journal of Pediatric Surgery*, **17**, 144–148.

4 Filston, H. C., Chitwood, R. R., Schkolne, B. & Blackmon, L. R. (1982) The Fogarty balloon catheter as an aid to the management of the infant with esophageal atresia and tracheoesophageal fistula complicated by severe respiratory distress syndrome or pneumonia. *Journal of Pediatric Surgery*, **17**, 149–151.

5 Freeman, N. V. (1969) Oesophageal atresia and tracheo-oesophageal fistula. In *Neonatal Surgery* (Ed.) Rickham, P. P. & Johnston, J. H. pp. 198–223. London: Butterworths.

6 Holder, T. M. & Ashcraft, K. W. (1981) Developments in the care of patients with oesophageal atresia and tracheoesophageal fistula. *Surgical Clinics of North America*, **61**, 1051–1061.

7 Jolley, S. G., Herbst, J. J., Johnson, D. G. *et al.* (1981) Esophageal pH monitoring during sleep identifies children with respiratory symptoms from gastro-esophageal reflux. *Gasteroenterology*, **80**, 1501–1506.

8 Jolley, S. G., Johnson, D. G., Herbst, J. J. & Matlak, M. E. (1981) The significance of gastroesophageal reflux patterns in children. *Journal of Pediatric Surgery*, **16**, 859–865.

9 Orringer, M. B. (1977) in discussion of Randolph, J. G., Altman, R. P. & Anderson, K. D. Selective management based upon clinical status in infants with oesophageal atresia. *Journal of Thoracic and Cardiovascular Surgery*, **74**, 335–342.

10 Replogle, R. L. (1963) Esophageal atresia. Plastic sump catheter for drainage of the proximal pouch. *Surgery*, **54**, 296–297.

11 Schey, W. L., Meus, P., Levinsky, R. A. *et al.* (1981) Esophageal dysmotility and the sudden infant death syndrome. *Radiology*, **140**, 73–77.

12 Schey, W. L., Replogle, R., Campbell, C. *et al.* (1981) Esophageal dysmotility and the sudden infant death syndrome. Clinical experience. *Radiology*, **140**, 67–71.

13 Waterston, D. J., Bonham-Carter, R. E. & Aberdeen, E. (1962) Oesophageal atresia. Tracheo-oesophageal fistula. *Lancet*, **i**, 819–822.

PHYSIOLOGY

MUSCLE AND MOTOR NERVES

The muscle of the pharyngeal wall, cricopharyngeus, and upper three centimetres of the oesophagus is striated, with motor end-plates connected to medullated nerves from the medulla (IX, X, XI). Tone or contraction is achieved and maintained by a stream of impulses discharged from the medulla. Relaxation requires the cessation of this discharge. The pharynx is a flaccid airway kept open by the pterygoid plates and the wings of the hyoid and thyroid cartilages except during a swallow. Oesophageal striated muscle is flaccid except for the duration of the passage of a peristaltic wave. By contrast the cricopharyngeus is contracted continuously by a stream of impulses which is interrupted for a fraction of a second to allow relaxation during the swallowing sequence.

Swallowing

A normal swallow sequence starts with the collection of the liquid or solid to form a bolus between the back half of the tongue and the hard palate. Loss of the front half of the tongue causes dysarthria but not dysphagia. The bolus is propelled into the pharynx by the back of the tongue, which is pulled upwards and backwards by the styloglossus. Once this movement is achieved the remainder of the swallowing sequence continues. The tongue and bolus push the soft palate against the posterior pharyngeal wall to close off the nose. The epiglottis bends backwards to provide a slipway for the bolus into the hypopharynx and to form a protective lid over the laryngeal vestibule which closes to prevent the bolus reaching the vocal cords. These also close to stop spill into the trachea.

Loss of part of the back of the tongue or loss of motor power or coordination by upper or lower motor neurone disease results in failure to propel the bolus into the pharynx and may result in inability to initiate the swallow sequence. A syndrome of failure to form and propel the bolus by the tongue without other neurological lesions results in an inability to swallow solids and to drink except in sips. The cause is unknown. If a solid bolus enters the pharynx without a swallow sequence being initiated the bolus is not propelled into the oesophagus and closure of the larynx does not occur. There is spill into the larynx and there may be spill into the nose.

Upper oesophageal sphincter

The upper closing mechanism is unexplained.[1] It appears to be 3–5 cm long from manometric studies; by radiology it extends about 2 cm, starting at the cricopharyngeus muscle, which is 5–7 mm long. Proximal to the cricopharyngeus the hypopharynx is closed by the elastance of the neck tissues holding the thyroid and cricoid cartilages against the vertebral column. Distal to the cricopharyngeus, radiological studies indicate that there is a closed segment 2 cm long which is outlined when air accumulates at the upper end of the oesophagus. The muscle fibres are not obviously different here, and this closure is probably maintained by the elastance of the neck tissues.

So-called 'reflex cricopharyngeal spasm'

Patients with an obstruction at the oesophagogastric junction may feel it is at the thyroid cartilage level. Some patients without any obstruction feel that they have a lump in the throat or that food sits in the neck. The sensation occurs when the bolus reaches the obstruction and not when it passes the cricopharyngeus. Those with a sensation but no obstruction have paraesthesia. In both instances the cricopharyngeus behaves normally.

Peristalsis

The body of the oesophagus and the lower oesophageal sphincter consist of plain (smooth) muscle, excited by postganglionic neurones whose cell bodies lie in Auerbach's intermuscular plexus and synapse with the ends of preganglionic neurones arising in the oesophageal plexus or in the medulla.[10] The postganglionic neurones of the oesophagus are the only ones attacked in achalasia, but in Chagas' disease all postganglionic neurones are damaged. There is no basal electrical activity or pacesetter in the body of the oesophagus, but the peristaltic sequence is precisely and constantly timed from the pharynx to its end in the cardiac sphincter segment. The peristaltic wave can jump a gap produced by transection of the oesophagus, suggesting that the sequence is determined in the medulla and not by myogenic activity or Auerbach's plexus.

Primary peristalsis follows the initiation of a swallow sequence by the tongue and is propagated from the pharynx into the cardiac sphincter. Although the wave is strong enough to close the lumen to make a gas and liquid-tight joint it often fails to propel a solid or semi-solid bolus.

Small flattened objects such as tablets and coins may not be moved by repeated dry swallows, but require a bolus of liquid to distend the oesophagus so that they fall down. They tend to stay just proximal to where the aortic arch or the left bronchus indent the oesophagus. Oesophagitis or stricture may develop if tablets are corrosive as they disintegrate.

Secondary peristalsis is a sequential contraction of the smooth muscle initiated in the oesophagus by a reflex within the oesophageal plexus activated by stretching the oesophagus. The wave starts at the point of distension. It is probably not important clinically. Tablets up to 15 mm diameter do not provoke secondary peristalsis, and a food bolus may have to wait for a primary wave. Small volumes of reflux do not provoke it, but gross reflux often does. In achalasia a constant writhing movement is common suggesting that contraction in one place displaces barium to another; this stretches the wall there and induces a contraction. This reciprocal movement is more likely to be a response of denervated plain muscle to stretch than a reflex.[2, 8, 9]

Lower oesophageal sphincter

The lower oesophageal sphincter has three states of tone – basal, relaxed and 'after-swallow' contraction. It is now doubtful that basal tone is controlled by circulating polypeptides or by a known cholinergic–adrenergic system. It may have its own basal electrical activity with a pacesetter. When a swallow sequence is initiated the basal tone progressively falls within two seconds reaching zero in four to five seconds, recovers in three to four seconds, to be followed by a contraction to about twice basal level in three to four seconds and a fall to normal basal tone in a further three to four seconds. This control is exerted by the medulla through the oesophageal plexus and continues after transection or atresia of the upper oesophagus in man. The neurogenic changes are not modified by therapeutic doses of drugs enough to be detectable clinically or to cause symptoms; for example, patients on ganglion-blocking agents or beta-blockers do not have dysphagia.[7]

LOWER OESOPHAGEAL VESTIBULE AND OTHER PHENOMENA

Examination of the oesophagogastric junction region yields observations which depend on the method used. Different descriptions with different names for similar structures have confused the literature. Understanding of barium shadows has reduced the structures to (a) the body of the oesophagus, which is flaccid at rest but supports the peristaltic wave when stimulated, and (b) the lower oesophageal sphincter, which forms the lowest 18 mm of the tube before it joins the bag of the stomach. The sphincter is contracted at rest and flaccid when stimulated.

Effect of loss of the peristaltic wave

Poor peristaltic activity or a dilated oesophagus is commonly seen at a radiological examination in the absence of relevant symptoms. A cardiomyotomy for achalasia removes the dysphagia, but does not restore the peristaltic wave. In systemic sclerosis the patient rarely has dysphagia until a peptic stricture develops at the oesophagogastric junction, causing obstruction. In both systemic sclerosis and postmyotomy achalasia the oesophagus does not empty completely because there is no closing force upon the lumen, and the difference in pressure between abdomen and thorax has to be overcome by hydrostatic pressure.

Effect of oesophagitis, corrosives, idiosyncratic reactions and neoplastic infiltrations

Peptic strictures and the deep ulcers of columnar epithelium do not disturb the capacity of the peristaltic wave or sphincter to close the lumen; fibrosis only reduces the capacity to stretch. Circular muscle, Auerbach's plexus and longitudinal muscle may be destroyed or temporarily damaged by swallowed corrosives. Any persistence of the peristaltic wave can be determined radiologically. Superficial lesions may stop peristalsis for days or the wave may be permanently lost. Postintubation strictures are an idiosyncratic reaction to the tube. A violent inflammatory and sometimes fibrotic reaction may extend through the whole thickness of the wall, stenosing the lumen. Peristalsis is lost initially. If it returns recovery is likely. Circumferential infiltration of the muscle wall and Auerbach's plexus by neoplasm stops radiologically visible local movement of the wall, but does not always prevent a peristaltic contraction below the tumour.

ELASTANCE AND COMPLIANCE

Compliance

The wall of the body of the oesophagus is flaccid except where a peristaltic wave is passing, and the circumference of the oesophagus while eating and drinking is about 45 mm (45 F. bougie). Dysphagia for solids occurs if it is less than 40 mm. The compliance of the achalasic sphincter is half that of a normal sphincter and offers no perceptible resistance to a bougie. Nevertheless, it causes severe obstruction to liquid and solids because the oesophageal force is inadequate to open it. The normal hiatus is compliant enough to expand to about 40 mm circumference when food is swallowed. The wall is contractile but compliant, and if sewn up too tight during a hiatal repair it may allow a bougie to pass easily but will obstruct food and liquid as in achalasia. In some peptic strictures and the perioesophagitis after a vagotomy, the compliance may be much less. Some surgeons define a stricture as something which obstructs a bougie; the patient defines it as something which obstructs food. The best assessment is by suitable radiological demonstration of the compliance to swallowed liquid and solid food.

Elastance

Compliance is the resistance to stretch of the tissue: elastance is the force tending to return the wall to its original length after it has been stretched. All obstructions in the pharynx, oesophagus and hiatus have some elastance. If the obstruction is caused by contraction of muscle, the lumen returns immediately to its previous size after dilatation. If inflammatory, fibrous or neoplastic tissue is the cause the lumen usually returns rapidly almost to its predilatation size. In a few peptic strictures the lumen does not return to its previous size.

THE ANTI-REFLUX MECHANISMS

There are two current concepts about the anti-reflux mechanism. One is that the lower oesophageal sphincter is the only component. A good sphincter is said to stop reflux both when the sphincter and some stomach are herniated and when the sphincter is in its normal position in the hiatal canal and partly in the abdomen. The good sphincter responds to the challenge of a changing intra-abdominal pressure by simultaneously contracting more than the challenge. This mechanism is thought to be mediated via the vagus and to be impaired by atropine.

There are many reasons why the 'sphincter alone' hypothesis is inadequate.[6] The alternative hypothesis suggests there are two components to the anti-reflux mechanism, one physiological and one anatomical. Correspondingly there are two kinds of reflux: physiological, which is normal, and anatomical, which is abnormal and responsible for the majority of reflux problems.

THE PHYSIOLOGICAL MECHANISM

The lower oesophageal sphincter has a squeeze of about 15 mmHg (2 kPa). Intragastric pressure is zero most of the time because the contraction which occurs is of a ring of muscle, with relaxation of the remaining part of the wall. Occasionally, and regularly after meals, intragastric pressure rises for a few seconds to 10–15 mmHg (1.3–2.0 kPa). If stomach squeeze (produced by contraction of the stomach wall against resistance to outflow and the remaining wall) exceeds sphincter squeeze, reflux could occur. An indwelling pH electrode shows that normal subjects reflux small amounts regularly after meals. Sphincter squeeze may have fallen or stomach squeeze risen, or both, resulting in *physiological* reflux.[3, 4] In this hypothesis the sphincter has a greater squeeze than *stomach* squeeze nearly all the time. In normal people reflux cannot be provoked by bending or lying or increasing *intra-abdominal* pressure, and cannot be seen in an X-ray examination.

THE ANATOMICAL MECHANISM

The anatomical, or hiatal, component of the anti-reflux mechanism, seems to be designed to protect the sphincter from being challenged by increased *intra-abdominal* pressure. That part of the sphincter that lies in the abdomen will be subjected to the same intra-abdominal forces as act upon the stomach. When the abdominal wall contracts, intra-abdominal pressure will not rise unless the diaphragm also contracts, and this also squeezes the gut going through the hiatus. The greater the intra-abdominal pressure the more will the hiatus squeeze its contents unless it is too wide to do so. As long as the hiatus is a narrow slit it will appose the walls of the tube of gut going through it so that they form a 'flutter valve' as the tube passes through the slit from a zone of high to lower ambient pressure.

These two mechanisms, the physiological and the anatomical, give rise to the two kinds of reflux. *Physiological reflux* is commonly normal but would be abnormal if there was an abnormally low sphincter squeeze, for example in systemic sclerosis, or an abnormally high stomach squeeze, for example in pyloric obstruction. *Anatomical* or *mechanical reflux* is always abnormal and depends on the degree of failure of the hiatal mechanism. This failure may be caused by naturally occurring enlargement of the hiatus, by tearing of the oesophageal attachments to the hiatus or by damage to the hiatal structures by a surgeon. Drugs which increase sphincter squeeze do so by 1.5–2 times and usually increase stomach squeeze. An increase in sphincter squeeze of 6–8 times is needed to protect the sphincter from raised intra-abdominal pressure.

RUMINATION

In some people the volume of refluxate or the force with which it occurs is greater than normal. Food repeatedly returns to the mouth after meals when standing or sitting. There is no capacity to herniate stomach or sphincter, the hiatus has a normal size and the reflux or regurgitation cannot be induced voluntarily by increasing intra-abdominal pressure on bending or lying; nor is it seen during a barium examination. Rumination seems to be an exaggeration of a normal phenomenon.

OTHER MOTOR MECHANISMS

Belching and aerophagy

Belching is the release of gas from the stomach, while aerophagy is the inflow of air from the mouth to the oesophagus and its immediate return. Belching is a mystery. It is not under voluntary control in its initiation, stopping or prevention. When a large volume of gas is released into the stomach neither swallowing, which relaxes the sphincter, nor deep inspiration, which obliterates the angle of entry, will provoke release.

Aerophagy has no connection with belching, although the subject has a paraesthesia or false sensation that there is some wind to get up. The stimulus and the receptor are unknown but there is commonly disease of the oesophagus or gallbladder or gastroduodenal pathology. Anxiety may enhance the sequence – patients may aerophage violently at the beginning of a consultation, ceasing as they become relaxed – but primary neurotic aerophagy is uncommon. 75–250 ml of air is sucked into the oesophagus by intrathoracic pressure in a fraction of a second. This is expelled abruptly as a belch or more slowly for oesophageal speech. The mechanism of opening the upper closing mechanism is the mystery. The air is not swallowed.

Clamping a cork between the teeth to stop the swallowing process, and holding the chin onto the chest to reduce mylohyoid activity will not stop aerophagy.

The air rarely enters the stomach unless the hiatus is enlarged; nor is there any flow of gas or liquid from the abdominal stomach with the belch unless there is hiatal abnormality. Some patients pump air into the stomach, distending it so that air enters the duodenum and is propelled into the colon, where it collects at the sigmoid flexure.

Vomiting

All necessary motor power comes from contraction of the abdominal parietes including the diaphragm and the pelvic floor, which preserves continence. Section of the vagus at the cardia does not stop vomiting or nausea. Barium may seem to move from the antrum to the fundus with the movements of retching but these movements are due to extragastric forces. The stomach has a passive role as a reservoir. Radiologically, retching is accompanied by a temporary herniation of the sphincter and a small loculus of stomach. This minor herniation may explain the small mucosal tears which occur in this region in severe vomiting (Mallory–Weiss Syndrome). How the anti-reflux mechanism is breached is not explained. The speed of events is that of striated, not smooth muscle.

Accessory movements of the jaw, neck, pharynx, tongue, and chest muscles are included in the motor discharge of vomiting. Closure of the nasal and laryngeal openings has been described, but vomit may come down the nose as well as through the mouth. The entry of vomit into the trachea is unusual and is then often by aspiration with inspiration after the emesis. The body of the oesophagus seems to be passive. Retching is movement of muscles without expulsion; nausea is sensation without movement. 'Projectile' vomiting occurs when there is not enough warning or control to direct it, but non-projectile vomiting is usually regurgitation 'in disguise'.

Patients use the term 'vomit' to describe the return of solid or liquid to the mouth, whether this is a powered projection by contraction of the abdominal wall, postprandial rumination, a gross failure of the anti-reflux mechanism during bending or lying, or regurgitation from an obstructed oesophagus.

The sensory input to the vomiting centre is not well understood. The 'chemoreceptor trigger zone' is sensitive to undefined circulating agents in biochemical disorders, inflammatory processes, and the effects of ionizing radiation, and to defined circulating agents such as drugs and oestrogen. The neural pathways mediating afferent impulses from visceral and somatic tissues and from pain endings are known to exist but are not defined. Distension of the stomach is not enough, because the patient with pyloric obstruction only vomits occasionally and the patient with bloat, whose stomach is tightly distended with air, does not vomit at all. Emetic agents and drugs which cause retching or vomiting as a side-effect act in different ways, on the nodose ganglion, the chemoreceptor trigger zone, and on afferent nerve endings in the mucosa of the stomach or duodenum and elsewhere. Control of vomiting and nausea is rarely possible but some reduction can be achieved by centrally acting drugs. The antiemetic phenothiazine derivatives appear to decrease the sensitivity of the chemoreceptor trigger zone. Drugs with sedative or depressant action on the nervous system may diminish nausea from agents acting on the afferent or central nervous system.

Distension, pseudo-bloat, hiccup, diaphragmatic tic and flutter

The diaphragm has a basal or postural tone, which can be over-ridden voluntarily and upon which is superimposed repetitive discharges from the respiratory centre causing the movements of respiration. The position of the anterior abdominal wall is varied by changing the postural level of the diaphragm without change in the volume of the contents of the abdomen; or by a change in volume with a fixed postural level; or a combination of both. Patients who complain of 'distension' rarely have any significant change in the volume of the abdominal contents. Those whose girth increases must reset the postural level of the diaphragm with a change in the postural length of the anterior abdominal wall which exhibits receptive relaxation.

Hiccup
Hiccup is a slow (about ten per minute) rhythmic discharge of motor impulses to either or both leaves of the diaphragm which cause an abrupt contraction whatever the phase of respiration or the postural tone. If unilateral it is caused by irritation of the phrenic nerve or the diaphragm. Commonly the contraction is bilateral; the discharge is then from the medulla and is accompanied by a synchronous contraction of

additional muscle units in most of the respiratory muscles. Blocking one or both phrenic nerves will only partially reduce the amount of movement. The cause of prolonged hiccup is usually central stimulation.

Diaphragmatic tic and flutter
Flutter is the manifestation of very fast rhythmic (about 200 per minute) discharges from the respiratory centre. In tic they are irregular in time and amplitude but average about 30 per minute. Both superimpose a contraction of the diaphragm and accessory muscles of respiration. The vigour of diaphragmatic movement upsets body posture causing writhing and twitching movements and a bizarre distressing appearance. Flutter may produce upper abdominal pain, and hiccup and tic may cause regurgitation, usually described as vomiting by patients. With each contraction, if hiatal herniation can occur, a loculus is blown into the chest together with a spray of gastric contents into the oesophagus. Gross oesophagitis may develop. The superimposed contraction causes erratic speech and ventilation.

THE SENSORY SYSTEM

Sensory endings are presumed to be present in the subepithelial layer of the oesophagus but have not been demonstrated with certainty.[10] The sensations attributed to the oesophagus are:
a   that called heartburn,
b   discomfort or pain when a bolus is obstructed,
c   discomfort or pain when the flow of liquid is obstructed and the subject drinks too fast,
d   the spontaneous pain of achalasia,
e   'tender oesophagus' pain,
f   'non-specific chest pain', 'oesophageal spasm', 'super peristalsis', 'symptomatic peristalsis',
g   paraesthesias of (i) food sticking or sitting or (ii) a 'lump' or (iii) 'having swallowed a boiled sweet',
h   'spasm' pain,
i   pain provoked by swallowing,
j   summation pain.

Distribution of sensations
All sensations are referred, either over a wide area similar in distribution to pain attributed to the myocardium, or to part of this area, or are highly localized. Even when localized, the site of referral does not correspond to the surface marking of the receptors except by chance.[5]

Heartburn

This term is used to indicate a sensation arising from oesophageal mucosal receptors stimulated by refluxing gastric contents. The receptors are not defined, but are not sensitive to radial pressure or stretch, osmotic pressure, human bile or most substances that go over them. They are sensitive to acids of pH 2.2 or less, alcohol stronger than 5–7%, potassium ions, emepronium bromide, some other substances in tablets at sufficient concentration, and probably to heat.

Bolus obstruction

A sense of food sticking may occur when food impacts at an obstruction, and there may be mild discomfort or a severe pain. Tablets and capsules do not usually provoke a sensation when they stick. A bolus of bread swallowed on top of the tablet may fail to push it through and not provoke a sensation. If a drink of water follows and fails to push anything through, the subject is aware of potential regurgitation.

Distension by food or liquids

When the outflow of liquid from the oesophagus is obstructed in achalasia, post-vagotomy dysphagia, a too-tight hiatal repair or neoplastic obstruction, drinking faster than the outflow causes a pain which persists until the contents of the oesophagus are reduced. A patient can distinguish this pain by character and distribution from other pains. The receptors are not known but are likely to be stimulated as a result of the distension of the oesophagus to its limit of compliance. Pain induced by distending a balloon in the oesophagus does not develop until the diameter of the balloon is 3.5–4 cm.

Spontaneous pain of achalasia

Occurs in 75% of patients with achalasia, commonly starting before the dysphagia. The receptors and stimulus are unknown. The distribution is often wide, from chest to ears, teeth and fingers; the duration is minutes to hours and it may occur at any time of day or night. It is not related to eating, drinking, posture or reflux. It is commonly relieved by drinking cold water and commonly but not always reduced in severity and frequency by cardiomyotomy. There is no good evidence that it is caused by muscle contraction.

'Tender oesophagus'

Which endings are stimulated and why are unknown. The whole or only a part of the oesophageal wall is sensitive either to stretch or mild pressure. The patient complains that swallowing lumps causes pain which characteristically persists for minutes to hours after the bolus has passed. Oesophagitis is not present but sometimes the oesophagus is heat-sensitive. Drinking may be painful, but slow sipping with small swallows is not. Distending a balloon to 1–2 cm diameter provokes the discomfort in the sensitive area.

'Non-specific chest pain'

This is a not uncommon syndrome of severe pain felt retrosternally, spreading out laterally, sometimes to the neck, shoulders and arms, lasting minutes to hours and usually attributed to myocardial ischaemia initially. Identifiable causes of chest pain such as myocardial conditions, gastro-oesophageal reflux, achalasia, diffuse spasm, costochondritis, cervical spondylosis, Tietze's syndrome and pericarditis are presumed to have been excluded by appropriate tests. Pope has described 'super peristalsis' as a cause, and Vantrappen and Hellemans call this 'symptomatic peristalsis';[11] others have attributed it to oesophageal 'spasms'. Nevertheless, the subject is able to eat and drink at the time of the pain without dysphagia or any effect on the pain. Although it is fashionable to attribute such unidentified pain to abnormal muscle contraction in the oesophagus, the case is not proven. 'Non-specific chest pain' seems a better name.

Paraesthesias

These are sensations that something is happening when or where it is not. For example, patients may feel that food is sitting in their chest like a lump of lead, that they have swallowed a boiled sweet that was too big, that they have a lump in their neck which makes them want to swallow or that there is something in their throat which is stuck and cannot be swallowed or washed away. Almost always these sensations are not hysterical, psychogenic or 'functional'. The stimulus, the site of the receptors and the pathway to the sensation are unknown. The sensation that food is sitting in the chest comes on 10–110 minutes *after* eating or drinking and is removed by eating or drinking. The 'swallowed a boiled sweet' sensation is present all the time but waxes and wanes in intensity spontaneously. It is momentarily lost, not aggravated, during eating and drinking. The 'lump in the throat which cannot be swallowed away' does not interfere with and is not aggravated or lessened by eating or drinking. 'Globus hystericus' is restricted to a transient sensation or reality of being unable to initiate a swallow, or a strange need to swallow during a moment of emotion, especially fear, or when distraught.

'Spasm' pain

'Spasm', either as excessive or inappropriately timed contraction or as a failure to relax belongs to the folklore of the oesophagus. It is supposed to be responsible for obstruction and for pain. The only inappropriate muscle contraction which causes obstruction is that of the sphincter in achalasia. Disorganized, spontaneous and stretch-induced contractions of the wall in achalasia and so-called 'diffuse spasm' occur most of the time and can be induced, but are not associated with pain and do not cause obstruction.

Pain provoked by swallowing

Pain provoked by a dry swallow may be synchronous with the pharyngeal phase; in this case it is caused by the remains of trauma, by acute thyroiditis or by inflammatory lesions attached to the pharynx or oesophagus, infected lymph glands, pharyngitis, and upper monilial oesophagitis. If the onset of pain is delayed after the pharyngeal phase it is caused by the movement of the peristaltic wave down the oesophagus, so that the duration of delay gives an indication of the level of the lesion.

Summation pain

Because the areas of referral of pain from the myocardium and the oesophagus are almost identical, subliminal stimulation of both is said to summate to a sensation in some patients with disease of both organs. The concept is clinically seductive but not proven.

THE MUCOSA

The epithelial lining is stratified squamous from the pharynx to the junction with a monolayer of columnar epithelium. This junction is a wavy line, commonly within 2 cm of the anatomical junction of the oesophagus and stomach, within the cardiac sphincter. The distribution of the lining epithelium is independent of the motor activity of the overlying muscular wall. This monolayer of columnar cells extends over the edge of the cardiac orifice and becomes continuous with the fundal epithelium about 1 cm from the orifice. The upper limit of the columnar layer may very rarely be within 1–2 cm of the pharynx, is occasionally up to the aortic arch, and more commonly in the lower third above the sphincter. When severe oesophagitis affects the squamous epithelium, tongues of columnar cells extend upwards from the normal 'Z-line' junction and are thought to be migrating cells replacing damaged squamous germinal epithelium.

Squamous cells are damaged by gastric juice, and scanning electron microscopy shows that acid will destroy the linkages between the surface squames so that they separate more easily. Bile has been claimed to damage squamous epithelium, although it is less active as a detergent at a low pH than at a high pH. The columnar cells are not damaged by gastric juice. They have a transmucosal electrical potential difference of about ten millivolts. Squamous cells do not have a transmucosal difference. This difference may be used to identify the squamocolumnar junction experimentally.

Peptic strictures always start at the squamocolumnar junction. If squamous epithelium is obtained from both sides of a stricture, the stricture is almost certainly not caused by reflux oesophagitis. Strictures are very rarely congenital; nearly always they are traumatic, caused by a tablet with corrosive contents (see p. 69) or by an idiosyncratic reaction to a nasogastric tube. The Schatzki-Kramer ring stricture always occurs at the squamo-columnar junction and is only 1–2 mm long, with a lumen between 7 mm and 15 mm in diameter (see p. 67). An increased resistance to stretch by food causes total bolus obstruction, but the ring is compliant enough to allow a bougie up to 20 mm diameter to be passed easily. It is not caused by muscle contraction, and is rarely if ever associated with histological oesophagitis or symptoms of oesophagitis.

Venous plexuses and haematomas

A submucosal venous plexus behind and below the cricoid cartilage may be damaged and bleed. A longitudinal or encircling haematoma may form, causing temporary dysphagia. Submucosal fibrosis develops as a sleeve in a zone about 15 mm long below the pharyngo-oesophageal junction. The cause is uncertain but it may be a result of bleeding from the venous plexus. Submucosal haematomas of the lower oesophagus tend to be longitudinal. These are distinct from varices, which are also longitudinal and submucosal.

SECRETION

Secretion by the oesophageal mucosa is minimal. Mucus glands occur under the lining epithelium, usually deep to the muscularis mucosae, with a single duct and multiple acini.

They may become infected with monilia (*Candida*), dilate and fill with barium during a barium swallow, giving the appearance called intramural diverticulosis. The infection with monilia may be secondary and not a cause of dilatation. Adenocarcinoma may arise in these cells. Exclusion surgery of the oesophagus does not usually produce a mucocoele. Mucus regurgitated from an obstructed oesophagus is mostly swallowed saliva which contains a thick mucus component as well as a serous component. 'Waterbrash' is hypersalivation, not a regurgitation of oesophageal mucus.

TECHNICAL PROBLEMS AND PITFALLS OF MANOMETRY

Manometry has been an essential tool in the past and there is still much use for it in research by those who do it themselves and know what they are doing. To make an intelligent and useful interpretation of a manometry tracing requires considerable knowledge and understanding of (a) how the oesophagus works, (b) what manometry can and cannot do and (c) the precise circumstances of the recording. It is neither necessary nor desirable for routine diagnostic use. The same knowledge and understanding applied to the radiological examination of the oesophagus will provide all the clinically necessary information that manometry might provide, and a good deal more besides. The interpretation of a manometry tracing should be checked by radiology.

Manometry is liable to artifacts and limitations of interpretation. Pressures in the pharyngo-oesophageal region during swallowing are impossible to determine because the pressure-sensitive holes of the manometer are fixed while the wall of the lumen moves 10–20 mm up and down over them in a fraction of a second. The cardiac sphincter moves 5–20 mm during respiration. Measured by radiology and at operation the cardiac sphincter is about 18 mm long but by manometry it is 35–40 mm. To detect peristalsis, two or more recording points are necessary. If the oesophagus contains liquid or gas a contraction of the wall produces the same change of pressure in all channels so no peristaltic activity will be recorded. Lesions causing obstruction to liquid, for example achalasia, carcinoma, post-vagotomy perioesophagitis, a too-tight hiatus after repair, benign circumferential ulceration of the cardiac orifice of the stomach or extrinsic pressure on the oesophagus or oesophagogastric junction, have non-peristaltic high-basal-pressure tracings. Failure of the cardiac sphincter zone to show a relaxation response to a swallow may be caused by carcinomatous infiltration as well as by achalasia.

There are many variables influencing a manometry tracing. 'Statistically significant' differences should not be accepted between groups of 10–20 subjects: several hundred are needed to determine if a pattern is clinically discriminative. If manometry is to be used as a diagnostic tool, the incidence of false-positives and false-negatives and the repeatability of the interpretation must be determined for each laboratory on a population of patients in whom the diagnoses are unknown but suspected. Such figures have not yet been published, but sphincter tone, for example, does not separate likely from unlikely refluxers in spite of earlier claims.

The greatest hazard of manometry is the production of man-made syndromes by the separation of a group of patients into a new disease entity by their specific pattern of pressure on a manometric record. The distinction between symptomatic diffuse oesophageal spasm and achalasia is man-made and not a natural event.

REFERENCES

1 Asoh, R. & Goyal, R. K. (1978) Manometry and electromyography of the upper oesophageal sphincter in the opossum. *Gastroenterology*, **74**, 514–520.
2 Christensen, J. (1976) The controls of oesophageal movement. *Clinics in Gastroenterology*, **5**(1), 15–28.
3 Dodds, W. J., Hogan, W. J., Helm, J. F. & Dent, J. (1981) Pathogenesis of reflux oesophagitis. *Gastroenterology*, **81**, 376–394.
4 Edwards, D. A. W. (1961) The mechanism at the cardia. *British Journal of Radiology*, **34**, 478–487.
5 Edwards, D. A. W. (1976) Discriminatory value of symptoms in the differential diagnosis of dysphagia. *Clinics in Gastroenterology*, **5**(1), 49–57.
6 Edwards, D. A. W. (1982) The anti-reflux mechanism, its disorders and their consequences. *Clinics in Gastroenterology*, **11**(3), 479–496.
7 Goyal, R. K. & Rattan, S. (1978) Progress in gastroenterology. Neurohumoral, hormonal and drug receptors for the lower oesophageal sphincter. *Gastroenterology*, **74**, 598–619.
8 Hellemans, J. & Vantrappen, G. (1974) Physiology. In *Diseases of the Esophagus* (Ed.) Vantrappen, G. & Hellemans, J. pp. 40–102. New York & Heidelberg: Springer-Verlag.
9 Meyer, G. W. & Castell, D. O. (1982) Physiology of the oesophagus. *Clinics in Gastroenterology*, **11**(3), 439–451.
10 Smith, B. (1976) The autonomic innervation of the oesophagus. *Clinics in Gastroenterology*, **5**(1), 1–14.
11 Vantrappen, G. & Hellemans, J. (1982) Oesophageal spasm and other muscular dysfunction. *Clinics in Gastroenterology*, **11**(3), 453–477.

MOTOR DISORDERS

The oesophagus may be considered as a muscular tube, closed at both ends by sphincteric mechanisms. The main function of the oesophagus is to transport swallowed boluses of food into the stomach and to clear the oesophageal lumen of any material that is left over after a swallow or has refluxed into the gullet. The active transport of a swallowed bolus is brought about by primary peristaltic contractions that begin as a centrally programmed sequence of contractions of pharyngeal and upper oesophageal striated muscles and progress down the oesophagus by a complicated and incompletely understood interplay of central and peripheral neural mechanisms, in which the myenteric Auerbach's plexus has an essential role. Lesions of the central nervous system, therefore, will affect mainly the function of the pharynx and the upper oesophageal sphincter (UOS), whereas disorders of motor activity of the tubular oesophagus are usually produced by lesions in the myenteric plexus.

The sphincters function as anti-reflux barriers. The UOS prevents reflux of oesophageal contents into the pharynx and, hence, aspiration into the airways. The lower oesophageal sphincter (LOS) has an important role in the prevention of gastro-oesophageal reflux. The mechanism of tone of the LOS is poorly understood but probably results from the integrated action of intrinsic myogenic characteristics and modulating nervous and hormonal factors.

These various motor functions are performed by the coordinated action of two different types of muscles: striated muscle in the UOS and the upper few centimetres of the gullet, and smooth muscle in the remaining part of the oesophagus and the LOS. Therefore, motor disorders of the oesophagus may be caused by striated muscle disease as well as by conditions affecting smooth muscle.

From a clinical point of view, normal oesophageal motility is characterized by normal peristaltic contractions, a normal LOS tone and complete LOS relaxation on swallowing. So far, manometric examination has proved to be the best, but still imperfect, way to study these events and to determine the degree of abnormality. A normal peristaltic contraction progresses in an orderly way down the entire gullet at a velocity of 3–4 cm/s in the lower half of the oesophagus.[36] The height of the deglutitive pressure waves depends on the recording system and the nature (whether dry or not) of the swallow. If miniature intraoesophageal pressure transducers are used deglutitive pressure peaks in the lower two-thirds of the oesophagus reach mean values of 70 mmHg (9.3 kPa) with dry swallows and 123 mmHg (16.4 kPa) with a water bolus.[42, 43] The duration should be less than 7.5 seconds (mean + 2 s.d. of normal value).[4, 59]

The LOS pressure is even more difficult to quantify because it depends on the location and radial orientation of the sensing probe in the sphincter. The normal value of the LOS pressure, as measured by conventional methods, is about 20 mmHg (2.6 kPa) above the fundic pressure. Complete relaxation of the LOS means that the sphincter pressure decreases to the level of the pressure in the gastric fundus. The fall in pressure begins within one to two seconds of swallowing and lasts until the arrival of the peristaltic contraction at the sphincter.

These three indices of normal oesophageal motility (peristalsis, sphincter tone and sphincter relaxation) may be disturbed in several ways in oesophageal motility disorders.[86] The peristaltic nature of the contraction wave may become lost. This often results in pressure waves which develop simultaneously or in a nonsequential way at different levels of the oesophagus and, therefore, have lost much of their propulsive force. The contraction may also be too strong and last too long, resulting in painful spasm or dysphagia. Contractions that are too weak will have little or no propulsive force. Other manifestations of disordered motility are 'spontaneous' motor activity (not elicited by swallowing) and repetitive contractions in response to a single swallow. Sphincters may be hypotensive and relax inappropriately, thus allowing reflux. They may be hypertensive and produce pain, or they may fail to relax sufficiently, so that dysphagia ensues and stasis develops proximally. In most cases of disordered motility, several of these abnormalities are combined. However, the combination is not always sufficiently typical and specific to be pathognomonic.

Oesophageal motility disorders have been classified as primary and secondary. In primary motor disorders the oesophagus is the site of major involvement; this group includes achalasia, diffuse oesophageal spasm and related motor disorders, as well as the conditions termed presbyoesophagus and symptomatic (or hypertensive) peristalsis (nutcracker oesophagus). In secondary motor disorders the oesophageal abnormalities are due to more generalized nervous, muscular, or systemic diseases, to metabolic disturbances, or to inflammatory or new growth lesions of the oesophageal wall.

PRIMARY OESOPHAGEAL MOTOR DISORDERS

Achalasia

Typical achalasia (also called achalasia of the cardia) may be defined as a disease of unknown aetiology characterized by aperistalsis in the body of the oesophagus and defective relaxation of the lower oesophageal sphincter, which is often hypertonic. Loss of propulsive peristaltic contractions together with defective sphincter relaxations cause stasis of food in a progressively dilating gullet. The oesophageal stasis is the common factor in most of the symptoms and complications of achalasia.

INCIDENCE

The incidence of achalasia is in the range of 1 per 100 000 population per year. The disease can occur at any age, but only 5% of the patients have onset of symptoms before the age of 14 years.

PATHOLOGY AND PATHOPHYSIOLOGY

The pathology of achalasia is still incompletely understood. Lesions have been demonstrated in the dorsal vagal nucleus,[13] in the vagal nerve fibres,[11] in Auerbach's plexus and in the oesophageal muscle.[80] There is pharmacological evidence of denervation.[50] Direct cholinergic stimulation by methacholine (mecholyl) results in a strong contractile reaction in both the oesophageal body and the LOS. The denervation, however, cannot be complete because a cholinesterase inhibitor (edrophonium) will increase the pressure in the LOS.[17] There is also pharmacological evidence that the non-adrenergic, non-cholinergic inhibitory postganglionic nervous system is impaired in achalasia patients. This system mediates sphincter relaxation in the opossum and may also have a role in the peristaltic progression of the oesophageal contractions.[22, 32]

SYMPTOMS

Dysphagia, regurgitation, weight loss and pain are the most important symptoms.[83] Characteristically, the patient has dysphagia for liquids as well as solids from the onset of the disease. This 'functional dysphagia' differs from organic dysphagia, which is initially for solids, and only later for both solids and liquids. The degree of swallowing difficulty varies considerably from

day to day, but tends to get worse with time. Prandial or postprandial regurgitation is often mistaken for vomiting. Retention of large quantities of food in a dilated gullet may lead to regurgitation when the patient is in the recumbent position or to aspiration in the airways and bronchopulmonary complications. The degree of weight loss is related to the severity of the dysphagia. Retrosternal pain occurs more often in the younger age groups and in patients with vigorous achalasia which is characterized by strong and often repetitive deglutitive contractions and by 'spontaneous' activity (not elicited by swallowing).[71] The frequency of these various symptoms is summarized in Figure 2.4.

DIAGNOSIS

The diagnosis can be made in most instances by radiological examination. Manometry, however, allows a better appreciation and a quantitative evaluation of the diagnostically important motor disorders. In doubtful cases a methacholine (mecholyl) test may be used.[50]

Radiology
Cineradiography may visualize the absence of peristaltic contraction waves and the disorganized and non-propulsive nature of the contractions. Because the lower oesophageal sphincter fails to open normally following deglutition, the head of the barium column takes a smoothly tapered 'bird's beak' appearance (Figure 2.5). The oesophageal body gradually becomes dilated and eventually elongated and tortuous; the gastric air bubble disappears. In approximately 20% of patients there is a symmetrical or asymmetrical dilatation in the narrowed sphincter zone that may simulate an ulcer niche.

Manometry
On manometric examination the deglutitive pressure peaks develop shortly after swallowing and occur simultaneously throughout the oesophageal body (Figure 2.6). In some patients progressive contractions still occur in the upper few centimetres of the gullet, corresponding to the striated muscle portion. According to the classical description the presence of normal peristaltic waves, even if rare, excludes the diagnosis of achalasia. However, it is possible that manometry within a dilated oesophagus may overestimate the incidence of non-peristaltic contractions. It is possible that weak peristaltic contractions produce simultaneous pressure peaks in a widely dilated gullet. After treatment the oesophageal diameter decreases in nearly

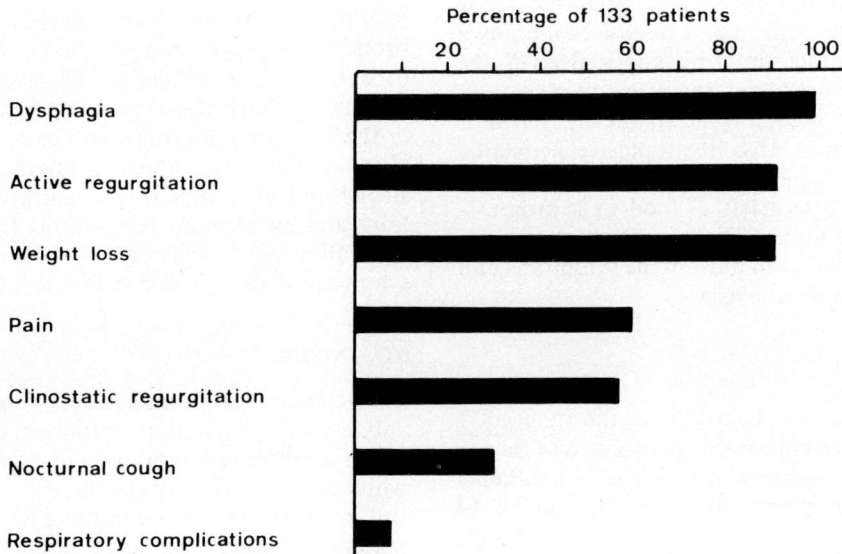

Fig. 2.4 Frequency of symptoms of achalasia.

one-third of the patients and peristaltic contractions may reappear.[89] These patients may represent the initial stages of the disease.

The amplitude of the pressure waves decreases when the oesophagus becomes dilated and they assume a typical broad-based shape. When there is 'vigorous achalasia'[71] the amplitude of the contraction waves is high, the pressure waves are repetitive, and spontaneous contractions occur. The motility of the oesophageal body and some clinical features of vigorous achalasia resemble the pattern of symptomatic diffuse oesophageal spasm. However, peristaltic waves are not seen, and the sphincteric relaxations are defective.

The resting pressure of the lower oesophageal sphincter is increased in achalasia.[16] Pressures above 30 mmHg (4 kPa) have been measured in 40%[6] to 90%[16] of patients. Furthermore, sphincter relaxation upon swallowing is incomplete (about 30% relaxation), in contrast to the normal sphincter, which relaxes completely. The residual sphincter pressure seems responsible for the obstruction to the passage from the oesophagus into the stomach.

DIFFERENTIAL DIAGNOSIS

A megaoesophagus with a smooth distal narrowing has been found in children with familial dysautonomia (Riley–Day syndrome), but in these patients oesophageal peristalsis is preserved.[46] Amyloidosis may cause a megaoesophagus which resembles achalasia both on radiological and on manometric examination; bulbar paralysis and intestinal pseudoobstruction can also cause an atonic oesophagus. In these instances extra-oesophageal manifestations will point to the diagnosis. In scleroderma the skeletal muscle portion of the oesophagus is usually not involved, some degree of peristalsis may be preserved in the smooth muscle portion, the oesophageal contractions are weak and the tone of the LOS is decreased. Barium is readily evacuated in the upright position but not in the recumbent position.

Carcinoma of the cardia may pose a difficult diagnostic problem. Oesophagoscopy with biopsy may be necessary to rule out carcinomatous involvement of the distal oesophagus. Endoscopy is also the best way to recognize car-

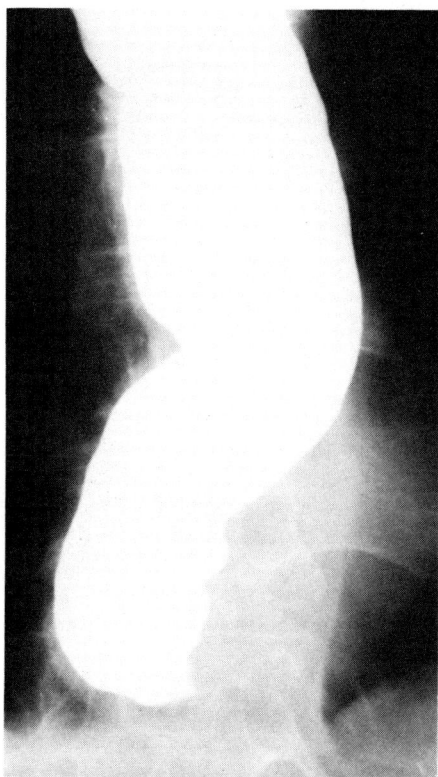

Fig. 2.5 X-ray picture of classical achalasia.

cinomatous change (usually in the body of the oesophagus), which may complicate long-standing achalasia.

Pancreatic, bronchial and gastric cancer and lymphoma of the distal oesophagus may produce an achalasia-like picture.[49, 81] The manometric features are identical to those in idiopathic achalasia, but the clinical history is slightly different. Patients are usually more than 50 years old, have a short duration of dysphagia (less than one year) and weight loss is prominent. The mechanism of this type of secondary achalasia is unknown.

TREATMENT

Drug treatment

Current treatment of achalasia is palliative and aims at improving oesophageal emptying by reducing the resistance at the cardia sufficiently to allow aboral flow but not gastro-oesophageal reflux. Several drugs, including anticholinergics, short-acting nitrites and gastrointestinal hormones, have been tried but are of doubtful value. The calcium entry blocker, nifedipine (30–40 mg/day) gave 70% excellent or good results in a group of 20 patients who were followed for 6 to 18 months.[8] Trials in larger groups of patients

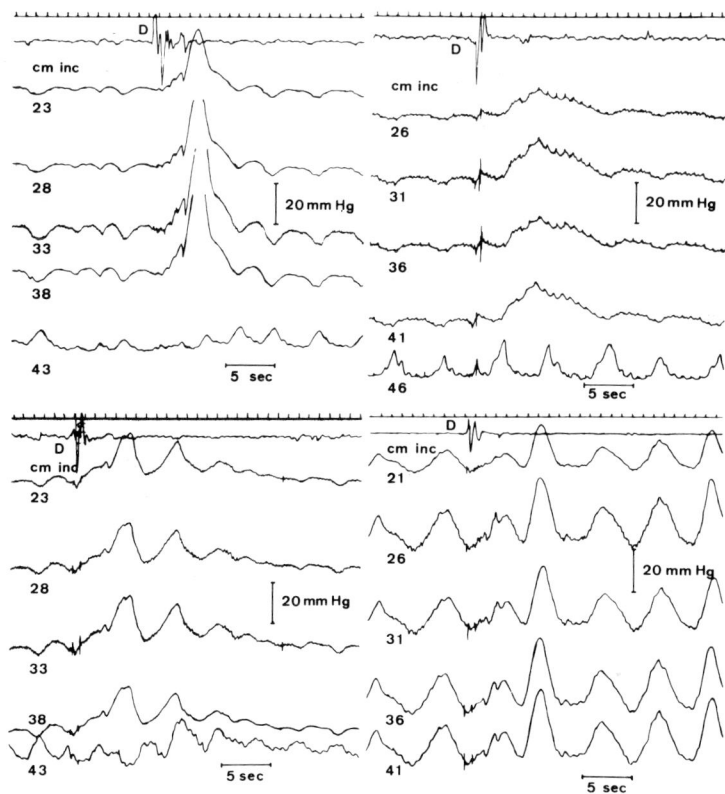

Fig. 2.6 Manometric patterns in achalasia (D, deglutition): (upper left) simultaneous waves of normal amplitude; (upper right) simultaneous waves in dilated oesophagus; (lower left) simultaneous repetitive waves; (lower right) vigorous achalasia.

Table 2.1   Late results of forcible dilatation in achalasia.

	Number followed up	Follow-up (years)	Symptomatic results (%)			
			Excellent	Good	Fair	Poor
Single hydrostatic dilatation						
Olsen, Harrington, Moersch and Anderson[63]	452	4–16	68.2		30.2	
Sanderson, Ellis and Olsen[63]	313	2.5	28.2	37	16	19
Progressive pneumatic dilatation						
Vantrappen and Hellemans[70]	403	7.8	37.5	39.5	8.7	14.4

and over longer periods of time are required to clarify whether drug therapy has a place alongside the two currently accepted forms of therapy, forcible dilatation and myotomy.

Dilatation
Most authors report excellent to good results in about 67% of the patients after a single dilatation with a hydrostatic or pneumatic bag of fixed diameter, while about 18% are not improved (Table 2.1). Treatment by repeated dilatations with bags of progressively larger diameter yields excellent to good results in 77% of the patients, whereas 7% are not improved.[86] The technique of progressive pneumatic dilatation consists of a series of two to four dilatations with bags of diameters of 3 cm to 4.5 cm. Disappearance of dysphagia, ease in emptying the oesophagus on fluoroscopy and, particularly, a substantial reduction of the LOS pressure are used as a guide to the required number of dilatations.[87] Contraindications to pneumatic dilatation are (a) poor patient cooperation because of young age or psychosis, (b) inability to exclude an organic stenosis, (c) the presence of lesions of the cardia or the stomach that make surgery mandatory, such as carcinoma, and (d) the occurrence of an epiphrenic diverticulum, which increases the risk of perforation.

The major immediate complication of progressive forcible dilatation is perforation at the lower end of the oesophagus. In the experience of the author this occurred in 13 of 570 patients (2.3%).[86] Conservative treatment with antibiotics and total parenteral alimentation produced complete healing in 10 of the 13 patients. Two other patients were treated by surgical drainage, and one patient died. The late results were excellent or good in 80% of this subgroup of patients.

Myotomy
The modified Heller procedure yields excellent to good results in 65% to 88% of the patients (Table 2.2).[86] The incidence of reflux and reflux oesophagitis (3–52%) has been sufficiently high for many surgeons to combine the Heller myotomy with an anti-reflux procedure. Excellent to good results are reported in 54–100% of patients treated in this way. Because the follow-up period of this type of surgery has not been sufficiently long and the number of patients so treated not sufficiently large, it is too early to draw firm conclusions on its value. Table 2.3 compares the results the Mayo Clinic group obtained by a Heller myotomy with the results obtained by progressive pneumatic dilatations in Leuven, Belgium. From these data it would

Table 2.2   Late results of surgery in achalasia.

	Number followed up	Follow-up (years)	Symptomatic results (%)			
			Excellent	Good	Fair	Poor
Myotomy						
Okike *et al.*[62]	456	6, 6.5	50	35	9	6
Akuamoa[1]	84	6	53.6	17.8	16.7	11.9
Black, Vorbach and Collis[7]	53	4	67.9	15.1		17
Barker and Franklin[3]	30	1	93.3	3.3		3.3
	14	10–20	35.7	28.6	35.7	
Myotomy + anti-reflux procedure						
Black, Vorbach and Collis[7]						
+ anterior suture	44	4	54.5	38.7		6.8
+ formal repair	11	4	100	0	0	0
Ribet, Callafi and Hamon[67]	45	2–10	38	41	21	

Table 2.3 Comparison of myotomy and forcible dilatation.

	Myotomy (Mayo Clinic)	Progressive dilatation (Leuven)
Number of patients with follow-up	427	403
Duration of follow-up	6 years; 6.5 years	7.8 years
Results: excellent or good	85%	77%
fair	9%	8.7%
poor	6%	14.4%
improved	94%	93%
Early morbidity (surgical oesophageal leak; perforation)	1%	2.6%
Mortality	0.21%	0.17%
Late stricture	3%	0.7%

seem reasonable to perform forcible dilatations as the initial treatment (provided that there are no contraindications) and to reserve cardio-myotomy (with or without an anti-reflux procedure) for those patients who failed to benefit from dilatation.

Symptomatic diffuse oesophageal spasm

Symptomatic diffuse oesophageal spasm (SDOS) is characterized by clinical symptoms of intermittent chest pain, dysphagia or both in the absence of a demonstrable organic lesion, and by abnormal non-peristaltic contractions on manometry or radiological examination.[23, 28, 31] Motor disturbances in asymptomatic subjects may resemble closely those found in SDOS. It is not known in what way the symptomatic subjects are different, and to what extent the motor disorders in both groups can be distinguished, so the term 'asymptomatic diffuse spasm'[53, 69] should be used with caution. The relationship between diffuse oesophageal spasm and acid sensitivity of the oesophagus remains to be established. The distinction between 'asymptomatic diffuse spasm' and 'presbyoesophagus' is also difficult to make (see below).

INCIDENCE

Typical diffuse spasm is a rare disorder, being less than one-fifth as frequent as achalasia. It can occur in either sex and at any age, but is more common in individuals over 50.

PATHOLOGY

The pathology of diffuse oesophageal spasm is incompletely understood. Although ganglionic cells are present in Auerbach's plexus,[69] there is a local infiltrate of chronic inflammatory cells in and sometimes around the plexus.[61] Electron-microscopic examination of four patients with severe diffuse spasm showed Wallerian degeneration in the oesophageal branches of the vagus nerves and generalized degenerative changes of the Wallerian type in many axons.[12] The differences between achalasia and diffuse oesophageal spasm may be quantitative rather than qualitative.

PATHOPHYSIOLOGY

The oesophageal motility disorders of patients with diffuse oesophageal spasm are less severe than those of achalasia patients. The oesophagus has not completely lost the capacity to produce normal peristaltic contractions and normal LOS relaxation. In the typical patient peristalsis progresses in a normal way from the pharynx along the oesophagus over a length of several centimetres. Once in the middle third of the gullet the peristaltic contraction is replaced by 'tertiary contractions', which develop simultaneously over the entire length of the remaining distal oesophagus. The tertiary contractions of diffuse oesophageal spasm often produce pressure waves of high amplitude and longer duration. Not infrequently deglutition results in repetitive contractions (several waves in response to a single swallow).[19] Sometimes the peristaltic progression is interrupted in a segment of several centimetres and reappears in the more distal part of the oesophagus.

The propulsion of the swallowed bolus may be hindered by 'spastic' tertiary contractions that obliterate the lumen prior to the passage of the bolus. This is one mechanism for dysphagia, another being defective relaxation of the LOS. Pain is probably produced by strong contractions following deglutition or occurring 'spontaneously'.

Sphincter disorders can occur as apparently isolated motor abnormalities in patients with clinical symptoms of retrosternal pain or dysphagia. Several abnormalities have been described including a hypertensive sphincter[15, 88] and hyper-reacting sphincter.[29] However, the peristaltic amplitude of the oesophageal contraction has not been measured accurately in most of these patients.

SYMPTOMS

Most patients have both pain and dysphagia; these occur intermittently and vary from being mild and occasional to severe and daily. The pain is precipitated by a meal in approximately 50% of patients, is often associated with dysphagia, and may worsen during periods of emotional stress. However, the pain may be unrelated to meals, occur at night and mimic pain of myocardial origin. Both types of pain are relieved by glycerol trinitrate (nitroglycerin).

The dysphagia is of variable severity and lacks the persistence seen in achalasia or organic stenosis. One of the main problems is the relation between symptomatic diffuse oesophageal spasm and acid sensitivity. Both conditions may coexist. Twenty-four-hour pH and pressure monitoring may prove to be useful for the recognition of pain of oesophageal origin and for the identification of spasm or gastro-oesophageal reflux as the cause of pain.

DIAGNOSIS

The diagnosis of SDOS is based on a combination of clinical symptoms and a poorly defined complex of manometric abnormalities

(Figure 2.7) in a gullet which has not completely lost its capability to produce peristaltic contractions and LOS relaxations.

MANOMETRY

There are no uniform, generally accepted criteria for the manometric diagnosis of diffuse oesophageal spasm. The following criteria have been proposed.

1 Thirty per cent of the deglutitive responses should consist of simultaneous waves of high amplitude and long duration.[23, 59] A mean duration of 7.5 seconds has been proposed as the definition of prolonged contractions, because this value is greater than the mean + 2 s.d. in normal subjects.[4, 59] The concept of 'high amplitude' has not yet been well defined. However, with intraluminal transducers or a low compliance perfusion system and wet swallows, pressure peaks of 100 mmHg (13 kPa) or more are generally considered to be of high amplitude.
2 Repetitive waves (several pressure peaks in response to a single swallow) are seen in the majority (56–95%) of patients,[31, 69] and 'spontaneous' contractions (not induced by swallows) occur in more than half of these patients.[59]
3 Interrupted peristalsis was observed in 7 of 12 patients with diffuse oesophageal spasm, and abnormally slow distal progression (0.8–1.5 cm/s) occurred in 6.[47]

RADIOLOGY

The radiological appearance of symptomatic diffuse oesophageal spasm (Figure 2.8) is described as 'curling', 'segmental spasm', 'ladder spasm', 'rosary bead oesophagus', 'spastic pseu-

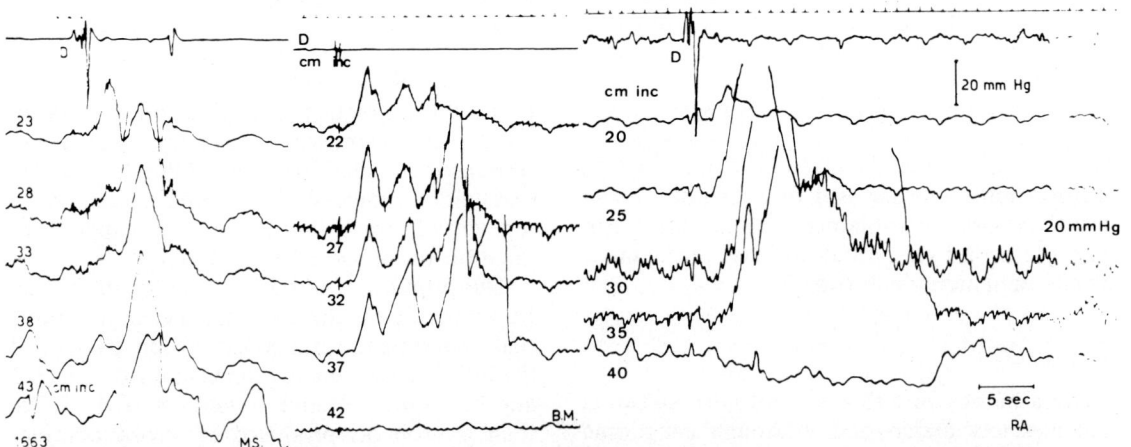

Fig. 2.7 Manometric patterns in diffuse oesophageal spasm (D, deglutition): (left) peristaltic waves becoming simultaneous in the distal oesophagus; (centre) repetitive waves; (right) peristaltic 'giant' waves.

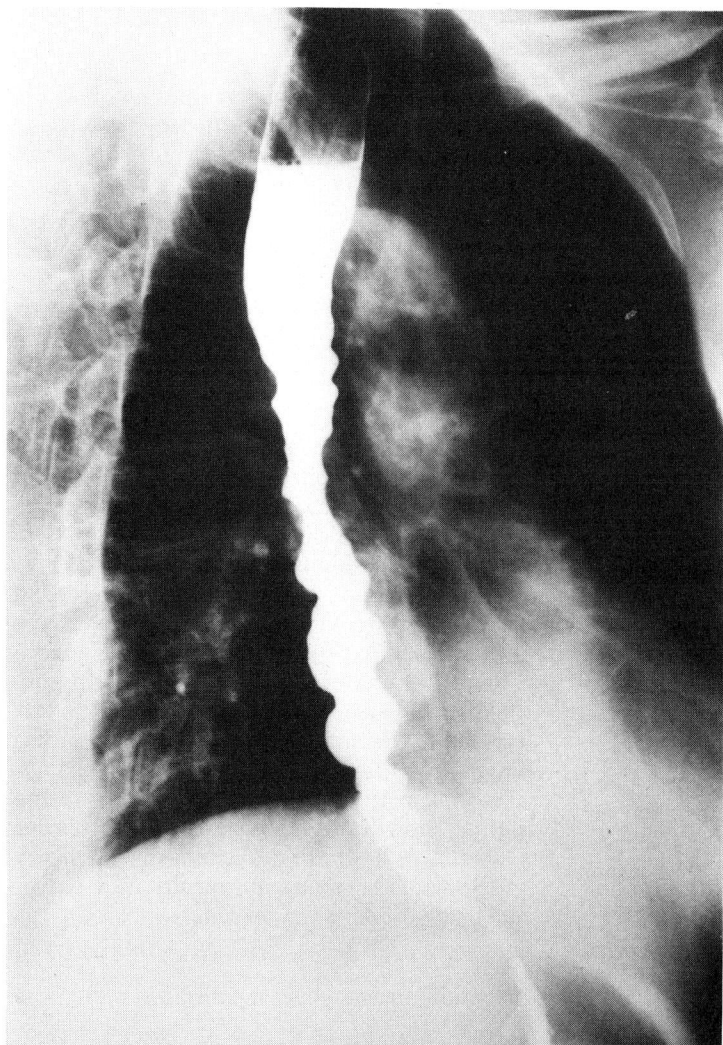

Fig. 2.8　X-ray pictures of diffuse oesophageal spasm.

dodiverticulosis', 'corkscrew oesophagus', and so on. These terms refer to segmental, non-peristaltic contractions, which may trap the barium and push it back and forth. This is best demonstrated when the patient is in the recumbent position. A second, but less common, picture is a tight contraction of the oesophagus over a length of several centimetres or a slight diffuse narrowing of the lower half of the oesophagus with a slightly dilated upper segment.[84] Marked dilatation of the oesophagus and prolonged stasis of food and fluids are rare in diffuse spasm.

The extent and severity of the radiological abnormalities may vary widely from patient to patient and from one time to another in the same patient.[5] The severity of the radiological changes correlates poorly with the clinical, manometric or pathological findings. Patients with diffuse oesophageal spasm may appear normal on routine radiological examination, and 'typical' radiological pictures may occur in asymptomatic patients (mainly the elderly) or in patients with diffuse spasm at a symptom-free moment.

DIAGNOSTIC TESTS

The lack of strict diagnostic criteria and the need to distinguish diffuse spasm from achalasia on the one hand and from non-specific or asymptomatic motor disorders on the other, make provocation tests highly desirable. The oesophagus of many patients with symptomatic diffuse oesophageal spasm is hypersensitive to cholinergics such as methacholine (mecholyl)[53] and bethanechol[59] and is also hypersensitive to the cholinesterase inhibitor edrophonium chloride.[59] The methacholine test, however, is also positive in patients with primary achalasia, those with Chagas' disease and in some patients with carcinomatous infiltration of Auerbach's plexus.[40] The test can be useful to distinguish diffuse spasm from asymptomatic similar motor disorders[51] and from reflux-related spasm.[59] The oesophagus of patients with diffuse spasm has been reported to be supersensitive to pentagastrin or gastrin administration.[26, 54] In later studies the pentagastrin test proved to be disappointing because it was often negative in patients with symptomatic diffuse oesophageal spasm and positive in patients with achalasia[64] and in some elderly patients.[34]

Ergometrine (ergonovine) maleate, an alpha-adrenergic agonist, has been used as a provocative test for coronary artery spasm[41] and for oesophageal spasm.[21] However, serious side-effects may occur and the test should not be used in routine medicine.

TREATMENT

The drug treatment of symptomatic diffuse oesophageal spasm is disappointing; anticholinergics, nitrites and calcium entry blockers have been used with moderate success. If patients with severe symptoms fail to respond to medical therapy, pneumatic dilatations may be performed but this is less successful than in achalasia,[86] and influences the dysphagia rather than the pain. Severely affected patients may benefit from a long oesophago-myotomy,[39, 55] but here again the results cannot equal those obtained in achalasia. The myotomy can be complemented by an anti-reflux procedure. However, some reservations have been expressed about the routine addition of an anti-reflux procedure, except in cases of hiatal hernia.[55]

Primary oesophageal motility disorders of the intermediate type

Although achalasia and symptomatic diffuse oesophageal spasm have distinctive properties, a number of patients do not fit into this simple classification. Some patients who would otherwise fit the criteria have occasional peristaltic waves or sphincter relaxations. Up to 24% of those with motility disorders severe enough to justify treatment with dilatation do not fit well into the two classic categories.[89] Furthermore, after dilatation as many as 45% of the patients fell into the intermediate category. These patients presented with either complete absence of peristalsis and the presence of (at least some) normal lower oesophageal sphincter relaxations, or with some degree of peristalsis and complete absence of normal lower oesophageal sphincter relaxation. These observations suggest that the primary oesophageal motility disorders constitute a spectrum of motor disorders composed of achalasia, diffuse spasm and intermediate types (Figure 2.9).[89] Moreover, transition from symptomatic diffuse oesophageal spasm to achalasia has been documented,[51, 89] although most patients with diffuse spasm remain unchanged over long periods of time. Radiological examination shows an oesophagus that resembles achalasia rather than diffuse spasm. Treatment with pneumatic dilatation results in a success rate comparable to that of achalasia.

Symptomatic oesophageal peristalsis

The development of measurement systems able to pick up rapid pressure rises has enabled different investigators to identify patients with

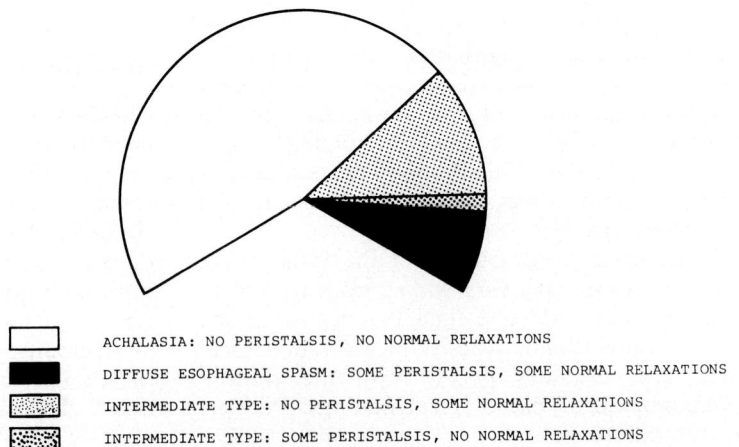

Fig. 2.9 Spectrum of primary oesophageal motility disorders.

☐ ACHALASIA: NO PERISTALSIS, NO NORMAL RELAXATIONS

■ DIFFUSE ESOPHAGEAL SPASM: SOME PERISTALSIS, SOME NORMAL RELAXATIONS

▨ INTERMEDIATE TYPE: NO PERISTALSIS, SOME NORMAL RELAXATIONS

▨ INTERMEDIATE TYPE: SOME PERISTALSIS, NO NORMAL RELAXATIONS angina-like chest pain that is caused by peristaltic contractions of increased amplitude or duration. Brand, Martin and Pope examined 43 patients with chest pain but no evidence of coronary heart disease.[9] Of 14 patients with pain of oesophageal origin one had achalasia and three met the criteria of diffuse spasm, but nine had disorders of amplitude and one a disorder of duration of peristalsis. Increased amplitude and duration occurred together in most patients. These abnormalities may be present only intermittently, for example during an episode of chest pain.

The criteria proposed for the diagnosis of symptomatic oesophageal peristalsis are a mean amplitude above 120 mmHg (16 kPa) in the lower third of the oesophagus or a peak pressure above 200 mmHg (27 kPa).[4, 66] A reasonable criterion for prolonged contraction is a duration time that equals or exceeds the normal mean + 2 s.d. (i.e. 7.5 seconds).[59] The relationship of symptomatic oesophageal peristalsis to reflux and to symptomatic diffuse oesophageal spasm has still to be defined. Some patients develop a manometric tracing consistent with symptomatic diffuse oesophageal spasm after acid perfusion or improve with antacids. However, as long as the mechanism of pain is not clearly defined, it is confusing to include patients with chest pain and 'giant' simultaneous waves characteristic of diffuse oesophageal spasm in this category. It would seem wise to limit the term 'symptomatic oesophageal peristalsis' to patients with vigorous peristalsis without vigorous tertiary contraction. Ergometrine (ergonovine), by acting via an alpha-adrenergic receptor, precipitates the pain in these patients. These pain attacks are related to the time of occurrence of high-amplitude and long-duration peristaltic waves.[9]

Treatment is not very satisfactory. Clinical improvement has been obtained with nitrates, hydralazine and calcium entry blockers. The results, however, are disappointing.

Presbyoesophagus

Manometric studies of elderly subjects have shown an increase in non-peristaltic contractions after deglutition.[45, 92] Many deglutitions are followed by repetitive waves, and spontaneous contractions may occur independently of swallowing.[37, 76] These abnormalities are found mainly in the lower third of the oesophagus and to a lesser degree in the middle third. Older people, however, show an increased incidence of diabetes mellitus, neuropathies, gastro-oesophageal reflux and neurological disorders, all of which can affect oesophageal motility. It has not yet been firmly established to what degree these motor abnormalities are due to the advanced age itself or to associated conditions.

SECONDARY OESOPHAGEAL MOTOR DISORDERS

Various generalized diseases may cause motor disorders of the oesophagus (Table 2.4), but only some of these will be discussed here.

Systemic sclerosis and other collagen diseases

The oesophagus is abnormal in 50–80% of patients with scleroderma;[38] the degree of oesophageal involvement bears no relation to the degree of involvement of other organs. Sometimes the skin lesions improve while the oesophageal involvement progresses. Histological studies of the oesophagus show that the smooth muscle layers are atrophied with some fibrous replacement while the striated muscle fibres are remarkably well preserved.[2, 20, 25, 79] Inflammatory and fibrous changes also occur in the mucosa and submucosa. At least some of the mucosal lesions are due to gastro-oesophageal reflux. Intraluminal pressure measurements indicate that peristalsis usually remains normal

Table 2.4 Diseases causing oesophageal motility disorders.

Collagen diseases	*Central nervous system diseases*
Systemic sclerosis	Brainstem lesions
Systemic lupus erythematosus	Poliomyelitis
Polymyositis–dermatomyositis	Motor neurone disease
	Extrapyramidal disturbances
Muscle diseases	Stiff-man (Moersch–Woltmann) syndrome
Myotonic dystrophy	Dysautonomia
Ocular and oculopharyngeal myopathy	Intestinal pseudo-obstruction
Myasthenia gravis	
	Peripheral neuropathies
	Diabetic neuropathy
	Alcoholic neuropathy

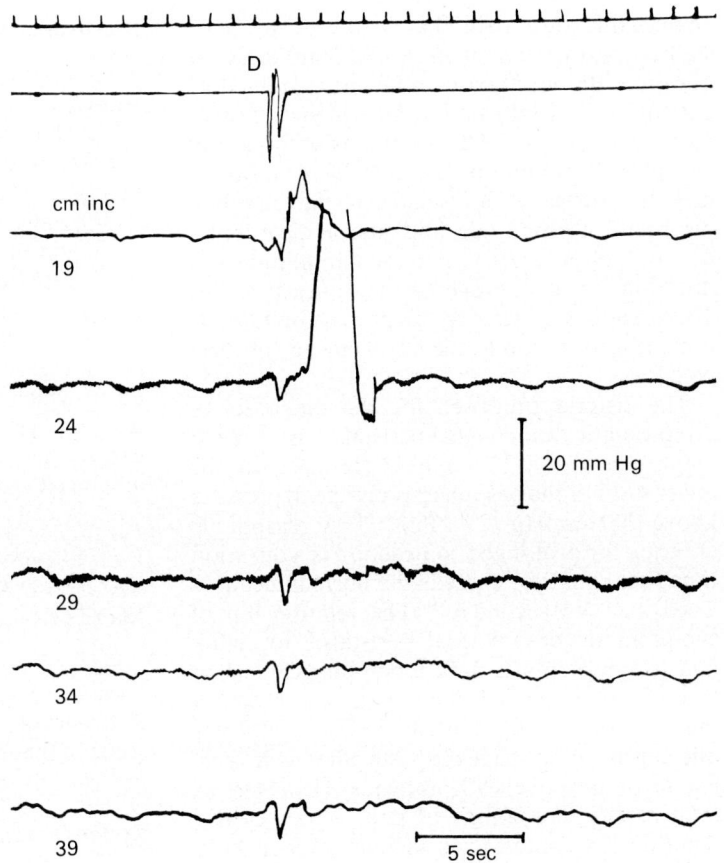

Fig. 2.10 Manometric pattern of oesophageal motility in scleroderma. Normal peristaltic contractions in the upper part; absence of deglutitive response in the lower part.

in the upper, striated portion of the gullet, whereas in the smooth muscle portion the contractions are often non-peristaltic, weak and may eventually disappear completely (Figure 2.10).[30, 82] The LOS pressure is frequently lower than normal, which may lead to gastro-oesophageal reflux and oesophagitis. The loss of coordinated peristalsis in the distal oesophagus is fairly well correlated with the development of Raynaud's phenomenon.[77] Dysfunction of Auerbach's plexus is assumed to be the cause of this coordination. The loss of contractile strength of the LOS and distal oesophagus is unrelated to Raynaud's phenomenon.

It is unlikely that muscle atrophy is responsible for the motor disturbances in the early stages of the disease. In cases of aperistalsis the sphincter muscle contracts normally on direct stimulation but responds poorly to edrophonium. Although in most patients the intramural ganglion cells appear normal, the loss of peristaltic progression, the occurrence of motor disorders without muscle atrophy and the pharmacological observations suggest that neural dysfunction has a role.[18] In advanced cases

radiological examination reveals a slightly dilated gullet, often with a patulous LOS and gastro-oesophageal reflux. The contractions are weak and frequently non-peristaltic and emptying is delayed in the recumbent position.

The oesophagus is involved in 10–25% of patients with systemic lupus erythematosus. The motility disorders resemble those of systemic sclerosis but are less pronounced.[77]

More than 60% of patients with dermatomyositis or polymyositis complain of high dysphagia.[14, 24, 65] The degree of dysphagia parallels the course and severity of the muscle involvement. Initially the motility disturbances are most prominent in the pharynx and upper oesophagus; later, smooth muscles are involved as well. Weakness of oesophageal contractions often leads to tracheal aspiration and nasal reflux. Radiological examination reveals an atonic upper oesophageal sphincter, and pooling of barium in the valleculae and pyriform sinuses. When the lower oesophagus is involved the contractions become weak and non-peristaltic and the LOS pressure decreases, which may lead to reflux oesophagitis.

Muscle disease

Myotonia dystrophica, myotonic dystrophy or Steinert's disease is a familial disease characterized by the continued active contraction of a muscle, persisting after the cessation of voluntary effort or stimulation, and by muscle weakness and wasting. The disease affects mainly the muscles of the hands and feet and the facial, ocular and oropharyngeal muscles. The most telling symptom is a slowness of relaxation after a forceful contraction such as a handshake. Lesions of striated muscles of the pharynx and oesophagus have been observed in virtually all cases examined, while dysfunction of the smooth oesophageal musculature is found in at least half of the patients.[35, 74]

About half of the patients with *ocular myopathy* have swallowing difficulties, which often develop a few years after the initial sign of the disease (usually ptosis). In patients with *oculopharyngeal dystrophy* the swallowing difficulties are more prominent and may precede, as well as follow, the ptosis.[10, 68, 90] Initially, the pharynx and upper oesophagus are involved; later the entire oesophagus may show weak contractions and disordered peristalsis. The pharynx and oesophagus are frequently involved in *myasthenia gravis*, when the resting pressure in the upper oesophageal sphincter is decreased and the contraction waves of pharynx, sphincter and upper oesophagus are weak.[27, 52, 60] The strength of the contractions rapidly decreases upon repeated deglutitions, as in other involved muscles. The dysfunction can be partially corrected by the administration of 2–8 mg of edrophonium, a drug with anticholinesterase activity.[60] The smooth muscles of the gullet may be involved and are not improved by edrophonium.

Lesions of the central nervous system

Unilateral *cerebrovascular accidents* in the brain stem (as in the Wallenberg syndrome) may produce swallowing difficulties with asymmetric passage of the bolus through the throat. *Pseudobulbar palsy* generally develops in patients with multi-infarction dementia. This syndrome may produce a disturbed swallowing act, weak peristaltic contraction, forceful simultaneous contractions and a weak lower oesophageal sphincter.[27]

In *bulbar poliomyelitis* laxity of the hypopharyngeal walls and impaired movements of tongue and palate hinder bolus formation and passage. This results in nasal reflux, pooling of

secretions and spill-over in the pharynx. Although radiological examination suggests persistent closure of the upper oesophageal sphincter, relaxations are observed on manometry.[52]

Amyotrophic lateral sclerosis and the syndromes related to it (progressive muscular atrophy) may affect tongue, pharynx, oesophagus and even stomach. *Multiple sclerosis* may cause dysphagia and uncoordinated oesophageal contractions. Patients with *Parkinson's disease* experience dysphagia and a difficulty in initiating swallowing which may improve on levodopa (L-dopa) therapy.[44, 48] Parkinson's disease not only produces depigmentation of cells in the substantia nigra and the locus coeruleus but also affects the dorsal nucleus of the vagus. The latter involvement may be the cause of the oesophageal motor disorders found on manometric and radiological examination.[75] The *stiff-man (Moersch–Woltmann) syndrome* appears to affect the striated muscle portion of the oesophagus, and leaves the motility of the distal oesophagus intact.[78] In *familial dysautonomia (Riley–Day syndrome)*, sucking and swallowing difficulties are usually present from birth.[58] The radiological picture of the oesophagus may mimic achalasia and in two cases a cardiomyotomy had been performed. The intramural plexuses were described as normal.[56]

The oesophagus appears to be abnormal in idiopathic *intestinal pseudo-obstruction*.[72, 73] At least two different forms are observed. In one variety familial intestinal pseudo-obstruction is the presenting manifestation of an as yet unclassified neurological disease characterized by gait ataxia, dysarthria, anhydrosis and absent deep tendon reflexes. The oesophagus lacks peristaltic contractions, contracts spontaneously and is hypersensitive to methacholine (mecholyl). The myenteric plexus is degenerated, and degenerative cytoplasmic changes are found in the brain. The smooth muscle is normal. It is not clear whether this syndrome is related to familial dysautonomia. In the second variety the myenteric plexus is normal, but the smooth muscle degenerates. Oesophageal peristalsis is absent, and the methacholine test is negative. The interdigestive motor complex may be absent in the small intestine.

Peripheral neuropathies

Some patients with diabetes mellitus have markedly disordered motility both of the oesophagus and of other parts of the gastrointestinal tract.[57]

Only a few of a series of diabetics preselected on the basis of symptoms of neuropathy–gastroenteropathy had clinical oesophageal symptoms. Therefore, dysphagia in the diabetic should not be ascribed to neuropathy unless other well-known causes have been excluded first.[33]

In patients with *peripheral neuropathy secondary to chronic alcoholism* non-peristaltic contractions occur frequently in the distal oesophagus, whereas the lower oesophageal sphincter functions normally.[91]

REFERENCES

1   Akuamoa, G. (1971) Achalasia oesophagi. *Acta Chirurgica Scandinavica*, **137**, 782–788.

2   Atkinson, M. & Summerling, M. D. (1966) Oesophageal changes in systemic sclerosis. *Gut*, **7**, 402–408.

3   Barker, J. R. & Franklin, R. H. (1971) Heller's operation for achalasia of the cardia. A study of the early and late results. *British Journal of Surgery*, **58**, 466–468.

4   Benjamin, S. B., Gerhardt, D. C. & Castell, D. O. (1979) High amplitude peristaltic esophageal contractions associated with chest pain and/or dysphagia. *Gastroenterology*, **77**, 478–483.

5   Bennett, J. R. & Hendrix, T. R. (1970) Diffuse esophageal spasm: a disorder with more than one cause. *Gastroenterology*, **59**, 273–279.

6   Berger, K. & McCallum, R. W. (1981) The hypertensive lower esophageal sphincter: a clinical and manometric study. *Gastroenterology*, **80**, 1109.

7   Black, J., Vorbach, A. N. & Collis, J. L. (1976) Results of Heller's operation for achalasia of the esophagus. The importance of hiatal repair. *British Journal of Surgery*, **63**, 949–953.

8   Bortolotti, M. & Labo, G. (1981) Clinical and manometric effects of nifedipine in patients with esophageal achalasia. *Gastroenterology*, **80**, 39–44.

9   Brand, D. L., Martin, D. & Pope, C. E. (1977) Esophageal manometrics in patients with angina-like chest pain. *Digestive Diseases*, **22**, 300–304.

10 Bray, G. M., Kaarsoo, M. & Ross, R. T. (1965) Ocular myopathy with dysphagia. *Neurology*, (Minneapolis), **15**, 678–684.

11 Cassella, R. R., Ellis, F. H. Jr & Brown, A. L. (1965) Fine-structure changes in achalasia of the esophagus. I. Vagus nerves. *American Journal of Pathology*, **46**, 279–288.

12 Cassella, R. R., Ellis, F. H. Jr & Brown, A. L. (1965) Diffuse spasm of the lower part of the esophagus. Fine structure of esophageal smooth muscle and nerve. *Journal of the American Medical Association*, **191**, 379–382.

13 Cassella, R. R., Brown, A. L. Jr, Sayre, G. P. & Ellis, F. H. Jr (1964) Achalasia of the esophagus: pathologic and etiologic considerations. *Annals of Surgery*, **160**, 474–486.

14 Christianson, H. B., Brunsting, L. A. & Perry, H. L. (1956) Dermatomyositis: unusual features, complications, and treatment. *Archives of Dermatology* (Chicago), **74**, 581–589.

15 Code, C. F., Schlegel, J. F., Kelley, M. L. Jr, Olsen, A. M. & Ellis, F. H. Jr (1960) Hypertensive gastroesophageal sphincter. *Proceedings of the Mayo Clinics*, **35**, 391–399.

16 Cohen, S. & Lipshutz, W. (1971) Lower esophageal sphincter dysfunction in achalasia. *Gastroenterology*, **61**, 814–820.

17 Cohen, S., Fisher, R. & Tuch, A. (1972) The site of denervation in achalasia. *Gut*, **13**, 556–558.

18 Cohen, S., Fisher, R., Lipshutz, W. *et al.* (1972) The pathogenesis of esophageal dysfunction in scleroderma and Raynaud's disease. *Journal of Clinical Investigation*, **51**, 2663–2668.

19 Creamer, B., Donoghue, F. E. & Code, C. F. (1958) Pattern of esophageal motility in diffuse spasm. *Gastroenterology*, **34**, 782–796.

20 d'Angelo, W. A., Fries, J. F., Masi, A. T. & Shulman, L. E. (1969) Pathologic observations in systemic sclerosis (scleroderma). *American Journal of Medicine*, **46**, 428–440.

21 Dart, A. M., Alban Davies, H., Lowndes, R. *et al.* (1980) Oesophageal spasm and 'angina': diagnostic value of ergometrine provocation. *European Heart Journal*, **1**, 91–95.

22 Diamant, N. E. & El-Sharkawy, T. Y. (1977) Neural control of esophageal peristalsis. A conceptual analysis. *Gastroenterology*, **72**, 546–556.

23 DiMarino, A. J. Jr & Cohen, S. (1974) Characteristics of lower esophageal sphincter function in symptomatic diffuse esophageal spasm. *Gastroenterology*, **66**, 1–6.

24 Donoghue, F., Winkelmann, R. & Moersch, H. (1960) Esophageal defects in dermatomyositis. *Annals of Otology*, **69**, 1139–1145.

25 Dornhorst, A. C., Pierce, J. W. & Whimster, I. W. (1954) The esophageal lesion in scleroderma. *Lancet*, **i**, 698–699.

26 Eckhardt, V. F., Krüger, J., Holtermüller, K. H. & Ewe, K. (1975) Alteration of esophageal peristalsis by pentagastrin in patients with diffuse esophageal spasm. *Scandinavian Journal of Gastroenterology*, **10**, 475–479.

27 Fischer, R. A., Ellison, G. W., Thayer, W. R. *et al.* (1965) Esophageal motility in neuromuscular disorders. *Annals of Internal Medicine*, **63**, 229–248.

28 Fleshler, B. (1967) Diffuse esophageal spasm. *Gastroenterology*, **52**, 559–564.

29 Garrett, J. M. & Godwin, D. H. (1969) Gastroesophageal hypercontracting sphincter. *Journal of the American Medical Association*, **208**, 992–998.

30 Garrett, J. M., Winkelmann, R. K., Schlegel, J. F. & Code, C. F. (1971) Esophageal deterioration in scleroderma. *Mayo Clinic Proceedings*, **46**, 92–96.

31 Gillies, M., Nicks, R. & Skyring, A. (1967) Clinical, manometric and pathological studies in diffuse oesophageal spasm. *British Medical Journal*, **ii**, 527–530.

32 Goyal, R. K. & Rattan, S. (1978) Neurohumoral, hormonal and drug receptors for the lower esophageal sphincter. *Gastroenterology*, **84**, 589–619.

33 Goyal, R. K. & Spiro, H. M. (1970) Esophageal function in diabetes mellitus. *Annals of Internal Medicine*, **72**, 281–282.

34 Guelrud, M., Simon, C., Gomez, G. & Villalta, B. (1981) Pentagastrin supersensitivity of the lower esophageal sphincter (LES) in the elderly. *Gastroenterology*, **80**, 1165.

35 Harvey, J. C., Sherbourne, D. H. & Siegel, C. I. (1965) Smooth muscle involvement in myotonic dystrophy. *American Journal of Medicine*, **39**, 81–90.

36 Hellemans, J. & Vantrappen, G. (1974) Physiology. In *Diseases of the Esophagus* (Ed.) Vantrappen, G. & Hellemans, J. pp. 40–102. Berlin, Heidelberg & New York: Springer-Verlag.

37 Hellemans, J. & Vantrappen, G. (1974) Presbyesophagus. In *Diseases of the Esophagus* (Ed.) Vantrappen, G. & Hellemans, J. pp. 372–378. Berlin, Heidelberg & New York: Springer-Verlag.

Motor Disorders 39

38 Hellemans, J. & Vantrappen, G. (1974) Motor disorders due to collagen diseases. In *Diseases of the Esophagus* (Ed.) Vantrappen, G. & Hellemans, J. pp. 383–393. Berlin, Heidelberg & New York: Springer-Verlag.

39 Henderson, R. D. & Pearson, F. C. (1976) Reflux control following extended myotomy in primary disordered motor activity (diffuse spasm) of the esophagus. *Annals of Thoracic Surgery*, **22**, 278–283.

40 Herrera, A. F., Colon, J., Valdes-Dapena, A. & Roth, J. L. A. (1970) Achalasia or carcinoma? The significance of the mecholyl test. *American Journal of Digestive Diseases*, **15**, 1073–1081.

41 Heupler, F. A. Jr, Proudfit, W. L., Razavi, M. *et al.* (1978) Ergonovine maleate provocative test for coronary arterial spasm. *American Journal of Cardiology*, **41**, 631–640.

42 Hollis, J. B., Levine, S. M. & Castell, D. O. (1972) Differential sensitivity of the human esophagus to pentagastrin. *American Journal of Physiology*, **222**, 870–874.

43 Humphries, T. J. & Castell, D. O. (1977) Pressure profile of esophageal peristalsis in normal humans as measured by direct intraesophageal transducers. *Digestive Diseases*, **22**, 641–645.

44 Hurwitz, A. L., Nelson, J. A. & Haddad, J. K. (1975) Oropharyngeal dysphagia: manometric and cineesophagographic findings. *American Journal of Digestive Diseases*, **20**, 313–324.

45 Ingelfinger, F. J. (1958) Esophageal motility. *Physiological Reviews*, **38**, 533–584.

46 Joseph, R. & Job, J. C. (1963) Dysautonomie familiale et mégaoesophage. *Archives françaises de Pédiatrie*, **20**, 25–33.

47 Kaye, M. D. (1981) Anomalies of peristalsis in idiopathic diffuse oesophageal spasm. *Gut*, **22**, 217–222.

48 Kaye, M. D. & Hoehn, M. M. (1975) Esophageal motor dysfunction in Parkinson's disease. In *Proceedings of the 5th International Symposium on Gastrointestinal Motility* (Ed.) Vantrappen, G. pp. 393–399. Herentals: Typoff-Press.

49 Kolodny, M., Schrader, Z. R., Rubin, W. *et al.* (1968) Esophageal achalasia probably due to gastric carcinoma. *Annals of Internal Medicine*, **69**, 569–573.

50 Kramer, P. & Ingelfinger, F. J. (1951) Esophageal sensitivity to mecholyl in cardiospasm. *Gastroenterology*, **19**, 242–253.

51 Kramer, P., Harris, L. D. & Donaldson, R. M. Jr (1967) Transition from symptomatic diffuse spasm to cardiospasm. *Gut*, **8**, 115–119.

52 Kramer, P., Atkinson, M., Wyman, S. M. & Ingelfinger, F. J. (1957) The dynamics of swallowing. II. Neuromuscular dysphagia of pharynx. *Journal of Clinical Investigation*, **36**, 589–595.

53 Kramer, P., Fleshler, B., McNally, E. & Harris, L. D. (1967) Oesophageal sensitivity to mecholyl in symptomatic diffuse spasm. *Gut*, **8**, 120–127.

54 Lane, W. H., Ippoliti, A. F. & McCallum, R. W. (1979) Effect of gastrin heptadecapeptide (G17) on oesophageal contractions in patients with diffuse oesophageal spasm. *Gut*, **20**, 756–759.

55 Leonardi, H. K., Shea, J. A., Crozier, R. E. & Ellis, F. E. Jr (1977) Diffuse spasm of the esophagus. Clinical, manometric and surgical considerations. *Journal of Thoracic and Cardiovascular Surgery*, **74**, 736–743.

56 Linde, L. M. & Westover, J. L. (1962) Esophageal and gastric abnormalities in dysautonomia. *Pediatrics*, **29**, 303–306.

57 Mandelstam, P., Siegel, C. I., Lieber, A. & Siegel, M. (1969) The swallowing disorder in patients with diabetic neuropathy–gastroenteropathy. *Gastroenterology*, **56**, 1–12.

58 Margulies, S. I., Brunt, P. W., Donner, M. W. & Silbiger, M. L. (1968) Familial dysautonomia. A cineradiographic study of the swallowing mechanism. *Radiology*, **90**, 107–112.

59 Mellow, M. (1977) Symptomatic diffuse esophageal spasm. Manometric follow-up and response to cholinergic stimulation and cholinesterase inhibition. *Gastroenterology*, **73**, 237–240.

60 Moldow, R. E. & Cohen B. R. (1971) A disorder of esophageal smooth muscle in myasthenia gravis (abstract). *Gastroenterology*, **60**, 787.

61 Nicks, R., Gillies, M. & Skyring, A. (1968) Diffuse muscular spasm. (Diffuse muscular hypertrophy of the oesophagus.) *Bulletin de la Société internationale de chirurgie*, **6**, 637–648.

62 Okike, N., Payne, W. S., Neufeld, D. M. *et al.* (1979) Esophagotomy versus forceful dilators for achalasia of the esophagus: results in 899 patients. *Annals of Thoracic Surgery*, **28**, 100–102.

63 Olsen, A. M., Harrington, S. W., Moersch, H. J. & Anderson, H. A. (1951) The treatment of cardiospasm analysis of a twelve-year experience. *Journal of Thoracic Cardiovascular Surgery*, **22**, 164–167.

64 Orlando, R. C. & Bozymski, E. (1979) The effects of pentagastrin in achalasia and diffuse esophageal spasm. *Gastroenterology*, **77**, 472–477.

65 Pearson, C. M. (1969) Polymyositis and related disorders. In *Disorders of Voluntary Muscle* 2nd edn (Ed.) Walton, J. N. pp. 501–539. London: Churchill.

66 Pope, C. E. (1976) Abnormalities of peristaltic amplitude and force – a clue to the etiology of chest pain. In *Proceedings of the 5th International Symposium on Gastrointestinal Motility* (Ed.) Vantrappen, G. pp. 380–386. Herentals: Typoff-Press.

67 Ribet, M., Callafi, R. & Hamon, Y. (1975) Mégaoesophage idiopathique. Résultats et séquelles de son traitement chirurgical. *Archives françaises des maladies de l'appareil digestif*, **64**, 629–637.

68 Roberts, A. H. & Bamforth, J. (1968) The pharynx and esophagus in ocular muscular dystrophy. *Neurology* (Minneapolis), **18**, 645–652.

69 Roth, H. P. & Fleshler, B. (1964) Diffuse esophageal spasm. *Annals of Internal Medicine*, **61**, 914–923.

70 Sanderson, D. R., Ellis, F. H. Jr & Olsen, A. M. (1970) Achalasia of the esophagus: results of therapy by dilatation. 1950–1967. *Chest*, **58**, 116–121.

71 Sanderson, D. R., Ellis, F. H. Jr, Schlegel, J. F. & Olsen, A. M. (1967) Syndrome of vigorous achalasia: clinical and physiologic observations. *Diseases of the Chest*, **52**, 508–517.

72 Schuffler, M. D. & Deitch, E. A. (1980) Chronic idiopathic intestinal pseudo-obstruction. *Annals of Surgery*, **192**, 752–761.

73 Schuffler, M. D. & Pope, C. E. II (1976) Esophageal motor dysfunction in idiopathic intestinal pseudo-obstruction. *Gastroenterology*, **70**, 677–682.

74 Siegel, C. I., Hendrix, T. R. & Harvey, J. C. (1966) The swallowing disorder in myotonia dystrophica. *Gastroenterology*, **50**, 541–550.

75 Silbiger, M. L., Pikielny, R. & Donner, M. W. (1967) Neuromuscular disorders affecting the pharynx: cineradiographic analysis. *Investigative Radiology*, **2**, 442–448.

76 Soergel, K. H., Zboralske, F. F. & Amberg, J. R. (1964) Presbyesophagus: esophageal motility in nonagenarians. *Journal of Clinical Investigation*, **43**, 1472–1479.

77 Stevens, M. B., Hookman, P., Siegel, C. I. *et al.* (1964) Aperistalsis of the esophagus in patients with connective-tissue disorders and Raynaud's phenomenon. *New England Journal of Medicine*, **270**, 1218–1222.

78 Sulway, M. J., Baume, P. E. & Davis, E. (1970) Stiff-man syndrome presenting with complete esophageal obstruction. *American Journal of Digestive Diseases*, **15**, 79–84.

79 Treacy, W. L., Baggenstoss, A. H., Slocumb, C. H. & Code, C. F. (1963) Scleroderma of the esophagus. A correlation of histologic and physiologic findings. *Annals of Internal Medicine*, **59**, 351–356.

80 Trounce, J. R., Deucher, D. C., Kauntze, R. & Thomas, G. A. (1957) Studies in achalasia of the cardia. *Quarterly Journal of Medicine*, **28**, 433–443.

81 Tucker, H. J., Snape, W. J. Jr, & Cohen, S. (1978) Achalasia secondary to carcinoma: manometric and clinical features. *Annals of Internal Medicine*, **89**, 315–318.

82 Turner, R., Lipshutz, W., Miller, W. *et al.* (1973) Esophageal dysfunction in collagen disease. *American Journal of Medical Sciences*, **265**, 191–199.

83 Vantrappen, G. & Hellemans, J. (1974) Achalasia. In *Diseases of the Esophagus* (Ed.) Vantrappen, G. & Hellemans, J. pp. 287–354. Berlin, Heidelberg & New York: Springer-Verlag.

84 Vantrappen, G. & Hellemans, J. (1976) Diffuse muscle spasm of the oesophagus and the hypertensive lower oesophageal sphincter. *Clinics in Gastroenterology*, **5**, 59–72.

85 Vantrappen, G. & Hellemans, J. (1979) Motility. In *Scientific Foundations of Gastroenterology* (Ed.) Sircus, W. & Smith, A. N. pp. 227–253. London: Heinemann Medical.

86 Vantrappen, G. & Hellemans, J. (1980) Treatment of achalasia and related motor disorders. *Gastroenterology*, **79**, 144–154.

87 Vantrappen, G. & Hellemans, J. (1981) Achalasia. In *Therapeutic Endoscopy and Radiology of the Gut* (Ed.) Bennett, J. R. pp. 73–86. London: Chapman & Hall.

88 Vantrappen, G., Van Derstappen, G. & Vandenbroucke J. (1960) The syndrome of the hypertonic gastroesophageal sphincter. *Proceedings of the International Congress of Gastroenterology, Leiden, 1960.* pp. 377–384. Amsterdam: Excerpta Medica.

89 Vantrappen, G., Janssens, J., Hellemans, J. & Coremans, G. (1979) Achalasia, diffuse esophageal spasm, and related motility disorders. *Gastroenterology*, **76**, 450–457.

90 Walton, J. N. (1964) Muscular dystrophy: some recent advances in knowledge. *British Medical Journal*, **i**, 1271–1274.

91 Winship, D. H., Caflisch, C. R., Zboralske, F. F. & Hogan, W. J. (1968) Deterioration of esophageal peristalsis in patients with alcoholic neuropathy. *Gastroenterology*, **55**, 173–178.

92 Zboralske, F. F., Amberg, J. R. & Soergel, K. H. (1964) Presbyesophagus: Cineradiographic manifestations. *Radiology*, **82**, 463–467.

OESOPHAGITIS

REFLUX OESOPHAGITIS

Definition and causation

If digestive juices frequently reflux from the stomach the mucosa of the lower oesophagus may become inflamed by their irritant effect (reflux oesophagitis) giving rise to symptoms such as pain and dysphagia and complications such as haemorrhage or stricture.

This simple definition has to be qualified. Reflux of gastric juice into the oesophagus is normally prevented by barrier mechanisms, which include the anatomical arrangements at the diaphragmatic oesophageal hiatus, and the lower oesophageal sphincter (gastro-oesophageal sphincter, GOS). The barrier mechanism is necessarily incomplete as it has, at least, to allow belching and vomiting. Reflux of gastric contents across the barrier into the lower oesophagus occurs in everyone several times a day, the errant juices being quickly returned to the stomach by gravity, by primary peristalsis induced by swallowing or by secondary peristalsis triggered by oesophageal distension. To produce reflux oesophagitis, with visible mucosal inflammation, or symptoms (or both), one or more other factors must be involved. Compared with normal subjects, therefore, patients with reflux oesophagitis may have:

a more frequent episodes of reflux;
b greater volume of reflux;
c slower oesophageal emptying ('reduced clearance');
d more irritant juice;
e diminished mucosal resistance.[4, 20]

The importance of each factor varies from patient to patient, and may do in any individual patient from time to time. An element of self-perpetuation may be present, as the presence of reflux oesophagitis may itself promote poorer clearing, diminish mucosal resistance and even reversibly weaken the gastro-oesophageal sphincter.

Frequency of reflux

The elements in the normal barrier to reflux are shown in Figure 2.11. It is impossible to determine the contribution of each fixed structure, but in some patients deficiency of one or more may be a major contribution to reflux.

The gastro-oesophageal sphincter exists as a band of specialized muscle squeezing the oesophageal lumen. Factors which may adversely influence sphincter tone and contribute to reflux oesophagitis are shown in Table 2.5.

Until recently it was believed that reflux forced its way through a weakened sphincter at rest, but it has been suggested that the sphincter may relax 'inappropriately' (that is, not in response to swallows),[19] or that reflux occurs when the sphincter relaxes after swallowing.[14]

Gastro-oesophageal barrier

Fixed strictures

Gastro-oesophageal sphincter
controlled by:
    myogenic influences
    neural influences
    hormonal influences

Compression
  diaphragmatic pinch-cock
  liver tunnel
  right diaphragmatic sling

Valvular
  mucosal flap
  flutter valve
  oesophago-gastric angle
  gastric sling

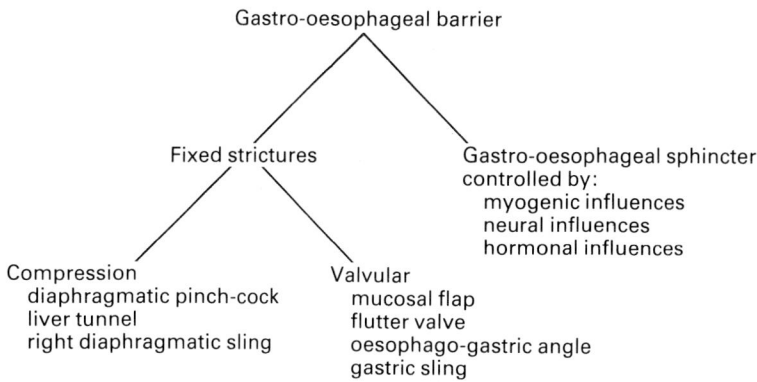

Fig. 2.11 Normal mechanisms for preventing gastro-oesophageal reflux

Table 2.5 Factors diminishing gastro-oesophageal sphincter tone and increasing reflux

Myogenic	Systemic sclerosis[12]
	Oesophagitis[21]
	After achalasia therapy[5, 37]
Neural	Early systemic sclerosis[12]
	Smoking[18, 32]
Hormonal	Menstruation[35]
	Pregnancy[36]
	Fat/chocolate eating[28]
	Coffee[34]

Hiatal hernia. Early descriptions of gastro-oesophageal reflux stressed its relationship with herniation of the stomach through the oesophageal hiatus of the diaphragm, but it is now known that if stressful manoeuvres are applied a hiatal hernia may be produced transiently in most normal individuals; furthermore, reflux of barium into the oesophagus is dependent upon radiological technique. A hiatal hernia is not the most important causative factor in gastro-oesophageal reflux, and the radiological demonstration of a hernia is not the best way to confirm the diagnosis of reflux oesophagitis. The term 'hiatal hernia' should not be used as a diagnostic label in patients with reflux symptoms.

Volume of refluxed material
This is assumed to be related to the volume available for reflux, itself determined by (a) gastric secretion, (b) gastric emptying, (c) duodeno-gastric reflux, and (d) volume ingested as food and drink. Gastric secretion in reflux oesophagitis has been the subject of many studies, with discrepant findings. It is usually little different from that in normal subjects. Gastric emptying is probably slower, especially for solids, in some, but not all, patients with gastro-oesophageal reflux,[27] while duodeno-gastric reflux occurs more commonly in patients with reflux oesophagitis. Gastric reflux is commonest after meals, but factors other than volume ingested may be involved. However, many patients notice heartburn to be worse after large meals.

Oesophageal clearance
The rate at which the oesophagus empties itself of refluxed material is one of the determinants of contact time with the mucosa. Clinically, oesophageal aperistalsis (as in systemic sclerosis or achalasia) predisposes to severe oesophagitis, and a variety of abnormalities of oesophageal motor function have been described in oesophagitis. More swallows are required to raise an acid pH in the oesophagus to a neutral level in patients with reflux oesophagitis than in normal subjects,[9] but this may be as much due to neutralization by saliva as to peristaltic adequacy.

Composition of refluxed juice
The constituents of refluxed juice chiefly responsible for epithelial damage are acid, pepsin and bile; the contribution of pancreatic enzymes is uncertain. Oesophagitis may occur in achlorhydric subjects and even after total gastrectomy, but in most patients acid and pepsin are probably important.

Mucosal sensitivity (tissue resistance)
Hydrogen ions can penetrate the squamous mucosa, a process increased by pepsin, bile or alcohol. The inflamed mucosa is more susceptible to painful stimuli, its potential difference alters, as does its cellular enzymatic content, and its structure – both microscopic and ultramicroscopic – changes in a characteristic manner. The mucosa may be more susceptible to chemical damage in some subjects than in others, or may become so under certain environmental influences. Equally, the pain-sensitivity of the oesophagus varies between individuals.

Symptoms of gastro-oesophageal reflux

INFANTS

Regurgitation occurs in infants quite commonly; this is sometimes known as chalasia. There is frequent vomiting, which may lead to poor nutrition, and carries the hazard of aspiration and pulmonary complications. It is usually short-lived and responds to thickening of the feeds and keeping the infant propped up when sleeping rather than flat, but occasionally it causes pain, and on rare occasions goes on to severe oesophagitis, leading to haemorrhage or stricture formation.[15]

ADULTS

Heartburn (pyrosis)
This is the commonest symptom of gastro-oesophageal reflux and is thought to be due to direct mucosal irritation by refluxed juice. Discomfort or pain, usually burning in character, is felt behind the sternum; it often appears to rise from the epigastrium towards or into the throat, sometimes radiating into the back, and occasionally, entirely in the throat or in the epigastrium. Heartburn is an intermittent symptom, occurring particularly within 30 minutes of meals, on exercise, after bending or on lying down; it may waken patients from sleep. A large meal, particularly with excess fat or alcohol, is particularly likely to precipitate heartburn. The discomfort often disappears quickly on drinking water or milk, or after taking an antacid. If heartburn occurs frequently it can interfere with the patient's way of life, particularly work or pleasure involving lying or bending, including gardening and sexual intercourse.

Many people who are considered healthy have experienced heartburn from time to time. Only when it becomes frequent, or sufficiently easily precipitated to interfere with normal life, need it be considered abnormal. Heartburn occurs in about two-thirds of all pregnant women especially in the second and third trimesters.

Other oesophageal pain
The oesophagus may give rise to pain other than heartburn, probably by motor changes ('spasm'). This may be of any character, but is often described as 'gripping' or 'knife-like'. These pains are usually central-sternal in origin, but may radiate widely to abdomen, back, neck and arms. The pain may be severe. The character, radiation and severity may cause diagnostic difficulty, readily simulating cardiac, biliary or duodenal pain. As many as one-third of patients admitted to hospital with a provisional diagnosis of cardiac pain may turn out to have only oesophageal disease.[6]

Sometimes oesophageal pain is experienced entirely in the epigastrium, when it may mimic peptic ulceration.

Regurgitation and vomiting
Fluid may be regurgitated into the mouth when the patient lies down, bends or strains, and may even wake him at night. The fluid may taste bitter (bile) or sour (acid). There may be vomiting, and in some patients with gastro-oesophageal reflux the predominant symptom is frequent, effortless vomiting.

Odynophagia
This term describes a transitory discomfort, usually of burning character, felt behind the sternum when food or fluid (usually hot or alcoholic drinks, but also citrus fruit juices) is swallowed. It is characteristic and diagnostic of reflux oesophagitis.

Dysphagia
A sensation of delay at the lower end of the sternum as food is swallowed may be experienced in reflux oesophagitis. If it is more than mild and occasional it suggests that a stricture is present or that there is an associated motor abnormality.

Haemorrhage
Overt bleeding from reflux oesophagitis accounts for about 4% of all gastrointestinal haemorrhage. Occult bleeding is also uncommon. Identification of the oesophagus as the sole site of haemorrhage can only be achieved by gastrointestinal endoscopy. 'Hiatal hernia' diagnosed radiologically is not a satisfactory explanation for overt or occult gastrointestinal bleeding, and endoscopic confirmation of a site of bleeding is essential; if there is no visible abnormality the remaining gastrointestinal tract must be investigated.

Oesophageal ulcers or gastric ulcers in the intrathoracic portion of a herniated stomach bleed more often than uncomplicated oesophagitis.

Respiratory symptoms
Some individuals with chronic bronchitis, recurrent pneumonia or asthma may be shown to have gastro-oesophageal reflux, and in some of

these radio-opaque contrast medium swallowed at night has been demonstrated in the lung next morning. The frequency with which reflux *causes* respiratory problems is uncertain; sometimes the conditions must be coincidental, and the intrathoracic pressure changes caused by respiratory disease may predispose to gastro-oesophageal reflux. However, reflux is worth searching for in any patient with a recurrent pulmonary problem where there is no other likely causative factor; if there is free reflux the patient may benefit from anti-reflux surgery, though at present no preoperative test offers a satisfactory prediction of outcome.

Diagnosis of reflux oesophagitis

In many patients the diagnosis is easy (Figure 2.12) and is based on the characteristic symptoms outlined above. In such individuals tests are unnecessary, though follow-up is desirable to ensure that appropriate therapy has given relief, and that no new symptom has arisen.

If the symptoms arise unexpectedly, are less typical, are associated with epigastric pain or dysphagia, or if typical symptoms fail to respond to treatment, then a barium meal or, preferably, upper gastrointestinal endoscopy is desirable, not only to confirm reflux oesophagitis, but particularly to seek a peptic ulcer or carcinoma of cardia or pylorus, which may cause reflux symptoms.

More careful assessment is required if chest pain is not typically oesophageal in character, especially if it resembles cardiac pain, using tests to provoke oesophageal pain, and to measure reflux quantitatively.

BARIUM SWALLOW AND MEAL

This is simple and relatively comfortable for the patient, and will discover most peptic ulcers or gastric carcinomas. It may also demonstrate oesophageal anatomy and reveal a hiatal hernia. However, demonstration of a hiatal hernia does not in itself mean that there is gastro-oesophageal reflux, or that reflux is the cause of a patient's symptoms. The demonstration of reflux depends to some extent on the technique used by the radiologist. Barium radiology will not usually show any abnormality due to oesophagitis unless there is an ulcer or a stricture: its main value is in ruling out alternative causes of disease.

UPPER GASTROINTESTINAL ENDOSCOPY

Although more uncomfortable, and slightly more hazardous to the patient, endoscopy gives more information than radiology in patients with oesophageal symptoms. It will detect peptic ulcers and carcinomas at least as well, but enables a visual assessment of oesophagitis to be made, as well as permitting mucosal biopsies.

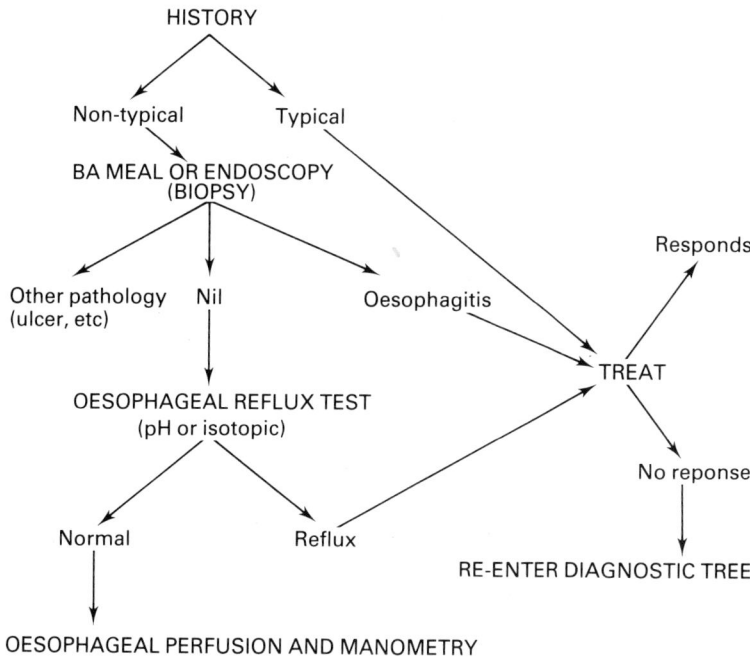

Fig. 2.12 Methods for making a diagnosis of gastro-oesophageal reflux

The mucosal assessment of oesophagitis is subject to much observer variation. Descriptions of changes should be detailed, and may best be referred to by the grading system of Savary and Miller.[30]

Grade I   Single or non-confluent multiple mucosal lesions; erythema and/or superficial erosions.

Grade II   Confluent erosions, not including the whole circumference of the oesophagus.

Grade III Confluent erosions including the whole oesophageal circumference, but with no stenosis.

Grade IV   Chronic lesions
           – ulcers
           – stenosis
           – short oesophagus
           – gastric mucosa in oesophagus (Barrett's syndrome)

OESOPHAGEAL BIOPSY

Some patients with undoubted reflux symptoms who do not have oesophagitis as judged endoscopically may be shown to have mucosal abnormalities on histological examination of mucosal biopsies. Conventional histological changes of inflammation are not always present, but alteration of the squamous mucosa with basal cell hyperplasia and elongation of papillae towards the surface are characteristic.[24]

A biopsy should be taken 5 cm above the gastro-oesophageal mucosal junction for interpretation by the above criteria if reflux oesophagitis is suspected and the oesophageal mucosa looks normal through the endoscope, although the small biopsies taken through fibre-optic endoscopes may pose interpretative problems.[25]

OESOPHAGEAL PERFUSION

In almost all patients with pain from reflux oesophagitis, the discomfort can be precipitated or reproduced by dripping 0.1 mol/l hydrochloric acid into the oesophagus.[8] With the patient sitting, a nasogastric tube is passed to about 5 cm above the cardia (40 cm from the nose). Bottles of 0.9% saline and 0.1 mol/l hydrochloric acid are connected to the tube by a three-way connection, all hidden from the patient.

0.9% saline is dripped at 10 ml/min for ten minutes and at 20 ml/min for five minutes as control. Without the patient's knowledge 0.1 mol/l hydrochloric acid is substituted and per-fused at 10 ml/min for 15 minutes and 20 ml/min for 15 minutes. If pain occurs with acid the solution is changed to saline until the pain disappears, then the procedure is repeated. Alternatively, 0.1 mol/l sodium bicarbonate may relieve the discomfort more quickly. The patient should be able to compare any induced discomfort with his or her spontaneous pain. The pain of reflux oesophagitis is usually precipitated by acid but not by saline, though in a few 'hyper-reactors' saline also causes pain. Some patients have substernal burning generated by acid which is different from their spontaneous pain; this is termed a 'positive unrelated response' and indicates that their spontaneous pain is probably not oesophageal. This test is particularly useful in differentiating between oesophageal and cardiac pain.[7, 16]

INTRALUMINAL pH MEASUREMENT

Although acid is not the entire cause of reflux oesophagitis, acid does reflux abnormally frequently in the great majority of patients with the disorder. Thus, measuring the frequency with which acid enters the lower oesophagus using a small glass pH electrode is a relatively simple way of quantifying reflux. This has been done in various ways; the best-known short test (sometimes known as the Standard Acid Reflux Test, SART) is to have the subject perform a series of provocative movements, such as coughing or Valsalva's manoeuvre, in different positions, normal subjects causing three or four spurts of acid in 12 manoeuvres. This test is specific but insensitive.[3] Oesophageal pH can be monitored continuously over 12 to 24 hours, using a fixed recording system or a mobile tape-recorder. Various measurements, such as the frequency of acid spurts, their mean duration, or the proportion of recording time under pH 4 or pH 5 may be measured and compared with results obtained in normal subjects. Almost everyone has a few episodes of acid reflux every day; in patients with reflux oesophagitis their frequency and duration are increased.[10, 17, 33]

OESOPHAGEAL SCINTISCAN

An isotope-labelled substance such as $^{99}Tc^m$-labelled sulphur colloid instilled into the stomach can be detected by a gamma-camera. If standard provocation such as an abdominal binder or postural manoeuvres are used, reflux of the isotope can be detected and quantified. This seems a sensitive test, and is comparable to pH monitoring in accuracy.[26]

DYE TEST

Gastro-oesophageal reflux in infants and children may be demonstrated by recovering from an oesophageal tube methylene blue or brilliant blue previously placed in the stomach. This may be as sensitive as pH electrode monitoring.[22]

OESOPHAGEAL MANOMETRY

Pressure recording in the oesophagus allows measurement of lower oesophageal sphincter tone and assessment of oesophageal peristalsis. However, it is of small value in the *diagnosis* of gastro-oesophageal reflux because, although gastro-oesophageal sphincter tone tends to be lower in reflux subjects, there is considerable overlap with the normal population, and the test therefore has poor discrimination. Manometry may be helpful in assessing patients who respond poorly to treatment, or as a preliminary to surgery in ensuring that oesophageal peristalsis is normal. It will detect aperistalsis (as in systemic sclerosis, in which reflux oesophagitis is common), or motor abnormalities such as diffuse oesophageal spasm which may themselves cause oesophageal pain in the absence of gastro-oesophageal reflux.

Differential diagnosis of reflux oesophagitis

PEPTIC ULCER

Gastro-oesophageal reflux often complicates or coexists with peptic ulceration, probably because of changes in gastric motility and the acid and bile content of the gastric juice. In a patient with reflux symptoms an ulcer may be suggested by unusually rapid progress of the symptoms, epigastric pain as well as heartburn, or periodicity (of the duodenal ulcer type). A peptic ulcer should be sought radiologically or endoscopically in most patients with reflux oesophagitis.

CARDIAC PAIN

Characteristic heartburn with postural and postcibal aggravation is unlikely to be confused with cardiac pain. However, some patients with gastro-oesophageal reflux experience more severe pain, which may simulate cardiac pain, sometimes even radiating into the arms or jaws, and occurring particularly during or after exercise. Conversely, cardiac pain is occasionally of burning character, and sometimes predominantly postcibal or nocturnal. Occasionally,

electrocardiograms, perhaps after exercise, and tests for reflux oesophagitis may be needed. Acid perfusion of the oesophagus is helpful. Ischaemic heart disease and reflux oesophagitis are both common conditions in the middle-aged, and patients may have pain from both causes. This can give rise to problems with therapy if the patient has difficulty in differentiating between the two pains.[6]

FLATULENT DYSPEPSIA

The syndrome of flatulent dyspepsia embraces a number of symptoms, including upper abdominal fullness, nausea, easy satiety, anorexia, morning vomiting, belching, and also heartburn. Although this condition is not fully understood it may be due predominantly to disordered antral and duodenal motility with duodeno-gastric reflux. Although the heartburn may partly respond to appropriate anti-reflux measures, the other symptoms will not. Anti-reflux surgery should be avoided in such patients, for they respond poorly.

There is little purpose in a 'routine' search for gallbladder disease in patients with reflux oesophagitis, but if a patient with gallstones has significant reflux oesophagitis consideration may be given to performing an anti-reflux procedure at the same time as cholecystectomy.

Management of gastro-oesophageal reflux

Many patients who experience intermittent heartburn find quick relief from any antacid preparation; others require more treatment. As reflux oesophagitis is usually caused by a number of interacting abnormalities treatment should be directed at one or other of these factors.

Frequency of reflux
Certain foods reduce lower oesophageal sphincter tone and should be avoided – particularly fat, chocolate, coffee, alcohol and spices. Cigarette smoking, which markedly weakens the sphincter and allows reflux, should be stopped.

The lower oesophageal sphincter may be strengthened (i.e., its resting tone increased) by metoclopramide, domperidone or bethanechol. However, all these drugs produce a rise in pressure proportional to the resting tone, so that the weakest sphincters are helped least. Moreover, reflux may be due not to weakness of the resting sphincter, but rather to inappropriate relaxation (especially during sleep), or to spurts of reflux when the sphincter relaxes in response to a

swallow. Compounds containing sodium alginate and antacids are commercially available. On
contact with gastric acid these produce a floating, viscous foam which diminishes the frequency and duration of acid reflux. Several
surgical anti-reflux operations markedly diminish reflux.

Volume of reflux
This can be diminished by lowering the volume
of gastric contents. Meals should be small in
volume, and gastric emptying may be accelerated by metoclopramide or domperidone.
Gastric secretory volume is lowered by histamine H_2 blocking drugs.

Oesophageal emptying
Any refluxed juices should be cleared from the
oesophagus as quickly as possible to shorten
contact with the mucosa. Swallowing induces
primary peristalsis and may be encouraged by
antacids given as chewable tablets, which also
stimulate secretion of alkaline saliva. Peristaltic
pressure is increased by metoclopramide and
domperidone. At night, having the bed-head
propped up 20 cm increases clearance.

Constituents of refluxed juice
The acid content can be neutralized by antacids,
or reduced by histamine H_2-blocking or other
antisecretory drugs. At present no effective agent
is available to lower concentrations of pepsin or
bile salts, though the amount of duodeno-gastric
reflux of bile may be lessened by metoclopramide or domperidone. Drugs such as corticosteroids or non-steroidal antirheumatics may be
particularly irritant to the oesophagus and
should be stopped if possible, or reduced to the
minimum practicable dose.

Mucosal sensitivity
Local anaesthetic agents have been used to
diminish mucosal pain-sensitivity, but have not
been shown to be effective. Carbenoxolone combined with alginate may increase healing of
oesophagitis.

A PRACTICAL APPROACH TO TREATMENT

Any overweight should be removed. Most clinicians believe this helps, though the mechanism is
uncertain. Smoking should stop, and fat, chocolate, alcohol and coffee should be discouraged.
Meals should not be taken late at night. An
antacid–alginate compound is prescribed after
meals and at bedtime, supplemented by antacid
tablets sucked frequently (every 1–2 hours

between meals). If symptoms persist, a histamine
H_2-blocking drug may be given, and metoclopramide or domperidone added. If improvement
is still inadequate the bed-head should be elevated on 20 cm blocks.

Most patients will respond to this regimen,
which should be maintained for about 12 weeks.
One measure at a time may be withdrawn, any
recurrence of symptoms indicating its restitution. In this way the minimum maintenance
treatment may be determined. If improvement is
inadequate, or can only be maintained at the
cost of continuous irksome measures, surgery
should be considered, but only if it is certain that
the symptoms are due exclusively to gastro-
oesophageal reflux. Acid-reducing operations
such as vagotomy alone are inadequate but they
may be combined with an anti-reflux procedure
if there is evidence of hypersecretion or associated peptic ulceration. The most widely used
effective anti-reflux procedure is the Nissen fundoplication or one of its variants. The earlier
anatomical repairs of the oesophageal hiatus
were associated with a high incidence of radiological and symptomatic recurrence. A silicone
ring (the Angelchik prosthesis) tied round the
lower oesophagus below the diaphragm[1] has
produced good results. Bile diversion, using a
Roux-en-Y anastomosis, may relieve heartburn
dramatically, especially when oesophagitis has
followed gastric surgery or a Heller's cardiomyotomy or if the cardia is inaccessible for technical reasons.

OESOPHAGEAL ULCER

An ulcer may complicate reflux oesophagitis.
Such ulcers usually occur at the junction
between oesophageal squamous mucosa and the
distal mucosa, be this true columnar gastric epithelium or some transitional form in Barrett's
syndrome. The symptoms of reflux oesophagitis
do not necessarily change when an ulcer occurs,
but many patients report a pain in the lower
sternal region which is more persistent, penetrating and severe than before. Dysphagia is
usually present, even if there is no demonstrable
stricture.

An oesophageal ulcer only occasionally
causes haematemesis, and spontaneous perforation rarely occurs. Oesophageal ulcers may be
caused by corrosives, particularly tablets; in
such cases the patient notices the rapid or
sudden onset of substernal pain and dysphagia,
which may be total. The ulcer may be seen endoscopically, and usually heals quickly if the
offending medication is stopped.

BARRETT'S SYNDROME

Barrett described a condition of the oesophagus in which the lower part is lined not with the normal stratified squamous epithelium but with columnar epithelium similar to that found in the stomach.[2] Ulcers develop in this columnar epithelium, usually just below the mucosal junction. Migration of columnar epithelium up the oesophageal lumen, replacing ulcerated squamous epithelium, has been recorded. The reason why the epithelial change occurs is unknown, but it may be a response to reflux, since columnar epithelium is more resistant to acid–peptic digestion. Furthermore, there is provisional evidence that the process might be reversible, either by surgical cure or by medical control of gastro-oesophageal reflux.

Symptoms are no different from those in patients with oesophagitis, oesophageal ulcers or stricture. There is general agreement that there is a greater incidence of carcinoma supervening in a Barrett's oesophagus than in a normal oesophagus, and Barrett's epithelium can be considered as a premalignant condition. The diagnosis of Barrett's syndrome is often open to dispute, depending as it does on the demonstration of a gastric type of epithelium inside a tube which is oesophagus and not simply a tubular hernia of the stomach. For this reason the exact incidence of carcinoma associated with this anomaly is uncertain. However, it seems desirable to advise regular surveillance, such as an annual endoscopy with multiple biopsies, in such patients.

The epithelium distal to most oesophageal strictures is abnormal, and is usually described as transitional. Whether, in fact, all strictures are a minor form of Barrett's syndrome, or have an entirely different causation awaits elucidation. There is a higher than expected likelihood of malignancy occurring in previously undoubted benign strictures, so that annual surveillance is equally desirable.

To avoid confusion it seems best to use the term Barrett's syndrome only where columnar epithelium is histologically demonstrated within a tubular segment which clearly has the motility characteristics of oesophagus, as shown either by radiological screening or, preferably, by intraluminal manometry.

OESOPHAGEAL STRICTURES

Definition

An oesophageal stricture is a narrowing of the lumen caused by an abnormality of the oesophageal wall. Strictures other than those caused by carcinoma are due to inflammation, usually with mucosal ulceration and fibrous scarring. In this, the oesophagus behaves like other parts of the alimentary tract, which may likewise respond to mucosal damage by cicatricial narrowing.

Narrowing of the oesophagus may, however, be transient, may disappear after being stretched, or after removal of an irritant agent, or may be visible radiologically yet cause no obstruction to the passage of food or an endoscope. Such abnormalities are rarely removed surgically or explored at autopsy, so their nature remains in doubt. They are sometimes called 'elastic strictures', with the implication that circular muscle fibre spasm is responsible (though this can rarely be demonstrated by pressure measurements), or 'webs' or 'rings'. Their relation, if any, to fibrous strictures is unclear.

Causes

CORROSIVE STRICTURES

Diffuse corrosion
Strong alkali or strong acid damages oesophageal mucosa, and if the concentration, volume and duration of contact are sufficient, oesophageal inflammation results.

The necrosis of the wall which follows may be deep and extend over a considerable area, sometimes leading even to full thickness necrosis and perforation. Within three weeks fibrous scarring appears and readily leads to stricture formation. Such strictures may be graded as:

Grade I   Shelf strictures, involving a short segment but not circumferential.
Grade II   Annular strictures, less than one centimetre in length.
Grade III Dense annular strictures, less than one centimetre long extending through all layers.
Grade IV   Tubular strictures with peri-oesophageal adhesions.

Local corrosion
Various tablets are known to cause oesophagitis locally if they adhere to the mucosa. Among those recognized as implicated are Clinitest (a diagnostic solution-tablet containing copper sulphate), emepronium bromide (Cetiprin), potassium chloride, and tetracycline and related antibiotics.[13]

Chemical damage is considered further later in this chapter (p. 59).

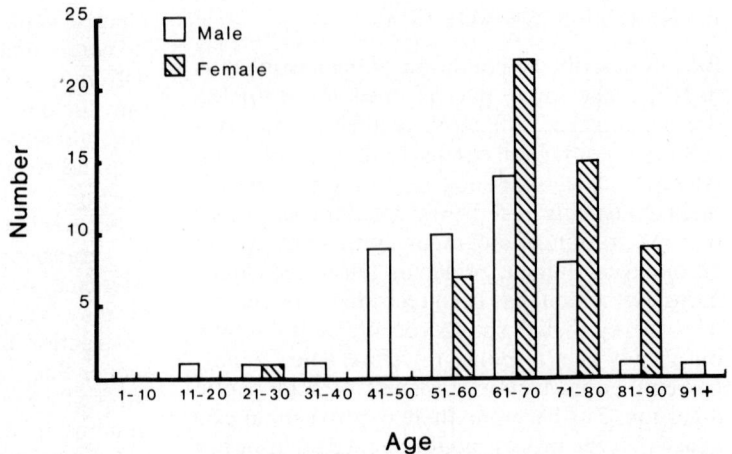

Fig. 2.13 Age distribution of patients with oesophageal strictures seen at Hull Royal Infirmary, 1970–1980

GASTRO-OESOPHAGEAL REFLUX

Fibrous oesophageal strictures result from reflux changes, but how they do so is less certain. Severe, prolonged oesophagitis, with mucosal and penetrating ulceration, is likely to lead eventually to a stricture, but strictures are found in patients who deny any previous symptoms of reflux, and occur particularly in the elderly (Fig. 2.13). Sometimes strictures appear very quickly, for example after a period of recumbency or the prolonged placement of a nasogastric tube. It is hard to see how a fibrous cicatrix can evolve so quickly if the usual explanation of recurrent ulceration and associated fibrous reaction is accepted, unless there has been pre-existing painless oesophagitis, and the intubation or recumbency has simply caused a major exacerbation.

In Britain almost all oesophageal strictures are due to reflux oesophagitis, as corrosive swallowing is rare. An association with the ingestion of non-steroidal antirheumatic drugs has been observed.[23]

WEBS AND RINGS

These are discussed later in this chapter (p. 56).

Symptoms

The symptom of an oesophageal stricture is dysphagia, a feeling of food 'sticking' or being delayed in its passage through the oesophagus. Corrosive strictures, especially if long, often lead to severe dysphagia affecting even liquids, and may obliterate the lumen completely. Benign 'peptic' strictures usually have a slow onset, with dysphagia often developing gradually over

several years. Dysphagia often only affects solids, even when the strictures are quite advanced, and it is rare for a benign stricture to cause difficulty in drinking liquids, unless a solid particle becomes impacted. There may also be pain on drinking hot liquids or strong alcohol because of the associated mucosal changes. A history of heartburn or reflux for some years previously may be present but is denied by up to half the patients.

Malignant disease should be suspected if the dysphagia progresses rapidly or leads to complete hold-up for fluids as well as solids, or if a solid bolus impacts with pain due to strong secondary peristalsis.

Radiology

Radiological screening of swallowed radio-opaque medium should be the first step in the investigation of a known or suspected oesophageal stricture. Barium is customarily used unless perforation is suspected. Radiology is not an essential preliminary to endoscopy, which is, however, mandatory. The purpose of radiology is to demonstrate (a) if there is a stricture, (b) its site (c) its length and (d) its nature.

A stricture will be demonstrated best if the oesophagus is well distended by a large volume of swallowed barium with the patient prone. Barium should be allowed to pass through the stricture into the stomach. By tipping the patient head-down the oesophagus may then be filled from below, demonstrating the lower limit of the stricture and hence its length, and possibly helping to decide whether the tube below it is stomach or columnar-lined oesophagus. It is not always easy to decide whether the stricture is benign or malignant. Distension and complete filling aid differentiation by demonstrating the abrupt transition to normal, distensible oesophagus ('shouldering'), and the irregularity of the channel through a carcinoma, whereas a benign stricture shows a smooth tapering.

The diameter of the stricture may be measured by comparing the width of the barium stream with a radio-opaque ruler placed behind the patient, or by asking the patient to swallow a series of radio-opaque balls of increasing size until one impacts. Such balls can be made of wax which will soon melt at body temperature.

Endoscopy

Any patient with dysphagia requires endoscopy whether or not a lesion has been shown radiologically. If a stricture is visible by X-ray its nature needs elucidation by inspection and biopsy; if no abnormality is seen radiologically a stricture may still be detectable by the endoscope.

The purpose of endoscopy is (a) to confirm the presence of a stricture, (b) to assess its bore, (c) to assess its nature from its appearance, (d) to obtain biopsies and cytology specimens and (e) occasionally to dilate by bougienage.

PRESENCE OF THE STRICTURE

Narrowing of the stream of swallowed barium seen radiologically does not always mean that a constant luminal obstruction is present. The endoscope may pass freely through, particularly in the case of 'webs' and 'rings' but also where there are apparent strictures. The mucosal appearances may be normal, or there may be oesophagitis or hiatal hernia. This apparent disappearance may be caused by the rapid progress of the endoscope stretching the narrowing without the operator realizing it, but on other occasions even a careful and gentle introduction with detailed scrutiny shows no sign of narrowing, which had presumably been due to a temporary motor phenomenon.

ASSESSMENT OF THE BORE

A stream of barium gives a fair indication of the lumen through a stricture, but there is often an elastic component, which is best assessed by having the patient swallow a series of radio-opaque spheres of increasing diameter. A measuring device may be used endoscopically but tapering of the lumen usually leads to under-assessment by this method.

ASSESSMENT OF THE NATURE OF THE STRICTURE

Characteristically, a benign stricture is smooth, not very narrow, sometimes with associated oesophagitis or mucosal peptic ulceration. A malignant stricture is usually irregular with polypoid projections, friable and haemorrhagic with some necrotic areas, and may be very narrow; but appearances may be misleading. Severe oesophagitis near a benign stricture may render it oedematous, haemorrhagic and friable, simulating the appearances of malignancy, while a malignant stricture may be relatively smooth and not friable. A particular problem is gastric fundal carcinoma spreading into the cardia submucosally. This may cause a symmetrical narrowing which is completely smooth because it is covered by normal epithelium.

Upper oesophageal webs and lower oesophageal rings may be invisible to the endoscopist, either because rapid passage of the instrument stretches them easily, or because inadequate distension of the lumen with air fails to demonstrate these slender structures, whose bore is usually wide. If seen, and displayed by distension with air, the appearance is of a thin, featureless ring of normal mucosa. Biopsies show no abnormal histological features, but it will be found that the mucosa immediately below a lower oesophageal ring is columnar in type.

An uncommon but important differentiation is between achalasia and a stricture, particularly in a patient known to have had achalasia treated in the past, either by surgery or dilatation. In this difficult problem, manometry and the endoscopic appearance are the only bases for diagnosis. In achalasia, with a sphincter of abnormally high tone, the endoscope will usually pass through with slight pressure, the pliable sphincter opening before it. A stricture will be appreciated as a firm obstruction which will either not yield or does so abruptly as the fibrous tissue is stretched. Although these strictures are due to reflux, the characteristic mucosal changes of oesophagitis are not always obvious in the endoscopic view.

BIOPSIES AND CYTOLOGY SPECIMENS

Tissue specimens for histology and exfoliated cells for cytology should always be taken except when there is known corrosive stricture or an obvious mucosal ring or web. Specimens for cytology are best obtained by brushing the lumen of the stricture, or through the stricture if it looks smooth. Ideally, biopsies of the narrowest part of the stricture are taken from each quadrant, plus two specimens taken by passing the forceps through the stricture. The tangential approach of the forceps to the lumen may make specimens hard to obtain, but crocodile-toothed or spiked biopsy forceps may help. The combination of cytology and biopsies should lead to a correct distinction between benign and malignant strictures in over 95% of patients.

Therapy

CORROSIVE STRICTURE

Local strictures due to corrosive tablet ingestion are usually short, not dense, easily dilated and may require only one course of bougienage. A few, caused by Clinitest, have necessitated surgical removal.

Strictures caused by liquid corrosives are dealt with according to their grade. Grades I, II and most of III can be treated by intermittent bougienage, beginning three weeks after the burn. Bougienage carried out earlier has a high incidence of perforation. At first, weekly dilatations are performed with lengthening intervals according to response. If the intervals between dilatations cannot be lengthened to a convenient period, the patient may be taught self-bougienage using Hurst's or Maloney's mercury bougies.

Those strictures of grade III which are tough, and most of the long grade IV strictures, may be difficult and hazardous to dilate. However, this is hard to predict and a trial of bougienage is always justified. If dilatation by bougies is impossible, or if it is required too frequently, surgery should be recommended, provided the patient is fit enough. Short strictures can be excised with re-anastomosis but long ones can be dealt with only by excision and replacement by colon or jejunum.

REFLUX (PEPTIC) STRICTURES

The choices of therapy are medical alone, medical plus intermittent bougienage or surgery (with bougienage).

Up to a third of patients will require no other treatment if the medical measures to treat reflux oesophagitis are applied, presumably because of reduction in oedema, diminution of spasm and improvement in oesophageal motor function. However, even if the stricture resolves or is alleviated, the propensity for reflux continues and it is therefore necessary to maintain the medical regimen permanently.

Bougienage
Several techniques for bougienage are available. The most desirable is to introduce a guide wire through the stricture using a fibre-optic endoscope in a sedated patient. Bougies of the Eder–Puestow or Celestin type may be passed over this guide wire, with radiological screening if desired. For benign strictures known to be smooth, central and regular, mercury-weighted bougies (Hurst or Maloney) may be swallowed by the patient.[11, 29]

Dilatation of the stricture is likely to be necessary at least once whether medical or surgical treatment is employed, but many patients require recurrent dilatation. A second dilatation may be performed one to two weeks after the first, in association with the medical regimen, but unless the stricture is clearly narrowing down rapidly the intervals between dilatation can quickly be prolonged. After the first six months few patients should need more than two or three dilatations a year and many will find them unnecessary.

It is desirable that cytology and biopsy specimens should be taken from the stricture once a year at the time of dilatation because of the possibility of malignant transformation.

Surgery
Although many patients may retain relatively trouble-free swallowing by medical treatment plus bougienage, the need for more than occasional dilatation is irksome, and not completely without hazard. Surgical treatment should be recommended for younger, fit patients if control of dysphagia is imperfect by bougienage. Unless oesophagitis and peri-oesophagitis has so damaged the oesophagus that its replacement by a segment of intestine is desirable an operation to prevent gastro-oesophageal reflux, or to modify the nature of the refluxed material, is usually combined with preoperative dilatation of the stricture and, if necessary, postoperative bougienage. Such surgery is not easy and carries a certain morbidity and mortality. Operation should not be considered as the first choice for treating a condition which predominantly affects the middle-aged and elderly, intermittent bougienage offering them the best long-term outcome. However, if operative treatment is necessary, fundoplication is generally recommended for short-segment strictures and a Roux-en-Y diversion for more extensive strictures. Resection causes a high mortality and should be avoided whenever possible.

REFERENCES

1 Angelchik, J. P. & Cohen, R. (1979) A new surgical procedure for the treatment of gastro-oesophageal reflux and hiatal hernia. *Surgery, Gynecology and Obstetrics*, **148**, 246–248.

2 Barrett, N. R. (1957) The lower esophagus lined by columnar epithelium. *Surgery*, **41**, 881–894.

3 Behar J., Biancini, P. & Sheahan, D. G. (1976) Evaluation of esophageal tests in the diagnosis of reflux esophagitis. *Gastroenterology*, **71**, 9–15.

4 Bennett, J. R. (1978) Medical management of gastro-oesophageal reflux. *Clinics in Gastroenterology*, **5**, 175–185.

5 Bennett, J. R. (1980) Treatment of achalasia, a review. *Journal of the Royal Society of Medicine*, **73**, 649–653.

6 Bennett, J. R. (1983) Chest pain – heart or gullet? *British Medical Journal*, **286**, 1231–1232.

7 Bennett, J. R. & Atkinson, M. (1966) Oesophageal acid perfusion in the diagnosis of precordial pain. *Lancet*, **ii**, 1150–1152.

8 Bernstein, L., Fruin, R. & Pacini, R. (1962) Differentiation of esophageal pain from angina pectoris. *Medicine*, **41**, 143–162.

9 Booth, D. J., Kemmerer, W. D. & Skinner, D. B. (1968) Acid clearing from the distal esophagus. *Archives of Surgery*, **76**, 732–734.

10 Branicki, F. J., Evans, D. F., Ogilvie, A. L. et al. (1982) Ambulatory monitoring of oesophageal pH in reflux oesophagitis using a portable radiotelemetry system. *Gut*, **23**, 992–998.

11 Celestin, L. R. & Campbell, W. B. (1981) A new and safe system for oesophageal dilatation. *Lancet*, **i**, 74–75.

12 Cohen, S., Fisher, R. & Lipschutz, W. (1972) The pathogenesis of esophageal dysfunction in scleroderma and Raynaud's disease. *Journal of Clinical Investigations*, **51**, 2663–2668.

13 Collins, F. J., Matthews, H. R., Baker, S. E. & Strakava, J. M. (1979) Drug-induced oesophageal injury. *British Medical Journal*, **i**, 1673–1676.

14 Corazziari, E., Bontemp, I., Anzini, F. & Torsoli, A. (1982) Motility of the distal esophagus and gastroesophageal reflux. *First European Symposium on Gastrointestinal Motility*.

15 Curci, M. & Dibbins, A. (1982) Gastroesophageal reflux in children: an under-rated disease. *American Journal of Surgery*, **143**, 413–416.

16 Davies, H. A., Jones, D. B. & Rhodes, J. (1982) 'Esophageal angina' as the cause of chest pain. *Journal of the American Medical Association*, **248**, 2274–2278.

17 De Meester, J. R. & Johnson, L. F. (1976) The evaluation of objective measurements of gastro-esophageal reflux and their contributions to patient management. *Surgical Clinics of North America*, **56**, 39–53.

18 Dennish, G. W. & Castell, D. O. (1971) Inhibitory effect of smoking on the lower esophageal sphincter. *New England Journal of Medicine*, **284**, 1136–1137.

19 Dent, J., Dodds, W. J., Friediman, R. H. et al. (1980) Mechanism of gastro-oesophageal reflux in recumbent asymptomatic human subjects. *Journal of Clinical Investigation*, **65**, 256–267.

20 Dodds, W. J., Hogan, W. J., Helm, J. F. & Dent, J. (1981) Pathogenesis of reflux oesophagitis. *Gastroenterology*, **81**, 376–394.

21 Eastwood, G. L., Castell, D. O. & Higgs, R. H. (1975) Experimental oesophagitis in cats impairs lower oesophageal sphincter pressure. *Gastroenterology*, **69**, 146–163.

22 Girardi, G., Vial, L., Fritis, E. et al. (1978) Diagnosis of gastro-oesophageal reflux in infants and children by methylene-blue test. *Lancet*, **i**, 1236–1237.

23 Heller, S. R., Fellows, I. W., Ogilvie, A. L. & Atkinson, M. (1982) Non-steroidal anti-inflammatory drugs and benign oesophageal stricture. *British Medical Journal*, **ii**, 167–168.

24 Ismil-Beigi, F., Horton, P. E. & Pope, C. W. II (1970) Histological consequence of gastroesophageal reflux in man. *Gastroenterology*, **58**, 163–169.

25 Kaboyoshi, S. & Kasugai, T. (1974) Endoscopic and biopsy criteria for the diagnosis of esophagitis with a fibreoptic esophagoscope. *Digestive Diseases*, **19**, 345–353.

26 Malmud, L. S. & Fisher, R. S. (1978) Quantitation of gastroesophageal reflux before and after therapy using the gastroesophageal scintiscan. *Southern Medical Journal*, **71**, 10–15.

27 McCallum, R. W., Berkowitz, D. T. & Lerner, E. (1981) Gastric emptying in patients with gastroesophageal reflux. *Gastroenterology*, **80**, 285–291.

28 Nebell, O. T. & Castell, D. O. (1977) Lower esophageal sphincter changes after food ingestion. *Gastroenterology*, **63**, 778–783.

29 Price, J. D., Stanciu, C. & Bennett, J. R. (1974) A safer method of dilating oesophageal strictures. *Lancet*, **i**, 1141–1142.

30 Savary, M. & Miller, G. (1978) *The Esophagus*. Switzerland: Gassman.

31 Schatzki, R. & Carey, J. R. (1953) Dysphagia due to a diaphragm-like localised narrowing in the lower esophagus. *American Journal of Roentgenology*, **70**, 911.

32 Stanciu, C. & Bennett, J. R. (1972) Smoking and gastro-oesophageal reflux. *British Medical Journal*, **ii**, 793–795.

33 Stanciu, C., Hoare, R. C. & Bennett, J. R. (1977) Correlation between manometric and pH tests for gastro-oesophageal reflux. *Gut*, **18**, 536–540.

34 Thomas, F. B., Sterbough, J. T., Frankes, J. J. et al. (1980) Inhibitory effect of coffee on lower esophageal sphincter pressure. *Gastroenterology*, **79**, 1262–1266.

35 Van Thiel, D. H., Gavaler, G. S. & Stremple, J. F. (1979) Lower esophageal sphincter strength during the menstrual cycle. *American Journal of Obstetrics and Gynecology*, **134**, 64–67.

36 Van Thiel, D. H., Gavaler, G. S., Joshi, S. N. et al. (1977) Heartburn of pregnancy. *Gastroenterology*, **72**, 666–668.

37 Vantrappen, G. & Hellermans, J. (1980) Treatment of achalasia and related disorders. *Gastroenterology*, **79**, 144–154.

TUMOURS

Malignancy dominates the tumour pathology of the oesophagus, for benign lesions are uncommon and account for only 1% of all neoplasms. Both benign and malignant tumours can be intramural or intraluminal; this has a bearing on radiology as well as endoscopy.

BENIGN LESIONS

These can be conveniently classified as epithelial, mesodermal and cysts.

Tumours of epithelial origin

Only two epithelial types are met: papillomas and adenomas. They are very rare and their only relevance is the disputed belief that they may be potentially malignant.

Papillomas are small squamous cell lesions very similar to those found in the mouth and may occur anywhere in the oesophagus. They are usually single but may occasionally be multiple.[74] They cause no symptoms and are discovered at endoscopy or autopsy. They rarely bleed and forceps biopsy will eradicate them.

Adenomas usually take the form of pedunculated or sessile polyps and have a predilection for the lower oesophagus.[46, 71] They may be associated with oesophagitis, when the origin may be inflammatory. Rare cases have been described in the upper oesophagus, and have had stalks long enough for them to be regurgitated into the mouth.[68] They resemble gastric polyps and may occasionally bleed or cause dysphagia. As a rule they are asymptomatic.

Tumours of mesodermal origin

The leiomyoma is the commonest benign tumour of the oesophagus, accounting for 65% of all benign solid tumours.[67] The remainder include lipoma, fibroma, haemangioma, neurofibroma, lymphangioma, eosinophilic granuloma and ectopic glandular tissue.

Leiomyoma

Less than 10% of alimentary tract leiomyomas occur in the oesophagus.[15] They are found in the distal two-thirds, that is, the smooth muscle portion. No age is exempt, but they are rare under the age of 20. They may be single or multiple (9%) and may undergo calcification.[29] The tumours are usually intramural and project into the lumen or into the mediastinum as they enlarge. When derived from the circular layer of muscle they become horseshoe-shaped, partially encircling the oesophagus, or annular, wholly encircling it. They are usually small, tend to be smooth rather than lobulated, and shell out easily. Leiomyomas, like other solid benign oesophageal tumours, are unlikely to progress to malignancy.[23] They grow very slowly, are covered by an intact mucosa, and the majority are found at autopsy (Figure 2.14).

Small growths are asymptomatic; large ones can cause dysphagia which is usually progressive and of long duration. Pain is recorded in half

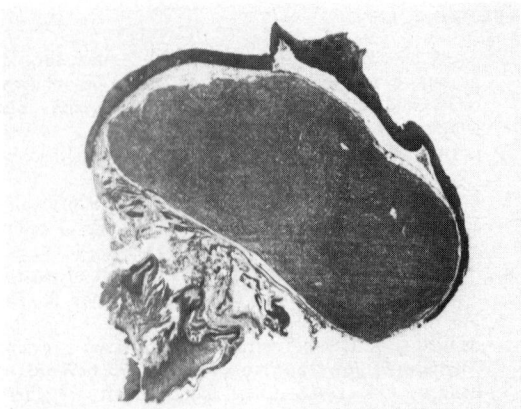

Fig. 2.14 Low-power section of a leiomyoma. The lesion is intramural, uniform in appearance, and is covered by an intact mucosa. (Courtesy of Dr N. Ibrahim.)

the cases. Oesophageal leiomyomas, in contrast to those elsewhere in the alimentary tract, rarely ulcerate or bleed. The size of the tumours correlates neither with symptoms nor with duration, and their location cannot be defined by the patient.

Cysts

Cysts rank second to solid tumours in their frequency of occurrence. They may be congenital or acquired. Congenital cysts are foregut duplication cysts. They are seen more often in children and are tubular mucosal structures that may extend the whole length of the oesophagus, and may communicate with other viscera. Their excision is a matter for the specialized surgeon.

Acquired cysts are mostly mucus retention cysts that occasionally become infected and cause pain. They may be multiple and mimic a leiomyoma in their extramucosal spread. When large they cause dysphagia and are treated similarly to leiomyomas.[68]

Investigation of benign tumours

Radiology and *endoscopy* are the mainstay of diagnosis. The radiological characteristics are those of a smooth ovoid or crescentic filling defect either projecting into the lumen on a wide base (Figure 2.15) or being obviously pedunculated. There is little proximal luminal dilatation. Leiomyomas and cysts, when small, move with the act of swallowing; when large they may project into the mediastinum. There are no precise differentiating features between the various types of tumours.

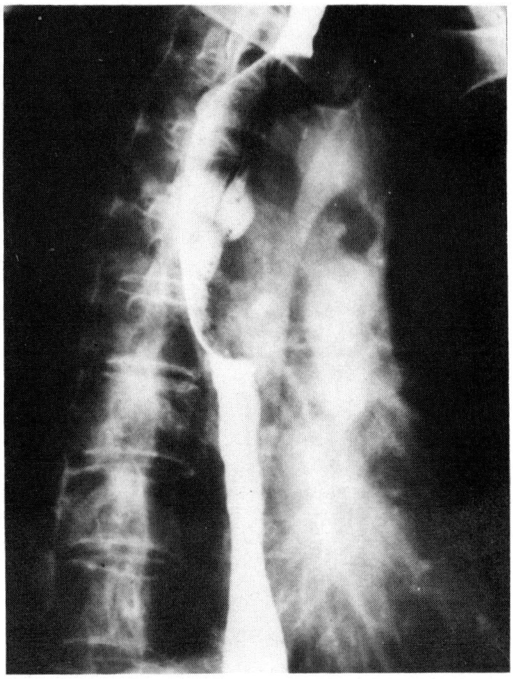

Fig. 2.15 Barium swallow appearance of an unusually large leiomyoma of the middle third of the oesophagus. Dysphagia was the presenting symptom.

Endoscopy completes the diagnosis. It clearly defines the lesion as being mucosal or intramural, sessile or pedunculated, ulcerating or angiomatous. A biopsy establishes the diagnosis of a mucosal lesion. An angioma should not be biopsied unless facilities for immediate diathermy are at hand. Intramural lesions with an unbroken overlying mucosa are best not biopsied, because breaching the mucosa fouls the surgical field for subsequent enucleation, turning it into a 'contaminated' procedure.

Treatment policy

Pedunculated lesions can be snared by diathermy via an endoscope and retrieved. Sessile lesions and those pedunculated on a broad stalk should not be snared, because the oesophageal wall may be transgressed or left exposed and bleeding can be brisk. Such lesions, as well as intramural lesions, are locally excised or enucleated transpleurally via a suitable thoracotomy without entering the lumen. Oesophageal resection is seldom required unless the lesion is large or encircles the viscus. Frozen section has been advised at difficult enucleation to exclude a mistaken diagnosis of sarcoma.

MALIGNANT TUMOURS

Tumours of the oesophagus can be primary or secondary, or the result of direct invasion by a tumour from adjoining structures. Malignant lesions are on the increase throughout the world. Primary malignant disease is by far the commonest and may be a carcinoma, a sarcoma or a carcinosarcoma (that is, a mixed epithelial and mesenchymal lesion). The latter two growths are very rare, accounting for 0.5% of all oesophageal neoplasms. Of the sarcomas, leiomyosarcomas are more commonly encountered than rhabdomyosarcomas and fibrosarcomas.[62] They are slow-growing and metastasize late, unlike carcinomas. Carcinosarcomas can be truly mixed, or they may arise from the divergent differentiation of a single stem, or they may be a 'collision' tumour.[73] These tumours are almost always polypoidal; they are less malignant than carcinomas and produce metastases that are sarcomatous in character.

Types of carcinoma

Four types of epithelial neoplasms may arise from the oesophagus: squamous cell carcinoma, adenocarcinoma, melanocarcinoma, and oat cell carcinoma. The latter three account for no more than 5% of all oesophageal cancers.

Squamous cell carcinomas and *melanocarcinomas* may affect any part of the oesophagus. There is no good evidence that the sites of predilection of the former are at points of 'physiological' narrowing, as was once believed.[31, 33]

Adenocarcinomas arise in areas lined by gastric epithelium or from submucous gastric glands[4] and are usually found in the lower oesophagus or in the Barrett type of oesophageal lesion (see p. 47). They must not be confused with growths at the cardia of gastric origin; although recognition of these as two separate entities is of long standing[53] this has frequently been ignored in reported series or in cancer statistics. These gastro-cardial adenocarcinomas are not considered in this section.

Oat cell carcinoma. This is considered to be a malignant APUDoma. It is argyrophilic, and is characterized on electron microscopy by dense core granules typical of the peptide-secreting tumours of the gastrointestinal tract. Although formerly believed to be more prevalent in Japan it has been described frequently in the West.[65]

Associated conditions

An association with certain disorders has been recorded, but it is not certain whether these are premalignant. In achalasia, where stasis oesophagitis may be a factor, cancer occurs eight times more frequently than in the general population,[77] and is usually present in the middle oesophagus. A similar increase in incidence has been noted in reflux oesophagitis and may account for the association of cancer with hiatal hernia[70] and peptic strictures.[6] The lesion can be either squamous or adenomatous and is closely related to the hernia (Figure 2.16).

Carcinoma has been described after mucosal damage by chemical agents such as lye.[22] The only genetic association with carcinoma is the inherited skin disorder of tylosis.[69] The hyperkeratosis of the palms and soles is first noticed at about four years of age, with the carcinoma appearing later on in life.[27]

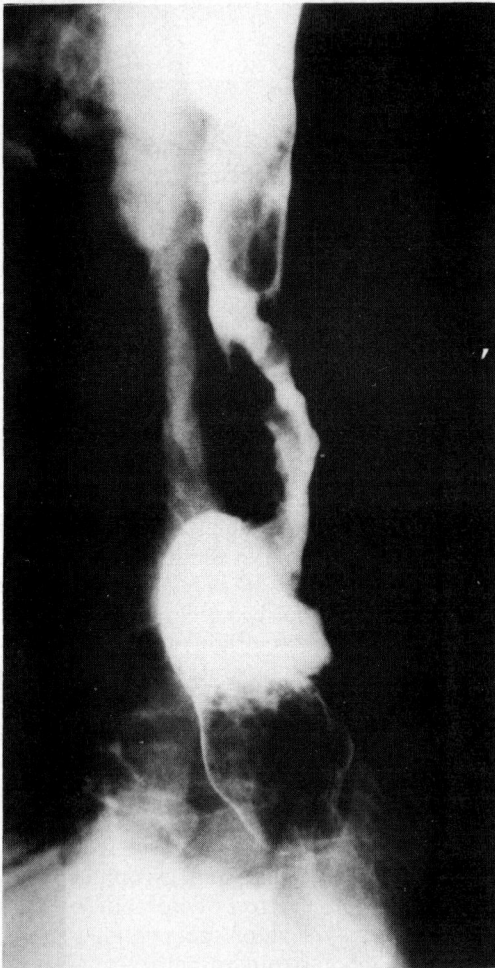

Fig. 2.16 Adenocarcinoma arising in the distal oesophagus in a patient with a long-standing hiatal hernia.

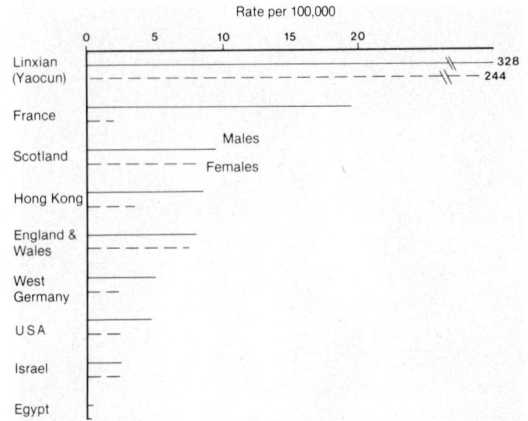

Fig. 2.17 Oesophageal cancer mortality in various countries. Note the great variation in the incidence of oesophageal cancer. In Linxian, China, it is 160 times commoner than in Israel.

Incidence

The striking feature of oesophageal squamous cell carcinoma is the great variation in incidence, not only across the world (Figure 2.17) but also within a single country, giving rise to clustering. This suggests a major environmental factor. There are also areas, such as France, where the male predominance is very marked and others where it is totally reversed, as in parts of Iran. Marked differences exist between southwest and north-east England.

Precursor states and causative agents

Studies on animal models, and surveys in high-risk populations, have defined more clearly the aetiological forces at work and suggest that at least three different factors may be involved, singly or in combination, to initiate malignant changes in an epithelium which is in a 'precursor' state. Precursor states include the Paterson–Kelly (Plummer–Vinson) syndrome, affecting the upper oesophagus in females, chronic oesophagitis of the middle and lower oesophagus, and the columnar-lined or Barrett's mucosa of the lower third. Because only a small proportion of the population with these predisposing conditions goes on to develop cancer, other factors must be selectively at work: three main circumstances are recognized – nutritional deficiencies, mutagenic initiators and chemical promoters.

Nutritional deficiencies

These include deficiencies of vitamins A, B, C and E, riboflavin and niacin, of animal protein, and of trace elements such as iron, zinc or molybdenum in the diet or the soil. These deficiencies may sustain or facilitate the oesophagitis induced by agents such as abrasive foods, hot drinks or strong spirits.

Mutagens

Certain mutagens are found repeatedly in the daily environment of high-risk populations, and whereas a high exposure may be required to induce changes in a normal epithelium, a smaller dose may be sufficient in chronic oesophagitis. Thus a high level of nitrosamines has been identified in pickled vegetables in China,[78] and chickens fed on such vegetables have a marked incidence of hypopharyngeal cancer. Tannins have been implicated in oesophageal carcinoma.[49] They are polyhydrophenols found naturally as glucosides of gallic acid and of catechol. They are components of the catechu nut and of 'tar' in cigarettes; they are extracted in the brewing of remedial 'tea', and are used in making home-made alcoholic drinks. There is a good correlation between oesophageal cancer, smoking and the drinking of dry red wine,[61] and tannin has induced cancer in animals.[37]

In non-human primates 1-methyl-1-nitrosourea (MNU) is highly carcinogenic, producing the full range of precancerous and precursor phases seen in man.[1] A similar process occurs in rats fed N-methyl-N-nitrosoaniline.[52]

Promoters

The third aetiologic group is that of promoters, compounds which are not carcinogenic on their own, but which act as catalysts to enhance the effect of mutagens. While tannins may also belong to this group those agents most implicated are alcohol and the phorbol esters. The former coexists with tannin in poorly prepared red wines, the latter in some folk remedies or 'teas'.

The chronic oesophagitis referred to above is different from reflux oesophagitis, being characterized by an oedematous, hyperaemic friable mucosa with areas of leucoplakia and none of the ulceration or bleeding found in reflux oesophagitis. Whereas the latter involves the supracardial region of the oesophagus, chronic oesophagitis involves the middle and contiguous portion of the lower third. It is not associated with a hiatal hernia and does not affect the most distal segment of the oesophagus.

The progression is thus from a normal mucosa to chronic oesophagitis with atrophy resulting from failure of cell maturation and associated with abnormal keratinization and papilloma formation. The normal epithelial architecture is destroyed, to be replaced by atypical cells which usher in dysplasia. A precancerous state has developed and is followed by carcinoma in situ and eventually frank malignancy. These steps are all encountered in the animal models and have been studied in epidemiological surveys in areas of high prevalence.[13]

Aspects of epidemiology

Two well-defined populations emerge in the epidemiological survey of oesophageal squamous cell malignancy: a *high-risk* population showing epidemic overtones, for example in Iran, China, the Transkei region of South Africa and the black male population of the USA, and a *low-risk* population including the white population of the USA and most of the nations of the Western World. Between exists a less well-defined group in parts of Japan, Argentina, Curaçao and the spirit-drinking northern areas of France.

In the high-risk areas, chronic oesophagitis of the middle and lower third of the oesophagus is found in over 80% of the subjects,[13, 66] most of whom are under 40 years of age, while the prevalence of dysplasia is as high as 18% in some groups[51] and 5% in the general population. By contrast, in a low-risk area the peak incidence of cancer is beyond the seventh decade (Figure 2.18), dysplasia is observed in 0.2% of the population,[60] and oesophagitis is of the reflux variety.[63]

In Gonbach, on the Caspian Sea in Iran, the male/female ratio of incidence is reversed, being 206/100 000 for males and 263/100 000 for females; individuals have a 1-in-6 chance of developing cancer before the age of 65. Neither

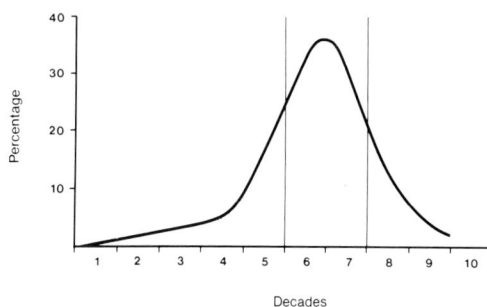

Fig. 2.18 Cancer of the oesophagus: age distribution. The peak prevalence in the low-risk areas is between the ages of 60 and 80.

alcohol nor tobacco is implicated here. Lack of fresh vegetables, riboflavin deficiency, mucosal abrasion from silica particles in bread and the ingestion of tar from opium pipes have all been suggested as causes.

In the Transkei, a multiplicity of other factors appear to operate. Much locally brewed drink is made from contaminated maize; the soil is poor in molybdenum, which increases the nitrate contents of vegetables and predisposes them to fungal infection, with the formation of nitrosamines; milk is curdled using a solanaceous fruit with a high content of dimethylnitrosamine; and the residue of tobacco pipes is chewed and swallowed. In a similar manner, molybdenum soil deficiency and nitrosamines are factors in Linxian in China, together with nutritional deficiencies. Beverages are drunk very hot in China, a factor also suggested in Argentina and Singapore, which have similar prevalence to Japan. In the Soviet Union, both hot drinks and strong liquor are possible initiators, while in parts of Brittany and Normandy males, who are heavy consumers of cider and calvados (apple brandy), have an incidence of 65/100 000, which is thirtyfold that in females.

Curaçao is of special interest: there the oesophageal cancer is associated with the plant *Croton flavens* from which a drink with a high content of phorbol esters is made.[26] These are also present in remedial 'teas', which are drunk very hot.[49]

Pathology

There are three main morphological types. The first, *fungating* or *polypoidal*, projects as a soft bulky mass into the lumen (Figure 2.19). Adenocarcinomas present in this way more frequently than do squamous cell cancers. The second type, *ulcerating* lesions with everted edges, may involve only part of the circumference, freely infiltrating the submucosa and penetrating the oesophageal wall to produce a large extramural mass (Figure 2.20). Finally, the *scirrhous* type encircles the lumen early, causing stenosis and producing as a result a very short segmental lesion (Figure 2.21).

Dissemination is principally by direct invasion of the mediastinum and its many vital structures, because the oesophagus has no serosa. The tumour extends widely under the mucosa, which may appear normal at endoscopy. By the time the mediastinal, cervical and gastric lymph nodes have become involved the growth is advanced. Liver metastases are a late

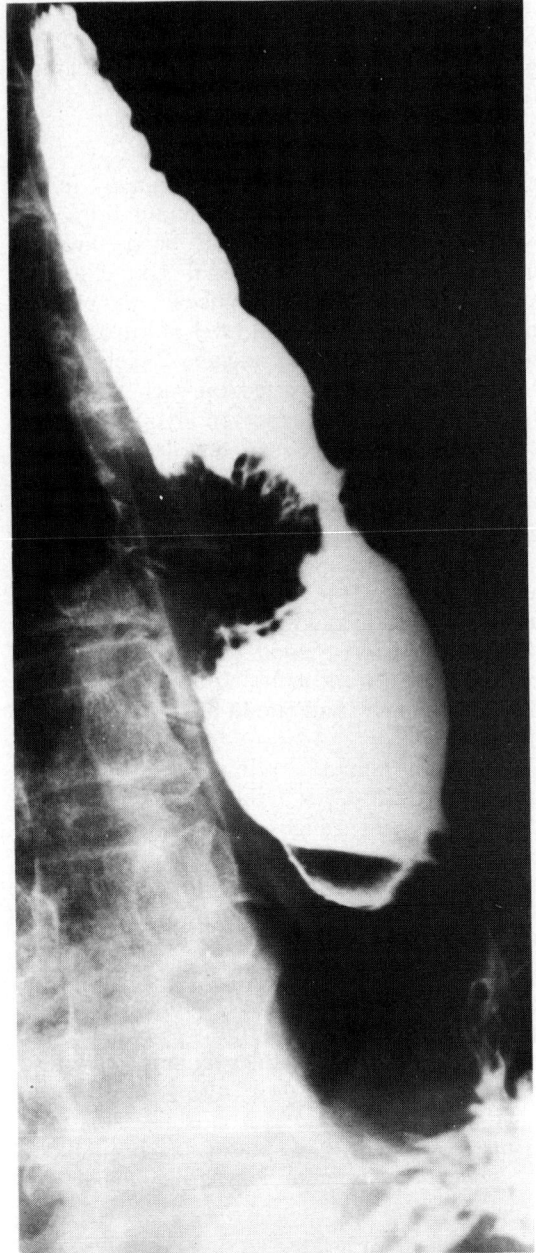

Fig. 2.19 Barium swallow showing polypoidal or fungating lesion of the lower third of the oesophagus, characteristic of an adenocarcinoma.

event. Death follows the erosion of a vital organ by a localized tumour. This usually occurs in a bronchus, leading to a fistula or to mediastinitis, or in the aorta, causing massive bleeding. Death may result from the cachexia caused by wide dissemination. In the final stages of the disease cardiopulmonary complications, jaundice and hepatorenal failure are common.

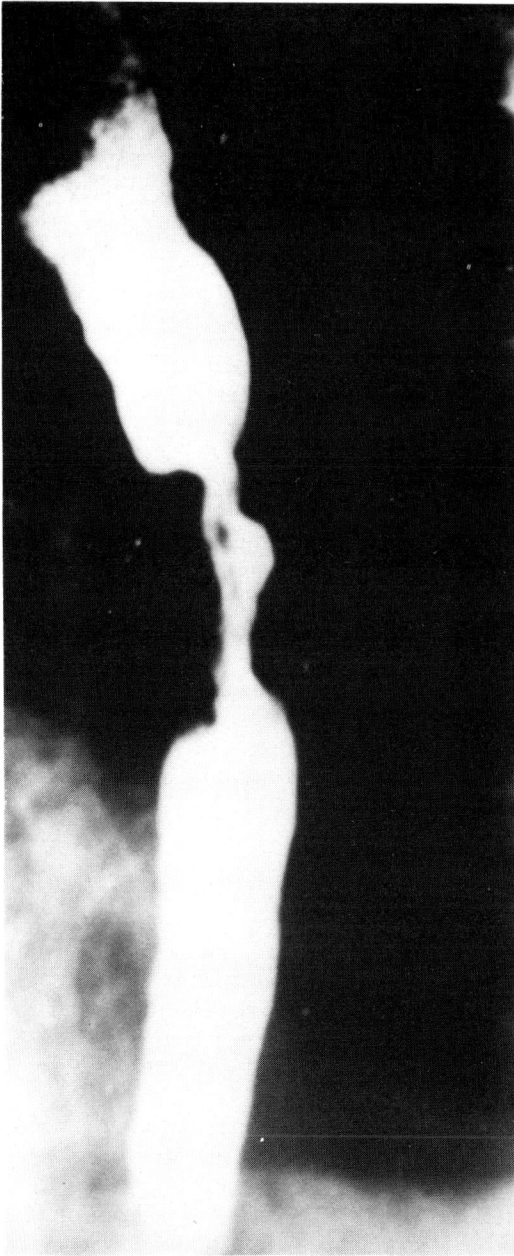

Fig. 2.20 Barium swallow showing an ulcerating squamous cell carcinoma. Note the angulation of the axis of the oesophagus due to a large extramural mass causing anterior displacement.

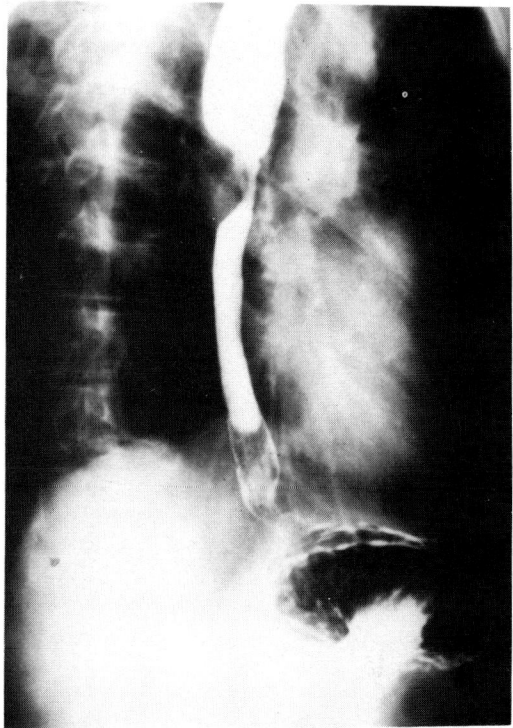

Fig. 2.21 Barium swallow showing scirrhous squamous cell lesion of the middle third, encircling and stenosing the oesophagus at an early stage.

Clinical features

These reflect the pathology. Dysphagia is the most prominent symptom. At first only for solids, it progresses relentlessly to liquids and by the time it is total the lumen of the tumour is only 4 mm in diameter. By then weight loss is marked. Pain is the next commonest symptom.

It may occur only on eating, but it may be persistent in late cases with mediastinal invasion; it is rarely due to bony metastases. Sialorrhoea occurs occasionally and may contribute to the presenting symptoms of aspiration cough or chest infections. Lymph nodes may be palpable in the neck, while invasion of the recurrent laryngeal nerve may cause hoarseness. Invasion of the phrenic causes paralysis of the diaphragm and invasion of the vagus produces pyloric hold-up. Hepatomegaly is a late sign. Anaemia from slow blood loss, low plasma proteins from inanition and a depressed lymphocyte count reflecting immunological disturbances can be present.

Investigations

Radiology and endoscopy are imperative. In doubtful cases cytology is invaluable. A barium swallow will yield a diagnosis in 90% of patients, and is a useful outpatient tool. The majority show a clearly demarcated constriction with shouldering or a tortuous lumen (Figure 2.22). Very early cases may elude radiology. Chest screening should always be done.

An endoscopy and tissue biopsy must follow in all patients. Fibre-optic endoscopy is now generally available and has the advantage of

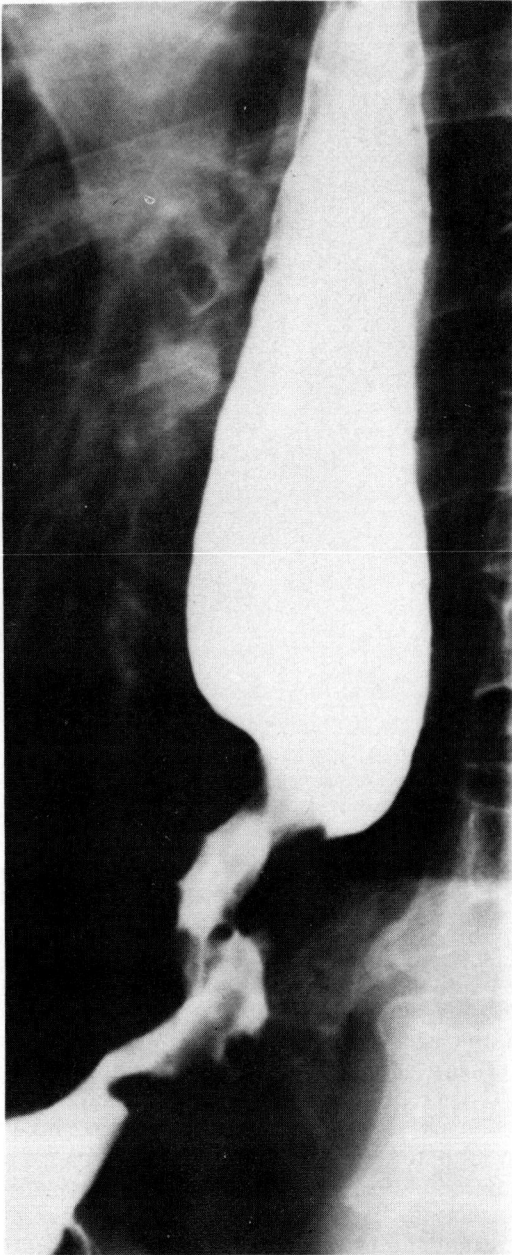

Fig. 2.22 Typical radiological appearance of a carcinoma. Note the shouldering and the tortuosity of the lumen, with proximal dilatation.

accurately defining the site of the lesion, the extent of the circumferential involvement and, after dilatation, the length. These are all important discriminants both in treatment and in prognosis. Upper and middle third lesions require in addition a bronchoscopy, while laparoscopy will reveal subdiaphragmatic spread to lymph nodes or liver.

CT scanning has been shown to be useful in defining the volume of the tumour and the extent of lymphatic spread; radioisotope labelling (thallium and cobalt-57) of squamous cell lesions has been equally useful.

Full blood count, liver function tests, simple tests of immunocompetence, and tests of nutritional status must be undertaken, because they will all influence management policy and outcome.

Factors influencing treatment policy and prognosis

Three sets of factors overlap: those relating to the tumour proper, general factors, and those relating to the type of operation offered.

Factors relating to the tumour itself
High lesions have a poorer outcome than the lower ones. Adenocarcinomas have a worse prognosis than squamous cell carcinomas at a similar site. Tumours longer than 5 cm show a significantly greater dissemination than shorter ones, and at 10 cm are virtually inoperable. Similarly, tortuosity, angulation of the oesophageal axis (Figure 2.20), and circumferential involvement reflect to some extent the invasiveness of a tumour and are poor prognostic features.

General factors
Distant metastases obviously carry a hopeless prognosis, but lymph node involvement is not always synonymous with short survival[75] and should not be a bar to resection.

Age is very relevant. The older the patient, the higher the operative mortality rate (Figure 2.23), and surgery is best avoided in patients over 75 years old.

Loss of weight and the presence of strongly positive occult blood in the stools are poor prognostic indicators. A loss of weight over 20% precludes major surgery, and the suggestion that correction of a major nutritional deficiency by preoperative feeding improves the surgical outcome[48] may not be correct.[5] Impaired cardiopulmonary function adversely affects the outcome, while studies of immunocompetence suggest that host reaction is markedly depressed in oesophageal cancer and may be an important factor against successful operability.[55]

Factors relating to the operation
Curative surgery is rational only if the operative mortality is below the five-year survival rate; palliation should aim at quality rather than quantity of life. Operative techniques have a bearing on results. A one-stage operation is

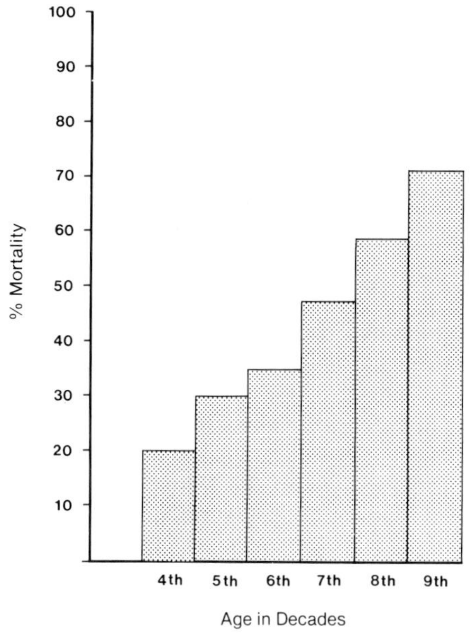

Fig. 2.23 Effect of age on operative mortality. This rises rapidly with advancing age.

When all these factors are taken into account a general treatment policy emerges; this is summarized in Table 2.6.

Results

The literature reveals a confusing picture, with mixing of histological types in records and a failure to separate gastro-oesophageal lesions from purely oesophageal ones. A thorough and comprehensive review of the subject has been compiled recently.[16] Figure 2.24 is a flow-chart of the overall outcome in round figures.

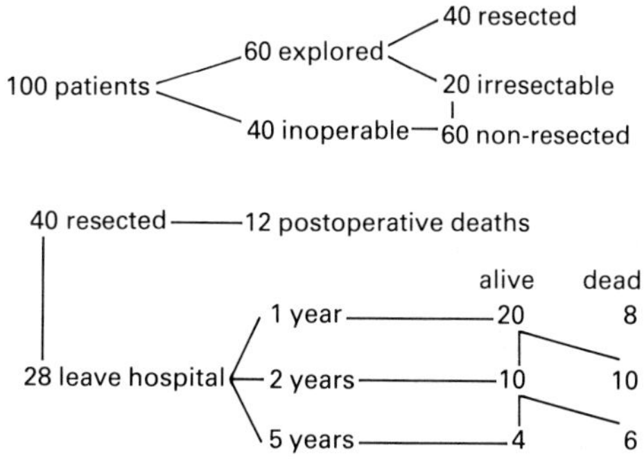

Fig. 2.24 Survival of patients with oesophageal carcinoma.[16]

accompanied by a shorter postoperative morbidity but a greater mortality rate. Multiple stage procedures reduce mortality but prolong hospitalization. Similarly, an intrathoracic approach carries a heavier toll of life than an extrathoracic approach; the latter however, is tedious and long, and may lead to a lesser quality of swallowing. A compromise is to 'strip' the oesophagus without opening the chest, but it is too early as yet to judge this operation. Oesophagectomy is an easy procedure, whereas reconstruction of the upper alimentary tract is daunting.[12] Hence, many techniques have been evolved to obtain a wide clearance of submucosal infiltration on the one hand, and a sound patent anastomosis on the other.[30]

Careful selection and good techniques have, in the best series, yielded five-year survival figures of 10%,[32, 38, 41] with an average resectability rate of 60% and an operative mortality rate of 24%, although single-figure mortality rates have been obtained in some series.[19, 45] If, however, stage 1 (T_1 N_0 M_0) tumours are evaluated[28] the operative mortality falls to 2.5%, with a five-year survival of 86%. Less favourable tumours have a mortality rate of 3.2% and a five-year survival rate of 50%.[58] Thus, early detection followed by radical surgery is promising, particularly in high-risk

Table 2.6 Summary of treatment policy in oesophageal carcinoma.

Aim	Treatment	Extent of lesion	Results
'Curative'	Radical resection with or without pre- or postoperative radiotherapy	Localized	Best
	'Radical' radiotherapy	With lymphatic spread	Long survival
Palliative			
Local tumour control	Resection Radiotherapy with or without intubation Chemotherapy	With or without liver or lymphatic node secondaries	Limited survival with freedom from local morbidity
No local tumour control	By-pass procedures Intubation Pain control Sedation	Unfit for any major surgical procedure	Short survival with relief of dysphagia

communities. It is essential that dysphagia, however slight, should be investigated aggressively. Detection must be in the symptom-free period if possible, because by the time oesophageal cancer is symptomatic it is disseminated and cannot be cured by the surgeon.

Treatment modalities

SURGERY

The three most popular approaches are: (a) the left thoracico-abdominal approach for lesions at the cardia, as a one-step procedure, (b) abdominal mobilization followed by a right thoracotomy in two steps, used mostly for middle and lower third lesions, (c) the three-step operation for a subtotal oesophagectomy. In all instances the stomach is fully mobilized but its right gastric and epiploic blood supplies are preserved. Because a total vagal section is necessary some surgeons perform a pyloroplasty. The spleen has to be removed in lower lesions and where gastrosplenic lymph nodes are involved; otherwise it is retained. Occasionally, the tail of the pancreas requires resection. Excision of the lesser curve of the stomach en bloc with the left gastric pedicle may provide greater lymphatic clearance without impairing the vascularity of the stomach. Once fully mobilized, the stomach can be brought up to the neck if required. If the anastomosis is made to the partially excised oesophagus via a left thoracotomy the stomach will be placed alongside the heart; this may embarrass cardiac function. There is much to recommend a right thoracotomy approach even for cardial lesions, and this approach also permits a higher clearance of the oesophagus with a reduced chance of recurrence at the anastomosis.

An anastomotic leak is the commonest cause of postoperative death in excisional surgery, so it is wise to perform the anastomosis outside the chest, namely in the neck. This is the rationale behind a three-step operation. First, the stomach is fully mobilized via an abdominal approach, then the oesophagus is mobilized through a right thoracotomy and finally the neck is opened for a high anastomosis of the cervical oesophagus to the stomach. The use of stapling devices has reduced anastomotic leaks but may have increased the incidence of stricture.

Sepsis remains the most severe complication of surgery, causing anastomotic breakdown or pulmonary complications. It is enhanced by both the catabolism accompanying the disease and the surgery, while impaired immuno-competence also adversely influences the outcome. This has led to the exploration of less catabolic methods of relieving dysphagia.

INTUBATION

The occurrence of subtotal or total dysphagia in an inoperable patient requires urgent relief by intubation. Gastrostomy or jejunostomy are to be condemned because they solve only inanition and prolong the agony. Intubation, however popular, must not be a substitute for surgery and must remain an ultimate but worthwhile palliation with the humane purpose of protecting the patient from the terror of an awareness of death from starvation. No more than 60% of all patients should come to intubation. Indications for intubation are quite clear-cut:

a in obstructive lesions from growths that are inoperable and irresectable or due to invasion by extraoesophageal lesions or in stubborn postoperative or post-irradiation strictures.
b as an adjunct to primary treatment, either for preoperative nutrition or with radiotherapy in total circumferential involvement.
c to minimize oesophageal wall contact with food and saliva when there are perforations or fistulas.

Stringent tube design based on physiological concepts is necessary to prevent the tube being experienced as an intraluminal foreign body; a safe method of introduction is also necessary. The major complications of intubation are perforation, pressure necrosis of the oesophageal wall, migration of the tube and blockage. There has been much commercial exaggeration about fragmentation of latex. Its occurrence is probably less than 1 in 500. By comparison, the lowest reported instrumental perforation rate is 11% and the overall rate is 18%.[54] Perforation was not uncommon in the days of pulsion intubation with a rigid endoscope. This led to the evolution of *traction* intubation by open surgery,[8, 50] which not only reduced instrumental transgression but also allowed fixation of the tube to the lesser curve, preventing migration. Wound infection and cardiopulmonary disorders were the commonest, though avoidable, complications of this method.

The advent of fibre-optic endoscopy and the use of guide wires reopened the way to safe pulsion intubation, and the Celestin traction tube has been modified to produce a pulsion tube[9, 10] with its own anti-retrograde-migration device easily detected on X-ray screening

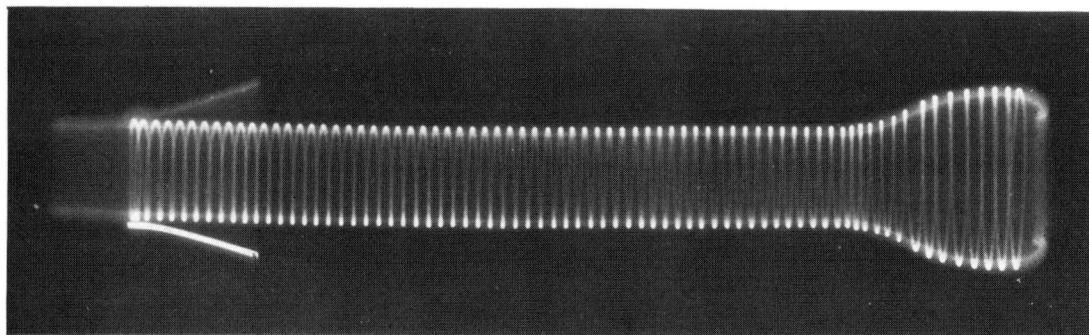

Fig. 2.25 The Celestin pulsion tube. Note the ink-welling of the tulip-shaped funnel, the radio-opacity of its nylon reinforcing spiral and the inverted 'skirt' at the lower end to prevent retrograde migration.

(Figure 2.25). A version of this traction tube, less elegant than the derived pulsion one, was used by others for a similar purpose.[3]

The commonest causes of perforation are instruments without a fail-safe device such as introducers of the coiled wire variety and rigid rammers. Flexible plastic mandrels using an inflated balloon that friction drive the prosthesis but slip if too high a pressure is used, seem to give the least instrumental perforation rate.[11] The safest and most elegant way of intubating is to use the fibre-optic endoscope as a mandrel over which the prosthesis is slid into position under direct vision.[14, 20] Regardless of the method used the essential first step to effortless and successful intubation is adequate dilatation.

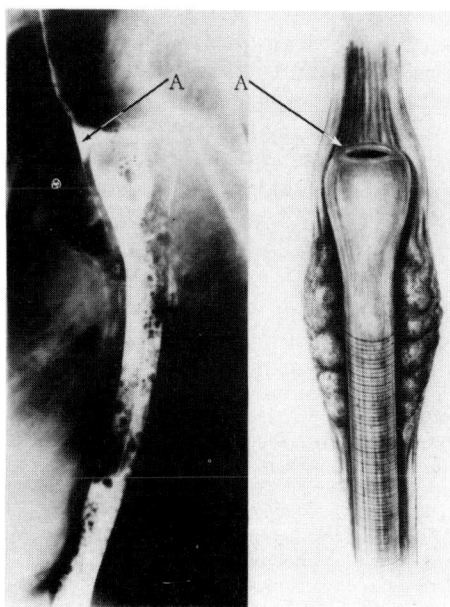

Fig. 2.26 An artists impression alongside an X-ray study of the funnel of a Celestin pulsion tube. Note the all-important pressure-free angle at A. (Courtesy of Medoc Ltd.)

Pressure necrosis of the oesophageal wall is a serious and fatal late complication which is prevented by using a funnel moulded on the form of a truncated bolus and thus 'physiological' in shape.[8] Not only does this offer a pressure-free angle between funnel and oesophageal wall (Figure 2.26) but it is oval in cross-section like the lumen of the oesophagus. Cylindrical or V-shaped funnels carry a high incidence of pressure necrosis and late perforation, particularly if their antero-posterior diameter is greater than 25 mm or their latero-lateral diameter is greater than 28 mm. These points should be looked for in the choice of a prosthesis.[18]

Blockage is minimized by inviting the patient to drink frequent sips of aerated water during meals. Intubated patients should be reviewed at regular intervals in order to achieve good results; otherwise, the method will fall into disrepute.

LASER FORAGE

The place of boring or 'forage' by laser in short tumours is being studied and attempts are being made to vaporize the mass to create an adequate channel. This may need repeating at intervals of three months or less, but this should not be a major objection to what seems an attractive though very sophisticated technique.

SURGICAL BYPASS

Surgical bypass to palliate dysphagia in advanced lesions is still widely used in endemic areas. Since the quality of swallowing is better than after intubation the most widely used procedure is to bring the mobilized stomach to the cervical oesophagus through the presternal or retrosternal route.

RADIOTHERAPY

Since 1956 kilovoltage irradiation has been superseded by megavoltage therapy, which has allowed more accurate dose distribution. More recently CT scanning has provided an important tool not only in planning the treatment but in following the rate and degree of tumour regression, and this should influence the incidence of recurrence. Whereas surgery offers ablation in length, radiotherapy offers one in width in addition, most particularly in those tumours which encroach on the vital structures, as for example in the upper reaches of the oesophagus.

Radiotherapy can be used as an adjunct to surgery either pre- or postoperative or as a primary method of treatment. Postoperative therapy is given in the hope that irradiation will complete what surgery has not been able to eradicate. There is little evidence that radiotherapy improves the prognosis. Preoperative radiotherapy in doses of 24–60 Gy (2400–6000 rad) may improve the results,[2, 25, 42] but none of the reported series were controlled and randomized. The prospective and randomized trial of Launois *et al.* shows no short-term or long-term advantage from the use of 40 Gy given preoperatively.[39a] It seems, therefore, that the combined modality of surgery and radiotherapy confers as yet no conclusive benefits on the patient. At present there is no prospective controlled randomized trial comparing surgery and radiotherapy as primary methods of treatment, but the evidence suggests that there is little to choose between the two methods, with the balance weighing possibly in favour of radiotherapy. The world-wide results of irradiation give figures of 18% survival at one year and 6% at five years, no different from those of surgery.[17] The best results are five-year survival figures of 20%.[24, 40, 56, 76] Radiotherapy has the advantage of treating lesions at all levels equally, whereas surgery favours lesions in the lower third. The improved radiotherapy results obtained in the upper third are due to the fact that the female population principally involved is a young one.

Radiotherapy has several advantages over surgery. The mortality rate is low and it has lower morbidity in the aged, in patients with cardiopulmonary disorders, and in those with associated conditions accentuating surgical catabolism such as cirrhosis. The patient retains a normal cardia and stomach, and in high lesions a normal larynx, so normal weight is regained more quickly and lung function can be well preserved.

Radiotherapy has complications, but these compare favourably with those of surgery. Radiation osteitis has been reported in up to 10% of all patients over a three-year period, but the symptoms are not pronounced.[56] Local recurrence is a problem in about half of the patients, and stricture formation requiring dilatation is not uncommon. The stricture is not a malignant lesion but hard and fibrotic owing to the replacement of radiolytic tissue by fibrous tissues, mostly in the totally circumferential lesions, and it may split on dilatation. This can be avoided by elective pre-irradiation intubation. Extubation six months later leaves a good euphagic channel which has retained its lumen.

CHEMOTHERAPY

Chemotherapy should be the treatment of choice since neither surgery nor radiotherapy have altered significantly the overall prognosis of this disease, and the majority of patients present with disseminated lesions. Most compounds tested do not have an effective antitumour effect, while their toxicity is at times distressing, and few reliable trials have been reported.

Bleomycin may be given intramuscularly and intravenously[64] but has little appreciable benefit. The same is true of methotrexate or fluorouracil given singly.[21] The same authors have reported unfavourably on doxorubicin,[21] while others observed encouraging partial responses.[39] Combinations of cisplatin with either bleomycin or vindesine[34, 35] or both[36] are the most promising therapy, while the dual modality of radiation and chemotherapy has been held to produce complete eradication of lesions.[72]

REFERENCES

1 Adamson, R. H., Krolokowski, J. P., Correa, P. *et al.* (1977) Carcinogenicity of 1-methyl-1-nitrosourea in non-human primates. *Journal of the National Cancer Institute,* **59,** 415–422.
2 Akakura, I., Nakamura, Y. & Kakegawa, I. (1970) Surgery of carcinoma of the esophagus with preoperative radiation. *Chest,* **57,** 47–57.
3 Atkinson, M., Ferguson, R. & Parker, G. C. (1978) Tube introducer and modified Celestin tube for use in palliative intubation of oesophagogastric neoplasms at fibre-optic endoscopy. *Gut,* **19,** 669–671.
4 Azzopardi, J. G. & Menzies, T. (1962) Primary oesophageal adenocarcinoma. Confirmation of its existence by the finding of mucous gland tumours. *British Journal of Surgery,* **49,** 497–506.

5 Belghiti, J., Langonnet, F., Wessely, J. Y. & Fékété, F. (1981) Faut-il corriger la dénutrition des malades ayant un cancer de l'oesophage ou du cardia en période pré-operatoire? *Nouvelle Presse Médicale*, **10**, 2273–2279.

6 Benedict, E. B. (1941) Carcinoma of the esophagus developing in benign stricture. *New England Journal of Medicine*, **224**, 408–412.

7 Carrie, A. (1950) Adenocarcinoma of the upper end of the oesophagus arising from ectopic gastric epithelium. *British Journal of Surgery*, **37**, 474.

8 Celestin, L. R. (1959) Permanent intubation in inoperable cancer of the oesophagus and cardia. *Annals of the Royal College of Surgery of England*, **25**, 165–170.

9 Celestin, L. R. (1976) Esophageal tumors and cysts. In *Surgery of the Alimentary Tract* (Ed.) Shackelford, R. T. p. 748. Philadelphia: W. B. Saunders.

10 Celestin, L. R. (1978) New techniques for intubation of the Celestin oesophageal pulsion tube. *Abstracts of the 4th World Congress of Digestive Endoscopy, Madrid, 1978*, p. 97.

11 Celestin, L. R., Etienne, J., Raimbert, P. et al. (1980) Traitement endoscopique des sténoses oesophagiennes par prothèse de Celestin. *Nouvelle Presse Médicale*, **9**, 2155–2157.

12 Chassin, J. L. (1978) Oesophagogastrectomy: data favouring end-to-side anastomosis. *Annals of Surgery*, **188**, 22–26.

13 Crespi, M., Grassi, A., Amiro, G. et al. (1979) Esophageal lesions in Northern Iran: a premalignant condition. *Lancet*, **ii**, 217–221.

14 Den Hartog, Jager, F. C., Bartelsman, J. F. W. M. & Tytgat, G. N. J. (1979) Palliative treatment of obstructing esophagogastric malignancy by endoscopic positioning of a plastic prosthesis. *Gastroenterology*, **77**, 1008–1014.

15 Dillow, B. M., Neis, D. D. & Sellers, R. D. (1970) Leiomyoma of the esophagus. *American Journal of Surgery*, **120**, 615–619.

16 Earlam, R. & Cunha-Melo, J. R. (1980) Oesophageal squamous cell carcinoma. I. A critical review of surgery. *British Journal of Surgery*, **67**, 381–390.

17 Earlam, R. & Cunha-Melo, J. R. (1981) Oesophageal squamous cell carcinoma. II. A critical review of radiotherapy. *British Journal of Surgery*, **67**, 457–461.

18 Earlam, R. & Cunha-Melo, J. R. (1982) Malignant oesophageal strictures: a review of techniques for palliative intubation *British Journal of Surgery*, **69**, 61–68.

19 Ellis, F. H. Jr & Gibb, S. P. (1979) Oesophagogastrectomy for carcinoma. *Annals of Surgery*, **190**, 699–705.

20 Etienne, J. & Celestin, L. R. (1979) Oesophageal intubation: past and present. *Acta Endoscopica*, **9**, 235–243.

21 Ezdinli, E., Gelber, R., Desai, D. et al. (1980) Chemotherapy of advanced esophageal carcinoma. *Cancer*, **46**, 2149–2153.

22 Gerami, S., Booth, A. & Pate, J. W. (1971) Carcinoma of the esophagus engrafted on lye stricture. *Diseases of the Chest*, **59**, 226–227.

23 Gray, S. W., Skandalis, J. E. & Shepard, D. (1961) Smooth muscle tumors of the esophagus. *International Abstracts of Surgery*, **113**, 205–220.

24 Gunderson, L. L. (1976) Cancer of the GI tract. Radiation therapy: results and future possibilities. *Clinical Gastroenterology*, **5**, 743–776.

25 Hambraeus, G. M., Merche, C. E., Hamman, E. et al. (1981) Surgery alone or combined with radiation therapy in esophageal carcinoma. *Cancer*, **48**, 63–68.

26 Hecker, E. (1981) Co-carcinogens and tumour promoters of the diterpene ester type as possible carcinogenic risk factors. *Journal of Cancer Research and Clinical Oncology*, **99**, 103–124.

27 Howell-Evans, A. W., McConnell, R. B., Clarke, C. A. & Sheppard, P. M. (1958) Carcinoma of the oesophagus with keratosis palmaris and plantaris (tylosis) A study of two families. *Quarterly Journal of Medicine*, **27**, 413–429.

28 Huang, K. C. (1981) Diagnosis and treatment of early esophageal carcinoma. In *Medical and Surgical Problems of the Esophagus* (Ed.) Stipa, S. Belsey, R. H. R. & Moraldi, A. London, New York, Toronto: Academic Press.

29 Huddy, P. & Griffiths, G. (1972) Leiomyoma of the esophagus with calcification. *British Journal of Surgery*, **59**, 239–242.

30 Inberg, M. V., Linna, M. I., Scheinin, T. M. et al. (1971) Anastomotic leakage after excision of oesophageal and high gastric carcinoma. *American Journal of Surgery*, **122**, 540–544.

31 Jackson, C. (1925) Carcinoma and sarcoma of the esophagus: a plea for early diagnosis. *American Journal of Medical Sciences*, **169**, 625–630.

32 Kasai, M., Mori, S. & Watanabe, T. (1978) Follow-up results after resection of thoracic oesophageal carcinoma. *World Journal of Surgery*, **2**, 543–551.

33 Kaufmann, E. (1929) *Pathology for Students and Practitioners* Vol. 1, p. 638. London: H. K. Lewis. Translated by S. P. Reimann.

34 Kelsen D. P., Cvitkovic R., Bains M. S. & Golbey R. (1978) Cis-dichlorodiammine platinum (II) and bleomycin in the treatment of esophageal carcinoma. *Cancer Treatment Reports*, **62**, 1041–1046.

35 Kelsen, D. P., Bains, M. S., Cvitkovic, E. & Golbey, R. (1979) Vindesine in the treatment of esophageal carcinoma: a phase II study. *Cancer Treatment Reports*, **63**, 2019–2021.

36 Kelsen, D. P., Bains, M. S., Chapman, R. & Golbey, R. (1981) Cisplatin, vindesine and bleomycin combination chemotherapy of esophageal carcinoma. *Cancer Treatment Reports*, **65**, 781–785.

37 Kirby, K. S. (1960) Induction of tumours by tannin extracts. *British Journal of Cancer*, **14**, 147–150.

38 Kock, N. G., Lewin, E. & Pettersson, S. (1967) Carcinoma of the thoracic esophagus. A review of 146 cases. *Acta Chirurgica Scandinavica*, **133**, 375–380.

39 Kolaric, K., Maricic, Z., Roth, A. & Dujmovic, I. (1977) Adriamycin alone and in combination with radiotherapy in the treatment of inoperable esophageal cancer. *Tumori*, **63**, 485–491.

39a Launois, B., Delarue, D., Campion, J. P. & Kerbaol, M. (1981) Prospective randomised trial of preoperative radiotherapy in the management of esophageal carcinoma. *Surgery, Gynecology and Obstetrics*, **153**, 690–692.

40 Lawrence, W. (1976) Surgical management of gastrointestinal cancer. *Clinical Gastroenterology*, **5**, 703–742.

41 LeRoux, B. T. (1961) An analysis of 700 cases of carcinoma of the hypopharynx, the oesophagus and the proximal stomach. *Thorax*, **16**, 226–255.

42 Marks, R. D., Scraggs, H. T. & Wallace, K. M. (1976) Pre-operative radiation therapy for carcinoma of the esophagus. *Cancer*, **38**, 84–89.

43 McDonald, G. B., Brand, D. L. & Thorning, D. R. (1977). Multiple adenomatous neoplasms arising in columnar lined (Barrett's) esophagus. *Gastroenterology*, **72**, 1317–1321.

44 McKeown, F. (1952) Oat-cell carcinoma of the oesophagus. *Journal of Pathology and Bacteriology*, **64**, 889–891.

45 McKeown, K. C. (1979) Carcinoma of the oesophagus. *Journal of the Royal College of Surgeons of Edinburgh*, **24**, 253–274.

46 Moersch, H. J. & Broders, A. C. (1935) Adenoma of the oesophagus. *Archives of Otolaryngology*, **21**, 168–170.

47 Moertel, C. G. (1976) Chemotherapy of gastrointestinal cancer. *Clinics in Gastroenterology*, **5**, 777–793.

48 Moghissi, K., Hornshaw, J. & Teasdale, P. R. (1977) Parenteral nutrition and carcinoma of the oesophagus treated by surgery: nitrogen balance and clinical studies. *British Journal of Surgery*, **64**, 125–128.

49 Morton, J. F. (1968) Plants associated with oesophageal cancer cases in Curaçao. *Cancer Research*, **28**, 2268–2271.

50 Mousseau, M., LeForestier, J., Barbin, J. & Hardy, M. (1956) Place de l'intubation à demeure dans le traitement palliatif du cancer de l'oesophage. *Archives des Maladies de l'Appareil Digestif*, **45**, 208–214.

51 Muñoz, N., Crespi, M., Grassi, A., Qiong, S. *et al.* (1982) Precursor lesions of oesophageal cancer in high-risk populations in Iran and China. *Lancet*, **i**, 876–879.

52 Napalkov, N. P. & Pozharisski, K. (1969) Morphogenesis of experimental tumors of the oesophagus. *Journal of the National Cancer Institute*, **42**, 922–940.

53 Notkin, L. J. (1928) Gastro-oesophageal carcinoma: its diagnosis. *Canadian Medical Association Journal*, **19**, 96–99.

54 Ogilvie, A. L., Dronfield, M. W., Ferguson, R. & Atkinson, M. (1982) Palliative intubation of oesophagogastric neoplasms at fibreoptic endoscopy. *Gut*, **23**, 1060–1067.

55 Oka, Masaaki. (1981) Immunological studies on esophageal cancer. *Archives of Japanese Surgery*, **50**, 29–44.

56 Pearson, J. G. (1978) Prognostic factors in oesophageal cancer. In *Carcinoma of the Oesophagus* (Ed.) Silber, W. pp. 449–455. Cape Town & Rotterdam: Balkema.

57 Pearson, J. G. (1981) Radiotherapy for carcinoma of the esophagus. In *Medical and Surgical Problems of the Esophagus* (Ed.) Stipa, S. Belsey, R. H. R. & Moraldi, A. pp. 368–373. London & New York: Academic Press.

58 Peix, J. L., Burnon, D., Baulieux, J. *et al.* (1981) Les petits cancers de l'oesophage. *Lyon Chirurgical*, **77**, 345–348.

59 Poleynard, G. D., Marty, A. T. & Birnbaum, W. B. (1977) Adenocarcinoma in the columnar-lined (Barrett's) esophagus. *Archives of Surgery*, **112**, 997–1000.

60 Postlethwaite, R. W. & Wendell. Musser, A. (1974) Changes in the esophagus in 1000 autopsy specimens. *Journal of Thoracic and Cardiovascular Surgery*, **68**, 953–956.

61 Pottern, L. M., Morris, L. E., Blot, W. J. *et al.* (1981) Esophageal cancer among black men in Washington DC. I: Alcohol, tobacco and other risk factors. *Journal of the National Cancer Institute*, **67**, 777–783.

62 Rainer, W. G. & Brus, R. (1965) Leiomyosarcoma of the esophagus. Review of the literature and report of 3 cases. *Surgery*, **58**, 343–350.

63 Rasmussen, C. W. (1976) A new endoscopic classification of chronic esophagitis. *American Journal of Gastroenterology*, **65**, 409–415.

64 Ravry, M., Moertel, C. G., Schutt, A. J. *et al.* (1973) Treatment of advanced squamous cell carcinoma of the gastrointestinal tract with bleomycin. *Cancer Chemotherapy Reports*, **57**, 493–495.

65 Reid, H. A. S., Richardson, W. W. & Cossin, B. (1980) Oat cell carcinoma of the esophagus. *Cancer*, **45**, 2342–2347.

66 Rose E. F. (1981) A review of factors associated with cancer of the esophagus in the Transkei. In *Cancer Amongst Black Populations* (Ed.) Mettkin, C. & Murphy, G. P. pp. 67–75. New York: Liss.

67 Seremetis, M. C., Lyons, W. S., DeCuzman, V. C. & Peabody, J. W. (1976) Leiomyomata of the oesophagus. Analysis of 838 cases. *Cancer*, **38**, 2166–2177.

68 Schmidt, H. W., Clagett, O. T. & Harrison, E. G. (1961) Benign tumours and cysts of the esophagus. *Journal of Thoracic and Cardiovascular Surgery*, **41**, 717–732.

69 Schwindt, W. D., Bernhardt, L. C. & Johnson, S. A. M. (1970) Tylosis and intrathoracic neoplasms. *Diseases of the Chest*, **57**, 590–597.

70 Smithers, D. W. (1955) The association of cancer of the stomach and oesophagus with herniation at the oesophageal hiatus of the diaphragm. *British Journal of Radiology*, **28**, 554–564.

71 Spin, F. P. (1973) Adenomas of the oesophagus: case report and review of the literature. *Gastrointestinal Endoscopy*, **20**, 26–27.

72 Steiger, Z., Franklin, R., Wilson, R. *et al.* (1981) Complete eradication of squamous cell carcinoma with combined chemotherapy and radiotherapy. *American Surgery*, **47**, 95–98.

73 Talbert, J. L. & Cantrell, J. R. (1963) Clinical and pathologic characteristics of carcinosarcomas of the oesophagus. *Journal of Thoracic and Cardiovascular Surgery*, **45**, 1–12.

74 Waterfall, W. E., Somers, S. & Desa, D. J. (1978) Benign oesophageal papillomatosis: a case report with a review of the literature. *Journal of Clinical Pathology*, **31**, 111–115.

75 Watson, A. (1982) A study of the quality and duration of survival following resection, endoscopic intubation and surgical intubation in oesophageal carcinoma. *British Journal of Surgery*, **69**, 585–588.

76 Watson, T. A. (1963) Radiation treatment of cancer of the esophagus. *Surgery, Gynecology and Obstetrics*, **117**, 346–354.

77 Wychulis, A. R., Woolam, G. L., Andersen, H. A. & Ellis, F. H. Jr. (1971) Achalasia and carcinoma of the esophagus. *Journal of the American Medical Association*, **215**, 1638–1640.

78 Yang, C. S. (1980) Research on oesophageal cancer in China: a review. *Cancer Research*, **40**, 2633–2644.

OTHER CONDITIONS

CRICOPHARYNGEAL DISORDERS

Reported disorders of the cricopharyngeus are summarized in Table 2.7. The upper oesophageal sphincter is formed by the cricopharyngeus muscle and probably by the circular fibres of the uppermost portion of the oesophageal muscle coat. The cricopharyngeus acts as a muscle sling and the cricoid cartilage forms the anterior aspect. The sphincter plays an important part in preventing entry of oesophageal contents into the pharynx and entry of air into the pharynx during inspiration. Its function is coordinated with that of the oesophagus below and with the pharynx above. As it consists of striated muscle it reacts much more quickly than the smooth muscle of the lower oesophagus: during swallowing it opens for only a second to allow the passage of the bolus. The sphincter

Table 2.7 Reported disorders of the cricopharyngeus

Disorders of resting tone	
Increased	Gastro-oesophageal reflux
	Residual food in oesophagus (achalasia)
	Globus syndrome
Reduced	Myasthenia gravis
	Dermatomyositis
	Dystrophia myotonica
	Bilateral recurrent laryngeal palsy
	Post-laryngectomy
Disorders of deglutition	
Incomplete relaxation	Gastro-oesophageal reflux
Delayed relaxation	Familial dysautonomia
Premature closure	Pharyngeal pouch

remains closed at rest and the resting tone is maintained by a stream of impulses coming down the vagus; this stream is interrupted temporarily during swallowing to allow the muscle to relax.

Variations in cricopharyngeal tone

Increased pressures in the upper oesophageal sphincter have been found in some patients with gastro-oesophageal reflux, where it is believed that the increased tone might be performing a protective function,[14] and also in patients with globus hystericus, where the sphincter does relax normally on swallowing.[24]

Hypotonicity of the sphincter is found in myasthenia gravis, dystrophia myotonica, dermatomyositis and some other neuromuscular disorders, but remarkably the sphincter often remains unaffected by bulbar poliomyelitis and motor neurone disease in spite of widespread paralysis of the pharyngeal constrictor muscles. This suggests that its innervation is derived not from the nucleus ambiguus, which is attacked by these diseases, but from the dorsal vagal nucleus.

Incoordination of cricopharyngeal function

Abnormalities of cricopharyngeal function during swallowing have been described, but their pathogenesis is largely uncertain. Failure of the sphincter to relax completely occurs in some patients with gastro-oesophageal reflux, and in some of these biopsies revealed pathological changes in the cricopharyngeal muscle with increased mitochondria and nemeline rods, suggesting that direct muscle damage is caused by refluxed gastric contents.[12] Incoordination of relaxation occurs after bilateral recurrent laryngeal nerve damage and is rarely seen in poliomyelitis and motor neurone disease.

Premature closure of the cricopharyngeus

Premature closure of the sphincter has been suggested as a cause of pharyngeal pouch (Zenker's diverticulum), which is a pulsion diverticulum of mucosa through the posterior pharyngeal wall immediately above the cricopharyngeus. (see below).

Delayed relaxation of the cricopharyngeus during swallowing occurs in familial dysautonomia (Riley–Day syndrome), in which there is congenital aplasia of peripheral autonomic neurones causing feeding difficulties in infancy.[16]

Cricopharyngeal bar

This is an indentation of the posterior aspect of the pharyngo-oesophageal junction seen on barium swallow and sometimes associated with dysphagia but often symptomless. Beyond occasional muscle hypertrophy no pathological changes have been shown and since the bar is difficult to identify endoscopically, it appears to represent muscle contraction. Although relief of dysphagia has been reported to follow cricopharyngeal myotomy this operation should not be undertaken lightly for such an ill-defined disorder.

DIVERTICULA OF THE PHARYNX AND OESOPHAGUS

Pharyngeal pouch (Zenker's diverticulum)

Anatomy
This diverticulum occurs through a triangular area on the posterior pharyngeal wall between the middle pharyngeal constrictor muscles and the cricopharyngeus (Killian's dehiscence). It varies from a slight bulge to a large pear-shaped diverticulum behind and to the left of the upper oesophagus. Pharyngeal pouches are commoner in the presence of gastro-oesophageal reflux,[23] possibly because of cricopharyngeal dysfunction. It seems probable that premature closure of the sphincter before pharyngeal contraction is complete, which generates high pressures in the pharynx, is at least in part responsible for the development of these diverticula.[4]

The disorder is commonest in elderly men, and when asymptomatic presents a hazard of perforation to the unwary endoscopist. Early symptoms include halitosis, a gurgling sensation on swallowing and nocturnal regurgitation of stale food material into the mouth and sometimes into the respiratory tract, but dysphagia from oesophageal compression is the usual presenting symptom. Large diverticula are usually palpable in the left side of the neck.

Radiologically, diverticula are easily demonstrable on the lateral radiograph and the degree of oesophageal compression can be assessed by this means. Filling defects in the pouch caused by retained food material are often visible. Carcinoma may develop in untreated pharyngeal pouches.[17]

Treatment

All pharyngeal pouches should be treated because of the risks of carcinoma and aspiration of pouch contents into the respiratory tree. Surgical excision with or without cricopharyngeal myotomy is the treatment of choice, but leakage at the suture line and even a cutaneous fistula may ensue. Furthermore, the recurrence rate is high. The Dohlman procedure of endoscopic division of the musculomembranous septum between the pouch and the oesophageal lumen, which of course includes the cricopharyngeus muscle, should be limited to those patients unfit for excision.

Oesophageal diverticula

Traction diverticula from fibrosis of adherent tuberculous mediastinal glands are now rare, as are diverticula following oesophageal trauma such as endoscopic perforation. The majority of oesophageal diverticula result from motor disturbances generating high intraluminal pressure and pushing out the mucosa through weak spots in the musculature of the wall. They occur most commonly in the middle and lower oesophagus and those in the epiphrenic region are often large. Diffuse oesophageal spasm is the usual underlying basis for these pulsion diverticula, and epiphrenic diverticula have been related to a hypertonic lower oesophageal sphincter. Diverticula rarely complicate achalasia. Oesophageal spasm secondary to gastro-oesophageal reflux is the basis for some diverticula which occasionally disappear after successful antireflux therapy.

Oesophageal diverticula are a hazard of endoscopy but the risk is small with the modern forward-viewing instruments. Endoscopy is necessary to detect signs of reflux oesophagitis and monilial infection in the diverticula. Oesophageal motility studies are helpful in assessing the underlying motor disorder.

Few oesophageal diverticula cause symptoms and most can safely be left alone. Dysphagia and regurgitation more frequently result from associated disease than from the diverticulum itself and spontaneous perforation is rare. Treatment should be aimed at correcting associated motility disorder and dealing with any associated moniliasis.

OESOPHAGEAL WEBS

Sideropenic dysphagia (Paterson–Kelly syndrome)

This disorder is virtually confined to women over the age of 25, but it is not invariably associated with evidence of iron deficiency and may persist long after iron repletion. It is related to atrophic changes in the upper oesophageal epithelium, with basal cell hyperplasia and hyperchromatic cell nuclei.[5] Thin, almost diaphanous webs stretch across the upper oesophagus, and the mucosa in this area is often inflamed. Intermittent dysphagia and choking may result from mechanical obstruction from the web itself, but since endoscopic rupture of the web does not invariably provide relief, it is probable that muscular spasm caused by upper oesophagitis often induces symptoms.

Evidence of iron deficiency is usually present, and a smooth tongue, angular stomatitis and koilonychia are frequently associated. The syndrome is recognized to occur in association with reflux oesophagitis and after gastric surgery. Diagnosis is usually made by radiology and the webs are easily overlooked by the endoscopist. The disorder carries a clear risk of carcinoma of the upper oesophagus, so endoscopic surveillance with biopsy and cytology is advisable.

Rarely, webs are discovered lower in the oesophagus, associated with no other disease and thought to be congenital in origin. They may cause dysphagia with bolus obstruction which is often intermittent.

OESOPHAGEAL RINGS

These may be indistinguishable from oesophageal webs but differ in forming a concentric narrowing of the whole of the lumen of the oesophagus. With the exception of the lower oesophageal ring (Schatzki–Kramer ring) they are extremely rare and probably of congenital origin, as for example those caused by developmental anomalies of the great vessels.

Schatzki–Kramer ring

This annular diaphragm-like narrowing of the lower oesophagus, with squamous epithelium on its upper and columnar epithelium on its lower aspect, was originally thought always to be a muscular contraction, but is now recognized often to be caused by a fibrous stricture in the submucosa.[8, 13] It is 1–2 mm long, with a lumen 7–15 mm in diameter. Its increased resistance to stretch causes total bolus obstruction, but unless tight the stricture is demonstrable on examination only if the oesophagus is distended. A bougie up to 20 mm can be passed easily. The ring may or may not be associated with hiatal hernia, but it is commonly accompanied by endoscopic evidence of reflux oesophagitis, which is its most probable cause. Lower oesophageal rings cause intermittent dysphagia with bolus obstruction often superimposed on symptoms of gastro-oesophageal reflux. They are easily dilated at endoscopy and usually require the institution of measures to combat gastro-oesophageal reflux.

INFECTIONS OF THE OESOPHAGUS

Monilial oesophagitis

Candida albicans seldom causes oesophagitis in the absence of other disease. It complicates obstructive lesions such as achalasia and carcinoma and it occurs in oesophageal diverticula. Endoscopic surveys show that oesophageal moniliasis is commoner in patients with gastric carcinoma and in the presence of chronic gastric ulcer.[21] Debility, immunosuppressive therapy and long-term antibiotics predispose to monilial oesophagitis, but it appears to be surprisingly rare in diabetes mellitus.

Although monilial oesophagitis may be a chance endoscopic finding, the usual presenting symptom is one of acute and painful dysphagia. Visible oral lesions may suggest the diagnosis and the radiological outline of the oesophagus appears shaggy because of ulceration and adherent membrane (Figure 2.27). The oesophagoscopic appearance of whitish plaques on a friable

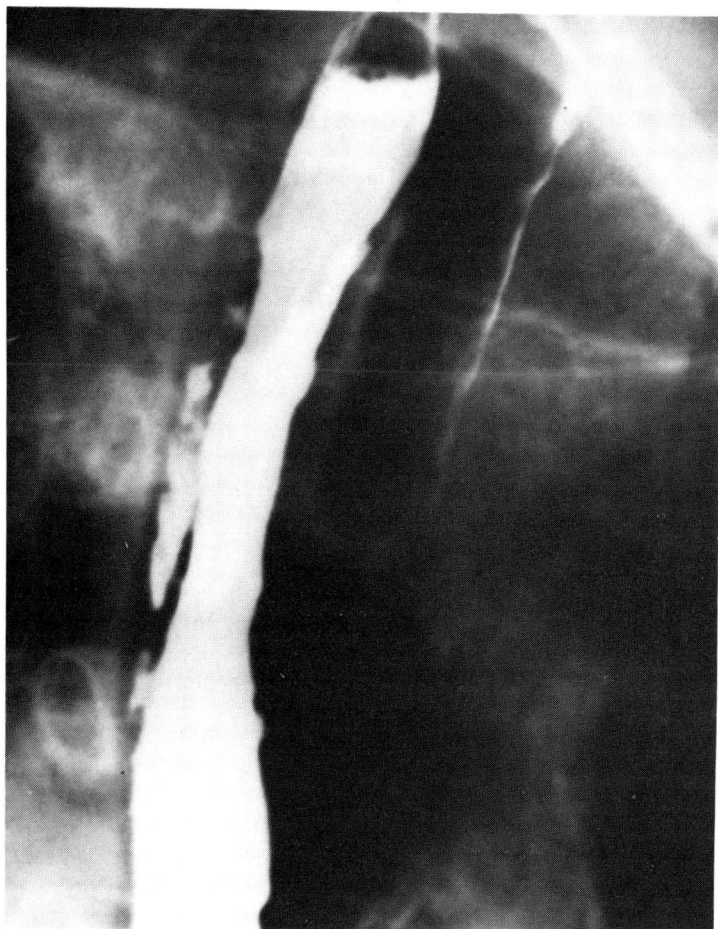

Fig. 2.27 Monilial oesophagitis showing ulceration of upper oesophagus. (Courtesy of Dr S. S. Amar.)

mucosa is not pathognomonic and may be seen in reflux oesophagitis. The essential diagnostic criterion is biopsy evidence of infiltration of tissue by hyphae and yeasts; inflammatory changes are often inconspicuous.

Oesophageal moniliasis, although usually a consequence of other disease, nevertheless aggravates and perpetuates mucosal damage. For this reason antifungal therapy with oral nystatin in liquid form or amphotericin (amphotericin B) lozenges should always be instituted and continued until the infection is eradicated.

Viral oesophagitis

Viral oesophagitis is commoner in immunocompromised patients and is caused by varicella/zoster, herpes simplex or cytomegalovirus.

Varicella not infrequently involves the mouth and throat; vesicular lesions of the oesophagus are probably not uncommon although seldom diagnosed.

Herpes simplex oesophagitis has long been recognized as complicating immunosuppressive therapy, but there is increasing evidence that it occurs in the absence of other disease and may be transmitted by direct contact with an infected person.[19] The disease causes abrupt and severe odynophagia associated with fever and persistent retrosternal pain. It is often preceded by an upper respiratory tract infection, by labial herpes or sore throat. The endoscopic appearances are characteristic, with discrete herpetic ulcers coalescing in severe cases to form larger areas of ulceration with haemorrhage. Eosinophilic intranuclear inclusions are found in biopsy specimens, but secondary bacterial infection of the ulcers commonly occurs, making histological diagnosis more difficult. A rising titre of antibodies to herpes simplex characterizes acute but not relapsing infections.

Treatment for herpes simplex oesophagitis is symptomatic using topical anaesthetics such as oxethazaine as in Mucaine. The value of topical antiviral agents such as idoxuridine remains to be proven and the outlook depends ultimately upon the nature of any underlying disease.

FOREIGN BODIES IN THE OESOPHAGUS[20]

Foreign bodies may lodge in the oesophagus at any age but children under 10 years and the mentally handicapped are the most likely to swallow such objects. Bones and coins are the most frequent but a fuller list is given in Table 2.8. Rarely the foreign body enters the oesophagus as a consequence of a medical procedure or a war injury. The majority of foreign bodies swallowed are small enough to pass through the alimentary tract without symptoms. In children the object often lodges in the upper oesophagus at or near the cricopharyngeus, causing pain, salivation, refusal to eat and occasional breathing difficulties. In adults larger objects tend to lodge in the mid or lower oesophagus, causing pain and dysphagia. Sharp objects that penetrate the oesophageal wall present with mediastinal abscess or torrential bleeding from one of the great vessels; this may also follow erosion of a prosthetic endo-oesophageal tube placed through a neoplastic stricture.[18]

Table 2.8 Foreign bodies in the oesophagus

Swallowed objects	
Food material	Chicken, fish and meat bones
	Fruit stones
	Unchewed boluses of meat, orange segments or other vegetable matter
Toys	Marbles
	Lead or plastic figures
Personal effects	Dentures
	Hairgrips & hair
	Razor blades
Household objects	Coins
	Pins, needles & safety-pins
	Cutlery
	Nuts, bolts, screws and nails
Medical	Large tablets and capsules
	Thermometers
	Hypodermic needles
	Dental drills
Other objects	Surgical sutures
	Prosthetic tubes
	Shrapnel

Every patient suspected of having ingested a foreign body must be investigated with posteroanterior and lateral radiographs of the neck, chest and abdomen. If the object is not metallic it will probably not be visible, but air in the tissues of the neck or mediastinum indicates perforation. For a swallow a contrast medium like propyliodone (Dionosil) is preferable to barium because it does not obscure the view at any subsequent endoscopy.

Endoscopy is needed in most patients in whom a foreign body is lodged in the upper alimentary tract, first to confirm the nature of the object and its lie and secondly for its possible retrieval. It must be decided whether to wait for the spontaneous passage of the foreign body or to attempt its removal; this will depend upon its size and position and whether it is embedded in the oesophageal wall.

It is now possible to deal with most objects lodged in the oesophagus by endoscopic means, by breaking up food boluses to allow their onward passage or by removing objects with the large armamentarium of grasping forceps and snares that are currently available for endoscopic use. Great care must be taken not to cause further damage to the pharynx or oesophagus during the procedure, and sharp objects such as open safety-pins should be grasped and pulled into an over-tube passed over the outside of a fibre-optic endoscope, before removing the whole assembly. Prophylactic antibiotic cover is used when there is a risk of oesophageal damage and mediastinitis, and repeat radiographic examination after the procedure is advisable to identify air in the tissues. Large foreign bodies, particularly those that have penetrated the wall of the oesophagus, need surgical removal, but this is fortunately rare.

PERFORATION OF THE OESOPHAGUS

This may occur spontaneously or as a result of trauma sustained from a foreign body or during an endoscopic procedure.

Spontaneous perforation[15]

This occurs during acute retching or vomiting, although such a history is not invariably present. Perforations occur in the lower oesophagus, most often on the left posterior wall just above the cardia. Their pathogenesis is related to that of Mallory–Weiss mucosal tears just below the cardia, in that the tear occurs when the pressure gradient across the wall is high, with the greatly raised abdominal pressure transmitted through the cardia opposed to the relatively low external intrathoracic pressure. Spontaneous oesophageal perforation presents with acute and severe chest pain often accompanied by dyspnoea, shock, fever and signs of surgical emphysema or pleural effusion. The risk of mediastinitis is high because food material enters the peri-oesophageal tissues and often the pleural cavity. Urgent operation, with closure of the tear and chest drainage, is essential and spontaneous tears should not be treated conservatively.

Perforation at endoscopy

Oesophageal tears are most likely to occur during the course of endoscopic therapy for obstructive oesophageal lesions. The majority happen in elderly patients undergoing endoscopic intubation for neoplasms of the oesophagus or cardia and occasionally during dilatation of fibrous oesophageal strictures.[18] Unlike spontaneous perforations, these do well with conservative management, so long as the tear does not extend to the pleural cavity and provided it is recognized early, before food material or barium has been allowed to enter the mediastinal tissues. Before commencing an endoscopic procedure carrying a high risk of perforation, the patient should receive a dose of a broad-spectrum antibiotic to provide a high level in the tissues in case tearing should occur. After the procedure radiographs of the neck, chest and abdomen should be taken to search for air in the tissues, and the ingestion of food or barium is avoided until a tear has been excluded. Conservative management for an oesophageal tear consists of parenteral antibiotic therapy and the withholding of any intake by mouth while maintaining nutrition by parenteral means. After 10 to 14 days a propyliodone swallow is undertaken to assess whether leakage is still occurring; if not, oral feeding with a soft diet is recommenced. Such measures have reduced the mortality of endoscopic oesophageal perforation to less than 10%.[9]

CHEMICAL AND PHYSICAL OESOPHAGEAL DAMAGE

Corrosive poisons

In some developing countries the ingestion of corrosives such as caustic soda, taken either accidentally (usually by children) or with suicidal intent, is still one of the commonest forms of poisoning.[1] Clinitest tablets (diagnostic reagent tablets containing copper sulphate), paint strippers and denture cleansers also contain caustic alkalies. Cresol-and-soap solution (e.g. Lysol) and concentrated acids may also cause oesophageal burns. Within a few minutes of ingestion, burns of the buccal, pharyngeal and oesophageal mucosa cause severe pain in the throat and chest, usually accompanied by vomiting, pallor and shock. Perforation of the oesophagus or stomach occurs in severe cases and carries a high mortality.

Early treatment consists of intravenous fluids, broad-spectrum antibiotics and hydrocortisone.

The maintenance of patency of the oesophagus is imperative because scarring develops within a week or two and the resulting strictures often involve virtually the whole length of the oesophagus (Figure 2.28) causing complete obstruction. Early endoscopy has been shown to be safe, and gentle dilatation should be used to maintain luminal patency.[1]

Established fibrotic strictures following the ingestion of corrosives are much more difficult to treat by endoscopic dilatation than peptic strictures. Furthermore, there is a considerable risk of squamous carcinoma of the oesophagus developing after 15 to 30 years. For these reasons oesophagectomy and oesophageal replacement by a colonic or jejunal loop is the treatment of choice for extensive corrosive strictures refractory to endoscopic dilatation.

Drug-induced oesophageal damage

In recent years an increasing number of drugs have been reported to cause direct oesophageal damage from mucosal contact with consequent ulceration or aggravation of pre-existing reflux oesophagitis.[2] Radiological studies reveal that tablets may remain in the normal oesophagus for periods of up to 90 minutes and the delay in transit is greatest when tablets are ingested by elderly patients in the recumbent position without an accompanying draught of fluid.[6] These are just the conditions which apply when an elderly patient afraid to drink because of urinary difficulties takes a tablet on retiring at night. Gastro-oesophageal reflux often impairs oesophageal clearing, and if it has caused a fibrous stricture delay is even more likely. Systemic sclerosis, achalasia and diffuse oesophageal spasm are all associated with delay in oesophageal transit and increase the probability of drug-induced damage.

Oesophageal ulceration has been described after a wide variety of drugs (Table 2.9). It often

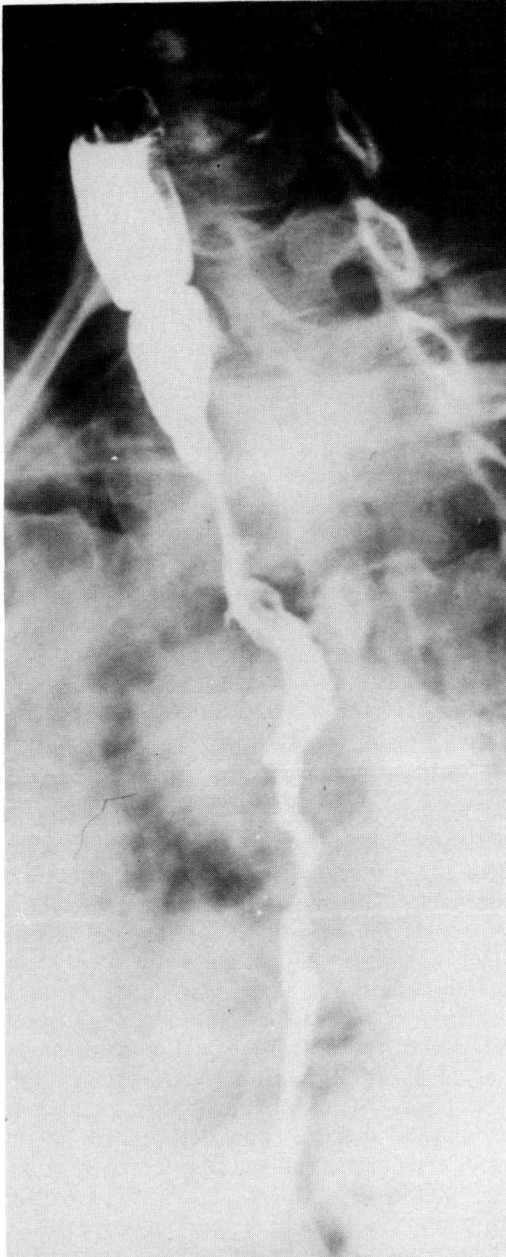

Fig. 2.28 Extensive oesophageal stricture after ingestion of caustic soda 25 years previously.

Table 2.9 Drugs which cause oesophageal damage

Emepronium bromide (Cetiprin)
Tetracycline, doxycycline, clindamycin
Potassium tablets
Non-steroidal anti-inflammatory drugs
Cytotoxic drugs, fluorouracil

involves the mid or upper oesophagus and may be mistaken for neoplasm. Fibrous strictures may follow healing (Figure 2.29), but these readily respond to endoscopic dilatation once their cause has been recognized. The regular ingestion of non-steroidal anti-inflammatory drugs, particularly in patients suffering from gastro-oesophageal reflux, is probably an important factor in causing stricture formation.[11] Extreme care is needed if these drugs are to be given orally in the presence of reflux oesophagitis.

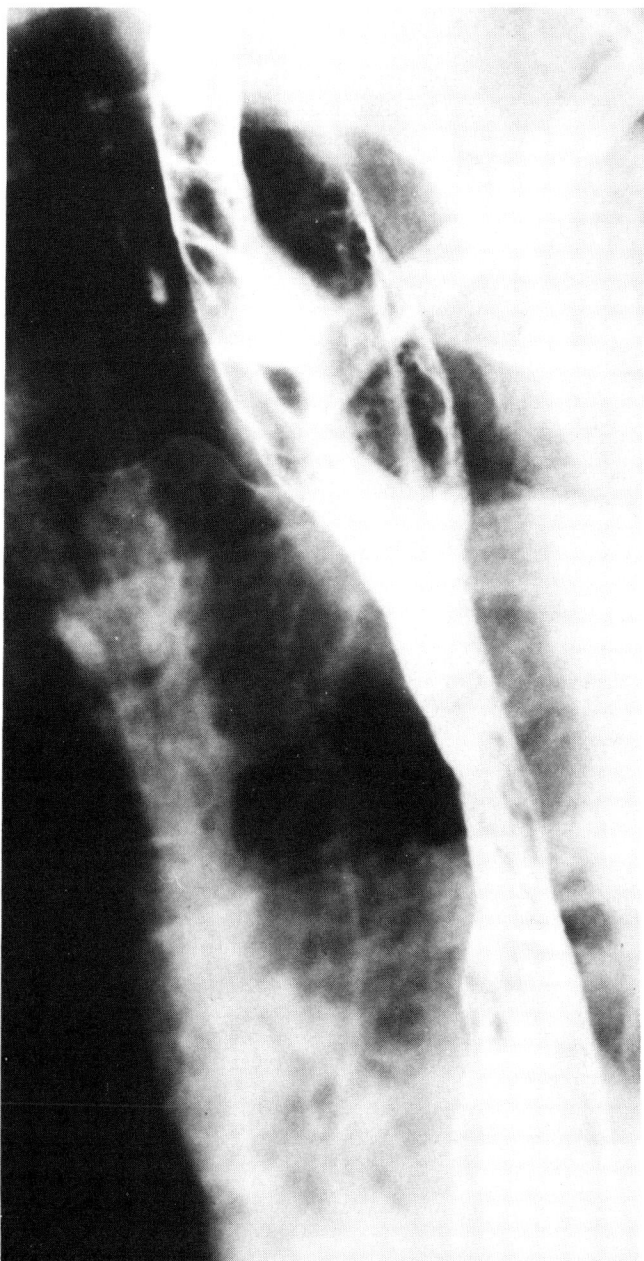

Fig. 2.29 Oesophageal ulceration and fibrous stricture induced by emepronium bromide.

Radiation-induced oesophageal damage

High-dosage mediastinal irradiation induces localized oesophagitis which is usually self-limiting and causes temporary odynophagia. However, if severe, the oesophagitis may progress to stricture formation with persistent dysphagia, and rarely a fistula develops to the bronchial tree. There is some evidence that the concomitant administration of cytotoxic drugs such as doxorubicin lowers the radiation threshold for oesophagitis from 40–60 Gy (4000–6000 rad) to as little as 5 Gy.[7]

OESOPHAGEAL INVOLVEMENT BY SYSTEMIC DISEASE

Motility disturbance

Muscle disorders such as dystrophia myotonica, myasthenia gravis and dermatomyositis affecting striated muscle disrupt the pharyngeal phase of swallowing, as do bulbar disorders such as poliomyelitis and motor neurone disease. Difficulty in initiating swallowing occurs in some patients with Parkinson's disease. Disturbance of motility of the lower oesophagus and lower oesophageal sphincter is found in systemic sclerosis and other collagen diseases, while autonomic neuropathy may disrupt motility in the diabetic, the alcoholic and in other disorders associated with peripheral neuropathy. These and other motor disturbances are dealt with above, in the section on motor disorders of the oesophagus.

Granulomatous oesophagitis

Crohn's disease[3]
Oesophageal symptoms are rare in Crohn's disease, but silent lesions such as localized mucosal thickening and aphthous ulcers with giant cell granulomas on biopsy are more frequently detectable in the oesophagus at endoscopy in patients suffering from the disease. The most characteristic feature is multiple intramural fistulous tracks, occasionally extending outside the oesophagus and often causing fibrotic narrowing leading to dysphagia. In these patients endoscopic dilatation may be required but otherwise treatment is that of the Crohn's disease elsewhere.

Sarcoidosis
This disease very rarely involves the oesophagus but it can cause granulomatous and fibrotic lesions.

Tuberculosis
Tuberculosis is almost always secondary to open pulmonary disease and causes oesophageal ulceration.

Miscellaneous disorders

Skin disorders

Bullous lesions of the oesophageal mucosa have been reported in pemphigus and in a rare disorder known as benign mucous membrane pemphigoid.[10] Dystrophic epidermolysis in its recessive form involves the buccal and oesophageal mucosa in infancy, causing haemorrhagic bullae. In each of these disorders dysphagia results from fibrosis and stricture formation.

Behçet's syndrome
In this chronic relapsing disorder ulceration may extend beyond the mouth into the oesophagus and healing of these lesions can cause fibrotic oesophageal stricture.

Tylosis (keratosis palmaris et plantaris)
In this hereditary (mendelian dominant) disorder thickening of the skin of the soles and palms with fissuring and flaking begins early in life and is associated with an increased incidence of oesophageal ulceration, stricture and squamous cell carcinoma.[22]

Neoplastic disease
Oesophageal involvement by tumours arising in the lung or mediastinal glands causes dysphagia and fistulas into the respiratory tree. Lymphoma rarely involves the oesophagus directly, but antimitotic therapy may cause severe oesophagitis with or without opportunistic monilial or herpetic infection.

REFERENCES

1 Balsegaram, M. (1975) Early management of corrosive burns of the oesophagus. *British Journal of Surgery*, **62**, 444–447.
2 Collins, F. J., Matthews, H. R., Baker, S. E. & Strakova, J. M. (1979) Drug-induced oesophageal injury. *British Medical Journal*, **i**, 1673–1676.
3 Cynn, W. S., Chon, H. K., Gureghian, P. A. & Levin, B. L. (1975) Crohn's disease of the oesophagus. *American Journal of Roentgenology*, **125**, 359–364.
4 Ellis, F. H., Schlegel, J. F., Lynch, V. P. & Payne, W. S. (1969) Cricopharyngeal myotomy for pharyngoesophageal diverticulum. *Annals of Surgery*, **170**, 340–349.
5 Entwistle, C. C. & Jacobs, A. (1965) Histological findings in Paterson–Kelly syndrome. *Journal of Clinical Pathology*, **18**, 408.
6 Evans, K. T. & Roberts, G. M. (1976) Where do all the tablets go? *Lancet*, **ii**, 1237–1239.
7 Goldstein, H. M., Rogers, L. F., Fletcher, G. H. & Dodd, G. D. (1975) Radiological manifestations of radiation-induced injury to the normal upper gastrointestinal tract. *Radiology*, **117**, 135–140.
8 Goyal, R. K., Glancy, J. J. & Spiro, H. M. (1970) Lower oesophageal ring. *New England Journal of Medicine*, **282**, 1298–1305.
9 den Hartog-Jager, F. C. A., Bartelsman, J. F. W. M. & Tytgat, G. N. J. (1979) Palliative treatment of obstructing oesophagogastric malignancy by endoscopic positioning of a plastic prosthesis. *Gastroenterology*, **77**, 1008–1014.
10 Hardy, K. M., Perry, H. O., Pingree, G. C. & Kirby, T. J. Jr. (1971) Benign mucous membrane pemphigoid. *Archives of Dermatology*, **104**, 467–475.
11 Heller, S. R., Fellows, I. W., Ogilvie, A. L. & Atkinson, M. (1982) Non-steroidal anti-inflammatory drugs and benign oesophageal stricture. *British Medical Journal*, **285**, 167–168.
12 Henderson, R. D., Wedad, H., Marryatt, G. V. & Kando, M. (1983) Reflux-induced cricopharyngeal dysphagia – pathological change on muscle biopsies. *Gut*, **24**, A467.
13 Hendrix, T. R. (1980) Schatzki ring, epithelial junction and hiatal hernia: an unresolved controversy. *Gastroenterology*, **79**, 584–585.
14 Hunt, P. S., Connell, A. M. & Smiley, T. B. (1970) The cricopharyngeal sphincter in gastric reflux. *Gut*, **11**, 303–306.

15 Leading Article (1977) Management of oesophageal perforation. *British Medical Journal*, **ii**, 540.
16 Margulies, S. I., Brunt, P. W., Donner, M. W. & Silbiger, M. L. (1968) Familial dysautonomia – a cineradiographic study of the swallowing mechanism. *Radiology*, **90**, 107–112.
17 Nansen, E. M. (1976) Carcinoma in a long-standing pharyngeal pouch. *British Journal of Surgery*, **63**, 417–419.
18 Ogilvie, A. L., Dronfield, M. W., Ferguson, R. & Atkinson, M. (1982) Palliative intubation of oesophagogastric neoplasms at fibre-optic endoscopy. *Gut*, **23**, 1060–1066.
19 Owensby, L. C. & Stammer, J. L. (1978) Esophagitis associated with herpes simplex infection in an immunocompetent host. *Gastroenterology*, **74**, 1305–1306.
20 Schiller, K. F. R. (1981) Foreign bodies of oesophagus or stomach. In *Therapeutic Endoscopy and Radiology of the Gut*. (Ed.) Bennett, J. R. p. 89. London: Chapman Hall.
21 Scott, B. B., & Jenkins, D. (1982) Gastro-oesophageal candidiasis. *Gut*, **23**, 137–139.
22 Shine, A. P. R. (1966) Carcinoma of the oesophagus with tylosis (keratosis palmaris et plantaris). *Lancet*, **i**, 951–953.
23 Smiley, T. B., Caves, P. K. & Porter, D. C. (1970) Relationship between posterior pharyngeal pouch and hiatus hernia. *Thorax*, **25**, 725–731.
24 Watson, W. C. & Sullivan, S. N. (1974) Hypertonicity of the cricopharyngeal sphincter; cause of globus sensation. *Lancet*, **ii**, 1417–1418.

Chapter 3
Diaphragmatic Hernia

J. Spencer

The common diaphragmatic hernia of adult life is the sliding hernia through the oesophageal hiatus. Rolling (or paraoesophageal) hernias are less common, but clinically important. Other hernias of adult life are associated with traumatic rupture or incision of the diaphragm or, most rarely, are due to late presentation of hernias through congenital defects.

Congenital diaphragmatic hernias occur either through the posterolateral space of Bochdalek (Figure 3.1) or anteriorly through the foramen of Morgagni (Figure 3.2).

CONGENITAL DIAPHRAGMATIC HERNIA

POSTEROLATERAL HERNIA

This occurs through the posterolateral pleuroperitoneal canal of Bochdalek. This canal may remain open, with pleura and peritoneum in direct continuity, in which case there is no true hernia sac. More commonly pleura and peritoneum are present, but muscle is absent; in such cases a sac is seen. Bochdalek hernias are twice as common on the left side, and present in the perinatal period, usually with respiratory distress. A true overall incidence is difficult to obtain, as they are mostly seen in autopsies on still-births, usually in association with other congenital defects. Such hernias, however, constitute the bulk of congenital diaphragmatic hernias, and the overall incidences reported range from 1:1000 to 1:12000 births. Several reports give an incidence of around 1:1500 live births.

Those diagnosed early have a worse prognosis, indicating more severe associated problems. Thus mortality in infants diagnosed within one hour of delivery is 70% and in those diagnosed within the first day is 44–65%, whereas almost all diagnosed after 24 hours survive. Most deaths are in infants with Apgar scores of less than 6; some are inevitable, occurring in infants with multiple congenital defects. The uncomplicated hernias which are diagnosed late present no therapeutic problem for they can be repaired by a transabdominal approach with low morbidity and zero mortality. Between these extremes lie hernias that are diagnosed early and which present the greatest therapeutic challenge. Considerable progress has been made in understanding the problems and management of these infants.

A few cases have been diagnosed very early when amniocentesis has revealed 'high-risk' lecithin/sphingomyelin ratios known to be associated with immaturity. The principal problem in such infants is pulmonary hypoplasia and the status in this regard must be determined early. Infants with minimal hypoplasia do not require pharmacological support, whereas those with bilateral hypoplasia cannot be helped; infants with unilateral changes may respond to aggressive therapy.

The initial diagnosis is made by plain radiographs on the basis of clinical suspicion. Collins[9]

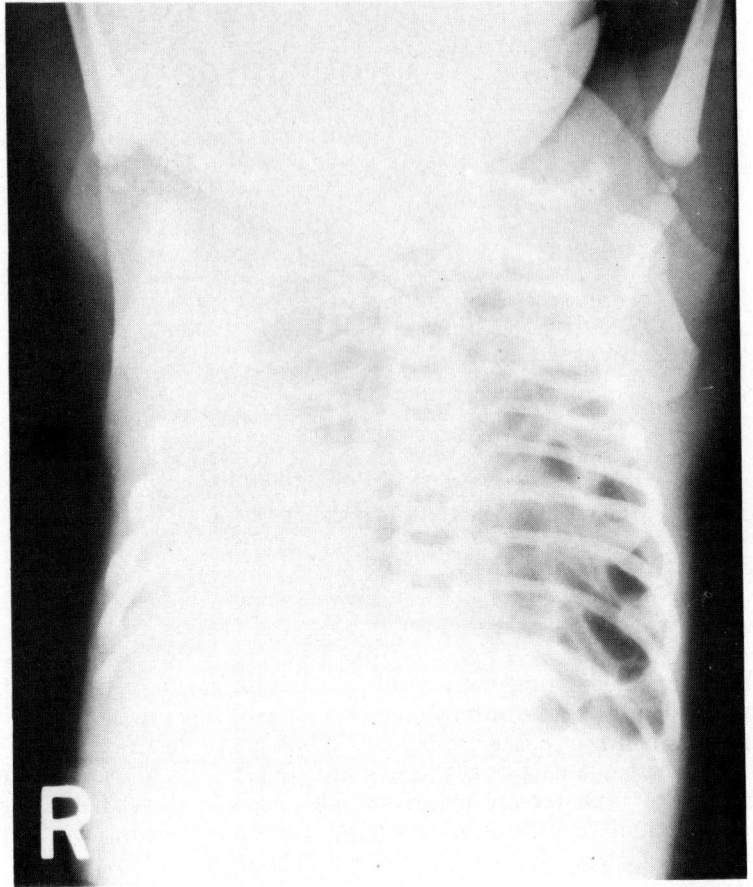

Fig. 3.1 Bochdalek hernia in a
neonate; coarctation of the aorta
was also present.

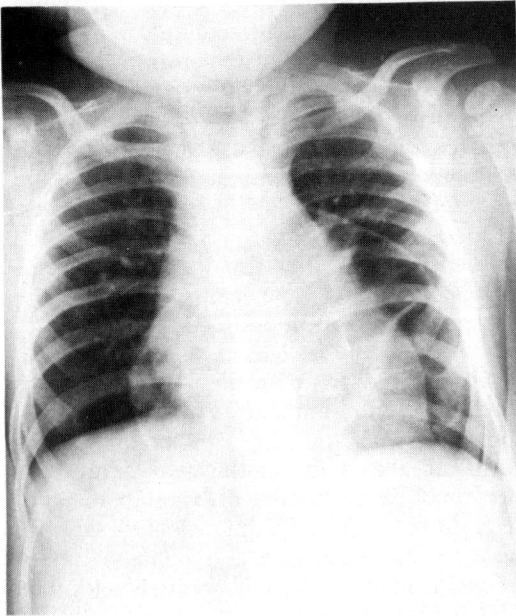

a

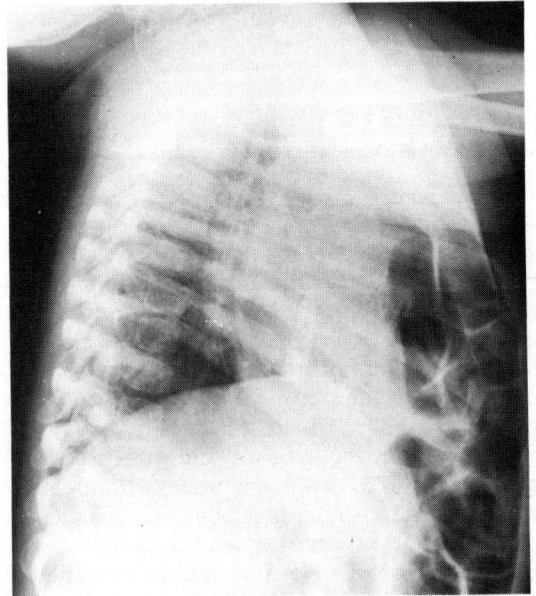

b

Fig. 3.2 Morgagni hernia. Bowel loops are well seen in the posteroanterior view; the lateral reveals the defect to be anterior.

postulated that increased pulmonary vascular resistance, with a persisting fetal circulation and right-to-left shunt was the main reason for death in neonatal Bochdalek hernias. His management comprised initial resuscitation, surgical repair of the defect, cardiac catheterization with balloon blockade of the ductus where indicated, intensive-care-unit monitoring, and pharmacological support.

A similar regimen has been adopted by Sumner and Frank[27] with considerable success. If a hernia is diagnosed within six hours they proceed as follows:

1 Immediate transabdominal repair.
2 Postoperative ventilation and paralysis.
3 Arterial blood pressure and gas monitoring.
4 Correction of acidosis with 8.4% $NaHCO_3$.
5 If a transitional circulation develops (right-to-left shunt) then a tolazoline bolus (1–2 mg/kg) is given over five minutes; tolazoline is then infused at the rate of 1–2 mg/kg an hour until the blood gases have been stable for 12 hours.
6 The baby is weaned to positive airways pressure and extubated.

Tolazoline is an alpha-adrenergic blocker, and also a non-adrenergic direct relaxant to vascular muscle, and is directly cardiotonic. It does, however, have many serious side-effects and must be used carefully. Such approaches have produced a dramatic improvement in the results of repair in a well-defined group of potentially curable neonates.

Bochdalek hernias may present later in childhood or even in adult life, when they may be asymptomatic or present as strangulation. Then they must be differentiated from post-traumatic hernias, which occur through a severed or ruptured diaphragm.

ANTERIOR HERNIA

Between 1% and 5% of congenital hernias are anterior, occurring through the foramen described by Morgagni (1761) as lying 'betwixt the fibres that come from the xiphoid cartilage, and the neighbouring fibres'. The hernias are seen more commonly on the right side; rarely they are bilateral. Usually they are an incidental finding and cause no symptoms, but they may present with symptoms or signs in the neonatal period, in infancy or later in life. A review of patients admitted to a large children's hospital revealed only eight such hernias in a 20-year period.[28] Four presented soon after birth, three because of respiratory distress and one on a chest radiograph done for other reasons. Four older infants were investigated for recurrent chest infections or vomiting.

These hernias may present with intermittent chest pain in adult life. Of 50 adults with such hernias, 14 were symptomatic.[11] In early adult life they occur more often in males than females; later in life this tendency is reversed.

The diagnosis of Morgagni hernias is radiological and includes contrast studies if viscera are involved. Liver scanning is used to confirm herniation of the liver.

The treatment is surgical, and in children repair should be advised. There is a difference of opinion about whether a symptomless hernia in adults should be left untreated. Operative repair presents no difficulties although a few deaths have been reported in neonates who developed a postoperative pneumo-pericardium. An abdominal approach excludes the possibility of overlooking a coexisting contralateral hernia, which, although rare, has caused the death of one patient following transthoracic herniorrhaphy.

SLIDING HIATAL HERNIA

Sliding hernias of the stomach occur through the oesophageal hiatus of the diaphragm, and are 'axial' hernias; that is to say the oesophagus–cardia–stomach axis remains intact but the cardia is elevated above the diaphragm. By contrast, in a paraoesophageal or rolling hernia the cardia remains below the diaphragm and the fundus of the stomach herniates through the hiatus alongside the oesophagus. The term 'sliding' is by analogy with sliding inguinal hernia: in both situations an organ herniates out of the abdomen carrying with it an anterior sac of peritoneum.

Herniation through the hiatus occurs during vomiting and eructation. It must therefore be considered, in its intermittent form, as a physiological phenomenon. Extreme manoeuvres sometimes employed by radiologists can produce herniation of the stomach on screening, indicating a mobility of the cardia which is not necessarily of clinical significance. These observations add fuel to the controversy over what is 'significant' herniation.

Aetiology and natural history

Little is known of the aetiology of herniation. Much of the past literature has discussed ways in which the stomach may be forced up into the chest, but this concept ignores a dominant anatomical feature, namely the longitudinal muscle of the oesophagus. This powerful muscle, attaching the cardia, via the median raphe of the pharynx, to the base of the skull, elevates the cardia when it contracts. Appropriate, and ill-understood, reflexes control elevation of the cardia during eructation and emesis, eliminating the intra-abdominal oesophagus and permitting reflux. Basic research in the 1930s and 1940s indicated that stimulation of intra-abdominal organs such as the gallbladder induced such contraction of the oesophagus. This, and much clinical evidence assembled by Johnson,[19] suggest that hernias are produced by an excessively frequent or forceful exercise of this reflex, the stomach being actively drawn into the chest. Such a hypothesis explains the association of reflux and heartburn with other upper abdominal disease, and the common association between gallstones and hiatal hernia. Clinical measurement of longitudinal muscle function presents difficulties which have hampered useful investigation of such phenomena.

Significant clinical reflux, with or without herniation, may be a transient phenomenon, particularly in pregnancy. Although it is tempting to attribute this to increased abdominal pressure, such an increase does not occur except as a direct hydrostatic effect on the hiatus in the supine position, and hormonal effects are almost certainly of much greater importance. Obesity contributes to reflux and herniation in a way which is reversible.

Small hernias associated with minimal symptoms may remain unchanged for years. Those with more marked symptoms tend to worsen if not actively treated. Observed hernias tend to enlarge with the passage of time.

A clinical assumption often made is that patients with mild oesophagitis will inevitably progress to severe inflammation and stricture if not treated; in fact, this rarely occurs. The majority of strictures, especially in the elderly, are of sudden onset, often with absent or minimal preceding symptoms.

The association between herniation and reflux is the cause of much debate, amidst which some loose thinking is often in evidence. In a classic paper in 1971 Cohen and Harris demonstrated in large groups of selected subjects that whether or not a hernia was present, symptoms occurred only if an incompetent sphincter barrier could be demonstrated,[8] and these data have been used as an indication that the hernia is irrelevant. Prevention of reflux is normally dependent on two main factors. The first is the existence of an intra-abdominal segment of oesophagus. Surgically creating and maintaining such a segment, or a substitute for it, prevents reflux. The second factor is the lower oesophageal sphincter (LOS), the activity of which is determined neurally and hormonally. The effects of hormones on the sphincter are readily demonstrable, but the doses needed tend to be pharmacological rather than physiological. Various drugs increase the tone of the LOS, but only metoclopramide has an effect which could be considered therapeutically useful.

It is possible that a hiatal hernia may follow a sequence of events initiated by gastro-oesophageal reflux. An initiating factor stimulates longitudinal muscle contraction of the oesophagus so that the intra-abdominal oesophagus is eliminated for varying periods of time. This enables reflux into the oesophagus to occur, causing irritation of the oesophageal mucosa. The irritation provokes further contraction and the intra-abdominal oesophagus is eliminated for longer periods. The cardia eventually becomes elevated above the diaphragm. Depending on the interplay of the factors involved, various courses are now possible: herniation may be increased; inflammation may be increased, with stricture formation; or volume and reflux may be increased, causing mechanical reflux symptoms to dominate.

The nature of the refluxed material is probably of crucial significance, particularly the presence of bile: this causes a much more severe oesophagitis than acid reflux alone. The bile salts have been implicated in this: at low pH conjugated bile salts cause oesophagitis, but at neutral pH deconjugated salts are more damaging. In some animal models pancreatic juice causes severe oesophagitis. Salo found that in acid-free conditions deoxycholate and cheno-deoxycholate together with trypsin caused severe damage in rabbits.[25] In man it is known that anastomosis of the oesophagus to small bowel after total gastrectomy in a way that permits bilio-pancreatic reflux causes severe oesophagitis.

Oesophageal clearance is a factor which helps determine the contact time between refluxed material and the mucosa. It is affected by gravity and salivation as well as by motility. The latter is disordered in oesophagitis and especially in scleroderma.

Clinical features

Most sliding hernias are probably asymptomatic. Many produce mild symptoms which are easily controlled and do not demand extensive investigation. Although many symptoms and sequelae are described, only four are commonly important: heartburn (pyrosis), reflux, respiratory symptoms and dysphagia. Other less frequent complications include anaemia and the possibility of oesophageal carcinoma if oesophagitis persists over a long period. The incidence of the latter progression is low and varies in different reports.

Heartburn is the most common symptom associated with reflux. It is characteristically burning and most often associated with bile in the oesophageal aspirates. The sensation appears to arise in the oesophageal mucosa, and can be reproduced by acid perfusion of the gullet as described by Bernstein and Baker.[4] It does, however, occur commonly in patients with gall-bladder disease and duodenal or gastric ulcer, possibly implying that reflux occurs in these patients and might be prevented by treating the primary disease. The severity of pyrosis is not related directly to the degree of inflammation in the oesophagus, though histological changes exist which are characteristically associated with the existence of reflux.[18] These consist of a thinning of the epidermis, with a thickened basal cell layer and more deeply penetrating dermal pegs (papillae). Such changes are often wrongly referred to as 'oesophagitis'; strictly speaking, they are changes associated with reflux, which appear to precede the appearance of inflammation. It has been suggested that thinning of the epithelium brings sensitive nerve endings nearer to the surface, making painful an acid insult which would not be noticed by a normal individual.

Reflux may be the dominant symptom in some patients, who experience the regurgitation of bitter fluid into the throat or mouth, especially on exertion or postural change. The symptom may or may not be associated with pyrosis. Clinical experience suggests that prolonged reflux of low volumes of gastric juice may be sufficient to sensitize the mucosa to produce pyrosis and oesophagitis. The dominance of reflux itself as a symptom implies a larger volume of refluxed material. This is a symptom complex that is less readily managed medically, except in the obese if weight can be lost and at the end of a pregnancy, and it therefore has logistic implications as regards therapy.

Chest infections are a consequence of overspill of refluxed material. In the adult infection seems less frequent in patients with gastro-oesophageal reflux than in those with achalasia, unless stricture formation occurs. In infants, however, evidence is emerging that asthma may well be initiated by gastro-oesophageal reflux, and that in some individuals a lifetime of asthma and bronchitis begins with reflux of this kind. Indeed, it is now postulated that surgical correction of reflux in infancy may avert life-long pulmonary problems in many individuals.

Dysphagia associated with reflux occurs in two forms. Clinical observation reveals that patients with dysphagia, contrary to much previous teaching, are very poor indicators of the true site of obstruction. The major discrepancy is due to food sticking in the cricopharyngeal area, the only radiological pathology being the existence of a sliding hiatal hernia with reflux. Manometric evidence is being produced, albeit not all consistent, that there is pharyngo-cricopharyngeal dyscoordination in these subjects. Most patients once described as having a 'globus hystericus' are now thought to have such a cricopharyngeal syndrome, and in many this is associated with reflux. It is not yet certain whether all patients respond to therapy directed towards the lower end of the oesophagus, though most do.

The more readily recognized dysphagia is that associated with oesophagitis, with or without stricture. As in other parts of the alimentary canal, inflammatory narrowing has three components – spasm, oedema and fibrosis. It is not often appreciated how much the first two components contribute to peptic oesophageal 'strictures'. Such strictures are remarkably reversible if the causative factors are relieved. Dysphagia of any kind is likely to be associated with overspill causing respiratory symptoms.

Rarely, a sliding hiatal hernia is present without reflux, and causes aching discomfort in the epigastrium or left hypochondrium which may be relieved by eructation. This appears to be analogous to the pain occurring in other abdominal hernias, and is relieved by operative repair.

Diagnosis

In the majority of patients with clinically significant sliding hiatal hernias there is no difficulty in diagnosis. Clinical suspicion leads to a request for a barium 'swallow and meal' during which the diagnosis is confirmed.

The existence of a hernia is confirmed if the radiologist can recognize the gastro-oesophageal junction lying above the diaphragm. The site of the hiatus is usually indicated by its compression on the herniated stomach; it may be surprisingly above or below the projected curve of the diaphragmatic dome. The mucosal pattern usually separates oesophagus and stomach readily, and a sphincter zone can be identified. Sometimes this is ring-like as described by Schatzki; if dilatation of such a ring is limited to a diameter of 12 mm or less then dysphagia is usual. The existence of free reflux without undue provocation is of great clinical significance, and probably more important than the documentation of an anatomical hernia. Double-contrast techniques permit the detection of quite early changes in oesophagitis. In more severe inflammation ulceration may be seen. Strictures due to peptic digestion are almost always short, but may appear long as the portion below the stricture cannot be distended with contrast medium. One exception is the stricture associated with nasogastric intubation in sick, and especially in comatose, patients; such strictures are long and tapering and occur in the lower third of the oesophagus. High strictures, usually at the level of the aortic arch, are seen associated with the Barrett's columnar-lined gullet.

Inflammatory strictures often occur in the elderly, and may present as dysphagia with little in the way of previous symptoms. A significant event must have occurred in these subjects. This may be a change in the nature of previously refluxing gastric juice, perhaps by the addition of *bile*. This is pure hypothesis at the moment.

Endoscopy has an important role in the diagnosis of dysphagia, being mandatory in every patient with this symptom. Fibre-optic examination is a simple outpatient procedure permitting biopsy of the oesophageal mucosa and of strictures. Cytological brushings should be obtained. If repeated biopsies do not exclude malignancy in doubtful cases, rigid endoscopy under anaesthesia permits more accurate and much larger biopsies.

The Bernstein acid-perfusion test has been widely used in the diagnosis of reflux oesophagitis. Hydrochloric acid (0.1 mol/l) is infused through an oro-oesophageal tube so that it perfuses the lower third of the oesophagus; the symptomatic effects of this are compared with those of a similar infusion of normal saline as a control. This is basically a pain-reproduction test. In most patients a good clinical history will tell everything that a Bernstein test can reveal.

Table 3.1 Bernstein oesophageal perfusion test: incidence of positive results in 140 subjects.

Diagnosis	n	Positive results	
Normal	11	2	(18%)
Peptic ulcer	17	5	(29%)
Gallstones	3	2	(67%)
X-ray negative			
Dyspepsia	27	10	(37%)
Hiatus hernia	82	40	(49%)

The greatest disadvantage of the test, however, is its poor specificity, the test often being positive, for example, in subjects with gallstones (see Table 3.1). If there remains any clinical use for this test, it is in the differentiation of cardiac and oesophageal pain in the occasional difficult patient. Other clinical features help in this differentiation, especially the persistence of pain after exercise has ceased.

Oesophageal pH measurements may be helpful in the diagnosis of difficult patients but have no routine value except as a research tool. The *pH profile* across the cardia is of little value; it may be less precise in the presence of a 'refluxing' hernia but is no reliable guide. *Stress tests*, in which a pH probe is left in the lower oesophagus during prescribed manoeuvres, have been standardized as the SART (standard acid reflux test).[26] This has at least been defined clearly so that pre- and postoperative tests can be done in a useful manner, but the results are not as reproducible as one would like. *Prolonged pH recordings* over periods of up to 24 hours have a valuable research application but are not very practical in routine clinical circumstances. They have been made simpler by developments in radiotelemetry and in digital recording techniques.

Acid-clearing tests are a development in which a pH probe is used to determine the time taken for the oesophageal muscle to clear away an instilled acid bolus. This technique demonstrates that oesophagitis is associated with diminished peristaltic efficacy, which may produce a vicious circle leading to worsening of the oesophagitis.

Oesophageal manometry is a well established method of assessing motility and sphincter tone. It is perhaps more accurate to refer to sphincter 'squeeze' rather than 'pressure'. In clinical practice manometry usually reveals fairly precisely what could be predicted from careful radiology; rarely does unexpected information emerge. On the other hand, measurements of sphincter function before and after therapy give a good indication of response and it is important that, in some centres at least, objective measurements of this kind are made.

Treatment of gastro-oesophageal reflux

CONSERVATIVE TREATMENT

All patients with documented reflux oesophagitis should be treated conservatively without surgical operation in the first instance. Table 3.2 lists the most useful measures in conservative management, which is discussed in greater detail in the section on reflux oesophagitis in Chapter 2. There are three main elements to such non-surgical treatment: weight loss, postural treatment and drug therapy.

Weight loss. Sliding hiatal hernias become symptomatic in people who become overweight. Although this is commonly attributed to increased abdominal pressure associated with obesity, such an increase has not been well documented. There is, however, a fat pad on the oesophagus which needs to be dissected away during operation. It appears to be a lubricating layer on which the cardia slides more readily than usual through the hiatus, and it is possible that this deposit of fat, as part of a more generalized deposition as obesity develops, predisposes to the formation of such a hernia.

Postural treatment. Patients are advised to avoid unnecessary bending. Advice about posture at night is most important: sleeping propped up on pillows is ineffective because patients fall off the pillows during the night and wake up crouched uncomfortably in a position which promotes reflux. Blocking of the head end of the patient's bed is necessary so that a more comfortable sleeping position can be combined with a slope that diminishes reflux.

Drug therapy. Agents used in the conservative medical treatment of reflux can be divided into those which form a mechanical barrier, those which reduce the acid load on the oesophageal mucosa, those which strengthen the resistance of the gastric mucosa, and those which increase sphincter tone and possibly have additional effect by increasing gastric emptying.

SURGICAL TREATMENT

Indications for surgery
Most patients are treated initially by conservative means. The decision as to which patients should be operated upon remains at the moment more a matter of art than science. There are so many areas of imprecision in assessment of this particular disease that fully objective assessment is not possible. Even if objective measurements such as pH recording give the same results, the reactions of different patients to given mechanical situations will be quite different, influencing the necessity for surgical intervention. The rather arbitrary nature of this decision has one important result, namely that in no two surgical series will the patients be strictly comparable. The aggressiveness of a particular surgeon, his attitude towards the importance of certain endoscopic criteria, his approach to stenosing oesophagitis, and many other such factors will influence the choice of patients for operation and produce a series with a unique blend of patients and situations, which he then treats in his own individual style.

The principal indication for surgery, however difficult it is to define, is the failure of conservative treatment. That is to say, symptoms which are severe and persistent in spite of therapy should be treated by an operation. There is no clear indication at present that oesophagitis, as seen endoscopically, is an urgent indicator of the need for operation; but contrary views are often

Table 3.2 Conservative management of reflux.

1 Weight loss	
2 Posture: blocking of bed	
3 Applied pharmacology	
Mechanical barriers	Gaviscon, Gastrocote, Pyrogastrone
Reduction of acid	antacids
	H_2 antagonists
Increase mucosal resistance	carbenoxolone
Increase sphincter tone	metoclopramide
4 Other factors:	
Stop smoking	
Timing of meals	
Eliminate tight clothing	

expressed. It is surprising how reversible such oesophagitis can be, though frequent and careful assessment in such a situation is clearly necessary if the disease is not to progress too far in a patient who is otherwise fit for operation.

There are, however, certain factors which will indicate the possible need for early operation.

The first is what may be called 'volume reflux'. There are patients with reflux oesophagitis whose symptoms are largely due to the oesophagitis. Their symptoms are predominantly heartburn, retrosternal pain and so on. On the other hand, there are those whose symptoms are predominantly reflux, and in these the ready reflux of large volumes of gastric juice on lying down, or on necessary bending makes life very difficult. These latter symptoms are much less likely to respond to conservative measures, and will therefore be important in deciding on an operation. Similarly, severe oesophagitis in a fit patient is an indication for a short well-controlled course of medical treatment, but an indication to go on to operation if this is seen not to be working.

Surgical objectives

The major surgical objective is to produce an intra-abdominal oesophagus. This may be achieved by repositioning of the cardia to produce a long intra-abdominal portion of the patient's oesophagus, or by the production of an oesophageal substitute. What is clear is that all the operations which prevent reflux have one major factor in common, namely that they produce an intra-abdominal oesophagus.

The surgical approach is a matter of great argument. The original recognition of the reflux syndrome by a thoracic surgeon led to the almost routine treatment of this disease by the transthoracic approach. In the 1960s the increasingly wide use of vagotomy in the treatment of duodenal ulcer created a generation of abdominal surgeons who were increasingly familiar with exposure and manipulation of the intra-abdominal oesophagus. There is no question that this new familiarity predisposed to the development of abdominal repair techniques. The same phenomenon has been witnessed in the planning of operations for achalasia of the cardia, which are now undertaken as commonly from below the diaphragm as from above. It probably does not matter in the majority of hiatal hernias whether the surgeon approaches the problem from above or below. The patient with severe oesophagitis may well benefit from a superior approach, which enables more mobilization of the thoracic oesophagus. Certainly

the surgeon who treats this disease with any regularity must be familiar with both approaches, and be able to adapt his approach to the needs of the individual patient.

Over the last decade there have been three commonly used operations for uncomplicated hernias. These are the Belsey mark IV repair, the Hill gastropexy and the Nissen fundoplication. Belsey described a transthoracic approach, by which the hernia can be reduced and a partial fundoplication performed, fixing the gastric fundus to the oesophagus and reducing it into the abdomen.[3] Hill's operation consists of reduction of the hernia, closure of the hiatus and suture of the intra-abdominal oesophagus, cardia and upper lesser curve to the pre-aortic fascia, with the subsequent addition of an anterior plication across the cardia. Over the last few years the plication has been quantified by the use of intraoperative manometry.[17] Nissen's fundoplication was originally performed abdominally by wrapping the fundus around the lower oesophagus and suturing fundus not only to fundus, but to oesophagus as well. More recently it has become popular to omit the sutures which go into the oesophagus allowing a short and loose plication to prevent the troublesome complication of the gas-bloat syndrome.[22]

A fourth contender has been the Boerema operation, which originated in Holland[5] and consists of reduction of the hernia and fixation of the cardia within the abdomen by suturing the lesser curve of the stomach to the anterior wall behind the right rectus muscle. This technique has been used with considerable success by one group in the United Kingdom[12] but has not been as popular as the other procedures.

Because of the disappointing incidence of bloating when the standard Nissen procedure is employed, a partial fundoplication, in which the fundus is wrapped around the intra-abdominal oesophagus and sutured to it, but not through a full 360 degrees, has been my usual choice of operation. A similar procedure has been used by Refsum in Oslo[24] and Ein in Toronto.[14]

A number of other modern techniques have been modified for use in hiatal hernia repair. In the United States automatic stapling devices are now widely used and these devices have encouraged surgeons to insert rows of staples in a variety of ways to produce a gastroplasty not unlike that originally described by Collis,[10] though in this new modification it can remain uncut, the staples producing a tunnel of 'new intra-abdominal oesophagus' which will prevent reflux. Alternatively, the gastroplasty can be cut and the newly formed and extended fundus may be used to perform any kind of fundoplasty that is desired. These new procedures are under investigation and results are awaited with interest. Henderson's total fundoplication gastroplasty has also given impressive results.[16]

Synthetic devices have now been produced which may be used in hiatal hernia repair. The Angelchik prosthesis from Phoenix, Arizona, is now being widely tried in the United States. It can be quite simply applied around the cardia after reduction of the hernia, and no further procedure is required.[1] Good results are claimed from early series, and controlled trials comparing it with other procedures are already under way in the United Kingdom. In the short term a good manometric high pressure zone is produced by this procedure.

Results of surgery

In order to give an overall impression of the results of surgery for gastro-oesophageal reflux, data from many series of patients have been collected. The surprising result is that in all the major series between 85% and 92% of operations performed give good or satisfactory results. Against this it must be said that assessment is not always objective or well-defined, and is not often made independently. There are virtually no data comparing different operations under similar circumstances with a satisfactory follow-up period. What is apparent, however, is that whichever operation is used the outcome claimed is about the same. This suggests very strongly that it is perhaps more important to choose an operation and learn to do it well, than to search endlessly and perhaps fruitlessly for a perfect procedure.

Some comparative data are available, but these are technical in nature, rather than clinical. Thus, the excellent study reported by De Meester and colleagues[13] compared three groups of 15 patients who underwent either a Nissen fundoplication, a Hill gastropexy or a Belsey procedure. A short time after these operations, objective measurements were made of gastro-oesophageal reflux by the use of the well-attested SART. This indicated that the full Nissen fundoplication gave the greatest control of reflux. It should not be assumed that this necessarily indicates that this particular operation is clinically superior. It may well be that the formation of a complete anti-reflux barrier produces as many problems as it solves. This may explain the high incidence of gas-bloat after this particular operation, which makes some surgeons seek a less complete repair.

Whilst medical therapy has its place, it is reassuring to note the results of the excellent controlled study reported by Behar et al.[2] In this study, patients with similar initial symptoms were randomized to receive either medical or surgical treatment. They were followed up and studied at the end of one year. The results indicate that sphincter tone is increased at the end of one year by an operation, but medical treatment, though reducing symptoms intermittently, has no effect on sphincter tone. The overall clinical results were better in this study in those who underwent operation. Reflux, as assessed by oesophageal pH recording, continued in spite of prolonged medical treatment but was reduced or abolished by surgery.

Morbidity and mortality

If an operation gives superior results, why should we not operate more readily on patients with hiatal hernias? The answer is that surgery is not without its complications. All operations carry some risk, and complications such as subphrenic abscess and even gastric fistula are reported after repair. The study of Franklin et al[15] contains an unusually large number of patients who underwent incidental splenectomy during fundoplication. Table 3.3 indicates that

Table 3.3 Incidence of complications after splenectomy with or without fundoplication.[15]

	n	Postoperative complications	No complications
Spleen removed	52	24	28
Spleen intact	36	7	29
Total	88	31	57

$X^2 = 9.63\ P < 0.01$.

in this series morbidity was significantly greater in those who underwent splenectomy. In particular, thromboembolic disease was a feature, and it is very important that splenectomy should be avoided if possible during hiatal hernia repair.

The mortality is very low in most surgical series, though a mortality of over 6% has been reported. The striking feature is the increase in mortality with age. Most of the postoperative deaths occur in patients over 60, and for this reason operations for hiatal hernia should be kept to a minimum in the elderly.

Recurrence of the hernia may occur after operation. This is a difficult area, because anatomical recurrence, if sought radiologically, may be seen to have occurred without any development of symptoms. Recurrent hernias are difficult to manage and particularly high complication rates have been reported after repair.

Overall, however, about 90% of patients report good results, which fully justifies operative treatment of hiatal hernias, and would seem to refute the pessimism with which many surgeons approach the subject of hiatal herniorrhaphy. Belsey has indicated that experience may be important. In his own series the recurrence rate was 15% when the operation was performed by a surgeon in training, and 6% when done by a senior, more experienced surgeon.

Special techniques

The subject of vagotomy when applied to hiatal hernia repair has been much discussed over the years. Table 3.4 indicates that patients with hiatal hernia have normal gastric acid secretion.

Table 3.4 Acid secretion and hernia.

	n	Basal acid output	Maximal acid output
Control	20	1.3 ± 0.35	21.6 ± 3.08
Hernia	29	1.2 ± 0.19	22.3 ± 2.00

The problem in these patients is not that they secrete too much acid, but that the acid secreted is reaching the oesophagus. There would therefore seem to be little logic in adding vagotomy. In one retrospective study satisfactory results were obtained in 99% of patients undergoing hiatal hernia repair, but in only 74% of patients who had an added vagotomy.[29] As vagotomy worsens the resu'.., it cannot be recommended.

However, the complications of vagotomy described by Vansant and Baker[29] may not apply to the proximal gastric (highly selective) operation. Several authors have recommended the addition of proximal gastric vagotomy to hiatal hernia repair. This is ilogical, for the reasons given above, and one might expect it to add complications of its own. Kennedy has reported an unusually high incidence of lesser curve necrosis in patients undergoing a combination of proximal gastric vagotomy and fundoplication.[20]

The use of intraoperative manometry has been mentioned above, and time alone will tell whether it improves the results.

One of the problem areas in hiatal hernia repair is that of the shortened oesophagus which does not permit adequate reduction of the cardia into the abdomen. One solution to this has been transverse oesophageal myotomy. Mullard[21] has described this, and though it does not always prevent problems in these very difficult patients, it is an area which needs further exploration. In experimental situations, division of the longitudinal muscle permits great prolongation of the oesophagus, without subsequent development of problems.

OESOPHAGEAL STRICTURES

The development of a stricture usually involves inflammation and spasm as well as fibrosis. The inflammatory element dominates in most cases, and the process is remarkably reversible in many patients. This fact, and their occurrence principally in the elderly, indicates conservative treatment in most patients. This consists of active medical treatment, as outlined earlier, together with endoscopic biopsy, cytology brushings and dilatation.

Dilatation is easily achieved, even in the elderly, under topical anaesthesia, usually as an outpatient procedure. The Eder–Puestow dilators are very effective and may be used repeatedly with safety. In a series of patients treated effectively by this method the mean interval between necessary dilatation was seven months – a surprisingly long response to so simple a treatment. Moreover, a significant weight gain was achieved after dilatation. Some prefer to use the Celestin dilators, which have stepwise increases in diameter and permit greater dilatation with less trauma. Balloon dilatation under radiological control is a new technique which needs careful prospective evaluation.

In younger patients or those with less responsive strictures, surgical treatment is indicated. This is usually an anti-reflux procedure, following which dilatation soon becomes unnecessary as oesophagitis resolves. In the irreducible hernia the situation is more complex and several surgical alternatives exist. First, duodenal diversion is a useful technique in the elderly. As illustrated in Figure 3.3, the procedure consists of an antrectomy and Roux loop procedure; a vagotomy should be added if at all possible. The most striking early effect of this procedure is the elimination of heartburn as a symptom; oesophagitis then becomes easy to control. In young or fitter patients the oesophagus can be lengthened by oesophago-gastroplasty to produce an intra-abdominal segment: a long gastroplasty will permit the addition of

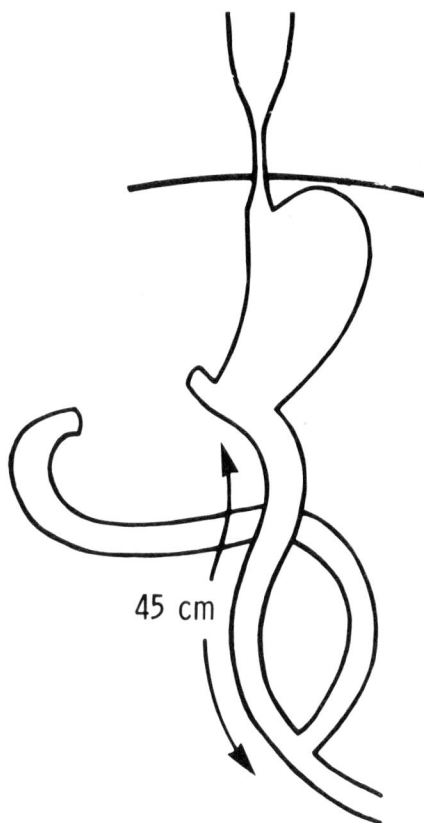

Fig. 3.3 Diagrammatic representation of the antrectomy reconstruction used for duodenal diversion in severe oesophagitis.

fundoplasty or fundoplication in addition. Good anti-reflux control may be obtained by such procedures, or by interposition of a jejunal or colonic loop after resection of the strictured oesophagus. The use of intrathoracic oesophago-gastric anastomosis after resection in younger patients is no longer justified for benign strictures.

PARAOESOPHAGEAL (ROLLING) HERNIA

A paraoesophageal hiatal hernia is quite different from a sliding hernia. There is herniation of the stomach through the oesophageal hiatus, the cardia remaining in its normal anatomical position below the diaphragm. One school of thought claims that such hernias are variants of Bochdalek's hernia, there sometimes being residual tissue indicating that the hernia did not originally occur through the oesophageal hiatus; in most, this tissue is atrophied, or destroyed unnoticed at operation. The majority

opinion is that the herniation is through the true oesophageal hiatus. Most often the gastric fundus herniates first. There may be progressive herniation of the stomach, usually with volvulus, so that the greater curve becomes uppermost, and eventually colon or other organs may be involved. A complete peritoneal sac is present.

These hernias are usually seen late in life, often as a finding on chest X-ray or else on a barium meal examination. Symptoms are often vague, with retrosternal or hypochondrial discomfort, nausea or fullness after meals. Vomiting is not common, and heartburn is not a feature. Dysphagia is not usual.

Mild symptoms may persist for years, but a rolling hernia is dangerous and not amenable to any conservative therapy. The major complications are (a) bleeding from gastritis or gastric ulcer, (b) gastric volvulus and (c) incarceration or strangulation.

Anaemia due to bleeding is common, one series indicating an incidence of 30%. The so-called 'riding ulcer' seen adjacent to the hiatus in these patients may be intractable until herniorrhaphy, implying mechanical factors in its causation.

An intra-abdominal gastric volvulus may be organo- or mesentero-axial. Organo-axial volvulus is more frequent and is commonly associated with rolling hernia, with much or all of the stomach lying in the chest. Acute presentation of such volvulus is characterized by a triad described by Borchardt in 1904:[2]

1 Severe epigastric pain or distension.
2 Vomiting, followed by retching with inability to vomit.
3 Difficulty in passing a nasogastric tube.

This triad suggests initial blockage of the pylorus followed by cardiac obstruction and gastric dilatation. Acute strangulation may follow.

In a series of 25 patients with acute gastric volvulus[7] 18 were associated with paraoesophageal hernia, 3 with traumatic damage to the diaphragm, 2 with eventration of the diaphragm and one with a Bochdalek hernia. Only one was not associated with a diaphragmatic defect of some kind.

Because of the high incidence and the severity of complications, all paraoesophageal hernias would ideally be treated surgically; in practice, however, they are seen most often in the extremely aged, often as an incidental finding. In patients who are considered fit for operation, an abdominal approach usually permits reduction of the hernia; anterior approximation of the crura to narrow the hiatus prevents recurrence.

TRAUMATIC DIAPHRAGMATIC HERNIA

Rupture of the diaphragm may follow either thoracic or abdominal trauma; iatrogenic trauma consists of surgical incisions in the diaphragm (Figures 3.4 and 3.5). Herniation may occur through resulting defects soon after the trauma or many years later; to confuse the issue further, early herniation may be symptomless and cause later complications. Presumably because of males' predisposition to trauma there is a 6 : 1 male : female ratio in incidence of traumatic diaphragmatic hernias.[18] The aetiology in any series is determined largely by social factors. Thus, crushing injuries due to car accidents are a common cause, and penetrating wounds are important where stab wounds are common. Rupture due to crushing requires considerable force, and is associated with a high incidence of other injuries. Lower thoracic stab wounds are commonly associated with diaphragmatic trauma.

Crushing trauma damages the left diaphragm more commonly than the right. This may be largely because of the presence of the liver on the right side, but cadaver studies have also demonstrated a relative weakness in the posterior part of the left diaphragm. Traumatic herniation must be considered in all patients with lower thoracic or upper abdominal trauma. Pain and dyspnoea occur and may be exacerbated by meals. Bowel sounds heard in the chest are an important sign. Examination of the chest reveals dullness and poor air entry. Chest radiographs may reveal bowel in the chest, elevated or indis-

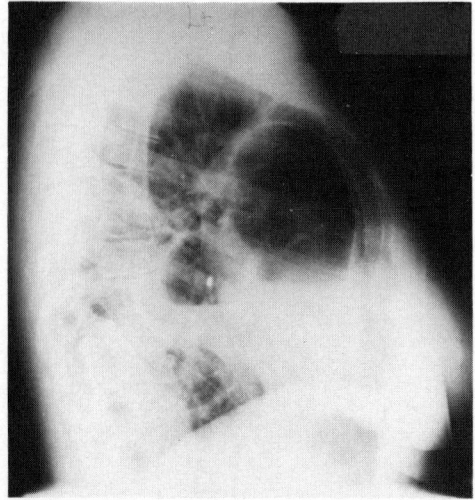

Fig. 3.5 Incisional hernia through the diaphragm, occurring through a surgical incision in the left dome. The whole stomach and splenic flexure of the colon lie in the chest.

tinct diaphragm, or effusion. Barium studies may be necessary to confirm the diagnosis.

In both acute and chronic traumatic herniation the treatment is surgical. Laparotomy, reduction and repair of the diaphragm is performed. In long-standing hernias thoracotomy may be preferred because the adhesions may bleed on division; a high incidence of empyema has been reported following repair of such hernias from below.

REFERENCES

1 Angelchik, J.-P. & Cohen, R. (1979) A new procedure for the treatment of gastroesophageal reflux. *Surgery, Gynecology and Obstetrics*, **148**, 246–248.

2 Behar, J., Sheahan, D. G., Biancani, P. *et al.* (1975) Medical and surgical management of reflux esophagitis. *New England Journal of Medicine*, **293**, 263–268.

3 Belsey, R. (1977) Mark IV repair of hiatal hernia by the transthoracic approach. *World Journal of Surgery*, **1**, 475–483.

4 Bernstein, L. M. & Baker, L. A. (1958) A clinical test for esophagitis. *Gastroenterology*, **34**, 760–781.

5 Boerema, I. (1969) Hiatus hernia: repair by a right-sided, subhepatic, anterior gastropexy. *Surgery*, **65**, 884–893.

6 Borchardt, M. (1904) Zur Pathologie und Therapie des Magnevolvulus. *Archiv für klinische Chirurgie*, **74**, 243.

7 Carter, R., Brewer, L. A. & Hinshaw, D. B. (1980) Acute gastric volvulus. A study of 25 cases. *American Journal of Surgery*, **140**, 99–106.

8 Cohen, S. & Harris, L. D. (1971) Does hiatus hernia affect the competance of the gastroesophageal sphincter? *New England Journal of Medicine*, **284**, 1053–1056.

9 Collins, D. L., Pomerance, J. J., Travis, K. W. *et al.* (1977) A new approach to a congenital posterolateral diaphragmatic hernia. *Journal of Pediatric Surgery*, **12**, 149–156.

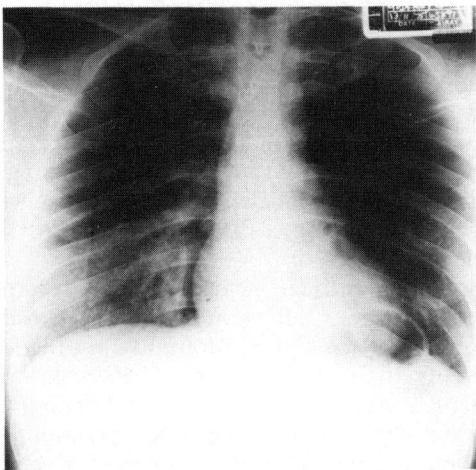

Fig. 3.4 Traumatic diaphragmatic hernia after a motorcycle accident. Stomach is seen in the chest.

10 Collis, J. L. (1961) Gastroplasty. *Thorax*, **16**, 197–206.

11 Comer, T. P. & Clagett, O. T. (1966) Surgical treatment of hernia of the foramen of Morgagni. *Journal of Thoracic and Cardiovascular Surgery*, **52**, 461–468.

12 Davies, C. J. (1975) A survey of the results of the Boerema anterior gastropexy for hiatus hernia over a 4-year period. *British Journal of Surgery*, **62**, 19–22.

13 De Meester, T. R., Johnson, L. F. & Kent, A. (1974) Evaluation of current operations for the prevention of gastroesophageal reflux. *Annals of Surgery*, **180**, 511–523.

14 Ein, S. H., Shandling, B., Stephens, C. A. & Simpson, J. S. (1979) Partial gastric wrap-around as an alternative procedure in the treatment of hiatal hernia. *Journal of Pediatric Surgery*, **14**, 343–346.

15 Franklin, R. H., Iweze, F. I. & Owen-Smith, M. S. (1973) Fundoplication for hiatus hernia. *British Journal of Surgery*, **60**, 65–69.

16 Henderson, R. D., Track, N. S., Hui, M. & Marryatt, G. (1980) The gastroplasty tube and its role in reflux control: an experimental and clinical study. *Canadian Journal of Surgery*, **23**, 63–66.

17 Hill, L. D. (1967) An effective operation for hiatal hernia: an eight-year appraisal. *Annals of Surgery*, **166**, 681–692.

18 Ismail-Beigi, F., Horton, P. F. & Pope, C. E. (1970) Histological consequences of gastroesophageal reflux in man. *Gastroenterology*, **58**, 163–174.

19 Johnson, H. D. (1968) *The Cardia and Hiatus Hernia*. London: Heinemann.

20 Kennedy, T., Magill, P., Johnston, G. W. & Parks, T. G. (1979) Proximal gastric vagotomy, fundoplication and lesser curve necrosis. *British Medical Journal*, **i**, 1455–1456.

21 Mullard, K. S. (1972) The surgical treatment of diaphragmatic oesophageal hiatus hernia. *Annals of the Royal College of Surgeons*, **50**, 73–91.

22 Nissen, R. & Rosetti, M. (1963) Surgery of the cardia ventriculi. *Ciba Symposium 11*, pp. 195–223.

23 Payne, J. H. & Lellin, A. E. (1982) Traumatic diaphragmatic hernia. *Archives of Surgery*, **117**, 18–24.

24 Refsum, S. & Nygaard, K. (1979) Repair of hiatus hernia by an abdominal semi-fundoplication technique. *Acta Chirurgica Scandinavica*, **145**, 39–44.

25 Salo, J. A. & Kivilaakso, E. (1983) Role of bile salts and trypsin in the pathogenesis of experimental alkaline eosophagitis. *Surgery*, **93**, 525–532.

26 Skinner, D. B. & Booth, D. J. (1970) Assessment of distal esophageal function in patients with hiatal hernia and/or gastroesophageal reflux. *Annals of Surgery*, **172**, 627–637.

27 Sumner, E. & Frank, J. D. (1981) Tolazoline in the treatment of congenital diagphragmatic hernias. *Archives of Diseases in Childhood*, **56**, 350–353.

28 Thomas, G. G. & Clitheroe, N. R. (1977) Herniation through the foramen of Morgagni in children. *British Journal of Surgery*, **64**, 215–217.

29 Vansant, J. H. & Baker, J. W. (1976) Complications of vagotomy in the treatment of hiatal hernia. *Annals of Surgery*, **183**, 629–635.

Chapter 4
The Stomach and Duodenum

EMBRYOLOGY AND ANATOMY

Embryology and attachments

The stomach develops as a fusiform dilatation towards the caudal end of the foregut. The left gastric wall becomes the anterior wall as axial rotation carries the ventral border (lesser curvature) to the right and the dorsal border (greater curvature) to the left (Figure 4.1). The right wall becomes the posterior wall, the ventral mesentery becomes the lesser omentum, the dorsal mesentery becomes the greater omentum and these three structures become the roof of the lesser peritoneal sac. The same rotation of the junctional segment of foregut and midgut, which becomes the duodenum, is accompanied by migration of the distal stomach and duodenum to the right upper quadrant. The

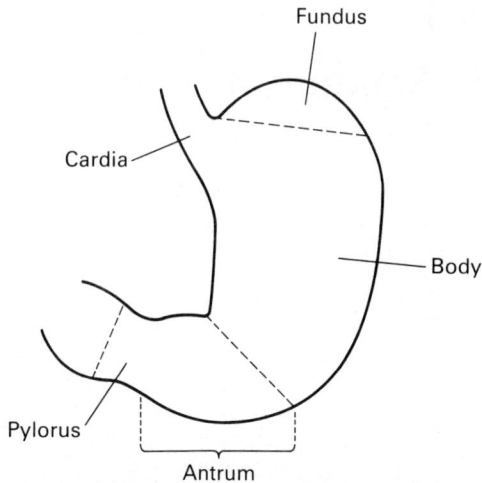

Fig. 4.1 Subdivisions of the stomach. From Weinshelbaum, E. I. (1974) in *Gastroenterology*, vol. 1 (Ed.) Bockus H. L. pp. 389–404, with kind permission of the author, the editor and the publisher, W. B. Saunders.

right surface of the dorsal mesentery of the duodenum, which contains the developing pancreas, fuses with the posterior parietal peritoneum; this results in the pancreas and most of the duodenum becoming retroperitoneal and fixed. The gastro-oesophageal junction is normally fixed by its attachments to the diaphragm. The stomach, pylorus and duodenal cap between these two points of fixation are enveloped in peritoneum. The lesser curvature is attached to the porta hepatis by the lesser omentum and the greater curvature is attached to the diaphragm, spleen and transverse colon by the gastrophrenic, gastrosplenic and gastrocolic portions of the greater omentum.

Macroscopic structure

The stomach may vary greatly in size and shape depending on the volume of its contents and the posture of the patient. The muscular wall has outer longitudinal, inner circular and innermost oblique layers of smooth muscle. The pylorus, a true physiological sphincter, consists of a thickening of the circular muscle layer with a contribution from the longitudinal layer. The incisura angularis shows great variability in its appearance and location and is not a reliable indicator of the junction of body and antrum.[4] The thick mucosal lining of the empty stomach lies in longitudinal folds on a well developed and loose submucosa.

The duodenum has outer longitudinal and inner circular smooth muscle layers. Its first portion (5 cm) passes anterior to the common bile duct and portal vein. The second portion (7 cm) curves downwards on the right side of the head of the pancreas. The papilla of Vater is usually located half way down the postero-medial wall, and the opening of the accessory pancreatic duct, if present, is approximately 2 cm proximal to the papilla. The third portion (10 cm) is crossed anteriorly by the superior mesenteric vessels. The fourth portion (3 cm) terminates as the jejunum. The mucosa of the first 2 cm of the duodenum (duodenal cap) is smooth and thin. The remainder of the duodenum has a thick villous mucosa with numerous circular folds (valvulae conniventes).

Microscopic structure

The two main functional divisions of the gastric mucosa are the parietal cell mass and the antrum. The parietal cells occur in the upper two-thirds of the stomach. Tubular glands secreting acid and pepsin open via the mucosal crypts onto the surface layer of tall mucus-secreting cells. Glands producing alkaline mucus predominate immediately distal to the oesophago-gastric junction. Parietal cells, secreting hydrochloric acid, extend from the oesophago-gastric junction to the corpus–antrum junction, which cannot be precisely identified macroscopically. This junction is identifiable microscopically as a transitional area which may be up to 2.0 cm in width.[6] The position of this mucosal junction may vary so greatly that a large antrum may extend high up the lesser curvature and be accompanied by a small parietal cell mass and a small antrum may extend for only 4–5 cm from the pylorus along both lesser and greater curvatures and be accompanied by a large parietal cell mass.[6] Parietal cells are scarce or absent in the antral mucosa, which contains only glands of the alkaline mucus-secreting type.

The tubular glands of the duodenum open into crypts between long slender villi. Columnar epithelium containing many goblet cells lines the villi. Starting abruptly at the pylorus the submucosa is packed with Brunner's glands, which secrete an alkaline mucus. These glands become less abundant as the duodenojejunal flexure is approached.

Endocrine cells are present between glands in the gastric and duodenal mucosa. These cells are sparse in the upper part of the stomach but are abundant in the antrum where the gastrin-secreting 'G cell' predominates. G cells are less abundant in the duodenal mucosa.[9]

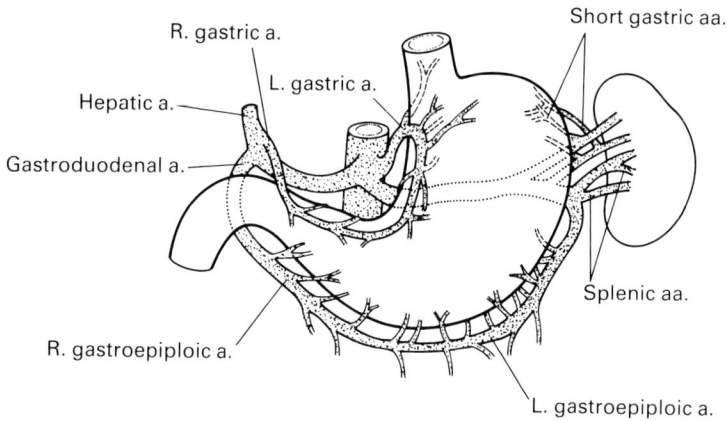

Fig. 4.2 Arteries of the stomach. From Weinshelbaum, E. I. (1974) in *Gastroenterology*, vol. 1 (Ed.) Bockus, H. L. pp. 389–404, with kind permission of the author, the editor and the publisher, W. B. Saunders.

Blood supply and venous drainage

The left gastric artery originates from the coeliac axis and a branch ascends on the right side of the cardio-oesophageal junction to anastomose with the descending thoracic oesophageal supply (Figure 4.2). The two descending branches of the left gastric artery run close to the lesser curvature of the stomach and anastomose with branches of the right gastric artery, which originates from the hepatic artery close to the pylorus. The hepatic artery also gives origin to the gastroduodenal artery which passes posterior to the first portion of the duodenum before it divides into the right gastroepiploic and superior pancreaticoduodenal arteries. The latter artery divides into anterior and posterior branches which pass distally in the concavity of the duodenum and anastomose with similar branches ascending from the superior mesenteric artery. These anterior and posterior arcades provide branches to the duodenum and the head of the pancreas. The right gastroepiploic artery passes upwards between the leaves of the greater omentum approximately 1 cm from the greater curvature of the stomach and anastomoses with the left gastroepiploic artery (from the splenic artery). A variable number of short gastric arteries, branches of the splenic artery, pass in the gastrosplenic ligament to the fundic portion of the greater curvature, which they supply in addition to anastomosing with the descending thoracic oesophageal blood supply.

Many small arteries pass from the gastric and gastroepiploic arteries through the muscularis propria and into the rich submucosal plexus,[2] which sends small arterioles to the gastric mucosa. The mucosa of the lesser curvature has a poorer blood supply than the remainder of the stomach.[1] Contrary to earlier reports[8] arterio-

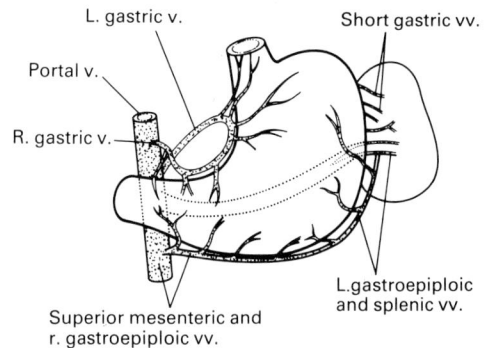

Fig. 4.3 Veins of the stomach. From Weinshelbaum, E. I. (1974) in *Gastroenterology*, vol. 1 (Ed.) Bockus, H. L. pp. 389–404, with kind permission of the author, the editor and the publisher, W. B. Saunders.

venous fistulas are not present in the submucosal plexus of the stomach.[7]

The veins from the stomach and duodenum follow the course of the arteries (Figure 4.3).

Lymphatic drainage

Lymphatics from the gastric mucosa enter the submucosal lymphatic plexus, which communicates freely with the submucosal plexus in the oesophagus. The submucosal plexus in the duodenum is less well developed. Lymphatics from the submucosal plexus pass through the muscularis propria into the subserosal plexus, which anastomoses freely with the subserosal plexus of the duodenum.[10]

Lymph flows away from the stomach in four directions (Figure 4.4). The upper lesser curvature drains to the left (superior) gastric nodes. The lower lesser curvature drains to the right gastric suprapyloric nodes and then to nodes behind the first part of the duodenum and along the hepatic artery to the coeliac nodes. The

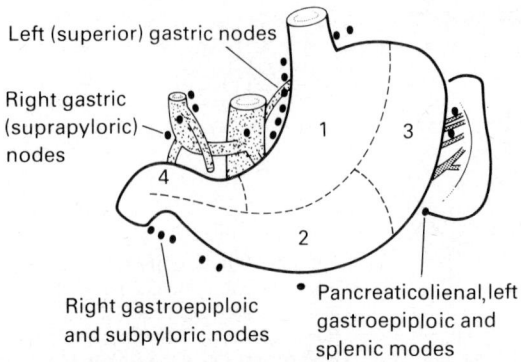

Fig. 4.4 Zones of lymphatic drainage of the stomach. Modified from Weinshelbaum, E. I. (1974) in *Gastroenterology*, vol. 1 (Ed.) Bockus, H. L. pp. 389–404, with kind permission of the author, the editor and the publisher, W. B. Saunders.

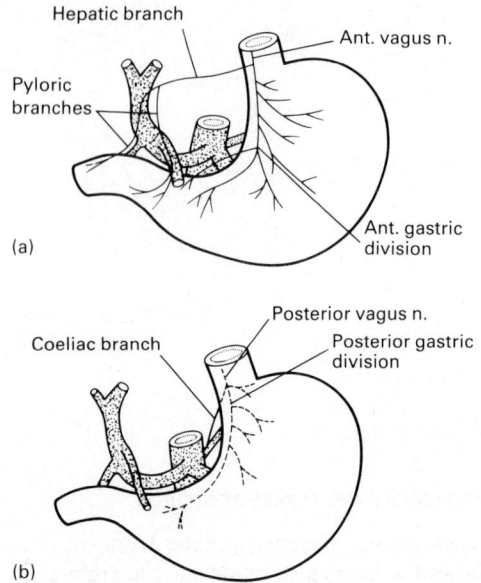

Fig. 4.5 Innervation of the stomach: (a) anterior vagus nerve; (b) posterior vagus nerve. Small coeliac branches of the anterior vagus and hepatic branches of the posterior vagus are omitted. Modified from Weinshelbaum, E. I. (1974) in *Gastroenterology*, vol. 1 (Ed.) Bockus H. L. pp. 389–404, with kind permission of the author, the editor and the publisher, W. B. Saunders.

fundus and upper greater curvature drain along the course of the short gastric vessels (pancreaticolienal nodes) and left gastroepiploic vessels to nodes in the hilum of the spleen and then along the splenic artery via retropancreatic nodes to the coeliac nodes. The lower greater curvature drains to nodes in the gastrocolic omentum along the course of the right gastroepiploic artery (inferior gastric nodes) and then to nodes behind the first portion of the duodenum and along the hepatic artery to the coeliac nodes. Lymph from the proximal portion of the duodenum drains to the subpyloric nodes and lymph from the distal portion of the duodenum and head of the pancreas drains to the superior mesenteric nodes. Lymph from the coeliac nodes passes via the cisterna chyli into the thoracic duct.

Nerve supply

Preganglionic sympathetic efferent fibres from the spinal levels T6 to T10 travel in the splanchnic nerves to the coeliac ganglia from which postganglionic fibres accompany the arteries to the stomach and duodenum. Sympathetic afferents (visceral pain perception) follow the reverse course, but without synaptic interruption.

The parasympathetic innervation of the foregut and midgut is provided by the left and right vagus nerves which form a plexus around the lower oesophagus and emerge as the anterior and posterior vagal trunks (Figure 4.5). The anterior trunk becomes the anterior nerve of Latarget (anterior gastric division) after hepatic branches have passed towards the porta hepatis in the lesser omentum. The posterior trunk becomes the posterior nerve of Latarget (posterior gastric division) after the origin of the

coeliac branch which descends to the coeliac ganglia. The nerves of Latarget descend within the lesser omentum close to the lesser curvature of the stomach and terminate in multiple branches to the antrum and pylorus. The proximal stomach is supplied by obliquely descending branches of the nerves of Latarget. Some fibres originating from the vagal trunks as high as 6 cm above the gastro-oesophageal junction may pass to the gastric wall within or posterior to the oesophagus.[3, 5]

REFERENCES

1 Barlow, T. E., Bentley, F. H. & Walder, D. N. (1951) Arteries, veins and arterio-venous anastomoses in the human stomach. *Surgery, Gynecology and Obstetrics*, **93**, 657–671.
2 Brown, J. R. & Derr, J. W. (1952) Arterial blood supply of human stomach. *Archives of Surgery*, **64**, 616–621.
3 Grassi, G. (1975) Highly selective vagotomy with intraoperative acid secretive test for completion of vagal section. *Surgery, Gynecology and Obstetrics*, **140**, 259–264.
4 Grossman, M. I. (1958) The names of the parts of the stomach. *Gastroenterology*, **34**, 1159–1162.
5 Lee, M. (1969) A selective stain to detect the vagus nerve in the operation of vagotomy. *British Journal of Surgery*, **56**, 10–13.
6 Oi, M., Oshida, K. & Sugimura, S. (1959) The location of gastric ulcer. *Gastroenterology*, **36**, 45–56.
7 Piasecki, C. (1974) Blood supply to the human gastroduodenal mucosa with special reference to the ulcer-bearing areas. *Journal of Anatomy*, **118**, 295–335.

8   Sherman, J. L. & Newman, S. (1954) Functioning arteriovenous anastomoses in the stomach and duodenum. *American Journal of Physiology*, **179**, 279–281.

9   Solcia, E., Vassallo, G. & Capella, C. (1969) Studies on the G cells of the pyloric mucosa, the probable site of gastrin secretion. *Gut*, **10**, 379–388.

10 Zinninger, M. M. & Collins, W. T. (1949) Extension of carcinoma of the stomach into the duodenum and oesophagus. *Annals of Surgery*, **130**, 557–566.

CONGENITAL ABNORMALITIES

Stomach

Reduplication

Reduplication of the entire stomach is rare[1] but smaller segments may be duplicated, especially at the pyloric end of the stomach. These reduplications hardly ever communicate with the gut. Reduplications most commonly present because of local pressure effects causing obstruction on neighbouring structures.

Aberrant pancreas

Aberrant pancreatic tissue may be found within the stomach, usually near the pylorus. The lesion is often not well defined and can undergo ulcerations with bleeding and stenosis.

Ectopic mucosa

Oesophageal mucosa may be found in the stomach. Conversely, gastric mucosa can be present at many other sites: in the oesophagus, in thoracic or abdominal cysts (minor duplications), in the mucosa of the small intestine, in the vitello-intestinal duct and even in the proximal colon.

Teratomas

Teratomas of the stomach have been described. They are rare and may be cured by surgical excision.

Congenital hypertrophic pyloric stenosis

Congenital pyloric stenosis is the commonest abnormality of the stomach in infants, affecting 1 in 200 male births and 1 in 1000 female births. Congenital pyloric stenosis develops in fetal life.[6, 10] There is a hypertrophy mainly affecting the circular muscle layer which sometimes results in a tumour of about 2 cm in diameter. The cause is not yet known, but genetic factors may be involved since there is a 15-fold increased risk in siblings. There is also an increased risk in winter births, in blood groups O and B, in babies with a high birth-weight and in first pregnancies. Only 10% of children with this condition have other congenital abnormalities. Stress during pregnancy has been thought to be a factor. There is almost complete absence of one type of ganglion cells in the pyloric tumour.[3] There is marked proximal dilatation of the stomach, often with quite severe mucosal inflammation or ulceration. Severe progressive projectile vomiting after feeds is usually seen, associated with visible peristalsis, typically beginning between the third and sixth week of life. It is rare after four months. Clinical or ultrasound demonstration of the tumour, together with careful preoperative intravenous rehydration and electrolyte replacement and washing-out of the stomach, should achieve an operative mortality below 1%.[5] Surgical treatment is by dividing the hypertrophied muscle down to, but not including, the mucosa – Ramstedt's operation. Medical treatment is only advised in mild cases, where the volume of gastric residue is small, using atropine methonitrate before feeds.

Pyloric atresia

Localized gastric atresia can simulate hypertrophic pyloric stenosis[8] but is at least 100 times less common and accounts for less than 1% of all atresias of the alimentary tract;[7] furthermore, it is extremely uncommon in the pyloric area. Variants of atresia may be subdivided into aplasia, atresia and diaphragms, the latter often being perforated and thus causing incomplete obstruction.

Congenital diaphragmatic hernia

Congenital diaphragmatic hernias are discussed in Chapter 3. They can be classified anatomically into four groups: (a) foramen of Bochdalek (posterolateral), (b) congenital abscence or hypoplasia of diaphragm, (c) foramen of Morgagni (anterior) and (d) paraoesophageal. Of these, the first is by far the most common, occurring in about 1 in 2200 births.[4] The neonate presents with cyanosis, dyspnoea, tachypnoea or vomiting. There is usually absence of breath sounds, and the diagnosis can usually be confirmed by radiology. Urgent surgical treatment is always indicated since mortality is still encountered due to pulmonary hypoplasia and other associated abnormalities. Mortality is inversely proportional to age.[2, 11] Plication of the hypoplastic diaphragm is the usual treatment of the central defect. Gastro-oesophageal reflux may be seen with or without a hiatal hernia and is an important differential diagnosis in pyloric stenosis.

Duodenum

Duodenal stenosis

Duodenal stenosis may be due to congenital atresia or congenital stenosis, the commonest site for such a lesion being the ampulla. Congenital stenosis is due to failure of the foregut and midgut to fuse. More commonly, however (1/6000 births) duodenal stenosis is due to a thin band of pancreatic tissue encircling the second part of the duodenum – the *annular pancreas*. This abnormality is probably due to a bifid ventral pancreatic bud which fuses with the dorsal bud, forming a ring. In the majority of cases there is a biliary opening into the duodenum proximal to this constriction, leading to bile-stained vomiting. There is commonly an association with Down's syndrome and other congenital abnormalities. After resuscitation surgical management used to be by duodeno-jejunostomy, but duodeno-duodenostomy is now regarded as a preferable method of treatment. Mortality in this condition (around 30%) is much greater than in pyloric stenosis, but is related to the presence of associated disease and other prognostic variables.[9]

Annular pancreas in adults is discussed in Chapter 18.

Malrotation causing duodenal obstruction

Duodenal obstruction may also occur in association with malrotation and is commonly associated with Ladd's bands. This is a remediable cause of duodenal obstruction, and it is important to recognize that it may not present until later in life.

REFERENCES

1 Abrami, G. & Dennison, W. M. (1961) Duplications of the stomach. *Surgery*, **49**, 794.
2 Adelman, S. & Benson, C. D. (1976) Bochdalek hernias in infants: factors determining mortality. *Journal of Paediatric Surgery*, **11**, 569.
3 Benson, C. D. (1969) Pre-pyloric and pyloric obstruction. In *Paediatric Surgery*, Vol. 2 (Ed.) Mustard, W. T., Ravitch, M. W., Snyder, W. H. *et al.* p. 795. Chicago: Year Book Medical Publishers.
4 Butler, N. & Claineux, A. E. (1962) Congenital diaphragmatic hernia. *Lancet*, **i**, 659.
5 Cook, K. R. C. M. & Rickham, P. P. (1978) Gastric outlet obstructions. In *Neonatal Surgery* (Ed.) Rickham, P. P., Lister, J. & Irving, I. M. pp. 335–351. London: Butterworth.
6 Donnovan, E. J. (1946) Congenital hypertrophic pyloric stenosis. *Annals of Surgery*, **124**, 709.
7 Gerber, B. C. (1965) Pre-pyloric diaphragm: an unusual abnormality. *Archives of Surgery*, **90**, 472.
8 Ghent, E. N. & Denton, M. D. (1974) Mucosal diaphragm of the gastric antrum: A case report and review of the literature. *Canadian Journal of Surgery*, **17**, 274.
9 Irving, I. M. & Rickham, P. P. (1978) Duodenal atresia and stenosis; annular pancreas. In *Neonatal Surgery* (Ed.) Rickham, P. P., Lister, J. & Irving, I. M. pp. 335–370. London: Butterworth.
10 Laurence, K. M. (1963) Hypertrophic pyloric stenosis. *Lancet*, **i**, 224.
11 Raphally, R. C. & Downes, J. J. Jr (1973) Congenital diaphragmatic hernia: prediction of survival. *Journal of Paediatric Surgery*, **8**, 815.

PHYSIOLOGY AND ABNORMAL SECRETION AND MOTILITY

GASTRIC SECRETION

Normal secretory physiology[20, 21, 22]

ACID SECRETION

In the body of the stomach the parietal cells secrete acid and intrinsic factor and the zymogen chief cells secrete pepsinogens, which are converted by acid into pepsins. The surface epithelial and mucous neck cells of the body of the stomach, and the pyloric cells of the antrum, secrete an alkaline mucus. Acid and intrinsic factor are secreted by the same cell, and the number of chief cells is correlated with the number of parietal cells, so that with few exceptions measurement of acid alone provides an expression of gastric secretory capacity.

There are three interconnected phases of gastric secretion: cephalic, gastric and intestinal. These phases overlap in time and are also mutually interrelated in a complicated nervous and hormonal system. Not all the complexities have been unravelled, nor can it be certain that each of the separate mechanisms has a role in normal physiology (Figure 4.6.)

The cephalic phase begins with the expectation, thought, sight and smell, and perhaps ingestion and chewing of food stimulating vagal centres via the hypothalamus. The vagus nerves send preganglionic cholinergic efferent fibres to the nerve plexuses of many parts of the alimentary system. Postganglionic nerves from these plexuses stimulate the stomach and intestines directly, as well as potentiating indirectly their response to other stimuli. Thus the vagi stimulate the exocrine cells of the body of the stomach by direct cholinergic stimulation and by cholinergic potentiation of other stimuli, such as gastrin. The vagi stimulate the endocrine cells of the antrum of the stomach by direct cholinergic stimulation of gastrin release and by cholinergic potentiation of gastrin release by other stimuli, including distension and the chemicals in food.

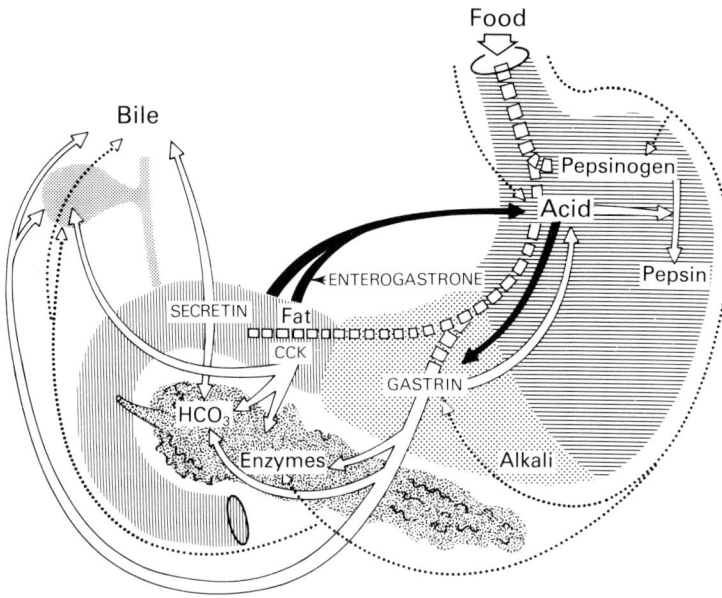

Fig. 4.6 The regulation of gastric acid secretion. Names in capitals are hormones. Names in lower case are alimentary secretions. The body of the stomach (parietal cell mass) is represented by horizontal shading, and the pancreas by stippling. The vagus nerves are shown as dotted lines. Stimulation is indicated by open arrows, and inhibition by solid arrows. From Baron (1971),[5] with kind permission of the editors of the *Proceedings of the Royal Society of Medicine*.

The gastric phase begins with food entering the stomach, where it stimulates stretch receptors and possibly chemoreceptors in the body of the stomach, eliciting local and vagovagal distension reflexes which evoke acid secretion. Food soon reaches the antrum of the stomach, where its bulk stimulates stretch receptors and its peptides and amino acids stimulate chemoreceptors in the pyloric gland area. The hormone gastrin is then released from specialized G cells in the mucosa of the antrum. Gastrin is carried by the bloodstream and stimulates the parietal cells of the body of the stomach to secrete acid. The antrum has an important pH-dependent negative feedback system by which acid in contact with the mucosa causes inhibition of further release of gastrin.

The intestinal phase of gastric secretion begins when food and its digestive products enter the intestine where neuroreceptors may be stimulated and intestinal gastrins and other hormones released. Acid secretion can also be inhibited by acid and fat entering the duodenum and intestine (see Chapter 8, p. 345).

Thus a meal entering the stomach elicits, by neural and endocrine mechanisms, neuroendocrine secretions of acid and pepsins, which acidify and partly digest the meal, producing chyme. When this reaches the antrum and duodenum it is partly neutralized by the alkaline secretion of the pyloric glands, duodenum, pancreas and bile, and it also causes inhibition of

further acid secretion. The now liquefied and partly digested meal is at the correct pH for intestinal digestion and absorption.

TESTS OF ACID SECRETION

There are at least three physiological stimulants of acid secretion: *neurocrine* (acetylcholine from postganglionic neurones), *endocrine* (gastrin from G cells) and *paracrine* (histamine from mast cells). However, it is not clear how many of these have specific receptors on parietal cells or how these receptors interact.

There are three principal tests of gastric secretion, all of which can be performed in the intubated fasting subject. The stomach is emptied and the gastric juice aspirated continually and measured for volume, pH and titratable acidity:

volume (l) × acidity (mmol/l) = acid output (mmol)

Basal interdigestive acid output is usually collected for one hour (or in four 15-minute samples) in the morning, as it is inconvenient to measure 12-hour overnight secretion. Maximal acid output is collected in four 15-minute samples after a maximal dose of pentagastrin, 6 µg/kg i.m. Vagal stimulation used to be measured after insulin 0.2 u/kg i.v. (taking eight 15-minute samples), but for comfort and safety sham feeding with a tasty meal is now preferred (six 10-minute samples are taken). Acid outputs are best represented as *peak* acid output, that is twice the sum of the two highest consecutive 15-minute collection periods, expressed as mmol/h, but may be expressed as the 'maximum' acid output – the total output in the hour after the stimulant. The methodology of these tests, of intravenous infusions, and corrections for gastroduodenal loss and reflux are detailed elsewhere.[2, 3, 9, 18, 23]

Tubeless tests of acid secretion with dyes, telemetry capsules and isotopic scans are not sufficiently reliable for clinical use. Gastric and duodenal acidity throughout the 24 hours can be studied by repeated aspiration, or by continuously recording from in situ pH electrodes.

PEPSINS[9]

About 99% of the pepsinogens pass into the lumen of the stomach where they are split by acid into their respective pepsins. Gastric pepsin is rarely measured because it is unusual for pepsin secretion not to follow acid secretion. Pepsins and pepsinogens can be separated by chromatography or electrophoresis. Samloff has separate radioimmunoassays for the fundic I and antroduodenal II pepsinogens.

A mere 1% of the pepsinogens pass from the chief cells into the blood (*serum pepsinogens*). Serum pepsinogen I (PG I) is normally between 50 ng/ml and 175 ng/ml, is correlated with basal and peak acid output, and is the first tubeless test which may reliably represent the gastric secretory capacity.

The fundic (I) pepsinogens, but not the antroduodenal (II) pepsinogens, are excreted as *urine pepsinogens* (uropepsin). Urine pepsinogen is an approximate indicator of the chief cell mass and is correlated with acid output and serum pepsinogen.

THE GASTRINS[9]

There are at least six different gastrins secreted by the G cells of the gastric antrum and duodenum. These are G34 'big gastrin' (MW 3839), G17 'little gastrin' (MW 2098) and G14 'mini gastrin' (MW 1851). Each exists in two forms: gastrin I without, and gastrin II with, a sulphated tyrosine.

Other gastrins of uncertain status include big–big gastrin, component I and the N-terminal 13 amino acids of G17.

Assay
All radioimmunoassayists now use synthetic human G17-I both for antiserum and for standard. These assays involve many technical difficulties; although there are relatively specific antibodies none are totally specific for one molecular species of gastrin, and different laboratories obtain different results from samples of the same plasma. It is convenient to express gastrin in pmol/l G17 equivalents irrespective of assay: 1 pmol/l G17 equivalent = 2.1 pg/ml.

Activity
The biological activity of gastrin resides in its carboxy-terminal portion. The half life of human G17 is 6 minutes, while that of G34 is 40 minutes, so G34 evokes a more sustained secretion. In terms of molar concentrations in the blood, the potency of G17 is four to eight times that of G34. In the human antrum 90% of the gastrin is G17, but in the duodenum half is G34 and half is G17.

Fasting serum gastrin is mostly G34, but most of the postprandial acid-stimulatory activity is G17. The calculated total gastrin output after a meal is correlated with fasting serum gastrin, so either may indicate the size of the functional G cell mass.

The G cells can be stimulated cholinergically by the vagus, but there may also be vagal inhibitory fibres. Serum gastrin is increased by hypercalcaemia and by adrenaline (epinephrine). Gastrin release is inhibited by acidification of the antral G cells, with 80% inhibition at pH 2.5 and complete suppression at pH 1.

Gastrins are removed from the circulation by the kidneys, the small intestine and the body of the stomach.

MUCOSAL RESISTANCE[1, 15, 16, 19, 26–29]

Hollander proposed two principal barriers: the superficial mucus and the mucosal cell layer, with its rapid turnover of four to six days. Mucus is a viscous mixture of the secretions of gastric mucous glands, cell fragments, leucocytes and salts. More than 90% by volume is water with a matrix of glycoprotein. Mucus is a partial barrier between acid and pepsin in the lumen and the cells of the mucosa. At the same time mucus allows the passage of bicarbonate secreted by surface mucous cells into the gastric lumen (possibly enough to neutralize 10% of maximal acid output). This bicarbonate may be confined in the unstirred layer of mucus as a high-concentration barrier to acid, rather than being released into the lumen generally, where it would be relatively ineffective against the greater mass of acid (Figure 4.7).

The physical and chemical methodology for studying mucus are only now improving and we lack data on whether there is quantitative or qualitative deficiency of mucus or the mechanical, neural (sympathetic and parasympathetic),

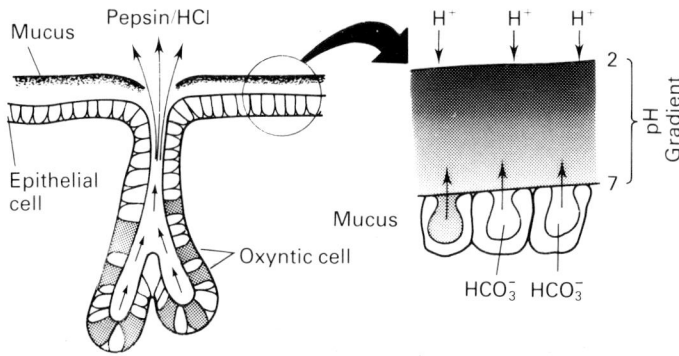

Fig. 4.7 The 'mucus–bicarbonate' barrier. Diagrammatic representation of the gastric epithelium, illustrating the interaction between hydrogen and bicarbonate ions within the mucus gel layer. Hydrogen ions diffusing from the lumen are neutralized by bicarbonate ions secreted by the surface cells, thus creating a pH gradient across the mucus interface. From Rees and Turnberg (1982),[27] with kind permission of the authors and the editors of *Clinical Science*.

chemical, hormonal (secretin) and paracrine (prostaglandins) factors stimulating mucus in peptic ulcer disease.

Prostaglandin E_2 (PGE_2) is normally to be found in gastric mucosa and secretions. Pharmacologically, PGE_2 inhibits gastric acid secretion, increases mucus, and both prevents and heals peptic ulceration. Robert's group pointed out that prostaglandins can prevent damage to the gastric mucosa either when given in doses which do not reduce gastric secretion or when given together with an exogenous acid.[28] Jacobson called this property *cytoprotection* and this term has since been applied to other drugs. 'Cytoprotection' is sometimes used synonymously with 'mucosal resistance'.

Abnormal secretory physiology[20–22]

GASTRITIS AND HYPOSECRETION[7]

Acid

Basal and maximal acid output are correlated with the histology of the mucosa of the body of the stomach. In the early stages of superficial gastritis there may be a hypersecretory phase, but acid output is usually below normal later. Patients with atrophic gastritis and intestinal metaplasia have marked hyposecretion, and those with gastric atrophy show anacidity. (Anacidity is defined as a pH not less than 7.0 even after maximal stimulation. This definition is preferable to the old and imprecise terms achlorhydria and 'no free acid', which were often re-interpreted as meaning pH > 3.5.)

Gastritis may be found, together with B_{12} malabsorption and a reduction in acid and pepsin secretion, in patients with pernicious anaemia. In some patients with iron or folate deficiency anaemia, the mucosa and secretions may improve after appropriate therapy. In patients with autoimmune type A gastritis and pernicious anaemia (but not in the type B non-immune gastritis, associated with gastric ulcer and carcinoma) acid and intrinsic factor, as well as actual parietal cells, may be restored by corticosteroids.

Intrinsic factor

Tests of secretion can be useful in patients with macrocytic anaemia or a megaloblastic marrow to distinguish between a gastric and an intestinal cause of anaemia. If an adult is capable of secreting acid, his intrinsic factor secretion is adequate: he therefore does not have pernicious anaemia, but probably has intestinal malabsorption. If an adult has anacidity and gastric atrophy exists, this is not proof of pernicious anaemia unless intrinsic factor is also absent. However, in clinical practice today measurements of serum B_{12} and B_{12} absorption make acid tests largely superfluous in the diagnosis of pernicious anaemia. If desired, gastric intrinsic factor production can be measured directly by radioimmunoassay and may provide a better index of the histological state of the secretory cells than measurement of either acid production or B_{12} absorption.

Gastrin

Patients with anacidity may have very high levels of serum gastrin if their antral mucosa, and thus their negative feedback system, are intact (type A gastritis). If the antrum is also involved in the gastritis (type B) then serum gastrin will be low.

GASTRIC ULCER[3, 7, 9, 17]

Most patients with gastric ulcer have normal basal and maximal acid outputs (Table 4.1), corresponding to the normal number of parietal cells in their stomachs, but ulcers at different sites are associated with different secretory patterns (Figure 4.8). Gastric ulcers almost always occur in pyloric mucosa, and only rarely in

Table 4.1 The mean (and range) of basal and maximal[a] acid output (mmol/h) in normal subjects and patients with peptic ulcer[2, 3]

	Normal		Duodenal ulcer		Gastric ulcer	
	Basal	Peak	Basal	Peak	Basal	Peak
Men	1 (0–5+)	22 (<1–45)	4 (0–15+)	42 (15–100+)	1 (0–5+)	23 (3–40)
Women	1 (0–5+)	12 (<1–30)	2 (0–5+)	32 (15–100+)	1 (0–2+)	10 (1–30)

[a] Maximal acid output is expressed in terms of peak output, as defined in the text.

TYPE 1   TYPE 2   TYPE 3

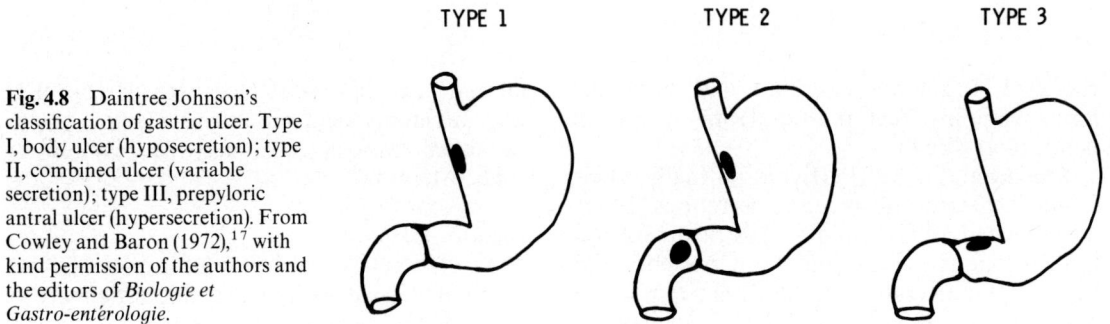

Fig. 4.8 Daintree Johnson's classification of gastric ulcer. Type I, body ulcer (hyposecretion); type II, combined ulcer (variable secretion); type III, prepyloric antral ulcer (hypersecretion). From Cowley and Baron (1972),[17] with kind permission of the authors and the editors of *Biologie et Gastro-entérologie*.

fundic mucosa. In general a peptic ulcer has parietal cells only above it (cephalad, nearer to the cardia), so that there is a theoretical gradient for maximal acid output: duodenal ulcer > prepyloric gastric ulcer > (incisural) angulus gastric ulcer > body (corpus) gastric ulcer. This gradient has been confirmed by measurements of maximal acid output and urinary pepsinogen.

The hypoacidity of a patient with an ulcer in the body of the stomach seems principally to be due to a reduction in the numbers of parietal cells producing acid, and these acid-secreting cells may return after the ulcer heals. The volume of acid parietal component in gastric ulcer disease runs parallel to acid output, but patients with gastric ulcer may secrete more alkaline non-parietal component than normal. Thus their stomachs may have fewer than normal parietal cells, because many of them have been replaced by alkaline-secreting pyloric type cells either before (and predisposing to) the gastric ulceration, or after (and secondary to) the ulceration.

There is often excessive reflux of alkali from the duodenum into the stomach. Less important factors include excess salivary contamination and acid back-diffusion from the lumen through the abnormally inflamed gastric mucosa associated with gastric ulcer (Figure 4.9).

Thus secretory tests are of little diagnostic value in distinguishing patients with gastric ulcer from normal subjects. Values of peak acid

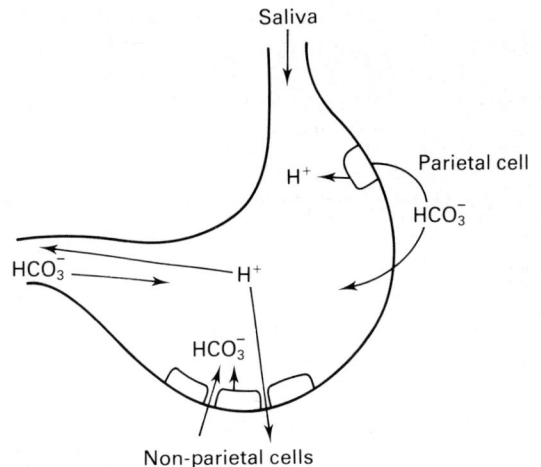

Fig. 4.9 Five possible causes of hypoacidity. From Baron (1977),[7] with kind permission of the editors of *Rendiconti di Gastroenterologia*.

output above the upper limit of normal suggest a prepyloric or duodenal ulcer. Because of the very low acid outputs of some patients with gastric ulcer, with pH values as high as 6.1 for body ulcers and 3.7 for antral ulcers, it is impossible to say that a particular patient does not have a gastric ulcer unless there is absolute anacidity, and even then there are a few well documented case reports of benign gastric ulcers occurring in patients whose stomachs could not secrete acid.

CARCINOMA[9]

Patients with carcinoma of the stomach usually secrete less acid than either normal subjects or patients with simple benign gastric ulcers. Many attempts have been made in the last hundred years to diagnose a patient's gastric lesion as malignant by secretion tests.

While absolute anacidity is found almost exclusively in patients with carcinomatous gastric ulcers, it occurs in only about one in five of such patients. More than 20 mmol/h is secreted by 5% of patients with gastric carcinoma, so that there is no upper limit of acid output above which carcinoma does not exist, and could therefore be excluded in diagnosis. Some doctors measure acid in the hope of being able to diagnose even one in five carcinomas. However, those carcinomas that can be picked out by associated anacidity are probably advanced, large or infiltrating, obvious by other diagnostic methods, and likely to be incurable. Measurements of concentrations or outputs of chloride, pepsinogen, intrinsic factor, beta-glucuronidase, lactate dehydrogenase, protein, mucus, lactic acid and nitrite have all shown differences from normal, alone or in combination. However, none of them are used in clinical practice because endoscopy with biopsies and cytology are sufficiently accurate by themselves.

DUODENAL ULCER[4–6, 8–12, 14, 15, 24, 25, 30–33]

At the local level the duodenal mucosa is inflamed and ulcerated by abnormally frequent bursts of acidity. There are also some failures of duodenal defences, but most attention has been paid to excessive or prolonged basal and/or maximal secretion of acid and pepsin. Abnormalities of meal-stimulated secretion, and of emptying, are discussed elsewhere later in this chapter (p. 105) and in Chapter 8.

Acid

The hypersecretory model proposed twenty years ago is still useful in classification and causation (Figure 4.10). The proportions of patients with a duodenal ulcer having a *maximal*, pentagastrin-stimulated, acid output above the upper limit of normal vary in different series. In the original studies about a third of patients with duodenal ulcer were hypersecretors and most reports since then have suggested a similar fraction. These findings apply whatever the route of stimulation, and however the data are analysed, even with corrections for losses from

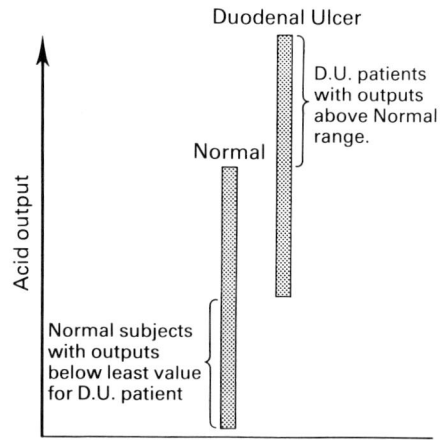

Fig. 4.10 The ranges of peak acid output in normal subjects and in patients with duodenal ulcer. From Baron (1963),[4] with kind permission of the editors of *Clinical Science*.

the stomach into the duodenum, for duodeno-gastric reflux and for height, weight or lean body mass. Maximal acid secretion is an expression of the number of parietal cells in the stomach. For example, 10^9 parietal cells can produce a response to maximal stimulation of about 20 mmol/h in dogs, 23 mmol/h in Scots and 25 mmol/h in Chinese. Gastric hypersecretion in duodenal ulcer disease is presumably due to an increased parietal cell mass (Figure 4.11), the cause of which is obscure. The majority opinion

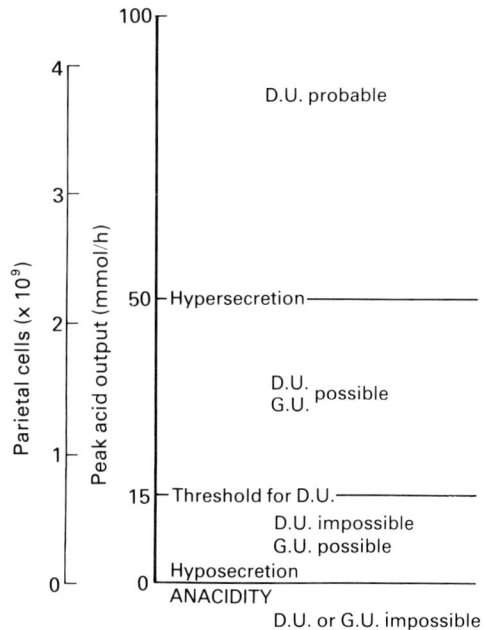

Fig. 4.11 Postulated parietal cell mass, peak acid output and the secretory situation in duodenal gastric ulcer. From Baron (1972),[6] with kind permission of the publishers, Butterworth.

favours the hypothesis that hypersecretion precedes and predisposes to duodenal ulceration, rather than the alternative hypothesis that hypersecretion is due to the duodenal ulcer itself, for example by impairment of normal duodenal inhibitory mechanisms. Gastric acid hypersecretion is probably partly genetically determined, but the experimental evidence for this assumption is weaker than that for a genetic basis for hypersecretion of pepsin.

The other component of the 1960s model was that there was a threshold for maximal acid output below which patients with duodenal ulcer were rarely seen; this threshold value was about 15 mmol/h for peak acid output and 12 mmol/h for maximum acid output. The pathophysiology of the approximately two-thirds of patients with duodenal ulcer who are normosecretors remains obscure. However, the threshold hypothesis means that there is a proportion of normal subjects with acid outputs below the least value of acid secretion of patients with duodenal ulcer, and the corollary to this is that medical or surgical acid-lowering treatments should reduce the secretions of patients with duodenal ulcer below the threshold and keep them in that non-ulcer range.

About one third of patients with duodenal ulcer have *basal* hypersecretion, and this can be explained merely on the basis of an increased parietal cell mass. It is tempting to postulate that there is an increased drive (vagal/hormonal) on the parietal cells of the stomach, but there are no convincing data. It is 40 years since Dragstedt introduced vagotomy based on the concept of an excess vagal drive on the stomach, as manifested by excess basal acid, and nocturnal acid in particular. Not only are the morning basal acid data neutral in this argument, but the earlier suggestions of there being brief periods of acid hypersecretion at night with simultaneous bouts of rapid eye movements during sleep (associated with dreaming) have not been confirmed. There has also been a claim that vagal activity can be estimated from plasma levels of pancreatic polypeptide (PP) and that there is a correlation between fluctuations in spontaneous acid secretion and fluctuations in pancreatic polypeptide. However, very few patients with duodenal ulcer do have high pancreatic polypeptide levels after stimulation with insulin, meals or sham feeding. Even the suggestion that a few patients with duodenal ulcer might have increased vagal tone is of uncertain value, because later studies have not found any significant correlation between acid and plasma pancreatic polypeptide.

Pepsins

There is an approximate correlation between the output of gastric acid and pepsin, depending on the respective parietal and chief cell masses. There is a long-standing suggestion that some patients with duodenal ulcer can be classified as vagal because they have a relative excess of pepsin, whereas others with higher acid but lower pepsin outputs are antral. Indeed, the discriminative capacity of the calculated maximal response (V_{max}) for pepsin stimulated by intravenous pentagastrin is better than that for acid.

However, measurements of gastric total pepsin output, or urine or plasma total pepsinogen, have given no additional pathological insight into the aetiology of duodenal ulcer. There have been considerable advances in pepsin chemistry and Taylor's group has found their pepsin 1 present in increased frequency and concentration in the gastric juice of patients with peptic ulcer. Samloff's group I pepsinogens (PG I) represent fundic pepsinogens 1–5 and were abnormally high in two-thirds of patients with duodenal ulcer.

Gastric control factors

Most studies suggest that patients with duodenal ulcer have parietal cells with an increased sensitivity to infused pentagastrin or exogenous or endogenous gastrin. This sensitivity, where demonstrated, has naturally been attributed to increased vagal tone. Cholinomimetics such as carbacholine or urecholine increase the sensitivity of the parietal cells of the normal stomach towards the hypersensitivity of parietal cells from patients with duodenal ulcer. In contrast, these drugs do not affect the sensitivity of the parietal cells of patients with unoperated duodenal ulcer. The position remains obscure.

It seems likely that the antrum becomes distended by meals. Experimental distension of the antrum actually inhibits basal, pentagastrin-stimulated and betazole-stimulated acid output in healthy subjects, but in patients with duodenal ulcer there is increased secretion. In normal subjects there is a non-hormonal, non-beta-adrenergic, non-dopaminergic ganglionic inhibitory reflex which is absent in patients with duodenal ulcer. It is important to distinguish the site of the distension in the stomach, because fundic distension, unlike antral distension, seems as potent a stimulus for gastric acid secretion in healthy subjects as it is in patients with duodenal ulcer. The mechanism for this is suppressable by atropine and vagotomy and probably involves short intramural and long vago-vagal paths.

When the antrum is acidified by exogenous acid, patients with duodenal ulcer fail to show the normal pH-sensitive acid-inhibitory feedback and may require a pH as low as 1 for complete suppression of meal-stimulated acid and gastrin. Similarly, endogenous acid stimulated by insulin is resistant to inhibition by antral acidification in patients with duodenal ulcer. Furthermore, the inverse relationship in normal subjects between the percentage increase in gastrin response and maximal acid output is absent. Control factors in the duodenum are discussed in Chapter 8.

Gastrins

Gastrins are indisputably physiological stimulators of gastric acid secretion, but it is still unclear whether they are primarily abnormal in the majority of patients with duodenal ulcer disease. About one in a thousand patients with duodenal ulcer has an underlying gastrinoma, and a few have G cell hyperplasia (see below).

There are often abnormally high and more sustained postprandial rises in serum gastrin in patients with duodenal ulcer, but there are conflicting results on the proportions of the G17 and G34 components which are in excess. In some studies normosecretors had higher than normal mean peak integrated postprandial gastrin levels, but levels in hypersecretors were normal. Smoking and exercise raise plasma adrenaline and could produce abnormally high serum gastrin levels in patients with duodenal ulcer.

Most estimates of the absolute numbers of G cells in the human antrum have suggested a twice-normal G cell population in patients with duodenal ulcer. In this disease acid and gastrin secretion are interrelated and both are determined by parietal cell and G cell mass. However, the control of the G cell population is unknown. Possible mechanisms include a deficiency of D cells producing inhibitory paracrine somatostatin, primary hyperbombesinaemia and lack of urogastrone, acting either as a gastric inhibitor or as an epidermal growth factor.

Histamine

The amount of stored histamine in biopsies of the gastric mucosa of hypersecretors, such as patients with duodenal ulcer, is abnormally low. This low histamine content is presumed to be due to an increased rate of formation and turnover in the mast cells, but the control factors are unknown.

DUODENAL ULCERATION AND DUODENITIS

It is difficult to produce a working conceptual model of the abnormalities of gastric secretion and duodenal acidity in the duodenal ulcer diathesis. It is impossible at present to understand what determines the occurrence, presentation, healing and recurrence of a duodenal ulcer. Patients with duodenal ulcers which are clinically active may or may not have increased basal acid output and maximal acid output is similar in patients with active and inactive ulcers. However, patients with duodenal ulcer who do not have active symptoms produce less than 15 mmol/h in response to a broth meal. The mean acid output in response to broth as a percentage of the response to histamine in patients with inactive ulcers is 32% (close to the normal ratio of 35%); this ratio is more than doubled (78%) in patients with active ulcers. This increased antral activity in response to the broth meal could be a response to the chemical constitution of the meal or to a distension of the antrum.

Antral activity is influenced by vagal cholinergic tone, which may also influence ulcer activity by another mechanism, because patients with active ulcers have higher gastric outputs of pepsin and pepsin 1.[30, 31, 32, 33]

Duodenitis as defined endoscopically, radiologically or preferably histologically may be the precursor of ulceration in those with the constitutional diathesis. Duodenitis without ulceration may also produce symptoms in its own right, since the inflamed duodenum (unlike that of normal subjects) is painful when perfused with 0.1 mol/l hydrochloric acid (but not saline). In the Cardiff series the mean maximal acid output of patients with coarse duodenal folds (44 mmol/h) was similar to that for all duodenal ulcer (42 mmol/h), and was the same whether or not the coarse folds were accompanied by an ulcer (47 mmol/h and 42 mmol/h respectively). Very coarse duodenal folds are associated with even higher acid outputs. Coarse gastric folds are also associated with hypersecretion of acid, and some of these patients have hypertrophic hypersecretory gastropathy (see 'Ménétrier's disease', p. 238).

GASTRIC HYPERSECRETION AND HYPERGASTRINAEMIA

Zollinger–Ellison syndrome

The Zollinger–Ellison syndrome of intractable peptic ulcer, gastric hypersecretion and pancreatic tumour is more clearly defined as 'gastric hypersecretion and hypergastrinaemia', due either to excess secretion of gastrin from a gastrinoma, to antral G-cell hyperplasia, or to a retained gastric antrum. Rarely, hypergastrinaemia may be due to hypercalcaemia, renal failure, resection or exclusion of the small intestine, or liver disease. The following results of acid tests are used to diagnose this syndrome:

a basal acid output more than 15 mmol/h in the unoperated, or more than 5 mmol/h in the operated stomach;
b 12-hour overnight acid secretion more than 100 mmol;
c basal acidity more than 100 mmol/l in the unoperated, or 70 mmol/l in the operated stomach;
d basal acid output/maximal acid output ratio of more than 60%;
e basal/peak acidity ratio of more than 60%;
f a disproportionate increase in gastric acidity compared with pepsin concentration.

Unfortunately, these acid criteria are not reliable and may give false-positive or false-negative diagnoses. Patients with suspicious clinical pictures or suspicious gastric hypersecretion (e.g. basal acid output more than 10 mmol/h) or both should have their serum gastrin measured. Serum gastrin should also always be measured in patients with recurrent ulceration after gastric operations. If the fasting serum gastrin is very high, a gastrinoma can be reliably diagnosed. If serum gastrin is in the intermediate range a stimulation test with secretin or calcium may help. This condition is also discussed in Chapter 18.

Antral G-cell hyperplasia
Gastric hypersecretion and high levels of fasting gastrin may be due, not to a gastrinoma, but to hyperplasia of the G cells of the gastric antrum, as demonstrated by immunofluorescence studies of preoperative biopsies or of the whole antrum after antrectomy. This hyperplasia is probably an extreme of the range of the number of G cells in the duodenal ulcer population. As in gastrinomas, the hypergastrinaemia is not inhibited by antral acidification. However, the hypergastrinaemia of patients with antral G-cell hyperplasia may increase further after a meal, remain unchanged after calcium and decrease after secretin, whereas the hypergastrinaemia associated with gastrinomas is unchanged by a meal and increased by secretin and calcium.

Retained antrum
A retained gastric antrum after Billroth II partial gastrectomy is a third possible cause of hypergastrinaemia, gastric hypersecretion and recurrent ulceration. This hypergastrinaemia is due to continued stimulation by food and alkali from the isolated antral tissue in the afferent loop, and may be inhibited by secretin.

RECURRENT ULCER

Recurrence is all too common after partial gastrectomy or vagotomy. Gastric secretion tests may be helpful because the commonest cause of recurrence is inadequate reduction of gastric acid secretion.

Partial gastrectomy
After partial gastrectomy secretion tests are difficult because of the need to position the tip of the tube in the gastric remnant, and there is a problem of preventing, or correcting for, loss or reflux through the stoma. Recurrent ulcer is rare if peak acid output is less than 1 mmol/h, but there is no lower limit of peak acid output (except zero) below which a recurrent ulcer can be excluded. Basal acid outputs more than 5 mmol/h are found only in cases of recurrent ulcer but occur in only about one-fifth of such patients. Peak acid outputs more than 15 mmol/h are unusual except in recurrent ulcer, where they are present in about half of the patients.

Not only may acid hypersecretion indicate a recurrent ulcer but it may also suggest a cause and a rational policy of revision surgery. A high basal acid output little increased by maximum stimulation may be due to increased gastrin (see above). A low basal and high peak acid output indicates a large parietal cell mass and would suggest the need for a higher gastric resection or the addition of a vagotomy.

Assessment of vagal innervation[14]
Each phase of gastric secretion is markedly reduced after any type of vagotomy. Although parietal cells are less sensitive to pentagastrin and histamine after vagotomy, it has not been possible in man to restore their preoperative output, however high the dose of stimulants used. After vagotomy there is probably no reduction in the number of parietal cells because a cholinergic stimulus can increase maximal histamine-stimulated acid output back to the preoperative level.[14]

Unfortunately, glycopenic stimulation of the hypothalamus produces both parasympathetic and sympathetic responses, and hypoglycaemia may also affect the gastric parietal and antral G cells as well as the adrenals.

The adrenal–sympathetic system may be a neural non-vagal pathway, so that part of the acid response after vagotomy may be due to sympathetic factors rather than to inadequate vagal section. Even though there is no general agreement on how to perform the insulin test or how to interpret the results, it is still widely used. The old statement 'The insulin test is positive' implied that vagal denervation was incomplete and was based on various criteria, both qualitative (concentration of acid) and quantitative (output of acid). The Hollander positive criterion of an incomplete vagotomy ($\Delta[H] > 20$ mmol/l, or $\Delta[H] > 10$ mmol/l if $[H]_{basal} = 0$) was qualitative and arbitrary, as were the divisions into early and late positive results.

Many gastroenterologists still expect an insulin test to yield a positive or negative answer to tell them that vagal innervation is either present or absent. Today we should no longer assume that a surgeon cuts either all or none of the vagal fibres to the stomach, and these terms and criteria should be abandoned.

The current quantitative approach uses basal and peak outputs after pentagastrin and insulin. No secretory value can be defined as an absolute dividing line between an incomplete and a complete vagotomy: the higher the peak acid output the more parasympathetic fibres remain. This quantitative estimate of vagal completeness is only presumptive in man but has experimental support. The modified sham feeding (chew and spit) test gives every sign of being equally valid or even better than the insulin test, and may eventually replace it. It is uncertain whether pepsin measurements provide additional useful data, and tubeless tests such as serum gastrin or pancreatic polypeptide measurements are of no clear value either.

Tests may be done routinely after vagotomy to assess the acid-lowering efficiency of surgery, and thus the likelihood of recurrent ulceration. In patients with dyspepsia after vagotomy, tests may suggest recurrent ulceration, and if so whether there is still substantial vagal innervation which needs exploration and division.

Acid tests as a method of audit
Acid output measurements are of great value to trainee and trained vagotomists in assessing the efficiency of their technique of denervation. In one centre patients operated on by general sur-geons produced more than twice as much acid in response to insulin than the patients operated on by gastrointestinal surgeons; the incidence of recurrent ulceration was five times higher in the hands of general surgeons.

Prognosis of the patient
Measurements of gastric function after vagotomy can be compared only with the incidence of subsequent recurrent duodenopyloric or gastrojejunal ulcer, because the numbers of uncut vagal fibres are unknown. Hobsley's group assess insulin-stimulated secretion after correcting juice volume (V_G) for pyloric loss and duodenal reflux.[23] After vagotomy, half of the men whose V_G is still more than 140 ml/h have developed recurrent ulcers, whereas all those with V_G reduced below 140 ml/h have remained symptom-free. The discriminant for conventional peak acid output is 8 mmol/h.

Acid tests to evaluate postoperative dyspepsia
In patients with dyspepsia after vagotomy absolute anacidity excludes a diagnosis of recurrent ulceration. A low basal, with a low insulin-stimulated, but high pentagastrin-stimulated, acid output suggests that the patient has a very large functional parietal cell mass, even if there is no obvious vagal or gastrin drive. A high basal secretion and a high peak acid (and pepsin) output after insulin suggests not only that recurrent ulceration is likely, but also that it is associated with significant remaining vagal innervation, needing repeat vagotomy, whether or not antrectomy is performed. A high basal secretion with a low peak acid (and pepsin) output, especially in relation to the pentagastrin-stimulated output, suggests that any recurrent ulceration is unlikely to be due to inadequate vagotomy, but is probably due either to excess antral gastrin, needing antrectomy, or to extragastric gastrin secretion, which needs appropriate investigation.

Clinical value of gastric secretion tests

The demonstration of anacidity (indicating gastric atrophy) is rarely necessary today to help support or exclude a diagnosis of pernicious anaemia or to support the carcinomatous nature of a suspicious gastric ulcer, because there are now newer and better tests of the specific pathological process involved.

Acid tests are occasionally helpful in patients with X-ray-negative, endoscopy-indefinite, ulcer-like dyspepsia, in that they may suggest that a particular patient probably has, or probably does not have, duodenal ulcer disease.

Basal secretion and pentagastrin-stimulated acid output should be measured in all patients before all operations for duodenal ulcer and, together with serum gastrin, in patients with dyspepsia after gastrectomy. These acid tests together with sham feeding (or insulin) stimulation should be performed routinely in all patients after vagotomy as part of the assessment of the vagotomist rather than to predict prognosis for the patient. Basal secretion pentagastrin and sham feeding (or insulin) tests and serum gastrin measurements should be done in patients with dyspepsia after vagotomy to seek a cause for their recurrent ulceration and to help plan revision operations.

REFERENCES

1 Allen, A. (1982) Structure and function of gastrointestinal mucus. In *Physiology of the Gastrointestinal Tract* (Ed.) Johnson, L. R. pp. 617–639. New York: Raven.
2 Baron, J. H. (1963) Studies of basal and peak acid output with an augmented histamine test. *Gut*, **4**, 136–144.
3 Baron, J. H. (1963) An assessment of the augmented histamine test in the diagnosis of peptic ulcer. *Gut*, **4**, 243–253.
4 Baron, J. H. (1963) The relationship between basal and maximum acid output in normal subjects and patients with duodenal ulcer. *Clinical Science*, **24**, 357–370.
5 Baron, J. H. (1971) Physiological control of gastric acid secretion. *Proceedings of the Royal Society of Medicine*, **64**, 739–741.
6 Baron, J. H. (1972) Aetiology. In *Chronic Duodenal Ulcer* (Ed.) Wastell, C. pp. 19–52. London: Butterworth.
7 Baron, J. H. (1977) Gastric secretion and diseases of the mucosal barrier. *Rendiconti di gastroenterologia*, **9**, 41–46.
8 Baron, J. H. (1978) Gastric secretion in duodenal ulcer disease. In *Aspects of Peptic Ulceration* (Ed.) Murphy, J. E. pp. 21–38. Northampton: Cambridge Medical Publications.
9 Baron, J. H. (1978) *Clinical Tests of Gastric Secretion: History, Methodology and Interpretation*. London: Macmillan.
10 Baron, J. H. (1981) Pathophysiology of gastric acid and pepsin secretion. In *Magen und Magenkrankheiten* (Ed.) Domschke, W. & Wormsley, K. G. pp. 131–149. Stuttgart: Thieme Verlag.
11 Baron, J. H. (1982) Current views on pathogenesis of peptic ulcer. *Scandinavian Journal of Gastroenterology*, **17** (supplement 80) 1–10.
12 Baron, J. H. (1984) Gastric secretion tests. In *Surgery of the Stomach and Duodenum – 4* (Ed.) Nyhus, L. M. & Wastell, C. Boston: Little, Brown.
13 Baron, J. H., Langman, M. J. S. & Wastell, C. (1980) Stomach and duodenum In *Recent Advances in Gastroenterology – 4* (Ed.) Bouchier, I. A. D. pp. 23–86. Edinburgh: Churchill Livingstone.
14 Baron, J. H., Alexander-Williams, J., Allgower, M. *et al.* (Ed.) (1982) *Vagotomy in Modern Surgical Practice* London: Butterworths.
15 Carter, D. C. (1980) Aetiology of peptic ulcer. In *Scientific Foundations of Gastroenterology* (Ed.) Sircus, W. & Smith, A. N. pp. 344–357. London: Heinemann.
16 Carter, D. C. (1981) Cytoprotection and its possible role in the pharmacology of gastric mucosa. In *Gastric Secretion. Basic and Clinical Aspects* (Ed.) Konturek, S. J. & Domschke, W. pp. 97–108. Stuttgart: Thieme Verlag.
17 Cowley, D. J. & Baron, J. H. (1972) Aetiological mechanisms in gastric ulcer. *Biologie et Gastroenterologie*, **5**, 117–126.
18 Elder, J. B. & Ganguli, P. C. (1979) Gastric function. In *Chemical Diagnosis of Disease* (Ed.) Brown, S. S., Mitchell, F. L. & Young, D. S. pp. 663–688. Amsterdam, Oxford & New York: Elsevier.
19 Fromm, D. (1981) Gastric mucosal barrier. In *Physiology of the Gastrointestinal Tract*. (Ed.) Johnson, L. R. pp. 733–748. New York: Raven.
20 Grossman, M. I. (1967) Neural and hormonal stimulation of gastric secretion of acid. In *Handbook of Physiology*, vol. II, section 6, pp. 835–863. (Ed.) Code, C. R. Washington DC: American Physiology Society.
21 Grossman, M. I. (1978) Control of gastric secretion. In *Gastrointestinal Disease*, 2nd edn (Ed.) Sleisenger, M. B. & Fordtran, J. S. pp. 640–659. Philadelphia: Saunders.
22 Grossman, M. I. (1980) Peptic ulcer: the pathophysiological background. In *Symposium on Pathophysiology and Drug Therapy of Peptic Ulcer* (Ed.) Myren, J. & Schrumpf, E. *Scandinavian Journal of Gastroenterology*, **15** (supplement 58), 7–14.
23 Hobsley, M. (1980) Tests of gastric secretory function. In *Scientific Foundations of Gastroenterology* (Ed.) Sircus, W. & Smith, A. N. pp. 316–332. London: Heinemann.
24 Hobsley, M. (1981) *Disorders of the Digestive System*. London: Edward Arnold.
25 Malagelada, J. R. (1979) Pathophysiology of duodenal ulcer. In *Peptic Ulcer Disease and its Treatment – Present Situation and Future Prospects* (Ed.) Walan, A. *Scandinavian Journal of Gastroenterology*, **14** (supplement 55), 39–48.
26 Piper, D. W. (1980) Mucus, chemistry and characteristics. In *Scientific Foundations of Gastroenterology* (Ed.) Sircus, W. & Smith, A. N. pp. 333–343. London: Heinemann.
27 Rees, W. D. W. & Turnberg, L. A. (1982) Mechanisms of gastric mucosal protection: a role for the mucus-bicarbonate barrier. *Clinical Science*, **62**, 343–348.
28 Robert, A. (1981) Current history of cytoprotection. *Prostaglandins*, **21** (supplement), 89–96.
29 Schrager, J. & Oates, M. D. G. (1978) Relation of human gastrointestinal mucus to disease states. *British Medical Bulletin*, **34**, 79–82.
30 Wormsley, K. G. (1974) The pathophysiology of duodenal ulceration. *Gut*, **15**, 59–81.
31 Wormsley, K. G., (1977) *Duodenal Ulcer 1976*. Montreal: Eden.
32 Wormsley, K. G. (1979) *Duodenal Ulcer 1977*. Edinburgh: Churchill Livingstone.
33 Wormsley, K. G. (1983) *Duodenal Ulcer – 3*. Montreal: Eden.

GASTRODUODENAL MOTILITY

Gastric emptying

NORMAL PHYSIOLOGY

On ingestion of a solid or liquid meal the body and fundus of the stomach dilate to accommodate the meal with little increase in intragastric pressure. This 'receptive relaxation' begins at the commencement of the act of swallowing and is maximal when the bolus reaches the stomach.[1]

The regulation of liquid emptying depends on the intraduodenal concentrations of the various products of digestion. These slow gastric emptying by excitation of duodenal receptors either by their osmotic pressure (e.g. monosaccharides and amino acids) or by a specific action (e.g. salts of fatty acids). The inhibition of gastric emptying is rapidly mediated, suggesting a neural effector mechanism. The degree of inhibition of gastric emptying that is produced by food products is proportional to their nutritive density (that is, energy content per unit volume). However, the slowing of gastric emptying by a meal of high nutritive density is not sufficient to prevent an increased rate of delivery of energy to the duodenum when such a meal is ingested.[10] It has therefore been postulated that obese patients may eat meals that have higher energy density than normal; hence, emptying of energy content is more rapid in the obese and satiety periods are shorter.[11]

The volume of liquid ingested at any one time does not affect the overall rate at which emptying occurs, although the early phase of emptying is relatively more rapid with larger meals.[8] Posture has little effect on liquid gastric emptying in normal individuals.[12]

Normal meals contain a liquid component and solid particles of different sizes and constitution. The gastric emptying of solid particles has been studied using radioisotopes to label the food and external detection of the gamma radiation. In normal individuals the stomach processes large particles of radiolabelled chicken liver into a slurry of particles mostly smaller than 1 mm in diameter before emptying them into the small bowel.[20] Smaller particles of liver empty more rapidly than larger particles, and different solid foodstuffs in the same meal have been shown to empty at differing rates.[24]

ABNORMALITIES IN DUODENAL ULCER, GASTRIC ULCER AND GASTRO-OESOPHAGEAL REFLUX

Abnormalities of gastric emptying have been suggested as possible pathogenetic factors for both duodenal ulceration (faster emptying) and gastric ulceration (slower emptying). However, the majority of studies of patients with duodenal ulcer disease have shown no difference between their gastric emptying and that of normal controls. There are, however, a few reports suggesting that solid foodstuffs do empty more rapidly in duodenal ulcer disease. In gastric ulceration gastric emptying is the same as in normals.

Delayed gastric emptying of liquids and solid food has been reported in patients with gastro-oesophageal reflux. The presence of food and secretions in the stomach for prolonged periods could be a contributory factor in the pathogenesis of gastro-oesophageal reflux and its symptoms.

ABNORMALITIES AFTER GASTRIC OPERATIONS

A number of the side-effects of gastric operations are associated with abnormalities of gastric emptying. The most common abnormalities are very rapid emptying of liquids (associated with early dumping symptoms and diarrhoea) and delayed emptying of solids (producing food vomiting, distension and foul eructations). These two abnormalities may coexist in the same patient.[3]

After both truncal vagotomy and proximal gastric vagotomy receptive relaxation is abolished by denervation of the body and fundus of the stomach. There is therefore an increase in the rate of liquid emptying as no accommodation is provided for the incoming fluid. The addition of a pyloroplasty increases the abnormality and the majority of a liquid meal empties during ingestion of the meal. Posture has a major influence, liquid emptying being more rapid when seated than when lying down.[18] The typical effects of vagotomy with or without a pyloroplasty upon liquid gastric emptying in the seated position are shown in Figure 4.12.[2] In the individual patient symptoms of dumping or diarrhoea are only likely when the abnormality is severe; consequently vagotomy and pyloroplasty produces more of such side-effects than proximal gastric vagotomy alone.

Increased liquid emptying is also seen after partial gastrectomy. Although innervation of the body and fundus is preserved, there is a reduction in gastric capacity and a wider than normal gastric outlet.

Drainage procedures were introduced into gastric surgery because it was found that a large number (30–50%) of patients who underwent truncal vagotomy developed severe symptoms of gastric retention. After proximal gastric vagotomy, drainage is unnecessary as the gastric emptying of solid food is almost normal. After gastric resections symptomatic gastric retention is uncommon. It may, however, occur if a truncal vagotomy is also performed and a gastroduodenal reconstruction is used.[3]

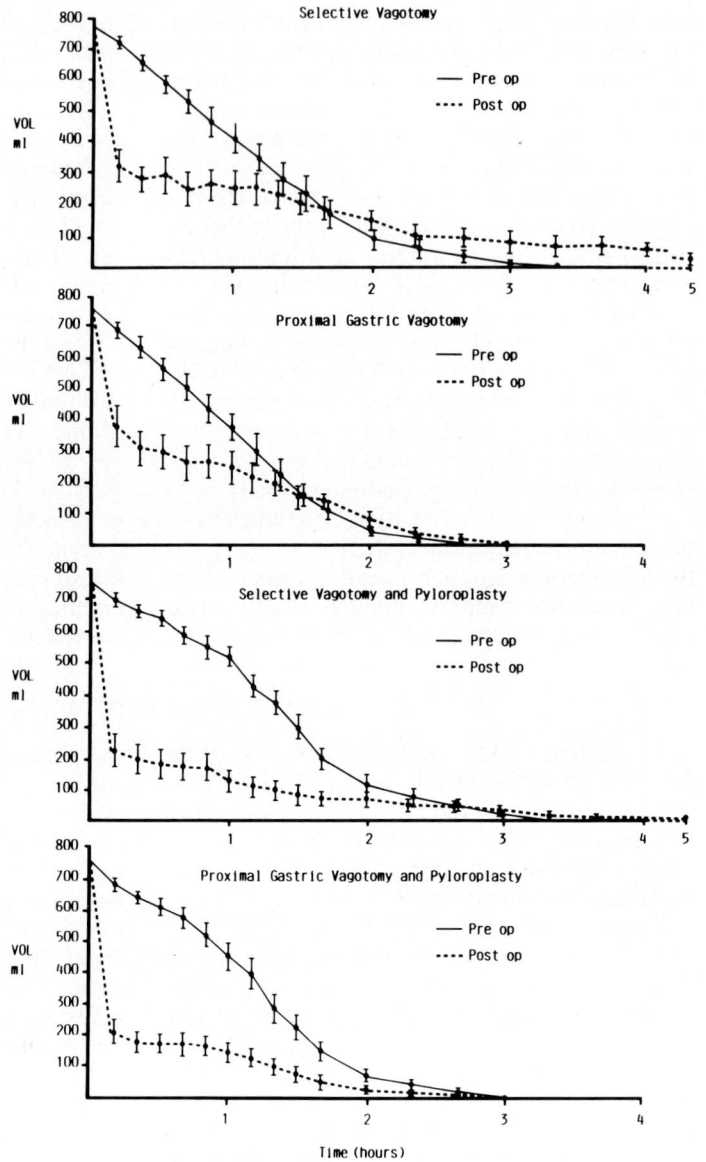

Fig. 4.12 Gastric emptying of 750 ml of 10% dextrose solution before and after proximal gastric vagotomy and selective vagotomy with and without pyloroplasty. From Clarke and Alexander-Williams (1973)[2], with kind permission of the authors and the editor of *Gut*.

METHODS OF MEASURING GASTRIC EMPTYING

The Serial Test Meal[9] has been used to obtain information in volunteers about the physiology of the gastric emptying of many different solutions. However, as it requires repeated nasogastric intubation over several days, it is not suitable for use in clinical practice.

The double-sampling dye-dilution technique[6] enables the gastric emptying of a liquid meal to be studied in its entirety after one intubation. A marker is added to the stomach contents, and after mixing the degree of dilution is used to calculate stomach volume; the procedure is repeated at intervals. Thorough mixing is essential and cumulative errors may occur which can only be overcome by cumbersome modifications of the technique.[13]

External scanning of radiolabelled food is used to measure the emptying of solids. A variety of different labels have been used[14] and investigators must base their choice on their particular needs. If it is desired to measure the emptying of a particular food particle size, then $^{99}Tc^m$-labelled chicken liver is the most valid material.[19] However, this is a complicated method, and for useful clinical data on the emptying of solids, a label that is distributed throughout the meal is satisfactory (e.g. $^{113}In^m$-DTPA).[3]

More than one isotope label can be used in the same meal[24] and it is easy to use a radioisotope to label liquid meals. Imaging is best performed with a gamma camera rather than a scanner, and for accurate quantitation corrections for scatter and the inevitable imperfections of collimation are required.[4, 24]

Interpretation of gastric emptying data requires at least two indices,[9] one to measure early emptying behaviour (especially important after gastric surgery) and the other to interpret the rest of the emptying process.[3] A number of the inconsistencies in the literature are due to differing methods of data interpretation, but standardization is not easy to achieve.[5a]

Duodenogastric reflux

NORMAL PHYSIOLOGY AND ASSOCIATION WITH ULCER

Duodenogastric reflux occurs in normal subjects both when fasting and after meals. Reflux is an intermittent phenomenon, and the incidence and quantity of reflux reported in normals and in disease varies widely (in normals from nil to 60%, in duodenal ulcer disease from nil to 88% and in gastric ulcer disease from 3% to 100%). Despite a wealth of theory, no definite pathogenetic relationship between the occurrence of duodenogastric reflux and disease has been established.

The amount of duodenal content found in the stomach depends on two factors: the amount refluxing and the rate at which it is cleared from the stomach. Reflux is produced by retrograde peristalsis from the duodenum into the stomach. In the fasting state it occurs mainly during phase II (irregular activity) of the interdigestive motor complex. The subsequent phase III motor activity then clears the refluxed material from the stomach.[15] Disorders of the phase III ('intestinal housekeeper') motor activity could therefore lead to prolonged contact between refluxed duodenal contents and gastric (and oesophageal) mucosa in the fasting state.

ENTEROGASTRIC REFLUX AFTER GASTRIC OPERATIONS

After gastric operations some patients develop a symptom complex which is improved by diversion of the duodenal contents from the gastric remnant. However, enterogastric reflux occurs in asymptomatic patients after gastric operations as well as in symptomatic patients. The decision to perform a bile diversion procedure therefore largely depends on the clinical history of bile vomiting and epigastric or retrosternal pain in the absence of recurrent peptic ulceration. Quantitative assessment of bile reflux is of debatable value, although the amount of bile acids collected from the stomach in the fasting state has been found to be a useful discriminant by some.[7] There is also some evidence that symptoms due to enterogastric reflux are more likely to occur in patients in whom the operation has produced severe abnormalities of gastric emptying.[5]

It has been suggested that postoperative symptoms are associated with gastritis as a consequence of bile reflux. However, superficial gastritis is common after gastric operations and its incidence does not appear to be related to the degree of bile reflux since it is not reversed by Roux-en-Y diversion operations.

METHODS OF MEASURING ENTEROGASTRIC REFLUX

Reflux can be measured either from the concentration in the stomach of substances normally present in the duodenum or from intragastric concentration of markers that have been introduced into the duodenum, either directly or indirectly by intravenous injection and subsequent biliary excretion.

The measurements of endogenous bilirubin, bile acids, bicarbonate, lysolecithin and trypsin are all affected by pH, and sodium ions are secreted by the gastric mucosa in varying amounts in addition to being present in the duodenal contents.[17] Consequently, none of these endogenous substances can be relied upon as quantitative markers of reflux. Furthermore, reflux can only be detected if the marker is available in the duodenum to reflux: bile, for example, is normally present only intermittently. Absolute amounts of a detected substance can be related from one study to another, but it is impossible to express the amount found in an individual as a percentage of the unknown quantity of substance available for reflux from the duodenum.

A variety of exogenous markers have been introduced into the duodenum through transpyloric tubes, including sulphobromophthalein, polyethylene glycol and phenol red. Estimation of the amount of substance has been aided by radiolabelling (^{14}C-PEG, ^{35}S-phenol red), and the amount retrieved from the stomach via a

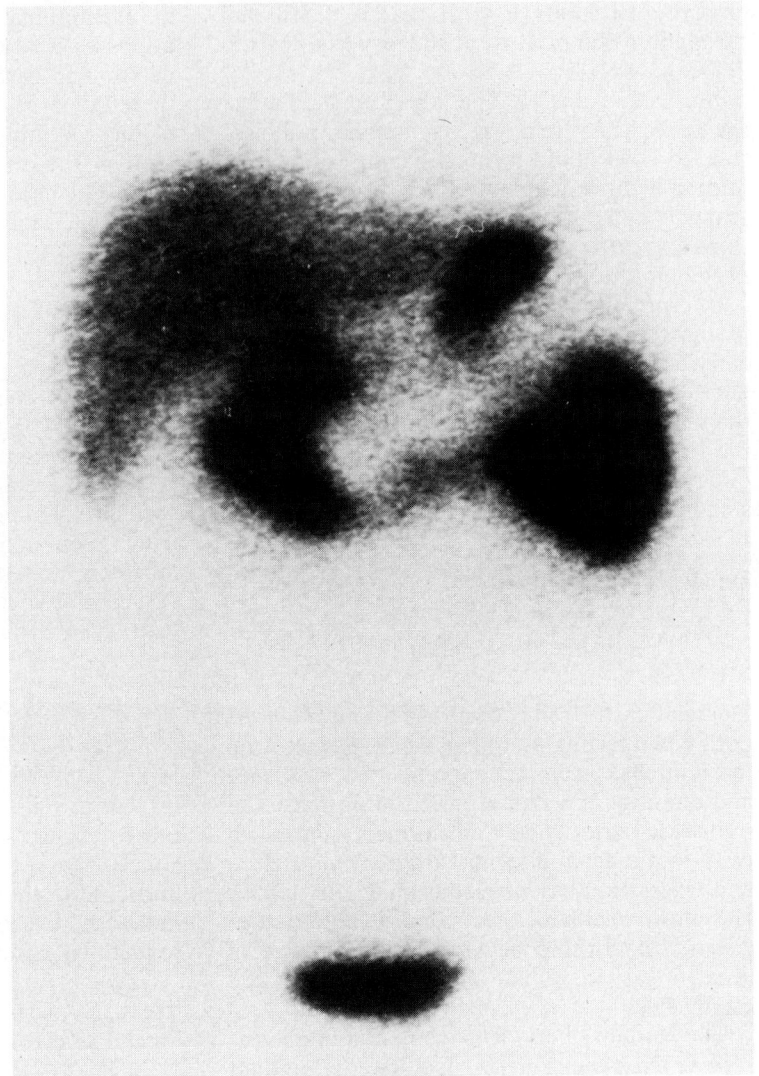

Fig. 4.13 Photograph of oscilloscope display from gamma camera after radiolabelled HIDA injection. The stomach is clearly seen adjacent to the left lobe of the liver. A proportion of the radiopharmaceutical is excreted in the urine, so the bladder is outlined inferiorly. The remainder of the HIDA excreted by the liver is in the duodenum and upper jejunum below the stomach.

nasogastric tube can be related to the amount instilled into the duodenum. There is a possibility of inducement of reflux by the transpyloric and nasogastric tubes, but if thin, pliable tubes are used the error is minimal.[21]

External scanning with a gamma camera allows detection of reflux without interfering with the normal physiology. Various lignocaine derivatives (such as diethyl-HIDA and BIDA) labelled with technetium-99m are now available. After intravenous injection these are excreted by the liver into the bile. A stimulus for gallbladder contraction is necessary, such as a fatty meal or cholecystokinin, and the study can only be of a limited duration. However, it is possible to quantitate the number of counts detected over the stomach as a proportion of the injected dose of radioisotope or as a proportion of the isotope excreted by the liver.[23] More simply, visual interpretation of the scans may be used to quantify the percentage of the study time during which reflux was present. Visual interpretation of the gamma camera display is usually straightforward (see Figure 4.13).

Electromyography

Two types of electrical activity can be recorded from the smooth muscle of the stomach: a 'slow wave', which forms the basic electrical rhythm, and 'action potentials', which give rise to a muscular contraction when associated with a slow wave. The pacemaker for the gastric slow wave is situated in the mid-position of the body of the stomach around the greater curvature and the potentials occur at a frequency of about three per minute in the fasting state. The slow wave propagates towards the pylorus rather than upwards towards the proximal stomach.

Slow waves spread across the pylorus from the antrum into the duodenum, augmenting duodenal slow waves. This coordination is abolished by transection of the pylorus suggesting that the conduction is myogenic rather than neurogenic. The propagation probably occurs in the longitudinal muscle layer.

Motor activity in the fasting human stomach is cyclical, with a periodicity of around 100 minutes but with considerable individual variation around this mean. The cycle consists of a period of quiescence (phase I), which is followed by a period of irregular motor activity (phase II) associated with an increase in gastric acid output and also an increase in pancreatic and biliary secretion into the duodenum.[15] Immediately following phase II there is a regular propulsive phase of motor activity (phase III), which migrates slowly from the lower oesophageal sphincter to the terminal ileum. Phase III has been described as the 'intestinal housekeeper' as it clears the fasting stomach of its contents – large inert solid particles, gastric juice and refluxed duodenal contents.

Feeding interrupts this fasting electrical activity: action potentials, which are seen with only a small percentage of slow waves in the fasting state $(11–33\%)$[22] occur with every antral slow wave. In the duodenum action potentials occur whenever antral slow waves coincide with duodenal slow waves.

The muscle contractions produced by this electrical activity are responsible for mixing and trituration as well as for propulsion of the intraluminal contents. Consequently, no direct correlation exists between the occurrence of electrical events and the rate of transit of intraluminal contents.

CHANGES IN ELECTRICAL ACTIVITY IN GASTRODUODENAL DISEASE

In gastric ulcer, duodenal ulcer and gastric cancer the frequency of gastric slow waves is greater than in patients with gallstones but no gastroduodenal disease.[16] In gastric cancer the frequency of slow wave activity is very variable. This behaviour is also seen to a lesser extent in patients with benign gastroduodenal disease. However, the changes in electrical activity are not sufficiently constant to characterize any specific disease for diagnostic purposes or to indicate any pathogenetic relationship.

CHANGES IN ELECTRICAL ACTIVITY AFTER GASTRIC OPERATIONS

Gastric slow wave activity is not affected by operations in the upper part of the peritoneal cavity which do not directly involve the stomach. Any form of vagotomy temporarily disorganizes antral myoelectrical activity, the effects being more marked with truncal vagotomy than with proximal gastric vagotomy. Truncal vagotomy also permanently reduces the amplitude of the slow waves and alters their shape from a triphasic to a sinusoidal form. Proximal gastric vagotomy does not alter the waveform and produces only a minimal reduction in amplitude of the slow waves.[22] In the presence of grossly delayed gastric emptying after vagotomy slow wave activity has been found to be absent, being replaced by disorganized and weak antral electrical activity.

REFERENCES

1 Cannon, W. B. & Lieb C. W. (1911) The receptive relaxation of the stomach. *American Journal of Physiology,* **29,** 267–273.

2 Clarke, R. J. & Alexander-Williams, J. (1973) The effect of preserving antral innervation and of a pyloroplasty on gastric emptying after vagotomy in man. *Gut,* **14,** 300–307.

3 Donovan, I. A. (1976) The different components of gastric emptying after gastric surgery. *Annals of the Royal College of Surgeons,* **58,** 368–373.

4 Donovan, I. A. (1977) Radio-isotope measurement of gastric emptying. In *Proceedings of the Fifth International Symposium on Gastrointestinal Motility* (Ed.) Vantrappen, G. pp. 258–262. Leuven: Belgium.

5 Donovan, I. A., Keighley, M. R. B., Griffin, D. W. *et al.* (1976) The association of duodeno-gastric reflux with dumping and gastric retention. *British Journal of Surgery,* **63,** 349–351.

5a Elashoff, J. D., Reedy, T. J. & Meyer, J. H. (1982) Analysis of gastric emptying data. *Gastroenterology,* **83,** 1306–1312.

6 George, J. D. (1968) New clinical method for measuring the rate of gastric emptying. *Gut,* **9,** 237–242.

7 Hoare, A. M., McLeish, A., Thompson, H. & Alexander-Williams, J. (1978) Selection of patients for bile diversion surgery: use of bile acid measurement in fasting gastric aspirates. *Gut,* **19,** 163–165.

8 Hunt, J. N. & MacDonald, I. (1954) Influence of volume on gastric emptying. *Journal of Physiology,* **126,** 459–474.

9 Hunt, J. N. & Spurrell, W. R. (1951) The pattern of emptying of the human stomach. *Journal of Physiology,* **113,** 157–169.

10 Hunt, J. N. & Stubbs, D. F. (1975) The volume and energy content of meals as determinants of gastric emptying. *Journal of Physiology,* **245,** 209–225.

11 Hunt, J. N., Cash, R. & Newland, P. (1975) Energy density of food, gastric emptying and obesity. *Lancet,* **ii,** 905–906.

12 Hunt, J. N., Knox, M. T. & Oginski, A. (1965) The effect of gravity on gastric emptying with various test meals. *Journal of Physiology,* **178,** 92–97.

13 Hurwitz, A. (1981) Measuring gastric volumes by dye dilution. *Gut*, **22**, 85–93.

14 Horowitz, M., Cook, D. J., Collins, P. J. *et al.* (1982) The application of techniques using radionuclides to the study of gastric emptying. *Surgery, Gynecology and Obstetrics*, **155**, 737–744.

15 Keane, F. B., Dimgno, E. P. & Malagelada, J. R. (1981) Duodenogastric reflux in humans. Its relationship to fasting antroduodenal motility and gastric, pancreatic and biliary secretion. *Gastroenterology*, **81**, 726–731.

16 Kwong, N. K., Brown, B. H., Whittaker, G. E. & Duthie, H. L. (1970) Electrical activity of the gastric antrum in man. *British Journal of Surgery*, **57**, 913–916.

17 Lewin, M. R., Pifano, E., Daniel, R. D. *et al.* (1983) Effect of sodium taurocholate on gastric secretion in patients with duodenal ulceration. *Gut*, **24**, 28–32.

18 McKelvey, S. T. D. (1970) Gastric incontinence and post-vagotomy diarrhoea. *British Journal of Surgery*, **57**, 741–747.

19 Meyer, J. H., MacGregor, I. L., Gueller, R. *et al.* (1976) 99mTc tagged chicken liver as a marker of solid food in the human stomach. *American Journal of Digestive Diseases*, **21**, 296–304.

20 Meyer, J. H., Ohashi, H., Jehn, D. & Thomson, J. B. (1981) Size of liver particles emptied from the human stomach. *Gastroenterology*, **80**, 1489–1496.

21 Muller-Lissner, S. A., Fimmel, C. J., Will, N. *et al.* (1982) Effect of gastric and transpyloric tubes on gastric emptying and duodeno-gastric reflux. *Gastroenterology*, **83**, 1276–1279.

22 Stoddard, C. J., Waterfall, W. E., Brown, B. H. & Duthie, H. L. (1973) The effects of varying the extent of the vagotomy on the myoelectrical and motor activity of the stomach. *Gut*, **14**, 657–664.

23 Tolin, R. D., Malmud, L. S., Stelzer, F. *et al.* (1979) Enterogastric reflux in normal subjects and patients with Billroth II. *Gastroenterology*, **77**, 1027–1033.

24 Weiner, K., Graham, L. S., Reedy, T. *et al.* (1981) Simultaneous gastric emptying of two solid foods. *Gastroenterology*, **81**, 257–266.

GASTRITIS

ACUTE GASTRITIS AND ACUTE ULCER

These two diseases are considered together because they represent the gastric mucosal responses to acute injury.

Acute gastritis consists of two entities: acute superficial gastritis and acute phlegmonous gastritis.

Acute superficial gastritis is a diffuse lesion localized to the mucosa or submucosa. Depending on the cause, there are varying degrees of mucosal necrosis and inflammatory reaction. This is the entity referred to when the term *acute gastritis* is used and discussed in detail below.

Acute phlegmonous or suppurative gastritis is rare, and fatal if untreated. It involves the whole thickness of the stomach wall and is due to bacterial invasion, usually by Gram-positive cocci or *Escherichia coli*, in a patient with a pre-existing mucosal lesion such as cancer, ulcer or a postoperative lesion. The patient presents with evidence of an acute bacterial infection, with chills, fever, malaise, severe toxaemia and leucocytosis. There are also gastrointestinal symptoms: nausea, vomiting (occasionally purulent), epigastric pain and tenderness. This entity is very rare; it will be discussed further later in this chapter (p. 244).

Acute superficial gastritis

AETIOLOGY

The causes are several and include:
a the ingestion of drugs, including alcohol, large doses of analgesic drugs and cytotoxic drugs;
b gastric irradiation and freezing;
c staphylococcal food poisoning and other less common severe gastrointestinal infections such as salmonella infections (a histological abnormality in this group has not been established);
d accidental or suicidal ingestion of corrosive substances, including acids, alkalis, fixatives such as formaldehyde and softeners such as lye. This results in a more severe form (corrosive gastritis).

SYMPTOMS

After exposure to the aetiological agent, there is a rapid onset of abdominal discomfort, anorexia, nausea and vomiting. The clinical state is limited to a few hours or days and recovery is complete. It is emphasized that even though patients may have symptoms consistent with acute gastritis, the gastric mucosa may be histologically normal.[20]

In acute corrosive gastritis the condition is more severe, with epigastric pain, retching and vomiting (often bloody). Shock may develop in the acute phase and survivors may develop gastric outlet obstruction.

DIAGNOSIS

This is entirely clinical. The diagnosis of acute gastritis firstly involves the exclusion of other diseases that may be accompanied by anorexia, nausea, vomiting and abdominal pain such as acute appendicitis, intestinal obstruction, pyelonephritis and systemic toxicity due to drugs. Secondly, it is important to elucidate the cause as far as possible.

TREATMENT

In most patients the management of acute gastritis is expectant, with control of symptoms and replacement of any fluid or electrolyte loss.

The gastritis resulting from ingestion of a corrosive substance is more serious. Nasogastric suction with a flexible double-lumen tube, large doses of antacids (60 ml of aluminium magnesium hydroxide gel every two hours) and fluid replacement are advised. Skilled endoscopy using an end-viewing fibre-optic instrument is required. If necrosis (i.e., blackened mucosa) is seen, gastric resection is advised.[2, 3, 13, 17] Survival after heavy corrosive ingestion will probably only be achieved by such aggressive measures.

Acute ulcer

An ulcer is a circumscribed defect in the wall of the stomach or duodenum. These lesions may penetrate varying distances through the stomach or duodenal wall; if they do not extend deep in the muscularis mucosae, they are sometimes called *erosions*. The latter term is probably best avoided because of the problems of defining ulcer depth at endoscopy.

Ulcers are conventionally divided into acute and chronic. An acute ulcer is a disease of sudden onset and short duration, whereas a chronic ulcer is of prolonged duration. Both lesions provoke an inflammatory reaction and have the potential to provoke a fibrotic reaction. An ulcer superficial to the muscularis mucosae (i.e. an erosion) heals by epithelial regeneration without scar formation. In a deeper lesion, the amount of fibrosis produced is a reflection of the duration of the lesion. Most acute ulcers therefore heal leaving little fibrotic reaction, whereas this may be marked in the case of a chronic ulcer. The problems of definition are well discussed by Ivy, Grossman and Bachrach.[7]

Acute ulcers may be single or multiple; if multiple they are often termed areas of *acute haemorrhagic* or *erosive gastritis*, but the term gastritis is probably best avoided in this context. If multiple, they occur predominantly in the body of the stomach.

RELATIONSHIP OF ACUTE ULCER TO CHRONIC ULCER

Very few acute ulcers progress to a chronic ulcer.[4, 8] It is impossible to conceive, however, that a chronic ulcer does not start with a lesion resembling an acute ulcer. An acute ulcer produced by biopsy heals rapidly. The factors that determine chronicity are largely unsolved. Exposure to acid and pepsin is essential for ulcer formation, but why some lesions persist or recur and others heal is not known.

AETIOLOGY

The aetiological factors in acute ulcer are extreme physical stress, drugs and possibly viral infection (see also p. 129). There may be other, so far unidentified, factors.

Stress ulceration
After the Second World War, the association of acute ulcer with serious injury and hypovolaemic shock became well documented. After the introduction of fluid and blood replacement and antibiotic therapy, patients who would previously have died of hypovolaemic shock, renal failure, pulmonary failure or subsequent multiple organ failure survived to develop acute stress ulcers in the second or third week after injury.[10] Acute stress ulcers are multifactorial in origin and those that perforate or bleed represent only a small fraction of the total number of cases.[11] Factors that are of *major* aetiological significance include (a) hypovolaemic shock, (b) sepsis, (c) kidney, liver and lung failure, (d) severe injuries (predominantly involving intra-abdominal or thoracoabdominal trauma), (e) neurological injury and (f) bile reflux.[10, 16]

Drug-induced ulceration
Analgesic and anti-inflammatory drugs may evoke several gastric responses. These include *chronic blood loss* (microbleeding) and *acute ulcer*. Most patients taking aspirin lose 3–6 ml of blood per day. This is usually not clinically important. However, some lose more, resulting in iron-deficiency anaemia. The topic of bleeding from drug-induced gastric mucosal injury is reviewed in detail elsewhere.[15] Bleeding usually results from rupture of small blood vessels just below the surface epithelium.[14]

Acute ulcer can be produced by aspirin ingestion in dogs and man.[11, 12, 18] This lesion is generally larger than the lesion that causes microbleeding because of peptic digestion of the microscopic lesion.

The association between analgesic ingestion and acute upper gastrointestinal bleeding is controversial; the evidence indicates that any association is not causal but appears by chance. Hence, despite numerous studies, there is no conclusive epidemiological evidence of an association between aspirin ingestion and bleeding.[15] Although aspirin can cause acute mucosal lesions, these lesions have not been shown to produce massive haemorrhage. Furthermore, those patients who bleed following ingestion of aspirin do not rebleed on challenge. Approximately one-third of patients with massive upper gastrointestinal haemorrhage have an acute ulcer,[9] and in the majority of cases no cause is identified.

Virus infection

Unlike chronic ulcer, where a viral aetiology has been postulated,[6] there is no evidence of a viral aetiology for acute gastric ulcer.

SYMPTOMS AND DIAGNOSIS OF ACUTE PEPTIC ULCER

The uncomplicated acute ulcer rarely produces symptoms. The diagnosis of an acute ulcer when it is complicated by haemorrhage or perforation in an otherwise well patient is usually simple. By contrast, in the acute stress ulcer syndrome diagnosis may be difficult since the patient is ill and often confused, shock may be attributed to other causes, and symptoms such as pain may be distorted by analgesics given for other reasons and by organic disease of the nervous system.

In the acute stress ulcer the diagnosis depends upon three sequential procedures:

1 The recognition of the group at risk.
2 The admission of such patients to an intensive care ward of a major referral hospital.
3 The initiation of measures that will detect bleeding or perforation at an early stage. This includes continuous gastric aspiration in the search for blood loss and careful observation of patients in the search for perforation; if doubt exists, repeated X-rays of the abdomen are indicated.

When bleeding occurs, endoscopy should be performed as soon as the patient has been resuscitated.

TREATMENT

The acute ulcer needs no specific treatment as healing is rapid. Ideally, endoscopy should be performed after four weeks to confirm healing. If the acute ulcer is complicated by bleeding, management in an intensive care ward of a major hospital equipped with staff to monitor central venous pressure accurately is essential (see Chapter 6). There is some evidence that prostaglandins should be administered as soon as an

acute ulcer is complicated by haemorrhage.[19] If the bleeding continues or becomes recurrent early operation is advised, preferably by oversewing the ulcer and vagotomy.

Conventional doses of antibiotics may not be appropriate because of organ failure, so the serum level of the appropriate antibiotics should be checked daily. Total parenteral nutrition must also be considered for therapy in the debilitated, wasted and infective patients.

REFERENCES

1 Caruso, I. & Bianchi Porro, G. (1980) Gastroscopic evaluation of anti-inflammatory agents. *British Medical Journal*, **i**, 75.
2 Chong, G., Beahrs, O. & Payne, W. (1974) Management of corrosive gastritis due to ingested acid. *Mayo Clinic Proceedings*, **49**, 861.
3 Chung, R. & Den Besten, L. (1975) Fibreoptic endoscopy in the treatment of corrosive injury of the stomach. *Archives of Surgery*, **110**, 725.
4 Clarke, A. D. & Piper, D. W. (1976) Acute upper gastrointestinal haemorrhage with negative barium meal x-ray findings: follow-up investigation. *Medical Journal of Australia*, **2**, 637–638.
5 Croft, D. N. & Wood, P. H. N. (1967) Gastric mucosa and susceptibility to occult gastrointestinal bleeding caused by aspirin. *British Medical Journal*, **i**, 137.
6 Editorial (1981) Virus and duodenal ulcer. *Lancet*, **i**, 705.
7 Ivy, A. C., Grossman, M. I. & Bachrach, W. H. (1950) In *Peptic Ulcer* pp. 3–19. Philadelphia & Toronto: Blakiston.
8 Jones, F. Avery, Read, A. E. & Stubbe, J. L. (1954) Alimentary bleeding of obscure origin. *British Medical Journal*, **i**, 1138.
9 Kang, J. Y. & Piper, D. W. (1980) Improvement in mortality rates in bleeding peptic ulcer disease. *Medical Journal of Australia*, **1**, 213–215.
10 Lucas, C. E. (1981) Stress ulceration: the clinical problem. *World Journal of Surgery*, **5**, 139–151.
11 McElwee, H. P., Sirinek, K. R. & Levine, B. A. (1974) Cimetidine affords protection equal to antacids in prevention of stress ulceration following thermal injury. *Surgery*, **86**, 620.
12 Muir, A. & Cossar, I. A. (1961) Aspirin and gastric bleeding: further studies of calcium aspirin. *American Journal of Digestive Diseases*, **6**, 1115–1125.
13 Nicosia, J., Thornton, J., Folk, F. & Saletta, J. (1974) Surgical management of corrosive gastric injuries. *Annals of Surgery*, **180**, 138.
14 Pfeiffer, C. J., Harding, R. K. & Morris, G. P. (1982) Ultrastructural aspects of salicylate-induced damage to the gastric mucosa. In *Drugs and Peptic Ulcer, Volume 2. Pathogenesis of Ulcer Induction Revealed by Drug Studies in Humans and Animals* (Ed.) Pfeiffer, C. pp. 110–126. Boca Raton, Florida: CRC Press.
15 Piper, D. W., Gellatly, R. & McIntosh, J. (1982) Analgesic drugs and peptic ulcer. Human studies. In *Drugs and Peptic Ulcer, Volume 2. Pathogenesis of Ulcer Induction Revealed by Drug Studies in Humans and Animals* (Ed.) Pfeiffer, C. pp. 76–94. Boca Raton, Florida: CRC Press.
16 Ritchie, W. P. (1981) Role of bile acid reflux in acute haemorrhage gastritis. *World Journal of Surgery*, **5**, 189–198.

17 Shaw, A., Garvey, J. & Miller, B. (1964) Lye burns requiring total gastrectomy and colon substitution for oesophagus and stomach. *Surgery*, **64**, 837.

18 Weiss, A., Pitman, E. R. & Graham, E. C. (1961) Aspirin and gastric bleeding. Gastroscopic observations with a review of the literature. *American Journal of Medicine*, **31**, 266–278.

19 Weiss, J. B., Pesking, G. W. & Isenberg, J. I. (1982) Treatment of haemorrhagic gastritis with 15(R)-15-methyl prostaglandin E$_2$: report of a case. *Gastroenterology*, **82**, 558–560.

20 Widerlite, L., Trier, J. S., Blacklow, N. R. & Schreiber, D. S. (1975) Structure of the gastric mucosa in acute non-bacterial gastroenteritis. *Gastroenterology*, **68**, 425–430.

CHRONIC GASTRITIS

Definition and classification

Chronic gastritis can be defined as any diffuse chronic inflammatory process involving the mucosal lining of the stomach. This definition encompasses both specific and non-specific chronic gastritis (Table 4.2). Specific forms of chronic gastritis are associated with distinctive disease processes and include established infections, granulomatous inflammation, eosinophilic gastritis and Ménétrier's disease. These disorders are presented elsewhere and will not be discussed further here. Pernicious anaemia (PA), in which severe chronic gastritis leads to failure of intrinsic factor secretion and vitamin B$_{12}$ malabsorption, is also described elsewhere (see Chapter 9). Some aspects of this disease will be reviewed that have relevance to our understanding of the nature and management of non-specific chronic gastritis (NSCG). The conventional classification of NSCG is based on pathological observations of biopsy samples of the gastric mucosa, as described by Whitehead, Truelove and Gear.[59] This classification includes the *grade* of gastritis (superficial or atrophic), its *activity* (quiescent or acute or chronic inflammation), the *mucosal type* affected (pyloric, body, cardiac, junctional or intermediate), and the presence and type of *metaplasia* (intestinal or pseudopyloric). A number of additional terms describing subtypes

of NSCG are in wide use. These terms emphasize specific clinical (e.g., post-gastrectomy, alcoholic), aetiological (e.g., alkaline reflux, bile), or endoscopic (e.g., erosive) features. Since the majority of patients showing NSCG cannot be assigned to such categories, it seems more appropriate to retain the descriptive morphological scheme. A simplified form of this scheme is useful and appears practical when applied to biopsy studies of random population samples. The three major pathological patterns observed are superficial gastritis, atrophic gastritis and gastric atrophy.

Pathological features

Superficial gastritis

This lesion is characterized by inflammatory cell (lymphocytes, plasma cells) infiltration confined to the pit or foveolar regions of the mucosa (Figure 4.14). On occasions, polymorphonuclear leucocyte infiltration is also observed. Reactive epithelial cell changes, including cuboidal cells, mucus depletion, increased basophilia and mitotic figures, are apparent. The glandular portion of the mucosa is unaffected. Intestinal metaplasia is slight and infrequently observed.

Atrophic gastritis

Here, inflammatory cell infiltration similar in type to that seen in superficial gastritis encroaches into the glandular zone of the mucosa and is accompanied by variable loss of the specialized cells (parietal and chief cells) lining the glands. If only one or two groups of glands within a mucosal section have disappeared, it is classified as mild atrophy (Figure 4.15). Loss of most or all glands is classified as severe atrophy (Figure 4.16), and all appearances between these extremes are classed as moderate atrophy. Intestinal and pseudopyloric metaplasia are usual in atrophic gastritis.

Gastric atrophy

The mucosal width is strikingly reduced, inflammation of the lamina propria is absent, and the gastric glands and their specialized cells are

Table 4.2 Classification of chronic gastritis.

Specific	Non-specific
Chronic infections (tuberculosis, syphilis)	Superficial gastritis
Granulomatous inflammation (Crohn's disease, sarcoid)	Atrophic gastritis
Eosinophilic gastritis	Gastric atrophy
Ménétrier's disease	corpus-predominant (Type A)
	antral-predominant (Type B)
	Pangastritis

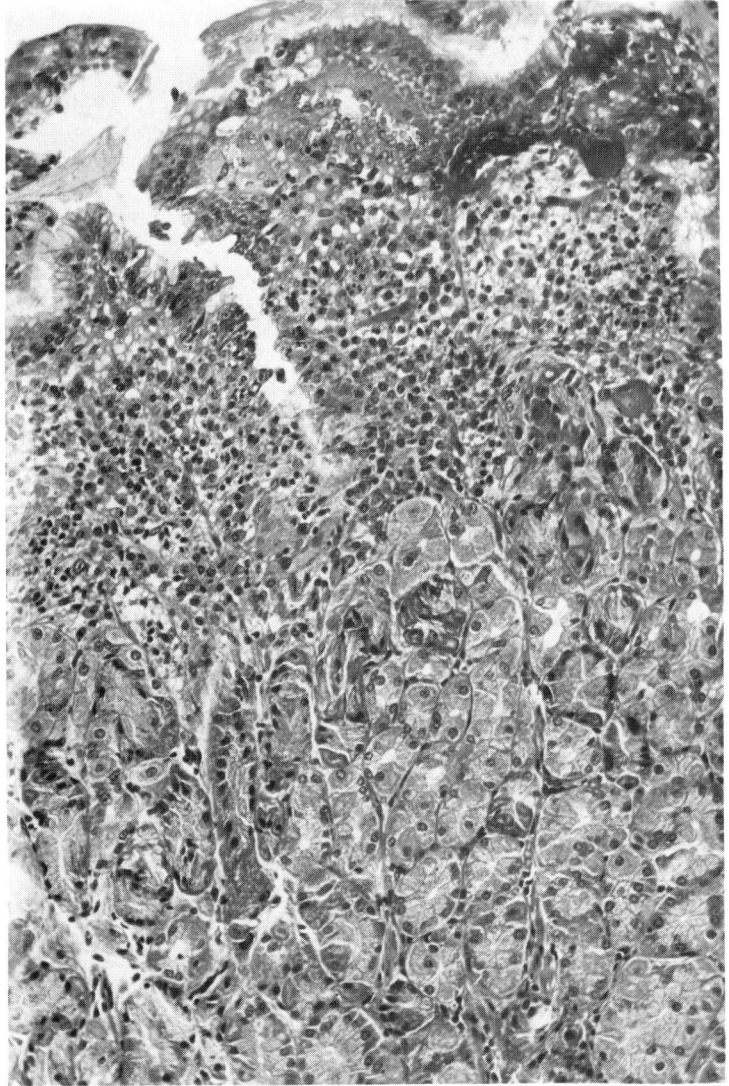

Fig. 4.14 Chronic superficial gastritis of corpus mucosa. There is acute and chronic inflammation confined to the foveolar region. Superficial mucosal haemorrhage and reactive epithelial cell changes are also present (× 200).

reduced or entirely absent (Figure 4.17). Metaplasia is extensive and always present.

Location and distribution

These three major patterns of NSCG may be variably distributed within the gastric mucosa. Thus, antral mucosa, corpus (body and fundus) gland mucosa, or both regions may be affected. When the changes are generalized, they are usually more severe in one region.[54] This variability in location and distribution of chronic gastritis was first emphasized by Strickland and Mackay.[48] In a selected series of patients with atrophic gastritis, we suggested that two major groups of patients could be identified: one, designated type A, with corpus-predominant atrophic gastritis, the other, designated Type B, with antral-predominant atrophic gastritis. To

these may be added a third type of distribution in which gastritis is generalized–pangastritis. The differing morphological patterns observed in this study were associated with important aetiological and clinical differences.

Prevalence of non-specific chronic gastritis

A number of recent biopsy studies in randomly selected population samples from different parts of Europe all indicate that NSCG is common (Table 4.3). These studies have also confirmed the increasing prevalence of gastritis in both corpus and antral regions with advancing age. It should be emphasized, however, that a majority of the subjects in these studies displayed the

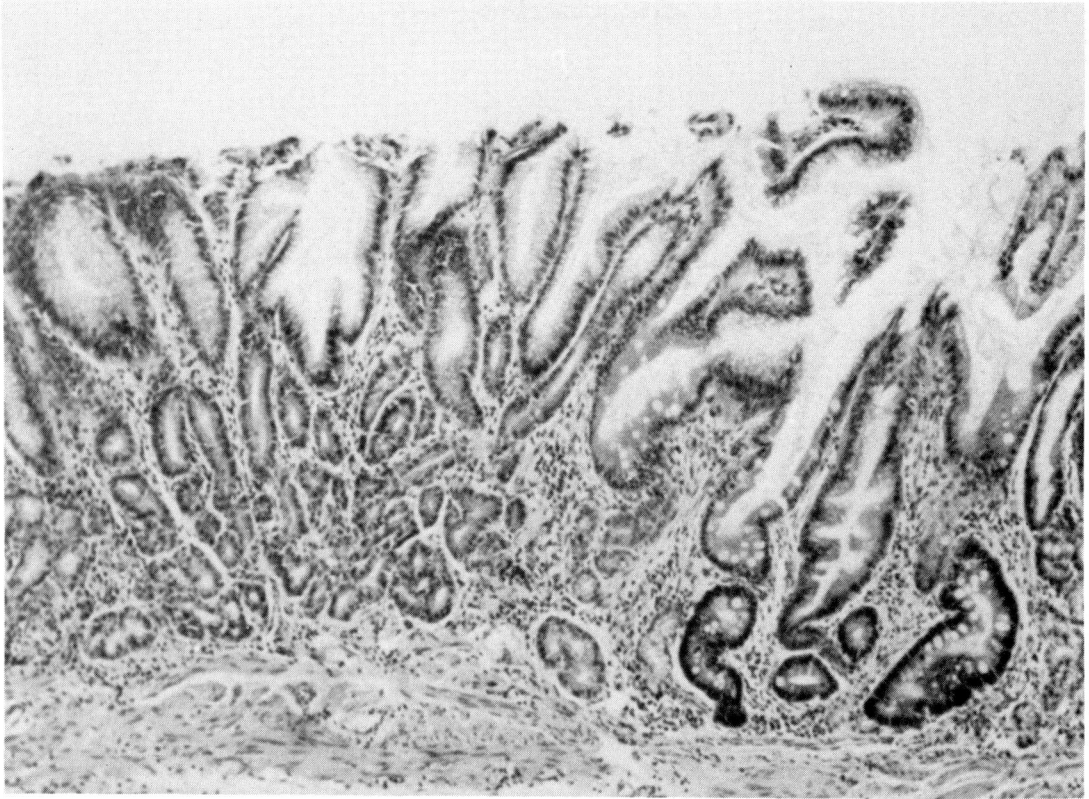

Fig. 4.15 Mild atrophic gastritis of corpus mucosa. There is chronic inflammation of foveolar and glandular regions, focal loss of normal glands and intestinal metaplasia (× 85).

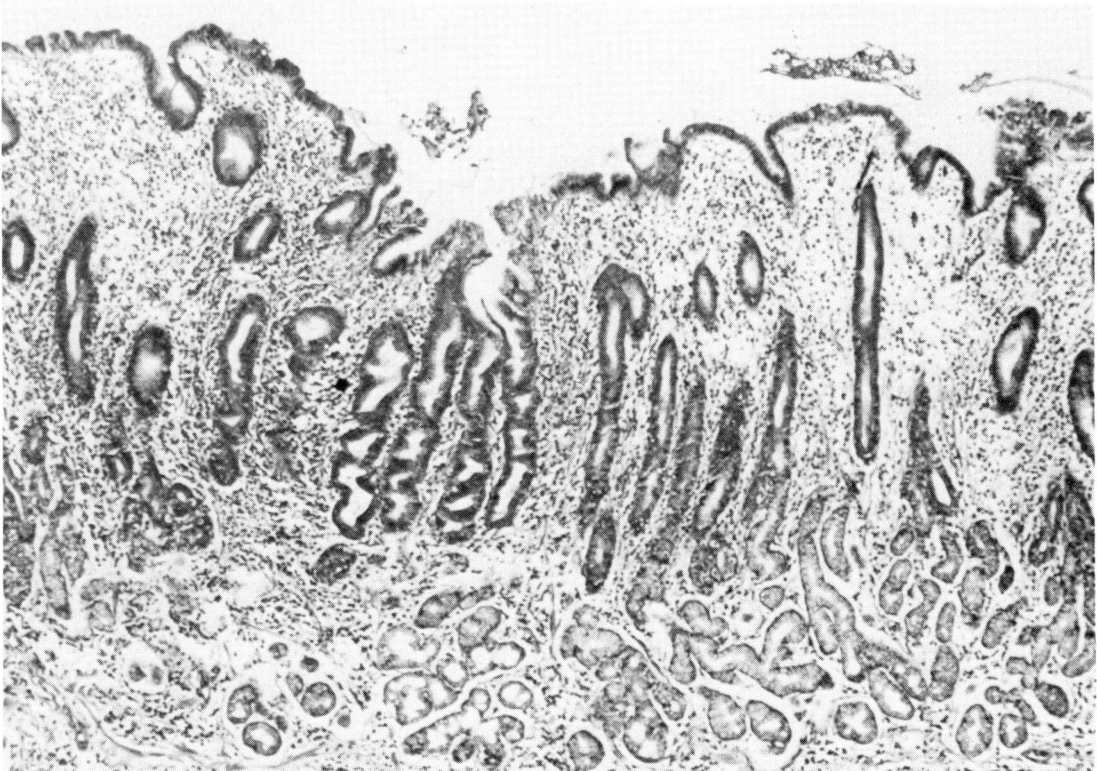

Fig. 4.16 Severe atrophic gastritis of corpus mucosa. Chronic inflammation and loss of normal glands is generalized. There is prominent pseudopyloric metaplasia (× 65).

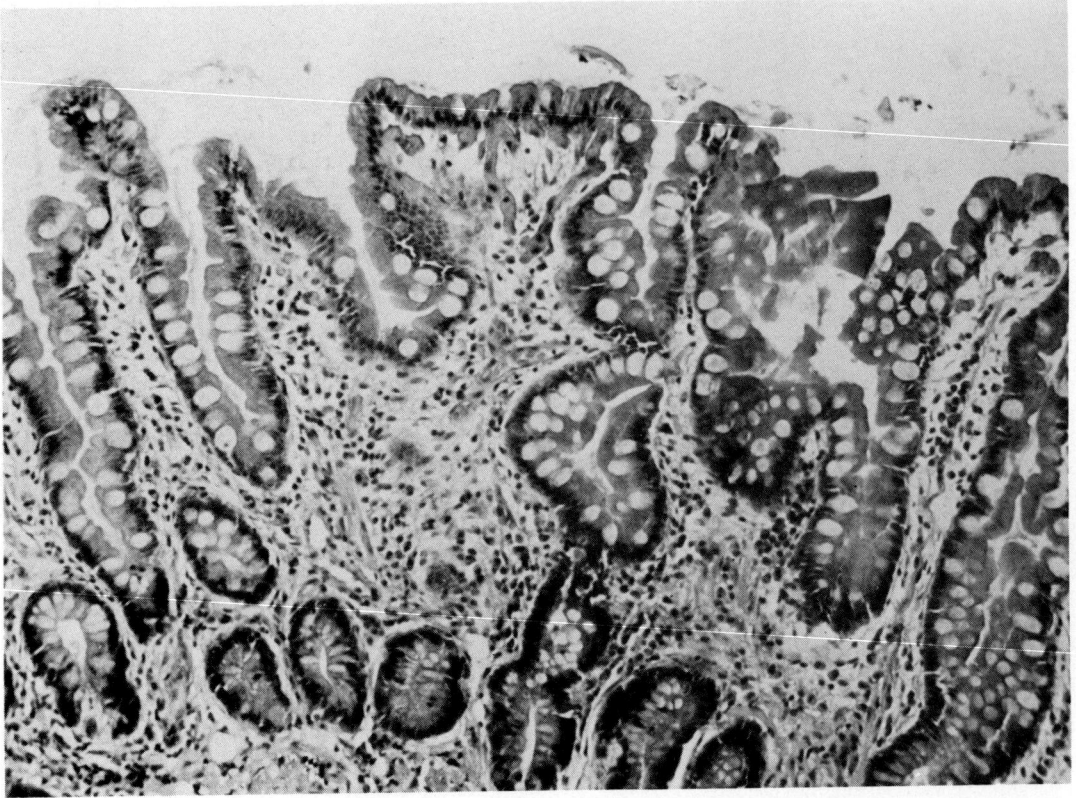

Fig. 4.17 Gastric atrophy of corpus mucosa. The mucosa is thinned and gastric glands have completely disappeared. Inflammation is not striking. There is generalized intestinal metaplasia (× 240).

Table 4.3 Prevalence of non-specific chronic gastritis in randomly selected populations.

Region	Number of subjects	Age range	Biopsy technique	Superficial gastritis (%)	Atrophic gastritis (%)
Pornainen, Finland[42]	142	16–65	Peroral	25 (C)	28 (C)
Kambja, Estonia[54]	155	16–69	Endoscopic	25 (C) 39 (A)	20 (C) 29 (A)
Genòa, Italy[4]	100	20–79	Endoscopic	26 (C + A)	22 (C + A)
Jaszbereny, Hungary[4]	100			36 (C + A)	37 (C + A)
Kingissepa, Estonia[55]	227	15–69	Endoscopic	25 (C) 30 (A)	37 (C) 34 (A)

C = corpus; A = antrum.

milder grades of gastritis, and severe atrophic gastritis was observed in less than 5%. Siurala, Varis and Kekki[40] have applied a stochastic mathematical model to cross-sectional data obtained from such defined populations in order to describe the progression of gastritis. The results suggest that on a population level chronic gastritis is a progressive disease and that superficial gastritis evolves into atrophic gastritis over many years. Recent application of this model by Villarko *et al.* suggests that antral and corpus gastritis behave differently.[55] Antral-predominant gastritis has an earlier onset and slower progression, whereas corpus-predominant gastritis, once established, progresses more rapidly. This analysis, if correct, would support the concept proposed by Strickland and Mackay[48] of the existence of fundamentally different disease subsets within the broad group of patients with NSCG.

Table 4.4 Aetiology of non-specific chronic gastritis.

Aetiological factor	Comments
Genetic	Established for severe Type A gastritis in pernicious anaemia relatives; possible for severe gastritis in gastric carcinoma relatives
Immunological Autoimmunity	Strong evidence for role in Type A gastritis, possible factor in minority of Type B gastritis patients
Immune deficiency	Likely factor in pangastritis of common variable immunodeficiency.
Allergic	Unproven but possible factor in chronic erosive gastritis
Ageing	Significant association with Type A and Type B gastritis. Nature unclear.
Luminal factors Exogenous Food, drug and thermal 'irritants'	Unproven, but possible
Infectious agents	Instances of 'epidemic hypochlorhydria' suggestive
Alcohol	High frequency of Type B or pangastritis in chronic alcoholics
Endogenous Components of duodenal secretion (? bile acids, ? lysolecithin)	Likely factor in post-gastrectomy gastritis. Probable factor in de novo Type B gastritis

Aetiology (Table 4.4)

GENETIC FACTORS

Biopsy studies of the gastric mucosa reveal an increased prevalence of severe atrophic gastritis in relatives of probands with pernicious anaemia (PA)[53] or gastric adenocarcinoma.[22] The evidence for these occurrences being due to a genetic rather than a common environmental factor is stronger amongst PA relatives. In particular, gastritis which mimics that seen in the probands, severe corpus gastritis with relative antral sparing, or Type A gastritis, is significantly more common in PA relatives than in control subjects. The nature of the inherited factor or factors and the mode of inheritance are not established. There is evidence that in PA families there may be an inherited susceptibility to gastric autoimmunity as defined by the presence of parietal cell antibodies.[51] This feature does not at present appear to be due to factors associated with the histocompatibility gene complex, since associations between established PA and a number of HLA-A, B and DR antigens do not extend to patients who have Type A atrophic gastritis but not PA.[60] Gastric autoimmunity is not involved in the occurrence of chronic gastritis in gastric carcinoma families and the putative genetic factor is completely unknown.

IMMUNOLOGICAL FACTORS

Two seemingly different immunological processes are associated with NSCG. These are gastric autoimmunity and primary immunodeficiency.

Gastric autoimmunity

Circulating autoantibodies to gastric parietal cells are detectable in some patients with NSCG. The actual prevalence of parietal-cell antibody in an unselected population with NSCG is uncertain, although it is clearly a minority and probably less than 20%. More certain is that this autoantibody is significantly correlated with corpus-predominant, Type A gastritis.[48] Intrinsic factor antibodies, so prevalent in pernicious anaemia, are rarely (in less than 2%) detected in NSCG. When present, they usually denote severe Type A gastritis. The role of parietal-cell and intrinsic-factor antibodies and of cellular immune reactions to gastric antigens in the actual causation of chronic gastritis remains conjectural. Experimental observations in animals injected repeatedly with semi-purified preparations of human parietal cell antibody,[50] intrinsic factor antibody,[23] or crude mucosal antigens[1] do support such a role, however. Recently, autoantibodies to gastrin-producing cells were described by Vandelli *et al.* in a small proportion of patients (8 of 106) with NSCG affecting the antral mucosa.[52] It is possible that such patients have an autoimmune variant of Type B gastritis.

Immunodeficiency

Approximately 40% of patients with the common variable form of primary immunodeficiency display NSCG.[20] Pan-hypogammaglobulinaemia and repeated bacterial infections are consistent features in this disorder. The gastric lesion is usually a severe pangastritis with equivalent involvement of both antral and corpus mucosa.[21] Plasma cells are conspicuously absent from the inflammatory infiltrate and circulating gastric autoantibodies are not detected. The pathogenesis of this uncommon form of chronic gastritis is not established. A report of circulating lymphocyte sensitization to gastric antigens in patients with common variable immunodeficiency[25] suggests that cellular immunological reactions may be important despite the absence of gastric autoantibodies.

Thus, there is evidence that immunological factors may participate in the causation of NSCG. It remains uncertain whether they are the sole cause of chronic mucosal injury, and an interaction between environmental and immunological factors seems more likely.

AGE

As already indicated, NSCG is more frequent in older population groups than in younger ones. Although this lesion is associated with advancing age, its relationship to the ageing process itself is uncertain, since the gastric mucosa can be normal in old age. Gastric autoimmune reactions also increase with advancing age,[47] but this mechanism could account for only a small proportion of the total incidence of chronic gastritis in older subjects. Other factors, such as prolonged exposure to luminal irritant factors, are likely to be involved.

LUMINAL FACTORS

A variety of exogenous and endogenous agents can cause chronic gastric mucosal injury by a number of mechanisms initiated within the lumen of the stomach.[10, 26] Exogenous agents so implicated include certain foods, hot beverages, nicotine, drugs, alcohol and infectious agents. Suggested mechanisms include direct and repeated mucosal injury (by drugs, alcohol, hot chillies, pickles and spices), IgE-mediated allergic reactions (to foodstuffs and drugs) and

mucosal invasion by microorganisms. With regard to the latter possibility, a recent report of 'epidemic hypochlorhydria' is of interest.[34] Although no organisms were isolated from these patients, the reversible nature of the 'chronic gastritis' is strongly suggestive of an infectious aetiology. The evidence that alcohol causes chronic gastritis is based solely on studies of the gastric mucosa in chronic alcoholic populations, where the incidence of NSCG may be as high as 80%. Similar though less well-studied associations of chronic gastritis are recorded in other populations, such as cigarette smokers or those ingesting hot beverages or foods for prolonged periods. The possibility of allergy as a cause of chronic gastritis is suggested by the work of Lambert *et al.* in which patients with chronic erosive (varioliform) gastritis displayed large numbers of IgE immunocytes in the gastric mucosal inflammatory infiltrate.[27]

The role of endogenous substances in the production of chronic gastric mucosal injury has been studied more systematically. The principal factor so far implicated is some component (or components) of duodenal secretions. Experiments in dogs have suggested that prolonged contact of the gastric mucosa with bile alone or bile and pancreatic juice in the presence of continued acid peptic secretion results in chronic gastritis.[28] The substance or substances in such secretions that are injurious to the mucosa have not been identified, but both bile salts and lysolecithin have been implicated. It is probable that, in man, duodenogastric reflux occurring either in the intact stomach or following disruption of the normal pyloroduodenal barrier by gastric surgery may be responsible for chronic gastritis through prolonged contact with duodenal secretions.

Diagnosis (Table 4.5)

It is evident from histopathological studies of the gastric mucosa in random population samples that NSCG, particularly in its less severe forms, is entirely compatible with normal health. However, the more severe grades of chronic gastritis (atrophic gastritis and gastric atrophy) and, probably, early-onset disease are associated with morbidity.

CLINICAL DIAGNOSIS

There is no single clinical feature predictive of NSCG. Many patients, even those with advanced chronic gastritis, are asymptomatic. On the other hand, symptoms may coexist with

Table 4.5 Diagnosis of non-specific chronic gastritis.

Method	Comments
Clinical	Poor correlation between symptoms and mucosal pathology. Some clinical features helpful in subtypes of gastritis
Laboratory	
acid secretion	Lacks discriminative value in superficial, mild atrophic gastritis
gastric autoantibodies	Parietal cell antibody identifies a subset with the likelihood of Type A atrophic gastritis
serum gastrin	Marked elevation in Type A atrophic gastritis
serum pepsinogens (PG-I and PG-II)	Potential non-invasive test for diagnosis of all forms of chronic gastritis
Radiology	Non-diagnostic in most patients with chronic gastritis. Chronic erosive gastritis has characteristic features
Endoscopy	Visual appearances are non-diagnostic except chronic erosive gastritis
Biopsy	Stepwise endoscopic biopsies provide the only definitive method for identification of chronic gastritis

histopathological evidence of chronic mucosal damage. Recent observations in post-gastrectomy patients serve to illustrate this enigma.[30] Upper gastrointestinal symptoms were commonly reproduced by instilling autologous intestinal secretions into the gastric pouch. The results of this provocative test support the hypothesis that post-gastrectomy symptoms are often due to duodenogastric reflux. Chronic gastritis thus accompanies, but is not the cause of, abdominal symptoms.

In patients with chronic erosive gastritis, relapsing upper gastrointestinal symptoms appear to be a consistent feature, and recent weight loss may lead one to suspect gastric malignancy.[16] There are other clinical associations with chronic gastritis, including a family history of pernicious anaemia, insulin-dependent diabetes mellitus, thyroid disease, hypoparathyroidism, hypoadrenalism, or vitiligo.[46]

Unexplained chronic iron deficiency may also lead one to suspect chronic gastritis.[6] The presence of chronic gastritis is frequent in patients with benign peptic ulcer, gastric polyps or carcinoma, or a history of previous gastric surgery.

LABORATORY INVESTIGATIONS

Acid secretion
There is a progressive decrease in maximum acid output with increasingly severe gastritis of the corpus mucosa. However, the discriminant value of maximum acid output in less severe forms, such as superficial gastritis, is poor, and there is also marked variability in acid secretion rates in patients with antral-predominant Type B gastritis, probably depending on the extent and degree of associated involvement of the corpus mucosa.

Gastric autoantibodies
The presence of circulating parietal-cell antibodies is generally diagnostic for chronic gastritis,[63] although some exceptions have been noted. There is also a correlation between the presence of parietal-cell antibodies and corpus-predominant, Type A, gastritis.[48] However, the severity of gastritis cannot be predicted, and as indicated earlier, the majority of unselected subjects with NSCG are antibody-negative. In other words, the presence of parietal-cell antibodies is predictive of only a small subset of the total population with chronic gastritis.

Serum gastrin
Fasting serum gastrin levels are greatly elevated in 75–80% of patients with pernicious anaemia.[14] This is because of the distribution of the gastritis: the antral mucosa is relatively spared in a majority of patients, leading to continued gastrin release which is uninhibited because of gastric achlorhydria. Hyper-gastrinaemia is also observed in a proportion of patients with NSCG. Most patients with hypergastrinaemia show a corpus-predominant, Type

A, distribution of atrophic gastritis, with circulating parietal-cell antibodies.[48] In antral-predominant, Type B, gastritis and severe pangastritis, gastrin levels are usually normal even if there is total achlorhydria.[49] Normogastrinaemia and achlorhydria are also seen in the severe gastritis that accompanies common variable immunodeficiency.[21] Absence of gastrin elevation in these circumstances is due to destruction of G-cells by severe antral gastritis. This mechanism probably also accounts for the small proportion of patients with pernicious anaemia or Type A gastritis who are normogastrinaemic. Thus, as with parietal cell antibodies, the discriminant value of gastrin levels in the diagnosis of NSCG is poor.

Serum pepsinogens
Two immunochemically distinct groups of pepsinogens have been identified in the gastric mucosa, and reproducible radioimmunoassays have been described for their measurement in human serum.[37] Group I pepsinogens (PG-I) are derived from chief cells in the corpus mucosa, whilst group II pepsinogens (PG-II) are present in chief and mucus neck cells in the corpus mucosa, in pyloric glands in the antral mucosa and in Brunner's glands of the duodenal mucosa. A recent study of first-degree relatives of patients with pernicious anaemia who had all undergone endoscopic biopsies suggests that serum measurements of PG-I and PG-II are useful in the diagnosis of NSCG and in the assessment of its severity.[38] Thus, PG-I and PG-II levels are increased in superficial gastritis, and the relative rise in PG-II exceeds that in PG-I. In mild to moderate atrophic gastritis PG-I levels are unaltered but PG-II is increased, and in severe atrophic gastritis PG-I is markedly decreased and PG-II is normal. Discriminant function analysis of these data revealed that the PG-I/PG-II ratio in combination with the absolute level of PG-I correctly assigned 70% of the subjects to the four categories: normal, superficial gastritis, mild to moderate atrophic gastritis and severe atrophic gastritis. This was a significant improvement over that achieved by acid-secretory tests in these subjects.

These data suggest that serum PG-I and PG-II measurements may provide a non-invasive test for the diagnosis of NSCG in most patients. However, the above findings relate only to observations of the corpus gland mucosa, and studies of their use in unselected population groups are needed to validate these initial observations.

The appearances of the gastric mucosa as displayed by double-contrast upper GI X-rays or upper endoscopy have very little place in the diagnosis of NSCG. Rugal fold size on X-ray and fold appearance or mucosal colour change seen on endoscopy are too imprecise to diagnose chronic gastritis and should not be substituted for mucosal biopsy. In the relatively uncommon syndrome of chronic erosive gastritis, however, these techniques may be diagnostic:[12] antral or generalized multiple small (3–10 mm) mucosal nodules with central superficial ulcerations are distributed along the rugal folds.

MUCOSAL BIOPSY

For many years, blind biopsy of the gastric mucosa with one of several peroral suction biopsy tubes was the definitive technique for the diagnosis of chronic gastritis. Much information about the nature and natural history of chronic gastritis was obtained by this method.[62] Most peroral biopsy samples, however, are from the corpus mucosa, and studies using this technique gave little or no information about the state of the antral mucosa. This technique has now largely been superseded by endoscopic biopsy of the gastric mucosa. This approach allows multiple target biopsies from different areas of the stomach, providing a more accurate assessment of the degree and extent of the gastritic process.[57] One disadvantage of endoscopic biopsy relates to the size of the mucosal samples, which are smaller than those obtained with a suction biopsy instrument, and a proportion (10–20%) of them may be uninterpretable because of shallowness or distortion. Endoscopic biopsies for assessment of chronic gastritis should involve stepwise sampling of both curvatures or walls of the antrum, body, and fundus. It is essential to document accurately the sites in the stomach where biopsies are obtained in order that the pathologist can give a rational histological diagnosis.

Sequelae (Table 4.6)

Current knowledge of the natural history of NSCG is entirely based on longitudinal studies of selected rather than random groups with this disorder. Whether predictions based on epidemiological mathematical models in randomly selected populations with chronic gastritis provide an accurate assessment of the course of this disorder remains to be seen. It seems clear,

Table 4.6 Course and natural history of non-specific chronic gastritis.

Category	Course	Comment
Gastritis in asymptomatic random populations	Uncertain	Stochastic models predict progression. Regression possible in some
Superficial gastritis in selected populations	Clinically silent progression to atrophic gastritis	More prospective studies needed
Atrophic gastritis in selected populations	Significant sequelae, which appear to vary according to pattern of gastritis	Additional studies required
Type A	Vitamin B_{12} malabsorption	2% incidence per year of follow-up
	Chronic iron deficiency	20% incidence over eight-year follow-up
Type B	Recurrent upper GI symptoms	Cause and effect relationship unproved
	Predisposition to acute gastric mucosal injury	Drug-related, or spontaneous
	Gastric polyps, adenocarcinoma	10% with 15-year follow-up
Pangastritis	Vitamin B_{12} malabsorption	Established in common variable immunodeficiency
	Gastric adenocarcinoma	Associated with common variable immunodeficiency

however, that NSCG is an extremely heterogeneous disorder. Thus, the idea that chronic gastritis is a progressive disease is not universally accepted. Certain forms of chronic gastritis may even be reversible.[35] Nevertheless, there are subsets of patients with NSCG in whom significant sequelae may develop with long-term follow-up. Those groups who are likely to develop sequelae include those with moderate or severe atrophic gastritis and corpus-predominant (Type A), antral-predominant (Type B), pangastritis.

Some patients with atrophic gastritis and initially normal vitamin B_{12} absorption will progress to latent or overt pernicious anaemia with frank vitamin B_{12} malabsorption (see Chapter 9). Two studies have indicated that this course is characteristic of patients with corpus-predominant, Type A, gastritis frequently associated with parietal cell autoantibodies.[24, 48] Fifteen to twenty per cent of the patients in these two studies developed vitamin B_{12} malabsorption over eight to ten years of follow-up. The mechanism leading to vitamin B_{12} malabsorption is uncertain but probably involves progression of gastritis and intrinsic factor secretory failure and perhaps an in vivo effect of intrinsic-factor antibodies. Patients with antral-predominant, Type B, atrophic gastritis do not appear to display progression to vitamin B_{12} malabsorption with any frequency.[48] In patients with common variable immuno-deficiency and pangastritis there is, however, an increased risk of developing pernicious anaemia.

The presence of atrophic gastritis also appears to be a risk factor for the development of iron deficiency.[48] Occult gastrointestinal bleeding, hypochlorhydria with malabsorption of food iron and enhanced iron loss through increased gastric epithelial cell turnover all contribute to the development of iron deficiency in this setting. Overt upper gastrointestinal haemorrhage is sometimes observed in patients with atrophic gastritis, either spontaneously or in relation to intake of ulcerogenic drugs or alcohol. Atrophic mucosa has an enhanced susceptibility to acute damage induced by such agents.[5, 9]

There is substantial indirect evidence linking atrophic gastritis to the occurrence of gastric adenocarcinoma. Long-term follow-up studies of patients with atrophic gastritis indicate a highly significant increased incidence (approximately 10%) of gastric cancer.[4, 41, 56] The actual risk, however, is probably lower than these estimates, since the follow-up studies so far reported have been on selected rather than random populations. There appear to be differences in the relative risk of gastric malignancy amongst the different subtypes of atrophic gastritis. In our own series, all the gastric cancers seen in follow-up occurred in patients with antral-predominant, Type B, gastritis. No instances of gastric carcinoma were observed in Type A gastritis. Irvine, Cullen and Mawhinney have made similar observations in their series of patients with Type A gastritis followed for up to ten years.[24] However, the enhanced risk of gastric cancer in established pernicious anaemia[11] would suggest that with prolonged follow-up such differences may disappear. Patients with common variable immuno-deficiency reportedly have a high incidence of gastric carcinoma,[20] and a relationship to the pangastritis occurring in this disorder seems likely.

Post-gastrectomy subjects, who display a high incidence of atrophic gastritis in the residual stomach, are also reported to have an increased incidence of carcinoma in the gastric stump.[44] The risk appears to begin 10 to 15 years after surgery and rises thereafter.

Gastric polyps also develop with increased frequency in patients with atrophic gastritis.[42] These include both hyperplastic (inflammatory) and, less commonly, true neoplastic (adenomatous) polypoid lesions.

Neoplastic transformation of the gastric mucosa in atrophic gastritis appears to involve a process of de-differentiation from intestinal metaplasia to epithelial dysplasia and then to early gastric adenocarcinoma.[58] The clinical implications of this process are currently unclear. This particularly applies to the problem of gastric epithelial dysplasia. Recognition of this change is currently hampered by the lack of a standard nomenclature and difficulties in distinguishing dysplasia from reactive inflammatory change. In addition, reports of spontaneous regression of even severe dysplasia[33] argue for a conservative approach if dysplasia is the sole indication of possible gastric malignancy.[31] The initiating factors in the process of neoplastic transformation are poorly understood. However, enhanced gastric epithelial cell proliferation often accompanies NSCG.[61] In addition, the milieu of the stomach in patients with atrophic gastritis favours bacterial overgrowth and intragastric N-nitrosation from bacterial reduction of nitrate-containing food.[36]

The association between NSCG and benign peptic ulcer is almost universal, irrespective of the ulcer site. The distribution of gastritis is antral-predominant, Type B. It is mild and superficial in duodenal ulcer and more extensive and severe (atrophic) in gastric ulcer. Certain studies in patients with gastric ulcer suggest that the gastritis precedes ulceration,[15] and may be related to pyloric dysfunction and duodeno-gastric reflux.[8] Although attractive, this sequence is not proven, and the actual relationship between NSCG and peptic ulceration remains uncertain.

Treatment

Since there is no agent known to be capable of reversing or improving the histopathological changes of NSCG, management is largely symptomatic; it includes careful follow-up and early detection of sequelae. One problem is that increasing numbers of patients with NSCG are being identified as a result of wider use of endoscopy.

A reasonable approach, based on the data presented in preceding sections, involves (a) clear definition of the distribution of gastritis, (b) evaluation of the degree of gastritis and (c) assessment of possible aetiology. With this information, it is suggested that patients with severe gastritis (moderate to severe atrophic gastritis) deserve careful follow-up. The nature of the follow-up should be based on the type of gastritis.

'SYMPTOMATIC' NON-SPECIFIC GASTRITIS

In practice, such patients are treated in a similar fashion to those with established peptic ulcer disease, including elimination of potential gastric irritants and the use of antacids. There is no firm scientific basis yet for administration of antisecretory drugs, surface-active agents such as sucralfate or cytoprotective drugs such as prostaglandin analogues.

Uncontrolled studies in small series of patients with chronic erosive gastritis have claimed therapeutic effects with cimetidine, disodium cromoglycate[2] and even prednisolone.[13]

A number of therapeutic measures have been proposed in reflux gastritis following gastric surgery. Cholestyramine, aluminium hydroxide or both have been recommended in this setting, with the aim of binding bile salts; however, a controlled trial did not confirm efficacy of cholestyramine.[29] Metoclopramide has been helpful in some patients with reflux gastritis, but the observations were uncontrolled.[7] Surgical therapy aimed at diverting duodenal content away from the stomach by Roux-en-Y reconstruction has also achieved variable success.[19] A recent study has indicated symptomatic improvement from administration of urso-deoxycholic acid;[45] presumably this approach alters the quantity or quality of endogenous bile salts reaching the gastric mucosa.

In my experience, symptomatic patients with isolated NSCG usually show a suboptimal or non-sustained response to most therapeutic approaches.

NUTRIENT DEFICIENCIES

Patients with atrophic gastritis should be intermittently evaluated for iron deficiency, and replacement therapy with iron supplements should be initiated if necessary. Tests of vitamin B_{12} absorption are indicated in patients with Type A atrophic gastritis perhaps on an annual or biannual basis. If vitamin B_{12} malabsorption is demonstrated, vitamin B_{12} replacement therapy should be given indefinitely.

SURVEILLANCE FOR GASTRIC CANCER

There is currently insufficient data to allow a firm statement on specific follow-up directed towards detection of early gastric cancer in patients with atrophic gastritis. One suggested approach is that of annual endoscopy with cytology and multiple mucosal biopsies of all major regions of the stomach. The use of radiographic and endoscopic examinations in asymptomatic subjects residing in high gastric cancer prevalence areas, such as Japan, has been extremely successful in the detection of early gastric cancer and has led to impressive five- and ten-year survival figures. Recent studies in Western countries have shown that early gastric cancer exists there also,[17] but the proportion of patients diagnosed early remains very low. Since the overall prevalence of gastric cancer is low and decreasing in these regions, mass screening is inappropriate. However, patients with atrophic gastritis would appear to represent the high-risk subset of Western populations who could benefit from such surveillance methods. Cost–benefit and risk–benefit ratios of such an approach, however, remain uncertain. What are needed most in screening for gastric cancer are reliable gastric juice or serum markers. Many such markers have been described, including levels of gastric juice lactate dehydrogenase and β-glucuronidase[39] and fetal sialoglycoprotein antigen[18] and, in serum, group I pepsinogen.[32] However, all these markers are reported in patients with atrophic gastritis in the absence of cancer and their use in screening remains to be established.

REFERENCES

1 Andrada, J. A., Rose, N. R. & Andrada, E. C. (1969) Experimental autoimmune gastritis in the rhesus monkey. *Clinical Experimental Immunology*, **4**, 293–310.

2 Andre, C., Mouliner, B., Lambert, R. & Bugnon, B. (1976) Gastritis varioliforms, allergy and disodium cromoglycate. *Lancet*, **i**, 964–965.

3 Cheli, R., Santi, L., Ciancamerla, G. & Canciani, G. (1973) A clinical and statistical follow-up study of atrophic gastritis. *Digestive Diseases*, **18**, 1061–1066.

4 Cheli, R., Simon, L., Aste, H. et al. (1980) Atrophic gastritis and intestinal metaplasia in asymptomatic Hungarian and Italian populations. *Endoscopy*, **12**, 105–108.

5 Chowdhury, A. R., Malmud, L. S. & Dinoso, V. P., Jr. (1977) Gastrointestinal plasma protein loss during ethanol ingestion. *Gastroenterology*, **72**, 37–40.

6 Coghill, N. F. (1960) The significance of gastritis. *Postgraduate Medical Journal*, **36**, 733–742.

7 Davidson, E. D. & Hersh, T. (1975) Bile reflux gastritis. *American Journal of Surgery*, **130**, 514–518.

8 Delaney, J. P., Cheng, J. W. B., Butler, B. A. & Ritchie, W. P. (1970) Gastric ulcer and regurgitation gastritis. *Gut*, **11**, 715–719.

9 Dinoso, V. P. Jr, Meshkinpour, H. & Lorber, H. (1973) Gastric mucosal morphology and faecal blood loss during ethanol ingestion. *Gut*, **14**, 289–292.

10 Edwards, F. C. & Coghill, N. F. (1966) Aetiological factors in chronic atrophic gastritis. *British Medical Journal*, **ii**, 1409–1415.

11 Elsborg, L. & Mosbech, J. (1979) Pernicious anaemia as a risk factor in gastric cancer. *Acta Medica Scandinavica*, **206**, 215–318.

12 Elta, G. H., Fawaz, K. A., Dayal, Y. et al. (1983) Chronic erosive gastritis – a recently recognized disorder. *Digestive Disease and Sciences*, **28**, 7–12.

13 Farthing, M. J. G., Fairclough, P. D., Hegarty, J. E. et al. (1981) Treatment of chronic erosive gastritis with prenisolone. *Gut*, **22**, 759–762.

14 Ganguli, P. C., Cullen, D. R. & Irvine, W. J. (1971) Radioimmunoassay of plasma-gastrin in pernicious anaemia achlorhydria without pernicious anaemia, hypochlorhydria, and in controls. *Lancet*, **i**, 155–158.

15 Gear, M. W. L., Truelove, S. C. & Whitehead, R. (1971) Gastric ulcer and gastritis. *Gut*, **12**, 639–645.

16 Green, P. G., Fevre, D. I., Bassett, P. H. et al. (1977) Chronic erosive (verrucous) gastritis. *Endoscopy*, **9**, 74–78.

17 Green, P. H. R., O'Toole, K. M., Weinberg, L. M. & Goldfarb, J. P. (1981) Early gastric cancer. *Gastroenterology*, **81**, 247–256.

18 Hakkinen, I. P. T. (1974) A population screening for fetal sulfoglycoprotein antigen in gastric juice. *Cancer Research*, **34**, 3069–3072.

19 Halpern, N. B., Hirschowitz, B. L. & Moody, F. G. (1973) Failure to achieve success with corrective gastric surgery. *American Journal of Surgery*, **124**, 108–115.

20 Hermans, P. E., Diaz-Buxo, J. A. & Stobo, J. D. (1976) Idiopathic late-onset immunoglobulin deficiency: clinical observations in 50 patients. *American Journal of Medicine*, **61**, 221–237.

21 Hughes, W. S., Brooks, F. P. & Conn, H. O. (1972) Serum gastrin levels in primary hypogammaglobulinemia and pernicious anemia – studies in adults. *Annals of Internal Medicine*, **77**, 746, 750.

22 Ihamaki, T., Varis, K. & Siurala, M. (1979) Morphological, functional and immunological state of the gastric mucosa in gastric carcinoma families. *Scandinavian Journal of Gastroenterology*, **14**, 801–812.

23 Inada, M. & Jerzy Glass, G. B. (1975) Effect of prolonged administration of homologous and heterologous intrinsic factor antibodies on the parietal and peptic cell masses and the secretory function of the rat gastric mucosa. *Gastroenterology*, **69**, 396–408.

24 Irvine, W. J., Cullen, D. R. & Mawhinney, H. (1974) Natural history of autoimmune achlorhydric atrophic gastritis: a 1–15-year follow-up study. *Lancet*, **ii**, 482–485.

25 James, D., Asherson, G., Chanarin, I. et al. (1974) Cell-mediated immunity to intrinsic factor in autoimmune disorders. *British Medical Journal*, **iv**, 494–496.

26 Jerzy Glass, G. B. & Pitchumoni, C. S. (1975) Atrophic gastritis – structural and ultrastructural alterations, exfoliative cytology and enzyme cytochemistry and histochemistry, proliferation kinetics, immunological derangements and other causes, and clinical associations and sequelae. *Human Pathology*, **6**, 129–150.

27 Lambert, R., Andre, C., Moulinier, B. & Bugnon, B. (1978) Diffuse varioliform gastritis. *Digestion*, **17**, 159–167.

28 Lawson, H. H. (1964) Effect of duodenal content on the gastric mucosa under experimental conditions. *Lancet*, **i**, 469–472.

29 Meshkinpour, H., Elashoff, J., Steward, H. & Sturdevant, R. A. L. (1977) Effect of cholestyramine on the symptoms of reflux gastritis – a double-blind, crossover study. *Gastroenterology*, **73**, 441–443.

30 Meshkinpour, H., Marks, J. W., Schoenfield, L. J. *et al.* (1980) Reflux gastritis syndrome: Mechanism of symptoms. *Gastroenterology*, **79**, 1283–1287.

31 Morson, B. C., Sobin, L. H., Grundmann, E. *et al.* (1980) Precancerous conditions and epithelial dysplasia in the stomach. *Journal of Clinical Pathology*, **33**, 711–721.

32 Nomura, A. M. Y., Stemmermann, G. N. & Samloff, M. (1980) Serum pepsinogen I as a predictor of stomach cancer. *Annals of Internal Medicine*, **93**, 537–540.

33 Oehlert, W., Keller, P., Henke, M. & Strauch, M. (1979) Gastric mucosal dysplasia: What is its clinical significance? *Frontiers of Gastrointestinal Research*, **4**, 173–182.

34 Ramsey, E. J., Carey, K. V., Peterson, W. L. *et al.* (1979) Epidemic gastritis with hypochlorhydria. *Gastroenterology*, **76**, 1449–1457.

35 Rosch, W., Demling, L. & Elster, K. (1979) Is chronic gastritis a reversible process? Follow-up study of gastritis by stepwise biopsy. *Acta Hepatogastroenterologica*, **22**, 252–255.

36 Ruddell, W. S., Bone, E. S., Hill, M. J. *et al.* (1976) Gastric-juice nitrite: a risk factor for cancer in the hypochlorhydric stomach? *Lancet*, **ii**, 1037–1039.

37 Samloff, I. M. (1982) Pepsinogens I and II: purification from gastric mucosa and radioimmunoassay in serum. *Gastroenterology*, **82**, 26–33.

38 Samloff, I. M., Varis, K., Ihamaki, T. *et al.* (1982) Relationships among serum pepsinogen I, serum pepsinogen II, and gastric mucosal histology. *Gastroenterology*, **83**, 204–209.

39 Simon, L. & Figus, I. A. (1972) Diagnostic value of determination of lactate dehydrogenase and β-glucuronidase activity of gastric juice. *Digestion*, **7**, 174–182.

40 Siurala, M., Varis, K. & Kekki, M. (1980) New aspects on epidemiology, genetics, and dynamics of chronic gastritis. *Frontiers of Gastroenterology Research*, **6**, 148–166.

41 Siurala, M., Varis, K. & Wiljasalo, M. (1966) Studies of patients with atrophic gastritis: a 10–15-year follow-up. *Scandinavian Journal of Gastroenterology*, **1**, 40–48.

42 Siurala, M., Lehtola, S. M. & Ihamaki, T. (1974) Atrophic gastritis and its sequelae. *Scandinavian Journal of Gastroenterology*, **9**, 441–446.

43 Siurala, M., Isokoski, M., Varis, K. & Kekki, M. (1968) Prevalence of gastritis in a rural population: bioptic study of subjects selected at random. *Scandinavian Journal of Gastroenterology*, **3**, 211–223.

44 Stalsberg, H. & Taksdal, S. (1971) Stomach cancer following gastric surgery for benign conditions. *Lancet*, **ii**, 1175–1177.

45 Stefaniwsky, A. B., Tint, G. S., Speck, J. & Salen, G. (1982) Ursodeoxycholic acid (UDCA) reduces pain, nausea and vomiting in patients with bile acid reflux gastritis. *Gastroenterology*, **82** (abstract), 1188.

46 Strickland, R. G. (1975) Gastritis. In *Frontiers of Gastrointestinal Research* (Ed.) Van der Reis, L. pp. 12–48. Basel: Karger.

47 Strickland, R. G. & Hooper, B. (1972) The parietal cell heteroantibody in human sera: prevalence in a normal population and relationship to parietal cell autoantibody. *Pathology*, **4**, 259–263.

48 Strickland, R. G. & Mackay, I. R. (1973) A reappraisal of the nature and significance of chronic atrophic gastritis. *Digestive Diseases*, **18**, 426–440.

49 Strickland, R. G., Bhathal, P. S., Korman, M. G. & Hansky, J. (1971) Serum gastrin and the antral mucosa in atrophic gastritis. *British Medical Journal*, **iv**, 451–453.

50 Tanaka, N. & Jerzy Glass, G. B. (1970) Effect of prolonged administration of parietal cell antibodies from patients with atrophic gastritis and pernicious anemia on the parietal cell mass and hydrochloric acid output in rats. *Gastroenterology*, **58**, 482–494.

51 te Velde, K., Abels, J., Anders, G. J. P. A. *et al.* (1964) A family study of pernicious anemia by an immunologic method. *Journal of Laboratory and Clinical Medicine*, **64**, 177–187.

52 Vandelli, C., Bottazzo, G. F., Doniach, D. & Franceschi, F. (1979) Autoantibodies to gastrin-producing cells in antral (type B) chronic gastritis. *New England Journal of Medicine*, **300**, 1406–1410.

53 Varis, K., Ihamaki, T., Harkonen, M. *et al.* (1979) Gastric morphology, function, and immunology in first-degree relatives of probands with pernicious anemia and controls. *Scandinavian Journal of Gastroenterology*, **14**, 129–139.

54 Villako, K., Tamm, A., Savisaar, E. & Ruttas, M. (1976) Prevalence of antral and fundic gastritis in a randomly selected group of an Estonian rural population. *Scandinavian Journal of Gastroenterology*, **11**, 817–822.

55 Villako, K., Kekki, M., Tamm, A. *et al.* (1982) Epidemiology and dynamics of gastritis in a representative sample of an Estonian urban population. *Scandinavian Journal of Gastroenterology*, **17**, 601–607.

56 Walker, I. R., Strickland, R. G., Ungar, B. & Mackay, I. R. (1971) Simple atrophic gastritis and gastric carcinoma. *Gut*, **12**, 906–911.

57 Weinstein, W. M. (1981) The diagnosis and classification of gastritis and duodenitis. *Journal of Clinical Gastroenterology*, **3** (supplement 2), 7–16.

58 Whitehead, R. (1979) Mucosal biopsy of the gastrointestinal tract. In *Major Problems in Pathology*, volume 3, (Ed.) Bennington, J. L. pp. 36–50. Philadelphia: W. B. Saunders.

59 Whitehead, R., Truelove, S. C. & Gear, M. W. L. (1972) The histological diagnosis of chronic gastritis in fibreoptic gastroscope biopsy specimens. *Journal of Clinical Pathology*, **25**, 1–11.

60 Whittingham, S., Youngchaiyud, U., Mackay, I. R. *et al.* (1975) Thyrogastric autoimmune disease: Studies on the cell-mediated immune system and histocompatibility antigens. *Clinical Exploratory Immunology*, **19**, 289–299.

61 Winawer, S. J. & Lipkin, M. (1969) Cell proliferation kinetics in the gastrointestinal tract of man. IV. Cell renewal in the intestinalized gastric mucosa. *Journal of National Cancer Institute*, **42**, 9–17.

62 Wood, I. J. & Taft, L. I. (1958) *Diffuse Lesions of the Stomach*. London: Arnold.

63 Wright, R., Whitehead, R., Wangel, A. G. *et al.* (1966) Autoantibodies and microscopic appearance of gastric mucosa. *Lancet*, **i**, 618–621.

DUODENITIS

The clinical importance of duodenal inflammation in the absence of chronic ulceration remains controversial. The most important advances relate to the development of fibre-optic endoscopy. This allows direct visualization of the duodenal mucosa with target biopsies of suspicious areas and repeat examinations.[21, 32, 41]

Aetiology

The exposure of the proximal duodenum to the potentially damaging effects of gastric acid produces pathological changes closely resembling those found in the stomach or distal oesophagus. The most notable change is peptic ulceration, which usually but not invariably results in dyspepsia. In experimental animals both duodenitis and duodenal ulceration can be produced by pantothenic acid deficiency[20] and gastric secretagogues.[24]

Duodenal inflammation occurs in specific conditions such as tuberculosis, Crohn's disease, septicaemia, giardiasis and ankylostomiasis.[7, 13, 33] It has been associated with duodenal diverticulosis, fistula, Brunneroma, gastritis, liver disease, biliary and pancreatic disease and chronic renal failure.[16, 32, 34]

Peptic duodenitis is defined as an inflammatory condition of the proximal duodenum, usually with maximum involvement of the bulb, showing certain histopathological changes and often but not invariably associated with dyspeptic symptoms occurring in the absence of a chronic duodenal ulcer.[23] This is frequently referred to as 'chronic non-specific duodenitis'.

Inflammatory changes are known to be present in the mucosa surrounding peptic ulcers in the duodenum and similar qualitative changes may be found in the proximal duodenum of patients with severe dyspepsia in the absence of frank duodenal ulceration. These changes may represent a stage in the development or regression of chronic duodenal ulceration.

Symptoms and signs

It is common to encounter patients with symptoms suggestive of peptic ulceration in whom no definite ulcer is revealed on barium meal examination.[9] The pain is burning in nature, occurs in the epigastrium or right upper quadrant of the abdomen and has the periodicity and chronicity seen in patients with duodenal ulceration. Epigastric bloating is often a presenting symptom.[39] Smoking, alcohol and spices aggra-

vate the pain and antacids sometimes, but not invariably, relieve it. Clinical examination usually shows nothing remarkable.

Investigations

RADIOLOGY

As the inflammatory changes almost exclusively affect the mucosa, radiological features are not diagnostic of the condition. An irritable duodenal bulb with rapid emptying, and a comb or star appearance due to mucosal hyperplasia are described. Other features include the presence of erosions and fine superficial ulcers in the duodenal bulb.[14, 37] These changes are only found in advanced disease.[28] Chronic pancreatitis or carcinoma may be associated with these changes and a nearby duodenal ulcer may be missed by the radiological investigation. Comparison of conventional barium meal with endoscopy shows that in half the patients diagnosed by endoscopy the barium meal is normal.[23]

Hypotonic duodenography, cineradiology and double-contrast barium meal undoubtedly improves visualization of the duodenum and the diagnostic accuracy in duodenal ulceration. Radiological diagnosis alone is probably of no value in establishing the presence or absence of duodenitis.[5]

FIBRE-OPTIC ENDOSCOPY

Endoscopy is required to confirm the diagnosis and exclude the presence of a duodenal ulcer. Hirschowitz[21] first reported, and others have agreed on, the endoscopic features of duodenitis. These are described as areas of haemorrhage, hyperplasia and oedema of the mucosal folds.[3, 8, 18] The lesions are frequently focal in nature, appearances may change rapidly, and observer error requires a quantitative assessment and biopsy evidence. The duodenal architecture has been studied in endoscopic biopsy specimens taken from both normal mucosa and areas of duodenitis: crypt hyperplasia with villous atrophy and increase in mitotic figures per crypt were demonstrated in both non-specific and ulcer-associated duodenitis, suggesting a similar disease process.[19]

The following endoscopic grading is based on appearances and does not necessarily imply that one grade progresses to the next: grade O – normal duodenal mucosa, grade I – oedema with increased thickening of the mucosal folds, grade II – reddening of the mucosa (inflammation including contact bleeding), grade III – petechial haemorrhages, grade IV – erosions which are often associated with petechial haemorrhages, giving rise to the so-called 'salt and pepper' or 'salami' duodenum. During endoscopy, it is important to exclude other causes of GI disease. These include oesophagitis, gastritis and gastric ulcer. Duodenogastric reflux is frequently found in the presence of duodenitis, especially in those patients with atrophic gastritis and duodenal ulcers.[27] Not infrequently, a duodenal ulcer with a wide surrounding area of inflammation is observed. Endoscopic assessment alone is inadequate for diagnosing and grading the severity of duodenitis; multiple target biopsies are required for histological examinations.[12] Endoscopic trauma must be avoided.

HISTOLOGY

There is a wide range of appearances of the duodenal mucosa which might be found in asymptomatic individuals. Kreuning *et al.* reported the histological and immunohistochemical changes found in 50 healthy volunteers. This study showed abnormalities in 64% of individuals with chronic inflammation in 12%.[26] Changes ranged from an increase in the cellularity of the lamina propria, through variations in the size and shape of the villi to gastric metaplasia with Brunner's glands above the muscularis mucosae. A suggested classification includes: (a) chronic non-specific duodenitis, (b) silent chronic non-specific duodenitis, and (c) active chronic non-specific duodenitis, with scoring of the degrees of the duodenitis from 0 to 4 and expressing it as a 'duodenitis index'.[26] Studies have correlated endoscopic appearances, histological changes and clinical symptoms. The results show mucosal congestion and oedema, epithelial atypia and syncytial changes in symptomatic patients with duodenitis. Neutrophil infiltration, indicating active duodenitis, and increased round cell infiltration, indicating chronic duodenitis, are also found. Villous atrophy and gastric metaplasia are common. There seems to be an excellent correlation between endoscopic duodenitis (grades II to IV) and the histological features. However, in patients with minimal duodenitis (grade I) there is a poor correlation between endoscopic appearances and histology.[23] In severe duodenitis, there is increased mucosal cell proliferation, either alone or associated with duodenal ulceration.[4]

Morphometric quantification has been attempted to overcome the problems of subjective grading of duodenitis,[43] but is too time-consuming for routine use. Electron microscopy does not help in the diagnosis.

Dyspepsia, duodenitis and duodenal ulceration

Dyspepsia is a common symptom and peptic ulceration, gastroduodenitis and functional dyspepsia can all present in a similar manner.[10, 40] Gastric and duodenal ulceration, reflux oesophagitis and pancreatico-biliary disorders including cholelithiasis may be responsible for the dyspeptic symptoms. Duodenitis with gastric metaplasia is frequently found in patients with alcohol-associated chronic pancreatitis. Once the appearances suggestive of duodenitis[36] have been shown endoscopically, the diagnosis should be confirmed by light microscopy. Only then can the clinician infer that the duodenal inflammation is responsible for the dyspepsia.[5] The pain provocation test may help in this regard.[22]

The pathological sequence of hyperchlorhydria, duodenitis and duodenal ulcer was proposed long ago,[25, 29, 38] but not all investigators agree with this hypothesis.[1, 6] Thomson *et al.* found that half of their patients presenting with endoscopic and symptomatic duodenitis subsequently developed duodenal ulcers and underwent surgery.[41] On the basis of acid secretory data and basal immunoreactive gastrin levels, it is suggested that duodenitis may not be a variant of duodenal ulcer disease.[11] We feel that peptic duodenitis can cause symptoms and may represent a part of the pathophysiological spectrum of the duodenal disease, including duodenal ulceration, rather than being a separate entity.[41, 42]

Treatment

When there is a specific factor causing the inflammation, this primary cause must be treated. Chronic non-specific duodenitis is more difficult to treat as the underlying aetiological factors are not definitely known. Cessation of smoking, avoidance of salicylates and other inflammatory drugs and abstinence from alcohol are recommended. Anticholinergics, antispasmodics and sedatives have a minor role to play in therapy, and during an acute exacerbation of pain liberal use of antacids is advised.

Cimetidine therapy, besides healing the chronic duodenal ulcers, also improved symptoms and the endoscopic duodenitis.[9] Relapses during maintenance therapy for duodenal ulcers were associated with worsening of the duodenitis.[2]

A double-blind study on dyspeptic patients with endoscopically proven duodenitis and without chronic ulceration showed that cimetidine (1 g/day) for six weeks caused a significant improvement in symptoms and in the endoscopic appearance of duodenitis when compared with the placebo group. This was not associated, however, with any change in the histological grading of the duodenitis.[30] It is thought that the newer H_2-receptor antagonists will have a similar beneficial effect.

Pirenzepine therapy produces healing of endoscopically diagnosed gastroduodenitis with improvement in clinical symptomatology without side-effects.[15, 35] As yet, no studies have been performed using prostaglandins.

Information relating to the effect of vagotomy in duodenitis is unreliable, and the wisdom of such operative intervention is questionable.

REFERENCES

1 Aronson, A. & Norfleet, R. (1962) The duodenal mucosa in peptic ulcer disease: a clinical pathological correlation. *American Journal of Digestive Diseases*, **7**, 506–514.

2 Bardhan, K. D., Saul, D. M., Edwards, J. L. et al. (1969) Double-blind comparison of cimetidine and placebo in the maintenance of healing of chronic duodenal ulceration. *Gut*, **20**, 158–162.

3 Belber, J. P. (1971) Endoscopic examination of the duodenal bulb: a comparison with X-ray. *Gastroenterology*, **61**, 55–61.

4 Branson, C. J., Boxer, M. E., Palmer, K. P. et al. (1981) Mucosal cell proliferation in duodenal ulcer and duodenitis. *Gut*, **22**, 277–282.

5 Cheli, R. & Aste, H. (1976) *Duodenitis*, 1st edn. Stuttgart: George Thieme. 96 pp.

6 Classen, M., Koch, H. & Demling, L. (1970) Duodenitis: significance and frequency. In *Inflammation in Gut. Bibliotheca Gastroenterologica, Vol. 9* (Ed.) Maratka, Z. & Ottenjann, R. pp. 48–49. Basel: Karger.

7 Corachan, M., Oomen, H. A. & Sutorius, F. J. (1981) Parasitic duodenitis. *Transactions of the Royal Society of Tropical Medicine and Hygiene*, **75**, 385–389.

8 Cotton, P. B., Price, A. B., Tighe, J. R. & Beales, J. S. M. (1973) Preliminary evaluation of 'duodenitis' by endoscopy and biopsy. *British Medical Journal*, **iii**, 430–433.

9 Danielsson, A., Ek, B., Nyhilin, H. & Steen, L. (1983) The relationship between active peptic ulcer, endoscopic duodenitis and symptomatic state after treatment with cimetidine. *Annals of Clinical Research*, **12**, 4–12.

10 DeLuca, V. A., Winnan, G. G., Sheahan, D. G. et al. (1981) Is gastroduodenitis part of the spectrum of peptic ulcer disease? *Journal of Clinical Gastroenterology*, **3**, 17–22.

11 Donovan, I. A., Green, G., Dykes, P. W. et al. (1975) The pathophysiology of duodenitis (abstract). *Gut*, **16**, 395.

12 Forrester, A. W., Joffe, S. N. & Lee, F. D. (1979) The endoscopic and histological features of peptic duodenitis. *Scandinavian Journal of Gastroenterology* (Supplement), **14**, 18–22.

13 Frandsen, P. J., Jarnum, S. & Malmstrum, J. (1980) Crohn's disease of the duodenum. *Scandinavian Journal of Gastroenterology*, **15**, 633–638.

14 Fraser, G. M., Pitman, R. G., Lawrie, J. H. et al. (1964) The significance of the radiological findings of coarse mucosal folds in the duodenum. *Lancet*, **ii**, 979–982.

15 Gasbarrini, G., Giorgi-Conciato, M., Donchino, M. et al. (1979) Pirenzepine in the treatment of benign gastroduodenal diseases. A double-blind controlled clinical trial. *Scandinavian Journal of Gastroenterology* (Supplement), **14**, 25–31.

16 Gerlovin, E. S. H., Reiskanen, A. V. & Iakhontova, O. I. (1980) Ultrastructural changes in the epithelial cells of the small intestine mucosa in chronic liver diseases. *Arkhiv Patologii*, **42**, 27–31.

17 Gomez-Maganda, Y., Silva, T., Garcia-Carrisosa, R. et al. (1981) Duodenitis caused by *Giardia lamblia*. *Revista de gastroenterologia de Mèxico*, **46**(1), 11–15.

18 Gregg, J. A. & Garabedian, M. (1974) Duodenitis. *American Journal of Gastroenterology*, **61**, 177–184.

19 Hasan, M., Ferguson, A. & Sircus, W. (1981) Duodenal mucosal architecture in non-specific and ulcer-associated duodenitis. *Gut*, **22**, 637–641.

20 Henrich, M. (1979) Duodenal lesions produced by pantothenic acid deficiency in animal experiments. *Research in Experimental Medicine*, **176**, 107–116.

21 Hirschowitz, B. J. (1962) Gastroduodenal endoscopy with the fibrescope'. In *Current Gastroenterology* (Ed.) MacHardy, P. pp. 158. New York: Harper & Row.

22 Joffe, S. N. & Primrose, J. N. (1983) Pain provocation test in peptic duodenitis. *Gastrointestinal Endoscopy* (in press).

23 Joffe, S. N., Lee, F. D. & Blumgart, L. H. (1978) Duodenitis. *Clinics in Gastroenterology*, **7**, 635–650.

24 Joffe, S. N., Gaskin, R., Barros D'Sa, A. A. J. & Baron, J. H. (1977) Secretagogue-produced duodenal ulcers in the rat. *British Journal of Surgery*, **64**, 218–220.

25 Judd, F. S. & Nagel, G. (1927) Excision of ulcer of duodenum. *Surgery, Gynecology and Obstetrics*, **45**, 17–23.

26 Kreuning, J., Besman, F. T., Kuiper, G. et al. (1978) Gastric and duodenal mucosa in 'healthy' individuals. *Journal of Clinical Pathology*, **31**, 69–77.

27 Koelsch, K. A., Herms, G. & Kuhne, C. (1981) Duodenogastric-reflux-favouring behaviour of the pylorus in patients with gastritis and duodenitis. *Deutsche Zeitschrift für Verdauungs- und Stoffwechselkrankheiten*, **41**, 18–20.

28 Kunstlinger, F. C., Theoni, R. F., Grendell, J. F. et al. (1980) The radiographic appearance of erosive duodenitis. *Journal of Clinical Gastroenterology*, **2**, 205–211.

29 MacCarty, W. C. (1924) Excised duodenal ulcers: a report of four hundred and twenty-five specimens. *Journal of the American Medical Association*, **83**, 1894–1898.

30 MacKinnon, M., Willing, R. L. & Whitehead, R. (1982) Cimetidine in the management of symptomatic patients with duodenitis: a double-blind controlled trial. *Digestive Diseases and Sciences*, **27**, 217–219.

31 Maratka, Z., Kocianova, J., Kurdrmann, J. et al. (1979) Hyperplasia of Brunner's glands – radiology, endoscopy and biopsy. *Acta Hepato-Gastroenterologica*, **26**, 64–69.

32 Maruyama, M., Uech, M., Otsubo, C. et al. (1975) Endoscopic study of duodenitis. *Japanese Journal of Gastroenterology*, **17**, 719–728.

33 Mazumdar, T. N., Tandon, R. K. & Bajaj, J. S. (1978) Hookworm duodenitis – an endoscopic and gastric secretory study. *Journal of the Association of Physicians of India*, **26**, 35–40.

34 Mitchell, C. J., Jewell, D. P., Lewin, M. R. et al. (1979) Gastric function and histology in chronic renal failure. *Journal of Clinical Pathology*, **32**, 208–213.

35 Morelli, A., Narducci, F., Pelli, M. A. & Spadacini, A. (1979) A double-blind, short-term clinical trial of pirenzepine in duodenal ulcer. *Scandinavian Journal of Gastroenterology* (Supplement), **14**, 45–49.

36 Piubello, W., Vantini, I., Souro, L. A. *et al.* (1982) Gastric secretion, gastroduodenal histological changes and serum gastrin in chronic alcoholic pancreatitis. *American Journal of Gastroenterology*, **77**, 105–110.

37 Rhodes, J., Evans, K. T., Lawrie, J. H. & Forrest, A. P. M. (1968) Coarse mucosal folds in the duodenum. *Quarterly Journal of Medicine*, **37**, 151–169.

38 Rivers, A. B. (1931) 'Clinical study of duodenitis, gastritis and gastro-jejunitis'. *Annals of Internal Medicine*, **4**, 1265–1281.

39 Sankar, M. Y. (1981) A profile of dyspepsia in Bangalore. *Karnataka Medical Journal*, **XLVI**, 91–96.

40 Sankar, M. Y., Jayanth, C. K., Menon, R. & Gowda, S. (1982) Preliminary report of the incidence of duodenitis in South India. *Abstracts of Collegium Internationale Chirurgiae Digestivae (CICD), 1982*, vol. 1, p. 549.

41 Thomson, W. O., Joffe, S. N., Robertson, A. G. *et al.* (1977) Is duodenitis a dyspeptic myth? *Lancet*, **i**, 1197–1198.

42 Vitaxu, J. & Paolaggi, J. A. (1979) Ulcers of the bulb of the duodenum and duodenitis (author's translation). *Nouveau Presse Medicale*, **8**, 3803–3806.

43 Whitehead, R., Roca, M., Meikle, D. D. *et al.* (1975) The histological classification of duodenitis in fibreoptic biopsy specimens. *Digestion*, **13**, 129–136.

CHRONIC PEPTIC ULCER

AETIOLOGY

The cause of peptic ulceration is unknown. Gastric and duodenal ulcers behave as separate entities, but failure to distinguish between them has led to much confusion in the literature. Still further subdivision of their sites may be needed if the various causes are ever to be determined. Both diseases, however, probably result from an interplay of genetic and environmental hazards and their description under one heading facilitates comparison and contrast.

Genetic aspects

Several pieces of evidence support the probability that there is a strong genetic component to increased susceptibility to peptic ulcer.

FAMILY STUDIES

The first-degree relatives of patients with peptic ulcers show a more than two-fold excess of ulcers compared with similar relatives of unaffected people.[10] Moreover the parents, siblings and children of gastric ulcer patients tend to have gastric ulcers while the relatives of duodenal ulcer patients tend to have duodenal ulcers.[11] The combination of gastric and duodenal ulcers in the same patient is also accompanied by both types of ulcer together in relatives more commonly than would be expected by chance.

TWIN STUDIES

The concordance rates for the presence of a peptic ulcer in monozygotic (identical) twins consistently exceed those in dizygotic twins. The ulcer site is usually concordant when both members of the pair are affected.[41] Gastric and duodenal ulcers therefore appear to be independent from the point of view of heredity.

ASSOCIATIONS WITH INHERITED CHARACTERISTICS

Blood group O

The chance of developing a peptic ulcer was found to be 35% greater among people of blood group O than among those of groups A, B or AB in a survey of more than 3000 patients from London, Manchester and Newcastle.[1] In Liverpool blood group O was commoner in duodenal ulcer patients than in controls, but in gastric ulcer patients the ABO distribution was normal.[5] In later series blood group O seemed to be associated with duodenal ulcers and with ulcers in the antrum and pyloric region but not with those in the body of the stomach.[25] This apparent association of blood group O with gastric ulcers may be due to a bias of ascertainment, since group O patients have a greater tendency to bleed. The association between duodenal ulcer and group O is strong, however, even in non-bleeding cases.[27]

Non-secretion of A, B and H substances

Secretion of A, B and H substances into body fluids is a dominantly inherited characteristic which is independent of ABO group. There is an excess of non-secretors among duodenal ulcer patients,[6] but not among patients with gastric ulceration.

The relative risk (RR) that a person of group O will develop a duodenal ulcer compared with persons of groups A, B or AB is 1.35. The risk for non-secretors compared with secretors is 1.5, and that for group O non-secretors is 2.5. The reason for these findings is not known. A protective effect of blood group substances in gastric juice seems unlikely and no consistent relationships with gastric acid secretion or serum pepsinogen levels have been found.

Pepsinogen phenotypes

There are two immunologically distinct human serum pepsinogens. Pepsinogen I contains five electrophoretically distinct components. All five bands are present in phenotype A while phenotype B lacks the slowest-moving component and is inherited as an autosomal recessive character. Since type I pepsinogens are excreted in urine the phenotype can be determined from urine samples. Ellis and McConnell have recently confirmed that phenotype A is commoner in males with duodenal ulcer (RR 1.74).[13] Elevated serum levels of pepsinogen I are found in about half of unrelated duodenal ulcer patients. In certain families this characteristic may be dominantly inherited.[44] How these observations relate to pepsinogen phenotypes, and how pepsinogen I and its phenotypes influence duodenal ulcer development remain to be explained.

Other associated polymorphic characteristics

There is a weak association of both gastric and duodenal ulcers with rhesus D positivity and with alpha-1-antitrypsin deficiency. Duodenal ulcer is perhaps commoner in people with the dominantly inherited ability to taste phenylthiocarbamide and related compounds. There is an association between glucose-6-phosphate dehydrogenase deficiency and duodenal ulceration in Sardinian men.

Human leucocyte antigens (HLA)

No confirmed associations between specific HLA antigens and either gastric or duodenal ulcers have been found. Positive associations with duodenal ulcer have been reported from California (B5: RR 2.9), Liverpool (B12: RR 2.1) and Leeds (BW35: RR 2.7).[14, 15, 43] No associations were found in three other studies, the second of which included patients with gastric ulcers.[17, 18, 29]

FAMILIAL SYNDROMES ASSOCIATED WITH PEPTIC ULCERATION

Multiple endocrine adenopathy type I (MEA I)

Hyperplasia or malignant change of pituitary, parathyroid and pancreatic endocrine tissue can be familial, the inheritance pattern being autosomal dominant. The Zollinger–Ellison syndrome of fulminant peptic ulceration associated with a gastrin-secreting pancreatic islet tumour may occur as part of this syndrome or in isolation. It is uncertain whether the increased peptic ulcer incidence described in hyperparathyroidism is due to hypercalcaemia or reflects a coexistent pancreatic endocrine tumour. MEA I is discussed in more detail in Chapter 9.

Rare syndromes

Constellations of abnormalities which include an unusually high incidence of peptic ulceration or an unusual mechanism of ulcerogenesis have been described in small numbers of families.[41] These include familial amyloidosis; essential tremor, nystagmus and narcolepsy syndrome; stiff skin syndrome; gastrocutaneous syndrome; and pachydermoperiostitis. A possible increase in duodenal ulcer prevalence in porphyria cutanea tarda patients requires confirmation. Familial systemic mastocytosis may lead to peptic ulceration because of excessive tissue histamine concentrations.

Mode of inheritance of peptic ulcers

While the above evidence supports a genetic component in ulcerogenesis, no simple Mendelian patterns are evident for the majority of patients. It was therefore suggested that the inheritance pattern was polygenic – the greater the number of abnormal genes present the greater the susceptibility. The concept of *genetic heterogeneity* has recently gained ground. This implies that many patterns of inheritance will emerge when all the different kinds of peptic ulcer which are currently grouped together have been separated using different genetic markers.

Psychological factors

There is a widely held belief that personality traits and mental stress make important contributions to the milieu in which peptic ulcers thrive. Premorbid personality traits leading to ulcer formation are not well-defined, however. Male duodenal ulcer patients are not different from controls in terms of childhood factors which might affect subsequent personality.[19] Likewise, stressful events such as illness, family bereavement or financial difficulty occur no more frequently prior to exacerbations of gastric or duodenal ulceration in patients than they do in matched control subjects.[33] The emotional response to a stressful event, however, can be very variable and there seems no doubt that some cases of ulceration may be precipitated by severe anxiety.[31]

Physical stress

Peptic ulceration may occur in association with severe illness in three main clinical settings (see also the discussion of acute ulceration on p. 111).

Burns

Posterior duodenal ulcers as originally described by Curling (1842) are probably rare after burns. Acute gastric ulceration seems much more common and has led to confusion in terminology. Ulcers requiring surgery were recorded in only 18 of 32 500 patients treated in various burns units in Great Britain.[28] A much higher incidence in the United States has been related in part to associated sepsis.[35]

Disease of the central nervous system

Multiple gastric or duodenal ulcers were originally described by Cushing (1932) following cerebellar or midbrain operations. These 'neurogenic' ulcers have also been ascribed to the presence of intracranial tumours, trauma, infection, haemorrhage and ischaemia. These lesions may differ from other 'stress' ulcers in involving the full thickness of the stomach or duodenal wall.[46]

Trauma and surgery

Patients recovering from injury or operation whose course is complicated by hypotension, sepsis, jaundice, renal failure or respiratory failure are at particular risk of developing ulcers in the stomach and duodenum. Incidence figures are not available and it is not clear whether the stress ulcers arising in these situations occur by the same or different mechanisms.

Association with other diseases

Descriptions of peptic ulcers complicating the course of other diseases are common but often anecdotal.[23, 53] Langman and Cooke find no compelling evidence for true associations except in the following conditions:[23] chronic renal failure (especially patients undergoing haemodialysis or following transplantation), hyperparathyroidism (possibly because of associated gastrinoma), cirrhosis (alcoholic and non-alcoholic), cardiovascular disease (excluding hypertension) and chronic respiratory disease. It is uncertain whether there is a truly raised incidence of duodenal ulcer in patients with chronic pancreatitis, Crohn's disease or carcinoid syndrome. It is impossible to reach conclusions about rheumatoid arthritis because of concurrent drug therapy.

Immune disorders

No evidence exists to implicate immune mechanisms in the cause of gastric ulcers. Two observations, however, link altered immunity with duodenal ulcers: first, high antibody titres against secretory IgA have been found in duodenal ulcer patients, and secondly, in some patients gastric acid hypersecretion may be caused by IgG antibodies acting as autoimmune secretagogues.[42]

Miscellaneous hypotheses

Anatomical factors put forward to account for the localization of ulcers at certain sites include malrotation of the duodenum,[16] muscle spasm[38] and end-arteriolar blood supply increasing the risk of ischaemia.[32]

Environmental agents

Smoking

The incidence of smoking is higher in both gastric and duodenal ulcer patients than in non-ulcer subjects. A history of smoking among students is associated with the development of peptic ulcers later in life. The risk of developing peptic ulceration is perhaps doubled for smokers compared with non-smokers and increases with the number of cigarettes smoked. Critics conclude that the evidence available to associate smoking with peptic ulceration is weak.[22, 52] The important practical point is that none of the reports conclude that smoking is safe in the present context and wisdom dictates abstention.

Alcohol

No epidemiological evidence exists to incriminate alcohol consumption as a cause of either gastric or duodenal ulceration.

Coffee

Little information is available on this subject. Habitual coffee-drinking by Californian students shows an association with the development of peptic ulcer (site unspecified) in later life.[30]

Diet

There is no definite evidence that any specific item of food taken regularly or any persistent dietary deficiency will lead to gastric or duodenal ulceration. Hypotheses have linked pickled food with the high incidence of gastric ulceration in Japan,[24] sloppy diets with the high prevalence of duodenal ulcer in southern India[26] and the introduction of refined carbohydrates with duodenal ulceration throughout the world.[7]

Drugs

Many drugs have been suspected to cause peptic ulceration, but the evidence for this is generally poor.

Aspirin. An association between heavy analgesic ingestion and chronic gastric ulceration, particularly in young women, has been recognized in Australia for more than twenty years, and this has been confirmed in the United States. A causal relationship with aspirin seems likely. However, this is still an area of controversy: some believe that the risk of aspirin has been exaggerated,[40] while others believe that quite small doses of aspirin taken regularly can cause gastric ulceration.[21]

Paracetamol (Acetaminophen). A surprising association between chronic ingestion of paracetamol and the presence of chronic gastric ulcer has recently been reported from Australia.[34] Paracetamol is universally regarded as a safe alternative to aspirin in this context and there is no proof of a causal relationship.

Non-steroidal anti-inflammatory drugs (NSAID). The clinical impression that NSAIDs cause chronic peptic ulceration awaits confirmation by large-scale longitudinal surveys.

Corticosteroids. Conn and Blitzer reviewed the literature and found no proof that these drugs cause chronic peptic ulceration.[9] Important conclusions may have been concealed, however, because it was impossible to consider gastric and duodenal ulcers separately.

Environmental pollutants
Little attention seems to have been paid to the possibility that pollution of food or the environment contributes to peptic ulceration in man. Limited evidence from animal experiments suggests that this may be a useful area for research.[48]

Infectious agents

Viruses. There are some similarities in behaviour between duodenal ulcers and herpes simplex lesions. *Herpes simplex virus type I* antibody titres are higher in duodenal ulcer patients than in controls but the meaning of this finding is not known.[39, 50]

Nematodes. The fish parasite *Eustomatum rotundum* causes chronic gastric ulcers in people who eat raw fish.[45]

Naturally occurring ulcers in animals
Both genetic and environmental mechanisms appear important in animals too. An inbred strain of NZB mice, susceptible to autoimmune

disease, has a very high incidence of duodenal ulcer. Certain strains of pig are also prone to gastric ulceration.[41] According to Sircus,[45] the Californian seal develops ulcers because it swallows stones, and nematodes nest in the traumatized mucosa. Both sheep and cows develop peptic ulcers after the winter.

EPIDEMIOLOGY

It may be argued that the best method for the diagnosis of active peptic ulceration is endoscopy. It follows that the best estimate of the *prevalence* of active ulceration will result from endoscopy of the entire population of a defined community. Estimation of the *incidence* of peptic ulcers would demand repeat endoscopy of the same population after a suitable interval. Obviously this is impossible. Surveys have had to depend on alternative methods of ascertaining ulcer prevalence such as an appropriate history of ulcer pain, single contrast barium radiology, hospital discharge figures, operation rates for a complication of peptic ulcer or post-mortem examination. Inevitably such methods give only approximate estimates and painless ulcers will not be regularly detected. Figures obtained in different places, or in the same place at different times, may not be comparable because of the methods used to obtain or express these data.

Prevalence

In London the overall prevalence of past or present ulceration was found to be 5.8% in men and 1.9% in women between the ages of 15 and 64 years.[12] In Leeds, review of 13 000 necropsies performed between 1930 and 1949 showed a much higher overall prevalence of active or inactive ulcers. Chronic duodenal ulcers were found in 11.6% of men and 4.8% of women; chronic gastric ulcers occurred in 3.9% of men and 2.9% of women.[51] The hospital admission rates for peptic ulcers and their complications have altered greatly in recent years, suggesting a change in prevalence.[8]

Duodenal ulcer. In 1958 the admission rate for non-perforated duodenal ulcer was almost four times greater in men than in women. After 1969 the admission rate for men steadily declined and had nearly halved by 1977. In contrast, there was only a slight fall in admissions for non-perforated ulcer in women and perforated ulcers in women actually increased. This suggests that there has been a sharp decline in duodenal ulcer prevalence in men. It is important to realise that the onset of these changes antedated any major impact of the histamine H_2-antagonists.

Gastric ulcer. The male admission rate for gastric ulcer also halved between 1958 and 1977. The most striking reduction has been in the number of young men admitted with perforated gastric ulcer, who now number less than 10% of those twenty years ago. In contrast, female non-perforated gastric ulcers decreased only slightly and perforated ulcers not at all.

These changes clearly illustrate the independent behaviour of gastric and duodenal ulcers, but the reasons for the observed changes are obscure.

Incidence

There have been few longitudinal surveys to find the rate at which new ulcers occur. In York between 1952 and 1963 the annual incidence rates for duodenal ulcer per 1000 people at risk were around 3 for men (falling to 1.5 at the end of the survey) and 0.6 for women. The rates for gastric ulcer were 0.5 for men and 0.3 for women.[37] In Copenhagen County between 1963 and 1968 the annual incidence per 1000 at risk aged 15 years and over for duodenal ulcer was 1.83 in men and 0.84 in women.[3] The corresponding incidence rates for gastric ulcer were 0.51 and 0.38.[2]

Factors affecting the incidence of peptic ulcer

Age

In the nineteenth century young women were especially prone to gastric ulceration. Now, both gastric and duodenal ulcers predominantly affect the older age groups. Overall incidence figures conceal this variation due to age. Age-adjusted incidence rates in the Copenhagen survey clearly show that for both gastric and duodenal ulcer there is a steady increase with age, reaching a maximum in those aged 70 years

or more. Susser and Stein[47] suggested that the increasing age of duodenal ulcer patients was a *cohort* phenomenon: that is, people born about the turn of the century were exposed to a risk which increased their susceptibility throughout life. This theory does not, however, explain the increase in perforated duodenal ulcers in women aged 45 years or more during the past twenty years.

Sex

There is a preponderance of males in both gastric and duodenal ulcer patients, this being more marked for duodenal ulcer (Table 4.7).

Social and economic factors

Mortality statistics suggest that in the early 20th century duodenal ulcer was more prevalent in the higher social classes while gastric ulcer was a disease of the less privileged. Doll, Avery Jones and Buckatszch found an excess of gastric ulcers in social classes IV and V, but duodenal ulcer was evenly distributed throughout the population.[12] Langman finds evidence that both types of ulcer are now commoner in the lower socioeconomic groups but not all authorities accept this.[22]

Geographical variations

The prevalence of peptic ulcer varies greatly in different places. In Great Britain duodenal ulcer is several times more common in Scotland than in the south of England, while no clear pattern of variation is seen for gastric ulcers.[4] In Denmark and Sweden the duodenal ulcer prevalence does not appear to be falling as it is in Britain. In North America gastric ulcer is less common than in Europe. In India duodenal ulcer is much more common in the south than in the north and the male-to-female ratio is higher than in Britain. In Africa, too, there are areas in which duodenal ulcer prevalence is recognized to be greatly increased.[49]

Racial factors

Very little information relates to racial, as opposed to geographical, variations in ulcer prevalence. Even where differences are shown

Table 4.7 Sex ratios in peptic ulcer disease.

	Incidence ratios (male : female)	
	Gastric ulcer	Duodenal ulcer
York – Pulvertaft, 1959[36]	1.7 : 1	3.5 : 1
Copenhagen – Bonnevie, 1975[2, 3]	1.3 : 1	2.2 : 1

between the indigenous population of a particular country and an immigrant group, cultural factors may be just as important as genetic ones in causing the difference. No major difference between United States whites and non-whites seems likely.[20] Emigrants from southern India to Durban, South Africa, appear to have taken their increased susceptibility to duodenal ulcer with them. Other differences between races living in the same area include higher peptic ulcer prevalences among Chinese in Java than among indigenous Javanese and among Indians and Europeans in Fiji than among native Fijians. Unfortunately, these observations have not helped to divine the cause of ulcers.

Areas of increased gastric ulcer prevalence
In most parts of the world the ratio of duodenal to gastric ulcers is three to one or greater. Again for no clear reason, there are areas where this ratio is reversed because of a greater prevalence of gastric ulcer. These include Sri Lanka, Chile, France, Japan, some islands off northern Norway, high altitudes in Peru, and Turkey.

The literature on peptic ulcer is already extensive and modern treatment is very effective – so why pursue the cause? Continuing economic, diagnostic and therapeutic burdens speak for themselves. Although numerous associations with peptic ulceration have been described, many require confirmation and all need explanation.

The cause of peptic ulceration remains unknown.

REFERENCES

1 Aird, I., Bentall, H. H., Mehigan, J. A. & Roberts, J. A. F. (1954) The blood groups in relation to peptic ulceration and carcinoma of colon, rectum, breast, and bronchus. *British Medical Journal*, ii, 315–321.

2 Bonnevie, O. (1975) The incidence of gastric ulcer in Copenhagen county. *Scandinavian Journal of Gastroenterology*, 10, 231–239.

3 Bonnevie, O. (1975) The incidence of duodenal ulcer in Copenhagen county. *Scandinavian Journal of Gastroenterology*, 10, 385–393.

4 Brown, R. C., Langman, M. J. S. & Lambert, P. M. (1976) Hospital admissions for peptic ulcer during 1958–1972. *British Medical Journal*, i, 35–37.

5 Clarke, C. A., Cowan, W. K., Edwards, J. W. et al. (1955) The relationship of the ABO blood groups to duodenal and gastric ulceration. *British Medical Journal*, ii, 643–646.

6 Clarke, C. A., Edwards, J. W., Haddock, D. R. W. et al. (1956) ABO blood groups and secretor character in duodenal ulcer. *British Medical Journal*, ii, 725–731.

7 Cleave, T. L. (1974) Peptic ulcer. In *The Saccharine Disease*. pp. 138–174. Bristol: John Wright.

8 Coggon, D., Lambert, P. & Langman, M. J. S. (1981) 20 years of hospital admissions for peptic ulcer in England and Wales. *Lancet*, i, 1302–1304.

9 Conn, H. O. & Blitzer, B. L. (1976) Nonassociation of adrenocorticosteroid therapy and peptic ulcer. *New England Journal of Medicine*, 294, 473–479.

10 Doll, R. & Buch, J. (1950) Hereditary factors in peptic ulcer. *Annals of Eugenics*, 15, 135–146.

11 Doll, R. & Kellock, T. D. (1951) The separate inheritance of gastric and duodenal ulcers. *Annals of Eugenics*, 16, 231–240.

12 Doll, R., Avery Jones, F. & Buckatzsch, M. M. (1951) Occupational factors in the aetiology of gastric and duodenal ulcers, with an estimate of their incidence in the general population. *Medical Research Council Special Report Series No. 276*. London: HMSO.

13 Ellis, A. & McConnell, R. B. (1982) Duodenal ulcer and urinary pepsinogen phenotypes. *Gastroenterology*, 83, 1261–1263.

14 Ellis, A. & Woodrow, J. C. (1979) HLA and duodenal ulcer. *Gut*, 20, 760–762.

15 Gough, M. J., Rajah, S. M. & Giles, G. R. (1982) HLA antigens in relationship to duodenal ulceration, gastric acid secretion and the clinical result following vagotomy. *British Journal of Surgery*, 69, 105–107.

16 Gravgaard, E. (1980) Malrotation of the duodenum. In *Symposium on Duodenal Ulcer* (Ed.) Kronborg, O. & Caldwell, A. D. S. *Scandinavian Journal of Gastroenterology*, 15 (Supplement 63), 16–20.

17 Hammond, M. G. & Moshal, M. G. (1980) HLA and duodenal ulcer in South African Indians. *Tissue Antigens*, 15, 508–509.

18 Heschl, R. & Tilz, G. P. (1976) Untersuchungen über die Verteilung der HL-A-Antigene bei Patienten mit Zwölffingerdarmgeschwüren. *Acta Medica Austriaca*, 3, 80–82.

19 Kellock, T. D. (1951) Childhood factors in duodenal ulcer. *British Medical Journal*, ii, 1117–1120.

20 Kurata, J. H. & Haile, B. M. (1982) Racial differences in peptic ulcer disease: fact or myth? *Gastroenterology*, 83, 166–172.

21 Kurata, J. H., Elashoff, J. D. & Grossman, M. I. (1982) Inadequacy of the literature on the relationship between drugs, ulcers and gastrointestinal bleeding. *Gastroenterology*, 82, 373–376.

22 Langman, M. J. S. (1979) Peptic ulcer. In *The Epidemiology of Chronic Digestive Disease*. pp. 9–39. London: Edward Arnold.

23 Langman, M. J. S. & Cooke, A. R. (1976) Gastric and duodenal ulcer and their associated diseases. *Lancet*, i, 680–683.

24 MacDonald, W. C., Anderson, F. H. & Hashimoto, S. (1967) Histological effect of certain pickles on the human gastric mucosa: a preliminary report. *Canadian Medical Association Journal*, 96, 1521–1525.

25 McConnell, R. B. (1966) The genetics of gastrointestinal disorders. In *Oxford Monographs on Medical Genetics*. pp. 76–111. Oxford: Oxford University Press.

26 Malhotra, S. L. (1964) Peptic ulcer in India and its aetiology. *Gut*, 5, 412–416.

27 Mourant, A. E. & Kopeć, A. C. & Domaniewska-Sobczak, K. (1978) Blood groups and diseases. A study of associations of diseases with blood groups and other polymorphisms. In *Oxford Monographs on Medical Genetics*. pp. 29–30. Oxford: Oxford University Press.

28 Muir, I. F. K. & Jones, P. F. (1976) Curling's ulcer: a rare condition. *British Journal of Surgery*, 63, 60–66.

29 O'Brien, B. D., Thomson, A. B. R. & Dossetor, J. B. (1979) HLA and peptic ulcer. *Digestive Diseases and Sciences*, 24, 314–315.

30   Paffenbarger, R. S., Wing, A. L. & Hyde, R. T. (1974) Chronic disease in former college students. XIII. Early precursors of peptic ulcer. *American Journal of Epidemiology*, **100**, 307–315.

31   Peters, M. N. & Richardson, C. T. (1983) Stressful life events, acid hypersecretion, and ulcer disease. *Gastroenterology*, **84**, 114–119.

32   Piasecki, C. (1977) Role of ischaemia in the initiation of peptic ulcer. *Annals of The Royal College of Surgeons of England*, **59**, 476–478.

33   Piper, D. W., McIntosh, J. H., Ariotti, D. E. *et al.* (1981) Analgesic ingestion and chronic peptic ulcer. *Gastroenterology*, **80**, 427–432.

34   Piper, D. W., McIntosh, J. H., Ariotti, D. E. *et al.* (1981) Life events and chronic duodenal ulcer: a case control study. *Gut*, **22**, 1011–1017.

35   Pruitt, B. A. Jr, Foley, F. D. & Moncrief, J. A. (1970) Curling's ulcer: a clinico-pathological study of 323 cases. *Annals of Surgery*, **172**, 523–539.

36   Pulvertaft, C. N. (1959) Peptic ulcer in town and country. *British Journal of Preventive and Social Medicine*, **13**, 131–138.

37   Pulvertaft, C. N. (1968) Comments on the incidence and natural history of gastric and duodenal ulcer. *Postgraduate Medical Journal*, **44**, 597–602.

38   Qvist, G. (1974) Muscle spasm in the etiology of chronic peptic ulcer. *Proceedings of the Royal Society of Medicine*, **67**, 365–369.

39   Rand, K. H., Jacobson, D. G., Cottrell, C. R. *et al.* (1982) Relationship of herpes virus Type 1 (HSV-1) infection to duodenal ulcer. *Gastroenterology*, **82**, 1154.

40   Rees, W. D. W. & Turnberg, L. A. (1980) Reappraisal of the effects of aspirin on the stomach. *Lancet*, **ii**, 410–413.

41   Rotter, J. I. (1980) The genetics of peptic ulcer: more than one gene, more than one disease. In *Progress in Medical Genetics, Vol. IV The Genetics of Gastrointestinal Disease.* (Ed.) Steinberg, A. G., Bearn, A. G., Motulsky, A. G. & Childs, B. pp. 1–58. Philadelphia: Saunders.

42   Rotter, J. I. & Heiner, D. C. (1982) Are there immunologic forms of duodenal ulcer? *Journal of Laboratory and Clinical Medicine*, **7**, 1–6.

43   Rotter, J. I., Rimoin, D. L., Gursky, J. M. *et al.* (1977) HLA-B5 associated with duodenal ulcer. *Gastroenterology*, **73**, 438–440.

44   Rotter, J. I., Sones, J. Q., Samloff, I. M. *et al.* (1979) Duodenal ulcer disease associated with elevated serum pepsinogen I. *New England Journal of Medicine*, **300**, 63–66.

45   Sircus, W. (1979) The enigma of peptic ulcer. *Scottish Medical Journal*, **24**, 31–37.

46   Skillman, J. J. & Silen, W. (1976) Stress ulceration in the acutely ill. *Annual Review of Medicine*, **27**, 9–22.

47   Susser, M. & Stein, Z. (1962) Civilization and peptic ulcer. *Lancet*, **i**, 115–119.

48   Szabo, S. & Reynolds, E. S. (1975) Structure–activity relationships for ulcerogenic and adrenocorticolytic effects of alkyl nitriles, amines, and thiols. *Environmental Health Perspectives*, **11**, 135–140.

49   Tovey, F. I. & Tunstall, M. (1975) Duodenal ulcer in black populations in Africa south of the Sahara. *Gut*, **16**, 564–576.

50   Vestergaard, B. F. & Rune, S. J. (1980) Type-specific herpes-simplex-virus antibodies in patients with recurrent duodenal ulcer. *Lancet*, **i**, 1273–1274.

51   Watkinson, G. (1960) The incidence of chronic peptic ulcer found at necropsy. *Gut*, **1**, 14–30.

52   Wormsley, K. G. (1978) Smoking and duodenal ulcer. *Gastroenterology*, **75**, 139–142.

53   Wormsley, K. G. (1980) The association between duodenal ulcer and other diseases. In *Symposium on Duodenal Ulcer* (Ed.) Kronborg, O. & Caldwell, A. D. S. *Scandinavian Journal of Gastroenterology*, **15** (Supplement 63), 27–35.

CHRONIC GASTRIC ULCER

Clinical features

Over the past few years there has been a renewed interest in the symptoms of peptic ulcer disease. As physical examination does not usually help the physician to arrive at the correct diagnosis, there has been a critical analysis of the pattern of symptoms in upper gastrointestinal disease. From this improved data base it is hoped that the accuracy of clinical diagnosis can be so improved that the demands on radiology or endoscopy can be reduced. In a recent paper on the analysis of dyspeptic symptoms Horrocks and de Dombal commented that the clinical features of peptic ulcer disease as presented in many textbooks do not stand up to critical review.[36] The following description of the clinical features of gastric ulcer disease is therefore based principally on a paper published in 1968 by Edwards and Coghill in which they carefully recorded and analysed the symptoms of 84 patients with gastric ulceration.[24]

Age. Gastric ulceration is a disease of late middle age: the median age is reported to be between 50 and 60 years.

Sex. Although men usually outnumber women (1.27 : 1), some recent studies have shown a trend towards equality or even a female dominance.

Pain. Pain is the most common presenting symptom (90%) and is often more severe than in duodenal ulcer disease.

Site. In almost half the patients the pain is epigastric in position (46%) with the left hypochondrium as the second most common site (19%).

Radiation. In one-third of the patients there is no radiation of the pain, but in the others the pain radiates either through to the back (30%) or to other abdominal sites (48%).

Character. Many patients find pain a difficult symptom to describe. However, the most common description was that of an aching, nagging or cramp-like discomfort (33%). The two other main descriptions were an acute or cutting pain (18%) or a gnawing or hunger-like pain (13%).

Pattern. In the majority of patients the pain came in attacks lasting usually less than eight weeks (85%) with periods of freedom varying from one to three months. One-third of the patients had no set pattern of attacks.

Relationship to food. The expected symptom of pain either precipitated or aggravated by food was found in only 24% of the patients and in 12% the pain was not related to meals.

Nocturnal pain. Almost a half (43%) were woken regularly from sleep by pain.

Additional symptoms. Over half the patients complained of flatulence (65%), abdominal distension (55%) or nausea (54%). Between a third and a half complained of belching (48%), loss of appetite (46%), acid regurgitation (43%), vomiting (38%) or waterbrash (33%). Approximately a quarter suffered from either constipation (29%) or weight loss (24%).

From this description it can be seen that gastric ulcer disease most commonly affects men between the ages of 50 and 60 who complain of epigastric pain after food and at night; this is eased by antacids. A large proportion will also complain of flatulence, abdominal distension and nausea.

PATHOPHYSIOLOGY OF GASTRIC ULCERATION

In gastric ulcer disease, acid and pepsin secretion is usually within normal limits or reduced, suggesting that the fundamental defect is a reduction in mucosal resistance.

The mucosal barrier
The mucosal barrier consists of epithelial cells and the overlying mucus layer. These cells are viable for two to six days and are replaced by new ones migrating from the neck of the gastric glands. The integrity of the mucosa also depends on an adequate blood supply.

The mucus that coats these cells is in the form of a gel, which is constantly being broken down by the action of food and pepsin. It must therefore be replenished at a rate sufficient to produce an adequate depth and concentration of mucus.

The gastric mucosa also secretes bicarbonate. Although this is small in amount when compared with the maximal acid output, it is secreted in high concentration into the mucosal side of the mucus layer, where it is trapped. Any hydrogen ion entering the mucus layer is opposed by the increasing bicarbonate gradient and is thus neutralized.

In gastric ulcer disease, gastric epithelial cell turnover is increased, and not only do these immature cells secrete a smaller than normal amount of mucus but the mucus they do secrete is abnormal. This abnormal mucus and the reduced quantity lead to reduced mucosal resistance.

Duodenogastric reflux
Reflux of duodenal contents into the stomach will occur when a duodenal contraction wave coincides with an open pylorus. This is usually followed by antral peristalsis, which rapidly clears the stomach of duodenal contents. An incompetent pyloric sphincter, abnormal duodenal activity, or reduced antral clearing will increase bile reflux and allow time for it to damage the gastric mucosa, producing either a gastritis or gastric ulceration.

Bile reflux is known to be increased in patients with gastric ulceration, and experimentally it can be shown that bile can break the gastric mucosal barrier and allow the back-diffusion of hydrogen ions. Duodenal reflux occurs mainly along the lesser curvature of the stomach, damaging the parietal cells. The parietal cell mass is reduced, as is the overall acid-secreting capacity. Bile reflux has also been shown to stimulate acid secretion, and the remaining parietal cells produce a locally high concentration of acid that bathes the already damaged mucosal cells. Gastric ulceration, therefore, often occurs just distal to the junction zone between the fundal parietal cells and the non-acid-secreting mucosa.

Ulcers that occur close to the pylorus are usually associated with high gastric acidity. As bile reflux damages the parietal cells and these are replaced by a non-acid-secreting mucosa, the boundary zone between the two types of gastric mucosa moves proximally up the lesser curvature, so an ulcer lying on the high lesser curvature is usually associated with a reduced parietal cell mass and hyposecretion of acid.

Investigation and diagnosis

DIFFERENTIAL DIAGNOSIS

The differential diagnoses include non-ulcer dyspepsia, duodenal ulcer, gastric carcinoma and hiatal hernia. The overlap in symptoms of these different conditions is considerable and many studies have concluded that it is not possible to separate gastric from duodenal ulcer disease by

Table 4.8 Pattern of symptoms[a] in 360 patients with gastric and duodenal ulcer, gastric cancer and non-ulcer dyspepsia.[36]

		Gastric ulcer	Duodenal ulcer	Gastric cancer	Non-ulcer dyspepsia
Age: Proportion over 50		62	28	90	45
Sex ratio (male: female)		1 : 0.47	1 : 0.25	1 : 0.74	1 : 1.7
Pain					
Site:	epigastric	66	86	54	52
Radiation to:	shoulder	8	3	4	8
	back	34	26	**10**	28
Pattern:	continuous pain	12	8	**27**	6
	episodic pain[b]	16	56	**0**	35
	continuing attacks[c]	64	34	72	56
Relationship to food:	immediate	20	**0**	18	14
	delayed more than 20 minutes	45	50	31	**19**
	not related	35	50	51	**7**
Eased by	antacids	36	39	**9**	26
	food	2	**20**	1	4
Nocturnal		32	**70**	16	32
Proportion with symptoms for less than one year		50	18	**90**	34
Symptoms					
Anorexia		57	36	**90**	36
Weight loss (>3.2 kg in one month)		61	44	**82**	32
Dysphagia		5	4	**19**	8
Nausea		70	59	77	60
Vomiting		73	57	66	**34**

[a] Apart from the sex ratios, the figures are percentages.
[b] Episodic pain: pain that comes on for a few weeks, with periods of freedom for weeks or months.
[c] Continuing attacks: attacks of pain occurring for an hour or two at frequent intervals.

analysis of the patient's symptoms alone. Table 4.8 summarizes the clinical presentation of 360 patients with dyspepsia.[36] No one symptom satisfactorily separates the four listed disorders: more often it is the pattern of symptoms which will guide the physician to the correct diagnosis.

DIAGNOSIS FROM ANALYSIS OF SYMPTOMS

In 1975 Horrocks, Jane and de Dombal showed that very few clinicians were able to make a correct diagnosis following the initial patient interview, and that the average accuracy was only 50%.[35] If, however, a structured history using pre-defined terms was taken, the clinician's diagnostic accuracy could be improved by some 20–30%. This difficulty in correctly diagnosing patients with dyspepsia is highlighted in our own department of radiology, where a recent review has shown that almost 80% of all barium meal investigations were normal. There may be several reasons for this. A clinician who has correctly diagnosed non-ulcer dyspepsia may feel that the patient can be better reassured with a normal barium study. During the delay between booking and the actual examination an ulcer may have healed, giving a false-negative result. Finally, the investigation may be inap-

propriate: for instance, a barium meal may be requested for a patient with gallstones.

It would therefore be of great benefit if patients with either ulcers or a cancer could be separated from those with non-ulcer dyspepsia by simple analysis of their symptoms. Over the past two years we have been using the techniques pioneered by de Dombal to try and place dyspeptic patients into risk groups. Ideally, a low-risk group would contain mainly patients with non-ulcer dyspepsia, who could be treated initially with antacids and only referred for investigation if their symptoms failed to settle. The medium-risk group should contain mainly patients with duodenal ulcer disease who could then be referred for investigation in the normal way. The high-risk group would contain most of the patients with gastric ulcers or cancer, and these patients could have their investigations expedited.

A non-medically-trained research assistant interviewed patients with dyspepsia who presented either to our dyspepsia clinic or to a general practitioner's surgery. Having taken a structured case history, the data were entered into a microcomputer. This compared the clinical features of the patient with several hundred similar patients in its memory and from this produced a risk prediction. The preliminary results are shown in Table 4.9.

Table 4.9 Computer prediction based on case history and clinical features compared with the final diagnosis in 904 patients with dyspepsia.

Final diagnosis	Computer prediction			Total
	Low risk	Medium risk	High risk	
Normal	207	202	140	549
Hiatal hernia	48	31	36	115
Duodenal ulcer	18	114	30	162
Gastric ulcer	4	18	19	41
Gastric cancer	1	2	25	28
Cancer – not gastric	—	—	6	6
Other findings	2	—	1	3
Total	280	367	257	904

Just over 900 patients have been studied, and the results show that the medium- and high-risk groups contain all but 11% of the diagnosed ulcers, and all but 3% of the cancers. Such a screening program could reduce demand for barium meal studies or endoscopy. Such analysis will still not separate gastric ulcer from duodenal ulcer, so all medium- and high-risk patients must be investigated by either radiology or endoscopy.

LOCATION OF ULCERS

Benign gastric ulcers occur mainly on the lesser curve of the stomach, usually proximal to the angulus. The second most common site is the prepyloric region. Prepyloric ulcers or gastric ulcers associated with duodenal ulcer disease are often associated with a high acid output, and thus behave more like duodenal ulcers than gastric ulcers. A 1980 study of 228 benign ulcers indicated the following distribution:[58]

- 45% on the lesser curve proximal to the angulus;
- 19% in the prepyloric region;
- 12% on the anterior or posterior wall;
- 8% in the antrum;
- 7% on the angulus;
- 5% on the greater curve;
- 4% at other sites.

RADIOLOGICAL DIAGNOSIS

The single-contrast barium meal has been the standard method for investigation of patients with dyspepsia for over 60 years and has the advantages of being both cheaper and safer than endoscopy. The high incidence of gastric cancer in Japan led in the mid 1960s to the development and wide use of the double-contrast barium meal in their mass screening programmes. This technique allows better mucosal detail and aids the differentiation between benign and malignant ulcers. The stomach is distended with gas and its inner wall coated with a thin layer of high-density barium, which allows the recognition of fine mucosal detail. Originally air was used to distend the stomach, but now an effervescent drink or effervescent tablet is used. The results can be further improved by paralysing the stomach with a smooth muscle relaxant such as hyoscine (scopolamine) butylbromide (Buscopan) or glucagon. The mucosal detail seen with these techniques allows such lesions as erosions, linear ulcers and ulcer scars to be demonstrated.

Acute and chronic ulcers
Most ulcers are round or oval in shape with clear-cut margins and project beyond the margin of the stomach wall. There is sometimes a collar of oedematous mucosa that projects into the lumen of the stomach, but this will disappear as the ulcer heals. The floor of a chronic ulcer is often irregular in shape.

Multiple ulcers
Multiple gastric ulcers occur in between 2% and 5% of patients. The ulcer crater is often difficult to demonstrate, but they usually produce a characteristic deformity of the stomach.

Linear ulcers
In Japan 30% of gastric ulcers are linear in shape and are usually found running across the lesser curve near to the angulus. Linear ulcers are less common in the West and often result from either the coalescence of a group of small ulcers or from the healing of a large ulcer.

Gastric ulcer – benign or malignant?
After many studies all over the world it is now accepted that between 5% and 10% of apparently benign gastric ulcers will turn out to be

malignant. Most of these represent the early stage of an ulcerating cancer and less than 1% will be a true ulcer cancer – that is, a carcinoma developing within an existing chronic gastric ulcer. The five-year survival with an early ulcerating cancer or an ulcer cancer may be two to three times as high as with the usual proliferative cancer.

It used to be taught that malignancy was unusual if the ulcer was sited away from the greater curvature of the stomach, if it was associated with a duodenal ulcer or if it healed with medical therapy. It is now well recognized that malignant ulcers are not confined to the greater curvature and that the site of an ulcer is thus of no assistance in excluding a cancer. Ulcer healing is also an unreliable indicator, as many malignant ulcers can undergo healing, either spontaneously or as the result of drug therapy, and are later followed by re-ulceration.

Radiological signs favouring a benign ulcer

1 A smooth, sharply defined ulcer crater that projects beyond the margin of the stomach wall (Figure 4.18a).
2 Smooth intact mucosal folds that radiate towards the base of an ulcer.
3 Normal areae gastricae surrounding the ulcer.
4 Normal peristaltic activity passing through the ulcer area.

Radiological signs favouring a malignant ulcer

1 The ulcer is often irregular in outline with a raised, rolled margin that projects within the stomach lumen (Figure 4.18b).
2 Rigidity or nodularity of the adjacent mucosa with thickening, widening, clubbing, irregularity or loss of the mucosal folds adjacent to the ulcer.
3 Loss of the normal areae gastricae surrounding the ulcer crater.
4 Reduction or absence of peristalsis in the area of the ulcer suggesting underlying infiltration.

Having diagnosed a gastric ulcer by radiology, what action should be taken? In the past, ulcers with stigmata of gastric cancer were referred direct for surgery, and the remainder were treated medically. If the ulcer was not significantly smaller after six weeks' treatment (60%), or if it was unhealed after three months' treatment, an operation was recommended.

In two recently published studies, standard radiological techniques failed to separate malignant from benign gastric ulcers in 31% and 40% respectively.[58, 68] Although it is claimed that the double-contrast barium meal in expert radiological hands will successfully separate most benign from malignant gastric ulcers, most experts still recommend that all patients with a proven gastric ulcer be referred for endoscopy coupled with biopsy and cytology of the ulcer.

ENDOSCOPIC DIAGNOSIS

With the advent of slimmer, wider angled instruments, endoscopy has made a major impact on the investigation of gastric ulcer disease. In spite of these improvements, endoscopy still remains an invasive technique, and although the risks are small there is still a definite morbidity and mortality. However, this is more than outweighed by the ability to take biopsies and brush cytology of gastric lesions.

Endoscopic signs favouring a benign ulcer. A benign gastric ulcer should have a regular, punched-out appearance with a smooth margin. The shape of an ulcer can be round, oval, or even linear in shape. The floor or base of the ulcer is covered with white fibrinoid material. The folds of the surrounding mucosa radiate towards the ulcer crater rather like the spokes of a wheel.

Endoscopic signs favouring a malignant ulcer. The ulcerating gastric cancer usually has an irregular, nodular margin, often with step formation. On biopsy the edge of the ulcer is often felt to be rigid, the biopsy site bleeds easily and may fragment and the surrounding mucosal folds lose their stellate appearance, are often thickened and distorted, and fail to reach the ulcer edge. Ulcers more than 2 cm in diameter have approximately four times as high a risk of being malignant as smaller ulcers. However, since 95% of ulcers are benign, most large ulcers will still be benign. Endoscopists relying on the appearance only in differentiating between benign and malignant ulcers can expect to be correct in up to 94% of patients.

Endoscopic biopsy

It is now standard practice for all ulcerating gastric lesions to be biopsied. Most papers recommend that biopsies should be taken from the edge of an ulcer on all four quadrants, as well as from the ulcer base. In practice it is very

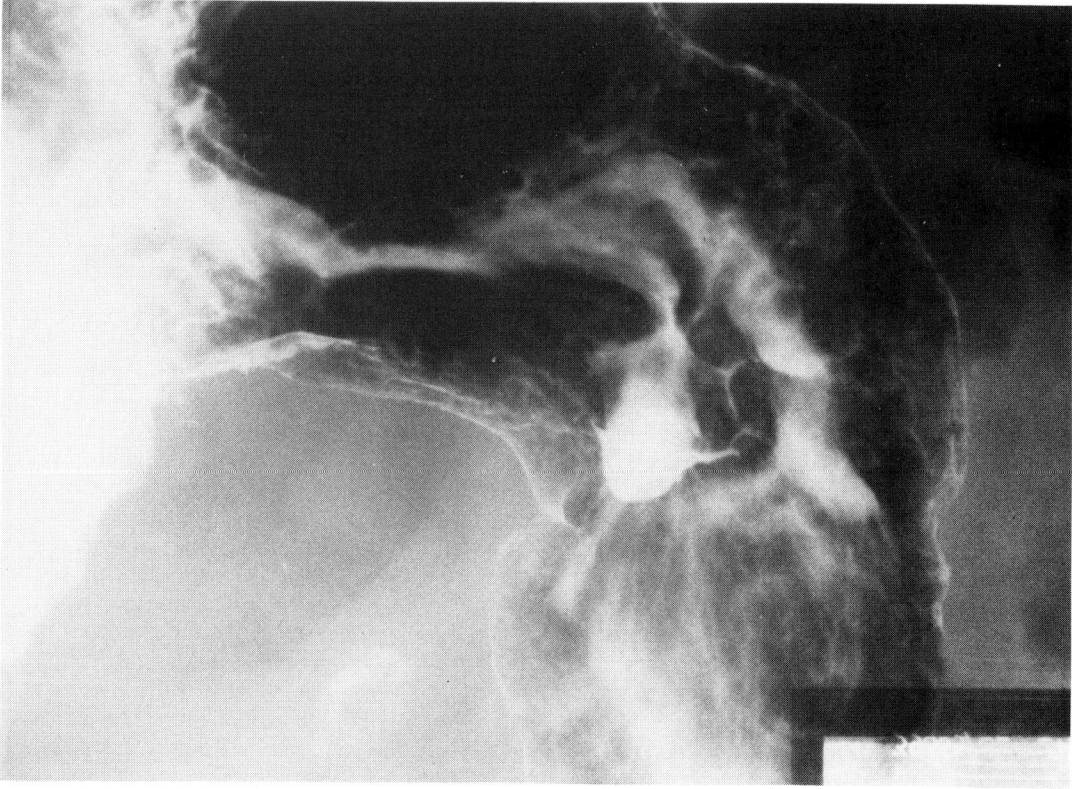

b

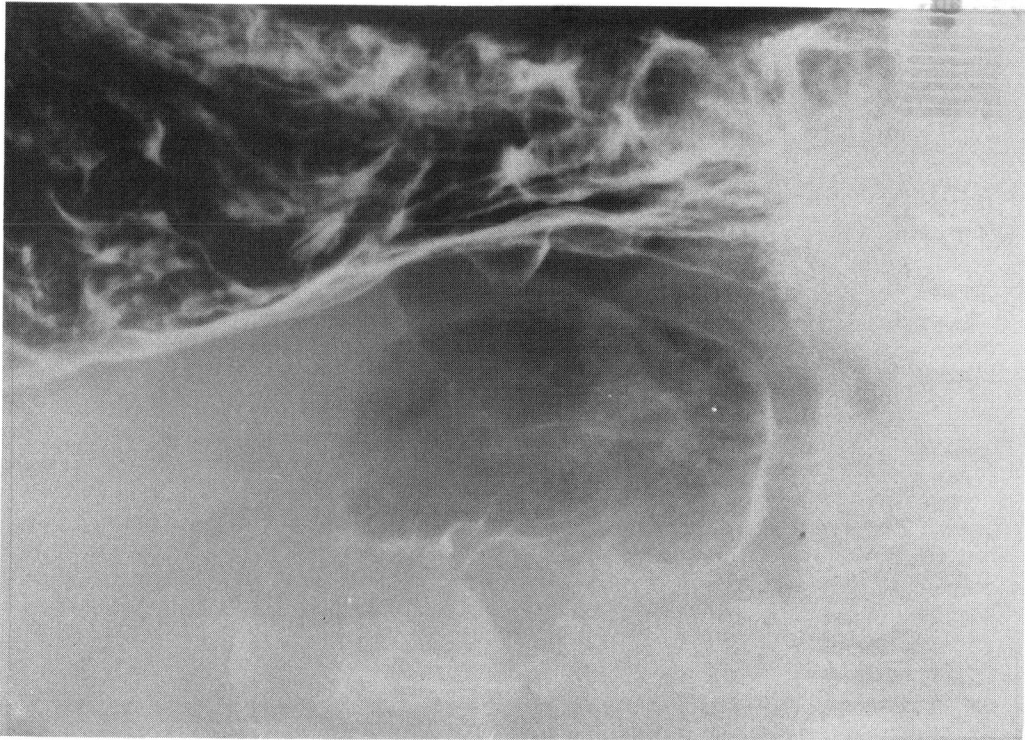

a

Fig. 4.18 (a) Radiograph showing benign, cone-shaped penetrating ulcer on the posterior wall of the mid body of the stomach. (b) Radiograph showing malignant gastric ulcer on posterior wall with an irregular and raised margin.

difficult to obtain biopsies from all four quadrants of an ulcer with a forward-viewing endoscope, and some endoscopists therefore suggest that a side-viewing instrument should also be used. However, provided at least six biopsies are taken from the ulcer edge, there appears to be little reduction in overall accuracy.[11] Two or three biopsies should also be taken from the ulcer base so that a type 2c (Japanese classification) mucosal cancer may not be missed.

Once the biopsies are taken, some endoscopists attempt to orientate them with a dissecting microscope so that histological sections can be cut in the right plane. Many centres will also take serial sections through the biopsy if any suspicious changes are encountered. For the best results the endoscopist and pathologist should review the endoscopic specimens together: in this way a correct diagnosis can be made in approximately 98% of all ulcers that are biopsied.

Cytology

There is now good evidence that cytology will complement both the visual appearance and the biopsy results. If all three parameters are used a diagnostic accuracy rate of almost 100% can be obtained. Most endoscopists now use a disposable brush to take cytological specimens, but it should be appreciated that the ulcer must be brushed vigorously enough to rub off cells rather than just the surface mucus.

Medical treatment

NON-SPECIFIC MEASURES

Doll and Pygott first showed in 1952 that a period of bed-rest in hospital resulted in more rapid ulcer healing than outpatient therapy.[18] However, with the advent of specific drug treatment the same or even better rates of ulcer healing can be achieved without bed-rest or hospital admission. Doll also showed that the speed of ulcer healing could be further improved if smoking was discouraged.[19] In the past patients with gastric ulceration were advised to take small frequent bland meals, but clinical trials have failed to show any relationship between diet and ulcer healing. Most of these gastric diets contained milk and it is now known that milk is a strong stimulant of acid secretion and is not even a particularly good neutralizing agent. Likewise, small frequent meals have little buffering effect, perhaps owing to the more continual stimulation of gastric acid secretion. Coffee and alcohol were likewise banned for ulcer patients. The stimulating effect of caffeine has, however, been shown to be small, and alcohol may even inhibit gastric acid output. Ulcer patients should, therefore, be allowed to choose their own diets and enjoy their meals.

ANTACID THERAPY

In a recent review on antacids and peptic ulcer, Morris and Rhodes[57] point out that in the United Kingdom in 1976 the total cost of antacid therapy was about £20 million. It is therefore surprising that most clinical studies have shown little, if any, effect of antacid therapy on the healing rate of gastric ulcers. Isenberg *et al.* have recently performed a study in which cimetidine at a dose of 1.2 grams per day was compared with low-dose antacid therapy and placebo.[37] They found that cimetidine, when compared with placebo at both the 8-week and the 12-week assessment period, significantly hastened gastric ulcer healing, but low-dose antacid therapy had no such effect. In 1978 two American studies were published in which cimetidine was compared with high-dose antacid therapy.[22, 25] In one, an average of 228 millimoles of in-vitro buffering capacity per day was employed and in the other 279 millimoles per day. Analysis of the healing rates for both studies showed a trend in favour of cimetidine when compared with this high-dose antacid therapy, but in neither case did this reach statistical significance. Very high-dose antacid therapy may therefore hasten ulcer healing, but the side-effects of such treatment were high, with approximately 40% of the patients complaining of either mild or moderate diarrhoea.

Side-effects. Most antacid mixtures now contain a combination of magnesium and aluminium salts. If taken in high dose, there is appreciable absorption of both aluminium and magnesium, although patients do not develop the type of systemic alkalosis observed with large doses of sodium bicarbonate. Although most proprietary preparations of antacids contain balanced amounts of aluminium and magnesium, the mixtures usually tend to cause diarrhoea. This tendency can be balanced by providing the patient with an aluminium hydroxide suspension which will cause constipation.

H$_2$-RECEPTOR ANTAGONISTS

One of the many actions of histamine is its role as the final common mediator of gastric acid

Table 4.10 Classification of histamine receptors.

H_1 receptor functions	H_2 receptor functions
Contraction of smooth muscle within the gastrointestinal tract Contraction of smooth muscle in the respiratory tract	Relaxation of contracted uterine smooth muscle Increased rate of contraction of cardiac muscle Stimulation of gastric acid secretion

and pepsin secretion. Antihistamines block most of the other actions of histamine but have no effect on gastric acid secretion. It was therefore postulated that there were two receptor sites: those which were blocked by the antihistamines were called H_1 receptors and those which were not, non-H_1 receptors. In 1964 Black first started to search for a compound that would block the non-H_1 receptors, and in 1972 he characterized the H_2 receptor (Table 4.10).

Black then produced the H_2-receptor antagonist burimamide followed by metiamide and finally cimetidine. Although gastric ulceration is usually associated with normal or low gastric output, the resulting reduction in acid secretion from H_2 receptor antagonist therapy is still sufficient to promote ulcer healing.

Cimetidine
Cimetidine was first introduced in 1976 and has now become the most commonly used drug in the treatment of peptic ulceration. It is estimated that by the end of 1982 it had been taken by over two million patients in 133 countries.[79] This has been made possible by the very low incidence of adverse reactions associated with its use.

Mechanism of action. Cimetidine is a histamine H_2 receptor antagonist which competitively blocks the action of histamine on the parietal cell's H_2 receptors.[29] Cimetidine causes a dose-related inhibition of gastric acid secretion. In humans normal doses of oral cimetidine (200–400 mg) cause an approximately two-thirds reduction of stimulated gastric acid secretion, whatever the stimulant. Cimetidine has a plasma half-life of approximately two hours: four doses a day are required to provide a relatively smooth 24-hour decrease of intragastric acidity (Figure 4.19). Perhaps surprisingly, a twice-daily regimen with cimetidine promotes duodenal ulcer healing despite considerable intragastric acidity in the late afternoon.[23]

Prescribing data. Initially the oral dose was 200 mg three times a day and 400 mg at night, but recently there has been a move to simplify the treatment regimen and clinical trials are now

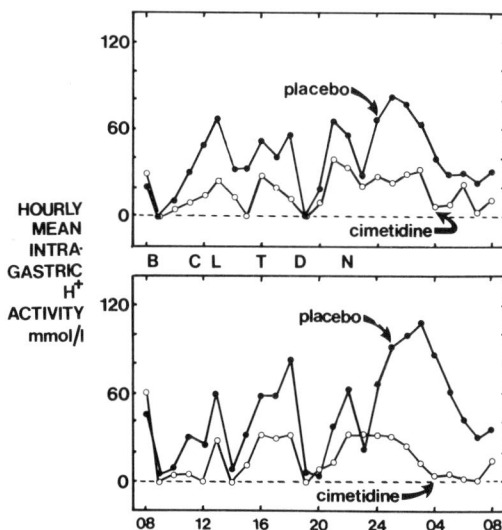

Fig. 4.19 Hourly mean intragastric acidity in duodenal ulcer patients. Cimetidine 200 mg three times a day, with 400 mg at bedtime, produces a smooth decrease of 24-hour intragastric acidity.[65] Letters indicate meals.

testing cimetidine at a dose of 400 mg twice a day. It may also be given by intramuscular or slow intravenous injection 200 mg every four to six hours with a maximum daily dosage of two grams.

Side-effects. In clinical practice cimetidine appears to be an extremely safe drug with a very low incidence of side-effects.

Burland has recently published a review of the side-effects encountered in 2182 patients treated with cimetidine for a period of between four and eight weeks, and 884 patients on placebo therapy.[12] The results are shown in Table 4.11

Table 4.11 Incidence of side-effects occurring in more than 1% of patients on short-term cimetidine therapy.[12]

Symptom	Cimetidine	Placebo
Diarrhoea	1.8%	1.0%
Tiredness	1.7%	1.6%
Dizziness	1.3%	1.0%
Drowsiness	1.3%	0.9%
Rash	1.2%	1.0%

and it can be seen that there is little difference in the overall occurrence of minor side effects between the cimetidine and placebo treated groups. Such side effects that do occur are often transient.

A further review of 1124 patients on long-term maintenance cimetidine treatment or placebo for periods up to a year were presented (Table 4.12). The reported side effects were again

Table 4.12 Incidence of side-effects of long-term cimetidine therapy.[12]

Symptom	Cimetidine	Placebo
Tiredness	3.5%	0.9%
Musculoskeletal pain	2.2%	1.3%
Rash	1.7%	0.8%
Constipation	1.5%	1.2%
Heartburn	1.1%	0.9%
Flatulence	1.1%	0.4%
Depression	1.1%	0.2%

generally mild and transient. Headache, dizziness, nausea and vomiting were more frequent among placebo treated patients than among patients treated with cimetidine. These data show that the pattern of side effects is similar to that seen during short-term therapy and that the overall incidence is low. Treatment was discontinued in only 2.1% of cimetidine treated patients because of adverse effects compared with 1.7% of placebo treated patients.[12]

Uncommon side-effects. Even though cimetidine has no H_1 receptor activity, it does bind to other receptor sites quite unconnected with the histamine system.

Cimetidine and gastric malignancy. There is no evidence that cimetidine treatment may predispose to the development of gastric malignancy.[21]

The theoretical sequence of events is that cimetidine, like ranitidine or successful gastric surgery, decreases intragastric acidity. A stomach that does not contain acid may allow bacterial proliferation in the gastric contents. Certain bacteria may act to facilitate the conversion of dietary nitrate to nitrite, which in turn could react with dietary amines to form nitrosamides and nitrosamines. In experimental animals nitroso compounds can act as topical or systemic carcinogens.

Cimetidine does not cause enough decrease of acidity in duodenal ulcer patients to allow sustained intragastric proliferation of bacteria.

Duodenal ulcer patients receiving cimetidine 1 g/day normally have only a mild shift of intragastric pH. Intragastric bacteria may survive at a pH of 4, but they only proliferate at a pH of approximately 5, or above. Physiological investigations show that neither bacteria nor nitrosamines accumulate in the cimetidine-treated stomach of patients taking a normal diet.[50]

If a decrease of intragastric acidity were associated with any risk, similar problems would be seen in patients who have received either gastric surgery or are receiving ranitidine. Treatment with cimetidine is different in only one way: cimetidine itself could theoretically be converted to nitrosocimetidine. When this substance was synthesized in the laboratory and fed to animals, there was no excess of gastric or systemic malignancy.[32]

Drug interaction. Cimetidine appears to partly inhibit the liver enzyme cytochrome P_{450}, and this can prolong the elimination of certain drugs including benzodiazepines, propranolol, warfarin, phenytoin and theophylline. Only the effect on warfarin, phenytoin and theophylline appeared to be of clinical significance, and drug dosages may need to be reduced.

Endocrine effects. It has been shown that an intravenous bolus of cimetidine will produce a transient rise in prolactin levels, but this appears to be of no clinical significance. Cimetidine has also been shown to compete with dihydrotestosterone at its binding sites, thereby causing a slight alteration in the oestrogen : testosterone ratio; this can occasionally produce gynaecomastia. In a post-marketing study undertaken in the United States 18 out of 9907 patients (0.18%) developed gynaecomastia, which resolved spontaneously once therapy was discontinued. In a double-blind placebo-controlled study in normal adult volunteers, a six-month course of cimetidine was shown to have no effect on either sperm production or the biological activity of the sperm.

Central nervous system. Reversible confusional states have been reported, usually in the elderly or already very ill patients, and are thought to be due to the action of cimetidine on undefined receptors lying within the brain tissue. Usually cimetidine does not cross the blood–brain barrier, but in uraemic, elderly or very ill patients, the blood–brain barrier may become 'leaky', and cimetidine has been found in the cerebrospinal fluid.

Cardiovascular system. It is known that H_2 receptors are present in both the heart and blood vessels, but oral cimetidine appears to have no effect on cardiovascular function either at rest or during exercise. Rapid intravenous bolus injection of cimetidine can produce an increase in pulse rate which is short-lived.

Miscellaneous side-effects. There have been occasional reports of reversible liver damage, interstitial nephritis and acute pancreatitis.

Clinical evaluation. Cimetidine has been used in more clinical trials than any other ulcer healing agent. The individual results are somewhat difficult to interpret as many of the trials have small numbers of patients and, like all gastric ulcer studies, report a very varied placebo healing rate. In two American studies in which cimetidine was found to be no more effective than placebo in healing gastric ulcers it was estimated that the average daily intake of antacids in one study was 279 mmol/day and in the other, 345 mmol/day. This high-dose antacid therapy may well have been responsible for the high placebo healing rate. Even allowing for the very varied placebo healing rate, the majority of published trials do show that cimetidine is more effective than placebo in promoting gastric ulcer healing.[55] In a recent review of the worldwide use of cimetidine, the results of eight double-blind placebo-controlled four-week healing studies and eight six-week studies are given.[79] The very varied placebo healing rate is evident: at four weeks between 20% and 78% of ulcers had healed. If, however, the results of the trials are amalgamated, after four weeks' treatment 68% of the ulcers (74 out of 109) had healed, compared with 38% (35 out of 93) in the placebo group. In the six-week assessment studies, 72% (157 out of 217) of the cimetidine-treated ulcers had healed, compared with only 43% (92 out of 215) of the placebo group.

Summary. The results from a large number of clinical studies confirm that cimetidine is both safe and an effective agent for healing gastric ulcers. It is now deservedly the standard therapy for gastric ulceration against which all other drugs must be measured for both healing rates and drug safety.

Ranitidine

Ranitidine is a new H_2 receptor antagonist which was first introduced into clinical practice in 1982 and is between five and ten times more potent than cimetidine.

Mechanism of action. Ranitidine, like cimetidine, is a histamine H_2-receptor antagonist.[10] It competitively inhibits all forms of stimulated gastric acid secretion, but it is several times more potent than cimetidine. A 150 mg dose of ranitidine is equivalent to at least 600 mg of cimetidine. Thus in terms of 24 hour intragastric acidity in duodenal ulcer patients, whereas cimetidine 1 g/day decreases acidity by raising median pH from 1.4 to 1.7, ranitidine 300 mg/day causes a more profound decrease in acidity: a median pH of 2.4 (Figure 4.20).

Ranitidine has a short plasma half-life of approximately two hours and 150 mg taken by mouth twice a day does not provide 24-hour control of intragastric acid. In the late afternoon there is a normal surge of acid secretion.[76]

Side-effects. Ranitidine appears to be a more specific competitive H_2 receptor antagonist than cimetidine and therefore has fewer side-effects. It has no effect on prolactin secretion and no anti-androgenic property. Although very small amounts do cross the blood–brain barrier, mental confusion has not been described. At therapeutic doses there is little binding of ranitidine with cytochrome P_{450} and it therefore does not alter the metabolism of such drugs as warfarin, diazepam, propranolol, phenytoin and theophylline. The adverse effects so far reported with ranitidine have been minor, and have usually resolved without having to discontinue drug therapy. Simon, Muller and Dammann compared the side-effects recorded in a group of 4532 patients treated with either ranitidine, cimetidine or placebo (Table 4.13). There was no significant difference in the incidence of side-effects between either ranitidine or cimetidine therapy and placebo.[70]

Table 4.13 Incidence of side-effects of ranitidine and cimetidine therapy.[70]

Symptom	Ranitidine (4532)	Cimetidine (908)	Placebo (1364)
Headache	1.8%	1.5%	1.8%
Tiredness	1.5%	3.5%	1.2%
Diarrhoea	1.1%	1.3%	1.2%
Constipation	0.8%	1.4%	0.7%
Rash	0.5%	0.6%	0.2%

Prescribing data. The recommended oral dose is 150 mg twice daily until ulcer healing has been achieved. It can also be given by a slow intravenous injection or infusion.

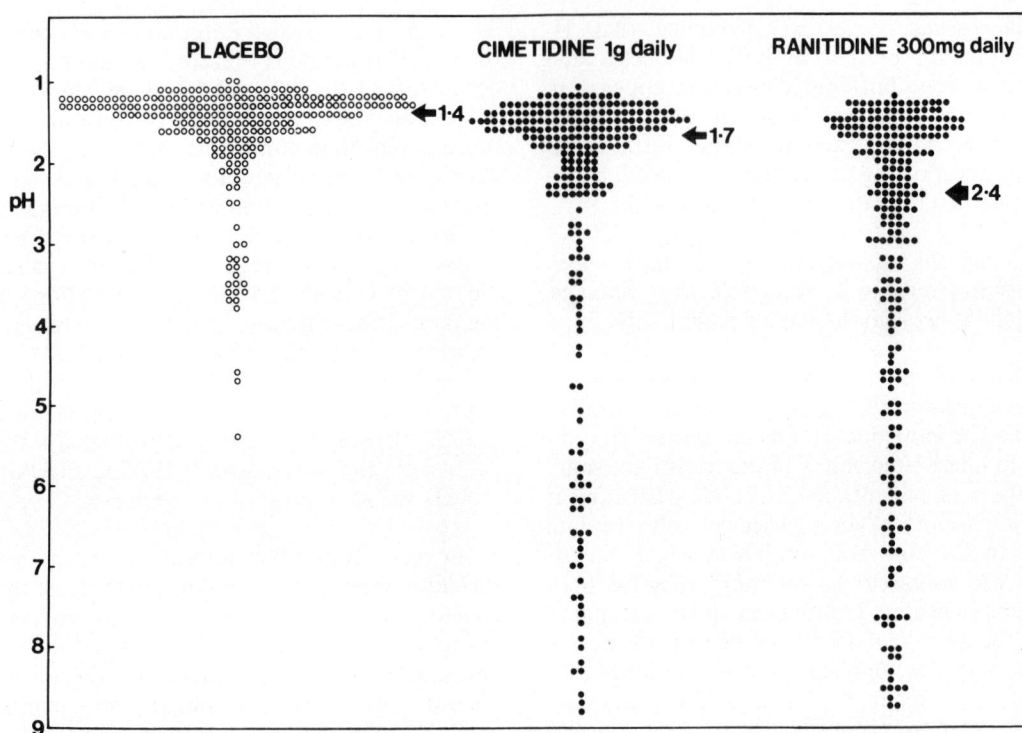

Fig. 4.20   Hourly intragastric pH in ten duodenal ulcer patients. Each patient was studied for three 24-hour periods, before and during treatment with cimetidine or ranitidine. The arrows indicate median 24-hour intragastric pH.[76]

Clinical evaluation. As ranitidine has been available for clinical trials for a relatively short time, the clinical trial data is less extensive than with cimetidine. The main studies published so far are listed in Table 4.14. Takemoto *et al.* have reported a 69% healing rate after six weeks and 87% at the end of eight weeks.[72] Ryan's double-blind placebo-controlled study was divided into three geographical areas: (a) Poland, (b) Canada, Italy and the United Kingdom and (c) Norway. Ranitidine was shown to be superior to placebo.[67]

Ashton's group from the United Kingdom also showed ranitidine to be superior to placebo.[1] Those patients with unhealed ulcers at four weeks were entered into an open study with ranitidine. At the end of a total of two months' treatment, 88% of all gastric ulcers treated with ranitidine were healed, and this rose to 97% at the end of three months.[1] In the study by Cockel's group ranitidine was compared with both cimetidine and placebo therapy.[16] Although there was a trend in favour of ranitidine, this did not reach statistical significance when compared with placebo. In the continuing Belgium multicentre study, there was no statistically significant difference between ranitidine and cimetidine therapy, but the authors state that the groups were not evenly matched for age, sex and ulcer size, and the results are therefore difficult to interpret.[5]

In a study from South Africa ranitidine and cimetidine were equally effective in producing ulcer healing.[80] It was also noted that both large ulcers and prepyloric ulcers had a lower healing rate. Barbara *et al.* have recently reported the results of an Italian multicentre study for gastric ulcers conforming to Johnson's type I classification.[2] There was no difference in healing rate between ranitidine and cimetidine.

Summary. The clinical trials to date have shown that ranitidine is both safe and effective for the treatment of gastric ulceration. Studies have shown its superiority over placebo therapy and healing rates that are very similar to those obtained for cimetidine, its main competitor. Sixty-six per cent (203/309) of all gastric ulcers are healed with ranitidine after four weeks' therapy and 85% (112/131) are healed after six weeks' treatment. Ranitidine, being a more selective H_2 receptor antagonist, has none of the potential side-effects of cimetidine, but in clinical practice this may not be very important because the incidence of such unwanted side effects are very low. The true place of ranitidine in the treatment of gastric ulcer will become clear as further clinical studies are reported.

Table 4.14 Healing rates in trials of ranitidine (150 mg twice daily) in gastric ulcer.

Authors	Ranitidine group (150 mg twice daily)						Control group						
	No. of patients	% healing at week					Treatment	No. of patients	% healing at week				
		3	4	6	8	12			3	4	6	8	
Takemoto et al. (Japan)[72]													
Pilot study	104	—	50	69	82	—	Open study						
Main study	413	—	42	69	87	—	Open study						
Ryan (Poland)[67]	44	75	—	—	—	—	Placebo	49	45	—	—	—	P < 0.01
Ryan (Canada, Italy and UK)[67]	123	—	65	—	—	—	Placebo	75	—	44	—	—	P < 0.01
Ryan (Norway)[67]	25	—	—	88	—	—	Placebo	20	—	—	20	—	P < 0.001
Ashton, Holdsworth, Ryan & Moore (UK)[1]	21	—	76	—	—	—	Placebo	17	—	29	—	—	P < 0.01
	17	—	73	—	88	97	Open study						
Cockel, Dawson & Jain (UK)[16]	14	—	71	—	79	86	Placebo	17	—	35	—	53	NS
							Cimetidine 1 g/day	16	—	63	—	75	NS
Belgian multicentre study[5]	79	—	66	83	—	—	Cimetidine 1 g/day	65	—	67	90	—	NS
Wright et al. (South Africa)[80]	32	—	58	91	—	—	Cimetidine 1 g/day	33	—	57	79	—	NS
Barbara et al. (Italy)[2]	18	—	50	—	93	—	Cimetidine 1 g/day	17	—	41	80	—	NS

PIRENZEPINE

Anticholinergics have been used in the treatment of peptic ulcer disease to produce a medical vagotomy. At a dose necessary to produce a therapeutic inhibition of acid and pepsin secretion, side-effects from the anticholinergic action at receptor sites other than the stomach become troublesome.

Mode of action. Pirenzepine is claimed to be a selective antagonist acting only on the muscarinic receptors in the stomach and so reducing unwanted side-effects. It is a complex tricyclic compound derived from the benzodiazepine group of drugs. It has hydrophilic properties, so its penetration through biomembranes is limited, and although it is rapidly absorbed only approximately a quarter of the oral dose reaches the peripheral circulation. Maximal blood levels are reached within two to three hours of oral therapy and the plasma half-life is approximately 12 hours. About 10% of circulating pirenzepine is bound to plasma proteins and this appears to be independent of drug dosage, so drug interreaction effects with more strongly bound drugs such as warfarin are unlikely. No enzyme induction or accumulation has been seen in animal experiments. The drug is metabolized to a slight extent only, and approximately 80% is excreted unchanged, mainly in the bile and only to a limited extent (10–20%) in the urine. At therapeutic doses pirenzepine reduces basal acid output by approximately a half, pentagastrin-stimulated acid secretion by a third, insulin-stimulated acid secretion by 45% and secretion stimulated by sham feeding by between 45% and 60%. Its anti-pepsin activity is said to be greater than that of the H_2 antagonists. This reduction in acid output is achieved with few of the usual side-effects associated with anticholinergic drugs.

Prescribing data. Although most clinical studies have been performed using doses of either 75 mg or 150 mg per day, a daily dose of 100 mg is now recommended. As food will reduce absorption of pirenzepine it is suggested that it is taken twice daily and at least half an hour before meals.

Side-effects. At therapeutic doses some clinical studies have reported mild problems with a dry mouth. However, it has little effect on the smooth muscle of the gut. There is an approximately 15% inhibition of oesophageal peristalsis with the patient in a recumbent position and little effect on gastric emptying, but colonic motility is reduced and in some studies patients have reported occasional problems with constipation. As the drug is hydrophilic, it does not easily pass the blood–brain barrier and is therefore unlikely to cause mental confusion. Like-

Table 4.15 Healing rates in trials of pirenzepine in gastric ulcer.

Authors	No. of patients	% healing at week				Treatment	No. of patients	% healing at week				
		4	6	8	12			4	6	8	12	
Pirenzepine 150 mg daily												
Bianchi and Dal Monte (Italy)[6]	5	—	88	—	—	Ranitidine 300 mg daily	8	—	88	—	—	NS
	15	—	73	—	—	Carbenoxolone 300 mg daily for 7 days then 150 mg daily	14	—	47	—	—	NS
Morelli, Pielli, Narducci & Spadacini (Italy)[53]	10	—	90	—	—	Placebo	10	—	40	—	—	$P < 0.05$
Ishimori & Yamagata (Japan)[38]	155	—	—	76	81	Gefarnate 300 mg daily	166	—	—	52	61	$P < 0.05$
Pirenzepine 100 mg daily												
Bown et al. (UK)[8]	6	—	50	—	—	Cimetidine 1 g daily	8	—	88	—	—	
Pirenzepine 75 mg daily												
Oselladore, Chierichetti, Norberto & Vibelli (Italy)[60]	10	60	—	—	—	Carbenoxolone 300 mg daily	9	67	—	—	—	NS
Pirenzepine 75 mg daily for 10 days then 50 mg daily												
Gasbarrini et al. (Italy)[30]	11	64	—	—	—	Carbenoxolone 300 mg daily for 10 days then 200 mg daily	11	70	—	—	—	NS

wise, it has little effect on accommodation, pupil diameter and intra-ocular pressure. Unlike other anticholinergic drugs it has been reported to decrease heart rate occasionally and has little, if any, action on bladder function.

Clinical evaluation. This is summarized in Table 4.15. There have been five clinical studies from Italy. In three studies it has been compared with carbenoxolone,[6, 30, 60] in a fourth against ranitidine[6] and in a fifth against placebo.[53] There was no significant difference between pirenzepine, carbenoxolone or ranitidine therapy, but pirenzepine was significantly better than placebo in promoting ulcer healing. Bown's group have reported preliminary results from a continuing United Kingdom study in which pirenzepine was compared with cimetidine, but at the moment numbers are too small to comment on the difference between the two drugs.[8] Ishimori from Japan in a large study found that pirenzepine produces significantly better results than gefarnate.[38]

Summary. The results from the drug trials reported so far suggest that pirenzepine will turn out to be an effective drug for the treatment of gastric ulceration but further large-scale studies are required. In spite of its selective action, some anticholinergic side-effects have been reported (a mildly dry mouth, transient blurred vision or diplopia and difficulty in micturition). The incidence of such side-effects will ultimately determine its place in the treatment of gastric ulcer disease.

TRI-POTASSIUM DI-CITRATO BISMUTHATE (COLLOIDAL BISMUTH SUBCITRATE, DE-NOL)

Mode of action. Tri-potassium di-citrato bismuthate is thought to coat the gastric mucosa with a protective mucin-like layer formed by the combination with mucoproteins. At an acid pH such as is usually found within the stomach a precipitate of bismuth oxychloride and citrate is formed; this precipitate has a special affinity for granulation tissue and forms a layer over the ulcer base, protecting it from acid and pepsin digestion. The coating action has been confirmed by a histochemical study in experimentally induced chronic gastric ulcer in rats. After histochemical staining with Castel's reagent the bismuth precipitate was found to be adherent to the ulcer base as a layer of orange-red precipitate, but it had no affinity for the adjacent normal mucosa. Finally, tri-potassium di-citrato bismuthate may also speed ulcer healing by an inhibitory effect on pepsin activity.

Prescribing data. Five millilitres of De-Nol liquid is diluted with 15 ml of water and taken 30 minutes before the three main meals, and two hours after the last meal of the day. A course of treatment usually lasts for four to eight weeks. A reformulation of De-Nol in tablet form is due to be introduced shortly. No liquids should be taken for at least half an hour before and after taking De-Nol. As the action of De-Nol depends upon acid pH within the stomach, De-Nol therapy should not be combined with an H_2 receptor antagonist or antacids.

Side-effects. The side-effects seen in clinical practice are minor but include the unpleasant ammoniacal odour and metallic taste of the liquid preparation. The newer tablet formulation is more acceptable but still produces blackening of the tongue, teeth and stools. The latter may be confused with melaena, so the patient should be warned of this when the drug is prescribed. Some patients may also complain of constipation. At therapeutic doses it is said that it is not absorbed. However, at high doses in the rat there is good evidence for its absorption and bismuth is found in many tissues including the brain. The major concern with all bismuth salts is the possibility of neurotoxicity;[11] however, this has not been observed in patients treated with short-term courses of tri-potassium di-

citrato bismuthate. Encephalopathy has been seen with bismuth subgalate and this resulted in its withdrawal from the Australian market. Serum bismuth concentrations rise during treatment with tri-potassium di-citrato bismuthate, and urinary bismuth excretion shows a profound increase during treatment which is sustained for some weeks after cessation of therapy. This accumulation of bismuth could be the reason for the reported prolonged beneficial effect of a short course of treatment.[48] It is recommended that it should be used with caution in patients with renal impairment. Because of the theoretical risks of bismuth accumulation, it has not been recommended for maintenance therapy.

Clinical evaluation. Many of the trials reporting on the use of De-Nol in gastric ulceration have been either open studies, or have contained very small numbers of patients. The main studies are listed in Table 4.16. The five studies in which De-Nol was compared with placebo all showed a statistically significant difference in favour of De-Nol. The four-week healing rates for three of these studies were remarkably high (86–90%). The two studies in which De-Nol was compared with cimetidine showed that both drugs were equally effective.

Summary. The clinical trials have shown that De-Nol is an effective drug for the treatment of gastric ulceration. An amalgamation of the results from the main clinical studies shows that 79% (100/127) of ulcers are healed after four weeks of therapy. The number of good clinical

Table 4.16 Healing rates in trials of De-Nol in gastric ulcer.

Authors	De-Nol group No. of patients	% healing at week 4	6	Control group Treatment	No. of patients	% healing at week 4	6	
Lee & Nicholson (Australia)[44]	20	90	—	Placebo	17	35	—	$P < 0.05$
Tanner, Cowlishaw, Cowen & Ward (Australia)[73]	30	—	66	Cimetidine 1 g daily	27	—	63	NS
Boyes et al. (UK)[9]	10	90	—	Placebo	10	30	—	
Sutton (UK)[71]	25	72	—	Placebo	25	36	—	$P < 0.02$
Koo, Lam & Ong (Hong Kong)[40]	24	87	—	Placebo	27	30	—	$P < 0.005$
Tytgat & van Bentem (Holland)[75]	28	61	—	Placebo	22	18	—	$P < 0.01$
				Cimetidine 1 g daily	30	43	—	NS

studies is, however, limited and further large-scale studies are required. The main problems are that it has poor palatability and that it cannot be recommended for maintenance therapy.

SUCRALFATE

Sucralfate is a basic aluminium salt of sucrose octasulphate and has little or no effect on blood coagulation.

Mode of action. In the presence of the acid pH of the stomach sucralfate becomes a highly condensed viscous adhesive substance with a low acid-neutralizing capability. This reaction with acid, however, is very slow, unlike antacids which act rapidly. However, since sucralfate adheres to the gastric mucosa, this acid-buffering capacity may still be important, because the interaction occurs close to the mucosal surface rather than in the lumen of the stomach. Experimental studies in animals using fluorescent staining techniques and ^{14}C-labelled material have demonstrated that sucralfate has an affinity for the granulation tissue at the ulcer base and forms a protective layer. Sucralfate inhibits peptic activity by direct adsorption of the enzyme itself. Bile salts are also adsorbed as well as forming insoluble bile complexes.

Prescribing data. Sucralfate is given at a dose of one gram four times a day to be taken one hour before meals and at night.

Side-effects. In a study involving 1663 patients who were treated with sucralfate, side-effects were noted in only 2.6%.[27] The only significant side-effects were constipation and nausea. Studies have shown that sucralfate is only minimally absorbed and less than 5% of the dose appears in the urine, but the manufacturers have suggested that sucralfate be used with caution in patients with renal impairment.

Clinical evaluation. The number of gastric ulcer studies is small but the main ones are shown in Table 4.17. In a study by Fixa and Komarkova ulcer healing was assessed by either radiology or endoscopy, and this is the only placebo-controlled study to report a significant difference between sucralfate and placebo.[28] In the other two placebo-controlled studies there was a trend in favour of sucralfate which with larger patient numbers might well have reached statistical significance.[59, 66] The four studies in which sucralfate was compared with cimetidine showed that both drugs were equally effective in promoting ulcer healing.[43, 47, 49, 63] The study by Pop's group from Belgium was remarkable as the four-week healing rate for sucralfate was extremely low, at 19%, but by the end of six weeks' treatment this had risen to 72%.[63]

Summary

Sucralfate appears to be safe and may be an effective drug in the treatment of gastric ulceration. After four weeks of treatment approximately 55% of all gastric ulcers are healed (58/105) and after six weeks of treatment this rises to 67% (36/54). More large-scale clinical trials are required to confirm these initial results. Sucralfate has the advantage over colloidal bismuth that it can be used for maintenance therapy.

Table 4.17 Healing rates in trials of sucralfate (four grams daily) in gastric ulcer.

| Authors | Sucralfate group (4 g daily) | | | | | Control group | | | | | |
| | No. of patients | % healing at week | | | | Treatment | No. of patients | % healing at week | | | |
		4	6	8	12			4	6	8	12	
Fixa & Komarkova (Czechoslovakia)[28]	24	71	—	—	—	Placebo	14	40	—	—	—	P < 0.05
Rhodes, Mayberry, Williams & Lowrie (UK)[66]	16	50	—	—	—	Placebo	12	17	—	—	—	NS
Orchard & Elliot (UK)[59]	13	62	—	—	—	Placebo	8	25	—	—	—	NS
Marks et al. (South Africa)[47]	27	—	63	—	88	Cimetidine 1 g daily	28	—	75	—	89	NS
Lahtinen et al. (Finland)[43]	20	48	—	82	—	Cimetidine 1 g daily	20	52	—	74	—	NS
Pop et al. (Belgium)[63]	27	19	72	—	—	Cimetidine 1 g daily	30	43	83	—	—	NS
Martin, Farley, Gagnon & Poitras (Canada)[49]	12	50	—	75	—	Cimetidine 1.2 g daily	13	54	—	77	—	NS

CARBENOXOLONE SODIUM

Carbenoxolone is derived from the hydrolysis of glycyrrhizic acid after its extraction from liquorice root and has been shown to be an effective drug for the treatment of gastric ulcer.[20]

Mode of action. Carbenoxolone is absorbed through the gastric mucosa and is excreted in the bile then reabsorbed in the small intestine. It is thought that its mode of action is in part a local one on the gastric mucosa. In patients with gastric ulceration it has been shown that there is defective synthesis and secretion of glycoproteins within the gastric mucosa. This is due to an increased epithelial-cell turnover, which shortens the time during which mucus can be synthesized and secreted. Carbenoxolone increases the lifespan of the rapidly proliferating gastric epithelial cells, leading to increased mucus production, a normalization of the mucus composition and strengthening of the mucus barrier. This, in turn, decreases the back-diffusion of hydrogen ions.

Prescribing data. Carbenoxolone sodium (Biogastrone) is usually given at a dose of 100 mg three times a day after meals for one week, then reduced to 50 mg three times a day until ulcer healing is achieved.

Side-effects. The main problem encountered with carbenoxolone therapy is salt and water retention. This occurs especially in those patients with cardiorespiratory disease and also in the elderly. Carbenoxolone is highly protein-bound. It has been shown that in the elderly plasma albumin levels fall so that the number of available binding sites is reduced. The side-effects of carbenoxolone in the elderly are thought to be caused partly by this reduced protein binding, leaving more free drug in the active unbound form and partly by reduced hepatic clearance. Carbenoxolone has also been shown to alter the binding of aldosterone to subcellular fractions of kidney tissue, and a local tissue effect therefore seems likely as the main mechanism of its aldosterone-like activity. Patients treated with carbenoxolone require careful follow-up to detect any fluid retention, congestive heart failure, hypertension and hypokalaemia.

Clinical evaluation. Many clinical trials over the years have shown that carbenoxolone is more effective than placebo in healing gastric ulcers. Table 4.18 summarizes the results of six recent studies. The two studies from the USA were not endoscopically controlled; in one carbenoxolone was shown to be superior to placebo[31] and in the other there was a trend in favour of carbenoxolone but this did not reach statistical significance.[39] In the three studies in which carbenoxolone was compared with cimetidine there was a trend in favour of cimetidine but in none of these studies did the difference reach statistical significance.[42, 61, 64] Oedema and hypokalaemia were problems in all three studies, and two of the authors have suggested that cimetidine should now replace carbenoxolone in the treatment of gastric ulcer disease.

Summary. Carbenoxolone has for many years been the drug of choice in the treatment of gastric ulceration. About 64% (58/90) of gastric

Table 4.18 Healing rates in trials of carbenoxolone in gastric ulcer

Authors	Carbenoxolone group					Control group					
	No. of patients	% healing at week				Treatment	No. of patients	% healing at week			
		4	5	6	8			4	5	6	8
Carbenoxolone 300 mg per day for one week then 150 mg daily											
Gilbert (USA)[31]	33	—	67	—	—	Placebo	36	—	44	—	—	$P < 0.05$
Lorber (USA)[45]	26	36	—	—	64	Placebo	39	33	—	—	47	NS
Schwamberger & Reissigl (Australia)[69]	20	—	—	60	—	Placebo	20	—	—	25	—	$P < 0.05$
Porro & Petrillo (Italy)[64]	26	—	—	72	—	Cimetidine 1 g daily	25	—	—	77	—	NS
Petrillo, Porro, Valentine & Dobrilla (Italy)[61]	17	—	—	77	—	Cimetidine 1 g daily	22	—	—	86	—	NS
Carbenoxolone 250 mg for one week then 200 mg daily											
La Brooy et al. (UK)[42]	27	—	—	52	—	Cimetidine 1 g daily	27	—	—	78	—	NS

ulcers can be expected to be healed after six weeks' treatment. The newer generation of drugs may not have improved the speed of ulcer healing much, but they are certainly safer to use in clinical practice and thus carbenoxolone is no longer recommended.

DEGLYCYRRHIZINIZED LIQUORICE

Deglycyrrhizinized liquorice (DGL) contains less than 3% of glycyrrhizinic acid and because of this does not have the fluid-retaining properties and risk of hypokalaemia associated with carbenoxolone.

Mode of action. Deglycyrrhizinized liquorice is thought to have the same effect as carbenoxolone on the gastric mucosa. It stimulates or accelerates the differentiation to glandular cells in the gastric mucosa as well as mucus formation and secretion. DGL has also been shown to increase gastric mucosal blood flow and so increase the ability of the gastric mucosal defence mechanisms to withstand injury.

Prescribing data. Caved-S is a compound tablet containing DGL plus a mixture of antacids including aluminium hydroxide mixture, light magnesium carbonate and sodium bicarbonate.

The dose is two tablets three times a day to be chewed between meals.

Side-effects. As DGL has no mineral corticoid-like action, Caved-S may be safely used in the elderly patient. A few patients complained of its liquorice taste and also of its mild laxative effect.

Clinical evaluation. The main studies are listed in Table 4.19. Our two trials[22, 59] and the one by Bardhan[3] were endoscopically controlled. The other studies have relied upon radiology to confirm ulcer healing. The study by Engqvist and colleagues showed a remarkably low healing rate for Caved-S and there was therefore no difference between it and placebo therapy.[26] The two studies in which Caved-S was compared with carbenoxolone showed no significant difference in healing rates. In our two studies, in which Caved-S was compared with cimetidine, the healing rates were similar. The first smaller study only contained patients over the age of 60 but in the second large study patients of all ages were included. Bardhan compared Ulcedal with placebo and could find no statistical difference.[3]

Summary. By combining the results listed in Table 4.19 it can be shown that 42% of all gastric ulcers treated are healed within four

Table 4.19   Healing rates in trials of deglycyrrhizinized liquorice (Caved-S and Ulcedal) in gastric ulcer.

Authors	Deglycyrrhizinized liquorice groups					Control group					
	No. of patients	% healing at week				Treatment	No. of patients	% healing at week			
		4	6	8	12			4	6	8	12
Caved-S											
Turpie, Runcie & Thompson (UK)[74]	16	44	—	—	—	Placebo	17	6	—	—	—	P < 0.001
Engqvist, von Feilitzen, Pyk & Reichard (Sweden)[26]	20	20	—	—	—	Placebo	18	28	—	—	—	NS
Montgomery & Cookson (UK)[52]	29	45	—	—	—	Carbenoxolone 300 mg daily for 1 week, then 150 mg/day	29	41	—	—	—	NS
Wilson (UK)[78]	20	45	—	—	—	Carbenoxolone 300 mg daily for 1 week then 150 mg/day	17	65	—	—	—	NS
Morgan *et al.* (UK)[55]	19	47	—	79	95	Cimetidine 1 g daily	20	45	—	85	100	NS
Morgan, McAdam, Pacsoo & Darnborough (UK)[56]	50	—	60	—	88	Cimetidine	50	—	66	—	94	NS
Ulcedal											
Bardhan, Cumberland, Dixon & Holdsworth (UK)[3]	42	48	—	—	—	Placebo	44	39	—	—	—	NS

weeks. This value is lower than with other ulcer healing agents, but if treatment is continued satisfactory healing rates are obtained at six, eight and 12 weeks. Caved-S has the advantage over many drugs in being remarkably free of any side-effects.

PROSTAGLANDIN THERAPY

The healing of an ulcer depends on the balance between the aggressive factors such as acid and pepsin, and the mucosal defence mechanisms. The main thrust of peptic ulcer treatment has been either to reduce acid and pepsin secretion (H_2 receptor drugs and pirenzepine) or to protect the ulcer from attack by acid and pepsin (sucralfate and colloidal bismuth). Both carbenoxolone and Caved-S strengthen the mucosal defence mechanism. Prostaglandins are naturally produced by the stomach and duodenum and appear to stimulate the mucosal defence mechanisms. These include a reduction in acid secretion, an increase in the proliferative activity of the mucosal epithelial cells, and a strengthening of the bicarbonate/mucus barrier. Clinical trials have shown that the cytoprotective action of the prostaglandins can be of use clinically in healing peptic ulcers. Oral PGE_2, which has cytoprotective actions but no acid inhibitory action, has been shown in placebo-controlled trials to promote the healing of gastric ulcers. However, synthetic analogues of PGE_2 with both cytoprotective and acid inhibitory actions are now undergoing clinical trials. If these studies show that the drugs are safe and free of side-effects then such cytoprotective agents may well play a major role in the treatment of peptic ulcer disease.

COMBINATION THERAPY

The drugs now available can heal most gastric ulcers if treatment is continued for periods ranging from 8 to 12 weeks. The speed of ulcer healing in gastric ulcer disease is, however, much slower than in duodenal ulcer disease. This raises the question of whether combination therapy, perhaps with an H_2 receptor antagonist and a drug such as carbenoxolone or deglycyrrhizinized liquorice, which will increase gastric mucosal resistance, would speed ulcer healing. The results of two such studies are shown in Table 4.20. Minoli and Terruzzi compared cimetidine with cimetidine plus carbenoxolone.[51] The study is still under way and although at the moment there is a trend in favour of combination therapy, it has not yet reached statistical significance. The second study is also still going on and gives the results at the half-way stage. Ranitidine has been compared with ranitidine plus Caved-S.[54] As can be seen, effective healing has been achieved, but with no difference between the two treatment regimens. Further work on such drug combinations is obviously required, but at the moment it looks as if any improvement in healing rates may only be marginal. Such drug combination regimens are certainly more difficult for patients to take and are more expensive.

SUMMARY OF MEDICAL TREATMENT

The H_2 receptor antagonists are the principal drugs used in the treatment of gastric ulceration. There are more clinical data supporting their use than with any other therapy. The safety profile for both cimetidine and ranitidine is good and the treatment regimens are easy to

Table 4.20   Results of combination therapy in gastric ulcer disease.

Authors	Drug	\% healing at week				
		3	4	6	8	12
Minoli *et al.* (Italy)[51]	Cimetidine 1 g daily (28 patients)	29	—	71	—	—
	v.					
	Cimetidine 1 g daily Carbenoxolone 300 mg daily for one week then 150 mg daily (28 patients)	50	—	86	—	—
Morgan, McAdam & Pacsoo (UK)[54]	Ranitidine 150 mg daily (25 patients)	—	60	—	88	92
	v.					
	Ranitidine 150 mg daily Caved-S six tablets daily (25 patients)	—	56	—	84	92

NS (Minoli study), NS (Morgan study)

follow. Time alone will show whether the more specific selectivity of ranitidine will be an advantage in clinical practice. Pirenzepine has a higher incidence of side-effects when compared with either cimetidine or ranitidine, and more clinical data is required before its place in treatment of gastric ulceration can be decided. Colloidal bismuth (De-Nol) has the disadvantage of poor palatability and a rather cumbersome treatment regimen and unlike sucralfate it cannot be used for maintenance therapy. Sucralfate appears to be a safe drug, but further large-scale trials are required, as at the moment it appears to be less effective than De-Nol or the H_2 receptor antagonists.

Carbenoxolone, because of its unpredictable and potentially serious side-effects, should no longer be used in the treatment of gastric ulcer disease. Caved-S is cheap and has an excellent safety record stretching over many years. The clinical trial data are rather sparse, but in our hands at least it appears to be as effective as cimetidine.

ULCER RECURRENCE AND MAINTENANCE THERAPY

Gastric ulcers behave rather like duodenal ulcers as approximately half of those patients in whom ulcer healing has been achieved will have a further recurrence within a period of two years – most within the first six months (Tables 4.21 and 4.22). It has also been shown that large ulcers heal more slowly and have a higher risk of subsequent relapse.

A case can be made for maintenance therapy if:
1 the gastric ulcer healed but then rapidly recurred,
2 if the patient
   (a) is over the age of 60,
   (b) has other chronic medical problems, or
   (c) will require further anti-inflammatory drug therapy.

The importance of anti-inflammatory drug therapy has been highlighted in our unit after a recent four-year study in which it was found that almost a quarter of the patients with newly diagnosed gastric ulceration were on such drug therapy at the time of initial diagnosis. These patients with drug-induced ulcers were slightly older, mainly female and had a higher risk of being admitted with acute gastrointestinal bleeding (47% compared with 16%) from a large ulcer (47% compared with 24%) (Simmonds, Acomb and Morgan, unpublished data). Similar findings were reported by Cooke and Thompson.[17]

For maintenance therapy to be a viable alternative to surgery, the following conditions are required:
a Drug therapy has to be effective.
b Long-term therapy must be safe.
c Patient compliance must be good; this requires a simple treatment regimen and a palatable drug.
d The cost of therapy must be reasonable.

Results of maintenance therapy
The main trials published so far are listed in Table 4.22. The number of good double-blind studies are few and patient numbers are often small.

Five of the placebo-controlled studies showed statistical significance in favour of either cimetidine or ranitidine,[7, 16, 34, 39, 46] and in the other two studies there was a trend in favour of active therapy, but this did not reach statistical significance.[4, 42] Porro and Petrillo also used cimetidine, at a dose of 400 mg at night, but had rather disappointing results with a 30% recurrence after a years' treatment.[64] The recurrence rate on carbenoxolone (47%) may well be no better than on placebo. From these results it would

Table 4.21 Gastric ulcer recurrence following complete ulcer healing.

| Authors | No. of patients | \% recurrence at | | | | |
		3 months	6 months	1 year	2 years	4 years
Hanscom & Buchman (USA)[33]	370	—	21	—	42	—
Piper, Shinners Greig & Thomas (Australia)[62]	83	—	—	—	28	47
Sutton (UK)[71]	29	27	31	34	41	—
Morgan, McAdam, Pacsoo & Darnborough (UK)[56]	54	—	24	33	44	—

Table 4.22 Results of maintenance studies in gastric ulcer disease.

Author	Drug/dosage	No. of patients	% recurrence rate at month			Drug/dosage	No. of patients	% Recurrence rate at month			
			6	7	12			6	7	12	
Kang, Canalese & Piper[39]	Cimetidine 400 mg twice daily	15	—	—	0	Placebo	16	33	—	47	$P < 0.02$
Birger Jensen et al.[7]	Cimetidine 400 mg twice daily	10	—	—	0	Placebo	9	—	—	44	$P < 0.025$
La Brooy et al.[41]	Cimetidine 200 mg four times a day	15	13	—	—	Placebo	14	21	—	—	NS
Machell et al.[46]	Cimetidine 1 g daily	11	—	—	18	Placebo	14	—	—	86	$P < 0.002$
Barr, Kang, Canalese & Piper[4]	Cimetidine 400 mg twice daily	24	—	8	—	Placebo	25	—	36	—	NS
Cockel, Dawson & Jain[16]	Ranitidine 150 mg at night	19	6	—	—	Placebo	20	42	—	—	$P < 0.05$
Hellier et al.[34]	Ranitidine 150 mg/100 mg at night	32	6	—	—	Placebo	12	33	—	—	$P < 0.05$
Morgan, McAdam, Pacsoo & Darborough[56]	Cimetidine 400 mg at night	41	—	—	10	Caved-S 2 tabs twice daily	34	—	—	12	NS
Porro & Petrillo[64]	Cimetidine 400 mg at night	19	—	—	37	Carbenoxolone 100 mg at night		—	—	47	NS
Classen et al.[13]	Sucralfate 1 g twice daily	30	37	—	—	Placebo	25	44	—	—	NS

seem that ulcer recurrence can be reduced by either cimetidine, ranitidine or Caved-S therapy.

Our own two-year maintenance study has shown a higher recurrence rate during the second year of treatment and a rapid recurrence once therapy is discontinued (Table 4.23). The high recurrence rate seen in patients initially treated with cimetidine suggests that if an H_2 receptor antagonist is used maintenance therapy should be for life.

Risks of long-term maintenance therapy
It is still debated whether long-term H_2 receptor antagonist therapy could result in an increased risk of gastric cancer. The alternative to such

therapy is surgery, but this still carries an increased mortality and morbidity. A partial gastrectomy may also increase the long-term risk of developing gastric cancer (5–10% after ten years).

The place of surgical treatment
The problem with a gastric ulcer is that if unhealed it may bleed or, more rarely, perforate. Furthermore, a persisting gastric ulcer may have been wrongly diagnosed as benign when in fact it is malignant. Surgical treatment should therefore always be recommended if after two courses of medical therapy the ulcer remains unhealed. Earlier consideration should be given to surgical

Table 4.23 Results of maintenance therapy with Caved-S and with cimetidine, and subsequent relapse after stopping treatment.[47]

Treatment group	% recurrence during maintenance therapy		% recurrence during first four months *off* treatment
	1st year	2nd year	
Caved-S (40 patients)	12%	20%	9% (2/22)
Cimetidine (42 patients)	10%	17%	30% (7/23)

treatment if the ulcer has previously bled or if the patient has had a past history of an ulcer causing symptoms for a long time. The indication that the ulcer might be malignant must always be borne in mind and negative biopsies or brush cytology should not lull the clinician into a false sense of security, as they may be wrong.

Summary

The results of maintenance therapy with cimetidine, ranitidine or Caved-S in gastric ulcer disease appear to be promising, but further large-scale long-term studies are required. The optimum drug dosage is at the moment unknown, as is the optimum duration of such therapy.

Surgery is recommended for those patients who develop an ulcer recurrence whilst on maintenance therapy or who develop complications.

REFERENCES

1 Ashton, M. G., Holdsworth, C. D., Ryan, F. P. & Moore, M. (1982) Healing of gastric ulcers after one, two and three months of ranitidine. *British Medical Journal*, **284**, 467–468.

2 Barbara, L., Corinaldesi, R., Porro, G. B. *et al.* (1982) Ranitidine versus cimetidine in the short treatment of gastric ulcer. *Scandinavian Journal of Gastroenterology*, **17** (supplement 78) (abstract 386) 97.

3 Bardhan, K. D., Cumberland, D. C., Dixon, R. A. & Holdsworth, C. D. (1978) Clinical trial of deglycyrrhizinised liquorice in gastric ulcer. *Gut*, **19**, 779–782.

4 Barr, G. D., Kang, J. Y., Canalese, J. & Piper, D. W. (1982) Prolonged maintenance cimetidine and gastric ulcer relapse. *Scandinavian Journal of Gastroenterology*, **17** (supplement 79) (abstract 622) 156.

5 Belgium Peptic Ulcer Study Group (1982) An interim report on a single-blind comparative study of ranitidine and cimetidine in patients with gastric ulcer. In *The Clinical Use of Ranitidine* (Ed.) Misiewicz, J. J. & Wormsley, K. G. pp. 206–214. Oxford: Medicine Publishing Foundation Symposium Series 5.

6 Bianchi, P. G. & Dal Monte, P. R. (1982) Pirenzepine for treatment of gastric ulcer. Results of two double-blind trials. *Symposium: Advances in Gastroenterology with the Selective Antimuscarinic compound Pirenzepine, Stockholm, 1982* (A48) Amsterdam, Oxford & Princeton: Excerpta Medica.

7 Birger Jensen, K., Møllmann, K. M., Rahbek, I. *et al.* (1979) Prophylactic effects of cimetidine in gastric ulcer patients. *Scandinavian Journal of Gastroenterology*, **14**, 175–176.

8 Bown, S. G., Pounder, R. E., Rampton, D. S. *et al.* (1982) Comparison of pirenzepine and cimetidine in gastric ulcer. *Symposium: Advances in Gastroenterology with the selective Antimuscarinic Compound Pirenzepine. Stockholm, 1982* (A54) Amsterdam, Oxford & Princeton: Excerpta Medica.

9 Boyes, B. E., Woolf, I. L., Wilson, R. Y. *et al.* (1975) Treatment of gastric ulceration with a bismuth preparation. *Postgraduate Medical Journal*, **51** (supplement 5), 29–31.

10 Brogden, R. N., Carmine, A. A. & Heel, R. C. *et al.* (1982) Ranitidine. *Drugs*, **24**, 267–303.

11 Buge, A., Rancunel, G. & Dechy, H. (1978) Encephalopathies bicmuthiques: données étiologiques et pharmacologiques. *Nouvelle Press Medicale*, **7**, 3531–3534.

12 Burland, W. L. (1982) *Worldwide Tagamet Experience*, pp. 141–142. Philadelphia: Smith, Kline & French International.

13 Classen, M. & Roesch, W. (1974) Gastroscopy biopsy and cytology in early detection of stomach cancer. In *Early Gastric Cancer. Current States of Diagnosis* (Ed.) Grundmann, E., Grunze, H. & Witte, S. pp. 113–117. Berlin: Springer-Verlag.

14 Classen, M., Bethge, H., Brunner, G. *et al.* (1982) Effect of sucralfate on peptic ulcer recurrence. A placebo controlled double-blind German Austrian multicentre study. *Scandinavian Journal of Gastroenterology*, **17** (supplement 78) (abstract 2212), 550.

15 Classen, M., Bethge, G., Brunner, B. *et al.* (1982) Effect of sucralfate on peptic ulcer recurrence. A placebo controlled double-blind German–Austrian multicentre study. *2nd International Sucralfate Symposium 7th World Congress of Gastroenterology, Stockholm, 1982.*

16 Cockel, R., Dawson, J. & Jain, S. (1982) Ranitidine in gastric ulceration. *Scandinavian Journal of Gastroenterology*, **17** (supplement 78) (abstract 616) 155.

17 Cooke, P. & Thompson, M. R. (1981) Old ladies, drugs and gastric ulceration. *Gut*, **22** (Abstract A) 430.

18 Doll, R. & Pygott, F. (1952) Factors in rate of healing of gastric ulcers – admission to hospital, phenobarbitone and ascorbic acid. *Lancet*, **i**, 171–175.

19 Doll, R., Jones, F. A. & Pygott, F. (1958) Effect of smoking on the production and maintenance of gastric and duodenal ulcers. *Lancet*, **i**, 657–662.

20 Doll, R., Hill, I. D., Hutton, C. & Underwood, D. J. (1962) Clinical trial of a triterpenoid liquorice compound in gastric and duodenal ulcer. *Lancet*, **ii**, 793–796.

21 Drug and Therapeutics Bulletin (1983) Cimetidine and gastric cancer. *Drug and Therapeutics Bulletin*, **21**, 65–67.

22 Dyck, W. P., Belsito, A., Fleshler, B. *et al.* (1978) Cimetidine and placebo in the treatment of benign gastric ulcer. *Gastroenterology*, **74**(2), 410–415.

23 Eckardt, V. (1981) Cimetidine: twice daily administration in duodenal ulcer – results of a European multicentre study. In *Cimetidine in the 80s* (Ed.) Baron, J. H. pp. 14–20. Edinburgh: Churchill Livingstone.

24 Edwards, F. C. & Coghill, N. F. (1968) Clinical manifestations in patients with chronic atrophic gastritis, gastric and duodenal ulcer. *Quarterly Journal of Medicine*, **37**, 337–360.

25 Englert, E., Freston, J. W., Graham, D. Y. *et al.* (1978) Cimetidine, antacid and hospitalization in the treatment of benign gastric ulcer. *Gastroenterology*, **74**, 416–425.

26 Engqvist, A., von Feilitzen, F., Pyk, E. & Reichard, H. (1973) Double-blind trial of deglycyrrhizinated liquorice in gastric ulcer. *Gut*, **14**, 711–715.

27 Fisher, R. S. (1981) Sucralfate. A review of drug tolerance and safety. *Journal of Clinical Gastroenterology*, **3** (supplement 2), 181–184.

28 Fixa, B. & Komarkova, O. (1981) Aluminium sucrose sulphate in the treatment of gastric and duodenal ulcer. In *Duodenal Ulcer, Gastric Ulcer. Sucralfate, A New Therapeutic Concept* (Ed.) Caspary, W. F. pp. 80–84. Baltimore: Urban & Schwarzenberg.

29 Freston, J. W. (1982) Cimetidine. *Annals of Internal Medicine*, **97**, 573–580 and 728–734.

30 Gasbarrini, G., Giorgi-Conciato, M., D'Anchino, M. *et al.* (1978) Pirenzepine in the treatment of benign gastroduodenal diseases. *Scandinavian Journal of Gastroenter-*

ology, **14** (supplement 57), 25–31.

31 Gilbert, J. A. L. (1976) Multicentre Canadian double-blind study of carbenoxolone (Biogastrone) in the treatment of gastric ulcer. In *North American Symposium on Carbenoxolone* (Ed.) Beck, I. T. pp. 85–92. Princeton & Amsterdam: Excerpta Medica.

32 Habs, M., Eisenbrand, G., Habs, H. & Schmähl, D. (1982) No evidence of carcinogenicity of *N*-nitrosocimetidine in rats. *Hepato-gastroenterology*, **19**, 265–266.

33 Hanscom, D. H. & Buchman, E. (1971) The Veterans Administration Co-operative Study on Gastric Ulcer: the follow-up period. *Gastroenterology*, **61**, 585–591.

34 Hellier, M. D., Gent, A. E., Walker, J. et al. (1982) Ranitidine in the treatment of gastric ulcers. Healing and maintenance. *Scandinavian Journal of Gastroenterology*, **17** (supplement 79) (abstract, 61), 155.

35 Horrocks, J. C. & de Dombal, F. T. (1975) Diagnosis of dyspepsia using data collected by a physician's assistant. *British Medical Journal*, **ii**, 421–423.

36 Horrocks, J. C. & de Dombal, F. T. (1978) Clinical presentation of patients with dyspepsia. *Gut*, **19**, 19–26.

37 Isenberg, J., Elashoff, J., Sandersfeld, M. & Peterson, W. (1982) Double-blind comparison of cimetidine and low-dose antacid versus placebo in the healing of benign gastric ulcer. *Gastroenterology*, **82**(5), 1090.

38 Ishimori, A. & Yamagata, S. (1982) Double-blind controlled study of pirenzepine on gastric ulcer and duodenal ulcer. *Symposium: Advances in Gastroenterology with the Selective Antimuscarinic Compound Pirenzepine. Stockholm, 1982* (A46) Amsterdam, Oxford & Princeton: Excerpta Medica.

39 Kang, J. Y., Canalese, J. & Piper, D. W. (1979) The use of long-term cimetidine in the prevention of gastric ulcer relapse – double-blind trial. In *Annual Science Meeting. Gastroenterology Society of Australia, Brisbane* (abstract A9).

40 Koo, J., Lam, S. K. & Ong, G. B. (1972) Tri-potassium dicitratobismuthate (De-Nol) in the treatment of gastric ulcer. *Scandinavian Journal of Gastroenterology*, **17** (supplement 78) (abstract 613), 154.

41 La Brooy, S. J., Taylor, R. H., Ayrton, C. et al. (1980) Cimetidine in the maintenance treatment of gastric ulceration. In *Hepatogastroenterology Supplement Proceedings of the 11th International Congress of Gastroenterology, Hamburg* (abstract E26 : 5).

42 La Brooy, S. J., Taylor, R. H., Hunt, R. H. et al. (1979) Controlled comparison of cimetidine and carbenoxolone in gastric ulcer. *British Medical Journal*, **i**, 1308–1309.

43 Lahtinen, J., Aukee, S., Miettinen, P. et al. (1982) Sucralfate and cimetidine for gastric ulcer. A single-blind endoscopically controlled randomized study. *2nd International Sucralfate Symposium. 7th World Congress of Gastroenterology, Stockholm, 1982.*

44 Lee, S. P. & Nicholson, G. I. (1977) Increased healing of gastric and duodenal ulcers in a controlled trial using tripotassium dicitrato-bismuthate. *Medical Journal of Australia*, **1**, 808–812.

45 Lorber, S. H. (1976) US trial of carbenoxolone (Biogastrone) in gastric ulcer. In *North American Symposium on Carbenoxolone* (Ed.) Beck, I. T. pp. 93–97. Princeton & Amsterdam: Excerpta Medica.

46 Machell, R. J., Farthing, M. J. G., Ciclitira, P. J. et al. (1979) Cimetidine in the prevention of gastric ulcer relapse. *Postgraduate Medical Journal*, **55**, 393–395.

47 Marks, I. N., Wright, J. P., Denyer, M. et al. (1980) Comparison of sucralfate with cimetidine in the short term treatment of chronic peptic ulcer. *South African Medical Journal*, **57**, 567–573.

48 Martin, D. F., May, S. J., Tweedle, D. E. F. et al. (1981) Difference in relapse rate of duodenal ulcer after healing with cimetidine or tri-potassium di-citrato bismuthate. *Lancet*, **i**, 7–10.

49 Martin, F., Farley, A., Gagnon, M. & Poitras, P. (1982) Comparative healing capacity of sucralfate and cimetidine in short term treatment of peptic ulcer. A double-blind randomized study. *Scandinavian Journal of Gastroenterology*, **17** (supplement 78) (abstract 2207), 548.

50 Milton-Thompson, G. J., Lightfoot, N. F., Ahmet, Z. et al. (1982) Intragastric acidity, bacteria, nitrate and *N*-nitroso compounds before, during and after cimetidine treatment. *Lancet*, **i**, 1091–1095.

51 Minoli, G., Terruzzi, V., Ferrara, A. et al. (1982) The association of cimetidine and carbenoxolone in the treatment of gastric ulcer. *Scandinavian Journal of Gastroenterology*, **17** (supplement 78) (abstract 401), 101.

52 Montgomery, R. D. & Cookson, J. B. (1972) The treatment of gastric ulcer. *Clinical Trials Journal*, **9**(1), 33–36.

53 Morelli, A., Pelli, A., Narducci, F. & Spadacini, A. (1979) Pirenzepine in the treatment of gastric ulcer. *Scandinavian Journal of Gastroenterology*, **14** (supplement 57), 51–55.

54 Morgan, A. G., McAdam, W. A. F. & Pacsoo, C. (1983) A double-blind controlled trial of combination therapy in the treatment of gastric ulcer. In preparation.

55 Morgan, A. G., McAdam, W. A. F., Pacsoo, C. et al. (1978) Cimetidine: an advance in gastric ulcer treatment? *British Medical Journal*, **ii**, 1323–1326.

56 Morgan, A. G., McAdam, W. A. F., Pacsoo, C. & Darnborough, A. (1982) Comparison between cimetidine and Caved-S in the treatment of gastric ulceration, and subsequent maintenance therapy. *Gut*, **23**, 545–551.

57 Morris, T. & Rhodes, J. (1979) Progress report. Antacids and peptic ulcer – a reappraisal. *Gut*, **20**, 538–545.

58 Mountford, R. A., Brown, P., Salmon, P. R. et al. (1980) Gastric cancer detection in gastric ulcer disease. *Gut*, **21**, 9–17.

59 Orchard, R. & Elliot, C. (1981) A double-blind placebo controlled study of sucralfate in the treatment of gastric ulcer. In *Duodenal Ulcer, Gastric Ulcer. Sucralfate, A New Therapeutic Concept* (Ed.) Caspary, W. F. pp. 85–88. Baltimore: Urban & Schwarzenberg.

60 Osalladore, D., Chierichetti, S. M., Norberto, L. & Vibelli, C. (1979) Pirenzepine in severe duodenal ulcer and in gastric ulcer. *Scandinavian Journal of Gastroenterology*, **14** (supplement 57), 33–39.

61 Petrillo, M., Porro, G. B., Valentine, M. & Dobrilla, G. (1979) Cimetidine and carbenoxolone sodium in the treatment of gastric ulcer. An open study. *Current Therapeutic Research*, **26**(6), 990–994.

62 Piper, D. W., Shinners, J., Greig, M. et al. (1978) Effect of ulcer healing on the prognosis of chronic gastric ulcer. *Gut*, **19**, 419–424.

63 Pop, P., Nikkels, R. E., Dorrestein, G. C. M. et al. (1982) A study of the comparative healing rates of sucralfate and cimetidine in a short term treatment of duodenal and gastric ulcers. A single-blind randomized controlled Dutch–Belgian multicentre study. *2nd International Sucralfate Symposium. 7th World Congress of Gastroenterology, Stockholm, 1982.*

64 Porro, G. B. & Petrillo, M. (1979) Short and long treatment of gastric ulcer – a controlled trial comparing cimetidine and carbenoxolone sodium. In *Second National Symposium on Cimetidine Brussels, 1979* (Ed.) Dresse, A. 161–170. Amsterdam: Excerpta Medica.

65 Pounder, R. E., Williams, J. G., Milton-Thompson, G. J. & Misiewicz, J. J. (1975) Twentyfour-hour control of

intragastric acidity by cimetidine in duodenal ulcer patients. *Lancet*, **ii**, 1069–1070.

66 Rhodes, J., Mayberry, J. F., Williams, R. A. & Lowrie, B. W. (1981) Clinical trial of sucralfate in the treatment of gastric ulcer. In *Duodenal Ulcer, Gastric Ulcer. Sucralfate, A New Therapeutic Concept.* (Ed.) Caspary, W. F. pp. 101–104. Baltimore: Urban & Schwarzenberg.

67 Ryan, F. P. (1982) A comparison of ranitidine and placebo in the acute treatment of gastric ulcer. In *The Clinical Uses of Ranitidine (Proceedings of the Second International Symposium on Ranitidine)* (Ed.) Misiewicz, J. J. & Wormsley, K. G. pp. 201–206. Oxford: Medicine Publishing Foundation.

68 Schulman, A. & Simkins, K. C. (1975) The accuracy of radiological diagnosis of benign primary and secondary malignant ulcers and their correlation with three simplified radiological types. *Clinical Radiology*, **26**, 317–325.

69 Schwamberger, K. & Reissigl, H. (1980) Carbenoxolone patients with gastric ulcer. In *Carbenoxolone Symposium, 11th International Congress of Gastroenterology, Hamburg* (Ed.) Sir Avery Jones, Hunt, T. C. & Reed, P. I. *Scandinavian Journal of Gastroenterology*, **15** (supplement 65) 59–60.

70 Simon, B., Muller, P. & Dammann, H. G. (1982) Safety profile of ranitidine. *Scandinavian Journal of Gastroenterology*, **17** (supplement 78) (abstract 359), 90.

71 Sutton, D. R. (1982) Gastric ulcer healing with tripotassium dicitrato-bismuthate and subsequent relapse. *Gut*, **23**, 621–624.

72 Takemoto, T., Okita, K., Namiki, M. *et al.* (1982) Clinical studies on gastric ulcer in Japan – pilot and extended open studies. In *The Clinical Uses of Ranitidine (Proceedings of the Second International Symposium on Ranitidine)* (Ed.) Misiewicz, J. J. & Wormsley, K. G. pp. 222–231. Oxford: Medicine Publishing Foundation.

73 Tanner, A. R., Cowlishaw, J. L., Cowen, A. E. & Ward, M. (1979) Efficacy of cimetidine and tri-potassium dicitrato-bismuthate (De-Nol) in chronic gastric ulceration. *Medical Journal of Australia*, **1**, 1–2.

74 Turpie, A. G. G., Runcie, J. & Thompson, T. J. (1969) Clinical trial of deglycyrrhizinised liquorice in gastric ulcer. *Gut*, **10**, 199–302.

75 Tytgat, G. N. & van Bentem, N. (1982) Double-blind study with colloidal bismuth subcitrate, cimetidine and placebo in the treatment of gastric ulcer. *De-Nol Symposium, 7th World Congress of Gastroenterology, Stockholm, 1982.*

76 Walt, R. P., Male, P. J., Rawlings, J. *et al.* (1981) Comparison of the effects of ranitidine, cimetidine and placebo on the 24-hour intragastric acidity and nocturnal acid secretion in patients with duodenal ulceration. *Gut*, **22**, 54–59.

77 Walt, R. P., Gomes, M. de F. A., Wood, E. C. *et al.* (1983) Profound decrease of 24-hour intragastric acidity by daily oral omeprazole. *British Medical Journal*, **287**, 12–14.

78 Wilson, J. A. C. (1972) A comparison of carbenoxolone sodium and deglycyrrhizinated liquorice in the treatment of gastric ulcer in the ambulant patient. *British Journal of Clinical Practice*, **26**(12), 563–566.

79 *Worldwide Tagamet Experience*. Philadelphia: Smith, Kline & French International. pp. 62–75.

80 Wright, J. P., Marks, I. N., Mee, A. S. *et al.* (1982) Ranitidine in the treatment of gastric ulcer disease. In *The Clinical Uses of Ranitidine (Proceedings of the Second International Symposium on Ranitidine)* (Ed.) Misiewiez, J. J. & Wormsley, K. G. pp. 214–221. Oxford: Medicine Publishing Foundation.

Surgical treatment

While controversy still surrounds the best surgical procedure to perform for duodenal ulcer most surgeons regard Billroth I gastrectomy as the most satisfactory operation for patients with gastric ulcer. This is partly because of the reported results of gastrectomy[37] and partly because few surgeons deal with enough cases to evaluate any alternative procedures fully. Here, the various alternative procedures that have been used to treat gastric ulceration will be discussed, with a review of their rationale and results. Before doing so it is important to define the 'types' of gastric ulcer that occur.

Johnston suggested that gastric ulcers should be subdivided into three types (Figure 4.21):[21]

Type I A chronic ulcer situated proximal to the gastric angulus (incisura) without any macroscopic evidence of duodenal, pyloric or prepyloric abnormality.

Type II A chronic ulcer proximal to the gastric angulus associated with an ulcer or scar of the duodenum or pylorus.

Type III A chronic ulcer occurring in the prepyloric area (within 3 cm of the pylorus) with or without associated duodenal ulceration or scarring or a type I gastric ulcer.

Johnston showed a difference between these types of ulcer with respect to (a) the patient's 12-hour and over-night secretion, (b) blood groups and (c) physical characteristics; he therefore suggested that they might need to be treated differently from one another.[22] Using a combined pentagastrin/insulin secretion test with estimate of loss we have found a variation in acid and pepsin output between individual patients which far outweighs any differences between the three types (Figure 4.22). We therefore doubt the wisdom of deciding the method of surgical treatment entirely on the basis of gastric ulcer type. This scepticism is borne out by the poor results that have been reported when type III ulcers are treated by proximal gastric vagotomy.[1]

INDICATIONS FOR SURGERY

The indications for surgical therapy have been refined by fibre-optic endoscopy, which has enabled repeat examinations of the ulcer with biopsy to be performed, and by more effective medical therapy.

Failure to heal the ulcer
Ulcer healing is of particular importance in gastric ulceration. This is because gastric ulcers

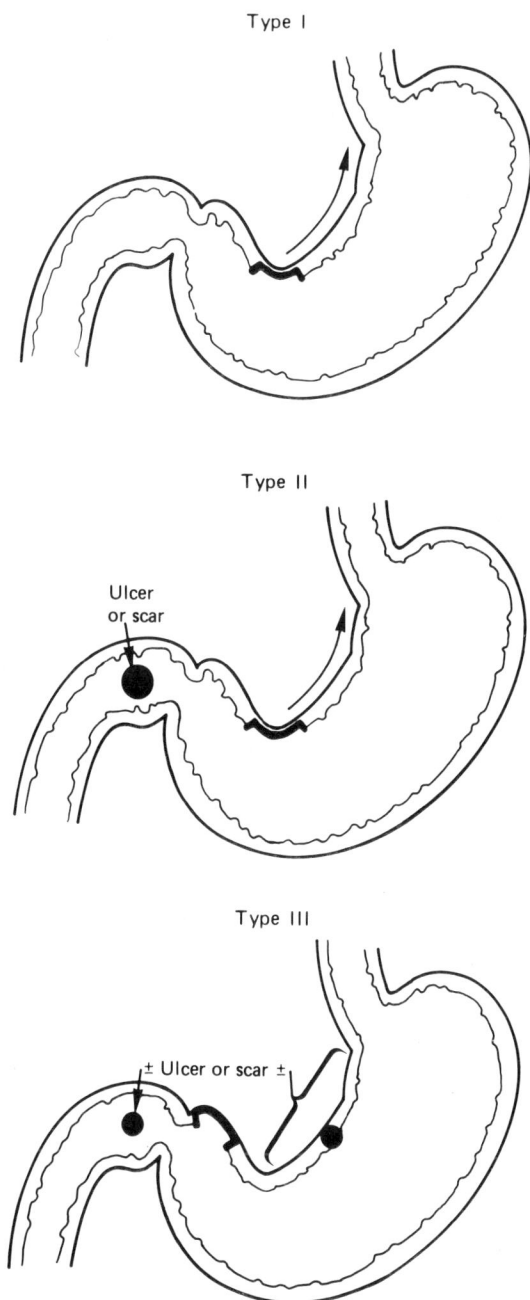

Type I

Type II

Ulcer
or scar

Type III

± Ulcer or scar ±

Fig. 4.21 Types of gastric ulcer as described by Johnston (arrows indicate area where ulcer may occur).

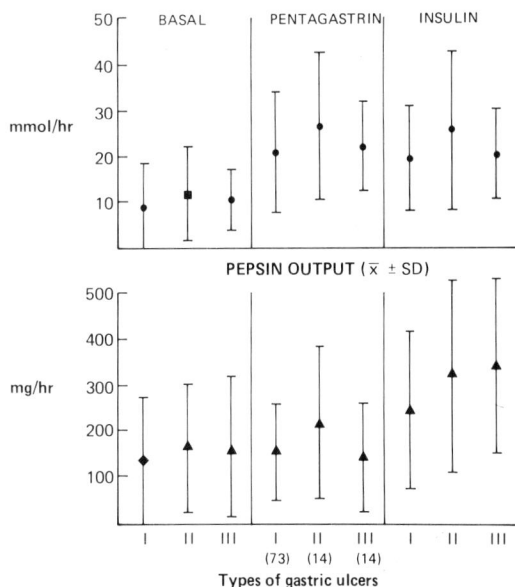

Fig. 4.22 Mean basal, pentagastrin- and insulin-stimulated acid and pepsin outputs ($\pm$ standard deviation) recorded in 73 type I, 14 type II and 14 type III gastric ulcer patients studied in Newcastle.

ulcer that has remained unhealed on endoscopic examination for a period of over three months on an effective medical therapy (usually an H_2 receptor antagonist).

Failed 'long-term control'
As with all chronic peptic ulcers gastric ulcers have a tendency to recur. We have found that these recurrences are more often asymptomatic than those in duodenal ulceration. We have therefore adopted the policy of placing all gastric ulcer patients upon 'maintenance' therapy with H_2 receptor antagonists. Results of therapy are monitored by repeat endoscopic examinations if symptoms recur or, if asymptomatic, after six months and then annually. This regimen has the advantages of detecting asymptomatic recurrences and checking the benign nature of the ulcer. Surgery is recommended if long-term control with such 'maintenance' therapy is ineffective.

Side effects or poor compliance
Operation is sometimes indicated if the patient is an erratic taker of medications or has serious side-effects that prevent successful control of the gastric ulcer.

Complications of gastric ulcer
These include perforation, haemorrhage and severe fibrosis. Their management will be discussed elsewhere.

are more likely to bleed than duodenal ulcers, they often occur in an older age group, who tolerate complications less well, they may be misdiagnosed and they can undergo malignant change. In addition, our own studies of long-term medical treatment have shown that gastric ulcers are more likely to remain 'asymptomatic' even when unhealed. For this reason we advise surgical treatment for any patient with a gastric

Suspected malignancy/dysplasia

All gastric ulcers should be regarded as malignant until proved otherwise. For this reason patients on medical therapy should have regular and multiple biopsies of the ulcer base and edges to exclude malignant changes. Should a biopsy show severe dysplasia or malignant change then operation should be recommended.

Social reasons

There are some patients for whom, because of their occupation or place of abode, it is safer to perform an operation than to embark upon a long period of medical treatment.

RATIONALE OF SURGICAL THERAPY

The surgeon has a very limited range of options for therapy: either the physiological control of gastric secretion can be altered or varying amounts of stomach can be resected, affecting secretion and removing potentially abnormal mucosa.

Gastric ulceration occurs when the balance between the erosive properties of gastric juice and the mucosa's intrinsic ability to resist digestion is altered. The surgeon can influence this balance by reducing the gastric secretion or by removing diseased mucosa.

Alteration of the physiological control of secretion

Vagotomy. This will reduce the neural control of acid secretion by reducing the amount of acetylcholine released from submucosal nerve endings in response to central stimulation. It also reduces the parietal and chief cells' sensitivity to other stimuli. Vagotomy reduces 'basal' acid secretion and the response of the stomach to external stimuli such as pentagastrin. Division of the vagal nerves at the oesophageal hiatus (truncal vagotomy) also involves denervation of the remainder of the intestinal and pancreatico-biliary systems, which results in side-effects. Antral denervation impairs gastric emptying and removes any vagal stimulation of gastrin release from the antral mucosa. Proximal gastric vagotomy (parietal cell vagotomy or highly selective vagotomy) divides only the nerve supply to the secretory mucosa and is without these effects, reducing the incidence of dumping, diarrhoea and bile vomiting.

Antrectomy. Gastrin is mainly produced by the antral mucosa, so removal of this mucosa by antrectomy significantly reduces the amount

available. Dragstedt proposed that gastric ulceration was caused by impaired gastric emptying resulting in an increased release of gastrin and thus causing acid hypersecretion. While this theory may explain occasional cases of gastric ulceration (for example, a gastric ulcer associated with pyloric stenosis), it has not been confirmed by investigation in most gastric ulcer patients.

Removal of diseased mucosa

There are several reasons for believing that the antral mucosa is abnormal or damaged in gastric ulceration. Severe chronic gastritis is present in the mucosa of the antrum and lesser curve in many patients with gastric ulceration. The extent of these changes appears to be related to the site of the gastric ulcer and they frequently persist even when the ulcer is healed. Hence, these changes are 'primary' and not 'secondary' to the ulcer. The cause of these changes is not established with certainty, but the most popular theory is that they are due to 'bile reflux'. Gastric ulceration is associated with increased amounts of bile in the gastric lumen[9, 33] and duodenal reflux is frequently observed during radiological investigation.[4] Furthermore, gastric mucosa affected by chronic gastritis is more liable to ulceration.[34] For these reasons the surgeon should try to reduce or eliminate bile reflux after operative treatment.

Recent studies have shown that the mucus lining the surface of the antral mucosa is mainly of an incomplete molecular form.[40] The gastric mucus in gastric ulcer patients provides a poor defence against autodigestion as its viscosity is reduced and it lacks the normal structural integrity. Measurements of the electrical potential resistance and hydrogen ion loss from the lumen also indicate that the gastric mucosa in gastric ulcer patients is less resistant to autodigestion. It is likely that the antral mucosa of patients with gastric ulceration is diseased and it is logical that the patients might benefit from its removal.

TYPES OF OPERATION (Figure 4.23)

Gastric resection only

Billroth I gastrectomy. This remains the most popular operation for gastric ulcer. There is still no agreement about how much of the stomach should be resected; good results have been reported when only 3–4 cm of antrum have been removed.[28] However, most surgeons believe that the whole of the antral mucosa, including the ulcer crater, should be removed, preserving the latter situation the use of a 'Pauchet manoeuvre', in which the ulcer is excised with a narrow tongue of the lesser curvature, may avoid sacrifice of an excessive amount of the stomach with the risk of long-term metabolic sequelae.[14] Following resection a new lesser curvature is constructed and an end-to-end anastomosis between the gastric remnant and the duodenum is then performed.

Billroth II (Polya) gastrectomy. Few surgeons would perform this procedure in gastric ulceration from choice. It is usually done because the gastric remnant is too small to reach the duodenum without tension or because the duodenum is severely distorted by previous ulceration or surgery. The major disadvantage of this procedure is the increased amount of bile reflux that is an inevitable consequence. Excessive bile reflux is undesirable in gastric ulcer disease as it can cause 'bile vomiting' and, possibly, an increased risk of malignancy.

Pylorus-preserving gastrectomy. This procedure was first described by Maki *et al.*[27] The operation is performed in a similar way to a Billroth I gastrectomy; the principal difference is that the pylorus plus 1.5 cm of antrum is preserved. It is clearly not an appropriate operation for type III ulcers but has been used for type I ulcers with good long-term results.[36]

Vagotomy and excision of ulcer (Figure 4.24)
There is now wide agreement that if vagotomy is to be used to treat gastric ulceration then it must be combined with total excision of the ulcer as well. At one stage it was thought that four-quadrant biopsy of the ulcer was sufficient, but follow-up studies have shown that there is still a risk of missing an early gastric carcinoma with this technique and that total excision is safer. Various techniques for excision of the ulcer have been described either using a transgastric approach[5] or external excision with various manoeuvres to prevent excessive narrowing around the oesophageal hiatus.[42]

Truncal vagotomy and drainage. This is performed in an identical manner to that for duodenal ulceration, the only addition being excision of the ulcer. Theoretically, pyloroplasty should be used as the drainage procedure rather than gastroenterostomy as there is less bile reflux.

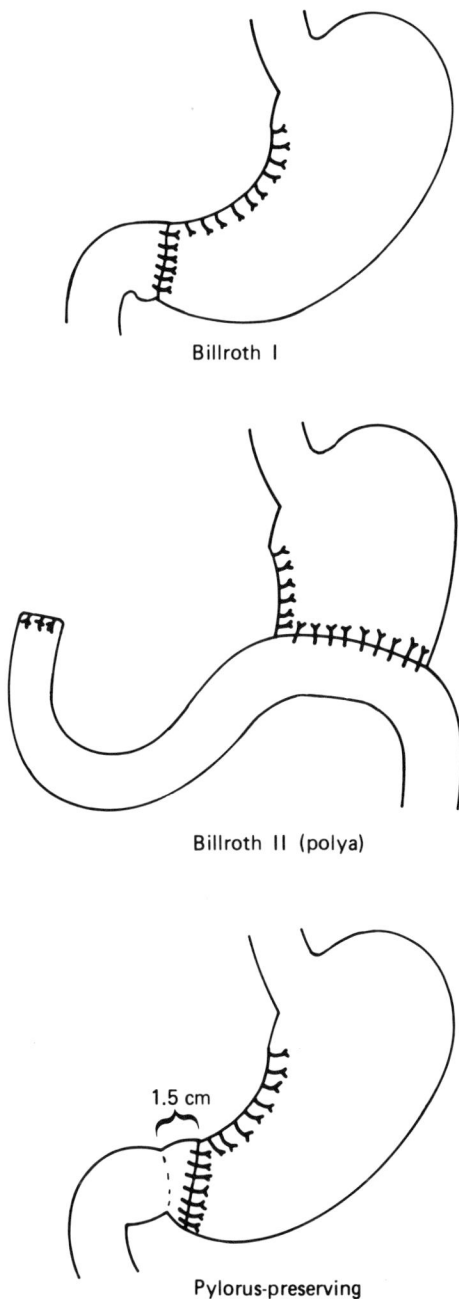

Fig. 4.23 Diagrammatic representation of types of gastric resection used in gastric ulcer management.

as much of the body mucosa as possible. Jensen *et al.* suggested that intraoperative testing to establish that all the antral mucosa had been resected would lead to improved results and that ulcer recurrence could be completely avoided.[17] When the ulcer is situated in the middle of the lesser curvature resection is relatively straightforward, but it can become very difficult when the ulcer is close to the oesophageal hiatus. In

Truncal vagotomy +
pyloroplasty +
ulcer excision

Proximal gastric vagotomy +
ulcer excision

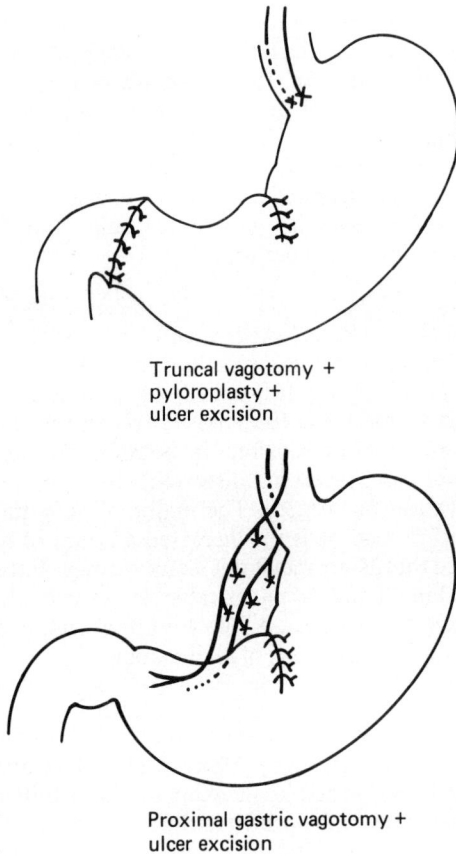

Fig. 4.24 Diagrammatic representation of vagotomy procedures used in gastric ulcer management.

Proximal gastric vagotomy. In gastric ulceration this procedure is complicated by the amount of scarring and oedema that may be present in the lesser omentum. Johnston *et al.* suggested that the lesser curve dissection should start at the site of the ulcer rather than at the point where the nerve of Latarget crosses the antrum.[19] They have reported good results using this technique,[19] but have cautioned that although the incidence of side-effects is low there is an increased risk of lesser curve necrosis when this operation is used to treat gastric ulcer and a higher mortality than after Billroth I gastrectomy.[12]

RESULTS OF OPERATION

The ideal operation would be one that offered certain 'cure' of the gastric ulcer without any operative mortality risk and with no short-term or long-term side-effects. Obviously no operation can fully match all these objectives.

Type I gastric ulcer
These are the commonest form of gastric ulcer and, therefore, their response to treatment is the best-known. For these patients the principal choice lies between gastric resection and some form of vagotomy with ulcer excision.

Clearly, the best way of identifying the best operation is by surgical 'controlled trials', where patients are randomly allocated to one or other procedure. Three such trials have been published (Table 4.24), two using truncal vagotomy and pyloroplasty and one using proximal gastric vagotomy. Unfortunately, these trials include relatively small numbers of patients and it is, therefore, necessary to turn to other large series, where only one operation has been tried, for further evidence.

These studies show that Billroth I gastrectomy is the better curative operation for type I gastric ulcers but carries twice the operative mortality of vagotomy.

Type II gastric ulcer
The incidence of this type of ulcer varies from 15% to 25% of all gastric ulcers. They usually occur in a younger age group, have a higher male-to-female ratio and have many of the clinical features of duodenal ulcer patients.[7] For these reasons it has been argued that ulcers should be treated by the same surgical procedures as are used for duodenal ulceration, the only difference being the need to excise the gastric ulcer for histological examination. Patients with these ulcers seem to respond much better to vagotomy than those with type I ulcers (Table 4.25).

Type III gastric ulcer
At one stage it was argued that these ulcers were but a variant of duodenal ulceration and should, therefore, be treated in an identical manner. Over the last few years there has been increasing evidence that this is not the case. Firstly, it is recognized that prepyloric ulcers seem to respond differently to treatment with H_2 receptor antagonists. In our studies we have had several patients where duodenal ulcers have been seen in association with prepyloric ulcers and while the duodenal ulcer has healed on cimetidine therapy the gastric ulcer has not. Secondly, it has been shown that prepyloric ulcers are particularly liable to recur after treatment by proximal gastric vagotomy (Table 4.26).

The best operation for type III gastric ulcers is still unresolved. My own practice is to treat such ulcers by Billroth I gastrectomy and to add

Table 4.24   Results of surgery for type I[a] gastric ulcer.

Authors	Number of patients	Mortality (%)	Recurrence (%)
Billroth I gastrectomy			
Salzer[35]	631	4	2
Hollender et al.[16]	228	3	0
Nielsen et al.[31]	97	6	5
Pichlmayr et al.[32]	109	0.7	5
Thomas et al.[37]	144	0.7	3.5
Madsen et al.[26]	**20**[b]	**4**	**0**
Duthie & Kwong[11]	**50**[b]	**0**	**4**
Duthie & Bransom[10]	**30**[b]	**0**	**7**
Totals	1309	4	2
Truncal vagotomy and pyloroplasty			
Kronborg[24]	123	2	13
Kraft et al.[23]	103	3	5
De Miguel[28]	73	0	19
Eastman & Gear[13]	58	0	8
Cade & Allen[3]	65	4	4.5
Madsen et al.[26]	**23**	**0**	**13**
Duthie & Kwong[11]	**50**	**0**	**10**
Proximal gastric vagotomy			
Duthie & Bransom[10]	**26**	**0**	**15**
Johnston & Axon[18]	104	1	5
Muller[30]	52	5	4
Totals	677	2	9

[a] Johnston's classification: see text.[21]
[b] Randomized controlled trial.

Table 4.25   Results of surgery for type II[a] gastric ulcer.

	Number of patients	Type of operation	Recurrence
Kronborg[24]	16	Truncal vagotomy and pyloroplasty	0
Johnston et al.[19]	25	Proximal gastric vagotomy	0
Pichlmayr et al.[32]	16	Billroth I gastrectomy	7%
Pichlmayr et al.[32]	5	Proximal gastric vagotomy	20%
Douglas & Duthie[7]	39	Truncal vagotomy and pyloroplasty	0

[a] Johnston's classification: see text.[21]

Table 4.26   Results of surgery for type III[a] gastric ulcer.

	Number of patients	Type of operation	Recurrence
Anderson et al.[1]	59	Proximal gastric vagotomy	22%
Becker & Siewert[2]	40	Proximal gastric vagotomy	20%
Pichlmayr et al.[32]	15	Billroth I gastrectomy	0
Pichlmayr et al.[32]	32	Proximal gastric vagotomy	25%
Kronborg[24]	78	Truncal vagotomy and pyloroplasty	6%

[a] Johnston's classification: see text.[21]

truncal vagotomy if there is an associated active duodenal ulcer or secretion studies shows a high acid and pepsin secretion.

COMPARISON OF SIDE-EFFECTS

Short-term effects

As far as the immediate postoperative period is concerned vagotomy is superior to gastrectomy. In all controlled trials there were significantly more complications in the gastrectomy group. These included postoperative bleeding, anastomotic dehiscence and hold-up, intra-abdominal sepsis and pulmonary embolus.

After discharge from hospital, the vagotomy patients fair slightly worse as temporary dysphagia and diarrhoea occur more often after vagotomy than after gastrectomy. However, after gastrectomy there is an increased risk of vomiting.

Medium-term effects

These include such well-recognized side-effects as dumping, vomiting, diarrhoea and heartburn. For the last 15 years our group has run a regular gastric surgery follow-up clinic. We have compared the results following Billroth I gastrectomy for gastric ulcer (Figure 4.25) with those in duodenal ulcer patients after truncal

vagotomy and pyloroplasty. Symptoms seldom occur in more than 15% of patients at any interval of follow-up after Billroth I gastrectomy. There is also a tendency for many of these symptoms to become less common with time.[38]

Our findings do seem to parallel those found in the 'controlled trials', where there was no significant difference between the clinical results of Billroth I gastrectomy and those of vagotomy and pyloroplasty for gastric ulcer.[11, 26]

We have not attempted to use the popular Visick grading system in our studies, believing like Hall *et al.*[15] that it is too subjective. However, it is our impression that patients are far happier after Billroth I gastrectomy than after vagotomy and pyloroplasty. This view is also supported by the study of Thomas *et al.*, who showed that 84% of their patients fell into Visick 1 and 2 at a mean follow-up period of 9.4 years after Billroth I gastrectomy.[37]

Finally, mention should be made of pylorus-preserving gastrectomy (the Maki operation), as it has been claimed that this operation removes some of the problems associated with loss of the pyloric sphincter (for example, dumping).[36] Unfortunately, only a few other groups have attempted this operation,[25, 41] so there is insufficient evidence on which to evaluate this operation at present.

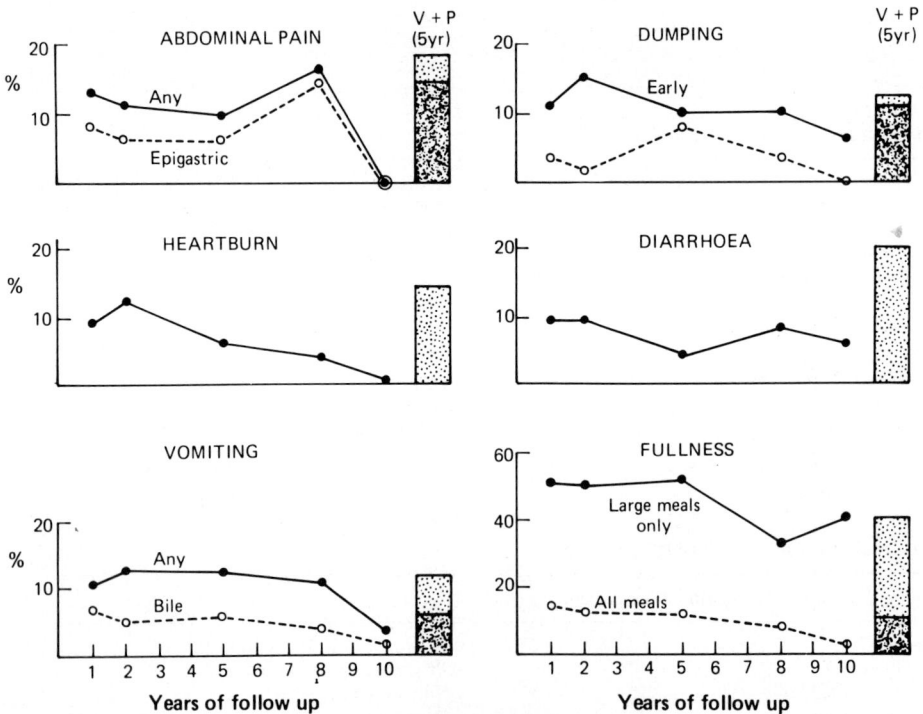

Fig. 4.25 Prospective symptomatic results recorded in our gastric follow-up clinic in 99 patients treated by Billroth I gastrectomy for chronic gastric ulcer (28 followed up for at least 10 years). Results are compared with incidence of the same symptoms following vagotomy and pyloroplasty at five-year follow-up.

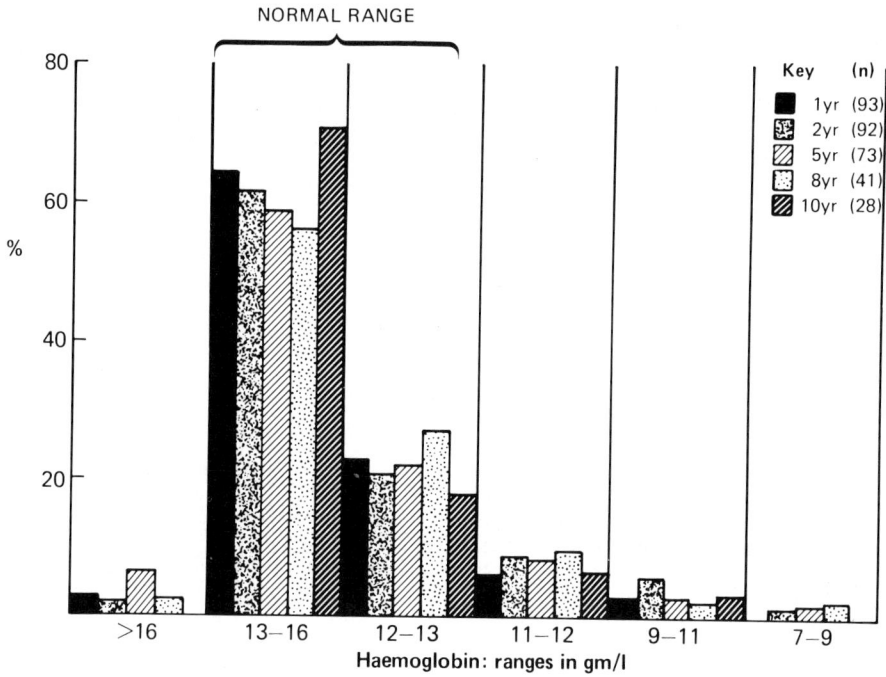

Fig. 4.26 Analysis of results of haemoglobin measurements in our prospective studies of Billroth I gastrectomy. Results are expressed as the percentage of patients whose haemoglobin falls within the defined ranges at each follow-up interval.

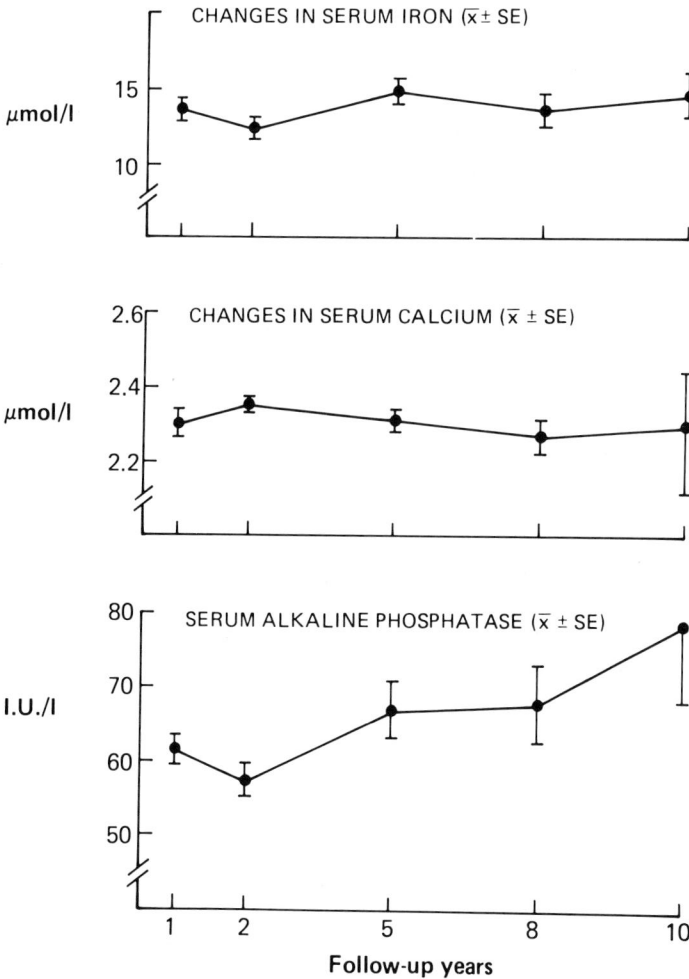

Fig. 4.27 Mean ± standard error of serum iron, calcium and alkaline phosphatase at each follow-up interval in our prospective studies of Billroth I gastrectomy for gastric ulcer.

Long-term effects

Surprisingly, there are few studies of the long-term results of gastric surgery for gastric ulcer. A recent one is that of Thomas *et al.*, who reviewed 144 patients treated previously by Billroth I gastrectomy at a mean follow-up interval of 9.4 years (range 3–15 years).[37] They reported that there was little evidence of any serious metabolic consequences. The patients weight had risen by an average of 4.4 kg over their pre-operative weights and only 8% of the patients had haemoglobin levels below 120 g/l. In addition, biochemical assessment failed to reveal any evidence of metabolic bone disease.

These findings are supported by our own prospective data (Figures 4.26 and 4.27). There is no evidence in our studies that there is any increase in the incidence of anaemia or any fall in serum iron. In addition, the small rise in alkaline phosphatase is less marked than we have previously recorded after vagotomy and pyloroplasty for duodenal ulceration.[39]

REFERENCES

1 Andersen, D., Høstrup, H. & Amdrup, E. (1978) Aarhus County Vagotomy Trials II: an interim report on reduction in acid secretion and ulcer recurrence following parietal cell vagotomy and selective gastric vagotomy. *World Journal of Surgery*, **2**, 91–100.

2 Becker, H. D. & Siewert, J. R. (1980) Advances in ulcer disease. In *Excerpta Medica* (Ed.) Holtermuller, K. H. & Malagelada, J. R. pp. 516–526.

3 Cade, D. & Allan, D. (1979) Long term follow-up of patients with gastric ulcers treated by vagotomy, pyloroplasty and ulcerectomy. *British Journal of Surgery*, **66**, 46–47.

4 Capper, W. M., Airth, G. R. & Kilby, J. O. (1966) A test of pyloric regurgitation. *Lancet*, **ii**, 621–623.

5 Chung, R. S. (1981) Transgastric approach to posterior juxta-esophageal gastric ulcer. *American Surgeon*, **47**, 247–250.

6 Domellof, L. & Janunger, K. G. (1977) The risk for gastric carcinoma after partial gastrectomy. *American Journal of Surgery*, **134**, 581–584.

7 Douglas, M. C. & Duthie, H. L. (1971) Vagotomy for gastric ulcer combined with duodenal ulcer. *British Journal of Surgery*, **58**, 721–724.

8 Dragstedt, L. B. (1956) A concept of the aetiology of gastric and duodenal ulcers. *Gastroenterology*, **30**, 208–220.

9 DuPlessis, D. J. (1965) Pathogenesis of gastric ulceration *Lancet*, **i**, 974–978.

10 Duthie, H. L. & Bransom, C. J. (1979) Highly selective vagotomy with excision of the ulcer compared with gastrectomy for gastric ulcer in a randomised trial. *British Journal of Surgery*, **66**, 43–45.

11 Duthie, H. L. & Kwong, N. K. (1973) Vagotomy or gastrectomy for gastric ulcer. *British Medical Journal*, **iv**, 78–81.

12 DuToit, D. F. & Kemp, C. B. (1979) Lesser curve necrosis following PGV for GU. *South African Medical Journal*, **55**, 98–100.

13 Eastman, M. C. & Gear, M. W. L. (1979) Vagotomy and pyloroplasty for gastric ulcers. *British Journal of Surgery*, **66**, 238–241.

14 Gebhardt, C., Moschinski, D. & Usmiani, J. (1977) Die Behandlung des Kardianahen Ulcus Ventriculi *Langgenbecks Archiv für Chirurgie*, **243**, 313–318.

15 Hall, R., Horrocks, H. C., Clamp, S. E. & deDombal, F. T. (1976) Observer variation in assessment of results of surgery for peptic ulcer. *British Medical Journal*, **i**, 814–816.

16 Hollender, L. F., Bur, F., Peteghem, R. P. *et al.* (1978) Hat die Resektion nach Billroth I Beim Magengeschwur an Bedeutung verloren. *Zentralblatt für Chirurgie*, **103**, 329.

17 Jensen, H. E., Badskaer, J., Andersen, B. N. & Johansen, A. (1979) Precise antrectomy. *World Journal of Surgery*, **3**, 765–773.

18 Johnston, D. & Axon, A. T. R. (1980) Long-term results of HSV in the treatment of benign gastric ulcer. *Gut*, **21**, A455.

19 Johnston, D., MacDonald, R. C. & Axon, A. T. R. (1982) Highly selective vagotomy with ulcer excision. In *Vagotomy in Modern Surgical Practice* (Ed.) Baron, J. H. *et al.* pp. 197–201. London: Butterworths.

20 Johnston, D., Humphrey, C. S., Smith, R. B. & Wilkinson, A. R. (1972) Treatment of gastric ulcer by highly selective vagotomy without a drainage procedure: an interim report. *British Journal of Surgery*, **59**, 787–792.

21 Johnston, H. D. (1957) The classification and principles of treatment of gastric ulcers. *Lancet*, **ii**, 518–520.

22 Johnston, H. D., Love, A. H. G., Rogers, N. C. & Wyatt, A. P. (1964) Gastric ulcer, blood groups and acid secretion. *Gut*, **5**, 402–411.

23 Kraft, R. O., Myers, J., Overton, S. & Fry, W. J. (1971) Vagotomy and gastric ulcer. *American Journal of Surgery*, **121**, 122.

24 Kronborg, O. (1982) Truncal vagotomy and drainage for gastric ulcer. In *Vagotomy in Modern Surgical Practice* (Ed.) Baron, J. H. *et al.* pp. 195–197. London: Butterworths.

25 Liaväg, I., Roland, M. & Broch, A. (1972) Gastric function after pylorus-preserving resection for gastric ulcer. *Acta Chirurgica Scandinavica*, **138**, 511–516.

26 Madsen, P., Kronborg, O., Hart-Hansen, O. & Pedersen, T. (1976) Billroth I gastric resection versus truncal vagotomy and pyloroplasty in the treatment of gastric ulcer. *Acta Chirurgica Scandinavica*, **142**, 151–153.

27 Maki, T., Shiratori, T., Hatafuku, T. & Sugawra, K. (1967) Pylorus-preserving gastrectomy as an improved operation. *Surgery*, **61**, 838–845.

28 Miguel, J. de (1975) Recurrence of gastric ulcers after selective vagotomy and pyloroplasty for chronic uncomplicated gastric ulcer. *British Journal of Surgery*, **62**, 875–878.

29 Miguel, J. de (1979) Pylorectomy and pre-pyloric antrectomy for gastric ulcer. *British Journal of Surgery*, **66**, 48–50.

30 Muller, C., Stadler, G. A. & Allgower, M. (1979) Die proximale selective Vagotomie biem Ulcus Ventriculi selective proximale Vagotomie. In *Gastroenterologischer Symposium: Koln, 1978*. Stuttgart: Georg Thieme Verlag.

31 Nielsen, J., Amdrup, E., Christiansen, P. *et al.* (1973) Gastric ulcer II: surgical treatment. *Acta Chirurgica Scandinavica*, **139**, 460–465.

32 Pichlmayr, R., Lohlein, D. & Kujat, R. (1982) Vagotomy or partial gastric resection as elective treatment for gastric ulcer. In *Vagotomy in Modern Surgical Practice* (Ed.) Baron, J. H. *et al.* pp. 205–212. London: Butterworths.

33 Rhodes, J., Barnado, D. E., Phillips, S. F. *et al.* (1969) Increased reflux of bile into the stomach in patients with gastric ulcer. *Gastroenterology*, **57**, 241–252.

34 Ritchie, W. P. & Delaney, J. P. (1968) Pathogenesis of gastric ulcer: an experimental model. *Surgical Forum*, **19**, 312–313.

35 Salzer, G. (1967) Indikationen zur Resektion nach Billroth I und Billroth II Einschlieblich des Hochsitzenden ulcus. *Klinische Medizin*, **22**, 13.

36 Sekine, T., Sato, T., Maki, T. & Shiratori, T. (1975) Pylorus-preserving gastrectomy for gastric ulcer: one to nine year follow-up study. *Surgery*, **77**, 92–99.

37 Thomas, W. G., Thompson, M. H. & Williamson, R. C. N. (1982) The long term outcome of Billroth I partial gastrectomy for benign gastric ulcer. *Annals of Surgery*, **195**(2), 189–195.

38 Venables, C. W., Wheldon, E. J. & Cranage, J. D. (1980) Adverse effects of gastric surgery for peptic ulceration. *Journal of the Royal College of Physicians*, **14**, 173–177.

39 Venables, C. W., Wheldon, E. J. & Johnston, I. D. A. (1982) The long-term metabolic sequelae of truncal vagotomy and drainage. In *Vagotomy in Modern Surgical Practice* (Ed.) Baron J. H. *et al.* pp. 288–293. London: Butterworths.

40 Younan, F., Pearson, J., Allen, A. & Venables, C. W. (1982) Changes in the structure of the mucous gel on the mucosal surface of the stomach in association with peptic ulcer disease. *Gastroenterology*, **82**, 827–831.

41 Zakrys, M. & Pawlowski, A. (1977) Pylorus preserving gastrectomy in the treatment of gastric ulcer. *Annales Universitatis Mariae Curie-Sklodowska*, **32**, 9–13.

42 Zhaoying, C., Weihan, L. & Qunying, C. (1980) Management of high-lying gastric ulcers. *Chinese Medical Journal*, **93**, 293–296.

CHRONIC DUODENAL ULCER

Clinical features

Duodenal ulceration is, for most patients, a chronic illness characterized by episodes of abdominal discomfort with intervening periods of symptomatic remission.

Since 1976, with the availability of effective medical treatment for acute ulcers and the possibility of prophylactic maintenance treatment, the rates of ulcer healing and relapse have changed. However, it remains uncertain whether the chronicity of duodenal ulcer disease has been influenced despite new advances in medical therapy.

Fry, in a study of duodenal ulcer patients in his South London general practice, suggested that most patients were free of symptoms 10 years after initial diagnosis; however, 16% of his patients had required surgical intervention by that stage.[16] The suggestion that duodenal ulcers tend to get less aggressive with time has not been confirmed by two studies from Denmark. In the first, only 37% of duodenal ulcer patients were symptom-free after a 13-year follow-up and a further 22% had required surgical treatment.[17] In the second, only 20% of patients were symptom-free after 18 to 33 years of follow-up, but 43% had been treated surgically and 7% had died from complications of ulcer disease.[46] For the majority of patients duodenal ulceration is a chronic illness causing symptoms and complications over many years.

Placebo-treated duodenal ulceration

During the development of modern ulcer-healing drugs, carefully monitored clinical trials have documented not only the effectiveness of many new agents, but also the short-term characteristics of placebo-treated duodenal ulcer. Since placebo controls are no longer ethical for trials of therapy in duodenal ulcer, this evidence may be the last record of the natural history of untreated duodenal ulceration.

It has been entertainingly, but unconvincingly, argued that placebo is an 'ideal anti-ulcer drug'.[7] Duodenal ulcer healing rates, assessed by endoscopy after four to six weeks of placebo treatment, show considerable variation around the world. The overall rate of ulcer healing in 18 trials involving 1068 patients who received placebo treatment for four to six weeks was 43%, ranging from 20% to 70% in different centres.[38] The reason for this wide range is not clear. It might be explained on the grounds that duodenal ulceration is a heterogeneous illness. Other possible factors include the influence of cigarette smoking, the availability of antacids and the speed that patients enter a trial after the onset of symptoms. Even the personality of individual physicians can influence ulcer healing.

Duodenal ulcers successfully treated with placebo tend to remain healed in the short-term, but most trials have exhausted placebo-treatment by a maximum of approximately eight weeks, at that stage switching the placebo-treated patients to an active treatment.

The relapse rate of healed duodenal ulcers has also been observed in recent clinical trials. During placebo treatment there is an inevitable relapse rate. At the end of one year of placebo therapy approximately two-thirds of healed ulcers will have recurred.[11] However, there is a similar relapse rate during a one year course of cimetidine 400 mg twice a day (Figure 4.28).[19] Furthermore, the rate of relapse is virtually identical after the first or second course of full-dose cimetidine for acute ulceration.[3] Hence, although modern agents achieve short-term healing of ulcers they seem to have very little influence on the natural history of the underlying disease.

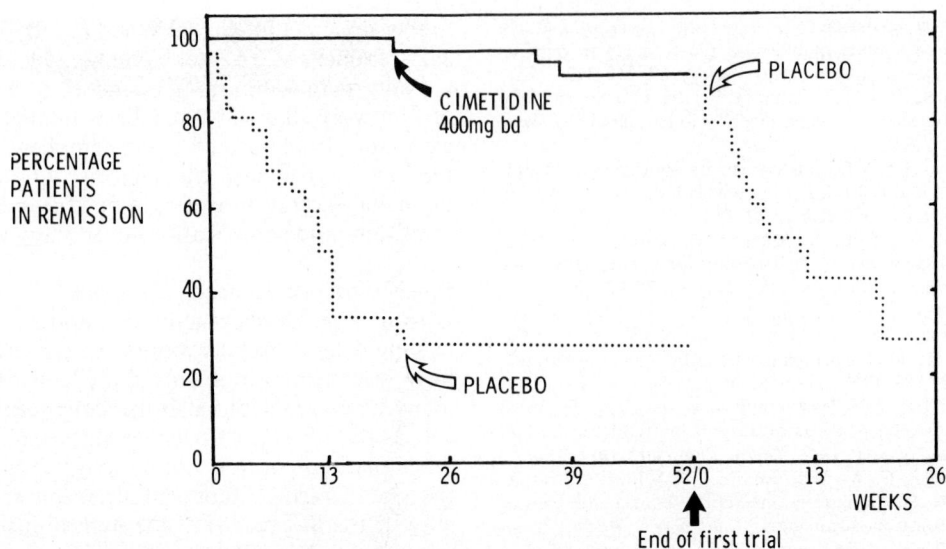

Fig. 4.28 Maintenance treatment of 59 healed duodenal ulcer patients. The rate of duodenal ulcer relapse during placebo treatment is unchanged by one year of treatment with cimetidine 400 mg twice daily.[19]

The results from acute and maintenance trials of placebo therapy for duodenal ulceration indicate that 83% of a group of duodenal ulcer patients on placebo therapy are likely to be in remission at any one time.[38]

THE SYMPTOMS OF DUODENAL ULCERATION

Epigastric pain is the principal feature of uncomplicated duodenal ulceration. An ulcer causes no other specific symptoms, unless there is bleeding, perforation or pyloric stenosis.

The classical stereotype of duodenal ulcer pain is that it is relieved by food or antacids, and is particularly troublesome in the early hours of the morning. This description is by no means universal: certain foods may precipitate discomfort, and 40% of patients state that eating aggravates the ulcer pain.[13] The place of symptomatic response to antacids in the typical clinical picture has now been taken by a history of response to H_2 receptor antagonists. Most duodenal ulcer patients report a prompt response to initial exposure to H_2 receptor antagonists. However, duodenal ulcer is not the only disease which may respond to these drugs: others include gastric ulcer, gastric cancer and oesophagitis. Even waking in the night with indigestion or heartburn does not provide reliable evidence of duodenal ulceration. Such pain has been reported by 70–88% of duodenal ulcer patients; although it is a very sensitive symptom

it is not specific, since a third of patients with non-ulcer dyspepsia have reported similar nocturnal symptoms.[25]

The location of duodenal ulcer pain is not a reliable means of diagnosis: although 86% of duodenal ulcer patients give a history of epigastric pain, so did 52% of patients with functional dyspepsia, 66% of gastric ulcer patients, 54% of patients with gastric cancer, and 25% of patients with gallstones.[25] Nausea, vomiting and anorexia are commonly reported by duodenal ulcer patients (59%, 57%, and 36%, respectively), a proportion that is virtually identical to that reported by patients with other causes of dyspepsia.[25]

It is clear that symptoms do not provide any basis for the confident clinical diagnosis of duodenal ulcer. It is possible that computer-assisted discriminant analysis may add precision to the clinical history,[12] but there is no recent report of such a system in everyday clinical use.[24]

Duodenal ulcer pain
It is not known why certain patients with duodenal ulceration suffer from pain, nor why an individual's pain waxes and wanes. For years it has been recognized that patients may actually perforate a duodenal ulcer yet have no preceding ulcer pain.

Recent clinical trials have documented an imprecise relationship between the presence of endoscopically-proven duodenal ulceration and typical symptoms. In a trial comparing cimetidine with antacid therapy, at the end of six weeks 18% of patients had symptoms, yet only one-third of these had active duodenal ulceration. Conversely, of the 82% who were asymptomatic, one in six still had an ulcer when reviewed at endoscopy.[18] During a one-year maintenance trial comparing cimetidine with placebo, 27% of symptom-free patients receiving placebo were found to have an active ulcer at endoscopy, whereas only 10% of the cimetidine-treated patients were ulcerated.[11]

It has always been considered that it is the duodenal acidity, acting on an ulcerated duodenal mucosa, that causes ulcer pain. This explains the prompt relief of pain by antacids or food, and the nocturnal pain which occurs when there is no food to buffer gastric acidity. However, this concept is eroded as placebo antacid provides as much acute pain relief as a genuine antacid.[45] In addition, instillation of acid into the stomach does not reliably provoke ulcer pain in patients with endoscopically-proven duodenal ulceration and a history of recent spontaneous ulcer pain.[23]

Investigation and diagnosis

RADIOLOGICAL DIAGNOSIS

A barium meal is the traditional investigation for duodenal ulceration. Radiologists identify three features of duodenal ulcer disease: the ulcer niche or crater, enlarged duodenal folds, and deformity of the duodenal bulb (Figure 4.29). The usual evidence of active ulceration is the collection of barium in a crater, which should be apparent in several films. If the duodenum is scarred, deformity may either obscure active ulceration or produce the illusion of an ulcer. Alternatively, a small ulcer in a normal duodenal cap, particularly if less than 3 mm in diameter, may escape the radiologist's attention, especially if a single-contrast study is performed.[30]

The main problem with a barium meal is inaccuracy. When endoscopy was used as the definitive diagnostic procedure, one study found that single-contrast or double-contrast meals were equally effective, but they only detected 60% of duodenal ulcers. However, when the radiologist reported a 'duodenal ulcer', one report in five was falsely positive.[31]

Although barium meal examination is relatively expensive, it is usually well tolerated, is safe and provides a permanent record of the anatomy of the stomach and duodenum.

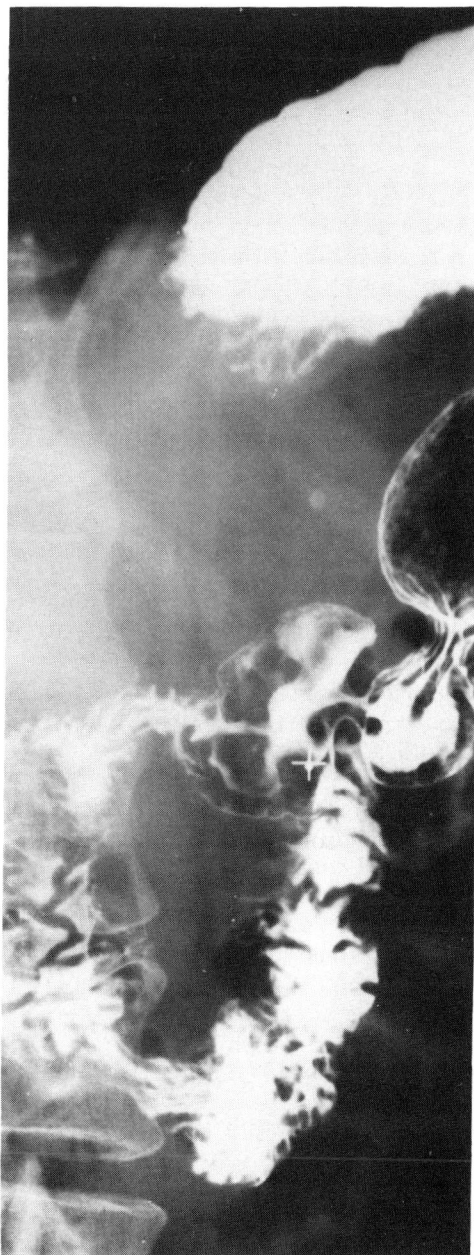

Fig. 4.29 Double-contrast barium meal: duodenal ulcer. The ulcer crater is in the first part of the duodenum above the X-ray marker.

ENDOSCOPIC DIAGNOSIS

With modern instruments most endoscopists can usually inspect the entire duodenal mucosa. If there is considerable oedema of the pyloric canal or if there is pyloric stenosis the endoscope may not enter the duodenum. However, a distant view of an ulcer may still be possible.

It is probably acceptable to use endoscopy as 'the definitive diagnostic procedure' for duodenal ulceration.[31] One group was able to compare endoscopy with a double-contrast barium meal within five days of surgery for duodenal ulceration.[10] Surgery and endoscopy agreed in 88% of patients, surgery and radiology in 82%, and endoscopy and radiology in 78%. Endoscopy would therefore appear to be more accurate than radiology.

Upper gastrointestinal endoscopy is a relatively safe procedure, which is tolerated by most patients. However, there may be a small risk of respiratory depression during sedation and there is often no permanent visual record of the endoscopic appearances. When performed in a salaried service the costs of endoscopy and double-contrast radiology are similar. Endoscopy becomes more expensive when performed in the private sector.

ENDOSCOPY VERSUS RADIOLOGY

If a patient has symptoms that warrant investigation, it is sensible to order the investigation that will produce the most accurate result.

The majority of patients presenting with indigestion do not have a duodenal ulcer. Hence, when ordering a barium meal for such patients there is a very high chance that the barium meal will be 'normal'. However, a negative barium meal examination is so unreliable that, if the patient is still symptomatic, further investigation by endoscopy is usually necessary. It is for this reason that it is sensible to recommend endoscopy as a primary procedure, except for the cardio-respiratory cripple or the young patient unable to tolerate an endoscope.

TESTS OF GASTRIC ACID SECRETION

Although patients with duodenal ulceration have a tendency to secrete more acid than healthy controls, there is no need to measure gastric acid secretion in the duodenal ulcer patient with an uncomplicated history.[4]

Similarly, there is no need to measure the fasting plasma gastrin concentration in patients with uncomplicated duodenal ulceration. However, if the duodenal ulceration is unusually aggressive, or does not respond to conventional doses of an H_2-receptor antagonist, it is prudent to eliminate the Zollinger–Ellison syndrome by this simple investigation.

PHYSICAL EXAMINATION

Physical examination of the patient with duodenal ulceration provides an opportunity to localize the epigastric discomfort accurately. If a patient spontaneously points with an index finger towards the epigastrium, it is quite likely that the patient has a duodenal ulcer.[12] Although the patient with a duodenal ulcer may have some epigastric discomfort on deep palpation, this does not discriminate between duodenal ulceration and other causes of dyspepsia. A succussion splash may be present if the patient has pyloric stenosis. Anaemia is a rare finding.

DIFFERENTIAL DIAGNOSIS

The differential diagnosis will include: oesophagitis, benign and malignant ulceration of the stomach, gastritis and duodenitis, pancreatic disease, biliary disease, the irritable bowel syndrome and alcohol-induced symptoms. These conditions can only be eliminated by investigation of the patient.[12]

Pathological hypersecretion of gastric acid, due to the Zollinger–Ellison syndrome or systemic mastocytosis, may produce aggressive duodenal ulceration. Normal gastric acid secretion may not be buffered, as in the patient with pancreatic exocrine failure, causing extensive duodenal ulceration.

Ulceration in the duodenum may not be due to peptic ulceration: tuberculosis, Crohn's disease, lymphoma, primary malignancy of the duodenal mucosa and secondary malignancy eroding into the duodenal mucosa may also present as apparently simple duodenal ulceration. All these groups may be identified by appropriate histology: bizarre or non-healing duodenal ulceration may warrant target biopsies during endoscopy.

ASSOCIATED DISEASES

Although there are a number of conditions that are traditionally associated with duodenal ulceration (for example, chronic lung disease, chronic renal failure, hyperparathyroidism, or cirrhosis), there are reasons to believe that these associations are coincidental rather than causal.[29]

Medical treatment

The aims of modern medical treatment are threefold: they are to relieve the patient's symptoms, to heal the duodenal ulceration, and to prevent recurrence of duodenal ulceration.

Patients with uncomplicated duodenal ulceration present to the doctor because of their dyspeptic symptoms. If the episode of pain can be eliminated, the patient will be happy even if he or she continues to have a silent ulcer.

The endoscopist can determine whether treatment has actually resulted in the healing of the duodenal ulcer. A completely healed ulcer means that there is no risk of any of the complications of duodenal ulceration. However, this risk is only eliminated while the ulcer can be seen to be healed, since ulceration may return (perhaps without symptoms) within days or weeks.

For most patients, duodenal ulceration is a chronic illness. There is no non-infectious chronic medical illness that can be cured by a course of tablets, and modern medical management provides only a treatment and not a cure for duodenal ulceration.

The majority of patients will be satisfied by prompt relief of ulcer symptoms, followed by asymptomatic remission of variable length. A minority of these patients will continue to have endoscopic duodenal ulceration, and hence are vulnerable to complications. However, the risk to the whole group is so small that it does not merit routine endoscopic follow-up of the duodenal ulcer patient. The natural history of duodenal ulceration is not apparently influenced by medical treatment: when people stop taking the treatment there is usually return of active ulceration.

Control of the patient's symptoms is a realistic, practical objective for the everyday management of the duodenal ulcer patient.

ACUTE MEDICAL TREATMENT

General advice
Although many ulcer patients, and some physicians, believe that relapse of duodenal ulceration may be precipitated by stress,[15, 36] it is difficult for most patients to manipulate or avoid their environmental or emotional stresses. As stress can cause hypersecretion of gastric acid, the prophylatic use of an anti-secretory drug in the ulcer-prone patient may be more successful than the use of tranquillizers. Phenobarbitone (phenobarbital) or diazepam can no longer be recommended as routine treatment for the ulcer patient.

With modern medical treatment there is no need to admit the uncomplicated duodenal ulcer patient to hospital for bed-rest[28] or to advise the patient to rest at home away from work.

An ulcer diet is expected by many patients, and this expectation is sometimes fulfilled by their physician. There is no evidence that a soft or sloppy diet, taken frequently throughout the day, offers either effective neutralization of gastric acidity, symptomatic relief or ulcer

healing. Such treatment may even be harmful since a bedtime snack will tend to stimulate nocturnal gastric acid secretion. Any drink stimulates acid secretion and the most potent stimulant is milk.[33]

The deleterious effects of cigarette smoking on ulcer healing remain controversial. In clinical trials of patients receiving a placebo, cigarette smokers' ulcers undoubtedly heal less frequently than non-smokers, but this effect is usually overcome by treatment with an effective anti-ulcer drug.[27] This does not mean that smoking is causally related to the delayed healing of duodenal ulceration. However, it is good general advice that patients should stop smoking cigarettes.

Avoidance of non-steroidal anti-inflammatory drugs, such as aspirin, is also recommended to most patients, but this advice is again controversial.[37, 43] Aspirin, like alcohol, can cause acute gastric mucosal damage, but much less is known about duodenal mucosal damage. It is probably prudent to advise a moderate alcohol intake, particularly as continued heavy drinking has been associated with failure of medical treatment.[21]

ULCER HEALING DRUGS CURRENTLY AVAILABLE

A wide range of drugs are now available for the treatment of patients with acute duodenal ulceration. All of these drugs have been demonstrated to be superior to placebo in double-blind endoscopically controlled clinical trials. Ulcer healing has usually been observed in approximately 70–80% of duodenal ulcer patients after four weeks of treatment with an active drug.[1, 8, 9, 14, 39, 44] These results should be compared with an average healing rate for placebo of approximately 40% in four weeks. The longer the patients are treated with the active drug, the more ulcers tend to heal. However, trials involving substantial numbers of patients never report the healing of every ulcer.

The reasons for failure of medical treatment are unclear, but the following factors may be relevant.
1 Compliance is a problem for any form of medical treatment, but regular medication is encouraged by improvement in symptoms for many ulcer patients.
2 In a clinical trial, the endoscopist may underestimate duodenal ulcer healing. The second endoscopy must be thorough to check whether the ulcer has healed; the endoscopist may over-report mucosal irregularity as continuing ulceration.

3 The aetiology of duodenal ulceration may be multifactorial. Hence, the main problem for some patients may not be excess acid but a poor mucosa; such patients may never respond to antisecretory drugs. Conversely, some gastric hypersecretors may never respond to the mucosal-protecting drugs.

4 As far as is known, none of the 'ulcer-healing' drugs actually heal ulcers. These drugs alter the environment of the ulcer so that ulcer healing may take place. A month is a long time for such a small mucosal defect to repair itself. Perhaps conventional drugs are not sufficiently strong to overcome the adverse effects which sustain the ulceration.

In terms of ulcer-healing trials, there is no one drug that stands out as being more efficient at ulcer healing than any of the other agents. Hence, the decision to choose an individual drug has to be based upon experience, safety and cost.

Mechanisms of action of the following drugs, and their side-effects, have been discussed in the section on gastric ulcer (pp. 140–156).

Cimetidine

Dosage. When cimetidine was introduced in Europe in 1976 the recommended dosage for duodenal ulcer patients was 200 mg three times a day with meals, with 400 mg at bedtime. This dosage provides a smooth, approximately two-thirds, decrease of 24-hour intragastric acidity. In the Americas, the recommended dosage is 300 mg four times a day, which causes a similar decrease of intragastric acidity. Recent studies have shown that even 400 mg twice a day, in the morning and at bedtime, is as effective as one gram a day in four divided doses; perhaps this low-dose regimen gains in compliance what it loses in pharmacological inhibition of gastric acid secretion.[14]

Ranitidine

Dosage. The oral dose of ranitidine is 150 mg twice a day, taken in the morning and at bedtime. Higher doses are not needed for uncomplicated duodenal ulceration.

Tri-potassium di-citrato bismuthate

Clinical evaluation

One preliminary report suggests that the electron-microscopic appearance of the duodenal mucosa returns to normal after acute treatment with tri-potassium di-citrato bismuthate, an improvement not seen during prolonged treatment with cimetidine.[35]

Another study reported that symptomatic relapse of duodenal ulceration was significantly more common after ulcer healing with cimetidine than after treatment with tri-potassium di-citrato bismuthate.[32] This is the only study which suggests that an acute course of any medical treatment for duodenal ulceration has a long-lasting influence on the rate of recurrence of this chronic illness.

Dosage. Tri-potassium di-citrato bismuthate can be given either as four liquid doses, or as four tablets, taken half an hour before meals and also at bedtime.[22] The dose is 5 ml of liquid diluted in 15 ml of water, or one tablet chewed in the mouth. The bismuth should not be taken with an antacid or an anti-secretory drug, as either may change the acid pH necessary for the formation of bismuth–protein complexes. The drug should not be taken with food, as the bismuth may combine with the protein in the meal rather than that in the base of the ulcer. The liquid has an unpleasant ammoniacal odour which may reduce compliance.

Treatment should be for four to eight weeks, but maintenance treatment is not recommended. The drug should not be given to patients with acute or chronic renal failure because of possible bismuth retention.

Sucralfate

Dosage. The usual dose of sucralfate is one gram four times a day. The tablet should be taken an hour before meals and at bedtime. The usual course of treatment is four to six weeks.

Safety. Apart from constipation, sucralfate appears to be well-tolerated. Approximately 5% of the oral dose is absorbed, but there are no reports of systemic complications.

Carbenoxolone

Dosage. Traditionally, carbenoxolone is prescribed for the duodenal ulcer patient in a 'position-release' capsule. This capsule is supposed to discharge its contents over the first part of the duodenum. Whether the action of carbenoxolone is due to its topical or systemic activity is unclear; the benefit of this capsule formulation may not outweigh the cheaper and easier-to-swallow carbenoxolone tablet.

The dosage of carbenoxolone for duodenal ulceration is 50 mg four times a day before meals – a different dose to that recommended for gastric ulceration. Treatment may be continued for six to twelve weeks.

Pirenzepine

Dosage. The recommended dose of pirenzepine in the United Kingdom is 50 mg twice a day, taken in the morning and at bedtime. The dose may be increased to 50 mg three times daily.

Antacids

If sufficient amounts of a potent antacid are given it is possible to neutralize intragastric acidity.[20] Conventional use of antacids has probably been as a placebo, as they were given neither in sufficient volume nor with sufficient frequency to achieve effective neutralization of acid.

In the United Kingdom antacids are marketed not primarily in terms of their acid-neutralizing activity but more in terms of general superlatives. Although tables comparing the relative activities of different antacids have been prepared,[5] these tables soon become invalid as the manufacturers change the formulation of the antacid mixtures.

The problem is further complicated by the discovery that immediate relief of duodenal ulcer pain does not depend upon the neutralizing capacity of an antacid mixture.[45] It is quite possible that immediate pain relief is actually due to the carminative effect of the peppermint flavouring added to the antacid mixture.[34]

Regular treatment with a high-dose antacid, for example 30 ml of a potent antacid one and three hours after every meal, can significantly decrease intragastric acidity during the daytime. However, even if a large dose is taken at bedtime, this is soon either neutralized or emptied from the stomach, leaving considerable acidity for the majority of the night.

Frequent doses of a potent antacid in the daytime, with a small dose of an H_2 antagonist at bedtime, offers relatively cheap and effective control of 24-hour intragastric acidity which is particularly suitable for Third World health care.

Dosage. If an antacid is to be given to heal duodenal ulcers high-dose therapy using approximately eight litres of potent antacid per month is required.[44] It is reassuring to know that such dramatic therapy will achieve healing, but it is clearly irrelevant for modern treatment.

FUTURE MEDICAL TREATMENT

Prostaglandins

Prostaglandins have for some years offered tantalizing glimpses of a new era in the treatment of peptic ulceration.[43, 48] Not only may they stop gastric acid secretion, but they may also stimulate gastric mucus secretion, and may stimulate bicarbonate secretion into the base of that layer of mucus. At the moment, clinical trials in duodenal ulceration are incomplete.

Omeprazole

Omeprazole is the first of a new class of antisecretory drugs (substituted benzimidazoles) to enter clinical trials for duodenal ulceration. Omeprazole is a hydrogen-potassium-ATPase inhibitor and it is capable of causing a complete inhibition of stimulated gastric acid secretion in humans. For the first time, there is a drug which causes a profound decrease of intragastric acidity that is sustained throughout the 24 hours (Figure 4.30).[47] It remains to be seen whether this inhibition does indeed speed duodenal ulcer healing.

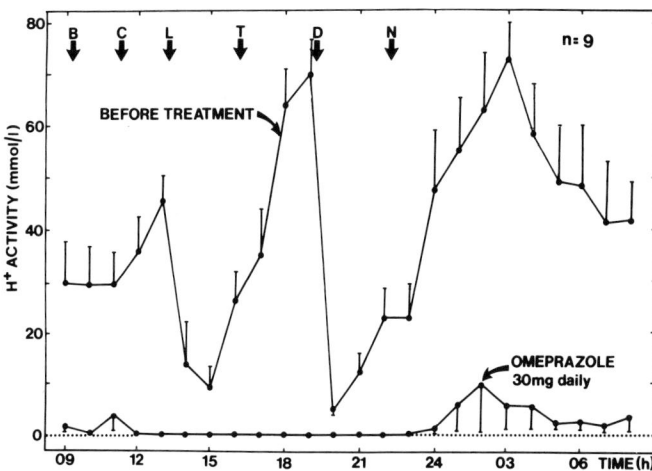

Fig. 4.30 Hourly mean intragastric acidity in duodenal ulcer patients before treatment and at the end of one week's treatment with omeprazole 30 mg daily.[60] Arrows indicate meals.

DUODENAL ULCERATION THAT DOES NOT RESPOND TO MEDICAL TREATMENT

The majority of duodenal ulcers respond promptly to medical treatment, such that four out of five patients are symptom-free at the end of six to eight weeks of treatment. However, a minority of patients do continue to have symptoms after an apparently adequate course of medical treatment.

If a patient continues to complain of dyspeptic symptoms despite full-dose treatment with an effective drug for six to eight weeks, it is important to determine whether the continuing symptoms are due to active duodenal ulceration. The only way to determine this is to perform an endoscopy, as distortion due to a scarred duodenal cap may obscure an intact mucosa on barium meal examination.

Approximately half of these 'failures' will be found to have a normal duodenal mucosa, and the physician then has to find another reason for the continuing dyspepsia.

The remaining half of the patients will be genuine failures who have continuing duodenal ulceration despite medical treatment. Four steps should then be considered.

1 It is worth re-interviewing the patient to make sure that an appropriate course of medical treatment has been prescribed and that the recommended dose has been taken.

2 The patient's duodenal ulceration may continue despite successful medical treatment to control acid secretion. The patient who has failed on H_2-antagonist treatment may be better treated by changing to either tri-potassium di-citrato bismuthate or sucralfate, rather than continuing with even longer courses of treatment with an H_2-antagonist. Alternatively, the antisecretory effect of an H_2-antagonist can be augmented by the addition of pirenzepine. This synergistic combination virtually eliminates all acid secretion.

3 It is prudent to perform an estimation of fasting serum plasma gastrin concentration in any patient with aggressive duodenal ulceration, in case the patient has the Zollinger–Ellison syndrome.

4 Should the patient have an operation? If a full dose of cimetidine or ranitidine has failed to heal a duodenal ulcer, it is quite possible that gastric surgery may be equally ineffective. The data are conflicting, but some surgeons believe that this type of patient has an equally poor response to technically successful surgery.

MAINTENANCE MEDICAL TREATMENT

There is no chronic medical illness that is cured by a single course of treatment with tablets. H_2-antagonists are a treatment for duodenal ulceration and not a cure.[38] When cimetidine was first introduced, many doctors expected that it would provide a cure for duodenal ulceration – an unrealistic expectation for any form of medical treatment.

The placebo-controlled maintenance trials using cimetidine have provided evidence that duodenal ulceration is a relapsing condition.[12] Studies have shown the same tendency to relapse after a second acute course of cimetidine,[2] and even after one year of full-dose treatment with cimetidine.[23] The majority of duodenal ulcer patients stay healthy whilst taking H_2 antagonists, but as soon as they stop treatment they display a tendency to relapse that is unaffected by previous treatment.

Maintenance treatment with H_2 antagonists

Extensive clinical trials have been performed comparing cimetidine with placebo for short-term maintenance therapy. Most of these trials, although lasting a year, must be considered short-term within the lifespan of most duodenal ulcer patients' illnesses.

The results of these studies show considerable variation around the world,[3, 6, 11] but treatment with an H_2 antagonist is associated with a lower incidence of ulceration than placebo treatment (Figure 4.31). Most of these studies have used a 400 mg dose of cimetidine, taken either at bedtime or twice a day. There is some evidence that the twice-a-day regimen may be slightly

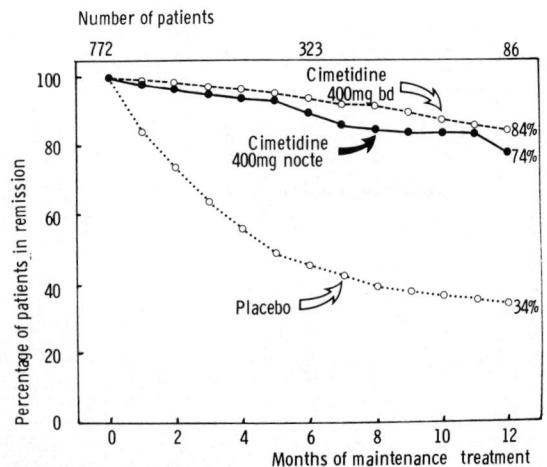

Fig. 4.31 Double-blind maintenance treatment of duodenal ulcers with either placebo, cimetidine 400 mg twice daily (bd) or cimetidine 400 mg at bedtime (nocte).

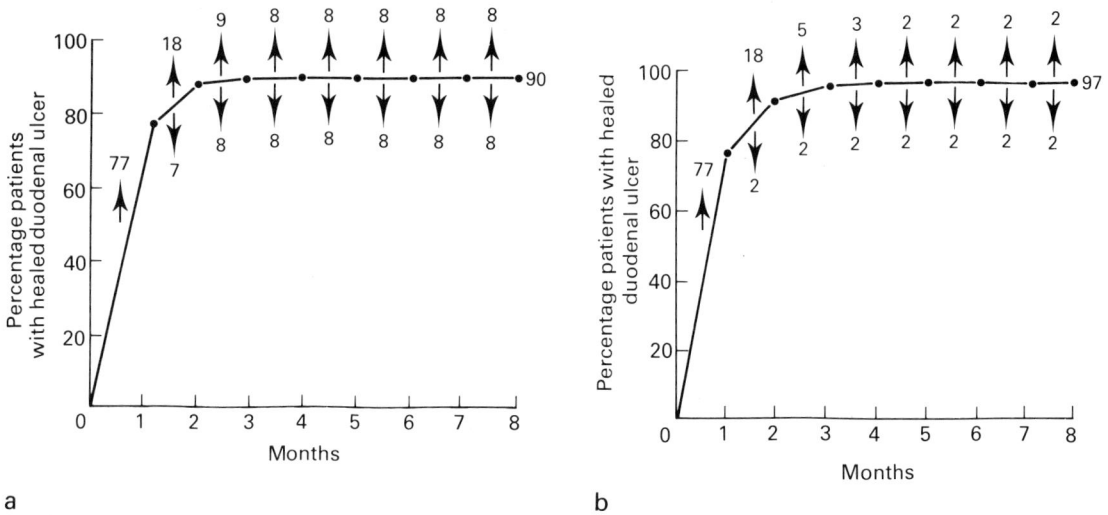

Fig. 4.32 Model of duodenal ulcer treatment in 100 patients. 77% of acute ulcer patients are cured by H_2-antagonist treatment each month; the number cured during each month is shown by an upward arrow. 8.5% of patients on placebo maintenance treatment relapse each month, whereas 2.5% of patients on H_2-antagonist maintenance treatment relapse; the number relapsing is denoted by the downward arrow, (a) If an H_2 antagonist is used to treat acute ulceration only, eight patients relapse every month. (b) If an H_2 antagonist is used for maintenance as well as acute treatment, only two patients relapse each month.[40]

more effective than the low-dose bedtime treatment.[6] Very similar results have been observed during maintenance treatment with ranitidine 150 mg at bedtime.[26]

The type of clinical trial that has been used to evaluate H_2 antagonists has used ulcer relapse as the end-point. When relapse was diagnosed, the patients were withdrawn from the clinical trial. However, the return of ulceration in a patient who is already receiving maintenance treatment with an H_2-antagonist does not mean an absolute and irrevocable treatment failure. The majority of these patients respond to an increased dose of an antisecretory drug and can later return to low-dose treatment.

The prevalence of active duodenal ulceration has never been reported in a population of patients receiving treatment with an H_2 antagonist, but models can be developed to predict the probable outcome of different treatment strategies.[39, 40] In a population of 100 duodenal ulcer patients receiving placebo treatment it can be expected that there will be 17 patients with active duodenal ulceration at any one time; if 100 patients receive treatment with an H_2 antagonist during acute episodes of ulceration only, it can be expected that 10 patients will have active ulceration at any one time (Figure 4.32a). The benefit of H_2-blockade is seen only when the patients receive maintenance treatment with high-dose treatment during episodes of relapse, when, in a population of 100 patients,

only three would be expected to have active ulceration at any one time (Figure 4.32b).

It is clear that, for the majority of duodenal ulcer patients, maintenance treatment with an H_2 antagonist can provide effective long-term treatment. Physicians are prepared to treat many chronic medical conditions with long-term medical treatment – for example, sulphasalazine for ulcerative colitis or propranolol for hypertension – so why should duodenal ulcer patients be denied the opportunity of effective medical treatment that will keep them free of pain for most of the year?

ON-DEMAND TREATMENT

The traditional methods of using histamine H_2-receptor antagonists for duodenal ulceration have been to provide the patient with either intermittent treatment, usually for four to six weeks, or maintenance treatment. A third possibility is to allow the patient to use an H_2 antagonist on demand.

The patient could start full-dose treatment at the very first sign of any symptoms, perhaps arresting the development of ulceration. The patient could then stop treatment when the symptoms have resolved, perhaps taking treatment for two further weeks to encourage complete healing of a, by then, asymptomatic ulcer. This strategy has never been tested by clinical trial, although in practice many patients use H_2-antagonists in just this way.

Clinical trials have shown that approximately four out of five ulcers are healed at four weeks during treatment with effective medical therapy. There must be many patients who do not require the full four weeks of treatment – whose ulcers heal after a much shorter time-scale.

The advantages of on-demand treatment are that it provides the patient with very prompt relief of symptoms with a minimal exposure to medication. However, it will not provide such an effective decrease in the prevalence of active ulceration as continuous treatment with an H_2 blocker. The reason for this failure is that whereas maintenance treatment with cimetidine has been shown to decrease asymptomatic ulceration,[11] on-demand treatment only controls the patient's symptoms. However, the risk of asymptomatic ulceration must be small for the majority of patients.

A STRATEGY FOR THE MEDICAL MANAGEMENT OF DUODENAL ULCERATION

1   When a clinical diagnosis of duodenal ulceration is first made, this impression must be confirmed by investigation. The ideal investigation is upper-gastrointestinal endoscopy, although a barium meal can be used to provide evidence of damage to the duodenum. Further investigation is not required in the majority of patients; in particular there is no need to reinvestigate later episodes of ulcer relapse which cause typical symptoms for that patient.
2   The physician has a choice of effective acute medical treatments for the acute phase of the illness. When choosing any drug, the physician should consider efficacy, cost and safety. The majority of duodenal ulcer patients are treated with cimetidine, which is known to be effective, has a well-defined safety profile and is relatively inexpensive.[39] However, all of the other treatments have their particular advantages.

To make sure that the majority of patients are healed there should be a second consultation before six weeks have passed. It may be convenient for the physician to provide six weeks' supply of treatment to be taken even if symptoms resolve within a few days. Alternatively, a more economical approach may be to advise the patient to take full-dose treatment until all symptoms have resolved, and then to take a further two weeks of treatment with the full dose. Using this regimen, a patient whose symptoms resolve after one week of treatment would need to receive only three weeks of full-dose treatment.

There is no need to perform follow-up investigations in the asymptomatic patient to prove that an ulcer has healed. All duodenal ulcer patients should be told to stop smoking. No dietary advice is required, and they should be encouraged to continue at work.
3   If symptoms do not resolve after six to eight weeks of full-dose medical treatment, the patient should be reinvestigated.
4   If a patient suffers from recurrent ulceration, a strategy must be devised for long-term medical treatment. If the relapses are rare, the patient may be suitable for intermittent treatment; ideally, the patient should be provided with a supply of tablets to start treatment at the first sign of relapse. If the patient's symptoms return within days of stopping treatment, continuous bedtime treatment is required.

Medical versus surgical treatment
Medical treatment can provide effective relief of symptoms for the majority of patients. Although some patients are troubled by side-effects from the drugs, these are rare and reversible. It is not known how long patients will require medical treatment and it is only reasonable to assume the worst – that they may require treatment for life.

Surgery provides the opportunity of cure, but is unpredictable. There is a small risk of death. There is a more appreciable, but unpredictable, risk of recurrent ulceration or side-effects. Indeed, there is a positive correlation between the cure rate of a surgical procedure and incidence of side-effects due to that procedure.

The principal indications for surgical treatment are chronic dyspeptic symptoms which have not responded to intensive medical therapy in a patient who had a proven duodenal ulcer before therapy and complicated disease. If there have been repeated episodes of bleeding which have not required emergency surgery in a patient with chronic dyspepsia, an elective operation would be strongly advised. If the patient has had a perforated ulcer which was not treated by definitive operation, an operation would also be advised if there was a long history of dyspepsia. Duodenal stenosis, particularly if complicated by vomiting, dehydration and electrolyte abnormalities, is an indication for operation. It is the chronic dyspeptic who poses the greatest dilemma. However, the possibility of operation must always be borne in mind for a well motivated male subject who is losing time from work and whose symptoms are not controlled by H_2 antagonists.

REFERENCES

1 Avery Jones, F. A., Langman, M. J. S. & Mann, R. D. (1978) *Peptic Ulcer Healing: Recent Studies on Carbenoxolone.* Lancaster: MTP.

2 Bardhan, D. K. (1980) Intermittent treatment of duodenal ulcer. *British Medical Journal*, **281**, 20–21.

3 Bardhan, K. D. (1982) The short- and medium-term treatment of duodenal ulcer with cimetidine. In *Peptic Ulcer Disease* (Ed.) Bianchi Porro, G. & Bardhan, K. D. pp. 85–106. Verona: Cortina International.

4 Baron, J. H. (1978) *Clinical Tests of Gastric Acid Secretion. History, Methodology, Interpretation.* London: Macmillan.

5 Barry, R. E. & Ford, J. (1978) Sodium content and neutralising capacity of some commonly used antacids. *British Medical Journal*, **i**, 413.

6 Bianchi Porro, G., Petrillo, M., Lazzaroni, M. & Sangletti, O. (1982) The longer-term treatment of duodenal ulceration with cimetidine. In *Peptic Ulcer Disease* (Ed.) Bianchi Porro, G. & Bardhan, D. K. pp. 107–113. Verona: Cortina International.

7 Blum, A. L. (1982) Is placebo the ideal anti-ulcer drug? In *Peptic Ulcer Disease* (Ed.) Bianchi Porro, G. & Bardhan, D. K. pp. 57–61. Verona: Cortina International.

8 Brogden, R. N., Pinder, R. M., Sawyer, P. R. *et al.* (1976) Tri-potassium di-citrato bismuthate: a report on its pharmacological properties and therapeutic efficacy in peptic ulcer. *Drugs*, **12**, 401–411.

9 Brogden, R. N., Carmine, A. A. & Heel, R. C. *et al.* (1982) Ranitidine. *Drugs*, **24**, 267–303.

10 Brown, P., Salmon, P. R. & Burwood, R. J. (1978) The endoscopic, radiological and surgical findings in chronic duodenal ulceration. *Scandinavian Journal of Gastroenterology*, **13**, 557–560.

11 Burland, W. L., Hawkins, B. W. & Beresford, J. (1980) Cimetidine treatment for the prevention of recurrence of duodenal ulcer; an international collaborative study. *Postgraduate Medical Journal*, **56**, 173–176.

12 Crean, G. P., Card, W. I., Beattie, A. D. *et al.* (1982) Ulcer-like dyspepsia. *Scandinavian Journal of Gastroenterology*, **17** (supplement 79), 9–15.

13 Earlam, R. (1978) A computerized questionnaire analysis of duodenal ulcer symptoms. *Gastroenterology*, **71**, 314–317.

14 Eckardt, V. (1981) Cimetidine: twice daily administration in duodenal ulcer – results of a European multicentre study. In *Cimetidine in the 80s* (Ed.) Baron, J. H. pp. 14–20. Edinburgh: Churchill Livingstone.

15 Feldman, E. K. & Sabovitch, K. A. (1980) Stress and peptic ulcer disease. *Gastroenterology*, **78**, 1087–1089.

16 Fry, J. (1964) Peptic ulcer – a profile. *British Medical Journal*, **ii**, 809–812.

17 Griebe, J., Bugge, P., Gjorup, T. *et al.* (1977) Long-term prognosis of duodenal ulcer: follow-up study and survey of doctors' estimates. *British Medical Journal*, **ii**, 1572–1574.

18 Grossman, M. I. (Ed.) (1982) *Peptic Ulcer, a Guide for the Practicing Physician.* p. 56. Chicago: Year Book Medical Publishers.

19 Gudmand-Hoyer, E., Birger, J. K. & Krag, E. (1978) Prophylactic effect of cimetidine in duodenal ulcer disease. *British Medical Journal*, **i**, 1095–1097.

20 Halter, F. (1981) *Antacids in the Eighties.* Munich: Urban & Schwarzenberg.

21 Hasan, M. & Sircus, W. (1981) The factors determining success or failure of cimetidine treatment of peptic ulcer. *Journal of Clinical Gastroenterology*, **3**, 255–229.

22 Hamilton, I. & Axon, A. T. R. (1981) Controlled trial comparing De-Nol tablets with De-Nol liquid in treatment of duodenal ulcer. *British Medical Journal*, **282**, 362.

23 Harrison, A., Isenberg, J. I., Senapira, M. & Hagic, L. (1982) Most patients with active symptomatic duodenal ulcers fail to develop ulcer-type pain in response to gastroduodenal acidification. *Journal of Clinical Gastroenterology*, **4**, 105–108.

24 Horrocks, J. C. & de Dombal, F. T. (1975) Diagnosis of dyspepsia from data collected by physician's assistant. *British Medical Journal*, **iii**, 421–423.

25 Horrocks, J. C. & de Dombal, F. T. (1978) Clinical presentation of patients with 'dyspepsia'. Detailed symptomatic study of 360 patients. *Gut*, **19**, 19–26.

26 Hunt, R. H., Walt, R. P., Trotman, I. F. *et al.* (1982) Comparison of ranitidine, 150 mg nocte, with cimetidine, 400 mg nocte, in the maintenance treatment of duodenal ulcer. In *The Clinical Use of Ranitidine* (Ed.) Misiewicz, J. J. & Wormsley, K. G. pp. 192–195. Oxford: Medicine.

27 Korman, M. G., Shaw, R. G., Hansky, J. *et al.* (1981) Influence of smoking in the healing rate of duodenal ulcer in response to cimetidine or high dose antacid. *Gastroenterology*, **80**, 1451–1453.

28 Kurata, J. H., Honda, G. D. & Franki, H. (1982) Hospitalization and mortality rates for peptic ulcers: a comparison of a large health maintenance organization and United States data. *Gastroenterology*, **83**, 1008–1016.

29 Langman, M. J. S. (1979) Peptic ulcer. In *The Epidemiology of Chronic Digestive Disease.* pp. 30–33. London: Edward Arnold.

30 Laufer, I. (1976) Assessment of the accuracy of double contrast gastroduodenal radiology. *Gastroenterology*, **71**, 874–878.

31 Lavelle, M. I., Venables, C. W., Douglas, A. P. *et al.* (1976) A prospective endoscopically controlled trial of double contrast against single contrast barium meals. *Gut*, **17**, 396–397.

32 Martin, D. F., May, S. J., Tweedle, D. E. F. *et al.* (1981) Difference in relapse rate of duodenal ulcer after healing with cimetidine or tri-potassium di-citrato bismuthate. *Lancet*, **i**, 7–10.

33 McArthur, K., Hogan, D. & Isenberg, J. I. (1982) Relative stimulatory effects of commonly ingested beverages on gastric acid secretion in humans. *Gastroenterology*, **83**, 199–203.

34 Morris, T. & Rhodes, J. (1979) Antacids and peptic ulcer – a reappraisal. *Gut*, **20**, 538–545.

35 Moshal, M. G. (1979) Does the duodenal cell ever return to normal? *Scandinavian Journal of Gastroenterology*, **14**, 48–51.

36 Peters, M. N. & Richardson, C. T. (1983) Stressful life events, acid hypersecretion and ulcer disease. *Gastroenterology*, **84**, 114–119.

37 Piper, D. W., McIntosh, J. H., Ariotti, D. E. *et al.* (1981) Analgesic ingestion and chronic peptic ulcer. *Gastroenterology*, **80**, 427–434.

38 Pounder, R. E. (1981) Model of medical treatment for duodenal ulcer. *Lancet*, **i**, 29–30.

39 Pounder, R. E. (1981) Maintenance treatment – cost–effectiveness. In *Cimetidine in the 80s* (Ed.) Baron, J. H. pp. 89–94. Edinburgh: Churchill Livingstone.

40 Pounder, R. E. (1982) The economics of long-term duodenal ulcer treatment. In *Topics in Gastroenterology 10* (Ed.) Jewell, D. P. & Selby, W. S. pp. 117–124. Oxford: Blackwell.

41 Pounder, R. E., Williams, J. G., Milton-Thompson, G. J. & Misiewicz, J. J. (1975) Twenty-four hour control of intragastric acidity by cimetidine in duodenal ulcer patients. *Lancet*, **ii**, 1069–1070.

42 Rees, W. D. W. & Turnberg, L. A. (1980) The stomach and aspirin. *Lancet*, **ii**, 410–416.

43 Rees, W. D. W. & Turnberg, L. A. (1981) Biochemical aspects of gastric secretion. *Clinics in Gastroenterology*, **10**, 521–554.

44 Peterson, W. L., Sturdevant, R. A. L., Frankl, H. D. *et al.* (1977) Healing of duodenal ulcer with an antacid regimen. *New England Journal of Medicine*, **302**, 426–428.

45 Sturdevant, R. A. L., Isenberg, J. I., Secrist, D. & Ansfield, J. (1977) Antacid and placebo produce similar pain relief in duodenal ulcer patients. *Gastroenterology*, **72**, 1–5.

46 Viskum, K. (1976) A comparison of the course of the disease among patients with gastric ulcer, duodenal ulcer and ulcer dyspepsia without ulcer demonstrable by x-ray. *Danish Medical Bulletin*, **23**, 129–136.

47 Walt, R. P., Gomes, M. de F. A., Wood, E. C. *et al.* (1983) Profound decrease of 24-hour intragastric acidity by daily oral omeprazole. *British Medical Journal*, **287**, 12–14.

48 Whittle, B. J. R. (1981) Antisecretory actions of prostacyclin and its analogues on the gastric mucosa. In *Clinical Pharmacology of Prostacyclin* (Ed.) Lewis, P. J. & O'Gredy, J. pp. 219–232. New York: Raven Press.

Surgical treatment

Preservation of the integrity of the pyloric sphincter and the antral mill has been the major advance in the surgical treatment of peptic ulceration in the past 15 years. This has been made possible by the use of highly selective vagotomy (HSV; otherwise known as parietal cell or proximal gastric vagotomy), which confines the vagal denervation to the acid- and pepsin-secreting part of the stomach, leaving the gastric antrum innervated by the nerves of Latarget. There is now wide agreement that HSV is the safest operation, produces the fewest side-effects such as dumping and diarrhoea and is followed by the fewest metabolic sequelae. Debate focuses on the incidence of recurrent ulceration, which in the hands of some surgeons is low but has been as high as 20% or even more in other series. This wide variation in recurrent ulceration is unrelated to preoperative factors such as acid output, age of the patient or length of ulcer history, but is related to the surgeon who operates, to the operative technique used and to incomplete vagotomy.

CHOICE OF THERAPY: MEDICAL TREATMENT OR SURGERY?

In this era of effective medical therapy with drugs such as cimetidine, ranitidine, De-Nol (tripotassium di-citrato bismuthate), pirenzepine and even antacids, one might well ask if *any* patients need surgical treatment; some physicians are now suggesting that they do not. Most surgeons would regard this view as a trifle extreme, but perhaps they are biased! It should be emphasized that surgical treatment is more effective than medical treatment in curing peptic ulcers, and also that HSV is more specific in its action than is medical treatment.

Effectiveness

When 100 patients with active duodenal ulceration are treated medically by the most modern methods, about 10–15% of the ulcers remain unhealed.[101] After almost any form of surgical treatment the incidence of recurrent ulceration is only 1–2% in the first postoperative year. If we now consider 100 patients whose duodenal ulcers have been healed by a course of cimetidine or ranitidine and who are not given maintenance treatment, the incidence of recurrent ulceration within six months is about 70%.[4,70] In contrast, vagotomy, once done, is always present, and could be regarded as being equivalent to life-long therapy with an H_2-receptor antagonist in full dosage. Hence, whereas the recurrence rate in the absence of maintenance therapy is 70% with medical treatment, it is still only 1–2% after vagotomy. Such comparisons, though to some extent artificial, have some validity, since most physicians prefer to treat their patients with intermittent courses of H_2-receptor antagonists in full dosage rather than giving them continuous maintenance therapy.

A minority of physicians, however, treat the ulcer by full dosage therapy and then give maintenance therapy indefinitely, or at least for several years. Even with such aggressive medical therapy, however, about 10% of ulcers will fail to heal and a further 10% will recur within a year, so that the cumulative incidence of failure after one year is about 20%.[4] After vagotomy, the comparable figure is 2%.

These recurrences during medical therapy are not innocuous. Some recurrent ulcers cause pain and some are 'silent', but all of them are inevitably accompanied by progression of the pathological process: the ulcer continues to penetrate the wall of the stomach or duodenum, further fibrosis takes place, and life-threatening perforation, haemorrhage or gastric outlet obstruction are ever-present risks. Whilst it would be wrong to exaggerate the extent of such dangers, they must not be ignored, and now that the mortality of elective vagotomy for duodenal ulcer is as low as 0.2–0.3%, it is possible that medical treatment, prolonged over many years, may carry a greater risk to life than does surgical treatment but this remains to be studied by appropriate clinical trials.

Specificity

H$_2$-receptor antagonists affect not only the stomach, but also other systems of the body (see p. 141). A highly selective vagotomy, on the other hand, while transiently unpleasant, is specific to the proximal three-quarters of the stomach and has no ill effects on other parts of the body. Moreover, HSV has been with us for 15 years, whereas many of the modern drugs have only been widely used for two or three years, so the full extent of their side-effects and potential dangers is not yet known.

Other considerations

Peptic ulceration is a chronic disease characterized by remissions and exacerbations, and prolonged medical therapy implies that the patient must take pills for many years, which many find irksome. Hence, compliance with medical therapy leaves much to be desired, and this probably accounts for a proportion of the recurrences. Surgical treatment, in contrast, is permanent in its effect. Moreover, after surgical treatment there is no necessity to keep attending the doctor's office or the hospital, whereas with repeated courses of medical treatment or with long-term maintenance therapy the patient's life is more likely to be dominated and distorted by the presence of the ulcer and the fear that it may recur. In addition, some physicians evince unbounded zeal in checking on the healing of the ulcer by means of repeated endoscopies, which are unpleasant to the individual patient and expensive to the state, the patient or the insurance company. Hence, although in the short term a surgical operation is expensive, in the long run it may be cheaper than medical therapy.[80]

Despite the above remarks we believe that most patients with duodenal ulcer or benign gastric ulcer should be treated medically in the first instance. Our only plea is that such medical therapy should not be continued for so long that the ulcer enlarges, to create pathological havoc and clinical danger. There will, of course, always be the category of elderly, unfit patients in whom prolonged maintenance therapy is entirely logical because of the risks of surgery. For the remainder, we feel that if, despite good medical treatment, the patient continues to be troubled by painful exacerbations of the ulcer that interfere with work, sleep or general enjoyment of life, he should be considered for surgical treatment. If, in addition, the ulcer has previously bled or perforated, that would tip the balance in favour of an operation.

In short, the indications for surgical intervention remain the traditional ones, namely failure of medical treatment or the occurrence of life-threatening complications. What precisely constitutes 'failure of medical treatment' remains a matter for debate.

In selecting patients for surgical treatment, it is desirable to avoid or forestall surgical failure. There are three main causes of such failure: recurrent ulceration, side-effects of the operation and selection of unsuitable patients for surgical treatment. The last group should, if possible, be identified before operation and surgery withheld. The difficulty, of course, is that this group tend to do badly both with medical and with surgical treatment. Identification of such patients is difficult and controversial. Our practice is to avoid operating on patients who smoke and drink to excess and who ignore advice to moderate these habits. We believe that the postoperative 'albatross syndrome' – in other words, continuing to plague the surgeon with distressing abdominal complaints after the operation – can be predicted with some confidence in young-to-middle-aged people who smoke and drink heavily, are tattooed, and (taking into account the current difficulties with employment) show little interest in holding down a steady job. Such patients are frequently young, underweight males. A history of psychiatric upset is also a relative contraindication. We would not utterly deny such patients the potential benefits of surgery, but we certainly try hard to avoid operating on them, being prepared instead to offer them prolonged maintenance treatment with a variety of the newer anti-ulcer drugs in the hope that they may obtain a cure or modify their lifestyle. These patients spoil any surgical series, because even if they do not develop recurrent ulceration they complain of numerous symptoms at the gastric follow-up clinic and so end up being classed as Visick grade IV, the category of failure.

CHOICE OF ELECTIVE OPERATION

This is, and always has been, a compromise – a kind of Odyssean steering between the Scylla of total gastrectomy, which would be 100% effective but crippling and dangerous, and the Charybdis of sham laparotomy, which is safe, with few side-effects, but ineffectual. Of course in practice the spectrum of operations available is not so unethically wide, but it still varies greatly, between gastric resection with or without vagotomy at the one extreme and highly selective vagotomy at the other. Vagotomy combined with antrectomy is almost completely effective in curing peptic ulcers, because it removes both the vagal drive on the parietal cells and the principal source of gastrin, but by the same token it brings with it the side-effects and sequelae of both gastric resection and vagotomy. HSV, on the other hand, is less effective, but considerably safer, produces few side-effects and has minimal metabolic sequelae.

Certain operative procedures, formerly widely used in the treatment of duodenal ulcer, can be virtually omitted from consideration. Partial gastrectomy, for example, is rapidly falling into disuse even in countries like Germany where it held sway for a century, because not only is the patient four times as likely to die as after HSV, but it also produces significantly more side-effects (such as dumping), more weight loss and anaemia in the long term, and probably increases the risk that gastric carcinoma will develop 20 to 25 years later. Selective gastric vagotomy combined with a drainage procedure, while an important milestone in the historical development of surgery for peptic ulcer, has now been virtually abandoned, because it still involves vagal denervation of the gastric antrum together with a pyloroplasty or gastroenterostomy. Most surgeons feel that if they are going to take the trouble to perform a selective type of vagotomy, they might as well perform a highly selective vagotomy that keeps the antral mill innervated and the pyloric sphincter intact. Thus in Britain today the choice lies between HSV and truncal vagotomy with a drainage procedure (TV + D), while in North America vagotomy combined with antrectomy still has its staunch adherents. Fortunately, the results of some excellent prospective trials that compare HSV with vagotomy and drainage and vagotomy and antrectomy are now available, and will be described later.

HIGHLY SELECTIVE VAGOTOMY AND TRUNCAL VAGOTOMY: A 'PHYSIOLOGICAL' COMPARISON

When Dragstedt reintroduced truncal vagotomy in his classic paper in 1943,[24] he described truncal vagotomy (TV) alone, without a drainage procedure. Later, however, it was found that 30–50% of the patients who were treated by TV developed gastric retention, so destruction of the pylorus by means of a pyloroplasty or its bypass by gastroenterostomy became an integral part of the operation. Truncal vagotomy was thought to heal the duodenal ulcer partly by abolishing the direct vagal drive to the parietal cell mass

and partly by diminishing vagal release of gastrin from the antrum. The addition of a drainage procedure was regarded with equanimity, because it was believed that gastric reservoir function was still preserved after vagotomy with drainage, and that the sequelae of partial gastrectomy such as dumping and bilious vomiting could be avoided, especially when pyloroplasty was used as the drainage procedure. Finally, it was thought that severance of the vagal fibres to the liver, gallbladder, bile ducts, pancreas and small intestine – an integral part of truncal vagotomy – was of minor importance and would not produce side-effects. All these assumptions about truncal vagotomy are now known to be false. It is because truncal vagotomy is physiologically unsound that in controlled prospective trials its clinical results have been found to be somewhat inferior to those of gastric resection with or without vagotomy.[36, 59, 79]

Serum gastrin. Gastrin levels in man are no higher when the gastric antrum is left innervated, as in HSV, than when it is vagally denervated, as in TV.[41] Both types of vagotomy lead to a significant increase in serum gastrin compared with preoperative levels. Since the stomach has been found to empty satisfactorily through an intact pylorus when the antrum is left innervated,[2, 11, 46] these findings are of great importance, because truncal vagotomy is clearly illogical and the performance of a pyloroplasty or gastroenterostomy is unnecessary. Hence, those well-known side-effects of gastric surgery – dumping, diarrhoea and bilious vomiting – which are attributable in large measure to loss of the pylorus, can now be virtually eliminated.

Lower oesophageal sphincter. The necessity of mobilizing the distal 5–6 cm of oesophagus and clearing it of all vagal fibres is common to both truncal and highly selective vagotomy. Both types of vagotomy are followed by symptoms of heartburn in 10–20% of patients. What is not often recognized, however, is that 60% of patients complain of heartburn before vagotomy and in most of them heartburn is either absent or greatly improved after operation. Neither TV + D nor HSV lowers pressure in the resting lower oesophageal sphincter,[94, 95] so surgical manoeuvres designed to increase the competence of the lower oesophageal sphincter in the course of vagotomy for duodenal ulcer are probably unnecessary. On the other hand, if heartburn is a prominent preoperative symptom, and especially if it is accompanied by the presence of a large hiatal hernia or severe oesophagitis, it is probably advisable to add an anti-reflux procedure to the vagotomy.

Gastric secretion. Both TV and HSV diminish secretion of acid and pepsin to a similar extent. Basal acid output is reduced by an average of 70–80% and maximal acid output by about 60%.[39] After both types of vagotomy an increasing proportion of patients develop positive responses to the insulin test,[34, 57, 71] as time passes, but these positive responses show little correlation with recurrent ulceration. It seems likely that many patients have a slightly incomplete, but still adequate, vagotomy. There is little rationale in performing routine preoperative acid secretion tests, which are disliked by patients. However, routine determination of basal serum gastrin levels before operation seems advisable, because the assay is easy to perform and permits the occasional case of Zollinger–Ellison syndrome to be detected before operation. After vagotomy, there again seems little point in routinely testing gastric function, unless a new type of vagotomy is being introduced, or some form of quality control is warranted to monitor the efficiency of the surgeon. Whether this 'quality control' should be intraoperative, in the form of the Burge electrical-stimulation test[8] or the Grassi test,[37] or postoperative, in the form of a Hollander insulin test[43] or a modified sham-feeding test,[28, 63, 64, 68] is still a matter for debate.

Gastric motility, intragastric pressure and gastric emptying. Both TV and HSV impair receptive relaxation and accommodation to distension by a meal, with the result that postprandial intragastric pressure is higher after vagotomy than before operation.[89] This rise in pressure produces a sensation of fullness or discomfort, which is experienced by 20% to 40% of patients after any type of vagotomy and causes them to reduce the size of their meals. The symptom is very mild in most patients and only a few are seriously inconvenienced. The elevation of intragastric pressure after both TV and HSV leads to accelerated gastric emptying of liquids, a feature that is more marked after TV + D than after HSV. Thus, while dumping can occur after both types of vagotomy, it is significantly more common after truncal vagotomy with a drainage procedure. It has been shown by several authors that the stomach behaves as an incontinent organ (for liquids) after TV + D, and that the fluid cascading out of the stomach in the early minutes after a meal gives rise not only to dumping but also to rapid intestinal transit and

diarrhoea in susceptible individuals.[13, 75] Gastric emptying of solid food is virtually normal after HSV,[7, 14, 16, 44, 45, 68] whereas after truncal vagotomy it may be slow, excessively fast or normal. Myoelectrical activity in the stomach is disorganized after TV, whereas after HSV the regular three-per-minute rhythm of electrical activity in the antrum is maintained with a normal waveform.[92, 92a] As time passes, these abnormalities diminish, but even in the long term, gastric myoelectrical activity, motility and emptying are much closer to the normal after HSV than after truncal vagotomy.

When a hypertonic test meal of glucose solution is given orally to patients after HSV or TV + D, significantly more dumping, diarrhoea and hypotension are produced in the patients who had undergone TV + D than in those who have undergone HSV.[48] Clinically, too, episodic diarrhoea occurs in about 25% of patients after truncal vagotomy (2–4% being severely afflicted), whereas after HSV only about 4% of patients develop diarrhoea, and this is always mild.[56] While gastric incontinence followed by rapid intestinal transit of fluids is partly responsible for 'post-vagotomy' diarrhoea, preservation of the hepatic and coeliac branches of the vagus, as in HSV, is also of value, because diarrhoea is significantly more common after TV + D than after selective vagotomy with a drainage procedure.[61, 67]

Duodenogastric reflux. In normal people the pylorus provides a relatively effective barrier against reflux of what Silen has termed 'malevolent gall' into the stomach. Bile salts and perhaps other constituents of the duodenal contents such as lysolecithin damage the gastric mucosal barrier and so facilitate acid–peptic attack, for example in patients with gastric ulceration.[19, 52] Dewar and his colleagues have shown that the stomach concentrations of bile acids before operation are significantly elevated both in patients with duodenal ulcer[20] and in patients with gastric ulcer.[21] As might be expected, these levels increase still further after both TV + D and partial gastrectomy. After HSV, however, duodenogastric reflux is found to be significantly diminished, presumably because the elevated intragastric pressure and the presence of an intact pylorus combine to minimize such reflux. These findings may be important, because duodenogastric reflux predisposes to the development of gastritis[9, 25, 29, 60, 69, 82] and perhaps to gastric carcinoma.[22, 86, 90] The carcinoma of the gastric stump that develops after partial gastrectomy is not evenly distributed in the gastric mucosa, but appears near the stoma, where the concentration of bile salts is presumably highest. Again, in patients with benign gastric ulcer it seems illogical to employ an operation such as partial gastrectomy or vagotomy with drainage that increases duodenogastric reflux, when it is known that such reflux damages the gastric mucosa by rendering it more susceptible to the action of endogenous acid and pepsin.

Liver and biliary tract. After truncal vagotomy in dogs, bile flow diminishes and the bile becomes more lithogenic in composition.[15, 30, 33] In man, the volume of the resting gallbladder increases significantly after truncal vagotomy,[51, 83] whereas it does not change after selective or highly selective vagotomy.[49, 78] Shields and colleagues[5] have shown recently that truncal vagotomy with pyloroplasty (TV + P) leads to significant delay in gallbladder emptying after a meal and to disturbance of the normal integration of gastric emptying and gallbladder emptying. Although in their review article in 1969 Fletcher and Clark concluded that the connection between truncal vagotomy and gallstones was 'not proven',[31] 15 years later papers by Clave and Gaspar,[12] Csendes et al.,[18] Tompkins et al.[96] and Sapala et al.[84] leave little doubt that the incidence of gallstones is significantly increased after truncal vagotomy. In fact, the mean incidence of gallstones seems to be about 20% within five years of truncal vagotomy. We have recently concluded a review of the incidence of gallstones in 100 patients who were followed up for a mean period of nine years after HSV and found an incidence of 11%, which, as far as we could calculate, did not differ significantly from the expected incidence in our area in people of similar age and sex distribution. The question of a possible connection between vagotomy and the subsequent development of gallstones is important clinically for two reasons. First, it is obviously undesirable that an operation designed to cure one benign condition should give rise to another painful and potentially hazardous condition that often necessitates operative treatment. Secondly, severe episodic diarrhoea is a complication of truncal vagotomy and drainage in only 2–4% of patients, but when cholecystectomy is added to TV + D the incidence of diarrhoea may be as high as 50%, and between 10% and 20% of patients experience severe diarrhoea.[93, 98] It follows that when patients who have both duodenal ulceration and gallstones come to operation, truncal vagotomy should be avoided.

Even in the absence of gallstones, the possibility that truncal vagotomy might predispose to the subsequent development of gallstones is a relative contraindication to the performance of this type of vagotomy.

Pancreas. It used to be taught that truncal vagotomy did not impair pancreatic function in man, but such statements were based on the results of unsophisticated tests of pancreatic function in which secretion was often stimulated by unphysiological amounts of secretin and pancreozymin, given intravenously. When a more physiological stimulus is used, such as a meal, or amino acids perfused through the duodenum, it becomes clear that pancreatic exocrine secretion is diminished by about 50% after truncal vagotomy,[74] whereas after HSV no such impairment is found.[68, 81, 88] We have also shown that pancreatic endocrine function is altered after truncal vagotomy.[47] In normal people and in patients who have undergone HSV, glucose given by mouth elicits a much greater secretion of insulin than the same amount of glucose given intravenously. After truncal vagotomy, however, we find that insulin secretion after oral glucose is no greater than insulin secretion after intravenous glucose. Hence truncal vagotomy in man seems to interfere with the entero-insulin axis, perhaps by modifying nervous reflexes or the release of some endocrine substance from the mucosa of the upper small intestine.

Faecal fat excretion and long-term effects on nutrition. After HSV, faecal fat excretion is normal,[26] whereas after TV + D it is significantly increased and about 40% of patients develop steatorrhoea,[17, 99] though the degree of steatorrhoea is mild and asymptomatic in the majority. However, in 10–20% of patients after TV + D, faecal fat output increases to ten grams per day or more (> 30 mmol/day) and malabsorption may contribute to nutritional deficiency in the long term. Certainly, long-term studies by Wheldon and her colleagues in Newcastle, England,[97, 100] suggest that there is significant weight loss and iron deficiency anaemia after truncal vagotomy with a drainage procedure. We have studied 100 patients for more than ten years after HSV in Leeds, England, and so far have found no evidence of iron-deficiency anaemia and no evidence of weight loss. Indeed, after HSV there is a significant gain in weight during the first postoperative year, after which body weight remains constant and does not differ significantly from the ideal body weight for height.

CLINICAL RESULTS OF HIGHLY
SELECTIVE VAGOTOMY FOR
DUODENAL ULCER IN LEEDS

One of us (DJ) first introduced HSV into clinical practice in Leeds in January 1969[54, 55] and has used it in the elective surgical treatment of a virtually consecutive series of patients with duodenal ulceration ever since. In 1970, we considered performing a prospective trial of HSV versus vagotomy combined with antrectomy (V + A), but the trial was not carried out for a variety of reasons, including the death of one patient who was subjected to vagotomy with antrectomy in another centre which was to take part in the trial, and also the occurrence of severe postoperative gastric stasis in a few patients who were included in a pilot study of vagotomy with antrectomy in this hospital. It thus became clear that the patients who would be assigned to vagotomy with antrectomy in the trial would be placed at greater risk of dying and would also suffer from more postoperative morbidity. Since the results of HSV continued to be excellent, with a low incidence of recurrent ulceration, the proposed trial was abandoned. In consequence, we are unable to present any controlled, comparative data from Leeds.

Follow-up of the many hundreds of patients who have undergone HSV has been undertaken in the gastric follow-up clinic by methods that have been described previously.[36] This clinic is also attended by many patients who have undergone operations other than HSV. Various modifications of HSV have been used in Leeds. Goligher, for example, in 1974[35] described a modification whereby 10–11 cm of prepyloric stomach was left innervated rather than the 5–7 cm described originally by Johnston in 1970.[55] G. L. Hill[42] also described an anterior highly selective, posterior truncal vagotomy, without pyloroplasty, but since the philosophy of this differs fundamentally from HSV, the results of Hill's operation are not included. Obesity of the patient was not a contraindication to the use of HSV, although it obviously made the procedure more difficult and prolonged. The mean age of the patients was 44 years, their mean weight 68 kg, and the mean length of ulcer history before operation was nine years. All ulcers were treated by HSV alone unless the patient had clinical symptoms of gastric outlet obstruction before operation.

The preoperative acid-secretory characteristics of these patients did not differ from those of patients in similar series in Europe and North America. This series of patients is therefore fairly typical of patients coming to elective surgery for duodenal ulcer in Britain during the 1970s, and the lessons derived from our experience are probably widely applicable.

Operative mortality. There was no mortality. Furthermore, there has been no ulcer-related mortality during follow-up.

Postoperative morbidity. Postoperative morbidity has been minimal. In fact, the patients' postoperative progress has been so smooth and their gastric emptying, in particular, so satisfactory, that our custom is to nurse them with neither a nasogastric tube nor an intravenous drip from the time of operation. All patients over the age of 40 received prophylactic subcutaneous heparin before operation and for at least five days after operation. Most patients were fit for discharge from hospital five to seven days after operation.

Splenectomy for trauma was required at the time of HSV in 0.7% of patients. The incidence of non-fatal pulmonary embolism was 0.7%. Three per cent of patients developed wound infection and 2% an incisional hernia. Reoperation in the early postoperative period was required by 1% of patients for wound dehiscence, ileus, intestinal obstruction and, in one case, peritonitis. This case of peritonitis was of particular interest, because for the first 11 years after the introduction of HSV no case of lesser curve necrosis was encountered, but in the 12th year this patient was found at re-operation to have a perforation of the lesser curvature just proximal to the incisura.

Side-effects of operation. HSV succeeded in its aim of significantly diminishing the incidences of dumping, diarrhoea and bilious vomiting. The virtual abolition of diarrhoea by the use of HSV and the large reduction in dumping was first documented by us in 1972.[56] As the years have passed, the large differences that exist between vagotomy with drainage or gastric resection on the one hand and HSV on the other have persisted. Moreover, this advantage in favour of HSV has not been bought at the price of any corresponding increase in the incidence of other side-effects such as heartburn, vomiting or dysphagia (Table 4.27). Although the data shown in Table 4.27 are not based on any prospective trial, they have been confirmed by randomized trials in other centres.

Recurrent ulceration. Here, recurrent ulceration is defined as any peptic ulcer causing symptoms

Table 4.27 Percentage incidence of side-effects after different elective operations for duodenal ulcer.

Symptom	Polya partial gastrectomy[a] (n = 107)	Truncal vagotomy with antrectomy[a] (n = 116)	Truncal vagotomy with gastro-jejunostomy[a] (n = 119)	Truncal vagotomy with pyloroplasty[a] (n = 161)	Selective vagotomy with drainage[b] (n = 85)	Highly selective vagotomy (n = 212)
Early dumping	22	9	18	12	20	2
Diarrhoea	7	23	26	22	16	5
Bilious vomiting	13	14	15	10	7	3
Epigastric fullness	37	36	40	37	38	23
Nausea	23	17	13	18	26	9
Food vomiting	6	10	4	4	—	2
Late dumping	1	4	6	2	—	2
Flatulence	20	23	18	20	—	9
Heartburn	8	16	20	13	14	18
Dysphagia	0	0	1	1	2	2

[a] From papers by Goligher *et al.* (1968, 1972).[36, 36a]
[b] Johnston and Goligher (1976);[53a] the drainage procedure was pyloroplasty in 68 and gastrojejunostomy in 17.
All patients were male except in the selective vagotomy with drainage group, of whom 24 were female.
The interviewing panel did not know which type of vagotomy had been performed.

that develops after HSV. However, recurrent ulceration may occur without producing symptoms, and in centres where patients have undergone routine endoscopy after HSV, the incidence of silent or asymptomatic recurrence was 30–50% of the incidence of symptomatic recurrence.[76]

After 5 to 14 years of follow-up in Leeds, 237 (82% of all patients) were reviewed. Approximately half of the missing patients had either died of causes unrelated to peptic ulceration or had emigrated, while half were lost to follow-up. The patients who were lost to follow-up did not differ significantly from those who attended for review.

The *incidence* of recurrent ulceration after 5 to 14 years was 11.8%. Of the 40 patients who have developed recurrence (after 0–14 years of follow-up), 22 (55%) presented within three years of operation and 29 (73%) within five years, but there were occasional recurrences up to nine years after operation.

The *site* of recurrent ulceration was duodenal in 27 patients and pyloric or gastric in the remainder. The mean interval between operation and the diagnosis of recurrence was 3.8 years.

Six of the 40 patients presented as emergencies, one with perforation and five with haemorrhage. Thirty-four patients complained of recurrent pain. Four of the six emergency cases were treated by partial gastrectomy with good results, while the other two fared well with conservative management. Of the 34 patients who presented with pain, 7 underwent re-operation and 27 have been treated medically,

mainly with cimetidine or ranitidine. There was no mortality among these 40 patients, either from the re-operations or from the recurrent ulcers themselves. Approximately two-thirds of the patients treated with H_2-receptor antagonists have achieved good results and many of them are doing well at present without any treatment whatsoever. Thus, only 2% of patients who underwent HSV for duodenal ulcer in Leeds have come to re-operation for recurrent peptic ulceration.

Long term metabolic sequelae

Body weight. The net effect in 140 patients who were followed up for a mean of ten years after HSV was a small but significant weight gain during the first year after operation only. Weight loss of more than 3 kg was recorded in 34% of patients after TV + P (Figure 4.33), compared with 13% of patients after HSV (Figure 4.34); weight gain of more than 3 kg was recorded in 52% of patients after HSV but in only 25% of patients after TV + P (both these differences are statistically significant: $P < 0.01$).

Anaemia. Only one of 90 patients who were studied a mean of nine years after HSV was found to be anaemic, and she had menorrhagia.

Tuberculosis was diagnosed in only one patient after HSV.

Carcinoma of the stomach has not been diagnosed in any patient after HSV for duodenal ulcer.

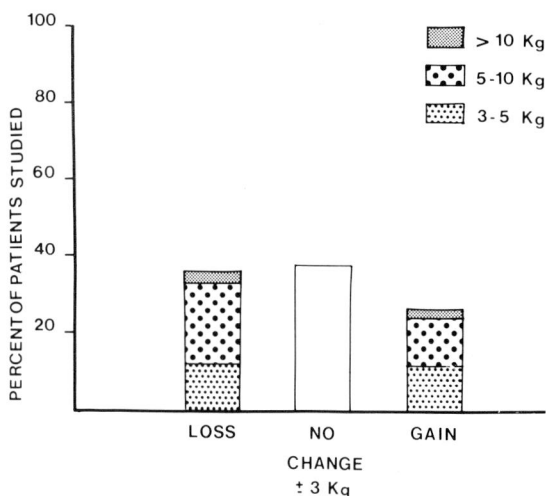

Fig. 4.33 Change in body weight after truncal vagotomy and pyloroplasty for duodenal ulcer in 67 male patients.

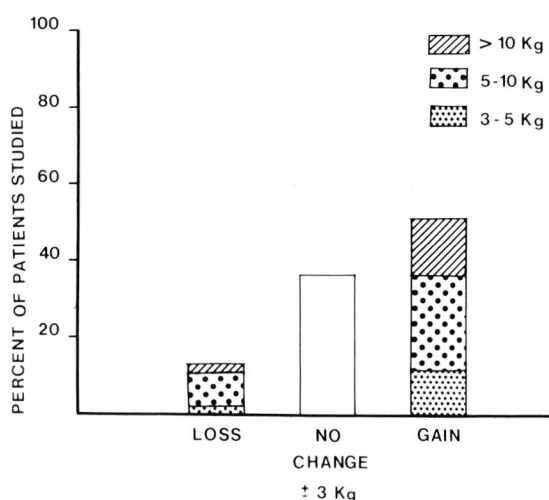

Fig. 4.34 Change in body weight after highly selective vagotomy for duodenal ulcer in 103 male patients.

These results from the University Department of Surgery at Leeds General Infirmary show that over a 14-year period, elective HSV for duodenal ulcer had no operative mortality and little postoperative morbidity, produced few side-effects such as dumping, diarrhoea and bilious vomiting, and did not lead to metabolic deficiency of any kind in the long term. The incidence of recurrent ulceration after five to eight years of follow-up was 10%, which should be compared with a figure of 8% after TV + P and 11% after selective vagotomy and drainage in the same department.

RESULTS OF HSV WORLDWIDE AND RESULTS OF PROSPECTIVE CONTROLLED TRIALS

The operative mortality, Visick grades and incidences of recurrent ulceration after HSV in a number of surgical centres are shown in Table 4.28. The operation is extremely safe, most centres recording no mortality whatsoever. In a survey of the operative mortality of elective HSV Johnston reported 17 deaths after 5257 operations, a mortality of 0.3%.[53] It can also be seen that 80% to 90% of patients were classified

Table 4.28 Clinical results of highly selective vagotomy for duodenal ulcer (review of the literature).

Authors	Number of patients	Operative mortality (%)	Length of follow-up (years)	Visick I + II (%)	Recurrent ulceration (%)
Dorricott *et al.* (1978)	116	0	1	82	4.3
Van Heerden *et al.* (1981)	194	0	0.5–6	—	5.2
Makey, Tovey & Heald (1979)	115	0	1–5	91	5.1
Stoddard, Vassilakis & Duthie (1978)	64	0	1–5	93	6.0
Kennedy *et al.* (1975)	50	0	1–4	96	2.0
Christiansen *et al.* (1981)	83	0	2–5	72	16.0
Sawyers, Herrington & Burney (1977)	86	1.2	1–4	96	3.5
Grassi (1977)	298	0	2–7	95	1.5
Koffman *et al.* (1983)	77	0	2.5–5.5	72	21.0
Andersen, Høstrup & Amdrup (1978)	273	0.7	2–5	83	9.8
Jordan (1979)	35	0	5	—	11.4
Hedenstedt, Schayah & Moberg (1980)	78	0	5	96	3.8
Fraser, Brunt & Matheson (1982)	69	0	5	87	1.5
Storey *et al.* (1981)	120	0	5	—	20.4
Wastell *et al.* (1977)	52	0	3–7	92	6.0
Liavåg & Roland (1979)	182	0	5–7	88	10.0
Goligher *et al.* (1978)	117	0	5–8	75	4.0
Jensen & Amdrup (1978)	100	0	5–8	86	9.0
Madsen & Kronborg (1980)	50	0	5–8	—	26.0
De Miguel (1982)	158	0.6	5–9	86	9.1

in Visick grades I and II. However, the incidence of recurrent ulceration ranged from 1.5% to 26%. The period of follow-up in several of these papers was fairly short, and in the Manchester study reported by Koffman,[65] for example, the recurrence rate has now risen to 21%. The wide range of recurrence will be noted and cause speculation as to why it should be so.

HSV compared with vagotomy and drainage

There have been several trials of HSV versus selective vagotomy and drainage (SV + D),[3, 62, 72, 85] the results of which have tended to favour HSV, mainly because the incidence of dumping after SV + D ranged from 20% to 40%, whereas after HSV it was 3–8%. Diarrhoea and vomiting were also less common after HSV than after SV + D. In Kronborg and Madsen's trial no fewer than 22% of patients developed recurrent ulceration after HSV, and yet 78% of patients (all the others) were in Visick grades I or II after HSV, whereas only 68% of patients were placed in Visick grades I or II after SV + P.

Truncal vagotomy and drainage compared with HSV

One of the earliest trials of this kind was conducted by Stoddard and colleagues in Sheffield, England. The incidence of side-effects in the two groups is shown in Table 4.29. Side-effects were significantly more common after TV + P than

after HSV. These authors concluded that HSV was superior to TV + P. Follow-up in that series now ranges from five to nine years, and the results continue to favour HSV.

A large multicentre trial of HSV versus TV + P was carried out in Manchester, England, by Koffman and his colleagues.[65] The results were much less favourable to HSV, the incidence of recurrent ulceration being 21%, compared with 8% after TV + P. However, no form of quality control, either intraoperative or postoperative, was used. The results serve as a warning of what may happen when a new operative technique such as HSV is introduced within a short space of time and employed by a large number of surgeons.

Undoubtedly the most elegant prospective trial of TV + P versus HSV has been carried out by Matheson and his colleagues in Aberdeen.[32] All 140 patients were operated upon by one experienced surgeon and subsequently reviewed by two independent physicians who were not aware of which operation had been performed. Follow-up was virtually 100% and the mean follow-up was five years. There were no deaths in either group of patients, but side-effects were significantly more common after TV + P than after HSV (Table 4.30). Four of 70 patients developed recurrent ulceration after TV + P, whereas only 1 of 69 patients developed recurrence after HSV. The overall clinical results were good to excellent in 87% of patients after HSV and in 70% of patients after TV + P. Matheson

Table 4.29 Percentage incidence of side-effects in a prospective trial of highly selective vagotomy and truncal vagotomy and pyloroplasty.[a]

Symptom	Highly selective vagotomy (*n* = 56)	Truncal vagotomy with pyloroplasty (*n* = 55)	Significance of difference *P*
Early dumping	2	17	<0.01
Late dumping	4	17	<0.05
Flatulence	20	42	<0.01
Bile vomiting	4	18	<0.02
Postprandial distension	21	44	<0.02
Diarrhoea	7	13	NS
Nausea	13	24	NS
Heartburn	16	18	NS
Dysphagia	5	5	NS
Food vomiting	7	11	NS

[a] From the prospective randomized trial in Sheffield by Stoddard, Vassilakis and Duthie (1978).[91] Patients were male and were followed up for 6 to 66 months. NS = not significant.

The interviewer did not know which type of operation had been performed.

Table 4.30 Percentage incidence of side-effects in a prospective randomized trial of highly selective vagotomy and truncal vagotomy and pyloroplasty.[a]

Symptom	Truncal vagotomy with pyloroplasty (% of 68)	Highly selective vagotomy (% of 69)	Significance of difference *P*
Diarrhoea	39	7	<0.001
Severe diarrhoea	6	0	
Epigastric fullness	39	15	<0.01
Dumping	13	4	NS
Bile vomiting	17	7	NS
Heartburn	28	25	NS
Weight loss >2 kg	35	13	<0.001

[a] From the prospective randomized trial in Aberdeen, Scotland, by Fraser, Brunt and Matheson (1983).[32]

Patients were followed up for 20 to 97 months (mean 61 months). NS = not significant. Results assessed independently by two physicians who did not know which type of operation had been performed.

and his colleagues concluded that highly selective vagotomy, although technically more demanding than truncal vagotomy and drainage, yielded superior clinical results.

HSV compared with vagotomy and antrectomy

Such trials are of particular interest because they compare the most conservative procedure with the most aggressive. Furthermore, even before the trial has begun it can be confidently predicted that vagotomy with antrectomy (V + A) will emerge as superior with regard to recurrent ulceration, because surgical ablation of both the vagal and the gastrin influence on the parietal cells results in a recurrence rate of 1%. By contrast, when antrectomy is omitted, the incidence of recurrent ulceration after any type of vagotomy is usually between 5% and 15%. The question, then, is whether the predictable superiority of V + A with respect to recurrence is outweighed by HSV's advantages in terms of operative risk, side-effects and metabolic consequences.

Three excellent prospective trials of HSV and V + A have been performed, by Jordan in Houston, Texas,[58] by Sawyers, Herrington and Burney in Nashville, Tennessee,[85] and by Dorricott and his colleagues in a multicentre study in Birmingham (England), London and Rotterdam.[23] The incidences of side-effects of operation and the Visick grades in some of these studies are shown in Tables 4.31, 4.32 and 4.33. The results of the three trials are in close agreement: postoperative morbidity and gastric retention is significantly greater after V + A than after HSV. Dumping, diarrhoea and vomiting are significantly more common after V + A than after HSV, and loss of weight is significantly greater after V + A than after HSV. Fewer patients return to full-time work after V + A than after HSV. Recurrent ulceration is

Table 4.31 Overall clinical evaluation in a prospective trial of highly selective vagotomy (HSV) versus truncal vagotomy with Billroth I antrectomy (TV + A) or selective vagotomy with pyloroplasty (SV + P).[a]

Clinical grading	HSV (n = 49)	vs	TV + A (n = 50)	HSV (n = 37)	vs	SV + P (n = 37)
Visick I	86[b]		56	78		73
Visick II	10		38	16		11
Visick III	0		0	3		13
Visick IV	4		6	3		3

[a] From the prospective randomized controlled trial of Sawyers, Herrington and Burney (1977).[85] Figures are the percentage of patients in each grade.
[b] Significant difference: $P < 0.01$.

Table 4.32 Postoperative sequelae in a prospective randomized trial of highly selective vagotomy (HSV) versus truncal vagotomy with Billroth I antrectomy (TV + A) or selective vagotomy with pyloroplasty (SV + P).[a]

Symptom	HSV (n = 49)	vs	TV + A (n = 50)	HSV (n = 37)	vs	SV + P (n = 37)
Dumping	0[b]		22	3		22
Diarrhoea	2[b]		18	0		3
Reflux gastritis	0		4	3		5
Epigastric fullness	8		0	8		8

[a] From the study by Sawyers, Herrington and Burney (1977).[85] Figures are the percentage incidence of each symptom.
[b] Significant difference: $P < 0.05$.

Table 4.33 Incidence of side-effects one year after operation in a prospective trial of highly selective vagotomy versus truncal vagotomy with antrectomy (Billroth I).[a]

Symptom	Highly selective vagotomy (n = 82)	Truncal vagotomy with antrectomy (n = 78)	P
Dumping	2	9	NS
Diarrhoea	5	14	<0.05
Vomiting	7	19	<0.05
Epigastric fullness	10	36	<0.0005
Heartburn	10	23	<0.05
Abdominal pain	11	12	NS
Dysphagia	0	4	NS

[a] From a multicentre randomized trial of HSV and TV + A (B1) carried out in Birmingham (England), London and Rotterdam by Dorricott et al. (1978).[23] Figures are the percentage incidence of each symptom.
The interviewer did not know which type of operation had been performed.

more common after HSV than after V + A, but the number of re-operations is about the same after either procedure, because more patients require re-operation for the relief of gastric stasis after V + A than after HSV. During the early years after operation, the overall clinical results (Visick grades) are better after HSV than after vagotomy and antrectomy.

RECURRENT ULCERATION AFTER HIGHLY SELECTIVE VAGOTOMY, AND HOW TO PREVENT IT

HSV is in many respects the ideal operation for duodenal ulcer – safe, with few side-effects or metabolic consequences. Its potential 'Achilles' heel', however, is the incidence of recurrent ulceration, which in the hands of some surgeons has been as low as 1–2% after five years of follow-up, whereas others have reported recurrence rates of 21–26% after shorter periods of follow-up.

It is possible that ulcer recurrence may be related to preoperative acid output, to stasis of food in the antrum after operation, or to factors such as completeness of the vagotomy. Should those patients who have gross hypersecretion of acid receive an antrectomy? Is there any test that could be used during operation to prove that the vagotomy is 'adequate'?

In Leeds, data on 40 patients with recurrent ulceration after HSV were compared with data on 399 patients who did not develop recurrence. Recurrence was unrelated to the patient's sex, age, length of ulcer history or previous history of perforation or haemorrhage. Postoperative gastric emptying of solid and liquid meals was the same in those with recurrence as in those without recurrence.

Preoperative basal (BAO) and peak (PAO) acid outputs were the same in patients who developed recurrence as in those who did not. Preoperative hypersecretors of acid were no more likely to develop recurrence after HSV than were normosecretors. This finding has been confirmed in the Aarhus County Vagotomy Trial.[1] Hence 'tailoring' the magnitude of the operation to pre-operative acid output does not seem logical.

Postoperative acid outputs, in contrast, were significantly greater in patients who were destined to develop recurrent ulceration than in patients who did not develop recurrence (Table 4.34). Basal and insulin-stimulated acid outputs were significantly greater in those with recur-

rence than in those without, whereas 'maximal' acid response to pentagastrin differed only slightly between the two groups of patients. Hence the pentagastrin test is much less useful in predicting recurrence than is the insulin test (or perhaps, than the modified sham feeding test). The greatest percentage difference was in BAO. When the insulin test one week after HSV was 'positive' by Hollander's criteria the chances that recurrent ulceration would subsequently develop were one in four (25%); when the test was 'negative' the chances of recurrence were 1 in 16 (6.7%). In short, the cause of recurrent ulceration is to be sought at the time of operation. Before operation, patients who will develop recurrence and patients who will not are indistinguishable; after operation they differ significantly with respect to acid output (Figure 4.35). Thus, recurrence is usually caused by incomplete vagotomy and is due, presumably, to faulty operative technique.

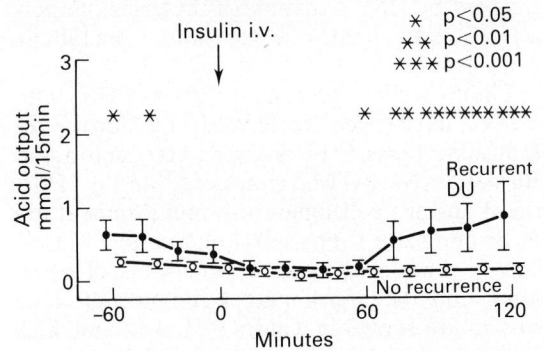

Fig. 4.35 Mean acid outputs (± 1 s.e. (mean)) in response to insulin one week after highly selective vagotomy for duodenal ulcer in 17 patients who subsequently developed recurrent duodenal ulcer and in 100 patients who did not develop recurrence.

Table 4.34 Acid outputs in patients with and without recurrent ulceration after highly selective vagotomy (HSV) for duodenal ulcer at Leeds General Infirmary.

		Number of patients	Acid output (mmol/h)		
			Before HSV	One week after HSV	More than one year after HSV
Basal acid output	Recurrence	28	7.2	1.5	**4.3**[a]
	No recurrence	90	7.6	0.8	**1.4** ($n = 44$)
Pentagastrin stimulated peak acid output	Recurrence	28	49	24	27
	No recurrence	100V47	23	23	($n = 44$)
Insulin stimulated peak acid output	Recurrence	28	—	**2.1**	**9.8**
	No recurrence	100	—	**0.6**	**4.7** ($n = 44$)

[a] Bold figures indicate a significant difference ($P < 0.01$) between patients with and without recurrent ulceration.

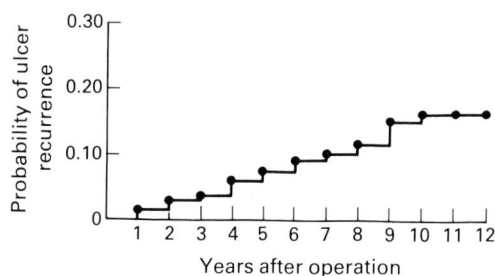

Fig. 4.36 Probability of developing a recurrent ulcer during follow-up after highly selective vagotomy for duodenal ulcer.

The next question is whether HSV carries an inevitable recurrence rate or is recurrence variable, depending on the surgeon and the adequacy of the vagotomy performed. In Figure 4.36 is shown the cumulative probability that a patient will develop recurrent ulceration after HSV in Leeds. However, the real answer to the question lies in the data shown in Figure 4.37, where it can be seen that the mean incidence of recurrence (12%) after HSV is meaningless without the knowledge that one surgeon has an incidence of recurrence of 3%, while another has an incidence of recurrence of 28%.

How to achieve a 'complete' HSV and a low incidence of recurrent ulceration
Good exposure of the operative field with a 'head-up' tilt and the use of a special substernal retractor to expose the oesophagus are of prime importance. In patients with duodenal ulcer, the parietal cell mass is extensive, often reaching

within 6 cm of the pylorus. Hence, vagal denervation must go far enough distally, to within 5–7 cm of the pylorus, if the distal portion of the acid-secreting mucosa is to be vagally denervated. Between incisura and cardia, the vagotomy is bound to be complete, because the lesser omentum with its neurovascular bundle is separated completely from the lesser curvature. It is important to spend about 20–30 minutes thoroughly mobilizing the oesophagus and clearing the distal 5–6 cm of all nerve fibres.[35, 40] At the same time, the upper 3–4 cm of the greater curvature are mobilized. When performed in this way, HSV is usually complete, as shown by the insulin test one week later, and the incidence of recurrent ulceration is 2% at five years and 3–4% after ten years.

We have conducted prospective controlled trials of the Burge electrical stimulation test and the Grassi test (both used at operation after HSV was completed) to see whether completeness of vagotomy was thereby improved, but no convincing evidence in favour of either test was found, compared with the results that were obtained in a 'control' group of patients whose HSV was performed in the usual way.[6, 27, 87] However, Johnson and Baxter,[50] and Allgöwer's group[77] have produced persuasive evidence in favour of the use of the Grassi and the Burge test, respectively, so the question of intraoperative testing remains open. Certainly some of the lowest recurrence rates after HSV have been reported by surgeons who do not use such tests:

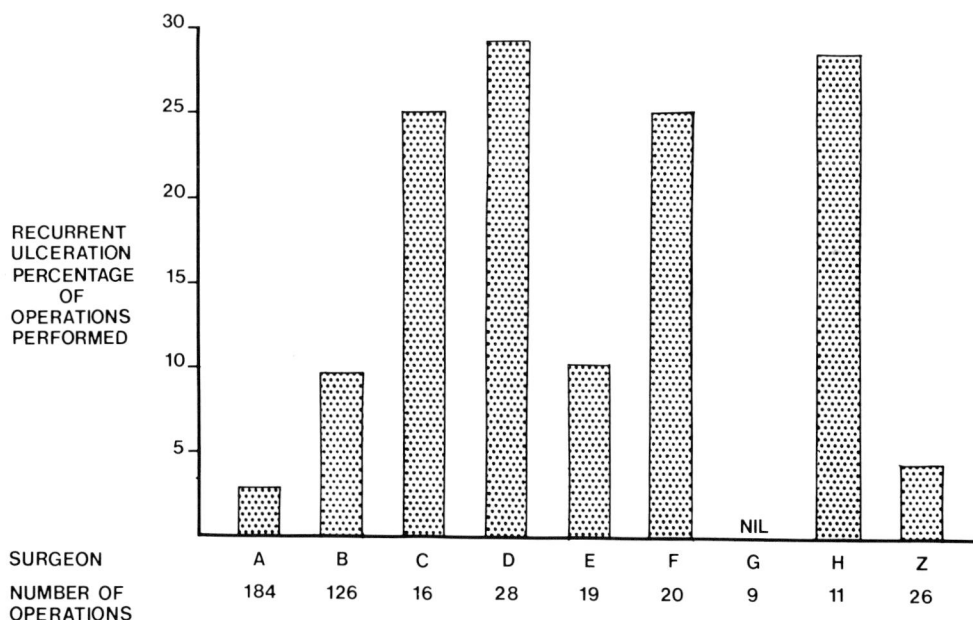

Fig. 4.37 Incidence of recurrent ulceration after highly selective vagotomy for duodenal ulcer expressed as a percentage of the number of operations performed by individual surgeons.

it remains to be seen whether the use of these tests helps surgeons with high recurrence rates to improve their results, or assists those learning to use the technique to achieve 'complete' vagotomy of the parietal cell mass regularly.

REFERENCES

1 Amdrup, E., Andersen, D. & Høstrup, H. (1978) The Aarhus County Vagotomy Trial I. An interim report on primary results and incidence of sequelae following parietal cell vagotomy and selective gastric vagotomy in 748 patients. *World Journal of Surgery*, **2**, 85–90.

2 Amdrup, E., Jensen, H.-E., Johnston, D. *et al.* (1974) Clinical results of parietal cell vagotomy (highly selective vagotomy) two to four years after operation. *Annals of Surgery*, **180**, 279–284.

3 Andersen, S., Høstrup, H. & Amdrup, E. (1978) The Aarhus County Vagotomy Trial II. An interim report on reduction of acid secretion and ulcer recurrence rate following parietal cell vagotomy and selective gastric vagotomy. *World Journal of Surgery*, **2**, 91–100.

4 Bardhan, K. D. (1981) Long-term management of duodenal ulcer – a physician's view. In *Cimetidine in the 80s* (Ed.) Baron, J. H. pp. 95–112. Edinburgh: Churchill Livingstone.

5 Baxter, J. N., Grime, J. S., Critchley, M. & Shields, R. (1983) The effect of truncal vagotomy and pyloroplasty on the relationship between gastric emptying and gall bladder emptying. *British Journal of Surgery* (in press).

6 Blackett, R. L., Baltas, B., King, R. F. G. J. *et al.* (1983) Does the Grassi test lead to more complete vagotomies? A prospective randomized trial (PRT). *British Journal of Surgery*, **70**, 294.

7 Buckler, K. G. (1967) Effects of gastric surgery upon gastric emptying in cases of peptic ulceration. *Gut*, **8**, 137–147.

8 Burge, H. & Vane, J. R. (1958) Method of testing for complete nerve section during vagotomy. *British Medical Journal*, **i**, 615–618.

9 Capper, W. M., Airth, G. R. & Kilby, J. O. (1966) A test for pyloric regurgitation. *Lancet*, **ii**, 621–623.

10 Christiansen, J., Jensen, H.-E., Ejby-Poulsen, P., *et al.* (1981) Prospective controlled vagotomy trial for duodenal ulcer. Primary results, sequelae, acid secretion and recurrence rates. *Annals of Surgery*, **193**, 49–55.

11 Clarke, R. J. & Alexander-Williams, J. (1973) The effect of preserving antral innervation and of a pyloroplasty on gastric emptying after vagotomy in man. *Gut*, **14**, 300–307.

12 Clave, R. A. & Gaspar, M. R. (1969) Incidence of gall bladder disease after vagotomy. *American Journal of Surgery*, **118**, 169–174.

13 Cobb, J. S., Bank, S., Marks, I. N. & Louw, J. H. Gastric emptying after vagotomy and pyloroplasty. Relation to some post-operative sequelae. *American Journal of Digestive Diseases*, **16**, 207–215.

14 Colmer, M. R., Owen, G. M. & Shields, R. (1973) Pattern of gastric emptying after vagotomy and pyloroplasty. *British Medical Journal*, **ii**, 448–450.

15 Cowie, A. G. A. & Clark, C. G. (1972) The lithogenic effect of vagotomy. *British Journal of Surgery*, **59**, 363–367.

16 Cowley, D. J., Vernon, P., Jones, T. *et al.* (1972) Gastric emptying of solid meals after truncal vagotomy and pyloroplasty in human subjects. *Gut*, **13**, 176–181.

17 Cox, A. G., Bond, M. R., Podmore, D. A. & Rose, D. P. Aspects of nutrition after vagotomy and gastrojejunostomy. *British Medical Journal*, **i**, 465–469.

18 Csendes, A., Larach, J. & Godoy, M. (1978) Incidence of gallstone development after selective hepatic vagotomy. *Acta Chirurgica Scandinavica*, **144**, 289–291.

19 Davenport, H. W. (1969) Gastric mucosal haemorrhage in dogs. Effects of acid, aspirin and alcohol. *Gastroenterology*, **56**, 439–449.

20 Dewar, P., King, R. & Johnston, D. (1982) Bile acid and lysolecithin concentrations in the stomach in patients with duodenal ulcer before operation and after treatment by highly selective vagotomy, partial gastrectomy or truncal vagotomy and drainage. *Gut*, **23**, 569–577.

21 Dewar, E. P., King, R. F. G. & Johnston, D. (1983) Bile acid and lysolecithin concentrations in the stomach of patients with gastric ulcer before operation and after treatment by highly selective vagotomy, Billroth I partial gastrectomy and truncal vagotomy and pyloroplasty. *British Journal of Surgery*, **70**, 401–406.

22 Domellof, L., Eriksson, S. & Janunger, K. G. (1975) Late precancerous changes and carcinoma of the gastric stump after Billroth II resection. *Acta Chirurgica Scandinavica*, **141**, 292–297.

23 Dorricott, N. J., McNeish, A. R., Alexander-Williams, J. *et al.* (1978) Prospective randomised multicentre trial of proximal gastric vagotomy or truncal vagotomy and antrectomy for chronic duodenal ulcer: interim results. *British Journal of Surgery*, **65**, 152–154.

24 Dragstedt, L. R. & Owens, F. M. (1943) Supradiaphragmatic section of the vagus nerves in the treatment of duodenal ulcer. *Proceedings of the Society of Experimental Biology & Medicine*, **53**, 152–154.

25 Du Plessis, D. J. (1965) Pathogenesis of gastric ulceration. *Lancet*, **i**, 974–978.

26 Edwards, J. P., Lyndon, P. J., Smith, R. B. & Johnston, D. (1974) Faecal fat excretion after truncal, selective and highly selective vagotomy for duodenal ulcer. *Gut*, **15**, 521–525.

27 Eltringham, W. K., Thompson, M. H., Davies, P. W. *et al.* (1982) The Grassi test and acid secretion. In *Vagotomy in Modern Surgical Practice* (Ed.) Baron, J. H., Alexander-Williams, J., Allgöwer M. *et al.* pp. 91–95. Sevenoaks, Kent: Butterworths.

28 Feldman, M., Richardson, C. T. & Fordtran, J. S. (1980) Experience with sham feeding as a test for vagotomy. *Gastroenterology*, **79**, 792–795.

29 Fisher, R. & Cohen, S. (1973) Pyloric-sphincter dysfunction in patients with gastric ulcer. *New England Journal of Medicine*, **288**, 273–276.

30 Fletcher, D. M. & Clark, C. G. (1969) Changes in canine bile-flow and composition after vagotomy. *British Journal of Surgery*, **56**, 103–106.

31 Fletcher, D. M. & Clark, C. G. (1968) Gall-stones and gastric surgery. A review. *British Journal of Surgery*, **55**, 895–899.

32 Fraser, A. G., Brunt, P. W. & Matheson, N. A. (1983) A comparison of highly selective vagotomy with truncal vagotomy and pyloroplasty – one surgeon's results after 5 years. *British Journal of Surgery*, **70**, 485–488.

33 Fritz, M. E. & Brooks, F. P. (1963) Control of bile flow in the cholecystectomized dog. *American Journal of Physiology*, **204**, 825–828.

34 Gillespie, G., Elder, J. B., Gillespie, I. E. *et al.* (1970) The long term stability of the insulin test. *Gastroenterology*, **58**, 625–632.

35 Goligher, J. C. (1974) A technique for highly selective (parietal cell or proximal gastric) vagotomy for duodenal ulcer. *British Journal of Surgery*, **61**, 337–345.

36 Goligher, J. C, Pulvertaft, C. N., DeDombal, F. T., *et al.* (1968) Five-to-eight-year results of Leeds/York controlled trial of elective surgery for duodenal ulcer. *British Medical Journal,* **ii,** 781–787.

36a Goligher, J. C., Pulvertaft, C. N., Irvin, T. T. *et al.* (1972) Five-to-eight-year results of truncal vagotomy and pyloroplasty for duodenal ulcer. *British Medical Journal,* **i,** 7–13.

37 Grassi, G. (1971) A new test for complete nerve section during vagotomy. *British Journal of Surgery,* **58,** 187–189.

38 Grassi, G. (1977) The results of highly selective vagotomy in our experience (787 cases). *Chirurgia Gastroenterologica,* **11,** 51–58.

39 Greenall, M. J., Lyndon, P. J., Goligher, J. C. & Johnston, D. (1975) Longterm effect of highly selective vagotomy on basal and maximal acid output in man.' *Gastroenterology,* **68,** 1421–1425.

40 Hallenbeck, G. A., Gleysteen, J. J., Aldrete, J. S. & Slaughter, R. L. (1976) Proximal gastric vagotomy: effects of two operative techniques on clinical and gastric secretory results. *Annals of Surgery,* **184,** 435–442.

41 Hansky, J. & Korman, M. G. (1973) Immunoassay studies in peptic ulcer. *Clinics in Gastroenterology,* **2,** 275–291.

42 Hill, G. L. & Barker, M. C. J. (1978) Anterior highly selective vagotomy with posterior truncal vagotomy: a simple technique for denervating the parietal cell mass. *British Journal of Surgery,* **65,** 702–705.

43 Hollander, F. (1948) Laboratory procedures in the study of vagotomy (with particular reference to the insulin test). *Gastroenterology,* **11,** 419–425.

44 Howlett, P. J., Ward, A. S. & Duthie, H. L. (1964) Gastric emptying after vagotomy. *Proceedings of the Royal Society of Medicine,* **67,** 836–838.

45 Howlett, P. J., Sheiner, H. J., Barber, D. C. *et al.* (1976) Gastric emptying in control subjects and patients with duodenal ulcer before and after vagotomy. *Gut,* **17,** 542–550.

46 Humphrey, C. S. & Wilkinson, A. R. (1972) The value of preserving the pylorus in the surgery of duodenal ulcer. *British Journal of Surgery,* **59,** 779–783.

47 Humphrey, C. S., Dykes, J. R. W. & Johnston, D. (1975) Effects of truncal, selective and highly selective vagotomy on glucose tolerance and insulin secretion in patients with duodenal ulcer. *British Medical Journal,* **ii,** 112–116.

48 Humphrey, C. S., Johnston, D., Walker, B. E. *et al.* (1972) Incidence of dumping after truncal and selective vagotomy and pyloroplasty and highly selective vagotomy without drainage procedure. *British Medical Journal,* **iii,** 785–788.

49 Inberg, M. V. & Vuorio, M. (1969) Human gallbladder function after selective gastric and total abdominal vagotomy. *Acta Chirurgica Scandinavica,* **135,** 625–633.

50 Johnson, A. G. & Baxter, H. K. (1977) Where is your vagotomy incomplete? Observations on operative technique. *British Journal of Surgery,* **64,** 583–586.

51 Johnson, F. E. & Boyden, E. A. (1952) The effect of double vagotomy on the motor activity of the human gall bladder. *Surgery,* **32,** 591–601.

52 Johnson, A. G. & McDermott, S. J. (1974) Lysolecithin: a factor in the pathogenesis of gastric ulceration. *Gut,* **15,** 710–713.

53 Johnston, D. (1975) Operative mortality and postoperative morbidity of highly selective vagotomy. *British Medical Journal,* **iv,** 545–547.

53a Johnston, D. & Goligher, J. C. (1976) Selective, highly selective or truncal vagotomy? *Surgical Clinics of North America,* **56,** 1313–1334.

54 Johnston, D. & Wilkinson, A. (1969) Selective vagotomy with innervated antrum without drainage procedure for duodenal ulcer. *British Journal of Surgery,* **56,** 626.

55 Johnston, D. & Wilkinson, A. R. (1970) Highly selective vagotomy without a drainage procedure in the treatment of duodenal ulcer. *British Journal of Surgery,* **57,** 289–296.

56 Johnston, D., Humphrey, C. S., Walker, B. E. *et al.* (1972) Vagotomy without diarrhoea. *British Medical Journal,* **iii,** 788–790.

57 Johnston, D., Wilkinson, A. R., Humphrey, C. S., *et al.* (1973) Serial studies of gastric secretion in patients after highly selective (parietal cell) vagotomy without a drainage procedure for duodenal ulcer. II. The insulin test after highly selective vagotomy. *Gastroenterology,* **64,** 12–21.

58 Jordan, P. H. (1979) An interim report on parietal cell vagotomy versus selective vagotomy and antrectomy for treatment of duodenal ulcer. *Annals of Surgery,* **189,** 643–652.

59 Jordan, P. H. & Condon, R. E. (1970) A prospective evaluation of vagotomy-pyloroplasty and vagotomy-antrectomy for treatment of duodenal ulcer. *Annals of Surgery,* **172,** 547–563.

60 Keighley, M. R. B., Asquith, P. & Alexander-Williams, J. (1975) Duodenogastric reflux: a cause of gastric mucosal hyperaemia and symptoms after operations for peptic ulceration. *Gut,* **16,** 28–32.

61 Kennedy, T., Connell, A. M., Love, A. H. G. *et al.* (1973) Selective or truncal vagotomy? Five-year results of a double-blind prospective, randomised, controlled trial. *British Journal of Surgery,* **60,** 944–948.

62 Kennedy, T., Johnston, G. W., MacRae, K. D. & Spencer, E. F. A. (1975) Proximal gastric vagotomy: interim results of a randomised controlled trial. *British Medical Journal,* **ii,** 301–305.

63 Knutson, U. & Olbe, L. (1973) The gastric acid response to sham feeding in duodenal ulcer patients after proximal selective vagotomy. *Scandinavian Journal of Gastroenterology,* (supplement) **20,** 16.

64 Knutson, U. & Olbe, L. (1973) Gastric acid response to sham feeding in the duodenal ulcer patient. *Scandinavian Journal of Gastroenterology,* **8,** 513–522.

65 Koffman, C. G., Hay, D. J., Ganguli, P. C., *et al.* (1983) A prospective randomized trial of vagotomy in chronic duodenal ulceration: 4-year follow up. *British Journal of Surgery,* **70,** 342–345.

66 Kronborg, O. & Andersen, D. (1980) Acid response to sham feeding as a test for completeness of vagotomy. *Scandinavian Journal of Gastroenterology,* **15,** 119–121.

67 Kronborg, O., Malmstrom, J. & Christiansen, P. M. (1970) A comparison between the results of truncal and selective vagotomy in patients with duodenal ulcer. *Scandinavian Journal of Gastroenterology,* **5,** 519–524.

68 Lavigne, M. E., Wiley, Z. D., Martin, P., *et al.* (1979) Gastric, pancreatic and biliary secretion and the rate of gastric emptying after parietal cell vagotomy. *American Journal of Surgery,* **138,** 644–651.

69 Lawson, H. H. (1964) Effect of duodenal contents on the gastric mucosa under experimental conditions. *Lancet,* **i,** 469–472.

70 Leading article (1978) Cimetidine for duodenal ulcer. *Lancet,* **ii,** 1237–1238.

71 Lyndon, P. J., Greenall, M. J., Smith, R. B. *et al.* (1975) Serial insulin tests over a five-year period after highly selective vagotomy. *Gastroenterology,* **69,** 1188–1195.

72 Madsen, R. & Kronborg, O. (1980) Recurrent ulcer

$5\frac{1}{2}$–8 years after highly selective vagotomy without drainage and selective vagotomy with pyloroplasty. *Scandinavian Journal of Gastroenterology*, **15**, 193–199.

73 Makey, D. A., Tovey, F. I. & Heald, R. J. (1979) Results of proximal gastric vagotomy over 1–5 years in a district general hospital. *British Journal of Surgery*, **66**, 39–42.

74 Malagelada, J. R., Go, V. L. W. & Summerskill, W. H. S. (1974) Altered pancreatic and biliary function after vagotomy and pyloroplasty. *Gastroenterology*, **66**, 22–27.

75 McKelvey, S. T. D. (1970) Gastric incontinence and postvagotomy diarrhoea. *British Journal of Surgery*, **57**, 741–747.

76 Mühe, E., Muller, C., Martolini, S., *et al.* (1982) Five-years' results of a prospective multicentre trial of proximal gastric vagotomy. In *Vagotomy in Modern Surgical Practice* (Ed.) Baron, J. H., Alexander-Williams, J., Allgöwer, M. *et al.* pp. 176–186. Sevenoaks, Kent: Butterworths.

77 Muller, C., Martolini, S. & Allgöwer, M. (1982) The vagometer electrotest (modified Burge test) for completeness of vagotomy. In *Vagotomy in Modern Surgical Practice* (Ed.) Baron, J. H., Alexander-Williams, J., Allgöwer, M. *et al.* pp. 77–85. Sevenoaks, Kent: Butterworths.

78 Parkin, G. J. S., Smith, R. B. & Johnston, D. (1973) Gall bladder volume and contractility after truncal, selective and highly selective (parietal cell) vagotomy in man. *Annals of Surgery*, **178**, 581–586.

79 Postlethwait, R. W. (1973) Five year follow-up results of operations for duodenal ulcer. *Surgery, Gynecology & Obstetrics*, **137**, 387–392.

80 Pounder, R. (1981) Maintenance treatment, part 3 – cost effectiveness. In *Cimetidine in the 80s* (Ed.) Baron, J. H. pp. 89–94. Edinburgh: Churchill Livingstone.

81 Ramus, N. I., Williamson, R. C. N., Oliver, J. M. & Johnston, D. (1982) Effect of highly selective vagotomy on pancreatic exocrine function and on cholecystokinin and gastrin release. *Gut*, **23**, 553–557.

82 Rhodes, J., Barnardo, D. E., Phillips, S. F. *et al.* (1969) Increased reflux of bile into the stomach in patients with gastric ulcer. *Gastroenterology*, **57**, 241–252.

83 Rudick, J. & Hutchison, J. S. F. (1964) Effects of vagal nerve section on the biliary system. *Lancet*, **i**, 579–581.

84 Sapala, M. A., Sapala, J. A., Resto Soto, A. D. & Bouwman, D. L. (1979) Cholelithiasis following subtotal gastric resection with truncal vagotomy. *Surgery, Gynecology & Obstetrics*, **148**, 36–38.

85 Sawyers, J. L., Herrington, J. L. & Burney, D. P. (1977) Proximal gastric vagotomy compared with vagotomy and antrectomy and selective gastric vagotomy and pyloroplasty. *Annals of Surgery*, **186**, 510–515.

86 Schrumpf, E., Stadaas, J., Myren, J. *et al.* (1977) Mucosal changes in the gastric stump 20–25 years after partial gastrectomy. *Lancet*, **ii**, 467–469.

87 Shorey, B. A., Owens, C., Davies, P., *et al.* (1977) Which is the best test of completeness of vagotomy – the Burge, the Grassi or the insulin test. *British Journal of Surgery*, **64**, 298.

88 Smith, R. B., Edwards, J. P. & Johnston, D. (1981) Effect of vagotomy on exocrine pancreatic and biliary secretion in man. *American Journal of Surgery*, **141**, 40–46.

89 Stadaas, J. & Aune, S. (1970) Intragastric pressure/volume relationship before and after vagotomy. *Acta Chirurgica Scandinavica*, **136**, 611–612.

90 Stalsberg, H. & Taksdal, S. (1971) Stomach cancer following gastric surgery for benign conditions. *Lancet*, **ii**, 1175–1177.

91 Stoddard, C. J., Vassilakis, J. S. & Duthie, H. L. (1978) Highly selective vagotomy or truncal vagotomy and pyloroplasty for chronic duodenal ulceration: a randomized prospective clinical study. *British Journal of Surgery*, **65**, 793–796.

92 Stoddard, C. J., Brown, B. H., Whittaker, G. B. *et al.* (1973) Effects of varying the extent of vagotomy on the myoelectrical and motor activity of the stomach in man. *British Journal of Surgery*, **60**, 307.

92a Stoddard, C. J., Smallwood, R., Brown, B. H. & Duthie, H. L. (1975) The immediate and delayed effects of different types of vagotomy on human gastric myeloelectric activity. *Gut*, **16**, 165–170.

93 Taylor, T. V., Lambert, M. E., Qureshi, S. & Torrance, B. (1978) Should cholecystectomy be combined with vagotomy and pyloroplasty. *Lancet*, **i**, 295–298.

94 Temple, J. G., Goodall, R. J. R., Hay, D. J. & Miller, D. (1979) The effect of highly selective vagotomy and truncal vagotomy on the lower oesophageal sphincter. *British Journal of Surgery*, **66**, 360.

95 Thomas, P. A. & Earlam, R. J. (1973) The gastro-oesophageal junction before and after operations for duodenal ulcer. *British Journal of Surgery*, **60**, 717–719.

96 Tompkins, R. E., Kraft, A. R., Zimmerman, E. *et al.* (1972) Clinical and biochemical evidence of increased gallstone formation after complete vagotomy. *Surgery*, **71**, 196–200.

97 Venables, C. W., Wheldon, E. J. & Johnston, I. D. A. (1982) The long-term metabolic sequelae of truncal vagotomy and drainage. In *Vagotomy in Modern Surgical Practice* (Ed.) Baron, J. H., Alexander-Williams, J., Allgöwer, M. *et al.* pp. 288–294. Sevenoaks, Kent: Butterworths.

98 Ward, M. W. N., Clark, C. G. & Karamanolis, D. (1982) Cholecystectomy and vagotomy – an unhappy combination. *Gut*, **23**, A900.

99 Wastell, C. & Ellis, H. (1966) Faecal fat excretion and stool colour after vagotomy and pyloroplasty. *British Medical Journal*, **i**, 1194–1197.

100 Wheldon, E. J., Venables, C. W. & Johnston, I. D. A. (1970) Late metabolic sequelae of vagotomy and gastroenterostomy. *Lancet*, **i**, 437–440.

101 Wormsley, K. G. (1981) Short-term treatment of duodenal ulceration. In *Cimetidine in the 80's* (Ed.) Baron, J. H. pp. 3–8 Edinburgh: Churchill Livingstone.

COMPLICATIONS OF CHRONIC PEPTIC ULCER

Duodenal and gastric ulcers share three principal complications: perforation, stenosis and bleeding. Both can penetrate adjacent structures and cause intractable symptoms, but the factor that distinguishes the management of gastric ulcer throughout is the difficulty of excluding malignancy. It might be argued that the outlook of carcinoma of the stomach is so poor that the distinction is theoretical, but this is not so, for the outlook is very good for the rare ulcer that undergoes malignant change, or the carcinoma alongside an ulcer that is being carefully monitored.

In a study of 1457 patients with duodenal ulcer, there was little change in the proportion of patients who bled as duration of symptoms increased, whereas the proportion with perforation decreased and the proportion with stenosis increased with prolonged symptoms.[16] The association between these three main complications is interesting: bleeding with perforation is twice as common as bleeding with stenosis and six times as common as perforation occurring with stenosis. This is not surprising when the pathological processes are analysed since bleeding and perforation may come from two different ulcers.

In the account which follows there is no discussion of bleeding, as this is considered in Chapter 6.

Intractability

Intractability implies a failure to respond to drug treatment. In a duodenal ulcer this may be a failure to respond at all, when the initial diagnosis should be doubted, or a second pathology, such as carcinoma of the pancreas, should be considered. Alternatively, it may mean that the ulcer becomes refractory to treatment after several courses of drugs. At present it is impossible to predict from early treatment which patients' ulcers will become refractory,[2] and it is still difficult to be sure if the intractable ulcer not responding to drugs will respond to vagotomy. There is evidence that many refractory ulcers will respond to vagotomy or vagotomy and antrectomy, but the criteria to select these have not been established. The response may be due to a more profound and persistent reduction in acid secretion[12] or to the effect of vagotomy on motility or some other mechanism not yet well understood. There is a suggestion that duodenal ulcers that do not respond to cimetidine or ranitidine, rather than those that recur after treatment, may need more aggressive surgery than proximal gastric vagotomy.[20]

Figure 4.38 is a guide to the treatment of the intractable duodenal ulcer.

Intractability in gastric ulcer should alert the clinician to malignant change, especially when the symptoms have originally been intermittent and responsive to treatment and then become continuous and unresponsive. However, response to treatment does *not* mean that the gastric ulcer is always benign. Intractability, even with negative biopsies, is probably an indication for operation and excision of the ulcer with vagotomy or resection. Ulcers should always be examined endoscopically after treatment and apparent healing. Brush cytology has the advantage over biopsy that the whole surface of the ulcer can be examined, whereas multiple biopsies always leave some areas unsampled. Figure 4.39 gives a scheme for the management of gastric ulcer.

Perforation

Perforation implies leakage of gastric or duodenal contents into the peritoneal cavity, but there need not be general peritonitis. A gastric ulcer may perforate into the lesser sac and a duodenal perforation may be walled off by liver, gallbladder, colon or omentum, leading to a local abscess (Figure 4.40). Characteristically there is sudden, severe pain, which may occur in the epigastrium or be felt generally in the abdomen. A brief period of stabilization and improvement is followed by further abdominal pain as generalized peritonitis develops. There will be tachycardia and hypotension and the patient will be cold, clammy and shocked. At this stage the abdomen is tender with guarding and rigidity and an ileus is present. Reduced

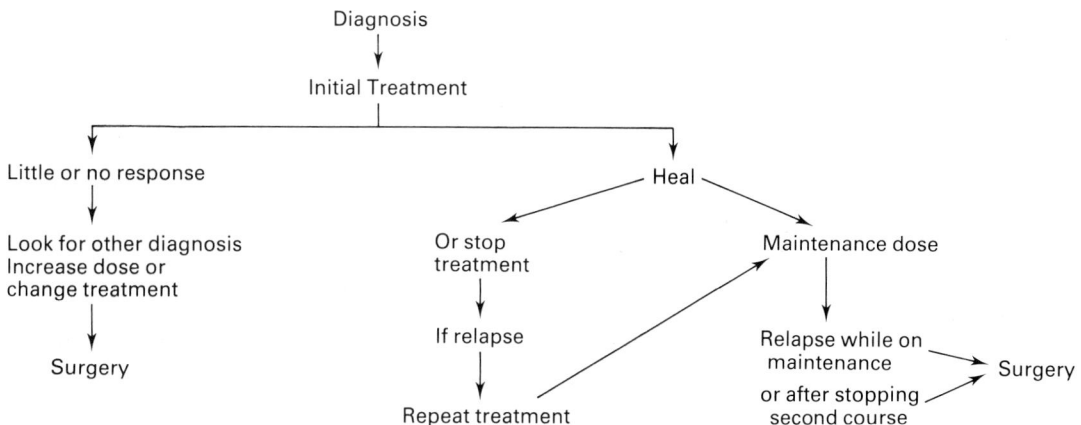

Fig. 4.38 Management of duodenal ulcer.

Diagnosis and Biopsy
↓
Initial Treatment

If not healed
by 8 weeks

Rebiopsy

Surgery

Rebiopsy

Heal
↓
Regastroscope and rebiopsy
↓
Maintenance dose

Relapse while on
maintenance
or after stopping
second course

Stop
↓
Relapse

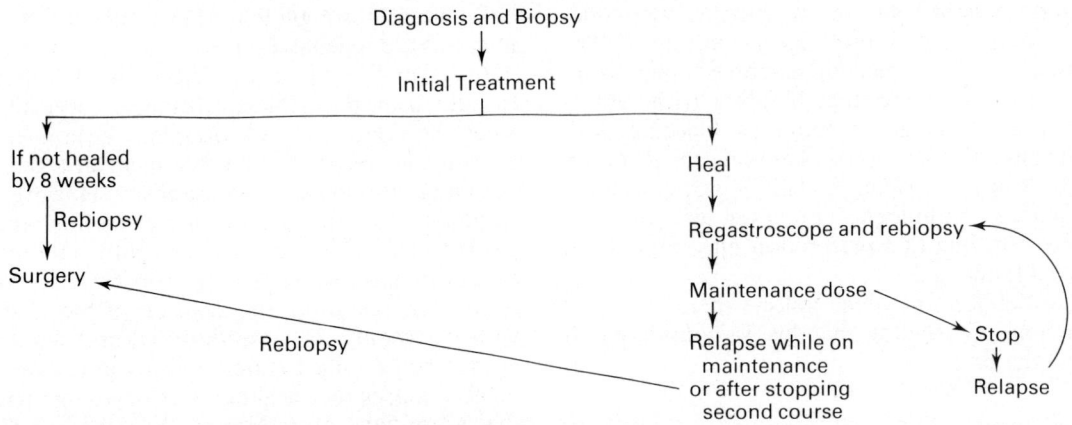

Fig. 4.39 Management of gastric ulcer.

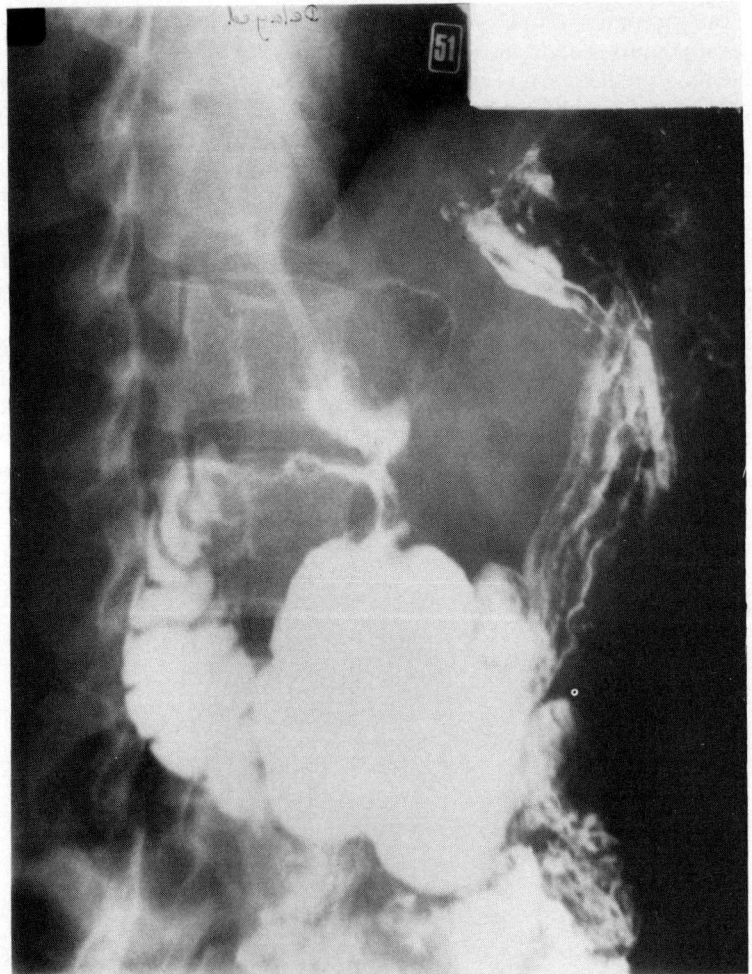

Fig. 4.40 Barium meal X-ray showing a walled-off perforation of a duodenal ulcer.

liver dullness may be present clinically but the diagnostic feature is air under the diaphragm seen on a plain X-ray of the abdomen taken in the erect position. A leucocytosis is present. Any delay in treatment results in ileus, shock, septicaemia and renal failure, with an appreciable mortality.

PROBLEMS OF DIAGNOSIS

The elderly patient may be confused and give a poor history. Poor muscle tone and possibly degeneration of peritoneal nerves, are responsible for absence of the standard signs of guarding and rigidity.

It has been said that the most dangerous place to have a perforation is in a medical ward. Felix and Stahlgren[10] found that the mortality of in-hospital perforation was 89%. Thirty-one (25%) of 126 patients with perforation presenting in hospital died without a diagnosis being made. The majority of patients were elderly males with duodenal ulcer and no previous ulcer history. All had serious associated disease and 50% suffered from neuropsychiatric disturbances. Shock and gastrointestinal bleeding were the main presenting signs and the usual signs of peritonitis were often absent. Two-thirds had tenderness or abdominal distension and nine bled from the same ulcer that perforated.

Retroperitoneal perforation is a rare form, involving a retroperitoneal leak which may arise from a posterior duodenal or gastric ulcer. Wulsin[21] reviewed four cases, in which there were three deaths. Slight extravasation may occur more often than is thought.

Perforation with a hiatal hernia may be associated with an atypical history and lead to a mediastinal abscess. A straight X-ray of the chest should show free air outlining the sac or mediastinal gas shadows.

Steroid therapy may make it difficult to diagnose a perforation. The clinician must be aware of this possibility. If the patient does vomit, a few flecks of blood or 'coffee grounds' are suggestive of the diagnosis, which must be confirmed by plain X-ray.

Differential diagnosis from a myocardial infarction and early leak from an aortic aneurysm must not be forgotten.

PERFORATION IN DUODENAL ULCER

Investigations

Only about 60% of patients with a perforated peptic ulcer show air under the diaphragm on plain X-ray (Figure 4.41). Some are too ill to stand or sit erect, in which case a lateral decubitus view is appropriate. Air in the peritoneal cavity may outline the intestinal wall because there is air on both sides. A posterior perforation in the lesser sac may give a fluid level. Ultrasound is helpful in detecting a walled-off abscess and excluding gallstone cholecystitis as a cause (Figure 4.42). If there is doubt about the diagnosis a radiograph of the stomach and duodenum should be performed using a water-soluble contrast medium with the patient rolled onto the right side. This will define the perforation in a high proportion of doubtful cases. Serum amylase should be measured to exclude acute pancreatitis, but can be moderately raised in perforation, probably as a result of absorption of pancreatic enzymes released into the peritoneal cavity. In fit patients little harm is done by operating, even if acute pancreatitis is found, if there is still real doubt about the diagnosis.

Management

Resuscitation with fluid replacement is the first priority. Patients may compensate well for many hours and then suddenly pass into circulatory collapse. It is essential that all patients should have an adequate urine output before operation. Even though the peritoneal cavity is sterile in 70% of patients, antibiotics should be given just before the operation preferably by the intravenous route. When there has been a long delay from the time of perforation or if there is severe respiratory disease, broad-spectrum antibiotics are indicated as soon as the patient is seen. Once the diagnosis is confirmed and treatment policy decided, analgesics should be given as it is quite unnecessary to leave the patient in severe pain while waiting for operation.

The place of non-operative treatment. There is no doubt that patients can survive a perforation without operation and that ulcers seal spontaneously with adherent omentum, gallbladder or liver. The problem lies in predicting those which will survive. Donovan *et al.* recommend giving a water-soluble contrast medium to confirm a sealed perforation by the absence of obvious extravasation.[7] In the past, some cases of suspected localized perforation may have been cholecystitis, but this confusion should now be avoided with the help of ultrasound and radionuclide scanning. In hospitals with good surgical and anaesthetic facilities conservative treatment only has a place in patients who have a very high operative risk from other medical

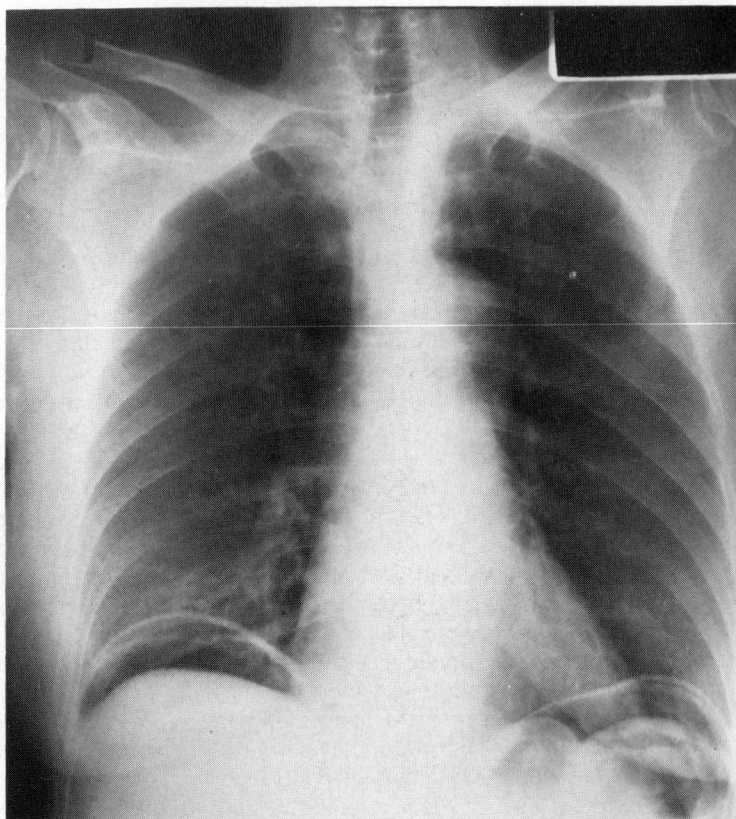

Fig. 4.41 Erect chest X-rays in a patient with perforated duodenal ulcer, showing free air under diaphragm.

conditions and, even then, only in those with localized signs or radiographic evidence that the perforation has sealed.

Operative treatment. The majority of patients should be treated by operation as soon as fluid and electrolyte balance has been restored. Delay after this stage merely increases the operative risk and complications.

The main controversy in the surgery of perforated ulcer is whether the surgeon should be content with closure of the ulcer with an omental patch, followed by a definitive ulcer operation at a later date if necessary, or whether a definitive operation should be performed initially. Many have written on this subject and devised criteria for selection of patients for definitive operation, but there have been few controlled trials. Boey *et al.*, however, randomly allocated patients with chronic duodenal ulcer to (a) simple closure, (b) truncal vagotomy and drainage and (c) proximal gastric vagotomy with closure but no drainage.[6] They excluded patients over 70 years of age or those with pre-operative shock, poorly-controlled concurrent illness, laparotomy more than 24 hours after the

onset of symptoms and gross peritoneal contamination, as well as patients with acute drug ingestion, acute ulcers or previous ulcer surgery. At 39 months' follow-up recurrent ulcer rates were as follows: closure, 63%; truncal vagotomy with drainage, 12%; proximal gastric vagotomy, 4%. Jordan reports no operative mortality in 60 patients with proximal gastric vagotomy and omental patch, with one recurrent ulcer in a 1–8 year follow-up.[13] Donovan *et al.* had a policy of simple closure for perforation of acute ulcers and definitive surgery for perforation of chronic ulcers if the patient was considered fit.[7] There was no mortality in those having definitive surgery. The overall mortality due to perforation was 16% for acute ulcer and 2–4% for chronic; however, all deaths were in patients with severe associated disease.

From a review of the literature, the following selective policy for treatment of perforated duodenal ulcer would be advised; the final decision must depend on the length of history, the fitness of the patient and the experience of the surgeon.

1 Perforation of an acute ulcer with no history may be treated by simple closure with omental patch, especially if the perforation has been

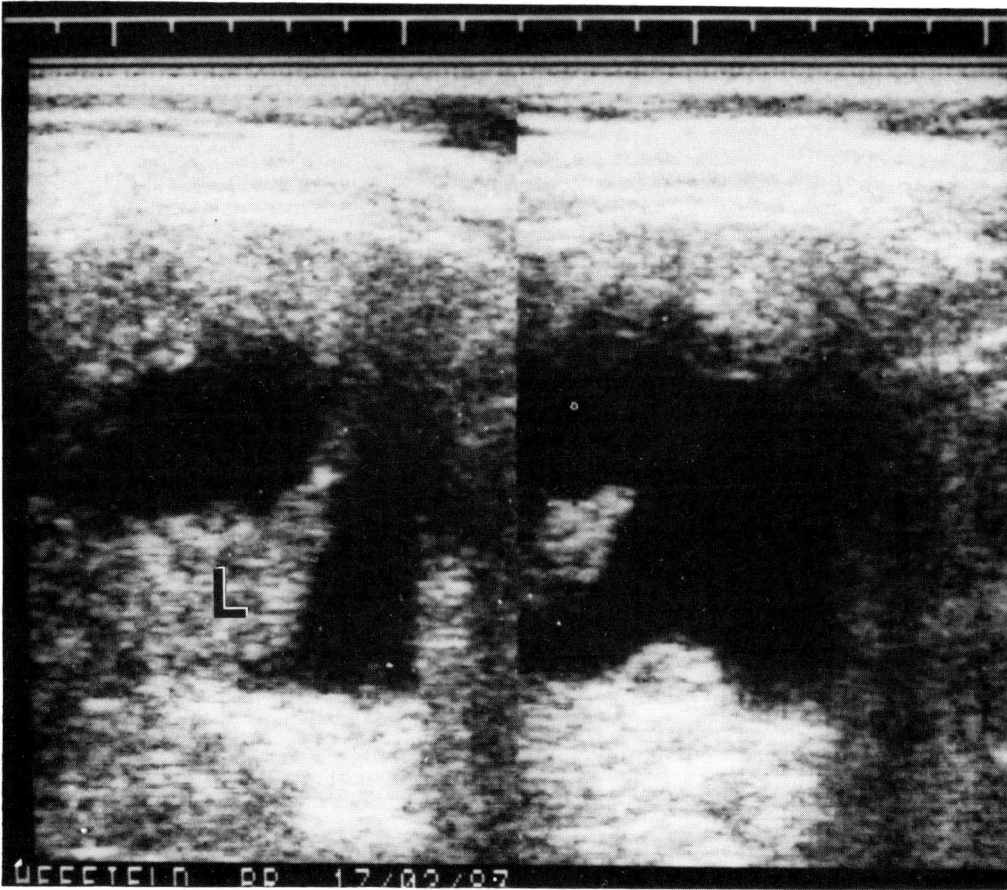

Fig. 4.42 Ultrasound examination of abscess around inflammed gallbladder in patient suspected of having a perforated duodenal ulcer (L = edge of liver).

present for more than 24 hours and is accompanied by extensive peritoneal soiling. The patient is then treated with H_2-receptor antagonist drugs in the same way as any other patient with a newly diagnosed duodenal ulcer.

2 Perforation of chronic ulcers, especially in the younger patient with a short time interval from the perforation to diagnosis, should be treated by definitive ulcer surgery, either truncal vagotomy with pyloroplasty or proximal gastric vagotomy with an omental patch. However, this policy only applies when the surgeon is experienced in these techniques. Surgeons who have not performed an adequate number of elective operations should not do them in the emergency situation and should be content with simple closure.

3 In the patient with additional serious medical conditions which increase the risk of operation, conservative therapy with gastric aspiration and intravenous fluids may be used, particularly if the perforation is shown to be sealed by contrast radiology.

PERFORATION IN GASTRIC ULCER

Simple suture is not associated with good results in type I gastric ulcer (see above) and there is a real risk that the apparently benign ulcer is a perforated carcinoma.

Resection of the distal stomach together with the ulcer and a margin of normal tissue is the treatment of choice, with either a Billroth I or a Polya (Billroth II) reconstruction. In a difficult high ulcer, excision and closure, with vagotomy and pyloroplasty is a satisfactory alternative provided the ulcer is examined carefully by histology. If the ulcer should prove malignant, an elective radical resection should be performed later. Perforated prepyloric ulcers (type III) may be biopsied and treated in the same way as for duodenal ulcers.

COMPLICATIONS OF PERFORATION

Death

The mortality from perforated peptic ulcer depends on a variety of high-risk factors including preoperative shock, perforation of more than 48 hours' duration and concurrent illnesses. Age, gross peritoneal soiling and length of ulcer history do not seem to affect mortality.[4]

Sepsis

Once the patient has survived the operation the main late complications are due to infection. In a study of 184 patients operated on for acute perforated peptic ulcer 13 infections occurred in eight patients (4.3%), despite the use of a cephalosporin which was started before the operation and continued for seven days.[5] In only four of the patients was there septic shock and an intra-abdominal abscess. Infection was more common in perforations that had been present for more than 48 hours and in the elderly. Nevertheless, cultures of peritoneal fluid were sterile in two-thirds of patients, probably because the gastric and duodenal contents of patients with an active duodenal ulcer are also usually sterile.[8]

Stenosis

Although the incidence of perforation and bleeding has not changed since the introduction of H_2-receptor antagonists, it is uncommon to see a severe pyloric stenosis nowadays. This may be because ulcers are treated earlier and their progress observed more closely, rather than because of the effect of the drugs. However, ulcers that were apparently completely stenotic have been shown to resolve with H_2-receptor antagonists.

The clinical feature of stenosis, or gastric outflow obstruction, is persistent vomiting. There may be little pain. Initially, when the gastric muscular tone is good, the vomiting is frequent and the vomitus contains recently ingested food. Subsequently gastric atony develops and vomiting is infrequent, occurring only once a day or less often. At this stage it is of a large volume, unpleasant in odour, and contains undigested food from meals eaten some days previously. Characteristically the vomitus contains no bile. The patient has anorexia, loses weight and is constipated. Physical examination may reveal a distended stomach and a succussion splash. Prolonged vomiting induces a metabolic alkalosis because of the loss of hydrochloric acid, sodium and potassium. The hypochloraemia is accompanied by an accelerated sodium–potassium and sodium–hydrogen exchange in the kidneys. The altered tubular function causes a rise of the bicarbonate threshold and a negative potassium balance. Tetany may be present.

DUODENAL ULCER

The expression 'pyloric stenosis' is ingrained in the medical literature, but it must be remembered that the pyloric canal may not be the site of stenosis in duodenal ulcer.[14] When there is much oedema round an ulcer it may be difficult at operation to distinguish it from a carcinoma of the pylorus.

Direct assessment of stenosis

Complete stenosis is easily diagnosed from the presence of a large stomach (sometimes extending into the pelvis), visible peristalsis and vomiting of unchanged food. The stomach has a remarkable capacity to dilate and adapt before causing symptoms. However, lesser degrees of stenosis are important to assess when deciding if a drainage procedure is necessary. External assessment at operation is unreliable.[14] The stomach would need to be opened to check the diameter, but this is undesirable because of the risks of sepsis. Preoperative endoscopy after the stomach has been well washed out is a simple method of assessment. If the standard, thin gastroscope can be passed through the lesion the stenosis can be ignored.

Assessment by gastric emptying studies

When planning an operation we are concerned not with small differences in gastric emptying but with gross delay. Barium sulphate is not physiological, but on the other hand it is not practical to submit many patients to dye-dilution or scintigraphic techniques. Stempien, Tester and Degradi devised the 'six-hour food and barium retention test', in which a standard meal was mixed with barium and a drainage procedure was only used for those with slow emptying.[19] Kreel and Ellis[15] use the following radiological criteria for stenosis:[15]

a   the presence of excessive fasting gastric juice,
b   excessive peristalsis (in the compensatory phase),
c   large atonic stomach (in the uncompensated phase),
d   delay in emptying of barium – more than 50% retention at six hours.

It is unwise to give barium preoperatively to patients with gross stenosis as it may be difficult to wash out and is dangerous if inhaled. However, only those with gross degrees of retention need a drainage procedure. It is now much more reliable to assess stenosis endoscopically than by radiology, particularly as biopsy can exclude a pyloric carcinoma.

Treatment

In established pyloric stenosis, it is imperative to restore fluids intravenously and correct the hypochloraemic alkalosis by infusing physiological saline with potassium. H_2-receptor blocking drugs may overcome an apparently complete obstruction by reducing oedema. There is little point in giving metoclopramide or domperidone to speed gastric emptying when there is already visible peristalsis, but good results have been obtained with metoclopramide in patients with pyloric diameters up to 5 mm.[22] Patients with complete stenosis who fail to respond to medical therapy need an urgent operation. It is also important to pass a wide-bore nasogastric tube to aspirate the stomach, and lavage with isotonic saline may be necessary to clear food residue. This manoeuvre is an essential for meaningful endoscopy. Gastric contents in the obstructed patient are often heavily colonized by pathogenic bacteria so prophylactic broad-spectrum antibiotics are advised, particularly as the stomach will be opened at operation.

Surgery

The best operation for most cases of benign pyloric stenosis is a truncal vagotomy and gastroenterostomy. This avoids a difficult pyloroplasty through grossly scarred tissue, and the stomach returns to its normal size and function.[9] A posterior gastroenterostomy at the most dependent part of the stomach is the treatment of choice, although Tanner's juxtapyloric anterior gastroenterostomy is effective if placed very close to the pylorus (Figure 4.43). If a pyloroplasty is chosen, the Finney type is better than the Heineke Mikulicz, but such procedures are best avoided in the huge atonic stomach of advanced stenosis. Proximal gastric vagotomy can be used together with a duodenoplasty in those patients whose scarring is beyond the pylorus. Proximal gastric vagotomy with digital dilatation of the stenosis through a gastrostomy was advocated,[18] but later follow-up showed it to be far from satisfactory.[3]

GASTRIC ULCER

Gastric ulcers may occur as a result of stenosis at the pylorus (type II) or may themselves cause stenosis in the body of the stomach. Type II ulcers will not be cured unless the pyloric and duodenal problem is also resolved. A proximal gastric vagotomy may cure both, but the results are not as good as in type I ulcers. Usually a vagotomy and drainage procedure or vagotomy and antrectomy are required.

The hour-glass stomach is a rare deformity, but lesser degrees are frequently seen (Figure 4.44). It is important to distinguish fibrosis from an infiltrating carcinoma. Figure 4.45 shows a stenosis on barium meal which was very suspicious of carcinoma but which proved to be benign at operation. In established stenosis a gastric resection including the stenosed segment is advisable.

Penetration

The commonest site of penetration for both duodenal and gastric ulcers is posteriorly into the pancreas, resulting in back pain. This is deep-seated and the patients complain of pain

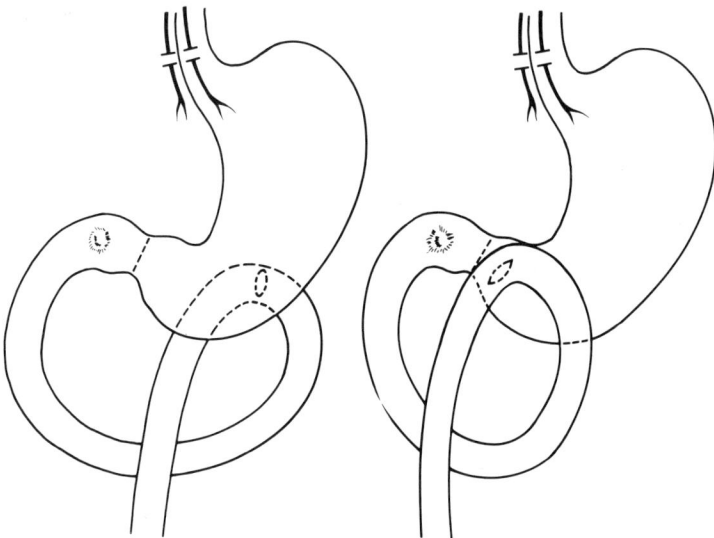

Fig. 4.43 Diagrams of (left) posterior and (right) anterior (juxtapyloric) gastroenterostomy with vagotomy.

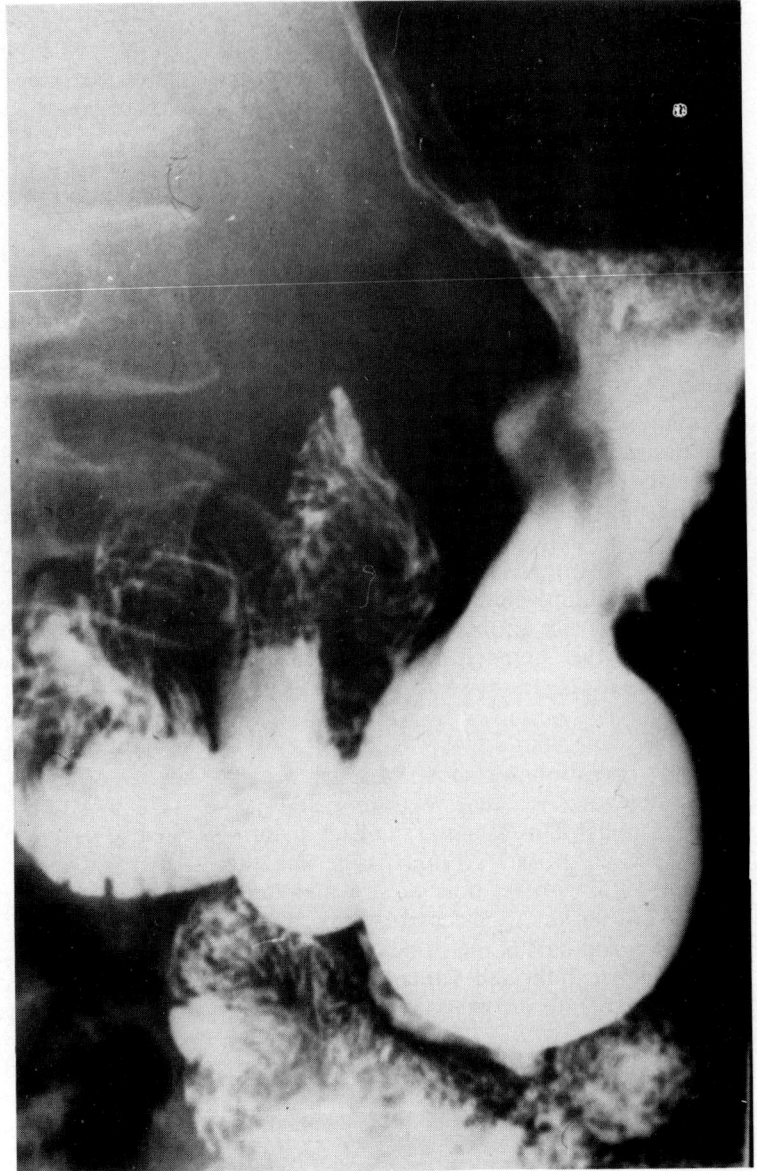

Fig. 4.44 Barium meal X-ray, showing early hour-glass deformity from large lesser-curvature gastric ulcer.

moving 'through' to the back. Other features suggestive of penetration are an alteration in the character of the regular ulcer pain, which becomes continuous and less responsive to medical treatments. It is usually the posterior, penetrating ulcer that bleeds. When back pain is a prominent symptom, it is important to exclude other conditions such as pancreatitis, aortic aneurysm and carcinoma of the pancreas. Sometimes an ulcer penetrates into an adjacent viscus, forming a fistula.

Gastrocolic fistula

It is rare for a primary benign ulcer to form a fistula into the colon. Most gastrocolic fistulas are due to carcinoma of the stomach and nearly a third to carcinoma of the colon, benign gastric ulcer accounting for the rest.[1] There is some evidence that steroids and aspirin therapy predispose to this complication. The symptoms are pain, faeculent vomiting and profuse diarrhoea or gastrointestinal haemorrhage and peritonitis. A barium enema will demonstrate the fistula and a barium meal and gastroscopy will show the underlying gastric lesion.[17] If the fistula is large, the gastroscope may be passed through it into the colon. Standard surgical management is to raise a proximal colostomy, thereby allowing the contamination of gastric juice by faecal bacteria to resolve, followed by a resection.

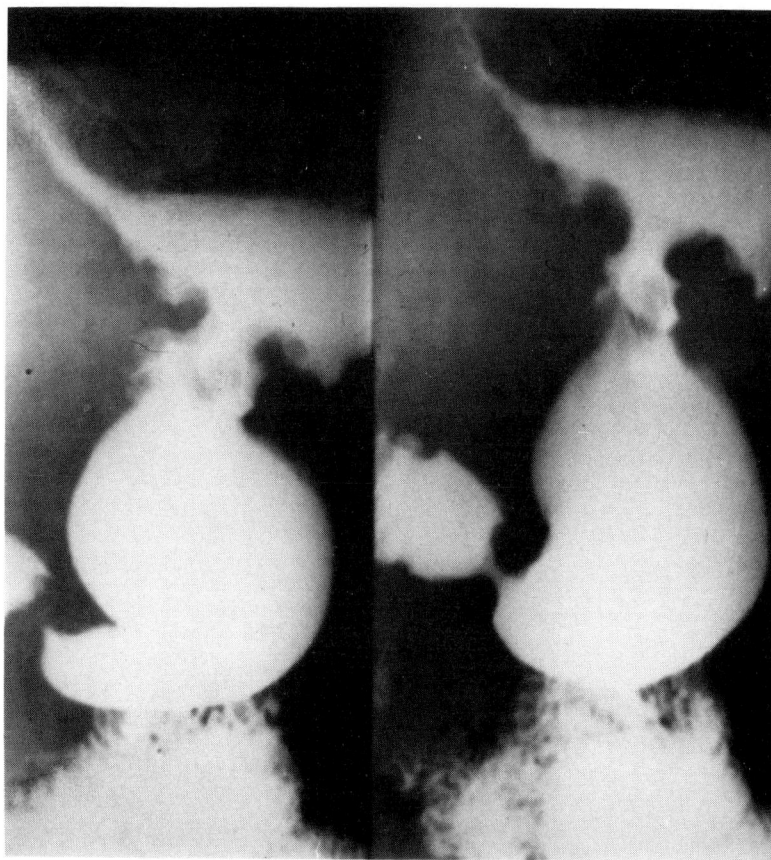

Fig. 4.45 Barium meal X-ray, showing gross hour-glass deformity suggestive of malignancy but found to be benign on resection.

However, with antibiotic cover and adequate preoperative bowel preparation, the fistula may be resected as part of an ulcer-curing operation.

Gastrojejunocolic fistula
This is a complication of a recurrent ulcer at a gastrojejunostomy whether the initial operation was a vagotomy and drainage or a Polya (Billroth II) partial gastrectomy. The symptoms are similar to a gastrocolic fistula, and gastroscopy is essential to confirm the recurrent ulcer, which may be just round the corner through the anastomosis and difficult to see. Surgical management used to include a proximal colostomy but this is rarely performed today. It is essential to correct any electrolyte abnormalities. If the original anastomosis was retrocolic, the dissection and identification of the fistula may be difficult. However, most fistulas occur after an antecolic gastrojejunostomy because the anastomosis adheres closely to the front of the colon.

Duodenobiliary fistula
Ninety per cent of biliary enteric fistulas are between the gallbladder and the duodenum and are caused by gallstones. Some of the fistulas are associated with gallstone obstruction in the terminal ileum. However, many of the rarer, choledochoduodenal fistulas are caused by duodenal ulcers.[11] Symptoms may be those of the underlying ulcer and the demonstration of a fistula may be an incidental X-ray finding. Alternatively, there may be recurrent cholangitis. The diagnosis is made by demonstrating air in the biliary tree on plain X-ray in the preoperative patient or by detecting barium refluxing up the bile ducts during a barium meal (Figure 4.46).

The correct management is to treat the ulcer and allow the fistula to close as the ulcer heals. H_2-receptor antagonists may heal the fistula. If an operation is required a vagotomy should be performed and the bile duct left alone. Occasionally, however, a bile duct stricture forms as the ulcer heals, producing obstructive jaundice with cholangitis. In this rare event, a Roux-en-Y choledochojejunostomy above the stricture is needed. Prophylactic broad-spectrum antibiotics are required when there is cholangitis.

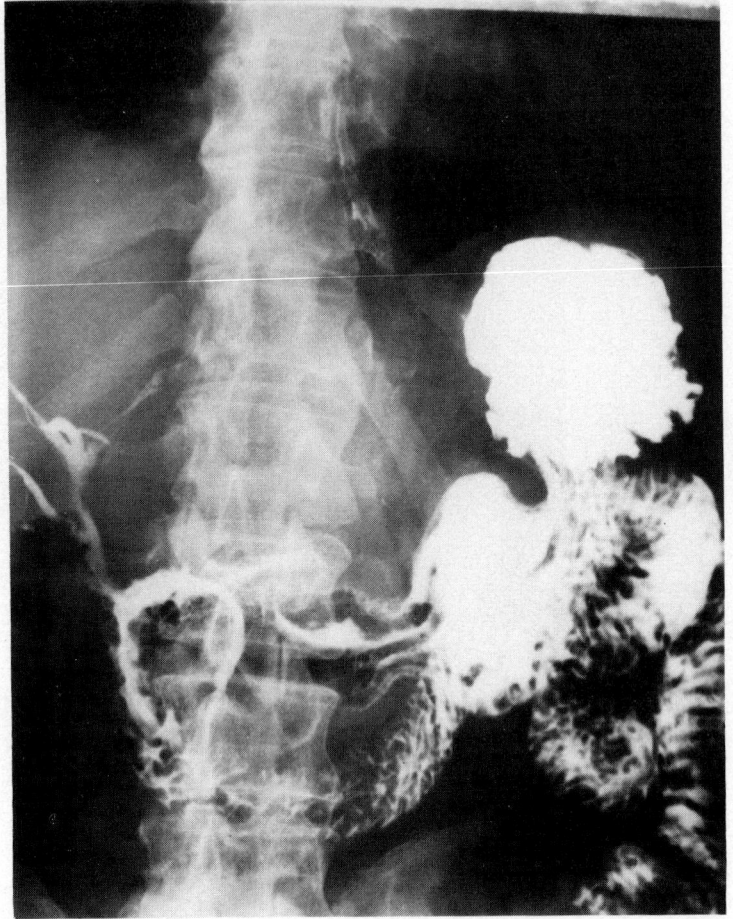

Fig. 4.46 Barium meal X-ray, showing biliary–enteric fistula from penetrating duodenal ulcer.

Malignant change

The risks of malignant changes in the gastric mucosa, particularly in the postoperative stomach, are considered in the next part of this chapter (p. 214). Here we are concerned with malignant change in a benign ulcer, an event which is very difficult to document because of the doubt that malignancy was excluded on the initial biopsies. Most cases of 'ulcer cancer' are cancers that have undergone secondary peptic ulceration, sometimes leaving only a small focus of malignancy. On the evidence of cases where there has been thorough histology and cytology, the risk of a benign gastric ulcer turning malignant is about 2%. The important lesson is that all gastric ulcers must be seen to have healed endoscopically, and any residual scar or mucosal irregularity should be biopsied even when healing is complete. It is also important to examine the rest of the stomach thoroughly each time and not just to concentrate on the site of the ulcer.

If conservative surgery is chosen for gastric ulcer it is safest to excise the whole ulcer from the mucosal aspects for histology. A recurrent gastric ulcer after medical or surgical treatment should be viewed with suspicion, especially after a Polya (Billroth II) partial gastrectomy.

The risk of a duodenal ulcer turning malignant is negligible and need not influence management policy. The occasional malignant ulcer in the duodenal cap is usually due to an ulcerating carcinoma of the pancreas. A primary carcinoma, however, may occur in the second and third parts of the duodenum and may give symptoms very similar to a duodenal ulcer. They can be missed when an endoscopy or barium meal is not continued far enough distally. The clinician should be alerted to this possibility if the changes in the duodenal cap do not match the symptoms or if there is vomiting or signs of obstruction with a normal or widely dilated pylorus.

ACKNOWLEDGEMENTS

I would like to thank Dr Bryan Ross (Consultant Radiologist), Mr Pat Elliott (Medical Artist), the staff of the Department of Medical Illustration and Mrs Carole Stenton (for the typescript).

REFERENCES

1 Allison, J. E. (1973) Gastrocolic fistula as a complication of gastric lymphoma. *American Journal of Gastroenterology*, **59**, 499–504.
2 Bardhan, K. D. (1981) Long-term management of duodenal ulcer – a physician's view. In *Cimetidine in the 80s* (Ed.) Baron, J. H. pp. 95–112. Edinburgh: Churchill Livingstone.
3 Blackett, R. J., Axon, A. T. R., Barker, M. C. et al. (1982) HSV with pyloric dilatation for pyloric stenosis due to peptic ulcer. *British Journal of Surgery*, **69**, 289.
4 Boey, J., Wong, J. & Ong, G. B. (1982a) A prospective study of risk factors in perforated duodenal ulcers. *Annals of Surgery*, **195**, 265–269.
5 Boey, J., Wong, J. & Ong, G. B. (1982b) Bacteria and septic complications in patients with perforated duodenal ulcers. *American Journal of Surgery*, **143**, 635–639.
6 Boey, J., Lee, N. W., Koo, J. et al. (1982) Immediate definitive surgery for perforated duodenal ulcers: a prospective controlled trial. *Annals of Surgery*, **196**, 338–344.
7 Donovan, A. J., Vinson, T. L., Maulsby, G. O. & Gewin, J. R. (1979) Selective treatment of duodenal ulcer with perforation. *Annals of Surgery*, **189**, 627–636.
8 Draser, B. S. & Hill, M. J. (1974) *Human Intestinal Flora*. London: Academic Press.
9 Ellis, H., Starer, F., Venables, C. & Ware, C. (1966) Clinical and radiological study of vagotomy and gastric drainage in the treatment of pyloric stenosis due to duodenal ulceration. *Gut*, **7**, 671–676.
10 Felix, W. R. & Stahlgren, L. H. (1973) Death by undiagnosed perforated peptic ulcer: analysis of 31 cases. *Annals of Surgery*, **177**, 344–351.
11 Feller, E. R., Warshaw, A. L. & Shapiro, R. H. (1980) Observations on management of choledochoduodenal fistula due to penetrating peptic ulcer. *Gastroenterology*, **78**, 126–131.
12 Hunt, R. H. (1981) Non-responders to cimetidine treatment, part 1. In *Cimetidine in the 80s* (Ed.) Baron, J. H. pp. 34–41. Edinburgh: Churchill Livingstone.
13 Jordan, P. H. Jr (1982) Proximal gastric vagotomy without drainage for treatment of perforated duodenal ulcer. *Gastroenterology*, **83** (1 pt 2), 179–183.
14 Kirk, R. M. (1970) The size of the pyloroduodenal canal: its relation to the cause and treatment of peptic ulcer. *Proceedings of the Royal Society of Medicine*, **63**, 944–946.
15 Kreel, L. & Elis, H. (1965) Pyloric stenosis in adults: a clinical and radiological study of 100 consecutive patients. *Gut*, **6**, 253–261.
16 Lam, S. K., Chan, P. K., Cheng, F. O. & Ong, G. B. (1978) The interrelationship between bleeding, perforation, and stenosis in duodenal ulceration. *Australia and New Zealand Journal of Surgery*, **48**, 152–155.
17 Laufer, I., Thornley, G. D. & Stolberg, H. (1976) Gastrocolic fistula as a complication of benign gastric ulcer. *Radiology*, **119**, 7–11.
18 McMahon, M. J., Greenall, M. J., Johnston, D. & Goligher, J. C. (1976) Highly selective vagotomy plus dilatation of the stenosis compared with truncal vagotomy and drainage in the treatment of pyloric stenosis secondary to duodenal ulceration. *Gut*, **17**, 471–476.
19 Stempien, S. J., Tester, R. J. & Dagradi, A. F. (1971) Six-hour food and barium retention test. *American Journal of Digestive Diseases*, **16**, 395–402.
20 Venables, C. W. (1980) Indications for surgery in duodenal ulcer nonresponders to cimetidine. In *H₂ Antagonists* (Ed.) Torsoli, A., Lucchelli, P. E. & Brimblecombe, R. W. pp. 16–23. Amsterdam: Excerpta Medica.
21 Wulsin, J. H. (1972) Peptic ulcer of the posterior wall of the stomach and duodenal with retroperitoneal leak. *Surgery, Gynecology and Obstetrics*, **134**, 425–429.
22 Zer, M. & Dintsman, M. (1975) The use of metoclopramide in acute pyloric obstruction. A clinical trial. *American Journal of Gastroenterology*, **63**, 232–239.

COMPLICATIONS OF GASTRIC SURGERY

Operations on the stomach, whether they are performed for tumour, trauma, bleeding or peptic ulceration, usually have few complications providing they are performed by technically competent, experienced surgeons and provided they are performed for the correct indications. Nevertheless, all gastric operations cause some alteration of the normal integrated physiological functions of the upper gastrointestinal tract, so to a lesser or greater degree they alter normal physiology.

Complications, when they do occur, may be the result of failures of operative technique or failure of the operation to cure the disease or be sequelae of altered physiology.[1]

Early complications are usually due to poor operative technique and occur while the patient is still in hospital. Intermediate complications occur within the first weeks or months of the operation when the patient fails to make a complete recovery. The late complications are usually the sequelae of the altered physiology or a recurrence of the original disease. Late sequelae may be further categorized as symptomatic, metabolic or 'predispotic'.

Early complications

Early complications are principally due to bleeding, leakage, gastric retention or complications within the biliary system or pancreas.

Bleeding

Bleeding from the gastrointestinal tract immediately after a gastric operation is usually from the suture line, either at the closure of the lesser curvature or at the gastroduodenal or gastrojejunal stoma. In my experience bleeding is a particular hazard after stapled anastomoses, particularly of the side-to-side variety. Although suture line bleeding is the commonest cause, it is important to consider the possibility of some abnormality of the bleeding or clotting mechanism. This is particularly important when the original gastric operation was performed for bleeding or if there has been a blood transfusion of more than four units (two litres). If the operation is performed for gastrointestinal bleeding and bleeding continues after operation it is essential to consider whether the true cause of bleeding was found at operation or whether the source of bleeding could still be present despite the operation; such a source might be angiodysplasia in the small or large bowel. Another possible cause of early postoperative bleeding is stress ulceration, particularly if the patient has another early postoperative complication leading to hypotension or septicaemia, or if the original gastric operation was not adequate to cure the ulcer diathesis.

It is uncommon for sudden profuse haemorrhage to occur immediately after operation. It is more common for the patient to present with vomiting of blood or melaena or with the aspiration of copious amounts of fresh or altered blood from a nasogastric tube. The patient may present with a progressively falling haemoglobin level with no overt sign of bleeding.

The nasogastric aspirate can provide much information. If the blood is fresh and copious the lesion is more likely to be in the stomach or oesophagus, whereas if there is only a small volume of altered blood in the stomach in the presence of obvious gross continued bleeding it is more likely that the bleeding lesion is distal to the stomach.

Upper gastrointestinal endoscopy is the most effective and direct means of investigating early postoperative bleeding, although there are dangers in distending the stomach with air soon after an operation. Conventional contrast radiology has little to offer in the assessment of this complication.

Angiography is usually considered only if there is a very strong suspicion that the bleeding lesion was missed at the first operation and that the true diagnosis is distal angiodysplasia.[34] Even under these rare circumstances I feel that it is wiser to perform endoscopy before selective angiography.

Isotopic labelling of red cells, followed by external scanning, has little or nothing to offer in the assessment of an immediate postoperative bleed.[34]

Treatment of bleeding may be medical or surgical. Pharmaceutical control is indicated when there is some detected abnormality of the bleeding or clotting mechanism. Some have advocated the empirical use of aminocaproic acid with the same rationale as that used for bleeding after prostatectomy but I have had no occasion to use it or recommend it.[72]

Pharmaceutical control of the bleeding may also be attempted with H_2-receptor antagonists if it is felt that the original operation has not controlled the ulcer diathesis. However, there is no evidence that H_2-receptor blockade is of any value in upper gastrointestinal bleeding other than for its prevention.[42]

Various methods of endoscopic control of postoperative bleeding have been proposed, from the spraying of clot-provoking drugs such as ancrod (pit viper venom), to electrocoagulation or laser coagulation. Reports of success are largely anecdotal and there are few well-controlled trials,[80] but bipolar electrode diathermy seems likely to prove the most practical method of local control.[51]

If some form of angiopathy is demonstrated the therapeutic options include angiographic control by pharmaceutical or embolic materials. Vasospastic drugs such as vasopressin appear to have the ability to halt bleeding temporarily but they have only a limited use in this clinical context.[23] Embolization as a control of bleeding seems to be potentially hazardous soon after an operation.[10, 15]

Knowing when to re-operate and suture the bleeding vessel often involves fine clinical judgement rather than scientific computation. Profuse continued bleeding requiring transfusion with more than four units (two litres) in 24 hours to maintain normal circulation is a strong indication for surgical reintervention, as is the endoscopic demonstration of an actively bleeding vessel that cannot be controlled by any of the aforementioned means. Immediately after operation it is probably less hazardous to reoperate on a patient to gain instant control by resuturing than it is to wait until the patient and the resources of blood are exhausted.

Leakage
Leakage may be due to unrecognized operative trauma, technical failure of the anastomosis, necrosis of either the suture line or part of the stomach or continued acute peptic ulceration.

Unrecognized trauma of the stomach or its adjacent organs is more likely to occur in the hands of the inexperienced surgeon. I have treated a number of patients in whom unsuspected trauma of the oesophagus had occurred during the course of a vagotomy. Often the surgeon had recognized that there was one tear in the oesophagus but had failed to recognize the second. Another type of damage to the oesophageal wall can occur with circular stapling devices, when the viscus is not pulled tightly over the head of the gun after the pursestring has been tightened.

Full-thickness damage can also occur when the greater curvature of the stomach is being dissected. The short gastric vessels can be included with part of the wall of the stomach in a clamp. As the stomach wall as well as the blood vessel is tied that portion of the stomach sloughs and a leak occurs.

Anastomotic failure can occur as a result of poor technique when part of the bowel wall is not incorporated in a continuous suture or when the suture is not pulled sufficiently tight. Another cause is the use of inappropriate suture material such as fine catgut, which can disintegrate rapidly in the interior of the stomach. The use of stronger, more slowly absorbed suture materials such as a polyglycolic acid and polygalactin has added strength and safety to intestinal anastomoses.

Intestinal stapling machines can allow leakage due to mechanical failures. They are more common if scrupulous attention is not paid to the detail of the technique. When circular stapling machines are used, if the head and anvil are not sufficiently closely approximated, the staples are not turned over adequately and leakage may occur. To avoid this risk many surgeons employ post-anastomotic air insufflation under tension to make sure that the anastomosis is air-tight.

Anastomotic or viscus ischaemia may cause leakage, which is often delayed for several days until the ischaemic segments slough. Mass ligature of vessels of the greater curvature has already been mentioned in this context. Too thorough a dissection of the blood supply to the duodenal stump sometimes results in avascular necrosis and leakage. Care must be exercised when performing a radical subtotal gastrectomy for carcinoma since flush ligation of the left gastric vessels places the gastric remnant in danger of becoming ischaemic, particularly if the splenic artery or the spleen is damaged. Under such circumstances it may be wiser to perform a total gastrectomy.

Lesser curvature necrosis once received much attention as a potential complication of proximal gastric vagotomy. Most of the early cases were probably caused by too vigorous a dissection and devascularization of the greater and lesser curvature. However, Johnston's exhaustive review proved this to be a rare complication and one that now seems to be disappearing from the surgical scene.[48]

After an 'ulcer-curative' operation continued peptic ulceration causing early postoperative perforation should arouse suspicion of a gastrinoma.

Leakage after a gastric operation may present as free perforation into the peritoneal cavity, as a perianastomotic abscess or as a fistula. Investigations will depend on the type of presentation. A free perforation will usually be detected by the physical signs of a sudden onset of peritonitis. However, immediately after operation the intense reaction of the whole peritoneal cavity to a perforation is suppressed and the classical board-like rigidity does not occur.

A postoperative pneumoperitoneum is seen soon after all gastric operations, but a sudden increase in the amount of intraperitoneal gas indicates a perforation. When there is a reasonable index of suspicion, a water-soluble-contrast X-ray examination is indicated.

A perigastric or perianastomotic abscess is suspected when there are clinical signs of sepsis with fever and leucocytosis. The diagnosis can sometimes be confirmed by an ultrasound scan, but this is often technically difficult in the early postoperative phase. A CT scan is more practical and accurate. However, this too may be difficult to interpret in the presence of early postoperative oedema. Perhaps the most sensitive method of detecting a localized upper abdominal abscess is gamma camera scanning for radiolabelled white cells.[83]

If the presentation suggests a fistula, the colour of the exudate, the presence of gas, and associated skin excoriation will establish the diagnosis. The oral ingestion of a coloured dye will give quick visual confirmation and a water-soluble-contrast X-ray will indicate whether the fistula is associated with a large intra-abdominal cavity. If there is a fistula it is best to stop oral intake and provide adequate continuous nasogastric aspiration (preferably with an air-bleed tube) and intravenous nutrition.[7]

If there is a leakage with free perforation soon after operation it is best to re-operate immediately, re-suture, decompress the stomach and drain. If the diagnosis has been delayed, if the patient is particularly ill or if there is a high degree of contamination in the upper gastrointestinal tract it may be unwise to re-suture. The best that then can be hoped for is to create a direct fistula with free drainage and no pocketing of leaking intestinal fluid. Refinements of surgical technique such as onlay omental patches or the onlay of jejunal loops are usually troublesome and rarely indicated.

The management of an established fistula is to ensure that there is direct drainage of the fistula with no intervening or satellite abscesses. Skin care is vitally important and requires the services of a stoma therapist.[7] To help prevent excoriation from an upper gastrointestinal fistula it may be helpful to prevent any residual acid secretion by a H_2-receptor antagonist. Obviously, such therapy is not indicated if the fistula output is not acid on pH testing.

When the presentation is that of a contained leak it is best to treat the patient initially by nasogastric aspiration and antibiotics. Reoperation is rarely indicated for a contained leak unless the abscess fails to drain into the alimentary tract. Occasionally, the contained leak forms an abscess that obstructs the normal intestinal tract and then may require reoperation or drainage.

Gastric retention

Possible causes of gastric retention are technical failures at the anastomosis, leak from the anastomosis, gastric motor malfunction and, rarely, failure of normal gastrointestinal propulsion resulting from prolonged preoperative gastric retention.

Technical failures include suturing the front of an anastomosis to the back, usually due to inexperience. More common is the inclusion of too large a 'bite' when suturing an intestinal anastomosis or too enthusiastic an inversion of a two-layer suture line.

Para-anastomotic abscess due to leakage is a common cause of prolonged delay in gastric emptying. This is often unrecognized and, in the past, has been erroneously labelled as fat necrosis or 'fibrous reaction'.[89]

Denervation of the motor part of the stomach is sometimes blamed for delay in gastric emptying. In particular it is believed that a total gastric vagotomy without a drainage procedure will frequently result in slow gastric emptying. It may, but it certainly does not always do so. We have performed two prospective randomized trials in which total gastric denervation without drainage was used.[21] In both of these trials we had no serious trouble from delayed gastric emptying and no indication to re-operate. Furthermore, we have conducted a trial with intraoperative testing of the completeness of proximal gastric vagotomy and have found that those patients who have apparently had a totally denervated antrum had no significant difference in their postoperative gastric emptying from those patients who had retained normal antral innervation.

It has been said that patients who have had prolonged gastric distension from ulcer stenosis will have a stomach that is slow to empty. Those who hold this view have suggested that, for patients with stenosis, pyloroplasty is an inadequate drainage operation and that such patients should have either a gastrojejunostomy or a partial gastric resection. We disagree with this view: it has been our policy to perform vagotomy and pyloroplasty or proximal gastric vagotomy and duodenal strictureplasty.[53] We have had no patient so treated in whom it was necessary to re-operate because of delayed gastric emptying. In our experience the only severe delays in postoperative emptying have been those associated with a para-anastomotic abscess due to leakage.

Delayed gastric emptying will become manifest either as vomiting or, if there is a nasogastric tube in place, as a persistent high-volume gastric aspiration. In some patients who have no nasogastric tube, gastric retention is not associated with vomiting, but the patient becomes distressed and exhibits tachycardia, sweating and even hypotension.

When the patient is not in too much discomfort it may be possible to elicit a gastric succussion splash.

The problem of postoperative gastric retention can be investigated by studying the character and volume of a nasogastric aspirate. The presence of obvious bile in the aspirate means that there is anatomical continuity between the ampulla and the aspirating tube and if the suspected obstruction is between these sites it is obviously incomplete. An aspiration of non-bile-stained fluid that is much greater than the volume of oral intake will indicate either inadequate nursing record-keeping or a complete block in the upper alimentary tract.

Plain or contrast radiography, endoscopy or isotope scanning can help in the assessment.

The principles of management of postoperative gastric retention are (a) to keep the stomach from becoming distended, (b) to provide adequate nutrition, (c) where indicated to give drugs to improve gastric emptying, (d) where possible to employ mechanical methods of bypassing the site of obstruction with a tube and (e) to know if and when to re-operate.

In the patient with postoperative gastric retention, it is important to minimize the distension in the stomach remnant proximal to the obstruction. The patient should be given nothing by mouth and the gut proximal to the obstruction should be aspirated. It must be remembered that if water is taken orally, even if

it is aspirated almost immediately it will be isotonic when aspirated and the patient will be constantly losing electrolytes.

If the delay in gastric emptying seems likely to
last for more than a week, adequate nutrition is
essential. It is often difficult to judge when to use
total parenteral nutrition, but it should be considered after four days and never delayed
beyond seven.

There is little scientific evidence of the efficacy
of stimulating drugs in the prevention of early
postoperative retention. However, there have
been a number of reports suggesting that
bethanechol may be beneficial.[91]

Mechanical aids to overcome postoperative
gastric retention should be considered. It may be
possible to pass a guide wire through the stenosis under radiological control and over this
thread a single- or double-lumen tube.

It requires considerable experience to know if
and when to re-operate. It is certainly unnecessary or unwise to rush into re-operation in the
early days or even weeks after the preliminary
gastric operation. It is often best to 'sit it out'
and provide the patient with adequate nutrition.
My tendency is to be as conservative as possible
and not to re-operate until the patient has had
the maximum opportunity for spontaneous
resolution.

When re-operating it is best to do the
minimum consistent with overcoming the obstruction. Sometimes a modified pyloroplasty
across a narrow gastroduodenal obstruction is
possible, but usually the obstructing mass is so
dense that a gastrojejunostomy is the safest
course, even if it has to be closed later when the
normal way reopens.

Biliary and pancreatic complications
Biliary and pancreatic complications are either
related to the disease, related to the operation or
are coincidental.

Disease-related complications occur when the
duodenal ulcer is either so deeply penetrating or
so far round in the duodenum that it affects the
biliary system. Perforation of an ulcer into the
common duct has occurred, and sometimes
biliary obstruction is caused by a perforation
through the wall of the duodenum with a para-
duodenal abscess. In the Zollinger–Ellison syndrome, ulcers often occur distal to the first part
of the duodenum but they rarely involve the
ampulla.

Operation-related complications include
damage to the common bile duct and gallbladder. This risk occurs particularly during dissection of a difficult duodenal stump during

gastric resection or when there is periduodenal
inflammation.

In the era of the Billroth II partial gastrectomy attempts to dissect out a penetrating
postero-inferior duodenal ulcer sometimes
resulted in damage to the main pancreatic duct.
Coincidental pre-existing biliary or pancreatic
disease may have been missed in the preoperative assessment of a patient; the pathology
may be reactivated by the ulcer operation and so
give rise to early postoperative cholecystitis or
pancreatitis.

It is surprisingly difficult to diagnose these
complications early after operation. They
usually present as one or more of the following
conditions: jaundice, septicaemia due to cholangitis, pancreatitis or bile leakage.

Immediate investigations of suspected biliary
and pancreatic disease include blood tests of
liver function, blood cultures and ultrasound or
CT scan to demonstrate the presence of dilated
ducts, paraduodenal swellings or collection of
fluid. Isotope-labelled white-cell scans may be
needed to localize abscesses.

Later investigations of persistent jaundice will
include ERCP, particularly if there has been a
Billroth I type of anastomosis or a pyloroplasty.
Less commonly a percutaneous transhepatic
cholangiogram is indicated. Both investigations
are better delayed until after the first two weeks
from operation. A pancreatic or biliary fistula
should always lead to the suspicion of an associated intra-abdominal abscess.

Persistence of a fistula will necessitate fis-
tulography to determine whether there is distal
obstruction.

Cholangitis or septicaemia are treated with
the appropriate antibiotics after identification of
the organism from blood culture or direct puncture of the biliary system.

It is wise to stop all oral intake and to aspirate
gastric contents to reduce the stimulus to biliary
and pancreatic secretion. Intravenous fluid and
electrolytes are always required and total parenteral nutritional support should be considered
if the complication seems unlikely to resolve
within three or four days;[7] there are few biliary
or pancreatic complications that resolve that
quickly.

If there is an abscess and/or a complex fistula
there should be early intervention to provide
adequate drainage. Otherwise there is little indication for immediate surgical intervention. If the
investigations suggest that there has been an
exacerbation of unsuspected biliary disease this
should be treated on its own merits and, providing the diagnosis is certain, early operation may

be required. If it is suspected that there are stones in the common bile duct then investigations by ERCP with a view to papillotomy may be considered after the first two weeks.

Biliary or pancreatic fistula should always initially be treated conservatively with nasogastric suction, skin protection and the provision of adequate parenteral nutrition. Operations to provide internal drainage of persistent fistula will only be considered after several weeks and the demonstration of an irremediable distal obstruction.[7]

Intermediate complications

Some of the early complications such as delayed gastric emptying and pancreatico-biliary complications can be most troublesome between the second and fourth post-operative week. However, the problems that present within the first few months in someone who has apparently made a good initial recovery are mechanical obstruction due to a variety of causes or persistent dyspeptic symptoms due to recurrent ulceration or failure to cure the primary ulcer (see later).

Mechanical obstruction
Any abdominal operation is likely to produce adhesions but gastric operations are no more likely than any others. Operations that do not alter the anatomical lie of the viscera are not particularly likely to produce obstruction, but operations such as gastrojejunostomy or subtotal or partial gastrectomy of the Billroth II type are particularly liable to this complication.

Internal herniation can occur through the hole in the mesocolon or around the gastrojejunostomy loop.[89] There are no prospective data to show that closing holes or fossae significantly reduces the risk of obstruction. One type of obstruction that is peculiar to gastrojejunal anastomoses is retrograde intussusception. This is a relatively uncommon, but dramatic, complication.[6] The intussuscepted jejunal mucosa becomes congested, will often bleed and occasionally become necrotic. Spontaneous reduction of an intussusception is said to be rare but, of course, it is not known how often self-reducing intussusceptions do occur. In the days of Billroth II gastrectomy, emphasis was placed on the rare mechanical complication of afferent loop obstruction. This was probably over-emphasized because it was confused with the symptoms produced by jejunogastric reflux of bile; it is a complication that is now rarely seen. The early literature on the mechanical complications of gastric operations also contained reports of mechanical obstruction due to bezoar.

The diagnosis of acute or subacute intestinal obstruction is rarely difficult. A plain radiograph of the abdomen will show gross distension of the stomach or small bowel and endoscopy will diagnose such uncommon conditions as bezoar and intussusception. Acute obstruction of the afferent loop due to internal herniation will often present as an acute emergency resembling pancreatitis for which it may be mistaken, particularly as the serum amylase is frequently raised. Indeed, afferent limb obstruction is probably a cause of pancreatitis after gastric resection. Ultrasound examination may help or may compound the difficulty, because a large cystic dilatation of the duodenum might be misinterpreted as a pseudocyst of the pancreas. In such an acute emergency the diagnosis may not be made until laparotomy; because of the potential dangers of high intestinal obstruction this should be considered early, rather than late. The treatment of the obstruction will depend on the cause.

Late complications

Late complications may be classified as symptomatic, metabolic or 'predispotic'.

SYMPTOMATIC COMPLICATIONS

Symptomatic complications include recurrent ulcer, incorrect assessment of the original symptoms and complications due to altered gastric physiology.

Recurrent ulcer
Surgery may fail to cure a peptic ulcer because it was due to an unrecognized gastrinoma with such profound gastric hypersecretion that nothing short of a total gastrectomy will cure the ulcer diathesis. The Zollinger–Ellison syndrome is such a rarity that most surgeons treating peptic ulcer do not routinely perform acid-secretory studies or serum gastrin estimations, and even those who do may occasionally miss the syndrome.

Another cause of recurrent ulceration due to continued hypergastrinaemia is the antral exclusion syndrome, when some gastrin-producing antral cells are left connected to the duodenum, and as there are no hydrogen ions in the lumen of the excluded antrum they are not subject to the normal inhibition of gastrin production.[38]

Inadequate resection of the acid-producing area may be a cause of recurrent ulcer, particularly when no vagotomy is performed. A 50% Billroth I or even Billroth II resection for duodenal ulcer is followed by a recurrence rate above 20%.[85, 87]

By far the commonest cause of recurrent ulceration or failure to cure the ulcer in contemporary surgical practice is inadequate vagotomy. Rarely an inexperienced surgeon may miss the whole of the posterior vagal trunk.[68] However, it is more likely that there is some anatomical anomaly where a number of secretory vagal fibres reach the stomach apart from the main vagal trunks. Experienced vagotomists can achieve a very high degree of vagal denervation of the acid-secreting part of the stomach and some have personal series with recurrence rates as low as 2%.[26] However, the average surgeon commonly experiences a recurrence rate around 10% irrespective of whether truncal or proximal gastric vagotomy is used.[29]

Many intraoperative tests have been devised to help surgeons achieve an adequate vagotomy. These are principally based on measuring the motor response of the stomach to electrical stimulation of the vagal fibres (Burge test)[19] or rely on the detection of acid-secretory responses to pentagastrin stimulation based on the premise that such a secretory response is abolished immediately the secretory vagal fibres are divided (Grassi test).[35]

There have been many studies comparing the efficacy of these intraoperative tests. Using an electrical stimulating apparatus based on the principle of the Burge test, surgeons have been able to achieve a recurrent ulcer rate as low as 2% using proximal gastric vagotomy.[65]

The diagnosis of recurrent or new ulceration in the upper gastrointestinal tract is made most reliably by endoscopy. When the ulceration is in the stomach or gastric remnant, biopsy is essential because of the risk of missing a gastric stump carcinoma.[66] Basal and pentagastrin-stimulated acid secretory measurements are important in the diagnosis of recurrent ulcer. The pH must fall below 3.5 before peptic digestion can occur, and most recurrent ulcers are associated with a pentagastrin-stimulated maximal acid output of greater than 15 millimoles per hour.[14] If the first operation has been a vagotomy, its incompleteness can be proven by demonstrating an enhancement of the acid output in response to insulin hypoglycaemia. However, the insulin provocation test is unpleasant and occasionally dangerous, and in my opinion it is not essential in the clinical management of a patient.

Serum gastrin should always be measured whenever a recurrent ulcer is diagnosed. A raised serum gastrin level may indicate a gastrinoma, a retained antrum and, less reliably, G-cell hyperplasia. Further refinements of serum gastrin estimations using stimulation with secretin or calcium are said to differentiate gastrinomas from hypergastrinaemia due to other causes.[55] Once hypergastrinaemia has been diagnosed it is investigated by selective venous sampling via a catheter introduced under radiological control through the liver into the portal vein.[9] If a gastrinoma is diagnosed, possible metastases should be sought by scanning techniques before planning treatment. These tests are only practical or even possible in highly specialized units where the facilities and expertise have been developed. There is good justification for referring all gastrinoma patients to such specialist centres for evaluation.

An important observation in the investigation of a recurrent ulcer is its response to therapy. An ulcer with associated symptoms that heals and disappears in response to H_2-receptor antagonists is obviously a true recurrent chronic peptic ulcer.[66] If a supposed recurrent ulcer fails to respond to adequate medical therapy it is reasonable to suspect that the ulcer might not be due to peptic digestion. Occasionally ulcers are seen in areas of severe reflux gastritis, in the presence of non-absorbed suture materials and at the site of a malignant lesion.[41]

After gastric surgery most recurrent ulcers can be managed medically with H_2-receptor antagonists. A few asymptomatic recurrent ulcers are discovered only on routine endoscopy, and in these cases it may be justifiable to withhold all treatment. In our experience patients with recurrent ulceration after proximal gastric vagotomy usually respond quite well to H_2-receptor antagonists. However, they often need constant therapy and, in some, re-operation may be an acceptable alternative.[43, 67]

Even patients with the Zollinger–Ellison syndrome can be managed successfully by H_2-receptor antagonists. However, in some patients, particularly those with a localized gastrinoma, surgical removal is indicated. In some such patients subtotal or distal pancreatectomy is curative. However, a gastrinoma is usually a malignant tumour and frequently metastasizes. At one time total gastrectomy was advised because the patients usually died as the consequences of their peptic ulceration before they died of disseminated tumour. However, there is now a tendency to manage disseminated gastrinoma with H_2-receptor antagonists.

In patients without gastrinoma who require

re-operation for recurrent ulcer there are two schools of thought; one favours detecting the precise cause for the failure of the first operation and simply correcting it (the logical approach), while the other school believes that someone who has had one failure from surgical treatment deserves the maximum surgical therapy to make sure that the problems do not recur again (the empirical approach).[87] The logical or minimal approach employs tests such as insulin hypoglycaemia to determine if there is an incomplete vagotomy, or basal and stimulated gastrin response to detect if the patient has G-cell hyperplasia. If the cause of the failure has been incomplete vagotomy, this is completed. If the problem is inadequate gastric resection and a vagotomy has not been performed, then a vagotomy is added. This philosophy can also be applied to patients with the antral exclusion syndrome who only need to have their antral remnant excised. Attractive though this logical method of management may be, in practice we have found that it has not been universally effective. We have had a poor experience with transthoracic vagotomy in patients whose symptoms were believed to be due to inadequate abdominal vagotomy. We have found other patients who have been cured of their recurrent peptic ulceration but still suffered symptoms such as dumping or bile regurgitation as a consequence of their antral resection.[67]

For these reasons we have tended to adopt the empirical or 'belt and braces' policy: to ensure that patients have no further recurrence they should have a re-vagotomy plus an antrectomy. Even this policy has a number of disadvantages, as we found when we treated our patients with re-vagotomy, antrectomy and a Billroth I anastomosis. Many of these patients, though cured of their recurrent ulcer, had quite severe postoperative symptoms principally related to duodenogastric reflux. Therefore, we have now adopted the policy of treating recurrent ulcers with re-vagotomy, antrectomy and a Roux-en-Y anastomosis. This maximum operation aims to prevent recurrent ulceration and bile reflux. Although symptomatically effective it does entail a large operation.

Incorrect assessment of the original symptoms

Incorrect assessment of the original symptoms is a common cause of failure after gastric operations. A patient who has symptoms due to the irritable bowel syndrome, chronic pancreatitis or biliary disease may have radiological stigmata of chronic duodenal ulcer seen on a barium meal examination and yet have an entirely quiescent or healed ulcer that is responsible for no symptoms. Naturally, if such a patient is treated by an ulcer-curative operation the original symptoms will not be improved. Therefore, it is important to ensure that an active peptic ulcer is the cause of the original symptoms before advising operation. Surgeons should also be wary of the patient who is reputed not to respond to adequate medical therapy, including H_2-receptor antagonists. Furthermore, when investigating patients with recurrent dyspepsia after a gastric operation it is important to try to determine how good the evidence was that a definite peptic ulcer existed initially. In the past we have designated this group of patients as having the 'phantom ulcer syndrome'. They probably never had an ulcer in the first instance.[44]

SYMPTOMS DUE TO ALTERED GASTRIC PHYSIOLOGY

Gastro-oesophageal reflux

The principal symptoms of gastro-oesophageal reflux are heartburn and dysphagia (see Chapter 2). Investigations of such symptoms include endoscopy, biopsy and oesophageal manometry by the pull-through technique, using fine-bore open-tip-perfused tubes. Monitoring of intra-oesophageal pH is also a useful test when there is residual acid-secretory capacity in the stomach. However, after gastric operations quite severe oesophagitis and symptoms can occur when the refluxate into the oesophagus is alkaline and contains bile acids and pancreatic enzymes; pH monitoring will not record these episodes of reflux. The separation of oesophageal from cardiac symptoms is best ensured by correlating symptoms with episodes of acid reflux. This is more reliable than the Bernstein test, which relies on provoking symptoms by perfusing 0.1 mol/l hydrochloric acid into the lower oesophagus.[2]

Heartburn associated with the reflux of acid into the oesophagus can usually be controlled readily by H_2-receptor antagonists. However, the reflux of bile into the oesophagus is much more difficult to manage. Patients with oesophageal reflux can usually help to minimize their symptoms by avoiding wearing tight clothing, smoking, being overweight, sleeping flat and eating shortly before going to sleep. Medical measures have a reasonable rate of success and should be tried energetically before considering surgical intervention. The severe cases of heartburn that do not respond well to medical treatment are due to the reflux of bile, and it is less effective to treat this symptom by restoring gastro-oesophageal competence than by diverting bile away from the stomach.

Some patients have dysphagia because they develop a stricture as a complication of reflux, others as a consequence of prolonged nasogastric intubation at an earlier operation, but most have oesophageal damage due to bile regurgitation. Strictures are best managed by endoscopic dilatation combined with attempts to cure the underlying cause; it is rarely ever necessary to perform a complicated gastroplasty. If re-operation is required because of severe oesophageal symptoms after a gastric resection that has bypassed or destroyed the antropyloric mechanism, it is better always to combine this with a bile-diversion procedure.[5, 54]

Duodenogastric reflux

The cardinal symptoms of duodenogastric reflux are nausea, bile vomiting, weight loss, heartburn and anorexia.

Duodenogastric reflux may be observed at endoscopy if bile-stained fluid is seen in the stomach or gastric remnant.[17] However, there are a number of problems if this diagnosis is based upon endoscopy alone, since bile reflux into the stomach can be detected as commonly in asymptomatic patients as in those with symptoms after ulcer surgery.[64] Furthermore, there appears to be a poor correlation between endoscopically diagnosed reflux and the presence of isotope-labelled bile in the stomach after a meal.[31] A more reliable method of assessing duodenogastric reflux is continuous aspiration of refluxed duodenal contents with measurement of bile pigment or bile acid. This has been shown to correlate well with the presence of symptoms and with histological abnormalities in the gastric mucosa. Furthermore, we have shown that the passage of a nasogastric tube does not increase the frequency or quantity of duodenogastric reflux.[94] A less invasive and more acceptable method of investigating duodenogastric reflux is by $^{99}Tc^m$-HIDA which is excreted by hepatocytes and cleared through the biliary system. It is also possible to quantify the amount of excreted HIDA that refluxes into the gastric area. However, in the absence of gallbladder contraction the quantity is very small and CCK stimulation may be needed as a provocation test. Unfortunately CCK also tends to affect the function of the pylorus.[86]

It is important to remember that bile reflux occurs commonly after all forms of gastric operation and in most patients it produces few or no symptoms. When it does they are usually a minor problem and often can be managed by dietary regulation, avoiding foods that provoke the symptoms. Drugs such as metoclopramide that speed gastric emptying will sometimes help patients who have duodenogastric reflux, and mild symptoms appear to be relieved by prescribing a bile-adsorbing agent such as hydrotalcite.[41]

Severe bile reflux can be corrected only by some form of bile-diversion operation. Many different types of operation have been devised but some are inadequate. It is inappropriate to convert a Billroth II to a Billroth I anastomosis because there is still a high incidence of bile reflux after a Billroth I operation. Similarly an enteroenterostomy between the two loops of a Billroth II operation is inadequate. In 1973 I reviewed our experience with 33 patients with bile vomiting: 15 of whom were treated by conversion from Billroth II to Billroth I with a 55% success rate and 18 treated by jejunal interposition with a 75% success rate.[4]

Since 1972 I have used the technically simpler Roux-en-Y conversion. Bile vomiting was cured in 51 of the 55 patients operated since then. The other two required re-operation to insert the Roux loop a further 50 cm distally. Despite this ability of the long Roux-en-Y operation to prevent bile reflux into the stomach the overall success rate in relieving all the patients' symptoms is only 65%. Furthermore, two of the 55 patients have died as a result of the operation.

Dumping and diarrhoea

Rapid gastric emptying and rapid intestinal transit are associated with a variety of symptoms, the best known of which is dumping. Dumping is due to large volumes of slowly absorbed hypertonic fluids present in the small bowel attracting fluid into the lumen and distending the bowel. The symptoms are probably mediated by vasoactive peptides liberated from the bowel wall (see below).[60] The symptoms characteristically include a feeling of faintness, palpitation and sweating, often associated with pallor and tachycardia. The symptom of epigastric distension that often accompanies dumping can also occur in association with duodenogastric reflux. The two mechanisms are difficult to disentangle and frequently occur together. Dumping is also often associated with diarrhoea, but the symptoms can occur independently. The outpouring of fluid into the lumen of the gut associated with the dumping syndrome can act as a saline cathartic and 'wash out' the distal bowel. Rapid gastric emptying undoubtedly plays some part in the genesis of postoperative diarrhoea, but this is not the only factor. There is reliable evidence that diarrhoea is more frequently associated with truncal vagotomy than with selective vagotomy, which preserves the small bowel nerve supply, or partial gastrectomy.[49, 55] Therefore, it must be something more than rapid gastric emptying that is responsible for the diarrhoea and it seems that parasympathetic denervation of the distal small bowel must be a factor. Other factors that have been implicated are alterations in bile acids, the incoordination of gastric and duodenal motility and, possibly, changes in intestinal microflora.[9, 10]

Dumping can be diagnosed and assessed by dumping-provocation tests using a hyperosmolar glucose solution, monitoring symptoms, and by serial measurements of the haematocrit before and for two hours after the test meal.[40, 78] Another method of evaluating patients with dumping is to measure the rate of gastric emptying of a liquid or a standard test meal labelled with a radioisotope such as $^{99}Tc^m$ or $^{113}In^m$.[28] In normal patients, the half-time of emptying of the stomach is 40–70 minutes, whereas after gastric operations it tends to be between 10 and 15 minutes. However, not all patients with a rapid rate of gastric emptying experience dumping.[84]

Hormone assays have been used in the investigation of the dumping syndrome, since some circulating hormone levels have been raised in patients with early dumping. These include gastric inhibitory polypeptides (GIP), motilin, vasoactive intestinal peptide (VIP) and 5-hydroxytryptamine. However, the measurement of these hormones is of no practical value in assessing an individual patient with dumping.

Diarrhoea after gastric operations is of two main types: (a) the episodic diarrhoea that occurs particularly after truncal vagotomy and is characterized by occasional unheralded attacks of profuse urgent diarrhoea with a relatively normal bowel habit between the attacks and (b) continuous diarrhoea, when there are frequent soft stools by day and sometimes by night.

The episodic, so called 'post-vagotomy' diarrhoea is not usually worth investigating. Although much research has been done into its cause no effective therapy has been devised.[61]

Continuous diarrhoea may be due to some abnormality which was not apparent before the gastric operation. Patients with an underlying gluten-sensitive enteropathy may have had no symptoms before their gastric operation and yet develop severe diarrhoea and even fat malabsorption and malnutrition after operation. Such patients can be identified by jejunal biopsy. Some patients have incipient pancreatic insufficiency before operation and become symptomatic after ulcer surgery. It is difficult to identify such patients before operating, but the presence of preoperative steatorrhoea indicates the need for a pancreatic function test. Another cause of continuous diarrhoea is the intestinal blind-loop syndrome in the afferent loop after a Billroth II type of gastrectomy. However, it is a rare event and there usually has to be some additional factor such as jejunal diverticulosis or partial small bowel obstruction. This syndrome can be investigated by measuring hydrogen excretion in the breath and fat absorption and by observing the response to antibiotic therapy.[9]

Dumping is rarely a serious problem and is never life-threatening. Also it is a symptom that tends to decrease in severity and frequency after the first postoperative year.

The treatment should be principally dietary. Many patients learn that drinks containing carbohydrates such as disaccharides or monosaccharides precipitate symptoms. Therefore, they learn to avoid sugars and to avoid drinking with their meals. Patients should be encouraged to take frequent small dry meals and, where possible, to lie down after a large meal. Drugs have been advocated, but in my experience, are rarely practical. Antiserotonin drugs such as cyproheptadine and methysergide maleate have been claimed to help those with motor symptoms, as have drugs that delay gastric emptying such as propantheline (Pro-Banthine). Others have advocated carbohydrate gelling agents.[47] A small proportion of patients with severe dumping will be resistant to medical treatment and will press for surgical relief, but such pressure should be resisted. Many of these patients are often unstable with a low threshold of tolerance of symptoms and are able to find new and even worse ones to substitute for any that are relieved. Surgical procedures that have been used to treat dumping include narrowing the gastrojejunal stoma or reconstructing a pyloroplasty, but they have not been universally successful.[20] Procedures that rely on re-routing diverted intestinal contents back from the jejunum into the duodenum, such as conversion from a Billroth II (Polya) to a Billroth I operation, have been singularly unsuccessful.[3] Others have advocated the interposition of an intestinal segment with reverse peristalsis between the stomach and the duodenum or the creation of a gastric reservoir pouch.[75] Although I have tried most of these procedures on a few occasions and have been impressed by their immediate good results, the long-term effects have never been encouraging and the patients who were once in Visick grade IV seemed to remain in Visick grade IV. I have had particularly bad experiences with the retroperistaltic interposed jejunal segment between the stomach and the duodenum. These patients substitute severe bile reflux and gastric retention for their dumping syndrome and are often worse than before.[3]

In my experience the only universally successful operative intervention for dumping has been in those patients who have a gastrojejunostomy. At one time I treated them by closing the gastrojejunostomy and substituting a pyloroplasty. Although the patients were undoubtedly improved they still had some of the sequelae of the pyloroplasty. Now I simply close the gastrojejunostomy and leave them without a pyloroplasty. As these patients usually have had a vagotomy many months or years before, the intrinsic gastric tone has returned to normal and they appear to be able to empty the stomach quite satisfactorily through their pylorus without the need for a pyloroplasty.[56]

Some of the remarks applicable to the medical management of the dumping syndrome also apply to the management of diarrhoea. Patients are often much less troubled if they have small frequent dry meals with few carbohydrates and more protein. The addition of carbohydrate gelling agents is also helpful. Antacids that contain aluminium salts and cholestyramine or hydrotalcite, which bind bile acids, are also helpful and are suitable for long-term administration. The most commonly used therapy is to give antidiarrhoeal agents such as loperamide or diphenoxylate or codeine; all help to reduce the frequency of watery stools. However, in patients with typical post-vagotomy diarrhoea the attacks are often unheralded and so preventative antidiarrhoeal agents are impractical. The patient who is only going to have one attack of loose, watery urgent stool each week will not wish to keep taking potent antidiarrhoeal drugs continuously.[13]

Nevertheless, it is fortunate that most patients with diarrhoea after gastric operations learn to control their symptoms, or their symptoms become less with the passage of time. Few if any, require surgical treatment, and even reversed ileal loops have rarely been successful for patients with continuing symptoms.

METABOLIC SEQUELAE

Malnutrition

Many patients who are undernourished at the time of their ulcer curative operation fail to regain their optimum weight and some lose more weight. The cause of the malnutrition may be failure to eat because of fear of provoking postoperative symptoms, poor appetite or a poor capacity.

Fear of provoking postoperative symptoms is an important cause of patients restricting their oral intake.[50] This applies particularly to those with severe bile-reflux oesophagitis. Patients soon find that the symptoms are brought on after almost any food, but they often find that they can drink without provoking much discomfort and many become alcoholics. Although alcohol can provide a reasonably high energy intake, such patients are particularly malnourished of protein and fat and have associated vitamin deficiencies.

Therapy is directed towards removing the unpleasant symptoms that the patients are seeking to avoid. There is a belief, but no proof, that bile-reflux gastritis and associated gastric atrophy contribute to a poor appetite. However, there are many patients who have had a total gastrectomy and some with advanced gastric atrophy who maintain a normal appetite. Some patients lose their appetite as they develop deficiencies of iron, folic acid or vitamin B_{12}. The detection of these deficiencies and their correction will often improve the appetite. The inability to eat a normal-sized meal is probably more related to anorexia than it is to the size of the stomach. It is well known that after extensive gastric resections the afferent loop becomes hypertrophied and food enters it rapidly, so that the effective volume of the reservoir can be little different from that of a normal stomach. It is also well known that after total gastrectomy many patients have a near-normal capacity for food. Therefore, any literal interpretation of the 'small stomach' syndrome is unjustifiable and there is little practical value in any objective assessment of gastric capacity. Nor does there seem to be any rational indication for operations designed simply to create a larger pouch.[32]

Malabsorption is a relatively uncommon cause of malnutrition. After gastric operations the small intestine has such a high capacity to absorb carbohydrates and proteins that gross disturbances are required to produce malabsorption. Gastric resections and vagotomy procedures in themselves are not enough to cause measurable malabsorption. A minor degree of malabsorption of fat is quite common after gastric resections, particularly the more major procedures involving gastrojejunal anastomosis. A faecal fat excretion of more than six grams (18 mmol) a day has been reported as occurring in 60–70% of patients after partial gastric resection. The majority of these patients have only mild steatorrhoea, and the disability is chemical rather than clinical. Patients who exhibit severe degrees of fat malabsorption and deficiencies of fat-soluble vitamins such as vitamin D usually have some additional abnormality such as gluten-sensitive enteropathy or pancreatic insufficiency.[39] A few patients with the intestinal blind loop syndrome also have severe fat malabsorption.[27] Patients with post-gastrectomy steatorrhoea warrant full evaluation including jejunal biopsy and, where possible, estimations of pancreatic function and quantitative upper gastrointestinal bacteriology.[16] In such a patient such conditions as an unsuspected gastrojejunocolic fistula or even the rare mistake of an inadvertent gastroileostomy should be excluded.

Any detected abnormalities require appropriate treatment, including a gluten-free diet for enteropathy and pancreatic enzyme substitution where deficiency is detected. For small intestinal bacterial overgrowth, tetracyclines or metronidazole with neomycin are the drugs of choice.

There is rarely, if ever, any indication to reoperate to treat malabsorption.[93]

Anaemia

Anaemia, which is a very common sequel of gastric resection, appears to be rare or non-existent after proximal gastric vagotomy. The types of anaemia that are seen after gastric resection are due to iron deficiency, folic acid deficiency and vitamin B_{12} deficiency.[52]

Iron deficiency is the commonest type and is found in between 33% and 50% of patients following partial gastric resection. The causes of iron deficiency are inadequate dietary intake, decreased availability of ingested iron, impaired absorption or increased loss.[46] Inadequate intake of iron has been thought by some to be an important factor, but detailed dietary histories have failed to provide evidence of impaired iron intake except in a very small proportion of patients – usually those with severe post-gastrectomy symptoms.

There is some evidence for a decreased ability of the patient to extract iron from its organic form in the diet and convert it rapidly into a ferric form. The proximal jejunum is the site for optimum iron absorption. There are many theoretical reasons why organic iron may have passed the proximal jejunum before it is converted into an absorbable form, but there is no irrefutable evidence to suggest that this is anything other than a minor contributory factor in producing iron deficiency after gastric resection.[11] It is certain that patients are able to absorb adequate amounts of therapeutic iron in the form of ferrous sulphate or similar compounds even after a subtotal gastric resection and Billroth II anastomosis.

It appears that the major factor leading to iron deficiency after gastric resection is the continued blood loss that occurs from a damaged, friable mucosa. This damage occurs principally around the gastrointestinal stoma, but occasionally around the lower oesophagus when there is reflux of acid or bile.[46]

Although iron deficiency is common it is not particularly difficult to treat with organic iron preparations and can almost certainly be prevented by regular small doses of iron supplements. However, this simple exercise in preventative medicine is honoured more in the omission than in the commission. Since gastric resection has been largely abandoned in favour of vagotomy with or without drainage, the need for iron supplementation after gastric operations has almost disappeared.

Investigations of the causes of iron deficiency are not particularly fruitful. Stomal gastritis can be confirmed endoscopically or histologically, and isotope labelling does permit accurate measurements of intestinal blood loss. However, these tests are of no practical value in the management of the patient. The pragmatic management of iron deficiency is to try simple oral iron supplements and to resort to parenteral iron administration only in the rare event of failure to respond. It is, of course, important to remember that patients who are anaemic after gastric operations could have coincidental intestinal bleeding lesions such as carcinoma of the right side of the colon. Such a combination of misfortunes is likely to defeat screening tests.

Folic acid deficiency is caused principally by poor intake.[25] It is virtually impossible for a gastric operation to so disturb upper small intestinal function as to impair folate absorption.

The poor intake of folic acid after gastric operations is due to the distaste some patients have for fresh vegetables. Some patients have such a strong fear of provoking postcibal pain that they take only alcohol or the blandest of carbohydrate diets. Impairment of folate absorption is so slight after gastric operations as not to contribute to the syndrome.

Although many patients have folate deficiency detected after gastric operations, there is no particular value in investigating them by folate absorption tests.

The presence of a macrocytic anaemia in the presence of a low serum folate and normal vitamin B_{12} level is an indication for permanent low-dose folic acid replacement therapy. Five milligrams of folic acid each day is easily tolerated and cures any deficiency.

Vitamin B_{12} deficiency can be due either to intrinsic factor deficiency caused by complete gastric mucosal atrophy or, less commonly, to the intestinal blind loop syndrome causing colonization of the upper gastrointestinal tract with organisms which impair normal vitamin B_{12} absorption.[81]

Gastric atrophy is particularly common after subtotal gastric resection with a Billroth II anastomosis. It is believed that the principal factor causing atrophy is the reflux of bile acids into the stomach. Gastric atrophy leads to a diminution and eventual disappearance of the most highly specialized secretory cells of the stomach. The acid- and pepsin-secretory cells probably disappear before the cells responsible for the production of intrinsic factor, but by the time gastric atrophy is well established patients may have a measurable defect in their ability to absorb vitamin B_{12}.[30]

If the patient is found to have a macrocytosis or a low serum vitamin B_{12} level it is easily investigated by liver scanning after the oral administration of radioactive labelled vitamin B_{12}. Failure to absorb the radioisotope can then be corrected by the simultaneous administration of oral intrinsic factor, thus confirming the presence of intrinsic factor deficiency. If intrinsic factor fails to correct the absorption defect the intestinal blind loop syndrome should be suspected; the patient is given antibiotics which should correct the absorptive fault and the test is repeated.[30]

Whether the problem is due to intrinsic factor deficiency or the blind loop syndrome, the treatment is simply to replace the poorly absorbed vitamin B_{12}. An injection of 250 µg of hydroxocobalamin every two months will correct the deficiency and prevent its recurrence.

Although there is evidence that oral administration of large doses of vitamin B_{12} will be associated with an adequate absorption, parenteral administration is more practical.

Bone disease

The two forms of metabolic bone disease that have been reported after gastric operations are osteomalacia and osteoporosis. There is no clear-cut differentiation between the two diseases but osteomalacia, the rarer of the two, is associated with a loss of calcium from bone due to vitamin D deficiency. Osteoporosis is due to a loss of normal bone tissue; the remaining thin bone is normally-calcified. Osteoporosis is a process that occurs normally with ageing and the normal ageing process seems to be accelerated by gastric resection.[69, 92]

Osteoporosis is associated with a higher susceptibility to fractures of the long bones and occurs commonly after gastric operations. It has been observed that fractures of the upper end of the femur occur significantly more commonly in patients who have had gastrectomy than in randomly selected controls.[71] One simple measure of osteoporosis is the relative thickness of the cortical bone as assessed by plain X-rays of long bones such as the femur or the metacarpal. In normal subjects this 'bone score' tends to remain relatively constant until the age of sixty, after which it gradually declines. This represents the common state of senile osteoporosis. After partial gastrectomy, the relative thickness of the cortex of the bone, as defined by the 'bone score', shows a gradual decline in cortical thickness that begins ten to twenty years earlier than normal.[62] Other workers have observed a greater than threefold increase in the incidence of fractures – the so-called 'fragility' fractures – in gastrectomized patients compared with matched controls.[58]

The cause of osteoporosis seems to be a gradual loss, associated with generalized malnutrition and inactivity, in the quantity of bone. On bone biopsy, an osteoporotic bone appears to have normally calcified osteoid seams.

Special investigations are of no particular value in the assessment of post-gastrectomy osteoporosis, but the 'bone score' is obtained from a simple long-bone X-ray.

Therapy is non-specific; general measures to improve overall nutrition and to increase activity will theoretically improve the strength of the bone and retard the pre-senile osteoporosis. However, there is no recorded evidence of any therapeutic success in the management of post-gastrectomy osteoporosis.

Osteomalacia, unlike osteoporosis, is a rare disease and a well-defined entity. It is reported to occur in about 2% of patients after subtotal gastric resection, with a much lesser incidence after a two-third partial gastrectomy and is almost non-existent after vagotomy and drainage procedures.[63] It has been recorded rarely after gastrojejunostomy.

The cause of osteomalacia is malabsorption of vitamin D, invariably associated with a generalized malabsorption of fat. The condition is recognized in its grossest form by the appearance of pseudofractures on X-ray. Bone biopsy surveys after gastrectomy have detected a high incidence of demineralized osteoid seams.[46] Also used as screening tests are serum levels of calcium, alkaline phosphatase and vitamin D. Serum calcium is often below normal and the serum alkaline phosphatase is elevated. Estimations of serum vitamin D are not available in all centres, but prospective studies have shown them to be significantly decreased in postgastrectomy patients.[82]

Osteomalacia is so uncommon after anything other than a major gastric resection that it is hardly worth while preventing it by prophylaxis. However, if a patient is malnourished after a partial gastric resection, it would be prudent to consider the possibility of osteomalacia and to prevent it by small doses of vitamin D. It is not usually necessary or advisable to give large doses of vitamin D. It is probably sufficient to give 40 000 units of vitamin D intramuscularly once a month and probably advisable to give 1–2 g of calcium orally per day. It is very important to be aware of the dangers of vitamin D overdose. Hypercalcaemia as a result of overdose of vitamin D is very much more dangerous than subclinical osteomalacia.

'PREDISPOTIC' SEQUELAE

Gastric operations are said to predispose to the development of biliary disease and to carcinoma in the gastric remnant.

Biliary disease

There have been many observations suggesting a higher incidence of cholelithiasis after gastric operations associated with vagotomy than in the control population.[22, 37, 59, 70] However, most of these observations constitute circumstantial evidence rather than direct proof. There have also been a number of reports incriminating vagotomy as a causal factor in cholelithiasis.[18, 24] However, most of the reports in the literature contain no control groups.

Approximately 20% of patients after vagotomy have been reported as developing biliary disease, but biliary disease is so common in the ageing population that an adequate control population is needed before vagotomy can be incriminated. It is, of course, theoretically possible that there might be a predisposition to cholelithiasis, because it can be shown that gallbladder contraction in response to fat is less after truncal vagotomy than before.[33, 74] There is some theoretical and practical data to suggest that a proximal gastric vagotomy, by retaining the nerve supply to the pylorus, antrum and the hepatobiliary system, will avoid any increased susceptibility to biliary disease.

Gastric remnant carcinoma

At one time it was thought that carcinoma arising in the gastric remnant was relatively uncommon,[12] but in recent years there have been a large number of reports of gastric remnant carcinoma. Up until 1975 about 300 cases of gastric remnant carcinoma had been reported.[88]

To qualify for the diagnosis of primary gastric remnant carcinoma it is necessary for the gastric operation to have been performed for histologically proven benign disease and for the carcinoma to develop at least five years later.

As the mean free interval between the primary gastric operation and the appearance of the gastric carcinoma is approximately 20 years it is easy to see why there have been no definitive prospective studies to determine the risk of malignant disease developing. However, retrospective studies have suggested that the gastric stump cancer rate varies between 0.8% and 2%.[73] Retrospective long-term studies after gastric resection for benign gastric ulcer show a malignancy risk of between 13% and 16%. On the other hand, there is evidence that approximately 10% of patients with conservatively treated gastric ulcer will develop a gastric cancer with long follow-up.[36, 75] If the gastric resection has been performed for duodenal ulcer the gastric stump cancer rate is much less.[36]

Apart from the higher incidence of cancer after operations for gastric ulcer as compared with duodenal ulcer, the risk factors include the residual pH of the gastric remnant, which is related to the number of microorganisms in the stomach. It also appears to be related to the amount of deconjugated bile acids found in the gastric remnant.[77] The risk of developing gastric cancer appears to be greater in those patients who have shown histological evidence of severe dysplasia on gastric biopsies. There is also a geographical variation in the prevalence of stump cancers, with an increased frequency where gastric cancer is common. It has not yet been shown whether it is worth while performing routine yearly endoscopy but a reasonably argued case has been made that regular surveillance of all post-gastric operation patients is not economically justifiable.[57] However, it is theoretically worth surveying patients who have had an operation for gastric ulcer and particularly those in whom one biopsy has shown severe dysplasia. There is so far no method known of preventing the dysplastic and metaplastic changes in the gastric remnant. However, as it seems that the mucosal changes only follow gastric resection, presumably the risk will slowly die out as patients are no longer being treated by major gastric resection and most patients with ulcer are being treated by proximal gastric vagotomy.

It has been said that the prognosis of resected gastric remnant carcinoma is so poor that it is not really worth the trouble to diagnose and treat. However, anecdotal evidence, including our own, suggests that long-term cure can follow diagnosis of gastric remnant carcinoma. Therefore, an entirely fatalistic attitude is not justified.[79, 90]

REFERENCES

1 Alexander-Williams, J. (1967) Post-gastrectomy problems. *British Medical Journal*, **iv**, 403–405.

2 Alexander-Williams, J. (1969) The disappointed patient. In *After Vagotomy* (Ed.) Alexander-Williams, J. & Cox, A. G. pp. 197–210. London: Butterworths.

3 Alexander-Williams, J. (1973) Gastric reconstructive surgery, *Annals of the Royal College of Surgeons of England*, **52**, 1–17.

4 Alexander-Williams, J. (1973) Pathogenesis and treatment of bile vomiting and dumping. In *Vagotomy on Trial* (Ed.) Cox, A. G. & Alexander-Williams, J. pp. 37–50. London: Heinemann.

5 Alexander-Williams, J. (1981) Duodenogastric reflux after gastric operations. *British Journal of Surgery*, **68**, 685–687.

6 Alexander-Williams, J. & Fielding, J. F. (1970) Recurrent retrograde intragastric intussusception. *Gut*, **11**, 840–842.

7 Alexander-Williams, J. & Irving, M. (1982) *Intestinal Fistulas*. Bristol: Wright.

8 Allan, J. G., Gerskowitch, V. P. & Russell, R. I. (1973) A study of the role of bile acids in the pathogenesis of post-vagotomy diarrhoea. *Gut*, **14**, 423–424.

9 Allan, J. G., Gerskowitch, V. P. & Russell, R. I. (1974) The role of bile acids in the pathogenesis of post-vagotomy diarrhoea. *British Journal of Surgery*, **61**, 516–518.

10 Athanasoulis, C. A., Waltman, A. C., Ring, E. J. *et al.* (1974) Angiographic management of post-operative bleeding. *Radiology*, **113**, 37–42.

11 Baird, I. McL. & Wilson, G. M. (1959) The pathogenesis of anaemia after partial gastrectomy. 2. Iron absorption after partial gastrectomy. *Quarterly Journal of Medicine*, **28**, 35–41.

12 Balfour, D. C. (1922) Factors influencing the life expectancy of patients operated on for gastric ulcers. *Annals of Surgery*, **76**, 405–408.

13 Barnes, A. D. & Cox, A. G. (1969) Diarrhoea. In *After Vagotomy*. (Ed.) Alexander-Williams, J. & Cox, A. G. pp. 211–219. London: Butterworths.

14 Baron J. H. (1973) The rationale of the different operations for peptic ulcer. In *Vagotomy on Trial* (Ed.) Cox, A. G. & Alexander-Williams, J. pp. 7–36. London: Butterworths.

15 Baum, S. & Nusbaum, M. (1971) The control of gastrointestinal haemorrhage by selective mesenteric arterial infusion of vasopressin. *Radiology*, **98**, 497–505.

16 Bond, J. H. & Levitt, M. D. (1977) Use of breath hydrogen (H_2) to quantitate small bowel transit time following partial gastrectomy. *Journal of Laboratory and Clinical Medicine*, **90**, 30–36.

17 Borg, I. (1959) Bile admixture in gastric juice in health and in peptic ulcer before and after operation according to Billroth I and Billroth II. *Acta Chirurgica Scandinavica*, **251**, 91–112.

18 Bouchier, I. A. D. (1970) The vagus, the bile and gallstones. *Gut*, **11**, 799–803.

19 Burge, H., & Vain, J. R. (1958) Method of testing for complete nerve section during vagotomy. *British Medical Journal*, **i**, 615–618.

20 Christiansen, T. M., Hart-Hansen, O. & Pedersen, T. (1974) Reconstruction of the pylorus for post-vagotomy diarrhoea and dumping. *British Journal of Surgery*, **61**, 519–520.

21 Clarke, R. J. & Alexander-Williams, J. (1973) The effect of preserving antral innervation and of pyloroplasty on gastric emptying after vagotomy in man. *Gut*, **14**, 300–307.

22 Clave, R. A. & Gaspar, M. R. (1969) Incidence of gallbladder disease after vagotomy. *American Journal of Surgery*, **118**, 169–176.

23 Conn, H. O., Ramsby, G. R., Storer, E. H. *et al.* (1965) Intra-arterial vasopressin in the treatment of upper gastro-intestinal haemorrhage. A prospective controlled clinical trial. *Gastroenterology*, **68**, 211–221.

24 Cowie, A. G. A. & Clarke, C. G. (1972) The lithogenic effect of vagotomy. *British Journal of Surgery*, **59**, 365–367.

25 Deller, D. J., Ibbotson, R. N. & Crompton, B. (1964) Metabolic effects of partial gastrectomy with special reference to calcium and folic acid. Part II. The contribution of folic acid deficiency to the anaemia. *Gut*, **5**, 225–229.

26 Dewar, P., Williams, N. S., Dixon, M. F. & Johnston, D. (1982) Vagotomy confined to the nerve supply of the gastric musculature. In *Vagotomy in Modern Surgical Practice* (Ed.) Baron, J. H., Alexander-Williams, J., Allgower, M. *et al.* pp. 137–140. London: Butterworths.

27 Donaldson, R. M. (1965) Studies on the pathogenesis of steatorrhoea in the blind loop syndrome. *Journal of Clinical Investigation*, **44**, 1815–1825.

28 Donovan, I. A. (1976) The different components of gastric emptying after gastric surgery. *Annals of the Royal College of Surgeons*, **58**, 368–373.

29 Dorricott, N. J., McNeish, A. R., Alexander-Williams, J. *et al.* (1978) Prospective randomised multi-centre trial of proximal gastric vagotomy or truncal vagotomy and antrectomy for chronic duodenal ulcer: interim results. *British Journal of Surgery*, **65**, 152–154.

30 Doscherholmen, A. & Swaim, W. R. (1973) Impaired assimilation of Co^{57} vitamin B_{12} in patients with hypochlorhydria and achlorhydria after gastric resection. *Gastroenterology*, **64**, 913–919.

31 Eyre-Brook, I. A., Holroy, A. M. & Johnson, A. G. (1983) Is bile reflux gastritis a meaningful endoscopic diagnosis? *Gut*, **24**, 460–461.

32 Fineberg, C., Templeton, J. Y. III, Wirts, C. W. & Gold-stein, F. (1973) The correction of post-gastrectomy malabsorption by jejunal interposition. *Surgical Clinics of North America*, **53**, 581–592.

33 Glanville, J. N. & Duthie, H. L. (1964) Contraction of the gallbladder before and after total abdominal vagotomy. *Clinical Radiology*, **15**, 350–354.

34 Gordon, R., Herlinger, H. & Baum, S. (1981) Arteriography and scintiscanning. In *Gastro-intestinal Haemorrhage* (Ed.) Dykes, P. W. & Keighley, M. R. B. pp. 209–231. Bristol: Wright PSG.

35 Grassi, G. (1971) A new test for the complete nerve section during vagotomy. *British Journal of Surgery*, **58**, 187–189.

36 Griesser, G. & Schmidt, H. (1964) Statistische Erhebungen über die Haufigkeit des Karzinoms nach Magenoperation wegen eines Geschwursleidens. *Medizinische Welt*, **35**, 1836–1840.

37 Griffith, J. M. T. & Holmes, G. (1964) Cholecystitis following gastric surgery. *Lancet*, **ii**, 780–782.

38 Harrison, R. C., White, T. T. & Heinbach, D. N. (1979) Late complications of gastric surgery. In *Re-operative Gastro-intestinal Surgery*. (Ed.) White, T. T. & Harrison, R. C. pp. 91–124. Boston: Little Brown.

39 Hedberg, C. A., Melnyk, C. S. & Johnson, C. F. (1966) Gluten enteropathy appearing after gastric surgery. *Gastroenterology*, **50**, 796–804.

40 Hinshaw, D. B., Thompson, R. J. & Branson, B. W. (1971) Pre and postoperative 'dumping studies' in patients with peptic ulcer. *American Journal of Surgery*, **122**, 269–274.

41 Hoare, A. M. & Alexander-Williams, J. (1977) Thread sutures seen on gastroscopy: do they cause ulcers or indigestion. *British Medical Journal*, **ii**, 996–997.

42 Hoare, A. M. & Bradby, G. V. H. (1981) Conservative therapy. In *Gastrointestinal Haemorrhage* (Ed.) Dykes, P. W. & Keighley, M. R. B. pp. 287–303. Bristol: Wright PSG.

43 Hoare, A. M., Jones, E. L. & Hawkins, C. F. (1978) Cimetidine for ulcers recurring after gastric surgery. *British Medical Journal*, **1**, 1325–1326.

44 Hoare, A. M., Keighley, M. R. B., Hawkins, C. F. *et al.* (1975) Non-ulcer dyspepsia and surgery. *Gut*, **16**, 397.

45 Hoare, A. M., McLeish, A., Thompson, H. & Alexander-Williams, J. (1977) Hydrotalcite in the treatment of bile vomiting. *British Journal of Surgery*, **64**, 849–850.

46 Holt, J. M., Gear, M. W. L. & Warner, G. T. (1970) The role of chronic blood loss in the pathogenesis of post-gastrectomy iron deficiency anaemia. *Gut*, **11**, 847–850.

47 Jenkins, D. J. A., Gassull, M. A., Leeds, A. R. *et al.* (1977) Effect of dietary fiber on complications of gastric surgery: prevention of postprandial hypoglycemia by pectin. *Gastroenterology*, **73**, 215.

48 Johnston, D. (1975) Operative mortality and postoperative morbidity of highly selective vagotomy. *British Journal of Surgery*, **62**, 160–164.

49 Johnston, D., Humphrey, C. S., Walker, B. E. *et al.* (1972) Vagotomy without diarrhoea. *British Medical Journal*, **iii**, 788–790.

50 Johnston, I. D. A., Welbourne, R. & Acheson, K. (1958) Gastrectomy and loss of weight. *Lancet*, **i**, 1242–1245.

51 Johnston, J. H., Jensen, D. M. & Mautner, W. A. (1978) A comparison of bipolar electrocoagulation and argon laser photocoagulation with coaxial CO_2 in the treatment of bleeding canine gastric ulcers. *Gastro-intestinal Endoscopy*, **24**, 200–201.

52 Jones, C. T., Williams, J. A., Cox, E. V. *et al.* (1962) Peptic ulceration. Some haematological and metabolic consequences of gastric surgery. *Lancet*, **ii**, 425–428.

53 Kennedy, T. (1976) Duodenoplasty with proximal

gastric vagotomy. *Annals of the Royal College of Surgeons of England*, **58**, 144–146.

54 Kennedy, T. & Green, R. (1978) Roux diversion for bile reflux following gastric surgery. *British Journal of Surgery*, **65**, 323–325.

55 Kennedy, T., Connell, A. M., Love, A. H. G. *et al.* (1973) Selective or truncal vagotomy? Five year results of a double-blind randomized, controlled trial. *British Journal of Surgery*, **60**, 944–948.

56 Kennedy, T., Johnston, G. W., Love, A. H. G. *et al.* (1973) Pyloroplasty versus gastro-jejunostomy. *British Journal of Surgery*, **60**, 949–953.

57 Logan, R. F. A. & Langman, M. J. S. (1983) Screening for gastric cancer after gastric surgery. *Lancet*, **ii**, 667–670.

58 Louyot, P., Mathieu, J. & Gaucher, A. (1961) L'osteose rareficante des gastrectomies. *Archives des Maladies de l'Appareil Digestif et des Maladies de la Nutrition*, **50**, 20–38.

59 Lundman, T., Orinius, E. & Thorsen, G. (1964) Incidence of gallstone disease following partial gastric resection. *Acta Chirurgica Scandinavica*, **127**, 130–133.

60 MacDonald, J. M., Webster, M. M., Tennyson, C. H. & Drapanas, T. (1969) Serotonin and bradykinin in the dumping syndrome. *American Journal of Surgery*, **117**, 204–213.

61 McKelvey, S. T. D. (1970) Gastric incontinence and post-vagotomy diarrhoea. *British Journal of Surgery*, **57**, 781–783.

62 Morgan, D. B. & Pulvertaft, C. N. (1969) Effects of vagotomy on bone metabolism. In *After Vagotomy* (Ed.) Alexander-Williams, J. & Cox, A. G. pp. 161–171. London: Butterworths.

63 Morgan, D. B., Patterson, C. R., Pulvertaft, C. N. *et al.* (1965) Search for osteomalacia in 1228 patients after gastrectomy and other operations on the stomach. *Lancet*, **ii**, 1085.

64 Mosimann, F., Sorgi, M., Wolverson, R. L. *et al.* (1983) Bile reflux after duodenal ulcer surgery: a study of 114 asymptomatic and symptomatic patients. *Scandinavian Journal of Gastroenterology* (in press).

65 Muhe, E., Muller, C., Martinoli, S. *et al.* (1982) Five years results of a prospective multicentre trial on proximal gastric vagotomy. In *Vagotomy in Modern Surgical Practice* (Ed.) Baron, J. H., Alexander-Williams, J., Allgower, M. *et al.* pp. 176–186. London: Butterworths.

66 Muller, C. (1982) Recurrent peptic ulcer after proximal gastric vagotomy. In *Vagotomy in Modern Surgical Practice* (Ed.) Baron, J. H., Alexander-Williams, J., Allgower, M. *et al.* pp. 312–318. London: Butterworths.

67 Muscroft, T. J., Taylor, E. W., Deane, S. A. & Alexander-Williams, J. (1981) Reoperation for recurrent peptic ulceration. *British Journal of Surgery*, **68**, 75–76.

68 Neustein, C. L., Bushkin, F. L., Weinshelbaum, E. I. & Woodward, E. R. (1977) Re-operation for post-surgical peptic ulcer recurrence: appraisal of ten years experience. *Annals of Surgery*, **185**, 169–174.

69 Nicolaysen, R. & Ragaard, R. (1955) Calcium and phosphorus metabolism in gastrectomized patients. *Scandinavian Journal of Clinical and Laboratory Investigation*, **7**, 298–299.

70 Nielsen, J. R. (1964) Development of cholelithiasis following vagotomy. *Surgery*, **56**, 909–911.

71 Nilsson, B. E. & Westlin, N. E. (1971) The fracture incidence after gastrectomy. *Acta Chirurgica Scandinavica*, **137**, 533–534.

72 Nilsson, I. M., Anderson, L. & Bjorkman, S. E. (1966) Epsilon-aminocaproic acid (E-ACA) as a therapeutic agent based on a five years' clinical experience. *Acta Medica Scandinavica*, **180** (supplement 448), 1–46.

73 Pack, G. T. & Banner, R. L. (1958) The late develop-

ment of gastric cancer after gastroenterostomy and gastrectomy for peptic ulcer and benign pyloric stenosis. *Surgery*, **44**, 1024–1033.

74 Parkin, G. J., Smith, R. B. & Johnson, D. (1973) Gallbladder size and contractability after truncal, selective and highly selective vagotomy in man. *Annals of Surgery*, **178**, 581–586.

75 Peitsch, W. & Becker, H. D. (1979) Frequency and prognosis of primary gastric stump carcinomas. *Frontiers of Gastrointestinal Research*, **5**, 170–177.

76 Poth, E. J. & Smith, L. B. (1966) Gastric pouches: their evaluation. *American Journal of Surgery*, **112**, 721–727.

77 Poxon, V. A., Youngs, D., Morris, D. *et al.* (1983) Deconjugation and degradation of bile acids after gastric resection. *Gut*, **24**, 466–467.

78 Ralphs, D. N. L. (1982) Dumping. In *Vagotomy in Modern Surgical Practice*. (Ed.) Baron, J. H., Alexander-Williams, J., Allgower, M. *et al.* pp. 255–259. London: Butterworths.

79 Saegesser, F. & James, D. (1972) Cancer of the gastric stump after partial gastrectomy (Billroth II principle) for ulcer. *Cancer*, **29**, 1150–1159.

80 Salmon, P. R. (1981) Therapeutic endoscopy. In *Gastrointestinal Haemorrhage* (Ed.) Dykes, P. W. & Keighley, M. R. B. pp. 304–318. Bristol: Wright PSG.

81 Schjonsby, H. (1974) The absorption of vitamin B$_{12}$ in the blind loop syndrome. *Scandinavian Journal of Gastroenterology* (supplement 9) 65–70.

82 Schoen, M. S., Lindenbaum, J., Roginsky, M. S. & Holt, R. R. (1978) Significance of serum level of 25-hydroxycholecalciferol in gastrointestinal disease. *American Journal of Digestive Diseases*, **23**, 137–142.

83 Segal, A. W., Arnot, R. N., Thakur, M. L. & Lavender, J. P. (1976) Indium-111-labelled leukocytes for localisation of abscesses. *Lancet*, **i**, 1056–1058.

84 Sigstad, H. (1970) A clinical diagnostic index in the diagnosis of the dumping syndrome. Changes in plasma volume and blood sugar after a test meal. *Acta Medica Scandinavica*, **188**, 479–486.

85 Small, W. P. (1964) The recurrence of ulceration after surgery for duodenal ulcer. *Journal of the Royal College of Surgeons of Edinburgh*, **9**, 255–278.

86 Sorgi, M., Wolverson, R. L., Mosimann, F. *et al.* (1983) Sensitivity and reproducibility of a bile reflux test using ^{99m}Tc HIDA. *Scandinavian Journal of Gastroenterology* (in press).

87 Stabile, B. E. & Passaro, E. (1976) Recurrent peptic ulcer. *Gastroenterology*, **70**, 124–135.

88 Stalsberg, H. & Taksdal, S. (1971) Stomach cancer following gastric surgery for benign conditions. *Lancet*, **ii**, 1175–1177.

89 Stammers, F. A. R. (1961) A clinical approach to the analysis and treatment of post-gastrectomy syndrome. *British Journal of Surgery*, **49**, 28–36.

90 Terjesen, T. & Erichsen, H. G. (1976) Carcinoma of the gastric stump after operation for benign gastroduodenal ulcer. *Acta Chirurgica Scandinavica*, **142**, 256–260.

91 Vasconez, L. O., Adams, J. T. & Woodward, E. R. (1970) Treatment of reluctant post-vagotomy stoma with bethanechol. *Archives of Surgery*, **10**, 693–694.

92 Williams, J. A. (1964) Effects of upper gastrointestinal surgery on blood formation and bone metabolism. *British Journal of Surgery*, **51**, 125–135.

93 Wirts, C. W., Templeton, J. Y., Fineberg, C. & Goldstein, F. (1965) The correction of post-gastrectomy malabsorption following a jejunal interposition operation. *Gastroenterology*, **49**, 141–149.

94 Wolverson, R. L., Sorgi, M., Mosimann, F. *et al.* (1983) Does gastric intubation cause enterogastric reflux? *Scandinavian Journal of Gastroenterology* (in press).

GASTRIC TUMOURS

BENIGN TUMOURS

Benign tumours of the stomach are much less frequent than malignant growths. However, in one respect they are more important because not only is there an opportunity to cure the patient but also to prevent the development of malignancy. The macroscopic features of gastric polyps have been classified:[18] they can be classified as sessile or pedunculated.

The two principal histological types of gastric polyp are hyperplastic or adenomatous. Although most pedunculated polyps are adenomatous, sessile polyps may be of either histological type.

Polypoid adenoma

This is the commonest benign gastric epithelial tumour. Its prevalence in the general population was assessed to be less than 1%[3] in a pathological study and 0.23% in an endoscopic study.[15] This is a true neoplasm, cell replication is unrestrained and the cells are incompletely differentiated. The histological appearance is similar to a colonic adenoma, with hyperchromatic elongated nuclei, nuclear atypia is common and there is an abrupt transfer to normal gastric mucosa at the edge of the polyp. Intestinal metaplasia of the gastric epithelium is commonly seen in association with both types of epithelial polyp. Adenomatous gastric polyps are usually single and most commonly occur in the antrum. These polyps are often an incidental endoscopic finding, although intussusception can occur.

In one series of 97 patients with gastric polyps, 35% were incidental findings in gastrectomy specimens for carcinoma whereas only 5% were found in gastric resections for peptic ulcer.[14] Carcinoma is quite common in situ in adenomatous polyps.

Management

The only means of obtaining an adequate biopsy is by examination of the entire polyp. This may be achieved for most patients by endoscopic polypectomy. Complications of this technique include bleeding and development of a peptic ulcer at the excision site. These risks may be reduced by the use of anti-ulcer treatment.[5]

Hyperplastic polyps
(regenerative or intestinal type)

Hyperplastic polyps are five times more common than the adenomatous polyp.[8] They are frequently multiple, usually smaller than 2 cm in diameter and occur typically in the body and fundus of the stomach. There is only a minor disturbance in the control of mitosis and no loss of cellular differentiation. They are not true neoplasms. Histological features include cystic dilatation of glands lined by normal gastric epithelial cells.

Management

The risk of developing carcinoma is much less than with adenomatous polyps, and is perhaps more closely related to the degree of underlying gastric epithelial change. Careful endoscopic follow-up with multiple biopsies is advocated. It is technically easy to remove such polyps by endoscopic biopsy.

Disorders associated with gastric polyps

In a follow-up of patients 10 years after partial gastrectomy, 9% were found to have gastric polyps,[4] the majority occurring around the stoma. Most of these polyps were of the hyperplastic type. There is an increased risk of hyperplastic gastric polyps in pernicious anaemia[2] and familial polyposis coli.[16] Gastroduodenal polyps occur in 40% of patients with Peutz-Jegher's syndrome and endoscopic removal is advocated both to prevent intussusception and the small risk of malignancy.[17] These familial syndromes are also discussed in Chapter 11.

Gastric polyps are also seen in Gardner's syndrome and may be either true adenomas or glandular cysts of the fundic mucosa.[1]

Leiomyoma

This is the commonest non-epithelial benign gastric tumour. Small nodular lesions may be found in almost 50% of autopsies.[7] Leiomyomas usually enlarge in their submucosal site to form intraluminal polypoid lesions, on the summit of which there are often multiple ulcers. Less commonly they grow out from the serosal surface of the stomach.

Clinical presentation is most commonly with haematemesis due to central ulceration.[6] Intussusception is rare, but necrosis and calcification may occur. Microscopically, most leiomyomas show well differentiated smooth muscle and hyalinized connective tissue. However, some tumours are very cellular and may display hyperchromatic nuclei, with round rather than spindle shaped cells. Differentiation from a leiomyosarcoma in such cases can be difficult

and should be based on the number of mitotic figures present.[11]

Management

Diagnosis of gastric leiomyomas is by double-contrast barium meal or endoscopy. Endoscopic biopsy is unlikely to provide a histological diagnosis unless taken from the ulcerated area. Whilst endoscopic removal of pedunculated leiomyomas has been described, local surgical excision with a cuff of normal stomach is to be advised.

Other benign gastric polyps

Other rare gastric polyps include carcinoid tumours, inflammatory fibroid polyps, neurofibromas and lipomas.

Benign duodenal tumours

Benign duodenal tumours are found in approximately 1% of duodenoscopic examinations.[10] Most tumours located in the first part of the duodenum are benign but the risk of malignancy increases as they become located more distally.[13] Adenoma is the commonest type[10] and gastrointestinal bleeding the commonest presentation. The risk of malignant change is not as clear as in gastric adenomas. Villous adenoma is more rare, usually solitary, and the tendency to bleed or undergo malignant change is much greater. Obstruction of the duodenum or ampulla can occur by benign villous adenomas and they may grow up the common bile duct.

Brunner's gland adenomas are rare and are usually confined to the fourth part of the duodenum; malignant change probably does not occur. Leiomyoma lipomas, inflammatory fibroid polyp[12] and carcinoid tumour[9] can also give rise to duodenal polypoid lesions.

REFERENCES

1　Eichenberger, P., Hammer, B., Gloor, F. *et al.* (1980) Gardner's syndrome with glandular cysts of the fundi mucosa. *Endoscopy,* **12,** 63–67.
2　Elsborg, L., Andersen, D., Myhre-Jensen, O. & Bastrup Madsen, P. (1977) Gastricmucosal polyps in pernicious anaemia. *Scandinavian Journal of Gastroenterology,* **12,** 49.
3　Grafe, W., Thorbjarnason, B. & Pearce, J. M. (1960) Benign neoplasms of the stomach. *American Journal of Surgery,* **100,** 561–571.
4　Janunger, K. G. & Domellof, L. (1978) Gastric polyps and precancerous mucosal changes after partial gastrectomy. *Acta Chirurgica Scandinavica,* **144,** 293–298.
5　Lanza, F. L., Graham, D. Y., Nelson, R. S. *et al.* (1981) Endoscopic upper gastrointestinal polypectomy. *American Journal of Gastroenterology,* **75** (5), 345–348.

6 Lee, F. I. (1979) Gastric leiomyoma and leiomyosarcoma – five cases. *Postgraduate Medical Journal*, **55**, 575–578.

7 Meissner, W. A. (1944) Leiomyoma of the stomach. *Archives of Pathology*, **38**, 207–209.

8 Ming, S. C. & Goldman, H. (1969) Gastric polyp. A histological classification of its relation to carcinoma. *Cancer*, **18**, 721.

9 Ott, D. J., Wu, W. C., Shiflett, D. W. & Pennell, T. C. (1980) Inflammatory fibroid polyp of the duodenum. *American Journal of Gastroenterology*, **73**, 62–64.

10 Reddy, R. R., Schuman, B. M. & Priest, L. R. J. (1981) Duodenal polyps: diagnosis and management. *Journal of Clinical Gastroenterology*, **3**, 139–145.

11 Rorchod, M. & Kempson, R. L. (1977) Smooth muscle tumours of the gastrointestinal tract and retroperitoneum. A pathologic analysis of 100 cases. *Cancer*, **39**, 255–262.

12 Saunders, R. J. & Axtell, H. K. (1964) Carcinoids of the gastrointestinal tract. *Surgery, Gynaecology and Obstetrics*, **119**, 369–380.

13 Stassa, G. & Klingensmith, W. C. (1969) 111 primary tumors of the duodenal bulb. *American Journal of Roentgenology*, **107**, 105–110.

14 Tomasulo, J. (1971) Gastric polyps. Histologic types and their relationship to gastric carcinoma. *Cancer*, **27**, 1346–1355.

15 Ueno, K., Oshiba, S., Yamayata, S. et al. (1976) Histochemical classification and follow up study of gastric polyp. *Contemporary Topics in Immunobiology*, **5**, 23–38.

16 Ushio, K., Sasagawa, M., Doi, H. et al. (1976) Lesions associated with familial polyposis coli. Studies of lesions of the stomach, duodenum, bones and teeth. *Gastrointestinal Radiology*, **1**, 67.

17 William, C. B., Goldblatt, M. & Delaney, P. V. (1982) Top and tail endoscopy and follow up in Peutz–Jegher's syndrome. *Endoscopy*, **14**, 22–34.

18 Yamada, T. (1966) Polypoid lesion in the stomach. *Stomach and Intestine (Tokyo)*, **1**, 43.

GASTRIC CARCINOMA

Epidemiology

The aetiology of cancer is still under intensive research. The most probable mechanism would be to postulate a two-stage mechanism of carcinogenesis. The first stage is the operation of 'initiators' on cell DNA, causing mutation (oncogene activation). The second phase is the exposure to 'promoters' causing dedifferentiation (perhaps due to oncogene amplification). The principal 'initiators' and 'promoters' have been searched for by intensive epidemiological studies.

CLASSIFICATION

Gastric cancer can be divided into two main types: 'diffuse' or undifferentiated and 'intestinal' or differentiated as described by Lauren.[13] The intestinal type usually arises from mucosa with intestinal metaplasia while the diffuse

variety stems from proper gastric mucosa. These two types show distinct epidemiological features and are sharply contrasted. Autopsy records on 10 494 patients dating from 1958 to 1967 in Japan were reviewed and classified into these two types, and distribution by sex and age were found to be quite different to each other.[6] The diffuse undifferentiated type is more predominant in females (42.3% of 3618 cases) than in males (29.1% of 6876 cases). It is also more frequent in younger age groups: under the age of 39 the predominance was 51.8% (of 1535 cases) between 40–59, 35.6% (of 4336 cases), and over 60, 25.8% (of 4623 cases). It is also more predominant in certain occupations.

MORTALITY

According to the National Vital Statistics for 1982 in Japan, 30 036 males and 18 974 females died from gastric cancer, the mortality rate per 100 000 population being 51.7 and 31.6, respectively. The corresponding rates for USA (1978) were 8.0 and 5.3, and for England and Wales (1978) were 28.0 and 19.1, respectively. The relative frequency or the percentage of gastric cancer to cancer of all sites in Japan was 30.3 for males and 26.7 for females in 1982. The corresponding percentage for the USA was 3.9 and 3.3, and for England and Wales, 9.8 and 8.2, respectively.

INCIDENCE

Based on data of population-based cancer registries in Miyagi (Japan), in Japanese in Hawaii, in Connecticut (USA) and in Birmingham (UK) the adjusted (to world population) incidence rates of gastric cancer per 100 000 in 1973–1977 were calculated in males as 88.0 for Japan, 34.0 for Japanese in Hawaii, 11.0 for the USA and 22.1 for the UK. In females the figures were 42.0 for Japan, 15.1 for Japanese in Hawaii, 5.1 for the USA and 10.1 for the UK.[10]

RISK FACTORS

Exogenous factors
Geography. There are marked variations in the incidence of gastric cancer between and within various countries. Sometimes even adjacent countries, prefectures or villages show striking differences as shown in cancer maps of the USA, China and Japan. Some of the variation in incidence of gastric cancer may be due to differences in the nitrate content of the local water supply.

High dietary nitrate may be converted to N-nitroso compounds in the presence of certain bacteria.[2]

Time trends. There is a uniform decline in the standardized stomach cancer death rate in almost all countries in the world, including Japan. This fall in frequency is believed to reflect certain essential changes in the factors governing the aetiology of the disease (Figure 4.47).[4, 7]

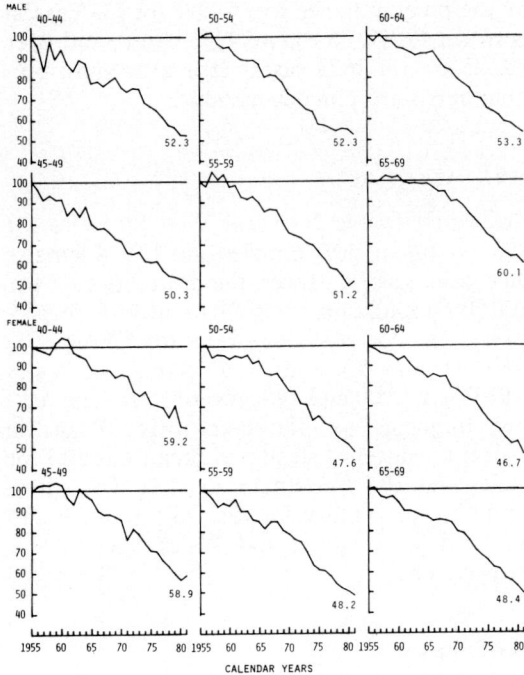

Fig. 4.47 Annual trend of age-specific death rate for stomach cancer in Japan, 1955–1981 (1955 = 100).

Changes in economic status, and in particular changes in diet, must be important factors. The introduction of electric refrigerators is believed to have played a major role in the falling frequency of stomach cancer since this method of

food preservation has replaced older methods (in particular, preservation by salting). Case-control studies conducted in Japan and in Hawaii showed that the frequency of gastric carcinoma was closely associated with the intake of highly salted food.

Soil type. A close association was observed between gastric cancer and soil type, acidic soil being associated with a greater frequency of the disease. The association may be connected with the intake of trace metals such as zinc as they are easily absorbed into vegetables, grains and eventually in animals and humans if soil is acidic.

Air pollution. The association between gastric cancer and air pollution was also suspected but supporting evidence is still limited.

Socio-economic status. In those countries where socio-economic studies have been conducted the disease has a tendency to be more common in the lower socio-economic strata.

Occupation. There is a higher risk of gastric cancer in certain occupations such as in metal workers.[8]

Smoking. In the current large scale prospective population study in progress in Japan (1966–81), the age standardized death rate per 100 000 for gastric cancer in males was 200.7 for daily smokers (1 035 833 person years) compared with 136.5 for non-smokers (248 155). In the case of females it was 96.9 for smokers (176 377) and 77.3 for non-smokers (1 431 798). The mortality ratio of smokers to non-smokers, was 1.47 for males ($P < 0.01$) and 1.25 for females ($P < 0.01$) (Figure 4.48).

Alcohol. No increased risk of stomach cancer was observed among daily drinkers of alcohol compared to non-daily drinkers in our prospective population study: 198.6 versus 194.1 in

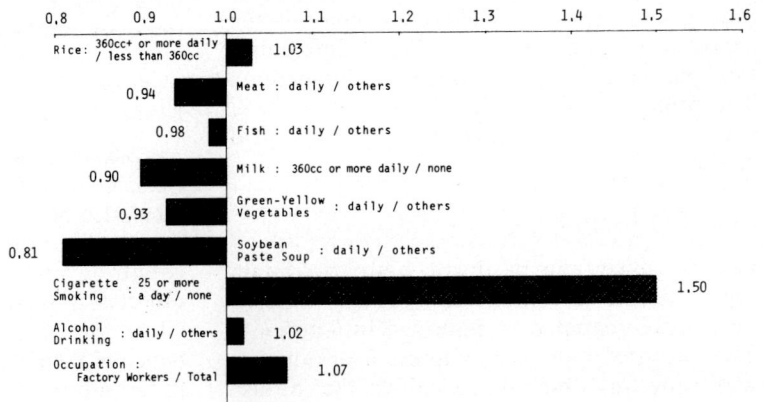

Fig. 4.48 Standardized mortality ratio for cancer of the stomach by selected risk factors. Prospective study, 1966–81, Japan.

males and 87.0 versus 84.9 in females respectively.

Diet. Dietary factors have long been suspected as risk factors in gastric cancer. The promoting effect of highly salted foods (particularly pickles and fish) and the protective effect of dairy products were observed by case-control studies conducted in Japan (Table 4.35).

Table 4.35 Effect of dietary factors on risk of gastric cancer in studies in Japan.

	Relative risk[a]	
	Males	Females
Highly salted food[b]	4.07	7.23
Dairy products[b]	0.22	0.29
Green–yellow vegetables[c]	0.65	0.59
Five-year increased intake[d]	0.73	
Soybean paste soup[e]	0.78	0.74

[a] Risk in group with daily intake of dietary factor relative to risk in group with no intake of dietary factor.
[b] Matched case-control study: 300 males and 154 females in each group.
[c] Prospective study.[10] 16 years follow-up of 265, 118 people aged 40 and above.
[d] Risk in those who increased their intake of yellow–green vegetables during the first five years of observation relative to risk in those who remained in the non-daily-intake group throughout the study.
[e] Cohort study.[9]

In addition, the intake of green-yellow vegetables was noted to lower the risk of stomach cancer significantly in our large-scale prospective study (Table 4.35). In this study those who increased their intake of green-yellow vegetables during the first five years of observation were found to show a lowered risk of gastric cancer in the course of a subsequent follow-up.[10] Thus improvement of diet might reduce the risk of gastric cancer. Soybean was also observed to lower the risk and daily intake of soybean paste soup was noted to carry a significantly lower mortality rate for gastric cancer in our cohort study (Table 4.35).[9]

Endogenous factors
Sex. A prominent epidemiological characteristic of this disease is the almost constant male–female ratio in mortality and morbidity, which is almost always about 60% higher in males than in females. This relationship is true for most countries, suggesting common factors that affect the occurrence of gastric cancer, e.g. a smoking habit which until recently prevailed in males.

Age. The linear rise in the rate of incidence when plotted on a logarithmic scale for age and death has long been discussed in testing models of carcinogenesis.

Blood groups. A slightly higher risk of gastric cancer has been observed in people with blood group A.

Heredity. Studies on the familial aggregation of gastric cancer in the literature are in close agreement. There is a two- to three-fold excess risk of gastric cancer among near relatives of gastric cancer patients. In case-control studies in six Japanese prefectures in 1963 the father had died of gastric cancer in 15 out of 148 cases of gastric cancer compared with four out of 153 controls under the age of 49. Similar frequencies for mothers were two and two, respectively. Thus a four-fold increased risk was observed in fathers of patients with gastric cancer but not in mothers. By contrast, in patients over 50 years, the father had died of gastric cancer in 44 out of 763 cases of gastric cancer compared with 31 out of 771 controls. The frequencies for mothers were 16 and 22, respectively. Again a significant risk was observed in fathers but not in mothers.[3]

Predisposing changes. Intestinal metaplasia (Figure 4.49) is the major predisposing factor in patients with the intestinal type of gastric cancer. Pernicious anaemia has been reported to coexist with the disease but this association is quite infrequent and is seldom observed as a factor. An association between gastric ulcers and the later development of cancer has often been postulated but supporting evidence is quite limited. There is evidence that persistent gastric hypochlorhydria and bile reflux may initiate areas of intestinal metaplasia and atrophic gastritis, which may be responsible for the increased risk of cancer after gastric resection.[14] The co-carcinogens which have been implicated in the postoperative stomach include N-nitroso compounds and free bile acids.[1, 15, 16] In summary, although many factors have been suspected and studied, one must recognize that dietary influence is apparently the most important factor in cancer of the stomach. The possibility of chemical carcinogens acting as both initiators and promoters is also high. Chemical factors have been suggested by animal experiments after feeding strong mutagens such as MNNG and also by the epidemiological observations of the associations of cancer with cigarette smoking and certain occupations.

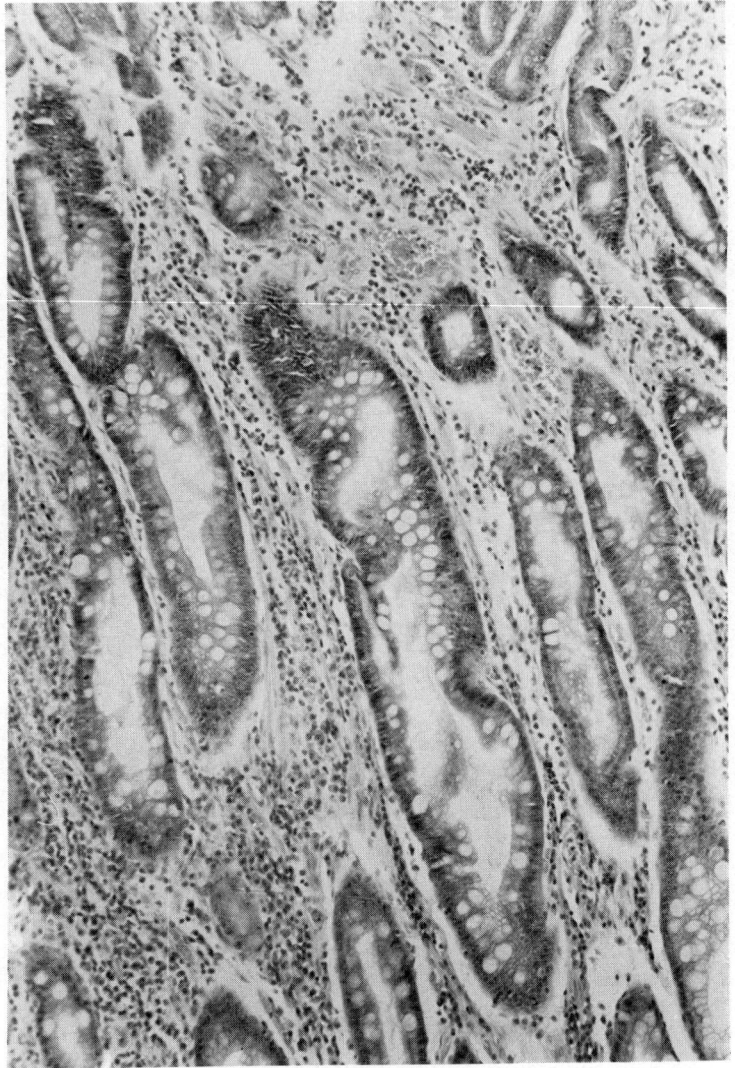

Fig. 4.49 Precancerous lesions: (a) intestinal metaplasia, (b) dysplasia. (Courtesy of Dr H. Thompson, Birmingham General Hospital).

a

Screening

Early detection programmes for gastric cancer by means of screening started in 1960 in Japan. A government subsidy was introduced from 1966 and helped the rapid spread of the programme. About three to four million people have been screened annually by mass gastrography in Japan in recent years. The number examined by mass radiography for gastric cancer and the number detected in 1981 were 4 350 479 and 4365. This programme is thought to have screened 9% of persons between 40–69 years of age and achieved a detection rate of 1.0 per 1000.

The age specific rates of annually screened persons per 1000 population are highest at 40–59 years of age in both men and women. The decline in deaths from gastric cancer is higher in the age groups where coverage by mass screening is most commonly performed (Figure 4.50). However, the decline in the death rate from gastric cancer was similar in both men and women, although the rate of mass screening was much higher in men than in women. This suggests that there is a fall in the overall incidence of the disease as well as earlier detection thanks to mass screening programmes.

Nearly 90% of the mass screenings are conducted by a mobile X-ray unit and the photofluorographic methods are well standardized. The patient is asked to swallow effervescent granules before the examination and six gastro-camera pictures are taken in various positions. Roll film 70–100 mm in width is used. It takes only three to four minutes to examine one

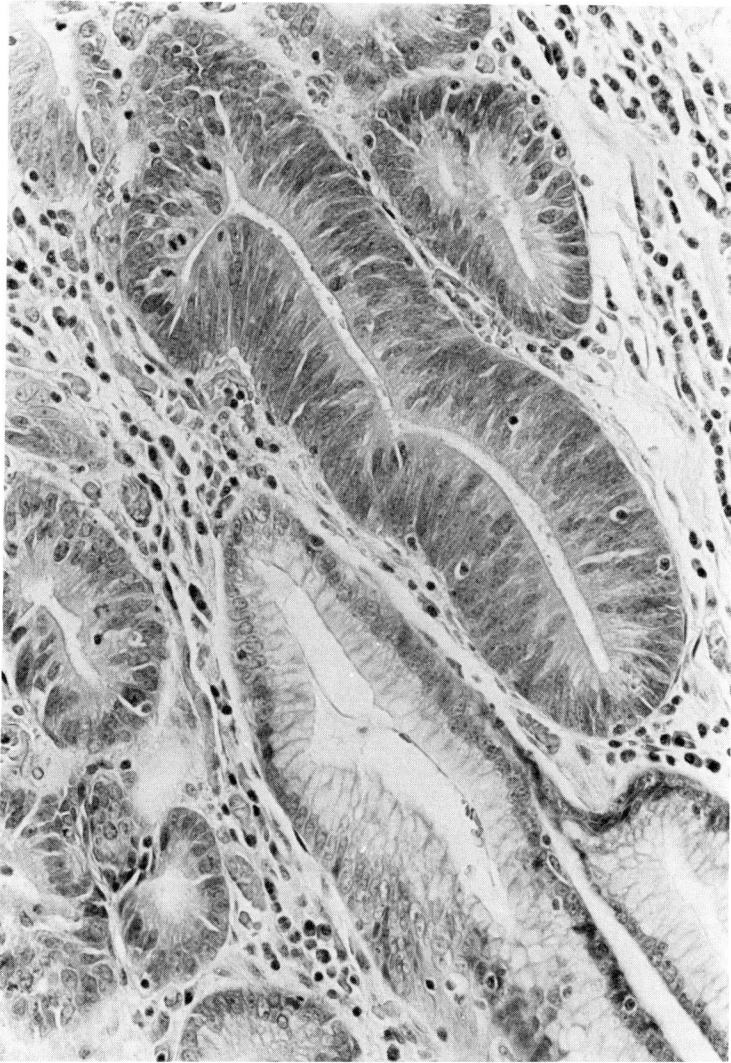

b

person by this method, covering 50 to 60 persons a day. This method is used for the purpose of economy and as a means of minimizing X-ray hazards without sacrificing diagnostic efficiency. The X-ray films thus taken are examined by two specialists independently and the cases which require further detailed examinations, such as fibre-optic gastroduodenoscopy and biopsy, are selected. A much higher proportion of early gastric cancers are found by such methods than with conventional diagnostic X-ray methods in outpatient departments. Of the cases of gastric cancer detected by screening in 1973–1975, 57.4% were without lymph node metastasis.[5]

The five- and ten-year survival rates for gastric cancer cases detected by mass screening are significantly higher than in patients detected in outpatient clinics. The results of follow-up in screened persons clearly shows a significantly lower gastric cancer adjusted death rate compared to unscreened persons: in males, this was 61.9 out of 38 377.5 screened person-years versus 137.2 out of 20 653.0 unscreened person-years, and in females, 28.1 out of 48 888.5 screened person-years versus 53.8 out of 21 579.5 unscreened person-years.[11] Similar results have been reported in other areas.

The change in gastric cancer death rate from 1969–1972 to 1973–1977 in 14 municipalities having an average screening rate of 17.7% was compared with that of 28 randomly selected comparable control municipalities having an average screening rate of 7.7%. The death rate from gastric cancer decreased by 25.5% in high screening areas (being 97.5 per 100 000 in 1969–

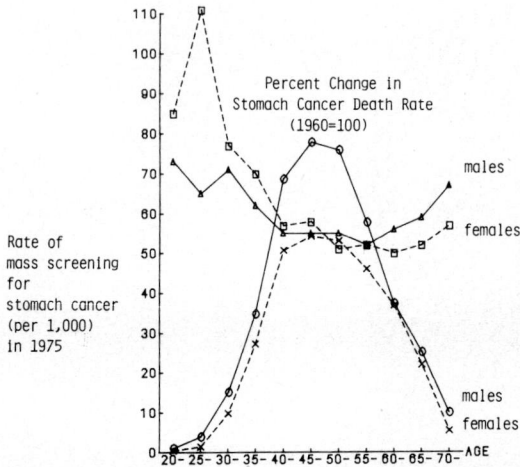

Fig. 4.50 Percentage change in stomach cancer death rate in 1960 and in 1981 and rate of mass screening for stomach cancer in 1975 by sex and age groups.

1972 and 73.0 per 100 000 in 1973–1977) compared to 0.7% in the low screening areas (P < 0.05) (death rates being 84.9 per 100 000 in 1969–1972 and 84.3 per 100 000 in 1973–1977).[12]

The following results of a natural history study of early gastric cancer also suggest the effectiveness of mass screening for prevention of deaths from gastric cancer. Forty-three cases in a total of 56 early gastric cancers detected in the Center for Adult Diseases in Osaka were followed up without performing surgical operations. Of the 43 cases, 27 progressed to clinical invasive cancer within six to 88 months (with a median of 27 months). It was also observed that 12 out of 34 early gastric cancer cases who did not receive surgical operation died from gastric cancer in the observation period, having a median survival of 77 months. These results suggested that detection and surgical resection of early gastric cancer would prevent death from gastric cancer.[17]

The observed effect of mass screening for gastric cancer may be influenced by lead-time or length bias. Furthermore, the influence of selection bias cannot be neglected in interpreting results, since none of the evaluations made so far are based on a randomized trial.

It has also been suggested that certain haematological and gastric juice markers might be used for screening. Such potential markers include carcinoembryonic antigen, α-feto protein and lactic dehydrogenase. In combination these markers might detect patients suitable for more invasive screening procedures, but their use in this field has not been confirmed.

REFERENCES

1 Domellof, L., Reddy, B. S. & Weisburger, J. H. (1980) Microflora and deconjugation of bile acids in alkaline reflux after partial gastrectomy. *American Journal of Surgery*, **140**, 291–295.
2 Hill, M. J., Hawksworth, G. & Tattersall, G. (1973) Bacteria, nitrosamines and cancer of the stomach. *British Journal of Cancer*, **28**, 256–262.
3 Hirayama, T. (1971) Epidemiology of stomach cancer. In *Early Gastric Cancer* (Ed.) Murakami, T. pp. 3–19. Gann Monograph on Cancer Research, 11.
4 Hirayama, T. (1975) Epidemiology of cancer of the stomach with special reference to its recent decrease in Japan. *Cancer Research*, **35**, 3460–3463.
5 Hirayama, T. (1978) Outline of stomach cancer screening in Japan. In *Screening in Cancer* (Ed.) Miller, A. B. pp. 264–278. UICC Technical Report Series, 40. Geneva: UICC.
6 Hirayama, T. (1979) The epidemiology of gastric cancer in Japan. In *Gastric Cancer* (Ed.) Pfeiffer, C. J. pp. 60–82. New York: Gerhard Witzstrick Publishing House.
7 Hirayama, T. (1980) *Cancer Risks by Site* (Ed.) Hirayama, T., Waterhouse, J. & Fraumeni, J. UICC Technical Report Series 41.
8 Hirayama, T. (1981) Proportion of cancer attributable to occupation obtained from a census population-based large cohort study in Japan. In *Quantification of Occupational Cancer* (Ed.) Peto, R. & Schneiderman, M. pp. 631–649. Banbury Report 9. New York: Cold Spring Harbor Laboratory.
9 Hirayama, T. (1982) Relationship of soybean paste soup intake to gastric cancer risk. *Nutrition and Cancer*, **3**(4), 223–233.
10 Hirayama, T. (1982) Does daily intake of green–yellow vegetable lower the risk of cancer in man? An example of application of epidemiological methods to identify individuals at low risk. *Proceedings of the Symposium on Host Factors in Human Carcinogenesis* (Ed.) Bartsch, H., Armstrong, B. & Davis, W. pp. 531–540. Lyon: IARC Scientific Publication 39.
11 Hisamichi, S. (1978) Prognosis of the patients with gastric cancer detected by mass survey. In *Principles and Practice in Gastric Mass Survey Examination*. pp. 91–96. Kanehara Shuppan, Tokyo (in Japanese).
12 Kuroishi, T., Hirose, K., Nakagawa, N. & Tominaga, S. (1983) Comparisons of trend in stomach cancer mortality between the model areas for stomach cancer screening and the control areas. *Journal of Gastroenterology Mass Survey*, **58**, 45–52 (in Japanese).
13 Lauren, P. (1965) The two main histological types of gastric carcinoma, diffuse and so-called intestinal type carcinoma. *Acta Pathologica et Microbiologica Scandinavica*, **64**, 31–49.
14 Nicholls, J. C. (1979) Stump cancer following gastric surgery. *World Journal of Surgery*, **3**, 731–736.
15 Reed, P. I., Smith, P. L. R., Haines, K. *et al.* (1981) Gastric juice N-nitrosamines in health and gastroduodenal disease. *Lancet*, **ii**, 550–552.
16 Schlag, P., Bockler, R., Ulrich, H. *et al.* (1980) Are nitrite and N-nitroso compounds in gastric juice risk factors for carcinoma in the operated stomach? *Lancet*, **i**, 727–729.
17 Tsukuma, H., Mishima, T. & Oshima, A. (1983) Prospective study of 'early' gastric cancer. *International Journal of Cancer*, **31**, 421–426.

Clinical features, diagnosis and treatment

Cancer of the stomach is the most common neoplasm of the upper gastrointestinal tract. Although there is epidemiological evidence that the incidence of adenocarcinomas is declining, there are still more than 10000 deaths a year from gastric cancer in the United Kingdom alone. There have been many advances in its management. The improvements of surgical and anaesthetic techniques have effectively reduced postoperative mortality from 50% in the last century to 5% in modern times. Similarly, developments in endoscopy and radiology have greatly facilitated diagnosis. The treatment remains primarily surgical and is stage-dependent. While most patients present with advanced disease, the identification of high risk groups and improved clinical awareness of the disease should increase the number of patients diagnosed with the favourable 'early' lesion. Also it is hoped that the cytotoxic effects of certain therapeutic agents might be translated into improvements in survival rates. The diagnosis and management of gastric cancer is multidisciplinary, requiring the expertise of gastroenterologists, radiologists, surgeons and oncologists.

Adenocarcinomas comprise 95% of all malignant diseases of the stomach, so this section will be concerned predominantly with the clinical features, diagnosis and treatment of this disease, although the less common epithelial and non-epithelial tumours will also be described. These are squamous cell carcinomas, carcinoids, lymphomas and leiomyosarcomas.

ADENOCARCINOMA OF THE STOMACH

Clinical features

The classical symptoms of 'advanced' gastric cancer are abdominal pain, dyspepsia, anorexia, anaemia, vomiting and dysphagia. 'Early' gastric cancer is a lesion in which the depth of penetration of the primary tumour is limited histologically to the submucosa of the stomach, irrespective of the presence or absence of lymph node metastases.[33] Approximately 30% of all patients with early gastric cancer have a long history of dyspepsia which is indistinguishable from chronic peptic ulcer disease. The five-year survival following surgical resection of this lesion is 90% in Japan. The difficulty for the physician is differentiating between the symptoms of benign upper gastrointestinal disorders and malignancy. It is important to identify the 'symptomatic at-risk' patients in whom it is essential to establish a precise diagnosis before initiating therapy.

Gastrointestinal bleeding occurs in about one-third of patients. It is usually occult, but occasionally massive. Acute perforation is rare.

Males develop gastric cancer more commonly than women in the ratio of 3 : 2. The highest incidence occurs between the ages of 55 and 65. Sex and age distribution are the same in both 'advanced' and 'early' gastric cancer.[13]

Particularly relevant is an analysis of the first symptoms of the disease. Detailed studies of the presenting symptoms[28, 43] have demonstrated that the first symptom of patients who later presented with advanced disease was similar to that found in patients with 'early' gastric cancer (Table 4.36). There is no typical dyspeptic syndrome that is diagnostic of gastric cancer, the symptoms may be typical of an ulcer or vague, such as abdominal discomfort or belching (Table 4.37).

By the time the patient is admitted to hospital, the clinical picture will have changed from that of the first symptom. The most striking feature is that 78% of patients have lost weight compared with only 18.9% of patients with 'early' gastric cancers. Similar findings have been reported by Green *et al.*[17] who made direct comparisons between early and advanced lesions, weight loss being significantly less common in patients with 'early' gastric cancer. It should be stressed that dyspepsia is a symptom

Table 4.36 Incidence of symptoms of gastric cancer.

	First symptom		Symptoms at presentation of 'early' gastric cancer
	UK: Radcliffe study[43]	Europe[28]	UK: West Midlands study[13]
Symptoms related to GI tract[a]	310 (83.6%)	678 (75.2%)	71 (82.6%)
Constitutional[b]	51 (13.7%)	187 (20.8%)	11 (12.8%)
Other	10 (2.7%)	36 (4.0%)	4 (4.7%)

[a] Dyspepsia, vomiting, abdominal pain, epigastric pain, indigestion, dysphagia, haematemesis, melaena.
[b] Weight loss, anaemia, weakness, lassitude, fever.

Table 4.37 Nature of early dyspeptic symptoms evaluated in 251 patients in the Radcliffe study.[43]

Mild[a]	21%
Ulcer-type	26.3%
Pain after meals (unrelieved by food and alkalis)	14.7%
Long history of vague dyspepsia	11.6%
Continuous pain	18.7%
Pyloric stenosis	7.6%

[a] Vague abdominal discomfort, fullness, belching, regurgitation.

and not a diagnosis and that no patient over the age of 40 complaining for the first time of dyspepsia should be treated until a definitive histological diagnosis has been established.

Physical examination is often unrewarding in gastric cancer, only 32% of patients having a palpable abdominal mass. However, there may be manifestations of metastatic disease, such as palpable lymph nodes, hepatic metastases or ascites. The presence of a palpable mass signifies advanced disease. Thus the absence of physical signs in a symptomatic patient does not exclude gastric malignancy. However, the presence of a mass does not indicate inoperability.

Diagnosis
The diagnosis of gastric cancer is made by radiology and fibre-optic endoscopy. These are complementary investigations and should not be considered mutually exclusive.

The only type of barium meal examination capable of diagnosing early gastric cancer (Figure 4.51) is a double-contrast study, preferably facilitated by inducing hypotonia and using compression. The fibre-optic endoscope allows a full macroscopic assessment of the gastric mucosa and enables biopsies and brush cytology to be obtained from a lesion. After macroscopic assessment of an abnormality at least six to eight biopsies should be taken. Repeated endoscopy and biopsy may be necessary to establish the diagnosis, especially if there is radiological or endoscopic suspicion of malignancy or if a benign appearing lesion fails to heal completely, or fails to remain healed. In addition, the healed area should always be biopsied on review endoscopy. Accuracy can be further increased by brushing all suspicious lesions for cytological examination. Using radiology and endoscopy in combination, the accuracy of diagnosis of gastric cancer is 98%.[35]

Preoperative investigations. Specific preoperative investigations to stage the disease or determine resectability usually prove unreliable. Angiography, liver function tests and radioisotope scans have all been evaluated and proven unreliable. Computerized axial tomography (CT scanning) has been valuable in the assessment of liver disease in colorectal cancer but has not been assessed for gastric neoplasms. Laparoscopy allows visualization and biopsy of metastatic disease, particularly the liver and peritoneal deposits, but is limited in its inability to visualize inaccessible areas (i.e. the lesser sac) and assess fixity.

Treatment
Surgery is the only effective treatment of adenocarcinoma of the stomach and none should be denied its possible benefit. Whilst investigations may give an indication of the stage of disease, most patients deserve a laparotomy unless prior laparoscopy has revealed extensive hepatic or peritoneal metastases or if the patient is otherwise unfit for operation. This general principle of operative assessment must be accepted for most patients because palliation is usually best achieved by surgery. The aim of the 'stage-appropriate' operation for gastric cancer must be to apply a treatment designed for maximal survival time while allowing patients to enjoy an optimal quality of life.

Surgical treatment must be related to the known pattern of spread and recurrence following resection, whether the extent of resection influences long-term survival, the postoperative mortality and the effect of the reconstructive procedure on long-term morbidity.

Gastric neoplasms may spread by: (a) direct extension, (b) lymphatic embolization, (c) lymphatic permeation, (d) blood stream embolization, and (e) transplantation.[6] Direct extension may penetrate surrounding organs (particularly the pancreas or submucosally) and into the oesophagus and duodenum; it is not true that the pylorus limits spread.[46]

Lymph node metastasis is common. The UICC[45] have classified lymph nodes as N1, N2 and N3 (Figure 4.52) and postoperative survival is related to the extent of node involvement. The Japanese, though using a more complicated system,[24] have reported a five-year survival rate for N1 involvement of 38.5%, with an N2 involvement of 22.8%, an N3 involvement of 11.1% and an N4 involvement of 8.5%. (The UICC classification combines N3 and N4 as N3.) Japanese gastroenterologists classify surgical resections according to the extent of the lymphadenectomy and are designated R0, R1, R2 and R3 (an R1 resection excises the N1 nodes, etc.). The corrected five-year survival rate

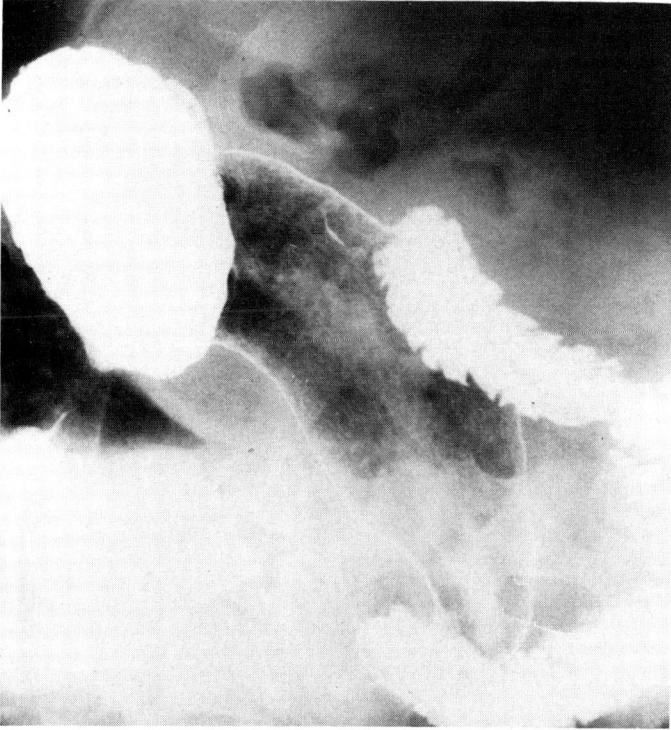

Fig. 4.51 Double-contrast barium studies demonstrating 'early' (a) and advanced (b–d) gastric carcinomas (see overleaf).

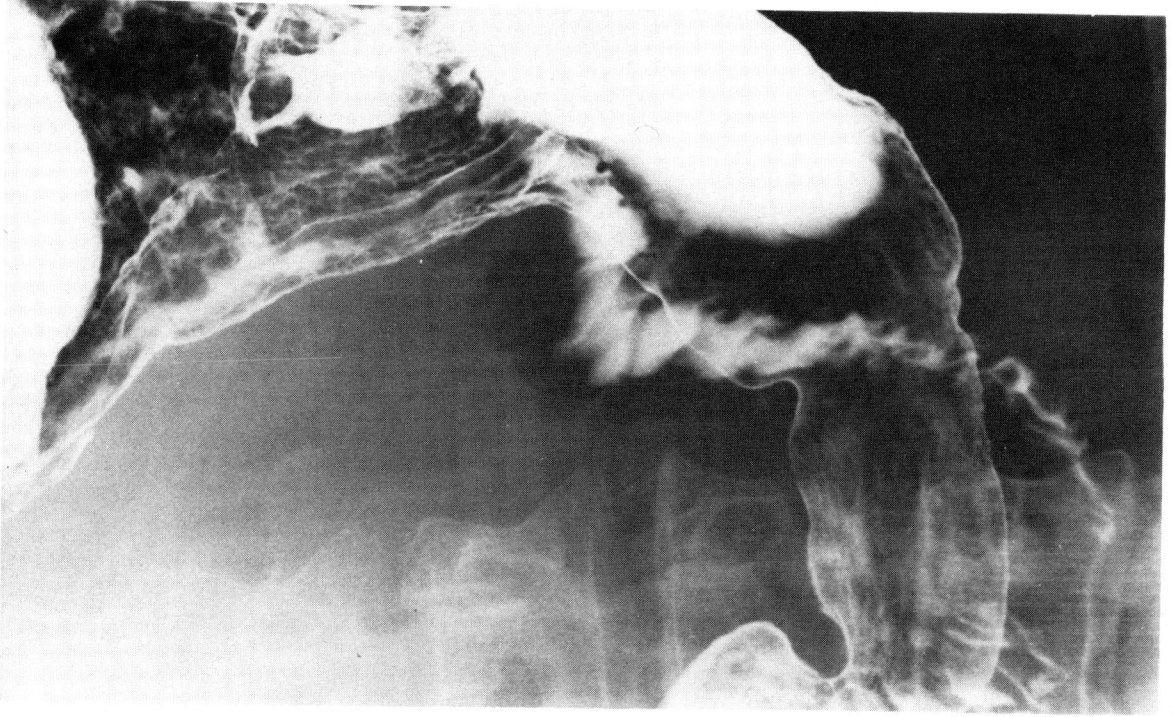

a

b

227

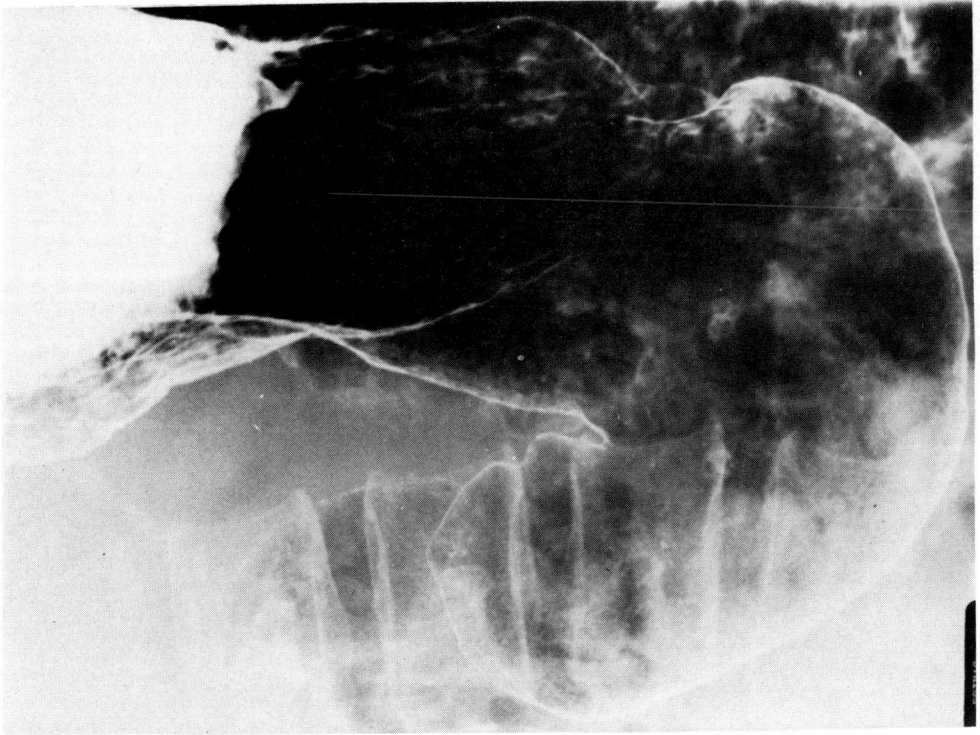

Fig. 4.51 (c–d) gastric carcinomas.

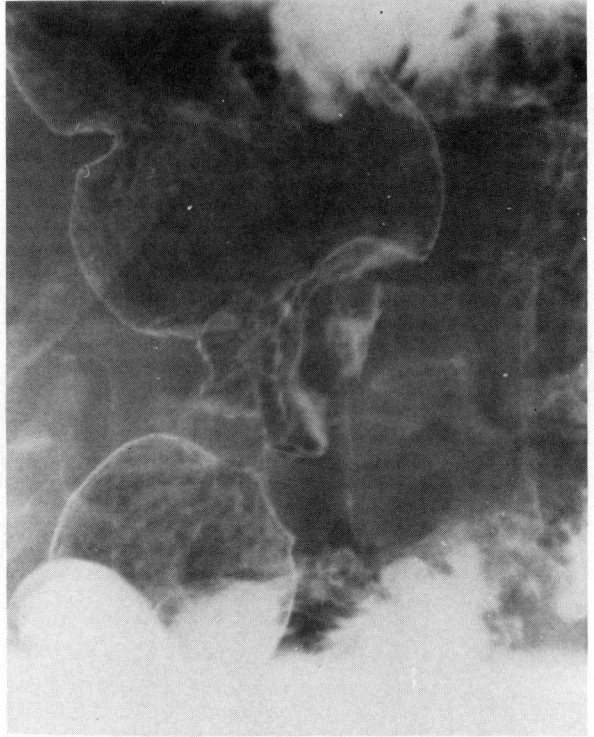

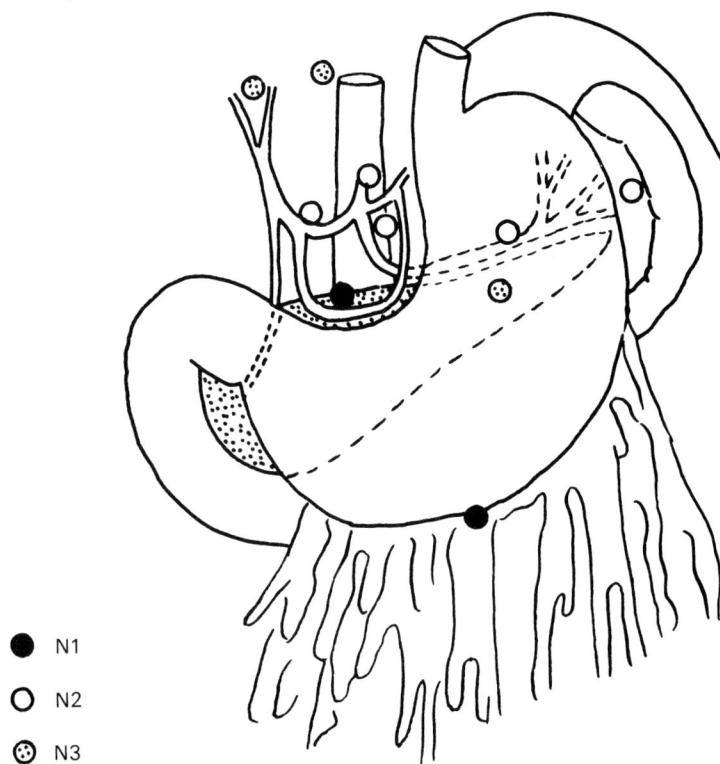

Fig. 4.52 TNM classification of tiers of lymph nodes. N1: nodes within 3 cm of the neoplasm. N2: nodes on lesser or greater curvature further than 3 cm from primary and nodes on the common hepatic artery, coeliac axis, left gastric artery, splenic artery and splenic hilum. N3: nodes at porta hepatis and para-aortic and retropancreatic nodes.

● N1
○ N2
◉ N3

following an R0 resection is 26%, R1 42.4%, R2 49.5% and R3 40%. In the light of these results, curative surgery is best reserved for patients whose extent of disease is limited to N2 involvement and the most appropriate resection would remove these nodes (R2).

The possible sites of recurrence of gastric carcinoma are in the gastric remnant, local residual lymph nodes and distant metastases. Remnant recurrence may occur in 10–15% and this has been used as an argument for total gastrectomy.[36] However, there is no evidence that this significantly increases survival. The necessity of the lymphadenectomy in curative operations for gastric cancer is supported by the increased survival of R2 resections. Further support is gained from the report of 59 patients with apparently benign gastric ulcers removed surgically which subsequently proved to be carcinomas by histological examination.[11] Twenty-four had a further operation to achieve a radical lymphadenectomy and the five-year survival rate in this group was 56% compared to 23% in the remainder. This supports the concept of wide surgical resection and lymphadenectomy as the treatment of choice for gastric cancer and suggests that surgical resection can influence the natural history of the disease.

The limiting factor to extensive resection is postoperative mortality. The overall mortality

of total gastrectomy is 21%, which is considerably higher than that of 4% following partial gastrectomy.[27] Similarly, extensive lymphadenectomies have been reported to effectively reduce the five-year survival rate from 28% to 17%.[16] Thus the most appropriate curative resection is a subtotal gastrectomy with an N2 lymphadenectomy.

In considering the method of reconstruction, all the factors related to benign disease must be considered. The reconstructive procedure, if badly conceived or badly constructed, may produce more severe symptoms than does the cancer itself. The reconstruction of a partial gastrectomy should be a modified Billroth I, Billroth II (Polya) or Roux-en-Y technique (Figure 4.53). The incidence of postgastrectomy problems, such as vomiting, diarrhoea, dumping, haematological and nutritional effects, is similar for the three anastomoses, but the Billroth and the Roux-en-Y techniques have the advantage of providing a wider stoma at a distance from the site of likely recurrence thus reducing the risk of postoperative obstruction due to recurrent disease. Furthermore, the Roux-en-Y reconstruction reduces the risk of troublesome bile reflux.

Total gastrectomy is occasionally associated with adverse long-term nutritional effects. Malabsorption of fat and protein occurs and the

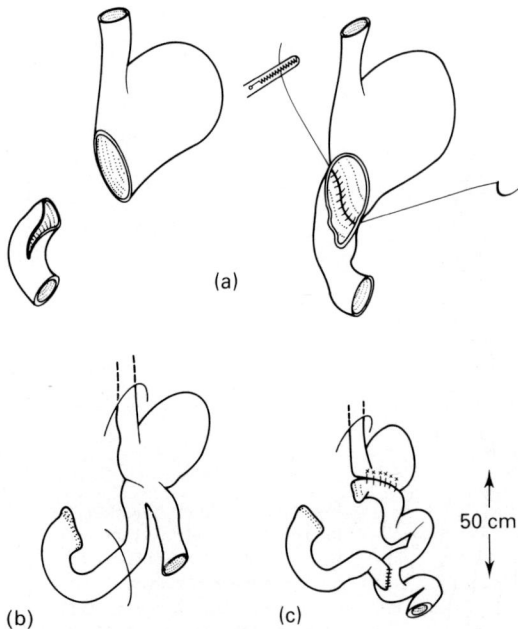

Fig. 4.53 Reconstructive procedures for a partial gastrectomy; (a) modified Billroth I; (b) Billroth II (Polya); (c) Roux-en-Y gastrojejunostomy.

absorption of glucose usually shows a pattern of early hyperglycaemia and late hypoglycaemia. As a consequence, many patients lose weight which can be corrected by dietary supplementation. Megaloblastic and iron-deficiency anaemia commonly occur warranting appropriate replacement therapy. The construction of a gastric pouch and the use of a jejunal segment to permit the passage of food through the duodenum have been used as reconstructive procedures,[29] but there is no evidence that they prevent the metabolic consequences. The most commonly employed reconstructions are the Roux-en-Y, Henley jejunal interpositions and the Omega loop (Figure 4.54). The incidence of post-gastrectomy syndromes, such as distension, dumping and diarrhoea is similar for all three methods, occurring in about 20% of all patients. In addition, bile reflux into the oesophagus is associated with significant morbidity and this can be prevented by constructing a 50 cm Roux-en-Y or 25 cm interposition.

At laparotomy, the first consideration is whether the tumour is resectable. Curative resection is impossible in the presence of peritoneal seedlings, distant metastases, extension to unresectable adjacent structures or involvement of N3 lymph nodes. Macroscopic assessment as to the presence of lymphatic metastases is unreliable. Therefore, in the presence of an apparently curative adenocarcinoma, N3 nodes

should be excised for immediate assessment of metastases, using either frozen section or imprint cytology.[32]

Radical gastrectomy. The definitive radical surgical operation is an R2 resection and should be reserved for patients in whom lymph node involvement does not extend beyond the N2 nodes. The first step is to detach the greater omentum from the transverse colon and mesocolon (Figure 4.55a). The right gastroepiploic artery is then ligated flush with the gastroduodenal artery. The next step includes the detachment of the lesser omentum from the under surface of the left lobe of the liver upwards to the oesophageal hiatus, and then the separation of the anterior leaf of the hepatoduodenal ligament downwards to the origin of the right gastric vessels. These vessels are divided and ligated, removing the appropriate lymph nodes.

The duodenum is divided and the distal stomach with the attached omentum is reflected over the left costal margin (Figure 4.55b). A portion of the duodenal cuff is excised for frozen section examination. Thereafter the lymph nodes of the hepatoduodenal ligament and those behind the pancreas are dissected en bloc from right to left through Winslow's foramen and the

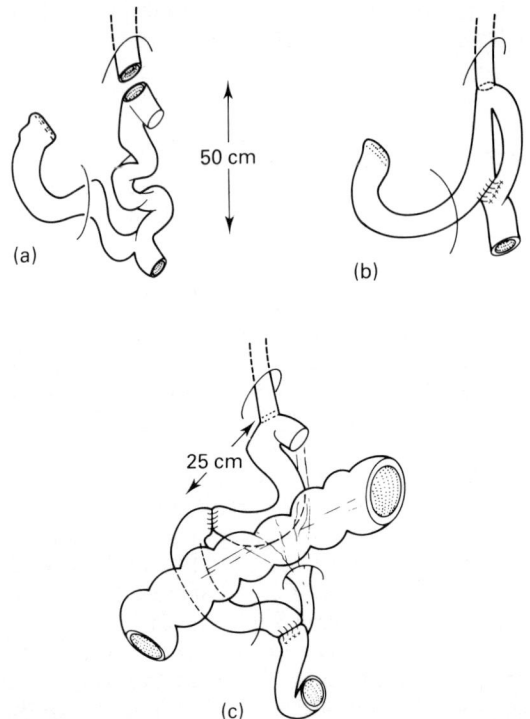

Fig. 4.54 Reconstructive procedures for a total gastrectomy; (a) Roux-en-Y; (b) Omega gastrojejunostomy; (c) Henley jejunal interposition.

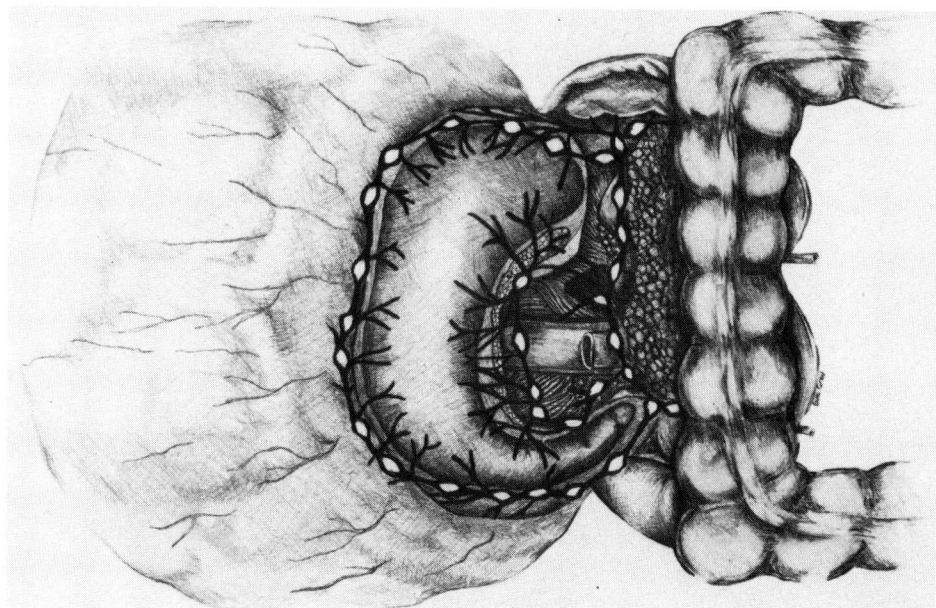

a

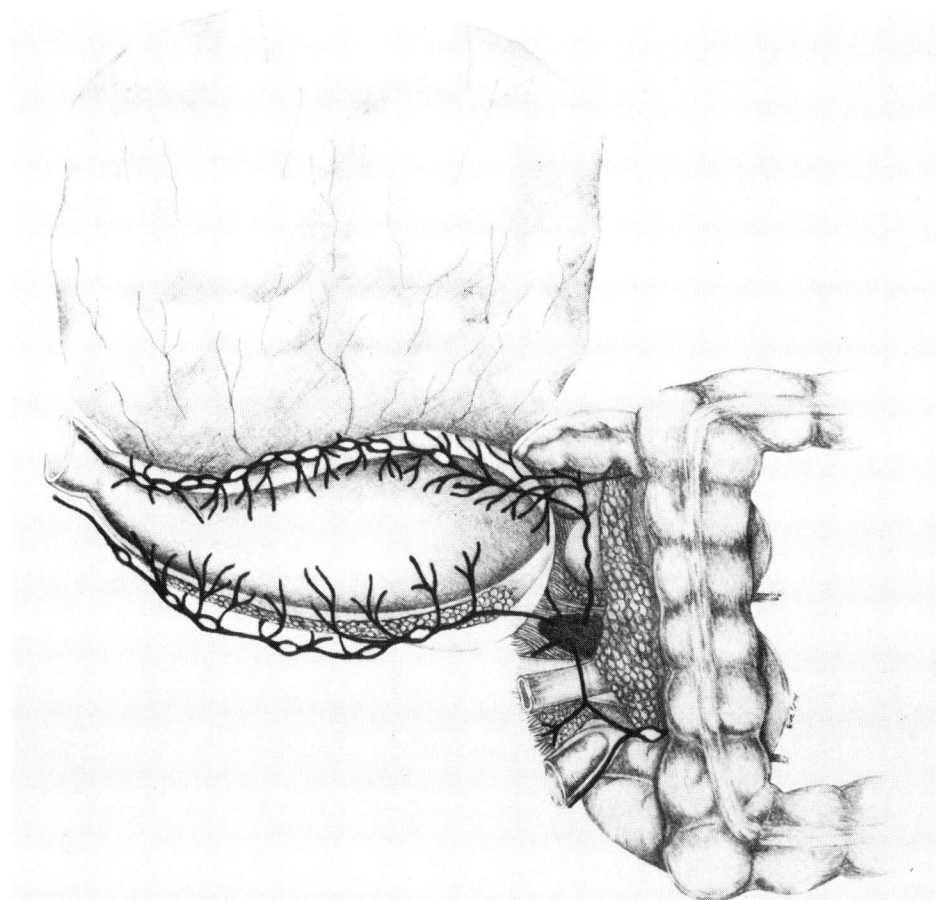

b

Fig. 4.55 (a) Radical gastrectomy (R2): the omentum has been dissected off the transverse colon and the N2 lymph nodes exposed. (b) Radical gastrectomy (R2): the N2 nodes have been dissected off the gastroduodenal artery, common hepatic artery, coeliac axis, splenic artery, left gastric artery and splenic hilum prior to dividing the stomach.

dissection is continued to the nodes along the common hepatic artery, gastroduodenal artery and those at the root of the coeliac axis. The left gastric artery is isolated, divided and ligated with removal of appropriate nodes. Then the lymph nodes along the splenic artery are dissected towards the splenic hilus. If the presence of pancreatic nodal metastases demands it, resection of the pancreas and spleen can be performed for complete clearance. The attachments of the right cardia to the oesophageal hiatus are separated, both the vagal nerves are divided and the lymph nodes of the right cardia are removed. This completes the mobilization of the stomach and the lymphadenectomy; a partial or total gastrectomy is then performed to ensure a 6 cm clearance of the primary. In a total gastrectomy the spleen is mobilized by dividing the lienorenal ligament; the splenic artery and vein and then the oesophagus are divided and the stomach removed.

Gastrointestinal continuity should be restored after a partial gastrectomy by either a modified Billroth I or Billroth II anastomosis and after a total gastrectomy by either a Roux-en-Y or jejunal interposition.

Palliative surgery. The ideal form of palliative treatment must be considered individually for each patient, evaluating the symptoms to be palliated and the quality of life afforded by the procedure. The symptoms most commonly requiring palliation are obstruction, pain and haemorrhage, and the procedures available are bypass, intubation, excision and resection (Figure 4.56). Pyloric obstruction may be palliated by resection or gastroenterostomy. Obstruction at the cardia is relieved by resection if feasible; if not, non-operative endoscopic intubation is preferred to operative intubation. Haemorrhage must be controlled by resection.

Pain is a frequent symptom. It may be intermittent like peptic ulcer pain or constant and related to the extragastric spread of the neoplasm. Resection of the carcinoma usually controls ulcer-type pain but that related to extra-gastric extension or metastatic disease is seldom relieved by resection. Symptomatic relief can often only be achieved by analgesics, although occasionally radiotherapy or chemotherapy might help. The best palliation follows resection[37] and the surgeon should always attempt this even if macroscopic disease cannot be completely removed.

Clinicopathological features

Staging. Clinicopathological features of gastric cancer are important for the accurate staging of tumours (Table 4.38). Clinically, the important factors are the extent of the disease, resectability and whether the resection is radical (curative) or palliative. Pathologically, the important microscopic factors are the depth of penetration of the

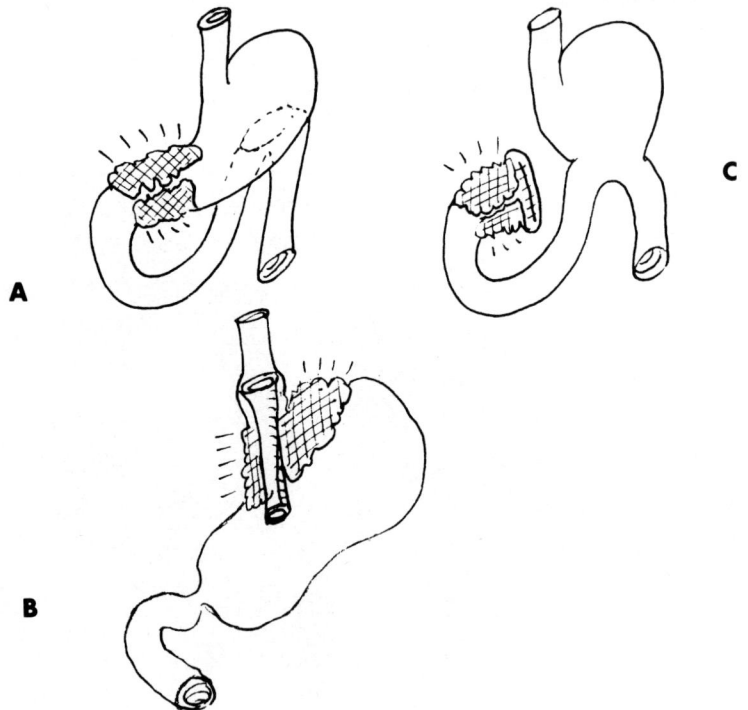

Fig. 4.56 Palliative procedures: (a) gastroenterostomy; (b) intubation; (c) exclusion.

Table 4.38 Staging system for gastric carcinoma.

Stage	Clinical	Pathology
I	Radical resection (T1 N0 M0)	Muscularis propria − Serosa − Node − (T1 N0 M0)
II	Radical resection (T2–4 N0 M0)	Muscularis propria + Serosa ± Node − (T2–4 N0 M0)
III	Radical resection (TX–4 N1–3 M0)	Muscularis propria ± Serosa ± Node + (TX–4, N1–3, M0)
IVA	Palliative resection (TX–4 NX–3 M0–1)	Residual disease (TX–4 N0–3 M0–1)
IVB	Inoperable (TX–4 NX–3 M0–1)	Positive histology (T4 N0–3 M0–1)

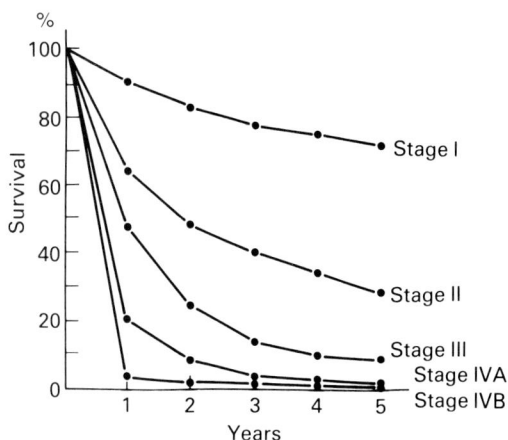

Fig. 4.58 Five-year-age-adjusted survival according to stage for gastric adenocarcinomas in the West Midlands (1960–1969).

primary lesion (Figure 4.57) and lymph node involvement (Figure 4.52). The age-adjusted five-year survival rates are 72.2%, 29.4%, 9.0%, 1.8% and 0.8% for stage I, II, III, IVA and IVB respectively (Figure 4.58).

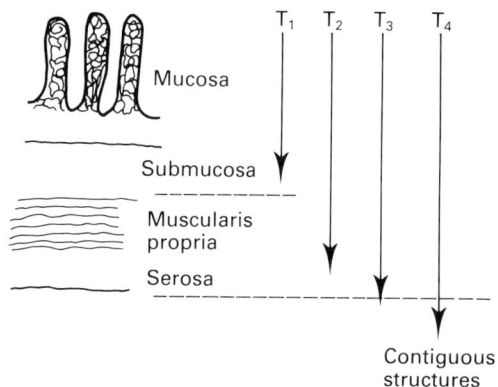

Fig. 4.57 The TNM classification of depth of penetration of the primary tumours.

Pathology. Gastric adenocarcinomas are most frequently found in the pyloric antrum: 49.8% of them are found here. 12.5% are found in the body, 18.4% in the lesser curvature, 10.4% in the cardia, 5.1% in the greater curvature, 0.1% on the anterior wall and 2.9% on the posterior wall.[4] Macroscopically, lesions can be described as ulcerative, polypoidal, diffuse scirrhous (linitis plastica) and superficial. The proportion of carcinomas in each group varies in different series. Berkson had 75%, 10% and 5% in each respective group.[3] More recently, particularly in Japan, the incidence of 'early' gastric cancers (superficial) has increased – to 30% in one report.[44] As a result of this, a macroscopic classification has been evolved for 'early' lesions (Figure 4.59).

Gastric carcinomas may be multicentric: at presentation 2.2% have more than one primary and on histological examination 22% are multicentric. Microscopically, the degree of differentiation can be graded according to Broder's

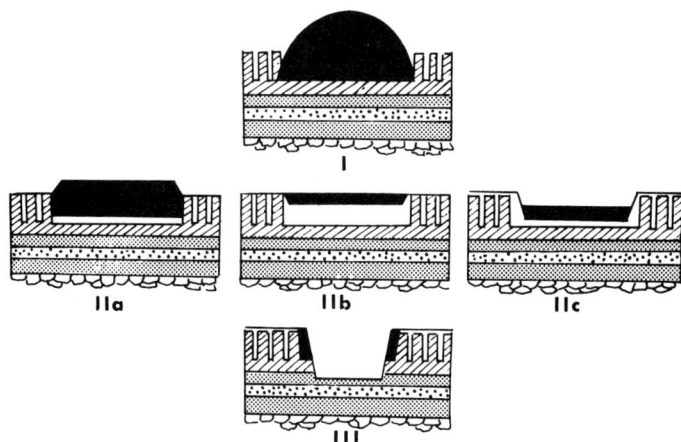

Fig. 4.59 Classification of early gastric cancer. Type I (protruded): protrusion into the gastric lumen. Type II (superficial): the surface is slightly uneven. Type II can be subdivided into the following three subtypes: type IIa (elevated) – the surface is slightly elevated; type IIb (flat) – hardly any noticeable elevation from or depression in the surrounding mucosa; type IIc (depressed) – slightly depressed surface. Type III (excavated: marked excavation in the gastric wall.

Table 4.39 An international comparison of the surgical treatment of gastric cancer.

		Laparotomy rate (%)	Resection rate (%)	Curative resection rate (%)	Overall five-year survival (%)
Europe					
Brookes et al. (1965)[4]	1950–1959	63.5	42.5	26.5	4.9
Desmond (1976)[10]	1944–1970	—	54.0	18.4	8.0
Svennevig and Nysted (1976)[42]	1959–1968	71.3	45.0	32.3	10.0
Inberg et al. (1975)[23]	1946–1955	53.9	21.1	17.1	3.7
	1956–1965	62.0	32.1	25.2	6.5
	1966–1972	69.3	45.1	23.6	10.8
USA					
Dupont et al. (1978)[12]	1948–1973	76.0	48.0	22.5	7.4
Cady et al. (1977)[5]	1940–1949	80.0	—	37.0	7.0
	1957–1966	94.0	58.0	44.0	11.0
Hoerr (1973)[21]	1950–1972	96.0	54.6	46.4	15.1
Adashek et al. (1979)[1]	1956–1965	71.0	39.0	24.0	8.0
	1966–1975	76.0	51.0	31.0	10.0
Japan					
Mine et al. (1970)[31]	1955–1963	93.2	63.2	52.3	14.4
Muto et al. (1968)[34]	1941–1961	98.7	79.4	—	19.0
Kajitani and Takagi (1979)[25]	1946–1970	97.7	—	67.0	33.3
Kajitani and Miwa (1979)[24]	1963–1966	94.3	63.4	44.7	16.4

classification from grade 1 (well differentiated) to grade 4 (undifferentiated). A more valuable classification is that of Lauren, who described lesions as either intestinal or diffuse (Figure 4.60).[26] The prognosis is better for the intestinal type. Also there are important associations with epidemiological findings. The intestinal type is common in areas of high incidence (such as Japan) and it is only the incidence of this lesion that has declined recently.

The earlier stage of disease and the higher incidence of intestinal cancer is probably the reason why the prognosis is apparently better in studies in Japan than in studies in other areas (Table 4.39).

Failure of surgery
Recurrent disease following radical resection is due to the progressive development of micro-metastases. The sites of recurrence are both local and distant. The local recurrences may be in the gastric bed, gastric stump or residual local lymph nodes. Distant metastases may occur at many sites, but most commonly in the liver or peritoneal cavity and more rarely in the lungs and bones. In a post-mortem study of 92 patients who had previously had subtotal gastrectomies McNeer et al. found some form of local recurrence in 80.5% and recurrence at distant sites alone in 15.2%.[30] Gunderson analysed the Minnesota patients who had had reoperations.[2] There was evidence of recurrent cancer in 80.4%, and the recurrence was entirely local in 53.7% of the group (Figure 4.61). The high incidence of recurrent disease following

surgery and the possibility that more extensive surgery might reduce this has already been explored. However, the inability of surgery to eradicate all disease and prevent the development of recurrence highlights the limitations of surgery as a single therapy in the management of gastric cancer. It is clear that adjuvant therapies must be evaluated in an attempt to improve control of this disease.

Chemotherapy
Cytotoxic agents have been evaluated in advanced disease and subsequently as an adjuvant to surgery. In advanced disease these agents have been used singly and as combinations, the latter showing marginally improved response rates (Table 4.40). A

Table 4.40 Cytotoxic agents in advanced gastric cancer.[8, 39, 41]

Agent	Response rate
Single agents	
Fluorouracil	22%
Mitomycin	30%
Carmustine (BCNU)	18%
Doxorubicin (Adriamycin)	24%
Combination chemotherapy	
Fluorouracil + Semustine(methyl-CCNU) + Doxorubicin	36%
Fluorouracil + Semustine	40%
Fluorouracil + Doxorubicin + Mitomycin	43%

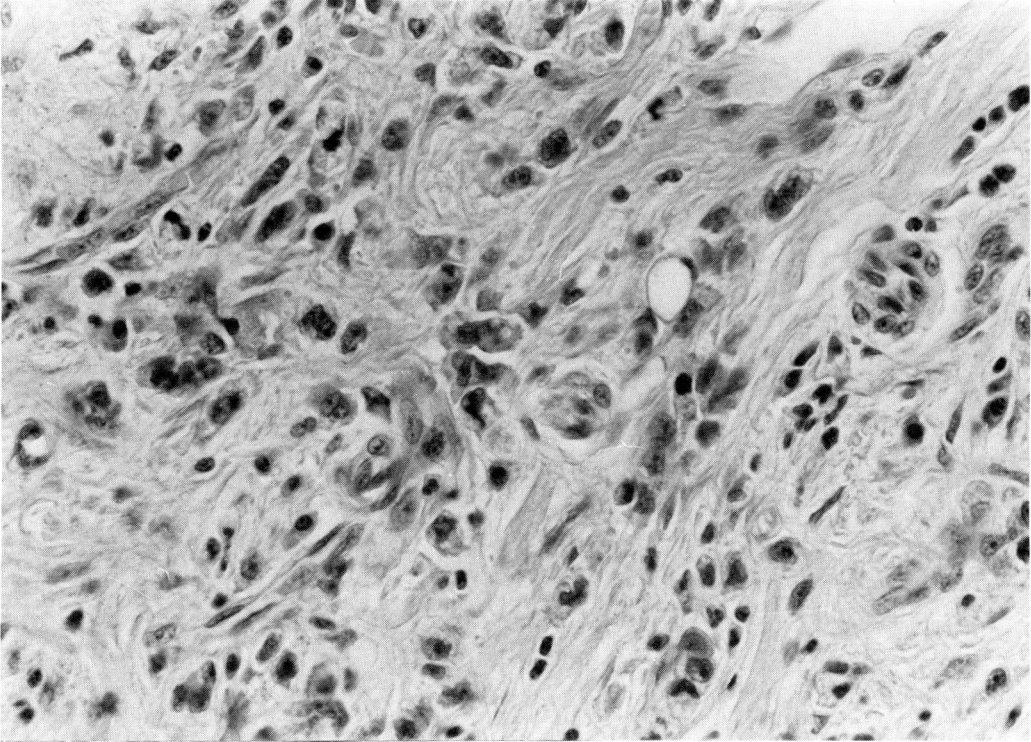

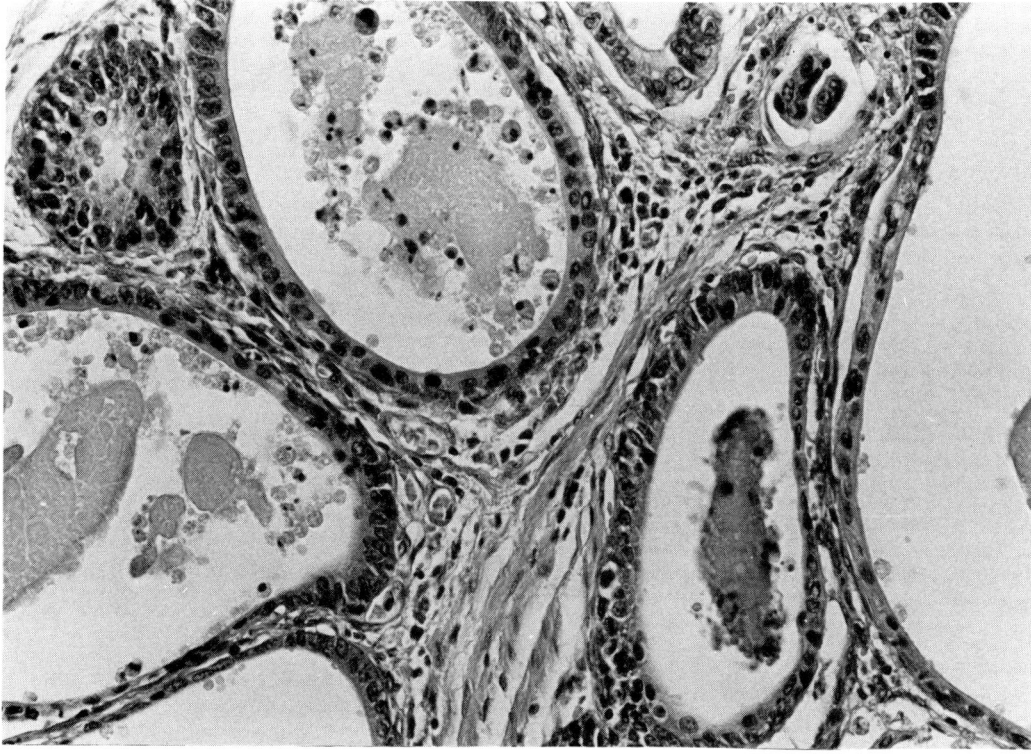

Fig. 4.60 Adenocarcinoma: (a) intestinal, (b) diffuse. (Courtesy of Dr H. Thompson, Birmingham General Hospital).

235

'response' is defined here as a reduction of at least 50% in the size of a measurable lesion. Chemotherapy may improve early survival,[39] but there is no evidence for higher long-term survival.

Cytotoxic agents should be most effective when the tumour burden is small, as after curative surgical resection. The results of adjuvant studies are conflicting. Imanaga and Nakazoto reported a controlled study of 2636 patients using mitomycin and demonstrated overall improvement of 13.5% at five years and 10% at ten years in the treated group. However, the British Stomach Cancer Group's controlled study of adjuvant fluorouracil and mitomycin in 411 patients has failed to show improvement in survival.[13] Similarly, Franz and Cruz and Higgins failed to show any benefit from adjuvant chemotherapy.[15, 19] However, the Gastro-Intestinal Tumour Study Group have reported a significant benefit from adjuvant chemotherapy.[9]

Whilst there is no convincing evidence from European and American studies to suggest that chemotherapy should be employed routinely, the fact that responses are obtained and that some studies have shown improved survival indicate that this type of treatment must continue to be evaluated in controlled prospective studies.

Radiotherapy

As many recurrences are local or regional and occur in an area that can be encompassed in a radiotherapy field (Figure 4.61), it is pertinent to consider the possible use of irradiation. The development of megavoltage radiotherapy has permitted radiation to be given without excessive damage to adjacent normal tissues. Robinson and Cohen demonstrated improved survival in patients receiving conventional postoperative irradiation, 40% surviving at two years compared to 20% in the group receiving no postoperative irradiation.[38] More work is now being done on the value of adjuvant radiotherapy after radical resections. Catterall *et al.* used fast neutron irradiation in 29 unselected patients, and in the 19 with a palpable epigastric lesion produced resolution in 16; 14 patients subsequently underwent a postmortem examination and 10 had no macroscopic evidence of tumour, although all but two had residual microscopic foci of malignant cells.[7] However, following neutron treatment, there was considerable damage to the stomach, and the authors recommended that gastrectomy should be performed routinely four to six months after irradiation.

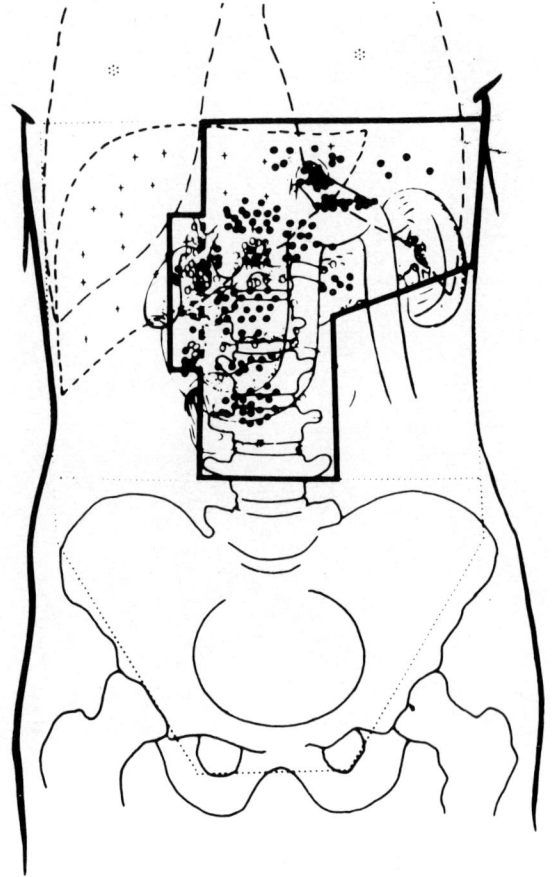

Fig. 4.61 Sites of recurrence after curative resection (Gunderson). * = lung metastasis; + = liver metastasis; △ = wound implant; ● = local failures in surrounding organs or tissues; ● = lymph node failure.

SQUAMOUS CELL CARCINOMA
AND CARCINOIDS

Squamous cell carcinomas are exceedingly rare (0.04–0.7% of all cancers), and four times as common in men as in women; their presentation is similar to that of adenocarcinoma. Similarly, argentaffinomas are not common, and the diagnosis is frequently only established at postmortem. They occur with equal frequency in men and women and the presenting symptoms are similar to adenocarcinomas, though they are often associated with a long preoperative history. Radiologically, carcinoids appear as polypoid neoplasms. If there is a small tumour with no evidence of metastasis it should be excised locally, but for neoplasms greater than 2 cm in diameter or with metastatic disease, the operation appropriate to the stage should be performed. The prognosis is good; among the 15 reported patients followed for more than five years, there have been 12 survivors. Amongst the

90 reported cases, six had the malignant carcinoid syndrome, producing large amounts of 5-hydroxytryptophan and histamine.

NON-EPITHELIAL TUMOURS

The most frequently encountered non-epithelial tumours are lymphomas and leiomyosarcomas.

Lymphoma

These account for between 0.5% and 8% of gastric cancers and about 60% of all sarcomas involving the stomach. Often gastric lymphoma is a manifestation of a generalized disease: 50% of lymphosarcomas have a gastric element, but only 4–6% have primary gastric involvement. The stomach is, however, the most common site of extranodal involvement.

Most frequently these are non-Hodgkin's lymphomas (usually lymphosarcoma or reticulum cell lymphomas); between 5–10% are Hodgkin's disease. Macroscopically, these lesions are difficult to differentiate from adenocarcinomas, and the diagnosis is usually only established by their characteristic histological appearance. Initially, the tumour may metastasize to the regional nodes, further dissemination may occur to distant nodes and can involve the peritoneum and liver.

The sexes are equally affected and though the mean age is in the 60s, it may occur in the young. The most common symptom is dyspepsia, which can have all the variable characteristics of symptoms associated with adenocarcinomas (Tables 4.36 and 4.37).

Preoperatively, the histological diagnosis is difficult to establish. Double-contrast radiology will be diagnostic of a gastric lesion, and the endoscopic findings are usually indistinguishable from those of adenocarcinoma. Because of the diffuse infiltration, endoscopic biopsy will only establish the diagnosis in 29% of patients.

Curative treatment is surgical, and for disease localized to the stomach without evidence of nodal metastasis resection has a 47% five-year survival rate. It is hoped that, in view of the efficacy of chemotherapy for non-Hodgkin's lymphomas, this survival may be further improved. Postoperative radiotherapy may be used as an adjuvant to surgical resection, but there is no evidence as yet that this improves survival.

Leiomyosarcoma

Leiomyosarcoma comprise 1–3% of all gastric tumours. The tumours are most commonly located on the anterior and posterior wall of the stomach. Macroscopically the tumours are bulky and vascular with multiple areas of ulceration. Microscopically, they originate from smooth muscle, and the frequency of mitotic figures is usually diagnostic. Direct spread is rare and lymph node involvement does not occur. At laparotomy, macroscopic dissemination is found in 10–45% of patients.

The incidence is approximately the same in men and women and the most frequent presenting symptom is bleeding, 75% having either haematemesis or melaena. There may also be associated epigastric symptoms, and on physical examination an abdominal mass is found in up to 60% of patients.

The diagnosis is established by a combination of endoscopy and radiology. Since they are usually located on the anterior or posterior wall, they can easily be missed if compression is not a routine part of the double-contrast study.

The curative treatment is surgical and involves a wide local excision without any lymphadenectomy. The prognosis is quite good, with a five-year survival rate ranging from 37% to 54%. Neither palliative nor adjuvant chemotherapy or radiotherapy has been shown to be of benefit.

REFERENCES

1 Adashek, K., Sangel, J. & Longmire, W. P. (1979) Cancer of the stomach. Review of ten year's intervals. *Annals of Surgery*, **189**, 6–10.

2 Aste, H., Amadori, D., Maltoni, G. *et al.* (1981) Early gastric cancer detection in four areas at different gastric cancer death rates. *Acta Endoscopica*, **11**, 123–132.

3 Berkson, J. (1964) Statistical summary. In *Cancer of the Stomach* (Ed.) Remine, W. H., Priestley, J. T. & Berkson, J. p. 207. Philadelphia: Saunders.

4 Brookes, V. S., Waterhouse, J. A. H. & Powell, D. J. (1965) Carcinoma of the stomach: 10 year survey of results and of factors affecting prognosis. *British Medical Journal*, **i**, 1577–1583.

5 Cady, B., Ramsden, D. A., Stein, A. & Haggitt, R. G. (1977) Gastric cancer. *American Journal of Surgery*, **133**, 423–429.

6 Carnett, J. B. & Howell, J. C. (1932) A case of coarctation of the aorta and gastric carcinoma with a discussion of the metastases. *Surgical Clinics of North America*, **12**, 1351–1362.

7 Catterall, M., Kingston, D., Lawrence, G. *et al.* (1975) The effects of fast neutrons on inoperable carcinoma of the stomach. *Gut*, **16**, 150–156.

8 Comis, R. & Carter, S. (1974) A review of chemotherapy in gastric cancer. *Cancer*, **34**, 1576–1586.

9 Gastrointestinal Tumour Study Group (1982) Controlled trial of adjuvant chemotherapy following curative results for gastric cancer. *Cancer*, **49**, 1116–1122.

10 Desmond, A. (1976) Radical surgery in treatment of carcinoma of stomach. *Proceedings of the Royal Society of Medicine*, **69**, 867–869.

11 Desmond, A., Nicholls, J. & Brown, C. (1975) Further surgical management of gastric ulcer with unsuspected

malignant change. *Annals of the Royal College of Surgeons*, **57**, 101–104.

12 Dupont, J. B., Lee Rillens, J., Burton, G. R. & Cohen, I. (1978) Adenocarcinoma of the stomach: review of 1497 cases. *Cancer*, **41**, 941–947.

13 Fielding, J. W. L., Ellis, D. J., Jones, B. G. *et al.* (1980) Natural history of 'early' gastric cancer: results of a 10-year regional survey. *British Medical Journal*, **281**, 965–967.

14 Fielding, J. W. L., Fagg, S. L., Jones, B. G. *et al.* An interim report of a prospective, randomised, controlled study of adjuvant chemotherapy in operable gastric cancer. *World Journal of Surgery*, **7**, 390–399.

15 Franz, J. L. & Cruz, A. B. (1977) The treatment of gastric cancer with combined surgical dissection and chemotherapy. *Journal of Surgical Oncology*, **9**, 131–137.

16 Gilbertson, V. A. (1969) Results of treatment of stomach cancer. *Cancer*, **23**, 1305–1308.

17 Green, P., O'Toole, K., Weinberg, L. & Goldfarb, J. (1981) Early gastric cancer. *Gastroenterology*, **81**, 247–256.

18 Gunderson, L. (1976) Radiation therapy: results and future possibilities. *Clinics in Gastroenterology*, **5**, 743–776.

19 Higgins, G. A. (1976) Chemotherapy, adjuvant to surgery, for gastrointestinal surgery. *Clinics in Gastroenterology*, **5**, 795–808.

20 Hirayama, T. (1981) Methods and results (cost effectiveness) of gastric cancer screening. In *Gastric Cancer – Advances in the Biosciences* (Ed.) Fielding, J. W. L., Newman, C. E., Ford, C. H. J. & Jones, B. G. Volume 32, pp. 77–84. Oxford: Pergamon.

21 Hoerr, S. O. (1973) Prognosis for carcinoma of the stomach. *Surgery, Gynaecology and Obstetrics*, **137**, 204–209.

22 Imanaga, H. & Nakazoto, H. (1977) Results of surgery for gastric cancer and the effect of adjuvant mitomycin C in cancer recurrence. *World Journal of Surgery*, **1**, 213–227.

23 Inberg, M. V., Heinonen, R., Rantakokko, V. & Viikari, S. J. (1975) Surgical treatment of gastric carcinoma. *Archives of Surgery*, **110**, 703–707.

24 Kajitani, T. & Miwa, K. (1979) Treatment results of stomach cancer in Japan, 1963–1966. *WHO cc Monograph, No. 2* (Ed.) Kajitani, T. & Miwa, K. Japan: WHO collaborating centre for evaluation of methods of diagnosis and treatment of stomach cancer.

25 Kajitani, T. & Takagi, K. (1979) Cancer of the stomach at Cancer Institute Hospital, Tokyo. *Gann Monograph on Cancer Research*, **22**, 77–87.

26 Lauren, P. (1965) The two main histological types of gastric carcinoma, diffuse and so-called intestinal type carcinoma. *Acta Pathologica et Microbiologica Scandinavica*, **64**, 31–49.

27 Longmire, W. P. (1980) Gastric carcinoma: is radical gastrectomy worth while? *Annals of the Royal College of Surgeons (England)*, **62**, 25–34.

28 Lundh, G., Burn, J. I., Kolig, G. *et al.* (1974) A co-operative international study of gastric cancer. *Annals of the Royal College of Surgeons (England)*, **54**, 219–228.

29 Lygidakis, N. J. (1981) Total gastrectomy for gastric carcinoma: a retrospective study of different procedures and assessment of a new technique of gastric reconstruction. *British Journal of Surgery*, **68**, 649–655.

30 McNeer, G., Vandenberg, H., Down, F. Y. & Boden, A. (1951) A critical evaluation of subtotal gastrectomy for cure of cancer of the stomach. *Annals of Surgery*, **134**, 2–7.

31 Mine, M., Majima, S., Harada, M. & Etani, S. (1970) End results of gastrectomy for gastric cancer. *Surgery*, **68**, 753–758.

32 Morris, D. L., Moore, J., Thompson, H. & Keighley, M. R. B. (1982) Accuracy of per-operative lymph node cytology in gastric carcinoma. *Clinical Oncology*, **8**, 219–221.

33 Murakami, T. (1979) Early cancer of the stomach. *World Journal of Surgery*, **3**, 685–692.

34 Muto, M., Maki, T., Majima, S. & Yamaguchi, I. (1968) Improvement in the end results of surgical treatment of gastric cancer. *Surgery*, **63**, 229–235.

35 Nagao, F. & Takahishi, M. D. (1979) Diagnosis of advanced gastric cancer. *World Journal of Surgery*, **3**, 693–700.

36 Pichlmayr, R. & Meyer, H. J. (1981) Patterns of recurrence in relation to therapeutic strategy. In *Gastric Cancer – Advances in the Biosciences* (Ed.) Fielding, J. W. L., Newman, C. E., Ford, C. H. J. & Jones, B. G. Volume 32, pp. 171–184. Oxford: Pergamon.

37 Remine, W. H. (1981) Preoperative assessment and palliative surgery. In *Gastric Cancer – Advances in the Biosciences* (Ed.) Fielding, J. W. L., Newman, C. E., Ford, C. H. J. & Jones, B. G. Volume 32, pp. 123–137. Oxford: Pergamon.

38 Robinson, E. & Cohen, Y. (1977) The combination of surgery, radiotherapy and chemotherapy in the treatment of gastric cancer. *Recent Results in Cancer Research*, **32**, 177–180.

39 Schien, R. S., Coffey, R. & Smith, F. P. (1981) Chemotherapy and combined modality treatment of gastric cancer. In *Gastric Cancer – Advances in the Biosciences* (Ed.) Fielding, J. W. L., Newman, C. E., Ford, C. H. J. & Jones, B. G. Volume 32, pp. 139–147. Oxford: Pergamon.

40 Sherman, R. S. & Snyder, R. E. (1960) Roentgenologic surveys for gastric neoplasms. *Journal of the American Medical Association*, **8**, 949–956.

41 Smith, F. P., Cambareri, R. J., Killen, J. Y. & Schein, P. S. (1980) Gastrointestinal Cancer. In *Cancer Chemotherapy: the EORTC Cancer Chemotherapy Annual* (Ed.) Pinedo, H. Volume 2, pp. 284–298. Amsterdam – Oxford: Excerpta Medica.

42 Svennevig, J. L. & Nysted, A. (1976) Carcinoma of the stomach. *Acta Chirurgica Scandinavica*, **142**, 78–81.

43 Swynnerton R. F. & Truelove, S. C. (1952) Carcinoma of the stomach. *British Medical Journal*, **1**, 287–292.

44 Takagi, K. (1981) Stages of gastric cancer and reconstruction after surgery. In *Gastric Cancer – Advances in the Biosciences* (Ed.) Fielding, J. W. L., Newman, C. E., Ford, C. H. J. & Jones, B. G. Volume 32, pp. 91–122. Oxford: Pergamon.

45 UICC (*International Union against Cancer*) (1978) TNM Classification of malignant tumours. 3rd edition, Geneva.

46 Zinninger, M. & Collins, W. (1949) Extension of carcinoma of the stomach into the duodenum and oesophagus. *Annals of Surgery*, **130**, 557–566.

MÉNÉTRIER'S DISEASE

Ménétrier's disease was first described in 1888, but in spite of more than 300 reported cases in the literature, the disease is almost as mysterious now as when it was first described. Ménétrier described two disorders – gastric polyposis and giant gastric rugae – but it is the latter which now bears his name. The eponymous name is more satisfactory than many other names given to the disorder as most are misleading pathologically.[4] The most satisfactory alternative would be hyperplastic gastropathy. The characteristic features of the disease are giant gastric rugae (folds), which are frequently associated with excessive gastric protein loss and hypoproteinaemia.

Aetiology[4]

The aetiology of Ménétrier's disease is unknown but it is probably an acquired disorder. Cytomegalovirus has been isolated from the gastric mucosa of two children and both tuberculosis and histoplasmosis can cause giant rugae but there is no good evidence to suggest an infective aetiology for Ménétrier's disease. The increased gastric epithelial cell turnover is similar to that seen in the Zollinger–Ellison syndrome and has led to speculation that a hormonal stimulus to the gastric mucosa is responsible. However, there is no evidence for an abnormality of hormone secretion, including gastrin. The most widely held view is that Ménétrier's disease is the result of a hypersensitivity response to dietary or other antigens.

Reported immunological abnormalities include peripheral blood eosinophilia, increased IgM plasma cell numbers in gastric fundal mucosa, increased fractional catabolic rate of IgM and impaired delayed hypersensitivity responses to BCG vaccine and *Candida*. However, studies are few and no patient has been shown to have all these abnormalities. Food antibodies have been reported but these probably reflect increased gastric permeability.

One group have shown increased gastric mucosal fibrinolysis in vitro,[12] and the antiplasmin drug tranexamic acid inhibited the fibrinolysis, improved symptoms and mucosal appearance and decreased gastric protein loss. Plasmin increases vascular permeability, so the idea of plasminogen activation being involved in aetiology is attractive. In the veterinary literature giant gastric rugae have been described in a number of species following different stimuli such as dithiothreitol in dogs, shale oil in monkeys, and parasites and fungal infections in snakes, monkeys and horses. This together with the limited human data suggests that Ménétrier's disease might represent a common response to a number of different endogenous or exogenous stimuli.

Clinical features

The disease can occur in adults of any age, with a peak in the fourth decade for females and in the sixth decade for males.[4] The male-to-female ratio is 3 : 1. The disease has been described in white Caucasians, American Negroes and Japanese, but this racial distribution probably reflects availability of advanced medical services rather than any racial predisposition. The onset is usually insidious. Acute onset has been described and may follow apparent hypersensitivity to foods or drugs. Usually there are no obvious precipitating factors. The duration of symptoms can vary from one week to 20 years. The important symptoms are epigastric pain (75%), weight loss (30–60%), vomiting (40%), peripheral oedema (40%) and diarrhoea (20%). The epigastric pain is variable in intensity and duration, may be cramp-like, burning or stabbing and is frequently dyspeptic with relief from food or antacids. Anorexia and some evidence of gastric blood loss are common. Severe gastric haemorrhage is rare but can be the presenting complaint, as can chronic iron-deficiency anaemia. The commonest signs are localized epigastric tenderness and peripheral oedema. Ascites, pleural effusion and epigastric mass have been reported.

Radiological features[4, 14]

No radiological feature is pathognomonic of the disease. The most characteristic feature is the thick uneffaceable gastric rugae, 1–2 cm in height, which can sometimes appear as polyps or mucosal masses (Figure 4.62). Between the rugae are deep sulci, into which barium may run, giving a spiculated appearance, which may mimic gastric ulceration. Barium often mixes with mucus in the lumen to give a characteristic reticulated appearance. The mucosal abnormalities may occur anywhere in the stomach, including the antrum, but they are most prominent along the greater curve.

Gastroscopic appearances[4]

The most striking abnormality observed during endoscopy is the thick, tortuous gastric rugae which do not flatten with intraluminal air. The mucosa may be dull, reddened, oedematous, cobblestoned, nodular or even polypoid. There may be patchy hyperaemia, haemorrhage or erosions. Chronic gastric ulcer is an occasional associated finding. Mucus is prominent, coating the mucosa tenaciously or lying free in the lumen.

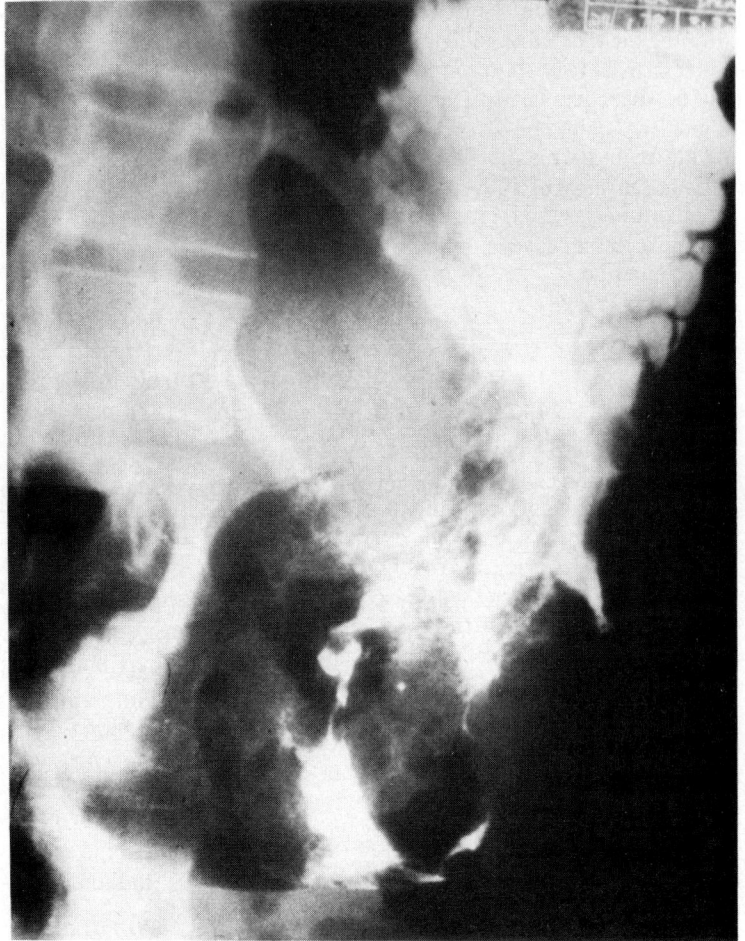

Fig. 4.62 Barium meal X-ray of a patient with Ménétrier's disease, showing huge gastric rugae that mimic mucosal masses and the characteristic appearance that results from barium and mucus mixing in the lumen.

Pathology

The large gastric folds, which are so prominent macroscopically, have been likened to the contours of the brain.[5] The stomach feels boggy and heavy and when palpated from the serosal side feels like a 'bag of worms'.[5] The demarcation line between involved and normal areas is very sharp.

The most important histological feature is hyperplasia of the mucus-producing cells in the gastric glands, leading to cystic change in the middle and deep thirds of the glands and to elongation of the pits and glands resulting in mucosal thickening (Figure 4.63).[2, 11] The cysts contain PAS-positive material. The glands may be relatively straight or very branched and tortuous. There is often a relative or absolute deficiency of parietal and peptic cells. In some patients, there is diffuse or patchy inflammation of the epithelium and lamina propria with infiltration by neutrophils, eosinophils, plasma cells or lymphocytes. Mucosal erosions may be seen. Intestinal metaplasia can occur in inflamed

areas. The lamina propria, muscularis mucosa and submucosa may be oedematous. There are two features which are virtually diagnostic of Ménétrier's disease but they are not seen in every case: these are (a) smooth muscle fibres extending from the muscularis mucosa through the lamina propria to the apices of the gastric glands (Figure 4.63) and (b) penetration of the muscularis mucosa by gastric glands which can balloon into the submucosa. This appearance may be misdiagnosed as carcinoma. On electron microscopy, the interepithelial cell spaces are dilated, there is intense micropinocytosis of the capillary endothelial cells beneath the mucus-producing cells[3] and tight junctions between gastric epithelial cells are widened.[10] These may be involved in the mechanism of protein loss.

Pathophysiology

Gastric secretion

Achlorhydria or hypochlorhydria are common in Ménétrier's disease, occurring in 50–70% of

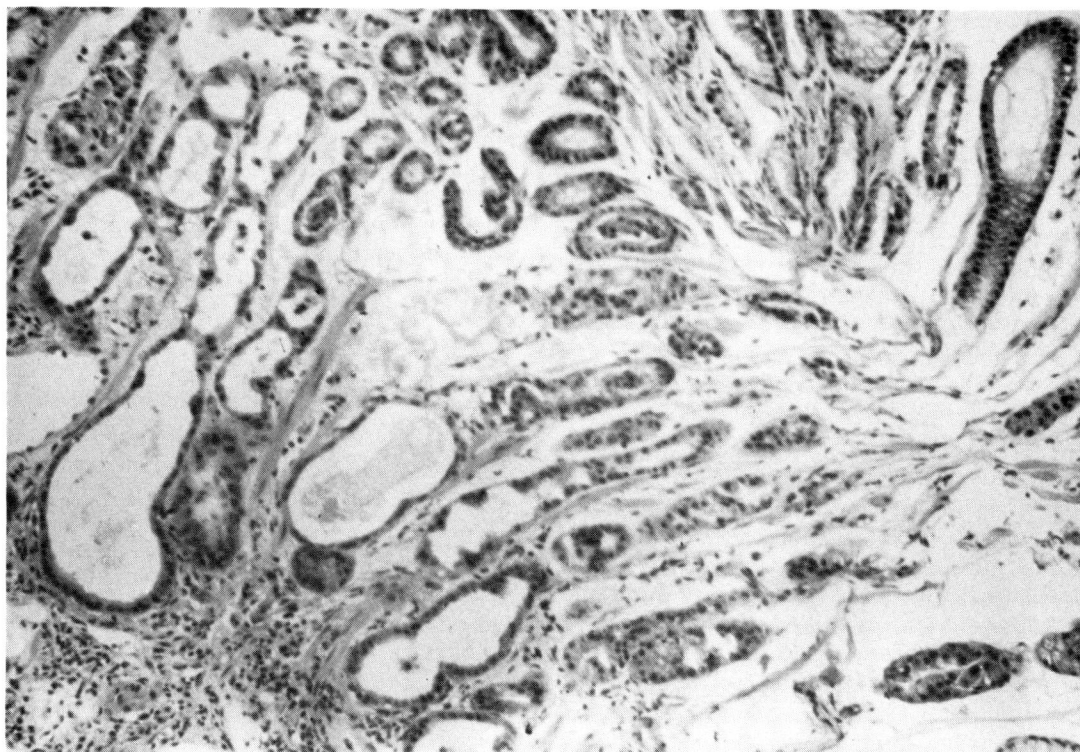

Fig. 4.63 Endoscopic biopsy in a case of Ménétrier's disease, showing elongated glands with cystic dilatation of the bases and smooth muscle fibres passing from the bases of the glands towards their apices.

cases.[4, 15] Serum gastrin is mildly elevated in approximately half the cases where it has been measured, and this probably reflects a diminished parietal cell mass. Little is known about pepsin secretion. Gastric secretory studies help to separate Ménétrier's disease from 'hypertrophic hypersecretory gastropathy', in which .thickened rugae, mucosal hyperplasia and acid hypersecretion occur, although a few cases have been described with features of both disorders.

Gastric protein loss
This is a cardinal feature of the disease: 80% of patients have a low serum albumin at presentation.[15] Protein loss has been confirmed by perfusion studies and it is completely abolished by total gastrectomy. Electrophoresis of gastric juice has shown increases in both albumin and the globulins, indicating a non-selective loss.[9] The protein loss can be demonstrated by any test for gastrointestinal protein loss such as the intravenous ^{51}Cr-labelled albumin test. Protein turnover studies have shown increased fractional catabolic rates for plasma proteins and normal or increased synthesis rates of plasma proteins.[9] Gastric protein loss probably results from alteration in the passive permeability of the gastric epithelium, and a recent study suggests

that protein loss is paracellular via widened gastric epithelial tight junctions and may be mediated by a cholinergic mechanism.[10] It is unlikely that the non-selective loss is explained by the excessive secretion of gastric mucus that occurs. There is no evidence for protein loss as a result of lymphatic blockage or mucosal ulceration.

Laboratory tests
Iron-deficiency anaemia is found in about 50% of Ménétrier's disease patients and peripheral blood eosinophilia in 12% of cases.[4] Intrinsic factor secretion is normal, but development of atrophic gastritis leads to vitamin B_{12} malabsorption.[6]

Diagnosis

The radiological and gastroscopic appearances suggest but do not confirm the diagnosis of Menetrier's disease, which can only be made if the typical histological appearances are found. To do this and to exclude other causes of large gastric rugae, an adequate gastric biopsy which includes the muscularis mucosa is necessary. Where this is not possible with an endoscopic or suction biopsy, a full-thickness biopsy at laparotomy is indicated.

Natural history

The natural history of this disorder is largely unknown, but the disease can be very chronic, as is indicated by reports of unrelieved symptoms for up to 20 years. In one review of 120 cases two-thirds of patients had some form of gastric resection, but the majority of the remainder had continued symptoms.[15] Nevertheless, there are well documented cases of spontaneous recovery three months to five years after diagnosis. In some of these cases, the gastric mucosa changed to atrophic gastritis.[1, 6]

Cancer risk

There have been many reports of patients with Ménétrier's disease and coexistent carcinoma of the stomach.[4] Whether Ménétrier's disease predisposes to carcinoma has been disputed. Carcinoma can cause large gastric rugae and the diagnosis of Ménétrier's disease in many of these cases was not based on histological criteria; however, patients with well-documented Ménétrier's disease have developed carcinoma of the stomach during follow-up. The carcinoma risk seems to be about 10%.[15] Circumstantial evidence for the association is the change to atrophic gastritis, which itself has a carcinoma risk, and the increased gastric epithelial cell proliferation rate, which may predispose to malignant change.

Ménétrier's disease in children

An apparently identical disease has been described in about a dozen children aged 3 to 14 years.[4] Characteristic features are a short history (1–12 weeks), peripheral blood eosinophilia and in most cases a spontaneous and permanent remission 16 days to 6 months after presentation.

Treatment

Treatment may be medical or surgical. As spontaneous remission occurs and some patients do seem to respond to medication, the older view that Ménétrier's disease must be treated by some form of gastric resection is no longer tenable. Medical treatment should always be tried first.

Medical treatment

A bland diet and antacids may help some cases. Nutritional support is important in most cases. Nutritional deficiency occurs because of anorexia and because the liver cannot synthesize enough protein to replace that lost from the stomach even though much of that protein is normally digested and reabsorbed. Initially a high-energy, high-protein diet is indicated, but if the nutritional state deteriorates enteral feeding may be required until remission or surgery takes place. Intravenous albumin is only of temporary value in relieving hypoproteinaemic oedema. The treatment of Ménétrier's disease is confused because many favourable responses to drugs could be explained by spontaneous remission. The effects of withdrawal and readministration of apparently beneficial drugs have rarely been reported. Anticholinergics may decrease protein loss and improve symptoms in some cases.[8] Tranexamic acid has been reported to lead to dramatic improvement,[12] but not in the author's own limited experience. Corticosteroids[16] and cimetidine[13] may have helped individual cases. Gastric irradiation has been tried but is not recommended. If a patient responds to treatment or remits spontaneously, life-long follow-up is mandatory because of the risk of carcinoma.

Surgical treatment

A full-thickness biopsy at laparotomy is necessary if endoscopic or suction biopsies fail to provide a definite histological diagnosis. Indications for gastric resection are intractable symptoms, severe or persistent hypoproteinaemic oedema, gastric bleeding or the presence of or high risk of carcinoma. Total gastrectomy leads to complete and permanent relief of symptoms[15] and is now less of a problem with modern surgical techniques and nutritional support. In the past partial gastrectomy with removal of all the diseased mucosa was favoured. This is not always technically possible and anastomoses involving diseased mucosa frequently break down. Moreover, recurrence in previously normal gastric mucosa is well documented after partial gastrectomy.[7] Vagotomy alone has benefited one patient but not another. If an operation is indicated the procedure of choice is probably total gastrectomy.

REFERENCES

1　Berenson, M. M., Sannella, J. & Freston, J. W. (1976) Ménétrier's disease. Serial morphological, secretory and serological observations. *Gastroenterology*, **70**, 257–263.

2　Butz, W. C. (1960) Giant hypertrophic gastritis. A report of 14 cases. *Gastroenterology*, **39**, 183–190.

3　Chambourlier, P., Pin, G., Treffot, M. J. *et al.* (1979) Syndromes oedémateux rélévateurs d'une maladie de Ménétrièr. *Semaine des hopitaux de Paris*, **55**, 684–688.

4　Cooper, B. T. & Chadwick, V. S. (1981) Ménétrier's disease. In *Butterworths International Medical Reviews:*

Foregut (Ed.) Baron, J. H. & Moody, F. G. pp. 141–191. London: Butterworths.

5 Feiber, S. S. (1955) Hypertrophic gastritis. Report of 2 cases and analysis of 50 pathologically verified cases from the literature. *Gastroenterology*, **28**, 39–69.

6 Frank, B. W. & Kern, F. (1967) Ménétrier's disease. Spontaneous metamorphosis of giant hypertrophy of the gastric mucosa to atrophic gastritis. *Gastroenterology*, **53**, 953–960.

7 Gold, B. M. & Meyers, M. A. (1977) Progression of Ménétrier's disease with postoperative gastrojejunal intussception. *Gastroenterology*, **73**, 583–586.

8 Gordon, M. N., Schaefer, E. J. & Finkel, M. (1976) Treatment of protein losing gastropathy with atropine. *American Journal of Gastroenterology*, **56**, 535–539.

9 Jarnum, S. & Jensen, K. B. (1972) Plasma protein turnover (albumin, transferrin, IgG, IgM) in Ménétrier's disease (giant hypertrophic gastritis): evidence of nonselective protein loss. *Gut*, **13**, 128–137.

10 Kelly, D. G., Miller, L. J., Malagelada, J. R. et al. (1982) Giant hypertrophic gastropathy (Ménétrier's disease): pharmacologic effects on protein leakage and mucosal ultrastructure. *Gastroenterology*, **83**, 581–589.

11 Kenney, F. D., Dockerty, M. B. & Waugh, J. M. (1954) Giant hypertrophy of gastric mucosa: a clinical and pathologic study. *Cancer*, **7**, 671–681.

12 Kondo, M., Ikezaki, M., Katu, H. & Masuda, M. (1978) Anti-fibrinolytic therapy of giant hypertrophic gastritis (Ménétrier's disease). *Scandinavian Journal of Gastroenterology*, **13**, 851–856.

13 Krag, E., Frederiksen, H. J., Olsen, N. & Henriksen, J. H. (1978) Cimetidine treatment of protein-losing gastropathy (Ménétrier's disease). A clinical and pathophysiological study. *Scandinavian Journal of Gastroenterology*, **13**, 636–639.

14 Reese, D. F., Hodgson, J. R. & Dockerty, M. B. (1962) Giant hypertrophy of the gastric mucosa (Ménétrier's disease): a correlation of the roentgenologic, pathologic and clinical findings. *American Journal of Roentgenology*, **88**, 619–626.

15 Scharschmidt, B. F. (1977) The natural history of hypertrophic gastropathy (Ménétrier's disease). *American Journal of Medicine*, **63**, 644–652.

16 Winney, R. J., Gilmour, H. M. & Matthews, J. D. (1976) Prednisolone in giant hypertrophic gastritis (Ménétrier's disease). *American Journal of Digestive Diseases*, **21**, 337–339.

OTHER GASTRODUODENAL DISORDERS

GASTRIC BEZOAR

Classification

In 1938, DeBakey and Ochsner reviewed 311 published cases of bezoar and proposed the classification shown in Table 4.41. Of the 126 phytobezoars in this series, 92 had resulted from eating persimmons and the term diospyrobezoar (from the botanical name of the fruit) has been coined for this common variety. The various unusual aggregates that are occasionally seen are grouped together as concretions.

Table 4.41 Classification of bezoars.[2]

	Composition
Trichobezoar	Hair
Phytobezoar	Vegetable matter
diospyrobezoar	Persimmon fibre and shibuol
Trichophytobezoar	Mixed hair and vegetable matter
Concretions	Various, including milk formulations and drugs

Aetiology

Trichobezoar

Trichobezoars arise from the chronic ingestion of hair; 80% of patients are in the first three decades of life and 90% are women. The underlying trichophagy may be a manifestation of a personality disorder, although only a small proportion of patients have overt features of psychiatric illness.

Phytobezoar

The persimmon contains large amounts of shibuol, which is coagulated by gastric acid into a form that efficiently binds vegetable fibre together. Studies of non-persimmon phytobezoars have demonstrated the presence of tannin monomers, which are probably polymerized in the stomach to form the necessary 'glue' for binding the vegetable matter.

Phytobezoars are especially common in people without teeth who cannot chew food thoroughly, and also in patients who have undergone gastric surgery, particularly vagotomy. Phytobezoars have been reported in diabetics with autonomic neuropathy and in a patient whose vagi had been destroyed by bronchial carcinoma, suggesting that gastric stasis and hypoacidity may be aetiological factors. Phytobezoars have arisen in patients receiving cimetidine.

Concretions

Many substances may aggregate in the stomach. An interesting example is the lactobezoar, which arises in premature infants fed on concentrated cow's milk formulations. Concretions of antacid preparations have also been described.

Presentation

A bezoar may present as a palpable epigastric mass, while its presence in the stomach can cause nausea, vomiting, anorexia, weight loss, gastritis, anaemia and peptic ulceration. All or part of a bezoar may pass into the small bowel and impact, so that the patient presents with intestinal obstruction.

Animal studies, in which rubber spheres were implanted in the stomachs of rats, indicate that there is hyperplasia of the muscle and mucosal lining of the stomach and an elevation in serum gastrin; these changes may contribute to the gastritis and ulceration which is seen in this condition.

Treatment

Large trichobezoars require surgical removal; smaller lesions have been retrieved intact using snares passed endoscopically, while others have been fragmented by endoscopic instrumentation, the remnants passing through the pylorus. Some patients need psychiatric advice and they should be followed-up, as recurrence may occur.

Phytobezoars have been dispersed enzymatically with instillations of 0.5% cellulase solution; satisfactory results have also been described with a mixture of cellulase, pepsin and ox bile, but operative removal is sometimes necessary.

Lactobezoars in premature infants often disperse if the concentrated feed is withheld, although some cases of gastric perforation requiring surgical intervention have been reported.

PHLEGMONOUS GASTRITIS (GASTRIC PHLEGMON)

Pathology

Phlegmonous gastritis is a bacterial infection of the muscularis mucosae and submucosa, with a polymorphonuclear lymphocytic and plasma cell infiltration. The mucosa is relatively unaffected. The inflammation does not extend beyond the cardia or the pylorus.

Incidence and aetiology

The condition is rare: Miller *et al.* were able to find only 23 cases in the American literature since World War 2, to which they added two more.[3] Bacteria were identified in 20 cases. In 15 they were Gram-positive organisms, *Streptococcus* spp. being isolated in nine. *Pneumococcus* spp., *Staphylococcus* spp., *Proteus vulgaris*, *Escherichia coli* and *Clostridium welchii* were also found. Two-thirds of these patients were aged over 40 years and 64% were women. Five were heavy drinkers and six had a recent history of pharyngitis.

Phlegmonous gastritis may arise as a complication of a systemic illness or following sepsis at a remote site; thus it has been reported after empyema, meningitis, pneumococcal endocarditis and measles, and after an infected hand wound. Gastric abnormalities, such as hypochlorhydria, gastritis, gastric ulcer, gastric cancer and previous gastric surgery have been indicated as predisposing factors.

Presentation

Acute phlegmonous gastritis can be difficult to diagnose, and many of the published cases have been recognized only at autopsy. The clinical course is a severe and rapidly progressive illness. Epigastric pain, nausea and vomiting are common symptoms, and signs of peritoneal irritation may be present. However, in some cases specific gastric symptoms have been absent or masked by coexisting disease.

A chronic form of phlegmonous gastritis with the clinical features of linitis plastica or chronic gastric ulcer has been described, but this appears to be extremely uncommon.

Investigation

Leucocytosis is a feature of many reported cases. The serum amylase is normal. Barium meal examination reveals gross mucosal thickening, often with rigidity of the antrum, and gastric dilatation may be observed. A few patients with this condition have been examined endoscopically: giant, purple, spongy mucosal folds were seen. As the mucosa is relatively spared, standard endoscopic biopsies will not reveal the pathology, but Bron *et al.* made a histological diagnosis from a snare biopsy obtained endoscopically.[1]

Treatment

Individual series of cases are small and no comparative studies of different treatment regimens have been published; however, surgical treatment is usually advised. For example, in the series described by Miller *et al.* nine of eleven patients survived after surgical treatment, while all 14 patients treated conservatively died.[3] The operative procedures ranged from gastrostomy to total gastrectomy, but partial gastrectomy was the one most widely used. A successful outcome has been reported by operative drainage of a gastric wall abscess followed by antibiotic therapy. The patient treated successfully by Bron *et al.* (see above) was managed conservatively and the authors speculated that the snare biopsy may have allowed the phlegmon to drain internally. Thus with early recognition and the use of broad-spectrum antimicrobial agents, possibly with endoscopic or open gastric wall drainage, resection may be avoidable.

CARCINOMA OF THE DUODENUM

Approximately half of all small bowel carcinomas arise in the duodenum; nevertheless, duodenal carcinoma is rare and accounts for only 0.3% of all gastrointestinal malignancies. No association has been found between duodenal carcinoma and previous peptic ulceration, but there is an increased incidence of duodenal carcinoma in patients with Crohn's disease and in Gardner's syndrome. The condition is most often seen in the sixth and seventh decades of life and is slightly more common in women.

The tumour carries a poor prognosis; in a series from the Mayo Clinic the mean survival time following diagnosis was 5.8 months. Initially, it is locally invasive and then spreads via the lymphatics. Metastases are common, being reported in 20–50% of cases. Local lymph nodes and the liver are the sites most often involved by metastases, but deposits have been recorded in the pancreas, the peritoneum, the ovary and the lung.

The majority of duodenal carcinomas arise in the periampullary region, the remainder being distributed fairly evenly above and below the ampulla.

Presentation

The mode of presentation depends upon the site of the malignancy: periampullary tumours can cause obstructive jaundice, whereas tumours above and below the ampulla produce symptoms of duodenal obstruction. Fluctuating jaundice and blood loss are suggestive of the condition. Steatorrhoea may occur if the pancreatic duct is occluded and the glucose tolerance test may be abnormal. Vomiting, marked weight loss and upper abdominal pain are common features of duodenal carcinoma, and a palpable mass may be present in 25% of patients.

Investigation

Barium meal examination may reveal the diagnosis, although tumours arising in the third part of the duodenum can be missed unless particularly sought. Endoscopic biopsy can provide a histological diagnosis, as can cytological examination of material obtained by duodenal aspiration.

Treatment

In appropriate cases, pancreaticoduodenectomy has been curative. However, extension of the malignancy into adjacent vital structures may make total excision difficult and metastatic disease often renders surgical cure impossible. Under these circumstances, palliative procedures to overcome biliary or duodenal obstruction may relieve symptoms. Both radiotherapy and chemotherapy have been employed in the treatment of duodenal carcinoma, but little evidence of benefit has been presented.

ACUTE DILATATION OF THE STOMACH

Acute dilatation of the stomach was at one time a common postoperative complication and was sometimes fatal. Fortunately, it is now rarely encountered, largely because of improved management of surgical patients.

Aetiology

Acute dilatation is a localized form of paralytic ileus. Although it most often occurs following upper abdominal surgery, it can also develop during debilitating illness and prolonged immobilization (such as in a plaster bed) and after trauma. It has been reported in cases of peritonitis, starvation, anorexia nervosa and diabetic ketoacidosis.

Presentation

The condition is characterized by a huge outpouring of fluid into the stomach, and in its most severe form may cause epigastric pain and hypotension, due to gastric distension, loss of circulating volume and compression of the inferior vena cava. Under such circumstances, myocardial infarction or pulmonary embolism may be erroneously diagnosed.

Complications of acute gastric dilatation include vomiting and aspiration, spontaneous rupture of the stomach and dehiscence of suture lines.

Diagnosis

The diagnosis can usually be made on clinical grounds. In addition to the features mentioned above, an epigastric mass may be palpable or even visible. If necessary, a plain abdominal radiograph will confirm the diagnosis.

Treatment

Many potential cases are prevented by awareness of the condition, with appropriate fluid replacement and nasogastric aspiration until gastric function returns. If acute gastric dilatation does occur the stomach is emptied by passing a large diameter nasogastric tube and aspiration is continued until the rate of secretion returns to normal. Rapid intravenous replacement of fluid and electrolyte losses is essential; physiological saline solution should be used, because the gastric aspirate contains large quantities of both sodium and chloride ions. Potassium is also lost in considerable amounts and this should be replaced. Once the patient has been resuscitated, treatment is continued until normal gastric emptying is restored.

REFERENCES

1 Bron, B. A., Deyhle, P., Pelloni, S. *et al.* (1977) Phlegmonous gastritis diagnosed by endoscopic snare biopsy. *American Journal of Digestive Diseases*, **22,** 729–733.
2 De Bakey, M. & Ochsner, A. (1938) Bezoars and concretions. *Surgery*, **4,** 934–963.
3 Miller, A. I., Smith, B. & Rogers, A. I. (1975) Phlegmonous gastritis. *Gastroenterology*, **68,** 231–238.

Chapter 5
Vascular Abnormalities of the Intestine

GENETIC AND CONGENITAL DISORDERS

The genetic and congenital vascular disorders of the intestine constitute an important group of conditions that may present to the gastroenterologist with either acute and massive or chronic, occult haemorrhage.

Table 5.1 is a classification of the various

Table 5.1 A classification of genetic and congenital vascular disorders of the intestine

---

Arteriovenous malformations (including angiodysplasia)

Multiple phlebectasia

Telangiectasia
  Hereditary haemorrhagic telangiectasia
    (Osler–Weber–Rendu disease)
  Telangiectasia associated with congenital syndromes
    e.g. Turner's syndrome

Haemangiomas
  Capillary
  Cavernous, simple or diffuse
  Mixed capillary–cavernous
  Peutz–Jeghers syndrome
  Blue rubber bleb naevus syndrome
  Klippel–Trenaunay–Weber syndrome

Disorders of connective tissue affecting blood vessels
  Pseudoxanthoma elasticum
  Ehlers–Danlos syndrome

---

vascular disorders that affect the intestine, based on the size of the lesion and the type of vessel affected. The important group of arteriovenous malformations or angiodysplasia is discussed later in this chapter and so little further reference will be made to these lesions here. Haemangiomas differ from all the other lesions since they can be identified as gross abnormalities on barium contrast examination, or by palpation of an intraluminal mass during surgery. Telangiectasia and phlebectasia may also be seen at laparotomy but these lesions, and arteriovenous malformations, usually require special angiographic and histopathological examination to be conclusively identified.

Although the occurrence and pathological characteristics of vascular lesions of the intestine have been recognized for many years,[26, 68] there have been significant advances in their pre- and intra-operative localization in the past two decades.

Preoperative localization of bleeding vascular lesions in the intestine is rarely achieved at upper gastrointestinal endoscopy or by barium contrast radiology because these lesions are often distal to the second part of the duodenum and (except for some haemangiomas) are not large enough to be detected by barium examination. It has been estimated that in patients

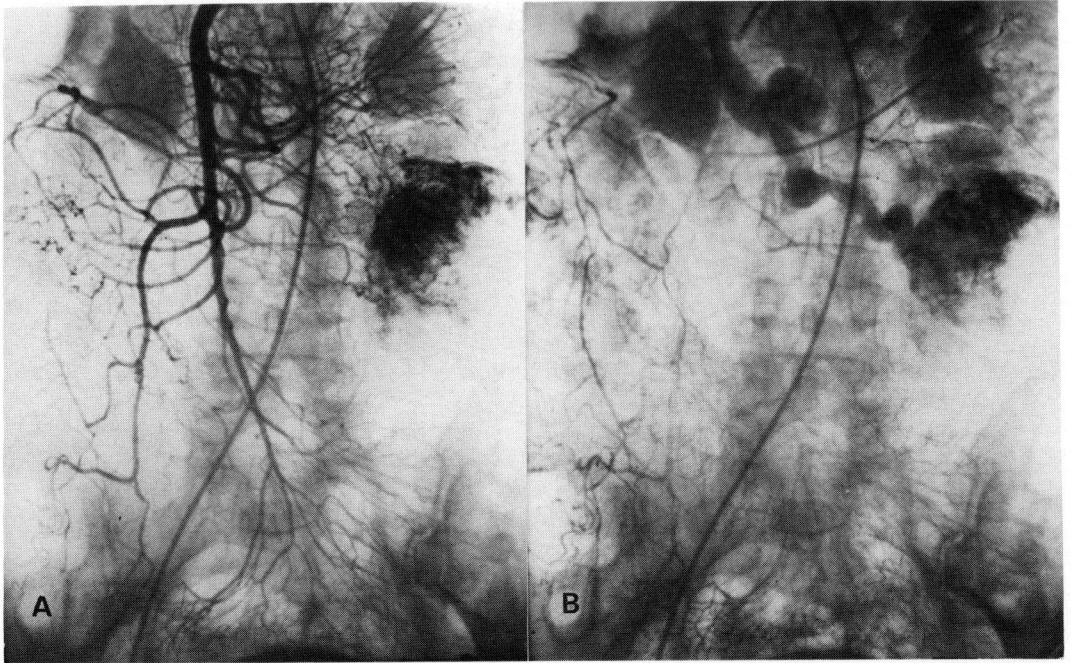

Fig. 5.1 Selective superior mesenteric arteriogram showing a large cavernous haemangioma in the jejunum. (A) Arterial phase. (B) Venous phase. (Courtesy of Dr D. J. Allison, Royal Postgraduate Medical School, London.)

who present with melaena without haematemesis, these investigations, applied early and aggressively, fail to localize the cause of bleeding in about 20% of cases.[42] Similarly with lower gastrointestinal bleeding, the cause was found in only 35–70% of patients in several series reviewed by Meyer *et al.*[55] Thus selective mesenteric arteriography (Figure 5.1) and [99]Tc[m]-labelled red cell scanning are often essential to localize vascular bleeding lesions in the intestine.[2, 53, 71, 83] The less sophisticated Einhorn string test[21] may contribute to the diagnosis by indicating the approximate level of the bleeding lesion but is now somewhat out-of-date. Since localization may only be achieved in 35–70% of patients even when using modern invasive techniques,[55] pharmacoangiography (using vasodilators, anticoagulants and fibrinolytic agents during selective angiography[75]) and intraoperative investigations have been devised to increase the diagnostic accuracy. The latter include: angiography with or without methylene blue injection,[6] endoscopy with transillumination of the intestinal wall[14, 30] and Doppler examination.[67] There is, as yet, no large series documenting the influence of these intraoperative investigations on the correct localization of vascular lesions in the intestine. However, the inclusion of these manoeuvres is essential in the evaluation of many patients since

the success of surgical excision, particularly of the macroscopically invisible arteriovenous lesions, depends on accurate localization. In the near future it is envisaged that digital subtraction angiography (DSA) using an intravenous injection of contrast medium will be used as a screening procedure for large vascular abnormalities or those with a large shunt and draining vein. The improved imaging and subtraction methods that have been developed to make DSA possible should also help to increase the diagnostic yield of selective arteriography.[57]

ARTERIOVENOUS MALFORMATIONS

These lesions (also known as angiodysplasia), which may be congenital, are described in detail later in this chapter (p. 259). Briefly, they consist of irregularly-shaped clusters of arteriolar, venular and capillary vessels located in the mucosa and submucosa of the intestine, most often in the right colon of elderly patients. Less commonly, lesions occur in the jejunum and stomach, and there have been several reports of such lesions causing gastrointestinal haemorrhage in younger patients, including adolescents.[4, 36, 55]

MULTIPLE PHLEBECTASIA

The term 'phlebectasia' refers to venous varicosities found in the gastrointestinal tract. There is some confusion in the literature of the first half of this century since this term was used to identify a small type of cavernous haemangioma.[26] The modern use of the term phlebectasia implies a non-neoplastic venous varicosity with a normal endothelial lining, and this would appear to be indistinguishable from Gentry's[26] phlebectasia type of cavernous haemangioma.

Phlebectasias are not uncommon in the oesophagus and rectum and may also be found infrequently in the small intestine. There are at least seven well described cases of multiple intestinal phlebectasia reported in the recent literature[65] and to these one must add the large number reported in the earlier literature[26] in which they accounted for a third of all benign vascular lesions of the intestine. In all cases, the greatest density of lesions occurred in the mid-small bowel with a fall off in distribution proximally and distally. The lesions vary from a few millimetres to several centimetres in diameter. Grossly, they appear as dark, bluish-red nodules that are soft and compressible. The lesions are located in the submucosa and have a normal endothelial lining.[65] Figure 5.2 shows the macroscopic and low power microscopic appearances of this lesion. The mucosa overlying these lesions may be extremely thin. Similar varicose vessels may be seen entering the intestine at its mesenteric attachment.[80]

Presentation and diagnosis

In the majority of cases, the diagnosis is made around the fifth or sixth decades, and the usual clinical presentations are occult bleeding or anaemia with alteration of stool colour.

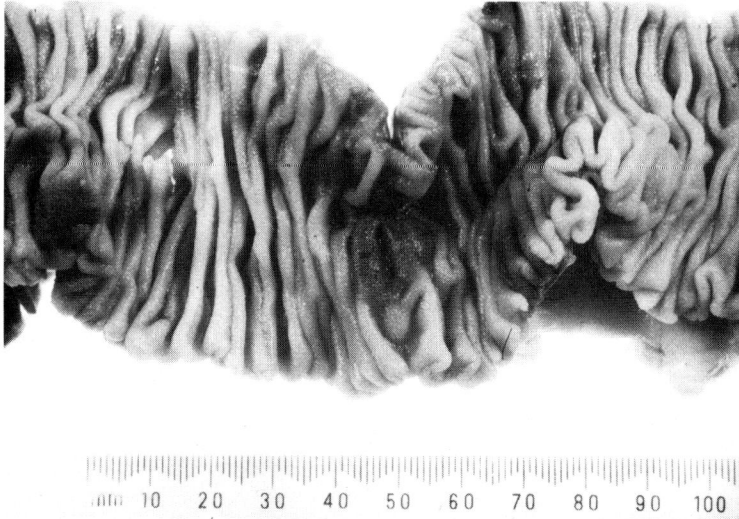

a

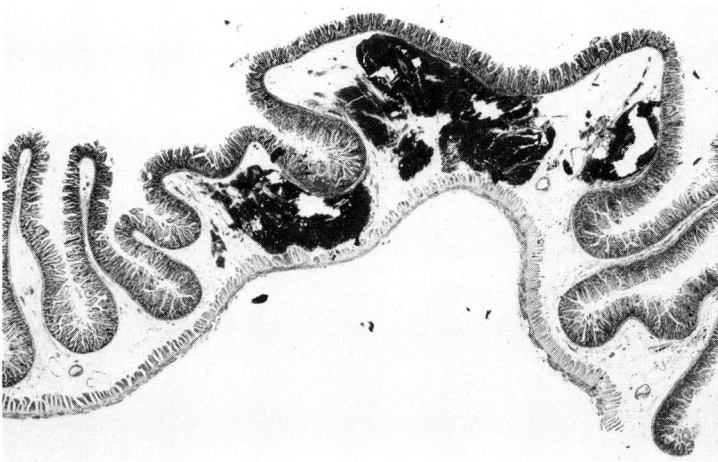

b

Fig. 5.2 (a) Macroscopic appearance of the mucosal surface of resected jejunum showing multiple phlebectasia. (b) Whole mount low power microscopy of lesion seen in (a). (Courtesy of Dr H. Hodgson, Royal Postgraduate Medical School, London.)

Although it has been stated that life-threatening haemorrhage does not occur in this condition,[65] we have seen this lesion presenting as massive gastrointestinal bleeding necessitating emergency laparotomy. It is striking that, although all preoperative diagnostic procedures have proved unsuccessful in the cases reported, in our patient abdominal scanning after intravenous injection of $^{99}Tc^m$ correctly localized bleeding to the jejunum.

Treatment

It is not surprising that reduction of the number of lesions by surgical excision of the mid-small bowel has not always been successful in stopping haemorrhage in every case. If surgical excision of all the lesions is not possible, intermittent blood transfusion and oral iron therapy are the mainstays of treatment.

TELANGIECTASIA

Hereditary haemorrhagic telangiectasia (Osler–Weber–Rendu disease)

Up to 1977, this disorder had been reported in around 1500 members of 300 families.[1] It is inherited as an autosomal dominant trait. Telangiectasias occur in the skin, mucous membranes and internal organs, resulting in recurrent haemorrhage. These lesions arise from simple dilatation of normal vascular structures. Congenital thinning of the arterial muscle coat[81] and absent elastin in arteriolar walls[65] may be responsible for the dilatation.

The telangiectasias are punctate, red to purple in colour, noncompressible and may be stellate or nodular.[81] Their size ranges from 1 to 4 mm and they occur on the face (Figure 5.3) and hands as well as the labial, buccal and nasal mucosae, and the conjunctiva. These mucocutaneous lesions usually appear in the second and third decades; the earliest haemorrhagic presentation is with repeated epistaxis in childhood. Bleeding from the gastrointestinal tract usually becomes manifest in the fourth decade[34] and occurs in about 15% of patients with this disorder.[65] Vascular abnormalities also occur in the lung, liver, uterus, kidney, bladder, meninges, spinal cord and eye.[1] One abnormality specific to the lung is the pulmonary arteriovenous fistula which may lead to cardiac failure and erythrocytosis.[34]

The gastrointestinal presentation is usually with chronic blood loss. Gastroscopy may reveal multiple punctate lesions in the stomach[63] and colonoscopy may also show typical lesions.[82] Selective mesenteric arteriography may be necessary to localize the precise bleeding site, and some cases have required peroperative enteroscopy to detect the bleeding lesion.[30] Although about 40% of patients require blood transfusions, death due to excessive blood loss rarely occurs.

A number of gastrointestinal vascular anomalies have been reported in association with congenital or acquired von Willebrand's disease. These include diffuse gastrointestinal telangiectasia[1, 17, 50, 74] similar to those of Osler–Weber–Rendu disease, and angiodysplasia consisting of masses of small tortuous, thin-walled blood vessels.[69] The inheritance of the coagulopathy was linked to that of the telangiectasia in three generations of one family studied by Conlon et al.[17] These authors suggested that an endothelial defect was responsible

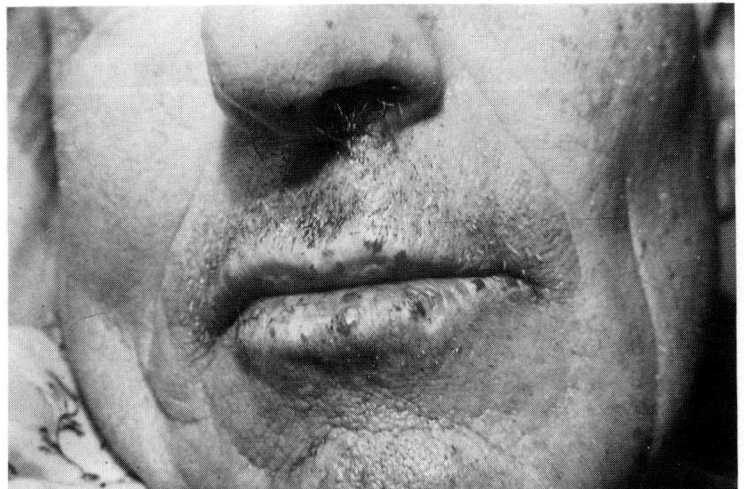

Fig. 5.3 Hereditary haemorrhagic telangiectasia.

for both disorders, resulting in inadequate synthesis of factor VIII and defective capillary structure. Ahr *et al.*,[1] in a review of the literature on hereditary haemorrhagic telangiectasia, found some cases where a second haemostatic defect was present, often demonstrated only by prolonged bleeding times particularly after ingestion of aspirin. In the acquired variety, an inhibitor to factor VIII (present in the IgG fraction of plasma and lacking precipitating properties) has been reported in some cases.[50] The presence of an associated clotting defect, or of disseminated intravascular coagulation, obviously increases the difficulty of managing acutely bleeding telangiectasia.[13]

Treatment
The management of patients with hereditary haemorrhagic telangiectasia should be conservative in the first instance. If bleeding continues despite blood transfusion, a search should be undertaken for an associated haemostatic defect and, failing this, selective mesenteric arteriography during active bleeding is mandatory to ensure localization and surgical excision of the bleeding telangiectasia. The role of hormonal therapy is still controversial. Some reports suggest that oestrogens are capable of stabilizing the brittle walls of blood vessels and may thus reduce the tendency to bleed;[54] however, a double-blind controlled clinical trial failed to show any benefit in terms of the frequency or intensity of bleeding or in the haemoglobin levels of patients with Osler–Weber–Rendu disease.[88]

Therapeutic embolization of affected blood vessels has been considered, and is certainly valuable for stopping bleeding from the upper respiratory tract in this condition.[3] However, when embolizing bleeding telangiectasia in the gut, the risk of causing infarction must be considered.

Telangiectasia associated with Turner's syndrome

Turner's syndrome is characterized by a variety of external somatic features as well as congenital malformations of internal organs, found in association with ovarian agenesis and a characteristic 45XO chromosome karyotype. The somatic features include infantilism, cubitus valgus, a webbed neck and shield-like chest. The congenital malformations include coarctation of the aorta, renal artery stenosis, septal defects in the heart, and lymphoedema.[31]

Turner's syndrome is associated with gastrointestinal haemorrhage due to vascular lesions in the intestinal wall.[46] These vascular anomalies have been described as haemangiomas, telangiectasias or dilated veins, and at laparotomy may be found throughout most of the small and large bowel and the mesentery but with a predilection for the small intestine. The incidence of gastrointestinal bleeding in Turner's syndrome is unknown. It occurred in 4 out of 56 patients in one series[31] but was not recorded in another series of 48 cases.[22]

Haemorrhage from these lesions is usually intermittent and often self-limiting, and death by exsanguination has only rarely been reported.[46] There are at least two well-documented reports suggesting that the vascular anomalies may spontaneously regress with time.[25, 79] Thus the clinical presentation of these patients is often with bleeding before 20 years of age; after 30 years of age bleeding tends to be intermittent and self-limited.[78] Preoperative demonstration of bleeding vascular anomalies is difficult. Rutlin *et al.*[77] have demonstrated telangiectatic lesions in the duodenal bulb, caecum and ascending colon by fibreoptic endoscopy, but in most of the previous reports, diagnosis was reached at laparotomy.

Treatment
Because of the strong impression, based on both clinical and pathological findings, that lesions undergo spontaneous regression after the age of 30, a conservative approach is warranted,[78] with intestinal resection restricted to small segments that include the bleeding lesions. Mesenteric arteriography may permit preoperative localization of both small or large intestinal bleeding lesions. It is possible that in the future, laser (or other) photocoagulation of bleeding lesions during upper gastrointestinal endoscopy, or colonoscopic diathermy or hot biopsy coagulation of colonic telangiectasia in patients with chronic anaemia may control haemorrhage in these patients as it has in those with caecal angiodysplasia.[36]

HAEMANGIOMAS

For the sake of accuracy, it must be stated that the lesions discussed in this section are better classified as hamartomas since they are congenital or appear soon after birth, they cannot be easily distinguished on histopathological grounds from other acknowledged vascular malformations, and they do not grow disproportionately or indefinitely as true neoplasms do; they grow *pari passu* with the surrounding tissues without involving a greater area than that originally affected.[89] The term 'haemangioma' is retained for uniformity with the literature. These lesions may be classified according to the size of vessel affected – (i.e. capillary, cavernous or mixed) or according to their association with cutaneous or other somatic abnormalities (e.g. Peutz–Jeghers syndrome, Klippel–Trenaunay–Weber syndrome).

Intestinal haemangiomas are rare and usually non-hereditary. In a review of 1.4 million case records at the Mayo Clinic, Gentry *et al.*[26] found 106 vascular lesions of the intestine; 60 other cases were detected by reviewing 10 000 autopsy reports over 20 years at the same institution. Haemangiomas constituted 98% of the benign vascular tumours in this study, and 86% of all benign vascular lesions reported in the literature till 1949.[26]

Intestinal haemangiomas account for around 10% of all benign small intestinal tumours.[16, 56, 73, 90] In River's review of 1399 cases in the literature,[73] it was shown that 5.4% of the tumours were solitary, localized lesions (3.7% being multiple or diffuse). In about half the cases, diagnosis was only reached at laparotomy. Wilson *et al.*[90] reviewed 1721 cases of benign small intestinal tumours from throughout the world and found 212 haemangiomas (the fifth commonest type of tumour). The distribution in the small intestine was predominantly in the jejunum (47%) and ileum (45%), with a minority in the duodenum (8%). Several authors[72, 90] stress the fact that most lesions are discrete, well circumscribed or encapsulated masses composed of blood vessels and are therefore hamartomas rather than true vascular neoplasms. The clinical presentations of 134 adequately documented small intestinal haemangiomas include haemorrhage (41%), abdominal pain (31%), and intussusception (13%). Rarely, abdominal masses are palpable (10%) and there may be evidence of weight loss.[90]

Presentation
Capillary haemangiomas usually present with haemorrhage, and occasionally obstruction or perforation often associated with intramural bleeding. The larger cavernous and mixed lesions are more likely to result in ulceration or obstruction of the intestine, although gut haemorrhage remains a common clinical presentation. Of 18 cases of mixed haemangiomas reviewed by Gentry,[26] eight developed subacute intestinal obstruction, six had prominent gastrointestinal haemorrhage (which was fatal in three

cases), and two were found incidentally at necropsy. Conversely, only 5% of cavernous haemangiomas are found incidentally at post mortem, the vast majority manifesting with haemorrhage (50%) or intestinal obstruction (35%).

Diffuse cavernous haemangiomas usually affect the colon and present with intermittent rectal bleeding (95%), often in childhood.

Diagnosis
Diagnosis of intestinal haemangiomas depends on a high index of suspicion in patients with haemorrhage particularly if associated with features that suggest subacute intestinal obstruction. Patients with cavernous haemangiomas may have calcified phleboliths in the region of the affected bowel on plain abdominal X-ray, a useful clue in children and young adults.[48] Mass lesions (single or multiple) may be visible on barium contrast examination by causing irregularity of the margins, stenosis or dilatations of intestinal loops.[61] Arteriography usually reveals the site of the vascular malformations by the appearance of contrast medium in vascular spaces in the bowel wall, often associated with slowing of the venous return from such lesions (in contrast to the early filling vein observed with angiodysplasia). Rarely, cavernous haemangiomas may be detected endoscopically in the duodenum.[38] However, the diagnosis of intestinal haemangiomas is often made at laparotomy in patients with intestinal obstruction or gut haemorrhage of unknown origin.

Capillary haemangiomas

These consist of small, closely packed blood vessels with a well differentiated hyperplastic endothelium which may obliterate the vascular space. They usually appear as single, discrete, encapsulated lesions, arising from the submucosal vascular plexus and enlarging towards the lumen of a hollow viscus. The lesions in the small intestine tend to be small plaques (around 1 cm^2) and constitute around 6% of vascular tumours in this organ.[26, 72] Surgical resection is possible in the majority of cases. There are a few reports of multiple intestinal capillary haemangiomatosis.[85]

Cavernous haemangiomas

Cavernous haemangiomas consist of large blood-filled spaces or sinuses lined by single or multiple layers of endothelial cells. These spaces are supported by scant connective tissue septa that may contain smooth muscle fibres. Coagulation of blood within these spaces may occur and is followed by organization of the thrombus, hyalinization and eventually calcification. This process accounts for the distinctive radiological features of these lesions. Cavernous haemangiomas may be *single* or *diffuse*.

The single lesions, which account for 18% of all benign vascular lesions of the intestine,[26] are usually polypoid and associated with the submucosal vascular plexus. They may enlarge and prolapse into the lumen of the viscus, resulting in ulceration, haemorrhage or intestinal obstruction; these manifestations occur in about 80% of patients with such lesions. The remainder are found incidentally at postmortem. The radiological features of these lesions are described above. Surgical excision was possible in about half the cases reviewed by Gentry.[26]

The multiple small simple cavernous haemangiomas described in the earlier literature are here classified as multiple phlebectasia.

Diffuse cavernous haemangiomas are characterized by great variation in size, shape and effect on the viscus in which they are located. Such lesions may involve 20–30 cm of one continuous segment of intestine, or there may be multiple lesions of this kind involving different segments of the gastrointestinal tract and surrounding viscera such as the urinary bladder. Diffuse cavernous haemangiomas account for 20% of all benign vascular lesions of the intestine. Their distribution appears to be equal for small intestine and colon. Their gross appearance on the luminal surface of the viscus is of a soft compressible, nodular, dark purple elevation under the mucosa. Microscopically they have the typical appearance of a cavernous haemangioma in most areas of the lesion; the periphery reveals numerous dilated tortuous vessels and an abundance of smooth muscle and connective tissue.

Overall this group has a very high mortality (about 30%) and morbidity, with continuing massive or chronic haemorrhage necessitating repeated transfusions of blood. Occasionally these diffuse lesions may spread to involve the urinary bladder and patients may present with haematuria.[26, 86] There have been isolated reports of diffuse cavernous haemangiomas associated with lymphangiomatosis,[86] as well as a protein-losing enteropathy which responded to surgical resection of a large segment of jejunum containing a diffuse lesion.[39] Extension of the haemangioma into the mesentery or retroperitoneum may result in haemorrhage at these sites. In a review of 47 cases of haemangiomas in the paediatric age group, 30 were of the cavernous variety (simple or diffuse) and the

average duration of symptoms before diagnosis was 16 years.[59]

Radical surgery, where possible, appears to offer the only hope for cure in cases of diffuse cavernous haemangiomatosis of the intestine. Radiotherapy and sclerosing injections have been unsuccessful in controlling haemorrhage.[59] Although high dose corticosteroids have been used successfully for large cutaneous angiomas[24] there is no experience of this therapy for intestinal haemangiomas.

Selective arterial embolization of lesions shown to be bleeding at arteriography may be considered, particularly if multiple areas of diffuse haemangiomas are demonstrated. The therapeutic plan must be tailored to the individual patient after considering the severity of bleeding, response to conventional resuscitation, and disease extent.

The prognosis of patients with diffuse cavernous haemangiomas therefore depends on the extent of residual diseased intestine. Malignant transformation of haemangiomas is said to be exceedingly rare and most malignant haemangio-endotheliomas are thought to arise *de novo*.[89] There is one report of a patient with multiple simple capillary haemangiomas of the small and large bowel who died of gastrointestinal haemorrhage and was found at necropsy to have multiple malignant tumours in the gut and one in the bladder, all apparently arising in pre-existing haemangiomas.[58]

Mixed capillary and cavernous haemangiomas

These lesions account for 6–12% of all vascular malformations in the intestine.[26, 72] They consist of solid areas of hyperplastic endothelial cells, partially obliterated vascular spaces and large blood-filled sinuses lined by a single endothelial cell layer. There is a variable amount of elastic and muscle tissue supporting these sinuses. The entire lesions tend to be encapsulated, and arise from submucosal vessels and enlarge towards the lumen of the viscus. They may eventually become peduculated or ulcerate through the overlying epithelium. Since many of the mixed haemangiomas tend to be single (usually polypoid, occasionally diffuse in a single segment of bowel), surgical excision is frequently possible.

Peutz–Jeghers syndrome

There have been at least three papers which record the presence of mucocutaneous pigmentation with intestinal haemangiomas in the

absence of polyposis, in the setting of a hereditary, dominantly-transmitted disease.

Jeghers *et al.*[40] described one patient with
characteristic pigmentation and gastrointestinal
bleeding without evidence of polyposis. Dormandy,[19] in a detailed study of five families
(with 21 cases), found that four of the patients
had pigmentation associated with gastrointestinal bleeding or abdominal pain but no
evidence of polyposis. Bandler[8] reported a
patient with mucocutaneous pigmentation and
cavernous haemangiomas of the entire small
intestine but no polyps. Two first-degree relatives of this patient also had haemangiomas of
the intestine but no pigmentation.

It appears that such cases represent sporadic
mutations and/or incomplete penetration of the
gene responsible for the Peutz–Jeghers syndrome.[19]

Blue rubber bleb naevus syndrome

This disorder is inherited as an autosomal
dominant trait,[12] although many reported cases
appear to be sporadic.[28] It is characterized by
cavernous haemangiomas of the skin, gastrointestinal tract and other viscera, including the
liver, lung, spleen and joints. The skin lesions
vary in number, may occur at any site including
the palms and soles, and are present at birth but
increase in number with age. They are typically
blue, often tender, range in size from 1 mm to 2
cm across and have a wrinkled surface (Figure
5.4). They empty on digital pressure leaving a
wrinkled blue sac that slowly refills over several
minutes. Histologically, the skin haemangiomas
consist of clusters of dilated capillary spaces
lined by cuboidal or flattened epithelium with a
variable amount of connective tissue stroma.[7]

Some reports also describe other elements
present with the vascular lesions, such as
smooth muscle cells and sweat glands.

The gastrointestinal tract lesions are usually
multiple, but may be solitary. The onset of gastrointestinal bleeding may be at any time from
early childhood to middle age. The small intestine is affected more frequently than the stomach
and colon, and the lesions may be picked up on
barium contrast examination as multiple mass
lesions that may be mistaken for polyps. Angiography demonstrates arteriovenous malformations and may help to identify the site of
bleeding, which is essential for surgical management of patients whose bleeding cannot be controlled medically.[7]

Klippel–Trenaunay–Weber syndrome

In 1900, Klippel and Trenaunay described a
non-hereditary, sporadic disorder of children
and young adults characterized by soft tissue
and bony hypertrophy, varicose veins and port-
wine haemangiomas, which are usually unilateral, often sharply demarcated, and involve a
lower extremity, but are occasionally bilateral
and affect the upper extremities, face or trunk.[45]
Enlargement of the soft tissues may be gradual
and may involve the whole limb, a portion of it,
or selected digits. An underlying vascular abnormality consisting of atresia, hypoplasia, or obstruction of the deep venous system was noted in
the 300 cases reported.[66] Parkes-Weber[64]
described patients who, in association with the
kind of abnormalities reported by Klippel and
Trenaunay, also had arteriovenous fistulas with
bruits over affected parts.

Other less frequent features of this syndrome
include intermittent claudication, varicose

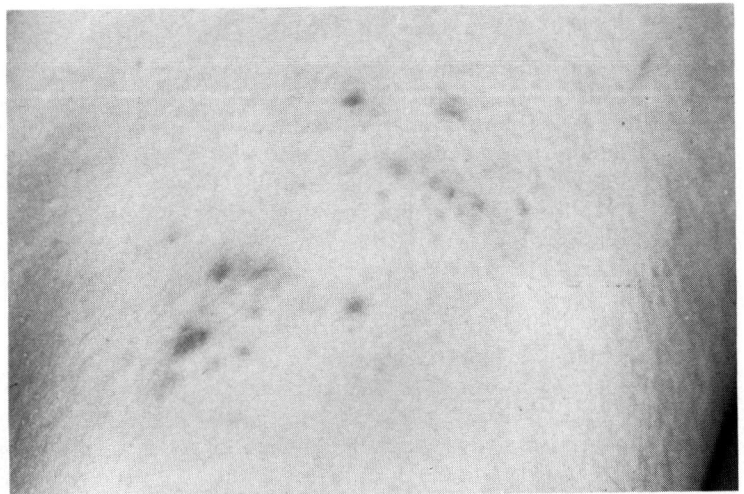

Fig. 5.4 Blue rubber bleb naevus
syndrome.

ulcers, gangrene of an extremity, thrombophlebitis, varicose pulmonary veins, diffuse hair loss,
dyskeratosis, altered sweating, lymphoedema,
cutaneous lymphangiomas, dislocation of joints
and gait abnormalities due to lower limb
inequality, congestive cardiac failure, and bleeding from the urinary and gastrointestinal tracts.

The earliest report of gastrointestinal bleeding
in association with limb hemihypertrophy is
that of Hulke.[37] Shepherd[81] reported a single
patient with this combination and reviewed the
previous report of Hulke. Both affected patients
were young boys (aged 7 and 5 years
respectively) who had unilateral limb hypertrophy, cutaneous naevi, and gastrointestinal
bleeding. Shepherd's patient was found to have
abnormal vessels on the serosal surface of the
small and large intestine, as well as in the mesentery. The bowel vascular malformations may be
mixed[51] or cavernous haemangiomas.

Plain abdominal radiographs reveal phleboliths in the anatomical location of the colon and
these increase in number and density with the
patient's age. At colonoscopy, the bowel lumen
is narrowed by multiple polypoid vascular
masses that collapse on pressure[27] and should
only be biopsied with caution.[11, 84] Similar
irregularity of the bowel and prominent folds
(resembling colonic varices) may be seen on
barium enema. Arteriography shows slow
venous drainage with contrast retained in vascular spaces in the colonic submucosa[27, 60, 66] and
similar changes are visible in studies of the
femoral artery.[27] Arterial embolization has been
considered by some authors[27] but may lead to
colonic infarction, especially since the majority
of lesions appear to affect the left side of the
colon and rectum. Treatment necessitates
primary resection of the affected intestinal

segment with a permanent colostomy or 'pull-
through' sphincter-saving procedure. This
necessitates adequate delineation of the extent of
bowel involvement with preoperative arteriography. Temporary relief may be obtained by
ligation of the vessels supplying the colonic
haemangioma.

Intestinal bleeding may be enhanced and
postoperative haemostasis impaired when there
is an associated consumptive coagulopathy
resulting from intravascular clotting within the
venous sinusoids of the cutaneous and visceral
haemangiomas.

DISORDERS OF CONNECTIVE TISSUE AFFECTING BLOOD VESSELS

Pseudoxanthoma elasticum

This disorder demonstrates genetic heterogeneity in that both recessive and dominant
modes of inheritance occur, and clinical variability is the rule.[18] Most cases are inherited as
autosomal recessive.[29] No primary biochemical
defect has been identified, although it is known
that elastin metabolism is deranged.[87] The disorder affects the skin, mucous membranes and
eyes, and the blood vessels of the gastrointestinal tract, heart and kidneys.[5] Prevalence
figures are from 1/160 000 to 1/70 000, although
these figures may be underestimating the true
prevalence since they are based only on the
number of reported cases.[18]

The skin changes are usually recognized in the
second decade and usually affect regions of
dermal stress, such as the neck, axillae and
groin. These areas develop a characteristic
yellowish, wrinkled appearance that simulates
the skin of a plucked chicken (Figure 5.5). The

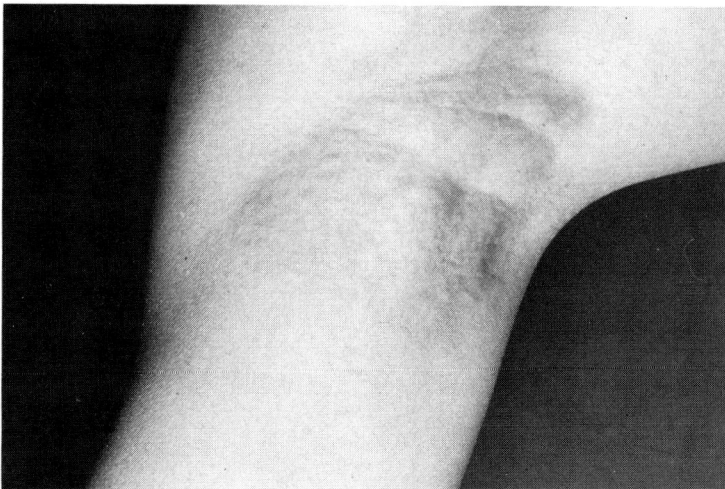

Fig. 5.5 Pseudoxanthoma
elasticum affecting axillary skin.
(Courtesy of Dr H. R. Vickers,
Royal Postgraduate Medical
School, London.)

skin eventually becomes lax and inelastic. Histologically there is a pathognomonic picture of clumping, fragmentation and calcification of elastic fibres in the mid- and deep dermis.

In the majority of patients, alteration of elastic fibres on the retina, with rupture of the unsupported Bruch's membrane, results in the formation of angioid streaks. Other ocular problems are epithelial retinal pigment disturbances, atypical drusen, and neovascularization. Visual acuity often progressively worsens, especially when the macula becomes involved.

Medium-sized arteries degenerate and calcify in this disorder; such changes may result in weak peripheral pulses, intermittent claudication, angina, or strokes, and may be detected using plain radiography. Peripheral arterial occlusion, often unsuspected, and usually affecting radial, ulnar or posterior tibial arteries, occurred in a significant number of patients in one series.[29]

Haemorrhage is the most common presentation of gut involvement, and has been reported to occur as early as five years of age.[21] There does appear to be a predilection for haemorrhage from the stomach.[18] Bleeding is thought to result from spontaneous vascular rupture and failure of calcified vessels to contract normally after injury, with resulting mucosal congestion and eventual erosion of the surface.[29, 41] Reports of the endoscopic appearance of the stomach describe a characteristic yellow, cobblestoned mucosa with a friable, oozing, eroded surface.[15, 29] Proctoscopic examination also shows marked redundancy of rectal mucosa that becomes folded upon itself, and yellowish plaques similar to those seen in the stomach.[29] Barium contrast studies fail to reveal any abnormality; arteriography is reported to show abnormal, tortuous, narrowed mesenteric vessels as well as vascular malformations within the gastrointestinal tract.[9, 15] This latter investigation may be necessary to demonstrate the site of bleeding if operative intervention is considered essential because of persistent haemorrhage. However, there has not, as yet, been a report of this technique during active bleeding. Fibreoptic endoscopy should be undertaken first, especially in view of the predilection for gastric bleeding.[18] Resected specimens of stomach show that gastric submucosal arteries are calcified and the internal elastic lamina is deficient.[23] There is no evidence that anastomotic or incisional healing is impaired. Some authors have suggested that selective arterial embolization may be used to stop bleeding in these patients.[18] Operative treatment is mandatory if haemorrhage cannot be controlled by such conservative means.

There is one report in the literature of coexistence of polyposis coli and pseudoxanthoma elasticum in one family.[62] Lesions such as peptic ulcer or hiatal hernia with oesophagitis may be more likely to bleed because of the underlying vascular abnormality in these patients.[47] The significance of the former association is uncertain, but it highlights the importance of considering other treatable conditions when patients who suffer from pseudoxanthoma elasticum present with gut haemorrhage.

Ehlers–Danlos syndrome (EDS)

This syndrome comprises a group of at least eight disorders.[43] It demonstrates genetic heterogeneity with documented kindreds showing autosomal dominant, autosomal recessive and sex-linked recessive patterns of inheritance. The spectrum of severity varies markedly from near normal to a life-threatening condition. The underlying aetiology is a defect in collagen synthesis, and the precise biochemical disorders are known for certain subgroups of the syndrome. There is a reduced content of type III collagen in subgroup IV of EDS, a deficiency of lysyl hydroxylase resulting in hydroxylysine deficiency in tissue collagen in subgroup VI, and deficiencies of lysyl oxidase and procollagen peptidase account for the disorder in subgroups V and VII.[35, 44, 52] Such biochemical markers are useful in distinguishing the various subgroups and provide a method for antenatal diagnosis which facilitates genetic counselling.[43]

The syndrome is characterized by joint hyperextensibility (occasionally causing hip dislocation and clubfoot), bruising, skin elasticity and fragility, and formation of paper-thin scars. Redundant chordae tendineae may result in cardiac valve cusp prolapse or valvular incompetence. The more severe forms may be complicated by spontaneous arterial or even visceral rupture, the latter being seen almost exclusively in subgroup IV.[52] Massive dilatation of the oesophagus, stomach, or the small or large bowel have also been reported,[32] and there is one well documented report of malabsorption due to bacterial overgrowth in a patient with EDS who had massive duodenal dilatation and multiple small intestinal diverticula.[33]

In a large series of 125 patients with this syndrome,[10] the gastrointestinal manifestations were haematemesis and melaena (6), jejunal intramural haemorrhage (1), colonic diverticular bleeding (2), colonic perforation (1), external piles (8) and skin splitting at the anal margin (5). Haematemesis and melaena were attributed to peptic ulceration in three, and a hiatal hernia in one patient, though no cause could be identified in two other patients. In view of the excessive tissue fragility, persistent haemorrhage and defective wound healing common in such patients, surgery should be avoided unless visceral rupture or uncontrollable haemorrhage supervene, and even angiography may be dangerous.

REFERENCES

1 Ahr, D. J., Rickes, F. R., Hoyer, L. W. *et al.* (1977) Von Willebrand's disease and hemorrhagic telangiectasia: association of two complex disorders of hemostasis resulting in life threatening hemorrhage. *American Journal of Medicine*, **62**, 452–458.

2 Alfidi, R. (1974) Angiography in identifying the source of intestinal bleeding. *Diseases of Colon and Rectum*, **17**, 442–446.

3 Allison, D. J. (1982) Therapeutic embolisation. *Spectrum International*, **25**, 22–25.

4 Allison, D. K., Hemingway, A. P. & Cunningham, D. A. (1982) Angiography in gastrointestinal bleeding. *Lancet*, **ii**, 30–32.

5 Altman, L. K., Fialkow, P. J. & Parkor, F. (1974) Pseudoxanthoma elasticum. An underdiagnosed genetically heterogenous disorder with protean manifestations. *Archives of Internal Medicine*, **134**, 1048–1054.

6 Athanasoulis, C. A., Moncuro, A. C., Greenheld, A. J. *et al.* (1980) Intraoperative localisation of small bowel bleeding sites: combined use of angiographic methods and methylene blue injection. *Surgery*, **87**, 77–84.

7 Baker, A. L., Kahn, P. C., Binder, S. C. & Patterson, J. F. (1971) Gastrointestinal bleeding due to blue rubber bleb naevus syndrome. A case diagnosed by angiography. *Gastroenterology*, **61**, 530–533.

8 Bandler, M. (1960) Hemangiomas of the small intestine associated with mucocutaneous pigmentation. *Gastroenterology*, **38**, 643–645.

9 Bardsley, J. L. & Koehler, P. R. (1969) Pseudoxanthoma elasticum: angiographic manifestations in abdominal vessels. *Radiology*, **93**, 559–562.

10 Beighton, P. H., Murdoch, J. L. & Votteler, T. (1969) Gastrointestinal complications of the Ehlers–Danlos syndrome. *Gut*, **10**, 1004–1008.

11 Bell, G. A., McKenzie, A. D. & Emmens, H. (1972) Diffuse cavernous haemangioma of the rectum: report of a case and review of the literature. *Diseases of the Colon and Rectum*, **15**, 377–382.

12 Berlyne, G. M. & Berlyne, N. (1960) Anaemia due to 'Blue-Rubber-Bleb' naevus disease. *Lancet*, **ii**, 1275–1277.

13 Bick, R. L. (1981) Hereditary haemorrhage telangiectasia and disseminated intravascular coagulation: a new clinical syndrome. *Annals of the New York Academy of Sciences*, **370**, 851–854.

14 Bowden, T. A. Jr, Hooks, V. H., III & Mansbergor, A. R. Jr. (1979) Intraoperative gastrointestinal endoscopy in the management of occult gastrointestinal bleeding. *Southern Medical Journal*, **72**, 1532–1537.

15 Cocco, A. E., Grayer, D. I., Walker, B. A. & Martyn, L. J. (1969) The stomach in pseudoxanthoma elasticum. *Journal of the American Medical Association*, **210**, 2381–2382.

16 Cohen, A., McNeill, D., Terz, J. J. & Lawrence, W. Jr. (1971) Neoplasms of the small intestine. *American Journal of Digestive Diseases*, **16**, 815–824.

17 Conlon, C. L., Weinger, R. S., Cimo, P. L. *et al.* (1978) Telangiectasia and von Willebrand's disease in two families. *Annals of Internal Medicine*, **89**, 921–924.

18 Cunningham, J. R., Lippman, S. M., Renie, W. A. *et al.* (1980) Pseudoxanthoma elasticum: treatment of gastrointestinal haemorrhage by arterial embolisation and observations on autosomal dominant inheritance. *Johns Hopkins Medical Journal*, **147**, 168–173.

19 Dormandy, T. L. (1957) Gastrointestinal polyposis with mucocutaneous pigmentation (Peutz–Jeghers syndrome). *New England Journal of Medicine*, **256**, 1093–1102.

20 Edward, H. (1958) Haematemesis due to pseudoxanthoma elasticum. *Gastroenterology (Basel)*, **89**, 345–346.

21 Edwards, M. H., Beairsto, E. B., Pessel, J. F. *et al.* (1955) Multiple jejunal phlebectasia as cause of melaena: localising value of the Einhorn String test. *Canadian Medical Association Journal*, **72**, 689–690.

22 Engel, E. & Forbes, A. P. (1965) Cytogenetic and clinical findings in 48 patients with congenitally defective or absent ovaries. *Medicine (Baltimore)*, **44**, 135–164.

23 Flatley, F. J., Atwell, M. E. & McEvoy, R. K. (1963) Pseudoxanthoma elasticum with gastric hemorrhage. *Archives of Internal Medicine*, **112**, 352–356.

24 Fost, N. C. & Estorly, N. B. (1968) Successful treatment of juvenile haemangiomas with prednisone. *Journal of Pediatrics*, **72**, 351–357.

25 Frame, B., Dhanwada, S. R., Ohorodnik, J. M. & Kwa, D. M. (1977) Gastrointestinal haemorrhage in Turner's syndrome. *Archives of Internal Medicine*, **137**, 691–692.

26 Gentry, R., Dockerty, M. B. & Clagett, O. T. (1949) Vascular malformations and vascular tumours of the gastrointestinal tract. *International Abstracts of Surgery*, **88**, 281–323.

27 Ghahremani, G. G., Kangarloo, H., Volberg, F. & Meyers, M. A. (1976) Diffuse cavernous haemangioma of the colon in the Klippel–Trenaunay syndrome. *Radiology*, **118**, 673–678.

28 Golitz, L. E. (1980) Heritable cutaneous disorders that affect the gastrointestinal tract. *Medical Clinics of North America*, **64**, 829–846.

29 Goodman, R. M., Smith, E. W., Paton, D. *et al.* (1963) Pseudoxanthoma elasticum. A clinical and histopathological study. *Medicine (Baltimore)* **42**, 297–334.

30 Greenberg, G. R., Phillips, M. J., Tovee, E. B. & Jeejeebhoy K. N. (1976) Fibreoptic endoscopy during laparotomy in the diagnosis of small intestinal bleeding. *Gastroenterology*, **71**, 133–135.

31 Haddad, H. M. & Wilkins, L. (1959) Congenital anomalies associated with gonadal aplasia. Review of 55 cases. *Pediatrics*, **23**, 885–902.

32 Harris, R. D. (1974) Small bowel dilatation in Ehlers Danlos syndrome: an unreported gastrointestinal manifestation. *British Journal of Radiology*, **47**, 623–627.

33 Hines, C. Jr & Davis, W. D. (1973) Ehlers Danlos syndrome with megaduodenum and malabsorption syndrome secondary to bacterial overgrowth: a report of the first case. *American Journal of Medicine*, **54**, 539–543.

34 Hodgson, C. H., Burchell, H. B., Good, C. A. & Clagett, O. T. (1959) Hereditary haemorrhagic telangiectasia and pulmonary arteriovenous fistula survey of a large family. *New England Journal of Medicine*, **261**, 625–636.

35 Hollister, D. W. (1978) Heritable disorders of connective tissue: Ehlers–Danlos syndrome. *Pediatric Clinics of North America*, **25**, 575–591.

36 Howard, O. M., Buchanan, J. D. & Hunt, R. H. (1982) Angiodysplasia of the colon. Experience of 26 cases. *Lancet*, **ii**, 16–19.

37 Hulke, J. W. (1876) *Lancet*, **ii**, 857. Referred to by Shepherd, J. A. (1953) *British Journal of Surgery*, **40**, 409–421.

38 Ikeda, K., Murayama, H., Takano, H. *et al.* (1980) Massive intestinal bleeding in haemangiomatosis of the duodenum. *Endoscopy*, **12**, 306–310.

39 Jackson, A. E. & Peterson, C. (1967) Haemangioma of the small intestine causing protein-losing enteropathy *Annals of Internal Medicine*, **66**, 1190–1196.

40 Jeghers, H., McKusick, V. A. & Katz, K. H. (1949) Generalised intestinal polyposis and melanin spots of oral mucosa, lips and digits: syndrome of diagnostic significance. *New England Journal of Medicine*, **241**, 993.

41 Kaplan, L. & Hartman, S. W. (1954) Elastica disease. Case of Gronblad–Strandberg syndrome with gastrointestinal haemorrhage. *Archives of Internal Medicine*, **94**, 489–492.

42 Katz, D., Douvres, P., Weisberg, H. *et al.* (1964) Sources of bleeding in upper gastro-intestinal haemorrhage: a re-evaluation. *American Journal of Digestive Diseases*, **9**, 447–458.

43 Krane, S. M. (1980) Understanding genetic disorders of collagen. *New England Journal of Medicine*, **303**, 101–102.

44 Krieg, T. (1981) Molecular defects of collagen metabolism in the Ehlers Danlos syndrome. *International Journal of Dermatology*, **20**, 415–425.

45 Lindenauer, S. M. (1965) The Klippel Trenaunay syndrome: varicosity, hypertrophy and haemangioma with no arteriovenous fistula. *American Surgeon*, **162**, 303–314.

46 Lisser, H., Curtis, L. E., Escamilla, R. F. *et al.* (1947) The syndrome of congenital aplastic ovaries with sexual infantilism, high urinary gonadotrophins, short stature and other congenital abnormalities. *Journal of Clinical Endocrinology*, **7**, 665–687.

47 Lombardo, P. C. (1969) Pseudoxanthoma elasticum. *Archives of Dermatology*, **99**, 370–372.

48 Marine, R. & Lattomus, W. W. (1958) Cavernous haemangioma of the gastrointestinal tract. *Radiology*, **70**, 860–863.

49 McCauley, R. G. K., Leonidas, J. C. & Bartoshesky, L. E. (1979) Blue rubber bleb naevus syndrome. *Radiology*, **133**, 375–377.

50 McGrath, K. M., Johnson, C. A. & Stuart, J. J. (1979) Acquired von Willebrand disease associated with an inhibitor to factor VIII antigen and gastrointestinal telangiectasia. *American Journal of Medicine*, **67**, 693–696.

51 McKay, E. R. & Clark, H. R. (1957) Mixed cavernous and capillary hemangiomatosis involving the large bowel. *Journal of International College of Surgeons*, **27**, 218–225.

52 McKusick, V. A. (1974) Multiple forms of the Ehlers Danlos syndrome. *Archives of Surgery*, **109**, 475–476.

53 McKusick, V. A., Froelich, J., Callahan, R. J. *et al.* (1981) ^{99m}Tc-labelled red blood cells for detection of gastrointestinal bleeding: experience with 80 patients. *American Journal of Roentgenology*, **137**, 1113–1118.

54 Menefee, M. G., Flessa, H. C., Glueck, H. I. & Hogg, S. P. (1975) Hereditary haemorrhagic telangiectasia (Osler–Rendu–Weber disease): An electron microscopic study of the vascular lesions before and after therapy with hormones. *Archives of Otolaryngology*, **101**, 246–251.

55 Meyer, C. T., Troncale, F. J., Galloway, S. & Sheahan, D. G. (1981) Arteriovenous malformations of the bowel: an analysis of 22 cases and a review of the literature. *Medicine (Baltimore)*, **60**, 36–48.

56 Miles, R. M., Crawford, D. & Duras, S. (1979) The small bowel tumour problem. An assessment based on a 20 year experience with 116 cases. *American Surgeon*, **189**, 732.

57 Mistretta, C. A., Crummy, A. B. & Strother, C. M. (1981) Digital angiography: a perspective. *Radiology*, **139**, 273–276.

58 Murray-Lyon, I. M., Doyle, D., Philpott, R. M. & Porter, N. H. (1971) Haemangiomatosis of the small and large bowel with histological malignant change. *Journal of Pathology*, **105**, 295–297.

59 Nader, P. R. & Margolin, F. (1966) Haemangioma causing gastrointestinal bleeding. *American Journal of Diseases of Children*, **111**, 215–222.

60 Nyman, U., Boijsen, E., Lindstrom, C. & Rosengren, J. E. (1980) Angiography in angiomatous lesions of the gastrointestinal tract. *Acta Radiologica Diagnosis (Stockholm)* **21**, 21–31.

61 Nys, A. & Buyssens, N. (1963) Diffuse cavernous haemangiomatosis of the small intestine. *Gastroenterology*, **45**, 663–666.

62 O'Helleran, M. & Merrell, R. C. (1981) Pseudoxanthoma elasticum and polyposis coli: a novel co-mutation. *Archives of Surgery*, **116**, 476–477.

63 Ona, F. V. & Ahluwalia, M. (1980) Endoscopic appearance of gastric angiodysplasia in hereditary haemorrhagic telangiectasia. *American Journal of Gastroenterology*, **73**, 148–149.

64 Parkes-Weber, F. (1918) Haemangiectatic hypertrophy of limbs: congenital phlebarteriectasis and so-called congenital varicose veins. *British Journal of Childrens Diseases*, **15**, 13.

65 Peoples, J. B., Kartha, R. & Sharif, S. (1981) Multiple phlebectasia of the small intestine. *American Surgeon*, **47**, 373–376.

66 Phillips, G. N., Gordon, D. H., Martin, E. C. *et al.* (1978) The Klippel–Trenaunay syndrome: clinical and radiological aspects. *Radiology*, **128**, 429–434.

67 Pinkerton, J. A. Jr. (1979) Intraoperative Doppler localisation of intestinal arteriovenous malformation. *Surgery*, **85**, 427–474.

68 Raiford, T. S. (1932) Tumours of the small intestine. *Archives of Surgery*, **25**, 122–177, 321–325.

69 Ramsay, D. M., Buist, T. A. S., Macleod, D. A. D. & Heading, R. C. (1976) Persistent gastrointestinal bleeding due to angiodysplasia of the gut in von Willebrand's disease. *Lancet*, **ii**, 275–278.

70 Redondo, D. & Swenson, O. (1967) Gastrointestinal bleeding associated with gonadal aplasia. *Surgery*, **61**, 285–287.

71 Reuter, S. & Bookstein, J. (1968) Angiographic localisation of gastrointestinal bleeding. *Gastroenterology*, **54**, 876–883.

72 Rissier, H. L. Jr. (1959) Hemangiomatosis of the intestine. *Gastroenterologia*, **93**, 357–385.

73 River, L., Silverstein, J. & Tope, J. W. (1956) Benign neoplasms of the small intestine: a critical comprehensive review with reports of 20 new cases. *International Abstracts of Surgery*, **102**, 1–38.

74 Rosborough, J. K. & Swaim, W. R., (1978) Acquired von Willebrand's disease, platelet release defect and angiodysplasia. *American Journal of Medicine*, **65**, 96–100.

75 Rösch, J., Keller, F. S., Wawrukiewicz, A. S. *et al.* (1982) Pharmacoangiography in the diagnosis of recurrent massive lower gastrointestinal bleeding. *Radiology*, **145**, 615–619.

76 Rosen, K. M., Sirota, D. K. & Marinoff, S. C. (1967)

Gastrointestinal bleeding in Turner's syndrome. *Annals of Internal Medicine*, **67**, 145–150.

77 Rutlin, E., Wisløff, E., Myren, J. & Serck-Hanssen, A. (1981) Intestinal telangiectasia in Turner's syndrome. *Endoscopy*, **13**, 86–87.

78 Schultz, L. S., Assimacopoulos, C. A. & Lillehei, R. C. (1970) Turner's syndrome with associated gastrointestinal bleeding: a case report. *Surgery*, **68**, 485–488.

79 Scott, T. (1968) Turner's syndrome and verniform phlebectasia of the bowel. *Transactions American Clinical Climatological Association*, **79**, 45–50.

80 Shandalow, S. L. (1956) Fatal massive gastrointestinal haemorrhage due to multiple phlebectasia of the small intestine. *Journal of the International College of Surgeons*, **24**, 445–447.

81 Shepherd, J. A. (1953) Angiomatous conditions of the gastrointestinal tract. *American Journal of Surgery*, **40**, 409–421.

82 Sogge, M. R. (1980) Detection of typical lesions of hereditary haemorrhagic telangiectasia by colonoscopy. *Gastroenterological Endoscopy*, **26**, 52–53.

83 Spechler, S. J. & Schimmel, E. M. (1982) Gastrointestinal tract bleeding of unknown origin. *Archives of Internal Medicine*, **142**, 236–240.

84 Stening, S. G. & Heptinstall, D. P. (1970) Diffuse cavernous haemangioma of the rectum and sigmoid colon. *British Journal of Surgery*, **57**, 186–189.

85 Storino, W. D. & Engel, G. H., (1973) Multiple capillary haemangiomatosis. Acquired case with adult onset. *Archives of Dermatology*, **107**, 739–740.

86 Taylor, T. V. & Torrance, H. B. (1974) Haemangioma of the gastrointestinal tract. *British Journal of Surgery*, **61**, 236–238.

87 Uitto, J. (1979) Biochemistry of the elastic fibres in normal connective tissues and its alterations in diseases. *Journal of Investigative Dermatology*, **72**, 1–8.

88 Vase, P. (1981) Estrogen treatment of hereditary hemorrhagic telangiectasia: a double-blind controlled clinical trial. *Acta Medica Scandinavica*, **209**, 393–396.

89 Willis, R. A. (1962) Hamartomas and hamartomatous syndromes. In *The Borderland of Embryology and Pathology* 2nd edn (Ed.) Willis, B. A. pp. 351–392. London: Butterworths.

90 Wilson, J. M., Melvin, D. B., Gray, G. & Thorbjarnarson, B. (1975) Benign small bowel tumour. *American Surgeon*, **181**, 247–250.

ANGIODYSPLASIA OF THE GUT

Vascular abnormalities of the gastrointestinal tract have attracted increasing interest in recent years. Although there have been numerous isolated reports in the literature since the first description by Phillips in 1839[34] of an erectile vascular tumour of the rectum, few series of patients with gastrointestinal bleeding have identified vascular malformations as a source of haemorrhage. As many as a quarter of patients with bleeding may go undiagnosed.[14] However, once diagnosed and the location and anatomical extent of a lesion are known, the management may be relatively easy.

The classification of vascular abnormalities of the gastrointestinal tract has become confused by the variety of terms which have been used synonymously to describe these malformations as mentioned earlier in this chapter (see Table 5.1). Problems of terminology have been compounded by a lack of conformity both within and between disciplines. In the recent literature, radiologists and endoscopists have often used terminology normally used in histopathology. Vascular lesions cause gastrointestinal bleeding when they involve the mucosa, but the abnormality may extend through the submucosa so that the term 'mucosal vascular abnormality' is open to criticism. I prefer the general term 'vascular abnormality' as an endoscopic or radiological description, reserving all others for a confirmed histological diagnosis.

This review is confined to the benign vascular lesion of the gut known as angiodysplasia; some classifications refer to it as 'non-hereditary telangiectasia'.[21] Some mention will also be made of hereditary telangiectasia and true haemangiomas, as clinically these may present in an identical fashion.

True angiomas are relatively rare in the gastrointestinal tract while telangiectasias are more common and often multiple. The most frequently recognized telangiectatic lesion is found in the right colon and commonly described as angiodysplasia,[8, 24, 38] arteriovenous malformation or vascular dysplasia. These lesions appear to be degenerative and the term vascular ectasia has been suggested by Mitsudo et al.[31] In contrast Weaver et al.[44] propose a spectrum of vascular lesions ranging from true hereditary haemorrhagic telangiectasia (HHT) through angiodysplasia to radiation associated telangiectasia. Mucosal vessels in angiodysplasia are small, ectatic and dilated, and similar to those seen in HHT, while haemangiomas show neovascularization with vessels of varying size displacing adjacent tissue.

Aetiology and pathology of angiodysplasia

The lesions of angiodysplasia (Figures 5.6 and 5.7) are most commonly seen in the caecum and ascending colon but their frequency in the population is not known. Some workers believe that the lesions are unique to the right colon[8] although others have reported similar lesions elsewhere in the colon[30] and in the stomach.[10, 15, 37, 38, 44]

Baum et al.[4] suggest that angiodysplasia is an acquired lesion resulting from mucosal ischaemia, secondary to arteriovenous shunting in

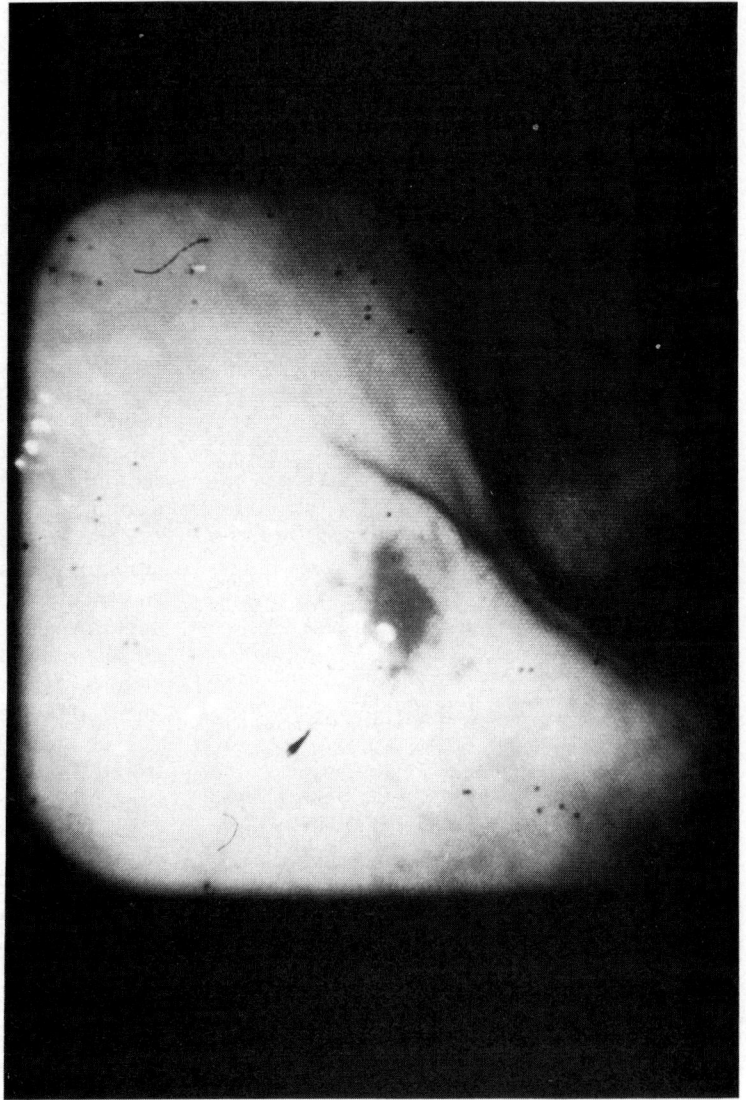

Fig. 5.6 Angiodysplasia lesion lying above the ileo-caecal valve. The lesion is cherry red, the dilated central vessel is under tension, with smaller radiating peripheral capillaries.

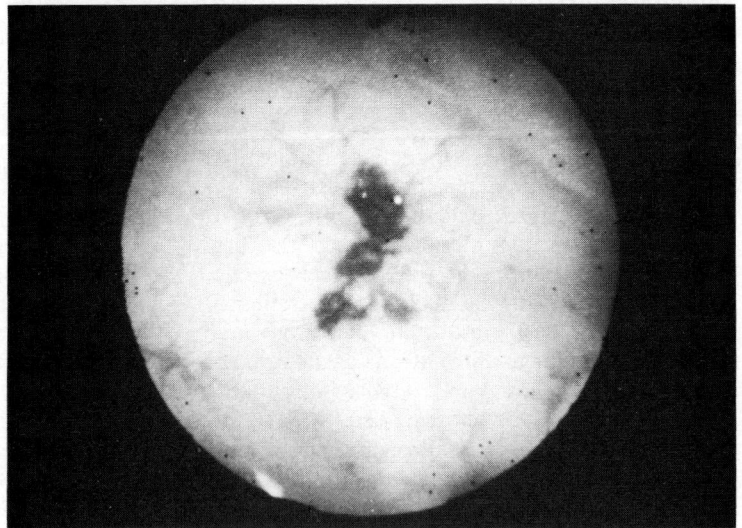

Fig. 5.7 Angiodysplasia lesion in the caecum. The lesion is bright red and the dilated irregular superficial vessels can be clearly seen.

the mucosa which occurs with changes in intra-colonic pressure.

Galloway *et al.*,[20] who confirmed earlier reports of an association with aortic stenosis, believe that the lesions develop as a consequence of decreased perfusion pressure in the terminal branches of the superior mesenteric artery, secondary to a decreased left ventricular output. A similar association with aortic valve disease and also chronic lung disease was noted by Rogers[38] whose patients were all diagnosed at colonoscopy. He has proposed that a lowered oxygen tension in the end-arterial vessels of the superior mesenteric artery results in capillary dilatation and proliferation, eventually leading to a vascular abnormality.

Boley *et al.*[7, 8, 31] hold the firm view that those lesions which occur in the right colon and caecum represent a separate and unique entity from other vascular lesions of the gastro-intestinal tract. They base their conclusions on the evidence obtained from elegant injection techniques and painstaking study of the histopathology of the lesions. They explain the aetiology by a chronic intermittent partial obstruction of the submucosal veins at the point where they pass through the longitudinal and circular muscle layers of the bowel. This occlusion of the low pressure veins occurs over many years and does not affect the higher pressure arterial inflow. The resulting pressure differential causes capillary vessel and later capillary ring dilatation with subsequent precapillary sphincter incompetence. Small arteriovenous malformations thus develop at the level of the mucosal capillaries. They attribute the frequency with which this lesion is now observed in the right colon to Laplace's law. When applied to the colon this states that the tension in the muscles of the bowel wall will be greater in that part of the colon with the greatest diameter, which is the caecum and right colon.[43] From their extensive work Boley *et al.*[7, 8] suggested that if angiodysplasia were due to ageing, lesions should be present in the colon of elderly patients who have not yet bled. They carried out injection and histopathological studies of the colon in a control group of 15 patients and identified mucosal ectasia in 27% and a large dilated submucosal vein in 53%.

In contrast Weaver *et al.*, who described lesions similar to angiodysplasia in the stomach[44] as well as the colon, have suggested a spectrum of vascular abnormalities of the gastrointestinal tract with the inherited Osler–Weber–Rendu lesions at one end and acquired lesions at the other.

The pathology of angiodysplasia of the right colon has been detailed by Mitsudo *et al.*[31] who have shown a spectrum from small early focal lesions to multiple large lesions. Superficial mucosal capillaries may or may not be dilated and mildly compress the lamina propria and communicate with a tortuous dilated submucosal vein. In more advanced cases, submucosal changes are more apparent and there is marked ectasia of mucosal vessels and the submucosal veins become increasingly tortuous and dilated while the arteries remain normal. The submucosal veins communicate with mucosal capillaries which are continuous with large or small groups of dilated vessels compressing the surrounding crypts. In severe cases, the capillary wall and attenuated epithelium are all that separate the capillary lumen from the colonic lumen (Figure 5.8). It is clear from these observations how easily the wall may rupture and result in severe colonic bleeding. A careful search by the histopathologist may reveal the site of bleeding (Figure 5.9).

Anatomical distribution of vascular abnormalities

Oesophagus

Haemangiomas may occur rarely in the oesophagus, accounting for about 2% of all benign oesophageal lesions in one series,[18] although only 29 cases are recorded in the literature. The lesions of hereditary haemorrhagic telangiectasia may be encountered in the oesophagus, but are less common than in the stomach or small and large bowel. It is wise not to biopsy suspect vascular lesions in the oesophagus.[18]

Stomach

Vascular lesions in the stomach may be localized or diffuse, the latter being increasingly recognized. A recent study has suggested a frequency of up to 1 in 285 upper gastro-intestinal endoscopies.[5] Apart from the lesions seen in hereditary haemorrhagic telangiectasia, an association has been suggested with previous abdominal radiation,[7] with the CRST (calcinosis, Raynaud's syndrome, sclerodactyly and telangiectasia) syndrome, and with von Willebrand's disease.[13, 28, 44]

Diffuse gastric antral vascular abnormality. Several reports have appeared in the last five years describing a gastric antral vascular abnormality radiating from the pylorus.[12, 15, 26, 45] To the inexperienced endoscopist this may appear as a linear gastritis with apparently normal

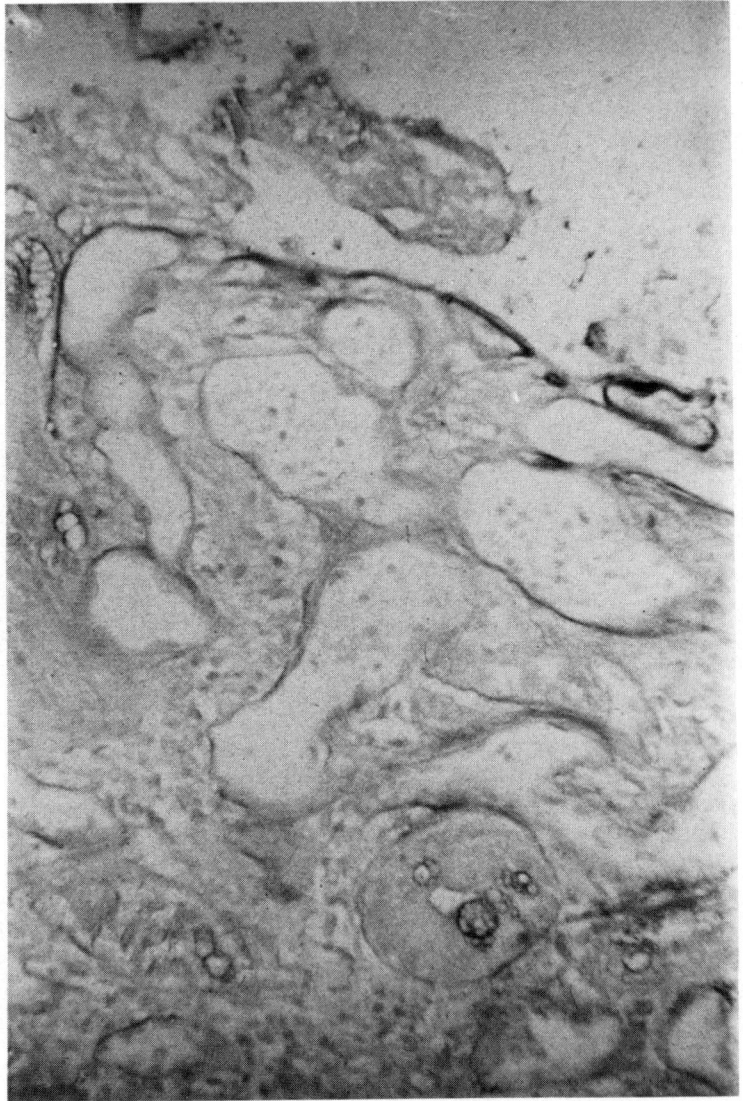

Fig. 5.8 Coagulation biopsy specimen (× 250). Dilated ectatic thin-walled superficial capillaries with effete red cells in the vessels. The vessel wall adjacent to the colonic lumen has no protective overlying mucosa.

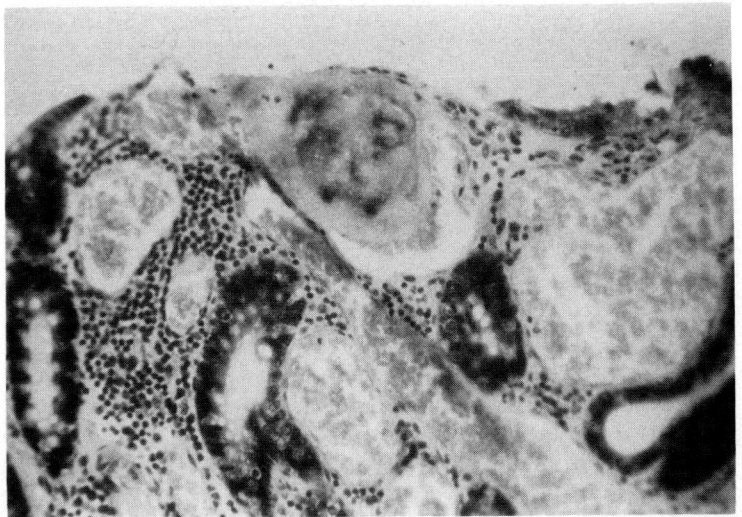

Fig. 5.9 Gross specimen (× 16). Shows tortuous submucosal vessels communicating with two areas of mucosal angiodysplasia (upper right and upper left). A platelet thrombus plugs the site of haemorrhage (upper right).

gastric mucosa between. Histology reveals a mass of tortuous dilated vessels.

Patients invariably present with recurrent anaemia, sometimes over many years. I have seen two such lesions, both in women with a histological diagnosis of primary biliary cirrhosis (although anti-mitochondrial antibodies were negative). One of these patients who had suffered from chronic anaemia ceased to bleed after oral corticosteroid therapy, a response which has also been reported by Calam and Walker.[12] These observations require confirmation, as partial gastrectomy is usually curative.

Gastric haemangioma. Gastric haemangiomas are rare; less than 50 cases have been published in the world literature. They usually present with chronic bleeding and may be polypoid in appearance, making differential diagnosis from other lesions initially difficult.

Duodenum and small bowel
Vascular abnormalities which affect the duodenal mucosa may be readily seen at endoscopy, but this is less readily available for small bowel lesions. Hereditary haemorrhagic telangiectasia usually affects the duodenum[32, 35] and frequently the small bowel. Non-hereditary telangiectasias and haemangiomas are also relatively common at these sites.

Blood loss may be mild, moderate or exsanguinating, and is more common from sessile lesions; polypoid haemangiomas more commonly produce partial or complete intestinal obstruction.

Developments in selective angiography and peroperative colonoscopy extended through to the small bowel have provided major clinical advances in the management of patients with bleeding from suspected vascular abnormalities in the small intestine.

Colon
Angiodysplasia of the right colon and caecum is the most commonly encountered vascular abnormality in the gastrointestinal tract. Lesions have been recognized by radiologists since the initial report by Margulis et al.[27] and the development of selective mesenteric angiography.[1, 3, 22, 42] Colonoscopic diagnosis of the lesions of angiodysplasia were first reported in 1976 by Skibba et al.[41] and by Rogers and Adler,[39] and are now recognized as an important cause of colonic bleeding which should be exhaustively sought by the colonoscopist.[24] Meticulous cleansing of the colon is essential when colonoscopy is performed in these cases.[33]

Diagnosis of angiodysplasia may be made at the time of operation immediately after segmental resection if a careful examination of the mucosal surface of the colon is made.[23] Although changes may be seen on the serosal surface of the colon at surgery with angiomatous lesions, this is not the case with angiodysplasia. This distinction emphasizes the importance of defining the extent of angiodysplasia by both colonoscopy and angiography when surgery is contemplated.

Clinical features

Vascular abnormalities of the gut may affect patients of all age groups, with hereditary telangiectasia and angiomas being more common in the younger patients while degenerative vascular ectasias are almost exclusively seen in the elderly. Sex incidence appears to be almost equal.

Patients usually present with anaemia which may be marked and many, especially those with mucosal angiodysplasia, will have experienced one or more episodes of overt gastrointestinal bleeding. This may vary from slow occult blood loss to massive haemorrhage with hypovolaemic shock.[24a] The pattern of bleeding may vary both within and between individuals but, even when severe, each episode is usually self limiting. Bleeding is often bright red or maroon-coloured from colonic or small bowel lesions, but a history of tarry stools may also be obtained. Typically patients with colonic vascular ectasias have often had one or more operations for a diagnosis such as duodenal ulcer or diverticular disease which had been thought to be the site of blood loss.[24a]

A careful history and physical examination should be taken in order to exclude the Osler–Weber–Rendu syndrome or von Willebrand's disease.[13, 28, 36, 44] It is not clear if the pathology of the vascular lesions associated with von Willebrand's disease correlate with the angiodysplasia lesions described by Mitsudo et al.[31]

Vascular abnormalities in the colon may be associated with aortic valve stenosis[7, 9, 38, 47] although few cases have been confirmed by cardiac catheterization. Aortic sclerosis, hypertension and other cardiovascular disorders are also common, although they may be chance associations due to ageing.

Diagnosis

Until recent years, vascular abnormalities in the gastrointestinal tract have been diagnosed almost exclusively by radiological means. With the widespread use of flexible fibreoptic endoscopy, more lesions are now diagnosed at routine upper gastrointestinal endoscopy or at colonoscopy.

A plain X-ray film of the abdomen may reveal calcification in a large angioma. Barium studies are seldom helpful unless lesions project into the lumen; most vascular abnormalities are flat or have a low profile and extend within the submucosa, making them invisible to these conventional investigations. The development of selective three-vessel angiography[1, 3, 4, 22, 42] has enabled the radiologist to identify the site and cause of bleeding. Further experience using subtraction film techniques has defined important radiological criteria for diagnosis. For angiodysplasia of the colon these include a vascular tuft, representing the mucosal capillary network, an early filling vein and a dense, slowly emptying vein (Figure 5.10).[7, 20] These features may be present alone or in combination.

In patients with a history of gastrointestinal bleeding, fibreoptic endoscopy should be undertaken before selective angiography is considered and will often provide the diagnosis, especially when the endoscopist has a high index of suspicion and makes a meticulous search for a lesion. Selective angiography may be valuable as a complementary investigation to confirm the extent of a lesion and exclude any additional lesions.

The endoscopic appearance of a vascular abnormality depends upon its nature. In the stomach, a diffuse antral vascular abnormality has been likened to an octopus with limbs which radiate from the pylorus. The surface is nodular with tortuous vessels which blanch on pressure with the biopsy forceps (Figure 5.11). Telangiec-

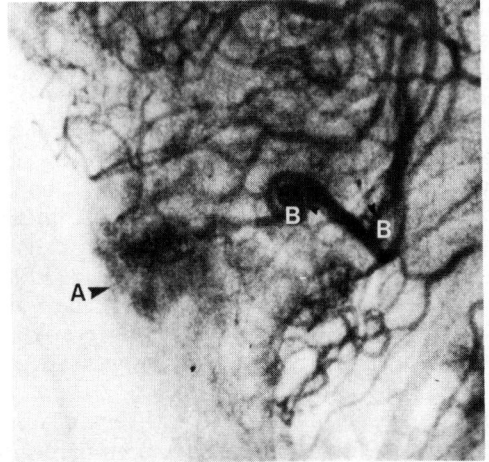

Fig. 5.10 Superior mesenteric angiogram in the arterial phase showing the vascular tuft of a large caecal angiodysplasia (A), and the dilated early draining vein (B). (Courtesy of Dr S. Somers.)

tasia in the stomach are more common in the fundus or body and are discrete, bright red lesions about 5 mm in diameter with a raised central bleb.

Angiodysplasia lesions in the right colon are similar to telangiectasia seen in the stomach. They are cherry-red in colour and usually about 5 mm in size (Figures 5.6 and 5.7), although they can be much larger (Figure 5.12). There is usually an elevated dilated central vessel, which is visibly distended, and radiating peripheral vessels.

Radionuclide studies are unhelpful in the diagnosis of vascular abnormalities unless there is active bleeding at the time of the study. technetium-99m sulphur colloid[2] or $^{99}Tc^m$-labelled red cells[29] have been successfully used as a screening test to see if the patient is bleeding

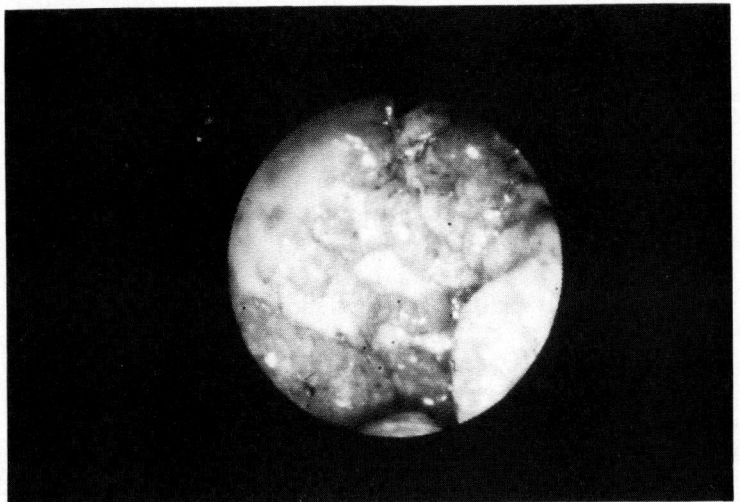

Fig. 5.11 Endoscopic view of the gastric antrum showing the angioma radiating from the pylorus which lies at the bottom right.

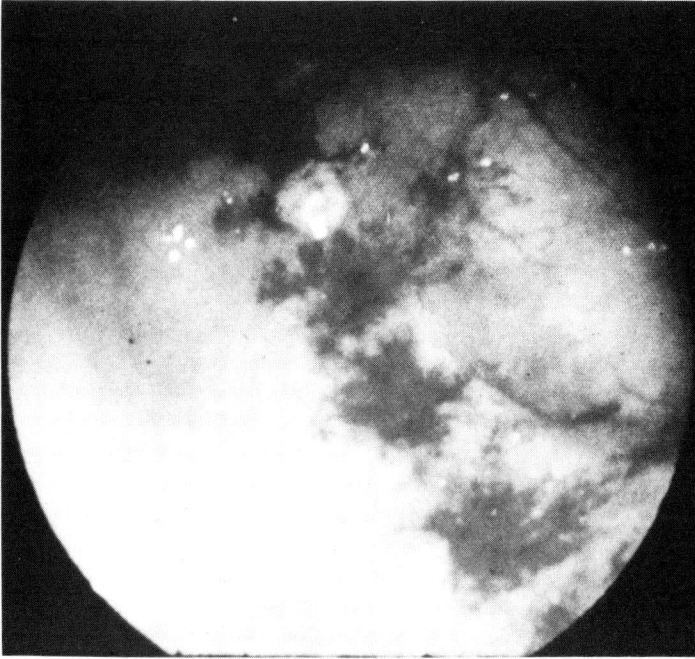

Fig. 5.12 Colonoscopic view of multiple angiodysplasia lesions in the caecum which follow the taenia coli. Ulceration of a lesion is seen in the upper part of the picture.

rapidly enough for formal angiography to identify the site of bleeding. technetium-99m sodium pertechnetate may be used to detect a Meckel's diverticulum.[25]

In the event that none of these investigations confirms a diagnosis, laparotomy is often considered if the patient shows evidence of continued blood loss, yet positive diagnosis is made at laparotomy in only half the cases in a paediatric series.[40] With modern diagnostic methods, most lesions may be detected without the necessity for surgery. Laparotomy is best reserved to manage life-threatening haemorrhage rather than to identify an otherwise undetected lesion.[6] If diagnostic laparotomy is performed, it is wise to consider the use of intraoperative endoscopy. Peroperative colonoscopy of the large bowel extended through to the small bowel may be valuable to transilluminate the intestinal wall in the search for vascular abnormalities. The surgeon views from the serosal aspect and pleats the bowel segments over the colonoscope, which is passed under direct vision by the endoscopist.[11, 17]

Treatment

When bleeding is severe, initial efforts are directed towards resuscitation before identifying the site and cause of bleeding. Although most vascular abnormalities can present as gastrointestinal bleeding, many episodes are self-limiting or lead to chronic blood loss.

Emergency surgery may be necessary for life-threatening haemorrhage, but with its increased morbidity and mortality it is not warranted until the diagnosis has been established and definitive surgery can be planned.

Most extensive vascular abnormalities will require resection, although limited angiodysplasia lesions in the caecum and right colon[24, 38] and telangiectasia in the stomach[15, 16, 44] have been treated at endoscopy by electrocoagulation using the Williams coagulation forceps,[24, 24a, 38, 46] a button electrode[15] or laser therapy.[19]

Results of these methods have been promising,[15, 24, 38, 44] especially for angiodysplasia of the right colon and caecum obviating the need for major surgery in an elderly high-risk population. For these lesions the coagulation forceps[24, 24a, 38, 46] are preferable to the button electrode which is more likely to result in perforation of the thin-walled caecum.

When vascular abnormalities are numerous or extensive, patients should undergo upper gastrointestinal endoscopy, colonoscopy and triple vessel angiography prior to surgery to assess the full extent of the lesion, and peroperative endoscopy may be useful to define the point of resection.

Conclusion

Patients with gastrointestinal vascular abnormalities may go undiagnosed for many years.

Successful diagnosis and management is dependent upon a high index of suspicion, an appreciation of the diversity of lesions and an awareness of the increasing importance of angiodysplasia in the older population.

REFERENCES

1 Allison, D. J., Hemingway, A. P. & Cunningham, D. A. (1982) Angiography in gastrointestinal bleeding. *Lancet*, **ii**, 30–33.

2 Alavi, A. & Ring, E. J. (1981) Localization of gastrointestinal bleeding: superiority of ^{99m}Tc sulfur colloid compared with angiography. *American Journal of Radiology*, **137**, 741–748.

3 Baum, S., Nusbaum, M., Blakemore, W. S. & Finkelstein, A. K. (1965) The preoperative radiographic demonstration of intra-abdominal bleeding from undetermined sites by percutaneous selective celiac and superior mesenteric arteriography. *Surgery*, **58**, 797–805.

4 Baum, S., Athanasoulis, C. A., Waltman, A. C. et al. (1977) Angiodysplasia of the right colon: a cause of gastrointestinal bleeding. *American Journal of Roentgenology*, **129**, 789–794.

5 Blankenstein, M., Van., Dees, J. & Tenkate, F. J. W. (1978) Bleeding arteriovenous malformations diagnosed by endoscopy. *Gut*, **19**, 432.

6 Boley, S. J., Brandt, L. J. & Frank, M. S. (1981) Severe lower intestinal bleeding. *Clinics in Gastroenterology*, **10** (1), 65–91.

7 Boley, S. J., Sprayregan, S., Sammartano, R. J. et al. (1977) The pathophysiologic basis for the angiographic signs of vascular ectasias of the colon. *Diagnostic Radiology*, **125**, 615–621.

8 Boley, S. J., Sammartano, R., Adamas, A. et al. (1977) On the nature and aetiology of vascular ectasias of the colon: degenerative lesions of aging. *Gastroenterology*, **72**, 650–660.

9 Boss, E. G. & Rosenbaum, J. M. (1971) Bleeding from the right colon associated with aortic stenosis. *American Journal of Digestive Diseases*, **16**, 269–275.

10 Bourdette, D. & Greenberg, B. (1979) Twelve year history of gastrointestinal bleeding in a patient with calcific aortic stenosis and haemorrhagic telangiectasia. *Digestive Disease and Sciences*, **24**, 77–82.

11 Bowden, T. A., Hooks, V. H. & Mansberger, A. R. (1979) Intraoperative gastrointestinal endoscopy. *Annals of Surgery*, **191**, 680–687.

12 Calam, J. & Walker, R. J. (1980) Antral vascular lesion, achlorhydria and chronic gastrointestinal blood loss. *Digestive Diseases and Sciences*, **25**, 236–239.

13 Cass, A. J., Bliss, B. P., Bolton, R. P. & Cooper, B. T. (1980) Gastrointestinal bleeding, angiodysplasia of the colon and acquired Von Willebrand's disease. *British Journal of Surgery*, **67**, 639–641.

14 Catem, W. S. & Jiminez, F. A. (1963) Vascular malformations of the intestines: their role as a source of haemorrhage. *Archives of Surgery*, **86**, 571–579.

15 Colin-Jones, D. G. (1984) Vascular malformations of the upper G.I. tract. In *Advances in Gastrointestinal Endoscopy*, (Ed.) Salmon, P. R. London: Chapman and Hall. (In press)

16 Farup, P. G., Rosseland, A., Stray, N. et al. (1981) Localised telangiopathy of the stomach and duodenum diagnosed and treated endoscopically. *Endoscopy*, **12**, 1–6.

17 Forde, K. A. (1981) Intraoperative colonoscopy. In *Colonoscopy Techniques, Clinical Practice and Colour Atlas*, (Ed.) Hunt, R. H. & Waye, J. D. pp. 189–198 London: Chapman and Hall.

18 Foster, C. A., Yomehiro, E. G. & Benjamin, R. B. (1978) Oesophageal haemangioma. *Ear, Nose and Throat Journal*, **57**, 455–459.

19 Fruhmorgen, P., Bodem, F., Reidenbach, H. D. et al. (1976) Endoscopic laser coagulation of bleeding gastrointestinal lesions with report of the first therapeutic application in man. *Gastrointestinal Endoscopy*, **23**, 73–75.

20 Galloway, S. J., Casarella, W. J. & Shimkin, P. M. (1974) Vascular malformations of the right colon as a cause of bleeding in patients with aortic stenosis. *Radiology*, **113**, 11–15.

21 Gentry, R. W., Dockerty, M. B. & Clagett, O. T. (1949) Vascular malformations and vascular tumours of the gastrointestinal tract. *International Abstracts of Surgery*, **88**, 281–323.

22 Giacchino, J. L., Geis, W. P., Pickleman, J. R. et al. (1979) Changing perspectives in massive lower intestinal haemorrhage. *Surgery*, **86**, 368–376.

23 Heald, R. J. & Ray, J. E. (1974) Vascular malformations of the intestine: an important cause of obscure gastrointestinal haemorrhage. *Southern Medical Journal*, **67**, 33–38.

24 Howard, O. M., Buchanan, J. D. & Hunt, R. H. (1982) Angiodysplasia of the colon: experience of 26 cases. *Lancet*, **ii**, 16–19.

24a Hunt, R. M. (1984) Angiodysplasia of the colon. In *Advances in Gastrointestinal Endoscopy*, (Ed.) Salmon, P. R. pp. 97–114. London: Chapman and Hall. (In press)

25 Jewett, T. C., Duszinski, D. O. & Allen, J. F. (1970) The visualization of Meckel's diverticulum with ^{99m}Tc pertechnetate. *Surgery*, **68**, 567–570.

26 Lewis, T. D., Laufer, I. & Goodacre, R. L. (1978) Arteriovenous malformation of the stomach. *Digestive Diseases*, **23**, 467–471.

27 Margulis, A. R., Heinbecker, P. & Bernard, H. R. (1960) Operative mesenteric arteriography in the search for the site of bleeding in unexplained gastrointestinal bleeding. *Surgery*, **48**, 534–539.

28 McGrath, K. M., Johnson, C. A. & Stuart, J. J. (1979) Acquired von Willebrand disease associated with an inhibitor to factor VIII antigen and gastrointestinal telangiectasis. *American Journal of Medicine* **67**, 693–696.

29 McKusick, U. A., Froelich, J., Callahan, R. J. et al. (1981) ^{99m}Tc red blood cells for detection of gastrointestinal bleeding: experience with 80 patients. *American Journal of Roentgenology*, **137**, 1113–1118.

30 Miller, K. D., Tutton, R. H., Bell, K. A. & Simon, B. K. (1979) Angiodysplasia of the colon. *Radiology*, **132**, 309–313.

31 Mitsudo, S. M., Boley, S. J., Brandt, L. J. et al. (1979) Vascular ectasias of the right colon in the elderly: a district pathological entity. *Human Pathology*, **10**(5), 585–600.

32 Moore, J. D., Thompson, N. W., Appelman, H. D. & Foley, D. (1978) Arteriovenous malformations of the gastrointestinal tract. *Archives of Surgery*, **111**, 381–389.

33 Nagy, G. S. (1981) Preparing the patient. In *Colonoscopy, Techniques, Clinical Practice and Colour Atlas*, (Ed.) Hunt, R. H. & Waye, J. D. pp. 19–26. London: Chapman and Hall.

34 Phillips, B. (1839) Surgical cases. *London Medical Gazette*, **23**, 514–517.

35 Posner, D. E. & Sampliner, R. E. (1978) Hereditary haemorrhagic telangiectasis in three black men. *American Journal of Gastroenterology*, **70**, 389–392.

36 Ramsay, D. M., MacLeod, D. A. D., Buist, T. A. S. & Heading, R. C. (1976) Persistent gastrointestinal bleeding due to angiodysplasia of the gut in Von Willebrand's disease. *Lancet*, **ii**, 275–278.

37 Roberts, L. K., Gold, R. E. & Routt, W. E. (1981) Gastric angiodysplasia. *Radiology*, **139**, 355–359.

38 Rogers, B. H. G. (1980) Endoscopic diagnosis and therapy of mucosal vascular abnormality of the gastrointestinal tract occurring in elderly patients and associated with cardiac, vascular and pulmonary disease. *Gastrointestinal Endoscopy*, **26**, 134–138.

39 Rogers, B. H. G. & Adler, F. (1976) Hemangiomas of the caecum. *Gastroenterology*, **71**, 1079–1082.

40 Shandling, B. (1965) Laparotomy for rectal bleeding. *Pediatrics*, **35**, 787–793.

41 Skibba, R. M., Hartong, W. A., Mantz, F. A. *et al.* (1976) Angiodysplasia of the caecum: colonoscopic diagnosis. *Gastrointestinal Endoscopy*, **22**, 177–179.

42 Tarin, D., Allison, D. J., Modlin, I. M. & Neale, G. (1978) Diagnosis and management of obscure gastrointestinal bleeding. *British Medical Journal*, **ii**, 751–754.

43 Wangensteen, O. H. (1955) *Intestinal Obstruction*, 3rd edn. Springfield, Illinois: C. C. Thomas.

44 Weaver, G. A., Alpern, H. D., Davis, J. S. *et al.* (1979) Gastrointestinal angiodysplasia associated with aortic valve disease: part of a spectrum of angiodysplasia of the gut. *Gastroenterology*, **77**, 1–11.

45 Wheeler, M. H., Smith, P. M., Cotton, P. B. *et al.* (1979) Abnormal blood vessels in the gastric antrum. *Digestive Diseases and Sciences*, **24**, 155–158.

46 Williams, C. B. (1973) Diathermy-biopsy: a technique of endoscopic management of small polyps. *Endoscopy*, **5**, 215–218.

47 Williams, R. C. Jr. (1961) Aortic stenosis and unexplained gastrointestinal bleeding. *Archives of Internal Medicine*, **108**, 859–863.

ACUTE ISCHAEMIA OF THE GUT

The response of the gut to ischaemia is the same whatever the underlying cause. However, the clinical presentation and management of individual cases do not share in this uniformity. These will alter according to aetiology, as well as to factors such as the magnitude, extent, and duration of circulatory deprivation. In this section, certain general elements common to all cases of acute ischaemia will be examined and the major aetiological categories discussed. In general terms, when cases diagnosed or suspected in premortem patients only are included, about half of all cases of mesenteric infarction will be non-occlusive in origin. Acute occlusion of the superior mesenteric artery or its branches, occlusion of the inferior mesenteric artery, venous thrombosis and small vessel thrombosis are the other major causes.[2, 16]

GENERAL CONSIDERATIONS

Anatomical factors

Three major arteries supply the abdominal part of the gastrointestinal tract. The *coeliac axis*, through the left and right gastric, short gastric and right gastroepiploic arteries, provides a relatively rich blood supply to the stomach. The anterior and posterior superior pancreaticoduodenal arteries provide a dual blood supply to the duodenum, being continuous with the inferior pancreaticoduodenal vessels from the superior mesenteric artery or its proximal branches. Additional collateral circulation occurs between the branches of the coeliac and the superior mesenteric arteries supplying the pancreas. The *superior mesenteric artery* supplies the jejunum, the ileum and the colon to the splenic flexure. Arcades connect its branches, the most peripheral of these constituting the marginal artery. The marginal artery gives rise to short end-arteries to the intestinal wall known as the vasa recti. The *inferior mesenteric artery*, a much smaller vessel, supplies the left and sigmoid colon, and most of the rectum. It anastomoses with the superior mesenteric artery through a common marginal artery, and with the middle and inferior haemorrhoidal arteries, which are branches of the hypogastrics. The relatively short length of intestine supplied by the coeliac axis, its rich collateral connections and the dual nature of its end branches makes ischaemic lesions of the stomach and duodenum very rare. The first two factors also apply to the inferior mesenteric artery, and there is, again, a relatively low incidence of occlusive lesions in its distribution.

The venous drainage parallels the arteries, except that the four major channels – the coronary, splenic, superior mesenteric and inferior mesenteric veins – combine in a single trunk, the portal vein. Collateral channels between the veins, and to the somatic venous system, are so numerous that infarction from thrombosis is rare unless the peripheral veins are involved.

Physiological factors

The normal arterial flow to the gut is about 10% of the cardiac output. It varies under conditions of both exercise and digestion, and the regulation of flow is complex. Not only is there control of flow at the arteriolar level by vasoconstriction and vasodilatation, but there is also autoregulation at the level of the vasculature in the villi.

Extramucosal shunting is a third important factor in the control of circulation at the mucosal level.[12]

Flow is shown to increase in the presence of nutrients in the intestinal lumen. Endogenous hormones such as secretin, gastrin and cholecystokinin perhaps mediate this response. The influence of the autonomic nervous system on flow has also been demonstrated, but is complex and variable.

Flow can decrease in response to muscular activity or an increase in intraluminal pressure. Catecholamines and angiotensin II are potent reducers of blood flow. Cardiac glycosides also cause a decrease in flow due to a direct action at the arteriolar level. Under some circumstances of diminished cardiac output, flow may become severely reduced. Arteriolar constriction and extramucosal shunting may play an important role in promoting mucosal ischaemia, and their pharmacological reversal sometimes offers a useful avenue of therapy.

Pathophysiology

The first response to a degree of ischaemia sufficient to cause cell damage is noted in the mucosal layers. The earliest evidence of injury is in the submucosa and may be observed by electron microscopy after a period of ischaemia as short as ten minutes.[6] By thirty minutes, light microscopy also reveals changes. These take the form of submucosal oedema and then haemorrhage. Plain X-rays and barium studies at this stage show mounds of fullness, often termed 'thumb-printing'. Mucosal slough follows, leading to ulceration and the release of blood into the lumen. With restoration of an adequate circulation, these changes are reversible and mucosal regeneration follows. This may be a prolonged process with recurrent bleeding and a transient period of impaired absorption. The muscular layers are more resistant to ischaemic injury. Initially muscle spasm occurs, but with the passage of time an atonic state develops. With moderate degrees of injury, fibrous strictures sometimes form, which usually become apparent two to six weeks later. More profound injuries lead to loss of integrity for the entire bowel wall. A characteristic foul, bloody transudate occurs in the early stages and frank perforation follows. The process may be hastened by the presence of digestive enzymes in the small bowel and by an inflammatory component in the colon. Serosal injury, especially in the colon, may lead to adhesive exudates preventing general soilage for a time. Details of the patho-

physiological process and its investigational background may be found in the review articles by Williams[22] and by Boley *et al.*[2]

The severity of intestinal injury reflects both the degree and the duration of the interruption of vascular flow. Extramucosal shunting and intraluminal pressure may worsen the injury. However, collateral flow in the arcades or marginal vessels distal to a site of arterial or venous occlusion and in intramural vessels may protect the peripheral portions of the bowel segment involved from injury. Both arterial spasm and a fall in cardiac output may contribute to the fall in perfusion; infarction may be precipitated by this means after a period of symptomatic ischaemia, even in the absence of worsening of the initial lesion. This is a major factor in producing the variety of clinical presentations so characteristic of mesenteric infarction.

Ischaemia may also cause abnormalities of motility and absorption, and intraluminal bleeding. With extensive tissue necrosis, metabolic acidosis and the systemic results of the release of vasoactive substances are sometimes observed.

Clinical presentation

Cases of acute intestinal injury, despite their varied aetiologies, are similar in clinical presentation. Though in many ways nonspecific, this presentation is characteristic, and will almost always suggest the diagnosis. The single most striking element is abdominal pain. In some cases this is the result of muscle spasm or perforation with peritonitis. In the majority of patients, however, the pain is visceral and caused specifically by the ischaemia. Such pain is dull rather than sharp, constant rather than colicky, and is rather poorly localized, though the region of referral bears some relationship to the site of the injury. It may range from mild to remarkably severe.

Ischaemic pain does not necessarily imply tissue necrosis. The pain observed in syndromes of chronic ischaemia supports this fact. Furthermore, some cases of mesenteric infarction are preceded by hours or even days of such pain before an actual ischaemic injury is sustained. Nevertheless, pain is the most reliable and, at times, the only symptom marking the onset of infarction.

Ischaemia may influence intestinal motility, resulting in nausea, vomiting, bloating or diarrhoea. These features are so unspecific as to be of little diagnostic value.

Finally, intestinal bleeding is a usual result of mucosal infarction, leading to gross or occult blood in the gastric and rectal contents in the majority of patients.

The combination of these nonspecific elements will in most patients suggest the diagnosis of mesenteric infarction. However, the diagnosis is sometimes elusive in the early stages, particularly in the presence of symptoms and signs of related or unrelated disorders. Later, with the appearance of peritonitis, the diagnosis is more obvious, but by then irreversible injuries are to be expected, and the likelihood of survival declines accordingly.

Diagnosis

Laboratory determinations have little value in establishing the diagnosis in mesenteric ischaemia or infarction. The white cell count may be elevated, the extent to some degree reflecting the volume of infarcted tissue. Thus counts in excess of $20 \times 10^9/l$ are frequently recorded, but in other cases of extensive infarction the count is normal. The serum amylase is elevated in about one half of patients, but seldom exceeds twice normal and rarely reaches the level expected in acute pancreatitis. Thus laboratory determinations are useful mainly in eliminating other causes of acute abdominal pain.

Plain X-rays of the abdomen are also seldom diagnostic.[21] In rare cases, spasm of the small bowel leads to a striking lack of bowel gas. The portal venous system may be filled with gas in late cases of extensive infarction. In the majority of cases, though, only dilatation of the bowel in a nonspecific pattern of ileus is observed. With acute superior mesenteric artery occlusion there may be dilatation of the small and proximal large bowel, suggesting obstruction of the transverse colon. On the whole, just as with laboratory tests, plain films are mainly useful for excluding other causes of abdominal pain.

Conversely, angiography offers a specific diagnosis in many cases. A lateral aortogram may demonstrate obstruction of the origin of the mesenteric vessels. Selective studies show more peripheral arterial blocks. Less specific findings may be noted in cases of venous occlusion and non-occlusive infarction. Angiograms are, therefore, perhaps most useful in the patient with appropriate symptoms and a suspected diagnosis of mesenteric occlusion. In cases where the diagnosis seems more certain and the study would impose more than a slight delay, a laparotomy is a better diagnostic measure. If peritonitis is already present, delay is never acceptable.

An additional potential value of angiograms in superior mesenteric artery occlusion is the provision of anatomical information that will aid the surgeon in selecting the best type of reconstruction.[15] Angiographic techniques also provide a potent means of relieving mesenteric spasm through the direct infusion of antispasmodic drugs. Under the proper circumstances this may restore sufficient arterial flow to limit or prevent infarction. The clinical application is in practice sometimes limited by difficulty in patient selection and in integrating perfusion with surgical intervention.[2, 3]

NON-OCCLUSIVE INFARCTION

The place of non-occlusive infarction in the general spectrum of mesenteric infarction is not readily defined. On the one hand, in large series upwards of one half of the patients investigated will have no macro-vascular occlusion;[2, 16] on the other hand, the finding of mucosal infarction after death from whatever cause is frequent. If these latter cases are eliminated, however, and only those patients included in whom infarction made a substantial contribution to the clinical illness, non-occlusive infarction still remains the most common cause of ischaemic bowel necrosis. The cases are far from uniform, with many causes, presentations and associated medical problems; the classification 'non-occlusive infarction' represents more a grouping than a specific aetiology. The common factor is the development of bowel infarction in the absence of a demonstrable major vascular occlusion. Infarction may be superficial or deep, patchy or extensive, and involve the small or large bowel and even other visceral structures including the stomach. Because of the underlying causes, rather than the extent or irreversibility of the mesenteric injury, mortality is very high.

Aetiology

Non-occlusive infarction is the end result of a factor or factors that decrease blood flow to the bowel wall. In about a quarter of cases these factors are not identifiable. Known factors include a diminished cardiac output, as in coronary or valvular heart disease or arrhythmias, and insufficient peripheral perfusion, as in hypovolaemic or septic shock. A second factor in many older patients is the presence of stenotic lesions due to atherosclerotic occlusive disease in the central or peripheral portions of the mesenteric vessels. These lesions cause a further decrease in flow, sometimes to the critical level that will lead to infarction. Thus some patients with chronic intestinal ischaemia will develop non-occlusive infarction with or without another factor such as heart failure. Finally, splanchnic artery spasm and shunting have an important role. These changes may reflect normal physiological shunting away from the splanchnic bed or a pathological degree of spasm. The latter may be in response to exogenous stimuli such as digitalis preparations or alpha-adrenergic agonists.

Clinical presentation

The clinical presentation differs from that in the general description only in that coexisting medical problems may tend to obscure the signs and symptoms. Abdominal pain and evidence of mucosal bleeding are present in the same proportion of patients, but may be overlooked in patients who are otherwise seriously ill. However, perforation with peritonitis is not missed so easily.

In a few patients a prior history of postprandial pain and weight loss will suggest a chronic ischaemic condition. The most helpful clinical symptom is abdominal pain. In a setting suggestive of ischaemia, this should lead to the presumptive diagnosis. Of course, pain from ischaemic bowel is probably relatively common in patients in intensive care settings and many do not develop infarction. The severity and persistence of the pain, as well as the presence of gastrointestinal bleeding and peritoneal signs, help to single out the patient with infarction.

Diagnosis

The clinical setting and symptoms will provide sufficient diagnostic evidence on which to base the practical elements of management. There are no direct measurements that are of value since there are no useful techniques for measuring in vivo mucosal blood flow. An increasing role for angiography in selected patients is advocated by some, their enthusiasm also reflecting the therapeutic value of angiographic techniques.[3] Given that the demands of proper management of associated and underlying conditions may preclude angiographic studies in many patients, indirect observation of splanchnic artery spasm and mural vascular changes may give clues to the diagnosis in an undetermined but substantial number of patients with non-occlusive infarction.[20] In practical terms, the presence of mesenteric emboli and the determination of the extent and location of atherosclerotic lesions will separate out those patients with an occlusive cause or contributing stenotic lesion from those with normal vessels.

Treatment

Measures to improve perfusion by treatment of the underlying central causes of decreased flow are essential. In many instances these measures will terminate symptoms of ischaemia or improve mural perfusion and limit infarction to the mucosal layers. The systemic use of drugs that may lead to splanchnic spasm may be unavoidable, but they should be eliminated when possible.

The development of peritoneal signs may dictate abdominal exploration, both to rule out some other cause such as cholecystitis or perforation of a peptic ulcer, and to resect segments of infarcted bowel. However, the latter does not greatly improve the chances of survival. The outcome is usually dictated by the underlying cause and, when this leads to bowel infarction, recovery is rare. The added burden of laparotomy may worsen the prognosis in some cases.

The use of local vasodilator drugs infused into the superior mesenteric artery through a percutaneously placed catheter will, in selected cases, lead to a marked increase in splanchnic perfusion. Papaverine is the drug frequently used for this purpose. Advocates of the technique point to a high incidence of survival compared with that observed in patients undergoing laparotomy. Although patient selection and treatment of patients who might have recovered without treatment cloud the evaluation of this approach, there is no question of its effectiveness in improving local perfusion.[3]

In patients in whom infarction has developed on a background of chronically compromised mesenteric arterial flow, restoration of flow will sometimes lead to patient survival.[18] This presupposes satisfactory reversal of any central cause of diminished circulation. The surgical considerations then do not differ from those of acute mesenteric thrombosis. In the absence of full thickness infarction, stenotic lesions may sometimes be managed by percutaneous transarterial dilatation. If satisfactory flow is restored, laparotomy may not be necessary or may be required in order to resect segments of non-viable intestine.

ACUTE SUPERIOR MESENTERIC ARTERY OCCLUSION

From a third to a half of all cases of mesenteric infarction are due to acute occlusion of the superior mesenteric artery or its branches. In many, perhaps the majority, the cause is an embolus.

As with other peripheral emboli, most originate from the heart, either from a postinfarction mural thrombus or in association with atrial fibrillation. A few are of mycotic origin, usually from valvular vegetations. Trauma to the inner surface of the aorta, either from the placement of clamps during operations or the passage of a catheter for diagnostic studies of the heart or aorta and its branches, is a rare iatrogenic cause of emboli. The resultant emboli of atheromatous material may be large enough to behave like other emboli. However, in some cases they are small and numerous. They may then cause not only infarction of the intestine, but also other visceral organs. Death in such patients usually results from renal failure due to renal emboli.[11, 15]

Large emboli typically lodge at or distal to the origin of the middle colic artery. With acute occlusion at this site, or more distal but within the main trunk, the area most severely affected is usually the terminal ileum. Insufficiency of collateral flow may modify this and, in many cases, infarction may develop in the entire area supplied by the vessel. When emboli pass into a major branch, ischaemic injury in the corresponding segment may develop or the collateral circulation may be sufficient to prevent actual infarction.

The other frequent cause of superior mesenteric artery occlusion is thrombosis. It tends to occur in an older age group and to involve almost exclusively the proximal few centimetres of the vessel. Thus infarction due to thrombosis also tends to be more extensive. The site of predilection reflects the pattern of visceral atherosclerotic narrowing, which usually affects the proximal portion of the major vessels.[17] More peripheral lesions are seen but seldom lead to infarction, even when acute thrombosis occurs.

A third and rare cause is dissection of the aorta. Most such dissections originate in the thoracic aorta and are associated with transient occlusion of other aortic branches.

Clinical presentation

Infarction due to superior mesenteric occlusion tends to present a less difficult diagnostic problem than that due to other causes. This reflects the usual relatively abrupt onset of symptoms with characteristically severe, early pain in the absence of other acute medical problems.

The collateral circulation in most instances is, theoretically, adequate to avoid infarction. Thus a period of ischaemic pain without infarction is seen in many patients. This may last for several hours to days with fluctuation in severity or even disappearance of the pain. Direct observation of the circulation at laparotomy during this stage may be deceptive in that viable intestine and even faint peripheral pulses may suggest some other cause for pain, and a favourable opportunity for timely restoration of arterial flow may thus be forfeited. Angiography during this pre-infarction stage is especially useful. Later infarction ensues in response to extension of the thrombus, arterial spasm, bowel distension, or a fall in perfusing pressure.

Diagnosis

In the early stages the diagnosis is relatively obscure; later with infarction and perforation it becomes obvious. Severe abdominal pain in the absence of abdominal findings on examination, and without other explanation, should suggest mesenteric ischaemia. The finding of occult blood in the gastric and rectal contents, a history of emboli, and a marked leucocytosis are all helpful; plain abdominal films usually are not.

Angiography is of considerable use in the management of selected patients. Not only can it suggest the diagnosis but, by localizing the site of occlusion, it may also point to the specific cause and aid the surgeon in planning a reconstruction. Whether it should be used in all cases in which evidence of peritonitis is absent, and where the diagnosis of mesenteric infarction is under serious consideration, is an unanswered question. The anticipated delay, the general condition of the patient and the probability of some other diagnosis all influence the urgency of laparotomy and the advisability of angiography.[10]

Treatment

Except in a few cases of peripheral emboli without peritoneal signs and in cases of aortic dissection, immediate laparotomy is the preferred approach in all cases of acute mesenteric artery occlusion unless the patient is moribund. The surgeon should be prepared not only to resect infarcted bowel, but also to restore the arterial circulation.

With peripheral emboli and infarction, resection alone produces excellent rates of survival. With more central sites of occlusion, however, even extensive resection is, by itself, seldom successful. Either the patient will have insufficient remaining small intestine for survival or the unresected segments may undergo infarction in the early post-operative period.[1, 15] Parenteral alimentation is a useful adjunct to management but cannot be used to maintain older patients after extensive small bowel resection.[8]

With central occlusion either from thrombosis or emboli, extensive areas of salvageable intestine will be found in about one half of patients requiring surgical exploration. Either an embolectomy for emboli, or a bypass for proximal thrombosis, may be performed. Embolectomy is almost always not only possible but also successful in restoring flow.[15, 19] Thromboendarterectomy usually fails, is technically difficult, and, in most instances, is inferior to an aortic or iliac to mesenteric bypass.[5, 15] Reconstruction is combined with resection when indicated. If segments of intestine are of questionable viability at the end of the operation, an elective laparotomy for further possible resection is advisable 12 to 24 hours later. The determination of viability intraoperatively may be aided by the use of fluorescein and observation of pulsatile mural blood vessels using a Doppler probe.[7] Postoperative complications of arterial reconstruction include thrombosis or re-embolization, bleeding from the arterial suture line, and bleeding from segments of bowel due to mucosal slough. Overall survival in cases of acute superior mesenteric artery occlusion remains poor, but is quite substantial in those cases successfully submitted to embolectomy.

VENOUS THROMBOSIS

Venous thrombosis, once regarded as a frequent cause of mesenteric infarction, is now thought to be responsible for 5–10% of cases.[9, 16] The clinical presentation of venous thrombosis does not differ from that of other causes of intestinal ischaemia. It is reported that a period of ischaemic symptoms, which may last several days, often precedes infarction. Patients are sometimes febrile during this prodromal stage and have vague abdominal pain and a disturbance of bowel function.

Aetiology

When an underlying cause is discovered, it will most commonly be cirrhosis, a hepatic tumour or some other cause of acute portal vein thrombosis. Occlusion of the portal vein alone usually does not cause infarction; where infarction has occurred, propagation of the thrombus into the mesenteric vein is found. Other cases are associated with hypercoagulability states, compres-

sion by tumours, sepsis, trauma, and the use of oral contraceptives. In over half the cases, no underlying cause is found, though there may be evidence of venous thrombosis in other areas such as the extremities.

Diagnosis

Only the presence of bloodstained peritoneal fluid distinguishes mesenteric venous thrombosis from arterial infarction. It is not known how often the diagnosis may be suspected from angiographic studies but, in some cases, indirect findings are noted. These include arterial spasm, delayed clearing of small arteries and failure to opacify the portal system. The uncertainty of the findings and the nonspecific signs and symptoms make preoperative diagnosis unusual.

Treatment

Thrombectomy seems to have little clinical application. This is because in most cases of infarction the thrombosis extends out to the edge of the bowel. It is this finding that gives rise to the rationale for a specific intraoperative diagnostic manoeuvre: when the mesentery of involved segments of bowel is incised, worm-like thrombus is extruded from the veins. Resection is the only successful approach to management.[16] The affected segment, usually the middle part of the small bowel, must be removed. A margin of normal bowel must be included, since infarction of the anastomosis is a common postoperative complication. Second look operations 12 to 24 hours after initial resection are probably indicated in most patients. Postoperative anticoagulation, though unproven, is a logical step in the prevention of further thromboses and infarction but anticoagulants in the early postoperative period increase the risk of intra-abdominal bleeding.

ISCHAEMIC COLITIS

Ischaemic lesions of the left colon deserve separate consideration because several aspects of their presentation and management are different to those of infarction at more proximal levels of the intestinal tract. By contrast, lesions of the right and transverse colon (usually the result of superior mesenteric artery occlusion, but sometimes non-occlusive in origin) are covered by the principles already related earlier in this section. The term ischaemic colitis will be used to designate the more distal colonic lesions. They may be the result of inferior mesenteric artery occlusion or be non-occlusive in aetiology. They tend to be of limited extent, to involve a single segment, to be reversible, and to present a distinctive clinical picture. Their management does not include arterial reconstruction, and delayed rather than early surgical intervention is the rule, if necessary at all.

Aetiology

Occlusion of the inferior mesenteric artery due to atheroma is common in older patients but mesenteric infarction is rare. This reflects the small size of the inferior mesenteric artery and the competence of the collateral supply to its distribution. In fact, many of the cases that are seen in clinical practice are the result of surgical ligation of the vessels in the course of colon resections or operations on the aorta. In the latter instance, a mucosal infarct that is centered in the distal sigmoid colon and extends from the descending colon to the rectum is produced. Although mucosal injuries are frequent, actual full thickness infarction is observed in only a small percentage of cases of ligation.

The more common cause is undefined non-occlusive infarction. Though underlying hypotension, cardiac failure, digitalis toxicity or a hypercoagulability state, including that observed in users of oral contraceptives, is seen in a few cases, in most, no such causative factor is apparent. Occlusion of small arteries and veins in the wall of the affected bowel is frequently seen but is thought to be a secondary manifestation.[4] The splenic flexure and the descending colon tend to be most commonly involved, though other segments may be affected. It is rare for more than a single isolated segment to be involved.[13, 14]

Clinical course

Whether the cause is non-occlusive infarction or inferior mesenteric artery occlusion, the presentation is similar. Onset is acute with bloody diarrhoea, and early signs of peritoneal irritation over the affected segment. Bacterial invasion following loss of mucosal integrity is an important element. Spontaneous recovery is seen in the majority of patients, though this may take several weeks. Rarely, a stricture develops. In patients with stricture, continued diarrhoea is observed, though the stricture is often not demonstrated until several weeks have elapsed. In a few patients, full thickness infarction or bacterial invasion may lead to perforation. Typically, this is delayed for a few days to up to three

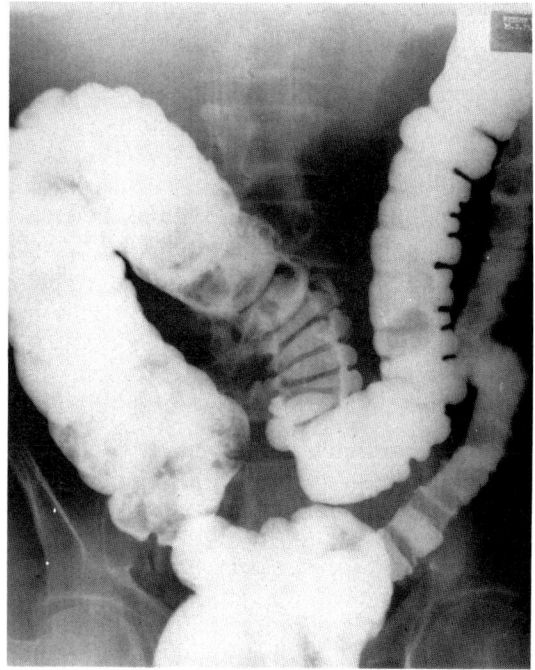

a

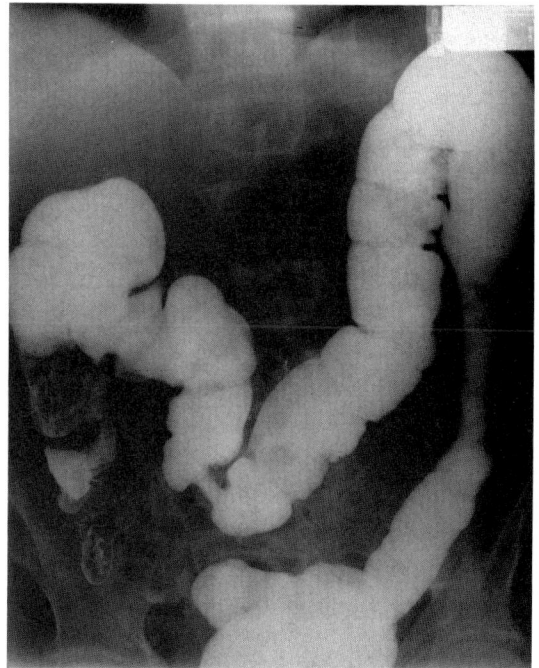

b

Fig. 5.13 (a) An 'instant' barium enema from a patient with acute left-sided abdominal tenderness and bloody diarrhoea due to ischaemic colitis. Narrowing, 'thumb-printing' and oedema are seen in the descending colon. (b) Repeat barium enema from the same patient ten weeks later. An ischaemic stricture of the descending colon is seen.

weeks after the onset of symptoms. Continued evidence of inflammation occurs during this interval.

The general presentation of ischaemic colitis leads to a clinical picture that must be differentiated from that of other acute forms of colitis, obstruction, and from perforated diverticular disease. Barium enema studies, sometimes repeated, are very helpful in this regard. Submucosal oedema and haemorrhage in an evolving pattern are characteristic of ischaemic colitis.

Treatment

The diagnosis should be confirmed by X-ray studies, except when a preceding surgical ligation of the inferior mesenteric artery makes the diagnosis obvious. Submucosal oedema and haemorrhage causing 'thumb-printing' may be diagnostic (Figure 5.13). If not, barium contrast studies should be performed. Without these findings, another diagnosis must be sought. When changes extend down into the rectum, sigmoidoscopy will show ischaemia and mucosal slough with ulceration. In most cases of non-occlusive infarction this will not be found.

When the diagnosis is sufficiently certain, management consists of close observation, intravenous fluids, restricting oral intake, and the use of parenteral antibiotics. Surgical intervention is reserved for cases in which perforation is suspected. Even when occlusion has occurred, inferior mesenteric artery reconstruction is not useful and is usually not possible. Worsening signs of sepsis and the development of a palpable mass are common indications for laparotomy. Free perforation with soilage of the peritoneal cavity is rare. Resection with a proximal colostomy is the preferred operation. If the rectum is not severely involved, and this is usually so, later restoration of the colon's continuity may be anticipated. When operation is not performed, follow-up X-ray studies should be obtained to ensure that mucosal abnormalities have resolved, and that a neoplasm or more chronic form of colitis has not been overlooked.[2]

REFERENCES

1 Bergan, J. J., Dean, R. H., Conn. J. Jr. & Yao, J. S. T. (1975) Revascularization in treatment of mesenteric infarction. *Annals of Surgery*, **182**, 430–438.
2 Boley, S. J., Brandt, S. J. & Veith, F. J. (1978) Ischaemic disorders of the intestine. *Current Problems in Surgery*, **15**, 1–85.
3 Boley, S. J., Sprayregan, S., Siegelman, S. S. & Veith, F. J. (1977) Initial results from an aggressive roentgenological and surgical approach to acute mesenteric ischemia. *Surgery*, **82**, 848–855.
4 Brandt, L. J., Gomery, P., Mitsudo, S. M. et al. (1976) Disseminated intravascular coagulation in non-occlusive mesenteric ischemia: the lack of specificity of fibrin thrombi in intestinal infarction. *Gastroenterology*, **71**, 954–957.
5 Brittain, R. S. & Early, T. R. (1963) Emergency thrombo-endarterectomy of the superior mesenteric artery. *Annals of Surgery*, **158**, 138–143.
6 Brown, R. A., Chu-Jeng, C., Scott, H. J. & Gurd, F. N. (1970) Ultrastructural changes in the canine ileal mucosal cell after mesenteric arterial occlusion. *Archives of Surgery*, **101**, 290–297.
7 Bulkley, G. B., Zuidema, G. D., Hamilton, S. R. et al. (1981) Intraoperative determination of small intestinal viability following ischemic injury. *Annals of Surgery*, **193**, 628–637.
8 Gusberg, R. & Gump. F. E. (1974) Combined surgical and nutritional management of patients with acute mesenteric vascular occlusion. *Annals of Surgery*, **179**, 358–361.
9 Hildebrand, H. D. & Zierler, R. E. (1980) Mesenteric vascular disease. *American Journal of Surgery*, **139**, 188–192.
10 Kaufman, S. L., Harrington, D. P. & Siegelman, S. S. (1977) Superior mesenteric artery embolization: an angiographic emergency. *Radiology*, **124**, 625–630.
11 Kealy, W. F. (1978) Atheroembolism. *Journal of Clinical Pathology*, **31**, 984–989.
12 Lanciault, G. & Jacobson, E. D. (1976) Gastrointestinal circulation. Progress in gastroenterology. *Gastroenterology*, **71**, 851–873.
13 Marcuson, R. W. (1972) Ischaemic colitis. *Clinics in Gastroenterology*, **1**, 745–763.
14 Marston, A., Pheils, M. T., Thomas, M. L. & Morson, B. C. (1966) Ischemic colitis. *Gut*, **7**, 1–15.
15 Ottinger, L. W. (1978) The surgical management of acute occlusion of the superior mesenteric artery. *Annals of Surgery*, **188**, 721–731.
16 Ottinger, L. W. & Austen, W. G. (1967) A study of 136 patients with mesenteric infarction. *Surgery, Gynecology and Obstetrics*, **124**, 251–261.
17 Reiner, L., Jimenez, F. A. & Rodriguez, F. L. (1963) Atherosclerosis in the mesenteric circulation: observations and correlations with aortic and coronary atherosclerosis. *American Heart Journal*, **66**, 200–210.
18 Russ, J. E., Haid, S. P., Yao, J. S. T. & Bergan, J. J. (1977) Surgical treatment of non-occlusive mesenteric infarction. *American Journal of Surgery*, **134**, 638–642.
19 Shaw, R. S. & Rutledge, R. H. (1957) Superior mesenteric artery embolectomy in the treatment of massive mesenteric infarction. *New England Journal of Medicine*, **257**, 595–598.
20 Siegelman, S. S., Sprayregan, S. & Boley, S. J. (1974) Angiographic diagnosis of mesenteric arterial vasoconstriction. *Radiology*, **112**, 533–542.
21 Tomchik, F. S., Wittenberg, J. & Ottinger, L. W. (1970) The roentgenographic spectrum of bowel infarction. *Radiology*, **96**, 249–260.
22 Williams, L. F. (1971) Vascular insufficiency of the intestines. Progress in gastroenterology. *Gastroenterology*, **61**, 757–777.

CHRONIC ISCHAEMIA OF THE GUT

Chronic intestinal arterial insufficiency may present in various ways. Often the presentation of chronic arterial disease is an acute, frequently lethal, episode of mesenteric infarction, without any premonitory symptoms. Whilst the symptoms described as 'intestinal angina' are the most characteristic of chronic ischaemia, they are also the rarest mode of presentation. Whether the presenting symptoms are acute or long-standing, the mesenteric circulation will usually show signs of chronic arterial disease. The clinical emphasis should be on early diagnosis, so that surgical intervention may be planned if indicated.

Since the beginning of this century, the clinical picture of chronic intestinal ischaemia has been fully recognized. Bacelli in 1904 introduced the term 'angor abdominalis',[10] but now the term 'intestinal angina' proposed by Mikkelsen is more universally accepted.[11]

In 95% of all cases the condition can be attributed to arteriosclerotic disease.[1, 10] There are usually multiple occlusions in the main arteries supplying the gastrointestinal tract (the superior mesenteric artery, the inferior mesenteric artery, and the coeliac artery.) Occlusions occur mainly in the proximal segments. There is a wide variety of other uncommon causes; these are listed in Table 5.2. They include the contentious condition of coeliac axis compression by

Table 5.2 Causes of intestinal ischaemia.

Intrinsic causes
Arteriosclerosis
Embolism
Arteritis
Medial hyperplasia
Prolongation of aortic dissection
Aortic aneurysm
Extrinsic causes
Coeliac axis compression
Retroperitoneal fibrosis
Haemodynamic causes
Mesenteric arterio-venous fistulas
Non-occlusive intestinal ischaemia

the median arcuate ligament, and idiopathic, neoplastic, or iatrogenic (e.g. caused by methysergide) retroperitoneal fibrosis.

Pathophysiology

Theoretically the three main gastrointestinal arteries (the coeliac artery, the superior mesenteric artery, and the inferior mesenteric artery) are end arteries. In fact, as Chiene demonstrated, obliteration of these three arteries can occur without intestinal infarction.[2] Numerous anastomoses develop between the three arteries, and there are also 'extra-gastrointestinal' arteries that can provide the gut with an adequate blood

supply, such as the internal mammary and inferior diaphragmatic arteries from above and the internal iliac system from below.

The pathophysiology of intestinal ischaemia has been described earlier in this chapter. It should be emphasized that, whilst all the three main visceral arteries supply the gut, the superior mesenteric artery is the most important because of the amount of blood it carries (800 ml/min) and its central position. The consequences of arterial blockage depend upon the position of the occlusion and on how rapidly it occurs. If the process is gradual, complete compensation may occur due to the development of a collateral circulation, which may involve both reverse flow and hypertrophy of the existing anastomotic circuits. Amongst the most important of these circuits are the 'Rio Branco' arcade between the coeliac axis and the superior mesenteric artery, and the 'Drummond' or 'Riolan' arcade joining the superior and inferior mesenteric arteries.

The consequences of chronic intestinal ischaemia may be transient or permanent and have been divided into several stages.

Stage 1. During this stage there is a total absence of any symptoms, as an efficient collateral circulation is present both at rest, during intense physical activity, and during digestion. However, at this stage there is a real risk of intestinal necrosis should an additional haemodynamic factor such as a low cardiac output supervene.

Stage 2. At this stage symptoms occur either during physical exertion or more commonly postprandially.

Stage 3. This stage is characterized by chronic, but non-necrotic, trophic lesions in the gut. They involve the mucosa, which becomes dystrophic, and then the muscular layers, which become hyperplastic, leading to strictures.

Stage 4. In this stage necrotic areas appear in the gut, leading to the events described earlier in this chapter as a consequence of acute ischaemia. It should be remembered that this stage may either be the first presentation of chronic arterial insufficiency, or occur after a well-defined period of symptoms corresponding to stage 2 or stage 3.[3]

No fixed anatomo-clinical correlation is apparent. Mikkelsen has emphasized that symptoms are more likely to occur when two main arteries are occluded.[11] However, it should also be remembered that the collateral circulation is extremely weak and the flow in it tends to be non-pulsatile, so that the blood flow is very sensitive to superimposed haemodynamic disturbances such as a fall in blood pressure.

Clinical aspects

There are a variety of manifestations of chronic ischaemia.

Intestinal angina

This syndrome is characterized by pain, weight loss, and an abdominal murmur. The pain is usually located in the epigastric area, is cramplike, and arises early after eating. Classically the patient will notice that pain occurs after eating a large meal. Weight loss, which may be very considerable (5–30 kg) stems directly from a self-imposed restriction of eating due to the fear of postprandial pain. The abdominal murmur is systolic and is usually found in a high position behind the xyphoid process; it reflects stenosis of the coeliac axis or the superior mesenteric artery. On occasions a continuous murmur may be heard over the left iliac fossa, corresponding to the dilated artery of Riolan. Rarely, a previously heard arterial murmur may disappear; this may herald acute intestinal ischaemia.[3] Such murmurs are not always present but have been reported in at least 40% of cases, and should be differentiated from those arising from the aorta, iliac or renal arteries.

Diagnosis is based on the history, on the negative results of conventional tests such as upper gastrointestinal endoscopy, barium X-rays, and ultrasound and CT scans, and usually on the evidence of arteriosclerotic disease in other areas. It is exceptional to have mesenteric ischaemia early in the course of arteriosclerotic disease; usually there is peripheral vascular occlusion as well as aneurysms in the abdominal aorta, and a history of myocardial infarction or angina pectoris, cerebral vascular disease, or hypertension.

The criteria for objective arteriographic proof are complex; they vary, for example, if the arteriographic findings are incidental or are found in the course of investigation of suspected mesenteric ischaemia. Abnormalities of the gastrointestinal arteries will be found using aortography in about 60% of patients with peripheral arterial occlusive disease. If an injection in the infra-renal aorta shows the Riolan artery arcade, no matter what its form or size, it should be considered as a sign of potential intestinal isch-

aemia. A further study should then be performed higher in the aorta at the level of T12 or L1, in both supine and lateral positions, in order to evaluate the ostia of the arteries.

When arteriography is being performed for complaints suggestive of gastrointestinal ischaemia, the aortogram is usually performed via the femoral route. Selective injections of the coeliac artery and superior mesenteric artery are not usually indicated since the lesions are commonly limited to the proximal segments of the arteries, and selective catheterization may aggravate pre-existing intestinal ischaemia. Care should be taken, however, to define the degree of stenosis and obstruction of the main arteries involved, and to evaluate the collateral circulation. The lateral projection is often of greater value. If intestinal angina is suspected, these investigations should be performed immediately, as a lethal acute ischaemic episode may occur at any time.

Malabsorption

Malabsorption due to intestinal ischaemia has been reported but is not extensively documented.[13] Steatorrhoea should be differentiated from diarrhoea, a frequent symptom in intestinal angina. During acute ischaemic necrosis of the gut, diarrhoea may occur and the mucosa may slough, leading to the passage of mucosal casts.

Intestinal obstruction

Intestinal obstruction may arise from ischaemic strictures caused by peripheral arterial occlusion in the territory of the superior mesenteric artery. The strictures are usually jejunal, but may occasionally be in the ileum, and are either single or multiple. Such strictures may be resected surgically,[12] but a period of conservative management is advised as repeat barium examination often shows them not to be fixed. Such studies may also show areas of ulceration of the mucosa of the small intestine, but they are rarer in this site than in the colon.

Premonitory signs

Dunphy[5] has pointed out that unrecognized premonitory signs occur in 75% of patients in whom intestinal infarction subsequently arises. This has led to the axiom that 'all functional digestive symptoms in a patient who has peripheral arterial occlusive disease must be considered as intestinal angina until proved to the contrary'.[3, 6, 7, 8] Thus both vascular surgeons and cardiologists should be alerted to complaints of weight loss or abdominal pain in their patients, and gastroenterologists should consider this diagnosis in the presence of cardiac or vascular abnormality.

Treatment

Until recently the treatment of this disease has been exclusively surgical, but transluminal angioplasty now represents an alternative means of treatment.[14] Whilst the operative technique lies outside the scope of this book, the following points should be noted. The large transperitoneal laparotomy incision needed will occasionally lead to the sacrifice of the collateral circulation and further impair the intestinal blood supply. The ischaemic gut does not usually appear 'like a dead leaf' or black, but is often merely greyish or yellowish with numerous hyperperistaltic waves. The precise vascular procedure depends upon which vessels are most seriously affected. Many authorities believe that the superior mesenteric artery is best reimplanted into the anterior aspect of the aorta below the level of the left renal vein (Figure 5.14 and 5.15),[4, 11] although occasionally a synthetic graft

may be required to form an aorto-superior mesenteric artery bypass. The precise operation will depend on the clinical picture and the presence of any co-existent disease. In intestinal angina the operation is normally directed at the superior mesenteric artery, and an additional procedure on the coeliac axis is required only if the liver appears ischaemic, or if the hepatic arterial pulse is weak after mesenteric revascularization.

It should be emphasized that the results of operation prior to an acute ischaemic episode are far better than those performed after gut ischaemia has supervened.[9, 10, 12] The operative mortality in our series of patients with chronic ischaemia has been less than 2% (1 out of 60), the only severe complication being the creation of lymphatic fistula requiring prolonged parenteral nutrition. Postoperatively, weight gain occurs and pain should completely disappear. In the follow-up of our series only one out of 60 patients subsequently developed intestinal infarction, although repeat operation was needed for two patients, both having a satisfactory outcome.

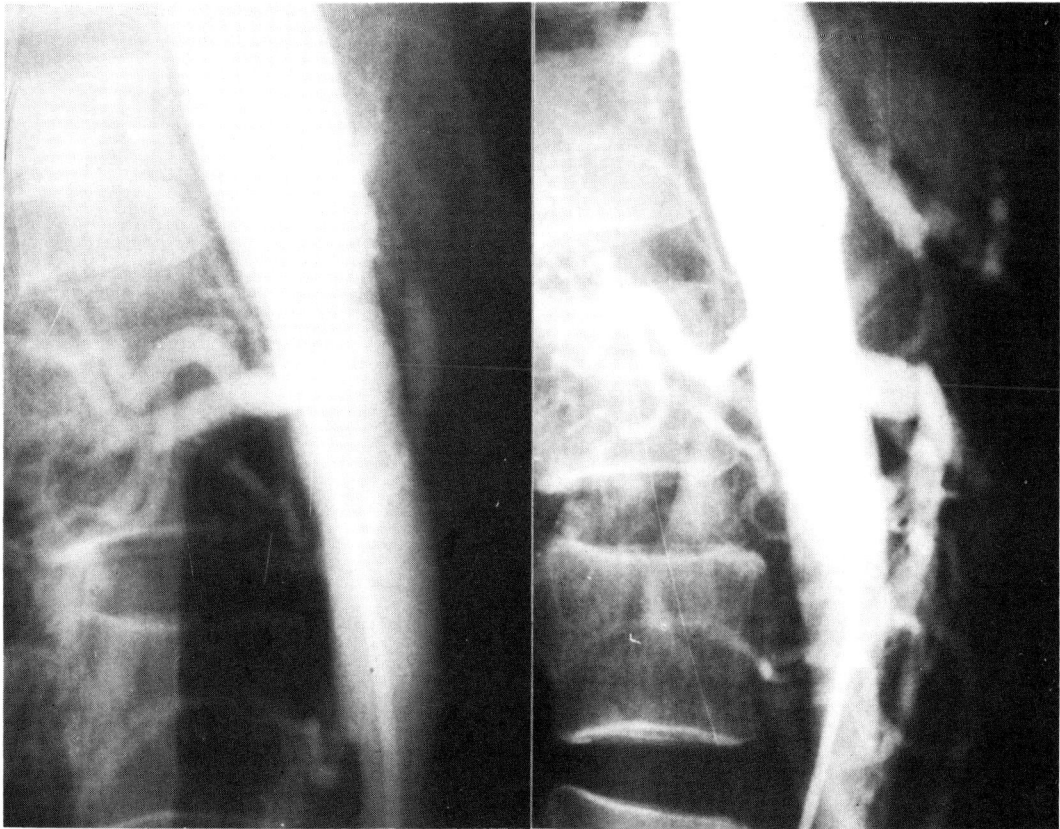

a   b

Fig. 5.14 Lateral aortogram. (a) Preoperatively: occlusion of the three main intestinal arteries. (b) Postoperatively: direct aorto-superior mesenteric artery reimplantation.

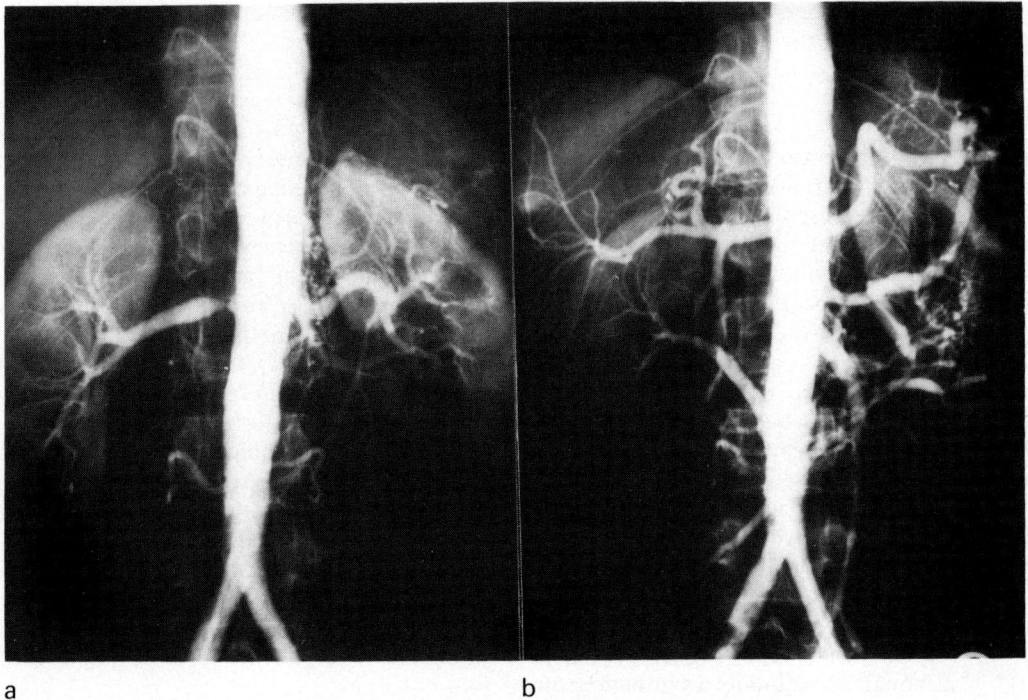

a　　　　　　　　　　　　　　　　　　b

Fig. 5.15 Antero-posterior view aortogram (same patient as in Figure 5.14). (a) Preoperatively: non visualization of the vessels of the gastrointestinal tract. Proximal stenosis of the right renal artery. (b) Postoperatively: evidence of all the vessels of the coeliac axis and mesenteric area after isolated superior mesenteric artery reimplantation. Aorto/right renal graft using autologous saphenous vein.

REFERENCES

1　Boley, S. J., Schwartz, S. S. & Lester, L. F. Jr (1971) *Vascular Disorders of the Intestine.* New York: Appleton-Century-Crofts.

2　Chiene, J. (1869) Complete obliteration of the celiac and mesenteric arteries: the viscera receiving their blood supply through the extrapyramidal system of the vessels. *Journal of Antomy and Physiology*, **3**, 65–72.

3　Cinqualbre, J., Wenger, J. J. & Kieny, R. (1981) Infarctus mésentérique: conduite à tenir. *La Revue du Praticien*, **31**, 2083–2105.

4　Descotes, J., Bouchet, A., Sisteron, A. & George, P. (1963) La réimplantation de l'artère mésentérique supérieure dans le traitement de l'insuffisance artérielle intestinale. Données anatomiques et chirurgicales. *Lyon Chirurgical*, **59**, 5–15.

5　Dunphy, J. E. (1936) Abdominal pain of vascular origin. *American Journal of Medical Sciences*, **192**, 109–111.

6　Kieny, R. & Cinqualbre, J. (1981) Chirurgie des artères digestives. In *Techniques chirurgicales*, 431050 Paris: Encyclopédie Médico-Chirurgicale.

7　Kieny, R., Cinqualbre, J., Eisenmann, B. & Tongio, J. (1976) Ischémie mésentérique chronique. *Annales de Radiologie*, **19**, 371–375.

8　Kieny, R., Cinqualbre, J., Wenger, J. J. & Tongio, J. (1978) *Ischémies intestinales aiguës.* Paris: L'expansion scientifique.

9　McCollum, C. H., Graham, J. M. & De Bakey, M. E. (1976) Chronic mesenteric arterial insufficiency: results of revascularization in 33 cases. *Southern Medical Journal*, **69**, 1266–1268.

10　Marston, A. (1977) *Intestinal Ischaemia.* London: Edward Arnold.

11　Mikkelsen, W. P. & Zaro, J. S. Jr (1959) Intestinal angina: report of a case with preoperative diagnosis and surgical relief. *New England Journal of Medicine*, **260**, 912–914.

12　Pokrovsky, A. V. & Kasantchjan, P. O. (1980) Surgical treatment of chronic occlusive disease of the enteric visceral branches of the abdominal aorta. Experience with 110 operations. *Annals of Surgery*, **191**, 51–56.

13　Shaw, R. S. & Maynard, E. P. Acute and chronic thrombosis of the mesenteric arteries associated with malabsorption. *New England Journal of Medicine*, **258**, 874–878.

14　Vflacker, R., Goldany, M. A. & Constant, S. (1980) Resolution of mesenteric angina with percutaneous transluminal angioplasty of a superior mesenteric artery stenosis using a balloon catheter. *Gastrointestinal Radiology*, **5**, 367, 1965.

COELIAC AXIS COMPRESSION SYNDROME

The coeliac axis compression syndrome describes abdominal pain or discomfort caused by complete or partial occlusion of the coeliac artery by the median arcuate ligament of the diaphragm, by the coeliac ganglia, or by a combination of these. Not all clinicians accept the existence of this entity, but well-documented cases have been reported.

Anatomy

The coeliac artery arises from the ventral surface of the aorta at the level of the twelfth thoracic and first lumbar vertebrae, distal to the median arcuate ligament of the diaphragm. After a short anterior course (about 1.5 cm) between the right and left coeliac ganglia and above the upper border of the pancreas, it divides into the left gastric, hepatic and splenic arteries. While this arrangement is fairly constant, variations are not uncommon and usually involve an alternative origin for one of the main branches. Important anastomotic channels connect the coeliac artery to the superior mesenteric artery, in particular the gastroduodenal artery and its pancreaticoduodenal branches.

Pathology

The main cause of the syndrome is compression of the coeliac axis by the median arcuate ligament of the diaphragm, either because of a higher-than-normal take-off of the artery, or a lower-than-normal position of the ligament. This causes a V-shaped indentation in the superior surface of the artery. Less frequently occlusion occurs due to lateral or circumferential compression of the vessel by the coeliac ganglion[13, 21] and periarterial fibrous tissue.[9] Mixed patterns also occur, and histology of the constricting tissue may show ganglion cells and ligamentous fibres.

Intrinsic occlusion of the coeliac artery by atherosclerosis, thrombosis, embolism, fibromuscular dysplasia and other pathologies may also be responsible for compression symptoms.

Clinical presentation

Diverse views are held as to whether or not coeliac axis compression is clinically significant. Some deny its existence[10, 12, 18, 22] and some large radiological series[2, 7] have shown a high frequency of coeliac axis compression in apparently normal subjects. However, in these two studies 36 out of 74 (49%) and 7 out of 17 (41%) of the subjects with compression had unexplained abdominal pain, and 5 of the 7 in Cornell's series[7] who had surgery for the compression improved. The presence of typical angiographic findings in asymptomatic subjects does not necessarily invalidate the syndrome,[6] since complete occlusion may occur without symptoms,[20] and occasionally patients may be asymptomatic even after occlusion of all three splanchnic vessels.[5, 20]

Other authors accept it as a real entity; surgical success rates of 75%,[23] 85%[16] and 100%[15, 20] have been reported.

The majority of patients are women and the average age is in the late 30's to early 50's. However, patients as young as 13, and as old as 80, have been reported.

SYMPTOMS

The main presenting symptom is abdominal pain, which may be restricted to the epigastrium or radiate to the right or left upper quadrants or to the back. The pain is variously described as stabbing, cramping or a dull ache. In most patients it is intermittent, but in some it is constant. It may be associated with eating (usually a large meal), but is not relieved by antacids or antispasmodics. Some patients complain of vague upper abdominal distension. Diarrhoea may occur in some patients and weight loss is not uncommon. Nausea and vomiting are infrequent.

It is clear that these symptoms are not diagnostically different from many other gastrointestinal disorders. Patients in whom the diagnosis of coeliac axis compression syndrome is ultimately made have usually had numerous negative routine investigations and have not responded to a variety of treatments which may have included psychiatric therapy; in other words, they fall into the category of unexplained abdominal pain.

SIGNS

The only diagnostic physical sign is an abdominal bruit, best heard in the epigastrium. However, epigastric bruits are not uncommon and have been variously reported as occurring in 6.5%,[12] 15.9%[14] and 31%[24] of normal or asymptomatic individuals. However, in coeliac axis compression, the murmur has certain characteristic features.[24] It is best heard in the mid-epigastrium, or slightly to the left or just above this point. It begins in early or mid-systole and has an ejection type of configuration. It is usually loud (grade 2 or 3 out of 3) and extends into early diastole. The diastolic component is much softer and must be listened for carefully. The murmur is best heard with the bell of the stethoscope (which needs to be directed at the acoustic axis of the murmur), varies with respiration (being loudest in expiration), and is very localized, becoming inaudible not more than 2 cm from the point of maximum intensity.

Occasionally patients with coeliac axis compression may have no murmur or the murmur may be faint because the artery is completely or almost completely occluded. In these patients, only a high index of clinical suspicion will lead to the definitive investigation of aortography.

Investigations

Routine investigations of abdominal pain, such as gallbladder and gastrointestinal radiology and endoscopy, are invariably negative. If they are not, an alternative diagnosis is made which should determine management until such time as it comes into question.

At present the only definitive investigation is aortography using the Seldinger technique via the femoral artery. Views should be taken in expiration and inspiration, and in anteroposterior and lateral positions, and whenever possible selective catheterization of the coeliac and superior mesenteric arteries should be attempted. If the coeliac axis stenosis is severe and close to the root of the vessel, selective catheterization may not be possible.

The purpose of radiology is threefold: firstly, to demonstrate the presence of coeliac artery compression; secondly, to determine the severity of the compression; and thirdly, to discover whether other major vessels (especially the superior mesenteric artery) are involved. The severity of the occlusion is assessed partly by the degree of compression (a percentage of the regular calibre of the vessel), the degree of post-stenotic dilatation, and the extent of the collateral filling (if any) from the superior mesenteric artery. Figure 5.16 shows a typical example of severe coeliac axis compression with retrograde filling from the superior mesenteric artery.

Pancreatic dysfunction sometimes occurs in patients with the coeliac compression syndrome. Incidences of 5 out of 22,[23] 1 out of 6[4] and 2 out of 15[17] have been reported. However, pancreatic function tests are not diagnostic for the syndrome.

Treatment

Whether patients are treated for the syndrome will depend on the personal opinion of the managing physician as to whether it is a real organic entity or not. If not, management continues as for any patient with chronic, undiagnosed abdominal pain.

Surgical relief of the arterial compression is safe and simple. It can be achieved in most patients by division of the median arcuate ligament, by dissection or excision of the encircling cuff of coeliac ganglia, or by a combination of both. If this approach is taken and the vessel does not pulsate, it may be dilated by a Fogarty catheter balloon inserted through an arteriotomy in the coeliac axis or one of its branches. A frequent consequence of this form of surgery is a periarterial sympathectomy.

Other surgical methods may be employed. Good results have been obtained by surgical bypass without correction of the compression. Lord et al.[15] found that in 8 of their 12 patients, the coeliac artery remained narrow after division of the compressing bands and they proceeded to arterial reconstruction. Curl et al.[8] advise inserting a graft or a bypass if a pressure gradient persists after the decompression. Others have resected the stenosed segment and reimplanted the artery elsewhere on the aorta.

THE RESULTS OF SURGERY

As mentioned earlier in this section, reported results of operation have ranged from good to poor[15, 16, 20, 23] and this is the main reason for a lack of consensus as to the validity of the syndrome. It is not easy to explain the discrepancy in the results on the grounds of patient selection, radiographic criteria, surgical technique or pathological findings. It would help to resolve the controversy if a controlled study could be performed, but no single series has been large enough, and a sham operation is unjustified.

The pain mechanism

If coeliac artery compression causes pain, the reason for it doing so is not clear. The pain is not necessarily ischaemic; angiograms usually show adequate collateral filling of the coeliac artery and its main branches. If the pain is ischaemic it may be due to a 'steal' from the superior mesenteric artery to the coeliac bed.[11, 19] If not, it may be due to neurogenic stimuli produced by throbbing of the compressed artery against the coeliac ganglion.[3, 16] Whatever causes the pain, its relief has been attributed either to restoration of normal coeliac blood flow or to extirpation or transection of the coeliac ganglia.

Summary

Coeliac axis compression is, in my opinion, a real anatomical and pathological entity. However, it is not universally recognized as being clinically significant. Even so, it seems reasonable to consider surgical decompression of the vessel in the small number of patients who are emotionally stable, who have distressing

The labels in the diagrams read:

(top diagram)
- Post-stenotic dilatation
- Coeliac artery
- Splenic artery
- L1

(bottom diagram)
- Splenic A
- Dorsal Pancreatic A
- Superior mesenteric A
- Common Hepatic A
- Ant Inf Pancreaticoduodenal A
- Gastro-Duodenal A
- R. Gastroepiploic A

a

b

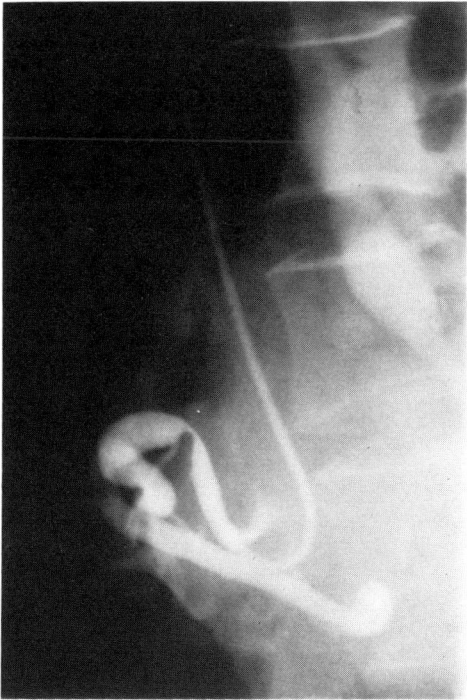

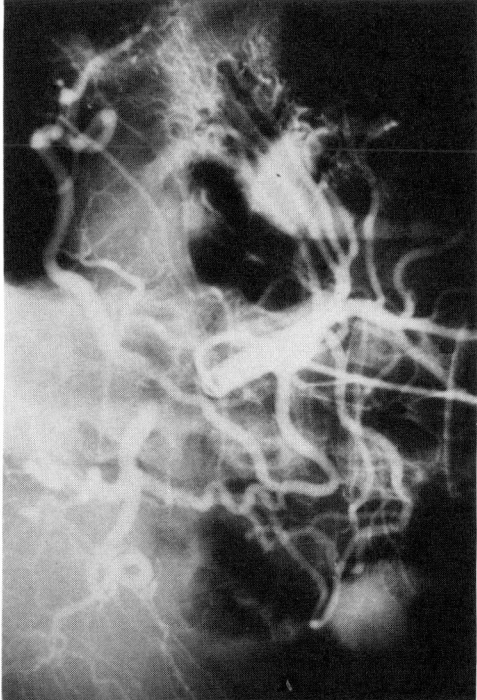

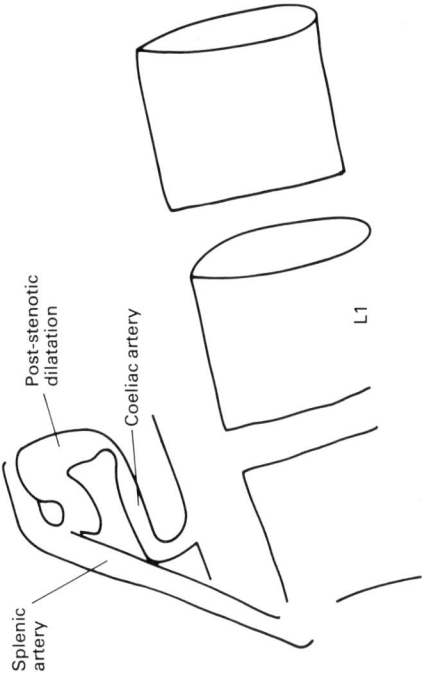

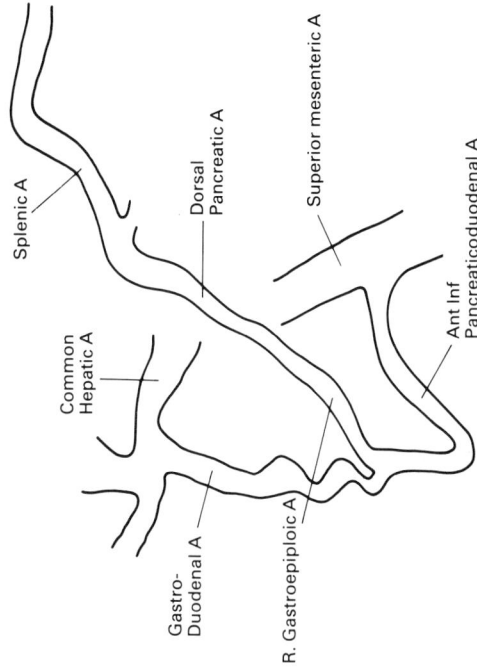

Fig. 5.16 (a) Very tight compression of the coeliac artery by the median arcuate ligament of the diaphragm in an unusually distal location. (b) Retrograde collateral filling of the hepatic and splenic arteries from the superior mesenteric artery. The prominent anastomosis between the right gastroepiploic and dorsal pancreatic arteries is also unusual. (These films are from a 45 year old male with a 25 year history of undiagnosed persistent epigastric pain and progressive weight loss.)

281

abdominal pain not explained by customary diagnoses and standard investigations, and who have not been helped by routine management including other kinds of surgery. The case is strengthened by such clinical features as weight loss, and pain which is aggravated by food, and not relieved by antacids or antispasmodics. This opinion is essentially similar to that of Brandt and Boley[1] which is based on a comprehensive review of the literature.

REFERENCES

1 Brandt, L. J. & Boley, S. J. (1978) Celiac axis compression syndrome. A critical review. *Digestive Diseases*, **23**, 633–640.

2 Bron, K. M. & Redman, H. C. (1969) Splanchnic artery stenosis and occlusion. Incidence, arteriographic and clinical manifestations. *Radiology*, **92**, 323–328.

3 Carey, J. P., Stemmer, E. A. & Connolly, J. E. (1969) Median arcuate ligament syndrome. Experimental and clinical observations. *Archives of Surgery*, **99**, 441–446.

4 Charrette, E. P., Iyengar, S. R. K., Lynn, R. B. *et al.* (1971) Abdominal pain associated with celiac artery compression. *Surgery, Gynecology and Obstetrics*, **132**, 1009–1014.

5 Chiene, J. (1869) Complete obliteration of the coeliac and mesenteric arteries: the viscera receiving their blood supply through the extra-peritoneal system of vessels. *Journal of Anatomy*, **3**, 65–72.

6 Colapinto, R. F., McLoughlin, M. J. & Weisbrod, G. L. (1972) The routine lateral aortogram and the celiac axis compression syndrome. *Radiology*, **103**, 557–563.

7 Cornell, S. H. (1971) Severe stenosis of the celiac artery. Analysis of patients with and without symptoms. *Radiology*, **99**, 311–316.

8 Curl, J. H., Thompson, N. W. & Stanley, J. C. (1971) Median arcuate ligament compression of the celiac and superior mesenteric arteries. *Annals of Surgery*, **173**, 314–420.

9 Di Marino, V., Tournigand, P., Adhote, B. & Mercier, C. (1972) A propos des compressions extrinsèques de tronc coeliaque. *Journal de Chirurgie*, **104**, 289–306.

10 Drapanos, T. & Bron, K. M. (1966) Stenosis of the celiac artery (editorial). *Annals of Surgery*, **164**, 1085–1088.

11 Dunbar, J. D., Molnar, W., Beman, F. M. & Marable, S. A. (1965) Compression of the celiac trunk and abdominal angina. Preliminary report of 15 cases. *American Journal of Roentgenology*, **95**, 731–744.

12 Edwards, A. J., Hamilton, J. D., Nichol, W. D. *et al.* (1970) Experience with coeliac axis compression syndrome. *British Medical Journal*, **i**, 342–345.

13 Harjola, P. T. (1963) A rare obstruction of the celiac artery. *Annales Chirurgiae et Gynaecologiae Fenniae*, **52**, 547–550.

14 Julius, S. & Stewart, B. H. (1967) Diagnostic significance of abdominal murmurs. *New England Journal of Medicine*, **276**, 1175–1178.

15 Lord, R. S. A., Stoney, R. J. & Wylie, E. J. (1968) Coeliac axis compression. *Lancet*, **ii**, 795–798.

16 Marable, S. A., Kaplan, M. F. & Beman, F. M. (1968) Celiac compression syndrome. *American Journal of Surgery*, **115**, 97–102.

17 Marable, S. A., Molnar, W. & Beman, F. M. (1966) Abdominal pain secondary to celiac axis compression. *American Journal of Surgery*, **111**, 493–495.

18 Mihas, A. A., Laws, H. L. & Jander, P. H. (1977) Surgical treatment of the celiac compression syndrome. *American Journal of Surgery*, **133**, 688–691.

19 Reuter, S. R. & Olin, T. (1965) Stenosis of the celiac artery. *Radiology*, **85**, 617–627.

20 Rob, C. (1966) Surgical diseases of the celiac and mesenteric arteries. *Archives of Surgery*, **93**, 21–32.

21 Snyder, M. A., Mahoney, E. B. & Rob, C. G. (1967) Symptomatic celiac artery stenosis due to constriction by the neurofibrous tissue of the celiac ganglion. *Surgery*, **61**, 372–376.

22 Szilagyi, D. E., Rian, R. L., Elliott, J. P. & Smith, R. F. (1972) The celiac artery compression syndrome: does it exist? *Surgery*, **72**, 849–863.

23 Watson, W. C. & Sadikali, F. (1977) Celiac axis compression. Experience with 20 patients and a critical appraisal of the syndrome. *Annals of Internal Medicine*, **86**, 278–284.

24 Watson, W. C., Williams, P. B. & Duffy, G. (1973) Epigastric bruits in patients with and without celiac axis compression. A phonoarteriographic study. *Annals of Internal Medicine*, **79**, 211–215.

Chapter 6
Gastrointestinal Tract Haemorrhage

ACUTE UPPER GASTROINTESTINAL HAEMORRHAGE

Bleeding from the gut is a continuing challenge to the gastroenterologist because of its dramatic presentation and its considerable mortality. It is also a problem which will be encountered not only by specialist gastroenterologists but by every general physician and surgeon. Occasionally the bleeding patient is admitted to a restricted unit under the care of specialist members of staff but on the whole the condition is dealt with on general medical wards under the care of physicians who have close liaison with surgical units.

Assessment of success in management can be made by the frequency of complications, units of blood transfused or length of hospital stay, but ultimately the only important criterion is mortality. Twentieth century literature abounds with mortality figures virtually all relating to the primary admission to hospital, and with few exceptions follow up has been neglected.

INCIDENCE

Gastrointestinal bleeding is a common problem and relates to many diseases. Analysis of data from the hospital inpatient inquiry of the United Kingdom Ministry of Health for the years 1956–1957 calculated an annual admission of 75 000 patients with peptic ulcer to hospitals in England and Wales, of which 12 300 were precipitated by gastrointestinal haemorrhage and of whom 1400 (11.4%) died.[25] Peptic ulceration is responsible for approximately 50% of all patients admitted with gastrointestinal bleeding and it is therefore reasonable to believe that approximately 25 000 patients are admitted annually to hospitals in England and Wales

with this problem. If the overall mortality remains at its present level of approximately 9% there must be well over 2000 deaths per year.

MORTALITY

Mortality is seldom considered in these overall terms now and must be related to individual causes for a meaningful study of the problem. None the less, the point has often been made in recent years of the notable failure to improve mortality rates despite the introduction of sophisticated investigative techniques and aggressive management policies. There was an impressive improvement in mortality between 1930 and 1950 mainly due to the introduction of blood transfusion, but in the last 30 years there has been little change in these overall figures. Two factors appear to have been responsible for this static mortality: the first is the rising mean age of these patients and the second is the increasing incidence of bleeding due to portal hypertension. Thus whereas in 1940 only 20% of patients were over the age of 60, current figures indicate that over 50% are over 60 years and it appears that this figure is still rising (Figure 6.1).

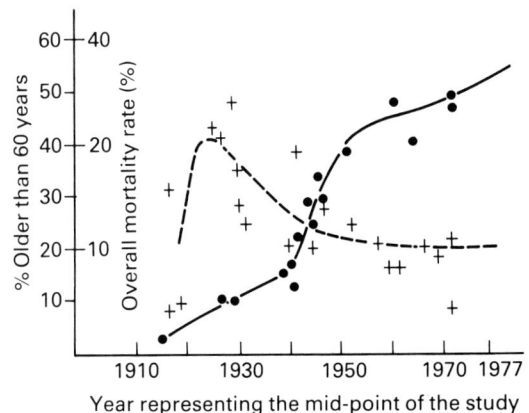

Fig. 6.1 The changing pattern of mortality (+) and age. The age is indicated as percentage of patients older than 60 years (●).

283

Table 6.1 Relative incidence of separate diagnoses at Birmingham General Hospital ten years apart.

	1970–73	1980–82
Total numbers	300	379
	Percentage incidence	
Duodenal ulcer	30	40
Gastric ulcer	19	17
Varices	2	8
Carcinoma	5	4
Erosions	17	12
Oesophagitis	4	8
Mallory–Weiss	2	2
Other	12	9
No diagnosis	9	0

Similarly, variceal bleeding is much more common and appears to be increasing rapidly. In a survey in the Birmingham General Hospital 1971–1973, 2% of 300 patients were found to be bleeding from varices, whereas in a similar group of 200 patients collected recently this figure has risen to 8% (Table 6.1).[82]

Although the majority of published data continues to show these rather depressingly steady mortality figures, there are a number of studies where mortality is substantially lower. It is important to separate defined peptic ulcer disease for such comparison, but there now exist some well documented mortality figures as low as 2% (Table 6.2).[11, 21, 52, 82, 91] The individual characteristics of these studies are listed but the common factor in all of them is an aggressive diagnostic and management policy.

It is gratifying to find that there are now very few patients in whom the source of bleeding is not found, and in fact our policy is never to accept a negative diagnosis but rather to repeat the endoscopy. Under these conditions we are almost never left with undiagnosed patients. Emergency endoscopy is too frequently carried out by an inexperienced member of staff and the

information presented from our own unit was obtained almost exclusively by two more senior members of staff dedicated to a gastrointestinal bleeding project. It is likely, therefore, that the so-called undiagnosed patient simply represents the ulcer that is more difficult to find or obscured by blood clot. Erosive bleeding has also been a source of confusion and its reported incidence varies widely. Erosions are rarely responsible for major bleeding, and if an ulcer is present the latter should be assumed as the site of haemorrhage.

REBLEEDING

Mortality rates depend on complications, which in turn are largely related to recurrent haemorrhage. Hence the current interest is in rebleeding rates and a search for indications which will define patients who are likely to rebleed. Attempts have therefore been made to define patients at risk of rebleeding by age and diagnosis, and by endoscopic signs of clot or exposed vessels in the ulcer base.

Similarly, the management of rebleeding is also under scrutiny and it should no longer be acceptable to urge clinicians to adopt a therapeutic policy without offering factual data to support it. Specialized units are therefore evaluating, by prospective controlled trials, the optimum timing of surgery, the value of H_2-receptor antagonist agents and other drugs on bleeding, the place of therapeutic endoscopy and the optimum approach to portal hypertension. Probably the greatest difficulty in running these trials is the relatively low overall mortality from bleeding peptic ulceration. It is therefore important to appreciate that death from bleeding peptic ulcer under the age of 60 is rare, and trials should probably be limited to patients over 60 years of age. Indices of therapeutic success must be easy to define, and the

Table 6.2 Series with low peptic ulcer mortality.

Ref.	Year	Cases of duodenal ulcer*	Cases of gastric ulcer*	Mortality (%)	Operation rate (%)	Study characteristics
91	1969	366 (6)	176 (6)	2.1	16	Mean age 41; aggressive policy
21	1973	50 (2)	59 (2)	3.3	37	Not consecutive; age not given
11	1977	30 (1)	17 (0)	2	53	All aged over 60; aggressive policy
52	1979	93 (2)	38 (0)	1.5	25	Centralized management; aggressive policy
82	1983	40 (1)	15 (0)	2	58	Centralized management; aggressive policy

* Numbers of deaths in parentheses.

only criteria which are of any value in monitoring success are rebleeding and mortality.

Thus, this section will concentrate on examining separate causes of bleeding, on methods of obtaining an early accurate diagnosis, and on reliable therapeutic data obtained from well-designed prospective randomized trials.

Oesophageal bleeding

Oesophageal sources of intestinal blood loss account for 10–20% of cases of haematemesis, largely comprising oesophageal varices, hiatal hernia and Mallory–Weiss tears of the oesophago-gastric junction.

HIATAL HERNIA AND REFLUX OESOPHAGITIS

Hiatal hernia is an extremely common condition found particularly in older sections of the community. It is frequently associated with the symptoms of acid reflux and sometimes with oesophagitis, but is a less common cause of gastrointestinal bleeding. Blood loss from oesophagitis and associated erosions is usually chronic and presents as iron deficiency anaemia of the elderly. None the less, severe haemorrhage does occur and accounts for approximately 10% of patients admitted because of bleeding from the gastrointestinal tract.

Oesophagitis first develops on the crests of mucosal folds above the cardia and therefore appears as linear red streaks often associated with lines of erosions. These may be seen to be bleeding and are associated with areas of adherent exudate. Care must be taken to inspect this area carefully on first passage of the endoscope, so as to avoid endoscopic trauma which may be mistaken for a cause of the bleeding. Severity of dyspeptic symptoms is not a good index of the presence of pathology and 30% of those patients admitted to hospital with oesophageal bleeding admit to no antecedent dyspepsia. Bleeding from oesophagitis may often be precipitated by irritants such as aspirin or potassium chloride which may remain in the oesophagus for long periods because of defective oesophageal motility.

Ulceration associated with hiatal hernia occurs on the gastric side of the oesophago-gastric junction and often at the level of the hiatus itself. Ulceration is much more commonly found in patients with a paraoesophageal rather than a sliding hiatal hernia and it has been estimated that up to 20% of such patients suffer a substantial haemorrhage.[5]

Barrett's syndrome is a particularly severe complication of this disorder, and is characterized by columnar epithelium lining the whole of the lower oesophagus.[8] The junction with normal oesophageal mucosa lies well above the cardia hence oesophagitis and stricture formation may occur in the mid-oesophagus. Major haemorrhage is due to chronic ulceration (Barrett's ulcer) of the gastric mucosa in the lower oesophagus. Such patients are usually elderly and management poses very serious problems.

MALLORY–WEISS SYNDROME

Tearing of the gastric mucosa at the level of the hiatus is an important cause of gastrointestinal bleeding. The tear usually occurs following violent diaphragmatic contraction during vomiting. It is believed that a small sliding hiatal hernia is usually present but as the oesophago-gastric mucosal junction normally lies above the level of the diaphragm, this is perhaps an irrelevant argument. This lesion is also relatively common as a cause of upper gastrointestinal haemorrhage and must be looked for with care during insertion of the gastroscope. It is of course necessary to invert the instrument and inspect the hiatus from below before excluding this as a cause of haemorrhage. The tears are linear, sited at or just below the mucosal junction, and extend into a submucosal plexus of thin-walled vessels. Occasionally the tear may occur in the mucosa of the distal oesophagus. Bleeding is usually minor and probably occurs in large numbers of patients who are never admitted to hospital.[45]

The characteristic clinical pattern is of retching and vomiting in alcoholics followed by haematemesis but may follow epileptic convulsions, status asthmaticus and paroxysms of coughing. However, this dramatic picture is not universal and bleeding may be the first symptom.

The tear rapidly becomes a linear ulcer and usually heals within a week to 10 days. Bleeding is usually mild, rebleeding is rare and surgical intervention is hardly ever necessary.

Peptic ulceration

Ulceration of the stomach and duodenum is the commonest cause of severe haematemesis and melaena. Although it occurs at any age, it appears to be increasingly a problem of the elderly, where it is particularly dangerous. There is little recent information on the liability of a given peptic ulcer to bleed, but in 1975 Emery and Munroe showed that of 1435 ulcer patients, 27% bled over a four-year period of observation.[32] Data from Sweden[120] later suggested that with a detailed history, this figure is probably higher. It would seem therefore that bleeding has probably twice the incidence of perforation. This information was obtained before modern medical and surgical therapy was introduced, and probably therefore reflects the true natural history of the illness. The current rates of bleeding may be lower, but as the main thrust of therapy shifts from surgery to drugs, so the number of patients at risk from bleeding is likely to increase.

Ulcers recurring after definitive surgical treatment are reported as being more liable to acute haemorrhage[35] and therefore to carry an increased morbidity. The siting of these ulcers has changed since the advent of vagotomy as the operation of choice, and anastomotic ulcers have given way to recurrent ulceration at the original site, commonly in the duodenum. Although bleeding after gastric operations may sometimes arise from haemorrhagic gastritis induced by bile reflux, major haemorrhage is usually due to a recurrent ulcer with its contained vessel which must be looked for.

CLINICAL FEATURES

A careful clinical history should, of course, always be taken and the occurrence of food and alkali-related epigastric pain is suggestive of peptic ulceration. However, this can be totally misleading and firm diagnostic information is necessary before any assumptions can be made as to the site of bleeding. Further, at least one in six ulcers will bleed in the absence of symptoms[53] and more recently it has been claimed that this incidence of haemorrhage from asymptomatic ulcers may be even higher.[21] Haemorrhage from asymptomatic ulcers has been shown to be much more common in gastric than in duodenal lesions confirming the need for early accurate diagnosis.

Longstanding ulcers are no more liable to rebleed than those of recent onset and in general the liability for haemorrhage is not related to the duration of the lesion. Stolte examined the histories of 333 ulcer patients and found the annual incidence of haemorrhage to be 8.4, 5.4, 5 and 5.9% for each of the four years after commencement of symptoms.[120] Others have confirmed this slightly greater tendency to bleeding within a year of diagnosis. It is likely that individual patients have a particular liability to haemor-

rhage in the presence of an ulcer as it has been shown that the incidence of further haemorrhage in patients who presented with bleeding was 75% whereas it was only 11% in those presenting with indigestion.[64]

The increasing age of patients with gastrointestinal bleeding has already been alluded to, and it seems likely that a given ulcer is more liable to bleed in an older person. Stolte again showed annual frequency rates of haemorrhage for each decade as 4% (under 20), 3% (30–40), 7% (40–50), 9% (50–60), 15% (60–70) and 20% (80+).[120] It also seems that this increased tendency to haemorrhage in the older patient applies to gastric and duodenal ulcers but not to mucosal erosions.[2]

MORPHOLOGY

Morphological aspects of bleeding peptic ulcers have attracted little recent interest, probably because these ulcers are seldom excised. Large blood vessels in the ulcer base have been described at endoscopy, particularly in ulcers liable to further haemorrhage.[36] It has been suggested that these vessels bleed from a saccular aneurysm, but the relationship between the life history of the ulcer and the supporting blood vessels in its base is very poorly understood.

EROSIVE DISEASE

Erosions are shallow, usually less than 5 mm in diameter and are oval or circular in shape. They are commonly multiple, have a tendency to be present in chains or clusters and are most commonly seen in the antrum.[46] The intervening mucosa is often congested and there may well be petechial haemorrhages or larger zones of confluent mucosal or submucosal bleeding.[85] Microscopically the dominant lesion is patchy inflammation with focal cell necrosis in an otherwise normal mucosa. The deeper mucosal layer is seldom involved, although local necrosis may lead to an acute penetrating ulcer.

Since Dupuytren recorded acute gastric erosions in burned patients many apparent precipitating factors have been proposed. Burns, head injury, cerebro-vascular accidents, infections, respiratory failure, metabolic derangements and severe infections have all been proposed as precipitating factors, together with drug and alcohol ingestion. In burned patients, Curling's ulceration appears to occur in two main forms: acute multiple ulcers developing within the first 48 hours in the fundal portion of the stomach and larger deeper erosions sited in the duodenum.[115] Ulcers associated with intracranial lesions (Cushing's ulcer) are also larger and deeper and may relate more to true gastric ulcers.

The role of drugs has been widely debated and caution should be exercised in relating bleeding to current drug therapy. There may well be interrelationships between separate drugs but the role of acid is considerable.

Patients with erosions are commonly to be found in intensive care units arising as a complication of a severe illness. Patients admitted directly to hospital with bleeding erosions usually have fairly limited haemorrhage and only rarely is the bleeding persistent and difficult to control.

Bleeding due to drug therapy

There has been much interest in the possible association between administration of aspirin and other anti-inflammatory drugs and the incidence of peptic ulceration and haemorrhage. Salicylates are undoubtedly gastric irritants and local exposure of the animal stomach to salicylates has regularly shown severe mucosal damage with the production of erosions and ulcers. Aspirin induces occult bleeding in 70% of recipients, the average daily blood loss being 5 ml.[111] Indomethacin has a similar but less marked effect, but the role of phenylbutazone and corticosteroids is less certain.[19] Prostaglandins have been shown to reduce the damage both in animals and humans and mucosal damage has been prevented with doses much less than those required to inhibit gastric acid secretion. Such cytoprotective doses of prostaglandins will also inhibit blood loss in man during aspirin and indomethacin therapy.[105]

Induction of chronic peptic ulceration itself is much more difficult to prove and can only be based on large series with statistically significant differences. Support for such an association with gastric ulceration has received strong support from Australian studies, where large scale consumption of analgesics has been found in middle-aged women.[30] Further support has been found for this observation in North America, and it appears that the association is limited to gastric rather than duodenal ulceration and to substantial doses of aspirin.

Although occult bleeding is a well established complication of aspirin administration, substantial haemorrhage is much less common and its demonstration requires great care in establishing satisfactory controlled populations. Many studies have been performed on hospital inpatient groups where an association has been established, particularly with a combination of anti-inflammatory drugs and anticoagulants.[56] In recent studies the selection of controls in non-hospital populations has been greatly improved and a link has been established between aspirin ingestion and bleeding both in North America and in Britain. Levy used the prehospital drug intake of non-bleeding patients and showed a higher proportion of heavy aspirin users (defined as at least four days a week for more than 12 weeks) among those admitted with acute bleeding than in the large control group.[70] Light aspirin intake was not associated with increased bleeding. A study in Nottingham has compared the recent drug intake of patients admitted with gastrointestinal bleeding against that of a random control population from general practice.[15] An association with aspirin-containing products was well shown but there was also a surprisingly similar association with paracetamol. It appears likely that the major phenomenon demonstrated in this study was the propensity of ill patients to take analgesics. There was, however, an increase of aspirin users over paracetamol particularly when the increasing use of paracetamol in the community was considered. It thus seems probable that the major association of analgesic drugs with acute gastrointestinal bleeding is a spurious one but that there is a small real effect associated with aspirin ingestion.

Unusual causes of intestinal bleeding

AORTO-INTESTINAL FISTULAS

Arterial fistula may occur from the aorta, most commonly to the fourth part of the duodenum.[42] It is usually a complication of an operation for abdominal aortic aneurysm but fistulas may also develop from the aorta or iliac artery into the ileum, sigmoid colon or rectum. The clinical course is not necessarily as fulminating as might be anticipated and patients may present with haematemesis and melaena which is difficult to diagnose. Characteristically an ulcer can be seen in the fourth part of the duodenum with an associated aneurysm or history of a previous aneurysmectomy.

HEREDITARY HAEMORRHAGIC TELANGIECTASIA

Gastrointestinal bleeding may occur in 13% of patients with the Osler–Weber–Rendu syndrome;[107] there is nearly always a family history and bleeding may occur from lesions of the stomach, small bowel or colon. Bleeding is characteristically intermittent and may well appear as recurrent iron deficiency anaemia. A careful search should be made on the face and the mouth for telangiectasia and the diagnosis is usually confirmed by endoscopy or angiography.

ARTERIOVENOUS MALFORMATION

Angiodysplasia has caused considerable interest in recent years[76] and malformations have been described almost anywhere in the gut.[103] Most of these, however, occur in the caecum and ascending colon and present as melaena or intermittent iron deficiency anaemia.

Liver disease

Bleeding is of grave significance in both acute and chronic liver disease. Of all patients admitted to hospital with a variceal bleed, only about one-third leave hospital alive, contrasting with figures of approximately 5% for peptic ulcer bleeding. The reason for the high death rate is related to the severe underlying liver disease and the patient dies as often from liver failure as from exsanguination. None the less, it is haemorrhage which has precipitated the catastrophe and prevention of haemorrhage would reduce mortality. Mortality relates directly to liver failure and nutritional deprivation[31] and there is little to be said for heroic measures in severely jaundiced patients with ascites.

The bleeding comes most commonly from oesophageal varices. The precise reason why the varices bleed is not known, but fluctuations in variceal pressure have been well described as have oesophageal erosions. Bleeding may also occur from widespread gastric erosions or duodenal ulceration and evidence is varied as to the proportion of patients where the bleeding arises from the gastric fundus. It is important to appreciate the possibility of gastric varices in the severely bleeding patient where the use of tamponade is being considered.

It is important to be aware of the many causes of chronic liver disease; previous hepatitis, Wilson's disease or schistosomiasis must all be considered along with chronic hepatitis and alcohol ingestion. In children, thrombotic and congenital anomalies of the portal venous system are not uncommon and are associated with perfectly normal hepatic histology.

An important though unusual cause of haematemesis is haemobilia where bleeding arises from the liver or biliary tree passing directly into the duodenum via the ampulla of Vater. Perhaps the commonest cause is liver biopsy but haemorrhage may also follow road accidents, previous biliary operations, vascular anomalies or anticoagulant therapy. Apart from haematemesis, the condition may present as biliary colic and the diagnosis is then established by unusual appearances on cholecystography or duodenoscopy. Bleeding may also occur into the pancreatic ducts.

Disordered haemostasis

Gastrointestinal bleeding occurs more commonly from defined lesions in the presence of haemostatic defects but may also occur spontaneously without previous pathological breaks in the mucosa. It is particularly important in liver disease where synthesis of coagulation factors is impaired.

THROMBOCYTOPENIA

Thrombocytopenic patients are more liable to bleed if the platelet count falls below $100 \times 10^9/l$ and the risk becomes great if this level drops below $30 \times 10^9/l$. Thrombocytopenia may occur as a failure of bone marrow production as in leukaemia, in the presence of decreased survival as in immunological defects and hypersplenism, or resulting from increased platelet consumption as in disseminated intravascular coagulation. Bleeding may occur at different platelet concentrations, partly because platelets produced from an active marrow are more effective than others produced in a leukaemic or cytotoxic marrow. A wide range of drugs affect platelet function and a history of ingestion of drugs, particularly non-steroidal anti-inflammatory, should be sought. The defect will last for the full life of the platelet and aspirin will therefore cause a prolonged bleeding time for a week or more. Renal failure may cause gastrointestinal bleeding because of platelet damage from retained metabolites[51] and platelets may also be damaged due to adsorption of immunoglobulin in myeloma.[94] Myeloproliferative disorders often show the paradoxical association of bleeding and a thrombotic tendency which can be aggravated by an increased incidence of peptic ulceration. Bleeding in leukaemia is mainly due to interference with platelet development and cytotoxic therapy, and leukaemic lesions have been found in the gut at necropsy. The hazard may be compounded because of coincident infection, particularly monilial oesophagitis.

DEFICIENCY OF COAGULATION
FACTORS

Bleeding may be the presenting feature in patients with haemophilia, von Willebrand's disease or Christmas disease. Von Willebrand's disease is most likely to produce gastrointestinal bleeding because of the combination of defects of coagulation, endothelial cells and platelet function.

Haemorrhage may also develop in patients on anticoagulant therapy, particularly where control becomes difficult, for example in the presence of unexpected liver disease or because of drug interactions. Prolongation of the prothrombin time beyond five-times the control value may precipitate spontaneous bleeding. Large doses of vitamin K render the patient refractory to further anti-coagulation but take two hours to be effective. Temporary correction may be achieved by coagulation factor concentrates, but the advice of a clinical haematologist should be obtained. Bleeding may also occur in the complex haemostatic abnormality of disseminated intravascular coagulation (DIC),[13] where it may arise from either the upper or lower alimentary tract and may be occult or massive.

Bleeding may also be affected by fibrinolytic agents present in the tissues and in the lumen of both stomach and colon, so tissue damage or inflammation may thus cause release of activator, generation of plasmin, fibrin digestion and bleeding. Activator and plasmin have been found in association with gastroduodenitis[86] and peptic ulceration.[23] We have carried out studies on fibrinolytic activity of gastric juice and found that the majority of the proteolytic activity in the stomach comes from trypsin.[84] Whether this activity plays a significant role in clot digestion and rebleeding is unresolved.

Bleeding in children

Acute gastrointestinal haemorrhage is less common in children but is much more alarming. It occurs most commonly in young infants, particularly neonates. At all ages rectal bleeding is more common than haematemesis.[77]

NEONATES

The commonest causes of true and apparent bleeding in neonates are the passage of swallowed maternal blood, haemorrhagic disease of the newborn and stress ulceration. Maternal and fetal blood can be distinguished chemically, and haemorrhagic disease of the newborn is both treatable and preventable by injection of vitamin K. Recent aggressive investigation has uncovered a substantial number of neonates with stress ulceration which can easily be missed by contrast radiography. Stress ulcers are commonest in the duodenum with a slight male preponderance.[116] Hiatal hernia has also been increasingly recognized and presents as persisting regurgitation in early infancy usually with only small quantities of blood. Melaena and rectal bleeding at this age are due to many causes including anal fissure, necrotizing enterocolitis, mid-gut volvulus and enteric duplication.

INFANTS AND YOUNG CHILDREN

Stress ulceration is the commonest cause of haematemesis although bleeding from oesophageal varices is commoner than in neonates. Extrahepatic portal hypertension is the commonest cause of variceal bleeding at this age, and is often due to umbilical sepsis, exchange transfusion and congenital anomalies of the portal vein.[132] None the less, no cause for the increased portal pressure is found in approximately 50% of patients. Blood in the stool at this age is usually due to Meckel's diverticulum or intussusception, and more rarely from polyps.

ADOLESCENTS

In the older child peptic ulceration is more common, and in the young teenager is nearly always duodenal and in males. A strong family history has been reported in up to 50% of patients.[27] The ulcers are often resistant to therapy.

The increasing use of endoscopy will undoubtedly clarify the nature and incidence of ulceration of the upper gastrointestinal tract and its relationship to such conditions as hiatal hernia. Fortunately the mortality of gastrointestinal bleeding in children is low but this will only remain so with continued vigilance and a high level of care.

DIAGNOSIS

Clinical

Full clinical details must be obtained speedily. It is now clear that a detailed evaluation of the patient's history of pain with its relationship to food and antacids is of little value[28] and the primary diagnostic aim at the bedside is to consider for exclusion the less common causes, which are easy to overlook. Thus the clinical history must include enquiry about any bleeding tendency, family history, drug and alcohol ingestion and previous surgery. Clinical examination should include a search for evidence of liver disease, of haemangiomas in the skin and mouth and changes in skin, subcutaneous tissue and joints, suggestive of rare connective tissue disorders (these are discussed in Chapter 9). Once these unusual causes have been looked for attention must concentrate on specialized investigation to obtain an accurate working diagnosis.

Investigation

The investigation of acute gastrointestinal bleeding has been so greatly improved over the past 20 years that early comparative studies are now of historical interest only. If dedication and skill are available, accurate diagnosis is nearly always practicable, whether by endoscopic or radiological techniques. Doubt has been expressed as to whether such accuracy carries any short term managerial benefit,[29] a view which must be strenuously resisted. Bleeding from complications of liver disease is becoming an increasingly important problem in this field and logical management is impossible until the source of bleeding has been defined. Judgement as to early surgical treatment of peptic ulcer disease is being increasingly affected by the risk of further haemorrhage, itself much higher in the presence of an obvious vessel seen at endoscopy. Thus the endoscopic findings must influence the decision as to whether surgery should be carried out urgently. Furthermore, it seems likely that endoscopic methods of coagulating small arteries will receive further attention in the next few years, and for this the diagnosis of the lesion and the morphology of its vessels is mandatory. Finally, most of the information relating to diagnosis has been obtained by units steadily improving their skills, and differences in mortality rates should not be expected in heterogeneous groups of patients with a 10–20% error in diagnostic rate. Investigation of acute gastrointestinal bleeding by whatever method represents the difficult edge of each diagnostic technique and should only be undertaken by those with sufficient skill and experience. Only when diagnostic rates achieve a high level of precision can therapeutic regimens and prognosis be meaningfully assessed and compared. It has been correctly said that 'the arguments for or against urgent endoscopy should now die; it clouds the real issue which concerns management'.[22]

OESOPHAGO-GASTRODUODENOSCOPY

The method of choice for investigating acute upper gastrointestinal bleeding depends on the skills available. The last 10 years have seen a proliferation of gastroenterologists well trained in endoscopy and few hospitals do not have emergency endoscopy available; this must now be the investigation of choice. Overall accuracy is generally claimed as 80–95%, but where the technique is assiduously pursued it is rare for the bleeding lesion to remain undiscovered. Much depends on the contents of the stomach and the endoscopist should be prepared to repeat the investigation 6–12 hours later if blood clot has prevented visibility. An ulcer should be carefully examined for the presence of thrombus and visible vessels as these have been shown to relate to rebleeding rates.[36] More recently this association has been shown to relate to the visible vessel, and not to clot.[47, 75] Washing ulcers or suspicious surfaces is not regarded as hazardous, and dislodgement of a clot from a potentially bleeding artery is unusual. Spurting vessels themselves are normally an indication for early surgery, but bleeding often stops spontaneously, as was shown in the control group of the argon laser trial.[127] None the less, presumption must play a role in assessment, and blood welling back through the pylorus reasonably implies the probability of a bleeding duodenal ulcer. Locally adherent clot in the stomach is also important, and even the limited information that there is no blood or bleeding site in the oesophagus can be of great importance to the surgeon choosing his approach. Usually it is possible to find an ulcer and often to find evidence of recent haemorrhage.

The diagnostic value of endoscopy depends greatly on its timing since too close a proximity to the episode of haemorrhage may result in obscured vision by clot; too long a delay, on the other hand, will remove important evidence of attached thrombus. Delay may also allow erosions to heal and on the whole it is recommended that endoscopy is performed between 6 and 18 hours after admission or recent haemorrhage. Sedation is desirable and lavage may occasionally be of benefit. The endoscopes have been greatly modified in recent years, and the ideal instrument now has end vision together with two wide channels in addition to the air and water supply. It is thus possible to carry out lavage and diathermy simultaneously and the more flexible end gives improved manoeuvrability.

RADIOLOGY

Contrast

The current preference for endoscopy as the first-line investigation in the acutely bleeding patient is partly a consequence of the indifferent results obtained by single contrast radiology. It is now believed that earlier claims of 70–80% accuracy were incorrect, and it is more likely that only 50% of patients are diagnosed correctly by this simple technique.[38] Use of the double contrast barium meal in skilled hands does, however, produce results comparable with those obtained by the best endoscopy units. Both techniques involve moving the patient to the investigator and adequate supervision must therefore be provided in seriously ill patients. Provided the patient is not clinically shocked there is no reason why the full technique cannot be applied, and after insertion of barium and air the patient is rotated several times in the prone and supine positions until satisfactory mucosal coating has been obtained. With care normal diagnostic techniques can be applied.[37]

Ulcers are demonstrated by their conventional appearances with radiating folds of scarred mucosa and round or linear craters. An ulcer may of course be filled with blood clot, but provided this is only partial the clot can still often be demonstrated, indicating that the ulcer has been responsible for the haemorrhage. Similarly careful radiology can sometimes show blood streaming from the ulcer surface. Mallory–Weiss lesions are well demonstrated with this technique and good mucosal patterns are not difficult to obtain at the lower end of the oesophagus. Demonstration of erosions, however, is exceedingly difficult and subject to error in interpretation. Often in the severely bleeding patient the radiologist may find it easy to demonstrate oesophageal varices even if the other potential bleeding lesions are not clear. However, radiology cannot be relied upon to define the source of bleeding.

Arteriography

The use of contrast material has always to be considered against the possibility that a patient may need arteriography. If the patient is bleeding severely, and the diagnosis has not been established by endoscopy, arteriography is sometimes the investigation of choice. However, this technique demands a skill and commitment only obtainable in certain units and is not recommended for the inexperienced. A skilled investigator can usually place the catheter in the appropriate vessel and inject adequate amounts of contrast material to obtain sometimes the most dramatically successful pictures of the bleeding lesion.[7] The technique has no place in the routine examination of the patient on admission but must be considered whenever the diagnosis has not been established and the patient continues to bleed. The bleeding is seen as a small blush or spurt associated with terminal vessels. This may appear at the time of maximal arterial filling or as a residue just after the venous blush has disappeared. In the majority of patients with gastric mucosal haemorrhage, bleeding arises from the left gastric artery and in the duodenum from the supraduodenal branch of the gastroduodenal artery. It is often necessary to cannulate the branches of the coeliac axis individually and it is apparent that this is a technique that requires very considerable experience and skill. Extravasation of blood cannot be demonstrated in the case of bleeding from oesophageal varices but these vessels will usually be demonstrable if careful pictures are taken during the venous stage. The technique is particularly valuable in patients with unusual causes of bleeding such as haemorrhage into the pancreas or the liver presenting as bleeding through the ampulla. Angiography is of most value in the demonstration of angiodysplasia, which is usually associated with repeated minor haemorrhages rather than acute upper gastrointestinal bleeding.

Scintigraphy

Another technique which has not been applied frequently enough, but is extremely promising, is scintigraphy. Radiolabelled material, such as $^{99}Tc^m$ sulphur colloid, is injected intravenously and bleeding recognized by the progressive accumulation of radioactivity at the bleeding site.[1] The reported accuracy of this technique is impressive and scanning correlates precisely with cessation of haemorrhage. This technique deserves further examination.

Portovenography

A further role for radiology in the diagnosis of gastrointestinal bleeding is by demonstrating the portal venous system. Although this can frequently be done best by observing the venous phase after mesenteric angiography, it is more usual to perform the examination by direct injection into the spleen if it is still present and there is no ascites. The technique is invasive and defects in blood coagulation often have to be corrected first. Many of the patients are extremely ill and an early decision should be taken as to whether resuscitation is feasible. If it is not, invasive procedures are irresponsible, and efforts should be concentrated on making the patient comfortable and keeping the relatives informed. Demonstration of the portal veins is of particular importance to the surgeon who is about to undertake decompressive procedures. Thus the use of portography is declining in parallel with the move away from emergency portacaval shunting.

ASSESSMENT OF RISK

Identification of the high-risk patient is one of the most important problems and is central to the evaluation of any new therapeutic procedure. Acute upper gastrointestinal haemorrhage can be a disastrous complication with the patient facing a mortality of over 50%, but it may also be a minor incident to a benign illness in a healthy young person. Avery Jones[6] first demonstrated in two retrospective studies a twelvefold increase in mortality in patients with recurrent haemorrhage following hospital admission. He also demonstrated that mortality increased with age, especially over the age of 60, and that it was higher in patients with chronic gastric ulcers than in those with acute lesions of the stomach or duodenum. The importance of age has become clear from almost every series published since then, and where death occurs under the age of 60 the management should always be closely examined.

The incidence of portal hypertension and bleeding from oesophageal varices is increasing and this condition is always associated with a high mortality. Thus overall mortality figures are not particularly valuable. Mortality is also increased in the presence of other associated medical disorders, especially cardiac, respiratory or liver disease.[81] The severity of the initial bleed is an important risk factor and is indicated by hypotension, low haemoglobin level, or a large volume of blood needed for transfusion. The severity of bleeding is indicated by the clinical presentation and haematemesis more commonly indicates the volume of blood lost than its site of origin.[89] Many of these factors are interrelated and the most important risk factor seems to be recurrent haemorrhage (Figure 6.2). Clearly if a patient never rebleeds the risks of violent circulatory changes are minimal and surgical complications eliminated. Rebleeding is much commoner in the presence of a chronic gastric ulcer or oesophageal varices[87] and also in a patient who has bled within two days of admission to hospital. There is conflicting evidence as to whether rebleeding is commoner over the age of 60. The endoscopic findings of a visible vessel and associated clot are also of great prognostic importance to patients bleeding from a peptic ulcer. Previous surgical operations also increase the risk of fatal haemorrhage in patients with peptic ulcer disease.

MEDICAL TREATMENT

Classically the physician's role in gastrointestinal haemorrhage has been to resuscitate the patient, watch carefully for rebleeding and select those patients for whom surgical treatment is necessary. There are no pharmacological agents proven to have a significant influence either on stopping bleeding or on preventing its recurrence. However, it is encouraging that the last decade has seen the commencement of critical evaluation of regimens of medical manage-

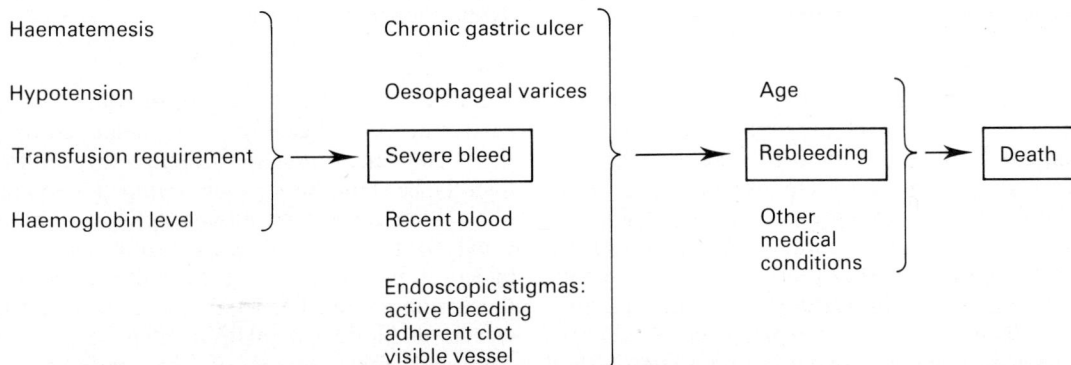

Fig. 6.2 Interrelationship between risk factors.

ment and the appearance of some drugs which show promise for the future.

Monitoring and general care

Attention should be given to the clinical state of the patient, to the appearance of further bleeding and to the patient's pulse and blood pressure. Management is easier if these patients are monitored on a special unit attached to a gastroenterological ward,[52] but of itself this is unlikely to reduce mortality. Patients with respiratory failure and those bleeding from oesophageal varices will often need the facilities of an intensive care unit. Urine output is particularly important and when this drops below 0.5 $ml \cdot kg^{-1} \cdot h^{-1}$, provided renal function was normal beforehand, it can be assumed that the patient has poor renal blood flow secondary to hypovolaemia. It may also be assumed that 20% of the blood volume has been lost and urgent resuscitation is necessary. Severe haemorrhagic shock occurs when more than 40% of the blood volume has been lost; in this situation there is inadequate perfusion of the heart and the brain. This seldom happens in modern hospitals but bleeding can be rapid in the elderly and in the patient with portal hypertension, and care must be taken to avoid irreversible circulatory damage. Changes in central venous pressure can be a useful guide to volume replacement, but venous pressure monitoring is usually only possible on a special unit.[88] The most important fluid for volume expansion is blood, but other fluids may be necessary, particularly at the moment of hospital admission. The fluid of choice on arrival at hospital is 0.9% sodium chloride or a balanced crystalloid solution. Care must be taken in transfusing saline, particularly in the elderly or in patients with heart disease, and it is contraindicated in patients with advanced liver disease. The expansion of blood volume is temporary but gives time for blood to be crossmatched, and the circulation is maintained adequately during this vital period. Colloids should be avoided at this stage, as leakage into the tissues provides problems for tissue lymphatics when the circulating blood volume has been re-established. Dextran is the most widely used of the colloids, and dextran 70 is the most effective. Its disadvantage in haemorrhagic shock is that it interferes with blood typing and may impair coagulation and immune mechanisms. Dextran 40 is relatively short-acting, but since it interferes less with blood typing it is to be preferred. Many plasma protein fractions are

also available and their use depends on availability and expense.

Bed rest

Bed rest has no therapeutic value per se and clearly depends on the clinical state of the patient. Once haemodynamic stability has been reached, bed rest has an adverse effect since thromboembolism is one of the most hazardous complications.[2] Low dose heparin reduces the incidence of fatal pulmonary embolism after surgery[3] but there is no reference to its use in non-operated patients with gastrointestinal bleeding.

Sedation

Mild sedation is desirable in a restless patient, but care should be taken because the restlessness is frequently due to hypovolaemia. Diazepam is probably the best drug available but it should be used cautiously in hepatic disease.

Oral intake

Starvation was the traditional treatment until Meulengracht[78] introduced early feeding and reported a reduced mortality. However, the reduced mortality was probably not due to feeding but to fluid replacement. Similar data were provided by Avery Jones[6] but again the results were probably due to adequate transfusion. In the absence of definitive evidence on the effects of volume, acid and proteolysis in the stomach, no definite recommendations can be made for feeding. Management must therefore depend on the state of the patient and the likelihood of endoscopy or surgery.

Nasogastric intubation

The passage of a nasogastric tube is of much less importance since the introduction of endoscopy because one of its main functions was simply to detect whether there was free blood in the stomach. Opinion at the moment is rather against leaving such a tube in the stomach in view of its well recognized tendency to induce erosions.[21] A nasogastric tube may play a role in the administration of drugs to the stomach, but otherwise its use should be discouraged.

Vasopressin and somatostatin

Vasopressin and somatostatin have been tried in non-variceal haemorrhage.[57] Vasopressin has been used particularly in association with oesophagitis, the Mallory–Weiss syndrome and gastric erosions but seems to be of little benefit since bleeding usually stops spontaneously. The role of somatostatin is currently unknown.[118] Antacids have been used extensively in upper gastrointestinal bleeding, mainly to relieve epigastric pain. There has also been the theoretical possibility that reduction of gastric acidity will reduce the activity of intragastric enzymes and prevent clot lysis in the base of the ulcer. Recent studies have shown that substantial amounts of alkali are necessary to neutralize gastric acid,[24] and a non-absorbable antacid is obligatory. Sixty millilitres of magnesium aluminium hydroxide is administered every 15 min to bring the pH of the gastric fluid above 5. There is evidence that such neutralization will reduce the incidence of rebleeding from erosive disease,[112] but a large-scale trial in patients with peptic ulcer is necessary. A similar effect can be obtained by the use of a milk–alkaline mixture given by continuous intragastric drip, but there is no evidence that this therapy reduces rebleeding rates.[114]

H₂-receptor antagonists

Cimetidine and ranitidine are valuable drugs in the reduction of gastric acidity. If reducing gastric acid is important in preventing clot lysis, it would be anticipated that these drugs would be helpful in reducing rebleeding rates. Extensive studies on cimetidine have failed to show an effect on overall rates of rebleeding from ulceration, but these agents may have a role in older patients and those more seriously ill who are bleeding from gastric ulcers.[50] A recent study with ranitidine has raised the possibility that rebleeding rates from duodenal ulceration may also be reduced.[26]

For the present, evidence is marginally in favour of the use of H₂-receptor antagonists in the prevention of rebleeding from peptic ulceration. Although intragastric titration of acidity with alkali may be more effective in neutralization, because intravenous infusion of cimetidine or ranitidine is so much easier, it is to be preferred. The hazards of these drugs are minimal except possibly in the elderly confused patient, and as the aim must be not only prevention of rebleeding but healing of ulceration it is logical to use these drugs from the moment the patient enters hospital. Cimetidine should be given in a dose of 200 mg, 4-hourly intravenously until the patient can take it orally;

then a more conventional dose of 400 mg orally, 8-hourly is given.

Anti-fibrinolytic agents

It has been suggested that excess fibrinolytic activity occurs in patients with bleeding peptic ulceration;[23] hence tranexamic acid has been suggested as a useful agent in preventing rebleeding.

Cormack *et al.*[20] performed a controlled trial of tranexamic acid against placebo in acute upper gastrointestinal haemorrhage in 150 patients and claimed a lower blood transfusion rate. In a larger study endoscopy was used as an index of assessment[9] and 1 g of tranexamic acid was given intravenously 8-hourly for 48 hours and 1 g orally from admission for five days. There was a significant reduction in emergency surgery and in transfusion requirements affecting all diagnostic groups, especially those with duodenal ulceration. Further recent studies have been carried out in the UK[66] and the evidence supports the possibility that this drug may be of value. However, the studies are by no means conclusive and the method of administration needs further examination.

Gastric cooling

Gastric acid secretion and activation of pepsinogen are markedly reduced at temperatures below 20°C and it has been suggested that hypothermia may prevent clot lysis.[134] This technique has been carefully examined using a double-lumen tube with a gastric balloon and the most popular agent for infusion has been a mixture of cooled alcohol and water. However, cooling is not without hazard[106] and is not to be routinely recommended. It is also complex to perform and should not be used unless well practised. There is at present no evidence that it reduces rebleeding significantly.

Treatment of erosions and stress-induced ulcers

Moderate haemorrhage from erosions usually stops with supportive treatment alone but a few patients have severe persistent bleeding for which they require surgery. There is no satisfactory evidence that any medication assists in the healing of erosions or in the control of haemorrhage. However, prophylactic cimetidine has been demonstrated to reduce haemorrhage in patients at risk of gastric erosions.[48] A controlled trial in patients with fulminating hepatic failure showed a reduction in gastrointestinal haemorrhage[73] but there was no influence on mortality.

SURGICAL TREATMENT

Oesophagus

Operation on the oesophagus is seldom necessary for gastrointestinal bleeding except when portal hypertension is present. Bleeding from hiatal hernia is nearly always chronic and sudden haemorrhage, if it occurs, is of short duration. Serious haemorrhage is usually due to ulcers which ride across the diaphragm; they may be quite deep and are sited on the lesser curvature. These ulcers however, are gastric ulcers, and the policy of management should be that used in the emergency treatment of bleeding peptic ulcers. Should surgery be necessary, excision of the ulcer and repair of the hernia are all that is necessary, although many surgeons will add a vagotomy to this approach.

Bleeding from Mallory–Weiss tears is usually self-limiting and minor, and surgical intervention is rarely necessary. When surgical treatment is required a high approach, possibly through an abdomino-thoracic incision, is sometimes necessary in order to provide adequate access. The mucosal tear is sutured and a hiatal repair should be added.

Stomach and duodenum

Surgery is often the best treatment for peptic ulcers that continue to bleed and it should not be regarded as a failure of management. It is generally believed that early surgery is associated with a lower mortality[33] and support for this view comes from a consecutive surgical series of 66 patients over the age of 60 years in which early surgery resulted in a mortality of only 2%,[11] a figure also arrived at by an Australian group whose policies were to centralize patients and offer early surgery.[52] Certainly operations carried out some time after hospital admission carry a much higher mortality rate than those undertaken within the first 24 hours. None the less, none of these studies were randomized or prospective and analysis of the causes of death has pointed to the close association between mortality and surgical complications.[2] The contrary view might be expressed, therefore, that older patients with coincident disease are at a very grave risk if emergency surgical procedures are necessary and hence surgery should be avoided.

A study from Nottingham of 908 patients admitted to two hospitals between 1975 and 1978 showed a reduction in operation rate over the second half of this period from 33 to 21%, but there was no associated change in mortality.[129] The mortality rates quoted of 9% for duodenal ulcer and 13% for gastric are high by modern standards and the comparisons were in fact made between two different hospitals and in two different time periods. This information must be received with caution. In a prospective randomized study in Birmingham 142 patients were included.[82, 84a] They were stratified according to age and diagnosis on admission and randomized into two groups. The indications for surgery in each group are listed in Table 6.3. We have now adopted the early-

Table 6.3 Indications for operation: surgery is performed if any of the criteria are met.

Group 1: early surgery
  2 litre blood transfusion for initial volume replacement
First rebleed
Endoscopic stigmata
Previous upper gastrointestinal bleed + >2 years dyspepsia

Group 2: late surgery
  4 litre blood transfusion for initial volume replacement
Second rebleed:
  6 litres of blood required in 48 hours
  8 litres required in 72 hours *and* continuing haemorrhage

surgery criteria for patients over 60 and the late-surgery criteria for patients under 60. The study on patients under the age of 60 was stopped because there were no deaths in the early-surgery group or in the late-surgery group, but the operation rate was found to be 53% for those randomized to early surgery as against 6% for those where surgical treatment was delayed. This big increase in operation rate was unreasonable, particularly as mortality rates would never seem likely to be affected and morbidity may well be higher in the surgical group. For patients over 60, however, there have been six deaths in the patients where surgery was delayed against one in the group who drew early aggressive surgery. In the latest analysis of this study the difference has reached a level of statistical significance for patients with peptic ulcer disease over the age of 60. The mortality for early surgery is 4%, compared with 16% for delayed operation. Thus, conclusive data are now available to answer the question of optimal timing of surgery. Patients under the age of 60 should not be operated on unless there is a clear failure of medical management. Over the age of 60, however, early surgical intervention is now advised. Far from surgery being contraindicated in older patients with coincident disease, it seems likely that these are the very patients where mortality rates rise to unacceptable levels if surgical treatment is delayed.

DUODENAL ULCER

Access to the bleeding site is provided through a longitudinal duodenotomy and the vessel responsible for haemorrhage should be exposed by removal of adherent clot with deliberate attempts to promote further bleeding. This is essential to enable the controlling 'figure-of-eight' suture to be sited in the right place;[130] vessel ligation alone is inadequate. Non-absorbable suture material must be used and the procedure should be associated with vagotomy and pyloroplasty. Under the conditions of operation it is perhaps inevitable that vagotomy is total, though even this may be difficult in the presence of obesity, hiatal hernia and hepatic enlargement. The incidence of recurrent ulceration is generally around 5–10%, which is acceptable, particularly since the main aim is to control bleeding and minimize mortality in dangerously ill patients. Johnston[62] has suggested that highly selective vagotomy (proximal gastric vagotomy) be used to control gastrointestinal haemorrhage. (This procedure is discussed by Johnston and Blackett in Chapter 4.) However, the operation is technically demanding, and we have not yet reached a situation where these seriously ill patients are operated upon by the most experienced surgeons. Recommendations for surgical management must therefore be seen in the realistic perspective of controlling blood loss and not necessarily the most appropriate ulcer curing operation.

Partial gastrectomy is still used in many centres for bleeding duodenal ulcers, particularly in the USA. It has been suggested that mortality for this operation is higher than vagotomy but a recent comparison of mortality rates from many centres failed to support this.[130] Nevertheless, most surgeons are trained in vagotomy and not partial gastrectomy and the least demanding operation should be chosen when operating to save life.

GASTRIC ULCER

The ulcer crater can usually be under-run or locally excised, and as some of these ulcers turn out to be malignant excision is desirable. The type of excision depends on the location of the ulcer. It is usually possible to perform a wedge excision of the ulcer; this is a rapid procedure but has the disadvantage that the ulcer is sometimes difficult to locate from outside the stomach. Such excision is accompanied by an ulcer curative operation such as vagotomy. Various forms of vagotomy have been used for

gastric ulceration and all carry a low complication rate. Truncal vagotomy and pyloroplasty has been used but wedge excision of an ulcer close to the cardia can be extremely difficult and the results in terms of ulcer healing are inferior to Billroth I gastrectomy.[113] Nevertheless, local excision for high gastric ulcers is much safer than Billroth I gastrectomy. Highly selective vagotomy has also been used but is subject to much the same disadvantages as in duodenal ulcer. An extensive trial of this procedure has not been published. Billroth I gastrectomy, on the other hand, has remained the operation of choice for definitive treatment of gastric ulceration and also for its complication of haematemesis. There is no evidence that mortality is any different between vagotomy with drainage or gastrectomy.

RECURRENT ULCER

The problem is more difficult when ulcer curative surgery has already been carried out and the patient is bleeding from recurrent ulceration. The surgical approach is largely dictated by technical practicalities in a situation where speed is important. Subtotal gastrectomy is usually the sensible approach if previous vagotomy has been undertaken because re-exploration of the hiatal area under these conditions can be hazardous. If, on the other hand, the patient has had a previous gastrectomy, truncal vagotomy and local suture of the bleeding site is recommended. Further resection of a large gastric remnant may also be indicated and it is important to ensure that no antrum is retained with the duodenal stump if a Polya type gastrectomy is performed.

GASTRIC EROSIONS

One of the most horrifying conditions to treat surgically is persistent bleeding from erosive gastritis, and published mortality rates are extremely high at around 50%.[14] Fortunately the condition is rare, and with improved medical management surgery should become obsolete. We have not needed to operate on such patients for several years and suspect that in some of these patients the problems may reflect poor management in the critical initial period. Partial gastrectomy and vagotomy is probably the procedure of choice if operation is necessary although total gastrectomy is sometimes required.

Complications

SEPSIS

The incidence of this important postoperative complication is greatly reduced by the administration of a single dose of a broad-spectrum antibiotic just prior to the operation.[49] This is to be recommended in all elderly patients where gastric resection will be performed. Breakdown of the anastomosis has become rare in these patients, largely because of the preference for vagotomy and pyloroplasty. Polya (Billroth II) gastrectomy may be complicated by leakage from the duodenal stump which can be a life threatening complication. If the patient has pre-existing malnutrition or requires prolonged nasogastric suction, nutritional support must be given, usually parenterally.

CARDIORESPIRATORY

Fatal complications are often related to cardio-vascular and pulmonary disease (Table 6.4). This is undoubtedly one of the most critical and difficult areas of management since operation is being increasingly recommended in older and more fragile individuals. Signs of heart failure and pneumonia should be sought and treatment with diuretics and antibiotics commenced promptly. The greatest dilemma is in patients with chronic respiratory disease and it is sometimes predictable that positive pressure respiration once started can never be withdrawn. Thromboembolic disease frequently occurs in these patients, particularly when there has been severe preoperative hypovolaemia. Low dose

heparin or dextran 70 infusions should be given from the time of operation. Provided there is no open ulcer or persistent bleeding vessel, there is no substantial danger of rebleeding despite the routine use of low dose subcutaneous heparin.

REBLEEDING

It has been suggested that rebleeding is commoner after vagotomy and local under-running of the ulcer than after gastrectomy[130] but this view has recently been disputed[33] partly because of improved technical expertise and the fact that many previous studies were based upon heterogeneous series including patients with bleeding gastric erosions. Rebleeding probably results from inadequate definition of the arterial source of haemorrhage in the base of an ulcer and the use of catgut suture ligation. A gastric ulcer must itself be excised. General considerations such as surgical delay, inadequate transfusion and postoperative sepsis are all contributory factors. Rebleeding is a potentially lethal complication and a second operation may be associated with a mortality of 50%.

LOCAL TREATMENT OF THE BLEEDING POINT

Treatment via the endoscope

The possibility that bleeding may be stopped or rebleeding prevented by an endoscopic technique is exciting. The volume of work currently in progress in this area is therefore understandable, but conclusions are still premature as to the general applicability of these techniques. None the less, data already exist to show clear benefit in skilled hands, and the most important questions relate to the best energy source, the hazard, the proportion of accessible ulcers, the necessary skill, the cost and transportability of the equipment (Table 6.5).

Table 6.4 Causes of death after operation for peptic ulcer (review of literature).[130]

Cause	No. of cases	% Total
Technical		
Repeat haemorrhage (or continued)	48	19.5
Anastomotic leakage	30	12.2
Septic complications	12	4.9
Pancreatitis	3	1.2
Total	93	37.8
Non-technical		
Cardiovascular complications	75	30.5
Pulmonary complications	37	15.0
Pulmonary embolus	16	6.5
Renal failure	5	2.0
Hepatic failure	5	2.0
Miscellaneous	15	6.1
Total	153	62.1
Overall total	246	100.0

Table 6.5 Methods of local treatment of the bleeding point.

Chemical	*Radiographic*
Clotting factors	Vasoconstrictor agents
Tissue adhesions	Vasopressin
Sclerotherapy	Particulate material
Physical energy	Autologous clot
Thermal probe	Gelfoam
Electrocoagulation	Polyvinyl alcohol
Monopolar	Steel coils
Bipolar	Glues
Liquid	Balloon catheters
Laser	
Argon	
Nd YAG	

CHEMICAL FACTORS

The introduction of clotting factors into the stomach is a method which has received new impetus from the development of the endoscope[71] and a similar approach has been the direct application of tissue adhesives, particularly those of the cyanoacrylate group. However, they are difficult to apply to the bleeding site[96] and as there is a substantial risk of toxicity present evidence is against these techniques being of clinical value. A more valuable method has been the development of sclerotherapy for variceal haemorrhage, and this is discussed below.

PHYSICAL ENERGY

Thermal probe

A probe has been developed to provide a small source of heat at the distal end of the endoscope[95] but the amount of energy deposited must be very variable. So far there has not been much development of this method apart from its application to 'hot biopsy forceps', and the technique has been overtaken by electrocoagulation and laser therapy.

Electrocoagulation

The possibility of applying surgical diathermy through the endoscope is attractive and has been developed in four ways. First, the most direct is the use of the monopolar electrode which is held in contact with the tissue. The returned current flows through the patient to a large ground plate. Several good pilot studies have given encouraging results[41, 92, 135] and data so far advanced suggest that bleeding can usually be stopped, rebleeding rates reduced and further haemorrhage controlled. Unfortunately, none of these studies was controlled and they included a substantial number of patients with erosions and Mallory–Weiss tears. Furthermore, the damage from the monopolar coagulation extends deeply and the electrode is often left attached to the lesion through the coagulum, thus inducing rebleeding on withdrawal. Second, in an attempt to overcome this last difficulty, the energy has been sparked across an air gap, but again the depth of tissue injury has proved unpredictable. The monopolar electrode does not at the moment seem promising for further development. Third, an alternative technique is bipolar coagulation, where the electrode is again in contact with the tissues, but current returns through the instrument and tissue damage is less extensive. Two pilot studies have

been reported[43, 83] but the information so far is inconclusive. The method does seem inherently more promising than monopolar coagulation; it is undoubtedly safer and it requires evaluation with studies comparable with those carried out with laser energy. Finally, there is the so-called liquid probe of a monopolar electrode through the centre of which is a continuous flow of saline. This maintains electrical contact and improves the predictability of energy deposition. The technique is inherently attractive and a pilot study reported permanent haemostasis in 11 out of 15 peptic ulcers.[40] Doubtless further information will be available in due course.

Laser coagulation

Lasers provide a means for delivering fairly precise amounts of energy to small defined areas of tissue without contact, and without the use of electrical diathermy. The word laser stands for Light Amplification by the Stimulated Emission of Radiation, and comprises high intensity light, polarized and of a single wavelength. There are two types of laser which give output beams of suitable power and light for endoscopic use; the argon ion laser (blue–green light) and the Nd YAG laser (infrared). With increasing amounts of energy absorbed in the tissues, the results are firstly warmth, secondly thermal contraction without damage, thirdly cell death and finally vaporization. As the tissue shrinks, small vessels may close, thus arresting haemorrhage and sometimes resulting in secondary thrombosis. Characteristically the energy is deposited in a hemisphere, centered on the site of administration. The radius of this sphere is 1 mm for argon and 5 mm for the Nd YAG laser system. Thus the argon laser produces superficial damage and seals vessels up to 1 mm in diameter, whilst the Nd YAG laser penetrates to a depth where perforation of the gut wall becomes a possibility and may seal vessels up to 1.5 mm diameter. Morphologically, the surface epithelium wrinkles and may detach, resulting in the creation of an ulcer, often covered with charred tissue. Histological changes appear with cell damage, clumping of connective tissue fibres, and vascular damage being the most prominent features. Fibrinoid medial necrosis of small arteries is followed by organizing thrombus and periarterial fibrosis. The deeper nature of the lesions produced by the Nd YAG laser is accompanied by a much slower evolution of the injury. Not only may ulcers take several days to become manifest, but healing may take up to a month. It is believed that haemostasis results from thermal contraction of the vessel walls and surrounding tissue, with thrombosis occurring later in the supplying vessels.

A number of well controlled laser studies have now been completed and reported, and a consistent pattern is emerging. The first trial carried out in Barcelona used the argon laser and stratified patients according to endoscopic stigmas of recent haemorrhage.[128] Overall results were unaffected by treatment, but there was a clear difference in rebleeding rates in patients shown to have a visible vessel in the ulcer base. In the other substantial study reported for argon lasers,[121] randomization was carried out only after accessibility for the treatment was established. Of 330 consecutive patients, 76 were found to have an ulcer with stigmas and were accessible for laser therapy. Rebleeding rates were minimal in all patients without a visible vessel. Of those where a vessel was seen, rebleeding occurred in 17 out of 28 control patients, but in only 8 out of 24 laser treated patients. These results achieved statistical significance, and all seven deaths occurred in the control group. However, the mortality in the control group was unusually high and this observation requires confirmation.

Information on Nd YAG laser therapy is available from five centres, but the study protocols are very different. Thus in a large Belgian study, stratification was on the basis of current bleeding with no subdivision as to diagnosis or ulcer appearance.[108] Similar stratification was carried out in other smaller European studies but from these three only the Belgians showed a difference of any statistical significance. Two British studies have stratified patients according to evidence of recent haemorrhage, a distinction which proved rewarding. Studies from London[122] and Glasgow[75] have confirmed that 'clean' ulcers or those with only coloured spots in their base have little tendency to rebleed and no advantage can be demonstrated from laser therapy. On the other hand, both studies showed a substantial reduction in rebleeding rates where vessels were observed in the ulcer base. In Glasgow, 16 such patients were evenly randomized and whereas only one laser treated patient required emergency surgery, this was necessary in all 8 controls, and two of these patients died. Thirty-seven such patients entered the study, where 12 out of 20 control patients re-bled against 3 out of 17 treated with lasers.

Consequently, results from Nd YAG laser administration are in broad agreement with those from the argon laser. Ulcers without visible vessels seldom rebleed and no advantage is likely from laser or indeed any other therapy.

However, the appearance of a visible vessel, whether or not it is actively bleeding, carries a high chance of rebleeding and current evidence suggests that laser therapy is an effective method of preventing this. The commitment and skill necessary to achieve this improvement is, however, very considerable, and even in highly sophisticated units there remain substantial numbers of patients in whom the ulcer was judged inaccessible. Although the technique of laser therapy has been demonstrated to be effective, its general applicability remains to be seen.

Radiographic therapy

The control of haemorrhage by radiographic means has been undertaken in two ways: clinically by injecting vasoconstricting agents and mechanically by occluding the vessel with particulate material. Vasopressin is an aqueous solution of the pressor amines from the posterior pituitary gland. It has an intense vasoconstrictive effect particularly on branches of the splenic artery, left gastric, gastroduodenal, superior and inferior mesenteric arteries. It is widely used in treatment of variceal haemorrhage (see below) but it has also been used for persistent bleeding from erosive lesions in the gut.[4] Under these conditions angiographic demonstration of the bleeding site is necessary and the drug can then be infused directly into the bleeding artery with minimal systemic effect.

Embolization of the vessel can be carried out by using particulate material of which the first and most primitive was the introduction of autologous blood clot. Unfortunately the clot is usually rapidly lysed. The embolic material now most widely used is gel foam, a slowly absorbed gelatin sponge. Small pieces of the sponge are soaked in contrast material, loaded into a small syringe and injected through the arterial catheter.[44] More complicated substances such as particles of polyvinyl alcohol, minute steel coils and rapidly setting glues have all been used. Finally, balloon catheters can provide temporary control of bleeding and in some centres with great radiological expertise these techniques have come into regular use. Control of gastrointestinal bleeding from the more common causes has not been as successful as with other therapeutic techniques but there are situations, such as secondary postoperative haemorrhage, bleeding from diffuse erosive gastritis and bleeding from vascular malformations of the mesenteric arteries, where the technique in skilled hands is of great value.

MANAGEMENT OF BLEEDING OESOPHAGEAL VARICES

Management of the ever increasing numbers of patients presenting with variceal haemorrhage is a major strain on resources and manpower. The complications of torrential haemorrhage and consequent hypovolaemia are compounded by those of advanced liver disease: disturbed coagulation, defective handling of fluid and electrolyte loads, and hepatic and renal failure.

There are no factors that indicate which patients are at risk of variceal haemorrhage, and there is no evidence to incriminate oesophageal trauma, gastro-oesophageal reflux or oesophagitis as precipitating factors. The relationship between portal pressure and risk of bleeding is unclear and although varices are rarely present, and probably pose little risk at portal pressure less than 10–12 mmHg (1.3–1.6 kPa), above this level there seems to be little correlation between increasing portal pressure and the risk of bleeding.[16, 67, 101, 131] The only way to diagnose unequivocally acute variceal bleeding is by urgent, early endoscopy performed by an experienced endoscopist under optimal conditions in a fully equipped endoscopy suite or theatre, ideally with an experienced anaesthetist on hand.

The problems in the acute management of bleeding varices fall into two broad categories: first, resuscitation, monitoring and general care of a patient with chronic liver disease, and second, specific therapy to control and prevent rebleeding.

General treatment

Initial resuscitation is undertaken with crystalloid solutions to restore blood volume, lower viscocity and resuscitate the microcirculation. Transfusion with fresh blood should nevertheless be started as soon as possible. To safeguard staff and equipment, hepatitis B screening is essential and all variceal bleeds should be considered to be B positive until proven otherwise. Patients should be nursed by experienced staff in a central gastrointestinal unit or in an intensive care area. Wherever possible patients should have accurate monitoring of central venous pressure and urine output. An arterial line is also often useful to facilitate pulse and blood pressure monitoring and repeated blood sampling, including arterial gases.

Variceal haemorrhage may be complicated by a number of problems:

Abnormal coagulation. All patients should receive parenteral vitamin K, and coagulation studies should be repeated. Close co-operation with a haematologist is recommended to ensure that, where required, platelet and clotting factor infusions are used efficiently.

Defective fluid and electrolyte handling. Failure to excrete a sodium load will lead to increasing ascites and peripheral oedema. Saline infusion should be restricted. Fluid overload will lead to hyponatraemia and daily monitoring of serum electrolytes and osmolality is required.

Hypoglycaemia. Hypoglycaemia may complicate hepatic failure and should be watched for.

Hepatic encephalopathy. The risk of encephalopathy is reduced by rapid elimination of blood from the gut, and nasogastric mannitol or 10% magnesium sulphate enemas are very efficient.

Oral neomycin (6 g daily) or oral lactulose (30 ml three times a day) reduce encephalopathy in 80–90% of patients and can be used over long periods.[18] Neomycin may however produce pseudomembranous colitis, ototoxicity and nephrotoxicity. Metronidazole 200 mg four times a day is as effective as neomycin in acute or chronic encephalopathy.[80] In resistant patients the combination of neomycin and metronidazole is worth trying.

Drug therapy

VASOPRESSIN

Vasopressin causes splanchnic and peripheral vasoconstriction. An intravenous injection produces a decrease in portal venous flow and portal venous pressure, probably by its action on splanchnic arterioles or on submucosal arterial venous anastomoses. In cirrhotic patients the reduction in portal venous flow may not be accompanied by an equivalent fall in portal pressure possibly due to the increased number of presinusoidal communications between the hepatic artery and the portal vein. Possible further action of vasopressin may involve compression of the lower oesophageal varices by contraction of the lower oesophageal sphincter.[57] An intravenous bolus injection of 20–40 units over 20 minutes will control variceal bleeding but bolus injections produce severe abdominal colic and diarrhoea, and the vasoconstriction may be so severe as to lead to angina, myocardial infarction and even infarction of the small bowel. The short half-life of 24 min necessitates repeating injections 2–3-hourly. Frequent injection is unfortunately subject to tachyphylaxis and a further disadvantage of vasopressin is the possible increase in thrombolytic activity due to vasopressin induced release of plasminogen activating factors. In an attempt to overcome these problems, low dose intra-arterial infusions have been tried and shown to be effective. The combined results of seven published clinical trials showed initial control of bleeding in 137 out of 170 patients.[109] The technique, however, requires considerable technical expertise. Two prospective, randomized clinical studies have compared intravenous and intra-arterial vasopressin infusion. Johnson et al,[57] infused a standard dose of 0.4 units/minute and controlled bleeding in 7 out of 14 patients with intra-arterial and 7 out of 11 with intravenous infusion. Two patients suffered major arterial damage. Chojkier et al,[12] controlled bleeding in 5 out of 10 patients with a variable intra-arterial dose of Pitressin (0.1–0.5 units/minute) and in 6 out of 12 patients with intravenous infusion (0.3–1.5 units/minute). Although the numbers in these trials are small and a type II error cannot be excluded, both groups felt that significant difference between the two infusion techniques was unlikely. Shields' group[110] have compared bolus intravenous injection (20 units over 20 minutes) with infusion (0.4 units/minute), finding that bolus injection controlled bleeding in 2 out of 16 episodes and intravenous infusion in 13 out of 15. In the light of these findings we recommend low dose intravenous infusion of Pitressin as the procedure of choice.

Triglycyl-lysine-vasopressin (glypressin) is an inactive agent which slowly releases active hormone in vivo following cleavage of the terminal amino acid residue and may maintain smooth muscle contraction for ten hours. A recent clinical trial comparing 2 mg of glypressin given as a six hourly bolus injection against vasopressin infusion (0.4 units/minute) suggested that glypressin was superior controlling initial haemorrhage in 7 out of 10 episodes compared with 1 out of 11 with vasopressin. This agent clearly warrants further study. However, the very low control rate with vasopressin is difficult to explain.[39]

Despite adequate initial control, 50% or more of patients will rebleed when vasopressin infusions are discontinued. Thus vasopressin usually only allows time to enable adequate resuscitation prior to more definitive therapy.

SOMATOSTATIN

It has been suggested that somatostatin used as a bolus or continual intravenous infusion lowers hepatic wedge pressure and portal venous flow without affecting peripheral cardiac output, blood pressure or vascular resistance, and hence this substance may be of value in controlling variceal haemorrhage.[10] This work has been disputed[119] and at present somatostatin cannot be recommended in standard management regimen.

PROPRANOLOL

Propranolol reduces portal venous pressure[68] probably by both reduction in cardiac output and blockade of splanchnic β_2-adrenoceptors.[137] The results of two major clinical trials are available. In the first,[69] 74 patients were randomized, 38 receiving a dose of propranolol sufficient to cause a 25% reduction in resting pulse rate, and 36 placebo. In the propranolol group only one patient rebled, from varices, and two died from septicaemia and liver failure. In the control group 16 patients rebled, 12 from varices and four from gastric erosions, four dying as a consequence of bleeding. The 12 months survival was 96% in the propranolol group and 50% in placebo. However, the majority of these patients were alcoholic cirrhotics in Child's category A and the general application of these findings has been seriously questioned in a recent study of 42 consecutive unselected patients.[133] No significant difference in rebleeding was found, seven in each group. There were three deaths all from recurrent variceal haemorrhage, two in the propranolol group and one in placebo. The authors specifically commented on the difficulty of resuscitation in patients receiving propranolol. Further studies are thus needed to clarify the role of propranolol in the management of variceal haemorrhage.

Obliteration of varices

BALLOON TAMPONADE

Should bleeding either fail to be controlled or recur during vasopressin infusion, balloon tamponade is essential, and must be readily available from the moment the patient is admitted to hospital. The four lumen 'Minnesota' tube with both gastric and oesophageal balloons and aspiration channels is the most satisfactory.[79] If the cheaper three lumen Sengstaken–Blakemore tube is used, a further nasogastric tube is essential to aspirate oesophageal secretions. Prior to

passing the tube 350 ml of air should be introduced into the gastric balloon and the pressure
measured using a sphygmomanometer. This
checks for leaks and in addition, by monitoring
balloon pressure during inflation, will reduce the
risk of oesophageal rupture should the balloon
fail to enter the stomach.

Although it is possible to pass a Minnesota
tube in an unsedated patient, a confused,
frightened and often actively bleeding encephalopathic patient requires sedation and we frequently elect to manage our patients
anaesthetized and with intermittent positive
pressure ventilation.

After insertion of the tube, the gastric balloon
should be inflated with air, and either placed on
gentle traction or taped firmly to the side of the
patient's face. The gastric balloon is often adequate to control haemorrhage, but if the oesophageal balloon is inflated, care must be taken
to apply pressure of no greater than 30–40
mmHg to the oesophageal wall. While the
balloon remains inflated the oesophagus must
be continually aspirated using low pressure
suction. The position of the tube must be
checked by plain abdominal and chest radiographs and care must be taken to ensure that the
position of the tube is not altered. Patients not
being ventilated may develop bronchial obstruction and, more frequently, bronchopneumonia.
Tubes should not remain in situ for more than
24 hours as there is a serious risk of pressure
necrosis of the oesophageal mucosa. Rebleeding
will occur in approximately 60% of patients following removal of the tube.[79]

INJECTION SCLEROTHERAPY

Neither vasopressin nor balloon tamponade are
definitive therapies for variceal bleeding. At best
they provide 24–48 hours to stabilize the patient
and to plan further therapy. Originally
described in 1939 and reintroduced to the UK
by MacBeth in 1955,[72] injection sclerotherapy
of varices is now accepted as an important
method of controlling haemorrhage and possibly in reducing the risk of rebleeding. Johnston
in 1973[61] reported his experience of injection
sclerotherapy carried out under general anaesthesia using a Negus oesophagoscope. In 117
patients with 194 admissions for variceal haemorrhage, bleeding was controlled in 177 with a
mortality of 18%.[61] In 1979 Terblanche[123]
reported equally encouraging results, acute variceal bleeding being controlled in 26 out of 36
admissions, with a mortality of 25% (nine
patients). In a small prospective controlled trial,
the rate of rebleeding was reduced in patients

undergoing repeated sclerotherapy, 7 episodes
in 11 patients compared with 39 in 13 patients in
the control group. There was no decrease in
mortality.[124] As a result of their experience over
five years, this group have concluded that a
combination of balloon tamponade and early
sclerotherapy is the initial treatment of choice
which should control up to 95% of acute bleeding episodes.[125]

The technique of rigid oesophagoscopy is difficult to acquire and associated with significant
morbidity, particularly the risk of oesophageal
perforation. Injection using a flexible fibre-optic
gastroscope is perhaps more widely available
and effective. The fibre-optic technique is facilitated by use of a flexible outer sheath passed
over the endoscope. The varix protrudes
through a small window in the sheath and rotation will allow sequential injection while maintaining compression of the varices.[139]

A recent prospective randomized trial using
the fibre-optic technique has shown that sclerotherapy not only reduces rebleeding but prolongs survival.[74] One hundred and seven
patients were randomized and of 51 patients
undergoing sclerotherapy rebleeding occurred
in 43%, mainly within three months of entry, 11
patients died, four of these from variceal haemorrhage. Of 56 controls, 75% rebled and 22 died,
17 as a direct result of haemorrhage. Life table
analysis showed a significant improvement in
survival in the sclerotherapy group at two years.

Although some European groups deliberately
inject outside the varix[93] most authorities
believe that effective control is best obtained by
direct injection into the vessels. However, it is
not clear whether prolonged compression with
an oesophageal balloon is required. Recent
pathological studies have shown that following
direct injection, variceal thrombosis occurs
rapidly within less than 24 hours, resulting in
fibrosis and more permanent clot organization
within one month.[34] A variety of sclerosants
have been used of which we favour 5% ethanol-
amine. Inducing thrombosis of all the varices is
difficult and may take as many as three or four
injection sessions spread over several weeks,
thus exposing the patient to the risk of early
rebleeding. Other complications are few and
perforation, usually associated with the use of a
rigid oesophagoscope, is rare. Strictures which
may occur can be safely dilated using either Celestin or Eder–Puestow techniques. The major
advantage of sclerotherapy is that it minimizes
the risk of rebleeding without altering liver
blood flow and increasing the risk of encephalopathy.

Transhepatic catheterization of varices with selected embolization using gel foam or thrombin has also proved effective at controlling acute variceal bleeding.[117] However, the technique is technically demanding with a high initial failure rate, is not advisable for repeated therapy and thus has limited application.

Surgical treatment

OESOPHAGEAL TRANSECTION

Variceal haemorrhage usually occurs from veins in the lower 5 cm of the oesophagus and a number of procedures aimed at devascularizing this area have been proposed. None of the early techniques have proved satisfactory.[58] The introduction of the circular stapling gun, either the Russian SPTU or American EEA has led to a reassessment of such procedures, and Johnston has recently reported encouraging results.[59, 60] In his study, the lower oesophagus is approached by an abdominal route and transection of the oesophagus carried out at or just above the oesophageal junction. Left gastric and paraoesophageal veins were also ligated. In 80 patients, treated by transection and all unfit for shunt surgery, the hospital mortality was 14%. In 19 patients, when used as an emergency procedure to stop bleeding, the technique had a high mortality of 32% and it is recommended that the patient should be stable for at least 48 hours before transection is carried out. Fifty-five patients (69%) survived with a mean follow up of nearly three years. The operation did not reduce portal blood flow and encephalopathy was uncommon. Rebleeding occurred in 14 patients, four from recurrent varices. Of the 14 late deaths: five resulted from haemorrhage, one from variceal bleeding, one from a source unknown, three from gastric erosions, and four patients died of liver failure, one each from hepatoma, laryngeal carcinoma, lung carcinoma, bronchopneumonia and cerebral vascular accident. Eleven patients developed easily dilatable strictures. This procedure appears to have major advantages compared with shunting in patients with poor liver reserve falling into Child's categories B or C and should be examined against sclerotherapy.

PORTO-SYSTEMIC SHUNTS

Prophylactic shunt operations have no role in the management of oesophageal varices. Two-thirds of patients with endoscopic evidence of varices will never bleed from them and the pro-

cedure does not prolong survival.[17, 54, 97] The question regarding the role of shunt operations centres around if or when shunts should be performed after an acute bleed. Orloff is the only major proponent of emergency shunt operations and in an unselected series of 180 patients, all shunted within eight hours of admission, he reported an operative mortality of 42%, with 31% of the surviving patients developing signs of encephalopathy. His five-year survival was 38%.[90] Thus emergency shunting is not a recommended procedure. Elective shunt operations undoubtedly reduce the risk of rebleeding,[55, 98, 100, 102] but in none of four controlled clinical trials was long-term survival significantly increased, although the combined results might suggest a benefit (Figure 6.3). However, these four studies can all be seriously criticized.

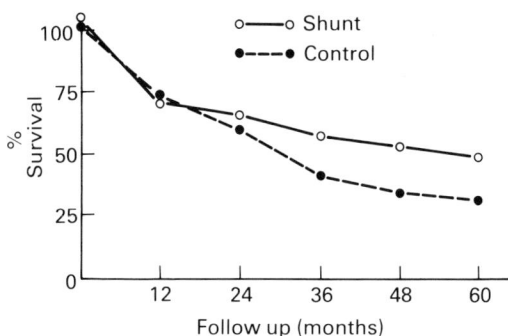

Fig. 6.3 Survival curves for shunt and control patients. Data from four controlled clinical trials of therapeutic portacaval shunt.

In the early studies, endoscopy was not routinely performed. Thus many of these patients may well have been bleeding from sources other than their oesophageal varices, a suggestion reinforced by the high proportion of patients who did not rebleed (22–35%). In the medical groups, many patients (16–37%) had shunt surgery which obviously biased the results. Also in the surgical groups a significant proportion of patients (9–28%) did not have an operation. There is therefore still room for further work and elective shunt operations cannot be ruled out as an effective option in managing variceal bleeding patients. The operative mortality in elective shunts should be less than 10% but there is a significant risk of encephalopathy (20–40% after total shunt, 5–20% after distal spleno-renal shunts). Although high risk patients can be identified by the use of Child's classification, there are no clear factors to select out a group who would clearly benefit from elective shunting. In view of mortality and morbidity, shunt operations should probably only be considered in patients in Child's group A, preferably those under the age of 50.[58] Many patients surviving their initial bleed can be converted from Child C to Child B or A with intensive medical inpatient management where total abstinence from alcohol can be maintained. In such patients elective shunts should be considered. The high rate of encephalopathy in patients with total shunting has led to the use of more selective procedures that lower pressure in the oesophageal varices but preserve blood flow to the liver. The most widely used and useful of these procedures is the distal spleno-renal shunt.[136] This procedure gives considerably lower rates of encephalopathy compared with conventional shunt[65, 99, 104] and will control variceal bleeding. Although it is suggested that patients with non-alcoholic liver disease do best with these procedures, alcoholics who stop drinking will have improved survival.[140] It seems likely that these shunts may become less selective over the years with the development of further collaterals between the high and low pressure regions in the portal system.[138] The

gradual transition may enable liver and brain to adapt, lessening the risk of encephalopathy. In the light of recent developments in local sclerotherapy and possible pharmacological control of recurrent bleeding with propranolol, the role of shunt surgery will need to be kept under constant review and further clinical trials are needed.

SUGGESTED OUTLINE OF MANAGEMENT

The approach to management of patients bleeding from oesophageal varices is shown schematically (Figure 6.4). Units dealing with unselected patients bleeding from varices can expect an often unavoidably high mortality. Close cooperation between physicians and surgeons is needed to improve mortality and such attention to detail is only possible in units with a particular interest in the problem. It is clear that there is much debate over the method of medium- to long-term management of these patients and it is

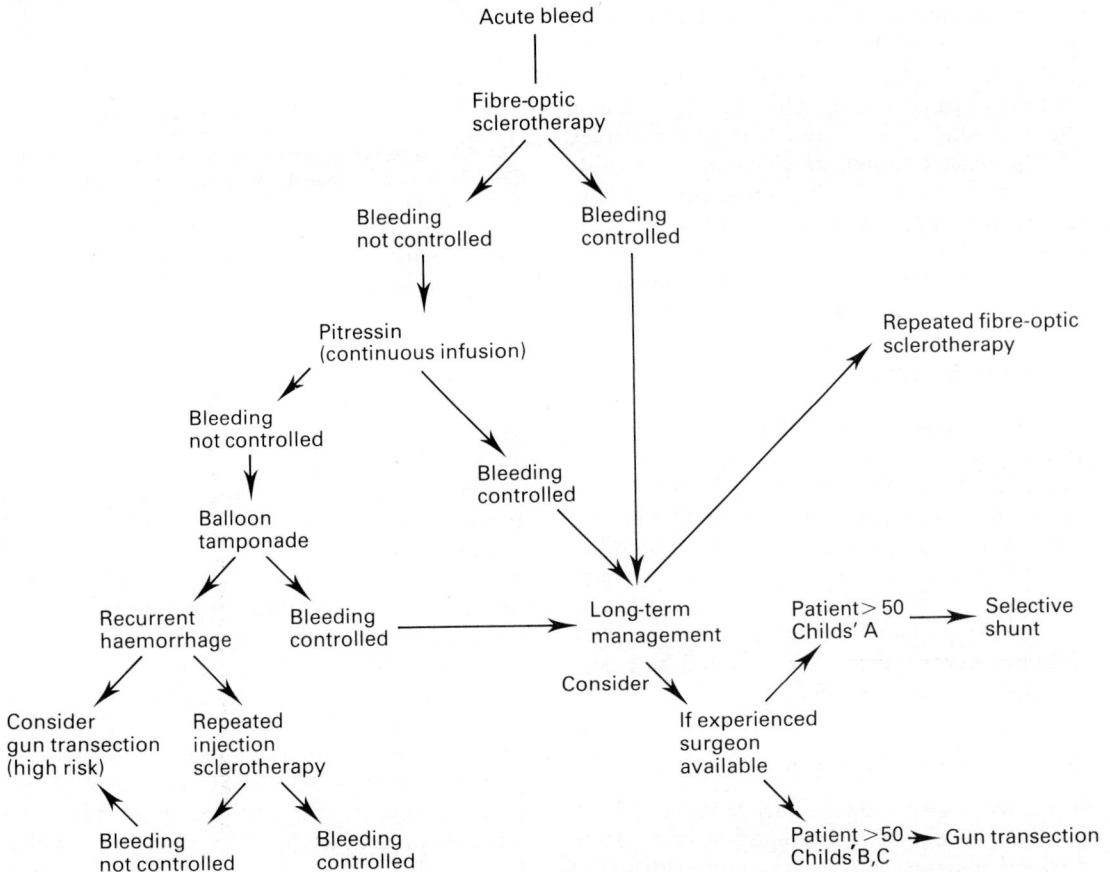

Fig. 6.4 Planned management of variceal haemorrhage.

only by carefully designed and rigorously assessed clinical trials that further improvements of management in these difficult patients will be made. None the less patients with liver disease complicated by bleeding varices are at serious risk, and it would be unrealistic to expect mortality rates to fall to levels found in bleeding peptic ulceration. The paramount consideration of all those dealing with such patients must be to save life where this is practicable but to avoid unseemly and unnecessary intervention in those in whom death is clearly inevitable.

REFERENCES

1   Alavi, A., Dann, R. W., Baunn, S. & Diery, D. M. (1977) Scintigraphic detection of acute gastrointestinal bleeding. *Radiology*, **124**, 753–756.
2   Allan, R. & Dykes, P. (1976) A study of the factors influencing mortality rates from gastrointestinal haemorrhage. *Quarterly Journal of Medicine*, **45**, 533–550.
3   An International Multicentre Trial. (1975) Prevention of fatal postoperative pulmonary embolism by low doses of heparin. *Lancet*, **ii**, 45–51.
4   Athanasoulis, C. A., Baum, S., Waltman, A. *et al.* (1974) Control of acute gastric mucosal haemorrhage. *New England Journal of Medicine*, **290**, 597–603.
5   Atkinson, M. (1981) Bleeding from the oesophagus. In *Gastrointestinal Haemorrhage* (Ed.) Dykes, P. W. & Keighley, M. R. B. pp. 23–33. Bristol: Wright PSG.
6   Avery Jones, F. (1943) Haematemesis and melaena with special reference to bleeding peptic ulcers. *British Medical Journal*, **i**, 689–691.
7   Athanasoulis, C. A., Waltman, A. C. & Novellin, R. A. (1976) Angiography, its contribution to the emergency management of gastrointestinal haemorrhage. *Radiologic Clinics of North America*, **14**, 265–280.
8   Barrett, N. R. (1950) Chronic peptic ulcer of oesophagus 'oesophagitis'. *British Journal of Surgery*, **38**, 175–182.
9   Biggs, J. C., Hugh, T. B. & Dodds, A. J. (1976) Tranexamic acid and upper gastrointestinal haemorrhage – a double blind trial. *Gut*, **17**, 729–734.
10 Bosch, J., Kravetz, D. & Rodes, J. (1981) Effects of somatostatin on hepatic and systemic haemodynamics in patients with cirrhosis of the liver: comparison with vasopressin. *Gastroenterology*, **80**, 518–525.
11 Chang, F. C., Drake, J. E. & Farha, G. J. (1977) Massive upper gastrointestinal hemorrhage in the elderly. *American Journal of Surgery*, **134**, 721–723.
12 Chojkier, M., Grossman, R. J. & Attenberg, C. E. (1979) A controlled comparison of continuous intra-arterial and intravenous infusion of vasopressin in haemorrhage from oesophageal varices. *Gastroenterology*, **77**, 540–546.
13 Clark, R., Borirakchanyavat, V., Gazzard, B. G. *et al.* (1973) Disordered hemostasis in liver damage from paracetamol. *Gastroenterology*, **65**, 788–795.
14 Cody, H. S. & Wichern, W. A. (1977) Choice of operation for acute gastric mucosal hemorrhage. *American Journal of Surgery*, **134**, 322–325.
15 Coggon, D., Langman, M. J. S. & Spiegelhalter, D. (1982) Aspirin, paracetamol and haematemesis and melaena. *Gut*, **23**, 340–344.
16 Conn, H. O. (1980) Varix-volcano connection. *Gastroenterology*, **79**, 1333–1337.

17 Conn, H. O. & Lindenmouth, W. W. (1968) Prophylactic portacaval anastomosis in patients with oesophageal varices. *New England Journal of Medicine*, **279**, 725–732.
18 Conn, H. O., Lee, V. Y., Vlagicevic, Z. R. *et al.* (1977) Comparison of lactulose and neomycin in the treatment of chronic porto-systemic encephalopathy. *Gastroenterology*, **72**, 573–583.
19 Cooke, A. R. (1973) Drugs and peptic ulceration. In *Gastrointestinal Disease* (Ed.) Sleisenger, M. H. & Fordtran, J. A. pp. 642–656. Philadelphia: Saunders.
20 Cormack, F., Chakrabarti, R. R., Jouhar, A. J. & Ferarnley, G. R. (1973) Tranexamic acid in upper gastrointestinal haemorrhage. *Lancet*, **i**, 1207–1208.
21 Cotton, P. B., Rosenberg, M. T., Waldram, R. P. L. *et al.* (1974) Early endoscopy of oesophagus, stomach and duodenal bulb in patients with haematemesis and melaena. *British Medical Journal*, **ii**, 505–509.
22 Cotton, R. B. (1981) Endoscopy – upper gastrointestinal bleeding. In *Gastrointestinal Haemorrhage*. (Ed.) Dykes, P. W. & Keighley, M. R. B. pp. 166–177. Bristol: Wright PSG.
23 Cox, H. T., Poller, L. & Thomson, J. M. (1967) Gastric fibrinolysis. A possible link with peptic ulcer. *Lancet*, **i**, 1300–1302.
24 Curtis, L. E., Simonian, S., Buerk, C. A. *et al.* (1973) Evaluation of the effectiveness of controlled pH in management of massive upper gastrointestinal bleeding. *American Journal of Surgery*, **125**, 474–476.
25 Daintree Johnson, H. (1962) Peptic ulcer in hospital. *Gut*, **3**, 106–117.
26 Dawson, J. & Cockel, R. (1982) Ranitidine in acute upper gastrointestinal haemorrhage. *British Medical Journal*, **285**, 476–477.
27 Deckelbaum, R. J., Roy, C. C., Lusier-Lazaroff, J. *et al.* (1974) Peptic ulcer disease: a clinical study in 73 children. *Canadian Medical Association Journal*, **111**, 225–228.
28 de Dombal, F. T., Morgan, A. G., Staniland, J. R. & Ohmann, C. (1981) Clinical features – computer analysis. In *Gastrointestinal Haemorrhage* (Ed.) Dykes, P. W. & Keighley, M. R. B. pp. 155–165. Bristol: Wright PSG.
29 Dronfield, M. W., Langman, M. J. S., Atkinson, M. *et al.* (1982) Outcome of endoscopy and barium radiography for acute upper gastrointestinal bleeding: controlled trial of 1039 patients. *British Medical Journal*, **284**, 545–548.
30 Duggan, J. M. (1974) Aspirin use in patients with major gastrointestinal bleeding and peptic ulcer disease. *New England Journal of Medicine*, **290**, 1158–1162.
31 Elias, E. (1981) Liver disease. In *Gastrointestinal Haemorrhage* (Ed.) Dykes, P. W. and Keighley, M. R. B. pp. 75–92. Bristol: Wright PSG.
32 Emery, E. S. & Monroe, R. T. (1935) Peptic ulcer. *Archives of Internal Medicine*, **55**, 271–292.
33 Esselstyn, C. B. (1976) Surgical management of actively bleeding duodenal ulcer. *Surgical Clinics of North America*, **56** (6), 1387–1393.
34 Evans, D. M. D., Jones, D. B., Cleary, B. K. & Smith, P. M. (1982) Oesophageal varices treated by sclerotherapy – a histopathological study. *Gut*, **23**, 615–620.
35 Forrest, J. A. H., Finlayson, N. D. C. & Shearman, D. J. C. (1974) Endoscopy in gastrointestinal bleeding. *Lancet*, **ii**, 394–397.
36 Foster, D. N., Milorzewski, K. J. A. & Losowski, M. S. (1978) Stigmata of recent haemorrhage in diagnosis and prognosis of upper gastrointestinal bleeding. *British Medical Journal*, **i**, 1173–1177.

37   Fraser, G. M. (1978) The double contrast barium meal in patients with acute upper gastrointestinal bleeding. *Clinical Radiology*, **29**, 625–634.

38   Fraser, G. M. & Simpkins, K. C. (1981) Contrast radiology. In *Gastrointestinal Haemorrhage*. (Ed.) Dykes, P. W. and Keighley, M. R. B. pp. 186–208. Bristol: Wright PSG.

39   Freeman, J. G., Cobden, I., Lishman, A. H. & Record, C. O. (1982) Controlled trial of Terlipressin (Glypressin) versus vasopressin in the early treatment of oesophageal varices. *Lancet*, **ii**, 66–68.

40   Fruhmorgen, P., Matek, W. & Demling, L. (1981) The difficult bleeder – recent advances. *Proceedings of the 3rd Congress 'Growing Points in Endoscopy'*, London.

41   Gaisford, W. D. (1979) Endoscopic electrohemostasis of active upper gastrointestinal bleeding. *American Journal of Surgery*, **137**, 47–53.

42   Garrett, H. E., Beall, A. C., Jordan, G. L. *et al.* (1963) Surgical considerations of massive haemorrhage caused by aorto-duodenal fistula. *American Journal of Surgery*, **105**, 6–12.

43   Gilbert, D. A., Verhoeven, T., Jessen, K. *et al.* (1982) A multicenter clinical trial of the bicap probe for upper gastrointestinal bleeding. *Gastrointestinal Endoscopy*, **28**, 2150 (A).

44   Gordon, R. & Baum, S. (1981) Radiographic therapy. In *Gastrointestinal Haemorrhage*. (Ed.) Dykes, P. W. and Keighley, M. R. B. pp. 310–329. Bristol: Wright PSG.

45   Graham, D. Y. & Schwartz, J. T. (1977) The spectrum of the Mallory–Weiss tear. *Medicine (Baltimore)*, **57**, 307–318.

46   Green, P. H. R., Fevere, D. I. & Barrett, P. J. (1977) Chronic erosive (verrucous) gastritis. *Endoscopy*, **9**, 74–78.

47   Griffiths, W. J., Neumann, D. A. & Welsh, J. D. (1979) The visible vessel as an indicator of uncontrolled or recurrent gastrointestinal hemorrhage. *New England Journal of Medicine*, **300**, 1411–1413.

48   Halloran, L. G., Zfass, A. M., Gayle, W. E. *et al.* (1980) Prevention of acute gastrointestinal complications after severe head injury: a controlled trial of cimetidine prophylaxis. *American Journal of Surgery*, **139**, 44–48.

49   Hares, M. M., Hegarty, M. A., Warlow, J. *et al.* (1981) A controlled trial to compare systemic and intraincisional cefuroxime prophylaxis in high risk gastric surgery. *British Journal of Surgery*, **68**, 276–280.

50   Hoare, A. M., Bradby, G. V. H., Hawkins, C. F. *et al.* (1979) Cimetidine in bleeding peptic ulcer. *Lancet*, **ii**, 671–673.

51   Horowitz, H. I., Stein, I. M., Cohen, B. D. *et al.* (1970) Further studies on the platelet-inhibitory effect of guanidinosuccinic acid and its role in uremic bleeding. *American Journal Medicine*, **49**, 336–345.

52   Hunt, P. S., Hanksy, J. & Korman, M. G. (1979) Mortality in patients with haematemesis and melaena; a prospective study. *British Medical Journal*, **i**, 1238–1240.

53   Ivy, A. C., Grossman, M. I. & Backrach, W. H. (1950) Complications in relationship to pathogenesis. In *Peptic Ulcer* (Ed.) Backrach, W. H., Grossman, M. I. & Ivy, A. C. pp. 538–603. London: Churchill.

54   Jackson, F. C., Perrin, E. B., Smith, A. G. *et al.* (1968) A clinical investigation of the portocaval shunt 2 survival analysis of the prophylactic operation. *American Journal of Surgery* **115**, 22–44.

55   Jackson, F. C., Perrin, E. B., Felix, R. & Smith, A. G. (1971) A clinical investigation of the portocaval shunt v. survival analysis of the therapeutic operation. *Annals of Surgery*, **174**, 672–701.

56   Jick, H. & Porter, J. (1978) Drug induced gastrointestinal bleeding. *Lancet*, **ii**, 87–89.

57   Johnson, W. C., Wildrich, W. C., Ansell, J. E. *et al.* (1977) Control of bleeding varices by vasopressin. *Annals of Surgery*, **186**, 369–376.

58   Johnston, G. W. (1981) Stapled oesophageal transection. In *Gastrointestinal Haemorrhage* (Ed.) Dykes, P. W. & Keighley, M. R. B. pp. 409–415. Bristol: Wright PSG.

59   Johnston, G. W. (1981) Bleeding oesophageal varices and the management of shunt reject. *Annals of the Royal College of Surgeons, England*, **63**, 3–8.

60   Johnston, G. W. (1982) Six years experience of oesophageal transection for oesophageal varices using a circular stapling gun. *Gut*, **23**, 770–773.

61   Johnston, G. & Rodgers, H. W. (1973) A review of 15 years experience in the use of sclerotherapy in the control of acute haemorrhage from oesophageal varices. *British Journal of Surgery*, **60**, 797–800.

62   Johnston, D., Lyndon, P. J., Smith, R. B. & Humphrey, C. S. (1973) Highly selective vagotomy without a drainage procedure in the treatment of haemorrhage, perforation and pyloric stenosis due to peptic ulcer. *British Journal of Surgery*, **60**, 790–797.

63   Jones, F. A. (1956) Haematemesis and melaena: with special reference to causation and to the factors influencing the mortality from bleeding peptic ulcers. *Gastroenterology*, **30**, 166.

64   Jordan, S. M. & Kiefer, E. D. (1934) Complications of peptic ulcer: their prognostic significance. *Journal of the American Medical Association*, **103**, 2004–2007.

65   Langer, B., Rotstein, L. E. & Stone, R. M. (1980) A prospective randomised trial of the selective splenorenal shunt. *Surgery, Gynaecology and Obstetrics*, **150**, 45–48.

66   Langman, M. J. S. (1983) Personal communication.

67   Lebrec, D., DeFleury, P., Reuff, B. *et al.* (1980) Portal hypertension, size of esophageal varices and risk of gastrointestinal bleeding in alcoholic cirrhosis. *Gastroenterology*, **79**, 1139–1144.

68   Lebrec, D., Nouel, O., Corbic, M. & Benhamou, J. D. (1980) Propranolol. A medical treatment for portal hypertension. *Lancet*, **ii**, 180–182.

69   Lebrec, D., Poynard, T., Hillon, P. & Benhamou, J. D. (1981) Propranolol for prevention of recurrent gastrointestinal bleeding in patients with cirrhosis. A controlled study. *New England Journal of Medicine*, **305**, 1371–1374.

70   Levy, M. (1974) Aspirin use in patients with major gastrointestinal bleeding and peptic ulcer disease. *New England Journal of Medicine*, **290**, 1158–1162.

71   Linscheer, W. G. & Fazio, T. L. (1979) Control of upper gastrointestinal haemorrhage by endoscopic spraying of clotting factors. *Gastroenterology*, **77**, 642–646.

72   MacBeth, R. (1955) Treatment of oesophageal varices in portal hypertension by means of sclerosing injection. *British Medical Journal*, **ii**, 877–880.

73   MacDougall, B. R. D., Bailey, R. J. & Williams, R. (1977) H_2 receptor antagonists and antacids in the prevention of acute gastrointestinal haemorrhage in fulminant hepatic failure. *Lancet*, **i**, 617–618.

74   MacDougall, B. R. O., Westaby, D., Theodosi, A. *et al.* (1982) Increased long term survival in variceal haemorrhage using injection sclerotherapy. *Lancet*, **i**, 124–126.

75   MacLeod, I. A., Mills, P. R., MacKenzie, J. F. *et al.* (1983) Neodymium yttrium aluminium garnet laser photocoagulation for major haemorrhage from peptic

ulcers and single vessels: a single blind controlled study. *British Medical Journal*, **286**, 345–348.

76 Marx, F. W., Gray, R. K., Duncan, A. M. *et al.* (1977) Angiodysplasia as a source of intestinal bleeding. *American Journal of Surgery*, **134**, 125–130.

77 McNeish, A. S. (1981) Bleeding in children. In *Gastrointestinal Haemorrhage* (Ed.) Dykes, P. W. and Keighley, M. R. B. pp. 126–145. Bristol: Wright PSG.

78 Meulengracht, E. (1947) Fifteen years experience with free feeding of patient with bleeding peptic ulcer: fatal cases. *Archives of Internal Medicine*, **80**, 697–708.

79 Mitchell, K., Silk, D. B. A. & Williams R. (1980) Prospective comparison of two Sengstaken tubes in the management of patients with variceal haemorrhage. *Gut*, **21**, 570–573.

80 Morgan, M. H., Read, A. E. & Speller, D. C. E. (1982). Treatment of hepatic encephalopathy with metronidazole. *Gut*, **23**, 1–7.

81 Morgan, A. G., McAdam, W. A. F., Walmsley, G. L. *et al.* (1977) Clinical findings, early endoscopy, and multivariate analysis in patients bleeding from the upper gastrointestinal tract. *British Medical Journal*, **ii**, 237–240.

82 Morris, D. L. (1983) Early or delayed surgery for gastrointestinal haemorrhage. MD Thesis, University of Birmingham.

83 Morris, D. L., Hawker, P. C., Keighley, M. R. B. & Dykes, P. W. (1982) Bipolar endoscopic electrocoagulation. *Gut*, **23**, A916.

84 Morris, D. L., Dykes, P. W., Davies, J. & Stuart, J. (1983) Fibrinolytic activity of gastric juice. (Unpublished data).

84a Morris, D. L., Hawker, P. C., Brearley, S. *et al.* (1984) *British Medical Journal*, **288**, 1277–1280.

85 Morson, B. P. & Dawson, I. M. P. (1979) *Gastrointestinal Pathology*. London: Blackwell.

86 Nilsson, I. M., Bergentz, S. E., Hedner, U. *et al.* (1975) Gastric fibrinolysis. *Thrombosis et Diathesis Haemorrhagica*, **34**, 409–418.

87 Northfield, T. C. (1971) Factors predisposing to recurrent haemorrhage after acute gastrointestinal bleeding. *British Medical Journal*, **ii**, 237–240.

88 Northfield, T. C. & Smith, T. (1970) Central venous pressure in clinical management of acute gastrointestinal bleeding. *Lancet*, **ii**, 584–586.

89 Northfield, T. C. & Smith, T. (1971) Haematemesis as an index of blood loss. *Lancet*, **i**, 990–991.

90 Orloff, M. J., Bell, R. H., Hyde, P. V. & Skivolocki, W. P. (1980) Longterm results of emergency portacaval shunt for bleeding oesophageal varices in unselected patients with alcoholic cirrhosis. *Annals of Surgery*, **192**, 325–337.

91 Palmer, E. D. (1969) The vigorous diagnostic approach to upper-gastrointestinal tract haemorrhage. *Journal of the American Medical Association*, **207**, 1477–1480.

92 Papp, J. P. (1979) Endoscopic electrocoagulation of actively bleeding arterial upper gastrointestinal lesions. *American Journal of Gastroenterology*, **71**, 516–521.

93 Paquet, K. J. & Oberhammer, E. (1978) Sclerotherapy of bleeding oesophageal varices by means of endoscopy. *Endoscopy*, **10**, 7–12.

94 Perkins, H. A., Mackenzie, M. R. & Fudenberg, H. H. (1970) Hemostatic defects in dysproteinemias. *Blood*, **35**, 695–707.

95 Protell, R. L., Rubin, C. E., Auth, D. C. *et al.* (1978) The heater probe – a new endoscopic method for stopping massive gastrointestinal bleeding. *Gastroenterology*, **74**, 257–262.

96 Protell, R. L., Silverstein, F. E., Gulacsik, C. *et al.* (1978) Failure of cyanoacrylate tissue glue to stop bleeding from experimental canine gastric ulcers. *American Journal of Digestive Disease*, **23**, 903–908.

97 Resnick, R. H., Chalmers, T. C., Ischihara, A. *et al.* (1969) A controlled study of the prophylactic portacaval shunt. *Annals of Internal Medicine*, **70**, 675–688.

98 Resnick, R. H., Iber, F. C., Ischihara, A. M. *et al.* (1974) A controlled study of the therapeutic portacaval shunt. *Gastroenterology*, **67**, 843–857.

99 Retchie, F. A., Fahmy, W. F. & Golsorkhis, M. (1979) Prospective comparative trial with distal splenorenal and mesocaval shunts. *American Journal of Surgery*, **137**, 13–21.

100 Reuff, B., Prandi, D., Degos, F. *et al.* (1976) A controlled study of the therapeutic portocaval shunt in alcoholic cirrhosis. *Lancet*, **i**, 655–659.

101 Reynolds, T. (1980) Interelationship of portal pressure, variceal size and upper gastrointestinal haemorrhage. *Gastroenterology*, **79**, 1332–1333.

102 Reynolds, T. B., Donovan, A. J., Mikkelson, W. P. *et al.* (1981) Results of a 12 year randomised trial of portocaval shunt in patients with alcoholic cirrhosis. *Gastroenterology*, **80**, 1005–1011.

103 Richardson, J. D., Marx, M. H., Flint, L. M. *et al.* (1978) Bleeding vascular malformations of the intestine. *Surgery*, **84**, 430–436.

104 Rikkers, L. F., Rudman, D., Galembos, J. *et al.* (1978) A randomised controlled trial about the distal splenorenal shunt. *Annals of Surgery*, **188**, 271–282.

105 Robert, A. (1979) Cytoprotection by prostaglandins. *Gastroenterology*, **77**, 761–767.

106 Rodgers, J. B., Older, T. M. & Stabler, E. V. (1966) Gastric hypothermia; a critical evaluation of its use in massive upper gastrointestinal bleeding. *Annals of Surgery*, **124**, 1010–1022.

107 Russell Smith, C., Bartholomew, L. C. & Cain, J. C. (1963) Hereditary haemorrhagic telangiectasia and gastrointestinal haemorrhage. *Gastroenterology*, **44**, 1–6.

108 Rutgeerts, P., Vantrappen, G., Broeckhaert, L. *et al.* (1982) Controlled trial of YAG laser treatment of upper digestive haemorrhage. *Gastroenterology*, **83**, 410–416.

109 Sagar, S. & Shields, R. (1981) Vasopressin. In *Gastrointestinal Haemorrhage* (Ed.) Dykes, P. W. & Keighley, M. R. B. pp. 385–391. Bristol: Wright PSG.

110 Sagar, S., Harrison, I. D., Brearley, R. & Shields, R. (1979) Emergency treatment of variceal haemorrhage. *British Journal of Surgery*, **66**, 824–826.

111 Salter, R. H. (1968) Aspirin and gastrointestinal bleeding. *American Journal of Digestive Disease*, **13**, 38–58.

112 Simonson, S. J., Stratoudakis, A., Iswerence, M. *et al.* (1976) Non-surgical control of massive acute gastric mucosal haemorrhage with antacid neutralization of gastric content. *Surgical Clinics of North America*, **56**, 21–27.

113 Schiller, K. F. R., Truelove, S. C. & Williams, D. G. (1970) Haematemesis and melaena with special reference to factors influencing the outcome. *British Medical Journal*, **ii**, 7–13.

114 Scobie, B. A. (1969) Milk drip therapy for upper gastrointestinal bleeding. *Medical Journal of Australia*, **1**, 1028–1029.

115 Sevitt, S. (1967) Duodenal and gastric ulceration after burning. *British Journal of Surgery*, **54**, 32–41.

116 Sherman, N. J. & Clatworthy, H. W. (1967) Gastrointestinal bleeding in neonates: a study of 94 cases. *Surgery*, **62**, 614–619.

117 Smith-Laing, G., Scott, J., Long, R. G. *et al.* (1981)

Role of percutaneous transhepatic obliteration of varices in the management of haemorrhage from gastro-oesophageal varices. *Gastroenterology*, **80**, 1031–1036.

118 Sonnenberg, A. & West, C. (1983) Somatostatin reduces gastric mucosal blood flow in normal subjects but not in patients with cirrhosis of the liver. *Gut*, **24**, 148–153.

119 Sonnenberg, G. E., Keller, U., Peruchoud, A. *et al.* (1981) Effect of somatostatin on splanchnic hemodynamics in patients with cirrhosis of the liver and in normal subjects. *Gastroenterology*, **80**, 526–532.

120 Stolte, J. B. (1944) The frequency of manifest bleeding in peptic ulcer with regard to the duration of the disease and to the age of the diseased. *Acta Medica Scandinavica*, **116**, 584–600.

121 Swain, C. P., Bown, S. G., Storey, D. W. *et al.* (1981) Controlled trial of argon laser photocoagulation in bleeding peptic ulcer. *Lancet*, **ii**, 1313–1316.

122 Swain, C. P., Bown, S. G., Salmon, P. R. *et al.* (1982) Controlled trial of Nd YAG laser photocoagulation in bleeding peptic ulcers. *Gut*, **23**, A915.

123 Terblanche, J., Northover, J. M. A., Bornman, P. *et al.* (1979a). A prospective evaluation of injection sclerotherapy in the treatment of acute bleeding from oesophageal varices. *Surgery*, **85**, 239–245.

124 Terblanche, J., Northover, J. M. A., Bornman, P. *et al.* (1979b) A prospective controlled trial of sclerotherapy in the long term management of patients after oesophageal variceal bleeding. *Surgery, Gynaecology and Obstetrics*, **148**, 323–333.

125 Terblanche, J., Yakoom, H. I., Bornman, P. C. *et al.* (1981) A five year prospective evaluation of tamponade and sclerotherapy. *Annals of Surgery*, **194**, 521–530.

126 Trunkey, D. D., Crass, R. & Cello, J. P. (1981) Management of haemorrhagic shock. In *Gastrointestinal Haemorrhage* (Ed.) Dykes, P. W. & Keighley, M. R. B. pp. 265–283. Bristol: Wright PSG.

127 Vallon, A. G., Cotton, P. B., Laurence, B. H. *et al.* (1981) Randomised trial of endoscopic argon laser photocoagulation in bleeding peptic ulcers. *Gut*, **22**, 228–233.

128 Vallon, A. G., Cotton, P. B., Lawrence, B. H. *et al.* (1982) Randomised trial of endoscopic argon laser photocoagulation in bleeding peptic ulcers. *Gut*, **22**, 228–233.

129 Vellacott, K. D., Dronfield, M. W., Atkinson, M. & Langman, M. J. S. (1982) Comparison of surgical and medical management of bleeding peptic ulcers. *British Medical Journal*, **284**, 549–550.

130 Venables, C. W. (1981) Gastroduodenal surgery. In *Gastrointestinal Haemorrhage* (Ed.) Dykes, P. W. & Keighley, M. R. B. pp. 337–356. Bristol: Wright PSG.

131 Viriel, J. P., Cassigneul, J., Louis, A. *et al.* (1982) Significance of portohepatic gradients in cirrhosis. *Surgery, Gynaecology and Obstetrics*, **155**, 347–352.

132 Walia, B. N. S., Mitra, S. K. & Chandra, R. K. (1979) In *The Liver and Biliary System in Infants and Children* (Ed.) Chandra, R. K. pp. 276–295. Edinburgh and London: Churchill Livingstone.

133 Walt, R. P., Burroughs, A. K., Dunk, A. A. *et al.* (1982) Propranolol for prevention of recurrent variceal bleeding in cirrhotic patients. *Gut*, **23**, A908.

134 Wangensteen, O. H., Root, H. P., Jenson, C. B. *et al.* (1959) Depression of gastric secretion and digestion by gastric hypothermia: its clinical use in massive haematemesis. *Surgery*, **44**, 265–274.

135 Wara, P., Hojsgaard, A. & Amdrup, E. (1980) Endoscopic electrocoagulation – an alternative to operative haemostasis in active gastroduodenal bleeding? *Endoscopy*, **12**, 236–240.

136 Warren, W. D., Salam, A. A., Huston, D. *et al.* (1974) Selective distal splenorenal shunt. Technique and results of operation. *Archives of Surgery*, **108**, 306–314.

137 Westaby, D., Gimson, A. E. S., Bihari, D. *et al.* (1982) Selective and non-selective β blockade in the reduction of portal hypertension. *Gut*, **23**, A889.

138 Wildrich, W. C., Robbins, A. H., Johnson, W. C. *et al.* (1980) Longterm follow-up of distal splenorenal shunts. Evaluation by arteriography, shuntography, transhepatic portal venography and cinefluography. *Radiology*, **134**, 341–345.

139 Williams, K. G. D. & Dawson, J. C. (1979). Fibre optic injection of oesophageal varices. *British Medical Journal*, **ii**, 766–767.

140 Zeppa, R., Hensley, G. I., Levi, J. U. *et al.* (1978) Comparative survival of alcoholics versus non-alcoholics after distal splenorenal shunt. *Annals of Surgery*, **187**, 510–514.

ACUTE COLONIC HAEMORRHAGE

Acute rectal blood loss is a frequent cause of hospital admission and will usually present problems in both diagnosis and management. In our experience the most successful outcome is achieved by a team which includes: gastroenterologist/endoscopist, radiologist and gastroenterological surgeon, who see the patient together and formulate management on the basis of joint discussions. Most cases of acute colonic bleeding can be managed conservatively[10] but between 10 and 20% will require emergency surgery.[10, 21, 52] However, the source of bleeding is often difficult to identify at laparotomy. Mortality in these patients has been much higher than in patients undergoing emergency colonic surgery for other indications[20, 43] and may rise to 50 per cent.[21] Primary segmental resection of an area obviously affected by diverticular disease was common practice[24] but often failed to control haemorrhage. The place of 'blind' subtotal colectomy has also been questioned as this will not stop bleeding from sites proximal or distal to the resected colon.[30]

For this reason some surgeons advocate total colectomy with an ileo-rectal anastomosis in patients who are desperately ill from colonic bleeding.[21, 31, 52, 66] However, diagnostic techniques are now available which alone or in combination may define the site and the nature of the bleeding. These include emergency upper gastrointestinal endoscopy, colonoscopy, nuclear imaging techniques and emergency three vessel angiography. The introduction of these diagnostic techniques has emphasized the importance of disease other than diverticular disease as a cause of major colonic haemorrhage and operation should not be contemplated until rigorous attempts have been made to identify the site and source of blood loss.

SYNDROMES OF ACUTE LOWER GASTROINTESTINAL BLEEDING

The causes of acute lower gastrointestinal bleeding are listed in Table 6.6 and emphasize the variations that occur with age. All of the listed conditions may also present as chronic intermittent bleeding. Episodes of bleeding from whatever cause may differ in character both within and between individuals.

The most common causes of lower gastrointestinal bleeding in children include hamartomatous or juvenile polyps. Sporadic instances of solitary adenoma do occur in childhood, but are uncommon. Inflammatory bowel disease may present with diarrhoea and bleeding, as in the adult, and parasitic or bacterial infections may occur, but massive bleeding is unusual in these conditions. Meckel's diverticulum is also commonly seen in this younger age group. When vascular abnormalities are found in the younger patient they usually lie above the reach of the rigid sigmoidoscope and are almost always haemangiomas.

In the adult patient adenomatous polyps and carcinoma are important causes of rectal bleeding[63] but bleeding is seldom massive from these lesions. Inflammatory bowel disease is usually associated with some bleeding but acute severe blood loss is unusual. Diverticular disease is typically associated with bleeding of variable severity and occasionally this may be massive, especially from an isolated diverticulum in the right colon.[18] However, angiodysplasia is increasingly recognized as a cause of massive

Table 6.6 Causes of severe lower intestinal haemorrhage.

Children and young adults	*Adults over 60 years*
Meckel's diverticulum	Angiodysplasia
Juvenile polyps	Diverticular disease
Inflammatory bowel disease	Polyps
Adults	Cancer
Diverticular disease	Ischaemic colitis
Inflammatory bowel disease	*Less common causes*
Polyps	Infections
Cancer	Rare tumours
Arteriovenous malformation	Coagulopathies
	Drug induced ulceration
	Vascular abnormalities
	Varices

haemorrhage, especially in elderly patients, and usually affects the caecum and right colon; the lesion is rare in patients under 50 years of age.

Bleeding syndromes

MECKEL'S DIVERTICULUM

Meckel's diverticulum, or rarely other intestinal duplication, may cause acute blood loss per rectum. Meckel's diverticulum occurs in 1–4% of the population, with an equal sex incidence, but symptoms are more common in males. In the infant the diverticulum lies about 30 cm proximal to the ileo-caecal valve but may be up to 90 cm proximal in adults. The diverticulum represents the proximal end of the vitello-intestinal duct and is between 2 and 8 cm in length. It is lined by heterotopic gastric epithelium occasionally associated with duodenal, colonic or pancreatic tissue.

Complications of bleeding occur in 10–20% of cases. Secretion of acid and pepsin may lead to ulceration in adjacent ileal mucosa causing haemorrhage or perforation. A Meckel's diverticulum is the cause of bleeding in almost half of all children with gastrointestinal bleeding. Bleeding may be accompanied by abdominal pain and is usually maroon in colour. The diverticulum may fill during a double contrast barium enema if there is reflux into the terminal ileum or may be demonstrated by small bowel enema. Diagnosis during acute bleeding is best made by selective mesenteric angiography or a Technetium-99m sodium pertechnetate isotope scan.[38]

INFLAMMATORY BOWEL DISEASE

Rectal bleeding is common in inflammatory bowel disease[63] especially in ulcerative colitis but is much less frequent in Crohn's disease. Up to 10% of patients who undergo colonoscopy for persistent bleeding after a 'normal' sigmoidoscopy and barium enema are found to have inflammatory bowel disease.[33]

Massive bleeding is usually only seen as a complication of severe extensive ulcerative colitis but may be a presenting feature of a localized Crohn's ulcer in the young. Radiation can result in ulcerative damage to the large or small bowel and intestinal damage may occur as long as 20 to 30 years after radiation treatment.[48] In the acute stage the mucosa is friable – in more advanced disease multiple telangiectasia may be seen and can be confused with angiodysplasia. A correct diagnosis is important in the female patient who has undergone irradiation for pelvic carcinoma in order to exclude a possible pelvic recurrence or primary bowel tumour.[65] Endometriosis, which may also present with intestinal bleeding, should also be distinguished from radiation enteritis.

ISCHAEMIC COLITIS

Ischaemic colitis usually occurs in patients over the age of 50 and may be divided into gangrenous and non-gangrenous types.[17, 42] Ischaemic colitis may be associated with rectosigmoid carcinoma.[11, 42]

An ischaemic episode may occur with or without abdominal pain. The patient has diarrhoea mixed with bright or altered blood, and the onset is usually sudden with no previous history. Emergency colonoscopy when bleeding has ceased may reveal fresh blood in the lumen with superficial serpiginous ulceration, mucosal oedema and reduced colonic motility.[33] Biopsies at this stage show clearly demarcated ulceration of the mucosa with oedema and dilated capillaries packed with blood.[35] Later healed ischaemic strictures may be diagnosed at colonoscopy,[36] when histology then shows haemosiderin deposition within macrophages.[48]

Until the advent of colonoscopy and selective angiography, barium enema was the main method of diagnosis. Characteristic changes include thumb-printing, pseuodopolyposis and mucosal irregularity with tubular narrowing and sacculation.[39]

SOLITARY ULCER

Solitary ulcer of the rectum[41, 59] commonly presents with bright red rectal bleeding accompanying the stool. Occasionally heavy bleeding may occur.[59] Solitary non-specific ulcers may occur elsewhere in the colon and often present with rectal bleeding. Such lesions are more likely to be due to ischaemia. More recently isolated right colon and caecal ulcers have been described in association with immunosuppressive therapy and cytomegalovirus infection in renal transplant patients. These cases invariably present with acute or subacute lower gastrointestinal bleeding.[46, 64]

DIVERTICULAR DISEASE

Diverticular disease is common in Western countries and occurs in 10% of patients over the age of 40 and in 35% of patients over the age of 60.[48] Bleeding may occur from diverticula anywhere in the colon and lead to mild, moderate or massive blood loss. In more than 5000 patients with diverticular disease Rigg and Ewing[55] reported bleeding in 15% of patients.

Massive bleeding is claimed to occur more frequently from the right side of the colon[18] but in our experience (unpublished data, 1983) 78% of cases are left sided. Bleeding is probably caused by recurrent trauma at the origin of a diverticulum which may lead to sudden rupture of a submucosal artery towards the lumen of the diverticulum at the antemesenteric margin.[45]

CANCER AND ADENOMATOUS POLYPS

Most cancers of the colon bleed at some time and overt bleeding is frequently reported by the patient.[40, 63] Adenomatous polyps also bleed although less predictably than carcinoma. Up to 20% of cases of severe rectal haemorrhage may be due to malignant disease, especially when advanced, and up to 10% are due to polyps.[58]

VASCULAR ABNORMALITIES

Vascular abnormalities constitute an uncommon but increasingly recognized cause of bleeding from the gastrointestinal tract. Before the availability of selective mesenteric angiography or colonoscopy a definitive diagnosis was not achieved in as many as 27% of patients with gastrointestinal haemorrhage.[19] A proportion of these patients are now found to have angiodysplasia of the colon (this is discussed in more detail in Chapter 5).

The literature has tended to use the terms angioma and angiodysplasia synonymously which has caused some confusion.[7, 54, 57, 61, 69] The majority of patients give a history of one or more episodes of bleeding which can vary from massive haemorrhage and hypovolaemic shock to slow occult blood loss presenting only as anaemia. The pattern of bleeding varies but is usually self limiting, which permits investigation to take place as soon as there is evidence that bleeding has ceased. Bleeding is usually bright red although maroon stools or melaena may occur.[32, 34] Lesions may be associated with aortic stenosis[15, 56, 68] or chronic pulmonary disease.[56]

Angiodysplasia is most frequently described in the right colon and caecum in elderly patients[12, 32, 56] and the nature of these lesions have been clarified by Boley and his colleagues.[13, 47] They have shown that the lesions of angiodysplasia are vascular ectasias which are degenerative in origin. By contrast, the term 'angioma' should probably be reserved for hamartomatous lesions.

The larger lesions of angiodysplasia may be diagnosed by angiography[5, 12, 28, 29, 50] (Figure 6.5) but it is probable that most early mucosal lesions will not be seen by these techniques and only be detectable by careful colonoscopy.[32, 34] At colonoscopy the angiodysplasia lesion is seen as a cherry red, slightly elevated meshwork of superficial capillary vessels (Figure 6.6).

MANAGEMENT OF ACUTE LOWER INTESTINAL BLEEDING

Lower intestinal bleeding occurs from any site in the gastrointestinal tract below the ligament of Treitz to the anus. The steps in management of acute or massive lower intestinal bleeding are shown in Table 6.7. The majority of patients who present with acute rectal bleeding cease to bleed spontaneously. Initial assessment and active resuscitation must precede any attempt to localize the site of haemorrhage. Once the patient's condition has stabilized active investigation to detect the source of haemorrhage should proceed. The techniques available for diagnosis include: endoscopy, radioisotope scan and emergency three vessel angiography. In some cases treatment of haemorrhage can be achieved by endoscopic or angiographic techniques. Occasionally barium studies may be used when these investigations have failed, but they should always be avoided in acute bleeding because barium in the bowel prevents investigation by endoscopy or angiography and may make subsequent surgery difficult.

The first investigation of choice and the order in which other procedures are used depends on the presentation and condition of the patient and is decided after joint discussions by the management team.

ENDOSCOPY

A bleeding site in the oesophagus, stomach or duodenum should be excluded by upper gastro-intestinal endoscopy.[37] After digital rectal examination a rigid procto-sigmoidoscope should be passed. This permits exclusion of local anorectal lesions and removal of blood and clots which tend to collect in the region of the rectal ampulla. If bleeding has ceased fibre-optic sigmoidoscopy or colonoscopy should be attempted.[37, 58] After severe colonic haemorrhage stool is evacuated by the cathartic effect of the blood. Further blood or clots may be removed by tap water enemas before the procedure is started or by oral purgation. In the presence of continued bleeding useful information may still be obtained regarding the segment of bowel from which haemorrhage is arising although the nature of the bleeding lesion may not be determined. This is especially important in the case of angiodysplasia or diverticular disease.

Emergency endoscopic treatment of a bleeding lesion may be possible using the polypectomy snare, electrofulguration techniques or laser therapy.[26] Snare polypectomy is the most appropriate treatment for those rare cases when there has been massive bleeding from a polyp. The technique may also be used for bleeding from a fungating carcinoma. When there is active bleeding the procedure may be facilitated by advancing beyond the lesion and snaring on withdrawal. The lesions of angiodysplasia may be difficult to see in the presence of active bleeding but haemorrhage usually ceases spontaneously allowing elective colonoscopy during this interval, when electrocoagulation may be undertaken.[32, 34, 56, 65] The lesions of angiodysplasia, Osler–Weber–Rendu and small angiomas are probably best managed by laser therapy.[27]

Table 6.7 Steps in management of acute or massive lower intestinal haemorrhage.

Diagnostic protocol
Nasogastric aspiration
Sigmoidoscopy
Coagulation profile
Blood urea nitrogen

Active bleeding	*Bleeding ceased*
Endoscopy	Colonoscopy/barium enema
Upper GI	Pertechnetate-99m scan
Colonoscopy	Selective angiography
Technetium-99m scan	
Pertechnetate-99m scan	
Selective angiography	
Barium enema	
Upper GI/small bowel series	

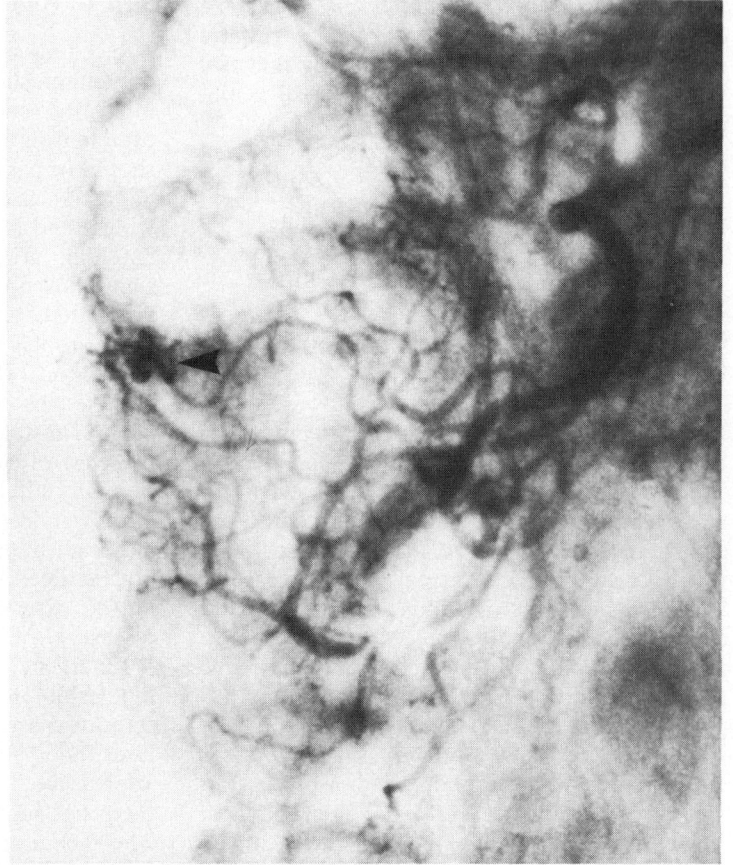

Fig. 6.5 Angiodysplasia seen at angiography in the arterial phase showing the vascular tuft (arrowhead).

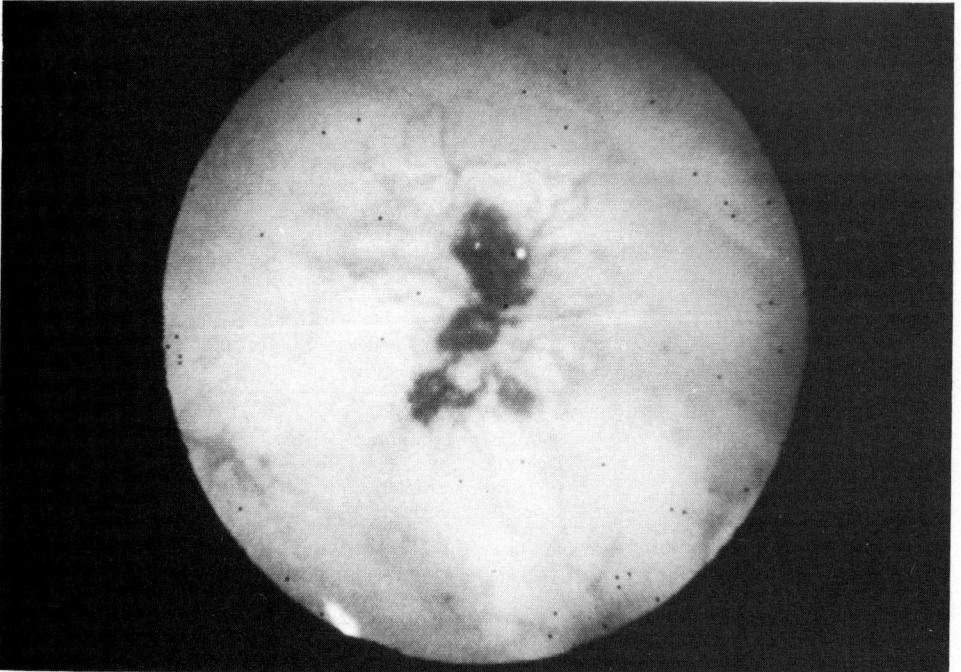

Fig. 6.6 Angiodysplasia lesion seen at colonoscopy in the caecum of an elderly patient who presented with acute massive haemorrhage. The lesion is cherry red in colour and the dilated capillary network can clearly be seen.

RADIOLOGICAL AND RADIOISOTOPE
INVESTIGATIONS

If endoscopy fails to identify the source of haemorrhage, or in the few patients where there is
persistent active bleeding, emergency three
vessel abdominal angiography is the single most
useful investigation. The site of bleeding can be
identified using this technique in about 80% of
patients.[9, 18, 25, 28, 50, 51, 53] However, the procedure requires a skilled team and is associated
with a morbidity particularly in shocked
patients with an already compromised circulating blood volume.

Although elective angiography may detect a
tumour blush or vascular ectasia it is principally
of benefit during active bleeding and requires a
flow rate from the bleeding lesion of about
0.5–1.0 ml/min to demonstrate extravasation.
Recent work suggests that two radioisotope
techniques are considerably more sensitive than
angiography,[1, 44] detecting bleeding rates as low
as 0.05–0.1 ml/min. Technetium-99m sulphur
colloid is easily prepared and has the advantage

that scanning can be performed immediately
after intravenous injection. Technetium-99m
labelled red cells take longer to prepare and
background counts are high. However, the
labelled red cells survive in the circulation for up
to 24 hours after injection so that this technique
allows repeat scanning to be performed if the
patient has recurrent bleeding.[44, 62]

Radioisotope scans are unable to accurately
identify the site of bleeding but may be useful as
an initial screening investigation to indicate
whether bleeding is present and if angiography
is likely to be successful.[8]

In patients who have had an acute episode of
lower gastrointestinal haemorrhage and where
a Meckel's diverticulum is suspected, a confident
diagnosis can usually be made by a technetium-
99m sodium pertechnetate isotope scan[38, 60, 67]
(Figure 6.7). A Meckel's diverticulum may
occasionally fill with barium during a double
contrast enema if there is reflux into the terminal
ileum or by small bowel enema. Diagnosis can
also be made at angiography if the vitelline
artery is identified or if extravasation of contrast
is observed (Figure 6.8)

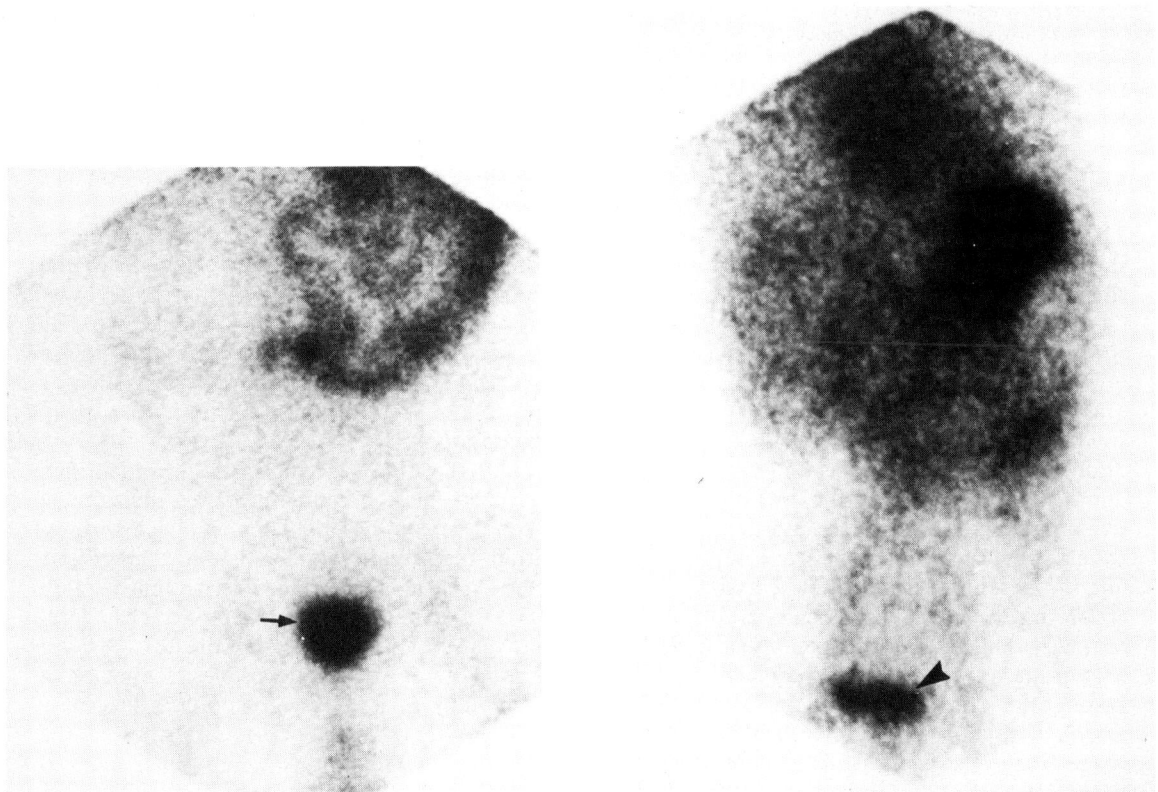

a   b

Fig. 6.7a, b Meckel's diverticulum seen on a technetium-99m pertechnetate scan showing the increased activity in the region
of ectopic gastric mucosa (arrows). (Courtesy of Dr G. Coates.)

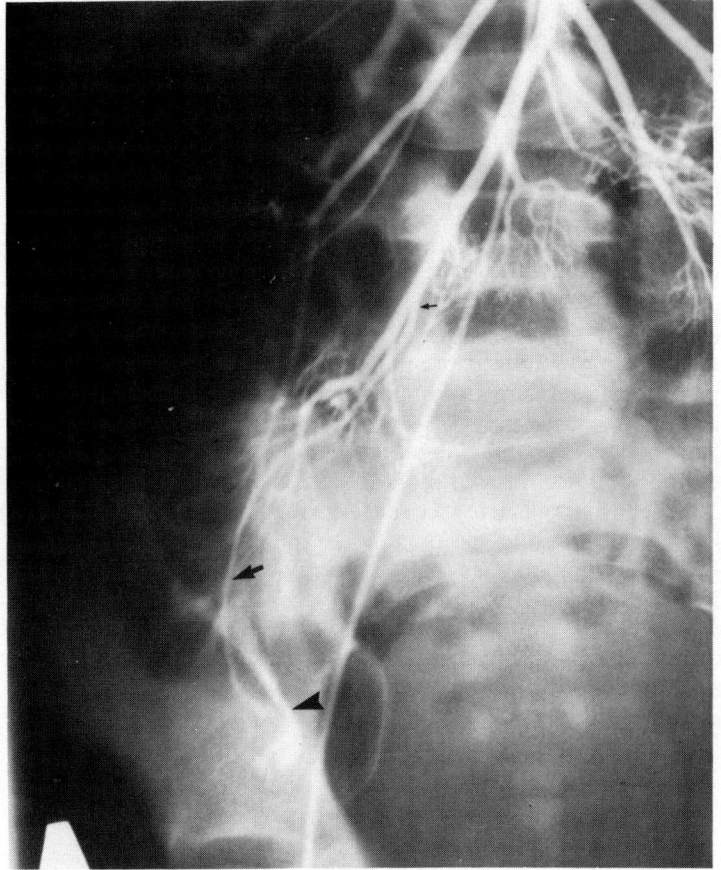

Fig. 6.8 Bleeding Meckel's diverticulum seen at angiography in the arterial phase showing extravasation of contrast (arrowhead) and vitelline artery (large arrow) arising proximally (small arrow) from a major branch of the superior mesenteric artery (Courtesy of Dr R. J. Tuttle.)

ABDOMINAL ANGIOGRAPHY

The usual sequence for abdominal angiography starts with the superior mesenteric artery. If the site of bleeding is not identified on either the regular or subtraction films, a magnification study of the right colon, caecum and distal small bowel with subtraction is performed. The magnification and subtraction films often show small angiodysplastia lesions with early venous drainage which may not be seen on the regular films (Figures 6.9 and 6.10)). If this study is negative, a selective inferior mesenteric arteriogram should be performed. A negative superior and inferior mesenteric angiogram necessitates a selective injection into the coeliac trunk and its branches. The middle colic artery which supplies part of the transverse colon may be an aberrant vessel and arise from the dorsal pancreatic artery. If this artery is not opacified, haemorrhage from this vessel will be missed.[4] Also, a pancreatic tumour or abscess, or an aneurysm of the splenic artery, may erode into the transverse colon causing lower gastrointestinal haemorrhage. A coeliac axis injection will also ensure

that a bleeding upper gastrointestinal lesion was not missed at earlier endoscopy.

The use of vasodilators such as papaverine or tolazoline (Priscoline) may be valuable in the identification of the site of haemorrhage, especially if the bleeding is slow. If bleeding has stopped and a vascular tumour or angiodysplasia is suspected, the use of a vasodilator with magnification films enhances the early draining veins.

Once the site of bleeding has been identified treatment may be attempted by infusion of vasopressin or by embolization. Haemorrhage within the territory of the inferior mesenteric artery such as a bleeding diverticulum (Figure 6.11), appears to respond well to peripheral intravenous infusion of vasopressin.[4, 8, 49] If there is no response to peripheral infusion a direct infusion into the mesenteric artery may be attempted. Bleeding from branches of the superior mesenteric artery only responds to direct infusion into the major vessel. The response to therapy should be checked by arteriography 20 min after the initial infusion has been started.

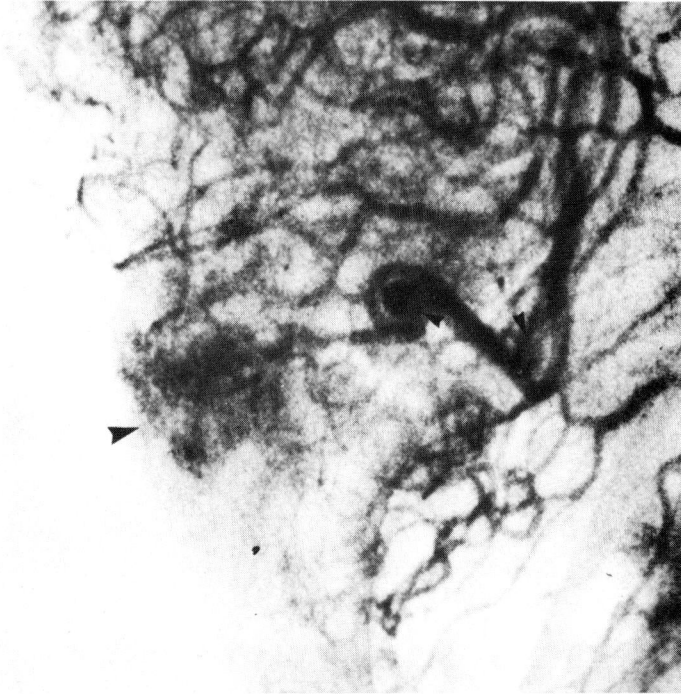

Fig. 6.9 Angiodysplasia in the early capillary phase showing vascular tuft (large arrowhead) and early draining vein (small arrowhead).

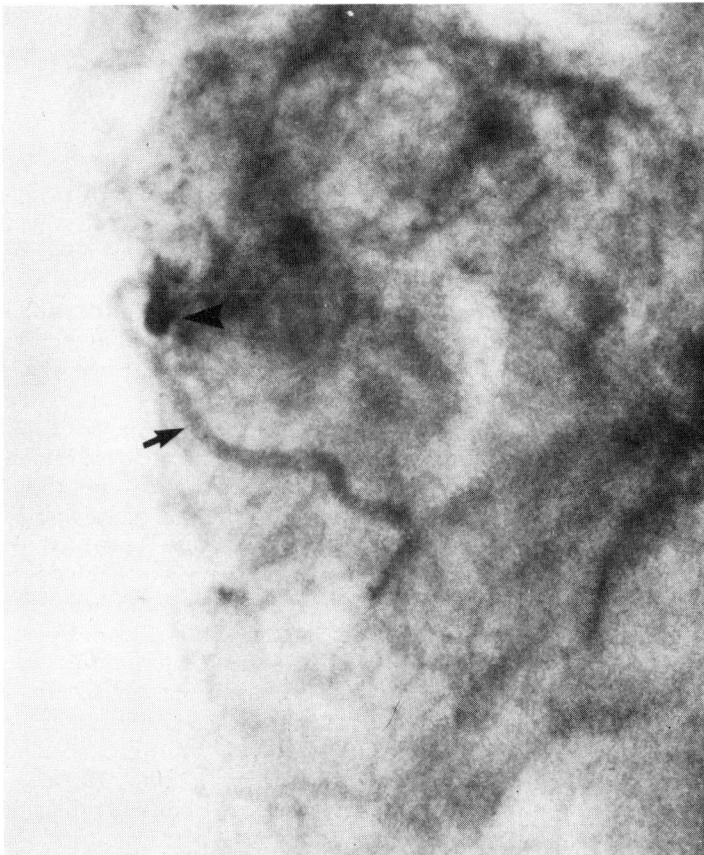

Fig. 6.10 Angiodysplasia showing the vascular tuft (arrowhead) with the early draining vein (arrow).

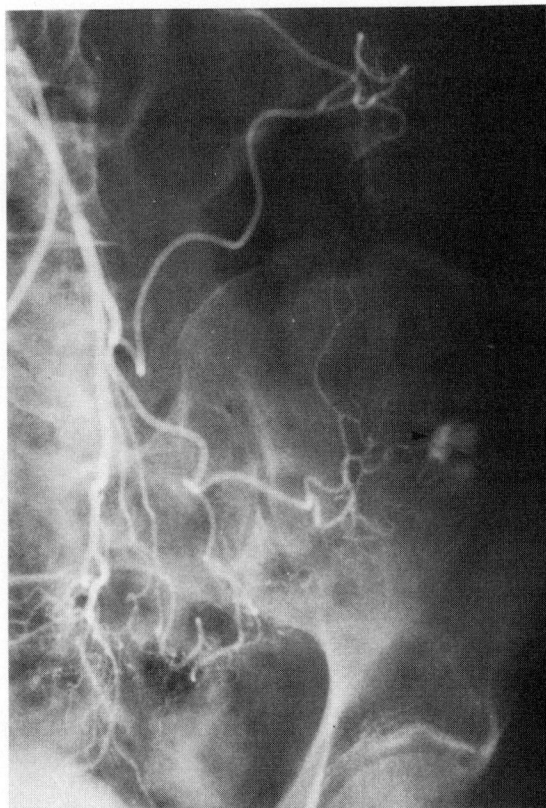

a

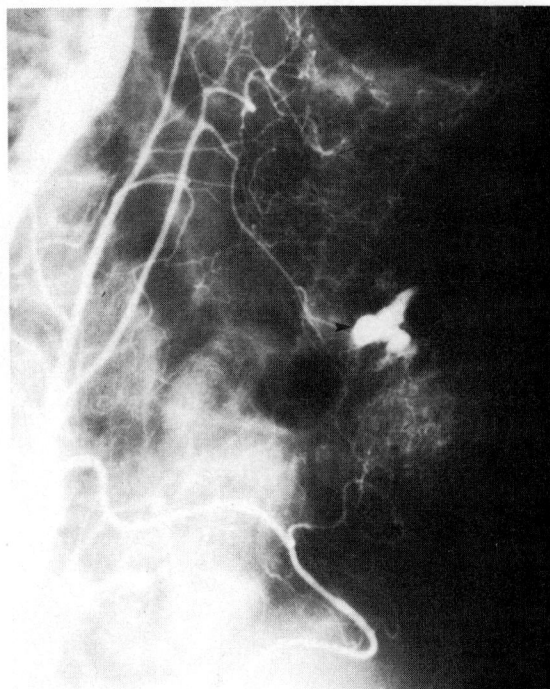

b

Fig. 6.11a, b   Bleeding diverticulum in the left colon seen at angiography with extravasation of contrast at the bleeding site (arrowhead).

It may be possible to embolize some bleeding sites by the transcatheter route. In order to embolize a bleeding vessel, the artery has to be subselected and the embolus deposited at the site of extravasation or in a vessel leading directly to the lesion. If this is not possible embolization should not be attempted as severe ischaemia may occur in several segments of the bowel. Disadvantages of this technique when compared with vasoconstriction are the lack of control and the fact that treatment is irreversible. Rebleeding may arise from sites with a dual blood supply and it is not always possible to place the catheter close to the bleeding lesion. Materials used for embolization currently include Gelfoam, Oxycel, Ivalon and cyanoacrylate. Gelfoam usually lyses within a few weeks to several months while Oxycel and Ivalon produce a longer occlusion. Ivalon frequently produces permanent occlusion as does cyanoacrylate but the latter is much more difficult to handle.

Once an active bleeding site or an arteriovenous malformation has been identified at angiography, it may be extremely difficult to find the lesion at laparotomy, particularly in disorders of the small bowel. The radiologist can assist the surgeon by subselecting the vessel of interest prior to surgery and this is made easier with a coaxial catheter system. Once the bowel has been exposed at laparotomy 1 ml of methylene blue is injected through the catheter which has been left in place; this readily identifies the segment of bowel to be resected.[6] When it has not been possible to identify the site or nature of the bleeding, and haemostasis has not been satisfactorily achieved by endoscopic or radiological means, emergency surgery is required. In such circumstances it is always worth considering intraoperative colonoscopy[23] and hence the patient should be placed in the Lloyd–Davies (Trendelenburg) position. Enterotomy and endoscopy should be available, especially if there is any suspicion that the bleeding might be arising in the small bowel or from a small mucosal angiodysplastia lesion. However, intraoperative endoscopy is technically difficult if there is active haemorrhage.[16, 23]

CONCLUSION

It should now be possible using the methods outlined to identify the source of intestinal haemorrhage in 90% of patients. Nevertheless, there is still a need in some patients to resort to urgent laparotomy. The source of bleeding, such as a caecal ulcer, a Meckel's diverticulum or a Crohn's stricture, may be immediately obvious. If not, intraoperative endoscopy after on-table whole bowel lavage will frequently identify the bleeding source. If there remains real doubt about the origin of bleeding, a loop ileostomy and loop sigmoid colostomy are wiser procedures than a blind intestinal resection. The source of bleeding should then become apparent in the postoperative period allowing detailed investigation and definitive resection. For patients who have stopped bleeding and where a diagnosis has been made by endoscopy or angiography rebleeding is an indication for a localized segmental resection. When the source of bleeding has not been defined, subtotal colectomy should only be considered as a last resort.

REFERENCES

1 Alavi, A. & Ring, E. J. (1981) Localisation of gastrointestinal bleeding – superiority of ^{99m}Tc sulphur colloid compared with angiography. *American Journal of Roentgenology*, **173**, 741–748.

2 Alavi, A., Ring, E. J. & Baum, S. (1979) Radiographic demonstration of acute intestinal bleeding. *Journal of Nuclear Medicine*, **20**, 631.

3 Alavi, A., Dann, R. W., Baum, S. & Berry, D. N. (1977) Scintigraphic detection of acute gastrointestinal bleeding. *Radiology*, **124**, 753–756.

4 Athanasoulis, C. A. (1982) Lower gastrointestinal bleeding. In *Interventional Radiology* (Ed.) Athanasoulis, C. A., Pfister, R. C., Greene, R. E., Robertson, G. H. Philadelphia: Saunders.

5 Athanasoulis, C. A., Galdabini, J. J., Waltman, A. C. *et al.* (1978) Angiodysplasia of the colon: a cause of rectal bleeding. *Cardiovascular Radiology*, **1**, 3–13.

6 Athanasoulis, C. A., Moncure, A. C., Greenfield, A. J. *et al.* (1980) Intraoperative localisation of small bowel bleeding sites with combined use of angiographic methods and methylene blue injection. *Surgery*, **87**, 77–84.

7 Bartelheimer, W., Remmele, W. & Ottenjann, R. (1972) Colonoscopic recognition of haemangiomas in the colon ascendens. *Endoscopy*, **4**, 109–114.

8 Baum, S. (1982) Angiography and the gastrointestinal bleeder. *Radiology*, **142**, 569–572.

9 Baum, S., Athanasoulis, C. A. & Waltman, A. C. (1974) Angiographic diagnosis and control of large bowel bleeding. *Diseases of the Colon and Rectum*, **17**, 447–453.

10 Behringer, S. E. & Albright, N. L. (1973) Diverticular disease of the colon. A frequent cause of bleeding. *American Journal of Surgery*, **125**, 419–423.

11 Boley, S. J. & Schwarz, S. (1971) *Vascular Disorders of the Intestines.* New York: Appleton-Century-Crofts.

12 Boley, S. J., Sprayregan, S., Sammartano, R. J. *et al.* (1977). The pathophysiological basis for the angiographic signs of vascular ectasias of the colon. *Radiology*, **125**, 615–621.

13 Boley, S. J., Sammartano, R., Adams, A. *et al.* (1977) On the nature and aetiology of vascular ectasias of the colon: degenerative lesions of aging. *Gastroenterology*, **72**, 650–656.

14 Bookstein, J. J., Naderi, M. J. & Walter, F. W. (1978) Transcatheter embolisation for lower gastrointestinal bleeding. *Radiology*, **127**, 345–349.

15 Boss, E. G. & Rosenbaum, J. M. (1971) Bleeding from the right colon associated with aortic stenosis. *American Journal of Digestive Diseases*, **16**, 269–275.

16 Bowden, T. A., Hooks, V. H. & Mansberger, A. R. (1980) Intra-operative endoscopy. *Annals of Surgery*, **191**, 680.

17 Brown, A. R. (1968) Diagnosis and management of non-gangrenous ischaemic colitis. *Gut*, **9**, 937–938.

18 Casarella, W. J., Kanter, I. E. & Seaman, W. B. (1972) Right sided colonic diverticula as a cause of acute rectal haemorrhage. *New England Journal of Medicine*, **286**, 450–453.

19 Catem, W. S. & Jiminez, F. A. (1963) Vascular malformations of the intestine: their role as a source of haemorrhage. *Archives of Surgery*, **86**, 571–579.

20 Drapanas, T., Pennington, G. & Kappelman, M. (1973) Emergency subtotal colectomy: the preferred approach to the management of massively bleeding diverticular disease. *Annals of Surgery*, **177**, 519–526.

21 Eaton, A. C. (1981) Emergency surgery for acute colonic haemorrhage – a retrospective study. *British Journal of Surgery*, **68**, 109–112.

22 Forde, K. A. (1979) Intraoperative colonoscopy. *Diseases of the Colon and Rectum*, **22**, 508.

23 Forde, K. A. (1981) Intraoperative colonoscopy. In *Colonoscopy: Techniques, Clinical Practice and Colour Atlas* (Ed.) Hunt, R. H. & Waye, J. D. pp. 189–198. London: Chapman & Hall.

24 Fraenkel, C. J. (1954) Rectal bleeding and diverticulitis. *British Journal of Surgery*, **41**, 643–645.

25 Frey, C. F., Reuter, S. R. & Bookstein, J. J. (1970) Localization of gastrointestinal hemorrhage by selective angiography. *Surgery, Gynecology and Obstetrics*, **67**, 549–553.

26 Fruhmorgen, P. (1981) Therapeutic colonoscopy. In *Colonoscopy: Techniques, Clinical Practice and Colour Atlas* (Ed.) Hunt, R. H. & Waye, J. D. pp. 199–253. London: Chapman and Hall.

27 Fruhmorgen, P., Bodem, F., Reidenbach, H. D. *et al.* (1976) Endoscopic laser coagulation of bleeding gastrointestinal lesions with report of the first therapeutic application in man. *Gastrointestinal Endoscopy*, **23**, 73–75.

28 Galloway, S. J., Casarella, W. J. & Shipkin, P. M. (1974) Vascular malformations of the right colon as a cause of bleeding in patients with aortic stenosis. *Radiology*, **113**, 11–15.

29 Giacchino, J. L., Geis, W. P., Pickleman, J. R. *et al.* (1979) Changing perspectives in massive lower intestinal hemorrhage. *Surgery*, **86**, 368–376.

30 Gianfrancisco, J. A. & Abcarian, H. (1982) Pitfalls in the treatment of massive lower gastrointestinal bleeding with 'blind' subtotal colectomy. *Diseases of the Colon and Rectum*, **25**, 441–445.

31 Heald, R. J. & Ray, J. E. (1972) Bleeding in diverticular disease of the colon. *Proceedings of the Royal Society of Medicine*, **65**, 779–780.

32 Howard, O. M., Buchanan, J. D. & Hunt, R. H. (1982) Angiodysplasia of the colon – experience of 26 cases. *Lancet*, **ii**, 16–19.

33 Hunt, R. H. (1978) Rectal bleeding. *Clinics in Gastroenterology*, **7**, 719–740.

34 Hunt, R. H. (1984) Angiodysplasia of the colon. In *Advances in Gastrointestinal Endoscopy* (Ed.) Salmon, P. R. pp. 97–114. London: Chapman and Hall (in press).

35 Hunt, R. H. & Buchanan, J. D. (1978) Transient ischaemic colitis – colonoscopy and biopsy in diagnosis. *Journal of the Royal Navy Medical Service*, **65**, 15–19.

36 Hunt, R. H., Teague, R. H., Swarbrick, E. T. & Williams, C. B. (1975) Colonoscopy in management of colon strictures. *British Medical Journal*, **iii**, 360.

37 Jensen, D. M., Machicado, G. A. & Tapia, (1983) Emergent colonoscopy in patients with severe hematochezia. *Gastrointestinal Endoscopy*, **29**, 177.

38 Jewett, T. C., Duszniski, D. O. & Allen, J. F. (1970) The visualization of Meckel's diverticulum with ^{99m}Tc pertechnetate. *Surgery*, **68**, 567–570.

39 Lea Thomas, M. (1972) Plain films and barium studies of the ischaemic bowel. *Clinics in Gastroenterology*, **1**, 581–597.

40 Leicester, R. J., Lightfoot, A., Millar, J. *et al.* (1983) Accuracy and value of the haemoccult test in symptomatic patients. *British Medical Journal*, **286**, 673–674.

41 Madigan, M. R. & Morson, B. C. (1969) Solitary ulcer of the rectum. *Gut*, **10**, 871–881.

42 Marcuson, R. W. (1972) Ischaemic colitis. *Clinics in Gastroenterology*, **1**, 745–765.

43 McGuire, H. H. & Haynes, B. W. (1972) Massive haemorrhage from diverticulosis of the colon: guidelines for therapy based on bleeding patterns in 50 cases. *Annals of Surgery*, **178**, 847–852.

44 McKusick, K. A., Frohlich, J., Callaghan, R. J. *et al.* (1981) ^{99m}Tc red blood cells for the detection of gastrointestinal bleeding: experience with 80 patients. *American Journal of Roentgenology*, **137**, 1113–1118.

45 Meyers, M. A., Alonso, D. R., Gray, G. F. & Baer, J. W. (1976) Pathogenesis of bleeding colonic diverticulosis. *Gastroenterology*, **71**, 577–583.

46 Mills, B., Zuckerman, G. & Sicard, G. (1981) Discrete colon ulcers as a cause of lower gastrointestinal bleeding and perforation in end stage renal disease. *Surgery*, **89**, 548–552.

47 Mitsudo, S. M., Boley, S. J., Brandt, L. J. *et al.* (1979) Vascular ectasias of the right colon in the elderly: a distinct pathological entity. *Human Pathology*, **10**, 585–600.

48 Morson, B. C. & Dawson, I. M. P. (1979) *Gastrointestinal Pathology*. 2nd Edition. Oxford: Blackwell Scientific Publications.

49 Naderi, M. J. & Bookstein, J. J. (1978) Rectal bleeding secondary to fecal disimpaction: angiographic diagnosis and treatment. *Radiology*, **126**, 387–389.

50 Nusbaum, M. & Baum, S. (1963) Radiographic demonstration of unknown sites of gastrointestinal bleeding. *Surgical Forum*, **14**, 374–375.

51 Nusbaum, M., Baum, S. & Blakemore, W. S. (1969) Clinical experience with the diagnosis and management of gastrointestinal haemorrhage by selective mesenteric catheterisation. *Annals of Surgery*, **170**, 506–514.

52 Ramanath, H. K. & Hinshaw, J. R. (1971) Management and mismanagement of bleeding colonic diverticula. *Archives of Surgery*, **103**, 311–314.

53 Reuter, S. R. & Bookstein, J. J. (1968) Angiographic localization of gastrointestinal bleeding. *Gastroenterology*, **54**, 876–883.

54 Richardson, J. D., McInnis, W. D., Ramos, R. & Aust, J. B. (1975) Occult gastrointestinal bleeding: an evaluation of available diagnostic methods. *Archives of Surgery*, **110**, 661–665.

55 Rigg, B. M. & Ewing, M. R. (1966) Current attitudes on diverticulitis with particular reference to colonic bleeding. *Archives of Surgery*, **92**, 321–332.

56 Rogers, B. H. G. (1980) Endoscopic diagnosis and therapy of mucosal vascular abnormalities of the gastrointestinal tract occurring in elderly patients and associated with cardiac, vascular and pulmonary disease. *Gastrointestinal Endoscopy*, **26**, 134–138.

57 Rogers, B. H. G. & Adler, F. (1976) Hemangiomas of the cecum. Colonoscopic diagnosis and therapy. *Gastroenterology*, **71**, 1079–1082.

58 Rossini, F. P. & Ferrari, A. (1981) Emergency colonoscopy. In *Colonoscopy: Techniques, Clinical Practice and Colour Atlas* (Ed.) Hunt, R. H. & Waye, J. D. pp. 289–299. London: Chapman and Hall.

59 Rutter, K. R. P. & Riddell, R. H. (1975) The solitary ulcer syndrome of the rectum. *Clinics in Gastroenterology*, **4**, 505–530.

60 Sfakianakis, G. N. & Conway, J. J. (1981) Detection of ectopic gastric mucosa in Meckels' diverticulum and other observations by scintigraphy. II Indications and methods – a ten-year experience. *Journal of Nuclear Medicine*, **22**, 732–738.

61 Skibba, R. M., Hartong, W. A., Mantz, F. A. *et al.* (1976) Angiodysplasia of the cecum: colonoscopic diagnosis. *Gastrointestinal Endoscopy*, **22**, 177–179.

62 Som, P. Oster, Z. H., Atkins, H. C. *et al.* (1981) Detection of gastrointestinal blood loss with ^{99m}Tc-labelled heat treated red blood cells. *Radiology*, **138**, 207–209.

63 Staniland, J. R., Ditchburn, J. & de Dombal, F. T. (1976) Clinical presentation of diseases of the large bowel (a detailed study of 642 patients). *Gastroenterology*, **70**, 22–28.

64 Sutherland, D. B. R., Chan, F. Y., Foucar, E. *et al.* (1979) The bleeding cecal ulcer in transplant patients. *Surgery*, **86**, 386–403.

65 Swarbrick, E. T. & Hunt, R. H. (1981) Rectal bleeding. In *Colonoscopy: Techniques, Clinical Practice and Colour Atlas* (Ed.) Hunt, R. H. & Waye, J. D. pp. 267–288. London: Chapman and Hall.

66 Tagart, R. E. B. (1974) General peritonitis and haemorrhage complicating colonic diverticular disease. *Annals of the Royal College of Surgeons (England)*, **55**, 175–183.

67 Treves, S., Grand, R. J. & Evalkis, A. J. (1978) Pentagastrin stimulation of Technetium-99m uptake by ectopic gastric mucosa in Meckels' diverticulum. *Radiology*, **128**, 711–712.

68 Williams, R. C. (1961) Aortic stenosis and unexplained gastrointestinal bleeding. *Archives of Internal Medicine*, **108**, 859–863.

69 Wolff, W. I., Grossmann, M. B. & Shinya, H. (1977) Angiodysplasia of the colon: diagnosis and treatment. *Gastroenterology*, **72**, 329–333.

CHRONIC GASTROINTESTINAL HAEMORRHAGE

Gastrointestinal haemorrhage may be chronic and recurrent rather than acute; such bleeding may be overt or occult. Chronic overt bleeding is defined as obvious haematemesis, melaena, or bright red rectal haemorrhage, not requiring massive blood replacement and not associated with signs of circulatory embarrassment. Occult gastrointestinal haemorrhage is characterized by positive tests for occult blood in the stools, usually associated with accompanying chronic iron deficiency anaemia. Occasionally such patients may have recurrent but brief episodes of more severe haemorrhage.[3, 41]

Chronic gastrointestinal haemorrhage frequently presents a formidable diagnostic challenge since many standard investigations will not provide the diagnosis. Birke and Engstedt[7] studied 1252 patients with chronic haemorrhage and found that a definitive diagnosis of the source of bleeding could not be made in 15%. However, in this early study endoscopy was not used. Douvres and Glass,[16] in a series of 800 patients in whom endoscopy was available, found that 15.5% remained undiagnosed.

It is always unsatisfying when the diagnosis of the source of bleeding is obscure, but how far is it important to pursue an accurate diagnosis in patients with chronic gastrointestinal haemorrhage? Birke and Engstedt[7] followed, for 4–14 years, 109 patients in whom a firm diagnosis had not been made and found that 45% never rebled, although 46% were subsequently correctly diagnosed because of recurrent bleeding. Douvres and Glass[16] found that one-third of their undiagnosed patients returned with recurrent haemorrhage and that in patients presenting with melaena only, the frequency of an undiagnosed source of bleeding was as high as 43%. Some of these patients have malignant tumours, amenable to radical treatment, or benign lesions which may also be satisfactorily treated. It is therefore desirable to pursue a diagnosis in these patients with vigour, using all the diagnostic techniques currently available.

AETIOLOGY

There are many causes of chronic gastrointestinal haemorrhage and these are listed in Table 6.8. Most relate to disorders of the gastrointestinal tract but others include vascular malformations, haematological disorders, collagen diseases, inherited disorders of connective tissue, infections or infestations, and drug induced gastrointestinal lesions. There have been a number of papers on the pathogenesis of haemorrhage particularly in the more obscure causes.[23, 46] Although many of the causes listed are more likely to present as acute rather than chronic gastrointestinal bleeding, all may appear with chronic or occult blood loss.

Oesophageal and gastro-oesophageal disorders

Most of these conditions are more likely to give rise to acute and overt bleeding rather than chronic or occult haemorrhage. Of this group hiatal hernia, often accompanied by reflux oesophagitis, is perhaps the disorder most likely to be associated with chronic gastrointestinal haemorrhage. Surprisingly, chronic gastrointestinal bleeding can occasionally be due to a Mallory–Weiss tear and oesophageal or gastric varices (see p. 300). The occurrence of gastric mucosa in the oesophagus (Barrett's syndrome) is a frequent cause of ulceration and chronic haemorrhage in this group.

Disorders of the stomach

Gastric ulcer, haemorrhagic gastritis and gastric erosions, often associated with drug or alcohol abuse are the commonest causes of chronic bleeding in this group. Benign or malignant tumours of the stomach may also cause chronic or occult bleeding and must always be considered in the differential diagnosis.

Disorders of the small intestine

Duodenal ulceration is a common cause of chronic gastrointestinal haemorrhage. Jejunal or ileal ulceration is less frequent and may be associated with the ingestion of potassium chloride preparations or coeliac disease, in which there may be persistent severe intestinal ulceration.

Tumours of the small intestine are relatively rare, the commonest being lymphomas which may be a complication of coeliac disease. Adenocarcinoma of the small intestine is also a rare cause of intestinal blood loss. Adenomatous polyps may occur in the small intestine, the best known being the Peutz–Jeghers syndrome where multiple polyps of the small intestine occur in association with melanin pigmentation around the mouth and face (Figure 6.12). Such patients may present with chronic gastrointestinal haemorrhage, although severe colicky abdominal pain and intermittent intestinal obstruction due to intussusception are perhaps more common. Juvenile polyps also occur in the small intestine and may cause chronic bleeding.

Crohn's disease of the small intestine can occasionally present with chronic gastrointestinal haemorrhage, although anaemia in Crohn's disease is more commonly associated with malabsorption and infection.

Table 6.8 Classification of causes of chronic gastrointestinal haemorrhage

Oesophageal and gastro-oesophageal disorders
  Oesophageal ulceration and Barrett's syndrome
  Oesophagitis
  Hiatal hernia
  Tumours of oesophagus
  Oesophageal diverticula
  Mallory–Weiss syndrome
  Oesophageal and gastric varices

Disorders of the stomach
  Gastric ulcer
  Stomal ulcer
  Haemorrhagic gastritis and gastric erosions
  Tumours of stomach
    Malignant tumours
    Benign tumours and polyps
    Adenoma, leiomyoma, haemangioma
  Gastric diverticula

Disorders of the small intestine
  Duodenal ulcer
  Stomal ulcer
  Jejunal ulceration
  Tumours of small intestine
    Lymphoma
    Adenocarcinoma
    Benign tumours
      Leiomyoma, haemangioma, lipoma
      Peutz–Jeghers syndrome
  Crohn's disease
  Tuberculosis
  Radiation damage
  Intussusception
  Small intestinal diverticula
    Duodenal and jejunal diverticula
    Meckel's diverticulum
  Enteric duplication cyst
  Small intestinal ischaemia

Disorders of the large intestine
  Ulcerative colitis
  Crohn's disease
  Rectal ulcer
  Anal fissure
  Haemorrhoids
  Tumours of large intestine
    Malignant tumours
    Benign tumours
      Adenoma, haemangioma
      Adenomatous and villous polyps
      Familial polyposis of the colon
  Tuberculosis
  Radiation damage
  Diverticular disease of colon
  Ischaemic colitis
  Endometriosis
  Angiodysplasia (see vascular malformations)

Disorders of the liver and gallbladder
  Primary hepatic tumours
  Hepatic cirrhosis
  Viral hepatitis
  Hepatic abscess
  Hepatic cyst
  Aneurysm of hepatic artery
  Calculi
  Tumours of bile ducts or gallbladder
  Haemorrhagic cholecystitis

Disorders of the pancreas
  Acute pancreatitis
  Chronic pancreatitis
  Pancreatic pseudocyst
  Tumours of pancreas
  Splenic artery aneurysm

Vascular malformations
  Arteriovenous malformations
    Angiodysplasia
    Hereditary haemorrhagic telangiectasia
      (Osler–Weber–Rendu syndrome)
  Aneurysms and aorto-enteric fistulas
  Haemangiomas
    Blue naevus bleb syndrome

Haematological disorders
  Haemophilia
  Christmas disease
  von Willebrand's disease
  Thrombocytopenia
  Purpuras
  Leukaemias
  Lymphoma
  Disseminated intravascular coagulation
  Polycythaemia rubra vera
  Haemolytic anaemias
  Aplastic anaemia
  Myelomatosis

Collagen disorders
  Systemic lupus erythematosus
  Polyarteritis nodosa
  Dermatomyositis
  Progressive systemic sclerosis
  Rheumatoid arthritis
  Henoch–Schönlein purpura

Inherited disorders of connective tissue
  Pseudoxanthoma elasticum (Groenblad–Strandberg
    syndrome)
  Ehlers–Danlos syndrome

Infections and infestations
  Amoebic colitis
  Bacillary dysenteric infection
  Pseudomembranous colitis
  Hookworm disease

Drugs
  Acetylsalicylic acid
  Indomethacin
  Phenylbutazone
  Oxyphenbutazone
  Benorylate
  Piroxicam
  Naproxen
  Ibuprofen
  Aloxiprim
  Flufenamic acid
  Anticoagulants
  Ethanol
  Ethacrynic acid
  Potassium chloride (Slow-K)
  Emepronium bromide (Cetiprin)

Miscellaneous
  Primary amyloidosis
  Uraemia
  Renal carcinoma
  Aortic stenosis

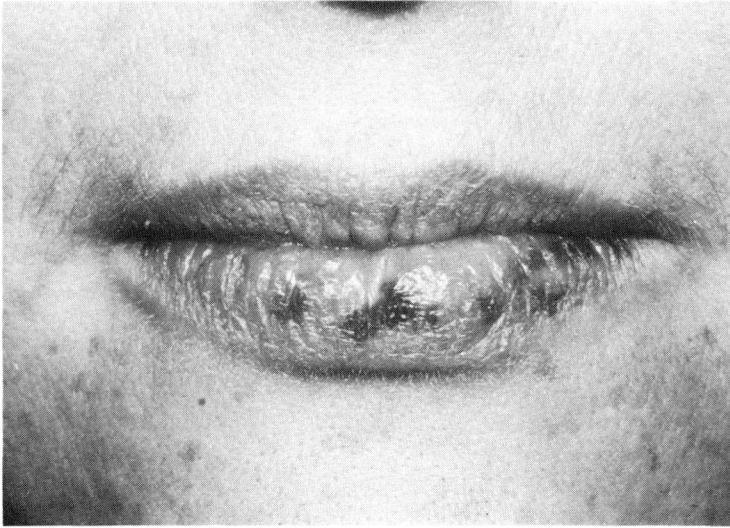

Fig. 6.12 Peutz–Jeghers syndrome.

Small intestinal diverticula are fairly common and tend to decrease in frequency as the intestine is traced downwards, being most marked in the region of the duodeno-jejunal flexure. Meckel's diverticulum is the most frequent congenital anomaly of the gastrointestinal tract, although a relatively uncommon cause of gastrointestinal tract bleeding. While only 16% of Meckel's diverticula contain gastric mucosa, gastric mucosa and peptic ulceration are present in virtually all those Meckel's diverticula which bleed. Haemorrhage from a Meckel's diverticulum is usually acute with major blood loss and rarely presents as chronic anaemia.

Enteric duplication cysts share a common wall and blood supply with the adjacent segment of the gastrointestinal tract and may sometimes be lined by gastric epithelium which may ulcerate and bleed.

Disorders of the large intestine

Patients with ulcerative colitis usually have overt haemorrhage although it may also be chronic. Patients with colonic Crohn's disease rarely bleed, but chronic haemorrhage may occur. Solitary rectal ulcer, unrelated to the presence of inflammatory bowel disease, may cause chronic gastrointestinal haemorrhage and is usually also associated with the passage of mucus, rectal pain and disturbance of bowel habit.

Benign and malignant tumours are a common cause of chronic bleeding. Familial polyposis of the colon frequently presents with bleeding, which is generally chronic and may be associated with diarrhoea, mucus, and later with abdominal pain and weight loss.

Colonic diverticula are one of the commonest causes of bleeding from the lower gastrointestinal tract; bleeding may be acute, chronic or occult. Chronic bleeding may also be associated with ischaemic colitis. A rare cause of chronic gastrointestinal haemorrhage is endometriosis involving the lower part of the bowel, usually the rectosigmoid, terminal ileum or caecum.

Disorders of liver and gallbladder

Liver disease should always be considered as a possible, although rare, cause of chronic gastrointestinal haemorrhage, particularly in conditions such as hepatoma, hepatic cirrhosis, viral hepatitis, abscesses, cysts and aneurysms.

Bleeding in the biliary tract (haemobilia) is uncommon but is an important cause of undiagnosed intestinal haemorrhage. It may be due to calculi, haemorrhagic cholecystitis, tumours of bile duct and gallbladder or an arteriovenous malformation in the liver. Arteriovenous malformations are rarely congenital and are more frequently due to trauma or previous biliary surgery.

Disorders of the pancreas

Acute pancreatitis, chronic pancreatitis, pancreatic pseudocysts and tumours of the pancreas are all rare causes of chronic gastrointestinal haemorrhage. Chronic pancreatitis should be considered in obscure cases of gastrointestinal bleeding, particularly when it is associated with excess alcohol ingestion and left sided upper quadrant or epigastric pain.[19] Bleeding down the pancreatic duct may occasionally be due to a splenic artery aneurysm.

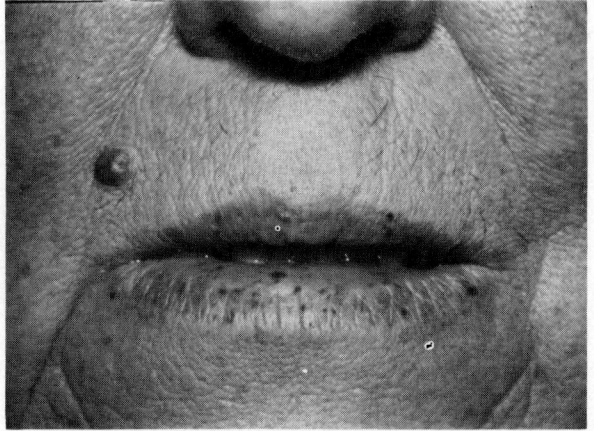

Fig. 6.13   Hereditary telangiectasia.

Vascular malformations

ARTERIOVENOUS MALFORMATIONS

These are dilatations or malformations of existing vascular structures.[46] They have been classified into three groups by Moore and his colleagues:[33]

Angiodysplasia, vascular ectasia and dysplasia of the colon. These are important causes of chronic lower gastrointestinal bleeding, especially in older patients, and 20–25% of these patients have aortic stenosis.[26] They are frequently multiple and occur principally in the right colon; they are small (< 5 mm in diameter) and are difficult to identify, even using modern diagnostic methods.

Congenital lesions. These may occur anywhere in the alimentary tract, are larger than angiodysplastic lesions and generally present with chronic haemorrhage at a younger age.

Hereditary haemorrhagic telangiectasia (Osler–Weber–Rendu syndrome). This is a rare disorder inherited as an autosomal dominant trait. Telangiectasias may be found throughout the gastrointestinal tract and generally present with chronic gastrointestinal bleeding. Most patients have a family history of the disorder and more than 90% have visible telangiectasias of the face (Figure 5.3), oral and nasopharyngeal mucosae, or upper extremities (Figures 6.13 and 6.14). This syndrome is discussed in more detail in Chapter 5 (p. 250).

ANEURYSMS AND AORTOENTERIC FISTULAS

These may occur spontaneously or as a late complication of aortoiliac reconstructive surgery; leakage of aneurysms may occur into any part of the gastrointestinal tract but occult bleeding is often down the bile or pancreatic ducts.[24]

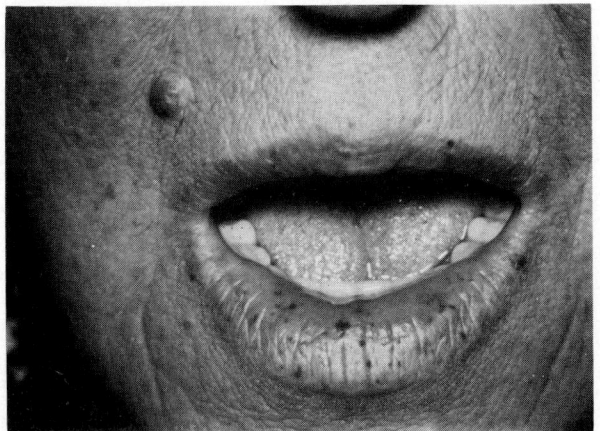

Fig. 6.14   Hereditary telangiectasia.

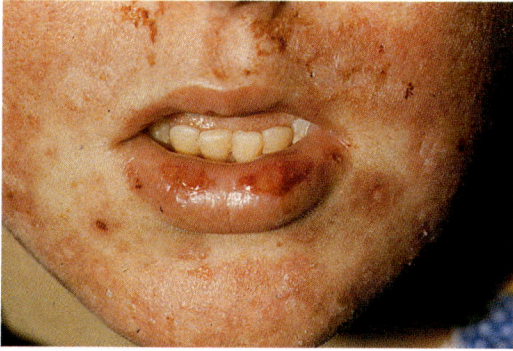

Plate 7.1   Crusting of lips in patient with erythema multiforme.

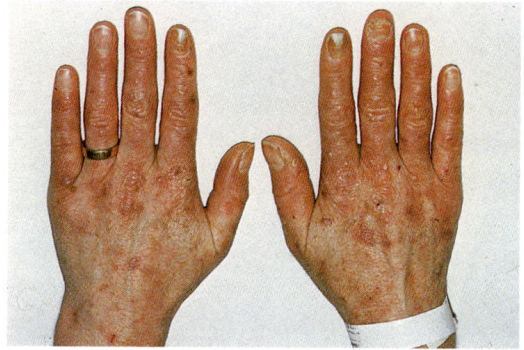

Plate 7.2   Light-exposed skin of patient with variegate porphyria, showing blisters, milia (horn cysts) and scars.

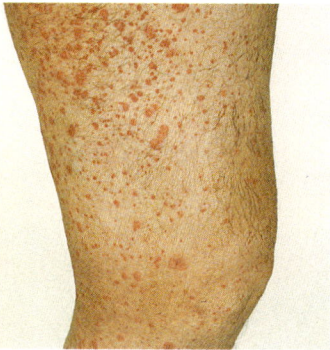

Plate 7.3   Palpable purpuric lesions in patient with Henoch–Schönlein disease.

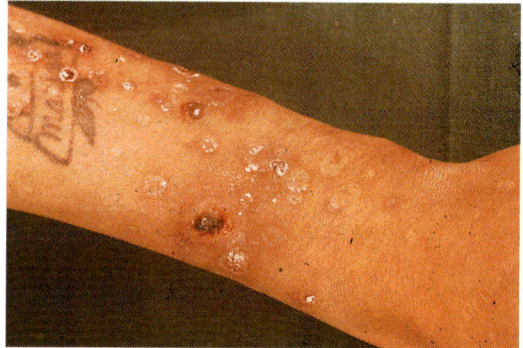

Plate 7.4   Scars of vasculitic ulcers in patient with malabsorption due to chronic mesenteric vessel disease.

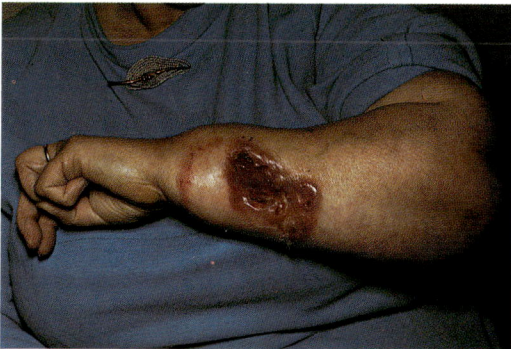

Plate 7.5   Pyoderma gangrenosum.

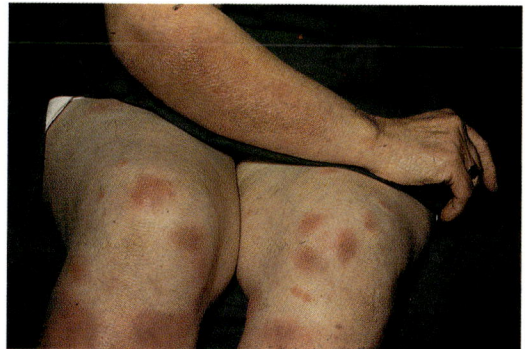

Plate 7.6   Erythema nodosum.

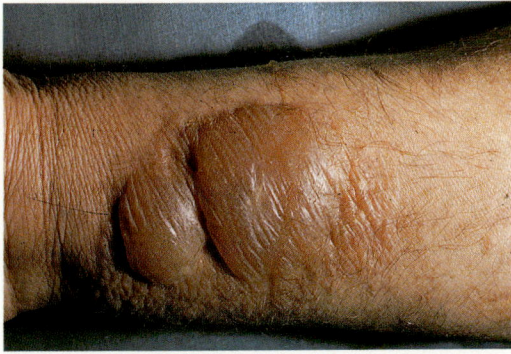

Plate 7.7 Grouped blisters on elbow in patient with dermatitis herpetiformis.

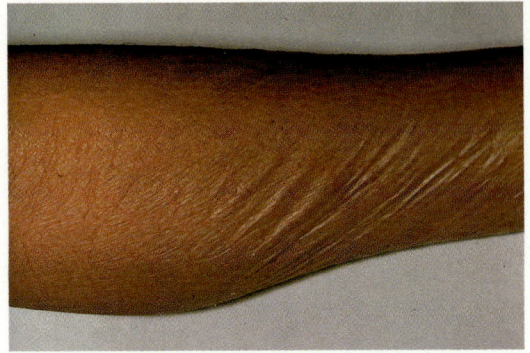

Plate 7.8 Acquired ichthyosis and wrinkling of skin in patient with uncontrolled coeliac disease.

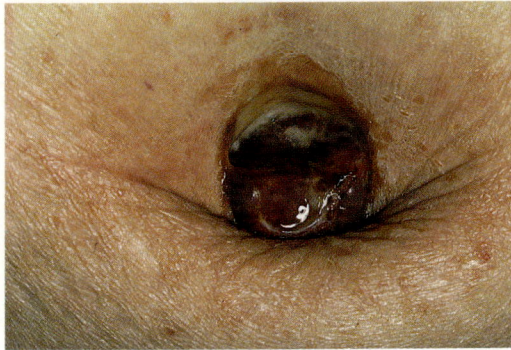

Plate 7.9 Metastatic deposit in umbilical skin from adenocarcinoma of colon.

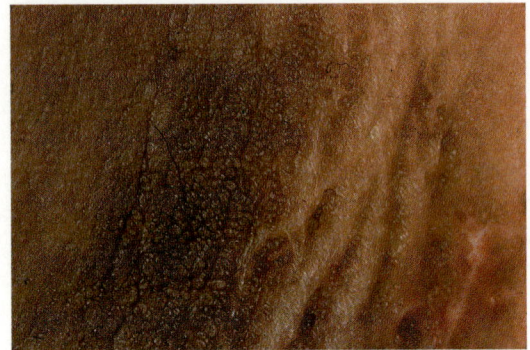

Plate 7.10 Velvety axillary skin in patient with acanthosis nigricans.

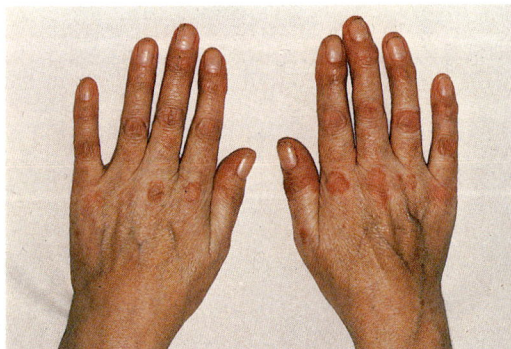

Plate 7.11a Glucagonoma: rash on hands.

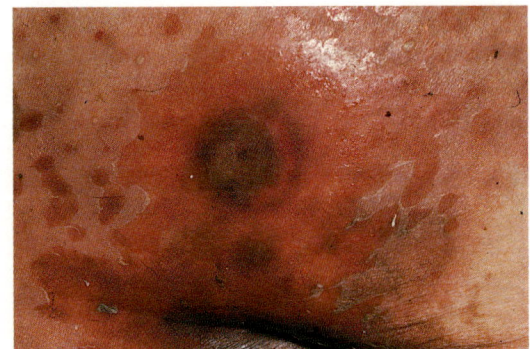

Plate 7.11b Glucagonoma: close-up view of necrolytic migratory erythema.

HAEMANGIOMAS

Haemangiomas may occur as isolated lesions anywhere in the gastrointestinal tract (Figure 6.15). Patients with the rare blue naevus bleb syndrome generally have both cutaneous and visceral haemangiomas.

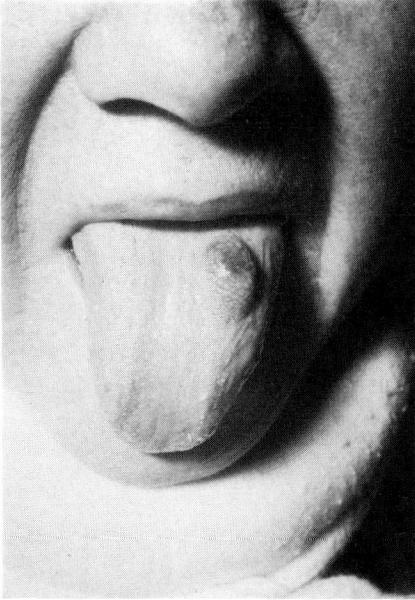

Fig. 6.15 Haemangioma on tongue associated with similar lesions in gastrointestinal tract giving rise to chronic gastrointestinal haemorrhage.

Haematological disorders

A wide range of haematological disorders may be associated with chronic gastrointestinal haemorrhage. These include clotting disorders, leukaemias, lymphomas, and haemolytic and aplastic anaemias. In polycythaemia rubra vera, chronic gastrointestinal haemorrhage may result from thrombosis leading to local infarction and ulceration of the gut.

Collagen disorders

Collagen disorders, such as systemic lupus erythematosis, polyarteritis nodosa, dermatomyositis and rheumatoid arthritis, may be associated with visceral vasculitis which may cause chronic gastrointestinal haemorrhage. In polyarteritis nodosa, involvement of the visceral vessels may result in gastrointestinal bleeding which is generally chronic and often occult.[10] In progressive systemic sclerosis, chronic gastrointestinal bleeding may be due to ischaemia and infarction of the gut.

In Henoch–Schonlein purpura there is a vasculitis of the small vessels associated with non-thrombocytopenic purpura of the lower extremities, polyarthritis, glomerulonephritis, localized subcutaneous oedema, abdominal discomfort and chronic gastrointestinal bleeding.[15]

Inherited disorders of connective tissue

Pseudoxanthoma elasticum (Groenblad–Strandberg syndrome) is a rare hereditary disorder in which there is an accumulation of abnormal elastic tissue throughout the body.[29] Angioid streaks are present in the retina, xanthomatous papules appear on the skin and chronic or recurrent gastrointestinal haemorrhage may occur from rupture of a blood vessel in the stomach or small intestine. The diagnosis is generally suspected from the characteristic finding of lax skin in the neck, axilla and groin.

The Ehlers–Danlos syndrome is a generalized defect in the organization of connective tissue characterized by hyperextensibility of the skin and hypermobility of the joints.[30] Gastrointestinal tract bleeding is relatively rare and may result from associated colonic diverticula or the rupture of visceral arteries.

Infections and infestations

Chronic gastrointestinal haemorrhage may be due to infection such as amoebic colitis, bacillary dysentery and hookworm disease. Pseudomembranous colitis, due to *Clostridium difficile*, is also a rare cause of chronic gastrointestinal haemorrhage, bleeding being an unusual feature of this disease.

Drugs

Many drugs have been incriminated as a cause of gastrointestinal bleeding. The precise association between ingestion of any particular drug and the causation of chronic gastrointestinal haemorrhage is difficult to determine and the inadequacy of the data available has recently been highlighted.[25]

A wide range of anti-inflammatory drugs have been associated with chronic gastrointestinal haemorrhage, notably acetylsalicylic acid,[27] indomethacin and phenylbutazone. However, the whole range of non-steroidal anti-inflammatory drugs are all liable to cause chronic or occult gastrointestinal haemorrhage.[43] Multiple complex mechanisms are probably associated with such gastrointestinal damage and have been the subject of much research in recent years.

It is claimed that in man the corticosteroids increase the prevalence of peptic ulcer or the incidence of upper gastrointestinal haemorrhage, but the evidence is conflicting.[13]

Other drugs which may be associated with chronic gastrointestinal haemorrhage are ethacrynic acid, potassium chloride preparations, emepronium bromide, anticoagulants and alcohol.

Miscellaneous

Chronic gastrointestinal haemorrhage may occur in association with primary amyloidosis; localized ulceration may occur in the small intestine affected by amyloid.

Chronic renal insufficiency and uraemia may cause bleeding from the duodenum or colon, often in patients undergoing renal dialysis. Recurrent duodenal haemorrhage has also been reported in patients with renal carcinoma.

Chronic or occult gastrointestinal haemorrhage may occur in patients with aortic stenosis, which may be associated with angiodysplasia[12]; solitary ulcer of the caecum is also a rare cause of acute or chronic intestinal blood loss.

CLINICAL PRESENTATION

Evidence of haemorrhage. The patient with chronic gastrointestinal haemorrhage which is clinically evident will usually present because of the bleeding. Patients with occult gastrointestinal haemorrhage will generally be unaware of the occurrence of bleeding and present because of the clinical features of chronic anaemia, or with the features of a systemic disorder if one is present.

Clinical features of chronic iron deficiency anaemia. The typical features of anaemia may be present in these patients: fatigue, malaise, pallor, tachycardia, dyspnoea on exertion and oedema.

Clinical features of an underlying disease which has led to chronic gastrointestinal blood loss. These may be very varied in accordance with the wide range of possible diagnoses. Symptoms which may be present include heartburn, flatulence, abdominal discomfort, alteration in bowel habit, weight loss, anorexia and other non-specific features. In patients with occult haemorrhage, the presenting symptoms may not necessarily indicate that the gastrointestinal tract is the source of pathology and a positive faecal occult blood test may be the only indicator of gastrointestinal disease.

INVESTIGATIONS

The investigations available to identify the cause of chronic gastrointestinal haemorrhage are listed in Table 6.9. The common causes of chronic haemorrhage ought to be excluded and may sometimes be missed, even by advanced diagnostic techniques; hence repeat of standard diagnostic investigations is often appropriate.

Table 6.9 Investigation of chronic or occult gastrointestinal haemorrhage.

Detailed history and clinical examination
Laboratory tests
Haematology
Biochemistry
Faecal studies
Confirmation of faecal blood loss
Quantitation of faecal blood loss – ^{51}Cr studies
Radiology
Barium swallow and meal
Barium enema
Small bowel enema
Angiography
Endoscopy
Sigmoidoscopy
Upper gastrointestinal endoscopy
Colonoscopy
Fluorescein string test
Small bowel intubation – aspiration and testing for blood
Radionuclide scanning techniques
Laparotomy

In the patient in whom bleeding is continuing, oral iron therapy or repeated blood transfusions may be required during the course of these investigations. If the bleeding has either stopped or slowed to such an extent that oral iron therapy is sufficient to maintain normal haemoglobin levels, conservative management should be continued but the patient maintained under careful observation. If bleeding becomes more severe the patient should be thoroughly reinvestigated.

The identification of a gastrointestinal tract lesion is not necessarily proof of it being the cause of blood loss. Thus Palmer,[36] studying 1400 patients with upper gastrointestinal tract haemorrhage, found that 50.9% had lesions not considered to be responsible for the bleeding episode.

The investigative approach to patients with chronic gastrointestinal haemorrhage is as follows:

Detailed history and clinical examination

Many of the most common causes of chronic bleeding will be suggested by a detailed history and clinical examination of the patient. These include hiatal hernia, peptic ulceration, diverticular disease and tumours. A history of previous bleeding episodes and haemorrhage from other sites, or a family history of bleeding, suggests the possibility of one of the rarer hereditary conditions. A detailed history of drug ingestion is also very important.

Characteristic features on physical examination may suggest the diagnosis of hereditary telangiectasia, angiomas, pseudoxanthoma elasticum and the Ehlers–Danlos syndrome. The presence of spider naevi, palmar erythema or jaundice suggests hepatic disease and abdominal examination may reveal evidence of hepatomegaly, splenomegaly or masses suggesting neoplasia. A rectal examination is essential and may immediately provide evidence for haemorrhoids, rectal ulcer, fissure or a polyp. Examination of the stool for parasites may also be valuable.

Laboratory tests

Standard haematological and biochemical tests should be performed and may provide a guide to the diagnosis. A complete blood count and blood film will determine if blood loss has been sufficient to cause anaemia and if the blood film suggests iron deficiency, confirmation will be obtained by determining the amount of stainable iron in the bone marrow. Platelet count, prothrombin time, bleeding time and partial thromboplastin time will detect clinically significant clotting defects in more than 90% of patients. An increased white cell count, if persistent, may suggest a neoplastic lesion or infection complicating colonic diverticula. Eosinophilia may point to hookworm disease, and thrombocythaemia suggests polycythemia rubra vera.

Routine biochemical tests, such as blood urea, electrolytes, sugar, albumin, globulin, calcium, magnesium, alkaline phosphatase, bilirubin and transaminases, may provide evidence of hepatic disease, inflammatory bowel disease or uraemia.

Faecal studies

Confirmation of faecal blood loss
Blood loss in the faeces may be obvious, depending upon the amount present or the site of blood loss. Thus, a distal source of chronic blood loss is more likely to give red blood in the stools than a proximal site, although this is not always the case. The presence of occult blood may be confirmed by a number of chemical tests which depend on the oxidation of a phenolic compound to a quinone structure by hydrogen peroxide catalysed by the peroxidase activity of haemoglobin.[22] Tests for faecal occult blood tend to be either highly sensitive (such as the formerly widely used benzidine and orthotolidine tests) or relatively insensitive (guaiac test). The highly sensitive tests tend to be positive after the shedding of 0.5–1.9 ml of blood in the gastrointestinal tract and a large number (over 70%) of false positive reactions occur on an unrestricted diet. The relatively insensitive tests provide a positive result after passing 2–15 ml of blood and provide false positive results in less than 25% of patients on a normal diet, but may give a false negative reaction in up to 50% of patients. The interpretation of faecal occult blood tests is thus complicated by the loss of 'normal' small amounts of blood in the gastrointestinal tract, variations in the sensitivity of the chemical tests available, and the possibility that substances other than haemoglobin may be capable of producing a positive reaction, particularly with the 'sensitive' tests. False positive results may occur with dietary meat or haemoglobin in poorly cooked meat and drugs containing bromide, iodide, potassium permanganate but not iron.

The present slide tests available, using either Haemoccult (guaiac) and Haemastix (orthotolidine), have recently been compared as screening procedures for occult gastrointestinal haemorrhage.[4] In a study of 438 patients, a false positive rate of 22.9% was found with Haemastix, compared with 3.4% with Haemoccult. It was considered that the false positive rate with Haemastix made this method unacceptable as a screening test, particularly in outpatients, although a test of greater sensitivity than Haemoccult may be needed in the investigation of hospital patients. Haemoccult may be too insensitive to detect lesions, particularly in the colon, which may be bleeding slowly or intermittently, but may be useful as a screening test in outpatients. In all patients suspected of chronic or occult gastrointestinal haemorrhage, repeated faecal occult blood tests may be necessary before occasional positive tests may provide confirmation of bleeding.

The test which is most commonly used at present is the relatively insensitive Haemoccult test which is less liable to provide false positive results, may not routinely need dietary restriction before being applied, but if positive provides valuable confirmation of gastrointestinal bleeding.

Quantitation of faecal blood loss

The amount of blood lost in the stools can be determined quantitatively by labelling the patient's circulating red blood cells with radioactive chromium (^{51}Cr), collecting the faeces and measuring the amount of faecal radioactivity.[11, 32] Venous blood (20 ml) is drawn and after labelling with ^{51}Cr is injected intravenously into the patient. The stools are collected for five days and after preparation the amount of radioactivity is determined by means of a scintillation counter. Using this method an average daily blood loss of 0.3–1.3 ml has been found in normal subjects. The value of the technique is to confirm abnormal faecal blood loss in patients suspected of having gastrointestinal bleeding but in whom faecal occult blood tests have been negative or equivocal, and to determine the amount of blood loss. The technique can also be used to calculate red cell survival.

Radiology

Contrast radiology of the gastrointestinal tract

By and large, standard radiological evaluation of oesophagus, stomach, small intestine and colon is relatively unsuccessful in defining sources of chronic haemorrhage. Bleeding lesions may be too superficial for radiological detection, and even when a lesion such as a peptic ulcer is demonstrated, this does not prove that it is the source of haemorrhage.[3] Improvements in techniques, such as double contrast radiology, have provided greater accuracy of diagnosis, particularly in identifying superficial mucosal lesions in the stomach and colon. The technique of small bowel enema has also been an advance in the radiology of small intestinal lesions. However, all these methods have been disappointing in identifying the cause of bleeding, and often demonstrate spurious abnormalities.[14, 50] However, such procedures are worthwhile in patients being investigated for chronic gastrointestinal haemorrhage as they may in individual patients identify a hitherto unrecognized pathological entity which might have been the source of bleeding.

Angiography

Selective arteriography or angiography has become an important technique in the diagnosis of chronic gastrointestinal haemorrhage.[35] For successful visualization, however, the patient must be bleeding at a minimum rate of 0.5 ml per minute; under these circumstances extravasation of contrast material may provide evidence of the site of haemorrhage.[5] However, some lesions will escape detection, especially if they are small in size, in the small intestine, not primarily vascular and not bleeding rapidly. Chronic gastrointestinal bleeding is frequently intermittent, and angiography will not be helpful if the study is performed between bleeding episodes. The technique used, together with an assessment of its value and risks, have recently been reviewed.[5, 8]

Sheedy, Fulton and Atwell[42] found that there is a 45% chance of finding an angiographically identifiable lesion which may have been the site of haemorrhage. In half of the patients with a positive diagnosis, the lesion was an arteriovenous malformation of the bowel. Half of the malformations were located in the caecum or the ascending colon. However, the incidence of false negative examinations was relatively high.

The value of angiography in diagnosing angiodysplasia as a cause of chronic haemorrhage has also been reported.[6] Thirty-four patients were studied with intermittent or chronic gastrointestinal haemorrhage in which angiography demonstrated angiodysplasia of the caecum or right colon; in all patients repeated barium enema and endoscopy were normal. Right colectomy was performed on 17 patients and after a seven year follow up, four were found to have re-bled; two of these had angiographic evidence of related lesions in other parts of the colon and terminal ileum. Even if an area of angiodysplasia is found, a careful search should be made to exclude other lesions such as a tumour which may be the cause of haemorrhage since angiodysplasia may be only an incidental finding. The arterial branch which supplies the angiodysplasia should be identified in order to determine its exact location in the bowel. When an area of angiodysplasia is detected in a patient with recurrent occult bleeding, the involved segment of bowel should be removed. (An example demonstrated by angiography is shown in Figure 6.16.) The angiodysplastic lesion is soft and submucosal and so the mucosa may appear normal, or at the most slightly reddened. The specific pathological bleeding lesions, amongst a tangle of dilated submucosal vessels, can be identified by injecting Microfil or barium into the resected specimen which, after tissue clearing techniques, may facilitate pathological identification of the lesions.[47]

As a result of the increased use of angiography in patients with chronic haemorrhage, angiodysplasia and other similar lesions are being demonstrated with increasing frequency as a cause of haemorrhage in patients presenting with chronic or occult gastrointestinal bleeding.

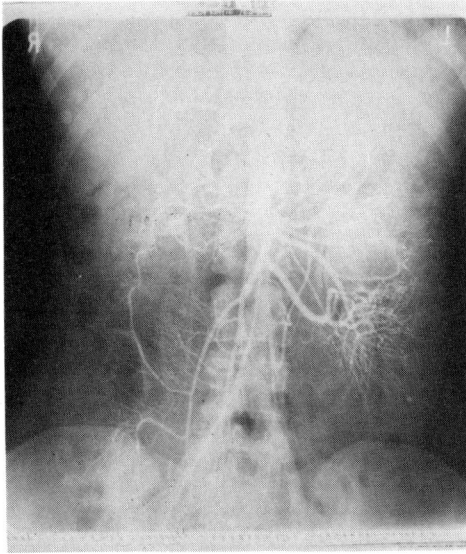

Fig. 6.16 Angiography demonstrating angiodysplasia.

Endoscopy

Sigmoidoscopy
Sigmoidoscopy is an essential investigation in all patients presenting with chronic gastrointestinal haemorrhage. Rectal and sigmoid lesions such as ulceration, inflammation, or tumours can easily be diagnosed in this way.

Upper gastrointestinal endoscopy
All patients with chronic or occult gastrointestinal bleeding require upper gastrointestinal endoscopy to exclude an upper alimentary cause for the haemorrhage such as hiatal hernia or peptic ulceration.

Colonoscopy
Colonoscopy is valuable in the investigation of the patient with chronic lower intestinal haemorrhage, especially when the barium enema is unhelpful. Tedesco et al.[49] found that colonoscopy detected neoplasms (cancer or polyps) greater than 5 mm in diameter which were not demonstrated by single contrast barium enema examinations in 75 out of 304 (25%) patients studied because of rectal haemorrhage. Similar results were obtained by Teague, Salmon and Read,[48] who found that of 75 patients with occult bleeding, 21 patients had small cancers or polyps and 15 had inflammatory bowel disease. Colonoscopy has also been reported of being of value in diagnosing angiodysplasia of the large intestine (Figure 6.17).[44]

All endoscopic techniques have an important potential advantage over conventional radiology in that actual bleeding may be identified.

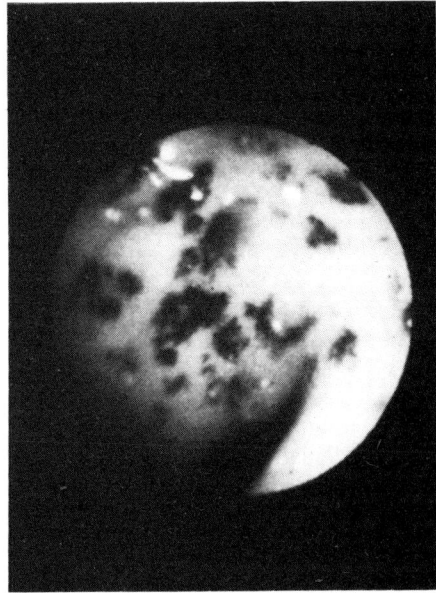

Fig. 6.17 Angiodysplasia of colon demonstrated at colonoscopy.

Fluorescein string test

This test was specifically devised to determine the site of chronic upper gastrointestinal blood loss.[21] The patient swallows a long string with radiopaque markers at regular intervals (usually 10 cm) along its length, with a weight attached to facilitate swallowing and passage through the pylorus. When the string has reached the desired position, 10–20 ml of fluorescein sodium is injected intravenously and the string removed 5 min later. The string is then examined under ultraviolet light for areas of fluorescence which correspond to sites where bleeding has occurred. Comparison with a straight X-ray film taken just before the string is removed will possibly demonstrate the approximate site of chronic haemorrhage.

The test has been shown to be of some value when other diagnostic tests such as barium meal and endoscopy were unhelpful[38] but has the disadvantage of being difficult to position at the desired part of the upper gastrointestinal tract within a reasonable time. This problem has been resolved aided by the introduction of a rapid-entry radiopaque tube horizontally marked with a radiopaque filament, and covered by a sheath of white non-fluorescent cotton material.[39] Although this method reduced the technical problems of the test to some extent, angiographic, endoscopic and radionuclide developments have replaced this test and it is now rarely performed.

Small bowel intubation

The passage of a long intestinal tube with step-wise aspiration of intestinal contents may be useful occasionally in confirming the presence and determining the site of chronic gastro-intestinal haemorrhage.[34, 46] The position at which the aspirate becomes stained with blood or changes from negative to positive for occult blood may correspond to the site of the lesion, and radiological demonstration of this lesion may be possible by injecting barium through the tube at a point slightly proximal to where the blood-stained aspirate is obtained.

A modification involves the intravenous injection of red cells labelled with ^{51}Cr; recovery of radioactivity in the aspirate confirms fresh bleeding and may aid in localizing the lesion.[37] Measurement of stool radioactivity may also be valuable. Radioactivity in the intestinal aspirate in the absence of faecal radioactivity may suggest bleeding originating proximal to the caecum, whereas faecal radioactivity in the absence of radioactivity in the aspirate suggests that the site of bleeding is in the colon.

Radionuclide scanning techniques

Various radionuclide techniques have been considered to be of value in identifying the site of chronic gastrointestinal haemorrhage. There are two principal approaches: first, the use of substances that are rapidly extracted from the blood, demonstrating the activity extravasated into the lumen of the bowel during the relatively brief transit of the material; and second, the imaging of non-diffusible intravascular indicators, which concentrate at the bleeding site over a period of time.[20] The first approach has been successfully used with ^{99}Tc^{m}-sulphur colloid[1, 2] and bleeding rates as low as 0.05 ml/min have been detected using this method. However, active bleeding is required for this technique to be successful and as the compound is taken up by the liver, this organ may mask a bleeding site in the right upper quadrant.

The second approach has been used successfully with ^{99}Tc^{m}-labelled red cells.[9, 28, 45] The patient's red cells are prepared 'in vivo' by injecting ^{99}Tc^{m}O$_4^-$. This produces significant quantities of free ^{99}Tc^{m}O$_4^-$, which is extracted and secreted by the gastric mucosa, and this may lead to a false positive intraluminal accumulation. This can be avoided either by continuous nasogastric aspiration or by using an 'in vitro' labelling technique which results in very little

free TcO$_4^-$.[28] The advantage of labelled red cells over sulphur colloid is that the material circulates continuously, allowing monitoring over at least 24 hours and thereby identifying slow and intermittent bleeding lesions.[45] Markisz and his colleagues[28] found that 47% of their patients only became positive after six hours, suggesting that an acute colloid study would have been negative. In addition, 40% of bleeding patients in whom both studies were performed consecutively had negative colloid studies and positive red cell studies.[9]

These radionuclide techniques have been shown to be of practical value in diagnosing the cause of chronic haemorrhage.[18] The technique of Markisz with 'in vitro' labelling may be of value as an investigative screening technique before angiography, providing possible specific vessel localization before angiography.

Other red cell labels have been used, notably indium-111[17] and further work is required to determine the most convenient specific label for these techniques.

Other blood-pool labels have also been developed, such as ^{99}Tc^{m}-labelled albumin, but have not so far been studied extensively because of cost, inconvenience and instability.[31]

Laparotomy

In a few patients in whom the judicious and planned use of investigations has not demonstrated a site of haemorrhage, laparotomy may still be indicated. The development of modern radiological, endoscopic and radionuclide techniques have tended to make the use of laparotomy unnecessary in the majority of patients, but it should still be considered when other investigations have proved to be negative. The value of laparotomy in the diagnosis of chronic or occult gastrointestinal haemorrhage was reviewed by Retzloff, Hagedorn and Bartholomew[40] some years before many of the more modern investigative methods were developed. In their study 100 patients underwent surgical exploration but only 30% showed a definite site of haemorrhage and in 17% a possible site was considered; in 53% no lesion was found. Laparotomy is thus of little value in many patients and should be reserved for those patients with severe recurrent blood loss in whom less invasive diagnostic techniques have repeatedly failed to establish a diagnosis and who require frequent blood transfusions. By and large, the diagnostic yield of surgery in patients with chronic or occult gastrointestinal blood loss is small.

INDIVIDUAL ASSESSMENT OF PATIENTS

This section has provided an account of the investigations which may be of value in the diagnosis of chronic or occult gastrointestinal haemorrhage, but all of these investigations may not of course be necessary in every patient. Following a detailed history and clinical examination there may be pointers to a likely cause (such as a history of drug ingestion, physical features of a hereditary disease, etc). Basic blood examinations including haematology and biochemistry will determine the severity of anaemia and possibly provide other clues as to the cause. Faecal studies of occult blood will confirm the presence of faecal blood loss, and the amount of blood loss can be estimated by means of ^{51}Cr studies.

The investigative programme should then continue with routine radiology (barium swallow and meal, barium enema, small bowel enema) and endoscopy (sigmoidoscopy, upper gastrointestinal endoscopy, colonoscopy).

Modern radionuclide scanning techniques and angiography will be the next line of investigation. A scan may be of value as a screening procedure before angiography. If a red cell scan is negative, angiography is unlikely to be helpful. If the scan is positive, angiographic localization should direct the catheter to the specific vessel, thus allowing a greater chance of angiographic success.

If the site of haemorrhage has still not been determined by these methods, the fluorescein string test and small bowel intubation should be considered, followed, if necessary, by diagnostic laparotomy.

TREATMENT

The principal aspects of management of patients with chronic gastrointestinal haemorrhage relate to the accurate identification and treatment of specific bleeding lesions. In the majority of patients the site of gastrointestinal bleeding should be identified by the judicious use of the investigations outlined. Treatment thereafter consists of specific therapy for the condition which has led to bleeding by appropriate medical or surgical techniques. Diseases such as peptic ulceration, hiatal hernia, colonic diverticular disease, and benign and malignant tumours, are managed by standard methods. In addition iron therapy, possibly preceded by blood transfusion, may be necessary to correct

anaemia. Areas of arteriovenous fistulas or angiodysplasia should be treated by surgical resections but diffuse lesions such as telangiectasia are not amenable to resection and these patients may require long-term therapy with iron supplements and transfusions.

In patients for whom a diagnosis of the source of chronic gastrointestinal haemorrhage has not been made, a conservative course is justified if bleeding has stopped since the majority of such patients either have no further problem or will have a benign disorder which is likely to be diagnosed and treated if further haemorrhage occurs. If bleeding continues, attempts to identify the site must be continued, while maintaining the patient's therapy for blood loss with iron supplements or blood transfusion if necessary.

REFERENCES

1 Alavi, A. & MacLean, G. (1980) Radio-isotopic detection of gastrointestinal bleeding: an integrated approach with other modalities. In *Nuclear Medicine Annual* (Ed.) Freeman, L. W. & Weisman, H. S. pp. 177–218. New York: Raven Press.

2 Alavi, A. & Ring, E. J. (1981) Localisation of gastrointestinal bleeding: superiority of ^{99m}Tc sulphur colloid compared wtih angiography. *American Journal of Radiology*, **137**, 741–748.

3 Balint, J. A., Sarfeh, I. J. & Fried, M. B. (1977) *Gastrointestinal Bleeding – Diagnosis and Management*. New York, London: John Wiley.

4 Barrison, J. A., Primavesi, J., Gilmore, I. T. *et al.* (1981) Screening for occult gastrointestinal bleeding in hospital patients. *Journal of the Royal Society of Medicine*, **74**, 41–43.

5 Baum, S. (1982) Angiography and the gastrointestinal bleeder. *Radiology*, **143**, 569–572.

6 Baum, S., Athanasoulis, C. A., Galdabrini, J. *et al.* (1977) Angiodysplasia of the right colon: a cause of gastrointestinal bleeding. *American Journal of Roentgenology*, **129**, 789–794.

7 Birke, G. & Engstedt, L. (1956) Melaena and haematemesis – a follow-up investigation with special reference to bleeding of unknown origin. *Gastroenterologia (Basel)*, **85**, 97–115.

8 Boijsen, E. & Tylén, U. (1978) Gastrointestinal angiography. *Clinics in Gastroenterology*, 7(2), 431–452.

9 Bunker, S. R., Brown, J. M., McAuley, R. J. *et al.* (1982) Detection of gastrointestinal bleeding sites – use of 'in vitro' technetium Tc^{99m}-labelled RBC. *Journal of the American Medical Association*, **247**, 789–792.

10 Cabal, E. & Holtz, S. (1977) Polyarteritis as a cause of intestinal haemorrhage. *Gastroenterology*, **61**, 99–105.

11 Cameron, A. D. (1960) Gastrointestinal blood loss measured by radioactive chromium. *Gut*, **1**, 177–182.

12 Cody, M. C., O'Donovan, T. P. B. & Hughes, Jr, R. W. (1974) Idiopathic gastrointestinal bleeding and aortic stenosis. *American Journal of Digestive Diseases*, **19**, 393–398.

13 Conn, H. O. & Blitzer, B. L. (1976) Non-association of adrenocorticosteroid therapy and peptic ulcer. *New England Journal of Medicine*, **294**, 473–479.

14 Cooley, R. N. (1961) The diagnostic accuracy of upper gastrointestinal radiological studies. *American Journal of Medicine,* **242,** 628–650.

15 Cream, J.J., Gumpel, J. M. & Peachey, R. D. G. (1970) Schonlein–Henoch purpura in the adult: a study of 77 patients with anaphylactoid or Schonlein–Henoch purpura. *Quarterly Journal of Medicine,* **39,** 461–484.

16 Douvres, P. A. & Glass, G. B. J. (1970) Cryptogenic gastrointestinal bleeding. In *Progress in Gastroenterology 2* (Ed.) Glass, G. B. J. New York and London: Grune and Stratton.

17 Ferrant, A., Dehasque, N., Leners, N. & Meunier, H. (1980) Scintigraphy with In-111 labelled red cells in intermittent gastrointestinal bleeding. *Journal of Nuclear Medicine,* **21,** 844–845.

18 Gordon, I. (1980) Gastrointestinal haemorrhage unrelated to gastric mucosa diagnosed on ^{99}Tc^{m} pertechnetate scans. *British Journal of Radiology,* **53,** 322–324.

19 Hall, R. I., Lavelle, M. I. & Venables, C. W. (1982) Chronic pancreatitis as a cause of gastrointestinal bleeding. *Gut,* **23,** 250–255.

20 Hattner, R. & Engelstad, B. L. (1982) An advance in identification and localisation of gastrointestinal haemorrhage. *Gastroenterology,* **83,** 484–492.

21 Haynes, W. F., Pittman, F. E. & Christakis, G. (1960) Location of site of upper gastrointestinal tract haemorrhage by the fluorescein string test. *Surgery,* **48,** 821–827.

22 Irons, G. V., Jr & Kirsner, J. B. (1965) Routine chemical tests of the stool for occult blood; an evaluation. *American Journal of Medical Science,* **249,** 247–260.

23 Jones, F. A. (1969) Problems of alimentary bleeding. *British Medical Journal,* **ii,** 267–273.

24 Kiernan, P. D., Pairolero, P. C., Hubert, J. P., Jr *et al.* (1980) Aortic graft-enteric fistula. *Mayo Clinic Proceedings,* **55,** 731–738.

25 Kurata, J. H., Elashoff, J. D. & Grossman, M. I. (1982) Inadequacy of the literature on the relationship between drugs, ulcers and gastrointestinal bleeding. *Gastroenterology,* **82,** 373–382.

26 Lancet – Editorial (1981) Angiodysplasia. *Lancet,* **ii,** 1086–1087.

27 Leonards, J. R., Levy, G. & Niemczura, R. (1973) Gastrointestinal blood loss during prolonged aspirin administration. *New England Journal of Medicine,* **289,** 1020–1022.

28 Markisz, J. A., Front, D., Royal, H. D. *et al.* (1982) An evaluation of ^{99m}Tc-labelled red blood cell scintigraphy for the detection and localization of gastrointestinal bleeding sites. *Gastroenterology,* **83,** 394–398.

29 McKusick, V. A. (1972a) Pseudoxanthoma elasticum. In *Heritable Disorders of Connective Tissue* 4th Edition. pp. 475–520. St Louis: C. V. Mosby.

30 McKusick, V. A. (1972b) The Ehlers–Danlos syndrome. In *Heritable Disorders of Connective Tissue* 4th Edition. pp. 292–371. St Louis: C. V. Mosby.

31 Miskowiak, K., Nielsen, S. L., Munck, O. *et al.* (1979) Acute gastrointestinal bleeding detected with abdominal scintigraphy using technetium-99m labelled albumin. *Scandinavian Journal of Gastroenterology,* **14,** 389–394.

32 Mollison, P. L. & Veall, N. (1955) The use of the isotope ^{51}Cr as a label for red cells. *British Journal of Haematology,* **1,** 62–74.

33 Moore, J. D., Thompson, N. W. & Appleman, H. D. (1976) Arteriovenous malformations of the gastrointestinal tract. *Archives of Surgery,* **111,** 381–388.

34 Netterville, R. E., Hardy, J. D. & Martin, R. S. (1968) Small bowel haemorrhage. *Annals of Surgery,* **167,** 949–957.

35 Nusbaum, N. & Baum, S. (1963) Radiographic demonstration of unknown sites of gastrointestinal bleeding. *Surgical Forum,* **14,** 374–375.

36 Palmer, E. D. (1969) The vigorous diagnostic approach to upper gastrointestinal haemorrhage: a 23-year prospective study of 1400 patients. *Journal of the American Medical Association,* **207,** 1477–1480.

37 Pillow, R. P., Hill, L. D., Ragen, P. A. *et al.* (1962) Newer methods for localisation of obscure small bowel bleeding. *Journal of the American Medical Association,* **179,** 23–26.

38 Pittman, F. E. (1964) The fluorescein string test. An analysis of its use and relationship to barium studies of the upper gastrointestinal tract in 122 cases of gastrointestinal tract haemorrhage. *Annals of Internal Medicine,* **60,** 418–429.

39 Pittman, F. E. (1965) A rapid-entry tube for use in fluorescein string test. *Lancet,* **i,** 1308–1309.

40 Retzloff, J. A., Hagedorn, A. B. & Bartholomew, L. G. (1961) Abdominal exploration for gastrointestinal bleeding of obscure origin. *Journal of the American Medical Association,* **177,** 104–107.

41 Reuter, S. R. & Redman, H. C. (1977) Gastrointestinal bleeding. In *Gastrointestinal Angiography.* 2nd Edition. pp. 218–268. London, New York: W. B. Saunders.

42 Sheedy, P. F., Fulton, R. E. & Atwell, D. T. (1975) Angiographic evaluation of patients with chronic gastrointestinal bleeding. *American Journal of Roentgenology,* **123,** 338–347.

43 Simon, L. S. & Mills, J. A. (1980) Nonsteroidal anti-inflammatory drugs. *New England Journal of Medicine,* **302,** 1179–1185, 1237–1243.

44 Skibba, R. M., Hartong, W. A., Mantz, F. A. *et al.* (1976) Angiodysplasia of the caecum; colonoscopic diagnosis. *Gastrointestinal Endoscopy,* **22,** 177–179.

45 Smith, R. K. & Arterburn, J. (1980) Detection and localisation of gastrointestinal bleeding using Tc-99m-pyrophosphate in vivo labelled red blood cells. *Clinical Nuclear Medicine,* **5,** 55–60.

46 Spechler, S. J. & Schimmel, E. M. (1982) Gastrointestinal tract bleeding of unknown origin. *Archives of Internal Medicine,* **142,** 236–240.

47 Tarin, D., Allison, D. J., Modlin, I. M. & Neale, G. (1978) Diagnosis and management of obscure gastrointestinal bleeding. *British Medical Journal,* **ii,** 751–754.

48 Teague, R. H., Salmon, P. R. & Read, A. E. (1973) Fibreoptic examination of the colon: a review of 255 cases. *Gut,* **14,** 139–142.

49 Tedesco, J., Waye, J. D., Raskin, J. B. *et al.* (1978) Colonoscopic evaluation of rectal bleeding: a study of 304 patients. *Annals of Internal Medicine,* **89,** 907–909.

50 Theoni, R. F. & Cello, J. P. (1980) A critical look at the accuracy of endoscopy and double contrast radiography of the upper gastrointestinal tract in patients with substantial upper gastrointestinal haemorrhage. *Radiology,* **135,** 305–308.

Chapter 7
Skin Disease and the Gut

J. M. Marks

Skin clues to gastrointestinal disease are, for the most part, easy to obtain with no more complicated apparatus than a good light. Additional help in diagnosis may come from histological and immunofluorescence studies on the skin, but interpretation of the findings requires dermatological expertise.

There are a number of reasons for examining the skin in any gastroenterological consultation. Occasionally, skin signs are present before any others and exceptionally, for example in malignant disease, this may result in vital early intervention. In emergencies such as gastrointestinal bleeding and pain, particularly in the case of rarer diseases, skin phenomena may enable a diagnosis to be made before operation. Nearly always they are of great interest.

The finding of dermatological abnormalities in gastrointestinal disease does not necessarily mean that the gastrointestinal disorder is primary[27] and establishing the relationship between the disease of the two systems is important in planning treatment.

MOUTH ULCERS AND DYSPHAGIA IN SKIN DISEASE (Table 7.1)

Aphthous ulcers
Patients with aphthous ulcers are often sent to dermatologists, but the lesions may be the presenting feature of coeliac disease (CD),[1] ulcerative colitis (UC)[6] and Crohn's disease.[4]

Table 7.1 Mouth ulcers and dysphagia and the skin.

Aphthous ulcers in coeliac disease, ulcerative colitis and Crohn's disease
Rash extending on to mucosae, e.g. blisters, lichen planus
Oro-occulo-genito-cutaneous syndromes, i.e. Stevens–Johnson and Behçet's
Collagen–vascular disease of oesophageal wall or muscles of swallowing, especially systemic sclerosis and dermatomyositis
Tylosis, dermatitis herpetiformis, koilonychia, arsenical keratoses in carcinoma of oesophagus

In addition, severe aphthous ulcers occur in Behçet's disease. In this oro-occulo-genito-cutaneous syndrome of unknown aetiology the small intestine is occasionally involved. Skin lesions include trivial pustules at venepuncture sites and superficial thrombophlebitis.

Candida albicans infection
This is a rare cause of mouth ulceration and dysphagia. The gut acts as a reservoir for the organism even in some healthy individuals. Skin lesions may help in making the diagnosis, and the demonstration of the yeast in skin usually indicates that it is pathogenic. The flexures are often involved and nails are deformed as a result of chronic paronychia. In those with immunosuppression and endocrinopathies granulomas and deep invasion of tissues occur.

Stevens–Johnson syndrome

Crusting and blistering of the lips (Plate 7.1) and ulceration of the mouth and pharynx interfere with eating and swallowing in this acute febrile disease, which is usually caused by an infection or a drug. The characteristic skin lesions are concentric circles of redness, oedema, blistering and purpura – the 'iris' or 'target' lesions of erythema multiforme.

Lichen planus

This most commonly presents as a rash with bluish, flat-topped, shiny papules. In the majority of cases symptomless lesions appear, forming a white, lacy network on the lips, tongue, cheeks and gums. Rarely, there are symptoms due to ulceration and scarring, and the pharynx and the oesophagus can be involved. Most cases are idiopathic but drugs are occasionally responsible and a similar rash occurs as a late manifestation of the graft-versus-host reaction.

Acquired blistering diseases

Blisters in the mouth often burst and present as superficial ulcers. Diagnosis is easy if the skin is involved, for characteristic clinical, histological and immunological features are present in pemphigus, pemphigoid and dermatitis herpetiformis (DH). Rarely, the oesophagus is involved. It is possible for mucosal lesions to predate skin lesions by weeks or months.

Epidermolysis bullosa

This is a group of genetically determined blistering diseases, and the worst oesophageal involvement occurs in the recessive dystrophic form. Blisters in the oesophagus interfere with feeding, and the scarring which follows leads to strictures. The skin signs are blistering, destruction of nails, and acquired syndactyly. Very large doses of corticosteroids followed by reconstructive surgery have enabled some of these children to survive.[22] The condition can now be diagnosed in utero.

Collagen–vascular diseases

These cause dysphagia due to fibrotic changes in the oesophageal wall or myopathy of the muscles of swallowing. The first mechanism is commonest in systemic sclerosis and the second in dermatomyositis.

Systemic sclerosis (SS)

Radiological or manometric abnormalities in the oesophagus can be detected in up to 70% of patients, not all of whom have symptoms.[29] The basis of the oesophageal abnormalities, which result in decreased peristalsis, dilatation and stricture formation, is thought to be fibrosis. Skin changes include tight skin, beaked nose, thin lips and sclerodactyly. Additional skin signs of vasculitis, such as nail-fold haemorrhages and infarcts, also occur, but these are found in other collagen–vascular diseases besides SS. Occasionally, gastrointestinal changes occur without skin changes, and occasionally other collagen–vascular diseases produce identical gastrointestinal abnormalities. Antinuclear antibodies are detectable in the serum in almost all patients with SS as well as in those with systemic lupus erythematosus.

Dermatomyositis

Characteristically in this collagen–vascular disease, and occasionally in the others, the muscles of swallowing may be affected along with the proximal skeletal muscles. The typical rash which occurs is oedematous and is heliotrope in colour; it often presents round the eyes and on the back of the hands. Antinuclear factor is negative. A number of adults who develop dermatomyositis have an underlying neoplasm (see below).

Carcinoma of the oesophagus

Tylosis

This genetically determined, warty thickening of palms and soles is on rare occasions associated with carcinoma of the oesophagus. In two families described the tylosis started between the ages of 5 and 15 years, while the cancer occurred from 30 years upwards; it was confined to those who had tylosis, and long-term follow-up of one family showed it to occur in 95% of such patients.[12]

Dermatitis herpetiformis (DH)

The strong association of this disease with coeliac disease (see below) suggests that it too may carry with it increased risk of carcinoma of the oesophagus.[13] The author's one patient with DH who died of carcinoma of the oesophagus was diagnosed as having DH and coeliac disease 17 years previously and these had been controlled well by a gluten-free diet.

GASTROINTESTINAL BLEEDING (Table 7.2)

Vascular abnormalities

Hereditary haemorrhagic telangiectasia

The raised vascular dilatations that characterize the disease occur on skin and on oral, gastro-

Table 7.2 The skin and gastrointestinal bleeding.

Blood vessel abnormalities, e.g. hereditary haemorrhagic telangiectasia, blue rubber bleb naevi, Kaposi's sarcoma

Inherited connective tissue defects, i.e. Ehlers–Danlos syndrome and pseudoxanthoma elasticum

Vasculitis

Polyposis syndromes

Skin signs of malignant gastrointestinal disease

Skin signs of ulcerative colitis and Crohn's disease

intestinal, and other mucosae. Although the condition is inherited as an autosomal dominant trait, lesions may not be apparent until young adult life.

Blue rubber bleb naevus syndrome
This is inherited as an autosomal dominant trait. The skin haemangiomas look and feel exactly as their name suggests, and in the bowel project as submucous tumours into the lumen, particularly of the small intestine.

Kaposi's sarcoma
This is an acquired vascular tumour, in which reddish-blue papules and nodules occur, usually on the legs, but rarely the condition involves the bowel and results in bleeding. This aggressive variant of the disease was only seen in young African men until recently, when it was reported in immunosuppressed individuals and homosexuals with the acquired immune deficiency syndrome.

Inherited defects of connective tissue

The pattern of inheritance of these varies from one type to another, and collagen or elastic fibres are involved.

Ehlers–Danlos syndrome
There are at least eight types of this disease, probably representing different enzyme defects. Many organs may be involved. In type IV there is a deficiency of the type of collagen which is normally present in skin and gastrointestinal tract.[24] The physical signs are hyperextensible fragile skin and hypertrophic scars, as well as rupture of blood vessels and perforation of gut.

Pseudoxanthoma elasticum
This is a similar group of diseases which affects elastic fibres.[23] The skin lesions consist of yellow papules, thought to resemble plucked chicken skin, on the neck and in the flexures, and

'angioid streaks' are seen on ophthalmoscopy. Gastrointestinal bleeds and signs of blockage of the major arteries occur.

ABDOMINAL PAIN

Herpes zoster
Pain may predate blisters, which are usually of 'root' distribution (T7–L1). Involvement of the sacral roots can produce, in addition, difficulty with defecation.[15]

Porphyria
Skin lesions and abdominal signs occur together only in the rarer variegate porphyria and hereditary coproporphyria; these forms cannot be excluded by 'screening' tests and formal estimations of urinary delta-aminolaevulinic acid and porphobilinogen and faecal coproporphyrin and protoporphyrin are necessary. The main skin signs are blisters and friable skin, on light-exposed areas (Plate 7.2). The abdominal signs are pain, vomiting and constipation. A number of drugs, including alcohol, barbiturates, anticonvulsants and oestrogens, precipitate attacks and must therefore be avoided. Rarely, primary hepatocellular cancers produce porphyrins and the patients can present with clinical porphyria.

Fabry's disease
In this rare deficiency of the enzyme α-galactosidase A, which is inherited as a sex-linked recessive trait, unexplained pains are frequent. The skin lesions do not appear till adolescence; classically they are small vascular tumours with a warty centre and occur particularly on the penis and scrotum. Vomiting and diarrhoea may be explained on the basis of deposition of lipid in the myenteric plexus.

VASCULAR DISEASE OF INTESTINAL VESSELS

Anaphylactoid purpura
This leucocytoclastic vasculitis is manifested by palpable purpura, especially on the legs and buttocks, joint swellings, haematuria and abdominal bleeds and colic (Plate 7.3).

Collagen–vascular diseases
Acute involvement of different-sized vessels in the small and large intestine can occur. More gradual obliteration of small intestinal vessels results in malabsorption (Plate 7.4).[3]

Malignant atrophic papulosis (Degos' disease)
The histological findings of endarteritis and thrombosis are said to be diagnostic of the condition. The scars in the skin resemble porcelain, and the patient usually dies from vascular disease or perforation of the bowel.[11]

POLYPOSIS

True polyps are adenomatous tumours which are commonest in the colon and rectum and have malignant propensity. Hamartomatous and inflammatory polyps occur in all parts of the gut.[2]

Gardner's syndrome[9]
Adenomatous polyps with a high risk of malignancy occur in association with multiple sebaceous cysts, fibromas, lipomas and osteomas. The syndrome is inherited as an autosomal dominant trait.

Peutz–Jeghers syndrome[14]
Hamartomatous polyps occur mainly in the small intestine. The risk of malignancy is small. Dark freckles are seen round the mouth, on the lips, fingers and toes; patchy pigmentation occurs inside the mouth, and this may be the only remaining skin abnormality when the patient gets older. The syndrome is inherited as an autosomal dominant trait, but some members of the families seem to have either the skin or the intestinal changes alone.

Cronkhite–Canada syndrome
In this rare acquired disease inflammatory polyps are present in the stomach as well as the bowel. Diarrhoea is prominent; the cause is not always clear, but may be related to fat, protein and carbohydrate malabsorption. The cutaneous features are hyperpigmentation, hair loss and nail atrophy.[5]

ULCERATIVE COLITIS AND CROHN'S DISEASE

A number of skin complications occur which are common to both conditions. However, pyoderma gangrenosum is rare in Crohn's disease and granulomas are rare in ulcerative colitis.

Pyoderma gangrenosum (PG)
Small papules, pustules or haemorrhagic blisters enlarge rapidly and break down to form ulcers (Plate 7.5). Half the patients with PG have ulcerative colitis; other causes include rheumatoid arthritis and myeloma. In contrast, less than 10% of patients with ulcerative colitis have PG. It has been suggested that the underlying mechanism in PG is a Schwartzmann reaction. As a rule, the ulcers heal as the bowel responds to treatment, but this is not invariably so. In the absence of a clear cause for PG the bowel should be investigated because a number of patients sent to dermatology clinics with this condition have no bowel symptoms and yet are found to have ulcerative colitis on endoscopic or radiological examination.

Erythema nodosum
Ulcerative colitis and Crohn's disease should be considered if more common causes are absent (Plate 7.6).

Aphthous ulcers
These are considered at the beginning of this chapter.

Granulomas
Granulomatous lesions which may have a cobblestone appearance in the mouth or present as diffuse thickening of the lips are features of Crohn's disease. Granulomas also occur round the anus, at ileostomy and colostomy sites, in abdominal scars and at skin sites remote from the bowel.[20]

Sinuses and fistulas
These are common in Crohn's disease; they are often in the perineum or abdominal wall and may be lined with granulomatous tissue.

Malnutrition
Various specific and non-specific deficiencies can arise as a result of extensive bowel disease or of the elemental diets used in treatment.

SKIN DISEASE AND MALABSORPTION

Many skin changes occur in association with malabsorption; some are the result of it, some are due to a disease process which affects the bowel as well as the skin, and some occur because of a genetic 'susceptibility' to the two different diseases; in addition, skin disease can actually cause malabsorption.

Dermatitis herpetiformis (DH)
This is a distinctive rash and usually easy to recognize (Plate 7.7, Table 7.3). It has an association with coeliac disease but with no other

Table 7.3 Diagnosis of dermatitis herpetiformis.

Children and adults affected

Itchy papules and blisters, especially on extensor surfaces

Histology – subepidermal blisters; papillary tip microabcesses

Immunofluorescence of clinically uninvolved skin shows IgA, usually in a granular pattern in upper dermis

Rapid response of rash to dapsone

HLA type usually includes B8

forms of malabsorption. Because of the implication of the diagnosis it is important that it should not be made in the absence of its special features. About 1% of patients with coeliac disease have dermatitis herpetiformis. The percentage of patients with DH who are considered to have coeliac disease depends upon the definition of coeliac disease used: clinical coeliac disease occurs in a few, but histological changes in small intestinal mucosa occur in about 80%.[7, 18, 19] Immunofluorescence of skin is probably the most useful single diagnostic test but it needs special expertise and experience in interpretation. The enteropathy is due to gluten, and the rash almost certainly is too, though the mechanism by which the latter is produced is particularly poorly understood: it is not due to malabsorption for it can occur without any evidence of bowel involvement, and the responses of skin and gut to a gluten-free diet may occur independently of one another.[8]

The skin lesions respond rapidly to dapsone. In most patients they also respond to a gluten-free diet but the improvement is very slow, often taking years, and many patients prefer to take dapsone.

Dapsone has no effect on the mucosal abnormality: a gluten-free diet is necessary and should be instituted if there are clinical or biochemical signs of coeliac disease. Where there are histological abnormalities alone management is much more difficult; when malignant disease occurs in DH it is usually in conjunction with coeliac disease, and with the present uncertainty about whether a gluten-free diet can protect against malignancy it is difficult to insist that it should be used in those patients with DH who are quite fit apart from their rash. However, other authorities hold that an abnormal mucosa might eventually cause nutritional upsets and a gluten-free diet should therefore be recommended in an attempt to restore normal mucosal morphology.

Aphthous ulcers
Although these can be the presenting features of coeliac disease, our own efforts to find coeliac disease by jejunal biopsy in a group of patients sent to a skin clinic with severe aphthous ulceration have failed in all cases.

Eczematous rashes due to malabsorption
These occur with coeliac disease and tropical sprue,[30] and are the consequence of the malabsorption; they disappear when this is corrected. No specific deficiency has been identified but similar rashes have been described in essential fatty acid deficiency, and linoleic acid has been shown to be therapeutically effective in patients with rashes after intestinal resection.[25] Clinically, the skin is dry (acquired ichthyosis), eczematized and hyperpigmented (Plate 7.8).

Zinc deficiency and acrodermatitis enteropathica
Zinc deficiency can occur from malabsorption in coeliac disease and inflammatory bowel disease. It was relatively common in the early days of elemental feeds, which were deficient in zinc.

A genetic abnormality of zinc absorption, acrodermatitis enteropathica is rare, but is extremely important because it is eminently treatable. It presents, usually at the time of weaning, with a rash on hands and feet and round the mouth and anus. Alopecia and failure to thrive are other features, and all are reversed by administering zinc by mouth. The precise defect is unknown but it is possible that in affected infants dietary zinc is chelated in the bowel by an abnormal small-molecular-weight substance.[21]

Jejuno-ileal bypass
Dryness of the skin and hair loss occur, and a number of unexplained inflammatory skin lesions have also been reported.[16]

Systemic sclerosis
In addition to malabsorption from ischaemia, changes in the gastrointestinal tract wall similar to those in the skin and oesophagus cause malabsorption due to bacterial overgrowth in a bowel with poor peristalsis.

Dermatogenic enteropathy[28]
A number of patients with extensive eczema and psoriasis develop malabsorption. The steatorrhoea responds rapidly to topical treatment of the rash; it is not related to gluten sensitivity, and structural changes, if they occur at all, are minimal. Its mechanism is unknown. Symptoms are rare, but confusion can occur if the pheno-

menon is not recognized for what it is in patients with a rash and malabsorption. A gluten-free diet is neither necessary nor effective and should not be given.

MALIGNANT DISEASE OF THE GASTROINTESTINAL TRACT

Some skin signs of these processes are specific to a particular tumour, some indicate malignant disease in general, and others are common to many wasting diseases (Table 7.4).

Table 7.4 The skin in malignant gastrointestinal disease.

Signs of wasting
Acquired ichthyosis, fine skin, excessive sweating, poor hair and nails, hyperpigmentation

Signs of malignant disease
Secondary deposits in skin (or primary skin tumour with metastasis in gut), dermatomyositis, acanthosis nigricans

Signs of specific tumours
Tylosis, dermatitis herpetiformis, koilonychia (oesophagus)
Carcinoid flush (tumour non-intestinal or spread to liver)
Urticaria pigmentosa (mastocytosis)
Necrolytic migratory erythema (glucagonoma)
Gardner's syndrome (colon)
Skin signs of ulcerative colitis (colon)
Dermatitis herpetiformis (intestinal lymphoma)

Metastases
The skin, especially the scalp, is a common site for secondary tumours, which present as nodules or vascular tumours (Plate 7.9).

Dermatomyositis
The association of dermatomyositis with malignancy is confined to adults, where 7–52% of patients with dermatomyositis are reported to show such an association, particularly with common cancers, including gastric and colonic cancers. Dermatomyositis may be a relatively early sign of malignant disease and can regress after removal of the tumour.

Acanthosis nigricans
The clinical lesions are dark velvety plaques in the axillae and groins (Plate 7.10). The mouth may be involved, as may the palms, which, from their appearance and feel are known as 'tripe hands'. Acanthosis nigricans also occurs as a congenital condition in children and in obesity and in endocrinopathies, but in the absence of any of these it should be assumed that the cause is malignant. Eighty to ninety per cent of the

patients have well established malignant disease when the rash appears. Adenocarcinoma, often of the stomach, is the usual tumour.

Carcinoid flush
The flush is not seen in carcinoid tumours confined to the gastrointestinal tract, because the vasoactive substances responsible are metabolized by the liver and do not reach the systemic circulation; when carcinoid tumours arise from other tissues, for example the bronchus, and when liver metastases are present, there may be dermatological features. The pharmacology of the carcinoid flush is still not fully understood:[10] serotonin is the main culprit and diagnosis can be made by finding an excess of 5-hydroxy-indole-acetic acid in the urine although initially the excretion may be intermittent.

Mastocytosis
Certain varieties of cutaneous mastocytosis, particularly urticaria pigmentosa, can involve internal organs. Very occasionally mastocytosis occurs without involvement of the skin. Release of histamine from skin mast cells, for instance after bathing, can have pharmacological effects on the gastrointestinal tract, causing colic and diarrhoea. Infiltration of the gut can produce malabsorption and occasionally coeliac disease coexists.[26]

Glucagonoma
A characteristic rash has been described as occurring with glucagonoma of the pancreas.[17] It is commonest round orifices and in the flexures, where it is seen as a blistering, erythematous plaque which spreads and heals with hyperpigmentation (Plate 7.11).

Intestinal lymphoma
The relationship of this to dermatitis herpetiformis seems to be through coeliac disease for nearly all the patients who have been described have had coeliac disease as well as dermatitis herpetiformis.

REFERENCES

1 Asquith, P. & Basu, M. (1978) Aphthous ulceration – the incidence of coeliac disease and gluten sensitivity. In *Perspectives in Coeliac Disease* (Ed.) McNicholl, B., McCarthy, C. F. & Fothrell, P. F., pp. 315–321. Lancaster: MTP.
2 Bussey, H. & Morson, B. (1978) Familial polyposis coli. In *Gastrointestinal Tract Cancer* (Ed.) Lipkin, M. & Good, R. pp. 275–294. New York: Plenum Medical.
3 Carron, D. B. & Douglas, A. P. (1965) Steatorrhoea in vascular insufficiency of the small intestine. *Quarterly Journal of Medicine,* **34,** 331–340.

4   Croft, C. B. & Wilkinson, A. R. (1972) Ulceration of the mouth, pharynx and larynx in Crohn's disease of the intestine. *British Journal of Surgery*, **59**, 294.

5   Cunliffe, W. & Anderson, J. (1967) Case of Cronkhite–Canada syndrome with associated jejunal diverticulosis. *British Medical Journal*, **iv**, 601–602.

6   Edwards, F. C. & Truelove, S. C. (1964) The course and prognosis of ulcerative colitis. *Gut*, **5**, 1–15.

7   Fry, L., Kier, P., McMinn, R. M. H. *et al.* (1967) Small intestinal structure and function and haematological changes in dermatitis herpetiformis. *Lancet*, **i**, 557–561.

8   Fry, L., Leonard, J., Swain, F. *et al.* (1982) Long-term follow up of dermatitis herpetiformis with and without gluten withdrawal. *British Journal of Dermatology*, **107**, 631–640.

9   Gardner, E. J. (1951) A genetic and clinical study of intestinal polyposis: predisposing factor for carcinoma of colon and rectum. *American Journal of Human Genetics*, **3**, 167–176.

10 Graham-Smith, D. D. (1970) The carcinoid syndrome. *Gut*, **11**, 189–191.

11 Hall-Smith, P. (1969) Malignant atrophic papulosis (Degos' disease). *British Journal of Dermatology*, **81**, 817–822.

12 Harper, P. S., Harper, R. M. & Howell-Evans, A. W. (1970) Carcinoma of the oesophagus with tylosis. *Quarterly Journal of Medicine*, **39**, 317–333.

13 Harris, O., Cooke, W. T., Thompson, H. & Waterhouse, J. (1967) Malignancy in adult coeliac disease and ideopathic steatorrhoea. *American Journal of Medicine*, **42**, 899–912.

14 Jeghers, H., McKusick, V. & Katz, K. (1949) Generalised intestinal polyposis and melanin spots of the oral mucosa, lips and digits. *New England Journal of Medicine*, **241**, 1031–1036.

15 Jellinek, E. H. & Tulloch, W. S. (1976) Herpes zoster with dysfunction of bladder and anus. *Lancet*, **ii**, 1219–1222.

16 Kennedy, C. (1981) The spectrum of inflammatory skin disease following jejuno-ileal bypass for morbid obesity. *British Journal of Dermatology*, **105**, 425–436.

17 Mallinson, C. N., Bloom, S. R., Warin, A. P. *et al.* (1974) A glucagonoma syndrome. *Lancet*, **ii**, 1–5.

18 Marks, J. (1977) Dogma and dermatitis herpetiformis. *Journal of Clinical and Experimental Dermatology*, **2**, 189–207.

19 Marks, J., Shuster, S. & Watson, A. (1966) Small-bowel changes in dermatitis herpetiformis. *Lancet*, **ii**, 1280–1282.

20 McCallum, D. I. & Kinmont, P. D. C. (1968) Dermatological manifestations of Crohn's disease. *British Journal of Dermatology*, **80**, 1–8.

21 Moynahan, E. (1974) Acrodermatitis enteropathica: a lethal inherited human zinc-deficiency disorder. *Lancet*, **ii**, 399–400.

22 Moynahan, E. (1982) The treatment and management of epidermolysis bullosa. *Clinical and Experimental Dermatology*, **7**, 665–672.

23 Pope, F. M. (1974) Autosomal dominant pseudoxanthoma elasticum. *Journal of Medical Genetics*, **11**, 152–157.

24 Pope, F. M., Martin, G., Lichtenstein, J. *et al.* (1975) Patients with Ehlers–Danlos syndrome type IV lack type III collagen. *Proceedings of the National Academy of Sciences*, **72**, 1314, 1316.

25 Prottey, C., Hartop, P. & Press, M. (1975) Correction of the cutaneous manifestations of essential fatty acid deficiency in man by application of sunflower seed oil to the skin. *Journal of Investigative Dermatology*, **64**, 228–234.

26 Scott, B. B., Hardy, D. I. & Losowsky, M. S. (1975) Involvement of the small intestine in systemic mast cell disease. *Gut*, **16**, 918–924.

27 Shuster, S. (1967) The gut and the skin. In *Third Symposium on Advanced Medicine, Royal College of Physicians, London* (Ed.) Dawson, A. M. pp. 349–361. London: Pitman.

28 Shuster, S. & Marks, J. (1965) Dermatogenic enteropathy – a new cause for steatorrhoea. *Lancet*, **i**, 1367–1368.

29 Weihrauch, T. R. & Korting, G. W. (1982) Manometric assessment of oesophageal involvement in progressive systemic sclerosis, morphoea and Raynaud's disease. *British Journal of Dermatology*, **107**, 325–332.

30 Wells, G. (1962) Skin disease and malabsorption. *British Medical Journal*, **ii**, 937–943.

Chapter 8
The Small Intestine

ANATOMY

From duodenojejunal flexure to ileocaecal valve, the small intestine measures approximately 6 m in length. This refers to measurements at autopsy, after resection of the mesentery, and in life the muscular tone of the intestine results in a considerably shorter length. The upper two-fifths of the small intestine are jejunum, the lower three-fifths ileum. Although in general the jejunum is thicker and wider than the ileum, and the transverse folds of the mucosa are considerably more prominent, there is no definite point of transition from jejunum to ileum. Usually, the jejunum occupies the left upper quadrant of the abdominal cavity and the ileum the right lower area.

The fixed relation of the small intestine is the root of the mesentery, which is attached caudally to the left of vertebra L2, and runs down and to the right to finish to the right of L4/5, in the area of the right sacro-iliac joint. The mesentery itself is fat-laden, particularly that of the ileum, and contains lymph nodes, lacteals and blood vessels. The arcades of arteries from the superior mesenteric artery tend to be single in the jejunum, but to have three or four levels by the time the terminal ileum is reached.

The small intestine is a highly evolved hollow muscular tube, designed for one major purpose – absorption of nutrients from the lumen. Consequently, the epithelial lining of the intestine becomes the focus of greatest attention, but the mucosa also consists of the lamina propria, which is an underlying vascular and reticular stroma, generally containing lymphocytes and their plasma cell derivatives. Beneath this is a strip of smooth muscle, the muscularis mucosae. The mucosa also contains large aggregates of lymphoid tissue called Peyer's patches. The submucosa is a fibrous connective tissue layer which bears blood vessels and lymphatics for the mucosa, while beneath the submucosa is the muscularis propria, with its inner layer of circular muscle and outer longitudinal layer. The adventitia, a layer of loose connective tissue, covers the muscularis propria, and there is also a mesothelial lining of peritoneum, the serosa.

Since the main function of the small intestine is absorption, there are numerous specializations designed to increase the surface area of the mucosa: the mucosa, with the submucosa, is thrown into circular or spiral folds called plicae circulares. These folds are thickest in the jejunum, and may at their greatest be 0.75 cm in height. In the ileum they are fewer as well as less prominent. The mucosa shows numerous finger- or leaf-shaped projections, measuring 0.5 to 1.5 mm in length, called villi, which are covered with epithelium and have a core of lamina propria. Opening between the villi are the orifices of the vestibules, into which open the simple tubular crypts of Lieberkühn (Figure 8.1).

The villous architecture of the small intestine is usually studied using the stereomicroscope, and this procedure is generally regarded as essential in the interpretation of mucosal appearances in small intestinal diseases. There is, however, no general agreement concerning what is normal, and the range of normality does vary considerably with the locality. Morphological terms which are used to describe villous appearances include 'fingers', 'leaves' (narrow and broad), 'tongues', linear and curvilinear 'ridges', and 'convolutions'. While most of these terms are self-explanatory, the word 'convolution' is usually used to denote complex villous forms in which two consecutive angles exceeding 180° can be discerned. Although convolutions may be dismissed among an indigenous population in tropical or subtropical areas, most observers in temperate climates would regard their presence as abnormal, while the other villous shapes would raise no comment. However, some authors have described convolutions in small intestinal biopsies from what were regarded as 'a control population'.[10] Wright et al[17] classified jejunal biopsies into several groups according to their content of convolutions: those with only a few convolutions set among leaves and ridges showed essentially no histological abnormality.

In most species, probably including man,[18] there is a distinct tendency for villi to be largest in the proximal small intestine, and to decrease in size with distance from the pylorus.[15] Varia-

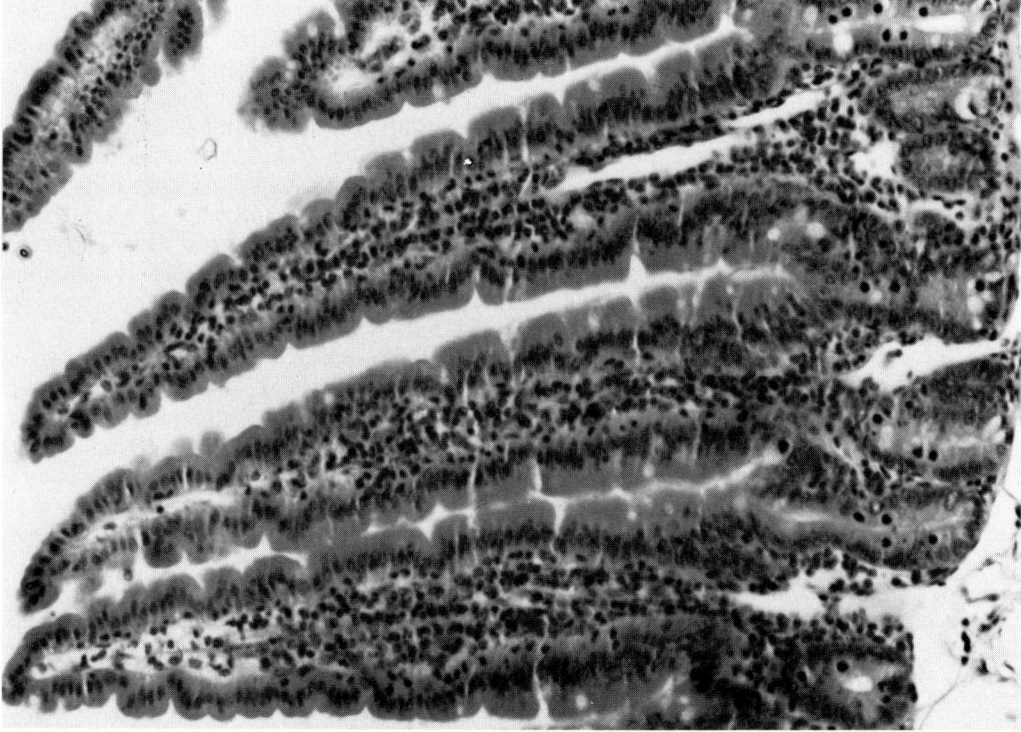

b

(b) A small intestinal crypt in semi-thin section: note the basal Paneth cells, darkly stained goblet cells and crypt mitoses.

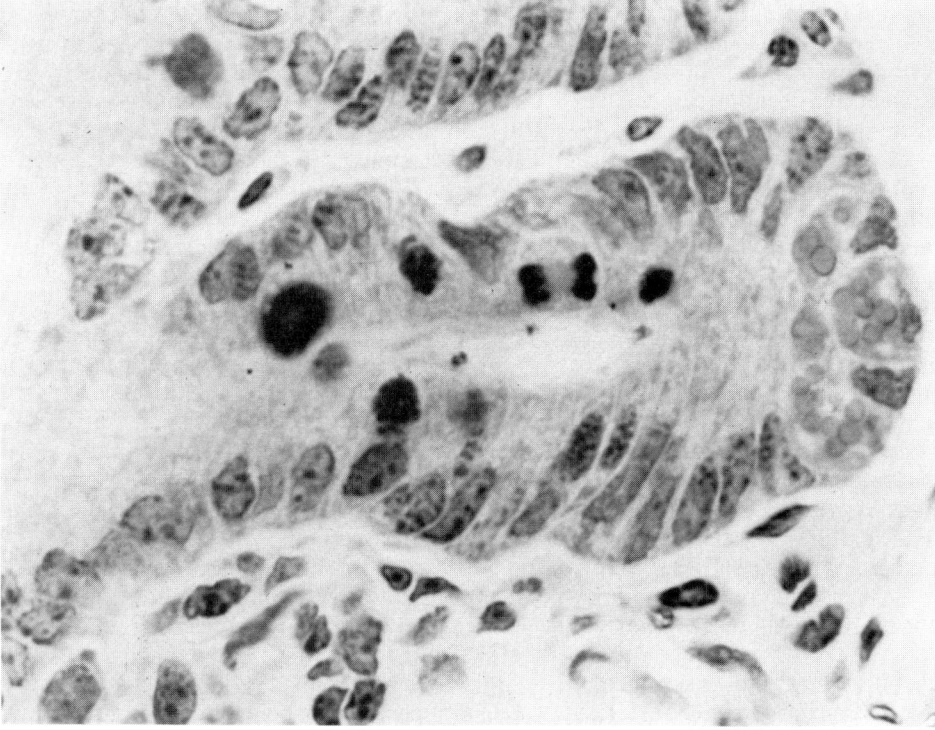

a

Fig. 8.1 (a) A general view of the small intestinal mucosa showing the relationships of crypts to villi (haematoxylin and eosin × 200).

tions in shape with site in the intestine are also described, with duodenal and jejunal villi having a more finger-like or narrow leaf format, while ileal villi are stubbier and foreshortened. There is no such similar variation in the size of the crypts in the small intestine, but there are variations in the number of crypts associated with each villus, with a distinct tendency for the crypt : villus ratio to decrease with distance from the pylorus.[5, 15, 18]

The crypts constitute the proliferative area of the small intestinal epithelium, cells migrating from the crypts upwards to form, and cover, the villous projections. The migration of cells is rapid – approximately 48–72 hours – and during this migration the cells mature, synthesizing brush border enzymes such as sucrase, and losing proliferative enzymes such as thymidine kinase. Many of the pathological appearances of the intestinal mucosa, such as subtotal villous atrophy, are in fact associated with a hyperproliferative mucosa with enhanced crypt cell production rates.

The mere fact that each villus is supplied by in excess of one crypt means that the interrelationships at the level of the crypt : villus junction are complex. The highly detailed study of Cocco *et al*,[6] made using serial sections, shows that in the human jejunal mucosa, several crypts open together into shallow depressions between the villi; these are called vestibules, and, at a slightly higher level, these vestibules coalesce to form the circumvillous basin, which runs around the villous base, and is continuous with the intervillous space above. This arrangement means that any sequence for cell migration is likely to be very complex indeed.[14] Of direct relevance to the evolution of abnormal mucosae are the scanning electron microscope studies of Loehry and Creamer[9]: running between adjacent villi are small elevations called intervillous ridges. In hyperplastic states, these intervillous ridges increase in size, indicating that increased cell traffic directly influences ridge size. In human jejunal biopsies displaying mucosal abnormalities of varying degree, it was noted that increasing abnormality correlated with increasing ridge size, and that the evolution of the surface features of the flat avillous mucosa of coeliac disease could be explained on the basis of intervillous ridge hypertrophy. From a practical viewpoint, it should be recalled that the holes one sees on the surface of a flat avillous mucosa are not crypt orifices, but the openings of the vestibules.

As extreme variation in villous and crypt architecture occurs in disease, it is not surprising that investigators have attempted to apply some form of quantitative measure to jejunal biopsy appearances. By far the commonest procedures are simple linear measurements made in histological sections with the aid of a calibrated eyepiece graticule, giving the villus height and the crypt depth. However, it has been shown that linear measurements only correlate with villus population size in situations where the villi are *all* normal in shape – in human work, a most unlikely finding, and even in 'normal' individuals, correlation between villous height and population is very poor.[18] In critical work, if the villous population size must be measured, then the only accurate way is to microdissect, squash and count the epithelial cells,[1] but such techniques are for research rather than clinical purposes. Other methods which have been used to quantify mucosal appearances include measurement of the surface : volume ratio by a cuts and hits procedure using random lines[7] and the use of the image analysing computer.[12]

The villi are clothed by absorptive columnar cells, which are tall and cylindrical and rest on a thin basal lamina. The cells have complex lateral interdigitations, prominent terminal bars and a terminal web, and the apical surface bears numerous microvilli with a distinct glycocalyx. The microvilli are approximately 1 μm in length and 0.1 μm in diameter. Mitochondria are plentiful and the Golgi apparatus is supranuclear. These cells are mainly involved in the absorption of nutrients from the bowel lumen; the nucleus is centrally placed, with dense chromatin masses.

The crypts contain columnar cells of different types (see Figure 8.1b).[4] At the bottom of the crypt are the crypt base columnar cells, which have basal nuclei, a distinct nucleolus and diffuse chromatin. There are numerous free ribosomes, but little rough endoplasmic reticulum, small Golgi and few mitochondria. Scattered apical microvilli are evident, but well-formed junctional complexes are seen. It is highly likely that these cells are 'stem cells' for all the different types of cell seen in the small intestinal mucosa.[4] The mid-crypt columnar cells are taller, with larger Golgi and more mitochondria, while the crypt-top columnar cells contain many more mitochondria and fewer ribosomes; lateral interdigitations become more marked.

Goblet cells are found mainly on the villi, but also in the upper half of the crypt; early goblet cell forms begin to accumulate membrane-bound mucin droplets above the nucleus, and, as these increase in amount, mucin fills the supra-nuclear cytoplasm, and the cells acquire the rounded contours of the goblet. The mucous glycoprotein is synthesized in the rough endo-plasmic reticulum, and the final product is col-lected in the Golgi membranes. Finally the secretion is released in an apocrine manner, and the mucin flows into the bowel lumen.

In the base of the crypt lie the enigmatic Paneth cells, pyramidal in shape, with hyaline, RNA-rich cytoplasm, containing abundant rough endoplasmic reticulum; in the supra-nuclear region are conspicuous refractile gran-ules, which contain lysozyme. Paneth cell function remains unknown, although the pre-sence of such abundant cytoplasmic lysozyme might suggest a role in the regulation of the local bacterial flora, and there is some evidence that Paneth cells may be actively phagocytic for crypt lumen bacteria.

Endocrine cells, variously called argentaffin, APUD, entero-endocrine, and many other appellations, are also found in the small bowel mucosa. There has been considerable debate concerning the origin of these cells, but most current opinion is in favour of the hypothesis that they are of strictly local origin, and are in fact progeny of the undifferentiated crypt base columnar cell.[16] Though in some cases the apices of these endocrine cells can reach the crypt or intestinal lumen, most endocrine cells have no contact with the bowel lumen. These cells are characterized by their numerous neuro-secretory granules, often concentrated in the infranuclear region ('basal granulated cell'). Classification of these cells is difficult, and has been based mainly on the electron-microscope appearance of the secretory granules, combined with cytochemical characteristics such as argen-taffinicity and argyrophilia – the Weisbaden classification.[13] As cytochemical methods have become more reliable, this classification has become outmoded, and it is perhaps best to clas-sify these cells on the basis of the polypeptides they produce.[2]

We have already seen that there are numerous lymphoid cells in the lamina propria of the small intestine. Moreover, numerous lymphocytes are found in among the epithelial cells clothing the villi – the so-called intra-epithelial lymphocytes. There has been considerable debate concerning the importance of these cells and their number in the diagnosis of gluten sensitivity; there is little doubt that the method of counting the cells has a direct influence on the results obtained. More recently, attention has been focused on the

number of such intra-epithelial lymphocytes which are in mitosis, i.e. in the process of trans-forming;[11] this concept certainly deserves more attention.

CONGENITAL ABNORMALITIES

The complex embryological development of the intestine offers a background for a variety of congenital abnormalities. The central, complex phenomenon concerned is the process of rota-tion of the intestine. At about six weeks of embryonic life, the midgut extends as a pro-longed loop into the umbilical cord, whilst the superior mesenteric vessels form the axis of this loop. At approximately three months the loop of intestine begins to rotate around this arterial axis – counterclockwise as the abdomen of the fetus is viewed from the front. The lower limb thus passes upwards so that its future deriv-atives, the colon and ileum, come to lie above and in front of the upper limb, from which the duodenum and jejunum will derive. Subse-quently, as the gut returns from the cord to within the abdomen, a further 90° rotation takes place, carrying the caecum to the right lower quadrant of the abdomen.

ROTATION

Incomplete rotation commonly leaves the caecum high on the right side of the abdomen beneath the liver; when more marked, the rota-tion of the jejunum *to* the left upper quadrant of the abdomen, or of the caecum and transverse colon *out of* the left side of the abdomen, may not have occurred. Whilst minor or even major degrees of incomplete rotation may be entirely asymptomatic, complications may occur either because the process is associated with persist-ence of developmental bands, which may initiate obstruction, because incomplete development of the mesentery predisposes to volvulus, or because internal hernias develop, usually para-duodenal or paracaecal. Precise classifications of rotatory anomalies encompass:

A Non-rotation: with a right-sided small intes-tine and left-sided colon.
B Reversed rotation: when a clockwise 90° rotation leaves the small bowel superficial to the transverse colon, which often passes through the small intestinal mesentery.
C Malrotation: failure to complete the normal rotatory process.

DUPLICATIONS

The duodenum, the ileum and more rarely the jejunum may contain duplications – partial or complete doubling of a length of bowel, which may possess its own mesentery or be included in the mesentery of the normal small bowel. Similar developmental aberrations may give rise to diverticula (except Meckel's, see below) and enterogenous cysts. The diverticula are usually outpouchings of the whole bowel wall, and often contain heterotopic gastric or other gastro-intestinal mucosae. Enterogenous cysts may lie submucosally, intramuscularly or subserosally. Although these anomalies are often asymptomatic, they can give rise to obstruction, intus-susception, bleeding, perforation or volvulus, requiring surgical intervention.

MECKEL'S DIVERTICULUM

When the embryonic midgut extends into the umbilical cord, at the apex of the loop is the omphalomesenteric duct communicating with the yolk sac. Persistence of this duct as a diverticulum gives rise to Meckel's diverticulum; this may on occasion be connected to the umbilicus by a fibrous cord, or else isolated cysts may lie along this pathway.

As an anatomical finding Meckel's diverticulum is common. The English mnemonic of 2% of the population, 2 inches long, 2 feet from the ileocaecal valve is parochial in its units, but a fair approximation. In fact the diverticulum may arise anywhere from 2 to 200 cm from the ileo-caecal valve; it lies on the antimesenteric border, and contains all normal layers of intestine. In a very high percentage of cases heterotopic mucosa is present within the diverticulum – gastric mucosa in about one third, pancreatic in about one tenth. The presence of acid-producing mucosa predisposes to the development of symptoms and complications from a Meckel's diverticulum – bleeding or perforation from ulceration of the adjacent ileal-type mucosa. Obstruction of the ileum or acute diverticulitis mimicking appendicitis are other presentations. Whilst commoner in children, bleeding Meckel's diverticula have been reported in elderly patients.

Diagnosis is rarely a problem when complications requiring surgery arise; dilemmas usually arise in the context of recurrent gastro-intestinal bleeding. Small bowel radiology rarely identifies the diverticulae. An isotope-scanning technique based on the concentration of ^{99}Tc^m-pertechnetate in heterotopic, as well as ortho-topic, gastric mucosa has been advocated.[8] Anecdotally, this is less impressive than the published experience.

REFERENCES

1 Bramble, M., Zucoloto, S., Wright, N. A. & Record, C. (1983) Early changes in the human small intestine after gluten challenge in coeliac patients in remission. *Gut*, submitted.

2 Buchan, A. M. J. & Polak, J. M. (1980) The classification of human gastroenteropancreatic endocrine cells. *Investigative and Cell Pathology*, **3**, 51–71.

3 Cheng, H. (1974) Origin, differentiation and renewal of the four main epithelial cell types. II. Mucous cells. *American Journal of Anatomy*, **141**, 481–502.

4 Cheng, H. & Leblond, C. P. (1974) Origin, differentiation and renewal of the four main epithelial cell types in the mouse small intestine. V. Unitarian theory for the origin of the four epithelial cell types. *American Journal of Anatomy*, **141**, 537–562.

5 Clarke, R. (1970) Mucosal architecture and epithelial cell production rate in the small intestine of the albino rat. *Journal of Anatomy*, **107**, 519–532.

6 Cocco, A. E., Dohrmann, M. J. & Hendrix, T. R. (1966) Reconstruction of normal jejunal biopsies: three dimensional histology. *Gastroenterology*, **51**, 24–31.

7 Dunnill, M. S. & Whitehead, R. (1972) A method for the quantitation of small intestinal biopsy specimens. *Journal of Clinical Pathology*, **25**, 243–246.

8 Kilpatrick, Z. M. & Aseron, C. A. (1972) Radioisotope detection of Meckel's diverticulum causing acute rectal haemorrhage. *New England Journal of Medicine*, **287**, 653–654.

9 Loehry, C. A. & Creamer, B. (1969) Three dimensional structure of the human small intestinal mucosa in health and disease. *Gut*, **10**, 6–12.

10 Marks, J. M. & Shuster, S. (1970) Small intestinal mucosal abnormalities in coeliac disease – fact or fancy? *Gut*, **11**, 281–291.

11 Marsh, M. N., Mathan, M. & Mathan, V. I. (1983) Studies of intestinal lymphoid tissue. VII. The secondary nature of lymphoid cell 'activation' in the jejunal lesion of tropical sprue. *American Journal of Pathology*, **112**, 302–312.

12 Meinhard, E. A., Wadbrook, D. G. & Risdon, R. A. (1975) Computer morphometry of jejunal biopsies in childhood coeliac disease. *Journal of Clinical Pathology*, **28**, 85–92.

13 Solcia, E., Pearse, A. Ge., Forssman, W. G. & Creutz-feldt, W. (1970) Weisbaden classification. In *Origin, Chemistry and Pathophysiology of the Gastrointestinal Hormones* (Ed.) Creutzfeldt, W. pp. 71–82. Stuttgart: Schattauer Verlag.

14 Wilson, G., Ponder, B. & Wright, N. A. (1983) How epithelial cells move in sheets; pathways of villus cell migration in the small intestine. *Journal of Anatomy*, in press.

15 Wright, N. A. & Irwin, M. (1982) The kinetics of villus cell populations in the mouse small intestine. 1. Normal villi: the steady state requirement. *Cell and Tissue Kinetics*, **15**, 595–609.

16 Wright, N. A. & Alison, M. R. (1984) *The Biology of Epithelial Cell Populations*. Oxford: Oxford University Press.

17 Wright, N. A., Appleton, D. R., Marks, J. & Watson, A. J. (1979) Cytokinetic studies of crypts in convoluted human small intestinal mucosa. *Journal of Clinical Pathology*, **32**, 462–470.

18 Zucoloto, S., Bramble, M., Record, C. & Wright, N. A. (1984) The measurement of villus and crypt population sizes in the human small intestine. *Gut*, submitted.

THE GUT RESPONSE TO A MEAL AND ITS HORMONAL CONTROL

THE NORMAL HUMAN DIET

The human diet is extraordinarily varied. Even if one only considers the dietary habits prevalent in the Western World, where some common standards are identifiable, the range of foods and beverages consumed by adults is very wide. Therefore, it is difficult to define a physiological meal or even establish its limits. Nevertheless, it is important to recognize that the human gastrointestinal tract handles ingested elements in different ways, adapting its response to the different characteristics of the foods consumed. Ordinary meals are physically and chemically heterogeneous; they are composed of both solid and liquid substances and contain more than one essential nutrient such as protein, fat or carbohydrate.[56, 62]

Physiological meals usually contain, or decompose intragastrically into, different physical phases: aqueous, solid, and oil (fats that are liquid at body temperature). Water constitutes the largest mass in the typical meal. It may be taken as plain water or in other liquid beverages. Water may also be released intragastrically from certain foods and, conversely, may be adsorbed by some elements of the meal, such as pectins and other fibre components.

Two classes of solid foods can be recognized – digestible and non-digestible solids. Digestible solids (e.g. cooked meat, liver, egg, starch-based tubers) tend to be broken down into fine particulate matter by gastric grinding contractions and largely hydrolysed by luminal gut enzymes as a prelude to their absorption. In contrast, nondigestible solids (typically dietary fibre derived from the cell wall of plants) are impervious to both the mechanical forces and enzymatic action, and thus tend to progress along the upper gastrointestinal tract as solid particles; this progression is dependent on particular types of physiological motor activity.

Fat exists in different physicochemical forms. Ninety percent of the fat in the American diet is composed of triglycerides containing fatty acids with 16 to 18 carbon molecules. Shorter chain fatty acids are found in milk and vegetable oils. Some fats (e.g. butter) are liquefied at body temperature; others (e.g. olive oil) are ingested in liquid form. Animal fat that remains solid at body temperature is probably handled by the stomach in the same way as the meat which is usually intimately associated with it.

Carbohydrate can also be ingested in different physical forms; this may greatly influence its effect on gastric emptying and its absorption. Sucrose, which constitutes about a quarter of the total carbohydrate intake, and other soluble carbohydrates are partly dissolved in the intragastric aqueous phase, if they are not already ingested in solution. Starch, which constitutes about 50% of dietary carbohydrate, is largely found in grains and vegetables (particularly tubers and legumes), in association with pectins and other structural fibre. The extent to which such foods are susceptible to trituration and mixing varies a great deal. Some are soft, easily digestible solids, whereas others are so protected by structural fibre as to be virtually unavailable for hydrolysis.

Most dietary protein is animal protein that is ingested in solid form such as meats, fish and cooked egg. About one third of dietary protein may be provided by vegetable protein in foods such as cereal grains, nuts and peanuts. Unlike fats and the majority of carbohydrates, protein is subjected not only to mechanical trituration in the stomach but also to chemical hydrolysis by pepsin. (Some hydrolysis of carbohydrate also occurs before the duodenum due to the action of salivary amylose.)

HORMONAL CONTROL OF GUT RESPONSES TO A MEAL: GENERAL CONCEPTS

The gastric, pancreatic, biliary and intestinal responses to a meal are carefully regulated by hormonal and neural mechanisms (Figure 8.2). The way in which these mechanisms regulate and integrate digestive functions to permit 'normal' handling of the meal is just beginning to be understood. It is important to recognize that every function of every digestive organ is affected, both positively and negatively, by neural input and by hormones. The net response of an organ at any point in time in the postprandial period is a summation of the many agonis-

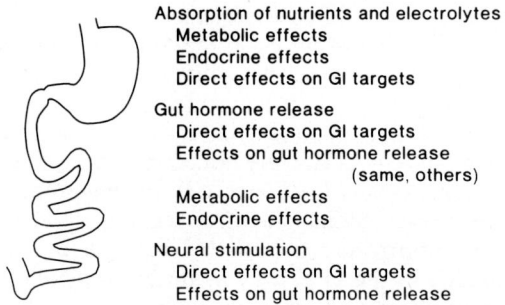

Absorption of nutrients and electrolytes
   Metabolic effects
   Endocrine effects
   Direct effects on GI targets

Gut hormone release
   Direct effects on GI targets
   Effects on gut hormone release
                              (same, others)
   Metabolic effects
   Endocrine effects

Neural stimulation
   Direct effects on GI targets
   Effects on gut hormone release

Fig. 8.2 Regulation of digestive function. Major aspects of neurohormonal regulation and postabsorptive effects are listed.

tic, antagonistic and potentiating effects of all the regulatory substances which affect it.

To gain insight into the role of hormones in this process, we must first understand the location of the gastrointestinal endocrine cells and their stimuli for secretion. Each peptide is synthesized and secreted by a distinct cell type which is found in a characteristic area of gut. These have been very successfully mapped morphologically using immunocytochemistry and antisera directed against the peptides themselves. Our understanding of the stimulation of the cells is more indirect since, because the endocrine cells are scattered amongst enterocytes which are of similar size and density, it has been very difficult to successfully isolate them for in vitro study. Understanding of these functions is, therefore, derived from 'black box' type experiments, in which a particular luminal stimulus is given and peripheral blood levels of hormones are measured. Using various approaches, such as feeding whole meals, feeding parts of meals, perfusing the bowel, perfusing segments of the bowel, and superfusion experiments, the stimuli which cause release of each peptide have been elucidated.

The major regulator of secretion of most gastrointestinal hormones is the composition of the intestinal chyme at that level of the bowel associated with each particular endocrine cell type. This is complicated by a differential gastric emptying of liquids and solids and of different nutrients, non-uniformity of bowel transit, and differential nutrient absorption rates. All of this results in a constantly changing milieu in the bowel, with the composition of the chyme at any given level of the bowel constantly changing in the postprandial period. The gastrointestinal hormone profile reflects this. Combining an understanding of luminal events with an understanding of gastrointestinal endocrine cell location and function permits correlation of various events.

Although there are many possible gastrointestinal hormones, with new candidates being discovered at a rapid pace, we will concentrate here on the hormones which are well-established. The most proximal hormone is *gastrin*, which is located primarily in the stomach and the very proximal duodenum. Duodenal and upper small bowel hormones include *cholecystokinin* (CCK), *secretin*, *gastric inhibitory polypeptide* (GIP) and *motilin*. *Enteroglucagon* (GLI) and *neurotensin* are lower intestinal hormones. Each of these hormones affects multiple gastrointestinal target cells (Figure 8.3). They also directly or indirectly affect classical endocrine and metabolic functions. These effects may be mediated by the absorption of nutrients or fluid and electrolytes, as well as by direct interaction between gastrointestinal hormones and endocrine organs. Thus, there are many interactions going on at any point in time in the postprandial period.

GASTRIC SECRETION AFTER A MEAL

The gastric secretory response to a meal is characterized by a rapid increase in secretory rate which begins when a person starts eating (or even earlier if he psychically anticipates appetizing food). Peak rates are reached between 30 to 60 minutes after ingestion of the meal. Thereafter, gastric secretion rapidly decreases towards basal rates; a low plateau is frequently observed during the third or fifth hour after meals, with some food still remaining in the stomach. Thus the gastric secretory response to a meal is characterized by two phases – acceleration followed by deceleration (Figure 8.4).

The initial accelerating phase corresponds to a predominance of stimulatory forces over inhibitory forces; the converse is true for the decelerating phase. Peak acid output occurs at the transition point between these two phases. When many individuals with a wide range of secretory capacities are studied, a statistically significant correlation is observed between responses to exogenous secretagogues and luminal stimuli.[20, 47] However, even during the period of peak secretion, a balance between stimulatory and inhibitory mechanisms is also likely to be occurring; therefore, the latter should not be assumed to be identical to 'maximal acid output' as measured after administration of high doses of exogenous secretagogues. In addition, gastric secretory capacity varies enormously, even among apparently

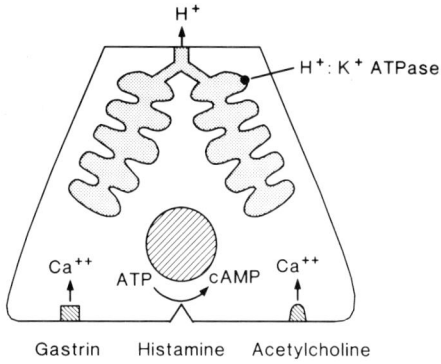

a

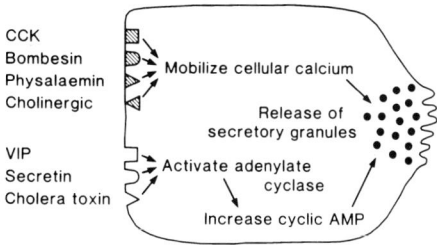

b

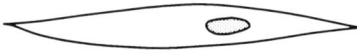

Excitatory	Inhibitory
Acetylcholine	VIP
Cholecystokinin	Pancreatic polypeptide
Gastrin	
Secretin (Potentiates CCK)	
Bombesin (? indirect - mediated by CCK)	

c

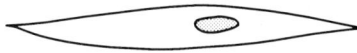

Excitatory	Inhibitory	
Acetylcholine	Norepinephrine	↓plateau potential
Gastrin	Neurotensin	↓contractile force
CCK	VIP	↓electro-mechanical coupling

d

Fig. 8.3 Prototypes of regulation of cellular function in the digestive tract. (a) Parietal cell. (b) Pancreatic acinar cell. (c) Gallbladder smooth muscle cell. (d) Antral smooth muscle cell.

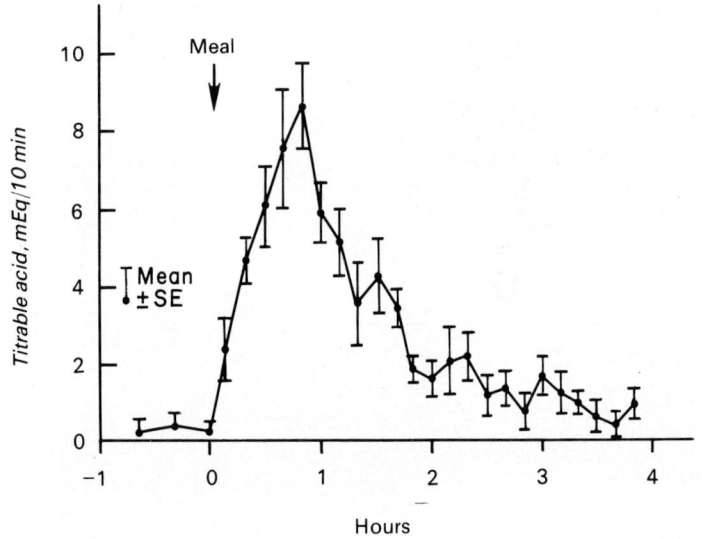

Fig. 8.4 Postprandial gastric acid output in man. The biphasic profile of the normal secretory response to a meal is shown. From Malagelada, J.-R., *et al.* (1976),[44] with kind permission of the authors and the editor of *Gastroenterology.*

healthy individuals. Extensive studies of gastric acid secretion during basal conditions and in response to secretagogues[3] show that 'maximal' acid secretion rates ranging from less than 5 to over 60 mEq/hour are found in unselected populations. Although fewer individuals have been studied in response to meals, there is similar variation.

The stimulatory phase of postprandial gastric secretion

There is little doubt about the importance of cephalic stimulation during the early period of postprandial gastric secretion. Unlike in the dog, in which sham feeding stimulates gastric secretion to the same level achieved by injection of maximally stimulating doses of exogenous histamine or gastrin,[57] sham feeding achieves only partial stimulation in man (Figure 8.5).

Richardson *et al.*[61] and Mayer *et al.*,[48] employing a modified sham feeding technique, found that the cephalic stimulation led to a response of about one-third of the maximal secretory capacity. In patients with duodenal ulcer in whom a true sham feeding technique was employed (that is, including actual swallowing of an appetizing meal), Knutson and Olbe[32] obtained about one-half the maximal acid response to pentagastrin. Cephalic stimulation of gastric acid secretion in humans is probably mediated by direct vagal stimulation of the parietal area and partially through vagal stimulation of gastrin release from the antrum.[70]

Another important part of the stimulus provided by a meal probably comes from gastric distension. It is thought to be mediated by vago-vagal and intramural cholinergic reflexes.[24] Hunt and MacDonald,[28] Cooke[9] and Richardson *et al.*[61] have measured the human gastric

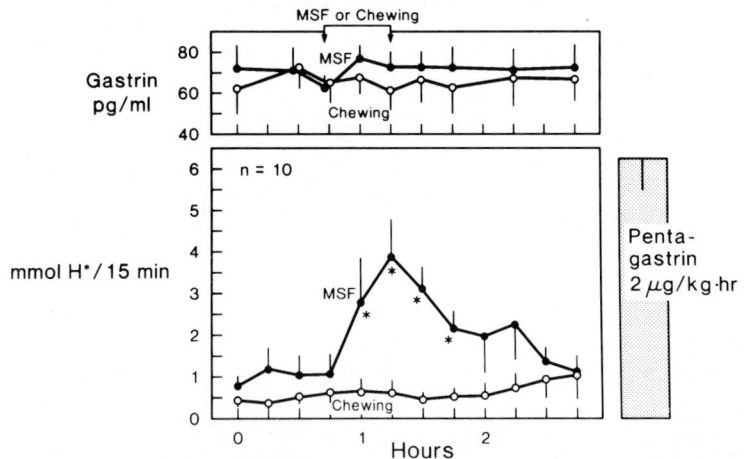

Fig. 8.5 Gastrin and gastric acid responses to modified sham feeding in health. Modified sham feeding (MSF) provides a standardized measurement of cephalic stimulation of gastric acid secretion in man. Note the absence of a rise in serum gastrin. Modified from Konturek, S. J. (1981). In *Gastric Secretion, Basic and Clinical Aspects,* (Ed.) Konturek, S. J. and Domschke, W. pp. 62–79. New York: Thieme Stratton.

response to distension with inert aqueous solutions, and agree that its magnitude amounts to one-third of the maximal response, and that it is probably responsible for about one-third of the response to a meal as well. Furthermore, gastric distension prolongs the response to cephalic stimulation, which otherwise is of short duration.

The third stimulatory component of the gastric secretory response to a meal is chemical stimulation of gastrin release from the antrum by certain polypeptides and amino acids, plus possible direct stimulation of the oxyntic gland area.[13] This component, according to calculations by Richardson et al.,[61] may account for the remaining one-third of the acid response to a meal.

Gastrin is the classical hormone most responsible for stimulation of gastric acid secretion. It is rapidly released after a meal. The main stimuli for gastrin release seem to be amino acids and peptides; thus, protein meals give rise to larger increases in serum gastrin than do meals rich in carbohydrates or fats. The vagus also seems to play a role in the release of gastrin; its stimulatory effect occurs during the cephalic phase of gastric secretion. Calcium is another stimulant of gastrin release.

It appears that, unlike in the dog, gastrin release in man probably does not participate in the distension-mediated effects on secretion. Although gastrin's main effect seems to be stimulation of gastric acid secretion, it also has effects on smooth muscle in the stomach and surrounding sphincters as well as a trophic influence on various gastrointestinal tissues. Its trophic effects on parietal cell mass may explain the reduction in gastric secretory response observed in individuals receiving total parenteral nutrition for prolonged periods of time.[33]

The quantitative importance of the intestinal phase of postprandial gastric secretion is less well defined. Unlike the cephalic and gastric phases, which early in the postprandial period are overwhelmingly stimulatory, during the intestinal phase net inhibition or net stimulation may occur, depending on a variety of factors. In two separate studies of diversion of chyme at the ligament of Treitz performed in our laboratory in healthy individuals, we observed opposite effects with different liquid meals: potentiation of the gastric secretory response occurred with diversion of chyme after one meal,[7] and a reduction in the secretory response occurred with another type of meal.[53] The proportions of energy provided by carbohydrate, protein and

fat were similar with both meals, but the sources of these nutrients and gastric emptying were different. Thus, many variable factors may determine the net effect on gastrin secretion during the intestinal phase.

Gastric secretion can be stimulated at a level of the intestine where there is no gastrin to mediate this response. The nutrient which has been shown to be responsible for this is in the protein and amino acid family. A hypothetical hormone, *entero-oxyntin*, has been implicated. However, this hormone has not been characterized on a biochemical level and the cell responsible for its secretion has not been identified.

A postabsorptive effect of amino acids and peptides in stimulating gastric acid secretion has also been described. This appears not to be mediated by gastrin, and may be a direct effect of the nutrient on the gastric parietal cells.

The inhibitory phase of postprandial gastric secretion

As indicated earlier, gastric secretion peaks around one hour after ingestion of food and declines rather rapidly afterward, reflecting a predominance of inhibitory over stimulatory factors.[44] This occurs not only because of increasing inhibitory forces but also because the stimulatory forces are decreasing. First, the effects of cephalic stimulation are reduced since the visual and olfactory stimuli of the food are gone, chewing and swallowing no longer occur, and a feeling of satiety develops. Second, gastric distension diminishes as the volume of the gastric contents begins to decline by the end of the first hour or earlier (Figure 8.6). The only stimulatory factors that remain are the chemical action of food in the stomach and, depending on the type of meal, perhaps some stimulation from the intestine.

The decline in stimulatory activity coincides with a strengthening of inhibitory forces, the most important of which appears to be acidification of gastric contents.[80] In most normal individuals, acidification of gastric contents proceeds until a pH of about 2.0 is reached; the secretory rate then markedly declines. This luminal pH is optimum for peptic activity and, therefore, it makes teleological sense that gastric secretion would be inhibited when it is reached. Probably gastric and duodenal pH-sensitive mechanisms are involved, but the neuro-hormonal mechanisms by which gastric and duodenal acidification inhibit postprandial gastric secretion are poorly understood. Dimi-

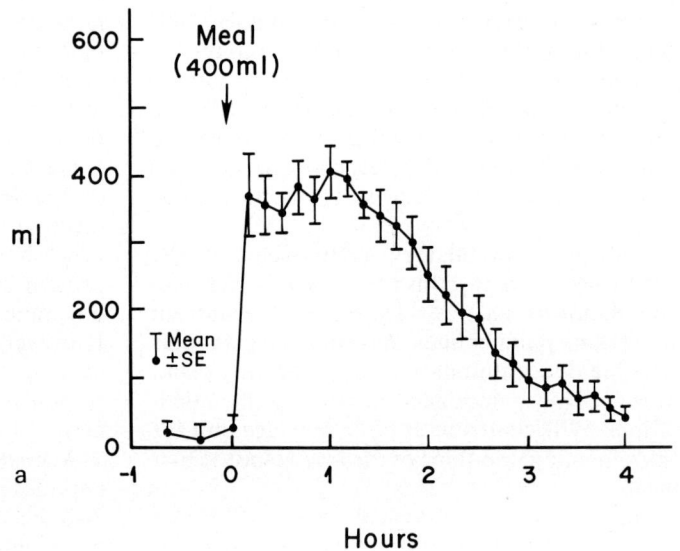

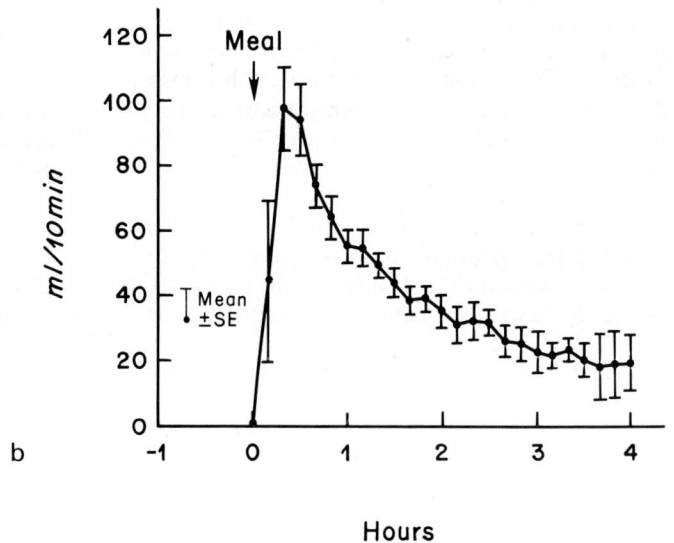

Fig. 8.6 (a) Postprandial volume of gastric contents. (b) Volume of gastric contents emptied into the duodenum after meals in health. Intragastric volume during the first postprandial hour is relatively stable. During this period gastric secretory activity and emptying rates peak and offset each other. When secretory rates decline intragastric volume also falls. From Malagelada, J.-R., *et al.* (1976),[44] with kind permission of the authors and the editor of *Gastroenterology*.

nution of antral and duodenal gastrin release by low pH may be important.[12, 80] There is also the possibility of a paracrine effect of the vagal release of somatostatin at low antral pH.[75] Bulbogastrone,[2] a humoral agent released from the acidified duodenal bulb in experimental animals, has not been evaluated in humans to assess its physiological status. Secretin appears to be released after meals and probably plays a physiological role in stimulating the exocrine pancreas and hepatic secretion of bicarbonate.[6, 66] Whether it plays a physiological role in regulating postprandial gastric acid secretion is unknown.

Other hormones in the small bowel seem to be primarily inhibitory to gastric acid secretion. In fact, lipid and carbohydrates infused into any part of the small intestine will inhibit acid secretion, and even protein will inhibit acid secretion when it is infused into the distal small bowel. Which hormones are mediating these effects is not well understood.

Cholecystokinin (CCK) is released in response to protein, fat, acid, and calcium. Its main effects are in stimulating gallbladder contraction, stimulating pancreatic enzyme secretion, augmenting the action of secretin on pancreatic secretion, and decreasing the tone in the body of the stomach; it also has a trophic influence on the pancreas. More recently, this peptide has been postulated to play a role in augmenting satiety; however, this activity has not been fully characterized.

Gastric inhibitory polypeptide (GIP) is secreted in response to protein, fat, and carbohydrate. Its main physiological action seems to be as an incretin. Although this hormone received its name because of its activity in inhibiting gastric acid secretion in the rat, in man it seems to have little or no activity to do this.

Motilin is released in response to intestinal acid. This peptide seems to have its major physiological effect during the interdigestive period in stimulating the initiation of the migrating myoelectric complex. No effect on postprandial digestive function has been attributed to this peptide.

Neurotensin and enteroglucagon (GLI) are hormonal markers for the distal small bowel. Postprandially, in health, these hormones do not have a major regulatory effect on digestive function. They have been implicated, however, in playing a role in pathological states such as the dumping syndrome.

THE MOTOR RESPONSE OF THE UPPER GUT TO A MEAL

The fasting motor pattern

Fasting gut motility is characterized by cyclic periods of activity alternating with quiescence. These cycles consist of three identifiable phases: motor quiescence (phase I), irregular but persistent contractions (phase II), and a short burst of rhythmic contractions (phase III).[8, 71, 78] In studies carried out in healthy volunteers in our laboratory[60] the range of duration of each cycle (measured as the interval between two consecutive phase III's) varied from 53 to 136 minutes, depending on the individual studied. The duration of interdigestive cycles also varied considerably within each individual (in one healthy person cycles varied in duration from 49 to 149 minutes).

Cyclic electrical and motor activity usually originates in the stomach or upper small intestine and is propagated distally from the upper gut to the terminal ileum, taking approximately the same period of time as the inter-cycle interval. Motilin and pancreatic polypeptide increase just before or during the most intense motor activity (phase III) arrives at the level of the upper gut. On the other hand, gastrin, GIP, glu-

cagon, insulin and GLI remain low and constant in the interdigestive period and do not vary at all with the interdigestive motor activity. Although gastrin and cholecystokinin have been shown to inhibit interdigestive motor activity, these hormones are not present at a level adequate to cause this effect during the interdigestive period. Ingestion of a meal abolishes the interdigestive activity and elevates the concentrations of these hormones.

Postprandial motor activity

Ingestion of a meal modifies interdigestive motor activity in several ways. Assuming it is eaten at an ordinary pace, the volume of the meal (ranging from 400 to 800 ml for most meals), plus the volume of gastric secretion and swallowed saliva, far exceeds the gastric emptying rate (Figure 8.6). The expansion of intragastric volume during the early postprandial period with minimal increase in intragastric pressure is an expression of the 'reservoir' function of the stomach. Receptive relaxation and accommodation are largely a function of the proximal stomach and are partially mediated through vagal reflexes, perhaps in close association with those stimulating gastric secretion in response to fundal distension.[1, 5, 31, 69] It is not surprising, therefore, that early satiety and postprandial epigastric fullness are a common complaint of patients after vagotomy. Relaxatory vagal fibres are probably nonadrenergic and noncholinergic.[29]

The motor responses of the stomach to a meal are determined in part by the physicochemical composition of the meal. Studies in our laboratory have shown that ingestion of 400 ml of 0.15 mol/l saline (an inert, isotonic solution) does not usually disturb the ongoing fasting motor activity.[59] In contrast, ingestion of a liquid meal containing nutrients inhibits the characteristic fasting cyclic activity and replaces it with an irregular pattern of intestinal pressure activity termed the 'fed pattern'. In the antrum, very little phasic pressure activity occurs after a liquid meal. When most of the liquid has been emptied from the stomach, characteristic interdigestive migrating motor complexes reappear. Carbohydrate- or protein-containing meals interrupt the interdigestive motor pattern for a shorter time than lipid meals or mixed meals containing all essential nutrients; the duration of the interruption approximately coincides with the duration of gastric emptying for each meal.

Ingestion of a solid or solid and liquid meal is associated with a pattern of gastric motor activity different from that for inert and nutrient-containing liquid meals. Shortly after ingestion of solid food, vigorous contractions take place in the distal antrum, which cause phasic increases in pressure often reaching over 100 mmHg.[58] These contractions occur at or close to the maximal rate (established by the gastric pacemaker) of 3/minute, and are most apparent in the terminal antrum. The antral pressure waves may persist for several hours, evolving later into a migrating phase III which signals the re-establishment of the interdigestive motor pattern. Therefore, meals of different physical characteristics and composition differ in the types of antral pressure response they elicit in the stomach, but the intestinal motor fed pattern shows no such differences on visual inspection (Figure 8.7).

The mechanism responsible for postprandial inhibition of interdigestive cyclic motility may be both neuronal and hormonal.[72, 73] Protein and mixed meals release gastrin, which has been shown to inhibit interdigestive motor activity in both dog and man.[25, 45, 81] However, gastrin release is not responsible for the interruption of gastric motor activity after lipid and carbohydrate meals. Numerous other hormones, including cholecystokinin, secretin and insulin,[4, 55] may also be important, but their physiological role in switching the gut from a fasting to a fed motor pattern requires further study.

Gastric emptying

As indicated earlier, intragastric contents after a physiological meal separate into three phases – aqueous, solid and oil – which are emptied by the stomach at different rates. Plain water or isotonic aqueous solutions with low nutrient content leave the stomach most rapidly and are continuously replaced by gastric secretion.[39] Fluids of high osmolality or soluble nutrient content, or both, have slower emptying rates than water, allowing for gradual adjustment of the chyme osmolality to isotonicity in the upper intestine (Figure 8.8). Fats which are liquid at body temperature (the oil phase) and solids leave the stomach much more slowly than the aqueous phase.

There is evidence that different mechanisms and regions of the stomach are involved in the emptying of the solid and liquid components of gastric contents. Experimental studies suggest that tonic fundal activity is primarily responsible for the emptying of fluids, whereas the antrum is mostly concerned with the emptying of solids.[26] This concept represents a departure from the earlier view that an 'antral pump' was the main determinant of gastric emptying of all kinds of contents. In the case of digestible solids, the antrum plays an important role in reducing the size of the ingested solids to fine particulate matter and suspending them in fluid. This grinding–mixing process is accomplished

Fig. 8.7 Antral and duodenal motor responses to different types of meals in man. The top tracings illustrate the typical response to ingestion of a small amount of water or saline, which cause no perceptible change in the interdigestive migrating motor pattern. The middle tracings illustrate the response to liquid food. Antral phasic pressure activity disappears until the majority of the meal has been evacuated from the stomach. In the duodenum, irregular activity characteristic of the fed pattern is observed. The bottom tracings illustrate the response to a solid meal, which causes intense distal antral phasic pressure activity. The duodenal fed pattern is similar to that observed after liquid food. From Malagelada, J.-R. (1981). In *Physiology of the Gastrointestinal Tract (Volume 2)*, (Ed.) Johnson, L. R. pp. 893–924, with kind permission of the publishers, Raven Press.

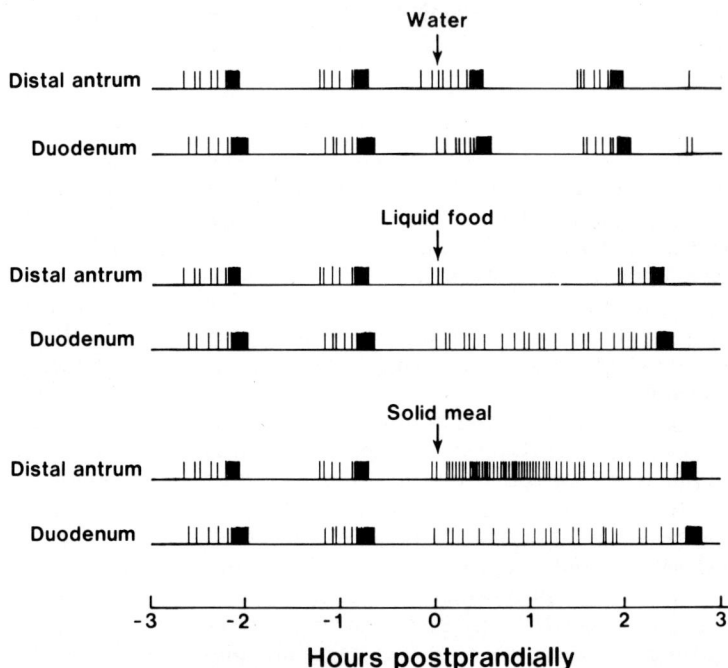

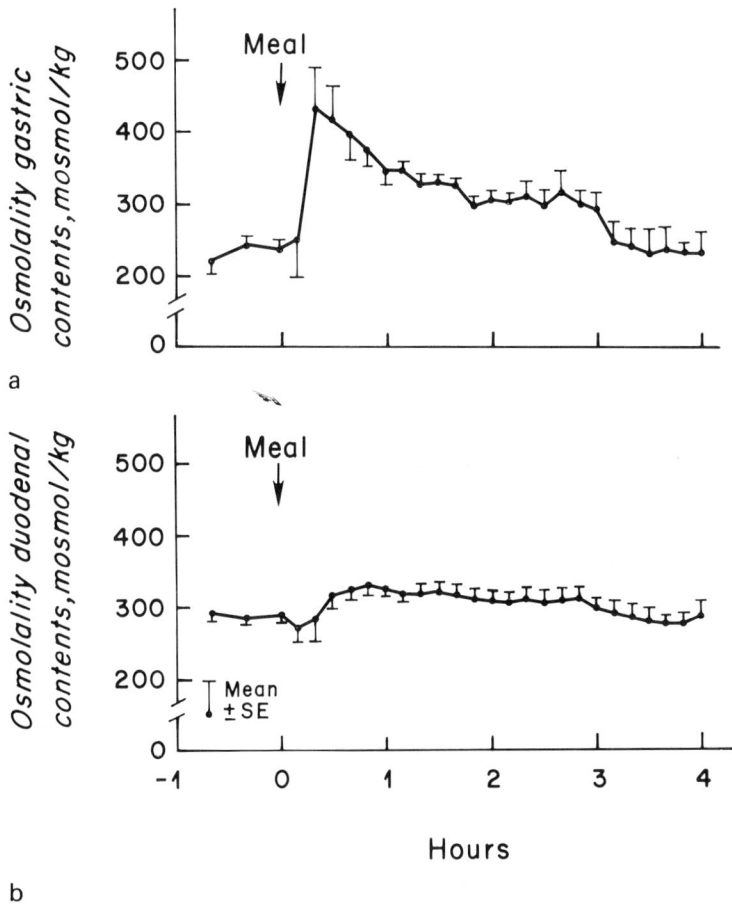

Fig. 8.8 Osmolality of gastric and duodenal contents after a meal in health. (a) Osmolality of gastric contents. (b) Osmolality of duodenal contents aspirated at the ligament of Treitz. Note the gradual decrease in gastric osmolality as the meal becomes more diluted with gastric juice and food is emptied from the stomach. In the duodenum, large fluctuations in osmolality are prevented by mechanisms regulating gastric emptying and through dilution of chyme in the duodenum by biliary and pancreatic secretions. Modified from Malagelada, J.-R. *et al.* (1979).[40]

by rhythmic and powerful antral contractions described earlier. Solid particles and some liquid are propulsed forward, and then backwards by the terminal antropyloric contraction, which allows some liquid to pass through but retains most solid particles in the stomach until they have been finely broken down. Meyer *et al.*,[51] for instance, have shown in the dog that only liver particles of less than 1 mm are allowed to pass into the duodenum. In summary, in this process of emptying of digestible solids, three interacting functions are important: the grinding pressure waves of the distal antrum, the discriminatory mechanism that allows small suspended particles to leave with the liquids and retains large particles for further grinding in the stomach, and the propulsive forces, mostly fundal, that push the fluids (and the small suspended solid particles) into the duodenum.

Non-digestible solids, such as the fibrous, cell-wall structures of plants, are rather impervious to mechanical grinding by antral contractions. As a result, the larger nondigestible solid particles in a meal probably remain in the stomach until the rest of the food has left. However, the return of the interdigestive migrating motor complexes propels them across the pylorus. This mechanism may explain the development of fibrous bezoars in patients with gastric motility disorders in which gastric interdigestive migrating motor complexes are frequently absent.

The regulation of gastric emptying

Mechanisms regulating gastric emptying have gradually been characterized through several decades of experimental work. They can be divided into central and peripheral mechanisms. Central mechanisms are intimately related with the emetic centre in the medulla oblongata and, indeed, inhibition of gastric emptying is observed preceding vomiting and in response to a variety of nauseating stimuli. Psychological and emotional factors may affect emptying as well, but the mechanisms involved are not well characterized.

The peripheral mechanisms are located on both sides of the pylorus. The gastric mechanisms are largely stimulatory and are triggered by distension of the stomach. Their regulatory role was probably overestimated by early experimental work carried out with simple crystalloid solutions. With complex, nutrient-containing meals, the intragastric volume is probably not the primary determinant of gastric emptying. The gut mechanisms, which are inhibitory, are probably more important. The key factors are the pH, osmolality and nutrient content of the material being emptied into the duodenum. If the duodenal load or the characteristics of the emptied material are not adequate, inhibitory mechanisms will reduce gastric emptying, even at the expense of an expanding intragastric volume. It is impossible to dissociate postprandial gastric emptying from gastric secretion in a physiological context since the gut regulatory mechanisms 'see' the whole of the gastric contents, which includes the meal itself and two to three times its volume in gastric juice,[39] pass through the pylorus.

Distal to the pylorus, inhibitory mechanisms appear to be arranged in a 'priority system', which sometimes allows stimulation of one receptor to override the effect on others. Volume and osmolality are probably more important factors than acidity, which exerts a more obvious inhibitory effect on gastric secretion than on emptying. The nutrient composition and load are also important. Protein, carbohydrates and lipids are all inhibitory for gastric secretion and, at least for liquid meals, there appears to be an inverse relationship between the energy content of the duodenal load and the rate of gastric emptying. The osmotic receptors are thought to reside in the duodenum, whereas the main acid-sensitive mechanisms are located in the first 5 cm of the duodenum.[10] The nutrient-sensitive areas extend much more distally into the jejunum. Therefore, nutrient load may be more important than initial concentration since a larger load means the nutrients are spread over a longer portion of the intestine where inhibitory mechanisms are located.

PANCREATIC SECRETION AFTER MEALS

Physiological concepts

It is estimated that each day the exocrine pancreas secretes about 1 litre of isotonic, alkaline juice containing 5 to 8 g of protein, most of which is digestive enzymes. Phospholipases and proteases are secreted as inactive precursors; other enzymes are secreted in active form. The functional reserve of the pancreas is enormous. Eighty to ninety per cent of the functional acinar mass must be absent before clinical evidence of malabsorption appears;[15] therefore, normal digestion of a meal occurs in a comfortable abundance of pancreatic enzymes. Most of the acinar mass of the pancreas is located in the head of the gland and drains into the proximal 40% of the main pancreatic duct, and accessory duct if one is present.[16]

The exocrine pancreas also secretes water and electrolytes, which have an important digestive function. The isotonic pancreatic juice increases duodenal flow and helps to solubilize nutrients at a concentration optimal for digestion and absorption. Its high bicarbonate content neutralizes acidic gastric chyme emptied into the duodenum and helps maintain luminal pH in the optimal range for most pancreatic enzymes to act. Small amounts of calcium, magnesium and zinc are also secreted by the pancreas, but their significance in relation to digestive function is unknown.

Fasting and postprandial patterns of exocrine pancreatic secretion

The secretory activity of the pancreas varies a great deal, as does gastric secretion, at different times of the day. During fasting, interdigestive motor complexes are synchronously associated with increased pancreatic secretion of enzymes, bicarbonate and water.[30, 79] Ingestion of an ordinary meal breaks the interdigestive motor–secretory cycles and produces a rapid increase in pancreatic secretion. As assessed by measuring duodenal enzyme output,[40] the pancreatic response to a meal begins as soon as the individual starts eating, reaches its peak within the first hour, plateaus and then gradually declines as the input of nutrients into the duodenum declines. This profile is quite monotonous and varies little for a wide range of meals and individuals (Figure 8.9). 'Maximal' pancreatic enzyme secretion is consistently caused by a wide range of meals (e.g. liquid formula meals, homogenized mixed meals, ordinary meals), as long as they contain protein and lipid, which are the main dietary stimuli to pancreatic enzyme secretion.[40, 52, 63] The main difference in enzyme response among these meals is in the duration rather than the magnitude of the response. On the other hand, responses to crystalloid test meals not containing nutrients have not exceeded 50% of the maximal pancreatic response.[34, 49]

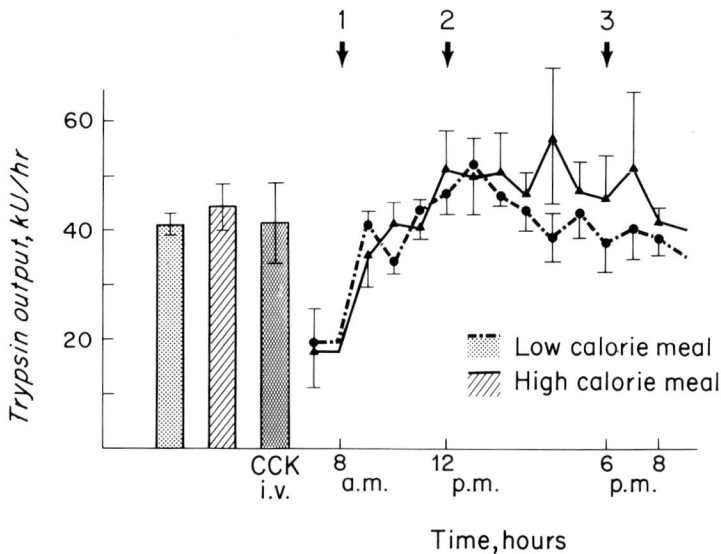

Fig. 8.9 Hourly output of trypsin during three liquid meals in healthy individuals. Ingestion of relatively low calorie meals (each 20 cal/kg body weight) and high calorie meals (each 40 cal/kg body weight) resulted in similar pancreatic enzyme responses. Modified from Brunner, H., *et al.* (1974) *Mayo Clinic Proceedings*, 49, 851–860.

Control of the pancreatic exocrine response to a meal

The physiological control of pancreatic secretion is overwhelmingly stimulatory, appears to lack a fine tuning system, and seems primarily directed to assuring an excess of enzymes whenever food reaches the duodenum. The pancreatic response to a meal is controlled by interacting neurohormonal mechanisms, whose relative contributions are poorly known. The hormones which physiologically affect pancreatic function seem to be the stimulatory hormones, cholecystokinin and secretin, and the inhibitory hormone, pancreatic polypeptide. Cholecystokinin is the most potent stimulant of pancreatic secretion. There also appears to be a potentiating interaction between secretin and cholecystokinin. Since cholecystokinin is situated in the upper gastrointestinal tract and is released by protein and lipid, it seems ideal that it should also act as messenger to stimulate pancreatic enzyme secretion for the digestion of these nutrients.

Secretin seems to have its primary effect on the ductal systems of the pancreas in stimulating bicarbonate secretion. This is important to generate the proper intraluminal pH for the activity of pancreatic enzymes, as well as for enteric enzymes. The importance of this action is illustrated in gastric hypersecretion, such as that which occurs in the Zollinger–Ellison syndrome, when intraduodenal pH may be reduced to a very low level; maldigestion and malabsorption can become so severe that they constitute the presenting complaint of the patient.

Sight, smell, taste and chewing of food generate a 'cephalic phase' of some importance in humans,[65] possibly accounting for a quarter to a third of the maximal response. It is mediated by the vagus nerve, in part through the release of antral gastrin. When food reaches the stomach, further stimulation of pancreatic secretion occurs. Gastropancreatic reflexes, such as those described in the dog,[76] and gastrin release may participate in this gastric phase of pancreatic response to a meal, but their relative contributions to postprandial secretion remains unknown.

When chyme reaches the upper small bowel, an intestinal phase of pancreatic secretion takes place. Whereas hormonal stimulation has long been thought to be the primary stimulatory mechanism, enteropancreatic vagovagal reflexes are now being recognized as being of major importance. Interruption of these reflexes may explain the diminished pancreatic response to intraluminal stimuli observed after vagotomy.[67, 68] Enteropancreatic reflexes may be critical in obtaining a rapid pancreatic response as chyme begins to flow into the duodenum, with hormonal mechanisms providing a sustained subsequent stimulus.

Inhibitory neural and hormonal mechanisms may also come into play in the regulation of postprandial pancreatic secretion. Glucagon,[17] whose serum concentration rises in the postprandial period, and other hormones and active peptides (vasoactive intestinal peptide, pancreatic polypeptide and somatostatin) have been shown to influence pancreatic secretion. It is impossible at this time to determine which of these mechanisms plays a physiological role in humans. Even less is known about the significance of neural inhibitory mechanisms.

The inter-relationships between gastric emptying, nutrient composition of chyme and the pancreatic response to a meal

Duodenal acid load is an important determinant of the volume and bicarbonate content of pancreatic secretion after a meal. The acid load is mostly gastric hydrochloric acid, but weak acids, such as fatty acids, may play a part.[50] Pancreatic enzyme secretion after meals depends largely on stimulation by protein, fat, and possibly calcium. Human perfusion studies have established the relative potency of luminal digestive products in stimulating pancreatic enzyme output (Figure 8.10). Fat appears to be the most potent stimulus, fatty acids and monoglycerides being the active components.[41, 42] With long-chain (C18) to medium-chain (C8) fatty acids, there is an inverse relationship between carbon chain length and potency to stimulate pancreatic secretion.[41] In humans, protein is another potent stimulus[18, 22, 42] because of the essential amino acids it contains (phenylalanine, valine, methionine and tryptophan). In our experience, luminal protein can achieve only about 60% of maximal pancreatic enzyme output.[42]

Calcium is also a potent stimulus to human enzyme secretion; magnesium has a weaker but significant effect. Both minerals exert significant stimulatory effects at duodenal concentrations above 6 mmol/l.[27, 43] It is questionable whether such luminal concentrations of ionic minerals are reached postprandially. Dextrose is ineffective as a stimulus; it is unlikely that the carbohydrate content influences the pancreatic response to a meal. The effects of alcohol inges-

tion on pancreatic secretion are confusing. Depending on the amount of alcohol administered and the experimental conditions, either net stimulation[37, 74] or net inhibition[46, 54] may be observed. The stimulatory effect of alcohol may be mediated through release of antral gastrin and stimulation of gastric acid output.[37, 74]

Accepting the premise that intestinal mechanisms are important in the control of postprandial pancreatic secretion, it is appropriate to investigate what segment and length of intestine are required to stimulate and sustain a normal response. Our studies[52] suggest that stimulation of the stomach and duodenum is sufficient to elicit a normal pancreatic enzyme response to a meal. It also corroborates the clinical observation that patients with malabsorption secondary to short-bowel syndrome do not generally benefit from enzyme therapy, since their malabsorption is not compounded by secondary pancreatic insufficiency.

BILIARY SECRETION AFTER MEALS

Physiological concepts

The complex structure of the biliary tract seems intended to obtain efficient utilization of a relatively small pool of bile acids. The enterohepatic circulation of bile acids is a conserving mechanism whose integrity is required for bile acids to reach physiological concentrations in the upper gut during digestion. The gallbladder exerts both reservoir and concentrating functions. A fraction of the bile flow is diverted into the gallbladder during fasting and is stored there until required. The biliary excretory system also has a distal sphincter (the sphincter of Oddi) whose function is poorly understood, but it is probably

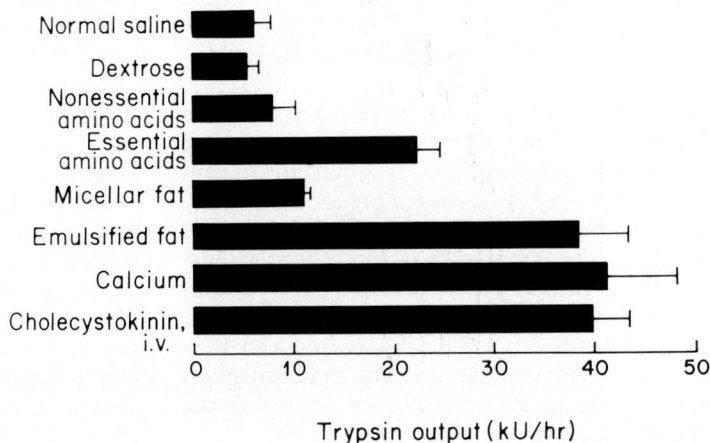

Fig. 8.10 Trypsin output during intraduodenal perfusion of digestive products in health. The stimulatory effect of emulsified fat and calcium is comparable to that of 'maximal' intravenous cholecystokinin. In contrast, nonessential amino acids and dextrose lack significant stimulatory effects. Micellar fat and essential amino acids lead to intermediate responses.

important in the regulation of bile flow into the intestine. The biliary system, unlike the excretory systems of other digestive glands such as the pancreas, depends on motor mechanisms as well as secretory mechanisms for the fulfilment of its physiological role.

Fasting and postprandial patterns of biliary secretion

During fasting, the cyclic changes seen in both the interdigestive motor activity and its secretory counterpart also involve the biliary system. In experimental animals and in humans, duodenal outputs of bile acids and bilirubin increase during phase II of the interdigestive motor cycle, reach peak values just prior to phase III activity, and decrease again to low levels during phase I.[30, 77] The storage capacity of the gallbladder is about 30 ml; up to 10 ml of gallbladder bile may be discharged into the duodenum with each interdigestive motor–secretory cycle, which occurs every one to two hours. Phase III probably propels fasting intestinal contents in the aboral direction;[78] therefore, interdigestive motor–secretory cycles probably coincide with an acceleration of the enterohepatic circulation of bile acids.

Ingestion of a meal disrupts the fasting cyclical pattern of motor and secretory activity and replaces it with the more continuous, although irregular, fed motor pattern. Secretory activity by the digestive glands also markedly increases postprandially. Both motor and secretory responses contribute to a rapid discharge of bile into the duodenum after meals. Contraction of

the gallbladder begins within a few minutes of the ingestion of food and reduces its volume by about two-thirds. After reaching a peak within the first postprandial hour, bile acid output usually remains at a high plateau, or declines slightly, until gastric emptying of the meal has been completed, at which time it returns to basal level. If the profile of duodenal bilirubin output is analysed rather than bile acid output, the early postprandial peak tends to be somewhat sharper; otherwise it is similar to that of bile acid output.

Control of the biliary response to a meal

Much of what is known about biliary discharge into the duodenum in response to intraluminal stimuli in humans has been gathered from perfusion studies. In response to single intraluminal nutrients, such as fatty acids or essential amino acids, duodenal outputs of bilirubin and bile acids rise sharply as the gallbladder contracts and discharges its contents, but then output drops quickly to a low plateau (Figure 8.11).[23, 41, 42] In contrast, after meals biliary output of bile acids is more sustained, reflecting the accelerating effect of feeding on the enterohepatic circulation of bile acids.[35, 36]

The similarity observed between luminal stimulation of pancreatic enzyme and biliary outputs is due to the fact that both systems share a number of neurohormonal stimulatory mechanisms, chiefly CCK; this causes gallbladder contraction,[38] produces relaxation of the sphincter of Oddi[21] and, as mentioned earlier, plays an important role in the stimulation of pancreatic

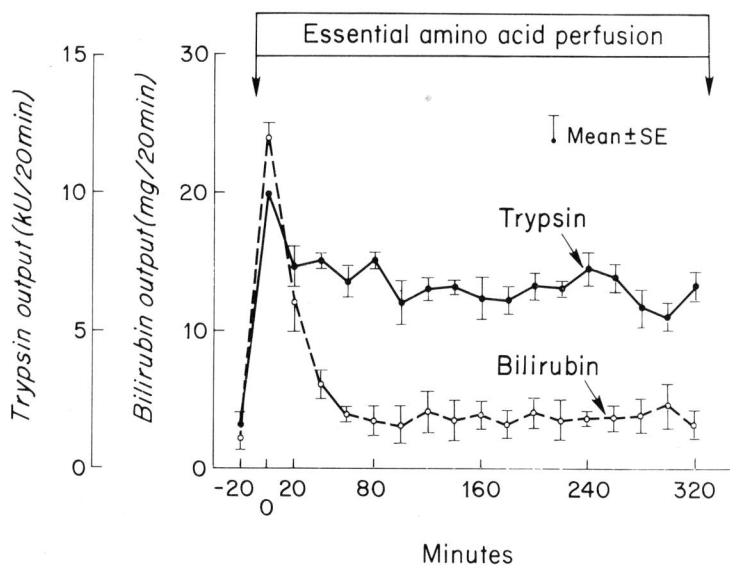

Fig. 8.11 Gallbladder and pancreatic response to essential amino acid perfusion in the duodenum in health. Gallbladder contraction at the onset of perfusion causes a sharp peak in bilirubin output followed by a low plateau. The pancreatic enzyme response is more stable since it depends largely on new synthesis and release of enzymes.

enzyme secretion. Secretin increases biliary flow by stimulating secretion of water and electrolytes (mainly bicarbonate) from both the pancreas and the biliary system. Secretin and glucagon may inhibit gallbladder contraction, although it is not known whether this is a physiological effect. Neural mechanisms may also be shared, but they have not been as well characterized. Cholinergic agonists contract and β-adrenergic agonists relax gallbladder smooth muscle. Vasoactive intestinal peptide immunoreactivity has been demonstrated in close association with gallbladder nerve fibres and may point to neuropeptide mediation of relaxation impulses.[64]

Among the inhibitory mechanisms, the luminal bile acid concentration appears to be an important modulator of biliary response to digestive products, fatty acids and amino acids.[41, 42] This effect of bile acids, which is also observed for pancreatic enzyme secretion, is exerted in part through changes in the rate of absorption of nutrients, chiefly fatty acids, which determine the length of proximal small bowel exposed to luminal stimuli. Again, the parallel effect of bile acids on pancreatic enzyme and biliary responses to nutrients suggests that the pancreas and biliary system share common regulatory mechanisms.

The relationship between physical state, nutrient composition of meals and postprandial biliary secretion

There is a greater variation in the biliary response to meals than that manifested by the exocrine pancreas, although the range of meals tested so far is small. When comparing the effect of meals ingested either in ordinary solid and liquid form or after thorough homogenization,[40] the ordinary meal caused a lower early peak bile acid output into the duodenum, but a more prolonged response, than the homogenized meal. It seems likely that initial emptying of the liquid phase of the ordinary meal (predominantly water and soluble carbohydrates) may have provided insufficient luminal stimulus to fully contract the gallbladder. However, the response would last longer after the ordinary meal because of the more gradual emptying of protein (meat) and fat (butter), which maintain a high level of stimulation.[11, 39]

The sustained plateau of duodenal bile acid output which follows the early rise is due to continuing recirculation of the bile acid pool after initial gallbladder contraction. Under constant

stimulation by chyme flowing through the duodenum, the gallbladder is largely bypassed, and the sphincter of Oddi remains relaxed, allowing bile acids returning to the liver from the intestine to re-enter the gut.[19] Studies in healthy volunteers ingesting three liquid meals per day suggest that the entire bile acid pool recirculates up to two times per meal.[14] However, the number of times that the pool circulates will vary depending on the size and composition of the meal and its rate of emptying from the stomach (Figure 8.12). In turn, enterohepatic

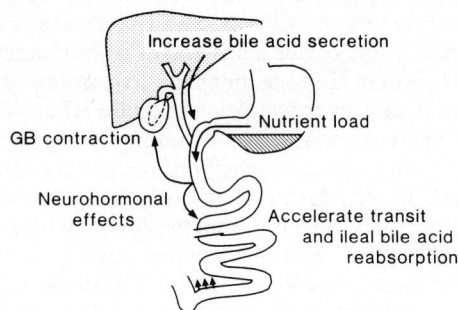

Fig. 8.12 Inter-relationships between nutrient load, neurohormonal stimulation of gallbladder contraction and small bowel transit, and biliary secretions of bile acids. Postprandial nutrient loads in the upper intestine cause gallbladder contraction and increase duodenal bile acid output. They also shorten transit along the small bowel with a corresponding increase in ileal bile acid reabsorption and acceleration of enterohepatic cycling. These effects are neurohormonally controlled.

bile acid recycling has significant effects on biliary lipid composition. Acceleration of the enterohepatic circulation of bile acids increases total biliary lipid secretion but, since the relationship between bile acid and cholesterol secretion is curvilinear, the molar percent of cholesterol in the bile, and hence its potential lithogenicity, decrease.

ACKNOWLEDGEMENTS

Dr Malagelada was the recipient of Research Career Development Award AM-00330 from the US National Institutes of Health. Dr Miller was supported by the Rappaport Foundation Clinical Investigator Award and by the Mayo Foundation.

REFERENCES

1   Abrahamson, H. (1973) The inhibitory nervous control of gastric motility. *Acta Physiologica Scandinavica* (Supplement), **390**, 1–38.
2   Andersson, S., Nilsson, G., Sjodin, L. & Uvnas, B. (1973) Mechanism of duodenal inhibition of gastric acid secretion. In *Nobel Symposium 16: Frontiers in Gastrointestinal Hormone Research* (Ed.) Andersson, S, pp. 223–238. Stockholm: Almqvist and Wiksell.

3 Baron, J. H. (1979) *Clinical Tests of Gastric Secretion.* New York: Oxford University Press.

4 Bueno, L. & Ruckebusch, Y. (1976) Evidence for a role of endogenous insulin on intestinal motility. In *Proceedings of the Fifth International Symposium on Gastrointestinal Motility* (Ed.) Vantrappen, G. pp. 64–69. Herentals, Belgium: Typoff-Press.

5 Carlson, H. C., Code, C. F. & Nelson, R. A. (1966) Motor action of the canine gastroduodenal function: a cineradiographic, pressure, and electric study. *American Journal of Digestive Diseases*, **11**, 155–172.

6 Chey, W. Y., Kim, M. S., Lee, K. Y. & Chang, T. (1979) Effect of rabbit antisecretin serum on postprandial pancreatic secretion in dogs. *Gastroenterology*, **77**, 1268–1275.

7 Clain, J. E., Malagelada, J.-R., Go, V. L. W. & Summerskill, W. H. J. (1977) Participation of the jejunum and ileum in postprandial gastric secretion in man. *Gastroenterology*, **73**, 211–214.

8 Code, C. F. & Schlegel, J. R. (1973) The gastrointestinal interdigestive housekeeper: motor correlates of the interdigestive myoelectric complex of the dog. In *Proceedings of the Fourth International Symposium on Gastrointestinal Motility* (Ed.) Daniel, E. E., *et al.* pp. 631–634. Vancouver: Mitchell Press.

9 Cooke, A. R. (1970) Potentiation of acid output in man by a distention stimulus. *Gastroenterology*, **58**, 633–637.

10 Cooke, A. R. (1974) Duodenal acidification: role of first part of duodenum in gastric emptying and secretion in dogs. *Gastroenterology*, **67**, 85–92.

11 Cortot, A., Phillips, S. F. & Malagelada, J.-R. (1981) Gastric emptying of lipids after ingestion of solid–liquid meal in humans. *Gastroenterology*, **80**, 922–927.

12 Csendes, A., Walsh, J. H. & Grossman, M. I. (1972) Effects of atropine and antral acidification on gastrin release and acid secretion in response to insulin and feeding in dogs. *Gastroenterology*, **63**, 257–263.

13 Debas, H. T. & Grossman, M. I. (1975) Chemicals bathing the oxyntic gland area stimulate acid secretion in dog. *Gastroenterology*, **69**, 654–659.

14 DiMagno, E. P., Go, V. L. W. & Summerskill, W. H. J. (1972) Impaired cholecystokinin-pancreozymin secretion, intraluminal dilution, and maldigestion of fat in sprue. *Gastroenterology*, **63**, 25–32.

15 DiMagno, E. P., Go, V. L. W. & Summerskill, W. H. J. (1973) Relations between pancreatic enzyme outputs and malabsorption in severe pancreatic insufficiency. *New England Journal of Medicine*, **288**, 813–815.

16 DiMagno, E. P., Go, V. L. W. & Summerskill, W. H. J. (1973) Intraluminal and postabsorptive effects of amino acids on pancreatic enzyme secretion. *Journal of Laboratory and Clinical Medicine*, **82**, 241–248.

17 Dyck, W. P., Texter, E. C., Lasater, J. M. & Hightower, N. C. (1970) Influence of glucagon on pancreatic exocrine secretion in man. *Gastroenterology*, **58**, 532–539.

18 Ertan, A., Brooks, F. P., Ostrow, J. D. *et al.* (1971) Effect of jejunal amino acid perfusion and exogenous cholecystokinin on the exocrine pancreatic and biliary secretions in man. *Gastroenterology*, **61**, 686–692.

19 Everson, G. T., Lawson, M. J., McKinley, C. *et al.* (1983) Gallbladder and small intestinal regulation of biliary lipid secretion during intraduodenal infusion of standard stimuli. *Journal of Clinical Investigation*, **71**, 596–603.

20 Fordtran, J. S. & Walsh, J. H. (1973) Gastric acid secretion rate and buffer content of the stomach after eating: results in normal subjects and in patients with duodenal ulcer. *Journal of Clinical Investigation*, **52**, 645–657.

21 Geenan, J. E., Hogan, W. J., Dodds, W. I. *et al.* (1980) Intraluminal pressure recording from the human sphincter of Oddi. *Gastroenterology*, **78**, 317–324.

22 Go, V. L. W., Hofmann, A. F. & Summerskill, W. H. J. (1970) Pancreozymin bioassay in man based on pancreatic enzyme secretion. *Journal of Clinical Investigation*, **49**, 1558–1564.

23 Go, V. L. W., Hofmann, A. F. & Summerskill, W. H. J. (1970) Simultaneous measurements of total pancreatic, biliary, and gastric outputs in man using a perfusion technique. *Gastroenterology*, **58**, 321–328.

24 Grotzinger, U., Bergegarth, S. & Olbe, L. (1977) The effect of fundic distension on gastric acid secretion in man. *Gut*, **18**, 105–110.

25 Hellemans, J., Vantrappen, G., Janssens, J. & Peeters, T. (1978) Effect of feeding and of gastrin on the interdigestive myoelectric complex in man. In *Proceedings of the 6th International Gastrointestinal Motility Symposium* (Ed.) Duthie, H. L. pp. 29–30. Lancaster, England: MTP Press.

26 Hinder, R. A. & Kelly, K. A. (1977) Canine gastric emptying of solids and liquids. *American Journal of Physiology*, **233**, E335–E340.

27 Holtermuller, K. H., Malagelada, J-R., McCall, J. T. & Go, V. L. W. (1976) Pancreatic, gallbladder, and gastric responses to intraduodenal calcium perfusion in man. *Gastroenterology*, **70**, 693–696.

28 Hunt, J. N. & MacDonald, I. (1952) The relation between the volume of a test meal and the gastric secretory response. *Journal of Physiology*, **117**, 289–302.

29 Jahnberg, T., Abrahamsson, H., Jansson, G. & Martinson, J. (1977) Gastric relaxatory response to feeding before and after vagotomy. *Scandinavian Journal of Gastroenterology*, **12**, 225–228.

30 Keane, F. B., DiMagno, E. P. & Malagelada, J.-R. (1980) Role of the migrating motor complex and its secretory counterpart on duodenogastric reflux in man. *Gastroenterology*, **78**, 1192 (abstract).

31 Kelly, K. A. (1970) Effect of gastrin on gastrin myoelectric activity. *American Journal of Digestive Diseases*, **15**, 399–405.

32 Knutson, U. & Olbe, L. (1973) Gastric acid response to sham feeding in the duodenal ulcer patient. *Scandinavian Journal of Gastroenterology*, **8**, 513–522.

33 Kotler, D. P. & Levine, G. M. (1979) Reversible gastric and pancreatic hyposecretion after long-term parenteral nutrition. *New England Journal of Medicine*, **300**, 241–242.

34 Krawisz, B. R., Miller, L. J., DiMagno, E. P. & Go, V. L. W. (1980) In the absence of nutrients, pancreatic–biliary secretions do not exert feedback control of human pancreatic or gastric function. *Journal of Laboratory and Clinical Medicine*, **95**, 13–18.

35 LaRusso, N. F., Korman, M. G., Hoffman, N. E. & Hofmann, A. F. (1974) Dynamics of the enterohepatic circulation of bile acids. *New England Journal of Medicine*, **291**, 689–692.

36 LaRusso, N. F., Hoffman, N. E., Korman, M. G. *et al.* (1978) Determinants of fasting and postprandial serum bile acid levels in healthy man. *American Journal of Digestive Diseases*, **23**, 385–391.

37 Llanos, O. L., Swierczek, J. S., Teichmann, R. K. *et al.* (1977) Effect of alcohol on the release of secretin and pancreatic secretion. *Surgery*, **81**, 661–667.

38 Makhlouf, G. M. (1979) Transport and motor function of the gallbladder. *Viewpoints on Digestive Diseases*, **11**, 1–4.

39 Malagelada, J.-R. (1977) Quantification of gastric solid–liquid discrimination during digestion of ordinary meals. *Gastroenterology*, **72**, 1264–1267.

40 Malagelada, J.-R., Go, V. L. W. & Summerskill, W. H.

J. (1979) Different gastric, pancreatic and biliary responses to solid–liquid or homogenized meals. *Digestive Diseases and Sciences*, **24**, 101–110.

41 Malagelada, J.-R., DiMagno, E. P., Summerskill, W. H. J. & Go, V. L. W. (1976) Regulation of pancreatic and gallbladder functions by intraluminal fatty acids and bile acids in man. *Journal of Clinical Investigation*, **58**, 493–499.

42 Malagelada, J.-R., Go, V. L. W., DiMagno, E. P. & Summerskill, W. H. J. (1973) Interactions between intraluminal bile acids and digestive products on pancreatic and gallbladder function. *Journal of Clinical Investigation*, **52**, 2160–2165.

43 Malagelada, J.-R., Holtermuller, K. H., McCall, J. T. & Go, V. L. W. (1978) Pancreatic, gallbladder and intestinal responses to intraluminal magnesium salts in man. *American Journal of Digestive Diseases*, **23**, 481–485.

44 Malagelada, J.-R., Longstreth, G. F., Summerskill, W. H. J. & Go, V. L. W. (1976) Measurement of gastric functions during digestion of ordinary solid meals in man. *Gastroenterology*, **70**, 203–210.

45 Marik, F. & Code, C. F. (1975) Control of the interdigestive myoelectric activity in dogs by the vagus nerves and pentagastrin. *Gastroenterology*, **69**, 387–395.

46 Marin, G. A., Ward, N. L. & Fisher, R. (1973) Effect of ethanol on pancreatic and biliary secretions in humans. *American Journal of Digestive Diseases*, **18**, 825–833.

47 Marks, I. N. & Shay, H. (1960) Augmented histamine test, Ewald test meal and Diagnex test. *American Journal of Digestive Diseases*, **5**, 1–23.

48 Mayer, G., Arnold, R., Feurle, K. *et al.* (1974) Influence of feeding and sham feeding upon serum gastrin and gastric acid secretion in control subjects and duodenal ulcer patients. *Scandinavian Journal of Gastroenterology*, **9**, 703–710.

49 Meeroff, J. C., Go, V. L. W. & Phillips, S. F. (1975) Control of gastric emptying by osmolality of duodenal contents. *Gastroenterology*, **68**, 1144–1151.

50 Meyer, J. H. (1975) Release of secretin and cholecystokinin. In *Gastrointestinal Hormones* (Ed.) Thompson, J. C. pp. 475–490. Austin: University of Texas Press.

51 Meyer, J. H., Thomson, J. B., Cohen, M. B. *et al.* (1979) Sieving of solid food by the canine stomach and sieving after gastric surgery. *Gastroenterology*, **76**, 804–813.

52 Miller, L. J., Clain, J. E., Malagelada, J.-R. & Go, V. L. W. (1979) Control of human postprandial pancreatic exocrine secretion: a function of the gastroduodenal region. *Digestive Diseases and Sciences*, **24**, 150–154.

53 Miller, L. J., Malagelada, J.-R., Taylor, W. F. & Go, V. L. W. (1981) Intestinal control of human postprandial gastric function: the role of components of jejuno-ileal. chyme in regulating gastric secretion and gastric emptying. *Gastroenterology*, **80**, 763–769.

54 Mott, C. B., Sarles, H., Tiscornia, O. & Gullo, L. (1972) Inhibitory action of alcohol on human exocrine pancreatic secretion. *American Journal of Digestive Diseases*, **17**, 902–910.

55 Mukhopadhyay, A. K., Thor, P. J., Copeland, E. M. *et al.* (1977) Effect of cholecystokinin on myoelectric activity of small bowel of the dog. *American Journal of Physiology*, **232**, E44–E47.

56 Pike, R. L. & Brown, M. L. (1975) *Nutrition: An Integrated Approach*, 2nd edn. New York: Wiley.

57 Preshaw, R. M. (1970) Gastric acid output after sham feeding and during release or infusion of gastrin. *American Journal of Physiology*, **219**, 1409–1416.

58 Rees, W. D. W., Go, V. L. W. & Malagelada, J.-R. (1979) Antroduodenal motor response to solid–liquid and homogenized meals. *Gastroenterology*, **76**, 1438–1442.

59 Rees, W. D. W., Go, V. L. W. & Malagelada, J.-R. (1979) Simultaneous measurement of antroduodenal motility, gastric emptying and duodenogastric reflux in man. *Gut*, **20**, 963–970.

60 Rees, W. D. W., Malagelada, J.-R., Miller, L. J., & Go, V. L. W. (1982) Human interdigestive and postprandial gastrointestinal motor and gastrointestinal hormone patterns. *Digestive Diseases and Sciences*, **27**, 321–329.

61 Richardson, C. T., Walsh, J. H., Cooper, K. A. *et al.* (1977) Studies on the role of cephalic-vagal stimulation in the acid secretory response to eating in normal human subjects. *Journal of Clinical Investigation*, **60**, 435–441.

62 Robinson, C. H. (1968) *Normal and Therapeutic Nutrition.* New York: Macmillan.

63 Ruppin, H., Bar-Meir, S., Soergel, K. H. & Wood, C. M. (1979) Effects of liquid diets on proximal gastrointestinal function. *Gastroenterology*, **77**, 1231 (abstract).

64 Ryan, J. & Cohen, S. (1977) Effect of vasoactive intestinal peptide on basal and cholecystokinin-induced gallbladder pressure. *Gastroenterology*, **73**, 870–872.

65 Sarles, H., Dani, R., Preselin, G., Souville, C. & Figarella, C. (1968) Cephalic phase of pancreatic secretion in man. *Gut*, **9**, 214–221.

66 Schaffalitzky de Muckadell, O. B. & Fahrenkrug, J. (1978) Secretion pattern of secretin in man: regulation by gastric acid. *Gut*, **19**, 812–818.

67 Solomon, T. E. & Grossman, M. I. (1977) Cholecystokinin and secretin release are not affected by vagotomy or atropine. *Gastroenterology*, **72**, 1134 (abstract).

68 Solomon, T. E. & Grossman, M. I. (1979) Effect of atropine and vagotomy on response of transplanted pancreas. *American Journal of Physiology*, **236**, E186–E190.

69 Stadaas, J. & Aune, S. (1970) Intragastric pressure-volume relationship before and after vagotomy. *Acta Chirurgica Scandinavica*, **136**, 611–615.

70 Stenquist, B. (1979) Studies on vagal activation of gastric acid secretion in man. *Acta Physiologica Scandinavica* (Supplement), **465**, 7–31.

71 Szurszewski, J. H. (1969) A migrating electric complex of the canine small intestine. *American Journal of Physiology*, **217**, 1757–1763.

72 Thomas, P. A. & Kelly, K. A. (1979) Hormonal control of the interdigestive motor cycle of the canine proximal stomach. *American Journal of Physiology*, **237**, E192–E197.

73 Thomas, P. A., Schang, J. C., Kelly, K. A. & Go, V. L. W. (1980) Can endogenous gastrin inhibit canine interdigestive gastric motility? *Gastroenterology*, **78**, 716–721.

74 Tiscornia, O. M., Gullo, L., Mott, C. B. *et al.* (1973) The effects of intragastric ethanol administration upon canine exocrine pancreatic secretion. *Digestion*, **9**, 490–501.

75 Uvnas-Wallensten, K., Efendic, S. & Luft, R. (1977) Vagal release of somatostatin into the antral lumen of cats. *Acta Physiologica Scandinavica*, **99**, 126–128.

76 Vagne, M. & Grossman, M. I. (1969) Gastric and pancreatic secretion in response to gastric distension in dogs. *Gastroenterology*, **57**, 300–310.

77 Vantrappen, G. R., Peeters, T. L. & Janssens, J. (1979) The secretory component of the interdigestive migrating motor complex in man. *Scandinavian Journal of Gastroenterology*, **14**, 663–667.

78 Vantrappen, G., Janssens, J., Hellemans, J. & Ghoos, Y. (1977) The interdigestive motor complex of normal subjects and patients with bacterial overgrowth of the small intestine. *Journal of Clinical Investigation*, **59**, 1158–1166.

79 Vidon, N., Hecketsweiler, P., Butel, J. & Bernier, J. J. (1978) Effect of continuous jejunal perfusion of elemental and complex nutritional solutions on pancreatic enzyme secretion in human subjects. *Gut*, **19**, 194–198.

80 Walsh, J. H., Richardson, C. T. & Fordtran, J. S. (1975) pH dependence of acid secretion and gastrin release in normal and ulcer subjects. *Journal of Clinical Investigation*, **55**, 462–468.

81 Weisbrodt, N. W., Copeland, E. M., Kearley, R. W. *et al.* (1974) Effects of pentagastrin on electrical activity of small intestine of the dog. *American Journal of Physiology*, **227**, 425–429.

DIGESTION AND MALABSORPTION OF NUTRIENTS

DIGESTION AND MALABSORPTION OF CARBOHYDRATE

Carbohydrates make up at least half of the energy intake of western man, and a greater proportion of dietary energy in underdeveloped countries. The important dietary carbohydrates are starch, sucrose and lactose. These compounds are not absorbed whole, but are first digested by intestinal enzymes to their constituent monosaccharides, which are the only form of carbohydrate which is absorbed in nutritionally significant amounts. Monosaccharides, which are absorbed only in the small bowel, enter the mucosal cells by specific transport mechanisms and thereafter gain entry to portal blood. The specificity of the digestive enzymes is limited and many ingested sugars cannot be cleaved to monosaccharides and thus are unabsorbable. These unabsorbable sugars include cellulose, the major constituent of plant cell walls, and simpler plant sugars such as raffinose and stachyose; these are now generally termed dietary fibre.

Physiology of digestion and absorption of carbohydrates

Assimilation of carbohydrate proceeds in three stages: luminal hydrolysis, mucosal (brush border) hydrolysis, and mucosal transport of monosaccharides.

LUMINAL HYDROLYSIS

Starch is a glucose polymer, of which 10–20% (depending on the source) is an α1-4 linked straight chain polymer known as amylose. The remainder, known as amylopectin, consists of α1-4 linked glucose chains with α1-6 cross links occurring about every 25 glucose units (Figure 8.13).

Digestion is initiated by salivary α-amylase in the mouth, but is rapidly halted by the low pH in the stomach. The bulk of starch is hydrolysed in the intestinal lumen by pancreatic α-amylase. α-Amylase can degrade only α1-4 bonds, and has lower affinity for α1-4 links adjacent to the ends of the glucose chains or to α1-6 cross links. The final products of luminal digestion of starch by amylase are therefore maltose, maltotriose, and five to eight unit glucose polymers containing both α1-6 and α1-4 bonds known as α-limit dextrins (Figure 8.13). Very little free glucose is released by the action of amylase. Pancreatic α-amylase is primarily a luminal enzyme, but some may bind to the mucosal surface and act with the brush border enzymes.

MUCOSAL BRUSH BORDER HYDROLYSIS

Since only monosaccharides can be absorbed actively, or to any nutritionally relevant extent, further degradation of ingested saccharides is necessary. The brush border enzymes involved are glucoamylase, sucrase–isomaltase, maltase, lactase, and trehalase. These enzymes are glycoproteins and have a large hydrophilic head portion containing the catalytic site orientated towards the intestinal lumen (Figure 8.14), and a

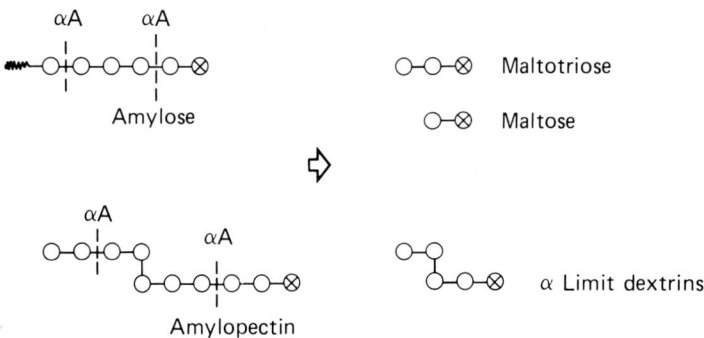

Fig. 8.13 Luminal digestion of starch by pancreatic α-amylase (αA). ○ = glucose units, ⊗ = reducing glucose unit. Horizontal links indicate α1-4 bonds, vertical links indicate α1-6 bonds.

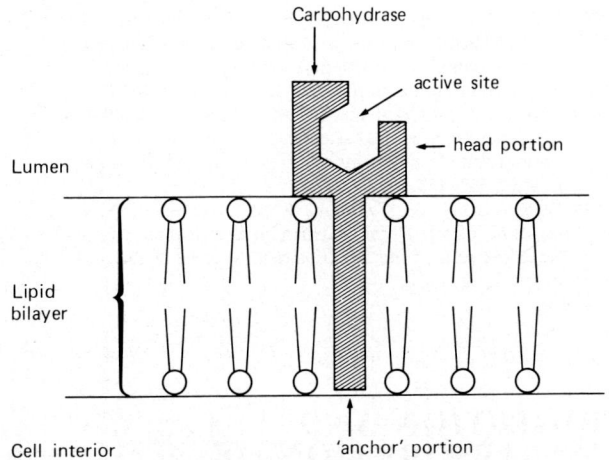

Fig. 8.14 Diagrammatic representation of the integration of brush border carbohydrases into the lipid cell membrane. Most of the molecule is the hydrophilic head portion containing the active site. The 'tail' anchors the head portion into the membrane.

smaller hydrophobic anchor intercalated into the brush border membrane. These brush border membrane carbohydrases are in a state of dynamic equilibrium maintained by the antagonistic actions of synthesis and degradation, the latter probably being effected to a large extent by pancreatic proteases.[2] As a result of these processes the half-life of brush border sucrase in the rat is as short as 2.5–6 hours.[24]

Glucoamylase can degrade linear α1-4 glucose chains from the non-reducing ends, liberating free glucose. All the α-glucosidases except trehalase can hydrolyse maltose to yield glucose and are therefore 'maltases'. Sucrase and isomaltase exist as a hybrid molecule composed of two non-identical subunits joined by disulphide bonds. This dimer is responsible for about 80% of the 'maltase' activity of the intestine and for more than 90% of the isomaltase activity. α-Limit dextrins are hydrolysed by the sequential action of glucoamylase and the sucrase–isomaltase complex[19] (Table 8.1 and Figure 8.15). Lactase (a β-glucosidase) hydrolyses lactose to release

the monomers glucose and galactose, and trehalase liberates glucose from trehalose.

Luminal and brush border enzymes act together to effect rapid hydrolysis of dietary carbohydrate to monosaccharides. This hydrolytic process occurs primarily in the upper and mid-jejunum. It is the capacity of the monosaccharide transport pathways, rather than enzymatic hydrolysis, which forms the rate-limiting step in absorption of most carbohydrates in health. Lactose, however, is exceptional because it is relatively slowly hydrolysed and lactase activity is the rate limiting step.[18] Despite the very rapid rate of hydrolysis of most carbohydrates, large amounts of monosaccharides do not accumulate in the intestinal lumen, suggesting feedback regulation of the hydrolytic enzymes by their products.[1] This mechanism is important in preventing the osmotic flux of fluid into the intestine which would occur in the presence of large quantities of unabsorbed intraluminal monosaccharides.

Table 8.1 Brush border hydrolysis of carbohydrates.

Carbohydrate	Enzyme	Action	Product
Sucrose	Sucrase	Hydrolysis of α1-4 link	Glucose, fructose
Maltose and maltotriose	Glucoamylase or sucrase	Sequential removal of glucosyl residues from non-reducing end	Glucose
α-limit dextrins	Glucoamylase or isomaltase	Initial removal of α1-4 linked glucosyl residues from non-reducing end	Glucose and oligosaccharide with terminal α1-6 linked glucose
	Isomaltase	Cleavage of α1-6 linked glucose residue	Glucose and malto-oligosaccharide
	Sucrase or glucoamylase	Hydrolysis of released malto-oligosaccharides (see Figure 8.15)	Glucose
Lactose	Lactase	Hydrolysis of β1-4 linkage	Glucose and galactose

Modified from Gray, G. M. (1981),[17] with kind permission of the author and the publishers, McGraw-Hill.

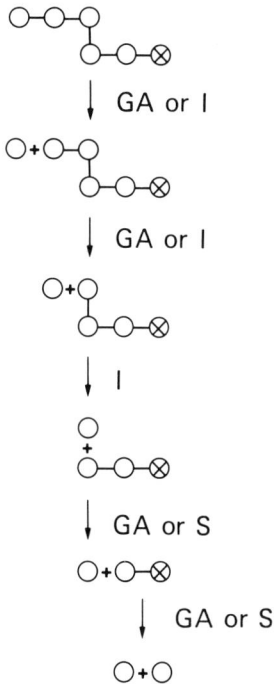

Fig. 8.15 Hydrolysis of an α-limit dextrin by sequential co-operative action of brush border carbohydrases. GA = glucamylase, I = isomaltase, S = sucrase. Other symbols as in Figure 8.13. The α-dextrin is degraded by sequential removal of glucose units from the non-reducing end. Adapted from Gray, G. M. (1981).[17]

MUCOSAL TRANSPORT

Glucose and galactose enter the mucosal cells via an active carrier system located in the brush border membrane first postulated by Crane.[7] Absorption is powered by an electrochemical gradient of sodium ions, such that the diffusion of sodium down its concentration gradient into the cell drives a carrier molecule which also transports glucose or galactose. The gradient of sodium across the cell membrane is maintained by the independent action of sodium–potassium ATPase in the basolateral portion of the cell wall (Figure 8.16). The energy required for this process is derived from the hydrolysis of adenosine triphosphate (ATP). Although the glucose transport molecule has not been isolated from the brush border membrane, studies with isolated brush border membrane vesicles[22] and artificial lipid vesicles into which brush border components have been inserted[8] provide strong evidence for their existence.

Fructose enters the mucosal cells by facilitated diffusion using a stereo-specific, sodium-independent carrier in the brush border.[40] Sugars probably leave the cell by facilitated dif-

fusion into the lateral intercellular spaces and thence into the portal blood.

Special, relatively sodium-independent carrier systems for monosaccharides liberated at the brush border by disaccharidase activity – so called 'hydrolase-related transport' – have been suggested in animals in vitro.[31] Such privileged transport would have the advantage of presenting high concentrations of monosaccharides for transport and would also minimize back-diffusion of monomers into the intestinal lumen. Although theoretically attractive, recent in vitro work suggests that the explanation for this effect is that liberation of monosaccharides by brush border enzymes achieves greater local concentrations at glucose transport sites than can be achieved by a random diffusion of the glucose through the unstirred water layer.[43] Indeed, no evidence for hydrolase-related transport has ever been produced in man.[12, 23]

Symptoms of carbohydrate malabsorption

The consequences of carbohydrate malabsorption are essentially the same whatever the defect in assimilation. If there is a defect in mucosal hydrolysis or transport, unabsorbed oligosaccharides and/or monosaccharides accumulate in the intestinal lumen. These molecules cause osmotic shifts of fluid and electrolytes from the plasma into the small bowel lumen. The stimulation of water and sodium absorption by sugar absorption is also reduced. The consequent dilatation of the small bowel is associated with crampy abdominal pain, and intestinal transit is accelerated.[26] Thus excessive amounts of fluid and sugar enter the large bowel. Volatile short-chain fatty acids, hydrogen and carbon dioxide are generated in the colon by bacterial fermentation. Colonic dilatation may contribute to the abdominal discomfort. The volatile fatty acids are osmotically active and the acid pH of the large bowel contents inhibits colonic absorption of water and electrolytes.[6] The combination of increased ileal inflow and impaired colonic absorption of water and electrolytes is sufficient to account for the diarrhoea of carbohydrate malabsorption.

Patients with carbohydrate malabsorption often present in childhood with failure to thrive, diarrhoea, distension, colicky abdominal pain, and sometimes vomiting after ingestion of the offending sugars. In infants, the stools are acid and watery (they may be mistaken for urine) and cause perianal excoriation. Free reducing sugars may be detectable in the stool using Clinitest tablets[25] or by chromatography. Fresh stool

Brush border
membrane

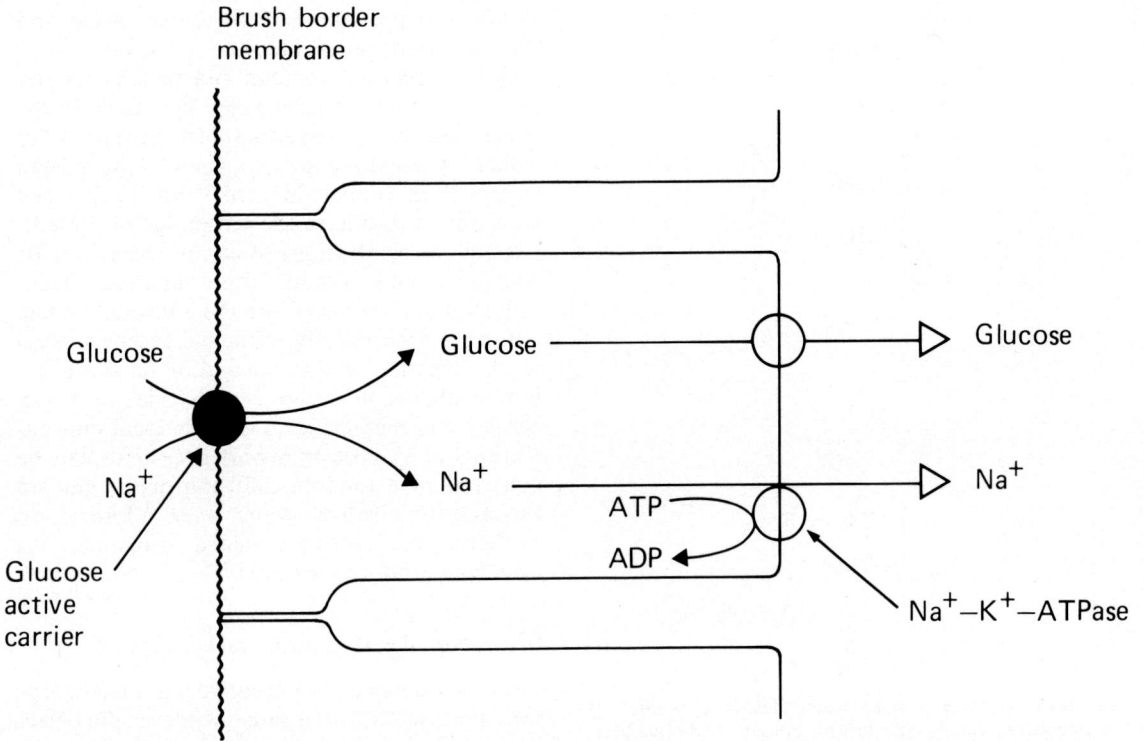

Fig. 8.16 Model of active transport of glucose across intestinal epithelial cells. Glucose enters the cell by an Na^+-dependent carrier molecule in the brush border, and leaves via a separate Na^+-independent carrier in the basolateral membrane. The energy needed to operate the brush border carrier is derived from the gradient of Na^+ across the cell membrane which is maintained by Na^+–K^+ ATPase.

must be tested since the sugars are rapidly destroyed by bacterial action. Severe dehydration and death may result from excessive loss of fluid and electrolytes.

Symptoms in adults are generally much milder because they have learnt to avoid the offending sugars. The timing of symptoms after ingestion of the particular sugar varies. Abdominal pain usually starts 5 to 60 minutes later and diarrhoea usually occurs after 30 minutes to 5 hours. In adults, a dose of at least 10 g of the poorly tolerated sugar is usually required to produce symptoms.

Specific disorders

Defective carbohydrate digestion secondary to pancreatic amylase deficiency is discussed in Chapter 17.

SUCRASE–ISOMALTASE DEFICIENCY
(ASUCRASIA)

Congenital deficiency of sucrase and isomaltase[45] is rare in adult practice in the United Kingdom. It has been said to occur in 0.2% of North Americans[36] and as many as 10% of Greenland Eskimos.[33] Its mode of inheritance is probably autosomal recessive.[3]

The severity of symptoms varies greatly. There may be severe and life-threatening diarrhoea, starting usually at about four weeks of age when sucrose is introduced into the diet. Symptoms in adults, however, may be mild and intermittent with flatus, abdominal griping and loose stools, which may be easily dismissed as the 'irritable bowel syndrome'. The relation to ingestion of sucrose should alert suspicion, but the patient or his parents may not volunteer or even be aware of this crucial information. Diagnosis is by demonstration of low or absent levels of sucrase in jejunal biopsy specimens. Levels of total maltase are also reduced to about 20% of normal, but all other brush border enzymes are normal, as is light microscopy of the specimen. Unless prior hydrolysis of sucrose has occurred in the colon, reducing sugars will be absent from the stools as sucrose itself is non-reducing. Treatment is by permanent avoidance of sucrose. There is no need to restrict starch because of the relatively small quantities of α-limit dextrins and isomaltase that result from its hydrolysis. The apparent increase in tolerance of sucrose with age is due to unconscious sucrose restriction.

The precise nature of the defect, whether enzyme deletion[19, 37] or functional abnormality of the enzyme molecule[13] is not known and, indeed, may not be the same in all affected subjects.

TREHALASE DEFICIENCY

Trehalose is an uncommon dietary sugar in man. It occurs in many insects, some worms and many lower plants, of which young mushrooms are most commonly eaten. In older mushrooms the trehalose is converted to glucose. Only one affected family has been described in whom autosomal dominant inheritance was suggested.[30]

LACTASE DEFICIENCY

Two forms of lactase deficiency are recognized. One is termed *congenital* or *infantile*, and the other *adult* or *acquired*, though the latter is probably also genetically determined.

Infantile lactase deficiency[21]
Infants affected by this rare defect present with diarrhoea and dehydration on introduction of milk feeds, leading to death if milk is not withdrawn. These children tolerate feeds containing monosaccharides, but have explosive diarrhoea if given lactose. The clinical history is, therefore, usually highly suggestive, but the definitive diagnosis is made by the demonstration of isolated severe hypolactasia in jejunal biopsy specimens.[27] Inheritance is probably by an autosomal recessive gene.[16]

A recent study of brush border lactase activity in infantile lactase deficiency has shown traces of lactase activity in some patients.[13] They found low levels of lactase in three out of four subjects, with reduced amounts of lactase protein, and absent enzymic activity and protein in the fourth. They suggested that this 'congenital' form of lactase deficiency is due to a defect in the regulation of lactase protein synthesis.

Congenital lactose intolerance[11] is an entirely different clinical and pathological condition which is mentioned here to avoid confusion. In this very rare condition there is excessive absorption of lactose possibly from the stomach rather than from the small bowel.[4] Lactosuria also occurs which is not a feature of lactase deficiency. Often familial, the illness is characterized by vomiting, failure to thrive and some diarrhoea with acidosis and aminoaciduria. Intestinal lactase activity is normal. Symptoms remit after treatment with a lactose free diet, and lactose tolerance returns to normal, usually between 12 and 18 months of age.

Adult lactase deficiency
The majority of adults worldwide have 'hypolactasia', but in caucasians lactase activity remains high in adult life and they are, therefore, in a sense the 'abnormal' group. Population studies have shown 'hypolactasia' in 50–90% of non-caucasians, but in only 2–30% of caucasians.[16] Brush border lactase activity does not appear in substantial amounts in utero until the 28th week of gestation and is therefore often low in premature infants. Lactase activity is highest in early infancy, decreasing during weaning to about one tenth of the maximum, at which level it remains throughout life. In caucasians the infantile level is preserved. The residual brush border enzyme in adult hypolactasia has the same molecular weight, optimum pH, and kinetic characteristics as the normal enzyme. Furthermore, it shares immunological determinants with normal lactase. Reduced amounts of enzyme protein have been detected on polyacrylamide gel electrophoresis[8, 13] and immunologically, using crossed immunoelectrophoresis.[41] In the latter study, enzymatic activity and the amount of lactase protein detected immunologically correlated well, suggesting that the low enzyme activity is due to a decreased amount of normal enzyme protein. The regulatory mechanism is unknown. Both adaptive and genetic theories have been proposed to explain the variation between populations.[38] Although prolonged feeding of large amounts of lactose can induce lactase activity in rats,[5] the effect is relatively small. Furthermore, in man, abstinence from milk does not reduce previously normal lactase levels[15] and lactose feeding does not increase intestinal lactase activity.[9] The evidence thus favours a genetic mechanism.

Symptoms in childhood are generally mild and in our experience are usually absent in adults because they avoid milk. It is therefore unwise to ascribe diarrhoea in adults to hypolactasia unless all other causes have been excluded, the symptoms are reproduced by normal amounts of dietary lactose, and the patient responds to a lactose-free diet.

Firm diagnosis is made by quantitative measurement of mucosal lactase activity in small bowel biopsy material. As little as 3 mg of a normal 10–25 mg biopsy is sufficient for diagnosis.[42] Stool pH may be a useful pointer to lactose intolerance in children,[44] but is normal in affected adults.[32] Oral lactose tolerance tests have a high incidence of false positive results when venous glucose levels are measured (a rise in venous glucose of less than 20 mg/100 ml after 50 g of lactose). The false positive rate can be reduced by infusing lactose into the duodenum and using capillary blood. Abdominal discomfort, borborygmi and diarrhoea after oral lactose are considered diagnostic.[10] Reduced quantities of $^{14}CO_2$ in the breath after ingestion of 50 g of ^{14}C-lactose,[39] and increased amounts of hydrogen in the breath after oral lactose,[28] due to bacterial fermentation of unabsorbed lactose in the colon are indirect measurements of lactase activity. They are probably more sensitive than measurement of serum glucose levels after lactose ingestion[35] and in particular the breath hydrogen test, which involves no isotopes, may be useful for population screening. These tests do not, however, substitute for the measurement of enzyme activity in biopsy material, although it must be remembered that hypolactasia in adults is usually asymptomatic.

CONGENITAL GLUCOSE–GALACTOSE MALABSORPTION[29]

The very existence of this condition is strong evidence for the validity of the concept of a carrier molecule for glucose and galactose in the mucosal cell brush border. In this rare condition the postulated glucose–galactose transporter appears to be defective or absent. Affected subjects present in infancy with severe diarrhoea and acid, glucose-containing stools following the first milk feed. Glycosuria may also be present. Unless glucose and galactose are withdrawn from the diet, the infant usually succumbs rapidly to diarrhoea and dehydration. Tolerance to carbohydrate is said to increase with age, although the transport defect persists and there is no evidence of development of 'hydrolase-related transport' of glucose.[12, 23] In vivo and in vitro studies have shown markedly impaired or absent sodium-coupled mucosal glucose uptake. Absorption of fructose, xylose and all amino acids so far tested are normal, as are brush border disaccharidase activities and light microscopy of the jejunal mucosa.[12, 23, 34, 45] The diagnosis of monosaccharide intolerance in an infant with a normal small bowel biopsy can be made by sugar tolerance tests, together with the finding of glucose in the stools after an oral glucose load. In vitro incubation studies[45] or in vivo perfusion studies[12, 23] may also be

employed. Treatment is by initial rehydration and correction of electrolyte abnormalities, followed by life-long avoidance of glucose- and galactose-containing foods. Dietary carbohydrate is supplied as fructose, which is absorbed normally.

REFERENCES

1 Alpers, D. H. & Cote, M. N. (1971) Inhibition of lactose hydrolysis by dietary sugars. *American Journal of Physiology,* **221,** 865–868.
2 Alpers, D. H. & Tedesco, F. J. (1975) The possible role of pancreatic proteasis in the turnover of intestinal brush border proteins. *Biochimica et Biophysica Acta,* **401,** 28–40.
3 Ament, M. E., Perera, D. R. & Esther, E. J. (1973) Sucrase–isomaltase deficiency – a frequently misdiagnosed disease. *Journal of Paediatrics,* **83,** 721–727.
4 Berg, N. O., Dahlquist, A., Lindberg, T. & Von Studnitz, W. (1969) Severe familial lactose intolerance – a gastrogenic disorder? *Acta Paediatrica Scandinavica,* **58,** 525–527.
5 Bolin, T. D., McKern, A. & Davis, A. E. (1971) The effect of diet on lactase activity in the rat. *Gastroenterology,* **60,** 432–437.
6 Christopher, N. L. & Bayless, T. M. (1971) Role of the small bowel and colon in lactose-induced diarrhoea. *Gastroenterology,* **60,** 845–852.
7 Crane, R. K. (1960) Intestinal absorption of sugars. *Physiological Reviews,* **40,** 789–825.
8 Crane, R. K., Menard, D., Preiser, H. & Eerda, J. J. (1976) The molecular basis of brush border membrane disease. In *Membranes and Diseases: International Conference on Biological Membranes* (Ed.) Botz, L., Hoffmann, J. F. & Leaf, A. pp. 229–241. New York: Raven Press.
9 Cuatrecasas, P., Lockwood, D. H. & Caldwell, J. R. (1965) Lactase deficiency in the adult. *Lancet,* **i,** 14–18.
10 Dawson, A. M. (1970) *Modern Trends in Gastroenterology.* (Ed.) Card, W. I. & Creamer, B. London: Butterworths.
11 Durand, P. (1958) Lattosuria idiopatica in cena paziente con diarrea cronica ed acidosi. *Minerva paediatrica,* **10,** 706–711.
12 Fairclough, P. D., Clark, M. L., Dawson, A. M. *et al.* (1978) Absorption of glucose and maltose in congenital glucose–galactose malabsorption. *Paediatric Research,* **12,** 1112–1114.
13 Freiburghaus, A. V., Dubs, R., Hadorn, B. *et al.* (1977) The brush border membrane in hereditary sucrase isomaltase deficiency: abnormal protein pattern and presence of immunoreactive enzyme. *European Journal of Clinical Investigation,* **7,** 455–459.
14 Freiburghaus, A. M., Schimitz, J., Schindler, M. *et al.* (1976) Protein patterns of brush border fragments in congenital lactose malabsorption and in specific hypolactasia of the adult. *New England Journal of Medicine,* **294,** 1030–1032.
15 Gilat, T. (1971) Lactase – an adaptable enzyme. *Gastroenterology,* **60,** 346–347.
16 Gray, G. M. (1978) Intestinal disaccharidase deficiencies and glucose–galactose malabsorption. In *The Metabolic Basis of Inherited Diseases,* 4th edn. (Ed.) Stanbury, J. B., Wyngaarden, J. B. & Fredrickson, D. S. pp. 1526–1536. New York: McGraw-Hill.
17 Gray, G. M. (1981) Carbohydrate absorption and malabsorption. In *Physiology of the Gastrointestinal*

Tract, (Ed.) Johnson, L. R. pp. 1063–1072 New York: Raven Press.

18 Gray, G. M. & Santiago, N. A. (1969) Disaccharide absorption in normal and diseased intestine. *Gastroenterology*, **51**, 489–498.

19 Gray, G. M., Conklin, K. A. & Townley, R. R. W. (1976) Sucrase–isomaltase deficiency. Absence of an inactive enzyme variant. *New England Journal of Medicine*, **294**, 750–753.

20 Gray, G. M., Lally, B. C. & Conklin, K. A. (1979) Action of intestinal sucrase–isomaltase and its free monomers on α-limit dextrin. *Journal of Biological Chemistry*, **254**, 6038–6043.

21 Holzel, A., Schwartz, V. & Sutcliffe, K. W. (1959) Defective lactose absorption causing malnutrition in infancy. *Lancet*, **i**, 1126–1128.

22 Hopfer, U., Nelson, K., Perrotto, J. & Isselbacher, K. J. (1973) Glucose transport in isolated brush border membrane from rat small intestine. *Journal of Biological Chemistry*, **248**, 25–32.

23 Hughes, W. S. & Senior, J. R. (1975) The glucose-galactose malabsorption syndrome in a 21 year old woman. *Gastroenterology*, **68**, 142–145.

24 Kaufman, M. A., Korsmo, H. A. & Olsen, W. A. (1980) Circadian rhythm of intestinal sucrase activity in rats: mechanism of enzyme change. *Journal of Clinical Investigation*, **65**, 1174–1181.

25 Kerry, K. R. & Anderson, C. M. (1964) A ward test for sugar in faeces. *Lancet*, **i**, 1981.

26 Launiala, K. (1968) The mechanism of diarrhoea in congenital disaccharide malabsorption. *Acta Paediatrica Scandinavica*, **57**, 425–432.

27 Launiala, K., Kuitunen, P. & Visakorpi, J. K. (1966) Disaccharidases and histology of duodenal mucosa in congenital lactose malabsorption. *Acta Paediatrica (Uppsala)*, **55**, 257–263.

28 Levitt, M. D. & Donaldson, R. M. (1970) Use of respiratory hydrogen (H_2) excretion to detect carbohydrate malabsorption. *Journal of Laboratory and Clinical Medicine*, **75**, 937–945.

29 Lindquist, B., Meeuwisse, G. W. & Melin, K. (1962) Glucose–galactose malabsorption. *Lancet*, **ii**, 666.

30 Madzarovova-Nohejlova, J. (1973) Trehalase deficiency in a family. *Gastroenterology*, **65**, 130–133.

31 Malathi, P., Ramaswamy, K., Caspary, W. F. & Crane, R. K. (1973) Studies on the transport of glucose from disaccharides by hamster small intestine in vitro. I. Evidence for a disaccharidase-related transport system. *Biochimica et Biophysica Acta*, **307**, 613–626.

32 McMichael, H. B., Webb, J. P. W. & Dawson, A. M. (1965) Lactase deficiency in adults: a cause of 'functional diarrhoea'. *Lancet*, **i**, 717–720.

33 McNair, A., Gudmand-Hoyer, E., Jarnum, S. & Orrild, L. (1972) Sucrose malabsorption in Greenland. *British Medical Journal*, **ii**, 19–21.

34 Meeuwisse, G. W. & Dahlquist, A. (1968) Glucose–galactose malabsorption: a study with biopsy of the small intestinal mucosa. *Acta Paediatrica Scandinavica*, **57**, 273–280.

35 Newcomer, A. D., McGill, D. B., Thomas, P. J. & Hofmann, A. F. (1975) Prospective comparison of indirect methods for detecting lactase deficiency. *New England Journal of Medicine*, **293**, 1232–1236.

36 Peterson, M. L. & Herber, R. (1967) Intestinal sucrase deficiency. *Transactions of the American Association of Physicians*, **80**, 275–283.

37 Preiser, H., Menard, D., Crane, R. K. & Cerda, J. J. (1974) Deletion of enzyme protein from the brush border membrane in sucrase–isomaltase deficiency. *Biochimica et Biophysica Acta*, **363**, 279–282.

38 Rosensweig, N. S. (1971) Adult lactase deficiency: genetic control or adaptive response? *Gastroenterology*, **68**, 431–436.

39 Sasaki, Y., Iio, M., Kameda. H. *et al.* (1970) Measurement of ^{14}C-lactose absorption in the diagnosis of lactase deficiency. *Journal of Laboratory and Clinical Medicine*, **76**, 824–835.

40 Sigrist-Nelson, K. & Hopfer, U. (1974) A distinct D-fructose transport system in isolated brush border membrane. *Biochimica et Biophysica Acta*, **367**, 247–254.

41 Skovberg, H., Gudmand-Hoyer, E. & Fenger, H. (1980) Immunoelectrophoretic studies on human small intestinal brush border proteins: amount of lactase protein in adult-type hypolactasia. *Gut*, **21**, 360–364.

42 Walter, W. M. & Gray, G. M. (1968) Enzyme assay of peroral biopsies. Storage conditions and basis of expression. *Gastroenterology*, **54**, 56–59.

43 Warden, D. A., Fannin, F. F., Evans, J. O. *et al.* (1980) A hydrolase-related transport system is not required to explain the intestinal uptake of glucose liberated from phlorizin. *Biochimica et Biophysica Acta*, **599**, 664–672.

44 Weijers, H. A., Van De Kamer, J. H., Dicke, W. K. & Ijsseling, J. (1961) Diarrhoea caused by a deficiency of sugar splitting enzymes. *Acta Paediatrica*, **50**, 55–71.

45 Weijers, H. A., Van De Kamer, J. H., Mossel, D. A. & Dicke, W. K. (1960) Diarrhoea caused by deficiency of sugar-splitting enzymes. *Lancet*, **ii**, 296–297.

46 Wimberley, P. D., Harries, J. T. & Burgess, E. A. (1974) Congenital glucose–galactose malabsorption. *Proceedings of the Royal Society of Medicine*, **67**, 755–756.

DIGESTION AND MALABSORPTION OF FAT

The normal human gut is capable of absorbing efficiently at least four times the average fat intake.[35] This large functional reserve means that absorptive mechanisms may be considerably impaired without causing overt problems.

The basic mechanisms may be summarized thus. Fat, usually ingested as triglycerides, is emulsified by mechanical action of the stomach. The emulsified fat is then broken down enzymatically (lipolysis) into free fatty acids and monoglyceride. These are rendered soluble in water as micelles by combination with bile acids, thereby being aided to cross the unstirred water layer to come into contact with enterocyte microvillous membranes. Diffusion of lipid across lipid membranes is passive. Once in the enterocyte, triglycerides are resynthesized by energy-dependent processes. Triglycerides are then enveloped in lipoprotein membranes and excreted into lymphatics as chylomicrons.

Variations in and details of these basic mechanisms are discussed below.

DIETARY FATS

The average daily dietary intake of fat in Britain is around 70 g. Most of this is in the form of

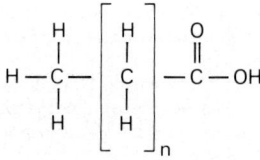

Fig. 8.17 A triglyceride molecule.

long-chain (hydrophobic) fatty acids combined with glycerol as triglycerides (Figure 8.17).

Some fatty acids – especially those derived from vegetables – have double carbon bonds. These are unsaturated fats perhaps of relevance to cholesterol metabolism and atheroma formation. From the point of view of absorption, they are largely indistinguishable from saturated fatty acids.

When there are eight, ten or twelve carbon atoms (i.e. n > 6, 8 or 10) in a fatty acid, they are classified as medium-chain fatty acids and triglycerides (MCT). The shorter hydrocarbon chain allows these fats (oils) to be soluble in water so their mechanism of absorption differs very significantly from long-chain fats. They are present in milk.

Shorter chain (volatile) fatty acids are water soluble, readily absorbed and are found mainly as a result of bacterial breakdown, especially of carbohydrate residues. In man, they are produced in the colon and are absorbed efficiently, at least in adults. They will not be discussed further.

Phospholipids are ingested in small quantity. Secretion by the liver is probably a major source of intestinal phospholipid.

Sterols are highly complex fats based on the cholesterol molecule (Figure 8.18). They are incorporated into micelles and chylomicrons. Vitamin D – in its various forms – is a substituted sterol. Clinically, sterols may be less well absorbed than other dietary fats in marginal malabsorption situations – for example causing osteomalacia – while absorption of other fats is generally efficient.

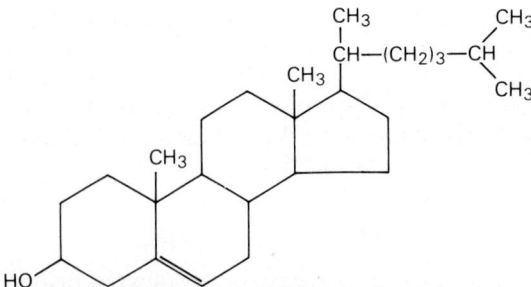

Fig. 8.18 A cholesterol molecule.

There are a few unusual fatty acids which may occur in the diet. For example, Brazil nuts contain a complex branched fatty acid which is rather poorly absorbed in man. It may be postulated that such a complex fatty acid fits poorly into the physical structure of a micelle.

INTRALUMINAL PHASE

Lingual and gastric lipases
There is unequivocal evidence of secretion of a lingual lipase.[21] This enzyme is present in the oesophageal pouch of neonates with oesophageal atresia. It is active in the absence of bile acids. Its pH optimum is 2.5–6.0 and therefore it may be active in the stomach, particularly in neonates. Fat absorption is not very efficient in neonates[12] since pancreatic lipase[59] and hepatic production of bile acids[56] are deficient at this time; lingual lipase may consequently be of some significance in neonates and especially in premature infants. It is particularly active in breaking down MCT, which comprise about 10% of human milk fat but up to 60% of the fat of some synthetic milk formulations for premature infants. It seems unlikely that lingual lipase is of functional significance in adults.

The work of Levy[30] has demonstrated – at least in the neonatal rat – that there is also lipase of gastric origin which differs in its biochemical characteristics from both lingual and pancreatic lipase. It is strongly activated by bile acids and so it may aid digestion in both the stomach and small bowel in the neonate. Like lingual lipase, it is particularly active with MCT.[22] In three infants with pyloric stenosis, one third of lipolysis took place in the stomach. Nasogastric feeding of premature babies causes less steatorrhoea than nasojejunal feeding.[38] By six to twelve months of age pancreatic function is sufficiently developed that gastric lipase is probably of no further physiological significance. However, both preduodenal lipases may be relevant in the presence of severe pancreatic insufficiency.

Emulsification
Lipase is active at water–fat interfaces. Breakdown of fat into fine particles is advantageous to lipolysis by increasing the area of the interface. The active motility of the gastric antrum is the major emulsifier.[36] Phospholipids aid emulsification. Those secreted by the liver are relatively resistant to hydrolysis compared with dietary phospholipids.

Bile acids have been thought to play a role in emulsification. However, they do not have true emulsifying action[31] and their role in facilitating lipolysis has other interpretations (see under Lipolysis, below).

Much theory of fat digestion and absorption is based on a two-compartmental model of an aqueous and a lipid phase in intestinal contents,[24] fat globules being acted on by a lipase, which releases fatty acids and monoglyceride which then enter the aqueous phase in micelles. Patton and Carey[39] observed a (liquid) crystalline phase of soap formation and a further phase – designated 'viscous isotropic phase' – containing unionized fatty acids. These latter two phases may be of relevance in removing the products of hydrolysis prior to micelle formation. Various attempts are being made to increase understanding of the physicochemical events during lipolysis.

Lipolysis

Gastric emptying following a meal stimulates pancreatic secretion and gallbladder contraction. For its efficient action, pancreatic lipase requires the presence of bile acids, colipase and a controlled pH. Bile acid metabolism will be discussed later (see Micelle formation). Interpretation of lipolysis studies is difficult and complex.[2, 19] For example, removal of hydrolysed fatty acids from the water–fat interface may be rate limiting, as indicated by the observation that albumin, added to an in vitro incubation medium as a fatty acid receptor, greatly increases the rate of lipolysis. Rates of mixing an in vitro incubation medium are important. Bile acids, by aiding micelle formation and fatty acid removal, increase lipolysis – but are thought to have other effects also. Colipase is extremely important for the binding of lipase to the fat–water interface, and much work prior to about 1973 was done with lipase 'contaminated by' colipase. Colipase and bile acids also prevent irreversible binding and inactivation of lipase on fat surfaces. Each of these effects may be different at differing pHs and furthermore differ with different chain lengths of substrate.

Colipase.

Colipase is a small protein, molecular weight about 11 000, secreted by the pancreas as a precursor, which is activated by trypsin. Optimally, it should be present in equimolecular concentration with lipase. Isolated colipase defects have not been described. There are probably two colipases.[11] It probably increases the rate of lipolysis by at least threefold.[57]

Pancreatic lipase. This is a protein of molecular weight about 52 000. Several children with apparently isolated pancreatic lipase deficiency have been studied.[53] In the presence of colipase and a physiological concentration (4 mmol/l) of bile acids, lipase is active over a pH range of 6–8, with a rapid fall-off in activity below pH 5 and irreversible inactivation below pH 4. The presence of bile acids without colipase drastically reduces its activity. Calcium ions probably increase lipolysis by aiding intermediate soap formation.

Lipase hydrolyses preferentially the outer (1: and 3:) fatty acids. Its action on 2:monoglycerides is weak, and this is probably advantageous in providing a mechanism for the entry of glycerol into the cell, where it is required for re-esterification.

Dietary phospholipid may be hydrolysed completely, but, when only partially hydrolysed, the fatty acid is mainly in the 1: position and this is probably of importance in the subsequent formation of chylomicrons.[5] Phospholipids of hepatic origin are relatively resistant to hydrolysis[3] so that there appears to be an enterohepatic circulation of bile phospholipids.

About 20% of dietary cholesterol is esterified and these esters are hydrolysed by a specific pancreatic enzyme.

MCT is readily hydrolysed by pancreatic lipase. Since medium-chain fatty acids are already water soluble, digestion and absorption are independent of bile acids.

Causes of deficient lipolysis. Disturbance of bile acid metabolism will be discussed later. Other causes of deficient lipolysis may be classified as impaired stimulation of the pancreas, obstruction of pancreatic secretions, and generalized or specific deficiency of pancreatic function.

Release of pancreatic secretions is stimulated by secretin and cholecystokinin (CCK, pancreozymin). Secretin is released by the small intestine in response to a pH of less than 4.5 and is responsible mainly for the release of bicarbonate (which prevents inactivation of lipase). CCK is released mainly from the duodenal and jejunal mucosa in response to amino acids, fat and an acid pH. It stimulates release of pancreatic enzymes including lipase and also stimulates gallbladder contraction, resulting in bile flow. Release of these hormones may be deficient in patients with small intestinal mucosal damage, for example coeliac disease.[7]

Obstruction of the pancreatic duct(s), for example by cancer of the head of the pancreas or ampulla of Vater, causes impaired pancreatic secretion. This is usually clinically associated with impaired bile flow, which is of equal relevance to fat absorption.

Pancreatic function may be lost due to resection, chronic pancreatitis of any aetiology, distal carcinoma (without main duct obstruction), cystic fibrosis or the Shwachman syndrome. The rare congenital lipase deficiency has already been referred to. Pancreatic secretions are reduced by vagotomy.[33] The acid inactivation of lipase is relevant in the Zollinger–Ellison syndrome. It is also relevant when administering pancreatic supplements therapeutically, their effectiveness being greatly increased by measures to reduce the acid medium of the stomach.[10]

Effects of deficient lipolysis. In the children with congenital lipase deficiency, about 50% of ingested fat is absorbed – and nutritional problems do not occur. Significant lipolysis takes place in the stomach, and pancreatic esterases other than lipase may play a role.

The physiological reserve of pancreatic exocrine function is great. About 70% of the pancreas can be resected without causing malabsorption.[27, 28] When 95% of human pancreas is resected, lipase activity is about 10% of normal and bicarbonate output is restricted, but absorption of fat remains at about 80% on a normal diet. This fits in with the observation that fat lipolysis is physiologically almost complete by the duodenojejunal junction.[25]

Micelle formation

A micelle is a molecular complex with a very variable 'molecular' weight of the order of 30 000, comprising bile acids, fatty acids, monoglycerides, and often phospholipid, cholesterol and fat-soluble vitamins. It is the bifacial structure of bile acids – one hydrophilic and one hydrophobic face – that enables micelles to disperse fatty molecules in the aqueous phase of intestinal contents.[24]

Why solubilize? The ability of bile acids to form micelles to disperse fats is important for the following reasons:

1 Lipolysis is impaired if the liberated fatty acids have no 'receptor' (see above). The natural in vivo receptor is the micelle, which accepts the liberated fatty acids and monoglycerides from the fat–water interface into the aqueous medium.
2 Drops of oil undispersed would make contact only with very small areas of intestinal mucosa.

3 Energy changes during absorption in experiments increasing mixing and stirring[58] indicate that the diffusion across the unstirred water layer is rate-limiting for fat absorption. Hofmann[24] has calculated that micelle solubilization increases the diffusion flux through the unstirred layer by a factor of 100–200. The micelle solubility of various fats will therefore determine the capacity of the gut to absorb that fat.

Physicochemical considerations.[24] There is a minimum concentration of bile acids required for micelle formation – the 'critical micelle concentration' – which is around 4 mmol/l.

Fatty acid chain length has an inverse logarithmic effect on solubility in water; for example an increase in chain length from eight to fourteen results in a decrease in solubility of some 10 000-fold. MCT (of chain length eight to twelve) may be absorbed without micelle formation.

Longer chain fatty acids are also less soluble in bile acid solution (micelles) but the solubility change between chain lengths eight and fourteen is merely 10-fold. Ionization aids micelle solubility but long-chain saturated fatty acids are largely unionized. On the other hand, long-chain unsaturated fatty acids have an apparent pK of about 6.5 and thus a significant proportion of these fatty acids will be ionized at normal intestinal pH (but less so if the jejunum is acid, as in Zollinger–Ellison syndrome or associated with pancreatic insufficiency). Soaps are infinitely soluble in micelles.

Monoglycerides are more micelle soluble than free fatty acids and they compete with fatty acid solubilization. Di- and triglycerides are relatively insoluble.

Cholesterol dissolves in the centre of a micelle, and its solubility is increased by the presence of fatty acid and monoglyceride – explaining in part the increase in blood cholesterol levels associated with high fat diets.

The rate of flux of fats between the micelle and aqueous phases is not known. It seems likely that micelles come into direct contact with the lipid enterocyte membrane before releasing the fats for absorption.

Physiology of bile acids[18]

Hepatic synthesis and secretion. Bile acids are synthesized from cholesterol in the liver by the addition of one or two hydroxyl groups, removal of the double bond and addition of a side-chain. The rate-limiting step is the addition of a hydroxyl group in the 7α position. 7α-Hydroxylase activity increases or decreases as the pool size decreases or increases respectively, although the mechanism for this feedback has not been determined. The bile acids are conjugated with glycine or taurine in a ratio of about 3 : 1. The main bile acids synthesized are cholic acid (CA) and chenodeoxycholic acid (CDCA).

The appearance of bile acid in the duodenum usually follows gallbladder contraction; CCK stimulates gallbladder contraction but also appears to stimulate hepatic flow of bile.

Bile acid absorption and enterohepatic circulation. Bile acids are absorbed actively from the lower small bowel. The efficiency of absorption is about 95%. It is an active, saturatable mechanism and there is competition between related bile acids.[29] There is also some absorption of bile acids from the colon.

Bacteria – mainly in the colon but also in the distal ileum in health – dehydroxylate bile acids at the 7 position, producing deoxycholic acid (DCA) from CA and lithocholic acid (LCA) from CDCA. DCA and LCA are known as secondary bile acids. LCA is sulphated by the liver and the sulphated form is very poorly reabsorbed, so it is rapidly excreted in the stool. Some details of the differential efficiency of the absorption of various bile acids have been described by Hepner, Hofmann and Thomas[23] and these lead to the components of the body pool of bile acids varying significantly from the respective rates of hepatic synthesis. Twice as much CA is produced as CDCA but the latter is reabsorbed more efficiently. CA makes up about 45% of the pool, CDCA about 33%, DCA about 18% and LCA about 4%, the total pool size being around 2.5 g. Bile acids (except LCA) remain in the body an average of three to four days, with five to ten cycles per day. The pool size varies inversely with the frequency of enterohepatic cycling,[32] reflecting the 5% loss of bile acids with each cycle. Coeliac patients, with sluggish CCK release, have a large pool, while cholecystectomized patients have a small pool. In disease involving loss of bile acids, the liver may increase its rate of synthesis ten- to twenty-fold.[26]

Causes of deficient bile acids. Deficiency of bile acids may result from deficient hepatic synthesis or impaired flow or recycling.

One infant has been described[42] with a congenital deficiency (but not absence) of bile acid synthesis. Premature infants have low intraluminal bile acid levels[47] probably due to low hepatic synthesis.

Steatorrhoea is common in patients with chronic liver disease, and is greater than 15–20 g per day in 15–20% of such patients. The mechanism is not clear. Some of the affected patients may be alcoholics with concomitant pancreatic disease. CA production is markedly reduced while CDCA synthesis is generally maintained.[55] Renal clearance of bile acids is greater in patients with liver disease, related to increased sulphation,[49] and shunting of bile acids away from the liver causes markedly elevated systemic blood levels, increasing renal loss. However, renal loss accounts for only about 5% of hepatic synthesis in cirrhotic patients. Impaired gallbladder contraction in response to CCK in cirrhotic patients has been shown by Turnberg and Grahame,[54] but they concluded that the alterations in bile acid metabolism and flow were insufficient to account for the observed steatorrhoea. Cholestasis, intra- or extrahepatic, causes intraluminal bile acid deficiency.

The most important long-term cause of disturbance of the enterohepatic recycling of bile acid arises from loss of functioning ileum, usually from bypass, resection or involvement with Crohn's disease. Ileal resections of greater than 100 cm are likely to be associated with greatly increased faecal bile acid loss and gross steatorrhoea, in spite of a ten- to twenty-fold increase in hepatic synthesis rates.

Overgrowth of many bacterial species in the small intestine, from whatever cause, results in dehydroxylation of bile acids, rendering them insoluble and, therefore, ineffective in the aqueous medium of the small intestine.[50] Other bacteria deconjugate bile salts, thereby facilitating their reabsorption in the jejunum. The very low intraluminal pH associated with the Zollinger–Ellison syndrome[17] and administration of neomycin[52] may also cause precipitation of bile salts.

Effects of deficient bile acids. Children with total biliary obstruction absorb 50% of ingested fat.[14] Bile fistula rats absorb long-chain fats rather efficiently, but most of it is absorbed into the portal vein.[13] In one adult with a bile fistula, 70% of ingested fat was absorbed.[41] In more complex adult clinical situations, patients with extensive distal small bowel resections usually absorb 75% more of ingested fat in spite of disturbance of bile acids and loss of absorptive surface.[26]

MEMBRANE PHASE

Physiology

Micelle formation and dispersion through the aqueous medium of the intestinal lumen increases the diffusion rate of fats through the unstirred layer by 100- to 200-fold.[24] Wilson, Sallee and Dietschy[58] have argued convincingly that diffusion through the unstirred layer is the rate-limiting step for fat absorption in their in vitro system. This is probably also true physiologically, at least for those fats which enter easily into micelles.

Absorption across the lipid surface of the enterocyte is passive, and is not changed by a reduction of temperature from 37°C to 0°C (although this temperature difference greatly affects the intraluminal fate of the fat).

The old story that pinocytosis occurs through the enterocyte membrane is dead. The evidence for this was based on very rare electron microscopy pictures, but these pictures proved extremely difficult to obtain in spite of the absorption of large amounts of fat. Lipid can diffuse through lipid, and there is no need to postulate any other mechanism.

One question – as yet unanswered – is how the micelle breaks up, allowing free bile acids to return through the unstirred layer to the main lumen, at least in the upper small intestine from which bile acid absorption is slow. It may be that the fat emerges readily when the micelle is in physical contact with the enterocyte membrane. At any rate, there is nothing to suggest that such a step is rate limiting or energy dependent.

Pathology

The observation of Masterton, Lewis and Widdowson,[35] that healthy man can absorb efficiently (more than 96%) some 260 g ingested fat per day indicates that there is a large functional reserve. There is good evidence in animals that the ileum adapts to the presence of intraluminal fat.[34] A large part of the upper small intestine may therefore probably be lost – for example by resection or functionally by coeliac disease – without causing significant net malabsorption. However, the faecal fat output may sometimes be raised, depending on variables such as the fat content of individual meals or intestinal hurry. (Coeliac disease also affects gallbladder function – see above.) Loss of or damage to the distal small intestine will cause problems related to bile acid absorption but the patient also loses some of the mucosal reserve capacity.

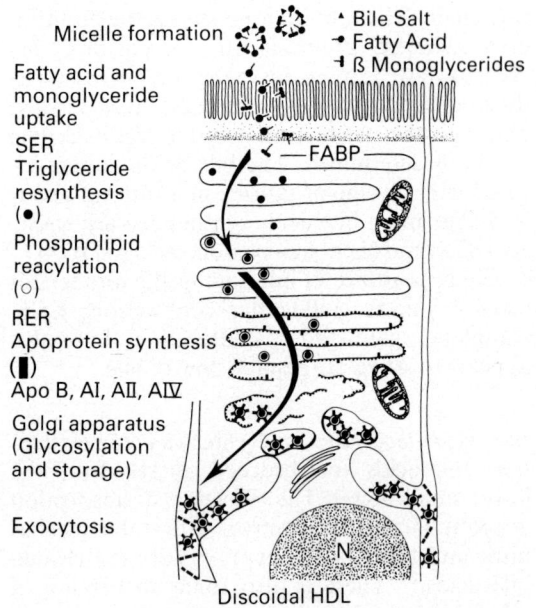

Fig. 8.19 Schematic representation of an intestinal epithelial cell during fat absorption. FABP = Fatty acid binding protein. From Glickman, R. and Ley, J. R. (1979), *American Journal of Medicine*, 67: 984, with kind permission of the authors and the editor.

ENTEROCYTE PHASE (FIGURE 8.19)

Fatty acid binding protein

Substances which cross membranes by simple diffusion can diffuse in both directions. While bile acid concentrations may not be optimal on the luminal side of the enterocyte membrane for removal of fat into the lumen, nonetheless some fat exsorption would be expected, for example in the post-prandial state, in the absence of a 'capturing' mechanism. (Some exsorption occurs from gastric cells.)

Such a tendency in the small bowel is greatly reduced by fatty acid binding protein (FABP). It is a protein (or proteins) of molecular weight about 12 000 found in the cytosol of human (and rat) enterocytes, as well as in other tissues such as liver, myocardium, kidney and adipose tissue. Its role[37] is to bind absorbed fatty acids and to transport them to the smooth endoplasmic reticulum where re-esterification takes place. It has further been shown that, due to reduction in free energy when fatty acids adsorb to the enterocyte membrane, energy would be required to desorb it if there were no carrier present.[45]

Whereas long-chain fatty acids at this stage enter a metabolic and spatial pathway in the enterocyte, MCT being water soluble appears to diffuse through the cytosol. Various of the enzymes concerned in the long-chain fatty acid pathway have been shown to have reduced affinity for MCT. This may apply to FABP.

Cholesterol is probably not bound by FABP. It is released only slowly from the enterocyte membrane and much is 'lost' back into the lumen, partly by desquamation but also perhaps by diffusion.

Re-esterification. Following a meal, droplets of triglycerides are first identified in the smooth endoplasmic reticulum in the apical portion of the enterocyte below the microvillous membrane.[6] The fatty acid esterases have been localized chemically to the same site. Re-esterification helps to maintain a concentration gradient for fatty acids across the enterocyte membrane by acting as a receptor from FABP.

The re-esterification of fatty acids goes by way of acyl-CoA and requires two high-energy bonds. In the absence of monoglyceride, pathways are present for the synthesis of triglycerides via glycerol phosphate or dihydroxyacetone phosphate. These substrates can also be converted to phospholipids if the latter are not being absorbed. (Phospholipids are required later for chylomicron synthesis.)

Chylomicron formation
Chylomicrons form in the Golgi apparatus. The transport of triglycerides from the smooth endoplasmic reticulum, however, appears to depend on lipoproteins and phospholipids (constituents of chylomicrons), which themselves are synthesized in the rough endoplasmic reticulum.[4] Morphologically, with time triglycerides pass slowly through the endoplasmic reticulum, but, apart from the importance of lipoproteins and phospholipids, nothing is known of the mechanism, nor of the initial complex of lipoproteins, phospholipid and fat.

Chylomicrons, which contain about 1% protein, do not form in patients with a beta-lipoproteinaemia or in animals in which protein synthesis has been inhibited. In patients with beta-lipoprotein deficiency, triglyceride remains primarily at the cell apex.[8] There are suggestions from animal work that alpha-lipoproteins are not essential for chylomicron formation, although they are normally the major protein component.

There is great interest currently in intestinal synthesis of lipoproteins since the gut contributes greatly to those proteins with which cholesterol is transported. The interrelationship is complex,[20] but beta-lipoproteins are identified with very-low-density and low-density lipoproteins and alpha-lipoproteins with high-density lipoproteins. However, at least three different

alpha-lipoproteins and others designated C and E have been described. Although the liver and other tissues also synthesize these proteins, the gut is a significant site of synthesis.[15] Gut synthesis of these proteins is impaired in kwashiorkor leading to accumulation of fat within the enterocyte.[51] Aspects of lipoprotein metabolism are discussed elsewhere (p. 689).

The elegant study of Glickman, Perrotto and Kirsch[16] suggests that chylomicrons are transferred from the Golgi apparatus to the laterobasal membrane via the microtubular system. Electron microscopic studies suggest that the chylomicrons fuse with the membrane and are then discharged into the intercellular space by reverse pinocytosis.

In intact man, long-chain fatty acids are absorbed predominantly by this route and thereafter pass into the lymphatics. Nonetheless, some long-chain fats are absorbed into the portal vein, and work in rats[13] suggests that the portal vein route may be of increased importance in states of bile acid deficiency.

Medium-chain triglycerides are absorbed without chylomicron formation into the portal vein. Little is known of the mechanism but simple diffusion is probably dominant.

SOME GENERAL CONSIDERATIONS

The process of fat absorption is highly complex, requiring the co-operation and integration of gut motility, pancreatic and biliary secretions, and uptake and re-export by the enterocyte. At many stages this complicated mechanism may be upset, particularly by pancreatic or small intestinal mucosal disease. In addition a number of other factors are relevant.

Severe malnutrition with protein starvation causes poor enterocyte structure, enzyme deficiency and reduced lipoprotein formation, resulting in fat malabsorption. Acute starvation leads to a decrease in many enzymes associated with the enterocyte phase, while high-fat diets increase the relevant enzyme activities, particularly in the ileum.[5] Ileal adaptation occurs when jejunum is resected. Various drugs can interfere: neomycin interferes with micelle formation, probably through its polybasic structure.[52] Cholestyramine is also polybasic, and is used therapeutically to bind bile salts. Its effect in preventing bile acid catharsis in patients with small ileal resection is thus usually associated with a modest increase in fat excretion. Alcohol has multiple effects on the enterocyte both structurally and enzymatically.[1] Hormonal effects are also apparent: hypophysectomy decreases bile acid turnover rates, and growth hormone deficiency causes decreased intraluminal bile acid levels.[40]

Despite the complexities outlined in this article, it is relevant to note again that in man the process of fat absorption has a large functional reserve, so that considerable impairment of the mechanisms may occur before steatorrhoea results.

REFERENCES

1 Baraona, R., Pirola, R. C. & Lieber, C. S. (1975) Acute and chronic effects of ethanol on intestinal lipid metabolism. *Biochimica et Biophysica Acta*, **388**, 19–28.

2 Borgstrom, B. (1975) On the interactions between pancreatic lipase and colipase and the substrate, and the importance of bile salts. *Journal of Lipid Research*, **16**, 411–417.

3 Boucrot, P. (1972) Is there an entero-hepatic circulation of the bile phospholipids? *Lipids*, **7**, 282–288.

4 Brindley, D. N. (1974) The intraluminal phase of fat absorption. In *Biomembranes, Intestinal Absorption* Volume 4B (Ed.) Smyth, D. H. pp. 621–671. London, New York: Plenum Press.

5 Brindley, D. N. (1977) Absorption and transport of lipids in the small intestine. *Excerpta Medica*, **391**, 350–362.

6 Cardell, R. R., Badenhausen, S. & Porter, K. R. (1967) Intestinal triglyceride absorption in the rat – an electron microscopical study. *Journal of Cell Biology*, **34**, 123–155.

7 Di Magno, E. P., Go, V. L. W. & Summerskill, W. H. J. (1972) Impaired cholecystokinin–pancreozymin secretion, intraluminal dilution, and maldigestion of fat in sprue. *Gastroenterology*, **62**, 25–32.

8 Dobbins, W. O. (1966) An ultrastructural study of the intestinal mucosa in congenital β-lipoprotein deficiency with particular emphasis upon the intestinal absorptive cell. *Gastroenterology*, **50**, 195–210.

9 Dobbins, W. O. (1968) Drug-induced steatorrhea. *Gastroenterology*, **54**, 1193–1195.

10 Durie, P. R., Bell, L., Linton, W. *et al.* (1980) Effect of cimetidine and sodium bicarbonate on pancreatic replacement therapy in cystic fibrosis. *Gut*, **21**, 778–786.

11 Erlanson, C. M., Charles, M., Astier, M. & Desnuelle, P. (1974) The primary structure of co-lipase II. *Biochimica et Biophysica Acta*, **359**, 198–203.

12 Fomon, S. J., Ziegler, E. E., Thomas, L. N. *et al.* (1970) Excretion of fat by normal full-term infants fed various milks and formulas. *American Journal of Clinical Nutrition*, **23**, 1299–1313.

13 Gallagher, N., Webb, J. & Dawson, A. M. (1965) The absorption of ^{14}C oleic acid and ^{14}C triolein in bile fistula rats. *Clinical Science*, **29**, 73–82.

14 Glasgow, J. F. T., Hamilton, J. R. & Sass-Kortsak, A. (1973) Fat absorption in congenital obstructive liver disease. *Archives of Diseases in Childhood*, **48**, 601–607.

15 Glickman, R. M. & Green, P. H. R. (1977) The intestine as a source of apolipoprotein A_1. *Proceedings of the National Academy of Sciences*, **74**, 2569–2573.

16 Glickman, R. M., Perrotto, J. L. & Kirsch, K. (1976) Intestinal lipoprotein formation: effect of colchicine. *Gastroenterology*, **70**, 347–352.

17 Go, V. L. W., Poley, J. R., Hofmann, A. F. & Summerskill, W. H. J. (1970) Disturbances in fat digestion induced by acidic jejunal pH due to gastric hypersecretion in man. *Gastroenterology*, **58**, 638–646.

18 Goldman, M. A., Schwartz, C. C., Swell L. & Vlahcevic, Z. R. (1979) Bile acid metabolism in health and disease. *Progress in Liver Diseases*, **6**, 225–241.

19 Granon, S. & Semeriva, M. (1980) Effect of taurodeoxycholate, colipase and temperature on the interfacial inactivation of porcine pancreatic lipase. *European Journal of Biochemistry*, **111**, 117–124.

20 Green, P. H. R., Glickman, R. M., Saudek, C. D. *et al.* (1979) Human intestinal lipoproteins. Studies in chyluric subjects. *Journal of Clinical Investigation*, **64**, 233–242.

21 Hamosh, M. (1979) The role of lingual lipase in neonatal fat digestion. *Ciba Foundation Symposium*, **70**, 69–98.

22 Helander, H. F. & Olivecrona, T. (1970) Lipolysis and lipid absorption in the stomach of the suckling rat. *Gastroenterology*, **59**, 22–35.

23 Hepner, G. W., Hofmann, A. F. & Thomas, P. J. (1972) Metabolism of steroid and amino acid moieties of conjugated bile acids in man. II. Glycine-conjugated dihydroxy bile acids. *Journal of Clinical Investigation*, **51**, 1898–1905.

24 Hofmann, A. F. (1976) Fat digestion: the interaction of lipid digestion products with micellar bile acid solutions. In *Lipid Absorption: Biochemical and Clinical Aspects* (Ed.) Rommel, K. & Bohmer, R. pp. 3–18. Maryland, Baltimore: University Park Press.

25 Hofmann, A. F. & Borgstrom, B. (1964) The intraluminal phase of fat digestion in man: the lipid content of the micellar and oil phase of intestinal content obtained during fat digestion and absorption. *Journal of Clinical Investigation*, **43**, 247–257.

26 Hofmann, A. F. & Poley, J. R. (1972) Role of bile acid malabsorption in pathogenesis of diarrhea and steatorrhea in patients with ileal resection. *Gastroenterology*, **62**, 918–934.

27 Hotz, J., Goberna, R. & Clodi, P. H. (1973) Reserve capacity of the exocrine pancreas. Enzyme secretion and fecal fat assimilation in the 95% pancreatectomized rat. *Digestion*, **9**, 212–223.

28 Kalser, M. H., Leite, C. A. & Warren, W. D. (1968) Fat assimilation after massive distal pancreatectomy. *New England Journal of Medicine*, **279**, 570–576.

29 Krag, E. & Phillips, S. F. (1974) Active and passive bile acid absorption in man. Perfusion studies of the ileum and jejunum. *Journal of Clinical Investigation*, **53**, 1686–1694.

30 Levy, E., Goldstein, R., Freier, S. & Shafrir, E. (1981) Characterisation of gastric lipolytic activity. *Biochimica et Biophysica Acta*, **664**, 316–326.

31 Linthorst, J. M., Bennett Clark, S. & Holt, P. R. (1977) Triglyceride emulsification by amphipaths present in the intestinal lumen during digestion of fat. *Journal of Colloid and Interface Science*, **60**, 1–10.

32 Low-Beer, T. S. & Pomare, E. W. (1973) Regulation of bile salt pool size in man. *British Medical Journal*, **ii**, 338–340.

33 Malagelada, J. R., Go, V. L. W. & Summerskill, W. H. J. (1974) Altered pancreatic and biliary function after vagotomy and pyloroplasty. *Gastroenterology*, **65**, 22–27.

34 Mansbach, C. M. & Tyor, M. P. (1970) Effect of reduced luminal pH in the proximal small intestine on fat absorption in the hamster. *Gastroenterology*, **59**, 222–233.

35 Masterton, J. P., Lewis, H. E. & Widdowson, E. M. (1957) Food intakes, energy expenditures and faecal excretions of men on polar expedition. *British Journal of Nutrition*, **11**, 346–358.

36 Meyer, J. H., Thomson, J. B., Cohen, M. B. *et al.* (1979) Sieving of solid food by the canine stomach and sieving

after gastric surgery. *Gastroenterology*, **76**, 804–813.

37 Ockner, R. K. & Manning, J. A. (1976) Fatty acid binding protein. Role in esterification of absorbed long chain fatty acid in rat intestine. *Journal of Clinical Investigation*, **58**, 632–641.

38 Olivecrona, T., Billstrom, A., Fredrikzon, B. *et al.* (1973) Gastric lipolysis of human milk lipids in infants with pyloric stenosis. *Acta Paediatrica Scandinavica*, **62**, 520–522.

39 Patton, J. S. & Carey, M. C. (1979) Watching fat digestion. *Science*, **204**, 145–148.

40 Poley, J. R. (1976) Fat digestion and absorption in lipase and bile acid deficiency. In *Lipid Absorption: Biochemical and Clinical Aspects* (Ed.) Rommel, K. & Bohmer, R. pp. 151–199. Baltimore, Maryland: University Park Press.

41 Porter, H. P., Saunders, D. R., Tytgat, G. *et al.* (1971) Fat absorption in bile fistula man. A morphological and biochemical study. *Gastroenterology*, **60**, 1008–1019.

42 Powell, G. K., Jones, L. A. & Richardson, J. (1973) A new syndrome of bile acid deficiency – a possible synthetic defect. *Journal of Pediatrics*, **83**, 758–766.

43 Riley, J. W. & Glickman, R. M. (1979) Fat malabsorption – advances in our understanding. *American Journal of Medicine*, **67**, 980–988.

44 Rommel, K. & Bohmer, R. (1976) (Ed.) *Lipid Absorption: Biochemical and Clinical Aspects*. Baltimore, Maryland: University Park Press.

45 Sallee, V. L. (1975) Permeation coefficients for long chain fatty acids in rat intestine. *Federation Proceedings*, **34**, 310 (Abstract).

46 Singh, A., Balint, J. A., Edmonds, R. H. & Rodgers, J. B. (1972) Adaptive changes of the rat small intestine in response to a high fat diet. *Biochimica et Biophysica Acta*, **260**, 708–715.

47 Signer, E., Murphy, G. M., Edkins, S. & Anderson, C. M. (1974) Role of bile salts in fat malabsorption of premature infants. *Archives of Diseases in Childhood*, **49**, 174–180.

48 Smyth, D. H. (1974) (Ed.) Intestinal absorption. *Biomembranes*, Volume 4B. London, New York: Plenum Press.

49 Stiehl, A., Earnest, D. L. & Admirand, W. H. (1975) Sulfation and renal excretion of bile salts in patients with cirrhosis of the liver. *Gastroenterology*, **68**, 534–544.

50 Tabaqchali, S. (1970) The pathophysiological role of small intestinal bacterial flora. *Scandinavian Journal of Gastroenterology* (Supplement) **6**, 139–163.

51 Theron, J. J., Wittmann, W. & Prinsloo, J. G. (1971) The fine structure of the jejunum in kwashiorkor. *Experimental and Molecular Pathology*, **14**, 184–199.

52 Thompson, G. R., Barrowman, J., Gutierrez, L. & Dowling, R. H. (1971) Action of neomycin on the intraluminal phase of lipid absorption. *Journal of Clinical Investigation*, **50**, 319–323.

53 Trompeter, R. S., McCollum, J. P. K., Muller, D. P. R. & Harries, J. T. (1975) Studies in congenital isolated pancreatic lipase deficiency. *Gut*, **16**, 838 (Abstract).

54 Turnberg, L. A. & Grahame, G. (1970) Bile salt secretion in cirrhosis of the liver. *Gut*, **11**, 126–133.

55 Vlahcevic, Z. R., Prugh, M. F., Gregory, D. H. & Swell, L. (1977) Disturbances of bile acid metabolism in parenchymal liver cell disease. *Clinics in Gastroenterology*, **6**, 25–43.

56 Watkins, J. B. (1974) Bile acid metabolism and fat absorption in newborn infants. *Pediatric Clinics of North America*, **21**, 501–512.

57 Wieloch, T., Borgstrom, B., Pieroni, G. *et al.* (1981) Porcine pancreatic procolipase and its trypsin-activated form. *Febs Letters*, **128**, 217–220.

58 Wilson, F. A., Sallee, V. L. & Dietschy, J. M. (1971) Unstirred water layers in intestine: rate determinant of fatty acid absorption from micellar solutions. *Science*, **174**, 1031–1033.

59 Zoppi, G., Andreotti, G., Pajno-Ferrara, F. *et al.* (1972) Exocrine pancreas function in premature and full term neonates. *Pediatric Research*, **6**, 880–886.

DIGESTION AND MALABSORPTION OF PROTEIN

The aim of this section is to review our current knowledge of the physiology of digestion and absorption of dietary protein, to discuss the specific inherited disorders of nitrogen absorption, and to briefly highlight the common alimentary disorders that can be associated with clinically significant abnormalities of protein digestion and absorption.

The digestion of dietary and endogenous protein

DAILY PROTEIN INTAKE

In order to maintain nitrogen balance, a daily protein intake of 0.5–0.7 g/kg of body weight is necessary for the adult. Dietary protein is derived from animal and vegetable sources and constitutes 11–14% of the average daily energy intake. In addition to dietary protein, proteins derived from endogenous sources also enter the intestinal lumen. These endogenous proteins are derived from gastric, biliary, pancreatic and intestinal secretions and consist of secretory glycoproteins (mucins) and digestive enzymes. Protein derived from desquamated mucosal epithelial cells and small quantities of plasma proteins also enter the intestinal tract. The total amount of endogenous protein entering the small intestine daily is not known with any precision, but it has been estimated to be in the region of 35–130 g in the adult. The healthy adult excretes 1–2 g of faecal nitrogen per day (equivalent to 6–12 g of protein), indicating that the processes involved in the digestion and absorption of both dietary and endogenous proteins are very efficient.

GASTRIC PROTEOLYSIS

Dietary protein is hydrolysed within the stomach by pepsins, a group of proteolytic enzymes secreted by gastric mucosa. They are active in the acid milieu of the stomach, and hydrolyse internal peptide bonds (CO—NH) between amino acids in the protein chains. They are most active on bonds involving leucine and the aromatic amino acids phenylalanine and tyrosine. Negligible amounts of free amino acids are released, the products of gastric proteolysis consisting predominantly of medium- and long-chain polypeptides. Extensive or total gastrectomy rarely leads to significant impairment of protein absorption, so the contribution of the stomach to the overall assimilation of dietary protein is thought to be of minor importance only.

PANCREATIC PROTEOLYSIS

The hydrolysis of dietary proteins mainly occurs in the lumen of the duodenum and proximal jejunum and is primarily due to the concerted actions of pancreatic proteolytic enzymes. These enzymes – trypsin, chymotrypsin, elastase, and the carboxypeptidases – which are synthesized in the pancreatic acinar cells, are secreted as inactive precursors via the pancreatic ducts into the upper duodenal lumen where activation occurs by specific splitting of the protein molecules.

The first step in the activation of these proenzymes is the conversion of trypsinogen to trypsin by the action of enterokinase, an enzyme which is now thought to be an intrinsic constituent of small upper intestinal mucosal microvillus membranes. However, as enterokinase is also found in a soluble form in the intestinal lumen, it is probable that the lumen is the actual site of proenzyme activation. Following conversion of trypsinogen to trypsin, the other proenzymes are then activated by trypsin. Trypsin, chymotrypsin and elastase are endopeptidases, and attack internal peptide bonds; they differ functionally from each other only in their specificity for particular amino acids. The carboxypeptidases are exopeptidases, and act on terminal peptide bonds at the carboxyl (COOH) end of the polypeptide chains. The action of these enzymes,[16] as well as that of the freely soluble intraluminal intestinal mucosal aminopeptidases, results in the production of a mixture of free amino acids and small peptides (chain length two to six amino acid units). These are the final products of luminal protein digestion and are presented to the intestinal mucosa for absorption.

Absorption of the products of luminal protein digestion

Although brush border hydrolysis together with the monosaccharide transport system is the pre-dominant method of absorption of the luminal products of carbohydrate digestion in man, it now appears certain that, in the absorption of the luminal products of protein digestion, two major mechanisms are involved: transport of liberated free amino acids by group-specific active amino acid transport systems, and uptake of unhydrolysed peptides by mechanisms independent of the specific amino acid entry mechanisms.

Much of the more recent work leading to the basic concepts of peptide transport has already been reviewed in detail.[3, 12, 23, 24, 25, 33, 35]

FREE AMINO ACID TRANSPORT

As with glucose transport, active amino acid transport in vitro depends on a gradient of sodium ions across the brush border membrane of intestinal epithelial cells. In man, steady state perfusion techniques have shown saturation of the transport systems with increasing solute concentration, suggesting the existence of carrier-mediated mechanisms.[1] Also, different affinities of different free amino acids for these mechanisms are indicated by variations in the absorption rate of individual amino acids when perfusion studies were performed using equimolar mixtures of different acids.[1] Sodium dependency of amino acid transport has been difficult to demonstrate in man,[35] although methodological problems are the most likely cause for this.

The results of competition studies in animals have indicated the likely existence of three major group-specific active transport systems:[23]

a Monoamino monocarboxylic (neutral) amino acids.
b Dibasic amino acids and cystine.
c Dicarboxylic (acidic) amino acids.

The subject is complicated by species differences and by the fact that certain amino acids may be transported by more than one mechanism. Thus, studies of iminoglycinuria have suggested the existence of a group-specific system responsible for mediating the transport of glycine, proline and hydroxyproline, which may also be transported by system *a*. Studies of amino acid transport in Hartnup's disease and cystinuria have firmly established the existence of systems *a* and *b* in man.

TRANSPORT OF UNHYDROLYSED PEPTIDES

Animal experiments performed in the late 1950s and early 1960s suggested that dipeptides could be taken up intact by intestinal mucosa.

However, the concept of intact peptide uptake as a second mode of protein absorption, although not disputed, was not thought to be quantitatively significant, as it seemed much more likely that absorption of peptides, like that of disaccharides, would involve brush border hydrolysis with subsequent absorption of the released amino acids by amino acid transport systems.

Modern knowledge of peptide absorption stems from the results of oral load experiments carried out by Craft *et al.*[9] in man. They found that a given quantity of glycine was absorbed faster when administered orally as the dipeptide or tripeptide than in the free form. It was concluded that the glycine peptides were transported unhydrolysed into the mucosal cell since, if hydrolysis had preceded uptake then, at best, the net rates of glycine transport of the free and peptide forms would have been the same. In the light of recent in vivo perfusion data showing more rapid transport of glucose from maltose,[20] their data was perhaps somewhat over-interpreted, but their conclusions provided a powerful stimulus for further research in this area, which has subsequently provided unequivocal evidence for the existence in man of peptide transport systems which are distinct from those used by free amino acids.

Evidence for intestinal transport of unhydrolysed peptides

Of all the experimental data available in favour of dipeptide transport in the human intestine, the most persuasive is derived from experiments performed in patients with Hartnup's disease and cystinuria. As described later, Hartnup's disease involves an intestinal transport defect for neutral amino acids; cystinuria involves a transport defect for dibasic amino acids.[26] Despite these transport defects, the 'affected' amino acids were shown to be absorbed normally or near normally if presented to the mucosa in the form of homologous or mixed dipeptides.[5, 6, 38]

If any of the dipeptides administered to these patients had been hydrolysed to a substantial degree in the gut lumen or by brush border peptidases, before transport of released amino acid by specific active transport processes, then absorption of the affected amino acids would not have occurred. This was clearly not the case in these experiments.

Additional evidence supporting the existence of intact dipeptide transport in human small intestine includes the following facts. First, the known competition between free amino acids for mucosal uptake is absent or much reduced when solutions of dipeptides instead of corresponding free amino acid mixtures are presented to the mucosa for absorption.[24, 35] Second, in most studies of peptide transport, faster rates of uptake of at least one of the constituent residues have been observed for dipeptides than for corresponding free amino acid solutions.[3, 24, 25, 33] This line of evidence is open to some criticism because the same phenomenon has been observed with disaccharides[21] which are hydrolysed at the brush border and not transported intact. However, the kinetic advantage conferred by dipeptides on amino acid transport has been a consistent finding of much greater magnitude, and has been observed during perfusion of dipeptide substrates known to have a low affinity for human brush border peptidases.

Mucosal hydrolysis of dipeptides

A consistent finding during in vivo and in vitro uptake experiments with dipeptides has been the detection of free amino acids in the media bathing the mucosal preparations.[3, 24, 25, 33, 35] The rate of appearance of free amino acids during assimilation of different dipeptides varies[2, 37] and substantially faster rates of appearance have been observed during ileal, as compared with jejunal, experiments.[2, 40]

Although there are two distinct groups of mucosal peptidases, one located within the cytoplasmic compartment and the other at the brush border membrane of the cell,[22, 30] experimental data have shown that the appearance of free amino acids during dipeptide transport correlates well with the specific activities of the brush border, and not the cytoplasmic, peptidases.[36] Thus those dipeptides with a high affinity for brush border peptidases seem likely to undergo significant hydrolysis at the brush border and to be transported as free amino acids, whereas dipeptides with a low affinity for the surface enzymes are absorbed intact in an unhydrolysed form.

TRIPEPTIDE AND TETRAPEPTIDE ASSIMILATION

All the evidence suggests that tripeptides are handled in a similar fashion to dipeptides. Thus those with a low affinity for brush border peptidases are absorbed intact, whereas those with a higher affinity for the surface enzymes undergo proportionally greater degrees of hydrolysis and are absorbed as free amino acids or dipeptides.

Intestinal uptake of few tetrapeptides has been studied. All but one have been shown to be transported only after surface hydrolysis to free amino acid and tripeptide components have taken place.[8] However, significant proportions of the tetrapeptide Leu—Gly—Gly—Gly appeared to be transported intact and hydrolysed by cytoplasmic rather than brush border peptidases.[8] Further work is therefore needed to elucidate whether it is the molecular structure of peptides (the length of molecule and/or width of side chains) or the presence of cytoplasmic peptidase activity that dictates whether the intact peptide transport apparatus is utilized during the assimilation of tetra- and higher peptides.

THE CHARACTERISTICS OF DIPEPTIDE AND TRIPEPTIDE TRANSPORT

Although the kinetics of peptide transport have not been extensively investigated in man, mainly on account of the expense of purchasing sufficient amounts of model peptides, animal studies have shown that uptake of unhydrolysed dipeptides and tripeptides is mediated by an energy- and sodium-dependent saturable carrier mechanism. The question as to whether all dipeptides and tripeptides are transported by one common or multiple peptide transport systems has recently been discussed.[34] The work of Taylor *et al.*[44] suggests the existence of a single peptide carrier, whereas the other data point towards the existence of at least two or more.[34]

The nutritional importance of peptide transport

The kinetic advantage conferred by individual dipeptides, tripeptides, and tetrapeptides on the intestinal assimilation of amino acid residues has been a consistent finding in most experiments, and has suggested the possibility that there could be nutritional implications for peptide transport in normal human subjects. In addition, the kinetic advantage conferred by two particular dipeptides on the intestinal assimilation of their amino acid residues has been shown in patients with untreated coeliac disease with subtotal villous atrophy of the small intestinal mucosa,[4, 39] suggesting nutritional implications in patients with impaired gastrointestinal absorptive function. As there are 400 possible dipeptides and 8000 possible tripeptides, it clearly has been impossible to assess the overall nutritional importance of peptide transport by studying the absorption characteristics of each

in turn. As an alternative means of investigating the problem, native proteins have been hydrolysed by enzymic methods under controlled in vitro conditions to yield final mixtures consisting predominantly of oligopeptides, with smaller quantities of free amino acids. Equivalent free amino acid mixtures whose composition and molar pattern simulated those of the partial enzymic hydrolysates of protein have also been prepared. Comparisons have been made in humans of the extent of absorption of amino acid residues from the partial enzymic hydrolysates of whole protein and their respective equivalent free amino acid mixtures, using a steady state in vivo perfusion technique. Results have consistently showed a greater absorption of α-amino acid nitrogen from the protein hydrolysates than from the equivalent free amino acid mixtures. Moreover, the data highlighted the extreme variability in the extent of absorption of amino acid residues from the free amino acid mixtures.

As shown in Figure 8.20, this variability in amino acid uptake is not nearly so marked during perfusion of the protein hydrolysates, as those amino acids which were poorly assimilated from free amino acid solutions were absorbed to a greater extent from the protein hydrolysate solution.[41]

Two important points emerge from these perfusion experiments. The first concerns the finding of a 'more even' absorption of amino acid residues during perfusion of the protein hydrolysates. It has been suggested that more efficient protein synthesis is induced when amino acids are presented to the tissues at even, rather than different, rates. If this is indeed the case, then there could be advantages in administering peptides rather than amino acid mixtures, since in the case of amino acid mixtures there was a marked variation in the extent of absorption of the individual amino acids.

The second point relates to the fact that in studies using casein and lactalbumin hydrolysates, greater proportions of infused α-amino nitrogen were absorbed during perfusion of the hydrolysate preparations than during perfusion of the respective free amino acid mixtures. If maximally effective absorption is required in the clinical situation, such as in patients with exocrine pancreatic insufficiency or loss of absorptive surface area due to coeliac disease or intestinal resection, there would appear to be a significant advantage in administering protein hydrolysates containing oligopeptides rather than free amino acid mixtures.

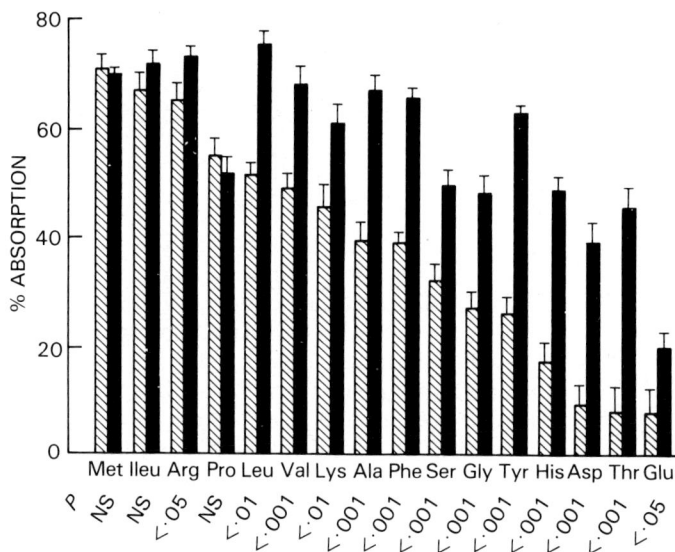

Fig. 8.20 Absorption of individual amino acid residues from an amino acid mixture simulating a casein soy lactalbumin protein mixture and a partial papain hydrolysate of the casein soy lactalbumin protein mixture. The total height of each column represents the mean value (n = 6) and the SE is represented by a vertical bar. Where the difference between absorption was significant, the level and significance (P) are indicated. ▨ Free amino acids. ■ Enzyme hydrolysate.

Inherited disorders of intestinal amino acid absorption (Table 8.2)

IMINOGLYCINURIA

Joseph et al.[21] have reported a child with convulsions, high cerebrospinal fluid protein and increased amounts of proline, hydroxyproline and glycine in the urine. More recently, Whelan and Scriver[46] have described several healthy individuals with a similar transport defect. Data on intestinal transport have been scanty. One case has been shown to have decreased proline absorption, but normal glycine absorption, after oral loading, and one patient has been described with an increased faecal excretion of proline and glycine after oral loading. When either proline,

hydroxyproline or glycine were given orally, the faecal excretion of the other two amino acids increased, which supports the existence of a group-specific amino acid transport system for all three amino acids. As neither proline, hydroxyproline or glycine are nutritionally essential, it is not surprising that none of the patients studied has symptoms or any recognizable disability. It is not known whether the affected amino acids are absorbed normally when presented as peptides.

HARTNUP'S DISEASE

This is a rare autosomal recessive disease, named by Baron et al.[7] after the surname of the first affected family. Since then over 60 cases have been reported.[47]

The transport defect

In this condition the basic abnormality is a reduced efficiency of neutral amino acid transport by the proximal renal tubular cells of the kidney.[27] Although earlier workers thought that the kidneys alone were affected in this disorder, Milne et al.[27] felt that a more generalized defect may occur, possibly involving neutral amino acid transport in all body cells. To test this hypothesis they have, over the years, investigated neutral amino acid transport in the gut. In 1960 they reported that faecal excretion of tryptophan and its metabolites was increased in three patients with Hartnup's disease after these patients had been fed tryptophan orally.[27]

Table 8.2 Inherited disorders of intestinal amino acid absorption.

Disease	Amino acid affected by transport defect
Iminoglycinuria	Glycine, proline, hydroxyproline
Hartnup's disease	Neutral amino acids
Cystinuria	Dibasic amino acids, cystine
Lysinuric protein intolerance (LPI)	Lysine, arginine, ornithine
Blue diaper syndrome	Tryptophan
Oast house syndrome	Methionine
Lowe's syndrome	Arginine, lysine (partial)

From Silk, D. B. A. (1982) *Clinics in Gastroenterology, 11,* 47–72.

Later, using an oral tolerance technique, they found no significant change in the plasma level of histidine, phenylalanine and tryptophan when these amino acids were fed orally to patients with Hartnup's disease.[5, 6] These results confirmed the presence of a severe intestinal transport defect for these neutral amino acids in this condition.

A curious anomaly was thought to exist in Hartnup's disease since, despite the group-specific transport defect for absorption of essential amino acids, these patients did not have any severe nutritional defects. The reason for this is now clear as it has been shown that the 'affected' amino acids are absorbed normally or near normally when presented as dipeptides.[5]

CYSTINURIA

Cystinuria is a complex autosomal recessive inherited disorder characterized by abnormalities in the transport of cystine, lysine, ornithine and arginine in both the intestinal tract and the renal tubule. If it were not for the relative insolubility of cystine in urine, resulting in the formation of cystine calculi, this disorder would only be a metabolic curiosity.

The transport defect
The basic defect in this condition is a reduced efficiency of the transport of dibasic amino acids and cystine by the proximal tubular cells of the kidney. In 1954 Dent *et al.* demonstrated that blood levels of cystine were low in patients with homozygous cystinuria after the oral administration of 5 g of cystine.[13] Milne *et al.* later showed that, after oral administration of 20 g of lysine or 10 g of ornithine, the levels of lysine, ornithine and arginine in the faeces of patients with cystinuria were elevated, as were the levels of cadaverine and putrescine, the diamines of lysine and ornithine.[28] These results strongly suggested that in homozygous cystinuria an intestinal transport defect exists for the dibasic amino acids and cystine. Subsequently, it was shown in vitro that there is a defect of active carrier-mediated transport of the dibasic amino acids and cystine by jejunal mucosa obtained from patients with cystinuria.[45] Later, in vitro and in vivo experimental data indicated that at low concentrations (below the K_t for lysine) a transport defect for free lysine exists throughout the small intestine, but at higher concentrations free lysine is absorbed normally, presumably by passive diffusion or via other transport mechanisms. At all concentrations tested, however, there is an intestinal transport defect for free arginine and cystine in cystinuria.[18]

As in Hartnup's disease, patients with cystinuria do not become severely malnourished because the 'affected' amino acids are absorbed normally or near normally when presented as dipeptides.[38]

LYSINURIC PROTEIN INTOLERANCE

Lysinuric protein intolerance (LPI) is an autosomal recessive defect of dibasic amino acid transport. Unlike cystinuria and Hartnup's disease, LPI is associated with severe symptoms which include failure to thrive, vomiting, diarrhoea, protein aversion, severe growth retardation, hepatosplenomegaly, and sometimes mental retardation. A transport defect for the dibasic amino acids has been demonstrated in the proximal renal tubules and uptake in liver slices is also impaired.[42] The characteristic hyperammonaemia and protein aversion is thought to arise on account of the hepatocyte transport defect, which in turn gives rise to a deficiency of the dibasic intermediates of the urea cycle.

Recent oral load studies have shown that LPI homozygotes have an intestinal transport defect for lysine, arginine and ornithine, whereas citrulline uptake is normal. Unlike the situation in Hartnup's disease and cystinuria, where 'unabsorbed' amino acids are absorbed normally or near normally when presented as dipeptides, no significant absorption of dipeptide-bound lysine occurs in LPI.[31] In this study, lysylglycine was administered orally and normal absorption of glycine but not lysine was noted. This interesting observation suggested that the defect for lysine uptake exists at the site of the basolateral membrane, a suggestion that has been subsequently confirmed in vitro, when lysine fluxes across jejunal epithelium obtained from patients with LPI were studied.[14] Prior to this latter study, little was known about the mechanism of transport of amino acids across the basolateral membrane, although earlier work had implied the existence of a facilitated transport system that is independent of sodium. The genetically determined basolateral membrane transport demonstrated for lysine in LPI highlights, therefore, the existence of a special transport system for amino acids across the basolateral membrane, and it may be inferred that this is a different process to that responsible for the translocation of amino acids across the microvillous membrane, and under different genetic control.

BLUE DIAPER SYNDROME

This rare inherited disorder presents in newborns with failure to thrive, recurrent unexplained fever, infections, irritability, constipation and a bluish discoloration of the nappies (diapers). Hypercalcaemia and nephrocalcinosis are present, and are presumed to be secondary to increased calcium absorption. The stools contain markedly increased amounts of indoles and tryptophan as well as tryptamine and indolic acid. On the basis of this it was assumed that there is a malabsorption of tryptophan in this condition. To support this, low plasma levels were seen after oral loading with tryptophan, and the indoles disappeared from the stool and urine following neomycin administration. Unabsorbed tryptophan is converted by bacterial enzymes to indoles in the intestine which are then absorbed and converted to indoxyl sulphate (indican) by the liver. The bluish discoloration of the nappies is due to the presence of indigotin (indigo blue), an oxidation product of indican excreted into the urine. Renal excretion of amino acids appears to be normal, so thus far there is no evidence that this disorder affects the kidneys as well as the intestine.

METHIONINE MALABSORPTION (OAST HOUSE SYNDROME)

Hooft *et al.*[19] have described a patient with severe mental deficiency, in whom they demonstrated an isolated defect of methionine absorption in the urine and kidney. The bacterial breakdown product of methionine – α-hydroxybutyric acid – was isolated from the urine and faeces following oral loading with methionine. When the patient was treated with a methionine-free diet, the diarrhoea and convulsions subsided and the mental state improved.

LOWE'S SYNDROME

Unlike the other disorders of transport, Lowe's syndrome is inherited as a sex-linked trait. It is characterized by mental retardation, ataxia, cataracts, glaucoma, renal disease, metabolic acidosis, proteinuria, generalized hyperaminoaciduria and organic aciduria. The disease usually results in renal failure in late childhood or adolescence.

Intestinal absorption and renal transport of lysine and arginine is impaired in Lowe's syndrome. It is not known whether or not peptide-bound arginine and lysine transport is impaired in this condition, and the significance of the intestinal transport defect in relationship to the clinical syndrome is unclear.

Clinical protein deficiency due to impaired digestion and absorption

Many common alimentary disorders are associated with significant abnormalities of protein digestion and absorption, and severe clinical protein deficiency can result. As can be seen from Table 8.3, different disease processes may exert a deleterious effect at different stages during the digestion and absorption of protein.

Table 8.3 Clinical protein deficiency due to impaired digestion and absorption.

Stage in protein absorption	Abnormality
Gastric phase	Gastric surgery
Pancreatic proteolysis	Enterokinase deficiency
	Diseases of the pancreas
	Cancer of the pancreas
	Acute pancreatitis
	Chronic pancreatitis
	Hereditary pancreatitis
	Cystic fibrosis
	Shwachman's syndrome
	Prematurity
Mucosal hydrolysis (?)	All mucosal disorders
Mucosal uptake	Abnormalities of intestinal mucosa
	Coeliac disease
	Dermatitis herpetiformis
	Tropical sprue
	Whipple's disease
	Immunodeficiency syndromes
	Lymphoma
	Transient protein intolerance of infancy
Loss of absorptive surface	Intestinal resection
	Fistulas
	Jejunal-ileal bypass
Adverse luminal interactions	Blind loop syndrome
	Parasitic infection

From Silk (1980) Disordered protein metabolism. In *Scientific Foundations of Gastroenterology* (ed.) Sircus, W. & Smith, A. N., pp. 408–426, with kind permission of the publisher, William Heinemann Medical Books.

GASTRIC SURGERY

Severe clinical protein deficiency is well documented following gastric surgery. However, this is not an invariable consequence even of total gastrectomy which suggests that the stomach only plays a minor role in the overall assimilation of dietary protein. The Hammersmith Group reported on a group of patients who developed severe clinical protein deficiency after gastric surgery.[17] Described as having 'post gastrectomy kwashiorkor', all the patients studied were found to have co-existing disorders of the alimentary tract. Thus, gastric surgery *per se* is not a primary cause of protein malabsorption, and co-existing disorders may contribute to the clinical protein deficiency that occurs in some of these patients.

PANCREATIC PROTEOLYSIS

Enterokinase deficiency
As mentioned earlier, enterokinase is an intrinsic intestinal mucosal microvillus enzyme which is responsible for the conversion of trypsinogen to trypsin. As all other pancreatic enzymes are activated by trypsin, enterokinase plays a key role in protein digestion. It is not surprising, therefore, that in the absence of this enzyme, severe clinical protein deficiency results. Several cases of intestinal enterokinase deficiency have been described.[29] Patients usually present during the first few months of life with diarrhoea, failure to thrive, and hypoproteinaemia. Severe anaemia with evidence of haemolysis is usually a prominent, early feature. Diagnosis depends on the initial finding of low or absent levels of trypsin, chymotrypsin and carboxypeptidases in duodenal contents which markedly increase when enterokinase is added. Mucosal enterokinase activity is absent, but this condition is not a primary mucosal disorder as intestinal morphology, as judged by light and electron microscopy, is normal. It has been suggested that intestinal enterokinase deficiency is an inherited congenital defect as it has recently been described in two siblings. During the early phase of the disease, when patients suffer from hypoproteinaemia, they also show more generalized malabsorption. Most have been found to have steatorrhoea, and levels of lipase and amylase are low in duodenal juice. In addition, disaccharidase activities of duodenal mucosa are low. These changes are probably secondary to the protein malnutrition, as similar changes have been found in kwashiorkor.

Diseases of the pancreas
These are an important group of alimentary disorders associated with clinical protein deficiency. In adults, clinical evidence of protein deficiency is seen most commonly in patients with cancer of the pancreas, chronic pancreatitis, and after pancreatic resection. In children, it is most common in patients with cystic fibrosis, but may occur in hereditary pancreatitis and the Shwachman syndrome (pancreatic insufficiency with bone marrow dysfunction). Although oral protein tolerance tests in patients with pancreatic disease show that mean levels of plasma and amino nitrogen are lower, and post

absorption curves flatter than in controls,[32] it is remarkable how often nutrition is reasonably well preserved in patients with severe pancreatic exocrine deficiency. Indeed significant (20–50%) protein digestion and absorption have been shown in two patients after total pancreatectomy.[10] Another surprising finding is that protein deficiency is seen less commonly in patients with chronic exocrine pancreatic insufficiency than in coeliac disease.[15] In this study, faecal nitrogen excretion in the two groups were similar. In retrospect it was found that the patients with chronic pancreatitis had ravenous appetites with increased food intake when compared with the patients with coeliac disease, the majority of whom complained of anorexia and abdominal distension, and had a markedly reduced food intake.[15] It appears, therefore, that in patients with chronic pancreatitic exocrine deficiency, development of severe clinical protein deficiency may in part be prevented by increasing dietary protein intake. Two other aspects of alimentary physiology may also explain the absence of invariable protein malnutrition in pancreatic disease. Firstly significant disappearance of uniformly labelled ^{14}C protein from rat Thiery-Vella loops with total deficiency of pancreatic proteolytic enzymes has been found; the rates of disappearance are enhanced if the protein is pre-digested in vitro with either pepsin at acid pH, or acid alone.[11] It seems unlikely that absorption of whole protein, or even large polypeptide chains, could explain these results, but the subsequent demonstration by the same group that the brush border fraction of intestinal mucosa contains endopeptidase activity against un-denatured protein and large polypeptides (Kim, personal communication) suggests that the small intestinal mucosa may be able to digest whole proteins.

DISORDERS OF MUCOSAL UPTAKE

It is not surprising that diseases leading to structural alteration or damage to the intestinal epithelial cells are associated with malabsorption of protein digestion products. Table 8.3 lists the common alimentary disorders that are characterized by structural abnormalities of the intestinal mucosa. Clinical protein deficiency, which may often be very severe in these conditions (e.g. coeliac disease and tropical sprue) has been attributed in most cases to a combination of anorexia, malabsorption of protein digestion products, and excessive loss of endogenous protein (protein losing enteropathy).

LOSS OF ABSORPTIVE SURFACE

Clinical protein deficiency is liable to develop in any condition in which the absorptive area of the small intestine is reduced. Loss of absorptive surface most commonly results from massive small intestinal resection, performed usually because of Crohn's disease or vascular lesions (e.g. strangulated hernias, acute thrombosis or embolus in the superior mesenteric artery, and thrombosis of the superior mesenteric vein). Fistula formation (e.g. gastro-colic due to cancer; gastro-ileal due to inadvertent gastro-ileal enterostomy during Polya gastrectomy; jejuno-cutaneous, jejuno-ileal, or jejuno-colic in Crohn's disease) may result in marked loss of absorptive surface. More recently, many patients have been seen with clinical protein deficiency following intestinal bypass operations for hyperlipidaemia and morbid obesity.

Protein losing enteropathy

The qualitative detection of albumin, gamma globulin and other serum proteins in the gastro-intestinal secretions by electrophoretic and immunological techniques confirms the role of the gastrointestinal tract in the physiological degradation of serum proteins. Latest figures suggest that 5–15% of the normal turnover of albumin and gamma globulin can be accounted for by enteric protein loss. In protein losing enteropathy there is an excessive loss of serum proteins into the gastrointestinal tract. Despite the fact that these proteins are rapidly digested and reabsorbed, patients may develop hypo-proteinaemia and clinical protein deficiency. The reason for this is that resynthesis rates are, at best, only twice normal and thus are often insufficient to counteract severe enteric protein loss.

REFERENCES

1 Adibi, S. A. (1969) The influence of molecular structure of neutral amino acids on their absorptive kinetics in the jejunum and ileum of human intestine in vivo. *Gastroenterology*, **56**, 903–911.

2 Adibi, S. A. (1971) Intestinal transport of dipeptides in man: relative importance of hydrolysis and intact absorption. *Journal of Clinical Investigation*, **50**, 2266–2275.

3 Adibi, S. A. (1976) Intestinal phase of protein assimilation in man. *American Journal of Clinical Nutrition*, **29**, 205–215.

4 Adibi, S. A., Fogel, M. R. & Agrawal, R. M. (1974) Comparison of free amino acid and dipeptide absorption in the jejunum of sprue patients. *Gastroenterology*, **67**, 586–591.

5 Asatoor, A. M., Bandoh, J. K., Lant, A. F. *et al.* (1970) Intestinal absorption of carnosine and its constituent amino acids in man. *Gut*, **11**, 250–254.

6 Asatoor, A. M., Cheng, B., Edwards, K. D. G. *et al.* (1970) Intestinal absorption of two dipeptides in Hartnup disease. *Gut*, **11**, 380–387.

7 Baron, D. N., Dent, C. E., Harris, H. *et al.* (1956) Hereditary pellagra-like skin rash with temporary cerebellar ataxia, constant renal amino acid uria and other bizarre biochemical features. *Lancet*, **ii**, 421–428.

8 Chung, Y. C., Silk, D. B. A. & Kim, Y. S. (1979) Intestinal transport of a tetrapeptide, L-leucylglycylglycylglycine, in rat intestine in vivo. *Clinical Science*, **57**, 1–11.

9 Craft, I. L., Geddes, D., Hyde, C. W. *et al.* (1968) Absorption and malabsorption of glycine and glycine peptides in man. *Gut*, **9**, 425–437.

10 Crane, C. W. (1969) Some aspects of protein absorption and malabsorption. In *Malabsorption*, Girdwood, R. H. & Smith, A. N. p. 33. Edinburgh: Edinburgh University Press.

11 Curtis, K. J., Kim, Y. S., Perdomo, J. M. & Whitehead, J. S. (1978) Protein digestion and absorption in the rat. *Journal of Physiology*, **274**, 409.

12 Das, M. & Radhakrishnan, A. N. (1976) Role of peptidase and peptide transport in the intestinal absorption of proteins. *World Review of Nutrition and Dietics*, **24**, 58–87.

13 Dent, C. E., Heathcote, J. G. & Joran, G. E. (1954) The pathogenesis of cystinuria. I Chromatographic and microbiological studies of the metabolism of sulphur containing amino acids. *Journal of Clinical Investigation*, **33**, 1210–1215.

14 Desjeux, J. F., Ragantie, J., Simell, O. *et al.* (1980) Lysine fluxes across the jejunal epithelium in lysinuric protein intolerance. *Journal of Clinical Investigation*, **65**, 1382–1387.

15 Evans, W. B. & Wollaeger, E. E. (1966) Incidence and severity of nutritional deficiency states in chronic exocrine pancreatic insufficiency. Comparison with nontropical sprue. *American Journal of Digestive Diseases*, **11**, 594.

16 Gray, G. M. & Cooper, H. L. (1971) Protein digestion and absorption. *Gastroenterology*, **61**, 535–544.

17 Haworth, J. C., Hadorn, B., Gourley, B. *et al.* (1975) Intestinal enterokinase deficiency. Occurrence in two sibs and age dependency of clinical expression. *Archives of Diseases in Childhood*, **50**, 277.

18 Hellier, M. D., Holdsworth, C. D. & Perrett, D. (1973) Dibasic amino acid absorption in man. *Gastroenterology*, **65**, 613–618.

19 Hooft, C. J., Timmermans, J., Snoeck, J. *et al.* (1964) Methionine malabsorption in a mentally defective child. *Lancet*, **ii**, 20–21.

20 Jones, B. J. M., Beavis, A. K., Edgerton, D. & Silk, D. B. A. (1980) Intestinal absorption of glucose polymers in man. *Gut*, **21**, A450.

21 Joseph, R., Ribierre, M., Job, J. C. & Girault, M. (1958) Maladie familiale associent des convulsions à début très précoce, une hyperalbuminorachie et une hyperaminoacidurie. *Archives Francaises de Pédiatrie*, **15**, 374–387.

22 Kim, Y. S. (1977) Intestinal mucosal hydrolysis of proteins and peptides. In *Peptide Transport and Hydrolysis. Ciba Foundation Symposium 50 (New Series)*, pp. 159–176.

23 Matthews, D. M. (1971) Protein absorption. *Journal of Clinical Pathology*, **5** (Supplement 24), 29–40.

24 Matthews, D. M. (1975) Intestinal absorption of peptides. *Physiological Reviews*, **55**, 537–608.

25 Matthews, D. M. & Adibi, S. A. (1976) Peptide absorption. *Gastroenterology*, **71**, 151–161.

26 Milne, M. D. (1971) Disorders of intestinal amino acid

transport. *Journal of Clinical Pathology*, **24** (Supplement 5), 41–44.

27 Milne, M. D., Asatoor, A. M., Edwards, K. D. G. & Loughridge, L. W. (1961) The intestinal absorption defect in cystinuria. *Gut*, **2**, 323–337.

28 Milne, M. D., Crawford, M. A., Girao, C. B. & Loughridge, L. W. (1960) The metabolic disorder in Hartnup disease. *Quarterly Journal of Medicine*, **29**, 407–421.

29 Neale, G., Antcliff, A. C., Welbourn, R. B. *et al.* (1967) Protein malnutrition after partial gastrectomy. *Quarterly Journal of Medicine NS*, **36**, 469.

30 Nicholson, J. A. & Peters, T. J. (1979) Subcellular localisation of peptidase activity in human jejunum. *European Journal of Clinical Investigation*, **9**, 349–354.

31 Ragantie, J., Simell, O. & Perheentupa, J. (1980) Basolateral membrane transport defect for lysine in lysinuric protein intolerance. *Lancet*, **i**, 1219–1221.

32 Richmond, J. & Girdwood, R. H. (1962) Observations on amino acid absorption. *Clinical Science*, **22**, 301.

33 Silk, D. B. A. (1974) Peptide absorption in man. *Gut*, **15**, 494–501.

34 Silk, D. B. A. (1982) Disorders of nitrogen absorption. *Clinics in Gastroenterology*, **11**, 47–72.

35 Silk, D. B. A. & Dawson, A. M. (1979) Intestinal absorption of carbohydrate and protein in man. *International Review of Physiology. Gastrointestinal Physiology III, Volume 19*, (Ed.) Crane, R. K. pp. 151–204. Baltimore: University Park Press.

36 Silk, D. B. A., Nicholson, J. A. & Kim, Y. S. (1976) Relationships between mucosal hydrolysis and transport of two phenylalanine dipeptides. *Gut*, **17**, 870–876.

37 Silk, D. B. A., Perrett, D. & Clark, M. L. (1973) Intestinal transport of two dipeptides containing the same two neutral amino acids in man. *Clinical Science and Molecular Medicine*, **45**, 291–299.

38 Silk, D. B. A., Perrett, D. & Clark, M. L., (1975) Jejunal and ileal absorption of dibasic amino acids and an arginine-containing dipeptide in cystinuria. *Gastroenterology*, **68**, 1426–1432.

39 Silk, D. B. A., Kumar, P. J., Perrett, D. *et al.* (1974) Amino acid absorption in patients with coeliac disease and dermatitis herpetiformis. *Gut*, **15**, 1–8.

40 Silk, D. B. A., Webb, J. P. W., Lane, A. E. *et al.* (1974) Functional differentiation of human jejunum and ileum: a comparison of the handling of glucose, peptide and amino acids. *Gut*, **15**, 444–449.

41 Silk, D. B. A., Fairclough, P. D., Clark, M. L. *et al.* (1980) Uses of a peptide rather than free amino acid nitrogen source in chemically defined 'elemental' diets. *Journal of Parenteral and Enteral Nutrition*, **4**(6) 548–553.

42 Simell, O., Perheentupa, J., Rapola, J. *et al.* (1975) Lysinuric protein intolerance. *American Journal of Medicine*, **59**, 229–240.

43 Smithson, K. W. & Gray, G. M. (1977) Intestinal assimilation of a tetrapeptide in the rat. Obligate function of brush border membrane amino peptidase. *Journal of Clinical Investigation*, **60**, 665–674.

44 Taylor, E., Burston, D. & Matthews, D. M. (1980) Influx of glycylsarcosine and L-lysyl-L-lysine into hamster jejunum in vitro. *Clinical Science*, **58**, 221–225.

45 Thier, S. O., Segal, S., Fox, M. *et al.* (1965) Cystinuria: defective intestinal transport of dibasic amino acids and cystine. *Journal of Clinical Investigation*, **44**, 332–448.

46 Whelan, D. T. & Scriver, C. R. (1968) Cystathioninuria and renal iminoglycinuria in a pedigree. *New England Journal of Medicine*, **278**, 924–927.

47 Wilcken, B., Yu, J. S. & Brown, D. A. (1977) Natural history of Hartnup disease. *Archives of Disease in Childhood*, **52**, 38–40.

ABSORPTION AND MALABSORPTION OF MINERALS

The Oxford dictionary defines a mineral as a 'substance obtained by mining', a definition which considerably overlaps with the term 'trace element'. Biologically important minerals include the elements copper (Cu), phosphorus (P), chlorine (Cl), potassium (K), sulphur (S), sodium (Na) and magnesium (Mg) as well as the trace elements (Table 8.4) which, in addition to being minerals, also have the distinction of being essential to life while being present in the body in only trace amounts. Recent experiments using total parenteral nutrition (TPN) to maintain life for prolonged periods have provided a great impetus to our understanding of the importance of such elements. Limitations of space will only permit us to concentrate on the absorption of the relatively well-researched cations Mg^{2+}, Zn^{2+} and Cu^{2+}; Ca^{2+} and Fe^{3+} will be discussed later in this chapter. Although knowledge of the precise daily requirements is far from complete in man, deficiency syndromes have been described for most of these elements (Table 8.4), mainly in severe malabsorption requiring long term TPN.

Table 8.4 Trace elements considered to be essential in man.

Element	Daily requirements	Deficiency syndrome in man
Iron	10–18 mg	Anaemia, lethargy
Iodine	10–20 µg	Myxoedema
Cobalt	1.5–40 µg	Vitamin B_{12} deficiency
Zinc	3–15 mg	Eczema, hypogonadism, dwarfism, poor wound healing, anorexia (Prasad *et al.*[23])
Selenium	100–200 µg	Cardiomyopathy (Fleming *et al.*[13])
Copper	0.3–0.5 mg	Anaemia, leucopenia (Cordano & Graham[8]), bony abnormalities
Chromium	50–200 µg	Impaired glucose tolerance, neuropathy (Jeejeebhoy *et al.*[18])
Molybdenum	150–500 µg	Amino acid intolerance (Abumrad[1])
Manganese	2–3 mg	
Vanadium	—	Salt and water retention (Golden & Golden[14])

Table 8.5 Dietary intake of certain minerals in an average Western diet.

Mineral	Intake (mg/day)	Minimum requirements (mg/day)	Sources
Mg^{2+} (Davidson et al.[10])	200–400	160–250	Green vegetables, cereals
Zn^{2+} (Spencer et al.[27])	12–15	8–12	Meat, cereals, beans
Cu^{2+} (Sternbieb[28])	3–5	0.3–0.5	Vegetables, fish, meat

Dietary intake and body stores of Mg^{2+}, Zn^{2+} and Cu^{2+} (Table 8.5)

The wide distribution of magnesium in many foods, together with a substantial total body content (25 g for a 70 kg man) means that deficiency is rare apart from in chronic malabsorption and alcoholism, where longstanding inadequate intake together with alcohol-induced renal magnesium wasting leads to symptomatic deficiency.

Unlike magnesium, zinc body stores are much smaller (2.5 g) and the dietary intake is often marginal especially when requirements are increased such as during growth spurts. Thus symptomatic zinc deficiency has been described not only in malnourished children in the rural poor of the Middle East[23] but also in middle class, apparently well-nourished children in Denver, USA.[16] Given the normal borderline intake of zinc, it is apparent that dietary factors altering the bioavailability of ingested zinc may well determine whether or not frank deficiency develops.

As shown in Table 8.5, copper is superabundant in most diets and dietary deficiency is exceedingly rare in man, being only described in very small (< 1500 g) premature neonates[8] and in a few adult patients on long-term TPN. Premature neonates have low hepatic copper stores, and poor copper intake (milk is relatively low in copper) renders them vulnerable to symptomatic copper deficiency which is often precipitated by a diarrhoeal episode with increased faecal loss.

Luminal factors influencing absorption (Table 8.6)

Mg^{2+}, Zn^{2+} and Cu^{2+} ions all form insoluble, and hence non-absorbable, precipitates in the presence of phosphate and Ca^{2+} when the luminal pH rises from 5.5 to 7.0.[17, 26] These cations are absorbed largely in the upper small intestine of man, where the pH often fluctuates within these limits. Thus a delicate balance exists, and absorption of each cation can be substantially altered both by endogenous secretions and by simultaneously ingested foodstuffs and minerals. Furthermore, the atomic configuration of Zn^{2+} and Cu^{2+} means that they readily form stable complexes with chelating agents which include some important dietary components, namely amino acids, oligopeptides, the hydroxyl groups of carbohydrates such as cellulose, phosphates, especially mesinositol hexaphosphate (phytate),[24] bile salts,[20] and specific cation binding proteins such as have been described for zinc in pancreatic secretions.[12]

Table 8.6 Factors influencing the absorption of certain minerals.

Mineral	Dietary factors Inhibitory	Dietary factors Stimulatory	Luminal interactions Inhibitory	Luminal interactions Stimulatory	Adaptive increase in absorption in deficiency
Mg^{2+}	Cu^{2+} (Alcock & MacIntyre[4]) PO_4^{3-} (Smith & McAllan[26])	—	pH > 7.0 (Smith & McAllan[26]) Steatorrhoea	—	Yes
Zn^{2+}	Cu^{2+} (Hockstru[17]) Phytate (Reinhold et al.[24]) Cellulose Clay	Protein	—	Zinc binding protein (Evans et al.[12])	Yes
Cu^{2+}	—	—	Bile salts (Lewis[20])	—	?

Ingested   200-400 mg

Plasma
(65% free Mg^{2+})

80-160 mg

Intestinal
fluxes

8-16 mg

Renal excretion

72-144 mg

Faecal   48-336 mg
excretion

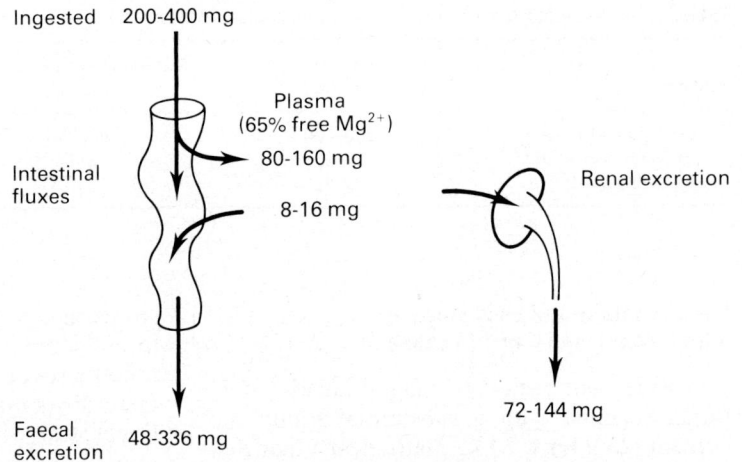

Fig. 8.21 Daily magnesium
balance. Hypothetical balance in
normal man, derived from Aikawa
et al.[3] and Graham *et al.*[15]

Sites and mechanisms of absorption and excretion

MAGNESIUM (FIGURE 8.21)

Magnesium salts are ionized and water soluble, and are readily absorbed, on average about 40% of an oral dose being taken up. Radioisotope studies in man show that orally ingested magnesium appears in the circulation within one hour, suggesting that uptake occurs mainly in the upper small intestine.[15] There is uncertainty as to whether active magnesium absorption occurs, but in vivo most is absorbed by passive diffusion down its electrochemical gradient.[5] The adaptive increase in net absorption in magnesium depletion appears to be largely due to a reduction in the magnesium level in duodenal and pancreatic secretions; normally a considerable amount of magnesium is found in these secretions. After absorption, 65% of magnesium in the plasma is present as free magnesium ions and only 35% is bound to albumin. This ensures

a very rapid renal clearance and alteration in tubular magnesium reabsorption is the main physiological mechanism for maintaining magnesium balance. On a low magnesium diet, urinary excretion can fall to 1 mg/24 h which, when combined with the decrease in magnesium secretion via the gut, usually ensures metabolic equilibrium. Renal compensation fails not only in renal tubular disease, e.g. acute tubular necrosis, but also under the influence of diuretics and alcohol, both of which impair magnesium absorption and can be associated with symptomatic magnesium deficiency. Gut malabsorption is frequently accompanied by increased faecal magnesium due to the formation of insoluble magnesium soaps and in the long term this often leads to magnesium depletion.

ZINC (FIGURE 8.22)

Compared with magnesium, zinc salts are much less soluble; zinc ions are often firmly bound to dietary protein and carbohydrate groups. As a

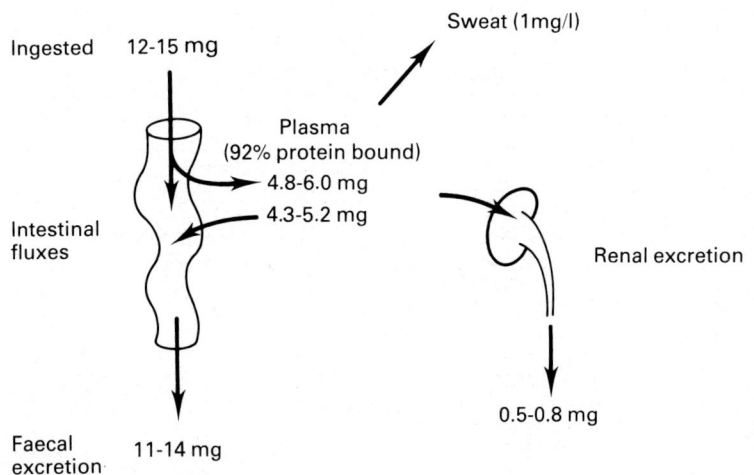

Sweat (1mg/l)

Ingested   12-15 mg

Plasma
(92% protein bound)

4.8-6.0 mg

Intestinal
fluxes

4.3-5.2 mg

Renal excretion

0.5-0.8 mg

Fig. 8.22 Daily zinc balance.
Hypothetical balance in normal
man, derived from Evans *et al.*[11]
and Spencer *et al.*[27]

Faecal   11-14 mg
excretion

result, a normal man will absorb only about 15% of dietary zinc, though in zinc depletion this may rise to 45%. Active uptake has been demonstrated in everted intestinal segments at all levels of the rat small intestine[19] and radio-isotope studies with ^{65}Zn in man show that blood levels peak 2–3 h after oral dosing[6] suggesting that most uptake occurs in the duodenum and jejunum. Once absorbed, zinc is transferred to albumin and α_2-macroglobulin which account for 66% and 30% of circulating zinc. This high degree of protein binding results in a low renal clearance, and urinary excretion is only a small fraction of daily zinc flux. Most zinc is excreted in the faeces, derived from gastro-intestinal secretions and cells, though in hot countries appreciable amounts of zinc can be lost in the sweat. Perhaps because of its low dietary levels and relative lack of toxicity there are no clear pathways for excreting toxic loads of zinc; high zinc intakes usually lead to a positive zinc balance for at least several months.

COPPER (FIGURE 8.23)

Free copper ions are highly reactive, and hence toxic, so that copper in vivo is usually found firmly complexed to carrier proteins. Radioisotope studies indicate that like Mg^{2+} and Zn^{2+}, uptake is in the upper small intestine, about 40% of an oral dose of ^{64}Cu being absorbed. After an early rise in plasma copper which is loosely bound to albumin, there is rapid clearance by the liver and after 24–48 h ^{64}Cu appears tightly and irreversibly bound to caeruloplasmin[28] (molecular weight 150 000). This distribution ensures that little copper is filtered by the glomeruli; urinary excretion is less

than 10% of dietary intake.[2] The main route of excretion of this potentially highly toxic element is in the bile, in which it is excreted as a bile salt–lecithin–copper complex. In this form copper is unavailable for absorption and thus safely excreted.[21] Diseases of the bile duct which impede bile flow, in particular primary biliary cirrhosis, are often associated with hepatic copper accumulation which may contribute to the hepatic fibrosis which follows. This is the logic behind the recent trials of penicillamine in primary biliary cirrhosis; penicillamine is a chelating agent which has been notably successful in removing accumulated hepatic copper in Wilson's disease. The latter condition is inherited as an autosomal recessive trait (prevalence 1/200 000) and is characterized by a life-long deficiency of caeruloplasmin and an accumulation of copper in the liver owing to a defect in biliary excretion.[29] The steady rise in total body copper ultimately leads to a rise in plasma free copper with toxic manifestations, particularly in the brain, eyes and liver. Even rarer is a recently described genetic syndrome of copper deficiency – 'Menkes kinky hair syndrome' – in which oral copper fails to be absorbed although intravenous copper is handled normally.[9] Neonates affected by this syndrome have low plasma and hepatic copper associated with severe, and ultimately fatal, neurological and connective tissue damage. The kinky hair appears to be due to a lack of di-sulphide linkages which normally stabilize keratin, a very similar lesion to that found in sheep grazing on copper deficient pastures. It is suggested, though unproven, that there is a lack of a copper enzyme responsible for creating these linkages.

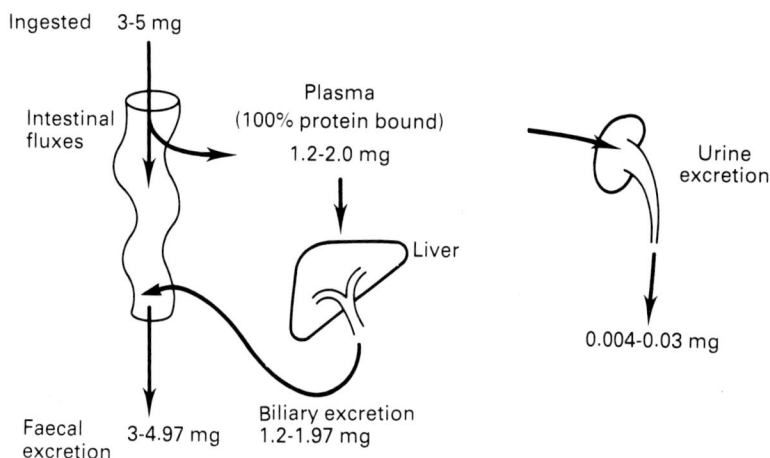

Fig. 8.23 Daily copper balance. Hypothetical balance in normal man, derived from Adelstein & Vallee,[2] Mistilis & Farrer[21] and Steinbieb.[28]

Specific clinically significant interactions leading to malabsorption

MAGNESIUM

Animal studies in both the rat[4] and calf[26] have shown that the presence of Cu^{2+} and PO_4^{3-} lower the concentration of ionized Mg^{2+} if the pH rises above 6.0, and human studies have confirmed that a high Ca^{2+} intake will lower Mg^{2+} absorption.[7] This may be clinically important in neonates fed on cow's milk since its high PO_4^{3-} and Ca^{2+} content may cause transient hypomagnesaemia even in the presence of an entirely normal gut. In diseases accompanied by steatorrhoea, luminal Ca^{2+} and Mg^{2+} ions form insoluble soaps and Mg^{2+} lost in the faeces can be increased by both Ca^{2+} and fat loading.[7] Interestingly, this loss can be reduced by substituting normal dietary fat with medium chain triglycerides (MCTs) since Mg^{2+} salts formed with short chain fatty acids are more soluble than those formed with long chain fatty acids. There does seem to be some mucosal adaptation to Mg^{2+} depletion since in both rats[22] and man[15] there is a compensatory increase in intestinal absorption as depletion increases.

ZINC

Although only recently described, human zinc deficiency is not uncommon, especially in areas such as the Middle East where a major part of the diet consists of unleavened, high-fibre, phytate-rich bread. Both in vitro[25] and in vivo[24] studies have shown strong binding of zinc ions to this bread, and in a prolonged balance study a negative zinc balance was induced in healthy Westerners merely by adding the local bread to their diet. Geophagia, the custom of ingesting finely powdered clay, is also thought to play a part in zinc deficiency in parts of Iran, since clay is capable of complexing with zinc and rendering it unabsorbable. Like magnesium, zinc faecal loss is increased in association with steatorrhoea, presumably because of the formation of insoluble zinc soaps. The level of protein intake may be important in determining the overall effect of these dietary differences, since in vitro at least[25] protein hydrolysates facilitate the release of fibre-bound zinc, probably by forming more soluble amino acid and oligopeptide zinc complexes. Another agent which stimulates zinc absorption is found in rat pancreatic secretions and is a low molecular weight ligand[12] which facilitates zinc mucosal uptake. Exclusion of pancreatic secretions in the rat lowers zinc absorption from an aqueous solution, pointing to another mechanism for zinc deficiency in malabsorption secondary to exocrine pancreatic insufficiency.

REFERENCES

1   Abumrad, N. W. (1981) Amino acid intolerance during prolonged total parenteral nutrition reversed by molybdenum. *Clinical Research,* **27**, 621A.

2   Adelstein, S. J. & Vallee, B. L. (1961) Copper metabolism in man. *New England Journal of Medicine,* **265**, 892–897.

3   Aikawa, J. K., Gordon, G. S. & Rhoades, E. L. (1960) Magnesium metabolism in human beings: studies with Mg^{28}. *Journal of Applied Physiology,* **15**, 503–507.

4   Alcock, N. & MacIntyre, I. (1962) Interrelation of calcium and magnesium absorption. *Clinical Science,* **22**, 185–193.

5   Aldor, T. A. & Moore, E. W. (1970) Magnesium absorption by everted sacs of rat intestines and colon. *Gastroenterology,* **59**, 745–753.

6   Andersson, K. E., Bratt, L., Dencker, H. & Lanner E. (1976) Some aspects of the intestinal absorption of zinc in man. *European Journal of Clinical Pharmacology,* **9**, 423–428.

7   Booth, C. C., Hanna, S., Babouris, N. & MacIntyre, I. (1963) Incidence of hypomagnesaemia in intestinal malabsorption. *British Journal of Medicine,* **iii**, 141–144.

8   Cordano, A. & Graham, G. C. (1966) Copper deficiency complicating severe chronic intestinal malabsorption. *Pediatrics,* **38**, 596–604.

9   Danks, D. M., Campbell, P. E., Walker-Smith, J. *et al.* (1972) Menkes' kinky hair syndrome. *Lancet,* **i**, 1100–1103.

10 Davidson, S., Passmore, R., Brock, J. F. & Trusswell, A. S. (1979) *Human Nutrition and Dietetics.* 7th edn. New York: Churchill Livingstone.

11 Evans, G. W., Grace, C. C. & Hahn, C. (1973) Homeostatic regulation of zinc absorption in the rat. *Proceedings of the Society of Experimental Biology and Medicine,* **143**, 723–725.

12 Evans, G. W., Grace, C. I. & Votava, H. J. (1975) A proposed mechanism for zinc absorption in the rat. *American Journal of Physiology,* **228**, 501–505.

13 Fleming, C. R., McCall, J. T., O'Brien, J. F. *et al.* (1982) Selenium deficiency and fatal cardiomyopathy in a patient on home parenteral nutrition. *Gastroenterology,* **83**, 689–693.

14 Golden, M. H. & Golden, B. E. (1981) Trace elements. Potential importance in human nutrition with particular reference to zinc and vanadium. *British Medical Bulletin,* **37**, 31–36.

15 Graham, L. A., Caesar, J. J. & Burgen, A. S. V. (1960) Gastrointestinal absorption and excretion of Mg^{28} in man. *Metabolism,* **9**, 646–659.

16 Hambridge, K. M., Hambridge, C., Jacobs, M. & Baum, J. D. (1972) Low levels of zinc in hair, anorexia, poor growth and hypogeusia in children. *Pediatric Research,* **6**, 868–874.

17 Hockstru, W. G. (1964) Recent observations on mineral interrelationships. *Federation Proceedings,* **23**, 1068–1076.

18 Jeejeebhoy, K. M., Chu, R., Marliss, E. B. *et al.* (1975) Chromium deficiency, diabetes and neuropathy reversed by chromium infusion in a patient on total

parenteral nutrition (TPN) for $3\frac{1}{2}$ years. *Clinical Research*, **23**, 636A.

19 Kowarski, S., Blair-Stuneck, C. S. & Schacter, D. (1974) Active transport of zinc and identification of zinc-binding protein in rat jejunal mucosa. *American Journal of Physiology*, **226**, 401–407.

20 Lewis, K. W. (1973) The nature of the copper complexes in bile and their relationship to the absorption and excretion of copper in normal subjects and in Wilson's disease. *Gut*, **14**, 221–232.

21 Mistilis, S. P. & Farrer, P. A. (1968) The absorption of biliary and non-biliary radio copper in the rat. *Scandinavian Journal of Gastroenterology*, **3**, 586–592.

22 Petith, M. M. & Scheldl, H. P. (1978) Effects of magnesium deficiency on duodenal and ileal magnesium absorption and secretion. *Digestive Diseases*, **23**, 1–5.

23 Prasad, A. S., Miale, A., Farid, Z. *et al.* (1963) Biochemical studies on dwarfism, hypogonadism and anaemia. *Archives of Internal Medicine*, **iii**, 407–428.

24 Reinhold, J. G., Lahimgarzadek, A., Nasr, K. & Hedayati, H. (1973) Effects of purified phytate and phytate-rich bread upon metabolism of zinc, calcium, phosphorus and nitrogen in man. *Lancet*, **i**, 283–288.

25 Reinhold, J. G., Pursu, A., Karimian, N. *et al.* (1974) Availability of zinc in leavened and unleavened whole meal wheaten bread as measured by solubility and uptake by rat intestine in vitro. *Journal of Nutrition*, **105**, 976–982.

26 Smith, R. H. & McAllan, A. B. (1966) Binding of magnesium and calcium in the contents of the small intestine of the calf. *British Journal of Nutrition*, **20**, 703–718.

27 Spencer, H., Osis, D., Krumer, L. & Norris, C. (1976) Intake, excretion and retention of zinc in man. In *Trace Elements in Human Health and Disease*, Volume 1. (Ed.) Prasad, A. S. & Oberleas, D. pp. 345–362. London: Academic Press.

28 Sternlieb, I. (1967) Gastrointestinal copper absorption in man. *Gastroenterology*, **52**, 1038–1041.

29 Sternlieb, I., Morrell, A. G., Bauer, C. D. *et al.* (1961) Detection of the heterozygous carrier of the Wilson's disease gene. *Journal of Clinical Investigations*, **40**, 707–715.

ABSORPTION AND MALABSORPTION OF VITAMINS

This section deals with the absorption and malabsorption of the fat soluble vitamins A, E and K, and the water soluble vitamins thiamine, pyridoxine, riboflavin, niacin, biotin, ascorbic acid and pantothenic acid. Vitamins D and B_{12} and folate are discussed elsewhere.

Clinical vitamin deficiency is uncommon in the Western World because of the adequacy of the diet, the vast reserve absorptive capacity of the normal intestine and the relatively small amounts of vitamins needed for normal metabolism. Probably because of these factors, relatively little information is available about the absorption of many vitamins, most of which have, until recently, been regarded as being absorbed by purely passive mechanisms.[26]

Fat soluble vitamins

VITAMIN A

The term 'vitamin A' encompasses all compounds, other than the carotenoids, which exhibit the biological activity of retinol. Retinol (vitamin A alcohol) is essential for normal vision, a derivative being an integral part of the visual pigment rhodopsin. Vitamin A is also required for the maintenance of epithelial integrity and reproductive function, and in young animals for growth and neurological development. It is present mainly as esters in animal products and fish. Plants contain carotenoids which themselves have no vitamin A activity, but can be converted to retinol in the intestine; 0.3 µg of retinol is equivalent to 6 µg of carotene or 12 µg of dietary carotenoids. Daily requirements are of the order of 1000 µg of retinol equivalents, and come mainly from dairy products such as butter, egg yolk or fortified margarine, and from plant carotenoids. The liver is the major site of storage in man, where $3–5 \times 10^6$ iu of vitamin A are stored as retinyl esters.

Only 67% of orally administered retinol acetate and between 6.7 and 41% of retinol appeared in thoracic duct lymph in man.[11] Although some absorption probably takes place via the portal vein, absorption of vitamin A appears incomplete. Hydrolysis of dietary retinyl esters by pancreatic retinyl hydrolase is obligatory for absorption. Since vitamin A is very hydrophobic, micellar solubilization is also important. Although little is known of the exact mechanisms of transport of any of the fat soluble vitamins, movement of vitamin A from the lumen into the cell is probably by passive diffusion. Retinol within the cell is re-esterified with long chain fatty acids, usually palmitic (C16 : 0) and exported in chylomicrons via the lymph. Dietary β-carotene is hydrolysed to two molecules of retinal (retinaldehyde) within the intestinal cells. The retinaldehyde is then converted to retinol, esterified, and exported in chylomicrons as before.

Retinoic acid is a metabolite of vitamin A which cannot be converted to retinol or retinal and will not perform the ocular or fertility functions of retinol, but apparently will substitute in all other respects. This compound is absorbed via the portal system, but is not stored in the liver.[13]

World-wide, vitamin A deficiency almost always arises because of dietary inadequacy and is a common cause of blindness, particularly in childhood, in underdeveloped countries.

Patients with prolonged steatorrhoea due to severe small bowel disease, intraluminal bile salt deficiency or exocrine pancreatic insufficiency (particularly cystic fibrosis) and patients with intestinal fistulas or liver disease may develop low blood levels of vitamin A. Frank clinical deficiency is, however, very rare in the West where the diet contains adequate amounts of the vitamin.

The earliest and most consistent sign of deficiency is defective dark adaptation resulting in night blindness. Severe deficiency produces xerophthalmia with Bitot's spots, white spots on the retina (Uyemura's syndrome), keratomalacia, and blindness. Epithelial surfaces become dry and thickened, and infants fail to grow and develop normally.

VITAMIN E

Vitamin E is a term used to describe a family of tocopherols and tocotrienols of which α-tocopherol is the most biologically active. The functions of vitamin E in man are uncertain. It appears to act as a biological antioxidant, and is probably required for normal neurological function. Although vitamin E deficient female rats are infertile, an effect on fertility has not been shown in man. The daily requirement is also uncertain, but is probably 10–30 mg. Requirements are often expressed in international units (iu); 1 iu is equivalent to 1 mg of *dl-α-*tocopherol. Body stores are probably large since deficiency takes years to develop on a deficient diet. The most concentrated dietary sources are grains, seed-germ oils and nuts.

Ingested vitamin E esters can be absorbed, but are probably hydrolysed by pancreatic enzymes to free tocopherols which are better absorbed. Even so, absorption is incomplete, being only 20–40% of the dietary intake. Maximal absorption occurs in the proximal small bowel. Micellar solubilization is important for absorption which takes place at the brush border, probably by passive diffusion. Absorbed tocopherols are not re-esterified within the cell and appear unchanged in chylomicrons in the thoracic duct lymph. Absorption directly into the portal vein is possible but unquantified.[12]

Low serum levels of vitamin E occur in any situation associated with prolonged fat malabsorption, such as prolonged cholestasis, chronic exocrine pancreatic insufficiency, intestinal lymphangiectasia and coeliac disease.[22] The degree of malabsorption of α-tocopherol correl-

ates roughly with the faecal fat excretion.[17] Low serum levels are found consistently in cystic fibrosis patients with exocrine pancreatic insufficiency. These patients may have evidence of tissue deficiency in the form of abnormal sensitivity to haemolysis by peroxide and accumulation of brown lipofuscin pigment in the tissues. The severest deficiencies arise in abetalipoproteinaemic subjects, who develop a peroxide-sensitive haemolytic state with acanthocytosis and a neurological syndrome consisting of areflexia, cerebellar ataxia and loss of position sense, usually occurring within the first decade of life. The neurological sequelae also occur in adults with longstanding cholestasis. Treatment of abetalipoproteinaemic patients with supramaximal doses of α-tocopherol acetate (100 $mg \cdot kg^{-1} \cdot day^{-1}$) certainly delays, and may prevent, the development of neurological complications. In patients with established lesions, vitamin E analogues can arrest or even reverse the neuropathy.[21]

VITAMIN K

Vitamin K is present in many plant foods as phylloquinone (vitamin K_1). A bacterial product, menaquinone (K_2) can be synthesized by intestinal bacteria and in some circumstances may be available to the host. Menadione (K_3) is a purely synthetic molecule which lacks the long side chain of K_1 or K_2 and is never a normal dietary constituent. Vitamin K is involved in the biosynthesis of clotting factors in the liver, principally prothrombin (factor II) and factors VII, IX, and X. Daily requirements are uncertain but are of the order of 50–150 μg in adults. Deficiency causes a defect in the clotting mechanism manifest by skin ecchymoses and purpura, gum bleeding, haematuria, and gastrointestinal bleeding. Stores of the vitamin, which are held in the liver, are relatively small; prolongation of the plasma prothrombin time occurs within weeks of dietary deprivation.

Absorption of the natural fat soluble vitamin in man is only 40–50% of an oral dose whether measured by recovery in thoracic duct lymph[5] or by faecal excretion.[27] Absorption of the vitamins K_1 and K_2 depends on micellar solubilization with subsequent uptake into the intestinal cells, probably by passive diffusion. Vitamin K is transferred to the lymphatics without esterification[5, 27] and appears in the chylomicrons unchanged. Absorption of natural vitamin K may also occur via the portal vein as with vitamins A and E, but again the quantitative importance of this is unclear. Menaquinone synthesized in the colon is probably not available to man, since vitamin K deficiency in adults cannot be corrected by intracolonic phylloquinone.[33] Whether sufficient menaquinone is manufactured in the normal human small gut to materially effect vitamin K supply is unknown but seems unlikely. Menadione (K_3) is much more water soluble than K_1 or K_2 and is absorbed directly into the portal vein where it is bound to albumin.[19]

Deficiency of vitamin K is clinically and biochemically much easier to detect than deficiency of the other fat soluble vitamins. The liver stores are smaller, and it is therefore much more common than deficiency of the other fat soluble vitamins. Malabsorption occurs in chronic intraluminal bile salt deficiency such as chronic cholestasis and after prolonged therapy with cholestyramine.[34] Malabsorption may also occur in any disease of the small intestine associated with a decrease in functional surface area or with intestinal lymphatic obstruction.

Water soluble vitamins

L-ASCORBIC ACID (VITAMIN C)

Humans have an absolute dietary requirement for vitamin C because they are deficient in the enzyme gulonolactone oxidase which enables most other species to synthesize ascorbic acid. Vitamin C is required in many tissues, predominantly as a reducing agent or as a source of peroxide. It is particularly important in collagen biosynthesis. The recommended daily intake is 60 mg in adults, which is usually easily supplied by fresh fruit, vegetables, and liver. In man, liver stores last four to five months before clinical deficiency is apparent.

Absorption in both man and the guinea pig appears to be by an active sodium dependent mechanism confined to the ileum.[18, 28] Passive absorption of large doses may, however, occur by diffusion.

Deficiency almost always arises because of dietary insufficiency, either self-induced or obligatory. Deficiency due to loss of the ileal absorptive mechanism has not been recorded. Deficiency gives rise to the clinical syndrome of scurvy, with malaise, weakness, and lassitude, progressing to dyspnoea, bone pain, and perifollicular haemorrhages with hyperkeratotic hair follicles and fragmented, coiled hairs. In the late stages petechiae and ecchymoses occur with the characteristic enlarged, spongy, and bleeding gums. Leucocyte ascorbic acid levels, normally 20–30 mg/100 ml, correlate quite well with clinical deficiency, which occurs at levels of 0–2 mg/100 ml.

THIAMINE (VITAMIN B_1)

Thiamine is required as a co-enzyme in the decarboxylation of α-keto acids and in the formation of α-ketols. It occurs in cells largely as the active co-enzyme thiamine pyrophosphate. The daily requirement of 1–2 mg is easily supplied by most diets since thiamine is widely distributed in foods.

Dietary deficiency arises only on extremely restricted diets – classically those consisting almost entirely of polished rice. The major storage site is the liver where about 30 mg are sequestered. These stores last only a few weeks if thiamine is absent from the diet.

Absorption of thiamine is by an active sodium dependent mechanism[10] and takes place mainly from the proximal small bowel. Maximal absorption is about 8 mg from a single oral dose.[31] Alcohol in either the blood or intestinal lumen impairs absorption and there is some evidence that chronic malnutrition may also interfere with absorption.[32] These two factors, plus dietary inadequacy, account for the frequency of thiamine deficiency in alcoholics.

Absorption is possibly reduced in a number of malabsorptive states including adult coeliac disease,[30] but clinical deficiency due to malabsorption is very rare. Most deficient subjects are alcoholics or patients with protracted vomiting. Because of the frequency of thiamine deficiency in alcoholics, thiamine supplementation of alcoholic beverages has been suggested.[7] Recognized deficiency diseases include beriberi, either with predominantly neurological or predominantly cardiac manifestations, and the Wernicke–Korsakoff syndrome. Subjects developing the Wernicke–Korsakoff syndrome may be predisposed to clinical deficiency by a genetic defect in the binding of thiamine pyrophosphate to transketolase.[4] Less well-recognized manifestations of thiamine deficiency include anorexia, nausea, impaired gastrointestinal motility, vague muscle pains, paraesthesia and heaviness of the legs, personality disturbance, altered behaviour, and hypotension. This sort of presentation may be much more common than is generally realized, particularly in patients with malabsorption.[25] The best test for deficiency is probably measurement of red cell transketolase activity and its response to thiamine pyrophosphate.[9]

PYRIDOXINE

Pyridoxal phosphate is a cofactor for many enzymes involved in the synthesis, catabolism and transport of amino acids, and in the metabolism of glycogen and unsaturated fatty acids. It occurs in foodstuffs as pyridoxamine phosphate and pyridoxal phosphate in animal products, and as pyridoxine in plants.

Absorption is probably by passive diffusion both in man and the rat; absorption appears linearly related to concentration.[6] Absorption in patients with distal small intestinal resection was almost normal, but was reduced in 6 out of 13 patients with coeliac disease. In the coeliac patients there was, however, no correlation between other parameters of malabsorption and malabsorption of the tritiated vitamin.[6] The commonest causes of pyridoxine deficiency are probably INAH treatment and dietary deficiency; deficiency due to malabsorption is rare. Secondary deficiency of nicotinic acid is common because of failure of nicotinic acid synthesis from tryptophan in the absence of pyridoxine. Pure pyridoxine deficiency such as occurs with isoniazid (INAH) treatment causes a peripheral neuropathy. Pyridoxine deficiency occurring in infants fed a proprietary formula rendered deficient in pyridoxine by the sterilization process employed caused restlessness and irritability, and some infants developed convulsions.[8] The most reliable test for deficiency is probably measurement of urinary xanthenuric acid excretion after an oral tryptophan load.[1]

NIACIN

Niacin (nicotinic acid and nicotinamide) forms an essential part of pyridoxine co-enzymes such as nicotinamide-adenine dinucleotide (NAD), which is required for oxidoreductases necessary for tissue respiration, glycolysis and fat synthesis. The normal daily requirement is 10–20 mg of niacin, or 60 times as much tryptophan, from which approximately 50% of niacin requirements are normally synthesized. Diets containing animal or good quality vegetable protein contain enough tryptophan to prevent deficiency even when niacin intakes are low. Major sources of preformed niacin are yeast, liver, meat, peanuts, and vegetables. Deficiency is traditionally associated with maize diets because maize has a low content of both tryptophan and niacin.

Absorption in the rat jejunum has been shown to be sodium dependent and reduced by structural analogues, features which are in favour of a specific carrier mediated transport.[23]

Deficiency causes pellagra, which consists of a photosensitive pigmented, keratinized skin condition with a sore, swollen and scarlet tongue. In severe deficiency, dementia and acute encephalopathy may also occur. The cause is usually dietary insufficiency, either obligatory or in association with alcoholism, in which case other vitamin deficiencies usually co-exist. Although pellagra has been reported in association with almost every gastrointestinal disease,[25] many of the associations are probably false. Deficiency in these cases is usually due mainly to dietary deficiency or vomiting rather than to a true association with a particular disease. Acute nicotinamide encephalopathy responding dramatically to parenteral vitamin administration has been reported in a patient with jejunal diverticulosis.[29] Pellagra also occurs in Hartnup's disease and in the carcinoid syndrome.

RIBOFLAVIN

This vitamin forms the active prosthetic group of flavoproteins concerned in oxidative processes. The daily requirement is 1–2 mg; it is found mainly in milk, liver, eggs, meat, and in many green and yellow vegetables.

Riboflavin is rapidly absorbed after oral administration. Peak levels in urine are achieved after 2 hours, suggesting absorption takes place in the proximal small intestine.[20] The mode of transport in man has not been examined, but it is known that bile salts facilitate absorption.[15]

Although poorly absorbed from the rectum,[16] synthesis by colonic bacteria with subsequent absorption appears adequate to prevent deficiency in some circumstances.[24]

Body stores of flavonoids appear to be large because deficiency does not develop for many months and is usually precipitated by stress such as pregnancy, lactation, or infection. Deficiency is usually dietary, and is commonly associated with niacin and protein deficiency. Mild dietary deficiency is common among the Third World poor. More severe deficiency is usually associated with pellagra and kwashiorkor. In the West, alcoholics and patients after partial gastrectomy, or with chronic debilitating diseases or chronic severe small intestinal disease, are the usual candidates for deficiency. Symptoms and signs of deficiency include sore, burning lips, mouth and tongue, with angular stomatitis and glossitis, photophobia, lacrimation, and burning and itching of the eyes. The 'burning feet syndrome' has sometimes been ascribed to riboflavin deficiency, but not all such patients respond to riboflavin.[25]

BIOTIN

This vitamin is important in the enzymatic transfer and incorporation of carbon dioxide. Biotin is synthesized by intestinal bacteria and deficiency cannot therefore easily be induced by dietary deprivation. Clinical deficiency can be induced by consumption of large amounts of raw egg-white which contains the biotin-binding protein avidin. Deficiency is characterized by scaly dermatitis, pallor, lassitude, anorexia, muscle pains, insomnia, precordial pain, and anaemia. There is no information on the absorption of biotin in man. In hamster intestine in vitro, absorption appears to be sodium dependent and inhibited by structural analogues suggesting a carrier mediated mechanism of absorption.[3]

PANTOTHENIC ACID

This vitamin is a vital constituent of acetyl coenzyme A on which acylation and acetylation depend. It is so widely distributed in plant and animal tissues that deficiency does not occur spontaneously. A daily intake of 5–10 mg is probably adequate. Experimental deficiency induced by feeding the metabolic antagonist omega-methyl pantothenic acid together with a deficient diet resulted in overt deficiency within a few months.[2, 14] An interesting feature of the deficiency state was reduced antibody formation. In malnourished alcoholics, a neuropathy has been associated with low serum pantothenic acid levels but this is more likely to be multifactorial. No reliable information is available on the absorption of pantothenic acid, and malabsorption has not been documented.

REFERENCES

1 Baker, E. M., Canham, J. E., Nunes, W. I. et al. (1964) Vitamin B_6 requirement for adult men. *American Journal of Clinical Nutrition*, 15, 59–66.
2 Bean, W. B. & Hodges, R. E. (1954) Pantothenic acid deficiency induced in human subjects. *Proceedings of the Society for Experimental Biology and Medicine*, 86, 693–698.
3 Berger, E., Long, E. & Semenza, G. (1972) The sodium activation of biotin absorption in hamster small intestine in vitro. *Biochimica et Biophysica Acta*, 255, 873–887.
4 Blass, J. P. & Gibson, G. E. (1977) Abnormality of a thiamine-requiring enzyme in patients with Wernicke–Korsakoff syndrome. *New England Journal of Medicine*, 297, 1367–1370.
5 Blomstrand, R. & Forsgen, L. (1968) Vitamin K_1-^{3}H in man. Its intestinal absorption and transport in thoracic duct lymph. *Internationale Zeitschrift für Vitamin-Forschung*, 38, 45–64.
6 Brain, M. & Booth, C. C. (1964) The absorption of tritium-labelled pyridoxine HCl in control subjects and in patients with intestinal malabsorption. *Gut*, 5, 241–247.
7 Centerwall, B. S. & Criqui, M. H. (1978) Prevention of Wernicke–Korsakoff syndrome. *New England Journal of Medicine*, 299, 285–289.
8 Coursin, D. B. (1964) Vitamin B_6 metabolism in infants and children. *Vitamins and Hormones*, 22, 755.
9 Dreyfus, P. M. (1962) Clinical application of blood transketolase determinations. *New England Journal of Medicine*, 267, 596–598.
10 Ferrari, G., Ventura, U. & Rindi, G. (1971) The Na^+ dependence of thiamine intestinal transport in vitro. *Life Sciences*, 10, 67–75.
11 Forsgren, L. (1969) Studies on the intestinal absorption of labelled fat-soluble vitamins (A, D, E and K) via the thoracic duct lymph in the absorption of bile in man. *Acta Chirurgica Scandinavica*, Supplement 399.
12 Gallo-Torres, H. E. (1980) Absorption (of Vitamin E). In *Vitamin E: a comprehensive treatise*. (Ed.) Machlin L. J. pp. 170–192. New York: Marcel Dekker Inc.
13 Goodman, D. S. (1979) Vitamin A and retinoids: recent advances. *Federation Proceedings*, 38, 2501–2503.
14 Hodges, R. E., Bean, W. B., Ohlson, M. A. & Bleiler, R. (1959) Human pantothenic acid deficiency produced by omega-methyl pantothenic acid. *Journal of Clinical Investigation*, 38, 1421–1425.
15 Jusko, W., Levy, G., Yaffe, S. & Gorodischer, R. (1970) Effect of probenecid on renal clearance of riboflavin in man. *Journal of Pharmacological Science*, 59, 473–477.
16 Levy, G. & Jusko, W. (1966) Factors affecting the absorption of riboflavin in man. *Journal of Pharmacological Science*, 55, 285–289.
17 MacMahon, M. T. & Neale, G. (1970) The absorption of α-tocopherol in control subjects and in patients with intestinal malabsorption. *Clinical Science*, 38, 197–210.
18 Mellors, A., Nahrwold, D. C. & Rose, R. C. (1977) Ascorbic acid fluxes across mucosal border of guinea pig and human ileum. *American Journal of Physiology*, 233, E272–E278.
19 Mezick, J. A., Tompkins, R. K. & Cornwell, D. G. (1968) Absorption and intestinal lymphatic transport of ^{14}C-menadione. *Life Sciences*, 7, 153–158.
20 Morrison, A. B. & Campbell, J. A. (1960) Vitamin absorption studies: I. Factors involving the excretion of oral test doses of thiamine and riboflavin by human subjects. *Journal of Nutrition*, 72, 435–440.
21 Muller, D. P. R., Lloyd, J. K. & Wolff, O. (1983) Vitamin E and neurological function. *Lancet*, i, 225–227.
22 Muller, D. P. R., Harries, J. T. & Lloyd, J. K. (1974) The relative importance of the factors involved in the absorption of vitamin E in children, *Gut*, 15, 966–971.
23 Myers, L. A., Nahrwold, D. C. & Rose, R. C. (1981) Quoted in: Rose, R. C. (1981) Absorption of water-soluble vitamins. In *Physiology of the Gastrointestinal Tract*, volume 2, p. 1236, (Ed.) Johnson, L. R. New York: Raven Press.
24 Najjar, V., Johns, G., Medairy, G. et al. (1944) The biosynthesis of riboflavin in man. *Journal of the American Medical Association*, 126, 357–358.
25 Pallis, C. A. & Lewis, P. D. (1974) Other vitamin deficiencies. In *The Neurology of Gastrointestinal Disease*. pp. 98–123. London: W. B. Saunders.
26 Rose, R. C. (1981) Transport and metabolism of water-soluble vitamins in intestine. *American Journal of Physiology*, 3, G97–G101.
27 Shearer, M. J., Barkhan, P. & Webster, G. R. (1970) Absorption and excretion of an oral dose of tritiated

vitamin K_1 in man. *British Journal of Haematology*, **18**, 297–308.

28 Stevenson, N. (1974) Active transport of L-ascorbic acid in the human ileum. *Gastroenterology*, **67**, 952–956.

29 Tabaqchali, S. & Pallis, C. A. (1970) Reversible nicotinamide-deficiency encephalopathy in a patient with jejunal diverticulosis. *Gut*, **11**, 1024–1028.

30 Thomson, A. D. (1966) The absorption of radioactive sulphur-labelled thiamine hydrochloride in control subjects and in patients with intestinal malabsorption. *Clinical Science*, **31**, 167–179.

31 Thomson, A. D. & Leevy, C. M. (1972) Mechanism of thiamine absorption. *Clinical Science*, **43**, 153–163.

32 Thomson, A. D., Baker, H. & Leevy, C. M. (1970) Patterns of ^{35}S-thiamine HCl absorption in the malnourished alcoholic patient. *Journal of Laboratory and Clinical Medicine*, **76**, 34–45.

33 Udall, J. A. (1965) Human sources and absorption of vitamin K in relation to anticoagulation stability. *Journal of the American Medical Association*, **194**, 127–129.

34 Visintine, R. E., Michaels, G. D., Fukayama, G. *et al.* (1961) Xanthomatous biliary cirrhosis treated with cholestyramine: a bile acid adsorbing resin. *Lancet*, **ii**, 341–343.

ABSORPTION AND MALABSORPTION OF HAEMATINICS

Vitamin B_{12}
(see also p. 685)

DIETARY SOURCES

Vitamin B_{12} was originally isolated as cyanocobalamin but is now known to consist of a group of compounds, known as cobalamins, each with a nucleotide portion (composed of the base 5,6-benzimidazole attached to the sugar, ribose) and a planar corrin ring with a cobalt atom at its centre. In the four compounds found in human tissues a methyl-, deoxyadenosyl- (ado-), hydroxyl- or cyano- group is attached to the cobalt atom. Cyanocobalamin has a molecular weight of 1355. The two main naturally occurring compounds are methyl-B_{12} and ado-B_{12} but light rapidly oxidizes them to hydroxocobalamin which is therefore the main form eaten by man. Traces of cyano- and other minor cobalamins are also eaten, as well as nonphysiological B_{12} analogues with an altered or absent nucleotide moiety or with different substitutions in the corrin ring. Ado-B_{12}, which is a coenzyme for methylmalonyl coenzyme A mutase, is the major form in human cells whereas methyl-B_{12}, which is a coenzyme for methylation of homocysteine to methionine, dominates in plasma but forms only about 20% of tissue B_{12}.

A normal Western diet contains 7–30 µg B_{12} daily; it is present in foods of animal origin and absent from cereals, nuts, vegetables and fruits. Micro-organisms can synthesize the vitamin; thus bacterial synthesis in the gut may provide a supply (e.g. in sheep) or B_{12} animal food or food contaminated by micro-organisms may be eaten (e.g. in humans). The foods richest in B_{12} are liver, kidney, and red meats. Daily losses, and thus requirements, in adults are 1–2 µg; stores are 2–3 mg, i.e. enough for two to four years if dietary supplies are completely cut off. The body does not degrade the vitamin and there are no well documented syndromes of B_{12} deficiency due to increased B_{12} utilization.

ABSORPTION OF B_{12}

All B_{12} in nature is tightly bound to protein and it is released by cooking and by peptic digestion within the stomach. B_{12} then binds, one molecule to one molecule, with the glycoprotein, intrinsic factor (IF) with a molecular weight of approximately 45 000. IF is secreted by the gastric parietal cells, stimulated by histamine and regulated by cyclic nucleotides. The IF–B_{12} complex has a smaller diameter than free IF and is more resistant to digestion in the small intestine. The nucleotide portion of B_{12} is innermost and the CH_3-, CN-, OH or ado- group on the outside. The complex subsequently attaches to specific receptor molecules on the brush border surface of the terminal ileum. This process requires calcium ions and a neutral pH. The receptors are macromolecular (molecular weight $> 1 \times 10^6$) lipoproteins with two subunits, one (α) facing the lumen and the other (β) facing into the ileal cell.[17] The number of receptors is limited (0.3–4.9×10^{12} molecules/g of mucosa) so that only a few micrograms of B_{12} can be absorbed from a single large dose of IF–B_{12} complex. Thus, from 1 µg of B_{12}, 0.5–0.8 µg are normally absorbed, but with smaller doses proportionately more is absorbed and with larger doses proportionately less. This is relevant to the interpretation of results from absorption tests using radioactive B_{12}. Following a single dose of IF–B_{12} complex the ileum is refractory to further B_{12} absorption for three to four hours.

The exact fate of the IF which attaches to the brush borders is unknown; it is probably digested inside the cell in lysosomes, implying uptake of the complex by a pinocytic process.[15] Alternative suggestions have included digestion at the brush border or in mitochondria.[20] B_{12} itself appears, after a delay of several hours during which transfer across the mucosal cell occurs, in the portal blood, attached to a polypeptide transport protein, transcobalamin (TC) II. There is some evidence that this TCII is synthesized in the ileal cell itself.[6] Because of the delay in dietary B_{12} reaching the ileum and the subsequent slow absorptive process, the peak level in systemic blood is only reached 8–12 hours after a single oral dose in man.

Some dietary B_{12} attaches in the stomach to a second B_{12} binding protein present in gastric juice, a so-called 'R' protein (similar to TCI). This does not facilitate cellular uptake of B_{12}. This 'R' protein-bound B_{12} (perhaps 30% of normal dietary B_{12}) is released by digestion of the 'R' protein by pancreatic trypsin and is then available for absorption after subsequently binding to IF. Low gastric pH favours IF and 'R' protein binding of B_{12} equally, but the combination of an alkaline pH and trypsin in pancreatic secretion favours transfer of B_{12} from 'R' protein to IF.[1] The main function of gastric (and salivary) 'R' proteins, however, is probably to bind non-physiological analogues of B_{12} and make them unavailable for absorption. IF itself does not bind these analogues.

Normally the stomach secretes a vast excess of IF. By definition, one unit of IF binds 1 ng of B_{12} and so only about 1000 units of IF are needed for absorption of the normal daily requirements of B_{12}. In response to maximal pentagastrin stimulation, however, the normal adult male stomach secretes 1000–3000 units of IF in one hour (females secrete about half this, due to a smaller volume of gastric juice). Following histamine or pentagastrin stimulation, there is initially wash-out of preformed IF but after 15 minutes secretion of newly formed IF reaches a plateau which may last for several hours with continuous maximal stimulation. Although H_2 antagonists block acid secretion by parietal cells, IF secretion is not specifically inhibited, although the fall in volume of gastric juice results in a proportionate fall in total IF secreted.

B_{12} absorption is not increased in response to B_{12} deficiency. Indeed, severe B_{12} deficiency may actually reduce ileal uptake of IF–B_{12} complex by damaging the mucosal cells. On the other hand, adaptation of the ileum to an upper intestinal resection may lead to an increased number of ileal receptors and thus increased capacity for B_{12} absorption. In the absence of IF, about 1% of an oral dose of crystalline B_{12} is passively absorbed, mainly through the upper small intestine but also through the buccal and gastric mucosae. This absorption is rapid and occurs by diffusion in contrast to the active IF-mediated normal physiological absorption.

Entero-hepatic circulation of B_{12} occurs and is variably estimated to be from 1 to 43 µg of B_{12} daily. This B_{12} is reabsorbed by the IF mechanism. The bile may be a route for excretion of unwanted B_{12} analogues which have either been absorbed or have been produced by degradation of endogenous B_{12} and carried to the liver by the plasma 'R' protein (transcobalamin I).

Tests of B_{12} absorption

Since malabsorption is the major cause of B_{12} deficiency, tests of absorption of B_{12} are important. These all use radioactive (^{57}Co or ^{58}Co) labelled cyano-cobalamin. Five techniques are available: whole-body, liver uptake, faecal excretion, urinary excretion, or plasma radioactivity measurement. In practice, the urinary excretion (Schilling) test is the most widely used. This involves feeding an oral dose of 1 µg of crystalline, labelled B_{12}, and simultaneously giving an intramuscular 'flushing' injection of 1 mg of unlabelled B_{12} to saturate body B_{12} binding sites. This allows absorbed, labelled B_{12} to largely remain unbound and to be excreted after glomerular filtration in the urine. This is collected for 24 hours or, in more accurate techniques, for 48 hours. The test may be repeated giving an active preparation of IF with the oral labelled B_{12}, to test whether any malabsorption of the vitamin detected is due to a gastric or intestinal cause; if an intestinal lesion is likely, the test is repeated after a course of antibiotics to reduce the intestinal bacterial flora. In the 'Dicopac' test, free and IF-bound B_{12}, labelled with ^{57}Co and ^{58}Co respectively, are given simultaneously and differential counting is performed. Some exchange of isotope occurs, however, and the results do not give such a wide separation of results in pernicious anaemia as when the two tests are carried out separately. The Schilling test gives abnormal results in renal failure and also depends on complete urine collection. Whole-body counting is a more accurate technique which does not require a flushing dose, but in order for unabsorbed labelled B_{12} to be excreted, 7 days must be allowed after ingestion of the test dose before the follow-up whole-body count is performed to estimate amount of labelled B_{12} absorbed.

B_{12} absorption tests using protein (e.g. egg ovalbumin) bound B_{12} have been used to provide a better test of food B_{12} absorption, e.g. in conditions such as atrophic gastritis or following partial gastrectomy. However, they are not widely used.

MALABSORPTION OF B_{12}

This is due to gastric or intestinal causes (Table 8.7). By far the most common cause in Western communities is acquired (Addisonian) pernicious anaemia (PA) in which there is an auto-immune gastritis with achlorhydria and failure of IF secretion, which is usually undetectable or secreted at the rate of only a few units/hour. IF antibodies in the gastric juice may block the action of any residual IF. Total gastrectomy and congenital lack of, or abnormality of, IF are other gastric causes of B_{12} malabsorption. Following partial gastrectomy, subsequent IF secretion and thus B_{12} absorption depends largely on the size of the gastric remnant, but a stagnant loop syndrome may also develop. A wide variety of intestinal lesions may lead to malabsorption of the vitamin. These usually affect the ileal cell surface or involve bacterial contamination of the upper small intestine. They also include two rare congenital

Table 8.7 Causes of vitamin B_{12} malabsorption.

Gastric causes
  * Pernicious (Addisonian) anaemia
  * Total gastrectomy
  * Partial gastrectomy
    Corrosive gastritis
  * Congenital absent or abnormal IF

Intestinal causes
  * Intestinal stagnant loop syndrome
      e.g. jejunal diverticulosis
          ileo-colic fistula
  * Tropical sprue
  * Ileal resection
  * Specific malabsorption with proteinuria
      (Imerslund–Gräsbeck syndrome)
  * Fish tapeworm
  * Transcobalamin II deficiency
    Adult coeliac disease
    Pancreatic disease
    Zollinger–Ellison syndrome
    Giardiasis
    Scleroderma
    Whipple's disease
    Radiation damage
    Drugs
        e.g. neomycin
            phenformin
          * metformin
            alcohol
            anticonvulsants
            slow release potassium chloride
            cholestyramine
            colchicine
    Deficiencies
        e.g. folate
            vitamin B_{12}
            protein

---

* Severe B_{12} deficiency causing megaloblastic anaemia or B_{12} neuropathy has been reported to occur with these causes of B_{12} malabsorption.

defects, one of ileal uptake or ileal transport (selective malabsorption of B_{12} with proteinuria), the other being a congenital deficiency of transcobalamin II. In pancreatic disease, there is failure of release of dietary B_{12} from its binding with the 'R' protein secreted by the stomach.[1] As indicated in Table 8.7, many causes of B_{12} malabsorption rarely, if ever, lead to B_{12} deficiency of sufficient severity to cause megaloblastic anaemia or B_{12} neuropathy.

Folate

NATURAL FORMS

Folate was initially crystallized from spinach as folic (pteroylglutamic) acid, but most foods contain folates, the highest content being in liver, kidney, yeast, nuts, and green vegetables. An average Western diet contains about 600 µg daily and daily requirements are about 100–200 µg. Stores of 12–15 mg are sufficient for only 4 months if supplies are completely cut off. However, the body is able to degrade folates by splitting the C_9–N_{10} bond, and this may be increased in conditions of increased cell turnover such as severe haemolytic anaemia or malignant diseases.

Folates occur naturally as a variety of compounds which differ from the parent structure, pteroylglutamic acid, by being reduced to di- or tetrahydro- forms, or by having additional single carbon units (e.g. methyl, formyl, methylene, methenyl, or formimino) attached at the N_5 or the N_{10} position and having additional glutamate residues linked in a chain by γ-carboxypeptide bonds, the usual number in foods being four to seven. In general, folates are not tightly bound to proteins in natural materials and cooking may destroy them by oxidation (particularly if ascorbate has already been destroyed by preheating) with cleavage of the C_9–N_{10} bond; folates are also easily extracted by large volumes of water. The effects of storage of food at various temperatures on folate content vary from food to food.

ABSORPTION OF FOLATE[8, 11, 23]

Absorption takes place largely in the duodenum and jejunum, with conversion of all folates to the single, fully reduced, monoglutamate derivative, 5-methyl tetrahydrofolate (methyl THF), which enters the portal blood.[19] Reduction and methylation occur in the cytoplasm of the enterocyte. The exact site of deconjugation still remains controversial. The enzyme folate conjugase ('pteroylpolyglutamate hydrolase' or 'γ-

glutamyl caboxypeptidase') is present in pancreatic juice and succus entericus at low concentrations. Higher concentrations are present in the enterocytes, largely in lysosomes. At all these sites, the enzyme has an optimum pH of 4.6 with little activity at neutral pH. Studies in rats and humans have suggested, but not proven, that an additional enzyme with an optimum pH near neutral is present in the brush borders of the small intestinal mucosa; it has been proposed that this may be responsible for deconjugation of dietary folates at or near the brush border.[10] Alternatively, a microclimate of lower pH than in the lumen has been considered to be present at the small intestinal surface and this may allow deconjugation by the low pH enzyme.[18] Folic (pteroylglutamic) acid, itself, when used therapeutically in large (5 mg) doses, is largely absorbed into the portal blood unchanged because it is a poor substrate for the reducing enzyme dihydrofolate reductase. It then enters the liver and other tissues, and displaces methyl THF into the plasma. Folate in the plasma is only loosely and non-specifically bound to protein, and is easily dialysed away. Apart from methyl THF, trace amounts of 10-formyl THF and other minor components have also been identified, but their physiological significance is unknown.

The proportion of natural folates absorbed depends partly on the length of the polyglutamate chain; monoglutamates are almost completely absorbed whereas only 50–80% of higher polyglutamates is absorbed. The more folate eaten, the more is absorbed, with no saturation of the absorptive mechanism. Folate absorbed in excess of the body's needs is largely excreted in the urine, either unchanged or as breakdown products. An enterohepatic circulation exists, the folate concentration in bile ranging from 60 to 90 μg daily. This, and folate in sloughed enterocytes, is largely reabsorbed.

Absorption of folates from the lower small intestine is substantially less than from the jejunum, and folates are not absorbed from the large intestine. Bacteria synthesize folates and, if present in the upper small intestine, as in the stagnant loop syndrome, produce folate which is absorbed and can lead to excessively high serum, red cell and urine folate levels.

MALABSORPTION OF FOLATE

Malabsorption of folates is common, but is only the major cause of deficiency in a few conditions, particularly gluten-induced enteropathy and tropical sprue (Table 8.8). In conditions of

Table 8.8 Causes of folate malabsorption.

Major causes
  Gluten-induced enteropathy (child or adult)
  Dermatitis herpetiformis
  Tropical sprue
  Congenital specific malabsorption of folate

Minor causes
  Partial gastrectomy
  Jejunal resection
  Intestinal lymphoma
  Systemic infections
  Inflammatory bowel disease

Drugs
  Salazopyrine
  Cholestyramine
  Methotrexate
  ? Anticonvulsants
  ? Oral contraceptives
  ? Alcohol

minor degrees of folate malabsorption, alone or combined with conditions of increased cell turnover, severe folate deficiency can occur if there is reduced dietary folate intake. Tests of folate absorption, using either tritium labelled folate and urinary or faecal excretion techniques or unlabelled folate with measurement of the rise in plasma folate, are not widely used and are only performed in special centres, often for research purposes only.

Iron

ABSORPTION OF IRON

The human body controls its iron content mainly by regulating iron absorption. With increasing amounts of oral iron, the proportion absorbed falls; there is, nevertheless, some increase in absorption so there is no absolute 'mucosal block' to absorption. The amount of iron in the daily diet is generally well in excess of the body's daily needs·to make up for iron losses or needs for growth, so normally only a small proportion (5–10%) of the iron in food is absorbed. This may be increased in some situations (Table 8.9), but if losses of iron, e.g. by chronic haemorrhage, are substantial, iron deficiency will result. It is convenient to consider iron absorption in two phases.

Table 8.9 Causes of increased absorption of iron.

Iron deficiency
Pregnancy
Increased erythropoiesis
Reducing substances, e.g. vitamin C
Low molecular weight chelating agents, e.g. amino acids, sugars
Primary haemochromatosis

Intraluminal events

Iron in food is largely in the Fe(III) state as iron hydroxides, bound to proteins, or in an organic porphyrin or haem complex. Peptic digestion releases inorganic iron which binds to muco-proteins in the gastric and small intestinal juice and subsequently is largely transformed to low molecular weight chelating substances such as sugars, amino acids or vitamin C. Reduction to the more soluble Fe(II) state by gastric acid or vitamin C favours absorption whereas alkaline pancreatic secretion has the opposite effect, Fe(III) tending to polymerize and form insoluble hydroxides. Inorganic iron is best absorbed in the fasting state, as food generally inhibits absorption by raising the pH and forming insol-uble iron complexes, e.g. with phytates or phos-phates. Less than 50% of the iron in most foods is released by peptic digestion and in general iron is better absorbed from some foods, parti-cularly those of animal origin such as liver and meat, than from other foods such as vegetables or eggs. Specific inhibitors or activators of iron absorption have been postulated to exist in gastric juice but have not been proven.

In general, haem iron is less well absorbed than inorganic iron. It is less affected than inor-ganic iron by other substances present in the lumen; some haem enters the intestinal mucosa intact to be digested there by haem oxygenase, some is broken down to release inorganic iron in the lumen. A specific mucosal receptor for haem has been described.[9] The iron released from haem in the mucosa forms a common pool with absorbed inorganic iron for subsequent transfer to portal blood.

Mucosal uptake

Absorption of small amounts of inorganic iron, largely from its low molecular weight chelates, appears to be an active, carrier-mediated process partly related to body needs. The first stage consists of rapid uptake by the brush border; the second involves transfer across the cell, possibly by combination with low molecu-lar weight chelates or with a specific transferrin-like carrier protein.[13, 16, 21] The second stage appears to be active and dependent on oxidative phosphorylation, but there is controversy as to whether the initial uptake is by simple or facili-tated diffusion, or by an active receptor medi-ated process.[7] Some of the absorbed iron enters cell organelles, particularly mitochondria, or binds with apoferritin to form ferritin. Iron des-tined to enter portal plasma rapidly, however, remains in the soluble cytoplasmic fraction of the cell. Iron trapped in the cell, e.g. as ferritin, is

shed into the gut lumen when the cell reaches the tip of the intestinal villus; this is one impor-tant control mechanism (or 'block') of the amount of iron absorbed. Iron leaving the serosal cell surface binds to transferrin in the portal blood, although in vitro everted loop experiments have shown that this protein is not essential for this transfer. The overall amount of iron entering the portal plasma increases with the amount of iron presented to the mucosa, but the percentage absorption falls. Control mecha-nisms within the intestinal epithelial cell are still not completely understood, but may include the amount of free carrier present, the amount of apoferritin and ferritin present, or the amount of iron required by the intestinal cell for its own haem synthesis. Intestinal macrophages and goblet cells[22] have also been thought to be involved in excretion of ferritin iron or transferrin-bound iron. The amount leaving the serosal surface of the cell is related not only to body stores of iron but also to body iron turn-over for erythropoiesis, and it is postulated that plasma iron turnover may partly indicate to the mucosa how much iron to release into portal blood. The concept of two different iron binding sites on transferrin, differentially affecting iron absorption, is not established, nor are other spe-cific control signals. Cavill *et al.*[4] have suggested that serosal iron transfer from the absorptive cell is similar to the normal exchange of iron between plasma and exchangeable iron in tissues.

MALABSORPTION OF IRON (TABLE 8.10)

It has been estimated that it takes up to 8 years for an adult male, starting with normal iron stores, to develop iron deficiency anaemia solely due to absent dietary iron or to impaired iron absorption. This is because iron stores (mainly as haemosiderin and ferritin in the reti-

Table 8.10 Causes of iron malabsorption.

Dietary factors and drugs
 Phytates
 Phosphates
 Alkalis
 Tea
 Desferrioxamine

Gastric causes
 Achlorhydria
 Atrophic gastritis
 Partial or total gastrectomy

Intestinal causes
 Gluten-induced enteropathy
 Chronic infections
 Iron overload
 Decreased erythropoiesis

culoendothelial cells) of about 1500 mg are large compared to the daily losses of iron (approximately 1 mg); also, as iron stores are reduced, these small losses become even less. Thus, although many factors may reduce iron absorption, iron deficiency anaemia solely due to malabsorption of iron is unusual; excess iron loss as haemorrhage, or increased needs as in growth are generally more important factors. Tests of iron absorption are thus not used routinely in the investigation of patients with iron deficiency.

Reduced absorption of dietary iron occurs with ingestion of foods containing large amounts of phytates or phosphates. Tea has also been shown to reduce absorption of inorganic iron, possibly by forming insoluble iron–tannin complexes. Gastric atrophy and achlorhydria, and antacids such as aluminium hydroxide or magnesium trisilicate also reduce absorption. Iron overload, for example due to multiple transfusions for refractory anaemia, or decreased erythropoiesis as in aplastic anaemia, also reduce iron absorption, as do chronic infections.

Diseases which reduce absorption of iron largely affect the stomach or small intestine. Gastric atrophy, as in pernicious anaemia, impairs iron absorption but it is remarkable how few of these patients develop severe iron deficiency on long-term follow-up unless another cause of iron deficiency such as menorrhagia or carcinoma of stomach is present. Absorption of iron in food is reduced following partial gastrectomy because of reduced acid secretion, chronic gastritis in the remnant with failure of peptic digestion, and because of rapid by-pass of the duodenal mucosa. Absorption of iron is also reduced in gluten-induced enteropathy of children and adults, but it is difficult to know whether reduced absorption of dietary iron or increased loss of mucosal iron is the main cause of iron deficiency in this condition. Other diseases of the upper small intestine may also impair iron absorption, but haemorrhage is usually present in those patients who develop severe iron deficiency anaemia.

Iron absorption is increased in iron deficiency and pregnancy, and if there is increased plasma iron turnover due to increased erythropoiesis, e.g. in some chronic haemolytic anaemias such as thalassaemia intermedia and in some cases of hereditary spherocytosis and sideroblastic anaemia. Iron absorption is also inappropriately raised in relation to body stores in the hereditary disorder primary haemochromatosis, but the mechanism for this remains controversial.

REFERENCES

1 Allen, R. H., Seetharam, B., Podell, E. & Alpers, D. H. (1978) Effect of proteolytic enzymes on the binding of cobalamin to 'R' protein and intrinsic factor. *Journal of Clinical Investigation*, **61**, 47–54.
2 Björn-Rasmussen, E. (1983) Iron absorption: present knowledge and controversies. *Lancet*, **i**, 914–916.
3 Bothwell, T. H., Charlton, R. W., Cock, J. D. & Finch, C. A. (1979) *Iron Metabolism in Man*. Oxford: Blackwell Scientific Publications.
4 Cavill, I., Worwood, A. & Jacobs, A. (1975) Internal regulation of iron absorption. *Nature*, **256**, 328–329.
5 Chanarin, I. (1979) *The Megaloblastic Anaemias*, 2nd Edn. Oxford: Blackwell Scientific Publications.
6 Chanarin, I., Muir, M., Hughes, A. & Hoffbrand, A. V. (1978) Evidence for intestinal origin of transcobalamin II during vitamin B_{12} absorption. *British Medical Journal*, **i**, 1453–1455.
7 Cox, T. M. & Peters, T. J. (1979) The kinetics of iron uptake in vitro by human duodenal mucosa. Studies in normal subjects. *Journal of Physiology*, **189**, 469–478.
8 Folic Acid (1977) *Biochemistry and Physiology in Relation to the Human Nutrition Requirement*. Washington, D.C.: National Academy of Sciences.
9 Gräsbeck, R., Majuri, R., Kuovonen, I. & Tenhumen, R. (1982) Spectral and other studies on the intestinal haem receptor of pig. *Biochimica et Biophysica Acta*, **700**, 137–142.
10 Halsted, C. H. (1979) The intestinal absorption of folates. *American Journal of Clinical Nutrition*, **32**, 846–855.
11 Hoffbrand, A. V. (1975) Synthesis and breakdown of natural folates (folate polyglutamates). In *Progress in Hematology*, volume IX (Ed.) Brown, E. B. pp. 85–105. New York: Grune & Stratton.
12 Hoffbrand, A. V. (1982) Vitamin B_{12} and folate metabolism. In *Blood and its Disorders*, 2nd Edn. (Ed.) Hardisty, R. M. & Weatherall, D. J., pp. 199–263. Oxford: Blackwell Scientific Publications.
13 Huebers, H., Huebers, E., Rummel, W. & Crichton, R. R. (1976) Isolation and characterisation of iron-binding proteins from rat intestinal mucosa. *European Journal of Biochemistry*, **66**, 447–455.
14 Jacobs, A. & Worwood, M. (1982) Iron metabolism, iron deficiency and overload. In *Blood and its Disorders*, 2nd Edn. (Ed.) Hardisty, R. M. & Weatherall, D. J. pp. 149–197. Oxford: Blackwell Scientific Publications.
15 Jenkins, W. J., Empson, R., Jewell, D. P. & Taylor, K. B. (1982) The subcellular localization of vitamin B_{12} during absorption in guinea pig ileum. *Gut*, **22**, 617–623.
16 Johnson, G., Jacobs, P. & Purves, L. R. (1983) The iron binding proteins of iron absorbing rat intestinal mucosa. *Journal of Clinical Investigation*, **71**, 1467–1476.
17 Kuovonen, I. & Gräsbeck, R. (1981) Topology of the hog intrinsic factor receptor in the intestine. *Journal of Biological Chemistry* **256**, 154–158.
18 Lucas, M. L., Cooper, B. T., Lei, F. H. et al. (1978) Acid microclimate in coeliac and Crohn's disease: a model for folate malabsorption. *Gut*, **19**, 735–742.
19 Perry, J. & Chanarin, I. (1970) Intestinal absorption of reduced folate compounds in man. *British Journal of Haematology*, **18**, 329–339.
20 Peters, T. J. & Hoffbrand, A. V. (1970) Absorption of vitamin B_{12} by the guinea pig. I. Subcellular localisation of vitamin B_{12} in the ileal enterocyte during absorption. *British Journal of Haematology*, **19**, 369–382.

21 Pollack, S. & Lasky, F. D. (1976) A new iron-binding
    protein isolated from intestinal mucosa. *Journal of
    Laboratory and Clinical Medicine*, **87**, 620–629.
22 Refsum, S. B. & Schreiner, B. (1980) Iron excretion from
    the goblet cells of the small intestine in man. An addi-
    tional regulative mechanism in iron homeostasis in
    man. *Scandinavian Journal of Gastroenterology*, **13**,
    1013–1020.
23 Rosenberg, I. H. (1976) Absorption and malabsorption
    of folates. *Clinics in Haematology*, **5**, 589–618.

CALCIUM, VITAMIN D AND METABOLIC BONE DISEASE

Calcium homeostasis is maintained by the regulatory actions of parathyroid hormone (PTH) and vitamin D metabolites on gut, bone, and kidney. In health, man can adapt successfully to a wide range of dietary calcium intake and to the increased mineral requirements of growth, pregnancy and lactation. However, chronic negative calcium balance may occur in gastrointestinal disorders and may be associated with significant bone disease. The purpose of this chapter is to describe the normal metabolism of calcium and vitamin D with regard to the gut and the adverse effects of disordered gastrointestinal absorption, and to outline a rational approach to prophylaxis and therapy.

Clarification of vitamin D nomenclature

Endogenous (i.e. skin-synthesized) vitamin D is cholecalciferol or D_3. Vitamin D_2, ergocalciferol, is used to fortify some foodstuffs as well as therapeutically. D_2 and D_3 have been considered to be of approximately equal potency, but this concept is currently being re-evaluated.

Plasma calcium regulation

Plasma calcium homeostasis is the result of a balance between calcium absorption from the gut and its excretion into urine and faeces. This is complicated by an approximately balanced uptake and release of calcium from bone (Figure 8.24). In the event of a negative external calcium balance, homeostatic negative feedback mechanisms are activated. A fall in plasma calcium increases the secretion rate of PTH, which mobilizes calcium from bone surfaces and increases the hydroxylation of 25-hydroxyvitamin D (25(OH)D) to 1,25-dihydroxycholecalciferol (1,25-DHCC) in the kidney. In turn, 1,25-DHCC acts on the gut to increase calcium absorption and potentiates the action of PTH on bone. A prolonged hypocalcaemic stimulus of several weeks or months

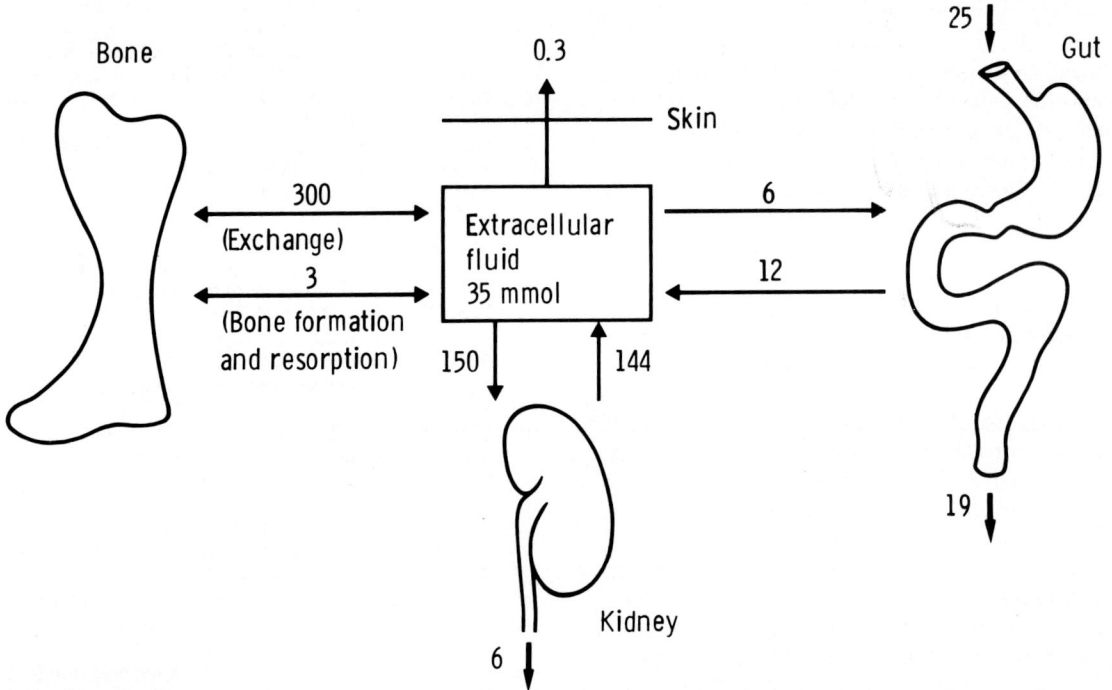

Fig. 8.24 Principle fluxes of calcium in normal adult man. Figures are in mmol of calcium/day. Note that there is significant loss of endogenous calcium in the faeces which in some diseases may exceed true calcium absorption, which makes slow loss of body calcium stores inevitable. Most transfer of calcium between blood and bone occurs at resting bone surfaces and is independent of bone formation and resorption. Such exchange contributes to the rapid adjustment of plasma calcium under the influence of PTH. Cortical bone turnover is probably as little as 5% replaced annually, with trabecular bone being renewed at approximately four times this rate.

duration leads to chronic secondary hyperparathyroidism. This results in the additional response of increased bone turnover, with increased numbers of osteoclasts and osteoblasts seen on bone biopsy, and net loss of bone.[3, 11]

Mechanisms of calcium absorption

Dietary calcium exists as complexes and salts of varying solubility, so that solubilization must precede transport across the intestinal mucosa. Short term in vivo studies on the effects of foodstuffs which complex calcium (e.g. phytate and uronic acid) have been difficult to interpret because of the phenomenon of adaptation, by which the gut can take a surprisingly long period of time (sometimes many weeks) to increase its ability to transport calcium in response to a reduction in availability of substrate.[36] Similar considerations apply to claims that dietary fat, protein and carbohydrate influence calcium bioavailability. Moreover, the un-ionized fraction of dietary calcium may be subsequently released by digestion of the complexing ion (e.g. phytate) in the gut lumen.[43] Further ionization may be achieved by the operation of simple chemical equilibria as the ionized fraction is taken up by the mucosa.[1]

ACTIVE AND PASSIVE TRANSPORT OF CALCIUM

Much attention recently has been directed to the transport of calcium across the mucosal cell. The kinetics of calcium absorption in vivo resemble those of sodium and phosphate in that all three ions are most rapidly absorbed within 30 to 45 minutes of passing the pylorus, suggesting that absorptive activity is at its highest in the duodenum and jejunum. In contrast, magnesium absorption continues for longer (Figure 8.25). Active transport of calcium occurs across the enterocyte, but this mechanism is saturated at relatively low intraluminal calcium concentrations.[30] At higher concentrations nonsaturable passive processes, unaffected by metabolic inhibitors, can be demonstrated.[15]

THE CONTROL OF CALCIUM ABSORPTION BY 1,25-DHCC (FIGURE 8.26)

Both active and passive calcium absorption is reduced in vitamin D deficiency and can be stimulated by vitamin D.[30] The active hormone is 1,25-dihydroxycholecalciferol (1,25-DHCC),[3, 11] but the molecular basis of its action on the intestine remains controversial.

Single injections of 1,25-DHCC into D deficient rats produce a biphasic increase in calcium

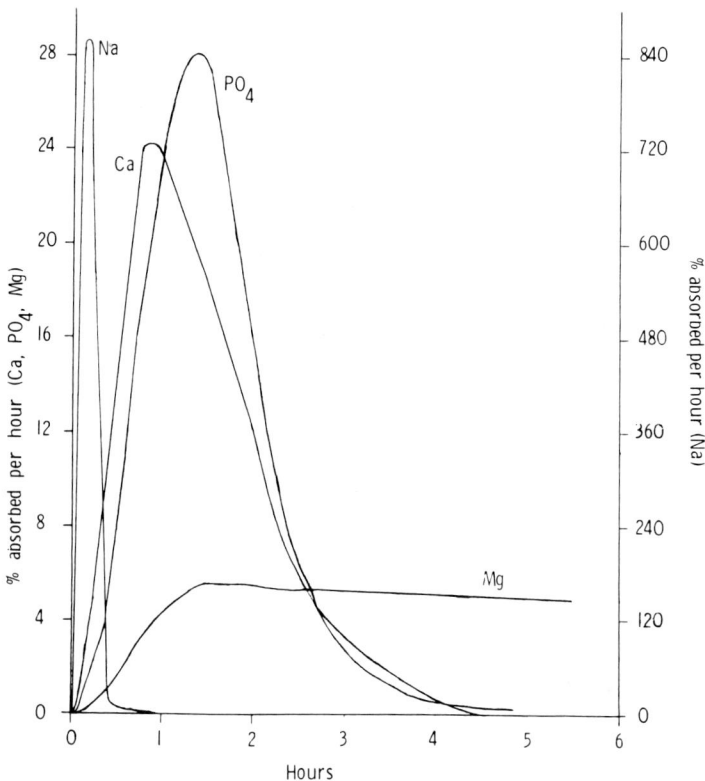

Fig. 8.25 Rates of absorption of four mineral ions from the whole gut in normal man. Note the much larger ordinate scale for sodium absorption, which is rapidly and almost completely absorbed in a pattern similar to ^{133}Xe, a blood flow indicator.[35] In contrast, the absorption of Ca^{2+}, Mg^{2+} and PO_4^{3-} are clearly not limited by gut blood flow. Whereas Mg^{2+} shows a time course of absorption suggesting that ileal absorption rates may be similar to those seen more proximally,[24] Ca^{2+} and PO_4^{3-} normally reach their peak rates of absorption within the first two hours of ingestion, following which the unabsorbed residue is absorbed at a rate which declines much more rapidly.[37, 52]

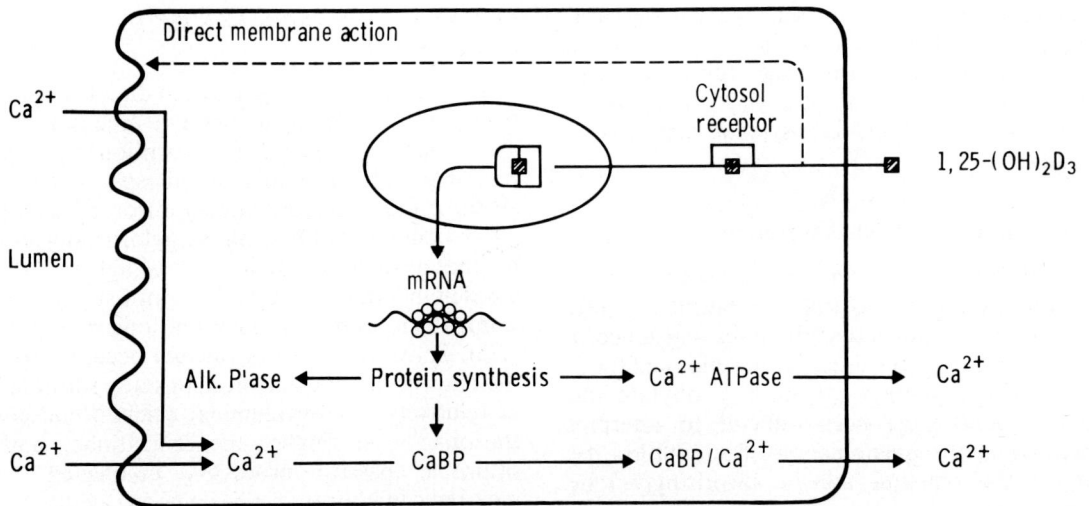

Fig. 8.26 A model of some of the current ideas concerning the mechanism of action of 1,25-DHCC on the enterocyte.

transport, with a brisk response after two hours peaking at six hours and then declining before a slower rise occurs which is sustained for some days. High resolution autoradiographic studies show uptake of 1,25-DHCC by the nuclei of mature villus cells and undifferentiated crypt cells within 30 minutes. A receptor molecule of high specificity for 1,25-DHCC has been identified in cytosol fractions of the mucosa.[12]

Following nuclear uptake, 1,25-DHCC induces the synthesis of several mucosal cell proteins including alkaline phosphatase, calcium activated ATPase (CaATPase) and calcium binding protein (CaBP).[4, 30, 33] The second phase of 1,25-DHCC-promoted calcium absorption is synchronized with increased CaBP synthesis.[6, 12] CaBP may act to prevent the build-up of toxic intracellular concentrations of ionic calcium during its absorption.[3, 4]

An alternative explanation for the action of 1,25-DHCC in increasing calcium transport is an alteration of the phosphatidylcholine content of membrane phospholipids and hence their permeability. These changes in lipid structure precede or parallel increases in calcium transport and are not blocked by cyclohexamide.[49]

Other mucosal proteins induced by vitamin D

The roles of other proteins (CaATPase, alkaline phosphatase) induced by the action of 1,25-DHCC are less certain but they appear to correlate with the second phase increase in calcium transport.[12, 14] CaATPase is located exclusively in the basolateral portions of the cell membrane, suggesting its role lies in extrusion rather than uptake.[22]

ADAPTIVE CHANGES IN CALCIUM ABSORPTION

It is established that fractional calcium absorption is increased on low calcium diets although absolute calcium uptake is reduced.[1, 30] Adaptation parallels increases in mucosal CaBP content as measured in isolated loop experiments.[45] The location of active transport sites appears to be extended in calcium deficiency to include the whole of the small gut in experimental animals.[1, 30] Similar increases in calcium absorption occur during pregnancy and lactation in animals and humans.[1, 30]

The molecular basis for these adaptations is unclear. Although increased 1,25-DHCC levels are found during pregnancy and lactation and the simultaneously increased prolactin levels are known to increase 1α-hydroxylation of 25(OH)D, DeLuca *et al.* have shown that pregnancy and lactation occur normally in D deficient rats.[12] Exogenous prolactin increases calcium absorption rapidly in non-pregnant D deficient rats in the absence of detectable serum 1,25-DHCC.[12, 44] Similarly, PTH has been suggested to have a D-independent role in stimulating calcium absorption in some species.[30] Growth hormone has been reported to increase calcium absorption, and somatostatin may decrease it.[17, 30] Evidence is still scanty that other metabolites of vitamin D (e.g. 24,25-DHCC) in normal plasma concentrations have a role in calcium absorption in man.[3, 11, 12]

The absorption of phosphate

In animals, phosphate absorption takes place against an electrochemical gradient, is inhibited by metabolic inhibitors and shows carrier saturation consistent with an active process.[14] In contrast, perfusion studies in man show a linear relationship between intraluminal phosphate concentration and net phosphate movement over the range 1.2–70 mmol/l and uptake is stimulated by 1,25-DHCC.[14]

The absorption of vitamin D

Vitamin D is lipid soluble and therefore incorporated into micelles. The more polar metabolites are relatively more water soluble and their absorption may be partially independent of fat absorption. The absorption of vitamin D is enhanced by bile salts, fatty acids and monoglycerides.[3, 30] The vitamin is transported to the liver for conversion to 25(OH)D, the circulating form of the hormone. However, in healthy individuals 90% of circulating 25(OH)D is derived from endogenous vitamin D synthesized in the skin by the action of the ultra-violet component of sunlight on 7-dihydroxycholecalciferol;[3, 11, 30] in Britain this only occurs between April and October. The storage of 25(OH)D is largely in adipose tissue and the plasma, bound to vitamin D binding globulin which is also synthesized in the liver. It is 1α-hydroxylated to the active 1,25-DHCC by the kidney. The details of this and other metabolic conversions of vitamin D have recently been extensively reviewed.[3, 11, 30]

ENTEROHEPATIC CIRCULATION OF VITAMIN D

The enterohepatic circulation of bile salts is well known and, since both vitamin D and bile salts are derived from cholesterol, it has been suggested that vitamin D and its metabolites are also recycled. A proportion of intravenously administered tritiated D_3 may be recovered as polar metabolites in bile drained by a T-tube, and about one third of intravenous 25(OH)D appears in the duodenum within 24 hours compared with only 3% recovered from the faeces.[2, 23, 39] Radioisotope experiments have provided evidence of enterohepatic recycling of perhaps 50% of 25(OH)D, 1,25-DHCC and 24,25-DHCC in animals and man.[23, 32, 42, 59]

Very little of the biliary vitamin D metabolites are found in their free forms, but a substantial fraction appear to be conjugated, e.g. as the glucosiduronate.[23] These conjugates are probably physiologically inert but it is proposed that they may be deconjugated before or during reabsorption, and hence regain biological activity.[23, 42]

Bone disease in gastrointestinal disorders

The cause of bone disease in disorders of the gut is multifactorial and many possible mechanisms can be envisaged, some of which are listed below; however, in most cases their relative importance is not known and often no direct evidence of any particular mechanism is present.

1 Endogenous production of vitamin D in the skin forms the main source of active metabolites, so reduced sun exposure, perhaps due to ill health, may be important in some patients.

2 Inadequate diets are common, and lack of absorptive surface due to resection or disease, rapid gut transit times, loss of gastric acid and bile salts and alteration in pH may all reduce the availability of exogenous vitamin D and calcium. Steatorrhoea is associated with malabsorption of vitamin D, 25(OH)D and calcium, although faecal fat excretion does not correlate well with 25(OH)D levels.[1, 39]

3 The importance of disordered enterohepatic circulation of vitamin D metabolites has still to be fully evaluated in man. However, reabsorption of deconjugated metabolites may be affected by damaged mucosa, resection or bacterial overgrowth.[23, 39]

4 Liver disease frequently coexists with gastrointestinal diseases. Although in advanced cholestatic or hepatocellular cirrhosis the evidence for serious failure of 25(OH)D synthesis is conflicting, osteoporosis is often found in these conditions and in alcoholic liver disease.[39]

5 Low magnesium levels associated with diarrhoea may produce refractory hypocalcaemia due to inhibition of PTH release.

6 It has been suggested that end organ resistance to 1,25-DHCC may occur in coeliac disease.[46]

7 The effects of drugs which affect calcium and vitamin D absorption, e.g. steroids and cholestyramine, must be borne in mind.[15, 39]

POSTGASTRECTOMY STATES

Low serum calcium and 25(OH)D are common in patients after gastrectomy. Reduced intake and malabsorption of calcium and vitamin D have been observed in relation to rapid gastric emptying, poor mixing and steatorrhoea.[15, 21, 29, 30, 39, 55] Phosphate binding antacids may contribute by causing hypophosphataemia although serum phosphate levels are usually normal.[29, 39] The correction of postgastrectomy vitamin D deficiency by antibiotics has been reported[55] and, since bacterial dehydroxylation of cholesterol is known to occur, similar effects on D metabolites may disrupt their enterohepatic circulation.

In histological surveys, partial or total gastrectomy and, to a lesser extent, gastrojejunostomy have been associated with osteomalacia, secondary hyperparathyroidism and osteoporosis in about 30% of patients – a much higher frequency than noted clinically or radiologically, and probably increasing with time from surgery.[5, 14, 16, 19, 39] The cause of the osteoporosis is unclear, unless it is due to calcium malabsorption. In this context it should be borne in mind that not all patients who are biochemically deficient in vitamin D have exuberant, thick osteoid seams on bone biopsy and it seems possible that if osteoblast activity is very reduced it may mask histological osteomalacia in bone biopsies by reducing osteoid formation.

INTESTINAL BYPASS SURGERY

Low serum calcium, phosphate, 25(OH)D and 1,25-DHCC are common, and increased immunoreactive PTH (iPTH) with low urinary calcium and increased cAMP have been reported, reflecting secondary hyperparathyroidism.[8, 14, 39, 41, 56] Malabsorption of calcium and vitamin D metabolites is known to occur and loss of mucosal surface and steatorrhoea are presumably involved; it is interesting that the biochemical abnormalities tend to decrease with time from surgery, probably due to hypertrophy of the remaining bowel.[39, 56] Secondary hyperparathyroidism will contribute to the low phosphate by enhancing its renal excretion, but in those patients with reduced PTH after surgery, hypomagnesaemia may underlie the hypocalcaemia.[39] Disruption of enterohepatic recycling could theoretically be important in these patients and it is interesting that ileal resections may cause more disruption of calcium metabolism than those involving the jejunum.[1] Liver disease is reported to complicate bypass surgery, but whether it causes reduced production of 25(OH)D or prevents re-secretion into bile is unknown.[39]

In one series, histological osteomalacia was found in 50% of patients, with frequent secondary hyperparathyroidism.[8] Other reports stress the progressive loss of bone with time from surgery, with osteoporosis being the more common lesion.[48] Even in patients with increased osteoid, iliac trabecular bone volume is reduced.[27]

COELIAC DISEASE

Serum calcium levels and urine calcium excretion are depressed in coeliac disease and these patients are often in negative calcium balance. Presumably malabsorption plays a major part, consequent on mucosal damage, vitamin D deficiency and steatorrhoea.[14, 39, 57] Most coeliac patients with osteomalacia have hypophosphataemia, contributing factors being phosphate malabsorption, D deficiency and increased renal clearance due to secondary hyperparathyroidism.[14, 26, 39, 57]

25(OH)D levels are low in coeliacs and malabsorption of vitamin D has been documented in radiotracer experiments;[57] there are suggestions that there may be differential absorption of vitamin D and its metabolites.[10] Although the malabsorption can theoretically be explained by mucosal damage and steatorrhoea, severe osteomalacia may occur as the sole clinical feature of the disease without steatorrhoea.[26] The observation of increased plasma clearance and faecal loss of radiolabelled intravenous 25(OH)D suggests that the main problem might be reduced enterohepatic recycling,[39] or perhaps increased renal 1α-hydroxylase activity in compensation for end organ resistance. In the rare patient who also has primary biliary cirrhosis, aggressive osteoporosis may also be expected.

Histologically, osteomalacia, secondary hyperparathyroidism and osteoporosis may all be seen.[14, 39]

CROHN'S DISEASE

Calcium absorption is usually normal in patients with Crohn's disease uncomplicated by extensive resection or corticosteroid therapy[31] and 25(OH)D levels were reduced in only 4 out of 37 patients who had not been operated on, all of whom had ileitis.[54] After bowel resection, low 25(OH)D levels are much more common.[7] Apart from the potential mechanisms already discussed above, protein losing enteropathy has been suggested to cause loss of bound vitamin D metabolites, in a way analogous to the nephrotic syndrome.[39]

The reported incidence of bone disease varies widely, reflecting the techniques used and the extent of bowel resection. In patients with inflammatory bowel disease, 70% show reduced bone mineral content in the forearm[20] while only 8% have clinical disease with pain and fractures.[9] Histological osteomalacia has been reported in 30% of patients with bowel resection, while in a small group of seven patients with Crohn's disease and low 25(OH)D levels, all had osteoporosis and five had osteomalacia.[13] The incidence of secondary hyperparathyroidism in biopsies is said to be low; it is not known if this reflects hypomagnesaemia.[13]

PANCREATIC DISEASE

Steatorrhoea commonly complicates pancreatic exocrine insufficiency; low 25(OH)D levels are reported in such patients[57] and in 36% of patients with cystic fibrosis, who also show secondary hyperparathyroidism and reduced bone mineral content.[25] Although the reported incidence of clinical bone disease is low, in a careful study of four patients with chronic alcoholic pancreatitis, all showed histological evidence of osteomalacia.[39]

Metabolic bone disease

INVESTIGATION

Biochemistry
The development of osteomalacia is accompanied by a fall in the plasma calcium and a rise in the plasma alkaline phosphatase. Frequently, the plasma phosphate is also low, but this is not a reliable index. In the elderly, the alkaline phosphatase also becomes unreliable.[28] There is little correlation between the degree of hypocalcaemia and the severity of histological osteomalacia. Few routine laboratories can distinguish between alkaline phosphatase of bone and liver (or placental) origin; when co-existent liver pathology is possible, 5-nucleotidase and γ-glutamyl transpeptidase estimations can be helpful. In pregnancy, placentral alkaline phosphatase is often present in sufficient amounts to make this investigation of little value in detecting early osteomalacia.

Plasma PTH and 25(OH)D concentrations are available in some centres. PTH is measured by immunoassays which detect both the functional (intact) molecule and inactive cleavage products. The 'carboxyterminal' immunoassays are still most commonly used, but they have the disadvantage that they detect a locus on the PTH molecule that is rather remote from the bioactive locus that binds to the cell membrane receptor. Inactive carboxyterminal fragments accumulate in even mild states of renal impairment, which leads to difficulties of interpretation in patients suspected of renal osteodystrophy

and in the elderly because of the normal reduction of GFR with ageing. 'Aminoterminal' immunoassays detect loci which are closer to, but probably rarely identical to, the receptor binding site. PTH levels are increased in the secondary hyperparathyroidism associated with hypocalcaemia. If this is prolonged, gland hypertrophy ensues, which allows PTH levels to go even higher. Hypomagnesaemia causes functional hypoparathyroidism in the presence of hypocalcaemia. Otherwise, a low PTH in the presence of a low calcium usually indicates parathyroid gland damage. Hypomagnesaemia also causes potassium wasting by the kidney, which is readily reversed on magnesium repletion. Over-enthusiastic repletion of magnesium and potassium together has been known to cause hyperkalaemia.

The nutritional status of a patient with respect to vitamin D can be assessed by estimating the 25(OH)D level. However, an adequate 25(OH)D concentration is no guarantee of an adequate 1,25-DHCC level, which depends on an adequate functioning renal tubular 'mass' and PTH levels, among other factors.

Urine biochemistry can also be helpful. The 24 hour urine calcium is reduced in osteomalacia. The renal transport maximum of inorganic phosphate[58] is also reduced in conditions leading to raised PTH levels, although some tumours also have the same effect.

In osteoporosis uncomplicated by other bone pathology, all these biochemical indices are characteristically normal, except that the fasting calcium : creatinine ratio in the urine is sometimes raised.

Imaging
Radiography can be diagnostic in osteomalacia. The characteristic pseudo-fractures or Looser's zones are practically never seen in other bone disorders. Eighty per cent of pseudo-fractures can be detected on a combination of a chest and a pelvic X-ray. They are, however, often difficult to detect in the ribs and the scapulae, two commonly involved sites. A pseudo-fracture is usually a small, incomplete fissure fracture which fails to show signs of healing (sclerosis). Another useful, if late, sign is 'cod-fishing' of the vertebral bodies, which become bi-concave. Isotope bone scanning (e.g. with $^{99}Tc^m$-methylene diphosphonate) often reveals further pseudo-fractures (as 'hot' spots) and increased tracer clearance into the skeleton from the circulation (low soft tissue 'background'). Tracer retention after 24 hours is increased in osteomalacia.

In osteoporosis, conventional radiography can be misleading in the assessment of bone density. Fine (industrial) grade films of the hands can be used to assess cortical thickness, but routine films are not advised for this purpose. Vertebral crush fractures can be assessed by lateral views of the dorsal and lumbar spine. Vertebrae may be wedged, completely crushed, or merely show end plate infractions. When the disc herniates through into the vertebral body, this is termed a Schmorl's node. If aortic calcification (common in older osteoporotic patients) and intervertebral discs are both denser than the vertebral body, the patient probably does have axial osteoporosis. Quantification of bone loss in the axial skeleton is a research procedure for which dual photon absorptiometry or quantitative axial computed tomography are required. Isotope bone scans reveal relatively recent (within six months) crush fractures as symmetrical band-shaped areas of increased uptake in one or more vertebral bodies showing loss of height. Asymmetrical uptake, unaccompanied by radiological evidence of degenerative disease, should alert to the possibility of metastases, or possibly Paget's disease.

Histology

When a firm diagnosis cannot be made on other grounds, it may be helpful to obtain a bone biopsy from the iliac crest, although no useful information will be obtained if the laboratory decalcifies the specimen, unless the patient has metastatic disease. To simply determine whether the patient has an excess of thick osteoid to make a diagnosis of osteomalacia, a vertical biopsy is sometimes adequate, although for the assessment of osteoporosis and the more detailed assessment of osteomalacia and other bone disorders, an 8 mm trans-iliac biopsy including both cortices is required, preferably after two short courses of demethylchlortetracycline to allow the dynamic characteristics of osteoid mineralization to be established. The laboratory must have facilities for embedding and cutting calcified bone samples. Iliac biopsies can be taken under local anaesthetic; adequate infiltration of both periosteal surfaces prior to a trans-iliac biopsy is essential to minimize pain and discomfort. The standard site for trans-iliac biopsies is 2.5 cm inferior and 2.5 cm posterior to the anterior superior iliac spine. Previous biopsy sites must be avoided. The scope and usefulness of bone biopsies has recently been clearly reviewed by Meunier[40] and practical and technical aspects are also dealt with in a recent monograph edited by Recker.[50]

MANAGEMENT

The main pharmacological treatments in current use include vitamin D, 1,25-DHCC (calcitriol) and its analogue 1α-hydroxycholecalciferol (1α-OHD) (alfacalcidol). Calcium supplements may also be necessary.

It is worth emphasizing that vitamin D in small doses (up to 200 µg daily, 8000 iu) requires further well regulated transformation for metabolic activation.[3, 11] Other metabolites such as 24,25-DHCC are synthesized during these transformations and will not therefore be available if 1α-OHD or 1,25-DHCC are given. As yet the importance of these other metabolites in preserving bone is uncertain.[3, 11] The major problem with the direct use of 1α-OHD and 1,25-DHCC is the narrow therapeutic range (usually 0.25–1.0 µg/day) that results from having bypassed the normal metabolic control mechanisms. Fortunately, any hypercalcaemia so resulting is very rapidly reversible, unlike that caused by the use of vitamin D in large doses. Interestingly, there is evidence that vitamin D given to deficient patients will produce supra-normal serum 1,25-DHCC levels which may convey a therapeutic advantage not provided by using 1,25-DHCC itself.[38, 46] Whatever form of treatment is used, regular biochemical monitoring is essential to document the therapeutic response and, if an active metabolite or doses of vitamin D in excess of 250 µg/day are used, regular checks on plasma calcium are required for the duration of the treatment.

PROPHYLAXIS

Patients who develop hypocalcaemia or low 25(OH)D levels should be treated with vitamin D and usually calcium supplements as well. Oral vitamin D in daily doses of 100–300 µg (4000–12 000 iu) is usually adequate in patients with steatorrhoea or liver disease,[53] while in simple vitamin D deficiency in otherwise normal subjects, 10 µg (400 iu) should suffice. Occasionally, patients respond poorly to vitamin D; the use of 1α-OHD or 1,25-DHCC may then be justified but may also fail, sometimes due to poor patient compliance. In such cases, intramuscular doses of calciferol may be given at infrequent intervals (e.g. 100 000 units every 4 to 12 weeks).

TREATMENT OF ESTABLISHED BONE DISEASE

Many different regimens have been shown to reverse osteomalacia associated with digestive diseases. Histological improvement in osteomalacia associated with primary biliary cirrhosis has been observed with intramuscular vitamin D_2, and oral 25(OH)D (calcifidiol), 1α-OHD (alfacalcidol), and 1,25-DHCC (calcitriol).[34] Two-thirds of patients with osteomalacia following intestinal bypass surgery heal histologically with alfacalcidol. Low dose oral vitamin D therapy can return 25(OH)D levels to normal and induce a clinical response in patients with intestinal resection.[10]

Further trials are necessary to assess the most effective sequence of therapeutic measures in the treatment of osteomalacia associated with digestive disorders. Any of the established regimens may be used in the treatment of osteomalacia, but a reasonable approach is to initially use oral vitamin D in doses up to 300 µg (12 000 iu) daily. If this proves ineffective then larger parenteral doses of calciferol, or alternatively oral alfacalcidol or calcitriol at a dose of up to 2 µg daily are justified. Higher doses than these may result in excessive bone resorption. Patients treated with active metabolites (alfacalcidol, calcitriol) and larger parenteral doses of vitamin D should have regular serum calcium, phosphate, alkaline phosphatase and, in the latter case, if possible 25(OH)D estimations.

Neither 25(OH)D (calcifidiol) nor calcitriol results in substantial improvement of established osteoporosis[51] and this parallels the experience in primary osteoporosis in larger trials.[18] Nevertheless, maintenance of a normal calcium absorptive capacity may well prevent the development of osteoporosis or its exacerbation, and the prophylactic role of vitamin D metabolites in gastrointestinal disorders which lead primarily to osteoporosis needs further evaluation.

On the other hand, the usefulness of calcium supplements in the treatment of osteomalacia is undisputed but frequently forgotten. Patients on optimal treatment for privational osteomalacia may often go into positive calcium balance to the extent of 12 mmol (480 mg) per day. In patients with problems of gastrointestinal absorption, the value of readily absorbable calcium supplements (e.g. three calcium galactogluconate tablets to give 30 mmol calcium daily between meals) for healing at an optimal rate should be obvious, particularly in view of the importance of the predominantly passive absorption mechanisms and low dietary calcium intakes frequently seen in these patients.

REFERENCES

1 Allen, L. H. (1982) Calcium bioavailability and absorption: a review. *American Journal of Clinical Nutrition*, **35**, 783–808.

2 Arnaud, S. B., Goldsmith, R. S., Lambert, P. W. & Go, V. L. W. (1975) 25-Hydroxyvitamin D_3: evidence of an enterohepatic circulation in man. *Proceedings of the Society for Experimental Biology and Medicine*, **149**, 570–572.

3 Bikle, D. D. (1982) The vitamin D endocrine system. *Advances in Internal Medicine*, **27**, 45–71.

4 Bikle, D. D., Zolock, D. T., Morrissey, R. L. & Herman, R. H. (1978) Independence of 1,25-dihydroxyvitamin D_3 mediated calcium transport from de novo RNA and protein synthesis. *The Journal of Biological Chemistry*, **253**, 484–488.

5 Bordier, P., Matrajt, H., Hioco, D. *et al.* (1968) Subclinical vitamin D deficiency following gastric surgery: histologic evidence in bone. *Lancet*, **i**, 437–440.

6 Bronner, F., Lipton, J., Pansu, D. *et al.* (1982) Molecular transport effects of 1,25-dihydroxyvitamin D_3 in rat duodenum. *Federation Proceedings*, **41**, 61–65.

7 Compston, J. E., Ayers, A. B., Horton, L. W. L. *et al.* (1978a) Osteomalacia after small intestinal resection. *Lancet*, **i**, 9–12.

8 Compston, J. E., Laker, M. F., Woodhead, J. S. *et al.* (1978b) Bone disease after jejuno-ileal bypass for obesity. *Lancet*, **ii**, 1–4.

9 Cooke, W. T., Mallas, E., Prior, P. & Allan, R. N. (1980) Crohn's disease: course, treatment and long term prognosis. *Quarterly Journal of Medicine*, **49**, 363–384.

10 Davies, M., Mawer, E. B. & Krawitt, E. L. (1980) Comparative absorption of vitamin D_3 and 25-hydroxyvitamin D_3 in intestinal disease. *Gut*, **21**, 287–292.

11 DeLuca, H. F. (1981) Vitamin D revisited. *Clinics in Endocrinology and Metabolism*, **9**, 3–26.

12 DeLuca, H. F., Franceschi, R. T., Halloran, B. P. & Massaro, E. R. (1982) Molecular events involved in 1,25-dihydroxyvitamin D_3 stimulation of intestinal calcium transport. *Federation Proceedings*, **41**, 66–71.

13 Driscoll, R. H., Meredith, S., Wagonfield, J. W. & Rosenberg, I. H. (1977) Bone histology and vitamin D status in Crohn's disease: assessment of vitamin D therapy. *Gastroenterology*, **72**, 1051 (Abstract).

14 Duncombe, V. M. & Reeve, J. (1981) Calcium homeostasis in digestive disorders. *Clinics in Gastroenterology*, **10**(3), 653–670.

15 Duncombe, V. M., Watts, R. W. E. & Peters, T. J. (1980) In vitro calcium uptake by jejunal biopsy specimens from patients with idiopathic hypercalciuria. *Lancet*, **ii**, 1334–1336.

16 Eddy, R. L. (1971) Metabolic bone disease after gastrectomy. *American Journal of Medicine*, **50**, 442–449.

17 Favus, M. J., Berelowitz, M. & Coe, F. L. (1981) Effect of somatostatin on intestinal calcium transport in the rat. *American Journal of Physiology*, **241**, G215–G221.

18 Gallagher, J. C., Riggs, B. L. & De Luca, H. F. (1981) Effects of calcitriol in osteoporosis. In *Osteoporosis* (Ed.) de Luca, H. F. *et al.* pp. 419–423. Baltimore: University Park Press.

19 Garrick, R., Ireland, A. W. & Posen, S. (1971) Bone abnormalities after gastric surgery. A prospective histologic study. *Annals of Internal Medicine*, **75**, 221–225.

20 Genant, H. K., Mall, J. C., Wagonfield, J. B. *et al.* (1976) Skeletal demineralisation and growth retardation in inflammatory bowel disease. *Investigative Radiology*, **11**, 541–549.

21 Gertner, J. M., Lilburn, M. & Domenech, M. (1977) 25-Hydroxycholecalciferol absorption in steatorrhoea and postgastrectomy osteomalacia. *British Medical Journal*, **i**, 1310–1312.

22 Ghijsen, W. E. J. M., DeJong, M. D. & Van Os, C. H. (1980) Dissociation between Ca^{2+} ATPase and alkaline phosphatase activities in plasma membranes of rat duodenum. *Biochimica et Biophysica Acta*, **599**, 538–551.

23 Goldsmith, R. S. (1982) Enterohepatic cycling of

vitamin D and its metabolites. *Mineral and Electrolyte Metabolism*, **8**, 289–292.

24 Graham, L. A., Caesar, J. J. & Burgen, A. S. V. (1960) Gastrointestinal absorption and excretion of Mg^{28} in man. *Metabolism*, **9**, 646–659.

25 Hahn, T. J., Squires, A. E., Halstead, L. R. & Strominger, D. B. (1979) Reduced serum 25-hydroxyvitamin D concentration and disordered mineral metabolism in patients with cystic fibrosis. *Journal of Paediatrics*, **94**, 38–42.

26 Hajjar, E. J., Vincenti, F. & Salti, I. S. (1974) Gluten-induced enteropathy. Osteomalacia as its principal manifestation. *Archives of Internal Medicine*, **134**, 505–506.

27 Halverson, J. D., Teitelbaum, S. L., Haddad, J. G. & Murphy, W. A. (1979) Skeletal abnormalities after jejunoileal bypass. *Annals of Surgery*, **189**, 785–790.

28 Hodkinson, H. M. (1977) *Biochemical Diagnosis of the Elderly*. London: Chapman & Hall.

29 Imawari, M., Kozawa, K., Akanuma, Y. *et al.* (1980) Serum 25-hydroxyvitamin D and vitamin D binding protein levels and mineral metabolism after partial and total gastrectomy. *Gastroenterology*, **79**, 255–258.

30 Kenny, A. D. (1981) *Intestinal Calcium Absorption and its Regulation*. Boca Raton, Florida: CRC Press (monograph).

31 Krawitt, E. L., Beeken, W. L. & Janney, C. D. (1976) Calcium absorption in Crohn's disease. *Gastroenterology*, **71**, 251–254.

32 Kumar, R., Nagubandi, S., Mattox, V. R. & Londowski, J. M. (1980) Enterohepatic physiology of 1,25-dihydroxyvitamin D$_3$. *Journal of Clinical Investigation*, **65**, 277–284.

33 Lawson, D. E. M. (1978) Biochemical responses of the intestine to vitamin D. In *Vitamin D* (Ed.) Lawson, D. E. M. pp. 167–200. London: Academic Press.

34 Long, R. G. (1980) Hepatic osteodystrophy: outlook good but some problems unsolved. *Gastroenterology*, **78**, 644–647.

35 Love, A. H. G., Chen, L. C., Reeve, J. & Veall, N. (1977) The relative transfer rates for sodium and xenon from gut lumen to plasma in man. *Clinical Science and Molecular Medicine*, **52**, 249–254.

36 Malm, O. J. (1958) Calcium requirement and adaptation in adult man. *Scandinavian Journal of Clinical and Laboratory Investigation*, **10** (supplement 36), 1–290.

37 Marshall, D. H. (1976) Calcium and phosphate kinetics. In *Calcium, Phosphate and Magnesium Metabolism* (Ed.) Nordin, B. E. C., pp. 257–297. Edinburgh: Churchill Livingstone.

38 Mawer, E. B. (1980) Clinical implications of measurements of circulating vitamin D metabolites. *Clinics in Endocrinology and Metabolism*, **9**(1), 63–79.

39 Meredith, S. C. & Rosenberg, I. H. (1980) Gastrointestinal hepatic disorders and osteomalacia. *Clinics in Endocrinology and Metabolism*, **9**(1), 131–150.

40 Meunier, P. J. (1983) Histomorphometry of the skeleton. In *Bone Mineral Research, annual 1* (Ed.) Peck, W. A., pp. 191–222. Amsterdam: Excerpta Medica.

41 Mosekilde, L., Melsen, F., Hessov, I. *et al.* (1980) Low serum levels of 1,25-dihydroxyvitamin D and histomorphometric evidence of osteomalacia after jejunoileal bypass for obesity. *Gut*, **21**, 624–631.

42 Nagubandi, S., Kumar, R., Londowski, J. M. *et al.* (1980) Role of vitamin D glucosiduronate in calcium homeostasis. *Journal of Clinical Investigation*, **66**, 1274–1280.

43 Nicolaysen, R. & Njaa, L. R. (1951) Investigations on the effect of phytic acid on the absorption of calcium in rats, pigs and men. *Acta Physiologica Scandinavica*, **22**, 246–259.

44 Pahuja, D. N. & DeLuca, H. F. (1981) Stimulation of intestinal calcium-transport and bone calcium mobilization by prolactin in vitamin D-deficient rats. *Science*, **214**, 1038–1039.

45 Pansu, D., Bellaton, C. & Bronner, F. (1981) Effect of Ca intake on saturable and non-saturable components of duodenal Ca transport. *American Journal of Physiology*, **240**, G32–G37.

46 Papapoulos, S. E., Adami, S. & O'Riordan, J. L. H. (1980) Hormonal resistance in disorders of calcium homeostasis. *Annals of Clinical Research*, **12**, 254–263.

47 Papapoulos, S. E., Clemens, T. L., Fraher, L. J. *et al.* (1980) Metabolites of vitamin D in human vitamin D deficiency: effect of vitamin D$_3$ or 1,25-dihydroxycholecalciferol. *Lancet*, **ii**, 612–615.

48 Parfitt, A. M., Miller, M. J., Frame, B. *et al.* (1978) Metabolic bone disease after intestinal bypass for treatment of obesity. *Annals of Internal Medicine*, **89**, 193–199.

49 Rasmussen, H., Matsumoto, T., Fontaine, O. & Goodman, D. B. P. (1982) Role of changes in membrane lipid structure in the action of 1,25-dihydroxyvitamin D$_3$. *Federation Proceedings*, **41**, 72–77.

50 Recker, R. R. (1983) *Bone Histomorphometry: Techniques and Interpretation*. Boca Raton, Florida: CRC Press. (monograph).

51 Reed, J. S., Meredith, S. C., Nemchausky, B. A. *et al.* (1980) Bone disease in primary biliary cirrhosis: reversal of osteomalacia with oral 25-hydroxyvitamin D. *Gastroenterology*, **78**, 512–517.

52 Reeve, J., Hesp, R. & Veall, N. (1974) Effects of therapy on rate of absorption of calcium from gut in disorders of calcium homeostasis. *British Medical Journal*, **iii**, 310–313.

53 Sitrin, M., Meredith, S. & Rosenberg, I. H. (1978) Vitamin D deficiency and bone disease in gastrointestinal disorders. *Archives of Internal Medicine*, **138**, 886–888.

54 Sonnenberg, A., von Lilienfeld-Toal, H., Sonnenberg, G. E. *et al.* (1977) 25-hydroxycholecalciferol serum levels in patients with Crohn's disease. *Acta Hepatogastroenterologica*, **24**, 256–258.

55 Stamp, T. C. B. (1974) Intestinal absorption of 25-hydroxycholecalciferol. *Lancet*, **ii**, 121–123.

56 Teitelbaum, S. L., Halverson, J. D., Bates, M. *et al.* (1977) Abnormalities of circulating 25-OH vitamin D after jejunal-ileal bypass for obesity. *Annals of Internal Medicine*, **86**, 289–293.

57 Thompson, G. R., Lewis, B. & Booth, C. C. (1968) Absorption of vitamin D-^{3}H in control subjects and patients with malabsorption. *Journal of Clinical Investigation*, **45**, 94–102.

58 Walton, R. J. & Bijvoet, O. L. M. (1975) Nomogram for derivation of renal threshold phosphate concentrations. *Lancet*, **ii**, 309–310.

59 Weisner, R. H., Kumar, R., Seeman, E. & Go, V. L. W. (1980) Enterohepatic physiology of 1,25 dihydroxyvitamin D$_3$ metabolites in normal man. *Journal of Laboratory and Clinical Medicine*, **96**, 1094–1100.

INTESTINAL TRANSPORT OF FLUID AND ELECTROLYTES

Approximately 9 l of fluid containing about 50 g of sodium enter the gut each day. Of this, approximately 1.5 l comes from the diet. The remainder comes from salivary, gastric, pancreatic, biliary, and intestinal secretions. Most absorption of fluid and electrolyte (about 7.5 l) takes place in the small intestine, though some occurs in the large intestine (1.4 l); only a very small proportion is voided in the stool (0.1 l). If larger volumes enter the gut, the intestine is capable of absorbing considerably more than 9 l/day. Using the technique of whole gut perfusion, Love *et al.*[58] estimated that the human intestine can absorb between 15 and 20 l of isotonic saline per day. Moreover, the colon of normal subjects can itself absorb up to 6 l per day under conditions of steady state perfusion.[19] The rates of absorption and secretion at different parts of the gut are controlled so that almost complete absorption occurs despite widely differing fluid, electrolyte, and solute intakes. Any deficiency in absorption or excessive secretion, however, may result in diarrhoea with a net loss of water and electrolytes from the body. Thus, adequate salt and water absorption from the gut is essential for maintaining salt and water homeostasis.

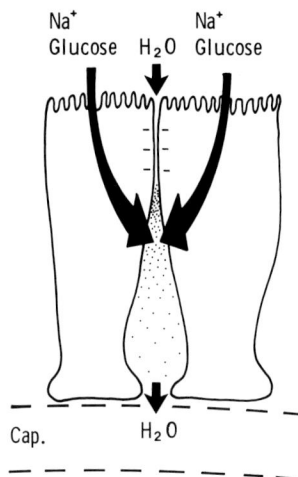

Fig. 8.27 A diagram of the standing gradient hypothesis for fluid absorption. The transport of sodium and non-electrolyte across the cell into the lateral intercellular space establishes a hyperosmotic gradient between the lateral space and the lumen, which encourages water to enter from the lumen. This increases the hydrostatic pressure in the lateral space so that fluid moves in the direction of least resistance towards the capillary.

MECHANISMS OF WATER ABSORPTION

Standing gradient hypothesis

Fluid absorption from the intestine occurs in response to osmotic gradients set up by the active transport of sodium and non-electrolytes such as hexose sugars and amino acids. According to the most widely held hypothesis,[21] the transport of sodium and non-electrolytes across the enterocyte establishes a hypertonic zone in the spaces between the cells (the lateral intercellular spaces). This encourages water to flow into these spaces, mainly through the so called 'tight' junctions (Figure 8.27), which connect adjacent cells at their mucosal poles. Distension of the lateral spaces by osmotic influx of water increases the hydrostatic pressure, and fluid moves in the direction of least resistance towards the capillary. Backflow into the lumen is restricted by the tight junctions between the cells. The observation that absorption of water can take place against an adverse lumen-to-plasma osmotic gradient, yet still employ osmotic forces,[6, 68] is compatible with this model as long as the osmolality and hydrostatic pressure in the lateral space is higher than in the submucosal compartment.

While the standing gradient hypothesis is reasonable for epithelia such as the gall bladder and colon, where the 'tight' junctions are relatively impermeable, one might expect the greater permeability of the jejunal tight junctions to allow water and electrolytes to leak back into the lumen.

Counter current hypothesis

An alternative hypothesis proposes that the zone of hypertonicity responsible for fluid absorption in the small intestine is situated in the lamina propria at the villus tip.[59] This hypertonic zone is maintained by the operation of a counter current multiplier, formed by the hairpin vascular loop configuration of the central artery and the subepithelial capillary network (Figure 8.28). Active transepithelial absorption of sodium establishes a sodium gradient between the peripheral capillary and the central artery. This results in a cross diffusion of sodium from the capillary to the artery, while water travels in the opposite direction from the artery to the capillary (Figure 8.28). This effect is multiplied towards the villus tip until very large osmotic gradients are built up.[39] The osmotic attraction of water into the tip of the villus will establish a hydrostatic gradient from villus tip to base which could force fluid down the central lymphatic vessel. This could explain why 50% of net water absorption takes place via the lymph, in spite of the fact that villus blood flow is 500 times larger than lymphatic flow.[3]

a   b

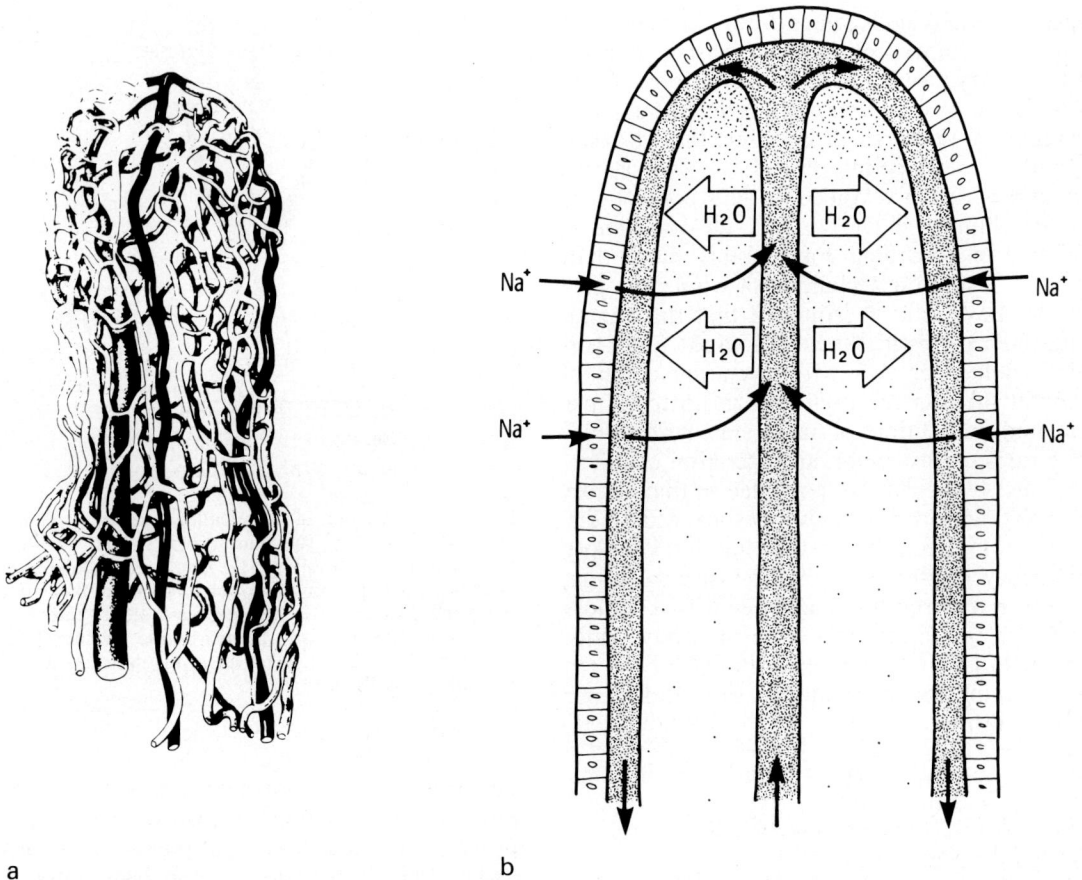

Fig. 8.28 (a) A drawing of the vascular arrangement in a cylindrical villus from the human jejunum. From Spanner, R. (1932),[82] with kind permission of the author and the publisher, Akademische Verlagsgesellschaft. (b) A diagram of the counter current hypothesis for fluid absorption from the small intestine. Active transepithelial absorption of sodium establishes a sodium gradient between the peripheral capillary and the central artery. This results in a cross diffusion of sodium from capillary to artery, while water travels in the opposite direction from artery to capillary. This effect is multiplied towards the villus tip until very large osmotic gradients are built up. From Hallback *et al.* (1978),[39] with kind permission of the authors and the editor of *Gastroenterology*.

Osmotically induced intestinal secretion

If the osmolality of the luminal contents is sufficiently high (a drink of pineapple juice may have an osmolality of 900 mosm/kg), one might expect it to oppose the effects of the high osmolality in the intercellular spaces or the villous tip, and cause secretion into the lumen. However, it is more difficult to cause fluid secretion than fluid absorption by osmotic mechanisms, because the hydraulic conductivity of the epithelium is higher during fluid absorption, when the lateral intercellular spaces are widely dilated, than during osmotically-induced fluid secretion when the lateral spaces are collapsed.[57] This mechanism presumably protects the organism against excessive fluid loss into the gut lumen after ingestion of hypertonic food materials.

Steep osmotic pressure gradients can exist across the epithelium even when the theoretical osmolalities are equal on either side. This is because the epithelium does not behave as a true semi-permeable membrane, but is permeable to a variety of small solutes. Thus, the effective or actual osmotic pressure of a given solute will be lower than its theoretical osmotic pressure by an amount which is directly related to its permeability through the epithelium.[83] The ratio of effective to theoretical osmotic pressures is known as the reflection coefficient. If the jejunum is perfused with a solution of mannitol which is isotonic with plasma, the effective osmotic pressure in the lumen will be higher than the effective osmotic pressure in the plasma because the epithelium is less permeable to mannitol than it is to sodium chloride.[51] The net result is fluid secretion.

Influence of hydrostatic forces

Hakim and Lifson[38] observed that pressures of only 6 cmH$_2$O applied to the serosal side of the canine epithelium in vitro inhibited absorption and induced secretion, while pressures of up to 22 cmH$_2$O applied to the mucosal side of the epithelium had no effect on absorption. The reason for this is that pressure applied to the serosal aspect of the epithelium distends the lateral spaces and increases hydraulic conductivity, while mucosal pressure does not affect the configuration of the lateral space or alter hydraulic conductivity. This mechanism prevents excessive fluid absorption which might occur during periods of enhanced intestinal motility or distension, and acts as a safety valve to release excessive increases in tissue pressure.

Secretion has been induced in experimental animals by acute volume expansion,[42, 45] though the portal venous pressure required to cause secretion from the canine small intestine (35 cmH$_2$O)[91] is well above the serosal pressure that induces secretion in vitro. Perhaps the high venous pressure is required to overcome the high tissue osmotic pressure caused by the operation of a counter current mechanism in vivo. This could partly explain why diarrhoea and intestinal secretion are uncommon in patients with portal hypertension.[67]

TRANSPORT OF ELECTROLYTES

Electrolytes can cross the intestinal epithelium, either propelled by active ion pumps requiring metabolic energy, or by diffusing passively down their electrochemical gradients or accompanying the movement of water in response to osmotic or hydrostatic forces (solvent drag).

Passive diffusion

The fact that water and water-soluble substances can be absorbed passively across the epithelium implies the existence of aqueous channels or pores. Frizzell & Schultz[33] studied the influence of electrical gradients on the influx of ions across the rabbit ileum and showed that 82% of the passive ion conductance in the rabbit ileum conformed to the laws of simple aqueous diffusion and occurred via aqueous channels, presumably at the sites of the 'tight' junctions and lateral intercellular spaces (paracellular shunt pathway). The observation that conductance to cations was greater than conductance to anions[33] suggests that the aqueous channels

are cation-selective, probably because they are lined by negative charges.

The limiting diameter of these aqueous channels has been assessed by exposing the mucosa to hypertonic solutions and measuring the reflection coefficient for a series of passively transported molecules of different molecular sizes.[56] Results indicate that the diameter of the aqueous channels in the human jejunum (0.7–0.9 nm) is larger than in the ileum (0.4 nm),[31] or in the colon (0.2 nm).[6] However, it is important to note that the diameter of the aqueous channels in the jejunum is larger during fluid absorption when the lateral spaces are distended (1.5 nm)[54] than during osmotically induced fluid secretion.

If there are equivalent numbers of pores per unit area in each region of the intestine, the larger diameter of the jejunal pores would allow more rapid absorption of fluid than in the remainder of the intestine, and would enable the major proportion of the absorption of sodium, potassium and small non-electrolytes such as urea to accompany the osmotic influx of water by the process of solvent drag.[28, 29] It would also explain the rapid osmotic equilibration of hypotonic or hypertonic solutions instilled into the lumen of the duodenum and jejunum. On the other hand, high fluid and electrolyte conductance means that active transcellular absorption of ions in the jejunum cannot take place against high electrochemical gradients or generate high transepithelial potential differences (PDs), because the actively transported ions would tend to leak back via the paracellular route.

The tighter aqueous channels in the ileum means that fluid cannot be absorbed as rapidly as in the jejunum, and solvent drag is a less important mechanism for absorption of electrolytes. However, sodium can be absorbed against higher concentration gradients than in the jejunum.[29]

In the colon, where aqueous channels are even tighter, and the paracellular pathways in man may be more selective for chloride than for sodium,[18] nearly all sodium is absorbed by the active transcellular route and continues to be absorbed even at luminal concentrations as low as 15 mmol/l (a tenfold plasma-to-lumen concentration gradient)[6, 20] and adverse electrical gradients of up to 80 mV. The tightness of the aqueous channels could also allow very high osmolalities to be generated within the lateral spaces, allowing water to be extracted from the faecal mass against steep transepithelial osmotic gradients.[6] Although this mechanism may not permit rapid absorption of water, faecal material usually remains in contact with colonic mucosa for several days, which is more than enough time to solidify the stool. Paracellular pathways appear to be less permeable to sodium and water in the distal colon compared to the proximal colon.[6, 18, 53] This would explain the more rapid absorption of salt and water in the proximal colon, and the greater ability of the distal colon to extract sodium from the stool.[24] Excision of the proximal colon is more likely to result in diarrhoea than excision of the distal colon.

Thus the properties of the tight junctions dictate that the more proximal regions of the intestine are adapted to the rapid absorption of a large quantity of fluid and electrolytes, while the more distal regions of the intestine are adapted for extraction of salt and water against high electrochemical and osmotic gradients.

Certain diseases may impair salt and water transport and cause diarrhoea via alterations in permeability. In coeliac disease, evidence suggests that aqueous channels in the small intestine are reduced in size.[30] This could contribute to the reduction in salt and water absorption and the diarrhoea seen in patients with this disease. Conversely, an increased permeability of the colonic epithelium, induced by unabsorbed bile acids[16] or hydroxy fatty acids[37] (produced by bacterial action on unabsorbed fat), and possibly also by inflammatory disease of the bowel, may lead to diarrhoea by preventing salt and water extraction against high osmotic or electrochemical gradients.

Transcellular ion transport

Most electrolytes can only cross the intestinal cells by an active process involving expenditure of energy. This is because intracellular ion concentrations are either much higher or much lower than the extracellular concentrations in the plasma and the lumen, and the cytosol is about 40 mV negative to plasma and luminal fluids.[76] Thus, although an electrolyte may be able to cross one membrane by passive diffusion, it requires an active mechanism to cross the other.

JEJUNUM

Absorption of salt and water from the jejunum is markedly increased in the presence of actively transported sugars, amino acids and peptides. Sodium interacts with the non-electrolyte in a common transport mechanism (carrier or pore)

on the mucosal membrane. The energy for the transfer of both into the cell is provided by the inwardly directed sodium gradient. Sodium is then pumped out of the cell into the lateral intercellular space by an ion exchange mechanism, thought to be coupled to a specific sodium/potassium dependent ATPase, while sugars or amino acids are transferred into the lateral space by a passive carrier-mediated mechanism. Both entry and exit mechanisms depolarize the cell membrane, causing a change in the transepithelial potential difference (electrogenic transport). The osmotic gradient set up by the transcellular passage of sodium and sugars of amino acids encourages water and more electrolytes to enter via the paracellular route. This mechanism accounts for the important therapeutic effect of glucose and electrolyte solutions in countering fluid losses and preventing fluid and electrolyte depletion in cholera and other secretory diarrhoeas.

In the absence of actively transported sugars and amino acids, active absorption of sodium in perfused loops of human and rat jejunum in vivo[69, 88] is thought to be electrically neutral and mediated via a sodium/hydrogen exchange pump at the mucosal membrane (Figure 8.29). According to this hypothesis, increasing the luminal concentration of bicarbonate encourages sodium absorption by neutralizing the hydrogen ion and increasing its diffusion gradient from cell to lumen. The increased exit of hydrogen from the cell is accompanied by the increased entry of sodium, and results in loss of bicarbonate from the lumen. Experiments carried out in vitro suggest that some sodium may also be absorbed independently of hydrogen via an electrogenic mechanism.[7]

ILEUM

In the ileum the coupling of active transcellular sodium transport with sugar and amino acid absorption does not result in the net transfer of sodium across the epithelium.[29] This can be explained by a tighter paracellular pathway, which not only allows less sodium to enter by solvent drag but also means that active sodium transport will generate a larger transepithelial potential difference (PD), which could result in the recycling of actively transported sodium back into the lumen via the paracellular route.[29] Thus unlike the jejunum, it seems likely that most sodium and water will be absorbed in the ileum by an electro-neutral mechanism not linked to the transport of non-electrolyte.

JEJUNUM ILEUM COLON

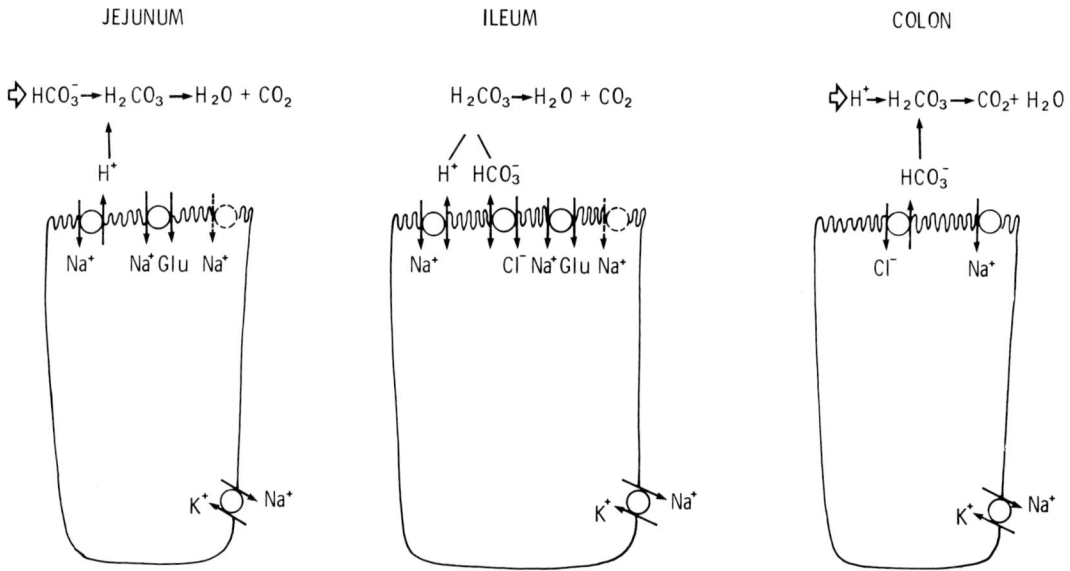

Fig. 8.29 Diagrams of the carrier-mediated mechanisms proposed to exist for the absorption of sodium, potassium and chloride across the mucosal and basolateral membranes in the human jejunum, ileum and colon.

Perfusion studies carried out in the human ileum[87] indicate that, in the absence of actively transported sugars and amino acids, electrolyte absorption occurs by a neutral double exchange process (Figure 8.29). Sodium is exchanged for hydrogen as in the jejunum, but this is coupled with the absorption of chloride in exchange for bicarbonate secretion.

Experiments carried out on short-circuited sheets of rat or rabbit ileum, however, suggest that, in the absence of sugar or amino acids, at least 50% of sodium is absorbed independently via an electrogenic route. The remainder of sodium absorption is linked to the absorption of chloride,[33] possibly through functionally coupled anion and cation exchange pumps[80] (Figure 8.29). It is possible that the presence of an intact blood supply and enhanced tissue metabolism favours the dominance of the double exchange process in vivo.

Congenital absence of the chloride/bicarbonate exchange mechanism in the ileum is thought by some to be responsible for the severe diarrhoea observed in congenital chloridorrhoea.[5] The absorption of sodium in exchange for hydrogen ion leads to luminal acidification, which may itself inhibit further sodium absorption and hence reduce water absorption. The net result is diarrhoea with alkalosis.

Transport of potassium across the small intestinal epithelium behaves as if it occurs by passive diffusion and solvent drag along the paracellular pathway.[86]

COLON

Ion transport studies carried out in vitro and in vivo suggest that the colon absorbs sodium and chloride and secretes bicarbonate against electrochemical gradients.[20, 53] Sodium is absorbed independently by an electrogenic mechanism in most species, though there is evidence in the rat for some coupled sodium and chloride absorption.[9, 24] The rate of sodium absorption in the human colon is not influenced by the intraluminal presence of glucose, amino acids or bicarbonate. It is, however, thought to be controlled according to body requirements by levels of circulating mineralocorticoids. Measurement of the rectal PD generated by active sodium transport has been suggested as a method of diagnosing hyperaldosteronism.[23]

The observations that bicarbonate secretion is reduced in the human colon when luminal chloride is replaced by sulphate[20] and that a reduced luminal pH stimulates chloride absorption[11] indicate the existence of a colonic chloride/bicarbonate exchange mechanism.

Although the human colon possesses no direct mechanism for absorbing sugars, unabsorbed carbohydrate is rapidly converted by bacteria to volatile fatty acids (VFA). While it seems likely that most VFA are absorbed by non-ionic diffusion, some may substitute for chloride and be absorbed by an ionic diffusion in exchange for bicarbonate.[60] The rapid absorption of VFA is an important mechanism for removing unabsorbed carbohydrate from the colonic lumen and so preventing the diarrhoea produced by the osmotic effects of unabsorbed sugars.

Potassium is the dominant cation of faecal fluid. The surprisingly large epithelial conductance to potassium (approximately ten times that of sodium and chloride) suggests the existence of specific channels selective to potassium in the epithelium,[35] while the accumulation of potassium in the colonic lumen is favoured, though not entirely explained, by the high electrical gradient set up by electrogenic sodium transport. It is possible that dead or damaged epithelial cells and mucus rich in potassium contribute to the high luminal potassium concentrations, though one cannot rule out the existence of active potassium secretion.[2]

To summarize, data, largely derived from perfusion experiments carried out in man, indicate that the jejunum, ileum and colon all contain a mechanism for the electrogenic entry of sodium into the cell (Figure 8.29). In the jejunum and ileum this is coupled to entry of sugars and amino acids. The jejunum and ileum also exhibit neutral entry of sodium in exchange for hydrogen, while the ileum and colon contain a neutral mechanism for absorption of chloride in exchange for bicarbonate secretion. Coupled sodium and chloride entry, which is well documented in experimental animals in vitro, has not been confirmed in man. Transport of potassium probably occurs by passive mechanisms, though active secretion may take place in the colon.

The exit of sodium at the basolateral pole of the enterocyte is mediated at all three regions of the intestine by an active sodium pump. This mechanism is probably linked to a specific sodium/potassium dependent ATPase and is thought to pump sodium out of the cell in exchange for potassium at a ratio of $3:2$.[76] Corticosteroids may increase salt and water absorption in the ileum and colon by increasing the activity of Na/K ATPase,[17] though the effects of corticosteroids on transport occur several hours ahead of a demonstrable change in activity of the enzyme.[8, 85]

ACTIVE SECRETION OF WATER AND ELECTROLYTES

Evidence suggests that secretogogues such as cholera toxin probably exert their major effect by increasing the permeability of the mucosal membrane to chloride, allowing it to leak from the cell.[34] Chloride can enter the cell from the serosal aspect by an active process linked to the entry of sodium down its electrochemical gradient. The sodium is then pumped into the lateral space by the sodium extrusion pump. The selective permeability of the tight junctions to cations is thought to inhibit the diffusion of sodium into the lumen, because this would set up an adverse electrical gradient which would discourage further movement. The opening up of chloride channels in the mucosal membrane removes the electrical brake on sodium movement and allows sodium and water to leak passively from the hypertonic lateral space (Figure 8.30). This could account for the collapse of the lateral intracellular spaces after treatment of isolated epithelium with cholera toxin. It is difficult, however, to see how this mechanism could cause continuous secretion from an epithelium in vivo unless there is also a mechanism which allows the lateral intercellular space to refill with fluid from the serosal side. For this it is necessary to suggest that secretogogues must increase capillary permeability, or capillary hydrostatic pressure (filtration pressure), or both.

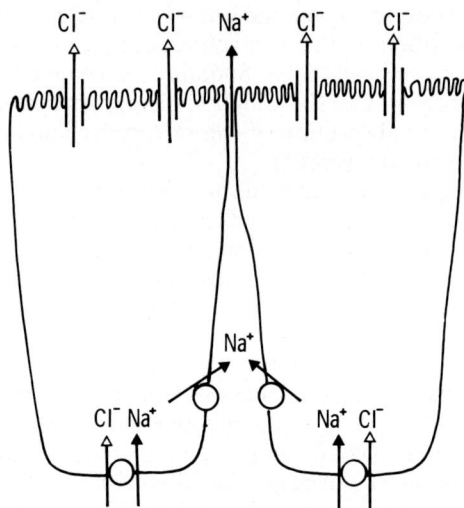

Fig. 8.30 A diagram of the ionic mechanism underlying the active secretion of salt and water from the intestinal epithelium.

The scheme outlined above does not discriminate between villous and crypt epithelia and allows all enterocytes to secrete and absorb fluid depending on the differential permeability of the anion and cation selective pathways. However, if secretion took place on the villi as well as the crypts, then it is difficult to see how administration of glucose and electrolyte mixtures to a secreting intestine could oppose net fluid secretion. Further observations that secretion remains unimpaired when villus cells are selectively damaged with hypertonic sodium sulphate[75] but is inhibited by selective damage to the crypts by cyclohexamide,[79] and that villous hyperosmolality persists in the presence of cholera secretion[40] suggests that the crypts are the predominant sites of active secretion.

The recent finding that perfusion of the lumen with hypotonic solution normally abolishes the villous hyperosmolality in the cat small intestine but fails to do so in the cholera-treated intestine[40] suggests the existence of a circuit whereby some sodium and chloride secreted in the crypts can be reabsorbed in the villous epithelium creating the hyperosmolality for fluid absorption (Figure 8.31). This mechanism could

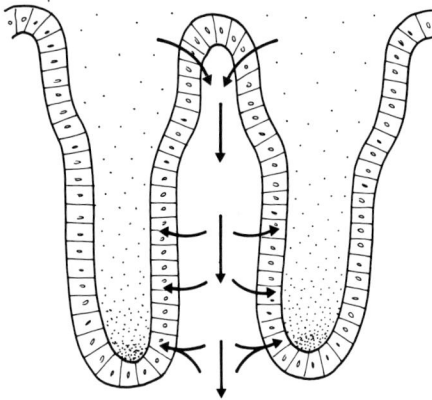

Fig. 8.31 A diagram of the proposed fluid circuit which could occur between actively secreting crypts and absorbing villous enterocytes. From Hallback *et al.* (1982),[40] with kind permission of the authors and the editor of *Gastroenterology.*

also explain why relatively more bicarbonate compared with chloride is secreted from the ileum than from the jejunum.[73] In the ileum, secreted chloride can be exchanged with bicarbonate at the mucosal surface of the villous enterocyte. The jejunum, however, does not contain a chloride/bicarbonate exchange mechanism.

The reason why enterocytes should have the capacity to secrete when in the crypts but develop absorptive mechanisms as they climb the villous escalator is unclear. It could be that as the enterocytes mature they lose their ability to respond to secretogcgues or that the permeability of the tight junctions and lateral intercellular spaces change. Alternatively, the neurohumoral environment in the crypt may facilitate secretion. In support of this is the dense

colonic innervation in the crypt region[48] and the recent evidence that prostaglandin E_2 is not only a more potent stimulator of adenylate cyclase in crypt enterocytes but also is less rapidly degraded at that site (L. A. Turnberg, personal communication).

The cellular control of intestinal secretion

The cellular action of intestinal secretogogues appears to be mediated by an increase in intracellular levels of calcium. Agents such as cholera toxin or vasoactive intestinal peptide (VIP) interact with a receptor on the cell surface, resulting in the activation of adenylate cyclase and formation of cyclic AMP. The latter is thought to release calcium from intracellular stores, but probably also increases calcium uptake into the cell from the extracellular fluid. Other secretogogues, such as serotonin or acetylcholine, do not act by increasing cyclic AMP. Instead they interact with a receptor to cause hydrolysis of phospholipid components within the cell membrane[63] and the opening of channels in the cell membrane to allow the entry of calcium (Figure 8.32). Calcium is then thought to activate a specific calcium dependent regulator protein, called calmodulin, which increases chloride permeability by mechanisms that are so far unknown. Neuroleptic agents such as trifluoperazine, pimozide and diazepam

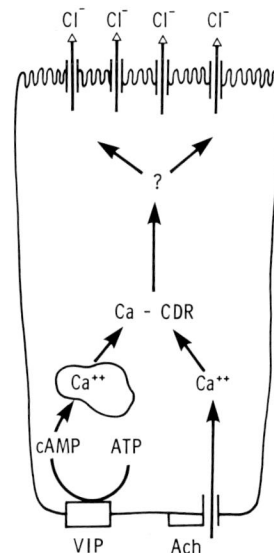

Fig. 8.32 A diagram of the proposed intercellular mechanism via which secretogogues exert their effects on the enterocyte.

prevent secretion by binding to the calcium/ calmodulin complex.[46] Chlorpromazine, a similar agent, has been used to treat cholera and other secretory diarrhoeas, though it appears to have only a relatively mild effect in reducing fluid losses.[49]

NEUROENDOCRINE CONTROL OF FLUID AND ELECTROLYTE TRANSPORT

When the small intestine of normal human subject is perfused with a plasma-like solution, it usually absorbs salt and water. However, the rate of absorption varies widely from subject to subject and in the same subject on different test days. Some apparently normal subjects (and animals) secrete fluid into the intestine rather than absorb it.[73, 87] The mechanisms responsible for this physiological variation are unknown, although it seems likely that the autonomic nervous system plays an important role. Histological studies have demonstrated dense cholinergic innervation of the cells in the crypt region.[48] Pharmacological studies suggest that cholinergic agents cause fluid and electrolyte secretion,[41, 48, 64] while adrenergic agents have the opposite effect and induce absorption of salt and water.[27, 64] The implication from these studies is that sympathetic stimulation induces fluid absorption while vagal stimulation induces fluid secretion. However, indirect vagal stimulation by sham feeding does not cause a significant change in intestinal fluid and electrolyte transport in man[72] although it increases gastric secretion, and vagotomy does not appear to cause any alteration in intestinal transport in man,[12] despite producing severe diarrhoea in some patients. One complicating factor is that the branches of the autonomic nervous system are not mutually exclusive. The release of acetylcholine from cholinergic nerves may be modulated by noradrenaline and vice versa[13, 84] and it is even possible that some enteric neurones may release both noradrenaline and acetylcholine.[13]

It is probable that much of the control of intestinal transport is mediated by local reflexes. It is known, for example, that distension of the lumen[14] or tactile stimulation[4] will induce intestinal secretion, and there is compelling evidence to suggest that part of the secretory response to cholera toxin may be mediated by a nervous reflex culminating in the release of vasoactive intestinal polypeptide (VIP).[15]

Action of transmitter substances in the intestinal mucosa

The list of polypeptides and other chemical transmitters which are present in the small intestinal wall and which can alter intestinal transport is long (Tables 8.11 and 8.12). Some of these substances (enkephalin, somatostatin and VIP) are found within nerves, while the remainder are found in cells within the mucosa or submucosa.

Table 8.11 Possible transmitter substances which may act on the intestinal epithelium to reduce absorption or increase secretion of fluid and electrolytes.

Muscarinic agonists	Neurotensin
Vasoactive intestinal polypeptide	ATP
Angiotensin (high dose)	Gastrin
Secretin	Cholecystokinin
Serotonin	Bradykinin
Bombesin	Histamine
Substance P	Prostaglandins

Table 8.12 Possible transmitter substances which may act on the intestinal epithelium to increase absorption or reduce secretion of fluid and electrolytes in man.

Catecholamines	Enkephalins
Dopamine	Somatostatin
Angiotensin (low dose)	Prostacyclin

If all of these agents do in fact regulate intestinal fluid and electrolyte transport, it seems surprising that this function requires so many different mediators. It is possible that some serve as transmitters at an interneurone site or act to modulate a secretory or absorptive mechanism, providing fine control.

Table 8.11 lists the transmitters which act on the intestinal mucosa to induce secretion or inhibit absorption.

Vasoactive intestinal polypeptide is found in enteric neurones, and can be released by vagal stimulation[25, 26] and by electrical field stimulation of intramural nerves.[44] It interacts with high affinity receptors on enterocytes and may be the major neurotransmitter mediating intestinal secretion. The rare patients who have VIP secreting ganglioneuromas or islet cell tumours of the pancreas exhibit considerable intestinal secretion and present with voluminous diarrhoea.

Histamine is found in large quantities in the intestinal epithelium and may induce net secretion by inhibiting chloride/bicarbonate exchange in the ileum[55] or by altering capillary permeability.[52] The actions of histamine may be of relevance in patients with food allergy and may be responsible for the severe diarrhoea seen in some patients with systemic mastocytosis.

Prostaglandins are produced from cell membrane components and act directly on the cell to stimulate intestinal secretion and increase production of cyclic AMP. They can be released by distension of the gut wall,[4] vagal stimulation, and mucosal injury. They probably mediate intestinal secretion induced by local stimuli, and may serve to amplify the effects of other secretogogues. They are thought to be responsible, at least in part, for the diarrhoea induced by inflammatory diseases of the bowel, by irradiation, and by certain endocrine tumours.

Serotonin (5-hydroxytryptamine) is found in enteric neurones and in enterochromaffin cells. Intestinal perfusion studies, carried out in the rabbit, suggest that it causes secretion by inhibiting sodium and chloride absorption in the ileum.[50] It is produced in large amounts in patients with the carcinoid syndrome, and the diarrhoea and intestinal secretion found in this condition have been inhibited by methysergide, a peripheral inhibitor of serotonin.[22] It may also be partly responsible for the intestinal secretion seen in coeliac disease.

Table 8.12 lists the transmitters that have been shown to act on the intestinal mucosa to inhibit intestinal secretion or enhance absorption. Of these, only catecholamines have been shown to act directly on the enterocyte (via two receptors). The remainder are thought to modulate the action of other transmitters.

Endogenous opiates are present in the myenteric and submucous nerve plexuses and probably act by inhibiting the release of transmitters, in particular acetylcholine, from postganglionic neurones, though some evidence supports a direct action on the enterocyte.[47] Recent studies have shown that morphine and opiate-like agents reverse intestinal secretion induced by a number of secretogogues.[77] This has led to speculation that the potent antidiarrhoeal action of these agents may be due to direct stimulation of fluid and electrolyte absorption and reversal of secretion, as well as inhibition of propulsive motility.

Action of bile acids and hydroxy fatty acids

Among substances which can alter intestinal fluid and electrolyte transport in the colon, perhaps the most important are the dihydroxy bile acids[62] and the hydroxy fatty acids.[1] These substances may be formed in the colon by bacterial degradation of unabsorbed bile acid and fat and are thought to be responsible for the diarrhoea following disease or surgical resection of the ileum. Evidence suggests that they impair colonic absorption and/or induce secretion by increasing the permeability of the epithelium[37] as well as stimulating production of cyclic AMP[10] and increasing propulsive motor activity.

Indirect action on intestinal transport

It is important to note that the action of transmitter substances on intestinal absorption and secretion may not only be mediated by a direct action on the enterocyte, but can also occur via an action on blood flow or intestinal motility.

Blood flow

The influence of intestinal blood flow upon absorption depends upon the permeability of the intestinal epithelium to the probe molecule.[89] The absorption of highly permeable substances such as small ions and some lipid soluble substances are limited by blood flow, whereas larger water soluble molecules are less influenced by blood flow. The absorption of permeable substances may be restricted to a certain extent by the operation of the counter current exchanger. If the blood flow is low, these molecules become trapped in the villous tip, increasing the osmolality and the efficiency of water absorption. If the blood flow is increased, the exchange is less efficient, permeable solutes are absorbed more rapidly, but water absorption is reduced.

The possibility that transmitter substances may influence transport via an effect on blood flow deserves further study. In particular, there is little insight into whether, and to what extent, secretion can be induced by diversion of blood flow to the crypts or by increases in capillary permeability or filtration pressure.

Motor activity

Motor activity may influence the absorption or secretion of salt and water in many ways.[71] Increases in intestinal motor activity may limit absorption by reducing intestinal blood flow[70] or by reducing the effective surface area for absorption.[61] Moreover, the inverse correlation between stool weight and mouth to anus transit time,[74] and between small bowel transit time and the wet weight and sodium content of ileostomy effluent[43] suggests that absorption of salt and water is related to the time that luminal contents remain in contact with the absorptive epithelium. This must, in turn, be inversely related to the degree of propulsive motility.

Finally, motor activity may enhance absorption by mixing food components. The role of the villous movements in mixing the environment close to the epithelium may be particularly important but remains unexplored.

ACKNOWLEDGEMENT

The author is grateful to Dr P. T. Hardcastle for his helpful comments.

REFERENCES

1 Ammon, H. V. & Phillips, S. F. (1973) Inhibition of colonic water and electrolyte absorption by fatty acids in man. *Gastroenterology*, **65**, 744–749.

2 Archampong, E. Q., Harris, J. & Clark, C. G. (1972) The absorption and secretion of water and electrolytes across the healthy and diseased human colonic mucosa measured in vitro. *Gut*, **13**, 880–886.

3 Barrowman, J. & Roberts, K. B. (1967) The role of the lymphatic system in the absorption of water from the small intestine of the rat. *Quarterly Journal of Experimental Physiology*, **52**, 19–30.

4 Beubler, E. & Juan, H. (1978) PGE released blood flow and transmucosal water movement after mechanical stimulation of the rat jejunal mucosa. *Naunyn Schmeidebergs Archives of Pharmacology*, **305**, 91–95.

5 Bieberdorf, F. A., Gordon, P. & Fordtran, J. S. (1972) Pathogenesis of congenital alkalosis with diarrhoea. Implications for the physiology of normal ileal absorption and secretion. *Journal of Clinical Investigation*, **51**, 1958–1968.

6 Billich, C. O. & Levitan, R. (1969) Effects of sodium concentration and osmolality on water and electrolyte absorption from the intact human colon. *Journal of Clinical Investigation*, **48**, 1336–1347.

7 Binder, H. J. (1974) Sodium transport across the isolated human jejunum. *Gastroenterology*, **67**, 231–236.

8 Binder, H. J. (1978) Effect of dexamethasone on electrolyte transport in the large intestine of the rat. *Gastroenterology*, **75**, 212–217.

9 Binder, H. J. & Rawlings, C. L. (1973) Electrolyte transport across isolated large intestinal mucosa. *American Journal of Physiology*, **225**, 1232–1239.

10 Binder, H. J., Filburn, C. & Volpe, B. T. (1975) Bile acid alteration of colonic electrolyte transport: role of cyclic adenosine monophosphate. *Gastroenterology*, **68**, 503–508.

11 Bown, R. L., Sladen, G. E., Rousseau, B. et al. (1972) A study of water and electrolyte transport by the excluded human colon. *Clinical Science*, **43**, 891–902.

12 Bunch, G. A. & Shields, R. (1973) The effect of vagotomy on the intestinal handling of water and electrolytes. *Gut*, **14**, 116–119.

13 Burnstock, G. (1979) Non-adrenergic, non-cholinergic nerves in the intestine and their possible involvement in secretion. In *Mechanisms of Intestinal Secretion*. (Ed.) Binder, H. J., pp. 147–174. New York: Alan R. Liss.

14 Caren, J. F., Meyer, J. H. & Grossman, M. I. (1974) Canine intestinal secretion during and after rapid distension of the small bowel. *American Journal of Physiology*, **227**, 183–188.

15 Cassuto, J., Jodal, M., Tuttle, M. & Lundgren, O. (1981) On the role of intramural nerves in the pathogenesis of cholera toxin-induced intestinal secretion. *Scandinavian Journal of Gastroenterology*, **16**, 377–384.

16 Chadwick, V. S., Gaginella, T. S., Carlson, G. L. et al. (1979) Effect of molecular structure on bile acid induced alterations in absorptive functions, permeability and morphology in the perfused rabbit colon. *Journal of Laboratory Clinical Medicine*, **94**, 661–664.

17 Charney, A. N., Kinsey, M. D., Myers, L. et al. (1975) (Na^+-K^+) activated adenosine triphosphatase and intestinal electrolyte transport. Effect of adrenal steroids. *Journal of Clinical Investigation*, **56**, 563–660.

18 Davis, G. R., Santa Ana, C. A., Morawski, S. G. & Fordtran, J. S. (1982) Permeability characteristics of human jejunum, ileum, proximal colon and distal colon. Results of potential difference measurements and unidirectional fluxes. *Gastroenterology*, **83**, 844–850.

19 Debongnie, J. C. & Phillips, S. F. (1978) Capacity of the human colon to absorb fluid. *Gastroenterology*, **74**, 698–703.

20 Devroed, G. J. & Phillips, S. F. (1969) Conservation of sodium, chloride and water by the human colon. *Gastroenterology*, **56**, 101–109.

21 Diamond, J. M. & Bossert, W. H. (1967) Standing gradient osmotic flow. A mechanism for coupling of water and solute transport in epithelia. *Journal of General Physiology*, **59**, 2061–2083.

22 Donowitz, M. & Binder, H. J. (1975) Jejunal fluid and electrolyte secretion in carcinoid syndrome. *American Journal of Digestive Diseases*, **20**, 1115–1121.

23 Edmonds, C. J. & Richards, P. (1970) Measurement of rectal electrical potential difference as an instant screening test for hyperaldosteronism. *Lancet*, **ii**, 624–627.

24 Edmonds, C. J. & Thompson, B. D. (1980) Absorption by the colon during prolonged infusions in conscious unrestrained rats. *Journal of Physiology*, **302**, 399–409.

25 Edwards, A. V., Bircham, P. M. M., Mitchell, S. J. & Bloom, S. R. (1978) Changes in the concentration of vasoactive intestinal polypeptide in intestinal lymph in response to vagal stimulation in the calf. *Experientia*, **34**, 1186.

26 Fahrenkrug, J., Galbo, H., Holst, J. J. & Schaffalitsky de Muckadel, O. B. (1978) Influence of autonomic nervous system on the release of vasoactive intestinal polypeptide from the porcine gastrointestinal tract. *Journal of Physiology*, **280**, 405–422.

27 Field, M. & McColl, I. (1973) Ion transport in rabbit intestinal mucosa. III. Effects of catecholamines. *American Journal of Physiology*, **225**, 852–857.

28 Fordtran, J. S. (1975) Stimulation of active and passive absorption by sugars in the human jejunum. *Journal of Clinical Investigation*, **55**, 728–737.

29 Fordtran, J. S., Rector, F. C. & Carter, N. W. (1968) The mechanisms of sodium absorption in the human small intestine. *Journal of Clinical Investigation*, **47**, 884–900.

30 Fordtran, J. S., Rector, F. C., Locklear, T. W. & Ewton, M. F. (1967) Water and solute movement in the small intestine of patients with sprue. *Journal of Clinical Investigation*, **46**, 287–298.

31 Fordtran, J. S., Rector, F. C., Ewton, M. F. et al. (1965) Permeability characteristics of human small intestine. *Journal of Clinical Investigation*, **44**, 1935–1944.

32 Frizzell, R. A. & Schultz, S. G. (1972) Ionic conductances of extracellular shunt pathway in rabbit ileum. Influence of shunt on transmural sodium transport and electrical potential difference. *Journal of General Physiology*, **59**, 318–346.

33 Frizzell, R. A. & Schultz, S. G. (1979) Models of electrolyte absorption and secretion by gastrointestinal epithelia. In *International Review of Physiology*. (Ed.) Crane, R. K. pp. 205–225. Baltimore: University Park Press.

34 Frizzell, R. A., Field, M. & Schultz, S. G. (1979) Sodium coupled chloride transport by epithelial tissues. *American Journal of Physiology*, **236**, F1–F8.

35 Frizzell, R. A., Koch, M. J. & Schultz, S. G. (1976) Ion transport by the rabbit colon: active and passive components. *Journal of Membrane Biology*, **27**, 297–316.

36 Fromter, E. & Diamond, J. M. (1972) Route of passive ion transport in epithelia. *Nature (New Biology)*, **235**, 9–13.

37 Gaginella, T. S., Chadwick, V. S., Debongnie, J. C. *et al.* (1977) Perfusion of the rabbit colon with ricinoleic acid: dose related mucosal injury, fluid secretion and increased permeability. *Gastroenterology*, **73**, 95–101.

38 Hakim, A. A. & Lifson, N. (1969) Effects of pressure on water and solute transport by dog intestinal mucosa in vitro. *American Journal of Physiology*, **216**, 276–284.

39 Hallback, D-A., Hulten, L., Jodal, M. *et al.* (1978) Evidence for the existence of a countercurrent exchanger in the small intestine of man. *Gastroenterology*, **74**, 683–690.

40 Hallback, D-A., Jodal, M., Sjoquist, A. & Lundgren, O. (1982) Evidence for cholera secretion eminating from the crypts. *Gastroenterology*, **83**, 1051–1056.

41 Hardcastle, P. T. & Eggenton, J. (1973) The effect of acetylcholine on the electrical activity of intestinal epithelial cells. *Biochimica et Biophysica Acta*, **298**, 95–100.

42 Higgins, J. R. & Blair, N. P. (1971) Intestinal transport of water and electrolytes during extracellular volume expansion in dogs. *Journal of Clinical Investigation*, **50**, 2569–2579.

43 Holgate, A. M. & Read, N. W. (1982) Can rapid small bowel transit limit absorption of a meal? *Gut*, **83**, A912.

44 Hubel, K. A., Gaginella, T. S. & O'Dorisio, T. M. (1978) Release of vasoactive intestinal polypeptide by electrical field stimulation of rabbit ileum. *Gastroenterology*, **74**, 1127.

45 Humphreys, M. H. & Earley, L. E. (1971) The mechanism of decreased intestinal sodium and water absorption after acute volume expansion in the rat. *Journal of Clinical Investigation*, **50**, 2355–2367.

46 Ilundain, A. & Naftalin, R. J. (1979) Role of Ca^{2+} dependent regulator protein in intestinal secretion. *Nature*, **279**, 446–449.

47 Ilundain, A. & Naftalin, R. J. (1981) Opiates increase chloride permeability of the serosal border of rabbit ileum. *Journal of Physiology*, **316**, 56P–57P.

48 Isaacs, P. E. T., Corbett, C. L., Riley, A. K. *et al.* (1976) In vitro behaviour of human intestinal mucosa. The influence of acetylcholine on ion transport. *Journal of Clinical Investigation*, **58**, 535–542.

49 Islam, M. R., Sack, D. A., Holmgren, J. *et al.* (1982) Use of chlorpromazine in the treatment of cholera and other severe acute watery diarrhoeal diseases. *Gastroenterology*, **82**, 1335–1340.

50 Kisloff, B. & Moore, E. W. (1976) Effect of serotonin on water and electrolyte transport in the in vivo rabbit small intestine. *Gastroenterology*, **71**, 1033–1038.

51 Krejs, G. J. & Fordtran, J. S. (1978) Physiology and pathophysiology of ion and water movement in the human intestine. In *Gastrointestinal Disease*. (Ed.) Sleisenger, M. H. & Fordtran, J. S. pp. 297–335. Philadelphia: W. B. Saunders.

52 Lee, J. S. & Silverberg, J. W. (1976) Effect of histamine on intestinal fluid secretion in the dog. *American Journal of Physiology*, **231**, 793–798.

53 Levitan, R., Fordtran, J. S., Burrows, B. A. & Ingelfinger, F. J. (1962) Water and salt absorption in the human colon. *Journal of Clinical Investigation*, **41**, 1754–1759.

54 Levitt, D. G., Hakim, A. A. & Lifson, N. (1969) Evaluation of components of transport of sugars by dog jejunum in vivo. *American Journal of Physiology*, **217**, 777–783.

55 Linaker, B. D., McKay, J. S., Higgs, N. B. & Turnberg, L. A. (1981) Mechanisms of histamine stimulated secretion in the rabbit ileal mucosa. *Gut*, **22**, 964–970.

56 Lindemann, B. & Solomon, A. K. (1962) Permeability of luminal surface of intestinal mucosal cells. *Journal of General Physiology*, **45**, 801–810.

57 Loeschke, K., Bentzel, C. S. & Csaky, T. Z. (1970) Asymmetry of osmotic flow in the frog intestine, functional and structural correlation. *American Journal of Physiology* **218**, 1723–1731.

58 Love, A. H. G., Mitchell, T. G. & Phillips, R. A. (1968) Water and sodium absorption in the human intestine. *Journal of Physiology*, **195**, 133–140.

59 Lundgren, O. & Svanik, J. (1977) Gastrointestinal circulation. In *International Review of Physiology*. (Ed.) Crane, R. K. pp. 1–34. Baltimore: University Park Press.

60 McNiel, N. I., Cummings, J. H. & James, W. P. T. (1978) Short chain fatty acid absorption by the human large intestine. *Gut*, **19**, 819–822.

61 Matuchansky, C., Huet, P. N., Mary, J. Y. *et al.* (1972) Effects of cholecystokinin and metoclopramide on jejunal movements of water and electrolytes and on transit time of luminal fluid in man. *European Journal of Clinical Investigation*, **2**, 169–175.

62 Mekhjian, H. S., Phillips, S. F. & Hoffman, A. F. (1971) Colonic secretion of water and electrolytes induced by bile acids: perfusion studies in man. *Journal of Clinical Investigation*, **50**, 1569–1577.

63 Michell, R. N. (1979) Phospholipids and cell surface receptor function. *Biochimica et Biophysica Acta*, **415**, 81–147.

64 Morris, A. I. & Turnberg, L. A. (1980) The influence of a parasympathetic agonist and antagonist on human intestinal transport in vivo. *Gastroenterology*, **79**, 861–866.

65 Morris, A. I. & Turnberg, L. A. (1981) Influence of isoproterenol and propranolol on human intestinal transport in vivo. *Gastroenterology*, **81**, 1076–1079.

66 Murer, H., Hopfer, U. & Kinne, R. (1976) Sodium proton transport in brush border membrane vesicles isolated from rat small intestine and kidney. *Biochemical Journal*, **154**, 597–604.

67 Norman, D. A., Atkins, J. M., Seelig, L. L. *et al.* (1980) Water and electrolyte movement and mucosal morphology in the jejunum of patients with portal hypertension. *Gastroenterology*, **79**, 707–715.

68 Parsons, D. S. & Wingate, D. L. (1961) The effect of osmotic gradients on fluid transfer across rat intestine in vitro. *Biochimica et Biophysica Acta*, **46**, 170–183.

69 Podesta, R. B. & Mettrick, D. F. (1977) HCO_3 transport in rat jejunum: relationship to NaCl and H_2O transport in vivo. *American Journal of Physiology*, **232**, E62–E68.

70 Pytowski, B. & Michalowski, J. (1977) Motility and blood flow: dependent absorption of amino acids in canine small intestine. *European Journal of Clinical Investigation*, **7**, 79–86.

71 Read, N. W. (1981) The relationship between intestinal motility and intestinal transport. In *Clinical Research Reviews*, vol. 1 (Supplement 1), 73–81. Janssen Research Foundation.

72 Read, N. W., Cooper, K. & Fordtran, J. S. (1978) Effect of modified sham feeding on jejunal transport and pancreatic and biliary secretion in man. *American Journal of Physiology*, **234**(4), E417–E420.

73 Read, N. W., Krejs, G. J., Barkley, R. M. *et al.* (1979) Spontaneous secretion from the dog small intestine in vivo. *Journal of Laboratory and Clinical Medicine*, **93**, 381–389.

74   Read, N. W., Miles, C. A., Fisher, D. *et al.* (1980) The transit of a meal through the stomach, small intestine and colon in normal subjects and the role in the pathogenesis of diarrhoea. *Gastroenterology*, **79**, 1276–1282.

75   Roggin, G. M., Banwell, J. G., Yardley, J. H. & Hendrix, T. R. (1972) Unimpaired response of rabbit ileum to cholera toxin after selective damage to villus epithelium. *Gastroenterology*, **63**, 981–989.

76   Rose, R. C. & Schultz, S. G. (1971) Studies on the electrical potential profile across rabbit ileum. Effects of sugars and amino acids on transmural and transmucosal electrical potential differences. *Journal of General Physiology*, **57**, 639–663.

77   Sandhu, B., Tripp, J. H., Candy, D. C. A. & Harries, J. T. (1979) Loperamide inhibits cholera toxin-induced intestinal secretion. *Lancet*, **i**, 689–690.

78   Savitch, V. V. & Sochestvensky, N. A. (1917) L'influence du nerf vague sur la secretion de l'intestin. *Comptes Rendus des Seances et Memoires de la Societe de Biologie*, **80**, 508–509.

79   Serebro, H. A., Iber, F. L., Yardley, J. H. & Hendrix, T. R. (1969) Inhibition of cholera toxin action in the rabbit by cyclohexamide. *Gastroenterology*, **56**, 506.

80   Sheerin, H. E. & Field, M. (1975) Ileal HCO_3 secretion: relationship to Na and Cl transport and effect of theophylline. *American Journal of Physiology*, **228**, 1065–1074.

81   Sjovall, H., Redfors, S., Jodal, M. & Lundgren, O. (1981) The effect of splanchnic nerve stimulation on jejunal water and sodium transport. *Proceedings of the European Intestinal Transport Group*. Berlin.

82   Spanner, R. (1932) Neue befinde uber die Blutwege der darmwand und ihre funktionelle bedentung. *Gegenbaurs Morphologisches Jahrbuch*, **69**, 394.

83   Staverman, A. J. (1951) The theory of measurement of osmotic pressure. *Recueil des Travaux Chimiques des Pays-Bas*, **70**, 344–372.

84   Tapper, E. J., Powell, D. W. & Morris, S. M. (1978) Cholinergic adrenergic interaction of intestinal ion transport. *American Journal of Physiology*, **235**, E402–E409.

85   Thompson, B. D. & Edmonds, C. J. (1974) Aldosterone, sodium depletion and hypothyroidism on the ATPase activity of rat colonic epithelium. *Journal of Endocrinology*, **62**, 489–496.

86   Turnberg, L. A. (1971) Potassium transport in the human small bowel. *Gut*, **12**, 811–818.

87   Turnberg, L. A., Bieberdorf, F. A., Morawski, S. G. & Fordtran, J. S. (1970) Inter-relationships of chloride, bicarbonate, sodium and hydrogen transport in the human ileum. *Journal of Clinical Investigation*, **49**, 557–567.

88   Turnberg, L. A., Fordtran, J. S., Carter, N. W. & Rector, F. C. (1970) Mechanism of bicarbonate absorption and its relationship to sodium transport in the human jejunum. *Journal of Clinical Investigation*, **49**, 548–556.

89   Winne, D. (1980) Influence of blood flow on intestinal absorption of xenobiotics. *Pharmacology*, **21**, 1–15.

90   Wright, R. D., Jennings, M. A., Florey, H. W. & Lium, R. (1940) The influence of nerves and drugs on secretion by the small intestine and an investigation of the enzymes in intestinal juice. *Quarterly Journal of Experimental Physiology*, **30**, 73–120.

91   Yablonski, M. E. & Lifson, N. (1976) Mechanism of production of intestinal secretion by elevated venous pressure. *Journal of Clinical Investigation*, **57**, 904–915.

MECHANISMS OF MALABSORPTION AND DIARRHOEA

Definitions

The term *malabsorption* is usually used to denote a failure to absorb exogenous nutrients or substances such as drugs, or to re-absorb endogenous substances such as bile acids. *Diarrhoea* may be defined as an increased frequency, fluidity or volume of bowel movements. In many instances, but not all, there is an increase in faecal water and electrolyte excretion with consequent increase in faecal weight. In other instances there is frequent passage of stools of normal consistency and weight, or of blood and pus (exudative diarrhoea). Malabsorption frequently results in diarrhoea but not necessarily so, but where absorption of nutrients is affected characteristic nutritional deficiencies usually develop eventually.

Physiological considerations

The normal handling of individual nutrients, fluid and electrolytes, and drugs by the intestinal tract is dealt with elsewhere in this chapter. The gut as a whole exhibits a homeostatic response to fluid and electrolyte depletion mediated by hormonal influences on the ileum and colon[8] and may be involved in the regulation of appetite and satiety. In contrast there is little or no evidence that absorption of nutrients from the lumen is regulated homeostatically, as is evident from the prevalence of obesity. Furthermore, the intestine plays little or no part in acid–base homeostasis, which is regulated by systemic buffering systems and the kidneys. While the part played by the gut in homeostasis is limited, it has a great capacity to absorb exogenous minerals and nutrients and to retrieve endogenously secreted hydrochloric acid, bicarbonate, bile salts, sodium chloride and water. For reabsorption of fluid, electrolytes, fat, protein, carbohydrate and bile salts, the gut operates with about 90–95% efficiency. A fall in the efficiency of absorption for one of these substances may or may not have immediate clinical consequences in the form of diarrhoea or longer-term consequences in the form of a nutritional deficiency. Under certain circumstances the gastrointestinal tract is stimulated to secrete greater than normal volumes of digestive secretions or fluids and electrolytes, and when inflamed secretes a protein rich exudate.

Thus, in simple terms, malabsorption results from a failure to absorb intestinal luminal solute, whereas diarrhoea may result either from failure to absorb solute, from increased secretion of fluids and electrolytes, or from production of an inflammatory exudate.

MECHANISMS OF MALABSORPTION

Malabsorption may occur as a result of excess ingestion of poorly absorbed solute, or when there is a defect of an essential step in digestion, mucosal uptake, processing or export from enterocyte to blood or lymph of a substance normally well absorbed. In addition, malabsorption may occur in the absence of a specific defect when the exposure time to such mechanisms is markedly reduced by rapid transit (e.g. post-vagotomy, diabetic autonomic neuropathy), inadequate mixing (e.g. gastroenterostomy), loss of functional gut (e.g. gut resection), or as a consequence of the metabolic activity of bacteria when bacterial overgrowth occurs in the small bowel lumen. In any clinical malabsorptive state, a disorder at one or more of these stages can be defined.

Ingestion of poorly-absorbable solute

Polyvalent ions such as magnesium, phosphate and sulphate are only slowly absorbed from normal intestine, as are certain disaccharides such as lactulose or sugar-alcohols such as mannitol. Ingestion of substantial amounts of these results in osmotic retention of fluid within the gut lumen, manifest as increased faecal fluid output. Unlike the inorganic ions, poorly absorbed carbohydrates may be susceptible to bacterial degradation with generation of osmotically active small molecular weight fatty acids such as acetate, butyrate, propionate and lactate. Colonic mechanisms for reabsorption of small fatty acids exist[41] so that diarrhoea will occur only if these mechanisms are stressed. The metabolic activity of gut bacteria may adapt to constant ingestion of organic anions such as tartrate (metabolized to bicarbonate)[7] so that initial purgation following ingestion may be replaced by entirely normal stool outputs. Similar mechanisms operate when defects in digestion and absorption of 'absorbable' carbohydrates such as lactose and sucrose occur (see later).

Failure of digestion

Fat

Conditions associated with defective lipolysis are shown in Table 8.13. Pancreatic lipase outputs must be below 10% of normal before steatorrhoea results[12] and complete failure of pancreatic secretion results in massive fat malabsorption, with faecal fat levels of 50–100 g/day. This is only seen with end-stage chronic pancreatitis, pancreatic atrophy, fibrocystic disease, complete duct obstruction by carcinoma, or after total pancreatectomy.

Table 8.13 Conditions causing defective lipolysis.

Failure of emulsification and mixing problems
  Gastric surgery
  Duodenal bypass

Reduced duodenal pH
  Gastrinoma

Impaired CCK response
  Coeliac disease

Pancreatic lipase deficiency
  Chronic pancreatitis
  Pancreatic cancer
  Congenital lipase deficiency

Luminal bile salt deficiency
  Cholestasis
  Acid hypersecretion
  Drugs (neomycin and cholestyramine)
  Ileal resection and disease

Functional pancreatic exocrine deficiency due to failure of cholecystokinin (CCK) release (e.g. in coeliac disease) is probably not clinically significant since cephalic stimulation via vagal efferents may produce up to 50% of maximal pancreatic secretory responses. After vagotomy, CCK-mediated pancreatic secretion may be more important and this may account for the frequent prevention of coeliac disease following vagotomy, when the failure of CCK secretion would result in functional pancreatic insufficiency and fat malabsorption.

Steatorrhoea in bile acid deficiency (e.g. total obstructive jaundice) is modest (10–15 g/day) although there is no micellar phase, suggesting that non-micellar lipid is reasonably well absorbed when the small intestine is healthy and complete. After substantial ileal resection (more than 100 cm) the combination of intraluminal bile salt deficiency and loss of intestinal surface area results in steatorrhoea which increases with the length of resected gut.[24] Loss of gut surface area alone (e.g. after jejunal resection) does not result in steatorrhoea, so that although pancreatic lipase, bile salts and healthy gut mucosa are all requirements for efficient fat absorption, substantial reserve capacity exists for partial failure of any of these components. Failure of two of these components, such as in severe coeliac disease where there is an extensive mucosal abnormality and a failure of gallbladder contraction after meals with poor bile salt delivery to the duodenum, frequently results in fat malabsorption. Luminal precipitation or destruction of bile acids by acid hypersecretion in the Zollinger–Ellison syndrome[22] or by bacterial deconjugation in bacterial overgrowth syndrome[26] is usually accompanied by deleterious effects of acid and bacterial toxins on gut mucosal function, again explaining the frequency and severity of steatorrhoea in these conditions. The absorption of fat soluble vitamins may be more critically dependent on micellar solubilization than is absorption of triglyceride itself, which may explain the frequency of vitamin D deficiency after gastric surgery and in cholestatic liver disease.

Protein and carbohydrate
Large polypeptides and polysaccharides are not absorbed well when pancreatic exocrine outputs are below 10% of normal. However, in contrast to fat, their independence from other intraluminal phases of digestion means that in many conditions malabsorption is less evident than for fat. However, the final stage of peptide and disaccharide digestion is at the mucosal brush border so that either congenital or acquired deficiencies of the brush border enzymes may result in malabsorption. In practice, peptidase deficiency is never clinically important, though disaccharidase deficiency may result in malabsorption and osmotic diarrhoea.

Failure of mucosal uptake and intracellular processing

Enterocyte damage
Prior to uptake across the microvillous membrane of the enterocyte, hydrophobic lipid molecules must cross the unstirred water layer. This process is greatly facilitated by incorporation of the lipid products of digestion in the micellar complex.[46] Thereafter, uptake of lipid is passive and depends on its solubility in the lipid components of the cell membrane. A sequence of intracellular events occurs, involving binding to a fatty acid binding protein, resynthesis to triglyceride on the smooth endoplasmic reticulum, and the addition of apoproteins to form chylo-

microns on the rough endoplasmic reticulum; these processes require normal structure and function of the enterocytes.[40] In coeliac disease and tropical sprue, enterocytes are obviously abnormal but their capacity for triglyceride resynthesis and apoprotein synthesis has not been evaluated. In these conditions and others (e.g. viral enteritis), there is an increased crypt cell production rate in response to increased villous cell loss or damage, and the enterocytes populating the villus are relatively immature. It seems likely, as has been demonstrated for salt and water transport (see later), that these cells will not have acquired the full biochemical apparatus for processing lipid. In abetalipoproteinaemia, defective apoprotein B synthesis results in accumulation of lipid within the enterocytes.[29] In coeliac disease this is not seen; it may be that mucosal uptake is more defective than intracellular processing in this and similar conditions. In contrast, where enterocyte morphology is well preserved as in bacterial overgrowth syndromes, a specific defect of triglyceride resynthesis in enterocytes has been postulated.

Enterocyte damage may have marked effects on the uptake and processing of minerals and vitamins, some of which in turn may further reduce enterocyte function. For example, folic acid absorption is diminished by alkalinization of the gut lumen, and it is believed that loss of the acid microclimate adjacent to the brush border reported in coeliac disease and Crohn's disease may have marked effects on folate uptake by the enterocytes.[31] Folate deficiency itself may secondarily impair mucosal structure and function, and many patients with tropical sprue show improvement in jejunal morphology and function following folate administration.[28]

Enterocyte deficit
Congenital absence of specific transport mechanisms for glucose–galactose, various amino acids, folate, and B_{12} have been reported.

Failure of exportation to lymph or portal blood

Lymphatic abnormalities
The major effects of congenital or acquired abnormalities of lymphatic drainage from the intestine is in impairing absorption of long chain fats. In these conditions[13] (primary and secondary lymphangiectasia), chylomicrons accumulate in dilated lymph channels clearly visible in the villous core. Rupture of dilated lymphatics into the bowel lumen results in loss of absorbed

lipid and apoproteins, and the other constituents of intestinal lymph (i.e. plasma proteins, immunoglobulins and lymphocytes). The magnitude of fat malabsorption and secondary protein and cell loss is dependent on the amount of ingested long chain triglyceride and the extent of the lymphatic abnormality.

Infiltrations in the lamina propria
Dense cellular infiltration in the lamina propria occurs in α-chain disease,[3] other types of intestinal lymphoma, and Whipple's disease.[27] In each case the villi may be effaced or grossly distended and misshapen by the accumulation of plasma cells, lymphocytes or PAS-positive macrophages. While the enterocytes are often morphologically normal, gross fat malabsorption is often seen in these conditions. Secondary lymphatic blockage is likely since gut losses of protein are also great in these conditions.

Composite mechanisms:
Small bowel bacterial overgrowth

The presence of bacterial overgrowth in the small intestine is usually suspected on the basis of a defined anatomical abnormality such as stricture, fistula, diverticulosis or a blind loop. Malabsorption of fat, protein, carbohydrate and vitamins may be profound, and yet the mucosal architecture of the small intestine shows little abnormality, with nearly normal brush borders and enterocytes and minimal cellular infiltration of the lamina propria.[2] However, the enterocytes may be functionally abnormal with swollen mitochondria and lipid accumulation suggesting defective intracellular processing.[14] Deconjugation of luminal bile salts reduces micellar solubilization of lipid, and 'free' bile salts may damage the enterocytes or reduce the function of the brush border disaccharidases and peptidases.

Luminal metabolism of proteins and carbohydrates by bacteria reduces the availability of these substrates. Bacterial generation of low molecular weight fatty acids, hydroxylated long chain fatty acids and deconjugated bile acids are thought to account for defective salt and water absorption in the small intestine and secretion of fluid and electrolytes into the colon; these effects probably account for the diarrhoea seen in this condition.

Thus the malabsorption and diarrhoea seen in small bowel bacterial overgrowth is due to a complex combination of enterocyte abnormality and the presence of osmotically active solutes and secretogogues in the lumen.

MECHANISMS OF DIARRHOEA

Approximately 7–8 l of fluid enter the upper small intestine daily as a result of ingestion of liquid and the digestive secretory response to nutrients. The small intestine itself secretes a substantial, but unknown, volume of fluid, but at the same time re-absorbs fluids, electrolytes and nutrients from the lumen, so that the volume of fluid passing the ileocaecal valve is only 1–2 l/day in healthy individuals.[36] An increased delivery of fluid and electrolytes to the colon can occur in a wide variety of conditions which compromise the re-absorptive capacity of the small intestine. Whether diarrhoea will result from an increased ileocaecal flow depends on the re-absorptive capacity of the colon. For simple isotonic saline solutions, flow rates above 6–8 ml/min exceed the reserves of the healthy colon,[35] whereas in many clinical disorders associated with increased ileocaecal flow, the presence of unabsorbed osmotically active food residues, or of fatty acids and bile acids which impair colonic absorptive function, will result in diarrhoea at lower fluid flow rates.[11] The diseased colon may secrete rather than absorb fluid and electrolytes or, if inflamed, secrete an exudate; this results in watery or exudative diarrhoea, respectively.

Thus, diarrhoea may be due to a failure to cope with normal volumes of fluid, the secretion of abnormally large volumes of fluid which exceed normal re-absorptive mechanisms, or to the production of an exudate in the distal colon (Table 8.14).

Reduced fluid re-absorption

Osmotic effects
Water absorption from the gut is passive and occurs in response to osmotic gradients generated by the active absorption of nutrients and electrolytes. An increase in the luminal osmolality will therefore result in net fluid accumulation in the lumen and may cause diarrhoea. The ingestion of inorganic salt laxatives (e.g. magnesium, sulphate, phosphate) or of poorly absorbed organic molecules (e.g. the disaccharide lactulose) are examples of how luminal osmolality may be increased.

Monosaccharide or disaccharide malabsorption due to transport or digestive defects are usually associated with diarrhoea. Fifty grams of unabsorbed disaccharide results in osmotic retention of some 500 ml of water in the small intestine in order to preserve isotonicity, and

Table 8.14 Mechanisms of diarrhoea in gastrointestinal disorders.

Reduced fluid absorption
 Osmotic effects
  Laxative ingestion
  Monosaccharide or disaccharide intolerance
  Congenital choloridorrhoea
 Mucosal defects
  Intestinal resections and bypass
  Intestinal mucosal diseases
 Motility effects
  Irritable bowel syndrome
  Vagotomy and gastrectomy
  Autonomic neuropathy
  Drugs and hormones

Increased fluid secretion
 Bacterial toxins
 Hormones
 Prostaglandins
 Neurotransmitters
 Bile acids and fatty acids in the colon
 Laxatives
 Viral enteritis
 Coeliac disease
 Intestinal obstruction

Exudative diarrhoea
 Rectal carcinoma
 Villous adenoma
 Colitis

osmotic activity is further increased by the bacterial metabolism of the malabsorbed carbohydrate to short chain fatty acids, with production of gas (CO_2 and H_2) in the colon.

Since the normal intestine has a finite capacity to digest and absorb carbohydrate, large loads of hypertonic sugars in the form of proprietary mixtures or elemental diets may provoke nausea, due to fluid distension of the small bowel, and osmotic diarrhoea. Any condition which speeds up gastric emptying, shortens gut transit time, or reduces functional surface area of intestine will impair tolerance to such mixtures.

Primary defects of electrolyte transport are rare; in congenital chloridorrhoea[45] the ileal and colonic chloride/bicarbonate exchange process is absent and the failure of chloride reabsorption results in osmotic diarrhoea and hypochloraemic alkalosis.

Mucosal defects

The most obvious example of this is bowel resection, the effects of which depend on the extent and region of resection, the state of the residual gut, the presence of adaptive changes in the residual gut and the diet presented to the intestine.[16] Jejunal resection does not result in diarrhoea because the ileum shows marked adaptive hyperplasia and the preservation of the ileal bile salt reabsorptive site maintains the enterohepatic circulation of bile salts. The ability to cope with normal intakes of fat, protein and carbohydrate is preserved. In contrast, ileal resection is frequently complicated by diarrhoea as a result of bile salt malabsorption (see later) and, when more than 100 cm has been removed, by fat malabsorption (see earlier). After total colonic resection, ileostomy outputs reach 800–1000 ml but malabsorption of nutrients is not evident. Smaller colonic resections lead to diarrhoea which is related to the extent of resection and usually diminishes with time due to adaptive mechanisms. In the so-called 'short bowel syndrome' diarrhoea is multifactorial in causation, but the main factors are a reduced capacity to digest and absorb dietary nutrients and a marked sensitivity to luminal osmotic loads.[23]

Extensive small gut mucosal abnormalities leading to malabsorption of nutrients are a major factor in the diarrhoea associated with coeliac disease, Crohn's disease, radiation enteritis, Whipple's disease and lymphoma. However, other mechanisms including increased fluid and electrolyte secretion from the diseased gut and colonic secretion in response to malabsorbed bile and fatty acids are also important in some of these conditions.

Motility defects

For intestinal absorption to occur with the maximal possible efficiency, the intestinal contents must be exposed to the absorptive surface area for a critical time period; exposure time is obviously dependent on the small gut transit time.[39] Furthermore, the contents must be adequately mixed with the digestive secretions. Transit time and mixing are dependent on coordinated small gut motility, an area of intestinal physiology which is still in its infancy. Various causes of disordered small bowel motility and transit time have been described and include thyrotoxicosis, medullary carcinoma of the thyroid, carcinoid syndrome, autonomic neuropathy (e.g. diabetic), post-vagotomy diarrhoea, and systemic sclerosis. Malabsorption of nutrients, such as fat and carbohydrate, and of bile salts has been described in these disorders but other diarrhoeagenic factors such as bacterial overgrowth (in diabetes and systemic sclerosis) and intestinal fluid and electrolyte secretion (in medullary carcinoma of the thyroid and carcinoid syndrome) may be as important as the altered exposure time for digestion and absorption.

In the colon the role of altered motility is also not well defined. The irritable bowel syndrome is associated with abnormal motility patterns which appear to be especially sensitive to luminal deoxycholate (a secondary bile acid).[19] Other factors such as ileal secretion in response to bile acids,[34] prostaglandin generation, and food intolerance[1] have also been implicated in the genesis of diarrhoea in this heterogeneous condition. Laxative drugs such as bisacodyl and ricinoleic acid produce marked changes in colonic motility,[44] but are also secretogogues.[20] Evidence is emerging that motility and secretion are to some extent coupled processes in the normal intestine and defining the primary mechanisms for diarrhoea in pathological states may be difficult.

Increased fluid secretion

Intracellular mediators of intestinal secretion
The concept that there might by a single final common pathway for intestinal secretion is an attractive one, but on current evidence there appear to be at least three agents: cyclic AMP, cyclic GMP, and calcium. Cyclic AMP inhibits sodium and chloride influx and activates chloride secretion.[17] Cyclic GMP has similar effects but its role is less certain, since some agents which stimulate cyclic GMP production do not cause secretion. Agents which increase intracellular calcium concentration such as calcium ionophores, cholinergic agonists, and serotonin, stimulate active chloride secretion by enterocytes. Calmodulin, a calcium-dependent regulatory protein, may be the mediator between calcium ions and the secretory process.[33] Postulated interactions between the cyclic AMP and calcium–calmodulin pathways have renewed interest in the possibility that the latter mediator could be the final common secretory pathway, since both cyclic AMP mediated and non cyclic AMP mediated secretion are inhibited by trifluoperazine (Stelazine),[25] which binds to the calcium–calmodulin complex.

Bacterial toxins
A variety of bacterial enterotoxins have been described which act as powerful stimuli for intestinal secretion (Table 8.15). The prototypic example is that of cholera toxin. A latent period of over 30 minutes occurs after exposure of the gut mucosa to the toxin before the onset of secretion, which is explained by the complex series of cellular reactions which mediate the secretory signal. These include binding of the toxin to the luminal brush border receptor,

Table 8.15 Enterotoxin-producing bacteria which lead to intestinal secretion.

Vibrio cholerae
Escherichia coli
Shigella dysenteriae, flexneri
Staphylococcus aureus
Clostridium perfringens (welchii)
Clostridium difficile
Pseudomonas aeruginosa
Yersinia enterocolitica
Bacillus cereus
Klebsiella pneumoniae
Aeromonas hydrophila

translation steps involving protein synthesis, and activation of the enzyme adenyl cyclase with generation of cyclic AMP within the cell. The secretory phase involves changes in mucosal permeability, and interactions with prostaglandins, calcium ions and neural pathways. *Escherichia coli* heat labile enterotoxin activates similar pathways, but the heat stable toxin of this organism acts in a different way, initially activating guanylate cyclase rather than adenylate cyclase. Secretory mechanisms for other enterotoxins are not defined. The multiple steps in cholera and *E. coli* enterotoxin secretory pathways have prompted attempts at pharmacological blockade of the secretory response. Thus chlorpromazine, nicotinic acid, colchicine, indomethacin and loperamide may all inhibit cholera toxin induced secretion to a greater or lesser extent.

Hormones and neurotransmitters
A variety of hormones and neurotransmitters stimulate intestinal secretion and the ones associated with clinical diarrhoeal disorders are listed in Table 8.16 together with their postulated cellular mechanisms.

Vasoactive intestinal peptide (VIP) is a powerful secretogogue in animal and human small intestine. Pancreatic apudomas or ganglioneuromas which secrete VIP cause severe watery diarrhoea and hypokalaemia. The secretory effect is predominantly on the small intestine, and fasting ileal flow rates exceeding the

Table 8.16 Agents producing intestinal secretion in clinical diarrhoeal disorders.

Agent	Cellular mechanism
Vasoactive intestinal peptide	Cyclic AMP
Calcitonin	?
5-Hydroxytryptamine	Calcium ions
Prostaglandin E	Cyclic AMP
Histamine	?

colonic reabsorptive capacity have been recorded.[32] *Calcitonin* is secreted by medullary thyroid carcinomas and promotes small intestinal secretion and decreases intestinal transit time.[10, 37] Diarrhoea evident during fasting is markedly increased during feeding, possibly due to fat, carbohydrate and bile acid malabsorption. A similar pattern of secretory and motor responses is seen in the carcinoid syndrome where *5-hydroxytryptamine (serotonin)* is the most important secretogogue.

Prostaglandins
Prostaglandins are a family of fatty acids which are generated by the cyclo-oxygenase pathway from arachidonic acid, a constituent of mucosal phospholipids. Some of them (E_2, $F_2\alpha$) are potent activators of adenylate cyclase in the gut, leading to cyclic AMP production. These prostaglandins are powerful secretogogues at all levels in the gut. Based on findings of elevated prostaglandins in gut luminal fluid in a variety of conditions[38] such as inflammatory bowel disease, small bowel obstruction, coeliac disease, carcinoid syndrome, and irritable bowel syndrome,[1] and reports of the beneficial effects of prostaglandin synthesis inhibitors in some of these conditions, a central role for prostaglandins in these diarrhoeal disorders has been proposed.

Bile salts and fatty acids
Dihydroxy bile acids and hydroxylated fatty acids[20] are potent stimuli for fluid and electrolyte secretion in the colon. Both these agents cause mucosal damage and stimulate mucus secretion at concentrations or exposure times less than those required to stimulate fluid secretion.[5] Since the detergent damage has marked effects in increasing mucosal permeability to ions,[6] it has been suggested that secretion occurs as a consequence of this altered permeability under the driving force of capillary hydrostatic pressure. Others have demonstrated increased mucosal cyclic AMP levels.[9] The relative importance of these proposed mechanisms is controversial.

Detergent laxatives
Ricinoleic acid (castor oil), a hydroxy fatty acid, and dioctyl sodium sulphosuccinate, a non-ionic detergent, have similar effects to bile acids and fatty acids on colonic morphology and function, and are believed to stimulate secretion by similar pathways.[4]

Immature enterocytes and secretion
A substantial amount of evidence suggests that immature crypt cells differ functionally from mature villous cells, particularly in relation to sodium transport.[21] These observations suggest that intestinal fluid and electrolyte secretion predominates in crypt cells and absorption in villous cells. In conditions such as coeliac disease, tropical sprue, viral enteritis and a variety of other disorders, villous cells are lost or damaged and the crypts show hyperplasia. The mucosa is thus populated by relatively immature cells with a propensity to secrete fluid and electrolytes. Perfusion studies in conditions associated with villous damage and crypt hyperplasia have shown a net secretion and an absence of glucose stimulation of sodium and water absorption, which is consistent with this hypothesis.

Exudative diarrhoea

Exudation of protein, mucus or pus from inflammatory sites, ulcers or villous tumours may cause diarrhoea. Prostaglandins have been implicated in the diarrhoea associated with ulcerative colitis[42] and villous adenomas.[43]

CONCLUSIONS

Mechanisms of malabsorption and diarrhoea are very diverse. In recent years the major advances have been in our understanding of the intracellular mediators and pathways involved in intestinal secretion. It seems likely that specific pharmacological blockade of these processes will soon be possible.

REFERENCES

1 Alun Jones, V., Shorthouse, M., McLaughlan, P. *et al.* (1982) Food intolerance: a major factor in the pathogenesis of irritable bowel syndrome. *Lancet,* **ii,** 1115–1117.
2 Ament, M. F., Shimoda, S. S. & Sanders, D. P. (1972) Pathogenesis of steatorrhoea in three cases of small intestinal stasis syndrome. *Gastroenterology,* **63,** 728–747.
3 Asselah, C. H. & Asselah, F. (1982) Alpha chain disease and intestinal lymphoma. In *Gastroenterology 2: Small Intestine* (Ed.) Chadwick, V. S. & Phillips, S. pp. 174–202. London-Butterworth.
4 Binder, H. J. (1977) Pharmacology of laxatives. *Annual Review of Pharmacology and Toxicology,* **17,** 355–367.
5 Camilleri, M., Murphy, R. & Chadwick, V. S. (1981) Dose-related effects of chenodeoxycholic acid in the rabbit colon. *Digestive Diseases and Science,* **25,** 433–438.
6 Chadwick, V. S., Phillips, S. F. & Hofmann, A. F. (1977) Measurement of intestinal permeability using low

molecular weight polyethylene glycols (PEG 400). II. Application to normal and abnormal permeability states in man and animals. *Gastroenterology*, **73**, 247–251.

7 Chadwick, V. S., Vince, A., Killingley, M. & Wrong, O. M. (1978) The metabolism of tartrate in man and the rat. *Clinical Science and Molecular Medicine*, **54**, 273–281.

8 Charney, A. N., Kinsey, M. D., Myers, L. *et al.* (1975) Na^+/K^+ activated adenosine triphosphatase and intestinal electrolyte transport. Effect of adrenal steroids. *Journal of Clinical Investigation*, **56**, 653–660.

9 Conley, D. R., Coyne, M. J. & Bonorris, G. G. (1976) Bile acid stimulation of colonic adenylate cyclase and secretion in the rabbit. *American Journal of Digestive Diseases*, **21**, 453–458.

10 Cox, T. M., Fagan, E. A., Hillyard, C. J. *et al.* (1979) Role of calcitonin in diarrhoea associated with medullary carcinoma of the thyroid. *Gut*, **20**, 629–633.

11 Debongnie, J. C. & Phillips, S. F. (1978) Capacity of the human colon to absorb fluid. *Gastroenterology*, **74**, 698–703.

12 DiMagno, E. P., Go, V. L. W. & Summerskill, W. H. J. (1973) Relations between pancreatic enzyme outputs and malabsorption in severe pancreatic insufficiency. *New England Journal of Medicine*, **228**, 813–815.

13 Dobbins, W. O. (1976) Electron microscopic study of the intestinal mucosa in intestinal lymphangiectasia. *Gastroenterology*, **51**, 1004–1017.

14 Donaldson, R. M. (1965) Studies on the pathogenesis of steatorrhoea in the blind loop syndrome. *Journal of Clinical Investigation*, **44**, 1815–1825.

15 Donowitz, M. & Binder, H. J. (1975) Jejunal fluid and electrolyte secretion in carcinoid syndrome. *American Journal of Digestive Diseases*, **20**, 1115–1122.

16 Dowling, R. H. (1982) Intestinal adaptation and its mechanisms. In *Topics in Gastroenterology*, vol. 10 (Ed.) Jewell, D. P. & Selby, W. S. pp. 135–156. Oxford: Blackwell Scientific.

17 Field, M. (1971) Ion transport in rabbit ileal mucosa. II. Effects of cyclic 3′,5′-AMP. *American Journal of Physiology*, **221**, 992–997.

18 Field, M., Graf, L. H., Laird, W. J. & Smith, P. L. (1978) Heat stable enterotoxin of *Escherichia coli*: In vitro effect on guanylate cyclase activity, cyclic GMP concentration, and ion transport in small intestine. *Proceedings of the National Academy of Sciences (USA)*, **75**, 2800–2804.

19 Flynn, M., Hammond, P., Darby, C. *et al.* (1979) Faecal bile acids and the irritable colon syndrome, *Gut*, **20**, A946.

20 Gaginella, T. S., Chadwick, V. S., Debongnie, J. C. *et al.* (1977) Perfusion of rabbit colon with ricinoleic acid: dose-related mucosal injury, fluid secretion, and increased permeability. *Gastroenterology*, **73**, 95–101.

21 Gall, G. D., Chapman, D., Kelly, M. & Hamilton, J. R. (1977) Na^+ transport in jejunal crypt cells. *Gastroenterology*, **72**, 452–456.

22 Go, V. L. W., Poley, J. R., Hoffmann, A. F. & Summerskill, W. H. J. (1970) Disturbance in fat digestion induced by acidic jejunal pH due to gastric hypersecretion in man. *Gastroenterology*, **58**, 638–646.

23 Griffin, G. E., Fagan, E. A., Hodgson, H. J. F. & Chadwick, V. S. (1982) Enternal therapy in the management of massive gut resection complicated by chronic fluid and electrolyte depletion. *Digestive Diseases and Sciences*, **27**, 202–208.

24 Hofmann, A. F. & Poley, J. R. (1972) Role of bile acid malabsorption in pathogenesis of diarrhoea and steatorrhoea in patients with ileal resection. *Gastroenter-

ology*, **62**, 918–934.

25 Ilundian, A. & Naftalin, R. J. (1979) Role of Ca^+ dependent regulator protein in intestinal secretion. *Nature*, **279**, 446–448.

26 Kim, Y. S., Spritz, N. & Blum, M. (1966) The role of altered bile acid metabolism in the steatorrhoea of experimental blind loop syndrome. *Journal of Clinical Investigation*, **45**, 956–962.

27 Kirkpatrick, P. M. Jr, Kent, S. P., Mihas, A. & Pritchett, P. (1978) Whipple's disease: a case report with immunological studies. *Gastroenterology*, **75**, 297–301.

28 Klipstein, F. A. & Falaiye, J. M. (1969) Tropical sprue in expatriates from the tropics living in the continental United States. *Medicine*, **48**, 475–491.

29 Levy, R. I., Fredrickson, D. S. & Laster, L. (1966) The lipoproteins and lipid transport in abetalipoproteinaemia. *Journal of Clinical Investigation*, **45**, 531–541.

30 Lindenbaum, J., Pezzimenti, J. F. & Shea, N. (1974) Small intestinal function in vitamin B_{12} deficiency. *Annals of Internal Medicine*, **80**, 326–331.

31 Lucas, M. L., Cooper, B. T. & Lei, F. H. (1978) Acid microclimate in coeliac and Crohn's disease: a model for folate malabsorption. *Gut*, **19**, 735–742.

32 Modigliani, R., Rambaud, J. C., Matuchanksy, C. & Bernier, J. J. (1979) Hormones, intestinal secretion and diarrhoea: human studies. In *Frontiers of Knowledge in the Diarrhoeal Diseases* (Ed.) Janowitz H. J. & Sachar, D. B. pp. 289–302. Raritan: Ortho Pharmaceutical Corporation.

33 Naftalin, R. J. (1981) The role of intracellular calcium in the induction of intestinal secretion. *Clinical Research Reviews*, **1** (Supplement 1), 63–71.

34 Oddson, E., Rask-Madsen, J. & Rask-Madsen, J. (1978) A secretory epithelium of the small intestine with increased sensitivity to bile acids in irritable bowel syndrome associated with diarrhoea. *Scandinavian Journal of Gastroenterology*, **13**, 408–416.

35 Palma, R., Vidon, N. & Bernier, J. J. (1981) Maximal capacity for fluid absorption in human bowel. *Digestive Diseases and Sciences*, **26** (10), 929–934.

36 Phillips, S. F. & Giller, J. (1973) The contribution of the colon to the electrolyte and water conservation in man. *Journal of Laboratory and Clinical Medicine*, **81**, 733–746.

37 Rambaud, J. C., Modigliani, R. & Matuchansky, C. (1981) Hormones and diarrhoea. *Clinical Research Reviews*, **1** (Supplement 1), 23–32.

38 Rask-Madsen, J. & Bukhave, K. (1981) The role of prostaglandins in diarrhoea. *Clinical Research Reviews*, **1** (Supplement 1), 33–48.

39 Read, N. W. (1981) The relationship between intestinal motility and intestinal transport. *Clinical Research Reviews*, **1** (Supplement 1), 73–81.

40 Riley, J. W. & Glickman, R. M. (1979) Fat malabsorption: advances in our understanding. *American Journal of Medicine*, **67**, 980–987.

41 Ruppin, H., Bar-Meir, S., Soergel, K. H. *et al.* (1980) Absorption of short-chain fatty acids by the colon. *Gastroenterology*, **78**, 1500–1507.

42 Sharon, P., Ligumsky, M., Rachmilewitz, D. & Zor, U. (1978) Role of prostaglandins in ulcerative colitis: enhanced production during active disease and inhibition by sulfasalazine. *Gastroenterology*, **75**, 638–640.

43 Steven, K., Lange, P., Bukhave, K. & Rask-Madsen, J. (1981) Diarrhoea in villous adenoma of rectum: effect of treatment with indomethacin. *Gastroenterology*, **80**, 1562–1566.

44 Stewart, J. J., Gaginella, T. S. & Bass, P. (1975) Actions of ricinoleic acid and structurally related fatty acids on the gastrointestinal tract. I. Effects on smooth muscle

contractility in vitro. *Journal of Pharmacology and Experimental Therapeutics*, **195**, 347–354.

45   Turnberg, L. A. (1978) Intestinal transport of salt and water. *Clinical Science and Molecular Medicine*, **54**, 337–348.

46   Wilson, F. A., Sallee, V. L. & Dietschy, J. M. (1971) Unstirred water layers in the intestine: rate determinant of fatty acid absorption from micellar solutions. *Science*, **174**, 1031–1033.

CLINICAL INVESTIGATION OF PATIENTS WITH MALABSORPTION AND DIARRHOEA

There are many different causes of diarrhoea and malabsorption (Table 8.17) and an even larger number of diagnostic tests and procedures available to the clinician. If the full spectrum of investigations were applied to every patient the cost would be enormous. Several investigators have attempted to devise algorithms based on a logical sequence of investigations with appropriate branch points so that, by following the diagnostic route map, successful diagnosis is assured. I have little faith in such systems and prefer a much more selective approach in which the primary aim is to define the anatomical location of the disease, its histological features and the agent or process responsible for the lesion.

A number of disorders producing diarrhoea are associated with normal intestinal anatomy, and a variety of tests are available to sort these problems out. The selection of appropriate radiological, endoscopic and biopsy procedures is based on the results of clinical history, physical examination, and stool, urine and blood tests. There is much debate about the role of intestinal function tests. They are rarely of diagnostic help and are never first line investigations in patients with diarrhoea, although tests for vitamin B_{12} malabsorption, lactose intolerance and pancreatic insufficiency are helpful in certain circumstances. A wider spectrum of function tests may be useful in the assessment of patients with gut resections and in monitoring the effects of therapeutic manoeuvres in more complicated cases.

Table 8.17   Causes of diarrhoea and malabsorption.

Gastric causes
  Resection
  Gastroenterostomy
  Vagotomy
  Gastrinoma

Pancreatic causes
  Resection
  Chronic pancreatitis
  Carcinoma
  Fibrocystic disease
  Hypoplasia (Schwachman's syndrome)
  Congenital enzyme defects

Hepatic causes
  Cholestatic liver disease

Small intestinal causes
  Resection or bypass
  Infections and infestations
  Bacterial overgrowth
  Tropical sprue
  Coeliac disease
  Crohn's disease
  Eosinophilic enteritis
  Radiation enteritis
  Whipple's disease
  Vasculitis
  Vascular insufficiency
  Lymphoma
  Lymphangiectasia
  Abetalipoproteinaemia
  Drugs, alcohol
  Systemic sclerosis
  Visceral myopathy
  Autonomic neuropathy
  Ulcerative ileojejunitis
  Immunodeficiency
  Graft versus host disease

Colonic causes
  Resection or bypass
  Infectious agents
  Ulcerative colitis
  Crohn's disease
  Radiation enteritis
  Immunodeficiency
  Purgative ingestion
  Irritable bowel syndrome
  Diverticular disease
  Carcinoma
  Villous adenoma
  Bile acid malabsorption
  Fat malabsorption
  Graft versus host disease

Extra-intestinal causes
  Hormones
  Prostaglandins
  Serotonin
  Histamine

ACUTE DIARRHOEA

The symptom complex of anorexia, nausea, vomiting, abdominal pain, and diarrhoea of sudden onset, often occurring within families or other groups, is loosely termed gastroenteritis. A variety of viruses, bacteria, protozoa or their toxic products may be implicated.[3] These disorders are commonly (though not always) short-lived and self-limiting, and the only problem is guarding against significant dehydration.

A specific diagnosis should be sought when there is a 'point' source for the outbreak, when it occurs in a nursery or geriatric unit, or when there is a marked fever and rectal bleeding. Faecal microscopy and culture, sigmoidoscopy and biopsy, and the taking of blood for serological tests is then advisable. Suspect food, milk or water supplies may need to be investigated. Diarrhoea due to preformed enterotoxins in food (such as those produced by *Staphylococcus aureus*, *Clostridium perfringens* (type A) and *Bacillus cereus*) is usually shortlived (less than 48 hours) while that due to enterotoxins formed in the gut lumen (by *Escherichia coli*, *Vibrio cholerae*, *Enterobacter*, *Citrobacter serratia* and *Pseuodomonas* spp.) are rarely of prolonged duration though may be very severe; none of these types produces inflammatory changes in the gut mucosa or cause significant fever. *Clostridium perfringens* and *Clostridium difficile* produce both enterotoxins causing intestinal secretion and cytotoxins which damage gut mucosa, the former species causing severe, sometimes fatal necrotizing enterocolitis[17] and the latter causing a severe colitis, often pseudomembranous.[2] Fever and a more prolonged course characterize these infections. Invasive organisms include viruses[5] such as rotaviruses, coronaviruses and adenoviruses, which damage small intestinal enterocytes (with sometimes severe fluid losses, but running a short-lived, self-limiting course), and bacteria such as *Salmonella*, *Campylobacter* and *Yersinia enterocolitica* spp.,[18] which predominantly affect the ileum and colon and may cause high fever, severe abdominal pain and diarrhoea with blood and pus. Ideally electron microscopy of jejunal mucosa and immune electron microscopy of stools should be used to detect viruses, but routine identification of viruses is impractical. In all but the most short-lived diarrhoeal illnesses, appropriate in vitro tests to detect faecal cytotoxins and the usual cultures for pathogens should be performed. It is important that the bacteriologist is provided with fresh faecal specimens so that microscopy for inflammatory exudate, protozoa (*Giardia* and amoebae) and parasites is optimal.

CHRONIC DIARRHOEA AND MALABSORPTION

When diarrhoea persists for more than a week or two it should be fully investigated. It is convenient to divide investigation into two stages as illustrated in Table 8.18. Stage one includes the

Table 8.18 Stages in investigation of chronic diarrhoea.

Stage one
History
Physical examination
Stool test
Screening blood tests
Stage two
Anatomical investigations
Gastrointestinal function tests
Special blood and urine tests

history, physical examination, and blood, stool and urine tests, and takes place in the outpatient clinic or consulting room. Stage two procedures are selected on the basis of findings in stage one, and the emphasis is on 'anatomical' studies, supported where necessary by tests of gut or pancreatic function. There should also be access to special blood and urine tests which are necessary in some disorders.

Stage one

HISTORY

Time–frequency relationships
The duration of symptoms of diarrhoea should be determined. Marked physical deterioration with weight loss and a short history of a few weeks or months suggests malignancy, severe inflammatory disease or severe malabsorption, and will rarely be a diagnostic problem. Intermittent symptoms extending over years with periods of normality may occur in organic disorders such as coeliac disease or Crohn's disease, but the irritable bowel syndrome may also present in this way. Diarrhoea occurring in the night almost always indicates organic disease. Normal bowel frequency is variable, but in the irritable bowel syndrome frequency rarely exceeds 3–4/day, commonly occurring in clusters in the early part of the day; a frequency of 5–10/day, especially if spread throughout the day, usually indicates organic disease.

Nature of the stools
The nature of the stools may be diagnostic in that passing oil per rectum indicates pancreatic insufficiency, whereas the very pale voluminous 'floating' stools of steatorrhoea indicate a gross disorder proximal to the ileocaecal valve such as extensive jejunoileal disease (coeliac disease, tropical sprue, diverticulosis, Crohn's disease, lymphoma) or pancreatic insufficiency. It is important to differentiate between bleeding associated with diarrhoea and blood loss accompanying otherwise normal stools. Colitis

and carcinoma may cause the former, whereas bleeding from a polyp, carcinoma, benign vascular malformation or haemorrhoids may give the latter pattern. Watery diarrhoea may occur with a wide variety of conditions affecting all levels of the gut and is the main problem in diagnosis. The presence of undigested food in the stools is a manifestation of rapid transit and is not of diagnostic importance. Sour smelling stools suggest carbohydrate malabsorption.

Abdominal pain
Colicky abdominal pain preceding bowel movements is common in most diarrhoeas. Small bowel colic is peri-umbilical and large bowel colic usually suprapubic in location. Severe colic following meals or associated with vomiting, temporary cessation of diarrhoea and flatus production suggests partial intestinal obstruction. Prolonged episodes of continuous abdominal pain occur in both organic and non-organic disorders. The typical dull continuous upper abdominal pain or back pain of chronic pancreatitis or pancreatic cancer, with frequent superimposed paroxysms of burning or boring discomfort forcing the patient to adopt a characteristic 'leaning forward' or crucifix position, clearly focus attention on the pancreas. Postprandial pain, remorseless in nature, which varies in severity in proportion to meal size, and is accompanied by freedom of pain on starvation (fear of eating) suggests mesenteric ischaemia. In general in organic disease the site and nature of the pain are consistent on repeated history taking, in contrast to the variable location, bizarre radiation and dramatic associations of psychogenic pain. The pain associated with the irritable bowel syndrome most commonly has the features of gut spasm, with an abrupt onset and often lasting several hours with a slow decline but with occasional pronounced exacerbations after bowel movements. Continuous pain in patients with inflammatory bowel disease suggests severe bowel ulceration, or complications such as abscess or perforation with peritonitis; in those with malignancy continuous pain suggests involvement of adjacent structures with neural infiltration or pressure.

Drugs
A wide variety of drugs produce diarrhoea (Table 8.19) and the relationship between starting the drug and onset of diarrhoea is crucial in diagnosis. Stopping the drug for a trial period under these circumstances is wise. Alcohol is a common cause of diarrhoea but usually patients are obviously heavy imbibers with other clinical,

Table 8.19 Drugs causing diarrhoea and proposed mechanisms.

Drug	Proposed mechanism
Laxatives	
Senna	Intestinal secretion
Phenolphthalein	Increased motility
Cascara	
Castor oil	
Magnesium salts	Osmotic
Lactulose	
Antibiotics	
Ampicillin	? altered gut flora occasionally haemorrhagic colitis
Tetracycline	? altered gut flora
Lincomycin ⎫ Clindamycin ⎭	Colitis (*Clostridium difficile* toxin)
Neomycin	Steatorrhoea and mucosal damage
Antimetabolites	
Methotrexate	
6-Mercaptopurine	Mucosal damage
Colchicine	
Sympathetic blockers	
Guanethidine	Increased motility
Ethanol	? mucosal damage

haematological and biochemical features of alcoholism. Occasionally diarrhoeal illnesses are empirically treated with neomycin-containing preparations which can themselves provoke diarrhoea.

Dietary factors
Patients often report that specific foods provoke diarrhoea but an allergic mechanism, though possible, is rarely defined. Initially these patients should be investigated for common organic disorders. Ingestion of milk leading to gaseous distension and diarrhoea suggests lactose intolerance and this is worth checking for in those individuals who might otherwise be classified as having irritable bowel syndrome. In my experience exclusion diets for conditions other than coeliac disease and lactose intolerance often produce temporary benefit but within a few weeks or months the patient returns with a recurrence of symptoms claiming intolerance to more and more dietary factors. The recent reports implicating food allergy in the irritable bowel syndrome[1] are interesting, but require confirmation before these findings are widely applied to clinical problems.

Other important historical facts
The presence of weight loss suggests organic disease. Diarrhoea dating from a surgical operation may be due to resection of bowel (terminal ileum resection leading to bile salt malabsorption, left hemicolon resection leading to loose

stools for a period of time); in the absence of substantial gut resection postoperative diarrhoea points to the possibility of a stricture, fistula or surgically created stagnant loop with bacterial overgrowth. Failure to thrive following weaning suggests coeliac disease; delayed growth and development or a history of unexplained anaemia suggest coeliac disease or inflammatory bowel disease. A history of foreign travel alerts one to the possibility of intestinal parasites or tropical sprue. A number of patients have diarrhoea lasting several months following an acute diarrhoeal illness on holiday (not always abroad). While a few of these will have Crohn's disease or even coeliac disease, many have minor abnormalities of blood tests and jejunal histology, and slowly recover to normality. This condition is conveniently classified as 'temperate sprue' though its pathophysiology is poorly understood. The time course of this condition is the main factor in making the diagnosis and a gradually improving symptomatology is reassuring.

Other points

A history of long-standing confirmed steatorrhoea with no diagnosis after hospital investigation suggests either small intestinal lymphangiectasia[24] or pancreatic hypoplasia (Schwachman's syndrome).[23] A history of severe watery diarrhoea previously investigated with no diagnosis suggests either an endocrine tumour associated diarrhoea (e.g. medullary carcinoma of the thyroid or vipoma),[19] or chronic purgative abuse. A history of 'pernicious anaemia' in a young adult with diarrhoea suggests immunoglobulin deficiency of the common variable type.[11]

PHYSICAL EXAMINATION

Obvious weight loss and anaemia suggest a chronic infective, inflammatory or neoplastic disorder. These symptoms also occur in severe malabsorption syndromes, when they are usually accompanied by abdominal distension and obvious steatorrhoea on rectal examination. Vascular insufficiency[12] or a systemic vasculitis[8] may be suspected if the history is typical and there is a prominent abdominal bruit or a cutaneous vasculitic rash.

Skin lesions are frequently associated with gastrointestinal disorders: dermatitis herpetiformis with coeliac disease, erythema nodosum with inflammatory bowel disease (*Yersinia* enteritis, Crohn's disease, and ulcerative colitis),

flushing and telangiectasia with carcinoid syndrome, pigmentation with chronic malabsorption and Whipple's disease, and pyoderma with colitis. Common disorders like lichen planus and psoriasis appear to be more common in patients with inflammatory bowel disease. Skin features of systemic sclerosis (scleroderma) are sometimes quite subtle, even though gut involvement may be severe.

Lymphadenopathy with splenomegaly suggest lymphoma, while hepatomegaly must raise the suspicion of malignancy. A careful search for abdominal and pelvic masses is mandatory. Peri-anal lesion such as piles or fistulas suggest Crohn's disease, and rectal examination and sigmoidoscopy should enable up to 70% of large bowel cancers to be diagnosed in the clinic or consulting room. The macroscopic appearances of severe inflammation and mucosal friability indicate a colitis, whereas discrete ulcers with patchy inflammation are found in Crohn's disease and amoebiasis. Frank 'pus' in the lumen should alert one to the possibility of venereal proctitis (gonococcal) and appropriate swabs for microscopy and culture should be taken. Very mild reddening of the mucosa without friability should not be labelled colitis in a patient with severe diarrhoea since this is not an uncommon finding in non-inflammatory disorders. Rectal biopsies should be taken routinely and processed for histology. Despite a normal mucosal appearance, pigmented macrophages may be seen in chronic purgative abuse and granulomas in Crohn's disease; amyloid or schistosoma ova may also be seen.

THE STOOL TEST

Visual inspection of the faeces at sigmoidoscopy or of a collected sample is vital. A simple classification into oily, steatorrhoeic, exudative (pus with or without blood), watery, or within normal limits will suffice. The presence of blood should be recorded and an occult blood test performed. A fresh stool sample should be looked at microscopically by a skilled person; the presence of large numbers of neutrophil leucocytes indicates inflammatory disease, eosinophils and Charcot–Leyden crystals suggest eosinophilic gastroenteritis, and a relative absence of cells is good evidence against either pathology. Mobile parasites (amoebae, *Giardia*), cysts (protozoa or nematodes) and ova (nematodes and trematodes) should be carefully searched for and if there is a high suspicion (e.g. a history of foreign travel or blood eosinophilia) several samples should be examined. Culture for specific organisms and, if suspected, assays for cyto-toxins should be performed. Ideally as a routine procedure, but particularly in all patients with diarrhoea previously investigated without a diagnosis, a fresh watery stool sample should be centrifuged and the supernatant pH determined; a pH below 6 indicates fermentation of unabsorbed carbohydrate to volatile fatty acids and prompts investigation of carbohydrate intolerance (lactose, sucrose–isomaltose). Stool supernatant osmolality is usually 280–340 mosmol/kg but is often much higher in carbohydrate malabsorption and during ingestion of osmotic purgatives. Stool water electrolytes measured in the supernatant or by the in vivo dialysis technique[25] permit calculation of the osmotic gap (Osmolality − $[(Na^+ + K^+) \times 2]$), which if more than 15 mosmol/kg suggests the presence of an additional cation such as magnesium (in magnesium salt purgative abuse). The Na/K ratio, which is high in colonic disorders and low in small bowel disorders, can also be calculated. Perfection in routine stool analysis is only achieved by attention to detail, and discussion and co-operation with the bacteriology department. In practice this relatively cheap investigation is badly performed on inadequate samples and therefore too often leads to multiple inappropriate investigations. As an example of this a patient with the rare condition of asucrasia comes to mind. He complained of passing 'sour, stinking stools' and of gross abdominal distension and flatulence. After multiple investigations he underwent exploratory laparotomy which revealed nothing abnormal. After many referrals a registrar finally made a careful examination of the stools and recorded a stool pH of 5.1 and a growth in culture of pure lactobacilli, which led to a series of disaccharide tolerance tests (which were positive for sucrose and starch) and finally a deficiency of sucrase–isomaltase was demonstrated in a peroral jejunal biopsy.[10]

SCREENING BLOOD TESTS

Table 8.20 lists the blood tests which are helpful in early evaluation of patients with diarrhoea and should be performed in all cases. These tests may provide positive clues which, taken together with the history, physical examination and stool test, point to the most direct diagnostic approach. In those individuals who have no worrying features in the history and who have a normal physical examination and stool test, a set of completely normal blood tests excludes all but a modest number of organic pathologies.

Table 8.20 Screening blood tests in chronic diarrhoea and malabsorption.

Nutritional
Haemoglobin, red blood cell indices
Serum and red cell folate
Serum B_{12}
Serum iron and transferrin
Serum calcium, phosphorus and alkaline phosphatase
Serum albumin

General
Erythrocyte sedimentation rate
C-reactive protein
Serum potassium

Iron deficiency anaemia always demands explanation in patients with diarrhoea. Bleeding from the gut is likely if the anaemia is associated with elevated reticulocyte and platelet counts and should lead to faecal occult blood tests. Malabsorption or dietary deficiency of iron produces a hypochromic microcytic anaemia with a low or normal reticulocyte count. The changes of hyposplenism (target cells and Howell–Jolly bodies) suggest coeliac disease. A macrocytic anaemia suggests folate or B_{12} malabsorption. A low serum or red blood cell folate suggests proximal small intestinal disease and may be the only abnormality in coeliac disease. A low serum B_{12} level points to a gastric lesion like pernicious anaemia, to ileal disease, or to bacterial overgrowth at any point in the small intestine. A low serum albumin may reflect protein losing enteropathy from a lesion in the stomach, small or large bowel.

Viewed as a whole, the pattern of results should point to the correct diagnostic pathway if this is not already clinically obvious. Thus, for example, a barium follow through and jejunal biopsy is indicated for diarrhoea in association with folic acid deficiency, iron deficiency with negative faecal occult bloods and stool test, and a low serum albumin with normal liver function and negative urine test for protein. Steatorrhoea without abnormalities of the nutritional blood tests is usually pancreatic, prompting a careful look for calcification on plain abdominal X-ray, and ultrasound or preferably CT scan to image the pancreas. Abnormalities of liver function prompt delineation of hepatic and pancreatic anatomy by scanning and ultrasound. A very low serum potassium with otherwise normal blood tests in a patient with severe watery diarrhoea and a normal stool test would prompt assays for peptide hormones and a search for a pancreatic apudoma or thyroid medullary carcinoma. Pattern recognition of this type requires careful attention to each aspect of investigation.

Abnormal blood tests must never be ignored; a diagnosis of irritable bowel syndrome or nervous diarrhoea must never be made unless the blood tests are normal and there is no suspicion of organic pathology in the history, physical examination or stool test.

If no abnormalities are found in stage one investigations, the physician must ask himself 'Should I do a barium enema now, or see the patient after four to six weeks and re-evaluate then?'. It is my policy to order a barium enema directly in all those over 30 years of age on the pretext that an early carcinoma might be discovered or, in more elderly subjects, diverticular disease. In younger subjects in the same category I review and if necessary repeat the screening tests. As a matter of policy I am never happy with a diagnosis of irritable bowel syndrome appearing for the first time in middle aged men since it is usually not correct – as in many branches of medicine, clinical instincts should lower one's threshold for definitive investigation.

Stage two

INVESTIGATIONS OF INTESTINAL ANATOMY

Table 8.21 illustrates the value of different diagnostic techniques.

Barium enema
Double contrast enemas are performed first in those patients with watery or exudative (pus with or without blood) diarrhoea and in those with 'change of bowel habit' or rectal bleeding. The diagnostic accuracy depends on adequate bowel preparation, radiological technical expertise and experienced reporting. These three criteria are not always optimal. Even under the best circumstances caecal carcinomas, polyps and low grade colitis are occasionally missed. Re-reporting of films in the light of further clinical information, repeat studies, or colonoscopy increase the diagnostic yield where there is any doubt. Studies from other hospitals may be acceptable, but if more than one to two months old may need to be repeated.

Colonoscopy
This is not a routine investigation for diarrhoea but is most helpful for defining the nature or extent of a lesion seen on barium enema. For example, a stricture in the transverse colon in a patient with Crohn's colitis could be inflammatory or neoplastic, or a caecal lesion could be carcinoma, amoeboma, Crohn's disease or tuberculosis; similarly bleeding could be coming

Table 8.21 Investigations of intestinal anatomy and their diagnostic value in chronic diarrhoea and malabsorption.

Anatomical investigation	Diagnosis
Barium enema	Carcinoma Ulcerative colitis Crohn's disease Diverticular disease Polyposis Fistulas Ischaemic colitis Tuberculosis Megacolon

Barium follow through	Non-specific
	  malabsorption
	  pattern (e.g. coeliac
	  disease)
	Crohn's disease
	Diverticulosis
	Stricture
	Stagnant loop
	Fistulas
	Lymphoma
	Tuberculosis
	Whipple's disease
	Lymphangiectasia
	Nodular lymphoid
	  hyperplasia

Sigmoidoscopy (colonoscopy) and rectal biopsy	Carcinoma Ulcerative colitis Crohn's disease Amoebiasis Melanosis coli Amyloid Lymphoma
Jejunal biopsy	Coeliac disease Tropical sprue Lymphoma Whipple's disease Alpha chain disease Giardiasis Lymphangiectasia Immunodeficiency syndromes Disaccharide deficiency
Endoscopic pancreatography	Carcinoma of the pancreas Chronic pancreatitis
Liver/spleen scan and liver biopsy	Carcinoma Carcinoid Lymphoma

from a small polyp, carcinoma or a vascular malformation. Colonoscopy is also essential for surveillance of the colon in individuals with long standing colitis to detect dysplasia[6] and other stigmata of incipient malignancy.

Barium follow through
This should be the first investigation in patients with steatorrhoea or watery diarrhoea with blood tests suggesting small intestinal pathology. Otherwise it usually follows the barium

enema. The interpretation of small bowel X-rays requires considerable experience and in many instances discussion with the radiologist who performed the study is essential to aid interpretation. An intubated follow through enables double contrast pictures of high quality to be obtained and is especially useful in detecting areas of narrowing and mucosal lesions which may be missed with conventional studies. Adequate visualization of the terminal ileum requires spot views and careful positioning of the patient and, where ileal loops are low in the pelvis, a lateral view may be helpful. It is important to realize that disease of the small intestine (e.g. coeliac disease, Crohn's disease) may be found even when small bowel X-rays appear normal. Abnormalities of the mucosal pattern may be characteristic of, for example, Crohn's disease but the possible differential diagnosis of lymphoma, vasculitis (e.g. Henoch–Schönlein purpura) with submucosal haemorrhage, or tuberculosis must be carefully considered.

Whenever possible histological confirmation of the diagnosis should be obtained and if reasonable doubt exists a laparotomy may be necessary. A decision to repeat a follow through examination should be taken whenever symptoms suggestive of intermittent small bowel obstruction occur or after an interval if the diarrhoea persists and no clear diagnosis has been made.

Indium-111 leucocyte scanning

This technique[21] involves taking a sample of venous blood, separating the polymorphonuclear leucocytes using centrifugation with percol or metrizamide plasma gradients, and labelling the cells with indium-111 using troponate as chelating agent. Labelled cells are re-injected intravenously and after 40 minutes abdominal scans are performed. A normal (negative) scan shows maximal activity in the spleen, lesser activity in the liver and least activity in the bone marrow (Figure 8.33), while the

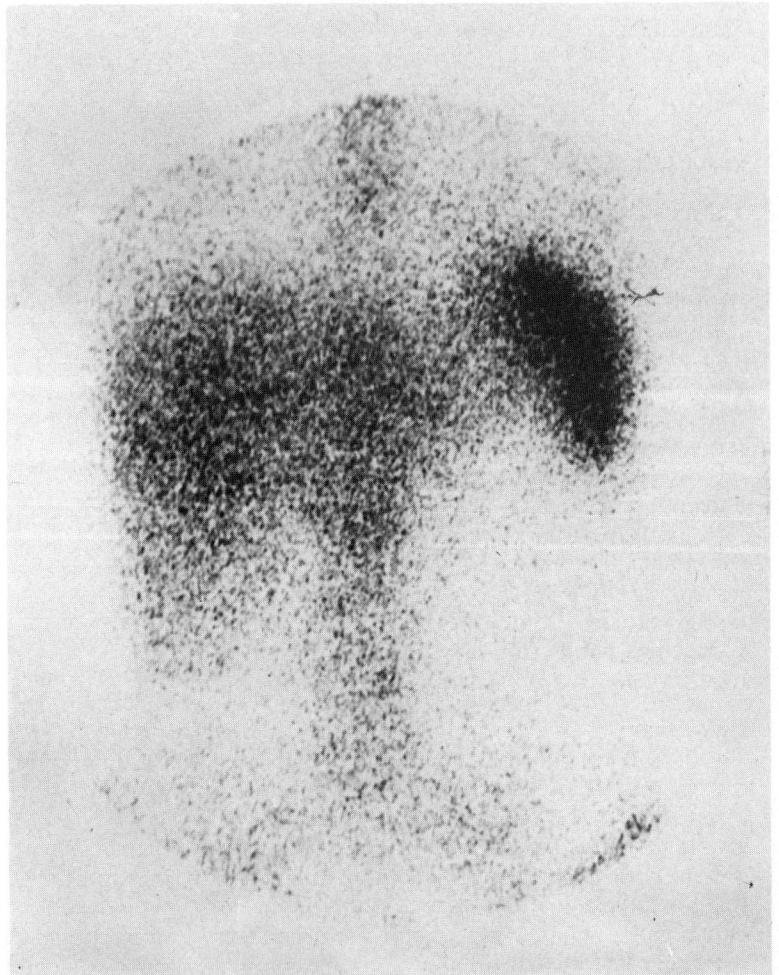

Fig. 8.33 Indium-111-labelled granulocyte scan in a normal subject obtained by external imaging at 40 minutes after re-injection of labelled cells. Note the normal appearance with uptake in liver, spleen, vascular pool, and the bone marrow of the spine and pelvis.

bowel does no image. Abnormal activity in the bowel loops is readily seen in early scans (Figure 8.34). In the colon the extent of acute inflammation and the presence of skip lesions is usually obvious[22] whereas in the small bowel, clearly defined inflamed bowel loops or more diffuse activity representing overlapping loops may be seen. Labelled cells rapidly migrate from diseased bowel wall to bowel lumen and later scans show a column of cells in transit through the bowel with clearance of activity at the diseased segment. Sequential scans thus distinguish bowel inflammation from an abscess, where activity persists at the original site of localiza-

tion for up to 48 hours (Figure 8.35). In patients with inflammatory disease, faecal collections and gamma counting of the stool permit calculation of the percentage excretion of labelled cells, which is a measure of disease severity.

The sensitivity of indium-111 scanning in detecting inflammation in bowel is substantially greater than radiology and in the colon is equivalent to colonoscopy and biopsy; in detecting abscesses it is superior to ultrasound. Although the technique is not yet widely available, it offers the potential for rapid diagnosis of inflammatory disease and assessment of activity and extent of disease in patients presenting with

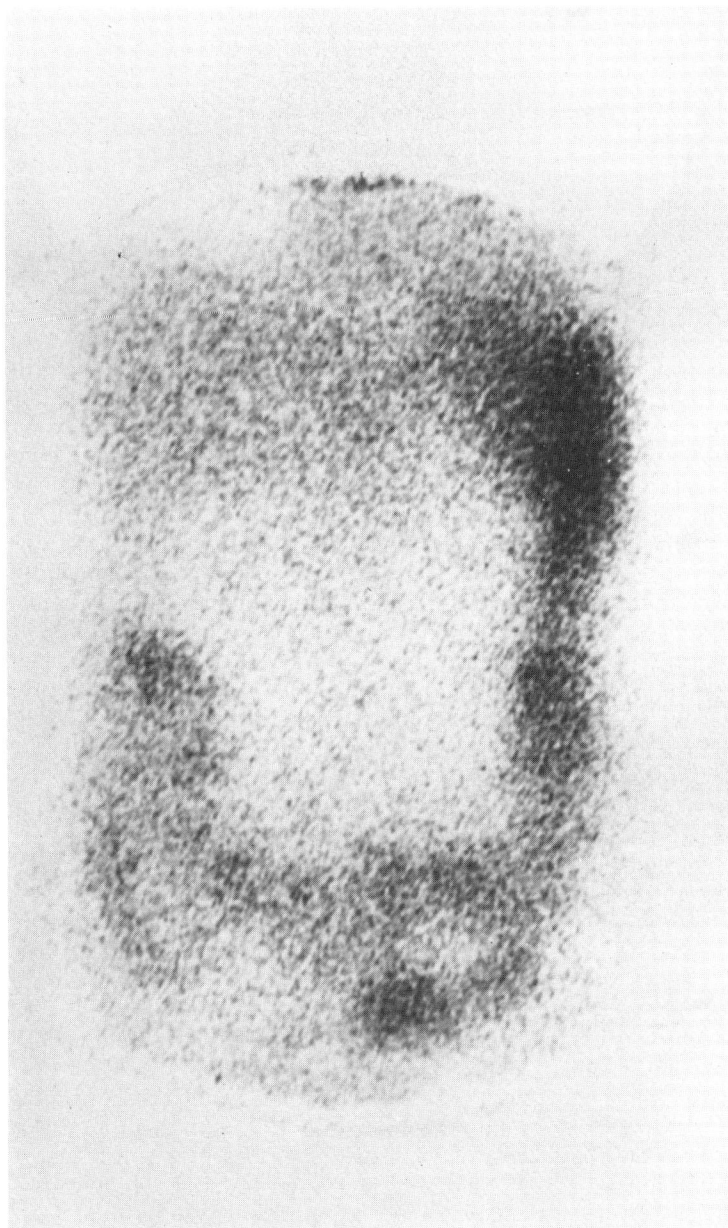

Fig. 8.34 Indium-111-labelled granulocyte scan at 40 minutes after re-injection of labelled cells. Note the accumulation of activity throughout the large intestine indicating pancolitis.

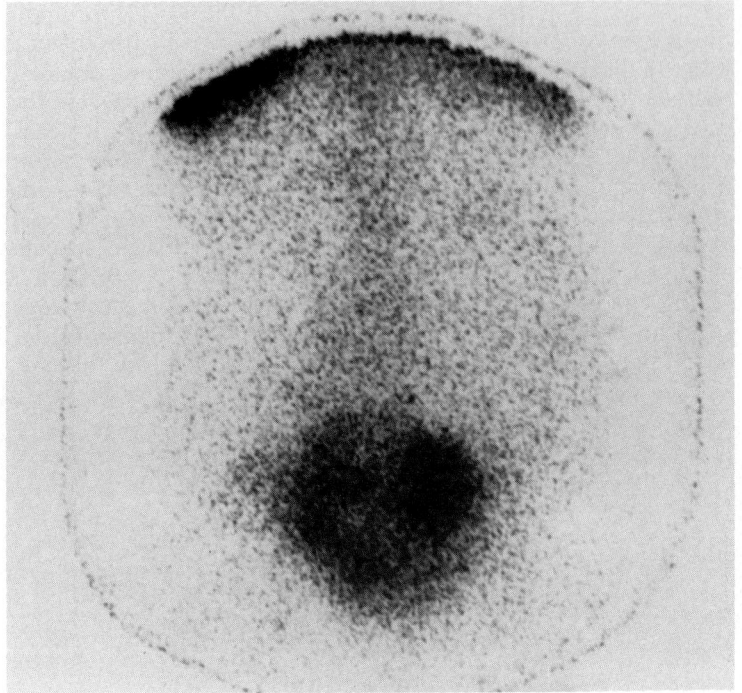

Fig. 8.35 Indium-111-labelled scan at 24 hours after re-injection of labelled cells. Note the dense persistent accumulation of activity in central part of lower abdomen and pelvis indicating an abscess at this site.

diarrhoea. No bowel preparation is required and it is therefore a suitable early investigation in the sick and elderly. The finding of normal faecal indium excretion (less than 2%) virtually excludes inflammatory disease as a cause of diarrhoea; gut carcinoma, coeliac disease, endocrine diarrhoea, diverticular disease and irritable bowel syndrome are associated with negative scans and normal faecal indium excretion. Positive scans and elevated faecal indium confirm inflammation but are not specific to any particular inflammatory process, so that Crohn's disease, ulcerative colitis, tuberculosis, pseudomembranous colitis and colitis due to other toxigenic or infective causes would all give a positive scan. Nevertheless the combination of these techniques with selective use of colonoscopy, biopsy techniques, and bacteriological studies represents a major advance in the assessment of patients with diarrhoea.

Jejunal biopsy
Jejunal biopsy should be performed in all patients with steatorrhoea, in those with watery diarrhoea and blood tests suggesting small bowel disease, in those with a radiological abnormality of the small intestine, and in those in whom a suspicion of parasitic disease of the small intestine is raised because of country of origin, foreign travel or immunodeficiency. It is

wise to perform barium studies first since the presence of single or multiple diverticula represent a risk of perforation should the biopsy capsule enter a diverticulum. Under these circumstances, duodenal biopsies via an endoscope would be safer. Examination of the biopsy under the dissecting microscope, and of the jejunal juice under dark ground illumination for motile parasites, is very valuable since a flat or convoluted appearance of the tissue may provisionally confirm suspicions of coeliac disease or tropical sprue, and the finding of *Giardia* or *Strongyloides* permits rapid institution of therapy. Histological confirmation of the diagnosis is, of course, essential. The problem of patchy mucosal abnormalities in jejunal Crohn's disease or dermatitis herpetiformis has led several authorities to stress the need for multiple biopsies. In practice this is rarely routinely necessary, providing the size of the biopsy is adequate and it is correctly oriented so that an adequate assessment of villous morphology is possible.

Attempts to biopsy more distal regions of the small intestine are unnecessary and I cannot think of a single example where this has provided a definite diagnosis. This means that a clear pathological diagnosis of a lesion in the lower small intestine demonstrated radiologically is not possible except at laparotomy. In practice, for Crohn's disease, classical radiological appearances together with abnormalities in biopsies from more accessible sites (e.g. rectum, colon, or terminal ileum at colonoscopy) may suffice or, for an ileitis, the finding of positive serological tests for *Yersinia* may confirm the diagnosis. In other instances laparotomy may be necessary.

Gastroscopy and endoscopic pancreatography
Gastroscopy is advisable in all patients with diarrhoea who have upper gastrointestinal symptoms or abnormalities of the oesophagus, stomach or duodenum on barium X-ray. In several units it is now performed in all patients with diarrhoea and malabsorption. The frequency of gastric abnormalities in patients with Crohn's disease have recently been emphasized, though the biopsy appearances are rarely diagnostic.

Typical appearances of effacement of circular folds and absence of villi under magnification are recognized in coeliac disease, and stippling and club-shaped villous enlargement due to lymphatic distension are seen in Whipple's disease. Visible enlargement of lymph vessels may also be seen in intestinal lymphangiectasia. Duodenal villous morphology is variable and therefore, to confirm partial or total villous atrophy, conventional jejunal biopsy is often necessary. In patients who cannot swallow, a jejunal biopsy capsule can be introduced via an endoscope (the tubing is passed retrogradely up the biopsy channel) and advanced to the jejunum under fluoroscopic control. Aspiration of duodenal fluid for microbiological studies is also useful.

Endoscopic pancreatography (*ERP*) may define the characteristic duct abnormalities of chronic pancreatitis. In patients with steatorrhoea, with or without diabetes, in whom blood tests, X-rays and jejunal biopsy have excluded small bowel disease, pancreatic insufficiency is likely. If such patients have obvious pancreatic calcification on plain X-ray or CT scan then ERP is unnecessary. A pancreatic function test in these circumstances is convenient, useful and safe. In the absence of calcification or suggestive abnormalities on ultrasound or CT scan, it is wise to examine the duct anatomy using ERP and to obtain cytology for malignant cells.

INTESTINAL AND PANCREATIC FUNCTION TESTS

Small gut function tests
Table 8.22 illustrates the pattern of abnormal function tests to be expected with disease in different anatomical locations. It has already been stressed that these are not first line investigations for diarrhoea.

The jejunum, pancreas and colon are accessible to the anatomical diagnostic approach previously outlined, but the ileum is relatively inaccessible and, in the absence of obvious

Table 8.22 Intestinal function tests in chronic diarrhoea and malabsorption.

Disease location or type	Intestinal function tests
Jejunal disease	Reduced xylose and glucose absorption Normal or increased faecal fat
Ileal disease	Normal xylose and glucose absorption Increased faecal fat (with greater than 100 cm of disease or resection) Schilling test abnormal Increased faecal bile salt excretion ^{14}C bile acid breath test positive
Pancreatic insufficiency	Normal xylose absorption Diabetic glucose tolerance Increased faecal fat and nitrogen Abnormal pancreatic function test
Small bowel bacterial overgrowth*	Normal glucose absorption Reduced xylose absorption Increased faecal fat Schilling test abnormal Normal faecal bile salt excretion ^{14}C bile acid breath test positive Bacterial counts greater than 10^5 in jejunal fluid
Colonic disease	Normal faecal fat, absorption and breath tests High sodium/potassium ratio in stool

* Normalized after antibiotics.

radiological abnormality, a sensitive function test may exclude or suggest significant ileal disease. Furthermore, to confirm bacterial overgrowth in those patients with an anatomical basis (e.g. stricture, fistula, diverticulosis, dilated gut) or in those with immunodeficiency, function tests before and after antibiotics are useful. Although of limited value in diagnosis, function tests may be repeated at intervals as a parameter of treatment response or to assess functional reserve after gut resection (e.g. Schilling test after ileal resection). Finally carbohydrate tolerance tests are convenient ways of demonstrating lactose and sucrose intolerance which should have been suspected on the basis of history and a low faecal pH.

The *measurement of faecal fat* is extremely unpopular among biochemists for obvious reasons, though it is an established and sensitive test. Reliable results depend on adequate fat intake so that, on an outpatient basis, supplements in the form of cream must be given to ensure a fat intake of more than 70 g/day. Since the normal coefficient of fat absorption is 5%, a young male adult who may eat up to 200 g of fat in a day will have a normal faecal fat excretion of about 10 g. For inpatients, dietary supervision excludes these obvious pitfalls. A two day run-in period is usually followed by a five day collection period. Faecal markers to estimate recovery are useful but not essential. Attempts have been made to replace the faecal fat test with radio-isotopic breath tests. The ^{14}C *triolein test*, for example, detects all patients with steatorrhoea but gives no assessment of the severity of fat malabsorption.[20] It is obvious that a decrease in efficiency of fat absorption from 95% to 90% will increase faecal fat excretion by 100% but change fat absorption by only 5% so that any test based on events reflecting variable absorption and subsequent metabolism is intrinsically less sensitive than measurement of the fraction appearing in faeces. In my view the tests proposed as alternatives to faecal fat estimation have not been beneficial in clinical diagnosis and I suggest there is no role for a screening test for fat malabsorption. Clinicians should limit the number of requests for faecal fat determination by following the diagnostic approach outlined in this chapter, but must ensure this test is available to them for specific situations.

Of the other 'tubeless' isotopic function tests, the *Schilling test* remains popular and is useful providing it is correctly carried out and there is a complete urine collection. Modifications of the Schilling test to detect pancreatic insufficiency[7] mean that it is possible to use this test to detect pernicious anaemia, ileal disease, bacterial overgrowth and pancreatic disease.

The ^{14}C *cholyl glycine breath test*[15] is usually positive in patients with bacterial overgrowth of the small intestine, but quantitative faecal ^{14}C excretion is essential to differentiate between bacterial overgrowth (faecal excretion less than 10% of the dose) and ileal disease or resection with bile acid malabsorption (faecal excretion greater than 10% with or without increased breath $^{14}CO_2$ output). Faecal ^{14}C counting is difficult and requires expensive combustion apparatus. As a test of ileal function, total body counting at seven days after administration of SeHCAT (a selenium labelled bile acid) may be more useful in those institutions with whole body gamma counters.[14]

Non-radioisotopic breath tests based on hydrogen excretion[9] after administration of glucose (for bacterial overgrowth), lactose (for lactose malabsorption), or lactulose (for small intestinal transit time or bacterial overgrowth) are simple to perform and the newer H_2 analysers are useful additions to the gastrointestinal function laboratories. It should be remembered that lactose intolerance may be due to organic disease of the small intestine and tests to exclude such disorders are mandatory before a diagnosis of primary hypolactasia is made.

Pancreatic function tests

Tubeless pancreatic function tests are increasingly popular (e.g. PABA test, fluorescein dilaurate test, modified Schilling test). They are useful in assessing pancreatic function in patients with steatorrhoea but not sensitive enough for detection of pancreatic disease in the absence of severe exocrine deficiency.[13] Of the intubation tests, the Lundh test is widely used in clinical gastroenterology, but the secretin or secretin–cholecystokinin test using a continuous intravenous infusion of hormones and a duodenal perfusion system to measure outputs of bicarbonate and enzymes is probably the only test which offers the potential for measurement of lesser degrees of pancreatic insufficiency. The main value of pancreatic function tests in investigation of diarrhoea is that they can define exocrine deficiency as the cause of steatorrhoea. In some instances this will obviate the need for endoscopic retrograde pancreatography, which is not always available, may fail to visualize the ducts, may provoke acute pancreatitis, and may introduce infection. In units with appropriate expertise and low complication rates, however, visualization of pancreatic duct anatomy by ERP is the most definitive procedure.

Other function tests

Recently several groups have suggested that the measurement of intestinal permeability is clinically useful in screening for, or monitoring the response to therapy in, small gut disorders such as coeliac disease and Crohn's disease. These tests depend on the administration of molecules of different sizes by mouth and assess gut permeability by the ratio of concentrations excreted in urine. For example, in coeliac disease the mannitol to cellobiose ratio is markedly reduced compared to normal, reflecting the decreased absorption of mannitol (due to loss of surface area) and the increased absorption of cellobiose (due to increased permeability). Ratios return towards normal with treatment.[16] The use of single probes such as ^{51}Cr-EDTA has demonstrated increased absorption in coeliac disease and small bowel Crohn's disease.[4] While interesting, these tests have not been evaluated prospectively in patients presenting with diarrhoea and their sensitivity and specificity are not known. They need further evaluation before being applied in clinical diagnostics.

Tests of small and large bowel transit time, while of research interest, have no obvious role to play in the diagnosis or management of patients with diarrhoea.

SPECIAL BLOOD, STOOL AND URINE TESTS

Endocrine causes of diarrhoea

Table 8.23 illustrates the endocrine causes of diarrhoea and the diagnostic tests most appropriate in each case. Thyrotoxicosis and the Zollinger–Ellison syndrome should be suspected on clinical history or physical examination,

Table 8.23 Endocrine causes of diarrhoea and diagnostic tests.

Endocrine syndromes	Diagnostic tests
Thyrotoxicosis	Plasma T_3 and T_4 Thyroid scan
Medullary carcinoma of thyroid	Plasma calcitonin Thyroid and bone scans CT scan
Zollinger–Ellison syndrome	Plasma gastrin Acid secretion studies Pancreatic angiography CT scan
Vipoma (pancreatic cholera or WDHA syndrome)	Plasma vasoactive intestinal peptide (VIP) Mesenteric angiography Transhepatic portal venous sampling CT scan
Carcinoid syndrome	Urinary 5-HIAA excretion Liver scan and biopsy

while obvious flushing is always, in my experience, associated with the diarrhoea of the carcinoid syndrome. The vipoma syndrome (Verner–Morrison or WDHA syndrome) should be suspected when severe watery diarrhoea occurs in any patient who has a negative stool test (normal microscopy, culture and pH), hypokalaemia (usually marked) as the only abnormal blood test (except for minor abnormalities of serum calcium and abnormal liver tests when there are widespread hepatic secondaries), and normal intestinal anatomy. The key investigation is the plasma vasoactive intestinal polypeptide (VIP) level which if elevated indicates a pancreatic tumour (children or adults) or a ganglioneuroma (usually children). Pancreatic imaging (ultrasound and CT scan) may show the tumour, but selective pancreatic angiography is the most sensitive test.

Medullary carcinoma of the thyroid causes a usually persistent, painless diarrhoea, watery in nature, and is the main differential diagnosis of the vipoma syndrome. The mechanism of diarrhoea is not completely understood, but it is clearly different from that in patients with vipomas. Diarrhoea persists during fasting but is much greater when feeding. Stool tests during fasting show normal osmolality and pH but, unlike Vipomas, osmolality increases and pH falls during feeding suggesting malabsorption (possibly secondary to fast transit). Hypokalaemia is less marked, though usually present, and again intestinal anatomy is normal. In the absence of an obvious tumour in the neck or elsewhere, diarrhoea usually indicates a substantial tumour mass, and mediastinal lymph nodes, bones, and liver are likely sites. If the clinical picture fits, a plasma calcitonin is the key investigation and other tests are useful to assess location of the tumour and its metastases.

Endocrine tumour related diarrhoeas are rare, and in units which act as referral centres occasional patients are seen with a clinical picture resembling the vipoma syndrome but in whom VIP levels are normal (including repeat measurements). These patients do not usually have a tumour, but a careful search in the pancreas, lung and liver should be made. There is little point in performing laparotomy on the basis of reports in the literature to date, but careful assessment and surveillance is warranted. The possibility of small tumours secreting uncharacterized secretogogues exists.

Chronic purgative abuse

This condition, which is almost confined to females, may be difficult to diagnose. Patients with diarrhoea who have obvious melanosis coli on sigmoidoscopy or pigment-laden macrophages on rectal histology are almost certainly taking anthraquinone purgatives (e.g. Senokot). Phenolphthalein purgatives may be detected by the development of a red colouration on alkalinization of the stool supernatant and sometimes the urine, and magnesium salt purgatives by the high stool osmolality, high ionic gap and high faecal magnesium concentration. It is important to try and identify any purgatives the patient may have with them; locker searches, although of questionable ethics, may reveal the nature of the purgative. Discharging a patient home for the weekend is usually helpful if stool and urine samples for analysis are obtained immediately on return to hospital. This sometimes overcomes the problem of diminishing diarrhoea and negative tests during hospital confinement, possibly due to the patient not having access to purgatives in the hospital ward. A variety of anatomical, blood test and function test abnormalities may be found in patients with surreptitious laxative ingestion in addition to those already mentioned. The barium enema may show variable dilatation and loss of haustral pattern, there may be an elevated ESR and a low serum potassium, and mild abnormalities of xylose, vitamin B_{12} and fat absorption.

Conclusion

The diagnostic approach to patients with chronic diarrhoea has been outlined. In order to avoid unnecessary tests and inordinate expense, emphasis is placed on the value of clinical features and screening blood and stool tests. Careful assessment of these permits selection of the further investigations necessary to make a firm diagnosis in almost all patients.

REFERENCES

1   Alun Jones, V., Shorthouse, M., McLaughlan, P. *et al.* (1982) Food intolerance: a major factor in the pathogenesis of irritable bowel syndrome. *Lancet*, **ii,** 1115–1117.
2   Bartlett, J. G., Chang, T. W., Taylor, N. S. & Onderdonk, A. B. (1979) Colitis induced by clostridium difficle. *Reviews of Infectious Diseases,* **1,** 370–378.
3   Bishop, R. F. (1982) Spectrum of infectious agents in acute diarrhoea. In *Gastroenterology 2: Small intestine* (Ed.) Chadwick, V. S. & Phillips, S. pp. 319–331. London: Butterworths.
4   Bjarnason, I., Peters, T. J. & Veall, N. (1983) A persistent defect in intestinal permeability in coeliac disease demonstrated by a ^{51}Cr-labelled EDTA absorption test. *Lancet*, **i,** 323–325.

5   Blacklow, N. R. & Cukor, G. (1981) Viral gastroenteritis. *New England Journal of Medicine,* **304,** 397–406.
6   Blackstone, M. D., Riddell, R. H., Rogers, B. H. G. & Levin, B. (1981) Dysplasia-associated lesion or mass (DALM) detected by colonoscopy in long standing ulcerative colitis: an indication for colectomy. *Gastroenterology,* **80,** 366–374.
7   Brugge, W. R., Goff, J. S., Allen, N. C. *et al.* (1980) Development of a dual label Schilling test for pancreatic exocrine function on the differential absorption of cobalamin bound to intrinsic factor and R protein. *Gastroenterology,* **78,** 947–949.
8   Camilleri, M., Pusey, C. D., Chadwick, V. S. & Rees, A. J. (1982) Vasculitis and the intestine. In *Gastroenterology 2: Small intestine* (Ed.) Chadwick, V. S. & Phillips, S. pp. 227–248. London: Butterworths.
9   Caspary, W. F. (1978) Breath tests. *Clinics in Gastroenterology,* **7,** 351–374.
10 Cooper, B. T., Candy, D. C. A., Harries, J. T. & Peters, T. J. (1979) Subcellular fractionation studies of the intestinal mucosa in congenital sucrose–isomaltase deficiency. *Clinical Science,* **57,** 181–185.
11 Dawson, J., Hodgson, H. J. F., Pepys, M. B. *et al.* (1979) Immunodeficiency, malabsorption and secretory diarrhoea. A new syndrome. *American Journal of Medicine,* **67,** 540–545.
12 Dick, A. P. & McC.Gregg, D. (1972) Chronic occlusions of the visceral arteries. In *Clinics in Gastroenterology,* **1,** 689–706.
13 DiMagno, E. P. (1982) Diagnosis of chronic pancreatitis: are non-invasive tests of exocrine pancreatic function sensitive and specific? *Gastroenterology,* **83,** 143–145.
14 Fagan, E. A., Chadwick, V. S. & McLean Baird, I. (1983) SeHCAT absorption: a simple test of ileal dysfunction. *Digestion,* **26,** 159–165.
15 Fromm, H. & Hofmann, A. F. (1971) Breath test for altered bile acid metabolism. *Lancet*, **ii,** 621–625.
16 Hamilton, I., Cobden, I., Rothwell, J. & Axon, A. T. (1982) Intestinal permeability in coeliac disease: the response to gluten withdrawal and single-dose gluten challenge. *Gut,* **23,** 202–210.
17 Lawrence, G. & Walker, P. D. (1976) Pathogenesis of enteritis necroticans in Papua New Guinea. *Lancet*, **i,** 125–126.
18 Mark, M. I., Pai, C. H., Lafleur, L. *et al.* (1980) *Yersina enterocolitica* gastroenteritis: a prospective study of clinical, bacteriologic and epidemiologic features. *Journal of Paediatrics,* **96,** 26–31.
19 Modigliani, R. & Bernier, J. J. (1982) Pathophysiology of hormonal diarrhoea. In *Gastroenterology 2: Small intestine* (Ed.) Chadwick, V. S. & Phillips, S. pp. 265–279. London: Butterworths.
20 Newcomer, A. D., Hofmann, A. F., DiMagno, E. P. *et al.* (1978) Triolein breath test: a sensitive and specific test for fat malabsorption. *Gastroenterology,* **76,** 6–13.
21 Peters, A. M., Saverymuttu, S. H., Reavy, H. J. *et al.* (1983) Imaging of inflammation with indium-III troplolonate labelled leucocytes. *Journal of Nuclear Medicine,* **24,** 39–44.
22 Saverymuttu, S. H., Peters, A. M., Hodgson, H. J. F. *et al.* (1982) ^{111}Indium autologous leucocyte scanning: comparison with radiology for imaging the colon in inflammatory bowel disease. *British Medical Journal,* **285,** 659–666.
23 Shwachman, H., Diamond, L. K., Oski, F. A. & Khaw, K. T. (1964) The syndrome of pancreatic insufficiency and bone marrow dysfunction. *Journal of Paediatrics,* **65,** 645–663.

24 Strober, W., Wochner, R. D., Carbone, P. P. & Waldmann, T. A. (1967) Lymphangiectasia: a protein losing
enteropathy with hypogammaglobulinaemia, lymphocytopenia and impaired homograft rejection. *Journal of
Clinical Investigation*, **46**, 1643–1656.

25 Wrong, O., Morrison, R. B. I. & Hurst, P. E. (1961) A
method of obtaining faecal fluid by in vivo dialysis.
Lancet, **i**, 1208–1209.

THE CONSEQUENCES OF MALABSORPTION

This section describes the consequences of disorders causing generalized intestinal malabsorption, but not those features which are more
characteristic of individual disease states.
Firstly, general features which occur in the
context of malabsorption are considered, and
then osteomalacia, hyperoxaluria, hyposplenism, and effects on the absorption of
administered drugs are described.

The information available on most of these
topics is by no means authoritative. Systematic
studies on many aspects have not been conducted and in some cases would need to be very
extensive to allow firm conclusions to be drawn.
For example, in considering the incidence of
osteomalacia in coeliac disease there are factors
in the mechanisms of osteomalacia and in the
method of selection of patients which would
make any conclusions not generally applicable.
It is now recognized that many, perhaps most,
patients with coeliac disease present with minor
problems.[47] Such patients, presumably, either
have the disorder in a milder form or are recognized at an earlier stage. Other studies indicate
that although the classical features of weight loss
and gastrointestinal symptoms occur in a
minority, many patients present with established
complications.[28] Thus the incidence and severity of particular features in any series may not be
representative.

General features of malabsorption

The presenting features in a patient with malabsorption may be related to effects on general
health, to gastrointestinal symptoms, or to specific nutritional deficiencies.

Effects on general health

Of the general features, weight loss is perhaps
the most likely to be present.[4] Weight loss is
common in the classical descriptions of gross
disease, but in coeliac disease, for example, a
majority of patients now present in much more
subtle ways.[47] The weight loss is not solely due
to malabsorption; significant decrease in dietary
intake has been shown to occur in many subjects.[19] This may be due to anorexia, as in any
severe illness, but may also be due to discomfort
brought on by food, especially fatty food. In
some patients, however, more particularly in
association with pancreatic disease, an increase
in food intake (hyperphagia) occurs.[19, 22] Other
general symptoms and signs include lethargy
and easy fatiguability, short stature, depression,
amenorrhoea, and susceptibility to infections.

Gastrointestinal symptoms

Gastrointestinal symptoms loom large in
patients with severe disease, but are entirely
absent in many patients with coeliac disease and
in some patients with other disorders affecting
absorption. Abdominal pain is a major
symptom in Crohn's disease and is the presenting feature in a minority of patients with coeliac
disease. It is not rare for the diagnosis of coeliac
disease to be made following laparotomy, and
sometimes even gastric surgery, for a suspected
peptic ulcer. Abdominal distension can usually
be ascribed to impaired motility of the small
intestine but, in some diseases, may be due to a
degree of mechanical obstruction. Abnormality
of the stools, which become bulky, offensive,
semi-formed, and difficult to flush away, is a
useful indicator of steatorrhoea. It is important
to recognize, however, that steatorrhoea may be
present without visible abnormality of the stools
and that extensive small bowel or pancreatic
disease may be present without steatorrhoea.

Nutritional deficiencies

Symptoms and signs related to nutritional deficiencies are anaemia (iron, folate or B_{12}
deficient), oedema (with a low serum albumin),
haemorrhages (prolonged prothrombin time
due to vitamin K deficiency), glossitis and cheilosis (deficiency of B vitamins), polyneuritis
(sometimes unexplained), and features of
vitamin D deficiency including muscle cramps,
frank tetany, proximal myopathy, and bone
pains. These features are frequent in older
descriptions dealing with gross disease[5, 19, 50]
but some at least are much rarer today. Subclinical deficiencies are, however, still common.[26]
Nutritional deficiencies are commoner in
patients with severe steatorrhoea but cannot be
directly related to diagnosis or severity in the
individual patient. Some relationship can be
found between deficiency of fat soluble vitamins
and severity of steatorrhoea, but in pancreatic

steatorrhoea, which is often very severe, deficiencies are not as common as might be expected.[19, 26]

The mucosa of the small intestine constitutes a large amount of tissue with a rapid rate of turnover and thus makes considerable nutritional demands on the body. It has been well shown that in states of nutritional deficiency there are changes in the structure and function of the small intestine[20] and of the pancreas[41, 48] leading to malabsorption.[40] Thus there is the likelihood of a vicious circle with malabsorption causing malnutrition, which itself then exacerbates the malabsorption.

Osteomalacia

Osteomalacia in the adult, and rickets in the child, is now best defined as a defect in calcification of osteoid. In practice this is recognized histologically by staining or labelling of calcification fronts and comparison of the extent of the calcification front with that in control subjects. This feature is more specific than the recognition of increased osteoid, which remains a very valuable indication of osteomalacia but is not, in itself, sufficient to prove the diagnosis since excess osteoid occurs in other conditions. In an occasional patient osteoid excess is minimal or even absent, presumably because of recent development of the calcification deficit.

In the context of malabsorption, osteomalacia is due to a deficiency in the action of vitamin D metabolites. With increasing understanding of the metabolism of vitamin D, the suggested mechanisms, assessment and management of osteomalacia are continually being revised. In the normal adult probably the vast majority of vitamin D is provided by the effect of sunlight on the skin and a minority is obtained from the diet. Vitamin D in the body is first hydroxylated in the liver to 25-hydroxyvitamin D and then again hydroxylated in the kidney to 1,25-dihydroxyvitamin D, which is the main active form in the body. The main storage form, however, is 25-hydroxyvitamin D.

Clinical features

The patient with gross osteomalacia may complain of generalized bone pains or proximal muscle weakness. There may be symptoms due to a low serum calcium, with paraesthesiae or even occasionally tetany. There may be fractures after relatively minor trauma. These, however, are late developments and the diagnosis cannot be ruled out in the absence of symptoms.

The prevalence of osteomalacia is relatively high in gluten sensitive enteropathy,[30] although figures vary, and also in Crohn's disease,[17] jejunoileal by-pass,[11] and after resection of the small intestine.[10] The prevalence is probably relatively low in tropical sprue,[5] perhaps because of the access to sunlight. The prevalence is also thought to be low in the steatorrhoea associated with pancreatic disease[19] and after gastric surgery.[33]

Mechanisms

Osteomalacia associated with malabsorption is multifactorial.[31] Indisposition due to the disease may lead to the patient being relatively housebound and having less exposure to sunlight. This is probably important in view of the fact that normally most of the vitamin D is obtained in this way.

Dietary intake of vitamin D may be diminished either because of anorexia or because of the precipitation of abdominal symptoms by food and especially by fat. Furthermore, in some patients with malabsorption, low fat diets or lactose-free diets are prescribed, which lead to a diminished intake of vitamin D.

Malabsorption of vitamin D accompanies the malabsorption of fat; the mechanisms are similar and inter-related. Loss of small bowel surface available for absorption, due either to disease or to surgical resection, contributes to this, as does bile salt deficiency due particularly to dysfunction or resection of the terminal ileum, or to bacterial action in the small intestine. Lymphatic obstruction in some conditions is an added problem.

Certain drugs which are used in these conditions may worsen the situation. Since bile salts entering the colon cause diarrhoea, the resin cholestyramine is used to bind them and thus prevent their action ·on the colon. However, in so doing it carries bile salts into the stool and thus makes the steatorrhoea and the malabsorption of vitamin D worse. Corticosteroids have been shown to reduce calcium absorption, but probably cause osteoporosis rather than osteomalacia.

One of the important effects of vitamin D is to stimulate the absorption of endogenous and dietary calcium and, in the absence of normal intestinal function, vitamin D may be unable to produce this effect.

Deficiency of magnesium, which may occur in small bowel disease, leads to resistance to parathyroid hormone release and this may contribute to hypocalcaemia. It is possible that hypomagnesaemia, without deficiency of vitamin D, may be a cause of osteomalacia.

There are certain other factors which are thought to contribute to these problems. The enterohepatic circulation of vitamin D may be inefficient. In certain exudative conditions, such as Crohn's disease, there may be increased loss of vitamin D through the gut. In a period of rapid bone growth, perhaps associated with treatment such as the institution of a gluten-free diet in coeliac disease, the requirement for vitamin D may be increased; conversely it seems that severe malnutrition may protect against the expression of osteomalacia.

Diagnosis and assessment

Traditional biochemistry involves the estimation of serum calcium, phosphorus, and alkaline phosphatase. The total serum calcium may be low because of a low protein-bound fraction due to a low serum albumin. However, it is the ionized calcium fraction which is important, although this is not easily measurable. There are formulas available to adjust for albumin concentration, but this is clearly not very satisfactory. A low serum phosphate, due to secondary hyperparathyroidism, is suggestive of the condition but not diagnostic, although not all patients with osteomalacia have a low value. Serum alkaline phosphatase is so frequently abnormal for other reasons that it is of little discriminatory value and refinements measuring different phosphatase fractions have not proved to be as useful as might be expected.

Radiology is of value in demonstrating gross disease. Demineralization is difficult to assess unless gross and usually represents osteoporosis since bone mineral content in the axial skeleton may be normal in osteomalacia. Looser's zones are virtually pathognomonic when in well defined situations and symmetrical, but these occur only in gross disease.

The measurement of plasma 25-hydroxyvitamin D level gives the best index of vitamin D stores. This does not correlate entirely with histological osteomalacia since some patients have low levels without osteomalacia, presumably because the stores need to be exhausted for a considerable time before the histology becomes clearly abnormal. Measurements of 25-hydroxyvitamin D are not freely available.

A high plasma parathyroid hormone level indicates that homeostatic mechanisms are acting to maintain the ionized calcium level. The parathyroid hormone level may, however, not be increased in the very early stages of vitamin D deficiency, or if there is concurrent magnesium deficiency.

The cornerstone of the diagnosis of osteomalacia is histological assessment of bone biopsy. The biopsy can be performed as an outpatient procedure. A sample is usually taken from the region of the anterior superior iliac spine. The definitive criterion is a diminution in the calcification front, labelled either by tetracycline in vivo or toluidine blue in vitro. Techniques for quantitative assessment of the calcification front are not widely available since experience is needed in preparation and interpretation of the sections.

Treatment

Vitamin D is the basic requirement. Oral therapy is usually effective and most patients will respond to small doses. However, a very few patients appear to have great difficulty in absorbing vitamin D and for these parenteral administration is preferable. Whether the synthetic derivative 1α-hydroxycholecalciferol is effective by mouth in such patients remains to be established. Adequate calcium intake must be ensured during the time that vitamin D supplements are being given.

In coeliac disease the vitamin D may be relatively ineffective until the intestinal mucosa is improving on a gluten-free diet.

There may be some advantage in using 1α-hydroxycholecalciferol instead of the usual forms of vitamin D, since the effect of inadvertent overdose is more rapidly reversed.

Hyperoxaluria

Hyperoxaluria (excess oxalate in the urine) occurs in a number of conditions associated with malabsorption and may then be termed enteric hyperoxaluria. This has been described in Crohn's disease, tropical sprue, coeliac disease, pancreatic disease, in patients after ileal resection, in patients with jejunoileal bypass and in patients with stasis of the small intestine. The prevalence in these conditions depends on the extent and severity of disease, or the amount of ileum resected. It seems that a half to a third of patients with Crohn's disease may show hyperoxaluria.

Oxalate metabolism[18]

Oxalate is a metabolic end-product which is excreted largely in the urine. Of urinary oxalate, normally more than half comes from glyoxalate, more than a quarter from the oxidation of ascorbic acid, and only a small proportion from the food. Renal clearance is thought to be complete. The calcium salt is very insoluble in water.

The Small Intestine

Mechanisms of enteric hyperoxaluria

It has been shown that excess urinary oxalate in association with small bowel disease results from increased absorption of dietary oxalate. Although it seems likely that oxalate can be absorbed in the small intestine, the colon is the major site of absorption.[15]

Excessive absorption of oxalate correlates with faecal fat excretion.[29] It seems that fatty acids in the bowel lumen bind calcium, thus making it unavailable to form the insoluble, and hence unabsorbed, calcium oxalate. In addition, there is evidence to suggest that bile salts escaping into the colon, because of disease or resection of the terminal ileum, cause an increase in colonic oxalate absorption.[1]

Clinical effects

Most patients with hyperoxaluria suffer no ill effects. Some patients with jejunoileal bypass[16] and some with ileal disease[14] or resection[46] develop urinary oxalate stones. Patients with jejunoileal bypass frequently have oxalate crystallization in the renal tubules, occasionally leading to renal failure[16] and one such patient with Crohn's disease has been described.[27]

Urinary oxalate stones must be differentiated from the urinary uric acid stones which occur in certain patients with Crohn's disease. These latter stones occur in patients with an ileostomy and can be attributed to the low volume of urine (because of ileostomy fluid loss) which is relatively acid (because of bicarbonate loss); in contrast oxalate stones do not occur in patients with an ileostomy because oxalate absorption in the colon cannot occur.

Treatment

Treatment of the underlying disease to minimize the malabsorption of fat and bile salts is clearly the first major consideration. If this cannot be attained then a low fat diet will reduce faecal fat,[2] but at the expense of reducing the amount of fat absorbed and hence the calories and also the fat-soluble vitamins absorbed.

Cholestyramine binds oxalate and hence reduces its absorption, but probably has a greater effect in binding bile acids and hence reducing their effect on the colon. This drug, however, has a number of disadvantages. It is unpleasant to take, the fact that it increases faecal bile salt loss may make the steatorrhoea worse if there is an element of bile salt deficiency involved, and it also binds other drugs which the patient may require.

A high calcium intake has been recommended so as to bind the oxalate in the bowel lumen. There is, however, the theoretical disadvantage that this will cause an increase in urinary calcium and thus insoluble calcium oxalate. This is of particular concern when the urinary calcium is increasing due to treatment of the malabsorption.

A low oxalate diet can be attempted. Foods especially high in oxalate include spinach, rhubarb, tea, chocolate, cocoa, Ovaltine and some proprietary cola drinks. In desperation, in the occasional patient, colectomy and ileostomy might need to be considered.

It must be emphasized, however, that, with the possible exception of jejunoileal bypass,[16] in most patients the hyperoxaluria does not lead to any harm, and treatment should only be instituted if symptoms can be attributed to this condition.

Diminished splenic function

Diminished function of the spleen (hyposplenism) has been found in a number of diseases involving the small intestine. The best documented example is coeliac disease,[44] but hyposplenism is also well described in tropical sprue, Whipple's disease, non-specific ulcerative jejunoileitis[32] and Crohn's disease,[35] although in the latter the defect in splenic function appears to be more related to involvement of the large intestine.

Functions of the spleen[6]

Splenic function is important in the processing of erythrocytes. After leaving the bone marrow, reticulocytes are sequestered in the spleen and remodelled there by removal of a certain amount of membrane protein. The spleen is one of the major sites of removal of senescent red cells. It also removes abnormally shaped red cells from the circulation and removes various types of inclusion bodies, notably the nuclear remnants known as Howell–Jolly bodies, from the erythrocytes before returning them to the circulation.

In addition, the spleen sequesters platelets and plays a part in the regulation of the platelet count in small bowel disease. It is of importance in the immune response, particularly in the early immune responses to circulating organisms and antigens when specific antibody is not present.

There is a relationship between hyposplenism and autoantibody formation; it seems likely that this is because defective splenic function leads to the formation of autoantibodies and hence, potentially, to autoimmune disease.

Recognition of hyposplenism
Hyposplenism may be suspected from the blood film if Howell–Jolly bodies, giant platelets, or abnormally shaped red cells (acanthocytes) are found. All these features occurring together are a very specific indication of hyposplenism, but this is only seen when the defect in splenic function is severe.

The function of the spleen in removing abnormal red blood cells may be assessed by infusing autologous heat-damaged red blood cells and plotting the rate of removal. This is a sensitive test but requires meticulous technique. Similarly the rate of removal of colloid particles from the circulation may be followed.

When splenic function is deficient, interference phase microscopy shows an increased proportion of red cells with localized membrane defects which appear as 'pits'. This is a simple, reproducible and quantitative technique which requires only a drop of blood.

If the hyposplenism is associated with marked atrophy of the spleen, decrease in size of the organ can be demonstrated by isotopic scanning, ultrasound, or by computerized tomography. Hyposplenism can, however, occur with a normal sized spleen, or with an enlarged spleen if the spleen is infiltrated by disease deposits or if the reticuloendothelial function is blocked by increased activity.

The significance of hyposplenism
Long-term complications of splenectomy include reports of ischaemic and thrombotic disease[34, 43] and an increased susceptibility to severe and sometimes overwhelming infections, including pneumonia, meningitis and septicaemia.[23] The same problems might be expected in states of hyposplenism without splenectomy. However, the documentation of the long-term effects of hyposplenism without splenectomy is poor. The best documentation concerns the risks in patients with ulcerative colitis rather than in disease of the small intestine.

In the context of small bowel disease, most studies relate hyposplenism to coeliac disease. It seems likely that the prevalence of hyposplenism found in coeliac disease will depend upon patient selection, the stage of treatment, and the method used to demonstrate the hyposplenism. Hyposplenism in coeliac disease may, theoretically, be functional, due to blockage of the reti-

culoendothelial system by the uptake of immune complexes in the spleen, or may be structural, due to atrophy of the spleen with ensuing fibrosis for reasons which are not understood, but which may possibly be related to chronic loss of lymphocytes from the bowel. The functional element would be expected to be reversible when the coeliac disease was treated with a gluten-free diet, whereas the structural change would not.

In well-treated patients with coeliac disease about 1 in 3 have a smaller-than-normal spleen.[44] Moreover, in this series the incidence correlated with the age at diagnosis and hence with the duration of exposure to gluten, although this finding has not been confirmed by other workers. Views differ as to whether there is a reversible element in the hyposplenism of untreated coeliac disease.[49]

Although we have heard of overwhelming infection in coeliac disease with hyposplenism, this is not documented in the literature and careful studies of mortality and morbidity in relation to splenic function in coeliac disease are needed. Impaired immunity,[8] an increase in platelet count,[7] and an increase in autoimmunity[9] in relation to hyposplenism in coeliac disease are documented. It has been suggested that the splenic atrophy may itself be a result of an underlying failure of lymphocytic immune surveillance which also results in autoantibody formation and autoimmune disease.[51] The defect in immunity in hyposplenism does not appear to be associated with the development of malignancy in coeliac disease.[42]

Drug absorption

The general principles governing absorption of drugs and their potential effects are discussed later in this chapter. Here we shall briefly look at the alterations in absorption of specific drugs in malabsorption states.

Antibiotics
For most purposes the effect of an antibiotic depends on the blood levels achieved, particularly the peak blood level. Thus changes in absorption and other factors affecting the blood level may be of crucial importance.

The effects of malabsorption syndromes differ from one disease to another and from one antibiotic to another,[36] and some of the information available is contradictory. The amount of systematic information available is small and most relies on blood level measurements, so that precise information about absorption and the contribution of other factors cannot be deduced.

In coeliac disease there is evidence[13, 37] to suggest that after oral doses of phenoxymethyl-penicillin, amoxycillin and pivampicillin lower blood levels than normal are reached (taken to imply decreased absorption), while ampicillin and lincomycin show no changes from normal, and some other antibiotics, including cephalexin, clindamycin, fucidin, sulphamethoxazole and trimethoprim show higher blood levels (taken to imply increased absorption). It is suggested that absorption of rifampicin is delayed but not decreased. In the case of erythromycin, the effect appears to depend upon the particular compound, in that the absorption of erythromycin stearate seems unchanged from normal while the absorption of erythromycin ethylsuccinate appears increased.

In jejunal diverticulosis there seems to be increased absorption of sulphamethoxazole, clindamycin, and trimethoprim. In Crohn's disease there appears to be decreased absorption of trimethoprim and lincomycin, and increased absorption of sulphamethoxazole and clindamycin. Trimethoprim and sulphamethoxazole are often formulated together as co-trimoxazole, and an increase in the absorption of one constituent with a decrease in the absorption of the other might well affect the efficacy of the combination. It appears that in Crohn's disease the direction of change in absorption for some antibiotics is similar to that found in coeliac disease but this does not apply to all antibiotics. Since, however, the mechanisms of malabsorption in Crohn's disease are complex, and differ from one patient to another, such results are not surprising.

Propranolol

Recorded plasma levels following oral administration of propranolol in patients with coeliac disease vary in different studies.[25, 38, 45] One study showed higher than normal plasma propranolol concentrations in treated coeliac disease. Another showed no change from normal in plasma levels but a decrease in absorption of perfused drug from the proximal jejunum in untreated coeliac disease. Yet another study showed increased plasma propranolol levels in treated and untreated coeliac disease with no significant difference between the two groups.

Other drugs

Fragmentary information is available on the blood levels of other drugs in malabsorption syndromes.

From consideration of steady state levels it is suggested that the absorption of digoxin is less in malabsorption states due to disease of the small intestine, and is unchanged in pancreatic insufficiency.[24]

Plasma curves of prednisolone following oral absorption have been found to be no different from normal in treated or untreated coeliac disease.[39]

Blood ethanol levels have been shown to be decreased in untreated coeliac disease.[12]

Folic acid absorption, as judged by serum levels, is decreased in coeliac disease, whether treated or untreated.[25]

Practical considerations

Conclusions about drug absorption cannot be drawn from plasma levels alone since these also depend on other factors. Drug absorption in malabsorption syndromes is extremely variable and unpredictable. The information available is fragmentary, derived from small and heterogeneous groups of patients, and often contradictory.

In clinical practice, modifications of drug regimens for patients with malabsorption cannot be suggested on the basis of the present evidence. It is necessary, however, to bear in mind that blood levels may be higher or lower than normal. When it is clinically important, drug administration should, if possible, be varied according to blood levels, or by careful monitoring of clinical effects.

REFERENCES

1 Andersson, H. & Bosaeus, I. (1981) Hyperoxaluria in malabsorptive states. *Urologia Internationalis*, **36,** 1–9.
2 Andersson, H. & Jagenburg, R. (1974) Fat-reduced diet in the treatment of hyperoxaluria in patients with ileopathy. *Gut*, **15,** 360–366.
3 Back, D. J., Bates, M., Breckenridge, A. M. *et al.* (1980) Drug metabolism by gastrointestinal mucosa: clinical aspects. In *Drug Absorption* (Ed.) Prescott, L. F. & Nimmo, W. S. pp. 80–87. Australia: Adis Press.
4 Badenoch, J. (1960) Steatorrhoea in the adult. *British Medical Journal*, ii, 879–887 & 963–974.
5 Bossak, E. T., Wang, C. I. & Adlersberg, D. (1957) Clinical aspects of the malabsorption syndrome (idiopathic sprue): observations in 94 patients. *Journal of Mount Sinai Hospital*, **24,** 286–303.
6 Bullen, A. W. & Losowsky, M. S. (1979) Consequences of impaired splenic function. *Clinical Science*, **57,** 129–137.
7 Bullen, A. W., Hall, R., Brown, R. C. & Losowsky, M. S. (1977) Mechanisms of thrombocytosis in coeliac disease. *Gut*, **18,** A962.
8 Bullen, A. W., Hall, R., Cooke, E. M. & Losowsky, M. S. (1977) Immunity and the hyposplenism of coeliac disease. *Gut*, **18,** A961–A962.
9 Bullen, A. W., Hall, R., Gowland, G. & Losowsky, M. S. (1978) Relationship of hyposplenism, adult coeliac disease and autoimmunity. *Gut*, **19,** A438.

10 Compston, J. E., Horton, L. W. L., Ayers, A. B. *et al.* (1978) Osteomalacia after small-intestinal resection. *Lancet*, **i**, 9–12.

11 Compston, J. E., Horton, L. W. L., Laker, M. F. *et al.* (1978) Bone disease after jejuno-ileal bypass for obesity. *Lancet*, **ii**, 1–4.

12 Cotton, P. B. & Walker, G. (1973) Ethanol absorption after gastric operations, and in the coeliac syndrome. *Postgraduate Medical Journal*, **49**, 27–28.

13 Davis, A. E. & Pirola, R. C. (1968) Absorption of phenoxymethyl penicillin in patients with steatorrhoea. *Australian Annals of Medicine*, **17**, 63–65.

14 Dharmsathaphorn, K., Freeman, D. H., Binder, H. J. & Dobbins, J. W. (1982) Increased risk of nephrolithiasis in patients with steatorrhoea. *Digestive Diseases and Sciences*, **27**, 401–405.

15 Dobbins, J. W. & Binder, H. J. (1977) Importance of the colon in enteric hyperoxaluria. *New England Journal of Medicine*, **296**, 298–301.

16 Drenick, E. J., Stanley, T. M., Wayne, A. *et al.* (1978) Renal damage with intestinal bypass. *Annals of Internal Medicine*, **89**, 594–599.

17 Driscoll R. H., Jr., Meredith, S. C., Sitrin, M. & Rosenberg, I. H. (1982) Vitamin D deficiency and bone disease in patients with Crohn's disease. *Gastroenterology*, **83**, 1252–1258.

18 Earnest, D. L. (1979) Enteric hyperoxaluria. *Advances in Internal Medicine*, **24**, 407–427.

19 Evans, W. B. & Wollaeger, E. E. (1966) Incidence and severity of nutritional deficiency states in chronic exocrine pancreatic insufficiency: comparison with non-tropical sprue. *American Journal of Digestive Diseases*, **11**, 594–606.

20 Fleming, C. R. & Phillips, S. F. (1982) Response of the small intestine to nutritional deficiencies. In *Gastroenterology 2: Small Intestine* (Ed.) Chadwick, V. S. & Phillips, S. pp. 332–344. London: Butterworth Scientific.

21 George, C. F. (1976) Absorption, distribution, and metabolism of drugs: effects of disease of the gut. *British Medical Journal*, **ii**, 742–744.

22 Hall, R. J. C. & Creamer, B. (1974) Hyperphagia in intestinal disease. *Gut*, **15**, 858–861.

23 Heier, H. E. (1980) Splenectomy and serious infections. *Scandinavian Journal of Haematology*, **24**, 5–12.

24 Heizer, W. D., Smith, T. W. & Goldfinger, S. E. (1971) Absorption of digoxin in patients with malabsorption syndromes. *New England Journal of Medicine*, **285**, 257–259.

25 Kitis, G., Lucas, M. L., Bishop, H. *et al.* (1982) Altered jejunal surface pH in coeliac disease: its effect on propranolol and folic acid absorption. *Clinical Science*, **63**, 373–380.

26 Losowsky, M. S., Walker, B. E. & Kelleher, J. (1974) *Malabsorption in Clinical Practice*. Edinburgh: Churchill Livingstone.

27 Mandell, I., Krauss, E. & Millan, J. C. (1980) Oxalate-induced acute renal failure in Crohn's disease. *American Journal of Medicine*, **69**, 628–632.

28 Mann, J. G., Brown, W. R. & Kern, F. (1970) The subtle and variable clinical expression of gluten-induced enteropathy (adult celiac disease, non-tropical sprue). An analysis of twenty-one consecutive cases. *American Journal of Medicine*, **48**, 357–366.

29 McDonald, G. B., Earnest, D. L. & Admirand, W. H. (1977) Hyperoxaluria correlates with fat malabsorption in patients with sprue. *Gut*, **18**, 561–566.

30 Melvin, K. E. W., Hepner, G. W., Bordier, P. *et al.* (1970) Calcium metabolism and bone pathology in adult coeliac disease. *Quarterly Journal of Medicine (New Series)*, **39**, 83–113.

31 Meredith, S. C. & Rosenberg, I. H. (1980) Gastrointestinal-hepatic disorders and osteomalacia. *Clinics in Endocrinology and Metabolism*, **9**, 131–150.

32 Mills, P. R., Brown, I. L. & Watkinson, G. (1980) Idiopathic chronic ulcerative enteritis. *Quarterly Journal of Medicine (New Series)*, **49**, 133–149.

33 Morgan, D. B., Paterson, C. R., Woods, C. G. *et al.* (1965) Search for osteomalacia in 1228 patients after gastrectomy and other operations on the stomach. *Lancet*, **ii**, 1085–1088.

34 Nagasue, N., Inokuchi, K., Kobayashi, M. & Saku, M. (1977) Mesenteric venous thrombosis occurring late after splenectomy. *British Journal of Surgery*, **64**, 781–783.

35 Palmer, K. R., Sherriff, S. B., Holdsworth, C. D. & Ryan, F. P. (1981) Further experience of hyposplenism in inflammatory bowel disease. *Quarterly Journal of Medicine (New Series)*, **50**, 463–471.

36 Parsons, R. L. (1976) The absorption of drugs in malabsorption syndromes. *Hospital Update*, **2**, 221–232.

37 Parsons, R. L., Hossack, G. & Paddock, G. (1975) The absorption of antibiotics in adult patients with coeliac disease. *Journal of Antimicrobial Chemotherapy*, **1**, 39–50.

38 Parsons, R. L., Kaye, C. M., Raymond, K. *et al.* (1976) Absorption of propranolol and practolol in coeliac disease. *Gut*, **17**, 139–143.

39 Pickup, M. E., Farah, F., Lowe, J. R. *et al.* (1979) Prednisolone absorption in coeliac disease. *European Journal of Drug Metabolism and Pharmacokinetics*, **2**, 87–89.

40 Ramalingaswami, V. (1969) Interface of protein nutrition and medicine in the tropics. *Lancet*, **ii**, 733–736.

41 Regan, P. T. & DiMagno, E. P. (1980) Exocrine pancreatic insufficiency in celiac sprue: a cause of treatment failure. *Gastroenterology*, **78**, 484–487.

42 Robertson, D. A. F., Swinson, C. M., Hall, R. & Losowsky, M. S. (1982) Coeliac disease, splenic function and malignancy. *Gut*, **23**, 666–669.

43 Robinette, C. D. & Fraumeni, J. F., Jr. (1977) Splenectomy and subsequent mortality in veterans of the 1939–45 war. *Lancet*, **ii**, 127–129.

44 Robinson, P. J., Bullen, A. W., Hall, R. *et al.* (1980) Splenic size and function in adult coeliac disease. *British Journal of Radiology*, **53**, 532–537.

45 Sandle, G. I., Ward, A., Rawlins, M. D. & Record, C. O. (1982) Propranolol absorption in untreated coeliac disease. *Clinical Science*, **63**, 81–85.

46 Smith, L. H., Fromm, H. & Hofmann, A. F. (1972) Acquired hyperoxaluria, nephrolithiasis and intestinal disease. *New England Journal of Medicine*, **286**, 1371–1375.

47 Swinson, C. M. & Levi, A. J. (1980) Is coeliac disease underdiagnosed? *British Medical Journal*, **281**, 1258–1260.

48 Tandon, B. N., Banks, P. A., George, P. K. *et al.* (1970) Recovery of exocrine pancreatic function in adult protein-calorie malnutrition. *Gastroenterology*, **58**, 358–362.

49 Trewby, P. N., Chipping, P. M., Palmer, S. J. *et al.* (1981) Splenic atrophy in adult coeliac disease: is it reversible? *Gut*, **22**, 628–632.

50 Volwiler, W. (1957) Gastrointestinal malabsorption syndromes. *American Journal of Medicine*, **23**, 250–268.

51 Wardrop, C. A. J., Dagg, J. H., Lee, F. D. *et al.* (1975) Immunological abnormalities in splenic atrophy. *Lancet*, **ii**, 4–7.

COELIAC DISEASE AND RELATED DISORDERS

COELIAC DISEASE

Coeliac disease is the term most commonly used in the United Kingdom for the condition associated with an abnormal jejunal mucosa caused by gluten in the diet. Gluten-sensitive enteropathy is perhaps a more descriptive title but is not in common usage. In the USA coeliac sprue is the preferred terminology; there is no reason to continue to use such terms as non-tropical sprue, coeliac syndrome, idiopathic steatorrhoea or primary malabsorption. Dermatitis herpetiformis is a subepidermal blistering eruption; at least two thirds of those with this disease will have an abnormal jejunal mucosa.[62] This enteropathy is due to gluten sensitivity and improves on gluten withdrawal.[63] Only those features of dermatitis herpetiformis that differ from coeliac disease will be discussed here.

Booth[8] defined coeliac disease in the adult as a condition in which there is an abnormal jejunal mucosa which improves morphologically when treated with a gluten-free diet and relapses when gluten is reintroduced. This definition is brief and practical and has the advantage that it does not specify the exact nature of the histological abnormality and therefore includes patients with partial as well as subtotal villous atrophy. Gluten reintroduction into the diet followed by a further jejunal biopsy is included in this definition and, although not always performed in the typical case, it is essential to the diagnosis when a good clinical response does not occur. Whether the term coeliac disease should be used for the rare patients who have the typical histological lesion, but do not respond to a gluten-free diet, is very controversial and will be discussed later. A number of disorders can occasionally produce subtotal villous atrophy of the jejunal mucosa in adults (Table 8.24), but in clinical practice coeliac disease is the most likely diagnosis and gluten withdrawal should be instituted in the majority of cases.

Table 8.24 Disorders which can produce subtotal villous atrophy of the jejunal mucosa in adults.

Coeliac disease ⎫	
Dermatitis herpetiformis ⎬	Gluten sensitive
Zollinger–Ellison syndrome	
Giardiasis	
Tropical sprue	
Hypogammaglobulinaemia	
'Unresponsive coeliac disease'	

Incidence

This varies throughout the world, the disease being quite common in the United Kingdom with a frequency of about 1/2000. In the West of Ireland the incidence is very high at 1/300.[70] Coeliac disease has now been described in virtually all parts of the world. The true prevalence of the disease is unknown and difficult to study as many cases are asymptomatic.

Inheritance

There is an increased incidence of coeliac disease in the families of patients with 10–20% of siblings being affected.

In 1972, the genetic marker HLA-B8 was found in 80% of patients with coeliac disease compared with 20% in a control population.[22, 101] More recent work has shown coeliac disease to be strongly associated not only with the haplotype B8 but also with CW7, DR3/AW24, BW59 and DR3, and less strongly with AX-B12-DR7.[5] The incidence of these different genetic markers varies in people from different geographic regions and ethnic origins.[68] It now seems that coeliac disease is primarily associated with HLA-DR3, and the association with B8 is due to the linkage disequilibrium that normally exists between B8 and DR3. However, less than 0.2% of individuals with HLA-B8 and HLA-DR3 antigens will develop coeliac disease. This finding, and the lack of complete concordance for coeliac disease in identical twins, suggests that additional genetic loci such as the immunoglobulin heavy chain allotype locus[48] are involved, and that possibly some unidentified environmental factor plays a role.[78]

Mann *et al.*[60] found that coeliac disease was strongly associated with a specific B lymphocyte surface antigen recognized by maternal antisera. Pena *et al.*[78] found this B cell antigen in 70% of patients with coeliac disease compared with 6% of controls, and its presence was independent of HLA status. This finding has led to speculation that this cell surface antigen might be a receptor site for gluten on the surface of B lymphocytes resulting in cell activation after gluten exposure.

Pathology

Paulley[77] described the characteristic intestinal lesion of coeliac disease in surgical specimens obtained from two patients. Shiner[93] in the United Kingdom and Rubin *et al.*[87] in the USA demonstrated the classical findings in the intestinal mucosa using peroral suction biopsy instruments.

Coeliac disease predominantly affects the mucosa of the proximal small bowel. Mucosal damage gradually decreases in severity towards the ileum, but in a small number of patients the lesion extends into the ileum.[100] This distribution reflects the fact that gluten, or its 'toxic' fragment, is digested to non-toxic substances before reaching the distal small intestine. Rubin et al.[88] infused gluten into the ileum and rectum of coeliac patients and produced mucosal abnormalities. The jejunal mucosal lesions are usually confluent, but a patchy lesion can occasionally occur[90] and is typically found in dermatitis herpetiformis.

Under the dissecting microscope ($\times 40$) the characteristic finding is a flat mucosal surface without villi (Figure 8.36). A few small elevations in the epithelium are sometimes seen, giving a 'mosaic' pattern. There is a good correlation between the stereomicroscopic findings and those seen on light microscopy in a typical case, but both techniques should always be performed because difficulties of interpretation can arise when 'convolutions' are seen on stereomicroscopy. These convolutions are produced by short, broad villi, with some villi being fused to form long ridges. This finding may occasionally be seen in normal subjects and confirmation of villous atrophy must be obtained from histological examination. Scanning electron microscopy shows the flat mucosal surface, and crypt openings are easily seen.[66] This technique is not performed routinely.

Histological examination confirms the loss of normal villous architecture seen on stereomicroscopy. The mucosal surface is flat, the intestinal crypts are elongated, and there is infiltration with chronic inflammatory cells in the lamina propria (Figure 8.37). Subtotal villous atrophy has always been used to describe this lesion, but true atrophy of the mucosa is not present because crypt hypertrophy compensates for villous loss and thus mucosal thickness is normal or increased. A small percentage of patients have partial villous atrophy only; here the villi are stunted and club-shaped but still present. In dermatitis herpetiformis the mucosal lesion is usually not as marked as in coeliac disease, partial villous atrophy being the commonest finding. Normal villous architecture is seen in approximately 20% of cases. Weinstein et al.[109] showed that the mucosal damage could be increased in dermatitis herpetiformis by adding gluten to the diet.

The structure of the villi in the intestinal mucosa depends on new epithelial cells formed in the crypts migrating upwards towards the villous tip. This process, which normally takes 48–72 hours, leads to continual extrusion of cells at the villous tip. In untreated coeliac disease the rate of cell loss from the villous tip is increased six-fold[83] with compensatory increased cell proliferation in the crypts. The crypts are increased in length and girth and the cells show an increased rate of mitosis.[74] Goblet cells in the crypts are usually normal while Paneth cells are increased in number.[107] The function of the Paneth cells is unclear.

The normal columnar surface cells are usually replaced by cuboidal or squamous cells,[7] and the brush border is distorted and irregular with the number of microvilli on electron microscopy diminished. These morphological findings are paralleled by histochemical changes showing decreased levels of brush border disaccharidases and alkaline phosphatase.

Normal intestinal mucosa contains lymphocytes both in the lamina propria and the epithelium (6–40 lymphocytes: 100 epithelial cells). These intraepithelial lymphocytes (IEL) appear to be T cells that have migrated from the lamina propria. The ratio of intraepithelial lymphocytes

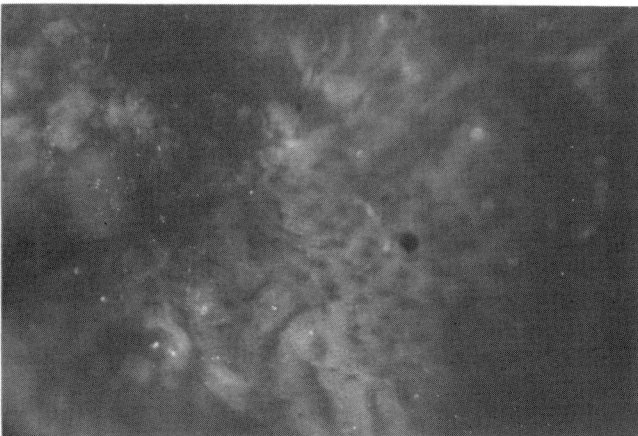

Fig. 8.36 Dissecting microscope appearance of jejunal mucosa in coeliac disease.

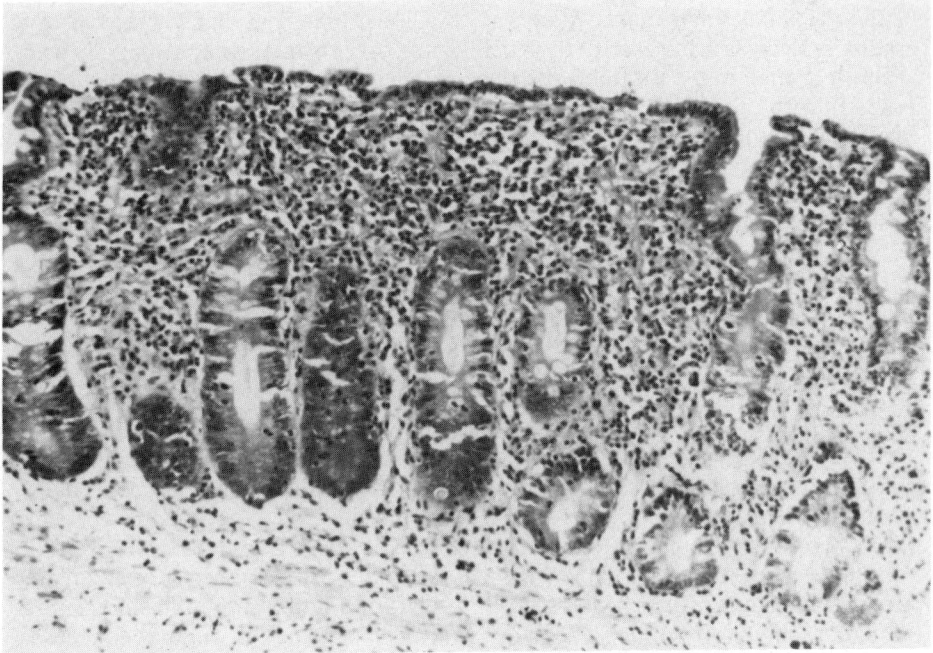

Fig. 8.37 Histological appearance of jejunal mucosa in coeliac disease.

to epithelial cells is raised (60–160 lymphocytes: 100 epithelial cells) in virtually all patients with coeliac disease.[28] The absolute number of lymphocytes within the epithelium is not increased. The increased ratio occurs because of the reduction in the number of epithelial cells resulting from loss of villi. The finding of an increased IEL count occurs in other small intestinal disorders, such as tropical sprue. A high mitotic index among these intraepithelial lymphocytes is, however, said to be exclusive to coeliac disease.[67] The pathogenetic importance of these intraepithelial lymphocytes is still uncertain. In dermatitis herpetiformis a raised intraepithelial lymphocyte count is found in over 95% of patients, irrespective of the macroscopic appearance of the mucosa.[32] It is suggested that the raised intraepithelial count is an early or more reliable sign of a damaged mucosa.

In the lamina propria there is an increase in all cell types, predominantly plasma cells and lymphocytes. In the normal intestinal mucosa IgA-producing cells are most abundant, but IgM-producing cells predominate in the coeliac mucosa. Polymorphonuclear leucocytes, eosinophils and mast cells are also increased in number.

The basement membrane of the epithelium cells is sometimes thickened and irregular. Subepithelial collagenization is seen in approximately one-third of patients with coeliac disease. The term 'collagenous sprue'[108] was used to describe patients with a thick collagen layer thought to be associated with a poor prognosis after treatment. This association, however, is unjustified as most patients with increased collagen respond normally to a gluten-free diet.[9]

Aetiology

Dicke *et al.*[19] observed that during the Second World War, children with coeliac disease improved when wheat and rye flour were in short supply. Van de Kamer *et al.*[104] subsequently showed that gluten was the substance that damaged the small intestinal mucosa of coeliac patients. Gluten is found in wheat, rye, barley and oats, all of which have been found to be toxic to the intestinal mucosa of susceptible individuals.

An aqueous extract of wheat flour consists mainly of starch and albumin, while the alcoholic extract (water-insoluble) contains gluten (Figure 8.38). Fraser *et al.*[31] showed that a peptic–tryptic digest of gluten was toxic to the intestinal mucosa. This digest (Fraser Fraction III) contained many different peptides of varying molecular size. Gliadin is the alcohol-soluble portion of gluten and is toxic to the intestinal mucosa of coeliac patients, while glutenin (alcohol-insoluble) is not. Gliadin proteins are divided into four groups – alpha, beta, gamma and omega – on the basis of their electrophoretic

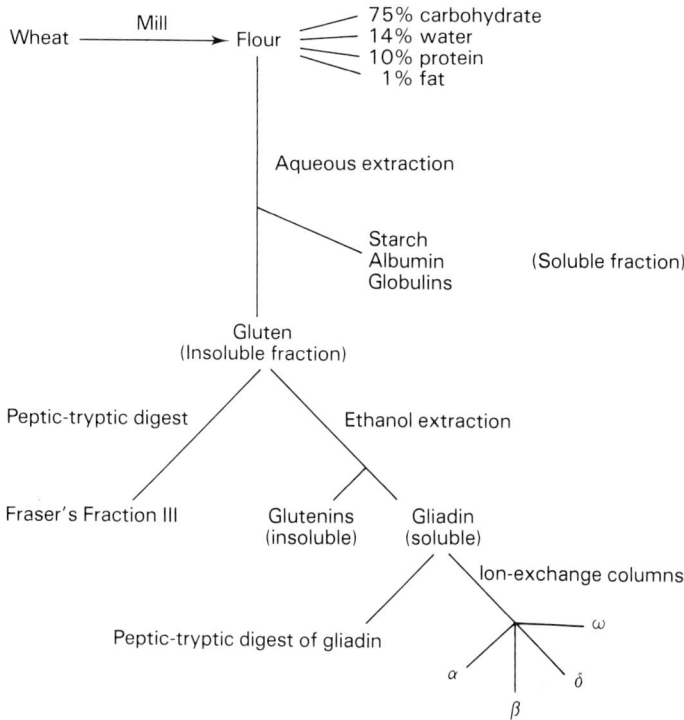

```
Wheat ──Mill──▶ Flour ⟨ 75% carbohydrate
                       14% water
                       10% protein
                        1% fat
```

Fig. 8.38   Fractionation of wheat.

mobility. Most studies have shown that only the alpha fraction is toxic,[37] although Jos et al.,[47] using an in vitro organ culture method, showed that all four gliadin fractions were toxic. This study highlights the difficulties in assessing toxicity: firstly, because of the different proteins in gliadin, separation techniques to produce pure substances are extremely difficult; secondly, there are discrepancies between results obtained by in vivo techniques instilling gliadin fractions into coeliac patients compared with in vitro techniques or organ culture.[85] Furthermore, many workers have used gliadin extracted from flour containing several varieties of wheat; these different wheats are likely to have different component proteins.[76] We are thus still not sure of the exact nature of the toxic compound.

It has been suggested by Phelan et al.[82] that the toxicity of gluten resides in the carbohydrate side-chain. They showed that removal of the carbohydrate side-chain from gliadin reduced its toxicity. This work has not been reproduced elsewhere.

The mechanism of how and why gluten damages the intestinal mucosa in susceptible individuals is not known. The possible mechanisms of mucosal damage following gluten ingestion include non-immunological mechanisms, such as a specific enzyme deficiency, and the more popular view of a primary local immunological reaction.

The idea that an intestinal peptidase deficiency was the primary abnormality in coeliac disease was first suggested by Fraser et al.[31] when he showed that digestion of gluten with fresh hog intestinal mucosa removed the toxicity. The absence of this postulated peptidase, and hence incomplete gluten digestion, suggested that accumulation of toxic material in the intestinal lumen or mucosa might cause the damage.[21] The levels of mucosal peptidase necessary for gliadin digestion are reduced in the mucosa of untreated coeliacs,[84] but following a gluten-free diet they return to normal,[80] suggesting that peptidase deficiency merely occurs as a consequence of the mucosal damage. Clearly, if a deficiency of a specific peptidase were the primary defect, the enzyme levels would have to be low in patients with a 'normal' mucosa on a gluten-free diet as well as in untreated patients.

More recently it has been proposed that gluten may act like a lectin and bind to a glycoprotein on the mucosal surface.[110] These workers were able to prepare a fraction of gluten which bound to the intestinal mucosa of patients with coeliac disease, but not to normal intestinal mucosa. This binding was interfered with by free carbohydrate which suggested that gluten might act in a way similar to plant lectins. This finding, if substantiated, implies that an abnormality of glycoprotein structure in the surface membrane is the primary abnormality.

The most popular theory to explain gluten toxicity is that the disease is due to an abnormal immunological reaction to gluten.[3] Many immunological abnormalities have indeed been demonstrated in patients with coeliac disease, but these return to normal after treatment, suggesting that most of them are secondary to the disease process itself rather than a primary defect. The strong association with a particular histocompatibility type, which in turn may be adjacent to an immune response locus, and the response to steroids[10] make the immune theory attractive.[64]

Humoral immune responses

Serum IgM levels are low in two-thirds of patients with untreated coeliac disease.[38] This low level appears to be due to decreased synthesis, but increased loss, mainly through the intestinal wall, also occurs. Serum IgA levels were initially reported as increased, but this has not been confirmed and in most cases of coeliac disease the serum level is normal. Serum IgG levels are sometimes low. All of these abnormalities return to normal on a gluten-free diet.

There is an increased incidence of selective serum IgA deficiency in patients with coeliac disease compared with the general population (1/50 compared with 1/700), and some patients with generalized hypogammaglobulinaemia and coeliac disease have been reported.[2]

Plasma cells found in the lamina propria of the jejunal mucosa contain IgA, IgG and IgM.[54] The IgM plasma cells and the IgA-containing cells in the lamina propria are increased in untreated coeliac disease. These cellular changes are reflected in the intestinal secretion, where there is an increased concentration of both IgA and IgM.[55]

Antibody response following primary immunization with a bacteriophage is impaired in coeliac patients, and after a further challenge the secondary response is further impaired. This secondary response shows a higher-than-normal production of IgM antibody, suggesting a failure to convert to IgG production. This degree of response was more marked in ill patients and those patients with splenic atrophy.[4] However, the results of immunization with tetanus toxoid and with polio vaccine are normal.[102]

Antibodies to a number of substances found in the diet, including gluten and milk proteins, are found in the serum of patients with coeliac disease.[13] These antibodies are, however, occasionally seen in normal subjects and in patients with other gastrointestinal diseases such as Crohn's disease.[1] The widespread nature of these antibodies to many dietary proteins other than gluten make it likely that they are not important as a primary mechanism, but are probably due to the damaged mucosa allowing increased permeability of dietary macromolecules. Indeed, these serum antibody levels correlate with the degree of intestinal mucosal damage in coeliac disease and dermatitis herpetiformis (Figure 8.39).[51]

Antireticulin antibodies are found in the serum in up to 75% of patients with coeliac disease.[93] These antibodies have been shown to also occur in 25% of patients with Crohn's disease and occasionally in other gastrointestinal diseases. Their significance is not known; the original suggestion that there was a cross-reactivity with gluten has not been confirmed and it is now generally considered that the increased level of antibody reflects increased absorption of dietary reticulin. An increased incidence of other autoimmune antibodies is also found, the most consistent being antibodies to thyroid and gastric parietal cells.[56] Antinuclear and smooth muscle antibodies are also found in higher proportions than in the general population. Patients with dermatitis herpetiformis have a higher percentage of gastric parietal cell antibodies associated with

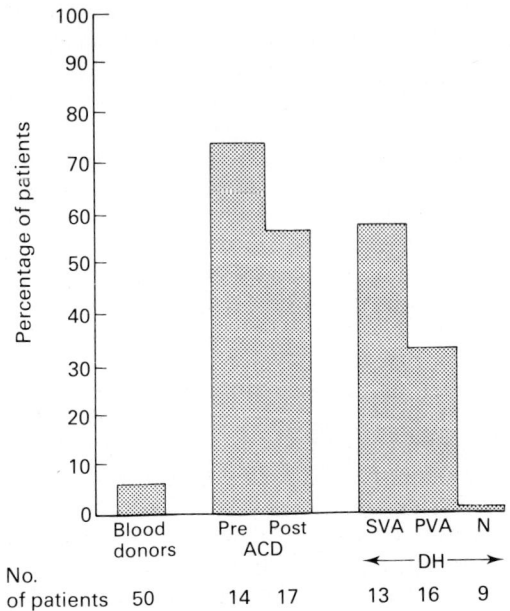

Fig. 8.39 Food antibodies in the serum of patients with coeliac disease (ACD) and dermatitis herpetiformis (DH): percentage of patients with one or more positive tests. SVA = subtotal villous atrophy; PVA = partial villous atrophy; N = normal mucosa. From Kumar, P. J., Ferguson, A., Lancaster-Smith, M. and Clark, M. L. (1976) *Scandinavian Journal of Gastroenterology, 11*, 5–9, with kind permission of the authors and the editor.

achlorhydria and gastric atrophy, and higher levels of immunoglobulins in jejunal juice than patients with coeliac disease.

In keeping with the finding of increased serum autoantibodies is an increased incidence of autoimmune diseases in patients with coeliac disease (Table 8.25). These include thyroid disease, diabetes and chronic liver disease.[89] In addition, an increased incidence of these diseases has been found in the relatives of patients with coeliac disease.[39] A number of patients with allergic alveolitis and coeliac disease have been found,[54] and precipitins to various avian antigens are found in the serum of 40% of patients.[69]

Table 8.25 Reported immunological disorders associated with coeliac disease.

*Endocrine**
  Thyroid
  Diabetes mellitus type 1
  Addison's disease

Pulmonary
  Fibrosing alveolitis
  Allergic alveolitis
  Sarcoidosis
  Idiopathic pulmonary haemosiderosis

Hepatic
  Chronic liver disease

Gastrointestinal
  Ulcerative colitis
  Pernicious anaemia
Rheumatic
  Systemic lupus erythematosus
  Rheumatoid arthritis
  Sjögren's syndrome
  Polyarteritis nodosa

Dermatological
  Cutaneous vasculitis
  Vitiligo

Miscellaneous
  Selective IgA deficiency
  Atopic diseases

* These are more common in dermatitis herpetiformis where the gut lesion is less severe.

Cellular immune responses

The total number of peripheral blood lymphocytes is reduced in untreated coeliac disease; the number of T cells is also reduced.[72] The most likely cause for this finding is loss of lymphocytes through the damaged mucosa. The cell counts return to normal on treatment with a gluten-free diet. The lymphocyte response to phytohaemaglutinin is depressed in coeliac disease,[90] and further evidence for a depression in T cell function is an impaired response when these cells are incubated with the Epstein–Barr virus.[59]

Splenic atrophy is found in patients with coeliac disease,[63] indicated by the presence of Howell–Jolly bodies on routine blood films and pitted red cells detected by interference phase microscopy.[16] Radioactive uptake studies show that two-thirds of patients with coeliac disease have splenic atrophy.[81] Originally splenic atrophy was thought to be irreversible,[103] but recent work suggests some reversibility on a gluten-free diet.[73] The mechanism of splenic atrophy is uncertain.

Immune complexes and complement

Circulating immune complexes were found in a group of coeliac patients, but the finding has not been confirmed, partly due to technical problems involved in their detection.[3] Lower C3 and C4 levels have been found in coeliac patients, and if patients are challenged with gluten the C3 levels fall and complement breakdown products can be detected.[20] Immunofluorescent studies have shown increased IgA and C3 deposition in the basement membrane of the jejunal mucosa of untreated coeliac patients.[95]

Specific immunological responses to gluten

Delayed hypersensitivity by skin testing was initially reported as being positive in coeliac disease when compared with a control population, but this has not been confirmed.[85] Lymphocytic activation by gluten subfractions in vitro is found by most workers, although the results are by no means uniform.[3] Gluten fractions have been shown to inhibit leucocyte migration, and this finding has been used as evidence of lymphokine production.[12] A reappraisal of this test[97] suggests that the inhibition caused by the gluten subfraction is not due to lymphokine production by sensitized lymphocytes, but is caused by a cytophilic antibody.

Trier and Browning[104] were the first to show that jejunal mucosa could be cultured in vitro. A number of studies have been performed since then to try and elucidate the mechanism of gluten toxicity, but technical difficulty has prevented uniform results.[42, 43] Falchuk *et al.*[23] measured the levels of the brush border enzyme alkaline phosphatase as an indicator of mucosal changes. In the jejunal mucosa of normal subjects, and patients with untreated or treated coeliac disease, the alkaline phosphatase levels rose during culture. When gluten peptides were added to the culture medium, the rise in enzyme activity was abolished in untreated coeliac mucosa but there was no effect on the mucosa of treated patients or of normal control subjects. It was possible, however, to inhibit the rise in alkaline phosphatase in the treated patients by co-culturing these biopsies with biopsies from untreated patients. This suggests that gluten peptides are not directly toxic but in some way they induce the mucosa to release a soluble factor that in turn damages the epithelial cells. Unfortunately, these studies have not been reproduced.[44]

Ferguson *et al.*[29] cultured jejunal mucosa in the presence or absence of gluten. The culture medium obtained from control subjects did not inhibit leucocyte migration, but inhibition was seen with material from patients with untreated coeliac disease.

All of the above evidence suggests that an abnormal response to gluten is important in the pathogenesis of coeliac disease. It depends on the presence of gluten in the upper gastrointestinal tract and a genetic predisposition to develop the disease. Gluten presumably in some way enters the mucosa either through the intestinal cell or by binding to a specific surface receptor. An immunological response then occurs, possibly producing a gluten antibody. However, no evidence has yet been found for the presence of an antibody in the jejunal epithelium, or for the existence of gluten antibodies that can cross-react with epithelial cell antigens. The formation of antigen–antibody complexes with fixation of complement components, followed by release of cytotoxic agents within the lamina propria, may then be responsible for the tissue damage.

Clinical features

Coeliac disease presents at any age (Figure 8.40), but only the presentation in adults will be discussed here. The peak incidence of this disease is in the third and fourth decades and there is a female preponderance.

The symptoms of adult coeliac disease are many (Table 8.26) and often non-specific; there may be no gastrointestinal symptoms.[14] A

Table 8.26 The symptoms of adult coeliac disease.

Symptoms	Percentage affected
Diarrhoea	81
Steatorrhoea	50
Weight loss	57
Lassitude	52
Abdominal pain	36
Anorexia	24
'Wind'	24
Mouth ulcers	23

number of vague symptoms, such as tiredness, lethargy and malaise, are often attributed to coeliac disease, but these symptoms probably occur in this disease no more frequently than in the general population. Some patients are completely asymptomatic as evidenced by relatives of patients with coeliac disease who have mucosal abnormalities without symptoms. Typically patients with dermatitis herpetiformis have no gastrointestinal symptoms and present because of their irritating blistering rash.

The commonest features are diarrhoea, abdominal discomfort and nutritional disturbances consisting mainly of weight loss and anaemia. Mouth ulcers and stomatitis are frequent and often tend to be intermittent.

Diarrhoea is found in 70–80% of patients and may be watery or typical of steatorrhoea. It can be intermittent, sometimes alternating with constipation, and can be a relatively mild feature. A history of diarrhoea in childhood is noted in less than a quarter of adult cases.

Generalized abdominal discomfort with distension and borborygmi is often present, but severe abdominal pain is unusual. There may be no weight loss, but occasionally severely emaciated patients are seen. The weight loss is mainly due to anorexia; the malabsorption that is present is trivial when compared to dietary intake.

The anaemia is predominantly caused by folate and iron deficiency; vitamin B_{12} deficiency is rare and only occurs when the ileum is

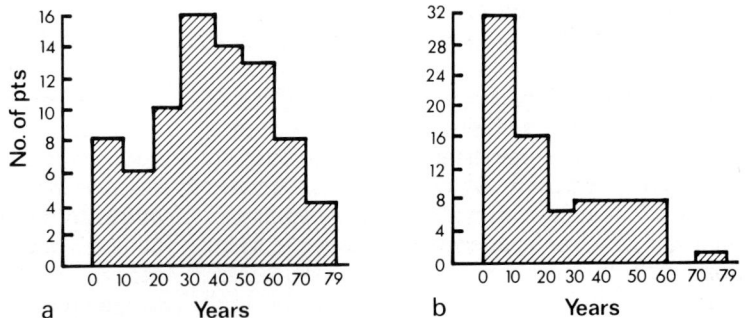

Fig. 8.40 (a) Age at diagnosis and (b) age of first symptoms of 79 patients with coeliac disease.

involved in the disease. Osteomalacia and tetany, which used to occur in up to 10% of patients with coeliac disease, are now much rarer. Rarely patients with dermatitis herpetiformis present with gross malabsorption, osteomalacia and anaemia.

Hypogonadism occurs in 5–10% of men with coeliac disease.[25] Reversible infertility has been described in both men and women with coeliac disease; improvement in semen quality and pregnancy in coeliac patients occurs after dietary gluten withdrawal. The mechanisms involved in the pathogenesis of this phenomenon are still obscure. Reversible androgen insensitivity occurs in men which in other situations has been associated with reduced sperm count.[26, 34] A disturbance of pituitary regulation of gonadal function is seen in some patients with coeliac disease and may be a contributory factor to endocrine abnormalities and infertility. It is possible that vitamin and/or trace element deficiency may be an additional factor in producing infertility.

A number of neurological symptoms have been described in coeliac disease[75] including muscle weakness, paraesthesiae, epilepsy and ataxia. A peripheral neuropathy may be demonstrated in some patients, and demyelination syndromes and cerebral atrophy have been described. Occasionally, these features are due to B_{12} deficiency, but often in these rare patients no specific deficiency is found, although deficiency of a number of vitamins and trace metals have been suggested. In most cases these neurological syndromes do not respond to a gluten-free diet.

A number of other diseases have been found in association with coeliac disease, in particular inflammatory bowel disease, chronic liver disease, thyroid disease and insulin-dependent diabetes. Allergic alveolitis due to exposure to birds (bird fancier's lung), fibrosing alveolitis and sarcoidosis have also been described, and in some series up to 20% of coeliac patients have evidence of another autoimmune disease.[89] Autoimmune diseases are seen slightly more frequently in dermatitis herpetiformis.

Physical signs

The physical findings if present are related to the anaemia and malnutrition; few signs are found in the abdomen. Some distension may be noted and there is occasionally ascites due to severe hypoalbuminaemia. Hepatomegaly occurs in some malnourished patients due to fatty infiltration.

The patient is often pale because of the anaemia and koilonychia may be present due to iron deficiency. Angular stomatitis, mouth ulcers and atrophic glossitis occur and may be due to vitamin deficiency.

In the severely ill patient, emaciation may be present with dependent oedema. The skin may be dry due to severe dehydration. Skin pigmentation and occasionally clubbing are seen. Spontaneous bruising due to vitamin K deficiency, and follicular hyperkeratosis due to vitamin A deficiency, are rare. A positive Chvostek's or Trousseau's sign is found with severe calcium and/or magnesium depletion. Bone tenderness and myopathy with spontaneous fractures are found with osteomalacia.

All of these latter findings are rare and are due to malabsorption and malnutrition and therefore are not specific for coeliac disease.

Investigations

Haematology

Anaemia occurs in approximately 50% of patients with coeliac disease, the varying incidence between different reported series often reflecting different referral patterns.[15] In some cases, although the haemoglobin may be normal, the mean corpuscular volume (MCV) is raised due to folate deficiency. Folate deficiency is almost invariably present in coeliac disease[40] and measurement of the red cell folate is a useful diagnostic indicator. Although malabsorption of folate can be demonstrated, a low folate intake due to anorexia is by far the most important cause of the deficiency. Vitamin B_{12} deficiency with low serum levels is confined to a small number of patients with more extensive disease involving the ileum. However, if investigated, some degree of vitamin B_{12} malabsorption is found in 75% of coeliac patients.[100] Iron deficiency anaemia is common due to some degree of malabsorption and increased iron loss in desquamated intestinal epithelial cells. Because of the mixed iron, folate, and occasionally B_{12} deficiency, the MCV may be normal, but the routine blood smear will show both micro- and macrocytosis with hypersegmented polymorphs and Howell–Jolly bodies. The finding of Howell–Jolly bodies in the absence of a splenectomy is almost diagnostic of coeliac disease. The bone marrow findings, because of the mixed deficiency pattern, varies from normoblastic with no stainable iron to a megaloblastic picture.[40] In dermatitis herpetiformis, the haemoglobin and blood picture are usually normal, but if abnormal, subtotal villous atrophy is almost invariably found on jejunal biopsy.

Leucopenia and thrombocytopenia are very rare. The prothrombin time may be prolonged due to malabsorption of vitamin K. Vitamin B_6 deficiency causing a sideroblastic anaemia has been described.[18]

Biochemistry

In most patients with coeliac disease, no abnormality is found in the routine biochemical tests normally performed. In severely ill patients with diarrhoea, serum potassium and magnesium may be low. A low serum calcium and low serum vitamin D level are found, and osteomalacia can be demonstrated on bone biopsy.[15] A raised serum alkaline phosphatase can be associated with osteomalacia, but in addition it may reflect liver dysfunction due to severe malnutrition (fatty liver). The serum albumin level is reduced in approximately 30% of patients due to protein loss from the gut and impaired albumin synthesis. Abnormal serum immunoglobulins are frequently found as discussed earlier; determination of reticulin[93] and gliadin antibodies[49] are sometimes useful. A number of gastrointestinal hormones have been measured in this disease. Reduced secretin and cholycystokinin/pancreazymin release is in keeping with the finding of reduced exocrine pancreatic function and a very sluggish gallbladder response to food.[11] A failure of gastric inhibitory polypeptide (GIP) release has also been demonstrated and serum enteroglucagon levels are elevated.[6]

Gastrointestinal function tests

In the uncomplicated case these tests are now superfluous and of academic interest only, as whenever coeliac disease is suspected a jejunal biopsy must be performed.

A number of oral tolerance tests have been used over the years where the test substance is given by mouth and either urinary or faecal excretion or blood levels are measured. The most popular have involved the carbohydrates glucose, lactose or xylose. The glucose tolerance test is affected by many things, so that xylose tolerance has been used more frequently.[99] In most patients with coeliac disease, either the serum level or the urinary excretion after an oral load of xylose is abnormal, but unfortunately some cases will be missed if this is the only test used for diagnosis.

Faecal fat estimation is still the best way to investigate a patient with suspected steatorrhoea, although it is only abnormal in half of the patients with coeliac disease (Figure 8.41). Measurement of the serum carotene is seldom per-

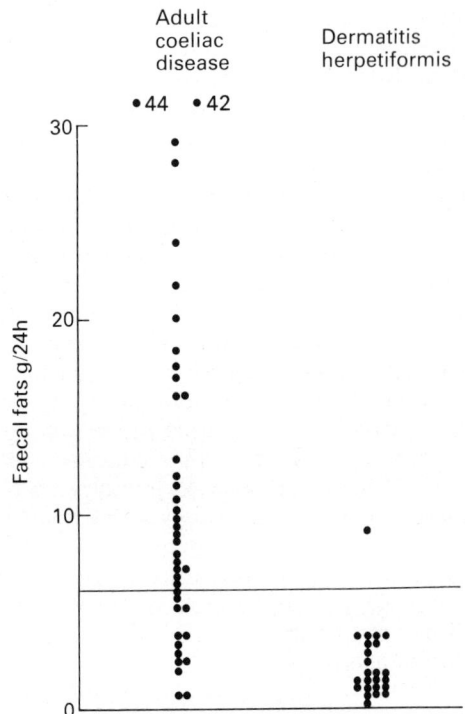

Fig. 8.41 Presence of steatorrhoea in coeliac disease and dermatitis herpetiformis.

formed; more recently measurement of ^{14}C-labelled lipid in blood or stools after an oral load has been advocated.

Tests of protein absorption are not usually performed. Protein loss can, however, be demonstrated by giving intravenous radioactive chromium chloride to label the circulating albumin in vivo. The faeces should contain little radioactivity unless there is excess protein loss.

Malabsorption of folate, B_{12} and iron are usually inferred from the serum levels, but absorption tests have been performed in some patients, and malabsorption of iron and folate are almost invariably present.

Vitamin B_{12} absorption, measured with a whole body counter or with a Schilling test, is used as a test of ileal function. Malabsorption of B_{12} occurs in approximately 75% of patients. Bacterial overgrowth due to intestinal stasis may rarely contribute to B_{12} deficiency.

Using intestinal perfusion techniques, malabsorption of glucose, amino acids and peptides can be demonstrated. Water and electrolyte secretion is seen in some patients when perfused with glucose bicarbonate solutions.[53] This secretory state may contribute to the diarrhoea seen in coeliac patients. Ileal adaptation in most cases will, however, compensate for the jejunal secretory state.[95]

The small intestinal mucosa of patients with untreated coeliac disease is abnormally permeable to large molecules such as lactulose and cellobiose. Tests of intestinal permeability using oral loads of sugar have been used both in diagnosis and in order to assess response to treatment.[35] In addition to their lack of specificity for coeliac disease, the difficulties in measuring the sugars has meant that this test has not had widespread use.

Radiology
In patients with mild coeliac disease, the small bowel appears normal radiologically in approximately 20%. The more severely ill the patient, the more widespread the intestinal involvement radiologically.[50]

Dilatation of the jejunum and, less frequently,

of the ileum can be seen (Figure 8.42). An abnormal fold pattern with flocculation of the barium can occur, partly due to excess intestinal secretion. None of these findings are specific and they have occasionally been seen in patients with no evidence of gastrointestinal disease but with hypoalbuminaemia.[24] Osteomalacia with pseudofractures may be seen if a skeletal survey is performed.

Jejunal biopsy
This is the definitive test for coeliac disease and must be performed in all suspected cases. It is unjustifiable to submit any patient of whatever age to a gluten-free diet unless a biopsy has been performed. There are a number of instruments used to obtain jejunal biopsies, the most common being used in this country is the

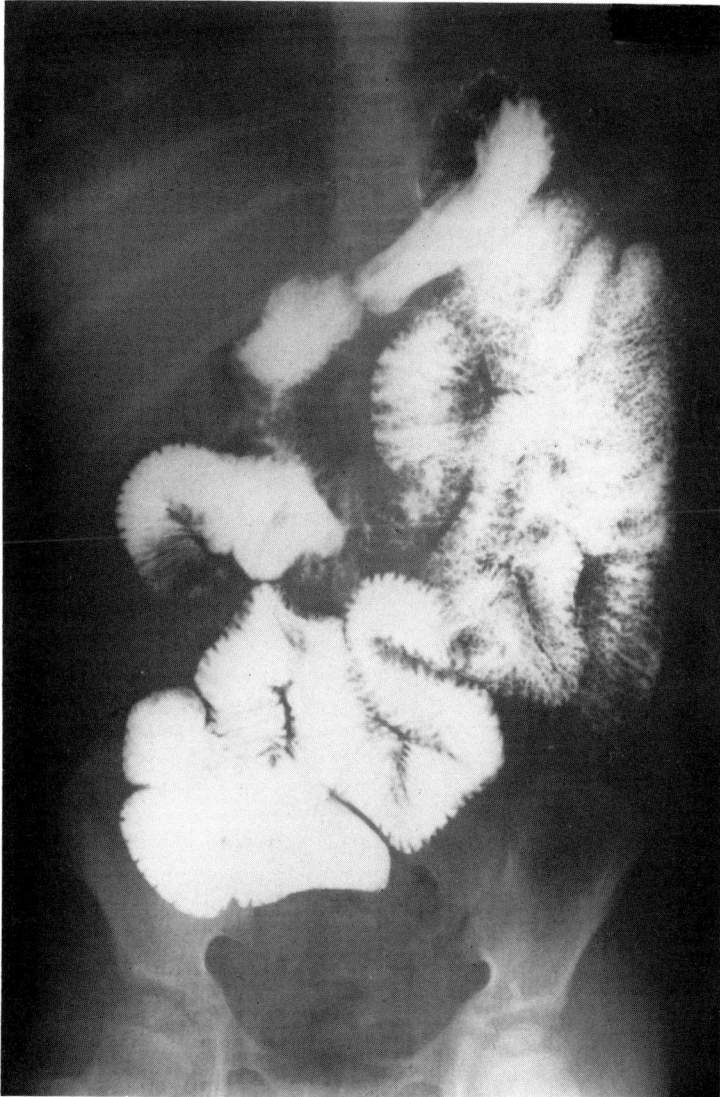

Fig. 8.42 Small bowel follow through in coeliac disease showing dilated loops of jejunum.

Crosby capsule.[17] This capsule is placed, under radiographic control, just distal to the duodeno-jejunal junction and a biopsy obtained. Correct orientation is necessary both for viewing under a dissecting microscope and for good histological assessment. If there is any doubt regarding the mucosal architecture, a repeat biopsy should be performed as the lesion may be patchy.

Diagnosis

If a patient is suspected of having small bowel disease by virtue of, for example, an anaemia or the presence of diarrhoea, it is essential to study the anatomy of the small bowel. An X-ray of the small bowel will show the gross anatomy and rule out blind loops, diverticula and Crohn's disease, and a jejunal biopsy will show the detailed structure of the jejunal mucosa. Very few conditions give a flat appearance with sub-total villous atrophy in the adult (Table 8.24), but if only partial villous atrophy is seen the differential diagnosis is more extensive. On some occasions it may be impossible to be sure of the diagnosis and a therapeutic trial of a gluten-free diet should be instituted, with repeat biopsies after about three months to assess the progress.

Treatment

The treatment for coeliac disease is a gluten-free diet, on which the patient's symptoms will improve and the biopsy will return to normal. Repeat biopsy is always indicated if the patient

does not respond clinically, but with a good clinical response a repeat biopsy is not always performed. In some patients a gluten challenge may be necessary for confirmation of the diagnosis; Figure 8.43 shows the results of a typical gluten challenge.

A gluten-free diet is difficult to maintain long-term and most patients do not stick absolutely rigidly to it. A conspiratorial relationship is then established with their doctors so that although both know that occasional lapses occur, a mutual pact of silence is agreed. It may well be that a number of patients could be kept asymptomatic on a low or very low gluten intake, but this has not yet been tried. Indeed most physicians advocate a strict gluten-free diet for life. This insistence on a strict gluten-free diet was instituted because of the risk of developing a malignancy. It has, however, not yet been shown that a strict gluten-free diet will prevent malignancies developing. Patients' sensitivity to gluten seems to vary, some developing symptoms after minute amounts of gluten.

A gluten-free diet is instituted with the help of a dietician who is then able to point out the less obvious foodstuffs that contain flour. In the UK, gluten-free flour, biscuits and pasta are available on National Health prescription and the Coeliac Society provides useful information on gluten-containing foods and has been instrumental in persuading manufacturers to provide gluten-free products. In the majority of patients no other treatment is required, but in patients who are ill, malnourished or who have evidence of severe deficiency, appropriate replacement therapy is

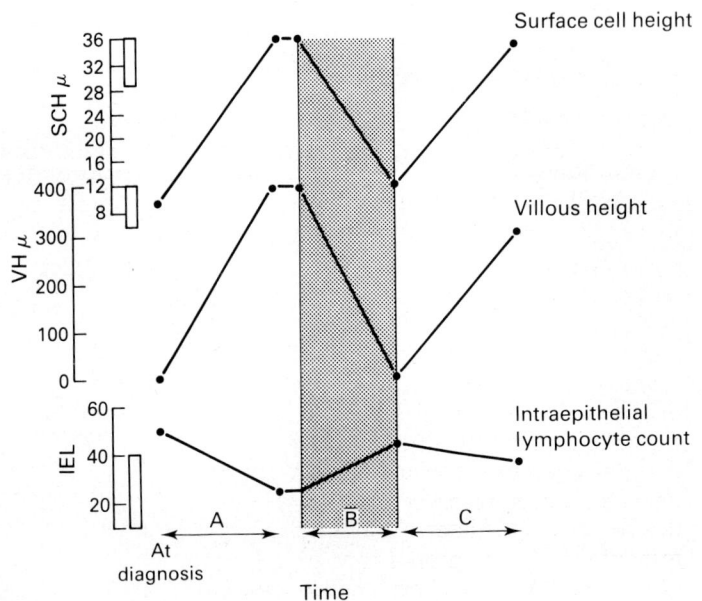

Fig. 8.43 Response to treatment followed by gluten challenge in a 40-year-old female patient with coeliac disease. A = gluten-free diet for eight months; B = normal diet for ten days; C = gluten-free diet for four months.

indicated. Iron, folic acid and occasionally vitamin B_{12} are necessary, but these can be discontinued as absorption returns to normal. Calcium and vitamin D should be given to patients with evidence of osteomalacia. Dapsone improves the skin lesions of dermatitis herpetiformis, but has no effect on the gut. A gluten-free diet improves both lesions,[33] but it can take many years before the dapsone can be discontinued.

Prognosis

This is usually excellent, most patients responding dramatically to a gluten-free diet. A few patients will not respond, and some will develop malignancies (see p. 465).

Failure to respond to a gluten-free diet
The commonest reason for a patient not to respond to a gluten-free diet is non-adherence to the diet. Patients who are initially virtually asymptomatic are reluctant to stick to a restricted diet. In a symptomatic patient who does not appear to be responding clinically a jejunal biopsy should be performed. A grossly abnormal jejunal mucosa will usually be found in these circumstances and a careful dietary history is then obtained. It appears that some patients are particularly sensitive to gluten and very small amounts can occasionally not only damage the intestinal mucosa but also produce symptoms. If a strict diet is adhered to, the number of unresponsive patients will be exceedingly small. A few patients, however, are completely unresponsive to a gluten-free diet. The mucosal abnormality in most of these patients is exactly the same as seen in typical coeliac disease. This makes it very difficult to decide whether the mucosal lesion is indeed due to sensitivity to gluten, sensitivity to some other unknown dietary constituent, or due to some other disease process as yet unidentified. By strict definition this condition cannot be termed coeliac disease as it does not respond to a gluten-free diet. Attempts have been made to separate these patients from typical coeliac disease and in some patients a hypoplastic mucosa[46] or thickened mucosal collagen[108] has been seen. No identifying features have, however, been found in all patients and hence these patients are usually referred to collectively as non-responsive coeliac disease. A few patients have been recorded who initially respond to the diet but later fail to maintain that response.[71] In a proportion of these non-responsive patients a clinical and morphological improvement will occur with corticosteroid therapy.[52, 106] Some patients, however, will not respond to this medication and a few will gradually deteriorate and die. More recently, azathioprine[36] has been used in this group and, although in most cases this agent is only useful for its steroid-sparing effect, it seems occasionally to be effective when corticosteroids have failed.[98] A few patients with non-responsive coeliac disease have been shown to have low serum zinc levels. It must be stressed that true unresponsive coeliac disease is rare, but undoubtedly some patients with all the typical features and mucosal abnormalities fail to respond to any therapy.

In a patient whose condition has deteriorated despite total gluten restriction, the addition of corticosteroids, and possibly azathioprine, the development of a malignancy must be considered. Malignancies occur frequently in coeliac disease[41] and are also found in dermatitis herpetiformis[57] (see p. 334). One further complication occasionally seen is ulcerative jejunoileitis (see p. 462). Only some of the reported cases seem to be true coeliacs who have responded to gluten withdrawal.[86] Ulceration and stricture of any part of the small intestine is found, leading to intestinal perforation, obstruction or gastrointestinal haemorrhage. The histology of the ulcers are non-specific and the associated mucosa shows subtotal villous atrophy; Isaacson believes that jejunoileitis occurs in patients with malignant histiocytosis rather than being a separate entity.[45]

REFERENCES

1 Alp, M. H. & Wright, R. (1971) Autoantibodies to reticulin in patients with idiopathic steatorrhoea, coeliac disease and Crohn's disease and their relation to immunoglobulins and dietary antibodies. *Lancet*, **ii**, 682–685.
2 Asquith, P. (1974) Immunology. *Clinics in Gastroenterology*, **3**, 213–234.
3 Asquith, P. & Haeney, M. R. (1979) Coeliac disease. In *Immunology of the Gastrointestinal Tract* (Ed.) Asquith, P. pp. 66–94. London: Churchill Livingstone.
4 Baker, P. G., Verrier-Jones, J., Peacock, D. B. & Read, A. E. (1975) The immune response to X 174 in man. III. Evidence for an association between hyposplenism and immunodeficiency in patients with coeliac disease. *Gut*, **16**, 538–542.
5 Betuel, H., Gebuhrer, L., Descos, L. *et al.* (1980) Adult coeliac disease associated with HLA-DRW3 & DRW7. *Tissue Antigens*, **15**, 231–238.
6 Bloom, S. R., Polak, J. M. & Besterman, H. S. (1978) Gut hormone profile in coeliac disease: a characteristic pattern of pathology. In *Perspectives in Coeliac Disease* (Ed.) McNicholl, B., McCarthy, C. F. & Fottrell, P. F. pp. 399–411. Lancaster: MTP Press.
7 Booth, C. C. (1970) Enterocyte in coeliac disease. *British Medical Journal*, **iii**, 14–17; **iv**, 725–731.

8   Booth, C. C. (1974) Definition of adult coeliac disease. In *Coeliac Disease, Proceedings of the Second International Coeliac Symposium* (Ed.) Hekkens, W. T., Th., J. M. & Pena, A. S. pp. 17–22. Leiden : Steinfert Kroese.

9   Bossart, R., Henry, K., Booth, C. C. & Doe, W. F. (1975) Subepithelial collagen in intestinal malabsorption. *Gut*, **16**, 18–22.

10 Brow, J. R., Parker, F., Weinstein, W. M. & Rubin, C. E. (1971) The small intestinal mucosa in dermatitis herpetiformis. I. Severity and distribution of the small intestinal lesion and associated malabsorption. *Gastroenterology*, **60**, 355–361.

11 Buchanan, K. D. & O'Connor, F. A. (1978) The role of the gastro-entero-pancreatic (GEP) hormones in coeliac disease. In *Perspectives in Coeliac Disease* (Ed.) McNicholl, B., McCarthy, C. F. & Fottrell, P. F. pp. 385–397. Lancaster : MTP Press.

12 Bullen, A. W. & Losowsky, M. S. (1978) Cell mediated immunity to gluten fraction III in adult coeliac disease. *Gut*, **19**, 126–131.

13 Carswell, F. & Ferguson, A. (1973) Plasma food antibodies during withdrawal and reintroduction of dietary gluten in coeliac disease. *Archives of Diseases of Childhood*, **48**, 583–586.

14 Cooke, W. T., Peeney, A. L. P. & Hawkins, C. F. (1953) Symptoms, signs & diagnostic features of idiopathic steatorrhoea. *Quarterly Journal of Medicine*, **22**, 59–77.

15 Cooke, W. T., Fone, D. J., Cox, E. V. *et al.* (1963) Adult coeliac disease. *Gut*, **4**, 279–291.

16 Corazza, S. R., Bullen, A. W., Hall, R. *et al.* (1981) Simple method of assessing splenic function in coeliac disease. *Clinical Science*, **60**, 109–113.

17 Crosby, W. H. & Kugler, H. W. (1957) Intraluminal biopsy of the small intestine : the intestinal biopsy capsule. *American Journal of Digestive Disorders*, **2**, 236–241.

18 Dawson, A. M., Holdsworth, C. D. & Pitcher, C. S. (1964) Sideroblastic anaemia in adult coeliac disease. *Gut*, **5**, 304–308.

19 Dicke, W. K., Weijers, H. A. & van de Kamer, J. H. (1953) Coeliac disease, presence in wheat of a factor having deleterious effect in cases of coeliac disease. *Acta Paediatrica*, **42**, 34–42.

20 Doe, W. F., Henry, K. & Booth, C. C. (1974) Complement in coeliac disease. In *Coeliac Disease* (Ed.) Hekkens, W. & Pena, A. S. pp. 189–196. Leiden : Stenfert Kroesse.

21 Douglas, A. P. & Booth, C. C. (1970) Digestion of gluten peptides by normal human jejunal mucosa and by mucosa from patients with adult coeliac disease. *Clinical Science*, **38**, 11–25.

22 Falchuk, Z. M., Rogentine, G. N. & Strober, W. J. (1972) Predominance of histocompatibility antigen HL-A8 in patients with gluten-sensitive enteropathy. *Journal of Clinical Investigations*, **51**, 1602–1605.

23 Falchuk, Z. M., Gebhard, R. L., Sessoms, C. & Strober, W. (1974) An in vitro mode of gluten-sensitive enteropathy. Effect of gliadin on intestinal epithelial cells of patients with gluten-sensitive enteropathy in organ culture. *Journal of Clinical Investigation*, **53**, 487–500.

24 Farthing, M. J., McLean, A. M., Bartram, C. I. *et al.* (1981) Radiologic features of the jejunum in hypoalbuminaemia. *American Journal of Radiology*, **136**, 883–886.

25 Farthing, M. J. G., Edwards, C. R. W., Rees, L. H. & Dawson, A. M. (1982) Male gonadal function in coeliac disease. 1. Sexual dysfunction, infertility and semen quality. *Gut*, **23**, 608–614.

26 Farthing, M. J. G., Rees, L. H., Edwards, C. R. W. & Dawson, A. M. (1983) Male gonadal function in coeliac disease. 2. Sex hormones. *Gut*, **24**, 127–135.

27 Ferguson, A. (1977) Intraepithelial lymphocytes of the small intestine. *Gut*, **18**, 921–937.

28 Ferguson, A. & Murray, D. (1971) Quantification of intraepithelial lymphocytes in human jejunum. *Gut*, **12**, 988–994.

29 Ferguson, A., MacDonald, T. T., McClure, J. P. & Holden, R. J. (1975) Cell mediated immunity to gliadin within the small intestinal mucosa in coeliac disease. *Lancet*, **i**, 895–897.

30 Fordtran, J. S., Rector, F. C., Locklear, T. W. & Ewton, M. F. E. (1967) Water and solute movement in the small intestine of patients with sprue. *Journal of Clinical Investigations*, **46**, 287–298.

31 Fraser, A. C., Fletcher, R. F., Ross, C. A. C. *et al.* (1959) Gluten-induced enteropathy. The effect of partially digested gluten. *Lancet*, **ii**, 252–255.

32 Fry, L., Seah, P. P., McMinn, R. R. M. & Hoffbrand, A. V. (1972) Lymphocyte infiltration of epithelium in diagnosis of gluten-sensitive enteropathy. *British Medical Journal*, **iii**, 371–374.

33 Fry, L., Leonard J. N., Swain, F. *et al.* (1982) Long term follow-up of dermatitis herpetiformis with and without dietary gluten withdrawal. *British Journal of Dermatology*, **107**, 631–640.

34 Green, J. R. B., Goble, H. L., Edwards, C. R. W. & Dawson, A. M. (1977) Reversible insensitivity to androgens in men with untreated gluten enteropathy. *Lancet*, **i**, 280–282.

35 Hamilton, I., Cobden, I., Rothwell, J. & Axon, A. T. R. (1982) Intestinal permeability in coeliac disease : the response to gluten withdrawal and single-dose gluten challenge. *Gut*, **23**, 202–211.

36 Hamilton, J. D., Chambers, R. A. & Wyn-Williams A. (1976) Role of gluten, prednisolone and azathioprine in non-responsive coeliac disease. *Lancet*, **i**, 1213–1215.

37 Hekkens, W. J. H., Haex, A. J. & Willighagen, R. G. J. (1970) Some aspects of gliadin fractionation and testing by a histochemical method. In *Coeliac Disease, Proceedings of the International Coeliac Symposium* (Ed.) Booth, C. C. & Dowling, H. pp. 11–19. Edinburgh and London : Churchill-Livingstone.

38 Hobbs, J. R. & Hepner, G. W. (1968) Immunoglobulins and alimentary disease. *Lancet*, **ii**, 47.

39 Hodgson, H. J. F., Davies, R. J., Gent, A. F. & Hodson, M. E. (1976) Atopic disorders and coeliac disease. *Lancet*, **i**, 115.

40 Hoffbrand, A. V. (1974) Anaemia in adult coeliac disease. *Clinics in Gastroenterology*, **3**, 71–89.

41 Holmes, G. K. T., Stokes, P. L., Sorahan, T. M. *et al.* (1976) Coeliac disease, gluten free diet and malignancy. *Gut*, **17**, 612–619.

42 Howdle, P. D. (1983) Organ culture in the study of the gastrointestinal tract : health and disease. *Clinical Science*, **65**, 105–110.

43 Howdle, P. D., Corazza, G. R., Bullen, A. W. & Losowsky, M. S. (1981) In vitro diagnosis of coeliac disease – an assessment. *Gut*, **22**, 939–947.

44 Howdle, P. D., Corazza, G. R., Bullen, A. W. & Losowsky, M. S. (1981) Gluten sensitivity of small intestinal mucosa in vitro : quantitative assessment of histological change. *Gastroenterology*, **80**, 442–450.

45 Isaacson, P. & Wright, D. H. (1980) Malabsorption and intestinal lymphomas. In *Recent Advances in Gastrointestinal Pathology* (Ed.) Wright, R. pp. 193–212. London : W. B. Saunders.

46 Jones P. E. & Peters T. J. (1977) DNA synthesis by

jejunal mucosa in responsive and non-responsive coeliac disease. *British Medical Journal*, **i,** 1130–1131.

47 Jos, J., Charbonnier, L., Moregenot, J. F. *et al.* (1978) Isolation and characterization of the toxic fraction of wheat gliadin in coeliac disease. In *Perspectives in Coeliac Disease* (Ed.) McNicholl, B., McCarthy, C. F. & Fottrell, P. F. pp. 75–89. Lancaster: MTP Press.

48 Kagnoff, M. F., Brown, L. S., Weiss, J. B. *et al.* (1983) Immunoglobulin allotype markers in gluten-sensitive enteropathy. *Lancet*, **i,** 952–953.

49 Kilander, A. F., Dotwall, G., Fallstrom, S. P. *et al.* (1983) Evaluation of gliadin antibodies for detection of coeliac disease. *Scandinavian Journal of Gastroenterology*, **18,** 377–384.

50 Kumar, P. J. & Bartram, C. (1979) The relevance of the barium meal follow-through examination in the diagnosis of adult coeliac disease. *Gastrointestinal Radiology*, **4,** 285–289.

51 Kumar, P. J., Ferguson, A., Lancaster-Smith, M. L. & Dawson, A. M. (1973) Relationship between dietary food antigen and jejunal mucosal morphology. *Gut*, **14,** 829–830.

52 Kumar, P. J., Silk, D. B. A., Marks, P. *et al.* (1973) Treatment of dermatitis herpetiformis with corticosteroids and a gluten-free diet: a study of jejunal morphology and function. *Gut*, **14,** 280–283.

53 Kumar, P. J., Silk, D. B. A., Rousseau, B. *et al.* (1974) Assessment of jejunal function in patients with dermatitis herpetiformis and adult coeliac disease using a perfusion technique. *Scandinavian Journal of Gastroenterology*, **9,** 793–798.

54 Lancaster-Smith, M. L., Joyce, S. & Kumar, P. (1977) Immunoglobulins in the jejunal mucosa in adult coeliac disease and dermatitis herpetiformis after reintroduction of dietary gluten. *Gut*, **18,** 887–891.

55 Lancaster-Smith, M., Kumar, P. J., Marks, R. *et al.* (1974) Jejunal mucosal immunoglobulin-containing cells and jejunal fluid immunoglobulins in adult coeliac disease and dermatitis herpetiformis. *Gut*, **15,** 371–376.

56 Lancaster-Smith, M. J., Perrin, J., Swarbrick, E. T. & Wright, J. J. (1974) Coeliac disease and autoimmunity. *Postgraduate Medical Journal*, **50,** 45–48.

57 Leonard, J., Tucker, W., Fry, J. & Fry, L. (1982) The incidence of malignancy in dermatitis herpetiformis. *British Journal of Dermatology*, **107** (Supplement 22) p. 27(Abstract).

58 Love, A. H. G., Elmes, M., Golden, M. K. & McMaster, D. (1978) Zinc deficiency and coeliac disease. In *Perspectives in Coeliac Disease* (Ed.) McNicholl, B., McCarthy, C. F. & Fottrell, P. F. pp. 335–342. Lancaster: MTP Press.

59 MacLaurin, B. P., Cooke, W. T. & Ling, N. R. (1971) Impaired lymphocyte reactivity against tumour cells in patients with coeliac disease. *Gut*, **12,** 794–800.

60 Mann, D. L., Katz, S. I., Nelson, D. L. *et al.* (1976) Specific B-cell antigens associated with gluten-sensitive enteropathy and dermatitis herpetiformis. *Lancet*, **i,** 110–111.

61 Marks, R. & Whittle, M. W. (1976) Results of treatment of dermatitis herpetiformis with a gluten-free diet after one year. *British Journal of Medicine*, **2,** 772.

62 Marks, J., Shuster, S. & Watson, A. J. (1966) Small bowel changes in dermatitis herpetiformis. *Lancet*, **ii,** 1280–1282.

63 Marsh, G. W. & Stewart, J. S. (1970) Splenic function in adult coeliac disease. *British Journal of Haematology*, **19,** 445–457.

64 Marsh, M. N. (1980) Studies of intestinal lymphoid tissue. III. Quantitative analyses of epithelial lymphocytes in the small intestine of human control subjects and of patients with coeliac sprue. *Gastroenterology*, **79,** 481–492.

65 Marsh, M. N. (1981) The small intestine: mechanisms of local immunity and gluten sensitivity. *Clinical Science*, **61,** 497–503.

66 Marsh, M. N. (1982) Studies of intestinal lymphoid tissue in gluten sensitive enteropathy. In *Basic Science in Gastroenterology Studies of the Gut* (Ed.) Polak, J. M., Bloom, S. R., Wright, N. A. & Daly, M. J. pp. 87–106. Norwich: Page.

67 Marsh, M. N. & Haeney, M. R. (1983) Studies of intestinal lymphoid tissue. VI. Proliferative response of small intestinal epithelial lymphocyte distinguishes gluten from non-gluten induced enteropathy. *Journal of Clinical Pathology*, **36,** 149–160.

68 Mearin M. L. Biemond I., Pena A. S. *et al.* (1983) HLA-DR phenotypes in Spanish coeliac children: their contribution to the understanding of the genetics of the disease. *Gut*, **24,** 532–538.

69 Morris, J. S., Read, A. E., Jones, B. *et al.* (1971) Coeliac disease and lung disease. *Lancet*, **i,** 754.

70 Mylotte, M. J., Egan-Mitchell, B., McCarthy, C. F. & McNicholl, B. (1973) Incidence of coeliac disease in the West of Ireland. *British Medical Journal*, **i,** 703–705.

71 Neale G. (1968) A case of adult coeliac disease resistant to treatment. *British Medical Journal*, **ii,** 678–684.

72 O'Donoghue, D. P., Lancaster-Smith, M., Johnson, O. D. & Kumar, P. J. (1976) Gastric lesion in dermatitis herpetiformis. *Gut*, **17,** 185–188.

73 O'Grady, J. G., Stevens, F. M., O'Gorman, T. A. & McCarthy, C. F. (1983) Hyposplenism of coeliac disease is largely reversible. *Gut*, **24,** A494.

74 Padykula, H. A., Strauss, E. W., Ladman, A. J. & Gardner, F. H. (1961) A morphologic and histochemical analysis of the human jejunal epithelium in nontropic sprue. *Gastroenterology*, **40,** 735–765.

75 Pallis, C. A. & Lewis, P. D. (1974) *The Neurology of Gastrointestinal Disease*. pp. 138–156. London: W. B. Saunders.

76 Patey, A. L. & Waldron, N. M. (1976) Gliadin proteins from Maris-Widgeon wheat. *Journal of Scientific Food Agriculture*, **27,** 838–842.

77 Paulley, L. W. (1954) Observations on the aetiology of idiopathic steatorrhoea. *British Medical Journal*, **ii,** 1318.

78 Pena, A. S. (1981) Genetics of coeliac disease. In *Topics in Gastroenterology*, vol. 9 (Ed.) Jewell, D. P. & Lee, E. pp. 69–81. Oxford: Blackwell Scientific.

79 Pena, A. S., Mann, D. L., Hague, N. E. *et al.* (1978) B-cell alloantigens and the inheritance of coeliac disease. In *Perspectives in Coeliac Disease* (Ed.) McNicholl, B., McCarthy, C. F. & Fottrell, P. F. pp. 131–136. Lancaster: MTP Press.

80 Peters, T. J., Jones, P. E., Jenkins, W. J. & Nicholson, J. A. (1978) Analytical subcellular fractionation of jejunal biopsy specimens from control subjects and patients with coeliac disease. In *Perspectives in Coeliac Disease* (Ed.) McNicholl, B., McCarthy, C. F. & Fottrell, P. F. pp. 423–436. Lancaster: MTP Press.

81 Pettit, J. E., Hoffbrand, A. V., Seah, P. P. & Fry, L. (1972) Splenic atrophy in dermatitis herpetiformis. *British Medical Journal*, **ii,** 438–440.

82 Phelan, J. J., Stevens, F. M., Cleere, W. F. *et al.* (1978) The detoxification of gliadin by the enzymic cleavage of a side chain substituent. In *Perspectives in Coeliac Disease* (Ed.) McNicholl, B., McCarthy, C. F. & Fottrell, P. F. pp. 33–39. Lancaster: MTP Press.

83 Pink, I. J., Croft, D. N. & Creamer, B. (1970) Cell loss

from small intestinal mucosa: a morphological study. *Gut*, **11**, 217–222.

84 Pitmann, F. E. & Pollitt, R. J. (1966) Studies of jejunal mucosal digestion of peptic-tryptic digests of wheat protein in coeliac disease. *Gut*, **7**, 368–371.

85 Rawcliffe, P. M. (1981) The toxic fraction of wheat gluten. In *Topics in Gastroenterology*, vol. 9 (Ed.) Jewell, D. P. & Lee, E. pp. 53–67. Oxford: Blackwell Scientific.

86 Robertson, D. A. F., Dixon, M. F., Scott, B. B. *et al.* (1983) Small intestine ulceration: diagnostic difficulties in relation to coeliac disease. *Gut*, **24**, 565–575.

87 Rubin, C. E., Brandborg, L. L., Phelps, P. C. & Taylor, H. C. Jnr (1960) Studies of coeliac disease. I. The apparent identical and specific nature of the duodenal and proximal jejunal lesion in coeliac disease and idiopathic sprue. *Gastroenterology*, **38**, 28–49.

88 Rubin, C. E., Brandborg, L. L., Flick, A. C. *et al.* (1966) Studies of coeliac sprue. III. The effect of repeated wheat instillation into the proximal lesion of patients on a gluten-free diet. *Gastroenterology*, **43**, 621–641.

89 Scott, B. B. & Losowsky, M. S. (1975) Coeliac disease: a cause of various associated diseases? *Lancet*, **ii**, 956–957.

90 Scott, B. B. & Losowsky, M. S. (1976) Depressed cell-mediated immunity: coeliac disease. *Gut*, **17**, 900–905.

91 Scott, B. B. & Losowsky, M. S. (1976) Patchiness and duodenal–jejunal variation of the mucosal abnormality in coeliac disease and dermatitis herpetiformis. *Gut*, **17**, 984.

92 Scott, B. B. & Losowsky, M. S. (1976) Cell-mediated autoimmunity in coeliac disease. *Clinical and Experimental Immunology*, **26**, 243–246.

93 Seah, P. P., Fry, L., Rossiter, M. A. *et al.* (1971) Anti-reticulin antibodies in childhood coeliac disease. *Lancet*, **ii**, 681–682.

94 Shiner, M. (1956) Jejunal biopsy tube. *Lancet*, **i**, 85.

95 Shiner, M. & Ballard, J. (1972) Antigen–antibody reactions in jejunal mucosa in childhood coeliac disease after gluten challenge. *Lancet*, **i**, 1202–1205.

96 Silk, D. B. A., Kumar, P. J., Webb, J. P. W. *et al.* (1975) Ileal function in patients with untreated adult coeliac disease. *Gut*, **16**, 261–267.

97 Simpson, F. G., Field, H. P., Howdle, P. D. *et al.* (1983) Leucocyte migration inhibition test in coeliac disease – a reappraisal. *Gut*, **24**, 311–317.

98 Sinclair, T., Kumar, P. J. & Dawson, A. M. (1983). Azathioprine responsive villous atrophy. *Gut*, **24**, 494.

99 Sladen, G. E. & Kumar, P. J. (1973) Is the xylose test still a worthwhile investigation? *British Medical Journal*, **iii**, 223–226.

100 Stewart, J. S., Pollock, D. J., Hoffbrand, A. V. *et al.* (1967) A study of proximal and distal intestinal structure and absorptive function in idiopathic steatorrhoea. *Quarterly Journal of Medicine, New Series*, **36**, (143), 425–445.

101 Stokes, P. L., Asquith, P., Holmes, G. K. T. *et al.* (1972) Histocompatibility antigens associated with adult coeliac disease. *Lancet*, **ii**, 162–164.

102 Thomas, H. C. & Jewell, D. P. (1979) *Clinical Gastrointestinal Immunology*. pp. 10–120. Oxford: Blackwell Scientific.

103 Trewby, P. N., Chipping, P. M., Palmer, S. J. *et al.* (1981) Splenic atrophy in adult coeliac disease: is it reversible? *Gut*, **22**, 628–632.

104 Trier, J. S. & Browning, T. H. (1970) Epithelial cell renewal in cultured duodenal biopsies in coeliac sprue. *New England Journal of Medicine*, **283**, 1245–1364.

105 van de Kamer, J. H., Weijers, H. A. & Dicke, W. K. (1953) Coeliac disease. IV. An investigation into the injurious constituents of wheat in connection with their action on patients with coeliac disease. *Acta Paediatrica*, **42**, 223–231.

106 Wall, A. J., Douglas, A. P., Booth, C. C. & Pearce, A. G. E. (1970). Response of the jejunal mucosa in adult coeliac disease to oral prednisolone. *Gut*, **11**, 7–14.

107 Watson, A. J. & Wright, N. A. (1974) Morphology and cell kinetics of the jejunal mucosa in untreated patients. *Clinics in Gastroenterology*, **3**, 11–31.

108 Weinstein, W. M., Saunders, D. R., Tytgat, G. N. & Rubin, C. E. (1970) Collagenous sprue – an unrecognised type of malabsorption. *New England Journal of Medicine*, **283**, 1297–1301.

109 Weinstein, W. M., Brow, J. R., Parker, F. & Rubin, C. F. (1971). The small intestinal mucosa in dermatitis herpetiformis: relationship of the small intestinal lesion to gluten. *Gastroenterology*, **60**, 362–369.

110 Weiser, M. M. & Douglas, A. P. (1976) An alternative mechanism for gluten toxicity in coeliac disease. *Lancet*, **i**, 567–569.

CHRONIC NON-SPECIFIC ULCERATIVE ENTERITIS

Chronic non-specific ulcerative enteritis (CNSUE), first described by Nyman in 1949,[15] is a rare disease with less than fifty published cases. It is characterized by multiple chronic benign small bowel ulcerations of unknown aetiology, without distinctive pathological findings, resulting in abdominal pain, fever, diarrhoea, malabsorption, and surgical complications. It carries a poor prognosis and no specific treatment is available.

Pathology

Ulcerations are multiple, and always involve the jejunum, usually the ileum and rarely the duodenum and the colon. Histologically, the ulcers vary in depth, penetrating frequently to the muscularis propria and sometimes to the serosa causing perforation (Figure 8.44). Submucosal oedema and fibrosis may be prominent, the latter causing stenosis in many cases. The ulcer base is infiltrated by lymphocytes, plasma cells, histiocytes and polymorphonuclear leucocytes. The mucosa adjacent to the ulcerations may have normal or atrophic villi; pyloric metaplasia is sometimes found. The intervening mucosa may be completely flat or show blunted or normal villi. Most importantly, no specific histological features are found anywhere (no tuberculoid granulomas, no sign of vasculitis or neoplastic disease). Mesenteric lymph node enlargement is often seen, but microscopical examination reveals only reactive hyperplasia.

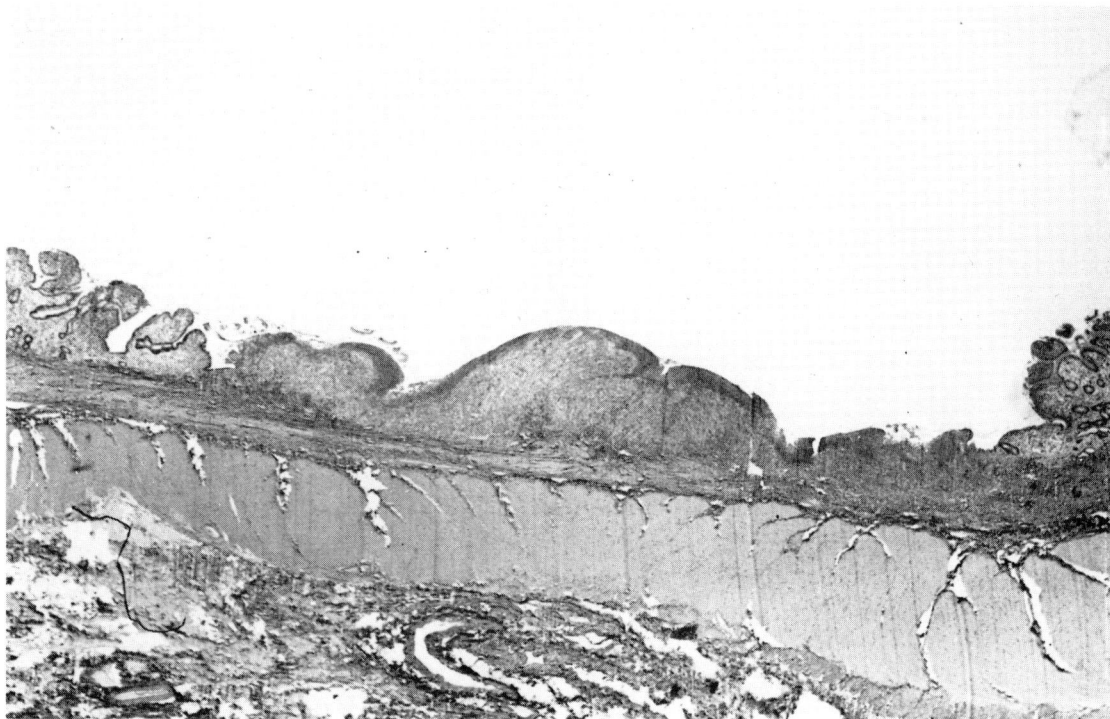

Fig. 8.44 Ileal resection specimen. Chronic ulceration surrounded by dystrophic mucosa. From Modigliani *et al.* (1979),[14] with kind permission of the authors and the editor of *Gut*.

Clinical features and diagnosis

The mean age at onset is 50 years (the range being 18–78 years) with a small majority (58%) of females.[13] Chronic diarrhoea with steatorrhoea, periumbilical or epigastric pain, and marked weight loss are almost constant features of the condition. Vomiting, fever, finger clubbing, wasting, and signs of multiple nutritional deficiencies are frequent. Laboratory findings are non-specific: anaemia, usually due to iron deficiency, is frequent; Howell–Jolly bodies and target cells have been rarely reported; neutrophil leucocytosis is found in one third of patients. Serum calcium, folate, iron and albumin are usually low. Serum immunoglobulins are frequently normal but an increased level of IgA may occur, or a deficiency of IgA[13] or IgG.[6] Malabsorption of xylose and fat is almost always present. Vitamin B_{12} absorption is variable. Small bowel X-rays are constantly, but not specifically, abnormal; the most suggestive appearance is a diffuse narrowing of the intestinal loops with total effacement of the mucosal pattern (moulage sign) (Figure 8.45). Mucosal folds may also be coarsened with spiculation of the intestinal margins. Duodenal or jejunal strictures may be seen, but X-ray documentation of ulceration is exceptional.[2, 17]

Blind peroral small bowel biopsies may show a diffuse or patchy subtotal villous atrophy or a normal mucosa (see below); this procedure, however, is of little use in making the diagnosis of CNSUE because it almost never shows ulceration, even when biopsies are taken at multiple levels and from areas ultimately shown to be ulcerated. The only histological clue to the diagnosis might be the discovery of a dystrophic mucosal pattern (variable villous height and shape, irregularity of crypt distribution, and sclerosis of the lamina propria) suggestive of scarred ulceration.[14] Jejunoscopy with biopsies has been rarely performed[4] and is a potentially useful tool to demonstrate the ulcerations, but does not preclude the need for laparotomy to establish their nature. Thus surgical exploration with biopsy-resection of the small bowel and mesenteric nodes is, at present, the only reliable diagnostic method. The usual findings are of small bowel thickening or oedema, and hyperaemia of the serosa; mesenteric lymph node enlargement has been often described. However, the serosa of the small intestine may look normal at operation. Peroperative enteroscopy is helpful in locating the ulcerations and guiding surgical sampling.[5]

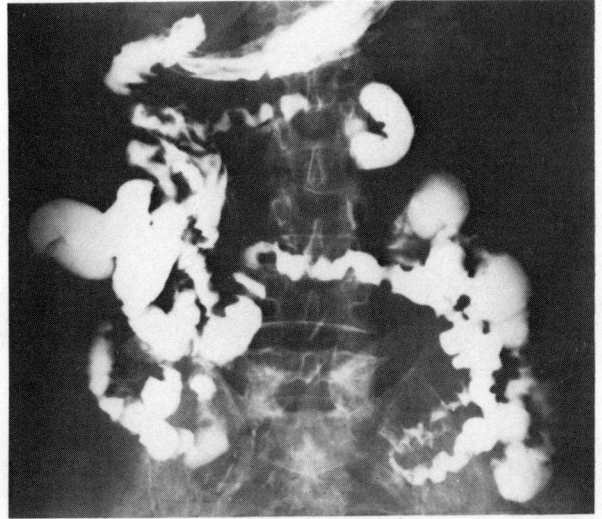

Fig. 8.45 Radiograph of upper gastrointestinal tract showing diffusely narrowed jejunum and effacement of the normal mucosal pattern. From Modigliani *et al.* (1979),[14] with kind permission of the authors and the editor of *Gut*.

Differential diagnosis and relationship with coeliac disease and intestinal lymphoma

Due to the absence of any available specific diagnostic criterion, the diagnosis of CNSUE can only be made after ruling out all other causes of secondary small bowel ulceration such as Crohn's disease, Zollinger–Ellison syndrome, tuberculosis, fungal infections, ingestion of enteric coated potassium tablets, small bowel malignancy (particularly lymphoma), and vascular diseases. Primary non-specific ulcer of the small intestine is different from CNSUE; usually the ulcer presents with a surgical complication, is not associated with diarrhoea or malabsorption, is single, and does not recur after surgical resection.

The relationship between CNSUE and coeliac disease has been extensively studied. Patients with CNSUE fall into three categories which occur with approximately similar frequency.[14]

1 CNSUE may be clearly associated with coeliac disease as demonstrated by the presence of the mucosal lesion characteristic of this disease in the intervening non-ulcerated mucosa of the proximal small bowel, and a clear-cut improvement on a gluten-free diet. Both diseases are often diagnosed simultaneously and ulcerations may be found distal to the area of total villous atrophy, at a site where the villous height is normal.[14] CNSUE may also supervene in patients with coeliac disease whose villous height has returned to normal after prolonged treatment with a gluten-free diet.[2, 14] Thus, the ulcerative process complicating coeliac disease does not seem to be directly related to villous atrophy nor to be gluten-induced.

2 The second group of patients only differs from the previous one in the failure of a gluten-free diet to improve intestinal villous height.[16, 17] The search for a family history of coeliac disease, HLA typing or organ culture of a jejunal biopsy specimen[12] may then be helpful in the diagnosis of coeliac disease.

3 In the third group of patients the histological pattern of the intervening non-ulcerated mucosa, with normal villi, or patchy villous atrophy with flat and strictly normal mucosa adjacent,[10] clearly rules out coeliac disease. A single peroral biopsy may falsely suggest coeliac disease by showing a flat mucosa; multiple small intestinal biopsies are thus necessary.

Relationship of CNSUE with intestinal lymphoma and malignant histiocytosis

The diagnosis of CNSUE obviously implies that an intensive search for lymphoma had been carried out and is negative. In a few cases, however, lymphomatous cells, especially of the histiocytic type, have been obscured by the inflammatory cells in the base of an ulcer and thus overlooked, leading to a false diagnosis of CNSUE.[1, 7] Furthermore, intestinal lymphoma may be preceded by, or associated with, truly benign small bowel ulcerations.[1] An intensive search for a lymphomatous process is therefore mandatory before diagnosing CNSUE. However, the suggestion that CNSUE 'is but a manifestation of malignant histiocytosis of the intestine'[9] is excessive.

Treatment and prognosis

There is no specific treatment for CNSUE. Most patients will require surgery either for a complication (obstruction, haemorrhage or perforation) or for diagnostic purposes. When feasible, surgical excision of the worst affected segment of small bowel is the most appropriate therapy. Gluten withdrawal may be beneficial to patients with associated coeliac disease, but only after the ulcerative process has been surgically controlled; it does not influence or prevent the ulcerative process itself. Corticosteroids have been useful in a limited number of patients.[8, 11] Exclusive parenteral nutrition can overcome severe nutritional deficiencies but our limited experience does not suggest it improves small intestinal function or morphology.[14]

The overall prognosis of CNSUE is poor; two-thirds of patients whose follow-up has been reported are dead at the time of publication,[14] with a mean survival period of 37 months (the range being 5–120 months) from the onset of the illness.[13] The cause of death is almost invariably related to a surgical complication of the ulceration, especially perforation. The prognosis seems to be slightly better in the group of patients with associated proven coeliac disease, and worst in those with normal villi or patchy villous atrophy.[14]

REFERENCES

1 Baer, A. N., Bayless, T. M. & Yardley, J. H. (1980) Intestinal ulceration and malabsorption syndromes. *Gastroenterology*, **79**, 754–765.

2 Bayless, T. M., Kapelowitz, R. F., Shelley, W. M. *et al.* (1967) Intestinal ulceration. A complication of celiac disease. *New England Journal of Medicine*, **276**, 996–1002.

3 Belaiche, J., Modigliani, R., Modigliani, E. *et al.* (1977) Jejuno-iléite ulcéreuse chronique non spécifique. Présentation d'un nouveau cas. *Gastroentérologie Clinique et Biologique*, **1**, 553–560.

4 Cerf, M., Gouerou, H., Marche, C. *et al.* (1977) Jéjunoiléite ulcéreuse diffuse: intérêt diagnostique de la jéjunoscopie. *Gastroentérologie Clinique et Biologique*, **1**, 571–576.

5 Conley, D. R., Feffer, M. & Cove, H. (1975) Duodenal jejunal ulcers and recurrent hemorrhage: diagnostic value of total enteroscopy. *American Journal of Digestive Diseases*, **20**, 876–881.

6 Corlin, R. F. & Pops, M. A. (1972) Nongranulomatous ulcerative jejunoileitis with hypogammaglobulinemia. Clinical remission after treatment with gammaglobulin. *Gastroenterology*, **62**, 473–478.

7 Freeman, H. J., Weinstein, W. M., Shnitka, T. K. *et al.* (1977) Primary abdominal lymphoma: presenting manifestation of celiac sprue or complicating dermatitis herpetiformis. *American Journal of Medicine*, **63**, 585–594.

8 Goulston, K. J., Skyring, A. P. & McGovern, V. J. (1965) Ulcerative jejunitis associated with malabsorption. *Australasian Annals of Medicine*, **14**, 57–64.

9 Isaacson, P. (1980) Malignant histiocytosis of the intestine: the early histological lesion. *Gut*, **21**, 381–386.

10 Jeffries, G. H., Steinberg, H. & Sleisenger, M. H. (1968) Chronic ulcerative (nongranulomatous) jejunitis. *American Journal of Medicine*, **44**, 47–59.

11 Jones, P. E. & Gleeson, M. H. (1973) Mucosal ulceration and mesenteric lymphadenopathy in coeliac disease. *British Medical Journal*, **3**, 212–213.

12 Klaeveman, H. L., Gebhard, R. L., Sessoms, C. & Strober, W. (1975) In vitro studies of ulcerative ileojejunitis. *Gastroenterology*, **68**, 572–582.

13 Mills, P. R., Brown, I. L. & Watkinson, G. (1980) Idiopathic chronic ulcerative enteritis. Report of five cases and review of the literature. *Quarterly Journal of Medicine*, **194**, 133–149.

14 Modigliani, R., Poitras, P., Galian, A. *et al.* (1979) Chronic non-specific ulcerative duodenojejunoileitis: report of four cases. *Gut*, **20**, 318–328.

15 Nyman, E., (1949) Ulcerous jejuno-ileitis with symptomatic sprue. *Acta Medica Scandinavica*, **134**, 275–283.

16 Shiner, M. (1963) Effect of a gluten-free diet in 17 patients with idiopathic steatorrhea. A follow-up study. *American Journal of Digestive Diseases*, **8**, 969–983.

17 Stuber, J. L., Wiegman, H., Crosby, I. & Gonzalez, G. (1971). Ulcers of the colon and jejunum in celiac disease. *Radiology*, **99**, 339–340.

THE MALIGNANT COMPLICATIONS OF COELIAC DISEASE

The occasional occurrence of lymphoma in patients presenting with steatorrhoea has been well recognized since the 1930s.[9] In 1962 a report from Bristol suggested that malignant lymphoma of the small intestine might be a complication of longstanding coeliac disease.[11] A later report from the same centre indicated that carcinomas, particularly of the fore- and mid-gut, might also complicate coeliac disease.[7] In a subsequent statistical study from Birmingham 29 out of 202 (14%) adult patients with coeliac disease observed over many years were reported to have developed malignancy.[12] Fourteen patients developed lymphoma compared to the expected rate of less than one, but there was also a statistically significant increase in the incidence of other malignancies, particularly carcinomas of the gastrointestinal tract. Further studies showed that carcinomas of oesophagus and pharynx are particularly associated with coeliac disease among men.[16] A report from Australia[26] confirmed the increased incidence of oesophageal carcinomas and also suggested an increased incidence of adenocarcinoma in the small intestine. Four cases of small intestinal adenocarcinoma have subsequently been reported in patients with coeliac disease attending clinics in Birmingham or Derby.[15]

The histological type of lymphoma most frequently associated with coeliac disease was initially described as either Hodgkin's disease or reticulum cell sarcoma.[4, 12] In 1978 it was suggested that the lymphoma was of histiocytic derivation and should be classified as a malignant histiocytosis.[18] The term 'malignant histiocytosis of the intestine' was proposed.[18, 19] A collaborative study involving more than 70 centres throughout the United Kingdom, based on the analysis of 235 patients with biopsy proven coeliac disease and histologically proven malignancy, confirmed that the predominant type of malignancy is a malignant histiocytosis, and that small intestinal adenocarcinoma, oesophageal carcinoma and pharyngeal carcinoma also occur more frequently than expected.[30]

Incidence

The recorded incidence of malignancy in coeliac disease has ranged from 11–14%,[12, 16, 26] rising with longer duration of follow-up.[16] The true incidence and prevalence of malignancy in all patients with coeliac disease is, however, unknown. Figures from special referral centres probably over-estimate the number of malignancies likely to be encountered among patients with coeliac disease in a District General Hospital, but there are probably also significant numbers of patients with undiagnosed coeliac disease in the community.[28]

Patients affected

Age and sex distribution
Malignancy is a complication of *adult* patients with coeliac disease. Both sexes are affected equally. A few patients give a history of coeliac disease in childhood, but the diagnosis is often not made until the fifth or sixth decade, when malignancy also most commonly develops.

The relationship between the diagnosis of coeliac disease and of malignancy
The diagnosis of malignancy in coeliac disease is most commonly made amongst patients who are already known to have coeliac disease. Individuals are recorded who have developed malignancy more than 30 years after the diagnosis of coeliac disease has been made, but half of those who develop malignancy do so within five years. Alternatively, symptoms of malignancy may serve to draw attention to previously undiagnosed coeliac disease, or symptoms of coeliac disease may develop after the diagnosis of malignancy has been made. In the UK collaborative study, 66% of the patients had previously diagnosed coeliac disease, in 19% the two diagnoses were made simultaneously, and in 15% coeliac disease was diagnosed later.

The relationship to gluten withdrawal
As is the case in other patients with coeliac disease, the majority of those who develop malignancy show histological improvement of their enteropathy if treated with a gluten-free diet. Malignancy may develop in those whose jejunal biopsy has previously returned to normal following gluten withdrawal. In such patients, malignancy is not accompanied by worsening of the jejunal biopsy appearance provided the patient maintains a gluten-free diet.

Types of malignancies

Approximately half the malignancies which occur in patients with coeliac disease are classified as malignant lymphomas. Of the remaining tumours, most are invasive tumours, and approximately half arise from the gastrointestinal tract.

Malignant lymphomas
The predominant type of lymphoma, accounting for approximately 90% of those which can be adequately classified, is a tumour of histiocytic cell origin. This tumour is called malignant histiocytosis of the intestine since it usually presents with a lesion in the small intestine and its pattern of dissemination closely resembles that of classical malignant histiocytosis.[8] The histiocytic origin of malignant histiocytosis of the intestine has been shown by marker studies on fresh tissue from three cases[21] and by immunoperoxidase staining of paraffin sections in these and numerous other cases.[20] It is thus distinct from the 'histiocytic' lymphomas in Rappaport's classification, the majority of which are B cell tumours. Malignant histiocytosis of the intestine rarely occurs in patients without coeliac disease, and so for practical purposes can be considered to be specifically associated with coeliac disease.

Other tumours
Approximately half of the other invasive malignancies encountered in patients with coeliac disease arise from the gastrointestinal tract. This proportion is significantly greater than that expected in the general population. This is accounted for principally by a large excess of small intestinal adenocarcinomas, but there is also a significant excess of oesophageal and pharyngeal squamous carcinomas (Figure 8.46). The proportion of tumours arising from lung and breast is smaller than expected, but this is, at least in part, accounted for by the distorting effect of the high proportion of small intestinal adenocarcinomas.

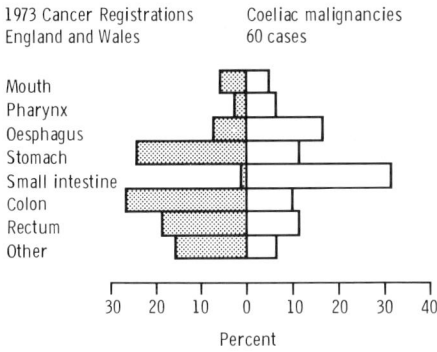

Fig. 8.46 The excess proportion of gastrointestinal tumours in patients with coeliac disease is accounted for principally by a large excess of small intestinal adenocarcinomas, but significantly more oesophageal and pharyngeal squamous carcinomas than expected also occur. These figures are adjusted for age.

Adenocarcinomas of the small intestine are rare tumours occurring in only 0.6–0.7/100 000 of the general population per year. The high observed relative risk of 82.6[30] thus only increases the expected incidence among patients with coeliac disease to approximately 50/100 000 per year. This is of the same order as for large intestinal cancer in the general population. The risk to an individual patient of developing oesophageal or pharyngeal carcinoma is also small. Only ten adequately documented cases of oesophageal and four of pharyngeal squamous carcinomas occurred in the whole of the recent national study.[30]

In patients with coeliac disease the clinical features of malignancy do not differ significantly from the same tumours seen in other patients; the pathological features are also similar. The principal difference is that, in patients with coeliac disease, approximately 60% of the small intestinal adenocarcinomas affect the jejunum and approximately 25% affect the duodenum, whereas in the general population, sites in the duodenum, jejunum and ileum are affected

equally.[6] The clinical picture of malignancy may, however, be complicated by symptoms and signs of inadequately treated or previously undiagnosed coeliac disease; in such cases villous atrophy is seen in the mucosa of the small intestine that is uninvolved by tumour.

Multiple malignancies
The majority of patients with coeliac disease and malignancy have single tumours, but approximately 8% have two. Occasional patients have more than two tumours. There is no evidence to suggest any particular combination of tumours occurs more frequently than expected by chance alone.

Malignant histiocytosis of the intestine

Age and sex distribution
Malignant histiocytosis of the intestine is seen most frequently in patients in their fifth or sixth decade. Men and women are affected equally.

Clinical presentation
Approximately 80% of patients present with a lesion in the small intestine (Figure 8.47). Of those presenting with tumour outside the gastrointestinal tract some are subsequently found to have intestinal involvement, but in a small number no such evidence is found.

The commonest initial symptoms are malaise, anorexia, marked weight loss, and diarrhoea, often accompanied by abdominal pain. In many patients these symptoms are accompanied by pyrexia. This may be the principal abnormal finding, but peripheral lymphadenopathy, skin rashes, hepatomegaly, splenomegaly, a palpable abdominal mass, pleural effusion, pericardial effusion, or ascites may all occur. Other patients present with an acute gastrointestinal emergency. Up to 50% of patients may require an

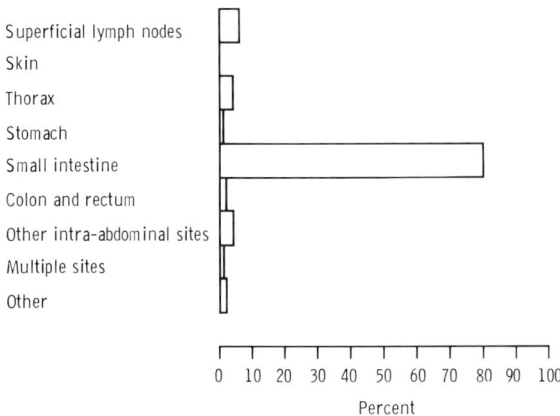

Fig. 8.47 Site of presenting manifestations of 84 cases of malignant histiocytosis diagnosed in life. Of 84 patients with malignant histiocytosis of the intestine, 67 (79.8%) presented because of a lesion in the small intestine. Of 14 patients who presented with tumour outside the gastrointestinal tract, three were subsequently shown to have extensive small intestinal involvement.

emergency laparotomy before diagnosis. Commonly this is for intestinal perforation or obstruction, but gastrointestinal haemorrhage may also occur. A small number of patients give a history of previous resection for apparently benign small intestinal ulcers or strictures some years earlier, or may have had a previously unexplained small intestinal perforation.

Diagnosis

The symptoms and signs at presentation often suggest coeliac disease, but the two particular features which should alert the clinician to the possibility of underlying malignant histiocytosis of the intestine are the prominence of abdominal pain and the presence of fever. Anaemia, abnormal liver function tests and hypoalbuminaemia are usually found.[14] Serum lysozyme levels have been shown to be significantly raised in patients with malignant histiocytosis of the intestine compared to controls and patients with uncomplicated coeliac disease.[13]

In patients with marked peripheral lymphadenopathy, lymph node biopsy may be diagnostic, but in the majority of patients in whom there is a high index of clinical suspicion, early laparotomy will often provide the most direct means of diagnosis. A barium meal and follow through may show a lesion but, even in patients who at subsequent laparotomy have a small intestinal lesion, it may show a non-specific malabsorption pattern or even be normal. Similarly lymphangiography may fail to show mesenteric lymph nodes which are involved with tumour.[14] Jejunal biopsy rarely shows frank tumour, but will confirm the diagnosis of coeliac disease in a patient not previously known to have the disorder. In some cases diagnosis may be made on needle aspiration of liver, but such biopsies may be difficult to interpret, even from cases where the liver is subsequently shown to be extensively involved. In some cases diagnosis may be made from bone marrow aspiration, but malignant cells are often difficult to see in a trephine preparation and may be missed unless a smear is done. At laparotomy, resection of any obviously involved intestine, multiple biopsies of mesenteric lymph nodes, wedge and core biopsies of liver, and splenectomy should enable the diagnosis to be made; whether or not to remove the spleen must be considered in the light of the increased operative risk to the patient.

Gross pathological appearances

Involvement of the gastrointestinal tract. Over 80% of patients who undergo laparotomy or come to post mortem examination have involvement of the gastrointestinal tract with macroscopic tumour. In the majority of cases the small intestine alone is affected but stomach and large bowel may be involved, either alone or in combination with other sites in the gastrointestinal tract.

Macroscopic features of small intestinal lesions. Tumour occurs in all parts of the small intestine, but most commonly in the jejunum. Approximately 70% of patients have some involvement of the jejunum, either alone or in combination with tumour at other sites. Only 45% of patients have some ileal involvement, and 3% some duodenal involvement. The majority of patients have multiple discrete lesions, but some have single lesions and a smaller number have complex lesions involving several loops of bowel. The most frequent type of lesion is a mass or plaque-like thickening. This can be localized, often near the mesenteric border, or it may surround the bowel wall in a circular fashion, narrowing its lumen and sometimes producing a hosepipe-like thickening extending over several centimetres. Another frequent type of lesion is an ulcer which is often indistinguishable macroscopically from benign causes of small intestinal ulceration (Figure 8.48). Some patients have strictures which are macroscopically identical to inflammatory strictures. Both mass lesions and strictures are frequently ulcerated, and a higher proportion are found to have perforated than is suspected clinically.

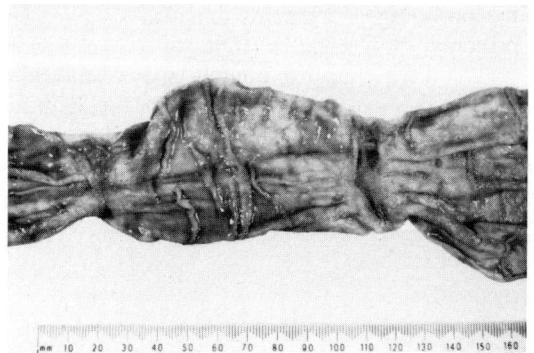

Fig. 8.48 Postmortem specimen from the small intestine of a patient with malignant histiocytosis of the intestine showing multiple ulcers and strictures which on histology were infiltrated by tumour. Courtesy of Professor P. Isaacson.

Associated changes in lymph nodes, liver and spleen. Mesenteric lymph nodes are usually enlarged, even in cases where no small intestinal lesion is visible macroscopically. The majority of patients have normal-sized livers, but some have hepatomegaly. The spleen is often of normal size or small and atrophic, reflecting the splenic atrophy that is a feature of coeliac disease. A few patients have splenomegaly.

Histology

Gastrointestinal tract lesions. The appearances of small intestinal lesions vary markedly in different patients and at different sites in the same patient. Characteristically there is a very pleomorphic picture, often with tumour giant cells (Figure 8.49). Tumour cells may often be seen invading blood vessels and lymphatics, and may produce a vasculitis-like lesion in the vessel wall. Phagocytosis of red cells, white cells and debris is also often present.

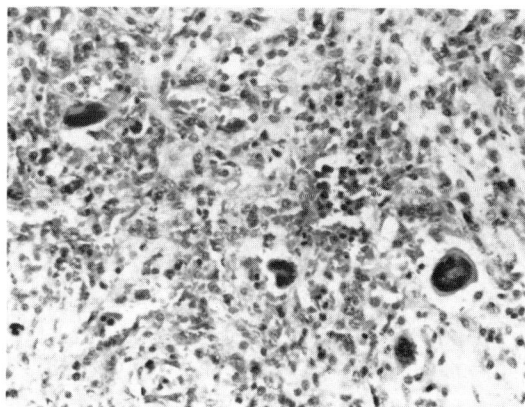

Fig. 8.49 Small intestine. In the lamina propria there is an infiltrate of large pleomorphic cells with many giant cell forms characteristic of malignant histiocytosis of the intestine (haematoxylin and eosin × 170).

In the majority of tumours there is a background of inflammatory cells, sometimes accompanied by fibrosis. An increased number of eosinophils may be present and in some cases these are particularly prominent, forming 'eosinophilic abscesses'. In other cases plasma cells are particularly prominent. Occasionally tumour cells are organized into fairly well-defined granulomas. In some lesions the inflammatory component may be so overwhelming that it is difficult to identify the malignant cells. In such cases examination of mesenteric lymph nodes, liver, spleen or bone marrow may be particularly helpful.

Villi in the region of a tumour may be flat or blunted by infiltration with tumour even when villi away from the tumour show histological improvement following a gluten-free diet. Away from the site of tumour early neoplastic lesions with aggregates of malignant histiocytes invading and destroying crypt epithelium may be seen. A further common feature is the presence of fissures extending from the mucosal surface deep into the lamina propria. Less commonly there may be associated benign ulceration or pyloric metaplasia indicative of previous ulceration.

In blood vessels, fibrinoid necrosis and thrombosis, sometimes associated with focal infarction and necrosis, may be seen in addition to the changes described above. Endarteritis may be seen in the base of ulcers.

Some patients without obvious tumour in the small intestine have microscopic lesions, but in a few no lesion can be found even when the entire small intestine is examined post mortem.

Lymph nodes, liver, spleen and bone marrow
Characteristically spread of tumour in lymph nodes is by sinusoidal infiltration of single cells, but this infiltrate later spreads into the medullary cords and eventually forms a solid tumour mass.

In the liver, spread of tumour is also typically by sinusoidal infiltration of single cells, but malignant cells are commonly also seen in portal tracts. Ill-defined granulomas, vasculitis-like lesions, and thrombosis of blood vessels may occasionally be seen.

In the spleen, single infiltrating malignant cells are most commonly seen in the red pulp, but the white pulp may also be affected. The bone marrow is best examined in the form of an aspirate smear rather than a trephine. Characteristically, bizarre phagocytic histiocytes are present.

Course
Approximately 20% of patients die before a diagnosis is made. Overall survival rate following diagnosis in life is 43% at six months, 36% at one year, and 10% at five years. Patients presenting with tumour outside the gastrointestinal tract appear to have a worse prognosis than those with gastrointestinal lesions, but only a small number of such patients have been studied.

Treatment
Because individual clinicians see relatively few cases, there are as yet no clear guidelines for treatment. Reports of effective chemotherapy for classical malignant histiocytosis are now emerging[2, 22, 24, 27] but it is not known whether similar regimens are effective in malignant histiocytosis of the intestine.

Relationship to classical malignant histiocytosis

The clinical features of malignant histiocytosis of the intestine differ from those of classical malignant histiocytosis.[25] Nevertheless intestinal involvement may occur in classical malignant histiocytosis;[1] there have been several recent case reports of patients presenting with intestinal involvement very similar to malignant histiocytosis of the intestine, although in none of the reports has the appearance of the uninvolved mucosa been described.

Relationship to ulcerative jejunitis

Some authors believe that ulcerative jejunitis is a manifestation of malignant histiocytosis of the intestine, perhaps representing the opposite end of the spectrum from those patients who present with disseminated disease without obvious small intestinal involvement; however, other authors disagree (see earlier in this chapter).

Identification of the patient at risk

The small number of patients who fail to respond clinically and histologically to a strict gluten-free diet may be at particular risk of developing malignant lymphomas,[5] but the majority of lymphomas develop in patients who show histological improvement following gluten withdrawal.

Other features which it has been suggested should alert the clinician to the development of lymphoma are a relative paucity of inflammatory infiltrate in the lamina propria and a low intraepithelial lymphocyte count on jejunal biopsy,[10] and a rising IgA level in a patient on a strict gluten-free and milk-free diet.[3] Occasional patients who develop malignant histiocytosis of the intestine have been shown on review to have early neoplastic lesions in jejunal biopsies taken up to five years before diagnosis.[17]

There are no differences in HLA type between patients with coeliac disease with and without malignancy to enable identification of the individuals particularly at risk.[29] The development of lymphoma is not related to splenic function.[23]

The role of a gluten free diet in prevention

No definitive answer can yet be given to the crucial question of whether adherence to a gluten-free diet reduces the risk to an individual of developing malignancy. Attempts to resolve the question have given conflicting answers.[12, 16] If a gluten-free diet does offer protection against malignancy this is most likely to become apparent from analysis of a large group of patients who have been prescribed a gluten-free diet from childhood, but it will be at least 20 years before the first group of treated children reach the age at which malignancy commonly develops. In the meantime the pragmatic course is to direct efforts to the early diagnosis of coeliac disease and encourage adherence to the diet.

Aetiology

Why patients with coeliac disease develop more malignancies than the general population is unknown. The mucosal lesion itself may predispose to malignant change. In coeliac disease there is a greatly increased epithelial cell turnover, and the epithelial cell damage may make the small intestine more susceptible to the effect of carcinogens. The epithelial cell damage may also increase access of antigens to lamina propria macrophages and the constant stimulation may make malignant change more likely. Altered immune responses in the small intestine and the general abnormalities of cellular immunity described in coeliac disease may also be important, perhaps by altering the response of the patient to an as yet unidentified oncovirus for malignant histiocytosis. Vitamin A deficiency, a frequent finding in coeliac disease, enhances the susceptibility of various epithelial tissues to chemical carcinogens as well as promoting metaplasia, and there is increasing evidence in both developing and Western countries of an association between multiple vitamin and mineral deficiencies and an increased risk for oesophageal carcinoma. The relative contributions of these various features to the development of malignancy in coeliac disease is unknown.

REFERENCES

1 Abele, D. C. & Griffin, T. B. (1972) Histiocytic medullary reticulosis: report of two cases and a review of the literature. *Archives of Dermatology*, **106**, 319–329.
2 Alexander, M. & Daniels, J. R. (1977) Chemotherapy of malignant histiocytosis in adults. *Cancer*, **39**, 1011–1017.
3 Asquith, P., Thompson, R. A. & Cooke, W. T. (1969) Serum immunoglobulins in adult coeliac disease. *Lancet*, **ii**, 129–131.
4 Austad, W. I., Cornes, J. S., Gough, K. R. *et al.* (1967) Steatorrhoea and malignant lymphoma. *American Journal of Digestive Diseases* (*New Series*), **12**, 475–489.
5 Barry, R. E. & Read, A. E. (1973) Coeliac disease and malignancy. *Quarterly Journal of Medicine* (*New Series*), **42**, 665–675.
6 Brookes, V. S., Waterhouse, J. A. H. & Powel, D. J. (1968) Malignant lesions of the small intestine: a ten-year survey. *British Journal of Surgery*, **55**, 405–410.

7 Brzechwa-Ajdukiewicz, A., McCarthy, C. F., Austad, W. *et al.* (1966) Carcinoma, villous atrophy and steatorrhoea. *Gut*, **7**, 572–577.

8 Byrne, G. E. & Rappaport, H. (1973) Malignant histiocytosis. In *Malignant Diseases of the Haemopoietic System* (Ed.) Akazak, T., Rappaport, H. & Berard, C. W. Gann monograph on cancer research 15. pp. 145–162. Tokyo: University of Tokyo Press.

9 Fairly, H. N. & Mackie, F. P. (1937) The clinical and biochemical syndrome in lymphoma and allied diseases involving the mesenteric lymph glands. *British Medical Journal*, **i**, 375–380.

10 Ferguson, R., Asquith, P. & Cooke, W. T. (1974) The jejunal cellular infiltrate in coeliac disease complicated by lymphoma. *Gut*, **15**, 458–461.

11 Gough, K. R., Read, A. E. & Naish, J. M. (1962) Intestinal reticulosis as a complication of idiopathic steatorrhoea. *Gut*, **3**, 232–239.

12 Harris, O. D., Cooke, W. T., Thompson, H. & Waterhouse, J. A. H. (1967) Malignancy in adult coeliac disease and idiopathic steatorrhoea. *American Journal of Medicine*, **42**, 899–912.

13 Hodges, J. R., Isaacson, P., Eade, O. E. & Wright, R. (1978) Serum lysozyme levels in malignant histiocytosis of the intestine. *Gut*, **19**, A933.

14 Hodges, J. R., Isaacson, P., Smith, C. L. & Sworn, M. J. (1979) Malignant histiocytosis of the intestine. *Digestive Diseases and Sciences*, **24**, 631–638.

15 Holmes, G. K. T., Dunn, G. I., Cockel, R. & Brookes, V. S. (1980) Adenocarcinoma of the upper small bowel complicating coeliac disease. *Gut*, **21**, 1010–1016.

16 Holmes, G. K. T., Stokes, P. L., Sorahan, T. M. *et al.* (1976) Coeliac disease, gluten-free diet and malignancy. *Gut*, **17**, 612–619.

17 Isaacson, P. (1980) Malignant histiocytosis of the intestine: the early histological lesion. *Gut*, **21**, 381–386.

18 Isaacson, P. & Wright, D. H. (1978) Intestinal lymphoma associated with malabsorption. *Lancet*, **i**, 67–70.

19 Isaacson, P. & Wright, D. H. (1978) Malignant histiocytosis of the intestine: its relationship to malabsorption and ulcerative jejunitis. *Human Pathology*, **9**, 661–676.

20 Isaacson, P. & Wright, D. H. (1980) Malabsorption and intestinal lymphomas. In *Recent Advances in Gastrointestinal Pathology* (Ed.) Wright, R. pp. 193–212. London: W. B. Saunders.

21 Isaacson, P., Jones, D. B., Sworn, M. J. & Wright, D. H. (1982) Malignant histiocytosis of the intestine: report of three cases with immunological and cytochemical analysis. *Journal of Clinical Pathology*, **35**, 510–516.

22 Lampert, I. A., Catovsky, D. & Bergier, N. (1978) Malignant histiocytosis: a clinico-pathological study of 12 cases. *British Journal of Haematology*, **40**, 65–77.

23 Robertson, D. A. F., Swinson, C. M., Hall, R. & Losowsky, M. S. (1982) Coeliac disease, splenic function, and malignancy. *Gut*, **23**, 666–669.

24 Ruuskanen, O., Kero, P., Rajamaki, T. *et al.* (1977) Malignant histiocytosis: histiocytic medullary reticulosis. *Acta Paediatrica Scandinavica*, **66**, 249–254.

25 Scott, R. B. & Robb-Smith, A. H. T. (1939) Histiocytic medullary reticulosis. *Lancet*, **ii**, 194–198.

26 Selby, W. & Gallagher, N. D. (1979) Malignancy in a 19-year experience of adult coeliac disease. *Digestive Diseases and Sciences*, **24**, 684–688.

27 Stein, R. S., Morgan, E. M. & Byrne, G. C. (1976) Malignant histiocytosis: complete remission with combination chemotherapy. *Cancer*, **38**, 1083–1086.

28 Swinson, C. M. & Levi, A. J. (1980) Is coeliac disease underdiagnosed? *British Medical Journal*, **281**, 1258–1260.

29 Swinson, C. M., Hall, P. J., Bedford, P. A. & Booth, C. C. (1983) HLA antigens in coeliac disease associated with malignancy. *Gut*, **24**, 925–928.

30 Swinson, C. M., Slavin, G., Coles, E. C. & Booth, C. C. (1983) Coeliac disease and malignancy. *Lancet*, **i**, 111–115.

TROPICAL SPRUE

Tropical sprue is a primary malabsorption syndrome occurring in residents of, or visitors to, certain tropical areas where the disease is endemic.[3, 15] The aetiology of this disease and the pathogenesis of malabsorption is not fully understood. The diagnosis of tropical sprue in the individual patient is therefore dependent on the demonstration of malabsorption of nutrients and the exclusion of conditions which can produce malabsorption by known pathogenic mechanisms (the secondary malabsorption syndromes). A comparison of the clinical features in patients described from different parts of the tropics suggests that the aetiology of the syndrome is likely to be multiple. As several factors which can damage the intestinal mucosa and produce malabsorption have been described, what is now described as the 'syndrome of tropical sprue' is likely eventually to be classified into several entities.

Historical aspects

Chronic diarrhoea associated with wasting was familiar to the physicians of India from at least 600 BC; they attributed this to the 'weakness of the digestive fire which only scorched the ingested food and did not allow it to contribute to the growth of the body'.[4] In English medical literature, the syndrome was first documented in Barbados by Hillary.[13] British and Dutch physicians described the clinical syndrome in great detail in expatriates from Europe in India and south-east Asia during the eighteenth and nineteenth centuries. These clinical descriptions emphasize the presence of anaemia and glossitis as well as wasting. It was generally thought at that time that the disease did not affect indigenous populations of tropical countries.[2] Reports from the Caribbean region, especially the detailed studies undertaken by the United States Army, emphasized the haematological abnormalities considered essential for diagnosis and for some time sprue was considered to be a primary haematological disease.[7] During the Second World War, tropical sprue occurred as epidemics in the Assam Theatre of War, and in the 1960s several epidemics of tropical sprue were reported from southern India.[1, 14, 31] After the mid-1950s, the availability of a variety of methods to study intestinal absorption and the ability to obtain intestinal mucosal biopsies established that tropical sprue was a gastro-intestinal disease and that the nutritional deficiencies seen are secondary to malabsorption. It was also shown that the syndrome was widely prevalent in the indigenous populations of many tropical developing areas.

Epidemiology and aetiology

Hillary[13] reported that two years after his arrival in Barbados, tropical sprue assumed epidemic proportions. On clinical and investigational grounds all patients with tropical sprue have malabsorption of unknown aetiology. However, on epidemiological grounds, it appears reasonable to divide patients into three groups:

a Tropical sprue in expatriates from temperate climates.
b Endemic tropical sprue in indigenous populations.
c Epidemic tropical sprue in indigenous populations.

Endemic tropical sprue in expatriates and in indigenous populations occurs sporadically without any temporal or spatial relationship with other known cases of tropical sprue. While the clinical manifestations are similar, it is possible that the aetiological factors are different. One particular group affected in this way are overland travellers from Europe to the Indian subcontinent who were detected to have malabsorption on return to their home countries.[28] A proportion of these patients had giardiasis, while others were considered to be cases of tropical sprue since no agent could be detected. In these patients, treatment with folic acid, vitamin B_{12} and tetracycline was very effective.

There are many reports of endemic tropical sprue from the Indian subcontinent and descriptions of the disease from different centres in the country appears to be similar.[9, 10, 11] In the Caribbean, although tropical sprue has been described from many of the islands, it has not been found in Jamaica. The reasons for this, or the low prevalence of tropical sprue in sub-Saharan Africa, are not clear.[27]

Epidemic tropical sprue was first described in detail in British and Indian troops and Italian prisoners of war during the Second World War. While malabsorption and its sequelae were present, no aetiological studies were carried out.

Subsequently, several large epidemics of tropical sprue have been described from southern India.[18, 19, 20] A high proportion of the population in affected villages is afflicted; the incidence is higher in adults than in children. Fifty percent of the subjects affected in an epidemic are symptom-free by the end of a month, but patients have been followed up for over 20 years after the first reported epidemic in 1960/61. There is temporal and spatial clustering of cases in villages and the evolution of an epidemic in a village usually takes one or two years, with secondary and tertiary waves of the epidemic appearing 5–10 years later. In subsequent waves of the epidemic, the age-specific attack rate is changed; those who had been asymptomatic at the time of the original epidemic in a village appear to be protected during the subsequent waves. The attack rate in children born after the first wave of the epidemic is significantly higher than would be expected in the secondary and tertiary waves. Available data suggests that these epidemics are likely to be caused by an infectious agent, but detailed bacteriological, virological and other studies thus far have failed to identify an agent.

The clinical features and natural history of tropical sprue reported from different regions suggest that there are regional differences and that the disease is a syndrome of multiple aetiology.[26] However, as yet no critical comparative study of patients evaluated according to a uniform protocol in different areas has been performed.

It is reasonable to consider this syndrome as the end result of damage to the intestinal absorptive cell. Nutritional deficiency, food toxins or infections have been considered as possible factors which could produce the intestinal mucosal damage. The majority of the people in many of the areas where tropical sprue is endemic live on marginal diets, but it has not yet been possible to identify a particular nutritional deficiency that can produce an enteropathy, or to 'cure' the intestinal lesion by giving physiological amounts of nutrients. It is, however, possible that deficiency states may be predisposing or perpetuating factors for enterocyte damage. Food toxins or an immunological response similar to coeliac disease has also been considered but has not been demonstrated. Immunological parameters are normal in tropical sprue[24] and the mucosal immunological alterations appear to be secondary to enterocyte damage.[22]

The study of epidemic tropical sprue gives the strongest support for an infectious aetiology but conventional techniques have failed to isolate an agent. In Puerto Rico, small bowel colonization by toxin-producing coliforms appear to be important in the aetiology,[16] but in southern India a similar situation was not found. An agent or agents which can produce persistent enterocyte damage have yet to be discovered.

Clinical features

HISTORY

Diarrhoea, of usually longer than two weeks duration, anorexia, and abdominal distension are the major symptoms. The symptoms of nutritional deficiency, including weight loss, pallor, weakness, sore tongue and mouth, oedema of the legs, and night blindness, are related to the duration of malabsorption and the antecedent nutritional status of the patient. Occasionally a patient may present with only a nutritional deficiency syndrome with no abdominal complaints and malabsorption is found only on investigation.

The exact time of onset of symptoms can be given by some patients, especially those who have been affected in epidemics of tropical sprue. In about a quarter of such individuals, fever, malaise and anorexia precede the onset of diarrhoea. In the early stages of the illness the symptoms are predominantly abdominal, the bowels are opened usually five to eight times a day, the stools being large in volume and watery or mushy in consistency. Less than 10% of patients may complain of small amounts of blood and mucus in the stool. During the first few weeks of illness the patients may have nausea and associated vomiting, although these symptoms tend to clear up while the anorexia and abdominal distension persist. In a few patients, severe diarrhoea during the early stage may produce significant dehydration and electrolyte imbalance leading to death. Early loss of weight may be a feature. The development of the nutritional sequelae of persistent malabsorption characterize the later or chronic stage of the illness. Diarrhoea may persist throughout the course of the illness, but usually there are repeated remissions and relapses. Mild abdominal pain, sometimes colicky in nature, is found in over half the patients at some point during the course of illness. Weight loss is progressive. Earlier textbooks describe the classic picture of chronic tropical sprue dominated by the secondary features of multiple nutritional deficiencies and wasting.

PHYSICAL FINDINGS

The findings on abdominal examination are usually minimal: mild abdominal distension, loud and irregular bowel sounds, and visible peristalsis, especially when the abdominal wall is thin due to weight loss. Marked dehydration and acidosis may be present in a small number of patients, especially in hot and dry climates.

The signs of nutritional deficiency dominate the clinical picture in the chronically ill patient. Severe megaloblastic anaemia is characterized by pallor and mild icterus. Other features of nutritional deficiency are glossitis, stomatitis, cheilosis, cutaneous and mucosal hyperpigmentation associated with vitamin B_{12} or folate deficiency, dependent oedema, exfoliation of the skin, and thin dyspigmented hair. Sigmoidoscopic examination is usually unremarkable, although in about a third of patients with chronic symptoms, internal haemorrhoids may be present as well as some hyperaemia of the rectal mucosa.

LABORATORY FINDINGS

Investigations of patients with tropical sprue should determine the severity and extent of malabsorption, exclude secondary malabsorption, and evaluate the extent of nutritional deficiency.

Stool examination
The volume and weight of stool passed in 24 hours is increased in patients with tropical sprue. Although the prevalence of intestinal parasites such as *Entamoeba histolytica*, *Giardia lamblia* and *Strongyloides stercoralis* in patients with tropical sprue is the same as in the general population, if any of these parasites are found in the individual patient, it would be advisable to give appropriate therapy to see if there is improvement in absorptive parameters and clinical status. However, these are not usually significantly altered by parasite eradication. The rate of isolation of bacterial pathogens from the stool in tropical countries in patients and control populations is similar. Examination of a Sudan III stained smear of the stool is useful for screening patients for steatorrhoea.

Tests of absorption
It is possible to test the absorption of water, electrolytes and a large number of nutrients by appropriate techniques. In the clinical situation, the absorption of fat, D-xylose and vitamin B_{12}

are usually tested; it is accepted that malabsorption of at least two of these three substances is necessary for the diagnosis of tropical sprue.

In most reported series, over 90% of the patients have steatorrhoea, the daily faecal fat excretion on a 50 g fat intake ranging from about 6 g to around 25 g. Malabsorption of D-xylose is found in almost 99% of patients, but its absence in an occasional patient does not invalidate the diagnosis. Vitamin B_{12} malabsorption has been reported in 60 to over 90% of patients in different regions. The highest prevalence of vitamin B_{12} malabsorption appears to be in expatriates from temperate countries and in the Caribbean area, while in India it is found in only about 60% of the patients. The absorption of vitamin B_{12} is usually not improved when additional intrinsic factor is given, but in a small number of patients vitamin B_{12} malabsorption improves or becomes normal with intrinsic factor, suggesting that there is also a gastric lesion in this condition.[30]

Tropical enteropathy – the presence of morphological abnormalities in the jejunal mucosa associated with malabsorption of one nutrient such as fat, xylose or vitamin B_{12} in apparently healthy asymptomatic individuals – which occurs in many tropical countries has to be taken into consideration when tests of absorption and jejunal mucosal biopsies are evaluated in indigenous populations.[5] Tropical enteropathy is probably an adaptation of the intestinal mucosa to the contaminated environment of the tropics.[21] The prevalence of tropical enteropathy varies in different parts of the world and is high in countries like southern India and Haiti. The results in an individual patient with chronic diarrhoea and malabsorption therefore have to be evaluated in the light of the normal background for the population being studied.

Intestinal mucosal morphology
The availability of peroral biopsy instruments since the mid-1950s has made it possible to undertake systematic studies of the intestinal mucosal morphology in patients with tropical sprue, and confirm the early findings from postmortem or laparotomy material.

The overall thickness of the mucosa in patients with tropical sprue is within normal limits, but the villi are shortened and the crypt height is increased (Figure 8.50). The surface epithelial cells are abnormal, low cuboidal or columnar, and at higher power cytoplasmic

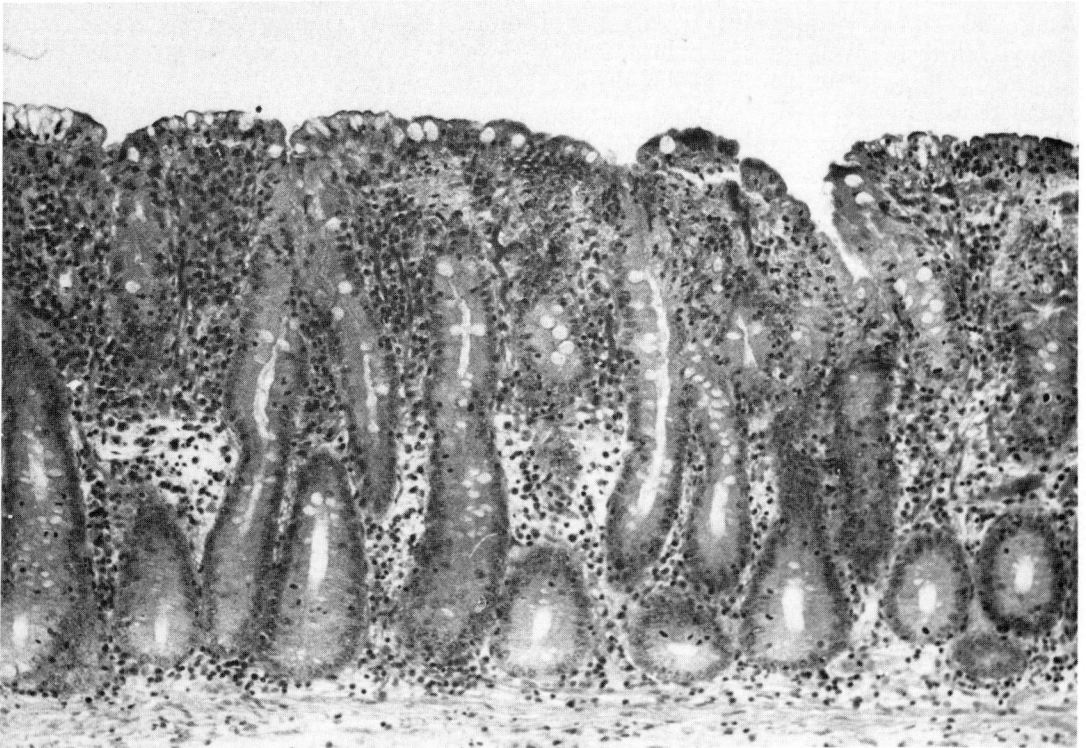

Fig. 8.50 Light micrograph of a paraffin-embedded jejunal biopsy from a patient with chronic tropical sprue showing a moderately severe lesion. The crypts occupy about three-quarters of the total mucosal thickness. Surface enterocytes are damaged and there is increased cellularity of lamina propria and the epithelial layer (× 275).

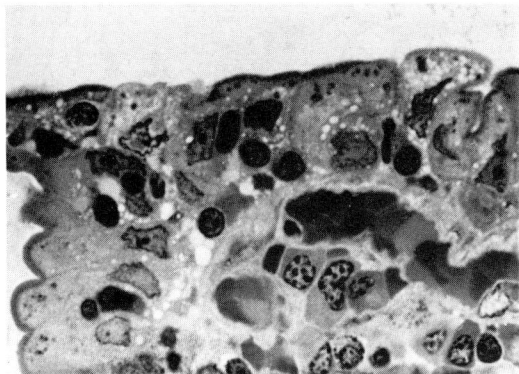

Fig. 8.51 Light micrograph of an epon-embedded jejunal biopsy sectioned 1 μm thick and stained with toluidene blue. The apical portion of a villus with intervillous enterocytes is on the left. Note the increased lysosomes, damaged cytoplasm and brush border, and loss of nuclear polarity. Epithelial lymphocytes are increased (× 1200).

damage can be recognized (Figure 8.51). Total villus atrophy as seen in coeliac disease is seldom found and the surface epithelial cell damage is less than in gluten sensitivity. The basement membrane is usually thickened. Fine droplets of fat may be present in the thickened basement membrane, in the surface epithelial cells, and free in the lamina propria even after 12 to 18 hours of fasting. Epithelial lymphocytes are significantly increased in the surface and crypt epithelium; this parallels the severity of the mucosal lesion.[24] There is also a moderate to marked increase in the cellularity of the lamina propria. In large groups of patients the severity of the jejunal mucosal abnormality correlates significantly with the severity of the malabsorption,[4] although occasionally severe malabsorption may be present with a relatively normal biopsy. This may be a reflection of the sampling error of jejunal biopsy.

Electron microscopic examination of jejunal mucosal biopsies has shown significant abnormalities in the epithelial cells, in both the crypt and the surface epithelium. Abnormalities of the microvilli, with shortening, sparsity and grouping, a marked increase in lysosomes, intracellular fat, and degenerative changes in the rough endoplasmic reticulum and mitochondria can all be found in individual cells. Such damaged cells are interspersed between apparently normal cells. The ultrastructural change in these cells (Figure 8.52) is similar to the changes described in coeliac disease but, unlike coeliac disease, such damaged cells are also present in crypts.[17] The damaged crypt cells resemble cells which have been described in radiation- or methotrexate-damaged small intestine. It is not

yet possible to say whether the presence of damaged enterocytes in the crypt is a characteristic and possibly diagnostic feature in tropical sprue.

Exclusion of secondary malabsorption

The secondary malabsorption syndromes are the result of deficient intraluminal digestion, damaged intestinal mucosa, or interference with transport from the gut. In the individual patient in whom tropical sprue is suspected, it is important to exclude these conditions. Apart from a careful history and physical examination, the investigations that are particularly useful are jejunal mucosal biopsy and careful radiology. Conditions such as agammaglobulinaemia with nodular lymphoid hyperplasia, parasites damaging the intestinal epithelium, Whipple's disease, coeliac disease, or diffuse intestinal lymphoma can often be diagnosed by peroral biopsy. Careful radiological examination of the small intestine using stabilized barium preparations and image intensification can show structural abnormalities such as blind loops, diverticula, fistulas, or strictures – conditions associated with bacterial overgrowth and the stagnant bowel syndrome. The radiological features of tropical sprue include altered peristalsis with slow transit of the barium column through the small intestine, dilatation of the loops of intestine, and thickening of the primary mucosal folds. These features are nonspecific and not of themselves diagnostic.[23] Other tests which are of importance are the detection of parasites in jejunal luminal fluid, the demonstration of bacterial overgrowth by appropriate sampling of the intestinal luminal contents, the detection of hypo- or agammaglobulinaemia, abetalipoproteinaemia or other metabolic abnormalities.

Assessment of nutritional status

In tropical sprue the prevalence and severity of nutritional deficiency states increases with the increasing duration of symptomatic diarrhoea.[4] Anaemia is the result of varying degrees of deficiency of iron, folic acid and vitamin B_{12}. Megaloblastic anaemia is found in over 60% of the patients, although in different regions the role of vitamin B_{12}/folate deficiency may differ. Since nutritional iron deficiency is widely prevalent in the normal population of many tropical developing countries,[6] the additional contribution of tropical sprue to iron deficiency anaemia in the tropics is difficult to assess. Reports from temperate climates suggest that megaloblastic anaemia is far more common in patients with tropical sprue than iron deficiency anaemia.

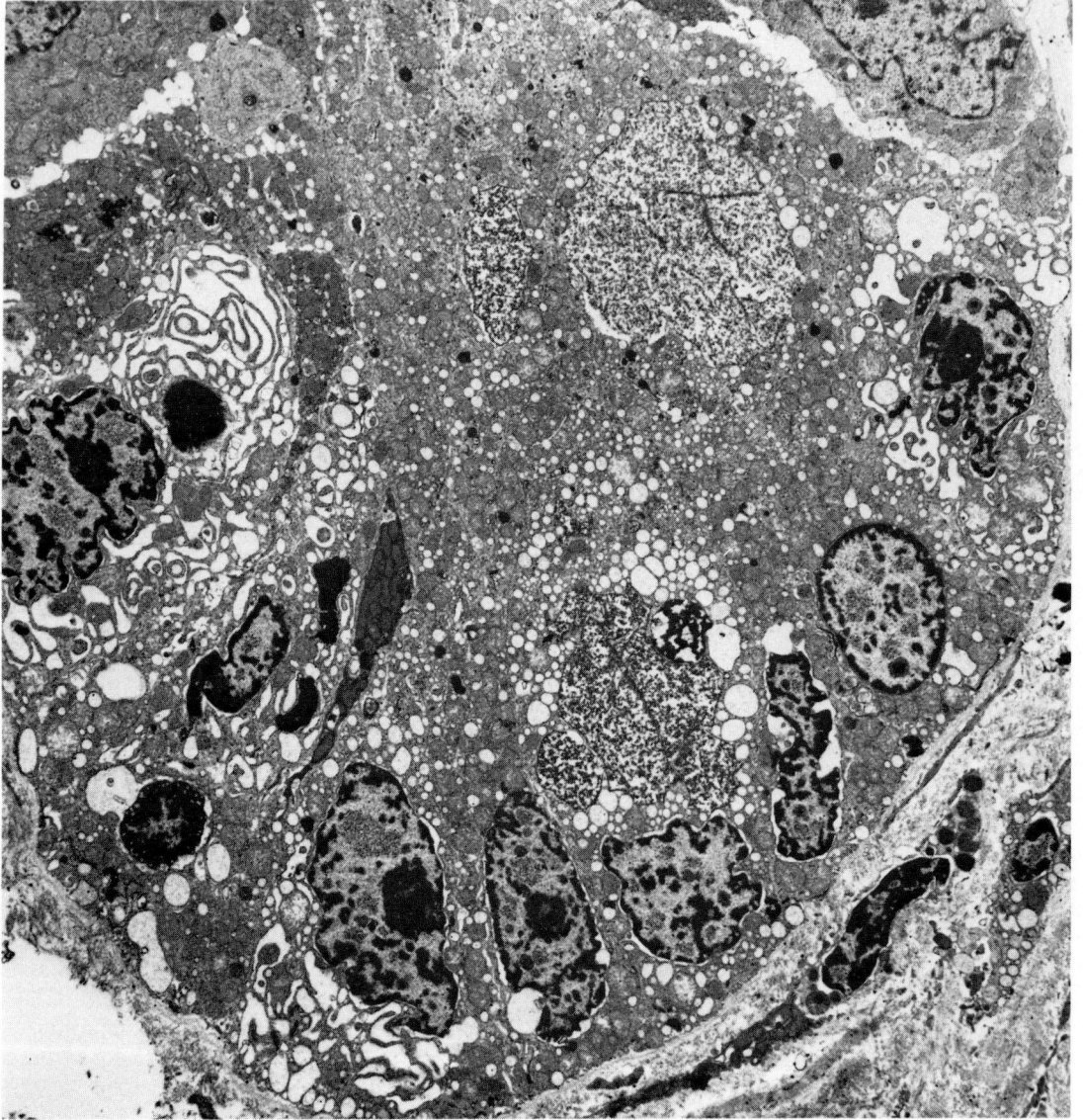

Fig. 8.52 Electron micrograph of enterocytes at the base of a crypt in a jejunal biopsy from a patient with chronic tropical sprue. Note the marked dilatation of the endoplasmic reticulum and perinuclear space (× 3800).

Hypoproteinaemia, with its sequelae of oedema and hair and skin changes, has been extensively documented. It has been suggested that the intestinal lesion is the result of a hypoproteinaemic enteropathy; however, critical analysis of available data does not support this but rather shows that hypoproteinaemia develops as a consequence of malabsorption. Protein losing enteropathy may also contribute to the hypoproteinaemia in this condition.[30] Dehydration associated with hypokalaemia, hyponatraemia and acidosis is a major complication in patients with large-volume, watery diarrhoea and is often a cause of death, espe-

cially in areas where adequate treatment is not available. Deficiency of other nutrients may also be present.

Diagnosis and differential diagnosis

In a patient presenting with chronic diarrhoea and signs of malnutrition or megaloblastic anaemia in the tropics, or with a history of having visited tropical regions, the diagnosis of tropical sprue should be considered.

In the chronic well-established case of tropical sprue, parasitic diseases that are of particular importance are giardiasis, strongyloidiasis and capillariasis. Since these parasites damage the upper small bowel, examination of the jejunal luminal fluid or jejunal mucosal biopsies may be necessary to exclude their presence. Rapid normalization of absorptive parameters following appropriate treatment of parasitic infestation will help to establish the diagnosis.

The most important condition to be considered in the differential diagnosis in tropical countries is intestinal tuberculosis producing secondary malabsorption by bacterial overgrowth. This, and other conditions which give rise to bacterial overgrowth and a stagnant bowel syndrome, can best be excluded by careful radiological examination, although laparotomy may occasionally be necessary. Quantitative bacteriological cultures of the intestinal luminal fluid have to be interpreted with caution since coliforms and bacteroides up to a concentration of 10^4/ml of luminal fluid can be cultured from healthy adults in the tropics.[8]

Coeliac disease is not widely prevalent in tropical countries and it was felt that this was primarily because wheat or rye were not part of the diet. The introduction of wheat to many traditional rice-eating populations was expected to produce a large number of cases of coeliac disease. However, in southern India, although wheat consumption has gone up significantly over the last ten years, no case of coeliac disease has been detected.

Primary disaccharidase deficiency as a cause of malabsorption can be diagnosed by low intestinal mucosal disaccharidase levels in the presence of morphologically normal biopsies. It is important to remember that many populations in tropical countries are lactase deficient.[25]

In early cases with symptoms of acute diarrhoea with or without small amounts of blood in the stool, especially in epidemic stituations, infectious diarrhoeal diseases have to be excluded by appropriate microbiological techniques. Most acute infectious diarrhoeas are of less than two weeks duration although some of them may lead to a post-dysenteric syndrome which may last longer (see later in this chapter). In epidemic tropical sprue, malabsorption is present even during the first few days of the illness.

Complications and mortality

The course of the illness is characterized by remissions and relapses. Prolonged follow up of patients in southern India for over 20 years did not show a higher incidence of small intestinal malignancy. The susceptibility to infections is increased and the prevalence of tuberculosis (usually pulmonary or nodal) is higher in groups of patients with tropical sprue. Mortality in the indigenous population and in those in whom the nutritional deficiency is not corrected is high and has been as much as 40% in the epidemic situation. However, there is a marked tendency towards spontaneous remissions; in epidemics nearly 90% are symptom-free by the end of the first year.

Treatment

Controlling the diarrhoea, correcting the nutritional deficiencies and attempting to cure the intestinal lesion are the major aims in the treatment of tropical sprue. A follow-up study of a large number of patients has shown that spontaneous recovery occurs in a significant proportion of the patients.[4]

Control of diarrhoea
Symptomatic control of the diarrhoea can usually be achieved using Lomotil (diphenoxylate and atropine) 2.5–5.0 mg three or four times a day, loperamide 5–10 mg three or four times a day, or mixtures of belladonna, opium, paregoric or bismuth salicylate. The dosages have to be tailored for the individual patient. While these measures make the patient feel more comfortable and may reduce the extent of fluid and electrolyte losses, it does not appear to shorten the duration or extent of the malabsorption.

Correction of deficiency states
In severely dehydrated patients, parenteral replacement of fluids may be necessary, although the majority of patients can be managed by oral maintenance of hydration; the glucose electrolyte solutions recommended for the treatment of acute diarrhoea have proved to be equally useful in tropical sprue. Maintenance of hydration in epidemics of tropical sprue has significantly reduced the mortality associated with this condition.[20] Therapeutic supplements of vitamins and trace nutrients may have to be given depending on the pattern of nutritional deficiency found. While iron and folic acid are satisfactorily absorbed when given orally in pharmacological doses, vitamin B_{12} should preferably be given parenterally.

The diet in patients with tropical sprue should ideally promote weight gain. Various types of experimental or elemental diets have been advocated, but there is no critical study showing a specific advantage for any of them. Any particular item of the diet which seems to aggravate the symptoms should be avoided. Patients should be encouraged to take at least 3000 calories/day with 1 g of protein/kg ideal body weight. The adequacy of the nutritional intake should be monitored by keeping a careful record of weight gain. The majority of patients gain weight satisfactorily, even though malabsorption is persistent, if sufficient calories are taken. Anorexia and abdominal distension are the major constraints in ensuring adequate nutritional intake.

Specific therapy

Since the aetiology of tropical sprue is unknown, there is as yet no rational therapy for the small intestinal lesion. Evaluation of treatment aimed at curing the lesion is difficult because of the spontaneous remissions that characterize the natural history of the disease. In the Caribbean islands, it is accepted that treatment with folic acid, vitamin B_{12} and tetracycline for up to six months is curative.[12] The reports that tropical sprue in the Caribbean islands is associated with colonization of the small intestine by a toxin-producing coliform provide the rationale for this treatment. In southern India, treatment with folic acid and vitamin B_{12}, with or without tetracycline, did not produce a rate of remission higher than in untreated controls,[4] although in an occasional patient there was a rapid and dramatic response to the institution of tetracycline therapy. While the situation in indigenous patients was not clear-cut, expatriates from temperate climates treated in southern India responded promptly to tetracycline and folic acid. It is not clear whether the difference in the response between the indigenous patient and the expatriate is related to differences in nutritional status, differences in aetiology, or due to secondary factors which could perpetuate the lesion.

Definitive treatment of patients with tropical sprue awaits the identification of aetiological agents and possible perpetuating factors but, with our present knowledge, it appears justifiable to treat patients by correcting the deficiencies and giving a course of tetracycline for up to six months.

ACKNOWLEDGEMENT

The author's work referred to here is supported by the Wellcome Trust, London.

REFERENCES

1 Ayrey, F. (1948) Outbreaks of sprue during the Burmah Campaign. *Transactions of the Royal Society of Tropical Medicine and Hygiene*, **41**, 377–382.

2 Bahr, P. H. (1915) *A report on research on sprue in Ceylon 1912–1914.* Cambridge: University Press.

3 Baker, S. J. and Mathan, V. I. (1968) Syndrome of tropical sprue in south India. *American Journal of Clinical Nutrition*, **21**, 984–993.

4 Baker, S. J. & Mathan, V. I. (1971) Tropical sprue in southern India. In *Tropical Sprue and Megaloblastic Anaemia. A Wellcome Trust Collaborative Study.* pp. 189–260. London: Churchill Livingstone.

5 Baker, S. J. & Mathan, V. I. (1972) Tropical enteropathy and tropical sprue. *American Journal of Clinical Nutrition*, **25**, 1047–1055.

6 Baker, S. J. Mathan, V. I. (1975) Prevalence, pathogenesis and prophylaxis of iron deficiency in the tropics. In *Iron Metabolism and its Disorders* (Ed.) Kief, H. pp. 145–158. Amsterdam: Excerpta Medica.

7 Bayless, T. M., Wheby, M. S. & Swanson, V. L. (1968) Tropical sprue in Puerto Rico. *American Journal of Clinical Nutrition*, **21**, 1030–1041.

8 Bhat, P. S., Shantakumari, D., Rajan, D. et al. (1972) Bacterial flora of the gastrointestinal tract in southern Indian control subjects and patients with tropical sprue. *Gastroenterology*, **62**, 11–21.

9 Chaudhuri, R. N. & Saha, T. K. (1963) Jejunal mucosa in malabsorption syndrome. *Journal of the Indian Medical Association*, **41**, 427–432.

10 Chuttani, H. K., Kasthuri, D. & Misra, R. C. (1968) Course and prognosis of tropical sprue. *Journal of Tropical Medicine and Hygiene*, **71**, 96–99.

11 Desai, H. G. & Jeejeebhoy, K. N. (1967) Jejunal mucosa and absorption studies in tropical malabsorption syndrome. *Indian Journal of Pathology and Bacteriology*, **10**, 107–122.

12 Guerra, R., Wheby, M. S. & Bayless, T. M. (1965) Long term antibiotic therapy in tropical sprue. *Annals of Internal Medicine*, **63**, 619–639.

13 Hillary, W. (1759) *Observations on the Changes on the Air and Concomitant Epidemical Diseases in the Island of Barbados*, pp. 277–297. London: Hitch and Hawes.

14 Keele, K. D. & Bound, J. P. (1946) Sprue in India: clinical survey of 600 cases. *British Medical Journal*, **i**, 77–81.

15 Klipstein, F. A. & Baker, S. J. (1970) Regarding the definition of tropical sprue. *Gastroenterology*, **58**, 717–721.

16 Klipstein, F. A., Holdeman, L. V., Corcino, J. J. & Moore, W. E. C. (1973) Enterotoxigenic intestinal bacteria in tropical sprue. *Annals of Internal Medicine*, **79**, 632–641.

17 Mathan, M., Mathan, V. I. & Baker, S. J. (1975) An electron microscopic study of jejunal mucosal morphology in control subjects and in patients with tropical sprue in southern India. *Gastroenterology*, **68**, 17–32.

18 Mathan, V. I. & Baker, S. J. (1968) Epidemic tropical sprue and other epidemics of diarrhoea in South Indian villages. A comparative study. *American Journal of Clinical Nutrition*, **21**, 1077–1087.

19 Mathan, V. I. & Baker, S. J. (1970) An epidemic of tropical sprue. *Annals of Tropical Medicine and Parasitology*, **64**, 439–452.

20 Mathan, V. I. & Baker, S. J. (1971) The epidemiology of tropical sprue. In *Tropical Sprue and Megaloblastic Anaemia. A Wellcome Trust Collaborative Study.* pp. 159–188. London: Churchill Livingstone.

21 Mathan, V. I., Mathan, M. & Ponniah, J. (1981) Tropical enteropathy: an adaptation of the small intestine to accelerated cell loss in contaminated environments. In *Mechanisms of Intestinal Adaptation.* (Ed.) Robinson, J. W. L., Dowling, R. H. & Riecken, E. O. pp. 609–610. Lancaster: MTP Press.

22 Marsh, M. N., Mathan, M. & Mathan, V. I. (1983) The secondary nature of lymphoid cell activation in the jejunal lesion of tropical sprue. *American Journal of Pathology*, **112**, 302–309.

23 McLean, A. M., Farthing, M. J. G., Kurian, G. & Mathan, V. I. (1982) The relationship between hypoalbuminaemia and the radiological appearance of the jejunum in tropical sprue. *British Journal of Radiology*, **55**, 725–728.

24 Ross, I. N. & Mathan, V. I. (1981) Immunological changes in tropical sprue. *Quarterly Journal of Medicine*, **50**, 435–449.

25 Swaminathan, N., Mathan, V. I., Baker, S. J. & Radhakrishnan, A. N. (1970) Disaccharidase levels in jejunal biopsy specimens from American and South Indian control subjects and patients with tropical sprue. *Clinica Chimica Acta*, **30**, 707–712.

26 The Wellcome Trust (1971) *Tropical Sprue and Megaloblastic Anaemia*. London: Churchill Livingstone.

27 Tomkins, A. (1981) Tropical malabsorption: recent concepts in pathogenesis and nutritional significance. *Clinical Science*, **60**, 131–137.

28 Tomkins, A. M., James, W. P. T., Cole, A. C. E. & Walters, J. H. (1974) Malabsorption in overland travellers to India. *British Medical Journal*, **iii**, 380–384.

29 Vaish, S. K., Ignatius, M. Baker, S. J. (1965) Albumin metabolism in tropical sprue. *Quarterly Journal of Medicine*, **34**, 15–32.

30 Vaish, S. K., Sampathkumar, J., Jacob, R. & Baker, S. J., (1965) The stomach in tropical sprue. *Gut*, **6**, 458–465.

31 Walters, J. H. (1947) Dietetic deficiency syndromes in Indian soldiers. *Lancet*, **i**, 861–864.

POST-INFECTIVE MALABSORPTION

Relatively little is known about the incidence and severity of malabsorption in acute infective conditions – viral, bacterial and parasitic – and the extent to which such malabsorption can continue after the specific organism has been eliminated from the intestinal lumen.

In this section, malabsorption following several infective conditions involving the small intestine – 'post-infective' malabsorption (PIM) is described. In some cases the initiating infective cause or causes may persist in a chronic form; a more precise term is therefore 'post-acute infective' malabsorption. As with many diseases, the spectrum varies markedly from subclinical cases to those with gross malabsorption. PIM is of particular clinical relevance in tropical countries. The infective conditions themselves are considered in more detail in Chapter 14.

There is obviously an area of considerable overlap between PIM and the tropical sprue syndrome (see earlier in this chapter) and in some cases the entities are probably synonymous. Much of this difficulty is associated with semantics. Manson first used the term tropical sprue in the English language in 1880.[15] It was then applied to all cases of malabsorption in tropical countries, undoubtedly including some of those caused by tuberculosis and parasites. Despite suggestions in early descriptions that chronic tropical diarrhoea had an insidious onset,[15] it is clear that the vast majority of cases present acutely. The picture is further complicated when acute epidemic cases of small intestinal infection with gross dehydration as well as malabsorption of xylose and fat are labelled tropical sprue.[4] The term 'tropical sprue' would be better reserved for a condition where the malabsorption of nutrients is quantitatively more important than that of water and electrolytes. Although the aetiology of tropical sprue remains in doubt (see below), it is known that most cases follow an acute small intestinal insult from either bacterial, viral or parasitic infection.

Overall, evidence for PIM after small intestinal infection is more complete for bacterial and parasitic infections; infections of viral origin might however be more important numerically. Lack of precise data may be attributed to some extent to the fact that virology remains an under-developed discipline in most developing Third World countries, where infections of all types are far more common than in the Western World. In a tropical setting it is likely that multiple intestinal infections of viral, bacterial and parasitic origins are responsible for the small intestinal changes, as demonstrated in preschool Guatemalan village children[50] ('tropical enteropathy', see below). However, many asymptomatic people in tropical countries have at least one pathogenic organism in the small intestinal lumen, which may be viral, bacterial or parasitic. Hence it is often difficult, or impossible, to incriminate a particular causative agent.

The effect of malabsorption syndromes following divergent small intestinal insults on nutritional status in the Third World is largely unknown;[77] children are especially at risk. The magnitude of energy loss is unknown;[78] one estimate is 10% of dietary energy, which is substantial in tropical populations subsisting on a marginal diet.[68] The role of anorexia in exacerbating the associated malnutrition is also under-explored.[38]

ACUTE INTESTINAL INFECTIONS PREDISPOSING TO PIM

Viral infections

Significant intestinal protein loss (with a mean of 1.7 g daily) and xylose malabsorption have been demonstrated in northern Nigerian children with measles;[23] approximately 25% also had lactose malabsorption. Other infections in children caused by entero- and herpes simplex viruses are also associated with diarrhoea and weight loss, and malnutrition may follow;[52] the mechanism is probably similar to that in measles. Volunteers infected with enteric viruses develop small intestinal morphological lesions which are not always associated with symptoms.[1]

Jejunal mucosal changes giving rise to severe malabsorption have been well documented in viral hepatitis;[14] these may persist for some time after resolution of the hepatic changes.

The Norwalk agent, a 27 nm picornavirus, can also produce mucosal damage and malabsorption.[69] Rotavirus infections[51, 67] give rise to morphological abnormalities and, especially in children, malabsorption.

These viral infections are therefore invasive, and the resulting diarrhoea and malabsorption are caused by enterocyte destruction. Malabsorption occurs after the virus has been shed into the intestinal lumen. The villi contain immature crypt-type enterocytes. In coronavirus infections in piglets, which resemble human rotavirus infections, glucose absorption is significantly impaired.[74] This has practical importance in management since sodium and water secretion cannot be reversed by glucose; oral rehydration fluids, commonly used in small intestinal diarrhoea, contain high sugar concentrations which overwhelm the limited absorptive capacity.

Baker *et al.*[5] have suggested that coronavirus infections are responsible for at least some cases of tropical sprue; however, the fact that some symptomatic individuals excrete these viruses need not necessarily indicate a cause–effect relationship.

Bacterial infections

Moderate to severe malabsorption is common during acute intestinal infections of bacterial origin,[48] and subnormal absorptive capacity persists for variable periods after termination of the diarrhoea and apparent clinical recovery. In one study in Bangladesh, approximately 70% of the patients still had evidence of xylose malabsorption one week after the diarrhoea had ceased; this was less common after cholera than shigella, salmonella and staphylococcal infections. Xylose and B_{12} malabsorption persisted for up to 378 and 196 days, respectively, after the diarrhoea had cleared. Although this was not the first study to demonstrate persistence of malabsorption after recovery from small intestinal bacterial disease, it emphasized that it is a relatively common entity.

Although many infective insults to the enterocyte are probably important in PIM, evidence for bacteria being responsible has more support than that involving other agents.

Escherichia coli

These organisms produce diarrhoea and malabsorption by enterotoxin production and mucosal invasion, which is similar to that caused by shigellae.[24] They are frequently food- or water-borne, and may cause outbreaks of gastroenteritis.[9, 73] Heat-labile (LT) enterotoxins exert their effect by activating adenylcyclase in the same way as *Vibrio cholerae*. Both heat-labile (LT) and heat-stable (ST) enterotoxins are probably important in traveller's diarrhoea (see below). A large pool of resistant organisms (often showing resistance to multiple antimicrobials) now exists in the community.[32] Enterotoxin production by *Escherichia coli* may be transferred simultaneously with antibiotic resistance.[26] In that study, 72% and 44% of enterotoxigenic *E. coli* isolated in south-east Asia were resistant to one or more and four or more antibiotics, respectively. Adhesiveness of *E. coli* to the enterocyte is also present with some strains[11] and that may be important in continuing colonization and subsequent malabsorption.[42] The relationship between adherence and Vero-toxin production is not yet clear.[45] Attachment of microorganisms to the enterocyte prevents them being cleared by peristaltic activity; such mucosal receptors may be genetically determined.[63] Ultrastructural studies have shown *E. coli* adherent to mucosal cells with flattening of the microvilli, loss of the cellular terminal web, and cupping of the plasma membrane around individual bacteria.[60] Intracellular damage was marked in the most heavily colonized cells. Histological improvement was demonstrated following clearing of the *E. coli* with neomycin and nutritional support. This mechanism can lead to protracted diarrhoea in infants.

In most cases, resultant malabsorption is short-lived. However, some cases of PIM are a long-term result of such infections (see below).

Traveller's diarrhoea

This disease accounts for large numbers of cases of transient diarrhoea in travellers to developing Third World countries.[16] Most cases of PIM in a tropical context probably begin with this disease; small intestinal colonization then persists and results in chronic malabsorption.[15] Enterotoxigenic serotypes of *E. coli* account for the majority of cases.[31, 62] The enterotoxin attaches to ganglionoside receptors on the small intestinal villi, adenylate cyclase is produced, and that in turn raises the luminal cyclic AMP concentration.[27] Other causative organisms are *Shigella, Campylobacter,* and the Reo- and Norwalk viruses. However, 25–30% of cases do not have a recognizable aetiological agent.[31]

Prophylaxis forms the basis of management, but symptomatic treatment is sometimes required. Diphenoxylate and loperamide, which inhibit peristalsis and inhibit secretions, encourage continuing small intestinal colonization. Antibiotics, which are often used both prophylactically and therapeutically, should be used selectively and not generally. Neomycin, doxycycline, co-trimoxazole (trimethoprim and sulphamethoxazole) and Streptotriad (streptomycin, sulphadimidine, sulphadiazine) and sulphathiazole are all effective prophylactically.[31] However, they should not be used indiscriminately because the causative organisms are frequently resistant and their widespread use encourages further resistant strains. There is no vaccine available.

Initiation of treatment early in the disease is the correct management in an established case. Many antibiotics have been used; trimethoprim, alone or in combination with sulphamethoxazole (as co-trimoxazole), has given satisfactory results.[25]

Salmonellosis
Malabsorption occasionally follows infection with *Salmonella* spp.[35] The incidence is unknown.

Campylobacter
Dysenteric disease has for long been known to predispose to tropical PIM;[15, 16] in addition to shigellosis it is clear that some cases of bloody diarrhoea are caused by *E. coli* (see above) and others by *Campylobacter.*

Although most cases of campylobacter infection are acute, present with gastroenteritis, and are self-limiting, the initial symptoms can be prolonged.[10, 44] The disease is a zoonosis; poultry are frequently contaminated. Most outbreaks have been traced to contaminated cow's milk. Dogs are also a source of infection.[34] Although the infection is self-limiting, erythromycin is occasionally required for severe cases. The carrier state is common. It is not clear how often the disease progresses to PIM.

'Pig bel' disease (enteritis necroticans)
This acute infection, which is more common in children than adults, occurs in some tropical countries, notably Papua New Guinea, Thailand and Uganda,[16] and can cause malabsorption. PIM may be associated with structural changes in the small intestine.

The disease is caused by the toxin of *Clostridium perfringens* (*welchii*), which is sometimes ingested in contaminated pork following pig feasts. The acute disease varies from an acute gastroenteritis to a haemorrhagic necrotizing jejunitis with severe dysentery; in the fulminant form, resection of devitalized small intestine may be necessary. The mortality rate is high.

Fluid and electrolyte replacement are essential. Penicillin and type C gas gangrene antisera are of value; laparotomy is often indicated. In Papua New Guinea, immunization against *Cl. perfringens* (type C) has given good results;[46] in a controlled trial a marked reduction in incidence and mortality was demonstrated in the treatment group.

Parasitic infections

Giardiasis
PIM resulting from infection with this flagellated protozoan has been well reviewed.[16, 18, 19, 20, 22] The reason why some individuals are prone to symptomatic giardiasis is not clear; size of infecting dose, strain variability, genetic predisposition, acquired immunity factors, achlorhydria, a local secretory IgA deficiency, and the presence of blood group A phenotype have all been considered. An increase in IgE and IgD cell numbers has been reported in the jejunal mucosa of 20 affected patients;[30] the former reversed after treatment, when an increase in IgA cell numbers was also recorded. The actual mechanism by which the trophozoites cause an absorption defect is also not clear. Injury to the mucosa with or without invasion, bacterial overgrowth in association with parasitization and bile salt deconjugation by bacteria and/or parasites have all been considered. Morphological changes in the jejunum vary widely.[82] There is a wide range of symptoms varying from subclinical cases to severe malabsorption and malnutrition.

Clinical presentation is usually between one and three weeks after infection; contaminated water and, less commonly, food are the usual sources of infection. It occurs both endemically and epidemically. The disease can be contracted from domestic animals. It is more common in male homosexuals. Diarrhoea of acute onset, flatus and weight loss may all be present; the stools have the characteristics of malabsorption. The disease is clinically indistinguishable from PIM in the absence of giardiasis; investigations also give similar results. Cysts may be found in a stool specimen; trophozoites can be detected in either a jejunal biopsy or jejunal fluid, or with the string test ('Entero test'). If mucosal changes and malabsorption exist, circulating antibodies to *G. lamblia* cysts are usually present.[55]

Treatment is with metronidazole 2 g daily on three consecutive days; alcohol should be avoided during the treatment period. A single dose of 2 g of tinidazole orally has been used with success. Two 5-nitroimidazoles – ornidazole and tinidazole (in a single dose of 1.5 g) – have been compared;[36] recurrence of the infection during the following two months was similar with both compounds (about 10%). Nimorazole has also been used.[83] Alternatively, mepacrine (100 mg three times a day for 10 days) usually gives a satisfactory result.

Other parasites

In addition to *G. lamblia*, several other parasitic infections can give rise to PIM. Although *Ascaris lumbricoides*, *Ancylostoma duodenale* and *Necator americanus* have at various times been implicated, there is as yet no definite evidence.[20] *Diphyllobothrium latum* infections are occasionally associated with a low serum B_{12} concentration; however, this is caused by uptake of B_{12} within the small intestinal lumen, and is not an example of malabsorption.

There is clear evidence that *Strongyloides stercoralis* is causally related to malabsorption.[16, 20] This helminth can survive in the human host for several decades; some 10–20% of ex-prisoners of war in south-east Asia during World War II (1939–45) are still infected.[29] Onset of diarrhoea is less acute than with *G. lamblia*. Larvae can be demonstrated by the string test and less well by jejunal biopsy. Both ova and larvae can occasionally be detected in stool specimens. Eosinophilia may be gross. The immunofluorescent antibody test (IFAT) is positive in approximately 70% of cases; however, cross-reaction with filaria is common. The enzyme-linked immunosorbent assay (ELISA) test has given promising results and is far more specific. Immunosuppressed patients often have negative results. Treatment is with thiabendazole 1.5 g twice daily on three successive days; repeated courses may be required. Mebendazole 100 mg twice daily for four days is less effective. In animal experiments, cambendazole has also

given encouraging results. Other *Strongyloides* species are important, especially in children. *S. fulleborni* has been implicated in the pathogenesis of severe PIM in Zambia and Papua New Guinea[2] where a significant mortality rate has been recorded.

In the northern Philippines and Thailand, *Capillaria philippinensis* has been causally associated with PIM. It occurs in epidemics. An acute onset of diarrhoea is followed by malabsorption and, if untreated, carries a substantial mortality rate. Protein-losing enteropathy may also be present. Treatment with mebendazole has given promising results.[70]

The protozoa *Sarcocystis hominis* and *Isospora belli*, usually conveyed by undercooked pork and beef, are further causes of malabsorption.[13, 83] These organisms replicate within the enterocyte. Pyrimethamine with sulphadiazine, and co-trimoxazole with nitrofurantoin, have been used with some success. A further protozoan infection, cryptosporidiosis, has recently achieved widespread attention.[71] It usually, though not always, occurs in immunosuppressed individuals, including some with AIDS. Treatment is unsatisfactory. Other parasitic infections, such as *Plasmodium falciparum* malaria (both acute and chronic) and visceral leishmaniasis (kala-azar) can also produce significant malabsorption.

CHRONIC INTESTINAL INFECTION PREDISPOSING TO PIM – INTESTINAL TUBERCULOSIS

This is a grossly underdiagnosed cause of malabsorption in a tropical context;[16] in many countries in the tropics and subtropics, including Saudi Arabia,[54] it is the most common cause. The condition should be suspected in immigrants from Africa and Asia in the UK who present with features of malabsorption (even after several years residence here) as well as people indigenous to Third World countries.

Presentation is with weight loss, low grade fever, anorexia, abdominal pain and diarrhoea.[47] Malnutrition may be severe enough to cause adult kwashiorkor. Generalized lymphadenopathy is occasionally present. Miliary spread, dissemination within the peritoneal cavity, and granuloma formation in the ileum and colon may complicate the picture. Clinically, a mass is sometimes palpable in the right iliac fossa.

Transverse ulcers with undermined edges in the ileum follow involvement of Peyer's patches; fibrosis and stenosis with stricture formation occur. The resulting malabsorption and steatorrhoea is largely a result of chronic bile salt loss, since these are normally reabsorbed in the terminal ileum. The direct effect of unabsorbed bile salts on the colon worsens the diarrhoea.

Barium meal and follow through, or barium enema, may show multiple ileal strictures; shortening of the ascending colon and caecum with loss of the normal ileocaecal angle are other features. Chest radiography is usually normal. *Mycobacterium tuberculosis* is rarely detected in a faecal specimen. Protein-losing enteropathy may also be present. Anaemia and hypoalbuminaemia are usual. Peritoneoscopy (and peritoneal biopsy) and laparotomy are often required for a positive diagnosis. Crohn's disease is an important differential diagnosis; however, vomiting, fever and menstrual disorders are more common and diarrhoea is less common in tuberculosis.

Treatment is with antituberculous agents.[28] Resection of ileal strictures and a right hemicolectomy are often required to deal with stricture formation.

TROPICAL ENTEROPATHY AND SUBCLINICAL MALABSORPTION

The small intestinal mucosa of people living in developing Third World countries has minor structural differences compared with that of those who have always lived in a temperate country.[16] It is not related to the clinical syndrome of tropical sprue.[37] Although the cause of these changes is not entirely clear, they seem to result from repeated viral and bacterial infections. The incidence is greater in lower socioeconomic groups.[75] Subclinical malabsorption exists in many people in Third World developing countries.[16, 77] Thus xylose and B_{12} malabsorption was present in 39% and 52%, respectively, of Peace Corps workers in Pakistan living under rural conditions.[49] Similarly, xylose and glucose malabsorption has been shown to be present in large numbers of people indigenous to tropical countries. Apart from repeated small intestinal infections, other factors seem to be important.[16] Xylose, glucose and folic acid absorption have been shown to be impaired in people with systemic bacterial infections such as pulmonary tuberculosis and pneumococcal pneumonia. There is also good evidence that dietary folate depletion causes malabsorption of xylose.[16] Although marginal malnutrition and pellagra have been suggested as causing subclinical malabsorption, the evidence is contradictory.

The practical importance of subclinical malabsorption is not clear. It seems likely that it significantly contributes to malnutrition in people in Third World countries who subsist on a marginal dietary intake, consisting largely of carbohydrate. Before any rigid conclusions are made, however, it must be appreciated that the small intestine has a substantial functional reserve, and that the role of the colon in absorption of carbohydrate (and other substances) is still unclear.

TROPICAL PIM

The clinical entity of PIM related to tropical exposure has been reviewed by Cook,[16, 21] Tomkins,[77] and Baker.[3]

The geographical distribution of the disease is of interest; although it is common in Asia and the Central Americas, it is a very unusual condition in tropical Africa. In the Middle East post-infective malabsorption is unusual[54] but does occur.[66]

Aetiology

Infection
In severe PIM (without parasites) bacterial colonization both within the jejunal lumen and in biopsy specimens has been demonstrated.[6, 40, 79] The importance of adhesive properties of bacteria in the pathogenesis of the disease is unclear; many bacteria, including *E. coli*, *Salmonella typhimurium* and *Vibrio cholerae*, have adhesive properties which are mediated by a transmissible plasmid. Tomkins, Drasar and James[79] have demonstrated a higher concentration of enterobacteria in relation to the enterocyte than in luminal fluid in tropical malabsorption. It seems likely that a variety of toxins released by these enterobacteria induce net water secretion and malabsorption.[41] It is of interest that in the blind loop syndrome, enterobacteria do *not* produce toxins.[39] In mild tropical malabsorption, Tomkins, Wright and Drasar[80] have reported on the intraluminal bacterial flora of the upper small intestine (mucosal biopsy or luminal fluid) several months after tropical exposure: 7 out of 11 patients had enterobacteria in numbers ranging from 10^3–10^8/g or ml. The most common organism was

Klebsiella pneumoniae; Citrobacter feundii, Serratia marcescens and *Pseudomonas* spp. were also detected. It seems likely that these organisms had been present since the tropical exposure. The origin of the overgrowth has not been adequately studied in tropical PIM. In patients in England with small intestinal bacterial overgrowth, faecal flora account for most of the organisms, and salivary flora are important in some cases.[33]

Although a predisposing immunological deficit has been postulated in tropical PIM, there is no satisfactory evidence for this; immunological changes (increased IgG, IgE, C4 and orosomucoid, gastric parietal cell antibodies, and lymphopenia with a low peripheral blood T cell count) are thought to be *sequelae* of mucosal damage.[61]

Small intestinal stasis

Small intestinal stasis in tropical PIM[15] may be a result of excessive enteroglucagon production in response to ileal mucosal injury[7,16] (see below). However, many patients with PIM have taken diphenoxylate or loperamide for acute diarrhoea; both of those agents produce relative small intestinal stasis.[43,65] They induce antiperistalsis as well as preventing prostaglandin-induced diarrhoea;[65] an inhibiting effect on small intestinal secretion also occurs. This stasis is of interest because peristalsis is usually *increased* by the presence of intraluminal bacteria.[16]

Gut hormones

Gut hormones have been studied in the fasting state and following a standard meal.[7] Fasting and postprandial concentrations of enteroglucagon and motilin were markedly elevated; the high enteroglucagon concentrations showed a significant correlation with small intestinal transit using the H_2 breath test. Both enteroglucagon and motilin concentrations fall after treatment.[21] Patients with PIM have a reduced postprandial rise in gastric inhibiting polypeptide; gastrin and pancreatic polypeptide were normal.

The role of the colon

Frequently the colon, in addition to the small intestine, is damaged in PIM. Few causes of diarrhoea are strictly confined to one or other of these sites; e.g. shigellosis frequently involves the small intestine, and campylobacter and salmonella infections, the colon.

Recent recognition of the importance of the colon in absorption is clearly relevant in PIM.

The normal colon can absorb 4–7 l of water/24 hours[58] together with 100–160 mmol carbohydrate as volatile fatty acids.[64] Thus failure of the diseased colon to 'salvage' the increased ileal effluent increases the intensity of diarrhoea.

Colonic abnormalities have been reported in 'tropical sprue;'[57] using a colonic perfusion system, impaired water and electrolyte absorption was demonstrated. These abnormalities might be the result of impaired fatty acid absorption and the effect of free fatty acids on the colonocyte.[76] Other suggested mechanisms are colonocyte damage, enterotoxin production by colonic bacteria, and local action of bile acids unabsorbed by the small intestine. Bile acids can be converted to deconjugated, dihydroxy-bile acids by colonic bacteria, and they can impair the colonic salvage of water and salt by stimulating colonic secretion and propulsion.[8,72] Colonic bacteria are able to convert long chain fatty acids to hydroxy-fatty acids, which stimulate colonic secretion,[8] modify colonic motility, and cause diarrhoea.

Colonic function has not been investigated in PIM seen in London.[16]

Clinical picture

The clinical picture is dominated by chronic diarrhoea with large, pale, fatty stools, and sometimes excessive flatulence, following an acute intestinal infection. Weight loss may be gross, but is probably related to anorexia as much as to the intestinal disease.[77] There is a wide range of clinical presentation from the very acute onset type, described by Baker and Mathan,[4] often occurring in epidemics (with vomiting and pyrexia in up to 50%) as seen at Vellore, India, to a far more chronic entity. Most other clinical features, such as glossitis, fluid retention, depression, apathy, amenorrhoea and infertility, occur only after considerable chronicity.

The condition must be differentiated from persisting bacterial overgrowth within the lumen of the small intestine, which should be treated early with antibiotics,[59] and giardiasis, which is sometimes difficult to diagnose and for which the correct treatment is metronidazole[12]

During, and immediately after, an acute small intestinal infection, xylose, glucose, fat, B_{12} and folate malabsorption frequently occur (see above). After four months or so, moderate or severe morphological changes occur in the jejunal mucosa, and serum folate and later B_{12} concentrations decline, often to very low concentrations.

Gastric acid secretion is often depressed but whether this precedes the initiating infection is unknown.[4] Secondary hypolactasia may be present.[16]

Investigation

Investigations should include D-xylose excretion after a 5 or 25 g loading dose, 72-hour faecal fat estimation, a Schilling test and jejunal biopsy; stool parasites should be excluded. Serum B_{12} and red blood cell folate concentrations should be estimated; after four months of illness, most patients have low folate concentrations. Serum albumin and globulin concentrations are of value. Monosaccharide absorption is impaired to a greater extent than that of amino-acids.[17] A barium meal and follow through shows dilated loops of jejunum with clumping of barium, and reduced transit rate.

Jejunal mucosal changes are variable, largely depending on the duration of the disease. By three or four months most biopsies are ridged and/or convoluted; a flat mucosa is very unusual and, if present, gluten-induced enteropathy should be suspected. Submucosal invasion with lymphocytes, predominantly T cells, and plasma cells is usually present.

Ultrastructural changes in jejunal biopsy specimens have been studied;[56] lysosomes, peroxisomes and mitochondrial enzymes are not depressed, but the organelles are more fragile. Endoplasmic reticulum is unchanged. A significant reduction in 5-nucleotidase in the basolateral (plasma) membrane is present which persists after recovery. The latter finding might reflect an underlying abnormality in the enterocytes of individuals susceptible to PIM.

Intestinal permeability has also been investigated;[53] abnormalities in urinary excretion of lactulose and rhamnose after an oral load are similar to results obtained in gluten-induced enteropathy.

Aetiology and treatment

A hypothesis to account for the aetiology of tropical PIM is given in Figure 8.53.[21] This vicious circle can be broken by (a) eliminating the bacterial overgrowth, and (b) aiding mucosal recovery with folic acid supplements. An adequate diet should be combined with tetracycline (250 mg three times a day for two weeks) and folic acid (5 mg three times a day for one month). Symptomatic treatment may be necessary in the acute stage of the disease; codeine phosphate (30 mg three times a day) or propantheline

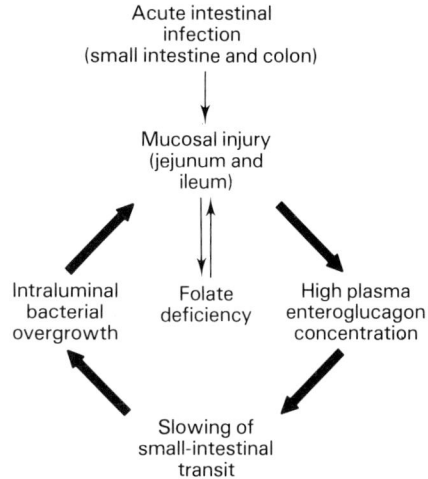

Fig. 8.53 Proposed aetiology of tropical post-infective malabsorption.

bromide (30 mg four times a day) are of value. Mild cases respond without treatment, but this may take several months. Recovery is usually straightforward.[3, 16] Evidence from south India[3] suggests that the response to antibiotics there is not as good; this is used in support of the hypothesis that a viral rather than a bacterial aetiology is likely.

CONCLUSION

The aetiology of PIM – especially that presenting in association with tropical exposure – is becoming clearer. However, it is probable that several primary insults to the enterocyte are involved. Whereas PIM resulting from most viral, bacterial and parasitic causes is usually self-limiting, the tropical sprue syndrome is not. The reason why only a minority of affected individuals who suffer acute small intestinal infections are involved is unknown, and the possibility of a genetic or ethnic basis for susceptibility has not been eliminated.

REFERENCES

1 Agus, S. G., Dolin, R., Wyatt, R. G. et al. (1973) Acute infectious non-bacterial gastroenteritis: intestinal histopathology. *Annals of Internal Medicine*, **79**, 18–25.
2 Ashford, R. W., Hall, A. J. & Babona, D. (1981) Distribution and abundance of intestinal helminths in man in western Papua New Guinea with special reference to *Strongyloides*. *Annals of Tropical Medicine and Parasitology*, **75**, 269–279.
3 Baker, S. J. (1982) Idiopathic small intestinal disease in the tropics. In *Critical Reviews in Tropical Medicine*, vol. 1 (Ed.) Chandra, R. K. pp. 197–245. New York and London: Plenum Press.

4   Baker, S. J. & Mathan, V. I. (1971) Tropical sprue in southern India. In *Tropical Sprue and Megaloblastic Anaemia.* A Wellcome Trust Collaborative Study. pp. 189–260. London: Churchill Livingstone.

5   Baker, S. J., Mathan, M., Mathan, V. I. *et al.* (1982) Chronic enterocyte infection with coronavirus. One possible cause of the syndrome of tropical sprue? *Digestive Diseases and Sciences,* **27,** 1039–1043.

6   Banwell, J. G. & Gorbach, S. L. (1969) Tropical sprue. *Gut,* **10,** 328–333.

7   Besterman, H. S., Cook, G. C., Sarson, D. L. *et al.* (1979) Gut hormones in tropical malabsorption. *British Medical Journal,* **ii,** 1252–1255.

8   Binder, H. J. (1980) Pathophysiology of bile acid and fatty acid induced diarrhoea. In *Secretory Diarrhoea* (Ed.) Field, M., Fordtran, J. S. & Schultz, S. G. p. 157. American Physiological Society.

9   Black, R. E., Merson, M. H., Rowe, B. *et al.* (1981) Enterotoxigenic *Escherichia coli* diarrhoea: acquired immunity and transmission in an endemic area. *Bulletin of the World Health Organization,* **59,** 263–268.

10   Blaser, M. J. & Reller, L. B. (1981) Campylobacter enteritis. *New England Journal of Medicine,* **305,** 1444–1452.

11   Boedeker, E. C. (1982) Enterocyte adherence of *Escherichia coli:* its relation to diarrhoeal disease. *Gastroenterology,* **83,** 489–492.

12   Bolin, T. D., Davis, A. E. & Duncombe, V. M. (1982) A prospective study of persistent diarrhoea. *Australian and New Zealand Journal of Medicine,* **12,** 22–26.

13   Bunyaratvej, S., Bunyawongwiroj, P. & Nitiyanant, P. (1982) Human intestinal sarcosporidiosis: report of six cases. *American Journal of Tropical Medicine and Hygiene,* **31,** 36–41.

14   Conrad, M. E., Schwartz, F. D. & Young, A. A. (1964) Infectious hepatitis – a generalized disease. *American Journal of Medicine,* **37,** 789–801.

15   Cook, G. C. (1978) Tropical sprue: implications of Manson's concept. *Journal of the Royal College of Physicians, London,* **12,** 329–349.

16   Cook, G. C. (1980) *Tropical Gastroenterology.* Oxford: Oxford University Press. pp. 228–229, 271–324, 325–339.

17   Cook, G. C. (1981) Jejunal absorption rates of glucose and glycine in post-infective tropical malabsorption. *Transactions of the Royal Society of Tropical Medicine and Hygiene,* **75,** 378–384.

18   Cook, G. C. (1984) In *Tropical Medicine and Parasitology* (Ed.) Goldsmith, R. S. & Heyneman, D. USA: Lange Medical Publications, in press.

19   Cook, G. C. (1984) In *Diseases of the Gut and Pancreas* (Ed.) Misiewicz, J. J., Pounder, R. E. & Venables, C. W. London: Grant McIntyre, in press.

20   Cook, G. C. (1984) In *Disorders of the Small Intestine* (Ed.) Booth, C. C. & Neale, G. Oxford: Blackwell, in press.

21   Cook, G. C. (1984) Aetiology and pathogenesis of post-infective tropical malabsorption (tropical sprue). *Lancet,* in press.

22   Desai, H. I. & Chandra, R. K. (1982) Giardiasis. In *Critical Reviews in Tropical Medicine,* vol. 1 (Ed.) Chandra, R. K. pp. 109–141. New York and London: Plenum Press.

23   Dossetor, J. F. B. & Whittle, H. C. (1975) Protein-losing enteropathy and malabsorption in acute measles enteritis. *British Medical Journal,* **ii,** 592–593.

24   Dupont, H. L., Formal, S. B., Hornick, R. B. *et al.* (1971) Pathogenesis of *Escherichia coli* diarrhea. *New England Journal of Medicine,* **285,** 1–9.

25   Dupont, H. L., Reves, R. R., Galindo, E. *et al.* (1982) Treatment of travelers' diarrhea with trimethoprim/ sulfamethoxazole and with trimethoprim alone. *New England Journal of Medicine,* **307,** 841–844.

26   Echeverria, P., Verhaert, L., Ulyangco, C. V. *et al.* (1978) Antimicrobial resistance and enterotoxin production among isolates of Escherichia coli in the Far East. *Lancet,* **ii,** 589–592.

27   Evans, N. (1979) Bacterial toxins and diarrhoea. *Tropical Doctor,* **9,** 10–15.

28   Findlay, J. M. (1982) Medical management of gastro-intestinal tuberculosis. *Journal of the Royal Society of Medicine,* **75,** 583–584.

29   Gill, G V. & Bell, D. R. (1982) Longstanding tropical infections amongst former war prisoners of the Japanese. *Lancet,* **i,** 958–959.

30   Gillon, J., André, C., Descos, L. *et al.* (1982) Changes in mucosal immunoglobulin-containing cells in patients with giardiasis before and after treatment. *Journal of Infection,* **5,** 67–72.

31   Gorbach, S. L. (1982) Travelers' diarrhea. *New England Journal of Medicine,* **307,** 881–883.

32   Gross, R. J., Ward, L. R., Threlfall, E. J. *et al.* (1982) Drug resistance among infantile enteropathogenic *Escherichia coli* strains isolated in the United Kingdom. *British Medical Journal,* **285,** 472–473.

33   Hamilton, I., Worsley, B. W., Cobden, I. *et al.* (1982) Simultaneous culture of saliva and jejunal aspirate in the investigation of small bowel bacterial overgrowth. *Gut,* **23,** 847–853.

34   Holt, P. E. (1981) Role of *Campylobacter* spp. in human and animal disease: a review. *Journal of the Royal Society of Medicine,* **74,** 437–440.

35   Iushchuk, N. D. & Abdullaev, Skh. (1981) Sostoianie vsasyvatel'noĭ funktsii tonkoi kishki pri sal'monelleze u deteĭ. *Pediatriia,* **7,** 23–24.

36   Jokipii, L. & Jokipii, A. M. M. (1982) Treatment of giardiasis: comparative evaluation of ornidazole and tinidazole as a single oral dose. *Gastroenterology,* **83,** 399–404.

37   Klipstein, F. A. (1979) Sprue and subclinical malabsorption in the tropics. *Lancet,* **i,** 277–278.

38   Klipstein, F. A. & Corcino, J. J. (1977) Factors responsible for weight loss in tropical sprue. *American Journal of Clinical Nutrition,* **30,** 1703–1708.

39   Klipstein, F. A., Engert, R. F. & Short, H. B. (1978) Enterotoxigenicity of colonising coliform bacteria in tropical sprue and blind-loop syndrome. *Lancet,* **ii,** 342–344.

40   Klipstein, F. A., Holdeman, L. V., Corcino. J. J. & Moore, W. E. C. (1973) Enterotoxigenic intestinal bacteria in tropical sprue. *Annals of Internal Medicine,* **79,** 632–641.

41   Klipstein, F. A., Horowitz, I. R., Engert, R. F. & Schenk, E. A. (1975) Effect of *Klebsiella pneumoniae* enterotoxin on intestinal transport in the rat. *Journal of Clinical Investigation,* **56,** 799–807.

42   *Lancet* Editorial (1981) Microbial adhesion, colonisation, and virulence. *Lancet,* **i,** 508–510.

43   *Lancet* Editorial (1981) Loperamide – what does it block? *Lancet,* **ii,** 1088–1089.

44   *Lancet* Editorial (1982) Campylobacter enteritis. *Lancet,* **ii,** 1437–1438.

45   *Lancet* Editorial (1983) Mechanisms in enteropathogenic *Escherichia coli* diarrhoea. *Lancet,* **i,** 1254–1256.

46   Lawrence, G., Shann, F., Freestone, D. S. & Walker, P. D. (1979) Prevention of necrotising enteritis in Papua New Guinea by active immunisation. *Lancet,* **i,** 227–230.

47   Lewis, E. A. & Kolawole, T. M. (1972) Tuberculous ileo-colitis in Ibadan: a clinico-radiological review. *Gut,* **13,** 646–653.

48   Lindenbaum, J. (1965) Malabsorption during and after

recovery from acute intestinal infection. *British Medical Journal*, **ii**, 326–329.

49 Lindenbaum, J., Kent, T. H. & Sprinz, H. (1966) Malabsorption and jejunitis in American Peace Corps volunteers in Pakistan. *Annals of Internal Medicine*, **65**, 1201–1209.

50 Mata, L. J., Kromal, R. A., Urrutia, J. J. & Garcia, B. (1977) Effect of infection on food intake and the nutritional state: perspectives as viewed from the village. *American Journal of Clinical Nutrition*, **30**, 1215–1227.

51 McCormack, J. G. (1982) Clinical features of rotavirus gastroenteritis. *Journal of Infection*, **4**, 167–174.

52 McKenzie, D., Hansen, J. D. L. & Becker, W. (1959) Herpes simplex virus infection: dissemination in association with malnutrition. *Archives of Disease in Childhood*, **34**, 250–256.

53 Menzies, I. S., Cook, G. C., Noone, C. *et al.* (1983) Comparison of intestinal sugar permeation following iso- and hyper-osmolar test solutions in coeliac disease and tropical sprue. *Proceedings of the 2nd Joint Meeting of the Belgian, Dutch, German and British Societies for Clinical Chemistry*. Newcastle-upon-Tyne.

54 Montgomery, R. D., Atiyeh, M., Seales, W. R. *et al.* (1982) Intestinal absorption in Saudi Arabia: an evaluation of the one-hour blood xylose test. *Transactions of the Royal Society of Tropical Medicine and Hygiene*, **76**, 25–28.

55 Moody, A. H., Ridley, D. S., Tomkins, A. M. & Wright, S. G. (1982) The specificity of serum antibodies to *Giardia lamblia* and to enterobacteria in gastrointestinal disease. *Transactions of the Royal Society of Tropical Medicine and Hygiene*, **76**, 630–632.

56 Peters, T. J., Jones, P. E., Wells, G. & Cook, G. C. (1979) Sequential enzyme and subcellular fractionation studies on jejunal biopsy specimens from patients with post-infective tropical malabsorption. *Clinical Science and Molecular Medicine*, **56**, 479–486.

57 Ramakrishna, B. S. & Mathan, V. I. (1982) Water and electrolyte absorption by the colon in tropical sprue. *Gut*, **23**, 843–846.

58 Read, N. W. (1982) Diarrhoea: the failure of colonic salvage. *Lancet*, **ii**, 481–483.

59 Read, N. W., Krejs, G. J., Read, M. G. *et al.* (1980) Chronic diarrhoea of unknown origin. *Gastroenterology*, **78**, 264–271.

60 Rothbaum, R., McAdams, A. J., Giannella, R. & Partin, J. C. (1982) A clinicopathologic study of enterocyte-adherent *Escherichia coli*: a cause of protracted diarrhoea in infants. *Gastroenterology*, **83**, 441–454.

61 Ross, I. N. & Mathan, V. I. (1981) Immunological changes in tropical sprue. *Quarterly Journal of Medicine*, **50**, 435–449.

62 Rowe, B., Taylor, J. & Bettelheim, K. A. (1970) An investigation of travellers' diarrhoea. *Lancet*, **i**, 1–5.

63 Rutter, J. M., Burrows, M. R., Sellwood, R. & Gibbons, R. A. (1975) A genetic basis for resistance to enteric disease caused by *Escherichia coli*. *Nature*, **257**, 135–136.

64 Saunders, D. K. & Wiggins, H. S. (1981) Conservation of mannitol, lactulose and raffinose by the human colon. *American Journal of Physiology*, **241**, G397–G402.

65 Sandhu, B. R., Tripp, J. H., Candy, D. C. A. & Harries, J. T. (1981) Loperamide: studies on its mechanism of action. *Gut*, **22**, 658–662.

66 Salem, A. A. & Allam, C. K. (1982) Tropical sprue: a case report from the Middle East. *American Journal of Gastroenterology*, **77**, 51–52.

67 Schoub, B. D. (1981) Enteric adenoviruses and rotaviruses in infantile gastroenteritis in developing countries. *Lancet*, **ii**, 925.

68 Schneider, R. E., Shiffman, M. & Faigenblum, J. (1978) The potential effect of water on gastrointestinal infections prevalent in developing countries. *American Journal of Clinical Nutrition*, **31**, 2089–2099.

69 Schreiber, D. S., Blacklow, N. R. & Trier, J. S. (1973) The intestinal lesion of the proximal small intestine in acute infectious nonbacterial gastroenteritis. *New England Journal of Medicine*, **288**, 1318–1323.

70 Singson, C. N., Banzon, T. C. & Cross, J. H. (1977) Mebendazole in the treatment of intestinal capillariosis. *American Journal of Tropical Medicine and Hygiene*, **24**, 932–934.

71 Sloper, K. S., Dourmashkin, R. R., Bird, R. B. *et al.* (1982) Chronic malabsorption due to cryptosporidium in a child with immunoglobulin deficiency. *Gut*, **23**, 80–82.

72 Snape, W. J., Shiff, S. & Cohen S. (1980) Effect of deoxycholic acid on colonic motility in the rabbit. *American Journal of Physiology*, **238**, G321–G325.

73 Taylor, W. R., Schell, W. L., Wells, J. G. *et al.* (1982) A foodborne outbreak of enterotoxigenic *Escherichia coli* diarrhea. *New England Journal of Medicine*, **306**, 1093–1095.

74 Telch, J., Shepherd, R. W., Butler, D. G. *et al.* (1981) Intestinal glucose transport in acute viral enteritis in piglets. *Clinical Science*, **61**, 29–34.

75 Thomas, G., Clain, D. J. & Wicks, A. C. B. (1976) Tropical enteropathy in Rhodesia. *Gut*, **17**, 888–894.

76 Tiruppathi, C., Balasubramanian, K. A., Hill, P. G. & Mathan, V. I. (1983) Faecal free fatty acids in tropical sprue and their possible role in the production of diarrhoea by inhibition of ATPases. *Gut*, **24**, 300–305.

77 Tomkins A. (1981) Tropical malabsorption: recent concepts in pathogenesis and nutritional significance. *Clinical Science*, **60**, 131–137.

78 Tomkins, A. (1983) Nutritional cost of protracted diarrhoea in young Gambian children. *Gut*, **24**, A495.

79 Tomkins, A. M., Drasar, B. S. & James, W. P. T. (1975) Bacterial colonisation of jejunal mucosa in acute tropical sprue. *Lancet*, **i**, 59–62.

80 Tomkins, A. M., Wright, S. G. & Drasar, B. S. (1980) Bacterial colonization of the upper small intestine in mild tropical malabsorption. *Transactions of the Royal Society of Tropical Medicine and Hygiene*, **74**, 752–755.

81 Tomkins, A. M., James, W. P. T., Walters, J. H. & Cole, A. C. E. (1974) Malabsorption in overland travellers to India. *British Medical Journal*, **3**, 380–384.

82 Vega-Franco, L., Alvarez, E. L. & Romo G. & Bernal, R. M. (1982) Absorción de proteinas en niños con giardiasis. *Boletin Medico Hospital Infantil de Mexico*, **39**, 19–22.

83 World Health Organization (1981) Intestinal protozoan and helminthic infections. Report of a WHO scientific group. *Technical Report Series*, No. 666. p. 150. Geneva: World Health Organization.

BACTERIOLOGY OF THE SMALL GUT AND BACTERIAL OVERGROWTH

The normal microbial flora of the lumen of the small intestine in healthy man has not been fully characterized and there is still much to be learned about its effect on structure and function. Pasteur believed that a bacterial flora was essential to life, but a wide range of species, and even man himself, have been successfully maintained in a 'germ-free' state. In contrast Mechnikoff[92] argued that indigenous microorganisms were antagonistic to the health of mammals, competing for factors essential to life. Certainly there are many animals, particularly ruminants, which benefit from the bacteria they carry in the upper gastrointestinal tract but in man this may not be the case.

THE NORMAL GUT MICROFLORA IN HUMANS

The germ-free state

A germ-free state can be maintained in humans only under the most stringent conditions in a plastic isolator;[62] even then the condition is relative, depending on the sophistication of the tests used to define microbial sterility.[24] Very interesting observations have been made on gut structure and function in the experimental germ-free animal: the epithelium of the small intestine is more regular, the mucosa and lamina propria are thinner, and the crypts of Lieberkühn are shallower and the enterocytes shorter-lived than in controls.[152] Man is germ-free only in utero and the manner by which colonization of gut occurs immediately after birth is important, particularly in sick, premature infants.

Colonization of the intestine after birth

Microbial colonization of the gut of the newborn infant occurs during and after birth and depends on a variety of factors (Table 8.27).

Table 8.27 Factors affecting colonization of the small intestine in the newborn.

Gestational age
Route of delivery
Degree of exposure to hospital environment
Mode of nutrition

Differences in gestational age, mode of delivery and type of feeding are associated with significantly different colonization patterns during the first week of life.

The inoculum of bacteria from the vagina is clearly important. By the end of 48 hours, 40% of stools in the normally delivered infant contain anaerobic bacteria and 70% contain aerobic bacteria, compared with 5% and 30% in the infant delivered by caesarean section.[82] Breast-

feeding leads to the subsequent predominance of bifidobacteria.[56] *Bacteroides fragilis* is slow to colonize, but at the end of one week can be isolated from the faeces of 60% of bottle-fed infants compared with only 20% of the breast-fed. The infrequent finding of *B. fragilis* does not appear to be related to the nature of the aerobic flora as isolation rates for aerobic Gram-negative bacilli and streptococci appear similar in both breast-fed and bottle-fed infants.[82]

The microflora of infant stools at one week is already extremely complex – over 100 species of anaerobic bacteria were isolated from a study of 196 neonates and the aerobic organisms were also fully represented, with *Escherichia coli*, *Klebsiella* spp., *Enterobacter* spp., *Proteus* spp., and group D streptococci predominating.[82] These data, of course, tell us nothing about what is occurring in the small intestine, but may be important in our understanding of necrotizing enterocolitis, in many cases of which there appears to be a delay in the normal bacterial colonization of the intestine.[77]

The established normal flora

The 'normal flora' of the small intestine refers solely to bacteria. Although viruses may be cultured from the gut of otherwise healthy children, a normal viral flora is generally believed not to exist in humans.[112]

There are two groups of bacteria to be considered: firstly those found in small intestinal fluid which largely reflect the microflora of swallowed saliva and which vary in a phasic manner with the ingestion of meals, and secondly the apparently more stable flora of the mucosal surface.

In the Western World, where most people eat either freshly cooked meals or bacteriologically clean food which has been stored under hygienic conditions, the luminal contents of the upper small intestine contain less than 10^4 (with an average of 10^2) viable organisms/ml of fasting aspirate; the organisms are predominantly aerobic and Gram-positive. Although published reports show considerable differences (Table 8.28) and although direct counts of bacteria in aspirates of jejunal fluid suggest that some bacteria are not being grown under standard laboratory conditions (Figure 8.54), most workers agree that the jejunum is not sterile but populated by 'transients' originating from the oral cavity. Streptococci, lactobacilli and veillonellae are the principal organisms recovered. After a light meal the concentration of microorganisms in the jejunum increases by about 100 times;

Table 8.28 Studies on normal flora of human small intestine. Results are expressed as $\log_{10}$ (numbers of viable organisms/ml).

Number of control samples studied	Sterile	Aerobic organisms (max.)	Coliform organisms (max.)	Anaerobic organisms (max.)	Bacteroides (max.)	Reference
Upper small intestine						
13	1 (8%)	3.5	—	3.9	—	Gorbach et al.[48]
25	17 (68%)	5	2	3	3	Drasar et al.[32]
12	0 (0%)	9.1	2.5	5.0	—	Hamilton et al.[58]
13	7 (54%)	5.5	—	6.0	—	Challacombe et al.[20]
22	4 (18%)	4.0	1.0	3.0	2.0[a]	Dickman et al.[27]
10[b]	2 (20%)	6.9	4.7	2.8	1.6	Bhat et al.[14]
Lower small intestine						
12	—	6.3	6.3	5.5	5.5	Gorbach et al.[48]
4	—	6	6	7	7	Drasar et al.[32]
6	—	9.1	8.1	7.8	7.8	Hamilton et al.[58]

[a] Only one specimen.
[b] One control excluded because of very high counts.

although more species may be isolated, enterobacteriaceae and *Bacteroides* spp. are rarely found.

In contrast, the flora of the small intestine close to the ileocaecal valve is dramatically greater and approximates to that found in the caecum (Table 8.28). There is little data to indicate the length of normal ileum carrying such a heavy load of bacteria, but it is probably no more than 50 cm.[48] Removal of the ileocaecal valve may allow an increased growth of bacteria.[55]

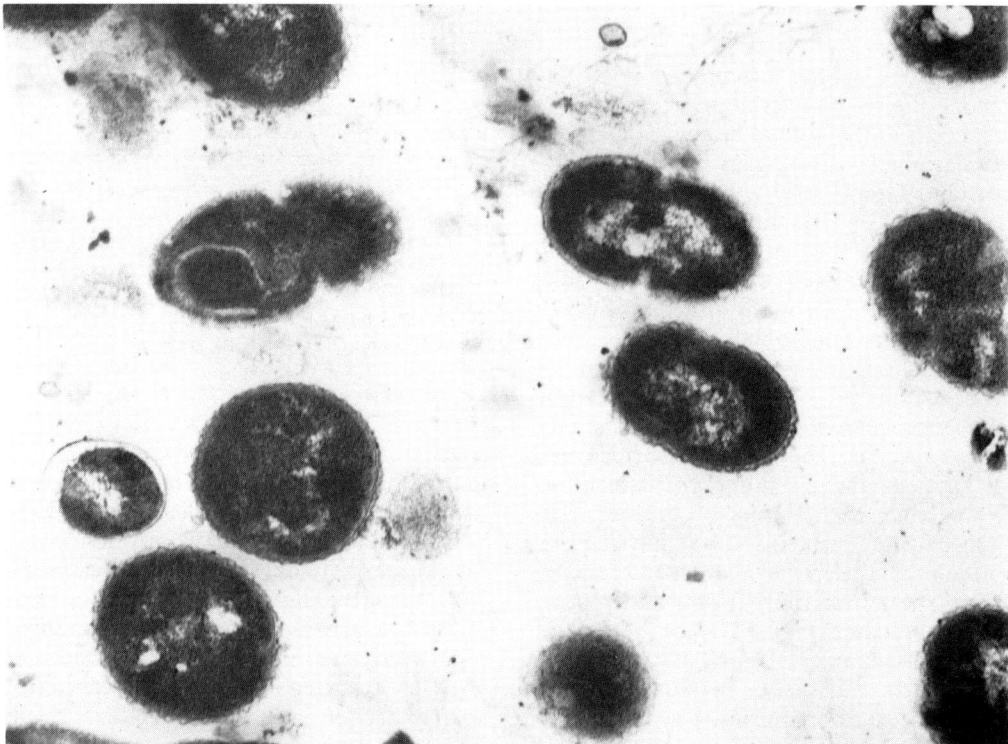

Fig. 8.54 Electronmicroscopic image of bacteria in centrifuged duodenal fluid aspirated from a patient with diverticulosis of the upper small intestine. This sample was one of an unpublished series collected by Dr A. Challen (MRC Dunn Nutrition Unit) and Dr J. Anderson (Department of Pathology, University of Cambridge). In this series up to 10^9 Gram-positive particles/ml of jejunal fluid aspirated were counted under the light microscope; by standard methods of aerobic and anaerobic culture the viable bacterial count did not exceed 10^5 organisms/ml.

Apparently healthy residents of tropical countries carry a richer microflora in the small intestine than their Western counterparts. Studies from India, south-east Asia and South America show that the jejunum often contains 10^4–10^5 coliform organisms/ml of fasting fluid. These findings may correlate with a lower normal range for the absorption of xylose and vitamin B_{12} than is accepted in the West.[19]

Maintenance of the bacterial flora

The bacterial population of fasting jejunal fluid is maintained at a low concentration by the peristaltic contractions of the normal gut. Colonization of the mucosal surface appears to depend on the capacity of the bacteria to adhere to epithelial cells. This property of adherence not only prevents the physical expulsion of microorganisms but may also stimulate their growth, since nutrients tend to concentrate at the cell surface.[89] The organisms are also subject to the effects of local immune systems, non-specific host antimicrobial agents, and variations in the biochemical and biophysical environment, and to the shedding of epithelial cells into the lumen of the intestine.

Bacterial properties
At present there is little information regarding the factors affecting bacterial adherence to the epithelial cells of the normal human small intestine. Occasionally histologists identify Gram-negative and Gram-positive bacteria in mucus on the mucosal epithelium of the small intestine,[102, 108] but the microbial population appears to be extremely sparse. This is quite unlike the situation in many other species. In particular intimate microbial–epithelial associations throughout the gut are readily demonstrated in rodents.[121] Adherence is mediated by species-specific microbial lectins complementary to host cell-specific receptors.[11] These microbial surface antigens are detectable on filamentous projections (pili or fimbriae) of the cell wall and react with proteins (albumin-like or glycoproteins) of the epithelial cell membrane.

In some species microorganisms adherent to the surface epithelium may influence the flora of intestinal contents in the fasting state,[84] but in man this seems unlikely. In South Indian studies, the range of organisms raised from cultures of jejunal aspirates was often very different from those obtained from cultures of jejunal biopsies. Anaerobic organisms were more commonly isolated from the mucosal surface[14] but, as with the luminal flora, there is almost certain-

ly a considerable variation between populations. In a study from Costa Rica the findings were similar to those described above,[64] whereas Plaut[108] in the USA obtained few or no bacteria from the mucosal surface.

It is possible to speculate on the density of bacteria adherent to jejunal mucosa by extrapolating from published data. The culture of 10^5 organisms/g of wet jejunal mucosa[14] sounds impressive, but a *milligram* of mucosal biopsy may carry 100 villi, each with something like 2000 surface cells. The cell population of the crypts is less than 10% that of the villi. Thus these figures suggest a bacterial concentration of perhaps one organism per villus, or not more than ten per crypt.

Little is known about the adherence of bacteria to the epithelium of the small intestine in chronic diarrhoeal illnesses. This may become an important topic following the demonstration of damage to brush borders associated with *Escherichia coli* overgrowth in the small intestine of man and experimental animals.[145]

Host mechanisms

Epithelial factors. Very little is known about host mechanisms and their effects on small intestinal flora (Table 8.29). Apart from intestinal

Table 8.29 Factors which may inhibit bacterial colonization of the epithelial surface.

Peristaltic flow of gut contents
Luminal mechanisms
Variations in pH and oxidation–reduction potential
Non-specific antimicrobial agents
Bile acids and volatile fatty acids
Surface mechanisms
Local immune systems
Epithelial cell turnover
Microbial competitors

motility, important control mechanisms exist at the epithelial surface. Specific secretory IgA provides an immunological barrier for unwanted organisms,[153] lysozyme hinders adherence by its steric properties,[63] and blood group reactive glycoproteins combine with and neutralize bacterial receptors.[152] It is also suggested that the growth of bacteria may be influenced by the availability of iron at the epithelial surface, which in turn is controlled by the production of iron-binding proteins.[17] The establishment of a resident normal flora on the epithelial surface might provide a barrier to colonization by other species.

Luminal factors. Within the lumen of the intestine the antibacterial activity of unconjugated bile acids may play a part by regulating the growth of anaerobic organisms.[15] In addition physicochemical factors such as pH and the oxidation–reduction potential will favour the growth of some microorganisms but not others.[95]

Exogenous factors

Exogenous influences of importance include age, diet, ingestion of microbes, the debilitation which accompanies serious disease, factors influencing gastrointestinal motility (e.g. pregnancy, drugs, emotional stress) and, probably the most potent influence of all, antimicrobial agents.

The effects of diet on the normal flora of the small intestine are virtually unknown, although they may explain, at least in part, the differences in the histological appearances of the small intestinal mucosa between normal subjects in the Western World eating a highly purified diet and the people of tropical countries who commonly consume large quantities of unprocessed food.

Serious illness undoubtedly alters the flora of the oropharynx with an increase in the prevalence of Gram-negative bacilli;[65, 66] similar findings are reported in both diabetics and alcoholics.[85, 86] At present one can only speculate on the effect that this may have on bacteria in the small intestine.

Viruses may also influence the normal flora. Again there is a paucity of data for the small intestine, but in the respiratory tract there is good evidence that viruses promote colonization of the upper respiratory tract by bacteria which are often pathogenic,[83] possibly by facilitating the adherence of these bacteria to epithelial cells.[38]

Stasis has a critical role in regulating the microbial population of the small intestine. Disruption of normal intestinal peristalsis allows bacteria to proliferate rapidly in the lumen of the intestine,[78] although again there is little data regarding the effect of this on the bacterial population of the epithelial surface. Emotional stress may disrupt the gastrointestinal microbial ecosystem; it has been suggested that this might influence the susceptibility of travellers to diarrhoeal illnesses.[121]

Antimicrobial agents not only kill or inhibit the growth of bacteria, but also may impair their adherence to cell surfaces even when present only in sub-inhibitory concentrations.[147] The alteration of membrane proteins of bacterial strains developing resistance to antimicrobial agents affects their ability to colonize surfaces.[106]

Finally inhibition of the growth of sensitive microbes may allow the rapid growth of an otherwise unimportant species in the overall microflora. The all-too-frequent development of candidiasis after suppression of the resident flora by broad-spectrum antibiotics suggests that the inhibitory mechanisms work against fungi as well as bacterial pathogens. Thus the presence of a normal flora is probably more important than the immune system in warding off overgrowth by *Candida*.[60]

Role of the normal flora

Nutrition

Most bacterial species in the small intestine are capable of synthesizing vitamins in excess of their own metabolic needs, especially vitamin K and constituents of the vitamin B group – riboflavin, pyridoxine, pantothenic acid, biotin, folic acid, and vitamin B_{12} – but the balance is often uncertain.[117] In disorders of the small intestine allowing bacterial overgrowth, the availability of vitamin B_{12} to the host is usually sharply reduced and nicotinic acid deficiency has also been described.[138] Ascorbic acid (vitamin C) may be broken down by bacteria, although possibly not in significant amounts.

The degradation of urea by the gut flora leads to the release of ammonia which may be absorbed and used for the synthesis of non-essential amino acids[45, 113] but this is estimated to account for no more than 1% of daily amino nitrogen requirements.[146] Moreover, in uraemic patients, the suppression of gut flora with broad-spectrum antibiotics improves nitrogen balance.[97]

Resistance to infection

There have been several studies of the methods by which the normal flora may act as a barrier to infection by preventing or limiting the colonization of the surface epithelium with pathogenic microorganisms (Table 8.29). However, the importance of these mechanisms as barriers to infection remains largely unproven. Some bacteria (e.g. *Streptococcus viridans*) have been shown to be capable of producing protein antibiotics (bacteriocins) which play a role in preventing bacterial overgrowth.[135] The metabolic end-products of anaerobic metabolism such as volatile fatty acids and deconjugated bile acids are toxic to some bacteria; the lowering of the oxidation–reduction potential may also be inhibitory.[121]

In some species the presence of a normal gastrointestinal flora has been shown to inhibit the passage of bacteria (e.g. indigenous *Escherichia coli*) through the epithelial mucosa into the lymphocytes and mesenteric lymph nodes. In germ-free animals this barrier is reduced.[12] The resident bacteria may even be capable of degrading the toxins of pathogenic bacteria, although this mechanism has so far been demonstrated only in animals with rumens.[2] Bacterial interrelationships also may be important in preventing invasion of epithelial surfaces, as has been demonstrated in mice infected with *Shigella*.[33]

Effect on immune mechanisms

The presence of intestinal bacteria primes the immune system and this state of readiness may be of marginal benefit to the host. For example, the resistance of germ-free mice to *Vibrio cholerae* after immunization is enhanced by the simultaneous colonization of the gut with intestinal flora obtained from conventional animals.[133] Conversely, the overall decrease in the cellular immune response in germ-free animals appears to decrease the mortality from viruses capable of causing hepatitis and lymphocytic chorio-meningitis.[109, 136]

Intestinal bacteria as a cause of systemic infection

The indigenous microflora of the gut can be a major source of disease. This is most clearly seen in immunosuppressed patients in whom the microorganisms of the intestine are a potent cause of opportunistic infections. The suppression of these bacteria by antibiotics may reduce the incidence of complications in susceptible subjects.[134]

Having a normal flora in the small intestine has other disadvantages: firstly, secondary bacterial invasion of the circulation in overwhelming strongyloidiasis is a life threatening state[130] and, secondly, the role of bacteria in maintaining or promoting the inflammatory process in chronic ulcerative conditions of the small intestine appears to be important in both experimental and clinical situations. Thus it is possible that the use of a bowel sterilization regimen is beneficial in the short term to patients with Crohn's disease.[70] This is supported by experimental evidence showing that the administration of antibiotics inhibits the development of intestinal ulceration in animals given carrageenan.[105]

Conclusion

The role of the normal microflora of the small intestine has not been fully explored. Under experimental conditions it is not a prerequisite for life; indeed if life-span is taken as a marker, germ-free animals often do better than animals reared under conventional conditions.[50] Nevertheless, in a world teeming with microorganisms, it has been suggested that bacteria residing on mucosal surfaces provide a degree of protection against infection by a range of other microorganisms including *C. albicans*, *V. cholerae* and salmonellae.[84] The effects on the nutritional state of the host appear to be marginal but the role of the intestinal microflora on the health and well-being of poorly-nourished people living in unhygienic environments warrants further study.

BACTERIAL OVERGROWTH

From the discussion above it is clear that there cannot be any absolute definition of bacterial overgrowth in the small intestine. For practical purposes the demonstration of viable bacteria in concentrations of more than 10^4–10^5 organisms/ml in the upper small intestine of the fasting subject is adequate evidence of bacterial overgrowth, especially if the flora contains coliform organisms and/or *Bacteroides* in concentrations of greater than 10^2–10^3/ml. These are the sort of results obtained in competent microbiological laboratories using accepted culture techniques, but there are no valid standards against which individual units can check the quality of their work (Table 8.28). The problem is compounded by difficulties in obtaining specimens from multiple sites in the small intestine, by the relative paucity of data for normal control subjects, by our incomplete understanding of factors which control bacterial growth, and, in some cases, by the poor correlation between microbiological data and the apparently adverse metabolic effects of bacteria in the small intestine.

For practical purposes the clinician may have to be content with:

a The demonstration of a lesion known to be associated with bacterial overgrowth.

b The finding of one or more metabolic disturbances which may occur as a result of bacterial action (classically the malabsorption of vitamin B_{12} and/or steatorrhoea) and a positive breath test to indicate bile salt deconjugation or carbohydrate breakdown in the upper gut.

c The reversal of such metabolic abnormalities by the oral administration of appropriate antibiotics.

Historical aspects

The combination of bacterial overgrowth and a demonstrable metabolic disturbance reversible by the administration of oral antibiotics has been called the blind loop syndrome,[7] the stagnant loop syndrome,[139] the small intestinal stasis syndrome,[36] and the contaminated small bowel syndrome.[51]

Nearly a century ago, in a review of patients dying with pernicious anaemia at Guy's Hospital, it was suggested that attention should be paid to the small number of patients with 'changes in the small intestine'.[150] Within the next decade four separate case reports of intestinal strictures and a 'pernicious anaemia' appeared in the Scandinavian medical literature.[36] Surgical cure of this rare syndrome was attempted successfully in 1924.[131] Shortly afterwards the use of liver therapy for pernicious anaemia was extended effectively to patients with a megaloblastic anaemia associated with a number of abnormalities of the small intestine including blind pouches and diverticulae (hence 'blind loop syndrome').[94] Steatorrhoea was demonstrated in many such patients and the major clinical features were summarized in a review by Barker and Hummel.[9] The syndrome was extended to patients with stasis of the contents of the small intestine without self-filling loops, and treatment with appropriate antibiotics was shown to be effective. More recently Gracey[51] used the term contaminated small bowel syndrome to cover patients with conditions in which stasis is not a necessary factor in the maintenance of bacterial overgrowth, such as cholangitis (in which the upper intestine is seeded with bacteria), immune deficiency states, and malnutrition.

The first experiments to produce bacterial overgrowth in the small intestine of animals were undertaken to try to find the cause of pernicious anaemia. Dogs were made anaemic by operations designed to produce intestinal strictures or blind loops.[131, 143] More detailed observations became possible when it was demonstrated that blind loops of small intestine could be produced satisfactorily in rats.[148] Much of our knowledge of the mechanisms of the metabolic disturbances arising from bacterial overgrowth in the small intestine stem from studies of this experimental model stimulated by observations on patients. The results of these studies have been extensively reviewed.[30, 52, 101, 137] Progress has been slow over the past 10 years and probably awaits new methods of studying the interaction between bacteria and the epithelial surfaces with which they are in close association. For example, there is now evidence to show that bacteria in the small intestine can survive on host cell glycoproteins[111] and that they secrete enzymes which damage the enzyme systems of epithelial cell brush borders.[115]

Aetiology and pathogenesis

The bacterial population in the lumen of the small intestine will depend on the rate of entry of viable organisms into the gut, their rate of reproduction, and the rate of clearance from the gut. Changes in one or more of these mechanisms may lead to bacterial overgrowth in the fluid contents of the fasted small intestine (Table 8.30). The normal phasic changes of luminal flora with meals probably become less pronounced, but the effect on the surface flora remains uncertain.[14] With the limited data available one cannot even be certain that the surface flora is more abundant in subjects with bacterial overgrowth in the lumen. Thus the pathogenetic mechanisms of disorders caused by bacterial overgrowth are discussed principally in relation to concentrations of viable bacteria isolated from aspirates of fluid from the intestine of fasting patients. In patients with bacterial overgrowth there is characteristically an increase in the concentration of organisms, especially those species normally confined to the lower small intestine and colon (Table 8.28).

Metabolic and nutritional consequences

Caloric undernutrition

It has not been shown that bacterial proliferation in the small intestine per se significantly impairs the supply of nutrients for energy production. Indeed ruminants obtain a major part of their nutrition in the form of volatile fatty acids from the fermentation of complex carbohydrates. However, young experimental animals with surgically created blind loops grow less well than control animals[96] or animals with an equivalent small intestinal resection.[91] The experimental evidence would suggest that growth impairment is largely related to diminished food intake and can be reversed by giving antibiotics. This may also be responsible for the failure of growth and infantilism described in children with the blind loop syndrome.[99] Nevertheless, there is also impairment of the absorption of fat and carbohydrate in patients with bacterial overgrowth in the small intestine.

Table 8.30 Conditions favouring bacterial overgrowth in the small intestine.

Excess bacteria entering the small intestine
  Heavily contaminated food (?)
  Impaired gastric barrier
    Achlorhydria (Drasar et al.[32])
    Gastrojejunostomy (Nygaard[104])
    Partial or total gastrectomy (Tabaqchali[137])
  Internal bacterial 'seeding' of the small intestine
    Cholangitis (Scott & Khan[129])
    Fistulae (Donaldson[31])
    Loss of ileocaecal valve (Mutch[98])

Conditions which may allow excess bacterial proliferation in the absence of readily demonstrable stasis
  With defined mechanisms
    Immune deficiency states (Parkin et al.[107])
    Bile salt deficiency (Floch et al.[40])
  Without clearly defined mechanisms
    Old age (Roberts et al.[116])
    Uraemia
    Malnutrition (Gracey et al.[54])
    Tropical sprue (Gorbach et al.;[49] Klipstein[74])
    Monosaccharide malabsorption (Gracey et al.[53])

Delayed clearance of bacteria from the lumen of the intestine
  Localized anatomical abnormalities
    Duodenal and jejunal diverticulosis (Cooke et al.[25])
    Strictures
      Congenital (Astley[6])
      Crohn's disease (Donaldson;[31] Rutgeerts et al.[118])
      Tuberculosis (Barker & Hummel[9])
      Caused by ulcers of varying aetiology
  Postoperative problems
    Afferent loop stasis (Wirts & Goldstein[155])
    Postoperative blind loops (Ellis & Smith;[36] Lennert[79])
    Jejunoileal bypass (Barry et al.[10])
    Entero-enterostomy (Donaldson[30])
    Continent ileostomy (Schjønsby et al.[126])
  Generalized disorders of the bowel wall
    Coeliac disease (rarely)
    Scleroderma (Salen et al.[119])
    Irradiation
    Amyloidosis (Tete et al.[141])
    Intestinal pseudo-obstruction (Maldonado et al.[87])
  Neurological disorders affecting motility
    Diabetes mellitus (Scarpello et al.[123])
    Vagotomy
    Degeneration of the myenteric plexus (Dyer et al.[34])

The relationship of malnutrition and diarrhoeal illnesses to the 'normal' flora of the small intestine in malnourished children of Third World countries is incompletely understood, but is of considerable potential importance. The polluted environment is probably the main determinant of bacterial overgrowth, but the role of impaired immune function secondary to malnutrition has not been adequately assessed. The high concentrations of jejunal bacteria, some of which may be enterotoxigenic, almost certainly play a key role in the diarrhoea and malabsorption which may accompany dietary malnutrition in childhood.[52]

Steatorrhoea

Malabsorption of fat is common in patients with bacterial overgrowth and is due primarily to the poor formation of micelles. The structured agglomeration of phospholipid, bile acid, monoglyceride and diglyceride is produced most efficiently by conjugated bile acids. Intestinal bacteria (especially bacteroides, veillonellae, clostridia and bifidobacteria) are capable of deconjugating and dehydroxylating conjugated bile salts which then become poorly soluble at the pH of the upper small intestine. As a result the total concentration of available effective bile acids may fall below the critical level for micelle formation. The importance of this mechanism has been supported by the direct estimation of bile salt concentrations in fluid aspirated from the contaminated small intestine of both patients and experimental animals, and by assessing the effect of feeding additional conjugated bile salts.[137] As might be expected, however, the clinical situation does not always appear to conform to this elegant mechanism. In some patients with steatorrhoea the concentration of conjugated bile acids does not appear to fall below the critical micellar concentration.

The adverse effect of bacteria on the ability of the epithelial cell to take up fat has not been adequately assessed, although there is increasing evidence of damage to brush border membranes.[115] In addition the presence of anaerobic bacteria in the small intestine does not necessarily lead to steatorrhoea. This is particularly true of bacterial overgrowth limited to the ileum and very localized lesions in duodenum (e.g. a solitary diverticulum).[47]

Production of hydroxy-fatty acids

Unabsorbed fat may be metabolized by intestinal bacteria to produce long chain hydroxy-fatty acids some of which are similar to ricinoleic acid, the major fatty acid in castor oil.[142] Unsaturated hydroxy-fatty acids may also be produced by the bacterially-mediated hydration of linoleic acid.[127] These fatty acids stimulate the gastrointestinal mucosa to secrete[4] and this, together with the increased concentration of intraluminal volatile fatty acids (see below), may contribute to the diarrhoea which is a prominent symptom in many patients with bacterial overgrowth in the small intestine.

Carbohydrate malabsorption

Several groups of workers have documented the malabsorption of carbohydrate in subjects with bacterial overgrowth in the small intestine,[30, 52] but some anomalies persist. For example, it has been shown that the transport of glucose by the intestinal mucosa is impaired in the presence of deconjugated bile salts both in vivo and in vitro, yet the standard glucose tolerance test administered to patients with bacterial overgrowth nearly always gives a normal result. The uptake of glucose from disaccharides may be more consistently depressed, although data regarding this is scanty. Certainly in experimental animals the creation of a blind loop depresses the disaccharidase activities of the mucosal brush border.[68]

It is generally agreed that the standard test for the absorption of D-xylose is abnormal in the majority of patients with bacterial overgrowth. Bacteria are capable of fermenting many carbohydrates, but the production of bacterial metabolites from xylose are difficult to demonstrate. It seems likely that there is a defect in transport superimposed on the effects of bacterial fermentation.[144]

The relatively small amount of unabsorbed carbohydrate provides an important substrate for the growth of bacteria. In addition it is readily converted into volatile fatty acids which are then available to the host for energy production.

In children severe bacterial contamination of the upper small intestine appears to be associated with temporary monosaccharide malabsorption. Bacterial damage to the jejunal mucosa has been postulated as contributing to the malabsorption of all carbohydrates, including the monosaccharides glucose, galactose and fructose. In turn these may provide an excellent substrate for bacterial growth.[18]

Protein malnutrition
Overt signs of protein–energy malnutrition are not commonly seen in patients with bacterial overgrowth in the small intestine,[100] but mild hypoalbuminaemia is a frequent finding. A number of factors may be responsible, including damage to the intestinal mucosa with protein loss, impaired uptake of peptides and amino acids, and the diversion of protein products into bacterial catabolic pathways.[71] Protein-losing enteropathy is much better documented in the experimental animal with a blind loop than it is in humans. In rats significant protein loss appears to occur not only from the blind loop but also from the contaminated adjacent small intestine. Reversal of the protein-losing state may require long-term treatment with antibiotics.[73] However, losses of protein into the gut appear to be small compared with the total catabolism of protein.[101]

Impaired uptake of amino acids, especially of the branched chain group (leucine, isoleucine and valine), correlates with the finding of reduced concentrations of circulating essential amino acids (Figure 8.55). In turn this may be

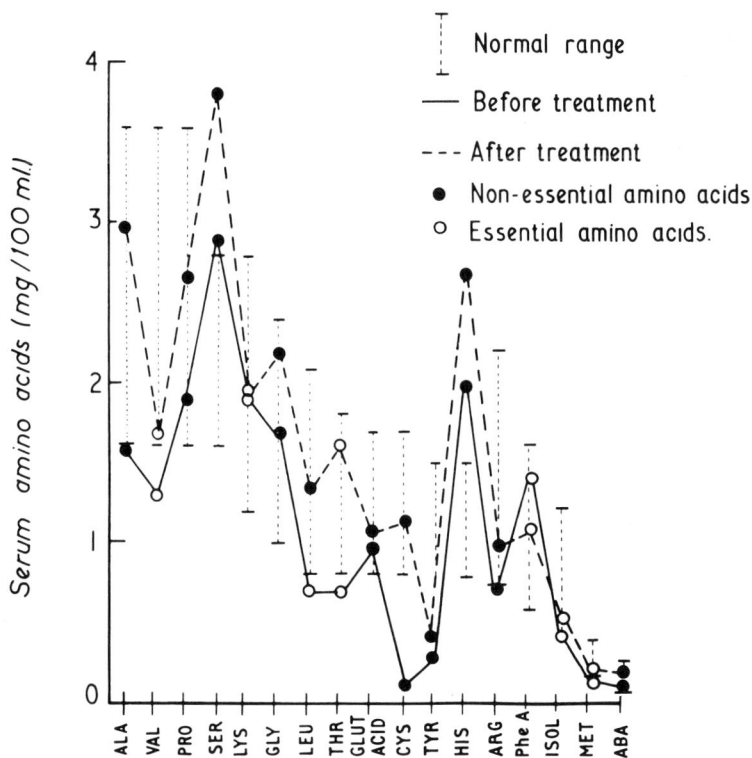

Fig. 8.55 Fasting circulating amino acid profile in a patient with protein–calorie malnutrition secondary to malabsorption associated with dual pathology (partial gastrectomy and jejunal diverticulosis). The concentrations of branched chain essential amino acids are low.

responsible for the impaired synthesis of proteins.[8, 68] Nevertheless some loose ends remain: the absorption of dipeptides containing branched chain amino acids is only minimally impaired[8] and, at least in animals with blind loops in the proximal small intestine, overall nitrogen absorption is delayed but not reduced.[26]

The effects of bacterial overgrowth on the metabolism of proteins has been studied in some detail.[72, 96] Many of the resulting metabolites are of no value to the host, including indole derivatives from L-tryptophan, volatile phenols from tyrosine, hippuric acid from phenylalanine, piperidine from lysine, and pyrollidine from arginine and ornithine. There is some evidence to suggest that the circulating concentrations of L-tryptophan may fall to such low levels that it becomes rate-limiting for protein synthesis.[68] It is estimated that as much as 60% of the dietary intake of L-tryptophan may be diverted into unavailable indolic compounds.[100]

Water and electrolytes

In the Western World, diarrhoea occurs in no more than one-third of patients with anatomical abnormalities of the small intestine leading to bacterial overgrowth. Stool volumes are usually not markedly increased unless there is severe steatorrhoea. In contrast, watery diarrhoea occurs commonly in tropical sprue especially at the onset of the illness. Some workers claim that the bacterial flora found in the bowel lumen of patients with tropical sprue is very different from that of patients with the classical blind loop syndrome.[75] In tropical sprue the coliform organisms (*Klebsiella*, *Enterobacter* and *Escherichia*) are of a limited range of serotypes or biotypes, and enterotoxigenic strains are commonly found. The toxin from these strains will induce water and salt secretion in perfused rat jejunum. In contrast, in the blind loop syndrome, coliform and anaerobic organisms can be cultured and enterotoxigenic bacteria have not been found. This elegant explanation of the symptomatic differences between patients with tropical sprue and those with the blind loop syndrome requires confirmation. Not all reported results are concordant. For example, anaerobic organisms could not be cultured from patients with 'tropical sprue' in the West Indies,[75] but were present in patients with 'sprue' in South India.[14]

Diarrhoea may also be induced by the effect of bacterial metabolites of fatty acids (short chain fatty acids, hydroxy-fatty acids) on the mucosa of the small and large intestine.[3]

Vitamin deficiencies

Fat-soluble vitamins. In patients with steatorrhoea the absorption of the fat-soluble vitamins will be impaired; however, there are few reported studies. Some data is available for vitamin D[23, 132] and the occasional case of osteomalacia is well documented.[124]

Vitamin K deficiency has not been described in the blind loop syndrome perhaps because of the ability of some intestinal bacteria (especially Gram-positive organisms) to synthesize menaquinones, but is not uncommon in some patients with severe tropical sprue.

Vitamin B group. Signs of vitamin B deficiency are not uncommon in malnourished patients with bacterial overgrowth in the small intestine, but they rarely progress to dramatic disease. The description of the patient with jejunal diverticulosis who developed an encephalopathic syndrome responding to an intravenous injection of nicotinic acid remains an isolated case report.[138] There is little good evidence that deficiency of vitamin B may occur as a result of competition by bacteria for a dietary substrate, but it is interesting that nicotinic acid may be the one element of the B group most required by intestinal bacteria.[42]

Vitamin B_{12}. Megaloblastic anaemia secondary to vitamin B_{12} deficiency may be regarded as the hallmark of long-term bacterial overgrowth in the small intestine. It dominates the early literature on the subject.[21] This is paradoxical because, although vitamin B_{12} is found in all animal tissues, it is synthesized solely by bacteria. Unfortunately vitamin B_{12} synthesized in the colon is not absorbed, thus in both animals and humans a clean vegetarian diet may lead to vitamin B_{12} deficiency, which explains the megaloblastic anaemia sometimes found in vegans.[21] Under natural conditions bacteria contaminate all foodstuffs and appear to be the natural source of vitamin B_{12} for herbivorous animals which are not coprophagic.

In patients with bacterial overgrowth in the small intestine tests for the absorption of vitamin B_{12}–intrinsic factor complex are often abnormal. Intestinal bacteria bind readily with the free vitamin. Furthermore most species will compete with intrinsic factor (IF) for vitamin B_{12}. There appear to be powerful binding sites in the cell walls of some bacteria,[43] especially of *Bacteroides*, which are capable of taking up most of the B_{12} from the B_{12}–IF complexes.[149] In clinical experiments it has been shown that more than 50% of orally administered labelled B_{12} is precipitated with the bacterial pellet when aspirates of fluid from the ileum of patients with bacterial overgrowth are centrifuged. In contrast, only 10% of the labelled B_{12} can be precipitated in the ileal fluid of control subjects or of patients shown to have bacterial overgrowth and given appropriate antibiotics.[125]

Bacteria are also capable of metabolizing both intrinsic factor and vitamin B_{12}. It is possible to impair the binding capacity of intrinsic factor by incubating neutralized gastric juice with enteric bacteria. This effect is probably not of great significance. In contrast, the bacterial conversion of vitamin B_{12} to physiologically inactive derivatives (cobamides) is of greater importance. These derivatives block both intrinsic factor and ileal receptors and may even displace vitamin B_{12} from hepatic stores.[16, 90]

Folic acid. Folic acid deficiency is uncommon in patients with bacterial overgrowth secondary to intestinal stasis. Indeed serum values are often abnormally high, which may be due in part to the absorption of folic acid synthesized by the bacteria and in part to the accumulation of folate compounds in the circulation occurring as a result of disordered folate metabolism. The absorption of folic acid is generally normal in the patient with an uncomplicated blind loop. Experimentally, elevated levels of serum folic acid can be produced by constructing blind loops in the proximal, but not the distal, small intestine of dogs.[21] Marked folate deficiency is rare, but may occur, and malabsorption of folic acid corrected by treatment with antibiotics has been described.[25]

Once again the situation is different for tropical sprue. In some studies 90% of patients are folate-depleted and, although this is usually ascribed to a poor dietary intake of food folates, malabsorption of folic acid is probably the more important factor.[21]

Presentation and diagnosis

Clinical
Patients with bacterial overgrowth in the small intestine often present with non-specific symptoms of lassitude and weight loss associated with evidence of disturbed intestinal function such as increased bowel sounds or diarrhoea (Table 8.31). Less frequently, nutritional disturbances are the major presenting feature, with glossitis and stomatitis, anaemia, hypoproteinaemic oedema, and rarely the muscle weakness or bone pain of vitamin D deficiency.

Table 8.31 Symptomatology of patients with jejunal diverticulosis.

Weight loss	75%
Nausea	50%
Vomiting	45%
Diarrhoea	45%
Diarrhoea/constipation	20%
Constipation	25%
No bowel disturbance	10%

Data from a study of 30 patients (mean age 63 years) referred to hospital (Cooke *et al.*[25]). More than half these patients were or had been anaemic (Hb less than 12 g/100 ml).

Laboratory tests
Laboratory screening tests often provide pointers, the most significant of which is red cell macrocytosis (usually, but not always, due to vitamin B_{12} deficiency), mild or moderate hypoproteinaemia, and steatorrhoea. One or more standard tests of intestinal absorption (D-xylose absorption, faecal fat excretion, and the Schilling test) will usually be abnormal and provide a baseline for assessing the response to treatment. In themselves they do not provide a diagnosis, but by this stage of the investigation the experienced clinician will have considered the possible aetiology and pathogenesis of the malabsorptive disorder. Often he can now arrange the diagnostic test, e.g. radiology of the small intestine, jejunal biopsy, or measurement of pancreatic function.

Radiology
Carefully performed radiological examination of the small intestine by straightforward barium follow through will usually identify sites of potential bacterial overgrowth. It is relatively easy to show anatomical abnormalities such as jejunal diverticulosis (Figure 8.56) and to delineate the extent of intestine involved in a known disorder (Figure 8.57). In addition, the radiologist should be alerted to the possibility of altered transit and motility, although this is difficult to assess with barium. Not all cases will be picked up on a barium follow through examination. In particular it is easy to miss those cases in which the basic problem is seeding of the small intestine with microorganisms such as may occur from the afferent limb of a Polya gastrectomy, from cholangitis, or from an entero–enteric fistula. Other imaging techniques may be helpful, such as cholangiography, HIDA scanning, and the infusion of barium into the small or large intestine (Figure 8.58).

In most cases it is not difficult to detect the presence of a structural disorder which will

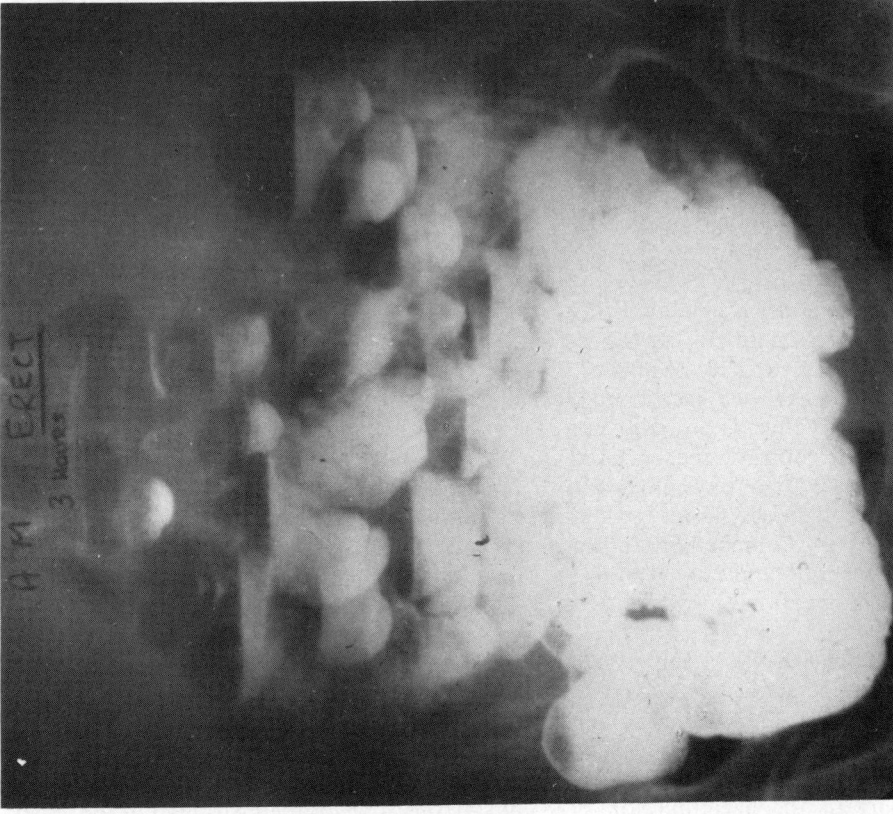

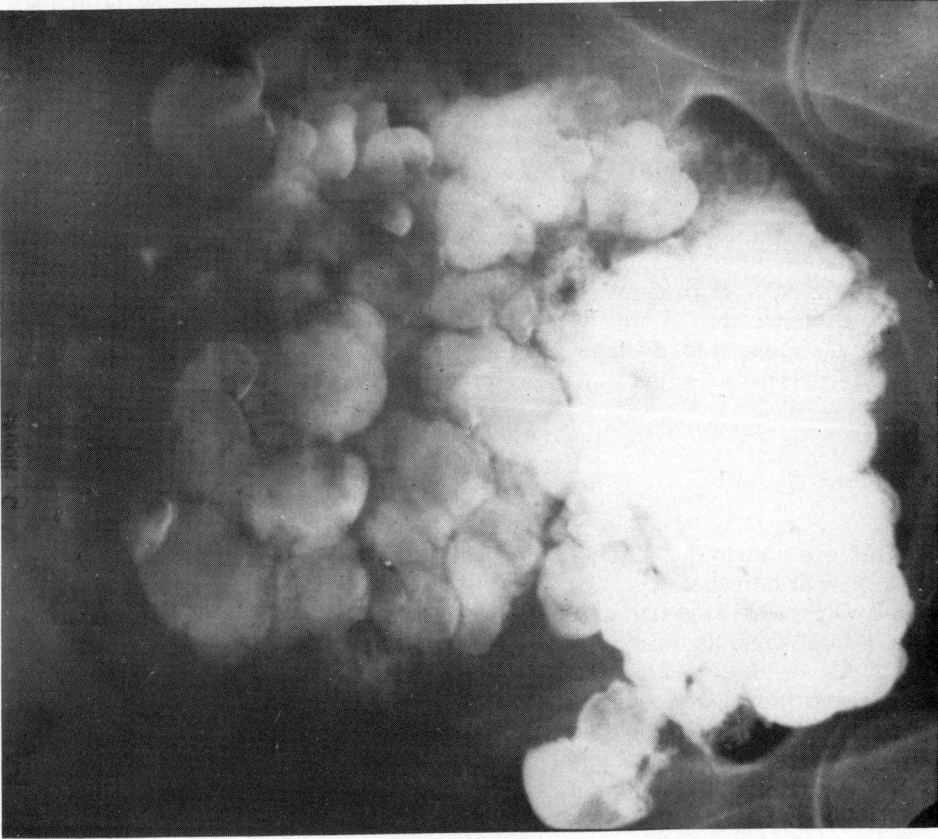

Fig. 8.56 Jejunal diverticulosis. Radiographs taken after the ingestion of barium with the subject (a) supine and (b) erect.

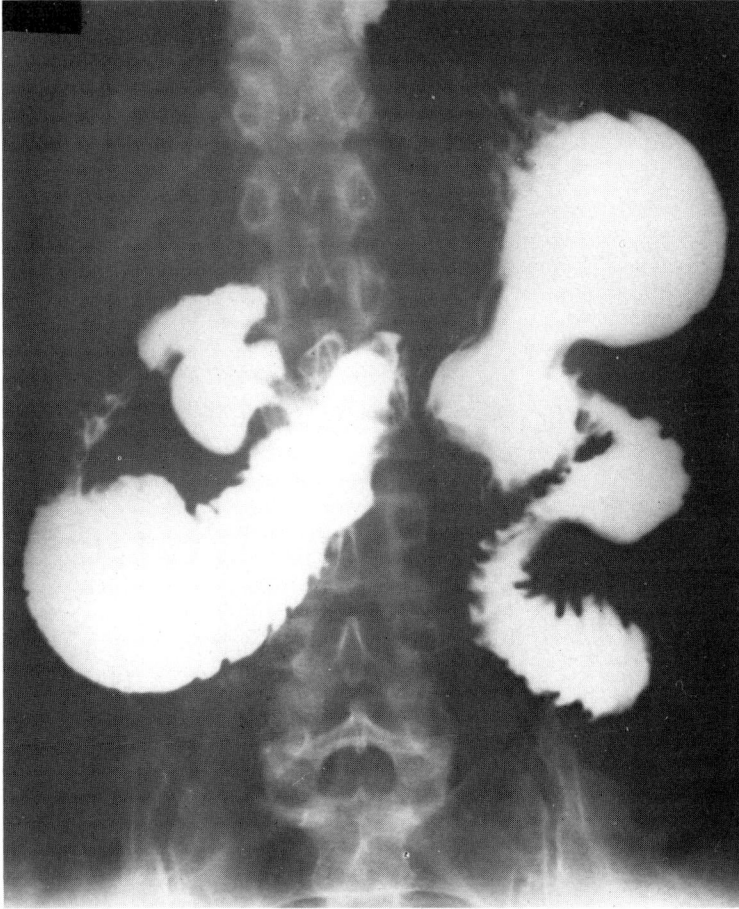

Fig. 8.57 Scleroderma. Barium follow through examination showing a dilated duodenum. Culture of fluid aspirated from the upper small intestine yielded 10^6 viable organisms/ml.

encourage bacterial overgrowth in the small intestine. In other cases there may be an alternative predisposing condition with the loss of a protective mechanism, such as may occur in the patient with hypogammaglobulinaemia.

Tests for bacterial overgrowth

At this stage of investigation the clinician needs clear evidence that bacterial overgrowth is present. Three approaches are available: one or more of the indirect tests of bacterial overgrowth may be applied; a sample of the contents of the small intestine may be aspirated and cultured; or the clinical and biochemical response to the administration of antibiotics may be assessed (Table 8.32).

These three approaches should be regarded as complementary. The indirect tests give evidence of the metabolic activities of bacteria and may be used in the long-term monitoring of the effects of therapy; culture of aspirated fluid, although rarely helpful in guiding the choice of

Table 8.32 Tests for bacterial overgrowth in the small intestine.

Indirect measures of the effects of bacterial metabolism
In the circulation
 Free bile acids
In urine
 Amino acid derivatives
 Indoles (from tryptophan)
 Phenols (from tyrosine)
 Hippuric acid (from phenylalanine)
 Piperidine (from lysine)
 Pyrrolidine (from arginine and ornithine)
In expired air
 $^{14}CO_2$ from: ^{14}C-labelled bile acids (glycocholic acid)
  ^{14}C-labelled carbohydrate (xylose)
  ^{14}C-labelled amino acid (taurine)
 Hydrogen from: absorbable sugar (glucose)
  non-absorbable sugar (lactulose)

Direct measures of bacteria and their metabolites in aspirates
 Viable bacterial counts
 Concentration of volatile fatty acids
 Presence of deconjugated bile acids

Response to therapy
 Improvement of clinical measurements of malabsorption (e.g. of fat, vitamin B_{12}, and xylose)

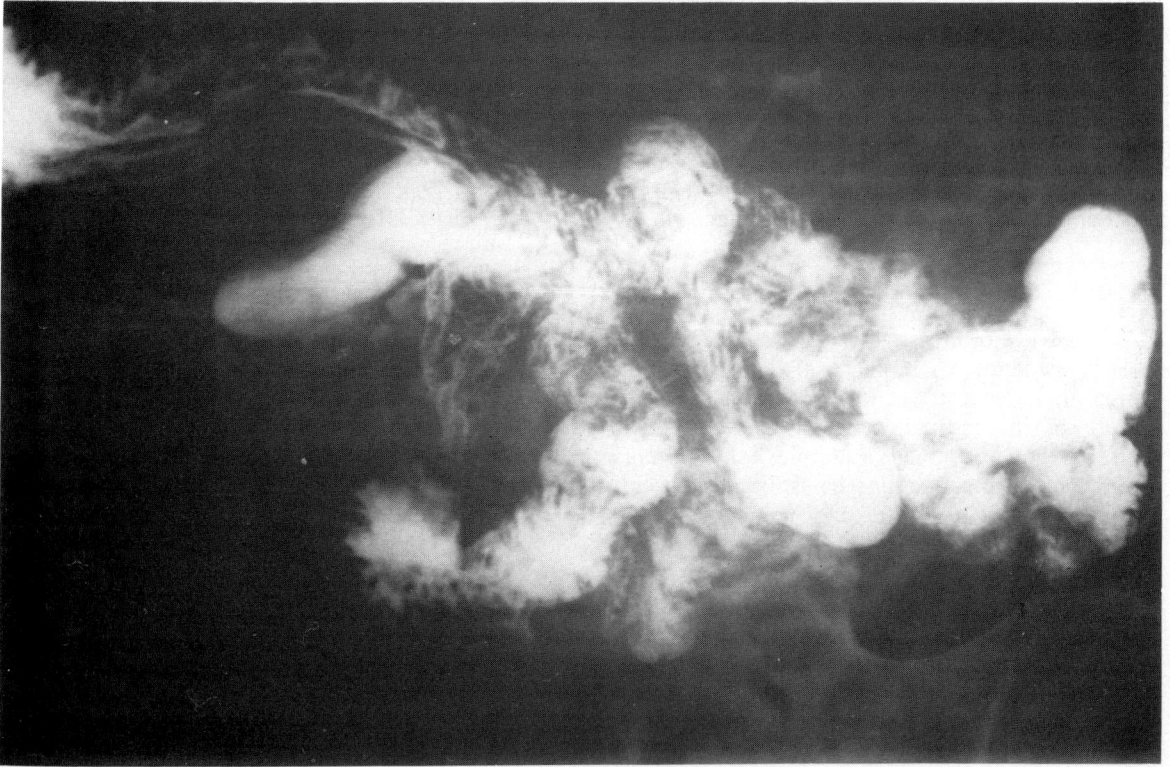

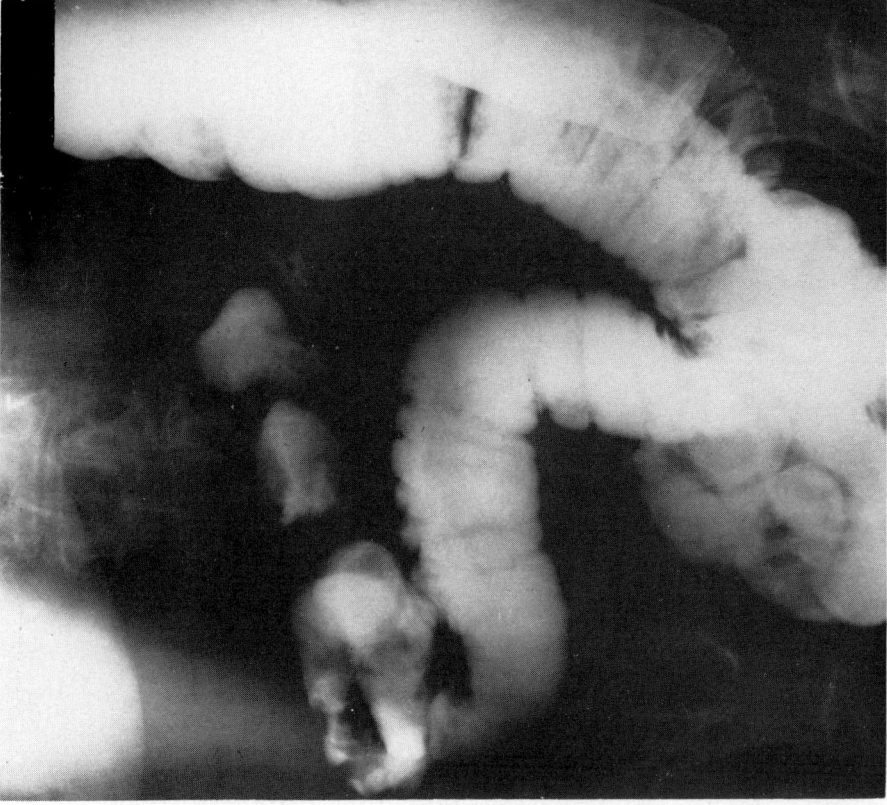

Fig. 8.58 Duodenocolic fistula. Barium studies of a 48-year-old woman who presented with a megaloblastic anaemia (serum vitamin B_{12} 40 pg/ml). (a) A normal barium follow through examination. (b) The fistula is revealed by barium enema. The patient was a seamstress and in the absence of other pathology it was thought that her duodenum was perforated by a swallowed pin. There were no symptoms other than those of anaemia and the diagnosis of fistula was made only after it was shown the impaired absorption of vitamin B_{12}–IF complex could be corrected by the oral administration of tetracycline.

antibiotics, provides a background for further clinical research; and monitoring the response to treatment with antibiotics or other forms of therapy is vital to the correct management of such patients.

Over the past 20 years a plethora of tests have been devised but they are not always well-validated (Table 8.32). The use of these tests will depend very much on the facilities available and on the skills and experience of the specialist staff. It is sensible to limit the range of tests available and to ensure that they are used intelligently. Much care is necessary to ensure good quality control. In particular considerable attention must be devoted to explaining procedures to patients and to ensuring the complete collection of samples. The clinician must be familiar with the methodology, must know the limits of accuracy of measurement, and must understand the sensitivity and specificity of each test before interpreting the results in relation to the clinical picture.

Indirect tests

Circulating free bile acids. In normal subjects the concentration of circulating bile acids in the fasting state is less than 10 μmol/l, whereas in patients with the stagnant loop syndrome levels of 13–52 μmol/l have been described.[80] This potentially useful test has not received much attention because of methodological difficulties. Moreover, abnormal results are also found in patients with an interrupted enterohepatic circulation as a result of ileal resection or ileal dysfunction.

Bacterial metabolites in urine. Intestinal bacteria may produce a number of metabolites which after absorption are excreted in the urine. The excretion of indoxyl sulphate (indican) derived from the essential amino acid L-tryptophan has been correlated with bacterial overgrowth, but cannot be used under routine ward conditions because of the many variables involved in the production of indicanuria. These include the quantity of dietary protein ingested, the efficacy of hydrolysis by proteolytic enzymes, the presence of malabsorption as a result of factors other than bacterial overgrowth, and the composition of intraluminal contents (e.g. the presence or absence of sugars, the hydrogen ion concentration).[101]

In a small series it has been shown that the measurement of both indican and phenol in urine is a reasonably reliable and specific method of providing support for the diagnosis of bacterial overgrowth in the small intestine.[1]

Nevertheless the measurement of urinary markers is of limited overall value, except perhaps in monitoring the response of a patient to treatment in a metabolic unit (Figure 8.59).

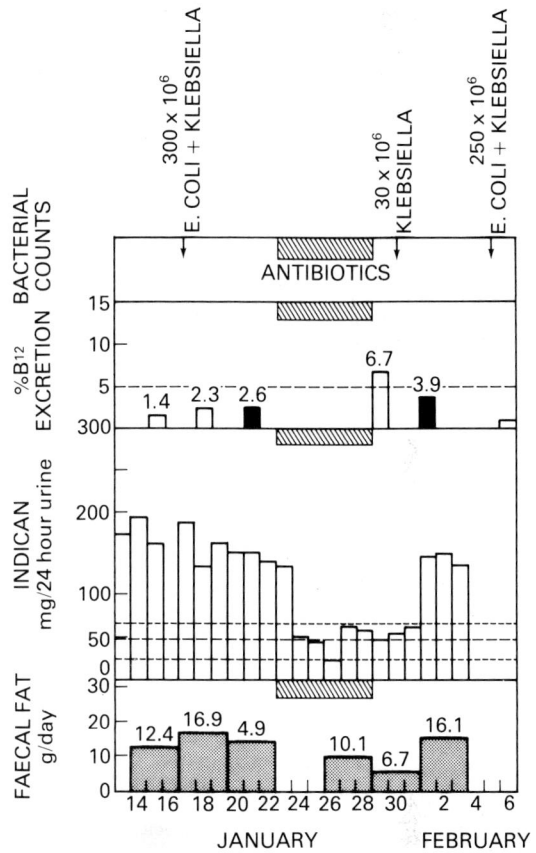

Fig. 8.59 Response to the administration of oral tetracycline in a patient with bacterial overgrowth secondary to jejunal diverticulosis. In this case viable bacterial counts in jejunal fluid can be assessed against measurements of B_{12} absorption (open columns = B_{12} given alone; closed columns = B_{12} + IF), indican excretion (dietary protein 70 g/day) and faecal fat (dietary fat 70 g/day).

Breath tests. The respiratory excretion of gases (carbon dioxide and hydrogen) produced by the metabolism of several substrates provides an elegant way of studying the effect of intestinal bacteria (Figure 8.60).[61] These tests are readily accepted by patients because they involve neither intubation nor the collection of urine and faeces. They are relatively easy to perform and to control, and the method of quantification is well within the scope of a department of nuclear medicine.

False negative results occur if there is delay in the ingested substrate reaching the site of bacterial overgrowth or if the bacteria present are incapable of metabolizing that particular substance. Breath tests will not localize the site of

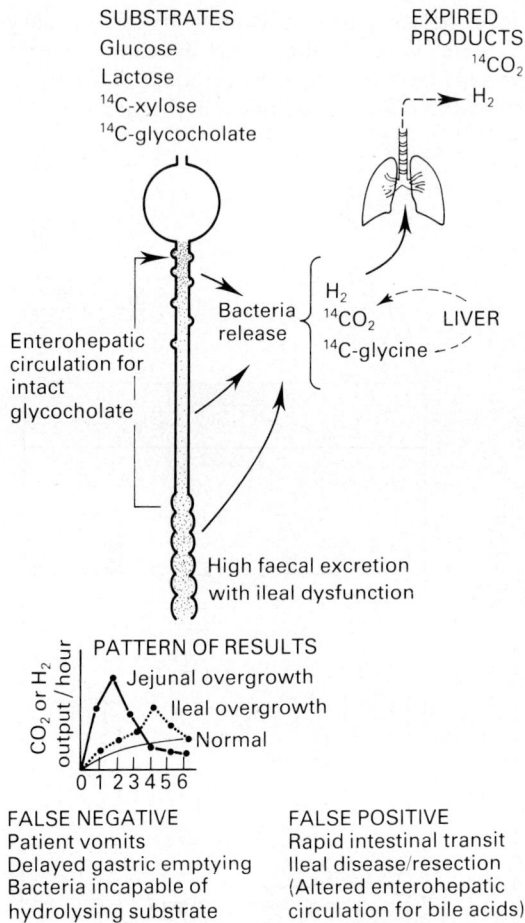

SUBSTRATES
Glucose
Lactose
^{14}C-xylose
^{14}C-glycocholate

EXPIRED PRODUCTS
$^{14}CO_2$
H_2

Enterohepatic circulation for intact glycocholate

Bacteria release

H_2
$^{14}CO_2$
^{14}C-glycine
LIVER

High faecal excretion with ileal dysfunction

PATTERN OF RESULTS
CO_2 or H_2 output/hour
Jejunal overgrowth
Ileal overgrowth
Normal

0 1 2 3 4 5 6

FALSE NEGATIVE
Patient vomits
Delayed gastric emptying
Bacteria incapable of hydrolysing substrate

FALSE POSITIVE
Rapid intestinal transit
Ileal disease/resection
(Altered enterohepatic circulation for bile acids)

Fig. 8.60 The principle of the breath test as used for the detection of bacterial overgrowth in the small intestine.

bacterial catabolism of the substrate, although this may be overcome to some extent by using a radiopaque or radiolabelled (^{99}Tc) marker and undertaking serial imaging at the same time as the breath test.[61, 128] This may be particularly important in patients with rapid transit of material to the colon.

The *bile acid breath test*, introduced for the diagnosis of altered bile acid metabolism,[41] has remained the one most commonly used in the diagnosis of bacterial overgrowth in the small intestine. The patient drinks a solution of glycocholic acid labelled with ^{14}C-1-glycine, and hourly samples of expired carbon dioxide are collected for six hours by trapping the gas in a measured quantity of an organic base. The patient must remain in a resting state to ensure a constant rate of CO_2 production. Under these circumstances the specific activity of expired $^{14}CO_2$ corrected for body weight gives a measure of the bacterial splitting of the amide bond linking ^{14}C-glycine to cholic acid.

The radiolabelled bile acid mixes with the bile acid pool and the rate of excretion of $^{14}CO_2$ reflects its fractional catabolic activity. Thus a high specific activity of expired CO_2 may reflect a decreased pool size (e.g. after cholecystectomy or ileal resection) as well as an absolute increase in breakdown of conjugated bile acids. A high specific activity also occurs in patients with ileal dysfunction sufficiently severe to allow bile acids to spill into the colon. This defect may be detected by the measurement of ^{14}C in the faeces.[122]

The value of the bile acid breath test is limited by the fairly high incidence of false positive (10%) and false negative (30%) results as judged by a careful analysis of more than 200 tests performed at the Mayo Clinic.[76] Thus, although the test is reasonably specific, it is only moderately sensitive, picking up no more than 70% of cases shown to have bacterial overgrowth by direct culture. It seems likely that no one biochemical test will pick up all cases of bacterial overgrowth because of the variable metabolic activities of the differing bacterial species.

Less information is available for the ^{14}C-*xylose breath test*, but it appeared to be more sensitive than the bile acid breath test in a small series reported by King *et al.*[72] There is as yet no evidence regarding its specificity.

The bacterial fermentation of carbohydrates may be monitored by measuring the excretion of released hydrogen in expired air using mass spectrometry. The sensitivity of the *hydrogen breath test* is similar to that of the bile acid breath test, but it is suggested that, taken together, the two tests are capable of providing a diagnosis in over 90% of patients with a contaminated small intestine.[93]

In all breath tests it is much easier to identify bacterial overgrowth in the upper than in the lower small intestine, and to some extent this may explain the variable sensitivity and specificity of reported results. Theoretically an unabsorbed sugar such as lactulose might be preferable to glucose for use in the test. In addition it has been suggested that one may identify the site of bacterial proliferation by combining a barium meal with the substrate,[39] but this method is cumbersome and the result not always easy to interpret.

Analysis of aspirates from the lumen of the small intestine

Ideally indirect evidence of bacterial overgrowth in the small intestine should be confirmed by intubating the gut and analysing fluid aspirated from an anatomically abnormal zone. This exercise needs careful attention to detail and the active participation of a microbiologist with an interest in gut bacteria.

The patient should be studied in the fasting state and before treatment with antibiotics. A variety of tubes with devices to prevent contamination from salivary bacteria have been described, but a simple single-lumen, open-ended sterile tube may provide satisfactory results. In practice it is easier to use a double lumen tube. The additional channel should be flushed with carbon dioxide or nitrogen to help drive gut fluid up to the aspirating syringe. It is not always easy to pass the tip of the tube to the appropriate segment of small intestine and a great deal of patience and encouragement is needed to obtain samples from the ileum. Throughout the period of intubation the patient is asked to spit out saliva and should not be given fluid by mouth unless the study is to include observations on the effects of feeding. It may be possible to recognize salivary contamination of jejunal fluid by comparing the results of cultures of saliva and jejunal fluid taken at the same time.[57]

Aspirated specimens are treated with oxygen-free nitrogen before being passed to the bacteriologist for culture under aerobic and anaerobic conditions. Aliquots should be analysed for bile acid and volatile fatty acid content (if necessary after storage at $-20°C$).

A full bacterial profile in the aspirate could be provided only by a research laboratory, but it should be possible for a good hospital service to quantitate viable anaerobic and aerobic organisms and to isolate coliform and bacteroides species. Although reports from the literature show a lack of agreement regarding the bacteriology of the upper small intestine of control subjects (Table 8.28), most microbiologists agree that total aerobic counts rarely exceed 10^4 organisms/ml and that *E. coli* are never present in more than very small numbers (less than 10^3). Anaerobic organisms (e.g. *Veillonella*) are usually less plentiful than aerobes, and representatives of the species *Bacteroides* are only rarely isolated.

Few clinicians will submit their patients to sampling of fluid from the distal ileum except for research purposes and the data on the flora of this segment of intestine in normal subjects is scanty (Table 8.28).

Biochemical study of aspirates. As indicated above, it is not always easy to get reliable results from the bacteriological analysis of fluid aspirated from the small intestine. Not only are there problems in culturing bacteria in the laboratory, but the clinician may not be able to exclude the possibility of contamination of the specimen, especially during a difficult intubation. Thus biochemical indices of bacterial activity in situ are valuable. Bile acids may be measured semi-quantitatively using simple thin layer chromatography. The presence of free cholic, deoxycholic, and chenodeoxycholic acids in the jejunum provide good evidence of the presence of bile acid splitting organisms.[139] These bile acids may be detected in aspirates from the upper ileum of normal subjects[103] in spite of only apparently small changes in the bacterial flora.

It is also useful to measure the concentration of volatile fatty acids in jejunal contents. The demonstration of acetate (more than 0.5 mmol/l), propionate (more than 0.1 mmol/l) and butyrate (more than 0.01 mmol/l) is reported to occur only in the presence of bacterial overgrowth.[22, 151]

Response to treatment
In some cases the response of metabolic tests to treatment with appropriate antibiotics may be sufficiently brisk to make this a useful method of diagnosis. In this respect the Schilling test for the absorption of vitamin B_{12} is particularly useful, and in some studies is as valuable in making a diagnosis as the bile acid breath test.[39] On the other hand the response to antibiotics may be unpredictable and frequently incomplete (Figure 8.59).

Selection of tests
Three general problems confront the clinician in testing patients for the possibility of bacterial overgrowth in the small intestine:
a A lack of absolute bacteriological criteria, especially in the consideration of those with apparently minor abnormalities of structure and function of the small intestine such as the elderly, patients with metabolic disease such as diabetes and uraemia, and malnourished people living in tropical and subtropical countries.
b A rather uncertain correlation between bacterial overgrowth and metabolic sequelae, again especially in those with minor abnormalities of structure and function of the small intestine.[140]
c The variable biochemical potential of intestinal microflora which means that only a proportion of metabolic tests may give abnormal results.

Thus members of a specialist gastroenterology unit should aim to be familiar with a carefully selected range of tests and should know their individual advantages and pitfalls. The logical and planned application of selected tests together with a sensible clinical assessment will provide more valuable information than haphazard attempts to obtain a complete profile.

Management

Many patients with bacterial overgrowth in the small intestine appear to suffer little harm. Minor degrees of diverticulosis of the small intestine are common in the elderly population and one suspects that the metabolic consequences are insignificant, although there are few published data to support this.

It is essential to characterize the underlying conditions of patients with suspected bacterial overgrowth and gastrointestinal symptoms or nutritional deficiencies as fully as possible. Obviously ill patients often have more than one disorder and the clinician must be aware of this possibility. Many of the patients are elderly and malnourished and protection against hypothermia may be necessary even under hospital conditions.[100] In such patients nutritional support is necessary before investigating the gastrointestinal disorder in detail.

The approach to management will depend on the cause of bacterial overgrowth and predisposing conditions. Ideally the cause should be removed and the predisposing conditions modified. Frequently this is not possible and the clinician will then consider how best to use antibiotics to minimize the metabolic consequences of bacterial overgrowth.

Surgical correction of 'blind loops'
Patients with certain anatomical abnormalities (e.g. stricture of the small intestine, enteroenteric fistula, and dilated afferent loop of a Polya partial gastrectomy) can be readily cured by appropriate gastrointestinal surgery.[36, 79] These patients must be selected with care because many of those who appear to have a correctable lesion have had previous surgery or have inflammatory disease of the bowel. In such situations surgery is often difficult and may culminate in the resection of otherwise useful lengths of small intestine.

Diverticulosis of the small intestine is rarely an indication for surgery, although the removal of a solitary large duodenal sac may be justifiable. Operations for pseudo-obstruction of the small intestine secondary to neuromuscular abnormalities or to scleroderma (Figure 8.57) are usually hazardous and unrewarding.

Modification of predisposing causes
Malnutrition is a predisposing cause of bacterial overgrowth in the intestine.[54] Correction of nutritional deficiencies may play an important part in the recovery of patients with tropical sprue and certain non-specific gastrointestinal disorders such as have been described in elderly subjects.[116]

Patients with primary immune deficiency frequently have episodes of diarrhoea which may be associated with malabsorption. Bacterial overgrowth and a degree of bile salt deconjugation has been described in such patients. Nevertheless the cause of the bowel disturbance is not clear cut as many of the patients have concomitant infection with *Giardia lamblia*,[107] and a proportion have significant abnormalities of the intestinal mucosa.

Treatment with antibiotics
In most patients with bacterial overgrowth in the small intestine it is not possible to correct the underlying defect and the clinician will wish to use antibiotics. Unfortunately detailed knowledge of the organisms present in the bowel does not help in the selection of the most appropriate drugs. Control of anaerobic organisms seems to be the most helpful step and this can be done using metronidazole or broad-spectrum antibiotics.[67] Tetracycline, which has little intrinsic activity against *Bacteroides*, is surprisingly effective (Figure 8.59), perhaps because it inhibits the growth of many organisms which act synergistically to favour the growth of anaerobes. Treatment for seven to ten days is usually sufficient to get a response which can be monitored clinically and by laboratory tests. Although the numbers and species of the luminal flora may return rapidly to pretreatment levels (Figure 8.59), clinical improvement is often sustained for months. There are no set rules regarding the best way of giving antibiotics; either long-term or intermittent treatment may appear to be more beneficial. In particular it often seems necessary to prolong treatment for patients with bacterial overgrowth in association with 'tropical malabsorption'. Tetracycline is given for several months before the functional defects are reversed and even then relapses are not infrequent.[114]

Prolonged remissions in the presence of renewed colonization of the small intestine are well documented[25, 58] but, as mentioned earlier, bacterial overgrowth in the small intestine is often not overtly harmful. Nevertheless careful follow up of patients who cannot be cured is desirable because of the risk of development of nutritional deficiencies.[52]

Nutritional support

The wide range of nutritional disorders which may occur in patients with bacterial overgrowth in the small intestine have been outlined earlier in this section. It is particularly important to avoid nutritional deficiencies in children because of the danger of irreversible impairment of growth.[52] Regular monthly injections of vitamin B_{12} are desirable not only to prevent the development of B_{12} deficiency but also to provide a means of keeping a check on the progress of the patient. It may also help to supplement the diet with calcium and the fat-soluble vitamins, especially in patients with persistent steatorrhoea. Supplements of preparations of medium chain triglycerides are sometimes prescribed as a means of enhancing the intake of calories without increasing the loss of fat in stools.

Special problems

Most of the early reports of the 'blind loop' syndrome concerned patients with intestinal strictures, of which more than a third were ascribed to tuberculosis.[9] Curiously diverticular disease of the small intestine was rarely mentioned,[7] possibly because it is largely a disorder of the elderly. Certain interesting aspects of this condition are described below.

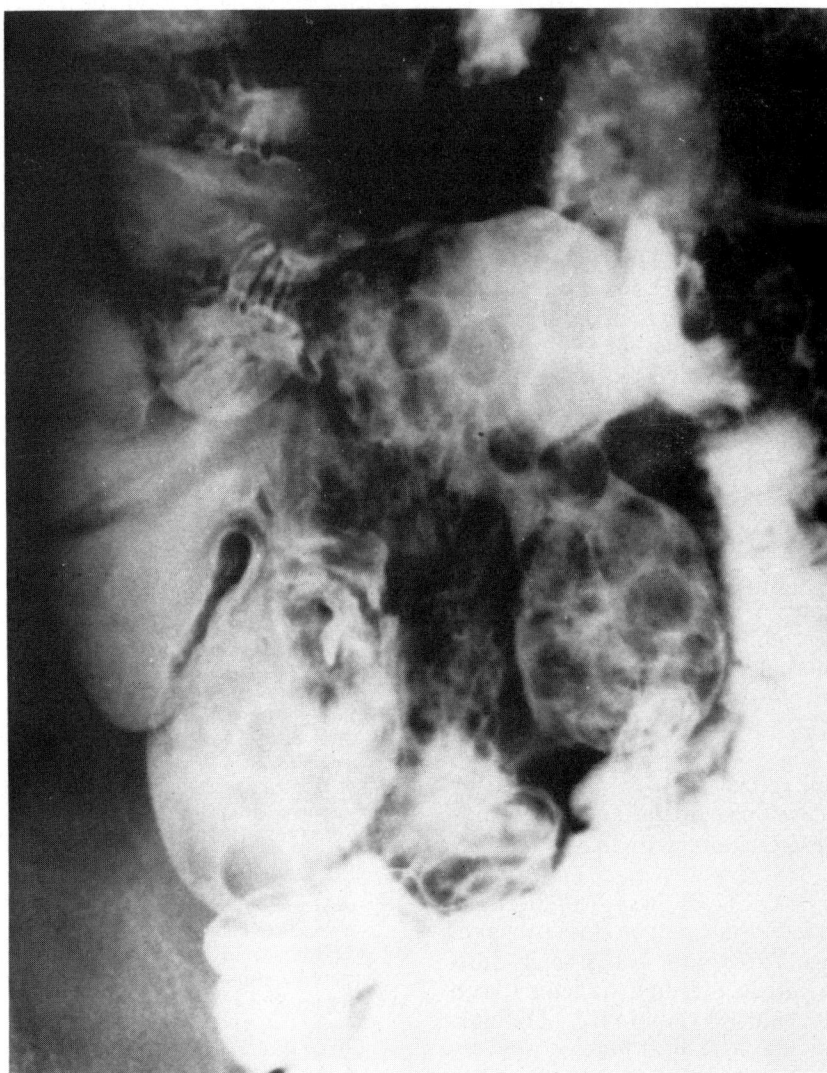

Fig. 8.61 Enteroliths in a blind loop. This patient had an operation in infancy for reduplication of the ileum. At 22 years, after a trouble-free childhood, he presented with anaemia secondary to blood loss from the intestine. This view of the ileocaecal region reveals a dilated terminal ileum with a pouch containing enteroliths. The patient felt completely well after correction of the anaemia, and his faeces became free of occult blood. He refused laparotomy and his progress is monitored by his family doctor. Courtesy of Dr A. H. Freeman.

Duodenal diverticula. Duodenal diverticula are usually benign lesions found by chance, but may cause serious symptoms including weight loss, bleeding and jaundice. Bacterial proliferation in a diverticulum close to the ampulla of Vater seems to predispose the patient to contamination of bile with the risk of cholangitis and pancreatitis.[35] Precipitated material in the diverticulum may lead to enterolith formation. In patients with recurring symptoms the administration of antibiotics is often not curative and diverticulectomy or a bypass procedure may be necessary.[88]

Jejunal diverticula. Diverticulosis of the jejunum may affect up to 5% of the elderly population.[25] The diverticula are usually small in size and number and frequently there are no symptoms. In younger people diverticulosis may be diffuse and affect the whole of the small and large intestine. There may be an association with congenital disorders of connective tissue.[59] The diverticula in these patients are not infrequently thin-walled and may perforate. On two occasions the author has seen young patients with intestinal perforation shortly after taking tetracycline tablets. It may be wise to give antibiotics in a liquid suspension to avoid the risk of erosion of the wall of the intestine by the hold-up of a tablet in a diverticulum. Spontaneous bleeding from a jejunal diverticulum is also a well recognized acute complication and it too may be precipitated by the administration of tetracycline. Other complications reviewed by Cooke *et al.*[25] include intestinal obstruction, cyst formation by occlusion of the mouth of a diverticulum, intussusception, diverticulitis, lodgment of foreign bodies, and enterolith formation. An enterolith may develop on a nidus of precipitated bile salts and may be seen in strictured intestine as well as in a diverticulum (Figure 8.61).

A further set of special problems are posed by two recently developed operations which may predispose to bacterial overgrowth.

Ileal reservoirs (Koch pouches). The bacterial growth in ileal reservoirs may be close to that of normal colon. There are occasionally disturbances of small intestinal function with malabsorption of fat and vitamin B_{12}. The morphological changes of the ileal mucosa are very variable. In some cases there is moderate to severe inflammation; in others the changes are minimal.[81] It is probable that malabsorption, when it occurs, is secondary to bacterial prolifer-

ation, and this is believed to be the mechanism of the commonly occurring increase in faecal bile acids.[5]

Jejunoileal bypass surgery. Although bypass surgery for obesity involves the creation of a long blind segment of small intestine, it was originally believed that its self-emptying nature would protect the patient against the dangers of bacterial overgrowth. However, this has not been the case. More than half the patients develop significant bacterial overgrowth in the jejunum,[110] and the degree of malabsorption is greater than that for an equivalent resection of small intestine.[91] Appetite appears to be diminished and bacterial metabolites may contribute to the occasionally life-threatening liver disease which may occur after jejunoileal bypass. Bacterial overgrowth has also been implicated in the development of pseudo-obstruction of the colon.[10]

ACKNOWLEDGEMENTS

I would like to thank members of staff of the Royal Postgraduate Medical School (especially Professor C. C. Booth, Dr S. Tabaqchali and Dr S. Gorbach) who made many of the observations reviewed in this section. I am indebted to the Department of Radiology, Hammersmith Hospital, for most of the radiographic illustrations. Dr Michael Marsh (Hope Hospital, Salford) provided data for the calculation of the density of bacteria adherent to jejunal mucosa. I am grateful to him and to my colleagues at Addenbrooke's Hospital for much helpful discussion.

REFERENCES

1 Aarbakke, J. & Schjønsby, H. (1976) Value of urinary simple phenol and indican determination in the diagnosis of stagnant loop syndrome. *Scandinavian Journal of Gastroenterology*, **11,** 409–414.
2 Allison, M. J., Maloy, S. E. & Mabon, R. R. (1976) Inactivation of *Clostridium botulinum* toxin by ruminal microbes from cattle and sheep. *Applied and Environmental Microbiology*, **32,** 685–688.
3 Ammon, H. V. & Phillips, S. F. (1973) Inhibition of colonic water and electrolyte absorption by fatty acids in men. *Gastroenterology*, **65,** 744–749.
4 Ammon, H. V., Thomas, P. H. & Phillips, S. F. (1974) Effects of oleic and ricinoleic acid on net jejunal water and electrolyte movement. *Journal of Clinical Investigation*, **53,** 374–379.
5 Andersson, H., Fasth, S., Filipsson, S. *et al.* (1979) Faecal excretion of intravenously injected ^{14}C-cholic acid in patients with a conventional ileostomy and in patients with a continent ileostomy reservoir. *Scandinavian Journal of Gastroenterology*, **14,** 551–554.
6 Astley, R. (1975) Radiology of the gastrointestinal tract. In *Paediatric Gastroenterology* (Ed.) Anderson, C. M. & Burke, V. p. 522. Oxford: Blackwell Scientific Publications.
7 Badenoch, J. (1958) The blind loop syndrome. In: *Modern Trends in Gastroenterology*. (Ed.) Jones, F. A., pp. 231–242. Butterworth: London.

8   Bark, S. (1981) Amino acid absorption after intestinal by-pass procedures. *International Journal of Obesity*, **5**, 527–530.

9   Barker, W. H. & Hummel, L. E. (1939) Macrocytic anemia in association with intestinal strictures and anastomoses. *Bulletin of the Johns Hopkins Hospital*, **46**, 215–254.

10 Barry, R. E., Chow, A. W. & Billesdon, J. (1977) Role of intestinal microflora in colonic pseudo-obstruction complicating jejunoileal bypass. *Gut*, **18**, 356–359.

11 Beachey, E. H. (1981) Bacterial adherence: adhesion-receptor interactions mediating the attachment of bacteria to mucosal surfaces. *Journal of Infectious Diseases*, **143**, 325–345.

12 Berg, R. D. & Owens, W. E. (1979) Inhibition of translocation of viable *Escherichia coli* from the gastrointestinal tract of mice by bacterial antagonism. *Infection and Immunity*, **25**, 820–827.

13 Bernstein, L. H., Gutstein, B., Efron, G. & Wager, G. (1975) Experimental production of elevated serum folate in dogs with intestinal blind loops. II. Nature of bacterially produced folate co-enzymes in blind loop fluid. *American Journal of Clinical Nutrition*, **28**, 925–929.

14 Bhat, P., Albert, M. J., Rajan, D. *et al.* (1980) Bacterial flora of the jejunum: a comparison of luminal aspirate and mucosal biopsy. *Journal of Medical Microbiology*, **13**, 247–256.

15 Binder, H. J., Filburn, B. & Floch, M. (1975) Bile acid inhibition of intestinal anaerobic organisms. *American Journal of Clinical Nutrition*, **28**, 119–125.

16 Brandt, L. J., Bernstein, L. H. & Wager, A. (1977) Production of vitamin B_{12} analogues in patients with small bowel bacterial overgrowth. *Annals of Internal Medicine*, **87**, 546–551.

17 Bullen, J. J., Rogers, H. J. & Griffiths, E. (1974) Bacterial iron metabolism in infection and immunity. In *Microbial Iron Metabolism – A Comprehensive Treatise* (Ed.) Neilands, J. B. pp. 517–551. New York: Academic Press.

18 Burke, V., Houghton, M. & Gracey, M. (1977) Effect of enteric microorganisms on intestinal sugar and fatty acid absorption. *Australian Journal of Experimental Biology and Medical Science*, **55**, 423–430.

19 Cain, J. R., Mayoral, L. G., Lotero, H. *et al.* (1976) Enterobacteriaceae in the jejunal microflora: prevalence and relationship to biochemical and histological evaluation in healthy Colombian men. *American Journal of Clinical Nutrition*, **29**, 1397–1403.

20 Challacombe, D. N., Richardson, J. M. & Anderson, C. M. (1974) Bacterial microflora of the upper gastrointestinal tract in infants without diarrhoea. *Archives of Diseases of Childhood*, **49**, 264–269.

21 Chanarin, I. (1979) Vitamin B_{12} deficiency and abnormal intestinal flora. In *The Megaloblastic Anaemias*, 2nd edn. pp. 406–419. Oxford: Blackwell Scientific Publications.

22 Chernov, A. J., Doe, W. F. & Gompertz, D. (1972) Intrajejunal volatile fatty acids in the stagnant loop syndrome. *Gut*, **13**, 103–106.

23 Clinicopathological Conference (1967) A case of osteomalacia, osteoporosis and hypercalcaemia. *British Medical Journal*, **i**, 219–223.

24 Coates, M. E. (1975) Gnotobiotic animals in research: their uses and limitations. *Laboratory Animal*, **9**, 275–282.

25 Cooke, W. T., Cox, E. V., Fone, D. J. *et al.* (1963) The clinical and metabolic significance of jejunal diverticula. *Gut*, **4**, 115–122.

26 Curtis, K. J., Prizont, R. & Kim, Y. S. (1979) Protein digestion and absorption in the blind loop syndrome. *Digestive Diseases and Sciences*, **24**, 929–933.

27 Dickman, M. D., Chappelka, A. R. & Schaedler, R. W. (1976) The microbial ecology of the upper small bowel. *American Journal of Gastroenterology*, **65**, 57–62.

28 Donaldson, R. M. Jr (1964) Normal bacterial populations of the intestine and their relation to intestinal function. *New England Journal of Medicine*, **270**, 938–945 and 1050–1056.

29 Donaldson, R. M. Jr (1965) Studies on the pathogenesis of steatorrhea in the blind loop syndrome. *Journal of Clinical Investigation*, **44**, 1815–1820.

30 Donaldson, R. M. Jr (1965) Malabsorption in the blind loop syndrome. *Gastroenterology*, **48**, 388–395.

31 Donaldson, R. M. Jr (1973) The blind loop syndrome. In *Gastrointestinal Disease* (Ed.) Sleisenger, M. H. & Fordtran, J. S. p. 928. Philadelphia: W. B. Saunders.

32 Drasar, B. S., Shiner, M. & McLeod, G. M. (1969) Studies on the intestinal flora. I. The bacterial flora of the gastrointestinal tract in healthy and achlorhydric persons. *Gastroenterology*, **56**, 71–79.

33 Ducluzeau, R., Ladire, M., Callut, C. *et al.* (1977) Antagonistic effect of extremely oxygen-sensitive clostridia from the microflora of conventional mice and of *Escherichia coli* against *Shigella flexneri* in the digestive tract of gnotobiotic mice. *Infection and Immunity*, **17**, 415–424.

34 Dyer, N. H., Dawson, A. M., Smith, B. F. & Todd, I. P. (1969) Obstruction of the bowel due to a lesion in the myenteric plexus. *British Medical Journal*, **i**, 686–689.

35 Eggert, A., Teichmann, W. & Wittman, D. H. (1982) The pathological implications of duodenal diverticula. *Surgery, Gynecology and Obstetrics*, **154**, 62–64.

36 Ellis, H. & Smith, A. D. M. (1967) The blind loop syndrome. *Monographs in Surgical Science*, **4**, 193–215.

37 Faber, K. (1895) Perniciøs Anaemia som Følge af Tarmlidelse. *Hospitalstidende*, **4**, 601–615.

38 Fainstein, V. & Musher, D. M. (1979) Bacterial adherence to pharyngeal cells in smokers, non-smokers and chronic bronchitis. *Infection and Immunity*, **26**, 178–182.

39 Farivar, S., Fromm, H. & Schindler, D. (1979) Sensitivity of bile acid breath test in the diagnosis of bacterial overgrowth in the small intestine with and without stagnant (blind loop) syndrome. *Digestive Diseases and Sciences*, **24**, 33–40.

40 Floch, M. H., Gershengoren, W. & Diamond, S. (1970) Cholic acid inhibition of intestinal bacteria. *American Journal of Clinical Nutrition*, **23**, 8–10.

41 Fromm, H. & Hofmann, A. F. (1971) Breath test for altered bile acid metabolism. *Lancet*, **ii**, 621–625.

42 Gall, L. S. (1970) Normal fecal flora of man. *American Journal of Clinical Nutrition*, **23**, 1457–1465.

43 Giannella, R. A., Broitman, S. A. & Zamcheck, A. (1971) Vitamin B_{12} uptake by intestinal microorganisms: mechanisms and relevance to syndromes of intestinal bacterial overgrowth. *Journal of Clinical Investigation*, **50**, 1100–1107.

44 Gibbons, R. J. & van Houte, J. (1975) Bacterial adherence in oral microbial ecology. *Annual Review of Microbiology*, **29**, 19–44.

45 Giordano, C. (1963) Use of exogenous and endogenous urea for protein synthesis in normal and uremic subjects. *Journal of Laboratory and Clinical Medicine*, **62**, 231–246.

46 Gorbach, S. L. (1971) Intestinal microflora. *Gastroenterology*, **60**, 1110–1129.

47 Gorbach, S. L. & Tabaqchali, S. (1969) Bacteria, bile and the small bowel. *Gut*, **10**, 963–972.

48 Gorbach, S. L., Plaut, A. G., Nahas, L. *et al.* (1967) Studies of intestinal microflora. II. Microorganisms of the small intestine and their relations to oral and fecal flora. *Gastroenterology*, **53**, 856–867.

49 Gorbach, S. L., Banwell, J. G., Jacobs, B. *et al.* (1970) Tropical sprue and malnutrition in West Bengal. I. Intestinal microflora and absorption. *American Journal of Clinical Nutrition*, **23**, 1545–1558.

50 Gordon, H. A & Pesti, L. (1971) The gnotobiotic animal as a tool in the study of host-microbial relationships. *Bacteriological Reviews*, **35**, 390–429.

51 Gracey, M. (1971) Intestinal absorption in the 'contaminated small bowel syndrome'. *Gut*, **12**, 403–410.

52 Gracey, M. (1979) The contaminated small bowel syndrome: pathogenesis, diagnosis and treatment. *American Journal of Clinical Nutrition*, **32**, 234–243.

53 Gracey, M., Burke, V. & Anderson, C. M. (1969) Association of monosaccharide malabsorption with abnormal small intestinal flora. *Lancet*, **ii**, 384–385.

54 Gracey, M., Suharjono, S. & Stone, D. E. (1973) Microbial contamination of the gut: another feature of malnutrition. *American Journal of Clinical Nutrition*, **26**, 1170–1174.

55 Griffen, W. O. Jr, Richardson, J. D. & Medley, E. S. (1971) Prevention of small bowel contamination by ileocaecal valve. *Southern Medical Journal*, **64**, 1056–1058.

56 György, P. (1953) Hitherto unrecognised difference between human milk and cow's milk. *Pediatrics*, **11**, 98–107.

57 Hamilton, I., Worsley, B., Shoesmith, J. G. *et al.* (1981) Salivary and jejunal flora in the normal and contaminated small bowel. *Gut*, **22**, A865.

58 Hamilton, J. D., Dyer, N. & Dawson, A. M. (1970) Assessment and significance of bacterial overgrowth in the small bowel. *Quarterly Journal of Medicine*, **39**, 265–285.

59 Hayakawa, A. (1982) Two cases of Ehlers–Danlos syndrome with gastrointestinal complications. *Gastroenterology* (Japan), **17**, 61–67.

60 Helstrom, P. B. & Balish, E. (1979) Effect of oral tetracycline, the microbial flora and the athymic state on gastrointestinal colonisation and infection of BALB/c mice with *Candida albicans*. *Infection and Immunity*, **23**, 764–774.

61 Hepner, G. W. (1978) Breath tests in gastroenterology. *Advances in Internal Medicine*, **23**, 25–45.

62 Hutchison, J. C. P., Gray, J., Flewett, T. H. *et al.* (1978) The safety of the Trexler isolator as judged by some physical and biological criteria: a report of experimental work at two centres. *Journal of Hygiene* (Cambridge), **81**, 311–319.

63 Iacono, V. J., Taubman, M. A., Smith, D. J. *et al.* (1976) In *Immunological Aspects of Dental Caries* (Ed.) Bowen, W. H., Genco, R. J. & O'Brien, T. C. Washington, DC: Information Retrieval Service.

64 Jarumilinta, R., Miranda, M. & Villarejos, V. M. (1976) A bacteriological study of the intestinal mucosa and luminal fluid of adults with acute diarrhoea. *Annals of Tropical Medicine and Parasitology*, **70**, 165–179.

65 Johanson, W. G., Pierce, A. K. & Samford, J. P. (1969) Changing pharyngeal bacterial flora of hospitalised patients: emergence of gram-negative bacilli. *New England Journal of Medicine*, **281**, 1137–1140.

66 Johanson, W. G., Jr., Pierce, A. K., Sanford, J. P. & Thomas, G. D. (1972) Nosocomial respiratory infections with gram-negative bacilli: the significance of colonisation of the respiratory tract. *Annals of Internal Medicine*, **77**, 701–706.

67 Joiner, K. A. & Gorbach, S. L. (1979) Antimicrobial therapy of digestive diseases. *Clinics in Gastroenterology*, **8**, 3–35.

68 Jonas, R., Flanagan, P. R. & Forstner, G. C. (1977) Pathogenesis of mucosal injury in the blind loop syndrome. Brush border enzyme activity and glycoprotein degradation. *Journal of Clinical Investigation*, **60**, 1321–1330.

69 Jones, E. A., Craigie, A., Tavill, A. S. *et al.* (1968) Protein metabolism in the intestinal stagnant loop syndrome. *Gut*, **9**, 466–469.

70 Kane, S. P. & Neale, G. (1976) Ileocolitis responding to bowel sterilisation. *Proceedings of the Royal Society of Medicine*, **69**, 266–267.

71 King, C., Lorenz, E. & Toskes, P. (1976) The pathogenesis of decreased serum protein levels in the blind loop syndrome: Evaluation including a newly developed ^{14}C-amino acid breath test. *Gastroenterology*, **70**, A43/901.

72 King, C., Toskes, P., Guilarte, T. & Lorenz, E. (1976) Advantages of the xylose breath tests over the bile salt breath test in diagnosis of the blind loop syndrome. *Gastroenterology*, **70**, A43/901.

73 King, C. E. & Toskes, P. P. (1981) Protein-losing enteropathy in the human and experimental rat blind-loop syndrome. *Gastroenterology*, **80**, 504–509.

74 Klipstein, F. A. (1981) Tropical sprue in travellers and expatriates living abroad. *Gastroenterology*, **80**, 590–600.

75 Klipstein, F. A., Engert, R. F. & Short, H. B. (1978) Enterotoxigenicity of colonising coliform bacteria in tropical sprue and blind loop syndrome. *Lancet*, **ii**, 342–344.

76 Lauterburg, B. H., Newcomer, A. D. & Hoffmann, A. F. (1978) Clinical value of the bile acid breath test. Evaluation of the Mayo Clinic experience. *Mayo Clinic Proceedings*, **53**, 227–233.

77 Lawrence, G., Bates, J. & Gaul, A. (1982) Pathogenesis of neonatal necrotising enterocolitis. *Lancet*, **i**, 137–139.

78 Lee, A. (1980) Normal flora of animal intestinal surfaces. In *Adsorption of Micro-organisms to Surfaces* (Ed.) Britton, G. & Marshall, K. C. pp. 145–173. New York: John Wiley.

79 Lennert, K. A. (1979) Das Dunndarmstase syndrom nach seit-zu-seit-anastomose. *Chirurg* (Berlin), **50**, 21–25.

80 Lewis, B., Panvelliwalla, D., Tabaqchali, S. & Wootton, I. D. P. (1969) Serum bile acids in the stagnant loop syndrome. *Lancet*, **i**, 219–223.

81 Loesche, K., Bolkert, T., Kiefhaber, P. *et al.* (1980) Bacterial overgrowth in ileal reservoirs (Kock pouch): extended functional studies. *Hepatogastroenterology*, **27**, 310–316.

82 Long, S. S. & Swenson, R. M. (1977) Development of anaerobic fecal flora in healthy newborn infants. *Journal of Pediatrics*, **91**, 298–301.

83 Mackowiak, P. A. (1978) Microbial synergism in human infections. *New England Journal of Medicine*, **298**, 21–26 and 83–87.

84 Mackowiak, P. A. (1982) The normal bacterial flora. *New England Journal of Medicine*, **307**, 83–93.

85 Mackowiak, P. A., Martin, R. M. & Smith, J. W. (1978) Pharyngeal colonisation by gram-negative bacilli in aspiration-prone persons. *Archives of Internal Medicine*, **138**, 1224–1227.

86 Mackowiak, P. A., Martin, R. M. & Smith, J. W. (1979) The role of bacterial interference in the increased prevalence of oro-pharyngeal gram-negative bacilli among alcoholics and diabetics. *American*

Review of Respiratory Diseases, **120**, 589–593.

87 Maldonado, J. E., Gregg, J. A., Green, P. S. & Brown, A. L. (1970) Chronic idiopathic intestinal pseudo-obstruction. *American Journal of Medicine*, **49**, 203–212.

88 Manny, J., Muga, M. & Eyal, Z. (1981) The continuing clinical enigma of duodenal diverticulum. *American Journal of Surgery*, **142**, 596–600.

89 Marshall, K. C. & Britton, G. (1980) Microbial adhesion in perspective. In *Adsorption of Micro-organisms to Surfaces* (Ed.) Britton, G. & Marshall, K. C. pp. 1–5. New York: John Wiley.

90 Mathan, V. I., Babcor, B. M. & Donaldson, R. M. (1974) Kinetics of the attachment of intrinsic factor-bound cobamides to ileal receptors. *Journal of Clinical Investigation*, **54**, 598–608.

91 McGouran, R. C. M., Goldie, A., Ang, L. & Maxwell, J. D. (1979) Weight loss after jejuno-ileal bypass and resection in the rat: food intake, faecal calorie loss and the effect of antibiotics. *Gut*, **20**, A946.

92 Metchnikoff, E. (1901) Sur la flore du corps humain. *Manchester Literary and Philosophical Society*, **45**, 1–38.

93 Metz, G., Gassull, M. A., Drasar, B. S. *et al.* (1976) Breath hydrogen test for small intestinal bacterial concentration. *Lancet*, **i**, 668–669.

94 Meulengracht, E. (1929) Pernicious anaemia in intestinal stricture (with one liver-treated case). *Acta Medica Scandinavica*, **72**, 231–240.

95 Meynell, G. G. (1963) Antibacterial mechanisms of the mouse gut. II. The role of Eh and volatile fatty acids in the normal gut. *British Journal of Experimental Pathology*, **44**, 209–219.

96 Miller, B., Mitchison, R., Tabaqchali, S. & Neale, G. (1971) The effects of excess bacterial proliferation on protein metabolism in rats with self-filling jejunal sacs. *European Journal of Clinical Investigation*, **2**, 23–31.

97 Mitch, W. E. (1978) Effects of intestinal flora on nitrogen metabolism in patients with chronic renal failure. *American Journal of Clinical Nutrition*, **31**, 1594–1600.

98 Mutch, W. M. Jr (1977) Stasis syndrome following abdominal colectomy. *Diseases of the Colon and Rectum*, **20**, 340–346.

99 Neale, G. (1968) Protein deficiency in temperate zones. *Proceedings of the Royal Society of Medicine*, **60**, 1069–1073.

100 Neale, G., Antcliff, A. C., Welbourn, R. B. *et al.* (1967) Protein malnutrition after partial gastrectomy. *Quaterly Journal of Medicine*, **36**, 469–481.

101 Neale, G., Gompertz, D., Schjønsby, H. *et al.* (1972) The metabolic and nutritional consequences of bacterial overgrowth in the small intestine. *American Journal of Clinical Nutrition*, **25**, 1409–1417.

102 Nelson, D. P. & Mata, L. J. (1970) Bacterial flora associated with the human gastrointestinal mucosa. *Gastroenterology*, **58**, 56–61.

103 Northfield, T. C., Drasar, B. S. & Wright, J. T. (1973) Value of small intestinal bile acid analysis in the diagnosis of stagnant loop syndrome. *Gut*, **14**, 341–347.

104 Nygaard, K. (1967) Changes in the intestinal flora after resections and bypass operations on the small intestine in rats. *Acta Chirurgica Scandinavica*, **133**, 569–583.

105 Onderdonk, A. B. & Bartlett, J. G. (1979) Bacteriological studies of experimental ulcerative colitis. *American Journal of Clinical Nutrition*, **32**, 258–265.

106 Onderdonk, A., Marshall, B., Cioneros, R. & Levy, S. B. (1981) Competition between congenic *Escherichia coli* K-12 strains in vivo. *Infection and Immunity*, **32**, 74–79.

107 Parkin, D. M., McClelland, D. B. L., Moore, R. R. O. *et al.* (1972) Intestinal bacterial flora and bile salt studies in hypogammaglobulinaemia. *Gut*, **13**, 182–188.

108 Plaut, A. G., Gorbach, S. L., Nahas, N. *et al.* Studies of intestinal microflora. III. The microbial flora of human small intestinal mucosa and fluids. *Gastroenterology*, **53**, 868–873.

109 Pollard, M. (1965) The use of germ-free animals in virus research. *Progress in Medical Virology*, **1**, 362–376.

110 Powell-Jackson, P. R., Maudgal, D. P., Sharp, D. *et al.* (1979) Intestinal bacterial metabolism of protein and bile acids: role in pathogenesis of hepatic disease after jejuno-ileal surgery. *British Journal of Surgery*, **66**, 772–775.

111 Prizont, R. (1981) Glycoprotein degradation in the blind loop syndrome. Identification of glycosidases in jejunal contents. *Journal of Clinical Investigation*, **67**, 336–344.

112 Reed, S. E. & Tyrrell, D. A. J. (1974) Viruses associated with the healthy individual. In *The Normal Microbial Flora of Man* (Ed.) Skinner, F. A. & Carr, J. G. pp. 255–257. New York: Academic Press.

113 Richards, P., Metcalfe-Gibson, A., Ward, E. E. *et al.* (1967) Utilisation of ammonia nitrogen for protein synthesis in man and the effect of protein restriction and uraemia. *Lancet*, **ii**, 845–849.

114 Rickles, F. R., Klipstein, F. W., Tomasini, J. *et al.* (1972) Long-term follow up of antibiotic treated tropical sprue. *Annals of Internal Medicine*, **76**, 203–210.

115 Riepe, S. P., Goldstein, J. & Alpers, D. H. (1980) Effect of secreted *Bacteroides* proteases on human intestinal brush border hydrolases. *Journal of Clinical Investigation*, **66**, 314–322.

116 Roberts, S. H., James, O. & Jarvis, E. H. (1977) Bacterial overgrowth syndrome without 'blind loop': a cause for malnutrition in the elderly. *Lancet*, **ii**, 1193–1195.

117 Rosebury, T. (1962) Distribution and development of the microbiota of man. In *Microorganisms Indigenous to Man*. pp. 310–384. New York: McGraw-Hill.

118 Rutgeerts, P., Ghoos, Y., Vantrappen, G. & Eyssen, H. (1981) Ileal dysfunction and bacterial overgrowth in patients with Crohn's disease. *European Journal of Clinical Investigation*, **11**, 199–206.

119 Salen, G., Goldstein, F. & Wirts, C. W. (1966) Malabsorption in intestinal scleroderma. Relation to bacterial flora and treatment with antibiotics. *Annals of Internal Medicine*, **64**, 834–841.

120 Savage, D. C. (1970) Associations of indigenous micro-organisms with gastrointestinal mucosal epithelia. *American Journal of Clinical Nutrition*, **23**, 1495–1501.

121 Savage, D. C. (1980) Colonisation by and survival of pathogenic bacteria on intestinal mucosal surfaces. In *Adsorption of Micro-organisms to Surfaces* (Ed.) Britton, G. & Marshall, K. C. pp. 175–206. New York: John Wiley.

122 Scarpello, J. B. & Sladen, G. E. (1977) Appraisal of the ^{14}C-glycocholate acid test with special reference to the measurement of faecal^{14}C excretion. *Gut*, **18**, 742–748.

123 Scarpello, J. B., Hague, R. V., Cullen, D. R. & Sladen, G. E. (1976) The ^{14}C-glycocholate breath test in diabetic diarrhoea. *British Medical Journal*, **ii**, 673–675.

124 Schjønsby, H. (1977) Osteomalacia in the stagnant loop syndrome. *Acta Medica Scandinavica* (Supplement) **603**, 39–41.

125 Schjønsby, H., Drasar, B. S., Tabaqchali, S. & Booth, C. C. (1973) Uptake of vitamin B_{12} by intestinal bac-

teria in the stagnant loop syndrome. *Scandinavian Journal of Gastroenterology*, **8**, 41–47.

126 Schjønsby, H., Halvorsen, J. F., Hofstad, T. & Hovdenak, N. (1977) Stagnant loop syndrome in patients with continent ileostomy (intra-abdominal ileal reservoir). *Gut*, **18**, 795–799.

127 Schroepfer, J. L. Jr, Niehaus, W. G. Jr & McCloskey, J. A. (1970) Enzymatic conversion of linoleic acid to 10D-hydroxy-Δ12-cis-octadenoic acid. *Journal of Biological Chemistry*, **245**, 3798–3801.

128 Sciaretta, G. (1977) Diagnosis of blind loop syndrome by x-ray – breath hydrogen test. *Lancet*, **i**, 310–311.

129 Scott, A. J. & Khan, G. A. (1968) Partial biliary obstruction with cholangitis producing a blind loop syndrome. *Gut*, **9**, 187–192.

130 Scowden, E. B., Schaffner, W. & Stone, W. J. (1978) Overwhelming strongyloidiasis: an unappreciated opportunistic infection. *Medicine* (Baltimore), **57**, 527–544.

131 Seyderhelm, R., Lehmann, W., & Wichels, P. (1924) Experimentelle intestinale perniziöse Anämie beim Hund. *Klinische Wochenschrift*, **3**, 1439–1445.

132 Sêze, S. de, Bernier, J.-J., Caroit, M. *et al.* (1972) Un cas d'osteomalacie par malabsorption de mécanisme inhabituel au cours d'un syndrome de l'anse borgne. *Revue du Rhumatisme et des Maladies Osteo-Articulares*, **39**, 297–303.

133 Shedlofsky, S. & Freter, R. (1974) Synergism between ecologic and immunologic control mechanisms of intestinal flora. *Journal of Infectious Diseases*, **129**, 296–303.

134 Spiers, A. S. D., Dias, S. F. & Lopez, J. A. (1980) Infection protection in patients with cancer: microbiological evaluation of portable laminar air flow isolation, topical chlorhexidine and oral non-absorbable antibiotics. *Journal of Hygiene* (Cambridge), **84**, 457–465.

135 Sprunt, K., Leidy, G. A. & Redman, W. (1971) Prevention of bacterial overgrowth. *Journal of Infectious Diseases*, **123**, 1–10.

136 Szeri, I., Anderlik, P., Bános, Z. & Rádnai, B. (1976) Decreased cellular immune response of germ-free mice. *Acta Microbiologica Academiae Scientarium Hungaricae* (Budapest), **23**, 231–234.

137 Tabaqchali, S. (1970) The pathophysiological role of small intestinal bacterial flora. *Scandinavian Journal of Gastroenterology*, **5** (Supplement 6), 139–163.

138 Tabaqchali, S. & Pallis, C. (1970) Reversible nicotinamide deficiency encephalopathy in a patient with jejunal diverticulosis. *Gut*, **11**, 1024–1028.

139 Tabaqchali, S., Hatzioannou, J. & Booth, C. C. (1968) Bile acid deconjugation and steatorrhoea in patients with the stagnant loop syndrome. *Lancet*, **ii**, 12–16.

140 Taylor, R. H., Argerinos, A., Taylor, A. J. *et al.* (1981) Bacterial colonisation of the jejunum: an evaluation of five diagnostic tests. *Gut*, **22**, A442.

141 Tete, R., Boyer, J. D., Slaoui, H. & Mas, R. (1979) Diarrhee chronique avec malabsorption par amylose intestinale secondaire à une polyarthrite rhumatoide au cours d'un diabete. *Lyon Medecin*, **242**, 283–288.

142 Thomas, P. J. (1972) Identification of some enteric bacteria which convert oleic acid to hydroxy-stearic acid in vitro. *Gastroenterology*, **62**, 430–435.

143 Tönnis, W. & Brusis, A. (1931) Veranderungen der morphologischen Blut bildes bei Skuter und chronischer Darminhaltsstaung. *Deutsche Zeitschrift fur Chirurgie*, **233**, 133–139.

144 Toskes, P. P., King, C. E., Spivey, J. C. & Lorenz, E. (1978) Xylose catabolism in the experimental rat blind loop syndrome. Studies including the use of a newly developed D-14C-xylose breath test. *Gastroenterology*, **74**, 691–697.

145 Ulshen, M. H. & Rollo, J. L. (1980) Pathogenesis of *Escherichia coli* gastroenteritis in man – another mechanism. *New England Journal of Medicine*, **302**, 99–101.

146 Varcoe, R., Halliday, D., Carson, E. R. *et al.* (1975) Efficiency of utilisation of urea nitrogen for albumin synthesis by chronically uraemic and normal man. *Clinical Science and Molecular Medicine*, **48**, 379–390.

147 Vosbeck, K., Handschin, H., Menge, E-B., & Zak, O. (1979) Effects of subminimal inhibitory concentration of antibiotics on adhesiveness of *Escherichia coli* in vitro. *Reviews of Infectious Diseases*, **1**, 845–851.

148 Watson, G. M., Cameron, D. G. & Witts, L. J. (1948) Experimental macrocytic anaemia in the rat. *Lancet*, **ii**, 404–408.

149 Welkos, S. L., Toskes, P. P. & Baer, H. (1981) Importance of anaerobic bacteria in the cobalamin malabsorption of the experimental rat blind loop syndrome. *Gastroenterology*, **80**, 313–320.

150 White, W. H. (1890) On the pathology and prognosis of pernicious anaemia. *Guy's Hospital Reports*, **47**, 149–194.

151 Whitehead, J. S., Kum, Y. S. & Prizont, R. (1976) A simple quantitative method to determine short chain fatty acid levels in biological fluids. *Clinica Chimica Acta*, **72**, 315–318.

152 Whitt, D. D. & Savage, D. C. (1980) Kinetics of changes induced by indigenous microbiota in the activity levels of alkaline phosphatase and disaccharidases in small intestinal enterocytes in mice. *Infection and Immunity*, **29**, 144–151.

153 Williams, R. C. & Gibbons, R. J. (1972) Inhibition of bacterial adherence by secretory immunoglobulin A: a mechanism of antigen disposal. *Science*, **177**, 697–699.

154 Williams, R. C. & Gibbons, R. J. (1975) Inhibition of streptococcal attachment to receptors on human buccal epithelial cells by antigenically similar salivary glycoproteins. *Infection and Immunity*, **11**, 711–718.

155 Wirts, C. W. & Goldstein, F. (1963) Studies of the mechanism of post-gastrectomy steatorrhea. *Annals of Internal Medicine*, **58**, 25–36.

WHIPPLE'S DISEASE

Although rare, Whipple's disease is well recognized as a condition affecting the small intestine in which infiltration with characteristic foam-laden macrophages leads to a severe and potentially fatal malabsorptive state. In recent years it has become clear that the condition may affect virtually any organ of the body, and frank intestinal disease may have been preceded by years of non-specific systemic complaints such as arthralgia or fever. The universal finding of rod-shaped bacilli in addition to the characteristic macrophages within the tissues of affected individuals, together with a usually good response to antibiotic therapy, has led to the classification of Whipple's disease as an infective process. Many questions regarding the nature of the infecting agent and the possible role of diminished host immunity remain to be answered.

Pathology

SMALL INTESTINE

In virtually every case of untreated Whipple's disease, diffuse small intestinal disease is present.[30] The jejunum and ileum, and sometimes the duodenum, are thickened and oedematous, and the mucosa shows either total loss of the villous pattern or clubbed, flattened villi (Figure 8.62). Ulceration is rare. The intestinal lacteals are dilated, and yellow lipid deposits may be seen in all layers of the small intestine beneath the epithelium in untreated cases at autopsy. This latter finding, together with irregular fat-filled cystic spaces in the enlarged mesenteric lymph nodes, led Whipple to coin the name 'intestinal lipodystrophy', for the condition, but these fatty deposits are probably merely the consequence of lymphatic damage and obstruction.[9]

Histologically the villi are distorted by the classical microscopic abnormality of Whipple's disease, the foam-laden macrophages. These are large cells, usually 20–30 μm across, and are often densely packed within the lamina propria, giving it a uniform appearance without any other marked inflammatory cell infiltrate (Figure 8.63). The foamy cells stain a dramatic magenta colour with periodic acid Schiff reagent; this PAS stain is diastase-resistant.[31] Occasional PAS-positive macrophages may be seen in the small intestine of normal individuals, and more commonly in normal colonic tissue, but differentiation from those of Whipple's disease can usually readily be made, based on the number present and the light microscopic appearances of the cells.[25]

Other histological features in the small intestinal mucosa include dilated lymphatics with a virtually normal enterocyte layer and normal numbers of intraepithelial lymphocytes; occasional acute inflammatory cells are occasionally seen. Aetiologically, the most interesting finding is the presence of bacilli. With both light and electron microscopy, bacilli are

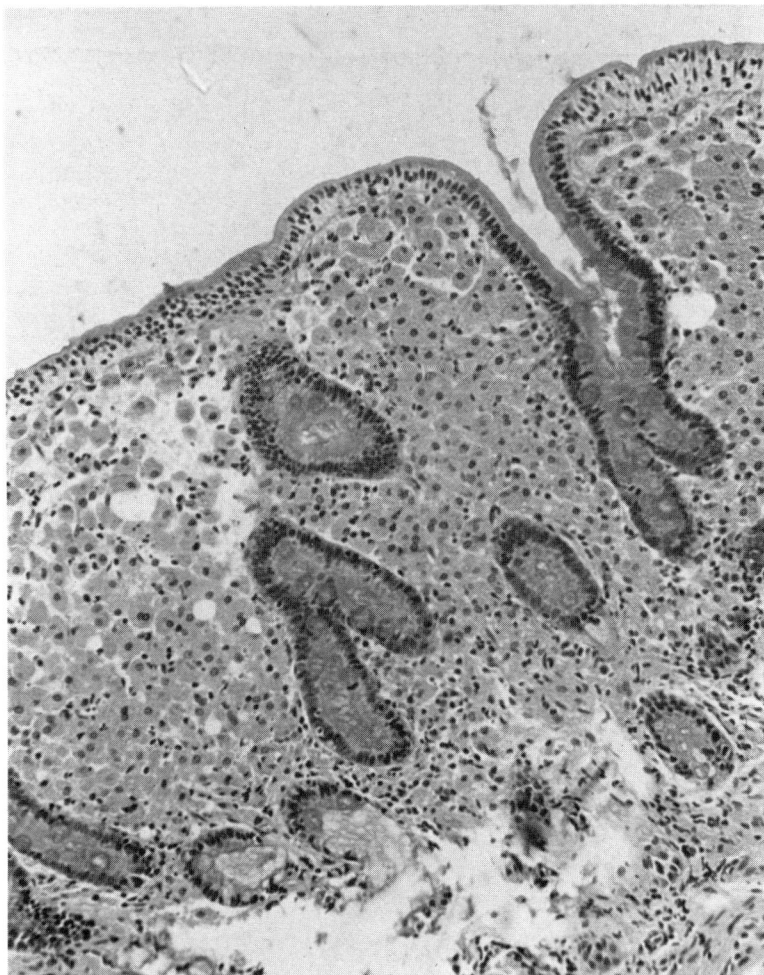

Fig. 8.62 Jejunal biopsy appearances of untreated Whipple's disease, showing villous atrophy, a well-preserved epithelial cell layer, and the uniform appearance of the lamina propria due to macrophage infiltration (haematoxylin and eosin × 150).

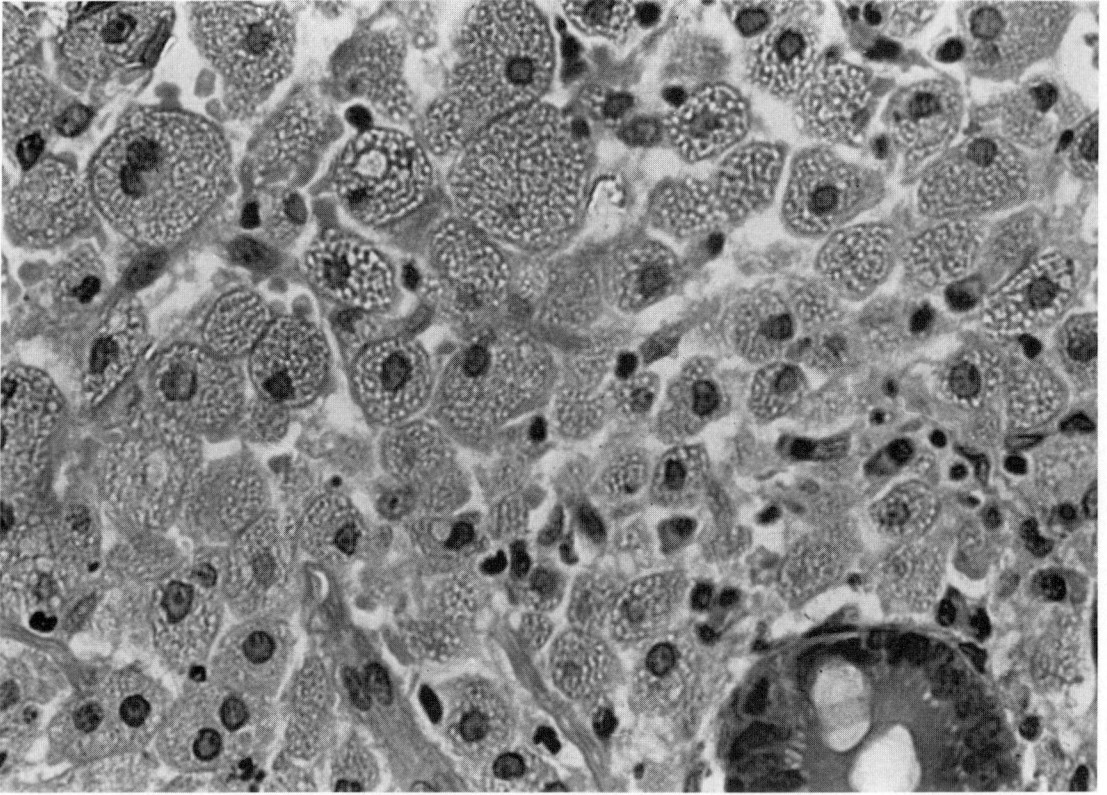

a

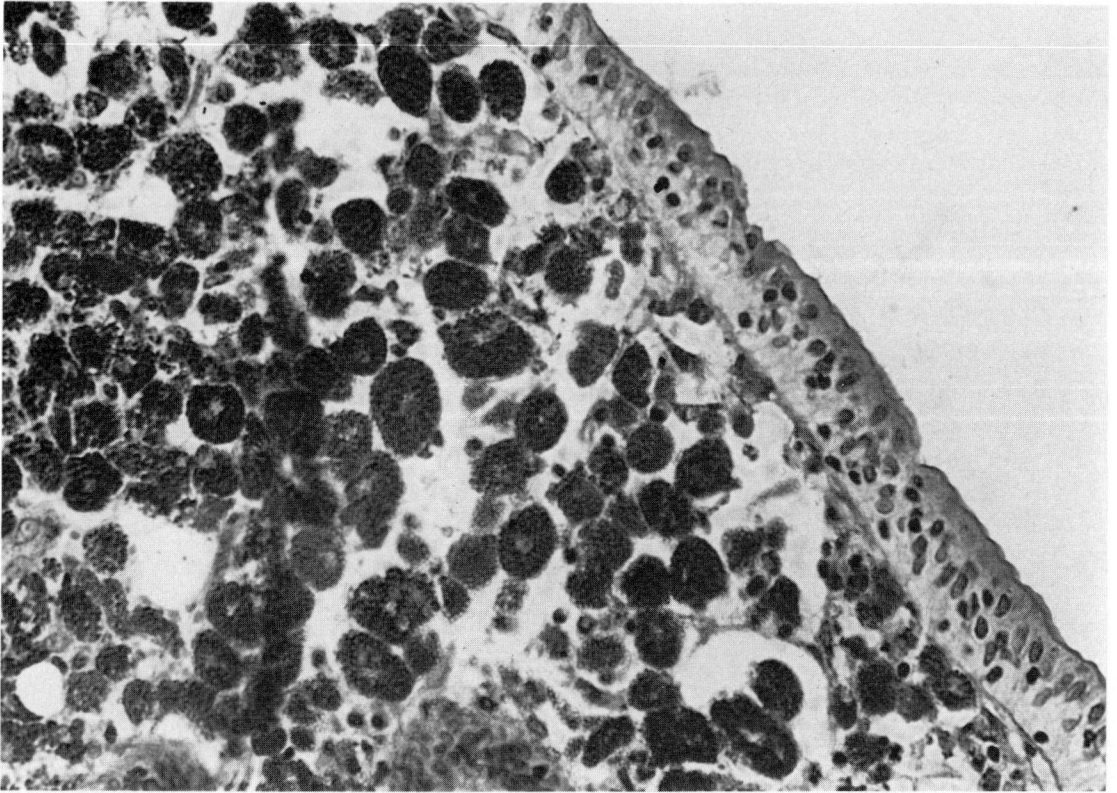

b

Fig. 8.63 (a) High power (× 400) of the lamina propria of the same tissue as Figure 8.62 demonstrating the foam-laden macrophages (haematoxylin and eosin). (b) PAS-staining of same tissue, demonstrating the typical glycoprotein material within the macrophages and also scattered within the lamina propria (× 400).

found within and between the foam-laden macrophages, and they also stain brilliant magenta with PAS.[5, 33] It seems probable that it is the presence of whole and degenerating bacteria, and of granules of membranous glycoprotein-rich material derived from bacteria, that explains the PAS-staining properties of the macrophages. The bacilli are similar in all reported cases. They are rods, 1–1.5 μm long and 0.25 μm across, and may occasionally be seen in division. In the small intestine they are most abundant just beneath the epithelial basement membrane and decrease in numbers towards the submucosa, perhaps supporting the concept of invasion from the luminal side. The evidence concerning the identity of these bacteria is discussed later.

OTHER PATHOLOGICAL FINDINGS

In advanced cases, mesenteric lymph nodes may be greatly enlarged, up to 3–4 cm across, with cystic fat-filled spaces and fibrosis apparent macroscopically. Histology confirms the presence of PAS-positive macrophages and bacilli, and granulomas are fairly frequently seen. Other intra-abdominal findings include peritoneal adhesions, thickening of the capsule of the liver and spleen, and ascites, which may be a transudate or chylous in nature.

Outside the abdomen, involvement of the heart, lung, brain and skin occurs. Valvular endocarditis occurred in one third of an autopsy series of patients, with a similar distribution of valve involvement to that seen in rheumatic endocarditis.[9] Fibrinous pericarditis, myocarditis, and coronary arteritis may also occur.[28] The respiratory system may be involved with pleural adhesions, pleural effusions, and nodular pulmonary involvement.[31] Approximately 10% of cases show involvement of the central nervous system at autopsy, with cortical atrophy, spongy demyelination, and areas of infarction.[10] Both macrophages and bacilli have now been identified in all these affected areas.[24]

Clinical features

The majority of patients are middle-aged males, presenting between the ages of 30 and 70.[20] However, affected women and infants have been reported. Most patients are caucasian, but affected negroes and indians have also been reported. Two sets of affected brothers have been recorded, but most of the cases are sporadic, and there is no obvious aetiological clue from geographical or occupational factors.

The disease is systemic and, as the pathological findings would suggest, symptoms and signs of involvement of almost any organ system may occur. Most patients, however, are not diagnosed until frank symptoms of gastrointestinal disease have developed, at which time routine investigation of a malabsorption state should lead to the diagnosis. Retrospectively a set of early symptoms, present for many years (anything from one to well over ten) before the development of symptoms of intestinal disease, can usually be recognized. These commonly include arthritis, fever, malaise, and pulmonary complaints; the challenge for the clinician is to make the diagnosis in this early stage.

Skin manifestations
Pigmentation is seen, particularly in exposed areas, in about half the patients. Non-specific cutaneous manifestations, similar to those seen in other malabsorptive states, are also seen, such as petechiae, ecchymoses, and follicular hyperkeratosis. Finger clubbing is unusual but can occur, and skin nodules with characteristic histology have been reported.[12] General examination may also reveal oedema.

Reticuloendothelial system
Peripheral lymphadenopathy occurs in about 50% of patients, but hepatomegaly and splenomegaly in less than 5%. Biopsy of lymph nodes may be diagnostic.[21]

Arthritis
Most patients have some history of arthritis – up to 90% in some series.[15] The arthritis is non-specific in nature and affects peripheral joints, either with frank swelling or, less commonly, with arthralgia alone. The symptoms are episodic, and affect the knees, ankles, wrists, hands and elbows most frequently, but virtually any joint can be involved. The arthritis may be symmetrical or asymmetrical, unilateral or bilateral. It is seronegative in type, does not cause abnormal radiological signs, and rarely leads to deformity. Sacroiliitis and spondylitis are also associated with Whipple's disease but occur much more rarely – probably in less than 10% of cases. Synovial biopsies have only rarely been performed, but both characteristic macrophages and bacteria have been identified in such material.[13]

Cardiac and pulmonary manifestations
Pericarditis is reported at some time in about 10% of cases, and may even lead to cardiac constriction. Myocarditis with conduction defects,

and valvular disease, mainly of the aortic and mitral valve, also occur; the combination of these may lead to presentation with cardiac failure. The diseased valves may subsequently be the site of conventional bacterial endocarditis; affected valves have been treated by the insertion of prostheses.[32] Pulmonary manifestations are very common; a recurrent cough, associated either with pleurisy or with pulmonary infiltrates, may be one of the early features of Whipple's disease and occurs in about 50% of cases.[31]

Central nervous system
Clinical central nervous system involvement is rare, occurring in perhaps 5% of cases. Most commonly it occurs after some years of systemic involvement. The manifestations of central nervous system involvement are non-specific, and include depression, apathy, dementia, fits, myoclonus, and dizziness. A variety of ocular manifestations occur, including supranuclear ophthalmoplegia, papilloedema, optic atrophy and scotomas, uveitis, and vitreous haemorrhages and opacities.[18] Meningitis, with PAS-positive cells in the CSF has also been reported.[27] In some patients, central nervous system disease has occurred after apparently adequate antibiotic treatment of intestinal Whipple's disease; presentation under these circumstances with apparent hypothalamic involvement, with insomnia, hyperphagia or polydipsia, has been reported.[10, 18] Such recurrences clearly have implications for the treatment and follow-up of patients with Whipple's disease.

Intestinal symptoms
Despite the historical concept of Whipple's disease as a disease of the small intestine, the clinical features of small gut involvement are non-specific. However, they are of great importance, as it is usually investigation of this organ that leads to the diagnosis. In advanced cases, diarrhoea, weight loss, abdominal pain and distension may occur. Investigation may show steatorrhoea, often of the order of 20–30 g/day, and a protein-losing enteropathy. Abdominal distension may be due to gas, ascites, or mesenteric node enlargement. Bleeding from ulcerations of the gastrointestinal tract rarely occur. In a few patients a diffuse colitis resembling ulcerative colitis has been reported.[14]

Investigations

Apart from the histological findings, there are no specific investigations in Whipple's disease.

Routine laboratory tests will show an elevated ESR, an anaemia which may show the combined effects of folate and iron deficiency, and chronic inflammation; B_{12} levels and absorption are usually normal. Thrombocytosis and an elevated white blood count may be seen.[22] The serum albumin may be very low, but globulin levels may be normal or elevated and serum IgA levels may be high.

Radiological investigation of the small gut often shows a characteristic pattern of dilatation and oedema (Figure 8.64), but in about 15% of patients the small bowel X-ray will be normal.[20] Endoscopic examination of the duodenum may show thickened folds and yellow-white areas, which on histology prove to be enlarged club-shaped villi; however, the duodenum is not infrequently spared.[29]

The cardinal investigation is a jejunal biopsy which, in virtually every case of untreated Whipple's disease, shows the characteristic histological abnormality. Very occasionally patchy changes occur and multiple biopsies are necessary, but in the majority the changes are diffuse. There are very rare cases in which Whipple's tissue has been found elsewhere in the body at a time when small intestinal disease has not been present. The best documented of such cases are those in which central nervous system relapse has occurred after the treatment of Whipple's disease involving the small intestine.[10]

Treatment

Early cases of Whipple's disease were fatal. A dramatic and sustained clinical response in a patient with Whipple's disease following chloramphenicol therapy was reported in 1952;[23] since the electron microscopic description of bacteria in the tissues, the central role of antimicrobial therapy has been recognized. Corticosteroids, initially advocated during the 1950s for the treatment of this condition, would seem now to have a very restricted role for the short-term support of desperately ill patients.

A variety of antimicrobial treatments have proved successful, although there have been no controlled trials. Penicillin, streptomycin, tetracycline, and sulphonamides have all been used, but there are also well documented instances in which one or other of these antibiotics has proved unsuccessful.[2] Treatment can be seen to be effective within a few days, with a rapid improvement in general condition, and cessation of fever, diarrhoea or arthritis; weight gain occurs over the ensuing few weeks. Occasionally an initial febrile Herxheimer-like reaction has

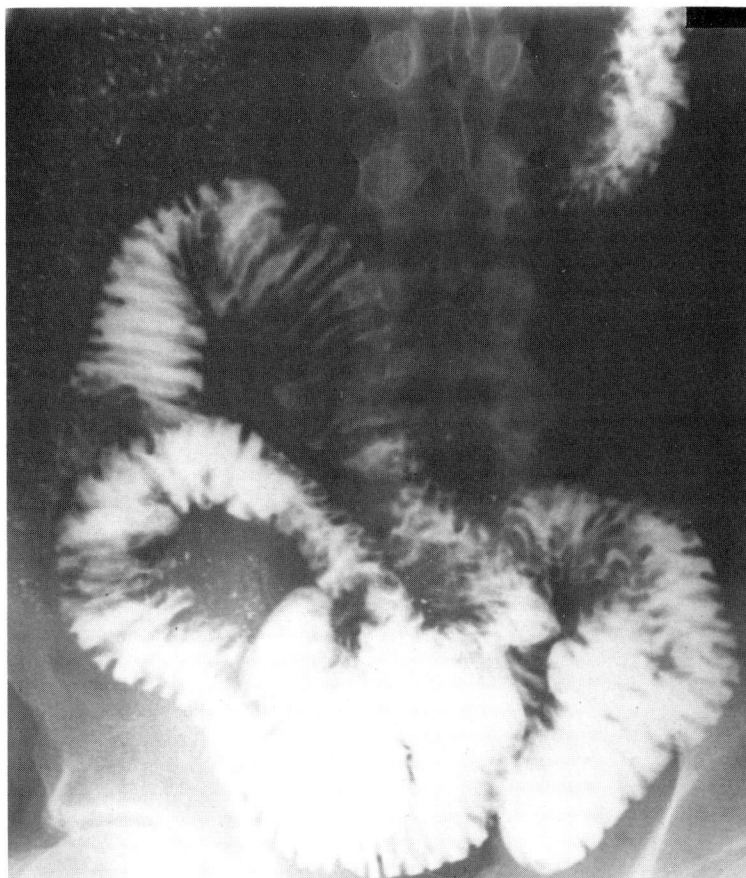

Fig. 8.64 Small bowel radiograph showing dilated oedematous intestine in Whipple's disease.

been reported. Follow-up biopsies of the small intestine show that the bacteria disappear within a few weeks, followed by restoration of the normal villus architecture, although occasionally PAS-positive macrophages may persist for some years.

Despite the good initial response to a wide variety of antibiotics, there is a high incidence of relapse after stopping treatment.[26] Probably up to one third of patients will relapse at some time, indicating the need for life-long follow-up. Interestingly, relapse may occur despite, and even during, long-term antibiotic therapy with a drug which was initially responsible for causing remission. Clinical relapse can be foretold by the reappearance of bacteria within serial small intestinal biopsies.[26] Clinical follow-up, including measurement of sedimentation rate and serum and red cell folate levels, may also be of value.

The appearance of relapses within the central nervous system, despite apparently successful treatment of intestinal disease some years before, is well recognized; it seems appropriate to commence treatment with high doses of par-

ental antibiotics in the hope that this will provide a sufficient concentration within the central nervous system. A regimen of 1.2 grams (2 mega units) of penicillin and 1 g of streptomycin daily for two weeks, followed by long-term tetracycline, has been recommended.[18]

Aetiology

The presence and distribution of bacteria within the body suggests that Whipple's disease is an infection, entering via the gastrointestinal tract. However, despite clear visualization within the tissues, the bacteria have not been clearly identified. This, together with the histological evidence of an abnormal response from the macrophage cell line, has led to the concept that pre-existing immunodeficiency in the host is a prerequisite for the development of Whipple's disease.

Bacteriology
The bacteria appear morphologically similar in all reported cases.[8] Culture of gut tissues has been disappointing due to a high incidence of

contaminated specimens; a wide variety of organisms have been grown from such tissues. These include corynebacteria, *Haemophilus*, *Klebsiella*, streptococci, *Nocardia*, and *Brucella*-like organisms.[19] Contamination is less likely in cultures of lymph node tissue; corynebacteria of at least two different strains,[4] and cell wall-deficient strains of streptococci[6] and enterococci have been isolated from this site. Some of these corynebacteria would now probably be classified as propionobacteria.

Encouraging results have recently been reported using immunofluorescent antisera to bacteria. Such antisera react mainly with the polysaccharide components of bacteria cell walls. However, the information they give is limited by the considerable cross-reactivity of grouping antisera between both species and genera. However, grouping antisera to streptococci of group A, B, and G, and *Shigella* B have reacted strongly with material in Whipple's macrophages, and fluorescence has also been observed with antisera and other groups of streptococci and propionobacteria. The findings of various workers have been similar, and suggest that a closely related group of organisms, whose surface carbohydrate is at least similar to those in streptococci and shigellae occur in Whipple's tissue.[16, 17] Further analysis with more specific antisera may eventually identify a specific or closely related group of bacteria.

Immunology
Even if the organism found in Whipple's tissue is identified, the ability of this bacteria to survive over years despite the host immune response requires explanation. Many authors have suggested that this is evidence of an immune deficiency in the host, and have provided evidence of this by describing a variety of immunological abnormalities in patients with active Whipple's disease.[7] These abnormalities have mainly affected cell-mediated immunity, and include decreased in vitro proliferative response of lymphocytes, decreased numbers of circulating lymphocytes, and abnormal delayed hypersensitivity. Whilst such observations have been fairly frequently made in untreated patients with active disease, investigations in treated patients, who should show a persistent defect if a primary immune deficiency is of importance, have been much less dramatic. Studies on HLA haplotypes, often used to explain a genetic predisposition to diseases associated with abnormal immune responsiveness, have been unremarkable. The B27 haplotype, strongly associated

with ankylosing spondylitis, may be more common in Whipple's disease, but is present in only about one third of patients.[11]

Conclusion

To the gastroenterologist, Whipple's disease is a treatable cause of malabsorption, and is particularly important because much systemic disease may be associated with it. To the general physician, the early presentation with arthritis, fever, pericarditis, central nervous system involvement, or ill defined collagenosis, offer an important diagnostic opportunity.

REFERENCES

1 Austin, L. L. & Dobbins, W. O. (1982) Intraepithelial leucocytes of the intestinal mucosa in normal man and Whipple's disease. *Digestive Diseases of Science*, **27**, 311–320.
2 Bayless, T. M. (1970) Whipple's disease – newer concepts of therapy. *Advances in Internal Medicine*, **16**, 171–189.
3 Black-Shaffer, B. (1949) Tinctorial demonstration of glycoproteins in Whipple's disease. *Proceedings of the Society for Experimental Biology and Medicine*, **72**, 225–227.
4 Caroli, J., Julien, C., Etévé, J. et al. (1963) Trois cas de maladie de Whipple. *Seminars Hopitaux de Paris*, **31**, 1457–1480.
5 Chears, W. C. & Ashworth, C. T. (1961) Electron microscopic study of the intestinal mucosa in Whipple's disease – demonstration of encapsulated bacilliform bodies in these lesions. *Gastroenterology*, **41**, 129–138.
6 Clancy, R. L., Tomkins, W. A. F., Muckle, T. J. et al. (1975) Isolation and characterization of an aetiologic agent in Whipple's disease. *British Medical Journal*, **ii**, 568–570.
7 Dobbins, W. O. (1981) Is there an immune deficit in Whipple's disease? *Digestive Diseases of Science*, **26**, 247–252.
8 Dobbins, W. O. & Kawanishi, H. (1981) Bacillary characteristics in Whipple's disease: an electron microscopic study. *Gastroenterology*, **80**, 1468–1475.
9 Enzinger, F. M. & Helwig, E. B. (1963) Whipple's disease – a review of the literature and report of 15 patients. *Virchows Archiv A Pathologische Anatomie*, **336**, 238–269.
10 Feurle, G. E., Volk, B. & Waldherr, R. (1979) Cerebral Whipple's with negative jejunal histology. *New England Journal of Medicine*, **300**, 907–908.
11 Feurle, F. E., Dörken, B., Schöpf, E. & Lenhard, V. (1979) HLA B27 and defects in the T cell system in Whipple's disease. *European Journal of Clinical Investigation*, **9**, 385–389.
12 Good, A. E., Beals, T. F., Simmons, J. L. & Ibrahim, M. A. H. (1980) A subcutaneous nodule with Whipple's disease – key to early diagnosis. *Arthritis and Rheumatism*, **23**, 856–858.
13 Hawkins, C. F., Farr, M., Morris, C. J. et al. (1976) Detection by electron microscopy of rod-shaped organisms in synovial membrane from a patient with the arthritis of Whipple's disease. *Annals of Rheumatic Diseases*, **35**, 502–509.

14 Hendrix, J. P., Black-Shaffer, B., Withers, R. W. & Handler, P. (1950) Whipple's intestinal lipodystrophy: report of 4 cases and discussion of possible pathogenic factors. *Archives of Internal Medicine*, **85**, 91–131.

15 Kelly, J. J. & Weisiger, B. B. (1963) The arthritis of Whipple's disease. *Arthritis and Rheumatism*, **6**, 615–632.

16 Kent, S. P. & Kirkpatrick, S. M. (1980) Whipple's disease. Immunological and histopathological studies of eight cases. *Archives of Pathology and Laboratory Medicine*, **104**, 544–547.

17 Keren, D. F., Weisburger, W. R., Yardley, J. H. *et al.* (1976) Whipple's disease: demonstration by immunofluorescence of similar bacterial antigens in macrophages from three cases. *Johns Hopkins Medical Journal*, **139**, 51–59.

18 Knox, D. L., Bayless, T. M. & Pittman, F. E. (1976) Neurologic disease in patients with treated Whipple's disease. *Medicine* (Baltimore) **55**, 467–476.

19 Kok, N., Dykbaer, R. & Rostgaard, J. (1964) Bacteria in Whipple's disease. *Acta Pathologica Microbiologica Scandinavica*, **60**, 431–449.

20 Maizel, H., Ruffin, J. M. & Dobbins, W. O. (1970) Whipple's disease. A review of 19 patients from one hospital and a review of the literature since 1950. *Medicine* (Baltimore) **49**, 175–205.

21 Mansbach, C. M., Shelbourne, J. D., Stevens, R. D. & Dobbins, W. O. (1978) Lymph node bacilliform bodies resembling those of Whipple's disease in a patient without intestinal involvement. *Annals of Internal Medicine*, **89**, 64–66.

22 Nuzum, C. T., Sandler, R. S. & Paulk, H. T. (1981) Thrombocytosis in Whipple's disease. *Gastroenterology*, **80**, 1465–1467.

23 Paulley, J. W. (1952) A case of Whipple's disease (intestinal lipodystrophy). *Gastroenterology*, **22**, 128–133.

24 Sieracki, J. C. (1958) Whipple's disease – observations on systemic involvement I. Cytologic observations. *American Medical Associations Archives of Pathology*, **66**, 464–467.

25 Sieracki, J. C. & Fine, G. (1959) Whipple's disease – observations on systemic involvement. II. Gross and histologic observations. *American Medical Associations Archives of Pathology*, **67**, 81–93.

26 Trier, J. S., Phelps, J. C., Eidelman, S. & Rubin, C. E. (1965) Whipple's disease. Light and electron microscopic correlation of jejunal mucosal histology with antibiotic treatment and clinical status. *Gastroenterology*, **48**, 384–407.

27 Thompson, D. G., Ledingham, J. M., Howard, A. J. & Brown, C. L. (1978) Meningitis in Whipple's disease. *British Medical Journal*, **ii**, 14–15.

28 Vliestra, R. E., Lie, J. T., Kuhn, W. E. *et al.* (1978) Whipple's disease involving the pericardium. Pathological confirmation during life. *Australian and New Zealand Journal of Medicine*, **8**, 649–651.

29 Volpicelli, N. A., Salyer, W. R., Milligan, F. D. *et al.* (1976) The endoscopic appearance of the duodenum in Whipple's disease. *Johns Hopkins Medical Journal*, **138**, 19–23.

30 Whipple, G. H. (1907) A hitherto undescribed disease characterised anatomically by deposits of fat and fatty acids in the intestinal and mesenteric lymphatic tissues. *Johns Hopkins Hospital Bulletin*, **198**, 382–391.

31 Winberg, C. D., Rose, M. E. & Rappaport, H. (1978) Whipple's disease of the lung. *American Journal of Medicine*, **65**, 873–880.

32 Wright, C. B., Hiratzka, L. F., Crossland, S. *et al.* (1978) Aortic insufficiency requiring valve replacement in Whipple's disease. *Annals of Thoracic Surgery*, **25**, 466–469.

33 Yardley, J. H. & Hendrix, T. R. (1961) Combined electron and light microscopy in Whipple's disease – demonstration of bacillary bodies in the intestine. *Johns Hopkins Hospital Bulletin*, **109**, 76.

RADIATION ENTEROPATHY

Radiation enteropathy, or radiation enteritis refers to a broad spectrum of structural and functional disturbances seen in the radiation-injured intestine.

The critical level of radiation which results in radiation enteropathy is 4500 rads. The average radiation dosage for therapy of abdominal neoplasms is listed in Table 8.33. At these dosages demonstrable enteropathy can be anticipated in up to 15% of patients undergoing therapy. The higher the dosage required for the control of the neoplasm, the higher will be the expected incidence of enteric sequelae. The combination of

Table 8.33 Average dosage schedules for common neoplasms.

Neoplasm	Average dosage (rads)	Organs injured
Oesophageal cancer	5000–6500	Oesophagus
Pancreatic cancer	5000–6000	Stomach, small intestine, colon
Hodgkin's disease	4000–4500	Small intestine, colon
Non-Hodgkin's lymphoma	3000–4500	Small intestine, colon
Retroperitoneal liposarcoma	5500–6500	Small intestine, colon
Testicular cancer		
Seminoma	3000	Small intestine, colon
Embryonal	4500–5000	Small intestine, colon
Ovarian cancer	4000–5500	Small intestine, colon
Uterine cancer		
Cervix	4500–8000	Small intestine, colon, rectum
Endometrium	4000–8000	Small intestine, colon, rectum
Bladder cancer	4000–6000	Small intestine, colon, rectum
Rectal cancer	4500–5500	Small intestine, rectum

Table 8.34 Comparative radiation tolerance.

Organ	Injury	Minimum tolerance dose (rads) (TD 5/5)	Maximum tolerance dose (rads) (TD 50/5)
Oesophagus	Ulcer, stricture	6000	7500
Stomach	Ulcer, perforation	4500	5000
Intestine	Ulcer, stricture	4500	6500
Colon	Ulcer, stricture	4500	6500
Rectum	Ulcer, stricture	5500	8000

Adapted from Rubin and Casarett.[15]

external beam and intracavitary radiation is especially likely to result in a high incidence of complications.

Dosage levels which induce injury have been quantified in terms of expected morbidity.[15] The 'minimum tolerance dose' (TD 5/5) is the dose at which up to 5% of patients will manifest radiation-induced damage within five years. The 'maximum tolerance dose' (TD 50/5) is that dose at which up to 50% of patients will manifest damage within five years.

The comparative sensitivity of different portions of the intestinal tract is listed in Table 8.34. The variation in sensitivity is a function of the cellular kinetics of each portion of the intestinal tract. The small intestine, which has the highest cellular turnover rate, is most vulnerable. Although the rectum is comparatively less vulnerable, rectal radiation injury is common because of the higher radiation dosage employed in pelvic neoplasms; the anatomical fixation of the rectum also predisposes it to injury. This section will principally discuss the small intestine, although radiation injury in other portions of the gastrointestinal tract will be briefly described.

Pathology

Excellent descriptions of the pathological changes occurring in radiation injury have been published by Warren and Friedman,[21] White,[23] and Berthrong and Fajardo.[1] A knowledge of these changes is basic to the understanding of the clinical syndromes associated with radiation enteropathy. The pathological changes commence within hours after the inception of radiation and continue throughout the individual's lifetime.

The earliest changes are those which affect the cytokinetics of replication in the intestinal mucosa. Within hours after an average therapeutic dose of irradiation (150–200 rads), cell necrosis occurs along the crypt walls. Although regeneration occurs rapidly from stem cells at the crypt base, overall cell turnover is dimin-

ished, with resultant flattening and blunting of the villi, mucosal atrophy, shortened crypts and focal ulceration (Figure 8.65). Regeneration and repair are impeded with each successive dose of radiation. It is in the initial phases of injury that the inflammatory component of enteropathy is greatest, with large numbers of polymorphonuclear leukocytes forming a surface syncytium with the desquamated mucosal cells. The acute inflammatory reaction subsides when the radiation treatment is stopped, although the inexorable progression of radiation-induced damage continues.

Subacute and chronic changes, which are more insidious in their development and more serious from the clinical point of view, affect the submucosa, the blood vessels, the muscularis propria, and the serosa. The submucosa exhibits oedema, progressive hyalinization, and deposition of dense masses of collagen containing bizarre, abnormal fibroblasts ('radiation fibroblasts') (Figure 8.66). The principal vascular changes are submucosal telangiectasia, hyalinization of vessel walls, alterations in endothelial cells, subendothelial swelling (foam cells), intimal plaque formation, and obliterative endarteritis. Veins show similar intimal and mural changes. The muscularis propria may show focal areas of fibrosis and may be secondarily involved in fissures or deep, penetrating ulcers. Damage to the basic structure of the muscularis, however, is not an important aspect of radiation enteropathy. The serosa exhibits diffuse or patchy hyalinosis with scattered, bizarre fibroblasts, telangiectasia of smaller vessels, and the vascular changes already mentioned in larger vessels (Figure 8.67). Grossly, this is manifest as a 'peel' of opaque greyish or grey-white tissue enveloping the intestinal wall (Figure 8.68). Dense adhesions between adjacent intestinal loops result in fusion of the abnormal serosal surfaces.

Warren and Friedman[21] have designated the primary criteria of radiation enteropathy as follows: hyalinization of connective tissue, abnormal fibroblasts, telangiectasia, and hyaline

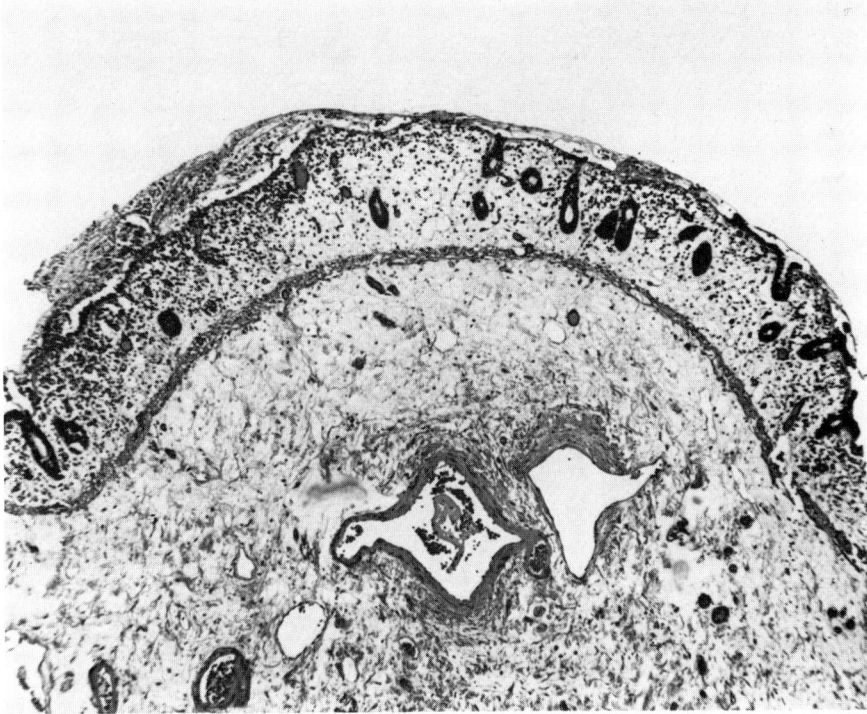

Fig. 8.65 Section of irradiated ileum showing distortion of villous architecture, vascular ectasia and perivascular hyalinosis (haematoxylin and eosin × 60).

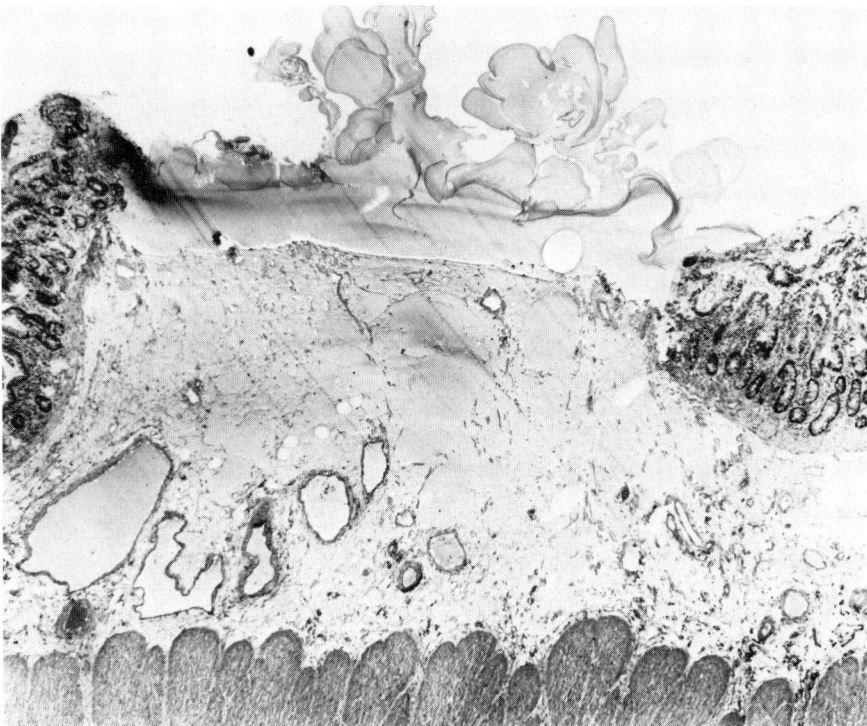

Fig. 8.66 Marked oedema of the submucosa in irradiated ileum, with focal ulceration and vascular ectasia (haematoxylin and eosin × 40).

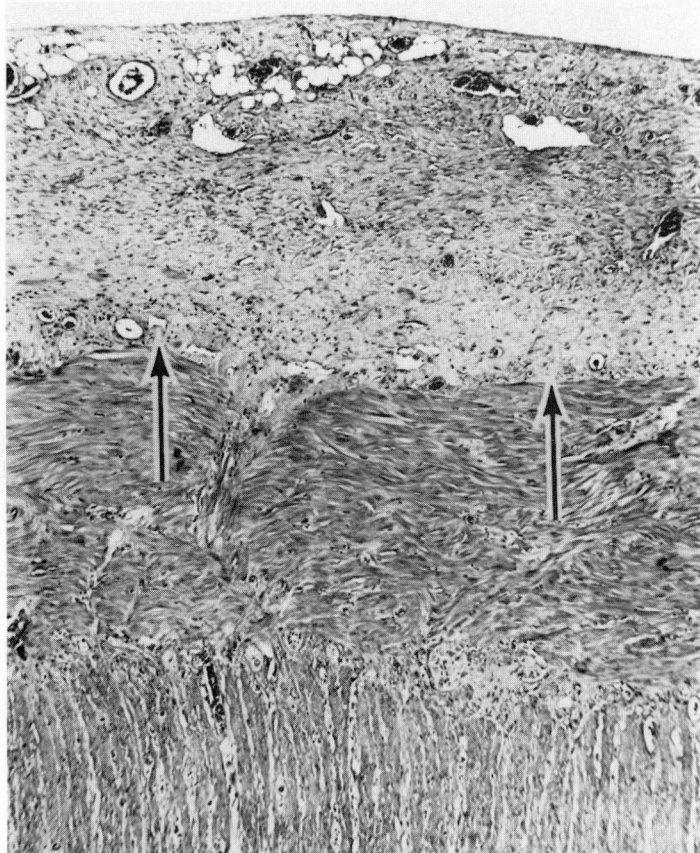

Fig. 8.67 Thickened serosa or peel (arrows) over irradiated ileal segment showing hyalinization and telangiectasia (haematoxylin and eosin × 60).

degeneration of vessel walls. Secondary criteria include the mucosal changes, endothelial abnormalities, phlebosclerosis, and changes in muscle fibres.

Changes at the microscopic level are reflected clinically in the occurrence of ulceration, haemorrhage, stricture, infarction, and perforation.

Clinical syndromes

Early

The acute or early effects of therapeutic irradiation are transient and non-specific. They include nausea, vomiting, abdominal cramps, and diarrhoea. Acute ulceration may occur but is rare.

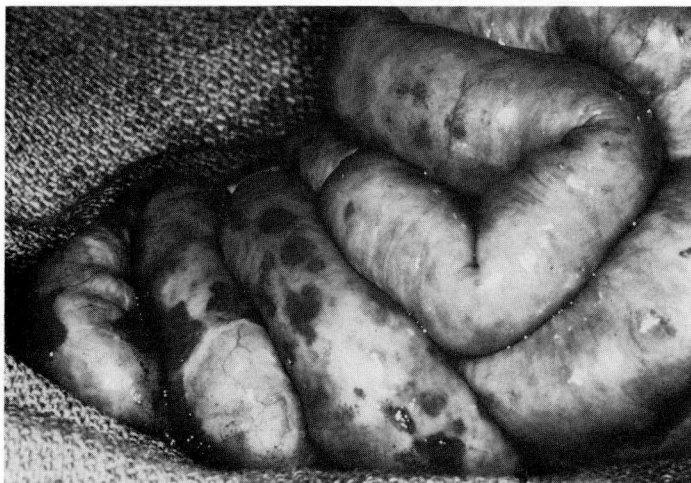

Fig. 8.68 Gross appearance at operation of late changes in irradiated obstructed ileum. Loops are oedematous and thick serosal peel over the chronically thickened bowel wall is evident. The haemorrhagic spots are due to handling.

X-ray studies performed at this time show evidence of oedema of bowel loops and hypermotility, but none of the specific features of radiation enteropathy. Signs and symptoms abate shortly after the radiation is stopped.

Delayed

Following the cessation of irradiation, a quiescent period ensues unless the dosage was unusually high. The average onset of late symptoms is shortly after the first year; primary or recurrent symptoms may then occur at any time thereafter for the lifetime of the individual.

Severe symptoms during the early phases of therapy or shortly following cessation of therapy may be predictors of the development of late sequelae.

Late sequelae

FUNCTIONAL

Varying degrees of malabsorption are common following therapeutic irradiation. Bile acid absorption has been shown to be impaired, as demonstrated by abnormal ^{14}C bile acid breath tests.[7] There is also impaired absorption of carbohydrate, fat and vitamin B_{12}. Significant protein loss may occur, particularly in the presence of severe steatorrhoea.

Disturbances in motility, apart from those due to altered absorption patterns, are due to the direct effect of radiation on the muscularis propria. Myofibrillar degeneration, muscle fibre atrophy, and patchy hyalinization are common histological findings. Effects on the intrinsic

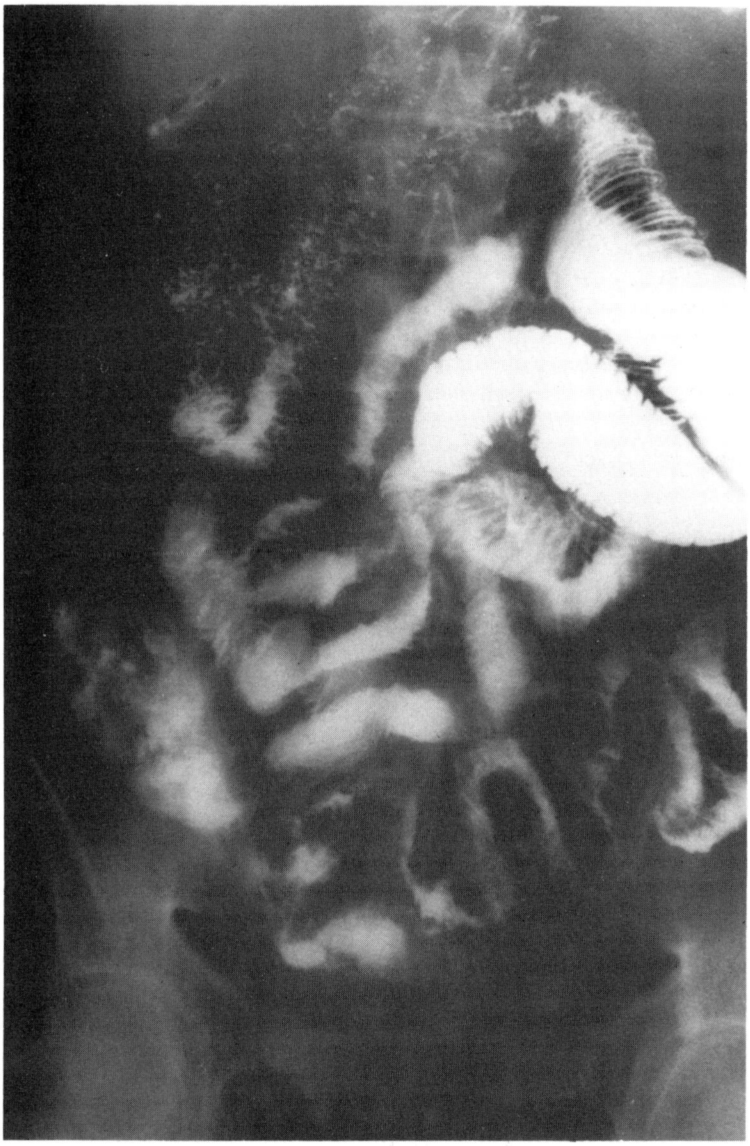

Fig. 8.69 Typical radiographical appearance in radiation enteropathy. Note obstructed dilated jejunal loop, distorted architecture, and narrowing and separation of distal loops.

neural mechanisms are not well documented. Characteristic X-ray findings are hypermotility, delayed segmental motility, 'feathering' of the mucosal pattern, separation of bowel loops, and a generalized distortion of the normal architecture (Figure 8.69). 'Pseudo-obstruction' has been reported by Conklin and Anuras,[3] referring to functional obstruction in the absence of a true obstructing lesion.

STRUCTURAL

The principal late clinical sequelae following radiation are obstruction, ulceration, haemorrhage, fistula formation, infarction and perforation.[4, 12, 24]

Obstruction
Acute and subacute intestinal obstruction is perhaps the most common mechanical clinical disorder caused by radiation injury. It is a manifestation of radiation-induced fibrosis, chiefly in the submucosa, as well as adhesion formation between bowel loops due to radiation-induced serositis (Figure 8.70). The obstructed bowel loops become heavy with oedema and intraluminal fluid, initiating the cycle of events leading to complete obstruction. The obstructed, distended loops are tender to palpation and may give rise to rebound tenderness even in the absence of infarction or perforation. Volvulus is not as common as is seen in simple adhesive

obstruction due to the thickening and foreshortening of the irradiated mesentery. Partial obstruction of varying degrees is more common than complete obstruction, since the obstructive mechanisms are strictures, stenotic segments and multiple adhesions, rather than the single fibrous bands usually seen in adhesive obstruction. Nevertheless, the progression to a picture of complete obstruction, if the partial obstruction is not treated early, is not uncommon.

Ulceration
Ulceration is probably the result of ischaemic changes induced by progressive vascular sclerosis. Ulcers may be shallow and scattered (Figure 8.71) or deeply penetrating through all layers (Figure 8.72). Deep penetrating ulcers may perforate, may cause obstruction by the cicatricial reaction they evoke, or may bleed. Although shallow ulcers heal with a thin layer of regenerative mucosa and a tendency to recurrence, deeper ulcers which traverse all layers rarely heal. If healing does occur, stricture and resultant obstruction are inevitable.

Haemorrhage
Bloody diarrhoea is not uncommon during the initial phases of radiation therapy, particularly in the higher dosage range, and it reflects diffuse mucosal damage. When bleeding occurs as a late phenomenon, it usually occurs as frank haematochezia due to a solitary ulcer or diffuse

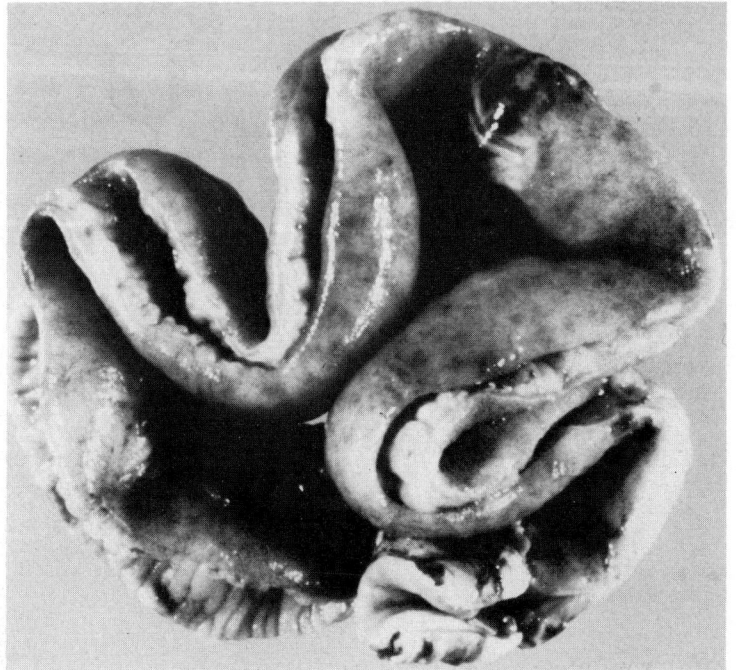

Fig. 8.70 Resected, obstructed segment of irradiated small intestine. Note thickness of wall, rigidity, opaque serosal peel, and intersegmental adhesions.

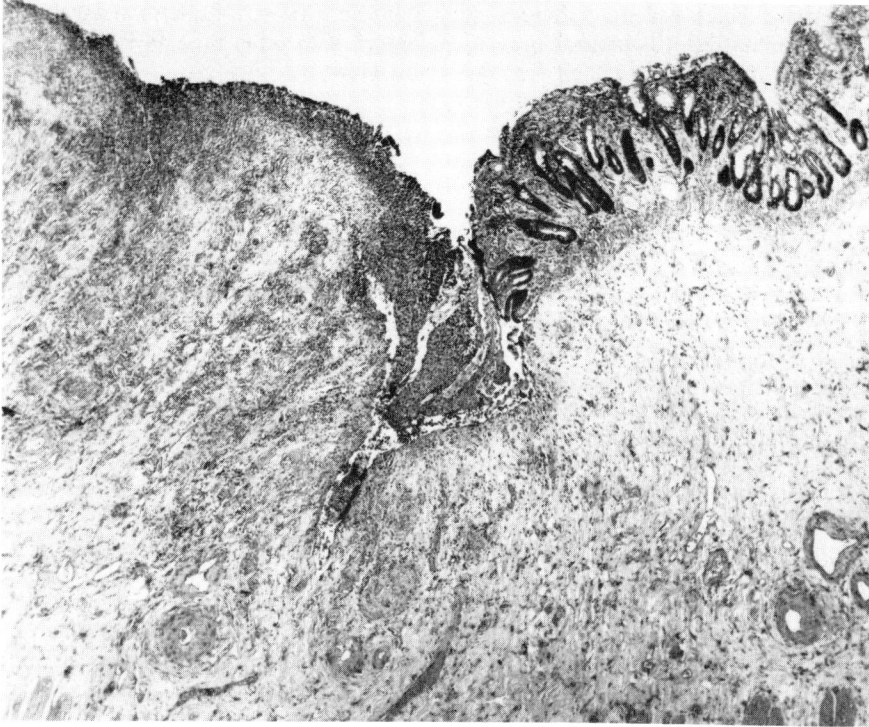

Fig. 8.71 Superficial mucosal ulceration. Note submucosal vascular sclerosis underlying ulcerated zone (haematoxylin and eosin × 45).

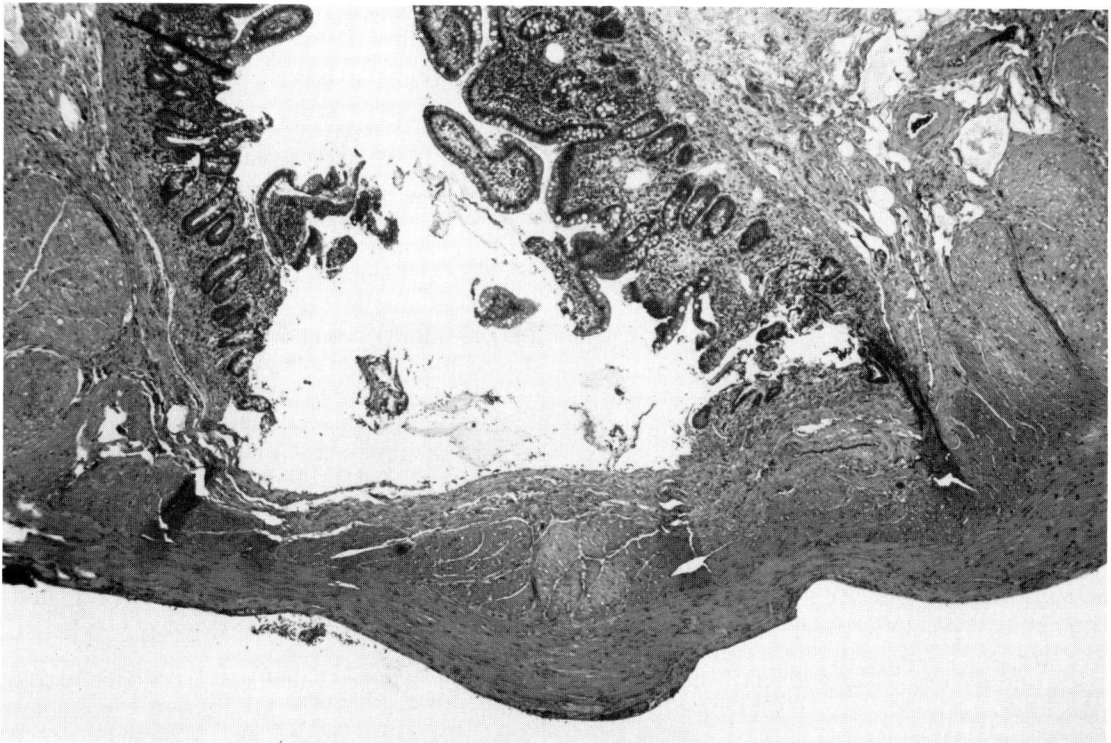

Fig. 8.72 Deeply penetrating ulcer in irradiated small intestine. Resection was necessary because of obstruction.

ulceration occurring over ectatic submucosal vessels.[20] Exsanguinating haemorrhage is uncommon. Occasionally mucosal haemorrhage may be exacerbated in the radiation-induced intestine by chemotherapeutic agents which have a radiomimetic action on the intestinal mucosa.

Fistula formation

Fistula formation is probably a late manifestation of a deeply penetrating ulcer or the commonly seen deep fissures which may traverse the wall of the radiation-injured bowel. Sometimes a dense adhesion will have sealed such a fistula at its serosal exit, and an overt fistula results only when the adhesion is severed. Fistulas seek a point of exit; they may do so through an adjoining loop of bowel, recent wounds, drain sites, or old scars. Lacking a point of exit, unsealed fistulas result in intra-abdominal abscesses.

Infarction

This disastrous and often lethal complication occurs rarely in end-stage enteropathy. It is a consequence of major vessel occlusion due to obliterative endarteritis. The infarction is segmental at times, involving multiple segments of irradiated bowel. The full thickness of intestinal wall is affected. Left unresected, free perforation occurs. The most common site for infarction, sometimes many years after the original injury, is the pelvic ileum. This region of the intestine often receives the brunt of the radiation injury. The usual clinical manifestation of infarction is the acute surgical abdomen, with tenderness, rigidity and rebound tenderness.

Perforation

Free perforation of the intestine into the peritoneal cavity is the ultimate catastrophe. It usually occurs as a consequence of infarction. Generalized peritonitis from free perforation is not as common as with other causes of free perforation since the radiation-injured bowel is enveloped in dense fibrous adhesions.

Malignancy

The late occurrence of malignancy in radiation-injured intestine deserves passing mention. Sandler and Sandler[16] have recently assessed the risk of radiation-induced cancers of the colon and rectum. They concluded that women who have received pelvic irradiation are more prone to develop colon cancer, the risk factor being 1.2–8 times that of the general population.

Manifestations of radiation injury in enteric sites other than the small intestine

Oesophagus

The oesophagus is relatively resistant to radiation injury. During the second or third week of therapy, oesophagitis is common, with dysphagia as the major symptom.

If radiation is given to an extremely radiosensitive neoplasm, acute haemorrhage and ulceration may ensue due to rapid radionecrosis of the neoplasm. Ulceration, abscess formation or even free perforation into adjacent structures or the pleural cavity may also occur.

The principal late complication is stenosis due to fibrosis.

Stomach

No significant sequelae occur in the irradiated stomach until the dose exceeds 2000 rads. All of the changes described in the small intestine occur in the stomach, albeit to a lesser degree. Radiation-induced acute gastritis subsides following cessation of therapy, but achlorhydria may persist for years. Purposely induced achlorhydria for the treatment of peptic ulcer with 2000 rads of external irradiation is an obsolete therapeutic procedure.

The late manifestation of radiation injury to the stomach is atrophic gastritis with attendant dyspepsia. Chronic ulceration may be superimposed on the atrophic gastritis, a situation in which healing is unlikely.

Colon

The transverse colon is vulnerable during irradiation of the upper abdomen. Bleeding, usually secondary to a radiation-induced ulcer, is the principal symptom. Later problems in the colon are related to fibrotic stenosis and partial obstruction.

The rectum is one of the most highly radioresistant portions of the alimentary tract. Some degree of radiation proctitis occurs at all dosages above 4000 rads and is manifested clinically by cramping, tenesmus and frequent stools. The late sequelae of radiation injury to the rectum are stenosis, ulceration, haemorrhage and fistulas. Rectovaginal fistula at the point of maximum injury on the anterior rectal wall usually results from combined intracavitary and external beam irradiation in excess of 6000 rads.

Factors which enhance radiation injury

Radiation injury from dosages in the average therapeutic range (around 4500 rads) is a rela-

tively unpredictable phenomenon in any individual patient. Certain factors, however, are known to predispose to radiation injury. Potish[13, 14] has summarized and quantified some of these predisposing factors, alone and in combination.

A thin physique increases the likelihood of radiation enteropathy, as does malnutrition and lean tissue loss. Diabetes and hypertension predispose to radiation injury due to the structural and functional microvascular abnormalities which exist in these disorders.

Adhesions which result in the abnormal fixation of normally mobile intestinal loops also predispose to radiation enteropathy.[9] Adhesions from prior pelvic infection or prior pelvic surgery are common in women subjected to pelvic irradiation. Prior abdominal surgery is common in patients being irradiated for lymphoma, retroperitoneal neoplasms, pancreatic carcinoma, bladder carcinoma and other miscellaneous neoplasms.

Simultaneous or post-irradiation chemotherapy may aggravate radiation injury.[11, 18] Among the principal chemotherapeutic agents which exert a radiomimetic effect on intestinal mucosa, and thus predispose to or aggravate previous radiation damage, are actinomycin D, 5-fluorouracil, methotrexate, and adriamycin. A quiescent radiation enteropathy may become actively symptomatic during chemotherapy.

Finally, misjudgements in administration of radiation may result in injury. Unusually high fractionation doses, overlap of portals, excessive total dosage (especially with combined intracavitary and external beam irradiation), and lack of attention to fixed anatomical structures can all be implicated in the induction of radiation injury.

Treatment

MEDICAL

Symptoms occurring during the early phases of radiation are treated with simple non-specific measures. The diet should be bland and low residue. Mild antiemetic, antispasmodic and sedative drugs will relieve the majority of acute radiation symptoms. If radiation proctitis is a problem in early phases of treatment, hydrophilic stool softeners, sitz baths, analgesics and, in more severe cases, steroid retention enemas are effective. More stringent medical measures in the acute treatment phases are rarely necessary.

In the intermediate and late stages of radiation enteropathy, there is a plethora of measures in the medical armamentarium, none of which are universally effective. The bland, lactose-free diet is often used in the management of small intestinal symptoms. In the recovery from an acute bout of intestinal obstruction, or to offset an impending obstruction, elemental diets have been used with some success. Anticholinergics, antispasmodics, and analgesics are of minimal value, but nonetheless may be useful. Prednisone is a lysozomal stabilizing agent and can be useful in small intestinal syndromes where bleeding is a prominent symptom. Cholestyramine, which binds excess bile salts, is useful for the more persistent diarrhoeal syndromes. Non-absorbed antibiotics, such as sulphasalazine, may also be helpful.

For radiation proctitis, dietary measures, hydrophilic stool softeners, and steroid retention enemas (administered nightly for 10 to 14 days) may give significant relief. Intractable bleeding rarely responds to purely medical measures and ultimately requires operation. Rectal fistulas do not respond to medical measures.

SURGICAL

Surgical intervention in patients with radiation enteropathy is reserved for acute life-threatening complications, such as obstruction, haemorrhage, infarction or perforation, or for chronic morbidity refractory to medical therapy, such as bleeding, fistula formation, ulceration, recurrent obstruction, intractable pain or incontinence. Radiation-induced carcinoma is, of course, an absolute indication for surgical intervention. Approximately 15% of patients with radiation enteropathy ultimately require operation. The indications and guidelines for surgical intervention have been well described by Localio et al.,[8] Morgenstern et al.,[10] and Schmitt and Symmonds.[17] The following principles are applicable to most operations for radiation enteropathy.

1 Avoid operations, if at all possible, in patients with radiation enteropathy.
2 In elective procedures, achieve optimal nutritional status before operation. This may require 7–14 days of total parenteral nutrition. Continue total parenteral nutrition for as long as necessary postoperatively.
3 Avoid incisions in heavily irradiated areas. Skin necrosis, infection and wound dehiscence may ensue.
4 In elective procedures involving the small intestine, insert a long tube (Cantor, Miller–Abbot) for decompression before operation.
5 Prepare the bowel with antibiotics preoperatively. The irradiated or obstructed bowel

is not bacteria-free. Continue broad-spectrum parenteral antibiotics for five days postoperatively.

6 Although bypass procedures may be safer and more expeditious in any individual patient, it is generally more effective to resect a diseased segment rather than bypass it. Bypassed segments may bleed, ulcerate, perforate or infarct.

7 Avoid extensive adhesiolysis, which may open sealed perforations. Instillation of methylene blue through the long intestinal tube aids in the detection of occult mural defects.

8 Remember that all anastomoses in irradiated bowel are precarious and require meticulous surgical technique. Avoid multiple anastomoses.

9 Mark anastomoses with identifiable metallic clips at the extremities of each anastomosis.

10 Avoid early postoperative oral feeding and continue long tube decompression for at least seven days. Study the anastomotic integrity radiographically before removing the tube.

11 Protect low colorectal anastomoses with a proximal transverse colostomy. The anastomotic leakage rate is high and can be lethal if the anastomosis is unprotected.

12 In the formation of stomas, avoid using irradiated bowel if possible. If use of irradiated bowel is unavoidable, exteriorize an ample segment. Sloughing, retraction and ulceration are common.

13 Fistulas do not respond to simple closure or diversion, particularly in the rectum. Resection of the diseased segment is nearly always necessary.

Prevention

Stewart and Gibbs[19] have provided a comprehensive summary of measures to prevent radiation injury in general. Unfortunately, no currently available preparations are radioprotective. Bounous[2] has proposed that elemental, hydrolysed protein diets administered during intensive radiation protect against radiation enteropathy. Green et al.[6] have described surgical measures to minimize small intestinal injury during pelvic irradiation. Perhaps the most promising measures lie in advances in radiotherapeutic technique. A technique recently described by Fowler,[5] utilizing hyperfractionated radiotherapy, shows promise, particularly in the prevention of late complications. Modifications in radiation dosage, fractionation and mode of delivery, especially in patients with known predisposition to injury, may possibly reduce the incidence of this condition.

REFERENCES

1 Berthrong, M. & Fajardo, L. F. (1981) Radiation injury in surgical pathology. Part II. Alimentary tract. *American Journal of Surgical Pathology*, **5**, 153–178.

2 Bounous, G., Le Bel, E., Shuster, J. et al. (1975) Dietary protection during radiation therapy. *Strahlentherapie*, **149**, 476–483.

3 Conklin, J. L. & Anuras, S. (1981) Radiation-induced recurrent intestinal pseudo-obstruction. *American Journal of Gastroenterology*, **75**, 440–444.

4 DeCosse, J. J., Rhodes, R. S., Wentz, W. B. et al. (1969) The natural history and management of radiation induced injury of the gastrointestinal tract. *Annals of Surgery*, **170**, 369–384.

5 Fowler, J. F. (1982) Non-standard fractionation in radiotherapy. *International Journal of Radiation Oncology, Biology, Physics*, **8**, 50 (Abstract).

6 Green, N., Iba, G. & Smith, W. R. (1975) Measures to minimize small intestine injury in the irradiated pelvis. *Cancer*, **35**, 1633–1640.

7 Kinsella, T. J. & Bloomer, W. D. (1980) Tolerance of the intestine to radiation therapy. (Collective review). *Surgery, Gynecology and Obstetrics*, **151**, 273–284.

8 Localio, S. A., Pachter, H. L. & Gouge, T. H. (1979) The radiation-injured bowel. *Surgery Annual*, **11**, 181–205.

9 LoIudice, T., Baxter, D. & Balint, J. (1977) Effects of abdominal surgery on the development of radiation enteropathy. *Gastroenterology*, **73**, 1093–1097.

10 Morgenstern, L., Thompson, R. & Friedman, N. B. (1977) The modern enigma of radiation enteropathy: sequelae and solutions. *American Journal of Surgery*, **134**, 166–172.

11 Phillips, T. L., Wharam, M. D. & Margolis, L. W. (1975) Modification of radiation injury to normal tissues by chemotherapeutic agents. *Cancer*, **35**, 1678–1684.

12 Poddar, P. K., Bauer, J., Gelernt, I. et al. (1982) Radiation injury to small intestine. *Mount Sinai Journal of Medicine*, **49**, 144–149.

13 Potish, R. A. (1980) Prediction of radiation-related small bowel damage. *Radiology*, **135**, 219–221.

14 Potish, R. A. (1982) Importance of predisposing factors in the development of enteric damage. *American Journal of Clinical Oncology: Cancer Clinical Trials*, **5**, 189–194.

15 Rubin, P. & Casarett, G. (1972) A direction for clinical radiation pathology: the tolerance dose. In *Frontiers of Radiation Therapy and Oncology*, Vol. 6 (Ed.) Vaeth, J. M. pp. 1–16. Baltimore: University Park Press.

16 Sandler, R. S. & Sandler, D. P. (1983) Radiation-induced cancers of the colon and rectum: assessing the risk. *Gastroenterology*, **84**, 51–57.

17 Schmitt III, E. H. & Symmonds, R. E. (1981) Surgical treatment of radiation induced injuries of the intestine. *Surgery, Gynecology and Obstetrics*, **153**, 896–900.

18 Shehata, W. M. & Meyer, R. L. (1980) The enhancement effect of irradiation by methotrexate: report of three complications. *Cancer*, **46**, 1349–1352.

19 Stewart, J. R. & Gibbs, Jr, F. A. (1982) Prevention of radiation injury: predictability and preventability of complications of radiation therapy. *Annual Review of Medicine*, **33**, 385–395.

20 Taverner, D., Talbot, I. C., Carr-Locke, D. L. & Wicks, A. C. B. (1982) Massive bleeding from the ileum: a late complication of pelvic radiotherapy. *American Journal of Gastroenterology*, **77**, 29–31.

21 Warren, S. & Friedman, N. B. (1942) Pathology and pathologic diagnosis of radiation lesions in the gastrointestinal tract. *American Journal of Pathology*, **18**, 499–513.

22 White, D. C. (1975) Esophagus and stomach. In *An Atlas of Radiation Histopathology* (Ed.) White, D. C. pp. 136–140. Technical Information Center, Office of Public Affairs, U. S. Energy Research and Development Administration.

23 White, D. C. (1975) Intestines. In *An Atlas of Radiation Histopathology* (Ed.) White, D. C. pp. 141–160. Technical Information Center, Office of Public Affairs, U.S. Energy Research and Development Administration.

24 Yoonessi, M., Romney, S. & Dayem, H. (1981) Gastrointestinal tract complications following radiotherapy of uterine cervical cancer: past and present. *Journal of Surgical Oncology*, **18**, 135–142.

SURGICAL CAUSES OF MALABSORPTION

JEJUNO-ILEAL BYPASS

Because of the very disappointing results of conservative treatment for gross obesity, many operations have been devised in an attempt to ameliorate the problem by a more radical approach. Until recently, apart from simply excising redundant adipose tissue, the only radical treatment to gain reasonably wide popularity was the operation of jejuno-ileal bypass, following the publication of their initial results by Payne and De Wind.[8] Earlier procedures, such as jejuno-colic anastomosis, produced dramatic weight loss but were associated with a high incidence of complications.

The original concept of jejuno-ileal bypass was to bypass 90% of the small intestine and so produce a state of profound malabsorption which would result in weight loss even in the presence of a large dietary food intake. Once the grossly obese patient reached normal weight, it was intended to restore normal intestinal continuity in the belief that the patient would find the subsequent maintenance of normal weight by dietary means considerably easier than weight reduction. However, the second operation to restore continuity was soon abandoned as it became apparent that patients soon returned to their preoperative obese state, and the operation was frequently refused by patients who had achieved normality.

Since the operation produces a state of malabsorption, the potential incidence of complications is high. Consequently, meticulous and conscientious long-term follow-up of the patient is essential following jejuno-ileal bypass. This burden has proved too great for some centres with the result that the popularity of this procedure is presently declining.

Indications for operation

To assess the indications for jejuno-ileal bypass objectively requires accurate knowledge of the risks of the operation which can then be compared with the risks of obesity. A large amount of literature is available to assess the operative and postoperative risks, but there is a surprising lack of information on the actual risks of obesity itself. Although the increased incidence of, for example, diabetes mellitus, hypertension and cholelithiasis, is well recorded, the mortality and morbidity from the complications of obesity are not. Even insurance company data are unhelpful since patients with gross obesity tend to be denied life insurance and therefore do not figure prominently in the statistics. Furthermore, the social, economic and emotional results of gross obesity cannot be objectively quantified.

However, some generally agreed principles may be stated although details vary considerably with individual opinion. Firstly, the patient should be sufficiently obese. This has been defined variably as being: over 135 kg (300 lb), more than 44 kg (100 lb) over 'ideal' body weight, greater than twice the 'ideal' weight, or having a body mass index (ponderal index) of greater than 30. Body mass index is given by:

$$\left(\frac{\text{weight (kg)}}{\text{height}^2 \text{ (m)}}\right).$$

The obesity should be long-standing and the patient should have failed in attempts at genuine, concerted and supervised conservative treatment regimens.

Youth (age less than 40) is often insisted upon and is clearly advantageous for medical and economic reasons.

Although diabetes mellitus, hypertension or resting hypoventilation may justifiably be considered as an indication for jejuno-ileal bypass, the presence of diabetic complications, ischaemic heart disease, or respiratory failure must be regarded as relative contraindications.

Psychiatric illness has been regarded both as an indication and as a contraindication for jejuno-ileal bypass. Certainly many grossly obese patients are seriously depressed. It can be extremely difficult to decide whether such depression is an effect or a contributory cause of the obesity. If doubt exists then expert help is strongly advised. However, it has been shown that the dramatic alteration of body image following jejuno-ileal bypass will often improve rather than compound any neurotic traits in properly selected patients.[4]

As in all operative procedures, the patient must give informed consent. This requires an

understanding of the inevitable effects and possible complications of jejuno-ileal bypass. Also (possibly more important), the patient should be sufficiently reliable to comply with the requirements of any long-term medication and long-term follow-up attendance.

The highest incidence of serious postoperative metabolic complications occurs in those patients with the highest rates of weight loss postoperatively. Since the patients with the highest weight preoperatively are also those who lose weight the fastest postoperatively, some patients are *too* obese to risk jejuno-ileal bypass. Unfortunately, the quantification of risks is too difficult to allow this upper limit of weight to be accurately defined.

In practice, these indications mean that relatively small numbers of patients are suitable for this form of radical treatment.

The operations

The precise details of lengths and regions of small intestine bypassed tend to vary from centre to centre but all aim to achieve a 90% exclusion of the small intestine. In practice this requires 50 cm of functioning small intestine to remain in continuity, and at least 10 cm of this must be ileal to prevent the very severe fluid and electrolyte loss which was experienced with the early jejunocolic anastomoses. An anastomosis of 40 cm of jejunum to 10 cm of terminal ileum, or 25 cm of jejunum to 25 cm of terminal ileum are most commonly used. The jejuno-ileal anastomosis may be end-to-side (Payne procedure),[8] in which the jejunum is transected 40 cm distal to the ligament of Treitz and the proximal end of the jejunum anastomosed to the side of the ileum 10 cm from the ileocaecal valve (Figure

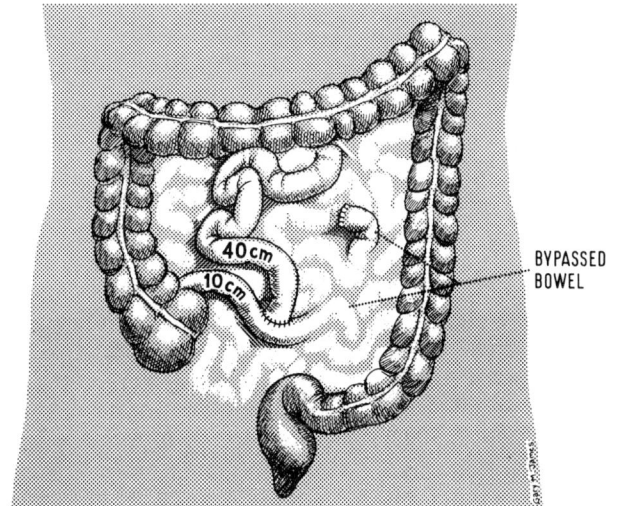

a

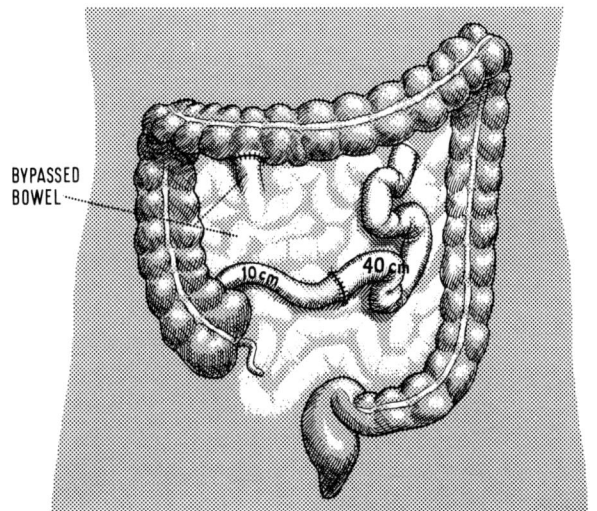

b

Fig. 8.73   (a) End-to-side jejuno-ileal bypass (Payne procedure). (b) End-to-end jejuno-ileal bypass (Scott procedure).

8.73a). The distal end of the transected jejunum is closed and tethered to prevent intussusception. More recently, attempts have been made to minimize postoperative bile salt depletion and catharsis by anastomosing this distal segment to the gallbladder as a cholecystenterostomy. Scott *et al.*[13] believe a more predictable weight loss is achieved by an end-to-end jejuno-ileal bypass, in which the proximal end of transected jejunum is anastomosed end-to-end to the transected terminal ileum (Figure 8.73b). In this procedure, the bypassed jejunum is closed at the proximal end as before and the distal end of the bypassed segment is drained by end-to-side anastomosis to the sigmoid or transverse colon.

Results of jejuno-ileal bypass

Very few patients with gross obesity achieve a weight loss of 18 kg (40 lb) or more on conservative treatment. Even this weight loss is small compared with the gross obesity for which jejuno-ileal bypass may be considered. Conservative treatment of gross obesity rarely achieves permanent weight reduction of sufficient degree to result in normal risk levels for conditions such as ischaemic heart disease and diabetes. Provided that the patient has been properly selected and the operation accurately performed, then the weight loss following jejuno-ileal bypass is both large and permanent.

Weight loss begins as soon as the immediate postoperative ileus resolves, and is most rapid in the early months after surgery. The total amount of weight which will be lost is difficult to predict; however, in general, the heavier the preoperative weight, the faster the rate of postoperative weight loss will be.

The immediate postoperative consequences of jejuno-ileal bypass are very similar to those of the short bowel syndrome. Diarrhoea is almost invariable but the severity is surprisingly variable. Diarrhoea tends to be most severe in the first few weeks following surgery but is rarely an important problem by six to twelve months postoperatively provided that the functional segments have been accurately determined. At operation, it is important to measure and mark the proposed functional segments immediately on gaining access to the peritoneum and before much handling of the small intestine has occurred, otherwise the subsequent contraction of bowel will result in incorrect estimation of the lengths to be used. Similarly, attempts at immediately preoperative weight reduction by starvation are to be avoided as similar errors in measurement may occur in the hypotonic and

hypoplastic bowel of the fasting subject.

The rate of weight loss usually begins to decline approximately six months after jejuno-ileal bypass but continues at a reduced rate for a further eighteen months to two years. By two years the weight lost is usually maximal and thereafter there is often a slow rise before reaching a plateau. This small rise can usually be controlled by mild dietary restriction even though preoperative dietary treatment had failed. The reasons for this cessation of weight loss are interesting, complex and insufficiently understood. There is no doubt that the malabsorption and steatorrhoea decrease with time. This may be related to the adaptive response of the small intestinal mucosa in the functioning (non-bypassed) segments,[2] a response which is well recorded in the small intestinal mucosa after massive intestinal resections.[5] The importance in quantitative terms of any functional (absorptive) adaptation is uncertain. But there can be no doubt that changes in oral food intake play an important role in weight loss.[10] It was noted early[3] that food intake is considerably decreased following jejuno-ileal bypass compared with the preoperative state in grossly obese subjects. This decreased intake far outlives any perioperative discomfort associated with eating. This is probably a true alteration in appetite or satiety, particularly since not only does food intake decrease but taste preferences also change towards a more normal pattern. Although this decreased food intake is prolonged, there is an upward trend after about two years. However, food intake does not again reach preoperative levels. The timing of the phenomenon tends to suggest that increasing intake may play a part in the arrest and slight reversal of the weight loss described above.

Anorexia is common in the months following jejuno-ileal bypass and may progress to nausea. In more extreme cases, vomiting may occur which may, when severe or prolonged, be a forerunner of metabolic complications, particularly 'bypass hepatitis'. Such patients tend to be those who are losing weight at the fastest rates. The optimal rate of weight loss in the first year should be less than 4.5 kg (10 lb)/month. If the rate of weight loss is significantly in excess of this, it is desirable to intervene with nutritional support before evidence of hepatic impairment becomes manifest.

Properly selected patients achieving normal weights after bypass may be expected to achieve economic and social rehabilitation. In addition to weight loss, there is a significant and permanent decrease in serum lipids and a decrease in arterial blood pressure.

Postoperative management

Fluid and electrolyte losses due to diarrhoea are considerable in the first few months following surgery, hence prophylactic supplements are essential. Provided patient compliance is good, normal electrolyte status can be maintained with supplements of potassium, magnesium and calcium. Potassium is best tolerated as effervescent potassium chloride. Magnesium is better taken as a parenteral dose at weekly intervals in the first few months to avoid osmotic catharsis. Calcium may be taken alone or incorporated in antidiarrhoeal mixtures (such as aromatic chalk with opium mixture) or in combination with vitamin D. Calcium supplements may also be important in preventing renal calculi as discussed later. Early use of vitamin D is desirable to promote calcium absorption and as prophylaxis against metabolic bone disease which can develop early and subclinically. However, the need for high potency vitamin D derivatives such as 1α-hydroxycholecalciferol has been questioned.[11]

Complications

All surgical procedures have an associated morbidity. Many metabolic sequelae have been described following jejuno-ileal bypass. Although some authors have included steatorrhoea or malabsorption in their data as part of the complications, this can hardly be regarded as a complication since it occurs by design. However, consequences of malabsorption such as deficiencies in fat-soluble vitamins can be fairly described as complications. Such deficiencies should not be allowed to develop as a result of an elective procedure.

Although the number of complications described in the literature is large, many of these only occur rarely, e.g. interstitial nephritis. Nevertheless, it can be extremely difficult from the literature to estimate the frequency with which some complications occur. This may reflect regional differences. For example, nephrolithiasis seems common in North America, but relatively rare in Scandinavia. Other complications, such as the varying incidence of thromboembolism or severe electrolyte disturbance, must reflect to some extent the quality of postoperative care.

The data presented in Table 8.35 are a composite of many published series and give an assessment of the lowest and highest rates which may be expected for the commoner or more serious complications listed.

Table 8.35 Complications of jejuno-ileal bypass.

Complication	Range of incidence
Direct surgical mortality	2–6%
Perioperative morbidity (e.g. thromboembolism)	4–13%
Renal and ureteric calculi	3–10%
Hepatic failure	0–14% (probably approximately 4%)
Arthralgia	7–15%
Abdominal distension ± pseudo-obstructive syndromes	13–100%
Electrolyte disturbance	Up to 80%
Metabolic acidosis	13–80%
Metabolic bone disease	Uncertain because of varied diagnostic criteria

Perioperative morbidity, even in the grossly obese, can be minimized by the usual precautions including *pre*operative physiotherapy, early mobilization and the judicious use of prophylactic subcutaneous heparin.

Renal calculi

Deaths from renal failure resulting from obstructive uropathy are well described. Ureteric calculi are usually oxalate in composition. Hyperoxaluria occurs following jejuno-ileal bypass, as with severe steatorrhoea of any cause. Its aetiology is multifactorial but may be related in part to increased absorption by the colonic mucosa and to the increased availability of oxalate for absorption as a consequence of steatorrhoea (see p. 441). An increased calcium intake is desirable following jejuno-ileal bypass to help prevent this increased oxalate absorption.

Poor hydration in the presence of diarrhoea, and postoperative urinary tract infections related to unnecessary catheterization or poor catheter technique, may be contributory factors to the precipitation of urinary tract calculi. Good hydration is particularly important to minimize crystal-induced renal parenchymal damage.

Liver disease

Although the incidence of liver disease following jejuno-ileal bypass is relatively small, the mortality from this complication is so high that it is probably the major reason for the recent decline in the popularity of this procedure. Deaths occur from hepatic failure which may be the end-stage of a cirrhotic process occurring months or years after jejuno-ileal bypass, or as a consequence of an acute or subacute hepatitic

illness. This 'bypass hepatitis' is histologically indistinguishable from alcoholic liver disease but occurs in the absence of alcohol. The hepatitis tends to occur relatively early after jejuno-ileal bypass and seems to occur in those patients losing weight at an excessive rate, and is sometimes associated with continued nausea and vomiting. Apart from this, the first sign of serious hepatitic disease may be the appearance of jaundice, by which time restorative surgery is contraindicated. Hepatocellular enzymes are commonly raised in the serum following jejuno-ileal bypass in the absence of serious liver problems and cannot, therefore, be used as an indicator of impending hepatic disease.

Although the cause of this hepatitic illness is obscure, there is no doubt it can be ameliorated by nutritional support. If necessary this can be provided by the intravenous route. A similar syndrome in dogs following jejuno-ileal bypass can be prevented by antibiotic treatment. However, the similarity to the human counterpart may only be superficial – in humans the incidence of this complication is approximately 4% but in dogs the liver failure is almost universal within a few months of jejuno-ileal bypass.

The occurrence of liver disease has been regarded as an indication for the restoration of normal intestinal continuity. However, if a further operation is performed at the time of hepatic insufficiency as manifested by jaundice, then the mortality is unacceptably high. Surgery should therefore be delayed until the hepatic failure has been controlled by nutritional support. However, cirrhosis may develop insidiously and be detectable only by sequential liver biopsies.

Arthropathy

Arthralgia is more common than overt arthritis following jejuno-ileal bypass, but a true reactive arthritis is well described. The larger joints tend to be affected more commonly. The condition is rarely severe but has on occasions necessitated restoration of normal intestinal continuity. The arthritis is transitory and non-destructive, appearing in exacerbations and remissions which tend to peter out. Circulating immune complexes with gut-derived antigens have been suggested as a cause.

Dermatological complications

Some degree of alopecia is almost universal during the period of rapid weight loss. Deficiency states may be manifested as skin rashes.

The incidence of tender red papular or pustular lesions caused by a cutaneous vasculitis may have been underestimated in the literature. Occasionally erythema nodosum occurs. Provided there is no evidence of large vessel vasculitis or haematuria then symptomatic treatment is recommended and usually sufficient. Spontaneous resolution is the rule.

'Gas/bloat syndrome'

Abdominal distension is caused by gas in the bypassed small intestine and has a wide spectrum of severity. Abdominal bloating, often associated with discomfort or colicky abdominal pain, is common. At the opposite end of the spectrum, distension can be extreme with severe pain, vomiting and obstipation, and is caused by intestinal ileus, apparently due to bacterial colonization of the bypassed intestine.[2] This syndrome of pseudo-obstruction is common in advanced systemic sclerosis and is well described in other conditions associated with small bowel bacterial colonization such as small intestinal diverticulosis.[9] In the acute phase, rapid relief is obtained from oral antibiotics effective against anaerobic organisms such as metronidazole.

Metabolic bone disease
The incidence and severity of metabolic bone disease is controversial, perhaps because of the varying diagnostic criteria used in different studies. It would, perhaps, be surprising if some osteopenia did not occur and this may be compounded by the commonly found mild, non-ion gap, metabolic acidosis. Routine supplements of vitamin D are widely employed and monitoring of the serum calcium and alkaline phosphatase is recommended.

Other forms of radical surgical treatment for gross obesity

In the decade following the introduction of jejuno-ileal bypass, large numbers of operations were performed, particularly in North America. The incidence and severity of the metabolic complications soon became obvious, with the result that the popularity of the procedure has declined and other forms of radical surgical treatment for gross obesity have been developed. Some, such as pancreatic-biliary diversion, have not yet been sufficiently well documented to allow an objective assessment of their role to be made. Two, however, have gained a limited acceptance – jaw-wiring and gastric partitioning procedures.

Jaw-wiring

In this procedure the mandible is firmly fastened to the maxilla by means of plastic splints to prevent the ingestion of solid food. Liquid feeds are taken by straw. Weight loss can be small, depending on the volume and energy content of liquids taken. However, median weight losses of 25 kg at six months have been achieved.[12] The major advantage of the procedure is its simplicity. Vomiting can be hazardous, despite precautions. Regular removal and reapplication of the splint is essential for dental care. The default rate is high (17%) but the major drawback is the very high relapse rate (66%) when the splints are removed.

Gastric partitioning procedures

Gastric bypass as a treatment for gross obesity was introduced by Mason.[7] The gastric partitioning procedures currently in use are developed from this concept.

The operations are designed to prevent large dietary intakes by decreasing the gastric reservoir space. This may be achieved by partial gastric bypass or various partitioning procedures in which a small fundal pouch is created by suturing or stapling across the gastric body and creating only a small aperture from this pouch into the rest of the body and antrum. These procedures have the attraction of a much lower rate of metabolic complications compared with jejuno-ileal bypass. However, at least in some procedures, there is a high operative morbidity because the operation is technically more difficult than jejuno-ileal bypass in the grossly obese. The procedure has been dogged by mechanical problems such as obstruction at the stoma, disruption of staple lines and stomal dilatation. Vomiting is common in all effective gastroplasties and bile-induced oesophago-gastritis is a problem in some.

The weight loss achieved by gastric partitioning can be comparable in the early months to that after jejuno-ileal bypass. However, progressively increasing stomal dilatation and distension of the gastric reservoir have resulted almost uniformly in a significant reaccumulation of weight in the longer term.

The most recent development in this area is the vertical gastroplasty, bound or banded with non-absorbable mesh to prevent expansion of the stoma (Figure 8.74). Its introduction is too recent to enable an assessment of its long-term efficacy.[6]

Whereas jejuno-ileal bypass is a simple operation, the recent gastroplasties are technically less easy. Gastroplasty produces quite good

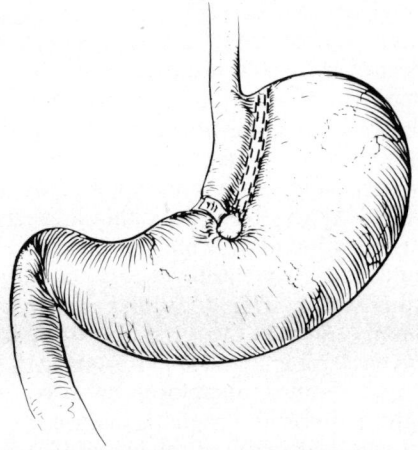

Fig. 8.74 Vertical banded gastroplasty. From Mason (1982),[6] with kind permission of the author and the editor of *Contemporary Surgery*.

weight loss in the short term but has been disappointing in the long term. In jejuno-ileal bypass, however, the weight loss is not only large but also permanent; however, the price of this operation is a high rate of metabolic complications.

REFERENCES

1   Barry, R. E., Chow, A. W. & Billesden, J. (1977) The role of intestinal microflora in colonic pseudoobstruction complicating jejuno-ileal bypass. *Gut*, **18**, 356–359.
2   Barry, R. E., Barisch, J., Bray, G. A. *et al.* (1977) Intestinal adaptation after jejunoileal bypass in man. *American Journal of Clinical Nutrition*, **30**, 32–42.
3   Bray, G. A., Barry, R. E., Benfield, J. R. *et al.* (1976) Intestinal bypass surgery for obesity decreases food intake and taste preferences. *American Journal of Clinical Nutrition*, **29**, 779–783.
4   Crisp, A. H., Kalucy, R. S., Pilkington, T. R. E. & Gazet, J.-C. (1977) Some psychosocial consequences of ileojejunal bypass surgery. *American Journal of Clinical Nutrition*, **30**, 109–119.
5   Dowling, R. H. (1976) Intestinal adaptation. In *12th Symposium on Advanced Medicine* (Ed.) Peters, D. K. pp. 251–261. London: Pitman Medical.
6   Mason, E. E. (1982) Evolution of gastric reduction for obesity. *Contemporary Surgery*, **20**, 17–23.
7   Mason, E. E. & Ito, C. (1967) Gastric bypass in obesity. *Surgical Clinics of North America*, **47**, 1345–1357.
8   Payne, J. H. & De Wind, L. T. (1969) Surgical treatment of obesity. *American Journal of Surgery*, **118**, 141–147.
9   Phillips, J. H. C. (1953) Jejunal diverticulosis: some clinical aspects. *British Journal of Surgery*, **40**, 350–354.
10 Pilkington, T. R. E., Gazet, J. C., Ang, L. *et al.* (1976) Explanations for weight loss after jejunoileal bypass in gross obesity. *British Medical Journal*, **i**, 1504–1505.
11 Rickers, H., Christiansen, C., Balslev, I. *et al.* (1983) Vitamin D and bone mineral content after intestinal bypass operation for obesity. *Gut*, **24**, 67–72.
12 Rodgers, S., Burnet, R., Goss, A. *et al.* (1977) Jaw wiring in the treatment of obesity. *Lancet*, **i**, 1221–1222.
13 Scott, H. W., Law, D. H. & Sandstead, H. H. (1970) Jejunoileal shunt in surgical treatment of morbid obesity. *Annals of Surgery*, **171**, 770–782.

SHORT GUT SYNDROME

Removal of part or all of the intestine may be necessitated by trauma or diseases such as regional enteritis, mesenteric vascular occlusion, mechanical obstruction with bowel infarction, and malignant tumour. While resection of short segments is usually well tolerated without any detectable consequences, more extensive resections may cause specific nutritional disturbances, or may be life-threatening if an alternate method of nutrition is not provided.

The outcome after intestinal resection will depend on the extent of the resection, the loss or preservation of the terminal ileum which has specific absorptive functions, the function of the remaining small bowel and preservation of the ileocaecal valve, and the ability of the shortened intestine to undergo morphological and functional adaptation.

Extent of resection

The length of the normal small intestine is quite variable. Moreover, great differences in length are found with different methods of measurement (Table 8.36). While the average length of the jejunoileum is 657 cm at autopsy (with loss of tone of smooth muscle), only 261 cm have been measured on peroral intubation due to telescoping of the intestine around tubing. Irrespective of the differences in mean length obtained by different methods, the range in each study is considerable (Table 8.36). Thus, knowledge of the length of the resected segment may not be meaningful in many instances. It is the length of the remaining intestine that is of importance, and this may be more informative if also expressed as a percentage of the original total length of small bowel.

In 1935, Haymond reviewed 257 cases of massive intestinal resection and concluded that a 33% resection of the small bowel is tolerated well, and that 50% was the limit of safety with respect to maintaining adequate nutrition from oral intake. Patients with more extensive resection have malabsorption problems; if less than 25% of small bowel remains, special management is required.

Area resected

The total surface area of the small bowel is estimated to be about 100 m[2].[66] Since the surface area decreases markedly from the proximal to the distal end, almost half of the total mucosal surface area is found in the proximal quarter of the small intestine. The jejunum is particularly important for the absorption of iron, calcium and folic acid. However, the ileum can absorb what is normally absorbed in the upper small bowel, and acts as a large functional reserve area if substances have escaped absorption more proximally. There is not a similar reserve area to take over ileal function after resection. Special transport mechanisms for active absorption of bile salts and vitamin B_{12} are localized in the ileum. Relatively small resections (50–80 cm) involving the ileum may therefore result in significant malabsorption of vitamin B_{12} and bile acids. Ileal resections interrupt the enterohepatic circulation of bile salts, and may result in several disturbances:

1 Bile acids can alter colonic water and electrolyte transport, reducing absorption or even stimulating secretion, and cause diarrhoea (bile acid diarrhoea).

2 If bile acid loss into the colon exceeds the capacity of the liver for accelerated bile acid synthesis, depletion of the bile acid pool will impair micellar fat absorption in the small bowel, resulting in steatorrhoea. This usually occurs with the loss of 100 cm or more of terminal ileum.[38]

3 Enhanced oxalate absorption in the colon, due to an increase in oxalate solubility and/or mucosal permeability caused by the abnormal presence of bile acids and long chain fatty acids, may result in hyperoxaluric urolithiasis.[22]

4 Bile may be lithogenic because of the decreased bile acid pool, and the incidence of gallstones appears to be significantly increased in these patients.[26]

Table 8.36   Length of the small intestine (jejunum and ileum).

Method	Mean length (cm)	Range (cm)	Number of observations	References
Measured with ruler at autopsy	657	305–1220	502	Treaves;[75] Lamb;[47] Dreike;[27] Bryant;[11] Underhill[77]
Measured with ruler during abdominal surgery	643	400–846	32	Backman & Hallberg[6]
	421	320–521	6	Cook & Carruthers[17]
Measured by peroral intubation	261	206–329	10	Hirsch *et al.*[37]

Function of the remaining bowel

It is obvious that concomitant disease of the remaining small bowel may lead to severe malabsorption and diarrhoea, even if the length of the remaining intestine would otherwise have been expected to provide normal absorption. Examples are the short bowel syndrome in Crohn's disease following multiple resections with active disease in the remaining bowel, or in scleroderma after resection of severely dilated segments with subsequent progression of the disease. Any concomitant disease such as chronic liver disease with some degree of portal hypertension or right-sided heart failure may be detrimental for a patient with intestinal resection. Mild lactose intolerance latent before resection may contribute to the diarrhoea following resection.

Functional integrity of the remaining bowel is also of importance, e.g., rapid transit may aggravate a malabsorptive state or even cause its manifestation. Diarrhoea seems to be less of a problem in patients in whom the ileocaecal valve is preserved. The reason for this may be protection from bacterial overgrowth of the colon by the valve. Bacterial overgrowth may cause diarrhoea by enhancing bile acid loss due to deconjugation and dehydroxylation.[38] Bacterial metabolism of vitamin B_{12} may also accelerate the development of deficiency of the vitamin.

A hemicolectomy (as is often required for Crohn's disease) or a total colectomy may significantly influence the outcome after small bowel resection. The absorptive capacity of the colon has probably long been underestimated. The normal colon is able to absorb up to 6 l of fluid/day.[20] Even in the setting of abnormal delivery of nutrients to the colon, significant absorption of short chain fatty acids (metabolic products of unabsorbed carbohydrates) may take place before osmotic diarrhoea occurs.[9] It has in fact been recognized that following small bowel resection, stool volume and frequency depend on the length of the remaining colon rather than the remaining small intestine.[14,19]

Adaptation

Morphological adaptation of the remaining small bowel

Morphological adaptation is difficult to investigate in man since it is almost impossible to perform the necessary studies for technical and ethical reasons. The effects of small bowel resection have, however, been studied extensively in various animal models, particularly the rat. Using morphometric methods, Dowling and Booth[25] showed that resection of the proximal and mid-small bowel results in a true increase in villous size in the remaining ileum. Hyperplasia of the epithelial cells with expansion of the proliferative zone out of the crypts occurs within two days following resection.[56] Following injection of tritiated thymidine, a significantly increased activity of DNA synthesis was found in the elongated crypts of rats with resection when compared with control animals. This increased cell proliferation probably leads to an absolute increase in number of enterocytes. However, because the life span of individual cells may be reduced by the increased turnover, it is not clear whether all cells become functionally mature and optimally subserve absorption.

Functional adaptation

Following extensive small bowel resection (less than 25% of the small intestine remaining), patients often can be weaned off intravenous hyperalimentation after prolonged periods of time. An improvement in nutrient absorption over months has been described.[84] Improved glucose absorption per unit length of jejunum has been suggested from follow-up studies using intestinal perfusion techniques.[24] On X-ray studies, an increase in calibre and length of the remaining small bowel may be observed after massive resection (Figure 8.75).[76]

Mechanisms of adaptation

From animal studies, several mechanisms have been suggested to mediate adaptation following small bowel resection.

Luminal nutrients. There is an impressive body of evidence suggesting that luminal nutrients are a major factor in intestinal adaptation after resection. Feldman *et al.*[30] showed that jejunectomized dogs developed mucosal hyperplasia and improved glucose absorption in the remaining ileum only if fed orally. Dogs that were fed intravenously and remained well nourished showed mucosal hypoplasia in the remaining ileum six weeks after resection. The role of high nutrient concentration is also obvious from experiments in rats in which, following ileojejunal transposition without resection, mucosal hyperplasia developed in the ileum while the transpositioned jejunum shows villous atrophy.[24] Likewise, mucosal hypoplasia has been observed in bypassed segments of small bowel; this phenomenon is fully reversible when the bypassed segment is put back into the

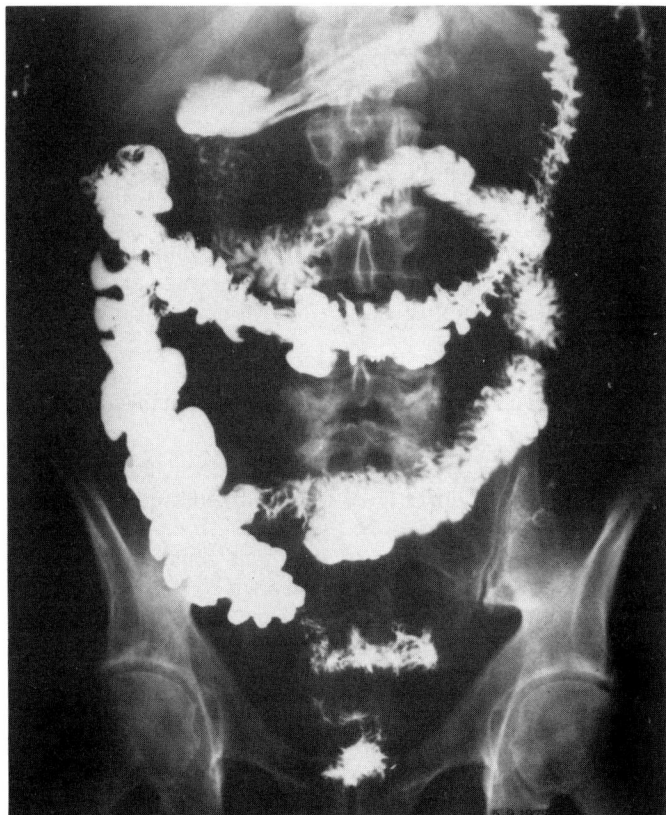

Fig. 8.75 Barium meal in a patient 12 months after massive small bowel resection for infarction due to mesenteric vein thrombosis. While barium is still in the stomach, some barium has already reached the rectum. The remaining loop of small bowel (about 40 cm in length) shows an increase in mucosal folds and dilation indicating adaptation with mucosal hyperplasia.

stream of luminal contents. Whether chyme has such an important trophic effect in humans has been questioned by Tomkins *et al.*,[74] since no evidence of widespread mucosal atrophy was found in two patients in whom a segment of intestine had been bypassed for several years. Mucosal atrophy, however, is the rule in ileal bladders, but this may be due either to the absence of chyme or to a direct effect of urine.[34]

It is also uncertain whether the nutrients themselves cause mucosal hyperplasia in the remaining gut, or whether the associated presence of stimulated bile and pancreatic secretions play a major role. Bile and pancreatic juice, if diverted into the ileum, stimulate mucosal growth even in the absence of chyme.[2] Thus, a trophic effect of bile acids and possibly pancreatic enzymes appears likely.

Endocrine factors. When amino acids are infused into the ileum of rats, mucosal hyperplasia occurs not only in the ileum, but also in the duodenum and proximal jejunum.[51] Since local luminal contact cannot explain these effects, a hormonal mechanism has been postulated. The trophic effects of gastrin on the intestinal tract have been well documented;[42]

however, high exogenous doses are necessary to obtain these changes. It is not clear whether circulating gastrin levels, which have been found to be elevated after intestinal resection (see below), are high enough to cause such changes. Moreover, in antrectomized rats, small bowel resection leads to mucosal growth in the remaining small intestine (shown by an increase in total DNA content), while serum gastrin concentration remains unchanged.[21] Since the pancreas shows a similar response (increased weight and DNA content), a humoral factor other than gastrin is postulated as the responsible 'enterotrophin'.[23]

Marked hypertrophy of the small intestine, particularly the jejunum, has been described in a patient with an enteroglucagonoma; the morphological changes were reversible after tumour resection.[33] In rats with a 75% small bowel exclusion, oral feeding resulted in significantly higher plasma enteroglucagon levels and crypt cell production rate in the excluded segment than did intravenous feeding.[64] Thus, it appears likely that enteroglucagon may be a mediator of adaptive responses. Cholecystokinin has also been implicated as a stimulus for mucosal growth,[44,88] while the role of secretin is uncertain.[29] In summary, numerous peptides have been shown to exert trophic effects on gastro-intestinal tissues. In order to identify the 'enterotrophin,' it may be necessary to show that levels of that peptide increase endogenously to levels sufficient to produce the effects caused by exogenous administration.[43]

Colonic adaptation

In rats, small bowel resection leads to cell proliferation and increased water and NaCl absorption in the colon.[55,78] Patients with small bowel resection absorb more calcium when the colon is preserved, and it has been suggested that colonic calcium absorption may be induced as an adaptive response.[39] In the rat colon, $1,25(OH)_2$ vitamin D_3 can induce active calcium absorption.[49]

Gastric hypersecretion following small bowel resection

Enhanced gastric acid secretion has been recognized in about 50% of patients with extensive small bowel resection, particularly during the postoperative period.[1,85] This phenomenon has been reproduced in animal models using rats, dogs, and rhesus monkeys.[13,54,83] Based on experimental and clinical observations, several explanations have been presented. The first is that clearance of gastrin from the circulation may be delayed, since there is some evidence that the small bowel extracts significant amounts of gastrin from the circulation.[7,73] Alternatively, as both fasting and meal-stimulated serum gastrin levels may be elevated in patients after resection, a humoral inhibitor of gastrin release may have been lost. This is at least in part supported by the observation that the increase in acid output after intestinal resection is less in dogs if antrectomy precedes the resection than after resection alone.[48] Little is known about the changes in plasma levels of other inhibitory hormones or hormone-like agents such as somatostatin and gastric inhibitory polypeptide (GIP). These two agents suppress gastric acid secretion, and reduction of their circulating levels could explain gastric acid hypersecretion. However, the opposite was found in the rhesus monkey where GIP was elevated following 50% resection.[54]

A morphological correlate for the finding of increased gastric acid secretion has been described by Seelig, Winborn and Weser,[68,69] who, while studying gastric mucosal cell kinetics, found a hyperplastic response with increased numbers of parietal, chief, and mucous cells. The involvement of peptic cells in the hyperplastic response suggests that gastrin may not be solely responsible for the gastric hyperplasia.

Completely different results were found in a recent study in dogs in which massive small bowel resection lead to gastric hyposecretion; acid secretion was measured by intragastric titration in the totally innervated stomach.[67] The discrepancy between this study and the ones listed above cannot be reconciled at the present time.

Clinical features and laboratory findings

Diarrhoea

During the first days and weeks after resection, watery diarrhoea is prominent, and daily stool volumes may be as high as 10 l.[8] Dehydration, electrolyte losses and acid base disturbances may pose severe problems.

Several mechanisms are responsible for diarrhoea following small bowel resection. First, due to significant loss of absorptive surface, the approximately 8–9 l of fluid that enter the jejunum every day overwhelm the transport capacity of the remaining small intestine, and a large fluid load is spilled into the colon. The colon has a high reserve capacity (it can absorb 6 l/day of an isotonic electrolyte solution);[20] however, many patients have had an additional resection of part or even all of their colon and therefore do not benefit from this compensating action of the large intestine. Second, dietary constituents that are usually completely absorbed in the small bowel are delivered to the colon. Carbohydrates may then be metabolized to short chain fatty acids by colonic bacteria, and cause diarrhoea by virtue of a high osmolar load and a low pH; this type of osmotic diarrhoea is otherwise seen in disaccharidase deficiency or lactulose therapy. Long chain fatty acids may enter the colon because of incomplete fat absorption, and by themselves may inhibit colonic absorption, particularly if hydroxylated by colonic bacteria.[4,71] Third, bile acids lost into the colon, particularly dihydroxy bile acids, are known to alter colonic absorptive function; bile acid-induced colonic secretion may be an additional factor.[52] Bile acid diarrhoea and steatorrhoea may also result from bacterial overgrowth of the remaining bowel due to loss of the ileocaecal valve. Finally, gastric hypersecretion may aggravate the diarrhoea.

Malabsorption

The malabsorption syndrome following small bowel resection may consist of a wide variety of symptoms including night blindness, tetany, osteomalacia, macrocytic anaemia, coagulopathy, neuropathy, and dermatitis due to zinc deficiency.

Other complications

D-lactic acidosis has been reported in a few patients with short gut syndrome. This is presumably due to colonic overgrowth of lactobacillus as a result of the high carbohydrate delivery to the colon which offers increased substrates for D-lactate production by colonic bacteria.[65]

Laboratory results

Impaired absorption of nutrients, vitamins, minerals and trace elements will result in deficiency states that are reflected by appropriate laboratory tests similar to other malabsorptive diseases that reduce mucosal surface area (such as coeliac disease). For assessing intestinal function the spectrum of tests may include tolerance tests, breath tests, balance studies and intubation techniques.[50] A checklist of laboratory tests and relevant results is given in Table 8.37.

Management

Postoperative period

During the postoperative period, meticulous parenteral fluid and electrolyte replacement is required to compensate for the losses associated with the voluminous watery diarrhoea. Intravenous alimentation is of greatest importance. All essential nutrients, dissolved in a readily tolerated fluid volume (2000–3500 ml/day), are administered slowly into a high flow vessel, usually the superior vena cava. Adequate energy is provided by sugar (glucose 20–50 g/dl) and fat (soybean oil [Intralipid] 10 g/dl). Amino acid mixtures provide nitrogen, and for optimal positive nitrogen balance, each gram of nitrogen needs to be given with 600–1000 kJ (150–250 kcal) in glucose and fat.

Oral feeding

Oral feeding will initially aggravate the diarrhoea and must therefore be resumed gradually and with great care. Since the rate of gastric emptying is positively correlated with intragastric volume, frequent meals of small size will help optimally utilize the remaining absorptive capacity of the small bowel. The patient should eat at least every two hours; ideally the patient should eat constantly at a very slow rate. Over the following days and weeks, the size of the meals is gradually increased. From dietary surveys later in the course of this condition, it is clear that many patients maintain their normal body weight by greatly increasing their energy intake.[14] Chemically defined liquid diets may be given early in the course of oral feeding.[79,87] However, the high osmolality of these preparations (often 800–900 mosmol/kg) may cause

Table 8.37 Checklist for laboratory tests and relevant findings in patients after small bowel resection.

Test	What to look for	Comments and management (other than replacement)
Complete blood count and blood chemistry	Anaemia, low serum iron and ferritin	
	Macrocytosis, low serum vitamin B_{12} and folate	
	Hypocalcaemia	Adequacy of calcium and vitamin D replacement may be judged from bone density measurements every 6 to 12 months
	Hypomagnesaemia	
	Hypokalaemia, metabolic acidosis	High faecal K and HCO_3 losses in response to high electrical gradient and low pH in colon
	Hypoproteinaemia	Sign of severe malnutrition, may indicate need for parenteral nutrition
	Low serum vitamin A (carotene) Prolonged prothrombin time Low serum zinc and copper	
Lactose tolerance test	Lactose intolerance	Lactose free diet
Quantitative stool collection	24-hour stool volume and daily faecal potassium loss	Provide replacement in excess of losses
	24-hour stool fat	MCT diet if steatorrhea severe
Urinary oxalate	Hyperoxaluria (upper limit of normal is 40 mg/day)	
Gastric acid analysis	Acid hypersecretion Hypergastrinaemia	H_2-antagonists

osmotic diarrhoea, and the bad taste is often poorly tolerated over prolonged periods of time. In a dilute form, these elemental diets may be administered at a slow rate via an intraduodenal or jejunal feeding tube, which also has been used successfully in paediatric patients.[60] Elemental diets with lower osmolality containing oligopeptides (rather than bad-tasting individual amino acids) are more promising. These di- and tri-peptides do not require hydrolysis prior to absorption. Total protein supplements may also be given and a number of preparations are commercially available.

Reduction of fat intake (down to 40 g/day) may significantly lower the stool volume in patients with small bowel resection if diarrhoea is a significant problem.[5,10,82] However, not all studies have supported this concept. Simko[70] showed that a high fat diet resulted in less diarrhoea in a patient with short gut syndrome. In a randomized study with cross-over design, Woolf et al.[86] did not find any difference in stool weight when eight patients were put on either a high-carbohydrate or high-fat diet. Hence, they did not recommend dietary restrictions in these patients.

Medium chain triglyceride (MCT) supplementation is a very rational dietary manipulation which is quite successful if tolerated by the patient.[8,84] Unfortunately, many patients will not comply with such a regimen because of the bad taste and the difficulties in cooking appetizing meals using MCT. Lactose tolerance should be evaluated, for lactose intolerance may have been latent prior to resection, and may subsequently contribute to osmotic diarrhoea. If hyperoxaluria is present (as shown by repeated analysis of 24-hour collections of urine during follow-up, with an upper limit of normal of 40 mg/24 h), high oxalate foods such as rhubarb, spinach, tea and chocolate need to be avoided.[22]

While awaiting intestinal adaptation in patients with significant fluid and electrolyte losses, sugar and salt solutions of the type which formed a major advance in the treatment of Asiatic cholera[58] may be helpful. These isotonic solutions are physiologically the most readily absorbed, contain 110 mmol/l NaCl and 80 mmol/l glucose, and are easily prepared by the patient himself. They may be given as oral supplementation in patients in whom replacement of fluid and electrolytes is more of a problem than satisfying the nutritional requirements.[18] In some patients, glucose electrolyte solutions may fail to provide a positive fluid and salt balance.[31] A more promising approach is the use of glucose polymers. These polymers consist of linear chains of four to ten glucose molecules attached by α-1,4-glucosidic bonds (average molecular weight of 1000), and are available as Caloreen in the UK and as Polycose in the USA. They are obtained from hydrolysis of cornstarch. Hydrolysis of glucose polymer in the intestine is so rapid that corresponding amounts of free glucose and glucose polymer lead to identical rises in blood sugar in healthy volunteers.[62] The use of glucose polymer electrolyte solutions allows administration of large amounts of glucose and salt while maintaining isotonicity of the solution. We have successfully used the following solution: glucose polymer 40 mmol/l, NaCl 90 mmol/l, $NaHCO_3$ 30 mmol, KCl 15 mmol/l, with an osmolality of 290 mosml/kg.[46] Griffin et al.[35] have also reported success in one such patient.

In the setting of a bypassed colon with a mucous fistula, Rodgers et al.[61] have successfully used instillation of an electrolyte solution into the otherwise unused colon for fluid and salt repletion.

Specific replacements
Some specific replacements will be required even after adequate energy intake by mouth has been achieved following a prolonged process of adaptation. Calcium and vitamin D replacement is almost always necessary to treat or prevent deficiency.[15,16] Magnesium replacement will also be required by most patients. If deficiency has developed, initial parenteral replacement should be given (e.g., 24 mmol of magnesium intramuscularly, daily for three days). It may also be necessary to supplement other fat-soluble vitamins (A, E, and K). Vitamin B_{12} should be given parenterally at regular intervals.

Drug treatment
Antimotility drugs are of great importance since prolongation of the transit time in the shortened bowel will increase the contact time of chyme with the mucosa and net absorption per unit surface area may be enhanced. Opiates have remained the drugs of choice, and initially parenteral codeine administration may be necessary. Oral agents should be tried alone or in combination, and these include loperamide, diphenoxylate, paregoric, and anticholinergics. If oral anticholinergics are not effective, parenteral self-administration may be successful in selected patients.[12]

In patients with ileal resection in whom bile acid-induced diarrhoea is causing significant problems, cholestyramine may be employed to bind bile acids to prevent their effect on the colon. While this often improves or stops the diarrhoea, steatorrhoea may be enhanced due to bile acid pool depletion. Once bound to the drug, bile acids are not available for micelle formation to subserve fat absorption.

If bacterial overgrowth is found (with a colony count in intestinal aspirate of more than 10^6/ml) or suspected, antibiotic treatment should be given (e.g. tetracyclines, lincomycin). On an empirical basis, pancreatic enzymes may be prescribed in an attempt to improve fat absorption.[80]

Prolonged parenteral nutrition
Transition period while intestinal adaptation is awaited. Considering the length of the remaining small bowel and anticipating adaptation, parenteral nutrition may appear necessary for several months or even for a year or two. In this situation, parenteral hyperalimentation may be planned on an outpatient basis. The patient may come to the hospital to get intravenous hyperalimentation over a period of several hours on alternate days (or daily if necessary). Solutions are administered either via an indwelling superior vena cava catheter, or an arteriovenous fistula (as is used for haemodialysis) with peripheral puncture and insertion of a venous cannula performed on each visit. Disadvantages of the arteriovenous fistula are the irritation of the venous wall by the highly concentrated infusates despite high flow, and the fact that it may be surgically difficult to construct the fistula. On a single visit, some 17 000 kJ (4000 kcal) may be given consisting of glucose, intralipid, and amino acids. Vitamins and trace elements are added as required. Simultaneous insulin administration may be necessary to avoid hyperglycaemia and a loss of energy due to glycosuria. In most patients, it will be possible to increase gradually the interval between visits for hyperalimentation. Maintenance of a normal, or at least acceptable, body weight should be the parameter on which the duration of intervals between visits should be determined. This is a good challenge for the patient to direct his utmost efforts toward improvement of his oral nutrition. If he maintains his body weight on oral feeding and supportive drug therapy, the programme of parenteral nutrition can be discontinued and the superior vena cava catheter can be removed or the arteriovenous fistula closed.

Permanent parenteral nutrition at home. If total or almost total enterectomy has been performed, plans for life-long intravenous alimentation should be made soon after surgery. This means a home treatment programme, and the number of patients leading an almost normal life with an 'artificial gut' is steadily increasing. The patient needs a superior vena cava or right atrial catheter that is brought out through the skin after a sufficient length of subcutaneous tunnelling. Correct surgical anchoring of the catheter is important, and so is the subsequent care of the area where the skin is penetrated. The patient needs to undergo careful instruction and must gather sufficient experience under supervision. However, a certain degree of intelligence, insight, technical understanding, physical fitness and manual dexterity is necessary and must be provided by the patient or by another person who is constantly available to the patient at home. The formula for the composition of the infusates has been described in detail.[28,41,59] A peristaltic pump is used for administration.

All nutrients, minerals, vitamins, and trace elements are provided in the infusate. A large body of experience has been gathered, sometimes on the basis of deficiency conditions that were practically unknown before the era of long-term parenteral alimentation. Examples are deficiency of zinc, copper, and essential fatty acids.

Surgical treatment of the short bowel syndrome
Reversal of a short segment (9–14 cm) of small bowel has been used in some cases, the rationale being an attempt to slow transit of chyme by the antiperistaltic segment creating a low grade obstruction.[57, 63] However, it is this author's impression that the risks of such intervention outweigh the possible benefits. Risks and disadvantages are the operative mortality, loss of surface at the anastomosis, stagnant loop syndrome, and operative morbidity which includes anastomotic leak, complete obstruction, and infarction of the reversed segment.

Treatment of other associated problems
Gastric hypersecretion early after resection with losses of 4–5 l of gastric juice (via nasogastric suction or gastrotomy tube) is not uncommon, and needs to be replaced diligently in parenteral therapy.[84] However, peptic ulcer disease and its complications rarely cause serious problems. H_2-receptor blockers may be preferred in this situation, since antacids may themselves increase or cause diarrhoea.[3,40] Ulcer surgery (no matter what method) should be avoided under all circumstances, since any of these surgical procedures may reduce the absorptive capacity of the upper small bowel and worsen

diarrhoea because of dumping, motility changes, and impaired mixing. Even in the rare situation of a bleeding ulcer, prolonged conservative treatment should be employed.

ACKNOWLEDGEMENTS

This work was supported by Grant Number 5-R01-AM28390-03 from the National Institute of Arthritis, Metabolism and Digestive Diseases, and Grant Number 5-M01-RR-00633 from the General Clinical Research Center.

REFERENCES

1 Aber, G. M., Ashton, F., Carmalt, M. H. B. & White-head, T. P. (1967) Gastric hypersecretion following massive small bowel resection in man. *American Journal of Digestive Diseases*, **12**, 785–794.
2 Altman, G. G. (1971) Influence of bile and pancreatic secretions on the size of the intestinal villi in the rat. *American Journal of Anatomy*, **132**, 167–178.
3 Aly, A., Barany, F., Kollberg, B. *et al.* (1980) Effect of an H_2-receptor blocking agent on diarrhoeas after extensive small bowel resection in Crohn's disease. *Acta Medica Scandinavica*, **207**, 119–122.
4 Ammon, H. V. & Phillips, S. F. (1973) Inhibition of colonic water and electrolyte absorption by fatty acids in man. *Gastroenterology*, **65**, 744–749.
5 Anderson, H., Isaksson, B. & Sjogren, B. (1974) Fat-reduced diet in the symptomatic treatment of small bowel disease. Metabolic studies in patients with Crohn's disease and in other patients subjected to ileal resection. *Gut*, **15**, 351–359.
6 Backman, L. & Hallberg, D. (1974) Small-intestinal length. An intraoperative study in obesity. *Acta Chirurgica Scandinavica*, **140**, 57–63.
7 Becker, H. D., Reeder, D. D. & Thompson, J. C. (1973) Extraction of circulating endogenous gastrin by the small bowel. *Gastroenterology*, **65**, 903–906.
8 Bochenek, W., Rodgers, J. B. & Balint, J. A. (1970) Effects of changes in dietary lipids on intestinal fluid loss in the short bowel syndrome. *Annals of Internal Medicine*, **72**, 205–213.
9 Bond, J. H. & Levitt, M. D. (1976) Fate of soluble carbohydrate in the colon of rats and man. *Journal of Clinical Investigation*, **57**, 1158–1164.
10 Booth, C. C., MacIntyre, I. & Mollin, D. L. (1964) Nutritional problems associated with extensive lesions of the distal small intestine in man. *Quarterly Journal of Medicine*, **131**, 401–420.
11 Bryant, J. (1924) Observations upon the growth and length of the human intestine. *American Journal of Medical Sciences*, **167**, 499–520.
12 Cameron, J. L., Gayler, B. W. & Hendrix, T. R. (1976) The use of intramuscular propantheline in the short bowel syndrome. *Johns Hopkins Medical Journal*, **138**, 91–95.
13 Caridis, D. T., Roberts, M. & Smith, G. (1969) The effect of small bowel resection on gastric acid secretion in the rat. *Surgery*, **65**, 292–297.
14 Compston, J. E. & Creamer, B. (1977) The consequences of small intestinal resection. *Quarterly Journal of Medicine*, **46**, 485–497.
15 Compston, J. E. & Creamer, B. (1977) Plasma levels and intestinal absorption of 25-hydroxyvitamin D in patients with small bowel resection. *Gut*, **18**, 171–175.
16 Compston, J. E., Horton, L. W. L., Ayers, A. B. *et al.* (1978) Osteomalacia after small-intestinal resection.

Lancet, **i**, 9–12.
17 Cook, G. C. & Carruthers, R. H. (1974) Reaction of human small intestine to an intraluminal tube and its importance in jejunal perfusion studies. *Gut*, **15**, 545–548.
18 Crow, R. M. & Meyer, G. W. (1978) 'Cholera solution' in short bowel syndrome. *Southern Medical Journal*, **71**, 1303–1304.
19 Cummings, J. H., James, W. P. T. & Wiggins, H. S. (1973) Role of the colon in ileal-resection diarrhoea. *Lancet*, **i**, 344–347.
20 Debongnie, J. C. & Phillips, S. F. (1978) Capacity of the human colon to absorb fluid. *Gastroenterology*, **74**, 698–703.
21 Dembinski, A. B. & Johnson, J. R. (1982) Role of gastrin in gastrointestinal adaptation after small bowel resection. *American Journal of Physiology*, **243**, G16–G20.
22 Dobbins, J. W. & Binder, H. J. (1977) Derangements of oxalate metabolism in gastrointestinal disease and their mechanisms. In *Progress in Gastroenterology*, vol. III (Ed.) Glass, G. B. J. pp. 505–520. New York, San Francisco, London: Grune & Stratton.
23 Dowling, R. H. (1982) Small bowel adaptation and its regulation. *Scandinavian Journal of Gastroenterology*, **17** (Supplement 74), 53–74.
24 Dowling, R. H. & Booth, C. C. (1966) Functional compensation after small bowel resection in man. *Lancet*, **ii**, 146–147.
25 Dowling, R. H. & Booth, C. C. (1967) Structural and functional changes following small intestinal resection in the rat. *Clinical Sciences*, **32**, 139–149.
26 Dowling, R. H., Bell, G. D. & White, J. (1972) Lithogenic bile in patients with ileal dysfunction. *Gut*, **13**, 415.
27 Dreike, P. (1894) Ein Beitrag zur Kenntniss der Länge des menschlichen Darmkanals. *Deutsche Zeitschrift für Chirurgie*, **40**, 43–89.
28 Dudrick, S. J. & Ruberg, R. L. (1971) Principles and practice of parenteral nutrition. *Gastroenterology*, **61**, 901–910.
29 Enochs, M. R. & Johnson, L. R. (1977) Hormonal regulation of gastrointestinal tract growth; Biochemical and physiological aspects. In *Progress in Gastroenterology*, vol. III (Ed.) Glass, G. B. J. pp. 3–28. New York, San Francisco, London: Grune & Stratton.
30 Feldman, E. J., Dowling, R. H., McNaughton, J. & Peters, T. J. (1976) Effects of oral versus intravenous nutrition on intestinal adaptation after small bowel resection in the dog. *Gastroenterology*, **70**, 712–719.
31 Gerson, C. D. (1972) Failure of oral glucose electrolyte therapy in short bowel syndrome. *Lancet*, **ii**, 353–355.
32 Gleeson, M. H., Cullen, J. & Dowling, R. H. (1972) Intestinal structure and function after small bowel bypass in the rat. *Clinical Sciences*, **43**, 731–742.
33 Gleeson, M. H., Bloom, S. R., Polak, R. M. *et al.* (1971) Endocrine tumor in kidney affecting small bowel structure, motility and absorptive function. *Gut*, **12**, 773–782.
34 Goldstein, M. J., Melamed, M. R., Grabstald, H. & Sherlock, P. (1967) Progressive villous atrophy of the ileum used as a urinary conduit. *Gastroenterology*, **52**, 859–864.
35 Griffin, G. E., Fagan, E. F., Hodgson, H. J. & Chadwick, V. S. (1982) Enteral therapy in the management of massive gut resection complicated by chronic fluid and electrolyte depletion. *Digestive Diseases and Sciences*, **27**, 902–908.
36 Haymond, H. E. (1935) Massive resection of small intestine: analysis of 257 collected cases. *Surgery, Gynecology and Obstetrics*, **61**, 693–705.

37 Hirsch, J., Ahrens, E. H. & Blankenhorn, D. H. (1956) Measurement of the human intestinal length in vivo and some causes of variation. *Gastroenterology*, **31**, 274–284.

38 Hofman, A. (1978) The enterohepatic circulation of bile acids. In *Gastrointestinal Disease* (Ed.) Sleisenger, M. & Fordtran, J. S. pp. 418–429. Philadelphia: W. B. Saunders.

39 Hylander, E., Ladefoged, K. & Jarnum, S. (1980) The importance of the colon in calcium absorption following small-intestinal resection. *Scandinavian Journal of Gastroenterology*, **15**, 55–60.

40 Hyman, P. E., Garvey, T. Q., Harada, T. & Ament, M. E. (1983) Ranitidine inhibits basal gastric acid hypersecretion in an infant with short bowel syndrome. *Gastroenterology*, **84**, 1193.

41 Jeejeebhoy, K. N., Zohrab, W. J., Langer, B. *et al.* (1973) Total parenteral nutrition at home for 23 months, without complication, and with good rehabilitation. A study of technical and metabolic features. *Gastroenterology*, **65**, 811–820.

42 Johnson, L. R. (1974) Effect of gut hormones on growth of gastrointestinal mucosa. In *Endocrinology of the Gut* (Ed.) Chey, W. Y. & Brooks, F. P. pp. 163–177. Thorofare, New Jersey: Charles B. Slack.

43 Johnson, L. R. (1982) Effect of exogenous gut hormones on gastrointestinal mucosal growth. *Scandinavian Journal of Gastroenterology*, **17** (Supplement 74), 89–92.

44 Johnson, L. R. & Guthrie, P. (1976) Effect of cholecystokinin and 16,16-dimethyl prostaglandin E$_2$ on RNA and DNA of gastric and duodenal mucosa. *Gastroenterology*, **70**, 59–65.

45 Keren, D. F., Elliott, H. L., Brown, G. D. & Yardley, J. H. (1975) Atrophy of villi with hypertrophy and hyperplasia of paneth cells in isolated (Thiry–Vella) ileal loops in rabbits. *Gastroenterology*, **68**, 83–93.

46 Krejs, G. J. (1983) Allgemeine Störungen nach Ileostomie. In *Therapie Postoperativer Störungen des Gastrointestinaltraktes.* (Ed.) Domschke, W. & Lux, G. pp. 229–236. Stuttgart: Georg Thieme.

47 Lamb, D. S. (1893) The Meckel diverticulum. *American Journal of Medical Sciences*, **105**, 633–641.

48 Landor, J. H. (1969) Intestinal resection and gastric secretion in dogs with antrectomy. *Archives of Surgery*, **98**, 645–646.

49 Lee, D. B. N., Walling, M. W., Gafter, U. *et al.* (1980) Calcium and inorganic phosphate transport in rat colon. Dissociated response to 1,25-dihydroxyvitamin D. *Journal of Clinical Investigation*, **65**, 1326–1331.

50 Levin, R. J. (1982) Assessing small intestinal function in health and disease in vivo and in vitro. *Scandinavian Journal of Gastroenterology*, **17** (Supplement 74), 31–51.

51 Loran, M. R. & Carbone, J. V. (1968) The humoral effect of intestinal resection of cellular proliferation and maturation in parabiotic rats. In *Gastrointestinal Radiation Injury* (Ed.) Sullivan, M. F. pp. 127–141. Amsterdam: Excerpta Medica.

52 Mekhjian, H. S., Phillips, S. F. & Hofmann, A. F. (1971) Colonic secretion of water and electrolytes induced by bile acids: perfusion studies in man. *Journal of Clinical Investigation*, **50**, 1569–1577.

53 Mitchell, J., Zuckerman, L. & Breuer, R. I. (1977) The colon influences ileal resection diarrhoea. *Gastroenterology*, **72**, 1103.

54 Moossa, A. R., Hall, A. W., Skinner, D. B. & Winans, C. S. (1976) Effect of fifty per cent small bowel resection on gastric secretory function in rhesus monkeys. *Surgery*, **80**, 208–213.

55 Nundy, S., Malamud, D., Obertop, H. *et al.* (1977) Onset of cell proliferation in the shortened gut. Colonic

hyperplasia after ileal resection in the dog. *Gastroenterology*, **72**, 263–266.

56 Obertop, H., Nundy, S., Malamud, D. & Malt, R. A. (1977) Onset of cell proliferation in the shortened gut. Rapid hyperplasia after jejunal resection. *Gastroenterology*, **72**, 267–270.

57 Pertsemlidis, D. & Kark, A. E. (1974) Antiperistaltic segments for the treatment of short bowel syndrome. *American Journal of Gastroenterology*, **62**, 526–530.

58 Pierce, N. F., Banwell, J. G., Mitra, R. C. *et al.* (1968) Effect of intragastric glucose-electrolyte infusion upon water and electrolyte balance in Asiatic cholera. *Gastroenterology*, **55**, 333–343.

59 Rault, R. & Scribner, B. H. (1977) Parenteral nutrition in the home. In *Progress in Gastroenterology* (Ed.) Glass, G. B. J. pp. 545–562. New York, San Francisco, London: Grune & Stratton.

60 Ricour, C. (1975) Constant rate enteral nutrition, a transition from total parenteral nutrition to voluntary intake. In *Total Parenteral Nutrition* (Ed.) Ghadimi, H. pp. 601–613. New York: J. Wiley.

61 Rodgers, J. B., Bernard, H. R. & Balint, J. A. (1976) Colonic infusion in the management of the short bowel syndrome. *Gastroenterology*, **70**, 186–189.

62 Ross Laboratories. (1977) Polycose. *Product Information.* pp. 3–4. Columbus, Ohio: Ross Laboratories.

63 Rygick, A. N. & Nasarov, L. U. (1969) Antiperistaltic displacement of an ileal loop without twisting its mesentery. *Diseases of the Colon and Rectum*, **12**, 409–411.

64 Sagor, G. R., Ghatei, M. A., Al-Mukhtar, M. Y. T. *et al.* (1983) Evidence for a humoral mechanism after small intestinal resection. *Gastroenterology*, **84**, 902–906.

65 Satoh, T., Narisawa, K., Konno, T. *et al.* (1982) D-lactic acidosis in two patients with short bowel syndrome: bacteriological analysis of the fecal flora. *European Journal of Pediatrics*, **138**, 324–326.

66 Schmidt, W. (1965) Morphologische Grundlagen der enteralen Resorption. *Naunyn-Schmiedeberg's Archiv für Pathologie*, **250**, 178–189.

67 Seal, A. M., Debas, H. T., Reynolds, C. *et al.* (1982) Gastric and pancreatic hyposecretion following massive small-bowel resection. *Digestive Diseases and Sciences*, **27**, 117–123.

68 Seelig, L. L., Winborn, W. B. & Weser, E. (1977) Effect of small bowel resection on the gastric mucosa in the rat. *Gastroenterology*, **74**, 421–428.

69 Seelig, L. L., Winborn, W. B. & Weser, E. (1978) Changes in gastric glandular cell kinetics after small bowel resection in the rat. *Gastroenterology*, **74**, 1–6.

70 Simko, V. (1980) Short bowel syndrome. *Gastroenterology*, **78**, 190–191.

71 Soong, C. S., Thompson, J. B., Poley, J. R. & Hess, D. R. (1972) Hydroxy fatty acid in human diarrhea. *Gastroenterology*, **63**, 748–757.

72 Straus, E., Gerson, C. D. & Yalow, R. S. (1974) Hypersecretion of gastrin associated with the short bowel syndrome. *Gastroenterology*, **66**, 175–180.

73 Temperly, J. M., Stagg, B. H. & Wylie, J. H. (1971) Disappearance of gastrin and pentagastrin in the portal circulation. *Gut*, **12**, 372–376.

74 Tomkins, R. K., Waisman, J., Watt, C. M. H. *et al.* (1977) Absence of mucosal atrophy in human small intestine after prolonged isolation. *Gastroenterology*, **73**, 1406–1409.

75 Treves, F. (1885) Lectures on the anatomy of the intestinal canal and peritoneum in man. *British Medical Journal*, **i**, 415–419.

76 Trier, J. S. (1978) The short bowel syndrome. In *Gastrointestinal Disease* (Ed.) Sleisenger, M. & Fordtran, J. S. pp. 1652–1655. Philadelphia: W. B. Saunders.

77 Underhill, B. M. L. (1955) Intestinal length in man. *British Medical Journal*, **ii**, 1243–1246.

78 Urban, E., Starr, P. E. & Michel, A. M. (1983) Morphologic and functional adaptations of large bowel after small-bowel resection in the rat. *Digestive Diseases and Sciences*, **28**, 265–272.

79 Voitk, A. J., Echave, V., Brown, R. A. & Gurd, F. N. (1973) Use of elemental diet during the adaptive stage of short gut syndrome. *Gastroenterology*, **65**, 419–426.

80 Weser, E. (1976) The management of patients after small bowel resection. *Gastroenterology*, **71**, 146–150.

81 Weser, E., Bell, D. & Tawil, T. (1981) Effects of octapeptide-cholecystokinin, secretin, and glucagon on intestinal mucosal growth in parenterally nourished rats. *Digestive Diseases and Sciences*, **26**, 409–416.

82 Weser, E., Fletcher, J. T. & Urban, E. (1979) Short bowel syndrome. *Gastroenterology*, **77**, 572–579.

83 Wickbom, G., Landor, J. H., Bushkin, F. L. & McGuigan, J. E. (1975) Changes in canine gastric acid output and serum gastrin levels following massive small intestinal resection. *Gastroenterology*, **69**, 448–452.

84 Winawer, S. J., Broitman, S. A., Wolochow, D. A. *et al.* (1966) Successful management of massive small-bowel resection based on assessment of absorption defects and nutritional needs. *The New England Journal of Medicine*, **274**, 72–78.

85 Windsor, C. W. O., Fejfar, J. & Woodward, D. A. K. (1969) Gastric secretion after massive small bowel resection. *Gut*, **10**, 779–786.

86 Woolf, G. M., Miller, C., Kurian, R. & Jeejeebhoy, K. N. (1983) Diet for patients with a short bowel: high fat or high carbohydrate. *Gastroenterology*, **84**, 823–828.

87 Young, E. A., Heuler, N., Russell, P. & Weser, E. (1975) Comparative nutritional analysis of chemically defined diets. *Gastroenterology*, **69**, 1338–1345.

CHRONIC DISEASES OF THE SMALL INTESTINE IN CHILDHOOD

Diseases of the small intestine account for the most frequently seen gastroenterological problems that occur in childhood. They can be divided into acute disorders such as gastroenteritis (by far the most important problem worldwide), and chronic disorders such as coeliac disease. In most of these there is some abnormality of the gut mucosa, i.e. a small intestinal enteropathy is present. In all, there is some degree of malabsorption; in the acute diarrhoeal syndromes of gastroenteritis this is principally of salt and water, but in the chronic conditions such as coeliac disease malabsorption of a wide variety of nutrients such as fat and folic acid also occurs. The most important of these chronic disorders occurring in children will be briefly reviewed here. In the past, in these chronic disorders the emphasis in diagnosis was to first establish the existence of malabsorption, e.g. fat malabsorption by faecal fat estimation, and then to consider the possible cause. Now the emphasis in the first instance is often upon diagnosis of the underlying disease process. Thus if on analysis of the clinical features coeliac disease appears likely, a small intestinal biopsy should be done; if cystic fibrosis is considered possible, sweat electrolytes are estimated first. In practice the initial clinical assessment of children presenting with gastrointestinal symptoms usually suggests two or three possibilities. Those tests that are most relevant to these possible diagnoses should be performed.

COELIAC DISEASE

The aetiology, incidence and pathogenesis of coeliac disease are discussed earlier in this chapter.

Clinical features

There is considerable variation in the age of onset of symptoms in children with coeliac disease. As Gee described in 1888,[8] symptoms present most often between the age of one and five years. There is usually a variable 'latent interval' between the introduction of gluten into the diet and the development of clinical manifestations, the explanation for which remains unknown. In some children the interval may be months and in others many years, as coeliac disease may present for the first time in adult life. Occasional infants may have symptoms immediately gluten is added to their diet.

Mode of presentation

Classical presentation aged 9–18 months. There is gradual failure to gain weight or loss of weight after introduction of cereals, the child having previously been well. There is also anorexia and chronic diarrhoea; typically the stools are softer, paler, larger, more offensive, and more frequent than usual.

Presentation in infants before nine months. Vomiting is frequent and may be projectile. Diarrhoea may be severe, especially with intercurrent infections (not necessarily gastroenteritis). Abdominal distension may not be marked.

Presentation with constipation. These children are often very hypotonic with marked abdominal distension.

Presentation at an older age. Short stature, iron-resistant anaemia, rickets and personality problems all may occur.

Presentation in children originating in the Indian Sub-Continent but now in Western countries. These present later, often with iron-resistant anaemia or rickets and/or short stature. Diarrhoea is not a prominent feature.

Presentation in asymptomatic siblings. After a case is positively diagnosed, siblings should have their clinical history and growth checked. If a suspicion of coeliac disease arises, a full blood count, serum folate, and red cell folate should be performed. A biopsy is then necessary if there is evidence of a deficiency state.

Physical findings

On physical examination these children characteristically have wasting of the proximal limb girdles with a protuberant abdomen. There may be some ankle oedema due to hypoproteinaemia and occasionally finger clubbing. Typically the child is very miserable. Measurements of height and weight are valuable, especially when serial observations are available, often showing a slowing of weight gain and then weight loss. If the disease has been present for some time there is also slowing of growth (Figure 8.76).

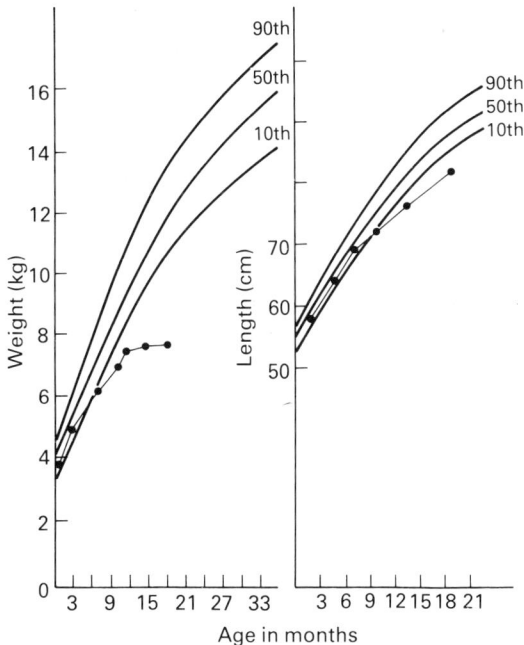

Fig. 8.76 Weight and growth chart for an infant with untreated coeliac disease. From Walker-Smith, J. A. (1979), *Diseases of the Small Intestine in Childhood*, 2nd edn., with kind permission of the publisher, Pitman Medical.

Diagnosis and differential diagnosis

The diagnosis of coeliac disease is based initially upon the demonstration of an abnormal small intestinal mucosa (usually flat) by small intestinal biopsy, and then upon a clinical response to the gluten withdrawal consisting of significant weight gain and relief of symptoms. The principal differential diagnoses are cystic fibrosis, giardiasis, toddler's diarrhoea, cow's milk protein intolerance, and the post-enteritis syndromes. Other causes of a flat mucosa are listed in Table 8.38. Reintroduction of gluten into the

Table 8.38 Causes of a flat small intestinal mucosa in childhood.

Coeliac disease
Gastroenteritis
Giardiasis
Cow's milk protein intolerance
Soya protein intolerance
Tropical sprue
Protein–energy malnutrition
Acquired hypogammaglobulinaemia

child's diet at a later date when the small intestinal mucosa has been shown to return to normal, followed by mucosal deterioration with or without a clinical relapse, is necessary before the diagnosis of coeliac disease may be said to have been definitively established (Figure 8.77). Most paediatricians recommend this for children presenting under two years of age. The relapse in mucosal appearance may not occur for up to two years after the reintroduction of gluten into the child's diet.

Complications

Most of these are due to malabsorption.

Growth retardation
Some children with coeliac disease may be asymptomatic apart from severe growth retardation. Nine out of thirteen children studied by Vanderschueren-Lodeweyckx[22] had low plasma growth hormone. Thus coeliac disease should be considered whenever a child with short stature has evidence of impairment of the release of growth hormone.

Anaemia
The incidence of anaemia in children with coeliac disease is variable. The most common type is a hypochromic microcytic anaemia due to iron deficiency. Megaloblastic anaemia only rarely occurs. Despite this, serum folate and red

Abnormal mucosa on biopsy

↓

Gluten-free diet
(two years or more)

Mucosa normal　　　　　　　　　　　　　　Mucosa still abnormal

↓　　　　　　　　　　　　　　　　　　　　　↓

'Gluten challenge'　　　　　　　　　　　? Lax diet — check
? Other pathology

Relapse　　　　　　　　　　　No symptoms

↓　　　　　　　　　　　　　↓

Biopsy after one week　　　Biopsy three months after challenge

↓

Abnormal mucosa　　　Abnormal mucosa　　　Normal mucosa

↓　　　　　　　　　↓　　　　　　　　　↓

Coeliac disease confirmed　　Coeliac disease confirmed　　Continue gluten challenge for two years

↓

Biopsy

Abnormal mucosa　　　Normal mucosa

↓　　　　　　　　　↓

Coeliac disease confirmed　　Coeliac disease excluded

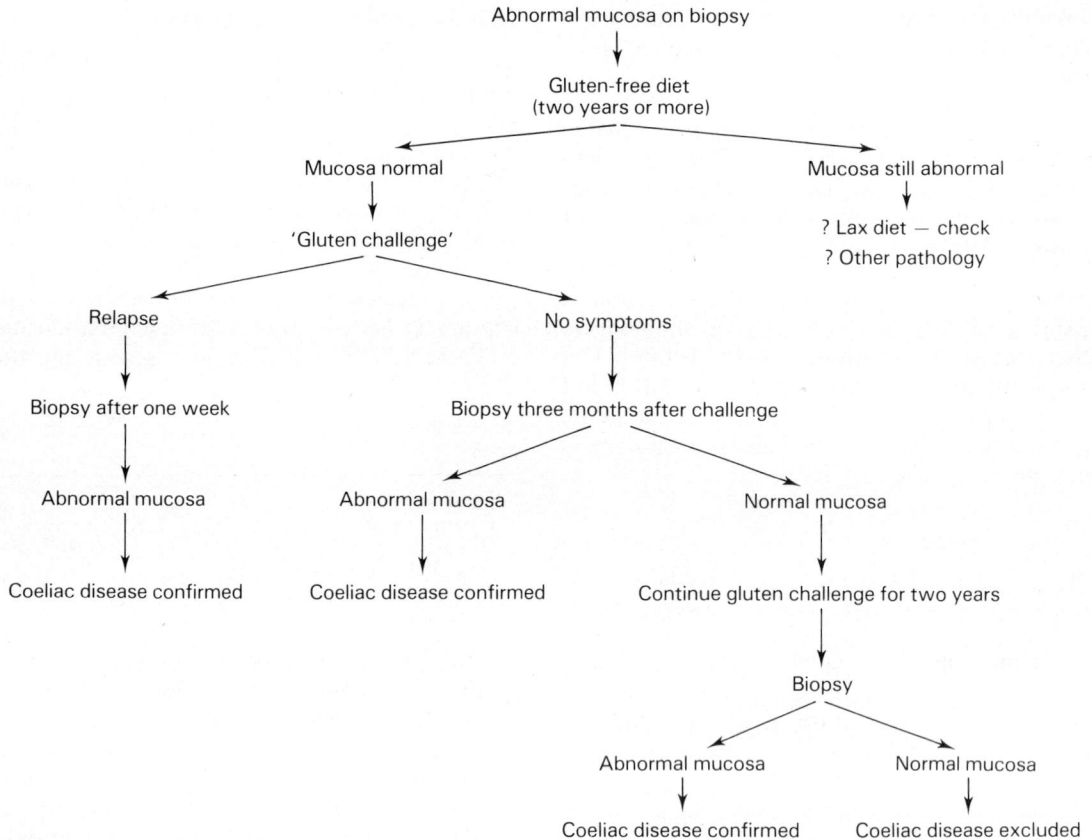

Fig. 8.77 Diagnostic criteria and investigation regimen for coeliac disease. From Walker-Smith, J. A. (1979), *Disease of the Small Intestine in Childhood*, 2nd edn., with kind permission of the publisher, Pitman Medical.

cell folate levels are usually reduced in children with untreated coeliac disease. Folate levels rapidly rise on a gluten-free diet and tend to fall, although not always to a pathological level, after a gluten challenge. Estimation of folate levels is thus a useful way to evaluate progress on a gluten-free diet of a child with coeliac disease.

Hypoproteinaemia
Hypoproteinaemia due to protein-losing enteropathy is a common complication of coeliac disease. When there is severe hypoproteinaemia, the child may present with generalized oedema mimicking the nephrotic syndrome. The oedema is relieved by treatment with a gluten-free diet.

Hypogammaglobulinaemia
Low levels of serum IgA and IgM have been described in some children with coeliac disease. The IgA deficiency is not reversible with a gluten-free diet, whereas IgM levels rise to normal. It is possible that pre-existing IgA deficiency predisposes to coeliac disease. On the other hand serum IgA levels are more commonly elevated in coeliac disease.

Hypoprothrombinaemia
An abnormal prothrombin time due to malabsorption of vitamin K may occur in coeliac disease, and estimation of prothrombin time and other parameters of coagulation before small intestinal biopsy has been recommended. Hypoprothrombinaemia is rapidly corrected by intramuscular vitamin K_1.

Treatment

Elimination of gluten from the child's diet usually leads to a dramatic and rapid clinical response, but this may sometimes be delayed. Weight gain and relief of emotional symptoms in the mother as well as the child usually occurs first, before cessation of diarrhoea and other signs of improvement. There is some disagreement as to precisely what constitutes a gluten-free diet. All authorities are agreed that wheat and rye should be eliminated from the diet, but some also recommend elimination of barley and oats, although it is still uncertain whether these two cereals are also toxic to children with coeliac disease.

Although secondary disaccharidase deficiency has been shown, by assay of small intestinal biopsies, to be present in virtually all children with untreated coeliac disease, clinical lactose intolerance is present in only 5%. Only when there is evidence of such intolerance, i.e. an abnormal amount of reducing substances in the stool and diarrhoea after a lactose load, is elimination of lactose from the diet indicated.

OTHER FOOD-RELATED DISORDERS

Apart from coeliac disease, all other food-related disorders associated with gastro-intestinal symptoms in children appear to be transient. Food intolerance comprises a wide range of abnormal reactions to food. Some of these categories clearly may overlap, for example allergy and enteropathy. An approach to the diagnosis of chronic diarrhoea in infancy which may be food-related is given in Figure 8.78.

Changes in the structure of the small intestinal mucosa, assessed by biopsy in response to ingestion of particular foods, provide clear objective evidence of food-sensitive disorders. Serial small intestinal biopsies related to dietary elimination and then to challenge have impli-

cated chiefly three foods in the production of small intestinal mucosal damage, possibly mediated via allergic mechanisms. These foods produce *cow's milk sensitive enteropathy* as part of cow's milk protein intolerance, *soy protein intolerance* and *transient gluten intolerance*. All are temporary disorders of early life and usually resolve clinically by the third year. In addition Vitoria et al.[23] have recently described an enteropathy related to fish, rice and chicken. Other food allergic disorders may or may not be associated with recognizable small intestinal mucosal damage or enteropathy; it is possible that in part at least their clinical manifestations are mediated through structural or functional abnormality of the small intestinal mucosa. These disorders are not yet well defined clinically but include multiple food allergy.

The features of small intestinal mucosa pathology which may provide evidence of local allergic reactions, based upon animal experiments, are illustrated in Figure 8.79. When a small intestinal biopsy in food allergy shows enteropathy characterized by crypt hyperplasia, villous atrophy and an increased number of intraepithelial lymphocytes, a cell-mediated immune reaction may be present. On the other hand a type I reaction in the gut, due to IgE antibody, is likely to produce virtually no structural abnormality on biopsy apart from oedema.

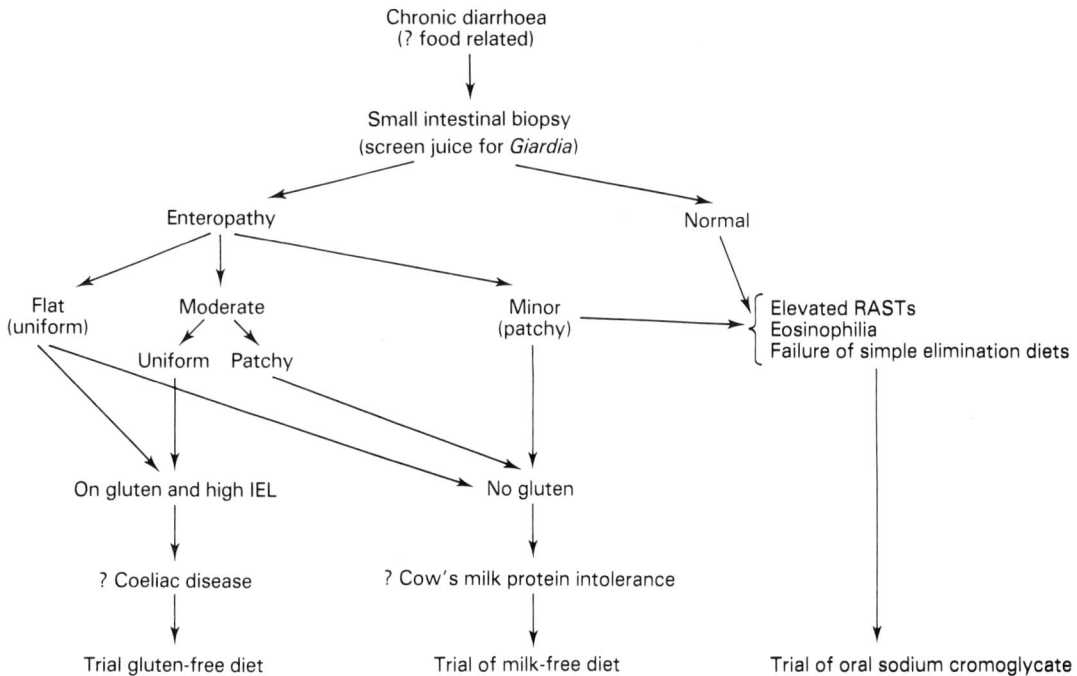

Fig. 8.78 The diagnosis of chronic diarrhoea in infancy which may be food related. A practical approach currently used at Queen Elizabeth Hospital for Children, London. High IEL: increased counts of intraepithelial lymphocytes.

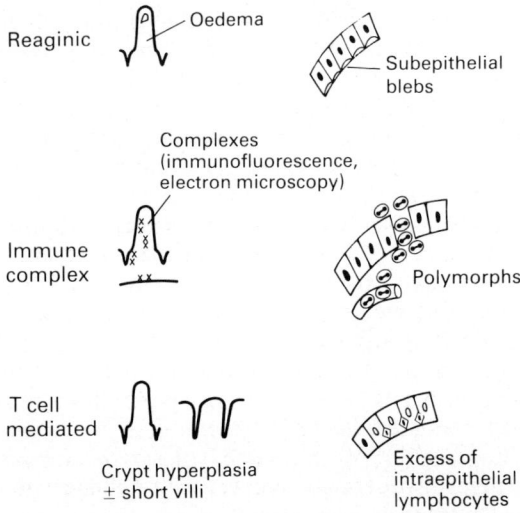

Fig. 8.79 Features of small intestinal mucosal pathology which (on the basis of experimental work in animals) may provide evidence of local allergic reactions. From Ferguson, A. (1980) Pathogenesis and mechanisms in the gastrointestinal tract. In *Proceedings of the First Fisons Food Allergy Workshop*, pp. 28–38. With kind permission of the author and the publishers, Medicine Publishing Foundation.

Cow's milk protein intolerance

Cow's milk protein intolerance is the clinical syndrome or syndromes resulting from the sensitization of an individual child to one or more proteins in cow's milk, presumably following absorption via a permeable small intestinal mucosa.

Pathogenesis

The pathogenesis of cow's milk protein intolerance is not clear. There appear to be two syndromes: a primary form in which there appears to be no predisposing factors, and a secondary form following acute gastroenteritis. Two factors may be important in both: firstly, the permeability of the small intestinal mucosa to the antigen, and secondly, the control of the antigen and the immune response to it once it has been absorbed. Primary cow's milk intolerance may be due to a primary disturbance of the local immune system for antigen control, particularly antigen exclusion. The secondary syndrome may be a sequel to primary gut damage due to gastroenteritis permitting excess antigen entry, perhaps coupled with a defect of local antigen control. An immunodeficiency state, such as transient IgA deficiency, may be an important predisposing factor for both syndromes. Figure 8.80 outlines an hypothesis for the pathogenesis of cow's milk protein intolerance and suggests a relationship between gastroenteritis and lactose intolerance.

Pathology

Most children with cow's milk protein intolerance who have gastrointestinal symptoms appear on biopsy to have an abnormal small intestinal mucosa at the time of initial diagnosis. However, unlike coeliac disease, this enteropathy is not an invariable finding on a single proximal biopsy, but is patchy and of variable severity. The mucosa is often thinner than in coeliac disease, although a mucosa indistinguishable from coeliac disease may be found; more often the mucosal abnormality is less severe. When present, the enteropathy can be shown to be sensitive to cow's milk by serial biopsies related to withdrawal of and challenge with cow's milk. After a positive milk challenge, alteration in the microvilli of the enterocyte may be seen in parallel with a fall in disaccharidase activity. Although the numbers of intraepithelial lymphocytes may rise after a positive milk challenge, the level reached is usually within the normal range.

Some children who are milk intolerant have a colitis which histologically is characterized by an increase in lamina propria eosinophils. This usually occurs independently of the small intestinal lesion.

Clinical features

Most children with gastrointestinal symptoms due to cow's milk protein intolerance have these symptoms commencing within the first six months of life, either acutely or insidiously. In

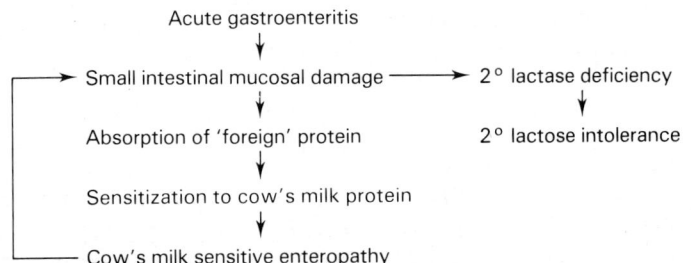

Fig. 8.80 An hypothesis for the relationship between gastroenteritis and lactose intolerance with cow's milk sensitive enteropathy. From Walker-Smith, J. A. (1979), *Diseases of the Small Intestine in Childhood*, 2nd edn., with kind permission of the publisher, Pitman Medical.

some children, there may be a family history of atopy or cow's milk protein intolerance, but often there is not. Such a history is usually absent when the syndrome occurs as a sequel to acute gastroenteritis.

The acute onset syndrome may be characterized by a sudden attack of vomiting and diarrhoea, which then becomes persistent. It may be impossible at first to distinguish such an illness from acute gastroenteritis, which is confusing as cow's milk protein intolerance may itself be a sequel to gastroenteritis. The acute onset syndromes may be subdivided as follows: firstly, there are those infants who appear to be so sensitive to cow's milk that they develop acute symptoms immediately on weaning onto cow's milk, although they are still being chiefly breast-fed; secondly, there are those infants who have an acute attack of symptoms after receiving cow's milk feedings for several months. In this latter group particularly, an attack of acute gastroenteritis is often implicated as a triggering event. Finally, another but fortunately rare acute onset syndrome is characterized by the sudden onset of vomiting, followed by pallor and an acute anaphylactic state of circulatory collapse (hypotension and altered consciousness) or significant upper airway obstruction (swelling of structures in the mouth or throat).

The chronic onset syndrome may manifest as chronic diarrhoea with failure to thrive and clinical features to suggest coeliac disease. It may also present as the intractable diarrhoea syndrome and must always be considered in the differential diagnosis of this condition. The colitis with increased lamina propria eosinophils, referred to above, presents with chronic bloody diarrhoea with many of the features of ulcerative colitis. This syndrome may present in the first few days of life and needs to be distinguished from necrotizing enterocolitis as well as chronic inflammatory bowel disease.

Diagnosis
Until recently, the only satisfactory way to make the diagnosis of cow's milk protein intolerance was clinical observation of the effects of repeated withdrawal of and challenge with milk as formulated by Goldman and colleagues in 1963.[9] However, serial small intestinal biopsies at the time of initial presentation, after a clinical response to milk withdrawal, and finally after the return of symptoms following a milk challenge, now permit a firm diagnosis of cow's milk-sensitive enteropathy to be made on the basis of one diagnostic milk challenge. This approach is only usually practical in a paediatric

gastroenterology unit but it has clearly established the existence of this syndrome. In practice a cow's milk challenge is often deferred until about the age of one year, both because the risk of anaphylaxis is greater under a year and because of the natural reluctance to prematurely change the feeding when an infant is doing well on cow's milk-free diet. Often, therefore, by the time of the challenge, the infant has recovered and post-challenge biopsy is not done. An initial biopsy, however, is indicated as part of the diagnostic investigation of an infant with chronic diarrhoea and failure to thrive.

Differential diagnosis
Cow's milk-sensitive enteropathy has to be distinguished from secondary lactose intolerance (occurring as a temporary sequel to acute gastroenteritis), coeliac disease, other forms of food allergy, toddler's diarrhoea, and even at times from normality. Small intestinal biopsy is the most useful diagnostic test to make this distinction, combined with clear knowledge of the child's precise dietary intake; the principal clinical feature is a clear response to a cow's milk-free diet.

Treatment
The obvious treatment for this condition is to eliminate cow's milk and all foods based on cow's milk from the child's diet. This latter point is most important as therapeutic failure is sometimes related to neglect of a restriction of cow's milk-based foods such as ice-cream, despite strict avoidance of cow's milk itself. It is usually necessary to provide a cow's milk substitute, and it is essential to ensure that the diet is nutritionally adequate.

The need for such dietary restriction of milk is nearly always temporary, although there is little documentation concerning the precise duration of this intolerance. On clinical grounds, most children over two years of age are apparently able to tolerate milk without any untoward sequelae. The timing of a re-challenge with cow's milk is arbitrary and varies from paediatrician to paediatrician.

A large number of substitute products are available and vary in nutritional adequacy for different age groups. They fall into three categories based on casein hydrolysate, soya protein, or goat's milk. A factor of key importance, especially in early infancy, is the osmolality of the formula. High osmolality feeds draw water into the gut and may increase any diarrhoea that is present. Casein hydrolysate feeds are often preferred for children with cow's milk-sensitive enteropathy, especially as such children can occasionally be sensitive to other proteins used in replacement feeds such as soya protein or goat's milk. Casein hydrolysate formulas appear to be very low in allergenicity. Pregestimil is especially suitable for the young infant because of its nutritional adequacy and the low osmolality of the current formulation. A number of soya 'milks' are available on the market but many are only a social replacement of milk without providing calcium, riboflavin and other nutrients provided by cow's milk. Several new soya infant formulas are available and appear to be safe nutritional alternatives to modified cow's milk feeds, e.g. Formula S Soya Food, Velactin, Prosobee, and Wysoy. The first two are solely of vegetable origin and so are acceptable to vegetarians and vegans.

Soya protein intolerance

A soya bean food prepared to resemble milk has been used in many countries since it was first recommended by Hill and Stuart in 1929[11] for infants with milk allergy. It has also been suggested that soya bean milk when used as a substitute for cow's milk could play an important role in the prevention of allergy to cow's milk in those who are at risk. Although soya bean has low antigenicity, over the past ten years there have been an increasing number of reports of intolerance to soya protein. Such reactions have varied from a dramatic anaphylactic response, to the onset of respiratory and gastrointestinal symptoms.

In 1972, Ament and Rubin[1] clearly documented soya protein intolerance in an infant by monitoring the clinical and small intestinal mucosal response to a soya protein challenge. Challenge produced a flat small intestinal mucosa indistinguishable from that found in untreated coeliac disease. The lesion was reversible and serial biopsies revealed that it disappeared within four days of withdrawal of soy protein, only to recur on further challenge. Varying degrees of small intestinal mucosal abnormality have been recognized by other workers.

Soya-free diets are almost as difficult to maintain as cow's milk-free diets, because of the extensive use of soya in manufactured food products.

Transient gluten intolerance

Transient gluten intolerance is recognized when a child with gastrointestinal symptoms and an abnormal small intestinal mucosa responds to a gluten-free diet, but subsequently thrives on a normal gluten-containing diet and after two years on such a diet is found to have a normal mucosa. In Holland in 1952, Dicke[4] described a transient wheat sensitivity in pre-school children after enteritis. In 1970, a child with transient gluten intolerance was described in Australia.[24] This child had an abnormal mucosa (a severe degree of partial villous atrophy) and responded clinically to a gluten-free diet. After one year, while he was still taking a gluten-free diet, a further biopsy revealed a normal mucosa. He was put back on a normal diet and 16 months later a further biopsy demonstrated a persistently normal mucosa. He has subsequently remained in excellent health.

Although a diagnosis of transient gluten intolerance was made retrospectively in this child, more recent criteria lay down stricter requirements for this diagnosis. These are firstly, the need to provide evidence that gluten toxicity was in fact present and that the apparent response to gluten restriction was not fortuitous,[14] and secondly, the need to demonstrate the presence of a normal small intestinal mucosa two years or more after the return to a normal diet.[16]

The precise criteria necessary to establish the existence of any form of transient intolerance to a dietary substance associated with small bowel mucosal abnormality have been outlined by McNeish[14] and are indicated in diagrammatic form in Figure 8.81.

Pathogenesis
Two explanations have been proposed to explain the development of this syndrome. Firstly, there may be a temporary depression of dipeptidase activity occurring in the small intestinal mucosa secondary to non-specific mucosal damage, such as may occur after gastroenteritis. Secondly, it is possible that a transient 'allergy' to gluten may occur in a similar and equally unknown manner to that suggested earlier in relation to cow's milk protein, possibly also secondary to mucosal damage. There is little evidence available so far to support either theory.

Pathology
The small intestinal mucosa is by definition abnormal, i.e. a thickened, ridged mucosa characterized histologically by partial villous atrophy or, sometimes, a flat mucosa. The demonstration of a flat mucosa should not ordinarily suggest this diagnosis, being characteristic of coeliac disease; the mucosal abnormality is

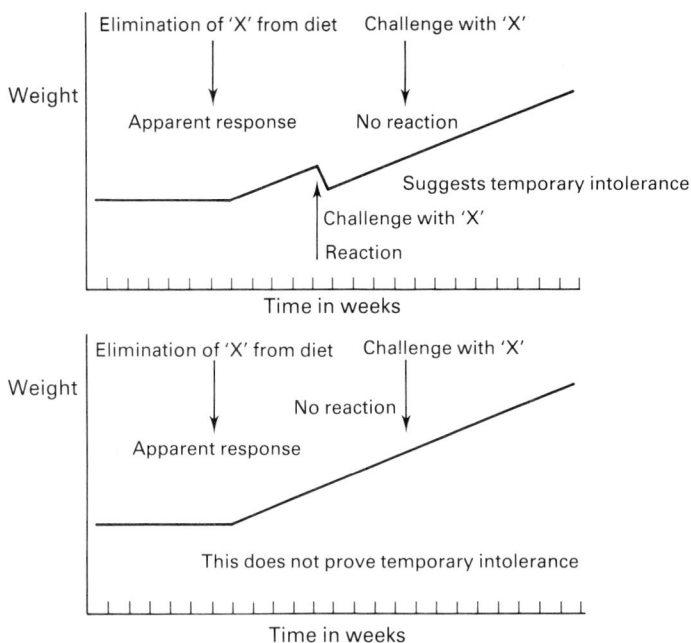

Fig. 8.81 Diagrammatic representation of the diagnostic criteria for transient gluten intolerance. From McNeish, A. S. (1974),[14] with kind permission of the author and the editor of *Acta Paediatrica Scandinavica*.

usually less severe than that found in coeliac disease. Only long-term follow-up with subsequent reinvestigation would allow the retrospective diagnosis of transient gluten intolerance to be made in a child with a flat mucosa who earlier has responded clinically to gluten withdrawal, but who is now thriving on a gluten-containing diet.

Clinical features

Transient gluten intolerance may accompany other forms of food intolerance, or occur on its own. The diagnosis should be considered in the infant who develops gastrointestinal symptoms when he first encounters wheat protein, especially when he appears to be intolerant to other food proteins such as milk and egg. It should also be considered in a child who fails to thrive following gastroenteritis in the presence of an abnormal small intestinal mucosa and the absence of other explanations, such as secondary lactose intolerance or secondary cow's milk protein intolerance.

Management

Initial management is as for coeliac disease; the diagnosis is inevitably retrospective after the child has been reinvestigated to establish the presence or absence of permanent gluten intolerance. Early challenge is not recommended routinely, so in most cases the diagnosis is not only retrospective but provisional as the initial response to a gluten-free diet is not definite

proof of gluten sensitivity. Whether any or all such children with transient gluten intolerance will ultimately relapse remains uncertain.

Sugar intolerance

Sugar intolerance is characterized by the development of diarrhoea and/or vomiting and failure to thrive in infants and children due to ingestion of sugar. Such a syndrome may be primary, for example glucose-galactose malabsorption, or it may be secondary to temporary damage to the small intestinal mucosa, as may occur, for example, following an acute rotavirus gastroenteritis. There are two principal syndromes – monosaccharide and disaccharide intolerance. The latter is often more severe and persistent. Causes of secondary lactose intolerance are listed in Table 8.39.

Table 8.39 Causes of secondary lactose intolerance.

Gastroenteritis
Coeliac disease
Giardiasis
Protein–energy malnutrition
Following neonatal surgery
Cow's milk protein intolerance
Immunodeficiency syndrome
Massive small intestinal resection

Diagnostic criteria

The simplest clinical way to make the diagnosis of sugar intolerance is to demonstrate the presence of excess amounts of reducing substances in diarrhoeal stools. The stools are typically watery, i.e. 1–5% only of solid matter. The importance of proper stool collection cannot be over-stressed. If there is some doubt about which feed may be responsible for the child's continuing diarrhoea (as may be the case when there has been a recent change of feed) stool chromatography may help identify the sugar present. More recently the breath hydrogen test has been used in the diagnosis of both monosaccharide and disaccharide intolerance. An increasing concentration of breath hydrogen reflects bacterial fermentation of carbohydrate reaching the colon; this test may be more reliable than stool reducing substances.

The second aspect of clinical diagnosis is the demonstration of a clinical response to the removal of the offending sugar from the diet. The formulas discussed earlier as being appropriate for cow's milk protein intolerance are also lactose-free, and so can be used in sugar intolerance.

POST-ENTERITIS SYNDROME

The post-enteritis syndrome describes the child who has had an attack of acute gastroenteritis followed by intermittent or chronic diarrhoea. There may or may not be failure to gain weight following the return to a normal diet.

Two main groups of problems cause delayed recovery after acute gastroenteritis in infancy. Firstly, there may be an acute intolerance to the increasing concentrations of milk, and secondly, there may be a more chronic problem with persistent diarrhoea and failure to thrive. An acute intolerance to milk leads to diarrhoea, which is often watery and copious and sometimes accompanied by vomiting. This is most often due to malabsorption of lactose and sometimes also of sucrose, but there may be intolerance to cow's milk protein. Sometimes, in addition, there may be temporary monosaccharide intolerance. The acute problem of sugar intolerance is usually easily dealt with, but the more chronic problem of persistent diarrhoea and failure to gain weight following gastroenteritis is more difficult to solve. The differential diagnosis of, for example, a child under two years in this state is as follows: post-enteritis syndrome, coeliac disease, cystic fibrosis, giardiasis, and cow's milk protein intolerance, as well as an anatomical abnormality of the small intestine producing obstruction. These also need to be distinguished from toddler's diarrhoea, in which there is chronic diarrhoea but no failure to thrive.

Sometimes long-term follow-up is the only way to establish the diagnosis definitively. In view of this, when symptoms have been present for three weeks or more after gastroenteritis, should there still be doubt about the diagnosis, a small intestinal biopsy should be performed to demonstrate whether there is any structural abnormality of the small intestinal mucosa. When the mucosa is flat, the diagnosis of coeliac disease must be considered if the child is eating gluten, even though it is known that gastroenteritis per se may cause a flat mucosa. However, unlike coeliac disease, intraepithelial lymphocytes are not increased in post-enteritis syndrome. More often a characteristic less severe patch enteropathy is present. Why such persistent mucosal damage occurs in only a minority of children after gastroenteritis is uncertain, but in some children at least it appears to be due to cow's milk-sensitive enteropathy or other food-sensitive enteropathy.

TODDLER'S DIARRHOEA

This disorder, variously known as toddler's diarrhoea, chronic non-specific diarrhoea, or the irritable colon syndrome,[3] is one of the commonest causes of chronic diarrhoea in childhood.

Pathogenesis

It seems most probable that this is a motility disorder. When small intestinal motility has been studied in normal individuals, there is a fasting pattern characterized by recurring migrating complexes which is disrupted within two minutes of eating and replaced by random segmenting activity known as the postprandial pattern. In children with toddler's diarrhoea, intraduodenal dextrose fails to disrupt the migrating motor complex. This could play a major role in the pathogenesis of this condition.[7] The small intestinal mucosa in these children is morphologically normal, although there is a significant increase in the specific enzyme activity of adenyl cyclase, and also of Na^+–K^+–ATPase in small intestinal tissue.[21] This increase could be the response of normal villous cells to crypt cell secretion which in turn may be mediated via prostaglandins, as high plasma prostaglandin F levels have been reported in children with this syndrome.[10] Whether the colon is also functionally abnormal is not yet clear.

Clinical features

Toddler's diarrhoea usually begins between the age of 6 and 24 months. Often, the child has previously been constipated and sometimes has had infantile colic. It may also be a sequel to acute gastroenteritis. In most children the diarrhoea ceases spontaneously between the ages of two and four years, sometimes earlier. The stool pattern is, typically, a large stool early in the day, formed or partly formed, followed by the passage of smaller looser stools containing undigested vegetable material and mucus. The passage of undigested food is characteristic; indeed, one popular name for the syndrome stemming from this observation is 'the peas and carrots syndrome'. A severe napkin rash may accompany the diarrhoea. Despite the diarrhoea, the child grows and develops completely normally. Psychosomatic factors may be important as suggested by the higher proportion of children coming from families of the professional classes. Often the mother may become preoccupied with every stool the child passes, the loose stools causing severe anxiety despite the child's evident general well-being. Sometimes these children are given complicated elimination diets which may even lead to weight loss and unnecessarily add to maternal anxiety.

Differential diagnosis

Detailed investigation such as small intestinal biopsies are indicated only when there is some doubt about the child's nutritional status or the presence of other symptoms. There is no evidence of malabsorption or enteric infection. However, giardiasis and sucrase–isomaltase deficiency can sometimes be confused with this disorder, and then biopsy and examination of duodenal juice is helpful. It is also important to differentiate toddler's diarrhoea from cow's milk-sensitive enteropathy, where the small intestinal mucosa is characteristically abnormal, and also from multiple food allergy where the mucosa may be normal or show only minor abnormality. In this disorder serum IgE is typically raised, specific radioallergosorbent (RAST) tests are positive, indicating the presence of IgE antibodies against specific foodstuffs, and there is often an eosinophilia.[20]

Toddler's diarrhoea should only be considered as the diagnosis when the child is otherwise thriving and in good general health. In some children this diarrhoea may be part of a spectrum of familial functional bowel disorders with continuing gastrointestinal complaints presenting later in life.

Treatment

Treatment at the moment ranges from reassurance and explanation to the prescription of drugs. Hamdi and Dodge[10] showed that loperamide gave symptomatic benefit to some children with this syndrome. It was as effective in those with raised prostaglandin levels as those without. The widespread use of antidiarrhoeal drugs in paediatrics is to be deplored, but occasionally a child with a severe form of this syndrome benefits from a course of loperamide (although it may be the mother who benefits the most). Such therapy should be given for a limited period only. Elimination diets of any kind are not indicated and their use in this syndrome is to be discouraged. As fruit and vegetables are recognizable in stools these are sometimes excluded, but restriction of these, or of total fat intake, is of no value.

REFERENCES

1 Ament, M. E. & Rubin, C. E. (1972) Soy protein – another cause of the flat intestinal lesion. *Gastroenterology*, **62**, 227.
2 Cohen, S. A., Hendricks, K. M., Mathis, R. K. *et al.* (1979) Chronic non-specific diarrhoea: dietary relationships. *Pediatrics*, **64**, 402–407.
3 Davidson, M. & Wasserman, R. (1966) The irritable colon of childhood (chronic non-specific diarrhoea syndrome). *Journal of Pediatrics*, **69**, 1027–1038.
4 Dicke, W. K. (1952) De subacute, chronische en recidiverende darmstoornis van de kleuter. *Nederlandsch Tijdschrift voor Geneeskunde*, **96**, 860.
5 Dormandy, K. M., Waters, A. H., & Mollin, D. L. (1963) Folic acid deficiency in coeliac disease. *Lancet*, **i**, 632.
6 Dowd, B. D. & Walker-Smith, J. A. (1974) Samuel Gee, Aretaeus and the coeliac affection. *British Medical Journal*, **ii**, 45.
7 Fenton, T. R., Harries, J. T. & Milla, P. J. (1983) Disordered small intestinal motility: a rational basis for toddler's diarrhoea. *Gut*, in press.
8 Gee, S. J. (1888) On the coeliac affection. *St Bartholomew's Hospital Reports*, **24**, 17.
9 Goldman, A. S., Anderson, D. W., Sellers, W. *et al.* (1963) Milk allergy. *Pediatrics*, **32**, 425.
10 Hamdi, I. & Dodge, J. A. (1978) Prostaglandins in non-specific diarrhoea. *Acta Paediatrica Belgica*, **31**, 106.
11 Hill, L. W. & Stuart, H. C. (1929) A soy-bean food preparation for feeding infants with milk allergy. *Journal of the American Medical Association*, **93**, 986.
12 Kenrick, K. G. & Walker-Smith, J. A. (1970) Immunoglobulins and dietary protein antibodies in childhood coeliac disease. *Gut*, **11**, 635.
13 Lloyd-Still, J. D. (1979) Chronic diarrhoea of childhood and the misuse of elimination diets. *Journal of Pediatrics*, **95**, 10–13.
14 McNeish, A. S. (1974) The role of lactose in cow's milk intolerance. *Acta Paediatrica Scandinavica*, **63**, 652.
15 McNeish, A. S., Rolles, C. J. & Arthur, L. J. H. (1976) Criteria for diagnosis of temporary gluten intolerance. *Archives of Disease in Childhood*, **51**, 275.
16 Meeuwissen, G. W. (1970) Diagnostic criteria in coeliac disease. *Acta Paediatrica Scandinavica*, **59**, 461.

17 Mortimer, P. E., Stewart, J. S., Norman, A. P. & Booth, C. C. (1968) Follow-up of coeliac disease. *British Medical Journal*, **ii**, 7.

18 Nelson, R., McNeish, A. S. & Anderson, C. M. (1973) Coeliac disease in children of Asian immigrants. *Lancet*, **i**, 348.

19 Rudd, P., Manuel, P. & Walker-Smith, J. (1981) Anaphylactic shock in an infant after feeding with a wheat rusk. A transient phenomenon. *Postgraduate Medical Journal*, **57**, 794–795.

20 Syme, J. (1979) Investigation and treatment of multiple intestinal food allergy in childhood. In *The Mast Cell* (Ed.) Pepys, J. & Edwards, A. M. pp. 438–443. Tunbridge Wells: Pitman Medical.

21 Tripp, J. H., Manning, J. A., Muller, D. P. P. *et al.* (1978) Abnormalities of intestinal transport systems in the postenteritis syndrome (PES) and toddler 'nonspecific' diarrhoea. *Acta Paediatrica Belgica*, **31**, 257.

22 Vanderschueren-Lodeweyckx, M., Wolter, R., Molla, A. *et al.* (1973) Plasma growth hormone in coeliac disease. *Helvetica Paediatrica Acta*, **28**, 349.

23 Vitoria, J. A., Camarero, C., Sojo, A. *et al.* (1982) Enteropathy related to fish, rice and chicken. *Archives of Disease in Childhood*, **57**, 44–48.

24 Walker-Smith, J. A. (1970) Transient gluten intolerance. *Archives of Disease in Childhood*, **45**, 523.

25 Walker-Smith, J. A. (1982) Cow's milk intolerance as a cause of postenteritis diarrhoea. *Journal of Pediatric Gastroenterology and Nutrition*, **1**, 163–175.

26 Walker-Smith, J. A., Kilby, A., and France, N. E. (1978) Reinvestigation of children previously diagnosed as coeliac disease. In *Perspectives in Coeliac Disease* (Ed. McNicholl, B., McCarthy, C. F., and Fottrell, P. F.) p. 267. Lancaster: MTP Press.

DRUGS AND THE SMALL INTESTINE

THERAPEUTIC CONSIDERATIONS

The small intestine plays a vital role in the absorption of nutrients, minerals and drugs used therapeutically. Its mucosa contains metabolic enzymes and its lumen contains bacteria which may alter the structure and function of a number of exogenous substances, presumably acting as a protective mechanism for the organism. Biliary secretion may represent a major route of elimination for some drugs and is particularly important for conjugated metabolites. Local hydrolysis in the gut lumen may then lead to the enterohepatic cycling of these drugs. All these processes may be altered in the presence of small bowel disease.

Drug absorption

The factors influencing the absorption of drugs from the upper gastrointestinal tract are complex (Table 8.40) and are governed by the physicochemical properties of the drug.[39]

Table 8.40 Factors influencing drug absorption.

Drug characteristics
Molecular size
Lipid–water partition coefficient
Degree of ionization
Formulation
Gut metabolism

Patient characteristics
pH at absorptive site
Gastric emptying time
Intestinal motility
Surface area of small intestine
Mesenteric blood flow
Gastrointestinal disease

Other factors
Large meal
Interacting drugs

Although absorption can take place throughout the gastrointestinal tract, all drugs are substantially absorbed in the upper small intestine; the absorptive area has been calculated to be equivalent to two full size tennis courts. The pH at the mucosal surface is approximately 5.4. Lipid-soluble drugs are rapidly absorbed across the mucosal cells by passive diffusion. Absorption of water-soluble drugs is slower and often incomplete. Acidic drugs such as aspirin, phenobarbitone and warfarin might be expected to be ionized in the alkaline contents of the small intestine and therefore less well absorbed (the un-ionized form will cross biological membranes less readily) but this is compensated for by the enormous absorptive surface area available. Strong acids or bases (e.g. neostigmine) are completely ionized in aqueous solution and therefore poorly absorbed from all regions of the gut.

The two most important factors affecting drug absorption are the small intestine surface area and the rate of gastric emptying. The latter dictates the rate at which drug reaches the major absorptive surface of the upper jejunum, which influences the time to, and extent of, the peak concentration. Absolute bioavailability is unaffected unless the drug is also metabolized or degraded in the gut lumen or gastric wall (Figure 8.82).

A number of disease states have been reported to affect drug absorption. As can be seen from Table 8.41, the amount of drug absorbed is simultaneously affected by many factors. Upper small bowel disease may change the pattern of absorption, so that more drug is absorbed further down the gastrointestinal tract.[38] This only has clinical relevance if a rapid high peak plasma concentration is important, such as with an antibiotic or analgesic. Gut oedema in patients in congestive cardiac failure may also

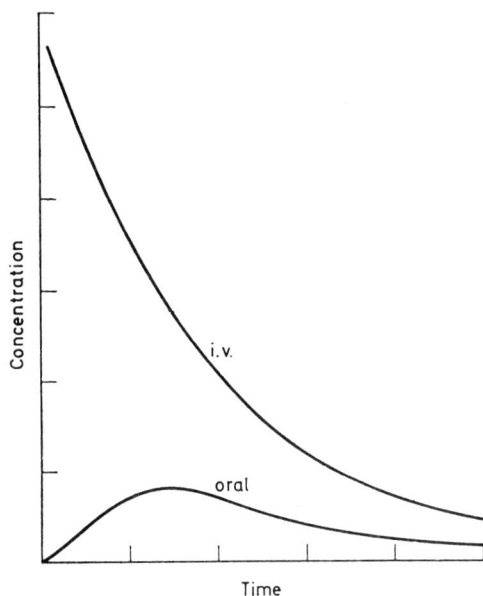

Fig. 8.82 A typical concentration time curve for a well-absorbed drug given orally. The time to, and extent of, the peak concentration can be decreased by reducing gastric emptying time and increased by accelerating gastric emptying. The absolute bioavailability of the drugs remains unaltered unless the drug is metabolized or degraded in the gastric wall or lumen.

ties of drugs and in the extent of disease in patients, it is difficult to predict drug malabsorption and in practice it is not usually necessary to alter dosage purely because absorption may be theoretically impaired in disease states. However, if a patient with gastrointestinal disease does not respond in the expected manner to his oral medication, drug malabsorption should be suspected.

Metabolism in the gastrointestinal tract

The gut provides a protective as well as digestive function. This is mediated by an active reticuloendothelial system together with a substantial metabolic component. Degrading enzymes are present in the gut lumen, within the gastrointestinal secretions, and also in the intestinal flora. The gastrointestinal wall itself contains a wide variety of metabolic enzymes responsible for the full range of chemical biotransformation reactions. Intestinal enzymes not only metabolize potentially toxic substances but also drugs given therapeutically. The extent of enzyme activity for a particular reaction can approach that of the liver on a weight for weight basis. For most drugs, gastrointestinal drug metabolism is apparent only when they are given orally or rectally.

Intestinal lumen
Enzymes in the gut lumen originate either from exocrine glands or shed mucosal cells. Many enzyme reactions, such as the hydrolysis of

reduce absorption. In general terms, lipid-soluble drugs continue to be well absorbed even in the face of extensive gastrointestinal disease, whereas the absorption of water-soluble substances is more likely to be impaired.[33] Because of the variability in the physicochemical proper-

Table 8.41 Factors affecting drug absorption in disease states.

Factor	Disease state	Drug absorption
Reduced gastric acid secretion	Pernicious anaemia	Normal or reduced
Reduced gastric emptying time	Gastric ulcer Migraine Myocardial infarction Chronic pain (Labour)	Normal or reduced
Increased gastric emptying time	Duodenal ulcer Gastrointestinal surgery	Normal, reduced or increased
Increased intestinal transit time	Gastroenteritis Crohn's disease	Normal or reduced
Reduced intestinal surface area	Coeliac disease Crohn's disease	Normal, reduced or increased
Steatorrhoea	Coeliac disease Chronic pancreatitis	Normal or reduced
Bacterial colonization	Blind loop syndrome Crohn's disease	Normal or increased
Reduced splanchnic blood flow	Congestive cardiac failure Mesenteric ischaemia	Normal or reduced
Reduced biliary flow	Cholecystitis Primary biliary cirrhosis	Normal or reduced

Sulphasalazine

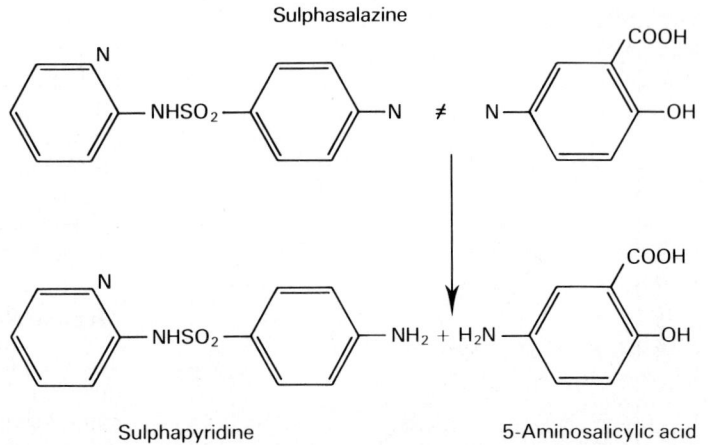

Fig. 8.83 Bacterial azo reduction of sulphasalazine to sulphapyridine and 5-aminosalicylic acid.

Sulphapyridine   5-Aminosalicylic acid

pivampicillin, can take place to some extent in the gut lumen.[41] Proteins such as insulin are also natural substrates for these enzymes.

Intestinal flora

The intestinal microorganisms represent a potent, diverse and adaptable metabolizing force for environmental xenobiotics and drugs. These are capable of performing a number of chemical functions such as hydrolysis, reduction, and deconjugation. Gut organisms are responsible for the breakdown of the now banned sweetener cyclamate to cyclohexylamine and the metabolism of the dubious anticancer agent, laetrile, with the release of cyanide.[35]

Sulphasalazine, used in the prophylaxis of inflammatory bowel disease, undergoes azo reduction in the gut lumen to the sulphonamide sulphapyridine and 5-aminosalicylic acid, which is thought to be the active moiety of the drug (Figure 8.83).[3] Bacterially mediated metabolic steps are involved in the breakdown of metronidazole, chloramphenicol and digoxin. This metabolism can be reduced by treatment with a broad-spectrum antibiotic.[24]

Gut wall

Drug metabolism is classically divided into phase 1 and phase 2 reactions involving oxidative and conjugating enzymes (Figure 8.84).

Phase 1 enzymes are responsible for oxidation, hydroxylation, dealkylation, reduction and hydrolysis, and have been shown to be present in the gut wall,[20] but the oxidative metabolic capacity in this site is less than that of the liver on a weight for weight basis. However, when conjugation mechanisms are considered, the activity of the gut wall may even exceed that of the liver for some reactions. Conjugation with glucuronide, sulphate, glutathione and glycine all take place.[9] N-acetylation and O-methylation reactions also occur, the latter being an important metabolic pathway for catecholamines.

The activity of these mucosal enzymes is not static but constantly changing under the influence of inducing substances in natural foodstuffs such as indoles in vegetables of the genus Brassica (e.g. brussels sprouts, cabbage, kale) and polycyclic hydrocarbons produced by cooking procedures such as charcoal broiling of meat. Cigarette smoke and enzyme-inducing drugs such as phenobarbitone also increase the synthesis of gastrointestinal enzymes.

The ability of the gut to perform some metabolic functions, particularly sulphation and glucuronidation, can be saturated by excess substrate since the availability of certain cofactors for these reactions is low in the enterocyte. Inhibition of conjugation can also occur due to competition from other substrates utilizing the

Lipid soluble ——————————————————→ Water soluble

Fig. 8.84 Stages of drug metabolism. The gut wall is particularly rich in conjugating enzymes.

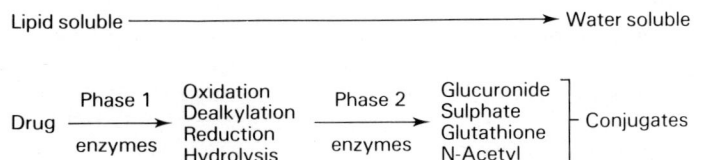

Drug →(Phase 1 enzymes)→ Oxidation Dealkylation Reduction Hydrolysis →(Phase 2 enzymes)→ Glucuronide Sulphate Glutathione N-Acetyl] Conjugates

same metabolic route. Dose-dependent metabolism can, therefore, occur and this may be responsible for the marked variability of the first-pass metabolism of drug substrates.

First-pass metabolism

For oral absorption a drug must pass through the gut wall, largely in the upper jejunum, and from there cross the liver via the portal circulation. A number of drugs undergo substantial biotransformation on the 'first pass' through to the systemic circulation. For most of these drugs, this presystemic elimination takes place in the liver but for a minority it occurs primarily in the gut wall. Some drugs are metabolised at both sites.[22] Aspirin is rapidly hydrolyzed by esterases to salicylic acid both in the gut wall and liver. The O-dealkylation of phenacetin to paracetamol can also take place in the gut wall and this may be accelerated by polycyclic hydrocarbons in charcoal-broiled beef and cigarette smoke.[32] Conjugation of the narcotic analgesics, morphine and pentazocine, and the oxidation of lignocaine also appear to have an intestinal component. The phase 2 metabolism of the sympathomimetic amines, such as isoprenaline, salbutamol and terbutaline, occurs largely in the intestinal epithelium,[19] and gut wall dopadecarboxylase may be responsible for the high presystemic elimination of levodopa.[2] This peripheral decarboxylation can be inhibited by the concomitant administration of a dopadecarboxylase inhibitor, such as carbidopa or benserazide, and these are now routinely included in combined preparations used to treat parkinsonism. Ethinyloestradiol, the most commonly used oestrogenic component of the oral contraceptive pill, is largely sulphated in the small bowel.[5] The dopaminergic antagonist chlorpromazine also undergoes substantial and variable first-pass metabolism in the gut wall.[36]

Tyramine, found in foodstuffs such as cheese, bananas, tomatoes, red wine and yeast extracts, is another substance which is extensively metabolized in the gut. The enzyme involved, monoamine oxidase (MAO) can be inhibited by concurrent administration of the antidepressant MAO inhibitors. This forms an important component of the 'cheese reaction' discussed later.

The synthesis of 'pro-drugs', which are themselves inert but are rapidly converted to the active parent compound within the body, is a pharmacologically attractive concept. Pivampicillin is one such compound which is rapidly hydrolysed to ampicillin largely in the intestinal mucosa.[25] This drug is 100% bioavailable as ampicillin. Other similar 'pro-antibiotics' include talampicillin, bacampicillin and pivmecillinam.

Biliary excretion of drugs

Excretion in bile plays a relatively minor role in the elimination of unmetabolized drugs, but is a major route for drug metabolites, particularly water-soluble conjugates. Small molecules can passively diffuse into bile and this may account for the elimination of 5–10% of the dose. An active transport system into the bile exists for substances of molecular weight greater than 300 which possess an ionic polar group. Conjugated drug metabolites tend to fulfil both these criteria. The biliary excretion of most antibiotics is generally low. The exception is rifampicin and this has led to a vogue for its use in biliary infection. Drugs which seem to have substantial biliary excretion include digitoxin, doxorubicin, steroid moieties and spironolactone.[37] Bile may also serve as an important alternative route of elimination in patients with renal failure. The biliary secretion of only a few drugs has been actively studied so far and recent advances in the methods of bile collection will undoubtedly increase the amount of available information.

A number of these conjugated drug metabolites, on entering the alimentary tract, undergo hydrolysis or deconjugation by enzymes in the gut wall and gastrointestinal flora to form the parent compound. The reconstituted drug is then reabsorbed. A drug taking part in such a cycle will persist in the body longer than expected from single dose kinetic studies and this mechanism will produce post-absorption peaks in concentration. This has been described for benzodiazepines, phenothiazines and some of the β-adrenergic antagonists.[14] Depending on the concentration gradient and membrane permeability, drugs can also diffuse from the general circulation back into the gastrointestinal lumen.

The effect of blocking the biliary excretion of a drug which is predominantly eliminated by this route will lead to accumulation of the drug. Interruption of the enterohepatic cycle of a drug may markedly reduce its biological half life. This is the mechanism by which activated charcoal increases phenobarbitone, carbamazepine and phenylbutazone elimination, suggesting a role for this substance in the management of poisoning with these drugs.[23] Similarly, cholestyramine will substantially reduce digitoxin clearance by binding it in the gut and preventing its enterohepatic circulation.[10] Biliary excretion of drugs will, of course, be impaired if the liver is diseased, particularly in cirrhosis.

UNDESIRABLE EFFECTS

Drugs may, of course, also produce unwanted effects in the small bowel. This may result in interference with the normal processes of absorption of fat, nutrients or other drugs. Rarely structural damage to the intestinal mucosa may be produced.

Iatrogenic malabsorption

Drugs may affect small intestinal function in a number of ways, but severe malabsorption only rarely occurs.[17] Colchicine and methotrexate affect mitotic activity and hence cell renewal, producing a malabsorption syndrome associated with morphological changes similar to those found in coeliac disease. Milder abnormalities in fat and carbohydrate absorption may be found in patients taking these drugs. Methyldopa and neomycin have also been reported to cause malabsorption with abnormal jejunal histology. Other drugs implicated in the production of steatorrhoea include phenindione, cholestyramine, anthraquinone cathartics, tetracycline[28] and allopurinol.[11]

Malnutrition

Pharmacological agents can produce nutritional deficiency by inhibiting the absorption of vitamins and minerals. As folic acid is not stored to any appreciable extent, malabsorption of this haematinic may rapidly produce marrow megaloblastosis. Alcohol, anticonvulsant drugs (particularly phenytoin and primidone), oral contraceptive agents, cycloserine and methyldopa have all been suggested to impair the bioavailability of folic acid. The mechanism of these effects is complex and generally ill-understood.[13]

The anion exchange resin cholestyramine and, to a lesser extent, the aminoglycoside neomycin can bind fat-soluble vitamins as well as bile salts, and deficiency syndromes involving vitamins D and K have been reported.[26] Impairment of folic acid and vitamin B_{12} absorption may also occur. Sodium aminosalicylate, colchicine and the biguanides, metformin and phenformin, interfere with the ileal transport of B_{12}.[17] The aluminium-containing antacids bind phosphate and may be given therapeutically to the uraemic patient when phosphate retention occurs.

Intestinal ulceration

Ulceration and perforation of the intestine is a well recognized adverse effect of slow release preparations in which the drug is incorporated into a wax or plastic matrix which is often eliminated intact once the drug has been released.[40] Patients with small bowel strictures such as in Crohn's disease are particularly at risk. Potassium chloride and iron preparations are most often implicated in this complication. Phenylbutazone is a rarer cause of small bowel ulceration, though recent 'improved' formulations may be more dangerous.[15]

Small intestinal ischaemia

Among the many cardiovascular complications of the contraceptive pill, small intestinal ischaemia is one of the least familiar. Prognosis is limited as there is much morbidity and a high mortality.[7] It is particularly associated with a high oestrogen content, although the progesterone component may also play a part in the aetiology of emboli.[27] Other drugs incriminated in a necrotic process in the gut include digitalis glycosides, gold therapy, corticosteroids and vasopressors.[17] In many cases a compromised splanchnic circulation antedates the event.

Drug bioavailability interactions

Drug absorption interactions are most likely to occur with drugs which are relatively poorly absorbed, particularly if they have a narrow therapeutic index (e.g. digoxin, phenytoin). There are three mechanisms by which such interactions can take place: luminal effects, changes in gastric emptying time, and damage to the gut wall.[8] Interference with the bioavailability of a drug can also be produced by modification of its intestinal first-pass metabolism.

Luminal effects
Chemical reactions between drugs in the upper gastrointestinal tract resulting in treatment failure are probably more common than is currently realized. The best known example is the mutual interaction between ferrous salts and tetracycline, with the absorption of both being reduced.[29] Antacids also bind tetracycline as well as other drugs such as digoxin, phenytoin, isoniazid[21] and prednisolone.[43] Antacids also increase gastric pH, thus delaying gastric emptying time. This effect may explain the few reports implicating cimetidine in the reduction of drug

absorption, although, with the exception of ketoconazole, these interactions seem not to occur to a predictable degree.[42] Malabsorption of acidic drugs such as digoxin, warfarin, penicillin and paracetamol are most likely to occur with concomitant administration of the basic anion exchange resin, cholestyramine, although more recently binding of this agent to basic drugs such as trimethoprim has also been reported.[33] Significant reduction of drug absorption can occur with kaolin–pectin mixtures and neomycin.[1] These interactions only occur if both drugs are present simultaneously in the same part of the gut and can generally be avoided by separating the doses by at least two hours.

A few patients given broad-spectrum antibiotics may show an increase in serum digoxin concentrations due to the elimination of digoxin-metabolizing bacteria in the gut lumen.[24] Bacterial interaction may occur in young women taking an oral contraceptive agent for whom an antibiotic is prescribed. A number of unwanted pregnancies have been described and it has been postulated that the antibiotic kills the gut flora which deconjugate ethinyloestradiol, thus interfering with its enterohepatic circulation.

Motility effects
A number of drugs, including anticholinergics, phenothiazines, tricyclic antidepressants and narcotic analgesics, can slow the rate of gastric emptying. This has been shown to modify the concentration/time profile of a single dose of a number of drugs, producing delayed and attenuated peak concentrations.[30] This effect has been known for some time although the mechanism has only been elucidated relatively recently. Thus Agatha Christie's Hercules Poirot knew that narcotic analgesics delayed the absorption of a fatal dose of strychnine in solving 'The Mysterious Affair at Styles'.[12] The total amount of drug absorbed is unaltered unless it is subject to biodegradation in the gut lumen (e.g. penicillin) or metabolism in the gastric wall (e.g. chlorpromazine, levodopa). This type of interaction has most relevance for therapeutic situations where an early high peak plasma concentration is important (e.g. with analgesics and antibiotics).

Conversely, if gastric emptying time is accelerated pharmacologically with the anti-emetic dopaminergic antagonist metoclopramide, earlier and higher peak concentrations of drug can be produced. Parenteral metoclopramide administration may reverse the gastric stasis in severe migraine restoring acceptable absorption of simple analgesics such as aspirin and paracetamol. Oral metoclopramide is ineffective as it has itself to reach the upper small bowel to be absorbed. The effect of both slowing and accelerating the gastric emptying time on the absorption of paracetamol in a single patient is demonstrated in Figure 8.85. Rapid gastrointestinal transit may enhance the pharmacological effect of a drug for which there is good evidence of a concentration–effect relationship, e.g. sedation with a benzodiazepine, or may reduce the effectiveness of formulations which have a slow dissolution time, e.g. digoxin or phenytoin.

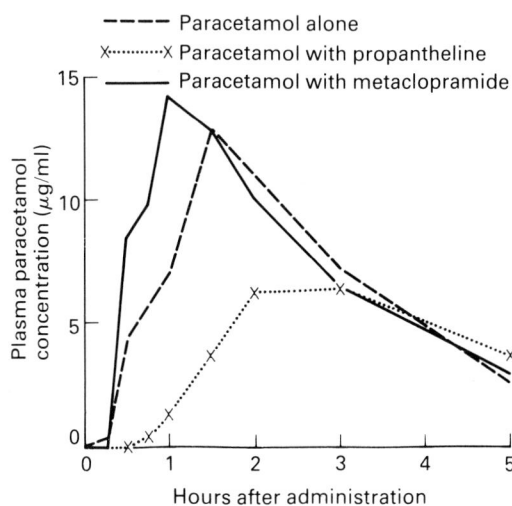

Fig. 8.85 The effect of propantheline and metoclopramide on paracetamol absorption in a 22-year-old man. From Nimmo, J. *et al.* (1973),[31] with kind permission of the authors and the editor of the *British Medical Journal*.

Enterotoxic effects
A number of drugs may themselves cause damage to the absorptive surface of the small intestine and thus reduce the bioavailability of other drugs. Although the number of reported interactions of this type is small, this must be a gross underestimate, particularly in patients receiving chemotherapy for malignant disease.[18] Neomycin, colchicine and the now superseded antituberculous agent para-amino salicylic acid (PAS) have also been implicated in this form of drug interaction.[33]

First-pass metabolism interactions
There is some evidence that drugs employing the same route of presystemic metabolism will compete for binding sites on the enzymes involved. Thus salicylamide has been found to

inhibit isoprenaline conjugation in the canine gut wall, increasing its systemic bioavailability.[6] Similarly in man, sulphate conjugation of ethinyloestradiol is inhibited by concomitant ascorbic acid administration.[4] Care, therefore, should be taken if combining two drugs metabolized by the same enzymes in the gut wall.

The first-pass metabolism of tyramine (found in foods such as cheese, tomatoes, bananas and chocolate), and phenylpropanolamine and pseudoephedrine (found in proprietary cough medicines) can be directly inhibited by monoamine oxidase inhibitors such as phenelzine and tranylcypromine. The substantial amounts of monoamine then reaching the systemic circulation stimulate the release of noradrenaline from storage granules in the sympathetic nerve endings. The resultant severe hypertension may produce subarachnoid haemorrhage in some patients.[34] Inhibition of intraneuronal monoamine oxidase may further increase the concentration of noradrenaline in the synaptic cleft.[16] When first described in the early 1960s this was known as the 'cheese reaction'.

ACKNOWLEDGEMENT

The author gratefully acknowledges the expert secretarial assistance of Carol Downes.

REFERENCES

1 Aarons, L. (1981) Kinetics of drug–drug interactions. *Pharmacology and Therapeutics*, **14**, 321–344.
2 Abrams, W. B., Coutinho, C. B., Leon, A. S. & Spiegal, H. E. (1971) Absorption and metabolism of levodopa. *Journal of the American Medical Association*, **218**, 1912–1914.
3 Azad Khan, A. K., Piris, J. & Truelove, S. C. (1977) An experiment to determine the active therapeutic moiety of sulphasalazine. *Lancet*, **ii**, 892–895.
4 Back, D. J., Breckenridge, A. M., MacIver, M. *et al.* (1981) Interaction of ethinyloestradiol with ascorbic acid in man. *British Medical Journal*, **282**, 1516.
5 Back, D. J., Breckenridge, A. M., MacIver, M. *et al.* (1982) The gut wall metabolism of ethinyloestradiol in humans. *British Journal of Clinical Pharmacology*, **13**, 325–337.
6 Bennett, P. N., Blackwell, E. W. & Davies, D. S. (1975) Competition for sulphate during detoxification in the gut. *Nature*, **258**, 247–248.
7 British Medical Journal Editorial (1978) Small-bowel ischaemia and the contraceptive pill. *British Medical Journal*, **i**, 4.
8 Brodie, M. J. (1982) Adverse drug interactions – mountain or molehill? *Journal of the Irish College of Physicians and Surgeons*, **11**, 151–154.
9 Caldwell, J. & Marsh, M. V. (1982) Metabolism of drugs by the gastrointestinal tract. In *Presystemic Drug Elimination*. (Ed.) George, C. F., Shand, D. G. & Renwick, A. G. pp. 29–42. London: Butterworth.
10 Caldwell, J. H., Bush, C. A. & Greenberger, N. J. (1971) Interruption of the enterohepatic circulation of digitoxin by cholestyramine. *Journal of Clinical Investigation*, **50**, 2638–2644.
11 Chen, B., Shapira, J., Ravid, M. & Lang, R. (1982) Steatorrhoea induced by allopurinol. *British Medical Journal*, **284**, 1914.
12 Christie, A. (1920) *The Mysterious Affair at Styles*. London: Pan Books.
13 Clark, F. (1981) Disorders of metabolism II. In *Textbook of Adverse Drug Reactions*. (Ed.) Davies, D. M. pp. 330–405. Oxford: Oxford University Press.
14 Curry, S. (1977) Disposition and fate. In *Drug Disposition and Pharmacokinetics*. pp. 62–64. Oxford: Blackwell Scientific.
15 Davies, D. R. & Brightmore, T. (1970) Idiopathic and drug-induced ulceration of the small intestine. *British Journal of Surgery*, **57**, 134–139.
16 Dollery, C. T. & Brodie, M. J. (1980) Drug interactions. *Journal of the Royal College of Physicians (London)*, **14**, 190–196.
17 Douglas, A. P. & Bateman, D. N. (1981) Gastrointestinal disorders. In *Textbook of Adverse Drug Reactions*. (Ed.) Davies, D. M. pp. 202–215. Oxford: Oxford University Press.
18 Fincham, R. W. & Schottelius, D. D. (1979) Decreased phenytoin levels in antineoplastic therapy. *Therapeutic Drug Monitoring*, **1**, 277–283.
19 George, C. F., Blackwell, E. W. & Davies, D. S. (1974) Metabolism of isoprenaline in the intestine. *Journal of Pharmacy and Pharmacology*, **26**, 265–267.
20 Hartiala, K. (1973) Metabolism of hormones, drugs and other substances by the gut. *Physiological Reviews*, **53**, 496–534.
21 Hurwitz, A. (1977) Antacid therapy and drug kinetics. *Clinical Pharmacokinetics*, **2**, 269–280.
22 Ilett, K. F. & Davies, D. S. (1982) In vivo studies of gut wall metabolism. In *Presystemic Drug Elimination* (Ed.) George, C. F., Shand, D. G. & Renwick, A. G. pp. 43–65. London: Butterworth.
23 Levy, G. (1982) Gastrointestinal clearance of drugs with activated charcoal. *New England Journal of Medicine*, **307**, 676–678.
24 Lindenbaum, J., Rund, D., Butler, V. P. *et al.* (1981) Inactivation of digoxin by the gut flora reversal by antibiotic therapy. *New England Journal of Medicine*, **305**, 789–794.
25 Lund, B., Kampmann, J. P., Lindahl, F. & Hansen, J. M. (1976) Pivampicillin and ampicillin in bile, portal and peripheral blood. *Clinical Pharmacology and Therapeutics*, **19**, 587–591.
26 Matsui, M. S. & Rozovski, S. J. (1982) Drug-nutrient interaction. *Clinical Therapeutics*, **4**, 423–440.
27 Meade, T. W., Greenberg, G. & Thompson, S. G. (1980) Progestogens and cardiovascular reactions associated with oral contraceptives. *British Medical Journal*, **280**, 1157–1161.
28 Mitchell, T. H., Stamp, T. C. B. & Jenkins, M. V. (1982) Steatorrhoea after tetracycline. *British Medical Journal*, **285**, 780.
29 Neuvonen, P. J., Pentikainen, P. J. & Gothoni, G. (1975) Inhibition of iron absorption by tetracycline. *British Journal of Clinical Pharmacology*, **2**, 94–96.
30 Nimmo, W. S. (1976) Drugs, diseases and altered gastric emptying. *Clinical Pharmacokinetics*, **1**, 189–203.
31 Nimmo, J., Heading, R. C., Tothill, P. & Prescott, L. F. (1973) Pharmacological modification of gastric emptying: effects of propantheline and metoclopramide on paracetamol absorption. *British Medical Journal*, **1**, 587–589.
32 Pantuck, E. J., Hsaio, K-C., Conney, A. H. *et al.* (1976) Effect of charcoal-broiled beef on phenacetin metabolism in man. *Science*, **194**, 1055–1057.

33 Parsons, R. L. (1977) Drug absorption in gastro-intestinal disease with particular reference to malabsorption syndromes. *Clinical Pharmacokinetics*, **2**, 45–60.

34 Pettinger, W. A. & Oates, J. A. (1968) Supersensitivity to tyramine during monoamine oxidase inhibition in man. *Clinical Pharmacology and Therapeutics*, **9**, 341–344.

35 Renwick, A. G. (1982) First-pass metabolism within the lumen of the gastrointestinal tract. In *Presystemic Drug Elimination* (Ed.) George, C. F., Shand, D. G. & Renwick, A. G. pp. 3–28. London: Butterworth.

36 Rivera-Calimlim, L., Castenada, L. & Lasagna, L. (1973) Effect of mode of management on plasma chlorpromazine in psychiatric patients. *Clinical Pharmacology and Therapeutics*, **14**, 978–986.

37 Rollins, D. E. & Klaassen, C. D. (1979) Biliary excretion of drugs in man. *Clinical Pharmacokinetics*, **4**, 368–379.

38 Sandle, G. I., Ward, A., Rawlins, M. D. & Record, C. O. (1982) Propanolol absorption in untreated coeliac disease. *Clinical Science*, **63**, 81–85.

39 Scott, A. K. & Hawksworth, G. M. (1981) Drug absorption. *British Medical Journal*, **282**, 462–463.

40 Shaffer, J. L., Higham, C. & Turnberg, L. A. (1980) Hazards of slow-release preparations on patients with bowel strictures. *Lancet*, **ii**, 487.

41 Shindo, H., Fukuda, K., Kawai, K. & Tanaka, K. (1978) Studies on intestinal absorption of pivampicillin and species differences in the intestinal esterase activity. *Journal of Pharmacobiodynamics*, **1**, 310–323.

42 Somogyi, A. & Gugler, R. (1982) Drug interactions with cimetidine. *Clinical Pharmacokinetics*, **7**, 23–41.

43 Uribe, M., Casian, C., Rojas, S. *et al.* (1981) Decreased bioavailability of prednisone due to antacids in patients with chronic active liver disease and in healthy volunteers. *Gastroenterology*, **80**, 661–665.

IMMUNOLOGICAL DISORDERS AFFECTING THE SMALL INTESTINE

BASIC GASTROINTESTINAL IMMUNOLOGY

Immune function

Immune function in vertebrates provides protection by a dual system that maintains two basic defences against foreign substances (toxins or antigens) and invaders (viruses, bacteria or parasites). Although both systems can potentially respond to a particular foreign substance, one type of response tends to predominate in any given situation. The first system – the humoral immune system – is mediated through antibodies synthesized by B lymphocytes. Individual B cells, when activated by recognition of a foreign substance, differentiate into plasma cells which secrete antibodies that bind specifically to the substance or agent and initiate a variety of elimination responses. The second

system – the cellular immune system – is primarily mediated by T lymphocytes. It is particularly effective against fungi, parasites, intracellular viral infections, cancer cells and foreign tissue. The two systems, which provide overlapping protection, interact and are to some extent interdependent. In addition to B and T lymphocytes, macrophages and mast cells, both of which are non-lymphoid accessory cells, are important to defence. These lymphoid and non-lymphoid components are present in the intestinal tract and at other locations in the body and operate together to protect the host from viruses, bacteria and antigenic substances.

Gastrointestinal-associated lymphoid tissues (GALT)

Lymphocytes are scattered throughout the lamina propria of the gastrointestinal tract and between the epithelial cells covering the intestinal villi. In addition, there are organized aggregates of lymphocytes associated with the gastrointestinal tract referred to as gastrointestinal-associated lymphoid tissues (GALT). The most frequently cited examples of GALT are Peyer's patches, the tonsils, and the appendix. It is generally considered that these aggregated lymphoid structures are the principal sites in the mucosa where interaction between antigens from the gut lumen and circulating lymphocytes takes place, whereas the cells in the lamina propria and epithelium are the effector cells which mediate immune responses.[20]

Peyer's patches, located in the ileum of man, consist of clusters of lymphoid follicles having well-defined structures.[13,29] Recent studies have demonstrated that specialized epithelial cells overlying the Peyer's patches, known as microfold or M cells, may facilitate the access of antigens to intestinal lymphoid tissues.[2,9,12] Morphologically these cells have a paucity of microvilli, a poorly developed glycocalyx and an absence of lysosomal organelles. Horseradish peroxidase has been used by Owen[21,22] to study antigen uptake by M cells (Figure 8.86). This marker is taken up into the specialized cells and rapidly released into the interstitial space where it is processed by lymphoid cells circulating through the Peyer's patches. This mechanism for antigen transport in the gut appears to represent an important specialized access route by which ingested antigens reach lymphoid tissues and thereby stimulate the local and distant immune systems. Intact macromolecules as well as viral particles appear to be processed by M cells.

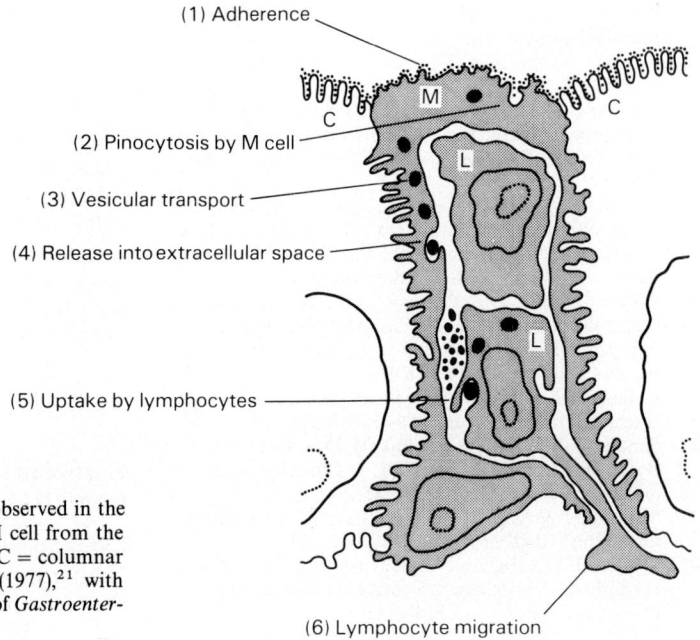

(1) Adherence

(2) Pinocytosis by M cell

(3) Vesicular transport

(4) Release into extracellular space

(5) Uptake by lymphocytes

(6) Lymphocyte migration

Fig. 8.86 Diagram summarizing the stages observed in the transport of horseradish peroxidase by the M cell from the intestinal lumen to the intraepithelial cell. C = columnar cells; L = lymphocytes. From Owen, R. L. (1977),[21] with kind permission of the author and the editor of *Gastroenterology*.

Wolf[35] inoculated reovirus into the intestinal lumen of mice and, using electron microscopy, noted that viruses were adherent to the surface of the intestinal M cells but not to other epithelial cells 30 minutes later. After one hour, virus particles were seen in M cell cytoplasm and were also associated with mononuclear cells in the adjacent intercellular space. The studies of Owen[21,22] and Wolf[35] indicate that these specialized M cells may be an important mechanism by which macromolecules and pathogens not digested or destroyed in the proximal small intestine gain access to the lymphoid tissue of the distal gut.

The most studied aspect of the mucosal defence mechanisms of GALT is the synthesis and release of a special form of the immunoglobulin A (IgA) – secretory IgA – which is the predominant immunoglobulin found in gastrointestinal secretions.[19] Secretory IgA acts to bind antigen (immune exclusion), thereby preventing its attachment to the epithelial cell surface.[8,31,32] It has been suggested that IgA may also coat the intestinal epithelium and prevent bacterial adhesion to the epithelial surface, thereby suppressing the growth of certain bacterial pathogens.[26,34,36] The quest for other potential actions of secretory IgA, such as opsonization and complement fixation, has been largely unsuccessful.[20]

Immunoglobulin A is produced by plasma cells in the lamina propria and transported into the gut lumen after linkage to secretory piece

which is a component of the epithelial cell surface.[19,30] Plasma cells in the small intestine which produce IgA have been shown to be derived from precursor cells initially stimulated in the distal ileum. The antigens absorbed via M cells participate in the activation of uncommitted lymphocytes which are modified on contact, released and then pass through the mesenteric nodes into the thoracic duct lymph, and ultimately can be identified as specific IgA antibody-producing plasma cells in the lamina propria (Figure 8.87). Pierce and Gowans[25] have studied this migration using cholera toxin in rats. They identified antitoxin-containing cells in thoracic duct lymph following the intraduodenal presentation of toxin. These cells eventually appeared in the lamina propria, particularly at sites where the antigen was first presented. Their studies and those of others demonstrate that cells stimulated by antigen to differentiate into IgA producers appear to 'home back' to the site where the antigen was originally present. This pattern of migrating cells from the gut back to the intestinal mucosal surface also occurs from the gut to the mucosa of the bronchus, and to mammary gland in the lactating animal.[11]

The 'homing' phenomenon is not completely understood. The hypothesis that factors other than antigen may be important to 'homing' is substantiated by recent experiments. When injected intravenously, mesenteric lymphocytes obtained from young mice 'home' to antigen-

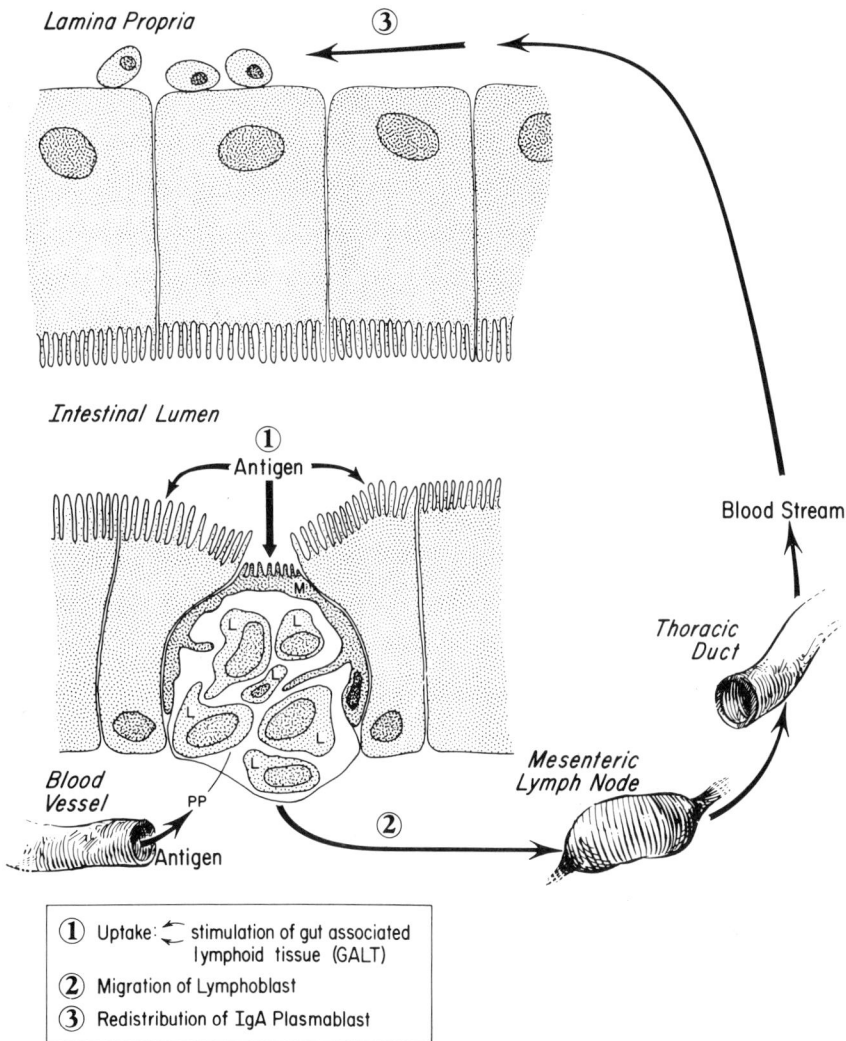

Fig. 8.87 Diagram depicting a lymphoblast (or lymphocyte) in a Peyer's patch which is exposed to an antigen. The lymphoblast (or lymphocyte) is transported to a mesenteric lymph node and then to the thoracic duct. It enters the blood and thereby returns to the intestinal tract. In the lamina propria it further differentiates into an IgA plasma cell. From Walker, W. A. and Isselbacher, K. J. (1977),[32] with kind permission of the authors and the editor of *New England Journal of Medicine*.

free fetal intestine located under the kidney capsule of an adult animal.[23] Cells committed to IgA synthesis may persist only at sites where there are sufficient IgA helper T cells.[1,5] T cell helper and suppressor activity for IgA synthesis varies for different tissues. Peyer's patches, although having a high level of non-specific suppressor activity, have increased amounts of specific IgA T lymphocyte helper activity compared to the spleen and peripheral lymph nodes.[5] Therefore, it is possible that antigenic stimulation in the Peyer's patches could induce a strong IgA response at the same time as IgG and IgM responses are suppressed. An additional explanation for why specific lymphocytes 'home' to the intestinal tract could relate to surface receptors on lymphocytes which interact with a specific component in the gastrointestinal tract.[1] Alternatively, random seeding of cells to the intestine followed by selective proliferation of lymphocytes due to factors such as secretory component may also contribute to this phenomenon.

The interaction of GALT with other lymphatic tissue has been investigated by McDermott and Bienenstock.[16] They have shown that lymphocytes from mesenteric lymph nodes not only 'home' to the lamina propria of the gut and bronchi, but a small number of cells migrate to peripheral nodes. Therefore there is support for the concept of integration of the mucosal and systemic lymphoid systems. This is strengthened by the experiments of Pierce and Gowans.[25] These investigators report that intraperitoneal primary immunization followed by oral challenge results in a large antigen-specific IgA plasmocyte response in the gut, indicating also that the systemic immune system interacts with GALT.

The liver may also contribute to intestinal mucosal barrier defences since it has been shown recently that the hepatocyte can transport free secretory IgA and immune complexes from the serum into the bile tract.[18,24,27,28] Ligation of the common bile duct has been shown to increase the concentration of secretory IgA in the serum. The hepatic transport of secretory IgA from serum to bile may not only be a means of eliminating antigen from the circulation, but it may also serve to bolster intestinal host defence by re-circulating IgA to the intestinal lumen. Recent evidence, however, indicates that this re-circulation is less prominent in humans than in animals.

The function of intestinal T lymphocytes has been studied less extensively than the function of intestinal B lymphocytes. However, there is some recent evidence that T cell lymphocytes migrate to mucosal surfaces in a similar manner to B cell lymphocytes.[7] Other than this finding, and the observation that IgA helper and suppressor activity is present in some subsets of T cells, little information is available concerning T cell function in the intestine. It is possible that the intestinal environment leads to the induction of clones of class-specific regulatory T cells which are vital to the expansion of the IgA/B cell system.

Tolerance

Macromolecules ingested by the host may stimulate the local immune system, resulting in secretory IgA production by B lymphocytes which have 'homed' to the lamina propria. Antigens may also penetrate the intestinal mucosal barrier and stimulate the systemic immune system resulting in the synthesis of specific circulating IgA antibodies. In addition or alternatively, ingested antigens may induce a state of unresponsiveness or tolerance, so that subsequent attempts to induce a systemic immune response, for example by injecting the antigen intraperitoneally, no longer result in antibody production. Immunological tolerance can be defined as a refractory state which is antigen-directed in that its development requires previous contact with a specific antigen.[33]

Over the past few years it has become obvious that there are diverse tolerant states, all having unresponsiveness as the end result, although this is attained by different mechanisms. Whether an immune response or tolerance develops following an antigen challenge depends on the age of the subject, and the quality and quantity of the antigen, as well as a number of other unappreciated factors. Additional studies are necessary to define the different mechanisms of tolerance better and to determine whether tolerance can be used advantageously to protect individuals predisposed to allergic or other immune-mediated disorders.

Macrophages and other cells

Although macrophages found in the lung, the peritoneal cavity, the spleen and the liver have been studied in great detail,[3,13] few studies have dealt directly with the origin, distribution and activity of macrophages in the gut. Intestinal macrophages are found associated with GALT, surrounding the crypts of Lieberkühn, and in the villous core. Although these macrophages are similar to macrophages in other parts of the body, they lack several characteristics, including a specific nuclear and lysosomal morphological appearance, phagocytic activity, and membrane receptors for complement and the Fc portion of the IgG molecule.[3,4,13]

Macrophages carry out diverse functions in the intestinal tract, including phagocytosis, secretion and participation in certain humoral and cellular immune responses. However, additional studies are necessary to better delineate the importance of phagocytosis and secretion by macrophages, and to characterize the role of macrophages in the immune function of the small intestine.

Recent evidence indicates that mast cells, a second type of non-lymphoid cell present in the intestine, may also be involved in immune function. There are at least two kinds of mast cells present in the gastrointestinal tract.[10] One type appears to be the typical connective tissue mast cell, and is confined to the submucosa. The second type has an atypical appearance and is present in the epithelium. Both cell types proliferate rapidly during certain parasite infections, have IgE receptors on their surface, and degranulate in response to antigen.[6,14,15,17]

We have much to learn about lymphoid and non-lymphoid cells of the gastrointestinal tract and are just beginning to appreciate the importance of intestinal immune function as a host defence mechanism. At the present time it is apparent that when functioning normally, the immune responses of the bowel act to protect the host from a diversity of foreign substances and agents. However, inadequate or abnormal immune function may be associated with a variety of gastrointestinal and/or systemic disease processes.

ACKNOWLEDGEMENTS

This work is supported in part by grants (HD-12437, AMDD-16269 and GM-21700) from the National Institute of Health. Dr Udall is the recipient of a Clinical Associate Physician Award (2-M01-RR-00088-18).

REFERENCES

1 Bienenstock, J. & Befus, A. D. (1980) Review: mucosal immunology. *Immunology*, **41**, 249–270.
2 Bockman, D. E. & Cooper, M. D. (1973) Pinocytosis by epithelium associated with lymphoid follicles in the bursa of Fabricius, appendix and Peyer's patches: an electron microscopic study. *American Journal of Anatomy*, **136**, 455–478.
3 Carr, I. (1973) The fixed macrophage. In *The Macrophage. A Review of Ultrastructure and Function.* pp. 20–40. London: Academic Press.
4 Carr, I. & Wright, J. (1978) The reticuloendothelial and mononuclear phagocyte systems and the macrophage. *Canadian Medical Association Journal*, **118**, 882–885.
5 Elson, C. O., Heck, J. A. & Strober, W. (1979) T-cell regulation of murine IgA synthesis. *Journal of Experimental Medicine*, **149**, 632–643.
6 Enerback, L. & Lundin, P. M. (1974) Ultrastructure of mucosal mast cells in normal and compound 48/80-treated rats. *Cell and Tissue Research*, **150**, 95–105.
7 Guy-Grand, D., Griscelli, C. & Vassalli, P. (1978) The mouse gut T lymphocyte, a novel type of T cell. *Journal of Experimental Medicine*, **148**, 1661–1677.
8 Heremans, J. F. (1974) Immunoglobulin A. In *The Antigens*, vol. II (Ed.) Sela, M. pp. 365–522. New York: Academic Press.
9 Kagnoff, M. F. (1977) Functional characteristics of Peyer's patch lymphoid cells. IV. Effect of antigen feeding on the frequency of antigen-specific B cells. *Journal of Immunology*, **118**, 992–997.
10 Kalinger, M. A. (1980) Is a mast cell a mast cell a mast cell? *Journal of Allergy and Clinical Immunology*, **66**, 1–4.
11 Kleinman, R. E. & Walker, W. A. (1979) The enteromammary immune system. An important new concept in breast milk host defense. *Digestive Diseases and Sciences*, **24**, 876–882.
12 Joel, D. D., Laissue, J. A. & LeFevre, M. E. (1978) Distribution and fate of ingested carbon particles in mice. *Journal of the Reticuloendothelial Society*, **24**, 477–487.
13 LeFevre, M. E., Hammer, R. & Joel, D. D. (1979) Macrophages of the mammalian small intestine: a review. *Journal of the Reticuloendothelial Society*, **26**, 553–573.
14 Mayrhofer, G. (1979) The nature of the thymus dependency of mucosal mast cells. I. An adaptive secondary response to challenge with *Nippostrongylus brasiliensis*. *Cellular Immunology*, **47**, 304–311.
15 Mayrhofer, G., Bazin, H. & Gowans, J. L. (1976) Nature of cells binding anti-IgE in rats immunized with *Nippostrongylus brasiliensis*: IgE synthesis in regional nodes and concentration in mucosal mast cells. *European Journal of Immunology*, **6**, 537–545.
16 McDermott, M. R. & Bienenstock, J. (1979) Evidence for a common mucosal immunologic system. I. Migration of B immunoblasts into intestinal, respiratory, and genital tissues. *Journal of Immunology*, **122**, 1892–1898.
17 Miller, H. R. P. & Jarrett, W. F. H. (1971) Immune reactions in mucous membranes. I. Intestinal mast cell response during helminth expulsion in the rat. *Immunology*, **20**, 277–288.
18 Nagura, H., Smith, P. D., Nakane, P. K. & Brown, W. R. (1981) IgA in human bile and liver. *Journal of Immunology*, **126**, 587–595.
19 Ogra, P. L. (1979) Ontogeny of the local immune system. *Pediatrics*, **64**, 765–774.
20 Ottaway, C. A., Rose, M. L. & Parrott, D. M. (1979) The gut as an immunological system. In *Gastrointestinal Physiology III, International Review of Physiology*, vol. 19 (Ed.) Crane, R. K. pp. 323–356. Baltimore: University Park Press.
21 Owen, R. L. (1977) Sequential uptake of horseradish peroxidase by lymphoid follicle epithelium of Peyer's patches in the normal unobstructed mouse intestine: An ultrastructural study. *Gastroenterology*, **72**, 440–451.
22 Owen, R. L. & Jones, A. L. (1974) Epithelial cell specialization within human Peyer's patches: An ultrastructural study of intestinal lymphoid follicles. *Gastroenterology*, **66**, 189–203.
23 Parrott, D. M. V. & Ferguson, A. (1974) Selective migration of lymphocytes within the mouse small intestine. *Immunology*, **26**, 571–588.
24 Peppard, J., Orlans, E., Payne, A. W. R. & Andrew, E. (1981) The elimination of circulating complexes containing polymeric IgA by excretion in the bile. *Immunology*, **42**, 83–89.
25 Pierce, N. F. & Gowans, J. L. (1975) Cellular kinetics of the intestinal immune response to cholera toxoid in rats. *Journal of Experimental Medicine*, **142**, 1550–1563.
26 Rogers, H. J. & Synge, C. (1978) Bacteriostatic effect of human milk on E. coli: the role of IgA. *Immunology*, **34**, 19–28.
27 Russell, M. W., Brown, T. A. & Mestecky, J. (1981) Role of serum IgA. Hepatobiliary transport of circulating antigens. *Journal of Experimental Medicine*, **153**, 968–976.
28 Socken, D. J., Simms, E. S., Nagy, B. R. *et al.* (1981) Secretory component-dependent hepatic transport of IgA antibody-antigen complexes. *Journal of Immunology*, **127**, 316–319.
29 Tomasi, T. B., Larson, L., Challacombe, S. & McNabb, P. (1980) Mucosal immunity: the origin and migration patterns of cells in the secretory system. *Journal of Allergy and Clinical Immunology*, **65**, 12–19.
30 Walker, W. A. (1976) Host defense mechanisms in the gastrointestinal tract. *Pediatrics*, **57**, 901–916.
31 Walker, W. A. (1978) Antigen handling by the gut. *Archives of Diseases in Childhood*, **53**, 527–531.
32 Walker, W. A. & Isselbacher, K. J. (1977) Intestinal antibodies. *New England Journal of Medicine*, **297**, 767–773.
33 Weigle, W. O. (1978) Immunological tolerance. In *Immunological Diseases* (Ed.) Samter, M. pp. 389–407. Boston: Little, Brown and Co.
34 Williams, R. C. & Gibbons, R. J. (1972) Inhibition of bacterial adherence by secretory immunoglobulin A: a mechanism of antigen disposal. *Science*, **177**, 697–699.

35 Wolf, J. L., Rubin, D. H., Finberg, R. *et al.* (1981) Intestinal M cells: a pathway for entry of reovirus into the host. *Science*, **212**, 471–472.
36 Wright, R. (1977) Normal immune responses in the gut and immunodeficiency disorders. In *Immunology of Gastrointestinal and Liver Disease.* (Ed.) Tuck, J. pp. 1–15. London: Edward Arnold.

IMMUNODEFICIENCY AND THE GUT

Immunodeficiency and gastrointestinal disease have complex interrelations. A primary defect in antibody-mediated immunity, or less commonly of cell-mediated immunity, can lead to gastrointestinal disease – frequently in the form of infection and infestation, but also of other types. Conversely primary disease of the gut can lead to losses of antibody or lymphocytes into the lumen, thus causing immunodeficiency and predisposing to systemic infections.

A further complexity is introduced by the specialized nature of the gut immune defences. The particular features of this have been outlined in the preceding section, notably the local protective action of secretory IgA, and also its role in inducing tolerance in the systemic immune system when antigens are presented via the gut. Thus a specific defect in the local immune system may allow ingress of antigens from the lumen, and initiate damaging generalized immune responses.

Classification of immunodeficiency states

Many types of immunodeficiency have now been described, often of considerable rarity, and active research is demonstrating further subgroups in each type. In broad terms immunodeficiency states may be classified as follows:
1 Primary specific immunodeficiencies – reflecting deficient antibody production, deficient T cell-mediated immunity, or both.
2 Primary non-specific immunodeficiencies – in which immunological memory is intact but there is a deficiency in the function of the mediators of the inflammatory response, such as the complement system or neutrophil polymorphonuclear leucocytes.
3 Secondary immunodeficiencies – such as those due to irradiation, immunosuppressive drugs, and neoplasm. Included in this group are the immunodeficiencies resulting from loss of immunoglobulin and lymphocytes into the gut lumen.

Table 8.42 shows a classification of the major immunodeficiency diseases. Most present in

Table 8.42 Major primary immunodeficiency syndromes.

B cell (antibody) defects
  X-linked (Bruton's) agammaglobulinaemia
  Common variable hypogammaglobulinaemia
  Selective IgA deficiency

T cell (cell-mediated) defects
  Di-George syndrome (thymic aplasia)
  Chronic mucocutaneous candidiasis

B and T cell defects
  Severe combined immunodeficiency
  Wiskott–Aldrich syndrome
  Ataxia telangiectasia
  Thymoma

Non-specific defects
  Chronic granulomatous disease
  Complement deficiencies

childhood. The only diseases commonly encountered by the specialist gastroenterologist in adults are selective IgA deficiency and, more rarely, common variable hypogammaglobulinaemia and intestinal lymphangiectasia. The latter condition is discussed on p. 605.

Antibody deficiency states

COMMON VARIABLE HYPOGAMMAGLOBULINEMIA

Patients with common variable hypogammaglobulinemia (CVH) have abnormally low serum immunoglobulin (Ig) levels and usually recurrent infections. The serum levels of all three main Ig classes – IgG, IgA and IgM – are low. The condition has a number of synonyms: common variable immunodeficiency,[13] idiopathic late onset immunoglobulin deficiency,[15] or primary acquired hypogammaglobulinaemia. These descriptive terms emphasize that the disease is frequently not manifest until adult life, that the serum levels of individual immunoglobulins may vary from time to time in individual patients, and that the condition is heterogeneous.

Aetiology
The aetiology of CVH is unclear. Functionally, there is inadequate production of immunoglobulin by cells of the B lymphocyte line. In a few rare individuals with strong family histories, this may be initiated by an infection with Epstein–Barr virus,[28] but this is now classified as a disorder separate from CVH, as a sex-linked recessive immunoproliferative disorder. There is no proof of a viral aetiology in most patients

with CVH. Some familial cases of CVH are reported, but different pedigrees suggesting autosomal dominant and recessive inheritance exist.

Immune defects
Studies of immunoglobulin production and other immune parameters in patients with CVH indicate that the low serum immunoglobulin levels may have a number of causes. In about 25% of patients, B lymphocytes, the precursors of immunoglobulin-producing plasma cells, are absent from peripheral blood;[19] in others B cells are present, but in culture they do not synthesize or release normal amounts of immunoglobulin. In some patients, but not all, this decreased production by B cells is attributable to the presence of an overactive regulatory suppressor T cell, removal of which permits normal immunoglobulin production by B cells.[31] Other immunological studies confirm the heterogeneity of CVH. About one third of patients have defective cell-mediated immunity demonstrable by in vivo or in vitro testing, and lymphopaenia may be present.[5] Further studies will undoubtedly subdivide CVH. Nonetheless, the similar clinical features and a common susceptibility to infections and a number of gastrointestinal conditions makes the establishment of a diagnosis of CVH useful.

Clinical features
The sex incidence of CVH is equal, with patients presenting at any age. The onset is taken as the time at which frequent infections begin; it is usually a supposition that serum immunoglobins become low at that stage, although there are well documented examples in whom a change from normal serum immunoglobulin levels has been demonstrated.

The majority of patients present with recurrent sino-pulmonary infections. There is a small minority in whom these are absent, and gastrointestinal symptoms are the only manifestations. In addition, patients are prone to meningitis, osteomyelitis and other severe systemic bacterial infections; other extraintestinal manifestations may include a sarcoid-like pulmonary infiltration, polyarthritis, haemolysis, neutropenia and thrombocytopenia.

Physical examination may reveal splenomegaly in 20–50% of individuals; lymphadenopathy is much rarer, and should prompt investigation to exclude lymphoma. In patients with severe intestinal disease, the physical signs of a malabsorptive state may be present.

Gastrointestinal disease
Between 60 and 90% of patients suffer gastrointestinal symptoms; the most common complaints being diarrhoea (intermittent or chronic), weight loss, and vomiting. Virtually every part of the gastrointestinal tract may be abnormal in CVH.[4]

Gastric disease. Achlorhydria, gastritis, and pernicious anaemia are all common. Approximately 50% of patients with CVH have pentagastrin-fast achlorhydria,[35] often, but not invariably, associated with intrinsic factor deficiency. The histological basis of this is atrophic gastritis, with a heavy mononuclear cell infiltrate, absent parietal and chief cells, and intestinal metaplasia. The atrophic inflammatory process tends to involve the whole stomach, without the antral sparing often found in Addisonian pernicious anaemia. This explains why the achlorhydria of CVH is not usually accompanied by a high serum gastrin level;[21] unlike the unaffected antrum of pernicious anaemia, the G cell-bearing area in CVH is atrophic.

The cause of the gastric atrophy is uncertain; as it occurs in the absence of autoantibodies, it cannot be due to an antibody-mediated autoimmune process. Cell-mediated autoimmunity may play a role, and circulating lymphocytes sensitized to parietal cells and intrinsic factor have been reported.[22]

A frank macrocytic anaemia due to B_{12} deficiency occurs in many patients with CVH but, as discussed below, it is apparently more frequently due to infestation of the small gut with *Giardia* than a consequence of intrinsic factor deficiency and gastritis.[4] A far more serious consequence of gastric atrophy is the development of gastric carcinoma; in one study 7 out of 50 patients with CVH were reported to have this complication.[15] This incidence is much higher than the incidence in Addisonian pernicious anaemia; the difference may reflect an additional defect in immunosurveillance against cancer, or differences in the extent and type of bacterial colonization of the stomach, leading to a higher concentration of carcinogenic or cocarcinogenic factors in CVH.[17] Whatever the explanation, the risk is high enough in CVH to justify surveillance endoscopy.

Small intestine. Between one third and two thirds of patients with CVH have chronic or recurrent attacks of diarrhoea. A number of causes have been documented, some occurring with and others without abnormal small intestinal morphology. Abnormalities of both small bowel structure and function may occur.

Nodular lymphoid hyperplasia occurs in between 20 and 60% of patients with CVH and diarrhoea. Small nodules of lymphoid cells, 1–3 mm in diameter, appear scattered through the lamina propria of the small intestine.[15] Whether the incidence is as high in patients without diarrhoea is unclear. The nodules are similar to normal lymphoid follicles or intestinal Peyer's patches, and may contain germinal follicles. Immunofluorescence studies have shown IgM present in some.[25] The normal villi of the small intestine may be stretched over the nodules. These nodules may be detected either by radiology (Figure 8.88) or on intestinal biopsy; in one series of patients with diarrhoea in whom biopsies showed nodules in 60%, only half showed the appearances on small bowel X-ray.[15] Much less commonly, similar nodules can be detected in the colon and the stomach.[7] Although giardiasis, the common parasitic infection of CVH, may be commoner when nodular lymphoid

hyperplasia is present, eradication of the giardiasis does not reverse the nodular lesion.

In addition to the nodular lymphoid hyperplasia, a spectrum of small intestinal findings occurs in patients with CVH known as *hypogammaglobulinaemic sprue*. The mucosa may show a normal villous architecture, with the only abnormality being an absence of plasma cells, or there may be varying degrees of lymphocytic infiltration, epithelial atrophy and villous blunting (Figure 8.89). Such inflammatory or atrophic changes were found on biopsy in one quarter of a series of patients with diarrhoea.[15] The abnormalities are rarely so severe as to warrant a description of subtotal villous atrophy; they are more commonly patchy, with normal villi present in adjacent areas or when multiple biopsies are taken. Frequently the changes may be shown to be a consequence of giardial infestation, returning to normal after eradication of the parasite, but in other cases

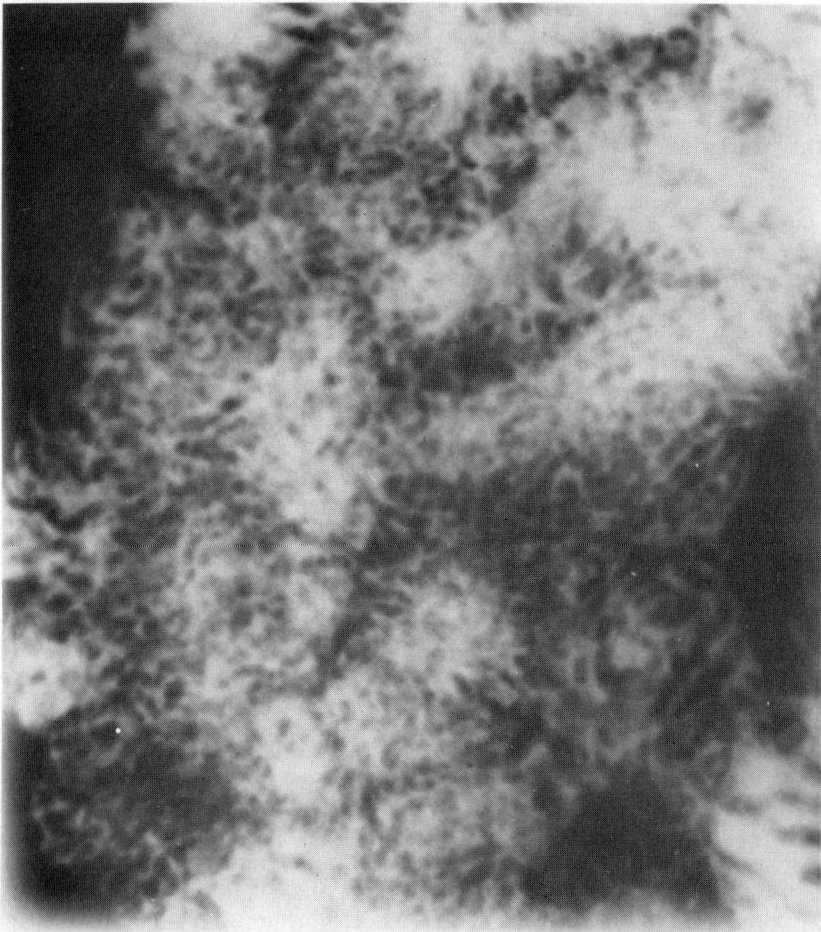

Fig. 8.88 Nodular lymphoid hyperplasia shown on small intestinal X-ray in a patient with CVH.

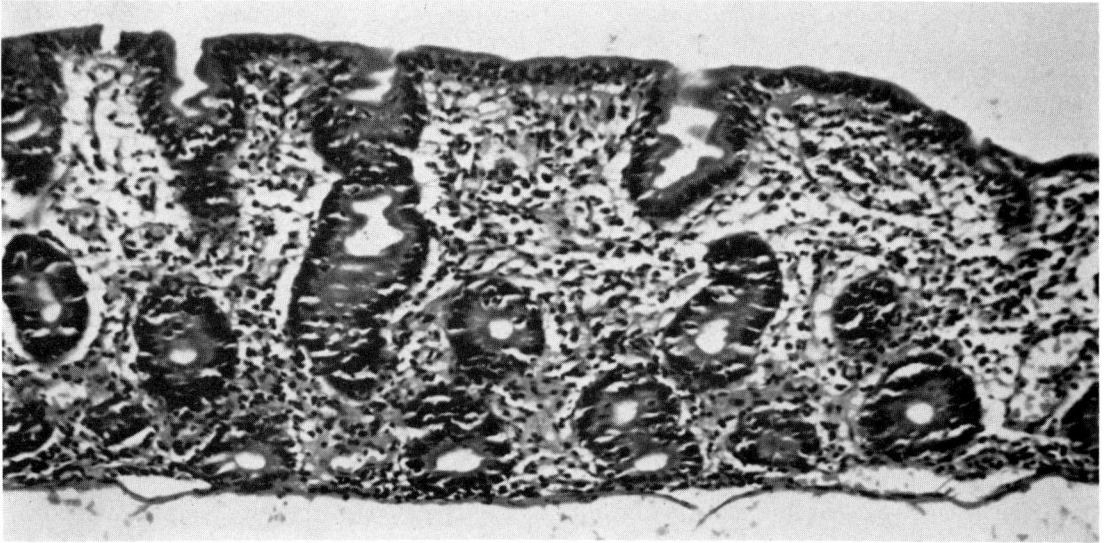

Fig. 8.89 Histological appearances of a small intestinal biopsy from a patient with CVH showing partial villous atrophy and crypt hyperplasia.

eradication causes no improvement.[4] Other infestations should then be sought, and the possibility of a gluten-sensitive enteropathy be considered, but often no cause other than hypogammaglobulinaemia will emerge.

Infections. The commonest gut infection in patients with CVH is giardiasis, which will be found in 60–80% of patients with diarrhoea, and occasionally but much less frequently (approximately 10%) in patients without gastrointestinal symptoms. The importance of using duodenal aspiration, biopsy and imprint techniques rather than simple stool examination to exclude infection has been emphasized.[16] Ament et al. have shown that giardiasis may cause not only diarrhoea, but also villous abnormalities, B_{12} and folate malabsorption, steatorrhoea, lactose intolerance, disaccharidase deficiency and protein-losing enteropathy. In 6 out of 10 patients with CVH, for example, B_{12} absorption returned to normal after treatment of the infection, and in all infested cases treatment resulted in improvement of the small intestinal mucosal damage.[4]

Other infections. Many other gut infections occur in CVH, although not as predictably as giardiasis. Bacterial overgrowth of the upper small intestine is common, with both aerobic and anaerobic organisms. This probably reflects both the achlorhydria and a loss of protective secretory immunoglobulin.[27] However, a high concentration of unconjugated bile acid, as would be expected were bacterial colonization of the duodenum and jejunum to contribute to malabsorption, is not found. Infection of the gut with *Salmonella* and *Campylobacter* is well documented.[27] Chronic viral infections such as with cytomegalovirus also occur.[12] The report of a fatal case of coccidial infection in CVH, and of severe infestations such as cryptosporidiosis in patients with childhood hypogammaglobulinaemia, emphasize that, in patients with immunodeficiency and severe malabsorptive states, parasites and other infective agents should be meticulously sought.

Other gastrointestinal diseases. An inflammatory colitis occurs in a minority of patients with CVH and diarrhoea – perhaps in 10%. In our experience the sigmoidoscopic appearances and rectal biopsy histology are those of mild ulcerative colitis, with crypt abscesses and a mixed neutrophil and lymphocyte infiltrate, although a severe colitis attributed to cytomegalovirus has been reported. Chronic *Campylobacter* infection may be the cause of a persistent colitis.

Cholelithiasis is common in CVH, with one series showing a 35% incidence of gallstones, perhaps reflecting either ileal disease or bacterial seeding of stones in the biliary tree.[15] Chronic pancreatitis may be more common, but this is poorly documented; some patients with familial pancreatic insufficiency of the Shwachman type also have hypogammaglobulinaemia, and this possibility should be considered.[8]

Mechanisms and management of diarrhoea in CVH

As already discussed, in the majority of cases diarrhoea in CVH is associated with giardiasis, and responds adequately to treatment with metronidazole or mepacrine; repeated courses may be necessary. In those in whom neither giardiasis nor any other clearly definable infection is present, the control of diarrhoea may be a formidable problem. The relative contributions of lactase deficiency, steatorrhoea, bile salt malabsorption,[4] bacterial overgrowth and colitis to the diarrhoea must be assessed; the possibility of a secretory diarrhoea, occasionally reported, must also be considered.[11] Colitis, in our experience, responds to conventional treatment for ulcerative colitis, with salicylazosulphapyridine or local corticosteroids. Symptomatic treatment of diarrhoea with a low fat, low lactose diet, with or without cholestyramine, may be successful. Very occasionally a true gluten-sensitive enteropathy may be present[36] but, in view of the patchy nature of hypogammaglobulinaemic sprue, it is difficult to be certain of the effects of dietary manipulation on villous architecture. There are occasional anecdotal reports of benefit from treatment with fresh frozen plasma infusions, colostral IgA by mouth, or high dose steroids. In a few unfortunate individuals persistent diarrhoea and malabsorption may be resistant to all treatment, and prove fatal.

The general management of CVH will involve parenteral immunoglobulin replacement to prevent systemic infections; this is rarely of help for the gastrointestinal disease.

OTHER CAUSES OF HYPOGAMMAGLOBULINAEMIA

Childhood, sex-linked (Bruton's) agammaglobulinaemia presents in male infants with recurrent bacterial infections. Gastrointestinal complications are far less common than in late onset hypogammaglobulinaemia, although minor villous abnormalities, giardiasis and bacterial overgrowth have all been reported. Investigations should follow the lines described for CVH.[5]

Thymomas are associated, in about 5% of cases, with hypogammaglobulinaemia, and in these patients diarrhoea may be a feature.[23]

SELECTIVE IMMUNOGLOBULIN A DEFICIENCY

Unlike the immunodeficiencies outlined above, selective IgA deficiency is a common state, often

asymptomatic, and frequently not meriting the term 'disease'. The incidence in the general population (estimated on blood donors) is approximately 1 in 500–700.[18] In some individuals serum IgA is virtually undetectable, in others it is persistently well below the lower limit of normal (approximately 0.7 g/l) but readily detectable. Occasionally IgA deficiency is familial, but more often sporadic; in a few patients, IgA deficiency follows therapy with drugs, notably phenytoin. Why one individual with IgA deficiency is symptomatic, but another not, is unclear, but a co-existing deficiency of the IgG_2 subclass of IgG has been suggested as a contributing factor.[26]

Clinical presentation

As already mentioned, most affected individuals are asymptomatic. Sino-pulmonary disease is the most obvious consequence of selective IgA deficiency, with repeated sinus and pulmonary infections.[3] Atopic disorders such as asthma, hay fever, and atopic eczema are common. It is tempting to interpret this latter fact in terms of a deficiency in mucosal immunity permitting increased ingress of antigens to the body, these antigens then initiating the production of IgE antibodies. It has also been suggested that atopic disorders in patients with normal immunoglobulin levels may be initiated in the same way – a delay in maturation of the IgA system at the mucosa permitting the development of IgE-mediated immune responses to common allergens.[32]

Autoimmune diseases, including Still's disease, rheumatoid arthritis, systemic lupus erythematosus, and autoimmune haemolytic anaemia are all associated with selective IgA deficiency.[3]

Gastrointestinal disease

The gastrointestinal disease associated with IgA deficiency is neither as common nor as dramatic as might be expected in view of the loss of the secretory IgA at the gut surface. Probably in such patients IgM plays an important protective role, for this immunoglobulin can also combine with secretory component at the mucosal surface and thus function as a secretory immunoglobulin. Nonetheless, food antibodies are relatively common in IgA deficiency, reflecting increased absorption of food protein.[10]

Infections. Giardiasis, and associated nodular lymphoid hyperplasia, have been reported in selective IgA deficiency, but are far less frequent than in common variable hypogammaglobulinaemia.[14] *Candida* overgrowth associated with decreased secretory IgA has been reported, but the immunoglobulin abnormality was not permanent and may have been secondary to the infection.[33]

Coeliac disease. IgA deficiency is far more common in patients with coeliac disease than the general population – approximately 1 in 50 compared with 1 in 500.[6] The coeliac disease is apparently identical to other cases with normal IgA, and responds to gluten withdrawal.[30] Again, one may speculate that diminished defences at the mucosa permit increased penetration of gluten or its elements, initiating damaging immune responses.

Crohn's disease. In virtually every series documenting immunoglobulin levels in patients with Crohn's disease, individuals with IgA deficiency are reported, with an overall incidence of approximately 1 in 70. Although this may suggest that individuals with IgA deficiency are more likely to develop or manifest Crohn's disease, the clinical features are indistinguishable in those with IgA deficiency from other patients with normal immunoglobulins.[17]

Other gastrointestinal disorders. There is an association between IgA deficiency and severe diarrhoea after gastric surgery, possibly mediated by bacterial overgrowth in the small intestine.[24]

Treatment
Immunoglobulin therapy is usually not required. Furthermore, although purified immunoglobulin preparations contain IgA, this is predominantly the monomer, which lacks the capacity to link with secretory component and thus appear at mucosal surfaces. A few individuals with total deficiency of IgA develop IgG antibodies to IgA, and in these patients administration of IgA or of plasma protein fractions may be dangerous.

Defects in cell-mediated immunity

Primary deficiencies in cell-mediated immunity are rarer than deficiencies of the antibody system; they usually present early in life. The deficiency may be limited to the T cell system, as in the Di-George syndrome, or be associated with B cell defects and hypogammaglobulinaemia, as in severe combined immunodeficiency. Gastrointestinal disease is often a feature, but poorly documented for obvious reasons in very sick infants. The following conditions are relatively well-defined.

Di-George syndrome
Afflicted infants present with the consequences of defective development of the third and fourth branchial arch, with absence of the thymus and parathyroid glands, and a selective loss of cell-mediated immune function. Presentation is usually with congenital heart disease, or due to hypocalcaemia. Apart from oral *Candida* infection or occasional associated developmental oesophageal defects, gastrointestinal manifestations are not prominent.

Severe combined immunodeficiency
This is a heterogeneous condition, presenting with recurrent viral, bacterial or fungal infections, failure to thrive, and diarrhoea.[20] Both small intestinal disease, with histological features of villous atrophy and of enlarged macrophages reminiscent of Whipple's disease, and a frank inflammatory colitis may occur. Candidiasis is also common. Untreated the disease may be rapidly fatal, but successful bone marrow transplantation is now possible.

Ataxia telangiectasia
This autosomal recessive condition appears to be due to a primary defect in ability to repair DNA. The clinical manifestations include cerebellar ataxia, telangiectasia, and recurrent infections; defective cell-mediated immunity is combined with IgA deficiency. There is a striking predisposition to malignancy, largely of the lymphoreticular system, and even in heterozygotes there is an increased incidence of gastric carcinoma.[28]

Wiskott–Aldrich syndrome
This sex-linked disorder affects males, and severe cases may present with bloody diarrhoea.[9] Other presentations include bleeding elsewhere, eczema, and recurrent infections; minor small intestinal morphological abnormalities have also been reported. Deficient cell-mediated immunity is associated with a platelet defect and high IgE levels.

Other primary immunodeficiencies

Chronic granulomatous disease
This condition results from a defect in the non-specific immune function of intracellular killing of phagocytozed material. The defect occurs in polymorphonuclear leucocytes and monocytes, and may be demonstrated by a failure of these

cells to reduce the dye nitroblue tetrazolium. The usual presentation is in infancy with multiple abscesses, lymphadenopathy and recurrent infections. A granulomatous involvement of the small and large intestine may mimic Crohn's disease;[2] perianal disease, severe mouth ulcers and gastric outlet obstruction due to inflammatory tissue also occur.

Chronic monocutaneous candidiasis

Chronic infection of the skin and mouth, and sometimes the oesophagus, may occur in a number of immunodeficiency states, either as a familial condition, or in association with hypoparathyroidism, or thymoma.[1] Treatment mainly involves antifungal agents, but attempts to boost cell-mediated immunity by, for example, transfer factor infusions or the drug levamisole have occasionally been successful.

Secondary immunodeficiencies

The growing aggression of medical treatment, with long-term immunosuppressive therapy for collagen–vascular disorders, and particularly with high-dose immunosuppressive or cytotoxic therapy in patients with leukaemia and those undergoing bone marrow transplantation, has demonstrated the importance of the gut as a portal of entry for infection. Oral treatment of such patients with non-absorbable antibiotics, for example 'FRACON' – framycetin, colistin and neomycin – reduces the incidence of septicaemia in such patients. Oral and systemic candidiasis develop easily in such patients, and also in patients with lymphoma or individuals whose immune function is debilitated by alcohol.

A particular risk applies to the parasite *Strongyloides* which, by autoinfection, may remain resident in the gastrointestinal tract for decades after leaving an endemic area. Hyperinfection leading to dilatation and subacute obstruction of the gut, and systemic strongyloidiasis due to invasion of brain, liver or lung, may be precipitated by immunosuppressive therapy; such patients also develop recurrent bacterial septicaemias as enteric bacteria are carried into the body by 'piggy-backing' on the invading larvae. Screening of patients from endemic areas is therefore strongly advised before immunosuppression.

REFERENCES

1 Ament, M. E. (1975) Immunodeficiency syndromes and gastrointestinal disease. *Pediatric Clinics of North America*, **22,** 807–825.

2 Ament, M. E. & Ochs, H. D. (1973) Gastrointestinal manifestations of chronic granulomatous disease. *New England Journal of Medicine*, **288,** 382–387.

3 Ammann, A. J. & Hong, R. (1971) Selective IgA deficiency. *Medicine (Baltimore)*, **50,** 223–236.

4 Ament, M. E., Ochs, H. D. & Davis, S. D. (1973) Structure and function of the gastrointestinal tract in primary immunodeficiency syndromes. *Medicine (Baltimore)*, **52,** 227–248.

5 Asherson, G. L. & Webster, A. D. B. (1980) *Diagnosis and Treatment of Immunodeficiency Diseases*. Oxford: Blackwell Scientific Publications.

6 Asquith, P., Thompson, R. A. & Cooke, W. T. (1969) Serum immunoglobins in adult coeliac disease. *Lancet*, **ii,** 129–131.

7 Bird, D. C., Jacobs, J. B., Silbiger, J. & Wolff, S. M. (1969) Hypogammaglobulinaemia with nodular lymphoid hyperplasia of the intestine. *Radiology*, **92,** 1535–1536.

8 Brueton, M. J., Mavromichalis, J., Goodchild, M. C. & Anderson, C. M. (1977) Hepatic dysfunction in association with pancreatic insufficiency and cyclic neutropenia. *Archives of Diseases in Childhood*, **42,** 147–157.

9 Cooper, M. D., Chase, M. P., Lowman, J. T. *et al.* (1968) Wiskott–Aldrich syndrome. An immunologic deficiency syndrome affecting the afferent limb of immunity. *American Journal of Medicine*, **44,** 499–513.

10 Cunningham-Rundles, C., Brandies, W. E., Good, R. A. & Day, N. K. (1979) Bovine antigens and the formation of circulating immune complexes in selective IgA deficiency. *Journal of Clinical Investigation*, **64,** 272.

11 Dawson, J., Hodgson, H. J. F., Pepys, M. B. *et al.* (1979) Immunodeficiency malabsorption and secretory diarrhoea. *American Journal of Medicine*, **67,** 540–546.

12 Freeman, H. J., Shnitka, T. K., Piercey, J. R. A. & Weinstein, W. M. (1977) Cytomegalovirus infection of the gastrointestinal tract in a patient with late onset immunodeficiency syndrome. *Gastroenterology*, **73,** 1397–1403.

13 Fudenberg, H. H., Good, R. A., Goodman, H. C. *et al.* (1971) Primary immunodeficiencies. *Bulletin of the World Health Organization*, **45,** 125–142.

14 Grybowski, J. D., Selft, T. W., Clemett, A. & Herskovic, T. (1968) Selective immunoglobin A deficiency and intestinal nodular hyperplasia. *Paediatrics*, **42,** 833–837.

15 Hermans, P. E., Diaz-Buxo, J. A. & Stobo, J. D. (1976) Idiopathic late-onset immunoglobulin deficiency. *American Journal of Medicine*, **61,** 221–237.

16 Hermans, P. E., Huizenga, K. A., Hoffmann, H. N. *et al.* (1966) Dysgammaglobulinaemia associated with nodular lymphoid hyperplasia of small intestine. *American Journal of Medicine*, **40,** 78–89.

17 Hodgson, H. J. F. & Jewell, D. P. (1977) Selective IgA deficiency and Crohn's disease. *Gut*, **18,** 644–648.

18 Holt, P. D. J., Tandy, N. P. & Anstee, D. J. (1977) Screening of blood donors for IgA deficiency. *Journal of Clinical Pathology*, **30,** 1007.

19 Horwitz, D. A., Webster, A. B. & Newton, C. (1977) B and T lymphocytes in primary hypogammoglobulinaemia. *Lancet*, **ii,** 823–825.

20 Horowitz, S., Lorenzsonn, V. W., Olsen, W. A. *et al.* (1974) Small intestinal disease in T cell deficiency. *Journal of Pediatrics*, **85,** 457–462.

21 Hughes, W., Brooks, F. & Conn, H. (1972) Serum gastrin levels in primary hypogammaglobulinaemia and pernicious anaemia. *American Journal of Medicine*, **77,** 746–750.

22 James, D., Asherson, G., Chanarin, I. *et al.* (1974) Cell-mediated immunity to intrinsic factor in autoimmune disorders. *British Medical Journal*, **iv,** 494–496.

23 Moffatt, R. E. (1976) Radiologic changes in the thymoma–hypogammaglobulinaemia syndrome. *American Journal of Radiology*, **126**, 1219.

24 McCoughlin, G. A., Bradley, J., Chapman, D. M. *et al.* (1976) IgA deficiency and severe post vagotomy diarrhoea. *Lancet*, **i**, 168–170.

25 Nagura, H., Kohler, P. F. & Brown, W. R. (1979) Immunocytochemical characterisation of lymphocytes in nodular lymphoid hyperplasia of the bowel. *Laboratory Investigation*, **40**, 66–70.

26 Oxelius, V. A., Laurell, A. B., Lindquist, B. *et al.* (1981) IgG subclasses in selective IgA deficiency. *New England Journal of Medicine*, **304**, 1476–1477.

27 Parkin, D. M., McClelland, D. B. L., O'Moore, R. R. *et al.* (1972) Intestinal bacterial flora and bile salt studies in hypogammaglobulinaemia. *Gut*, **13**, 182–188.

28 Purtilo, D. T. (1976) Pathogenesis and phenotypes of an X-limited recessive lymphoproliferative syndrome. *Lancet*, **ii**, 882–884.

29 Ruddell, W. S. J., Bone, E. S., Hill, M. J. *et al.* (1976) Gastric juice nitrate, a risk factor for cancer in the hypochlorhydric stomach. *Lancet*, **ii**, 1037–1039.

30 Savilhati, E. (1973) IgA deficiency in children. *Clinical and Experimental Immunology*, **13**, 395–400.

31 Siegal, F. P., Siegal, M. & Good, R. A. (1978) Role of helper, suppressor and B-cell defects in the pathogenesis of the hypogammaglobulinaemais. *New England Journal of Medicine*, **299**, 172–176.

32 Soothill, J. F. (1974) Immunodeficiency and allergy. *Clinical Allergy*, **3**, 511–519.

33 Strober, W., Krakauer, R., Klaerman, H. L. *et al.* (1976) Secretory component deficiency. A disorder of the IgA system. *New England Journal of Medicine*, **294**, 351–356.

34 Swift, M., Sholman, C., Perry, M. & Chase, C. (1976) Malignant neoplasms in families of patients with ataxia telangiectasia. *Cancer Research*, **36**, 209–216.

35 Twomey, J. J., Jordan, P. H., Laughter, A. H. *et al.* (1970) The gastric disorder in immunoglobin deficient patients. *American Journal of Internal Medicine*, **72**, 499–504.

36 Webster, A. D. B., Slavin, G., Skinner, M. *et al.* (1981) Coeliac disease with severe hypogammaglobulinaemia. *Gut*, **22**, 153–157.

LYMPHOMAS OF THE SMALL INTESTINE

The extent to which malignant lymphomas have been classified and re-classified, both pathologically and clinically, is notorious. In simple terms three main types of lymphoma involving the small intestine may be identified.

1 Primary small intestinal lymphoma, arising in a localized area of the small gut, in the absence of pre-existing diffuse mucosal disease. This group is sometimes described as the 'Western' type, as it is the most familiar to clinicians in Europe and the USA, and to distinguish it from 'Mediterranean' lymphoma.

2 Primary small intestinal lymphoma arising in a setting of diffuse mucosal disease. This includes the lymphoma associated with villous atrophy – presumed to be gluten-sensitive enter-

opathy; recent work has classified the malignancy arising in this setting as a malignant histiocytosis, and this is fully discussed on p. 465. The other example is the lymphoma arising in the setting of diffuse α-chain-containing plasma cell infiltration of the small intestine – the 'Mediterranean' lymphoma – part of the spectrum of immunoproliferative small intestinal disease. This is discussed later in this chapter.

3 Secondary small intestinal lymphoma, in which the gut is involved as part of a lymphomatous process initially manifest elsewhere.

Primary small intestinal lymphoma – 'western' type

The term primary implies that the lymphoma arises within the lymphoid tissue of the small intestine. In patients presenting with advanced lymphomatous disease, it is often not possible to define with certainty in which area the malignancy arose, and early studies therefore used restricted criteria so that only patients in whom the gut was definitely the site of origin were included. Dawson *et al.*[4] classified gastrointestinal lymphomas as primary when:

a There was no enlargement of intestinal or peripheral nodes.
b The peripheral white blood count was normal.
c There was a preponderance of alimentary tract lesions with only regional lymph node involvement.
d There was no liver or spleen involvement.

These criteria allow characterization of relatively early primary gut lymphomas, but it is clear that they are not met by many advanced tumours that are truly of primary gut origin. Lewin *et al.*[9] suggested an alternative definition, in which lymphomas are regarded as of primary alimentary tract origin if there is either obviously predominantly gut disease, or the patient initially presents with symptoms due to gastrointestinal lymphomatous involvement; those in whom gut involvement follows a diagnosis of extra-abdominal lymphomas are excluded. Such a definition is more likely to appeal to the clinical gastroenterologist as it effectively defines patients presenting to his or her care.

EPIDEMIOLOGY

Although neoplasms of all sorts in the small intestine are relatively rare, between 10–40% in different series are lymphomas.[15] However, primary gastrointestinal tract lymphomas are uncommon compared with nodal malignant lymphomas, usually comprising between 5 and 10% of reported cases.[6] In European and North American series, small intestinal lymphomas are about half as common as gastric lymphoma. Whilst incidence figures are difficult to find, in a well-defined area of Scotland with centralized medical facilities, and a population of just under half a million, Green *et al.* reported between two and three cases yearly.[5]

The peak incidence is in the fifth and sixth decade, with men affected approximately twice as often as women. Ileocaecal lymphomas, however, show a different pattern, with a peak incidence in the first decade and an even stronger male preponderance.

PREDISPOSING CAUSES

In the group of small intestinal lymphomas discussed here, which excludes those associated with diffuse mucosal disease, predisposing causes are usually absent. It is tempting to associate the ileocaecal lymphoma in children with the intense proliferation of lymphatic tissue seen in this region normally. There are rare examples of nodular lymphoid hyperplasia, in patients without immunodeficiency, being associated with jejunal lymphoma.[12] The association of ulcerative ileojejunitis (in which there may or may not be diffuse mucosal disease) and lymphoma is discussed on p. 464. The significance of the few reported cases of lymphoma in association with Crohn's disease is not clear.

PATHOLOGICAL FINDINGS

Macroscopic appearances
Lymphoma may arise at any level in the small intestine, although the ileocaecal preponderance in childhood has already been noted. Amongst adults also, tumours arc more frequent distally, again reflecting the normal distribution of intestinal lymphoid tissue, but in large series about one quarter are in jejunum or, less commonly, the duodenum.[3] The tumours vary in naked-eye appearance from diffuse infiltration over several or many centimetres to nodules or polypoid lesions, ulcerating masses, and 'aneurysmal' dilations in the intestine. In about one fifth of cases, multiple areas of involvement are found. Tumours may infiltrate locally and spread to mesenteric and distal nodes; when clinical progression has been documented, the commonest sites of spread are other sites in the gastrointestinal tract, liver, spleen, abdominal nodes

and kidney, but in over half of patients with progressive disease, the tumours eventually spread outside the abdomen, mainly to peripheral nodes and lung.[9]

Histological appearances
The classification of malignant lymphoma histologically is a rapidly moving field. The experiences of oncologists studying patients with nodal non-Hodgkin's lymphoma outside the gastrointestinal tract has shown strong implications for prognosis, both in natural history and response to therapy, in different histological types. Whilst it is far from clear that the histological type is of major prognostic significance in Western-type small intestinal lymphoma, similar classifications are used.

The classical Rappaport classification was based on histological appearances at light microscopy.[16] The Luke–Collins classification used cell markers to define the origins of lymphomatous cells as B cells, T cells or cells from the macrophage/monocyte line.[11] The Kiel classification uses a combination of surface markers and histological appearances.[8] Unfortunately, it is not possible to draw up a simple table interrelating these three major classifications; most information currently available on larger series of gastrointestinal lymphomas uses the now obsolete Rappaport system. The vast majority of small intestinal lymphomas are of the non-Hodgkin's type; most (approximately 60%) are classified as diffuse histiocytic, approximately one quarter as lymphocytic, and others mixed.[9] Under the Kiel classification, high grade malignancy is more common than low grade malignancy. Presumably further studies using more sophisticated cell markers will allow precise definition of the cell of origin in the future, with clearer implications for prognosis and therapy than current systems provide.[7]

CLINICAL STAGING

The clinical staging of disease extent is clearly related to prognosis. The original Ann Arbor system for classification of Hodgkin's disease is still used as the basis of most staging systems.[2] The stages for extranodal disease are:

I_E Disease in a single extralymphatic organ.
II_E Localized involvement of extralymphatic organ or site, and involvement of one or more lymph node regions on the same side of the diaphragm.
III_E Localized involvement of extralymphatic site, and involvement of lymph node regions on both sides of the diaphragm.

IV$_E$ Diffuse or disseminated involvement of more than one extralymphatic organ, with or without lymph node enlargement.

However, peculiarities of gastrointestinal lymphoma result in some anomalies in relating staging to prognosis. For example, local lymph node enlargement adjacent to the primary site appears not to worsen prognosis, whilst multiple sites of involvement of the small intestine indicate a worse prognosis. Perforation, particularly when complicated by peritonitis, is a poor prognostic sign. A number of modifications have been introduced, some of considerable complexity;[1] one useful concept is to divide Stage II thus:

II$_1$ Regional adjacent lymph node involvement (e.g. mesenteric).

II$_2$ Regional but non-confluent lymph node enlargement (para-aortic, para-iliac, para-inguinal).

Stage II$_1$ patients appropriately treated appear to do no worse than Stage I, whilst Stage II$_2$ is significantly poorer prognostically.[6] These stages should be defined after investigations including physical examination, an operative report, and studies such as bone marrow biopsy, liver biopsy, sometimes lymphangiography, and other radiology.

CLINICAL PRESENTATION AND INVESTIGATION

In an unselected series, nine out of fifteen patients presented as surgical emergencies with either perforation or, less commonly, obstruction.[5] Obstruction may be due to constricting tumour or intussusception. In large series of patients from cancer centres, the acute presentations are less common, and weight loss, vague abdominal pain, malaise and weakness are commoner presentations.[10] Symptoms may have been present from less than a month to over five years before diagnosis.[3] Nausea and vomiting, or diarrhoea, occur in about half the patients, and gastrointestinal bleeding less frequently. Abdominal masses are the most frequently found physical sign; peripheral lymphadenopathy, splenomegaly and clubbing of the fingers are very uncommon.

Investigation of a case of small intestinal lymphoma requires establishment of the histological diagnosis and clinical staging. The results of routine blood tests are non-specific, though the erythrocyte sedimentation rate is usually elevated and anaemia due to chronic disease or blood loss is common. Hypoproteinaemia from a protein-losing enteropathy is more common in extensive disease with lymphatic obstruction.

Small bowel radiology may show a variety of abnormalities, but fails to show any in perhaps 10% of cases. In about one third the affected area appears as a long dilated aperistaltic segment, either featureless and filled with diluted barium, or a site of nodular filling defects or ulcerations (Figure 8.90). Local perforations, and entero-enteric fistulas may occur (Figure 8.91). Other tumours may be annular and constricting, resembling a carcinoma. Non-specific appearances include areas resembling Crohn's disease, leiomyomas, or a malabsorption pattern with oedematous mucosa.[3]

Other imaging procedures, such as ultrasound or CT scanning, are unlikely to do more than confirm the presence of a mass lesion. Isotope scanning after ^{67}Ga-citrate administration should localize lymphomas, but abscesses and areas of inflammation will also take up this agent.

Since histological proof is required, and endoscopic access to the small intestine is limited, almost all patients will come to surgery, permitting a full clinical staging; some tumours, perhaps half, will be resectable. Routine biopsy of contiguous and distant lymph nodes should be performed, but there is no evidence that routine splenectomy, formerly advocated for assessment of nodal lymphomas, is beneficial. After surgical exploration, abdominal lymphangiography will rarely provide further information. Routine clinical examination and radiology should suffice to determine whether extra-abdominal spread has occurred.

PROGNOSIS AND TREATMENT

In treated cases, the outlook for patients with small intestinal lymphoma is variable. The two-year survival rate is around 40%;[6] after this the incidence of relapse is relatively low, and five and ten year survivals vary between 20 and 40%. Ileocaecal tumours may do particularly badly.[1]

In assessing prognostic features at presentation, and the effects of treatment, it is important to bear in mind that controlled therapeutic trials have not been performed. The addition, for example, of radiotherapy to surgical excision in a reported case may imply that residual disease was known to be present after resection. Furthermore, data from large collected series usually reflect experience with a selected group of patients who have survived long enough after

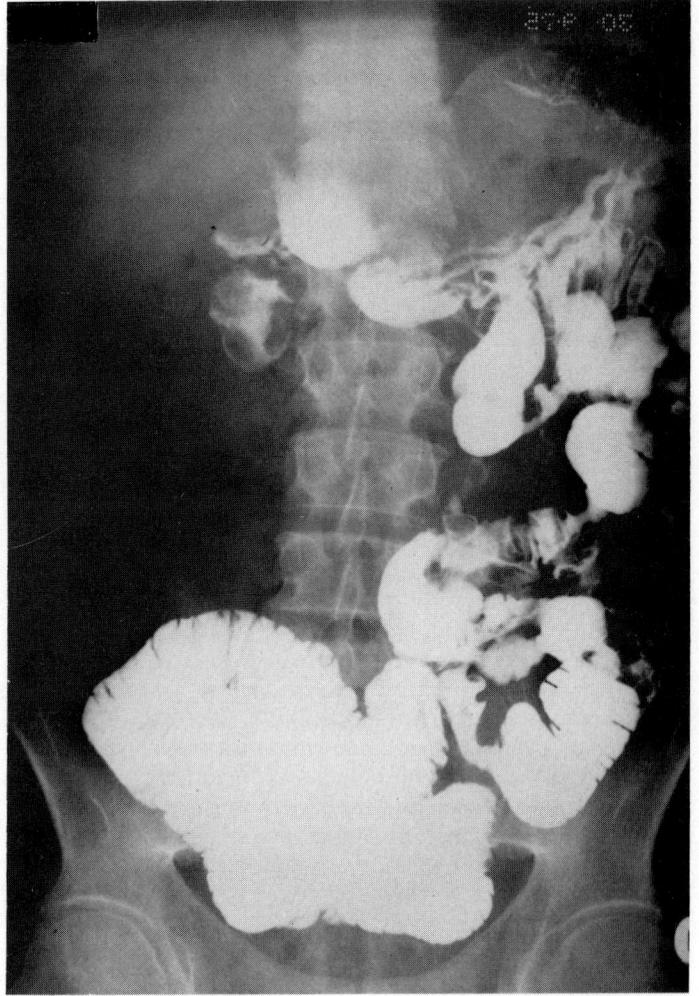

Fig. 8.90 Small bowel radiograph of jejunal lymphoma affecting approximately 1 m of gut, with areas of constriction, nodular filling defects and oedematous mucosa.

presentation to be adequately assessed in a major centre.

Certain findings, however, are clear. Most studies show relatively little impact of histological type on survival, although those with diffuse histiocytic disease may do a little worse.[6, 9] Relapse-free survival is significantly longer in Stage I disease compared with those in which there is nodal involvement, but the prognosis in merely adjacent node involvement (Stage II_1) is no worse than in Stage I – for example, survival is 70 months in Stages I and II_1 combined, compared with less than a year for Stage II_2.[6] There is, however, a tendency for small intestinal lymphomas to be diagnosed at a relatively late stage (less than half at Stages I or II, compared with over two thirds of primary gastric lymphomas).

The role for surgery, radiotherapy and chemotherapy still remain relatively undefined. Some authors emphasize the paramount impor-

tance of complete surgical excision as a determinant of survival, but patients in whom surgical excision is possible belong, by definition, in the prognostically good stagings; others have argued that in this group radiotherapy is as, or more, effective.[6] However, during radiotherapy some tumours may bleed or perforate, an additional argument in favour of surgery prior to radiotherapy.[14] The balance of opinion in Stage I and II disease is currently in favour of resectional surgery followed by radiation, but the arguments for chemotherapy rather than radiotherapy are increasingly being voiced.[6] Chemotherapy is indicated for disseminated disease, but in this group the five-year survival is usually less than 10%; whether adjuvant chemotherapy will prevent distant relapse in localized lymphoma is unclear.

Supportive therapy, including nutritional management, control of infection, and preven-

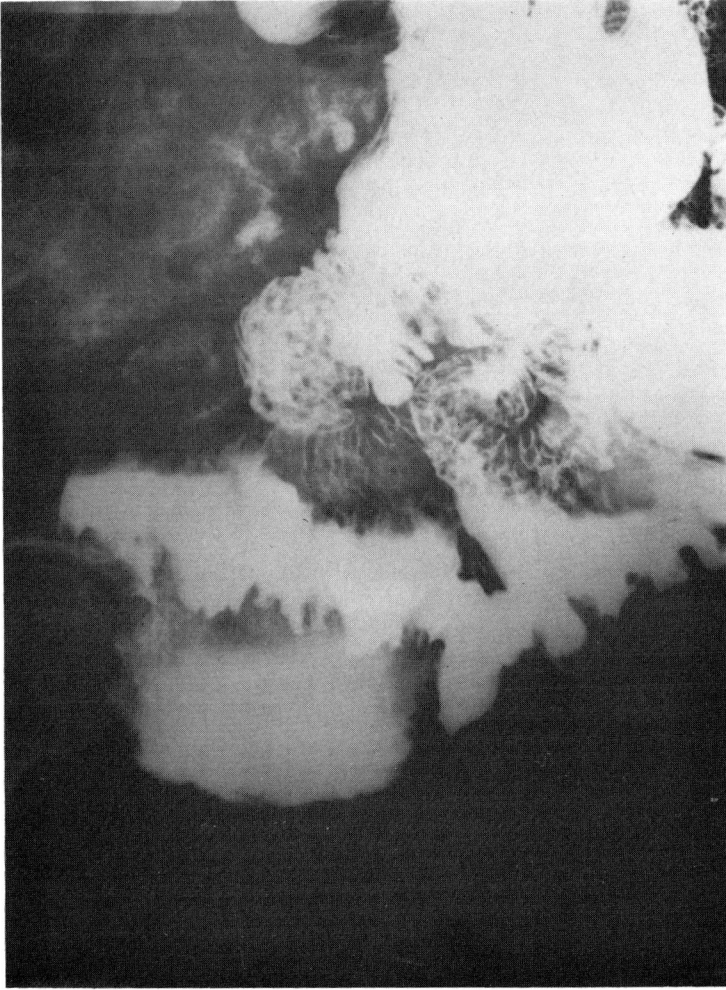

Fig. 8.91 Small bowel radiograph showing an irregular ulcerated area of ileum and barium filling an abscess cavity due to an associated perforation.

tion of the metabolic complications of tumour lysis by monitoring serum potassium levels and administering xanthine oxidase inhibitors, should be considered in addition.

Secondary lymphomatous involvement

Clinically, secondary gastrointestinal involvement in malignant lymphoma is uncommon – for example, it occurred in only 4% of over 800 patients with non-Hodgkin's lymphoma.[6] Clinical involvement usually appears several years after the initial presentation and, by definition, in patients who have responded poorly to treatment. Secondary small intestinal involvement is less common than secondary gastric involvement. A small proportion of these patients will still respond to further treatment with radiotherapy or chemotherapy, and prolonged survival has occasionally been achieved.

Unlike clinical gastrointestinal involvement, histological involvement is very common, and in patients dying of lymphoma nearly half will have autopsy evidence of this.

REFERENCES

1 Blackledge, G., Bush, H., Dodge, O. G. & Crowther, D. (1979) A study of gastrointestinal lymphoma. *Clinic Oncology*, **5**, 209–219.
2 Carbone, P. P., Kaplan, H. S., Musshof, K. *et al.* (1971) Report of the Committee on Hodgkin's disease staging classification. *Cancer Research*, **31**, 1860.
3 Cupps, R. E., Hodgson, J. R., Dockerty, M. B. & Adson, M. A. (1969) Primary lymphoma of the small intestine; problems of roentgenologic diagnosis. *Radiology*, **92**, 1355–1366.
4 Dawson, I. M. P., Cornes, J. S. & Morson, B. C. (1961) Primary malignant tumours of the intestinal tract. *British Journal of Surgery*, **49**, 80.
5 Green, J. A., Dawson, A. A., Jones, P. F. & Brunt, P. W. (1979) The presentation of gastrointestinal lymphoma:

a study of population. *British Journal of Surgery*, **66**, 798–800.

6 Herrmann, R., Panahon, A. M., Barcos, M. P. *et al.* (1980) Gastrointestinal involvement in non-Hodgkin's lymphoma. *Cancer*, **46**, 215–222.

7 Isaacson, P., Wright, O. H., Judd, M. A. & Mepham, B. L. (1979) Primary gastrointestinal lymphomas. A classification of 66 cases. *Cancer*, **43**, 1805–1819.

8 Lennert, K. (1981) *Histopathology of Non-Hodgkin's Lymphoma*. Berlin: Springer-Verlag.

9 Lewin, K. J., Ranchod, M. & Dorfman, R. F. (1977) Lymphomas of the gastrointestinal tract. *Cancer*, **42**, 693–697.

10 Loehr, W. J., Mujahed, Z. & Zahn, F. D. (1969) Primary lymphoma of the gastrointestinal tract: a review of 100 cases. *American Surgeon*, **170**, 232.

11 Lukes, R. J. & Collins, R. D. (1975) New approaches to the classification of the lymphomata. *British Journal of Cancer*, **31** (Supplement II), 1.

12 Matuchansky, C., Morichau-Beauchant, G. & Touchard, Y. (1980) Nodular lymphoid hyperphasia of the small bowel associated with primary jejunal malignant lymphoma. *Gastroenterology*, **78**, 1587–1592.

13 Musshoff, K. (1977) Klinische Stadieneinteilung der nicht-Hodgkin's lymphoma. *Strahlentherapie*, **153**, 218–221.

14 Narqui, M. S., Burrows, L. & Kark, A. E. (1969) Lymphoma of the gastrointestinal tract prognostic studies based on 162 cases. *Annals of Surgery*, **170**, 221–231.

15 Rambaud, J. (1983) Small intestinal lymphomas. In *Gastrointestinal and Hepatobiliary Cancer* (Ed.) Hodgson, H. J. F. & Bloom, S. R. pp. 229–250. London: Chapman & Hall.

16 Rappaport, H. (1966) Publication of the Armed Forces Institute of Pathology, **91**.

IMMUNOPROLIFERATIVE SMALL INTESTINAL DISEASE

The term immunoproliferative small intestinal disease (IPSID) has been proposed for a group of conditions which have certain features in common and are principally found in a few localized geographical areas.[25] These conditions arise from IgA-secreting B cells and some have the characteristic alpha or heavy chain in the blood and other fluids. Many other names have been used but none is comprehensive or accurate: Mediterranean lymphoma, Middle East lymphoma, primary upper small intestinal lymphoma (PUSIL) and alpha chain disease (ACD). The problems of nomenclature reflect the variety of the disease; the geographical distribution is not simple, the pathology is not always lymphomatous and the alpha heavy chain is not always present. The entity has only been recognized for twenty years and it is premature to write a definitive account.

IPSID covers a spectrum of conditions. At one end is a benign plasma cell hyperplasia in the small intestinal mucosa, while at the other end is a highly malignant lymphoma. In a few cases the disease has been observed to change from a benign hyperplasia with the alpha chain present in the blood into a lymphoma and it is widely assumed that this is the natural history. In practice most cases are lymphomatous at diagnosis and only about a third of these have detectable alpha chain, in contrast to plasma cell hyperplasia when it is always present. The balance of opinion is that they are all part of a single disease process. Rarely the plasma cell hyperplasia has been found outside the small intestine in the stomach and colon and in a few cases infiltration of the respiratory tract has also been reported.

GEOGRAPHICAL DISTRIBUTION

The majority of cases reported are from those countries that lie in the Middle East and North Africa, notably Israel, Iraq, Iran, Algeria and Tunisia.[16] Most attention has been focused in the Middle East,[23] but it is often overlooked that the first report came from Peru.[3] Since then it has been described in South Africa.[14] Sporadic cases have been recorded in other disparate places from the USA to Japan, and IPSID may well prove to be more widespread than originally thought. Few cases are seen in Britain and most are immigrants or visitors.[5]

There is no racial susceptibility; in all locations IPSID is predominant among the poor and undernourished. In Israel it occurs principally among immigrant non-Ashkenazy Jews and Arabs; in Iran it is seen mainly amongst village people. The cases from South Africa have been in the Cape Coloured group, while the Peruvian experience has been from the *mestizos*. It is of great interest that where living conditions and hygiene have improved, as in Israel, the disease has diminished. The overriding impression is of an environmental disease, and therefore, a preventable one.

AETIOLOGY

There has been much speculation but as yet precise proof is lacking as to the cause. However, the impoverished background of most patients, the site of the lesion (upper small intestine), the youth of most cases and the abnormal immunoglobulin fragment have encouraged hypotheses. Most workers see the plasma cell proliferation and mutation as the result of prolonged antigenic stimulation of IgA-secreting cells, probably due to repeated gastroenteritis.[16] In one Arab youth an abnormal chromosomal pattern $(D_{14}q9+)$ has been found.[9] Dutz argues that the seeds of IPSID are sown in infancy with a combination of malnutrition and gastrointestinal infections, which lead to immunosuppression and small intestinal mucosal damage.[6] Certainly thymic atrophy and depressed immune responses have been reported in young children with marasmus in Iran,[8] and many of these show small intestinal mucosal changes.[4] Patients with plasma cell hyperplasia and lymphoma have T-cell deficiency;[13] however, such changes are probably a widespread occurrence in underdeveloped countries,[19] while IPSID has curiously localized areas of occurrence. The search for another oncogenic factor has so far proved negative. Al-Saleem[2] has suggested that this might be the enterotoxin of *Vibrio cholerae* but this still defies the geographical pattern. It is this regional incidence that poses the most baffling problem.

PATHOLOGY

The commonest form of the disease at presentation is a frank lymphoma. Alpha heavy chain disease is comparatively rare.

Alpha heavy chain disease
This is a diffuse infiltration of the lamina propria of the mucosa, always of the upper small intestine and sometimes of the whole small intestine (Figure 8.92). The infiltration is sufficient to form a palpable thickening felt at laparotomy or autopsy. Microscopically this is usually composed of a dense sheet of mature plasma cells (Figure 8.93) but a mixture of lymphocytes and immature plasma cells can be found and these findings may vary at different levels of the intestine. Immunocytochemistry demonstrates the presence of IgA and alpha chains in the plasma cells and an in vitro study has shown that cells from both the intestine and lymph nodes produce heavy chain.[18]

The dense infiltrate distorts and may abolish the normal villous structure (Figure 8.94). Crypts are separated and villi become stunted or non-existent, giving the appearance of partial villous atrophy. The surface epithelium is usually columnar or cuboidal with an intact brush border.[1, 11, 16]

Lymphoma
The malignancy usually develops in a background of lymphoplasmocytic infiltration. The early foci are in the mucosa and are often multiple. The lymphomatous process spreads through the intestinal wall and affects the local lymph nodes. Macroscopically there is either diffuse thickening of the upper small intestine or localized tumour. Nodule formation is common with extension both into the lumen and through the wall. The tumour may ulcerate and also stenose the lumen with dilatation above the affected intestine and enlarged adjacent nodes which eventually form masses.

Microscopically the lymphoma is an immunoblastic sarcoma with mitotic activity but few multinucleate cells. Around lymphomatous foci are lymphocytes and immature plasma cells. Again immunocytochemistry may show the presence of alpha chains in the more differentiated plasma cells.

The villous structure is grossly distorted by the malignant tissue and ulceration is common. The surface epithelium is cuboidal and stretched over the tumour masses. However, an abnormal mucosal pattern has been demonstrated in areas not directly infiltrated by the lymphoma.[7]

Lymph node involvement usually parallels the intestinal change and infiltration of mesenteric nodes is the rule. Later para-aortic nodes are affected, but it is rare to find nodes affected outside the abdomen. Gross liver involvement is uncommon, but deposits in portal tracts may be discovered on histological examination. Splenic involvement is rare.[15]

IMMUNOGLOBULINS

The hyperplastic plasma cells secrete a fragment of IgA; this is an incomplete alpha or heavy chain about half to three-quarters the length of normal alpha chain. Minor variations in the N-terminal sequence occur in different cases. The absence of light chains and the need to postulate more than one genetic defect in alpha chain synthesis are ample evidence of a mutation.[22]

Detection of the abnormal alpha chain is technically difficult. Serum electrophoresis may show a band in the α_2 or β_1 positions if the chain is present in large amounts. Most workers have used immunoelectrophoresis with monospecific IgA, which usually reveals a precipitin line faster than and separate from normal IgA. However, in some cases there is no clear separation and it is now possible to separate light chains (and normal immunoglobulins) from heavy chains by 'rocket immunoselection'.[10] Essentially, plates are prepared with two sections, the one nearest the well with light chain antisera and the furthest with heavy chain antisera. During electrophoresis normal immunoglobulins containing light chains are precipitated in the first section while only free heavy chains reach the second and form a rocket-shaped precipitin line.

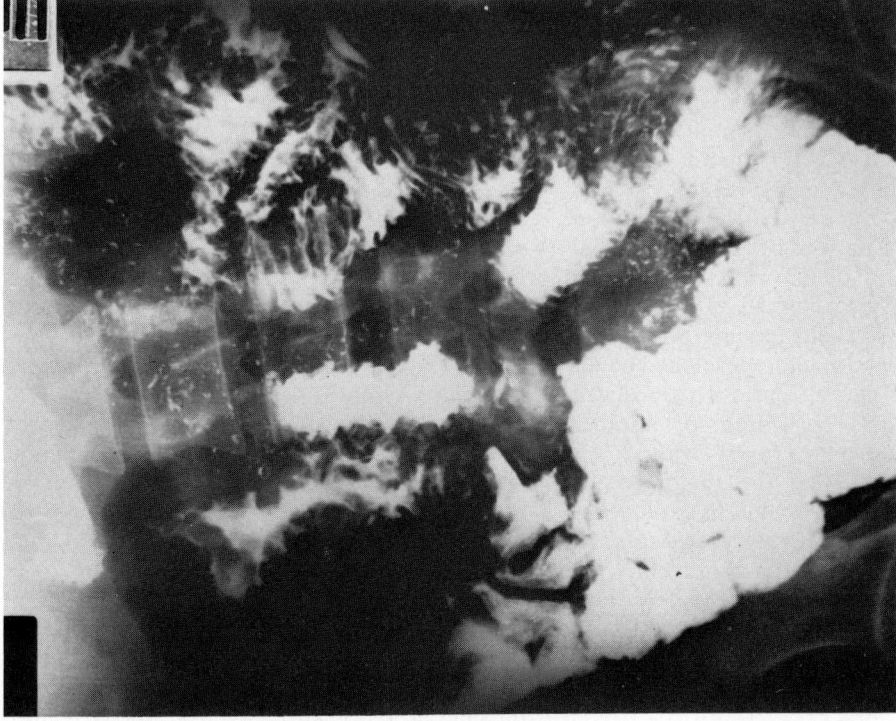

(b) Radiological appearance of the upper small intestine in same patient, showing diffuse oedematous mucosa with areas of nodular infiltration.

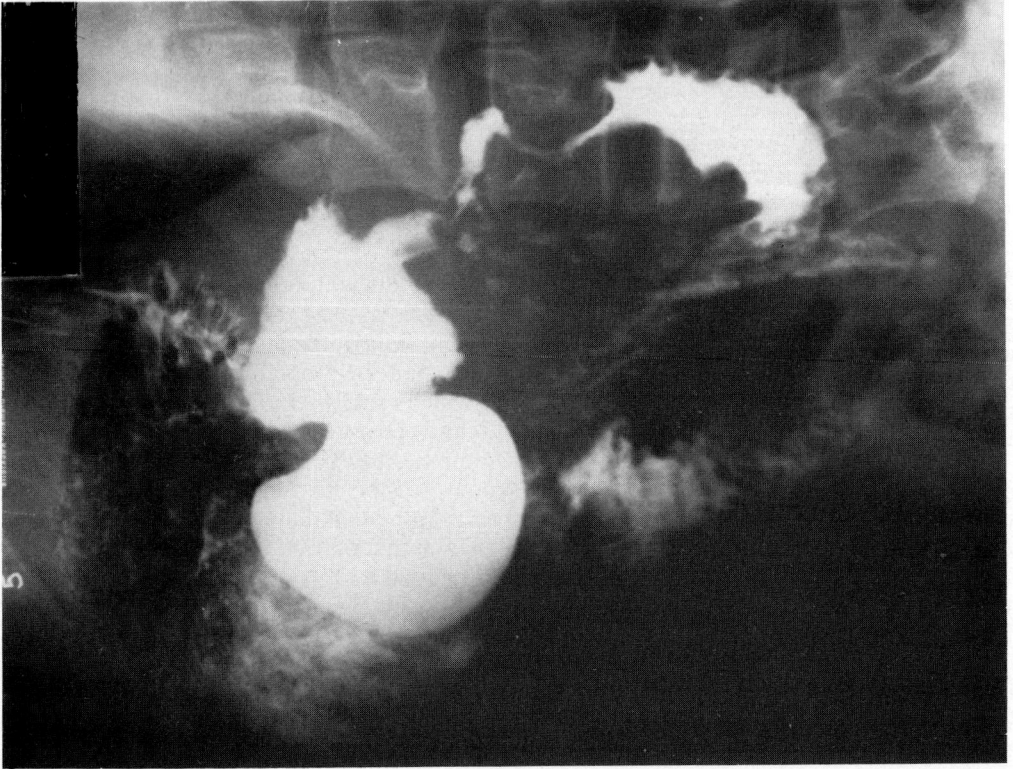

Fig. 8.92 (a) Radiological appearance of stomach and duodenum (oblique view) of a patient with duodenal obstruction due to lymphomatous deposit in alpha chain disease.

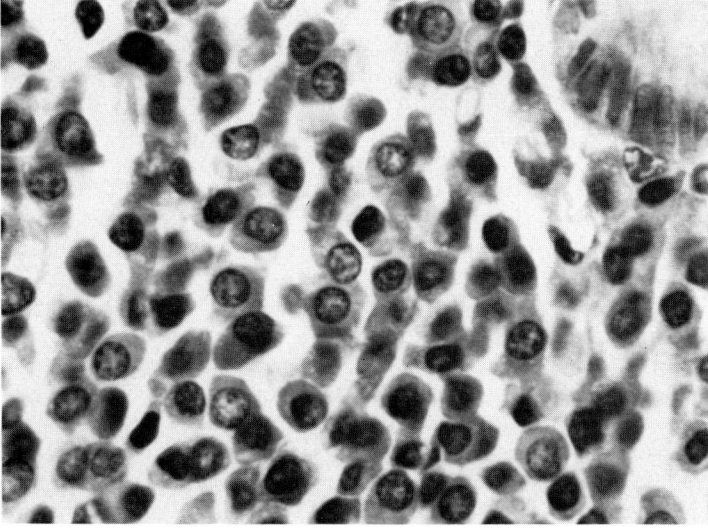

Fig. 8.93 Malignant alpha chain secreting plasma cells in the lamina propria of a patient with alpha chain disease (haematoxylin and eosin × 1100).

Serum is usually used for the detection of alpha chain although it can be found in jejunal juice and, sometimes, in saliva. Small amounts may be present in urine though Bence Jones proteinuria is never found.

Other immunoglobulins are normal in the blood but as the disease progresses may sink to low levels. Plasma albumen is frequently low.

PATHOPHYSIOLOGY

Widespread malabsorption is common in IPSID with steatorrhoea and diminished xylose excretion an almost constant finding. Almost every test of intestinal absorption has been used by various groups of workers and abnormalities found. The extensive mucosal infiltration and destruction is an obvious cause and also leads to exudative enteropathy, by which protein is lost. However, another potent cause of small intestinal malfunction is bacterial overgrowth, which has been repeatedly documented by jejunal intubation and by breath tests.[20] A dramatic reversal is obtained by antibiotics and in many instances absorption tests improved. *Giardia lamblia* infestation is present in about a quarter

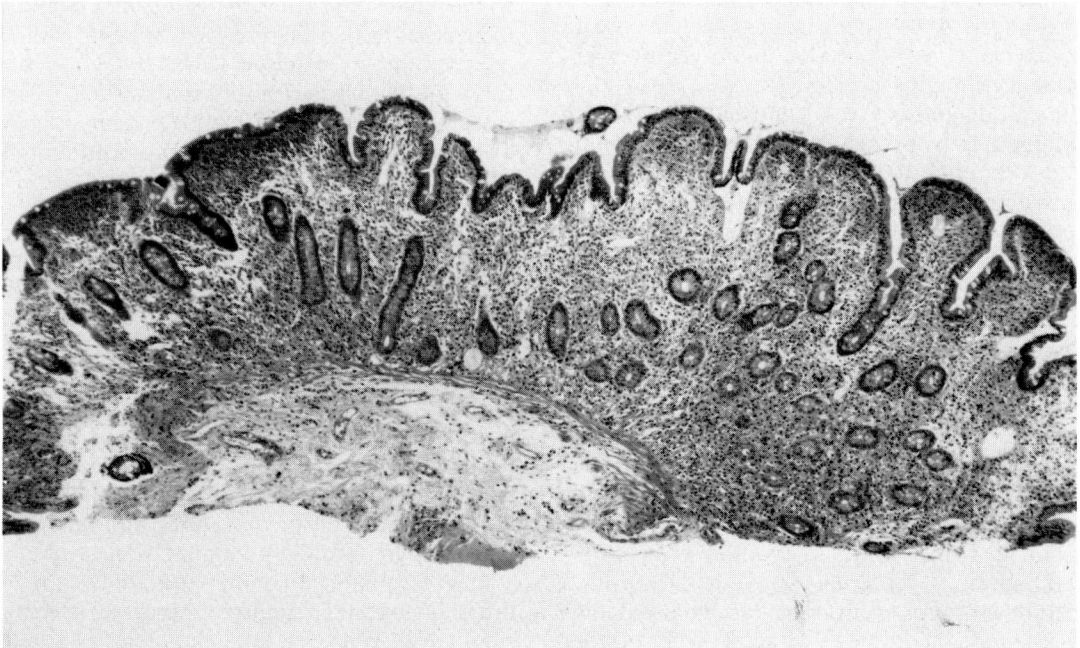

Fig. 8.94 Jejunal biopsy appearance in a patient with alpha chain disease, with partial villous atrophy and infiltration of lamina propria (haematoxylin and eosin × 54).

of patients studied but the significance of this is uncertain as symptomless giardiasis is common in these areas.

CLINICAL FEATURES

IPSID is uncommon even in endemic regions, and, not unexpectedly, patients present with similar symptoms due to other causes. There is little clinical difference between the various forms of IPSID and characterization depends upon investigation. The disease is principally seen in young people from the lower socio-economic classes with an age peak in the second and third decades. Young children are seen with IPSID as are some older people. The sex incidence is usually about equal, though some series show a male preponderance. Very occasionally more than one case in a family has been reported.

As the disease occurs in populations where diarrhoea and malnutrition are common, the early stages often go unnoticed. Most cases begin insidiously though there are a few reports of plasma cell infiltration with an abrupt onset. The picture is of abdominal pain, diarrhoea and weight loss. The pain is variable but may be colicky if there is an element of obstruction, and borborygmi are common. On examination the patients usually appear wasted and ill and finger clubbing is common. (Clubbing is a totally unexplained phenomenon.) About half the cases have a palpable abdominal mass. Other features are vomiting, hypoproteinaemic oedema and occasionally ascites. If the main features are present it may be possible to make a tentative clinical diagnosis. It is unusual to find an enlarged liver or spleen and palpable lymph nodes in extra-abdominal sites are rare. Fever may be present but is not usually a prominent feature.

In rural areas up to half the cases may present acutely through the surgical service with obstruction, perforation or haemorrhage. These cases usually come swiftly to operation when the diagnosis can be made.

Ordinary investigations reveal a modest anaemia; strangely, it is uncommon for anaemia to be severe. Hypoproteinaemia is common, which usually explains the hypocalcaemia. The most reliable investigation is small intestinal radiology, which nearly always shows an abnormal pattern.[24] This may be a malabsorption picture with prominent transverse mucosal folds and some dilatation. Frequently the tumour infiltrate shows as a nodular or pseudopolypoid pattern and more definite filling defects. Gross distortion and obstructing lesions with proximal dilatation occur in advanced cases.

The next stage of investigation is the search for the alpha chain in blood; other fluids are rarely examined in routine practice. If this is positive the diagnosis is virtually secure but histological proof is important, particularly as this is the only way plasma cell hyperplasia can be differentiated from lymphoma. Jejunal biopsy may reveal the diagnosis but the small and superficial sample usually leaves the picture incomplete. There are thus cogent reasons for laparotomy in most cases. Not only can a thorough search of the small intestine be made and biopsy performed, but relief of obstruction by resection or bypass attempted. A staging procedure has been advocated though there is little proof that this is of benefit in determining therapy. Certainly the spread of disease in intestine, glands and elsewhere can be mapped out with some precision.

TREATMENT

Much of the interest in IPSID is centred on a dramatic response to antibiotics in a comparatively few instances.

Plasma cell hyperplasia

This has been observed to regress completely in a few cases following treatment with tetracycline, usually 2 g daily for several weeks. Wellbeing returns, the alpha heavy chain disappears and jejunal biopsy returns to normal. Some of these cases have been observed for years without relapse, and it therefore seems that in certain cases the disease is curable at this stage. A few cases have also shown complete remission following chemotherapy without antibiotics.

Lymphoma

The outlook with lymphoma is completely different and an inexorable progress with some improvement on a temporary basis is the rule. Tetracycline undoubtedly makes these patients feel better and often improves gastrointestinal symptoms; it is usually given a long-term or repeated course regimen. More radical treatment is either with total abdominal radiotherapy or chemotherapy. Radiotherapy to a total of 30 Gy (3000 rads) is used in some centres with remission of masses and symptoms. Chemotherapy is usually a combination of prednisolone, cyclophosphamide and vincristine or other lymphoma regimens. Here again, remission can be obtained but relapse is the rule. In most areas follow-up has been found to be difficult.

PROGNOSIS

Apart from the few cases of plasma cell hyperplasia that respond to antibiotics the outlook is bad. Most cases relapse and few live more than three years from diagnosis. The outcome is recurrent disease with surgical complications or a remorseless wasting and death from malnutrition and infection.

REFERENCES

1 Al-Bahrani, Z., Al-Saleem, T., A.-Mondhiry, H. *et al.* (1978) Alpha heavy chain disease (report of 18 cases from Iraq). *Gut*, **19**, 627–631.

2 Al-Saleem, T. I. (1978) Evidence of acquired immune deficiencies in Mediterranean lymphoma. *Lancet*, **ii**, 709–712.

3 Barua, R. L. & Quintanillo, E. R. (1964) Control with antibiotics of diarrhoea and malabsorption in Whipple's disease and in diffuse lymphosarcoma of the small bowel: a connecting link between the two conditions. *Gastroenterology*, **46**, 521–522.

4 Creamer, B., Dutz, W. & Post, C. (1970) Small intestinal lesion of chronic diarrhoea and marasmus in Iran. *Lancet*, **i**, 18–20.

5 Doe, W. F., Henry, K., Hobbs, J. R. *et al.* (1972) Five cases of alpha-chain disease. *Gut*, **13**, 947–957.

6 Dutz, W. (1975) Immune modulation and disease patterns in population groups. *Medical Hypotheses*, **1**, 197–202.

7 Dutz, W., Asvadi, S., Sadri, S. & Kohout, E. (1971) Intestinal lymphoma and sprue: a systematic approach. *Gut*, **12**, 804–810.

8 Dutz, W., Kohout, E., Rossipal, E. & Vessal, K. (1976) Infantile stress, immune modulation and disease patterns. *Pathology Annual*, **2**, 415–454.

9 Gafter, U., Kessler, E., Shabtay, F. *et al.* (1980) Abnormal chromosome marker ($D_{14}q+$) in a patient with alpha heavy chain disease. *Journal of Clinical Pathology*, **33**, 136–144.

10 Gale, D. S. J., Versey, J. M. B. & Hobbs, J. R. (1974) Rocket immunoselection for detection of heavy-chain diseases. *Clinical Chemistry*, **20**, 1292–1294.

11 Haghshenas, M., Haghighi, P., Abad, P. *et al.* (1977) Alpha heavy chain disease in Southern Iran. *American Journal of Digestive Diseases*, **22**, 866–873.

12 Kharazmi, A., Haghighi, P., Haghshenas, M. *et al.* (1976) Alpha chain disease and its association with intestinal lymphoma. *Clinical and Experimental Immunology*, **26**, 124–128.

13 Kharazmi, A., Rezai, M. H., Abadi, P. *et al.* (1978) T and B lymphocytes in alpha-chain disease. *British Journal of Cancer*, **37**, 1–7.

14 Lewin, K. J., Kahn, L. B. & Novis, B. H. (1976) Primary intestinal lymphoma of 'Western' and 'Mediterranean' type, alpha chain disease and massive plasma cell infiltration: a comparative study of 37 cases. *Cancer*, **38**, 2511–2528.

15 Nasr, K., Haghighi, P., Bakhshandeh, K. *et al.* (1976) Primary upper small-intestinal lymphoma: a report of 40 cases from Iran. *American Journal of Digestive Diseases*, 313–323.

16 Rambaud, J. C. & Seligmann, M. (1976) Alpha-chain disease. *Clinics in Gastroenterology*, **5**(2), 341–358.

17 Ramot, B. & Hulu, N. (1975) Primary intestinal lymphoma and its relation to alpha chain disease. *British Journal of Cancer*, **11** (Supplement 31), 343–349.

18 Ramot, B., Levanon, M., Hahn, Y. *et al.* (1977) The mutual clonal origin of the lymphoplasmocytic and lymphoma cell in alpha-heavy chain disease. *Clinical and Experimental Immunology*, **27**, 440–445.

19 Ross, I. N. & Mathan, V. I. (1981) Immunological changes in tropical sprue. *Quarterly Journal of Medicine*, **200**, 435–499.

20 Russell, R. M., Abadi, P. & Ismail-Beigi, F. (1977) Role of bacterial overgrowth in the malabsorption syndrome of primary small intestinal lymphoma in Iran. *Cancer*, **39**, 2579–2583.

21 Seligmann, M. (1975) Immunochemical, clinical and pathological features of alpha-chain disease. *Archives of Internal Medicine*, **135**, 78–82.

22 Seligmann, M., Mihaesco, E. & Frangione, B. (1971) Studies on alpha chain disease. *Annals of the New York Academy of Sciences*, **190**, 487–500.

23 Seligmann, M., Danon, F., Hurez, D. *et al.* (1968) Alpha chain disease: a new immunoglobulin abnormality. *Science*, **162**, 1396–1397.

24 Vessal, K., Dutz, W., Kohout, E. & Rezvani, L. (1980) Immunoproliferative small intestinal disease with duodenojejunal lymphoma: radiologic changes. *American Journal of Radiology*, **135**, 491–497.

25 World Health Organization (1976) A memorandum: alpha chain disease and related small intestinal lymphoma. *Bulletin of the World Health Organization*, **54**, 615–624.

AMYLOIDOSIS AND THE GUT

Over the last decade there have been major advances in the understanding of the nature of amyloidosis and a number of recent extensive reviews have been written.[1, 7, 9, 13, 14] The gut is involved in the majority of cases of systemic amyloidosis and offers the easiest avenue to diagnosis in most patients. Gastrointestinal manifestations are protean, reflecting the widespread and variable effect of amyloid deposition.

The physical nature of amyloid

Amyloid appears as a hyaline, amorphous, eosinophilic, extracellular material on light microscopy. It has consistent light and electron microscopic features detailed in Table 8.43. The term amyloidosis embraces a heterogeneity of disorders which have in common the deposition, by different pathogenetic mechanisms, of proteinaceous substances resulting in these familiar microscopic and tinctorial properties. The major protein component (the amyloid fibril protein) of the deposits has different origins in the various types of amyloidosis, but always displays a β-pleated structure on X-ray diffraction and infrared spectroscopy, resulting in congo red binding and apple-green birefringence in polarized light. The class of protein appears to be predictable and typical, with few exceptions, for the clinical type of amyloidosis, and the

Table 8.43 Microscopic characteristics of amyloid deposits.

Characteristic	Physical or chemical correlate
Light microscopy	
Congo red or Sirius red binding with apple-green birefringence in polarized light	β-pleated structure of fibril protein
Crystal violet metachromasia	Associated mucopolysaccharides
Electron microscopy	
Fibrils (approximately 90% of the material) 5–15 nm wide, 60–800 nm long. Linear, non-branching and hollow. β-pleated sheet arrangement	Protein with different origins according to type of amyloidosis
'P' component (approximately 10% of the material). Stacked rods with pentagonal arrangement of five subunits on cross-section	Glycoprotein derived from specific glycoprotein in serum (common to all types of amyloidosis)

pathogenesis of amyloid deposition is slowly being clarified.

'Primary' amyloidosis is thought to be caused by an abnormality of immunocytes producing an excess of immunoglobulin light chains, and to be pathogenetically part of the spectrum that includes multiple myeloma. In these patients the amyloid fibril proteins, designated AL, have identical amino acid sequences to the variable portion of associated monoclonal light chains; peptic digestion in vitro of human Bence Jones proteins can create fibrils with the typical staining, X-ray diffraction and electron microscopic appearances of amyloid. Immunological cross-reactivity of antisera to AL fibril proteins and immunoglobulin light chains has been described. Not all monoclonal light chains can be converted to amyloid-like fibrils, perhaps explaining why only a minority of patients with myeloma develop amyloidosis.

In 'secondary' amyloidosis, the major amyloid fibril protein is designated AA, and this has also been partially characterized. It is related to an acute phase protein SAA, produced in response to inflammation which has α_1-globulin electrophoretic mobility. SAA protein can be dissociated into subunits (SAAL) which have amino acid sequences identical to AA protein. There appears to be chemical heterogeneity of different SAA proteins, again offering a possible explanation as to why only some patients with elevated SAA levels develop amyloidosis. The proteases likely to be responsible for the conversion of SAA to AA proteins have been identified on the surface of mononuclear cells.[17] The amyloid fibril protein in patients with familial Mediterranean fever is also the AA type. In only a minority of heredofamilial systemic amyloidoses has the amyloid fibril protein been identified. In the Portuguese neuropathic form, it appears to be derived from pre-albumin and is designated AF_p.

The organ-limited and senile types of amyloidosis will not be considered further. Localized amyloid 'tumours' occur occasionally and are probably associated with immunocytic lesions. It has been suggested that the terms primary and secondary amyloidosis should be discontinued, and the terms 'immunocyte dyscrasias with amyloidosis' (resulting in AL fibrils) and 'reactive systemic amyloidosis' (resulting in AA fibrils) adopted.[7] The various diseases responsible for reactive systemic amyloidosis are listed in Table 8.44.

Table 8.44 Causes of reactive systemic amyloidosis.

Chronic suppuration
  Osteomyelitis
  Paraplegia-associated infections
  Bronchiectasis
  Empyema/lung abscesses

Chronic granulomatous diseases
  Tuberculosis
  Lepromatous leprosy
  Crohn's disease
  Syphilis
  Schistosomiasis

Chronic inflammatory diseases
  Rheumatoid arthritis (and Still's disease)
  Ankylosing spondylitis
  Reiter's disease
  Psoriatic arthritis
  Dermatomyositis
  Scleroderma
  Behçet's syndrome
  Systemic lupus erythematosus

Neoplastic conditions
  Hodgkin's disease
  Hypernephroma
  Bladder carcinoma

The classification of amyloidosis

Based on these advances in the understanding of the physical nature of amyloid, a modern classification (Table 8.45), although incomplete, takes

Table 8.45   Classification of amyloidosis.

	Amyloid fibril protein	'Source' protein
Acquired systemic amyloidosis		
Immunocyte dyscrasias with amyloidosis		
Idiopathic ('primary')		
Multiple myeloma	AL	Immunoglobulin light chain
Waldenstrom's macroglobulinaemia		(variable portion)
Other immunocyte tumours		
Reactive systemic amyloidosis (see Table 8.44)		
Chronic suppuration		
Chronic granulomatous infections	AA	SAA protein (acute phase
Chronic inflammatory disorders		serum protein)
Non-immunocyte malignancies		
Heredofamilial syndromes		
Familial Mediterranean fever	AA	SAA
Portuguese neuropathic type (Andrade)	AF_p	Pre-albumin
Other neuropathic and non-neuropathic forms	?	?
Organ-limited and localized amyloidosis		
Endocrine		
Thyroid	AE_t	Calcitonin
Islets of Langerhans	AE	Insulin
Cutaneous	AD	?
Senile		
Heart	$ASc_1 \cdot ASC_2$	?
Brain	ASB	?
Other organs	?	?

into account both the presence of associated diseases and chemical analysis of the amyloid fibril protein. Differences in organ distribution of the various systemic amyloidoses, and differences in congo red avidity and precise initial histological siting of amyloid deposition, are now thought to be too inconsistent to provide a useful classification.

Histopathology

The precise location and degree of deposition is highly variable in systemic amyloidosis. Small amounts of amyloid in tissue may not be evident macroscopically. With heavier deposition the tissue becomes thickened and assumes a waxy appearance. Microscopically, the early deposition is perivascular, with a tendency toward 'pericollagen' (intimal) deposition in type AL amyloidosis, and 'perireticulin' (adventitial) in type AA amyloidosis.[11] Electron microscopy can be more sensitive in the diagnosis of amyloidosis when deposits are minimal.

In the gut the submucosal vessels are affected first, but with more extensive deposition the vessels in the lamina propria and subserosa are also involved, and amyloid becomes deposited between the muscle fibres of the muscularis mucosa and in the endothelial basement membrane. Amyloid does not invoke an inflammatory response, but is said to cause damage by 'pressure atrophy' and replacement of tissue. The lumen of affected vessels may become occluded with subsequent ischaemia and infarction of the mucosa, and ulceration of the mucosa may be evident. Partial villous atrophy is sometimes seen in association with small bowel amyloidosis. Damage to autonomic ganglia serving the gut and to the myenteric plexus within the bowel wall by amyloid deposits also occurs.

A promising, simple method to distinguish type AA amyloid from other forms has recently become popular: on incubation with potassium permanganate, AA amyloid tends to lose its affinity for congo red, although the specificity of this is not yet entirely established.[30]

Clinical features of systemic amyloidosis

GENERAL

Systemic involvement by amyloidosis can be manifest by a large variety of symptoms and clinical syndromes. When associated with other disease processes, the amyloid may easily be overlooked. Even with 'primary' amyloidosis, the diagnosis may not be made until necropsy – for example, in one recent series, the diagnosis was only made in 12 out of 20 patients premortem.[29]

The symptoms of weight loss, purpura (particularly 'pinch purpura'), paraesthesia, ankle swelling, light-headedness, chest pain and syncope should alert the clinician to the possibility of immunocyte-associated amyloidosis. This may also present as a number of 'syndromes' – carpal tunnel syndrome, peripheral neuropathies, orthostatic hypotension, congestive cardiac failure, heartburn, and nephrotic syndrome. Many of the cases of reactive systemic amyloidosis, and those associated with multiple myeloma, present with features of the primary diseases, although it must be emphasized that these may be quiescent when the amyloidosis becomes symptomatic. Cardiac, skin and neuronal involvement appear to be less common with reactive systemic amyloidosis than with the immunocyte-associated form. All types may present with gastrointestinal complications; these are considered below.

Physical examination may reveal purpura (often of the face and neck), macroglossia, hepatomegaly, splenomegaly, peripheral neuropathies, and cardiac failure. Periorbital purpura following proctoscopy (or Valsalva manoeuvres) is said to be typical.

There are no investigations other than biopsy that can positively identify amyloidosis. A careful search for monoclonal light chain in the serum and urine should always be made, but obviously can be present in the absence of amyloid.

GASTROINTESTINAL MANIFESTATIONS

In systemic amyloidosis, the gastrointestinal tract is usually involved diffusely. Any site can be affected, and there does not seem to be a consistent pattern with the type of amyloidosis. Amyloid deposits may also appear deceptively as 'tumours', which can be single or multiple, sessile or pedunculated, submucosal or ulcerated. Although reactive systemic amyloidosis involves the gastrointestinal tract almost as frequently as the forms associated with immunocyte dyscrasias, it is less commonly symptomatic.[29]

The mouth and pharynx
Diffuse deposition of amyloid in the tongue is particularly characteristic of amyloidosis associated with immunocyte dyscrasias.[15] Whilst often mild, the resultant macroglossia may be severe enough to interfere with deglutition and obstruct the oesophagus, leading to inanition. Haemorrhagic bullae in the mouth have also been described.

The oesophagus
Oesophageal involvement with amyloid is less well recognized, but may have profound effects. Dysphagia is the commonest manifestation, but occasionally more dramatic presentations such as perforation or haemorrhage are reported.[10] Barium and manometric studies do not show a consistent pattern. Manometric abnormalities similar to those found in scleroderma and diabetic neuropathy have been described. Cricopharyngeal sphincter abnormalities have not been reported, but variable alterations of peristaltic patterns in the body of the oesophagus, even aperistalsis, are probably common. The lower oesophageal sphincter resting pressure is either low or normal, and there may be impaired relaxation on swallowing.[23] Whether these abnormalities are primarily neurogenic, myogenic, or both is unknown. Portal hypertension with resultant oesophageal varices occurs rarely with heavy hepatic deposition of amyloid.

The stomach
Gastric stasis without obstruction is a common manifestation of gastric amyloidosis, and barium may be retained in the stomach for many hours. Both loss and increase in gastric rugae has been observed. Erosions seen in the presence of amyloidosis may be coincident, but there is no doubt that heavy amyloid deposition may ulcerate and mimic either benign ulcer disease or carcinoma. Amyloid deposits may also cause true pyloric obstruction.[24] Vitamin B_{12} deficiency has been attributed both to failure of production of intrinsic factor as well as ileal malabsorption of the B_{12}–intrinsic factor complex.

The small intestine
The clinical effects of small intestinal amyloidosis are variable and difficult to correlate with precise pathology. Motility disturbances are common, producing either constipation or diarrhoea. Small bowel transit is often greatly reduced and may be associated with dilatation of small bowel loops. Chronic intestinal pseudo-obstruction is a well described complication,[28] but again it is not clear whether it is neurogenic or myogenic in origin. The malabsorption syndrome is also well documented, occurring in 6 out of 103 patients in one series.[12] Steatorrhoea, low serum albumin, reduced D-xylose absorption, hypocalcaemia, and vitamin B_{12} deficiency have all been described. A number of mechanisms have been implicated (Table 8.46) and the relevant importance of each probably varies

Table 8.46 Possible factors in the production of malabsorption with small intestinal amyloidosis.

Luminal
  Small bowel overgrowth

Mucosal
  Partial villous atrophy
  Subendothelial amyloid band – 'diffusion block'

Vascular
  Vascular insufficiency – mucosal and mesenteric vessels

Motility disturbances
  Neurogenic involvement
    – intrinsic bowel plexuses
    – autonomic ganglia innervating bowel
  Myogenic involvement

Pancreatic
  Pancreatic insufficiency

Other associated diseases
  e.g. Crohn's disease, scleroderma

---

from case to case. For example, in one extensively investigated patient with 'primary' amyloidosis causing severe steatorrhoea, necropsy studies suggested the symptoms were almost entirely due to amyloid infiltration of the neural innervation of the gut.[4]

Amyloid-induced protein-losing enteropathies and small bowel perforations have also been reported.

The colon

Motility disturbances may occur in the colon as in other parts of the bowel. Amyloidosis of the colon is said to simulate a number of diseases including ulcerative colitis, Crohn's disease, and ulcerating colorectal cancer. Amyloidosis may also cause ischaemic colitis secondary to mesenteric vessel involvement. A diffuse haemorrhagic colitis may be seen at sigmoidoscopy.

Gastrointestinal bleeding

Gastrointestinal bleeding is not an uncommon manifestation of systemic amyloidosis, although its incidence varies widely in different series.[19] It can vary from occult bleeding resulting in iron deficiency anaemia to torrential haemorrhage, and may originate in any part of the gastrointestinal tract. Diffusely affected mucosa is often friable, resulting in a slow ooze of blood, but ulcerated amyloid deposits may erode vessels; amyloid deposition in larger vessels may occlude their lumen resulting in bowel ischaemia. Oesophageal varices secondary to hepatic involvement may also bleed. In some patients no actual bleeding site is found, and amyloidosis should be included in the differential diagnosis of obscure gastrointestinal bleeding. Various coagulopathies are occasionally

present and contribute to a bleeding tendency. Factor X deficiency is a relatively specific coagulation disorder in some patients with 'primary' amyloidosis.[5]

Hereditofamilial amyloidosis

There are a number of rare dominantly-inherited neuropathic familial amyloidosis syndromes in which gastrointestinal symptoms form a major part.[8] They include the Portuguese, Japanese and Swedish–American forms. The most studied is the Portuguese form, first described by Andrade, in which the initial symptoms are gastrointestinal in over 60% of patients. These symptoms include constipation, diarrhoea, vomiting and abdominal pain. As the disease progresses virtually all patients develop episodes of constipation and diarrhoea, thought to be mainly a result of amyloid deposition in the neural elements of the gut.

Gastrointestinal diseases associated with reactive systemic amyloidosis

A number of gastrointestinal diseases may give rise to amyloidosis, complicating the clinical picture and delaying diagnosis. These include tuberculosis, Behçet's syndrome and scleroderma, but inflammatory bowel disease probably results most commonly in diagnostic confusion. The fact that amyloidosis rarely, if ever, complicates ulcerative colitis, but is well recognized in Crohn's disease (up to 8% of cases) may help in the diagnosis.[25] This may be partially explained by the higher levels of SAA that occur in active Crohn's disease when compared with ulcerative colitis.[21] Resection of a segment of bowel affected by Crohn's disease has been reported to result in a regression of the associated amyloidosis,[3] but surgery is said to be hazardous in this situation and often complicated by renal failure.

Radiological appearances of systemic amyloidosis affecting the gut

No specific radiological patterns have been described. Ulcerated or tumour-like deposits may be demonstrated and motility disturbances, particularly severe delays in transit, are common. Diffuse involvement of the small intestine may result in thickened valvulae conniventes with areas of small bowel dilatation.[18] The changes may be segmental rather than generalized. Colonic appearances can simulate ulcerative colitis and Crohn's disease, or be typical of the associated ischaemic colitis. Few angiographic studies have been performed, but non-specific findings of attenuation, abrupt calibre changes and luminal irregularities of vessels have been noted.[26]

Diagnosis of amyloidosis

The diagnosis of amyloidosis depends on the demonstration of amyloid deposits in biopsy specimens. Deposition of amyloid in the gastro-intestinal tract is commonly quoted as 70% in 'primary' amyloidosis[27] and 55% in reactive systemic amyloidosis,[2] but the incidence is almost certainly higher and depends on the thoroughness of the search for amyloid and the use of electron microscopy for specimens with minimal deposition. In one series 68 out of 70 patients with a variety of types of systemic amyloidosis had gut involvement.[6] Consequently, biopsy of the gastrointestinal tract affords the easiest access for the diagnosis of amyloidosis. Rectal biopsy will be positive in the majority of patients (possibly greater than 80%), and complications are very rare. The biopsy material should be deep enough to include submucosa, and the pathologist should be warned in advance of the possible diagnosis. If negative for amyloid, other sites should be biopsied according to the clinical picture (Table 8.47). Gingival biopsy is less commonly positive than rectal biopsy, but is relatively safe and non-invasive.

Table 8.47 Sites used for biopsy in the diagnosis of systemic amyloidosis.

Rectum
Kidney
Gingiva
Small intestine
Stomach
Liver
Skin
Prostate gland
Endocardium
Subcutaneous fat (aspiration)
Spleen (aspiration)
Bone marrow (aspiration)

Small bowel biopsy will give a high yield. Percutaneous liver biopsy has a reputation, based on early case reports, for being unduly hazardous in amyloidosis, whereas percutaneous renal biopsy is believed to be safer and, although invasive, gives the highest yield of all methods.

Prognosis and treatment

The prognosis of systemic amyloidosis is poor and treatment far from satisfactory. Long sur-

vivors are reported in all types of systemic amyloidosis, but a mean survival of only 14 months was reported in one study of patients with 'primary' amyloidosis, and the prognosis of patients with amyloidosis associated with myeloma is even worse.[15] The mean survival of patients with reactive systemic amyloidosis may be somewhat better, but in most cases is still depressing. Control of the primary disease has been reported to cause a regression of the features of amyloidosis in a number of anecdotal cases, but it is to be remembered that nephrotic syndrome due to amyloidosis has also been reported to remit spontaneously. There is some enthusiasm for the use of cytotoxics in 'primary' amyloidosis, but the efficacy of these drugs is as yet unproven.[16] Colchicine inhibits casein-induced amyloidosis in mice, and may be beneficial to patients, especially with familial Mediterranean fever and amyloidosis.[22] There is also some hope that dimethylsulphoxide, which denatures amyloid, may reduce amyloid deposits but, because of its pungent odour, patient compliance is a problem.[20] The role for these various therapies should become clear over the next few years.

REFERENCES

1 Cohen, A. S. (1981) An update on clinical, pathologic and biochemical aspects of amyloidosis. *International Journal of Dermatology*, **20**, 515–530.

2 Dahlin, D. C. (1949) Secondary amyloidosis. *Annals of Internal Medicine*, **31**, 105–119.

3 Fitchen, J. H. (1975) Amyloidosis and granulomatous ileocolitis. Regression after surgical removal of the involved bowel. *New England Journal of Medicine*, **292**, 352–353.

4 French, J. M., Hall, G., Parish, D. J. & Smith, W. T. (1965) Peripheral and autonomic nerve involvement in primary amyloidosis associated with uncontrollable diarrhoea and steatorrhoea. *American Journal of Medicine*, **39**, 277–284.

5 Furie, B., Voo, L., McAdam, K. P. W. J. & Furie, B. C. (1981) Mechanism of factor X deficiency in systemic amyloidosis. *New England Journal of Medicine*, **304**, 827–830.

6 Gilat, T., Revach, M. & Sohar, E. (1969) Deposition of amyloid in the gastrointestinal tract. *Gut*, **10**, 98–104.

7 Glenner, G. G. (1980) Amyloid deposits and amyloidosis. The β-fibrilloses. *New England Journal of Medicine*, **302**, 1283–1292; 1333–1343.

8 Glenner, G. G., Ignaczac, T. F. & Page, D. L. (1978) The inherited systemic amyloidoses and localised amyloid deposits. In *The Metabolic Basis of Inherited Disease* (Ed.) Stanbury, J. B., Wyngaarden, J. B. & Fredrichson, D. S. pp. 1308–1339. Maidenhead: McGraw Hill.

9 Gorevic, P. D. & Franklin, E. C. (1981) Amyloidosis. *Annual Review of Medicine*, **32**, 261–271.

10 Heitzman, E. J., Heitzman, G. C. & Elliott, C. F. (1962) Primary esophageal amyloidosis. *Archives of Internal Medicine*, **109**, 595–608.

11 Heller, H., Missmahl, H., Sohar, E. & Gafni, J. (1964) Amyloidosis: its differentiation into perireticulin and pericollagen types. *Journal of Pathology and Bacteriology*, **88**, 15–41.

12 Herskovic, T., Bartholomew, L. G. & Green, P. A. (1964) Amyloidosis and malabsorption syndrome. *Archives of Internal Medicine*, **114**, 629–633.

13 Kyle, R. A. (1980) Amyloidosis. *International Journal of Dermatology*, **19**, 537–539.

14 Kyle, R. A. (1981) Amyloidosis. *International Journal of Dermatology*, **20**, 20–25; 75–80.

15 Kyle, R. A. & Bayrd, E. D. (1975) Amyloidosis: review of 236 cases. *Medicine (Baltimore)*, **54**, 271–299.

16 Kyle, R. A. & Greipp, P. R. (1978) Primary systemic amyloidosis: comparison of melphalan and prednisone versus placebo. *Blood*, **52**, 818–827.

17 Lavie, G., Zucker-Franklin, D. & Franklin, E. C. (1980) Elastase-type proteases on the surface of human blood monocytes: possible role in amyloid formation. *Journal of Immunology*, **125**, 175–180.

18 Legge, D. A., Carlson, H. C. & Wollaeger, E. E. (1970) Roentgenologic appearances of systemic amyloidosis involving the gastrointestinal tract. *American Journal of Roentgenology*, **110**, 406–412.

19 Levy, D. J., Franklin, G. O. & Rosenthal, W. S. (1982) Gastrointestinal bleeding and amyloidosis. *American Journal of Gastroenterology*, **77**, 422–426.

20 Osserman, E. F., Sherman, W. H. & Kyle, R. A. (1980) Further studies of therapy of amyloidosis with dimethylsulfoxide (DMSO). In *Amyloid and Amyloidosis. Proceedings of the Third International Symposium on Amyloidosis* (Ed.) Glenner, G. G., Pinho e Costa, P. & de Freitas, A. F. pp. 563–577. Excerpta Medica International Congress series No. 497.

21 Pepys, M. B. (1982) Goulstonian Lecture: C-Reactive protein, amyloidosis and the acute phase response. In *Advanced Medicine, No. 18* (Ed.) Sarner, M. pp. 208–229. London: Pitman.

22 Ravid, M., Robson, M. & Kedar (Keizman), I. (1977) Prolonged colchicine treatment in four patients with amyloidosis. *Annals of Internal Medicine*, **87**, 568–570.

23 Rubinow, A., Harris, L. D. & Cohen, A. S. (1980) Esophageal motor dysfunction in systemic amyloidosis. In *Amyloid and Amyloidosis. Proceedings of the Third International Symposium on Amyloidosis* (Ed.) Glenner, G. G., Pinho e Costa, P. & de Freitas, A. F. pp. 563–577. Excerpta Medica International Congress series No. 497.

24 Schnider, B. I. & Burka, P. (1955) Amyloid disease of the stomach simulating gastric carcinoma. *Gastroenterology*, **28**, 424–430.

25 Shorvon, P. J. (1977) Amyloidosis and inflammatory bowel disease. *American Journal of Digestive Diseases*, **22**, 209–213.

26 Shroeder, F. M., Miller, F. J. Jr, Nelson, J. A. & Rankin, R. S. (1978) Gastrointestinal angiographic findings in systemic amyloidosis. *American Journal of Roentgenology*, **131**, 143–146.

27 Symmers, W. St C. (1956) Primary amyloidosis: a review. *Journal of Clinical Pathology*, **9**, 187–211.

28 Wald, A., Kichler, J. & Mendelow, H. (1981) Amyloidosis and chronic intestinal pseudoobstruction. *Digestive Diseases and Sciences*, **26**, 462–465.

29 Wright, J. R. & Calkins, E. (1981) Clinical-pathologic differentiation of common amyloid syndromes. *Medicine (Baltimore)*, **60**, 429–448.

30 Wright, J. R., Calkins, E. & Humphrey, R. L. (1977) Potassium permanganate reaction in amyloidosis. A histologic method to assist in differentiating forms of this disease. *Laboratory Investigation*, **36**, 274–281.

FOOD ALLERGY

Nobody doubts that food allergy exists. Some people are predictably made ill by eating certain foods – urticaria following strawberries, and vomiting or diarrhoea after eating shellfish, are well known examples. Nevertheless, over recent years, many symptoms such as headaches, palpitations, vomiting, panic attacks and anxiety have been ascribed to food allergy[64, 74] and the reaction of the medical profession has been largely sceptical. The subject has become confused mainly because of a lack of firmly defined diagnostic criteria and a paucity of reliable diagnostic tests. Unfortunately, as symptoms are usually subjective, the differentiation of a true food allergy from psychiatric ill-health is often difficult.

Definition

Many foods are known to cause clinical symptoms on ingestion but these are not all necessarily due to an allergy and may be idiosyncratic. Allergy was initially defined as an acquired specific altered capacity of the tissues of the body to react to physical substances. This was rather a broad definition; most physicians now would reserve the term for phenomena resulting from immunological hypersensitivity mediated by immunoglobulin E (IgE), although IgG reactions may also be involved. Historically, the first clinical demonstration of the immunological basis of food allergy was in 1921 when Prauznitz transferred fish sensitivity from his friend Kustner[73a] to his own skin. Atopy is not an antigen-specific state; atopic subjects respond to a number of environmental inhalant and food antigens by an IgE response. As some patients show IgE antibodies and positive prick tests to foods, their food intolerance is presumably allergic. However, there are many other causes of food intolerance as shown in Table 8.48 and these will be considered in turn.

Table 8.48 Types of food intolerance.

Pharmacological
Chemical mediators
Toxic substance
Irritants
Idiosyncratic
Gastrointestinal (e.g. alactasia)
General (e.g. phenylketonuria)
Allergic
Gastrointestinal (e.g. cow's milk allergy)
General (e.g. eczema)

From Soothill, J. F. (1979),[81] with kind permission of the author and the publisher, Pitman Medical.

Firstly patients may be intolerant to a food because the food contains substances which themselves have a pharmacological action, like histamine in mackerel or canned foods, tyramine in certain cheeses, or caffeine.[9] Equally, foods may contain substances which release chemical mediators as, for example, histamine released by tomatoes or strawberries. Certain chemicals in foods may be toxic and produce clinical disease states; examples include hexachlorobenzene, used as a dressing for wheat in Turkey, which produced acquired porphyria[21] and acetanilide in rape-seed oil which results in respiratory failure.[86] Alternatively certain foods such as spices may be irritant to the gastrointestinal tract in some patients.

Idiosyncrasy to certain foods may be found associated with a deficiency of a particular enzyme involved in their degradation, e.g. milk-induced diarrhoea in patients with alactasia, or fava bean-induced haemolytic anaemia in patients with glucose-6-phosphate dehydrogenase deficiency.

Lastly a patient may be truly allergic to a food with evidence of an immunological hypersensitivity reaction. It would avoid confusion if the term 'food intolerance' were used to embrace the other reactions and the term 'food allergy' reserved for those cases where a food intolerance has a definite immunological basis.

Incidence and prevalence

Exact figures for the incidence and prevalence of food allergy are difficult to obtain. Food allergy presenting in childhood has been more clearly defined. The incidence is probably greatest in the first months and years of life and decreases with age, as most childhood food allergy has a natural tendency to recover.[26, 39] Infantile eczema, which is probably largely food allergic, affects 3% of infants[5] and infantile colic is said to be even more common.[49] Estimates of food allergy causing asthma and atopic dermatitis range from 3% to 40%.[46] Bleumink[12] estimated that foods may cause atopic symptoms in 0.2% of the general population.

Pathogenesis and mechanism

It is well known that antigenically-intact food proteins are absorbed across healthy gastrointestinal mucosa[94, 98] and, although the amounts absorbed may be nutritionally insignificant, it is sufficient to immunize and result in the production of antibodies. This immunological reaction, however, does not usually cause any clinical symptoms.

The exact mechanisms of the pathogenesis of food allergic disease is still unclear and several factors may be involved. These include the type and amount of antigen, the permeability of the gastrointestinal tract, the development of immune responses to the ingested antigen, both local and systemic, a genetic predisposition, and the effect on the end organ with the production of clinical symptoms.

Type of antigen
The nature of the allergens in particular foods is still uncertain. Some foods, like egg, milk, fish and wheat have a very strong tendency to sensitize,[84] while others are fairly innocuous. Equally, some substances can cross-sensitize, e.g. soya bean, which may not only sensitize patients to the various manufactured materials in which it is used, but also to related vegetables such as peas, beans and lentils.[36] For other foods, such as shrimp and cod,[1, 47] the reaction may be provoked by specific proteins. Milk is another example where, although there are more than 20 proteins, reactions are usually only observed with casein, α-lactalbumin, β-lactoglobulin and bovine serum albumin. Reactions are said to occur with two or more allergens,[40] and these may be denatured by heat.[35] Contaminating substances, e.g. penicillin must also be considered.[7] The response to some foods may be variable. Thus, some patients may get an enteropathy with gluten while others have been reported to have a gluten-sensitive diarrhoea without an enteropathy.[25]

In general, where a reaction is caused by very small amounts of a substance it is likely to have an allergic basis. However, reactions to food additives, e.g. monosodium glutamate,[59] colouring agents such as tartrazine, and preservatives such as benzoic acid[63] may be due to toxicity.

Permeability
The passage of antigens across the gastrointestinal mucosa is partly prevented by the tightly packed surface epithelial cells, the overlying mucus and the luminal secretory IgA. Nevertheless, antigens may cross the epithelium through defects in the gut, and the transport of large molecules across intact mature mucosa has been shown.[93]

In humans, gut mucosa is mature by full-term of pregnancy and there is evidence that gut closure occurs at about 30 weeks' gestation.[75] The immunological aspects of infant feeding are complex[82] but when a food is first eaten it appears in the blood and an antibody (usually IgA) is produced.[62] On subsequent ingestion of the antigen very little enters the blood due to a protective response (immune exclusion). Ingestion of an antigen also induces partial immunological tolerance to subsequent parenteral contact with the antigen.[22] It also appears that this tolerance, and possibly immune exclusion, can be influenced by nutrition.[85]

Maternal milk (colostrum) contains protective antibodies but may also contain antigens from the food that the mother has eaten[52] and these may trigger symptoms such as eczema in the already sensitized infant.

It has been suggested that IgA deficiency predisposes to food allergy by increasing gut permeability,[88] but these patients may also have other defective immunoregulatory processes.[30]

Immunological reactions
Local immunity. The gastrointestinal mucosa contains immunologically competent cells scattered in the lamina propria or in aggregates such as the Peyer's patches. It is thought that the most common allergic reactions to foods are caused by atopic phenomena (Type I) and the relevance of Type III (Arthus) and more rarely Type IV phenomena is uncertain. Secretory antibodies to a variety of foods have been demonstrated in the upper intestinal secretions.[31] Mucosal cell-mediated immunity to a dietary antigen may be the cause of intestinal damage in coeliac disease and cow's milk-sensitive enteropathy. There is some evidence that T cells can mediate damage similar to villous atrophy.[32] It is possible that local immune reactions may also contribute to malabsorption in some infants with intractable diarrhoea. In cow's milk allergy, deposition of complexes containing immunoglobulin, antigen, and complement may be seen in the submucosa.[78]

Hypersensitivity may be antibody-mediated or cell-mediated and tissue damage may involve a range of soluble factors, activated polymorphonuclear leucocytes, macrophages or direct effects on the cell membrane. The various types of hypersensitivity reactions may not be mutually exclusive and may occur at once or in sequence.

Systemic immunity. Most normal individuals have low titres of circulating antibody to food proteins.[57] Circulating immune complexes have been demonstrated in both healthy and food allergic subjects after ingestion of food.[72] In healthy subjects the immunoglobulin in these complexes is predominantly IgA,[61] whereas in the food allergic subjects the complexes may also contain IgG and IgE and may bind complement.[15, 16]

Genetic predisposition
A genetic predisposition is suggested by the familial tendency of some food allergies. The best documented is that of the association of coeliac disease with the tissue type HLA-A1, -B8, -DR W3.[80] Atopics presenting with eczema (usually a food allergy) also have an excess of HLA-A1 and -B8, whereas atopics with hay fever have an excess of HLA-A3 and -B7.[83] However there are other complex associations, as atopy may be associated with transient IgA deficiency[88] or defects in complement C2 and yeast opsonization.[91]

Other factors, such as environment, may well play a part, as concordance of atopic allergic disease in monozygotic twins is not 100%.[55] The type of feeding in infancy may be important as there is lower incidence of eczema in offspring of atopic parents fed breast milk when compared to those on artificial feeding.[66]

Miscellaneous factors
It has been suggested that some of the psychiatric changes seen in, for example, coeliac disease or schizophrenia, may be due to the direct toxic action of an antigen on brain cells. Klee *et al.*[54] have shown that some digests of dietary protein have opioid activity. These peptides, or exorphins, may act as opioids on central opiate receptors in the brain. Further studies are needed to establish whether there are any direct immunological or endocrine effects of foodstuffs on the central nervous system.

Prostaglandins have been put forward as causing the abdominal pain and diarrhoea in acute allergic gastroenteritis, and there is some evidence that raised stool and blood prostaglandin levels may be associated with gastrointestinal symptoms.[18]

Clinical features

A list of food allergic disorders is shown in Table 8.49. It should be emphasized that many patients presenting to gastrointestinal or allergy clinics with putative food allergies may have a food fad or a psychiatric problem. A careful history should always be taken.

Symptoms of allergy may be immediate or delayed. They may affect the patient with either a widespread systemic reaction, or produce predominantly gastrointestinal, dermatological, respiratory or some other symptoms. Immediate reactions, within minutes of eating certain foods,

Table 8.49   Diseases due to food allergy.

System affected	Proven diseases	Unproven diseases
Systemic	Anaphylaxis	Cot death
Gastrointestinal tract	Oral ulceration Coeliac disease Cow's milk protein enteropathy Ulcerative colitis (children)	Erosive gastritis Irritable bowel syndrome Crohn's disease
Respiratory tract	Rhinitis Nasal polyps Asthma Allergic alveolitis	
Skin	Urticaria, angioedema Atopic eczema Dermatitis herpetiformis	
Eye	Conjunctivitis	
Central nervous system	Migraine	Behavioural and affective disorders
Joints		Rheumatoid arthritis
Cardiovascular		

From Coombs, R. R. A. (1980),[24] with kind permission of the author and the publisher, Medical Education Services.

such as swelling of lips or tongue, vomiting, rhinorrhoea, urticaria or asthma are thought to be IgE-mediated. In these cases the total IgE is usually raised, a positive skin-prick test may be elicited or a positive radioallergosorbent test (RAST) obtained. In adults, such allergies are not often a clinical problem as patients learn to avoid the offending food. In infancy, however, such features as vomiting and anaphylactic shock can develop within minutes and may be provoked with less than a millilitre of milk.[77]

Late reactions, where symptoms develop over an hour after the food is ingested, are more of a diagnostic problem and evidence of an IgE reaction is less commonly found.

The clinical picture was studied by Lessof *et al.*[60] in 100 patients with food allergy and intolerance; they found that 64% developed asthma and eczema, 22% had urticaria, and gastrointestinal symptoms and rhinorrhoea were seen in only 14%. The foods provoking these symptoms are shown in Table 8.50.

Gastrointestinal symptoms
Nausea, vomiting, diarrhoea, abdominal pain, distension, constipation, malabsorption and a protein-losing enteropathy have all been attributed to food intolerance. Vomiting and abdominal pain are common manifestations of food allergy. Gastrointestinal symptoms due to allergic causes have mainly been described in children although they may persist or develop in adult life. A late onset of symptoms suggests that the route for sensitization may be alimentary rather than respiratory. Secondary symptoms,

Table 8.50   Food intolerances seen in 100 patients presenting to an allergy clinic.

Food	Number of patients
Milk	46
Egg	40
Nuts	22
Fish	22
Wheat	9
Chocolate	7
Artificial colours	7
Pork	7
Chicken	6
Tomato	6
Soft fruits	6
Yeast	3

From Lessof, M. H. *et al.* (1980),[60] with kind permission of the authors and the editor of *Quarterly Journal of Medicine.*

such as intestinal bleeding and iron deficiency anaemia,[97] hypoproteinaemia, and eosinophilia may occur.[92]

Aphthous ulceration occurs in up to 20% of the general population.[43] Although the aetiology is unknown, successful treatment with sodium cromoglycate[37] may suggest food allergy.

Allergic gastroenteritis is characterized by eosinophilic infiltration of the mucosa and there may be peripheral eosinophilia, an iron deficiency anaemia secondary to gastrointestinal blood loss, or a protein-losing enteropathy. The pathological classification is confused[51] and not all reports have a definite food allergic basis. Katz *et al.*[53] have described 6 children aged between 6 months and 15 years with eosinophilic infiltration of the gastric mucosa associated with protein and blood loss. There are reports of eosinophilic infiltration of the oesophagus[33] and stomach[53] in association with a history of food intolerance and response to food avoidance, and laboratory evidence of reaginic allergy.

Much of our knowledge of gastrointestinal food allergy comes from work on cow's milk protein intolerance in infancy.[28, 48] The syndrome results from the sensitization of a child to one or more proteins from cow's milk which results in damage to the gastrointestinal mucosa. Clinically, patients may present acutely with vomiting and a shock-like state or as a chronic syndrome with colic, diarrhoea or constipation and possibly malabsorption.[56] Urticaria and eczema or wheezing and asthma may also be present. Its reported prevalence varies from 3–12%,[23, 39, 41] presumably due to the use of different diagnostic criteria. With the advent of foods containing proteins other than cow's milk, other sensitivities such as those to soy protein have now been described. Soy sensitivity can cause various symptoms[3] and also can produce an enteropathy.[73] Coeliac disease is considered elsewhere (p. 448). A transient gluten intolerance with intestinal damage has been described in children[95] and possibly in adults.[58]

There is some evidence that certain conditions of the colon and rectum may be due to food sensitivity. An association between ulcerative colitis and cow's milk ingestion was postulated many years ago,[87] and Whorwell and Wright[96] favour an association between early ingestion of cow's milk protein and ulcerative colitis. Most cases of ulcerative colitis in infants below the age of one year are said to be due to food allergy[50] and a haemorrhagic proctitis can occur in patients with cow's milk intolerance.[17] Favourable responses to sodium cromoglycate in non-specific proctitis and ulcerative colitis[65] have been reported but corroborating reports are scanty. Non-specific anal disorders such as pruritis ani have also been associated with food allergies but with little supporting evidence.

Recently cases of the irritable bowel syndrome which improved on food exclusion diets have been reported[2] and remissions have been obtained in patients with Crohn's disease on elemental diets;[71] these studies again await confirmation.

Skin reactions

The main dermatological reactions associated with food allergic disorders are atopic eczema and urticaria or angio-oedema.

Atopic eczema. This is largely a disease of young children and affects at least 5% of all children at some time. It affects the face and limb flexures as an itchy red rash with scaling, vesiculation, exudation and crusting. Patients often have asthma, allergic rhinitis, a family history of atopy and a high serum IgE level.[10] Despite this, the slow evolution and eventual histological appearance are more suggestive of a delayed hypersensitivity reaction possibly due to cutaneous basophil hypersensitivity. These patients differ from those with asthma and hay fever by having a much higher frequency of positive immediate skin tests to foods[8] and much greater levels of circulating food-specific IgE (RAST).[90] Elimination diets have met with some success. In one study, two-thirds of the children improved after excluding milk and eggs from their diet.[5] The response of elimination diets in adults, however, is less dependable.

Urticaria. This consists of oedema and erythema of the skin; the lesions are itchy and last from 30 minutes to 72 hours. Histamine and possibly other mediators are involved in provoking urticarial reactions. Urticaria in children is provoked by food more often than in adults. Halpern[44] found that 44% of children with urticaria had a food intolerance and the foods producing urticaria were similar to those causing other clinical effects.

Synthetic food additives such as azo dyes (tartrazine, amaranth, coccine nouvelle, sunset yellow), preservatives (sodium benzoate) and other additives (fat antioxidants, sodium nitrate, sodium metabisulphite, tyramine and drugs such as penicillin, tetracycline, quinine and menthol) are thought to provoke a high percentage of the more resistant cases of urticaria.[6] Most patients who react to these substances also react to salicylates.[68]

The diagnosis of food-induced urticaria is not difficult if the patient can identify the provoking food eaten within one hour or two of the development of his symptoms. Recurrent attacks, however, may be difficult to analyse as urticarial rashes can be produced by other non-specific factors, like pressure and exercise. Recurrent challenges with capsules containing tartrazine, yeast, penicillin and placebo may be helpful, but laboratory investigations such as skin-prick tests or RASTs are often not helpful.

Respiratory effects

Food-induced rhinitis and asthma are well recognized and may be associated with other symptoms. Burr et al.[19, 20] found that 17% of his adult patients believed that a particular food could provoke an attack whilst this was only true in 3% of children. Asthma may be precipitated by inhalation of the antigen. However, the route of antigenic stimulation may vary from patient to patient – thus alcoholic drinks may provoke asthma whereas alcoholic fumes or intravenous alcohol are less likely to do so.[42] In some cases the congeners in spirits, or histamine in red and white wine may provoke the attack. Most patients with food-induced asthma have high IgE levels and often positive prick tests or RASTs. However, a subgroup with asthma and low IgE levels negative tests has been described.[60]

Symptoms of runny nose, sneezing and nasal obstruction may be caused by certain foods and are often part of a more generalized allergic reaction. Stimulation is caused not only by inhalation but has also been produced by nasogastric feeding of milk.[13] Nasal polyps may occur in adults. Other respiratory symptoms include chronic respiratory disease described in children with hypersensitivity to cow's milk; this may be followed by pulmonary haemosiderosis.[7]

Migraine

There are many reports suggesting that food can provoke migraine attacks.[69, 70] Hanington *et al.*[45] reported that one-third of their patients attending a migraine clinic related some of their headaches to specific foods. Chocolate, cheese, citrus fruits and alcohol seem to be the major precipitating factors. It has been suggested that foods containing tyramine may provoke headaches but this has not been confirmed. Sandler *et al.*[74] proposed that migraine is due to reduced phenylethylamine (contained in chocolate) and tyramine oxidation, and that one of the forms of platelet monoamine oxidase is defective. Phenylethylamine is thought to stimulate α-receptors and thus produce migraine.

Arthritis

Most clinical studies on the relationship between food and arthritis have been performed in an open and uncontrolled fashion. Wraith[99] has suggested that joint pains can be due to food sensitivity. Skoldstam *et al.*[79] performed a controlled dietary study in patients with rheumatoid arthritis and found reduced symptom scores during the fasting period. There is no evidence that palindromic rheumatism may be due to food allergies.

Psychiatric symptoms

This is perhaps the most controversial aspect of food allergic disorders. Many claims do not stand up to examination. Nevertheless, mental changes and depression are seen in patients with untreated coeliac disease, and irritability and behavioural disorders in the milk-allergic child disappear on a restricted diet. Current adult gastroenterological and allergy clinics are full of patients with food fads and obsessional neuroses, and it is important to distinguish these from patients with true food allergies.

The 'total allergy syndrome' has received much publicity. These patients are thought to be very sensitive to contaminants of the environment. Symptoms reported include weakness, lethargy, faintness, convulsions, blackouts, migraine, disorders of bowel and bladder, and aching joints. There is at present little to suggest that these patients have an allergic disease and they may well be suffering from anorexia nervosa or hysteria.

Diagnosis

The main problem is to identify the patient who warrants clinical and laboratory testing. A careful history may establish a direct relationship between the ingestion of a particular food and the development of symptoms on repeated occasions; this may be sufficient for diagnosis. Questions should be asked about the likes and dislikes of particular foods, foods taken in large quantities and atopic diseases in childhood and in the family. It may be possible to establish, on questioning, whether a patient has a true allergy, a food fad, or a personality or psychiatric problem.

Clinical testing

If a food has been delineated, the next most simple approach would be to eliminate it from the diet; most adult patients may already have done so. If the history is vague many practitioners would go on to try an elimination diet. These diets, however, are time-consuming and cumbersome and range from being very simple to extremely tedious. If multiple foods are involved it is suggested that elimination diets should not be undertaken unless the patient is atopic, has a high IgE and possibly positive RASTs.

A basic exclusion diet usually eliminates colourings, preservatives, milk, eggs, dairy products, fish and nuts, and empirically contains one meat, one vegetable and spring water. Many of these diets are being prescribed by clinical 'ecologists' and workers in fringe medicine.

The effect of dietary challenge is usually easier to evaluate when the patient has been symptom-free on an elimination diet. A 'challenge' can take various forms – it may be by a sublingual provocation test, by inhalation, by intragastric or duodenal instillation or by dietary introduction using capsules containing the particular food. If possible these should be performed in a double-blind fashion and the results assessed in terms of the symptoms produced. If the symptoms are predominantly respiratory, a peak flow reading may be helpful and, if gastrointestinal, a jejunal biopsy and the production of clinical symptoms of diarrhoea or pain may be helpful.

Laboratory testing
Laboratory testing, as with clinical testing, is usually of more help in the diagnosis of an immediate type of reaction. Tests should only be used as a diagnostic adjunct to clinical criteria.[34] A high IgE level may suggest an immediate type of hypersensitivity and this should be followed up by a food specific radioallergosorbent test (RAST). Although this test is now available in a kit form, there are many disadvantages. It is expensive, it is affected by the presence of IgG antibodies and it does not detect cell-bound IgE antibodies. There may also be interlaboratory variations and cross-reactivity problems. Because of the chemical limitations, a RAST can only be used to study allergens containing amino acids.

Skin-prick testing with a variety of common allergens may be an adjunct to the diagnosis of atopy. Unfortunately prick tests to foods may show a high proportion of false positives and have little correlation with the RAST test. Buisseret[17] found that only 31% of patients with cow's milk allergy (diagnosed by exclusion and challenge) had a positive skin test. However, tests for eggs, nuts and fish may be slightly more reliable.

Measurement of circulating immune complexes, leucocyte histamine release tests,[13] and organ culture tests[89] have all been performed in various conditions but are cumbersome, unreliable, and at the moment mainly used as research tools. Humoral antibodies against foods are also seen in normal individuals, but may be useful in assessing treatment in patients if antibody titres fall.

Treatment

Treatment is dependent, where possible, on antigen avoidance. Elimination of a suspect food – for example, strawberries or shellfish – presents no problems. However, more restrictive diets may present difficulties in ensuring adequate amounts of protein, calories, vitamins and calcium. The most common food problems are due to milk, egg, fish, nuts, spices and artificial colourings or preservatives. Having started a diet,[27, 60] a succession of new foods can be added one by one over a period of a few days. Alternatively, in severe cases, an elemental diet may be given. Hyposensitization to allergens has been tried with variable success.

Drugs used are either antihistamines or prostaglandin synthetase inhibitors. Antihistamines which do not contain artificial colourings include brompheniramine (Dimotane), mebhydrolin (Fabahistin), hydroxyzine (Atarax), azatadine (Optimine) and terfenadine (Triludan). Some of these drugs cause a degree of sedation.

Prostaglandin synthetase inhibitors such as aspirin and other non-steroidal anti-inflammatory drugs may be useful in the treatment of diarrhoea. Their action, however, may be non-specific.

Lastly, sodium cromoglycate, either inhaled or oral, has been used prophylactically in patients with IgE-mediated food allergy. Sodium cromoglycate, a mast cell stabilizer, has been very successful in the treatment of asthma but the oral preparation has yet to be evaluated.

REFERENCES

1   Aas, K. & Lundkvist, U. (1973) The radioallergosorbent test with a purified allergen from codfish. *Clinical Allergy*, **3**, 255–261.
2   Alun Jones, V., McLaughlan, P., Shorthouse, M. *et al.* (1982) Food intolerance: a major factor in the pathogenesis of irritable bowel syndrome. *Lancet*, **ii**, 1115–1117.
3   Ament, M. E. & Rubin, C. E. (1972) Soy protein – another cause of the flat intestinal lesion. *Gastroenterology*, **62**, 227–234.
4   Atherton, D. J. (1982) Atopic eczema. *Clinics in Immunology and Allergy*, **2**(1), 77–100.
5   Atherton, D. J., Sewell, M., Soothill, J. F. *et al.* (1978) A double-blind cross-over trial of an antigen avoidance diet in atopic eczema. *Lancet*, **i**, 401–403.
6   August, P. J. (1980) Urticaria. In *Proceedings of the First Food Allergy Workshop* (Ed.) Coombs, R. R. A. pp. 76–81. Oxford: Medical Education Services.
7   Bahna, S. L. & Heiner, D. C. (1980) *Allergies to Milk.* New York: Grune & Stratton.
8   Barnetson, R. St C. (1980) Hyperimmunoglobulinaemia E in atopic eczema is associated with 'food allergy'. In *International Symposium on Atopic Dermatitis*. (Ed.) Rajka, G. *Acta Dermatologica (Stockholm)*, Supplement 92, 94–96.
9   Barnetson, R. St C. & Lessof, M. H. (1983) Challenges to medical orthodoxy. In *Clinical Reactions to Food* (Ed.) Lessof, M. H. pp. 15–34. Chichester: John Wiley.
10 Barnetson, R. St C. & Merrett, T. G. (1980) Atopic eczema. In *Proceedings of the First Food Allergy Workshop* (Ed.) Coombs, R. R. A. pp. 69–75. Oxford: Medical Education Services.

11 Basomba, A. J. (1967) The role of food allergy in children's bronchial asthma. *Asthma Research*, **5**, 129–132.

12 Bleumink, E. (1979) Food allergy and the gastrointestinal tract. In *Immunology of the Gastrointestinal Tract*. (Ed.) Asquith, P. pp. 195–213. Edinburgh: Churchill Livingstone.

13 Bock, S. A., Buckley, J., Holst, A. & May, C. D. (1977) Proper use of skin tests with food extracts. *Clinical Allergy*, **7**, 375–383.

14 Bock, S. A., Lee, W-Y., Remigio, L. K. & May, C. D. (1978) Studies of hypersensitivity reactions to foods in infants and children. *Journal of Allergy and Clinical Immunology*, **62**, 327–334.

15 Brostoff, J., Carini, C., Wraith, D. G. & Johns, P. (1979) Production of IgE complexes by allergen challenge in atopic patients and the effect of sodium cromoglycate. *Lancet*, **i**, 1268–1270.

16 Brostoff, J., Carini, C., Wraith, D. C. *et al.* (1979) Immune complexes in atopy. In *The Mast Cell* (Ed.) Pepys, J. & Edwards, A. M. pp. 380–383. London: Pitman Medical.

17 Buisseret, P. (1978) Common manifestations of cow's milk allergy in children. *Lancet*, **i**, 304–305.

18 Buisseret, P. D., Youlten, L. J. F., Heinzelman, D. & Lessof, M. H. (1978) Prostaglandin synthesis inhibitors in the prophylaxis of food intolerance. *Lancet*, **i**, 906–907.

19 Burr, M. L., Eldridge, B. A. & Borysiewicz, L. K. (1974) Peak expiratory flow rates before and after exercise in school children. *Archives of Diseases in Childhood*, **49**, 923–924.

20 Burr, M. L., St Leger, A. S., Bevan, C. & Merrett, T. G. (1975) A community survey of asthmatic characteristics. *Thorax*, **30**, 663–668.

21 Cam, C. & Nigogosyan, G. (1963) Acquired toxic porphyria cutanea tarda due to hexachlorobenzene. *Journal of the American Medical Association*, **183**, 88.

22 Chase, M. W. (1946) Inhibition of experimental drug allergy by prior feeding of the sensitising agent. *Proceedings of the Society of Experimental Biology and Medicine*, **61**, 257.

23 Collins-Williams, C. (1956) The incidence of milk-allergy in paediatric practice. *Journal of Paediatrics*, **48**, 38–59.

24 Coombs, R. R. A. (1980) *Proceedings of The First Food Allergy Workshop*. p. 45. Oxford: Medical Education Services.

25 Cooper, B. T., Holmes, G. K. T., Ferguson, R. *et al.* (1980) Gluten-sensitive diarrhoea without evidence of coeliac disease, *Gastroenterology*, **79**, 801–806.

26 Danneus, A., Inganas, M., Johansson, S. G. O. & Foucard, T. (1979) Intestinal uptake of ovalbumin in malabsorption and food allergy in relation to serum IgG antibody and orally administered sodium cromoglycate. *Clinical Allergy*, **9**, 263–270.

27 Denman, A. M. (1980) Diagnostic methods and criteria. In *Proceedings of the First Food Allergy Workshop* (Ed.) Coombs, R. R. A. pp. 47–55. Oxford: Medical Education Services.

28 Eastham, E. J. & Walker, W. A. (1979) Adverse effects of milk formula and ingestion on the gastrointestinal tract. *Gastroenterology*, **76**, 365–374.

29 Ferguson, A. (1976) Coeliac disease and gastrointestinal food allergy. In *Immunological Aspects of the Liver and Gastrointestinal Tract* (Ed.) Ferguson, A. & MacSween, R. N. M. pp. 153–202. Lancaster: MTP Press.

30 Ferguson, A. (1983) Immunology and physiology of digestion. In *Clinical Reactions to Food* (Ed.) Lessof, M. H. pp. 59–86. Chichester: John Wiley.

31 Ferguson, A. & Carswell, F. (1972) Precipitins to dietary proteins in the serum and upper intestinal secretions of coeliac children. *British Medical Journal*, **i**, 75–77.

32 Ferguson, A. & Parrott, D. M. V. (1973) Histopathology and time course of rejection of allografts of mouse small intestine. *Transplantation*, **15**, 546–554.

33 Forget, P., Eggermont, E., Marchal, G. *et al.* (1978) Eosinophilic infiltration of the oesophagus in an infant. *Acta Paediatrica Belgica*, **31**, 91–93.

34 Freed, D. L. J. (1982) Laboratory diagnosis of food intolerance. *Clinics in Immunology and Allergy*, **2**(1), 181–203.

35 Fries, J. H. (1947) Milk allergy – diagnostic aspects and the role of milk substitutes. *Journal of the American Medical Association*, **165**, 1542–1543.

36 Fries, J. H. (1971) Studies on the allergenicity of soy bean. *Annals of Allergy*, **29**, 1–5.

37 Frost, M. (1973) Cromoglycate in aphthous stomatitis. *Lancet*, **ii**, 389 (Letter).

38 Gerrard, J. W. (1980) *Food Allergy – New Perspectives*. Springfield, Illinois: Charles C. Thomas.

39 Gerrard, J. W., MacKenzie, J. W. A., Goluboff, N. *et al.* (1973) Cow's milk allergy: prevalence and manifestations in an unselected series of newborns. *Acta Paediatrica Scandinavica*, Supplement 234, 2–21.

40 Goldman, A. S. & Heiner, D. C. (1977) Clinical Aspects of food sensitivity. Diagnosis and management of cow's milk sensitivity. *Pediatric Clinics of North America*, **24**, 133–135.

41 Goldman, A. S., Anderson, D. W., Sellers, W. A. *et al.* (1963) Milk allergy. I. Oral challenge with milk and isolated milk proteins in allergic children. *Paediatrics*, **32**, 425–443.

42 Gong, M., Tashkin, D. P. & Calvarese, B. M. (1981) Alcohol-induced bronchospasm in an asthmatic patient. *Chest*, **80**, 167–173.

43 Graysowski E. A., Barile, M. F., Lee, W. B. & Stanley, H. R. (1966) Recurrent aphthous stomatitis; clinical, therapeutic, histopathologic and hypersensitivity aspects. *Journal of the American Medical Association*, **196**, 637–644.

44 Halpern, S. R. (1965) Chronic hives in children: an analysis of 75 cases. *Annals of Allergy*, **23**, 589–593.

45 Hanington, E., Horn, M. & Wilkinson, M. (1970) Further observations on the effects of tyramine. In *Background to Migraine. Proceedings of the Third Migraine Symposium*, Chapter 2 (Ed.) Chochrane, A. L. London: Heinemann.

46 Hedström, V. (1958) Food allergy in bronchial asthma. *Acta Allergologica*, **12**, 153–185.

47 Hoffman, D. R., Day, E. D. & Miller, J. S. (1981) The major heat stable allergen of shrimp. *Annals of Allergy*, **47**, 17–22.

48 Hutchins, P. & Walker-Smith, J. A. (1982) The gastrointestinal system. *Clinics in Immunology and Allergy*, **2**(1), 45–48.

49 Jacobsson, I. & Lindberg, T. (1978) Cow's milk as a cause of infantile colic in breast-fed infants. *Lancet*, **ii**, 437–439.

50 Jenkins, H. R., Milla, P. J., Pincott, J. R., Soothill, J. F. & Harries, J. T. (1982) Food allergy: the major cause of infantile colitis. *Gut*, **23**, A924.

51 Johnstone, J. M. & Morson, B. C. (1978) Eosinophilic gastroenteritis. *Histopathology*, **2**, 335–348.

52 Kaplan, M. S. & Solli, N. J. (1979) Immunoglobulin E in breast-fed atopic children. *Journal of Allergy and Clinical Immunology*, **64**, 122–126.

53 Katz, A. J., Goldman, M. & Grand, R. J. (1977) Gastric mucosa biopsy in eosinophilic (allergic) gastroenteritis. *Gastroenterology*, **73**, 705–709.

54 Klee, W. A. & Iorio, M. A. (1977) Relationships between opiate receptor binding and analgetic properties of prodine-type compounds. *Journal of Medical Chemistry*, **20**(2), 309–310.

55 Konig, P. & Godfreys, S. (1974) Exercise-induced bronchial lability on monozygotic (identical) and dizygotic (non-identical) twins. *Journal of Allergy and Clinical Immunology*, **54**, 280–282.

56 Kuitenen, P., Visakorpi, J. K., Savilhati, E. & Pelkonen, P. (1975) Malabsorption syndrome with cow's milk intolerance. Clinical findings and course in 54 cases. *Archives of Diseases in Childhood*, **50**, 351–356.

57 Kumar, P. J., Ferguson, A., Lancaster-Smith, M. L. & Dawson, A. M. (1973) Relationship between dietary food antigen and jejunal mucosal morphology. *Gut*, **14**, 829–830.

58 Kumar, P. J., O'Donoghue, D. P., Stenson, K. & Dawson, A. M. (1979) Reintroduction of gluten in adults and children with treated coeliac disease. *Gut*, **20**, 743–749.

59 Kwok, R. H. M. (1968) Chinese restaurant syndrome. *New England Journal of Medicine*, **278**, 796.

60 Lessof, M. H., Wraith, D. G., Merrett, T. G. *et al.* (1980) Food allergy and intolerance in 100 patients – local and systemic effects. *Quarterly Journal of Medicine*, **195**, 259–271.

61 Levinsky, R. J., Paganelli, R., Robertson, D. M. & Atherton, D. J. (1981) Handling of food antigens and their complexes by normal and allergic individuals. In *The Immunology of Infant Feeding* (Ed.) Wilkinson, A. W. pp. 23–30, New York: Plenum Press.

62 Lippard, V. M., Schloss, O. M. & Johnson, P. A. (1936) Immune reactions induced in infants by intestinal absorption of incompletely digested cow's milk protein. *American Journal of Diseases of Childhood*, **51**, 562–574.

63 Lockey, S. D. (1972) Sensitizing properties of food additives and other commercial products. *Annals of Allergy*, **30**, 638–642.

64 Mackarness, R. (1976) *Not All in the Mind*. London: Pan Books.

65 Maini, V., Lloyd, G., Green, F. H. Y. *et al.* (1976) Treatment of ulcerative colitis with oral disodium cromoglycate. A double-blind controlled trial. *Lancet*, **i**, 439–441.

66 Matthew, D. J., Taylor, B., Norman, A. P. *et al.* (1977) Prevention of eczema. *Lancet*, **i**, 321–324.

67 Meara, R. H. (1965) Skin reactions in atopic eczema. *British Journal of Dermatology*, **67**, 60–64.

68 Michaëlsson, G. & Juhlin, L. (1973) Urticaria induced by preservatives and dye additives in food and drugs. *British Journal of Dermatology*, **88**, 525–532.

69 Monro, J. A. (1982) Food allergy and migraine. *Clinics in Immunology and Allergy*, **2**(1), 137–163.

70 Monro, J. A., Brostoff, J., Carini, C. & Zilkha, K. (1980) Food allergy in migraine. *Lancet*, **ii**, 1–4.

71 O'Morain, C., Segal, A. W. & Levi, A. J. (1980) Elemental diets in treatment of acute Crohn's disease. *British Medical Journal*, **iv**, 1173–1175.

72 Paganelli, R., Levinsky, R. J., Brostoff, J. & Wraith, D. G. (1979) Immune complexes containing food proteins in normal and atopic subjects after oral challenge and effect of sodium cromoglycate on antigen absorption. *Lancet*, **i**, 1270–1272.

73 Perkkiö, M., Savilahti, E. & Kuitunen, P. (1981) Morphometric and immunochemical study of jejunal biopsies from children with intestinal soy allergy. *European Journal of Paediatrics*, **137**, 63–69.

73a Prauznitz, C. & Kustner, H. (1921) Studien über die verbering Findlichkeit. *Zentralblatt für Bakteriologie, Parasitenkunde, Infektionskrankheiten und Hygiene, Abt. I, Orig. Reine A*, **86**, 160.

74 Randolph, T. G. (1962) *Human Ecology and Susceptibility to the Chemical Environment*. Illinois: Springfield.

75 Robertson, D., Paganelli, R., Dinwiddie, R. & Levinsky, R. J. (1982) Milk antigen absorption in the premature and term neonate. *Archives of Diseases of Childhood*, **57**, 369–370.

76 Sandler, M., Youdim, M. B. H. & Hanington, E. (1974) Conjugation defect in tyramine-sensitive migraine. *Nature*, **250**, 335–337.

77 Savilhti, E. (1981) Cow's milk allergy. *Allergy*, **36**, 73–88.

78 Shiner, M., Ballard, J. & Smith, M. E. (1975) The small intestinal mucosa in cow's milk allergy. *Lancet*, **i**, 136–140.

79 Sköldstam, L., Larsson, L. & Lindström, F. D. (1979) Effects of fasting and lactovegetarian diet on rheumatoid arthritis. *Scandinavian Journal of Rheumatology*, **8**, 249–255.

80 Solheim, B. G., Ek, J., Thune, P. O. *et al.* (1976) HLA antigens in dermatitis herpetiformis and coeliac disease. *Tissue Antigens*, **7**, 57–59.

81 Soothill, J. F. (1979) Food allergy. In *The Mast Cell* (Ed.) Pepys, J. & Edwards, A. M. pp. 367–376. London: Pitman Medical.

82 Soothill, J. F. (1983) Immunological aspects of infant feeding. In *Paediatric Clinical Immunology* (Ed.) Soothill, J. F., Haywood, A. R. & Wood, C. B. S. pp. 110–129. Oxford: Blackwell Scientific.

83 Soothill, J. F., Stokes, C. R., Turner, M. W. *et al.* (1976) Predisposing factors and the development of reaginic allergy in infancy. *Clinical Allergy*, **6**, 305–306.

84 Speer, F. (1973) Management of food allergy. In *Immunology in Children* (Ed.) Speer, F. & Dockhorn, R. J. pp. 397–402. Springfield, Illinois: Charles C. Thomas.

85 Swarbrick, E. T., Stokes, C. R. & Soothill, J. F. (1978) The absorption of antigens after oral immunisation and the simultaneous induction of specific systemic tolerance. *Gut*, **20**, 121–125.

86 Tabuenca, J. M. (1981) Toxic-allergic syndrome caused by ingestion of rape seed oil denatured with aniline. *Lancet*, **ii**, 567–568.

87 Taylor, K. B. & Truelove, S. C. (1961) Circulating antibodies to milk proteins in ulcerative colitis. *British Medical Journal*, **ii**, 924–929.

88 Taylor, B., Norman, A. P., Orgel, H. A. *et al.* (1973) Transient IgA deficiency and pathogenesis of infantile atopy. *Lancet*, **ii**, 111–113.

89 Trier, J. S. & Browning, T. H. (1970) Epithelial cell renewal in cultured duodenal biopsies in coeliac sprue. *New England Journal of Medicine*, **283**, 1245–1364.

90 Turner, M. W., Brostoff, J., Mowbray, J. F. & Skelton, A. (1980) The atopic syndrome: in vitro immunological characteristics of clinically defined subgroups of atopic subjects. *Clinical Allergy*, **10**, 575–584.

91 Turner, M. W., Mowbray, J. F., Harvey, B. A. M. *et al.* (1978) Defective yeast opsonization and C2 deficiency in atopic parents. *Clinics of Experimental Immunology*, **34**, 253–259.

92 Waldmann, T. A., Wochner, R. D., Laster, L. & Gordon, R. S. (1967) Allergic gastroenteropathy: a cause of excessive gastrointestinal protein loss. *New England Journal of Medicine*, **276**, 761–769.

93 Walker, W. A. (1982) Mechanisms of antigen handling by the gut. *Clinics in Immunology and Allergy*, **2**(1), 15–40.

94 Walker, W. A. & Isselbacher, K. J. (1974) Uptake and transport of macromolecules by the intestine: possible role in clinical disorders. *Gastroenterology*, **67**, 531–550.

95 Walker-Smith, J. A. (1970) Transient gluten intolerance. *Archives of Diseases of Childhood*, **45**, 523–526.

96   Whorwell, P. J. & Wright, R. (1979) Bottle feeding, early gastroenteritis and inflammatory bowel disease. *British Medical Journal*, **i**, 382.

97   Wilson, J. F., Heiner, D. C. & Lahey, M. E. (1964) Milk-induced gastrointestinal bleeding in infants with hypochronic microcytic anaemia. *Journal of the American Medical Association*, **189**, 568–572.

98   Wilson, S. J. & Walzer, M. (1935) Absorption of undigested proteins in human beings. IV. Absorption of unaltered protein in infants and in children. *American Journal of Diseases of Childhood*, **50**, 49–54.

99   Wraith, D. G. (1980) Respiratory Diseases. In *Proceedings of the First Food Allergy Workshop* (Ed.) Coombs, R. R. A. pp. 64–68. Oxford: Medical Education Services.

EOSINOPHILIC GASTROENTERITIS

Eosinophilic gastroenteritis has been recognized since 1937 as an uncommon disorder affecting one or more parts of the gut. It is characterized by gastrointestinal thickening with oedema and dense eosinophil infiltrates.[3, 7] It usually involves the gastric antrum and proximal small intestine.[11] The disease takes three main forms (Figure 8.95). The mucosal form may be associated with protein-losing enteropathy, anaemia and malabsorption and patients may have a history of allergic disorders with high IgE levels.

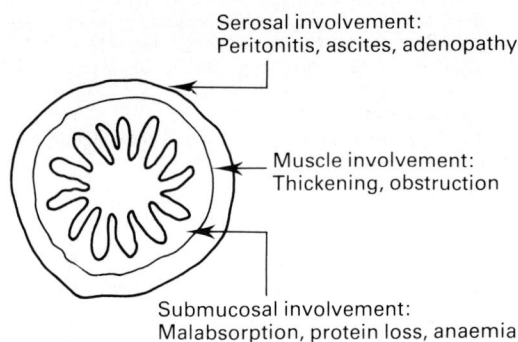

Serosal involvement:
Peritonitis, ascites, adenopathy

Muscle involvement:
Thickening, obstruction

Submucosal involvement:
Malabsorption, protein loss, anaemia

Lesions may be polypoid or diffuse

Fig. 8.95 The three main types of eosinophilic gastroenteritis are associated with involvement of different layers of the gut wall.

Muscle involvement produces thickening and obstruction which may require surgery, and occasionally bleeding or fistulas occur. Serosal disease gives rise to abdominal pain with peritonitis and ascites.

Eosinophilic gastroenteritis mainly occurs in young adults in their third decade. However it can occur in children[6] and in older people. Males appear to be affected twice as often as females. The incidence of the disease is hard to define, but may be as little as 1/10 000 hospital admissions.

The aetiology of eosinophilic gastroenteritis has not been determined. Food antigens are probably not involved, although 20% of patients have history of allergic diseases. In some patients it may be difficult to distinguish eosinophilic gastroenteritis from allergic gastroenteritis (see p. 590). However, in eosinophilic gastroenteritis the immunoglobulin content of the intestines is normal, in contrast to allergic gastroenteritis where tissue IgE and IgG levels are usually elevated.[2]

The role of eosinophils in this form of gastroenteritis has not been explained. Eosinophils commonly enter the small intestine, and this may be one of the main sites of eosinophil accumulation in normal individuals. The association of eosinophil infiltrates with a number of tissue lesions, including lesions which progress to fibrosis, has raised the possibility that eosinophils are actively involved in tissue damage in these patients.[3] This has not been tested directly but highly purified eosinophils in ascitic fluid from a patient with eosinophilic gastroenteritis showed many features consistent with an activated and fully functional state.[9] It is also of interest that some patients with eosinophilic gastroenteritis have associated chronic fibrotic lesions in the lungs, and fibrosis in areas of eosinophil infiltration in the gut has also been noted.

Clinical features

The disease may present as an acute illness with obstruction to the outflow of the stomach or with chronic abdominal pain, distension and ascites, and nausea and vomiting. Single episodes may occur, but some patients have a history going back many years.

Involvement of the stomach may be difficult to distinguish from peptic ulcer, adenomas or carcinomas, and helminths in the stomach may produce localized eosinophilic infiltrates. The differential diagnosis of small intestinal involvement includes Crohn's disease, diverticulitis and tropical sprue. Terminal ileal and caecal involvement may mimic Crohn's disease, amoebiasis or intestinal tuberculosis. Localized areas of eosinophilic gastroenteritis are similar in some respects to inflammatory fibroid polyps of the gastrointestinal tract.[8]

Localized forms of eosinophilic gastroenteritis
The stomach alone is involved in about 26% of patients with eosinophilic gastroenteritis

(eosinophilic gastritis). Lesions are often circumscribed and similar in appearance to eosinophilic granulomas of the stomach. The antrum is one of the main sites of involvement. A gastric mass may simulate a malignancy.[13]

About 50% of patients with eosinophilic gastroenteritis develop symptoms of obstruction even when there is evidence of diffuse involvement.[1] This may require surgery but wherever possible a trial of steroids should be given first.

Ileocolitis with narrowing and shortening of the caecum and ascending colon has been described and has led to hemicolectomy for intestinal obstruction,[16] but in the majority of patients eosinophilic gastroenteritis involves the *upper small intestine* where the disease is diffuse.

Fourteen patients with the *serosal* form of eosinophilic gastroenteritis have been described.[5, 12] These patients have ascites which contains up to 99% eosinophils. Protein in the fluid is usually an exudate. The discovery of eosinophils in ascitic fluid may suggest other diagnoses including vasculitic disorders, lymphomas, metastatic carcinomas and ruptured hydatid cysts. Peritoneal fluid can contain up to 40% eosinophils in about one third of patients having peritoneal dialysis, but this is not associated with increased eosinophils in the peripheral blood.

Eosinophilic gastroenteritis may also affect the oesophagus, liver and biliary system, or the large bowel and rectum. Oesophageal involvement can be associated with disorders of motor function;[10] this has also been seen in patients with allergic gastroenteritis. Eosinophilic gastroenteritis is a rare cause of eosinophilic hepatitis[4] and eosinophilic cholangitis and isolated rectal involvement have also been reported.

Investigations

Blood eosinophil counts are raised in only about 20% of patients with eosinophilic gastroenteritis. The counts may fluctuate and follow the course of the disease, but in many patients blood eosinophil counts remain normal throughout their illness. Radiology of the stomach demonstrates gastric antral rigidity with thickened folds and mucosal nodules. In the small intestine the circular folds and walls are thickened without evidence of ulceration or local abnormality.[15] The diagnosis is established by histology; endoscopic biopsies may well be adequate but the lesions may be patchy requiring multiple biopsies. Colonoscopy and fibre-optic sigmoidoscopy has occasionally demonstrated lesions in patients with distal gastrointestinal involvement.[14] Histologically, dense infiltrates of eosinophils are seen in localized or diffuse areas of the gut. There is no necrosis but there may be some fibrosis. Oedema is a constant feature, and where the serosal layer is involved this gives rise to ascites. Further investigations sometimes bring to light malabsorption and/or protein-losing enteropathy, which occurs in about 10% of patients. A full-thickness biopsy is rarely necessary but may be required in the serosal form of the disease, as superficial biopsies can fail to demonstrate the characteristic features of the disease.

Treatment

Correct diagnosis of eosinophilic gastroenteritis is rewarding as treatment is extremely effective. Surgery can usually be avoided, and a wide range of more sinister diagnoses can be eliminated. Steroids are the mainstay of treatment. Prednisolone 15–40 mg/day is usually given initially, with doses decreasing to alternate day therapy when symptoms and clinical signs have resolved. Occasionally disodium cromoglycate (Intal) has been used in patients who cannot take steroids. Some patients show spontaneous remission of their disease. However in others, relapses can occur; these usually also respond to treatment, even though it may have to be continued for many months.

Surgery is usually of little benefit and recurrence can occur even after partial gastrectomy in patients who have not received steroids.

The prognosis is usually excellent, providing the disorder is recognized and treated early. Occasional fatal cases have been reported in childhood. Since perforation and bleeding can also occur, some patients may need additional therapeutic measures.

Related disorders

A number of vasculitic and granulomatous diseases can also give rise to eosinophil infiltrations into the gastrointestinal tract.[17, 18] Patients with these disorders differ from those with eosinophilic gastroenteritis as they are usually older, frequently in their sixth decade. Of these patients, 40% have gastric involvement and 26% ileal involvement, but they may also present with epigastric pain, vomiting and obstruction; they may respond to treatment with steroids. The Churg–Strauss syndrome can affect the gut, producing areas of eosinophilic infiltration and focal necrotic lesions. The gut is also involved in some patients with the hyper-eosinophilic syndrome, which is characterized by high blood eosinophil counts of unknown cause, usually with characteristic lesions in other sites including the heart (eosinophilic endo-myocardial disease), skin and lung. These simi-larities between different eosinophilic disorders affecting the gastrointestinal tract raise the possibility that they are related, differing only in the sites where eosinophils localize and cause tissue injury. If eosinophilic gastroenteritis is part of a wider spectrum of hypereosinophilic disorders, it appears to be one of the most benign forms, with a good response to treatment with steroids, and an excellent prognosis in most patients.

REFERENCES

1   Caldwell, J. H., Mekhjian, H. S., Hurtubise, P. E. & Beman, F. M. (1978) Eosinophilic gastroenteritis with obstruction. Immunological studies of seven patients. *Gastroenterology*, **74**, 825–828.
2   Caldwell, J. H., Sharma, H. M., Hurtubise, P. E. & Colwell, D. L. (1979) Eosinophilic gastroenteritis in extreme allergy. Immunopathological comparison with non-allergic gastrointestinal disease. *Gastroenterology*, **77**, 560–564.
3   Cello, J. P. (1979) Eosinophilic gastroenteritis – a complex disease entity. *American Journal of Medicine*, **67**, 1097–1104.
4   Everett, G. D. & Mitros, F. A. (1980) Eosinophilic gas-troenteritis with hepatic eosinophilic granulomas. Report of a case with 30 year follow-up. *American Journal of Gastroenterology*, **74**, 519–521.
5   Harmon, W. A. & Helman, C. A. (1981) Eosinophilic gastroenteritis and ascites. *Journal of Clinical Gastroen-terology*, **3**, 371–373.
6   Hoefer, R. A., Ziegler, M. M., Koop, C. E. & Schnaufer, L. (1977) Surgical manifestations of eosinophilic gastro-enteritis in the paediatric patient. *Journal of Paediatric Surgery*, **12**, 955–962.
7   Johnstone, J. M. & Morson, B. C. (1978) Eosinophilic gastroenteritis. *Histopathology*, **2**, 335–348.
8   Johnstone, J. M. & Morson, B. C. (1978) Inflammatory fibroid polyp of the gastrointestinal tract. *Histopathol-ogy*, **2**, 349–361.
9   Klebanoff, S. J., Durack, D. T., Rosen, H. & Clark, R. A. (1977) Functional studies on human peritoneal eosinophils. *Infection and Immunity*, **17**, 167–173.
10 Landres, R. T., Kuster, G. G. & Strum, W. B. (1978) Eosinophilic esophagitis in a patient with vigorous achalasia. *Gastroenterology*, **74**, 1298–1301.
11 Marshak, R. H., Lindner, A., Maklansky, D. & Gelb, A. (1981) Eosinophilic gastroenteritis. *Journal of the Amer-ican Medical Association*, **245**, 1677–1680.
12 McNabb, P. C., Fleming, C. R., Higgins, J. A. & Davis, G. L. (1979) Transmural eosinophilic gastroenteritis with ascites. *Mayo Clinic Proceedings*, **54**, 119–122.
13 Milman, P. J. & Sidhu, G. S. (1978) Case report: eosino-philic gastritis simulating a neoplasm. *American Journal of Medical Science*, **276**, 227–230.
14 Partyka, E. K., Sanowski, R. A. & Kozarek, R. A. (1980) Colonoscopic features of eosinophilic gastroenteritis. *Diseases of the Colon and Rectum*, **23**, 353–356.
15 Schulman, A., Morton, P. C. & Dietrich, B. E. (1980) Eosinophilic gastroenteritis. *Clinical Radiology*, **31**, 101–104.
16 Schulze, K. & Mitros, F. A. (1979) Eosinophilic gastro-enteritis involving the ileocecal area. *Diseases of the Colon and Rectum*, **22**, 47–50.
17 Spry, C. J. F. (1982) The hypereosinophilic syndrome: clinical features, laboratory findings and treatment. *Allergy*, **37**, 539–551.
18 Suen, K. C. & Burton, J. D. (1979) The spectrum of eosinophilic infiltration of the gastrointestinal tract and its relationship to other disorders of angitis and granu-lomatosis. *Human Pathology*, **10**, 31–43.

PROTEIN-LOSING ENTEROPATHY

In 1957 Citrin[9] and his colleagues studied a patient with giant hypertrophy of the gastric rugae (Menetrier's disease) who had severe hypoalbuminaemia. Using metabolic turnover studies with radioiodinated albumin they deter-mined that this patient had an increased rate of albumin catabolism associated with a normal rate of albumin synthesis, and that he was excreting large amounts of intact (undegraded) albumin directly into the stomach. At about the same time, Steinfeld et al.[39] made similar obser-vations in patients with inflammatory bowel disease and hypoalbuminaemia. Here again metabolic studies with radioiodinated albumin disclosed an increased rate of albumin cata-bolism which, in this case, was associated with a normal or even increased rate of synthesis. In addition, an excessive amount of radioiodine was found in the stool, suggesting that there was loss of intact protein into the small intestine. These reports showing that hypoproteinaemia could be due to loss of protein into the gastro-intestinal tract ushered in a period of intense study of the phenomenon of protein-losing enteropathy (PLE). Subsequent investigation of this pathological process has involved firstly the search for better tools for measuring gastro-intestinal protein loss, and secondly the identifi-cation of PLE in a myriad of gastrointestinal conditions ranging from diseases in which PLE is a minor and incidental feature of the overall pathological picture to diseases in which PLE is the dominant abnormality. During the course of these studies, several new gastrointestinal syn-dromes have been identified, most notably intes-tinal lymphangiectasia and allergic gastro-enteropathy.

PLE is considered here first from a physio-logical point of view, emphasizing the basic fea-tures of serum protein metabolism and the methods used to measure both serum protein turnover and PLE. The range of diseases associated with PLE are then discussed, drawing attention to the major mechanisms responsible for this abnormality. Finally, intestinal lymphangiectasia is considered at length.

General features of serum protein metabolism

Protein-losing enteropathy (PLE) may be defined as the abnormal loss of serum proteins into the gastrointestinal tract resulting from a variety of gastrointestinal abnormalities and leading to reduced serum protein levels, particularly albumin levels. From a pathophysiological point of view, PLE is a disorder of serum protein metabolism and for this reason is best described by metabolic turnover studies utilizing radiolabelled proteins.

Protein turnover studies
Metabolically speaking, the body consists of a central intravascular compartment or pool which exchanges material with one or more extravascular compartments (Figure 8.96). Synthesis of serum proteins is followed by their rapid entry into the intravascular compartment. They then circulate there or move into one of the extravascular compartments. Catabolism of

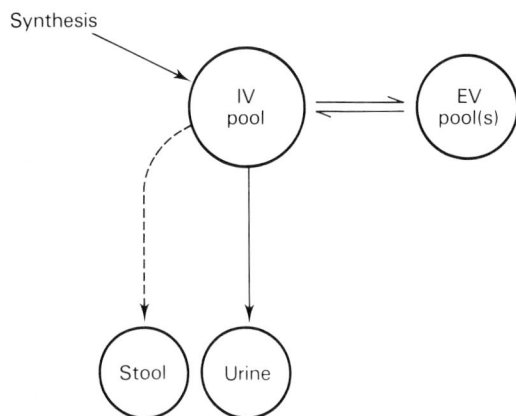

Fig. 8.96 Compartmental model of protein metabolism. Synthesis of serum protein is followed by its rapid introduction into the intravascular (IV) compartment or pool. The diagram shows that protein may circulate in this compartment, leave it temporarily by entering one or more extravascular (EV) compartments, or leave the IV pool permanently as a result of endogenous catabolism or loss of intact protein into the bowel (stool). The rate at which protein irreversibly leaves the IV pool can be expressed as a fractional catabolic rate – the fraction of the IV pool catabolized/unit time. In the diagram this is indicated by the vertical arrows leading into the urinary and stool compartments.

serum proteins occurs at sites which are in close relation to the intravascular compartment; it is quantitatively defined as the fraction of protein in the intravascular compartment that irreversibly leaves this compartment per unit time. Defined in this way, catabolism includes the protein degraded within the body (endogenous catabolism) as well as the protein lost to the outside via the gastrointestinal tract, kidney, lungs or skin. During steady-state (normal) conditions the intravascular compartment remains constant in size. This means that the amount of protein catabolized per unit time (i.e. the fraction of the intravascular pool catabolized/unit time × pool size) equals the synthetic rate. Thus during a steady state the pool size and hence the serum protein level is inversely proportional to the fractional catabolic rate.

The quantitative assessment of the metabolism of any given serum protein involves measuring various metabolic parameters defined above: the pool sizes, the intercompartmental transfer rates (which allow calculation of the percentage of the serum protein present in the intravascular compartment), and the fractional catabolic rate. These measurements are generally made by performing metabolic turnover studies using proteins labelled with radioactive tracers.[48] These are handled by the body in the same way as newly synthesized unlabelled protein, and allow the fate of a cohort of proteins to be followed. Radioiodine is the label of choice for metabolic turnover studies since it does not alter the metabolic characteristics of the protein to which it is attached, and it is not reincorporated into new protein after the protein to which it is bound is degraded, but is rapidly excreted into the urine (and thus cleared from the circulation).

In a typical metabolic turnover study, a purified radiolabelled protein such as ^{125}I-albumin is injected intravenously into the individual under study. Ten minutes after injection, when the radioiodinated protein has had time to be distributed evenly throughout the intravascular compartment but has not yet been catabolized and has not yet left the intravascular space, a sample is taken to estimate plasma volume (plasma volume equals counts injected divided by counts/ml in the 10 minute sample). The plasma volume (PV) can then be used to calculate the size of the intravascular protein compartment: PV multiplied by protein concentration is equal to the intravascular pool size.

The fractional catabolic rate and the intercompartmental transfer rates can be determined from the intravenous 'die-away' curve generated from radioactivity values in serum samples taken at intervals following radioiodinated protein injection. This 'die-away' curve is constructed by plotting the percentage of the 10 minute value remaining in serum samples against time on semilogarithmic paper (Figure 8.97). The reciprocal of the area under this die-away curve is equal to the fractional catabolic

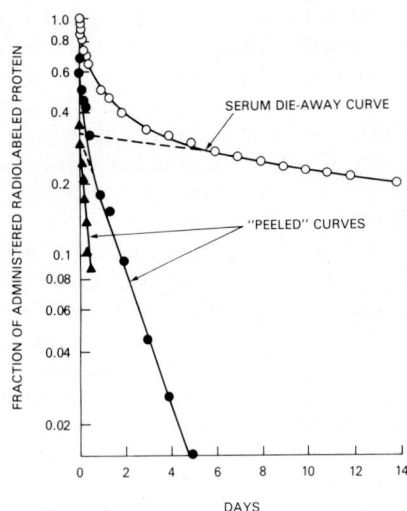

Fig. 8.97 Die-away curve of a radiolabelled protein (such as ^{125}I-albumin) following injection into the intravascular (circulating) protein pool. Die-away is initially very rapid because protein is lost from the pool as a result of transfer to extravascular compartments as well as because of endogenous catabolism. Later, when the labelled protein has entered the various compartments, the die-away curve assumes a straight-line (exponential) decline. The reciprocal of the area under the die-away curve is the fractional catabolic rate of the protein (see text for definition); it is obtained by 'curve peeling', i.e. obtaining the slope and intercept of the terminal exponential of the die-away curve, subtracting the latter from the die-away curve to obtain a new curve and repeating the process. The fractional catabolic rate is obtained from the expression

$$\frac{1}{\dfrac{C_1}{b_1} + \dfrac{C_2}{b_2} + \cdots + \dfrac{C_n}{b_n}}$$

where C_n and b_n are respectively the slope and intercept of the initial and peeled curves.

rate.[35] In more sophisticated metabolic turnover studies, serum die-away curves, urinary excretion data and other relevant information are analysed by complex computer programs which allow the metabolic data to be fitted to pre-selected compartment models. This is called compartmental analysis and provides a way of obtaining additional insight into the metabolic system under study.[6]

Serum protein metabolism in protein-losing enteropathy

When metabolic turnover studies are performed on patients with protein-losing enteropathy, several abnormalities are apparent. Most importantly, the fractional catabolic rate is invariably increased, indicating that protein is lost from the intravascular compartment at an increased rate either because of increased endogenous catabolism or because of excessive loss of intact protein into the gastrointestinal tract or urine.[23, 50] In addition, the synthetic rate is normal or increased, showing that the low protein level is due to a catabolic process rather than a defect in protein synthesis.

Metabolic turnover data obtained from patients with protein-losing enteropathy also indicate that the effect of the protein loss on serum protein concentration depends on the underlying metabolic characteristics of the protein.[41] Thus if the normal rate of catabolism of a particular serum protein is high, the addition of even a considerable extra catabolic pathway leads to only a small fractional change in that protein's total catabolism; however, if the normal rate of catabolism is low, a small additional catabolic pathway leads to a large fractional change in total catabolism. For example, if the normal fractional catabolic rate is low, say 10% of the intravascular pool/day (as it is for albumin) a gastrointestinal loss rate of 10% of the intravascular pool/day gives rise to a doubling of the fractional catabolic rate and, provided there is no increase in protein synthesis, a halving of the serum protein level. In contrast, if the normal fractional catabolic rate is high, say 25% of the intravascular pool/day (as it is for IgA immunoglobulin), a 10% protein-losing enteropathy would lead to only a 25% increase in total catabolism and a corresponding decrease in serum IgA concentration. Thus any level of protein-losing enteropathy will affect most acutely those proteins with relatively low fractional catabolic rates such as albumin and IgG, and even severe protein-losing enteropathy will have little impact on serum proteins with normally rapid rates of catabolism such as IgE.[21]

A second point that emerges from metabolic turnover data is that the loss process in protein-losing enteropathy is a 'bulk loss', i.e. proteins are lost regardless of size, charge or any other physical characteristics. This means that the increase in fractional catabolic rate accounted for by the gastrointestinal loss, expressed as the fraction of the intravascular pool lost/day, is the same for all serum proteins, regardless of their underlying fractional catabolic rate.[22, 41] In this way, protein-losing enteropathy differs from the urinary loss process encountered in the nephrotic syndrome, where proteins of intermediate and small size are more severely affected than larger proteins.

Finally, metabolic turnover studies provide important information on the capacity of the body to increase protein synthesis in the face of PLE. In general, such studies have disclosed that a low protein level per se is not a strong stimulus to protein synthesis and that gastrointestinal tract protein loss is not accompanied by large compensatory increases in the rate with which protein is added to the system.[55]

Measurement of protein-losing enteropathy

PLE can be identified and quantitated by measuring the excretion of circulating protein into the gastrointestinal tract. Since most proteins are digested in the gastrointestinal tract and are not, therefore, quantifiable after excretion, PLE is best measured with a radiolabelled protein labelled with a substance which survives the digestive process, i.e., a substance which is not broken down and/or absorbed. Another requirement for a label that is to be used in the estimation of PLE is that it must not be excreted into the gastrointestinal tract unless it is bound to protein; if this were otherwise, label freed from protein during endogenous catabolism would find its way into the lumen and the protein loss would be overestimated. Finally, it is useful, although not essential, for the label to be attached to the protein in a permanent and non-denaturing fashion; this allows the labelled protein to be used both in metabolic turnover studies such as those described above as well as in measurements of gastrointestinal protein loss.

Over the years a variety of labelled substances have been used to quantitate PLE. Radioiodinated proteins were among the first of such substances and offer the advantage that they are ideal for metabolic turnover studies. However, radioiodine released from protein during digestion within the gastrointestinal tract is readily reabsorbed; in addition, radioiodine released from protein during endogenous catabolism can be excreted into the gastrointestinal tract in a non-protein-bound form. For these reasons, radioiodinated proteins are clearly unsuitable for the measurement of PLE.

A series of other radiolabelled proteins (and non-proteins) have been used to measure PLE including ^{131}I-PVP, ^{59}Fe-dextran, [95]Nb-albumin, [67]Cu-caeruloplasmin, and ^{51}Cr-albumin (or [51]CrCl$_3$).[19, 23, 24, 50, 52] ^{131}I-PVP was the first radiolabelled compound to be successfully used to measure PLE,[19] but it is a non-physiological material which is rapidly cleared from the circulation; in addition, it can be broken down in the gastrointestinal tract and the ^{131}I released can be reabsorbed. [67]Cu-caeruloplasmin is, in many ways, the ideal radiolabelled compound for quantification of PLE;[52] the labelled copper is an integral part of the protein and thus is a non-denaturing label that remains with the protein throughout its biological life. However, [67]Cu-caeruloplasmin has a short chemical half life and is difficult to obtain, limiting its general use. In normal individuals, studies using this protein have shown that the gastrointestinal tract accounts for no more than about 10% of the total catabolism of caeruloplasmin, laying to rest the view that the gastrointestinal tract is normally an important site of degradation of caeruloplasmin and, by extension, other serum proteins.

A labelled material that has found widespread use in quantitating PLE is [51]chromium (^{51}Cr). This was initially, and to some extent still is, delivered to the patient under study as ^{51}Cr-albumin.[50] However, ^{51}Cr is not irreversibly bound to albumin and once in the circulation can dissociate from albumin and become attached to other serum proteins, particularly transferrin. Although this undermines the use of ^{51}Cr-albumin as a method of measuring albumin metabolism (^{51}Cr-albumin has a much shorter apparent half life than ^{125}I-albumin), it does not affect measurement of PLE because ^{51}Cr is excreted into the gastrointestinal tract only when it is attached to a serum protein. In addition, provided the excreted labelled protein has the same specific activity as the circulating labelled protein, the amount of ^{51}Cr excreted will reflect a similar fractional excretion rate (clearance) regardless of the protein to which it is attached. The recognition that the ^{51}Cr label in ^{51}Cr-albumin is dispersed to many proteins in vivo without compromise of its ability to measure PLE has led to the use of the more widely available [51]CrCl$_3$,[45] a ^{51}Cr preparation which, following intravenous injection, labels many proteins directly rather than residing initially with albumin. This material provides data equivalent to that obtained with ^{51}Cr-albumin (or with other labelled materials) thereby verifying the fact that a label used to measure PLE does not have to be attached to only one protein throughout the entire study. Finally, it should be noted that either ^{51}Cr-albumin or [51]CrCl$_3$ can be injected simultaneously with radioiodinated proteins to obtain a simultaneous measurement of protein metabolism and gastrointestinal tract protein loss because ^{51}Cr and ^{125}I have widely separate energy peaks which can be counted using appropriate detection devices in the presence of one another. Such dual isotope studies provide precise data on the extent to which an increase in protein catabolism is accounted for by protein-losing enteropathy.

There are two main methods of using ^{51}Cr-labelled proteins to quantitate PLE. In the first and simpler method, ^{51}Cr is injected, either as ^{51}Cr-albumin or as $^{51}CrCl_3$, and stool samples are collected for four days to determine the percentage of the injected dose excreted in that time. In normal individuals this four-day excretion value does not exceed 0.7% of the injected dose. This method provides a reliable 'yes or no' answer to the question of whether or not PLE is present, but does not provide a metabolically meaningful estimate of protein loss into the gastrointestinal tract. In the second and more quantitative method, ^{51}Cr clearance into the GI tract is measured in a manner similar to the determination of creatinine clearance. Clearance is calculated from the amount of ^{51}Cr excreted over a given period of time divided by the average number of counts in the serum during this period. In practice, the amount of ^{51}Cr excreted is obtained from the daily faecal excretion value of ^{51}Cr and the number of counts is obtained from the serum ^{51}Cr value obtained during the previous day, thus assuming a 24-hour delay in faecal excretion. A more exact measurement of clearance is obtained by pooling faecal excretion values over several days and dividing this value by the average serum value during this time (i.e. the reciprocal of the area under the ^{51}Cr die-away curve), thus avoiding errors introduced by faecal excretion delays. The clearance value is a measure of the volume of serum cleared into the gastrointestinal tract/unit time; by dividing this value by the plasma volume one obtains the fraction of the intravascular compartment cleared into the gastrointestinal tract/unit time. In normal individuals this value does not exceed 2%/day (Figure 8.98).

Recently, a new approach to the measurement of PLE has been developed. This involves the use of a non-labelled protein, α_1-antitrypsin, which is not broken down in the gastrointestinal tract (except in the stomach) so that its appearance in the stool is a measure of PLE.[17] When protein-losing enteropathy was measured in the same patient population using both α_1-antitrypsin and ^{51}Cr-labelled proteins, excel-

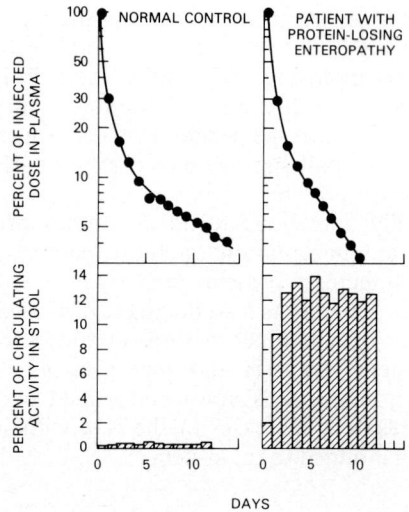

Fig. 8.98 ^{51}Cr-albumin study. The serum die-away curve of ^{51}Cr-albumin in a normal individual (left panel) and a patient with protein-losing enteropathy (right panel) is shown. This die-away is more rapid than that of ^{125}I-albumin even in a normal individual because the ^{51}Cr label does not remain with albumin but shifts to other, more rapidly degraded, proteins. Nevertheless, ^{51}Cr-albumin provides accurate data on protein loss into the GI tract (see text). Also shown is stool excretion data (expressed as a fractional loss rate); whereas ^{51}Cr excretion is almost non-existent in the normal control, it is quite considerable in the patient.

lent agreement in the clearance values was obtained. The normal clearance value for ^{51}Cr-albumin of 40 ml/day was lower than the normal clearance value for α_1-antitrypsin of 13 ml/day; this may be due to the fact that some α_1-antitrypsin is degraded in the stomach. The use of α_1-antitrypsin to measure PLE has some advantages over the use of ^{51}Cr-protein in that one avoids the use of a radioactive material and the need for specialized counting equipment. On the other hand, the ^{51}Cr-protein method may be easier to perform since one does not need to set up a protein quantification assay.

Pathological mechanisms responsible for protein-losing enteropathy

PLE has been found in numerous gastrointestinal and systemic diseases, and hypoproteinaemia occurring in the context of mucosal disease of the gastrointestinal tract may be assumed to be at least partially due to this abnormality. The various gastrointestinal diseases associated with PLE fall into several broad categories (Table 8.51). The first such category, dealt with at greater length below, comprises those disorders which lead to obstruction of

Table 8.51 Classification of diseases producing protein-losing enteropathy.

Disorders of intestinal lymphatics
 Idiopathic intestinal lymphangiectasia:
  Familial
  Sporadic
 Secondary intestinal lymphangiectasia due to:
  Cardiac disease (see Table 8.52)
  Inflammatory disease resembling lupus erythematosus
  Non-specific inflammatory disease, Crohn's disease
  Blockage of lymphatics by lipid filled macrophages, Whipple's disease, abetalipoproteinemia
  Blockage of lymphatics by neoplastic disease
  Specific infection involving mesenteric lymphatics, tuberculous peritonitis
  Non-specific or undefined infection involving mesenteric lymphatics, retroperitoneal fibrosis

Inflammatory and/or ulcerative diseases of the gastrointestinal mucosa
 Inflammatory bowel disease
 Specific infections of the GI tract
  Parasitic infections: roundworm, hookworm, amoebae
  Bacterial infections: Shigella
  Viral infections: GI viruses associated with diarrhoea, measles
  Fungal infections: histoplasmosis
 Non-specific infections of the GI tract associated with:
  Blind loop syndrome, stenotic and obstructive lesions, diverticula
  Immunodeficiency states especially common variable hypogammaglobulinaemia
 Ulcerative diseases
  Ulcerative gastritis, Zollinger–Ellison syndrome
  Carcinomas of oesophagus, stomach, small and large bowel
  Polypoid lesions, villous adenoma, Cronkhite–Canada syndrome
 Sprue syndromes
  Gluten-sensitive enteropathy (coeliac disease)
  Dermatitis herpetiformis
  Tropical sprue
  Ulcerative jejunitis (non-granulomatous jejunitis)
  Kwashiorkor
 Inflammation or ulceration caused by drug or physical agent
  Pseudomembranous colitis
  Chronic laxative ingestion
  Radiation enteritis
  Retained foreign body (intestinal tube)
 Vascular diseases of the bowel
  Vasculo-occlusive diseases, ischaemic bowel disease, diabetes mellitus
  Haemangiomas, angiomas
  Malrotation of the bowel
 Collagen–vascular diseases
  Henoch–Schönlein purpura
  Sjogren's syndrome
  Scleroderma
  Rheumatoid arthritis

Diseases associated with mediator-release and changes in vascular permeability
 Allergic gastroenteropathy, eosinophilic gastroenteritis
 Systemic mastocytosis
 Angioneurotic oedema
 Menetrier's disease (giant hypertrophy of the gastric rugae)
 Carcinoid syndrome

intestinal lymphatics. This includes congenital or idiopathic lymphatic abnormalities as well as lymphatic obstruction secondary to a large number of widely different pathological processes. It is in this category that one finds the most severe protein-losing states.

A second category of diseases associated with PLE are the inflammatory diseases of the gastrointestinal tract. This includes the various ulcerative diseases as well as the diseases in which the bowel wall contains an inflammatory infiltrate such as gluten-sensitive enteropathy, immunodeficiency states, specific infections of the bowel, and gastrointestinal damage caused by radiation or toxins. In addition, anatomical defects such as diverticulosis, stenotic lesions, fistulas, polyps, adenomas, blind loops and neoplasms also lead to PLE through an inflammatory pathway. The mechanism of PLE in inflammation of the bowel is not precisely defined; it seems reasonable to suggest, however, that it is due to loss of extracellular or inflammatory fluid that accumulates at the site of inflammation. The extent of protein loss in this category of PLE is generally mild and for this reason the PLE in these conditions is usually an incidental finding.

A final group of diseases characterized by protein-losing enteropathy are those associated with local release of mediators which lead to permeability changes and the outpouring of protein-rich fluid. The most well documented disease in this category is allergic gastroenteropathy, in which antigen–antibody interactions involving the IgE system lead to release of histamine and other substances which alter vascular permeability. This category also includes the PLE associated with Menetrier's disease where there again is some evidence for local release of mediators which alter vascular permeability.

All three mechanisms of PLE given above lead to accumulation of fluid (of vascular or lymphatic origin) in the interstitium of the mucosa. Munro has shown, in experimental PLE induced by reducing agents, that such fluid finds its way into the gastrointestinal lumen by passing between epithelial cells through the tight junctions rather than through the epithelial cells themselves. This fits well with the fact that PLE can occur when epithelial cells are intact.[32]

GASTROINTESTINAL DISEASES ASSOCIATED WITH PROTEIN-LOSING ENTEROPATHY

Gluten-sensitive enteropathy (coeliac disease)

Mild to moderate hypoalbuminaemia is a not infrequent accompaniment of gluten-sensitive enteropathy, particularly in adult patients with moderate to severe villous atrophy.[10] Studies of albumin metabolism in such patients frequently reveal abnormally low albumin synthesis rates, which is probably secondary to malabsorption of amino acids; this defect in synthesis appears to be mainly responsible for the low albumin level. Patients also have mild to moderate gastrointestinal protein loss as measured with $^{51}CrCl_3$; however, this does not directly correlate with the presence of hypoalbuminaemia, except when the latter is severe. Thus PLE probably plays only a minor role, if any, in causing the hypoalbuminaemia of gluten-sensitive enteropathy.

Although not proven, the PLE found in coeliac disease is probably inflammatory in origin due to infiltration of the lamina propria with inflammatory cells and the consequent release of substances which change mucosal

vascular permeability sufficiently to allow protein-rich fluid to leak into the lumen.

Malignancy

Hypoalbuminaemia is a frequent finding in all forms of malignancy and has a tendency to get worse as the neoplastic disease progresses.[49] In the majority of instances this is due to a defect in hepatic synthesis of albumin, even in those cancer patients without obvious liver disease or malabsorption, but can also be due to PLE. It can occur in patients harbouring a variety of tumours of the gastrointestinal tract or in patients with widespread metastatic disease. Thus, PLE has been demonstrated in oesophageal, gastric and pancreatic carcinomas, and in various polyposis syndromes; in addition, it has been observed in carcinoid syndrome, lymphomas, myelomas associated with amyloidosis of the bowel, and various metastatic carcinomas. PLE in most patients with malignancy is due to inflammation and ulceration of the bowel accompanied by loss of protein-rich exudate. In addition, disordered lymphatic channels can also cause PLE, particularly in patients with lymphomas, patients subjected to abdominal irradiation, and in patients with neoplasms associated with right heart failure (carcinoid syndrome).

Inflammatory bowel disease

Inflammatory bowel disease (ulcerative colitis and Crohn's disease), particularly when extensive, is frequently associated with hypoproteinaemia and hypoalbuminaemia. Albumin values in the 2.5–3.0 g/dl range are not uncommon and values below 2.0 g/dl are occasionally seen.[4, 40] Steinfeld et al.[40] showed that many patients with inflammatory bowel disease had normal or increased albumin synthesis values but decreased albumin survival (increased albumin fractional catabolic rates) associated with loss of ^{13}I-PVP into the stool. They thus concluded that the hypoalbuminaemia may be largely due to protein-losing enteropathy. Subsequently it was shown that clearance of ^{51}Cr-albumin (or $^{51}CrCl_3$) correlated better with the extent of radiological abnormalities than absorptive studies such as fat and D-xylose absorption.[4]

There are probably several causes of PLE in inflammatory bowel disease. Most importantly, the mucosa is ulcerated and inflamed and this, as discussed above, leads to exudation of protein-rich fluid into the lumen. In addition, lymphatic blockage can occur in Crohn's disease and therefore leakage of lymphatic fluid may contribute to the PLE.

Immunodeficiency states

In patients with immunodeficiency and associated gastrointestinal disease (see p. 564), hypoalbuminaemia and protein-losing enteropathy is a frequent finding.[47] However, in most cases, the PLE is not a prominent abnormality and the hypoalbuminaemia observed may be due to a defect in albumin synthesis as well as PLE. The mechanism of PLE is uncertain, although it seems reasonable to suggest that it is due to a low grade mucosal inflammatory process attributable to bacterial overgrowth.

Ménétrier's disease

Ménétrier's disease (giant hypertrophy of the gastric rugae, giant rugal hypertrophy) is a relatively uncommon abnormality of the gastric mucosa (see p. 238). As mentioned earlier, it was the first disease in which PLE was clearly demonstrated.[9] Hypoalbuminaemia occurs in about 70% of patients with Ménétrier's disease and, in all cases studied, this has been shown to be due to increased fractional catabolic rate of albumin.[26] The protein is lost chiefly, if not exclusively, into the stomach, so that strictly speaking Ménétrier's disease is a protein-losing gastropathy rather than a protein-losing gastroenteropathy.

Among the factors that may be responsible for this abnormality, release of vasoactive substances in the gastric mucosa is the best substantiated. Protein loss into the stomach was dramatically reduced in one patient with Ménétrier's disease by atropine and in another patient, by hexamethonium bromide.[22] Additionally, one group of investigators have noted reduced PLE in patients with Ménétrier's disease following administration of tranexamic acid, a substance said to act on plasminogen activators and thus indirectly on substances capable of stimulating kinin release.[30] The fact that PLE in Ménétrier's disease can be treated in this way places this form of PLE within the category of PLE-producing states due to changes in vascular permeability.

Allergic gastroenteropathy

Allergic gastroenteropathy is characterized by diffuse eosinophilia of the gastric mucosa associated with diarrhoea, abdominal pain and malabsorption (see p. 590). In addition, these gastrointestinal manifestations are associated with allergic symptoms and, at times, peripheral oedema.

That allergic mechanisms underlie allergic gastroenteropathy is supported by the fact that patients have high serum IgE levels and an increased number of IgE cells in the lamina propria of the mucosa. Also the gastrointestinal symptoms are usually accompanied by other allergic symptoms such as asthma, allergic rhinitis and eczema. However, only in occasional cases can a single allergen (most often milk protein) be identified; in most cases, patients seem to be sensitive to most foods and treatment with elimination diets are ineffective. This may be explained by the observation made in experimental animals that oral sensitization with one antigen can lead to sensitization to other antigens because of allergy-induced changes in mucosal permeability.

Patients with allergic gastroenteropathy are, in general, young individuals who display a somewhat variable clinical picture, ranging from diarrhoea, abdominal pain and malabsorption to peripheral oedema and anaemia. In the latter case, protein-losing enteropathy rather than malabsorption is a major pathological feature. This clinical spectrum is reflected in the small intestinal findings which can show a normal villous structure or mild to moderate villous atrophy reminiscent of gluten-sensitive enteropathy. In both instances, eosinophilic infiltration is prominent and gastric antrum biopsy shows epithelial cell damage and inflammation. The pathophysiological factors which determine these varying disease patterns are unknown. Whatever the clinical findings, most patients with allergic gastroenteropathy have positive ^{51}Cr-albumin tests and shortened survival of albumin associated with normal albumin synthesis rates.[27, 51] The protein-losing enteropathy thus revealed explains the immunoglobulin levels which, with the exception of IgE, are uniformly low.

The mechanism of protein-losing enteropathy in allergic gastroenteropathy is not precisely defined. Nevertheless, it is quite likely to be related to interactions between allergen and IgE bound to mast cells and subsequent release of vasoactive substances including histamine. Davenport has shown that chemically-induced histamine release caused by exposure of gastric mucosa to sulphydryl reagents is associated with vascular permeability changes and protein exudation into the lumen.[11] Thus, allergic sensitization of the mucosal surface probably leads to protein-losing enteropathy because of mediator release and subsequent changes in vascular permeability.

Intestinal lymphangiectasia

Intestinal lymphangiectasia (IL) is a distinctive and physiologically informative abnormality whose manifold clinical features have their origin in a central defect in the patency of the intestinal lymphatics. The protein-losing enteropathy of IL is distinguished in two ways: first, the protein loss is usually severe and therefore determines some of the most important symptoms; second, the protein loss is accompanied by lymphocyte loss and patients become lymphocytopenic and manifest immunodeficiency.

Historically, IL was recognized first by Waldmann et al.,[53] who showed that certain patients with idiopathic hypoalbuminaemia had a protein-losing enteropathy associated with dilated and presumably blocked intestinal mucosal lymphatics. From the first, it was recognized that IL could occur as a congenital and/or familial condition, as a variant of a generalized lymphatic abnormality (idiopathic lymphoedema). Indeed, many individuals with IL show obvious evidence of a peripheral lymphatic disorder. As time went on, however, it became apparent that IL could also occur as a secondary manifestation of a variety of diseases affecting the intestinal lymphatics. This has led to the current view that IL is either of unknown aetiology (primary or idiopathic IL) or is a syndrome complicating an array of diseases which affect the lymphatic system (secondary IL). It is among the cases with secondary IL that one can expect to achieve the most significant therapeutic effects.

The lymphatic abnormalities
Primary (idiopathic) IL, whether it be a genetic or an acquired defect, appears to be part of a spectrum of abnormalities of lymphatic development. At one end of the spectrum is idiopathic lymphoedema (including Milroy's disease) which is characterized by lymphatic abnormalities which affect mainly (if not exclusively) the extremities of the body.[29] Patients with idiopathic lymphoedema may, in fact, have disordered intestinal lymphatics: some 10–20% of such patients have abnormal ^{51}Cr-albumin tests.[15] However, by definition the intestinal abnormality is not clinically significant, otherwise the disease would be termed IL (see below). At the other end of the spectrum are patients with IL who have no peripheral lymphatic abnormalities and whose disease is limited to the intestine; such patients are similar to, and must be distinguished from, patients with secondary IL. Finally, an intermediate group exists with both peripheral and intestinal abnormalities; patients in this group are usually placed in the IL category since the intestinal abnormalities usually dominate the clinical picture.

The fundamental defect or group of defects leading to these various forms of primary lymphatic disease is unknown. Logically, one can postulate a defect of the lymphatic endothelium or the lymphatic supporting structures; however, no morphological or biochemical evidence indicating the presence of such a defect has been found. In one patient studied in our laboratories, a defect in fibroblast monolayer formation was observed, suggesting that in this patient cell–cell surface interactions are defective. Additional studies of this kind will be necessary to obtain an understanding of primary IL at a molecular level.

The cause of lymphatic blockage in secondary IL depends strictly on the nature of the primary disease present. Foremost among the latter are the reversible forms of IL, including systemic inflammatory disease resembling lupus erythematosus and various right-sided cardiac diseases. Inflammatory diseases probably lead to IL by causing inflammation and obstruction of the mesenteric lymphatic channels; however, this remains to be proven. Inflammatory disease may be responsible for certain cases of idiopathic IL since low grade lymphatic inflammation could well be clinically silent during an early phase and become manifest as lymphatic obstruction during a late fibrotic phase. This possibility finds some support in the occurrence of occasional cases of transient IL and IL due to frank mesenteric inflammation.[5, 36]

Cardiac diseases can lead to IL by causing restriction of lymphatic drainage into the venous system. In this instance the lymphatics are functionally rather than physically obstructed, accounting for the fact that IL secondary to cardiac disease can usually be reversed with correction of the cardiac lesion.

Other causes of secondary IL are the intestinal conditions marked by tissue infiltration which cause lymphatic obstruction as an incidental and sometimes inapparent by-product. These diseases include infections with known agents such as bacteria, fungi or parasites, nonspecific inflammations such as Crohn's disease, and Whipple's disease and hypolipoproteinaemia in which there is lymphatic obstruction by lipophages. Finally, IL can be secondary to neoplastic obstruction.

Clinical manifestations and course
IL is generally a disease of early life, with onset of symptoms occurring in the great majority of cases before the age of 30; when IL does occur later in life it is likely to be secondary to a cardiac, inflammatory or neoplastic condition.

In early-onset disease (i.e. during the neonatal period or during the first few months of life), IL can manifest as a severe illness characterized by massive oedema, diarrhoea, malabsorption and overwhelming infection; such patients usually die early. Next most devastating is the IL of childhood which affects growth, sexual development and emotional maturation. Finally, there is the most common pattern of disease, with onset in adolescence or early adulthood, in which chronic difficulties with oedema, excessive fatigue and various abdominal symptoms dominate the picture. Even in primary (idiopathic) IL, most affected individuals are without similarly affected family members. In an occasional case, however, a familial disease is evident, although never in a clearly definable genetic pattern.

The major symptom of IL is oedema. This may be asymmetrical, indicative of peripheral lymphatic abnormalities (Figure 8.99), or may be generalized, in which case it arises from hypo-albuminaemia and reduced tissue oncotic pressure. Fluid in the abdominal (or pleural) cavity is quite common (occurring in about 50% of patients) and is characteristically of a chylous nature arising from spillage of lymphatic fluid. In long-standing disease, such chylous fluid accumulation can give rise to peritoneal fibrosis and loculation of intestinal loops (intestinal 'cocooning'). Other manifestations related to fluid accumulation are macular oedema (causing reversible visual difficulties) and chronic stasis dermatitis which is sometimes associated with peripheral ulcer formation.

Gastrointestinal symptoms are quite frequent in IL but, particularly in later-onset disease, are usually mild. Diarrhoea is seen in only a minority of IL patients as a whole, but may be both more common and more severe in young children with the disease.[46] Clinically significant steatorrhoea is also relatively uncommon and tends to be more severe in those cases characterized by massive protein-losing enteropathy since both are attributable to blocked intestinal lymphatics. The cause of the steatorrhoea probably is not solely reduced lymphatic uptake of fat, since steatorrhoea may persist even when fat is completely removed from the diet; the latter argues for the presence of a 'fat-losing' enteropathy.[31]

Abdominal pain occurs in perhaps 15% of patients. Its cause is poorly understood, although it may be related to disturbances in intestinal motility. In some cases it may suggest the presence of intestinal obstruction; this consequence of intestinal fibrosis has been occasionally observed. Other symptoms attributable to gastrointestinal dysfunction include tetany secondary to hypocalcaemia, growth retardation due to malabsorption and recurrent thrombotic episodes, which may be due to intestinal loss of antithrombotic serum factors.[33]

As discussed later, patients with IL frequently, if not always, have an immunodeficiency state and may therefore have manifestations attributable to inadequate immune responses. These include persistent and generalized warts, presumably due to viral infection, infection with atypical mycobacteria, and various signs and symptoms arising from the presence of malignant disease.

Finally, another symptom of IL may occur, which is quite important from the patient's point of view, namely chronic fatigue. This is probably related to the huge intestinal fluid losses sometimes present in IL and may be severe enough to preclude a normal level of activity.

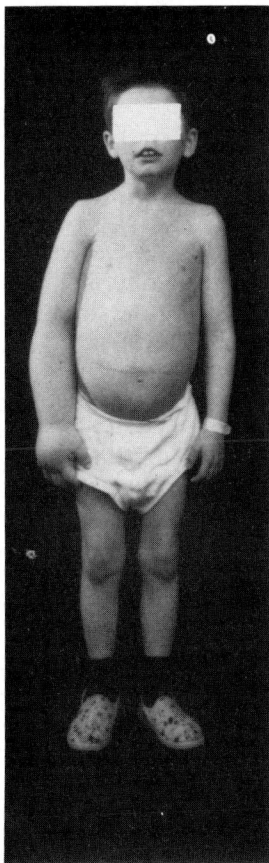

Fig. 8.99 An IL patient with asymmetrical oedema characteristic of fluid accumulation occurring as a result of a lymphatic abnormality. This patient also has abdominal distension due to the presence of chylous ascites.

The physical examination in primary IL is dominated by evidence of lymphatic abnormalities. This includes the characteristic physical finding of IL – asymmetrical oedema which is not necessarily dependent and which is resistant to diuretics (Figure 8.99). Such oedema in severe and chronic cases may be associated with lower limb stasis dermatitis, superficial skin weeping and ulceration, and local skin infection. Lymphatic blockage may also lead to peritoneal or pleural fluid accumulations; these can be quite massive and lead to respiratory difficulties. The peritoneal fluid is not associated with hepatomegaly or other evidence of liver disease. Finally, lymphatic abnormalities may also be associated with the occurrence of cutaneous or even intra-abdominal lymphangiomas.

The physical examination in secondary IL differs from that in the primary disease in that the fluid accumulation, due solely to the intestinal lymphatic dysfunction and protein-losing enteropathy, is uniform and dependent. In addition, patients may show evidence of an underlying abnormality, e.g. jugular venous distension in constrictive pericarditis, skin rash in systemic lupus erythematosus or pigmentation in Whipple's disease.

Laboratory abnormalities in IL are due chiefly to the protein-losing enteropathy or malabsorption that is present. Patients have markedly decreased total serum protein levels (the mean level in a group of our patients was 3.5 g/dl, the normal range being 6.0–8.0 g/dl) which, in turn, is due to low serum albumin levels (mean level of 1.8 g/dl, the normal range being 3.1–4.5 g/dl) and to low serum IgG levels (mean level of 4.5 ± 2.1 mg/ml, mean level in controls being 12.1 ± 2.7 mg/ml). The decrease in both albumin and IgG levels in IL is attributable to the fact that both of these are long-lived proteins which are most profoundly affected by a bulk loss process such as protein-losing enteropathy. The concentrations of serum proteins with intermediate half lives, such as IgA, IgM and transferrin, are only moderately decreased in IL, and the concentrations of proteins with short half lives, such as IgE and protein hormones, are virtually normal in IL.

The majority of patients have increased stool fat excretion, but in only a quarter of patients is fat excretion greater than 10% of ingested fat. This is in keeping with the observation, mentioned above, that steatorrhoea is rather uncommon in IL. Estimates of carbohydrate absorption in IL such as the D-xylose absorption test tend to be normal; this is not surprising as

intestinal epithelial cells in IL are morphologically intact. Finally, in the majority of IL patients, although total calcium levels are low (owing to low protein levels) ionized calcium levels are normal except in those patients with significant malabsorption, when ionized calcium levels are depressed.

Most patients with IL are not anaemic; on the contrary, many have a high haematocrit due to a reduced intravascular volume (due in turn to low oncotic pressure). However, for reasons that are not clear, an occasional patient with hypochromic anaemia associated with low serum iron is seen. In addition, patients with severe anaemia due to leakage of blood into the lymphatic system have been observed; this is thought to be due to abnormal connections between venous and lymphatic systems.[12]

Radiographic, lymphangiographic and endoscopic studies

Radiographic studies in IL show abnormalities that are found in other malabsorption states and are therefore not diagnostic of IL. In the X-ray study of a large IL group conducted at our hospital, 15 out of 20 patients showed abnormalities of various kinds, whereas 5 out of 20 patients showed no abnormalities.[38] Major abnormal features included enlargement of intestinal folds presumably due to oedema of the bowel wall (characteristically this was seen in the ileal region leading to so-called 'jejunization' of the ileum), dilution of the barium column unassociated with significant dilatation of bowel lumen, and mucosal nodularity and punctate radiolucencies attributable to lymphatic dilatation. In contrast to small bowel radiographs, X-ray studies of the oesophagus, stomach, duodenal bulb and colon were generally normal.

Lymphangiographic studies in IL have revealed a variety of abnormalities rather than one consistent or pathognomonic change.[7, 38] In patients with primary IL and asymmetrical oedema, one commonly finds hypoplastic or varicose peripheral lymphatics which may be accompanied by dermal back-flow. This finding is attributable to lymphatic obstruction and is also observed in idiopathic lymphoedema. In the abdominal area lymphatic blockage at a particular level (usually at the level of the cysterna chyli), tortuous lymphatic channels, absence of abdominal lymph nodes and obstruction or even absence of the thoracic duct may be seen. In occasional cases one may observe reflux of contrast material into the mesenteric lymphatics and entry of contrast material into the small bowel or into the peritoneal cavity; this finding usually signifies severe leakage of lymph fluid into the bowel lumen or even the presence of a frank lymphatico-duodenal fistula.[18] In patients with IL secondary to cardiac disease a somewhat different picture is seen; one may observe a dilated, tortuous thoracic duct, probably due to obstruction at the point of entry of the duct into the subclavian vein.

Endoscopic findings in IL are consistent with the morphological lesion present. Thus, on the jejunal surface one finds scattered white spots, which probably represent dilated lymphatics, white, swollen villi, and prominent intestinal folds. In addition, chylous fluid may be present.[3]

Morphological findings

Gross examination of the small intestine in IL, either at operation or at autopsy, reveals an oedematous bowel wall with prominent mucosal folds. The bowel may also have a brownish coloration because of lipofuscin pigment infiltration. Finally, dilated lymphatics may be seen on the serosal surface and these may be associated with yellow nodules representing local accumulations of fat-filled macrophages.

Light microscopic examination of IL intestinal tissue discloses dilated intestinal lymphatics, the virtually unique feature of the disease (Figure 8.100). These abnormal lymphatics are most in evidence at the tips of villi, but are often present in the submucosa as well. They may contain lymphocytes, foamy macrophages or proteinaceous material representing lymph fluid precipitated during tissue fixation. Generally speaking the dilated lymphatics are intact, thereby making it unlikely that protein leakage occurs because of frank rupture of the lymphatics. Finally, the abnormal lymphatics may have a patchy distribution, and it is clear that in many cases certain segments of bowel are much more heavily involved than others. Thus, failure to find dilated intestinal lymphatics in duodenal or jejunal biopsy specimens does not rule out the diagnosis of IL.

The villi have a normal length, but may appear clubbed because of the dilated lymphatics at their tips. On light microscopic examination, the epithelial cells have a normal morphology and there is generally no increase in lamina propria mononuclear cells. (One exception to this is IL secondary to Whipple's disease, where macrophage infiltration accompanies the lymphangiectasia.) The lack of epithelial cell abnormalities and mononuclear cell infiltration in IL generally distinguishes this disease from gluten-sensitive enteropathy and other malabsorptive states due to epithelial cell injury. Mesenteric nodes and other lymph nodes in IL show marked lymphocyte depletion (Figure 8.101), correlating well with the chronic and massive lymphocyte loss associated with the disease.

On electron microscopic examination of IL tissue one finds that the endothelial cells forming the walls of the dilated lymphatics have closed intracellular junctions and prominent intracellular filaments.[14] In addition, the lymphatic endothelium has a prominent basal

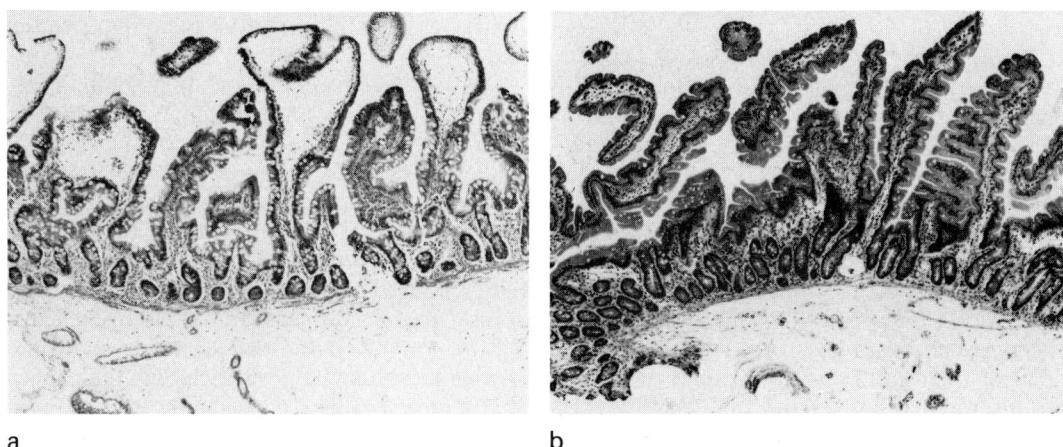

a   b

Fig. 8.100 Jejunal biopsies taken from a patient with intestinal lymphangiectasia due to constrictive pericarditis. (a) The typical lymphatic dilatation can be seen at the villous tips with lymphocytes visible in the dilated channels. (b) The normal histological picture obtained after cardiac surgery which resulted in resolution of the cardiac constriction and the intestinal lymphangiectasia.

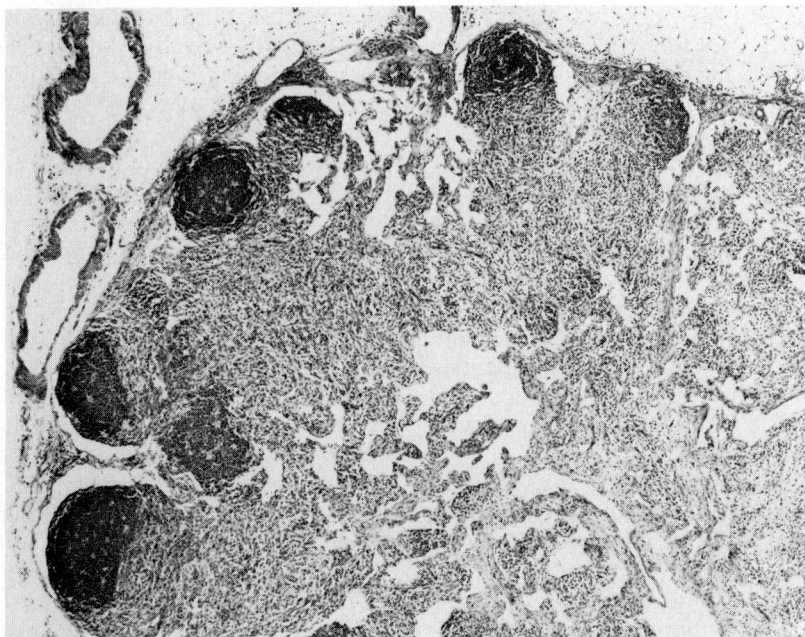

Fig. 8.101 Mesenteric lymph node obtained from a patient with intestinal lymphangiectasia. The B cell areas (germinal centres) have a normal cellularity whereas T cell areas (paracortical areas) are depleted of lymphocytes. This lymphoid histology indicates that the lymphocyte loss into the gastrointestinal tract drains the lymphoid tissue pool as well as the circulating pool of T cells.

lamina with increased numbers of supporting cells and collagen fibres. All this probably represents a secondary response to increased intralymphatic pressure. Another electron microscopic finding is the presence of lipid droplets (chylomicrons) at the base of absorptive cells, within the lymphatics and in the extracellular areas of the lamina propria. This is attributable to an 'exit-block' of absorbed lipid similar to that seen in abetalipoproteinaemia.

Protein-losing enteropathy associated with IL
Just as obstructed lymphatics are the major anatomical abnormality in IL, protein-losing enteropathy resulting from this lesion is the main physiological abnormality.

Studies of protein-losing enteropathy in our patients with IL conducted with ^{51}Cr-albumin showed that they excrete into the gastrointestinal tract 5–30% of the administered dose of ^{51}Cr within four days of its injection (normal four-day excretion is less than 1%) and 'clear' 5–40% of their intravascular volume into the gastrointestinal tract/day (normal loss by this route is less than 2%/day). Not surprisingly, study of IL patients with ^{125}I-labelled serum proteins (such as ^{125}I-albumin) discloses high fractional catabolic rates, which is the pathophysiological basis of the low levels of serum

proteins. The metabolic data described above indicate that the intestinal loss of protein in IL is both constant and, in many cases, massive, so that it cannot be treated by plasma infusions.

Immunological abnormalities
The loss process in IL is unique in that it includes cellular elements present in lymphatic fluid as well as the fluid itself. IL is therefore accompanied by an immunodeficiency which is marked by abnormalities of cellular immunity.[41]

Patients with IL almost invariably have a lymphocytopenia (mean count in our patients was 710 ± 34 cells/mm^3, the normal mean count being 2500 ± 600 cells/mm^3) and examination of lymphoid tissues shows lymphoid depletion, particularly of T cell areas (Figure 8.101). Also in vitro T cell responses of these patients are markedly reduced; this includes responses to mitogens, specific antigens and to allogeneic cells (HLA antigens). In vivo T cell responses of patients are also reduced, including the capacity to manifest delayed reactions to standard 'delayed' skin test materials or to reject skin allografts; the latter abnormality is particularly striking in that even second set grafts are not rejected (Figure 8.102).

The cells most at risk for loss in IL are the

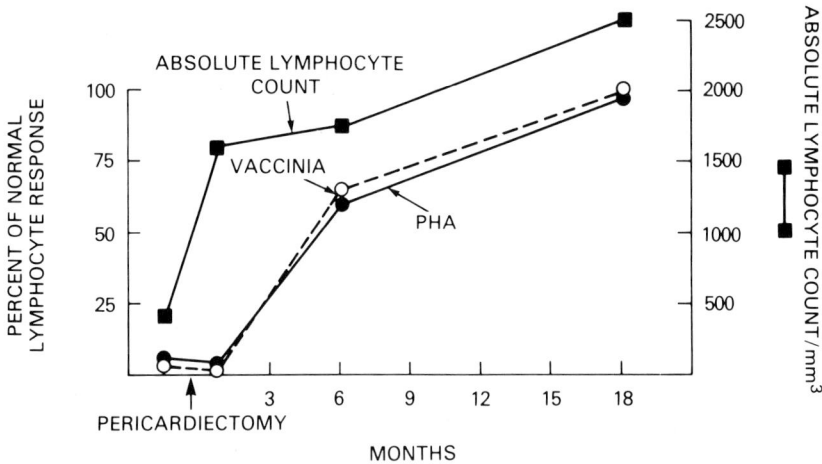

Fig. 8.102 Graph of recovery of cellular immune function after pericardiectomy in a patient with secondary intestinal lymphangiectasia due to constrictive pericarditis. It should be noted that lymphocyte levels and immune function return to normal rather slowly. (PHA = phytohaemagglutinin.)

long-lived cells which constantly recirculate through the lymphatic and vascular circulations.[54] These cells are, for the most part, T cells, and it is therefore not surprising that it is this lymphocyte subpopulation (rather than B cells) which is diminished in IL. The selective reduction of recirculating T cells explains the fact that in vitro proliferative responses are reduced in IL, since it is this population that contains the responsive cells. There is good evidence that IL patients have no intrinsic abnormality of lymphocyte production, i.e. the cellular immunodeficiency is entirely explained by the gastrointestinal loss. In support of this is the fact that treatment of secondary forms of IL which have no effect on the lymphoid system per se can nevertheless reverse the immunological abnormality.

Whereas the intestinal loss in IL has a major effect on cellular immunity, its effect on humoral immunity is relatively minor. Thus, in a large group of our patients, mean IgG levels were about 30% of normal levels and IgA and IgM levels were about 50% of normal. Such reductions are not usually low enough to result in an increased frequency of infections due to hypogammaglobulinaemia. Measurements of specific antibody responses in IL indicate that, while patients as a group have tangibly reduced responses, such responses are still substantial.

The question naturally arises as to whether or not patients are more susceptible to infection. Except perhaps for the very young (who have not had time to develop their immune systems), patients are not usually subject to excessive infections, although isolated instances of chronic infection with low-grade pathogens are encountered from time to time. This clinical picture reflects the fact that the immunodeficiency of IL is a partial abnormality, affecting only one part of the immune system.

Inflammatory IL

In recent years a secondary IL due to underlying inflammatory disease has been noted.[16] This form of IL occurs mainly in young women and is marked by oedema, hypoalbuminaemia and protein-losing enteropathy; in addition, in most cases, dilated lymphatics are seen on intestinal biopsy and some patients have chylous ascites. These patients can be distinguished from other patients with IL by the fact that they have elevated sedimentation rates, normal or even elevated immunoglobulin levels and, in many instances, positive serological tests for systemic lupus erythematosus (SLE). In addition, patients may have one or more clinical features normally associated with SLE such as carditis, glomerulonephritis, arthritis or skin rash. On the basis of this clinical picture, it is reasonable to suggest that the cause of inflammatory IL is blockage of critical lymphatic outflow channels serving the intestines by inflammation which is basically autoimmune in nature.

The importance of recognizing that inflammatory IL is an entity lies in the fact that this form of IL can often be successfully treated with steroids. Interestingly, such therapy not only leads to resolution of the extraintestinal features of the disease, but also the IL.

Table 8.52 Cardiac abnormalities associated with second-ary intestinal lymphangiectasia.

Constrictive pericarditis
  Idiopathic
  Secondary to lupus erythematosus
  Secondary to radiation

Congenital cardiac abnormalities
  Atrial septal defect (ASD)
  Lutembacher's syndrome (ASD, mitral stenosis)
  Noonan syndrome (ASD, pulmonary stenosis, cleft
  mitral valve)
  Pulmonary stenosis

Cardiomyopathy
  Familial
  Idiopathic, associated with generalized myopathy

Rheumatic heart disease
  Tricuspid regurgitation
  Mitral regurgitation

Metabolic/toxic cardiac disease
  Myxoedema
  Carcinoid syndrome

Post-surgical cardiac syndromes
  Glenn shunt (vena cava–right pulmonary artery shunt)
  Mustard procedure for transposition of the great
  vessels

IL due to cardiac abnormalities

Not long after the initial patients with primary (idiopathic) IL were described, it became apparent that IL could also occur as a secondary manifestation of certain forms of cardiac disease.[13] IL resulting from cardiac disease was first seen in patients with constrictive pericarditis, and indeed this condition remains the most frequent cardiac cause of dilated intestinal lymphatics and PLE. However, it is now recognized that a large number of cardiac lesions can lead to IL (Table 8.52).

The pathophysiological mechanism which accounts for IL secondary to cardiac disease undoubtedly involves the fact that lymphatic drainage into the venous system is impeded in the presence of right-sided cardiac disease associated with elevated venous pressures.[42] Increased lymph production may also play some pathogenical role, but cannot be the sole explanation of cardiac IL since dilated lymphatics and protein-losing enteropathy is slight or non-existent in patients with portal hypertension due to liver disease.[37] Finally, IL secondary to cardiac disease must also involve certain poorly defined local lymphatic factors, since the vast majority of patients with constrictive pericarditis or right-sided cardiac failure do not develop IL.[42]

When IL secondary to a cardiac abnormality occurs, a typical protein-losing enteropathy and lymphocytopenia ensues which leads, in turn, to a secondary immunodeficiency state.[34] The anergy that results may confuse certain diagnostic procedures such as skin testing with purified protein derivative (PPD) or other antigens in constrictive pericarditis. In several of our patients, successful surgical treatment of the constrictive pericarditis led to disappearance of the IL syndrome as well as the immunodeficiency[34] (Figure 8.102). Such cases provide dramatic evidence that the immunodeficiency of IL is secondary to the intestinal loss of lymphatic fluid, since treatment which eliminates the intestinal loss, but which has no direct effect on the lymphoid system, also leads to resolution of the immunological defect.

Cardiac lesions causing IL can be subtle and inapparent, and patients have been seen in whom cardiac disease was established only by cardiac catheterization. This emphasizes the need for careful cardiac evaluation in each new IL patient, so that a form of potentially treatable protein-losing enteropathy will not be overlooked.

Malignancy and IL

In common with many other immunodeficiency states, IL is associated with an increased incidence of lymphoid malignancy. Amongst our patients, three patients out of some 60 patients have had malignancy, two with lymphoma and one with reticulum cell sarcoma; in two of the three cases the neoplasm had its origin in the gastrointestinal tract. These malignancies cannot be considered the cause of the IL since they appeared long after its onset.

The association of IL with malignancy could stem from defective immunosurveillance and consequent impaired elimination of nascent neoplastic cell lines. An alternative explanation is that the chronic lymphocyte loss in IL, consisting mainly of T cells, leads to defective T cell regulation of B cell proliferation, and B cell malignancies emerge. This possibility is supported by the observation that one of our patients developed a monoclonal B cell malignancy.[8]

Diagnosis and differential diagnosis

The diagnosis of IL should be strongly suspected in a patient with oedema who has hypoalbuminaemia (usually less than 3.0 g/dl) associated with lymphocytopenia (usually less than 1500 cells/mm^3); these abnormalities suggest the presence of lymphocytopenic protein-losing gastroenteropathy. In primary IL one may also see evidence of systemic lymphatic abnormalities (asymmetrical oedema) as well as cutaneous lymphangiomas.

Two studies should be performed in potential IL patients to establish the diagnosis. The first is a protein-leak test to verify the presence of protein-losing enteropathy. This is usually performed with ^{51}Cr-labelled proteins but α_1-antitrypsin clearance can be measured instead. The second is a peroral biopsy of the jejunum to verify the presence of dilated intestinal lymphatics and rule out other intestinal diseases. Whilst dilated lymphatics are the hallmark lesion of IL, their absence does not exclude the diagnosis, as the blocked lymphatics may have a patchy distribution. It should be noted that dilated lymphatics also occur in Behçet's syndrome, a disease characterized by neurological abnormalities, aphthous ulcers of the mouth, eye inflammation and arthritis.[44] The cause of this disease is unknown, as is the reason for its association with dilated intestinal lymphatics. Interestingly, dilated lymphatics in Behçet's syndrome are not associated with protein-losing enteropathy.

Another diagnostic test of potential use in the diagnosis of IL is the lymphangiogram. However, while this test may provide useful adjunctive data about the lymphatic system in IL patients, it rarely, if ever, leads to a change in therapy. This, together with the fact that it is not without serious side effects, has led to its use only in cases where neoplasm is being seriously considered.

One normally encounters little difficulty in distinguishing IL from other protein-losing states and/or gastrointestinal disorders. Coeliac disease with hypoalbuminaemia may be differentiated by the biopsy appearances. Patients with allergic disease of the GI tract may have protein-losing enteropathy as severe as in IL, but lymphocytopenia and immunodeficiency are not present, diffuse oedema of the bowel wall sometimes associated with villous atrophy rather than dilated lymphatics is noted on biopsy, serum IgE levels are usually elevated, and there is a history of relation of symptoms to food ingestion.

Combined immunodeficiency, common variable hypogammaglobulinaemia and other immunodeficiency states may resemble IL in that they are sometimes associated with diarrhoea, protein-losing enteropathy and malabsorption; in addition, immunodeficiency patients have low immunoglobulin levels, lymphocytopenia, and anergy. Nevertheless, immunodeficiency states are usually distinguishable from IL in that the immunoglobulin levels are much lower than in IL, particularly the IgA and IgM levels, and the gastrointestinal disease is dominated by malabsorption rather than protein-losing enteropathy, reflecting the fact that villous atrophy, not dilated lymphatics, is the anatomical lesion present.

In summary, IL is a unique disease, and the main problem is to be aware of the possibility of its presence rather than its delineation from other diseases.

Treatment
The treatment of IL depends on whether the IL is primary (idiopathic) or secondary. In the former instance, treatment is largely supportive, since no definitive therapy is available to restore the disordered lymphatic channels. Surgical treatment of primary IL, by excising severely affected segments of bowel, has been attempted from time to time,[29] but this form of therapy is not decisively beneficial and may, in fact, lead to serious complications. Unless it can be clearly demonstrated that only a defined segment of bowel is involved, surgical therapy should not be attempted.

Supportive therapy in primary IL consists of diuretics and/or a low salt diet to control the oedema and ascites. In addition, a diet exceedingly low in fat (20 g/day) has led to increases in the albumin level of 0.5–1.0 g/dl.[25] The low fat intake probably works by reducing the load on the intestinal lymphatics, thereby reducing intralymphatic pressure and protein leaking. The low fat diet can be supplemented by medium chain triglycerides (MCT) since this form of fat is absorbed via the intestinal venous system rather than the lymphatics.[43] Protein repletion by albumin infusion is not generally useful, as the intestinal protein loss in IL (equivalent at times to a third to a half of the intravascular pool each day) precludes the possibility of meaningful protein replacement. It is, however, useful to provide patients with parenteral albumin during periods of crisis or prior to surgery.

In secondary IL, definitive therapy is frequently possible, depending on the underlying disease present. For instance, IL secondary to constrictive pericarditis can frequently be cured by pericardiectomy. Similarly, IL secondary to inflammatory disease may be effectively treated with relatively short-term steroid therapy. The possibility of cure in secondary IL is so important that every IL patient should be assumed to have this form of the disease until proven otherwise. In effect, this means that an exhaustive search for cardiac, inflammatory, infectious and neoplastic causes of IL should be conducted in every patient.

REFERENCES

1 Ament, M. E. & Ochs, H. D. (1973) Gastrointestinal manifestations of chronic granulomatous disease. *New England Journal of Medicine*, **288**, 382–387.

2 Ament, M. E., Ochs, H. D. & Davis, S. D. (1973) Structure and function of the gastrointestinal tract in primary immunodeficiency syndromes. A study of 39 patients. *Medicine*, **52**, 227–248.

3 Asakura, H., Miura, S., Morishita, T. *et al.* (1981) Endoscopic and histopathological study on primary and secondary intestinal lymphangiectasia. *Digestive Diseases and Sciences*, **26**, 312–320.

4 Beeker, W. L., Busch, H. J. & Sylvester, D. L. (1972) Intestinal protein loss in Crohn's disease. *Gastroenterology*, **62**, 207–213.

5 Belaiche, J., Vesin, P., Chaumette, M. T. *et al.* (1980) Intestinal lymphangiectasia associated with fibrosis of the mesenteric nodes. *Gastroenterologie Clinique et Biologique*, **4**, 52–58.

6 Berman, M., Shahn, E. & Weiss, M. F. (1962) The routine fitting of kinetic data to models: a mathematical formalism for digital computers. *Biophysical Journal*, **2**, 275–287.

7 Bookstein, J. J., French, A. B. & Pollard, H. M. (1965) Protein-losing gastroenteropathy: concepts derived from lymphangiography. *American Journal of Digestive Diseases*, **10**, 573–581.

8 Broder, S., Callihan, T. R., Jaffe, E. S. *et al.* (1981) Resolution of longstanding protein-losing enteropathy in a patient with intestinal lymphangiectasia after treatment for malignant lymphoma. *Gastroenterology*, **80**, 166–168.

9 Citrin, Y., Sterling, K. & Halsted, J. A. (1957) The mechanism of hypoproteinemia associated with giant hypertrophy of gastric mucosa. *New England Journal of Medicine*, **257**, 906–912.

10 Cluysenaer, O. J. J., Corstens, F. H. M., Hafkenscheid, J. C. M. *et al.* (1974) Mechanisms of hypoalbuminaemia in coeliac sprue. In *Coeliac Disease, Proceedings of the Second International Coeliac Symposium* (Ed.) Hekkens, W. Th. J. M. & Pena, A. S. pp. 386–396. Leiden: H. E. Stenfort Kroese B.V.

11 Davenport, H. W. (1971) Protein-losing gastropathy produced by sulfhydryl reagents. *Gastroenterology*, **60**, 870–879.

12 Davidson, J. D., Flynn, E. P. & Kirkpatrick, J. B. (1966) Protein-losing enteropathy and intestinal bleeding. *Annals Internal Medicine*, **64**, 628–635.

13 Davidson, J. D., Waldmann, T. A., Goodman, O. S. & Gordon, R. S. Jr (1961) Protein-losing gastroenteropathy in congestive heart failure. *Lancet*, **i**, 899–902.

14 Dobbins, W. O. (1966) Electron microscopic study of the intestinal mucosa in intestinal lymphangiectasia. *Gastroenterology*, **51**, 1004–1017.

15 Eustace, P. W., Gaunt, J. I. & Croft, D. N. (1975) Incidence of protein-losing enteropathy in primary lymphoedema using chromium-51 chloride technique. *British Medical Journal*, **iv**, 737.

16 Fliesher, T. A., Strober, W., Muchmore, A. V. *et al.* (1979) Corticosteroid-responsive intestinal lymphangiectasia secondary to an inflammatory process. *New England Journal of Medicine*, **300**, 605–606.

17 Florent, C., L'Hirondel, C., Desmazures, C. *et al.* (1981) Intestinal clearance of alpha-l-antitrypsin. A sensitive method for the detection of protein-losing enteropathy. *Gastroenterology*, **81**, 777–780.

18 Gold, R. H. & Youker, J. E. (1973) Idiopathic intestinal lymphangiectasia (primary protein-losing enteropathy). Lymphographic verification of enteric and peritoneal leakage of chyle. *Radiology*, **109**, 315–316.

19 Gordon, R. S., Jr (1959) Exudative enteropathy: abnormal permeability of the gastrointestinal tract demonstrable with labelled polyvinylpyrolidone. *Lancet*, **i**, 325–326.

20 Hermans, P. E., Diaz-Buxo, J. A. & Stobo, J. D. (1976) Idiopathic late-onset immunoglobulin deficiency. Clinical observations in 50 patients. *American Journal of Medicine*, **61**, 221–237.

21 Iio, A., Strober, W., Broder, S. *et al.* (1977) The metabolism of IgE in patients with immunodeficiency states and neoplastic conditions. *Journal of Clinical Investigation*, **59**, 743–755.

22 Jarnum, S. & Jensen, K. B. (1972) Plasma protein turnover (albumin, transferrin, IgG, IgM) in Menetrier's disease (giant hypertrophic gastritis): evidence of nonselective protein loss. *Gut*, **13**, 128–137.

23 Jarnum, S., Westergaard, H., Yssing, M. & Jensen, H. (1968) Quantitation of gastrointestinal protein loss by means of Fe^{59}-labelled iron dextran. *Gastroenterology*, **55**, 229–241.

24 Jeejeebhoy, K. N., Jarnum, S., Singh, B. *et al.* (1968) ^{95}Nb-labelled albumin for the study of gastrointestinal albumin loss. *Scandinavian Journal of Gastroenterology*, **3**, 449–457.

25 Jeffries, G. H., Chapman, A. & Sleisenger, M. H. (1964) Low fat diet in intestinal lymphangiectasia. *New England Journal of Medicine*, **270**, 761–766.

26 Jones, E. A., Young, W. B., Morson, B. C. & Dawson, A. M. (1972) A study of six patients with hypertrophy of the gastric mucosa with particular reference to albumin metabolism. *Gut*, **13**, 270–277.

27 Katz, A. J., Goldman, H. & Grand, R. J. (1977) Gastric mucosal biopsy in eosinophilic (allergic) gastroenteritis. *Gastroenterology*, **73**, 705–709.

28 Kinmonth, J. B. & Cox, S. J. (1974) Protein-losing enteropathy in primary lymphoedema: mesenteric lymphography and gut resection. *British Journal of Surgery*, **61**, 589–593.

29 Kinmonth, J. B., Taylor, G. W., Tracy, G. D. & Marsh, J. D. (1957) Primary lymphoedema. Clinical and lymphangiographic studies of series of 107 patients in which the lower limbs were affected. *British Journal of Surgery*, **45**, 1–10.

30 Kondo, M., Bomba, T., Hosokawa, K. *et al.* (1976) Tissue plasminogen activator in the pathogenesis of protein-losing gastroenteropathy. *Gastroenterology*, **70**, 1045–1047.

31 Mistilis, S. P., Skyring, A. P. & Stephen, D. D. (1965) Intestinal lymphangiectasia: mechanism of enteric loss of plasma protein and fat. *Lancet*, **i**, 77–80.

32 Munro, D. R. (1974) Route of protein loss during a model protein-losing gastropathy in dogs. *Gastroenterology*, **66**, 960–972.

33 Muntean, W. & Rossipal, E. (1979) Verlust von Inhibi-

toren des Gerinnungssystems bei der Exudativen Enteropathie. *Klinishi Pädiatrie*, **191**, 20–23.

34 Nelson, D. L., Blaese, R. M., Strober, W. *et al.* (1975) Constrictive pericarditis, intestinal lymphangiectasia, and reversible immunologic deficiency. *Journal of Pediatrics*, **86**, 548–554.

35 Nosslin, B. (1973) Analysis of disappearance time-curves after a single injection of labelled proteins. In *Protein Turnover. CIBA Foundation Symposium 9 (New Series)*. pp. 113–128. Amsterdam: Associated Scientific Publishers.

36 Orbeck, H., Larsen, T. E. & Honig, T. (1978) Transient intestinal lymphangiectasia. *Acta Paediatrica Scandinavica*, **67**, 677–682.

37 Petersen, V. P. & Ottosen, P. (1964) Albumin turnover and thoracic duct lymph in constrictive pericarditis. *Acta Medica Scandinavica*, **176**, 335–344.

38 Shimkin, P. M., Waldmann, T. A. & Krugman, R. L. (1970) Intestinal lymphangiectasia. *American Journal of Roentgenology, Radium Therapy and Nuclear Medicine*, **110**, 827–841.

39 Steinfeld, J. L., Davidson, J. D. & Gordon, R. S., Jr (1957) A mechanism for hypoalbuminemia in patients with ulcerative colitis and regional enteritis. *Journal of Clinical Investigation*, **36**, 931.

40 Steinfeld, J. L., Davidson, J. D., Gordon, R. S., Jr & Greene, F. E. (1960) The mechanism of hypoproteinemia in patients with regional enteritis and ulcerative colitis. *American Journal of Medicine*, **29**, 405–415.

41 Strober, W., Cohen, L. S., Waldmann, T. A. & Braunwald, E. (1968) Tricuspid regurgitation. A newly recognized cause of protein-losing enteropathy and immunologic deficiency. *American Journal of Medicine*, **44**, 842–850.

42 Strober, W., Wochner, R. D., Carbone, P. P. & Waldmann, T. A. (1967) Intestinal lymphangiectasia: a protein-losing enteropathy with hypogammaglobulinemia, lymphocytopenia and impaired homograft rejection. *Journal of Clinical Investigation*, **46**, 1643–1656.

43 Tift, W. L. & Lloyd, J. K. (1975) Intestinal lymphangiectasia. Long-term results with MCT diet. *Archives of Diseases in Childhood*, **50**, 269–275.

44 Tsuchiya, M., Hibi, T., Mizuno, Y. *et al.* (1976) Comparative, immunological studies on lymphangiectasia of the small intestine revealed in protein-losing gastroenteropathy and Behçet's disease. *Gastroenterologia Japonica*, **11**, 88–99.

45 Van Tongeren, J. H. M. & Reichert, W. J. (1966) Demonstration of protein-losing gastro-enteropathy: the quantitative estimation of gastrointestinal protein loss using ^{51}Cr-labelled plasma proteins. *Clinica Chimica Acta*, **14**, 42–48.

46 Vardy, P. A., Lekenthal, E. & Shevachman, H. (1975) Intestinal lymphangiectasia: a reappraisal. *Pediatrics*, **55**, 842–851.

47 Waldmann, T. A. & Laster, L. (1964) Abnormalities of albumin metabolism in patients with hypogammaglobulinemia. *Journal of Clinical Investigation*, **43**, 1025–1035.

48 Waldmann, T. A. & Strober, W. (1969) Metabolism of immunoglobulins. *Progress in Allergy*, **13**, 1–110.

49 Waldmann, T. A., Broder, S. & Strober, W. (1974) Protein-losing enteropathies in malignancy. *Annals of the New York Academy of Sciences*, **230**, 306–317.

50 Waldmann, T. A., Wochner, R. D. & Strober, W. (1969) The role of the gastrointestinal tract in plasma protein metabolism studies with ^{51}Cr-albumin. *American Journal of Medicine*, **46**, 275–285.

51 Waldmann, T. A., Wochner, R. D., Laster, L. & Gordon, R. S., Jr (1967) Allergic gastroenteropathy. A cause of excessive gastrointestinal protein loss. *New England Journal of Medicine*, **276**, 761–769.

52 Waldmann, T. A., Morell, A. G., Wochner, R. D. *et al.* (1967) Measurement of gastrointestinal protein loss using ceruloplasmin labeled with ^{67}copper. *Journal of Clinical Investigation*, **28**, 10–20.

53 Waldmann, T. A., Steinfeld, J. L., Dutcher, T. F. *et al.* (1961) The role of the gastrointestinal system in idiopathic hypoproteinemia. *Gastroenterology*, **41**, 197–207.

54 Weiden, P. L., Blaese, R. M., Strober, W. & Waldmann, T. A. (1972) Impaired lymphocyte transformation in intestinal lymphangiectasia. Evidence for at least two functionally distinct lymphocyte populations in man. *Journal of Clinical Investigation*, **51**, 1319–1325.

55 Wochner, R. D., Weissman, S. M., Waldmann, T. A. *et al.* (1968) Direct measurement of the rates of synthesis of plasma proteins in control subjects and patients with gastrointestinal protein loss. *Journal of Clinical Investigation*, **47**, 971–982.

TUMOURS OF THE SMALL INTESTINE

Malignant tumours of the small intestine are uncommon and account for only 1% of all gastrointestinal neoplasms. This is surprising in view of the high incidence of tumours in the adjacent stomach and large intestine and the relatively large surface area of the small intestine. The incidence of small bowel tumours in different parts of the world is closely related to the frequency of colonic cancer,[9] suggesting that similar causative factors may be operating. It is possible that the reduced bacterial flora of the small intestine compared with that of the large intestine may result in the formation of less carcinogen, which also has less contact with the mucosa because of rapid transit time. Accumulations of lymphoid tissues in the small intestinal wall and increased levels of immunoglobulins may also be protective; if damaged by immunosuppression for transplantation purposes, an increase in the incidence of small bowel tumours occurs.[36] If a patient has a small bowel tumour, the risk of developing a second primary elsewhere in the body is also increased.[31]

The main primary malignant tumours of the small intestine, in order of frequency, are adenocarcinomas, carcinoids, lymphomas and leiomyosarcomas. Malignant small bowel tumours are slightly more common in men than in women, with a peak age incidence in the sixth and seventh decades.[46]

Benign tumours of the small intestine are rare, the commonest being leiomyomas and lipomas.[46] They are often diagnosed as incidental findings at post mortem examination or during laparotomy for other reasons, whereas malignant tumours usually present with symptoms.[37]

Aetiology of malignant tumours

Crohn's disease
Many case reports of carcinoma complicating Crohn's disease of the small intestine have been reported. It occurs in a younger age group, and more frequently in the ileum, than carcinomas developing de novo.[8] Although the majority of patients have a long history of Crohn's disease, 17% of patients present within five years of the onset of symptoms.[13] Bypassed loops of bowel seem particularly prone to develop carcinoma,[14] and metachronous carcinoma complicating Crohn's disease has been reported[6] (see also Chapter 12).

Coeliac disease
Mucosal abnormalities, often with premalignant change, may be present in patients with untreated adult coeliac disease. The incidence of small bowel malignancy in patients suffering from adult coeliac disease is increased (see p. 465); the tumour is usually in the form of lymphoma but adenocarcinoma has also been described.[17] Carcinoma of the oesophagus and pharynx have been found more commonly in patients with coeliac disease than in the general population.[16]

Diseases of the immune system and immunosuppression
Lymphoma complicating immunosuppression for transplantation has been recognized for a number of years[36] and has now been reported following immunosuppression with cyclosporin A.[5] Small bowel lymphoma has also been reported as a complication of other diseases of the immunological system such as hypogammaglobulinaemia.[21]

Adenomas
Adenomas of the small bowel, although rare, are liable to undergo malignant change, especially in the duodenum; approximately 30% of duodenal villous tumours contain foci of invasive carcinoma at resection. Although less common, jejunal villous adenomas may also contain areas of invasive carcinoma.[23]

Peutz–Jeghers syndrome
Peutz–Jeghers syndrome, characterized by the development of hamartomatous polyps of the gastrointestinal tract and associated mucocutaneous pigmentation, is associated with a slightly increased risk of developing malignancy in the small intestine and duodenum,[29] though in the past the risk has been exaggerated due to mistaking the histology of the hamartomatous polyps for invasion of the muscle layers.[11]

Gardner's syndrome
In recent years there have been numerous reports of adenomatous polyps and adenocarcinomas occurring in the duodenum in Gardner's syndrome.[25] It is estimated that in patients with colorectal polyposis, the incidence of periampullary carcinoma is approximately 12%.[3] Adenomas of the ileum are a rare finding in Gardner's syndrome, and the risk of carcinoma of the small intestine distal to the duodenum appears to be very small.[15]

Therapeutic irradiation
A case of angiosarcoma developing in the terminal ileum following therapeutic irradiation has been reported.[7]

Adenocarcinoma

DUODENAL ADENOCARCINOMA

Approximately 40% of all adenocarcinomas of the small intestine arise in the duodenum, which is relatively much shorter than the other parts of the small bowel. The majority arise in the infra- or periampullary portion and only a small percentage in the supra-ampullary region.[34]

Symptoms and signs
The most common presenting symptoms are pain, anaemia, vomiting due to duodenal obstruction, and weight loss.[19] Jaundice may occur in those patients with a tumour in the periampullary region. Haematemesis and melaena, and a palpable mass are uncommon findings. Though massive haemorrhage is uncommon, occult bleeding is present in the majority of patients.[1, 38] Diagnosis is usually made by barium studies of the upper gastrointestinal tract; radiological findings include obstruction and ulceration with mucosal destruction, often with some degree of proximal dilatation. However, lesions are often missed by the initial barium examination[45] and a high index of suspicion is necessary. Hypotonic duodenography is valuable in identifying small lesions. Duodenoscopy is also a very valuable investigation and allows histological confirmation of the tumour. Care, however, must be taken not to miss infra-ampullary lesions by terminating the examination in the proximal duodenum.

Treatment

Curative surgical treatment is by pancreatoduo-denectomy or segmental resection, the latter procedure being usually only possible with small localized lesions in the infra-ampullary part of the duodenum. The five-year survival of patients undergoing pancreatoduodenectomy or segmental resection may be as high as 46%,[19] but the operative mortality of pancreatoduodenectomy is some three times that of segmental resection and in a series collected from the literature was 20–25%.[38] However, in many patients a curative resection is impossible and only a palliative bypass can be performed.

JEJUNAL AND ILEAL ADENOCARCINOMA

Approximately 40% of small intestinal carcinomas occur in the jejunum and 20% in the ileum.[30]

Symptoms and signs

Many patients present with epigastric discomfort, often postprandial, but the diagnosis is often not made until the later symptoms of colicky abdominal pain due to subacute obstruction, weight loss, and a palpable mass develop. Most carcinomas grow in an annular, constricting fashion, but occasionally a polypoid adenocarcinoma will cause an intussusception. Anaemia from gastrointestinal blood loss is occasionally found; perforation rarely occurs. Physical findings are not usually present until the disease is well advanced. The prognosis is directly related to the degree of spread of the tumour at the time of surgery, few patients surviving more than five years when positive nodes are identified in the specimen. Diagnosis is usually eventually made by barium follow through (Figure 8.103) or small bowel barium enema examination.[20] Adenocarcinomas may metastasize to the lymph nodes and liver; perineal carcinomatosis may also occur. Curative resection should be attempted unless widespread dissemination has occurred. An overall five-year survival in the region of 25% can be expected.[42]

Carcinoid tumours

Carcinoid tumours arise from the enterochromaffin cells of the gastrointestinal tract and may secrete 5-hydroxytryptamine. Eighty-five percent of small intestinal carcinoid tumours occur in the ileum, 10% in the jejunum and 5% in the duodenum. They are commonest in the sixth and seventh decades, men being affected more often than women. Carcinoid tumours and the carcinoid syndrome are considered in detail later in this chapter.

Malignant lymphomas

Malignant lymphomas of the small bowel are uncommon, representing about 20% of all small bowel neoplasms. They are discussed fully earlier in this chapter.

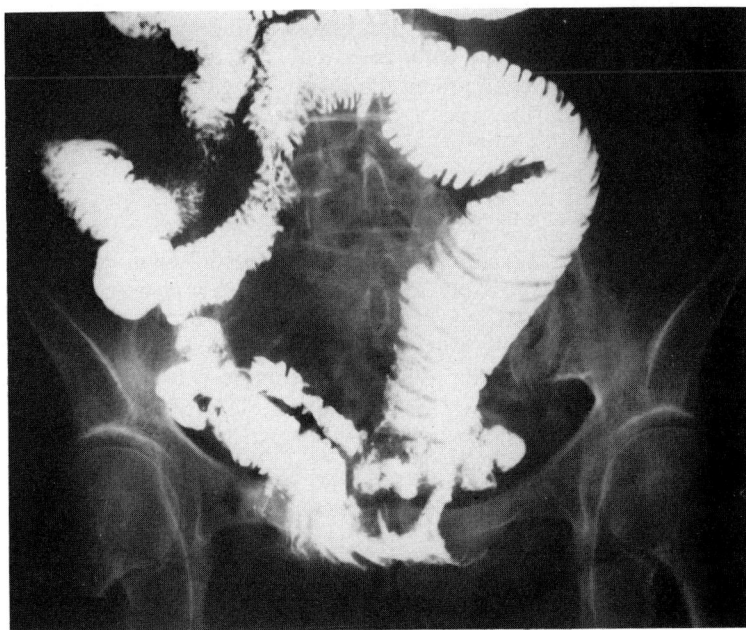

Fig. 8.103 Adenocarcinoma of the jejunum. Annular constricting lesion seen in the lower jejunum on barium follow through examination.

Leiomyosarcoma

These tumours, which arise from the circular or longitudinal muscle coats and rarely from the muscularis mucosa, represent about 10% of malignant small intestinal neoplasms. The average age at diagnosis is 50–60 years.

About 20% occur in the duodenum and 80% in the jejunum and ileum. They have been reported to occur in Meckel's diverticulum.[39] Most tumours are subserosal; however, they occasionally may grow towards the bowel lumen and become polypoid, when they assume a round or oval shape often with a central area of mucosal ulceration resulting in a high incidence of gastrointestinal bleeding. The diagnosis of malignancy is often difficult as tumours which histologically appear benign may produce metastases.[24] Large tumours with areas of necrosis or softening are usually malignant.

Symptoms and signs
One of the commonest presenting symptoms is melaena, which may have been present intermittently for many months, the blood loss being the result of mucosal ulceration of a slowly growing polypoid intraluminal tumour. Abdominal discomfort is commonly present, ranging from vague epigastric discomfort to the colicky abdominal pain of subacute obstruction, which is often due to intussusception of a polypoid tumour. An abdominal mass may be present. Leiomyosarcoma of the duodenum, more frequently found in the second and third parts,[26] rarely obstructs and usually presents with haematemesis. Unusual presentations include retroperitoneal haemorrhage, protracted fever and peritonitis.[28]

Treatment
Surgical treatment is by segmental resection of the bowel containing the tumour with the regional mesenteric lymphatic nodes. Although the two-year survival may be as high as 60%,[28] only 20% survive five years or more.

Neurogenic tumours of the small intestine

Neurogenic tumours of the small intestine are very uncommon and can be divided into nerve sheath tumours – neurilemomas and neurofibromas – and neuroblastic tumours of the sympathetic system – ganglioneuromas, sympathicoblastomas and paragangliomas. Neurofibromas similar to lesions seen in systemic neurofibromatosis (von Recklinghausen's disease) are found in the submucosa and muscle layers. They are commonest in the ileum and may present either with bleeding or intussusception. Paragangliomas are usually submucosal in site and vary in diameter from 1–4 cm, and present with either obstruction or gastrointestinal bleeding.

Adenomas

Adenomas of the small intestine are rare. In a review of 1721 benign tumours of the small intestine, Wilson *et al.*[46] found only 245 adenomas approximately equally distributed between the duodenum, jejunum and ileum. Obstruction, usually by intussusception, was the most common mode of presentation.

Villous adenomas are of particular interest because of their malignant potential. The majority have been reported in the duodenum.[23] The commonest presenting symptoms are epigastric discomfort associated with either occult or massive bleeding. Obstructive symptoms occur when the tumour is large.[35]

Small bowel adenomas may rarely be associated with familial colonic polyposis;[33] Gardner's syndrome is usually associated with the occurrence of duodenal adenomas and carcinomas.[25] Diagnosis can best be achieved by hypotonic duodenography and endoscopy.

Lipomas

Intestinal lipomas are well-circumscribed benign tumours arising within the submucosa and, when large, fat necrosis may be present within the tumour. A common method of presentation is the result of intussusception resulting in acute or subacute intestinal obstruction. Bleeding is less frequent than with other common tumours. The disease occurs more often in the older age groups.[46]

Angiomas

Discrete, well-circumscribed angiomas are probably hamartomatous arteriovenous malformations rather than true vascular neoplasms. They may also be associated with more widespread vascular disorders such as the inherited haemorrhagic telangiectasia or Rendu–Weber–Osler disease. They are discussed in full in Chapter 5.

REFERENCES

1 Blumgart, L. H. & Kennedy, A. (1973) Carcinoma of the ampulla of Vater and duodenum. *British Journal of Surgery*, **60**, 33–41.

2 Brookes, V. S. & Waterhouse, J. A. H. (1968) Malignant lesions of the small intestine. *British Journal of Surgery*, **55**, 405.

3 Bussey, H. J. R. (1972) Extracolonic lesions associated with polyposis coli. *Proceedings of the Royal Society of Medicine*, **65**, 294.

4 Calman, K. C. (1974) Why are small bowel tumours rare? An experimental model. *Gut*, **15**, 552–554.

5 Calne, R. Y., Rolles, K., Thiru, S. *et al.* (1979) Cyclosporin A initially as the only immunosuppressant in 34 recipients of cadaveric organs: 32 kidneys, 2 pancreases and 2 livers. *Lancet*, **ii**, 1033–1036.

6 Castellano, T. J., Frank, M. S., Brandt, L. J. & Mahadevia, P. (1981) Metachronous carcinoma complicating Crohn's disease. *Archives of Internal Medicine*, **141**, 1074–1075.

7 Chen, K. T. K., Hoffman, K. D. & Hendricks, E. J. (1979) Angiosarcoma following therapeutic irradiation. *Cancer*, **44**, 2044–2048.

8 Darke, S. G., Parks, A. G., Grogono, J. L. & Pollock, D. J. (1973) Adenocarcinoma and Crohn's disease: a report of 2 cases and analysis of the literature. *British Journal of Surgery*, **60**, 169–175.

9 Doll, R., Payne, P. & Waterhouse, J. (1966) *Cancer Incidence in Five Continents*, vol. 1. Geneve: International Union Against Cancer.

10 Dorman, J. E., Floyd, E. & Cohn, I. Jr (1967) Malignant neoplasms of the small bowel. *American Journal of Surgery*, **113**, 131.

11 Dozois, R. R., Judd, E. S., Dahlin, D. C. & Bartholomew, L. G. (1969) The Peutz–Jegher's syndrome. Is there a predisposition to the development of intestinal malignancy? *Archives of Surgery*, **98**, 509–517.

12 Ebert, P. & Zuidema, G. D. (1965) Primary tumours of the small intestine. *Archives of Surgery*, **91**, 452.

13 Fresko, D., Lazarus, S. S., Dotan, J. & Reingold, M. (1982) Early presentation of carcinoma of the small bowel in Crohn's disease ('Crohn's Carcinoma'). Case reports and review of the literature. *Gastroenterology*, **82**, 783–789.

14 Greenstein, A. J., Sachar, D., Pucillo, A. *et al.* (1978) Cancer in Crohn's disease after diversionary surgery. *American Journal of Surgery*, **135**, 86–90.

15 Hamilton, S. J., Bussey, H. J. R. Mendlesohn, G. *et al.* (1979) Ileal adenomas after colectomy in nine patients with adenomatous polyposis coli/Gardner's syndrome. *Gastroenterology*, **77**, 1252–1257.

16 Harris, O. D., Cooke, W. T., Thompson, H. & Waterhouse, J. A. H. (1967) Malignancy in adult coeliac disease and idiopathic steatorrhoea. *American Journal of Medicine*, **42**, 899–912.

17 Holmes, G. K. T., Dunn, G. I., Cockel, R. & Brookes, V. C. (1980) Adenocarcinoma of the upper small bowel complicating coeliac disease. *Gut*, **21**, 1010–1015.

18 Isaacson, P., Wright, D., Judd, M. A. & Mepham, B. L. (1979) Primary gastrointestinal lymphomas: a classification of 66 cases. *Cancer*, **43**, 1805–1819.

19 Joesting, D. R., Beart, R. W., Van Heerden, J. A. & Weiland, L. H. (1981) Improving survival in adenocarcinoma of the duodenum. *American Journal of Surgery*, **141**, 228–231.

20 Keddie, N. (1982) The value of the small bowel enema to the general surgeons. *British Journal of Surgery*, **69**, 611–612.

21 Lamers, C. B. H. W., Wagener, D. J. T., Assman, K. J. M. & Van Tongeren, J. H. M. (1980) Jejunal lymphoma in a patient with primary adult-onset hypogammaglobulinemia and nodular lymphoid hyperplasia of the small intestine. *Digestive Diseases and Sciences*, **25**, 553–557.

22 Lowenfels, A. B. (1973) Why are small bowel tumours so rare? *Lancet*, **i**, 24–26.

23 Mir-Madjilesse, S., Farmer, R. G. & Hawk, W. A. (1973) Villous tumours of the duodenum and jejunum. *Digestive Diseases*, **18**, 467–476.

24 Morson, B. C. & Dawson, I. M. P. (1979) *Gastrointestinal Pathology*, 2nd edn. Oxford: Blackwell Scientific.

25 Naylor, E. W. & Lebenthal, E. (1980) Gardner's syndrome. Recent developments in research and management. *Digestive Diseases and Sciences*, **25**, 945–959.

26 Olurin, E. O. & Solanke, T. F. (1968) Case of leiomyosarcoma of the duodenum and a review of the literature. *Gut*, **9**, 672–677.

27 Ostermiller, W., Jorgenson, E. J. & Weibel, L. (1966) A clinical review of tumours of the small bowel. *American Journal of Surgery*, **11**, 403.

28 Ranchod, M. & Kempson, R. L. (1977) Smooth muscle tumours of the gastrointestinal tract and retroperitoneum. *Cancer*, **39**, 255–262.

29 Reid, J. D. (1974) Intestinal carcinoma in the Peutz–Jegher syndrome. *Journal of the American Medical Association*, **229**, 833–834.

30 Reiner, M. A. (1976) Primary malignant neoplasms of the small bowel. *The Mount Sinai Journal of Medicine*, **43**, 274–280.

31 Reyes, E. L. & Talley, R. W. (1970) Primary malignant tumours of the small intestine. *American Journal of Gastroenterology*, **54**, 30.

32 Rochlin, D. B. & Longmire, W. P. Jr (1961) Primary tumours of the small intestine. *Surgery*, **50**, 586.

33 Ross, J. E. & Mara, J. E. (1974) Small bowel polyps and carcinoma in multiple intestinal polyposis. *Archives of Surgery*, **108**, 736–738.

34 Sakker, S. & Ware, C. C. (1973) Carcinoma of the duodenum: comparison of surgery, radiotherapy and chemotherapy. *British Journal of Surgery*, **60**, 867–872.

35 Schulten, M. F., Oyasu, R. & Beal, J. (1976) Villous adenoma of the duodenum. A case report and review of the literature. *American Journal of Surgery*, **132**, 90–96.

36 Sheil, A. G. R., Mahoney, J. F., Horvath, J. S. *et al.* (1979) Cancer and survival after cadaveric donor renal transplantation. *Transplantation Proceedings*, **11**, 1052–1054.

37 Silberman, H., Crichlow, R. W. & Caplan, H. S. (1974) Neoplasms of the small bowel. *Annals of Surgery*, **180**, 157–161.

38 Spira, I. A., Ghazi, A. & Wolff, W. I. (1977) Primary adenocarcinoma of the duodenum. *Cancer*, **39**, 1721–1726.

39 Starr, G. F. & Dockerty, M. B. (1955) Leiomyomas and leiomyosarcomas of the small intestine. *Cancer*, **8**, 101–111.

40 Steinberg, L. S. & Shieber, W. (1972) Villous adenoma of the small intestine. *Surgery*, **71**, 423.

41 Strauch, G. O. (1964) Small bowel neoplasms: elusive source of abdominal symptoms. *Surgery*, **55**, 240.

42 Treadwell, T. A. & White, R. R. (1975) Primary tumours of the small bowel. *American Journal of Surgery*, **130**, 749–755.

43 Tyers, G. F. O., Steiger, E. & Dudrick, S. J. (1969) Adenocarcinoma of the small intestine and other malignant tumours complicating regional enteritis. *Annals of Surgery*, **169**, 510.

44 Weaver, D. K. & Batsakis, J. G. (1964) Primary lymphomas of the small intestine. *American Journal of Gastroenterology*, **42**, 620.

45 Williamson, R. C. N., Welch, C. E. & Malt, R. A. (1983) Adenocarcinoma and lymphoma of the small intestine. *Annals of Surgery*, **197**, 172–178.

46 Wilson, J. M., Melvin, D. B., Gray, G. F. & Thorbjar-
    narson, B. (1974) Primary malignancies of the small
    bowel. A report of 96 cases and review of the literature.
    Annals of Surgery, **180**(2), 175–179.
47 Wilson, J. M., Melvin, D. B., Gray, G. & Thorbjarnar-
    son, B. (1975) Benign small bowel tumors. *Annals of
    Surgery*, **181**, 247–250.

CARCINOID TUMOURS AND THE CARCINOID SYNDROME

Carcinoids are solid tumours arising from enterochromaffin cells, usually of the gastrointestinal or respiratory tract. The characteristic histochemical properties of these tumours show them to be related to other tumours of neuroendocrine origin; they are probably derived embryologically from the neural crest (the APUD system). Carcinoid tumours of the gastrointestinal tract may arise in almost any region of the gut, but the appendix and the small intestine are the commonest sites. Although carcinoids in all sites are potentially malignant, the majority behave as benign tumours and are clinically insignificant. Thus most clinical attention attaches to the minority of carcinoid tumours that give rise to the carcinoid syndrome – characterized by flushing, diarrhoea and heart disease, and caused by elaboration and release of humoral factors by the tumour.

Incidence of carcinoid tumours

Carcinoid tumours are not uncommon, occurring as incidental findings in up to 1% of autopsies. In fact, carcinoids are the commonest ileal tumour. By contrast, the carcinoid syndrome is rare – one estimate being that two new cases would occur in a population of 250 000 over 10 years.[38]

Pathology of carcinoid tumours

Cell of origin

Enterochromaffin (EC) cells, like other cells of the diffuse neuroendocrine system, are scattered throughout the body. Within the gut the cells lie in the lamina propria, mainly near the base of the intestinal crypts; they were originally described as isolated granular cells of the intestine or Kulchitsky cells.[68] Similar cells also occur in the lungs – principally in the submucosal layers of the main bronchi and give rise to bronchial carcinoids and possibly oat cells carcinomas.[4, 5, 6] The term enterochromaffin refers to the fact that they stain with potassium chromate – a feature of cells which contain 5-

hydroxytryptamine. Thus other non-Kulchitsky cells which contain 5-hydroxytryptamine, such as mast cells, thyroid C (calcitonin-containing) cells and certain cells in pancreatic islets, the biliary tree, the ovary and the testis, may also give rise to a positive enterochromaffin reaction. Enterochromaffin cells are also stained by other reagents.[23, 68] They take up and reduce silver and are thus also termed argentaffin cells. Other closely related cells are stained by silver but do not reduce it spontaneously – argyrophilic cells; these may simply be argentaffin cells which do not store sufficient reducing material to give the appropriate staining reaction, but the precise relationship remains disputed. It has been suggested that application of enterochromaffin or argentaffin reactions directly under the electron microscope may be the most reliable method of identifying EC cells.[68]

The granules of these cells have a particular configuration, being rod-like or bi-concave in shape and heterogeneous in density, though granules in EC cells from the stomach, duodenum and distal small intestine may differ in morphology. Certain EC cells react with antisera to substance P, enkephalins and motilin.[69] Thus within the normal EC cell population there is a degree of histochemical heterogeneity reflecting different cell products, which may account for the heterogeneity of histochemical reactions in carcinoid tumours and clinical features seen in the carcinoid syndrome (Table 8.53).[67, 68]

Macroscopic appearance

The majority of carcinoid tumours arise in the appendix, with the small intestine, colon and stomach being the next most common sites[7] (Table 8.54). In the small intestine the tumours usually occur in the ileum, 80% of them within 60 cm (2 ft) of the ileocaecal valve. Tumours in this site are multiple in up to 30% of cases. Gastric carcinoids may also be multiple, though single tumours, usually situated in the antrum, are more common. Bronchial carcinoids are usually solitary and occur in the main bronchi, but in 15% of cases they are peripheral and multiple.[16, 56] When discovered, most gastrointestinal carcinoid tumours are less than 1 cm in diameter and only 5% are greater than 2 cm.[24, 48] The cut surface is yellow (but may vary from tan to grey) due to the high lipid content; necrosis is rare. Within the gut, tumours usually arise in the submucosa and spread outwards rather than involving the lumen. Ulceration of the mucosa is thus unusual, though it is more common in gastric tumours which may there-

Table 8.53 Characteristics of carcinoid tumours from various sites.

	Site of tumour		
	Foregut	Midgut	Hindgut
Histology	Trabecular	Solid mass of cells	Mixed
Cytoplasmic granules (EM)	Variable density, about 180 μm in size	Uniformly dense, about 230 μm in size	Variable density, about 190 μm in size
Silver staining	Argyrophil or negative	Argentaffin	Negative
Products			
Blood	5HTP, histamine	5HT	Negative
Urine	5HTP, 5HT, 5HIAA, histamine and others	5HT, 5HIAA	Negative
Metastasis to bone and skin	Common	Unusual	Common

Modified from Williams and Sandler[78] and Soga and Tazawa.[67]

fore bleed. MacDonald[40] has emphasized that all carcinoids are potentially malignant, but there are marked differences in the likelihood of these tumours producing metastases depending on their site of origin (see below). Local spread from the muscularis mucosa extends to the serosa, by which time the intramural lymphatics are usually involved. A striking feature that may occur at this stage is a dense fibrotic reaction occurring in the region of the primary tumour and sometimes extending into the mesentery. In cases of carcinoid syndrome, such fibrosis may be seen not only around the primary tumour but also in the heart and other sites (see below). Once regional lymph nodes are involved they often become much larger than the primary tumour, so that occasionally massive nodal deposits are found associated with a primary tumour that is only a few millimetres across. Hepatic involvement occurs after nodal involvement late in the disease. Deposits may occur in lung and in bone and rarely other tissues – metastases have been described in nearly every organ.[8]

Table 8.54 Carcinoid tumours: site of the primary, and the presence of metastases and the carcinoid syndrome.

	Number of cases	Percentage with metastases	Number of cases with carcinoid syndrome
Foregut			
Oesophagus	2	0	—
Stomach	84	23	8
Duodenum	115	20	4
Pancreas	5	20	1
Gallbladder	18	30	1
Bile duct	5	0	—
Ampulla	7	14	—
Larynx	4	50	—
Bronchus	2% of lung tumours	5	66
Thymus	74	25	0
Midgut			
Jejunum	56	35	} 91
Ileum	1013	35	
Meckel's diverticulum	44	19	6
Appendix	1687	2	6
Colon	89	60	5
Liver	4	—	—
Ovary	34	6	17
Testis	2	—	0
Cervix	33	25	0
Hindgut			
Rectum	573	18	1

Other rare primary sites included the middle ear, parotid, breast, kidney, bladder and prostate. None were associated with the carcinoid syndrome.
Modified from Cheek and Wilson,[7] with data from Mengel and Shaffer,[45] Hsu *et al.*,[30] Okike *et al.*,[56] Ricci *et al.*,[59] Riddle *et al.*,[60] Wick *et al.*,[77] Matsuyama *et al.*,[42] and Viteaux *et al.*[75]

Microscopic appearance

The microscopic appearance of carcinoids is usually characteristic, although on occasions metastases initially classified as an adenocarcinoma will be reclassified on review as neuroendocrine in origin. The tumours have no capsule and the cells are uniform in size and polygonal in shape with a centrally situated nucleus containing speckled chromatin and basal granules (Figure 8.104). Three major patterns of cellular arrangement have been described[67, 78] – alveolar clusters, ribbons or columns of cells; the rare scirrhous pattern may also occur. On electron microscopy, electron dense granules are seen (Figure 8.105) which may differ depending on the site of the primary tumour[67] (Table 8.53).

Histochemical reactions

The cells may stain red with eosin (eosinophilic), brown with potassium chromate (chromaffin), black with iron haemotoxylin (siderophilic), orange red with Erlich's diazo reaction, and brownish black with silver nitrate (argentaffin). Echoing the heterogeneity of the normal enterochromaffin cell population, different carcinoid tumours may exhibit different staining reactions to these and other agents. For example, tumours arising from embryological foregut (bronchus, oesophagus and stomach) do not usually give positive argentaffin reactions, but do stain with silver when reducing agents are also applied (argyrophilic). As with normal EC cells, application of histochemical techniques using the electron microscope may be useful (Figure 8.106).[67] Some workers have attempted to correlate the histochemical staining reactions with the embryological origin of the primary tumour and the clinical features of the carcinoid syndrome arising from tumours of different sites (Table 8.53).

In addition to these 'classical' histochemical reactions, the use of antisera to a number of peptides has expanded the concept of heterogeneity of substances produced by carcinoid tumours. By use of appropriate techniques particular carcinoids have been shown to contain a wide variety of biologically active products, including insulin, somatostatin, glucagon, cholecystokinin, substance P, enkephalins, gastrin, pancreatic polypeptide, ACTH, βMSH, parathyroid hormone, calcitonin, growth hormone, growth hormone releasing factor, dopamine or epinephrine and prostaglandins.[21, 37, 42, 70] Carcinoid tumours also give positive reactions with neurone specific enolase (Figure 8.107).

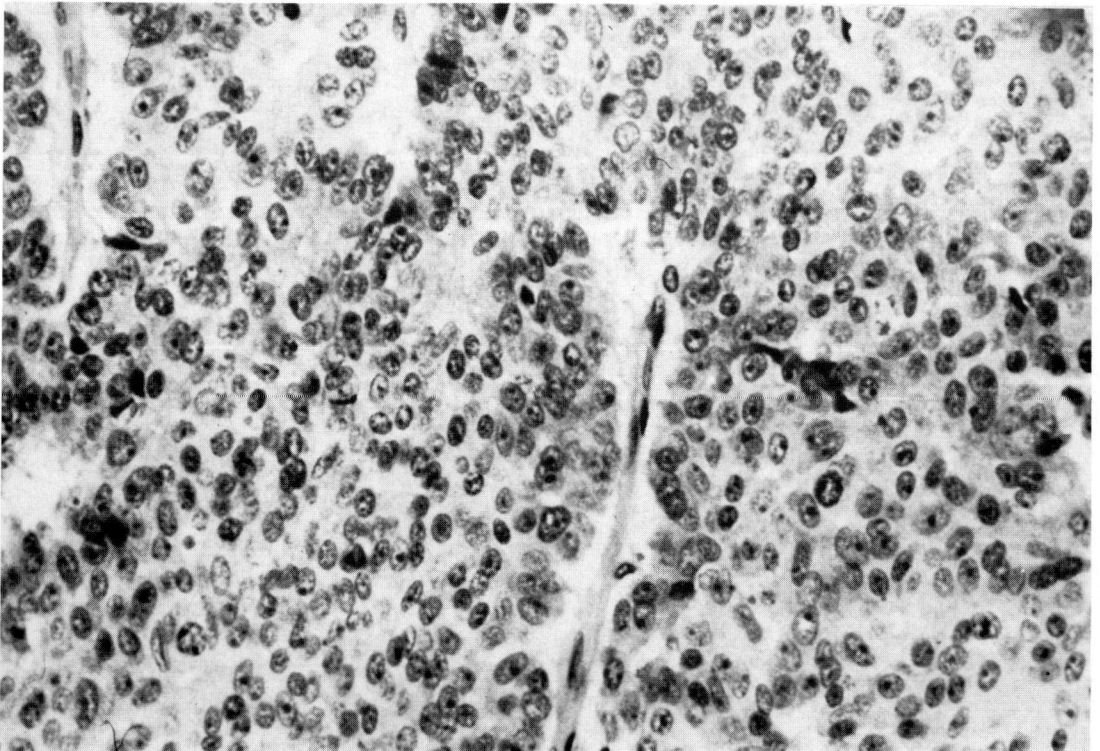

Fig. 8.104   Carcinoid of the gastrointestinal tract (haematoxylin and eosin, × 280). Courtesy of Dr J. Polak, RPMS.

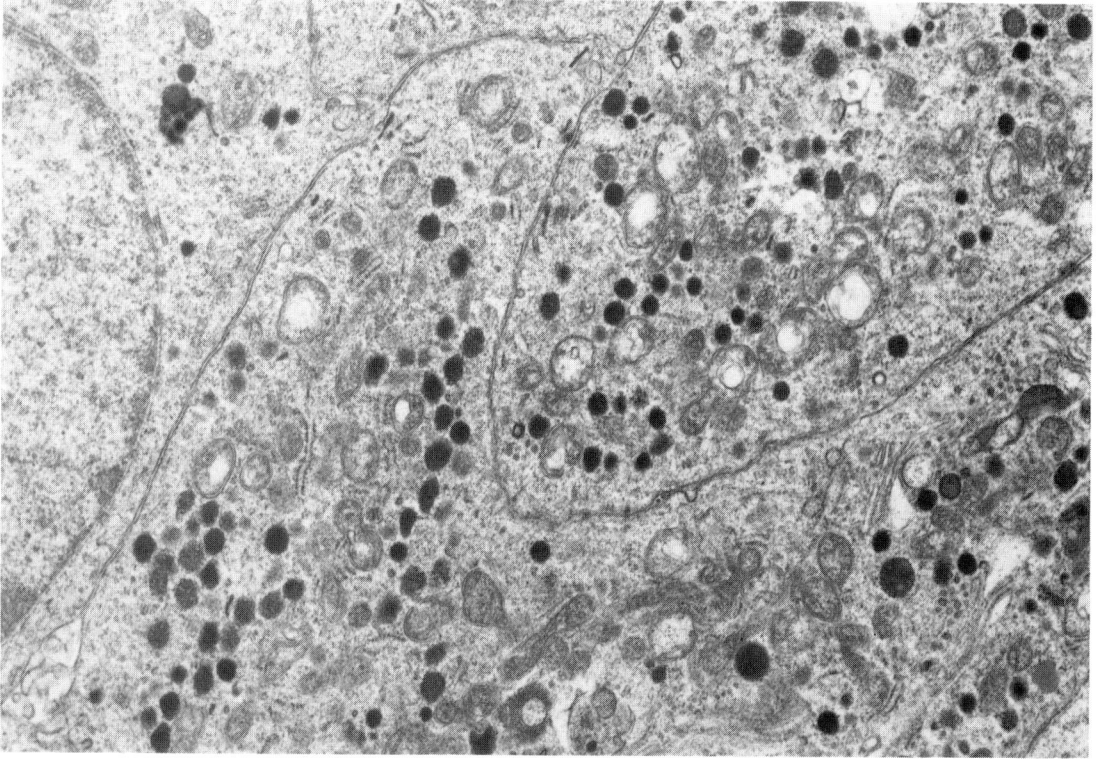

Fig. 8.105   Electron micrograph of carcinoid showing electron-dense polymorphic granules with a mean diameter of 280 nm (× 16 500). Courtesy of Dr J. Polak, RPMS.

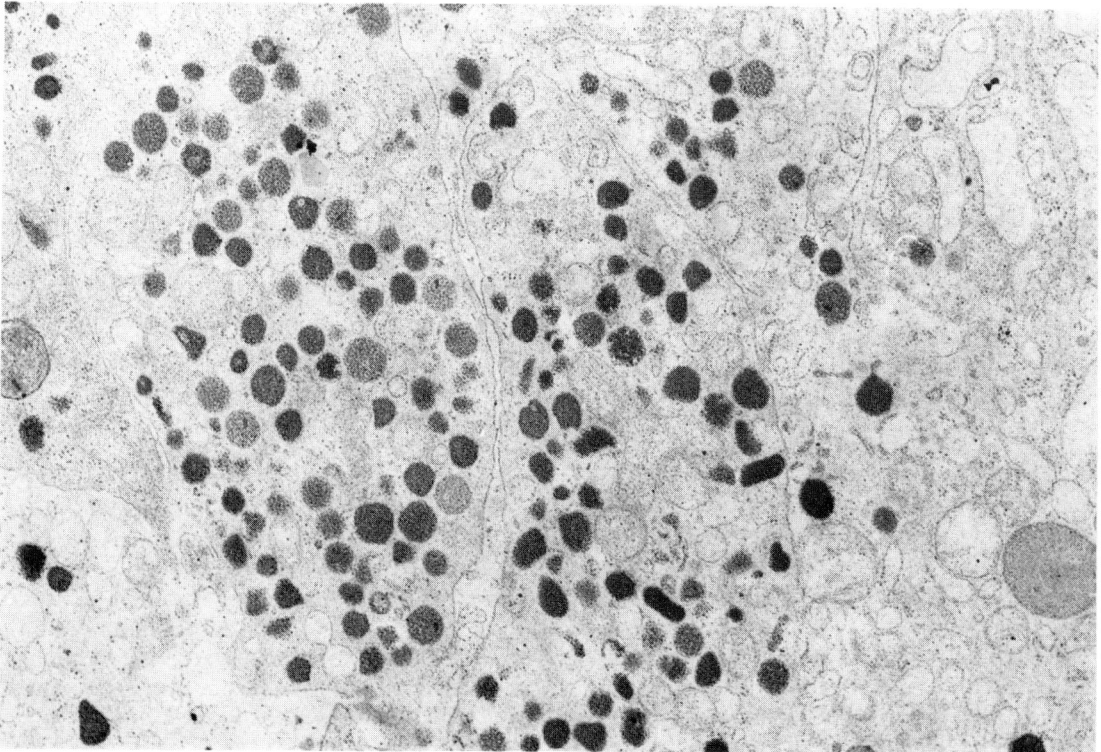

Fig. 8.106   Electron micrograph of carcinoid following application of the Masson–Fontana argentaffin reaction. Not counterstained (× 22 000). Courtesy of Dr J. Polak, RPMS.

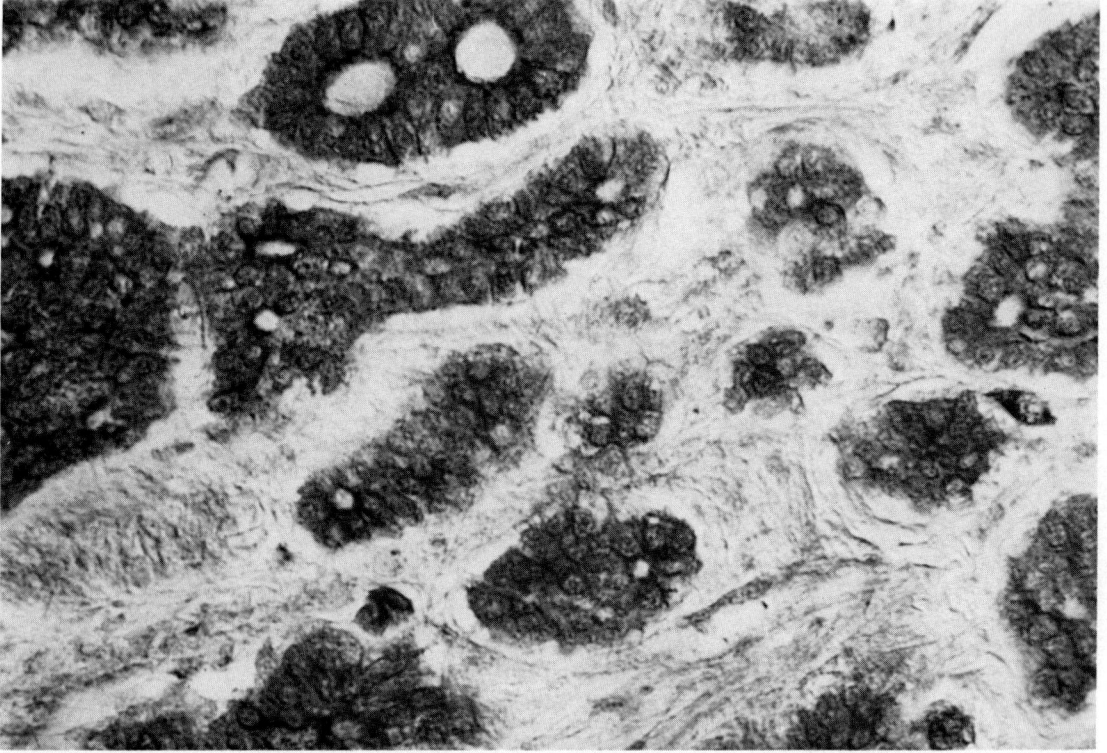

Fig. 8.107 Carcinoid of the gastrointestinal tract showing positive immunostaining for neuron specific enolase (NSE) (× 280). Courtesy of Dr J. Polak, RPMS.

The relationship between the primary tumour and the development of the carcinoid syndrome

The carcinoid syndrome occurs only when the tumour produces vasoactive and other substances which reach the systemic circulation. With gastrointestinal carcinoids, the presence of the syndrome is therefore associated with the presence of hepatic metastases in 95% of cases.[10] Occasionally, however, primary tumours in the gut or tumours with extensive nodal involvement and direct access to the systemic venous circulation will produce the syndrome.[10, 15] Carcinoid elements in ovarian teratomas can produce a syndrome in the absence of hepatic metastases, reflecting the direct venous drainage of these tumours into the systemic circulation.[76] Bronchial carcinoids can give rise to the syndrome in the absence of metastases, though in fact metastases are present in most cases.[59] In addition, rarely tumours of thyroid C cells may produce the carcinoid syndrome,[50] as may oat cell carcinomas of the lung.[23] Not all carcinoids produce the carcinoid syndrome when metastases are present. The approximate incidence of primary carcinoid

tumours, their propensity to metastasize and their ability to produce the carcinoid syndrome are shown in Table 8.54.

Clinical features of carcinoid tumours

Carcinoid tumours are usually unrelated to other disease processes, but there may be an apparent association with von Recklinghausen's neurofibromatosis (an autosomal dominant condition affecting tissues of neurocrest origin).[33] Multiple gastric carcinoids have been reported in a few patients with pernicious anaemia and diffuse hyperplasia of enterochromaffin cells,[28] and carcinoid tumours of lung, intestine or thymus or the carcinoid syndrome may arise as part of the multiple endocrine neoplasia syndrome Type 1.[2, 14, 77] Carcinoids have been described which not only contain but also secrete other hormones, including insulin,[66] growth hormone, ACTH, gastrin, calcitonin, ADH, βMSH and vasoactive intestinal polypeptide.[23, 37, 42] It seems that carcinoids of foregut origin are more likely to produce such peptides than are those from the midgut.

An association of carcinoids with other neoplasms in 17–53% of cases has been claimed.[23] Whether this is a true association, or only an apparent association occurring in a group of patients undergoing extensive investigation, is not clear.

Carcinoid tumours without systemic features

The presentation of carcinoid tumours that have not caused the carcinoid syndrome is diverse and related mainly to the site of origin. In the commonest position – the appendix – the majority of tumours are found at appendicectomy. In about 30% of these cases it is possible that the tumour may have led to the appendicitis by causing luminal obstruction, but usually the carcinoid represents a coincidental finding.[48] Similarly, in the small intestine the majority of carcinoids are asymptomatic, but a minority (possibly 20%) give rise to pain.[23] Usually this is related to subacute small intestinal obstruction by the tumour, although the fibrous reaction, mesenteric vascular occlusion, intussusception or direct tumour spread may also be responsible. Rarely perforation or haemorrhage occurs. Primary tumours within Meckel's diverticulum behave in a similar fashion to small intestinal rather than appendiceal primaries.[7]

Duodenal carcinoids may present as duodenal or biliary obstruction, but may be found during the investigation of pain suggestive of a duodenal ulcer.[7] Gastric carcinoids are often asymptomatic but pain or bleeding following surface ulceration may also occur. The rare oesophageal carcinoids present with dysphagia. Colonic carcinoids present like cancer of the colon with changes in bowel habit, obstruction or bleeding.[7]

The radiological features of gut carcinoids are non-specific but tumours impinging on the gut lumen may be seen during barium studies as a smooth swelling or polyp indistinguishable from other intestinal tumours, though multiple ileal polyps are highly suggestive of carcinoids.[3, 31] Mucosal irregularity may occur secondary to invasion, lymphatic obstruction or oedema. Mesenteric metastatic deposits may calcify. Bony deposits may be osteoblastic or osteolytic.[23] Angiography may demonstrate distorted stellate vessels in the region of the primary tumour and hepatic metastases are usually vascular.[22, 58] Computerized tomography may also be of assistance in identifying tumours.[65]

Bronchial carcinoids may present simply as a coin lesion on routine chest radiographs, or with cough, wheezing or haemoptysis together with symptoms of segmental obstruction and infection with bronchiectasis, pneumonia or anaemia.[36] Bronchoscopy may demonstrate a submucosal mass in one of the larger bronchi (as with the gut, much of the tumour spread may occur away from the lumen – a dumbell tumour). The mass may, of course, ulcerate. Lung carcinoids are very vascular; torrential bleeding may occur after a diagnostic biopsy.

Ovarian carcinoids present simply as a pelvic mass. Thymic carcinoids may be asymptomatic or present with the symptoms of an intrathoracic mass, with chest pain, dyspnoea and cough or superior vena caval obstruction. They may also present with Cushing's syndrome.[77]

Treatment of carcinoid tumours without systemic features

Management of carcinoid tumours, whether of the intestine or the bronchus, presenting without the syndrome is surgical – at least for disease which is not advanced.[7, 36, 59] Debate centres on two points: the management of large appendiceal tumours and the operative approach to apparently benign isolated intestinal carcinoids.

As noted above, appendiceal carcinoids are only infrequently malignant. Furthermore tumours may not be recognized at operation but only subsequently by the pathologist. The incidence of recurrent or metastatic tumour is very small even if apparent danger signals are present. In one series, even though there was serosal involvement in some 60% of cases and intramural lymphatics were involved in 90% of cases, there was no evidence of recurrent tumour after a simple appendicectomy.[48] It has been suggested therefore that a simple appendicectomy is adequate for most cases,[48] but some authors suggested a right hemicolectomy should be performed if the primary tumour is greater than 2 cm in diameter or if there is evidence of extensive local spread.[7]

Unlike appendiceal tumours, the incidence of metastatic spread with small intestinal and colonic carcinoids is high. It seems appropriate in cases without apparent metastases to undertake more radical surgery involving excision of the tumour with relatively wide margins and removal of adjacent lymph nodes and mesentery.[7, 71]

The optimal surgical policy for apparently solitary hepatic secondaries is unclear, but if metastases are surgically amenable then local hepatic resection may be appropriate. Radiotherapy and chemotherapy have been used in carcinoid tumours with widespread metastases but results have been disappointing.[25] An initial report suggesting benefit from external radiation in carcinoid tumours[19] was not borne out in a subsequent report from the same unit.[34] Hepatic embolization of massive tumour deposits causing severe pain may produce good symptom relief.

Clinical features of the carcinoid syndrome

General features
The syndrome affects both sexes equally, with the sixth decade being the most common time to present. All forms of temporal relationship to the appearance of the primary tumour have been reported, from an initial presentation with the syndrome in the absence of physical signs of primary or secondary tumour to presentation years after resection of a primary. However, over half the patients have physical signs of advanced metastatic disease at the time of presentation.

The cardinal features of the syndrome are flushing, diarrhoea and heart disease. The differing symptoms of individual patients reflect tumour origin and mass, the length of the history, and qualitative and quantitative differences in the release of tumour products. However, a patient with advanced disease is readily diagnosed at the bedside, being a weak cachectic individual with a continuous flush, plethora, facial and peripheral oedema, and marked knobbly hepatomegaly, often with an hepatic friction rub. As already stated, however, many patients lack one or more of these features.

Cutaneous manifestations
Flushing attacks affecting mainly the upper part of the body are the commonest manifestations of the syndrome, occurring in about 90% of patients. Flushes vary from patient to patient and may last from a few minutes to hours, and may be associated with a violaceous tinge, sweating, lacrimation, itching, facial and conjunctival oedema, palpitations, hypotension or diarrhoea. Whilst some patients are acutely disturbed by their flushes, others may be entirely unaware of them. The episodes may be spontaneous or precipitated by stress, alcohol, exertion, certain foods or abdominal palpation, and may be pharmacologically induced by infusions of noradrenaline (norepinephrine).[23] Grahame-Smith[23] has classified flushing into four clinical types, but only one of these is clinically distinctive: gastric carcinoids which produce histamine as well as other products may cause a specific pattern of a bright red geographical flush of the face and neck. However, there is a tendency for the flushing due to bronchial carcinoid to also follow a pattern, which is associated with salivation, lacrimation, hypotension, oedema, nausea, vomiting and diarrhoea.

As well as flushing, more permanent changes may occur in the skin including facial telangiectasia, morphoea-like thickening of the skin, and more rarely the syndrome may be complicated by the skin manifestations of pellagra.[73]

Gastrointestinal manifestations
Diarrhoea is common, occurring in about 70–80% of patients,[23, 73] but is said to be less evident with gastric carcinoids.[53] In some cases it seems clearly related to circulating products, the diarrhoea being episodic and associated with obvious hypermotility and borborygmi. Such episodes of diarrhoea may or may not be related to episodes of flushing. In some patients a secretory state may occur in the upper small intestine as demonstrated by perfusion studies,[13] whilst in others the diarrhoea may be related to rapid transit. Steatorrhoea may occur, though this is rarer than watery diarrhoea.[35] The abdominal symptoms and diarrhoea may, however, be due to other causes: subacute intestinal obstruction may occur associated with the primary tumour or fibrosis of the gut wall, whilst intestinal resection for a primary tumour, bile salt spillage, bacterial overgrowth and lymphatic obstruction may all contribute to the symptoms. Abdominal pain may reflect intestinal obstruction, spontaneous necrosis of hepatic metastasis, or rarely gut ischaemia due to fibrosis causing narrowing of mesenteric vessels.

Cardiac manifestations
Only a minority of patients (up to 40%) with malignant carcinoids and the carcinoid syndrome have heart disease;[23, 73] it seems to be less common in those with gastric tumours.[53] Unlike the flushing and diarrhoea which appear as immediate responses to released tumour products, the cardiac disease is due to a slowly developing, histologically unique form of fibrosis usually involving the endocardium of the right side of the heart.[62] This fibrosis mainly involves the ventricular aspect of the tricuspid valve and the associated chordae. Less commonly the pulmonary valve is also involved and left-sided cardiac fibrosis has also been described, though this seems to be more severe when the primary carcinoid tumour is situated in the lung and therefore drains directly into the

left side of the heart. By the time patients develop cardiac manifestations, other symptoms of the syndrome have usually been present for a number of years. The clinical signs of the cardiac disease include a raised venous pressure with obvious evidence of right ventricular hypertrophy, and the presence of right-sided cardiac murmurs indicative of tricuspid regurgitation or stenosis or pulmonary stenosis. Together with these findings there is evidence of cardiac failure. Peripheral oedema develops as the cardiac failure worsens. All cardiac signs may be more striking during episodes of flushing.

Other manifestations
A similar fibrosis to that seen in the heart and around primary ileal tumours may occur on the intima of the great veins, the coronary sinuses or the great arteries, and in the pleura or the pericardium, the latter causing constrictive pericarditis. Retroperitoneal fibrosis may cause ureteric obstruction and Peyronie's disease of the penis may occur.[23]

Wheezing occurs in about 10% of patients and late onset asthma may occasionally be the presenting feature of the syndrome. As well as true bronchoconstriction, some patients get episodes of hyperventilation during flushing attacks.

Confusional states may occur in the carcinoid syndrome for a number of reasons; during prolonged flushing episodes, particularly in patients with gastric or bronchial carcinoids; as a feature of liver failure in advanced disease; as a side effect of therapy, particularly if parachlorophenylalanine is used; as part of the pellagra syndrome, or possibly as a specific carcinoid encephalopathy.

Ophthalmic changes may occur in flushing attacks, with fundal changes of 'sludging' within retinal vessels sometimes leading to occlusion.[79]

A minority (about 10%) of patients suffer with arthralgia with stiffness and pain in the hands and minor periarticular changes in the hands may be seen on X-ray. Some reports also suggest a myopathy may occur.

Pathogenesis of the carcinoid syndrome

5-Hydroxytryptamine (5HT)
Midgut carcinoids secrete large amounts of 5HT (serotonin) which is responsible for several of the clinical features. 5HT markedly increases gastrointestinal motility[26] and probably induces a secretory state in the small intestine.[13] In addition it may affect the kidney, reducing blood flow and changing renal handling of salt and

water. Together with histamine, 5HT may be responsible for producing asthma[27] and seems to be involved in the fibrotic reactions that occur in the heart and elsewhere.[23]

Foregut tumours lack the decarboxylase enzyme (Figure 8.108) and thus secrete 5-hydroxytryptophan (5HTP), not 5HT, though circulating 5HTP may be decarboxylated by other tissues to product 5HT. 5HT secretion is therefore characteristic of the midgut carcinoids (Table 8.53), but not foregut carcinoids, and may account for the different clinical manifestations of these tumours.

5HT is metabolized principally by monoamine oxidase (MAO) (Figure 8.108). Certain carcinoid tumours contain MAO and may thus secrete 5HT metabolites into the circulation. Furthermore the liver contains large amounts of MAO and thus 5HT secreted by gastrointestinal tumours does not reach the systemic circulation unless hepatic metastases are present – accounting for the lack of symptoms in gastrointestinal carcinoids without metastases.

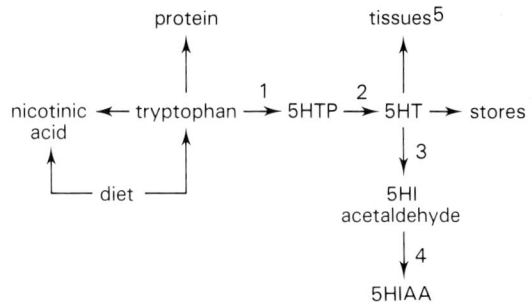

Fig. 8.108 Major pathways of tryptophan metabolism and the sites of action of drugs. 1 = hydroxylase (blocked by paracholorophenylalanine). 2 = aromatic 1-amino acid decarboxylase present in tissues and mid-gut carcinoids (partially blocked by methyldopa). 3 = monoamine oxidase present in liver and lung and some carcinoid tumours. 4 = aldehyde dehydrogenase. 5 = site of action of cyproheptadine and methysergide receptor antagonists.

Histamine
Primary gastric carcinoids produce histamine as well as tryptophan derivatives.[61] Histamine production seems to be associated with a distinctive flush (see above) and responds to combined histamine H_1 and H_2 blockade. Presumably the histamine production may also partially account for the reported increase in incidence of duodenal ulcer in the carcinoid syndrome.

Kallikrein
Carcinoids contain kallikrein, an enzyme which when released into the blood is capable of converting plasma kininogen to lysyl-bradykinin –

which in turn may be converted to bradykinin (Figure 8.109). These kinins are vasoactive and may be important in producing flushing in some, but not all, cases of the carcinoid syndrome.[55] Other actions of kinins include effects on intestinal motility and increased vascular permeability. Kallikrein release may be stimulated by sympathomimetic amines and may account for the precipitation of flushing by noradrenaline (norepinephrine) and alcohol.

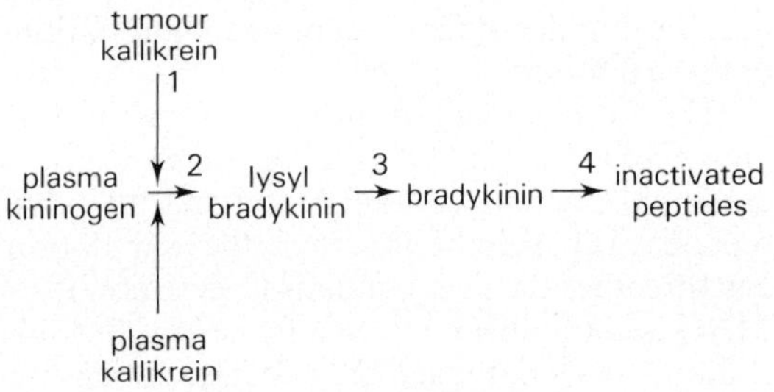

Fig. 8.109 Generation of bradykinin and the sites of action of drugs. 1 = release of tumour kallikrein promoted by norepinephrine and blocked by α-adrenergic antagonists. 2 = kallikrein, which is blocked by aprotinin. 3 = plasma amino peptidase. 4 = kininases.

Prostaglandins
Prostaglandins PGE and PGF (both of which are found within the normal gastrointestinal tract and which increase intestinal motility and induce fluid secretion) and other unidentified prostaglandins have been extracted from carcinoid tumours.[64] In addition, elevated serum concentrations of PGE and PGF have been found in patients with the syndrome. However, a review of these reports with an analysis of the response to prostaglandin synthesis inhibitors suggested that prostaglandins are unlikely to be major mediators of flushing and diarrhoea in most patients with the syndrome.[46]

Gastrointestinal hormones
Although somatostatin (which is known to reduce plasma concentrations of many peptide hormones) abolishes flushing and diarrhoea in the carcinoid syndrome,[18, 39] gastrointestinal peptides do not seem to be mediators of flushing or diarrhoea. When such symptoms were induced in patients with the carcinoid syndrome, there was no change in plasma concentrations of insulin, gastrin, pancreatic polypeptide, vasoactive intestinal polypeptide, gastric inhibitory peptide, somatostatin or neurotensin.[39]

Disturbed tryptophan metabolism
Even though not all patients with the carcinoid syndrome produce large amounts of 5HT, all

patients have disturbed metabolism of the essential amino acid tryptophan. Tryptophan is used for protein synthesis and as a precursor of the vitamin nicotinic acid, as well as being the precursor for 5HT. Normally only 1% of dietary intake of tryptophan is converted to 5HT, but in patients with the carcinoid syndrome, this may increase to 70% or more.[45] This diversion of tryptophan to 5HT synthesis reduces the availability of tryptophan to the rest of the body and may result in reduced protein synthesis with hypoalbuminaemia, and nicotinic acid deficiency with or without the clinical manifestations of pellagra (photosensitive dermatitis, neurological signs and diarrhoea).[72] These deficits of tryptophan and nicotinic acid may well be exacerbated by anorexia or malabsorption.

Other factors
Various cases of the carcinoid syndrome have been shown to produce a number of other biologically active peptides and amines (see above). In view of the rarity of these associations it seems unlikely that any of these substances are important in the pathogenesis of the features of the carcinoid syndrome.

Diagnosis of carcinoid syndrome

In most cases, once the suspicion has been raised, making the diagnosis of the carcinoid syndrome is not difficult. Urinary 5-hydroxyindol acetic acid (5HIAA) may be estimated quantitatively in a 24-hour urine sample. False positives can occur if patients are eating foods containing large amounts of 5-hydroxytryptamine, such as bananas, avocados, pineapples or walnuts, or taking drugs such as reserpine, acetanilide, mephenesin, methocarbamol, or cough medications containing glyceryl guaiacolate. Other drugs such as the phenothiazines interfere with the assay and may produce false negative answers. Mild elevations of urinary 5HIAA are also seen in the blind loop syndrome, Whipple's disease and coeliac disease – nevertheless, levels of greater than 30 mg (90 μmol)/24 hours are otherwise diagnostic.[23, 74] As already mentioned, foregut carcinoids tend to produce 5-hydroxytryptophan and not 5HT as they lack the appropriate decarboxylase. This can occasionally give rise to normal urinary 5HIAA excretion despite the presence of the carcinoid syndrome.[9] If there is a high degree of clinical suspicion, the urine may be screened for earlier metabolites of tryptophan by use of paper chromatography.[32] However, this is not usually necessary as even foregut carcinoids usually produce raised urinary 5HIAA excretion as the majority of circulating 5HTP is excreted as 5HIAA following metabolism by other tissues.[54]

Prognosis of the carcinoid syndrome

Primary carcinoid tumours grow only slowly and this is often true of the metastases. Patients with raised urinary 5HIAA levels may have only trivial symptoms of occasional mild flushing or mild diarrhoea for many years which requires no treatment. In one series, mean survival time in patients with the carcinoid syndrome was eight years, with some patients surviving up to 20 years.[57] However, in another series in which all patients had hepatic and/or bony metastases, survival was less than one year.[24] In the USA National Carcinoid Register containing 2837 cases the presence of the carcinoid syndrome was not specified, but in patients whose carcinoid tumours had metastasized widely, the relative five-year survival varied from zero for carcinoids of the stomach to 27% for appendiceal tumours (Table 8.55).[20]

Treatment of the carcinoid syndrome

The aims and mode of treatment will differ in different patients and may include removal of the primary tumour, blocking the effects or reducing the amounts of circulating agents by medical or surgical means, or simple palliation of advanced malignant disease.

Supportive and symptomatic therapy

The patients should be advised to avoid any factors known to precipitate carcinoid attacks, such as alcohol, provocative foods or physical activity. Particular attention should be taken to include sufficient nicotinamide in the diet. Heart failure should be treated with diuretics, and asthmatic attacks with aminophylline or salbutamol (this β_2-adrenergic stimulant does not precipitate flushing attacks). Codeine phosphate may be used to control the diarrhoea and potassium supplements may be necessary. If the patient has had an ileal resection for removal of the primary tumour with consequent bile salt spillage into the colon, cholestyramine may be of help.

DRUGS

Many drugs have been used to modify or inhibit the attacks of flushing and diarrhoea in the carcinoid syndrome. These act in a variety of ways: by inhibiting synthesis or blocking the peripheral actions of 5-hydroxytryptamine, by inhibiting release of tumour kallikrein, or by inhibiting the generation of vasoactive substances.

Inhibitors of 5-hydroxytryptamine synthesis

Parachlorophenylalanine. This agent has been shown to act by blocking the hydroxylase enzyme that converts tryptophan to 5-hydroxytryptamine (Figure 8.108). The major clinical effect is on gastrointestinal symptoms with a reduction in diarrhoea and abdominal pain, though there also seems to be some reduction in the flushing caused by foregut carcinoids. In some patients the drug markedly improves the patient's wellbeing, possibly due to its effect on gastrointestinal symptoms. The usual dose is up to 1 g four times daily. Side effects include tiredness, dizziness, anxiety, headache and psychic effects, including depression and hallucinations. Whether these are direct effects of the drug or secondary effects on brain 5-hydroxytryptamine concentrations is not clear.

Methyldopa. This agent partially blocks the conversion of 5-hydroxytryptophan to serotonin (Figure 8.108), but may also reduce catecholamine-stimulated release of flush-producing substances by the tumour. Methyldopa occasionally relieves flushing, but has little effect on gastrointestinal symptoms.

Table 8.55 Prognosis of carcinoid tumours.

| Site | Number of cases | Percentage with metastases | Age-adjusted 5-year survival rate (%) | |
			Local tumour only	Distant metastases present
Appendix	783	5	99	27
Small intestine	147	60	75	19
Stomach	19	55	93	0
Colon	33	71	77	17
Rectum	252	15	92	7
Lung and bronchus	151	21	96	11

Modified from Godwin.[20]

Prevention of release of substances by the tumour

Phenoxybenzamine. In some patients the flushes provoked by alcohol or catecholamines may be reduced by the α-adrenergic antagonist phenoxybenzamine in a dose of 10–20 mg four times daily, though patients seem to become refractory to its effects. β-Adrenergic antagonists do not seem to reduce flushing.

Phenothiazines. Phenothiazines may on occasion reduce flushing, possibly also through their action as α-adrenergic antagonists.

Inhibitors of kinin production

Aprotinin. In vitro evidence suggests that aprotinin inhibits the action of tumour kallikrein and thus prevents generation of bradykinin. However, it does not seem to be clinically useful in reducing flushing, and suffers from the disadvantage of needing to be administered by intravenous infusion.

5-hydroxytryptamine antagonists

Methysergide. This drug is a 5HT antagonist with mild vasoconstrictor actions. It frequently alleviates diarrhoea when used in doses of 3–8 g/day, but has little or no effect on flushing. Side-effects include heartburn, nausea, vomiting and abdominal pain, and it may cause diarrhoea as well as producing central effects including unsteadiness, drowsiness, confusion, insomnia, hallucinations and psychosis. Exacerbation of angina has also been reported. The major side-effect is, however, retroperitoneal fibrosis. Although this limits the usefulness of the drug in migraine, in the carcinoid syndrome (which may also lead to ectopic fibrosis) the benefits outweigh the risks.

Cyproheptadine. This agent blocks the actions of 5HT on smooth muscle and is therefore useful for the treatment of diarrhoea. It also has weak anticholinergic activity, is a histamine H_1 receptor blocker and is a mild central depressant. The usual dose is 4 mg four times a day.

Ketanserin. Recently serotonin S_1 and S_2 receptors have been identified and the S_2 blocker ketanserin has been used occasionally in the carcinoid syndrome. So far results from our own unit have been disappointing in all but one case, but there is a report of an apparently beneficial effect of ketanserin in reducing intestinal secretion and diarrhoea in one patient.[1]

Histamine antagonists

In patients with the carcinoid syndrome due to a gastric primary, a combination of histamine H_1 and H_2 receptor antagonists (diphenhydramine hydrochloride 50 mg six-hourly and cimetidine 300 mg six-hourly) seems to be uniquely effective in reducing the flushing and hypotension.[61]

Somatostatin

Infusions of somatostatin in doses of 500 µg/hour have been shown to abolish the flushing whether due to gastric or ileal carcinoids and whether these are induced by food, alcohol or pentagastrin.[18, 39] In addition diarrhoea is relieved.[12] Side-effects of this therapy include hypotension, bradycardia and severe rebound flushing on cessation of the infusion. It may be that in future analogues of somatostatin with a longer duration of action may prove to be useful.

Steroids

Prednisolone in doses of 20 mg/day has been reported as being effective in reducing flushing, facial oedema, diarrhoea and the hyperdynamic state associated with the carcinoid syndrome due to bronchial carcinoids. However, it seems to be ineffective in relieving symptoms due to gastrointestinal carcinoids.

SURGERY

Resection of an ovarian or bronchial carcinoid producing the syndrome is potentially curative. In the more common situation with hepatic metastases, surgery may be employed to reduce tumour mass either by partial hepatectomy[17, 71] (when deposits are confined to one lobe) or by shelling out metastases.[25, 43, 52, 80] Alternatively the hepatic artery may be ligated at laparotomy, but this has probably been superseded by hepatic arterial embolization because of more effective devascularization and lower morbidity.[44] Surgical procedures in patients with the carcinoid syndrome are potentially hazardous.[11, 51] Hyper- or hypotension, bronchial constriction, hyperpnoea, vomiting, diarrhoea, flushing and hyperglycaemia may all be encountered. The patient should be assessed carefully pre-operatively and given 5HT antagonists prior to the procedure (see earlier). Precipitants of flushing attacks should be avoided when possible and nerve blockers, acetylcholine, curare and morphine should all be used with care. Hypotensive attacks should be treated with transfusion and angiotensin (not catecholamines) and hypertensive episodes with hydrallazine.

Certain carefully selected patients have undergone tricuspid valve replacement when cardiac fibrosis and heart failure has been a major problem in patients who otherwise seemed quite well.[29]

RADIOTHERAPY

Although there is one report of radiotherapy inducing prolonged disease-free remission of carcinoid tumours with metastases,[19] a follow-up report from the same unit showed no benefit in the carcinoid syndrome.[34] Radiotherapy only has a place in producing symptomatic relief from metastases to bone and skin.

CHEMOTHERAPY

Several uncontrolled studies have shown a reduction in tumour size with a variety of chemotherapeutic regimens. Streptozotocin, alkylating agents and 5-fluorouracil seem to be the best single agents, with response rates of 30, 23 and 21%[25] (Table 8.56). Drug combinations seem to be more effective than single drug regimens and a combination of cyclophosphamide and methotrexate produced a 58% response rate in a small series. However in many cases

Table 8.56 Chemotherapy in carcinoid syndrome.

	Number of patients	Percentage response
Single agents		
Streptozotocin	23	30
Alkylating agents	39	23
5-Fluorouracil	29	21
Methotrexate	6	16
Dactinomycin	9	11
Mitomycin C	3	—
Doxorubicin	1	—
Dacarbazine	2	—
Combination therapy		
Cyclophosphamide and methotrexate	12	58
5-Fluorouracil and streptozotocin	53	38
Cyclophosphamide and streptozotocin	45	27
Doxorubicin and 5-fluorouracil	3	66
Cyclophosphamide and methyl CCNU	4	50
5-Fluorouracil, doxorubicin and methyl BCNU	2	—
5-Fluorouracil and BCNU	2	—

Single cases described with responses to streptozotocin and BCNU, cyclophosphamide and vincristine, cyclophosphamide, methotrexate and doxorubicin, and cyclophosphamide, vincristine and CCNU.
Modified from Mengel and Shaffer.[45]

'response' was merely a reduction in liver size and in general chemotherapy is not effective in producing symptomatic relief or prolonging life. Furthermore cytotoxic therapy may exacerbate symptoms,[47] presumably due to release of tumour products from necrotic cells. There is no evidence to support the suggestion that chemotherapy administered through a cannula into the hepatic artery is more effective than systemic administration.

HEPATIC ARTERIAL EMBOLIZATION

The advent of therapeutic introduction of emboli into the hepatic artery has offered a new approach to the management of the carcinoid syndrome. This procedure reduces tumour bulk and will produce amelioration of symptoms or even complete remission in most patients without the attendant risk of surgery, though its precise role in management has not yet fully been defined. As with chemotherapy, the destruction of hepatic deposits may release large amounts of tumour products causing severe symptoms, so blocking agents are used before and after the procedure.[41]

Forty eight hours prior to embolization cyproheptadine is given in a dose of 4 mg three times daily orally and 24 hours before the procedure parachlorophenylalanine is added in a dose of 500 mg three times daily. On the day of the embolization, the patient is premedicated with papaveretum (Omnopon) and scopolamine and broad-spectrum antibiotics (flucloxacillin 250 mg three times daily, tobramycin 80 mg three times daily, and metronidazole 200 mg three times daily). Just prior to the procedure, 1 g of methylprednisolone is administered, and an aprotinin infusion of 50 000 i.u./hour initiated.

Under local anaesthesia the coeliac axis is selectively cannulated via the femoral artery and the venous phase of the injection is studied to establish that the portal vein is patent. Having thus established that the liver will be viable even if the hepatic artery is completely embolized, the artery is selectively entered and an hepatic angiogram is performed. Once the site and distribution of the metastases has been identified, embolization of one or more branches of the hepatic artery is performed using sterile absorbable gelatin sponge (Sterispon) and human dura mata (Lyodura) in a solution containing gentamicin, followed by steel coils to segmental arteries. During the procedure fresh frozen plasma is available to treat hypotensive reactions and hydrallazine (10–15 mg intravenously) is available to treat hypertensive crises.

After the embolization, aprotinin (Trasylol), parachlorophenylalanine and cyproheptadine are continued for two to three days, and antibiotics for at least ten days or as long as the fever lasts to prevent infection of necrotic liver. Successful embolizations are manifest by fever, often up to 39°C, a leucocytosis and negative bacterial cultures. Aspartate aminotransferase (AST) levels rise often more than 20-fold, with a two or three fold rise in alkaline phosphatase. Bilirubin levels characteristically remain normal. Pain at the time of embolization is usually mild and an encouraging sign of tumour destruction. Abdominal friction rubs and right-sided pleural effusions occur on occasions.

One of our patients died from septicaemia after antibiotics were stopped on the seventh day, and one patient suffered necrosis of the gall-bladder requiring cholecystectomy – a recognized complication of hepatic arterial embolization since the cystic artery is a branch of the hepatic artery.

In eight of the first 12 patients treated in this way at out institution, flushing and abdominal pain were abolished; the other patients also responded but less dramatically. Diarrhoea was improved in all patients and urinary 5-HIAA levels fell significantly. Clinical remissions lasted from one to eighteen months and in two cases relapses were successfully treated with second embolizations with further remissions of up to six months. However, a third embolization in one of these two patients had no effect. Late deaths occurred due to heart disease or distant (non-hepatic metastases). The presence of bone or lung secondaries did not prevent remissions following hepatic embolization, presumably due to the reduction in tumour load. Whether long-term survival is affected by embolization is not yet clear.

SUMMARY

Patients with mild symptoms require no treatment other than avoidance of factors known to precipitate attacks. As symptoms become more severe a reasonable approach is to use cyproheptadine and codeine phosphate to control diarrhoea. Subsequently methysergide and parachlorophenylalanine may be needed. We have not found other agents to be useful (other than histamine blockers for gastric carcinoids) and find patients become resistant to pharmacological agents. At this point we proceed with hepatic arterial embolization, as it seems effective and carries a lower risk than surgery. Though we are prepared to embolize on more than one occasion, this decision should not be taken lightly as subsequent remissions are likely to be shorter than the first one.

REFERENCES

1 Antonsen, S., Hansen, M. G. M., Bukhare, K. & Rask-Madson, J. (1982) Influence of a new selective 5-HT$_2$ receptor antagonist (ketanserin) on jejunal PGE$_2$ release and ion secretion due to malignant carcinoid syndrome. *Gut*, **23**, A887.

2 Ballard, H., Frame, B. & Hartsock, R. J. (1964) Familial multiple endocrine adenoma-peptic ulcer complex. *Medicine*, **43**, 481–516.

3 Banks, N. H., Goldstein, H. M. & Dodd, G. D. (1975) The roentgenologic spectrum of small intestinal carcinoid tumours. *American Journal of Roentgenology*, **123**, 274–280.

4 Bensch, K. G., Corrin, B. & Pariente, R. (1960) Oat cell carcinoma of the lung and its relation to bronchial carcinoid. *Cancer*, **22**, 1163–1172.

5 Bensch, K. G., Gordon, G. B. & Miller, L. R. (1965) Studies on bronchial counterpart of the Kultschitzky (argentaffin) cell and innervation of bronchial glands. *Journal of Ultrastructural Research*, **12**, 668–686.

6 Bensch, K. G., Gordon, G. B. & Miller, L. R. (1965) Electron microscopic and biochemical studies on the bronchial carcinoid. *Cancer*, **18**, 592–602.

7 Cheek, R. C. & Wilson, H. (1970) Carcinoid tumours. *Current Problems in Surgery*, November, 4–34.

8 Davies, A. J. (1960) Carcinoid tumours (argentaffinoma). *Annals of the Royal College of Surgery*, **25**, 277–297.

9 Davis, R. B. & Rosenberg, J. C. (1961) Carcinoid syndrome associated with hyperserotoninaemia and normal 5-hydroxyindoleacetic acid excretion. *American Journal of Medicine*, **30**, 167–174.

10 Davis, Z., Moetel, C. G. & McIlrath, D. C. (1973) The malignant carcinoid syndrome. *Surgery, Gynecology and Obstetrics*, **137**, 637–644.

11 Déry, R. (1971) Theoretical and clinical considerations in anaesthesia for secreting carcinoid tumours. *Canadian Anaesthetists Society Journal*, **18**, 245–263.

12 Dharmsathaphorn, K., Sherwin, R. S., Cataland, S. *et al.* (1980) Somatostatin inhibits diarrhoea in the carcinoid syndrome. *Annals of Internal Medicine*, **92**, 68–69.

13 Donowitz, M. & Binder, H. J. (1975) Jejunal fluid and electrolyte secretion in carcinoid syndrome. *American Journal of Digestive Diseases*, **20**, 1115–1122.

14 Farid, N. R., Buehler, S., Russell, N. A. *et al.* (1980) Prolactinomas in familial multiple endocrine neoplasia syndrome Type 1. Relationship to HLA and carcinoid tumours. *American Journal of Medicine*, **69**, 874–880.

15 Feldman, J. M. & Jones, R. S. (1982) Carcinoid syndrome from gastrointestinal carcinoids without liver metastasis. *Annals of Surgery*, **196**, 33–37.

16 Felton, W. L., Liebow, A. A. & Lindskog, G. E. (1953) Peripheral and multiple bronchial adenomas. *Cancer*, **6**, 555–567.

17 Foster, J. (1970) Survival after liver resection for cancer. *Cancer*, **26**, 493–502.

18 Frohlich, J. C., Bloomgarden, Z. T. & Oates, J. A. (1978) The carcinoid flush: provocation by pentagastrin and inhibition by somatostatin. *New England Journal of Medicine*, **299**, 1055–1057.

19 Gaitan-Gaitan, A., Rider, W. D. & Bush, R. S. (1975) Carcinoid tumour – cure by irradiation. *International Journal of Radiation Biology*, **1**, 9–13.

20 Godwin, J. D. (1975) Carcinoid tumours: an analysis of 2837 cases. *Cancer*, **36**, 560–569.

21 Goedert, M., Otten, U., Suda, K. *et al.* (1980) Dopamine norepinephrine and serotonin production by an intestinal carcinoid tumour. *Cancer*, **45**, 104–107.

22 Goldstein, H. M. & Miller, M. (1975) Angiographic evaluation of carcinoid tumours of the small intestine: the value of epinephrine. *Radiology*, **115**, 23–28.

23 Grahame-Smith, D. G. (1972) *The Carcinoid Syndrome*. London: William Heinemann Medical Books.

24 Hajdu, S. I., Winawer, S. J. & Laird Myers, W. P. (1974) Carcinoid tumours: a study of 204 cases. *American Journal of Clinical Pathology*, **61**, 521–528.

25 Haskell, C. M. & Tompkins, R. K. (1980) In *Carcinoid Tumours in Cancer Treatment* (Ed.) Haskell, C. M. pp. 609–620. Philadelphia: W. B. Saunders.

26 Hendrix, T. R., Atkinson, M., Clifton, J. A. & Ingelfinger, F. J. (1957) The effect of 5-hydroxytryptamine on intestinal motor function in man. *American Journal of Medicine*, **23**, 886–893.

27 Herxheimer, H. (1953) Influence of 5-hydroxytryptamine on bronchial function. *Journal of Physiology*, **122**, 49P–50P.

28 Hodges, J. R., Isaacson, P. & Wright, R. (1981) Diffuse enterochromaffin-like (ECL) cell hyperplasia and multiple gastric carcinoids: a complication of pernicious anaemia. *Gut*, **22**, 237–241.

29 Honey, M. & Paneth, M. (1975) Carcinoid heart disease: successful tricuspid valve replacement. *Thorax*, **30**, 464–469.

30 Hsu, C., Ma, L., Wong, L. C. & Chan, C. W. (1981) Non-endocrine carcinoid tumour of the uterine cervix – aspects of diagnosis and treatment. *British Journal of Obstetrics and Gynaecology*, **88**, 1056–1060.

31 Hudson, H. L. & Margulis, A. R. (1964) The roentgen findings of carcinoid tumours of the gastrointestinal tract: a report of 12 recent cases. *American Journal of Roentgenology*, **91**, 833–839.

32 Jepson, J. B. (1955) Paper chromatography of urinary indoles. *Lancet*, **ii**, 1009–1011.

33 Johnson, L. & Weaver, M. (1981) Von Recklinghausen's disease and gastrointestinal carcinoids. *Journal of the American Medical Association*, **245**, 2496.

34 Keane, T. S., Rider, W. D., Harwood, A. R. *et al.* (1981) Whole abdominal radiation in the management of metastatic gastrointestinal carcinoid tumour. *International Journal of Radiation Oncology-Biology-Physics*, **7**, 1519–1521.

35 Kowlessar, O. D., Law, D. H. & Sleisenger, M. H. (1959) Malabsorption syndrome associated with carcinoid tumour. *American Journal of Medicine*, **27**, 673–677.

36 Lawson, R. M., Ramanathan, L., Hurley, G. *et al.* (1976) Bronchial adenoma: review of 18-year experience of the Brompton Hospital. *Thorax*, **31**, 245–253.

37 Leveston, S. A., McKeel, D. W. Jr., Buckley, P. J. *et al.* (1981) Acromegaly and Cushing's syndrome associated with a foregut carcinoid. *Journal of Clinical Endocrinology and Metabolism*, **53**, 682–689.

38 Linell, F. & Mansson, K. (1966) On the prevalence and incidence of carcinoids in Malmo. *Acta Medica Scandinavica*, **179** (Supplement), 377–382.

39 Long, R. G., Peters, J. R., Grahame-Smith, D. G. *et al.* (1980) Effect of somatastatin on flushing and gastrointestinal peptides in the carcinoid syndrome. *Clinical Science*, **59**, 9P.

40 MacDonald, R. A. (1956) A study of 356 carcinoids of the gastrointestinal tract. *American Journal of Medicine*, **21**, 867–878.

41 Maton, P. N., Camilleri, M., Griffin, G. *et al.* (1983) The role of hepatic arterial embolisation in the carcinoid syndrome. *British Medical Journal*, in press.

42 Matsuyama, M., Inoue, T., Ariyoshi, Y. *et al.* (1979) Argyrophil cell carcinoma of the uterine cervix with ectopic production of ACTH, βMSH, serotonin, histamine and amylase. *Cancer*, **44**, 1813–1823.

43 McDermott, W. V. & Hensle, T. W. (1973) Metastatic carcinoid to the liver treated by hepatic dearterialisation. *Annals of Surgery*, **180**, 305–308.

44 Melia, W. M., Nunnerly, H. B., Johnson, P. J. & Williams, R. (1982) Use of devascularisation and cytotoxic drugs in 30 patients with the carcinoid syndrome. *British Journal of Cancer*, **46**, 331–339.

45 Mengel, C. E. & Shaffer, R. D. (1973) The carcinoid syndrome. In *Cancer Medicine* (Ed.) Holland, J. F. & Frei, E. pp. 1584–1594. Philadelphia: Lea and Febiger.

46 Metz, S. A., McRae, J. R. & Robertson, P. R. (1981) Prostaglandins as mediators of paraneoplastic syndromes. Review and update. *Metabolism*, **30**, 299–316.

47 Moertel, C. G. (1975) Clinical management of advanced gastrointestinal cancer. *Cancer*, **36**, 675–682.

48 Moertel, C. G., Dockerty, M. B. & Judd, E. S. (1968) Carcinoid tumors of the vermiform appendix. *Cancer*, **21**, 270–278.

49 Moertel, C. G., Sauer, G., Dockerty, M. B. & Bagenstoss, A. H. (1961) Life history of the carcinoid tumor of the small intestine. *Cancer*, **14**, 901–912.

50 Moertel, C. G., Beahrs, O., Woolmer, L. B. & Tyce, G. M. (1965) 'Malignant carcinoid syndrome' associated with non-carcinoid tumours. *New England Journal of Medicine*, **273**, 244–248.

51 Murphy, D. M., Lockhart, C. H. & Burrington, J. D. (1975) Anaesthetic considerations in bronchial adenoma. *Canadian Anaesthetist's Society Journal*, **22**, 710–714.

52 Murray Lyon, I. M., Dawson, J. L., Parsons, V. A. *et al.* (1970) Treatment of secondary hepatic tumours by ligation of the hepatic artery and infusion of cytotoxic drugs. *Lancet*, **ii**, 172–175.

53 Oates, J. A. & Butler, T. C. (1967) Pharmacological and endocrine aspects of carcinoid syndrome. *Advances in Pharmacology*, **5**, 109–128.

54 Oates, J. A. & Sjoerdsma, A. (1962) A unique syndrome associated with secretion of 5-hydroxytryptophan by metastatic gastric carcinoids. *American Journal of Medicine*, **32**, 333–342.

55 Oates, J. A., Pettinger, W. A. & Doctor, R. B. (1966) Evidence for the release of bradykinin in carcinoid syndrome. *Journal of Clinical Investigation*, **45**, 173–178.

56 Okike, N., Berratz, P. E. & Woolner, L. B. (1976) Carcinoid tumours of the lung. *Annals of Thoracic Surgery*, **22**, 270–277.

57 Peskin, G. W. & Kaplan, E. L. (1969) The surgery of carcinoid tumours. *Surgical Clinics of North America*, **49**, 137–145.

58 Reuter, S. R. & Boijsen, E. (1966) Angiographic findings in two ileal carcinoid tumours. *Radiology*, **87**, 836–840.

59 Ricci, C., Patrassi, N., Massa, R. *et al.* (1973) Carcinoid syndrome in bronchial adenoma. *American Journal of Surgery*, **126**, 671–677.

60 Riddle, P. J., Font, R. L. & Zimmerman, L. E. (1982) Carcinoid tumours of the eye and orbit. *Human Pathology*, **13**, 459–469.

61 Roberts, L. J., Marney, S. R. & Oates, J. A. (1979) Blockade of the flush associated with metastatic gastric carcinoid by combined H_1 and H_2 receptor antagonists. Evidence for an important role of H_2 receptors in human vasculature. *New England Journal of Medicine*, **300**, 236–238.

62 Roberts, W. C. & Sjoerdsma, A. (1964) The cardiac disease associated with the carcinoid syndrome (carcinoid heart disease). *American Journal of Medicine*, **36**, 5–34.

63 Sandler, M. (1968) 5-hydroxyindoles and the carcinoid syndrome. *Advances in Pharmacology*, **6B**, 127–142.

64 Sandler, M., Karim, S. M. M. & Williams, E. D. (1968) Prostaglandins in amine-peptide-secreting tumours. *Lancet*, **ii**, 1053–1054.

65 Seigel, R. S., Kuhns, L. R., Borlaza, G. S. *et al.* (1980) Computed tomography and angiography in ileal carcinoid tumor and retractile mesenteritis. *Radiology*, **134**, 437–440.

66 Skrabanek, P. & Powell, D. (1978) Ectopic insulin and Occams razor: reappraisal of the riddle of tumour hypoglycaemia. *Clinical Endocrinology*, **9**, 141–154.

67 Soga, J. & Tazawa, K. (1971) Pathologic analysis of carcinoids. *Cancer*, **28**, 990–998.

68 Solcia, E., Capella, C., Buffa, R. *et al.* (1981) Endocrine cells of the digestive system. In *Physiology of the Gastrointestinal Tract* (Ed.) Johnson, L. R. pp. 39–58. New York: Raven Press.

69 Solcia, C., Polak, J. M., Larsson, L. I. *et al.* (1981) Update on Lausanne classification of endocrine cells. In *Gut Hormones*, 2nd edn. (Ed.) Bloom, S. R. & Polak, J. M. pp. 96–100. Edinburgh: Churchill Livingstone.

70 Sporrong, B., Falkmer, S., Robboy, S. J. *et al.* (1982) Neurohumoral peptides in ovarian carcinoids. *Cancer*, **49**, 68–74.

71 Strodel, W. E., Talpos, G., Eckhauser, F. & Thompson, N. (1983) Surgical therapy for small bowel carcinoid tumours. *Archives of Surgery*, **118**, 391–397.

72 Swain, C. P., Tavill, A. S. & Neale, G. (1976) Studies of tryptophan and albumin metabolism in a patient with carcinoid syndrome, pellagra and hypoproteinaemia. *Gastroenterology*, **74**, 484–489.

73 Thörson, A. (1958) Studies on carcinoid disease. *Acta Medica Scandinavica*, **334** (Supplement), 7–132.

74 Udenfriend, S., Weissbach, H. & Brodie, B. B. (1958) Assay of serotonin and related metabolites, enzymes and drugs. *Methods in Biochemical Analysis*, **6**, 95–130.

75 Viteaux, J., Salmon, R. J., Languille, O. *et al.* (1981) Carcinoid tumour of the common bile duct. *American Journal of Gastroenterology*, **76**, 360–362.

76 Waldenstrom, J. (1958) Clinical picture of carcinoidosis. *Gastroenterology*, **35**, 565–569.

77 Wick, M., Scott, R. E., Li C-Y. & Carney, J. A. (1980) Carcinoid tumor of the thymus. A clinico pathologic report of seven cases with a review of the literature. *Mayo Clinic Proceedings*, **55**, 246–254.

78 Williams, E. D. & Sandler, M. (1963) The classification of carcinoid tumours. *Lancet*, **i**, 238–239.

79 Wong, V. W. & Melmon, K. L. (1967) Ophthalmic manifestations of the carcinoid flush. *New England Journal of Medicine*, **277**, 406.

80 Zeegan, R., Rothwell-Jackson, R. & Sandler, M. (1969) Massive hepatic resection for the carcinoid syndrome. *Gut*, **10**, 617–622.

MOTILITY DISORDERS OF THE SMALL INTESTINE

The motor function of the small intestine ensures that the transit of food and secretions is regulated so that digestion and absorption are completed within its length and non-absorbable residues expelled into the colon. Neither the normal motor activity of the small bowel nor its derangement in disease are well understood for two main reasons: first, the length, complexity and inaccessibility of the small intestine are obstacles to systematic study; secondly, 'motility' is not a single entity susceptible to systematic study. 'Motility' is a term which embraces both the transit of material within the intestinal lumen and the movements of the intestinal wall which propel or retard the intestinal content. The relationship between wall movement and transit is complex; contractile activity of the wall may be propulsive or obstructive. Hence, terms such as 'increased motility' or 'decreased motility' are generally imprecise and unhelpful. For the clinician, it is disturbances of transit which are important, since it is these which will be reflected in dysfunction. For this reason, the classification of disorders of small intestinal motility is best considered in terms of disordered transit. There are few (if any) clinical tests for 'normal' or 'abnormal' motility which are both widely accepted and widely available; since investigation of suspected disorders of transit is often a matter of ingenuity and improvisation on the part of the physician, some understanding of the normal physiology is required.

Because the small intestine is a conduit between the stomach and the large intestine, it is not always easy or even possible to distinguish between 'primary' disorders of small bowel transit due to dysfunction in the wall of the small intestine itself, and 'secondary' disorders due to excessive fluid input from the stomach or obstructed output in the caecum; these 'secondary' disorders may be responsible for abnormal patterns of small intestinal movement which are indistinguishable from those caused by 'primary' disorders.

Normal motor activity of the small intestine

The motor activity of the small intestine is derived from the contractile activity of the inner circular layer and the outer longitudinal layer of smooth muscle. The property of contraction is inherent in the smooth muscle cells, but the occurrence of contractile activity in time and space is regulated by the extrinsic and intrinsic innervation of the small intestine, and probably modulated by local or humoral release of peptides (such as enkephalin and somatostatin) and amines (such as 5-hydroxytryptamine). The extrinsic nerve supply to the small intestine is from the autonomic nervous system and, as well as cholinergic and adrenergic components, it includes 'non-adrenergic non-cholinergic' nerves. The intrinsic innervation, increasingly known as 'the enteric nervous system'[10] consists of the myenteric (Auerbach's) plexus between the two muscle layers and the submucous (Meissner's) plexus deep to the mucosa. These plexuses are interconnected as well as being supplied by autonomic nerves. The intrinsic plexuses consist of a network of nerves connecting the ganglion cells, embedded in supporting glial cells. The neurotransmitters and neuro-modulators of the enteric nerves have not been fully described; neurones which show positive staining for a variety of substances, including enkephalin, somatostatin, vasoactive intestinal polypeptide (VIP), substance P and 5-hydroxytryptamine (5HT) have been reported.

There are three layers of smooth muscle – the longitudinal and the circular layer, and the muscularis mucosa. Virtually nothing is known about the movements of the latter. The longitudinal and circular layers consist of a syncytium of elongated cells orientated in the plane of the muscle layer. Junctional nexuses which are visible on electron microscopy appear to be the sites at which muscle cells are electrically coupled, so that the rhythmic electrical depolarization of the cells is virtually synchronous over an area of intestine. The cells with the fastest intrinsic frequency of depolarization, which are located close to the pylorus, act as a pacemaker zone. Electrical slow waves, generated at the pacemaker at a rate of 11/minute in man, rapidly traverse the longitudinal muscle layer, showing a frequency gradient declining to about 8/minute in the distal intestine. To this extent, the behaviour of the smooth muscle resembles that of the myocardium with regular, rhythmic and propagated depolarization. There is one important difference: contraction can only occur during depolarization (detected extra-cellularly as the electrical slow wave) but, except under particular circumstances, contraction is not seen with every cycle of depolarization. It is the neural control mechanisms which determine whether, at any given locus, depolarization will be associated with contraction. If the level of depolarization is sufficient, action potentials appear and contraction occurs. Because the cells are electrically coupled and synchronized, slow wave activity and 'spikes' which represent summed action potentials can be detected by a large volume electrode placed on the muscle mass. It is believed that the slow wave activity is in the longitudinal layer, while the spikes are derived from the circular muscle.

Co-ordinated and purposeful movement appears to be organized by the enteric nerves. Circular muscle contractions may be occlusive or non-occlusive, standing or propagated. When circular contractions are occlusive and propagated – almost always in an aboral direction – peristalsis will be seen and the luminal contents will be propelled along the intestine. Standing circular contractions separated by areas of relaxation will result in segmentation; these contractions and non-occlusive contractions serve to mix intestinal content by setting up turbulent flow. Contraction and relaxation of the longitudinal layer results in 'pendular' movements, which shorten or lengthen segments of bowel.

Physiological patterns of wall movement are usually abolished by anaesthesia and when the nerve supply is interrupted; thus our knowledge of physiological movement is derived from electromyographic studies in conscious animals and manometric studies in man. During fasting, the small intestine shows periodic activity.[5] A sensor at a single point will show a characteristic sequence of activity consisting first of a prolonged period of motor quiescence (about 40 minutes), followed by irregular contraction (for about 40 minutes), followed by a sequence of regular contractions at the frequency of the pacemaker; these regular contractions, which last for about seven minutes, are collectively known as the activity front, while the entire sequence is known as the motor complex. These complexes migrate (Figure 8.110) slowly down the entire small intestine, taking about 100 minutes or more to travel its length – hence the term 'migrating motor complex' or MMC.[8] Typically, activity fronts recur at 90-minute intervals,[7] but the repetition rate of MMCs in man is very variable (15–350 minutes),[6] although it is more regular during sleep.

When nutrient enters the small intestine, periodic activity ceases and only irregular contractions, representing a combination of mixing and propulsive movements are seen at all levels.[1] The return of interdigestive periodic activity appears to coincide approximately with the completion of gastric emptying.

The control of the MMC, and its abolition by food, is complicated.[9] The 'programme' for co-ordination of movement to produce the sequence and migration of the MMC appears to reside in the enteric nervous system; in the intact bowel, MMCs are initiated by a sequence which involves the release of the peptide motilin, but the onward propagation of the MMC through the small intestine is unaffected by motilin and unrelated to its release. The abolition of the

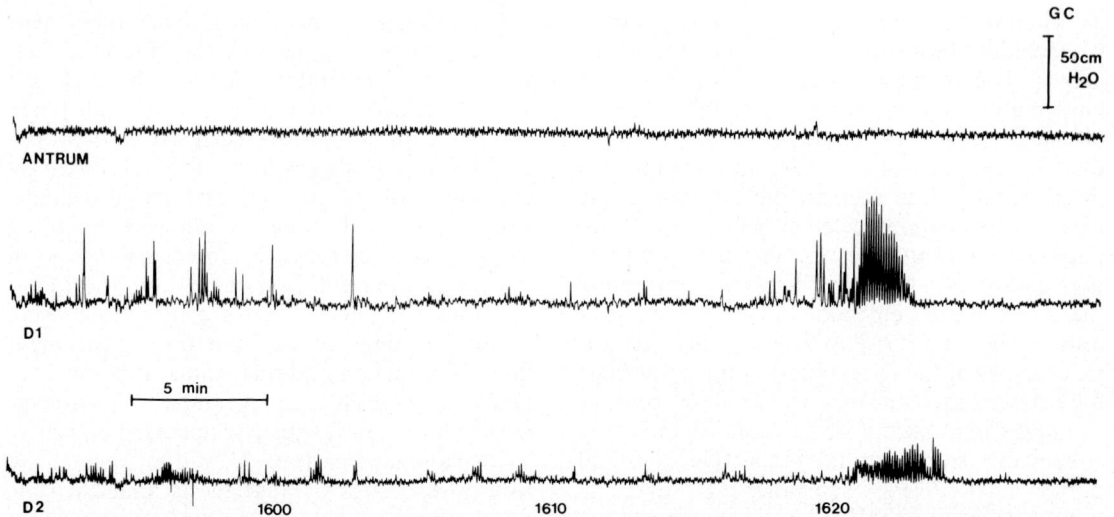

Fig. 8.110 Manometric study in a 23-year-old female, showing normal intestinal MMCs recorded from the duodenum (two lower traces). Irregular contractions followed by a burst of propagated regular contraction, followed by quiescence are seen. No contractions are seen in the antrum; in approximately 20% of MMCs, the antrum is quiescent. Failure to record antral activity can occur if the antral recording point is wrongly located at a more proximal gastric site. This recording was carried out as part of an investigation of florid symptoms including the inability to eat solid food, and the results confirmed the impression that the symptoms were hysterical.

MMC by food appears to be a neural event, probably initiated by duodenal chemoreceptors, and seems to be dependent upon vagal integrity.

The 'purpose' of the MMC is unknown but it is a fundamental property of the stomach and small intestine of most mammals (except the cat and, perhaps, the guinea pig). It has been suggested that it is an intestinal 'housekeeper', serving to clear debris and endogenous secretion along the fasted bowel and repel the orad migration of colonic flora. This is supported by some evidence that apparent absence of normal MMC activity is associated with bacterial overgrowth of the small intestine,[7] but while this may be true of man, it is certainly not true of ruminants; digestion in the ruminant small bowel is accomplished by bacteria even though they exhibit continuous periodic activity uninterrupted by feeding.

The clinical significance of normal motor activity
Because gross movements of the fasted small intestine filled with barium vary greatly, it is very difficult to be certain whether what can be observed in brief exposures to X-ray constitutes normal or abnormal motor activity. Manometric studies of fasted and fed motor activity have proved to be more helpful.

The *integrity of the muscle* can be deduced from the observation of contraction occurring at intervals, or multiples of intervals, corresponding to the slow wave frequency of the muscle. The *integrity of intrinsic innervation* is required for normal propagated periodic fasting activity. The *integrity of extrinsic innervation* is required for the abolition of periodic activity by food. While this may seem simple enough, other factors may invalidate these conclusions. In gastric stasis, for example, the rate of delivery of nutrient to the duodenum may be too slow to constitute an adequate stimulus for the normal postprandial abolition of MMCs even though the receptors and their afferent connections are normal.

Investigation of small intestinal motility

TRANSIT

Radiology
Observation of barium in the small bowel is the most widely used method of observing transit, but its value is limited. There is considerable evidence that the movements of the intestine in response to barium differ from those stimulated by a nutrient mixed meal, and so the transit of barium may be a poor guide to the transit of food. A more serious limitation is that the hazards of X-ray allow only very limited observation of barium transit. Even so, a follow through examination will give some indication of excessively rapid or grossly delayed transit.

Radioisotopes
Imaging of transit through the gut of a meal labelled with isotopes such as technetium and indium using gamma camera scanning has less to offer in the small intestine because of poor definition; overlapping bowel loops cannot be distinguished. These techniques, when normal values have been established, can give an *indirect* estimate of small bowel transit by comparing the kinetics of gastric emptying and caecal filling.

Breath tests
Detection of exhaled gases (hydrogen or $^{14}CO_2$) released by bacterial metabolism of substances in the colon can give an estimate of the arrival of a marker, such as lactulose, in the caecum. While useful in the study of normal physiology, such tests as the lactulose breath test are of limited value in disease states because obstructed or delayed transit is often associated with bacterial overgrowth of the small intestine.

MOVEMENT

Manometry
Manometry of pressure changes at multiple sites is the best method of detecting patterns of wall movement. Conventionally, this is carried out using an oro-intestinal tube with multiple lumens, connected to a pneumohydraulic water pump, through which water is slowly perfused; each lumen opens into the bowel. Pressure transducers attached to each lumen sense pressure changes in the fluid column transmitted from the bowel lumen. Recording over several hours is necessary to detect the expected periodic activity in fasting and its abolition on feeding (see above). The use of telemetric pressure-sensing 'radio-pills' stationed within the small bowel reduces the discomfort to the subject; however, this method is not widely used.

Electromyography
Numerous attempts have been made to record muscle activity by electrodes attached to an oro-intestinal tube. The problem of ensuring continuous electrical contact between the electrodes and the mucosa has not been adequately solved, and this technique has little to offer in clinical practice at present.

Disorders of intestinal motility

Since motility disorders of the small bowel present to the clinician as disorders of transit (rather than as disorders of wall movement) this offers a convenient basis for classification.

ACCELERATED TRANSIT

Aetiology

Primary or idiopathic. This is also known as 'intestinal hurry'.

Secondary. Causes include:
1 Post-surgical. Following surgery for peptic ulcer, accelerated transit may result either from rapid gastric emptying ('gastric incontinence') or an impaired motor response to food.
2 Gastrinoma (Zollinger–Ellison syndrome). Excessive transit may occur due to fluid overload as a result of hypersecretion.
3 Infective and post-infective. There is evidence from animal models that abnormal motility may be associated with infective diarrhoea; moreover, in some cases this may be a direct effect of a toxin on nerve or muscle rather than secondary to fluid secretion and distension of the lumen.
4 Carcinoid syndrome. Although not systematically studied, it is known that the diarrhoea associated with this syndrome is accompanied by altered motility. 5-Hydroxytryptamine is known to increase intestinal contractile activity and is implicated as a neurotransmitter in the enteric nervous system.
5 Diabetes mellitus. It is possible, but unproven, that some cases of diabetic diarrhoea may be due to accelerated transit caused by autonomic dysfunction, but it is more likely that most, if not all, cases are due to bacterial overgrowth of the small bowel.
6 Hyperthyroidism. Rapid transit with resultant diarrhoea may occur as a result of hyperthyroidism.

Investigation
A barium follow through examination may suggest rapid transit, but such examinations carried out on fasting patients may be deceptive. A lactulose or bile acid breath test may be more helpful. Manometry has not proved useful so far because the manometric patterns associated with accelerated transit have not been defined.

Management
Where the accelerated transit is secondary to other conditions, correction of the primary disorder, if possible, may remove the problem. The commonest cause of accelerated transit is following gastric surgery, usually as post-vagotomy diarrhoea. In such cases, surgical revision to treat 'gastric incontinence' may be helpful and the interposition of a reversed (antiperistaltic) loop has been advocated.

Opiates or opiate derivatives such as loperamide or diphenoxylate may be helpful in the long-term management. In most patients, diarrhoea due to accelerated transit is provoked by food, and modification of meal size, composition and timing may be helpful.

RETARDED TRANSIT

Aetiology

Primary. Chronic idiopathic intestinal pseudo-obstruction is a spectrum of rare disorders which are familial in some cases, sporadic in others. The pathology is varied, ranging from a generalized disorder of smooth muscle, often affecting the urinary tract with associated hydroureter and hydronephrosis, through mixed enteric nerve and muscle damage, to a pure enteric neuropathy. The condition presents as repeated episodes of subacute intestinal obstruction. The lesion may be generalized throughout the small and large bowel or confined to one area, as in cases of megaduodenum.[2, 4]

Secondary. Causes include:
1   Subacute and acute obstruction, as in Crohn's disease.
2   Paralytic ileus following surgery or associated with peritonitis.
3   Dysautonomias. Retarded transit may be associated with autonomic nerve damage, as in the Shy–Drager syndrome, diabetes mellitus and acute intermittent porphyria.
4   Scleroderma. Transit is delayed in progressive systemic sclerosis;[3] a patchy infiltrative myopathy is seen. Some cases of chronic idiopathic pseudo-obstruction show similar lesions confined to the bowel without evidence of the involvement of any other system.
5   Hypothyroidism. Slow intestinal transit with associated constipation is a common feature of myxoedema.
6   Chagas' disease. Infestation with *Trypanosoma cruzii* may affect the small intestine, although the oesophagus and colon are probably more commonly involved.

Investigation
The presentation of retarded small intestinal transit may be acute, as typical acute or subacute obstruction, or chronic, when the predominant feature is constipation. The investigation of the acute condition follows normal surgical management. The investigation of chronic cases is more difficult. Barium follow through studies will show slow transit and often dilated bowel loops with or without faecal obstruction may be seen. Since the problem may be secondary to colonic dysfunction, investigation of the colon by barium enema is important.

When it has become clear that the small intestine is involved, evidence of systemic disorders should be sought. If there is no evidence of contributory pathology outside the bowel, then manometric investigation of the small bowel is indicated. This is not always simple, since the retardation of transit may apply to the passage of a manometric tube; this can be solved by the introduction of a guide wire using a gastroscope along which a manometric tube may be threaded.

The motor abnormalities observed are usually of a bowel which is either hypotonic or hypertonic; the expected periodicity on fasting and its abolition by feeding may be absent (Figures 8.110 and 8.111). From the observed changes and a knowledge of the normal physiology, it may be possible to deduce whether the lesion is myopathic or neuropathic and, if the latter, which elements of the neural regulatory systems are involved. If surgery is required for diagnostic or therapeutic reasons, a full-thickness biopsy may be valuable; silver staining of the specimen will be required to demonstrate neuropathy.

Treatment
It is rarely possible to correct retarded transit, whether primary or secondary in origin; only myxoedema is readily treated. In the first instance management should be conservative, even though this rarely restores normal function. Osmotic purgatives such as lactulose may be helpful and some patients benefit from bulking agents such as ispaghula husk. Other patients benefit from dietary manipulation, but this must be a matter of trial and error in each case. Theoretically, surgery has more to offer by reducing the length of bowel which has to be traversed or by the surgical bypass of apparently obstructive areas. In practice, the data on which surgical procedures are based are usually scanty and often inadequate; operations often prove to be a disappointment to surgeon and patient alike. Surgery should not be undertaken lightly and procedures used should be capable of revision should they prove unsuccessful. A temporary ileostomy or jejunostomy may, if successful, be revised at a later date into an ileocolic or jejunocolic anastomosis, but bowel should not be removed unless patient and surgeon alike are satisfied that this will be beneficial. Each successive surgical intervention increases the risk of future problems from adhesions and, in particular, from declining morale in the patient.

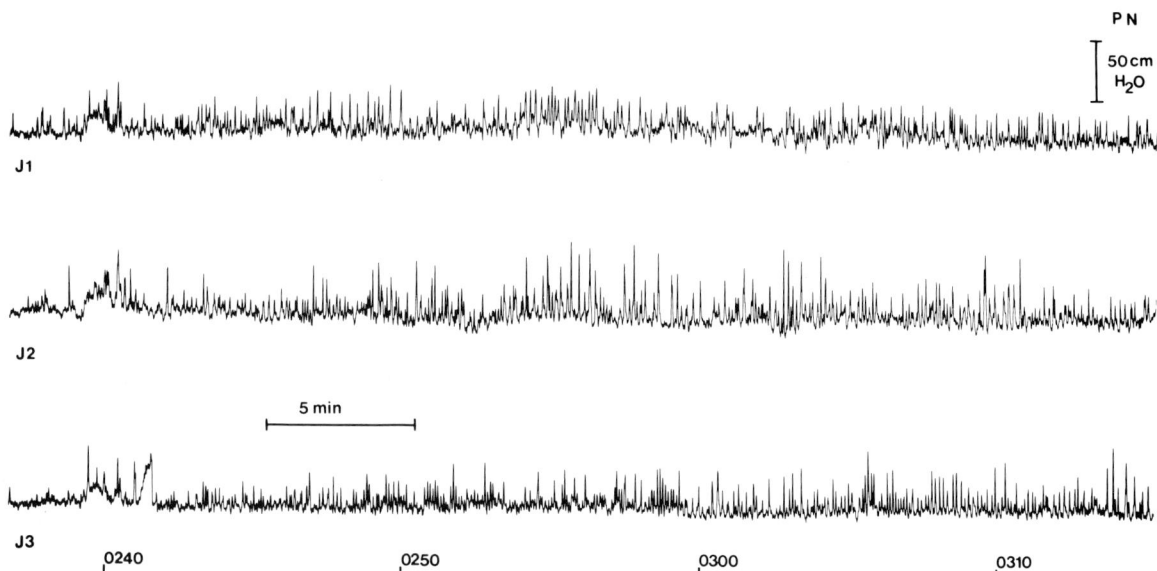

Fig. 8.111 Manometric study carried out in a 35-year-old female suffering from chronic intestinal pseudo-obstruction. In comparison with Figure 8.110, there is complete absence of periodic activity, with hyperactivity of the jejunum at all three recording sites. The small intestine was thus obstructed because of unco-ordinated hyperactivity; the cause, which was confirmed histologically, was acquired idiopathic degeneration of the myenteric plexus.

'FUNCTIONAL' DISORDERS OF TRANSIT

It is only in recent years that the normal motor physiology of the small intestine has been clarified; it has become clear that regulation of motility is complex, but also that the range of 'normality' is wide. While it is possible that some, or many, of the cases of 'functional disorders' of the bowel may be due to abnormal motor function of the small intestine, the incidence and nature of these cases remain to be defined. The systematic study of such patients on a large scale, which might answer these questions, remains to be performed and, until then, there is nothing of value to clinical practice which can be stated on the subject.

REFERENCES

1 Code, C. F. & Marlett, J. A. (1975) The interdigestive myoelectric complex of the stomach and small bowel of dogs. *Journal of Physiology*, **246**, 298–309.
2 Faulk, D. L., Anuras, S. & Christensen, J. (1978) Chronic intestinal pseudo-obstruction. *Gastroenterology*, **74**, 922–931.
3 Rees, W. D. W., Leigh, R. J., Christofides, N. D. *et al.* (1982) Interdigestive motor activity in patients with systemic sclerosis. *Gastroenterology*, **83**, 575–580.
4 Schuffler, M. D., Rohrmann, C. A., Chaffe, R. G. *et al.* (1981) Chronic intestinal pseudo-obstruction: a report of 27 cases and review of the literature. *Medicine*, **60**, 173–196.
5 Szurszewski, J. H. (1969) A migrating electric complex of the canine small intestine. *American Journal of Physiology*, **227**, 1757–1763.
6 Thompson, D. G., Wingate, D. L., Archer, L. *et al.* (1980) Normal patterns of human upper small bowel motor activity recorded by prolonged radiotelemetry. *Gut*, **21**, 500–506.
7 Vantrappen, G., Janssens, J., Hellemans, J. & Ghoos, Y. (1977) The interdigestive motor complex of normal subjects and patients with bacterial overgrowth of the small intestine. *Journal of Clinical Investigation*, **59**, 1158–1166.
8 Wingate, D. L. (1981) Backwards and forwards with the migrating complex. *Digestive Diseases and Sciences*, **26**(7), 641–666.
9 Wingate, D. L. (1983) Motility of the small intestine. In *A Guide to Gastrointestinal Motility* (Ed.) Christensen, J. & Wingate, D. L. pp. 128–156. Bristol: John Wright.
10 Wood, J. D. (1981) Physiology of the enteric nervous system. In *Physiology of the Gastrointestinal Tract* (Ed.) Johnson, L. R. pp. 1–37. New York: Raven Press.

Chapter 9
Systemic Disease and the Gut

VASCULITIC AND CONNECTIVE TISSUE DISORDERS

Involvement of the gastrointestinal tract may accompany the connective tissue disorders and explain a vast array of symptoms which suggest abnormal gastrointestinal function. On occasion, significant gastrointestinal symptoms may precede the clinical diagnosis of a specific connective tissue disorder. More commonly, gastrointestinal symptoms present late in the course of the disease. The literature is replete with information describing the different pat-terns of gastrointestinal involvement in progressive systemic sclerosis (PSS or scleroderma), systemic lupus erythematosus (SLE), polymyositis/dermatomyositis (PM/DM), polyarteritis nodosa (PAN) and rheumatoid arthritis (RA). Although all of these disorders involve connective tissue and vascular channels, each is probably distinct aetiologically and pathogenetically.

The gastrointestinal involvement of this group of diseases includes not only the entire visceral gastrointestinal tract extending from the mouth to the anus, but also some of the parenchymal organs such as the liver, biliary tract and pancreas. Scleroderma and polymyositis are prototypal diseases in which predominantly smooth and striated muscles, respectively, are involved. In contrast, the majority of the gastrointestinal manifestations due to PAN are associated with inflammation and occlusion of vascular channels.

This review will consider the organ distribution, associated symptoms, and treatment of the gastrointestinal manifestations of the major connective tissue disorders. Those at the more vasculitic end of the spectrum – polyarteritis nodosa and Henoch–Schönlein purpura – are also described. Although it would be convenient if each of these disorders were well-defined in its gastrointestinal involvement, readers will note that there are significant overlapping features which may lead to confusion.

PROGRESSIVE SYSTEMIC SCLEROSIS (SCLERODERMA)

The gastrointestinal tract is preceded only by the skin and joints in the frequency of organ system involvement in progressive systemic sclerosis (PSS).[5] Oesophageal involvement in PSS was initially described in 1903[8] with subsequent radiographic demonstration in 1916. Thereafter, changes in the small bowel were described by Kraus and by Rake[21] and colonic involvement by Hale and Schatzki.[10] While the earlier descriptions of gastrointestinal involvement by PSS used radiographic techniques, manometric methods for studying intraluminal pressures within gastrointestinal organs were first employed to study this disorder in 1954.[7] Subsequent physiological approaches have included the measurement of myoelectric activity[6] and scintigraphic quantitation of aboral movement of an ingested bolus.[29]

In general, clinical gastrointestinal manifestations of PSS occur late in its course.[6] This delay in presentation is probably related to the pathogenesis of the disease which presumably involves an initial vascular abnormality followed by physiological alterations progressing ultimately to tissue changes. Therefore, gastrointestinal studies in asymptomatic individuals with PSS will frequently yield evidence of altered physiology and provide a basis for preventive therapy (e.g. gastro-oesophageal reflux) leading to reduction in complications (e.g. stricture). Occasionally, however, PSS occurs in the absence of obvious skin manifestations and in these instances the gastrointestinal findings may predominate.[9, 25]

Oropharynx

Commonly, the skin around the mouth may become sclerotic, producing a characteristic appearance and restricting the introduction of food into the mouth. Hypertrophy of periodontal ligaments may cause characteristic changes around dental roots. The gums may become indurated, friable or even atrophic. In advanced cases, the buccal mucosa and tongue may appear atrophic. On occasion, aphthous ulcerations due to moniliasis may complicate the clinical picture. All of these disorders may contribute to feeding problems.

Oesophagus

In PSS, the oesophagus is the most commonly involved gastrointestinal organ, occurring in approximately 80% of patients.[26, 32] Raynaud's phenomenon occurs in 90 to 95% of these cases.[9, 31] In one-half of these patients, no symptoms referable to the oesophagus are present. With oesophageal involvement in PSS, changes are confined to the smooth muscle of the lower oesophageal sphincter and the distal two-thirds to four-fifths of the oesophageal body. These abnormalities are demonstrated best by manometric examination[28, 30] and include decreased resting lower oesophageal sphincter pressure and feeble non-progressive contractions in the smooth muscle portion of the oesophagus, but normal contractions in the proximal (striated muscle) portion of the oesophagus and the oropharynx (Figure 9.1). The radiologist may

Fig. 9.1 (opposite) Oesophageal manometric tracings from different segments of the oesophagus in a patient with progressive systemic sclerosis. Pressure recordings from proximal, middle and distal leads spaced at 5 cm intervals are shown in the top three tracings, respectively. Recordings of swallows and respiration are also shown. Dark squares represent 1 cm withdrawal of the tube assembly. (a) The tube assembly is withdrawn across the lower oesophageal sphincter (arrows). A mean pressure of approximately 6 mmHg (Normal 12–26 mmHg) is demonstrated. (b) Pressure recordings from the distal 10 cm of the oesophagus. Note that all oesophageal contractions are feeble and non-progressive. (c) Pressure recordings from the upper oesophageal sphincter, the proximal 5 cm of the oesophagus, and the mid-oesophagus 5 cm distally, respectively. A normal upper oesophageal sphincter with a normal resting pressure and complete post-deglutition relaxations is shown in the proximal pressure lead. In the middle lead, normal oesophageal contractions (arrows) from the proximal oesophagus are demonstrated. More distally, feeble oesophageal contractions are observed. In (c), the paper speed is faster than in (a) and (b).

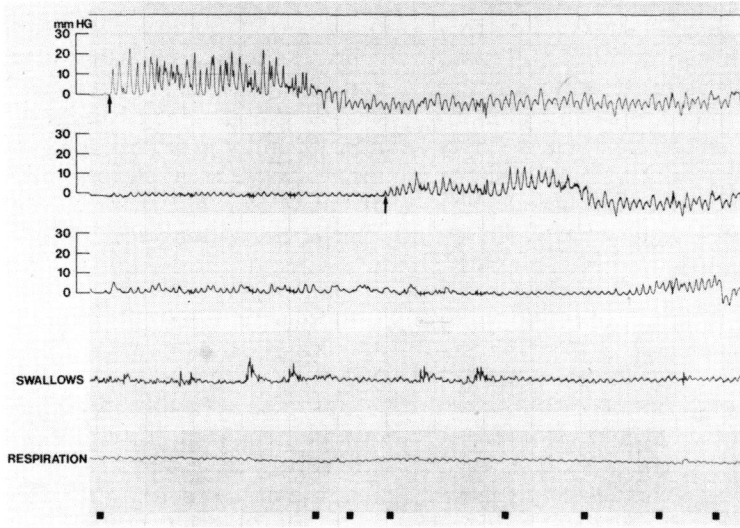

a

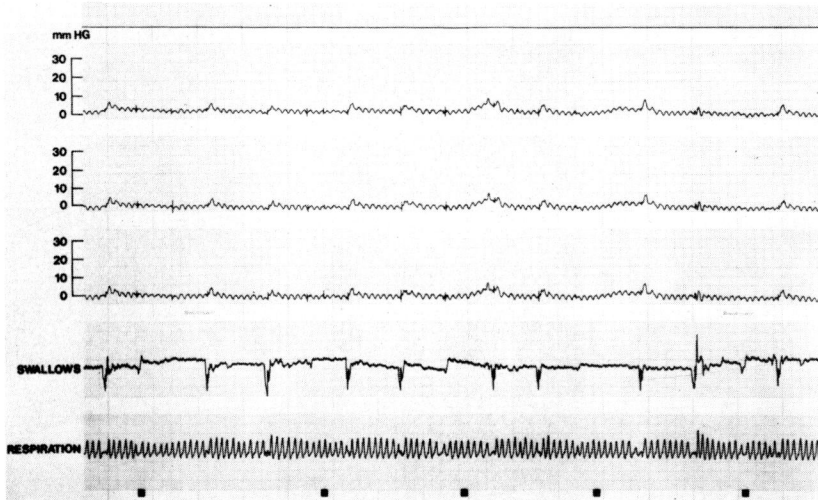

b

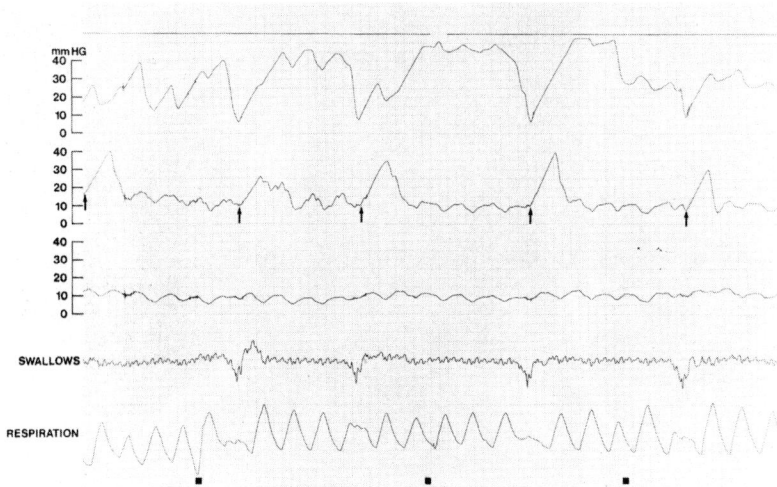

c

report feeble contractions in the distal oesophagus associated with poor emptying of swallowed barium. Care must be taken to examine
these patients in the prone or supine positions
because, if not, the force of gravity may empty
the contrast material into the stomach. Other
oesophageal radiographic findings include dilatation, widening of the diaphragmatic hiatus,
gastro-oesophageal reflux and strictures
(Figures 9.2 and 9.3). The body of the oesophagus may be dilated slightly or distension may
be so marked as to simulate achalasia. Differentiation from achalasia may be most difficult
when a benign distal oesophageal stricture complicates the picture. Significant gastro-
oesophageal reflux may be detected
fluoroscopically by acid reflux testing or using
gastro-oesophageal scintigraphy. The combination of gastro-oesophageal reflux and poor
oesophageal contractility may predispose to the

formation of benign oesophageal strictures.
Poor oesophageal emptying has been demonstrated recently using newer, quantitative oesophageal scintigraphic techniques.[29] Endoscopic
findings in oesophageal PSS range from a
normal oesophageal mucosa to severe mucosal
inflammation characteristic of oesophagitis.
Sometimes strictures can be visualized using the
endoscope.

Characteristic complaints attributable to
oesophageal PSS are: heartburn due to gastro-
oesophageal reflux of the gastric contents; dysphagia, usually for both solids and liquids; chest
fullness, especially after meals; and episodes of
nocturnal coughing associated with aspiration
of refluxed gastric contents while the patient is
in the supine or prone position during sleep.[17]

The typical histological findings associated
with oesophageal PSS are muscle atrophy
within the oesophageal mucosa with ultimate

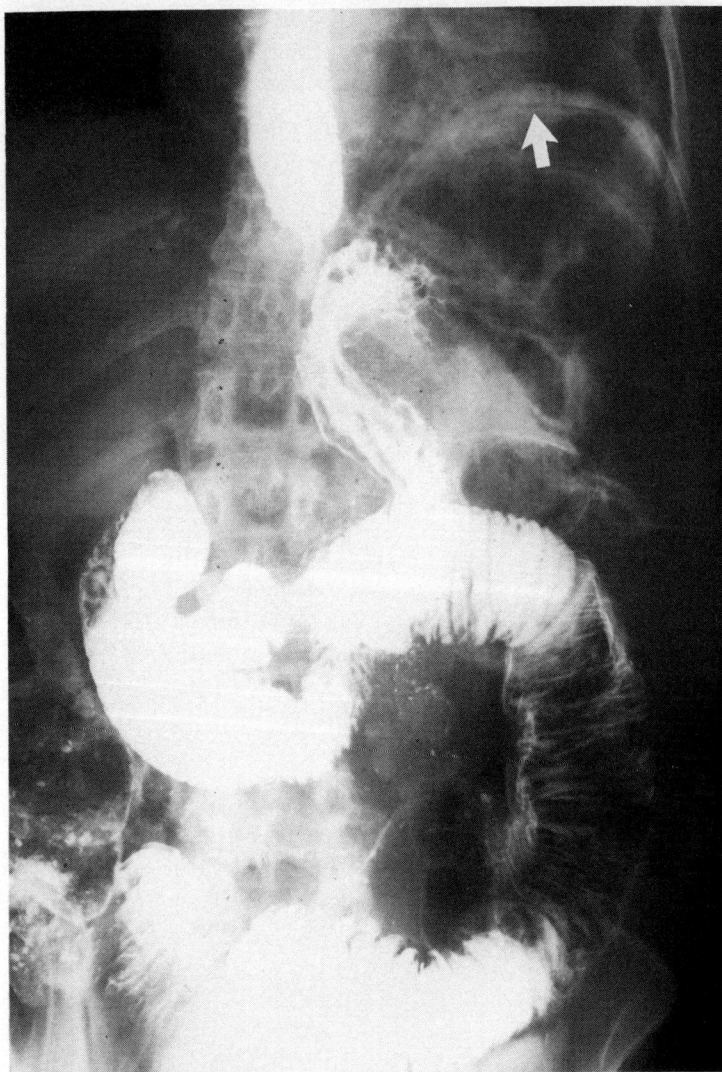

Fig. 9.2 Upper gastrointestinal
tract in a patient with scleroderma.
Note the focal dilatation of the
distal oesophagus with a stricture
at the gastro-oesophageal junction,
the dilatation in the second and
third portions of the duodenum
and the dilatation and prominent
valvulae conniventes resembling a
coiled spring in the jejunum. The
apparent free air under the left
diaphragm (arrow) represents
pneumatosis coli.

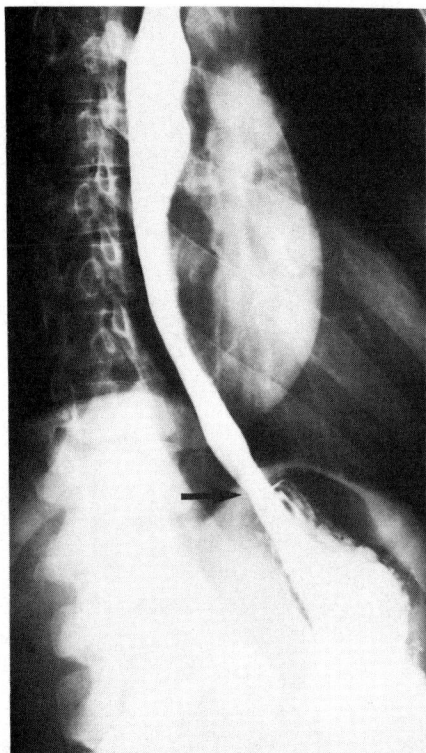

Fig. 9.3 Non-motile, non-dilated oesophagus of early scleroderma. The oesophago-gastric junction (arrow) is patulous.

replacement by fibrous tissue.[5] However, early in the course of disease, no fibrotic or atrophic histological abnormalities may be seen despite marked oesophageal motor dysfunction.[30] In such early cases of oesophageal PSS, the lower oesophageal sphincter pressure has been reported to increase in response to direct cholinergic stimulation but not in response to indirect cholinergic stimulation.[4] These findings suggest that a neural defect may be the earliest manifestation of gastrointestinal PSS. However, as time progresses, this physiological dysfunction is supplanted by muscle atrophy and fibrosis in the distal oesophagus, leading to dilatation and the other changes.

A vigorous anti-reflux regimen is the focus of treatment for oesophageal PSS.[20, 22] This includes: sleeping with the trunk of the body elevated in order to use the force of gravity to minimize reflux episodes; acid neutralization with common antacids or an alginic acid–antacid combination; anti-secretory treatment with H_2 receptor blocking agents; and specific anti-reflux treatment with cholinomimetic agents, such as bethanechol and metoclopramide, or the alginic acid–antacid combination which mechanically impedes gastro-esophageal

reflux. In very severe cases, anti-reflux surgery may be considered.[13] In view of the oesophageal motility dysfunction associated with PSS, surgery should be performed only as a last resort. In the case of PSS complicated by benign oesophageal stricture, treatment by an anti-reflux regimen and serial oesophageal bougienage (dilatation) is usually effective. On occasion, surgical correction of the stricture may be coupled with an anti-reflux procedure.

Stomach

Of the visceral gastrointestinal tract, PSS seems to involve the stomach least frequently (5%). Stomach involvement usually manifests itself as gastroparesis, i.e. delayed gastric emptying in the absence of a mechanical gastric outlet obstruction.[10] Delayed gastric emptying and gastric atony may be responsible for symptoms such as early satiety, postprandial nausea and vomiting, and epigastric pain. Gastroparesis may be demonstrated radiographically by a dilated stomach with retained barium for many hours. Recently, scintigraphic techniques have become the standard technique for measuring gastric emptying of solids and liquids simultaneously[11] and perhaps, if applied widely, sclerodermatous gastropathy will be found to be more frequent than has been recognized previously.

Small intestine

Small intestinal involvement has been reported in up to 50% of patients with PSS, usually in conjunction with oesophageal dysfunction.[5] Radiographic abnormalities involving the entire length of the small intestine have been described (Figures 9.2, 9.4 and 9.5). Dilatation and stasis are noted most prominently in the second and third portions of the duodenum and in the proximal jejunum.[2] In addition to dilatation, loops of the jejunum may appear thickened with an approximation of the valvulae conniventes resulting in a typical wire-spring configuration (Figures 9.2, 9.4 and 9.5).[15] Delayed small intestinal transit of contrast material and associated segmentation and flocculation of barium may be seen. At times the extensive dilatation of the sclerodermatous small bowel may simulate a mechanical obstruction (pseudo-obstruction).

While small intestinal involvement may be asymptomatic, the most striking symptoms associated with small intestinal PSS are diarrhoea, steatorrhoea, abdominal pain, abdominal distension and weight loss. These symptoms are

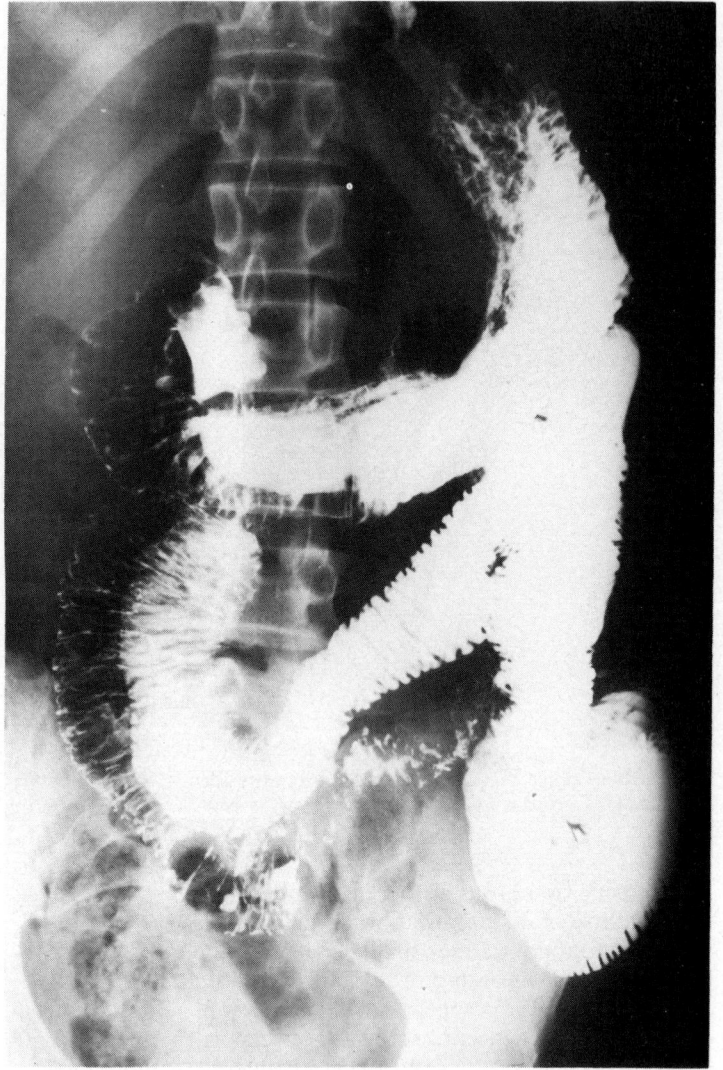

Fig. 9.4 Characteristic duodenal and jejunal pattern of scleroderma. Note the focal dilatation of the second and third portions of the duodenum. The jejunum is also dilated with a prominence of the valvulae conniventes resembling a coiled spring.

due to a combination of vascular obstruction, altered motility, impairment of the intestinal lymphatics and bacterial overgrowth. Of these, bacterial overgrowth is probably most important. Overgrowth may be associated with dehydroxylation and deconjugation of bile salts, coupled with direct damage to the small intestinal mucosa. These alterations may lead to fat malabsorption, decreased absorption of fat soluble vitamins, vitamin B_{12} deficiency, diarrhoea and weight loss. Less commonly, PSS involving the small intestine may present with more acute findings associated with true intestinal infarction, perforation, haemorrhage or ulcerations. There have been a number of reports of pneumatosis cystoides intestinalis with or without associated pneumoperitoneum resulting from obstruction, bacterial overgrowth of gas producing organisms and formation of

subserosal or submucosal cysts[18] (Figure 9.2). Histopathologically, muscle atrophy with little fibrosis is characteristic, but occasionally extensive collagen deposition has been observed. Nerve cells generally appear normal.

Physiological abnormalities have been recognized which may explain the clinical disorder of small bowel function noted in PSS. DiMarino *et al.*[6] evaluated duodenal myoelectric activity and observed small intestinal motor dysfunction analogous to that seen in the oesophagus. Rees *et al.*[23] found abnormal interdigestive motor activity in scleroderma patients with clinical evidence of small bowel involvement. Certainly, stasis of small bowel contents and its resultant complications could result from these defects.

The treatment of the small intestinal disorder of PSS requires awareness of the various complications. Bacterial overgrowth must be treated

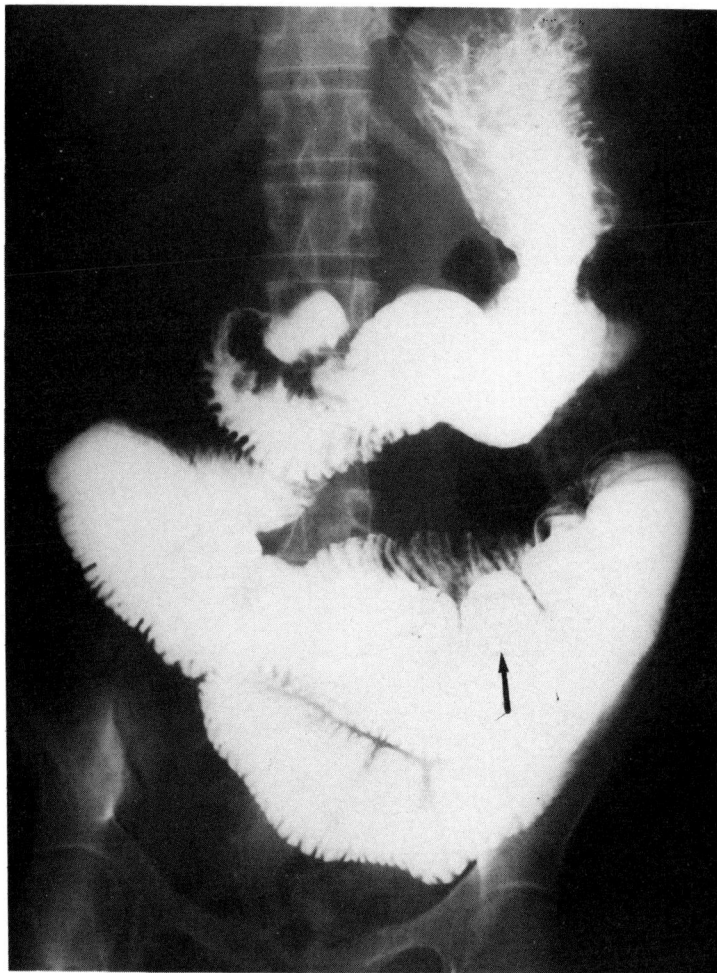

Fig. 9.5 Small bowel changes in scleroderma. Note dilated second and third portions of the duodenum and the sacculations of the jejunum (arrow) which closely resemble colonic haustrations.

aggressively with antibiotics (tetracycline 250 mg four times daily for 10 to 14 days initially) in order to correct maldigestion and malabsorption of fats and vitamins. The recognition of pseudo-obstruction is imperative in order to avoid unnecessary and ineffective surgical intervention. Conservative measures, including suction, bowel rest and hydration, are usually effective. Intravenous hyperalimentation may occasionally be used for the malnourished patient.

Colon

Although colonic involvement in patients with PSS is common (one-third of patients), symptoms referable to the large bowel are not often prominent. Usually, the colonic changes in PSS accompany other gastrointestinal involvement. Radiographic features of colonic PSS may be striking and include the virtually pathogno- monic wide-mouthed diverticula seen especially on the antimesenteric border of the transverse and descending colon (Figure 9.6). Wide-mouthed diverticula may be found also in the jejunum and ileum of PSS patients (Figure 9.5).[12, 19] Generalized dilatation may be present as well as hypomotility and loss of haustrations. The symptoms of colonic scleroderma may include abdominal bloating, a change in the calibre of the stools, diarrhoea, constipation and obstipation. Pathologically, atrophy and fibrosis of the colonic musculature may be found with colonic PSS. These changes are similar to those found in the oesophagus and small intestine. Complications of colonic PSS include pseudo-obstruction, perforation, infarction and volvulus. On occasion, mechanical obstruction may supervene due to a faecal impaction. Treatment of colonic involvement in PSS is non-specific, ranging from a high fibre diet and the use of various laxatives, to colonic resection in very severe cases.

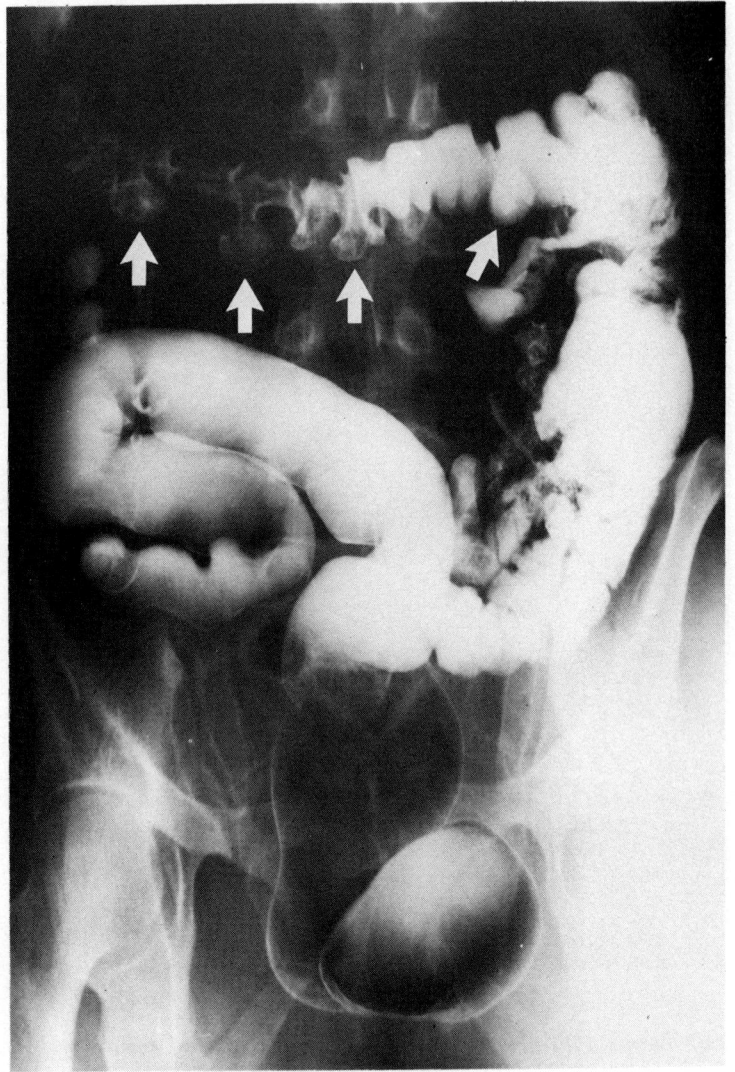

Fig. 9.6 Large bowel in a patient with scleroderma. Note the characteristic large mouth diverticula (arrows) primarily located in the transverse colon.

Studies of colonic motility in patients with PSS revealed findings similar to those found in the oesophagus and small intestine, i.e. a latent neural defect early in the disease and diminished muscle function in long-standing disease.[1]

Anal sphincter

In addition to constipation and diarrhoea, faecal incontinence may be encountered in patients with PSS. Impaired internal anal sphincter function has been observed[3, 14] and may account for significant constipation or faecal incontinence. Treatment of anal sphincter dysfunction is very difficult but behavioural techniques and electric stimulation may be helpful.

Liver

The association between primary biliary cirrhosis and progressive systemic sclerosis, particularly the CREST syndrome (Calcinosis, Raynaud's phenomenon, Esophageal dysmotility, Sclerodactyly and Telangiectasia) is well recognized.[24] The clinical presentation of these patients includes pruritus, jaundice, hepatomegaly, marked elevation of alkaline phosphatase and high titres of serum antimitochondrial antibodies in addition to the CREST features. In studying a group of 100 patients with primary biliary cirrhosis, three patients were noted to have the CREST syndrome.[27] In comparison, evaluation of 29 patients with CREST syndrome yielded 11 with evidence of primary biliary cirrhosis.[16]

REFERENCES

1 Battle, W. M., Snape, W. J., Jr, Wright, S. *et al.* (1981) Abnormal colonic motility in progressive systemic sclerosis. *Annals of Internal Medicine*, **94**, 749–752.

2 Bluestone, R., MacMahon, M. & Dawson, J. M. (1969) Systemic sclerosis and small bowel involvement. *Gut*, **10**, 185–195.

3 Cerulli, M., Nikoomanesh, P. & Schuster, M. M. (1976) Effect of progressive systemic sclerosis on electrical and motor activity of the internal anal sphincter. *Clinical Research*, **24**, 282.

4 Cohen, S., Fisher, R., Lipshutz, W. *et al.* (1972) The pathogenesis of esophageal dysfunction in scleroderma and Raynaud's disease. *Journal of Clinical Investigation*, **51**, 2663–2668.

5 D'Angelo, W. A., Fries, J. F., Masi, A. T. & Shulman, L. E. (1969) Pathologic observations in systemic sclerosis (scleroderma). *American Journal of Medicine*, **46**, 428–440.

6 DiMarino, A. J., Carlson, G., Myers, A. *et al.* (1973) Duodenal myoelectric activity in scleroderma. *New England Journal of Medicine*, **289**, 1220–1223.

7 Dornhurst, A. C., Pierce, J. W. & Whimster, I. W. (1954) The oesophageal lesion in scleroderma. *Lancet*, **i**, 698–699.

8 Ehrmann, S. (1903) Uber die Bezichung des sklerodermie zu den autotoxischen erythemen. *Wiener Medizinische Wochenschrift*, **53**, 1097–1102; 1159–1159.

9 Goldgraber, M. B. & Kirshner, J. B. (1957) Scleroderma of the gastrointestinal tract. *Archives of Pathology*, **64**, 255–265.

10 Hale, C. H. & Schatzki, R. (1944) The roentgenographic appearance of the gastrointestinal tract in scleroderma. *American Journal of Roentgenology and Radium Therapy*, **51**, 407–414.

11 Heading, R. C., Tothill, P. & McGloughlin, G. P. (1976) Gastric emptying rate measurement in man: a dual isotope scanning technique for simultaneous study of liquid and solid components of a meal. *Gastroenterology*, **71**, 45–50.

12 Heinz, E. R., Steinberg, A. J. & Sackner, M. A. (1963) Roentgenographic and pathologic aspects of intestinal scleroderma. *Annals of Internal Medicine*, **59**, 822–831.

13 Henderson, R. D. & Pearson, F. G. (1973) Surgical management of esophageal scleroderma. *Journal of Thoracic and Cardiovascular Surgery*, **66**, 686–692.

14 Hogan, W. J., Kahn, M. A., Nelson, J. W. & Winship, D. H. (1971) Impairment of anal sphincter function in progressive systemic sclerosis. *Clinical Research*, **19**, 394.

15 Horowitz, A. L. & Meyers, M. E. (1973) The 'hidebound' small bowel of scleroderma: characteristic mucosal fold pattern. *American Journal of Roentgenology, Radium Therapy and Nuclear Medicine*, **119**, 332–334.

16 Klatskin, G. & Kantor, F. S. (1972) Mitochondrial antibody in primary biliary cirrhosis and other diseases. *Annals of Internal Medicine*, **77**, 533–541.

17 Lorber, S. H. & Zarafonetis, C. J. D. (1963) Esophageal transport studies in scleroderma. *American Journal of Medical Sciences*, **245**, 654–667.

18 Meihoff, W. E., Hirschfield, J. S. & Kern, F. (1968) Small intestinal scleroderma with malabsorption and pneumatosis cystoides intestinalis. *Journal of the American Medical Association*, **204**, 854–858.

19 Meszaros, W. T. (1959) The colon in systemic sclerosis (scleroderma). *American Journal of Roentgenology, Radium Therapy and Nuclear Medicine*, **82**, 1000–1011.

20 Petrokubi, R. J. & Jeffries, G. H. (1978) Cimetidine versus antacid in scleroderma with reflux esophagitis. A randomized double blind controlled study. *Gastroenterology*, **74**, 1077–1080.

21 Rake, S. G. (1931) On the pathology and pathogenesis of scleroderma. *Johns Hopkins Hospital Bulletin*, **48**, 212–227.

22 Ramirez-Mata, M., Ibanez, G. & Alarcon-Segovia, D. (1977) Stimulatory effects of metoclopramide on the esophagus and lower esophageal sphincter of patients with progressive systemic sclerosis. *Arthritis and Rheumatism*, **20**, 30–34.

23 Rees, W. D. W., Leigh, R. J., Christofides, N. D. *et al.* (1982) Interdigestive motor activity in patients with systemic sclerosis. *Gastroenterology*, **83**, 575–580.

24 Reynolds, T. B., Denison, E. K., Frankl, H. D. *et al.* (1971) Primary biliary cirrhosis with scleroderma, Raynaud's phenomenon and telangiectasia. *American Journal of Medicine*, **50**, 302–312.

25 Rodnan, G. P. & Fennell, R. H., Jr (1962) Progressive systemic sclerosis sine scleroderma. *Journal of the American Medical Association*, **180**, 665–670.

26 Saladin, T. A., French, A. B., Zarafonetis, C. J. D. & Volland, H. (1966) Esophageal motor abnormalities in scleroderma and related diseases. *American Journal of Digestive Diseases*, **11**, 522–535.

27 Sherlock, S. & Scheuer, P. J. (1973) The presentation and diagnosis of 100 patients with primary biliary cirrhosis. *New England Journal of Medicine*, **289**, 674–678.

28 Stevens, M. B., Hookman, P., Siegel, C. I. *et al.* (1964) Aperistalsis of the esophagus in patients with connective tissue disorders and Raynaud's phenomenon. *New England Journal of Medicine*, **270**, 1218–1222.

29 Tolin, R., Malmud, L. S., Reilly, J. & Fisher, R. S. (1979) Esophageal scintigraphy to quantitate esophageal transit. *Gastroenterology*, **76**, 1402–1408.

30 Treacy, W. L., Baggenstoss, A. H., Slocumb, C. H. & Code, F. H. (1963) Scleroderma of the esophagus: correlation of histologic and physiologic findings. *Annals of Internal Medicine*, **59**, 351–356.

31 Tuffanelli, D. L. & Winklemann, R. K. (1961) Systemic scleroderma: a clinical study of 727 cases. *Archives of Dermatology*, **84**, 359–371.

32 Turner, R., Lipshutz, W. H., Miller, W. *et al.* (1973) Esophageal dysfunction in Collagen disease. *American Journal of Medical Sciences*, **265**, 191–199.

SYSTEMIC LUPUS ERYTHEMATOSUS

Gastrointestinal symptoms in patients with systemic lupus erythematosus (SLE) are common and include anorexia, dysphagia, nausea, vomiting, abdominal pain and diarrhoea.[3] Usually these symptoms are of limited significance and difficult to ascribe to specific organ involvement. Occasionally, however, gastrointestinal complications in SLE present as an acute surgical abdomen[4, 6] which may be secondary to a variety of problems including ulceration, haemorrhage, perforation, obstruction, or even sterile peritonitis.[5] In addition to the entire alimentary tract, involvement of the liver, spleen and pancreas may occur. The predominant lesion in the gastrointestinal tract appears to be an inflammatory vascular one while evidence for arteritis in the liver, spleen and pancreas is usually not present.

Alimentary tract

Clinical, radiographic[13] and manometric[7, 12] data indicate that oesophageal function may be altered in 25 to 35% of patients with SLE. Radiographic findings in the oesophagus include diffuse or focal dilatation and decreased aboral movement of contrast material. Oesophageal manometric studies have shown that the amplitude of oesophageal contractions may be decreased and contractions may be nonprogressive (i.e. aperistaltic). These abnormalities may be diffuse or they may be confined to specific segments of the oesophageal body. In some patients, the resting lower oesophageal sphincter pressure may be diminished. The relationship of the oesophageal dysfunction to Raynaud's phenomenon has been emphasized by Stevens *et al.*[12]

Oesophageal symptoms such as dysphagia are less common. The oesophageal findings in SLE may be similar to, but less severe than, those found in scleroderma. On occasion, the proximal or striated muscle portions of the oesophagus may be involved alone or in combination with the distal oesophagus. Pharmacological studies of the type performed in scleroderma have not been done; thus, the presence of a neural defect has not been suggested. Extensive pathological studies of the oesophagus are not available. Superimposed inflammatory or monilial oesophagitis may complicate SLE, particularly in view of the usual therapeutic programmes employed in these patients.

In regard to the stomach and small intestine, radiographic abnormalities may include a distended atonic stomach, frank ulceration in the stomach and duodenum, adynamic ileus involving any or all segments of the small intestine and true perforation of the small intestine. Reversible ischaemia of the small intestine in SLE has been noted and may be more common than clinically recognized.[11] Presumably, these findings are secondary to vascular lesions.[6] Malabsorption and protein losing enteropathy has been seen in SLE with evidence of immune deposits in intestinal vessels and basement membranes.[14]

Colonic involvement in SLE is well recognized and may present as perforation secondary to arteritis.[15]

Liver

Hepatic involvement secondary to SLE has been recognized relatively recently.[2, 9] Previously, liver disease found in SLE patients was most often ascribed to intercurrent illnesses or to pharmacological agents. While many drugs may produce hepatotoxicity, aspirin appears to be the most common offender in patients with SLE.[10] The liver toxicity is entirely reversible, however. Excluding drug-induced hepatotoxicity and other obvious causes, histological abnormalities such as fatty infiltration, chronic active hepatitis and even cirrhosis have been demonstrated in SLE.[2, 9] Both progression of SLE-related liver disease and death due to liver failure have been reported.[9] Subclinical and overt liver disease may be a more common concomitant of SLE than previously recognized.

Pancreas

Hyperamylasaemia is common in SLE[8] and has been most frequently attributed to corticosteroid therapy despite occasional recognition of arteritis as an aetiology.[1] Careful evaluation for pancreatitis as a cause of abdominal pain in SLE revealed that it was not a rare occurrence and that frequently it may be due to the inflammatory disease itself rather than any associated therapy such as corticosteroids.[8]

REFERENCES

1   Baron, M. & Brisson, M. (1982) Pancreatitis in systemic lupus erythematosus. *Arthritis and Rheumatism,* **25,** 1006–1009.
2   Gibson, T. & Myers, A. R. (1981) Subclinical liver disease in systemic lupus erythematosus. *Journal of Rheumatology,* **8,** 752–759.
3   Hoffman, B. I. & Katz, W. A. (1980) The gastrointestinal manifestations of systemic lupus erythematosus: a review of the literature. *Seminars in Arthritis and Rheumatism,* **9,** 237–247.
4   Matolo, N. M. & Albo, D. (1971) Gastrointestinal complications of collagen vascular diseases: surgical implications. *American Journal of Surgery,* **122,** 678–682.
5   Musher, D. R. (1972) Systemic lupus erythematosus: a cause of 'medical peritonitis'. *American Journal of Surgery,* **124,** 368–372.
6   Pollak, V. E., Grove, W. J., Kark, R. M. *et al.* (1958) Systemic lupus erythematosus simulating acute surgical conditions of the abdomen. *New England Journal of Medicine,* **259,** 258–266.
7   Ramirez-Mata, M., Reyes, P. A., Alarcon-Segovia, D. & Garza, R. (1974) Esophageal motility in systemic lupus erythematosus. *American Journal of Digestive Diseases,* **19,** 132–136.
8   Reynolds, J. C., Inman, R. D., Kimberly, R. P. *et al.* (1982) Acute pancreatitis in systemic lupus erythematosus: report of twenty cases and a review of the literature. *Medicine,* **61,** 25–32.

9 Runyon, B. A., LaBrecque, D. R. & Anuras, S. (1980) The spectrum of liver disease in systemic lupus erythematosus: report of 33 histologically proved cases and review of the literature. *American Journal of Medicine*, **69**, 187–194.
10 Seaman, W. E., Ishak, K. G. & Plotz, P. H. (1974) Aspirin-induced hepatotoxicity in patients with systemic lupus erythematosus. *Annals of Internal Medicine*, **80**, 1–8.
11 Shapeero, L. G., Myers, A., Oberkircher, P. E. & Miller, W. T. (1974) Acute reversible lupus vasculitis of the gastrointestinal tract. *Radiology*, **112**, 569–574.
12 Stevens, M. B., Hookman, P., Siegel, C. I. *et al.* (1964) Aperistalsis of the esophagus in patients with connective tissue disorders and Raynaud's phenomenon. *New England Journal of Medicine*, **270**, 1218–1222.
13 Tatelman, M. & Keech, M. R. (1966) Esophageal motility in systemic lupus erythematosus, rheumatoid arthritis and scleroderma. *Radiology*, **86**, 1041–1045.
14 Weiser, M. M., Andres, G. A., Brentjens, J. R. *et al.* (1981) Systemic lupus erythematosus and intestinal venulitis. *Gastroenterology*, **81**, 570–579.
15 Zizic, T. M., Shulman, L. E. & Stevens, M. B. (1975) Colonic perforations in systemic lupus erythematosus. *Medicine*, **54**, 411–426.

POLYMYOSITIS/ DERMATOMYOSITIS

Polymyositis/dermatomyositis (PM/DM) is a chronic disease characterized by degenerative and inflammatory changes in skeletal (striated) muscles. Associated characteristic dermal involvement occurs in 40% of cases. PM/DM is frequently associated with extramuscular disorders and gastrointestinal tract involvement is common.

Dysphagia for solid and liquid foods is the most common digestive symptom in PM/DM and occurs in about 60% of cases.[6] Most commonly dysphagia is due to involvement of the oropharynx; however, the proximal oesophagus is also frequently involved. Dysphagia may be associated with a nasal quality to the voice, regurgitation, and tracheal aspiration, related to weakness of pharyngeal and cricopharyngeal muscles.[2] Although PM/DM is regarded as a disease of the striated muscles,[7,8] several reports have suggested involvement of the distal (smooth muscle) oesophagus as well.[3,4,5] While some of the earlier reports represent misdiagnoses or overlapping syndromes between PM/DM and scleroderma, clearly some demonstrate true evidence of distal oesophageal disease. The relationship to Raynaud's phenomenon requires further study.

Radiographic studies may reveal pooling of contrast material in the vallecula, tracheal aspiration and/or decreased peristalsis. Studies in which oesophageal manometric examinations

have been performed have yielded conflicting results. Some have demonstrated decreased amplitudes of pharyngeal and oesophageal contractions confined to striated muscles, but others have shown abnormalities of both smooth and striated muscles. No studies utilizing pharmacological manipulation attempting to identify the lesion have been reported. Pathological examination of the oesophagus in PM/DM reveals infrequent evidence of smooth muscle atrophy or fibrosis as seen in scleroderma but mucosal ulceration is common.[4] Complicating oesophageal candidiasis may supervene.

A disturbing aspect of dermatomyositis (rarely polymyositis) is its association with cancer, especially in the lung and gastrointestinal tract.[1] Coexistent gastrointestinal cancers occur most commonly in the stomach, but have also been found in the gallbladder, colon, rectum, oesophagus and pancreas. Signs and symptoms of dermatomyositis may precede the discovery of the tumour by up to one year.

Treatment of the gastrointestinal manifestations of PM/DM relate mainly to the control of the myopathy for which corticosteroids are generally employed. Cricopharyngeal and proximal oesophageal involvement may lead to aspiration which must be protected against until control of the generalized disorder is achieved. Oesophageal ulceration may be inhibited by an antacid and anti-reflux programme.

REFERENCES

1 Barnes, B. E. (1976) Dermatomyositis and malignancy: A review of the literature. *Annals of Internal Medicine*, **84**, 68–73.
2 Bohan, A. & Peter, J. B. (1975) Polymyositis and dermatomyositis. *New England Journal of Medicine*, **292**, 344–347.
3 Creamer, B., Anderson, H. & Code, C. F. (1956) Esophageal motility in patients with scleroderma and related diseases. *Gastroenterology*, **86**, 763–775.
4 DeMerieux, P., Verity, M. A., Clements, P. J. & Paulus, H. E. (1983) Esophageal abnormalities and dysphagia in polymyositis and dermatomyositis. Clinical, radiologic and pathologic features. *Arthritis and Rheumatism*, **26**, 961–968.
5 Donoghue, F. D., Winkelmann, R. K. & Moersch, J. A. (1960) Esophageal defects in dermatomyositis. *Annals of Otolaryngology*, **69**, 1139–1145.
6 Pearson, C. M. (1979) Polymyositis and dermatomyositis. In *Arthritis and Allied Conditions* Ed. McCarty, D. 9th Edition, Chapter 52, pp. 740–761. Washington: Lea and Febiger.
7 Stevens, M. B., Hookman, P., Siegel, C. I. *et al.* (1964) Aperistalsis of the esophagus in patients with connective tissue disorders and Raynaud's phenomenon. *New England Journal of Medicine*, **270**, 1218–1222.
8 Turner, R., Lipshutz, W. H., Miller, W. *et al.* (1973) Esophageal dysfunction in collagen disease. *American Journal of Medical Sciences*, **265**, 191–199.

RHEUMATOID ARTHRITIS

While the gastrointestinal tract is frequently involved in connective tissue diseases, such as scleroderma, systemic lupus erythematosus, polyarteritis nodosa and polymyositis/ dermatomyositis, there have been few reports of such involvement in rheumatoid arthritis (RA). However, a variety of primary and secondary gastrointestinal problems may be seen in RA. In relation to the articular disorder itself, the temporomandibular joints are frequently involved, occasionally leading to impaired mastication of food. Studies documenting oesophageal involvement in RA are recorded and demonstrate diminished amplitudes of oesophageal contractions in the middle and distal segments of the oesophagus and decreased resting lower oesophageal sphincter pressure.[5] In many ways these alterations resemble those seen in scleroderma but in contrast to patients with scleroderma, dysphagia and heartburn are uncommon in patients with RA.

Acute erosive gastritis, chronic atrophic gastritis and frank gastric and duodenal ulcerations have been observed with a high prevalence in RA.[3, 5] Since the majority of patients with RA are under treatment with aspirin, other non-steroidal anti-inflammatory agents and/or corticosteroids, the role of these therapeutic agents in producing upper gastrointestinal erosion and/or ulceration must be taken into consideration. However, most would agree that the incidence of gastric and duodenal mucosal inflammatory lesions is increased in patients with RA, even in the absence of anti-inflammatory therapies.

Vasculitis or necrotizing arteritis is the most serious gastrointestinal complication of RA. Systemic vasculitis usually occurs in the setting of highly expressed RA (severe arthritis, subcutaneous nodules, neuropathy and high titre of rheumatoid factor) and patients with rheumatoid vasculitis are at risk for serious gastrointestinal complications such as massive haemorrhage, ischaemic ulceration, perforation and bowel infarction.[2]

Involvement of the liver in RA has been recognized increasingly, particularly in the presence of Felty's syndrome (triad of RA, leucopenia and splenomegaly). Histopathologically, nodular regenerative hyperplasia is typically seen and it frequently results in portal hypertension and even bleeding oesophageal varicies.[6] Consequently, screening of patients with Felty's syndrome for hepatic abnormalities and portal hypertension appears reasonable. Another significant liver disorder recognized in RA is salicylate-induced hepatotoxicity. It is usually associated with juvenile RA[1] but has also been observed in adult RA.[4] Like the salicylate-induced hepatotoxicity seen in SLE, the aetiology is unclear but the course is benign. In most RA patients, it is not necessary to discontinue salicylate therapy unless bleeding supervenes, since biochemical abnormalities normalize even on continued therapy.

REFERENCES

1 Athryea, B. H., Moser, G., Cecil, A. S. & Myers, A. R. (1975) Aspirin-induced hepatotoxicity in juvenile rheumatoid arthritis: a prospective study. *Arthritis and Rheumatism*, **18**, 347–352.
2 Bienenstock, H., Minick, R. & Rogoff, B. (1967) Mesenteric arteritis and intestinal infarction in rheumatoid disease. *Archives of Internal Medicine*, **119**, 359–364.
3 Marcolongo, R., Bayell, P. F. & Montagnani, M. (1979) Gastrointestinal involvement in rheumatoid arthritis: a biopsy study. *Journal of Rheumatology*, **6**, 163–173.
4 Saltzman, D. A., Gall, E. P. & Robinson, S. F. (1976) Aspirin-induced hepatic dysfunction in a patient with adult rheumatoid arthritis. *Digestive Diseases*, **9**, 815–520.
5 Sun, D. C. H., Roth, S. H., Mitchell, C. S. & England, D. W. W. (1974) Upper gastrointestinal diseases in rheumatoid arthritis. *American Journal of Digestive Diseases*, **19**, 405–412.
6 Thorne, C., Urowitz, M. B., Wanless, I. *et al.* (1982) Liver disease in Felty's syndrome. *American Journal of Medicine*, **73**, 35–40.

POLYARTERITIS

Polyarteritis is a systemic necrotizing vasculitis, with an inflammatory cell infiltrate and fibrinoid necrosis affecting vessel walls in many organs. Both arteries and veins may be involved. Polyarteritis can be subdivided into four subcategories: classical polyarteritis nodosa (PAN), the Churg–Strauss syndrome (CSS), a PAN–CSS overlap syndrome and microscopic polyarteritis (MPA). These groups can be defined pathologically, using the size of vessel affected and the presence or absence of granulomata histologically (Table 9.1); they present differing clinical patterns of disease activity, as discussed below. However, there is controversy

Table 9.1 Classification of polyarteritis.

Disease	Vessel size	Granulomas	Main organ affected
PAN*	Medium	Absent	Gut
CSS	Medium	Present	Lungs
MPA	Small	Absent	Kidneys

* PAN = Classical polyarteritis nodosa; CSS = Churg–Strauss syndrome; MPA = microscopic polyarteritis.

over the precise classification and definition of the varying disease groups in polyarteritis and the classification used here may turn out to be an over-simplification.[4]

Pathogenesis
The pathogenetic mechanisms occurring in polyarteritis are not fully delineated. It is generally thought to be an immune complex-mediated disorder, with inflammation brought about by complexes in the vessel wall, either deposited there from the circulation or formed in situ.[2] In fact assays for circulating immune complexes are positive in less than 50% of patients, but the assay techniques for these are relatively insensitive. Although there are good animal models of immune-complex disease with associated arthritis, nephritis and vasculitis, there is no direct evidence in man that vasculitis in general and polyarteritis in particular is the result of deposition or formation of immune complexes at the site of injury.

Classical PAN is the only type of polyarteritis which has been associated with an aetiological agent, namely hepatitis B antigen, and this antigen has been identified in circulating immune complexes, in cryoglobulins from the serum, and deposited in the walls of affected vessels.[3] In some areas of the world, this antigen may be implicated in up to 70% of cases, although a much lower incidence (less than 10%) has been found in Britain.

General clinical features
Polyarteritis affects a wide age range, with a peak incidence in middle age. Males are affected more than females. All forms of polyarteritis may be associated with severe constitutional upset causing malaise, fever and weight loss.

Classical, or macroscopic, polyarteritis

In addition to the general systemic features mentioned above, severe hypertension and multiple organ infarcts typically occur, reflecting the involvement of medium-sized muscular arteries with aneurysm formation at branching points (Figure 9.7). There are patients who on clinical grounds fit the pattern of classical polyarteritis, in whom aneurysms are not detected; aneurysms may also evolve and resolve with fluctuating disease activity. Aneurysms are also rarely to be found in other forms of vasculitis such as Wegener's granulomatosis, systemic lupus erythematosus and the Churg–Strauss syndrome.

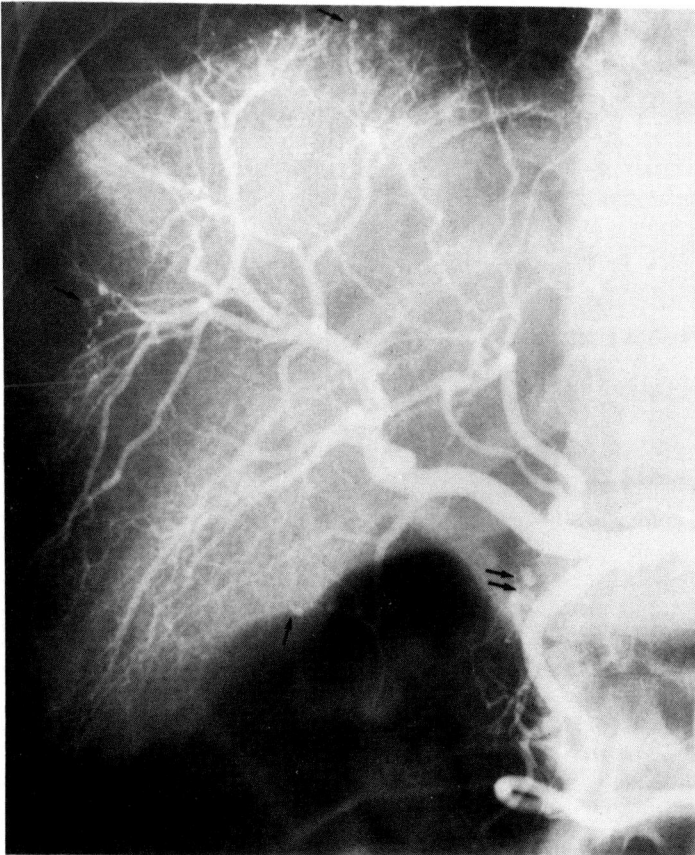

Fig. 9.7 Typical hepatic arteriogram of patient with necrotizing arteritis. Aneurysms (arrows) are seen in the pancreatico-duodenal, cystic and hepatic branches of the hepatic artery. Photograph courtesy of Drs R. S. Fisher and A. R. Myers.

GASTROINTESTINAL INVOLVEMENT

The gut involvement in polyarteritis is usually seen in the setting of an obvious systemic vasculitic illness, and isolated gastrointestinal disease is rare. Weight loss is common and may reflect only systemic upset, but nausea, vomiting and diarrhoea point to involvement of the gut. Such manifestations occur in 40–70% of patients. Infarction of a variety of organs may occur, including liver, gallbladder, pancreas or intestine, with the expected clinical manifestations. Intestinal infarction, with resulting intestinal perforation or massive gastrointestinal haemorrhage, occurs in about one in five patients with this type of polyarteritis. Diarrhoea may reflect either small intestinal or colonic involvement, either focally or diffusely. Steatorrhoea may occur with diffuse small intestinal involvement, with widespread inflammation mimicking coeliac or Crohn's disease, and in the colon a diffuse ulcerative colitis-like lesion may be seen.[7] In some patients, focal areas of vasculitis may give rise to discrete ulcers, visible with colonoscopy or sigmoidoscopy. Both acute and chronic pancreatitis are reported. Abdominal pain may also be of renal origin reflecting renal infarction.

The diagnosis of gastrointestinal disease is usually made when symptoms develop in the correct clinical setting. Although a histological diagnosis can be made on rectal, muscle or renal biopsy, histological proof is not always forthcoming. As would be expected, a wide variety of non-specific radiological abnormalities, or a normal finding, are seen with barium studies. In about 60% of patients visceral angiography shows the presence of aneurysms. The presence of pronounced persistent leucocytosis and an elevated ESR may be helpful clues.

OTHER CLINICAL FEATURES

The systemic symptoms of malaise, fever and weight loss have already been mentioned. Skin involvement is present in about a quarter of patients with polyarteritis and visceral involvement, which is a much lower frequency in classical polyarteritis than in the microscopic form discussed below. Nodules, ecchymoses, livedo reticularis and areas of cutaneous ulceration may appear. Glomerulonephritis is relatively unusual. The vasculitis may also affect the coronary circulation, and the central and the peripheral nervous system, the latter often as a mononeuritis multiplex.

The Churg–Strauss syndrome (allergic granulomatous angiitis)

This characteristically presents with fever, hyper-eosinophilia and severe asthma in young adults who have evidence of vasculitis active elsewhere in the body. The skin, heart, nerves, kidneys and gastrointestinal tract may be involved. There are abdominal manifestations in about 20% of patients with pain, bloody diarrhoea and perforation; occasionally the allergic granulomatous process may mimic a neoplasm.[6] Pathologically, in addition to vasculitis of small and medium sized vessels, there is eosinophilic infiltration and granuloma formation in connective tissue. Small venules may also be affected. A prominent pulmonary vasculitis is common, in contrast to classical PAN where such lung involvement is rare.

Microscopic polyarteritis

The clinical features of MPA tend to concentrate on the kidney. The capillaritis and arteriolitis produces a focal segmental necrotizing glomerulonephritis. Typically there is impairment of renal function with microscopic haematuria and proteinuria, occasionally severe enough to cause the nephrotic syndrome. Severe hypertension is unusual at presentation. There is always concurrent evidence of systemic vasculitic disease with myalgia, arthralgia, episcleritis, purpuric skin rashes and abdominal manifestations occurring frequently. As in the other polyarteritis syndromes, gastrointestinal involvement may cause non-specific colicky abdominal pains and diarrhoea, but such involvement is usually less prominent and severe than in PAN and CSS, and life-threatening infarction, perforation and haemorrhage are rare. Pulmonary involvement with asthma and pulmonary infiltrates is also rare in MPA in contrast to their invariable presence in CSS. Haemoptysis and lung haemorrhage may occur in MPA, as in CSS, and may be life-threatening.

There are many similarities between MPA and other vasculitis syndromes, such as Henoch–Schönlein purpura (see below) and Wegener's granulomatosis. The latter is characterized by involvement of the upper respiratory tract and lungs in a granulomatous process associated with a small vessel vasculitis. Again in this condition gastrointestinal disease can occur, but it is rare.

Prognosis and treatment

The prognosis in untreated polyarteritis is poor, with a 13% five-year survival rate in classical PAN. The use of corticosteroids improved this to 50–60% as the use of steroids became widely accepted, particularly in CSS. With cytotoxic drugs, notably cyclophosphamide and azathioprine, an 80% five-year survival rate can be achieved in severe systemic necrotizing vasculitis, and dramatic remissions can be obtained when high doses of corticosteroids have failed to control disease activity.[1] Relapses can occur in all types of polyarteritis but there is good evidence that cytotoxic agents can prevent or at least reduce their number.

Early deaths, within six months of presentation, are usually due to the effects of the vasculitis or to intercurrent infection in immunosuppressed patients. The mode of death may reflect the impact of the different types of polyarteritis on particular organ systems. Thus, bowel infarction and consequences of hypertension are seen most commonly in PAN, renal failure in MPA, status asthmaticus in CSS, and pulmonary haemorrhage in both CSS and MPA.

Treatment of gastrointestinal involvement
The major consequences of gut involvement – life threatening haemorrhage, perforation and peritonitis, and organ infarction – usually precipitate surgical intervention.[5] If no indication for surgical intervention exists the gut vasculitis will improve if the systemic vasculitic process responds to medical therapy. Treatment involves induction followed by maintenance of disease remission, initially using both high doses of corticosteroids, and either cyclophosphamide or azathioprine, to induce remission. In some centres plasma exchange is being used in addition, but further controlled evaluation of this method is required. Subsequently low-dose treatment with corticosteroids, together with cyclophosphamide or azathioprine, should be continued for at least a year if not longer.

General measures will include treatment of associated hypertension, and renal support by dialysis if required.

REFERENCES

1 Cohen, R. D., Conn, D. L. & Ilstrup, D. M. (1980) Clinical features, prognosis and response to treatment in polyarteritis. *Mayo Clin Proceedings*, **55**, 146–155.
2 Cupps, T. R. & Fauci, A. S. (1982) The vasculitic syndromes. In *Advances in Internal Medicine*. pp. 315–344. Year Book Medical Publishers.
3 Duffy, J., Lidsky, M., Sharp, J. *et al.* (1976) Polyarthritis, polyarteritis and hepatitis B. *Medicine (Baltimore)*, **55**, 19–37.
4 Fauci, A. S., Haynes, B. F. & Katz, P. (1978) The spectrum of vasculitis, clinical, pathologic, immunologic and therapeutic implications. *Annals of Internal Medicine*, **89**, 660–676.
5 Matalo, N. M. & Albo, D. (1971) Gastrointestinal complications of collagen vascular disease: surgical implications. *American Journal of Surgery*, **122**, 678–682.
6 Modigliani, R., Muschart, J. M., Galian, A. *et al.* (1981) Allergic granulomatous vasculitis (Churg–Strauss syndrome) Report of a case with widespread digestive involvement. *Digestive Diseases and Sciences*, **26**, 264–270.
7 Wood, M. K., Read, D. R., Kraft, A. R. & Barreta, T. M. (1979) A rare cause of ischaemic colitis: polyarteritis nodosa. *Diseases of the Colon and Rectum*, **22**, 428–433.

HENOCH–SCHÖNLEIN PURPURA

In the spectrum of multisystem vasculitic disease Henoch–Schönlein purpura (HSP) is the single best defined entity clinically and pathologically. The combination of purpuric skin lesions, characteristically involving the extensor surfaces of the limbs, colicky abdominal pain with occasional bloody diarrhoea, nephritis and arthralgias strongly favour the diagnosis clinically. Pathologically there are characteristic findings in the skin and the kidneys. Light microscopy of the skin shows a perivascular infiltration of polymorphonuclear leucocytes and monocytes around small blood vessels in the corium. In the kidney there is usually a focal glomerulonephritis with proliferation of cells within the glomerulus often a striking feature. Rarely an inflammatory necrotizing vasculitis may be seen affecting interlobular arteries and arterioles. Immunofluorescence examination of both skin and kidney show predominantly widespread deposition of IgA and this is helpful diagnostically (see below). In the skin IgA deposits may be found in capillary walls or at the dermo–epidermal junction and are not confined to areas affected clinically. In the glomerulus IgA deposits are not restricted to areas abnormal by light microscopy, but are generalized throughout the mesangium. Similar deposits are also to be found in vessels of the intestinal tract.

Pathogenesis
Development of HSP has often been related to a preceding upper respiratory tract infection. Organisms most frequently implicated have been β-haemolytic streptococci, mycoplasma and varicella. Other possible antecedent causes include drugs, insect bites and food allergies.

Raised IgA levels in serum are commonly found at an early stage in the disease and together with mesangial IgA deposits in the kidneys of patients with nephritis implicate IgA in the pathogenesis of HSP. The suggestion therefore is that an IgA-mediated immune response leads to immune complex formation with deposition of IgA immune complexes in the tissues. Ultrastructural studies of renal biopsy material have confirmed that immune deposits suggestive of immune complexes are present and that these may recur in an allografted kidney. Whether complement activation is involved in the pathogenesis of the disease is uncertain; development of HSP in patients genetically deficient in the second component of complement suggests that, if involved at all, activation is by way of the alternative pathway.

Clinical features

Most series have shown that males are twice as commonly affected as females. The peak incidence is in children aged between five and 15, and the onset of HSP is rare in adults.

Systemic manifestations

Usually HSP presents with a rash, starting as wheals on the extensor surfaces of the arms and legs, buttocks and lower back. The wheals change into dusky, red, non-blanching macules over the course of a few hours and persist for up to two weeks before eventually fading. Gastrointestinal involvement and joint symptoms are usually manifest at the same time as the rash, and the nephritis (present in about 50% of patients) is generally noticed at a later stage. Variations on this theme do occur, however, and may mislead the unwary. The rash may not always be purpuric; erythematous or urticarial lesions can occur in the early stages and in severe cases any surface of the body may be affected. In a few patients convulsions have been reported and pulmonary involvement is not unknown. Occasionally, nephritis is found before the purpura and can range in severity from transient proteinuria and haematuria to rapidly progressive renal failure. Sometimes hypertension is the only manifestation of renal involvement. The joint involvement is a transient non-migrating polyarthritis, usually affecting ankles, knees, wrists and elbows.

Gastrointestinal involvement[1, 3]

Clinical gut involvement occurs in one-quarter to two-thirds of affected individuals; the higher incidence is in children and young adults. The cardinal clinical feature is colicky abdominal pain, reflecting subacute obstruction from areas of submucosal oedema and haemorrhage in the small intestine. Nausea and vomiting occur in the majority of patients. Bleeding into the gastrointestinal tract can be detected by faecal testing in over threequarters of patients, but significant haemorrhage is less common. In some series, however, between 10 and 20% of individuals experienced haematemesis, melaena or rectal bleeding. Areas of submucosal haemorrhage or oedema may on occasion initiate intussusception[2] and perforation of the intestine rarely occurs. Vasculitic infarction of the gallbladder and pancreas may occur in adults.[5]

In approximately 14% of individuals, gastrointestinal disease may be the initial manifestation, without the diagnostically helpful rash or other features at that stage.

Clinical investigations may confirm the areas of vasculitis and oedema in the gastrointestinal tract. Gastritis and duodenitis are visible at endoscopy, with haemorrhage and necrosis, and either diffuse or perivascular inflammation on biopsy. Jejunal biopsies have shown a diffuse villous atrophy, but are usually not clinically indicated. Barium follow through examination may show easily recognizable 'thumb-printing' areas of oedema and haemorrhage, with areas of spasm, ulceration, or pseudo-tumour, but the appearances may also be non-specific, highly reminiscent of Crohn's disease, or unremarkable (Figure 9.8).[4] Hypoproteinaemia may reflect a combination of both urinary protein loss and protein-losing enteropathy.

Diagnosis can usually be made on clinical grounds as outlined above. In a patient with a multi-system disease, where doubt still exists, skin biopsy showing IgA deposition may be of help and if there is renal involvement the finding of mesangial IgA deposits restrict the diagnostic possibilities to HSP, subacute bacterial endocarditis or systemic lupus erythematosus.

Treatment

Unlike many other vasculitic conditions, HSP is usually a benign and self-limited disease, although there is a tendency to relapse. Importantly, the gastrointestinal involvement is reversible, as healing usually occurs without fibrosis and subsequent chronic subacute obstruction is very rare (though reported).[6] The major factor accounting for the morbidity and mortality of HSP is nephritis, but even in this group, over 90% of patients survive over 15 years.

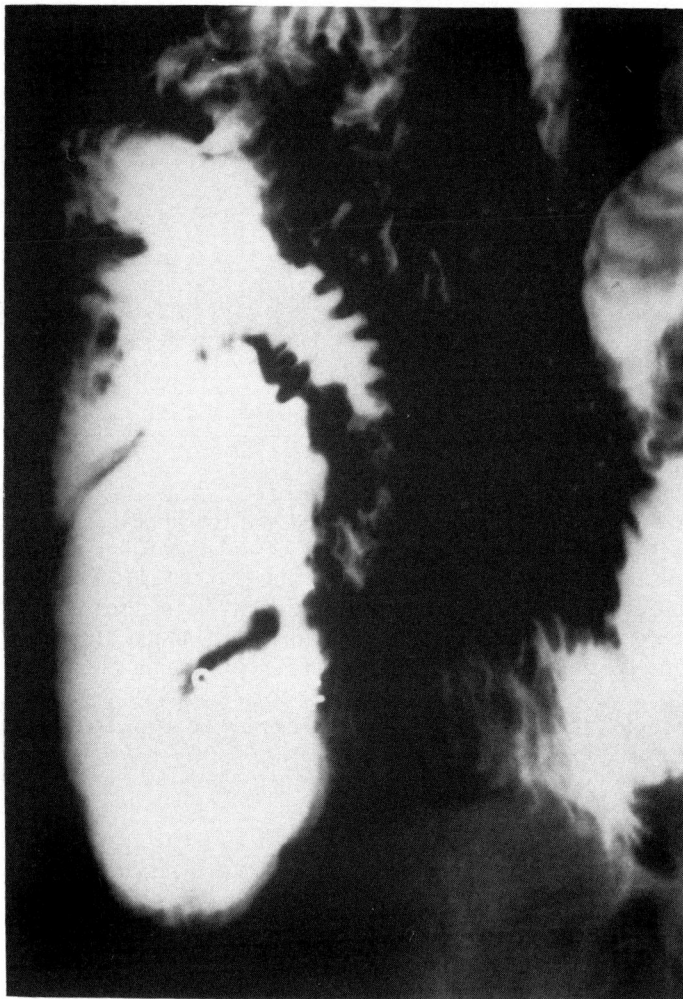

Fig. 9.8 Barium follow through examination showing terminal ileum and caecum in a case of Henoch–Schönlein purpura, with oedema and 'thumb-printing' of terminal ileal mucosa.

No specific form of therapy has gained acceptance in HSP. Anecdotally, high doses of steroids appear to be of benefit in patients with severe vasculitis. However, when the main manifestations are visceral, and local abdominal signs point to severe local inflammation which is potentially a site of bowel perforation, the decision to use corticosteroids is clinically taxing. With conservative management, the whole episode usually resolves within a couple of weeks to a month, although relapses are common. The possibility of perforation or intussusception should be borne in mind as these of course would indicate surgical intervention.

REFERENCES

1 Balf, C. L. (1951) The alimentary lesions in Henoch–Schönlein purpura. *Archives of Diseases in Childhood,* **26,** 20–27.
2 Brust, N. M. (1952) Ileo-ileal intussusception associated with Henoch–Schönlein purpura. *Archives of Paediatrics,* **69,** 212–218.
3 Feldt, R. H. & Stickler, G. B. (1962) The gastrointestinal manifestations of anaphylactoid purpura in children. *Staff meetings of Mayo Clinic,* **37,** 465–473.
4 Handle, J. & Swartz, G. (1957) Gastrointestinal manifestations of Henoch–Schönlein purpura. *American Journal of Roentgenology,* **78,** 645–652.
5 Puppala, A. R., Cheng, J. C. & Steinheber, F. U. (1978) Pancreatitis: a rare complication of Schönlein–Henoch Purpura. *American Journal of Gastroenterology,* **69,** 101–104.
6 Young, D. G. (1964) Chronic intestinal obstruction following Henoch–Schönlein disease. *Clinical Paediatrics,* **3,** 737–740.

BEHÇET'S SYNDROME

Behçet's syndrome is an uncommon and poorly understood multi-system disorder. The diagnosis is made exclusively by clinical criteria (Table 9.2); because it is not clear whether Behçet's syndrome is the result of a single pathological process or of several, most authors prefer to call it a syndrome rather than a disease.

Table 9.2 Diagnostic criteria for Behçet's syndrome.[36]

Major criteria:
  Buccal ulceration
  Genital ulceration
  Eye lesions
  Skin lesions

Minor criteria:
  Gastrointestinal lesions
  Thrombophlebitis
  Cardiovascular lesions
  Arthritis
  Central nervous system lesions
  Family history
Three major, or two major and two minor criteria, are
required for diagnosis

Table 9.3 Classification of Behçet's syndrome based on clinical patterns of disease.

Lehner's classification[26]
  Mucocutaneous: oral and genital ulcers with or without skin manifestations
  Arthritic: joints and two or more of the mucocutaneous manifestations
  Neurological: CNS involved and mucocutaneous or joint manifestations
  Ocular: uveitis and mucocutaneous, arthritic or neurological features

Japanese classification[57]
  Neuro-Behçet's ⎫ Defined by combination of major
  Intestinal-Behçet's ⎬ clinical criteria with predominantly
  Vasculo-Behçet's ⎭ neurological, intestinal, or vascular involvement

Pathological changes in Behçet's syndrome are non-specific; the central feature is vasculitis, predominantly of small vessels. Venous thrombosis is commonly found, and may dominate the clinical picture. Many immunological abnormalities have been described and these include elevated immunoglobulin levels, circulating immune complexes and tissue-specific autoantibodies. There are associations between different clinical features of Behçet's syndrome and a number of HLA antigens, suggesting that differing genetic susceptibilities may be involved. Popularity for the role of viruses as aetiological agents has waxed and waned over the last thirty years. Viruses are again in vogue with the finding that parts of the herpes genome are present and transcribed in the peripheral blood mononuclear cells of patients with Behçet's syndrome.[19]

Diagnosis

The most frequent clinical findings are orogenital ulceration, ocular inflammation and skin lesions. These form the major diagnostic criteria of Mason and Barnes[36] (see Table 9.2). The Behçet's Syndrome Research Committee of Japan have retained these major disease criteria and slightly modified the minor criteria; they suggest that Behçet's syndrome be termed 'complete' if all four major criteria are present and 'incomplete' if only three of the major criteria are fulfilled or if there is an especially characteristic finding (e.g. iritis with hypopyon) plus only one other major criterion.

These 'diagnostic' criteria are better viewed as classification criteria for the present; they are of greatest value in collecting groups of patients with similar clinical manifestations for analysis and for comparison.

An alternative approach to classification is taken by Lehner and his colleagues (reviewed in Lehner and Barnes)[29] and by some Japanese

workers[5] who classify Behçet's syndrome according to the predominant clinical manifestations (Table 9.3). Two lines of evidence support the value of this form of classification. Individual patients tend to have disease confined to a single pattern (e.g. mucocutaneous) and this may be of helpful prognostic value. Genetic evidence (reviewed below) suggests that different HLA antigens may be associated with different disease patterns.

Epidemiology

The incidence of Behçet's syndrome varies widely throughout the world. It is commonest in Japan and the Middle East; the prevalence was 1 in 1000 in Hokkaido, Japan,[2] only 0.064 in 10 000 in Yorkshire, U.K.[11] and the point prevalence was 0.033 in 10 000 per year in Olmsted County, Minnesota, USA.[42]

In most series there has been a predominance of male patients; 70% of 683 patients reviewed by Chajek and Fainaru[10] were male. Disease onset is commonest in the third decade.

Genetics

Only a small number of familial cases of Behçet's syndrome have been described which suggests that genetic influences do not play a major role. Aphthous ulceration is slightly commoner in consanguineous relatives than in a normal population.[12] There is an increased prevalence of the HLA antigen B5 (particularly the BW51 split of B5) in Japanese, Turkish, Israeli and French patients. Initial studies of British and American patients failed to find this association and this led Lehner and his colleagues[32] to study the associations of clinical subsets of disease with HLA antigens. In British patients they found that HLA–B5 was associated with the ocular form of Behçet's syndrome (see Table 9.3). Their most recent report[33] suggests that, in addition to the HLA–B5 associations, HLA–DR7 is increased in the ocular and neurological types and HLA–B12 and/or HLA–DR2 is increased in the mucocutaneous and arthritic types. Patients with recurrent oral ulcers alone show an increase in HLA–B12 and/or HLA–DR2. These findings have not yet been confirmed by other groups, and the role of particular HLA antigens (or of the products of other linked genes) in influencing the pattern of Behçet's syndrome is presently controversial.

Pathology

Vasculitis, predominantly of small vessels, is the major histopathological finding. Endothelial proliferation and swelling may result in obliteration of the lumen of small vessels. There is usually an accompanying mononuclear cell infiltrate. When these changes occur in larger veins they are frequently accompanied by thrombosis and may lead to the superficial thrombophlebitis, vena caval thrombosis, and Budd–Chiari syndrome that are characteristic clinical features of Behçet's syndrome. Changes affecting medium and large arteries are much rarer but fibrinoid necrosis of arteries and arterioles has been described in association with aneurysm formation and gangrene.

During periods of disease activity, the plasma levels of acute phase reactants (including C-reactive protein, alpha 1-antitrypsin and certain complement components) increase, accompanied by elevation of the ESR.

There is considerable evidence for immunological abnormalities in patients with Behçet's syndrome. Serum immunoglobulin levels are often raised. Immunofluorescent studies of blood vessels show deposition of immunoglobulins and complement components. Circulating immune complexes have been found by several different assays and their presence shown to correlate with disease activity. Lehner and his colleagues[32] found complexes mainly in patients with the ocular and arthritic forms.

Complement levels are usually normal or elevated, although an isolated report[50] described a fall in C4, C2 and C3 levels just preceding attacks of uveitis.

The predominance of mucosal lesions has stimulated many workers to study local mucosal immune responses. Oshima and his co-workers[45] found autoantibodies to oral mucosa. Lehner[27] confirmed these findings but showed that mucosal antibodies were also present in patients with recurrent oral ulceration alone. Lymphocyte cytotoxicity to cultures of gingival epithelial cells has also been found in individuals with isolated recurrent oral ulceration and those with oral ulceration and Behçet's syndrome (reviewed in Lehner).[28] Abdou and his colleagues[1] found a reduction in secretory component in saliva suggesting a disturbance of the mucosal IgA system.

Aspects of blood coagulation have been investigated by several groups; several studies show evidence of reduced fibrinolysis but little progress has been made towards understanding the pathological mechanisms resulting in thrombosis in these patients.

All attempts to isolate viruses from patients with Behçet's syndrome have failed. However, herpes simplex virus (HSV) failed to replicate in cultures of mononuclear cells from patients with several connective tissue diseases, including Behçet's syndrome,[15] which suggested pre-existing viral infection of these cells. Recently, Eglin, Lehner and Subak-Sharpe[19] have shown the greater capacity of HSV–1 DNA to hybridize with complementary RNA sequences in mononuclear cells from patients with the ocular and arthritic types of Behçet's syndrome, compared with controls. This demonstrates that at least parts of the HSV–1 genome are present and transcribed in these cells. Mononuclear cells from patients with minor aphthous ulceration also appeared to contain portions of the genome of HSV–1. Whether these findings are of pathogenetic significance is uncertain.

Clinical features

ORAL AND GENITAL ULCERATION

Recurrent oral ulceration is frequently the earliest symptom of Behçet's syndrome. Diagnosis at this stage, in the absence of other symptoms, is impossible as recurrent oral ulceration is common in most populations; several surveys of British people have recorded a prevalence of greater than 10%.

Oral ulcers are classified as major aphthous, minor aphthous and herpetiform (reviewed by Lehner[28] and Cooke[13]; see also Chapter 1) (Table 9.4). Recurrent major aphthous ulcers are a significant cause of morbidity. Their distribution includes the gums, palate and pharynx and they have a tendency to recur at the same sites. Treatment includes topical steroids, preferably initiated in the early prodromal phase of ulceration, chlorhexidine mouthwashes to help maintain dental hygiene, and dentistry to minimize

Table 9.4 Clinical features of recurrent oral ulcers (see Chapter 1).

	Prodrome	Size of ulcer	Duration of ulcer	Scarring	Crop size
Major aphthous	24–48 h	>1 cm	Several weeks	+ +	<10
Minor aphthous	24–48 h	<1 cm	Less than 14 days	–	<10
Herpetiform	24–48 h	0.1–0.2 cm	Less than 14 days	+	many; tend to coalesce

any dental trauma to the mucosa. The case for oral corticosteroids, levamisole and other systemic therapy is reviewed below.

Genital ulcers, distributed on the vulva and vagina or on the penis and scrotum, have the same appearances and clinical course as oral ulcers. They usually respond to local corticosteroids plus local antibiotics to prevent secondary infection. Although the prevalence of genital ulcers in women is higher than in men, vaginal and cervical ulcers may be painless and missed as a consequence. However, dyspareunia can be an important and distressing complication to both sexes. Ill repute surrounds genital lesions and sympathetic counselling may help to avoid the additional complication of the patient developing feelings of guilt.

SKIN INVOLVEMENT

Although a wide variety of rashes have been described, the most common are an acneiform rash distributed on the trunk and face and erythema nodosum. Especially characteristic (although not as specific as was once thought) is the formation of a sterile pustule at the site of a needle prick – the Behçetin reaction.

OCULAR DISEASE

In Japan and Turkey, Behçet's syndrome with ocular involvement is one of the commonest causes of blindness. Ocular Behçet's is much rarer in the UK; only 30 out of 1000 new patients with uveitis seen at Moorfields Eye Hospital had Behçet's syndrome[17] and 15 of these patients were from the Eastern Mediterranean. Signs of ocular involvement include iritis with hypopyon and posterior uveitis with prominent vascular changes (best seen by fluorescein angiography). Visual involvement is almost always bilateral. Dinning[17] reported that 51% of affected eyes had a visual acuity of less than 6/60 after four years. Late features of ocular involvement are optic nerve atrophy, secondary glaucoma and cataracts. A number of uncontrolled studies[18, 34, 35] have provided evi-

dence that early acute attacks of ocular disease may respond to corticosteroids with chlorambucil or azathioprine. The prospects for visual recovery in the late stages of ocular disease are gloomy.

OESOPHAGEAL INVOLVEMENT

Dysphagia complicating aphthous ulceration of the oesophagus is the commonest symptom of oesophageal involvement. Both stricture formation and perforation of the oesophagus have been described as rare but serious complications of ulceration. A unique case report documents a patient with dysphagia with features very similar to achalasia of the oesophagus from whom an aganglionic segment of the oesophagus was excised.[3]

INTESTINAL INVOLVEMENT

The nature of intestinal involvement in Behçet's syndrome is controversial. There are marked differences in the frequency of the reports of intestinal involvement between Japan where intestinal symptoms are said to be present in as many as half of the patients,[51] and European and American series in which intestinal symptoms are uncommonly noted. Indeed, up until 1982 there have only been 18 reports describing a total of 37 non-Japanese patients with severe intestinal involvement.

An epidemiological study[60] of 2520 patients with Behçet's syndrome in Japan found that 300 had intestinal involvement. Kasahara et al.[25] reviewed 136 patients who required surgical intervention for intestinal Behçet's and suggested that intestinal involvement requiring surgery was a rare complication which occurred in less than 1% of all cases of Behçet's syndrome. These figures contrast with those of Shimizu who reported intestinal symptoms in 50% of his series of 216 Japanese patients[51] and intestinal ulcers in 27%, of which nearly half perforated. It is likely that this latter series was not unselected.

Vomiting, abdominal pain, flatulence, diarrhoea and constipation are the most prominent gastrointestinal symptoms (reviewed in Shimizu et al.[52]). Patients with intestinal ulcers usually present with abdominal pain which may mimic appendicitis;[25] this is not surprising as ulceration most commonly affects the ileocaecal region. Other complications of ulceration are perforation (sometimes multiple) with peritonitis, or fistula formation and haemorrhage.

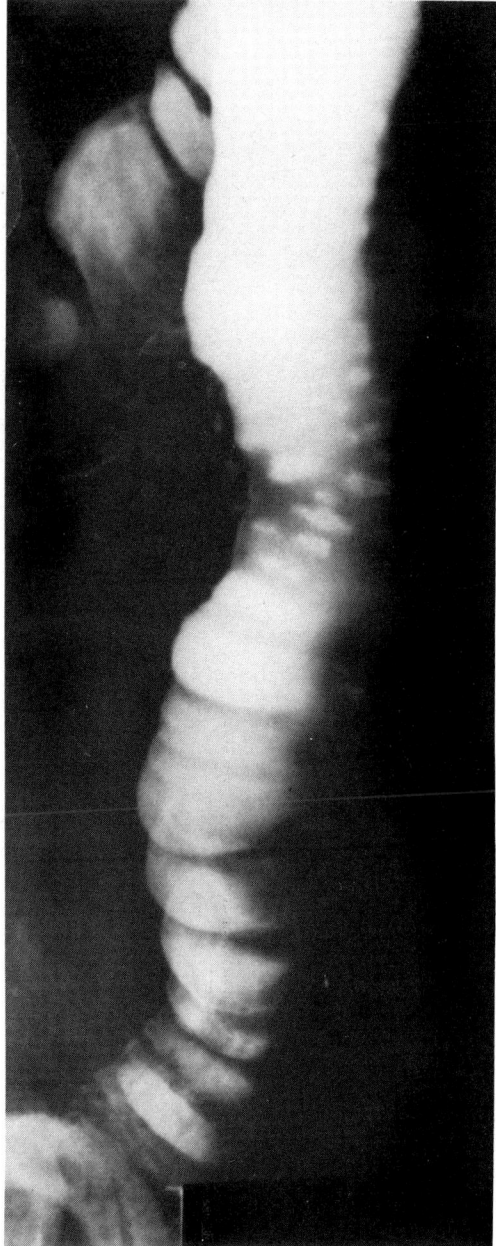

Fig. 9.9 Barium enema showing extensive ulceration of the large bowel. Courtesy of Dr R. Russell Jones.

Barium follow-through examination of 58 of Shimizu's patients[51] showed changes which included thickening of mucosal folds, flocculation of barium and dilatation of intestinal loops associated with reduced peristalsis; these changes were present more often during disease flares. Haustral markings are usually preserved in contrast to the appearances of ulcerative colitis.[5, 55] Ulcers have radiological characteristics (Figure 9.9) and colonoscopic appearances (Figure 9.10) very similar to those of peptic ulcers. Although the margins of the ulcers may be oedematous, the mucosa intervening between ulcers has a normal appearance – another feature that differentiates the lesions from those of ulcerative colitis. Surgical and pathological studies have shown that intestinal ulcers are usually multiple and located in the ileocaecal region[25] although a few patients have ulceration localized to other areas, ranging from the stomach to the rectum. A minority of patients have diffuse ulceration affecting large portions of the intestine. Obviously differentiation from Crohn's disease clinically may present difficulties.

Resected bowel specimens from these patients typically show multiple deep ulcers which extend to the serosal surface and sometimes cause multiple perforations of the bowel wall. Microscopic examination (Figure 9.11) shows non-specific changes with necrosis, infiltrates mainly composed of mononuclear cells, and obliteration of small vessels. Whereas some

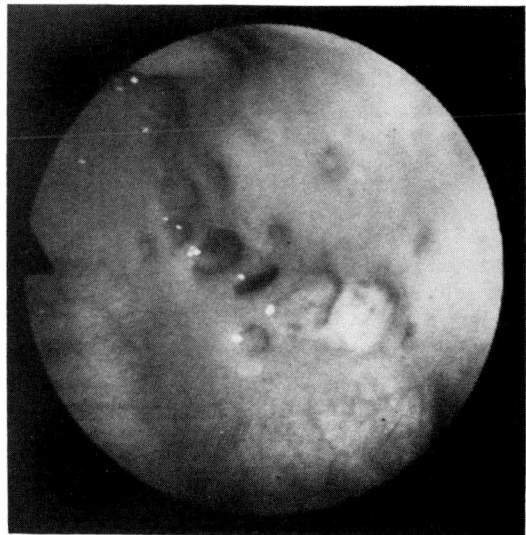

Fig. 9.10 Colonoscopic appearances showing discrete ulceration with apparently normal intervening mucosa. From Reuben, Russell Jones and Lovell (1980)[48] with kind permission of the authors and the editor of *Journal of the Royal Society of Medicine*.

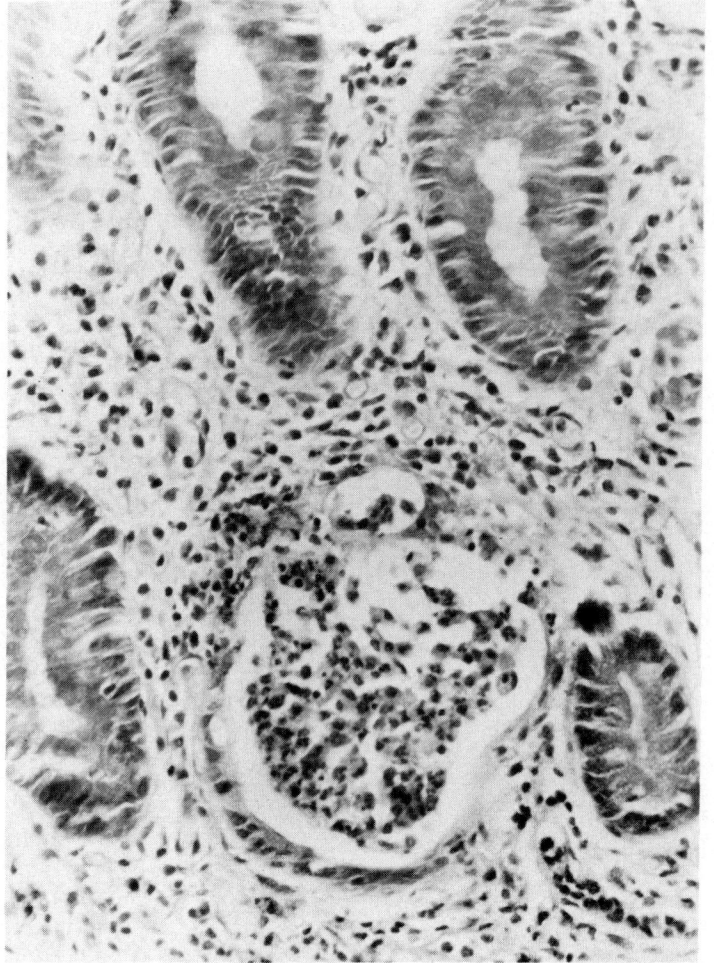

Fig. 9.11 Colonic biopsy showing crypt abscess formation with mucus and goblet cell retention in adjacent glands. From Reuben, Russell Jones and Lovell (1980)[48] with kind permission of the authors and the editor of *Journal of the Royal Society of Medicine*.

authors refer to the vascular changes as vasculitis[52] others have commented that they are not different from those seen in Crohn's disease, ulcerative colitis, or tuberculous enteritis[22] and suggest that they may be secondary changes.

Asakura and co-workers[4] studied jejunal biopsies from 15 patients with Behçet's syndrome and found marked lymphangiectasia in four. This was not accompanied by hypoproteinaemia or other evidence of malabsorption and its aetiology is unclear.

Treatment has been mainly surgical. Kasahara and his colleagues[25] reviewed 136 surgically treated cases reported in the Japanese literature. Postoperative recurrence of ulcers was common and it seemed possible that the frequency of this was related to the site and extent of bowel resection. Baba and co-workers[5] suggested that at least 60 cm of ileum from the ileocaecal valve should be resected at the time of hemicolectomy and Kasahara and his

colleagues[25] that a metre of ileum proximal to the area of ulceration should be removed. Prospective studies are needed to evaluate these suggestions.

It is interesting to compare the Japanese experience of intestinal Behçet's with the few reports of non-Japanese patients with apparent Behçet's syndrome affecting the intestine. Epidemiological studies suggest that intestinal involvement is rarer outside Japan. Sladen and Lehner[53] studied 70 patients with Behçet's syndrome attending Guy's Hospital, London. Eleven patients had gastrointestinal symptoms, which were mostly not severe. One of these patients developed perforation of an ulcer in the small intestine and four had rectal or anal aphthous ulcers. A single patient was found to have coexistent coeliac disease, a unique report of this association. Detailed studies including barium follow-through examination and jejunal biopsy performed on ten asymptomatic members of this series of patients showed no abnormalities.

In a general survey of 41 Israeli patients[10] no gastrointestinal involvement was reported.

The few reports of intestinal involvement in Behçet's syndrome in non-Japanese patients fall into two groups: those describing patients with similar intestinal involvement to that reported in Japan[20, 21, 48, 49, 53, 54, 55, 56] and those reporting patients with Behçet's syndrome and gastrointestinal involvement apparently indistinguishable from ulcerative colitis[8, 44] or Crohn's disease.[13] In view of the marked clinical overlap between certain features of Behçet's syndrome and extraintestinal manifestations of inflammatory bowel disease,[40, 59] some doubt must be cast on the precise diagnosis of this latter group of patients.

In summary, there appears to be a distinctive enteropathy associated with Behçet's syndrome, apparently commoner in Japanese than non-Japanese patients. It is characterized by localized areas of penetrating ulcers which are most commonly located in the ileocaecal region and frequently perforate. The mucosa between ulcers is normal and the histopathological changes in and around the ulcers are entirely non-specific. The clinical complications of these ulcers are serious and often require surgical intervention with resection of affected bowel and a wide margin of adjacent macroscopically normal bowel.

HEPATIC DISEASE

Primary liver involvement is rare. Oshima and colleagues[45] studied liver function in 17 patients and, apart from mild abnormal retention of sulphobromophthalein in three, found no abnormalities. Chajek and Fainaru[10] reported that hepatic biopsies from five of their patients were entirely normal.

Hepatic enlargement with abnormalities of liver function should suggest the possibility of the Budd–Chiari syndrome which has been described in five patients with Behçet's syndrome (reviewed by McDonald and Gad–Al–Rab[38]).

VASCULAR DISEASE

The vascular complications of Behçet's syndrome are protean in nature and bizarre vascular disease occurring in a young person should prompt questions about other manifestations of Behçet's syndrome. In the arterial system occlusion of major vessels may result in the infarction of organs or limbs; aneurysms occasionally develop and rupture leading to major haemorrhage.[52] In the venous system thrombophlebitis is particularly characteristic. Haim, Barzilai and Hazani[23] found thrombophlebitis in 12 out of 26 Israeli patients, which most commonly presented as recurrent superficial thrombophlebitis of the legs. Thrombosis of the venae cavae is a relatively common and serious complication.[24] Therapy for these vascular lesions has been empirical and anticoagulants and fibrinolytic agents have both been tried with only moderate results.

CENTRAL NERVOUS SYSTEM INVOLVEMENT

Between 10 and 20% of patients develop signs of central nervous system involvement.[43, 52] Pallis[46] reviewed the CNS manifestations in 42 patients; pyramidal signs were commonest, closely followed by organic confusional states. Other less common features included cranial nerve palsies, meningitis, fits, cerebellar and extrapyramidal signs. The cerebrospinal fluid may be normal or show a mild pleocytosis with or without elevation of protein levels. Pathological studies have demonstrated focal lesions, perivascular mononuclear cell infiltrates and demyelination. Brain stem lesions are most prominent but the cerebral hemispheres and spinal cord are also often involved.

ARTHRITIS

An inflammatory non-erosive arthropathy affects up to 50% of patients. It mainly involves the knees, ankles, elbows and wrists, and may be accompanied by synovial thickening and effusion. Some rheumatologists[40, 59] suggest that Behçet's syndrome should be classified among the seronegative spondyloarthritides, the other members of which are psoriatic arthritis, Reiter's disease, ulcerative colitis, Crohn's disease, Whipple's disease and ankylosing spondylitis. However, most surveys have found the prevalence of ankylosing spondylitis in Behçet's syndrome to be low (reviewed by Barnes[6]) with the exception of a series of Turkish patients described by Dilşen, Koniçe and Övül[16] in which it was 20%. Barnes[6] has suggested that the inflammatory arthropathy of Behçet's syndrome is clinically distinctive from that of the seronegative spondyloarthropathies.

OTHER ORGANS

Abnormalities apparently associated with Behçet's syndrome have been described in virtually all organs. Renal, cardiac and pulmonary disease seem to be very uncommon; the reviews of Oshima and colleagues[45] and of Chajek and Fainaru[10] provide a source of references for these and other rare manifestations of Behçet's syndrome.

Treatment

The large variety of therapies used to treat Behçet's syndrome testifies to the inefficiency or toxicity of most of the treatments currently in use (Table 9.5). The problems of objectively evaluating the effects of treatments are formidable in a rare condition with diverse clinical manifestations and variable prognosis.

Table 9.5   Current and recently fashionable (*) treatments for Behçet's syndrome.

Corticosteroids – local and systemic
Cytotoxic drugs: azathioprine,
  cyclophosphamide, chlorambucil
Colchicine
Levamisole
Fibrinolytic agents and anticoagulants
Transfusion of fresh blood*
Transfer factor*

The main principle of treatment of Behçet's syndrome is to minimize drug therapy unless vital organs are involved. There is no evidence for the prophylactic value of any drug in preventing the onset of new lesions.

Orogenital ulcers usually respond to a combination of local steroids and meticulous hygiene. Levamisole, an anthelmintic agent with ill-understood effects on the immune system, has been shown in a double-blind study to be effective in treating recurrent aphthous ulceration[31] and open studies in Behçet's syndrome[14, 30] have suggested that it may be efficacious in the treatment of mucocutaneous disease. The effects of levamisole on the haematological system require careful monitoring as neutropenia may be a dangerous side effect.

Japanese workers[37, 39] have claimed that colchicine may reduce the frequency and severity of ocular attacks. However, there are no controlled supporting data and the development of uveitis, with its poor prognosis for vision, is an indication for the administration of systemic corticosteroids and cytotoxic drugs.

Lessof and colleagues[34] have summarized the use of corticosteroids and cytotoxic drugs in Behçet's syndrome. The majority of patients with vital organ involvement or severe symptoms respond to oral corticosteroids. Although there is no evidence for the short-term effectiveness of cytotoxic drugs, most authorities agree that they have a longer-term effect and enable the reduction of corticosteroid dosage to levels that reduce side effects. Azathioprine,[34] chlorambucil[18] and cyclophosphamide[9] all have their advocates.

Intestinal ulceration probably responds to systemic corticosteroids, but rarely this treatment may predispose to silent perforation of ulcers and patients should be observed very carefully for this complication. Sulphasalazine has been administered on empirical grounds to a number of patients[48, 49, 54] with possible favourable results.

Prognosis

In the majority of patients the disease runs an indolent cause with much morbidity but low mortality. In Japan blindness occurs in over 50% of patients but mortality is only 3–4%.[52] Blindness is also common among Turkish patients but appears to be rarer in other caucasoid patients. Death is generally due to vascular, neurological and intestinal complications.

Conclusions

Although Behçet's syndrome is still rare in European and American populations, more cases will be diagnosed as its diverse features become more widely recognized. The gastrointestinal manifestations have distinctive characteristics that set them apart from other inflammatory bowel diseases. Fortunately only a small percentage of patients with Behçet's syndrome develop the major gastrointestinal complications which continue to represent a great clinical challenge.

REFERENCES

1   Abdou, N. I., Shumacher, H. R., Colman, R. W. *et al.* (1978) Behçet's disease: possible role of secretory component deficiency synovial inclusions and fibrinolytic abnormality in the various manifestations of the disease. *Journal of Laboratory and Clinical Medicine,* **91,** 409–422.

2   Aoki, K., Fujioka, K., Katsumata, H. *et al.* (1971) Epidemiological studies on Behçet's disease in Hokkaido district. *Japanese Journal of Clinical Ophthalmology,* **25,** 2239–2243.

3   Arma, S., Habibulla, K. S., Price, J. J. & Collis, J. L. (1977) Dysphagia in Behçet's syndrome. *Thorax,* **26,** 155–158.

4   Asakura, H., Morita, A., Morishita, T. *et al.* (1973) Histopathological and electron microscopic studies of lymphangiectasia of the small intestine in Behçet's disease. *Gut,* **14,** 196–203.

5 Baba, S., Maruta, M., Ando, K. *et al.* (1976) Intestinal Behçet's disease: report of five cases. *Diseases of the Colon and Rectum*, **19**, 428–440.

6 Barnes, C. G. (1979) Behçet's syndrome: joint manifestations and synovial pathology. In *Behçet's Syndrome: Clinical and Immunological Features* (Ed.) Lehner, T. & Barnes, C. G. pp. 199–212. New York, London: Academic Press.

7 Blumencrantz, Y. & Aviel, E. (1981) The diagnosis of Behçet's disease. *Metabolic and Pediatric Ophthalmology*, **5**, 89–97.

8 Bøe, J., Dalgaard, J. B. & Scott, D. (1958) Mucocutaneous ocular syndrome with intestinal involvement: a clinical and pathological study of four fatal cases. *American Journal of Medicine*, **25**, 857–867.

9 Buckley, C. E. & Gills, J. P., Jr (1969) Cyclophosphamide therapy of Behçet's disease. *Journal of Allergy*, **43**, 273–283.

10 Chajek, T. & Fainaru, M. (1975) Behçet's disease: report of 41 cases and a review of the literature. *Medicine (Baltimore)*, **54**, 179–196.

11 Chamberlain, M. A. (1977) Behçet's syndrome in 32 patients in Yorkshire. *Annals of the Rheumatic Diseases*, **36**, 491–499.

12 Chamberlain, M. A. (1979) Epidemiological features of Behçet's syndrome. In *Behçet's Syndrome: Clinical and Immunological Features* (Ed.) Lehner, T. & Barnes, C. G. pp. 213–221. New York, London: Academic Press.

13 Cooke, B. E. D. (1979) Oral ulceration in Behçet's syndrome. In *Behçet's Syndrome: Clinical and Immunological Features* (Ed.) Lehner, T. & Barnes, C. G. pp. 143–149. New York, London: Academic Press.

14 de Merieux, P., Spitler, L. E. & Paulus, H. E. (1981) Treatment of Behçet's syndrome with levamisole. *Arthritis and Rheumatism*, **24**, 64–70.

15 Denman, A. M. & Pinder, M. (1974) Assessment of immunological function in man: interaction between virus and human leukocytes. *Proceedings of the Royal Society of Medicine*, **67**, 1219–1221.

16 Dilşen, N., Koniçe M. & Övül, C. (1979) Rheumatic patterns in Behçet's disease. In *Behçet's Disease* (Ed.) Dilşen, N., Koniçe, M. & Övül, C. pp. 145–155. Amsterdam: Excerpta Medica.

17 Dinning, W. J. (1979) Behçet's disease and the eye: epidemiological considerations. In *Behçet's Syndrome: Clinical and Immunological Features* (Ed.) Lehner, T. & Barnes, C. G. pp. 179–189. New York, London: Academic Press.

18 Dinning, W. J. & Perkins, E. S. (1975) Immunosuppressives in uveitis. A preliminary report of experience with chlorambucil. *British Journal of Ophthalmology*, **59**, 397–403.

19 Eglin, R. P., Lehner, T. & Subak–Sharpe, J. H. (1982) Detection of RNA complementary to Herpes-simplex virus in mononuclear cells from patients with Behçet's syndrome and recurrent oral ulcers. *Lancet*, **ii**, 1356–1361.

20 Empey, D. W. (1972) Rectal and colonic ulceration in Behçet's disease. *British Journal of Surgery*, **59**, 173–175.

21 Eng, K., Ruoff, M. & Bystryn, J.-C. (1981) Behçet's syndrome: an unusual cause of colonic ulceration and perforation. *American Journal of Gastroenterology*, **75**, 57–59.

22 Fukuda, Y., Watanabe, I., Hayashi, H. & Kuwabara, N. (1980) Pathological studies on Behçet's disease. *Ryumachi*, **20**, 268–275.

23 Haim, S., Barzilai, D. & Hazani, E. (1971) Involvement of veins in Behçet's syndrome. *British Journal of Dermatology*, **84**, 238–241.

24 Kansu, E., Ozer, F. L., Akalin, E. *et al.* (1972) Behçet's syndrome with obstruction of the venae cavae: a report of seven cases. *Quarterly Journal of Medicine*, **41**, 151–168.

25 Kasahara, Y., Tanaka, S., Nishino, M. *et al.* (1981) Intestinal involvement in Behçet's disease: review of 136 surgical cases in the Japanese literature. *Diseases of the Colon and Rectum*, **24**, 103–106.

26 Lehner, T. (1967) Behçet's syndrome and autoimmunity. *British Medical Journal*, **i**, 465–467.

27 Lehner, T. (1969) Characterization of mucosal antibodies in recurrent aphthous ulceration and Behçet's syndrome. *Archives of Oral Biology*, **14**, 843–853.

28 Lehner, T. (1977) Oral ulceration and Behçet's syndrome. *Gut*, **18**, 491–511.

29 Lehner, T. & Barnes, C. G. (1979) Criteria for diagnosis and classification of Behçet's syndrome. In *Behçet's Syndrome: Clinical and Immunological Features* (Ed.) Lehner, T. & Barnes, C. G. pp. 1–9. New York, London: Academic Press.

30 Lehner, T. & Wilton, J. M. A. (1979) The therapeutic and immunological effects of levamisole in recurrent oral ulcers and Behçet's syndrome. In *Behçet's Syndrome: Clinical and Immunological Features* (Ed.) Lehner, T. & Barnes, C. G. pp. 291–305. New York, London: Academic Press.

31 Lehner, T., Wilton, J. M. A. & Ivanyi, L. (1976) Double blind, cross-over trial of levamisole in recurrent aphthous ulceration. *Lancet*, **ii**, 926–929.

32 Lehner, T., Batchelor, J. R., Challacombe, S. J. & Kennedy, L. (1979) An immunogenetic basis for the tissue involvement in Behçet's syndrome. *Immunology*, **37**, 895–900.

33 Lehner, T., Welsh, K. I. & Batchelor, J. R. (1982) The relationship of HLA–B and DR phenotypes to Behçet's syndrome, recurrent oral ulceration and the class of immune complexes. *Immunology*, **47**, 581–587.

34 Lessof, M. H., Jeffreys, D. B., Lehner, T. *et al.* (1979) Corticosteroids and azathioprine: their use in Behçet's syndrome. In *Behçet's Syndrome: Clinical and Immunological Features* (Ed.) Lehner, T. & Barnes, C. G. pp. 267–275. New York, London: Academic Press.

35 Mamo, J. G. (1976) Treatment of Behçet disease with chlorambucil. A follow-up report. *Archives of Ophthalmology*, **94**, 580–583.

36 Mason, R. M. & Barnes, C. G. (1969) Behçet's syndrome with arthritis. *Annals of the Rheumatic Diseases*, **28**, 95–103.

37 Matsumura, N. & Mizushima, Y. (1975) Leukocyte movement and colchicine treatment in Behçet's disease. *Lancet*, **ii**, 813.

38 McDonald, G. S. A. & Gad-Al-Rab, J. (1980) Behçet's disease with endocarditis and the Budd–Chiari syndrome. *Journal of Clinical Pathology*, **33**, 660–669.

39 Mizushima, Y., Matsumura, N., Mori, M. *et al.* (1977) Colchicine in Behçet's disease. *Lancet*, **ii**, 1037.

40 Moll, J. M. H., Haslock, I., Macrae, I. F. & Wright, V. (1974) Associations between ankylosing spondylitis, psoriatic arthritis, Reiter's disease, the intestinal arthropathias and Behçet's syndrome. *Medicine (Baltimore)*, **53**, 343–364.

41 O'Connell, D. J., Courtney, J. V. & Riddell, R. H. (1980) Colitis of Behçet's syndrome – radiologic and pathologic features. *Gastrointestinal Radiology*, **5**, 173–179.

42 O'Duffy, J. D. (1978) Summary of international symposium on Behçet's disease. *Journal of Rheumatology*, **5**, 229–233.

43 O'Duffy, J. D. & Goldstein, N. P. (1976) Neurologic involvement in seven patients with Behçet's disease. *American Journal of Medicine*, **61**, 170–178.

44 O'Duffy, J. D., Carney, J. A. & Deodhar, S. (1971) Behçet's disease: report of 10 cases, 3 with new manifestations. *Annals of Internal Medicine*, **75**, 561–570.

45 Oshima, Y., Shimizu, T., Yokohari, R. *et al.* (1963) Clinical studies on Behçet's syndrome. *Annals of the Rheumatic Diseases*, **22**, 36–45.

46 Pallis, C. A. (1966) Behçet's disease and the nervous system. *St John's Hospital Dermatological Society Transactions*, **52**, 201–206.

47 Raynor, A. & Askari, A. D. (1980) Behçet's disease and treatment with colchicine. *Journal of the American Academy of Dermatology*, **2**, 396–400.

48 Reuben, A., Russell Jones, R. & Lovell, D. (1980) Behçet's syndrome with colonic involvement and arterial thrombosis. *Journal of the Royal Society of Medicine*, **73**, 520–524.

49 Sawyer, A., Walker, T. M. & Terry, S. I. (1978) Behçet's syndrome with ileal involvement – the beneficial effect of sulphasalazine. *West Indian Medical Journal*, **28**, 218–221.

50 Shimada, K., Kogure, M., Kawashima, T. & Nishioka, K. (1974) Reduction of complement in Behçet's disease and drug allergy. *Medical Biology*, **52**, 234–239.

51 Shimizu, T. & Ogino, T. (1975) Clinico-pathological studies on the intestinal lesions in Behçet's disease – with special reference to entero-Behçet's syndrome. *Stomach and Intestine*, **10**, 1593–1600 (English summary).

52 Shimizu, T., Ehrlich, G. E., Inaba, K. & Hayashi, K. (1979) Behçet's disease (Behçet's syndrome). *Seminars in Arthritis and Rheumatism*, **8**, 223–260.

53 Sladen, G. E. & Lehner, T. (1979) Gastrointestinal disorders in Behçet's syndrome and a comparison with recurrent oral ulcers. In *Behçet's Syndrome: Clinical and Immunological Features* (Ed.) Lehner, T. & Barnes, C. G. pp. 151–158. New York, London: Academic Press.

54 Smith, G. E., Kime, L. R. & Pitcher, J. L. (1973) The colitis of Behçet's disease: a separate entity? *Digestive Diseases*, **18**, 987–999.

55 Stanley, R. J., Tedesco, F. J., Melson, G. L. *et al.* (1975) The colitis of Behçet's disease: a clinical-radiographic correlation. *Radiology*, **114**, 603–604.

56 Thach, B. T. & Cummings, N. A. (1976) Behçet's syndrome with 'aphthous colitis'. *Archives of Internal Medicine*, **136**, 705–709.

57 Tsukada, S., Yamazaki, T., Iyo, S. *et al.* (1964) Neuro-Behçet's syndrome: report of two cases and review of the literature. *Saishin-Igaku*, **19**, 1533–1541 (Japanese).

58 Williams, B. D. & Lehner, T. (1977) Immune complexes in Behçet's syndrome and recurrent oral ulceration. *British Medical Journal*, **i**, 1387–1389.

59 Wright, V. (1978) Seronegative polyarthritis: a unified concept. *Arthritis and Rheumatism*, **21**, 619–633.

60 Yamamoto, S., Toyokawa, H. & Matsubara, J. (1971) Nation-wide survey of Behçet's disease in Japan. *Japanese Journal of Ophthalmology*, **19**, 278.

OTHER VASCULITIC DISORDERS

Giant cell (temporal) arteritis can on rare occasions clinically affect intra-abdominal vessels;[2] the presentation then is usually as an abdominal emergency due to gut infarction, although chronic abdominal pain attributable to mesenteric ischaemia may occur.

Essential mixed cryoglobulinaemia has rarely been reported to give rise to intestinal vasculitis.[3] Conversely, however, a variety of intestinal diseases (notably coeliac disease but also possibly ulcerative colitis) have been reported to give rise to cryoglobulinaemia and a secondary vasculitis.[1]

After surgical relief of coarctation of the aorta, the response of the visceral vessels to a sudden increase in perfusion pressure and flow may result in dilatation, perivascular inflammation, and thrombosis of arterioles.[4] Symptoms develop within a few days of surgery in about 20% of patients who undergo this operation. The clinical picture may be mild, with some abdominal pain and distension, or the full picture of an intestinal infarction may result. If surgery is not required, conservative management will include resting the gut and control of hypertension.

Malignant atrophic papulosis (Kohlmeier–Degos disease)[5]

This is a very rare but recognizable condition in which a small vessel vasculitis involves the skin and gut. Most patients are young men, with only a quarter of reported patients being female. One pair of affected relatives – mother-son – has suggested a genetic basis for this disorder, but its aetiology is unknown.

The characteristic presentation is with scattered skin lesions, initially as pink papules, but evolving a characteristic 'porcelain-like' central area of atrophy, grey–white in appearance. They are from a few millimetres to 15 cm in diameter. The vasculitic process in the gut is mainly submucosal, and ischaemia and fibrosis lead to episodes of abdominal cramps or diarrhoea. Occasionally involvement of the retroperitoneum leads to chylous ascites from lymphatic obstruction and leakage. One-half of the reported patients died within three years, usually after intestinal perforation had occurred through a fibrotic plaque subserosally; both very rapid and much more indolent cases can occur. Vessels elsewhere in the body may also be involved and cerebrovascular disease may be prominent.

REFERENCES

1 Doe, W. F., Evans, D., Hobbs, J. R. & Booth, C. C. (1972) Coeliac disease, vasculitis and cryoglobulinaemia. *Gut*, **13**, 112–123.

2 Klein, R. G., Hunder, G. G., Stevenson, A. W. & Sheps, S. G. (1975) Large artery involvement in giant cell activity. *Annals of Internal Medicine*, **83**, 806–812.

3 Reza, M. J., Roth, B. E., Pops, M. A. & Goldberg, L. S. (1974) Intestinal vasculitis in essential mixed cryoglobulinaemia. *Annals of Internal Medicine*, **81**, 632–634.

4 Sealey, W. G., Harris, J. S., Young, W. H. & Callaway, H. A. (1957) Paradoxical hypertension following resection of coarctation of aorta. *Surgery*, **42**, 135–147.

5 Strole, W. E., Clark, W. H. & Isselbacher, K. J. (1967) Progressive arterial occlusive disease (Köhlmeier–Degos). *New England Journal of Medicine*, **276**, 195.

CHRONIC RENAL FAILURE

While the alimentary tract is always affected in the chronic forms of renal failure, the clinical syndromes are varied and indistinct. Traditionally, the stomach and colon have been thought to be most involved. Most characteristic are episodic vomiting in the early stages, and haemorrhagic superficially ulcerated mucosal lesions scattered throughout the gut in terminal (untreated) uraemia.[8]

Enterohepatic cycle of urea and ammonia

Urea normally enters the gut freely by diffusion from plasma and is largely hydrolysed to ammonia and carbon dioxide by bacterial ureases in the proximal colon (Figure 9.12). Since the colon is relatively impermeable to urea, the ureases act upon urea delivered intraluminally from the small intestine. Such urealysis, effected mainly by *Proteus spp.* or *Klebsiella spp.*, is the main source of urea degradation and it can be eliminated by intraluminal antibiotics.[15] Because of urealysis, urea is not detectable in the faeces of normal individuals. Patients with uraemia also have urea-free faeces or minimal concentrations.[17] The ammonia concentration and pH of the large bowel lumen may be increased in a minority, but the levels in the presence of diarrhoea, late in the course of chronic renal failure, are unknown.

It might be supposed that enterohepatic circulation of urea nitrogen is greatly increased in uraemia. Early claims that the urealysis rate in uraemia is twice normal or increased in proportion to the plasma urea concentration are now

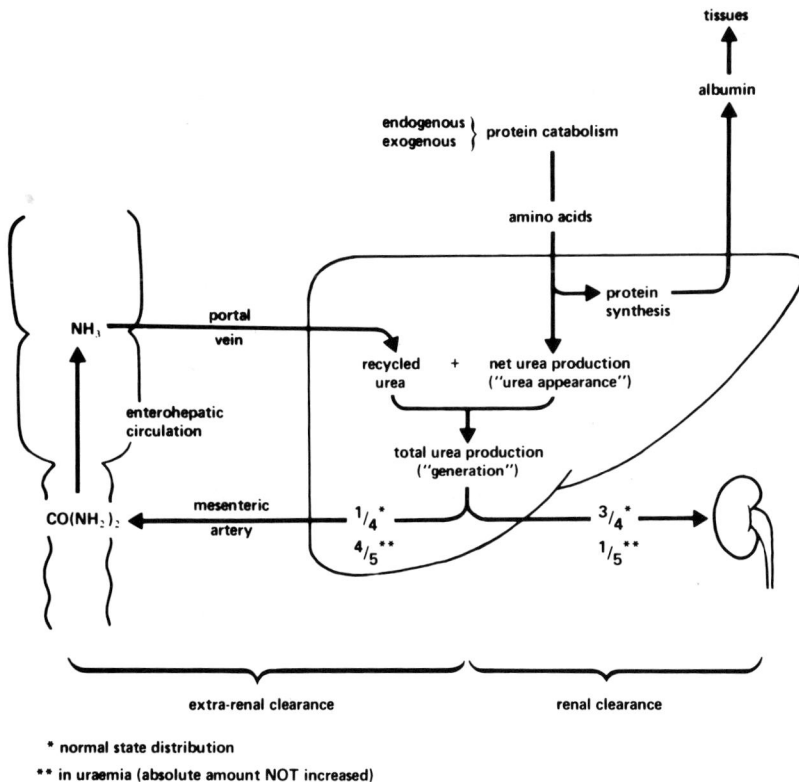

Fig. 9.12 The enterohepatic cycle of urea and ammonia, showing the relative proportions of renal and extrarenal clearance of urea under normal conditions and in uraemia.

contested. Walser[14] claimed that the absolute amount of urea converted to ammonia in the gut per day is usually similar to the amount so transformed in normal subjects. He inferred that some adaptation to azotaemia, possibly a decrease in permeability of the gut mucosa to urea or ammonia, may be involved. There is a conflict between the results of indirectly made (isotopic) measurements which show no increase in recycled urea and inference from a priori reasoning based on: first, the absence of urea in uraemic faeces; second, the assumed increased delivery of urea to the gut; and third, the presence of increased bacterial ureases in the uraemic colon.[3] The position in acute renal failure is more orthodox since rapid elevation of plasma urea does coincide with a corresponding increase in urea degradation by urealysis.[19] In chronic uraemia, peripheral blood ammonia is normal or even reduced reflecting reduced renal ammonia generation associated with kidney parenchymal destruction but the levels in portal venous blood are uncertain.

Pathogenesis of uraemic enterocolitis

Since urea and ammonia were assumed to be present in quantity within the gut of uraemics, these chemical factors have long been associated with the enterocolitis of end-stage renal failure.[13] Although a causal role for ammonia in the pathogenesis of uraemic colitis has not been demonstrated it does seem likely to be implicated. Bacterial action in the colon of uraemic animals is accompanied by high intraluminal pH, high total and free ammonia concentrations, and mucosal lesions, especially in the caecum.[2] Experimentally, the development of acute uraemic colitis in rats depends on the presence of microbial flora in the gut, and germ-free nephrectomized rats are protected. In man uraemic colitis is only an occasional component of the uraemic illness and may well represent an extreme near-terminal situation. The therapeutic role of urea-splitting enzyme inhibition does not appear to have been explored.

The role of urea and ammonia in the gastric and duodenal lesions is conjectural and unconvincing. Early experimental work is conflicting. Urea may directly damage the mucosal barrier in the stomach.[4]

Clinical syndromes

Nephrologists recognize the advent of symptomatic uraemia, signalled by nausea and vomiting, when the serum urea and creatinine are about 30 mmol/l and 900 µmol/l respectively. Initially, these symptoms are sharply episodic, often only in the early morning, but they become more frequent as the azotaemia progresses. The relationship between the level of azotaemia and the episodic nausea and vomiting is variable. Some patients are almost free of this feature until late in the illness. Absence of nausea and vomiting, and restoration of appetite, are features of the response to the high fat and carbohydrate but protein-restricted Giordano–Giovanetti diet. Although the relief of these uraemic symptoms parallels a decrease in endogenous protein catabolism and reduced build-up of nitrogenous waste substances, it is not known whether the effect is mediated via the gut luminal content or centrally on the brain stem. Phenothiazines only partly control uraemic vomiting, presumably by central action.

Even less constant in uraemia are a variety of other disturbances of the gut.

UPPER GASTROINTESTINAL SYNDROMES

Buccal cavity. Dry mouth, unpleasant metallic taste, and uriniferous odour (fetor) are usual in late renal failure. Occasionally, the buccal cavity is grossly abnormal with sordes or pseudomembranous ulceration, reminiscent of the mouth of agranulocytosis. These features clear readily with dialysis therapy.

Stomach and duodenum. Patients with long-standing renal failure, particularly those on maintenance haemodialysis treatment, seem prone to peptic, especially duodenal, ulceration.[5, 9] There is an associated gastric hypersecretory state characterized by both increased responsiveness to pentagastrin stimulation and high spontaneous secretion rates of acid[9] which may be prevented in some patients by coexistent chronic gastritis.[6]

Gastric hypersecretion in uraemia was at first attributed to the high basal serum gastrin levels. More recently, the 'hypergastrinaemia' has been shown to be heterogeneous with the less potent 'big gastrin' (G34) predominating. Basal gastrin levels were shown to be inversely related to maximum acid output in uraemia with high levels predicting hyposecretion.[12] Basal and meal-stimulated gastrin levels in uraemic patients with ulcers were comparable to the levels in uraemic patients without ulcers. The proneness to peptic ulceration is therefore of uncertain causation and is absent in some series.[11]

Liability of peptic ulcers to bleeding after renal transplantation is entirely unpredictable, since the duodenal or gastric ulceration is superficial, acute and of recent origin. Nevertheless, gastric assessment pre- and postoperatively is important. Dose-adjusted cimetidine is useful in the presence of ulcer symptoms. Although a pharmacologically mediated increment in serum creatinine occurs transiently, cimetidine responsiveness is essentially unchanged in patients with renal failure. Active upper gastrointestinal ulceration with haemorrhage and perforation have an almost 50% mortality in postrenal transplantation patients, and early surgical intervention is indicated.

Small intestine. Except for occasional late enterocolitis it has been assumed until recently that jejunoileal function was unaffected in uraemia. Some clinical investigations have shown morphological changes (shortening of villi, elongated crypts with Paneth's cells and plasma cell infiltration), decreased enzymic activity and no response to oral glucose loads. Others found no lesions. Experimental results in rats have been paradoxical in that small bowel morphology was unaffected and certain enzyme activities were increased.[10] Other circumstantial evidence also points, albeit inconclusively, to some malabsorption. The plasma amino acid pattern in clinical end-stage renal failure is characterized by reduced levels of most essential amino acids. This may reflect impaired intestinal absorption as has been shown directly with tryptophan.

While species difference may play a part in creating the observed difference between patients and rats, it seems important that the patients studied had been on conventional low protein diets while the rats were on normal rations. Barium contrast radiography has shown mucosal and valvular thickening of the jejunum in a minority of haemodialysed patients, there being no correlation with susceptibility to diarrhoea.

Questions about the adequacy of jejunoileal absorptive function in uraemia remain. Despite authenticated success in maintaining nitrogen balance, patients become wasted. The minimal changes observed to date may prove to be adaptive to dietary and other circumstances. No corresponding clinical syndrome has yet been demonstrated.

LOWER GASTROINTESTINAL SYNDROMES

Colon. Throughout most of the course of chronic renal failure, bowel actions are either undisturbed or constipated. Dietary restriction, oral aluminium-based phosphate binders in high dosage, ion-exchange resins and dehydration during dialysis all tend to constipate. Nevertheless, colitis is a characteristic but infrequent manifestation in late uraemia. It may involve only mucosal congestion or advance to pseudomembranous change or diffuse superficial ulceration indistinguishable from ulcerative colitis. A right-sided distribution is characteristic and is reflected in the experimental model.[2]

Constipation may lead to faecal impaction with obstruction or stercoral ulceration and perforation,[16] usually in the sigmoid but occasionally higher, even involving the caecum.

Discrete mucosal ulceration, usually solitary, may occur in the caecum or proximal colon of patients with chronic renal failure and lead on to gross bleeding or perforations. They appear to be linked to renal insufficiency, but are not unique to that state. In immunosuppressed patients after renal allografts, cytomegalovirus (CMV) infection may be causal, but before transplantation, suspicion rests on unrecognized stercoral impaction. Prophylaxis rests on the use of stool-softening agents and cathartics such as sorbitol.

Claims have been made that colonic diverticulitis, with perforation and resultant faecal peritonitis, is disproportionately common in haemodialysed patients who have polycystic kidney disease. It does seem clear that such diverticulitis may progress to perforation after allografting and prophylactic elective excision has been advocated.

The early postoperative period of the renal allografted patient is prone to major colonic disorders, all with a high mortality rate. In this setting renal insufficiency is compounded with immunosuppression, steroids, opportunistic infections and often graft rejection. Cytomegalovirus infection may present as a solitary ulcer manifested clinically by gross haemorrhage or perforation.[1] CMV particles have been demonstrated in the majority of these ulcers in one series. Alternatively, CMV or *Candida* may have opportunistically colonized a pre-existent ulcer of different causation.

Ischaemic colitis in renal transplant patients[7] may feature rectal haemorrhage or abdominal pain and ileus. Early surgical resection is necessary. The causative vascular lesion may be non-occlusive in basis, the result of blood redistribution with transient hypotension, especially during postoperative haemodialysis. The clinical features of these lower gut disorders (dyschezia, diarrhoea, rectal bleeding, lower abdominal pain and ileus) do not allow ready differentiation at the bedside. The inherent potential of the end-stage renal failure and especially of the postallograft situation for rapid deterioration warrants a policy of aggressive and necessarily invasive investigation linked to early surgical intervention. This would involve endoscopy and mesenteric arteriography for rectal haemorrhage, and contrast studies with water soluble media for lower abdominal pain and otherwise suspected early perforation.

Uncomplicated uraemic (entero-) colitis is said to respond within 24 hours to effective haemodialysis treatment. Persistence of lower bowel manifestations, including gross blood loss per rectum, suggests complicating factors.

ALIMENTARY HAEMORRHAGE

Bleeding time is prolonged in the later stages of uraemia and the extent of prolongation correlates with the risk of clinical bleeding. The haemorrhagic diathesis, mainly a platelet defect, is corrected by effective haemodialysis or peritoneal dialysis. Spontaneous epistaxis and covert oozing of blood into the alimentary tract is usual in chronic renal failure. When mucosal ulceration occurs, overt haematemesis or melaena may occur. Failure of hitherto successful conservation treatment by diet is signalled by the reappearance of mucosal bleeding, even in the absence of nausea and vomiting. However, gastrointestinal bleeding is more prominent in acute than chronic renal failure. Haemodialysis, which involves the use of heparinization, is more hazardous in the setting of overt alimentary bleeding than continuous or intermittent peritoneal dialysis. Haemodialysis can sometimes be undertaken with 'regional heparinization' to minimize systemic effects. Unfortunately, the technique is difficult to control and aggravated intestinal bleeding may result. Maintenance haemodialysis will largely, but not entirely, correct the low grade oozing of blood into the gut, possibly by the dialytic extraction of a diffusible plasma constituent, which disturbs platelet function.

Conclusions

It is likely, but as yet unproven, that in uraemia the lower gut is affected by a change in the urea–ammonia cycle. Enterocolitis may result but other concomitant states, diverticulitis, stercoral ulceration, ischaemic colitis, etc., call for decisive differentiation and intervention. Ulceration of stomach and duodenum is of unexplained causation in the uraemic patient although acute ulceration at these sites is 'stress-related' and occurs unpredictably in the early postrenal transplantation patient.

REFERENCES

1 Aldrete, J. S., Sterling, W. A., Hathaway, B. M. *et al.* (1975) Gastrointestinal and hepatic complications affecting patients with renal allografts. *American Journal of Surgery*, **129**, 115–124.

2 Bourke, E., Milne, M. D. & Stokes, G. S. (1966) Caecal pH and ammonia in experimental uraemia. *Gut*, **7**, 558–565.

3 Brown, C. L., Hill, M. J. & Richards, P. (1971) Bacterial ureases in uraemic men. *Lancet*, **ii**, 406–407.

4 Davenport, H. W. (1968) Destruction of the gastric mucosal barrier by detergents and urea. *Gastroenterology*, **54**, 175–181.

5 Doherty, C. C., O'Connor, F. A., Buchanan, K. D. *et al.* (1977) Treatment of peptic ulcer in renal failure. *Proceedings of the European Dialysis and Transplantation Association*, **14**, 386–395.

6 McConnell, J. B., Stewart, W. K., Thjodleifsson, B. & Wormsley, K. G. (1975) Gastric function in chronic renal failure. *Lancet*, **ii**, 1121–1123.

7 Margolis, D. M., Etheredge, E. E., Garza-Garza, R. *et al.* (1977) Ischemic bowel disease following bilateral nephrectomy or renal transplant. *Surgery*, **82**, 667–673.

8 Mason, E. E. (1952) Gastrointestinal lesions occurring in uremia. *Annals of Internal Medicine*, **37**, 96–105.

9 Shepherd, A. M. M., Stewart, W. K. & Wormsley, K. G. (1973) Peptic ulceration in chronic renal failure. *Lancet*, **i**, 1357–1359.

10 Sterner, G., Ash, N.-G., Dahlquist, A. *et al.* (1980) Small intestinal dipeptidases and disaccharidases in experimental uremia in rats. *Nephron*, **26**, 149–152.

11 Tani, N., Harasawa, S., Suzuki, S. *et al.* (1980) Lesions of the upper gastrointestinal tract in patients with chronic renal failure. *Gastroenterologica*, **15**, 480–484.

12 Taylor, I. L., Sells, R. A., McConnell, R. B. & Dockray, G. J. (1980) Serum gastrin in patients with chronic renal failure. *Gut*, **21**, 1062–1067.

13 Treitz, W. (1859) Ueber urämische darmaffectionen. *Vierteljahrsschrift für die praktische Heilkunde*, **64**, 143–198.

14 Walser, M. (1980) Determinants of ureagenesis, with particular reference to renal failure (Editorial Review). *Kidney International*, **17**, 709–721.

15 Walser, M. & Bodenlos, L. J. (1959) Urea metabolism in man. *Journal of Clinical Investigation*, **38**, 1617–1626.

16 Welch, J. P., Schweizer, R. T. & Bartus, S. A. (1980) Management of antacid infections in hemodialysis and renal transplant patients. *American Journal of Surgery*, **139**, 561–568.

17 Wilson, D. R., Ing, T. S., Metcalfe-Gibson, A. & Wrong, O. M. (1968) The chemical composition of faeces in uraemia, as revealed by in vivo faecal dialysis. *Clinical Sciences*, **35**, 197–201.

19 Wolpert, E., Phillips, S. F. & Summerskill, W. H. J. (1971) Transport of urea and ammonia production in the human colon. *Lancet*, **ii**, 1387–1390.

CARDIAC DISEASE

Patients suffering primarily from cardiac disease may present with symptoms or signs which either mimic those of gastroenterological disorders or which indeed reflect gastrointestinal pathology secondary to cardiovascular disease. This may arise as the result of disturbed haemodynamics associated with either heart failure or peripheral embolism, or as a side-effect of cardiovascular drug treatment.

Cardiovascular disease presenting gastroenterological symptoms

Heart failure may present as hepatomegaly. Most patients with cardiac failure in the Western World suffer from some form of left ventricular disease due to systemic hypertension, acquired valve disorder or coronary artery disease. The development of right-sided heart failure is, therefore, preceded by a period of pulmonary hypertension which causes dyspnoea so that when hepatomegaly develops the diagnosis is already well established. In certain cardiac disorders, however, right-sided heart failure is the presenting feature, as for example in constrictive pericarditis or in later life as a result of atrial septal defect. Such patients may present to their physician with a sensation of fullness in the upper abdomen as a result of hepatomegaly. Although clinically the aetiology of such hepatic enlargement is usually obvious, it is easy to be confused by the biochemical abnormalities resulting from hepatic venous congestion. A raised serum bilirubin, alkaline phosphatase and aspartate aminotransferase, due partially to central venous congestion and in part to reduced nutritional blood flow to the liver, may occur when the clinical signs of cardiac failure are only detectable with some difficulty or have been masked by effective diuretic therapy.[1] The classic picture of cardiac cirrhosis is rarely seen now, perhaps because modern diuretic therapy permits a near normal right ventricular filling pressure to be maintained in the presence of considerable impairment of cardiac function. The reduction in cardiac output will, however, be reflected in impaired hepatic and renal function.

Severe abdominal pain of sudden onset may represent mesenteric embolism. The splanchnic vascular bed is a common site for systemic embolism originating in the left atrium or ventricle. In patients with mitral stenosis atrial fibrillation usually precedes embolism, but its absence is no guarantee of immunity from this serious complication. Many cardiologists therefore recommend routine administration of oral anticoagulants to such patients. As rheumatic mitral valve disease declines in numerical importance, previously less common causes of thrombosis in the left heart assume greater significance. Mesenteric embolism secondary to thrombosis within the left ventricle after myocardial infarction, almost invariably extensive, is the commonest cause of severe abdominal pain three or four days after the onset of the acute illness. It is almost invariably fatal. The congestive or dilated cardiomyopathies are increasingly important causes of systemic embolism, whether or not the patient is in atrial fibrillation.

When the clinical picture of mesenteric embolism complicates a previously undiagnosed febrile illness, infective endocarditis is likely. Echocardiographic examination of the aortic and mitral valves may actually reveal evidence of vegetation. This is important in view of the high incidence of culture negative infective endocarditis as a result of previous inadequate antibiotic therapy. In an ageing population the source of infection is less frequently the mouth and may often be in the genitourinary tract so that enterococcal and coliform infections have become increasingly common. There is another link between infective endocarditis and gastroenterology in that the former may be caused by endoscopy. Bacteraemia follows endoscopy sufficiently often to justify the use of prophylactic antibiotics among patients at risk.[2]

The clinical presentation of mesenteric infarction may be mimicked by an aortic dissection. This is unlikely to pose a diagnostic problem when the origin of the dissection is in the ascending aorta, because involvement of vessels to the arm and brain, or involvement of the aortic valve and coronary arteries, render the diagnosis obvious. When the dissection originates in the region of the left subclavian, however, confusion may easily arise.

Gastroenterological disorder resulting from drug therapy

Since drug treatment of cardiovascular disease is sufficiently likely to cause gastrointestinal symptoms, a carefully taken history of current and recent medication is essential if this possibility is not to be overlooked. Nausea and vomiting are common side-effects of cardiovascular therapy and are classically associated with digitalis intoxication. This dramatic picture is less common than one of general malaise and loss of appetite, particularly among elderly patients who may be further exposed to digitalis toxicity by the use of diuretics and the presence of renal failure. Nausea and vomiting are also caused by several other commonly used cardiovascular drugs including spironolactone, mexiletine, verapamil, procainamide and tocainide (the more recently introduced orally effective analogue of lignocaine). Epigastric discomfort not infrequently occurs as a result of thiazide treatment and all diuretics can aggravate a tendency to constipation. The infrequently used ethacrynic acid, on the other hand, when given orally may occasionally result in very severe profuse diarrhoea.

Patients on diuretic therapy for heart failure are occasionally given potassium supplements, although in recent years there has been a tendency to use potassium sparing diuretics instead. When the passage of potassium containing tablets through the bowel is delayed, either as a result of intestinal stricture or even secondary to a hiatal hernia, high local concentration of potassium chloride may occur, particularly with slow-release preparations. This may result in local ulceration and subsequent fibrosis. Occasionally presentation of the condition is very dramatic and resembles acute gastrointestinal obstruction, occasionally accompanied by haemorrhage.

Many of the earlier antihypertensive drugs resulted in troublesome bowel symptoms as a result of interference with the normal balance of autonomic control. The ganglion blocking drugs which produced ileus have almost completely disappeared from the therapeutic scene; even guanethidine induced diarrhoea is rarely encountered now due to the gradual abandonment of the postganglionic adrenergic neurone blockers. Methyldopa occasionally results in hepatic damage particularly when there is pre-existing liver disease.

The β-adrenergic blocking agents are now the cornerstone of modern antihypertensive therapy. Practolol produced a diffuse fibrosing peritonitis as part of the oculo-mucocutaneous syndrome. Occasionally isolated reports of a plastic peritonitis have appeared in association with the administration of other β-adrenergic antagonists, but no consistent relationship has been established. The β-adrenergic antagonists are also employed in the treatment of angina; perhexiline is also sometimes used as an extremely effective antianginal drug but unfortunately it has a high incidence of side-effects, including a change in liver function tests to suggest hepatocellular injury.[3]

Confusion between heart and gastrointestinal disease

The classic diagnostic problem between gastroenterology and cardiology is of course, the distinction of angina from oesophageal pain. Few gastroenterologists would subscribe to the cardiological taunt that the diagnosis of angina is never confirmed until a barium swallow has shown oesophageal reflux! Unfortunately, the cost of failing to recognize the presence of angina pectoris is greater than that of failing to appreciate that central chest discomfort originates from the oesophagus. It is equally true to say, however, that the diagnosis of angina pectoris should not lightly be placed upon a patient for psychological reasons, quite apart from the practical difficulties of living with this diagnosis, including the threat that it poses to employment and insurance. Unfortunately, the tendency for angina to occur after meals and to result in belching often leads to confusion in the minds of both patient and doctor. Even prompt response of the pain to sublingual glyceryl trinitrate may reflect relaxation of oesophageal spasm, adding further to the confusion. Much depends upon obtaining a history of chest pain related to effort (other than bending) with rapid cessation of the discomfort on resting. Even so, recent concepts of coronary artery spasm to explain the occurrence of angina at rest or in the cold illustrate how difficult the differential diagnosis can be.[4] In the majority of patients a carefully taken history, followed where necessary by exercise electrocardiography and radioisotope myocardial perfusion studies, allows the correct diagnosis to be made. Occasionally, however, one encounters a patient in whom central chest pain has remained a major problem for some considerable time, often resulting in frequent hospital admission and conflicting opinions. Under these circumstances a coronary arteriogram is justified on a 'need to know' basis. In fact, in the majority of such patients the coronary arteries appear to be anatomically normal.

REFERENCES

1 Cohen, J. A. & Kaplan, M. N. (1978) Left sided heart failure presenting as hepatitis. *Gastroenterology*, **74**, 583–587.

2 Dickman, M. D., Farrell, R., Higgs, R. H. *et al.* (1976) Colonoscopy associated bacteraemia. *Surgery, Gynecology and Obstetrics*, **142**, 173–176.

3 Kopelman, P. & Morgan, P. G. M. (1977) Liver damage after perhexiline maleate. *Lancet*, **i**, 705.

4 Maseri, A. & Chierchia, S. (1982) Coronary artery spasm: demonstration, definition, diagnosis and consequences. *Progress in Cardiovascular Disease*, **25**, 169–192.

RESPIRATORY DISEASE

In the embryo the lungs arise as a pouch in the primitive foregut and a close anatomical relationship between the upper gastrointestinal and respiratory tracts remains in adult life. This close relationship explains the respiratory complications of certain gut diseases, notably those of the oesophagus, and there are equally obvious explanations for most of the others shown in Table 9.6. The explanation is often more obscure for other diseases affecting both systems and disease associations occurring between them. Certainly there are similarities between the gastrointestinal and respiratory tracts. Both have large epithelial surface areas for absorption and excretion which are constantly exposed to potentially noxious environmental agents. Both have comparable defence mechanisms, with a mucus lining, the ability to secrete immunoglobulins and non-specific antimicrobial substances into their lumina, and a similar arrangement of lymphoid tissue. In the lung this lymphoid tissue is found at the bifurcations of the bronchial tree, consists of follicular lymphoid aggregates beneath a modified epithelium devoid of cilia and is strikingly similar to the Peyer's patches of the gut.

In this brief review diseases affecting the gut and respiratory tract have been divided into three groups: (a) gut disease with respiratory tract complications (see Table 9.6); (b) infections with gut and respiratory tract manifestations; and (c) associated gut and respiratory disease.

Infections with gut and respiratory tract manifestations

It is well recognized that disease above and below the diaphragm may cause anatomically misleading symptoms and signs, and this is particularly true of basal pneumonias and subdiaphragmatic infections. Certain specific infections of either system may also produce confusing symptoms in the other. Thus diarrhoea is a feature of the prodromal illness of legionnaires' disease (*Legionella pneumophila*) and gastroenteritis may be suspected. Abdominal pain may occur in the course of Bornholm disease (Coxsackie B viruses), giving rise to an incorrect diagnosis of appendicitis, and pancreatitis has been reported in fulminant disease due to *Chlamydia psittaci*.[3] Conversely acute bronchitis may be an early manifestation of salmonellosis. Pulmonary eosinophilia (transient lung shadows with blood eosinophilia) can occur during the passage of certain parasites through the lungs and may be asymptomatic or associated with cough and wheeze. *Ascaris lumbricoides*, *Ancylostoma duodenale*, *Necator americanus*, *Strongyloides stercoralis*, *Toxocara canis*, *T. cati*, *Schistosoma mansoni* and *S. japonicum* are the responsible intestinal parasites. Embolization to the lungs of Schistosoma eggs (including those of *S. haematobium*) results in an endarteritis obliterans of the pulmonary vascular bed with the development of cor pulmonale, and granuloma formation around extravasated eggs is followed by fibrosis of lung parenchyma. A severe pneumonia may accompany the *Strongyloides stercoralis* hyperinfection syndrome.

Hepatic abscesses due to *Entamoeba histolytica* commonly cause a raised right hemidiaphragm and may be associated with a sympathetic right pleural effusion, or complicated by an amoebic empyema or lung abscess. Actinomycosis can occur in both the thoracic and abdominal cavities and spread from one to the other.

Table 9.6 Gut disease with respiratory tract complications.

Disease	Respiratory tract complications
Pharyngeal pouch Achalasia Familial dysautonomia	Aspiration pneumonia Recurrent pneumonia Lung abscess
Enterogenous cysts Diaphragmatic herniae	Routine chest x-ray findings
Oesophageal carcinoma	Oesophagobronchial fistula
Oesophageal rupture	Mediastinitis Pleural effusion
Metastatic carcinoma stomach Metastatic carcinoma pancreas	Lymphangitis carcinomatosa Nodular chest x-ray shadowing
Acute pancreatitis	Pleural effusion Adult respiratory distress syndrome
Whipple's disease	Pleurisy and pneumonia
Small bowel lymphoma	Pulmonary deposits
Metastatic carcinoid tumours	Asthma (as part of carcinoid syndrome)
Metastatic large bowel carcinoma	Nodular chest x-ray shadowing 'Cannon ball' secondary deposits

Finally tuberculosis must be considered in the differential diagnosis of granulomatous disease of the gut, particularly in patients from the Indian subcontinent.

Associated gut and respiratory disease

DISEASES INVOLVING BOTH SYSTEMS

The gut and respiratory tract may be involved in many systemic disorders but there is a heterogeneous group of diseases in which the major manifestations are in these two systems. One example is cystic fibrosis (Chapter 18). Although the aetiology of this disease remains unknown, a major feature is the production of an abnormally viscid mucus causing obstruction of bronchi and ducts of exocrine glands.

Familial Mediterranean fever (Chapter 20) is another autosomal recessive disorder affecting both systems. The aetiology of the polyserositis is obscure, but the peritoneum and pleura have a common embryonic origin and are histologically very similar.

Severe abdominal pain and vomiting may occur in association with respiratory symptoms in hereditary angioedema and the presence of such symptoms helps to distinguish the hereditary from the non-hereditary sporadic form of the disease. The abdominal pain is attributed to gastrointestinal oedema.

Recurrent chest infections and bronchiectasis occur in selective IgA deficiency, and acquired hypogammaglobulinaemia and gastrointestinal symptoms may develop in both. Infestation with *Giardia lamblia* may occur and the association between coeliac disease and IgA deficiency is well recognized.

It has been reported that patients with eosinophilic gastroenteritis may suffer from asthma and rhinitis, implying a common allergic response in the gut and respiratory tract.

Lastly, the development of pleural and peritoneal mesotheliomas following exposure to asbestos fibres illustrates an adverse effect of exposure of both organs to environmental agents.

INFLAMMATORY BOWEL DISEASE
(SEE ALSO CHAPTER 12)

An association between ulcerative colitis and severe chronic bronchial disease (bronchiectasis or chronic bronchitis) was first suggested in 1976[13] even though, as has recently been reported, smoking is less common in patients with ulcerative colitis than in control subjects or the general population.[6] The association was originally found in only 6 out of 1400 cases of ulcerative colitis but a strong temporal relationship was noted between the gut and respiratory symptoms. This was confirmed in a subsequent report of a further seven patients with severe bronchial disease in some of whom respiratory symptoms improved with systemic corticosteroids.[2] This strong temporal relationship has been cited as evidence that chronic bronchial disease is an extraintestinal manifestation of ulcerative colitis. Inhaled beclomethasone diproprionate was shown to relieve productive cough in the majority of another group of ten patients with ulcerative colitis who were non-smokers.[9] Bronchial biopsies were obtained in four of the patients and showed basal reserve cell hyperplasia, basement membrane thickening, submucosal inflammation and an overall increase in thickness of the epithelium. These non-specific inflammatory changes are seen in cigarette smokers and it has been suggested that the gut and respiratory tract epithelia may be responding similarly to an unknown systemic factor or have a heightened responsiveness to inhaled and ingested irritants.

An increased prevalence of atopic disorders, including asthma and allergic rhinitis, has been reported in a questionnaire survey of 300 patients with ulcerative colitis but this study did not include objective evidence of reversible airflow obstruction.[18] The finding at least of obstructive airways disease has been confirmed in a pulmonary function study of patients with inflammatory bowel disease, including Crohn's disease. Twenty-five percent of the patients in this series had a reduced transfer factor for carbon monoxide and in a quarter of these there was radiographic evidence of fibrosing alveolitis. However, it was not possible to exclude sulphasalazine therapy as a causative factor.[7] This drug is known to produce pulmonary eosinophilia as well as fibrosing alveolitis.

COELIAC DISEASE (SEE ALSO CHAPTER 8)

An increased prevalence of atopic disorders, including asthma and hay fever, has been reported in patients with coeliac disease and in their families.[10] It was suggested that either the damaged intestinal mucosa had become more permeable to antigen, allowing the subsequent development of atopic diseases, or that a local mucosal deficiency of IgA responses might be the cause since both atopy and coeliac disease have been associated with either quantitative or qualitative abnormalities in IgA production.

There have been several reports of interstitial lung disease occurring in association with coeliac disease. In a survey of 57 patients with this disorder, three were found to have lung disease considered to be cryptogenic fibrosing alveolitis,[15] but a larger survey revealed a much lower prevalence of 0.3%.[4] Whereas cryptogenic fibrosing alveolitis appears to be uncommon in coeliac disease, jejunal villous atrophy has been found in a high proportion of patients with features suggestive, but not diagnostic of, bird fancier's lung. All had diffuse shadowing on chest x-ray and a reduced transfer factor for carbon monoxide, but none had undergone specific inhalation tests to prove the diagnosis.[1] A later study of patients with bird fancier's lung proven on inhalation testing failed to confirm these findings.[8] The authors had previously reported that precipitating antibodies found in the serum of coeliac patients were not the same as those found in the serum of patients with bird fancier's lung but were directed against antigens from chicken egg. More recently jejunal villous atrophy has been reported in patients with a clinical diagnosis of farmer's lung and antibodies to farmer's lung antigens.[19] Although it is possible that jejunal villous atrophy may occur more commonly in patients with extrinsic allergic alveolitis compared to the normal population, this is not yet proven.

Coeliac disease has been reported in association with idiopathic pulmonary haemosiderosis, a syndrome of unknown aetiology in which spontaneous haemorrhage occurs in the lung but whether this is simply a chance association or not remains to be confirmed.[20]

HIATAL HERNIA (SEE ALSO CHAPTER 3)

An association between hiatal hernia and asthma was suggested as early as 1966[17] and more recently a high incidence of oesophageal dysfunction has been reported in asthmatic patients.[12] The hiatal hernia may be produced by changes in thoracic and intra-abdominal pressures, or asthma by inhalation of gastric contents, although a reflex mechanism resulting from stimulation of the vagus nerve in the oesophagus seems a more attractive hypothesis. Certainly instillation of 0.1 N hydrochloric acid into the oesophagus can produce bronchoconstriction.[16] Whatever the mechanisms, cimetidine therapy has been shown to significantly improve nocturnal asthma symptoms in a double-blind controlled study in a group of patients with both asthma and oesophageal reflux.[5]

OTHER DISEASES

An association between peptic ulcers and chronic airflow limitation has been noted in the past (e.g. Kroeker[14]). A recent epidemiological study failed to confirm this but did suggest an association between bronchial hypersecretion and a history of peptic ulcer which was independent of smoking habits.[11] Chronic obstructive lung disease has also been associated with pneumatosis cystoides intestinalis.

REFERENCES

1 Berrill, W. T., Fitzpatrick, P. F., Macleod, W. M. *et al.* (1975) Bird fancier's lung and jejunal villous atrophy. *Lancet*, **ii**, 1006–1008.

2 Butland, R. J. A., Cole, P., Citron, K. M. & Turner-Warwick, M. (1981) Chronic bronchial suppuration and inflammatory bowel disease. *Quarterly Journal of Medicine*, **197**, 63–75.

3 Byrom, P. N., Walls, J. & Mair, H. J. (1979) Fulminant psittacosis. *Lancet*, **i**, 353–356.

4 Cooper, B. T., Holmes, G. K. T. & Cooke, W. T. (1978) Coeliac disease and immunological disorders. *British Medical Journal*, **i**, 537–539.

5 Goodall, R. J. R., Earis, J. E., Cooper, D. N. *et al.* (1981) Relationship between asthma and gastro-oesophageal reflux. *Thorax*, **36**, 116–121.

6 Harries, A. D., Baird, A. & Rhodes, J. (1982) Non-smoking: a feature of ulcerative colitis. *British Medical Journal*, **284**, 706.

7 Heatley, R. V., Thomas, E. J., Prokipchuck, E. J. *et al.* (1982) Pulmonary function abnormalities in patients with inflammatory bowel disease. *Quarterly Journal of Medicine*, **203**, 141–150.

8 Hendrick, D. J., Faux, J. A., Anand, B. *et al.* (1978) Is bird fancier's lung associated with coeliac disease? *Thorax*, **33**, 425–428.

9 Higenbottam, T., Cochrane, G. M., Clark, T. J. H. *et al.* (1980) Bronchial disease in ulcerative colitis. *Thorax*, **35**, 581–585.

10 Hodgson, H. J. F., Davies, R. J., Gent, A. E. & Hodson, M. E. (1976) Atopic disorders and adult coeliac disease. *Lancet*, **i**, 115–117.

11 Kauffmann, F. & Brille, D. (1981) Bronchial hypersecretion, chronic airflow limitation and peptic ulcer. *American Review of Respiratory Disease*, **124**, 646–649.

12 Kjellen, G., Brundin, A., Tibbling, L. & Wranne, B. (1981) Oesophageal function in asthmatics. *European Journal of Respiratory Disease*, **62**, 87–94.

13 Kraft, S. C., Earle, R. H., Roesler, M. & Esterly J. R. (1976) Unexplained bronchopulmonary disease with inflammatory bowel disease. *Archives of Internal Medicine*, **136**, 454–459.

14 Kroeker, E. J. (1966) Pulmonary emphysema and peptic ulcer. *Medical Clinics of North America*, **50**, 479–486.

15 Lancaster–Smith, M. J., Swarbrick, E. T., Perrin, J. & Wright, J. T. (1974) Coeliac disease and autoimmunity. *Postgraduate Medical Journal*, **50**, 45–48.

16 Mansfield, L. E. & Stein, M. R. (1978) Gastro-oesophageal reflux and asthma: a possible reflex mechanism. *Annals of Allergy*, **41**, 224–226.

17 Overholt, R. H. & Ashraf, M. (1966) Esophageal reflux as trigger in asthma. *New York State Journal of Medicine*, **1**, 3030–3032.

18   Pugh, S. M., Rhodes, J., Mayberry, J. F. *et al.* (1979) Atopic disease in ulcerative colitis and Crohn's disease. *Clinical Allergy*, **9**, 221–223.

19   Robinson, T. J., Haire, M., McMillan, S. A. *et al.* (1981) Jejunal villous changes associated with farmer's lung. *Postgraduate Medical Journal*, **57**, 697–701.

20   Wright, P. H., Menzies, I. S., Pounder, R. E. & Keeling, P. W. N. (1981) Adult idiopathic pulmonary haemosiderosis and coeliac disease. *Quarterly Journal of Medicine*, **197**, 95–102.

NEUROLOGICAL DISORDERS

Interest in the neurological manifestations of gastrointestinal disease has developed steadily over the past decade. A comprehensive survey of this growing border zone between specialities hardly seems possible, and in an early monograph[36] only certain areas were selected for review. These were neurological aspects of gastrointestinal topics the general features of which are for the most part covered in this book, and included: (a) the pathophysiology of intestinal absorption with reference to neurologically significant dietary ingredients (Chapters 8 and 17); (b) paraneoplastic neurological disease related to intestinal tumours (Chapter 9); (c) amyloidosis involving both the gastrointestinal tract and the nervous system (Chapter 8); (d) Whipple's disease (Chapter 8); (e) neurological complications of infective diarrhoea (Chapter 14); (f) pseudoxanthoma elasticum (Chapter 7); (g) gastrointestinal disorders due to lesions of intrinsic bowel innervation, such as Hirschsprung's disease (Chapter 11) and Chagas' disease (Chapter 14); (h) pancreatic encephalopathy (Chapter 18); (i) smooth muscle involvement in diseases of voluntary muscle; (j) abetalipoproteinaemia; (k) central pontine myelinolysis; and (l) clioquinol neurotoxicity (subacute myelo-optical neuropathy; SMON). For information and comment on detailed neurological aspects of these topics, the interested reader is referred to the monograph of Pallis and Lewis.[36] In a brief supplementary review,[37] the pattern of neurological involvement in Whipple's disease was re-evaluated, reports of intestinal pathology in multiple sclerosis and other primary diseases of the nervous system were assessed, Fabry's disease was briefly discussed, and a conspectus of the rapidly evolving field of brain–gut peptides was presented. This last topic, touched upon repeatedly elsewhere in this book, has been comprehensively reviewed in numerous recent publications.[39, 40, 41]

Among the subjects discussed in detail by Pallis and Lewis[36] the neurological disorders associated with coeliac disease are of special interest. Recent years have seen several new clinical and laboratory reports, and it is appropriate here to re-examine this topic in the light of new suggestions about pathogenesis and treatment.

Nervous system involvement in coeliac disease (see also Chapter 8)

Patients with coeliac disease may rarely show evidence of severe neurological disease. This may take the form of encephalopathy, cerebellar dysfunction, myelopathy, peripheral neuropathy, or a combination of these. The available clinical and pathological evidence does not clearly indicate the cause of such neurological complications. However, data implicating dietary vitamin E deficiency will be considered. In a few cases direct involvement of the nervous system by histiocytic lymphoma, itself a complication of coeliac disease, may occur. In contrast to tropical sprue, the development of myopathy in coeliac disease is uncommon[36] though a number of reports[20, 22, 28, 34] describe a spectrum of features that may be encountered.

The early documentation of neurological manifestations in patients believed to have coeliac disease was either deficient in clinical detail or lacked pathological support. It was only with the important clinicopathological study of Cooke and Smith[5] that the existence of coeliac encephalomyeloradiculoneuropathy became certain.

Earlier reports had described three patients with non-tropical sprue with transient extensor plantar responses[18, 24, 49] or noted the finding of posterior column changes in autopsy material. In 1957 Sencer[44] described the neurological symptoms and signs in 94 patients with a malabsorption syndrome presumed to be due to coeliac disease. Forty-nine had features suggesting nervous system involvement. Twenty patients had evidence of tetany but no objective reflex or sensory changes. Ten patients had experienced paraesthesiae, and were found to be anaemic but had no abnormal neurological signs. A further 12 patients had reflex or sensory abnormalities on examination. There were two cases of severe myeloradiculopathy (referred to by the authors as 'pseudo-tabes'). In a review of 124 patients with 'non-tropical sprue' Green and Wollaeger[16] encountered six patients with neurological signs. Abnormalities included peripheral neuropathy, areflexia and (in one case) 'subacute combined sclerosis'.

The 16 patients described by Cooke and Smith[5] all had a definite jejunal biopsy-proven diagnosis of coeliac disease and all had severe neurological disease. Autopsy was performed in nine cases and data obtained on peripheral nerve or muscle biopsy in the other seven. Two patients were found to have 'neuropathy' at the time of original referral for their gastrointestinal symptoms. Four patients were referred on account of the neuropathy complicating their primary disorder and nine developed neurological complications while under treatment for adult coeliac disease.

The patients usually presented with symptoms affecting the lower limbs and sensory ataxia soon dominated the clinical picture in nearly all cases. Posterior column deficit and distal impairment of pain and tactile sense with absent ankle jerks were frequently encountered. Weakness was often marked but wasting relatively slight. One patient developed an extensor plantar response shortly before death, three had cerebellar signs and five had suffered from unexplained episodes of unconsciousness. One patient presented with neurological signs and symptoms suggestive of motor neurone disease, and probably had that condition.

In ten patients the 'neuropathy' proved steadily progressive, the rate of progression varying considerably from case to case. Of the nine fatal cases, 'neuropathy' was considered the main cause of death in four. Among the neurological findings reported were demyelination (often of spongiform type) of the posterior and lateral columns of the spinal cord, producing a subacute combined degeneration-like picture, dorsal column degeneration alone, and cerebellar cortical degeneration. Not surprisingly, in view of the rarity of the condition, there has been no comparable case-series to substantiate these dramatic findings, though several thorough and convincing case-studies with necropsy findings have since been published. Together with the nine autopsied cases of Cooke and Smith[5] these are summarized in Table 9.7.

An overview of these cases shows a mainly male preponderance (against a background of a higher incidence of coeliac disease in women) and again, in general, the development of neurological dysfunction years after the onset of coeliac disease. Unsteadiness of gait is a universal feature, with dementia, cranial nerve palsies and myoclonus being among the additional changes encountered. From the neuropathological standpoint two contrasting patterns of disease predominate. These are dorsal spinal column degeneration, of a type dissimilar to that encountered in subacute combined degeneration, and a diffuse cerebellar degeneration affecting mainly the cortical Purkinje cell population but also involving dentate nuclei.

Additional unusual pathological changes that may be found include malignant infiltration of spinal nerve roots in the cauda equina secondary to multiple histiocytic lymphomas in small and large bowel[4] and central pontine myelinolysis, a generally nutrition-related phenomenon.[3] This last point emphasizes the often posited but still unconfirmed role of dietary deficiency in the genesis of the encephalomyeloradiculopathy of coeliac disease. In the majority of affected patients the neurological disease progresses inexorably despite treatment with essential dietary trace constituents. However, the spinal disease may improve in subjects receiving vitamins A, B and E,[4] and obviously multivitamins and trace element supplementation should always be tried. Recent advances in the recognition of the clinical and pathological effects of vitamin E deficiency in man suggest that it may be reasonable to implicate lack of this dietary ingredient in the neurological complications of coeliac disease. The relationship of vitamin E malabsorption to disease of the nervous system will now be examined.

Vitamin E deficiency in gastrointestinal disease

Vitamin E was first discovered in 1922 when Evans and Bishop[11] demonstrated that a fat soluble nutritional factor was essential for normal reproduction in the rat. Despite the existence of a number of vitamin E deficiency syndromes in animals, the role of vitamin E in human nutrition is not clear, although it is generally accepted that deficiency may be associated with haemolytic anaemia in premature infants. It has only recently been recognized that vitamin E plays an important role in maintaining the integrity of the human nervous system. Nutritional deficiency of vitamin E in man is relatively rare; the average intake of α-tocopherol (the most biologically active and available tocopherol) in adults in the United States is 7 to 9 mg/day.[9] The naturally occurring tocopherols are synthesized by green plants. Rich dietary sources of the vitamin include dairy products, meat, fish, nuts, green vegetables, and vegetable and nut oils.

Table 9.7 Summary of clinicopathological data in thirteen autopsied cases of coeliac disease with involvement of the nervous system.

Source	Sex	Age at death	Onset of coeliac disease	Onset of neurological symptoms	Principal neurological symptoms and signs	Principal neurological findings
Cooke & Smith[5]						
Case 1	M	59	Childhood	57	Confusion; unsteady gait; limb ataxia; hyporeflexia	Hypothalamic changes suggestive of chronic Wernicke's encephalopathy. Necrotic foci in hypothalamus. Degeneration of posterior spinal columns.
2	M	36	34	36	Muscle weakness; ataxic gait	Cortical cerebellar degeneration. Degeneration of posterior and lateral spinal columns.
3	F	48	Childhood	48	Limb weakness and sensory loss; areflexia; left external rectus palsy	Spongiform degeneration of spinal cord reminiscent of SCD; demyelination of spinal nerve roots; anterior horn cell degeneration; widespread lymphoid infiltration; hypothalamic changes suggestive of Wernicke's encephalopathy.
4	M	47	Childhood	45	Muscle weakness, wasting and fasciculation	Degeneration of upper and lower motor neurones and of pyramidal tracts (i.e. motor neurone disease).
5	M	74	20	64	Unsteady gait	Demyelination of central parts of posterior columns, and anterior and posterior spinal nerve roots; focal atrophy and gliosis in cerebellar cortex; dentate atrophy.
6	M	65	Childhood	63	Distal paraesthesiae; ataxia	Myelin degeneration of anterior, lateral and posterior spinal columns; degeneration of dorsal root ganglia; focal Purkinje cell loss.
7	M	50	Childhood	48	Dysarthria; dysphagia; right facial weakness; absent ankle jerks; normal sensation	SCD-like changes in cord; anterior horn cell degeneration; midbrain changes resembling Wernicke's encephalopathy.

8	34	33	M	Weak legs; impaired micturition; spastic paraparesis; left vocal cord paralysis	SCD-like changes in cervical and dorsal cord; anterior horn cell loss; focal cortical scarring; left medullary degeneration with loss of normal structures and unusual astrocytic proliferation.
15	63	50	M	Ataxic gait; distal sensory loss; areflexia	Spongiform degeneration of posterior and lateral columns, with degeneration of anterior horn cells and nerve roots.
Case records[4]	50	35	M	Features of myelopathy and neuropathy; improvement after multivitamin treatment. Preterminal headache, neck stiffness, ataxia; distal sensory loss and areflexia	Histiocytic lymphomatous infiltration of cauda equina: loss of myelinated fibres in dorsal columns and roots, evidently a healed process.
Finelli et al.[13]	56	55	M	Ataxia; dysarthria; ophthalmoplegia; hyperreflexia; palatal myoclonus	Severe neuronal loss in cerebellar cortex (Purkinje cells) and dentate nuclei; myelin pallor of anterior and lateral corticospinal tracts.
Kinney et al.[27]	57	55	M	Dementia; dysarthria; ataxia; muscle wasting; distal sensory loss; diffuse myoclonus	Severe neuronal loss in cerebellar cortex (Purkinje cells) and dentate nuclei; demyelination in dorsal and lateral columns; cell loss in Clarke's column.
Camilleri et al.[3]	64	54	F	Right brainstem signs; lower limb weakness, sensory loss and areflexia; reduced bowel and bladder sensation	Central pontine myelin loss; dorsal column degeneration.

MECHANISMS OF VITAMIN E
MALABSORPTION

Vitamin E is a highly non-polar lipid which is dependent on adequate concentrations of bile salts in the small intestinal lumen and chylomicron formation for its solubilization and absorption.[31] It can therefore be expected that any pathological process deranging one or both of these factors may be associated with tocopherol deficiency. Low luminal concentration of bile salts results from cholestatic liver disease, with either intrahepatic or extrahepatic biliary obstruction. Bile salts are reabsorbed in the terminal ileum. Resection of this part of the intestine leads to interruption of the enterohepatic circulation and reduction in size of the bile salt pool. Other factors which affect the activity of bile salts are bacterial contamination of the intestine, which results in deconjugation, and increased pH of the gut contents. The latter may arise due to hypersecretion of gastrin following intestinal resection.[46] Increased acidity and deconjugation both lead to precipitation of bile salts, which renders them unavailable for micelle formation and solubilization of lipids, including vitamin E.

Disorders involving the absorptive surface of the small intestine giving rise to fat malabsorption, such as coeliac disease, are likely to be associated with a variable degree of vitamin E deficiency. More specifically, abnormal chylomicron formation is a potent cause of vitamin E malabsorption because lipid cannot be transported out of the mucosal cell into the gut lymphatic system.[31] This type of defect is exemplified by abetalipoproteinaemia.

EXPERIMENTALLY INDUCED VITAMIN E
DEFICIENCY

Early experimental studies of vitamin E deficiency in animals tended to stress the development of a chronic, necrotizing myopathy.[35, 38] A naturally occurring vitamin E deficiency state is associated with myopathy in the kwokka, a small marsupial found in Western Australia.[25]

In the central nervous system of the vitamin E deficient rat, axonal degeneration occurs in the posterior columns of the spinal cord which is most prominent in the cervical region. There is also degeneration of axons in the peripheral nerves and this is most marked distally. Lipopigment accumulates in neurones and central nervous system endothelial cells. These pathological findings are associated clinically with kyphoscoliosis, muscle weakness and ataxia in the deficient animals.[38, 51]

Nelson *et al*[35] described detailed neuropathological observations in vitamin E deficient monkeys. The most striking abnormality was loss of axons and myelin in the posterior columns which was more severe in the rostral part of the spinal cord. Degeneration of small numbers of neurones was seen in the dorsal root ganglia and there was slight fibre loss in the posterior roots. In the sural nerve there was marked loss of myelinated fibres, predominantly those of large calibre, which increased in severity in a proximal to distal direction. These observations in experimental animals suggest that vitamin E deficiency produces a 'dying-back' neuropathy in both centrally and peripherally directed fibres of the sensory neurones. Dying back appears to be more severe in the central nervous system, and it is possible that this is due to regenerative activity in the peripheral nerves partly compensating for axonal loss.[35]

Clinical features of vitamin E deficiency in man

CHRONIC LIVER DISEASE

As far as liver disease is concerned, neurological dysfunction secondary to vitamin E deficiency has been described most frequently in children with congenital biliary atresia.[10, 14, 17, 42, 47, 50, 52] Neurological symptoms, chiefly unsteadiness of gait and weakness, developed between the ages of 5 and 15 years, although depression or absence of the tendon reflexes may precede symptoms by a number of years.[42] Ptosis, failure of upgaze and limitation of eye adduction have been described in some children, as has dysarthria. Limb and gait ataxia were prominent features. The tendon reflexes were depressed or absent and the plantar responses often extensor. Proprioceptive and vibration sense loss was common and often severe. Some patients had generalized muscle weakness and lordosis.

The neurological syndrome varied somewhat in relation to progression. A few patients were unable to walk one year after the onset of gait ataxia but in others the disorder was more slowly progressive. Serum vitamin E levels were extremely low or undetectable in all these cases. Neurological dysfunction secondary to vitamin E deficiency has not been described in adults with liver disease, although serum vitamin E levels may be low in primary biliary cirrhosis.

CYSTIC FIBROSIS (SEE CHAPTER 18)

A neurological disorder similar to that described in biliary atresia has been reported in some patients with cystic fibrosis.[10, 52] Symptoms did not develop until the latter part of the second decade of life and these were relatively slowly progressive but disabling. Again, vitamin E levels were undetectable or extremely low. One of the patients described by Elias et al[10] improved considerably after starting vitamin E supplements; these had to be given intramuscularly.

Serum vitamin E concentration is significantly inversely correlated with faecal fat excretion in cystic fibrosis.[12] Excretion of bile salts from the gut is increased in this disease. Increasing survival is unfortunately associated with an increased incidence of hepatobiliary disease which further compromises the bile salt pool. Vitamin E deficiency is therefore more likely to arise in patients with abnormal liver function as well as chronic severe steatorrhoea.[9]

OTHER FAT MALABSORPTIVE STATES

Few adult patients with a spinocerebellar syndrome presumed due to vitamin E deficiency have been described.[2, 19] Of the cases reported by Harding and colleagues,[19] one had pseudointestinal obstruction and the other Crohn's disease; both had had extensive small bowel resections and chronic steatorrhoea with intermittent bacterial overgrowth in the gut. Neither developed neurological symptoms until 20 years or more after the onset of gastrointestinal disease. The first complaints were of unsteadiness of gait and clumsiness of the hands.

Both patients were dysarthric, had cerebellar ataxia in the limbs and of gait, mild proximal muscle weakness, absent tendon reflexes, and loss of joint position and vibration sense. Upgaze was defective in one and the other had extensor plantar responses. There was no evidence of vitamin B_{12} deficiency in either patient, but serum vitamin E levels were undetectable. The neurological disorder was slowly progressive; the older patient was just able to walk with a stick after seven years of symptoms. The younger patient improved neurologically after starting on oral vitamin E supplements. There was also electrophysiological evidence of improvement after four years of treatment.

It is perhaps surprising that neurological dysfunction secondary to vitamin E deficiency has rarely been described in adult patients with coeliac disease, as low circulating levels of vitamin E have been reported in affected children.[31] The report of Cooke and Smith[5] has already been examined in detail, and it seems likely that at least some of the cases described suffered from multiple nutritional deficiencies. Apart from the evident relationship of their malabsorption to the development of neurological disease, several patients showed arrest or even partial reversal of disability presumed to be due to myelopathy with multivitamin therapy. The possibility of vitamin E deficiency in these patients does not seem to have been adequately explored. Binder et al[2] described four males aged between 28 and 60 years who had chronic steatorrhoea, two as a result of coeliac disease, one with chronic pancreatitis and the other jejunal diverticulosis. Fat malabsorption had been present for periods ranging from 6 to 18 years prior to the development of neurological symptoms and signs. The latter included ophthalmoplegia, distal muscle wasting and weakness, areflexia, ataxia, and loss of vibration and joint position sense. The two patients with coeliac disease both had low serum vitamin E levels; the others were not investigated. The one with jejunal diverticulosis did not improve on vitamin E therapy, but this was only administered for one month. Other patients with jejunal diverticulosis, steatorrhoea, and neurological dysfunction have been reported.[6] Several of these had ataxia, rombergism, areflexia and proprioceptive loss which did not improve after treatment with vitamin B_{12}. It is quite possible that vitamin E deficiency was the cause of their neurological deficits.

ABETALIPOPROTEINAEMIA
(see also p. 690)

Abetalipoproteinaemia is an autosomal recessive disorder which is characterized clinically by mild steatorrhoea, night blindness due to pigmentary retinal degeneration, and a progressive spinocerebellar syndrome which resembles that found in Friedreich's ataxia. Acanthocytes are present in the peripheral blood. Plasma lipid concentrations are universally low, with absent low density lipoproteins and chylomicrons. Apoprotein B is undetectable in the plasma of patients with abetalipoproteinaemia and it may be that failure to synthesize this protein is the basic defect of the disorder.

Young children with abetalipoproteinaemia usually have fat intolerance and diarrhoea, but these symptoms may be mild and may subside with age. Neurological symptoms, of which the first tends to be ataxia, occur during the first decade of life in one-third of patients and by the age of 20 in the rest. The reflexes are often hypo-active before symptoms develop. The complete neurological picture consists of dysarthria, cerebellar ataxia of the limbs and of gait, areflexia, distal loss of vibration and joint position sense, pes cavus and scoliosis. Generalized muscle weakness is quite common. The plantar responses may be flexor or extensor. Ptosis and external ophthalmoplegia have been described. The disorder is progressive and relatively few patients are still ambulant after the age of 30.[23, 43]

Nocturnal amblyopia occasionally develops prior to ataxia but visual symptoms are very variable and may never arise. Pigmentary retinal degeneration has been seen in children aged ten years or less and it is usually evident during the second decade of life. The peripheral part of the retina contains hyperpigmented and depigmented areas with 'bone spicules'. These changes later spread to affect the macula with resulting loss of visual acuity. The visual fields become progressively restricted.[43]

Abetalipoproteinaemia represents the most severe vitamin E deficiency state known in man. The vitamin is absent from the serum of affected individuals from birth because of major defects in both absorption and transport.[26, 31] There is good evidence that vitamin E supplementation prevents the development of neurological symptoms if given in early childhood, and improves neurological function or prevents further deterioration if disability is present prior to starting treatment.[1, 30, 32] In Muller and colleagues'[32] series of eight cases, five received large oral doses (about $100 \, mg \cdot kg^{-1} \cdot day^{-1}$) of vitamin E in the first 18 months of life. They were all neurologically normal when aged between 10 and 14 years. The three older patients either improved or showed no further deterioration.[33]

Investigations and pathology

Patients with neurological dysfunction secondary to vitamin E deficiency usually have electrophysiological evidence of a mild peripheral sensory neuropathy. Sensory nerve action potentials are reduced in amplitude or absent.[2, 19, 30] Motor nerve conduction velocity is nearly always normal. Electromyography may show the changes of myopathy in proximal muscles, associated with elevation of the plasma creatine kinase, although myopathy is not a prominent feature of the neurological syndrome; some patients have been noted to have electromyographic evidence of denervation in distal muscles.[19, 30]

Somatosensory evoked potentials were performed in the two adult cases reported by Harding et al.[19] These showed central delay in conduction suggestive of an abnormality in the posterior columns. These findings are of interest in relation to the pathological abnormalities in vitamin E deficient animals referred to earlier. They again suggest that vitamin E deficiency produces a dying-back neuropathy in the centrally and peripherally directed fibres of sensory neurones, and that degeneration is more severe in the posterior columns than in the peripheral nerves.

This hypothesis is supported by the neuropathological abnormalities described to date in vitamin E deficient humans. In two children with biliary atresia, Rosenblum and colleagues[42] found degeneration of the posterior columns with some focal loss of nerve cells in the dorsal root ganglia at autopsy. There was mild loss of large myelinated fibres in the sural nerves, but the proximal nerve trunks were normal. In the older child there was also some degeneration of the spinocerebellar tracts. Sung and Stadlan[47] had earlier observed a high incidence of axonal dystrophy in the gracile nuclei of autopsied cases of biliary atresia.

In cystic fibrosis, degeneration of the posterior columns is more severe in the rostral part of the spinal cord and the lumbar and sacral segments are often spared.[15] Pathological evidence of a causal relationship between vitamin E deficiency and neurological disease was provided by Sung et al,[48] who observed a decrease in the incidence of axonal dystrophy in the gracile nucleus of patients with cystic fibrosis dying after 1970 compared with those who died between 1952 and 1969. This change coincided with the introduction of routine vitamin E therapy for patients with cystic fibrosis in the 1960s.

Degeneration of the posterior columns has also been reported in autopsied cases of abetalipoproteinaemia.[8, 45] In addition, there was loss of myelin in the spinocerebellar tracts and cerebellar white matter, and loss of Purkinje cells. Biopsies of the sural nerve show a reduced number of large myelinated fibres.[30]

Aetiology of neurological dysfunction in vitamin E deficiency

There is now evidence suggesting that vitamin E is essential for the normal function of the nervous system in man. This is based on the fact that vitamin E therapy prevents the neurological complications of abetalipoproteinaemia and can arrest or improve the neurological syndrome associated with deficiency of the vitamin caused by other fat malabsorptive states. In addition, the neuropathological changes seen in humans with vitamin E deficiency are similar to those found experimentally in vitamin E deficient animals. The mechanism of action of vitamin E in maintaining the integrity of the nervous system is unclear. It appears to have a stabilizing effect on biological membranes, and it acts as an antioxidant in vitro and probably in vivo. The phytyl side-chain of the vitamin E molecule interacts with polyunsaturated fatty acids, in particular arachidonic acid which is present in membrane phospholipids.[7] The molecule is therefore in an ideal position to inhibit peroxidation of the unsaturated lipids and to maintain other molecules in their correct oxidation state.[33] It may also facilitate molecular packing and thus maintain the stability of biological membranes.[29]

The neurological disease associated with vitamin E deficiency appears to be related to the duration and severity of the depletion. Neurological dysfunction was present consistently in patients with abetalipoproteinaemia prior to the use of vitamin E supplementation, and this condition represents the most severe deficiency of vitamin E known in man. Nevertheless, the neurological complications of abetalipoproteinaemia frequently do not develop until the second decade of life. Pigmentary retinal degeneration is common in untreated abetalipoproteinaemia but is rare in patients with other causes of vitamin E deficiency. The reason for this discrepancy is not clear.

In biliary atresia, fat malabsorption is also present from an early age and serum vitamin E levels are very low;[21] neurological signs may first be noted at any time between the ages of 2 and 15 years.[14, 42] Certainly neuropathological abnormalities antedate the onset of signs and symptoms in biliary atresia,[47] and the same probably applies to cystic fibrosis.[15] The prognosis of biliary atresia and cystic fibrosis, in terms of survival into adult life, has been poor until recent times. It is likely that many patients do not live long enough to develop neurological disease.

The relative paucity of reports of adult patients with fat malabsorption and neurological dysfunction might suggest that the developing nervous system is more sensitive to the effects of vitamin E deficiency. Again, patients with severe steatorrhoea of, for example, ten years or longer standing are somewhat infrequently encountered.

Treatment

It would seem reasonable to monitor serum vitamin E levels in all patients with chronic fat malabsorption, and to supplement those deficient with the aim of preventing neurological disability. It is assumed that investigation and replacement of other deficiencies, such as those of vitamin B_{12} and folic acid, are routinely undertaken in this context. Elias and Muller[9] and Muller et al[33] have stressed that vitamin E must be administered rationally. In abetalipoproteinaemia oral doses of about $100 \, mg \cdot kg^{-1} \cdot day^{-1}$ are required to achieve adequate serum levels. Many patients with very low concentrations of bile salts in the small intestine are unable to absorb vitamin E given orally and require intramuscular therapy. Absorption should be investigated by administering 1 to 2 g of tocopheryl acetate orally and measuring serum vitamin E levels over the next 24 hours. If there is absorption, large oral doses can be started; if not, intramuscular injections (of about 100 mg in adults) will be required once or twice weekly. In either case, serum levels should be monitored regularly to ensure that adequate concentrations are reached.[9]

REFERENCES

1 Azizi, E., Zaidman, J. L., Eshchar, J. & Szeinberg, A. (1978) Abetalipoproteinaemia treated with parenteral and oral vitamins A and E, and with medium chain triglycerides. *Acta Paediatrica Scandinavica*, **67**, 797–801.

2 Binder, H. J., Solitare, G. B. & Spiro, H. M. (1967) Neuromuscular disease in patients with steatorrhoea. *Gut*, **8**, 605–611.

3 Camilleri, M., Krausz, T., Lewis, P. D. et al. (1983) Malignant histiocytosis and encephalomyeloradiculopathy complicating coeliac disease. *Gut*, **24**, 441–447.

4 Case records of the Massachusetts General Hospital (1976) Case 48. *New England Journal of Medicine*, **295**, 1242–1248.

5 Cooke, W. T. & Smith, W. T. (1966) Neurological disorders associated with adult coeliac disease. *Brain*, **89**, 683–722.

6 Cooke, W. T., Cox, E. V., Fone, D. J. et al. (1963) The clinical and metabolic significance of jejunal diverticula. *Gut*, **4**, 115–131.

7 Diplock, A. T. & Lucy, J. A. (1973) The biochemical modes of action of vitamin E and selenium: a hypothesis. *FEBS Letters*, **29**, 205–210.

8 Dische, M. R. & Porro, R. S. (1970) The cardiac lesions in Bassen–Kornzweig syndrome. *American Journal of Medicine*, **49**, 568–571.

9 Elias, E. & Muller, D. P. R. (1983) Use of vitamin E for prevention and treatment of spinocerebellar disorders. *Comprehensive Therapy*, **9**, 56–60.

10 Elias, E., Muller, D. P. R. & Scott, J. (1981) Association of spinocerebellar disorders with cystic fibrosis or chronic childhood cholestasis and very low serum vitamin E. *Lancet*, **ii**, 1319–1321.

684   *Systemic Disease and the Gut*

11 Evans, H. M. & Bishop, K. S. (1922) On the existence of a hitherto unrecognised dietary factor essential for reproduction. *Science*, **56**, 650–651.

12 Farrell, P. M., Bieri, J. G., Fratantoni, J. F. *et al.* (1977) The occurrence and effects of human vitamin E deficiency: a study in patients with cystic fibrosis. *Journal of Clinical Investigation*, **60**, 233–241.

13 Finelli, P. F., McEntee, W. J., Ambler, M. & Kestenbaum, D. (1980) Adult celiac disease presenting as cerebellar syndrome. *Neurology*, **30**, 245–249.

14 Frydman, M., Rotter, J. I. & Kazimiroff, P. (1981) Neurologic syndrome in liver disease. *New England Journal of Medicine*, **305**, 108.

15 Geller, A., Gilles, F. & Scwachman, H. (1977) Degeneration of fasciculus gracilis in cystic fibrosis. *Neurology (Minneapolis)*, **27**, 185–187.

16 Green, P. A. & Wollaeger, E. E. (1960) The clinical behavior of sprue in the United States. *Gastroenterology*, **28**, 399–418.

17 Guggenheim, M. A., Ringel, S. P., Silverman, A. & Grabert, B. E. (1982) Progressive neuromuscular disease in children with chronic cholestasis and vitamin E deficiency: diagnosis and treatment with alpha tocopherol. *Journal of Paediatrics*, **100**, 51–58.

18 Hansen, K. & von Staa, H. (1936) *Die einheimische Sprue*. Leipzig: Thieme.

19 Harding, A. E., Muller, D. P. R., Thomas, P. K. & Willison, H. J. (1982) Spinocerebellar degeneration secondary to chronic intestinal malabsorption: a vitamin E deficiency syndrome. *Annals of Neurology*, **12**, 419–424.

20 Hardoff, D., Sharf, B. & Berger, A. (1980) Myopathy as a presentation of coeliac disease. *Developmental Medicine and Child Neurology*, **22**, 781–783.

21 Harries, J. T. & Muller, D. P. R. (1971) Absorption of vitamin E in children with biliary obstruction. *Gut*, **12**, 579–584.

22 Henriksson, K. G., Hallert, C., Norrby, K. & Walan, A. (1982) Polymyositis and adult coeliac disease. *Acta Neurologica Scandinavica*, **65**, 301–319.

23 Herbert, P. N., Gotto, A. M. & Fredrickson, D. S. (1978) Familial lipoprotein deficiency. In *The Metabolic Basis of Inherited Disease* (Ed.) Stanbury, J. H., Wyngaarden, D. S. & Fredrickson, D. S. pp. 544–588. New York: McGraw-Hill.

24 Hotz, H. W. & Lüthy, F. (1939) Funikuläre Spinalerkrankung bei einheimischer Sprue; Mitteilung eines Falles mit pathologisch-anatomischem Befund. *Helvetica Medica Acta*, **6**, 415–426.

25 Kakulas, B. A. (1982) *Man, Marsupials and Muscle*. Nedlands: University of Western Australia Press.

26 Kayden, H. J., Silber, R. & Kossmann, C. E. (1965) The role of vitamin E deficiency in the abnormal autohemolysis of acanthocytosis. *Transactions of the Association of American Physicians*, **78**, 334–342.

27 Kinney, H. C., Burger, P. C., Hurwitz, B. J. *et al.* (1982) Degeneration of the central nervous system associated with celiac disease. *Journal of Neurological Science*, **53**, 9–22.

28 Lundberg, A., Eriksson, B. O. & Jansson, G. (1979) Muscle abnormalities in coeliac disease: studies on gross motor development and muscle fibre composition, size and metabolic substrates. *European Journal of Pediatrics*, **130**, 93–103.

29 Maggio, B., Diplock, A. T. & Lucy, J. A. (1977) Interactions of tocopherols and ubiquinones with monolayers of phospholipids. *Biochemical Journal*, **161**, 111–121.

30 Miller, R. J., Davis, C. J. F., Illingworth, D. R. & Bradley, W. (1980) The neuropathy of abetalipoproteinaemia. *Neurology (NY)*, **30**, 1286–1291.

31 Muller, D. P. R., Harries, J. T. & Lloyd, J. K. (1974) The relative importance of the factors involved in the absorption of vitamin E in children. *Gut*, **15**, 966–971.

32 Muller, D. P. R., Lloyd, J. K. & Bird, A. C. (1977) Long term management of abetalipoproteinaemia: possible role for vitamin E. *Archives of Diseases in Childhood*, **52**, 209–214.

33 Muller, D. P. R., Lloyd, J. K. & Wolff, O. H. (1983) Vitamin E and neurological function. *Lancet*, **i**, 225–228.

34 Nanji, A. A., Freeman, H. J. & Anderson, F. H. (1982) Paralysis and rhabdomyolysis: a presenting feature of celiac disease. *Western Journal of Medicine*, **136**, 273–274.

35 Nelson, J. S., Fitch, C. D., Fischer, V. W. *et al.* (1981) Progressive neuropathologic lesions in vitamin E deficient rhesus monkeys. *Journal of Neuropathology and Experimental Neurology*, **40**, 166–186.

36 Pallis, C. A. & Lewis, P. D. (1974) *The Neurology of Gastrointestinal Disease*. London: Saunders.

37 Pallis, C. A. & Lewis, P. D. (1980) Neurology of gastrointestinal disease. In *Handbook of Clinical Neurology* Volume 39: Neurological manifestations of systemic disease (Ed.) Vinken, P. J. & Bruyn, G. W. Part II. pp. 449–468. Amsterdam: North Holland.

38 Pentschew, A. & Schwarz, K. (1962) Systemic axonal dystrophy in vitamin E deficient adult rats: with implication in human neuropathology. *Acta Neuropathologica*, **1**, 313–334.

39 Polak, J. M. & Bloom, S. R. (1982) Regulatory peptides in the gut and their relevance to disease. In *Disorders of Neurohumoral Transmission* (Ed.) Crow, T. J. pp. 83–104. London: Academic Press.

40 Polak, J. M., Bloom, S. R., Wright, N. A. & Daly, M. J. (Ed.) (1982) Autonomic nerves of the gut. *Scandinavian Journal of Gastroenterology*, **17**(Supplement 71).

41 Polak, J. M., Bloom, S. R., Wright, N. A. & Butler, A. G. (Ed.) (1983) Gut hormones in disease. *Scandinavian Journal of Gastroenterology*, **18**(Supplement 82).

42 Rosenblum, J. L., Keating, J. P., Prensky, A. L. & Nelson, J. S. (1981) A progressive neurologic syndrome in children with chronic liver disease. *New England Journal of Medicine*, **304**, 503–508.

43 Schwartz, J. F., Rowland, L. P., Eder, H. *et al.* (1963) Bassen–Kornzweig syndrome: deficiency of serum betalipoprotein. *Archives of Neurology (Chicago)*, **8**, 438–454.

44 Sencer, W. (1957) Neurological manifestations in malabsorption syndrome. *Journal of the Mount Sinai Hospital*, **24**, 331–345.

45 Sobrevilla, L. A., Goodman, M. L. & Kane, C. A. (1964) Demyelinating central nervous system disease, macular atrophy and acanthocytosis (Bassen–Kornzweig syndrome). *American Journal of Medicine*, **37**, 821–828.

46 Strauss, E., Gerson, C. D. & Yalow, R. S. (1974) Hypersecretion of gastrin associated with short bowel syndrome. *Gastroenterology*, **66**, 175–180.

47 Sung, J. H. & Stadlan, E. M. (1966) Neuroaxonal dystrophy in congenital biliary atresia. *Journal of Neuropathology and Experimental Neurology*, **25**, 341–361.

48 Sung, J. H., Park, S. H., Mastri, A. R. & Warwick, W. J. (1980) Axonal dystrophy in the gracile nucleus in congenital biliary atresia and cystic fibrosis (mucoviscidosis): beneficial effect of vitamin E therapy. *Journal of Neuropathology and Experimental Neurology*, **39**, 584–597.

49 Thaysen, T. E. H. (1932) *Non-tropical Sprue*. London: Oxford University Press.

50 Tomasi, L. G. (1979) Reversibility of human myopathy caused by vitamin E deficiency. *Neurology (NY)*, **29**, 1183–1185.

51 Towfighi, J. (1981) Effects of chronic vitamin E deficiency on the nervous system of the rat. *Acta Neuropathologica*, **54**, 261–268.

52 Umetsu, D. T., Couture, P., Winter, H. S. *et al.* (1980) Degenerative neurological disease in patients with acquired vitamin E deficiency. *Pediatric Research*, **14**, 512.

PERNICIOUS ANAEMIA

Definition

Pernicious anaemia (PA) is a disorder characterized by megaloblastic haemopoiesis and/or a neuropathy due to vitamin B_{12} deficiency, the result of severe atrophic gastritis.

Aetiology

The factors that lead to loss of the normal gastric mucosa in simple atrophic gastritis are also relevant in pernicious anaemia. Nevertheless, long-term follow up of patients with biopsy-proven atrophic gastritis indicates that very few proceed to develop PA, although the expected number develop a carcinoma of the stomach.[8]

Genetic and autoimmune factors are relevant in the transition from severe atrophic gastritis to PA. PA occurs with a high frequency in the races of Northern Europe and in these the frequency reaches 1% above the age of 60. It is a familial disorder with a history of an affected relative in 30% of patients. Those with a family history present at a younger age (mean 51 years) as compared to a mean age of presentation of 66 years in the absence of a family history.[5]

In these, too, there is a strong association with other disorders of autoimmune origin, namely hypo- and hyperthyroidism, insulin-sensitive diabetes mellitus, adrenal atrophy, vitiligo, etc. Even in the absence of manifest disease, patients and their healthy relatives have an unusually high frequency of serum antibodies against thyroid, gastric–parietal cells, adrenal gland, ovary, etc. Some 80% of patients with PA have demonstrable parietal-cell antibodies in serum and 57% have intrinsic factor antibodies. Others have demonstrable intrinsic factor (IF) antibody in gastric juice in the absence of serum antibody and others have lymphocytes in the stomach wall reacting with IF. Cell mediated immunity against gastric antigens are present in 80% of PA patients. It is in the formation of these antibodies (demonstrable in over 90% of patients) that those with PA differ from patients with simple atrophic gastric. Intrinsic factor antibodies, particularly IgA immunoglobulins produced in the gastric mucosa, are able to inactivate the small amount of residual IF available, leading to a negative vitamin B_{12} balance. Once this state is reached there a slow decline in B_{12} stores and eventually a failure of normal haemopoiesis and, in some, clinical neuropathy.

Clinical

Only 2% of patients are diagnosed before the age of 30 and only 11% under the age of 40. The mean age at diagnosis is about 60 years. The male to female ratio is 1 to 1.7. The onset is insidious, patients often being vaguely unwell for more than a year. Nevertheless there is surprisingly little correlation between duration of symptoms and degree of anaemia.

The common presenting symptoms are weakness, tiredness, dyspnoea on exertion, paraesthesia and sore tongue. Two-thirds have symptoms referable to the alimentary system including loss of appetite, sore mouth and/or tongue, loss of taste, less commonly dysphagia and aphthous ulcers. Flatulence is not uncommon and loose motions are present in about one-third. Numbness and tingling of extremities are present in one third of patients. Less common are abnormal skin pigmentation, impotence in males and difficulty with micturition. Infertility in the untreated state is the rule in younger patients.

Examination in the early case, will show little that is abnormal other than a smooth tongue. Some have a raw red tongue. There may be premature greying of hair in younger subjects and patches of vitiligo. Where severe, cases show slight icterus with pallor, evidence of cardiac failure and hepatomegaly. Splenomegaly is unusual.

Neurological examination may show impairment of superficial sensation and loss of vibration sense. Less commonly there may be exaggerated knee jerks and extensor plantars. Rarely a variety of other psychiatric and visual disturbances occur.

Increasingly, patients present to their doctors with very general symptoms of loss of well-being and the first indication of PA is an unexpected finding of slight macrocytosis in a blood count. Some patients present with a gastric carcinoma and at the same time are found to have the blood changes of PA.

Diagnosis

All patients must have either megaloblastic haemopoiesis or very rarely a neuropathy in the absence of blood changes. When anaemia is severe enough the blood changes are sufficient to diagnose a megaloblastic anaemia, but in the majority this must be done on marrow examination. Second, there must be evidence of B_{12} deficiency which in practice is a low serum vitamin B_{12} level. Third, the cause of the low B_{12} level is lack of IF, best demonstrated indirectly by showing impaired B_{12} absorption corrected by oral IF.

These are the minimum criteria for diagnosis. Elderly subjects with simple severe atrophic gastritis may have low serum B_{12} levels and may have impaired B_{12} absorption. They may continue in this state for many years without change.[9] The vast majority never develop evidence of PA. Only those who, in addition, have the blood changes of PA or the neuropathy should be so labelled. The term latent pernicious anaemia is not helpful and should not be used.

The difficulties in obtaining reliable B_{12} results when the assay is performed with many commercial kits sold for this purpose should always be borne in mind. The unreliability of tests based on urine collection in elderly patients in busy wards or on an outpatient basis, should always be considered in interpreting B_{12} absorption tests. An incomplete urine collection followed by a better effort when the test is repeated with IF is all too often the inadequate basis for a diagnosis of PA. Such tests should be accompanied by measurement of plasma radioactivity, the sample being collected about ten hours after the oral dose. These usually show normal plasma radioactivity while the urinary excretion is too low because of lost urine.

Laboratory tests

Blood count. This will show macrocytosis as assessed by the mean corpuscular volume (MCV). Neutropenia and thrombocytopenia are present in severely affected patients as well as hypersegmented nuclei in neutrophil polymorphs. The MCV will not be raised, however, if the patient also has a disorder which by itself is accompanied by small red cells, i.e. α- or β-thalassaemia trait, iron deficiency, or rarely the anaemia of chronic disorders.

Marrow is required to confirm megaloblastosis. There are a host of disorders giving rise to macrocytosis with a normoblastic marrow, including alcoholism, hypothyroidism, the use of a variety of drugs (particularly antimitotic drugs), disseminated neoplasia, and a reticulocytosis for whatever reason. This is an important reason why a marrow specimen is desirable as an early step of investigation.

Serum B_{12} level must be assayed and is always low.

Absorption tests. Impaired B_{12} absorption corrected by the addition of IF is present in PA as well as in postgastrectomy patients and otherwise healthy elderly subjects with severe atrophic gastritis. In one-third of PA patients, correction with IF falls short of the normal range. In some this is due to IF antibodies in gastric secretion but in others it indicates impaired ileal function which slowly improves over some three to nine months. Jejunal villi may be shortened and blunted in untreated PA, and the individual epithelial cells are wider and much larger than normal. There may be increased cellular infiltration and all this is reversed by treatment.[4] In addition impaired xylose absorption is present in 29% and impaired fat absorption in 9%.[6] Xylose absorption becomes normal two to three weeks after B_{12} treatment. Impaired iron absorption has been described but is probably related to achlorhydria.[2]

Biochemistry. The more severely affected patients have a raised bilirubin level and increased urinary urobilinogen. Serum iron is raised and transferrin saturation is increased. The serum iron level falls within hours of giving specific therapy. Many serum enzymes tend to be elevated, particularly lactate dehydrogenase and hydroxybutyrate dehydrogenase, and these return to normal levels within one week of specific therapy.[1]

Urine. Methylmalonic acid and formiminoglutamic acid excretion are increased in all but the mildest cases.

Serum gastrin levels are very high, reflecting achlorhydria.

The stomach

The changes are those of severe atrophic gastritis or gastric atrophy and involve the body of the stomach. In PA associated with hypogammaglobulinaemia the antrum is also atrophic and serum gastrin levels are not elevated. It is clear that endoscopy is not a very satisfactory way of recognizing atrophy and biopsy is necessary.

Gastric secretion. Pentagastrin-fast achlorhydria with small gastric juice volumes, and absent (or very low) IF secretion and low pepsin, is the rule.

Carcinoma. Some 6–8% of patients with PA ultimately die with a carcinoma of the stomach.[10] Gastric polyps are commonly seen on endoscopy in almost one in six patients.[3] They appear to remain benign.

Differential diagnosis of B_{12} deficiency states[1]

NUTRITIONAL

In nature B_{12} is only synthesized by microorganisms, and higher animals must strive to obtain their essential B_{12} supplies from such sources. Herbivores do so by absorbing B_{12} synthesized by the microorganisms in the gut rumen or, as in the cases of monkeys and fruit bats, by eating insects. Carnivores obtain B_{12} by eating herbivores. Vitamin B_{12} is absent from the plant kingdom and strict vegetarians (neither milk, nor eggs) obtain some B_{12} only from food that has acquired a bacterial flora. Trace amounts are present in some water supplies. Nutritional B_{12} deficiency should only be considered as a diagnosis in strict vegetarians such as Hindu Indians. The proof of diagnosis is a haematological response to daily *oral* B_{12}, either a solution supplying about 5 µg daily or tablets containing B_{12}. The absorption of B_{12} is generally normal in such patients. Megaloblastic anaemia due to nutritional B_{12} deficiency occurs at any age and with equal frequency in both sexes. Older patients, however, may have pernicious anaemia and hence adequate investigation is necessary.

Low serum B_{12} levels are the rule in Hindu vegetarians who are in normal health and who have normal blood pictures, and these levels may be as low as in some patients with untreated pernicious anaemia.

IMPAIRED B_{12} ABSORPTION

All other causes of acquired B_{12} deficiency are related to impaired intestinal absorption of B_{12}. Normal B_{12} absorption, irrespective of the serum B_{12} level in a subject taking a mixed diet, excludes a diagnosis of B_{12} deficiency.

Gastric causes

Total gastrectomy, if not followed by B_{12} injections, leads to megaloblastic anaemia due to B_{12} deficiency after two years but a few patients may not be diagnosed up to 12 years after operation. Peak time of diagnosis is five years.

Partial gastrectomy, removing not less than three-quarters of the body of the stomach, leads to a megaloblastic anaemia due to B_{12} deficiency in 5% of patients. The earliest time of diagnosis is five years after surgery. In these there is atrophy of the mucosa in the gastric remnant. Acid in the gastric secretion excludes diagnosis of megaloblastic anaemia due to B_{12} deficiency. As about one-half of postgastrectomy patients, if untreated at five years, have iron-deficiency anaemia the diagnosis may be complicated. Iron deficiency should be treated first and ensuing macrocytosis is a clue to an accompanying megaloblastic anaemia. Serum B_{12} assay is not decisive since some 30% of postgastrectomy patients may have low levels after five years and an equal proportion have impaired B_{12} absorption. But only one in six of these will develop a megaloblastic anaemia. Nevertheless a low B_{12} level accompanied by impaired B_{12} absorption is an indication for regular B_{12} injections and in some patients is accompanied by considerable clinical benefit despite still remaining normoblastic.

Gastroenterostomy of long standing may rarely be accompanied by megaloblastic anaemia. Investigation shows the feature of addisonian pernicious anaemia, i.e. there is impaired B_{12} absorption corrected by the addition of IF.

Corrosive gastritis, following ingestion of strong acid, has been followed by megaloblastic anaemia due to B_{12} deficiency.

Pancreatic causes

Impaired vitamin B_{12} absorption may occur in pancreatic disease, due to binding of B_{12} to 'R protein' rather than to intrinsic factor, when pancreatic enzymes are absent.[7]

Small intestinal causes

Abnormal flora. An abnormal resident intestinal bacterial flora may arise as a result of anatomical abnormalities that lead to stasis of intestinal contents or is due to impaired immunological capacity, or to the use of drugs that interfere with gut motility. Such disorders include surgically produced blind loops, strictures of the small gut, entero-enteric anastomoses, fistulas between gut segments, multiple diverticula, scleroderma, Whipple's disease, use of ganglion-blocking agents and hypogammaglobulinaemia. The abnormal flora removes B_{12} from the intestinal contents.

Clinical suspicion of this situation is a history of abdominal surgery, and symptoms that tend to be related to the abdomen (borborygmi, cramps, distension, bulky stools) rather than to anaemia. Often, however, the patient has megaloblastic anaemia apparently due to B_{12} deficiency but either acid is present in the gastric juice or there is no improvement in the impaired B_{12} absorption with added IF. These should point to an intestinal cause for B_{12} deficiency. Many such patients will have steatorrhoea and B_{12} malabsorption as the only evidence of abnormal gut function.

Tropical sprue. Residence at some time in an area where this disorder is endemic is essential for diagnosis. Vitamin B_{12} malabsorption is the rule usually with steatorrhoea and jejunal biopsy shows blunted villi.

Coeliac disease. With rare exceptions this is not a cause of megaloblastic anaemia requiring treatment with B_{12}. All patients with megaloblastic haemopoiesis require folate therapy for rapid restoration of a normal blood picture. The brunt of this disease is borne by the upper gut, and the ileum (which is the site of B_{12} absorption) is usually spared or mildly affected. Nevertheless, the B_{12} level is reduced in 42% of patients and B_{12} malabsorption present in 41% of patients.[1] Folate deficiency per se is accompanied by a secondary fall of the serum B_{12} level and folate therapy alone will restore the serum B_{12} level. The mechanism of this is unknown.

Gut resection. Generally when more than 180 cm of ileum are resected (following a volvulus, Crohn's or mesenteric embolus) B_{12} absorption is impaired but is generally normal if less than 60 cm is resected. There are many exceptions.

Ileal irradiation. Radiotherapy directed to the region of the pelvis, as in treatment of lesions of the uterine cervix or carcinoma of the bladder, is very likely to affect the ileal loops, and megaloblastic anaemia due to B_{12} deficiency may follow years later.

Fish tape worm (Diphyllobothrium latum). This tape worm is carried to man by larvae in fresh water fish primarily in Finland. The worm takes up B_{12} from the gut contents and the anaemia is cured either by B_{12} or by expelling the worm, preferably both. With PA, *D. latum* was the common cause of megaloblastic anaemia due to B_{12} deficiency in Finland. Pollution of the lakes and the relative scarcity of fresh fish seem to have diminished the problem.

HEREDITARY DISORDERS

These cause B_{12} deficiency in infancy and more rarely in older children or even young adults.

Congenital absence of IF. This differs from PA in that the gastric mucosa is normal, acid is present but IF is lacking. Some patients have an abnormal IF molecule reacting with an IF antibody but incapable of promoting intestinal absorption of B_{12}.

Congenital B_{12} malabsorption. (Imerslund–Gräsbeck) Gastric secretion is normal and there is an ileal defect which leads to isolated malabsorption of B_{12}. It is accompanied by proteinuria.

Transcobalamin II deficiency. This is the B_{12} carrier protein which transports the vitamin into cells and from the ileal cell into portal blood. In the absence of transcobalamin B_{12} is not absorbed. Its absence is accompanied by a severe megaloblastic anaemia responding only to massive parenteral doses of B_{12} given every few days. The absence of transcobalamin II can be demonstrated on column chromatography of serum with labelled B_{12} as a marker of B_{12} carrier proteins.

Prognosis

With treatment, women with PA have a normal life expectancy. Males, however, do not due to a higher frequency of carcinoma of the stomach.

Treatment

Once repletion of B_{12} stores has been achieved (1000 µg hydroxocobalamin for four to six doses), 250 µg B_{12} is given every four to eight weeks for life. It is impractical to survey for a gastric neoplasm other than when there is a clinical indication, such as dyspeptic symptoms or an elevation of ESR.

REFERENCES

1 Chanarin, I. (1979) *The Megaloblastic Anaemias.* Oxford: Blackwell.
2 Cook, J. D., Brown, G. M. & Valberg, L. S. (1964) The effect of achylia gastrica on iron absorption. *Journal of Clinical Investigation,* **43,** 1185–1191.
3 Elsborg, L., Andersen, D., Myhre-Jensen, O. & Bactrip-Madsen, P. (1977) Gastric mucosal polyps in pernicious anaemia. *Scandinavian Journal of Gastroenterology,* **12,** 49–52.
4 Foroozan, P. & Trier, J. S. (1967) Mucosa of the small intestine in pernicious anaemia. *New England Journal of Medicine,* **277,** 553–559.

5 Hippe, E. & Jensen, K. B. (1969) Hereditary factors in pernicious anaemia and their relation to serum-immunoglobulin levels and age at diagnosis. *Lancet*, **ii**, 721–724.

6 Lindenbaum, J., Pezzimenti, J. F. & Shea, N. (1974) Small intestinal function in vitamin B_{12} deficiency. *Annals of Internal Medicine*, **80**, 326–331.

7 Marcoullis, G., Parmentier, Y., Nicolas, J.-P. *et al.* (1980) Cobalamin malabsorption due to non-degradation of R-proteins in the human intestine. *Journal of Clinical Investigation*, **66**, 430–440.

8 Siurala, M., Lektola, J. & Ihamäki, T. (1974) Atrophic gastritis and its sequelae, results of 19–23 years' follow-up examinations. *Scandinavian Journal of Gastroenterology*, **9**, 441–446.

9 Whiteside, M. G., Mollin, D. L., Coghill, N. F. *et al.* (1964) The absorption of radioactive vitamin B_{12} and the secretion of hydrochloric acid in patients with atrophic gastritis. *Gut*, **5**, 385–399.

10 Zamcheck, N., Grable, E., Ley, A. & Norman, L. (1955) Occurrence of gastric cancer among patients with pernicious anemia at the Boston City Hospital. *New England Journal of Medicine*, **252**, 1103–1110.

LIPID ABNORMALITIES

LIPOPROTEIN PHYSIOLOGY (SEE ALSO CHAPTER 8)

The gastrointestinal tract plays an important role in the metabolism of plasma lipoproteins.[17] Dietary fat, mainly triglyceride, is first emulsified in the stomach and then undergoes hydrolysis by pancreatic lipase and solubilization by bile salts. The resultant fatty acids and mono-glycerides, together with some free cholesterol and lysophosphatidylcholine (lysoPC), become incorporated into mixed micelles and are then taken up by the jejunal mucosa, whereas bile salts get reabsorbed later in the ileum. Subsequent resynthesis of triglyceride, and partial re-esterification of cholesterol and re-acylation of lysoPC leads to the formation of chylomicrons, which comprise a core of triglyceride and cholesterol esters enclosed in a surface coat of free cholesterol, phosphatidylcholine (PC) and various apoproteins (apo). The latter include apoB48, apoA-I, apoA-II, apoA-IV and the apoC group of peptides. All are synthesized in the small intestine and are constituents both of chylomicrons and the similar but smaller particles in lymph known as intestinal very low density lipoprotein (VLDL). In addition apoA-I is a major constituent of high density lipoprotein (HDL) of intestinal origin, in contrast to HDL of hepatic origin which is rich in apoE.

After traversing the thoracic duct lymph chylomicrons enter the plasma and acquire apoE and additional apoC peptides from HDL, including apoC-II the activator of lipoprotein lipase. This enzyme is situated mainly in capillaries serving adipose tissue and muscle and effects the hydrolysis of chylomicron and VLDL triglyceride. During this process, chylomicrons decrease in size and lose much of their apoA-I, apoA-IV and apoC together with some of the polar lipids in their surface coat. The resultant chylomicron remnants are taken up by the liver, probably via apoE receptors, where they serve to regulate the activity of HMG-CoA reductase and thus control endogenous cholesterol synthesis. All the apoB48 gets removed from plasma but some free cholesterol and PC transfer from chylomicrons to HDL_3, promoting its conversion to HDL_2 by providing substrate for lecithin : cholesterol acyltransferase (LCAT). This enzyme functions in plasma to esterify free cholesterol with an unsaturated fatty acid derived from the 2-position of PC. HDL_3 is the major substrate for this reaction, which is activated by apoA-I.

Some of the free fatty acid released during peripheral lipolysis of chylomicrons is bound to albumin and transported to the liver, where it is converted into triglyceride and secreted back into plasma as VLDL of hepatic origin. The latter contains apoB100 and is hydrolysed in the periphery in a similar manner to chylomicrons, resulting in the formation of VLDL remnants which eventually get converted to low density lipoproteins (LDL), possibly via the action of hepatic lipase. VLDL remnants and LDL contain apoB100 but not apoB48 and interact with a receptor which recognizes both apoE and apoB100, the so-called LDL receptor. A simplified scheme of the various events which occur during lipoprotein metabolism is shown in Figure 9.13.

LIPOPROTEIN DISORDERS

The relation between abnormalities of lipoprotein metabolism and the gastrointestinal tract is complex. Primary, genetically determined defects of lipoprotein metabolism can lead to hypocholesterolaemia and malabsorption, as in abetalipoproteinaemia, or to severe hypertriglyceridaemia and acute pancreatitis, as in familial type I hyperlipoproteinaemia. More commonly, however, changes in serum lipids are secondary manifestations either of malabsorption caused by disease or surgical intervention, or of excessive alcohol intake. The changes in serum lipids which accompany diabetes will not be considered in this section. For the sake of

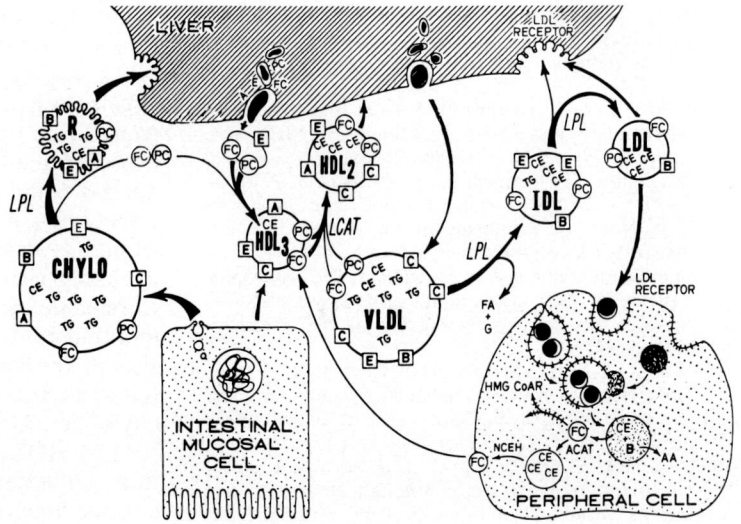

Fig. 9.13 A schematic diagram of lipoprotein metabolism. CHYLO = chylomicron, IDL = intermediate density lipoproteins, R = remnant, LPL = lipoprotein lipase, FC = free cholesterol, CE = cholesterol ester, TG = triglyceride, FA = fatty acid, G = glycerol, HDL = high density lipoprotein, LDL = low density lipoprotein; VLDL = very low density lipoprotein. A, B, C, E refer to respective apoproteins. From Davignon, Dufour and Cantin (1983),[8] with kind permission of the authors and McGraw-Hill.

clarity both primary and secondary abnormalities of lipoprotein metabolism have been subdivided according to whether they are primarily associated with malabsorption or with pancreatitis.

Malabsorption

PRIMARY HYPOLIPOPROTEINAEMIA

Abetalipoproteinaemia (see also p. 681)
This rare, recessively inherited disease is characterized by the onset during infancy of malabsorption and anaemia accompanied by the development in later childhood of progressively severe ataxia and of retinitis pigmentosa. Examination of the blood shows the presence of acanthocytosis and the absence from plasma of chylomicrons, VLDL and LDL. Serum cholesterol and triglyceride levels are both very low, usually in the range 0.5–2 mmol/l, and apoB is undetectable.[16] Nearly all the cholesterol in plasma is present as HDL, mainly as HDL_2. Serum phospholipids are also markedly decreased, as is the PC : sphingomyelin ratio. Postheparin lipolytic activity (which reflects mobilization of lipoprotein lipase and hepatic lipase) and LCAT activity are both reduced.

The clinical and biochemical features of this disorder have recently been reviewed by Herbert *et al.*[18] The majority of patients described seem to be males and at least half of them were the result of consanguineous unions. Obligate heterozygotes, however, show no signs of disease and have normal serum lipids. Homozygotes usually present with failure to grow and steatorrhoea in early childhood, with a differential diagnosis of either coeliac disease or cystic fibrosis of the pancreas. Jejunal biopsy shows the characteristic lipid-filled but otherwise normal looking villi.[19] Immunofluorescent studies have failed to demonstrate the presence of any apoB in the intestinal mucosa[13] or in the liver, which also contains excess fat. Thus it is assumed that the underlying defect is an inherited inability to synthesize both apoB48 and apoB100 and thus a failure to form either intestinal chylomicrons or hepatic VLDL.

Malabsorption of triglyceride, although less marked than that of fat-soluble vitamins, leads to decreases in the linoleate and arachidonate content of plasma lipids. Osteomalacia has been reported[20] but deficiency of vitamin D is less common than of vitamins A, E and K.[18] The fluidity and filterability of red cells is decreased and this has been attributed to an increase in the sphingomyelin : PC ratio of the red cell membrane. The central nervous system is severely affected in this disorder, especially the posterior columns which show patchy demyelination. It has been suggested that this could be caused by peroxidation of the unsaturated fatty acids present in myelin phospholipids, due to vitamin E deficiency.

Therapy for this disorder consists of a diet low in long-chain triglyceride, but containing 5–10 g linoleic acid daily, and supplements of vitamins A, E and K. Medium-chain triglyceride supplements are absorbed normally but have side-effects which limit their usefulness. Perhaps the most encouraging feature of therapy is the probability that large doses of oral vitamin E (100 $mg \cdot kg^{-1} \cdot day^{-1}$) given from an early age may prevent or modify the neurological and retinal complications of abetalipoproteinaemia.[22]

Familial hypobetalipoproteinaemia

In the homozygous form this disorder presents in a manner either identical to or as a milder version of abetalipoproteinaemia. It differs in that heterozygotes have hypocholesterolaemia and LDL levels which are about 25% of normal. Thus the disorder appears to be inherited in an autosomal dominant manner.[6] It has been suggested that heterozygotes are protected from coronary heart disease by their low LDL levels and that this leads to enhanced longevity.[15] Reduced synthesis of apoB has been demonstrated in such individuals.[31]

The distinction between homozygous hypobetalipoproteinaemia and abetalipoproteinaemia largely depends upon whether or not obligate heterozygote relatives have altered LDL levels. However, there does seem to be some overlap between the two conditions as illustrated by the description of an adult with steatorrhoea, typical fat-filled jejunal biopsy and ataxia in whom the plasma LDL-apoB was 35 mg/dl but whose first degree relatives all had normal values.[27]

Normotriglyceridaemic abetalipoproteinaemia

Malloy *et al.*[21] recently described a young girl with ataxia in whom VLDL and LDL were absent but who was able to absorb triglyceride normally and produce chylomicrons in response to dietary fat. Jejunal biopsy was normal. This disorder is of considerable interest in that it appears to represent selective deletion of the apoB100 gene but with maintenance of the ability to synthesize apoB48. The precise nature of the genetic defect and its relation to abetalipoproteinaemia and hypobetalipoproteinaemia remains to be established.

SECONDARY HYPOLIPOPROTEINAEMIA

Hypocholesterolaemia secondary to malabsorption ('sprue syndrome') was first described in adults by Adlersberg *et al.*[1] and similar findings were subsequently reported in children with coeliac disease.[25] Decreases in both LDL and HDL concentration in the face of normal or increased levels of VLDL were observed in a varied group of malabsorbers by Thompson and Miller[33] who noted that LDL levels were inversely correlated with the extent of steatorrhoea. These authors also observed changes in LDL composition, with a decreased proportion of cholesterol ester and a reciprocal increase in triglyceride. Such patients were subsequently shown to have reduced amounts of linoleic acid in lipoprotein lipids,[30] and in three instances overt essential fatty acid deficiency was documented following massive intestinal resection.[24] Decreased concentrations of LDL, HDL and linoleate have also been documented in children with pancreatic steatorrhoea due to cystic fibrosis.[34]

Hypocholesterolaemia was documented as a consequence of ileal resection by Buchwald,[3] who introduced partial ileal bypass as a means of treating patients with hypercholesterolaemia. This procedure results in a mean reduction in serum cholesterol of 40%[4] and appears to be especially useful in the treatment of patients with heterozygous familial hypercholesterolaemia in whom it lowers LDL levels by stimulating receptor-mediated LDL catabolism,[32] thus helping to counteract the underlying metabolic defect. Its superiority over anion exchange resins seems to be due to the more marked increase in bile acid excretion, and presumably bile acid synthesis, which results from the surgical procedure. Partial ileal bypass necessitates the administration of parenteral vitamin B_{12} on a life-long basis and may also decrease the absorption of calcium but promote that of oxalate.[10] Similar decreases in serum lipids accompanied the operation of jejuno-ileal bypass.

Pancreatitis

Although acute pancreatitis was originally thought to be the cause of the hyperlipaemia (i.e. gross hypertriglyceridaemia) which commonly accompanies it, evidence for this explanation is somewhat slender.[35] Studies by Cameron *et al.*[5] involving careful follow up of patients with acute pancreatitis and hyperlipaemia revealed defects in lipid metabolism which persisted long after their attack of pancreatitis had subsided, which suggested that hyperlipaemia was the cause rather than the consequence of acute pancreatitis. Most of their patients exhibited a type V lipoprotein phenotype (excess chylomicrons and VLDL) during the acute episode but subsequently this phenotype often changed, either to a type IV phenotype (excess VLDL) or, less commonly, to a type I (excess chylomicrons) or type III (excess chylomicron and VLDL remnants) phenotype.

The mechanism whereby extreme hypertriglyceridaemia induces acute pancreatitis is uncertain. One possibility is that some of the triglyceride undergoes hydrolysis by pancreatic lipase, with release of free fatty acids and consequent damage to the gland.[26] Alternatively it is possible that pancreatic ischaemia is caused by the hyperviscosity which results from the presence of high concentrations of chylomicrons and VLDL in plasma.[29]

PRIMARY HYPERLIPOPROTEINAEMIA

Familial lipoprotein lipase deficiency
This rare inherited disorder, also known as familial type I hyperlipoproteinaemia, is characterized by the onset in childhood of recurrent attacks of abdominal pain, acute pancreatitis and by eruptive xanthomas and hepatosplenomegaly. The condition is due to deficiency of lipoprotein lipase and a consequent inability to catabolize chylomicrons, which leads to marked hypertriglyceridaemia. Fasting chylomicronaemia is accompanied by normal or decreased levels of VLDL and by marked decreases in both LDL and HDL. The diagnosis depends upon establishing the presence in postheparin plasma of levels of lipoprotein lipase less than 10% of normal. Discrimination between lipoprotein lipase and the other lipases released into plasma by heparin, notably hepatic lipase, is essential and is best achieved by an immunochemical method or by affinity chromatography.

The condition is usually considered to be due to an autosomal recessive gene, although measurement of postheparin lipoprotein lipase levels in the siblings of affected patients shows bimodality.[23] The risk of acute pancreatitis is minimal as long as plasma triglyceride levels are kept below 15–20 mmol/l; this is best achieved by a < 50 g fat diet. Establishing the diagnosis of acute pancreatitis during an episode of acute abdominal pain is made difficult by the interference by triglyceride with the assay for serum amylase.

Familial apoprotein C-II deficiency
This rare recessively inherited disorder usually presents in adult life and is due to deficiency of apoC-II, the activator of lipoprotein lipase. Nineteen patients with this disorder have been described so far[23] among whom recurrent attacks of acute pancreatitis have been a common feature, in one instance progressing to chronic pancreatic insufficiency. The lipoprotein phenotype is type V and the diagnosis can be made by demonstrating absence of apoC-II on isoelectric focusing of delipidated VLDL.

The first report of apoC-II deficiency[2] described a man with a type V phenotype whose hypertriglyceridaemia improved dramatically after a blood transfusion. Further investigations revealed detectable amounts of lipoprotein lipase in postheparin plasma, which became evident only after addition of apoC-II in vitro. Infusions of normal plasma containing apoC-II dramatically reduce plasma triglyceride levels in affected subjects, albeit temporarily.

Familial type V hyperlipoproteinaemia
This disorder is characterized by the onset in adult life of attacks of abdominal pain, eruptive xanthomas and peripheral neuropathy. The abdominal pain can be due to pancreatitis, which occurs in 40–60% of patients,[23] or to hepatic or splenic enlargement. Hypertriglyceridaemia is due to a combination of chylomicronaemia and increased levels of VLDL, and is exacerbated by factors which promote triglyceride synthesis, notably oestrogens, alcohol and being male.

The disorder is probably inherited in an autosomal dominant manner. There is an increased prevalence of type IV phenotypes among first-degree relatives. The exact nature of the biochemical defect is uncertain; postheparin lipoprotein lipase levels are usually normal but the activity of this enzyme is often subnormal in adipose tissue and muscle, which is compatible with a defect of triglyceride clearance. However, turnover studies suggest that VLDL synthesis is increased which makes it difficult to know whether the accompanying decrease in fractional catabolic rate is a primary or secondary phenomenon. Glucose intolerance, often leading to frank diabetes, and hyperuricaemia are common accompaniments of type V hyperlipoproteinaemia.

Treatment of this disorder is difficult, necessitating reductions in both total calories and fat intake. Possibly the most useful drugs are oxandrolone in men and norethisterone acetate in women, both of which act by enhancing the activity of lipoprotein lipase. There have been several instances of patients with this condition in whom repeated attacks of acute pancreatitis eventually led to chronic pancreatic insufficiency.[11] It is debatable whether patients with type V hyperlipoproteinaemia have an increased prevalence of coronary heart disease, as has been claimed.

SECONDARY HYPERLIPOPROTEINAEMIA

Acquired type I hyperlipoproteinaemia has been described in systemic lupus erythematosus, due to the presence in plasma of an IgG antibody which blocked the release into plasma of lipoprotein lipase.[23] Oestrogens, given as replacement therapy[14] or as oral contraceptives,[7] can induce severe hypertriglyceridaemia and acute pancreatitis in patients with previously undiagnosed type IV or V hyperlipoproteinaemia. In one instance a similar effect has been attributed to β-blockers, which were shown to markedly impair triglyceride clearance.[9] But by far the commonest cause of secondary type V hyperlipoproteinaemia is alcohol, which was the precipitating factor in more than 50% of the patients with hyperlipaemia and acute pancreatitis reported by Cameron et al.[5] Alcohol is preferentially oxidized by the liver which results in increased amounts of free fatty acid becoming available for triglyceride synthesis, thus increasing VLDL synthesis. Whether the magnitude of the hypertriglyceridaemic response to alcohol is genetically determined remains to be seen. The recent discovery of apoE polymorphism and the apparent increase in the apoE$_4$ allele in type V patients[12] compared with normolipidaemic or type IV subjects, in whom the apoE$_3$ allele predominates, offers a potentially fruitful line of enquiry, especially in view of the well-established relationship between inheritance of the apoE$_2$ allele and type III hyperlipoproteinaemia.

REFERENCES

1 Adlersberg, D., Wang, C. I. & Bossak, E. T. (1957) Disturbances in protein and lipid metabolism in malabsorption syndrome. *Journal of the Mount Sinai Hospital,* **24,** 206.
2 Breckenridge, W. C., Little, A., Steiner, G. et al. (1978) Hypertriglyceridemia associated with deficiency of apolipoprotein C-II. *New England Journal of Medicine,* **298,** 1265–1273.
3 Buchwald, H. (1964) Lowering of cholesterol resorption and blood levels by ileal exclusion. *Circulation,* **XXIX,** 713–720.
4 Buchwald, H. & Varco, R. L. (1966) Ileal bypass in patients with hypercholesterolemia and atherosclerosis. *Journal of the American Medical Association,* **196,** 119–122.
5 Cameron, J. L., Capuzzi, D. M., Zuidema, G. D. & Margolis, S. (1974) Acute pancreatitis with hyperlipemia. Evidence for a persistent defect in lipid metabolism. *American Journal of Medicine,* **56,** 482–487.
6 Cottrill, C., Glueck, C. J., Leuba, V. et al. (1974) Familial homozygous hypobetalipoproteinemia. *Metabolism,* **23,** 779–791.
7 Davidoff, F., Tishler, S. & Rosoff, C. (1973) Marked hyperlipidemia and pancreatitis associated with oral contraceptive therapy. *New England Journal of Medicine,* **289,** 552–555.
8 Davignon, J., Dufour, R. & Cantin, M. (1983) Atherosclerosis and hypertension. In *Hypertension, Physiopathology and Treatment* (Ed.) Genest, G., Kuchel, O., Hamet, P. & Cantin, M. New York: McGraw-Hill (In press).
9 Durrington, P. N. & Cairns, S. A. (1982) Acute pancreatitis: a complication of beta-blockade. *British Medical Journal,* **284,** 1016.
10 Faegerman, O., Meinertz, H., Hylander, E. et al. (1982) Effects and side-effects of partial ileal by-pass surgery for familial hypercholesterolaemia. *Gut,* **23,** 558–563.
11 Fallat, R. W. & Glueck, C. J. (1976) Familial and acquired type V hyperlipoproteinemia. *Atherosclerosis,* **23,** 41–62.
12 Ghiselli, G., Schaefer, E. J., Zech, L. A. et al. (1982) Increased prevalence of apolipoprotein E$_4$ in type V hyperlipoproteinemia. *Journal of Clinical Investigation,* **70,** 474–477.
13 Glickman, R. M., Green, P. H. R., Lees, R. S. et al. (1979) Immunofluorescence studies of apolipoprotein B in intestinal mucosa. Absence in abetalipoproteinemia. *Gastroenterology,* **76,** 288–292.
14 Glueck, C. J., Scheel, D., Fishback, J. & Steiner, P. (1972) Estrogen-induced pancreatitis in patients with previously covert familial type V hyperlipoproteinemia. *Metabolism,* **21,** 657–666.
15 Glueck, C. J., Gartside, P., Fallat, R. W. et al. (1976) Longevity syndromes: familial hypobeta and familial hyperalpha lipoproteinemia. *Journal of Laboratory and Clinical Medicine,* **88,** 941–957.
16 Gotto, A. M., Levy, R. I., John, K. & Fredrickson, D. S. (1971) On the protein defect in abetalipoproteinemia. *New England Journal of Medicine,* **284,** 813.
17 Green, P. H. R. & Glickman, R. M. (1981) Intestinal lipoprotein metabolism. *Journal of Lipid Research,* **22,** 1153–1173.
18 Herbert, P. N., Assman, G., Gotto, A. M. & Fredrickson, D. S. (1983) Familial lipoprotein deficiency: abetalipoproteinemia, hypobetalipoproteinemia, and Tangier disease. In *The Metabolic Basis of Inherited Disease* (Ed.) Stanbury, J. B., Wyngaarden, J. B., Fredrickson, D. S. et al. 5th edition, pp. 589–621. New York: McGraw-Hill.
19 Isselbacher, K. J., Scheig, R., Plotkin, G. R. & Caulfield, J. B. (1964) Congenital β-lipoprotein deficiency: an hereditary disorder involving a defect in the absorption and transport of lipids. *Medicine (Baltimore),* **43,** 347.
20 Lamy, M., Frezal, J., Polonovski, J. et al. (1963) Congenital absence of beta-lipoproteins. *Pediatrics,* **31,** 277–289.
21 Malloy, M. J., Kane, J. P., Hardman, D. et al. (1981) Normotriglyceridemic abetalipoproteinemia. Absence of the B-100 apolipoprotein. *Journal of Clinical Investigation,* **67,** 1441–1450.
22 Muller, D. P. R., Lloyd, J. K. & Bird, A. C. (1977) Long-term management of abetalipoproteinaemia. *Archives of Diseases in Childhood,* **52,** 209–214.
23 Nikkila, E. A. (1983) Familial lipoprotein lipase deficiency and related disorders of chylomicron metabolism. In *Metabolic Basis of Inherited Disease* (Ed.) Stanbury, J. B., Wyngaarden, J. B., Fredrickson, D. S. et al. 5th edition, pp. 622–642. New York: McGraw-Hill.
24 Press, M., Kikuchi, H., Shimoyama, T. & Thompson, G. R. (1974) Diagnosis and treatment of essential fatty acid deficiency in man. *British Medical Journal,* **ii,** 247–250.
25 Rey, J. (1965) Modifications des lipides plasmatiques dans les troubles de l'absorption intestinale. *Revue Européene d'Etudes Cliniques et Biologiques,* **10,** 488.
26 Saharia, P., Margolis, S., Zuidema, G. D. & Cameron, J. L. (1977) Acute pancreatitis with hyperlipemia: studies with an isolated perfused canine pancreas. *Surgery,* **82,** 60–67.
27 Scott, B. B., Miller, J. P. & Losowsky, M. S. (1979) Hypobetalipoproteinaemia – a variant of the Bassen–Kornzweig syndrome. *Gut,* **20,** 163–168.
28 Scott, H. W., Dean, R. H., Younger, R. K. & Butts, W. H. (1974) Changes in hyperlipidemia and hyper-

lipoproteinemia in morbidly obese patients treated by jejunoileal bypass. *Surgery, Gynecology and Obstetrics*, **138**, 353–358.

29 Seplowitz, A. H., Chien, S. & Smith, F. R. (1981) Effects of lipoproteins on plasma viscosity. *Atherosclerosis*, **38**, 89–95.

30 Shimoyama, T., Kikuchi, H., Press, M. & Thompson, G. R. (1973) Fatty acid composition of plasma lipoproteins in control subjects and in patients with malabsorption. *Gut*, **14**, 716–722.

31 Sigurdsson, G., Nicoll, A. & Lewis, B. (1977) Turnover of apolipoprotein-B in two subjects with familial hypobetalipoproteinemia. *Metabolism*, **26**, 25–31.

32 Spengel, F. A., Jadhav, A., Duffield, R. G. M. *et al.* (1981) Superiority of partial ileal bypass over cholestyramine in reducing cholesterol in familial hypercholesterolaemia. *Lancet*, **ii**, 768–770.

33 Thompson, G. R. & Miller, J. P. (1973) Plasma lipid and lipoprotein abnormalities in patients with malabsorption. *Clinical Science and Molecular Medicine*, **45**, 583–592.

34 Vaughan, W. J., Lindgren, F. T., Whalen, J. B. & Abraham, S. (1978) Serum lipoprotein concentrations in cystic fibrosis. *Science*, **199**, 783–786.

35 Zieve, L. (1968) Relationship between acute pancreatitis and hyperlipemia. *Medical Clinics of North America*, **52**, 1493–1501.

HAEMOCHROMATOSIS

Pathological accumulation of iron in the tissues, with parenchymal injury and associated functional impairment, is known as haemochromatosis or iron-storage disease. Iron overload in tissues represents a failure of the normal control mechanisms of iron balance. The capacity to *excrete* incorporated iron is extremely limited and iron balance is regulated by the small intestinal mucosa which adjusts the net *absorption* to meet body requirements. Excess iron accumulates when the regulatory behaviour of the mucosa is disturbed or when overwhelming amounts of iron are administered. Whatever the pathway of iron accumulation, the clinical manifestations reflect widespread involvement of tissues throughout the body: hepatic fibrosis progressing to cirrhosis, cardiac failure and rhythm disturbance, polyarthropathy, dermal pigmentation, and pancreatic endocrine and exocrine disorder.

Pathophysiology

PRIMARY HAEMOCHROMATOSIS

Primary, or idiopathic, haemochromatosis is now recognized as an inborn error of metabolism transmitted by an autosomal recessive gene.[15] The estimated prevalence varies from 1 in 500 to 1 in 10 000 in different communities,[9] but in all groups so far studied there is a strong association with the HLA–A3 haplotype as well as certain B antigens (B7 and B14). Clinical haemochromatosis is only seen in homozygous individuals, although heterozygotes may manifest laboratory abnormalities of iron metabolism. The striking preponderance of male cases (up to 10 : 1) and variable age of presentation in adult life indicates that environmental factors, such as menstruation, pregnancy and diet, strongly influence expression of the disease in genetically predisposed individuals.

Iron absorption in primary haemochromatosis is either frankly increased or inappropriate for the level of body iron stores.[17] Storage iron is increased up to 100 fold in untreated patients, representing a burden of 15–60 g of iron in the tissues; this is compatible with estimates showing that the mean daily absorption of dietary iron is enhanced from about 1 mg to 3–5 mg in homozygous individuals,[8] leading insidiously over decades to the burden of accumulated iron in the tissues. Ferrokinetic studies have also demonstrated increased hepatic clearance of plasma radioiron, so that there may be a generalized disorder with enhanced tissue iron uptake in addition to avid incorporation by the intestine.[4,7]

SECONDARY HAEMOCHROMATOSIS

Haemochromatosis is also recognized when excess iron is ingested (in the form of medications or alcoholic drinks) or given parenterally (usually in the form of blood transfusions). Under these circumstances the body is simply overwhelmed by enormous iron loads. The iron content of beers prepared in metal pots by the Bantu and of some red wines is well known. Certain blood diseases are accompanied by a profound disturbance of the iron absorption. For example, anaemias where there is a large component of ineffective erythropoiesis (e.g. pernicious anaemia, sideroblastic anaemia and thalassaemia) are particularly associated with an inappropriate hyperabsorption of dietary iron.[10,13] However, haemochromatosis is also recognized as a complication of hereditary spherocytosis and even glucose-6-phosphate dehydrogenase deficiency. Transfusional loading, in addition to persistent hyperabsorption of dietary iron, contributes to the progressive iron storage disease which afflicts so many young patients suffering from the major thalassaemic syndromes and which frequently causes premature death. Each unit of blood contains about 250 mg of iron and since daily excretion of iron rarely exceeds 1 mg, transfusion treatment leads rapidly to severe iron overload.

MECHANISMS OF TISSUE INJURY AND PATHOLOGICAL FEATURES

Metal toxicity in iron storage disease is probably related to the electrochemical reactivity of iron. Alteration of the state of oxidation of iron atoms may facilitate formation of free oxygen radicals which could promote biological damage by accelerating peroxidation of unsaturated lipids in cellular membranes. Furthermore, iron deposition is accompanied by accumulation of haemosiderin and some ferritin in lysosomes which increases lysosomal fragility; disruption of these intracellular organelles may be associated with the development of tissue injury.[14]

Heavy deposits of iron in haemochromatotic tissues are generally accompanied by fibrosis and rust-like discoloration. In the abdomen, involvement of the liver, pancreas and lymph nodes is usually obvious. The enlarged liver is heavily pigmented and microscopically haemosiderin is found in all cell types but especially in the periphery of lobules where parenchymal degeneration gives way to formation of fibrous septa. In haemochromatosis secondary to dietary or transfusional iron overload, Kupffer cell siderosis reflects an early, but not exclusive, involvement of the reticuloendothelial system. The spleen is often enlarged, but severe portal hypertension is uncommon. The pancreas is grossly distorted by fibrosis and iron is found in ducts, acini and the B-cells of the islets.

There is a diffuse disorder of the myocardium where degeneration and hypertrophy accompany iron deposits and intermyocyte sclerosis. Heavy accumulation of haemosiderin is also found in salivary, sweat and Brunner's glands as well as the adenohypophysis, testis, thyroid, parathyroids and adrenal zona glomerulosa. Haemosiderin is deposited in the synovium and an asymmetrical destructive arthropathy of the small joints is frequent; chondrocalcinosis is usually demonstrable where larger joints are affected.

Clinical features

In contrast to findings on physical examination, the symptoms of haemochromatosis are fre-quently non-specific and difficult to recognize in the absence of overt endocrine disturbance or diabetes. In primary haemochromatosis the age of onset of symptoms is usually between 40 and 60 years. Asthenia, abdominal pain, weight loss, impotence or joint complaints may be long standing but often, unless there is a family history of iron storage disease or a pre-disposing blood disorder, the true nature of the complaint may go unsuspected for years.

In established haemochromatosis hepatomegaly, which may be tender, together with grey dermal pigmentation, occurs in more than 90% of patients. There may also be other physical signs: painful swelling of metacarpophalangeal joints, hypogonadism or koilonychia. Cardiac involvement may be inapparent, or shown only by minor arrhythmias on ECG monitoring. In more advanced disease, cardiac failure or pericardial constriction due to fibrosis may occur; in secondary haemochromatosis deaths due to cardiac arrhythmias, often in the second or third decade, are common. Pancreatic endocrine dysfunction, with overt diabetes mellitus, is relatively common and failure of the adrenal cortex, thyroid and parathyroid is also recognized. Pancreatic exocrine function is disturbed, but the hypersecretion of dilute pancreatic juice seen is of little clinical significance.[1]

Far advanced disease is usually unmistakable, but early presentation with non descript symptomatology and minimal physical signs is easy to overlook. In this connection, diabetics with liver abnormalities, alcoholics with pigmentation and patients with obscure myocardial disease or hypogonadism should all be screened for possible iron storage disease.

Investigations

In overt haemochromatosis radiological and laboratory investigations readily indicate widespread organ involvement. About one-third of patients have joint involvement with chondrocalcinosis and loss of joint spaces. Occasionally heavy iron deposition leads to decreased hepatic radiolucency on plain abdominal x-ray but more sensitive detection of increased liver iron in vivo has been achieved in early studies employing computed tomographic studies and nuclear magnetic resonance analysis. Each cardiac involvement may be revealed by spontaneous arrhythmias on ECG monitoring. Frank diabetes is common and serum levels of liver enzymes, especially transaminases, are often raised 2–4 fold above normal values.

DIAGNOSTIC EVIDENCE OF DISORDERED
IRON METABOLISM (TABLE 9.8)

In untreated haemochromatosis the serum iron
is raised and the transferrin saturation is greater
than 70%. In premenopausal females homozygous for idiopathic haemochromatosis these
tests are abnormal in more than 85% of cases
but in early precirrhotic disease some values
may be normal.[9] The serum ferritin level is
usually greatly elevated; again this is not invariable in full-blown disease and, moreover, serum
ferritin measurements are often normal in partially treated individuals. The serum ferritin may
also be increased in the presence of any cause of
liver necrosis and in malignant disease but
values greater than 1000 µg/l in the absence of
gross elevations of serum transaminases generally indicate significant iron overload. In haemochromatosis occurring in the context of
blood diseases, serum ferritin measurements correlate with the degree of transfusional iron
burden but do not indicate whether or not there
is severe parenchymal iron accumulation.
Additional information, useful particularly in
the follow up of patients with known
haemochromatosis, may be gained by carrying
out a chelation test; the 24-hour excretion of
more than 2 mg of iron following intramuscular
desferrioxamine (10 mg/kg body weight) is evidence for significant iron overload.

Chemical determination of tissue iron content
is a simple procedure and should always accompany histological examination of the liver in
cases of suspected haemochromatosis.[2] The iron
content of normal liver is less than 0.14% by dry
weight and in idiopathic or secondary haemochromatosis is generally greater than 1.5%; the
iron content of liver from alcoholic individuals is
usually less than 1% by dry weight but this criterion is not absolute.

Treatment and prognosis

Removal of iron and prevention of continuing
accumulation of this metal is beneficial to
patients with haemochromatosis. In primary

haemochromatosis iron may easily be removed
by phlebotomy and chelation therapy has no
place in management. Removal of 200–500 mg
iron by weekly or twice-weekly bleeding of 500
ml should be carried out until mild iron deficiency anaemia develops. This may take 1–2
years, and has been shown in a large series to
prolong mean life expectancy from 14 months at
the time of diagnosis to 70 months.[5] Despite
this, the risks of hepatoma development do not
appear to be reduced (this causes death in
15–35% of all patients with primary haemochromatosis and also frequently complicates
secondary iron storage disease).

Although iron depletion prolongs survival in
primary haemochromatosis, the quality of life
for many patients remains poor. Improvement
in liver, pancreatic and cardiac function are not
usually accompanied by improvement in diabetic control, impotence or disabling joint
disease – this latter may worsen during venesection treatment. Moreover, although iron depletion is associated with decreasing hepatic size
and resolution of fibrotic changes, death from
hepatoma and other coincident malignancies
remains common. Reaccumulation of iron can
be prevented by maintenance treatment
designed to remove about 2 g of iron annually
and long-term follow up with interval biopsy
and blood analysis is to be encouraged.

Management of primary haemochromatosis
is not complete without detailed pedigree
analysis. Non-invasive tests, such as serum iron
and ferritin, have not proved to be always definitive (especially in young women); HLA typing
provides additional information in terms of
disease risks[9] and may identify young individuals predisposed to develop iron overload at a
later date and who should be further evaluated.

In secondary haemochromatosis, chelation
therapy is used universally.[11] Desferrioxamine is
the only chelator in general clinical use, but it is
expensive and only useful when given parenterally. Regular injections can reduce tissue
iron concentrations and prevent progressing
hepatic fibrosis.[3] Currently, subcutaneous infusions of the drug have been found most suitable

Table 9.8 Laboratory measurements of iron status (range of values) in primary haemochromatosis.[9]

	Age (y)	Serum iron (µg/dl)	Transferrin saturation (%)	Serum ferritin (µg/l)	Hepatic iron (µg/100 mg wet tissue)
Normal males	2–86	30–192	10–58	3–675	2–34
Normal females	1–93	30–158	9–48	3–405	1–17
Male haemochromatotics	24–69	172–378	75–100	198–7300	211–1421
Female haemochromatotics	8–67	88–261	41–100	42–2600	47–1109

for chronic use; they are used in doses determined by individual experiment to be optimal for each patient. Administration for more than 12 hours daily using a pump system, has been advocated. Tolerance of the drug (up to 2 g/day) is usually good and limited only by local irritation. More serious complications, such as anaphylaxis or cataract formation, appear to be rare. Recently oral ascorbic acid has been shown to act synergistically with desferrioxamine in promoting iron excretion.[12]

Prospective controlled trials in thalassaemic children have shown that desferrioxamine treatment can reduce liver fibrosis and liver iron concentrations, although a diminution in cardiac iron content is clearly difficult to document. Prepubertal growth is enhanced and survival also appears to be improved in the treated group. These preliminary findings suggest that more aggressive and persistent chelation therapy may at least serve to prevent development of lethal iron storage disease as a complication of these chronic blood disorders.

REFERENCES

1 Althausen, T. L., Doig, R. K., Weiden, S. *et al.* (1951) Haemochromatosis: an investigation of twenty-three cases with special reference to nutrition, to iron metabolism, and to studies of hepatic and pancreatic function. *Archives of Internal Medicine,* **88,** 553–570.

2 Barry, M. & Sherlock, S. (1971) Measurement of liver-iron concentration in needle-biopsy specimens. *Lancet,* **i,** 100–103.

3 Barry, M., Flynn, D. N., Letsky, E. A. & Risdon, R. A. (1974) Long term chelation therapy in thalassaemia major: effect on liver iron concentration, liver histology and clinical progress. *British Medical Journal,* **i,** 16–20.

4 Batey, R. G., Pettit, J. E., Nicholas, A. W. *et al.* (1978) Hepatic iron clearance from serum in treated haemochromatosis. *Gastroenterology,* **75,** 856–859.

5 Bomford, A. & Williams, R. (1976) Long-term results of venesection therapy in idiopathic haemochromatosis. *Quarterly Journal of Medicine,* **XLV,** 611–623.

6 Bregman, H., Winchester, J. F., Knepshield, J. H. *et al.* (1980) Iron-overload-associated myopathy in patients on maintenance haemodialysis: a histocompatibility-linked disorder. *Lancet,* **ii,** 882–885.

7 Cox, T. M. & Peters, T. J. (1978) Uptake of iron by duodenal biopsy specimens from patients with iron-deficiency anaemia and primary haemochromatosis. *Lancet,* **i,** 123–124.

8 Crosby, W. H., Conrad, M. E. & Wheby, M. S. (1963) The rate of iron accumulation in iron storage disease. *Blood,* **22,** 429–440.

9 Edwards, C. Q., Dadone, M. M., Skolnick, M. H. & Kushner, J. P. (1982) Hereditary haemochromatosis. *Clinics in Haematology,* **11,** 411–435.

10 Erlandsen, M. E., Walden, B., Stern, G. *et al.* (1962) Studies on congenital haemolytic syndromes. IV. Gastrointestinal absorption of iron. *Blood,* **19,** 359–378.

11 Ley, T. J., Griffith, P. & Nienhuis, A. W. (1982) Transfusion haemosiderosis and chelation therapy. *Clinics in Haematology,* **11,** 437–464.

12 Pippard, M. J., Callender, S. T. & Weatherall, D. J. (1978) Intensive iron-chelation therapy with desferrioxamine in iron-loading anaemias. *Clinical Science and Molecular Medicine,* **54,** 99–106.

13 Pippard, M. J., Callender, S. T., Warner, G. T. & Weatherall, D. J. (1979) Iron absorption and loading in beta-thalassaemia intermedia. *Lancet,* **ii,** 819–821.

14 Seymour, C. A. & Peters, T. J. (1978) Organelle pathology in primary and secondary haemochromatosis with special reference to lysosomal changes. *British Journal of Haematology,* **40,** 239–253.

15 Simon, M., Bourel, M., Genetet, B. & Fauchet, R. (1977a) Idiopathic haemochromatosis. Demonstration of recessive transmission and early detection by family HLA typing. *New England Journal of Medicine,* **297,** 1017–1021.

16 Simon, M., Bourel, M., Genetet, B. *et al.* (1977b) Idiopathic haemochromatosis and iron overload in alcoholic liver disease: differentiation by HLA phenotype. *Gastroenterology,* **73,** 655–658.

17 Williams, R., Manenti, F., Williams, H. S. & Pitcher, C. S. (1966) Iron absorption in idiopathic haemochromatosis before, during and after venesection therapy. *British Medical Journal,* **ii,** 78–81.

INTERNAL PARANEOPLASTIC SYNDROMES ASSOCIATED WITH CANCER

Paraneoplastic syndromes are non-metastatic peripheral manifestations of malignancy. Their recognition is important since they are common modes of presentation of undiagnosed malignancies; they may cause significant symptoms in patients with gut cancer and disability out of proportion to the mass of tumour present; their control may improve the quality of life of the patient.[12]

The gastrointestinal tumours associated with these syndromes are shown in Table 9.9.[14] In this short section emphasis has been placed on the postulated mechanisms for the development of these disorders rather than their clinical presentations. The systemic effects of malignancy will not be discussed; the manifestations of 'classical' gut endocrine tumours, and genetic and acquired dermatological syndromes associated with gut cancer are discussed in Chapter 8.

Endocrine and metabolic syndromes

HYPERCALCAEMIA

The mechanisms of production of tumour-hypercalcaemia are still uncertain. Hypercalcaemia is present in 10% of patients with osteolytic secondaries; bone lysis may be due to

Table 9.9 Internal paraneoplastic syndromes and site of gastrointestinal tumour.

Syndromes	Adenocarcinoma						Squamous cell carcinoma – oesophagus	Hepatoma	Carcinoid	Other tumours
	St	SI	Colon	Pancreas	CBD	GB				
Endocrine/Metabolic										
Hypercalcaemia	+		+	+	+	+	+	+	+	Sarcomas, pancreatic islet tumours
Hypoglycaemia			+	+	+			+	+	Mesenchymal and β cell rest tumours
Ectopic ACTH			+	+	+	+	+	+	+	Pancreatic islet tumours
Inappropriate ADH		+		+			+			Gastric myosarcoma
Glycopeptides	+		+	+				+		Pancreatic islet tumour
Porphyria cutanea tarda			+					+		Gastric choriocarcinoma
Hyperlipidaemia								+		Hepatic adenoma and secondaries
Haematological and Cardiovascular										
MAHA	+		+	+				+		
Polycythaemia	+							+		
Leucocytosis	+							+		
Eosinophilia	+		+	+	+			+		
DIC	+		+	+	+					
Thromboembolism	+		+	+		+				
NBTE	+		+	+	+					
Renal										
Renal failure	+		+	+	+	+	+			
Nephrotic syndrome and glomerulo nephritis			+	+		+	+			
Renal tubular dysfunction			+	+		+		+		Histiocytic malignancy of small intestine
Neurological										
CNS	+		+	+						
PNS	+		+	+						
Muscle	+		+	+						
Rheumatic										
Arthritis	+		+	+						
PSS			+				+			

698

destruction by the tumour deposits or by prostaglandins released from tumour cells or monocytes around the deposits. A parathormone (PTH)-like material is produced by some tumours but this humoral agent has not been unequivocally established as the cause of hypercalcaemia.[20] Current radioimmunoassays for PTH may be detecting non-bioactive peptides produced by the tumour. Other bone-resolving factors have been identified in tumour dialysates and these include: osteoclastic activating factors associated with lymphomas; and prostaglandins (e.g. PGE_1, PGE_2) which stimulate lysis in animal tumour models, resorption of bone in vitro, and conversion of 1α-hydroxycholecalciferol to the more active 1,25-dihydroxycholecalciferol.

HYPOGLYCAEMIA

Various non-islet cell tumours may cause hypoglycaemia,[10] and numerous mechanisms have been postulated. The evidence for insulin production by non-islet tumours is weak, except for some carcinoid tumours. Stimulation of pancreatic insulin secretion is unlikely because plasma levels are normal and hypoglycaemia is not influenced by pancreatectomy. About 90% of the hypoglycaemic effect of plasma from patients with tumours is due to non-suppressible insulin-like activity (NSILA)[17] which consists of four peptides and several larger proteins. Increased levels of both smaller and larger peptide components of NSILA have been detected with non-islet tumour hypoglycaemia but require further evaluation.[11] Inhibition of hepatic glycogenolysis would explain the development of hypoglycaemia 2–10 months prior to death in patients with hepatoma, despite histological evidence of adequate glycogen stores. The evidence for other mechanisms such as inadequate gluconeogenesis, hepatic destruction and inadequate ACTH and glucagon secretion, is unconvincing.

ECTOPIC ACTH SYNDROME

The biological and immunological activities of tumour ACTH may be different from pituitary ACTH. Tumours that secrete ACTH may also secrete related peptides, such as β-lipotrophin, α- and γ-melanocyte stimulating hormone, and corticotrophin-like intermediate lobe peptide (CLIP), since all these peptides are transcribed from a single area on one chromosome.[15] However, other peptides that are not derived from this common precursor may also be secreted. For example, bronchial tumours may secrete calcitonin, gastrin, ADH and gonadotrophins.

INAPPROPRIATE ANTIDIURETIC HORMONE (ADH) SYNDROME

Tumour ADH appears to be similar to the pituitary hormone in its chemical properties and activity.[3] Other related peptides may also be produced by tumours and these include haemophysins and oxytocin. Antitumour therapy may result in disappearance of this syndrome.

GLYCOPEPTIDE HORMONES

Human chorionic gonadotrophin (HCG) and its component α or β (bioactive) chains are present in the plasma of 7–35% of patients with a variety of gut and islet cell tumours. Many tumours contain HCG-like immunoreactive material. However, this is often the asialo biologically-inactive form, and clinical features of circulating tumour HCG are rare, except with hepatomas and occasional gastric carcinomas.[5] The latter tumours may also convert oestrogen precursors to the active hormone. Hepatocellular cancer may cause gynaecomastia and sexual precocity in boys, apparently due to circulating HCG. Urinary 17-ketosterol and testosterone levels are elevated and not suppressed by dexamethasone.

Porphyria cutanea tarda (PCT)

Excessive porphyrin content of hepatocellular cancer (HCC) cells and excretion in urine and faeces is thought to be the mechanism of this metabolic disorder[22] and its development may be a marker of malignant transformation of cirrhosis since human HCC is commoner in cirrhotic patients with PCT than in alcoholic, macronodular or haemochromatotic cirrhosis.

Hyperlipidaemia

Markedly elevated cholesterol and triglyceride levels are rare in cases of HCC in the Western world whereas mild hypercholesterolaemia was present in 30% of Ugandan patients with HCC.[1] A defect in regulation of cholesterol synthesis appears to be the mechanism in animal HCC models and in studies of a single human HCC cell line in vitro.

Other metabolic and endocrine syndromes

Cystathioninuria (with or without hemi-hypertrophy) and osteoporosis occur in association with hepatoblastomas; some gut tumours also secrete other biologically-inactive peptides such as calcitonin immunoreactivity produced by gastric and pancreatic carcinoma, and hepatoma. Renin secretion is described below.

Haematological and vascular syndromes

ANAEMIA

Gastrointestinal tumours often cause anaemia due to blood loss, poor nutrition, bone marrow involvement or cytotoxic marrow suppression. Two other varieties of anaemia occur.

The anaemia of 'chronic disorders' is due to impaired re-use of iron, shortened red cell survival (due to an extracorpuscular defect and reticuloendothelial hyperplasia in response to tumour metabolites) and reduced erythropoietin responsiveness.

Microangiopathic haemolytic anaemia (MAHA) is usually due to primary haematological disease or renal failure; if these are excluded an internal malignancy is most likely. The association is particularly with mucin secreting adenocarcinomas and up to 50% of patients with MAHA have evidence of disseminated intravascular coagulation (DIC), the haemolysis resulting from shearing of erythrocytes on intraluminal fibrin strands. An alternative shearing effect may be caused by intraluminal embolic tumour cells or by changes in the pulmonary microvasculature reported with various gut tumours.[2]

POLYCYTHAEMIA

Polycythaemia occurs in men who develop HCC and may serve as a marker of neoplastic transformation in the presence of pre-existing cirrhosis. It is probably due to erythropoietin production by the tumour although positive assays are not invariable.[13] Prostaglandins produced by the tumour may enhance the effects of endogenous renal erythropoietin. Tumour production of an erythropoietin precursor has also been described. Failure to inactivate erythropoietin due to deposits in liver is unlikely to be important in view of simultaneous preservation of other hepatic functions.

LEUCOCYTOSIS

The mechanism of leucocytosis and leukaemoid reactions appears to be marrow 'irritation' by necrotic deposits or a granulopoietic factor. Eosinophilia may accompany disseminated malignancy, including carcinomas of colon, pancreas, biliary tree and stomach.

ABNORMAL PLATELET COUNT

Thrombocytopenia is the commonest cause of bleeding in cancer patients. It is usually due to marrow replacement but may also result from intrasplenic sequestration or consumption due to DIC (see below). Thrombocytosis may accompany any tumour and may contribute to a prothrombotic state.

COAGULOPATHY

A prothrombotic state occurs in patients with various cancers and is manifest in shortened blood clotting times (e.g. partial thromboplastin time and prothrombin time), elevated levels of clotting factors or fibrin degradation products and reduced anti-thrombin III levels. The most consistent defect is increased platelet and/or fibrinogen turnover.

Disseminated intravascular coagulation (DIC) is characterized by widespread deposition of altered fibrinogen and/or platelets in the microcirculation and a variable degree of activation of the fibrinolytic system. The relative activation of these two systems depends on the type of tumour and determines the clinical manifestations of the coagulopathy. Gut tumours are the commonest malignancies associated with chronic DIC, which is the mechanism responsible for a spectrum of cardiovascular and haematological complications of malignant disease, including MAHA, venous thrombosis, non-bacterial thrombotic endocarditis and arterial thromboembolism.[19]

The mechanisms responsible for the prothrombotic state include:
1 activation of the intrinsic pathway of coagulation by the abnormal vascular endothelial lining or infection;
2 activation of the extrinsic pathway by thromboplastins liberated after tumour destruction of normal tissue;
3 platelet tumour aggregation by cells; and
4 production of procoagulant factors (such as cancer procoagulant A, mucus glycoprotein and trypsin) which may activate an 'alternative' cellular pathway in coagulation distinct from the intrinsic and extrinsic pathways.[9]

Vascular thromboembolism. Thromboembolic complications are associated particularly with mucus secreting gastrointestinal and pancreatic adenocarcinomas and are often the cause of death in these patients.[19] The association between venous thrombosis and malignancy is rarer than commonly thought (4% in one large series) if all cases of thrombosis are considered, but migratory or multiple venous thromboses warrant a search for internal malignancy (with gut primaries accounting for about half the patients). Arterial emboli occurred in 25% of patients with chronic DIC and are usually associated with disseminated malignancy (the commonest primary being pancreatic carcinoma).[19]

VALVULAR HEART DISEASE

Carcinoid heart disease is described in Chapter 8. Non-bacterial thrombotic endocarditis (usually of the mitral and aortic valves) is associated with disseminated (usually mucus-secreting) gastrointestinal tumours, and may lead to embolization of the friable vegetations. An underlying chronic DIC is almost invariable.[19]

HYPERTENSION

There has been one report of adenocarcinoma of the pancreas producing active and inactive renin and causing hypertension. The levels of inactive renin in plasma are not seen in non-neoplastic conditions and may prove to be a useful marker of renin secreting tumours.[18]

Renal syndromes

Renal failure. Gastrointestinal tumours may be complicated by renal failure due to hypercalcaemia, renal vein thrombosis, or chronic DIC producing renal cortical necrosis. Rarely, renal tubular obstruction occurs due to formation of viscous casts of mucoproteins that are produced by pancreatic carcinoma.

Nephrotic syndromes and glomerulonephritis. Renal vein thrombosis causing nephrotic syndrome, may accompany cancer-associated coagulopathy or reactive systemic amyloidosis. The latter occurs rarely with carcinoma of the stomach, colon and gallbladder; the chemical nature of amyloid in these patients has not been studied, but in amyloidosis associated with Hodgkin's lymphoma and hypernephroma, the fibril protein is amyloid A protein.

Membranous glomerulonephritis is associated with various gut malignancies. The nephrotic syndrome due to such a glomerulonephritis associated with gastric carcinoma disappeared after resection of the tumour;[6] in two cases of colonic carcinoma[7, 8] the complexes deposited on the glomerular basement membrane contained tumour-specific antigens (one of which was carcinoembryonic antigen).[8] Though circulating immune complexes are reported in patients with various cancers, nephritis due to their deposition is not well established and this may be due to the size and solubility of the complexes associated with tumours.

Rarely, chronic DIC associated with colonic cancer may cause a glomerular microangiopathy resulting in the nephrotic syndrome.

Renal tubular dysfunction. Renal tubular acidosis has been reported with disseminated pancreatic carcinoma and hypokalaemia-induced renal tubular damage may occur with villous colonic tumours or the ectopic ACTH syndrome usually with carcinoid tumours.

Neurological syndromes

Central nervous system. Several of the metabolic abnormalities described above may lead to confusion, dementia and seizures. Cerebellar degeneration has been reported with gastric, pancreatic and colonic carcinomas. A necrotizing myelopathy has been described in at least six patients with gastric cancer, although the paraneoplastic nature is convincing in only one case.[16] Encephalomyelitis (with gastric carcinoma) and encephalomyeloradiculopathy (with histiocytic malignancies of the small intestine complicating coeliac disease) are rarer associations.

Peripheral nervous system. A mixed sensorimotor peripheral neuropathy is the commonest paraneoplastic neurological syndrome and occurs with gastric, colonic and pancreatic carcinoma. Characteristically it affects the longest peripheral nerves with variable degeneration of axons and myelin sheaths. A purely sensory neuropathy has been reported with a caecal carcinoma. A myasthenic syndrome has been associated with single cases of pancreatic and rectal cancers, although documentation in these reports is poor.

Muscle disorders. There appears to be a true association between polymyositis and dermatomyositis and internal malignancy, although the frequency of this association is disputed. Some cases (8.5%) with this muscle disorder have internal malignancies; in patients over 50 years of age, the incidence is 18%.[4] Gastric carcinoma is the commonest associated primary neoplasm (17% in one series).[23] Apart from an older age at presentation, and a dramatic initial remission after surgical excision of the tumour, the group of patients with tumour-associated polymyositis do not differ from the rest of the patients with the muscle disorder.[4]

Rheumatic syndromes

Arthritis. Carcinomatous arthritis may be the presenting manifestation of malignancies of the colon, liver and pancreas; the arthritis may resolve with treatment of the malignancy and relapse may occur with tumour recurrence. Pancreatic adenocarcinoma (usually of the acinous variety) may cause an arthropathy associated with skin fat necrosis. The monoarticular or polyarticular lesions are caused by periarticular fat necrosis induced by circulating pancreatic enzymes such as lipase, colipase, trypsin and possibly amylase.

Secondary gout may result from the effects of cytotoxic chemotherapy on gut malignancies.

OTHER RHEUMATIC SYNDROMES

Skin sclerosis may occur in the carcinoid syndrome (see Chapter 8). There is an association between progressive systemic sclerosis and tumours of the rectum, oesophagus and skin;[21] the gut tumours usually developed at sites that were involved before the malignancy became evident, suggesting that gut scleroderma may predispose to malignancy.

Other syndromes such as relapsing polychondritis with pancreatic carcinoma and a systemic lupus-like syndrome with gastric carcinoma may be chance associations.

REFERENCES

1 Alpert, M. E., Hutt, M. S. R. & Davidson, C. S. (1969) Primary hepatoma in Uganda. A prospective clinical and epidemiological study of forty six patients. *American Journal of Medicine*, **46**, 794–802.
2 Antman, K. H., Skarin, A. T., Mayer, R. J. *et al.* (1979) Microangiopathic haemolytic anaemia and cancer: a review. *Medicine (Baltimore)*, **58**, 377–384.
3 Bartter, F. C. (1973) The syndrome of inappropriate secretion of antidiuretic hormone. In *Endocrine and Non-Endocrine Hormone-Producing Tumours.* Chicago: Yearbook Medical Publishers.
4 Bohan, A., Peter, J. B., Bowman, R. L. & Pearson, C. M. (1977) A computer-assisted analysis of 153 patients with polymyositis and dermatomyositis. *Medicine (Baltimore)*, **56**, 253–286.
5 Braunstein, G. D., Vaitukaitis, J. L., Carbone, P. P. & Ross, G. T. (1973) Ectopic production of human chorionic gonadotrophin by neoplasms. *Annals of Internal Medicine*, **78**, 39–45.
6 Cantrell, E. G. (1969) Nephrotic syndromes cured by removal of gastric carcinoma. *British Medical Journal*, **ii**, 739–740.
7 Costanza, M. E., Pinn, V., Schwartz, R. S. & Nathanson, L. (1973) Carcinoembryonic antigen – antibody complexes in a patient with colonic carcinoma and nephrotic syndrome. *New England Journal of Medicine*, **289**, 520–523.
8 Couser, W. G., Wagonfeld, J. B., Spargo, B. H. & Lewis, E. J. (1974) Glomerular deposition of tumour antigen in membranous nephropathy associated with colonic carcinoma. *American Journal of Medicine*, **57**, 962–970.
9 Donati, M. B., Poggi, A. & Semeraro, N. (1981) Coagulation and malignancy. In *Recent Advances in Coagulation* (Ed.) Poller, L. Volume 3, pp. 227–259. London: Churchill Livingstone.
10 Frerichs, H. & Creutzfeldt, W. (1976) Hypoglycaemia I. Insulin secreting tumours. *Clinics in Endocrinology and Metabolism*, **5**, 747–767.
11 Gorden, P., Hendricks, C. M., Kahn, C. R. *et al.* (1981) Hypoglycemia associated with non-islet cell tumors and insulin-like growth factors. *New England Journal of Medicine*, **305**, 1452.
12 Hall, T. C. (1974) Introductory remarks. In *Paraneoplastic syndromes. Annals of the New York Academy of Sciences*, **230**, 5.
13 Hammond, D. & Winnick, S. (1974) Paraneoplastic erythrocytosis and ectopic erythropoietins. *Annals of the New York Academy of Sciences*, **230**, 219–227.
14 Maton, P. & Camilleri, M. (1983) Paraneoplastic syndromes. In *Gastrointestinal and Hepatobiliary Cancer* (Ed.) Hodgson, H. J. & Bloom, S. R. London: Chapman and Hall. pp. 377–419.
15 Orth, D. N., Guillemin, R., Ling, N. & Nicholson, W. E. (1978) Immunoreactive endorphins, lipotrophins and corticotrophins in a human non-pituitary tumour: evidence for a common precursor. *Journal of Clinical Endocrinology and Metabolism*, **46**, 849–852.
16 Pallis, C. A. & Lewis, P. D. (1974) Non-metastatic effects of gastrointestinal neoplasia in the nervous system and muscle. In *The Neurology of Gastrointestinal Disease. Major Problems in Neurology.* Volume 3, pp. 215–226. London: W. B. Saunders.
17 Poffenbarger, P. L. (1975) The purification and partial characterisation of an insulin-like protein from human serum. *Journal of Clinical Investigation*, **56**, 1455–1463.
18 Ruddy, M. C., Atlas, S. A. & Salerno, F. G. (1982) Hypertension associated with a renin-secreting adenocarcinoma of the pancreas. *New England Journal of Medicine*, **307**, 993–997.
19 Sack, G., Levin, J. & Bell, W. (1977) Trousseau's syndrome and other manifestations of chronic disseminated coagulopathy in patients with neoplasms. *Medicine (Baltimore)*, **56**, 1–37.
20 Skrabanek, P., McParthen, J. & Powell, D. (1980) Tumour hypercalcemia and 'ectopic hyperparathyroidism'. *Medicine (Baltimore)*, **59**, 262–282.
21 Talbott, J. A. & Barrocas, M. (1979) Progressive systemic sclerosis (PSS) and malignancy, pulmonary and non-pulmonary. *Medicine (Baltimore)*, **58**, 182–207.

22 Thompson, R. P. H., Nicholson, D. C., Farnan, T. *et al.* (1970) Cutaneous porphyria due to a malignant primary hepatoma. *Gastroenterology,* **59,** 779–783.

23 Williams, R. C. (1959) Dermatomyositis and malignancy: a review of the literature. *Annals of Internal Medicine,* **50,** 1174–1181.

GRAFT-VERSUS-HOST DISEASE

Following bone marrow transplantation for aplastic anaemia or leukaemia, recipients receive immunosuppressive drugs to prevent rejection of the graft. In such patients immunocompetent cells, particularly lymphocytes given in the graft, may react against the host giving rise to graft-versus-host disease (GVHD). This disease remains a major obstacle to the successful use of bone marrow transplantation.[12] Although the skin is the most commonly involved of the three main target organs, the severity of intestinal and liver involvement determines prognosis.[5] GVHD may be an acute or chronic process differing in time of onset after transplantation and relative degree of target organ involvement.

Acute intestinal GVHD

Acute intestinal GVHD occurs in up to 50% of allogeneic marrow recipients, almost invariably within the first 50 days after transplantation. It presents as watery diarrhoea, often producing several litres daily, usually accompanied by anorexia and cramping lower abdominal pain. The severity of intestinal GVHD is graded on daily stool volumes. The diagnosis is straightforward on clinical grounds in the typical patient; watery diarrhoea (> 500 ml/day) is associated with the red macular rash of skin GVHD and biochemical evidence of liver GVHD. In less typical cases, because of the known potential for chemoradiation and infection to cause diarrhoea post-transplantation, rectal biopsy, radiology and [111]Indium leucocyte scanning have all been used to aid diagnosis. Rectal biopsy is most useful diagnostically in early disease when the changes of individual crypt cell destruction, without widespread inflammation, is specific for acute intestinal GVHD.[2]

In more severe disease, rectal histology may show extensive changes, ranging from crypt abscess to complete epithelial denudation; however, these appearances are less specific as they can be caused by other destructive processes. Postmortem studies have shown that the whole of the gastrointestinal tract may be affected, with the maximum damage in the ileo-caecal region.[8] Although bowel radiology and [111]Indium leucocyte scanning have yet to be prospectively evaluated, both have confirmed extensive intestinal involvement in GVHD, with the severest changes in the ileum.[3] The diarrhoea in intestinal GVHD may reach volumes of up to 12 l/day and has both osmotic and secretory components. Although a variety of abnormalities of intestinal function have been described, including disaccharidase deficiency, fat malabsorption, protein losing enteropathy, rapid intestinal transit and crypt and villous damage, the relative contribution of these mechanisms are uncertain. In some patients there is a profuse secretory diarrhoea but negligible histological changes.

Extensive GVHD is associated with a high mortality, usually from infection. In addition to impaired resistance because of mucosal damage there is loss of immunoglobulins from inflamed bowel and depletion of mucosal IgA and IgM plasma cells, all of which predispose to enterally acquired infections.[1]

Supportive care is central to management, with early institution of total parenteral nutrition, adequate fluid and electrolyte replacement to cover enteral losses and prompt treatment of infections. Specific treatment of GVHD with anti-thymocyte globulin and conventional doses of prednisolone have been disappointing, but recently encouraging results have been reported using high-dose methylprednisolone.[6]

The pathogenesis of GVHD is unknown. Electron microscopic studies provide evidence for a cytotoxic lymphocyte mechanism, demonstrating point contact between lymphocyte and crypt cells which may represent the first stage of mucosal cell damage.[4] Other theories, based mainly on animal studies, suggest that antigenic cross-reactivity between bacterial and intestinal epithelial cells, or interactions between donor and host lymphocytes, are important. Approaches based on these mechanisms to prevent the development of acute GVHD are currently being evaluated. Promising results have been reported using a monoclonal antibody to deplete donor marrow of T cells potentially reactive against host antigens.

Acute hepatic GVHD

Hepatic involvement in acute GVHD presents as jaundice and hepatomegaly.[5] Although ascites may occur in severe disease, encephalopathy is rare. Liver function tests are abnormal, with the level of bilirubin, aspartate transaminase and alkaline phosphatase providing the basis of grading the severity of liver involvement. The clinical diagnosis of hepatic GVHD depends on demonstrating a temporal association of liver dysfunction with gut and skin GVHD. If this association is not present, the diagnosis is problematical because of the large number of potential causes of hepatic dysfunction in this group of patients. These include chemoradiation effects, veno-occlusive disease, viral hepatitis, opportunistic infection and drug toxicity. Needle liver biopsy is of limited diagnostic value because clotting abnormalities often preclude its use and it may miss the histological change of GVHD because of the patchy nature of this lesion.[10] Human and animal postmortem studies demonstrate that bile duct injury is the characteristic histological change of hepatic GVHD. Electron microscopic studies show intimate contacts between lymphocytes and bile duct epithelial cells, supporting a role for cytotoxic lymphocytes in disease pathogenesis. The prognosis of hepatic GVHD is related to severity and extent of other organ involvement. Treatment is similar to intestinal GVHD, but hepatic GVHD appears to respond less well than the gut to high dose methylprednisolone.[6]

Chronic GVHD

Chronic GVHD occurs after day 100 posttransplantation. In contrast to acute GVHD, the oesophagus is the most severely affected part of the gastrointestinal tract. Symptoms of dysphagia and chest pain are due to a desquamative oesophagitis and occasionally webs and strictures.[7] Although malnutrition is common, the cause is decreased calorie intake rather than malabsorption. Small or large bowel involvement has only rarely been documented – in four cases a peculiar extensive submucosal fibrosis was present at post mortem.

Liver involvement, recognized by a high alkaline phosphatase, is common in chronic GVHD but clinically is usually overshadowed by sclerodermatous skin lesions, contractures and a sicca-like syndrome.[9] Liver histology characteristically shows bile duct degeneration and destruction similar to primary biliary cirrhosis, but occasionally hepatocellular injury with piecemeal necrosis is present.

Oesophageal and liver involvement in chronic GVHD, in association with extensive skin disease, has a high mortality untreated but responds well to steroids in combination with azathioprine.[11] Isolated liver involvement, or with only localized skin disease, is nonprogressive and requires no treatment.

REFERENCES

1 Beschorner, W. E., Yardley, J. H., Tutschka, P. J. & Santos, G. W. (1981) Deficiency of intestinal immunity with graft vs host disease in humans. *Journal of Infectious Diseases*, **144**, 38–46.
2 Epstein, R. J., McDonald, G. B., Sale, G. E. *et al.* (1980) The diagnostic accuracy of the rectal biopsy in acute graft-versus-host disease: a prospective study of thirteen patients. *Gastroenterology*, **78**, 764–771.
3 Fisk, J. D., Shulman, H. M., Greening, R. R. *et al.* (1981) Gastrointestinal radiographic features of human graft-versus-host disease. *American Journal of Roentgenology*, **136**, 329–336.
4 Gallucci, B. B., Epstein, R., Sale, G. E. *et al.* (1982) The fine structure of human rectal epithelium in acute graft-versus-host disease. *American Journal of Surgical Pathology*, **6**, 293–305.
5 Glucksberg, H., Storb, R., Fefer, A. *et al.* (1974) Clinical manifestations of graft-versus-host disease in human recipients of marrow in HLA matched sibling donors. *Transplantation*, **18**, 295–304.
6 Kendra, J., Barrett, A. J., Lucas, C. *et al.* (1981) Response of graft-versus-host disease to high doses of methylprednisolone. *Clinical and Laboratory Haematology*, **3**, 19–26.
7 McDonald, G. B., Sullivan, K. M., Schuffler, M. D. *et al.* (1981) Oesophageal abnormalities in chronic graft-versus-host disease in humans. *Gastroenterology*, **80**, 914–921.
8 Sale, G. E., Shulman, H. M., McDonald, G. B. & Thomas, E. D. (1979) Gastrointestinal graft-versus-host disease in man: a clinicopathological study of the rectal biopsy. *American Journal of Surgical Pathology*, **3**, 291–299.
9 Shulman, H. M., Sullivan, K. M., Weiden, P. L. *et al.* (1980) Chronic graft-versus-host syndrome in man: a clinicopathological study of 20 long-term Seattle patients. *American Journal of Medicine*, **69**, 204–217.
10 Sloane, J. P., Farthing, M. J. G. & Powles, R. L. (1980) Histopathological changes in the liver after allogeneic bone marrow transplantation. *Journal of Clinical Pathology*, **33**, 344–350.
11 Sullivan, K. M., Shulman, H. M., Storb, R. *et al.* (1981) Chronic graft-versus-host disease in 52 patients: adverse natural course and successful treatment with combination immunosuppression. *Blood*, **57**, 267–276.
12 Thomas, E. D., Storb, R., Clift, R. *et al.* (1975) Bone marrow transplantation. *New England Journal of Medicine*, **292**, 832–843, 895–902.

SYSTEMIC ENDOCRINE DISORDERS

DIABETES MELLITUS

Patients with long-standing diabetes mellitus may have considerable derangement of gastrointestinal function which can lead to severe and intractable symptoms. Problems are usually seen in insulin-dependent diabetics, but are not unknown among those who do not require insulin. The mechanisms leading to these abnormalities are uncertain but suggested causes include autonomic neuropathy, micro-angiopathy, hyperglycaemia, electrolyte abnormalities and abnormalities in blood levels or release of insulin, glucagon or other hormones such as GIP or motilin. Acute diabetic ketoacidosis can also be associated with largely unexplained gastrointestinal problems.

Abdominal problems of diabetic ketoacidosis

Anorexia, nausea and vomiting occur in up to 75% of patients with ketoacidosis. Nasogastric aspiration is often recommended on the grounds that these symptoms reflect gastric stasis, but gastric emptying has never been properly studied during ketoacidosis. Acute gastric dilatation may occur but its frequency is unknown. During nasogastric aspiration, small amounts of blood are commonly seen, although frank haematemesis is rare. Bleeding usually results from acute erosions or acute haemorrhagic gastritis; endoscopy is not routinely necessary unless bleeding is severe or persists after correction of the metabolic derangements. The aetiology of the gastritis is unknown, but retention of acid or urea has been blamed.[15]

Severe abdominal pain, caused by ketoacidosis, occurs in about 8% of patients and is more common in diabetic children than in adults. It seems to be related to acidosis and settles with its correction. It may be severe enough to suggest an acute abdomen and differentiation may be difficult, especially as ketoacidosis is often associated with neutrophilia and hyperamylasaemia. Thus acute pancreatitis may either be missed, or incorrectly assumed to be present. A diabetic with ketoacidosis and abdominal pain should have the metabolic disorder treated and his abdomen closely observed, provided no obvious intra-abdominal catastrophe, such as perforation, has occurred. Early exploratory laparotomy without definite indications should be steadfastly avoided. Identification of isoamylases in diabetic ketoacidosis shows that in fact the elevated amylase is usually of the salivary type, rather than the pancreatic type associated with pancreatitis.[43]

Oesophagus in diabetes

Oesophageal abnormalities are not prominent in diabetes, but abnormal motility has been shown on cineradiography or manometry, usually in the absence of oesophageal symptoms.[19, 30] The amplitude of pharyngeal contractions may be diminished, primary oesophageal peristalsis may be decreased, infrequent or absent, and oesophageal emptying and relaxation of the lower sphincter may be delayed. A few patients have oesophageal dilatation while in others, tertiary spastic contractions are frequent. Rarely the appearance of the oesophagus may be similar to that in diffuse spasm.[19] Studies of resting lower oesophageal sphincter pressures are contradictory.[19, 39]

The prevalence of these abnormalities is unknown but they have been found in randomly selected insulin-dependent diabetics. There is no correlation between oesophageal dysfunction and symptoms, age of the patient or length of diabetic history. Most patients with oesophageal motor abnormalities are asymptomatic but some may have symptoms of gastro-oesophageal reflux. Dysphagia is very rare. If symptoms occur in a diabetic, other oesophageal disease should be excluded (see also Chapter 2).

The aetiology of these motility abnormalities is not certain but there is a strong association with the presence of neuropathy.[19, 39] Vagal damage and demyelination occur in diabetics with neuropathy and degeneration of the preganglionic parasympathetic fibres has been shown in the oesophagus of diabetics without oesophageal symptoms or neuropathy.[38] The exaggerated response to cholinergic drugs seen in achalasia or Chagas' disease does not occur and the few patients with symptoms may be helped by these as well as by the standard measures for gastro-oesophageal reflux. Bethanechol has been shown to improve oesophageal emptying and raise lower oesophageal sphincter pressure in diabetics.[39]

Oesophageal candidiasis is seen in poorly controlled diabetics or in diabetics with chronic renal failure. It may present with dysphagia or odynophagia and is readily diagnosed by barium swallow and endoscopy (see Chapter 2).

Gastric secretion, achlorhydria and chronic gastritis

In most diabetics basal acid output and maximal acid output in response to histamine or pentagastrin is normal, even in those with neuropathy.[12, 20] Similarly, food-stimulated acid secretion is normal.[12] However, gastric acid secretion is impaired in response to hypoglycaemia in long standing insulin-dependent diabetics most of whom will have evidence of neuropathy.[20] This suggests vagal dysfunction which is supported by impaired acid secretion to sham feeding.[12]

Most workers have found some diabetic patients with reduced or absent basal and stimulated acid secretion. Early workers found achlorhydria in 17–39% of patients studied. These figures are probably excessive but nevertheless achlorhydria is often found; Hosking *et al.*[20] found it in 2 out of eighteen diabetics studied. As in non-diabetic patients, achlorhydria is associated with the development of chronic atrophic gastritis[1] and it is widely believed that diabetics develop atrophic gastritis at a younger age than do normals.[24] The cause is unknown but may be immunological and related to the development of gastric antibodies, although it has also been suggested that diabetic microangiopathy could be responsible.[1] There is an increased incidence of gastric parietal cell and intrinsic factor antibodies in diabetics. The increase in parietal cell antibodies is most marked in young insulin-dependent diabetics but the increase in intrinsic factor antibodies is most striking in insulin-dependent females over the age of 40 years, 4% of whom have the antibody in their serum.[21] There is no relationship between neuropathy and the presence of antibodies, atrophic gastritis or achlorhydria. In spite of the known malignant potential of atrophic gastritis, diabetics do not appear to have an increased incidence of gastric carcinoma.

Pernicious anaemia and diabetes mellitus

A significant association between diabetes and pernicious anaemia seems to exist; the estimated incidence of pernicious anaemia among diabetics is 0.98% and of diabetes in pernicious anaemia is 2.1%. Latent cases of pernicious anaemia are often found; for example, six cases among nine diabetics with intrinsic factor antibodies and atrophic gastritis.[21]

Peptic ulcer and diabetes mellitus

The incidence of duodenal ulcer is reported to be reduced among diabetics.[11, 45] The data on which this conclusion is based are suspect and were collected before diagnosis by fibre-optic endoscopy. The view may be correct, especially as atrophic gastritis and achlorhydria may occur in diabetics, but it is unproven. In contrast, it is said that the incidence of gastric ulcer in diabetics is normal[11] but this is also unproven, as is the view that duodenal ulcer complications are more frequent and more severe in diabetics.[45]

Diabetic gastroparesis

In diabetics, gastroparesis barium studies show an atonic stomach with delayed emptying and few peristaltic waves.[23] Pyloric obstruction is excluded by the patulous appearance of the pylorus and by expression of barium into the duodenum manually. Retained gastric secretions may give the appearance of filling defects and duodenal dilatation may be seen.[46] Gastric motility studies in gastroparesis show abnormal interdigestive motor cycles, a marked decrease in sporadic motor activity[27] and, in particular, severely abnormal motor activity and diminished peristalsis in the antrum.[13]

Diabetic gastroparesis is a feature of severe insulin-dependent diabetes of longstanding in either sex and is usually seen in patients with evidence of neuropathy.[46] Patients may be asymptomatic and therefore the estimated incidence of 1 in 1000 diabetics[46] may be an underestimate. If symptomatic, patients present with unexplained weight loss, anorexia, vague epigastric or generalized abdominal pain and discomfort, nausea, epigastric bloating or fullness, or even halitosis. More severe cases may have severe or intractible vomiting. Vomit may contain food eaten more than 24 hours previously and bezoar formation is not uncommon. The clinical picture may mimic pyloric obstruction but a succussion splash does not often occur.[46] In most cases diabetic control has been poor in the past and good control is often difficult to achieve; indeed this may be the presenting complaint. A few cases may be complicated by gastric candidiasis or bacterial overgrowth.

Diagnosis of gastroparesis is usually made on a barium meal and the radiological appearances are strikingly similar to those of the vagotomized stomach, supporting the aetiological role of neuropathy. The stomach is normal endoscopically.[27] Treatment is unsatisfactory. Some improve symptomatically with good diabetic control and small, regular and frequent meals. Metoclopramide and bethanechol increase gastric motor activity and metoclopramide promotes gastric emptying.[5, 27] Most clinical reports are anecdotal but cholinergics (e.g. bethanechol or neostigmine), metoclopramide and domperidone have improved symptoms. Surgical procedures, such as pyloroplasty and partial gastrectomy, have not been helpful. Prognosis is poor; of 35 cases reported by Zitomer *et al.*[46] 12 died within three years of the diagnosis of gastroparesis. However, the deaths were due to vascular and renal complications of diabetes indicating that gastroparesis develops when diabetic complications are far advanced. Lesser degrees of gastric motor abnormalities have been reported in as many as 20–30% of diabetics, but this may be an overestimate; the results of recent studies have been discordant.[5, 35]

Constipation in diabetics

Constipation among diabetics is common. More diabetics (16%) reported constipation than normal controls (5%).[31] In one series of diabetics with neuropathy, 42% complained of constipation and 51% of these had severe constipation requiring regular enemas to prevent impaction.[34] Constipation, therefore, can be severe and disabling, can lead to symptoms mimicking large bowel obstruction and can cause stercoral ulceration. Radiological studies may reveal an atonic and often greatly dilated colon. Massive faecal retention with impaction may be seen. Diabetic microangiopathy has been demonstrated in rectal biopsies from severe diabetics but there is no evidence to link this directly with colonic motor abnormalities. Constipation is probably a further manifestation of autonomic neuropathy.[15, 31] Neostigmine or metoclopramide increase colonic motility in constipated diabetics, suggesting damage to the preganglionic nerve supply to otherwise normal colonic muscle and a possible therapy in difficult cases.[3] Domperidone has improved colonic motility and relieved symptoms in one badly constipated patient.

Diabetic diarrhoea

Diarrhoea is a relatively common complaint among diabetics; 7% of diabetics complained of it compared to 2% of non-diabetic controls.[31] True 'diabetic diarrhoea' is much less common, however; it describes the severe and occasionally disabling diarrhoea which is seen in severe diabetics and for which no cause is apparent apart from the diabetes itself. Diabetic diarrhoea occurs in adults at any age but is commonest in middle age and among men. It is typically seen in insulin-dependent diabetics of long standing. Poor control before the onset of diarrhoea is common. Rare cases of acute onset diabetes with diarrhoea have been recorded. At presentation, about 75% of patients have evidence of neuropathy, especially autonomic neuropathy, and 33% have retinopathy.[28] Diarrhoea is described in up to 20% of diabetics with neuropathy.[34]

Diarrhoea may be persistent or intermittent and may alternate with episodes of constipation. The stool is often watery, large in volume, and may contain undigested food. The diarrhoea may be explosive and incontinence may occur. Nocturnal diarrhoea is characteristic and in one series 50% of patients only had diarrhoea at night.[28] Attacks of diarrhoea may be preceded by abdominal distension, discomfort and rumbling but pain is rare. There is usually no obvious precipitating factor and attacks can last from several hours to months or even years. Diarrhoea persists in a few patients but in most cases, there is a tendency to spontaneous improvement over the years. Apart from the diarrhoea, patients are usually reasonably well.

Gastroparesis is seen in up to 30% of these patients and on barium follow-through intestinal transit may be normal, rapid or delayed. In most cases, the mucosal pattern is normal. Most diabetics with diarrhoea have no evidence of malabsorption, with normal faecal fat excretion, pancreatic function, serum vitamin B_{12}, iron and folate, and xylose absorption; however steatorrhoea does occur in perhaps one-third of patients with diabetic diarrhoea.[44] In these individuals, barium examination may show a nonspecific malabsorption pattern. Other causes of steatorrhoea (see below) must be excluded before ascribing it to diabetic diarrhoea. Patients with diabetic diarrhoea have normal jejunal biopsies whether or not they have steatorrhoea.[29]

AETIOLOGY OF DIABETIC DIARRHOEA

The most widely held view, that diabetic diarrhoea and steatorrhoea result from motility disturbances caused by autonomic neuropathy, is based on the frequent association of diarrhoea and neuropathy. Jejunal distension in patients with diabetic diarrhoea does not induce pain, suggesting afferent sympathetic nerve damage.[44] The small intestine responds normally to methacholine suggesting intact parasympathetic and efferent sympathetic pathways.[32, 44] An early autopsy study showed no evidence of autonomic nerve damage[4] but a more recent study showed giant sympathetic neurones and dendritic swelling of postganglionic neurones in the prevertebral and paravertebral ganglia of 3 patients with diabetic diarrhoea.[18] It has been suggested that glucagon might play a part in the small intestinal motor abnormalities of these patients.[15] Colonic motor abnormalities have also been described.

Other possible aetiological factors are bacterial overgrowth in the small intestine and bile salt malabsorption. Indirect evidence for the role of small intestinal bacterial overgrowth is provided by the relief of symptoms with antibiotics in some patients; for example, Malins and French[28] found that 16 out of 22 patients responded to chlortetracycline. The prevalence of bacterial overgrowth in diabetics with diarrhoea is unknown. Objective evidence for bacterial overgrowth has been gained from jejunal juice colony count,[14] ^{14}C-glycocholate breath test[36] and glucose hydrogen breath test.[9] However, Whalen, Soergel and Greenen found no evidence of overgrowth in 13 patients.[44] Reports of the relief of diabetic diarrhoea with cholestyramine have suggested that the diarrhoea might be caused by bile salt malabsorption. Some diabetics with diarrhoea have faecal bile acid loss and a small bile salt pool.[33]

There is no evidence that true diabetic diarrhoea is caused by pancreatic insufficiency since pancreatic function tests are normal in these patients even if they have steatorrhoea[44] and there is no response to pancreatic supplements. Early workers found flat jejunal biopsies in some patients with 'diabetic diarrhoea' but it is now realized that these patients had coexistent coeliac disease (see below). Sugar permeability studies have suggested that the small intestinal surface area may be reduced,[9] but jejunal sodium and water absorption is normal.[44]

STEATORRHOEA IN DIABETICS

Before concluding that steatorrhoea is caused by diabetic diarrhoea, other causes should be excluded, particularly pancreatic insufficiency and coeliac disease. It is now clear that coeliac disease and diabetes mellitus frequently coexist.[42] Both disorders are associated with the HLA-B8 haplotype. Crude figures suggest that coeliac disease is no more common in diabetics than in non-diabetics but that diabetes is three times more common among coeliacs than in the general population.[42] Clinical clues to coexisting coeliac disease are a family history of coeliac disease, frequent swings from hypo- to hyperglycaemia on small doses of insulin, a childhood history of diarrhoea, anaemia or failure to thrive, unexplained diarrhoea or anaemia before the onset of diabetes and features of malabsorption on physical examination. Infertility may be a problem in female coeliacs. Folate deficiency and hypoalbuminaemia are not features of diabetic diarrhoea and should suggest coeliac disease.[42] All diabetics with diarrhoea should have a jejunal biopsy to exclude coexistent coeliac disease but this can be a slow procedure because of the motility disturbances. Treatment with a strict gluten-free diet is usually effective in relieving symptoms and improving diabetic control, although daily insulin requirements usually increase.[42]

DIAGNOSIS AND TREATMENT OF DIABETIC DIARRHOEA

Diagnosis is by exclusion and investigation will include serum iron, vitamin B_{12} and folate, faecal fat excretion, plain abdominal radiography, barium follow-through, jejunal biopsy and pancreatic function tests.

Treatment is empirical and assessment of response to treatment is complicated by the tendency of the diarrhoea to occur in self limiting attacks and to improve with time. Strict diabetic control may help symptoms and should be vigorously applied in every case. Diets containing more or less fibre or carbohydrate have not been helpful. Treatment with constipating agents such as codeine phosphate may be helpful. Cholinergic drugs have helped some patients. Cholestyramine is worth trying in difficult cases, especially if bile salt malabsorption has been demonstrated, but it can precipitate or aggravate steatorrhoea. Symptoms in patients with steatorrhoea may improve with a low fat diet. Steroids have been tried in patients with and without steatorrhoea without conspicuous success and cannot be recommended. Antibiotics, such as tetracycline or metronidazole, are definitely indicated in patients with evidence of bacterial overgrowth on jejunal juice culture or breath test, and may be given as a therapeutic trial in severe cases. Treatment usually needs to be continued intermittently for many months or years.

Other gastrointestinal manifestations of diabetic neuropathy

Diabetic radiculopathy (diabetic plexus neuropathy), which is secondary to neuropathy involving the thoracic roots, is unique to diabetes.[26] It causes chronic severe abdominal pain which is often associated with weight loss and anorexia. The picture simulates malignancy, especially pancreatic carcinoma, so unnecessary diagnostic laparotomies are often performed. The patients are usually insulin dependent and have peripheral neuropathy. It is diagnosed by electromyography, the treatment is symptomatic and the symptoms often gradually subside over six to 20 months.

Diabetics with neuropathy have been described who get attacks of severe sharp epigastric pain with vomiting lasting a few hours to several days.[34] These are similar clinically to the gastric crises of tabes dorsalis. Postprandial facial sweating is said to be a specific manifestation of diabetic autonomic neuropathy, although this is disputed. It is most profuse after spicy food and may be treated by anticholinergics if troublesome.

Effect of diabetes and insulin on jejunal function

Perfusion studies in diabetics have shown that glucose absorption is either increased[41] or normal.[10] Sodium and water absorption[10] and brush border disaccharidase, peptidase and alkaline phosphatase activities[6] are normal. Blood insulin levels do not influence glucose, sodium or water absorption in diabetics or normal subjects.[10, 41]

Oral hypoglycaemic drugs and the gut

BIGUANIDES

These drugs inhibit glucose absorption from the small intestine. There are conflicting data on whether this inhibition is selective or not. Reports of inhibition of xylose absorption by metformin and sodium absorption by phenformin have not been confirmed by other studies. Metformin and (to a lesser extent) phenformin inhibit vitamin B_{12} absorption. Up to 30% of patients taking metformin for two or more years show vitamin B_{12} malabsorption,[40] although this rarely leads to megaloblastic anaemia. Vitamin B_{12} malabsorption may be a consequence of bacterial overgrowth secondary to poor intestinal motility caused by biguanides, since vitamin B_{12} absorption improves after antibiotic therapy and patients taking biguanides have evidence of bile salt deconjugation in the small intestine.[7]

Biguanides commonly cause anorexia, nausea, vomiting, abdominal pain and diarrhoea. As many as 25% of patients on phenformin complain of gastrointestinal disturbances. Phenformin has been blamed for causing acute pancreatitis, impaired pancreatic exocrine function and delayed gastric emptying.

SULPHONYLUREAS

These drugs do not affect glucose absorption but do cause minor nausea, epigastric pain and occasional vomiting.

Diabetes mellitus and the pancreas (see also Chapter 18)

PANCREATIC EXOCRINE FUNCTION

Abnormalities of pancreatic exocrine function have been found in 20–70% of all diabetics[8] although many of these patients may have had diabetes secondary to pancreatic disease. Reduced total volume, reduced amylase and bicarbonate concentrations have been found individually or together. Suggested causes include autonomic neuropathy, the wasting of uncontrolled diabetes, the inhibitory action of glucagon and the lack of stimulation by insulin. These abnormalities of pancreatic secretion are rarely severe and are not usually associated with steatorrhoea.

ACUTE PANCREATITIS

Hyperglycaemia occurs in 10–80% of patients with acute pancreatitis, but it is usually transient, lasting at most a few months and rarely requires specific treatment. Lasting diabetes mellitus is uncommon after an episode of acute pancreatitis, occurring in about 1% of cases. Confusion arises because diabetics with ketoacidosis may have transient hyperamylasaemia or even frank acute pancreatitis. Acute pancreatitis seems to be more common in diabetics than in non-diabetics and has a higher mortality.

CHRONIC PANCREATITIS

There is no evidence that chronic pancreatitis is more common among diabetics than normals. However chronic pancreatitis, particularly when associated with calcification, can lead to secondary diabetes mellitus when more than 90% of the gland is destroyed. In one series, 30% of patients with chronic pancreatitis had overt diabetes and a further 20% had impaired glucose tolerance.[2] If calcification was present, 70% of patients had diabetes and 20% had impaired glucose tolerance.

PANCREATIC CARCINOMA

Diabetes occurs in 25–50% of patients with carcinoma of the pancreas. The development of diabetes at the onset of symptoms related to carcinoma is a common occurrence or it can predate the onset of symptoms of carcinoma by a year or more. Some patients with carcinoma of the pancreas develop diabetes after the onset of symptoms related to the carcinoma.[22] Diabetes is most commonly manifested by abnormal glucose tolerance rather than glycosuria or hyperglycaemia. The diabetes may be unstable and the mechanism by which the carcinoma causes diabetes is unknown.[22] Pancreatic carcinoma should be considered in all new diabetics over 40 years of age, especially if they have no family history of diabetes, in deteriorating or unstable older diabetics or in older diabetics with abdominal symptoms.

This association has complicated the answer to the question of whether diabetes mellitus predisposes to pancreatic carcinoma. Kessler[25] reported the malignant deaths among 21 447 diabetics. The standard mortality ratio for pancreatic carcinoma was increased significantly for females at 2.13 and for males at 1.47. However, if cases where carcinoma developed within a year of the diagnosis of diabetes were excluded, the ratio was only significant for females.

PANCREATIC ISLET CELL TUMOURS
(SEE CHAPTER 18)

Glucagonomas and somatostatinomas cause hyperglycaemia which is usually mild but can occasionally require insulin. The syndrome of watery diarrhoea with hypokalaemia (Verner–Morrison syndrome) is associated with VIP-producing islet cell tumours. Some patients (15%) with VIPomas have hyperglycaemia which may require insulin. The mechanism of diabetes is unknown.

Diabetes mellitus and the biliary tract

In diabetics, the gallbladder on oral cholecystography tends to be large with poor filling and poor contraction after a fat meal, especially in those with autonomic neuropathy.[16] These findings have no clinical significance provided no gallstones are present.

The prevalence of gallstones among diabetics is about twice that of normals and the increase is due entirely to cholesterol stones. Maturity onset but not juvenile onset diabetics tend to have bile which is supersaturated for cholesterol but this is related to obesity rather than to the diabetes itself.[17]

In diabetics, acute cholecystitis is severe, tends to suppurate and has mortality of 10–20%.[37] Moreover, 20% of patients with emphysematous cholecystitis are diabetics. Early surgery is advisable but postoperative complications are still common. A strong case has been made for elective cholecystectomy in diabetics with asymptomatic gallstones since the operative mortality is not increased.[37]

REFERENCES

1 Angervall, L., Dotevall, G. & Lehmann, K. E. (1961) The gastric mucosa in diabetes mellitus. A functional and histopathological study. *Acta Medica Scandinavica*, **169**, 339–349.

2 Bank, S., Marks, I. N. & Vinik, A. I. (1975) Clinical and hormonal aspects of pancreatic diabetes. *American Journal of Gastroenterology*, **64**, 13–22.

3 Battle, W. M., Snape, W. J., Alavi, A. *et al.* (1980) Colonic dysfunction in diabetes mellitus. *Gastroenterology*, **79**, 1217–1221.

4 Berge, K. G., Sprague, R. G. & Bennett, W. A. (1956) The intestinal tract in diabetic diarrhoea. A pathologic study. *Diabetes*, **5**, 289–294.

5 Campbell, I. W., Heading, R. C., Tothill, P. *et al.* (1977) Gastric emptying in diabetic autonomic neuropathy. *Gut*, **18**, 462–467.

6 Caspary, W. F., Winckler, K. & Creutzfeldt, W. (1974) Intestinal brush border enzyme activity in juvenile and maturity onset diabetes mellitus. *Diabetologia*, **10**, 353–355.

7 Caspary, W. F., Zavada, I., Reimold, W. *et al.* (1977) Alterations of bile acid metabolism and vitamin B_{12} absorption in diabetics on biguanides. *Diabetologia*, **13**, 187–193.

8 Chey, W. Y., Shay, H. & Shuman, C. R. (1963) External pancreatic secretion in diabetes mellitus. *Annals of Internal Medicine*, **59**, 812–821.

9 Cooper, B. T., O'Brien, I. A. D., Ukabam, S. O. *et al.* (1983) Abnormal small intestinal permeability in patients with diabetic diarrhoea. *Clinical Science*, **64**, 16P.

10 Costrini, N. V., Ganneshappa, K. P., Wu, W. *et al.* (1977) Effect of insulin, glucose and controlled diabetes mellitus on human jejunal function. *American Journal of Physiology*, **233**, E181–E187.

11 Dotevall, G. (1959) Incidence of peptic ulcer in diabetes mellitus. *Acta Medica Scandinavica*, **164**, 463–477.

12 Feldman, M., Corbett, D. B., Ramsey, E. J. *et al.* (1977) Abnormal gastric function in long standing insulin dependent diabetic patients. *Gastroenterology*, **77**, 12–17.

13 Fox, S. & Behar, J. (1980) Pathogenesis of diabetic gastroparesis; a pharmacologic study. *Gastroenterology*, **78**, 757–763.

14 Goldstein, F., Wirts, C. W. & Knowlessar, O. D. (1970) Diabetic diarrhoea and steatorrhoea. Microbiologic and clinical observations. *Annals of Internal Medicine*, **72**, 215–218.

15 Goyal, R. K. & Spiro, H. M. (1971) Gastro-intestinal manifestations of diabetes mellitus. *Medical Clinics of North America*, **55**, 1031–1044.

16 Grodski, M., Mazurkiewicz-Rozinska, E. & Czyzyka, A. (1968) Diabetic cholecystopathy. *Diabetologia*, **4**, 345–348.

17 Haber, G. B. & Heaton, K. W. (1979) Lipid composition of bile in diabetics and obesity matched controls. *Gut*, **20**, 518–522.

18 Hensley, G. T. & Soergel, K. H. (1968) Neuropathologic findings in diabetic diarrhoea. *Archives of Pathology*, **85**, 587–597.

19 Hollis, J. B., Castell, D. O. & Braddon, R. L. (1977) Esophageal function in diabetes mellitus and its relation to peripheral neuropathy. *Gastroenterology*, **73**, 1098–1102.

20 Hosking, D. J., Moody, F., Stewart, I. M. & Atkinson, M. (1975) Vagal impairment of gastric secretion in diabetic autonomic neuropathy. *British Medical Journal*, **ii**, 588–590.

21 Irvine, W. J., Clarke, B. F., Scarth, L. *et al.* (1970) Thyroid and gastric auto antibodies in patients with diabetes mellitus. *Lancet,* **ii,** 163–168.

22 Karmody, A. J. & Kyle, J. (1969) The association between carcinoma of the pancreas and diabetes mellitus. *British Journal of Surgery,* **56,** 362–364.

23 Kassander, P. (1958) Asymptomatic gastric retention in diabetics (gastroparesis diabeticorum). *Annals of Internal Medicine,* **48,** 797–812.

24 Katz, L. A. & Spiro, H. M. (1966) Gastrointestinal manifestations of diabetes. *New England Journal of Medicine,* **275,** 1350–1361.

25 Kessler, I. I. (1970) Cancer mortality among diabetics. *Journal of the National Cancer Institute,* **44,** 673–686.

26 Longstreth, G. F. & Newcomer, A. D. (1977) Abdominal pain caused by diabetic radiculopathy. *Annals of Internal Medicine,* **86,** 166–168.

27 Malagelada, J. R., Rees, W. D. W., Mazzotta, L. J. & Go, V. L. W. (1980) Gastric motor abnormalities in diabetic and post vagotomy gastroparesis: effect of metoclopramide and bethanechol. *Gastroenterology,* **78,** 286–293.

28 Malins, J. M. & French, J. M. (1957) Diabetic diarrhoea. *Quarterly Journal of Medicine,* **26,** 467–480.

29 Malins, J. M. & Mayne, N. (1969) Diabetic diarrhoea. A study of 13 patients with jejunal biopsy. *Diabetes,* **18,** 858–866.

30 Mandelstam, P. & Lieber, A. (1967) Esophageal dysfunction in diabetic neuropathy-gastropathy. *Journal of the American Medical Association,* **201,** 582–586.

31 Mayne, N. (1965) Neuropathy in the diabetic and non-diabetic populations. *Lancet,* **ii,** 1313–1316.

32 McNally, E. F., Reinhard, A. E. & Schwartz, P. E. (1969) Small bowel motility in diabetics. *American Journal of Digestive Diseases,* **14,** 163–169.

33 Molloy, A. M. & Tomkin, G. H. (1978) Altered bile in diabetic diarrhoea. *British Medical Journal,* **ii,** 1462–1463.

34 Rundles, R. W. (1945) Diabetic neuropathy. General review with report of 125 cases. *Medicine (Baltimore),* **24,** 111–160.

35 Scarpello, J. H. B., Barber, D. C., Hague, R. V. *et al.* (1976) Gastric emptying of solid meals in diabetics. *British Medical Journal,* **ii,** 671–673.

36 Scarpello, J. H. B., Hague, R. V., Cullen, D. R. & Sladen, G. E. (1976) The ^{14}C-glycocholate test in diabetic diarrhoea. *British Medical Journal,* **ii,** 673–675.

37 Schein, C. J. (1969) Acute cholecystitis in the diabetic. *American Journal of Gastroenterology,* **51,** 511–515.

38 Smith, B. (1974) Neuropathy of the oesophagus in diabetes mellitus. *Neurology, Neurosurgery and Psychiatry,* **37,** 1151–1154.

39 Stewart, I. M., Hosking, D. J., Preston, B. J. & Atkinson, M. (1976) Oesophageal motor changes in diabetes mellitus. *Thorax,* **31,** 278–283.

40 Tomkin, G. H., Hadden, D. R., Weaver, J. A. & Montgomery, D. A. D. (1971) Vitamin B_{12} status of patients on long term metformin therapy. *British Medical Journal,* **ii,** 685–687.

41 Vinnik, I. E., Kern, F. J. & Sussman, K. E. (1965) The effect of diabetes mellitus and insulin on glucose absorption by the small intestine in man. *Journal of Laboratory and Clinical Medicine,* **66,** 131–136.

42 Walsh, C. H., Cooper, B. T., Wright, A. D. *et al.* (1978) Diabetes mellitus and coeliac disease: a clinical study. *Quarterly Journal of Medicine,* **47,** 89–100.

43 Warshaw, A. L., Feller, E. R. & Lee, K. H. (1977) On the cause of raised serum amylase in diabetic keto-acidosis. *Lancet,* **i,** 929–930.

44 Whalen, G. E., Soergel, K. H. & Greenen, J. E. (1969) Diabetic diarrhoea. A clinical and pathophysiological study. *Gastroenterology,* **56,** 1021–1032.

45 Wood, M. N. (1947) Chronic peptic ulcer in 94 diabetics. *American Journal of Digestive Diseases,* **14,** 1–11.

46 Zitomer, B. R., Gramm, H. F. & Kozak, G. P. (1968) Gastric neuropathy in diabetes mellitus: clinical and radiologic observations. *Metabolism,* **17,** 199–211.

PARATHYROID DISEASES

The four parathyroid glands secrete the 84 amino acid polypeptide hormone, parathyroid hormone. In the presence of a normal plasma magnesium, parathyroid hormone maintains the plasma calcium in the normal range of 2.05–2.55 mmol/l. When the plasma calcium is low, parathyroid hormone mobilizes calcium from bone, stimulates 25-hydroxy vitamin D 1-hydroxylase activity so that more dietary calcium is absorbed and causes decreased urinary calcium and increased urinary phosphate secretion. Experimentally raising the plasma calcium causes release of gastrin and raises basal gastric acid secretion; a fall in plasma calcium results in the converse. The rise in acid secretion is unaffected by atropine administration. A rise in plasma calcium to the supranormal range has an inhibitory effect on gut motility. These effects appear to be mediated directly through plasma calcium as parathyroid hormone infusions alone have no effect.

Primary hyperparathyroidism

The clinical state of primary hyperparathyroidism is changing as many patients are now identified with minimal or no symptoms when hypercalcaemia and hypophosphataemia are discovered on a multichannel biochemical analyser. Patients are therefore usually diagnosed much earlier than used to be the case and advanced cases with longstanding complications are rarely seen. The earlier diagnosis may also contribute to the current controversy over the previously accepted teaching that there was a strong association with peptic ulcer disease and pancreatitis.

The main gastrointestinal complications of primary hyperparathyroidism are thought to be peptic ulcers, acute and chronic pancreatitis and constipation. All are probably primarily related to the hypercalcaemia. The constipation may be very severe and reduced gastric emptying and small intestinal mobility along with colonic atony are reported. Other gastrointestinal symptoms include anorexia, nausea, vomiting, weight loss and diarrhoea. Obscure abdominal pain not due to peptic ulcer disease, pancreatitis or renal stones may also be a feature.[5]

PEPTIC ULCER DISEASE

The incidence of peptic ulcers in primary hyperparathyroidism has been estimated at 8–30% compared with about 2.5–3.2% in the normal population.[3] The increase is solely in duodenal ulcers, with no change in the incidence of gastric ulcer. The high incidence of duodenal ulcer is associated with raised plasma gastrin levels, and increased gastric acid and pepsin secretion; these all fall after successful parathyroidectomy. It has been suggested that the raised plasma gastrin levels are associated with increased antral G-cell numbers. The presence of an associated chronic pancreatitis with reduced pancreatic bicarbonate output might also contribute to the pathogenesis of duodenal ulcer. Recently Linos et al.[7] have suggested in a series of 46 patients that there is no association between ulcers and hyperparathyroidism, but as this was a retrospective study with small numbers, and in view of the previous evidence, a carefully controlled prospective study with larger patient numbers is needed to clarify the situation.

Duodenal ulcers associated with primary hyperparathyroidism should respond to H2 receptor antagonists. It has been shown that cimetidine may also reduce plasma parathyroid hormone levels so a double effect may be expected.[13] Despite this some patients may not respond to cimetidine but make a good response to excision of the parathyroid adenoma.[9]

A specific problem with duodenal ulcers and primary hyperparathyroidism is the possible presence of a coexistent gastrinoma as part of a multiple endocrine adenoma state. The release of gastrin from gastrinomas is highly sensitive to the serum calcium level, and after parathyroidectomy, plasma gastrin may return to normal despite a persisting gastrinoma. Under these circumstances a paradoxical rise in plasma gastrin with intravenous calcium or secretin suggests a gastrinoma. It is generally accepted that it is best to perform a parathyroidectomy as the first procedure. If the ulcer heals, and gastric acid secretion and the plasma gastrin levels are then normal (including with secretin or calcium provocation), it is reasonable to simply follow the patient. However, if the tests remain abnormal, attempts to localize a gastrinoma by gastroduodenoscopy, retrograde pancreatography,

selective pancreatic and duodenal arteriography and portal venous sampling should be considered.[6, 10]

PANCREATIC DISEASE

Both acute and chronic pancreatitis are thought to be associated with primary hyperparathyroidism. In the presence of an acute attack of pancreatitis the plasma calcium levels may become normal or even subnormal so it is important to estimate the plasma calcium after the patient has fully recovered. Possible aetiological factors include calcium stones in the pancreatic duct, increased trypsin activation because of increased pancreatic calcium secretion (trypsinogen conversion to trypsin is calcium dependent) and vasculitis; this latter hypothesis is based on the observation that experimental animals treated with parathyroid hormone have developed a thromboendarteritis. In some patients, pancreatic calcification seen on plain abdominal X-rays may be marked. The steatorrhoea, diabetes mellitus, pain and other complications should be treated in the standard manner (Chapter 18).

The association between primary hyperparathyroidism and pancreatitis is standard teaching but has recently been challenged. Bess, Edis and Van Heerden[1] retrospectively studied 1153 Mayo Clinic patients and found only 17 who had evidence of pancreatitis, 11 of whom had evidence for a gallstone and/or alcoholic aetiology. As this is similar to the incidence of pancreatitis in a control hospital population, they suggest that the association may not exist. An association between hyperparathyroidism and gallstones has also been claimed, but in a prospective study of Stockholm council workers 82 were found to have primary hyperparathyroidism and the frequency of cholelithiasis on oral cholecystography was the same in the patients as in 82 age and sex matched controls.[2] Clearly, a large prospective series is needed of hyperparathyroid patients without evidence of pancreatic endocrine tumours in whom full gastric and pancreatic assessment has been performed.

Secondary hyperparathyroidism

When there is chronic steatorrhoea, calcium and vitamin D malabsorption often ensue. This causes a reduction in the plasma calcium and parathyroid hormone is consequently secreted in large amounts from hyperplastic glands. Patients may then develop osteomalacia with the biochemical and bone changes of secondary hyperparathyroidism. Conditions associated with this problem include coeliac disease, Crohn's disease, postgastrectomy, the short bowel syndrome, jejunoileal bypass for morbid obesity and chronic cholestatic liver disease.[4, 11]

Clinically patients with severe disease may develop bone pains and pseudofractures. These along with radiological bone thinning indicate osteomalacia; subperiosteal resorption, particularly of the hand phalanges, suggests secondary hyperparathyroidism. Biochemical changes include a low or low normal fasting plasma calcium and phosphate, a low serum 25-hydroxy vitamin D and a raised plasma bony-type alkaline phosphatase isoenzyme level. Biochemical changes more specifically suggesting secondary hyperparathyroidism are raised plasma immunoreactive parathyroid hormone levels, raised plasma and 24 hour urinary hydroxy proline levels and evidence of increased phosphate excretion in the presence of hypophosphataemia (by demonstrating a reduced maximum tubular resorption of phosphate related to glomerular filtration rate). However, the most definite way of making a diagnosis is by bone biopsy including the examination of calcification fronts by in vivo tetracycline labelling. The changes of osteomalacia are increased osteoid tissue and reduced calcification fronts and of secondary hyperparathyroidism are increased osteoclastic resorption and increased fibrous tissue (osteitis fibrosa).

Treatment involves correction of the malabsorption, if feasible. In patients with coeliac disease, a careful gluten-free diet alone may allow full resolution. In other patients oral vitamin D supplements will allow resolution; increased exposure to ultraviolet light (from the sun or an ultraviolet lamp), vitamin D2 or D3 supplements and 1-alpha hydroxy vitamin D3 may all be effective. When there is biochemical evidence of magnesium or severe calcium deficiency, supplements of these ions may be helpful. Basic treatment monitoring can be done by estimating the plasma calcium and phosphate levels but the only accurate way is by bone biopsy, perhaps every 6 to 12 months, as many patients have normal biochemical and radiological markers but grossly abnormal bone histology.

Pseudohyperparathyroidism and tertiary hyperparathyroidism

Hypercalcaemia may result from parathyroid hormone-like substances produced by carcinomas, most commonly of the bronchus or pancreas; this is usually termed pseudo-hyperparathyroidism. In patients with secondary hyperparathyroidism an autonomous parathyroid hormone secreting adenoma may develop in the hyperplastic parathyroid glands and cause hypercalcaemia (tertiary hyperparathyroidism). The most common gastrointestinal complication of these problems is severe constipation. Treatment of the hypercalcaemia with tumour excision or by medical means (saline diuresis with frusemide, corticosteroids, calcitonin, diphosphonates or mithramycin) usually relieves the symptoms.

Hypoparathyroidism

The usual presenting symptoms of hypoparathyroidism are cramps, tetany and steatorrhoea. A familial association with Addison's disease, diabetes mellitus and hypothyroidism is described.[8] Some of these patients will have an immunodeficiency syndrome, which may initiate multiple causes of gastrointestinal disease (see Chapter 8). Biochemical changes include hypocalcaemia, hyperphosphataemia and unmeasurable immunoreactive parathyroid hormone levels. When the plasma calcium is less than 1.75 mmol/l, achlorhydria is usually present. Gastric acid secretion becomes normal as the plasma calcium is corrected.

The steatorrhoea is usually modest but may be very high, for example more than 352 mmol (100 g) daily. Reduced absorption of xylose, glucose and fat soluble vitamins is documented. The cause of the steatorrhoea which is corrected by successful treatment is controversial. Most small bowel biopsies have been reported as normal, but villous atrophy responding to treatment of the hypocalcaemia has been described.[12] Other suggested factors in the pathogenesis of the steatorrhoea are intestinal moniliasis, intestinal bacterial overgrowth and reduced bile acid secretion because of associated liver disease. Barium follow-through studies show delayed gastric emptying and small intestinal transit associated with dilated intestinal loops and flocculation of the barium; these changes resolve with successful vitamin D and calcium treatment. Pancreatic enzymes are unhelpful but medium-chain triglyceride supplements have been shown to improve calcium balance.

Pseudohypoparathyroidism is a rare X-linked dominant condition with similar symptoms and signs to hypoparathyroidism. However, plasma parathyroid hormone levels are high but may be suppressed by calcium infusions; the patients have a reduced response to exogenous parathyroid hormone indicating an increased peripheral resistance. Similar gastrointestinal problems might be expected to those seen with hypoparathyroidism but to date they are poorly documented.

REFERENCES

1 Bess, M. A., Edis, A. J. & Van Heerden, A. (1980) Hyperparathyroidism and pancreatitis – chance or a causal association. *Journal of the American Medical Association*, **243**, 246–247.

2 Christensson, T. & Einarsson, K. (1977) Cholelithiasis in subjects with hypercalcaemia and primary hyperparathyroidism detected in a health screening. *Gut*, **18**, 543–546.

3 Christiansen, J. (1974) Primary hyperparathyroidism and peptic ulcer disease. *Scandinavian Journal of Gastroenterology*, **9**, 111–114.

4 Compston, J. E., Horton, L. W. L., Laker, M. F. *et al.* (1978) Bone disease after jejuno-ileal bypass for obesity. *Lancet*, **ii**, 1–4.

5 Eversman, J. J., Farmer, R. G. & Brown, C. H. (1967) Gastrointestinal manifestations of hyperparathyroidism. *Archives of Internal Medicine*, **119**, 605–609.

6 Glowniak, J. V., Shapiro, B., Vinik, A. I. *et al.* (1982) Percutaneous transhepatic venous sampling of gastrin: value in sporadic and familial islet-cell tumours and G-cell hyperfunction. *New England Journal of Medicine*, **307**, 293–297.

7 Linos, D. A., Van Heerden, J. A., Abboud, C. F. & Edis, A. J. (1978) Primary hyperparathyroidism and peptic ulcer disease. *Archives of Surgery*, **113**, 384–386.

8 Lorenz, R. & Burr, I. M. (1974) Idiopathic hypoparathyroidism and steatorrhoea: a new aid in management. *Journal of Pediatrics*, **85**, 522–525.

9 McCarthy, D. M., Peikin, S. R., Lopatin, R. N. *et al.* (1979) Hyperparathyroidism – a reversible cause of cimetidine resistant gastric hypersecretion. *British Medical Journal*, **i**, 1765–1766.

10 McGuigan, J. E., Colwell, J. A. & Franklin, J. (1974) Effect of parathyroidectomy and hypercalcaemic hypersecretory peptic ulcer disease. *Gastroenterology*, **66**, 269–272.

11 Melvin, K. E. W., Hepner, G. W., Bordier, P. *et al.* (1970) Calcium metabolism and bone pathology in adult cocliac disease. *Quarterly Journal of Medicine*, **39**, 83–113.

12 Russell, R. I. (1967) Hypoparathyroidism and malabsorption. *British Medical Journal*, **3**, 781–782.

13 Sherwood, J. K., Ackroyd, F. W. & Garcia, M. (1980) Effect of cimetidine on circulating parathyroid hormone in primary hyperparathyroidism. *Lancet*, **ii**, 616–620.

THYROID DISEASES

Thyroxine and triiodothyronine are secreted by the thyroid gland and are normally under the control of thyroid stimulating hormone (TSH) from the anterior pituitary. The thyroid hormones have a major effect on gut motility, as well as other lesser effects, and consequently hyperthyroidism and hypothyroidism are associated with numerous gastrointestinal effects.[10] However, it should be stressed that it is very rare for gastrointestinal symptoms to be present without some of the other usual systemic symptoms and signs of thyroid disease.

An association between ulcerative colitis and a history of thyrotoxicosis, hypothyroidism and simple goitre has been demonstrated. A relationship between thyrotoxicosis and coeliac disease is also claimed. Under normal circumstances, the thyroid hormones are bound in plasma to thyroxine binding globulin (TBG) (75%), thyroxine binding prealbumin (15%) and albumin (10%). In protein-losing enteropathy states, levels of these proteins fall. In ulcerative colitis and Crohn's disease, there is evidence for iodine deficiency and reduced plasma albumin and prealbumin concentrations. Plasma TBG levels are raised in mild and moderate inflammatory bowel disease but fall with severe corticosteroid treated disease. In general, active ulcerative colitis is often associated with a small goitre but neither active ulcerative colitis nor Crohn's disease are associated with hyperthyroidism or hypothyroidism. However, thyroid uptake tests should be avoided in both conditions as iodine deficiency is common and results in increased uptake which suggests a misleading diagnosis of thyrotoxicosis.[8]

Hyperthyroidism

The most common gastrointestinal symptom of hyperthyroidism is diarrhoea, which occurs in about 25% of thyrotoxic patients. The symptom is usually modest and the patient notices only a slight increase in the frequency of bowel movements, along with some softening of the faeces. Profuse watery diarrhoea is unusual. On occasions patients may notice the yellow, floating, offensive stools of steatorrhoea. Rarely, when hypercalcaemia is marked in thyrotoxicosis, a tendency to constipation may occur. A large appetite along with hyperphagia usually occurs but some patients have severe anorexia which contributes to rapid weight loss. Nausea and vomiting may be prominent in the absence of hypercalcaemia and it has been suggested that this is a central effect.[11] Other rare symptoms are hyperbilirubinaemia (possibly reflecting hepatic fatty change or the unmasking of Gilbert's disease), abdominal pain and oedema which can be associated with either normal or low serum protein concentrations.

The gastrointestinal aspects of hyperthyroidism are usually modest. Final diagnosis rests on the usual thyroid function tests including serum thyroxine, triiodothyronine, thyroid uptake of radioiodine and a flat response of TSH to intravenous thyrotrophin releasing hormone (TRH). Investigation in the majority of patients shows a slight increase above the upper limit of normal of the faecal fats (18 mmol/24 h) but this is rarely above 90 mmol/24 h. There are numerous studies of the effect of hyperthyroidism on various parts of the gut and these are outlined below.

Proximal skeletal myopathy is well recognized and this effect is thought to occur sometimes in the oesophagus. There is a decrease in oesophageal propulsion and closure. Recurrent aspiration pneumonia due to oesophageal incoordination with tracheal overspill is reported; when the thyrotoxicosis was recognized and treated with carbimazole, there was no recurrence of the pneumonia.[9]

Gastric acid secretion varies greatly but mean acid outputs in thyrotoxic patients are reduced and gastric histology shows a marked gastritis. Initially, despite the hypochlorhydria, it was suggested that patients had an increased incidence of duodenal ulcers but subsequently this has been disproved. Wiersinga and Touber[14] have shown that high plasma gastrin levels occur in both Graves' disease and toxic nodular goitre and that they are associated with reduced acid secretion. In patients with hypochlorhydria the acid secretion and gastrin levels correct with treatment but in five patients with achlorhydria, only one recovered but the other four all had parietal cell antibodies.

The gastric emptying rate has been shown to be increased using barium sulphate and it has long been assumed that some of the malabsorption was exacerbated by rapid emptying of meals into the small intestine. Wiley *et al.*[15] used technetium-99m sulphur colloid-labelled chicken's liver in a mixed meal in four patients and suggested that physiological gastric emptying was similar in controls and hyperthyroidism. More patients need to be studied before this observation can be accepted.

Barium studies of small intestinal transit in thyrotoxicosis have suggested that transit times are greatly reduced due to increased peristaltic activity. In a rat experimental model of hyperthyroidism, it has been shown that small intestinal weight, villus height, total mucosal thickness, mucosal protein content and brush border enzymes are increased.[10] If this effect occurs in human hyperthyroidism, it explains

the minimal malabsorption seen in a situation where there is probably gross intestinal hurry. Thomas, Caldwell and Greenberger[12] found steatorrhoea in 60% of patients studied and related it to an increased fat intake (mean 873 mmol (248 g)/24 h) and increased intestinal hypermotility associated with a mild degree of malabsorption. Propranolol was shown to reduce faecal fat excretion by 50%. In contrast, glucose absorption is increased from isolated rat intestinal sacs by thyroxine administration and rapid absorption has been shown in thyrotoxic man. In thyrotoxicosis, the urinary D-xylose excretion is increased but this is a renal effect and is seen whether the xylose is given orally or intravenously and overall intestinal absorption appears normal. Other parameters of absorption and jejunal histology are normal.

Calcium malabsorption commonly occurs and there is a negative calcium balance associated with increased urinary and faecal loss. Some patients are also in negative phosphate balance. Bone histology shows osteoporosis with thin trabeculae and there is no evidence of osteomalacia or hyperparathyroidism. The negative calcium balance probably explains the osteoporosis. When the patients are treated with either drugs or radioiodine, the calcium balance becomes positive.[3]

Biliary and pancreatic function also change in thyrotoxicosis. Total bile acids are normal but there is an increase in the dihydroxy fraction, particularly taurochenodeoxycholic acid. The response of pancreatic bicarbonate to intravenous secretin is normal but trypsin output to a standard meal is reduced. This finding may be related to increased sympathetic activity as intravenous isoprenaline infusion has a similar effect and thyrotoxic steatorrhoea improves with propranolol.[15] The reduced trypsin output may indicate generalized pancreatic enzyme hyposecretion and this could also contribute to the pathogenesis of the steatorrhoea.

Hypothyroidism

Major gastrointestinal symptoms of hypothyroidism include reduced appetite without weight loss and mild to severe constipation. Some of the other non-gastrointestinal symptoms are nearly always present. Other symptoms include rectal prolapse, spurious diarrhoea because of faecal impaction and ascites. The ascites is a clear straw-coloured exudate with a protein electrophoretic strip pattern similar to plasma and occurs in the absence of cardiac, hepatic, renal or peritoneal disease; on occasions there may be concurrent pleural and pericardial effusions (see Chapter 20).

In the oesophagus, the peristaltic wave pressure and velocity are reduced and the peristaltic wave duration is prolonged in the distal three-quarters but normal in the proximal one-quarter. This shows that non-striated muscle is more affected than striated muscle. In some patients this can result in dysphagia and can be demonstrated by the majority of voluntary wet swallows producing non-propagated, simultaneous and repetitive contractions. These abnormalities disappear with treatment.[2]

Gastric acid secretion is variable but in general is normal, as are plasma gastrin levels. However, as a result of the association with pernicious anaemia, some patients have achlorhydria, hypergastrinaemia and positive parietal cell antibodies. Gastric histology usually shows gastritis and oedema of the mucosal muscles. Gastric emptying is markedly delayed.

The duodenum is the most affected part of the small intestine and in severe hypothyroidism may become dilated and atonic; rarely this may spread to the rest of the small bowel. On occasions frank intestinal obstruction with fluid levels may be seen. Histologically a diffuse mucoid infiltration, especially of the submucosa, is seen in duodenal, jejunal and colonic specimens. Jejunal biopsies may show subtotal villous atrophy and there may be associated mild steatorrhoea. Small bowel motility is reduced. Peroral radiotelemetry capsules in the jejunum have shown greatly reduced rhythm, wave amplitude and other indices of motility. A flat glucose tolerance curve is common and partially reflects slow gastric emptying. D-Xylose excretion is reduced when it is given intravenously and consequently D-xylose intestinal absorption is impossible to assess.

The colon is another major site of severe mucoid infiltration and atony, dilatation and sometimes a gross megacolon occur. Fluid levels are seen and if a diagnosis of obstruction is made, laparotomy may precipitate death. Histological examination of Auerbach's and Meissner's plexus is normal. Motility probes have been introduced into the colon and low motility indices found. If there is some response to parasympathetic stimulation with the muscarinic drug urecholine the prognosis for recovery with thyroxine is good but otherwise it is poor.[5]

Medullary carcinoma of the thyroid

These tumours are derived from thyroid parafollicular C cells which synthesize calcitonin and somatostatin. The commonest initial presentation is as a solid thyroid mass which may be bilateral. Macroscopically the tumours are grey and firm, usually lack a capsule and may diffusely infiltrate the local tissues. Histologically there are sheets of tumour cells with connective tissue septa forming nests; the number of mitoses varies and amyloid is often present. Metastases are initially to cervical lymph nodes and the mediastinum but later in the disease process may involve the lungs, liver, adrenals and bone. The tumours may occur sporadically or in families; the presence of familial cases in an area may raise the incidence of these tumours to about 10% of thyroid malignancies, but usually it is less than this. The familial cases may have raised plasma biochemical markers of a tumour (in particular, calcitonin) for many years before the tumour becomes palpable or symptomatic. The prognosis is very variable but total thyroidectomy and the general surgical excision of tumour mass may be very helpful; some patients survive for many years whereas others die within a year of diagnosis.

Numerous active substances have been found in the plasma and/or tumour extracts of patients with medullary carcinoma of the thyroid (Table 9.10). Calcitonin is a 32 amino acid polypeptide

Table 9.10 Active substances isolated from medullary carcinoma of the thyroid.

Calcitonin
Prostaglandin E_2
Prostaglandin $F_{2\alpha}$
Carcinoembryonic antigen
Histaminase
5-Hydroxytryptamine
Adrenocorticotrophic hormone
Kallikrein
Somatostatin
Neurotensin
β-Endorphin
Substance P

which lowers plasma calcium and phosphate levels and may play a role in preserving the skeleton and preventing osteoporosis; pharmacological infusions decrease gastrin levels and gastric acid secretion, and increase ileal secretion of sodium, chloride, potassium and water.[6] Calcitonin is always secreted by medullary carcinomas and plasma levels usually, but not always, correlate with the tumour mass.[13] Plasma calcitonin radioimmunoassay is widely used in patient diagnosis and follow-up and is particularly helpful in the management of presymptomatic familial cases. In doubtful situations, calcitonin provocation tests with whisky, pentagastrin or calcium may be useful. In some patients tumour mass may also be monitored by plasma prostaglandin, carcinoembryonic antigen or histaminase values, or 24 hour urinary 5-hydroxyindoleacetic acid levels. Rarely adrenocorticotrophic hormone secretion may result in the clinical and biochemical manifestations of Cushing's syndrome. The other listed substances do not have any definite clinical roles, or yet play a part in diagnosis or follow-up.

The main gastrointestinal symptoms of medullary carcinoma of the thyroid are dysphagia due to local cervical infiltration and diarrhoea which occurs at some stage in 30% of patients and may precede the presence of a palpable thyroid mass. Other occasional symptoms are weight loss, borborygmi and colicky abdominal pain. The diarrhoea may be modest or profuse and watery with more than one litre of stool daily, resulting in hypokalaemia. Steatorrhoea is usually minimal and rarely more than 50 mmol/fatty acid/day. Triple lumen tube studies in the jejunum have shown normal transport of electrolytes, and normal mucosal permeability and transit time, but in the ileum there is a failure to absorb sodium and chloride against a concentration gradient, an abnormal mucosal permeability and a rapid transit time.[7] The variability of the diarrhoea observed is probably dependent on the colonic ability to cope with the increased ileocaecal flow.

There is evidence that both calcitonin and prostaglandins play a role in the pathogenesis of the diarrhoea because infusions of both into healthy volunteers can cause intestinal secretion. When pharmacological doses of calcitonin are given to patients with Paget's disease, some 12% develop diarrhoea. Cox et al.[4] studied a patient with diarrhoea, increased distal ileal flow and very high plasma calcitonin concentrations. Large amounts of plasma were obtained by plasmapheresis and infused into dogs in whom an inhibition of small intestinal absorption was seen. These workers also showed that the diarrhoea is not associated with activation of the adenyl cyclase/cyclic AMP system since the mucosal cyclic AMP levels are normal and there is no response to anti-cyclic AMP drugs such as nicotinic acid and colchicine.

The evidence for prostaglandins mediating the diarrhoea is incomplete because many patients fail to respond to antiprostaglandin drugs. Exogenous F_2 alpha prostaglandin ($PGF_{2\alpha}$) infusion into normal volunteers can cause ileal secretion of sodium, chloride and water. It was initially shown that some patients with diarrhoea have raised plasma and/or tumour prostaglandin levels.[16] The diarrhoea of some patients responds to nutmeg (e.g. one teaspoonful nine times a day); this charmingly medieval substance, from *Myristica fragrans*, contains volatile oils, fats, myristin, elemicin and safrol, and has anticholinergic sympathomimetic and occasionally hallucinogenic, as well as antiprostaglandin, effects.[1] The more specific antiprostaglandin drug, indomethacin 25–50 mg three times a day, is effective in controlling diarrhoea in some patients but ineffective in most. It must be concluded that the precise pathogenesis of the diarrhoea in these patients is unknown.

REFERENCES

1   Barrowman, J. A., Bennett, A., Hillenbrand, P. *et al.* (1975) Diarrhoea in thyroid medullary carcinoma: role of prostaglandins and therapeutic effect of nutmeg. *British Medical Journal*, **iii**, 11–12.
2   Christensen, J. (1967) Esophageal manometry in myxedema (Abstract). *Gastroenterology*, **52**, 1130.
3   Cook, P. B., Nassim, J. R. & Collins, J. (1959) The effects of thyrotoxicosis upon the metabolism of calcium, phosphorus, and nitrogen. *Quarterly Journal of Medicine*, **28**, 505–529.
4   Cox, T. M., Fagan, E. A., Hillyard, C. J. *et al.* (1979) Role of calcitonin in diarrhoea associated with medullary carcinoma of the thyroid. *Gut*, **20**, 629–633.
5   Duret, R. L. & Bastenie, P. A. (1971) Intestinal disorders in hypothyroidism. Clinical and manometric study. *American Journal of Digestive Diseases*, **16**, 723–727.
6   Hunter, L. A. & Heath, H., III (1981) Calcitonin: physiology and pathophysiology. *New England Journal of Medicine*, **304**, 269–278.
7   Isaacs, P., Whittaker, S. M. & Turnberg, L. A. (1974) Diarrhoea associated with medullary carcinoma of the thyroid; studies of intestinal function in a patient. *Gastroenterology*, **67**, 521–526.
8   Jarnerot, G., Kagedal, B., von Schenck, H. & Truelove, S. C. (1976) The thyroid in ulcerative colitis and Crohn's disease. V. Triiodothyronine. Effects of corticosteroids and influence of severe disease. *Acta Medica Scandinavica*, **199**, 229–232.
9   Marks, P., Anderson, J. & Vincent, R. (1980) Thyrotoxic myopathy presenting as dysphagia. *Postgraduate Medical Journal*, **56**, 669–670.
10 Middleton, W. R. (1971) Thyroid hormones in the gut. *Gut*, **12**, 172–177.
11 Rosenthal, F. D., Jones, C. & Lewis, S. I. (1976) Thyrotoxic vomiting. *British Medical Journal*, **ii**, 209–211.
12 Thomas, F. B., Caldwell, J. H. & Greenberger, N. J. (1973) Diarrhoea in thyrotoxicosis. *Annals of Internal Medicine*, **78**, 669–675.
13 Trump, L., Mendelsohn, G. & Baylin, S. B. (1979) Discordance between plasma calcitonin and tumor-cell mass in medullary thyroid carcinoma. *New England Journal of Medicine*, **301**, 253–255.
14 Wiersinga, W. M. & Touber, J. L. (1980) The relation between gastrin, gastric acid and thyroid function disorders. *Acta Endocrinologica (Copenhagen)*, **95**, 341–349.

15 Wiley, Z. D., Lavigne, M. E., Liu, K. M. & MacGregor, I. L. (1978) The effect of hyperthyroidism on gastric emptying rates and pancreatic exocrine and biliary secretion in man. *American Journal of Digestive Diseases*, **23**, 1003–1008.
16 Williams, E. D., Karim, S. M. M. & Sandler, M. (1968) Prostaglandin secretion by medullary carcinoma of the thyroid: a possible cause of the associated diarrhoea. *Lancet*, **i**, 22–23.

PITUITARY DISEASES

The pituitary is divided into anterior and posterior parts and has been nicknamed the leader of the endocrine orchestra as its hormones (Table 9.11) control most adrenocortical,

Table 9.11 Pituitary hormones.

Anterior pituitary
Adrenocorticotrophic hormone (ACTH)
Thyrotrophin stimulating hormone (TSH)
Growth hormone (GH)
Follicle stimulating hormone (FSH)
Luteinizing hormone (LH)
Prolactin

Posterior pituitary
Arginine vasopressin

thyroid and gonadal hormone secretions as well as many other endocrine and metabolic functions. However, the term 'leader' is something of a misnomer because secretion of the anterior pituitary hormones is itself controlled by stimulatory hypothalamic peptides (e.g. corticotrophin releasing hormone, thyrotrophin releasing hormone and gonadotrophin releasing hormone) and in the case of growth hormone by both stimulatory and inhibitory hormones (growth hormone releasing hormone and somatostatin).

The pituitary hormones have major effects on the gut (see Chapter 8). Adrenocorticotrophic hormone (ACTH) stimulates cortisol secretion and enhances brush border enzyme activity and thyrotrophin stimulating hormone (TSH) causes thyroxine secretion with major effects on gut motility. Growth hormone causes intestinal villous growth and enhances absorption but there is no good evidence for the gonadotrophins having a physiological effect on the gut. In pregnancy and during lactation many animals develop intestinal mucosal growth and an increased absorptive capacity but evidence for prolactin, the obvious candidate, mediating this adaptive response has not been confirmed in experimental models of hyperprolactinaemia.[2]

Pituitary tumours

Pituitary tumours secrete ACTH (Cushing's disease), growth hormone (acromegaly) and prolactin (prolactinomas) while some appear non-secretory. They have two major types of effect, those due to the excessive hormone being secreted and those of secondary failure to excrete other hormones due to expansion of the tumour and loss of neighbouring normal cells. In general, the effects of hypersecretion appear to spare the gut. In acromegaly, increased intestinal mucosal growth occur and negative calcium balance is thought to be a factor in the pathogenesis of acromegalic osteoporosis, along with hypogonadism, muscle weakness and inactivity. A recent colonoscopic or double-contrast barium enema study in 17 acromegalics[1] found adenomatous polyps in five patients, hyperplastic polyps in three patients and unclassified polyps in one patient. The adenomatous polyps were small and varied in number from one to five; as no control group was included, this study needs expansion and confirmation before a clinically important association between acromegaly and adenomatous colonic polyps is accepted.

Hypopituitarism

This may occur because of an expanding primary or secondary tumour, a vascular accident, infection (e.g. tuberculosis) or a granulomatous process (e.g. sarcoidosis or Hand–Schüller–Christian syndrome). The gonadotrophins are usually the hormones lost first, and ACTH, TSH, prolactin and growth hormone follow; as a result, sexual dysfunction (amenorrhoea or impotence) is usually an early symptom. Subsequent common symptoms of hypopituitarism include lethargy, anorexia and weight loss; these symptoms are similar to those seen in some patients with anorexia nervosa and primary gastrointestinal problems such as inflammatory bowel disease and coeliac disease. Diarrhoea may be a major feature in hypopituitary patients and if treatment is not rapidly initiated death may ensue. Most of the symptoms can be reversed by standard physiological cortisone and thyroxine replacement therapy. In children growth failure is also present and growth hormone supplements are required.

REFERENCES

1 Klein, I., Parveen, G., Gavaler, J. S. & van Thiel, D. H. (1982) Colonic polyps in patients with acromegaly. *Annals of Internal Medicine*, **97**, 27–30.
2 Muller, E. & Dowling, R. H. (1981) Prolactin and the small intestine: effect of hyperprolactinaemia on mucosal structure in the rat. *Gut*, **22**, 558–565.

ADRENAL DISORDERS

The adrenal cortex secretes glucocorticosteroids and mineralocorticosteroids, and the adrenal medulla secretes primarily the catecholamines, noradrenaline and adrenaline. Glucocorticosteroids bind to specific cytoplasmic receptors on the enterocyte and the activated receptor–steroid complex is then translocated to the nucleus and causes new messenger RNA synthesis. They increase the absorptive capacity of the small intestine without increasing the number of cells. Studies of the ileum after jejunal resection in the rat have shown that the addition of pharmacological doses of prednisolone results in increased ileal epithelial cell DNA, RNA and brush border enzymes (i.e. α-glucosidase, leucyl-2-naphthylamidase and γ-glutamyl transferase), but there is no increase in cell numbers or in lysosomal and mitochondrial enzymes. Glucocorticosteroids, which are known to improve steatorrhea in patients with coeliac disease and diarrhoea in patients with the short bowel syndrome, therefore appear to act by enhancing brush border membrane digestive capacity.[6]

Cushing's syndrome

Cushing's syndrome may be due to Cushing's disease when there is an ACTH-secreting tumour in the pituitary, the ectopic ACTH syndrome when there is a tumour elsewhere (commonly in the bronchi or pancreas) secreting ACTH, or to benign and malignant tumours of the adrenal cortex secreting cortisol. Cushing's disease may be associated with multiple endocrine adenomatosis type I, and reported associations include gastrinoma, parathyroid adenoma, phaeochromocytoma and medullary carcinoma of the thyroid (see below).

The role of corticosteroid therapy in the pathogenesis of peptic ulcer disease remains controversial[2, 5] and there is currently no objective evidence for Cushing's syndrome being associated with an increased incidence of peptic ulcers. Theoretically absorption would be expected to be improved in Cushing's syndrome as a result of cortisol inducing brush border membrane enzymes but diarrhoea has been reported. In general the intestine appears little affected by Cushing's syndrome.

Adrenocortical insufficiency

Primary adrenal cortical failure (Addison's disease) is usually associated with autoimmunity or due to tuberculosis. The loss of weight, anorexia, dehydration, pigmentation, hypotension and hyponatraemia are features in common with severe coeliac disease and there is evidence that the two diseases may sometimes be associated. Other associations with Addison's disease include hypothyroidism, pernicious anaemia, hypoparathyroidism, diabetes mellitus, vitiligo and primary ovarian failure.

Adrenocortical insufficiency is associated with steatorrhoea, hypoglycaemia and normal jejunal histology. Faecal fats of up to 114 mmol (32.5 g) per day are reported but the values return to normal with glucocorticosteroid and mineralocorticosteroid replacement.[4] This response is compatible with the known effects of glucocorticosteroids on the small intestine.

Phaeochromocytoma

Phaeochromocytomas are catecholamine-secreting tumours of the adrenal glands and sympathetic chain. Reported gastrointestinal manifestations include nausea, vomiting, abdominal pain, diarrhoea or constipation, paralytic ileus and ischaemic colitis due to vasoconstriction. Phaeochromocytomas vary greatly in size and on occasions may be palpable as a large abdominal mass, for example mimicking a primary liver cell carcinoma. Catecholamines inhibit gut smooth muscle contraction and infusions do not cause diarrhoea. Phaeochromocytomas have been reported as sometimes secreting calcitonin[8] and enkephalin[7] and it is possible that hypersecretion of these two peptides may respectively contribute to the development of diarrhoea and constipation in some patients. The diagnostic exercise for a suspected phaeochromocytoma before surgery is complex and in most patients with high urinary 4-hydroxy-3-methoxymandelic acid (VMA) excretion should include plasma adrenaline and noradrenaline assays before and after pentolinium and abdominal computed tomography. In extra-adrenal cases, arteriography and venous sampling may also be needed.[1]

Ganglioneuroblastomas

Ganglioneuromas and ganglioneuroblastomas arise from similar anatomical sites to phaeochromocytomas but differ histologically. They most commonly present in childhood with an intra-abdominal mass and are found to have raised 24 hour urinary VMA concentrations. Profuse secretory diarrhoea has been recognized in some patients for more than 30 years but there is no correlation with catecholamine secretion. In 1973 it was shown that the diarrhoea was associated with high plasma and tumour vasoactive intestinal polypeptide (VIP) levels, and subsequently it has been shown that VIP causes secretory diarrhoea and most of the other features of this syndrome, including weight loss, abdominal colic, spontaneous cutaneous flushing, dehydration, hypokalaemic acidosis and reduced gastric acid secretion (see Chapter 18). In contrast to the usual bad prognosis of ganglioneuroblastomas, seven out of ten of our series of VIP-secreting tumours were successfully operated on and apparently cured[3] and consequently it must be concluded that this is an important diagnosis for gastroenterologists to make.

REFERENCES

1   Allison, D. J., Brown, M. J., Jones, D. H. & Timmis, J. B. (1983) Role of venous sampling in locating a phaeochromocytoma. *British Medical Journal*, **286**, 1122–1124.
2   Conn, H. O. & Blitzer, B. L. (1976) Nonassociation of adrenocorticosteroid therapy and peptic ulcer. *New England Journal of Medicine*, **294**, 473–479.
3   Long, R. G., Bryant, M. G., Mitchell, S. J. *et al.* (1981) Clinicopathological study of pancreatic and ganglioneuroblastoma tumours secreting vasoactive intestinal polypeptide (vipomas). *British Medical Journal*, **282**, 1767–1771.
4   McBrien, D. J., Jones, R. V. & Creamer, B. (1963) Steatorrhea in Addison's disease. *Lancet*, **i**, 25–26.
5   Messer, J., Reitman, D., Sacks, H. S., Smith, H. & Chalmers, T. C. (1983) Association of adrenocorticosteroid therapy and peptic ulcer disease. *New England Journal of Medicine*, **309**, 21–24.
6   Scott, J., Batt, R. M. & Peters, T. J. (1979) Enhancement of ileal adaptation by prednisolone after proximal small bowel resection in the rat. *Gut*, **20**, 858–864.
7   Sullivan, S. N., Bloom, S. R. & Polak, J. M. (1978) Enkephalin in peripheral neuroendocrine tumours. *Lancet*, **i**, 986–987.
8   Weinstein, R. S. (1980) Immunoreactive calcitonin in pheochromocytomas. *Proceedings of the Society for Experimental Biology and Medicine*, **165**, 215–217.

MULTIPLE ENDOCRINE ADENOMATOSIS

Multiple endocrine adenomatosis (MEA) is traditionally divided into two types, MEA I or Wermer's syndrome and MEA II or Sipple's syndrome (Table 9.12). However, occasionally the features of the two syndromes may overlap and the two types are not as distinct as was once thought. Both are usually inherited as an autosomal dominant trait with variable penetrance but sporadic cases are sometimes seen. Other features can include benign and malignant carcinoid tumours, multiple lipomas, schwannomas and thymomas.

Table 9.12 Basic details of multiple endocrine adenomatosis (MEA) types I and II.

MEA type I (Wermer's syndrome)
Pancreatic endocrine tumour
Pituitary tumour
Parathyroid tumour
MEA type II (Sipple's syndrome)
Medullary carcinoma of the thyroid
Phaeochromocytoma
Parathyroid tumour

Wermer's syndrome is more common than Sipple's syndrome. The pancreatic endocrine tumours may excrete one or more of insulin, pancreatic glucagon, gastrin, VIP somatostatin, pancreatic polypeptide, adrenocorticotrophic hormone and parathyroid hormone. The usual clinical presentation is as described in Chapter 18. The pituitary tumours may secrete growth hormone, prolactin or adrenocorticotrophic hormone or be apparently non-secretory. The parathyroid adenomas secrete parathyroid hormone and present with hypercalcaemia. The most common presentation of MEA I is with primary hyperparathyroidism and then subsequently other tumours become manifest.[1] It has been suggested that primary hyperparathyroidism in MEA I may have a more benign course than hyperparathyroidism alone but, in fact, MEA I patients appear to be younger, to have multiple glands involved more often and to have more recurrences.[3]

The diagnosis of pancreatic endocrine tumours can usually be made by making a clinical diagnosis and then measuring the appropriate regulatory peptide by radioimmunoassay. Pancreatic polypeptide secreting tumours are not associated with a specific metabolic syndrome but are usually co-secreted with other peptides which produce symptoms. Gastrinomas may be diagnosed by fasting hypergastrinaemia, high gastric acid output and inappropriate gastrin rises to intravenous calcium and secretin.[2] In patients at risk for MEA I, if one tumour arises it is usual for tumours to arise in the other characteristic sites later.[5] In the presence of any pancreatic endocrine tumour, it is always advisable to screen the pituitary radiologically and check the fasting plasma calcium and phosphate levels and, if there is any doubt, measure the hormone levels.

The treatment of MEA I must be considered individually for each case. In general the tumour producing the most symptoms should be treated first; the exception to this is a gastrinoma in the presence of primary hyperparathyroidism when the problems of the gastrinoma such as duodenal ulcers and diarrhoea usually settle with removal of the parathyroid adenoma.[4]

Sipple's syndrome (MEA II) can present with any of the three tumour types and because of the familial basis, early presymptomatic cases are often monitored biochemically and a gradual rise in the tumour marker seen. Some of the patients also have a marfanoid appearance with long limbs, poor muscular development, a high arched palate and pes cavus. Both the medullary carcinomas of the thyroid and the phaeochromocytomas may present with diarrhoea but occasionally a third cause of diarrhoea, constipation or intestinal obstruction, is seen; this is related to intestinal ganglioneuromas which may occur in all layers of the gut wall in some patients.

Medullary carcinoma of the thyroid should be monitored by plasma calcitonin levels (possibly with whisky, pentagastrin or calcium stimulation), phaeochromocytomas by 24 hour urinary 4-hydroxy-3-methoxymandelic acid (VMA) excretion and plasma adrenaline and noradrenaline levels before and after pentolinium, and parathyroid adenomas by plasma calcium, phosphate and parathyroid hormone values. If one tumour is present, it is important to screen for the other two types. Phaeochromocytomas in MEA II tend to secrete a very high proportion of adrenaline compared to noradrenaline and also to be bilateral in about 70% of cases.

If a phaeochromocytoma is present it is important to treat this first to avoid a hypertensive crisis. The patient is treated by α- and β-adrenergic blockade and after precise preoperative tumour localization, the tumour(s) is removed. The medullary carcinomas of the thyroid should be treated by total thyroidectomy and regional lymph node dissection when clinically indicated (some of the tumours are very slow growing) and the parathyroid adenomas should be localized by venous sampling, radioisotopic scanning or other methods[6] and excised.

REFERENCES

1 Betts, J. B., O'Malley, B. P. & Rosenthal, F. D. (1980) Hyperparathyroidism: a prerequisite for Zollinger–Ellison syndrome in multiple endocrine adrenomatosis Type I – report of a further family and a review of the literature. *Quarterly Journal of Medicine*, **73**, 69–76.

2 Lamers, C. B., Bois, J. T. & van Tongeren, J. (1977) Secretin-stimulated serum gastrin levels in hyperparathyroid patients from families with multiple endocrine adenomatosis Type I. *Annals of Internal Medicine*, **86**, 719–724.

3 Lamers, C. B. & Froeling, P. G. (1978) Clinical significance of hyperparathyroidism in familial multiple endocrine adenomatosis type I (MEA I). *American Journal of Medicine*, **66**, 422–424.

4 McCarthy, D. M., Peikin, S. R., Lopatin, R. N. *et al.* (1979) Hyperparathyroidism – a reversible cause of cimetidine-resistant gastric hypersecretion. *British Medical Journal*, **i,** 1765–1766.

5 Majewski, J. T. & Wilson, S. D. (1979) The MEA I syndrome: an all or none phenomenon. *Surgery*, **86**, 475–484.

6 Young, A. E., Gaunt, J. I., Croft, D. N. *et al.* (1983) Location of parathyroid adenomas by thallium-201 and technetium-99^m subtraction scanning. *British Medical Journal*, **286**, 1384–1386.

Chapter 10
The Acute Abdomen

INTESTINAL OBSTRUCTION AND ILEUS

Intestinal obstruction is one of the common causes of the 'acute abdomen' and afflicted patients require carefully conducted but energetic management. Inappropriate or ill-timed measures substantially increase the hazards of an already dangerous condition.

Intestinal obstruction implies a failure to propagate the intestinal contents. The method of obstruction, rapidity of onset and anatomical site in the intestine determine the presentation and likely consequences. It is the consequences of the obstruction which in turn determine the management. The distinction between obstruction and ileus is essentially one of degree since there is failure of propagation in both conditions. Ileus, however, implies a transient loss of normal myoelectrical activity such as occurs after operation, which reverts spontaneously or with a little therapeutic help. However, peristalsis is increased in true obstruction in an attempt to overcome the obstruction. The effects of ileus are usually less dramatic and dangerous than true obstruction but the important distinction between ileus and obstruction is that the latter may require urgent surgery.

PATHOPHYSIOLOGY

The pathophysiology of obstruction varies with the mechanism of obstruction and the site.

Mechanical obstruction

Acute obstruction to the passage of intestinal contents, whether it be from luminal or extraluminal causes, produces a progressive rise in luminal pressure and distension of the gut wall, with increase in bowel wall tension. The progressive rise of pressure and bowel wall tension is periodically punctuated by peristaltic waves which superimpose a sharp increase of pressure.

The increase in pressure is painful because of the increasing tension on the bowel wall. The background pain is in some measure proportional to the luminal pressure and to this is added the waves of colic which characterize small bowel obstruction. The periodicity and character of the colic reflects the site of the obstruction. For example, in high duodenal obstruction colic is slight because the stomach and duodenum do not produce closed segments ahead of a peristaltic wave. Further down the small intestine pain becomes progressively more severe as more segments become closed by peristalsis. Furthermore the frequency of the peristaltic waves is fairly rapid, in contrast to the large bowel where periodicity is relatively slow.

The increasing pressure and bowel wall tension affects mucosal and submucosal capillary blood flow and also mucosal secretion and absorption. Absorption is reduced relative to secretion with a net accumulation of luminal fluid and electrolytes. Failure of water and electrolyte transport may in part be due to reduced visceral blood flow, hypoxia and reduction of tissue ATP.[4] It may also be partly a direct response to increased luminal pressure.

The increase in luminal pressure progressively reduces bowel wall blood flow until the gut becomes so ischaemic that it infarcts. The mucosal villi are the most vulnerable to ischaemia. They are lost after about 1 hour of ischaemia, but will regenerate rapidly from the crypts if the ischaemia is relieved. After about 4 hours the whole wall becomes infarcted. Because of irregularities in the distribution of bowel wall tension, ischaemia and infarction tend to be patchy.

The rate at which these changes occur, in response to simple mechanical obstruction such as a band adhesion, is relatively slow because the intestine can decompress proximally for some time. A closed loop obstruction, such as an ileal volvulus round a band, produces a rapid rise in luminal pressure, hence early ischaemia. Consequently there is a greater risk of intestinal perforation and peritonitis.

The local changes in luminal pressure, fluid flux, intestinal blood flow and mucosal permeability induce profound systemic changes.

Failure of fluid and electrolyte absorption produces a progressive contraction of the extracellular compartment and circulating volume as the fluid accumulates within the lumen. Vomiting accentuates the fluid depletion. The visceral vascular volume also increases,[6] which further reduces cardiac output. These changes lead ultimately to hypovolaemic shock.

Changes in luminal permeability allow absorption of endotoxins and bacteria. Experimentally this is particularly marked in dogs, but there is considerable species variation and fortunately it is not so profound in man.[4] Nevertheless bacteraemia and endotoxaemia do occur, which potentiates the hypovolaemic shock and may precipitate renal failure.

With a closed loop obstruction, flux from the functional body spaces to the obstructed lumen are less pronounced because the volumes involved are proportionately smaller. However, the changes in intestinal permeability are more rapid. Endotoxaemia occurs early and is rapidly followed by spreading peritonitis and free perforation.

Similar changes are produced by acute mesenteric vascular occlusion (see Chapter 5).

Strangulation

When a piece of intestine passes through a narrow aperture, for example the neck of an inguinal hernia, or the paracolic space of an end left iliac fossa colostomy, there is a risk of vascular occlusion. The risk is increased if the intestine becomes fixed and irreducible. In these circumstances the veins become obstructed and even occluded, causing interstitial oedema and a rise in visceral tissue pressure. Ultimately the pressure is sufficient to prevent capillary flow and then obstruct the arterial supply. It is this progressive and sequential reduction of the blood supply which defines strangulation. The strangulated gut is ischaemic and will infarct unless the strangulation is relieved rapidly. The sequence is accelerated if the irreducibility is associated with luminal obstruction, which contributes to the rise in tension.

The effect of strangulating a loop of bowel within the abdomen is similar to a closed loop obstruction because the bowel wall rapidly becomes permeable, producing peritonitis. However, body fluid changes are usually relatively minor. When strangulation occurs in a hernial sac then the perforation produces local spreading cellulitis and abscess formation. Occasionally this may be complicated by synergistic gangrene of the groin.

Intussusception

Intussusception is an unusual form of luminal obstruction which occurs most commonly in children. Submucosal lymphoid aggregates may enlarge sufficiently to project into the lumen when infants are exposed to foreign antigens. This projection becomes caught in peristaltic waves and is propelled down the intestine invaginating the bowel wall as it goes. Occasionally a polyp may be at the head of an intussusception, particularly in adults. The most common intussusception is ileo-ileal, but ileocolic or colo-colic variants may also occur. While the intussusceptum causes obstruction the physiological changes are minor. Severe colic dominates the picture, not only because the gut is distended by the intussusceptum, but also because the mesentery is stretched and the intussusceptum rapidly becomes ischaemic. The engorged and ischaemic intussusceptum bleeds, producing redcurrant stools, which are the hallmark of this disorder.

Ileus

Ileus differs from mechanical obstruction in so far as there is a failure of organized peristalsis which is either complete or partial. Myoelectric potentials disappear, producing a failure of antegrade pacing and contraction. The intestine becomes flaccid and functionally obstructed.

Excess sympathetic activity has been suggested as a possible mechanism[21] particularly after surgery, major injury and burns. This may also explain the ileus which follows head injury, retroperitoneal haematomas and urinary extravasation. Vasopressin, which is released after injury, may be another cause of ileus. Experimentally infused vasopressin abolishes small bowel electrical activity and inhibits peristalsis. The intestine dilates and becomes flaccid.[18] Somatostatin has a similar effect on the ileum when infused intravenously. Somatostatin and other enteric hormones are released by injury and therefore may also be causes of ileus.[23]

Electrolyte disturbances, particularly hypokalaemia and hypomagnesaemia, are important causes or potentiators of ileus. Ileus or pseudo-obstruction may also be produced by anti-parkinsonian and anti-cholinergic drugs, as well as a number of other drugs.[2, 7]

Small bowel secretion is normal but absorption is reduced and fluid accumulates in the intestinal lumen. Because the fluid is evenly distributed throughout the intestine and peristalsis is absent or disorganized, the luminal pressure and bowel wall tension are relatively low. The vascular supply is therefore not so embarrassed and the risk of ischaemia and infarction is low. Pain is also rarely an important feature of ileus. However, the accumulation of fluids and electrolyte in the transcellular space not only causes vomiting but also reduces the functional extracellular compartment and blood volume. This produces dehydration, which may lead to shock and renal failure. Stasis also produces intestinal bacterial overgrowth, causing diarrhoea as motility returns. The toxaemia occasionally seen in cases with prolonged ileus may also be due to the bacterial overgrowth and endotoxin absorption.

Chronic obstruction

When obstruction occurs gradually, the pressure changes in the intestine, and its effect on the circulation is less dramatic than in acute obstruction. There is compensatory muscular hypertrophy which produces marked thickening of the bowel wall as well as visceral dilatation. Peristaltic activity appears to be increased producing recurrent colic and visible peristalsis, which are common clinical features. Intestinal dilation proximal to the obstruction reduces the net absorption of nutrients, fluid and electrolytes, which, combined with bacterial overgrowth, produces diarrhoea and malabsorption.

Examples of chronic small bowel obstruction are seen in patients with strictures from Crohn's disease, radiation enteritis or carcinoid tumours.

Persistent diarrhoea leads to dehydration and hypovolaemia and the kidneys compensate by maximally conserving salt and water. Malabsorption particularly of fat and protein often causes weight loss, sometimes to the point of obvious malnutrition. Malabsorption of specific factors such as folate and B_{12} produce anaemia, while zinc and magnesium produce rashes, ileus and aesthenia.[13, 27]

Chronic large bowel obstruction, such as stricture formation from recurrent sigmoid diverticulitis, produces a different clinical picture. Fluid and electrolyte disturbance is infrequent. Bowel disturbance dominates the picture. Nonetheless hypokalaemia may occur if the obstruction is due to a mucous-secreting carcinoma present in a villous adenoma.

Neonatal obstruction

Small and large bowel obstruction in neonates and infants is more dramatic than in adults. The pathophysiology is similar but the viscera are proportionally larger in the infant and have a correspondingly greater blood supply. The gut wall is less robust, more liable to ischaemia and, because of its immaturity, more permeable to toxins and bacteria. Consequently dehydration, circulatory collapse and septicaemia occur rapidly and require early recognition and appropriate management.

SYMPTOMATOLOGY

Neonates

Neonates with intestinal obstruction present a more dramatic picture than most adults. The period when they are restless, fractious, vomit and have abdominal distension is often short. Vascular collapse rapidly supervenes in an infant with sunken eyes, hypotension and tachycardia. Visible peristalsis in a distended abdomen is common when the obstruction is in the distal jejunum or ileum. The distension will only be epigastric in cases of duodenal atresia.

If the obstruction occurs in utero then there is no meconium in the rectum. In contrast, neonates with meconium ileus from mucoviscidosis or Hirschsprung's disease often have some meconium in the rectum, which is released after a digital examination. Bowel sounds are often absent for prolonged periods in neonatal obstruction and when present are more musical than in obstructed adults.

Infants

Infants with intussusception present with waves of colic initially interspersed with periods free from symptoms. The child may suddenly become pale, draw up the knees and cry out. As the symptoms progress the child may vomit and there may be signs of obstruction. A mass is often palpable in the right upper quadrant between bouts of colic. Blood or blood and mucus (redcurrant jelly) is passed per rectum once the intussusception is well established and the intussusceptum is ischaemic. Occasionally the intussusceptum is palpable per rectum.

Peritonitis supervenes if the condition is allowed to progress and the intussusceptum becomes gangrenous.

Adults

Adults with obstruction develop their symptomatic picture more gradually and therefore the signs are more obvious at presentation.

Proximal small bowel obstruction, particularly duodenal obstruction from such conditions as carcinoma of the pancreas, carcinoma of the hepatic flexure, or duodenal haematomas, is usually associated with little or no pain. Vomiting becomes progressive and copious. If the obstruction is distal to the ampulla, the vomit is bile stained and often contains undigested food particles from two or three earlier meals. Gastric distension is often marked, filling the upper abdomen, and this is associated with a succussion splash. Dehydration becomes obvious after two or three days with sunken eyes, lax skin and a dry mouth, when some 30% of the extracellular fluid is lost.

Associated symptoms such as steatorrhoea and progressive jaundice are common in patients with pancreatic carcinoma. Mid-gut obstruction anywhere from the mid-jejunum to the distal ileum differs in that colic precedes the vomiting. Pain is progressively more severe the further down the small bowel the obstruction occurs. Similarly vomiting is usually late in the clinical picture except in those circumstances when severe pain induces vomiting. When vomiting occurs, it rapidly becomes 'faeculent', brown and offensive due to bacterial contamination and fermentation.

Abdominal distension is also usually greater the more distal the obstruction. It is also greater and more gradual in onset with incomplete small bowel obstruction. The onset of dehydration is slower because the relatively unaffected proximal small bowel is capable of absorbing fluid and electrolytes. The extracellular space equilibrates with the enlarging intraluminal third space.

Bowel sounds are often very active in the early stages. This is followed by periods of silence interspersed by tinkles, as the fluid flows from one gas-filled segment to the next, or by rushes of borborygmi. Borborygmi are usually preceded and accompanied by a burst of colic and visible peristalsis migrating towards the right iliac fossa.

Constipation and lack of flatus are unreliable signs of small bowel obstruction since the colon initially contains faeces which in turn generates flatus. If the small bowel obstruction is incomplete then it may be accompanied by profuse diarrhoea, which is so often a feature of obstructing Crohn's disease. The symptoms in patients with a closed loop obstruction develop rapidly, often without much vomiting or distension. The colic has a crescendo pattern and as the loop becomes ischaemic so the pain becomes continuous. This is followed by signs of peritoneal irritation and endotoxaemia. If treatment is delayed, perforation occurs which leads to generalized peritonitis. The patient develops a thin, thready pulse, shallow respiration and a still, rigid, silent abdomen with percussion tenderness. It is vitally important to scrutinize the hernial orifices in any patient with the clinical features of obstruction. If a hernia is the cause of obstruction it is usually painful and there is often a tender swelling.

Inguinal, femoral and even para-umbilical hernias are often difficult to feel in the obese or when small. A knuckle of bowel may become caught, strangulating a small disc of the ileal wall, producing the so-called Richter's hernia. Obturator hernias are rare and seldom diagnosed preoperatively, but they may sometimes present with pain down the inner aspect of the ipsilateral thigh.

Large bowel obstruction

The onset of colonic obstruction is usually gradual, particularly when the cause is carcinoma, diverticular disease, ischaemia or Crohn's disease. However, large bowel obstruction is occasionally acute both in the disorders already considered but, more commonly, in volvulus of the sigmoid colon, caecum or, rarely, the transverse colon. The history is usually one of a change of bowel habit, either of progressive constipation or of diarrhoea culminating in absolute constipation and no flatus. The associated colic is normally of low periodicity on a background of lower abdominal discomfort and an urge to defecate. Abdominal distension is progressive and often impressive. Right iliac fossa pain and tenderness is a grave sign for it usually signifies caecal ischaemia and impending perforation, in the face of a competent ileocaecal valve. The caecum is at risk of perforation if the diameter exceeds 10 cm radiologically. The history is usually longer if the ileocaecal valve is incompetent since the colon is decompressed into the ileum.

Colonic volvulus occurs when the caecum or sigmoid is on a long mesentery and in the case of a sigmoid volvulus when the mesentery has a narrow base. A long sigmoid mesentery may be a congenital abnormality or it may be acquired with a megacolon. In contrast, a right colic mesentery is the result of a minor failure of intestinal rotation and fixation. Volvulus occurs suddenly with rapidly recurring pain in the right iliac fossa in the case of the caecum, and low on the left in the case of the sigmoid. Sigmoid volvulus is associated with an inability to pass faeces and flatus usually in the face of a strong desire to do so. Abdominal distension is massive. Sometimes spontaneous reduction occurs with an eruption of copious diarrhoea and an explosion of flatus which resolves the abdominal distension. Sigmoid volvulus is frequently intermittent and occurs commonly in subjects who take a very high fibre diet, for example, Africans. In the West it may occur in young women with a history of constipation,[30] in the elderly and, in particular, in those who are confined to mental institutions. The latter group of patients tend to acquire a megacolon from chronic constipation.

INVESTIGATION

Investigations are suitably divided into those which help confirm the diagnosis and those which facilitate management.

Diagnostic investigation

Plain abdominal radiographs are the most useful preliminary investigation and these often provide the final diagnosis. For example, the double bubble of gastric and duodenal distension in neonates is diagnostic of duodenal atresia. Similarly small bowel obstruction with the distal loops of ileum containing opaque meconium peppered with gas is typical of infants with meconium ileus.

Adults with small bowel obstruction show the ladder pattern of dilated loops of bowel with visible valvulae conniventes and multiple fluid levels on the erect film. The colon is relatively free of gas, in contrast to patients with prolonged ileus when the entire intestine is equally gas filled and the fluid levels are more numerous but smaller (Figure 10.1). Rarely large radiopaque gallstones may be visible in the right iliac fossa in elderly patients with gallstone ileus. In such cases the biliary tree may be outlined by gas from the duodenobiliary fistula. Free gas outside the bowel and under the diaphragm indicates perforation.

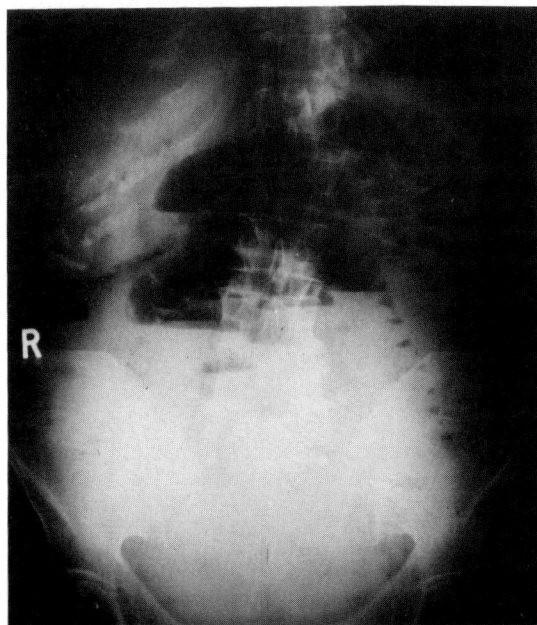

Fig. 10.1 An erect, plain abdominal radiograph of a female with complete small bowel obstruction. Note the gas-filled loops of small intestine with multiple fluid levels in the upper abdomen. Fluid fills the lower abdomen and there is no gas in the colon, in contrast to intestinal ileus. Radiograph courtesy of Dr D. J. Nolan.

The plain radiograph should include the pelvis, particularly in obese subjects. Gas shadows outside the pelvis in patients with obstruction may imply that a strangulated hernia is the cause of obstruction.

In patients with closed loop obstruction there is sometimes a single very dilated gas/fluid-filled loop in an otherwise normal abdominal radiograph.

Colonic obstruction is diagnosed by a grossly dilated colon with a normal small bowel pattern if the ileocaecal valve is competent. The caecum is sometimes grossly distended in comparison to the remaining colon. Occasionally there is a sharp cut off in the gas shadow, for example in the descending colon at the point where a carcinoma is causing obstruction. In these circumstances the rectum and distal colon contain little or no gas, but may contain visible faeces. Patients with colonic volvulus usually show a single loop of massively dilated colon, the apex of the loop directed to the right upper quadrant in sigmoid volvulus, whereas the axis for caecal volvulus is from the right iliac fossa to the left upper quadrant.

Free gas under the diaphragm, in the flanks or in the bowel wall are all signs of perforation or gangrene of the colon.

Occasionally the clinical picture of small bowel obstruction is not obvious. This is particularly so following abdominal irradiation, or postoperatively when the main differential diagnosis is a prolonged ileus, similarly when the obstruction is incomplete, or in cases of distal duodenal obstruction where pain is absent but vomiting is profuse. In such cases contrast radiology is most valuable and the best method is the small bowel 'enema'.[22] A careful examination will show the point of obstruction (Figure 10.2) and often gives the cause, such as a duodenal haematoma or Crohn's disease (Figure 10.3). Dilute barium above an obstruction rarely precipitates complete obstruction.

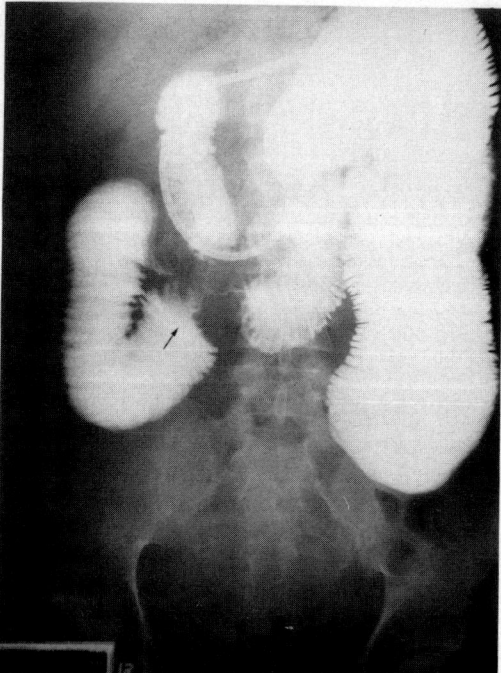

Fig. 10.3   A barium examination in a patient with duodenal obstruction. The third part of the duodenum is obstructed by a spontaneous duodenal haematoma (arrow). Note that the mucosal pattern within the stenosis is normal, signifying extrinsic compression. From Nolan, D. J. (1983) *Radiological Atlas of Gastrointestinal Disease*, with kind permission of the author and the publisher, John Wiley.

Similarly, in patients with a clinical diagnosis of colonic obstruction this can readily be confirmed by barium enema, which has the additional advantage of demonstrating the exact site of obstruction. This allows all the therapeutic options to be considered systematically rather than relying on an emergency laparotomy and a right upper quadrant colostomy.

Supplementary investigations

Some elementary investigations are necessary to enable a patient with obstruction to be managed adequately. The haemoglobin level, PCV and white cell count are important baseline measurements. A high haemoglobin and PCV with a correspondingly raised white cell count indicates dehydration and a reduction of extracellular fluid which requires correction before operation. A crude measure of the fluid and electrolyte replacement required for a 10% rise in haemoglobin is 10% of total body water, or about 4 litres in the average adult. Half of this volume should be of balanced electrolyte solution (Hartmann's) to replace the extracellular fluid and the remainder as dextrose to replace the intracellular fluid.

A disproportionate rise or fall in white cell count may signify septicaemia or toxaemia, which requires prompt administration of antibiotics.

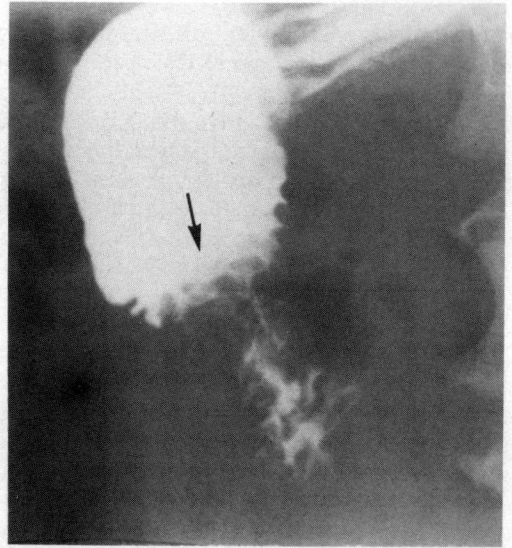

Fig. 10.2   A small bowel barium examination showing a narrowed area (arrow) in the jejunum which is producing sub-acute small bowel obstruction. From Nolan, D. J. (1984) in *Diagnostic Radiology* (Ed.) Grainger, R. G. & Allison, D. J., with kind permission of the author and the publisher, Churchill Livingstone.

Urea and electrolyte estimations are also important and, when possible, a creatinine level. Serum urea levels are frequently high, indicating dehydration and some prerenal failure. As with a high haemoglobin level, a rise in urea will indicate the amount of fluid replacement necessary, particularly when the creatinine level is normal. Electrolyte levels are frequently normal in the presence of dehydration but the potassium levels may be high if there is established renal failure or a metabolic acidosis. Hyponatraemia occurs with high intestinal obstruction where electrolyte-rich vomit is replaced by water.

Hypochloraemia follows pyloric stenosis and may be accompanied by an alkalosis, but there is seldom alteration of the acid–base balance when the obstruction is beyond the duodenum, the exception being when severe dehydration reduces tissue perfusion, which in turn produces lactic acidaemia and renal failure. In the very ill patient with obstruction it is therefore important to estimate blood pH and gases.

Sometimes patients present with obstruction and anaemia, for example from a long-standing carcinoma of the colon. If the anaemia is severe it will probably require replacement before or during surgery to relieve the obstruction. More commonly, occult anaemia is revealed by rehydration.

Urinalysis on admission is crucial. The urine should be concentrated and free of cells and casts in dehydrated patients who otherwise have healthy kidneys, but when tubular necrosis is occurring the specific gravity falls. Microscopic haematuria may occur in patients with ureteric obstruction, urinary extravasation and intestinal meteorism, which may mimic an acute abdomen and obstruction.[15]

Elderly patients require an ECG both for pre-operative anaesthetic assessment and to anticipate problems produced by rapid intravenous rehydration. A chest X-ray is also important for the same reasons, and to detect pulmonary metastases from a primary obstructing carcinoma or air under the diaphragm. The knowledge of pulmonary metastases obviously influences the subsequent management.

Less important investigations which may yield additional information in patients who are apparently obstructed are liver function tests, blood gases, blood film, mean cell volume (MCV), and tests of thyroid function. A raised MCV in an otherwise curiously unwell patient with a tender, distended but soft abdomen suggests a diagnosis of alcohol withdrawal. This would be supported by disordered liver function tests. Altered liver function tests may also signify

hepatic metastases, infection or malnutrition. Occasionally myxoedema presents with colonic pseudo-obstruction.

Blood culture is most important for patients with endotoxaemia or who are clinically septic.

MANAGEMENT

Superficially the management of a patient with obstruction is simple. The case is an emergency and the obstruction requires relieving surgically at the earliest opportunity to prevent perforation. This view has led to the widely held aphorism, 'Never let the sun set on a case of obstruction.' Enthusiastic adherence to this aphorism has lead many an eager but inexperienced surgeon to plunge into a pot of trouble in the middle of the night when calmer reflection might have circumnavigated the problems.

Nearly all patients presenting with obstruction are dehydrated, which will be increased both by operation and the failure of the intestine to absorb fluid postoperatively.[29] Operating in the face of dehydration is hazardous because the cardiovascular system becomes unstable under anaesthetic. If the blood pressure drops precipitously, cardiac, cerebral or renal damage may follow, making the postoperative course difficult.

Most of the patients are elderly and so a few hours are well spent rehydrating them as quickly as their cardiovascular systems will tolerate, and undertaking the simple initial investigations outlined. These few hours allow the patient to be reviewed clinically and a sound management policy to be followed.

Elderly, severely dehydrated or toxic patients are best catheterized, not only to obtain a urine sample but also to monitor the urine output hourly for the first 12–24 hours.

Similarly patients who are toxic or septic should receive a broad-spectrum antibiotic such as a second-generation cephalosporin and a 1 g metronidazole suppository (which is cheaper and almost as effective as i.v. metronidazole) after a blood culture has been taken.

It is best to take a longer view with adequate radiological assessment if the diagnosis of the obstruction is in doubt – for example postoperatively, after irradiation, or in patients receiving chemotherapy when there is some ileus.[2] Similarly pseudo-obstruction should be considered, and operation avoided, in patients suffering from diabetes, scleroderma, hypertension, Parkinson's disease and the rare idiopathic familial pseudo-obstruction.[7, 28] Also patients suffering an acute exacerbation of Crohn's disease should be given a trial of medical therapy, because there is hardly ever an indication for emergency operation in obstructive Crohn's disease.

Patients in whom the obstruction is mainly functional should be supported by parenteral nutrition while the ileus resolves or responds to therapy such as steroids in the case of Crohn's disease or triiodothyronine for myxoedema.[1] Parenteral nutrition should be started as soon as the fluid and electrolyte status has been corrected if it is anticipated that the ileus will last 7 days or longer, or if there is pre-existing clinical evidence of malnutrition, such as weight loss or hypoalbuminaemia. Alternatively if the ileus has not resolved after 5 days of conservative fluid therapy then total parenteral nutrition should be started. Parenteral nutrition is particularly valuable in subacute small bowel obstruction complicating Crohn's disease or radiotherapy. Patients with small bowel obstruction should have a fairly wide bore (14 FG) Ryle's tube passed into the stomach to alleviate repeated vomiting. This decompresses the stomach and the proximal small bowel and also minimizes the increase in intestinal distension.

It is important to empty the stomach if an anaesthetic is contemplated in order to reduce the risk of inhaling vomit on induction and subsequent inhalation pneumonia.

Long mercury-filled tubes are popular, particularly in America, to decompress the distended ileum either preoperatively or in an attempt to obviate operation.[3, 24] The method relies on the propagation of the mercury-tipped tube down the intestine while the tube is continually aspirated. Unquestionably it can be effective in decompressing the intestine in some cases but no controlled studies exist to compare this type of decompression against conventional nasogastric aspiration. In patients with subacute obstruction or ileus, for whom the mercury filled tube might be beneficial, they may also fail to propagate it sufficiently for decompression to be effective.

It must be stressed that it is best to avoid a laparotomy in patients with symptoms of obstruction who have received abdominal irradiation or recent anticancer chemotherapy, where the diagnosis is pseudo-obstruction, after recent abdominal surgery, or in patients with acute Crohn's disease, unless a definite and culpable mechanical abnormality can be demonstrated radiologically. Otherwise it is better to be prepared for a fairly protracted course and feed the patient parenterally. Oral intake should be restricted unless the stomach is decompressed by a nasogastric tube.

Mechanical obstruction

Patients who have a confident clinical diagnosis of a closed loop obstruction, strangulation, or an irreducible hernia require urgent surgery after a brief period of resuscitation and assessment. In contrast, patients with incomplete obstruction, or obstruction which can be decompressed orally, and those without symptoms or signs of peritonitis may be rehydrated more leisurely and operated upon the following day. Operations for intestinal obstruction can be difficult and are better performed during daylight when the surgeon and theatre staff are at their best. Nocturnal operations nearly always take longer than necessary, and more mistakes are made at night when the medical team are tired and there are fewer trained theatre staff available. These factors are responsible for a higher incidence of postoperative morbidity.

All patients who have a deliberate or unintentional enterotomy, or in whom the viability of intestine is doubtful, require prophylactic i.v. antibiotics during the operation and possibly a further dose 4 hours later.[14]

Inguinal hernia

When an inguinal hernia obstructs there is a risk of strangulation, perforation and severe spreading cellulitis. Operation should therefore be prompt. A standard incision is made, the hernial sac delivered and the neck of the sac enlarged laterally to allow reduction. If the viability of the intestine is doubtful, it is first reduced and then reinspected in 10 minutes or so when viability should be obvious. If the ileum is gangrenous then a resection with an end-to-end anastomosis is required. The hernia is subsequently repaired in the usual fashion.[17]

Femoral hernia

The best approaches for obstructed and possibly gangrenous femoral hernias are: (a) the preperitoneal approach (Nyhus), (b) the pararectal (McEvedy) approach, or (c) the lower midline (Henry) approach. The high approaches allow the femoral canal to be enlarged medially, the sac and intestine to be delivered and a resection to be performed if necessary. If there is a gangrenous Richter's hernia then a wedge excision of the necrotic segment and a two-layer closure is sufficient.[19]

An advantage of the Henry approach is that it readily allows both femoral orifices to be closed. The McEvedy incision allows the hernia to be approached first from below and, if the hernia can then be reduced and repaired without resection, an abdominal incision is avoided. This is a major advantage in elderly people, in whom femoral hernias are common, and who are also at risk of hypostatic pneumonia.

Umbilical hernias rarely cause obstruction but may do so when they are large. The neck of the hernia usually needs enlarging to reduce the obstructed bowel. Occasionally, in very ill and obese patients with respiratory difficulty, it is unwise to reduce and repair the hernia. In this situation the neck of the sac is enlarged to relieve the obstruction and the defect is left wide. Rare internal hernias such as the obturator, paraduodenal, para-ileostomy or paracolostomy hernias are seldom diagnosed preoperatively.

Intra-abdominal adhesive obstruction

A generous midline or paramedian incision is required for adhesive obstruction. The dilated obstructed bowel is delivered into the wound and followed to the point of obstruction. The ileum distal to the obstruction remains collapsed. The obstruction may simply be due to a single band adhesion which, when divided, releases the obstruction. A band may provide the pivot for a small bowel volvulus or form the neck of a closed loop obstruction. Again division of the band releases the obstructed bowel.

At the other extreme there may be dense adhesions producing progressive obstruction, for example after abdominal irradiation, multiple abdominal operations or severe peritonitis. Such circumstances lead to a long, tedious and often difficult operation. The adhesions require careful division until the entire small bowel is free from one end to the other. Sometimes this approach is too hazardous with the risk of numerous accidental enterotomies which may result in enterocutaneous fistula. Irradiated intestine is particularly prone to fistulate if damaged because of the compromised blood supply. When the risks of lysing the adhesions are too great then the obstruction is bypassed by anastomosing the proximal dilated bowel to a convenient collapsed loop of either ileum or colon. Occasionally it is more appropriate to resect the matted mass of small bowel and fashion an end-to-end anastomosis.

Intraoperative decompression and stenting the bowel postoperatively are two controversial techniques which are sometimes advocated. Decompression of the dilated intestine through an enterotomy, with a sucker, efficiently removes the copious stagnant fluid and gas from the lumen. This reduces the volume of the intes-

tine to manageable proportions and greatly facilitates the operation, particularly closure of the abdomen. However, the enterotomy converts a clean operation, with small risks of postoperative sepsis, into a potentially or frankly contaminated operation with substantially greater chances of infection even after prophylactic antimicrobial therapy. Aspiration of the intestinal contents increases mucosal secretion and therefore fluid and electrolyte loss from the functional extracellular fluid into the gut lumen.[12] This loss requires parenteral replacement.

Alternatively the gut may be decompressed by 'milking' the contents in a retrograde manner into the stomach, whence it is aspirated through a wide-bore nasogastric tube. This method is not particularly efficient and requires considerable handling of the intestine, which may prolong postoperative ileus. It is probably best to reserve decompression for the occasions when closure of the abdomen is going to be particularly difficult and then to do it effectively through an enterotomy.

Stenting the intestine in a ladder pattern of loops by means of long aspiration tube is popular with some surgeons.[5, 31] The tube is inserted through a proximal jejunal enterotomy and it is then fed down to the distal ileum. The intestine is then returned to the abdomen in regular loops which are held in place by the intraluminal tube. The proximal end of the tube is exteriorized through a stab incision. The technique is laborious and requires a lot of visceral handling. Although its value is unproven it is useful in cases which have had extensive dissection of adhesions and in particular when fistulas have to be closed. The bowel is not only stented in a position which is less likely to reobstruct, it is also decompressed by continuous aspiration. Stenting is clearly unnecessary for simple volvulus and band adhesion, and the risks of converting a clean into a contaminated operation must again be considered.

Intussusception

The principal investigation is also the method of treatment of early intussusception. Dilute barium is instilled into the rectum and outlines the 'snake's head' of the intussusceptum and demonstrates the obstruction.

If the duration of symptoms is 24 hours or less then an attempt is made to reduce the intussusception by barium enema.[26] The barium is infused using a pressure of no more than 100 cm H_2O, and the bowel screened. Provided the intussusception reduces easily the procedure is continued until normal anatomy is restored. Should the intussusception recur then the procedure may be repeated. When the history is between 24 and 36 hours or there has been copious 'redcurrant jelly' per rectum, barium reduction may be successful but there is a risk of perforation and the procedure is less likely to be successful.

Operation is essential if the history is longer than 36 hours, if there is peritonism, or if the intussusception fails to reduce easily. A laparotomy is performed and a gentle attempt is made to reduce the intussusception. Nothing further is required if this is successful, but if the gut is gangrenous or the reduction fails then a resection with end-to-end anastomosis is necessary.[25]

Large bowel obstruction

Large bowel obstruction presents some of the most difficult surgical problems because the burdens of major surgery on elderly patients are high and the consequences of failure are dangerous. The left colon is a particularly unforgiving structure and anastomoses in the obstructed colon are prone to leak, which is often fatal. Colonic obstruction is commonly an affliction of the elderly, hence it is important to have clear objectives before embarking on surgical treatment.

Right-sided colonic obstruction caused by carcinoma to the right of the mid-transverse colon or by a caecal volvulus which is gangrenous is simply treated by a right or extended right hemicolectomy with an end-to-end ileocolic anastomosis. Caecal volvulus without gangrene may be treated either by resection or, after reduction, by suturing the right colon to the right paracolic gutter. If a patient with obstruction is too ill for general anaesthesia, or if there is none available, then the caecum can be decompressed through a caecostomy under local analgesia.

Primary resection and colo-colic anastomosis is too dangerous for obstruction to the left of the mid-transverse colon. The traditional management is in three stages. A transverse colostomy is raised, then some 2 to 4 weeks later the obstruction is resected. Finally the colostomy is closed after a month or longer. Colostomies closed in less than a month appear to have a high morbidity.[8] While this multistaged approach is safe, it places an enormous burden on elderly patients who, in any event, have less than a 30% chance of surviving five years after resection of an obstructing carcinoma.[10] The stages can be reduced to two, either by closing the colostomy

at the same time as the resection, or performing the resection at the first operation and covering the anastomosis with a colostomy. The former is probably safer. Alternatively a Paul–Mickulicz resection with a double-barrelled colostomy may be carried out if the tumour can be delivered on sufficient mesentery. This operation is safe and the stoma is easily closed after applying an enterotome to the septum. An alternative to the two-staged operations is a total colectomy and ileorectal anastomosis.

Obstructing diverticulitis is difficult. The three-staged operation can be used but if there is a phlegmon then it is preferable to remove the diseased colon by Hartmann's operation.[11] Colonic continuity can be restored later either using a stapling gun or a sutured anastomosis. Occasionally it is possible to relieve the obstruction by a combined longitudinal and horizontal myotomy.[16]

Acute sigmoid volvulus is best deflated by passing a sigmoidoscope or a flatus tube. The aim is to open the twisted distal limb. Success is rewarded by a torrent of flatus and fluid faeces and the patient's abdomen deflates like a punctured balloon. Occasionally a colonoscope is useful and may succeed when the other methods have failed.[9] Recurrent volvulus usually requires elective resection and end-to-end anastomosis. If the volvulus cannot be deflated or the colon is gangrenous an emergency resection is necessary. A Mickulicz resection is adequate if the colon is viable but Hartmann's operation is safer if the colon is gangrenous.[20]

Hirschsprung's disease presenting as acute or chronic obstruction is treated initially by a colostomy (or ileostomy) through ganglionic bowel. When the child has recovered and grown, the defunctioned colon is prepared and the aganglionic segment is resected together with any atonic dilated but ganglionic colon. Continuity is restored by Duhamel's operation or a pull-through procedure.

REFERENCES

1   Batalis, T., Muers, M. & Royle, G. T. (1981) Treatment with intravenous triiodothyronine of colonic pseudo-obstruction caused by myxoedema. *British Journal of Surgery*, **68**, 439.
2   Bates, D. (1981) Drug-induced peripheral neuropathies. *Adverse Drug Reaction Bulletin*, **91**, 332–335.
3   Bizer, L. S., Liebling, R. W., Delaney, H. M. & Gliedman, M. L. (1981) Small bowel obstruction: the role of nonoperative treatment in simple intestinal obstruction and predictive criteria for strangulation obstruction. *Surgery*, **89**, 407–413.
4   Bounos, G., Hampson, L. G. & Gurd, F. N. (1964) Cellular nucleotides in hemorrhagic shock: relationship of intestinal metabolic changes to hemorrhagic enteritis

and the barrier function of intestinal mucosa. *Annals of Surgery*, **160**, 650–668.

5 Close, M. B. & Christensen, N. M. (1979) Transmesenteric small bowel plication or intraluminal tube stenting. Indications and contraindications. *American Journal of Surgery*, **138**, 89–96.

6 Derblom, H., Johansson, H. & Nylander, G. (1963) Vascular patterns of the intestinal villi in the obstructed small bowel of the rat. *Surgery*, **54**, 780–783.

7 Faulk, D. L., Anuras, S. & Christensen, J. (1978) Chronic intestinal pseudo-obstruction. *Gastroenterology*, **74**, 922–931.

8 Finch, D. R. A. (1976) The results of colostomy closure. *British Journal of Surgery*, **63**, 397–399.

9 Ghazi, A., Shinya, H. & Wolff, W. I. (1976) Treatment of volvulus of the colon by colonoscopy. *Annals of Surgery*, **183**, 263–265.

10 Gill, P. G. & Morris, P. J. (1978) Survival with colorectal cancer. *British Journal of Surgery*, **65**, 17–20.

11 Goligher, J. C. (1984) *Surgery of the Anus, Rectum and Colon*. 5th edition. London: Baillière Tindall.

12 Grace, R. H. (1971) The handling of water and electrolytes by the small bowel following the relief of intestinal obstruction. *British Journal of Surgery*, **58**, 760–764.

13 Jaun, D. (1982) Clinical review: the importance of hypomagnesemia. *Surgery*, **91**, 510–517.

14 Keighley, M. R. B. & Burdon, D. W. (1979) *Antimicrobial Prophylaxis in Surgery*. Tunbridge Wells: Pitman Medical.

15 Kettlewell, M., Walker, M., Dudley, N. & DeSouza, B. (1973) Spontaneous extravasation of urine secondary to ureteric obstruction. *British Journal of Urology*, **45**, 8–14.

16 Kettlewell, M. G. W. & Moloney, G. E. (1977) Combined horizontal and longitudinal colomyotomy for diverticular disease: preliminary report. *Diseases of the Colon and Rectum*, **20**, 24–28.

17 Maingot, R. (1980) Operations for inguinal hernia. In *Abdominal Operations*. 7th edition. (Ed.) Maingot, R. pp. 1573–1604. New York: Appleton Century Crofts.

18 Mitchell, A., Macey, D. J. & Collin, J. (1983) A scintigraphic method for the assessment of intraluminal volume and motility of isolated intestinal segments. *Journal of Nuclear Medicine*, **24**, 571–576.

19 Munro, A. K. (1980) Femoral hernia. In *Abdominal Operations*. 7th edition. (Ed.) Maingot, R. pp. 1605–1614. New York: Appleton Century Crofts.

20 Neely, J. (1970) The management of gangrenous sigmoid volvulus. *British Journal of Surgery*, **57**, 670–672.

21 Neely, J. & Catchpole, B. (1971) Ileus: the restoration of alimentary tract motility by pharmacological means. *British Journal of Surgery*, **58**, 21–28.

22 Nolan, D. J. & Marks, C. G. (1981) The barium infusion in small bowel obstruction. *Clinical Radiology*, **32**, 651–655.

23 Ormsbee, H. S., Koehler, S. L. & Telford, G. L. (1978) Somatostatin inhibits motilin induced interdigestive contractile activity in the dog. *Digestive Diseases and Sciences*, **23**, 781–788.

24 Peetz, D. J., Gamelli, R. L. & Pilcher, D. B. (1982) Intestinal intubation in acute, mechanical small bowel obstruction. *Archives of Surgery*, **117**, 334–336.

25 Raudkivi, P. J. & Smith, H. L. M. (1981) Intussusception: analysis of 98 cases. *British Journal of Surgery*, **68**, 645–648.

26 Ravitch, M. M. & McCune, R. M. (1950) Intussusception in infants and children. Analysis of 152 cases with a discussion of reduction by barium enema. *Journal of Pediatrics*, **37**, 153–173.

27 Sandstead, H. H. (1982) The nutritional role of zinc and effects of deficiency. *Current Concepts in Nutrition*, **11**, 97–124.

28 Schuffler, M. D. & Deitch, E. A. (1980) Chronic idiopathic intestinal pseudo-obstruction: a surgical approach. *Annals of Surgery*, **192**, 752–761.

29 Shields, R. (1964) Surgical aspects of the absorption of water and electrolytes by the intestine. *Monographs in Surgical Sciences*, **1**, 119.

30 Smith, R. B., Kettlewell, M. G. & Gough, M. H. (1977) Intermittent volvulus of the sigmoid colon. *British Journal of Surgery*, **64**, 106–109.

31 Weigelt, J. A., Snyder, W. H. & Norman, J. L. (1980) Complications and results of 160 Baker tube plications. *American Journal of Surgery*, **140**, 810–815.

ACUTE APPENDICITIS

More people in Western countries undergo appendicectomy than any other abdominal operation. In my unit serving a population of 60 000, there were 90 appendicectomies performed in 1982, compared with 53 cholecystectomies, 12 operations for peptic ulcer and 23 bowel resections for carcinoma. Yet is is less than 100 years since the first formal appendicectomy was performed.[3, 7]

The vermiform appendix was given that name by Andreas Vesalius in 1543, and John Hunter described a gangrenous appendix encountered at an autopsy he performed on Colonel Dalrymple in 1769.[8] Reginald Heber Fitz of Boston, USA, coined the name 'appendicitis' in a paper given at the inaugural meeting of the Association of American Physicians in 1886. He urged early appendicectomy, but this was not generally accepted for another 20 years.

ANATOMY

The lumen of the appendix is narrow and the muscular wall thick. Its size and position are variable – it may point down into the pelvis, up as far as the gallbladder, or medially either in front of, or behind, loops of ileum. It is capable of both independent and neurogenic contraction, and the diffuse colicky abdominal pain which heralds an attack of appendicitis is almost certainly due to its muscular contractions against an obstruction.

BACTERIOLOGY

The microorganisms found in the appendix are the same as those in the colon. By far the most numerous are *Bacteroides fragilis* and other members of the *Bacteroides* genus. Next in order of frequency is *Escherichia coli*, and then other Gram-negative enterobacteria. *Streptococcus faecalis* and other aerobic and anaerobic streptococci are common, and *Clostridium perfringens* is often found. The following bacterial species were recovered from a series of 474 appendicectomies in which the stump was swabbed: coliforms 76%, *B. fragilis* 40%, *Cl. perfringens* 28%, *Str. faecalis* 5%, and other aerobic and anaerobic streptococci 6%; 13% of the cultures were sterile. In this same series, parietal swabs were taken before skin closure. Sixty-five per cent of these were sterile, 23% showed a single species and 12% showed two or more species.

AETIOLOGY AND EPIDEMIOLOGY

Appendicitis is caused by the invasion of the walls of the organ by bacteria normally resident within its lumen and doing no harm there. Unfortunately we have no knowledge of what mechanism breaks down the mucosal barrier and allows bacterial invasion to occur.

Geographical distribution

Although acute appendicitis is found all over the world, it is much more common in Europe, North America and Australia than in Africa, South America or the Far East. In countries with a low incidence it is rarer in rural than in urban communities, and in poor than in rich people.

Racial factors

In Harare, Zimbabwe, in 1975, 604 white and 95 black people were admitted to hospital with appendicitis[4] and only 22 of the 95 black people came from rural communities. On the other hand, black and white people in the USA have a similar incidence of the disease; it seems probable that genetic factors play little part in the aetiology.

Familial factors

Siblings of a child who has had an operation for acute appendicitis are more likely than other children to come under the care of a surgeon because of suspected appendicitis. This, however, is likely to reflect parental anxiety not to overlook the significance of mild abdominal pain, rather than any inherited liability to the disease.

Dietary factors

The only hypothesis which fits most of the known epidemiological facts is that the disease is associated with a diet low in cellulose and high in meat and sugar. Arthur Rendle Short put forward this hypothesis over 60 years ago,[2] based on a survey of the incidence of acute appendicitis in boys and girls living in private boarding schools compared with those in orphanages. Dennis Burkitt[2] gave the following reasons for believing that removal of cellulose, lignin and other fibre from food is the main cause of appendicitis:

1 In Africa it is rare in blacks but common in white settlers.
2 It is rare in rural communities in developing countries.
3 Its incidence rises with economic development.
4 Its incidence is higher in those who enter educational establishments or migrate to towns.
5 Its incidence is higher in people from developing countries who emigrate to economically developed countries.

Role of obstruction of the lumen of the appendix

It has been customary to classify appendicitis as catarrhal or obstructive. This is of little value, and the disease is probably always due to obstruction of the lumen. Sometimes an obstructing faecolith is found at operation, but quite often the obstruction is due to swelling of the lymphoid tissue in the wall of the appendix (possibly occasioned by specific or non-specific enteritis). In favour of obstruction as the primary event are the facts that the caecal end of the appendix is never inflamed when the distal end is normal, that the inflammation usually stops short at the base of the organ, and that the initial ill-defined colicky abdominal pain is suggestive of a luminal obstruction.

PATHOLOGY

A breach in the mucosa of the appendix allows invasion by microorganisms from the lumen. The organisms first multiply in the submucosa and invade the muscle layers, reaching the peritoneum within a few hours. Further evolution of the disease depends on the adequacy of the inflammatory reaction, which in turn depends on an adequate supply of arterial blood. The usual outcome of an attack of acute appendicitis is resolution, with or without fibrosis, followed weeks or months later by another attack. If, however, the arterial blood supply is cut off by thrombosis, the appendix becomes gangrenous in part or as a whole and, in the absence of operation, perforates. In the meantime, fibrinous adhesions encourage adherence of the appendix to surrounding intestines and the omentum becomes attached, allowing a new blood supply to the gangrenous organ.

In favourable cases the inflammatory reaction digests and removes dead tissues and bacteria and, within a few days, the patient recovers. Subsequent operation shows that the tip of the appendix has disappeared, the stump being sealed off by fibrosis. In less favourable cases the walling-off process may fail, leading to general peritonitis or to a local abscess, which may enlarge and point either in the right iliac fossa, the rectum or the vagina, ultimately discharging its contents.

CLINICAL FEATURES

Uncomplicated acute appendicitis

The classical history of vague diffuse colicky central abdominal pain (accompanied by nausea, anorexia and constipation or diarrhoea), followed within a few hours by pain in the right lower quadrant of the abdomen, is found in only about half of all cases of acute appendicitis. Atypical presentations depend partly on the position of the organ – an inflamed pelvic appendix can simulate cystitis or pelvic inflammatory disease, whereas a high retrocaecal appendix can simulate cholecystitis. Presentation may also depend on the pain threshold of the patient. Patients may present with a fixed mass in the right iliac fossa due to a walled-off perforation of the appendix but deny any symptoms other than mild 'indigestion'.

Physical examination shows a patient who prefers to lie still; there is usually a mild pyrexia (37–38°C), a furred tongue and fetid breath, and tenderness with guarding in the right lower quadrant of the abdomen. There may be tenderness on rectal examination.

Laboratory investigations should not be allowed to take the place of clinical judgement, and should usually be confined to estimation of white cell count.

Perforated appendicitis

The incidence of appendiceal perforation relative to that of uncomplicated appendicitis varies considerably; it is higher in the very young and

very old (possibly because of diagnostic vacillation) and in places where there is a low incidence of appendicitis, and therefore a low incidence of clinical suspicion. In my own practice in 1982 only nine (10%) of the 90 appendicectomies were for perforated appendicitis.

There are three ways in which these patients can present. In the first, the patient may not feel ill enough to seek medical advice until he has an easily palpable fixed tender mass in the right lower abdomen. In the second type of presentation the patient is ill and examination shows tenderness and rigidity in the right lower abdomen. Under general anaesthesia the rigidity disappears and a mass can be felt. The third type of presentation is the very ill patient with generalized abdominal tenderness and rigidity indicative of general peritonitis. If such a patient is denied operation, and if he does not succumb to the infection, he may present later with residual intraperitoneal or extraperitoneal local or distant abscesses, with intestinal obstruction or even with pyrexia of unknown origin.

DIFFERENTIAL DIAGNOSIS

Non-specific abdominal pain and mesenteric adenitis

In children this is the most frequent diagnostic dilemma. On the one hand no surgeon wants to remove an uninflamed appendix, but, on the other hand, delay in removing an inflamed one may lead to the dangerous sequelae of gangrene and perforation. It is my policy to encourage the removal of the appendix from any child who complains of right-sided abdominal pain, but this results in 20% of the appendices removed being normal. I followed up 238 children after 5 to 11 years whose uninflamed appendices had been removed (mainly for recurrent abdominal pain), and compared their subsequent histories with those of 208 children whose acutely inflamed appendices had been removed. I found that 80% of the former and 92% of the latter had had no further attacks of abdominal pain.

Enteritis

Diarrhoea may be common in acute appendicitis and lead to dangerous diagnostic confusion with specific or non-specific enteritis. If a child does not respond rapidly to rehydration, and if he is tender on palpation in the right lower abdomen, he should have his appendix removed without waiting for the results of stool culture.

Crohn's disease and *Yersinia enterocolitica* infection

Acute Crohn's disease and *Yersinia* infection present a clinical picture which may be indistinguishable from acute appendicitis. If acute ileitis rather than appendicitis is found at operation, the abdomen should be closed without removing either appendix or ileum and right colon, since the disease in the terminal ileum nearly always resolves.

Acute pancreatitis and perforated peptic ulcer

In both these conditions, irritating fluid may leak into the paracaecal area and cause tenderness and rigidity indistinguishable from that caused by appendicitis.

Pelvic inflammatory disease

The symptoms and signs of pelvic appendicitis and salpingitis are very similar. If the patient's tongue is furred and the breath fetid, appendicitis is more likely.

TREATMENT

Acute appendicitis should normally be treated by early operation, except when a fixed mass is felt in the right lower abdomen, indicating a walled-off perforation. Such a patient is best treated conservatively, the appendix being removed a month or two later. Another possible exception is a mild attack of appendicitis under circumstances where the operation might be more dangerous than the disease. Most attacks of appendicitis will resolve and operation may be deferred until it can be performed with safety.

Antibiotics

Antibiotics should be used during the conservative management of an appendix mass or an appendix abscess. Antibiotics should also be used where there is diffuse peritonitis.

The most common complication following appendicectomy is wound infection, which is usually minor and occurs after discharge from hospital. Infection is distressing to the patient and its incidence can be considerably reduced by the administration of a single dose of an effective antibiotic. More prolonged antibiotic cover may be necessary if the appendix has perforated or is gangrenous.

The choice of antibiotic for prophylaxis and treatment remains controversial. There is evidence that *B. fragilis* acts synergistically with aerobic coliform organisms and that metronidazole is effective alone as a prophylactic agent. It is wiser, however, to give protection against both aerobic and anaerobic organisms, especially if the appendix has perforated.

Technique of appendicectomy

The 'grid-iron' muscle-splitting incision in the right iliac fossa is much to be preferred to a laparotomy. It is more comfortable for the patient, carries a low risk of wound infection and an even lower risk of incisional herniation. It can, if necessary, be extended to become a transverse muscle-cutting laparotomy. As for the appendix stump, it is traditional to bury it by means of an absorbable purse-string suture in the caecum, but this is sometimes impossible and patients seem to come to no harm if it is omitted.

THE USE OF DRAINS

Few surgeons still think that drainage of the peritoneal cavity is of any value in patients with general peritonitis, but a number do continue to leave drains in the right iliac fossa after removing a perforated appendix. A random control clinical trial in my unit,[5] however, showed that the insertion or omission of a transperitoneal drain made no difference to the incidence of postoperative septic complications.

THE QUESTION OF SKIN SUTURES

Many surgeons continue to approximate the skin with vertical mattress sutures of braided or monofilament man-made fibre after potentially contaminated abdominal operations. We have shown, however,[6] that the incidence of wound infection is significantly lower when the skin is approximated with metal clips, and clip closure is now our standard method.

When the abdominal wall is grossly contaminated, as it always is during an operation for bacterial peritonitis, it is advisable to leave the skin open and either close it secondarily or leave it to granulate and heal by second intention.[1]

COMPLICATIONS

Apart from the non-specific complications of any abdominal operation (pneumonia, thromboembolism, retention of urine, wound failure) the complications of appendicitis and appendicectomy are either septic or mechanical.

Septic complications

WOUND INFECTION

Division of the base of the appendix exposes the operation site to enteric bacteria, which may result in wound infection, nearly always minor; 79% of the 57 wound infections in my personal series of 474 appendicectomies manifested themselves after the patients had left hospital. In carefully documented series the incidence of wound infection lies between 7 and 12% (excluding perforated appendixes). It can be reduced by the use of appropriate prophylactic antibiotics and by the avoidance of vertical mattress skin sutures.

INTRAPERITONEAL ABSCESSES

Abscesses in the pelvis, right lower abdomen or elsewhere in the abdomen are much more common after removal of a gangrenous or perforated appendix, but may occur even after removal of a normal appendix in patients whose defences are impaired. Suspicion is aroused by persistence of pyrexia and usually confirmed by abdominal and rectal examination. In difficult cases, when neither examination reveals the site of an abscess, grey scale ultrasound examination or CT scanning are invaluable and may also be used to facilitate percutaneous aspiration of the abscess. Pelvic abscesses will usually discharge spontaneously into the rectum, and right iliac fossa abscesses discharge through the wound. Abscesses elsewhere need draining.

OTHER SEPSIS

Septicaemia, which may cause metastatic abscess in the liver, lungs, meninges or elsewhere, is rare but is usually caused by *E. coli* or *B. fragilis*.

Mechanical complications

PARALYTIC ILEUS AND INTESTINAL OBSTRUCTION

It is normal for intestinal function to be arrested when perforation of the appendix has caused general peritonitis. These patients require continuous aspiration through a nasogastric tube, with intravenous fluid and electrolyte replacement. Normally the volume of gastric aspirate falls sharply and ceases to smell foul after 24 to 48 hours. Oral fluids may then be given.

Sometimes, however, copious foul aspirate continues to drain for several days, indicating intestinal obstruction or persistent ileus. If there is evidence of mechanical obstruction, my own view is to wait for five days from the day of appendicectomy, and if by then the obstruction has not been relieved, I usually operate.

WOUND DEHISCENCE AND INCISIONAL HERNIA

Wound dehiscence is almost unknown after a grid-iron incision, but infection in the muscle layers may so weaken them that a hernia develops. This is sometimes not apparent until six months or even longer after the operation, and often requires repair.

REFERENCES

1 Brennan, S. S., Smith, G. M. R., Evans, M. & Pollock, A. V. (1982) The management of the perforated appendix: a controlled clinical trial. *British Journal of Surgery*, **69**, 510–512.
2 Burkitt, D. P. (1971) The aetiology of appendicitis. *British Journal of Surgery*, **58**, 697–699.
3 Cutler, E. R. (1889) Eleven cases of operation for appendicitis. *Boston Medical and Surgical Journal*, **120**, 554–556 (quoted by Williams *below*).
4 Friedlander, M. L. & Gelfand, M. (1981) Acute appendicitis, an urban disease in Africans. *Tropical Doctor*, **11**, 22–23.
5 Greenall, M. J., Evans, M. & Pollock, A. V. (1978) Should you drain a perforated appendix? *British Journal of Surgery*, **65**, 880–882.
6 Pickford, I. R., Brennan, S. S., Evans, M. & Pollock, A. V. (1983) Two methods of skin closure in abdominal operations: a controlled clinical trial. *British Journal of Surgery*, **70**, 226–228.
7 Senn, N. (1889) A plea in favor of early laparotomy for catarrhal and ulcerative appendicitis, with the report of two cases. *Journal of the American Medical Association*, **13**, 630–634.
8 Williams, G. R. (1983) A history of appendicitis with anecdotes illustrating its importance. *Annals of Surgery*, **197**, 495–506.

PERITONITIS

PHYSIOLOGY OF THE PERITONEUM

The peritoneal cavity is a potential space containing the viscera caudal to the diaphragm; it develops from the primitive coelom, and consists of flattened mesothelial cells lying on a connective tissue base, from which new peritoneum can be formed rapidly after an area is denuded of peritoneum. The primary function of the peritoneum is to provide a frictionless surface over which the abdominal viscera can move freely.

To aid this process the peritoneum secretes a fluid, of which 100 ml is normally present in the abdominal cavity. The constituents of this fluid vary in health and disease, and are dependent on the integrity of the lining membrane, through which water and solutes may move in either direction controlled largely by the osmolar gradient. Saline administered intraperitoneally is absorbed at the rate of 30 ml per hour, while hypertonic fluid can be associated with a water shift of 300–500 ml in one hour from the intravascular space into the peritoneal cavity. Blood, organisms and gas are also absorbed from this cavity. Exchange of many substances can take place through the peritoneal membrane, hence its increasing use in chronic ambulatory peritoneal dialysis.

The parietal peritoneum is richly supplied with nerves, and, when irritated, causes severe pain accurately localized to the affected area. The visceral peritoneum is poorly supplied with nerves, and irritation produces vague and poorly localized discomfort.

THE CONCEPT OF PERITONITIS

Peritonitis is inflammation of the peritoneum – it may be acute or chronic, septic or aseptic, primary or secondary, localized or diffuse, yet the term most usually refers to inflammatory change associated with contamination of the peritoneum secondary to some other event or disease process. Apart from the very rare primary peritonitis, it develops subsequent to and consequent upon another event or disease process. Peritonitis is but a name signifying that a primary disease process has reached a certain stage in its presentation such that the peritoneum has become involved in the process. As a result, the term has little more meaning as a diagnostic statement than the term abdominal pain. It is a holding diagnosis for the practising clinician awaiting, as a result of further evaluation, a more accurate diagnostic statement. Nevertheless, as a term, it has a value in communication because it signifies a severity of disease which requires action in the management of a patient. To make peritonitis a final diagnostic statement will lead to delay in the management of the primary disorder. The diagnosis or use of the term peritonitis indicates that there is an urgent need to continue the diagnostic process to determine the cause of the inflammatory change in the peritoneum. However, the diagnostic process should not be continued without treatment of the systemic effects of peritonitis,

namely the fluid and electrolyte changes associated with inflammation of the peritoneum.

Peritonitis is usually an acute process presenting as an abdominal emergency, but it can be chronic as in tuberculosis. It is either septic or aseptic, yet bacterial contamination of an aseptic peritonitis frequently ensues. Aseptic peritonitis is usually due to chemical or foreign body irritants. Chemical peritonitis follows leakage of sterile fluids into the peritoneum, for example bile, gastric juice and meconium or the release of enzymes from the pancreas as occurs in acute pancreatitis. Foreign body irritants are acquired through external trauma or at the time of operation, in the form of sutures, swabs or starch granules.

PATHOLOGY

The changes which occur in peritonitis vary according to the source of the infection or irritation, its severity, the age of the patient, his general condition and his resistance to infection. The initial response of the peritoneum is to become hyperaemic and oedematous with a secretion of fluid, which is at first serous, then turbid and finally purulent. The exuded fluid contains fibrin, which helps to localize the infection by causing coils of intestine and omentum to become stuck together, thereby walling off contaminated parts from the rest of the peritoneal cavity. This fibrinous exudate resolves completely unless ischaemia is present, in which case permanent adhesions may form. The mechanism of localization is ill-understood; the factors involved in resolution of the localized infection or abscess are unknown. The importance to the surgeon of this stage is paramount, because it determines whether or not an abscess will occur, whether obstructive adhesions will form or whether the peritonitis will become generalized with its ensuing toxicity.

After perforation of an organ, the peritoneal cavity may become totally or partially contaminated, depending on the ability to localize fluid. There appear to be barriers to the spread of fluid, which aid localization: the *longitudinal barrier*, consisting of the lumbar vertebrae, aorta, vena cava and mesentery, separates the right and left infracolic spaces with the transverse mesocolon acting as an *upper transverse barrier* and the pelvic brim, together with the psoas muscles and the iliac vessels, forming the *lower transverse barrier*. These barriers divide the abdomen into various compartments – supracolic, right and left infracolic and pelvic spaces – such that collections of fluid may be localized to one of these areas. Attention to these spaces during a laparotomy can limit contamination. The presence of localizing collections can be determined by noting the site of fibrinous exudate, which may aid localization by sealing mucosal defects.

TYPES OF PERITONITIS (Table 10.1)

Primary peritonitis

The term primary is used to signify that the inflammation of the peritoneal cavity is not related to intra-abdominal disease. True primary peritonitis without any predisposing cause is extremely rare.

Primary peritonitis occurs more commonly in children than in adults, and more often in females than in males. In children there are two peaks of incidence, one in the neonatal period and the second at the age of four to five years. Almost invariably there is a history of preceding

infection, often urinary tract disease, or the child is debilitated either by malnutrition or because of another disease, particularly that associated with immunosuppression such as occurs in hepatic and renal disease or as a result of chemotherapy for malignant conditions. With the advent of longer survival in patients with chronic hepatic or renal disease, adults frequently present with so-called primary peritonitis, especially if they are undergoing immunosuppressive therapy as part of a transplant programme or for treatment of malignant disease. The patient with a shunt draining into the peritoneal cavity is especially prone to so-called primary peritonitis. There have been many recent reports of patients undergoing chronic ambulatory peritoneal dialysis developing peritonitis. Removal of the offending foreign body invariably cures this form of peritoneal inflammation. Entry of organisms into the peritoneal cavity via the fallopian tubes is said to be a cause of peritonitis in young children, but like all forms of primary peritonitis this infection never occurs in the healthy and immunocompetent child. It is still reported to occur, particularly in malnourished communities, and is almost invariably associated with a pneumococcal or streptococcal infection. Gonococcal infections in the peritoneal cavity are being reported with greater frequency, and are probably related to the autoimmune deficiency syndrome.

Fungal and parasitic infections must also be included as a cause of primary peritonitis, for these organisms (usually in the presence of disseminated infection) have caused peritonitis associated with massive ascites. The commonest fungal infection is candidiasis, but many others have been reported. Amoebiasis may also be responsible for primary peritoneal inflammation either as a result of direct spread or by blood-borne transmission. Parasitic infection rarely leads to clinical peritoneal disease; its major importance lies in its ability to mimic peritoneal carcinomatosis or tuberculosis at laparotomy. Cases of granulomatous peritonitis caused by schistosomiasis have been reported, without other extra-intestinal involvement. Enterobiasis has been reported to give rise to granulomatous peritonitis in women by migrating through the upper female genital tract. Although most patients are asymptomatic, lower abdominal pain may be present.

Table 10.1 Causes of peritonitis.

Primary	
(a) Acute	Pneumococcus
	Streptococcus
	Gonorrhoea
	Candida
	Amoebiasis
	Schistosomiasis
	Enterobiasis
(b) Chronic	Tuberculosis
Secondary	
(a) Chemical irritants	Bile
	Gastric juice
	Meconium
	Blood
	Pancreatic enzymes
(b) Granulomatous disease	Sarcoid
	Crohn's disease
	Starch granules
(c) Inflammation of intestinal viscus	Diverticular disease
	Appendicitis
	Cholecystitis
	Crohn's disease
	Salpingitis
(d) Perforation of viscus	
(e) Foreign bodies	Sutures
	Swabs
	Peritoneal catheter
(f) Trauma	Blunt or perforating
(g) Postoperative	Anastomotic dehiscence
(h) Ischaemia	
(i) Spontaneous	Cirrhosis

Tuberculous peritonitis

Tuberculous peritonitis may be either secondary to intra-abdominal tuberculosis, such as ileal or salpingeal disease, or primary due to blood-stream spread. Although the majority of patients do not have clinical evidence of pulmonary or intestinal disease, these are invariably found at autopsy. Tuberculous peritonitis manifests either in a *dry* form with extensive adhesions and matting together of the intestines or in a *wet* form with massive ascites. The ascitic fluid is characterized by a specific gravity greater than 1.016 and a protein content greater than 35 g/l. Diagnosis is confirmed by peritoneal biopsy.

Secondary peritonitis

This is by far the commonest type of peritonitis, and is a complication of any abdominal condition whether it be traumatic, infective, obstructive or neoplastic. Postoperative peritonitis is a common if not uniform event following surgery; its severity depends on the degree of manipulation and whether organisms have been released into the peritoneal cavity to create a focus of infection. Leakage from an anastomosis is probably the most common form of peritonitis seen in hospital practice today. The infection can reach the peritoneum by any route – directly as occurs in perforation or in stab wounds, by local extension as occurs in appendicitis, or by transmigration through the intact and non-infected gut wall as occurs in ischaemic changes, such as strangulation. Infection may also occur by the bloodstream, by the lymphatics or by direct permeation across the diaphragm.

Secondary peritonitis, whether it be due to infection or as a result of a chemical injury such as occurs in pancreatitis, is a secondary and not a primary condition. Any inflammatory process within the abdominal cavity can give rise to a peritonitis, either local or diffuse; the diagnosis of the local condition or underlying disease is the prime objective in management, for any condition which incites an inflammatory reaction can give rise to peritonitis.

Haemoperitoneum

Blood in the peritoneal cavity, especially postoperatively, may elicit no inflammatory reaction; however, bleeding occurring in association with rupture of an organ, for example an ectopic pregnancy, does cause a mild peritoneal reaction, and should therefore be considered in the differential diagnosis of peritonitis. The reaction is mild, and thus the clinical signs are minimal. A haemoperitoneum should not be confused with an increase in the amount of peritoneal fluid which is blood stained. A true haemoperitoneum has a haemoglobin level within 5 g/l

of the blood while blood staining of the peritoneal fluid has a lower haemoglobin, and is associated with leakage of blood into the peritoneal cavity secondary to, for instance, an internal strangulation or haemorrhagic pancreatitis.

Meconium peritonitis

This condition occurs as a result of perforation of the gut prior to birth. Extravasation of sterile meconium into the fetal peritoneal cavity causes an intense chemical and foreign body reaction with characteristic calcification. There are many causes of perforation, the most common of which is obstruction, which will still require operative relief at the time of birth. There are four distinct varieties: (a) meconium pseudocyst, (b) meconium adhesive peritonitis, (c) meconium ascites, and (d) infected meconium peritonitis. The indications for operation are intestinal obstruction, persistent perforation with free gas on the plain abdominal X-ray, or an enlarging abdominal mass. Operation involves removing the underlying cause and preservation of as much intestine as possible. The results are good and more than 70% survive.

Granulomatous peritonitis

Sarcoidosis rarely affects the peritoneum, but can cause a granulomatous peritonitis and ascites. The diagnosis can be made only by exclusion with negative mycobacterial and fungal cultures, a positive Kveim test, and perhaps lack of response to antituberculous chemotherapy. A miliary form of Crohn's disease has been described in which there are non-caseating granulomas and minimal (but definite) abnormalities of the bowel wall. The principal importance of these conditions is in their differentiation from tuberculous peritonitis. Starch peritonitis is a granulomatous condition giving rise to a syndrome two to nine weeks after a previous operation. The condition usually presents with pain, tenderness, fever, nausea, vomiting and abdominal distension. The small bowel obstructs in about 25% of patients. At laparotomy, miliary peritoneal nodules, adhesions and ascites are found, giving an appearance similar to carcinomatosis. Pathologically, the lesions consist of granulomas with epithelioid cells, giant cells and an intense mononuclear infiltrate; starch granules identified by their characteristic Maltese cross confirm the diagnosis. The prognosis is usually good with spontaneous resolution. This condition must be distinguished from talc granulomas, since the silicone particles of these granulomas are birefringent.

Spontaneous bacterial peritonitis in cirrhotics

Peritonitis may appear in up to 10% of patients with overt cirrhosis and portal hypertension. It is probable that the organisms are enteric in origin in over 60% of patients. These patients have ascites and jaundice; the presence of peritonitis is indicated by abdominal pain which, if undiagnosed, will progress to increased ascites, hypotension and encephalopathy. Even with adequate treatment, the prognosis is poor.

BACTERIOLOGY (Table 10.2)

Peritonitis is caused by a polymicrobial contamination of the abdominal cavity. Such bacteria are either primarily aerobic or appear to function in an aerobic–anaerobic symbiosis. In one third of cases the organisms are purely aerobic or facultative anaerobes, principally Gram-negative rods. In the remaining two thirds there is a mixture of aerobic and anaerobic organisms varying in number from two to thirty different species. The synergism of aerobic and anaerobic bacteria is recognized as being more dangerous than pure aerobic infections. *Escherichia coli*, other Gram-negative rods and enterococci are the most prevalent aerobes. *Bacteroides fragilis* with its various subspecies, anaerobic streptococci and clostridia appear to

Table 10.2 Organisms isolated from non-specific peritonitis.

Aerobic bacteria	
Gram-positive	*Staphylococcus aureus*
	Staphylococcus albus
	β-Haemolytic streptococci
	Non-haemolytic streptococci
	Streptococcus milleri
	Streptococcus faecalis
Gram-negative	*Escherichia coli*
	Proteus spp.
	Klebsiella spp.
	Pseudomonas spp.
	Enterobacter spp.
	Serratia spp.
Anaerobic bacteria	
Gram-positive	*Peptococcus* spp.
	Peptostreptococcus spp.
	Clostridium spp.
Gram-negative	*Bacteroides fragilis*
	Bifidobacterium spp.
	Veillonella spp.
	Lactobacillus spp.
	Fusobacterium spp.

* Principal pathogens.

be the most commonly isolated anaerobic pathogens.

The site of origin of the contamination determines which species or combination of bacteria will reach the peritoneal cavity and thereby initiate the infection. In colon and rectal perforations, polymicrobial sepsis is likely; proximal gastrointestinal perforations are associated with anaerobic species. The stage of infection is important: early appendicitis is usually associated with Gram-negative rods with or without the enterococci. As the disease process advances, anaerobes join the polymicrobial flora and soon become the dominant pathogens.

Aerobic bacterial peritonitis, provided it is adequately treated, has a low mortality with a low incidence of wound infection if a laparotomy is performed. On the other hand, peritonitis due to a mixture of both aerobic and anaerobic organisms has a significantly greater mortality with an incidence of postoperative wound sepsis of up to 50%. In chronic ambulatory peritoneal dialysis, many organisms are encountered as a cause of peritonitis, including *Fusobacterium necrophorum*, *Haemophilus influenzae* and *Clostridium oedematiens*. The sporadic reports of these unusual organisms serve to emphasize that good bacteriology is essential, and careful choice of antibiotics is mandatory to achieve optimum results.

CLINICAL PRESENTATION

The response of the peritoneum to inflammation is hyperaemia and the formation of an exudate. The visceral peritoneum is poorly supplied with sensory nerves and pain fibres, while the parietal peritoneum is very sensitive to stimuli. Thus, inflammation of the visceral peritoneum gives rise to a dull aching discomfort which is poorly localized. On the other hand, inflammation of the parietal peritoneum causes well-localized pain, the intensity of which is related to the extent of involvement and the severity of the inflammatory response. The clinical signs of local or general tenderness, guarding and rigidity mirror this inflammatory process. The site of the pain, tenderness or guarding and its pattern of progression indicate the likely cause of the peritonitis.

The next stage in the inflammatory response, namely the stage of exudation, accounts for the secondary effects of peritonitis. Reabsorption of fluid from the inflamed peritoneum gives rise to dehydration and, if not corrected, tachycardia and hypotension. Pain decreases as the amount of exudate increases.

Finally, a stage of sepsis ensues, resulting in a paralytic ileus with further fluid reduction due to the loss of absorption and increased intestinal secretion. Eventually vomiting occurs with greater fluid loss. If sepsis remains uncontrolled, septicaemia develops, which is frequently fatal.

DIAGNOSIS

The diagnosis of peritonitis is largely clinical. This frequently leads to surprises at laparotomy, which remains the principal investigation and treatment of peritonitis. Improved accuracy in the diagnosis of the acute abdomen has been achieved by simple bayesian methods aided by microcomputers. The accuracy of computer-assisted diagnosis can be enhanced by investigations such as blood count, serum amylase, peritoneal four quadrant tap and plain X-ray of the abdomen. Such tests should be supplemented by specialized techniques. Bacteriology of the fluid from a peritoneal tap can be invaluable in the subsequent choice of antibiotics.

TREATMENT

The principles of treatment remain gastric decompression, fluid resuscitation, systemic antibiotics and closure, exteriorization or other definitive mechanical management of the source of contamination.[2] The role and value of adjunctive treatments have been most difficult to elucidate. Hudspeth[1] has advised radical surgical debridement of all fibrinous adhesions in the management of advanced generalized bacterial peritonitis. Although fibrin deposition lowers the early mortality in peritonitis by trapping the bacteria, this same protective role may become the source of subsequent life-threatening sepsis. A controlled trial comparing radical debridement with traditional management failed to show an advantage for the former.[3] Continuing peritoneal lavage in high-risk patients has its advocates: the peritoneal cavity is cleaned mechanically by repeated saline washing using three large drains in the hepato-renal pouch, subphrenic area and pelvic cavity. Lavage with antibiotics is continued over seven hours at the rate of one litre per hour.[3]

Since aerobic Gram-negative rods almost always participate, either as a primary pathogen or as a supportive member in a mixed aerobic–anaerobic flora, antibiotics are first selected according to their activity against these species. Aminoglycosides have been most effective despite their nephrotoxicity. However, aminoglycosides alone provide inadequate antimicrobial cover in approximately one half of patients. With a growing awareness of the importance of *Bacteroides* species, metronidazole is increasingly used with an aminoglycoside, and has been shown to be significantly more effective than either agent used alone. Nevertheless, this combination is not effective against many Gram-positive cocci, for which a broad-spectrum synthetic penicillin should be added. It has been claimed that some of the third-generation cephalosporins have a sufficient spectrum to encompass all usual peritoneal contaminants, but this remains unproven particularly with respect to the strict anaerobes. Good treatment requires good bacteriology, which must be monitored until a successful outcome has been achieved.[4]

REFERENCES

1 Hudspeth, A. S. (1975) Radical surgical debridement in the treatment of advanced generalized bacterial peritonitis. *Archives of Surgery*, **110,** 1233–1235.
2 Polk, H. C. (1979) Generalized peritonitis: a continuing challenge. *Surgery*, **86,** 777–778.
3 Polk, H. C. & Fry, D. E. (1980) Radical peritoneal debridement for established peritonitis. *Annals of Surgery*, **192,** 350–355.
4 Stone, M. H. & Fabian, T. C. (1980) Clinical comparisons of antibiotic combinations in the treatment of peritonitis and related mixed aerobic–anaerobic surgical sepsis. *World Journal of Surgery*, **4,** 415–421.

ABSCESS

Intra-abdominal abscesses constitute a major cause of surgical morbidity. Not infrequently this is because the clinical course of an abscess may be indolent, with late organ failure being the only indicator to the presence of a serious and unresolved septic process.[3] Consequently diagnosis is often delayed, resulting in an appreciable mortality.[12]

Accurate localization of intra-abdominal sepsis can be difficult, especially in the ill patient, but this has been greatly improved by new imaging techniques such as grey scale ultrasonography, computerized axial tomography (CT) and ^{111}In-labelled leucocyte scanning.[4] Treatment by drainage is now possible under X-ray control.

The clinical presentation has also been modified by the introduction of newer and more powerful antibiotics. These may obscure early symptoms and give the clinician a false sense of security; they have often become a substitute for prompt and adequate drainage. The guiding principle in the treatment of an abscess is to establish early dependent drainage. This is just as important now as it was in the pre-antibiotic era. The principal bacterial isolates from intra-abdominal abscesses are listed in Table 10.3.

Table 10.3 Bacteriology of intra-abdominal abscess in 72 patients.

Escherichia coli	40
Proteus spp.	18
Klebsiella spp.	16
Pseudomonas spp.	11
Streptococcus faecalis	10
Enterobacter spp.	9
Bacteroides fragilis	62
Clostridium spp.	45
Eubacterium spp.	23
Peptostreptococcus spp.	19
Fusobacterium spp.	17
Bacteroides melaninogenicus	13
Peptococcus spp.	8

After J. Bartlett.

CLASSIFICATION

Intra-abdominal abscesses can be divided into three groups by their anatomical location.[1]

Intraperitoneal abscess

A septic process anywhere in the abdomen may become walled off to form a localized abscess. Alternatively pus may track along natural tissue planes following generalized peritonitis, or after a postoperative anastomotic dehiscence, to become localized by omentum, visceral or parietal peritoneum or adjacent viscera and form an abscess in one of the classical dependent anatomical sites: the pelvis, the subphrenic space and the right or left paracolic gutter.

Retroperitoneal abscess

Sepsis which starts in the retroperitoneal space is often confined and it is very unusual for such an abscess to point and discharge into the peritoneal cavity. Much more commonly it may track from the retroperitoneum to be revealed as a fluctuant tender mass in the parietes. Thus, a perinephric abscess usually points in the loin and a psoas abscess complicating ileocaecal Crohn's disease may appear beneath the inguinal ligament in the femoral triangle.

Visceral abscess

An abscess may form in one of the abdominal viscera as a result of a pathological process in the affected organ; an example is empyema of the gallbladder. Others arise by local, lymphatic or haematogenous spread from another site. Examples of this are some liver abscesses, which are often multiple.

Four of the more common and clinically important abscesses will be considered individually.

PELVIC ABSCESS

This is the commonest type of intraperitoneal abscess.

Aetiology

Pelvic abscess can form as a result of gravitation of pus or infected material from anywhere in the abdominal cavity, but is usually a result of pathology in or adjacent to the pelvis (Table 10.4).

Table 10.4 Causes of pelvic abscess.

Common	Rare
Appendicitis	Foreign body perforation of viscera
Diverticular disease	Pelvic haematocoele
Tubo-ovarian abscess	Radiotherapy producing pelvic cellulitis
Generalized peritonitis	Crohn's disease
Rectal surgery	Pelvic tumour

Clinical features

A pelvic abscess often takes several days to become apparent after the initial infective event. The patient develops a fluctuating fever; there is tachycardia often accompanied by increased frequency of micturition and the passage of mucus per rectum. A palpable abdominal mass arising out of the pelvis may be present. Rectal examination reveals a hot, boggy and tender anterior rectal wall with a mass in the rectovesical or rectovaginal pouch. There may be mucus and blood on the finger stall. Blood count shows a polymorphonuclear leucocytosis. The clinical picture may be delayed if the patient has been treated with antibiotics[11] and the differentiation between pelvic cellulitis and pelvic abscess can be difficult.

Once formed a pelvic abscess rarely resolves without either discharging or being drained. It may burst into either the rectum, producing mucous diarrhoea, or the vagina, leading to a profuse offensive discharge. Alternatively it may discharge into the peritoneal cavity producing a generalized peritonitis. This is a grave and avoidable complication.

Treatment

Surgical drainage under a general anaesthetic is advised. At operation the location of the abscess should first be confirmed by needle aspiration, before the cavity is opened into either the rectum or posterior fornix of the vagina.

SUBPHRENIC ABSCESS

This is a collection of pus lying below but in contact with the diaphragm. A series of intraperitoneal and extraperitoneal spaces are classically described but the following simplified classification is more practical:[11]

Right anterior intraperitoneal
   (right subphrenic)
Right posterior intraperitoneal
   (right subhepatic)
Left anterior intraperitoneal
   (left subphrenic)
Left posterior intraperitoneal
   (left subhepatic – lesser sac)

Two further areas, the right extraperitoneal or bare area and the left extraperitoneal area, are much less important clinically as infections in these areas are rare.

Which intraperitoneal space becomes the site of abscess formation depends largely upon the organ from which the infection originates. The most frequent site is the right posterior or subhepatic space, following local or generalized peritonitis or as a complication of upper gastrointestinal surgery, particularly of the stomach, duodenum or biliary tract. Left anterior subphrenic abscess, which used to be quite common after splenectomy, is now relatively rare.

Clinical features

'Pus somewhere, pus nowhere, pus under the diaphragm.' This time-honoured aphorism still holds true, because there are often surprisingly few clinical manifestations of a subphrenic abscess. This diagnosis should be considered in any sick patient with a fever in whom no focus of intra-abdominal sepsis can be identified by clinical or rectal examination. Basal lung signs – pleural effusion or consolidation – are nearly always present. Abdominal examination is often non-contributory. The patient has a high swinging fever accompanied by leucocytosis. Plain abdominal and chest radiographs may confirm the basal lung changes and often show a raised and thickened diaphragm. Sometimes fluid levels are seen below the diaphragm on a penetrated film and, if present on the right side, are a strong indication of an abscess. The modern imaging techniques of ultrasound or CT scanning have almost completely eliminated the problem of locating a subphrenic abscess.

Treatment

Prompt drainage should always be carried out once the diagnosis has been made. Antibiotics will not allow resolution of an established abscess, and spontaneous perforation into the pleural cavity to produce an empyema is a serious complication which may follow neglected or delayed drainage. With the accurate localization techniques now available, planned open drainage should be undertaken early. However, percutaneous drainage under X-ray control, guided by ultrasound or screening techniques, is also becoming an accepted technique, particularly in the very ill postoperative patient.[7]

PSOAS ABSCESS

Chronic psoas abscess, traditionally due to tuberculosis of the spine, is not common except in areas with a large immigrant community. Acute non-tuberculosis psoas abscess, however, is increasingly being recognized. It commences in the retroperitoneal area, but usually points beneath the inguinal ligament in the femoral triangle.

Aetiology

The abscess usually originates by direct extension from an adjacent inflammatory process. On the right side they include:

A   Retrocaecal or retroileal appendicitis
B   Crohn's disease
C   Carcinoma of the caecum

On the left side:

A   Diverticular disease
B   Carcinoma of the left colon

On either side sepsis tracking from renal infection or from the lower dorsal or lumbar spine may present as a psoas abscess.

Clinical features

The original inflammatory episode may either be silent or have occurred and apparently resolved weeks or even months previously. The patient may then present with generalized signs of infection or, more commonly, with localized sepsis associated with exquisite tenderness just beneath the inguinal ligament in the femoral triangle. A fixed flexion deformity of the hip joint associated with a limp may result in a misdiagnosis of acute septic arthritis. X-ray will reveal a normal hip joint. As the organisms involved usually are of bowel origin, they are often gas forming so such abscesses may be detected radiologically by loculi of gas below the inguinal ligament.

Treatment

Although the abscess must be drained, the primary cause should be dealt with as well; failure to do so may result in a fistula or continuing sepsis.

LIVER ABSCESS

Liver abscesses are uncommon in the United Kingdom. Excluding amoebic abscesses and multiple liver abscesses found at post mortem after a terminal illness, pyogenic liver abscesses are seen approximately once a year in any average-sized general hospital.[13]

Most abscesses are not recognized at the time of initial presentation[6] and delay in diagnosis may lead to a fatal outcome in 40–65% of cases.[10]

Causes

The causes of pyogenic liver abscess are given (Table 10.5).

Table 10.5 Causes of pyogenic liver abscess.

1. Biliary obstruction
2. Portal pyaemia
3. Direct spread – from contiguous structures
4. Bacteraemia and septicaemia via hepatic artery
5. Trauma
6. Intrahepatic pathology
7. Hepatic infarction (therapeutic arterial embolization)
8. Cryptogenic

The overall incidence of pyogenic liver abscess is unchanged in the last fifty years.[2] However, portal pyaemia secondary to appendicitis in young people has become less common as a cause of liver abscess, while biliary obstruction in older patients has become much more common. The number of cryptogenic cases has also increased and now accounts for approximately 60% of all cases.[8, 9]

Distribution of pyogenic liver abscesses

Portal pyaemia is usually responsible for abscesses in the right lobe of the liver, whereas biliary obstruction and cholangitis give rise to multiple abscesses throughout both lobes. Unrecognized, and untreated, any abscess may eventually spread to involve adjoining organs, leading to the development of subphrenic abscess, pleural effusion, empyema, or pulmonary infection or abscess

Only rarely does a liver abscess burst into the peritoneal cavity to cause generalized peritonitis.

Clinical features

Diagnosis is often delayed because there are no specific signs or symptoms until the abscess is large and the patient is consequently very ill. Pain is eventually present in 80% of cases, often localized to the upper abdomen or referred to the corresponding shoulder tip. Pleuritic pain is experienced in 10–20% cases.[9] Most patients look ill with evidence of weight loss, fever and night sweating. Nausea, vomiting and diarrhoea become worse as the abscess progresses. Jaundice is a bad prognostic sign as it usually indicates underlying biliary disease and multiple abscesses, which have a mortality of 80%.[6] Basal lung signs are common. Most abscesses are fatal if left undiagnosed.[8]

It is important to exclude hydatid disease and amoebic abscess. Hydatid disease should be considered in sheep-farming communities; the appearance of the lesion on CT scan is usually diagnostic and complement fixation tests are strongly positive. Amoebic abscess is rare unless the patient has been resident abroad; diagnosis should be made on needle aspiration.

Investigations

Most patients are anaemic with leucocytosis and abnormal liver function tests. Vitamin B_{12} levels are reported to be very high in patients with liver abscesses but not in patients with extra-hepatic infection. However, this is a time-consuming investigation and is rarely helpful in critically ill patients. Plain radiographs may show a raised right diaphragm and changes at the lung base. Modern non-invasive imaging techniques are the most accurate means of diag-nosing a liver abscess. Radioisotope scanning will detect over 80% of cases, although its speci-ficity has recently been questioned.[8] In contrast, CT scanning is very accurate.[5] The diagnostic method of choice is undoubtedly ultrasound examination of the liver.[12] Other techniques such as biliary radiology, angiography and sple-noportography cause much greater discomfort, carry a greater risk and are now rarely used.

Treatment

Early drainage of pus is still the overriding prin-ciple of treatment. This needs to be emphasized even with the availability of powerful anti-biotics. For solitary abscesses, open drainage under antibiotic cover is very successful and will lead to resolution in 90% cases.[13] Recently, closed aspiration guided by ultrasound scanning combined with local installation of antibiotics and systemic antibiotic therapy has given excel-lent results,[5, 6, 8] with a considerable reduction in mortality, particularly in cryptogenic abscesses. Multiple abscesses are much more dif-ficult to treat. The patients are often very ill and, as these abscesses are usually due to biliary obs-truction, early decompression of the biliary tree is an important aspect of surgical management.

REFERENCES

1 Altemeir, W. A., Culbertson, W. R., Fullen, W. D. & Shook, C. D. (1973) Intra-abdominal abscesses. *American Journal of Surgery*, **125**, 70–79.
2 De La Maga, L. M., Naeim, F. & Berman, L. D. (1974) The changing etiology of liver abscess. Further obser-vations. *Journal of the American Medical Association*, **227**, 161.
3 Fry, D. E., Garrison, R. N., Heitsch, R. C. *et al.* (1980) Determinants of death in intra-abdominal abscesses. *Surgery*, **88**, 517–523.
4 Knochel, J. Q., Koehler, P. R., Lee, T. G. & Welch, D. M. (1980) Diagnosis of abdominal abscesses with com-puterised tomography, ultrasonography and ^{111}In leu-cocyte scan. *Radiology*, **137**, 425–432.
5 Kraulis, J. E., Bird, B. L. & Colapinto, N. (1980) Per-cutaneous catheter drainage of liver abscess: an alter-native to open drainage. *British Journal of Surgery*, **67**, 400–402.
6 Leading Article (1980) Pyogenic liver abscess. *British Medical Journal*, **i**, 1155.
7 MacEarlean, D. P., Owens, A. P. & Howibare, J. B. (1981) Ultrasound guided percutaneous abdominal abscess drainage. *British Journal of Radiology*, **54**, 394–397.
8 Northover, J. M. A., Jones, B. J. M., Dawson, J. L. & Williams, R. (1982) Difficulties in the diagnosis and management of pyogenic liver abscess. *British Journal of Surgery*, **69**, 48–51.
9 Shearman, D. J. C. & Finlayson, N. D. C. (1982) In *Diseases of the Gastro-intestinal Tract and Liver*. London: Churchill Livingstone.
10 Sheinfeld, A. M., Steiner, A. E., Rivkin, L. B. *et al.* (1982) Transcutaneous drainage of abscesses of the liver guided by computed tomography scan. *Surgery, Gyne-cology and Obstetrics*, **155**, 662–666.
11 Shepherd, J. A. (1968) *Surgery of the Acute Abdomen*. London: Livingstone.
12 Taylor, K. J. W., Wasson, J. F. Mc. I., De-Graaf, C. *et al.* (1978) Accuracy of grey-scale ultrasound diagnosis of abdominal and pelvic abscesses in 220 patients. *Lancet*, **i**, 83–84.
13 Young, A. E. (1976) The clinical presentation of pyo-genic liver abscess. *British Journal of Surgery*, **63**, 216–219.

OTHER CAUSES OF THE ACUTE ADDOMEN

ABDOMINAL TUBERCULOSIS

Abdominal tuberculosis may present as an acute abdomen but this is uncommon and only accounted for 2–17% of all cases of abdominal tuberculosis in two recent reports from the United Kingdom.[1, 2] The usual presenting symptom is abdominal pain localized to the right iliac fossa, which may mimic appendicitis or Crohn's disease. A mass may be present but this rarely develops into an abscess and simply represents adherent bowel in the ileocaecal region. Caseation of mesenteric glands to produce an abscess is rare. The other common form of presentation is as ascites, which may present as an acute abdomen.

Tuberculosis is considered in more detail in Chapter 14.

Diagnosis

In the United Kingdom the abdomen is usually the sole site of active disease, although the con-dition may be suspected if there are signs of tuberculosis elsewhere in the body. Laparoscopy and peritoneal biopsy, or the presence of a protein concentration over 2.5 g/dl accompa-nied by a cell count above $250/\text{mm}^3$ in ascitic fluid is usually diagnostic of the disorder.

Treatment

Antituberculous therapy is usually effective, but laparotomy may still be necessary if the diagnosis is in doubt. Fibrous strictures following successful medical treatment occasionally necessitate surgical resection, bypass or strictureplasty.

FOREIGN BODIES

Foreign bodies may be introduced into the abdomen in one of three ways:
1 via the alimentary tract;
2 via the genitourinary tract;
3 directly as a result of trauma.

Ingestion of foreign bodies is usually a problem in three groups of subjects: small children, elderly edentulous people, and psychiatric patients. The latter often deliberately ingest potentially dangerous objects such as pins, needles, nails and even razor blades. However, as these potentially dangerous objects are often found on X-ray to be lying in the stomach or small bowel in a patient who does not appear physically ill, the clinician should suspect that they have been well wrapped up in paper, tape or some other protective material. The best policy is to watch the progress of these objects by serial X-rays and operate only if the foreign body becomes obviously lodged or if there are signs of peritonitis or bleeding.

The variety of objects removed from the rectum is enormous. These may have been ingested orally or inserted anally, the latter usually as a result of deviant sexual practice. Removal of small foreign bodies can often be awaited naturally, but large objects may damage the rectum and require careful removal under general anaesthetic. If intraperitoneal injury has occurred, a proximal colostomy is mandatory.

Foreign bodies may also be introduced into the abdomen by a penetrating injury. The missile itself or the structure through which it passed are carried along the track into the abdomen. Any penetrating injury in the abdomen should be explored for foreign bodies.

An acute abdomen occurs only when a foreign body penetrates either the gastrointestinal or genitourinary tract to produce a local abscess or generalized peritonitis. The aim of early exploration is to prevent these complications.

BLUNT TRAUMA

Blunt trauma is damage produced by a crush injury. A blunt object compresses the anterior abdominal wall until it meets the resistance of the more rigid posterior abdominal wall. Any viscera which cannot be pushed aside by this force will be compressed and consequently contused or torn. Blunt trauma may damage the spleen, liver, pancreas, mesentery, major vessels, bladder or kidneys.

The management of such cases is based initially on vigorous and prompt resuscitation. Once resuscitation has been achieved, cases of blunt abdominal trauma can often be managed by careful and frequent observation. Provided the patient remains in a stable condition, exploration may be postponed and often avoided, but should any deterioration occur then laparotomy becomes mandatory. Modern management should include central venous pressure monitoring for hypovolaemia and peritoneal lavage with microscopic, biochemical and bacteriological examination of the resultant fluid to assist in determining the severity of any intra-abdominal injury. The examination can be repeated at intervals to aid evaluation of any extensive intra-abdominal blood loss, bowel perforation or damage to major retroperitoneal organs such as the pancreas.

REFERENCES

1 Kaufman, H. D. & Donovan, I. J. (1974) Tuberculous disease of the abdomen. *Journal of the Royal College of Surgeons Edinburgh*, **19**, 377–380.
2 Khoury, G. A., Payne, C. R. & Harvey, D. R. (1978) Tuberculosis of the peritoneal cavity. *British Journal of Surgery*, **65**, 808–811.

Chapter 11
The Large Intestine

EMBRYOLOGY AND ANATOMY

The large intestine extends from the caecum to the anorectal junction and is approximately 135 cm in length. It consists of the caecum and appendix, the ascending, transverse, descending and sigmoid colon, and the rectum (Figure 11.1). Its calibre is greatest at the caecum and diminishes distally towards the sigmoid colon. At the rectosigmoid junction it again dilates to become the rectum.

The general structure of the large intestine resembles that of the small intestine but there are several important differences in its external appearance. Throughout the greater part of the large intestine, the outer longitudinal layer of muscle is incomplete and takes the form of longitudinal bands known as taeniae coli. These are shorter than the colon itself giving rise to a sacculated appearance. These sacculations or haustrations can be readily seen at operation or during radiological examination. The taeniae coli coalesce in the appendix and lower sigmoid colon and rectum to give these areas a complete outer longitudinal coat. The large intestine can also be identified by the presence of the appendices epiploicae. These are small peritoneal sacs filled with fat and are most numerous in the sigmoid colon.

The caecum is a blind sac projecting downwards from the level of the ileocaecal junction. It is covered by peritoneum on its anterior and lateral surfaces. This peritoneal coat continues up behind the caecum for a variable distance before being reflected on to the floor of the right iliac fossa thus forming the retrocaecal recess. If the three taeniae coli are traced downwards on the caecum, they will be seen to coalesce at the base of the appendix. In infancy, the appendix lies at the apex of the caecum, but during growth the lateral wall of the caecum outgrows the medial wall so that the base of the appendix comes to lie on the posteromedial wall of the caecum about 2 cm below the ileocaecal junction. The appendix is attached to the small intestinal mesentery by a peritoneal fold – the meso-appendix. The appendicular artery passes through this fold to supply the appendix. The position of the tip of the appendix is very variable, the most common sites being behind the caecum, in the pelvis and behind the ileum.

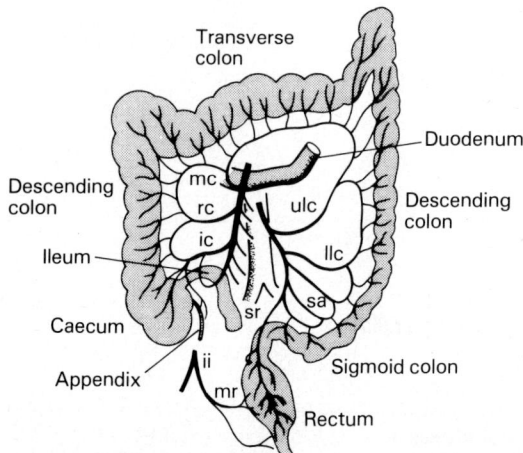

Fig. 11.1 The colon – its divisions and its arterial blood supply. The major branches of the superior mesenteric artery are the middle colic (mc), the right colic (rc) and the ileocolic (ic). The major branches of the inferior mesenteric artery are the upper left colic (ulc), the lower left colic (llc), the sigmoidal arteries (sa) and the superior rectal (sr). The rectal wall muscle is also supplied by the middle rectal branches (mr) of the internal iliac artery (ii). Modified from Hanbrich (1976) The anatomy of the colon. In *Gastroenterology*, vol. 2, 3rd edn (Ed.) H.L. Bockus, with kind permission of the author, the editor and the publisher, W.B. Saunders, Philadelphia.

The ileocaecal valve opens into the medial wall of the colon at the junction of the caecum with the ascending colon. It consists of upper and lower lips which project into the lumen of the bowel. It has no true valve and is controlled by a thickening of the circular muscle in the terminal 3 cm of the ileum.

The ascending colon extends from the ileocaecal junction to the hepatic flexure of the colon. It is retroperitoneal and lies in close contact with the ureter and gonadal vessels, the inferior pole of the right kidney and the second part of the duodenum.

The transverse colon lies between the hepatic and splenic flexures of the colon in a loop which is convex downwards. It is mobile, being suspended from the posterior abdominal wall by the transverse mesocolon. The greater omentum, a fatty apron rich in lymphatics, is attached to the convex surface and is particularly important in the adult in its capacity to localize intraperitoneal infection.

The descending colon, which again is retroperitoneal, passes directly downwards from the splenic flexure to the pelvic brim. The sigmoid colon extends from the pelvic brim to the upper margin of the rectum. It is mobile, of variable length and completely invested in peritoneum. It is attached to the posterior wall of the pelvis by a mesentery – the sigmoid mesocolon.

The rectum is a continuation of the sigmoid colon and starts at the level of the third sacral vertebra. It is about 12 cm long and curves downwards and forwards to the pelvic floor where it bends sharply downwards and backwards to form the anal canal. In its upper third, it is covered with peritoneum on its anterior surface and both sides. The middle third is in contact with peritoneum only on its anterior surface whereas the lower third lies below the peritoneal reflection. The interior of the rectum is divided into compartments by three crescentic horizontal shelves of circular muscle covered by mucosa. These are the rectal valves which can easily be seen at sigmoidoscopy.

Embryology

By the third week of intrauterine life, the alimentary canal is a simple tube suspended from the dorsal wall of the embryo by a dorsal mesentery. Three vessels leave the aorta and pass ventrally through this dorsal mesentery to supply the fore-gut, mid-gut and hind-gut of the digestive tube, respectively. As the digestive tube elongates, it forms a mid-gut loop which at its apex communicates with the yolk sac through the vitello-intestinal duct. The part of the mid-gut loop distal to this duct eventually becomes the terminal ileum and large intestine from the caecum to the splenic flexure. The remainder of the large intestine develops from the hind-gut. During the sixth week of intrauterine life, the mid-gut loop herniates through the poorly developed abdominal wall into the umbilical cord. It remains in this position until, by the tenth week of intrauterine life, the abdominal wall has grown enough to accommodate the abdominal contents. As the mid-gut loop returns to the abdominal cavity it rotates in an anticlockwise direction so that the distal limb goes upwards and to the left, while the proximal limb passes downwards and to the right. The last part of the mid-gut loop to return is the caecum which at first lies high up in the midline. It then grows to the right and descends to its definitive position in the right iliac fossa. As the mid-gut loop returns to the abdominal cavity, the hind-gut swings to the left on its dorsal mesentery. The layers of peritoneum behind the ascending colon and the descending colon fuse with the abdominal wall, leaving these two parts retroperitoneal. The dorsal mesentery of the transverse and sigmoid colon persist as the transverse and sigmoid mesocolon.

Blood supply

Arterial blood to the large intestine is supplied by branches of the superior and inferior mesenteric arteries (Figure 11.1). Close to the intestine, these branches anastomose with each other in such a way that they form a continuous anastomotic channel from ascending colon to the sigmoid colon. This is often termed the marginal artery.

The superior mesenteric artery arises from the front of the aorta at the level of the first lumbar vertebra. It passes downwards between the layers of the small intestinal mesentery to end at the ileum, approximately 50 cm from the ileocaecal junction. Three main branches arise from the right side of the superior mesenteric artery – the ileocolic, right colic and middle colic arteries. The ileocolic artery supplies the caecum, appendix and the lower ascending colon. The right colic branch supplies the ascending colon and hepatic flexure, while the middle colic artery passes through the transverse mesocolon to supply the transverse colon.

The inferior mesenteric artery supplies the left side of the colon from the splenic flexure to the anorectal junction. It arises from the aorta at the level of the third lumbar vertebra and passes to the left and enters the apex of the sigmoid mesocolon. It gives off upper and lower left colic branches which supply the descending colon with sigmoid branches to the sigmoid colon. After it enters the sigmoid mesocolon, the inferior mesenteric artery crosses the pelvic brim and enters the pelvis as the superior rectal artery to supply the rectum. The muscle of the rectal wall has an additional blood supply from the middle rectal branches of the internal iliac artery.

The venous drainage of the large intestine is into the portal venous system via the superior and inferior mesenteric veins. The superior mesenteric vein accompanies the artery and joins the splenic vein behind the neck of the pancreas to become the portal vein. The inferior mesenteric vein diverges from the artery and passes just to the left of the duodeno-jejunal junction to join the splenic vein.

Lymphatic drainage

The lymphatic drainage of the large intestine follows the main vessels. Lymphatic vessels in the wall of the intestine pass first to the epicolic lymph nodes. These are situated on the wall of the intestine often closely related to the appendices epiploicae. From these nodes, efferent lymphatics pass to the paracolic lymph nodes which lie on the medial side of the colon and thence to the intermediate lymph nodes alongside the main branches of the superior and inferior mesenteric arteries. These in turn drain to the preaortic lymph nodes around the origins of the main arteries.

Nerve supply

The large intestine is supplied by sympathetic and parasympathetic fibres of the autonomic nervous system. The sympathetic fibres enter the abdomen in the splanchnic nerves. These relay in the coeliac ganglion and then pass along the blood vessels to supply the whole of the large intestine. The source of parasympathetic fibres to the mid-gut and hind-gut differ. The mid-gut is supplied by parasympathetic fibres from the vagus nerve while the hind-gut is supplied by the pelvic parasympathetic nerves. These preganglionic fibres likewise pass along the blood vessels to relay in the wall of the intestine in cell bodies of the myenteric and submucosal plexuses.

HIRSCHSPRUNG'S DISEASE

Hirschsprung's disease, described by Hirschsprung in 1887[12] and termed 'congenital megacolon' by Mya in 1894,[25] is a condition where varying degrees of intestinal obstruction occur as a result of disordered propulsive activity in the gastrointestinal tract (Figure 11.2). This disordered activity is usually confined to the distal bowel, rectum and varying lengths of colon, but may extend into proximal colon and small bowel. It is associated with abnormalities of the myenteric plexuses (absent ganglion cells),[2, 41] with tortuous hypertrophied nerve trunks[40] and, in the distal large bowel, with abnormalities of innervation of the mucosa (excess acetylcholinesterase-staining nerve fibres)[15] and smooth muscle (excessive adrenergic innervation).[1] The affected bowel is usually of normal or reduced calibre. The proximal bowel shows secondary dilatation and hypertrophy, the degree depending on the severity of obstruction and the duration of the condition before presenting for treatment. The severity of the obstruction in the involved bowel varies not only with the length of the segment, the degree of hypertrophy in the proximal bowel, the consistency of the stool, but also with the severity of

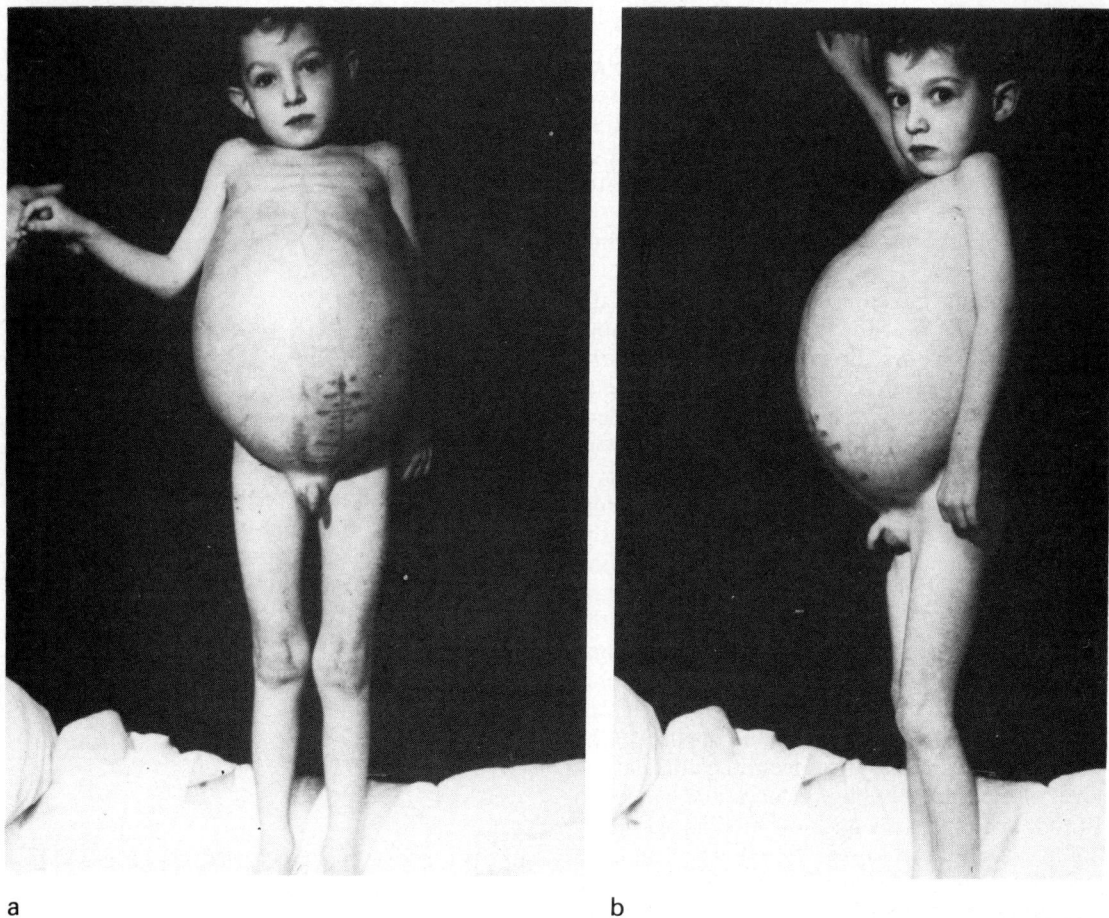

a   b

Fig. 11.2   Classical case of Hirschsprung's disease (1947).

the condition itself. Thus clinically the disease represents a disordered balance between propulsion and resistance.

Aetiology

The aetiology of Hirschsprung's disease is unknown. In a study of normal embryos, Okomoto and Ueda[26] showed that neuroblasts (precursors of the myenteric plexuses) appear in the head end of the gut tube during the fifth week. These neuroblasts migrate down the length of the intestinal tract to reach the developing anus by the twelfth week. They postulated an origin of these neuroblasts from the vagal nuclei and that the developing myenteric plexus obtained secondary connections from the sympathetic and parasympathetic systems. Failure of these connections accounted for the tortuous hypertrophied nerve trunks found in the distal bowel. Since a hold-up of this migration is the most likely explanation for Hirsch-

sprung's disease, a cause for this failure must be sought. A number of factors are involved. First, there are genetic factors, indicated by a familial tendency and association with Down's syndrome[28] and Waardenberg's syndrome.[23] Second, there may be environmental factors which would be expected to act on the embryo between the fifth and twelfth weeks. This theory of arrest of migration of ganglion cell precursors would not explain the very rare demonstration of skip lesions.

Degeneration of ganglion cells has been noted in the distal colon following gastrointestinal ischaemia, resulting from both clinical and experimental occlusion of vessels to the distal colon or injection of neurotoxic substances into these vessels. The resulting changes bear no resemblance to Hirschsprung's disease. A similar appearance has been produced in rats by the distension of an isolated segment of distal bowel with corrosive sublimate, which resulted in destruction of all neural elements and also, apparently, the mucosa.[14] In this experiment the distal segment remained contracted while there was proximal hypertrophy and dilatation.

The severity of the disease may correlate with the degree of the abnormal cholinergic positive innervation of the smooth muscle[10] of the distal segment.[13]

Pathology (Figure 11.3)

MACROSCOPIC

The distal bowel. The distal bowel is either small (newborn) or normal in external appearance and calibre.

The proximal bowel (Figures 11.4 and 11.5). The proximal bowel is dilated. The dilatation varies, from that associated with acute obstruction in the newborn to the massive hypertrophy and dilatation of the classic long standing case.

The cone (see Figure 11.5). Where the disease is confined to the bowel distal to the transverse colon, there will usually be a tapering from the dilated proximal bowel to the affected distal bowel. This is known clinically as the cone. It can be demonstrated radiologically and at operation, and usually corresponds to the 'transitional zone' histologically. Variants occur where there is a long 'transitional zone' and, in a few longstanding cases, where the dilatation may extend into the aganglionic segment (see Figure 11.4). No proper cone is formed if the aganglionic bowel extends proximal to the transverse colon.

Secondary changes
1 Colitic changes, stercoral ulcers and melanosis coli may be seen in the mucosa of the proximal bowel.
2 Areas of necrotizing enterocolitis and perforation may occur either in the bowel just proximal to the cone or in the caecum and ascending colon.
3 Diffuse superficial mucosal loss, widely distributed in the proximal and distal segment, can occur resulting in catastrophic diarrhoea with fluid and protein loss.[8] Rarely, a more protracted form results in mucosal changes very similar to ulcerative colitis.

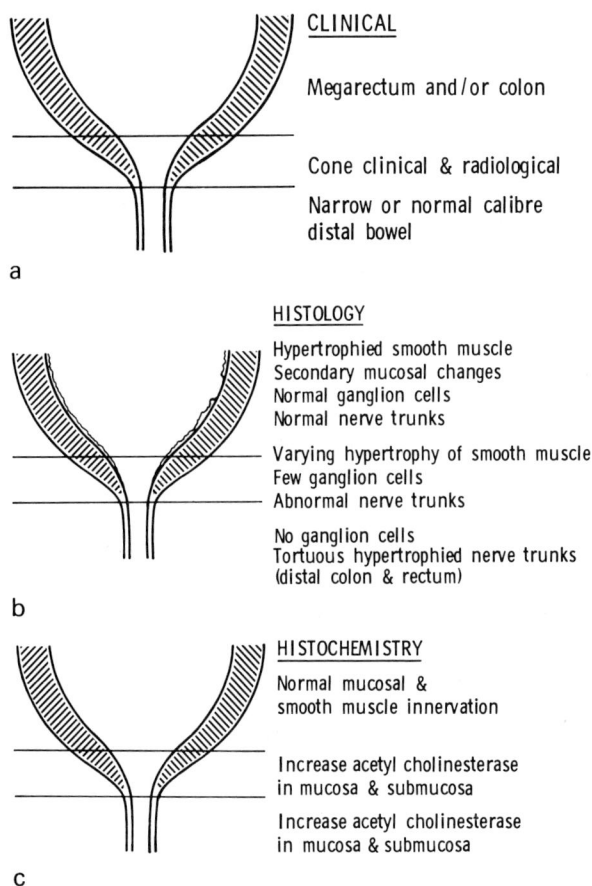

CLINICAL

Megarectum and/or colon

Cone clinical & radiological
Narrow or normal calibre distal bowel

a

HISTOLOGY

Hypertrophied smooth muscle
Secondary mucosal changes
Normal ganglion cells
Normal nerve trunks

Varying hypertrophy of smooth muscle
Few ganglion cells
Abnormal nerve trunks

No ganglion cells
Tortuous hypertrophied nerve trunks
(distal colon & rectum)

b

HISTOCHEMISTRY

Normal mucosal &
smooth muscle innervation

Increase acetyl cholinesterase
in mucosa & submucosa

Increase acetyl cholinesterase
in mucosa & submucosa

c

Fig. 11.3 (a) Clinical; (b) histological; and (c) histochemical findings in Hirschsprung's disease.

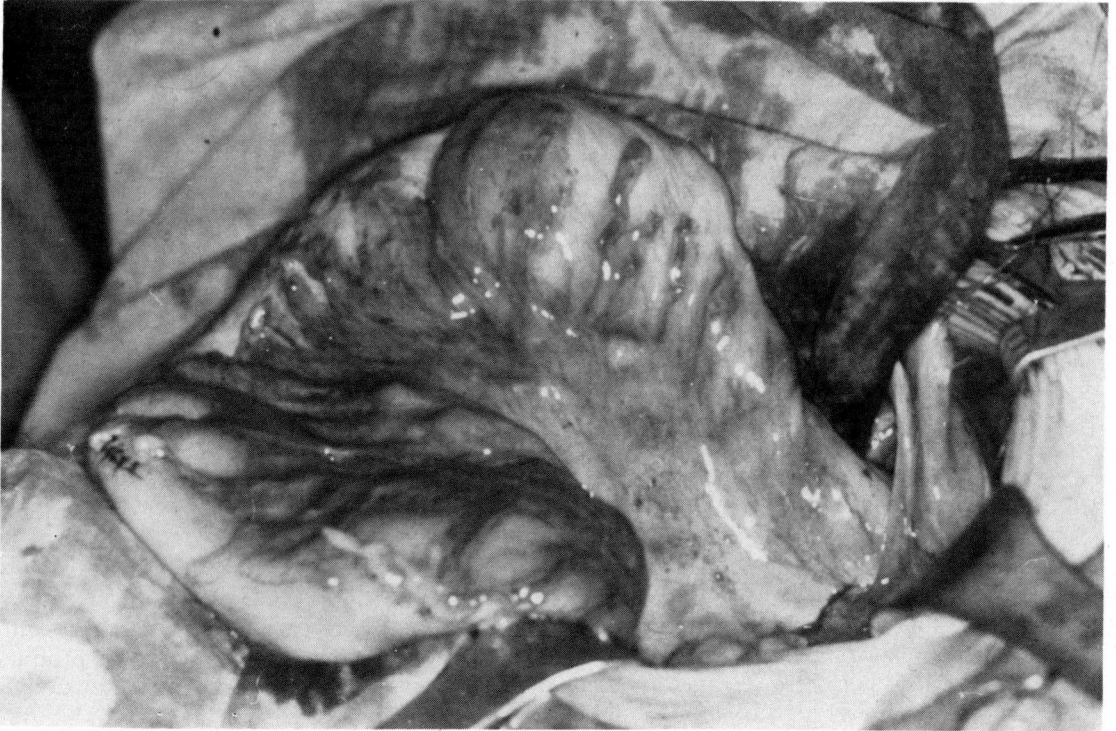

a

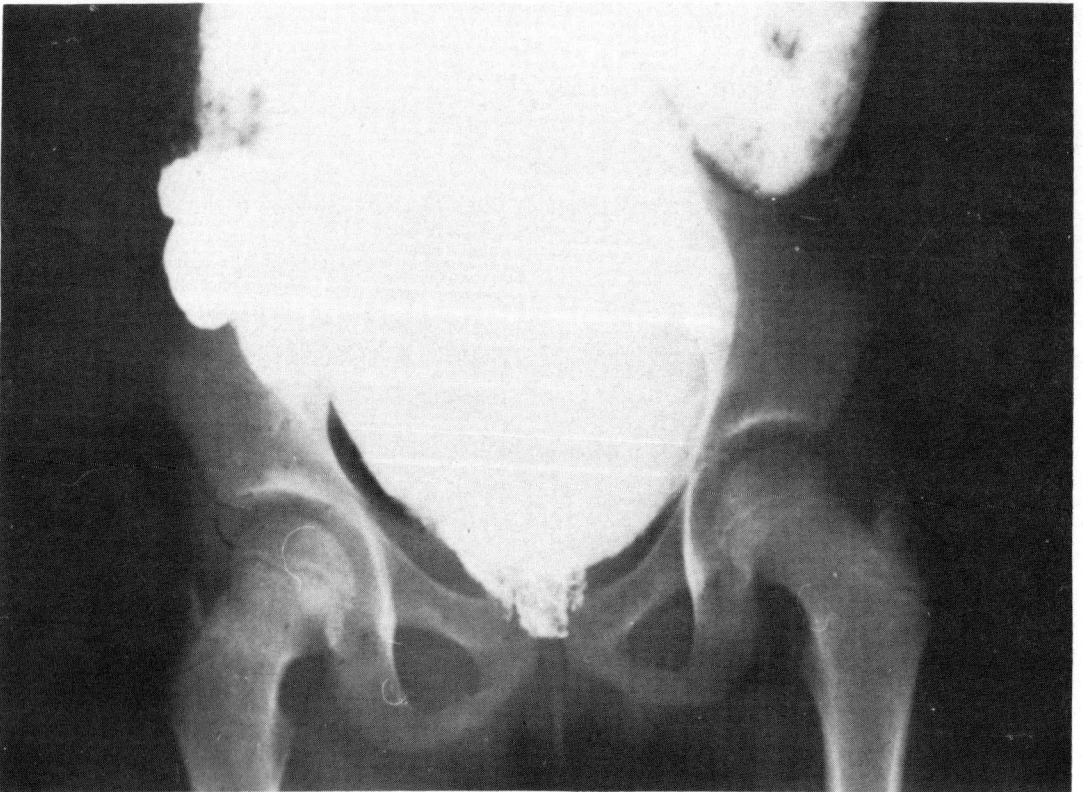

b

Fig. 11.4 Cone in rectum with massive dilatation and hypertrophy seen in classical Hirschsprung's disease: (a) bowel at operation (after decompression); (b) barium enema (dilatation extending into aganglionic segment).

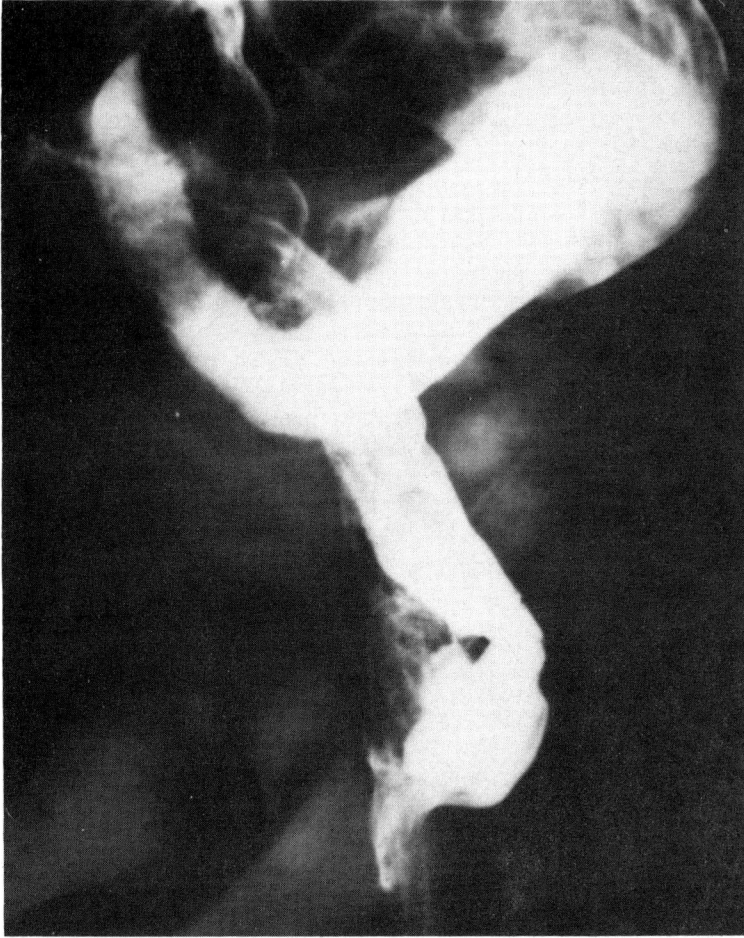

Fig. 11.5 Cone in pelvic colon in Hirschsprung's disease: (a) barium enema; (b) at operation.

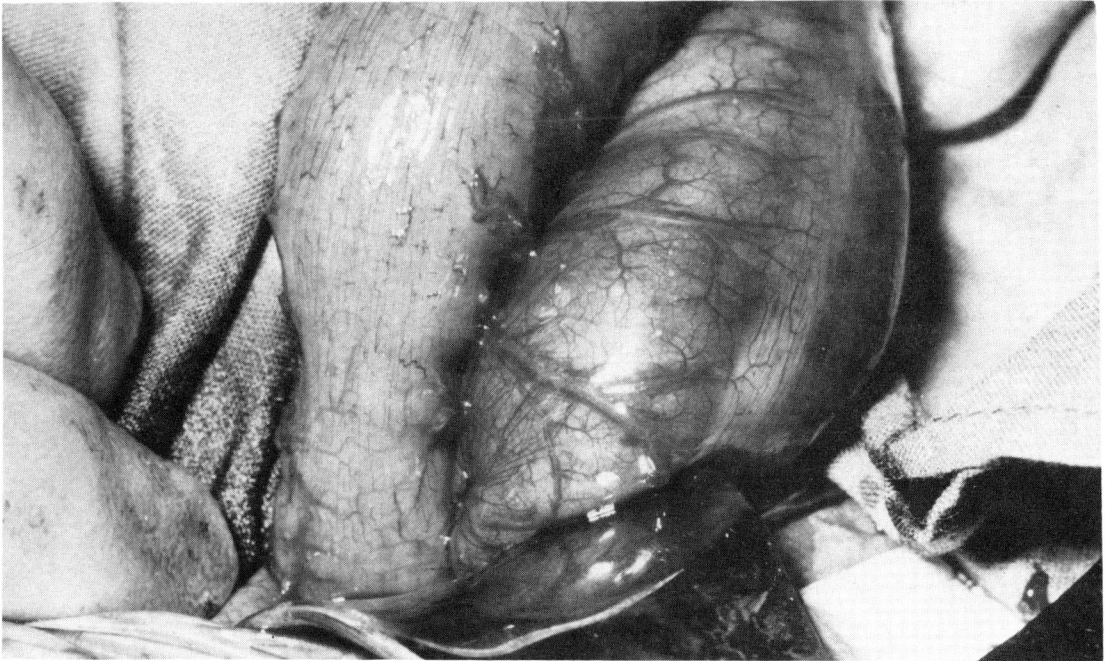

a

b

HISTOLOGY

The diagnosis of Hirschsprung's disease is based on the absence of ganglion cells and the presence of abnormal nerve trunks in the myenteric plexus of a distal segment. Biopsies need to be deep mucosal, or full thickness, if an accurate diagnosis is to be obtained using these criteria. Examination of the proximal bowel using haematoxylin and eosin staining confirms the hypertrophy of the muscle layers, the mucosal changes and normal innervation in most cases. Some degenerative change may occur in ganglion cells. The 'transitional zone' is characterized by fewer ganglion cells and abnormal nerve trunks, usually involving a matter of a few centimetres, but the changes may extend much further proximally. Excess ganglion cells,[24] particularly extending into the submucosa and muscle, indicate associated neuronal colonic dysplasia, more reliably demonstrated by acetylcholinesterase stains. In long segment disease the ganglion cells and nerve trunks are usually absent as in Zuelzer–Wilson syndrome.[41]

HISTOCHEMISTRY

Acetylcholinesterase stains.[16, 18] Acetylcholinesterase stains, demonstrating an excess of acetylcholinesterase staining nerve fibres in the mucosa and submucosa of the distal bowel (and the rare associated neuronal colonic dysplasia),[29] greatly facilitate the diagnosis of Hirschsprung's disease. Superficial mucosal suction biopsy has now become standard practice in most centres investigating this disease.

Formaldehyde-induced fluorescence of adrenergic fibres.[1, 9, 39] An increase in the number and the chaotic distribution of adrenergic fibres in the muscle layers of the affected distal large bowel can be demonstrated. This investigation appears to have limited clinical application.

Physiology: anorectal pressure studies
(Figure 11.6)

Disordered peristalsis has long been recognized in Hirschsprung's disease.[31] Since 1967, anorec-

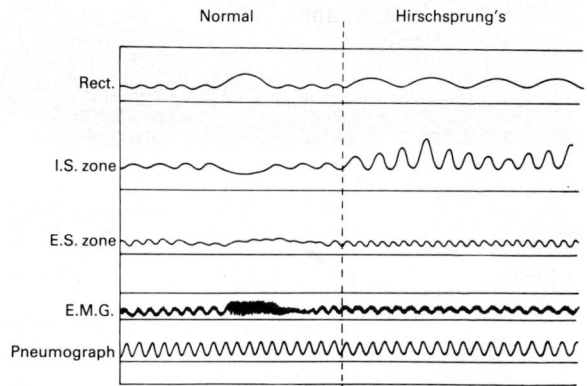

a

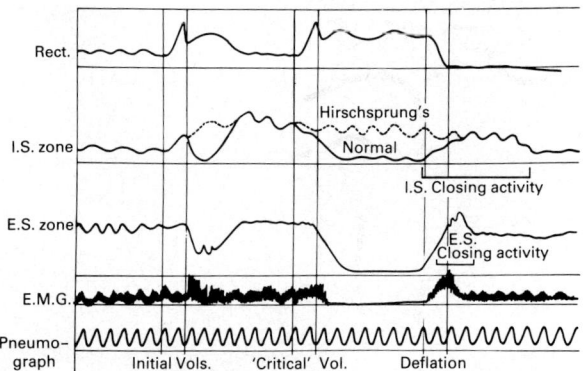

Fig. 11.6 Diagram representing the squeeze pressure changes in the normal anorectum and in Hirschsprung's disease: (a) Resting trace; (b) Response to rectal distension. Rect. = rectum; I.S. = internal sphincter; E.S. = external sphincter. From Lawson and Nixon (1967)[21] with kind permission of the editor of *Journal of Pediatric Surgery.*

b

tal pressure studies have been used both as an aid to diagnosis and for the measurement of residual segment and ultrashort segment disease.[19, 20, 21] The diagnosis of Hirschsprung's disease depends on:

1   The enhancement of rhythmical contraction waves seen in the smooth muscle of the anal canal and rectum, particularly in the former.
2   Loss of normal spontaneous contraction waves recorded from the rectum, where the recording balloon lies in the aganglionic segment.
3   The abnormal configuration of the rectal pressure trace when air is introduced into a rectal balloon lying in the aganglionic segment, or a hypertrophied stimulated wave recorded where the balloon lies above the segment.
4   The absence of the normal fall in pressure in the internal sphincter zone ('recto-anal reflex'). An actual increase in baseline pressure suggesting the more severe form of the disease; seen usually in the ultrashort segment disease or in cases with obstructive symptoms after definitive treatment (residual segment obstruction).[19] Occasional grossly abnormal mass contractions, with superimposed rhythmical waves which may be seen in the affected segment, can force the rectal balloon into the anal canal.

Length of aganglionic segment

In the majority of cases the 'transitional zone' or cone lies in the rectum or sigmoid colon (73–82%) in most large series (Figure 11.7a). Where the rectum has been reported separately the cone lies in the rectum in 45%. (Figure 11.7b).

These figures exclude ultrashort segment disease (segments under 5 cm long). Longer segments occur, with transitional zones demonstrated in the ascending colon and splenic flexure in 13.5–15%, transverse colon 2–4.2%, ascending colon and caecum 0.16–4% and extending into the small bowel in 3–8%. Fortunately total aganglionosis is rare, being reported in from none to 1.4% of cases.

Frequency

An increasing frequency has been noted since the end of the last century, when it was thought to be rare. By 1951 the frequency was 1 : 20 000 live births and in 1967 it was thought to be 1 : 5000 live births. It is certainly more common than this if ultrashort segment disease is included as it accounts for about 10% of children presenting with chronic constipation and soiling.[5]

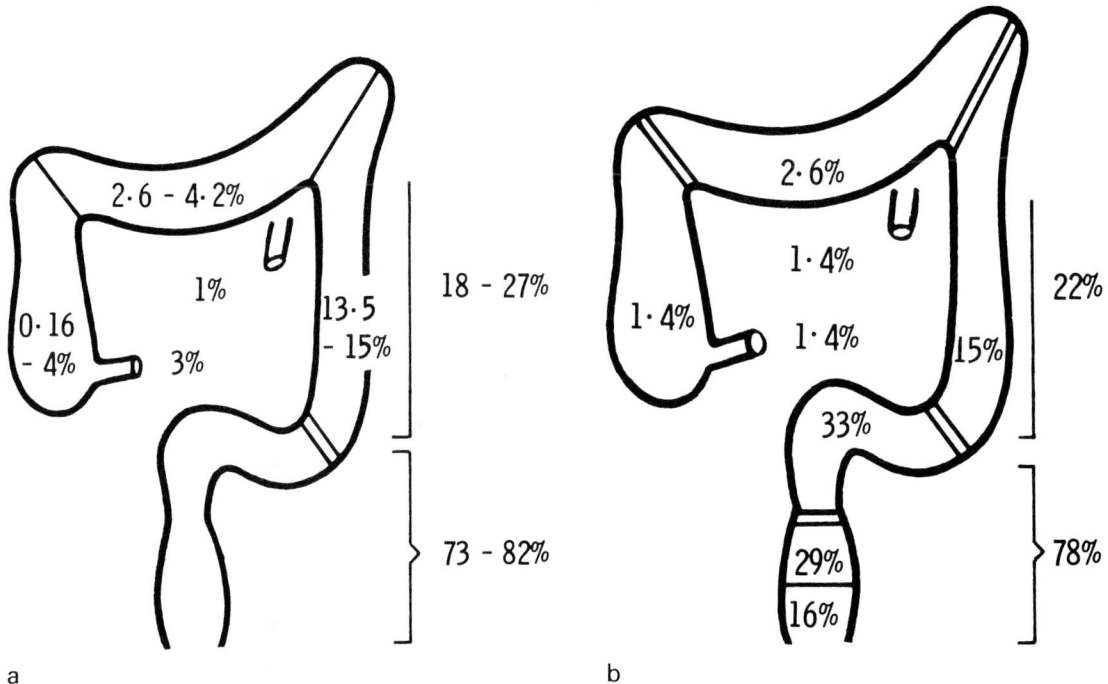

a   b

Fig. 11.7   (a) Distribution of transitional zone in 1175 cases of Hirschsprung's disease; (b) distribution of transitional zone (75 cases), including break-down of distribution in pelvic colon and rectum.

Sex ratio

An overall male preponderance is noted in Hirschsprung's disease. Recent reports suggest a 3.8 : 1 ratio.[17] The male preponderance is most marked in the distal colonic disease, the ratio increasing to 11.7 : 1, when the cone lies in the rectum. The preponderance becomes less marked in longer segment disease (2.8 : 1) and in disease extending beyond the sigmoid colon, and the ratio is 2.2 : 1 where the whole colon is involved. The figures for ultrashort segment disease suggest approximately equal frequency (1.5 : 1).[5] There is a 3 : 1 ratio when there is a family history of Hirschsprung's disease.

Race

Early reports of preponderance among Caucasian patients in the United States[36] has not been confirmed by a recent large series (1196 cases)[17] where the frequency was almost the same in black people as in whites.

Associated anomalies

In most studies there has been a low incidence of associated anomalies. The most consistent association has been with Down's syndrome, 3.2%[36] to 3.7%.[28] The two reports suggested that the overall frequency of other congenital anomalies was 13.5% and 4.4%; the former excludes 2% with mega-ureters. An association with Waardenburg's syndrome (white forelock, wide epicanthic distance, broad root of nose and congenital deafness) has been reported.[23]

Familial associations

A slight familial association appears to be related to the sex of the patient and the length of the segment. Early reports suggest a frequency of 3.6% (7.2% in families of female cases and 2.6% in families of male cases).[28] The recent American Academy of Pediatric Study[17] showed an overall frequency of 11%, with 8% for female and 6% for male patients. If the whole colon was involved, they found a family incidence of 21%. In one Mennonite family, diagnosed and presumptive cases were followed back through nine generations to the early 18th century.[6]

Clinical presentation

Hirschsprung's disease presents as intestinal obstruction of varying intensity. The degree of obstruction varies not only from patient to patient but also, in some cases, from time to time. It can be best understood if considered as a disorder of the balance between propulsive forces active above the aganglionic segment, and resistance afforded by the segment and the consistency of the bowel content.

The age of presentation can be subdivided broadly into those presenting: (a) in the neonatal period (first month of life); (b) in infancy (one month to one year) and early childhood; (c) in later childhood; and (d) in adult life.

Neonatal period (see Figure 11.8)

In the neonatal period, unremitting intestinal obstruction may be present until definitive colostomy or ileostomy is performed. However, obstructive symptoms and signs may settle temporarily following rectal examination or rectal wash-out, or may remit spontaneously. In the latter situation the remission is usually temporary (often occurring after an explosive passage of gas and fluid stool) and obstruction recurs within hours or days. On examination, apart from abdominal distension and increased bowel sounds, the anus and lower rectum may feel smaller than normal and may even present with anal stenosis.

Infancy and early childhood (Figure 11.9)

Patients in this age group present either with subacute or remitting symptoms which persist from the neonatal period, or have little in the way of symptoms, initially, and present later with increasing difficulty in defecation, accompanied by increasing abdominal distension. The symptoms usually commence at about the sixth month or at the end of the first year. The onset is related to changes in consistency of the stool, associated with weaning or increased physical activity. The distension may be intermittent. There may be episodes of diarrhoea and soiling, with semi-solid stool. There is often a marked failure to thrive, poor appetite and listlessness. On examination, varying degrees of emaciation and abdominal distension are noted; distension is often gross, with flaring of the ribs and visible loops of bowel. Rectal examination may be characteristic; the examining fingers enter a dilated bowel through what seems to be a long anal canal. The content is usually semi-solid or liquid and withdrawal of the finger may be followed by an explosive discharge of fluid stool and gas. The anal tone appears normal. The symptoms persist until definitive treatment, or colostomy, is carried out.

Later childhood

These include those patients with symptoms persisting from an earlier age and those presenting primarily with a history of refractory 'consti-

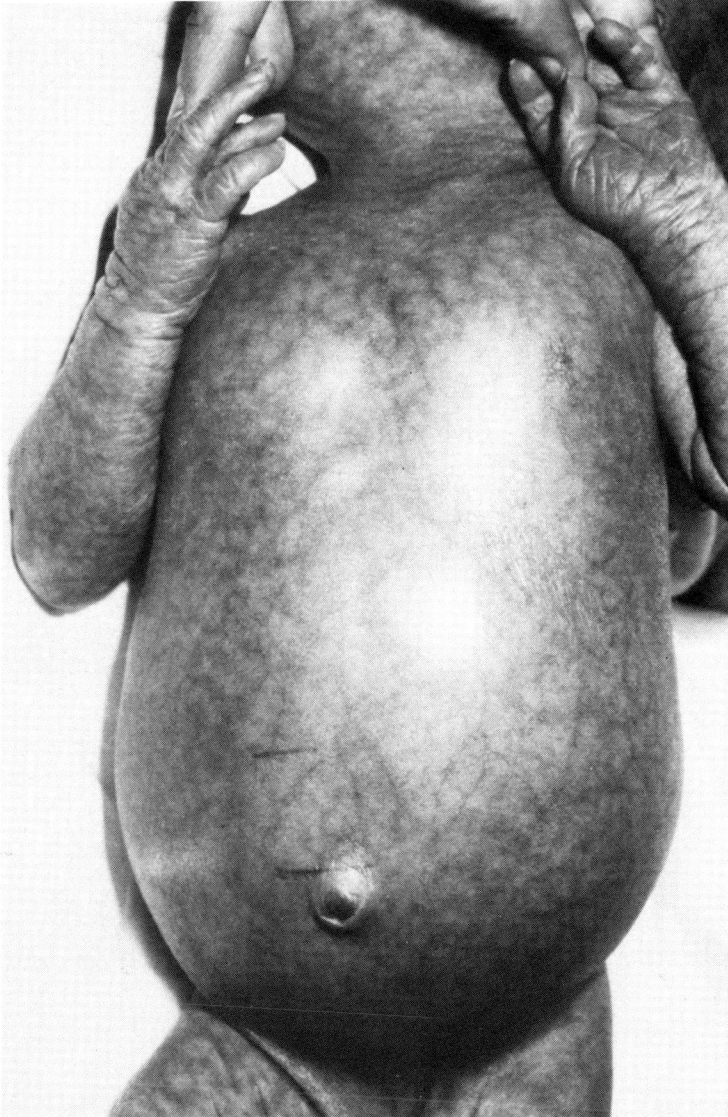

Fig. 11.8 Neonatal intestinal obstruction due to Hirschsprung's disease.

pation'. The complaint is one of difficulty in defecation, the child often experiencing difficulty in passing even soft or semi-solid stool. There is usually a history of failure to thrive, poor appetite and a poor school record. On examination the abdomen is distended, usually in excess of what would have been expected from the degree of faecal loading. Large loops of bowel may be seen through the abdominal wall. With rectal examination in short segment disease, the dilated rectum above the segment can sometimes be identified.

Adult life
Cases are noted into adult life even up to 65–75 years of age.

Diarrhoea and enterocolitis in Hirschsprung's disease

Diarrhoea as a terminal event was first noted by Hirschsprung[12] in his original presentation, and appears to have been the terminal event in 50–90% of the cases described in early reports.

There may be three causes of diarrhoea in children suffering from Hirschsprung's disease:
1 That associated with the relief of obstruction (spontaneous or induced).
2 The bloody diarrhoea associated with ischaemic enterocolitis which may culminate in septicaemia, ischaemic gangrene of the bowel and perforation.
3 The fulminating bloody diarrhoea with profound water, electrolyte and protein dis-

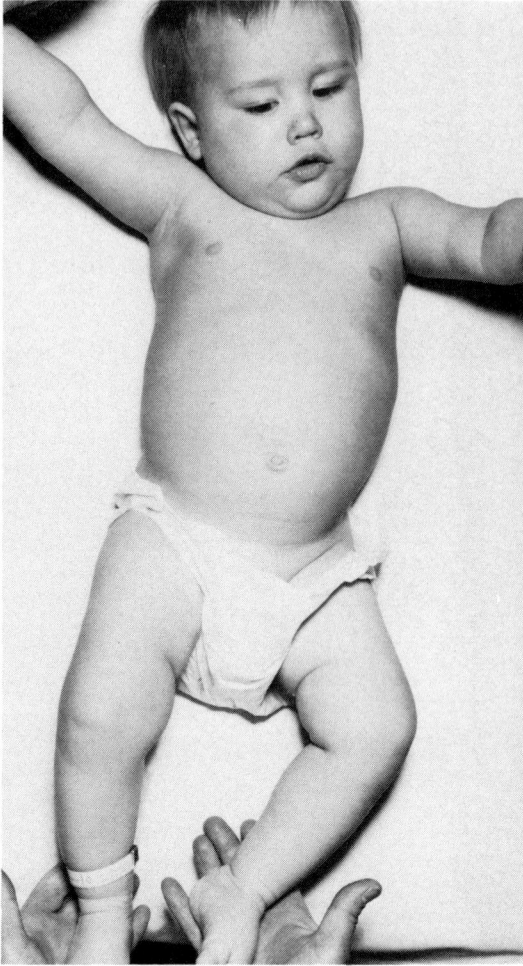
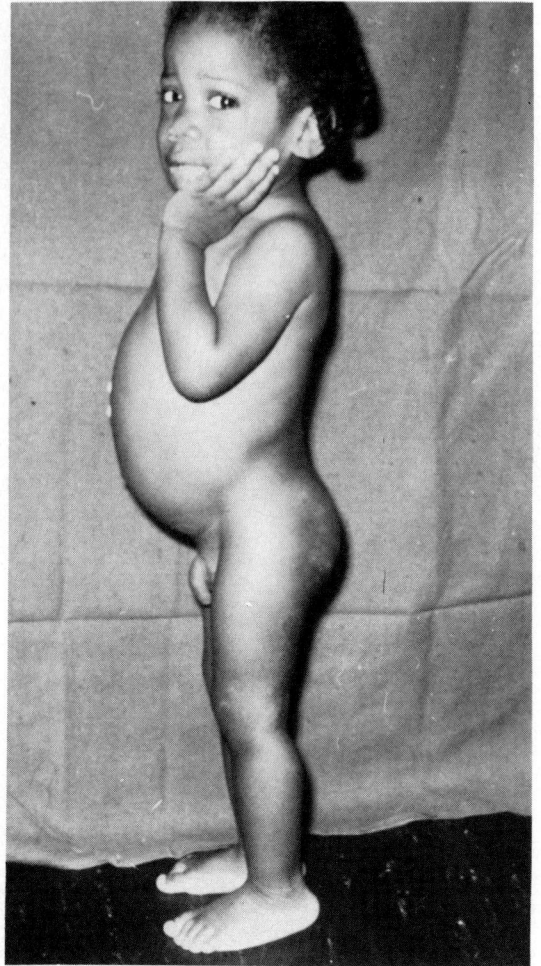

a   b

Fig. 11.9   (a) Hirschsprung's disease in infancy; (b) Hirschsprung's disease in early childhood.

turbance. These children are often moribund on presentation or die within a few hours of the onset of symptoms.[8]

Investigations

Radiology (Figures 11.4b, 11.5a and 11.10)

Plain film of abdomen. Supine and erect (or lateral decubitus in a sick child). To diagnose lower intestinal obstruction or to assess the degree of faecal retention.

Barium enema 'on unprepared bowel'. Introducing hypotonic solution into an enlarged bowel is a hazard.[11] Tap water enemas, or insoluble barium suspended in tap water,[35] have resulted in nausea, vomiting, fits and even death from water intoxication. This complication can be avoided by suspending barium in normal saline and by the technique of introducing very small quantities of barium into the unprepared bowel.[37] This technique also reduces the risk of proximal distension and risk of perforation.

Running small quantities of barium up the distal segment, until it spills into the distended proximal segment, facilitates the demonstration of the aganglionic segment and the cone. Lateral films of the pelvis are important to demonstrate short or ultrashort segment disease.

Anorectal physiology studies
The trace in Hirschsprung's disease is diagnostic. Traces can also be used to measure the segment in short and ultrashort segment disease.[19, 20, 21]

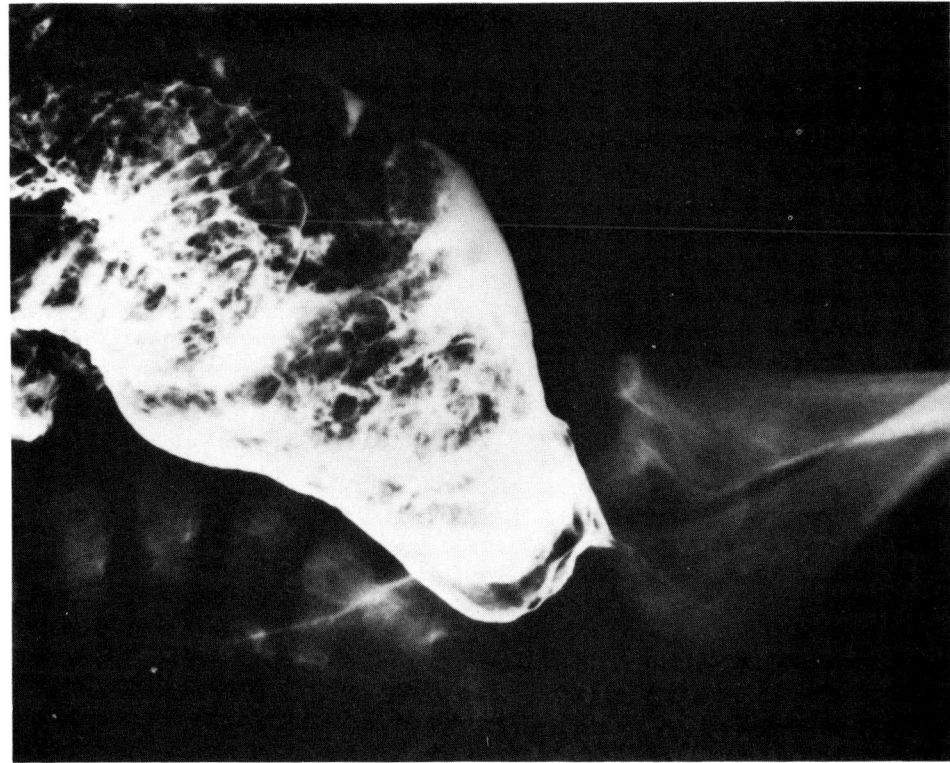

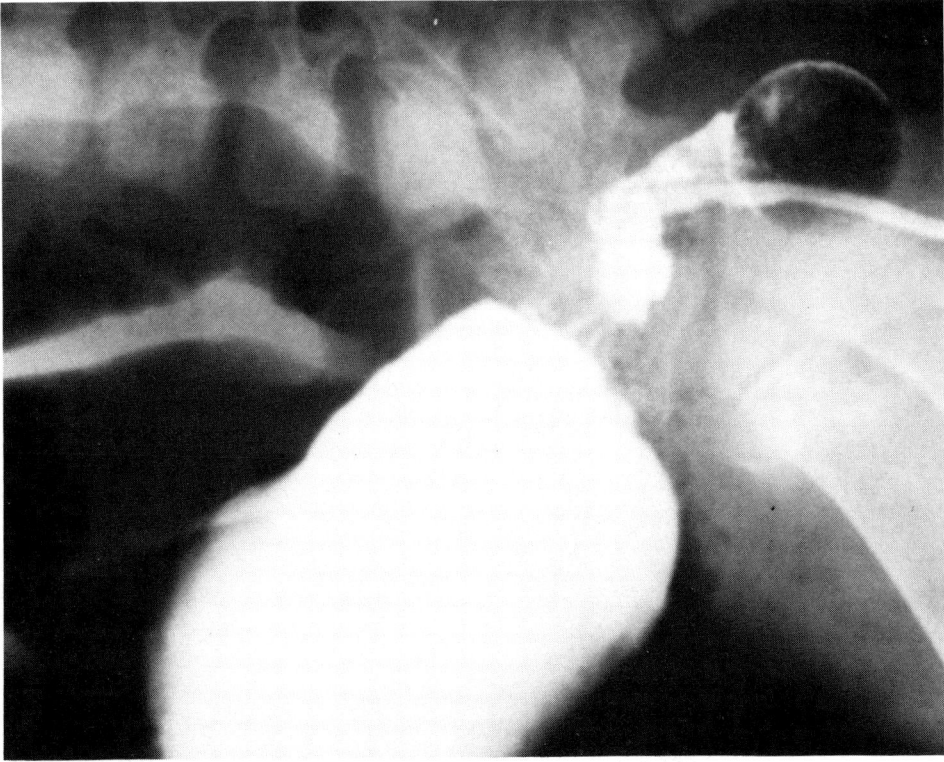

Fig. 11.10 Barium enema in Hirschsprung's disease: (a) ultrashort segment; (b) short segment; (c) long segment – overleaf.

a

b

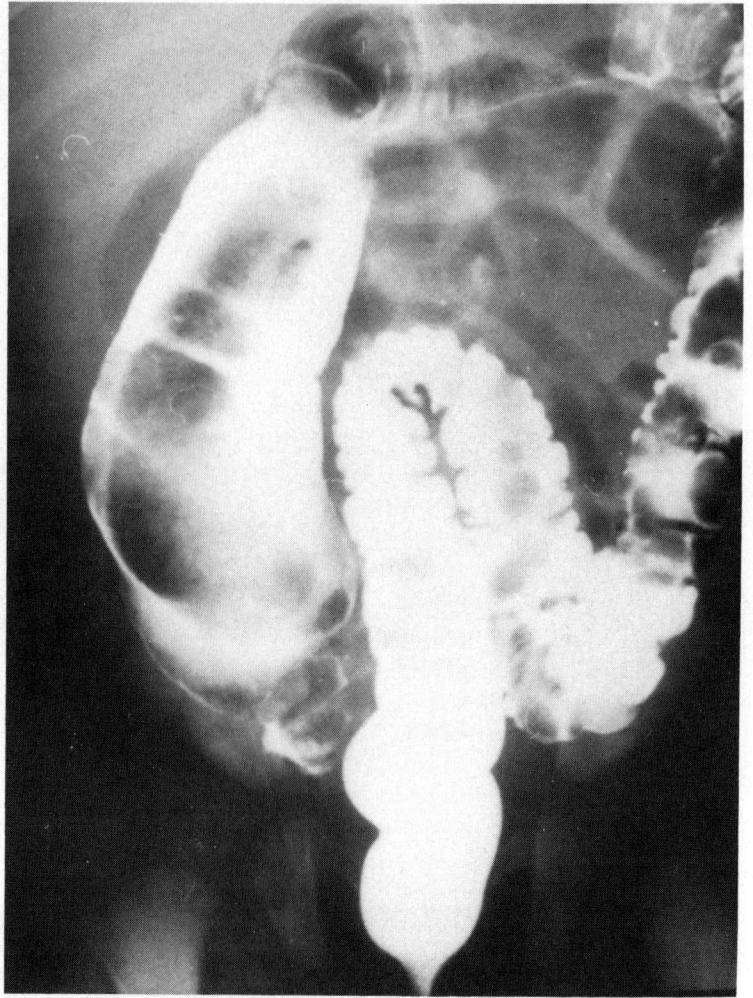

Fig. 11.10 (continued) Barium enema in Hirschsprung's disease: (c) long segment. The transitional zone extended 14 cm above the ileocaecal valve. There is apparent cone dilatation of the proximal colon and there are irregular contractions in the distal colon.

C

Biopsy

At laparotomy. Full thickness biopsies below and above the cone are important to assess the length of segment. This is both to decide on the level that a colostomy is to be established and to be sure that normally innervated bowel is used for the pull-through at definitive operation.

Rectal biopsy.[4] Mucosal or full thickness biopsy can be taken to establish the diagnosis. If histochemical stains are available the initial diagnosis can be made reliably by demonstrating an excess of acetylcholinesterase staining nerve fibres in the mucosa and submucosa. This enables serial suction biopsies to be carried out per anum without anaesthesia. Otherwise deep mucosal (to include muscularis mucosa) or full thickness biopsies are required to demonstrate the absence of ganglion cells and abnormal nerve trunks.

Treatment

The clinical presentation varies widely. Treatment will therefore vary with the mode and time of presentation. In general the more severe disease presents in the neonatal period, or early infancy, and will require more urgent treatment. A later presentation may allow for a fuller preoperative assessment.

Neonatal presentation

Laparotomy and colostomy (or ileostomy). Preoperative decompression of intestinal obstruction with saline rectal washouts is advisable where possible. At laparotomy a cone is identified if present. The level of transition from normal to abnormal innervation should be confirmed by frozen section biopsies. The latter is particularly important in the longer segment disease where a cone may not be apparent.

A defunctioning stoma is established proximal to the 'transitional zone'. In cases with a normal length segment this may be either a pelvic or transverse colostomy, the author favouring the latter. In the longer segment disease an ileostomy may be necessary.

Most paediatric surgeons favour a skin-bridge defunctioning loop colostomy; the loop is retained over a bridge of skin. An ileostomy is usually double ended.

Later presentation

In older children and adults, if the bowel can be adequately prepared a single stage definitive operation may be considered. In general, most of these cases will involve the distal large bowel and are better covered by a preliminary transverse colostomy.

DEFINITIVE OPERATIONS

Four main resection and pull-through procedures are currently in favour. In addition, short and ultrashort, segment disease may be treated per anum.

Rectosigmoidectomy, pull-through and colo-anal anastomosis with preservation of sphincters. Modification of the operation originally described by Swenson and Bill[36] (Figure 11.11).

Retro-rectal pull-through with colo-anal or ileo-anal anastomosis. Modification of the original operation described by Duhamel[7] (currently that described by Martin and Caudill[22] and Steichen, Talbert and Ravitch[34] (Figure 11.12).

Endorectal pull-through. The operation as described by Soave[32] or it's modification[3] (Figure 11.13).

Anterior resection to include dilated hypertrophied bowel.[33] This operation should include either forcible dilatation of the distal segment[30] or extended sphincterotomy (myotomy).[27]

Extended upper partial sphincterotomy (myotomy). In short or ultrashort segment disease, or in the residual segment disease where the segment can be approached per anum, an extended upper partial sphincterotomy, preserving only the lowermost fibres of the internal sphincter ani, can be carried out.[20]

Neuronal intestinal or colonic dysplasia (hyperganglionosis)[24]

This is a condition characterized by an excess of ganglion cells in the myenteric plexuses, and extending into the submucosa, associated with an increase in acetylcholinesterase staining

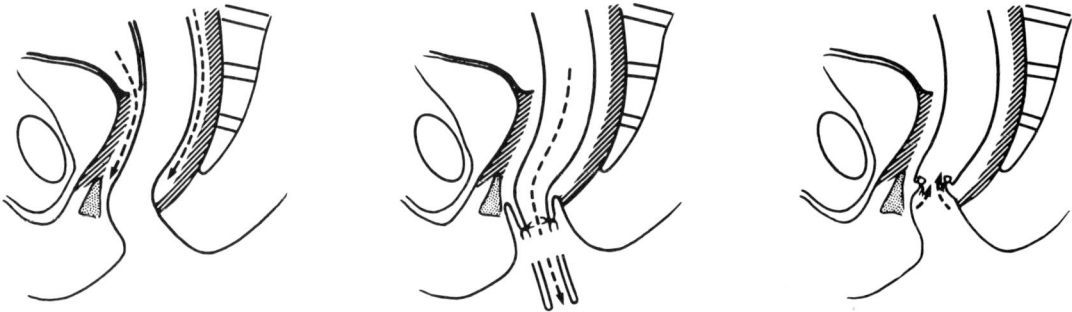

Fig. 11.11   Swenson's operation for Hirschsprung's disease.[36]

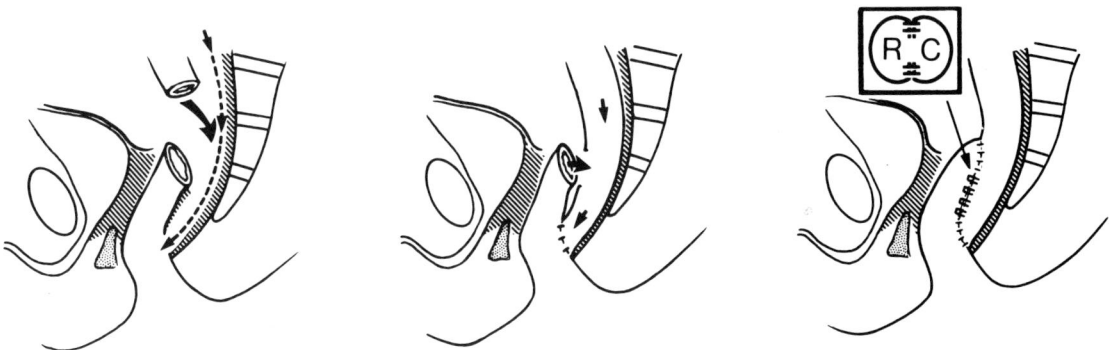

Fig. 11.12   Duhammel's operation for Hirschsprung's disease.[7, 22]

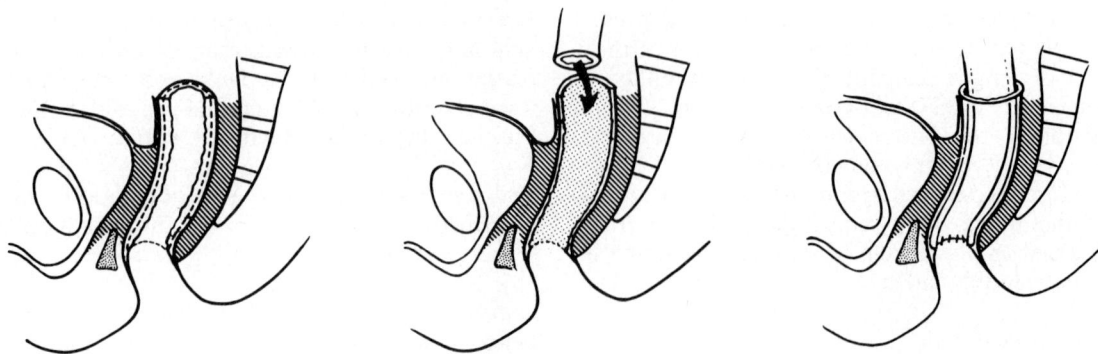

Fig. 11.13   Soave's operation for Hirschsprung's disease.[3, 32]

nerve fibres in the mucosa. It may be seen in association with Hirschsprung's disease[29] and has accounted for persistent obstruction following colostomy or a definitive operation.

REFERENCES

1 Bennett, A., Garrett, J. R. & Howard, E. R. (1968) Adrenergic myenteric nerves in Hirschsprung's disease. *British Medical Journal*, **i**, 487.

2 Bodian, M., Stephens, F. D. & Ward, B. L. H. (1949) Hirschsprung's disease and idiopathic megacolon. *Lancet*, **i**, 6.

3 Boley, S. J., Lafter, D. J., Kleinhaus, S. *et al.* (1968) Endorectal pull-through procedure for Hirschsprung's disease, with and without primary anastomosis. *Journal of Pediatric Surgery*, **3**, 258–262.

4 Campbell, P. E. & Noblett, H. R. (1969) Experience with rectal suction biopsy in the diagnosis of Hirschsprung's disease. *Journal of Pediatric Surgery*, **4**, 410–415.

5 Clayden, G. & Lawson, J. O. N. (1976) Investigation and management of long standing constipation in childhood. *Archives of Diseases in Childhood*, **51**, 918–923.

6 Cohen, J. J. & Gadd, M. A. (1982) Hirschsprung's disease in kindred: two possible clues to the genetics of the disease. *Journal of Pediatric Surgery*, **17**, 632–634.

7 Duhamel, B. (1956) Une nouvelle opération pour le mégacolon congenital: l'abaissement rétro-rectal et trans-anal du colon, et son application possible au traitement de quelques autres malformations. *Presse Medical*, **64**, 2249.

8 Fraser, G. C. & Berry, C. (1967) Mortality in neonatal Hirschsprung's disease: with particular reference to enterocolitis. *Journal of Pediatric Surgery*, **2**, 205–211.

9 Gannon, B. J., Noblett, H. R. & Burnstock, G. (1969) Adrenergic innervation of bowel in Hirschsprung's disease. *British Medical Journal*, **iii**, 338.

10 Garrett, J. R., Howard, E. R. & Nixon, H. H. (1969) Autonomic nerves in rectum and colon in Hirschsprung's disease. *Archives of Diseases in Childhood*, **44**, 406–417.

11 Hiatt, R. B. (1951) Pathologic physiology of congenital megacolon. *Annals of Surgery*, **133**, 313.

12 Hirschsprung, H. (1887) Stuhltragheit Neugeborener in Folge von Dilatation und Hypertrophie des Colons. *Jahresbericht Kuderheilkd*, **27**, 1.

13 Howard, E. R. & Garrett, J. R. (1970) Histochemistry and electron microscopy of rectum and colon in Hirschsprung's disease. *Proceedings of The Royal Society of Medicine*, **63**, 20.

14 Imamura, K., Yamamoto, M., Sato, A. *et al.* (1975) Pathophysiology of aganglionic colon segment: an experimental study on aganglionosis produced by a new method in the rat. *Journal of Pediatric Surgery*, **10**, 865.

15 Kamijo, K., Hiatt, R. B. & Koelle, G. B. (1953) Congenital megacolon. A comparison of the spastic and hypertrophied segments with respect to cholinesterase activities and sensitivities in acetylcholine, DFP and the barium ion. *Gastroenterology*, **24**, 173.

16 Karnovsky, M. J. & Roots, L. (1964) A 'direct-coloring' thiocholine method for cholinesterase. *Journal of Histochemistry and Cytochemistry*, **12**, 219.

17 Kleinhaus, S., Boley, S. J., Sheran, M. & Sieber, W. K. (1979) Hirschsprung's disease. A survey of the members of the surgical section of The American Academy of Pediatrics. *Journal of Pediatric Surgery*, **14**, 588.

18 Lake, B. D. (1976) A cholinesterase method for light and electron microscopy. *Proceedings of the Royal Microscopic Society*, **11**, 77.

19 Lawson, J. O. N. (1970) Structure and function of the internal anal sphincter. *Proceedings of the Royal Society of Medicine*, **63**, 84–89.

20 Lawson, J. O. N. (1972) Observations on 'residual segment obstruction' in treated Hirschsprung's disease. *Progress in Paediatric Surgery*, **4**, 129–164.

21 Lawson, J. O. N. & Nixon, H. H. (1967) Anal canal pressures in the diagnosis of Hirschsprung's disease. *Journal of Pediatric Surgery*, **2**, 544–552.

22 Martin, L. W. & Caudill, D. R. (1967) A method for elimination of the blind rectal pouch in the Duhamel operation for Hirschsprung's disease. *Surgery*, **62**, 951–953.

23 McKusick, V. A. (1973) Congenital deafness and Hirschsprung's disease. *New England Journal of Medicine*, **288**, 691.

24 Meier-Ruge, W. (1970) Hirschsprung's disease: it's aetiology pathogenesis and differential diagnosis. *Current Topics in Pathology*, Volume 59, pp. 131–179. Berlin, Heidelberg, New York: Springer-Verlag.

25 Mya, G. (1894) Due osservazioni di dilatazione ed ipertrofia congenita del colon. *Sperimentale*, **48**, 215.

26 Okamoto, E. & Ueda, T. (1967) Embryogenesis of intramural ganglia of the gut and it's relation to Hirschsprung's disease. *Journal of Pediatric Surgery*, **14**, 58.

27 Orr, J. D. & Scobie, W. G. (1979) Anterior resection combined with anorectal myectomy in the treatment of Hirschsprung's disease. *Journal of Pediatric Surgery*, **14**, 58–61.

28 Passarge, E. (1967) The genetics of Hirschsprung's disease. Evidence for heterogenous etiology and a study of sixty-three families. *New England Journal of Medicine*, **276**, 138.

29 Puri, P., Lake, B. D., Nixon, H. H. *et al.* (1977) Neuronal colonic dysplasia: an unusual association of Hirschsprung's disease. *Journal of Pediatric Surgery*, **12**, 681–685.

30 Rehbein, F. (1958) Intraabdominelle resektion oder recto-sigmoidektomie (Swenson) bei der Hirschsprungschen Krankheit? *Chirurgie*, **29**, 366.

31 Robertson, H. E. & Kernohan, J. W. (1938) The myenteric plexus in congenital megacolon. *Proceedings of Staff Meeting at the Mayo Clinic*, **13**, 123.

32 Soave, F. (1963) Die nahtlose colon-anastomose nach extramucoser Mobilierung und Herabziehung des Rectosigmoids zur chirurgischen Behandlung des M. Hirschsprung. *Zentralblatt fur Chirurgie*, **88**, 31.

33 State, D. (1952) Surgical treatment for idiopathic congenital megacolon (Hirschsprung's disease). *Surgery, Gynecology and Obstetrics*, **95**, 201.

34 Steichen, F. M., Talbert, J. L. & Ravitch, M. M. (1968) Primary side to side colorectal anastomosis in the Duhamel operation for Hirschsprung's disease. *Surgery*, **64**, 475–483.

35 Steinbach, H. L., Rosenberg, R. H., Grossman, M. & Nelson, T. L. (1955) Potential hazard of enemas in patients with Hirschsprung's disease. *Radiology*, **64**, 45.

36 Swenson, O. & Bill, A. H. (1948) Resection of rectum and rectosigmoid with preservation of the sphincter for benign spastic lesions producing megacolon: an experimental study. *Surgery*, **24**, 212.

37 Swenson, O., Neuhauser, E. B. D. & Pickett, L. K. (1949) New concept of etiology: diagnosis and treatment of congenital megacolon (Hirschsprung's disease). *Pediatrics*, **4**, 201.

38 Swenson, O., Sherman, J. O. & Fisher, J. H. (1973) Diagnosis of congenital megacolon. Analysis of 501 patients. *Journal of Pediatric Surgery*, **8**, 587–594.

39 Touloukain, R. J., Aghajanian, G. & Roth, R. H. (1973) Adrenergic hyperactivity of the aganglionic colon. *Journal of Pediatric Surgery*, **8**, 191.

40 Whitehouse, F. R. & Kernohan, J. W. (1948) Myenteric plexus in congenital megacolon. *Archives of Internal Medicine*, **82**, 75.

41 Zuelzer, W. W. & Wilson, J. L. (1948) Functional intestinal obstruction on congenital neurogenic basis in infancy. *American Journal of Diseases in Childhood*, **75**, 40.

ANORECTAL MALFORMATION

Anorectal malformations were noted in ancient times.[10] Accounts appear in Egyptian papyri (1600 BC) and in cuneiform tablets (650 BC). Empedocles, Democritus and Aristotle, writing in the 4th and 5th centuries BC, put forward theories for the aetiology of the condition, the latter noting that the disease was more common in males. Early treatment was recorded by the Soranos in the 2nd century AD, and accounts of treatment appear in Persian (Razes) and Arabic (Haliabbas) manuscripts dating back to the 9th century. The treatment seems to have been restricted to dilatation and dilatation following perineal incisions. It was not until 1793 that the first colostomy was successfully established, by Duret. The first sacroperineal pullthrough operation was carried out by Amussat in 1835. Abdomino-perineal pullthrough, performed as a single-stage operation, had to await the improvement of anaesthesia, and was first performed by Rhoads, Pipes and Randal in 1948.[7]

AETIOLOGY

Current theories of production of this malformation are based on the studies of Wood-Jones.[15] He attributed failure of formation of a permanent anus to a failure of communication between the postallantoic gut and the proctodaeum and attributed the fistulas to failure of separation of the hind-gut from the allantois.

CLASSIFICATIONS

The presence of two classifications – those of Keith[3] and Ladd and Gross[4] – has caused considerable confusion in the past. Following a meeting in Melbourne in 1970, there has been wide acceptance of an 'international classification' (Table 11.1).[8, 13] This classification is based on division into: (a) low deformities, where the bowel passes through the levator ani, (b) intermediate deformities, where the bowel enters the levator ani, and (c) high deformities, where the bowel ends above the levator ani. These are further divided into those that have an abnormal opening or fistula, and those that do not. Even this extensive classification does not include all the abnormalities, some of which are grouped under the heading 'miscellaneous deformities'.

CLINICAL FEATURES AND TREATMENT

Low abnormalities

In these the bowel extends below the levator ani, into or through voluntary sphincters.

Table 11.1 International classification of anorectal anomalies (1970).[8]

			Male	Female
Low deformities (translevator)				
1	At normal anal site			
	Covered anus – complete		2	13
	Anal stenosis		1	12
2	At perineal site			
	Anterior perineal anus		4	15
	Anocutaneous fistula (covered anus – incomplete)		3	14
3	At vulvar site			
	Female	vestibular anus		18
		anovulvar fistula		16
		anovestibular fistula		17
Intermediate deformities				
1	Anal agenesis:			
	Male	*without fistula:* anal agenesis	5	
		with fistula: rectobulbar	6	
	Female	*without fistula:* anal agenesis		19
		with fistula: rectovaginal – low		20
		rectovestibular		21
2	Anorectal stenosis		7	22
High deformities (supralevator)				
1	Anorectal agenesis			
	Male	*without fistula:* anorectal agenesis	8	
		with fistula: rectourethral	9	
		rectovesical	10	
	Female	*without fistula:* anorectal agenesis		23
		with fistula: rectovesical		26
		rectocloacal		25
		rectovaginal – high		24
2	Rectal atresia		11	27
Miscellaneous deformities, including:				
1	Imperforate anal membrane			
2	(a) Covered anal stenosis			
	(b) Anal membrane stenosis			
3	Vesico-intestinal fissure (cloacal exstrophy)			
4	Duplications of anus, rectum and genitourinary tract			
5	Combination of deformities from the basic list			
6	Perineal groove			
7	Perineal canal			

ABNORMALITIES IN WHICH THE BOWEL EXTENDS ALONG NORMAL LINE OF ANORECTUM TOWARDS NORMAL SITE

Covered anus (male and female: nos. 2 & 13)
The bowel extends down to its normal site, but is covered by an operculum (Figure 11.14). This covering consists of a layer of skin and a layer of mucosa (stratified cuboidal epithelium). Clinically, the membrane presents as a bulge at the normal anal site. There may be an anteroposterior bar or raphe with a thin membrane on either side.[1] Treatment consists of uncovering the anus by excising the membrane and anal dilatation. Some mucocutaneous sutures may be required, the suture line requiring digital dilatation for up to three months postoperatively.

Anal stenosis (male and female: nos. 1 & 12)
There is a small opening at the normal site (Figure 11.15). The size is between that of an

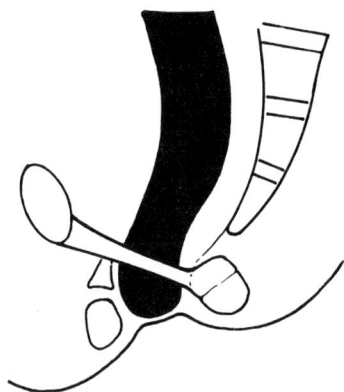

a

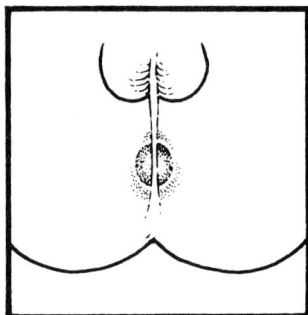

Fig. 11.14 Covered anus, complete (male *2* and female *13* – low anomaly): (a) diagram; (b) inversion film; (c) clinical appearance.

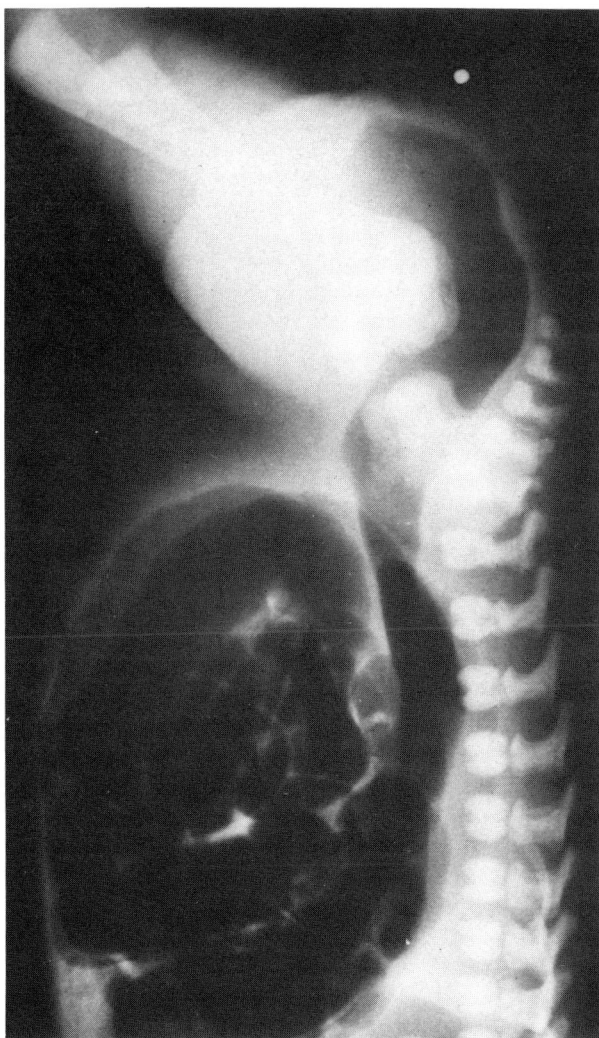

b

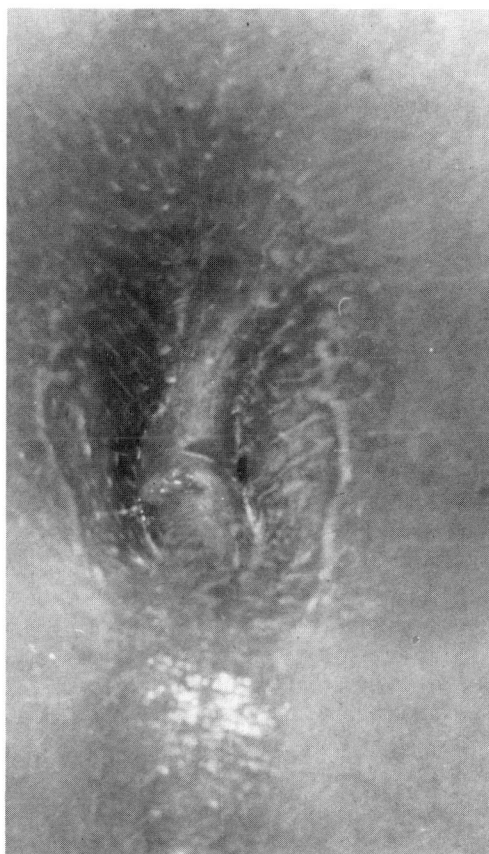

c

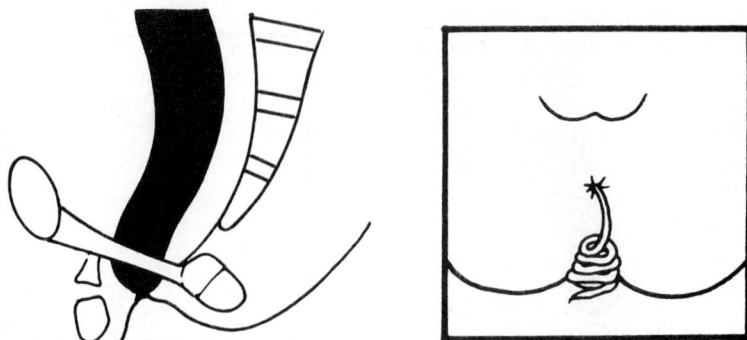

Fig. 11.15 Anal stenosis (male *1* and female *12* – low anomaly): (a) diagram; (b) clinical appearance; (c) 'ribbon' or 'toothpaste' stool.

a

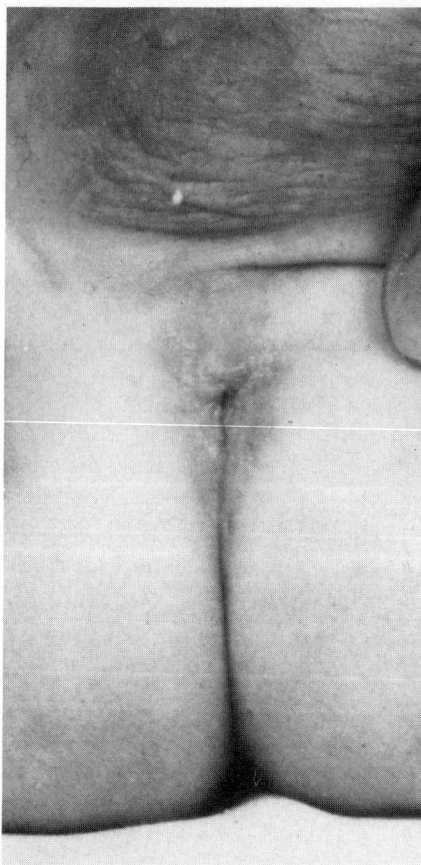

b

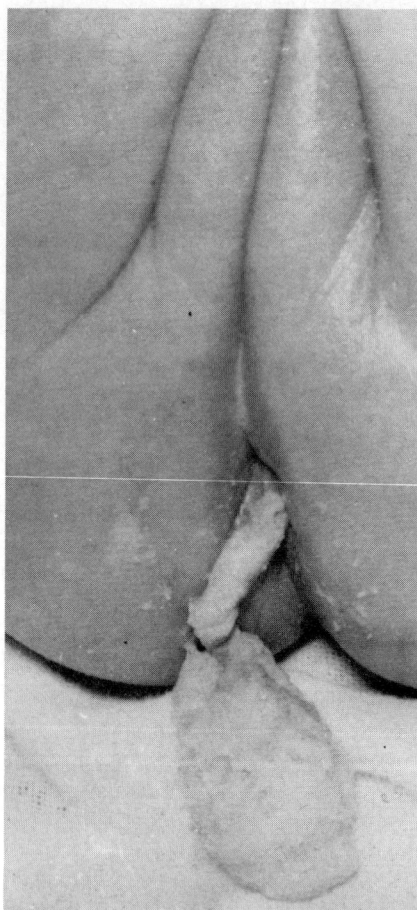

c

intravenous catheter and that of the distal phalanx of the fifth finger (in a full-term mature baby). Structurally this may consist of a thin mucocutaneous stricture or a stenotic segment, usually in the region of 0.5–1.0 cm in length. Histological study of the latter shows absence of the internal sphincter from the lower canal. The

muscle fibres between the mucosa and the voluntary muscle are predominantly arranged vertically.

These cases rarely present before the age of two or three months (Figure 11.15b). There is a history of straining, crying on defecation and sometimes blood in the stool and on the diaper.

If defecation has been witnessed, there may be a history of passage of a 'toothpaste' or 'ribbon' stool (Figure 11.15c). It is significant that the parents complaint that the child strains to defecate is often dismissed. Further, these children are liable to fulminating enterocolitis, comparable with that of Hirschsprung's disease, which may culminate in death.

The treatment is gentle graded dilatation, initially under general anaesthetic with Hegar's dilators, and subsequently progressive digital dilatation to the size of the index finger. This should be continued for three months. Vigorous dilatation may result in rupture of the stenosed segment with subsequent tendency to soil. As a result of the delay in diagnosis, this condition is usually associated with gross megarectum. The consequent constipation may require long-term treatment.

OPENINGS ON THE PERINEUM OTHER THAN THE NORMAL SITE

These openings vary in size; if adequate or near adequate, they are termed anuses, narrower openings being termed fistulas (nos. 4, 3, 15 & 14).

Anterior perineal anus (male and female: nos. 4 & 15)

This is an anteriorly placed anus, usually passing down in front of the annulus of the deep sphincter (Figure 11.16). There may be a dimple at the normal site, with or without a median raphe, with a palpable, contracting, voluntary sphincter around it. Even where the anus appears adequate, there may be a moderate mucocutaneous stenosis and, if associated with megarectum, a probe or finger passes back over a 'shelf' containing the voluntary sphincters (Figure 11.16c). Histologically, the internal sphincter can usually be shown to retain its normal relation to the bowel, which passes through the pelvic floor slings.

In males the abnormally placed anus, if not stenosed, may give little or no symptoms other than minimal incontinence of loose stools. If stenosed, it will present in the same way as anal stenosis.

In females clinical presentation will be similar to that in males, but in addition severe third-degree tears of the thin anovaginal septum (perineal body) may occur later during parturition.

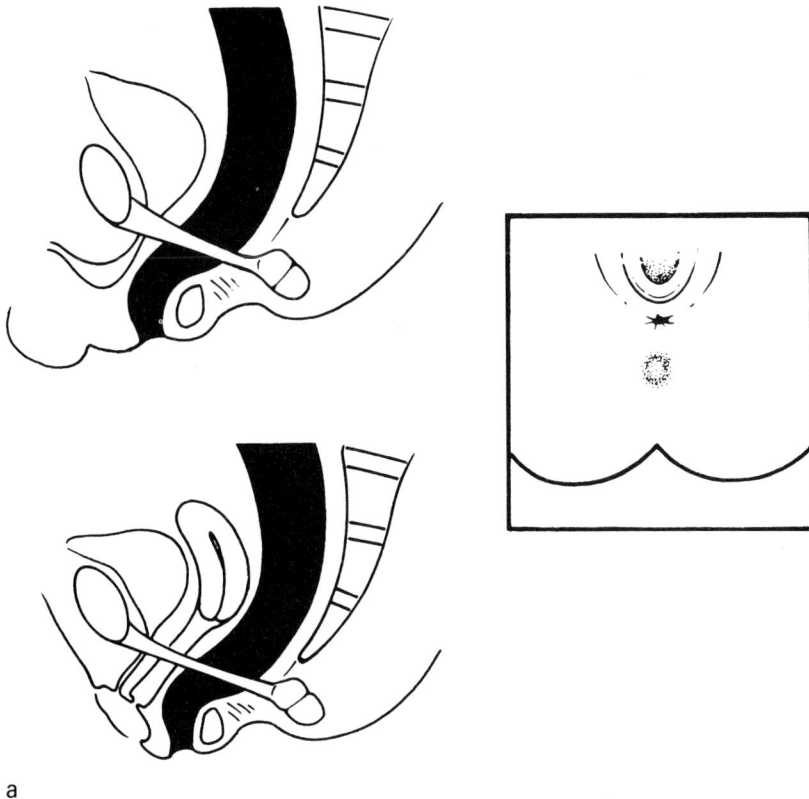

a

Fig. 11.16 Anterior perineal anus ('ectopic') (male *4* and female *15* – low anomaly): (a) diagram; (b) & (c), overleaf.

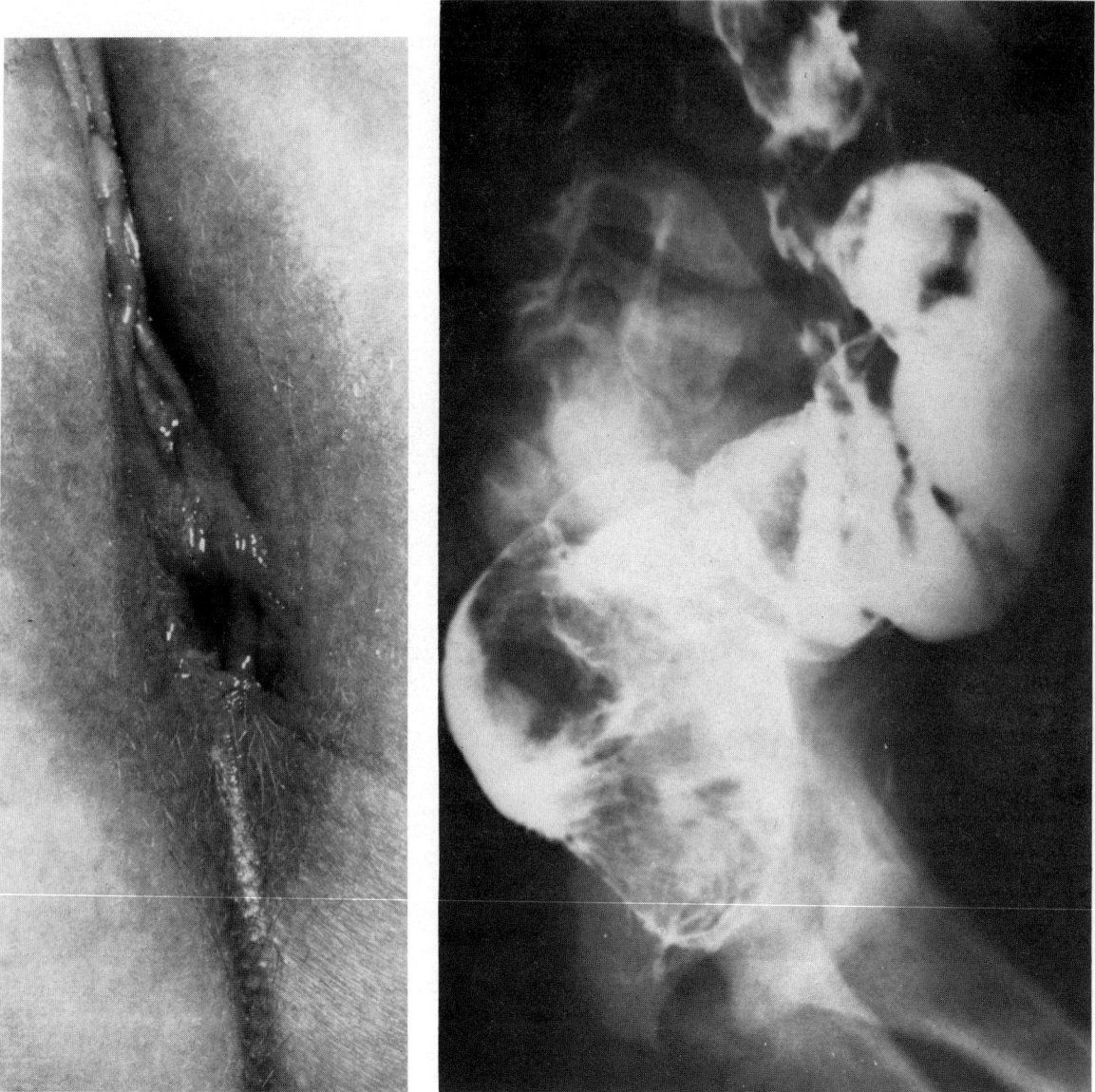

b   c

Fig. 11.16 (continued) Anterior perineal anus ('ectopic'): (b) clinical appearance; (c) barium enema, showing anterior opening and shelf over external sphincter.

When there is no stenosis, no treatment is required, except careful management of pregnancy and delivery in the female. Those presenting early with stenosis will require progressive anal dilatation, but if the presentation is delayed additional long-term management of constipation may be required. Some surgeons consider 'cut-back' to the 'shelf', but this may result in diminished continence.

Anocutaneous fistula (covered anus, incomplete)
(male and female: nos. 3 & 14)
Here the bowel passes down through the external sphincter ani (Figure 11.17a), but then turns

forward, being continued subcutaneously, as a fistulous track deep to the median raphe, to open anywhere from a point just in front of the normal anal site (Figure 11.17b) to the tip of the penis (Figure 11.17c) in males, and as far as the fourchette in females. If the fistula opens in front of the fourchette in a female it is termed an *anovulvar fistula* (Figure 11.18) (number 16; compare with anovestibular fistulas, considered below).

The abnormality appears to be associated with an over-migration of the internal sphincter. The thickened covering at the normal site usually contains the internal sphincter, which

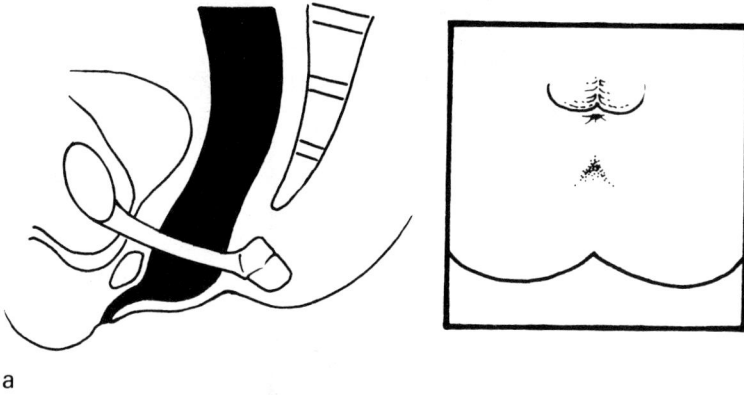

a

Fig. 11.17 Anocutaneous fistula (covered anus, incomplete) (male *3* – low anomaly): (a) diagram; (b) clinical appearance, fistula in front of anus; (c) clinical appearance, fistula extending forwards to tip of penis.

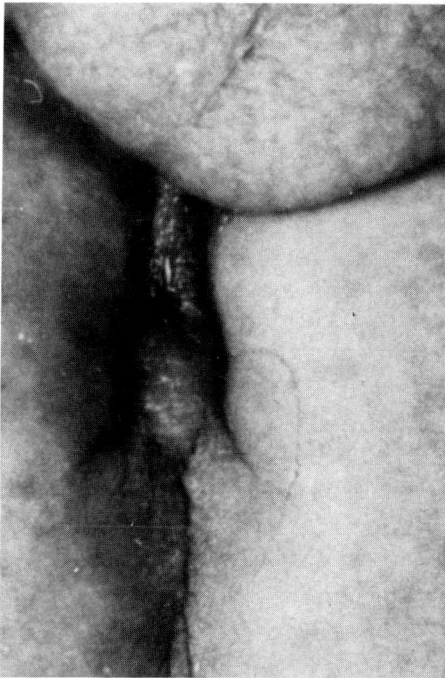

b

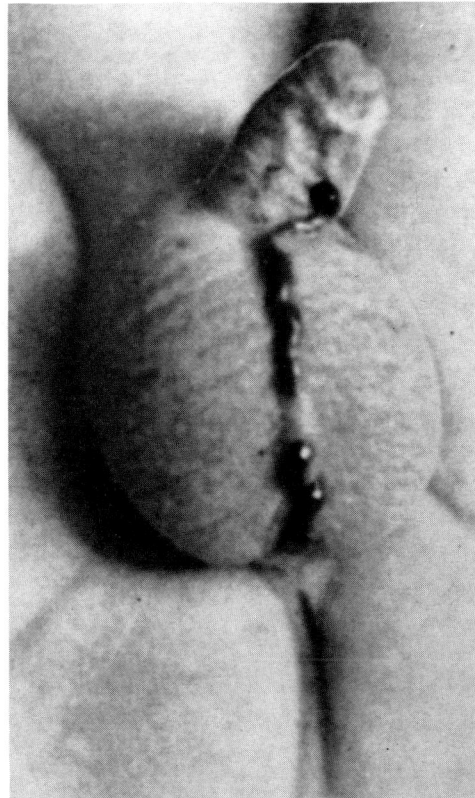

c

may be cut during the classical cut-back operation.

Clinically, most of the cases present as 'imperforate anus' in the newborn period. A few, with larger openings, present much later, usually with an associated gross megarectum. On examination there may be an appearance of an inverted 'V' over the normal anal site, and anterior to this a very superficial thin-walled tract extending forwards, coloured by the contained meconium, which discharges at the fistulous opening along the line of the median raphe.

OPENINGS AT VESTIBULAR SITES (BELOW THE HYMEN, BUT IN THE VESTIBULE OR INTROITUS)

Vestibular anus (no. 18) and anovestibular fistula (no. 17)

Here the lumen tracks more obliquely downwards and forwards, and may pass through the external sphincter to reach a vestibular opening (Figure 11.19). Where the opening is adequate the anus may contain an internal anal sphincter, but where it is fistulous the sphincter, if present, is attenuated.

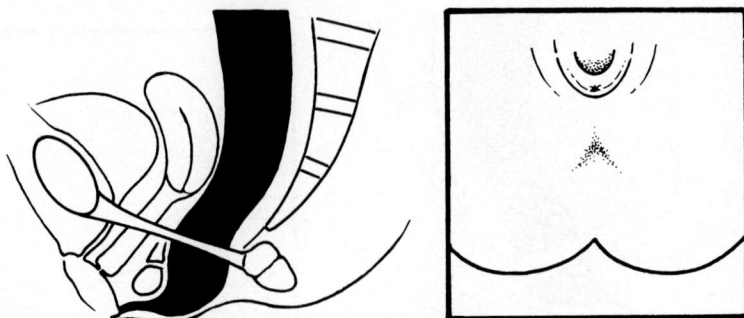

a

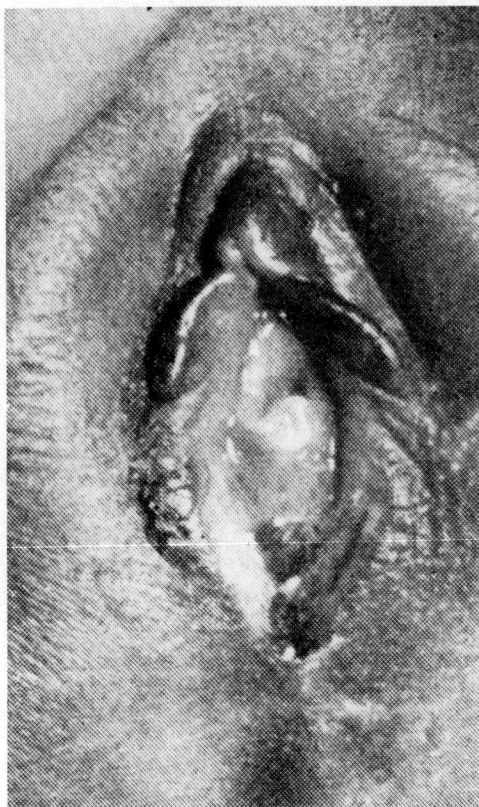

Fig. 11.18 Covered anus, incomplete, with anovulvar fistula (female *16* – low anomaly): (a) diagram; (b) clinical appearance.

b

Clinically, it is unusual for the diagnosis to be delayed, the abnormal appearance being noted at birth. Straining, abdominal distension and passage of 'toothpaste' or 'ribbon' stool may be noted. On examination the opening lies in front of the fourchette but below and behind the hymen. A finger or silver probe passes backwards and upwards from the abnormal opening. A varying degree of stenosis is usually present.

Initially, anal dilatation or modified cut-back is required. Later, anal transplant through a perineal or sacroperineal approach may be carried out.

Anovulvar fistula (*no. 16*)
This lesion is very similar to anocutaneous fistula (covered anus, incomplete) (see above). A probe introduced passes directly back to the normal anal site.

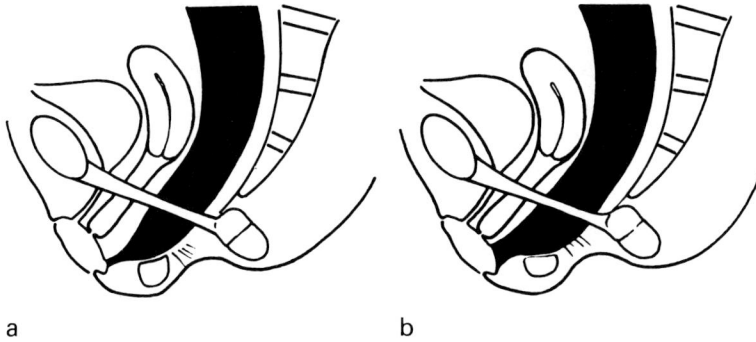

a

b

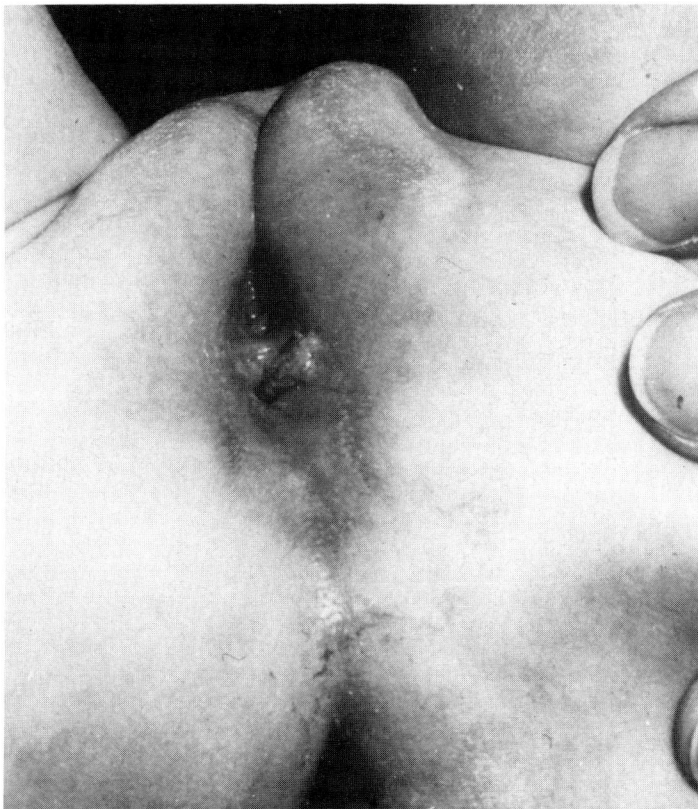

c

Fig. 11.19 Anovestibular fistula or vestibular anus (female – low anomaly): (a) anovestibular fistula *17*, diagram; (b) vestibular anus *18*, diagram; (c) anovestibular fistula, clinical appearance.

Intermediate abnormalities

Here the bowel extends into the levator ani but not through it.

ANAL AGENESIS

Anal agenesis without fistula (male and female: nos. 5 & 19)
Here the stump of the rectum extends into the pelvic floor and the blind end is lined with stratified cuboidal epithelium (Figure 11.20).

Macroscopically it is thrown into folds resembling anal columns. Simple tubular glands extend out into, or through, the internal anal sphincter.

On the initial examination this abnormality is indistinguishable from the high variants presenting as imperforate anus. Inversion (Wagenstein) films suggest the abnormality, and the expression cystoloopogram, in the male, and expression loopogram, in the female, will give the diagnosis.

Sacral and perineal approach gives adequate exposure for anoplasty.

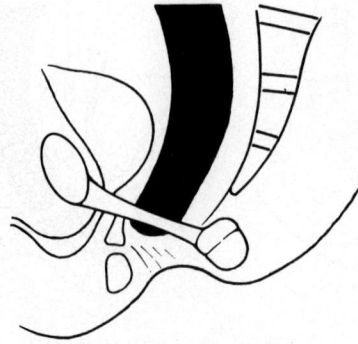

a

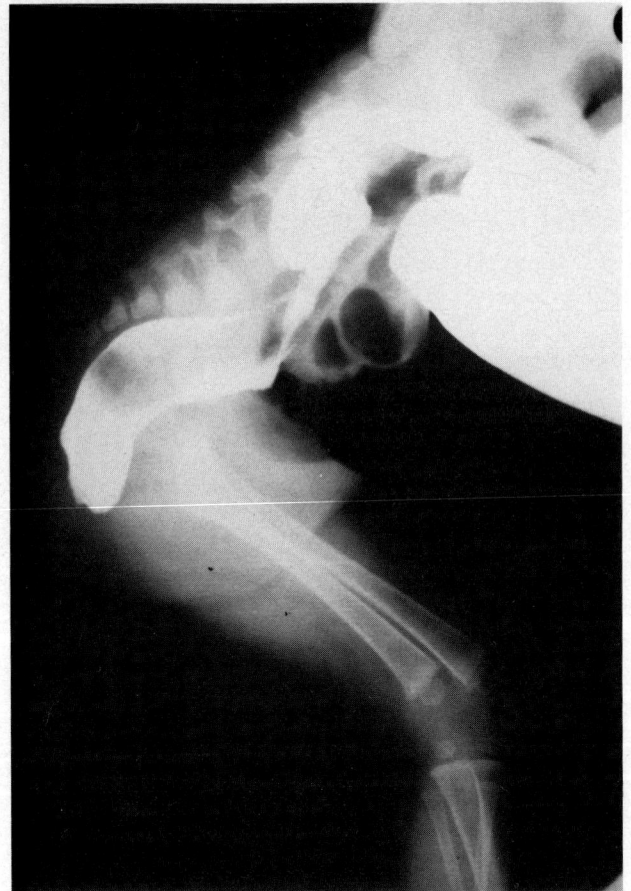

Fig. 11.20   Anal agenesis (male *5* and female *19* – intermediate anomaly): (a) diagram; (b) distal loop barium study.

b

Anal agenesis with fistula (male):
Rectobulbar fistula (no. 6)
This abnormality was considered intermediate at the Melbourne meeting. In many the fistula extends forwards, below the deep sphincter and perineal body and above the external sphincter and scrotum, to open into the bulb of the urethra (Figure 11.21).

Initially, this abnormality is clinically indistinguishable from the high variants. The passage of gas or meconium through the urethra may confirm the presence of a recto-urethral fistula. Inversion films may indicate that this is an intermediate, rather than a high variant.

Initial treatment is colostomy. Later, assessment with a cystoloopogram and

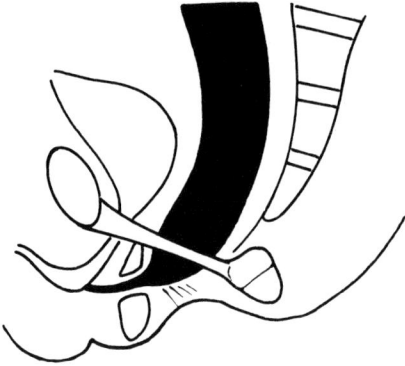

a

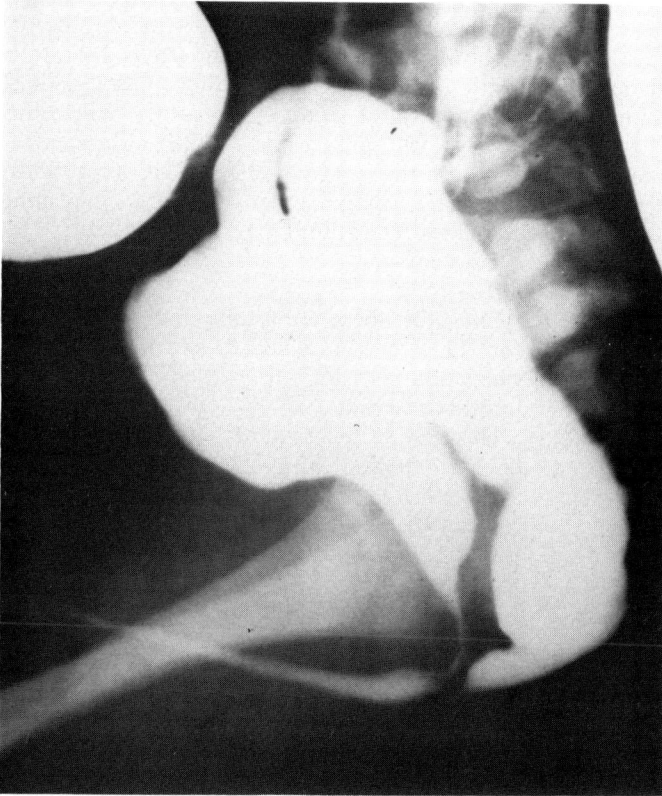

b

Fig. 11.21 Anal agenesis with rectobulbar fistula (male *6* – intermediate anomaly): (a) diagram; (b) cystoloopogram contrast studies.

cytourethroscopy is required to confirm bulbar fistulas (Figure 11.21b).

For mobilization and division of this fistula and anoplasty I approach through a transverse incision between dimple and scrotum, bringing the fistula and terminal bowel down through a cruciate incision at the normal anal site.

Anal agenesis with fistula (female):
Rectovaginal fistula (no. 21)
Rectovestibular fistula (no. 20)
In both of these the bowel extends into the pelvic floor, but in the former the fistula tracks horizontally forward and opens just above the hymen and in the latter it passes downwards and forwards obliquely through the perineal body to open below the hymen (Figure 11.22).

Diagnosis is usually made soon after birth, and is usually associated with a discharge of meconium from the vagina or vulva. The diagnosis is confirmed by probing the fistulous opening. In rectovaginal fistulas the probe passes into the fistula just above the hymen and passes almost directly backwards into the rectal stump. In rectovestibular fistulas entry is made below the hymen, and the probe passes

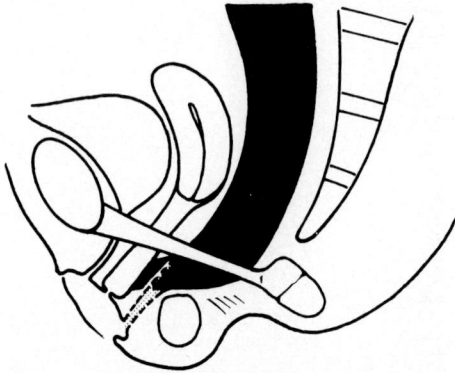

Fig. 11.22 Anal agenesis with rectovaginal (*21*) or rectovestibular (*20*) fistula (female – intermediate anomaly).

obliquely upwards through the perineal body. Inversion films may suggest the diagnosis but, as a result of the escape of gas, may not be helpful. Subsequent investigations, with expression loopogram, confirm the anatomical arrangement.

Most of these cases require initial colostomy to allow proper assessment. Treatment can usually be carried out through a sacroperineal approach, to bring the rectal stump down to the normal anal site.

Anorectal stenosis/atresia (male and female: nos. 7 & 22)
This consists of a fibrous narrowing at the level of the pelvic floor (Figure 11.23a) (higher in *rectal stenosis* or *atresia*) (nos. 11 & 27) (Figure 11.23b–e). The anus is of normal appearance, opening at the normal site, but a finger cannot be advanced up into the rectum. In my experience this is an extremely rare variant. The majority of cases referred to me with this diagnosis turn out to have Hirschsprung's

disease, spasm of the affected segment preventing the advancement of the examining finger into the rectum of a newborn.

High abnormalities

These are abnormalities in which the bowel ends above the levator ani.

ANORECTAL AGENESIS

Anorectal agenesis without fistula
(male and female: nos. 8 & 23)
In this abnormality the bowel ends above the pelvic floor (Figure 11.24). This group represents lesions of varying severity; in the most common the bowel extends down to the pelvic floor, to a position comparable with those cases with a rectourethral or rectovaginal fistula. Where the bowel is held up at a much higher level, even as high as the splenic flexure, it is usually associated with other severe congenital anomalies. The stump may be connected to the pelvic floor or to the back of the bladder by a fibrous cord.

Clinically, these are usually indistinguishable from the other intermediate and high variants. Meconium is not discharged through the urethra or vagina.

This condition requires colostomy in the newborn period and then assessment with expression cystoloopogram or loopogram. Later, abdominosacroperineal pullthrough will usually be required.

Rectal agenesis with fistula (male: no. 9/10)
Here the rectal stump lies above the levator ani, and is connected by the fistula with the posterior urethra (*9*), or higher with the bladder (usually the bladder neck) (*10*) (Figure 11.25).

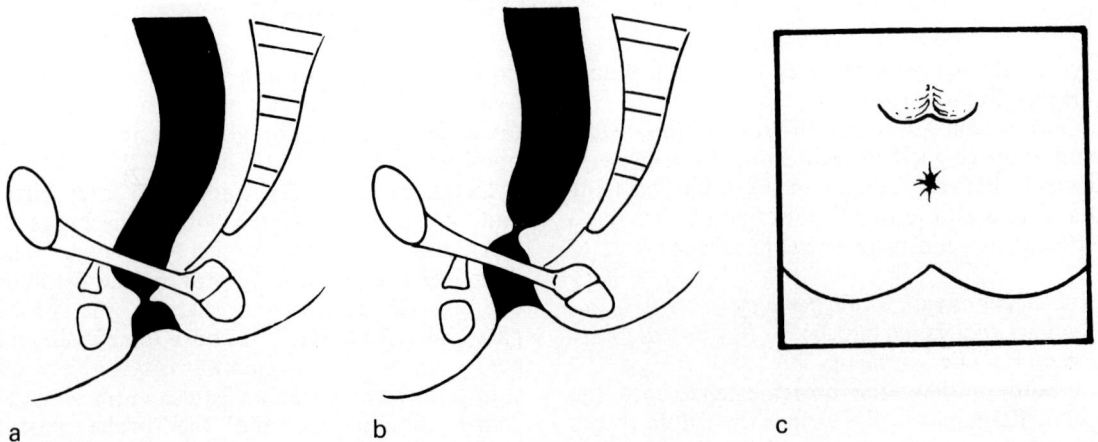

a

b

c

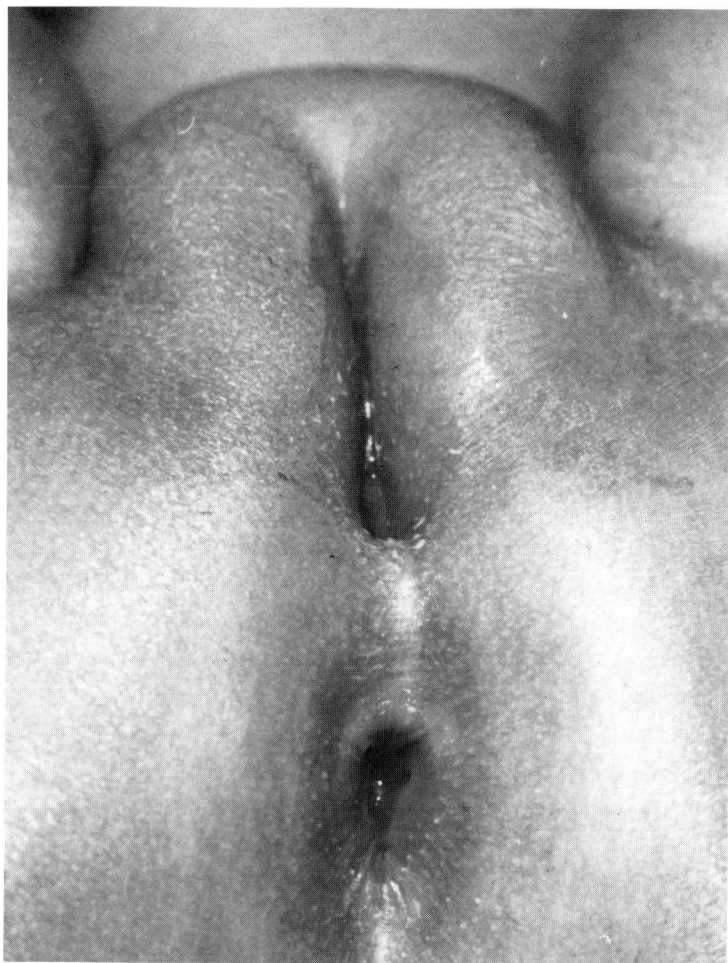

d

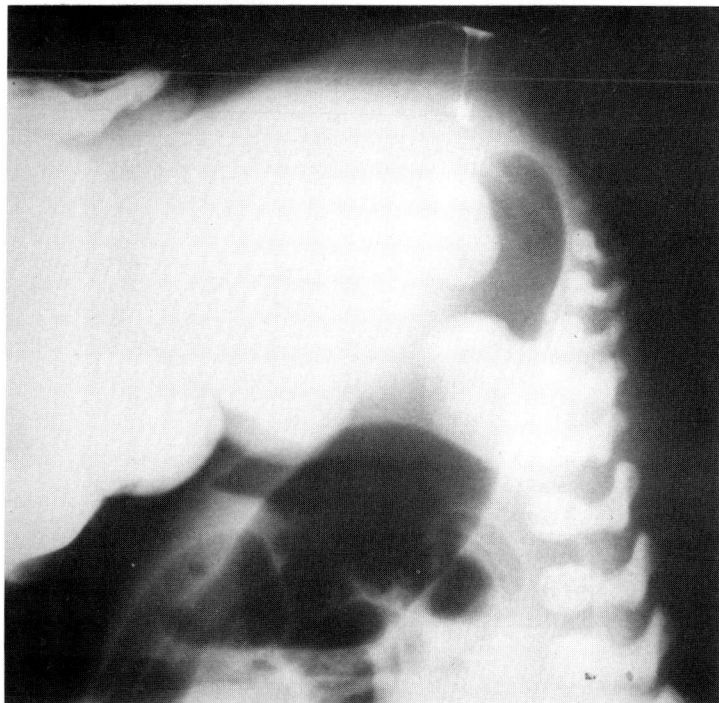

e

Fig. 11.23 (a, c, d, e) Anorectal stenosis or atresia (male *7* and female *22* – intermediate anomaly): (a, c) diagram; (d) clinical appearance; (e) inversion film with barium paste in anal canal. (b, c) Rectal stenosis or atresia without fistulas (male *11* and female *27* – high anomaly).

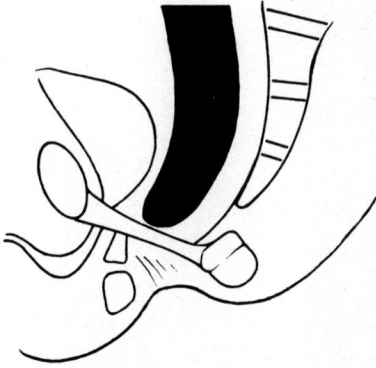

Fig. 11.24 Anorectal agenesis without fistulas (male *8* and female *23* – high anomaly).

Those extending into membranous urethra pass forwards below the apex of the prostate opening, most commonly, just below the verumontanum. Structurally these fistulas appear to represent the upper anal canal, with its lining of stratified cuboidal epithelium and circular smooth muscle, with the appearance of the upper internal anal sphincter. I have not seen a fistula entering the urinary tract higher than the bladder neck.

Clinically, these cases are indistinguishable from other high or intermediate cases until subsequent cystoloopogram and urethroscopy. Gas and meconium may be passed via the urethra.

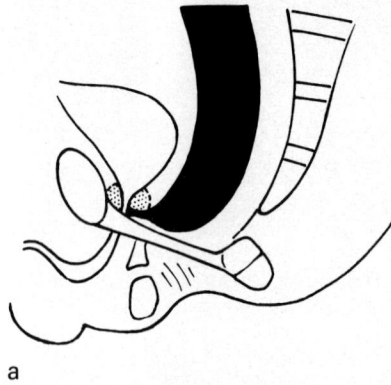

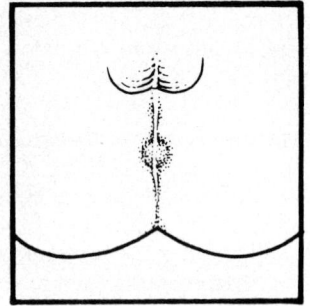

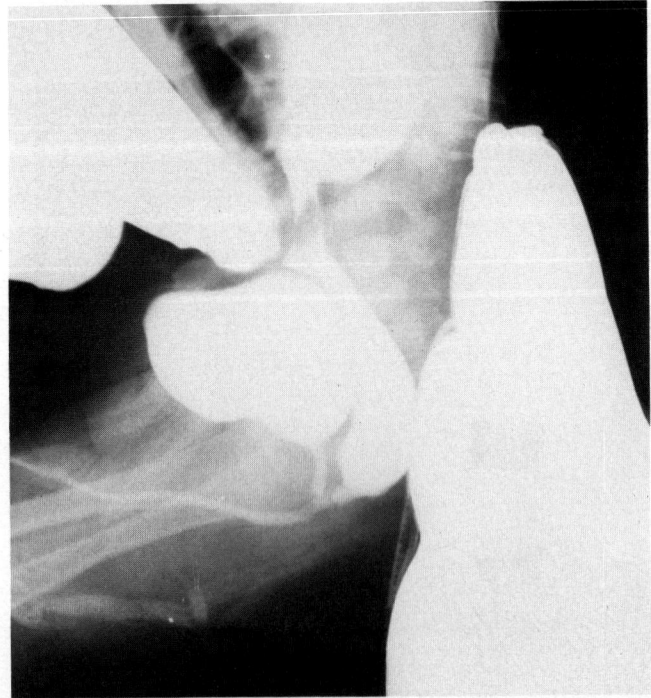

a

b

Fig. 11.25 Anorectal agenesis with recto-urinary fistula (male – high anomaly) – recto-urethral *9* (membranous or prostatic) or rectovesical *10*: (a) diagram; (b) 'cystoloopogram' contrast study, showing recto-urethral fistula.

Anorectal agenesis with fistula (female)

With rectovaginal fistula (no. 24). This is the commonest female high variant. The bowel ends above the levator ani and is connected to the vagina by a fistula which opens into the posterior wall, anywhere from the insertion of the pelvic floor, to as far up as the fornix of the vagina (Figure 11.26).

This abnormality presents in the newborn period with a variable degree of abdominal distension and usually discharge of gas or meconium from the vagina. It can be distinguished from the intermediate variant if a silver probe can be passed into the fistula. Inversion films may assist by indicating the level of air in the rectal stump.

Treatment is transverse colostomy in the newborn period and assessment with expression loopogram, followed later by abdominosacro-perineal pullthrough.

With rectovesical fistula (no. 26). Rectovesical fistulas in the female are very rare. In general, for a rectovesical fistula to be present in the female, there must be splitting of the mullerian cord and duplication of the resulting structures – the vagina and uterus.

Rectocloacal fistula (no. 25). Where there is an anorectal agenesis and fistula, and a urethra opening ectopically, high up, the cavity into which both open is known as a cloaca.

Clinically, these present in a similar fashion to the high and intermediate anomalies. It is important, when examining these children, to check that the urethral meatus is in the normal site. The anomaly is fortunately rare, representing about 1% of the anorectal anomalies. Its importance lies in the fact that many of these girls will be incontinent of urine.

RECTAL ATRESIA (nos. 11 & 27)

The findings in rectal atresia are comparable with those in anorectal atresia but the atresia is at a higher level (see 'anorectal stenosis/atresia' above and Figure 11.23).

Miscellaneous

There are numerous rare variants. Some form recognizable syndromes, such as vesicointestinal fissure (ectopia cloacae). Some of these anomalies are listed in Table 11.1.

INCIDENCE

The incidence appears to be somewhere between 1 in 3000 and 1 in 5000 live births,[5, 6] with a male preponderance of between 57% and 66%. The breakdown of the incidence between high, intermediate and low anomalies is difficult to ascertain, as the most recent figures antedate the international classification. There seems general agreement that the high abnormalities represent about 40%. It would appear that these figures fail to take into account all the cases of anal stenosis, many of whom will present later in childhood with chronic constipation.[2]

There is a high incidence of other congenital anomalies in cases of anorectal malformation. Prominent among these will be abnormalities of the genital and urinary tract, cardiovascular system and oesophagus.

INVESTIGATIONS

Initial investigation of anorectal malformation

As well as plain abdominal films in supine, erect or lateral decubitus positions (Figure 11.27), lateral inversion (Wagensteen) films[14] should be included, although the appearances should be interpreted with caution (Figures 11.14b, 11.23e and 11.28). The distance from a lead-shot marker on the perineum to the gas in the rectum is no longer considered reliable: the gas is now related either to a line drawn on the lateral film

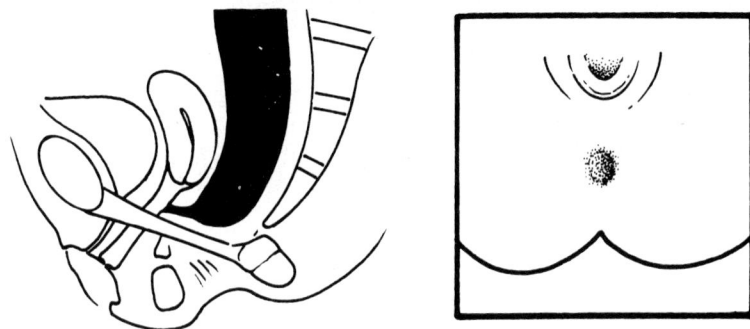

Fig. 11.26 Anorectal agenesis with rectovaginal fistula *24* (female – high anomaly).

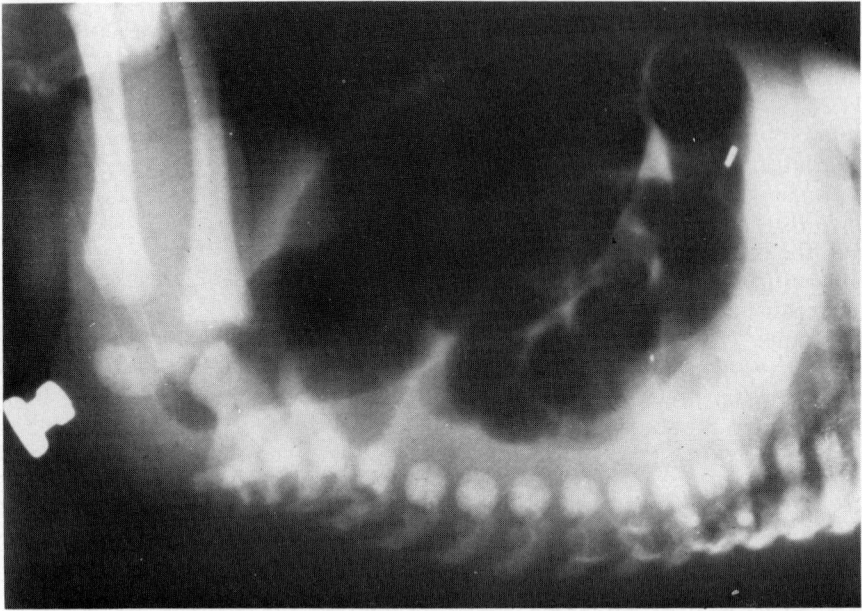

Fig. 11.28 Inversion (Wagensteen) film in low anomaly.

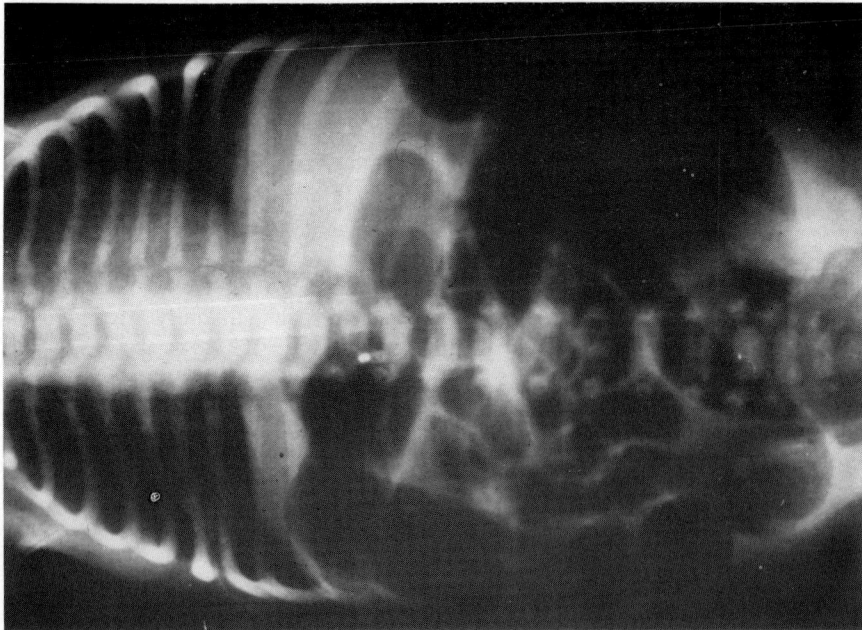

Fig. 11.27 Plain, supine, film of abdomen in imperforate anus, showing gaseous distension.

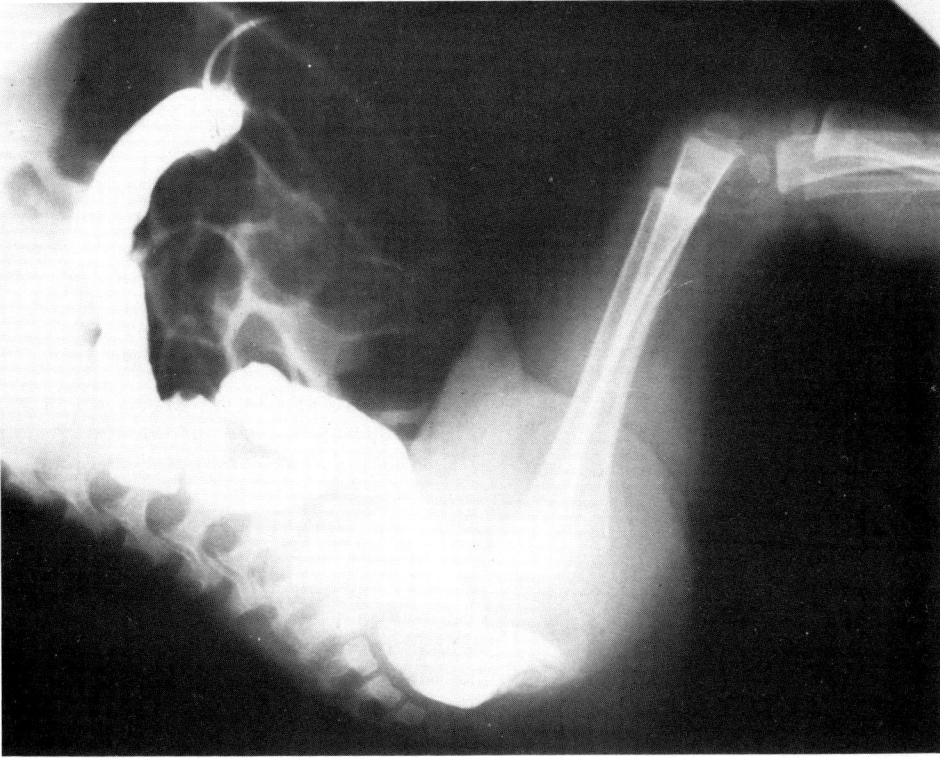

Fig. 11.30 Distal loop contrast study in female with anal agenesis without fistulous connection.

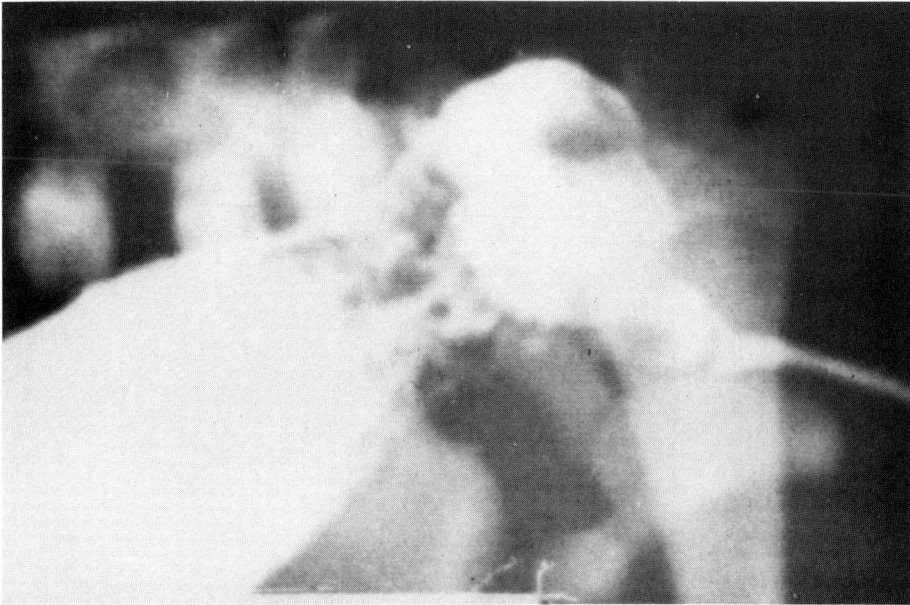

Fig. 11.29 Distal loop contrast study in male with anorectal agenesis and fistula to posterior urethra, barium being passed per urethra.

781

from the upper border of the pubis to the last ossified spinal segment (Stephen's line)[11] or to the distance the gas extends around the ossified ilium (Santulli's criterion.)[9] Meconium adherent to the stump and air escaping through a large rectourethral or rectovaginal fistula or the distal end of the stump gripped in the pelvic floor may give the appearance that the lesion is higher than it is.

Ultrasonic measurement of the distance between perineal skin and rectal gas suffers the same disadvantages as the original Wagensteen films.

Investigations after colostomy

Distal loop studies
Barium can be passed through the distal stoma of the double-barrelled colostomy to outline the rectal stump, and sometimes to pass through the rectovaginal or rectourethral fistula (Figures 11.20b and 11.29), in high lesions. In intermediate lesions the stump and fistula may not be outlined if the stump is gripped in the pelvic floor.

'Distaloopogram'
Distal-loop contrast studies can be augmented by pushing the barium in the colon and rectum down to the pelvis (Figure 11.30).

Expression cystoloopogram
In the male, an expression cystourethrogram will outline the urethra and demonstrate the angulation present at the site of a fistula. When this is combined with an expression loopogram, the entry of a fistula can be demonstrated with accuracy (Figures 11.21b, 11.25b and 11.31).

Cystourethroscopy
Cystourethroscopy can be carried out prior to definitive operation, to further identify the entry of the fistula into the bladder neck or urethra.

SUMMARY OF TREATMENT

With the multiplicity of variants, it is only possible to outline the principles of treatment. The aims of treatment are to provide an adequate opening at approximately the normal

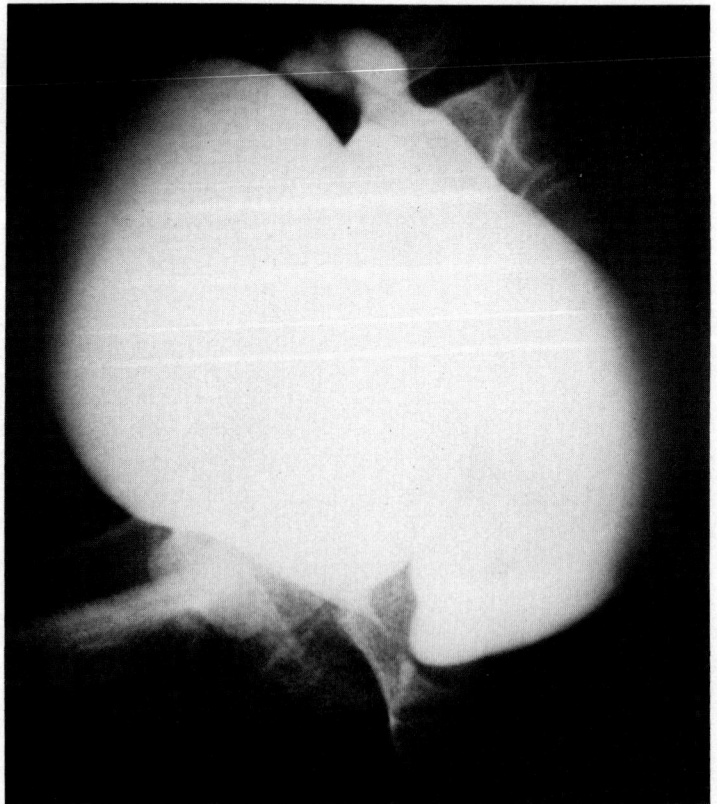

Fig. 11.31 Cystoloopogram contrast study showing anorectal agenesis without fistulous connection to urethra. (Older male child with faecolith in rectum.)

site and a mechanism that will enable the child to close this opening. The latter requires (a) adequate surrounding musculature, (b) adequate sensation of pending and urgent defaecation and (c) an adequate, but not excessive, reservoir for the retention of stool.

Surgical treatment of high and intermediate anomalies

Current surgical treatment, particularly of the high variants, represents a compromise between the need for adequate mobilization of the bowel and preservation of the voluntary sphincters and slings, on the one hand, and preservation of the nerve supply of the bowel, on the other.

The treatment of some of the intermediate and lower anomalies has already been mentioned. In the high anomalies and some of the intermediate ones there is a need for a more extensive procedure. After initial transverse skin-bridge colostomy most surgeons use a combined approach, involving a perineal or perineal and sacral approach with an abdominal approach, as in 'abdominosacralperineal pullthrough'[11] or 'rectoplasty'.[12] Many intermediate anomalies, particularly those without fistulas, may be approached via a sacral and perineal approach, without abdominal dissection.

Opinions on timing of the definitive operation differ. I aim to complete the definitive procedure and initial anal dilatations by six to seven months old.

Subsequent treatment

The new anus will require gentle progressive dilatation over the next few weeks, and then continued dilatation for about three months. It should be of an adequate size before the colostomy is closed.

Close observation over many years will be required to ensure that there is no obstruction at the site of anastomosis to cause rectal dilatation and further loss of sensation. Further anal dilatation or anoplasty may be required to ensure that this does not occur.

REFERENCES

1 Bill, A. H. & Johnson, R. J. (1953) Congenital median band of the anus. *Surgery Gynecology and Obstetrics*, **97**, 307–311.
2 Clayden, G. S. & Lawson, J. O. N. (1976) Investigation and management of long standing chronic constipation in childhood. *Archives of Disease in Childhood*, **51**, 918–923.
3 Keith, A. (1908) Malformation of the hind end of the body. *British Medical Journal*, **ii**, 1736–1741.
4 Ladd, W. E. & Gross, R. E. (1934) Congenital malformations of anus and rectum. *American Journal of Surgery*, **23**, 167–183.
5 Louw, J. H. (1965) Congenital abnormalities of the rectum and anus. *Current Problems in Surgery*. Chicago: Year Book Medical Publishers.
6 Nixon, H. H. (1972) Anorectal anomalies: With an international proposed classification. *Postgraduate Medical Journal*, **48**, 465–470.
7 Rhoads, J. E., Pipes, R. L. & Randal, J. P. (1948) A simultaneous abdominal and perineal approach in operations for imperforate anus with atresia of the rectum and rectosigmoid. *Annals of Surgery*, **127**, 552.
8 Santulli, T. V., Kiesewetter, W. B. & Bill, A. H. (1970) Anorectal anomalies: A suggested international classification. *Journal of Pediatric Surgery*, **5**, 281–287.
9 Santulli, T. V., Schullinger, J. N. & Amoury, R. A. (1965) Malformations of the anus and rectum. *Surgical Clinics of North America*, **5**, 1253–1271.
10 Scharli, A. F. (1978) Malformations of the anus and rectum and their treatment in medical history. *Progress in Pediatric Surgery*, **11**, 141–172.
11 Stephens, F. D. (1953) Congenital imperforate rectum, rectourethral and rectovaginal fistulae. *Australian and New Zealand Journal of Surgery*, **22**, 161–172.
12 Stephens, F. D. (1963) *Congenital Malformations of the Rectum, Anus, and Genito Urinary Tracts*. Edinburgh and London: E. & S. Livingstone.
13 Stephens, F. D. & Smith, E. D. (1971) *Anorectal Malformations in Children*. Chicago: Year Book Medical Publishers.
14 Wagensteen, O. H. & Rice, C. O. (1930) Imperforate anus: A method of determining the surgical approach. *Annals of Surgery*, **92**, 77–81.
15 Wood-Jones, F. (1904) The nature of the malformations of the rectum and urogenital passages. *British Medical Journal*, **ii**, 1630–1634.

PHYSIOLOGY AND SPHINCTER CONTROL

The principal functions of the colon are absorption of sodium and water. The rectum provides a reservoir for storing faeces prior to evacuation, while the final control of defecation depends upon normal sensory and motor function in the anal canal. This section considers the physiological mechanisms underlying these functions (Figure 11.32).

Normal colonic function

MOTILITY

Transit

Most studies of colonic motility are based upon radiological techniques using barium, but since barium is heavier than faeces these studies are not physiological and over-estimate normal

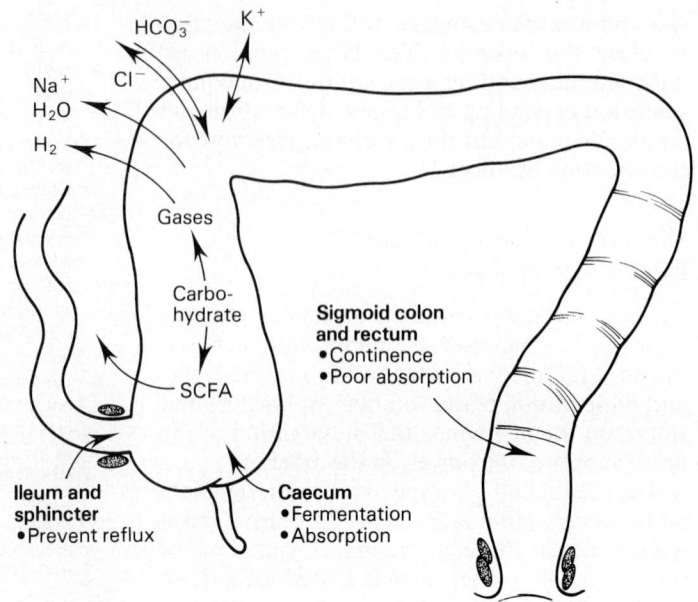

Fig. 11.32 Function of the large bowel (SCFA: short-chain fatty acids). From Kerlin. P. & Phillips, S.F. (1983) 'Absorption of fluids and electrolytes from the colon with reference to inflammatory bowel disease' in *Inflammatory Bowel Diseases* (Ed.) Allan, R., Keighley, M., Hawkins, C. & Alexander-Williams, J., with kind permission of the authors and the publisher, Churchill Livingstone.

transit times.[14] Small radiopaque pellets provide better information and indicate that transit from caecum to rectum takes about 12 hours; however, colonic transit is influenced by diet, physical exercise and drugs. More recent techniques for measuring transit include a swallowed pressure-sensitive radiotransmitter with a directional receiving aerial applied to the abdomen or the use of a radioisotope (^{51}Cr) incorporated in the capsule with a gamma scintillation counter to detect its position.[39] Movement of faeces throughout the colon does not proceed at a constant rate.[29] Progress is slow in the caecum and ascending colon. In the transverse and descending colon there are episodes of mass peristalsis which transmit the faeces rapidly to the rectum. This movement occurs two or three times a day and is a co-ordinated contraction over 10–20 cm of colon in a few seconds. Transit is also slow in the sigmoid and rectum.

Pressures
Movement in the colon is principally by segmentation, which churns the faecal material between closed segments and then delivers the contents from one segment to the next, and is associated with high intraluminal pressures. Segmentation slows colonic transit but encourages absorption by allowing greater time for mucosal contact.[22] Intraluminal pressure studies have been performed extensively in the sigmoid colon using open tipped perfused catheters but data on pressures in the right colon are generally lacking. Bursts of increased pressure

are observed after food and neostigmine. High pressure zones are common in the sigmoid in diverticular disease and these may be reduced by a high fibre diet.

Myoelectrical activity
Myoelectrical activity may be recorded in vivo by surface electrodes or from intraluminal suction electrodes. In vitro studies are usually from isolated muscle strips following short periods of refrigeration. In contrast to the observed constant electrical activity in the stomach or small bowel, the colon displays intermittent bursts of electrical activity which are present from 25% of the time in the sigmoid and up to 75% in the caecum and rectum[6] (Table 11.2). These slow waves have two ranges of frequency at 2–4 cycles/min and at 6–12 cycles/min. The faster waves are thought to be

Table 11.2 Colonic electrical activity percentage of recording time that regular slow waves are present (mean ± s.e.). From Taylor *et al.* (1975)[37] with kind permission of the authors and the editor of *Gut*.

Rectum	
5–9 cm from anus	71 ± 5
10–14 cm from anus	34 ± 3
15–19 cm from anus	31 ± 3
Sigmoid	
20–24 cm from anus	27 ± 3
25+ cm from anus	26 ± 3
Descending colon	37 ± 4
Transverse colon	70 ± 9
Ascending colon	71 ± 7

responsible for propulsive activity. The myoelectrical activity of the colon is increased by pentagastrin and cholecystokinin and inhibited by secretin and glucagon.[37] Acetylcholine causes contraction of isolated muscle strips whereas atropine and noradrenaline lead to relaxation.[9] Most prostaglandins as well as bradykinin and angiotensin cause smooth muscle colonic contraction whereas relaxation is usually observed after 5-hydroxytryptamine and histamine.

ABSORPTION AND SECRETION

Although colonic function does not seem essential, since ileostomy patients are capable of living an apparently normal existence, survival in adverse physiological circumstances is increased when the colon is intact and capable of normal function.

Assessment
There are various methods of assessing colonic absorption. The simplest is by a comparison of the composition of ileostomy and faecal effluent though there are chemical differences between the material entering the right colon and ileostomy fluid.[16] Assessment of absorption from isolated segments of colon provides direct measurement but in vivo studies are complicated by ethical considerations and patient compliance. The technique of rectal and colonic perfusion via a rectal catheter is more acceptable,[31] but the precise area of mucosal absorption is not known and the test solution may be lost from the test segment.[4] The most satisfactory perfusion technique is by placement of a per oral tube so that the tip lies in the caecum. This system allows assessment of bidirectional fluxes and can be used to study absorption in a variety of clinical situations. However, it is time consuming and unpleasant, the absorbing area is unknown and perfusion is usually at unphysiological rates. Finally it is not possible to evaluate the influence of motility, blood flow or bacterial flora on absorption. Hence no one technique is entirely satisfactory.

Normal maximum colonic function
The colon probably receives about 1500 ml of fluid a day from which it absorbs 1350 ml water, 200 mmol sodium, 150 mmol chloride and 60 mmol bicarbonate. The maximum daily capacity to absorb water is about 3 litres and the maximum sodium and chloride absorption is 450 mmol and 550 mmol respectively.[19] The majority of sodium and water absorption takes place in the ascending colon (Table 11.3).

Table 11.3 Rates of net transport and uni-directional flux of sodium, potassium and water in 11 healthy subjects. Data from Harris and Shields (1970).[12]

Direction of movement	Sodium (µmol/min)	Potassium (µmol/min)	Water (ml/min)
Net transport	+391 ± 148	−32 ± 4.0	+185 ±
Out of lumen	596 ± 108	11.5 ± 2.6	
Into lumen	206 ± 75	14.6 ± 5.0	

Sodium absorption
Sodium, the principal cation entering from the ileum, is the most important substance absorbed by the colon. Sodium is actively absorbed against electrical and concentration gradients. Sodium can be absorbed even when the luminal concentration is as low as 15 mmol/l. This active transport mechanism creates an electrical potential difference of 10–40 V (serosa being positive to lumen). The active sodium pump derives its energy from the hydrolysis of ATP by membrane bound ATPase. The absorption of sodium in the colon is not influenced by glucose, bicarbonate or amino acid concentrations. Sodium (as well as potassium and water) can move in both directions, i.e., out of the lumen – absorption, or into the lumen – secretion. The bidirectional flux for sodium is 3 : 1 or 4 : 1 in favour of absorption indicating that there is a tight barrier restricting back flow of sodium into the gut lumen (Figure 11.33).

Potassium chloride and water exchange
The human colon secretes small quantities of potassium by passive diffusion created by the sodium pump. The colon is capable of secreting up to 100 mmol/l but in practice normal secretion rates are much less than this. The majority of potassium secretion occurs in the right colon.[32] Chloride is passively absorbed until the luminal concentration is as little as 24 mmol/l. Chloride is rapidly absorbed, probably in exchange for bicarbonate ions by carbonic anhydrase which is present in high concentration in the colon. Water absorption by the colon is passive and secondary to the transport of sodium and chloride ions. This passive absorption is even possible from hypertonic intraluminal saline solutions where water is carried with saline via the intercellular space to the circulation.

Drugs
Mineralocorticoids stimulate sodium and water absorption but potassium secretion is increased. Low concentrations of angiotensin increase sodium absorption but antidiuretic hormone

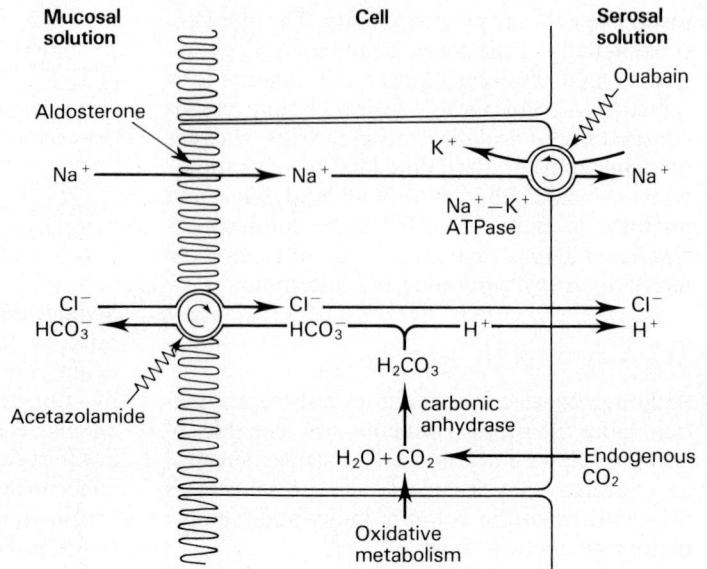

Fig. 11.33 Ion exchange across the colonic mucosal cell. From Kerlin, P. & Phillips, S.F. (1983) 'Absorption of fluids and electrolytes from the colon with reference to inflammatory bowel disease' in *Inflammatory Bowel Diseases* (Ed.) Allan, R., Keighley, M., Hawkins, C. & Alexander-Williams, J., with kind permission of the authors and the publisher, Churchill Livingstone.

(ADH) reduces sodium and water absorption. Neither pentagastrin nor prostaglandins seem to exert much influence on colonic absorption.

Abnormal colonic function

MOTILITY

Diarrhoea and constipation
Diarrhoea is associated with rapid colonic transit, flat pressure changes and slow wave myoelectrical activity. There are frequent bursts of mass peristalsis. Constipation is associated with slow transit times, excessive segmentation, accompanied by high pressure zones and excessive absorption of sodium and water.[39]

Diverticular disease
The principal changes are in the sigmoid colon and consist of increased segmentation, isolated high pressure compartments, increased transit times and a decrease in stool weight.[23] Colonic motor activity is greatly increased in diverticular disease particularly following neostigmine or after a meal. There are typical myoelectrical patterns in diverticular disease with a frequency of about 6 cycles/min which are not seen in normal subjects and which disappear after treatment with bran.[35]

Irritable bowel syndrome
Intracolonic pressures are generally increased in the irritable bowel syndrome, and so is the electrical activity of the colon especially in the frequency order of 3 cycles/min.[33]

ABSORPTION AND SECRETION

Inflammatory bowel disease
There is impaired absorption of sodium and water and increased secretion of potassium in ulcerative colitis and Crohn's disease.[27] These changes are probably due to a combination of a deficient sodium pump and increased mucosal permeability. In Crohn's disease even the apparently healthy small bowel contributes to this water and electrolyte depletion as a consequence of an impaired bidirectional flux of sodium and therefore an increased small bowel load to the colon. In diarrhoea of whatever cause there is excessive loss of sodium and water. The extent of electrolyte loss is proportional to stool flow rates. Losses of potassium are less than sodium. The electrolyte content of stool in severe diarrhoea approaches that of plasma.

Villous adenoma
There may be copious loss of fluid and electrolytes in patients with villous adenoma. Renal failure with excessive potassium loss is well recognized but there is no evidence for the selective secretion of potassium by these tumours. There is also disordered absorption of water and ions in patients with these tumours.[30]

Congenital chloridorrhoea
This is a rare congenital cause of watery diarrhoea and is a specific electrolyte transport defect. There is a loss of chloride in the faeces and a metabolic alkalosis. The faecal concentration of chloride ions is greater than the sum of

the faecal sodium and potassium values. There is secretion of chloride as a result of exchange for bicarbonate which is absorbed in excess.[38]

Altered mineralocorticoid secretion
In Addison's disease there is reduced sodium reabsorption and excessive faecal loss. In primary aldosteronism due to a hormone secreting tumour of the adrenal cortex, or in patients receiving excessive doses of corticosteroids, there is a reduction in the sodium/potassium ratio in faeces with excessive loss of potassium. Rectal transmucosal potential difference (which is increased due to increased sodium absorption) may be used as a screening test for aldosteronism.

Osmotic diarrhoea
If the lumen of the bowel contains osmotically active particles which are not absorbed there is excessive loss of sodium and water. This may explain the diarrhoea of disaccharidase deficiency and the electrolyte changes which accompany mannitol bowel preparation.[21]

Steatorrhoea
Impaired absorption of fat is often accompanied by diarrhoea. Bacterial action on unabsorbed fat in the colon produces hydroxy fatty acids, which act as cathartics in the colon.

Motility disorders
Increased colonic motor activity is associated with increased absorption of sodium and water, by increasing the duration of mucosal contact with luminal contents and by dispersing material from segment to segment in the colon. The result is the passage of hard small pelleted stools. On the other hand if the motility disorder is accompanied by excessive propulsion of its contents and increased transit times, diarrhoea is likely to occur.

Laxatives
Laxative abuse is sometimes responsible for chronic depletion of water and electrolytes. This may in turn stimulate aldosterone production which further increases the loss of potassium.[3] The mechanism of action of most stimulant laxatives is obscure; some act directly on intestinal smooth muscle whereas others have a direct effect on absorptive function.

Colorectal resection
Total excision of the colon and rectum with construction of an ileostomy enables patients to lead a normal life, though they may be subject to episodes of ileostomy flux. Hence while the colon is not necessary for fluid and electrolyte homeostasis, the ileostomy patient is in a more precarious state as far as water and electrolyte balance is concerned than patients with an intact normal colon. Even a patient with a well established ileostomy loses five to ten times the volume of normal faeces and is maintained in good health by compensatory retention of water and electrolytes. Despite this, ileostomy patients have lower levels of total body water and exchangeable sodium.

The right colon is capable of greater absorption than the rest of the large bowel so that preservation of the ascending colon and hepatic flexure are particularly important when considering resection for ileocaecal Crohn's disease. Similarly, excessive ileal resection should be avoided whenever possible since this impairs the enterohepatic circulation which leads to a loss of bile acids into the colon. Bacteria in the colon are then capable of forming secondary bile acids from this abnormal bile salt load. These secondary bile acids inhibit absorption of sodium, chloride and water, and exacerbate diarrhoea.[20]

Normal anorectal function

It is appropriate that the function of the rectum and anal canal should be considered together, particularly in any discussion of the causes of faecal incontinence. For instance, many patients with ulcerative colitis have episodes of urgency and incontinence despite a normal anal sphincter and pelvic floor because of a severe proctitis and small capacity hypersensitive rectal ampulla. Conversely, the rectal capacity is normal in patients whose incontinence is due to the descending perineal syndrome where the problem is a neuropathy of the pelvic floor. No division of large bowel function is entirely satisfactory since incontinence in patients with a weak external sphincter may be exacerbated by abnormal motor activity in the proximal colon.

ANATOMY

The rectum is approximately 10–12 cm long and terminates at the pelvic diaphragm. The anal canal is more variable in length (2–5 cm) and is usually closed. The anal canal is surrounded by two sphincters. The inner internal sphincter is an expanded continuation of the circular muscle coat of the rectum and is composed of smooth muscle. The external sphincter surrounds the internal sphincter and is formed of striated muscle; it is attached to the perineal body anteriorly and to the coccyx posteriorly. Above the external sphincter and continuous with it posteriorly is the levator ani. This inner component, the pubo-rectalis, forms a sling which is extremely important in the continence mechanism because it controls the anorectal angle and assists in the flutter valve mechanism which keep the anal canal empty. It is not always appreciated that the longitudinal axis of the anal canal is almost 90° to the posterior wall of the rectum.[34]

ANORECTAL SENSATION

Only extreme intraluminal distension of the sigmoid colon results in hypogastric pain and an impending desire to defecate.[10] The rectum, however, is much more sensitive to distension;[2] 20–30 cm³ of air introduced into a rectal balloon can usually be felt, but the sensation is transient, even when the balloon remains distended (threshold volume). Increasing volumes of air are later accompanied by a constant desire to defecate and this volume varies from 80–200 cm³ in normal subjects. With increasing balloon distension there is marked perineal pain, the desire to defecate becomes intolerable and the balloon is either evacuated or stool is passed (maximum tolerated volumes). The maximum tolerated volume is usually greater than 400 cm³ and reflects the distensibility of the rectum.[7] The rectal mucosa is insensitive to pain and light touch.

The entire anal canal is plentifully supplied with organized sensory nerve endings and is capable of acute appreciation of pain and touch throughout its length. The sensitive mucosa is not confined to the area below the dentate line.

MOTOR CONTROL MECHANISMS AND PRESSURE MEASUREMENTS

Our understanding of the physiology of continence is based upon manometric studies using either continuously perfused open-ended catheters or balloon probes.[5] Both techniques provide comparable results and pressure recordings are independent of the size of the recording balloon. Attempts to record internal and external sphincter activity independently using separate pressure recording probes is difficult and separation of the function of these muscles is only possible using electromyography.

Resting pressure
There is a zone of high resting anal canal pressure usually 1–3 cm from the anal verge which varies with age and sex, and remains between 60–100 mmHg until the sixth decade after which it progressively falls.[17] Resting pressure is 10–20 mmHg and is lower in women than men. Ultra-slow waves are noted in patients with high resting pressures as in anal fissure and in young patients with haemorrhoids. This high resting pressure is almost completely abolished by damage to the parasympathetic outflow as in lesions affecting the sacral outflow.[11] Conversely, resting anal canal pressures are only slightly reduced in patients with complete cord compression affecting the cervico-dorsal segments, after muscle relaxants or pudendal nerve block.[8]

Squeeze pressure
The activity of the external sphincter and pubo-rectalis can be measured by squeeze pressures, that is the highest pressure recorded after asking the patient to contract the control mechanism. The maximum squeeze pressure is also affected by age and sex and varies from 100–220 mmHg. The squeeze pressure is abolished by cord compression, muscle relaxants and pudendal nerve block.[40]

Reflexes
An involuntary reflex is elicited by distending a balloon in the rectum with 50 cm³ of air. The response is a transient rise followed by a profound fall in the resting anal canal pressure which lasts for 15–20 seconds.[15] This response is known as the 'sampling' reflex since it is probably important in initiating the control mechanism. Relaxation of the internal sphincter allows the faecal bolus to enter the sensitive upper anal canal. The bolus is recognized by the anal nerve endings and the voluntary control mechanism of the external sphincter and pubo-rectalis either contract, thus forcing the bolus back into the rectum, or relax to allow the bolus to be expelled. The sampling reflex is still present even after high cord compression, pudendal nerve block and following administration of muscle relaxants. The reflex is probably conveyed from the myenteric nerve plexus in the wall of the rectum and from sensory nerve endings in the levator ani since the response is well preserved after sleeve resection of the rectal mucosa and even after complete rectal excision with endo-anal anastomosis. Other reflexes include the 'accommodation' reflex whereby persistent distension of a rectal balloon is accompanied by a progressive fall in intraballoon pressure and a return to normal anal canal pressures. The 'defecation' reflex is produced by large volumes of air

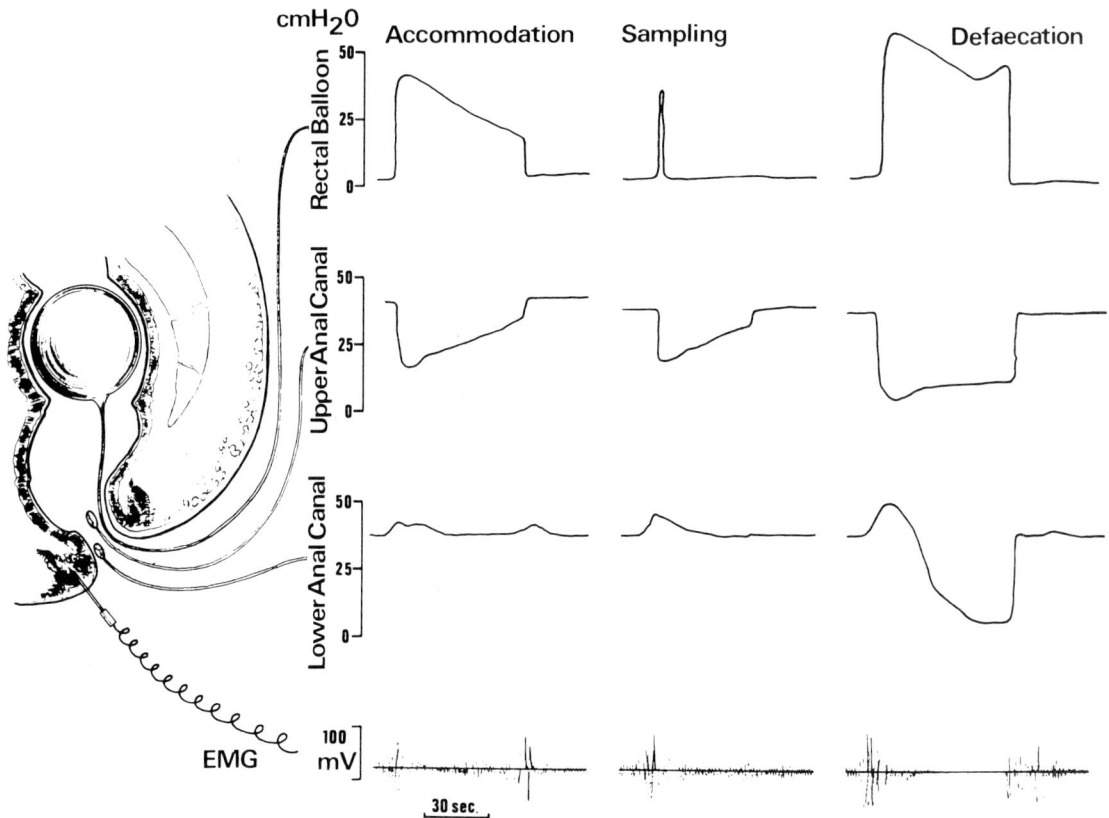

Fig. 11.34 Manometric measurements during rectal distension, sampling and defecation. From Duthie, H.L. (1979) 'Anorectal region' in *Scientific Basis of Gastroenterology* (Ed.) Duthie, H.L. & Wormsley, K., with kind permission of the author and the publisher, Churchill Livingstone.

in the rectal balloon, there is reflex relaxation of the pelvic floor accompanied by a fall in the anal canal pressures, the anorectal angle opens and the balloon is passed (Figure 11.34).

OTHER FACTORS AFFECTING CONTINENCE (Figure 11.35).

The consistency of the stool will influence continence. Fluid faeces associated with intestinal hurry may enter the upper anal canal so fast as to prevent the external sphincter contracting in time, even though anal sensation is normal. Conversely if the rectum is full of a solid faecal bolus, there is permanent relaxation of the internal anal sphincter with leakage of fluid material around the bolus. The capacity of the rectum is also important in the control of defecation. If the rectal capacity is reduced following resection, or as a result of disease, much smaller volumes can be accommodated. Reduced rectal capacity is associated with urgency and frequency. Failure of the anorectal angle to contract after a rise in intra-abdominal pressure may lead to incontinence. The flutter valve mechanism, maintained by contraction of the pubo-rectalis sling, is important in preserving continence during distension of the rectum. At rest the anal canal is kept closed by a combination of its physical characteristics and by the tonic activity of surrounding muscles. This tonic activity of the striated muscles of the external anal sphincter and levator ani helps to maintain the angle between the axis of the anal canal and rectum. If there has been damage to the anal canal or pelvic floor the anal canal is not completely closed and leakage of faecal material is a common symptom.

OTHER SPECIAL TESTS OF ANORECTAL FUNCTION

Radiology

Barium enema examination is important not only to exclude inflammatory bowel disease and neoplasia but also to define the configuration of the anorectum, particularly after operation. The

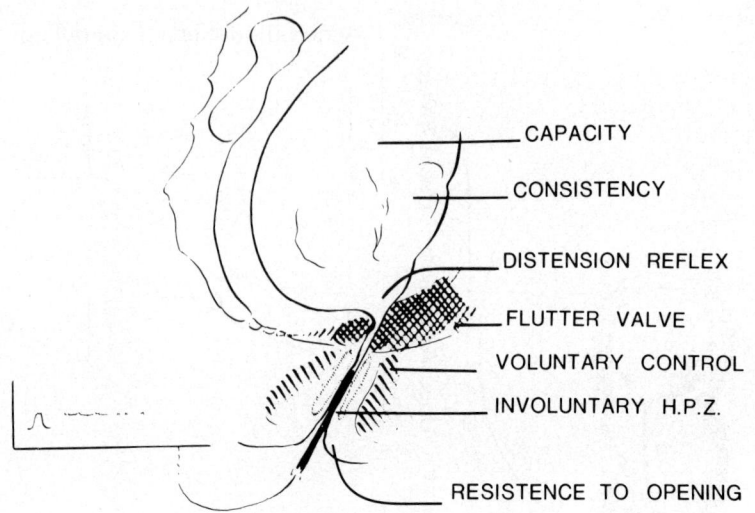

CAPACITY

CONSISTENCY

DISTENSION REFLEX

FLUTTER VALVE

VOLUNTARY CONTROL

INVOLUNTARY H.P.Z.

RESISTENCE TO OPENING

Fig. 11.35 Factors affecting continence.

lateral X-ray of the rectum has been used to judge rectal capacity. We have found interpretation is influenced by the degree of distension during air insufflation and the amount of contrast material introduced. Therefore the correlation between a radiological assessment of rectal capacity and the maximum tolerated volume has been poor (Table 11.4). Also the degree of proctitis as assessed by radiology may be misleading but severe stricture, postoperative fibrosis or altered anatomy are well displayed. Defecating proctograms have been used in the investigation of the descending perineal syndrome and rectal prolapse. The balloon proctogram is more valuable whereby 200 cm³ of a barium suspension is introduced into a rectal balloon. The anorectal angle is measured at rest and after contraction of the pelvic floor. The patient is then asked to pass the rectal balloon.

During this manoeuvre the degree to which the anorectal angle will open can be measured, and the ability of the patient to pass the balloon can be assessed.

Other tests of continence
The sensitivity of the rectum can be tested by perfusion with fluids at different temperatures. Continence for a solid sphere can be measured by inserting a smooth cork sphere into the rectum.[28] The weight required to displace the sphere from the rectum can be measured at rest and during voluntary contraction. Continence of liquids can be measured with the patient seated on a special chair. A solution containing 4 g/l of polyethylene glycol in saline is infused into the rectum at a rate of 60 ml/min. Measurements include the volume causing initial leakage and the total volume retained. Unfortunately the test is invalid if large volumes of liquid enter the proximal colon and if there is excessive absorption of saline.

Abnormal anorectal function

Sensory defects
Sensory defects resulting in urgency may occur when the rectum has been removed as in low anterior resection, but sensation is usually preserved if the levator ani remains intact. Sensory loss may be a factor responsible for incontinence in diabetic patients. Loss of the sampling reflex is often associated with impaired sensation in the anal canal. The reflex is absent in a variety of conditions particularly some patients with rectal prolapse, adult megacolon and in all children

Table 11.4 Correlation between maximum tolerated volume (MTV) and a radiological assessment of capacity and proctitis: 37 patients with Crohn's disease.

Radiology	MTV less than 150 cm³ (13)	MTV greater than 150 cm³ (24)
Assessment of capacity		
Severely reduced	7	4
Abnormal	2	3
Normal	4	17
Assessment of proctitis		
Severe	9	3
Abnormal	0	7
Normal	4	14

with Hirschsprung's disease.[1] Anal sensation may be impaired if the anal canal is incompletely closed as a result of scarring following anal surgery. Continence may be compromised following local anaesthetic suppositories. Repeated dilatation may be associated with loss of anal sensitivity and may be a factor contributing to incontinence in homosexual patients. Sensation may be inappropriate or confused in patients with coexisting anorectal pathology as in villous papilloma, carcinoma and particularly in rectal prolapse (see Table 11.5).

Table 11.5 Factors responsible for faecal incontinence (authors series of 325 patients: 1975–1980).

Central prolapsed disc	2
Diabetes mellitus and neuropathy	3
Descending perineal syndrome	16
Mucosal prolapse and idiopathic incontinence	6
Rectal prolapse	40
Inflammatory bowel disease	
Diverticular disease	12
Crohn's disease	37
Ulcerative colitis	21
Solitary rectal ulcer	3
Operation	
Ileorectal anastomosis	14
Colo-anal anastomosis	6
Low anterior resection	12
Surgical trauma	
Anal dilatation	8
Lateral subcutaneous sphincterotomy	3
Deroofing anal fistula	5
Haemorrhoidectomy	3
Fissurectomy	1
Trauma following road accident	3
Obstetric trauma	5
Imperforate anus	3
Villous papilloma	14
Carcinoma of rectum	104
Unknown cause	12

Motor defects
Autonomic control of the internal sphincter is from the sympathetic outflow (L1 and L2) via the hypogastric nerves to the perirectal plexus which is joined by sacral parasympathetics (S2, S3 and S4). Division of the sympathetics during vascular surgery and the parasympathetics during pelvic operations, however, rarely seems to compromise continence.

Voluntary control is mediated by the pudendal nerve (S2, S3 and S4) and an additional motor supply from S4 to the pubo-rectalis has recently been recognized. Division or anaesthesia of the pudendal nerve abolishes the ability to contract the voluntary control mechanism, but resting anal tone is preserved because the internal sphincter remains innervated. Damage

to the pudendal nerve by compression or traction occurs in the descending perineal syndrome.[24] Histochemical stains have shown that there is denervation in the external sphincter and pubo-rectalis in patients with this syndrome.[13, 25] Lesions of the cauda equina, central prolapsed disc and complete cord transection affecting the lumbo-sacral outflow result in complete incontinence and a patulous anus. Cervicodorsal cord transection abolishes the high control of defecation but the internal sphincter functions normally. Most of these quadraplegic patients are continent provided the colon is evacuated regularly with repeated enemas. Cortical control is impaired in the elderly, after extensive cerebral vascular disease and in the mentally retarded.

Stool consistency
The importance of a solid faecal bolus in the mechanism of continence has already been stressed. A fluid stool is more difficult to recognize, particularly if it arrives at speed. Diarrhoea exacerbates the incontinence seen in diabetes, inflammatory bowel disease and after ileorectal anastomosis. Gross constipation may also lead to incontinence. A large faecal mass in the rectum causes complete inhibition of the internal sphincter and liquid faeces leak around the solid bolus and into the anal canal.

Narrow or inflamed rectum
Reduced capacity of the rectum has already been considered and is an important cause of urgency in inflammatory bowel disease and after restorative rectal excision. Severe proctitis is also commonly associated with urgency.

Damage to the control mechanism

Obstetric trauma. Repeated labour may be associated with damage to the pelvic diaphragm and the external sphincter. Unless a well sited episiotomy is performed a complete posterior tear may result. In parts of the world not served by planned obstetric care, rectovaginal fistula is a common sequel to obstructed labour and results in complete incontinence.

Iatrogenic trauma. One of the commonest causes of incontinence results from over enthusiastic or repeated anal dilatation. Internal sphincterotomy may also precipitate incontinence. Haemorrhoidectomy, deroofing of a low fistula and excision of anal fissures may lead to scarring of the anal canal and is often accompanied by soiling. High anorectal fistulas usually result from damage during drainage of an ischiorectal abscess. Attempts to deroof these fistulas will lead to permanent faecal incontinence. Patients are often rendered incontinent in Crohn's disease because of attempts to treat perianal disease. Most patients with perianal Crohn's disease have very few symptoms; surgeons should be encouraged to leave the perineum alone whenever possible.

Other causes of trauma. Repeated dilatation may impair continence and is a feature of patients with various sexual motives for self dilatation. Trauma to the perineum may also occur following fractures to the pelvis and can be associated with complete destruction of the anorectal ring. Because of this trauma many of these patients have required amputations and some have sustained serious urethral or bladder neck injuries.

Rectal prolapse
Rectal prolapse is commonly associated with disordered anorectal function. A few of these patients have chronic constipation and difficulty with defecation because of an abnormal pelvic floor which fails to relax on straining. Some of these patients have a coexisting solitary rectal ulcer. The majority of patients with prolapse, however, complain of incontinence. In our experience 67 out of 100 patients with complete rectal prolapse gave a history of incontinence.[18] The incontinence is often associated with perineal descent, an absent sampling reflex, a patulous anus and pelvic floor neuropathy. Fortunately in over two-thirds of these patients continence is restored by repair of the rectal prolapse.

Imperforate anus
Defects of continence in children born with an imperforate anus depend upon the level of anorectal agenesis and the siting of the repaired anal canal. Low level defects are rarely associated with disordered development of the sphincters or levator ani, so that patients are continent provided the anal canal is routed through the sphincters. High defects are complicated by agenesis of the pelvic floor and continence is virtually never restored.[36]

Hirschsprung's disease
Congenital rectal aganglionosis is characterized by failure to defecate, a narrow rectal aganglionic segment which may be of variable length, and an absent sampling reflex. The diagnosis is confirmed by full thickness biopsies of the anorectum which characteristically contain no ganglion cells.

Adult megacolon
This curious condition may be a form of Hirschsprung's disease which only becomes manifest in late childhood or adult life. There is gross constipation and patients are usually incapable of evacuating the rectum unless given repeated enemas. There is dilatation of the colon or rectum, but full thickness biopsies reveal normal ganglia in the anorectum. The anal canal is often patulous. It has been suggested that the abnormality may be due to ultrashort segment aganglionosis but this seems unlikely.

Chagas' disease
Damage to the myenteric plexus affecting the rectum and oesophagus occurs in Chagas' disease.

Slow transit constipation
There is a group of young female patients who have delayed colonic transit (despite normal mouth to caecum motility as assessed by the hydrogen breath test), a flat sigmoid pressure trace which will often not respond to bisacodyl and a failure to defecate. Some of these subjects have damaged ganglion cells possibly from laxative abuse. These patients do not have a megacolon or megarectum and some are improved by colectomy.

Colorectal resections
Anorectal function is usually preserved provided the pelvic floor has not been disturbed and an adequate rectal ampulla has not been completely removed. Hence, although defects in the control of flatus may be common in the first few weeks after anterior resection this is usually transient and true incontinence is rare. Continence is even preserved after colo-anal sleeve resection and rectal excision with colo-anal anastomosis but continence is poor after pull-through operations. Continence is also preserved in the majority of patients having an ileo-anal anastomosis with a pelvic pouch, since a reservoir has been created and the levator ani preserved. Incontinence after ileorectal anastomosis suggests severe proctitis, rectal stricture or an intermittently obstructing ileal stenosis.

Drugs
There are many drugs which affect anorectal function. Colorectal stimulants may cause explosive uncontrollable colic, diarrhoea and incontinence. Bulking agents will influence continence by altering the consistency of the stool. Topical steroids or sulphasalazine may improve urgency if there is severe proctitis. Loperamide is said to have a specific action on the anal sphincters.[28]

REFERENCES

1 Aaronson, I. & Nixon, H. H. (1972) A clinical evaluation of anorectal pressure studies on the diagnosis of Hirschsprung's disease. *Gut*, **13**, 138–146.

2 Bennett, R. C. (1972) Sensory receptors of the anorectum. *Australian and New Zealand Journal of Surgery*, **42**, 42–45.

3 Cummins, J. H., Sladen, G. E., James, O. F. W. *et al.* (1974) Laxative induced diarrhoea: a continuing clinical problem. *British Medical Journal*, **i**, 537–541.

4 Devroede, G. J. & Phillips, S. (1969) Studies of the perfusion technique for colonic absorption. *Gastroenterology*, **56**, 92–100.

5 Duthie, H. L. (1971) Progress report and continence. *Gut*, **12**, 844–852.

6 Duthie, H. L. (1975) Colonic motility in man. *Mayo Clinic Proceedings*, **50**, 519–522.

7 Farthing, M. J. G. & Lennard Jones, J. E. (1978) Sensibility of the rectum to distension and the anorectal distension reflex in ulcerative colitis. *Gut*, **19**, 64–69.

8 Freckner, B. & Euler, C. V. (1975) Influence of pudendal block on the function of the anal sphincter. *Gut*, **16**, 482–489.

9 Cagnon, D. J., Devroede, G. & Belisle, S. (1972) Excitatory effects of adrenaline upon isolated preparations of human colon. *Gut*, **13**, 654–658.

10 Goligher, J. C. & Hughes, E. S. R. (1951) Sensibility of the rectum and colon. *Lancet*, **i**, 543–548.

11 Gunterberg, B., Kewenter, J., Peterson, I. & Stener, B. (1976) Anorectal function after major resections of the sacrum with bilateral or unilateral sacrifice of sacral nerves. *British Journal of Surgery*, **63**, 546–554.

12 Harris, J. & Shields, R. (1970) Absorption of water and electrolytes in Crohn's disease of the colon. *Gastroenterology*, **56**, 571–579.

13 Henry, M. M., Parks, A. G. & Swash, M. (1980) The anal reflux in idiopathic faecal incontinence; an electrophysiological study. *British Journal of Surgery*, **67**, 781–783.

14 Hinton, J. M., Lennard-Jones, J. E. & Young, A. C. (1969) A new method for studying gut transit times using radio opaque markers. *Gut*, **10**, 842–847.

15 Ihre, T. (1974) Studies on anal function in continent and incontinent patients. *Scandinavian Journal of Gastroenterology*, **9** (Supplement 25), 1–80.

16 Kanaghinus, T., Lubran, M. & Coghill, N. F. (1963) The composition of ileostomy fluid. *Gut*, **4**, 322–338.

17 Keighley, M. R. B. & Matheson, D. (1981) Results of treatment for rectal prolapse and faecal incontinence. *Diseases of the Colon and Rectum*, **24**, 449–502.

18 Keighley, M. R. B., Fielding, J. & Alexander-Williams, J. (1983) Results of Marlex Mesh abdominal rectopexy for rectal prolapse in 100 consecutive cases. *British Journal of Surgery*, **70**, 229–232.

19 Levitan, R., Fordtran, J. S., Burrows, B. A. & Ingelfinger, F. J. (1962) Water and salt absorption in the human colon. *Journal of Clinical Investigation*, **41**, 1754–1759.

20 Mekhjian, H. S., Phillips, S. F. & Hoffman, A. F. (1971) Colonic secretion of water and electrolytes induced by bile acids: perfusion studies in man. *Journal of Clinical Investigation*, **50**, 1569–1577.

21 Minervini, S., Alexander-Williams, J., Donovan, I. A. *et al.* (1980) Comparison of three methods of whole bowel irrigation. *American Journal of Surgery*, **140**, 400–404.

22 Misiewicz, J. J. (1975) Colonic motility. *Gut*, **16**, 311–314.

23 Painter, N. S. (1975) *Diverticular Disease of the Colon. A Deficiency Disease of Western Civilisation.* London: W. Heinemann.

24 Parks, A. G., Porter, H. H. & Hardcastle, J. (1966) The syndrome of the descending perineum. *Proceedings of the Royal Society of Medicine*, **59**, 477–482.

25 Parks, A. G., Swash, M. & Urich, H. U. (1977) Sphincter denervation in anorectal incontinence and rectal prolapse. *Gut*, **18**, 656–665.

26 Preston, D. M., Hawley, P. R. & Lennard-Jones, J. E. (1982) Results of colectomy for slow transit constipation. *Gut*, **23**, A903.

27 Rask-Madsen, J. (1973) Simultaneous measurement of electrical polarisation and electrolyte transport by the entire normal and inflamed human colon during in vivo perfusion. *Scandinavian Journal of Gastroenterology*, **8**, 327–336.

28 Read, N. W., Harford, W., Schmulen, A. C. *et al.* (1979) A clinical study of patients with faecal incontinence and diarrhoea. *Gastroenterology*, **76**, 747–756.

29 Ritchie, J. A. (1968) Colonic motor activity and bowel function. Pt. 1. Normal movement of contents. *Gut*, **9**, 442–456.

30 Shields, R. (1966) Absorption and secretion of electrolytes and water by the human colon with particular reference to benign adenoma and papilloma. *British Journal of Surgery*, **53**, 893–897.

31 Shields, R. & Miles, J. B. (1965) Absorption and secretion in the large intestine. *Postgraduate Medical Journal*, **41**, 435–439.

32 Sladen, G. E. (1975) Methods of studying intestinal absorption. In *Intestinal Absorption in Man* pp. 1–49. London: Academic Press.

33 Snape, W. J., Cartson, G. M. & Cohen, S. (1976) Colonic myoelectric activity in the irritable bowel syndrome. *Gastroenterology*, **70**, 326–330.

34 Tagart, R. E. B. (1966) The anal canal and rectum: their varying relationship and its effect on anal continence. *Diseases of the Rectum and Colon*, **9**, 449–452.

35 Taylor, I. & Duthie, H. L. (1976) Bran tablets and diverticular disease. *British Medical Journal*, **i**, 988–990.

36 Taylor, I., Duthie, H. L. & Zachary, R. B. (1973) Anal incontinence following surgery for imperforate anus. *Journal of Pediatric Surgery*, **8**, 497–503.

37 Taylor, I., Duthie, H. L., Cumberland, D. C. & Smallwood, R. (1975) Glucagon and the colon. *Gut*, **16**, 973–978.

38 Turnberg, L. A. (1971) Abnormalities in intestinal electrolyte transport in congenital chloridorrhoea. *Gut*, **12**, 544–551.

39 Waller, S. L. (1975) Differential measurement of small and large bowel transit times in constipation and diarrhoea: a new approach. *Gut*, **16**, 372–378.

40 Wheatley, I. C., Hardy, K. J. & Dent, J. (1977) Anal pressure studies in spinal patients. *Gut*, **18**, 488–490.

CONSTIPATION, FAECAL IMPACTION AND LAXATIVE ABUSE

Constipation is a symptom and not a disease. This complaint, which to the clinician may at first seem trivial, can indicate serious underlying disease or a motility disorder so severe that it destroys a patient's sense of well-being. The term constipation is used by patients in various ways that defy clear definition. It may mean difficulty in evacuating stool that is small or hard, a sensation of incomplete evacuation, infrequent defecation, or even a general sensation of abdominal fullness or 'wind'.

Stool size, consistency and frequency

Stool size, and the frequency of defecation can be measured to provide one objective definition of constipation. The average daily stool weight in Western society is 120 g[27] and 'normal' stool frequency varies from three per day to three per week.[7] However, such studies take no account of the amount of dietary fibre ingested and there are as yet no data on the range of bowel habit in a normal population on a standardized diet. Studies in rural African villages suggest that given a high residue vegetable diet most subjects will pass one or more soft stools daily with a total weight in excess of 400 g.[6] Though prolonged retention of faeces is not thought to be harmful, it is possible that Western stool size and frequency may be suboptimal in physiological terms. It is therefore impossible to define normality, but only to record the observed range in different communities in health.

Transit rate

In some patients an increased intake of dietary fibre does not relieve their symptoms. Delayed passage of faeces is best demonstrated by a whole gut transit study using an inert marker. Small polythene pellets with the same specific gravity as stool mix well and are excreted at an exponential rate. Healthy subjects in Europe and North America pass 80% of such markers within five days and failure to do so provides another objective definition of constipation.[13, 19]

Colonic size

Some patients with constipation develop massive enlargement of the colon. The normal range of colonic size is known and thus 'megacolon' can be defined, although recognition of a megacolon associated with constipation does not allow a definitive diagnosis to be made unless aganglionosis is demonstrated by rectal biopsy.

Inability to defecate

In many patients the complaint of constipation refers to difficulty in evacuating stool, which may be unduly hard or small, through a normal anus and rectum. In others the stool may be normal, or made soft by laxatives, yet still cannot be passed because of a disorder of the defecatory mechanism. Structural causes for this are well recognized, but the functional disorders and those possibly related to nerve damage such as the descending perineum syndrome are poorly understood. Disorders of defecation may be more important than is realized. Sir Arthur Hurst, who by his seminal radiological studies did more than anyone to classify constipation into 'colonic' and 'rectal' causes, changed his mind towards the end of his career and suggested that dyschezia was the most important factor in all cases of constipation.[15]

Investigation

History

A careful history of the complaint is essential and an attempt should be made to define the patient's complaint precisely. An estimate should be made of the frequency of defecation and of the amount of roughage in the diet. A drug history is important with particular attention to laxative use which may be minimized or concealed. If the complaint is longstanding, it is sometimes helpful to enquire into the reason for seeking medical advice. The onset of symptoms may give an important clue to the diagnosis. Constipation from birth in the absence of perianal soiling suggests congenital aganglionosis. Soiling from early childhood may indicate a congenital anorectal malformation or idiopathic megabowel. Symptoms developing in the late teens or early twenties suggest a functional bowel disorder whereas a change in bowel habit in middle-aged or elderly patients should raise suspicion of a neoplasm.

Examination

During the physical examination general medical causes of constipation, such as myxoedema and hypercalcaemia must be considered. Abdominal palpation may reveal faecal retention or a painful spastic sigmoid colon. There may be associated urinary retention in patients with neurological lesions. Rectal examination and sigmoidoscopy are mandatory and the perianal region should be examined for fissure, abscess, fistula formation and haemorrhoids. The patient should be asked to bear down, as if during defecation, to demonstrate any perineal descent. The anal reflex should be tested and digital examination of the lower rectum will show if there is faecal impaction or a rectal or pelvic tumour. On sigmoidoscopy the presence of blood or mucus in the lumen or a mucosal abnormality such as proctitis or melanosis should be noted and confirmed by rectal mucosal biopsy if indicated. Sigmoidoscopy also gives useful information about the size of the rectum and air insufflation may reproduce abdominal pain in patients with an irritable colon. If possible a stool sample should be inspected, both for the presence of blood or mucus, and also to get some indication of stool size. Small hard stools like rabbit droppings, or excessively thin stools, may suggest an irritable colon.

Is further investigation needed or can the patient be treated empirically for simple constipation? It is certainly undesirable and unnecessary to perform a barium enema on every young woman complaining of constipation and it should be reserved for those with intractable symptoms who do not respond to dietary manipulation, older patients or those with a recent change in bowel habit. A plain X-ray of the abdomen may demonstrate the degree of faecal retention, particularly in the obese where the colon is not easily palpable (Figure 11.36). In younger patients, if there is no evidence of faecal impaction or megacolon and no clue as to a primary cause for constipation, it is sufficient to recommend a high residue diet with or without an additional bulking agent such as bran or ispaghula. Some general advice should also be given about the importance of taking sufficient fluids and responding promptly to the call to stool.

Radiological contrast studies

In patients without megacolon a double-contrast barium enema after bowel preparation is the investigation of choice and can exclude a primary colonic cause for constipation such as diverticular stricture or carcinoma. In patients with palpable megacolon or faecal impaction, an unprepared water-soluble contrast (Gastrografin) enema is advisable. It gives a clearer picture of the degree of megacolon because, after faecal disimpaction, the radiologist may find that a grossly redundant colon is difficult to inflate adequately. The water-soluble contrast does not solidify and can be washed out afterwards. This technique may also show a distal narrowed segment which is strong evidence of Hirschsprung's disease, although this must be confirmed by rectal biopsy. A lateral view of the rectum is needed to demonstrate this narrowing (Figures 11.37 and 11.38).

Bowel transit studies

Some patients will complain of severe constipation which does not respond to dietary manipulation although there is no evidence of faecal impaction or megacolon. Some may have a psychological disorder and bowel transit studies are useful to confirm that bowel movements have not taken place.[13] The study should

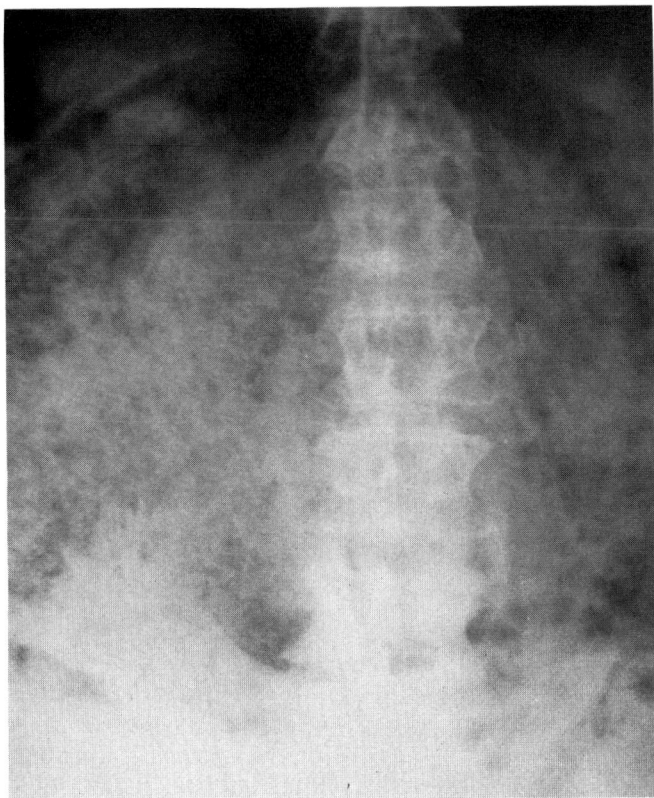

Fig. 11.36 Plain abdominal radiograph from an obese man complaining of chronic constipation. There is gross faecal retention due to a megacolon.

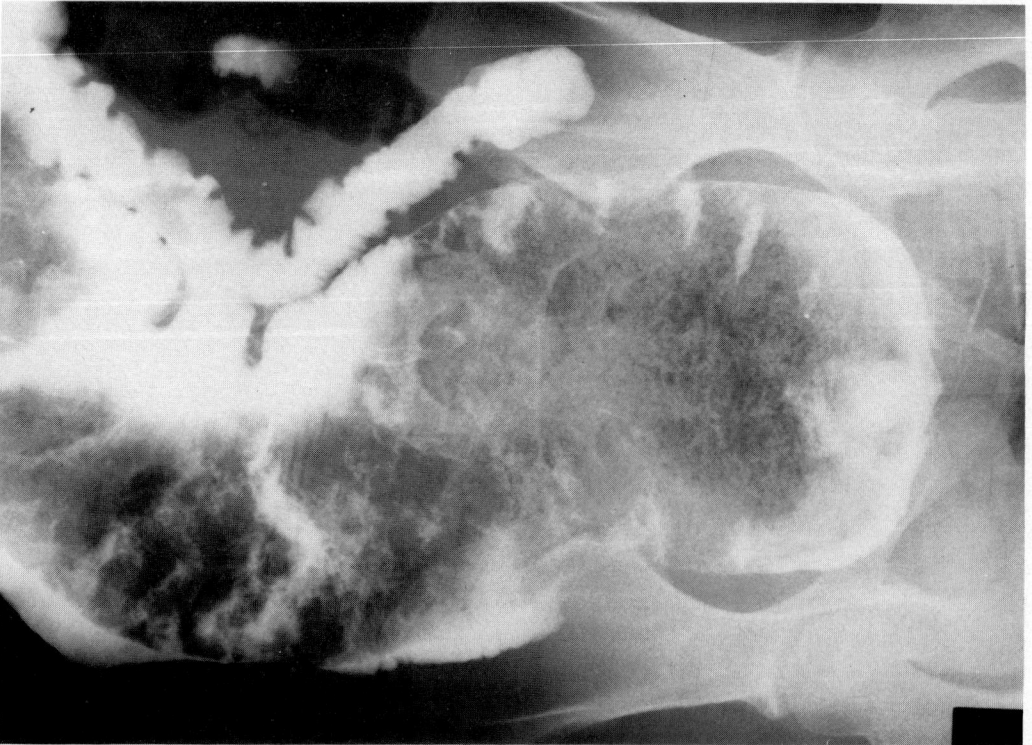

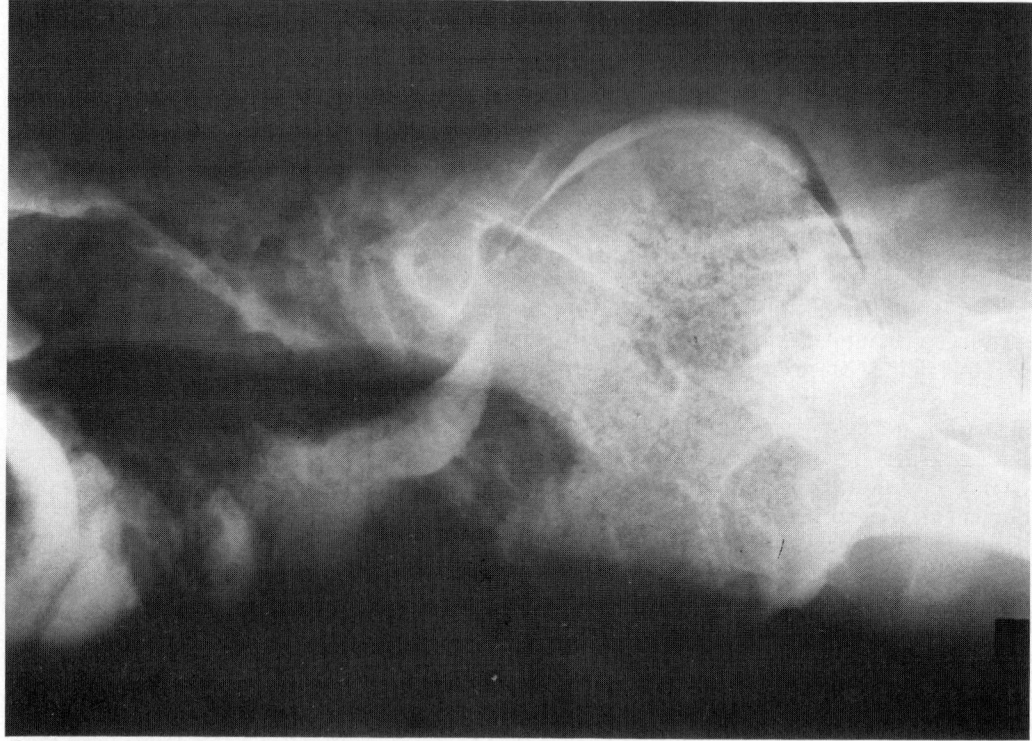

Fig. 11.37 Gastrografin enema on a young women with idiopathic megacolon. The gross faecal retention and dilatation of the rectosigmoid is outlined by the contrast (a) and on the lateral view (b) this dilatation is seen to extend down to the anal margin.

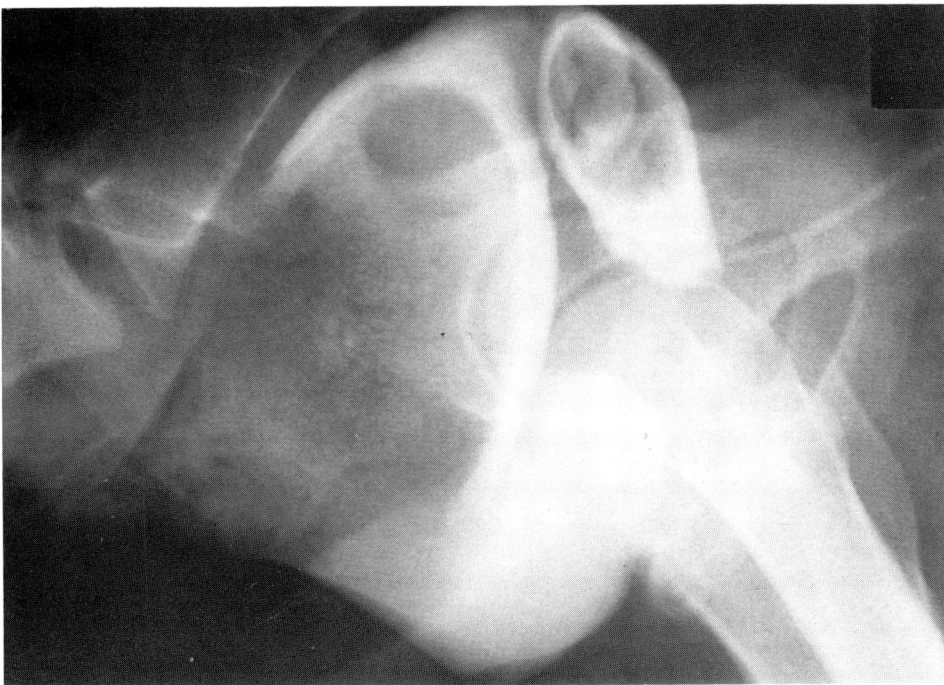

b

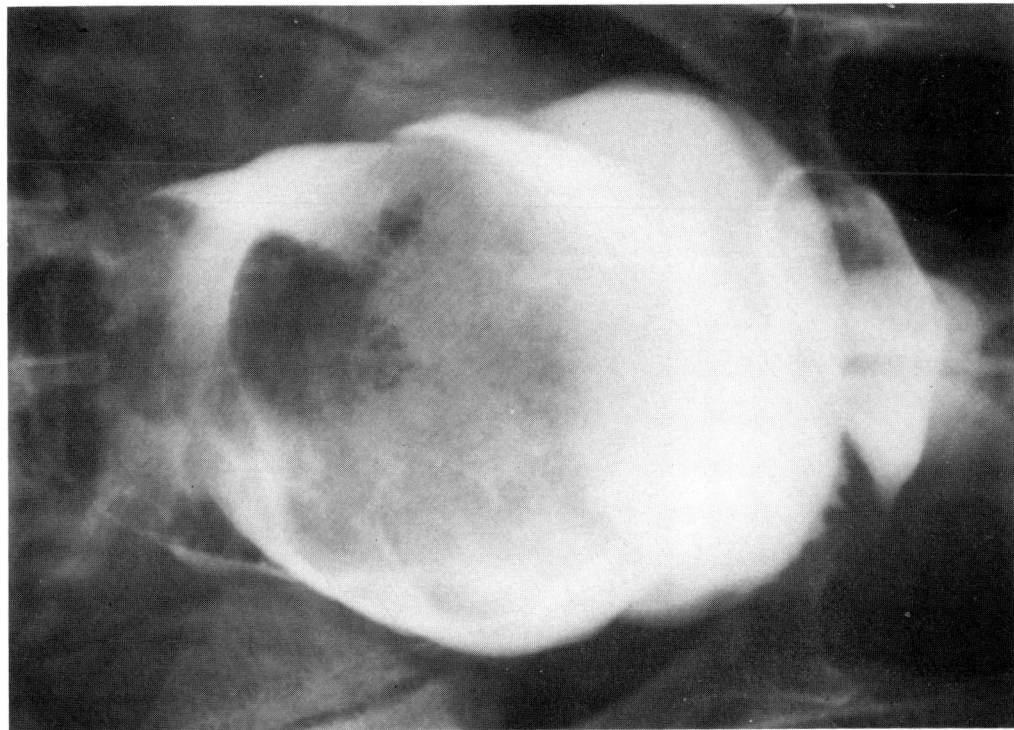

a

Fig. 11.38 Gastrografin enema on a young man with constipation caused by a short segment of aganglionosis in the rectum (Hirschsprung's disease). Dilatation of the rectum is apparent (a) but only the lateral view (b) demonstrated that this does not extend as far as the anal margin and that there is a distal narrowing.

be conducted after two weeks on a high residue diet, preferably with added fibre to ensure an adequate intake. The diet and any additional bulking agent should be continued throughout. Laxatives should be discontinued for 48 hours beforehand and must certainly be stopped during the study. On the first day, 20 inert polythene radiopaque markers are given with breakfast. A plain abdominal X-ray is taken after two and five days. Normal subjects excrete some of the markers within two days and at least 80% within five days. This transit rate is independent of age.[9] Delayed transit is shown by retention of all markers for more than five days (Figure 11.39). After all primary causes of constipation have been excluded such patients are described as having idiopathic slow-transit constipation. An alternative but less satisfactory method of estimating whole gut transit time is to collect and X-ray the stools and count the markers in each.

Colonic motility studies

The principal use of colonic motility studies is in research. Occasionally, an overactive trace with high pressure waves may be useful in helping to explain symptoms to a patient with irritable bowel syndrome, but the trace usually has no diagnostic value. Some patients who complain of constipation have a flat motility record with no response to stimulation with surface acting laxatives. This inactivity may reflect damage to the intramural nerve plexuses but the diagnostic value of this finding is not yet established.

Studies of defecation

Some patients with idiopathic constipation are unable to defecate. A defecating balloon proctogram may distinguish this group as well as demonstrating rectocoele or perineal descent in patients whose constipation is associated with a disorder of the pelvic floor.[23] The contribution of this apparent defecatory disorder to the

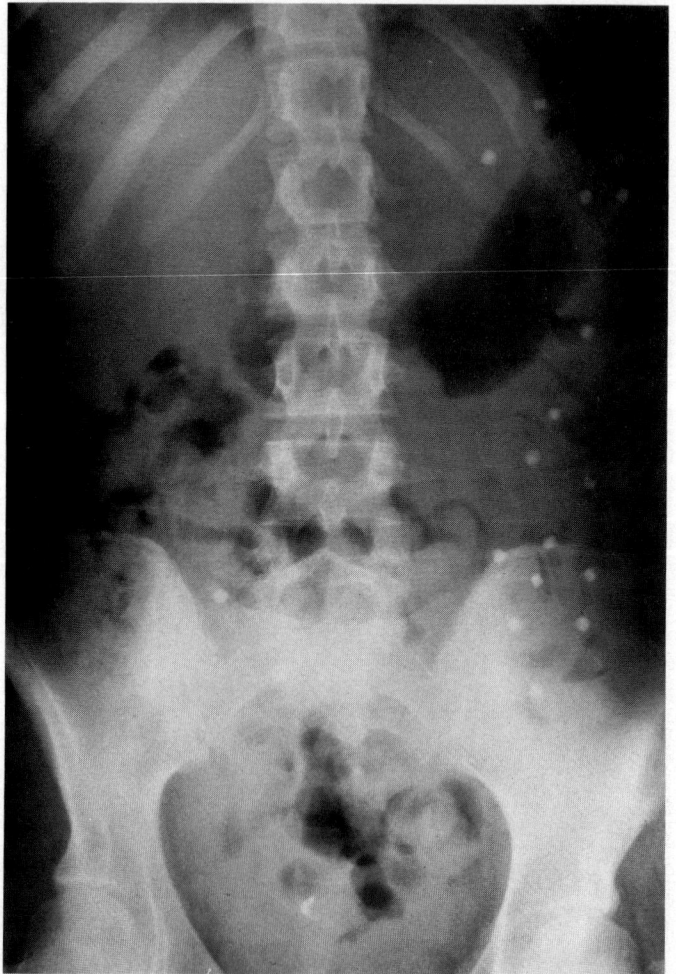

Fig. 11.39 Plain abdominal radiograph from a young girl with idiopathic slow-transit constipation. Five days after ingestion of 20 polythene markers the majority are seen distributed throughout the left side of the colon.

symptoms of patients with idiopathic constipation is still not clear.

Anorectal physiology

Measurement of anal canal pressure and its response to rectal distension is an important investigation that should be carried out in all patients with severe symptoms, even those without obvious megacolon. The anorectal inhibitory reflex is absent in Hirschsprung's disease and demonstration of a normal reflex excludes this condition (Figure 11.40).

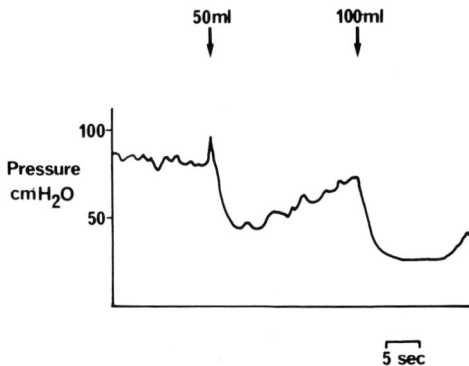

Fig. 11.40 Anorectal inhibitory reflex. Anal canal pressure 1·5 cm from the anal verge measured by distension of the lower rectum by an air-filled balloon (1 cmH$_2$O ≈ 98 Pa). Distension of the rectum causes an immediate reflex inhibition of the internal anal sphincter resulting in a fall in anal canal pressure.

Rectal biopsy

All patients with megacolon and an absent anorectal inhibitory reflex should have a full thickness rectal biopsy under general anaesthesia. Tissue should be taken from the low rectum down to the dentate line. Aganglionosis is diagnostic of Hirschsprung's disease and diagnostic changes may be seen in patients with other conditions causing megacolon, such as systemic sclerosis and amyloidosis.

Simple constipation (see Table 11.6)

This is the usual cause of symptoms in patients attending their general practitioner. Although the importance of fibre in the diet has been highlighted recently, many patients referred for specialist investigation at hospital have simple or dietary constipation. These patients will require a careful physical examination and reassurance, but some bowel retraining may be necessary for those who regularly take unnecessary laxatives.

Table 11.6 Differential diagnosis of constipation.

Primary or simple
  Low food intake
  Insufficient dietary fibre
  Lack of exercise
  Ignoring the call to stool

Secondary to known cause
  Anal disorders
    Painful anal lesion (e.g. fissure)
    Anal stricture
    Ectopic anus
    Pelvic floor dysfunction
  Colonic disorders
    Colonic stricture
    Carcinoma
    Sigmoid volvulus
    Systemic sclerosis
  Neurological disorders
    Intrinsic lesions
      Hirschsprung's disease
      Chagas' disease
      ? some forms of pseudo-obstruction
    Extrinsic lesions
      Autonomic neuropathy
      Spinal cord lesion
      Damage to sacral nerves
      Cerebrovascular accident
  Endocrine and metabolic disorders
    Hypothyroidism
    Hypercalcaemia
    Dehydration
    Hypopituitarism
    Porphyria
    Heavy-metal poisoning
    Amyloidosis
    Obstetric bowel
  Psychiatric disorders
    Depression
    Chronic schizophrenia
    Anorexia nervosa
    Purgative addiction
    Denied bowel action
  Drug-induced

Cause unknown
  Idiopathic slow-transit constipation
  Idiopathic megabowel
  Irritable bowel syndrome
  Pseudo-obstruction

Aetiology

The usual cause of simple constipation is a faulty diet. Foods with a high fibre content have hydrophilic properties which help to retain water in the bowel, and soften the faeces. Increased stool size is partly due to an increase in colonic bacteria which digest cellulose. Short chain fatty acids are produced as part of this metabolic process and they may stimulate colonic secretion and peristalsis. Many patients with simple constipation are young women which probably reflects their dietary habits, although fluctuations in levels of the reproductive hormones may play a part. Lack of exercise may also contribute as there is evidence that physical activity helps to stimulate colonic peristalsis.[14] Ignoring the call to stool contributes to the development of simple constipation. This may be partly due to environmental factors such as poor lavatory facilities and unfavourable working conditions, and partly due to hurry and a disorganized lifestyle. If the initial urge to defecate is resisted, the arrival of more stool in the rectum may fail to stimulate a suitable response. Studies with barium-impregnated pellets have shown that stool may even undergo retropulsion as far as the distal transverse colon if defecation is resisted.[12] Delay in evacuation results in progressive dehydration and hardening of the faeces so that defecation may become difficult or painful and thus reinforce the disordered bowel habit. Misuse of laxatives may play a part in the development or continuation of symptoms. Often proprietary laxatives bought over the counter are used to initiate defecation. Once the bowel has been artificially emptied in this way, it may take several days to fill with dietary residue. The absence of any bowel action may then be interpreted by the patient as constipation and a further dose of laxative is taken.

Treatment

If examination and routine biochemical investigations have shown no abnormality, patients with simple constipation require no more than a careful explanation of the nature of their disorder. Some patients benefit from a discussion with a dietitian and subsequent modification of their eating habits. If meals are taken away from home (e.g. in a works' canteen where choice may be restricted) it is sometimes helpful for patients to take a regular dose of Miller's bran, either with their morning cereal or mixed with soups or stews. Patients should be encouraged to answer the call to stool promptly. For those who have been using laxatives regularly, daily glycerine suppositories may be needed to empty the rectum and encourage a regular bowel habit.

Constipation secondary to anorectal or colonic disease

Local anal lesions

These produce constipation because of pain which causes difficulty in defecation. The deliberate suppression of the call to stool establishes a vicious circle, whereby the retained stool becomes harder and more difficult to pass, thus exacerbating the symptoms.

Pelvic floor disorders

Disorders of the pelvic floor may aggravate constipation or result in a sensation of incomplete evacuation. In the solitary ulcer syndrome there is a failure of the striated muscle of the pelvic floor to relax during defecation. The muscles of the pelvic floor are weak in patients with rectal mucosal prolapse or the descending perineum syndrome. The prolapsed rectal mucosa gives a continuous urge to defecate with a sensation of incomplete evacuation, or the whole perineum descends on straining making expulsion of stool difficult. Difficulty in defecation may follow pelvic surgery as a consequence of damage to the nerve supply to the pelvic floor muscles. Congenital disorders of the anorectal muscles such as an ectopic anus usually result in faecal retention and megacolon and were discussed earlier in this chapter.

Colonic lesions

Rarely carcinoma presents with constipation. Obstruction of the large bowel can be caused by a small annular growth or a large intraluminal polypoid lesion. An extrinsic tumour in the pelvis may also cause obstruction. Other causes of colonic stricture, such as ischaemia, Crohn's disease, endometriosis and diverticular disease, may induce obstructive symptoms.

Degeneration of colonic muscle is an uncommon cause of constipation with megacolon. The muscle may degenerate secondary to neurological damage associated with the cathartic colon. Systemic sclerosis is an important, though rare, cause of megacolon and must be distinguished from idiopathic megacolon. In some cases there are no skin changes, but a barium swallow and meal may show abnormal oesophageal motility or a dilated small bowel. The diagnosis can be made on full thickness rectal biopsy. Treatment is symptomatic and surgery should be avoided where possible.

Constipation secondary to disease of the nervous system

MYENTERIC PLEXUS ABNORMALITIES

The intramural nerve plexus of the colon is essential for normal peristalsis and for the initiation of the anorectal inhibitory reflex. Most patients in whom the myenteric plexus is damaged will have a megacolon, but rarely patients with congenital aganglionosis have involvement of the entire colon of normal calibre.

Hirschsprung's disease
Congenital aganglionosis of the rectum and colon usually presents in childhood but occasionally it may not be recognized until the second or third decade of life, and has been reported in patients over 70. Hirschsprung's disease has already been discussed in this chapter. It must be distinguished from idiopathic megacolon. Short segment Hirschsprung's disease cannot be excluded without a full thickness rectal biopsy.

Chagas' disease
This is an acquired form of aganglionosis due to a neurotoxin released by the parasite *Trypanosoma cruzi*. It is endemic in Brazil, particularly in the São Paulo region although the disorder is rarely seen outside South America. There is inflammation followed by degeneration and atrophy of the myenteric plexus throughout the gastrointestinal tract so that megaoesophagus and megacolon may occur. The heart may also be involved. In contrast to Hirschsprung's disease the aganglionic segment is dilated rather than normal and in severe cases the diseased portion of colon may need resection.[10]

Drug-induced plexus damage
A variety of drugs are associated with damage to the myenteric plexus of the bowel and can produce a megacolon. The best known of these are the anthracene derivatives (senna, cascara, aloes) which are used as colonic stimulants. In animals and in man administration of these causes degeneration and eventual destruction of the myenteric plexus.[32] Some patients with Parkinson's disease develop severe constipation and megacolon which may be secondary to drug therapy. These have anticholinergic effects and damage the myenteric plexus of the colon in animal experiments.[33] Many patients with chronic schizophrenia have megacolon, although there is anecdotal evidence that some are constipated before they have received phenothiazines. It seems likely that megacolon in these patients follows drug therapy. Phenothiazines such as chlorpromazine produce a megacolon secondary to destruction of the myenteric plexus in experimental animals.[38] The vinca alkaloids used as cytotoxic agents produce extensive neurological damage including destruction of the myenteric plexus which may result in a giant megacolon.[28]

EXTRINSIC NERVE LESIONS

Constipation is a common feature of neurological disorders affecting the spinal cord. If the lumbo-sacral cord has been destroyed so that reflex defecation is impossible, faecal impaction and megacolon usually ensue. Constipation can be a feature of disseminated sclerosis, tabes dorsalis and a cauda equina tumour. It also follows damage to the sacral outflow due to interference with the defecation reflex. Patients with a cerebrovascular accident or brain tumour can also be troubled by constipation either because of failure to answer the call to stool or because cortical damage affects colonic motility.

Management of constipation following spinal cord injury
Spinal injuries often cause irreversible damage to the cord and control of the bowels causes special problems. Following transection of the spinal cord in the lower cervical or thoracic area, patients will regain reflex control of bowel function after a period of spinal shock. With destruction of the lumbo-sacral cord or a cauda equina lesion no defecation reflex can be initiated.

In all spinal injuries there is little awareness of when faecal evacuation is pending but sometimes patients develop autonomic symptoms such as a tachycardia when the rectum is widely distended. Following acute spinal cord injury, the ileus may respond to neostigmine. Three to four days after the injury regular laxatives should be given, as well as suppositories each morning. A regular bowel action may then be achieved within a few days, although digital removal is sometimes necessary. After this a practical regimen should be initiated which makes minimum demands on the patient. The bowels should be evacuated every other day and a mild peristaltic stimulant may be needed. Spontaneous defecation may follow a meal. If this does not happen, pressing on the abdomen or digital stimulation of the anus will sometimes initiate the defecation reflex. A glycerine suppository also provides an effective stimulus. Those patients with lumbo-sacral segment disease will usually only respond to the introduction of suppositories or an enema, but with their greater mobility can be trained to administer their own suppositories.[11]

DISORDERS OF THE AUTONOMIC NERVOUS SYSTEM

The autonomic nerve supply to the bowel is extremely complex and the relationship between the sympathetic and parasympathetic system, and the peptidergic nervous system, has not been fully elucidated. Constipation or diarrhoea

with megacolon may be a feature of an autonomic neuropathy. The commonest cause in this
country is diabetic autonomic neuropathy, but a
neuropathy may occur secondary to drugs or in
rare congenital disorders such as the Shy–
Drager syndrome. Gastrointestinal crises may
develop with vomiting, abdominal distension
and massive dilatation of the small or large
intestine. Familial forms of autonomic neuropathy may be accompanied by generalized
hypotonia, decreased pain sensation, postural
hypotension and abnormal cardiovascular
response to exercise, as well as disturbances of
sweating.[4]

Constipation secondary to endocrine and metabolic disorders

Hypothyroidism is often missed because of its
gradual onset and thyroid function tests should
be performed routinely in all patients with constipation. In severe cases myxoedematous infiltration of the bowel wall causes megacolon
which returns to normal after treatment with
thyroxine.[3] Hypercalcaemia may be suggested
by associated symptoms of anorexia, thirst and
polyuria. Elevated serum calcium may follow
excess consumption of antacids, which can
themselves be constipating. Many diabetic
patients are constipated which may be as much
due to dehydration as to the effects of any autonomic neuropathy. Any disorder causing excess
fluid loss will eventually cause inspissation of
faeces. Vomiting and polyuria are the more
obvious causes, although dehydration commonly follows over-enthusiastic prescription of
diuretics. Constipation may be a feature of
patients with acute intermittent porphyria,
heavy metal poisoning, hypopituitarism and
phaeochromocytoma. Both primary and secondary amyloidosis can be associated with constipation and megacolon. In pregnancy,
constipation is probably due to hormonal
changes which impair gut smooth muscle tone.

Psychiatric disorders and constipation

Constipation can be the presenting symptom of
depression. However, a label of psychiatric
disease should not be used to shield our ignorance of the aetiology of many cases of constipation. Patients with anorexia nervosa may
become constipated, probably because of the
low food intake, although their emotional disturbance may alter the cortical effects on bowel
function. Constipation is a particular problem in
patients with chronic psychoses who are liable
to develop giant megacolon complicated by

sigmoid volvulus or megarectum with overflow
incontinence and bowel resection may be
needed.[36]

A few patients are addicted to laxatives often
initiated by mild constipation in adolescence
and followed by an obsession with their bowels.
Some patients deliberately take laxatives to lose
weight and this may be a variant of anorexia
nervosa. Such patients deliberately conceal
abuse of laxatives from their family and physician and may become dangerously ill from the
side-effects.

A few patients who complain of severe constipation are found by transit studies to be emptying their colon normally, although they firmly
deny having defecated. Some may be genuinely
mildly constipated, but the primary disorder is
psychological and psychiatric advice should be
sought.

LAXATIVE ABUSE

Serious laxative abuse and its more bizarre complications are now much less frequent with the
advent of the National Health Service and the
decline in sales of patent medicines. Some £22
million worth of laxatives are still sold annually
in the United Kingdom and most of these are
unnecessary. The spectrum of abuse ranges from
the habitual weekly purge to the addict who
may consume over 50 senna tablets daily and go
to great lengths to conceal this fact from family
and physician alike. A high index of suspicion is
needed in any patient presenting with unexplained diarrhoea.

Clinical features
Patients (who are nearly always female) present
with diarrhoea, weakness, abdominal pain and
occasionally vomiting. Weight loss may be
prominent and confusion arises because of the
features of malabsorption, such as peripheral
oedema, hypoproteinaemia, amenorrhoea,
hypokalaemia and iron deficiency anaemia,
which may be present. Hypocalcaemia and
hypomagnesaemia may also occur. Severe metabolic disturbance may be associated with a frank
psychosis, hallucinations, ataxia and epileptic
seizures. Less commonly there may be bone
pain, tetany, fever, clubbing and increased skin
pigmentation. Previous investigations may have
shown steatorrhoea, increased gastrointestinal
protein loss, abnormal renal function, abnormal
gastric and pancreatic function tests or a diabetic glucose tolerance curve. Not infrequently,
an unnecessary laparotomy is undertaken in
search of an elusive hormone-secreting tumour.[8]

Investigations

Once the diagnosis is suspected a barium enema and rectal biopsy should be done. Phenol-phthalein in the stool may be detected by alkalization which produces a red colour. Urine may be analysed for products of the anthraquinone-type laxatives. In about 20% of cases barium enema will show a dilated featureless colon without haustration sometimes with areas of narrowing or pseudo-stricture formation. These appearances may be confused with those of ulcerative colitis. Rectal biopsy may show melanosis coli which is diagnostic of recent and prolonged intake of laxatives (almost exclusively the anthraquinone group). A low serum potassium is found in nearly 50% of the patients and may be so low as to cause renal impairment. In patients with less severe disturbance the diagnosis may be difficult to establish. Admission to hospital for observation and a search of the patient's locker may be the only way of confirming the diagnosis.

Treatment

The prognosis is poor, particularly in those patients who have features suggestive of anorexia nervosa. The taking of laxatives is usually concealed, and it is difficult to decide whether to confront the patient once the diagnosis has been established. If confronted, patients may deny their use and discharge themselves from hospital. With psychiatric help some patients can be weaned off laxatives, and an attempt should be made to replace them with a high fibre diet and bulking agents. If constipation remains a problem an osmotic laxative should be used rather than stimulants which may damage the bowel. Occasional phosphate enemas or evacuant suppositories may be needed to supplement the oral regimen.

CATHARTIC COLON

This condition is now hardly ever seen, probably because of a decline in the sales of toxic proprietary laxatives. It refers to an extreme form of laxative abuse in which the colon has become permanently damaged, usually by prolonged use of anthraquinones. The mucosa of the colon becomes dark and shiny with an appearance like snakeskin. The patient who may have suffered all her life from constipation complains of intractable diarrhoea and may have hypokalaemia and dehydration.[2] Pathological studies in such cases have shown destruction of the myenteric plexus and atrophy of colonic

smooth muscle. Colectomy with caecorectal anastomosis offers the best chance of a return to a normal bowel habit.[34]

Drugs causing constipation

Constipation secondary to medication is very common. Some groups of drugs constipate in normal therapeutic doses including muscle paralysing drugs, some hypotensive agents and analgesics related to morphine. Other drugs may only constipate in high doses or when the patient is unduly susceptible. This group includes the diuretics, iron compounds and psychotropic agents. A list of drugs that may cause constipation is shown in Table 11.7.

Table 11.7 Drugs which cause constipation.

Type of drug	Example
Muscle relaxants	Tubocurarine
Ganglion blockers	Mecamylamine
Opiate analgesics	Morphine
Anticonvulsants	Phenytoin
Anticholinergics	Atropine
MAO inhibitors	Phenelzine
Antacids	Calcium carbonate/aluminium hydroxide
Psychotropic agents:	
Barbiturates	Phenobarbitone
Phenothiazines	Chlorpromazine
Benzodiazepines	Diazepam
Tricyclics	Amitriptyline
Diuretics	Frusemide
Haematinics	Ferrous sulphate
Cytotoxic agents	Vincristine

Idiopathic slow-transit constipation (idiopathic constipation)

This group of patients have severe constipation, confirmed by delayed passage of radiopaque markers around the colon, but have a normal calibre bowel without megacolon or megarectum.

Aetiology

The cause of this disorder is not known nor is it clear whether it is due to a disorder of colonic transport or of the defecatory mechanism. It occurs almost exclusively in women and although disorders of the reproductive hormones can often be demonstrated, there does not appear to be a causal relationship. Release of gastrointestinal hormones following an oral stimulus is reduced but this may be a secondary effect. Studies of colonic motility suggest that these patients have an inert colon, rather than the over-active colon often seen in patients with the irritable bowel syndrome who complain of constipation. Inactivity of the colon may play a part in producing symptoms. A few patients have a disorder of the myenteric plexus which may predispose to constipation, but it is not known if this is congenital or acquired.[25] Patients often complain that they have great difficulty in evacuating the stool and experimental studies using a water-filled balloon to simulate defecation have shown an apparent disorder of defecation. This inability to defecate may result from failure to relax the muscles of the pelvic floor, and could result from a neurological defect or suppression of the normal defecation reflex.[22]

Clinical features

Constipation in these women occurs at about the time of the menarche. A few develop symptoms before the age of five and identical symptoms are also seen in some older patients following pelvic surgery such as hysterectomy. They develop progressive reduction in bowel frequency complaining that their bowels open only once or twice a month. Gynaecological problems are common; many have menstrual disturbances and there is an increased incidence of hyperprolactinaemia, galactorrhoea and infertility. Gynaecological surgery is more commonly undertaken in this group of patients than in women without bowel symptoms and there is a high incidence of ovarian cysts.[24] There is also an increased incidence of epilepsy. Patients are usually prescribed a number of laxatives, all of which gradually lose their effect. Symptoms may be made worse by abdominal surgery, particularly appendectomy, but in some patients are relieved during menstruation.

Examination reveals an apparently healthy young girl, often fashionably dressed and well manicured. There are no palpable abdominal masses. There is no incontinence or perianal soiling. Rectal examination and sigmoidoscopy may paradoxically reveal an empty rectum; stool which is not defecated apparently returns to the sigmoid or descending colon. The rectum is of normal size and air insufflation is not painful. These findings help to distinguish this disorder from idiopathic megarectum and the irritable bowel syndrome. One curious feature in some patients is marked abdominal swelling in the absence of faecal accumulation or distension of the bowel with gas. This appears to be produced by spasm of the muscles of the lumbar spine, resulting in a lumbar lordosis. This spasm is involuntary and may persist for several days.

Under anaesthesia, however, it relaxes and the stomach becomes flat again.

Investigation

Barium enema in these patients shows a redundant colon with a long sigmoid loop. The lumen of the bowel is, however, of normal calibre. The rectosphincteric reflex is intact, although there is often some disturbance of rectal sensation. Radiopaque markers given by mouth may be retained for two weeks or more, depending on the frequency of defecation.

Treatment

Many patients will have adjusted to a life of chronic ill health and manage their symptoms either by taking vast doses of aperients or by using daily enemas; neither treatment is satisfactory. A high residue diet can make these patients worse by increasing dietary residue which they cannot evacuate. The best drug is an osmotic laxative such as magnesium sulphate. This should be given in large doses until the stool is liquid and diarrhoea results; the dose should then be gradually reduced and titrated against the patient's symptoms. It is important that the treatment is taken on a regular basis, otherwise the stool hardens again and cannot be passed. A few patients with more severe symptoms and those with myenteric plexus damage may need surgical treatment. The role of surgery in the treatment of constipation is discussed below.

Idiopathic megacolon and megarectum

Constipation associated with enlargement of the large bowel in the absence of any primary cause and with normal intramural ganglion cells is known as idiopathic megacolon. The distinction sometimes drawn between megarectum and megacolon may not be valid. The principal abnormality in both conditions is a grossly dilated rectum which extends to the anal margin. The dilatation may extend for a variable distance proximally and the condition in which the sigmoid alone is dilated (chronic sigmoid volvulus) should be regarded as a separate disease entity.

Aetiology

The cause of these conditions is not known. Megarectum is common in children where it may be related to psychological factors or follow an acute anal lesion such as fissure. Many children respond satisfactorily to treatment and it is not known whether adults who present with megacolon form a group who were not adequately treated in childhood or have a separate disorder. Some patients with adult megacolon give a history of faecal retention and soiling going back to childhood, but others may have no symptoms until adult life. The reservoir function of the rectum in these patients is abnormal so that even large amounts of faeces do not give rise to any defecation reflex, though the internal sphincter may be inhibited. The elasticity of the rectum is abnormal, but this may be a secondary phenomenon. Some studies suggest a defect of internal sphincter relaxation but it is difficult to interpret these tests when the rectum is so grossly dilated.[17]

Clinical features
The sex incidence is equal in adults, who usually present in their late teens or early twenties. Complaints may include constipation, abdominal swelling or pain, perianal irritation and soiling.[18] Many patients are of below average intelligence and may display a surprising lack of interest in their symptoms or be rather vague about the details of their bowel habit. Teenagers are not infrequently accompanied by a rather dominant parent who corrects their version of events during the interview.

If a history of childhood bowel training can be obtained from the parent, it may disclose difficulties from an early age with soiling of underclothes and defecation at inappropriate places. A history of several days constipation followed by the passage of a huge stool which is passed with great difficulty and blocks the lavatory is characteristic. Bowel frequency in the adult is variable; some patients having a daily bowel action which may result from spurious diarrhoea around a faecal mass in the rectum. With gross rectal distension the internal anal sphincter may be inhibited allowing soiling and seepage of mucus leading to perianal pruritus. A few patients are unaware of any bowel disturbance, and rare presentations of megabowel include pseudo-pregnancy and chronic anaemia secondary to stercoral ulceration.

Abdominal examination in cases of colonic enlargement shows a large mass, dull to percussion and firm on palpation. The anus is often dilated and the perianal skin soiled. Digital rectal examination will show a mass of soft stool distending the rectum down to the anal verge and the anal canal may feel rather short. Sigmoidoscopy is impossible when the rectum is impacted, but if the bowel has been emptied by enemas and laxatives the instrument may 'fall' into a cavernous rectum.

Investigation
The important differential diagnosis is from short-segment Hirschsprung's disease and full thickness rectal biopsy may be required. A Gastrografin enema should be performed first and will show gross dilatation of the lower rectum down to the anal margin. The rectosphincteric reflex is normal, but caution must be advised in the interpretation of physiological studies in the first few days after rectal disimpaction since the internal anal sphincter may be completely inhibited and take several days to recover its tone. Transit studies using radiopaque markers may be misleading if the markers progress normally around faecal masses with the flow of spurious diarrhoea. Biochemical tests should be carried out to exclude primary causes of megacolon (Table 11.8).

Table 11.8 Differential diagnosis of idiopathic megacolon in the absence of any obvious anatomical abnormality.

Cathartic colon
Autonomic neuropathy
Spinal cord lesion
Chagas' disease
Dystrophia myotonica
Systemic sclerosis
Amyloidosis
Hypothyroidism
Pseudo-obstruction (q.v.)
Drug-induced (especially antiparkinsonian agents and phenothiazines)

Treatment
The important aspect of treatment is to empty the rectum and to try and keep it empty. The patient must understand that normal rectal sensation is absent and defecation may have to be initiated using regular enemas or suppositories. The faecal accumulation must first be evacuated in hospital under anaesthesia at the same time as the rectal biopsy. Several kilograms of stool may be removed. If the mass recurs, it can sometimes be broken up by softening the impaction with olive oil, to be followed a day or two later by rectal washouts.

Surgical treatment of megacolon has uncertain results and an attempt should be made to find an acceptable medical regimen. About two-thirds of patients will respond to an osmotic laxative such as magnesium sulphate. This should be started in large doses after disimpaction until diarrhoea occurs. After this a regular prescription will keep the stool soft and defecation is encouraged at a regular time each day using glycerine or bisacodyl suppositories.

806   *The Large Intestine*

Bran and bulking agents are not helpful in patients with colonic enlargement as they tend to cause a recurrence of faecal impaction. In cases with megarectum alone increased dietary fibre can be helpful provided the rectum is kept empty.

STERCORAL ULCERATION

Stercoral ulcers result from pressure of an abnormally hard faecal mass on the mucosa of the colon or rectum. Such ulcers are quite often found at autopsy in elderly patients who have been confined to bed for a long time. They should be suspected in any patient with long-standing constipation associated with mega-rectum or megacolon who presents with abdominal pain, perforation and peritonitis, rectal bleeding or chronic anaemia.

MEGACOLON IN THE ELDERLY

Constipation is often a particular problem in elderly patients, perhaps because they are less active or bed-bound. Some elderly patients may be physically unable to get to the lavatory in time to answer the call to stool, or have their perception blunted by dementia. Faecal inconti-nence must be recognized as a sequel to rectal impaction because relief of this symptom may make the difference between the ability of a patient to live at home and the need for institu-tional care. The patient will usually give a history of constipation prior to the development of diarrhoea or incontinence, and the condition is sometimes referred to as the 'ball-valve' rectum (Figure 11.41).

Treatment of megarectum in the elderly is often effective. Diet is important and dentures should be checked to ensure that they can cope with the roughage in their diet. Drugs which cause constipation should be avoided and depression or hypothyroidism may need treat-ment. After the rectum has been emptied a laxa-tive will be required. Osmotic laxatives should be avoided as they can disturb water and elec-trolyte balance. Liquid paraffin should not be

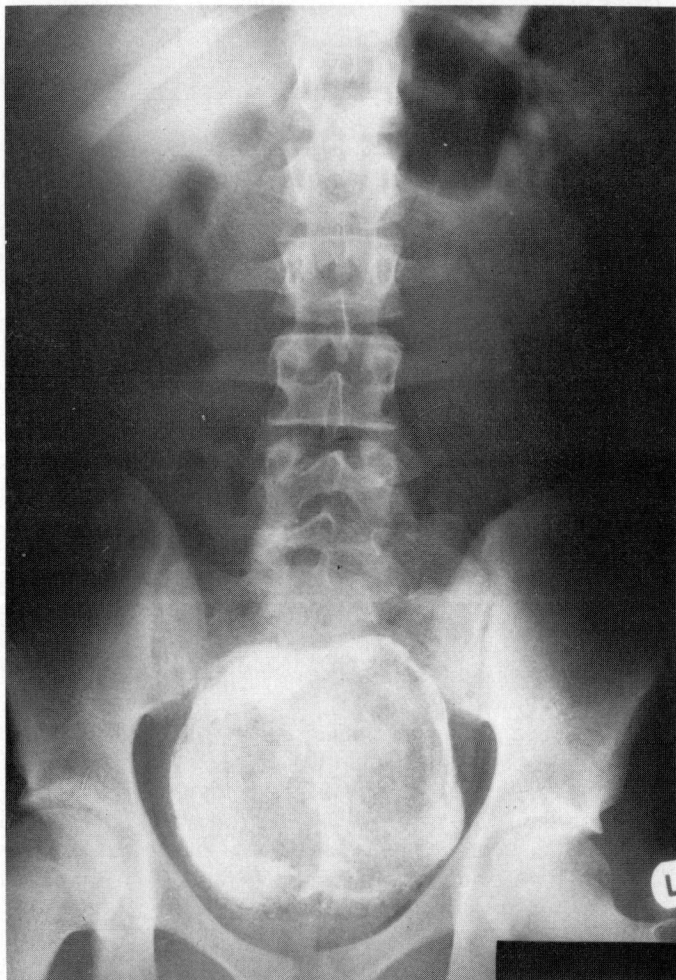

Fig. 11.41 Ball-valve rectum. Outline of a faecal mass in the rectum seven days after a barium enema. The impaction is solid and too large to be evacuated normally. Spurious diarrhoea leads to a presentation with faecal soiling and incontinence.

used because it may be inhaled. Senna or bisacodyl in regular small doses are effective and lactulose is a useful stool softener. Those patients who experience no call to stool will need regular suppositories or a twice-weekly enema under nursing supervision.

CHRONIC SIGMOID VOLVULUS

Some patients have a megacolon with a normal sized rectum. The sigmoid colon can become massively enlarged and produce a volvulus by rotating on its mesentery. The sex incidence is equal and the mean age at presentation in one series was 66 years.[29] There is a history of recurrent episodes of abdominal distension, colic, constipation and vomiting. Examination during one of these episodes will show marked abdominal distension associated with an empty rectum and a huge sigmoid loop on abdominal X-ray. When the diagnosis is made, flatus tube decompression should be attempted in acute cases. If this fails, emergency laparotomy is needed. The sigmoid colon is resected with a temporary colostomy. If flatus tube decompression is successful an outpatient barium enema should be arranged. This will show a normal size rectum leading to a grossly distended sigmoid loop (Figure 11.42). The enlarged sigmoid colon should be removed as an elective procedure and in most cases results in a complete cure. Occasionally a volvulus can occur in patients with idiopathic megacolon with dilatation down to the anal margin. In these patients there is a tendency for a proximal segment of bowel to distend with torsion at a later date if only the

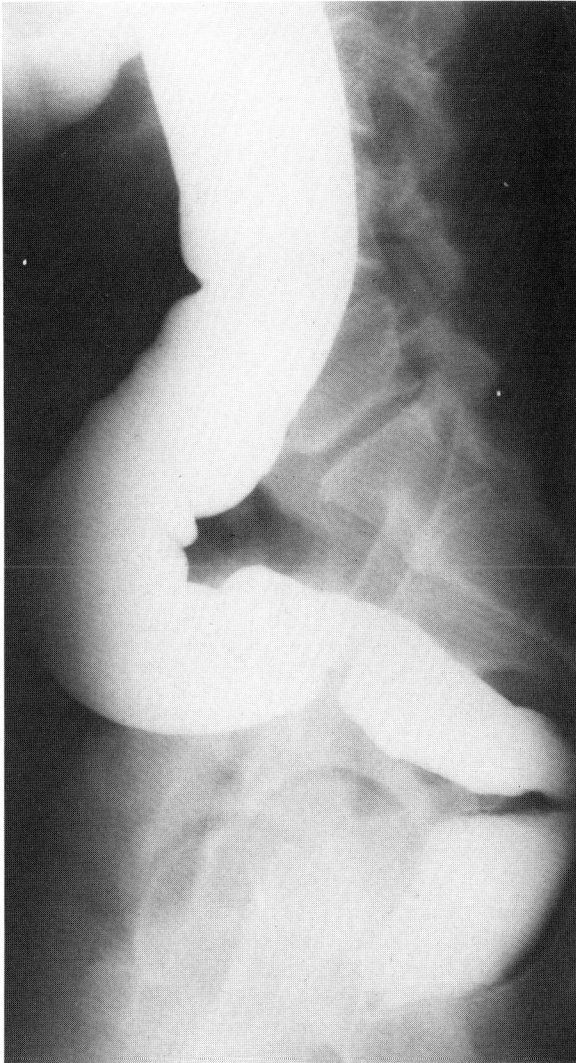

Fig. 11.42 Sigmoid volvulus. Barium enema has shown a normal sized rectum (a) leading to a massively enlarged and elongated sigmoid colon. Rotation of the sigmoid has resulted in a volvulus with the characteristic 'bird of prey' sign at the site of the torsion (b – overleaf).

a

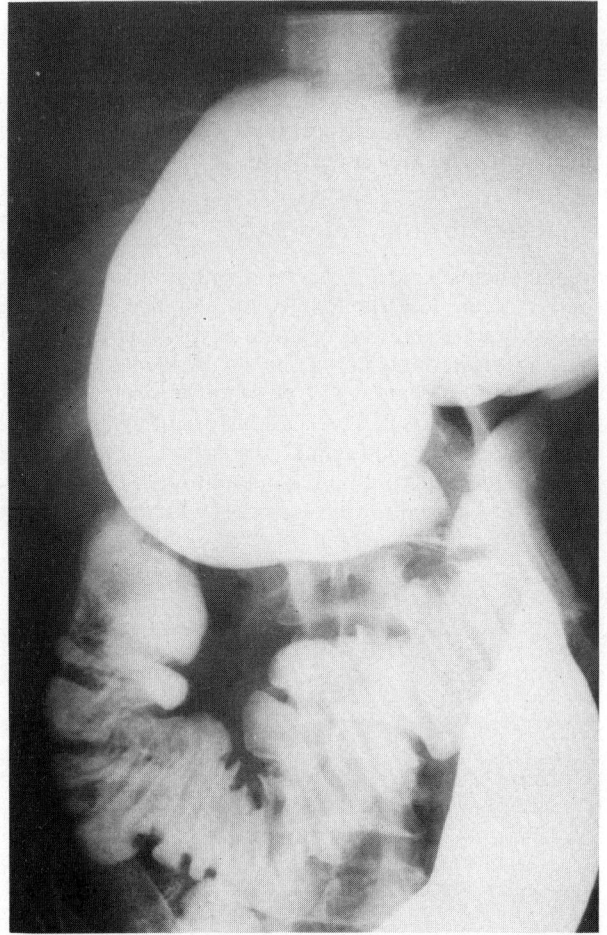

Fig. 11.42 (continued) Sigmoid volvulus. (b) Barium enema, showing the characteristic 'bird of prey' sign at the site of torsion.

b

sigmoid is removed. Such cases are probably best treated by subtotal colectomy with ileorectal anastomosis.

Constipation and the irritable bowel syndrome

The irritable bowel syndrome comprises a heterogeneous group of patients some of whom complain of constipation and abdominal pain, despite normal colonic transit times. It is discussed further later in this chapter (p. 867).

Aetiology

In these patients the colon and rectum may be unduly sensitive to distension and pain is experienced at lower volumes of distension than in controls. Colonic motility studies often show frequent high pressures which represent segmenting contractions. Excessive segmentation may result in fragmentation and dehydration of colonic content. The 'constipation' may relate to the size of the stool as some patients complain that they have difficulty in passing small, hard pellets. Alternatively their complaint may refer to a sensation of incomplete emptying which is a common feature of the irritable bowel syndrome.

Clinical features

Patients may be of either sex and any age, but women of middle or late middle age are more commonly affected. They usually make the physician's heart sink since they are totally absorbed in their symptoms. The usual complaint is of small hard pellety stools accompanied by the passage of mucus. Pain is experienced in the lower abdomen or left iliac fossa but may radiate to the epigastrium or back. The pain is colicky or continuous and may be either relieved or made worse by defecation.

Other symptoms include a sensation of incomplete evacuation and abdominal bloating. Because of the severity of their symptoms, most will have been investigated for other causes of abdominal pain and have often undergone abdominal surgery such as cholecystectomy, appendectomy or hysterectomy.

Examination usually shows a tense and introspective individual. Palpation of the abdomen is nearly always painful, particularly over the sigmoid and descending colon. Rectal examination is unremarkable but sigmoidoscopy with air insufflation will reproduce the abdominal pain.

Investigation

Barium enema should be carried out in this group to exclude a neoplasm. A bowel transit study using radiopaque markers is useful to confirm a normal gut transit rate. There are no specific diagnostic tests but distension of the rectum with a balloon is usually painful; these patients also tolerate a smaller rectal volume than normal subjects and other groups complaining of constipation.

Treatment

The management of this group of patients is a great challenge to the clinical gastroenterologist. The multiplicity of treatments available for the irritable bowel syndrome suggest that few, if any, are effective and patients with severe symptoms tend to move from one hospital to another undergoing repeated investigations or even exploratory laparotomy.

The most important step in management is to establish a good relationship and to accept that a number will require long-term support. Though psychological factors are important it does not help to suggest that the problem is all due to nerves or to probe the patient's past psychiatric history at the first interview. A careful history may reveal that the symptoms are brought on by a particular stress or, in some cases, by particular foods and the patients may be able to modify their lifestyle accordingly. Pain is the principal symptom and may be very severe. Antispasmodics, such as mebeverine, are helpful and can be combined with bran or a hydrophilic preparation such as Isogel or Celevac. Some patients will have a serious depressive illness requiring treatment. Although bowel transit time is normal with excess colonic activity, patients will often consume proprietary laxatives claiming that they relieve pain and bloating.

Pseudo-obstruction

Intestinal pseudo-obstruction is a syndrome in which there are signs and symptoms of intestinal obstruction in the absence of any mechanical cause. This may occur as an acute and transient disorder when it is really a form of paralytic ileus. Recurrent attacks may be secondary to systemic disease or due to a primary disorder of gut smooth muscle or of the myenteric plexus.

FAMILIAL PRIMARY CHRONIC INTESTINAL PSEUDO-OBSTRUCTION

A number of families have been reported whose members have postprandial abdominal pain, nausea and vomiting, abdominal distension, diarrhoea or constipation and urinary retention. Symptoms usually develop in the second decade of life and patients present with recurrent episodes of apparent intestinal obstruction. Abdominal X-rays show dilated loops of large and small bowel with fluid levels, but no cause is found at laparotomy.

Aetiology

In some families pathological studies have shown degeneration of smooth muscle and subsequent fibrosis affecting the whole gut and the urinary bladder. This condition has been called hereditary hollow visceral myopathy.[30] In another family there were additional neurological signs including an ataxic gait, irregular and poorly reactive pupils, dysarthria, absent deep tendon reflexes and impaired vibration and position sense. The smooth muscle in this group was normal but there was neuronal degeneration of the myenteric plexus throughout the bowel.[31] In other families no pathological abnormality has been demonstrated and some cases arise sporadically.

Treatment

Between attacks antibiotics may be needed to prevent intestinal bacterial overgrowth. During the acute phase treatment is supportive with intravenous fluids and nasogastric suction. Parenteral feeding may be required for prolonged ileus. In some families dilatation occurs in short segments only and these may be resected or drained.[1] In general, surgical interference should be avoided unless absolutely necessary. Medical treatment is disappointing, but the occasional patient will respond to regular neostigmine by mouth.

SECONDARY CHRONIC INTESTINAL PSEUDO-OBSTRUCTION

These patients present at a later age than the primary form and without a family history of recurrent abdominal pain. During assessment megacolon with faecal impaction or volvulus formation, giving rise to obstructive symptoms, must be excluded. Diseases reported as causing pseudo-obstruction include systemic sclerosis, systemic lupus erythematosis, dystrophia myotonica, diabetes mellitus, hypoparathyroidism, phaeochromocytoma, myxoedema, amyloidosis and porphyria. It may also be drug-induced.

ACUTE PSEUDO-OBSTRUCTION OF THE COLON (OGILVIE'S SYNDROME)

Acute large bowel pseudo-obstruction was first described secondary to a retroperitoneal neoplasm.[21] It is now most commonly seen secondary to severe metabolic disturbance in patients with renal, respiratory or cardiovascular disease. Treatment is of the primary disorder and the ileus is fortunately usually transient.

Treatment of constipation

MEDICAL TREATMENT

Laxatives
There have been advocates of a high roughage diet for over 2000 years, but the mechanism of its laxative action has only recently been studied. As well as cellulose, which absorbs water, plant fibre contains gums, pectins, phytic acid, lignin and other complex chemicals which alter cholesterol and bile salt metabolism. Increase in stool bulk is largely due to a rise in the numbers of colonic bacteria which digest fibre. The breakdown products of this process include volatile fatty acids which stimulate colonic secretion and motility, and gases produced may help to soften the stool.

Most patients are successfully treated by dietary manipulation. Use of a proprietary bulking agent may help to demonstrate how their symptoms can be relieved. These include synthetic cellulose and plant derivatives (Table 11.9).

Stool softeners may be needed in the elderly, the chronically sick or bedridden, and patients with structural abnormalities not amenable to surgery. Liquid paraffin is a traditional remedy but should not be used because of the danger of inhalation pneumonia. Other complications include interference with fat-soluble vitamin absorption and perianal seepage. It has now

Table 11.9   Classification of laxative agents.

Hydrophilic bulking agents
  Bran
  Synthetic cellulose ethers (e.g. methylcelluose)
  Mucilaginous seeds and seed coats (e.g. ispaghula)
  Mucilaginous gums (e.g. sterculia)
  Marine algae (e.g. agar)

Stool softeners and secretagogues
  Liquid paraffin
  Lactulose
  Dioctyl sodium sulphosuccinate
  Magnesium sulphate (Epsom salts)
  Magnesium hydroxide
  Sodium sulphate (Glauber's salt)
  Potassium sodium tartrate (Rochelle salt)

Stimulant laxatives
  Castor oil
  Polyphenolic laxatives
    Phenolphthalein
    Bisacodyl
    Sodium picosulphate
  Anthracene laxatives
    Senna
    Cascara
    Frangula
    Danthron

been replaced by osmotic laxatives and by the synthetic disaccharide, lactulose, which is not absorbed in the small bowel and provides a bacterial substrate in the colon. The saline laxatives are especially useful in treating patients with idiopathic megabowel and slow transit constipation. They attract a large volume of fluid into the gut increasing small bowel peristalsis and producing a large watery stool. They should be given with water to prevent dehydration. There are no long-term side-effects and unlike stimulant laxatives they do not damage the intrinsic nerves of the bowel.

Stimulant laxatives have been prescribed for many years but their long-term use is limited because of side-effects. The sale of these drugs in proprietary preparations should be discouraged. Their main use is in bowel preparation for surgical and radiological procedures, and in short courses when symptoms are short-lived or straining at stool is inadvisable – for example in the puerperium. Locally acting evacuants are useful in the elderly, those with megarectum and to help establish a normal bowel habit. Regular enemas may be needed in those who cannot defecate, either with functional disorders of the pelvic floor or neurological damage.

Behavioural retraining
Behavioural retraining techniques for the management of functional gut disorders have been highlighted recently.[37] Biofeedback was first

used to treat children with incontinence and has been successfully applied to children with constipation who were trained to increase intra-abdominal pressure to expel a stool.[20] Disorders of the pelvic floor muscles may play a part in development of some forms of adult constipation.[22] Failure to relax the pelvic floor during attempted defecation may be a 'habit' disorder possibly related to psychological stress. Relaxation techniques might therefore be useful in the management of some adults with chronic constipation, but have yet to be assessed.

SURGICAL TREATMENT

The surgical treatment of constipation is controversial. Clear indications exist for operation in Hirschsprung's disease and chronic sigmoid volvulus, or when constipation is secondary to a structural lesion such as carcinoma or benign stricture. Most would regard pseudo-obstruction and the irritable bowel syndrome as contraindications to surgery. Operation is sometimes undertaken in cases of functional constipation and secondary megacolon, but the results are not always satisfactory. The problem in assessing these results arises from our ignorance of the pathophysiology of the disorders and a failure to define them adequately.

Anorectal procedures
There is evidence of disordered anal sphincter function in patients with idiopathic megacolon and bowel dilatation could therefore be secondary. Colectomy in such cases may not deal with the primary disorder and some have suggested local operation on the anal sphincters. Internal sphincterotomy or anal stretch is used in children with megarectum with success. It may help adults with a short history of constipation secondary to anal fissure but not chronic cases. A more extensive sphincterotomy (anorectal myectomy) removes a 1 cm segment of the internal sphincter and a strip of the circular muscle of the lower rectum. This is a rational treatment for short segment Hirschsprung's disease[5] and has been suggested by some authors as a treatment for functional constipation including megacolon in adults; however, in this country its use has been disappointing. Partial division of the pubo-rectalis muscle as a treatment for constipation has been reported[35] but most surgeons are reluctant to interfere with the voluntary muscles because of the risk of causing incontinence.

Segmental colonic resection
Removal of part of the colon with Soave or Duhamel procedure is an accepted treatment for Hirschsprung's disease. Resection of the sigmoid colon in chronic sigmoid volvulus is also curative. There is no evidence that sigmoid or left hemicolectomy alters the symptoms of patients with functional constipation with or without megacolon.

Colectomy with ileo- or caecorectal anastomosis
This operation was popular in the early part of this century but has since fallen into disrepute. Any major procedure carries some risk and surgeons are understandably reluctant to remove a colon with no demonstrable structural abnormality. However, colectomy with caecorectal anastomosis has been shown to be a good treatment in cases where there is severe drug-induced nerve damage (cathartic colon).[34]

Faecal retention in megacolon can be so great as to endanger life, especially if there is a tendency towards volvulus formation. In severe cases refractory to medical treatment colectomy has been performed with variable results.[16, 18] Incontinence may result due to pre-existing anal sphincter damage after stretch or sphincterotomy. Alternatively, constipation may persist because the rectal enlargement is so great that it continues to be impacted or can generate no propulsive wave. In such cases an ileostomy is the only alternative. Despite the uncertain results, colectomy and ileorectal anastomosis seems justifiable before resorting to an ileostomy.

In patients with severe constipation without megacolon, colectomy and ileorectal anastomosis can give good results and restore normal bowel function. It should probably not be performed in those with pre-existing pelvic floor damage or those whose symptoms began after pelvic surgery.[26] Selection of patients for such radical surgery is hampered by our lack of knowledge of the causes of these disorders, but it seems unreasonable to deny possibly curative treatment to those whose symptoms are incapacitating and who fail to respond to medical measures.

REFERENCES

1 Anuras, S. & Christensen, J. (1981) Recurrent or chronic intestinal pseudo-obstruction. *Clinics in Gastroenterology*, **10**(1), 177–189.
2 Avery-Jones, F. (1967) Cathartic colon. *Proceedings of the Royal Society of Medicine*, **60**, 503–504.
3 Bacharach, T. & Evans, J. R. (1957) Enlargement of the colon secondary to hypothyroidism. *Annals of Internal Medicine*, **47**, 121–124.
4 Bannister, R. (1983) Autonomic failure. Oxford University Press.

5 Bentley, J. F. R. (1966) Posterior excisional ano-rectal myotomy in management of chronic faecal accumulation. *Archives of Diseases in Childhood*, **41**, 144–147.

6 Burkitt, D. P., Walker, A. R. P. & Painter, N. S. (1972) Effect of dietary fibre on stools and transit times and its role in the causation of disease. *Lancet*, **ii**, 1408–1411.

7 Connell, A. M., Hilton, C., Irvine, G. *et al.* (1965) Variation of bowel habit in two population samples. *British Medical Journal*, **ii**, 1095–1099.

8 Cummings, J. H. (1974) Progress report. Laxative abuse. *Gut*, **15**, 758–766.

9 Eastwood, H. D. H. (1972) Bowel transit studies in the elderly: radio-opaque markers in the investigation of constipation. *Gerontologia Clinica (Basel)*, **14**, 154–159.

10 Ferreira-Santos, R. (1961) Megacolon and megarectum in Chagas' disease. *Proceedings of the Royal Society of Medicine*, **54**, 1047–1053.

11 Guttmann, L. (1959) The regulation of rectal function in spinal paraplegia. *Proceedings of the Royal Society of Medicine*, **52**, 86–88.

12 Halls, J. (1965) Bowel content shift during normal defecation. *Proceedings of the Royal Society of Medicine*, **58**, 859–860.

13 Hinton, J. M., Lennard-Jones, J. E. & Young, A. C. (1969) A new method for studying gut transit times using radio-opaque markers. *Gut*, **10**, 842–847.

14 Holdstock, D. J., Misiewicz, J. J., Smith, T. & Rowlands, E. N. (1970) Propulsion (mass movements) in the human colon and its relationship to meals and somatic activity. *Gut*, **11**, 91–99.

15 Hurst, A. F. (1943) Constipation. *Medical Press and Circular*, **210**, 375–376.

16 Jennings, P. J. (1967) Megarectum and megacolon in adolescents and young adults: results of treatment at St Mark's Hospital. *Proceedings of the Royal Society of Medicine*, **60**, 805–806.

17 Lane, R. H. S. (1979) *The internal sphincter: its behaviour in normal subjects, chronic constipation and idiopathic megacolon*. M.S. Thesis, University of London.

18 Lane, R. H. S. & Todd, I. P. (1977) Idiopathic megacolon: a review of 42 cases. *British Journal of Surgery*, **64**, 305–310.

19 Martelli, H., Devroede, G., Arhan, P. *et al.* (1978) Some parameters of large bowel motility in normal man. *Gastroenterology*, **75**, 612–618.

20 Olness, K., McParland, F. A. & Piper, J. (1980) Biofeedback: A new modality in the management of children with fecal soiling. *Journal of Pediatrics*, **96**, 505–509.

21 Ogilvie, H. (1948) Large intestine colic due to sympathetic deprivation: a new clinical syndrome. *British Medical Journal*, **ii**, 671–673.

22 Preston, D. M. & Lennard-Jones, J. E. (1981) Is there a pelvic floor disorder in slow-transit constipation? *Gut*, **22**, A.890.

23 Preston, D. M., Lennard-Jones, J. E. & Thomas, B. M. (1983) The balloon proctogram. *British Journal of Surgery*, **70**, In Press.

24 Preston, D. M., Rees, L. H. & Lennard-Jones, J. E. (1983) Gynaecological disorders and hyperprolactinaemia in chronic constipation. *Gut*, **24**, A480.

25 Preston, D. M., Butler, M. G., Smith, B. & Lennard-Jones, J. E. (1983) The neuropathology of slow-transit constipation. *Gut*, **24**, A997.

26 Preston, D. M., Hawley, P. R., Lennard-Jones, J. E. & Todd, I. P. (1984) Results of colectomy for severe idiopathic constipation in women (Arbuthnot Lane's disease). *British Journal of Surgery*, **71** (In Press).

27 Rendtorff, R. C. & Kashgarian, M. (1966) Stool patterns of healthy adult males. *Diseases of the Colon and Rectum*, **10**, 222–228.

28 Rosenberg, R. F. & Caridi, J. G. (1983) Vincristine induced megacolon. *Gastrointestinal Radiology*, **8**, 71–73.

29 Ryan, P. (1982) Sigmoid volvulus with and without megacolon. *Diseases of the Colon and Rectum*, **25**, 673–679.

30 Schuffler, M. D. & Pope, C. E. (1977) Studies of idiopathic intestinal pseudo-obstruction. II. Hereditary hollow visceral myopathy: family studies. *Gastroenterology*, **73**, 339–344.

31 Schuffler, M. D., Bird, T. D., Sumi, S. M. & Cook, A. (1978) A familial neuronal disease presenting as intestinal pseudo-obstruction. *Gastroenterology*, **75**, 889–898.

32 Smith, B. (1968) Effect of irritant purgatives on the myenteric plexus in man and the mouse. *Gut*, **9**, 139–143.

33 Smith, B. (1972) *The Neuropathology of the Alimentary Tract*. London: Edward Arnold.

34 Todd, I. P. (1973) Cathartic colon: surgical aspects. *Proceedings of the Royal Society of Medicine*, **66**, 244–245.

35 Wallace, W. C. & Madden, W. M. (1969) Experience with partial resection of the puborectalis muscle. *Diseases of the Colon and Rectum*, **12**, 196–200.

36 Watkins, G. L. & Oliver, G. A. (1965) Giant megacolon in the insane: further observations on patients treated by subtotal colectomy. *Gastroenterology*, **48**, 718–727.

37 Whitehead, W. E. & Schuster, M. M. (1981) Behavioural approaches to the treatment of gastrointestinal motility disorders. *Medical Clinics of North America*, **65**(6), 1397–1411.

38 Zimmerman, G. R. (1962) Megacolon from large doses of chlorpromazine. *Archives of Pathology*, **74**, 47–51.

DIVERTICULAR DISEASE

Voigtel in 1804[43] was the first to describe diverticular disease of the colon and to recognize diverticula as acquired hernias of the large bowel. Diverticula were seen coincidentally at post mortem and surgery but full appreciation of the condition was not possible until the development of radiological methods for examining the colon. Until the widespread use of barium enemas, colonic diverticula were thus a pathological curiosity; it is just possible that the increased recognition of diverticular disease reflects the increased use of the barium enema in medicine rather than any increase in the prevalence of the condition. Radiology aids the definition of the disease and enables the symptoms and the complications to be differentiated from those caused by other disorders.[5]

It is debatable whether diverticular disease is, in its origin, a disease or a benign condition. The nomenclature has been somewhat complicated by the use of terms such as diverticulosis and diverticulitis. Diverticulitis implies that diverticula are both present and inflamed. It used to be assumed that colonic pain and other abdominal symptoms were caused by inflammation in the diverticula. However, it has been well demonstrated by Painter[27] that excessive segmentation of the sigmoid colon causes colicky pain. Morson[26] has also shown that when resected sigmoid colons are examined, histological evidence of inflammatory diverticulitis is often lacking. Painter[27] has used the term 'painful diverticular disease', which is particularly appropriate.

Epidemiology

Most patients with colonic diverticula are asymptomatic and so the true incidence of the condition is unknown. Evidence, however, is forthcoming from two types of studies, post mortem and radiological. In an autopsy survey in Australia Hughes[19] found that diverticula were rare before 30 years of age and their incidence rose to greater than 50% in those reaching the eighth and ninth decades of life. Radiological surveys, notably that of Manousos, Truelove and Lumsden[25] in Oxford, generally confirm this. The disease, however, is curiously rare in the Middle East, Africa and India,[29] except where there has been a Westernizing influence. In general, it appears true that the disease is less prominent in communities having a high fibre intake and this difference is highlighted where communities live close to one another with traditions in which dietetic differences are maintained. One example is the low incidence of diverticular disease in Chinese and Malays in Singapore,[23] which contrasts with the higher incidence among European residents. Nevertheless, where the cultural trend is to assume a similar diet, the incidence of diverticular disease converges. For example, the prevalence of diverticular disease, which was at first low among the blacks of the United States, has now risen to parity with the whites. The disease has also increased among Japanese migrating to Hawaii.[40] Curiously, the indigenous Japanese have a tendency to develop diverticular disease of the right colon, a type which often gives rise to haemorrhage.

It is now fairly well accepted that diverticular disease may be modified symptomatically by increasing the fibre intake. Epidemiological-type studies have been conducted to: (a) ascertain whether patients with diverticular disease consume different amounts of fibre from case-matched normal controls; (b) discover the prevalence of diverticular disease in selected groups of patients such as vegetarians who habitually consume a diet with a large amount of fibre; and (c) determine whether hospital admissions have

changed in the decade since 1974 when it became popular to increase the amount of fibre in the diet.

The studies with case-matched controls[4] showed that the intake of crude fibre was lower in diverticular disease subjects than in controls. Since the study was of patients with symptoms which could have led them to eat less fibre, the study was repeated in asymptomatic diverticular disease patients detected by radiological examination. In this group the habitual intake of dietary fibre was no different from controls. In vegetarians[14] the dietary fibre was lower in those with diverticular disease for an over 60-years-of-age group. The incidence of diverticular disease in vegetarians was 12%, in contrast to 33% in a control group. Vegetarians under 60 years of age did not have a significantly different intake of fibre from those with diverticular disease. There must, therefore, remain doubt about the causal relationship between diverticular disease and the amount of fibre in the diet.

Further assessment of the prevalence of diverticular disease has been made in Scotland which has a notoriously high incidence of all large bowel diseases. Eastwood[11] has shown that this disease varies not only throughout Scotland but within different districts of the City of Edinburgh. In a further study we examined whether the incidence of diverticular disease was influenced by the introduction of fibre therapy.[4a] Hospital discharges for diverticular disease in Scottish Hospitals were recorded by an analysis of Scottish Hospital Inpatient Statistics from 1968 to 1977; there was a progressive increase in the total number of cases seen throughout the entire decade under consideration. The increase was particularly marked where diverticular disease had been recognized as a subsidiary diagnosis. The increase was greater for females. 45% of the men with diverticular disease were under the age of 65, whereas 36% of the women were over 75 years. Nearly 75% were in general surgical units but relatively few had surgery, although 35% of the admissions were classed as emergencies (90/1000 total discharges compared with 60 for women). The highest operation rates occurred at the younger end of the age range. The female colectomy rate increased by 20% between the two periods examined: 1968–1972 and 1973–1977, i.e. in the 'bran era', with the male rate remaining constant. Mortality for diverticular disease in Scotland was relatively low (mean 40 males and 85 females per year in a population of five million). The discharge rate varied between health boards, the highest rate being from the predominantly rural Highland,

Grampian and Tayside regions. Throughout the period examined there was no evidence of any decrease in diverticular disease presenting in Scottish Hospitals.

However, although the Scottish incidence has not changed and may even be increasing, Hyland and Taylor[20] found that 91% of patients who had presented with diverticular disease in the Liverpool region and who were admitted to hospital remained symptom-free after bran had been prescribed. Fibre may also modify any remaining postoperative symptoms. When diverticular patients treated by resection were maintained on bran postoperatively colonic pressure remained low and patients were continuously free of symptoms, whereas in a control group the pressure was not altered, symptoms recurred and even further diverticula were detected.[35] However, few surgeons have chosen to modify the surgery required for complicated diverticular disease, avoiding resection by performing, for example, a defunctioning colostomy alone until the emergency episode is over. Theoretically it might be possible to close the colostomy and treat selected patients by bran. This is an area which may be exploited in the future.

Aetiology

Because colonic diverticula are acquired there has been considerable debate about whether diverticula are caused by high pressure in the bowel or result from a weakness in its wall. Painter[29] has discussed the theories which implicate a weakness of the colonic wall, obesity and the role of blood vessels. Diverticula in the colon usually appear between the taeniae on either side of the colon at the point weakened by the tunnel which contains the segmental blood vessels. Factors which further weaken the wall of the colon include arteriosclerosis and the distribution of fat around vessels as they enter the wall of the colon.

There are two ways of looking at the response of the colon to increasing pressure. On the one hand there is the inherent ability in the colonic musculature to respond to stress (i.e. its elasticity) but on the other hand pressure within the colon may increase if the colonic diameter stays the same. Painter has dismissed the concept of a change in the muscle wall saying that there is no evidence of muscle degeneration being the primary cause of diverticulosis. He holds the view that diverticulosis is primarily caused by prolonged increased intracolonic pressure.[29]

Pressure in the human colon causing diverticulosis

Arfwidsson[1] recorded intrasigmoid pressures with open ended tubes and showed that patients with diverticular disease generated greater pressure in the lumen of the diseased colon than did normal subjects. Painter and Truelove[30] confirmed the abnormal colonic pressure patterns and responses in patients with diverticular disease. They suggested that diverticula are the outward visible signs of a long standing abnormality of colonic motility. Painter[30] concluded that colonic luminal pressures are generated by local segmenting activity of the colonic musculature, contracting and partially occluding the colonic lumen. Therefore any stimulus which encourages segmentation will increase the intracolonic pressures and any drug which causes the colon to relax so that its lumen is widened will reduce the pressure. He pointed out that the colon functions as a series of little bladders or segments. Colonic diverticula are caused by intermittent functional obstructions of the outflow of the colonic segments and hence the increased pressure within the colon is the cause of the diverticula.[29]

Weakness of the colonic wall

Another factor in the pressure/stress equation is the tensile property of the musculature of the large intestine. This was determined in humans by Iwasaki and quoted by Yamada. The tensile breaking load per unit width shows age, anatomical site and direction differences. In the longitudinal and circular directions the breaking load is greatest between 10 and 19 years but by 60–89 years the ability to resist a breaking load decreases to 53% of its previous maximum value.[10] The tensile strength in the adult is greatest for the rectum followed by the ascending, descending and transverse colon, being between 66 and 80% in the colon to the rectum. It is interesting that in the longitudinal direction the breaking load is 1.1 times that in the circumferential direction for the ascending colon, 1.5 times for the transverse colon, 2.5 times for the descending colon and 1.6 times for the rectum. There were no significant sexual differences in tensile properties of the colon or rectum. Variations are seen in the expansive property of the large intestine with age so that at 70 to 90 years it is only 40% of its greatest strength in subjects in their 20s.

If the tensile properties of the large intestine are examined in the longitudinal and circular direction the tensile breaking load per unit width is greatest in dogs, next in cats and least in domestic fowls and rabbits. In each animal the breaking load in the circumferential direction is much greater than in the transverse direction. It is of interest that for animals tensile breaking load per unit width is between 154 and 255 g/mm for the dog, between 87 and 130 g/mm for the cat and between 32 and 60 for the rabbit. This is particularly significant because the only animal in which diverticula have been produced in the experimental situation is the rabbit. It is interesting that the two carnivores studied had a colonic musculature with a substantial tensile strength. On the other hand it has been shown in man that vegetarians develop diverticular disease much less readily than subjects eating a more mixed diet.

All of this makes for somewhat difficult interpretation. The two variables which seem to predispose to diverticula formation are, therefore, changes in the elasticity of the colon and prolonged high pressures generated within the colon, perhaps as the result of the low fibre containing diet.

Intestinal transit
An important property of ingested fibre is that it can absorb several times its weight of water. The bulking action of bran as opposed to fruit or vegetables is probably mostly related to this property and results in a softer and more readily passed stool. A characteristic which enforces this action is the particle size of the fibre.[22] The matrix of the coarse form allows more water to be retained in the inter- and intraparticulate spaces. Intestinal transit time is inversely related to the faecal bulk transit time. Spiller *et al.*[39] found that this relationship held till the faecal bulk became 150 g per day and that up to this point the relationship between transit time and faecal bulk was exponential, i.e. the product of the two was a constant.

Transit is also apparently influenced by the specific gravity of the intestinal contents. Kirwan and Smith[21] found that pellets of specific gravity of 0.9, 1.0 and 1.3 passed through the intestinal tract at different rates. They suggested that when the density of the markers was just slightly above or below that of the faeces, the lighter or heavier capsules passed more rapidly because they had separated from the gut contents and taken up a position closer to the bowel wall. Furthermore, there is the possibility that bran might be active in altering the transit time by a similar action on the specific gravity of the colon contents, either adding to the solids or by water binding. Studies on normal subjects and others with diarrhoea (cholerrhoeic

enteropathy) and constipation (diverticular disease) have shown that the solid and liquid phases of the faeces normally show an equal rate of transit through the intestinal tract.[13] The excretion patterns for diarrhoea and constipation are different, however, and show streaming in favour of the liquid phase in diarrhoea or the solid phase in constipation.

Intestinal transit has also been studied by making a comparison of the transit of radio-opaque shapes and that of an isotope capsule. These techniques have contributed information on the control of transit in the lower gastro-intestinal tract and the effect of dietary fibre. The isotope capsule method of Kirwan and Smith[21] is perhaps more applicable to diseases of the colon than any other part of the gastrointestinal tract because of its fairly constant topographical position at the 'periphery' of the abdomen. Fibre was shown to accelerate the transit of a capsule in all the segments of the colon. Delay in constipated subjects occurred not only at the rectosigmoid area but at the splenic flexure as well – bran reduced the delay at both of these intestinal segments in diverticular disease.

Cummings *et al.*[6] used intestinal transit markers under steady-state conditions. They administered serial markers over several days in order to overcome the difficulty of measurements based on a restricted number of markers. The ejection of the last of these markers tends to reflect delay in emptying the distal colon rather than a decreased rate of transit. Using this technique many of the variables of transit and fibre from various sources have been examined. Cabbage, carrot, apple and bran all affected transit but there was pronounced variation. Cummings was able to show day-to-day variations which were very great even on control diets. When fibre was added to the diet, those with the most prolonged mean transit time showed the most marked changes. A high fibre diet had a greater effect than had a low one.

The type II slower contractions in the distal colon probably reflect mixing of the contents and are non-expulsive in type. When exaggerated they may be the cause of the high intraluminal pressure which has been recorded in diverticular disease. These contractions may also explain the pain in diverticular disease if the motor activity associated with the contractions becomes mildly obstructive.[29] Early studies on diverticular disease were on patients who had symptoms and these generally established that they had a diminished faecal output, a delayed transit time and high intraluminal pressure. It is perhaps significant that these early studies were mainly done by surgeons and it seems likely that they were performed on patients showing the features of partial obstruction of the colon, and thus were likely candidates for operation. An alternative view is that the high pressure of diverticular disease is found only in the patients who have the combined features of the spastic colon as well as those of diverticular disease.

Studies on patients recruited from radiology and outpatient departments did not regularly show these features.[12] The range of values obtained for stool weight, transit time, faecal constituents (bile acids and fat) and the intraluminal pressure was considerably wide. Many of these results were similar to those obtained for normal volunteers. However, it could be argued that these volunteers were also exposed to the conditions which would environmentally create diverticular disease sooner or later. That apart, there was no evidence in this 'medically selected' group of diverticular disease patients of increased intracolonic pressure, a delayed transit or the diminished faecal output comparable to the former groups regarded as typical for diverticular disease.

Clinical features

Diverticular disease is essentially a benign condition, present in one-third of the population over 40 years of age and possibly over one-half of the population over 70 years of age.[25]

Complications of diverticular disease may present as symptoms of widespread abdominal pain, vomiting, tender palpable abdominal masses, or bleeding per rectum. Clearly the important differential diagnosis is the exclusion of carcinoma. Nausea, vomiting, flatulence, heartburn, coincidental gallstones, hiatal hernia and urinary symptoms may make the problem more complex and less easy to treat.

The commonest complication of diverticular disease is left-sided abdominal pain and an altered bowel habit, with passage of pellet- or toothpaste-like stool and relief of pain after the passage of this stool. This used to be called diverticulitis. There is no evidence that this is in fact an inflammatory change and there are strong indications that these symptoms coincide with a deficiency of fibre in the diet. However, the precise cause of the pain is not known.

Inflammation
When inflammatory change does take place this develops as peridiverticulitis or even a pericolic abscess. This may be recognized by the symptoms, the clinical examination, a raised white cell count and ESR, and radiological features of an ileus. Occasionally diverticula perforate and give rise to shock, widespread peritonitis and eventual subphrenic abscess. Important also in the medical treatment of a patient with diverticulitis is the treatment of the coincidental problems, such as fluid deficiency, cardiac failure, respiratory disease and the many complications which may be found in the older patient. A Gram-negative bacteraemia places the patient in grave danger and therefore blood culture examinations are of paramount importance. The type of antibiotic used ideally depends on the sensitivities of organisms grown from a blood culture. However, treatment has to be started before bacteriological results are available. Metronidazole should be given in combination with an aminoglycoside (tobramycin or gentamicin). When sensitivities are available the antibiotic regimen should be reconsidered. Subphrenic abscess and fistulas to the bladder or vagina can only be treated surgically. This may necessitate staged resection. The modern choice of operation for the emergency situation is Hartmann's procedure in which the inflamed bowel is removed, the upper end is exposed as a colostomy and the lower end closed off as a blind stump or as an exteriorized mucus fistula, until such time as re-anastomosis is capable at a second stage after resolution of the inflammatory process. If merely drained this focus of infection persists despite the administration of antibiotics because the abscess remains in communication with the bowel lumen through an area of necrotic diverticular disease. Operative resection is therefore required to overcome the continuous faecal soiling of the abscess resulting from a concealed fistula. A colovesical fistula should be considered in a patient with a persistent urinary tract infection who has been symptom free and who may, in addition, present with pelletty material (faecaluria) and bubbles of gas in the urine.

The patient may have an uncomplicated fistula as noted at operative resection of the pelvic colon. Some fistulas, however, develop because a pericolic abscess emptied into the bladder or some other portion of the urinary tract; this type usually requires a proximal colostomy before resection of the pelvic colon and later re-anastomosis and colostomy closure.

Haemorrhage
Mild haemorrhage may present with iron deficiency anaemia and is treated by iron therapy.

As always it is important to exclude carcinoma of the colon. However, if the bleeding persists surgical resection of the affected area may become necessary. Massive bleeding represents a considerable threat to the elderly patient, and transfusion and surgery are called for if more than 2–2.5 litres of blood are lost. Whilst urgent surgery is always desirable to arrest life threatening haemorrhage, the proportion of patients eventually requiring surgery by partial or even subtotal colectomy for bleeding from diverticular disease is low.

The identification of the bleeding site is not always easy. A combination of barium enema, colonoscopy and selective visceral angiography may be necessary to diagnose bleeding diverticula from the commonly occurring and more proximally distributed angiodysplasia. Careful preoperative assessment of the severely ill bleeding patients avoids repeat operations which carry an attendant mortality.

Pain
Pain is believed to be due to spasm in the colon and therefore the object of treatment is to reduce this localized colonic hypertension. One approach is the use of drugs. Relief of spasm and pain will accrue from the use of anticholinergic drugs. Merbeverine is useful in reducing intraluminal pressure since it acts directly on the muscle cells of the colon and does not affect normal peristalsis. Morphine has the undesirable effect of increasing intracolonic pressure and is therefore not recommended. It has even produced such dangerous effects as rupture of a diverticulum or of an abscess. Pentazocine decreases intraluminal colonic pressure and is of considerable value.

However, newer developments in our understanding of diverticular disease have resulted in a return to diet as a basis of therapy. It is now believed that if the volume of colonic contents increases the symptoms of pain, diarrhoea and constipation reduce. It must be said at the outset that some patients do not withstand pain easily and fail to comply with dietary advice. There is little value in persisting with dietary and bulking agents in such patients. Dietary fibre is not a vehicle for moral fibre! Therefore, in a patient who is not coping with severe pain, the diagnosis must be reviewed and if the diagnosis of diverticular disease with obstruction is upheld relief may be obtained by surgery. Modern surgery is capable of excellent results in elderly patients and resection of the offending area is still an advisable measure in some patients.

Faecal bulking

It is believed that by increasing stool weight it is possible to ameliorate the symptoms of pain on the left and right sides of the colon.[31] An understanding of the factors which contribute to stool weight leads to a more rational use of therapy.

Faeces are a complex mixture of microorganisms, dietary fibre residue, ions, organic compounds and water. The most important component of the stool is water. Almost regardless of the type or consistency of the stool, whether it be inspissated or liquid, the percentage of water seems to be constant at between 70 and 78% of the total wet weight.[16] The constancy of this proportion of water may be an important clue (as yet not understood) to the prime factors which determine the stool bulk.

Faecal dry material is a complex mixture of microorganisms (which probably constitute 40 to 50% of the dry weight) and dietary fibre (which comprises another 40%).[41] Clinicians and physiologists agree that, of the dietary constituents, fibre has a greater effect on stool volume than protein, fat and carbohydrate. The effect of fibre on stool weight varies with the fibre source, the response of the individual and the coincidental growth of bacteria.[41]

Scanning electron microscopy of stool shows a matrix structure of faeces which contains a large number of bacteria intermingled with smaller or amorphous particles of food residue. Some of the bacteria are grouped as colonies.[45] Within the faecal mass, fragments of plant cell residues are embedded. The bacteria are aligned on the outer coat of the fibre residues which suggests that extracellular bacterial enzymes are responsible for morphological and chemical changes in the fibre.

There have been several suggestions to identify the reason for the effect of fibre on stool weight. It has been suggested that fermentation of carbohydrate with the release of volatile fatty acid is important.[18] A second hypothesis suggests that the water holding capacity of fibre dictates stool weight.[7] A third suggestion is that stool weight is determined by the bacterial content of the stool.[41] As with many apparently conflicting hypotheses it is likely that all three factors are important and contributory.

Understanding the function of fibre in the colon is difficult, partly because of the diverse physical properties of the bulking agents and partly because of the diverse manner in which bacteria metabolize each fibre. Bacteria proliferate and increase their mass as a result of their metabolic activity in digesting dietary fibre.[42] Therefore the effect of any fibre source on stool weight will depend on the ability of the bacteria to grow while degrading a particular fibre source. Also of importance is how much fibre is left and the physical properties of this residual fibre after such bacterial metabolism.[7] The resistance of fibre to bacterial metabolism is also important.

Chemistry of fibre

Dietary fibre consists of a complex intermingling structure of water soluble and water insoluble polysaccharide materials. This structure results in a combination of surface and colloidal properties which change with the solution, temperature, pH, osmolality and with partial degradation by bacteria.

Some fibre sources (e.g. cellulose) are insoluble in water and act as surfaces. Other polysaccharides, such as pectins and guar, are very water soluble and slight chemical changes in the polysaccharide structure can have important consequences for faecal bulking properties.

Dietary fibre is plant cell wall material which consists predominantly of the polysaccharides cellulose, hemicellulose and pectins, but also the phenyl propane polymer lignin (Table 11.10).

Table 11.10 Dietary and pharmaceutical sources of fibre.

Sources of dietary fibre	
Cereal bran	Outer layer of bran
Fruit and vegetables	Leaves, stems, root, legumes, fruit
Pharmaceutical sources of bulking agents	
Gums	Guar
	Gum arabic
Mucilage	Ispaghula
Polysaccharide	Pectin
	Methylcellulose

These materials are resistant to hydrolysis by the digestive enzymes of man. There are chemical differences between species in cell wall composition which is also influenced by where the species grows. Each plant and fibre source will have a distinct chemical composition which may vary even in different parts of the same plant. The chemistry of fibre has been well reviewed by Southgate.[38]

Starch may be present in dietary fibre, depending on the degree of breakdown of the starch granules during cooking. It is possible for the starch to be retained in the interstices of the dietary fibre during preparation and such so-called 'retrograde' starch may be carried beyond the pancreatic outflow into the colon and digested in the colon, with production of gas and short chain fatty acids.

Sources of dietary fibre which are provided by the pharmaceutical industry include gums, which are produced by the plant as a response to a wound, mucilages, which prevent desiccation of seeds, and polysaccharide isolates from heterogeneous plant fibre sources (see Table 11.10).

The morphology of fibre

The differing function of fibre in the plant results in substantial differences from one fibre source to another. In fruit and vegetable sources of fibre the cellular structure is open. Cereal bran has two characteristic structures, one lignified and compressed, the other open and cellular. Bagasse, however, which is very fibrous and vascularized, does not show any evidence of cell structure and is compressed. Gum mucilages and polysaccharide isolates do not have a distinctive structure.[33]

The physical properties of fibre

The constituents of fibre each have their own function in the cell wall appropriate for anatomical and physiological function in the plant. These physical properties will influence their physiological effect in the gastrointestinal tract.

Fibre has a variety of actions along the gastrointestinal tract and it is not possible to understand why such different effects occur from current knowledge of the chemistry or morphology of fibre. One way of viewing fibre passing along the gut is to regard it as a sponge with defined physical properties. Such physical properties allow a better understanding of the physiological consequences of the ingestion of fibre on intestinal function along the colon. Fibre may act as a water binder, it has a cation exchange capacity, organic adsorptive ability, and exhibits a gel filtration phenomenon. These properties are a consequence of the chemistry of fibre. Probably the most important factor in influencing stool weight is the ability of a fibre source to bind water – the water holding capacity of the fibre. The methods of measuring water holding capacity are somewhat crude and include centrifugation, filtration and the ability of the fibre to hold water against an osmotic pressure gradient. The water associated with the fibre may be strongly held, as with a gel, or be loosely associated with it, as with cereal bran. However, these properties are modified by fermentation in the colon and also by the ability to hold water in the presence of a pressure difference generated by absorption of water from the colon.

Stool weight can be increased by the presence of fibre in the diet.[32] Cereal bran passes through the gut minimally affected by bacteria. The water holding capacity of the original bran is a good indicator of its efficacy in the colon, and hence its effect on stool weight.[9] The greater the water holding capacity of bran (which may be crudely recognized by the coarseness of bran) the greater the effect on stool weight. Cooking or baking bran reduces or modifies this property.[46] Other sources of fibre which have colloidal or gel properties behave somewhat differently. These gels are extensively metabolized. The result is that (a) volatile fatty acids are produced, so that the bacterial mass increases,[41] and (b) the residual fibre (which is mostly pentosans) will bind water. Both these affect stool weight. The volatile fatty acids are readily reabsorbed from the colon and therefore their role in influencing stool weight is not entirely clear.[24] It has been shown that there is a close relationship between the pentosan content of fibre of fruit and vegetable origin and its ultimate faecal bulking action.[6] The fibre which is digested contributes to bacterial growth. Whether this is by an increase in number or bacterial bulk is not known. This effect of fibre through metabolism by bacteria with subsequent proliferation is less direct than the water holding capacity of cereal bran. There is much more likelihood of individual variation.

What has bedevilled research in this field so far is the range of studies, the individual responses to a uniform enhancement by fibre and also the subtle differences in administered fibre. It is not even possible to obtain a clear picture of the consequences of feeding bran because of differences in preparation. Bran is affected, and even denatured, by cooking and other modes of preparation.[46] Another problem is that it is not known what constitutes a normal or even an ideal stool weight but it is known that there are differences in the normal or accepted stool weight between African and Western European communities.[29] However, within a European community itself the range of stool weight is considerable. In a survey conducted by the present authors, the range of stool weight in normal subjects ranged from 15 to 280 g per day and for each individual there was a substantial variation between individual stools during the week's collection. In a study of the diet of 63 normal English individuals, Bingham, McNeil and Cummings[2] showed that the range of intake

of nutrients was considerable and extended over the ranges that have been shown between dietary surveys for developed and underdeveloped countries.

Whichever source of fibre is used to increase stool weight, regardless of whether it acts by water holding capacity, as in bran, or to an increase in the bacterial population, as with vegetables, there is a proportional increase in held water which keeps the percentage of water at a relatively constant amount. The consequence of an enhanced faecal bulk increasing the water content of the stool is a reduction in the concentration of other faecal contents but this is not invariable, e.g. adding pectin to the diet results in an increase of faecal bile acids but not of stool weight. Generally, dietary fibre may have the property of diluting faecal constituents. It has been shown, for example, that giving 16 g of cereal bran daily for four weeks resulted in the concentration of faecal bile acids decreasing considerably.[9]

The treatment of symptoms of diverticular disease with fibre

There is no clear evidence that a high fibre diet prevents the development of diverticular disease. It has been claimed that the reason why so little diverticular disease is found in African and other groups is that they eat a high fibre diet.[29] Diverticular disease, however, is a disease of the elderly and it may be that insufficient numbers of Africans live to old age for diverticular disease to be a common problem.

However, the main role of fibre is to alleviate and prevent symptoms. There are considerable problems in interpretation of trials, partly because relatively few trials have been conducted on a double-blind basis. There are substantial problems associated with such studies, principally because it is difficult to give a placebo treatment. It is possible to study the problem by measuring intracolonic pressure and showing that a particular preparation reduces this pressure. The alternative is to study symptomatic relief with placebo control. Both of them have their shortcomings. On the other hand the difference between good trials and bad trials is often due to the mode by which the dietary fibre is prepared. There are trials in which the placebo has in fact contained a substantial amount of dietary fibre. This means that a trial is conducted comparing one form of treatment against another, rather than a comparison of placebo with treatment.

Pioneer studies by Painter on the effect of bran on patients with diverticular disease found that about 70% lost their symptoms with this agent; this has become the basis of management of the disease.[29] Brodribb[3] performed a crossover study from a high fibre to a low fibre diet using crispbread as the extra source of the fibre. The relief of symptoms was greatest with the high fibre regimen but there was a significant placebo effect of the low fibre regimen which took one month to disappear. The effect of the high fibre therapy was continuously maintained.

It has already been stated that raised pressure within the colonic lumen is a factor in producing the diverticulum or the degeneration in the colon wall. Can such processes be reversed by bran? Bran reduces the intraluminal pressure in the pelvic colon and rectum. The action is exerted on basal pressure and on stimulated pressure, whether effected by means of the gastrocolic reflex which follows the taking of food or cholinergic activity mimicked by neostigmine (Prostigmin). The effects were first described in 1974 for ordinary bran[13] but were later found to be greater for coarse bran; this has been generally confirmed by others.[32] The mechanism of the action of bran, however, is uncertain; the 'bolus' effect of bran may widen the diameter of the bowel lumen or the increased water binding of the fibre may dilute a spasmogen. The postcibal pressure after bran may even fall below that of basal non-stimulated pressure. There may be a degree of inhibition of smooth muscle tone in the distal gut, possibly as a result of release of an inhibitory factor such as glucagon or the antagonism of a stimulant of motility. A further means whereby a change in pressure might be registered within the bowel lumen is by an alteration in the viscosity of the bowel contents. Although the pressure is known to be reduced in the distal colon there is no information of whether there is a pressure change of note in the proximal colon, although there is a suggestion from clinical experience that the caecum and right colon dilates. A further factor which may be important in relationship to the pressure change is the dispersal of gas throughout the colon contents but this has not been studied before and after fibre treatments.

Few studies have been done on subjects in areas where diverticular disease is rare in contrast to the ones in areas where it is common. If the fibre 'presumption' is correct for diverticular disease, differences might be expected in areas where the dietary fibre intake is high because of the traditional ways of milling flour, or because the availability of other fibre sources is more plentiful than in the West. This should be capable of proof by the evidence of changes in faecal bulking, transit time and intraluminal pressure.

There has also been the suspicion that the fibre from various areas in the world may vary in its properties[34] perhaps because of intrinsic chemical and physical properties according to its source, growth, mode of preparation and cooking. The amount of lignin and other cellulose elements present might be different depending on its country of origin. Studies have shown that bran from wheat sources as far apart as France and Canada had effects which were dependent more upon the texture of the bran particles than the country of origin or the physical or chemical differences resulting from the country of origin.

Another paradox in diverticular disease is that while many agents lower the intraluminal pressure within the sigmoid colon a decrease has also been reported with placebo tablets.[44] Little is known of the specific changes in the wall of the bowel leading to the main symptom of pain and how this is influenced by fibre in the diet. Calcium ions in the lumen of the bowel may influence the concentration in the wall and since these ions are involved in nerve conduction this may influence the pain mechanism. Fibre binds calcium and there is a distinct difference between the calcium level in the faecal output in patients with diverticular disease in whom it is deficient and the greater amounts in those who have been given fibre to the point of becoming symptom-free and experiencing pressure changes.[8] In this study there was an inverse relationship between the motility index and the amount of calcium in the faeces of these patients; other faecal constituents (bile acids, fats, etc.) were not so related.

A change which suggests chronic damage to the wall is the altered compliance of the muscle wall in diverticular disease. This can be measured by balloon distension and it was found that the colon wall fails to oppose this as much as in normal subjects.[36] The change is present in vitro as well as in vivo. The reduced supportive property of the colonic wall does not change after successful bran treatment and although it is altered at first by resection it reverts to the former response. Perhaps one has to conclude from this evidence that there is a 'degenerative' component of diverticular disease in which the intrinsic mechanical properties of the intestinal wall alter. If this is so, this development cannot be restored by dietary fibre in the faecal luminal contents.

The stasis factor in diverticular disease may be one reason why agents like ispaghula (Fybogel),[12] which raise the luminal pressure, may be beneficial in alleviating the symptoms of diverticular disease, although any agent acting in this way is undoubtedly not desirable for the integrity of the diverticulum. Of the agents examined methylcellulose and sterculia reduce intraluminal pressure to much the same extent as bran, although ispaghula raises pressure and lactulose produces little change. Both bran and ispaghula can double stool weight in the elderly.[37]

One may sum up the action of fibre by saying that 'roughage' appears to be a necessary element of the action of dietary fibre by additional water binding in the fibre matrix or in the bacterial cell and that this produces a bulkier stool which lowers intracolonic luminal pressure. This may delay the effects of the 'wear and tear' changes which occur in the wall of the bowel and may correct the raised pressure which can damage it in established diverticular disease.

Relationship with the irritable bowel

The irritable bowel syndrome and diverticular disease have been linked in various ways. It has been shown that patients with an irritable colon not uncommonly develop diverticula,[17] but most of the studies are uncontrolled and such is the prevalence of the two conditions that overlap would readily occur especially in patients over forty years of age.

The faecal characteristics of patients with irritable colon and diverticular disease have been compared. No detectable difference in the faecal weights, whether dry or wet, or total bile acid secretion were found. Significantly less magnesium, potassium and calcium was found in both, unrelated to the age of the patients, suggesting a common aetiology for the disorders.[16] A further suggestion is that the irritable colon is an expression of a response of the large intestine to a fibre-less state and the condition is really that of an 'irritated' colon which has largely been created by the medical orthodoxy of former times who took many of their patients with a bowel problem off 'roughage' thus exposing their colonic function to the greater problem of dealing with faecal stasis.

Fast waves of a spasmogenic kind have been recorded in the irritable colon and appeared at first to differentiate it from diverticular disease. However, similar wave patterns have been recorded in diverticular disease and in normal subjects,[28] although the period of time occupied by the fast waves is greater in the irritable bowel syndrome than in the other groups. The typical changes in the motor activity of the distal bowel in the irritable colon are also similar to diverticular disease, namely, an exaggerated response to food and an elevated response to neostigmine. Whereas the basal pressure in diverticular disease is usually normal, in the irritable colon syndrome it is raised particularly when the patients are symptomatic. The motility effects in the irritable colon syndrome are reduced by the same spasmolytics that are given for diverticular disease and the bulk additives which influence the symptoms of diverticular disease are as effective in the irritable colon. Enriching the fibre in the diet with bran in both normal subjects and those with the irritable colon syndrome produced a dual effect. Those with a slow transit (over three days) had a considerable acceleration but in those in whom it was already fast (one day) transit slowed down. The new transit in each case was about two days which suggested that bran could produce a regulation of alimentary motor function in subjects who had marked deviation from the normal. Since it is a known feature that extremes of fast and slow transit are found in this condition, and since bran apparently corrects the abnormal transit times, the implication is that low residue diets may play an aetiological role in this condition.

Diverticular disease is a condition of increasing age and in the majority of individuals is symptomless. The majority of patients who are symptomatic have symptoms which result from increased intracolonic pressure and this is readily treated by increasing the stool weight and fibre content of the diet. A minority of patients do not respond to this treatment and require surgery. Surgery is also indicated for complicated inflammatory change and life threatening bleeding.

REFERENCES

1 Arfwidsson, S. (1964) Pathogenesis of multiple diverticula of the sigmoid colon in diverticular disease. *Acta Chirurgica Scandinavica* (Supplement), 342–345.

2 Bingham, S., McNeil, N. I. & Cummings, J. H. (1981) The diet of individuals: a study of a randomly chosen cross section of British adults in a Cambridgeshire village. *British Journal of Nutrition*, **45**, 23–27.

3 Brodribb, A. J. M. (1977) Treatment of symptomatic diverticular disease with a high fibre diet. *Lancet*, **i**, 664–666.

4 Brodribb, A. J. M. & Humphreys, D. M. (1976) Diverticular disease: three studies. *British Medical Journal*, **i**, 424–430.

4a Chalmers, K., Wilson, J. M. G., Smith, A. N. & Eastwood, M. A. (1983) Diverticular disease of the colon in Scottish hospitals over a decade. *Health Bulletin*, **41**(1).

5   Cummack, D. H. (1969) *Gastrointestinal X-Ray Diagnosis*. Edinburgh: E. & S. Livingston.

6   Cummings, J. H., Southgate, D. A. T., Branch, W. *et al.* (1978) Colonic response to dietary fibre from carrot, cabbage, apple, bran and guar gum. *Lancet*, **i**, 5–9.

7   Eastwood, M. A. & Mitchell, W. D. (1976) Physical properties of fibre: a biological evaluation. In *Fiber in Human Nutrition* (Ed.) Spiller, G. A. & Amen, R. J. pp. 109–129. New York, London: Plenum.

8   Eastwood, M. A. & Smith, A. N. (1980) Faecal characteristics and colonic intraluminal pressure in diverticular disease. *Digestion*, **20**, 399–402.

9   Eastwood, M. A., Brydon, W. G. & Tadesse, K. (1980) Effect of fiber on colon function. In *Medical Aspects of Dietary Fiber. Topics in Gastroenterology* (Ed.) Spiller, G. A. & Kay, R. M. pp. 1–26. New York: Plenum.

10 Eastwood, M. A., Watters, D. W. & Smith, A. N. (1982) Diverticular disease – is it a motility disorder? *Clinics in Gastroenterology*, **11**(3), 545–561.

11 Eastwood, M. A., Sanderson, J., Pocock, S. J. & Mitchell, W. D. (1977) Variation in the incidence of diverticular disease within the City of Edinburgh. *Gut*, **18**, 517–574.

12 Eastwood, M. A., Smith, A. N., Brydon, W. G. & Pritchard, J. (1978) Colonic function in patients with diverticular disease. *Lancet*, **i**, 1181–1182.

13 Findlay, J. M., Mitchell, W. D., Eastwood, M. A. *et al.* (1974) Intestinal streaming patterns in cholerrhoeic enteropathy and diverticular disease. *Gut*, **15**, 207.

14 Gear, J. S. S., Ware, A., Fursdon, P. *et al.* (1979) Symptomless diverticular disease and intake of dietary fibre. *Lancet*, **i**, 511–514.

15 Gordon, J. E. (1978) *Structures or Why Things Don't Fall Down*. England: Penguin Books.

16 Goy, J. A. E., Eastwood, M. A., Mitchell, W. D. *et al.* (1976) Faecal characteristics contrasted in the irritable bowel syndrome and diverticular disease. *American Journal of Clinical Nutrition*, **29**, 1480–1484.

17 Havia, T. & Mauner, R. (1971) The irritable colon syndrome. A follow-up study with special reference to the development of diverticula. *Acta Chirurgica Scandinavica*, **137**, 569–572.

18 Hellendoorn, E. W. (1978) Fermentation as the principal cause of the physiological activity of indigestible food residue. In *Topics in Dietary Fiber Research* (Ed.) Spiller, G. A. pp. 127–168. New York: Plenum.

19 Hughes, E. (1969) Post mortem survey of diverticular disease of the colon. *Gut*, **10**, 336–351.

20 Hyland, J. M. P. & Taylor, I. (1979) Diverticular disease: has its natural history altered? *Gut*, **20**, 441–442.

21 Kirwan, W. O. & Smith, A. N. (1974) Gastrointestinal transit estimated by an isotope capsule. *American Journal of Clinical Nutrition*, **30**, 659–661.

22 Kirwan, W. O., Smith, A. N., McConnell, A. A. *et al.* (1974) Action of different bran preparations on colonic function. *British Medical Journal*, **iv**, 187–189.

23 Kyle, J., Adesola, A. D., Tinckler, L. F. & De Beaux, J. (1967) Incidence of diverticulitis. *Scandinavian Journal of Gastroenterology*, **1**, 77–80.

24 McNeil, J. I., Cummings, J. H. & James, W. P. T. (1978) Short chain fatty acid absorption by the human large intestine. *Gut*, **19**, 819–822.

25 Manousos, O. N., Truelove, S. C. & Lumsden, K. (1967) Prevalence of colonic diverticulosis in general population of the Oxford area. *British Medical Journal*, **iii**,

762–763.

26 Morson, B. C. (1963) The muscle abnormality in diverticular disease of the colon. *Proceedings of the Royal Society of Medicine*, **56**, 798–803.

27 Painter, N. S. (1968) Diverticular disease of the colon. *British Medical Journal*, **iii**, 475–479.

28 Painter, N. S. (1972) Irritable or irritated bowel. *British Medical Journal*, **ii**, 46.

29 Painter, N. S. (1975) *Diverticular Disease of the Colon*. London: William Heinemann.

30 Painter, N. S. & Truelove, S. C. (1964) The intraluminal pressure patterns in diverticulosis of the colon, *Gut*, **5**, 201–213.

31 Painter, N. S., Almeida, A. Z. & Colebourn, K. W. (1972) Unprocessed bran in treatment of diverticular disease of the colon. *British Medical Journal*, **ii**, 137–140.

32 Report of the Royal College of Physicians (1980) *Medical Aspects of Dietary Fibre*. Tunbridge Wells: Pitman Medical.

33 Robertson, J. A. & Eastwood, M. A. (1981) An examination of factors which may affect the water holding capacity of dietary fibre. *British Journal of Nutrition*, **45**, 83–89.

34 Smith, A. N., Drummond, E. & Eastwood, M. A. (1981) The effect of coarse and fine Canadian Red Spring Wheat and French Soft Wheat bran on colonic motility in patients with diverticular disease. *American Journal of Clinical Nutrition*, **34**, 2460–2463.

35 Smith, A. N., Kirwan, W. O. & Shariff, S. (1974) Motility effects of operations performed for diverticular disease. *Proceedings of Royal Society of Medicine*, **67**, 1041–1043.

36 Smith, A. N., Shepherd, J. & Eastwood, M. A. (1981) Pressure changes after balloon distension of the colon wall in diverticular disease. *Gut*, **22**, 841–844.

37 Smith, R. G., Rowe, M. J., Smith, A. N. *et al.* (1980) A study of bulking agents in elderly patients. *Age and Ageing*, **9**, 267–271.

38 Southgate, D. A. T. (1976) The chemistry of dietary fiber. In *Fiber in Human Nutrition* (Ed.) Spiller, G. A. & Amen, R. J. pp. 31–72. New York: Plenum.

39 Spiller, G. A., Chernoff, M. C., Shipley, E. A. *et al.* (1977) Can faecal weight be used to establish a recommended intake of dietary fiber (plantix)? *American Journal of Clinical Nutrition*, **30**, 659–661.

40 Stemmerman, G. N. (1970) Patterns of disease among Japanese living in Hawaii. *Archives of Environmental Health*, **20**, 266–273.

41 Stephen, A. M. & Cummings, J. H. (1980) The microbial contribution to human faecal mass. *Journal of Medical Microbiology*, **13**, 45–56.

42 Stephen, A. M. & Cummings, J. H. (1980) Mechanism of action of dietary fibre in the human colon. *Nature*, **284**, 283–284.

43 Voigtel, F. G. (1804) *Handboch der Pathologischen. Anatomie*, volume 2. Halle.

44 Weinreich, J. (1978) Discussion statement at 3rd Kellogg Nutrition Symposium. In *Dietary Fibre: Current Developments of Importance to Health* (Ed.) Heaton, K. W. London: Libbey.

45 Williams, A. E., Eastwood, M. A. & Cregeen, R. (1978) SEM and light microscopy study of the matrix structure of human feces. *Scanning Electron Microscopy*, **II**, 707–712.

46 Wyman, J. B., Heaton, K. W., Manning, A. P. & Wicks, A. C. B. (1976) The effect on intestinal transit and the feces of raw and cooked bran in different doses. *American Journal of Clinical Nutrition*, **29**, 1474–1479.

TUMOURS

BENIGN TUMOURS – POLYPS AND POLYPOSIS

The word polyp is derived from the Latin *polypus* (literally 'many-footed') and is used in colloquial Greek and Italian to mean an octopus, which a stalked polyp resembles. A 'polyp' is the vernacular description of any elevation above the mucosal surface of the intestine and lacks precision unless qualified by its histological variety (e.g. metaplastic, adenomatous). It may be used to describe any lesion from a small tag of normal epithelium to a protuberant cancer. A polyp is nevertheless often the limit of the clinician's diagnosis and its histological nature is decided thereafter by the pathologist, except in the case of those few polyps with characteristic shapes such as the worm-like post-inflammatory polyps and the carpet-like villous adenomas. Polyps range in appearance from tiny, translucent and almost invisible 1–2 mm mucosal bumps, through stalked lesions with a diameter of 3–5 cm (Figure 11.43), to sessile growths which may reach 10–20 cm in extent. Polyps may be single, occur together in small numbers or carpet the colon in hundreds or even thousands as in some of the polyposis syndromes.

Many larger polyps, regardless of histological type, are stalked, particularly in the distal colon, where buffeting by formed stool and the activity of colonic musculature combines to exert traction. By contrast polyps such as lipomas or villous adenomas growing in the caecum or the fluid-filled ascending colon are seldom stalked. The stalk of a polyp is composed of normal epithelium overlying a core of connective tissue containing arteries and veins drawn up from submucosa; this makes snare polypectomy of the head easy and without risk of damage to the bowel wall.

The histopathology and clinical features of polyps

Although tumours can arise from any of the histological constituents of the intestine less than 1% derive from connective or lymphoid tissue and more than 95% from the epithelium; the latter is presumably related to its rapid cell turnover. The majority of developmental polyps (the hamartomas) are found in childhood or young adult life when neoplastic polyps (adenomas) are almost unknown. Careful necropsy studies show that almost half of the colons of elderly people contain one or more adenomas.[45] A classification of polyps and polyposis is given in Table 11.11. It is worth emphasizing that much of the older literature on polyps is confused by failure to differentiate between histological types, particularly between the common non-neoplastic metaplastic (hyperplastic) polyps and the adenomatous or neoplastic varieties. Occasionally careful histological assessment can demonstrate that small foci of neoplastic (adenomatous) tissue do occur in non-neoplastic polyps, and in a few patients there may be a chance coincidence of different polyp types.

NON-NEOPLASTIC POLYPS

Most non-neoplastic polyps are found coincidentally in the process of screening or diagnostic examinations for neoplastic or cancerous tumours. The exceptions are hamartomatous polyposis syndromes, post-inflammatory polyps

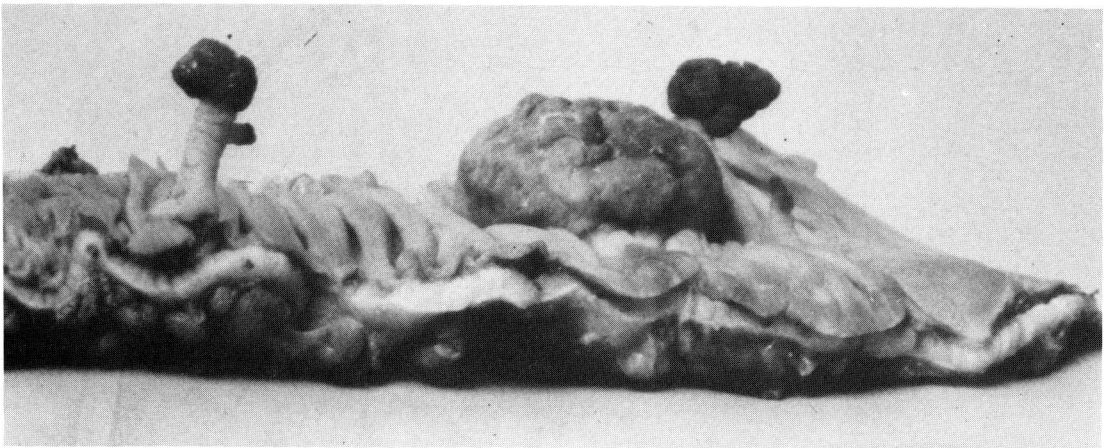

Fig. 11.43 Two stalked adenomas and a larger sessile adenoma in the sigmoid colon. A focus of carcinoma was present in the large polyp.

Table 11.11　Classification of colorectal polyps.

	Solitary	Multiple (polyposis syndromes)
Neoplastic		
	Adenoma	Familial adenomatous polyposis
	Tubular	
	Tubulovillous	
	Villous	
	Carcinoid	
		Malignant lymphoid polyposis
Non-neoplastic		
Hamartomas	Peutz–Jeghers	Peutz–Jeghers syndrome
	Juvenile	Juvenile polyposis
Inflammatory	Lymphoid	Benign lymphoid polyposis
	Inflammatory	
Miscellaneous	Metaplastic (hyperplastic)	Metaplastic polyposis
	Connective tissue polyps, e.g., fibroma, leiomyoma and lipoma	Cronkhite–Canada syndrome

and bleeding polyps in childhood. Non-neoplastic polyps are frequently covered by normal mucosa and thus look paler and more shiny than the larger neoplastic polyps, which have reddened, matt epithelium. Visual differentiation is uncertain, however, and representative polyps must always be submitted for a histopathological diagnosis.

METAPLASTIC (HYPERPLASTIC) POLYPS

The commonest polyp in the rectum is the 2–5 mm, pale or glistening, metaplastic polyp, which is almost a normal finding on sigmoidoscopy in the elderly, during which a score or more may be noticed in the distal 15 cm of the bowel (Figure 11.44). The incidence of metaplastic polyps

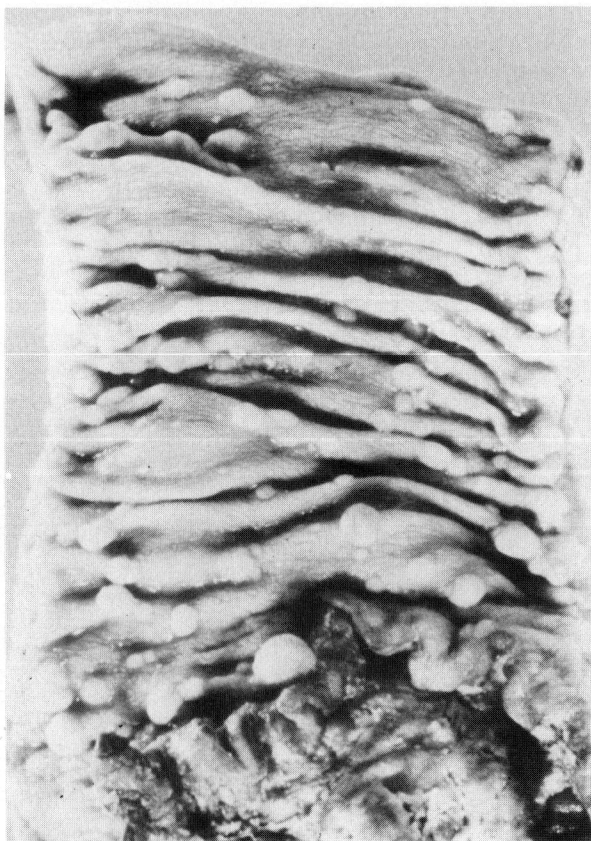

Fig. 11.44　Multiple metaplastic polyps clustered close to a rectal carcinoma.

increases with age, which partly explains the suggestion in some accounts that they are causally associated with cancer. In the colon, however, only 10% of small polyps prove to be metaplastic and the majority of even 2–5 mm polyps turn out to be adenomas.[20, 44] Larger metaplastic polyps are occasionally found in the colon, either semipedunculated or as a sessile mound of shiny tissue. Multiple metaplastic polyposis[48] is rare and can be indistinguishable to the naked eye from adenomatous polyposis. Histologically the differentiation is easy and important since the former requires no treatment (or merely follow-up) whereas the latter requires surgical treatment.

Microscopically the mucosal crypts within a metaplastic polyp are elongated with reduced numbers of goblet cells and characteristic sawtoothing of the lining epithelial cells producing a shallow papillary outline (Figure 11.45). There is no nuclear dysplasia and no malignant potential.[1] The description metaplastic, implying altered growth, has been encouraged instead of the commonly used term 'hyperplastic' which wrongly suggests abnormal nuclear activity and cellular regeneration.[48] Unlike the disorderly maturation and dedifferentiation in an adenomatous polyp, maturation is maintained but its regulation is disturbed. Mature forms are thus found deep within the crypts and 'hypermature' cells at the surface.

INFLAMMATORY POLYPS AND LYMPHOID POLYPS

Post-inflammatory polyps may be found as scattered worm-like or thread-like (filiform) tags of essentially normal mucosa and imply a previous severe attack of any form of colitis (ulcerative, Crohn's, amoebic, schistosomal or ischaemic) (Figures 11.46 and 11.47a). They are usually *not* inflamed, although some may show superficial ulceration of the tip with a characteristic covering of white slough at endoscopy. Larger inflammatory polyps occur which are composed mainly of granulation tissue (Figure 11.47) and may have a misleadingly sinister irregular appearance although their histology is entirely benign. Occasionally, especially after schistosomal colitis, the exudation from the numerous large inflammatory polyps may be sufficient to cause hypoproteinaemia. The description of post-inflammatory polyps as 'pseudo-polyps' seems unnecessary and arises only from the need to distinguish them from the neoplastic group. The postcolitic inflammatory polyps must not be confused with the 'plaque-like' polypoid areas of severe epithelial dysplasia (pre-cancer) which, although rare, can occur 8–10 years or more after the onset of ulcerative colitis. Post-inflammatory polyps themselves have no tendency to malignant change.

Benign enlargement of lymphoid tissue

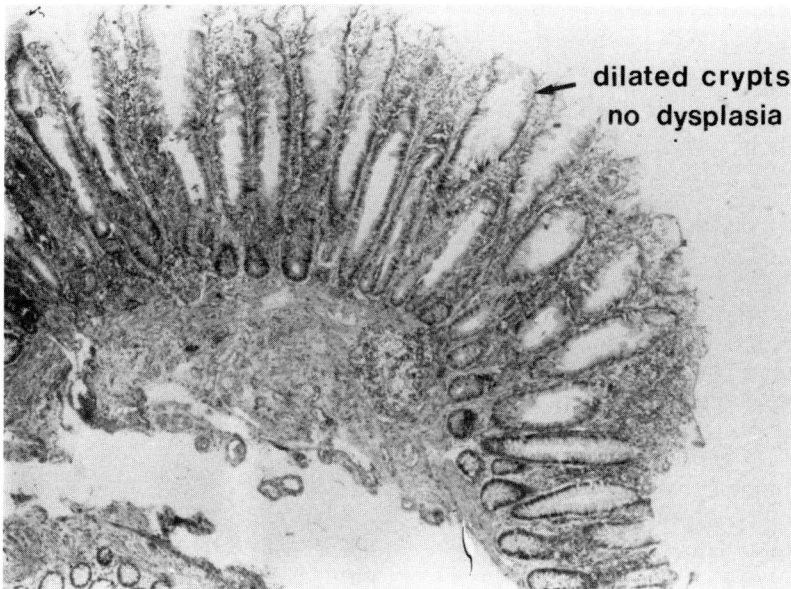

**dilated crypts
no dysplasia**

Fig. 11.45 A typical sessile metaplastic polyp. The absence of dysplasia is the important feature. Haematoxylin and eosin, × 30.

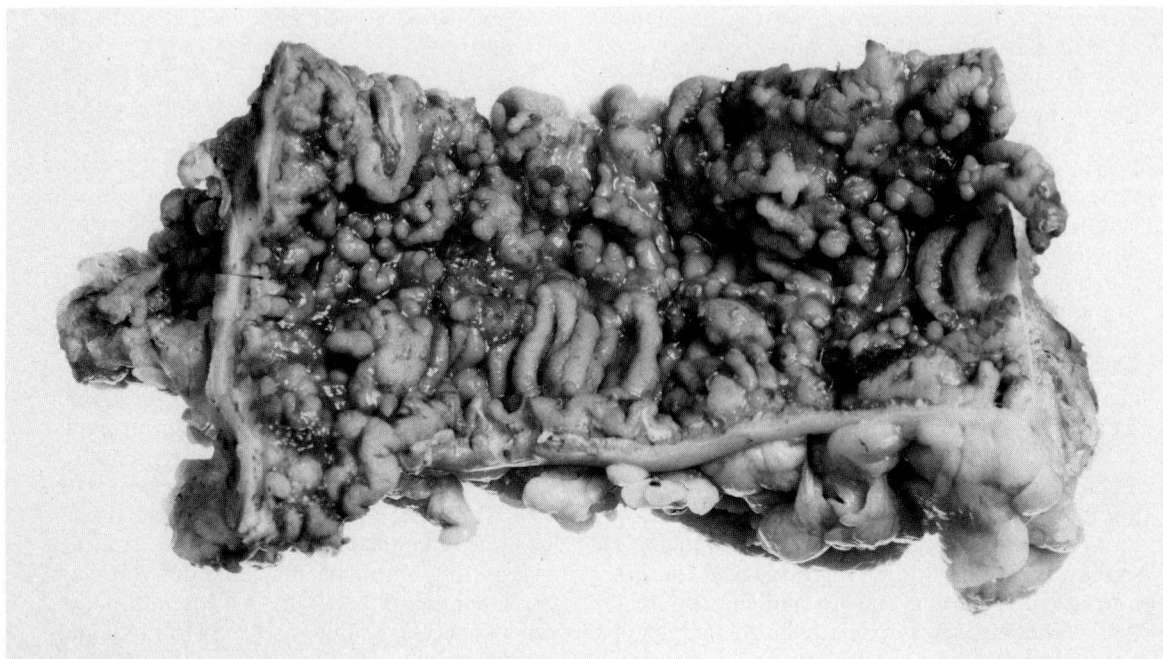

Fig. 11.46   A segment of transverse colon from a case of Crohn's disease showing multiple worm-like inflammatory polyps.

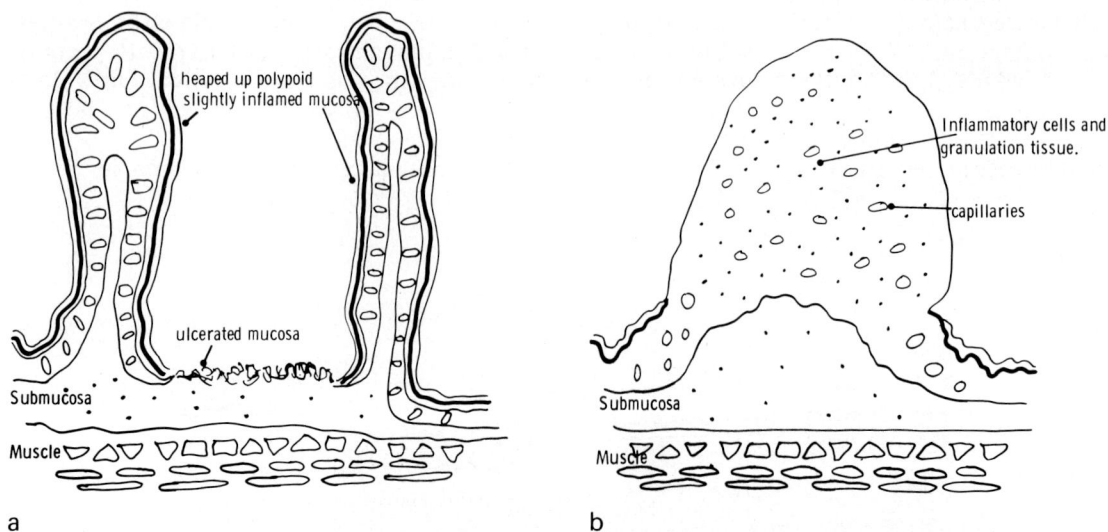

Fig. 11.47   The two patterns of inflammatory polyp: (a) a tag of almost normal mucosa, or (b) a polypoid excrescence of granulation tissue.

encompasses an entire spectrum of change from isolated polypoid follicular lesions (Figure 11.48) to diffuse lymphoid hyperplasia of the whole intestinal tract. The solitary benign lymphoid polyp of the rectum, occurring in young adults, is the commonest clinical entity.[36] Multiple benign lymphoid polyposis of the colon exists, but whether it is an exaggerated physiological reaction or a pathological entity is not clear. Minor degrees of diffuse lymphoid hyperplasia are well recognized in children as part of

the normal pattern. The importance of these changes is that they must not be confused with familial adenomatosis polyposis.

ENDOMETRIOSIS

Endometriosis, classified as heterotopic or misplaced tissue, is exceedingly rare in polypoid form; if the colon is involved the endometrial tissue is usually in the muscle layers or forms a submucosal mass mimicking cancer.

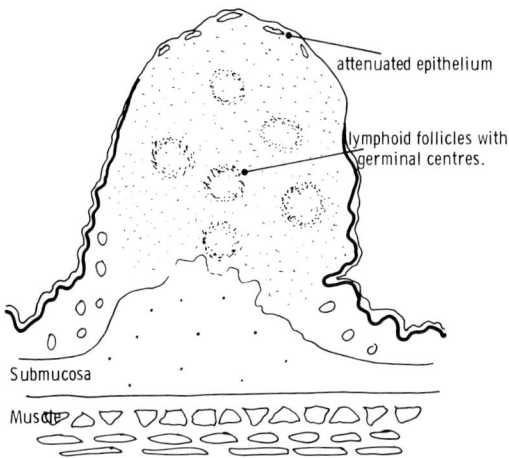

a

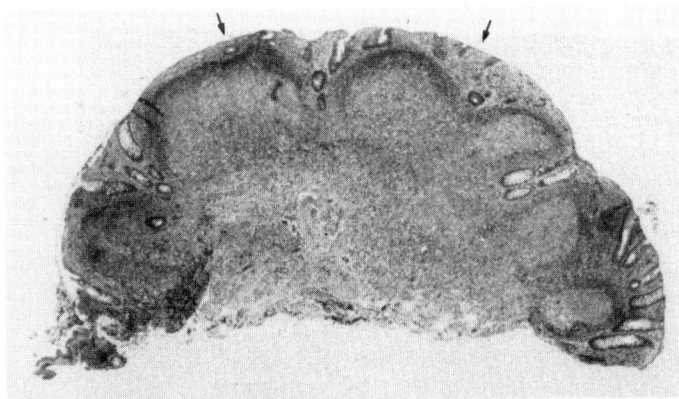

b

Fig. 11.48 (a) Diagram of a typical benign lymphoid polyp. (b) A lymphoid polyp with thinned mucosa over large lymphoid follicles (arrows) with germinal centres. Haematoxylin and eosin, ×9.

HAMARTOMAS

Hamartomas are localized tumour-like proliferations of normal tissues arranged in an abnormal and disorganized fashion. In the colon the juvenile and Peutz–Jeghers polyps fit this description.

Juvenile polyps are the characteristic polyps of children, although they may not present until adult life or middle age. They are sometimes referred to as mucus retention polyps because of the cystic inclusions of entrapped mucus (Figure 11.49a), which present a 'Swiss cheese' appearance on histological section. Typically they have a smooth surface and are 1–2 cm across. They may intussuscept or present at the anus. The stalk is short and does not usually include the muscularis mucosae. Because of this they may twist and auto-amputate – sometimes with massive haemorrhage. Several large polyps may occur in a small child and may be distributed anywhere in the colon, so that examination of

the whole colon is desirable if one is found distally.[13]

Although individual juvenile polyps have no malignant potential, families are recognized where juvenile polyposis (defined as ten or more juvenile polyps) is associated with a high risk of cancer due to the presence of adenomatous tissue included within some polyps.[5] The current recommendation, therefore, is that juvenile polyposis should be treated by subtotal colectomy with ileorectal anastomosis, whereas lesser numbers of juvenile polyps may be treated by snare polypectomy alone. With histological examination the crypts and cysts of juvenile polyps are seen to be lined by tall but otherwise normal cells (Figure 11.49b) and the polyp is covered by a single layer of normal colonic epithelium with mucus-secreting goblet cells. The surface is frequently ulcerated and the stroma usually shows marked inflammatory changes. Histologically similar multiple polyps of the colon may also occur as part of the Cronkite–

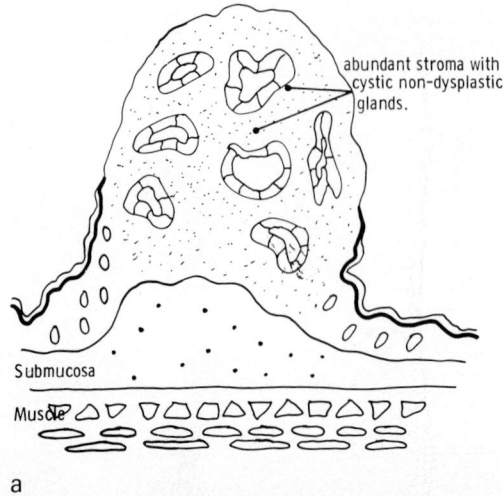

a

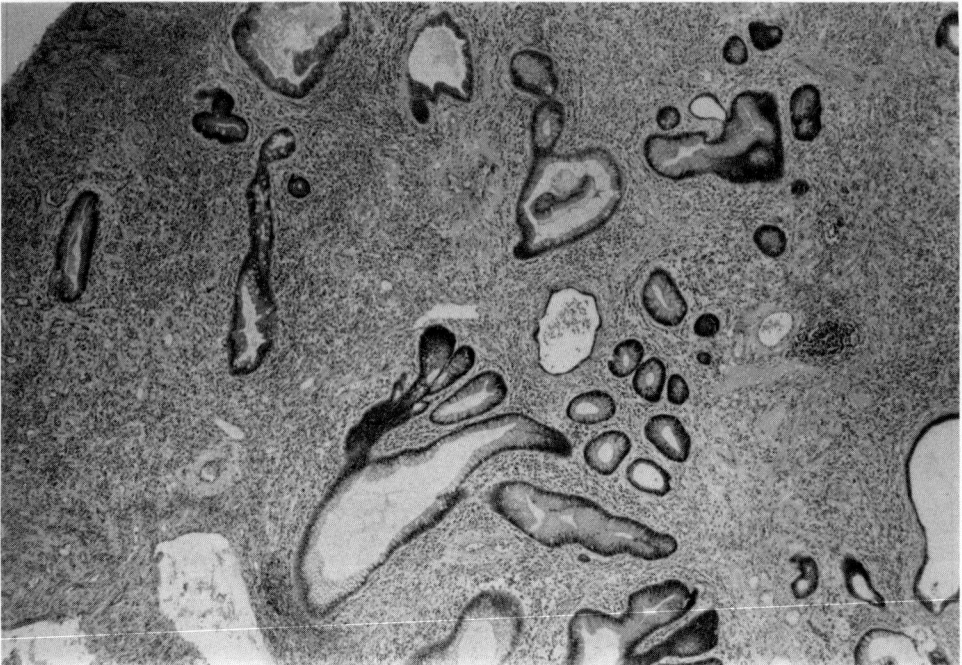

b

Fig. 11.49   (a) Diagram of a juvenile polyp. Note the absence of a stalk. (b) Detail from part of a juvenile polyp showing the abundant stroma and enlarged non-dysplastic cystic glands. Haematoxylin and eosin, × 61.

Canada syndrome, associated with alopecia, nail dystrophy and skin pigmentation.

Peutz–Jeghers polyps of the colon occur in the majority of those affected by the syndrome (mucocutaneous pigmentation, gastrointestinal polyposis and a Mendelian dominant inheritance). They are of secondary importance to those in the small intestine but can be a cause of blood loss and anaemia. Isolated Peutz–Jeghers polyps also occur without other features

of the syndrome. In the colon Peutz–Jeghers polyps appear to have negligible malignant potential although there is a small risk associated with those in the stomach and small intestine. The larger ones are probably best sought and removed at about two-yearly intervals in affected subjects to prevent blood loss.[46] Many of the smaller polyps disappear spontaneously and the tendency to polyp formation declines progressively after 25–30 years of age.

Histologically, Peutz–Jeghers hamartomas do not have the mucus cysts of juvenile polyps but show a branching framework of muscle fibres derived from the muscularis mucosa radiating between disorganized but otherwise normal mucosal crypts (Figure 11.50). As with any other colonic polyp liable to growth, ulceration or local haemorrhage, foci of epithelium can become misplaced into the stroma of the head and cause bizarre appearances (pseudo-invasion), but no dysplasia or true neoplastic tissue is present.[30]

OTHER MESODERMAL POLYPS

Lipomas are for some reason commonest in the right colon, sometimes as a fatty enlargement of the ileocaecal valve but usually as submucosal

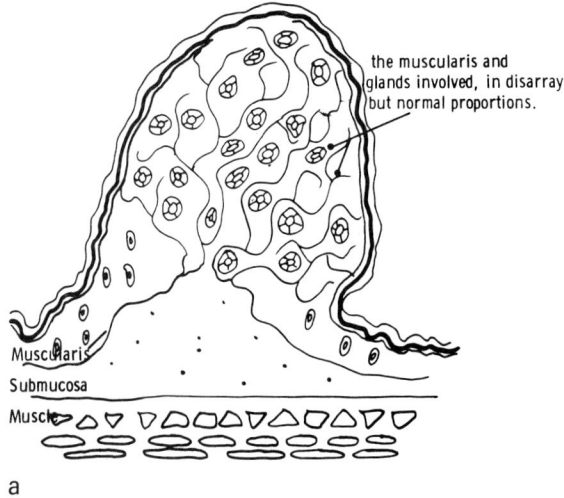

a

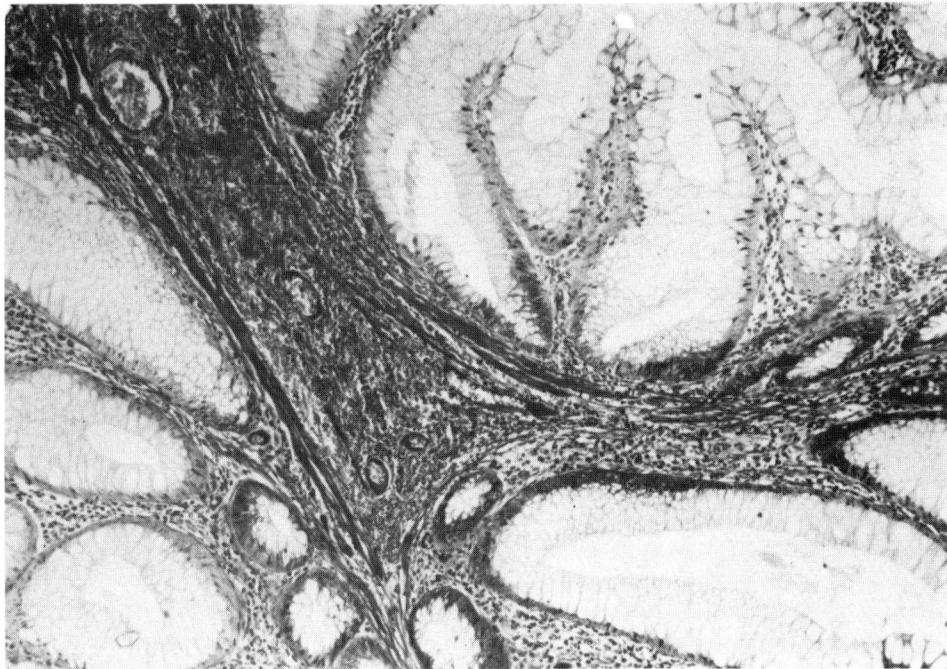

b

Fig. 11.50 Peutz-Jeghers polyp. (a) Schematic representation: the glands are not dysplastic and are intermingled with arborescent muscle fibres from the muscularis. (b) Detail of the histology to show the muscle fibres running between dilated glands. PTAH stain × 141.

rounded elevations and only rarely pedunculated. The shiny surface and the soft, cystic and pliable nature of the tumour is virtually diagnostic endoscopically.[10] Under the surface yellowish fat may be visible after repeated biopsy, but the fat, being loculated, will not run out. Polypectomy is not indicated once the diagnosis is made since lipomas are benign and symptomless.

Other tissue elements can rarely produce polyps, the exact diagnosis coming as a histological surprise after snare polypectomy. They include polypoid haemangiomas, neurofibromas and leiomyomas.

Neoplastic polyps – the adenomas

The 'adenoma' is the commonest colorectal neoplastic polyp and is the family name for polyps having a common and distinctive dysplastic epithelium but different architectural arrangements (Figures 11.51 and 11.52). Each type of adenoma may show varying degrees of epithelial dysplasia, which will influence the likelihood of

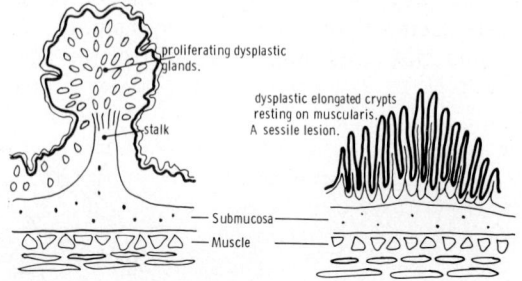

Fig. 11.51 The two main patterns of adenoma: tubular (left) and villous (right). The tubulo-villous adenoma has a structure combining both patterns.

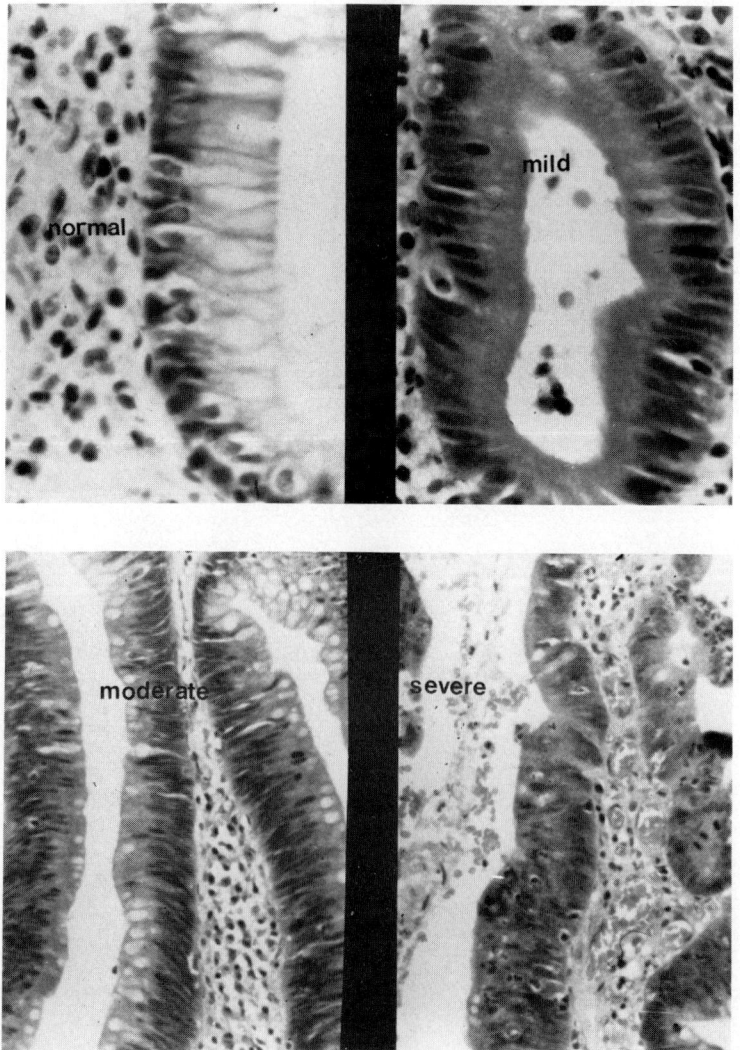

Fig. 11.52 The pathognomonic feature of an adenoma is the presence of dysplastic cryptal epithelium. The cytological grades of dysplasia are seen here. They are invariably accompanied by increasing architectural disorganization. Haematoxylin and eosin, × 460.

malignant change. Dysplasia is classified as mild, moderate or severe according to the degree of cytological and architectural abnormality.

The most frequent adenoma is the tubular variety, which is usually stalked. It has a relatively solid head divided into incomplete lobules which give a fissured appearance on gross inspection (Figure 11.53a). Histology demonstrates branching tubules most commonly lined by mildly dysplastic epithelium (Figure 11.53b). At the other end of the architectural spectrum is the villous adenoma (villous papilloma), which is often larger, sessile, and has a frond-like stroma covered usually by more severely dysplastic epithelium than the tubular variety (Figure 11.54). Between these types comes the tubulovillous (or villoglandular) adenoma, about 20–30% of most series, in which the structure is intermediate with both branching fronds and tubular elements.[19, 39]

Histological allocation of a particular polyp to one or other adenoma type is to some extent subjective so that the same pathologist may alter his classification on different occasions. The accuracy of classification will depend on the care with which it is examined and the number of histological sections taken, since if more than 20–25% of villous elements are present the polyp will be termed tubulovillous, whereas with only 15% present it will be called tubular.[30] The

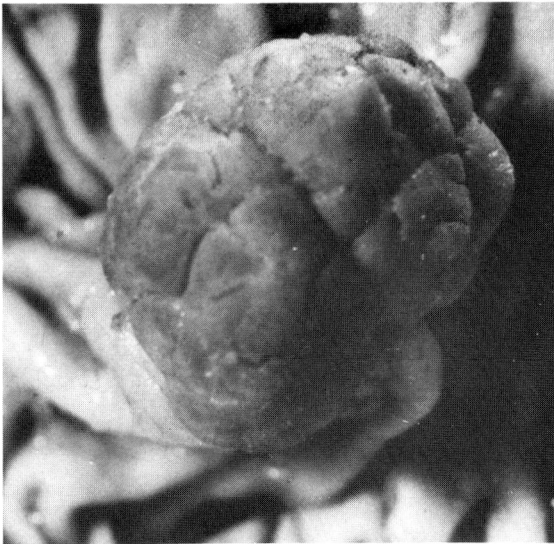

a

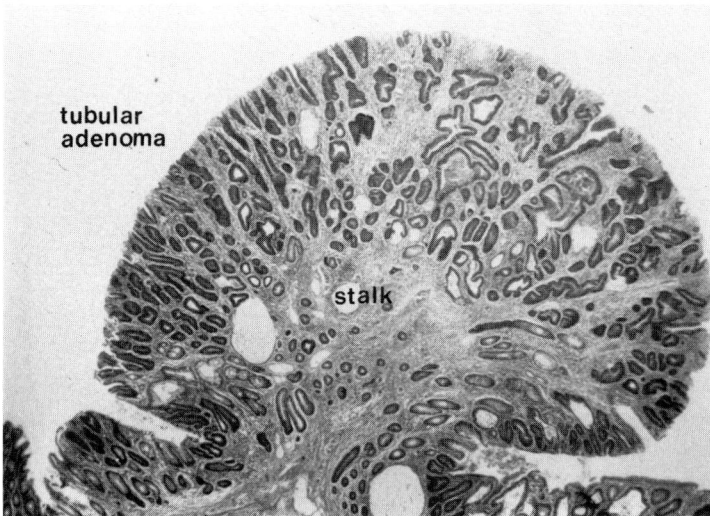

tubular
adenoma

stalk

b

Fig. 11.53 (a) A typical stalked lobulated tubular adenoma. (b) A tubular adenoma showing the dysplastic tubular epithelial pattern. Haematoxylin and eosin, × 27.

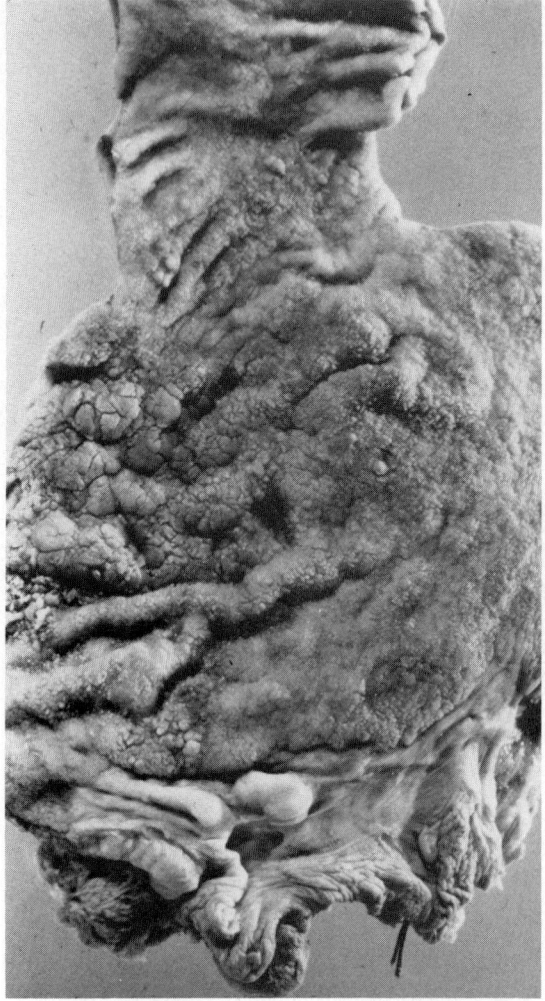

a

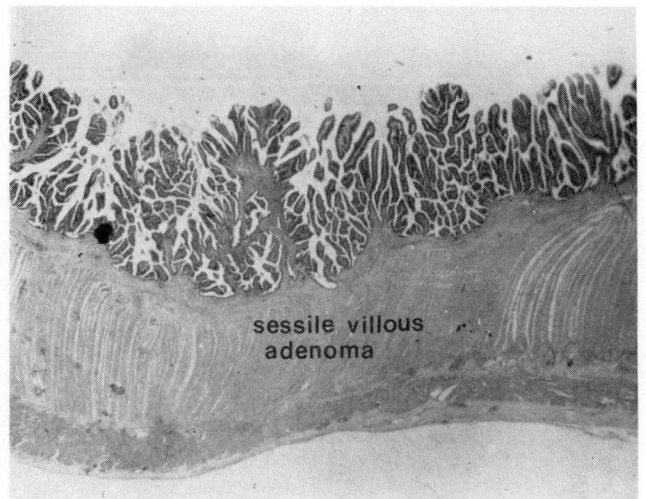

sessile villous
adenoma

b

Fig. 11.54   (a) The carpet-like pattern of a villous adenoma low down in the rectum. (b) The finger-like epithelial fronds of a villous adenoma. It is a sessile growth resting directly on the muscularis mucosae and deeper layers. Haematoxylin and eosin, × 12.

Table 11.12 Colorectal adenomas: relationship between histological type, size and frequency of carcinoma.

Histological type	Proportion of adenomas with carcinoma (%)							
	Surgical series[32]				Colonoscopic series[19]			
	<1 cm	1–2 cm	>2 cm	Total	<1 cm	1–2 cm	>2 cm	Total
Tubular (75%)	1%	10%	35%	5%	1%	3%	10%	2%
Tubulovillous (20%)	4%	7%	46%	23%	0%	4%	11%	6%
Villous (5%)	10%	10%	53%	4%	0%	5%	38%	18%
Overall proportion with carcinoma				10%				5%

tendency for tubular adenomas to be small and villous adenomas to be larger and the intermediate position of tubulovillous adenomas is shown in Table 11.12.

ADENOMAS, DYSPLASIA AND THE ADENOMA–CARCINOMA SEQUENCE

Histologically an area of severely dysplastic epithelium on the surface of an adenoma is very similar to the appearance of an infiltrating carcinoma and the cells of either will behave similarly in tissue culture; such severely dysplastic areas are thus sometimes referred to as 'carcinoma in situ' or 'focal carcinoma'. These terms should be avoided since they are clinically misleading, however attractive they may seem to the experimental pathologist. The point at issue is that until the dysplastic cells invade across the muscularis mucosae which divides the adenomatous epithelium of the head of the polyp from the submucosa and the lymphatic drainage in the stalk, the likelihood of distant metastasis is so remote that it can be ignored.[29] The diagnosis of carcinoma in an adenoma thus depends on the pathological demonstration of invasion across the muscularis mucosae (Figure 11.55). The benign phenomenon of 'misplaced epithelium' or 'pseudo-invasion' following local ulceration or infarction (which also occurs in hamartomatous polyps) may cause confusion; the misplaced epithelium is non-dysplastic and is surrounded by normal lamina propria rather than the fibrous (desmoplastic) reaction which occurs around carcinomatous tissue.

The risk of malignancy in adenomas is influenced not only by the severity of dysplasia (Table 11.13) and its morphological type but also by the size of the lesion (Table 11.12).[11, 19] The influence of size probably represents a statistical relationship between the mass of the polyp and the number of potentially cancerous cells present. Study of operation specimens from

patients with adenomatous polyposis give insight into the growth of adenomas from single dysplastic crypts to tiny polyps (Figure 11.56) which contain so few neoplastic cells that the likelihood of initiating carcinoma, although possible, must be extremely small. Malignancy is very rarely observed in tiny adenomas, although any adenomatous tissue would naturally be engulfed and destroyed by carcinoma at an early stage. This might explain the occasional report of 'de novo' colon cancer. The disparity between the malignancy rate reported in adenomas removed from surgical series[32] compared to an endoscopic series from the same department[19] may reflect selection bias. One explanation may be the inclusion of adenomas removed from cancer patients and the pre-endoscopic policy of delaying removal of colonic polyps until they showed suspicious appearances on serial barium enema examinations. Whatever the reason, endoscopic series uniformly find an overall malignancy rate for adenomas of about half the quoted figure of 10% for surgical series.[19, 33, 39]

There is much other direct and indirect evidence to support the concept of an adenoma–carcinoma sequence in the large bowel.[32] Cell culture lines from adenomas and carcinomas behave similarly and adenomatous cells show similar histochemical and chromosomal aberrations to those of cancer cells. Many early carcinomas show residual adenoma tissue within them, the percentage falling in the more advanced cancers where the initiating adenoma is presumed to have been destroyed. The distribution of adenomas and cancers is identical,

Table 11.13 Colorectal adenomas: grade of dysplasia and risk of carcinoma.[11, 19]

Grade of dysplasia	Percentage with carcinoma
Mild	6%
Moderate	18%
Severe	35%

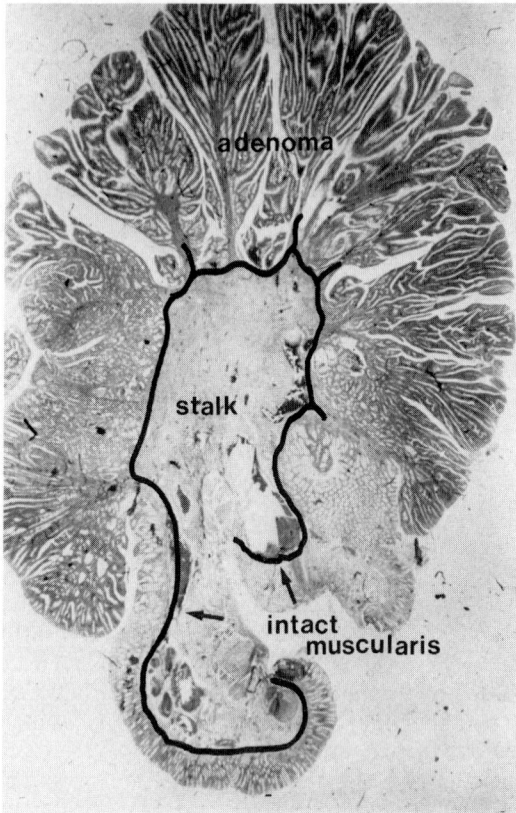

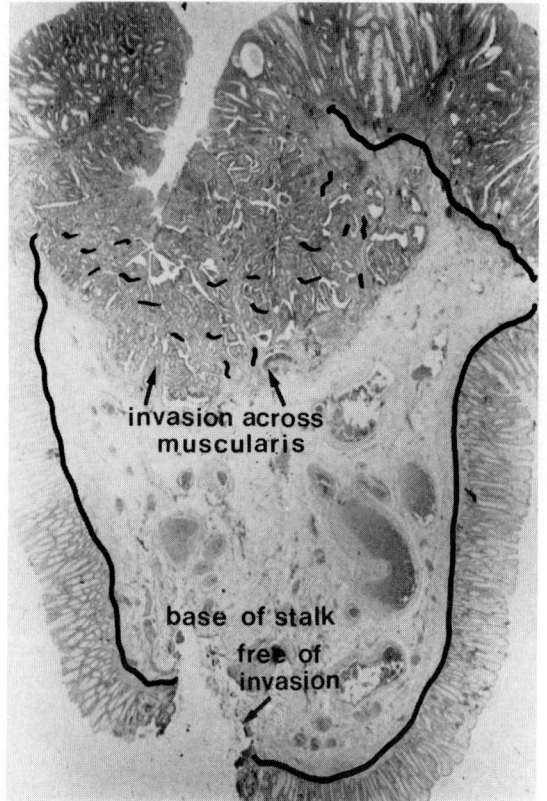

a   b

Fig. 11.55 (a) A *benign* tubulo-villous ademona. The feature to note is the intact muscularis mucosae outlined in black. (b) A *maligant* polyp, which in contrast to (a) shows the muscularis mucosae invaded by malignant epithelium. The broken black lines represent the disrupted muscularis, the arrows the infiltrating epithelium. (a, b): haematoxylin and eosin, × 13.

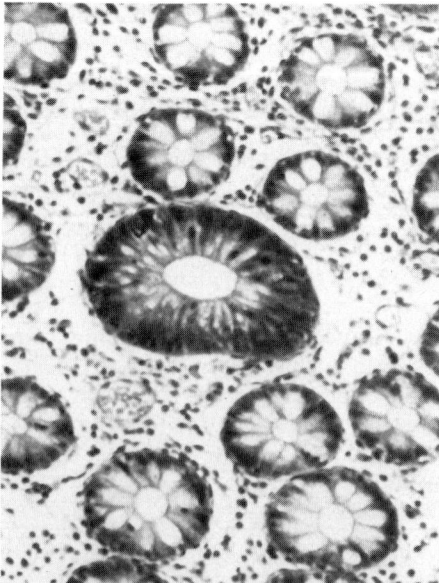

Fig. 11.56 A single dysplastic crypt, the seed of a potential adenoma, is seen in the centre. Courtesy of Dr H.J.R. Bussey. Haematoxylin and eosin, × 280.

predominately in the left colon but with a small increased incidence in the caecum; the latter is explained by an association with an increased incidence of sessile villous adenomas in the caecum.[2, 39] The world-wide geographic incidence of adenomas and carcinomas is also similar, both being rare in Africans and indigenous Japanese, but both common in Caucasians and 'Westernized' Japanese such as those living in Hawaii.

Synchronous adenomas are present in many patients with colorectal cancer and adenoma-bearing patients have a higher risk of developing colorectal cancer on follow-up than matched controls.[4] The risk of co-existent (synchronous) or subsequent (metachronous) cancer rises as the number of adenomas increases, with an incidence of 100% in adenomatous polyposis patients. Destruction of adenomas reduces the expected cancer incidence in the rectal stump of patients with adenomatous polyposis treated by colectomy[32] and in the rectum of normal subjects.[17]

The time taken to develop a 'significant size' of adenoma and the interval to cancer formation is merely conjectural, although figures have been given for the growth rate or doubling-time of polyps and cancers based on radiological observation.[14] Even cruder estimates have been based on anecdotal clinical data or the difference between the average age of clinical diagnosis of adenomas and colorectal cancer.[32] Morson[29] has suggested an average 5–7-year interval between an adenoma reaching 1 cm and the development of malignancy although the range is likely to be considerable. Colorectal cancer can occasionally be diagnosed in patients apparently normal when examined only a year or two previously, whereas the large adenomas found unexpectedly in some elderly patients may never become cancerous in the lifetime of the patient.[29]

AETIOLOGY AND GENETICS OF ADENOMA FORMATION

It seems that the aetiology of adenomas and colonic cancer are likely to be at least interrelated. Some of the geographic and epidemiological evidence has been discussed. Dietary factors are probably also important. Increased intake of meat and fat have been implicated and a low-fibre diet is another possible factor. Dietary factors may mediate their effect by modifying biliary metabolism with the production of toxic or carcinogenic substances by bacterial action in the colon. It is of interest that after ten years patients in whom the urinary stream has been diverted by ureteric implantation into the sigmoid colon (often because of congenital bladder defects) have an increased incidence of both adenomas and cancers in the colonic mucosa adjacent to the ureter.[40] The risk remains even if the urine flow is subsequently removed from the colon. This phenomenon could be explained by the production of nitrosamines (by bacterial action on urinary nitrites) which are known to be carcinogenic to intestinal mucosa.

The scanty evidence available suggests that in addition to environmental and dietary factors there may be a genetic factor involved in adenoma production. This could be a recessive gene predisposing to adenoma formation and present world-wide in low and high risk countries, the development of adenomas in predisposed persons being triggered by environmental factors. Conceptually, Veale and his coworkers have suggested adenoma-bearing subjects as being homozygous (*pp*) for the adenoma-

predisposing gene (*p*) whereas adenomatous polyposis subjects require only the dominant gene (*P*) to produce multiple adenomas.[6]

Diagnosis and treatment of polyps

The clinician makes a diagnosis of 'polyps' and although in most adults these will prove to be adenomatous, it is incorrect to assume this without histological examination. Even on endoscopy or radiology the different types of polyps can be indistinguishable. This section therefore considers polyps in general, although describing management based on the presumption that they will prove to be adenomas.

Colonic polyps only infrequently cause symptoms. The larger ones ($\geqslant 1$ cm) may bleed intermittently and if multiple may cause anaemia. Patients presenting with colorectal bleeding, however, often have obvious local causes for haemorrhage such as haemorrhoids, as well as the polyps found with further investigation. Since both lesions are promptly treated it is sometimes uncertain whether the polyps contributed to the bleeding or were a chance finding. In the authors' experience 60% of colonoscopically removed polyps occur in patients presenting with bleeding, 20% are found on follow-up examinations of symptomless patients and 20% in patients presenting with pain. Except for the remote possibility of traction or intussusception by a very large polyp, there is no mechanism by which a polyp can cause pain. This is usually due to coexisting functional bowel problems which precipitated the colonic examination.

Very large, usually sessile, villous adenomas may cause altered bowel habit, especially due to the production of copious quantities of mucus. Some may even cause mucoid diarrhoea and hypokalaemia but these are few compared to the numbers of villous adenomas (villous papillomas) presenting without electrolyte disturbance.

Rigid sigmoidoscopy or fibre sigmoidoscopy should diagnose a high percentage of colonic polyps since at least 30% occur within 25 cm of the anal canal and about 60% in the rectum and sigmoid colon, including most of the large or malignant lesions. It was thought that a higher percentage of polyps were within range of the rigid sigmoidoscope simply because clinicians did not know what they were missing proximally[26] until more accurate diagnostic techniques, such as colonoscopy or air-contrast barium enema, became available. Fibre sigmoidoscopy is likely to replace rigid tube examinations in screening for polyps since by visualizing more bowel the yield is about three times as high, and furthermore the examination may take only five minutes.[27] The relative ease and accuracy of fibre sigmoidoscopy is particularly important since this is the least accurate area for the barium enema. Except for reasons of size or in the case of multiple small polyps, the colonoscopist should aim to provide the pathologist with an 'excision biopsy'. Forceps biopsies do not allow an assessment of the polyp stalk, the crucial area required for the exclusion of malignancy (Figure 11.56). Since sigmoidoscopy and fibre sigmoidoscopy are usually performed after only limited bowel preparation, there is a serious explosion hazard during polypectomy and electrocoagulation from residual methane or hydrogen.[3, 38] Therefore an uninflammable gas such as carbon dioxide should be used if polypectomy is intended.

Barium enema examination has been the traditional investigation to identify polyps beyond the reach of the sigmoidoscope. Radiologists are increasingly turning to the more accurate air- or double-contrast barium enema technique.[15] This requires thorough bowel preparation and involves uncomfortable distension of the colon but should demonstrate 70–80% of significant sized polyps compared to the 50% seen on single-contrast enema (and over 90% on colonoscopy).[47] Barium enema is cheaper, quicker and safer than colonoscopy and as an initial screening investigation is usually the procedure of choice.[12, 15] It is relatively inaccurate in the sigmoid colon (due to overlapping folds or diverticular disease) and in the caecum (due to faecal residue). Barium enema also has the disadvantages of some doubtful or false-positive findings and if a polyp is found the patient must be cleared of barium prior to colonoscopy and polypectomy.

Colonoscopy[8] has the advantage of offering the option of immediate polypectomy and is more accurate, particularly in the left colon which is the site of most polyps. Unfortunately the colons of some patients, either because of fixation or undue mobility, are exceedingly difficult to intubate, so it is unrealistic to suggest total colonoscopy as the main diagnostic procedure for all patients. Colonoscopy is the logical procedure for high-risk patients, such as those with a family history of colon cancer or adenomatous polyposis and for the follow-up of patients where endoscopy was straightforward. If total colonoscopy is difficult the remaining colon can be examined immediately by barium enema as long as it has been evacuated of air. Combined examination of the whole colon by *both* techniques should give the greatest diagnostic accuracy and is justified in the examination of very high-risk patients, such as those with multiple polyps.

POLYPECTOMY

Once a polyp is found it must be removed,[39] allowing for the exceptions already mentioned such as typical post-inflammatory polyps or lipomas. Polyps within 10 cm of the anal verge (except for very small ones) are often removed under anaesthesia since this area is pain sensitive and also awkward for the fibre endoscope. Larger sessile polyps in the rectum are also surgically managed, preferably 'floating' them off the rectal wall by submucosal injection of adrenaline–saline solution to facilitate local scissor excision per anum. Over 95% of polyps proximal to the rectum are suitable for colonoscopic excision since few are too large or sessile. Surgery should never be resorted to without first attempting colonoscopic polypectomy, since some lesions that look sessile or malignant on X-ray prove to be on small stalks endoscopically. The colon is, except for its outer covering, devoid of sensory innervation and polypectomy is therefore painless and can be performed without sedation on an outpatient basis. Only stalked polyps with a head diameter of 2 cm or greater have any significant risk of haemorrhage and this is negligible if very low power coagulating current (15–30 watts equivalent) is used to cause heating and coagulation of the stalk before transection with the snare loop.[8] Polypectomy anywhere in the colon is usually quick and easy since 90% of polyps are under 2 cm diameter and have relatively thin stalks. Recovery of snared polyps means withdrawing the colonoscope with each one, if necessary using a split overtube through which the instrument is easily withdrawn and re-inserted. Small snared polyps can be aspirated through the biopsy channel with a mucus trap placed in the suction line.

Very small polyps (2–7 mm) can be snared but are usually biopsied and simultaneously destroyed by the so-called 'hot-biopsy' technique in which an electrocoagulating current is passed down insulated biopsy forceps. Large sessile polyps up to 3–4 cm diameter can sometimes be removed endoscopically by piecemeal snare polypectomy, repeated at several sessions if necessary.[7a] Whether this is justified depends on the operative risk in the individual and the configuration of the particular polyp.

MULTIPLE POLYPS AND POLYPOSIS SYNDROMES

A patient with a known diagnosis of Peutz–Jeghers syndrome, schistosomiasis or other non-neoplastic cause of polyposis can have 50 or more polyps snared in a single session since only one or two need be retrieved for histological review. Sporadic cases of unsuspected adenomatous polyposis occur, presumably by mutation, but multiple biopsies are sufficient to make this diagnosis and to exclude other forms of polyposis (such as metaplastic or lymphomatous polyps). The situation occasionally arises where, for example, a patient is found to have one or two polyps with sigmoidoscopy and barium enema and 10–15 additional smaller probable adenomas at endoscopy; before attempting multiple polypectomies it is logical to check first for the presence of other minute polyps because in such cases surgery might be considered as the first line of management. Visualization of polyps only 1–2 mm in diameter is much enhanced by the 'dye-spray technique' in which blue dye (0.3% indigo carmine or diluted writing ink) is sprayed onto the surface, causing any small polyps to protrude as pink islands against the blue background.[41] The identification of 20 or more additional polyps may, if they are shown to be adenomas, tip the balance towards surgery.

Familial adenomatous polyposis was often previously termed 'polyposis coli' but it is now recognized that it may involve the small intestine and stomach. Strictly speaking there must be at least 100 colonic adenomas to justify the term. The condition can be associated with benign mesodermal tumours such as osteomas and desmoids. The latter may present as large unresectable intra-abdominal masses involving the mesentery. The association with epidermoid cysts is known as Gardner's syndrome and with brain tumours, as Turcot's syndrome. The main risk of adenomatous polyposis is large bowel carcinoma but duodenal, ampullary or bile duct carcinomas are also reported, presumably arising from adenomas at these sites.

Symptoms are unusual in patients with adenomatous polyposis until the development of a cancer, usually in the second or third decade. Great efforts are made to diagnose the condition at the asymptomatic stage by contacting and examining all known relatives once one member of a family has been identified. The Mendelian dominant inheritance of the condition means that 50% of first-degree relatives should be affected and in practice about 43% are found to

be so.[6] The first screening fibre sigmoidoscopy should be at about 13 years of age, using the dye-spray technique to look for tiny polyps if none are obvious on initial examination. Examinations should be repeated every 2–3 years until the age of 30, by which time the diagnosis can reasonably be excluded. Affected patients may show hundreds or even thousands of polyps (Figure 11.57), although in the younger patients the small size of the polyps means that they can be easily overlooked (Figure 11.58) unless great care is taken.

Surgery is usually delayed until a socially convenient age (17–18 years) since there is no significant risk of cancer before this. If possible an ileorectal anastomosis is made to avoid ileostomy; however, this entails frequent and careful follow-up sigmoidoscopies to electrocoagulate rectal polyps and even so the risk of subsequent rectal cancer remains at 10% or more on long-term follow-up. As a result of this risk and the problem of occasional patients with unmanageable numbers of rectal polyps there is interest in new techniques of ileo-anal anastomosis, with or without a 'pelvic pouch', whereby all colorectal mucosa is removed with preservation of normal anatomy and sphincter control.

In addition to the management of identified patients the importance of contacting blood relatives (including cousins, nephews and nieces) cannot be overemphasized. 'Adenomatous polyposis' Family Registers of affected families are the prime example in modern medicine of the practical application of cancer prevention in high-risk patients.

TREATMENT OF MALIGNANT POLYPS

Endoscopically or radiologically it is often impossible to determine which polyps will be malignant. Signs of possible malignancy include a thick stalk and an ulcerated or indurated polyp head, but soft rounded polyps on thin stalks may contain cancer.[16] The histological diagnosis of malignancy may therefore come as a surprise several days after polypectomy. Providing the endoscopist is satisfied that his polypectomy satisfactorily removed the whole lesion, the principles of subsequent management depend entirely on the pathologist's assessment of the risk of spread to local lymph nodes. Well or moderately well differentiated carcinoma which has not invaded as far as the resection line in the polyp stalk (Figure 11.55) and which does not involve veins or lymphatics is exceedingly unlikely to have spread.[7, 16] The risk of early spread is much higher in poorly differentiated

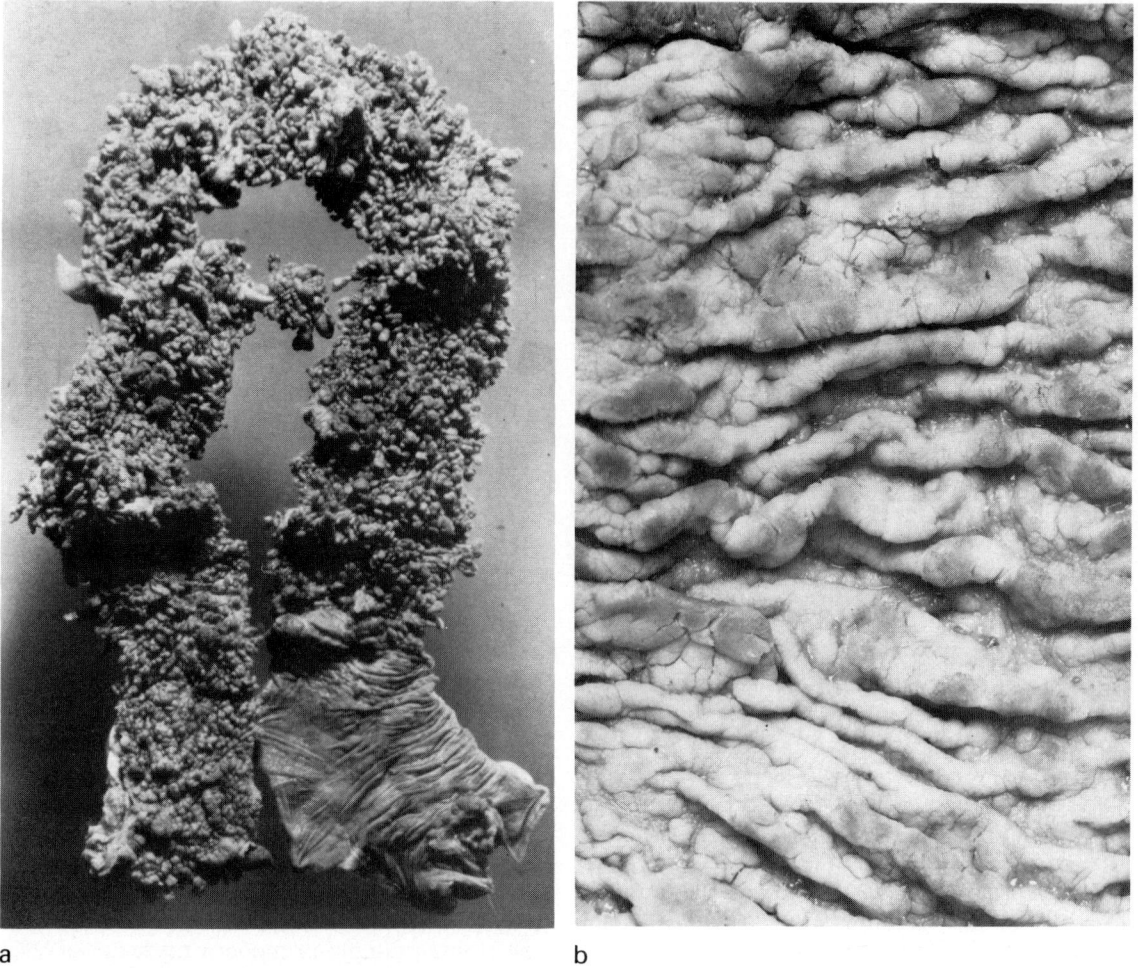

a   b

Fig. 11.57   Two patterns of familial adenomatous polyposis. (a) The whole of the colon except the caecum and proximal ascending colon is covered by adenomatous polyps. (b) Here the change is more subtle. Hundreds of tiny sessile polyps cover the mucosa giving it a cobblestone appearance. They resemble metaplastic polyps macroscopically.

anaplastic carcinoma, if involvement extends up to the resection line, or if the tumour involves vessels and lymphatics; any of these findings indicates surgery unless the patient is very infirm. By local resection in these at-risk patients the intention is to remove any local tumour extension or draining lymph nodes before distant metastases occur. The relatively high mortality of colonic surgery means that the lower-risk patients are likely to have a better prognosis by *not* proceeding to surgery, the locally malignant lesions being managed by endoscopic local excision alone.[24, 31] Clinical experience of endoscopists world-wide[7] and several series of patients followed for five years after polypectomy support this policy which can be applied equally to polypoid carcinomas meeting the same criteria.

Endoscopically, it is wise, if in doubt, to re-examine and biopsy the polypectomy site within days of the diagnosis of the malignancy being made since once healed it may be impossible to locate. A marker tattoo of 2 ml indian ink can be injected submucosally to identify the site for subsequent follow-up or to assist the surgeon in the event of resection.[35]

FOLLOW-UP OF ADENOMA PATIENTS

The exact future risk for a patient having had a previous adenoma removed must be re-defined now that more accurate diagnostic methods are available; some of the adenomas and cancers found in reported follow-up studies may simply represent lesions missed at the time of the first polypectomy. Nevertheless, the evidence sug-

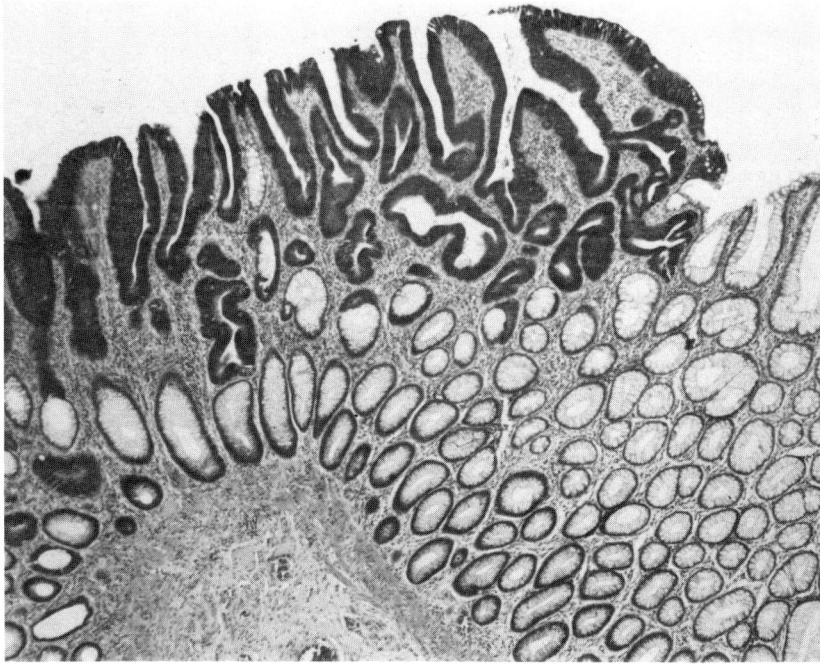

Fig. 11.58 The darker dysplastic epithelium is well seen in contrast to the normal mucosa in this case of adenomatous polyposis. However, the change is only producing a minor alteration in the surface mucosal contour and as seen in Figure 11.57b it is easy to overlook macroscopically. Haematoxylin and eosin, × 112.

gests that there is a significantly increased subsequent risk in adenoma patients and that they represent a high-risk group for development of colonic cancer.[4, 21, 22]

After a follow-up interval of about ten years, further adenomas (mostly small) can be expected in at least 20–30% of patients and carcinomas in 2–4%;[22] the only study with an age-matched control group of non-adenoma patients demonstrated only 7% with polyps and none with cancers at a similar follow-up interval.[4]

Follow-up examination must include the whole colon since many of the polyps and cancers occur proximally to the sigmoid colon.[9, 37] Rigid sigmoidoscopy alone gives a particularly low yield and should be abandoned as a follow-up procedure.[47] Occult blood tests also have no real role in follow-up since only some of the larger polyps bleed, and then intermittently.[25] Conventional practice is to advise colonoscopy or barium enema one year after the initial polypectomy,[43] with three-yearly total colonoscopy thereafter in those that are easy to examine; if colonoscopy was previously difficult, fibre sigmoidoscopy and double-contrast barium enema is an acceptable alternative but may miss some polyps in the right colon. There is good evidence that patients with more than one adenoma originally, especially those with

five or more, are at a higher risk still and older patients (over 55–60 years) are more at risk than younger ones. It may therefore be reasonable to examine a 50-year-old with one previous adenoma at only five-yearly intervals but to subject a 65-year-old with five adenomas to two-yearly checks. Whatever the follow-up routine adopted, there will always be some surprises; patients should thus be urged to attend earlier if suspicious symptoms occur, particularly bleeding. The problem of adenoma follow-up is essentially one of logistics;[23, 34] too frequent follow-up of the enormous numbers of adenoma bearing patients can easily make unreasonable demands on available diagnostic services. On the other hand, suitably managed, such patients present an opportunity for prevention or early diagnosis of colorectal cancer.

REFERENCES

1 Arthur, J. F. (1968) Structure and significance of metaplastic nodules in the rectal mucosa. *Journal of Clinical Pathology*, 21, 735–743.
2 Berge, T., Ekelund, G., Mellner, C. *et al.* (1973) Carcinoma of the colon and rectum in a defined population. *Acta Chirurgica Scandinavica* (Supplement), **438**, 1–86.
3 Bond, J. H. & Levitt, M. D. (1979) Colonic gas explosion – is a fire extinguisher necessary. *Gastroenterology*, 77, 1349–1350.

4 Brahme, F., Ekelund, G., Norden, J. G. & Wenckert, A. (1974) Metachronous colorectal polyps; comparison of development of colorectal polyps and carcinomas in persons with and without histories of polyps. *Diseases of the Colon and Rectum*, **17**, 166–171.

5 Bussey, H. J. R. (1983) Personal communication.

6 Bussey, H. J. R., Veale, A. M. O. & Morson, B. C. (1979) Genetics of gastrointestinal polyposis. *Gastroenterology*, **74**, 1325–1330.

7 Christie, J. P. (1978) Management of malignant colon polyps. *Gastrointestinal Endoscopy*, **24**, 193.

7a Christie, J. P. (1978) Colonoscopic removal of sessile colonic lesions. *Diseases of the Colon and Rectum*, **21**, 11–14.

8 Cotton, P. B. & Williams, C. B. (1982) *Practical Gastrointestinal Endoscopy*. Oxford: Blackwell Scientific.

9 Coller, J. A., Corman, M. L., Veidenheimer, M. C. (1975) Colonic polypoid disease: Need for total colonoscopy. *American Journal of Surgery*, **131**, 490–494.

10 De Beer, R. A. & Shinya, H. (1975) Colonic lipomas: An endoscopic analysis. *Gastrointestinal Endoscopy*, **22**, 90–91.

11 Deyhle, P. (1980) Results of endoscopic polypectomy in the gastrointestinal tract. *Endoscopy* (Supplement), 35–46.

12 Dodds, W. J., Stewart, E. T. & Hogan, W. J. (1977) Role of colonoscopy and roentgenology in the detection of polypoid colonic lesions. *American Journal of Digestive Diseases*, **22**, 646–649.

13 Douglas, J. R., Campbell, C. A., Salisbury, D. M. et al. (1981) Colonoscopic polypectomy in children. *British Medical Journal*, **281**, 1386–1387.

14 Figiel, L. S., Figiel, S. J. & Wietersen, F. K. (1965) Roentologic observations of growth rates of colonic polyps and carcinoma. *Acta Radiologica*, **3**, 417–429.

15 Fork, F. T. (1983) Reliability of routine double-contrast examination of the large bowel. A prospective study of 2590 patients. *Gut*, **24**, 672–677.

16 Gabriellson, N., Grandquist, S., Ohlsen, H. & Sundelin, P. (1978) Malignancy of colonic polyps. Diagnosis and management. *Acta Radiologica* (diagnosis section), **19**, 479–495.

17 Gilbertsen, V. A. & Nelms, J. M. (1978) The prevention of invasive cancer of the rectum. *Cancer*, **41**, 137–139.

18 Gilbertsen, V. A., McHugh, R., Schumann, L. & Williams, S. E. (1980) The earlier detection of colorectal cancers: a preliminary report of the results of the occult blood study. *Cancer*, **45**, 2899–2901.

19 Gillespie, P. E., Chambers, T. J., Chan, K. W. et al. (1979) Colonic adenomas – a colonoscopic survey. *Gut*, **20**, 240–245.

20 Grandquist, S., Gabriellson, N. & Sundelin, P. (1979) Diminutive colonic polyps – clinical significance and management. *Endoscopy*, **11**, 36–42.

21 Henry, L. G., Condon, R. E., Schulte, W. J. et al. (1975) Risk of recurrence of colon polyps. *Annals of Surgery*, **182**, 511–515.

22 Kirsner, J. B., Rider, J. A., Moeller, H. C. et al. (1960) Polyps of the colon and rectum: statistical analysis of a long-term follow-up study. *Gastroenterology*, **39**, 178–182.

23 Kronborg, D. (1980) Review: polyps of the colon and rectum. *Scandinavian Journal of Gastroenterology*, **15**, 1–5.

24 Langer, J. C., Cohen, Z., Taylor, B. R. et al. (1984) Management of patients with polyps containing malignancy removed by colonoscopic polypectomy. *Diseases of the Colon and Rectum*, **27**, 6–9.

25 Macrae, F. A. & St. John, D. J. B. (1982) Relationship of patterns of bleeding and haemoccult sensitivity in patients with colorectal cancers or adenomas. *Gastroenterology*, **82**, 891–898.

26 Madigan, M. R. & Halls, J. M. (1968) The extent of sigmoidoscopy shown on radiographs with special reference to the recto-sigmoid junction. *Gut*, **9**, 355–362.

27 Marks, G., Boggs, H. W., Castro, A. F. et al. (1979) Sigmoidoscopic examinations with rigid and flexible fiberoptic sigmoidoscopes in the surgeons office. *Diseases of the Colon and Rectum*, **22**, 162–168.

28 Mazier, W. P., Bowman, H. E., Sun, K. M. & Muldoon, J. P. (1974) Juvenile polyps of the colon and rectum. *Diseases of the Colon and Rectum*, **17**, 523–527.

29 Morson, B. C. (1978) In *The Pathogenesis of Colorectal Cancer. (Major Problems in Pathology No. 10)* (Ed.) Morson, B. C. Philadelphia: Saunders.

30 Morson, B. C. & Dawson, I. M. P. (1979) *Gastrointestinal Pathology*. Oxford: Blackwell Scientific Publications.

31 Morson, B. C., Whiteway, J. E., Jones, E. A. et al. (1984) Histopathology and prognosis of malignant colorectal polyps treated by endoscopic polypectomy. *Gut* (in press).

32 Muto, T., Bussey, H. J. R. & Morson, B. C. (1975) The evolution of cancer of the colon and rectum. *Cancer*, **36**, 2251–2270.

33 Nivatvongs, S. & Goldberg, S. M. (1979) Experience with colonoscopic polypectomy. Review of 700 polyps. *Minerva Medica*, **62**, 197–199.

34 Panish, J. F. (1979) State of the art: management of patients with polypoid lesions of the colon – current concepts and controversies. *American Journal of Gastroenterology*, **71**, 315–324.

35 Ponsky, J. L. & King, J. F. (1975) Endoscopic marking of colonic lesions. *Gastrointestinal Endoscopy*, **22** (1), 42–43.

36 Price, A. B. (1978) Benign lymphoid polyps and inflammatory polyps. In *The Pathogenesis of Colorectal Cancer (Major Problems in Pathology No. 10)* pp. 33–42. (Ed.) Morson, B. C. Philadelphia: Saunders.

37 Rhodes, J. B., Holmes, F. F. & Clark, G. M. (1977) Changing distribution of primary cancers in the large bowel. *Journal of the American Medical Association*, **238**, 1641–1643.

38 Rogers, B. H. G. (1974) The safety of carbon dioxide insufflation during colonoscopic electrosurgical polypectomy. *Gastrointestinal Endoscopy*, **20**, 115–118.

39 Shinya, H. & Wolff, W. I. (1979) Morphology, anatomic distribution and cancer potential of colonic polyps. An analysis of 7000 polyps endoscopically removed. *Annals of Surgery*, **190**, 679–683.

40 Stewart, M., Macrae, F. A. & Williams, C. B. (1982) Neoplasia and ureterosigmoidoscopy: a colonoscopy survey. *British Journal of Surgery*, **69**, 414–416.

41 Tada, M., Katoh, S., Kohli, Y. & Kawai, K. (1976) On the dye spraying method in colonfiberscopy. *Endoscopy*, **8**, 70–74.

42 Tedesco, F. J., Waye, J. D., Avella, J. R. & Villalobos, M. M. (1980) Diagnostic implications of the spatial distribution of colonic mass lesions (polyps and cancers). *Gastrointestinal Endoscopy*, **26**, 95–97.

43 Waye, J. D. & Braunfeld, S. (1982) Surveillance intervals after polypectomy. *Endoscopy*, **14**, 79–81.

44 Waye, J. D., Frankel, A. & Braunfeld, S. F. (1980) The histopathology of small colon polyps. *Gastrointestinal Endoscopy*, **26**, 80.

45 Williams, A. R., Balasooriya, B. A. W. & Day, D. W. (1980) Polyps and cancer of the large bowel: a necropsy study in Liverpool. *Gut*, **23**, 835–842.

46 Williams, C. B., Goldblatt, M. & Delaney, P. (1982) Top and tail endoscopy and follow-up in Peutz–Jeghers

syndrome. *Endoscopy*, **14**, 82–84.

47 Williams, C. B., Macrae, F. A. & Bartram, C. I. (1982) A prospective study of diagnostic methods in polyp follow-up. *Endoscopy*, **14**, 74–78.

48 Williams, G. T., Arthur, J. F., Bussey, H. J. R. & Morson, B. C. (1980) Metaplastic polyps and polyposis. *Histopathology*, **4**, 155–170.

MALIGNANT TUMOURS

Malignant disease of the large bowel was responsible for approximately 16 500 deaths in England and Wales in 1981 and is now second only to lung cancer as a cause of death from malignant disease.[166] The situation is similar in the USA, where colorectal carcinoma is now the commonest solid tumour except for the skin. While progress has been made in aetiology, in improving early diagnosis and in the development of new surgical techniques, the disease still remains a major challenge to physicians, surgeons and scientists alike.

Ninety-eight per cent of all malignant large bowel tumours are adenocarcinomas. The other epithelial tumours are carcinoid or squamous cell carcinoma. The latter nearly always arise from the anorectum and are considered elsewhere in this book. Tumours of mesenchymal origin (sarcomas and malignant melanoma) may also occur in the large bowel.

Adenocarcinoma

GEOGRAPHICAL DISTRIBUTION

The highest incidences of both colonic and rectal cancer are seen in Western Europe and North America, whereas intermediate rates prevail in Eastern Europe (Table 11.14). The lowest rates are seen in Asia, Africa and South America, excluding Argentina.[224] The incidence of rectal carcinoma varies less internationally than does cancer of the colon. Variations in incidence between countries are much larger than variations within each country, but the disease seems to occur more frequently in urban than in rural areas.[26, 224]

Some of the differences in geographical variation may be due to failure of detection in low incidence areas, where techniques for diagnosis are less sophisticated and patient tolerance of symptoms is high. However, this explanation probably only accounts for a small part of the variations and does not explain, for example, the marked differences in incidence between Denmark and Finland or the low rate recorded in Japan.[115]

AETIOLOGY

The basic processes underlying the development of carcinoma of the large bowel remain unknown. Nevertheless, there is new evidence which implicates new factors and suggests several hypotheses which might explain its development.

The high incidence of colorectal cancer in 'sophisticated' western society suggests that environmental factors are aetiologically more important than genetic factors. Further evidence to support this suggestion comes from studies involving migrants; the risk increases among

Table 11.14 Incidence of colorectal cancer in different countries.*

		Colonic	Rectal	Colorectal
Nigeria		1.3	1.2	2.5
India		4.6	4.4	9.0
Osaka (Japan)		6.3	6.9	13.2
East Germany		13.6	12.0	25.6
Vas (Hungary)		9.1	11.0	20.1
Connecticut (USA)		30.1	18.2	48.3
Detroit (USA)	White	26.2	16.0	42.2
	Black	24.5	13.8	38.3
Birmingham (UK)		16.5	16.1	32.6
Oxford (UK)		15.7	15.4	31.1
Ayrshire (UK)		16.6	14.0	30.0
Denmark		16.2	16.7	32.9
Finland		7.9	7.7	15.6
New Zealand	Maori	7.4	4.6	12.0
	Non-Maori	23.0	15.4	38.4
Hawaii	Japanese	22.4	16.3	38.7
	Caucasian	23.9	13.5	37.4
	Hawaiian	14.1	9.4	23.5

* Per 100 000 age-adjusted to world population.
Adapted from Waterhouse *et al* (1976).[224]

Japanese as they move from low-incidence Japan to high-risk United States.[91] The incidence of carcinoma among European Jews in Israel is higher than that among Asian and African-born Jews.[151] Similar observations have been made in Polish migrants moving to the USA and Australia.[200]

Dietary factors, bacteria and bile salts
Since epidemiological studies point to factors associated with Western society as being of aetiological importance, it is no surprise that diet has received most attention.

There is indirect evidence that a diet rich in animal fat is a major risk factor. The proportion of fat in the western diet is significantly greater than that in the diet of low-risk populations.[246] Some nutritional statistics on fat and meat consumption correlate positively with the incidence of colonic cancer[5, 45] and case-control studies support the association.[40, 92] Nevertheless, this view has recently been challenged. Enström[56] noted that a steady increase in the frequency of beef consumption in the USA from 1940 to 1970 was accompanied by stable or declining rates of incidence and mortality from colorectal disease. No association between fat intake and colorectal cancer was demonstrated when populations in Finland (low risk) and Denmark (high risk) were compared.[114] A carefully conducted case-control study performed as part of the Japan–Hawaii Cancer Study was also unable to confirm an association.[204]

The implication of fat as a possible aetiological factor is linked to the concept that the western diet favours the development of a bacterial flora containing organisms which are capable of degrading bile salts to carcinogens, possibly related to methylcholanthrene.[245] It has been suggested[106] that *Clostridium paraputrificum* is the responsible organism. Many studies comparing faecal flora in high and low risk populations have now been performed. Although certain organisms have been identified in the high-risk populations, no study has succeeded in linking a specific bacterium with colorectal cancer.[36, 38, 60, 77, 138, 140, 143] It is difficult to draw definite conclusions from studies of this sort since only small numbers of patients have been investigated and any individual may have up to 400 species of bacteria in the gut.

The role that bile acids play in the development of carcinoma is uncertain. Bile acids can promote colorectal cancer in animals.[104, 105] Human studies have involved epidemiological surveys which have compared populations at various levels of risk and have implicated bile acids in aetiology.[36, 103, 105] Case-control studies comparing faecal bile acid concentrations in bowel cancer cases and controls, however, have not shown such a clear relationship.[105] Nevertheless, there does seem to be a relationship between bile acids and benign adenomas, although further corroborative data are awaited.[103, 183, 227, 228]

The increased incidence of right-sided colonic neoplasm in patients who have previously undergone cholecystectomy[129, 218, 221] is of interest but remains to be established. This operation increases the production and turnover of degraded bile salts.[177]

In summary, therefore, although dietary fat, bacteria and bile salts have all been implicated in colorectal carcinogenesis, proof that any of them is directly involved is lacking.

A low intake of dietary fibre may also predispose the individual to carcinoma. The theory propagated by Burkitt[15] is that lack of fibre reduces faecal bulk, prolongs intestinal transit and allows faecal carcinogens a longer contact time with the mucosa than occurs with a diet rich in fibre. There is substantial indirect evidence to support this theory. Several case-control studies have shown a negative association between colorectal cancer and dietary intake of vegetables; the average weight of faeces is heavier in low-risk groups compared with high-risk groups.[204] Furthermore, higher fibre intake and more rapid intestinal transit have been recorded in high risk groups.[16] These studies can be criticized since the populations compared differed in various respects other than dietary intake. Only one large epidemiological study with adequate control data has demonstrated a low risk of colon cancer for those with a high fibre intake,[152] whereas several international surveys have been unable to do so.[5, 45]

Other dietary components have been implicated from time to time. Several authors[25, 247] have related high sugar intake to the development of the disease. Similarly, excessive beer consumption has been suggested as a possible risk factor[14] but controlled studies have not confirmed this impression.[113]

Adenomatous polyps
There is a relationship between benign polyps and carcinoma but this is not fully understood. The evidence that adenomas have malignant potential is based on several observations. Examination of operative specimens demonstrate that one or more adenomas are present in nearly one-third of cases with carcinoma.[161]

Furthermore, the remaining bowel in these patients is twice as likely to develop a second (or metachronous) tumour compared with patients who have no associated polyp.[18] Adenomas coexist in 75% of cases in which two or more carcinomas are present simultaneously. The finding of benign tissue in a colon carcinoma and vice versa lends weight to the argument.[162] Furthermore, many pathologists have shown a transition from a benign to a malignant neoplastic process on histological examination of polyps.[46, 52, 65, 133, 158, 225, 235] These observations are supported by the invariable development of carcinoma in patients with familial adenomatous polyposis. While benign polyps can undergo malignant change the proportion that will do so and which factors cause this transformation, are unknown. Some pathologists believe that most or all carcinomas develop from benign adenomatous polyps (the adenoma–carcinoma sequence). This concept is supported by Morson[159] who showed that of tumours confined to the submucosa alone, 60% had contiguous benign adenomatous tissue, whereas with carcinomas that extend into extramural fat this percentage was much reduced. Several pathologists have studied many hundreds of specimens[21, 57, 199] and failed to find any benign adenomatous tissue even in carcinomas of less than 2 cm in diameter.[198]

The malignant potential of villous papillomas is not disputed. The frequency of malignant change arising in these tumours varies between 6 and 75%[62, 64] with a median incidence of approximately 30%.[87, 209]

Inflammatory diseases
The colorectal cancer risk in patients with long standing ulcerative colitis is well appreciated while the relationship between Crohn's colitis and colonic carcinoma is less certain (see Chapter 12).

Although diverticular disease and carcinoma often coexist and make diagnosis difficult[205] there is no evidence to link the two disorders. Similarly although tumour-like granulomas of amoebiasis, tuberculosis or very rarely syphilis may be confused with a carcinoma, no case has yet been described in which carcinoma has been attributed to the underlying infection.

Schistosomiasis may be a precursor of carcinoma in China. Both diseases are endemic and frequently coexist. In addition the histological changes which precede the development of malignancy are similar to those in ulcerative colitis. Eradication of the infection reduces the incidence of carcinoma. Further studies are eagerly awaited.[22, 23]

Genetic factors
Although environmental factors play a primary role in colonic carcinogenesis, hereditary factors play a greater role than was previously appreciated. The familial incidence of colonic cancer in the general population is higher than that in the control groups. In addition, there is a significant increase in the number of deaths due to carcinoma among first degree relatives of index cases compared with the expected incidence.[135]

There are three variants of hereditary polyposis coli which eventually lead to the development of carcinoma. Familial polyposis coli (familial adenomatous polyposis) is an autosomal dominant disorder characterized by innumerable colonic and rectal adenomas.[35, 132] Fifty per cent of children of polyposis families are likely to inherit the disease. Carcinoma most frequently develops about 15 years after the commencement of symptoms at about 35 years of age. The risk of developing carcinoma is approximately 1% by 16 years of age, 50% by 28 to 30 years of age and 90% by 40 to 45 years of age.[17, 219, 220]

Gardner's syndrome is similar to familial polyposis coli and involves the same risks.[72] The colonic polyps are associated with sebaceous cysts, dermoid tumours, fibromas, facial bone osteomas and abnormal dentition. There is an increased susceptibility to other carcinomas including those of thyroid, the ampulla of Vater, the duodenum and the adrenal gland. Turcot's syndrome is the third variant in which tumours of the CNS occur with the colonic polyps.[216]

The 'cancer family syndrome' is a rare autosomal dominant condition characterized by the development of multiple primary carcinomas of colon and endometrium, but which is not associated with multiple colonic polyps.[137]

PATHOLOGY

Distribution of carcinoma within the large bowel
Variations in the classification of rectosigmoid growths create difficulties in determining the relative distribution of carcinoma of the colon and rectum. On balance, however, it seems that half the tumours of the large bowel are situated in the rectum. Within the colon approximately 50% occur in the sigmoid colon and 25% occur in the caecum and ascending colon. The remaining 25% are distributed in order of frequency as follows: transverse colon, splenic flexure,

descending colon and hepatic flexure.[68, 116, 121, 197] In the rectum approximately 70% occur in the upper and lower thirds in equal proportions.[78]

Multiple carcinomas

About 3% of patients will have two or more tumours present simultaneously, i.e. synchronous tumours.[80] In those patients without concomitant ulcerative colitis or polyposis coli, 75% will have associated benign adenomas.[96]

Macroscopic features

There are five varieties of colorectal cancer which can be identified by their gross appearance.

1 Polypoid or cauliflower lesion (Figure 11.59) protrudes into the lumen of the bowel, is often ulcerated over part of its surface and usually

does not exhibit extensive spread. Some of these tumours have a villous appearance; this occurs in about 7% of all carcinomas.

2 Ulcerative lesion (Figure 11.60) has a raised rolled everted edge with slough in its base. It tends to deeply infiltrate the bowel wall often distorting the lumen.

3 Annular lesion (Figure 11.61) is often referred to as the 'string' carcinoma and usually causes some degree of obstruction to the intestinal lumen.

4 Diffusely infiltrating scirrhous lesion. This is analogous to the linitis plastica type of gastric cancer but is a rare variant.[194] It is commonly a secondary manifestation of an occult carcinoma of the stomach rather than a true primary carcinoma.

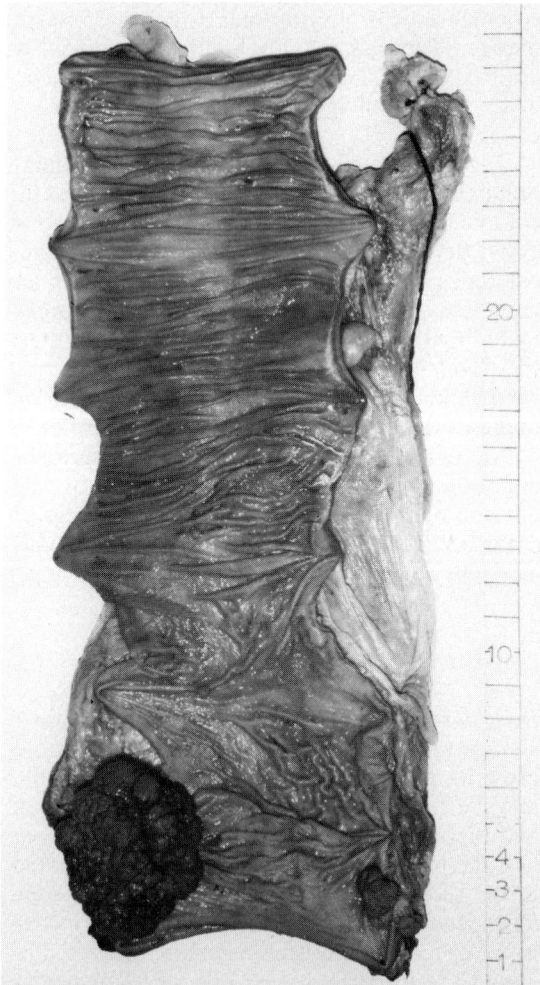

Fig. 11.59 Polypoid carcinoma in the upper rectum.

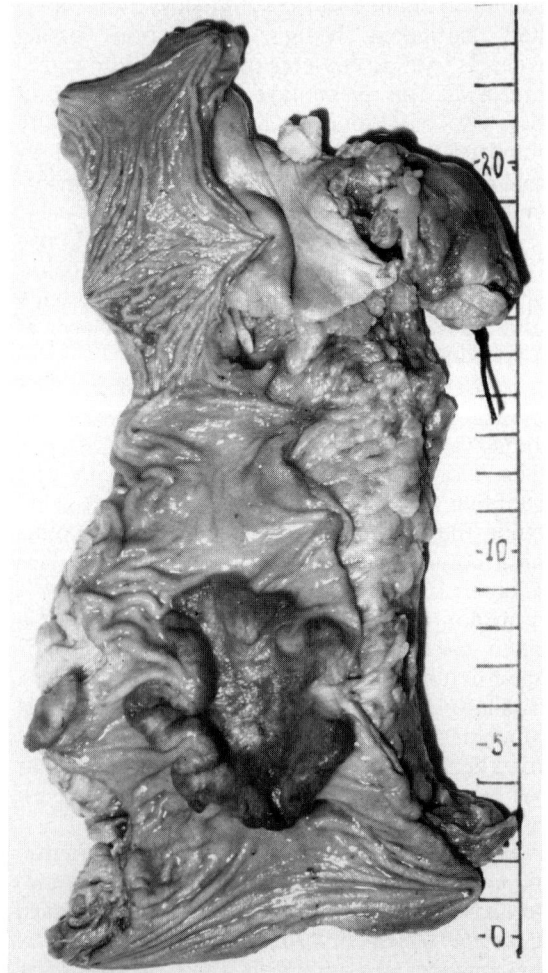

Fig. 11.60 Ulcerated carcinoma of the rectum.

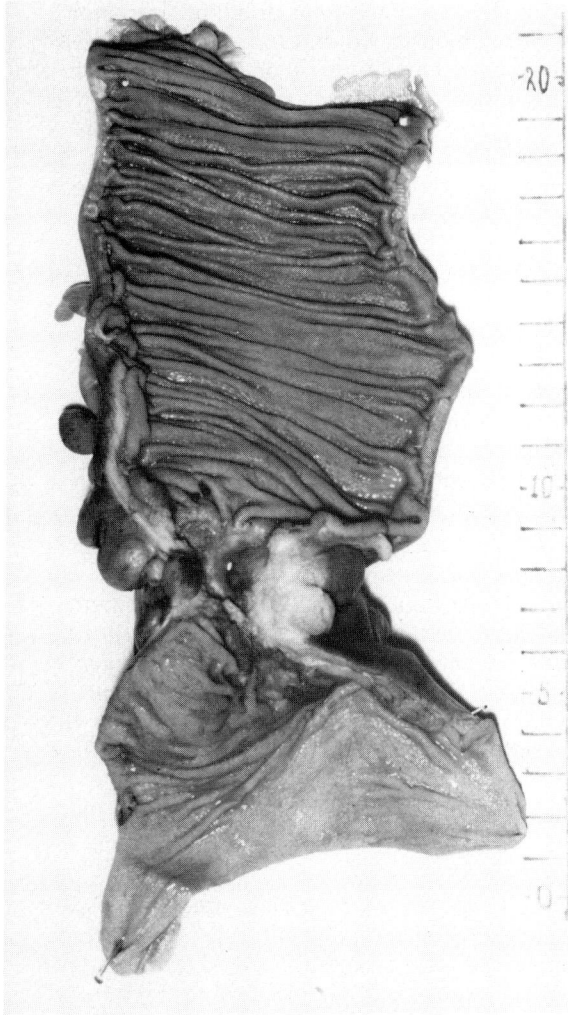

Fig. 11.61 Annular carcinoma of the colon.

5 *Colloid carcinoma.* Approximately 10% of tumours secrete large quantities of mucin which gives them a characteristic gelatinous appearance on their cut surface. They are usually bulky tumours which vary in their extent of infiltration.

Microscopic features and histological grading
The degree of differentiation of colorectal adenocarcinomas is extremely variable. Both Dukes[48] and Grinnell[83] introduced a system in which tumours were graded I to IV according to the relative degree of atypical cells. Grade I was well differentiated and Grade IV was anaplastic. Grade IV also included colloid tumours. The latter represent approximately 10 to 15% of all tumours and are characterized by the presence of large amounts of mucin either inside (signet ring) or outside the cell. Approximately 20% of tumours are well differentiated (low grade), 60% are moderately differentiated (average grade) and 20% are poorly differentiated (high grade or anaplastic). Grading is subjective and although modifications have been introduced to the original system[12] to obtain uniformity, variations from one pathologist to another are commonplace. In general the histological grade of the tumour is related to the ultimate prognosis, but the variability in reporting the degree of differentiation limits its value. This applies particularly to preoperative biopsies.[214]

Direct spread. The commonest mode of spread is in the transverse axis of the bowel wall itself. If allowed to progress it will eventually become circumferential. Complete encirclement of the rectum takes approximately two years.[148] Longitudinal spread within the bowel wall is rare but is important for the surgeon in order to determine the extent of resection. Distal intramural spread is particularly important in rectal carcinoma when the length of resection of macroscopic normal bowel may make the difference between the patient retaining the anal sphincter or being left with a permanent colostomy. Most of the studies suggest that distal spread is rare; when it does occur it is usually less than 1 cm, and in those cases where it exceeds this distance the tumour is advanced and the patient is very likely to die from widespread metastases.[11, 85, 180, 234]

With extension of the growth, penetration of the bowel wall takes place. The submucosa and muscle coats are first breached and gradually the tumour erodes through the serosa, involving the pericolonic or rectal fat and the peritoneum. If growth is allowed to continue, invasion of local structures will take place. In the rectum, if the growth is situated anteriorly below the peritoneal reflection, the prostate, seminal vesicles or bladder will be involved in the male and the posterior vaginal wall, cervix or uterus in the female. If the rectal growth is sited posteriorly below the pelvic peritoneum, spread will involve the fascia of Waldeyer and eventually the sacral plexus, sacrum and/or coccyx.

When the tumour lies above the peritoneal reflection, involvement of the ureters may occur in addition to invasion of the bladder, uterus, sigmoid colon or small bowel.

Lymphatic spread. Spread in the lymphatic system tends to follow the course of the blood vessels supplying the site of the carcinoma. The carcinoma spreads from node to node and in advanced growths, when the lymphatics are choked with metastases and lymph flow is blocked, metastases may occur in separate lymph node groups. This type of spread is referred to as retrograde lymphatic spread.[86]

When the carcinoma is situated in the colon, the epicolic and the paracolic lymph nodes are first involved, followed by the intermediate glands along either the ileocolic, right colic, middle colic or left colic arteries. Eventually spread reaches the para-aortic glands which surround the origin of the superior and inferior mesenteric vessels.

Carcinoma of the rectum was first thought to spread in three directions, upwards along the superior haemorrhoidal and inferior mesenteric vessels, laterally along the middle rectal vessels in the lateral ligaments to the internal iliac nodes, and downwards through the sphincter muscles into the ischiorectal fossa and perianal skin and finally to the inguinal nodes. It was considered that these three directions of spread were implicated no matter where the carcinoma was sited within the rectum.[147] This concept led to the adoption of the abdomino-perineal resection for the treatment of carcinoma since only this operation was considered to be radical enough to remove all of the pathways of spread. Careful research has since shown that although upward spread is most frequent, downward spread is rare and only occurs if the lymph flow along the superior rectal vascular pedicle is obstructed by metastases. Lateral spread is unusual with tumours of the intraperitoneal rectum but is more frequent with carcinomas below the peritoneal reflection.[47, 71, 222, 242] These findings have important implications for both surgeon and patient alike in view of the increasing popularity of sphincter saving resections for the treatment of low rectal cancer.

Blood-borne spread. Blood-borne spread occurs later than lymphatic spread, primarily to the liver. Pulmonary metastases occur in about 5% of cases[7] and the adrenal glands, kidneys and bones are affected in about 10% of cases.[235] Spread to the liver is via the portal vein and occurs in nearly one half of cases.[235] These data are obtained from postmortem studies. Not surprisingly the incidence of detectable liver metastases present at laparotomy is much lower (10 to 15%).[78] Recent studies which have performed serial ultrasound and computerized tomography of the liver during the postoperative period have identified 'occult' metastases not found at operation in a higher proportion of patients and the incidence of liver metastases present at the time of diagnosis is probably approximately 30%.[63]

Permeation of the veins draining a carcinoma can be demonstrated on careful section and histological examination of operative specimens. The presence of submucous venous spread has little or no effect on prognosis. Permeation of extramural veins on the other hand reduces the five-year survival by about 25%.[19, 210] The incidence of venous permeation varies between 17 and 38%.[8, 49]

Several investigators[155, 186] have demonstrated neoplastic cells in the circulation at the time of surgery. The viability of these cells is uncertain. It has not been shown that manipulation of the tumour at the time of operation increases the risk of metastases. It may be that although malignant cells are released they are unable to survive in the circulation.[28, 55, 66]

Transperitoneal spread. About 1 in 10 patients after a surgical resection for carcinoma will develop peritoneal deposits. The less differentiated the tumour the more likely the peritoneal involvement.[161] This mode of spread frequently involves the ovaries (so-called Krukenberg tumours). The peritoneal deposits stimulate the excretion of exudate which forms ascites. This form of spread is probably transcoelomic in nature although dissemination may take place via the subperitoneal lymphatics.[148]

Spread by implantation. The frequency with which exfoliated malignant cells can become implanted onto a raw surface and lead to a secondary deposit is debatable. There are reports of implantation metastases developing in anal fistulas, haemorrhoidectomy wounds, abdominal incisions and around colostomies.[44, 127] The concept that local recurrence at an anastomosis following resection was due to implantation of cells on the suture line is now disputed since it has not been possible to demonstrate viable cells within the lumen of the bowel at the time of surgery.[188] Similarly, although free malignant cells can be demonstrated in washings from the peritoneal cavity,[178, 179] attempts to grow them in tissue culture have failed.[156]

Staging of carcinoma

Staging of colorectal carcinoma has proved of some value in determining prognosis following treatment. The most widely used classification is that of Dukes:[47, 49]

Stage A. The carcinoma has not penetrated through the muscularis propria and there is no involvement of lymph nodes.

Stage B. The carcinoma has extended through the wall of the rectum and involved the perirectal tissues but has not produced lymph node metastases.

Stage C is subdivided into C_1, where nodes in the immediate vicinity of the tumour are involved but the most proximal node nearest the point of transection of the main vascular pedicle is free from tumour, and C_2, where nodes at the proximal margin of the vascular pedicle are involved.

Although Dukes did not originally include *Stage D*, this category is frequently used to describe patients in whom distant metastases are detected. Several variations in Dukes' classification have been described and these should be taken into account when comparing published data.[6, 119] Doubt has recently been cast on Dukes' staging, and its modifications, since they do not take into account the degree of fixity of the tumours at operation. This characteristic is important in determining prognosis. It has been shown[90, 243] that Dukes' B tumours, which are fixed or partially fixed, have a similar prognosis to mobile C tumours. In order to obtain some uniformity in staging, it has been suggested that a TNM classification should be introduced, similar to that used for breast carcinoma[10] but this has not been universally adopted yet.

CLINICAL FEATURES

Most patients with colorectal cancer are in the sixth to eighth decades of life. Approximately 200 patients per year in the UK below 35 years of age develop the disease and they tend to have a more favourable outlook than previously thought.[37, 167] Colon carcinoma occurs with equal frequency in men and women but rectal cancer seems to be rather more prevalent in men.[167]

In the early stage of development a colonic carcinoma rarely produces symptoms. At a later stage, one or more of the following is usually present:

1   Change in bowel habit, either constipation or diarrhoea or a combination of both.
2   Bleeding per rectum, often dark in colour.
3   Passage of mucus per rectum.
4   Abdominal pain.
5   Abdominal distension.
6   Borborygmi.
7   General malaise with loss of weight.

The site of the carcinoma often dictates the symptom complex. Carcinoma of the caecum and right colon are usually soft friable tumours and bleed easily. Patients complain of a non-specific deterioration in general health and are found to be anaemic. The passage of blood per rectum is unusual although occult blood may be detected by specific tests. Carcinoma in this region is often the cause of 'cryptogenic' iron deficiency anaemia. Some patients complain of abdominal pain and some have a palpable mass in the right iliac fossa.

When the tumour is situated on the left side, the clinical picture is usually different. The faecal contents are more solid, the calibre of the lumen is smaller and the tumours tend to be scirrhous and annular such that obstructive features are common. Constipation occurs in about half of the cases and is often accompanied by abdominal pain. The latter is usually diffuse and vague initially but gradually becomes more griping as the degree of obstruction increases. Bleeding and the passage of mucus per rectum are more common with tumours on the left side.

When the carcinoma is situated in the rectum the characteristic clinical picture is bleeding on defecation which may mimic the bright red bleeding which occurs with haemorrhoids or may be darker and more profuse. The bleeding is nearly always accompanied by a change in bowel habit. Sometimes constipation is present but more classically there is tenesmus in which the patient complains of frequent desire to defecate, with the passage of small amounts of faeces, blood or mucus. These symptoms are worse in the morning and tend to improve during the day.

Anorectal pain is not usually a feature of rectal cancer unless the tumour has invaded locally. Involvement of the sacrum and sacral plexus usually by a tumour on the posterior wall of the rectum will cause back pain and sciatica. Extension downwards into the anal canal can cause severe discomfort on defecation, symptoms which can mimic an anal fissure. Extension of the carcinoma into ureters, bladder or prostate can cause urinary tract symptoms, and involvement of the vagina may lead to a rectovaginal fistula.

Occasionally, rectal carcinoma may be entirely asymptomatic and only detected on routine digital examination.

DIAGNOSIS AND INVESTIGATIONS

The clinical history may well point to the diagnosis but further investigation is required.

A complete physical examination is essential and the findings will vary depending on the duration of the illness, the extent of spread and the presence of complications, ranging from a healthy appearance to severe cachexia. Abdominal palpation may detect a nodular enlarged liver suggestive of metastases. Palpation along the course of the colon may reveal the tumour itself. Its mobility will depend on the degree of local spread. If peritoneal metastases are present ascites may be present and, more rarely, a nodule of secondary tumour may be sited at the umbilicus (the so-called Sister Joseph's nodule). It is rare in colorectal cancer to detect enlarged peripheral lymph nodes.

Rectal examination may detect a mass and secondary deposits may be felt in the pelvic peritoneum. The findings in rectal carcinoma will vary depending on the macroscopic type of tumour, its size, its site within the rectum and the degree of spread. About 75% of all rectal cancers are within reach of the examining finger.[28, 208] Not all firm masses arising in the rectum are primary neoplasms. A rectal carcinoma can be confused with a carcinoma or diverticular mass of the sigmoid which becomes adherent to the pelvic floor and is palpable extrarectally. Similarly, a primary tumour of the cervix or prostate may be palpable outside the rectum. Either of the latter two neoplasms may invade the anterior rectal wall and it then becomes impossible, on digital examination, to differentiate them from a rectal cancer.

Proctoscopy and sigmoidoscopy
The appearance of a rectal carcinoma will depend on its macroscopic appearance. Often a polypoid tumour will completely fill the lumen so that its precise attachment cannot be identified. With an ulcerated growth, the observer first notices the lower extremity projecting into the lumen as a congested bleeding protrusion with a dull grey necrotic crater. Sometimes the endoscopist will find that the rectosigmoid junction is unduly fixed and difficult to negotiate due to a proximally adherent lesion. The distance of the lower margin of the tumour from the anal verge should always be noted to assist the surgeon in his decision as to the best operative approach. Although it is useful to examine the bowel lumen beyond the tumour, in practice this is often impossible and certainly so if the growth is of the annular variety. In those cases where a carcinoma is present beyond the reach of the sigmoidoscope, the presence of blood and mucus in the lumen should alert the endoscopist to this possibility.

In most outpatient clinics, the rigid sigmoidoscope is the only type of endoscopic instrument employed. The flexible sigmoidoscope may have considerable benefits. The instrument is 60 cm in length, thus increasing the length of bowel that can be examined. Patients find it more tolerable than the rigid instrument and the complication rate is low.[237] The main disadvantage is that the bowel needs to be prepared prior to examination. Nevertheless, the instrument is extremely useful in diagnosis and may reduce the number of patients requiring radiographic examination.[241]

Radiographic examination
Single contrast can be used but the double-contrast air inflation technique[226] has significantly improved the diagnostic yield of this investigation. Radiographic accuracy diminishes at the extremes of the large bowel (i.e. at the caecum or rectum). Difficulty in the precise delineation of a carcinoma in the caecum may result from unsatisfactory elimination of faecal material, a filling defect produced by an unusually prominent ileocaecal valve, deformity of the caecal wall by previous surgical manoeuvres (such as appendicectomy) and also the presence of adjacent disease in the ovary, appendix or terminal ileum. Although demonstration of a rectal carcinoma by radiography is rarely necessary, a barium enema is useful to rule out a synchronous tumour.

A colonic carcinoma is usually seen on barium enema examination as a filling defect and its exact configuration depends upon its size and macroscopic features. In many cases a constant stricture of 3 to 8 cm in length is seen. Such a stricture with characteristic shouldering is seen as an 'apple-core' deformity (Figure 11.62). If the carcinoma is an annular string-type neoplasm the narrowed segment will be much shorter. Another radiographic variant is produced by the presence of a bulky polypoid tumour which projects into the lumen and is seen as a filling defect with an irregular edge (Figure 11.63). Although large polypoid carcinomas are clearly evident on barium enema examination, difficulty may be experienced in detection of smaller lesions of this type. Radiographic features which suggest possible malignancy in a polyp include indrawing of the outline of the base when the polyp is sessile, an irregular surface, a large size or evidence of growth between consecutive radiographic studies (Figure 11.64). Any polyp greater than 2 cm in diameter should be regarded as a carcinoma until proved otherwise.[52, 248]

Carcinoma may be difficult to detect in loops of redundant colon and where the barium outlines of adjacent loops are superimposed. This particularly applies to the sigmoid segment and

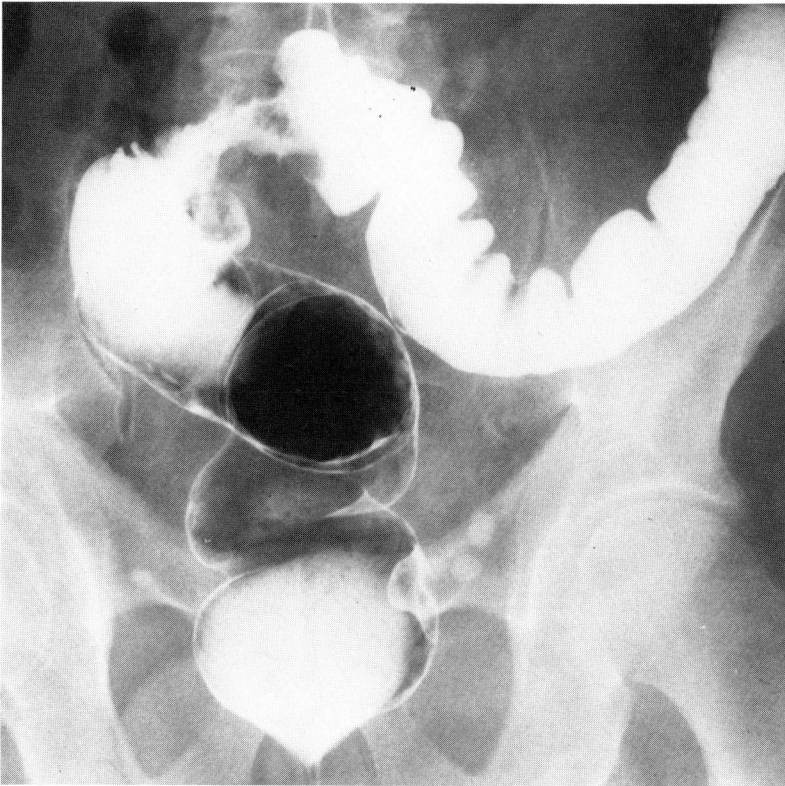

Fig. 11.62 Double-contrast barium enema showing annular carcinoma in the sigmoid colon – typical 'apple-core' deformity.

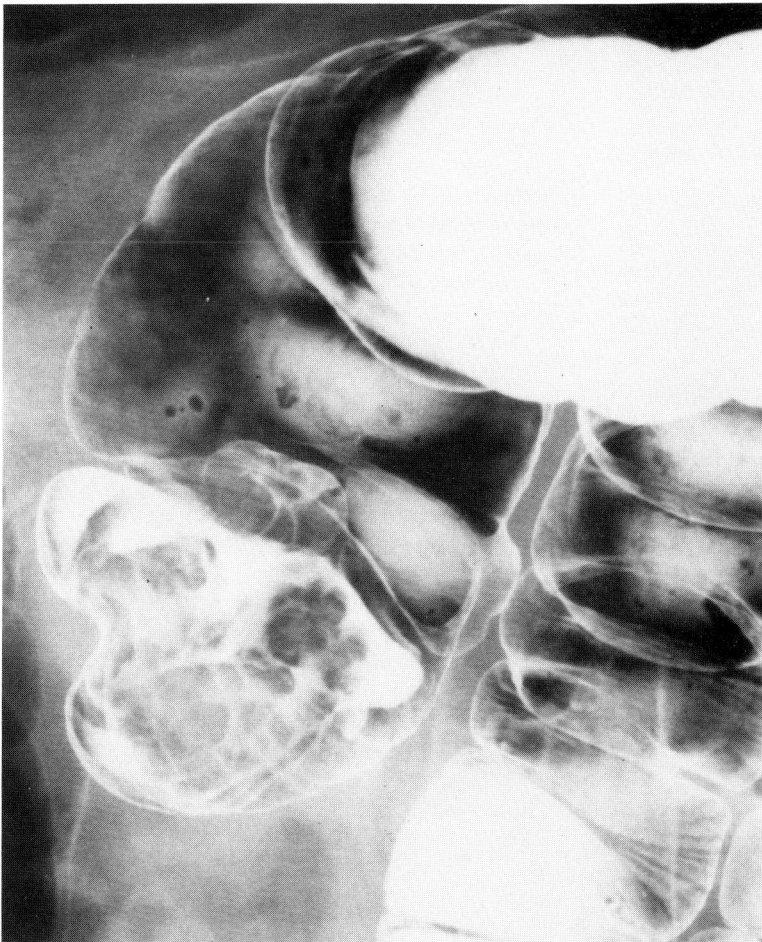

Fig. 11.63 Barium enema showing large polypoid carcinoma in the caecum.

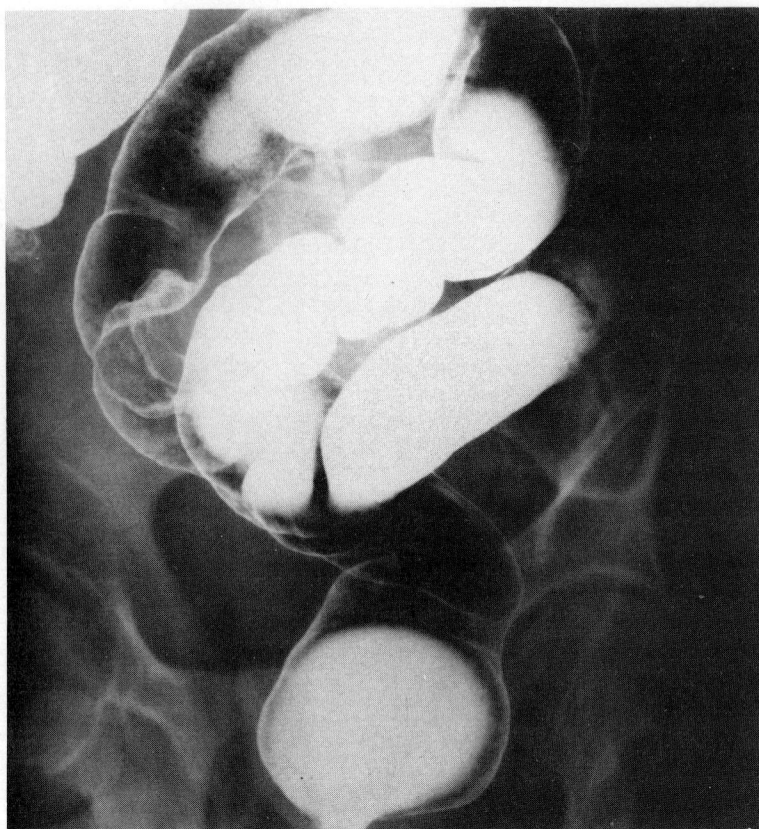

Fig. 11.64 Barium enema showing neoplastic polyp in sigmoid colon. It is 3 cm in diameter and has an irregular base which is drawn in.

to the hepatic and splenic flexures. Oblique views help to overcome this difficulty.

The accuracy of modern radiological techniques is high. The false positive rate at the Mayo Clinic for example was 0.8% and the false negative rate was 6.9%.[124] Nevertheless, if the study is negative or equivocal and the clinician is still suspicious, there should be no hesitation in proceeding to a colonoscopic examination.

Colonoscopy

Colonoscopy has substantially improved the accuracy of diagnosis in colorectal cancer. It enhances the sensitivity of barium enema throughout the colon but especially in the upper sigmoid, distal descending colon and caecum. A carcinoma of the sigmoid colon may be missed on barium enema in 8% of cases and more frequently if the growth is situated in the caecum.[30] Of 60 lesions missed on barium enema, and detected at colonoscopy, 17 were carcinomas.[213] Colonoscopy, however, is not a first line investigation. It needs to be performed under sedation, and the presence of adhesions, strictures or diverticular disease may make it impossible. In addition, there is a small risk of perforation even when performed for diagnostic purposes.[69a, 187]

SCREENING

Since colorectal tumours tend to be slow growing and are often asymptomatic at their onset, early detection depends on population screening. Screening can be divided into selective screening of high-risk groups and general screening of average risk patients. The high-risk group includes patients with long standing ulcerative colitis, a past history of adenoma of the colon or colon cancer, female genital cancer and perhaps those with a strong family history of the disease.[3, 42, 122, 137, 237] This group should undergo radiography and/or colonoscopy every one or two years. In patients with ulcerative colitis multiple biopsies should be taken since the finding of dysplasia, despite a negative colonoscopic investigation, is an important indication of impending carcinoma. Moderate dysplasia is associated with a colorectal cancer risk of approximately 30% and severe dysplasia with a risk of 50%. The presence of dysplasia should be confirmed by repeat biopsy.[43, 126] Those individuals who are at average risk of developing a carcinoma are men and women over 40 years of age with no underlying disease, past history or family history of bowel disease. It is in this large group that controversy exists concerning the cost–benefit of screening programmes. It is impractical to use endoscopic methods for detection since patient compliance will be low. Most interest has, therefore, focused on the detection of occult blood in the stool. The development of the impregnated guaiac slide test with stabilized reagent and the use of three to six slides has improved their value.[82] Several studies have now been performed in which the positive rate of detection has varied between 1.5 and 6%. The greater the number of positive tests the less the predictive value for neoplasm. It seems, however, that approximately one-third of patients with positive tests will eventually prove to have a neoplasm, either a polyp or less frequently a carcinoma. The more slides taken the greater the sensitivity.[13, 82, 238, 240] The population to be tested should preferably be on a meat-free diet since an unrestricted diet is associated with a high rate of false positives and negatives.[81]

Measurement of CEA both in blood and bowel washings has been used for screening purposes but this antibody has been found to be unreliable due to its lack of specificity.[239] The development of monoclonal antibodies may prove to be a more specific serum marker of the disease.[120]

Screening programmes are capable of detecting a higher percentage of localized cancer.[236] At present approximately 40% of patients with colorectal cancer have localized disease and since the latter has a better prognosis than non-localized disease it follows that screening should improve the general outlook. An additional benefit may be derived from the identification and removal of premalignant lesions, i.e. polyps. No screening study has yet demonstrated either a benefit in survival for individual patients or a benefit in mortality for the population.

COMPLICATIONS

Intestinal obstruction
Carcinomas of the left colon are more likely to cause obstruction than those of the right. The intestinal lumen is gradually obliterated by a constricting neoplasm. More rarely the tumour may cause obstruction by acting as the apex for either an intussusception or volvulus. Most commonly the patient complains of increasing constipation and the obstruction is thus classified as acute on chronic. The constipation gradually becomes worse and abdominal distension supervenes which is associated with discomfort.

Although nausea is common vomiting rarely occurs until late in the clinical course.

Occasionally, the clinical presentation is more acute with no preceding symptoms. This picture is seen more commonly with growths of the right colon. The patient complains of sudden acute colicky abdominal pain, absolute constipation, vomiting and abdominal distension. On examination dehydration may be present, the abdomen will be distended and if the ileocaecal valve remains competent a closed loop obstruction will be present; the right colon, particularly the caecum, may be grossly distended and tender on palpation. Visible peristalsis may be present and the abdomen is tense on palpation, the degree depending on the extent of distension. Bowel sounds will usually be hyperactive and borborygmi may be heard without recourse to a stethoscope. Rectal examination reveals an empty rectum which is often 'ballooned'. Rarely, a rectal carcinoma which is the cause of the obstruction is palpable. Sigmoidoscopy may be useful since the lower edge of the tumour in the sigmoid colon or upper rectum may be visible.

Erect and supine X-rays of the abdomen will often show gross dilatation of the colon proximal to the tumour with multiple fluid levels (Figure 11.65). There may also be fluid levels in the small bowel if the ileocaecal valve is incompetent. If the valve remains competent the distension of the closed loop may become so enormous that the appearances may mimic those of a volvulus of the sigmoid colon.

Occasionally, if time allows, a Gastrografin enema may be obtained to establish the diagnosis (Figure 11.66). Barium should not be used in these circumstances, since its removal from the bowel may be difficult and time consuming and may impede the subsequent surgical procedure.

Perforation
The carcinoma may perforate and cause either a generalized faecal peritonitis or a localized abscess. The latter may mimic a diverticular abscess on the left side or an appendix abscess on the right side.[174] Perforation of the colon may occur at a site distant from the carcinoma as a consequence of intestinal obstruction. Classically this occurs in the caecum when a closed loop obstruction exists or it can occur closer to the tumour through a stercoral ulcer. Patients who present with faecal peritonitis are usually in a state of extremis with abdominal distension, diffuse tenderness, vomiting and gross electrolyte disturbance. In this situation mortality rates are high.

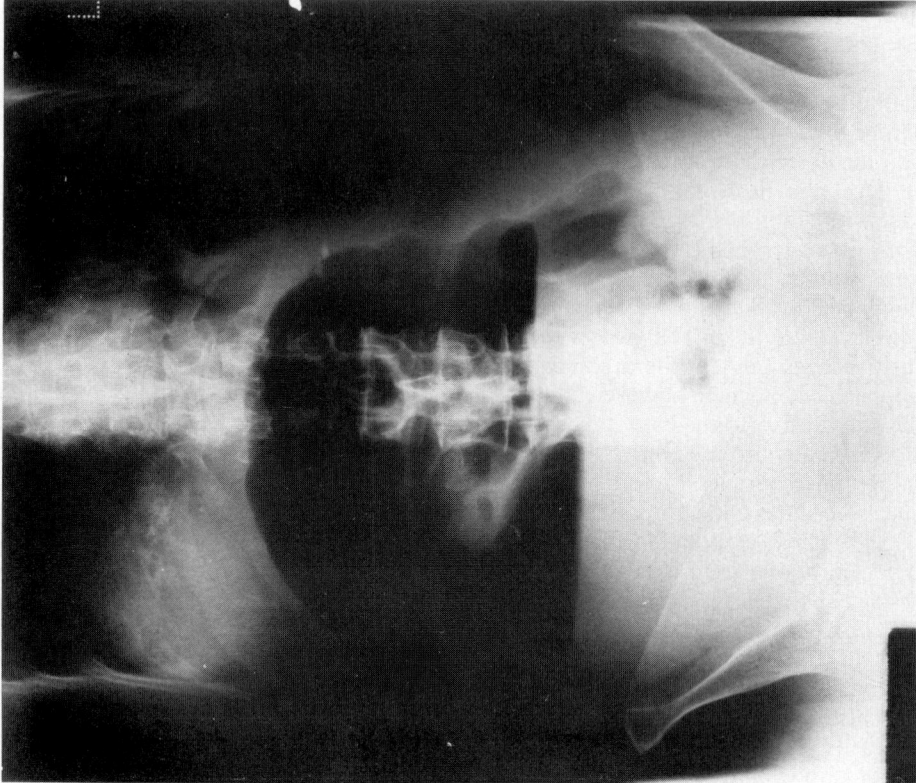

a

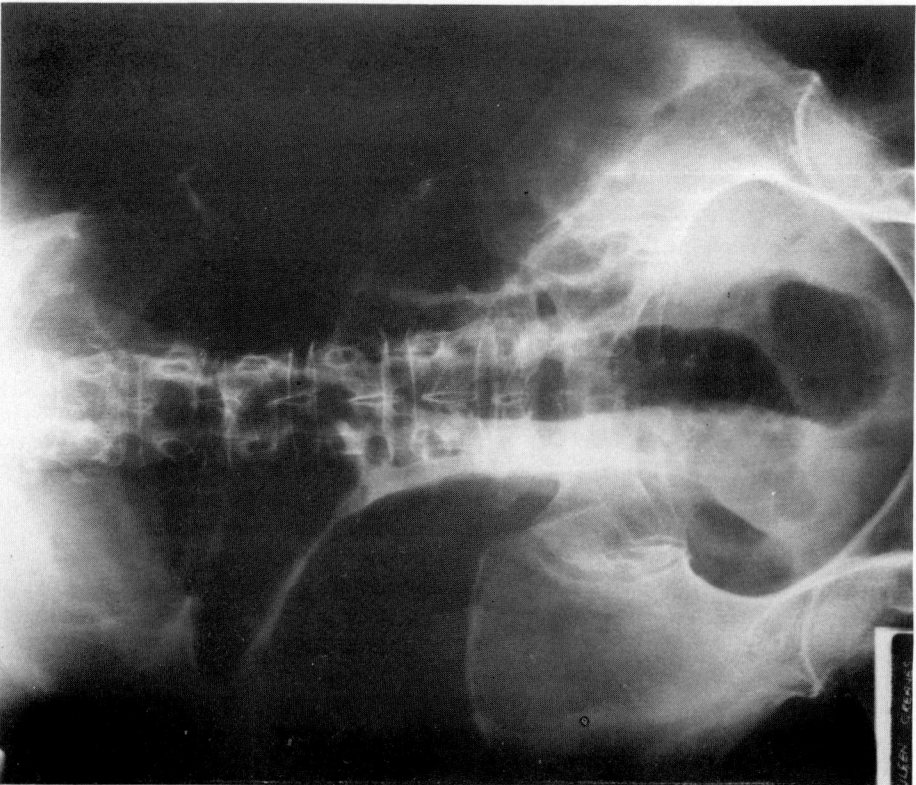

b

Fig. 11.65 (a) Supine and (b) erect straight abdominal X-rays of a patient with an obstructing carcinoma of the descending colon. The colon is grossly distended with multiple fluid levels.

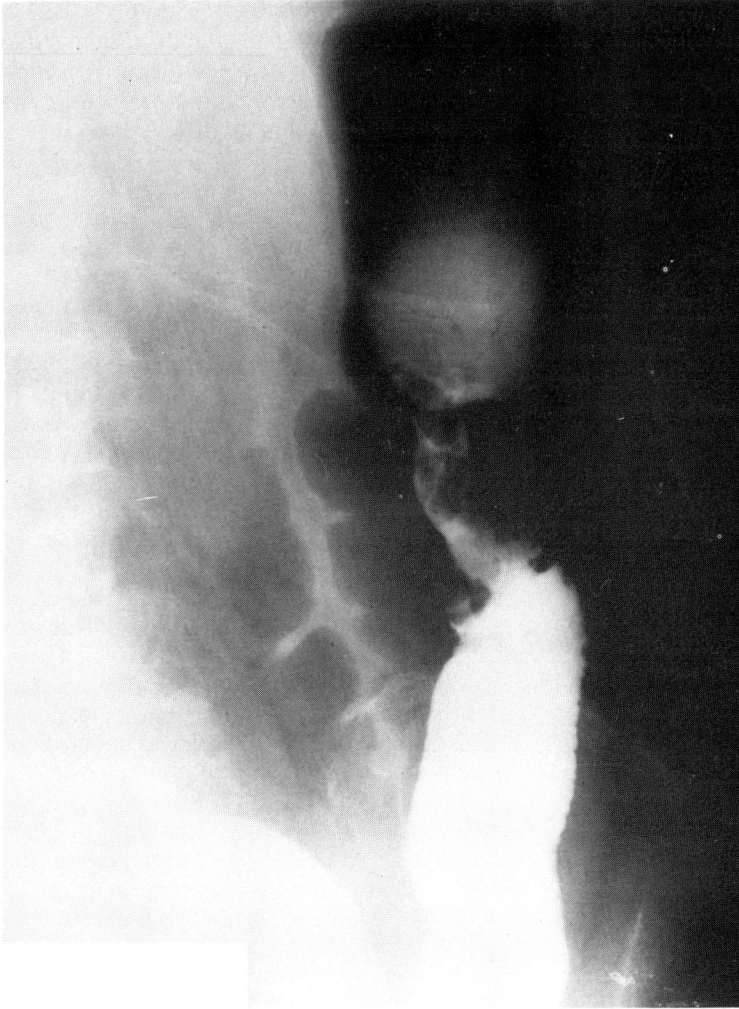

Fig. 11.66 Gastrografin enema (of patient in Figure 11.65) showing that the cause of the obstruction is a carcinoma in the descending colon.

Fistula formation

A carcinoma of colon or rectum may adhere to and eventually penetrate any abdominal organ. The bladder is most commonly involved and usually the carcinoma is in the sigmoid colon. The patient with a colovesical fistula may complain of pneumaturia but more often suffers from repeated bouts of cystitis. Men are affected more commonly than women. Diagnosis can be difficult since the fistula is rarely seen on cystoscopy. Carcinoma is second only to diverticular disease as the commonest cause of colovesical fistula.

A rectovaginal fistula may be the presenting feature of a rectal cancer. A fistula may also form between a transverse colon carcinoma and the stomach or duodenum. Rarely a tumour may present as an external spontaneous fistula, thus mimicking Crohn's disease. Initially a fistula may present as a subcutaneous abscess in the abdominal wall, the thigh or the perinephric region.[61, 141, 193]

Rarely, a caecal carcinoma obstructs the base of the appendix, and the patient presents with acute appendicitis.[58, 149] More than half of all intussusceptions of the large bowel in the adult are due to carcinoma.[189]

TREATMENT

Excision of the tumour should nearly always be attempted since even if the operation is palliative in nature, intestinal obstruction will be avoided and distressing symptoms alleviated. Many of these patients have coexistent medical problems which need treatment first.

Specific preoperative preparation

Until recently, sepsis has been a common problem. The primary source of infection is the endogenous bacteria in the bowel lumen. The bowel cannot be sterilized completely but a complete mechanical clearance of its contents is useful. The conventional method is a five-day course of purgatives, enemas and dietary restriction. More recently surgeons have practiced whole-gut irrigation, in which large volumes of a balanced electrolyte solution are given via a nasogastric tube until the fluid passed per rectum is clear. This method is quicker than a conventional preparation and produces better results.[24] Patients can avoid a nasogastric tube by drinking these solutions. These methods should not be used in the elderly or those with a history of cardiovascular or renal disease, or those who have a carcinoma which is causing obstruction.[99] Mannitol should not be used since it can produce explosive mixtures within the bowel.

The introduction of prophylactic antibiotic cover has reduced sepsis rates. Oral antibiotics which are not absorbed by the gut (e.g. neomycin, kanamycin or phthalylsulphathiazole) have some effect, but systemic antibiotics are of more value. A combination of antibiotics which are bactericidal to both aerobic and anaerobic organisms are most effective. Administration of either one dose with the premedication or three doses perioperatively reduces risks of drug resistance and side-effects whilst achieving maximum efficiency.[98, 117]

The nature of the surgery must be fully explained. This is particularly important if a colostomy is necessary. Patients who have needed a stoma often complain that they did not receive adequate counselling prior to surgery.[41] The best person to supply this information is either the stomatherapist or an experienced ward sister.

Principles and techniques of surgery

The colon. The type of operation depends on the site of the tumour. Since the lymphatic drainage accompanies the main blood vessels, the length of bowel resected is dependent on the extent of lymphatic clearance that is required. The aim of a radical operation is to remove the tumour with the whole of its appropriate lymphatic drainage. If, however, all tumour cannot be removed and a palliative procedure is planned it is only necessary to remove the minimum amount of tissue which will ensure relief of symptoms.

For cancer of the right colon (i.e. caecum, ascending colon, hepatic flexure and right half of the transverse colon, which are all supplied by

the superior mesenteric artery), resection involves ligation of the appropriate colic branches as close as possible to their origin from their parent vessel. The common types of resection are illustrated in Figure 11.67A, B, C.

For cancer of the left colon (i.e. the left half of the transverse colon, splenic flexure, descending and sigmoid colon), radical resection involves ligation of the appropriate colic branches of the inferior mesenteric artery (Figure 11.67D, E). Some surgeons believe that an even more radical excision is required for tumours of the left colon in which the inferior mesenteric artery is divided at its origin. The whole of the left colon is excised and an anastomosis is constructed between the distal transverse colon and upper rectum (Figure 11.67F). Colectomy with continuity restored by ileorectal anastomosis may be needed for multiple cancers or the presence of multiple polyps.

If the colonic tumour is invading or adherent to other organs (e.g. a loop of small intestine or uterus), as much of the adherent tissue as possible should be excised en bloc with the tumour. The adhesions are often inflammatory and not neoplastic and thus prognosis is better than anticipated.[29, 54, 112]

The rectum. There are two main types of operation for the treatment of carcinoma of the rectum: the abdomino-perineal excision of the rectum (APER) or one form of sphincter-saving resection (SSR). In all these operations the inferior mesenteric artery is divided as close to its origin as possible. In APER the whole of the rectum and sigmoid colon and their mesenteries are excised together with the anal sphincters, the ischiorectal fat and most of the levator ani muscles leaving the patient with a permanent colostomy (Figure 11.68). The procedure is usually conducted by two surgeons working simultaneously via the abdomen and perineum.

There are various types of sphincter-saving procedures but the principles are similar. The rectum containing the carcinoma is mobilized via the abdominal approach as for an APER. It is then divided at least 5 cm below the lower border of the cancer which is the margin usually recommended, although recent research suggests that this distance can safely be reduced.[79] Once the involved segment of bowel has been removed, an anastomosis between the anorectal stump and the colon, usually the descending part, is constructed. The anastomosis can usually be made via the abdominal approach using a one- or two-layered hand anastomosis. This procedure is referred to as an anterior

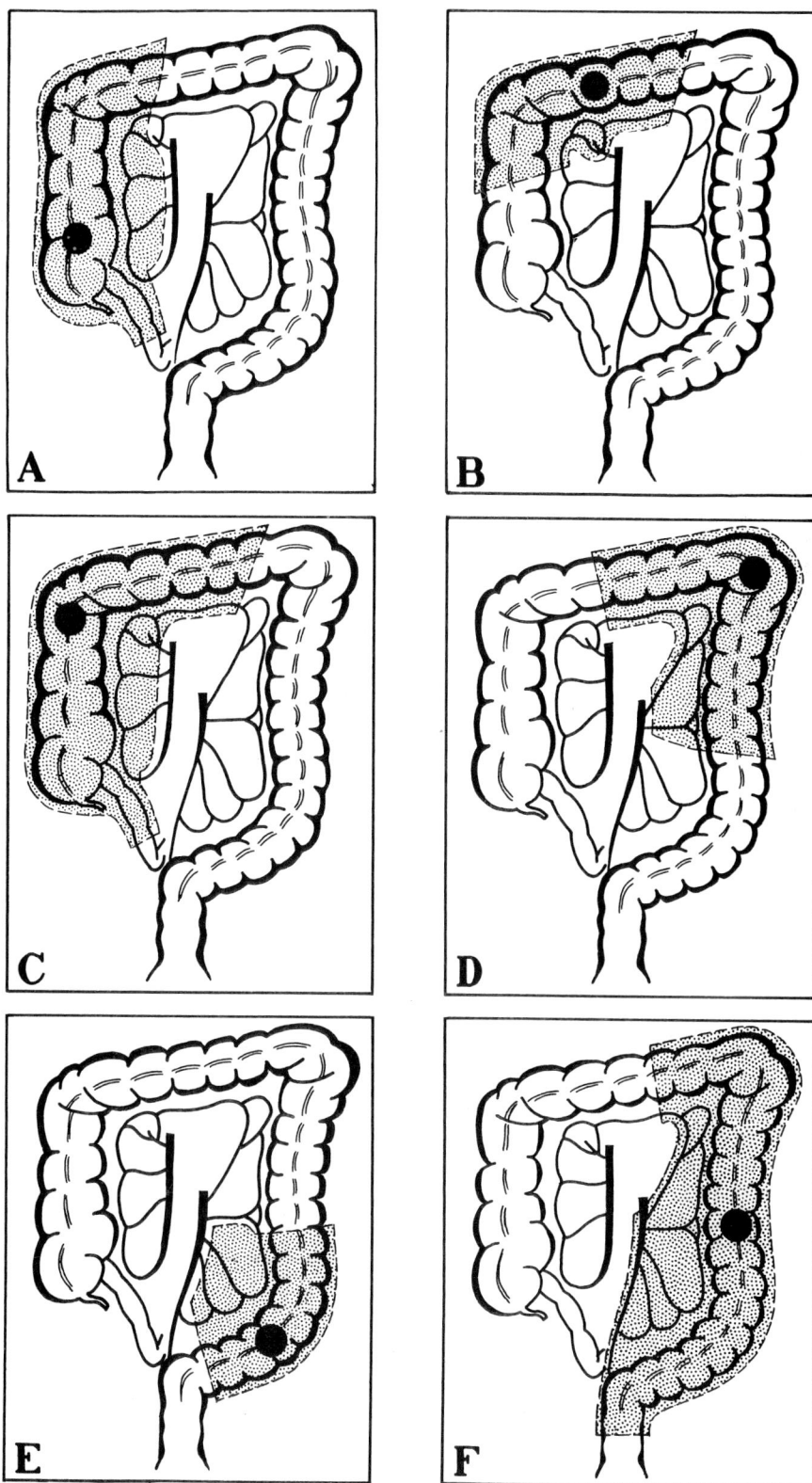

Fig. 11.67 Types of colonic resections. *A* Carcinoma of the caecum – right hemicolectomy; *B* Carcinoma of the transverse colon – transverse colectomy (this procedure is sometimes extended so as to include the splenic flexure); *C* Carcinoma of the ascending colon – extended right hemicolectomy; *D* Carcinoma of the splenic flexure – left hemicolectomy; *E* Carcinoma of the sigmoid colon – sigmoid colectomy; *F* Carcinoma of the descending colon – extended left hemicolectomy.

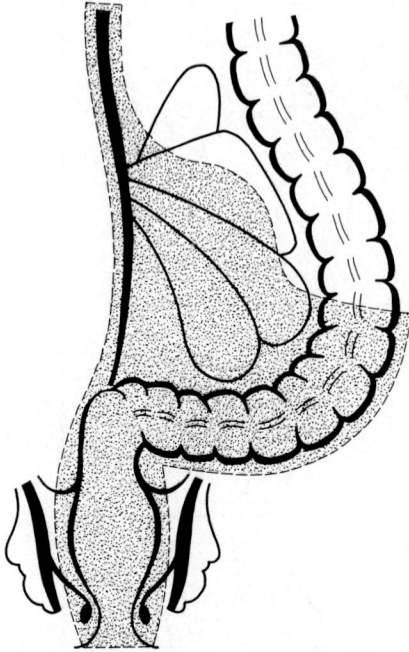

Fig. 11.68 Abdominoperineal resection. The structures within the shaded area are excised. The proximal colon is brought out in the left iliac fossa as an end colostomy.

resection. If the growth is too low or the pelvis too narrow, a conventional anterior resection cannot be performed. The simplest and most popular method to restore continuity is to use a stapling instrument or gun (Figure 11.69) of which there are two designs, one American (EEA),[182] the other Russian (SPTU).[59] The former is more popular since it utilizes two rows of staples and is supplied with a preloaded head. An abdominosacral operation can be used for a low anastomosis.[130] Access to the distal anorectum is achieved via the trans-sacral approach with the patient in the prone position (Figure 11.70). Another variation is the abdomino-transanal technique[172] in which after rectal excision the colon is drawn down through the anal canal and anastomosed to it via the trans-anal route (Figure 11.71). These techniques are associated with complete continence,[95, 123, 131] although this may take up to 18 months to be achieved.[232] Older methods, such as the abdomino-anal pull-through method[39] in which the anorectum is everted and anastomosis constructed externally, are rarely used since they often result in poor anorectal control.

It is generally agreed that carcinomas of the upper third of the rectum (above 13 cm from the anal verge) should be treated by anterior resection. Most surgeons also agree that tumours whose lower edge is 5 cm or less from the anal verge, as measured by sigmoidoscopy, should undergo APER with a permanent colostomy. The treatment of lesions between these two levels is debated. The new sphincter saving techniques result in a better quality of life than can be achieved after APER.[230] Apart from numerous psychosocial problems related to the colostomy,[41] patients who have undergone APER have a high incidence of bladder and sexual disturbances.[67, 230, 233] Since, however, less tissue is excised during an SSR than during an APER the fear is that recurrence and survival rates will be compromised. There is the theoretical risk

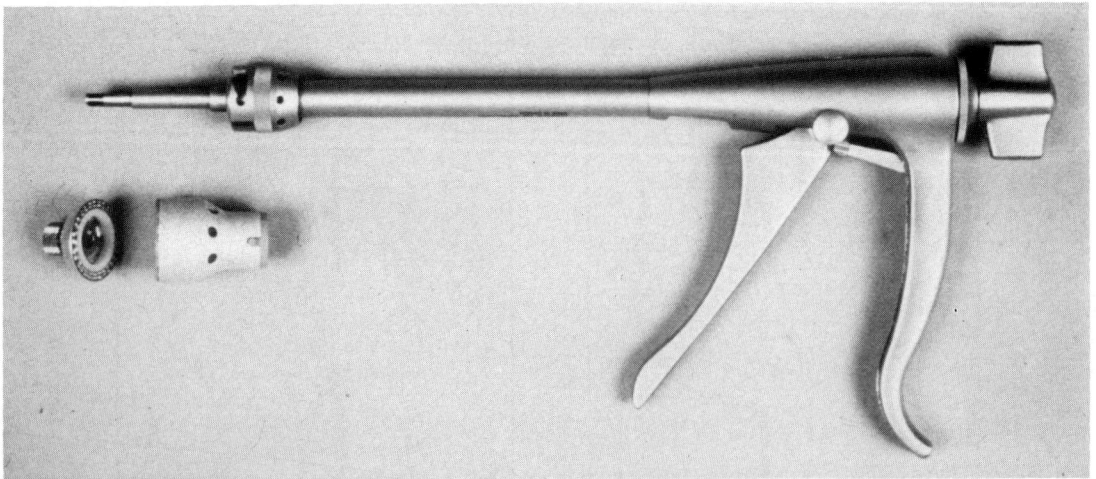

a

Fig. 11.69 (a) The American stapling 'gun' (EEA); (b) Anterior resection performed with the gun. The two ends of bowel, rectal stump and descending colon are racked together and when the gun is fired a circular knife cuts through the infolded bowel contained in the purse-string suture. Simultaneously the two ends of bowel are stapled together in two layers.

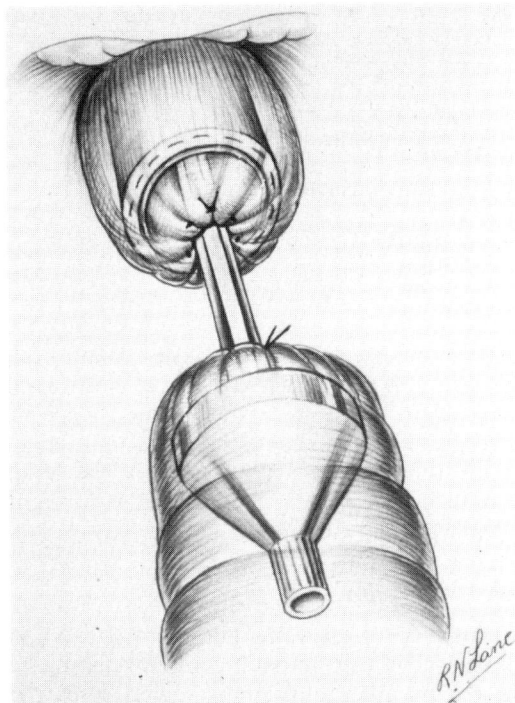

b

Fig. 11.69 (b)

that insufficient microscopic distal spread will be removed, and anastomotic recurrence will increase with transection of the rectum with a margin of clearance of less than the recommended 5 cm. Retrospective studies, however, suggest that survival and recurrence rates for carcinoma of the middle third of the rectum treated by either type of operation are similar.[145, 164, 231]

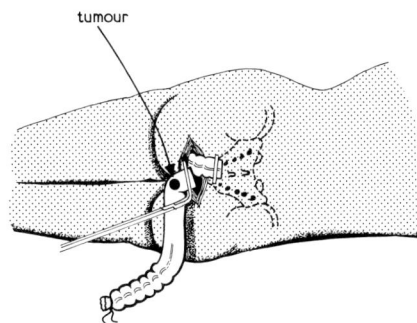

Fig. 11.70 Abdomino-trans-sacral anastomosis. The rectum and colon are mobilized via the abdomen and the trans-sacral route. After the tumour-bearing area has been resected, anastomosis is performed via the trans-sacral route.

Similarly, the incidence of local recurrence is not influenced by the margin of clearance.[176, 234]

If the tumour is well localized and mobile, and if it can be excised with a clearance of not less than 2 to 3 cm but preferably 5 cm, most surgeons perform a sphincter-saving procedure – an anterior resection with either hand or stapled anastomosis. When the tumour is more extensive, or is too low for either of these techniques, an APER is performed. In a few centres which have acquired special expertise, the ultralow lesions which are not accompanied by local spread are treated by either abdomino-transanal or abdomino-trans-sacral techniques.[97, 173]

Local treatment of rectal cancer. The techniques available for patients who are unfit for major surgery include electrocoagulation,[207] contact irradiation[171] or local excision.[34] These can relieve symptoms and are associated with very low mortality and morbidity rates.

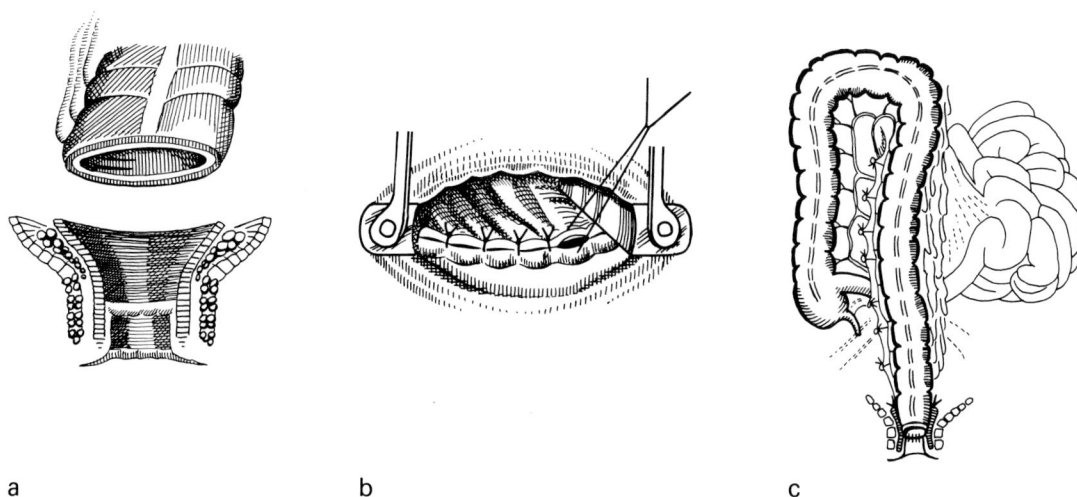

a   b   c

Fig. 11.71 After excision of the rectum and colon containing the tumour, the mucosa of the residual rectal stump is removed, and the colon brought down (a) and anastomosed to the anal mucosa (b) via the transanal route (c).

The Large Intestine

Occasionally, they can result in long-term cure, but there is no general support for their use as primary treatment as suggested by a few enthusiasts.[139]

Results of surgery

Carcinoma of colon. Over the last 30 to 40 years the proportion of colonic cancers amenable to resection has increased and the operative mortality rate has fallen, now being 70 to 80% and 5 to 10%, respectively. The overall crude five-year survival rate for patients treated by surgery in most centres ranges from 50% to 70%.[74, 84, 109, 181, 217] If all patients are included, the five-year survival rate is much lower (20 to 25% in the UK).[196, 223]

A number of factors influences the results of operative treatment. The most important is the extent of spread. Thus, the corrected five-year survival for Dukes' C lesions is 30 to 40% whereas that for Dukes' A and B lesions is 70 to 80%.[94] Younger patients may have a worse prognosis than older patients, and the shorter the history the worse the outlook.[32, 196] The development of complications, particularly perforation or acute obstruction, considerably decreases survival rates.[73, 110]

Carcinoma of rectum. The results of surgery for rectal carcinoma are similar to those described for colonic carcinoma. In specialized centres the proportion of tumours amenable to resection may be as high as 90%, with an operative mortality of approximately 5%.[134] The rate is much lower in other centres so that survival rates are worse (Table 11.15). The most obvious reason for this difference is the higher proportion of advanced and emergency cases which present to

Table 11.16 Crude 5-year survival rates after rectal excision for carcinoma according to Dukes' stage.

	A (%)	B (%)	C (%)
Whittaker and Goligher (1976)[229]	80	62	33
Slanetz, Herter and Grinnell (1972)[195]	84	55	35
Dukes (1957)[50] Men	80	61	26
Women	82	72	29

district general hospitals. The relationship between Dukes' stage and survival is shown in Table 11.16. Other factors which have a specific effect on survival include: the degree of mobility of the tumour;[90, 243] the height of the lesion from the anal verge;[75, 201] and females do slightly less well than men.[50, 144]

Adjuvant therapy

Radiotherapy. Adjuvant radiotherapy has been applied chiefly to patients with carcinomas of the rectum and rectosigmoid region. It may be given either before or after operation. Preoperative therapy aims to decrease the number of viable tumour cells to reduce the risk of dissemination at surgery. It may also enhance the immune response.[33] Preoperative therapy may be given in a low dose which allows the surgeon to proceed with the operation quickly and without prejudice to safety. A larger dose (about 60% of that normally used for curative radiotherapy) can be given over a three- to six-week period. This technique increases the risk of damage to other organs and delays surgery. High-dose radiation has been used particularly for fixed or partially fixed tumours.

Table 11.15 Absolute survival rate of patients with carcinoma of rectum.

Author	No. of cases	Submitted to rectal excision	Surviving 5 years or more (%)	Corrected 5-year survival rate (%)
Birmingham Regional Cancer Registry (1950–1961)[196]	5800	2900 (50%)	22	29
Bristol Cancer Registry (1961–1964)[223]	1346	857 (65%)	23	—
Leeds General Infirmary (1955–1965)[229]	550	498 (98.5%)	40	45
St Mark's Hospital (1948–1972)[134]	3163	2948 (93.2%)	47.1	56.6

3

Retrospective studies of the preoperative regimen used approximately 2000 rad (20 Gy) over 10 days and showed some benefit.[202] Carefully controlled prospective clinical trials have been unable to demonstrate a statistically significant improvement in survival[100, 185, 203] although in some series, Dukes' C lesions do better with irradiation therapy. All workers agree that irradiation treatment reduces the degree of local infiltration of tumours and the probability of regional lymph node involvement.

Postoperative radiotherapy has the advantage that it can be given after the extent of spread has been accurately defined and can be limited to those at high risk for developing recurrence. Several studies have suggested that when used in this way radiotherapy may be beneficial but there is considerable morbidity.[69, 146]

Chemotherapy. Patients with Dukes' A lesions have an excellent prognosis after resection and are unlikely to be helped by adjuvant chemotherapy. The prognosis of patients with obvious metastatic disease at the time of surgery is unlikely to be improved by adjuvant therapy. On the other hand patients with Dukes' B and C lesions who have undergone 'curative' resection might benefit most. Many of these patients will have circulating cancer cells which may develop into metastases. Indeed some of these patients will already have micrometastases undetected at operation which will lead to a fatal outcome.[63] Adjuvant therapy may intervene in this sequence of events and improve prognosis. There is little evidence so far to show that survival is prolonged in patients without metastases treated by adjuvant chemotherapy. Various drugs such as thiotepa[108] and 5-fluoro-2'-deoxyuridine (FUDR)[51] have been used but only 5-fluorouracil (5-FU) has been comprehensively investigated in randomized controlled trials. Although there are retrospective data to suggest that when 5-FU is given systemically prognosis is improved,[128] prospective studies have not borne this out.[101, 102, 153] The intraluminal route of administration has also been studied, but although this method, in combination with systemic therapy, might be beneficial in patients with Dukes' C lesions,[88] no study has demonstrated a significantly superior overall survival rate.[125] These disappointing results have led to studies using combinations of systemic agents. The most common additional agent is methyl-CCNU (semustine)[118] but mitomycin[20] is also being used. It is too early to draw any firm conclusions from these studies.

The most promising technique using adjuvant chemotherapy so far is perfusion of the liver via the portal vein with 5-FU in patients without macroscopic hepatic metastases. The idea is that since tumour cells reach the liver via the portal vein,[1, 211] perfusion with cytotoxic therapy will prevent the formation of micrometastases. The early results of this technique are encouraging[212] but longer follow up is required.

SURVEILLANCE

Follow up should be regular, at least annually, but more frequent in the first three years. Symptoms of general malaise, weight loss, anorexia, abdominal pain, alteration in bowel habit, bleeding or the passage of mucus, either per rectum or per colostomy, are suggestive of recurrence or the development of a metachronous tumour.[18, 76] Physical examination may reveal an abdominal mass, ascites, hepatomegaly or perineal nodules. Rectal and sigmoidoscopic examinations may demonstrate local recurrence either at the suture line or extrarectally. Metastatic disease may be detected on barium enema, colonoscopy, ultrasound or CT scan. However, by the time clinical features are apparent the disease is widely disseminated. More sophisticated techniques may detect recurrence at an earlier stage. Recent reports suggest that the CT scan may be very accurate in the detection of hepatic and pelvic recurrence.[63, 89, 111] Ultrasound may also have a role to play.

Elevated levels of CEA, particularly in combination with abnormal liver function tests, are indicative of widespread metastases,[31] but are not a reliable indicator of early recurrence,[27, 154] although some surgeons still regard a rise in CEA as an indication for a second-look laparotomy.[142]

Surgical cure of the patient with recurrence, no matter how early it is detected, is unlikely.[9] Early detection may, however, lead to more effective palliation.

Rare malignant tumours

Carcinoid

Carcinoid tumour, although only second in frequency to adenocarcinoma, is a rare tumour of the large bowel and only a proportion of these tumours are malignant. They are, like carcinoid tumours elsewhere, derived from the Kulchitsky cells of the crypts of Lieberkühn. Although these cells have the propensity to secrete 5-hydroxytryptamine, carcinoid tumours of the large bowel, even when accompanied by multiple hepatic metastases, are not usually associated with hypersecretion.[70, 175]

In their early stage they form polyps, often of a yellowish hue, which enlarge and become ulcerated. They are similar in appearance to adenocarcinomas.

Carcinoid tumours of the colon are more likely to be malignant than those of the rectum.[70, 206] The clinical presentation and treatment is identical to that of adenocarcinoma but the prognosis is often better.[169]

Primary malignant lymphoma

This tumour can occur in the large bowel but Goligher reported only two cases in a clinical experience of 1500 cases of malignant tumours.[79] Of 79 primary lymphomas in the gastrointestinal tract, Allen *et al.*[2] found that nine were in the colon or rectum. They occur more commonly in the caecum than the left colon or rectum[161] and this distribution is probably due to spread into the caecum from tumours arising in the terminal ileum. Primary lymphoma may complicate ulcerative colitis.[184] Their degree of malignancy depends on their cell type. All varieties of non-Hodgkin's lymphoma have been described. Classification is often difficult because of distortion resulting from ulceration and infection. Clinical presentation is usually indistinguishable from that of an adenocarcinoma. Although surgical excision is required, adjuvant chemotherapy and/or radiotherapy may be of particular benefit. The prognosis is rather better than adenocarcinoma.[244]

Secondary lymphoma

The large intestine may be infiltrated secondarily, the colon being more frequently involved than the rectum. The patient usually has obvious evidence of systemic disease.

Malignant lymphomatous polyposis

In this condition, the gastrointestinal tract is diffusely involved with polypoid thickening of the mucosa.[93, 193] Although the polyps may be pedunculated, the appearance is usually one of diffuse mucosal nodularity. The patients present with diarrhoea and malabsorption due to small bowel involvement. Splenomegaly and generalized lymphadenopathy are often present. The disease surprisingly tends to run a chronic course.

Leiomyosarcoma

These tumours originate from the muscle coat and project either into the bowel lumen or on the external surface of the bowel. They are usually large, rubbery, lobulated tumours. In about half of them, the overlying mucosa remains intact. The degree of differentiation varies and the pathologist may have difficulty in distinguishing between benign and malignant tumours.[163] They spread both by direct extension or by the blood stream. Lymphatic spread occurs rarely.[215] They are sited more frequently in the rectum than in the colon.[4] Symptoms are usually indistinguishable from other tumours although massive haemorrhage can occasionally occur.[190] Such a tumour should be suspected if on rectal or endoscopic examination the mucosa is intact. Although local excision has been attempted, the tumour usually recurs and a more radical procedure is required. Postoperative radiotherapy may be beneficial.

Fibrosarcoma, rhabdomyosarcoma, haemangiopericytoma, plasmacytoma and endothelioma[157, 165, 168, 170, 206] have all been reported.[157, 165, 168, 170, 206] Malignant melanoma and squamous cell carcinoma are tumours which invariably occur in the anorectal region and are described in detail elsewhere.

ACKNOWLEDGEMENTS

I would like to express my sincere thanks to the following who helped in the preparation of this section: Miss Ruth Bailey, Department of Medical Illustration; Mr Peter Hargreaves, Department of Photography; and Mrs Lorna McQuade, Department of Surgery, Leeds General Infirmary. Dr K. Simkins kindly allowed me access to his X-ray collection.

REFERENCES

1   Ackerman, N. B. (1972) Alteration of intrahepatic circulation due to increased tumour growth. *Proceedings of the VII Congress European Society Experimental Surgery*, 182.

2   Allen, A. W., Donaldson, G., Sniffen, R. C. & Goodale, F., Jr (1954) Primary malignant lymphoma of the gastrointestinal tract. *Annals of Surgery*, **140**, 428–433.

3   Anderson, D. E. & Ramsdahl, M. M. (1977) Family history: a criteria for selective screening. In *Progress in Cancer Research and Therapy. Genetics of Human Cancer* (Ed.) Mulvihill, J. J., Miller, R. W. & Fraumeni, J. F., Jr Volume 3. New York: Raven Press.

4   Anderson, P. A., Dockerty, M. B. & Buie, L. A. (1950) Myomatous tumours of the rectum (leiomyomas and myosarcomas). *Surgery*, **68**, 642–647.

5   Armstrong, B. K. & Doll, R. (1975) Environmental factors and cancer incidence and mortality in different countries with special reference to dietary practices. *International Journal of Cancer*, **15**, 167–172.

6   Astler, V. B. & Coller, F. A. (1954) The prognostic significance of direct extension of carcinoma of the colon and rectum. *Annals of Surgery*, **139**, 846–851.

7   Bacon, H. E. & Jackson, C. C. (1953) Visceral metastases from carcinoma of the distal colon and rectum. *Surgery*, **33**, 495–500.

8 Barringer, P. L., Dockerty, M. B., Waugh, J. M. & Bargen, J. A. (1954) Carcinoma of the large intestine: a new approach to the study of venous spread. *Surgery, Gynecology and Obstetrics*, **98**, 62–67.

9 Beart, R. W. & O'Connell, M. J. (1983) Post operative follow up of patients with carcinoma of the colon. *Mayo Clinic Proceedings*, **58**, 361–363.

10 Beart, R. W., Van Heerden, J. A. & Beahrs, O. H. (1978) Evolution in the pathologic staging of carcinoma of the colon. *Surgery, Gynecology and Obstetrics*, **146**, 257–262.

11 Black, W. A. & Waugh, J. M. (1948) The intramural extension of carcinoma of the descending colon, sigmoid and rectosigmoid: a pathologic study. *Surgery, Gynecology and Obstetrics*, **87**, 457–464.

12 Blenkinsopp, W. K., Stewart Brown, S., Blesovsky, K. et al. (1981) Histopathology reporting in large bowel cancer. *Journal of Clinical Pathology*, **34**, 509–513.

13 Bond, J. H. & Gilbertson, V. A. (1977) Early detection of colonic carcinoma by mass screening for occult stool blood. Preliminary Report. *Gastroenterology*, **72**, A-8/1031.

14 Breslow, N. E. & Enström, J. E. (1974) Geographic correlations between cancer mortality rates and alcohol–tobacco consumption in the United States. *Journal of the National Cancer Institute*, **53**, 631–639.

15 Burkitt, D. P. (1971) Epidemiology of cancer of the colon and rectum. *Cancer*, **28**, 3–13.

16 Burkitt, D. P., Walker, A. R. P. & Painter, N. S. (1972) Effect of dietary fibre on stools and transit times and its role in the causation of diseases. *Lancet*, **ii**, 1408–1411.

17 Bussey, H. J. R. (1975) Familial Polyposis Coli. Baltimore and London: John Hopkins University Press.

18 Bussey, H. J. R., Wallace, M. H. & Morson, B. C. (1967) Metachronous carcinoma of the large intestine and intestinal polyps. *Proceedings of the Royal Society of Medicine*, **60**, 208–213.

19 Carroll, S. E. (1963) The prognostic significance of gross venous invasion in carcinoma of the rectum. *Canadian Journal of Surgery*, **6**, 281–286.

20 Carter, S. K. & Friedman, M. (1974) Integration of chemotherapy into combined modality treatment of solid tumours. II. Large bowel carcinoma. *Cancer Treatment Reviews*, **1**, 111–115.

21 Castleman, B. & Krickstein, H. I. (1962) Do adenomatous polyps of the colon become malignant? *New England Journal of Medicine*, **267**, 469–474.

22 Cheng Ming-Chai, Chuang Chi Yuen, Chang Pei-Yu & Hu Jen-Chun (1980) Evolution of colo-rectal cancer in schistosomiasis. *Cancer*, **46**, 1661–1675.

23 Cheng Ming Chai, Chuang Chi Yuen, Wang Fu Pen et al. (1981) Colo-rectal cancer and schistosomiasis. *Lancet*, **ii**, 971–973.

24 Chung, R. S., Gurll, N. J. & Berglund, E. M. (1979) A controlled clinical trial of whole gut lavage as a method of bowel preparation for colonic operations. *American Journal of Surgery*, **137**, 79–81.

25 Cleave, T. L. (1974) *The Saccharine Disease*. Bristol: Wright.

26 Clemmesen, J. (1977) Statistical studies in the aetiology of malignant neoplasms. Volume V. *Trends and Risks in Denmark 1943–72.* Supplement 261. *Acta Pathologica, Microbiologica, et Immunologica Scandinavica*, Copenhagen: Munksgaard.

27 Cohen, A. M. & Wood, W. C. (1979) Carcinoembryonic antigen levels as an indicator for re-operation in patients with carcinoma of the colon and rectum. *Surgery, Gynecology and Obstetrics*, **149**, 22–27.

28 Cole, W. H., Packard, D. & Southwick, H. W. (1954) Carcinoma of the colon with special reference to prevention of recurrence. *Journal of the American Medical Association*, **155**, 1549–1554.

29 Cooke, R. V. (1956) Advanced carcinoma of the colon with emphasis on the inflammatory factor. *Annals of the Royal College of Surgeons of England*, **18**, 46–51.

30 Cooley, R. N., Agnew, C. H. & Rios, G. (1960) Diagnostic accuracy of the barium enema study in carcinoma of the colon and rectum. *American Journal of Roentgenology*, **84**, 31–35.

31 Cooper, E. H., Turner, R., Steele, L. et al. (1975) The contribution of serum enzymes and carcinoembryonic antigen to the early diagnosis of metastatic ano-rectal cancer. *British Journal of Cancer*, **31**, 111–116.

32 Copeland, E. M., Miller, L. D. & Jones, R. S. (1969) Prognostic factors in carcinoma of the colon and rectum. *Diseases of the Colon and Rectum*, **10**, 415–420.

33 Crile, G., Jr & Deodhar, S. D. (1971) Role of preoperative irradiation in prolonging concomitant immunity and preventing metastases in mice. *Cancer*, **27**, 629–634.

34 Cripps, W. H. (1880) *Cancer of the Rectum*. London: J. & A. Churchill.

35 Cripps, W. H. (1882) *Transactions of the Pathological Society (London)*, **33**, 165–170.

36 Crowther, J. S., Drasar, B. J., Hill, M. J. et al. (1976) Faecal steroids and bacteria and large bowel cancer in Hong Kong by socioeconomic groups. *British Journal of Cancer*, **34**, 191–196.

37 Cummings, J. H. (1983) *Recent Advances in Gastroenterology No. 5* (Ed.) Bouchier, I. A. D. Edinburgh, London, Melbourne & New York: Churchill Livingstone.

38 Cummings, J. H. (1978) Influence of diets high and low in animal fat on bowel habit in gastrointestinal transit time, faecal microflora, bile acid and fat excretion. *Journal of Clinical Investigation*, **61**, 953–958.

39 Cutait, D. E. & Figlioni, F. J. (1961) A new method of colo-rectal anastomosis in abdominoperineal resection. *Diseases of the Colon and Rectum*, **4**, 335–340.

40 Dales, L. G., Friedman, G. D., Ury, H. K. et al. (1978) A case control study of relationships of diet and other traits to colorectal cancer in American Blacks. *American Journal of Epidemiology*, **109**(2), 132–144.

41 Devlin, H. B., Plant, J. A. & Griffen, M. (1971) Aftermath of surgery for ano-rectal cancer. *British Medical Journal*, **iii**, 413–418.

42 Devroede, G. (1980) Risk of cancer in inflammatory bowel disease. In *Colo-rectal Cancer: Epidemiology and Screening. Progress in Cancer Research* (Ed.) Winawer, S. J., Sherlock, P. & Shottenfeld, D. New York: Raven Press.

43 Dobbins, W. O., III. & Appelman, H. D. (1980) Difficulties in interpretation of dysplasia. In *Colo-rectal Cancer: Epidemiology and Screening. Progress in Cancer Research* (Ed.) Winawer, S. J., Sherlock, P. & Shottenfeld, D. New York: Raven Press.

44 Dockerty, M. B. (1958) Pathologic aspects in the control of spread of colonic carcinoma. *Proceedings of the Staff Meetings of the Mayo Clinic*, **33**, 157–162.

45 Drasar, B. S. & Irving, D. (1973) Environmental factors and cancer of the colon and breast. *British Journal of Cancer*, **27**, 167–172.

46 Dukes, C. E. (1926) Simple tumours of the large intestine and their relation to cancer. *British Journal of Surgery*, **13**, 720–725.

47 Dukes, C. E. (1930) The spread of cancer of the rectum. *British Journal of Surgery*, **17**, 643–648.

48 Dukes, C. E. (1937) Histological grading of rectal cancer. *Proceedings of the Royal Society of Medicine*, **30**, 371–376.

49 Dukes, C. E. (1940) Cancer of the rectum; an analysis of 1000 cases. *Journal of Pathology and Bacteriology*, **50**, 527–532.

50 Dukes, C. E. (1957) Discussion on major surgery in carcinoma of the rectum, with or without colostomy, excluding the anal canal and including the rectosigmoid. *Proceedings of the Royal Society of Medicine*, **50**, 1031–1036.

51 Dwight, R. W., Humphreys, W. E., Higgins, G. A. & Keehn, R. J. (1973) FUDR as an adjuvant to surgery in cancer of the large bowel. *Journal of Surgical Oncology*, **5**, 243–248.

52 Ekelund, G. & Lindström, C. (1974) Histopathological analysis of benign polyps in patients with carcinoma of the colon and rectum. *Gut*, **15**, 654–659.

53 Ekelund, G., Lindström, C. & Rosengren, J. E. (1974) Appearances and growth of early carcinoma of the colon–rectum. *Acta Radiologica*, **15**, 670–679.

54 Ellis, H. (1971) Curative and palliative surgery in advanced carcinoma of the large bowel. *British Medical Journal*, **iii**, 291–296.

55 Engell, H. C. (1955) Cancer cells in the circulating blood: a clinical study on the occurrence of cancer cells in the peripheral blood and in venous blood draining the tumour area at operation. *Acta Chirurgica Scandinavica* (Supplement), 201.

56 Enström, J. E. (1975) Colo-rectal cancer and consumption of beef and fat. *British Journal of Cancer*, **32**, 432–437.

57 Enterline, H. T., Evans, G. W., Mercado-Lugo, R. *et al.* (1962) Malignant potential of adenomas of colon and rectum. *Journal of the American Medical Association*, **179**, 322–327.

58 Ewing, M. R. (1951) Inflammatory complications of cancer of the caecum and ascending colon. *Postgraduate Medical Journal*, **27**, 515–520.

59 Fain, S. N., Patin, C. S. & Morganstern, L. (1975) Use of mechanical suturing apparatus in low colo-rectal anastomosis. *Archives of Surgery*, **110**, 1079–1084.

60 Feingold, S. M., Sutter, V. L., Sugihara, P. T. *et al.* (1977) Faecal microbial flora in Seventh Day Adventist population and control subjects. *American Journal of Clinical Nutrition*, **30**, 1781–1786.

61 Feldman, M. A., Cotton, R. E. & Gray, M. W. (1968) Carcinoma of the colon presenting as left perinephric abscess. *British Journal of Surgery*, **55**, 21–26.

62 Ferguson, J. A. (1957) Management of villous tumours of the rectum. *Journal of the Kentucky Medical Association*, **55**, 996–1001.

63 Finlay, I. G., Meek, D. R., Gray, H. W. *et al.* (1982) Incidence and detection of occult hepatic metastases in colo-rectal carcinoma. *British Medical Journal*, **284**, 803–805.

64 Fisher, E. R. & Castro, A. F. (1953) Diffuse papillomatous polyps (villous tumours) of the colon and rectum. *American Journal of Surgery*, **85**, 146–151.

65 Fisher, E. R. & Turnbull, R. B., Jr (1952) Malignant polyps of rectum and sigmoid; therapy based on pathological considerations. *Surgery, Gynecology and Obstetrics*, **94**, 619–624.

66 Fisher, E. R. & Turnbull, R. B. (1955) The cytologic demonstration and significance of tumour cells in the mesenteric venous blood in patients with colo-rectal carcinoma. *Surgery, Gynecology and Obstetrics*, **100**, 102–107.

67 Fowler, J. W., Bremner, D. N. & Moffat, L. E. F. (1978) The incidence and consequences of damage to the parasympathetic nerve supply to the bladder after abdomino-perineal excision of the rectum for carcinoma. *British Journal of Urology*, **50**, 95–98.

68 Fraser, Sir John (1938) Malignant disease of the large intestine. *British Journal of Surgery*, **25**, 647–648.

69 Friedman, P., Park, W. C. & Afonya, I. I. (1978) Adjuvant radiation therapy in colo-rectal cancer. *American Journal of Surgery*, **135**, 512–517.

69a Frugmorgen, P. (1980) Colonoscopy. In *Endoscopy and Biopsy in Gastroenterology. Technique and Indications*. pp. 87–99. Berlin, Heidelberg & New York: Springer-Verlag.

70 Gabriel, W. B. & Morson, B. C. (1956) Carcinoid of rectum with lymphatic and liver metastases. *Proceedings of the Royal Society of Medicine*, **49**, 472–477.

71 Gabriel, W. B., Dukes, C. E. & Bussey, H. J. R. (1935) Lymphatic spread in cancer of the rectum. *British Journal of Surgery*, **23**, 395–400.

72 Gardner, E. G. (1951) A genetic and clinical study of intestinal polyposis, a predisposing factor for carcinoma of the colon and rectum. *American Journal of Human Genetics*, **3**, 167–172.

73 Gerber, A., Thompson, R. J., Reiswig, O. K. & Vannix, R. S. (1962) Experiences with primary resection for acute obstruction of the large intestine. *Surgery, Gynecology and Obstetrics*, **123**, 593–598.

74 Gilbertson, V. A. (1959) Adenocarcinoma of the large bowel: 1340 cases with 100 per cent follow up. *Surgery*, **46**, 1027–1032.

75 Gilchrist, R. K. & David, V. C. (1947) A consideration of pathological factors influencing 5-year survival in radical resection of the large bowel and rectum for carcinoma. *American Surgeon*, **126**, 421–426.

76 Ginzburg, L. & Dreiling, P. A. (1956) Successive independent (metachronous) carcinoma of the colon. *Annals of Surgery*, **143**, 117–119.

77 Goldberg, M. J., Smith, J. W. & Nicholls, R. L. (1977) Comparison of the faecal microflora of Seventh Day Adventists with individuals consuming a general diet. *Annals of Surgery*, **186**, 97–102.

78 Goligher, J. C. (1941) The operability of carcinoma of the rectum. *British Medical Journal*, **ii**, 393–398.

79 Goligher, J. C. (1980) *Surgery of the Anus, Rectum and Colon*. 4th Edition. London: Baillière Tindall.

80 Goligher, J. C., Dukes, C. E. & Bussey, H. J. R. (1951) Local recurrences after sphincter saving excisions for carcinoma of the rectum and rectosigmoid. *British Journal of Surgery*, **39**, 199–204.

81 Goulston, K. (1980) The role of diet in screening with faecal occult blood tests. In *Colo-rectal Cancer. Epidemiology and Screening. Progress in Cancer Research* (Ed.) Winawer, S. J., Sherlock, P. & Schottenfeld, D. New York: Raven Press.

82 Greegor, D. H. (1967) Diagnosis of large bowel cancer in the asymptomatic patient. *Journal of the American Medical Association*, **201**, 943–948.

83 Grinnell, R. S. (1939) The grading and prognosis of carcinoma of the colon and rectum. *Annals of Surgery*, **109**, 500–533.

84 Grinnell, R. S. (1953) Results in treatment of carcinoma of the colon and rectum. *Surgery, Gynecology and Obstetrics*, **96**, 31–36.

85 Grinnell, R. S. (1954) Distal intramural spread of carcinoma of the rectum and rectosigmoid. *Surgery, Gynecology and Obstetrics*, **99**, 421–430.

86 Grinnell, R. S. (1966) Lymphatic block with atypical retrograde lymphatic metastases and spread in carcinoma of the colon and rectum. *Annals of Surgery*, **163**, 272–277.

87 Grinnell, R. S. & Lane, N. (1958) Benign and malig-

nant adenomatous polyps and papillary adenomas of the colon and rectum. *International Abstracts of Surgery*, **106**, 519–524.

88 Grossi, C. E., Wolff, W. I., Nealand, T. F. *et al.* (1977) Intraluminal fluorouracil chemotherapy adjuvant to surgical procedure for resectable carcinoma of the colon and rectum. *Surgery, Gynecology and Obstetrics*, **145**, 549–554.

89 Guialdi, G. F., Poppalardo, G., Biase, C. D. & Pitasi, F. (1982) The use of computerised tomography in the study of recurrent pelvic malignancy after surgical treatment of the rectum. *Italian Journal of Surgical Sciences*, **12**, 33–38.

90 Habib, N. A., Peck, M. A., Sawyer, C. N. *et al.* (1983) Does fixity affect prognosis in colo-rectal tumours? *British Journal of Surgery*, **70**, 423–424.

91 Haenszel, W. & Carrea, P. (1971) Cancer of the colon and rectum and adenomatous polyps. *Cancer*, **28**, 14–24.

92 Haenszel, W., Berg, J. W., Segi, M. *et al.* (1973) Large bowel cancer in Hawaiian Japanese. *Journal of the National Cancer Institute*, **51**, 1765–1779.

93 Halkin, H., Meytes, D., Militeanu, J. & Ramot, B. (1973) Multiple lymphomatous polyposis of the gastrointestinal tract. *Israel Journal of Medical Sciences*, **9**, 648–653.

94 Hawley, P. R. (1981) quoted by Goligher, J. C. In *Results of Operations in Large Bowel Cancer* (Ed.) De Casse, J. J. Edinburgh: Churchill Livingstone.

95 Heald, R. J. (1980) Towards fewer colostomies – the impact of circular stapling devices in the surgery of rectal cancer in a district hospital. *British Journal of Surgery*, **60**, 198–208.

96 Heald, R. J. & Bussey, H. J. R. (1975) Clinical experience at St Mark's Hospital with multiple synchronous cancers of the colon and rectum. *Diseases of the Colon and Rectum*, **18**, 6–11.

97 Heald, R. J. & Leicester, R. J. (1981) The low stapled anastomosis. *British Journal of Surgery*, **68**, 333–337.

98 Herter, F. P. (1972) Preparation of the bowel for surgery. *Surgical Clinics of North America*, **52**, 859–870.

99 Hewitt, J., Rigby, J., Reeve, J. & Cox, A. G. (1973) Whole gut irrigation in preparation for large bowel surgery. *Lancet*, **iii**, 337–340.

100 Higgins, G. A., Jr (1978) The pros and cons of irradiation treatment of colo-rectal cancer. In *Surgery Annual* (Ed.) Nyhus, L. M. New York: Appleton-Century-Crofts.

101 Higgins, G. A., Dwight, R. W., Smith, J. V. & Keehn, R. (1971) Fluorouracil as an adjuvant to surgery in carcinoma of the colon. *Archives of Surgery*, **102**, 339–344.

102 Higgins, G. A., Humphrey, E., Juler, G. L. *et al.* (1976) Adjuvant chemotherapy in the treatment of large bowel cancer. *Cancer*, **38**, 1461–1466.

103 Hill, M. J. (1975) The role of colon anaerobes in the metabolism of bile acids and steroids and its relation to colon cancer. *Cancer*, **36**, 2387–2400.

104 Hill, M. J. (1981) Metabolic epidemiology of large bowel cancer. In *Gastrointestinal Cancer* (Ed.) De Cosse, J. & Sherlock, P. pp. 187–226. The Hague: Martinus Nijhoff.

105 Hill, M. J. (1983) Bile bacteria and bowel cancer. *Gut*, **24**, 871–875.

106 Hill, M. J. & Aries, V. C. (1971) Faecal steroid composition and its relationship to cancer of the large bowel. *Journal of Pathology*, **104**, 129–134.

107 Hill, M. J., Drasar, B. S., Williams, R. E. *et al.* (1971) Faecal bile acids and clostridia in patients with cancer of the large bowel. *Lancet*, **i**, 95–100.

108 Holden, W. D., Dixon, W. J. & Kuzma, J. W. (1967) The use of this topic as an adjuvant to the surgical treatment of colo-rectal carcinoma. *Annals of Surgery*, **65**, 481–486.

109 Hughes, E. S. R. (1966) Carcinoma of the right colon, upper left colon and sigmoid colon. *Australian and New Zealand Journal of Surgery*, **35**, 183–188.

110 Irvin, T. T. & Greaney, M. G. (1977) The treatment of colonic cancer presenting with intestinal obstruction. *British Journal of Surgery*, **64**, 741–746.

111 James, R. D., Johnson, R. J., Eddleston, B. *et al.* (1983) Prognostic factors in locally recurrent rectal carcinoma treated by radiotherapy. *British Journal of Surgery*, **70**, 468–472.

112 Jensen, H. E., Balslev, I. & Nielsen, J. (1970) Extensive surgery in treatment of carcinoma of the colon. *Acta Chirurgica Scandinavica*, **136**, 431–436.

113 Jensen, O. M. (1979) Cancer morbidity and causes of death among Danish brewery workers. *International Journal of Cancer*, **23**, 454–463.

114 Jensen, O. M. & MacLennan, R. (1979) Dietary factors and colo-rectal cancer in Scandinavia. *Israel Journal of Medical Sciences*, **15**, 329–334.

115 Jensen, O. M., Masbech, P., Salaspuro, M. & Ihumaki, T. (1974) A comparative study of the diagnostic basis for cancer of the colon and cancer of the rectum in Denmark and Finland. *International Journal of Epidemiology*, **3**, 183–186.

116 Judd, E. S. (1924) A consideration of lesions of the colon treated surgically. *5th Medical Journal of Nashville*, **17**, 75–80.

117 Keighley, M. R. B. (1977) Prevention of wound sepsis in gastrointestinal surgery. *British Journal of Surgery*, **64**, 315–340.

118 Killen, J. Y., Holyoke, E. D., Moertel, C. G. *et al.* (1981) Adjuvant therapy of adenocarcinoma of the colon following clinically curative resection: an interim report from the Gastrointestinal Tumour Study Group. In *Adjuvant Therapy of Cancer III* (Ed.) Jones, E. & Solman, S. E. New York: Grune & Stratton.

119 Kirklin, J. W., Dockerty, M. B. & Waugh, J. M. (1949) The role of peritoneal reflection in the prognosis of carcinoma of the rectum and sigmoid colon. *Surgery, Gynecology and Obstetrics*, **88**, 326–331.

120 Koprowski, H., Herlyn, M. & Steplewski, Z. (1981) Specific antigen in serum in patients with colon carcinoma. *Science*, **212**, 53–55.

121 Korte, W. (1900) Erfahrungen uber die operative Behandlung der malignen Dickdarm-Geschwulste. *Archiv. für Klinische Chirurgie*, **61**, 403–408.

122 Kussin, S. Z., Lipkin, M. & Winawer, S. J. (1979) Inherited colon cancer: clinical implications. State of the art. *American Journal of Gastroenterology*, **72**, 448–453.

123 Lane, R. H. S. & Parks, A. G. (1977) Function of the anal sphincter following colo-anal anastomosis. *British Journal of Surgery*, **64**, 596–597.

124 Lauer, S. D., Carlson, H. C. & Wollaeger, E. E. (1965) Accuracy of roentgenologic examination in detecting carcinoma of the colon. *Diseases of the Colon and Rectum*, **8**, 190–195.

125 Lawrence, W., Terz, J. J., Horsley, S. *et al.* (1975) Chemotherapy as an adjuvant to surgery for colo-rectal cancer. *Annals of Surgery*, **181**, 616–621.

126 Lennard-Jones, J. E., Morson, B. C., Ritchie, J. K. *et al.* (1977) Cancer in colitis: assessment of the individual risk by clinical and histological criteria. *Gastroenterology*, **73**, 1280–1289.

127 Le Quesne, L. P. & Thomson, A. D. (1958) Implantation recurrence of carcinoma of the rectum and colon. *New England Journal of Medicine*, **258**, 578–583.

128 Li, M. C. & Ross, S. T. (1976) Chemoprophylaxis for patients with colo-rectal cancer. *Journal of the American Medical Association*, **235**, 2825–2830.

129 Linos, D. A., O'Fallon, W. M., Beart, R. W. et al. (1981) Cholecystectomy and carcinoma of the colon. *Lancet*, **ii**, 379–381.

130 Localio, S. A. & Baron, B. (1973) Abdomino transsacral resection and anastomosis for mid rectal cancer. *Annals of Surgery*, **178**, 540–546.

131 Localio, S. A., Eng, K., Gouge, T. H. & Ransome, J. H. C. (1978) Abdominosacral resection for carcinoma of the mid rectum. Ten years experience. *Annals of Surgery*, **188**, 745–780.

132 Lockhart-Mummery, J. P. (1925) Cancer and hereditary. *Lancet*, **i**, 427–432.

133 Lockhart-Mummery, H. E. & Dukes, C. E. (1952) Surgical treatment of malignant rectal polyps with notes on their pathology. *Lancet*, **ii**, 751–756.

134 Lockhart-Mummery, H. E., Ritchie, J. K. & Hawley, P. R. (1976) The results of surgical treatment for carcinoma of the rectum at St Mark's Hospital from 1948–1971. *British Journal of Surgery*, **63**, 673–678.

135 Lovett, E. (1974) Familial factors in the aetiology of carcinoma of the large bowel. *Proceedings of the Royal Society of Medicine*, **67**, 751–752.

136 Lynch, H. T., Lynch, J. & Lynch, P. (1977) Management and control of familial cancer. In *Progress in Cancer Research and Therapy. Genetics of Human Cancer* (Ed.) Mulvihill, J. J., Miller, R. R. & Fraumeni, J. F., Jr. Volume 3. New York: Raven Press.

137 Lynch, H. T., Harris, R. E., Lynch, P. M. et al. (1977) Role of heredity in multiple primary cancers. *Cancer*, **40**, 1849–1854.

138 MacLennan, R. (1977) Dietary fibre transit time, faecal bacteria, steroids and colon cancer in two Scandinavian populations. *Lancet*, **ii**, 207–212.

139 Madden, J. L. & Kandalaft, S. (1971) Clinical evaluation of electrocoagulation in the treatment of cancer of the rectum. *American Journal of Surgery*, **122**, 347–352.

140 Maier, B. R., Flyren, M. A., Burton, G. C. et al. (1974) Effects of a high beef diet on bowel flora. *American Journal of Clinical Nutrition*, **27**, 1470–1475.

141 Mair, W. S. J., McAdam, W. A. F., Lee, P. W. R. et al. (1977) Carcinoma of the large bowel presenting as a subcutaneous abscess of the thigh: a report of 4 cases. *British Journal of Surgery*, **64**, 205–210.

142 Martin, E. W., Cooperman, M., King, G. et al. (1979) A retrospective and prospective study of serial CEA determinations in the early detection of recurrent colon cancer. *American Journal of Surgery*, **137**, 167–169.

143 Mastromarino, A. J., Reddy, B. S. & Wynder, E. L. (1978) Faecal profiles of anaerobic microflora of large bowel cancer patients and patients with non hereditary large bowel polyps. *Cancer Research*, **38**, 4458–4463.

144 Mayo, C. W. & Fly, O. A. (1956) Analysis of 5 years survival in carcinoma of the rectum and recto sigmoid. *Surgery, Gynecology and Obstetrics*, **103**, 94–99.

145 McDermott, F., Hughes, E. S. R., Pihl, E. et al. (1982) Long term results of restorative resection and total excision for carcinoma of the middle third of rectum. *Surgery, Gynecology and Obstetrics*, **154**, 833–837.

146 Mendiando, O. A., Wang, C. C., Welch, J. P. & Donaldson, G. A. (1976) Post-operative radiotherapy in carcinomas of the rectum and distal sigmoid colon. *Radiology*, **119**, 673–678.

147 Miles, W. E. (1910) The radical abdomino-perineal operation for cancer of the rectum and of the pelvic colon. *British Medical Journal*, **ii**, 941–946.

148 Miles, W. E. (1926) *Cancer of the Rectum*. London: Harrison.

149 Miln, D. C. & McLoughlin, I. S. (1969) Carcinoma of proximal large bowel associated with acute appendicitis. *British Journal of Surgery*, **56**, 143–148.

150 Minton, J. P., James, K. K., Hartubise, P. E. et al. (1978) The use of serial carcinogenic antigen determinations to predict recurrence of a carcinoma of colon and the second look operation. *Surgery, Gynecology and Obstetrics*, **147**, 208–213.

151 Modan, B. (1979) Patterns of gastrointestinal neoplasms in Israel. *Israel Journal of Medical Sciences*, **15**, 301–304.

152 Modan, B., Barell, V., Lubin, F. et al. (1975) Low fibre intake as an aetiological factor in cancer of the colon. *Journal of the National Cancer Institute*, **55**, 15 & 18.

153 Moertel, C. G. (1976) Fluorouracil as an adjuvant to colo-rectal cancer surgery. The breakthrough that never was. *Journal of the American Medical Association*, **236**, 1935–1940.

154 Moertel, C. G., Shutt, A. J. & Go, V. L. (1978) Carcinoembryonic antigen test for the detection of recurrent colo-rectal carcinoma – inadequacy for early detection. *Journal of the American Medical Association*, **239**, 1065–1070.

155 Moore, G. E., Sanberg, A. & Schuborg, S. R. (1957) Clinical and experimental observations on the occurrence and fate of tumour cells in the blood stream. *Annals of Surgery*, **76**, 755–760.

156 Moore, G. E., Sako, K., Kando, T. et al. (1961) Assessment of the exfoliation of tumour cells in the body cavities. *Surgery, Gynecology and Obstetrics*, **112**, 469–474.

157 Morgan, C. N. (1932) Endothelioma of the rectum. *Proceedings of the Royal Society of Medicine*, **25**, 1020–1025.

158 Morson, B. C. (1962) Precancerous lesions of the colon and rectum. *Journal of the American Medical Association*, **179**, 316–321.

159 Morson, B. C. (1966) Factors influencing the prognosis of early cancer of the rectum. *Proceedings of the Royal Society of Medicine*, **59**, 607–612.

160 Morson, B. C. (1970) Some leads to the aetiology of cancer of the large bowel. *Proceedings of the Royal Society of Medicine*, **64**, 959–963.

161 Morson, B. C. & Dawson, I. M. P. (1979) *Gastrointestinal Pathology*. 2nd. Edition. Oxford, London, Edinburgh & Melbourne: Blackwell Scientific Publications.

162 Muto, T., Bussey, H. J. R. & Morson, B. C. (1975) The evolution of cancer of the colon and rectum. *Cancer*, **36**, 2251–2270.

163 Nemer, F. D., Stoeckinger, J. M. & Evans, O. T. (1977) Smooth muscle rectal tumours. A therapeutic dilemma. *Diseases of the Colon and Rectum*, **20**, 405–410.

164 Nicholls, R. J., Ritchie, J. K., Wadsworth, J. et al. (1979) Total excision or restorative resection for carcinoma of the middle third of the rectum. *British Journal of Surgery*, **66**, 625–627.

165 Norbury, L. E. C. (1952) Specimen of endothelioma of rectum. *Proceedings of the Royal Society of Medicine*, **25**, 1021–1026.

166 *Office of Population Censuses and Surveys* (1981) Cancer statistics: incidence, survival and mortality in

England and Wales. Studies on medical and population subjects. No. 43. London: HMSO.

167 *Offices of Population Censuses and Surveys* (1981) Cancer statistics: registration 1976. London: HMSO.

168 Orda, R., Bawbik, J. B., Wiznitzer, T. & Schujman, E. (1976) Fibroma of the caecum. Report of a case. *Diseases of the Colon and Rectum*, **19**, 626–631.

169 Orloff, M. J. (1971) Carcinoid tumours of the rectum. *Cancer*, **28**, 175–180.

170 Pack, G. T., Miller, T. R. & Trinidad, S. S. (1963) Pararectal rhabdomyosarcoma: report of two cases. *Diseases of the Colon and Rectum*, **6**, 1–6.

171 Papillon, J. (1974) Endocavitary irradiation in the curative treatment of early rectal cancer. *Diseases of the Colon and Rectum*, **17**, 172–177.

172 Parks, A. G. (1972) Transanal technique in low rectal anastomosis. *Proceedings of the Royal Society of Medicine*, **65**, 975–976.

173 Parks, A. G. & Percy, J. P. (1982) Resection and sutured colo-rectal anastomosis for rectal carcinoma. *British Journal of Surgery*, **69**, 301–304.

174 Patterson, H. A. (1956) The management of caecal cancer discovered unexpectedly at operation for acute appendicitis. *Annals of Surgery*, **143**, 670–675.

175 Peskin, G. W. & Orloff, M. J. (1959) A clinical study of 25 patients with carcinoid tumours of the rectum. *Surgery, Gynecology and Obstetrics*, **109**, 673–678.

176 Pollett, W. G. & Nicholls, R. J. (1983) The relationship between the extent of distal clearance and survival and local recurrence rates after curative anterior resection for carcinoma of rectum. *Annals of Surgery*, **198**, 159–163.

177 Pomare, E. W. & Heaton, K. W. (1973) Alteration of bile salt metabolism by dietary fibre. *Gut*, **14**, 826–831.

178 Pomeranz, A. A. & Garlock, J. H. (1955) Postoperative recurrence of cancer of colon due to desquamated malignant cells. *Journal of the American Medical Association*, **158**, 1434–1439.

179 Quan, S. H. W. (1959) Cul de sac smears for cancer cells. *Surgery*, **45**, 258–263.

180 Quer, E. A., Dahlin, D. C. & Mayo, C. W. (1953) Retrograde intramural spread of carcinoma of the rectum and rectosigmoid. *Surgery, Gynecology and Obstetrics*, **96**, 24–30.

181 Rankin, F. W. & Olsen, P. F. (1953) The hopeful prognosis in cases of carcinoma of the colon. *Surgery, Gynecology and Obstetrics*, **56**, 366–371.

182 Ravitch, M. M. & Steichen, F. M. (1978) A stapling instrument for end to end inverting anastomosis in the gastrointestinal tract. *Annals of Surgery*, **189**, 791–797.

183 Reddy, N. S. & Wynder, E. L. (1977) Metabolic epidemiology of colon cancer: faecal bile acids and neutral steroids in colon cancer and patients with adenomatous polyps. *Cancer*, **39**, 2533–2539.

184 Renton, P. & Blackshaw, A. J. (1976) Colonic lymphoma complicating ulcerative colitis. *British Journal of Surgery*, **63**, 542–547.

185 Rider, W. D., Palmer, J. A., Mahoney, L. J. & Robertson, C. T. (1977) Pre-operative irradiation in operable cancer of the rectum: report of the Toronto trial. *Canadian Journal of Surgery*, **20**, 335–340.

186 Roberts, S., Johassan, O., Long, L. *et al.* (1961) Clinical significance of cells in the circulating blood: two to five years survival. *Annals of Surgery*, **154**, 362–367.

187 Rogers, B. H. G. (1981) Complications of hazards of colonoscopy. In *Colonoscopy: Techniques, Clinical Practice and Colour Atlas* (Ed.) Hunt, R. H. & Waye, J. D. pp. 237–264. London: Chapman and Hall.

188 Rosenberg, I. L., Russell, C. W. & Giles, G. R. (1978) Cell viability studies on the exfoliated colonic cancer cell. *British Journal of Surgery*, **65**, 188–193.

189 Sanders, G. B., Hazen, W. H. & Kinnaird, P. W. (1958) Adult intussusception and carcinoma of the colon. *Annals of Surgery*, **147**, 796–801.

190 Sanger, B. J. & Leckie, B. D. (1959) Plain muscle tumours of the rectum. *British Journal of Surgery*, **47**, 196–201.

191 Sellwood, R. A., Kaper, S. W. A., Burn, J. I. & Wallace, E. N. (1965) Circulating cancer cells; the influence of surgical operations. *British Journal of Surgery*, **52**, 69–74.

192 Sheahan, D. G., Martin, F., Baginsky, S. *et al.* (1971) Multiple lymphomatous polyposis of the gastrointestinal tract. *Cancer*, **28**, 408–413.

193 Shucksmith, H. S. (1963) Subcutaneous abscesses as the first evidence of carcinoma of the colon. *British Journal of Surgery*, **50**, 514–519.

194 Sizer, J. S., Frederick, P. L. & Osborn, M. P. (1967) Primary linitis plastica of the colon. *Diseases of the Colon and Rectum*, **10**, 339–344.

195 Slanetz, C. A., Herter, F. P. & Grinnell, R. S. (1972) Anterior resection versus abdomino-perineal resection for cancer of the rectum and rectosigmoid. An analysis of 524 cases. *American Journal of Surgery*, **123**, 110–117.

196 Slaney, G. (1971) Results of treatment of carcinoma of the colon and rectum. In *Modern Trends in Surgery 3* (Ed.) Irvine, W. T. London: Butterworth.

197 Smiddy, F. G. & Goligher, J. C. (1957) Results of surgery in treatment of cancer of the large intestine. *British Medical Journal*, **i**, 793–798.

198 Spratt, J. S. & Ackerman, L. V. (1962) Small primary adenocarcinomas of the colon and rectum. *Journal of the American Medical Association*, **179**, 337–342.

199 Spratt, J. S., Ackerman, L. V. & Moyer, C. A. (1958) Relationship of polyps of the colon to the development of colonic cancer. *Annals of Surgery*, **148**, 682–687.

200 Staszewski, J., McCall, M. G. & Stenhouse, N. S. (1971) Cancer mortality in 1962–1966 among Polish migrants to Australia. *British Journal of Cancer*, **25**, 599–604.

201 Stearns, M. W., Jr & Binkley, G. E. (1953) The influence of location on prognosis in operable rectal cancer. *Surgery, Gynecology and Obstetrics*, **96**, 368–373.

202 Stearns, M. J., Jr & Quan, S. H. W. (1959) Pre-operative roentgen therapy for cancer of the rectum. *Surgery, Gynecology and Obstetrics*, **109**, 225–230.

203 Stearns, M. W., Jr, Deddish, M. R., Quan, S. H. W. & Leeming, R. H. (1974) Preoperative roentgen therapy for cancer of the rectum and rectosigmoid. *Surgery, Gynecology and Obstetrics*, **138**, 584–589.

204 Stemmerman, G. N., Nomura, A. M. Y., Mower, H. & Glober, G. (1981) Clues to the origin of colo-rectal cancer. In *Large Bowel Cancer* (Ed.) DeCosse, J. J. Edinburgh, London, Melbourne & New York: Churchill Livingstone.

205 Stewart, M. J. (1931) Precancerous lesions of the alimentary tract. *Lancet*, **ii**, 565, 617, 669–674.

206 Stout, A. P. (1959) Tumours of colon and rectum (excluding carcinoma and adenoma). In *Diseases of the Colon and Ano-rectum* (Ed.) Turell, R. Volume 1. Philadelphia & London: W. B. Saunders.

207 Strauss, A. A., Strauss, S. F., Crawford, R. A. & Strauss, H. A. (1935) Surgical diathermy of carcinoma of the rectum; its clinical end results. *Journal of the American Medical Association*, **104**, 1480–1485.

208 Swinton, N. W. & Counts, R. L. (1956) Cancer of the colon and rectum: statistical study with end results.

Journal of the American Medical Association, **161**, 1139–1144.

209 Swinton, N. W., Neissner, W. A. & Soland, W. A. (1955) Papillary adenomas of the colon and rectum; a clinical and pathological study. *Archives of Internal Medicine*, **96**, 544–549.

210 Talbot, I. C., Ritchie, S., Leighton, M. *et al.* (1980) The clinical significance of invasion of veins by rectal cancer. *British Journal of Surgery*, **67**, 439–442.

211 Taylor, I., Bennett, R. & Sheriff, S. (1978) The measurement of blood flow into colo-rectal metastases. *British Journal of Cancer*, **36**, 749–754.

212 Taylor, I., Rowling, J. T. & West, C. (1979) Adjuvant liver perfusion for colo-rectal cancer. *British Journal of Surgery*, **66**, 833–838.

213 Teague, R. H., Salmon, P. R. & Read, A. E. (1973) Fibre optic examination of the colon; a review of 255 cases. *Gut*, **14**, 139–144.

214 Thomas, G. D. H., Dixon, M. F., Smeeton, N. C. & Williams, N. S. (1983) Observer variation in the histological grading of rectal carcinoma. *Journal of Clinical Pathology*, **36**, 385–389.

215 Thorlakson, R. H. & Ross, H. M. (1961) Leiomyosarcoma of the rectum. *Annals of Surgery*, **154**, 979–984.

216 Turcot, J., Després, J. P. & St Pierre, F. (1959) Malignant tumours of the central nervous system associated with familial polyposis of the colon. Report of two cases. *Diseases of the Colon and Rectum*, **2**, 465–470.

217 Turnbull, R. B., Jr, Kyle, K., Watson, F. R. & Spratt, J. (1967) Cancer of the colon: the influence of the no touch isolation technic on survival rates. *Annals of Surgery*, **166**, 420–425.

218 Turunen, M. J. & Kivilaakso, E. O. (1981) Increased risk of colo-rectal cancer after cholecystectomy. *Annals of Surgery*, **194**, 639–641.

219 Utsunomiya, J. (1977) Present status of adenomatous coli in Japan. In *Pathophysiology of Carcinoma in Digestive Organs* (Ed.) Forber, E. Tokyo: University Tokyo Press. Baltimore: Parks Press.

220 Veale, A. M. O. (1965) *Intestinal Polyposis*. London: Cambridge University Press.

221 Vernick, L. J. & Kuller, L. H. (1982) A case control study of cholecystectomy and right sided colon cancer. *American Journal of Epidemiology*, **116**, 86–101.

222 Villemin, F., Huard, P. & Montagne, M. (1925) Recherches anatomiques sur les lymphatiques du rectum et de l'anus: leurs applications dans le traitement chirurgical du cancer. *Revista Chirurgie (Paris)*, **63**, 69–74.

223 Walker, R. M. (1971) *Annual Report of South Western Regional Cancer Bureau*, UTF House, King Square, Bristol BS2 8HY.

224 Waterhouse, J. A. H., Muir, C. S., Carrea, P. & Powell, J. (Ed.) (1976) *Cancer Incidence in Five Continents*. Volume III. Lyon. *International Agency for Research in Cancer*. IARC Scientific Publications No. 15.

225 Welch, C. E., McKittrick, J. B. & Behringer, G. (1952) Polyps of the rectum and colon and their relation to cancer. *New England Journal of Medicine*, **247**, 959–964.

226 Welin, S. (1958) Modern trends in diagnostic roentgenology of the colon. *British Journal of Radiology*, **31**, 453–458.

227 Werf, S. D. J. van der, Nagengast, F. M., Henegouwan, G. P. van berge *et al.* (1982) Colonic absorption of secondary bile acids in patients with adenomatous polyps and matched controls. *Lancet*, **i**, 759–762.

228 Werf, S. D. J. van der, Nagengast, F. M., Henegouwan, G. P. van berge *et al.* (1983) Intracolonic environment and the presence of colonic adenomas in man. *Gut*, **24**, 876–880.

229 Whittaker, M. & Goligher, J. C. (1976) The prognosis after surgical treatment for carcinoma of the rectum. *British Journal of Surgery*, **63**, 384–388.

230 Williams, N. S. & Johnston, D. (1983) The quality of life after rectal excision for low rectal cancer. *British Journal of Surgery*, **70**, 460–462.

231 Williams, N. S. & Johnston, D. (1984) Survival and recurrence after sphincter saving resection and abdominoperineal resection of the rectum for carcinoma of the middle third rectum. *British Journal of Surgery* (In press).

232 Williams, N. S., Price, R. & Johnston, D. (1980) The long term effect of sphincter preserving operations for rectal carcinoma on the function of the anal sphincters in man. *British Journal of Surgery*, **67**, 203–208.

233 Williams, N. S., Neal, D. E. & Johnston, D. (1980) Bladder function after excision of the rectum for low rectal carcinoma. *Gut*, **21**, A453–454.

234 Williams, N. S., Dixon, M. F. & Johnston, D. (1983) Re-appraisal of the 5 centimetre rule of distal excision for carcinoma of the rectum; a study of distal intramural spread and of patients' survival. *British Journal of Surgery*, **70**, 150–154.

235 Willis, R. A. (1948) *The Pathology of Tumours*. London: Butterworth.

236 Winawer, S. J. (1981) Preventive screening and early diagnosis. In *Large Bowel Cancer* (Ed.) De Cosse, J. J. Edinburgh, London, Melbourne & New York: Churchill Livingstone.

237 Winawer, S. J., Sherlock, P., Schottenfeld, D. & Miller, P. G. (1976) Screening for colon cancer. *Gastroenterology*, **70**, 783–788.

238 Winawer, S. J., Fleisher, M., Green, S. *et al.* (1977a) Carcino embryonic antigen in colonic lavage. *Gastroenterology*, **73**, 719–722.

239 Winawer, S. J., Leidner, S. D., Miller, D. G. *et al.* (1977b) Results of a screening programme for the detection of early colon cancer and polyps using faecal occult blood testing. *Gastroenterology*, **72**, A-127. 1150–1155.

240 Winawer, S. J., Ginther, M., Weston, E. *et al.* (1978) Impact of modification in faecal occult blood test on screening programme for colo-rectal neoplasia. *Gastroenterology*, **74**, 1140–1145.

241 Winawer, S. J., Leidner, S. D., Boyle, C. & Kurtz, R. C. (1979) Comparison of flexible sigmoidoscopy with other diagnostic techniques in the diagnosis of recto-colon neoplasia. *Digestive Diseases & Sciences*, **24**(4), 277–281.

242 Wood, W. Q. & Wilkie, D. P. D. (1933) Carcinoma of the rectum. An anatomico pathological study. *Edinburgh Medical Journal*, **40**, 321–326.

243 Wood, C. B., Gillis, C. R., Hole, D. *et al.* (1981) Local tumour invasion as a prognostic factor in colo-rectal cancer. *British Journal of Surgery*, **68**, 326–328.

244 Wychulis, A. R., Beahrs, O. H. & Woolner, L. B. (1966) Malignant lymphoma of the colon. A study of 69 cases. *Archives of Surgery*, **191**, 169–174.

245 Wynder, E. L. (1975) The epidemiology of large bowel cancer. *Cancer Research*, **35**, 3388–3394.

246 Wynder, E. L. & Reddy, B. S. (1974) Metabolic epidemiology of colo-rectal cancer. *Cancer*, **34**, 801–806.

247 Yudkin, J. (1972) *Pure White and Deadly*. London: Davis.

248 Youker, J. E., Welin, W. & Main, G. (1968) Computer analysis in the differentiation of benign and malignant polypoid lesions of the colon. *Radiology*, **90**, 794–797.

IRRITABLE BOWEL SYNDROME

When a patient's symptoms clearly arise from disturbed motor function of his intestine but the intestine has no demonstrable disease a diagnosis is made of the irritable bowel syndrome (IBS). The term 'irritable bowel syndrome' suggests a single stereotyped set of symptoms but in reality the symptoms vary from one patient to another and, in the same patient, from one time to another. The term suggests a disease entity which can be diagnosed objectively and easily (such as Cushing's syndrome) but there are no objective tests for IBS and, apart from gastroenterologists, few doctors feel comfortable with the diagnosis. Even experienced gastroenterologists have to admit that it is an elusive entity. After treating many patients with IBS most doctors will agree with William Osler that 'it is much more important to know what sort of patient has a disease than what sort of disease a patient has'. Managing patients with IBS requires considerable patience and sympathy. It demands that the doctor practise the art as well as the science of medicine.

The standard definition of IBS as recurrent abdominal pain and/or disturbed bowel habit which is not due to organic disease is imperfect. It suggests that every patient needs extensive investigation to exclude organic disease, which is untrue. This definition would also include painless constipation in IBS but conventionally it is not included and constipation is discussed elsewhere in this book. Finally, some patients with undoubted IBS complain neither of pain nor of disturbed bowel habit but present with other symptoms of intestinal motor dysfunction such as bloating.

Definitions of IBS are not much help to the clinician. What is needed is a thorough knowledge of its symptoms – the symptoms of intestinal dysfunction. The clinician may be tempted to side-step a detailed history and concentrate on proving the absence of organic disease, but such an approach is inefficient, time-wasting, expensive and demoralizing to the patient, as well as unintelligent.

Varieties of IBS
The great majority of patients complain primarily of pain or discomfort in the abdomen. Such patients are often said to have colon spasm or a spastic colon because the pain is considered to come from powerful contractions of the colon. Bowel habit may be normal but is nearly always altered.

A much smaller group, perhaps 10%, have painless diarrhoea. The distinction between this and spastic colon is not absolute as the diarrhoea may alternate with constipation or at least with periods of one to three days with no bowel action.

Spastic colon syndrome

This is greatly underdiagnosed. One reason is that the pain can be felt in many and surprising places. Also, patients may be embarrassed to discuss their bowel habits – even now defecation is a taboo subject of conversation.

There are six cardinal symptoms (Table 11.17) which were identified by a systematic prospective comparison of the symptoms of patients ultimately diagnosed as IBS and those of patients found to have organic disease. All had been referred to physicians or surgeons with abdominal pain and/or altered bowel habit.[26]

Table 11.17 The six cardinal symptoms of the spastic colon syndrome.

Relief of pain with defecation
Onset of pain associated with more frequent defecation
Onset of pain associated with looser stools
Distension of the abdomen
Rectal dissatisfaction (feeling of incomplete evacuation)
Passage of mucus per rectum

Patients with organic disease usually had none, one, two or rarely three of these symptoms. IBS patients often had five or six of the symptoms and rarely less than three. Thus the greater the number of symptoms, the more likely was the diagnosis of IBS. The symptoms are all related to the large bowel and simply convey the message that there is dysfunction of the colon. This dysfunction can be caused by organic disease, especially colitis, and further assessment is generally needed to exclude an organic lesion. The six symptoms will be considered in detail.

Pain
Colonic pain can be felt anywhere in the abdomen. Inflating balloons in the colon has shown that pain arising from the sigmoid and descending colon is generally felt over expected sites (that is, suprapubically and in the left iliac fossa) but pain from the ascending and transverse colon is felt as often in the mid or upper abdomen as in the lower abdomen.[39] These studies also showed that the pain of IBS can

usually be reproduced by distending the colon. This was true even when the pain occurred in unusual sites, e.g. the back, the right lower ribs, the right shoulder, the left loin, the left sacroiliac region, the front of the left thigh and the perineum. Irritable bowel syndrome must be considered in the differential diagnosis of recurrent pain experienced anywhere between the nipples and the genitalia. Pain from the splenic flexure can even be felt in the left shoulder and down the left arm.[9]

The pain of IBS can be a mild discomfort or it can be severe enough to induce fainting. Commonly it lasts for hours or even days. It is often but not always eased by defecation; sometimes, paradoxically, it gets worse. Passage of flatus may also ease the pain but this is non-specific.

The pain of IBS is often made worse by eating, especially with large meals. This can induce such anxiety about eating that the patient loses weight, occasionally to such a degree that anorexia nervosa is suspected. More often, patients maintain their food intake, perhaps forcing themselves to eat 'to keep up their strength'. Irritable bowel syndrome patients often gain weight despite claims of having a poor appetite.

A helpful diagnostic point, though one seldom elicited by doctors, is the relationship between onset of pain and change in bowel habit. The doctor must enquire if there has been a change from constipation to a normal bowel habit which is a common occurrence in IBS but of which the patient will, quite understandably, not complain.

The term irritable colon syndrome has been abandoned by many gastroenterologists since in some patients functional abdominal pain can be traced to the small intestine (see below). However, this is an uncommon variant and the clinical picture is not well described. It is tempting to invoke a small bowel origin when the pain is provoked by eating but is not relieved by defecation and when it is not associated with a change in bowel habit.

Bowel disturbance

There can be constipation, diarrhoea, or alternating constipation and diarrhoea. The variations are many and a detailed bowel history must be elicited and recorded. Other symptoms related to defecation may be very distressing but not revealed without direct questioning. When constipation is present, the patient may spend 20–30 minutes at a time straining at stool; he may have resorted to manual evacuation or enemas; he may experience increasing bloating as the days go by without a bowel action; and he may by straining have induced haemorrhoids. When diarrhoea is present the desire to defecate may be almost continuous, defecation may be so urgent as to be socially crippling and faecal incontinence may cause great feelings of shame and depression.

The passage of ribbon-like stools may be interpreted by one patient as constipation but by another as diarrhoea. The same is true of the passage of frequent small hard lumps like rabbit droppings after which the desire to defecate persists.

Distension

Feelings of bloating or distension are very common. Sometimes the distension is visible: women may be accused of being pregnant and men have to loosen their trousers. Distension is often worst in the evening after the main meal of the day and may necessitate a change into looser clothing. These features suggest gaseous distension but it is not. The mechanism is unconscious hyperextension of the lumbar spine with contraction of the abdominal muscles or diaphragm.[2] This can cause a real increase in girth.

In patients with functional abdominal pain and bloating, even though they complain of too much gas, there is no excess of gas on X-ray, and the gas content of the intestines as measured by a washout technique is normal.[23] However, infused gas travels more slowly down the intestine and its passage was painful in patients but not controls. Thus, the complaint of gas or bloating may be due to abnormal awareness of slow moving intestinal gas.

Passage of mucus

Earlier this century physicians noted the large amount of mucus passed by some of their patients, which occasionally amounted to a cast of the colon; the condition was thus dubbed 'mucus colitis'. This extreme form is now rare and only a minority of patients admit to passing mucus at all. Those who answer 'Yes' to the question 'Do you pass slime?' may simply mean that their stools are unformed or slimy.

This symptom is poorly understood. There are no data on mucus output in health and disease. Analogy with other mucorrhoeas, such as chronic bronchitis, suggests that there is irritation of the rectal mucosa, presumably by the stool itself. If this is so, it might be a clue to the origin of the smooth muscle spasm which causes the pain of IBS.

Passage of blood cannot be attributed to IBS and a separate cause must be identified. The most common is haemorrhoids.

Dyspeptic symptoms

Patients with IBS often complain of symptoms suggesting gastric stasis (anorexia, nausea, belching, epigastric fullness or discomfort after meals) or oesophageal reflux (heartburn and acid regurgitation), and sometimes both stasis and reflux. In some cases it may be that the patient is anorexic because of anxiety or depression, possibly about his intestinal symptoms, and the dyspeptic symptoms arise from ingesting food that is not really wanted. Motility of the foregut may be abnormal at the same time as that of the hind-gut (see below). Certainly the dyspeptic symptoms often improve at the same time as the colonic complaints.

Other symptoms

Tiredness and lassitude are frequent complaints, as are headaches and dizziness. They are usually ascribed to anxiety or depression which are often present. It is conceivable, however, that they are secondary to gut dysfunction. Frequency of micturition is also common, especially in women.

Functional diarrhoea

Functional or painless diarrhoea is less common than the spastic colon syndrome. Typically the patient passes several stools in rapid succession, say, four times within an hour after rising in the morning ('the morning rush'), and then either has no further bowel actions that day or just defecates after meals. The first stool of the day is usually formed, the later ones mushy or watery. There may be much urgency and rectal dissatisfaction. Often the patient feels exhausted after the morning rush; he may say he feels scoured out. It is commonly accepted that the stool weight is normal (<200 g/day) and that large volume watery stools imply a secretory diarrhoea which must have an organic explanation, such as lactose intolerance or bile acid malabsorption. However, data are scanty and in one study male patients with functional diarrhoea excreted 230 ± 24 g stool per day.[5]

Physical examination and sigmoidoscopy

The patient is usually well nourished and although appearing physically well he/she may be tense, anxious or depressed. Nail biting, cold hands and excessive perspiration are common. In the abdomen, the colon can sometimes be felt as a firm, tender band or there may be widespread tenderness. Digital examination of the rectum may reveal hard, lumpy or pellety stools (scybala) even when the patient claims to have a normal bowel habit. Sigmoidoscopy is essential to exclude organic disease of the colon. Hyperaemia may be seen especially when there is diarrhoea, and excess mucus may make the rectal wall shiny or slimy. Obvious spasm or hypermotility may be seen. Above all, insufflating air may reproduce the familiar pain. The last sign is valuable in convincing the patient that his pain comes from the bowel. Testing the stool for occult blood (and finding none) is an essential part of the examination.

Association with other conditions

Barium enema examination in older patients with symptoms of IBS may reveal diverticular disease of the colon. This usually leads to the diagnosis of asymptomatic diverticular disease. However, there is now evidence that the presence of diverticula and of IBS in the same patient is purely coincidental.[45] Certainly, there is no evidence that IBS gets commoner with increasing age as diverticulosis does. It has been suggested that IBS may predispose to the later development of diverticular disease,[15] but the evidence is inconclusive.

Patients with ulcerative colitis have a high frequency of IBS symptoms, even when they are in remission.[20] This suggests there may be a link between the two conditions but its nature is obscure.

Irritable bowel syndrome in children

Neonatal colic is probably caused by colonic distension from swallowed air taken in during suckling. Constipation can occur in infants and be associated with colic. After six months of age there may be alternating constipation and diarrhoea or just diarrhoea as in adults. After the age of four years the commonest pattern is recurrent abdominal pain.[47]

Epidemiology

Since there is no objective marker or test for IBS its prevalence can be determined only by asking people if they suffer its symptoms. Systematic questioning along these lines has rarely been carried out. In Bristol, 14% of 301 apparently healthy people of all ages admitted to having recurrent attacks of abdominal pain relieved by defecation, 'recurrent' being defined as happening on at least seven days a year.[43] These people were prone to all the other symptoms of the spastic colon and there is no doubt that spastic colon would have been diagnosed if they had consulted a doctor. A further 4% had painless diarrhoea and another 6% painless constipation. Similar figures have been published in the USA[8] where IBS causes industrial absenteeism nearly as often as the common cold.[1] The common occurrence of IBS is obvious to all physicians (and surgeons) with a gastroenterological practice. One-third to one-half of all patients referred to them are given this diagnosis.[14] Two-thirds of the patients are women, but this sex difference is less obvious in the community.

Irritable bowel syndrome can occur at any age but seems commonest in young adults. In older people the diagnosis must always be made with particular caution.

Nothing is known of the prevalence of IBS in developing countries. In South Africa there is a strong impression that it is rare among the blacks, although the incidence may be increasing.[37]

Pathophysiology

There are considerable technical problems in studying intestinal motility and there is much disagreement among experts as to what is normal and what is abnormal.[29, 46] It has been suggested that 'the colon moves in ways too subtle and complicated to be accurately assessed by our primitive methods'.[42]

The search for a pathophysiological marker may be doomed to failure if, as Almy[1] suggests, 'qualitatively similar disturbances, differing only in intensity and in duration, occur from time to time in the vast majority of human beings as they adapt themselves to their environment'. In other words, the capacity to have IBS may be present universally. Nevertheless, the search has been and is being made.

The onset of pain in IBS often corresponds with a rise in intraluminal pressure. Pain can be reproduced by inflating a balloon in the colon. These two observations imply that IBS pain is due either to contraction or to distension of the bowel. The crucial question is whether pain is due to abnormal pressure (or stretch) or to a subnormal pain threshold. There are experimental data to support both possibilities. Some studies have shown that the normal increase in sigmoid motility after a meal (the 'gastrocolic reflex') is exaggerated in IBS patients. Otherwise, the abnormalities of colonic motility found in IBS largely reflect the presence of constipation or diarrhoea and are not specific to this disorder.[29]

When a balloon was placed within the pelvic colon and inflated with 60 ml of air, only 6% of normal subjects felt pain compared with 56% of patients with IBS.[34] Greater sensitivity of the rectum has also been reported. According to Fielding[11] pain can be provoked at rectal examination by tapping the posterior wall.

The electrical control activity of the colon has been studied extensively in recent years. Excessive slow-wave activity at a frequency of 3 cycles/min has been described[38] but this has also been noted in neurotic patients without gut symptoms;[24] hence its significance is uncertain.

It might be anticipated that patients with predominant constipation or diarrhoea could easily be distinguished by physiological measurements. In one study there were indeed obvious differences in daily stool weight and transit time[5] but in another study the groups were indistinguishable.[16] When motility was compared, patients with diarrhoea could be distinguished by a relative excess of fast contractions but there was no difference in slow contractions.[50]

Involvement of the small intestine is suggested by several findings: (a) pressure peaks detected by radiotelemetry may coincide with abdominal pain;[18, 41] (b) balloon distension of jejunum and ileum can reproduce the patient's pain;[28] and (c) small bowel transit tends to be fast in patients with predominant diarrhoea and slow in patients with predominant constipation.[5]

Involvement of the pylorus and lower oesophageal sphincter has also been reported. Endoscopically, bile reflux into the stomach has been noted twice as often as in non-IBS patients[3] but better documentation is needed. Lower oesophageal sphincter pressure appears to be low in many patients with IBS and other motility abnormalities of the oesophagus are common.[52] This may explain why IBS patients have a high incidence of oesophageal symptoms[49] but this high incidence has been disputed.[44]

Pathopsychology

Patients who are referred to hospital with IBS have a high prevalence of anxiety, depression and neurotic symptoms. Some meet the strict criteria for a psychiatric diagnosis.[50] In one series, depression was diagnosed in 49 out of 67 patients.[17] Recent stressful life events tend to occur more often than in the general population.[27] The significance of these findings is hard to evaluate. Chronic abdominal pain might well induce depression especially if, as often happens, it has been wrongly diagnosed or dismissed at previous consultations. Anxiety is unlikely to be an integral part of the syndrome if, as has been shown,[43] the majority of sufferers do not bother to seek medical advice. Anxiety spurs patients to consult their general practitioner. Referral to a specialist may be a sign of greater anxiety. To label the condition as psychosomatic is inconsistent in some patients who are well-balanced and cheerful and deny recent stress. Nevertheless, there is evidence from random telephone interviews in the general population that people who admit to frequent abdominal pain or distension and, therefore, probably have a spastic colon are prone to worry more than average about minor ailments, consult doctors more often and are more likely to have been pampered as children.[51] In other words, there is a high incidence of learned illness behaviour.

It is well established that acute stress alters colonic motility. Almy[1] observed that 'coping' behaviour, such as expressed hostility or resentment, defensive attitudes and feelings of self-sufficiency, is associated with heightened sigmoid contractions whereas 'giving-up' behaviour, such as expressions of helplessness, depression, grief, guilt and personal inadequacy, is associated with diminution of sigmoid contractions. Both reactions have been seen in the same patient, just as constipation (often associated with sigmoid hypermotility) and diarrhoea (often associated with sigmoid hypomotility) may occur alternately. Almy regards the disturbed motility of IBS as no more than bodily reflections of emotional stress. Others are less convinced,[29, 42] but most would accept that, in a susceptible person, stress can precipitate a bout of IBS. In some anxious people distress about bowel dysfunction may exacerbate and prolong it which, in turn, increases anxiety. There is certainly an important overlap between IBS and psychogenic abdominal pain.

Psychogenic abdominal pain

The bugbear of the gastroenterologist is the patient with abdominal pain or other abdominal symptoms which are certainly non-organic but are atypical of IBS (for example, the pain is not relieved by defecation) and which persist despite every form of treatment. In such patients depression or anxiety seem superficially to be the dominant problem. However, it is important to be aware that the patient may be a 'pain-prone person' who needs to have pain to express his (or more often, her) feelings of guilt or other psychological conflicts.[10] These patients constitute an important minority – 4% of all gastroenterological cases seen in Bristol.[14] Helpful points in diagnosing psychogenic pain are: (a) the location and timing of the pain are inconsistent with physiological principles and with recognized disease patterns; (b) the pain is described in dramatic terms yet the patient appears calm, even smiling; (c) there is often a history of multiple pains in other parts of the body in the past – these will have resisted diagnosis, though the patient may report disc lesions, gallbladder attacks, etc.; (d) the pain may have begun during a period of stress, especially one involving loss or bereavement or angry feelings towards a loved person resulting in feelings of guilt.[13]

Diagnosis and investigation

The diagnosis should be made positively on the characteristic history. This requires detailed and systematic questioning about bowel habit including the shape and consistency of the stools and the extent to which these and the frequency of defecation vary. It is especially important to establish whether the pain is eased with defecation, whether bowel habit changed or changes with the onset of a bout of pain, whether mucus is passed and whether the patient experiences abdominal distension or feelings of incomplete evacuation ('rectal dissatisfaction').

Assuming that physical examination and sigmoidoscopy are normal or show only the minor abnormalities mentioned above, is further investigation necessary? In a person under 40 years of age with a typical history of spastic colon going back over years, with no change in weight and no occult blood in the stools, it is unnecessary to undertake further investigation. Sometimes a barium enema is indicated to reassure the patient and/or the referring doctor. A barium enema is mandatory in older patients or if there is occult blood in the stool. The radiologist should not be expected to give positive diagnostic help. The old-fashioned single-contrast barium enema was sometimes held to show areas of spasm or hyper-haustration but this was never adequately documented and such findings cannot be expected with the double-contrast technique which involves giving drugs to relax the bowel muscle.

In patients with continuous diarrhoea, whether painful or painless, it is advisable to screen the patient for malabsorption and Crohn's disease, at least by a blood count and ESR or viscosity with perhaps a serum iron or red cell folate assay. In many cases a barium follow-through will be considered advisable. A

lactose–hydrogen breath test or lactose tolerance test and a therapeutic trial of cholestyramine for bile acid diarrhoea is often sensible.
When the symptoms are recent and follow travel
abroad, stool cultures should be done to exclude
amoebiasis, giardiasis and possibly for other
infestations.

When the patient admits to constipation part
or all of the time, or when the rectum contains
scybala, it is my practice to question them about
their diet and often to give them a diet diary in
which to record their food intake for a few days.
This prepares them for the dietary advice which
they are often given when they return to discuss
the results of the investigations.

Treatment (Table 11.18)

> *We retard what we cannot repel, we palliate
> what we cannot cure.*
>   Samuel Johnson, 1709–1784

Table 11.18 Treatment possibilities in irritable bowel syndrome.

Essential
  Explanation
  Reassurance

Conventional
  Treatment of associated anxiety, tension, depression
  High fibre diet or bulking agents (for constipation)
  Musculotropic drugs
  Anticholinergics

Unconventional
  Elimination diets
  Peppermint oil

Experimental
  Biofeedback

The essence of management is taking the patient
seriously. All too often the patient has not been
allowed to tell his whole story before or has been
too embarrassed to do so and, perhaps without
realizing it, the gastroenterologist helps the
patient as a detailed and sympathetic history is
taken.

Once the physician is reasonably confident of
the diagnosis (which in most cases should be at
the first visit) after the history, physical examination and sigmoidoscopy he should explain
what he believes to be the nature of the problem.
I always stress that it is not a disease but a mis-
behaviour of the bowel. I explain how spasm of
the bowel muscle can cause pain, just as cramp
in the calf muscles is painful. I emphasize that it
is a very real disorder, just like migraine or
asthma, that it is very common and, above all,
that it is harmless. This is a suitable moment to
enquire if the patient has been worried about

having any particular disease, naming cancer as
one. Cancerphobia is surprisingly common but
is usually dispelled quite easily. In summary, the
first two essentials of management are explanation and reassurance.

Subsequently management must be tailored
to the individual case. When symptoms are mild
or occasional no further action may be needed,
especially if the patient says he is quite happy to
live with them. More often there will ensue a
discussion of possible precipitating factors. The
patient may recognize that stress provokes pain
or diarrhoea. If so, the patient must either be
taught to accept this or be advised to reduce the
stress. Another patient may not recognize the
relationship but will admit to being unduly tense
or nervous. Possible measures include relaxation techniques (including meditation, yoga
and regular physical exercise) and tranquillizing
drugs. Future possibilities being investigated
include biofeedback or operant conditioning.

Diet

If the dietary history indicates a poor intake of
fibre-rich foods, and especially if there is any
element of constipation in the history or examination, the doctor can explain how the colon is
designed to cope with large amounts of undigested residue and how, in attempting to transport small hard stools, it generates excessive
pressures and hence pain. In this situation the
gastroenterologist can with some confidence
prescribe a high fibre diet, or better still request
the dietitian to discuss a high fibre diet with the
patient. This will be based on wholemeal bread,
wholegrain breakfast cereals and plentiful fruit
and vegetables. It will include bran if necessary
to obtain the desired effect, namely a soft stool
which is passed without effort.

Bran. During the wave of enthusiasm for bran
in the last decade, most British gastroenterologists recommended bran or a high fibre diet
routinely to IBS patients. This practice received
limited support from one randomized controlled
trial.[25] Fourteen patients allocated 20 g bran
daily or the equivalent in wholemeal bread experienced somewhat less pain, passed less mucus
and had less colonic motor activity than 12
patients allocated a low fibre diet. The low fibre
diet was essentially the same as the patients'
usual diet and may not have exerted as much
placebo effect as the bran diet. In a subsequent
comparison of placebo tablets and bran, symptoms were reduced equally by both treatments,
with the exception of constipation.[4] This trial
was short in duration but its results confirm the

clinical impression that bran is far from the panacea it first seemed. When bran is prescribed it should be introduced gradually to minimize bloating. If it is poorly tolerated the patient can usually take wholemeal bread. Alternatively, pharmaceutical bulking agents may be prescribed (see below).

Food intolerance seems to be a factor in some patients whose predominant symptom is diarrhoea. This has been demonstrated by both blind provocation of symptoms, when the food under test is administered via a nasogastric tube, and by a therapeutic response to an elimination diet.[22] The responsible foods in order of frequency are wheat products, corn products, dairy products, coffee, tea and citrus fruits. The mechanism of these food reactions is obscure but is a promising area of current research. The practical application is to encourage patients with resistant symptoms to try a diet which excludes the six foods mentioned. If improvement occurs each food is re-introduced in turn until the one which provokes symptoms is identified.

Drugs

Drug treatment should be kept to the minimum in a condition which is both benign and long-lasting with a good placebo response rate.[42] However, pharmaceutical bulking agents can be used freely. The choice is largely a personal one and lies between the ispaghula or psyllium products (Isogel, Fybogel, Metamucil, Regulan), sterculia gum (Normacol Special) and synthetic methylcellulose (Celevac). As with bran, the dosage should be adjusted to produce a soft and easily passed stool. When stubborn, constipation can be treated with lactulose syrup (which acts like bulking agents as a nutrient for colonic bacteria). Chemical laxatives should be used only in the last resort. The patient should be encouraged to respond to the call to defecate and allow adequate time for defecation after breakfast. These simple but neglected measures are often helpful.

Drugs used to relieve spasm include mebeverine and the anticholinergics. The efficacy of mebeverine, which seems to be specific for smooth muscle, has been demonstrated in controlled trials and is almost devoid of side-effects.[7, 40] It is of value but relatively few patients obtain complete remission of pain. The use of anticholinergic drugs is controversial.[21] They are widely prescribed but I rarely prescribe them. Tiresome side-effects are inevitable with effective cholinergic blockade.

Antidepressant drugs have their advocates[17] but, except in overtly depressed patients, they have few advantages over a placebo.[30]

Antidiarrhoeal drugs are often helpful of which loperamide is probably the most effective.

Triple therapy with a bulking agent, an antispasmodic and an anxiolytic drug was found to be more effective than a single drug or a combination of two by Ritchie and Truelove.[35, 36] The most effective combination was ispaghula, mebeverine and a mixture of fluphenazine and nortriptyline. However, most doctors will hesitate to prescribe four drugs at once unless all else has failed.

Peppermint oil relaxes smooth muscle. Capsules containing 0.2 ml were beneficial in a controlled trial of 16 patients.[33] Its safety is an attractive feature but in my experience it has proved disappointing.

Prognosis

The prognosis is good when IBS follows an intestinal infection, often acquired with foreign travel, or when it is precipitated by an isolated stressful event or a change in diet. It will often disappear within a few weeks or months. Otherwise patients referred to hospital tend to have persistent symptoms for years with perhaps only one-third becoming symptom-free.[6, 19, 48] Those with pronounced psychological problems or with psychogenic pain seem to do worst. Persistent symptoms can tempt the weary consultant or the inexperienced junior doctor to order fresh investigations but this is rarely profitable.[19] There is no substitute for a long-term supportive doctor–patient relationship. The doctor should normally be the general practitioner.

Aetiological factors

An attack of infective diarrhoea and a stressful life event can undoubtedly precipitate IBS. So too can a sudden change in diet, such as a 'crash' slimming diet. In many if not most patients it is impossible to identify a clear-cut cause from the history. This has led to a search for predisposing factors. On the psychological side, learned illness behaviour, hysteria, anxiety and depression have all come under scrutiny (see above). However, these may simply dictate that the patient complains to a doctor. It is hard to see how they can cause the disturbed motility which provides the basis of the complaint. When a quarter of the population admits to spastic colon symptoms, constipation or diarrhoea and no less than half experience feelings of incomplete evacuation[43] it suggests that the population as a whole may be exposed to environmental factors which can upset gut function. Much more epidemiological data must be collected before aetiological theories can be formulated. Should it be true that IBS is uncommon in developing and primitive communities, this would lend support to the view of Painter[31, 32] that a low intake of dietary fibre could be a factor. Certainly case-control studies have not consistently demonstrated a low intake of dietary fibre in patients with IBS.[12, 16] The variable benefit of a high fibre diet provides some support for this concept. Food intolerance may prove important when diarrhoea is predominant[22] but more data are needed to formulate a mechanism whereby such different foods as wheat and dairy products can provide the same end result.

Is IBS a disease at all or just a normal somatic response to stress? Is it one disease or several? These and many other questions remain to be answered.

REFERENCES

1 Almy, T. P. (1978) Irritable bowel syndrome. In *Gastrointestinal Disease* (Ed.) Sleisenger, M. H. & Fordtran, J. S. 2nd Edition, pp. 1585–1597. Philadelphia: W. B. Saunders.

2 Alvarez, W. C. (1949) Hysterical type of nongaseous abdominal bloating. *Archives of Internal Medicine*, **84**, 217–245.

3 Anderson, D. L. & Boyce, H. W. (1974) Duodenogastric reflux: association with irritable bowel syndrome. *Gastrointestinal Endoscopy (Denver)*, **20**, 112–114.

4 Cann, P. A., Read, N. W. & Holdsworth, C. D. (1984) What is the benefit of coarse wheat bran in patients with the irritable bowel syndrome? *Gut*, **25**, 168–173.

5 Cann, P. A., Read, N. W., Brown, C. *et al.* (1983) The irritable bowel syndrome: relationship of disorders in the transit time of a single solid meal to symptom patterns. *Gut*, **24**, 405–411.

6 Chaudhary, N. A. & Truelove, S. C. (1962) Irritable colon syndrome. A study of the clinical features, predisposing causes, and prognosis in 130 cases. *Quarterly Journal of Medicine*, **31**, 307–322.

7 Connell, A. M. (1965) Physiological and clinical assessment of the effect of the musculotropic agent mebeverine on the human colon. *British Medical Journal*, **ii**, 848–851.

8 Drossman, D. A., Sandler, R. S., McKee, D. C. & Lovitz, A. J. (1982) Bowel patterns among subjects not seeking health care. Use of a questionnaire to identify a population with bowel dysfunction. *Gastroenterology*, **83**, 529–534.

9 Dworken, H. J., Biel, F. J. & Machella, T. E. (1952) Supradiaphragmatic reference of pain from the colon. *Gastroenterology*, **22**, 222–231.

10 Engel, G. L. (1959) 'Psychogenic' pain and the pain-prone patient. *American Journal of Medicine*, **26**, 899–918.

11 Fielding, J. F. (1978) Clinical and radiological manifestations of the irritable bowel syndrome. *Journal of the Irish College of Physicians and Surgeons*, **8**, 11–15.

12 Fielding, J. F. & Melvin, K. (1979) Dietary fibre and the irritable bowel syndrome. *Journal of Human Nutrition*, **33**, 243–247.

13 Glaser, J. P. & Engel, G. L. (1977) Psychodynamics, psychophysiology and gastrointestinal symptomatology. *Clinics in Gastroenterology*, **6**, 507–531.

14 Harvey, R. F., Salih, S. Y. & Read, A. E. (1983) Organic and functional disorders in 2000 gastroenterology outpatients. *Lancet*, **i**, 632–634.

15 Havia, T. & Manner, R. (1971) The irritable colon syndrome. A follow-up study with special reference to the development of diverticula. *Acta Chirurgica Scandinavica*, **137**, 569–572.

16 Hillman, L. C., Stace, N. H., Fisher, A. & Pomare, E. W. (1982) Dietary intakes and stool characteristics of patients with the irritable bowel syndrome. *American Journal of Clinical Nutrition*, **36**, 626–629.

17 Hislop, I. G. (1971) Psychological significance of the irritable colon syndrome. *Gut*, **12**, 452–457.

18 Holdstock, D. J., Misiewicz, J. J. & Waller, S. L. (1969) Observations on the mechanism of abdominal pain. *Gut*, **10**, 19–31.

19 Holmes, K. M. & Salter, R. H. (1982) Irritable bowel syndrome – a safe diagnosis? *British Medical Journal*, **285**, 1533–1534.

20 Isgar, B., Harman, M., Kaye, M. D. & Whorwell, P. J. (1983) Symptoms of irritable bowel syndrome in ulcerative colitis in remission. *Gut*, **24**, 190–192.

21 Ivey, K. J. (1975) Are anticholinergics of use in the irritable colon syndrome? *Gastroenterology*, **68**, 1300–1307.

22 Jones, V. A., McLaughlan, P., Shorthouse, M. *et al.* (1982) Food intolerance: a major factor in the pathogenesis of irritable bowel syndrome. *Lancet*, **ii**, 1115–1117.

23 Lasser, R. B., Bond, J. H. & Levitt, M. D. (1975) The role of intestinal gas in functional abdominal pain. *New England Journal of Medicine*, **293**, 524–526.

24 Latimer, P., Sarna, S., Campbell, D. *et al.* (1981) Colonic motor and myoelectrical activity: a comparative study of normal subjects, psychoneurotic patients, and patients with irritable bowel syndrome. *Gastroenterology*, **80**, 893–901.

25 Manning, A. P., Heaton, K. W., Harvey, R. F. & Uglow, P. (1977) Wheat fibre and irritable bowel syndrome. A controlled trial. *Lancet*, **ii**, 417–418.

26 Manning, A. P., Thompson, W. G., Heaton, K. W. & Morris, A. F. (1978) Towards positive diagnosis of the irritable bowel. *British Medical Journal*, **ii**, 653–654.

27 Mendeloff, A. I., Monk, M., Siegel, C. I. & Lilienfeld, A. (1970) Illness experience and life stresses in patients with irritable colon and with ulcerative colitis. *New England Journal of Medicine*, **282**, 14–17.

28 Moriarty, K. J. & Dawson, A. M. (1982) Functional abdominal pain: further evidence that whole gut is affected. *British Medical Journal*, **284**, 1670–1672.

29 Murney, R. G. & Winship, D. H. (1982) The irritable colon syndrome. *Clinics in Gastroenterology*, **11**, 536–592.

30 Myren, J., Groth, H., Larssen, S.-E. & Larsen, S. (1982) The effect of trimipramine in patients with the irritable bowel syndrome. A double blind study. *Scandinavian Journal of Gastroenterology*, **17**, 871–875.

31 Painter, N. S. (1972) Irritable or irritated bowel. *British Medical Journal*, **ii**, 46.

32 Painter, N. S. (1979) High fiber treatment of the 'irritated' alias the 'irritable' bowel syndrome. *Practical Gastroenterology*, **3**, 46–53.

33 Rees, W. D. W., Evans, B. K. & Rhodes, J. (1979) Treating irritable bowel syndrome with peppermint oil. *British Medical Journal*, **iv**, 835–836.

34 Ritchie, J. (1973) Pain from distension of the pelvic colon by inflating a balloon in the irritable bowel syndrome. *Gut*, **14**, 125–132.

35 Ritchie, J. A. & Truelove, S. C. (1979) Treatment of irritable bowel syndrome with lorazepam, hyoscine butylbromide and ispaghula husk. *British Medical Journal*, **i**, 376–378.

36 Ritchie, J. A. & Truelove, S. C. (1980) Comparison of various treatments for irritable bowel syndrome. *British Medical Journal*, **281**, 1317–1319.

37 Segal, I. & Hunt, J. A. (1975) The irritable bowel syndrome in the urban South African Negro. *South African Medical Journal*, **49**, 1645–1646.

38 Snape, W. J., Carlson, G. M. & Cohen, S. (1976) Colonic myoelectrical activity in the irritable bowel syndrome. *Gastroenterology*, **70**, 326–330.

39 Swarbrick, E. T., Hegarty, J. E., Bat, L. *et al.* (1980) Site of pain from the irritable bowel. *Lancet*, **ii**, 443–446.

40 Tasman-Jones, C. (1973) Mebeverine in patients with the irritable colon syndrome: double blind study. *New Zealand Medical Journal*, **77**, 232–235.

41 Thompson, D. G., Laidlow, J. M. & Wingate, D. L. (1979) Abnormal small-bowel motility demonstrated by radiotelemetry in a patient with irritable colon. *Lancet*, **ii**, 1321–1323.

42 Thompson, W. G. (1984) The irritable bowel. *Gut*, **25**, 305–320.

43 Thompson, W. G. & Heaton, K. W. (1980) Functional bowel disorders in apparently healthy people. *Gastroenterology*, **79**, 283–288.

44 Thompson, W. G. & Heaton, K. W. (1982) Heartburn and globus in apparently healthy people. *Canadian Medical Association Journal*, **126**, 46–48.

45 Thompson, W. G., Patel, D. G., Tao, H. & Nair, R. (1982) Does uncomplicated diverticular disease cause symptoms? *Digestive Diseases and Sciences*, **27**, 605–608.

46 Tucker, H. & Schuster, M. M. (1982) Irritable bowel syndrome: newer pathophysiologic concepts. In *Advances in Internal Medicine* (Ed.) Stollerman, G. H. Volume 27, pp. 183–204. Chicago: Year Book Medical Publishers.

47 Turner, R. M. (1978) Recurrent abdominal pain in childhood. *Journal of the Royal College of General Practitioners*, **28**, 729–734.

48 Waller, S. L. & Misiewicz, J. J. (1969) Prognosis in the irritable-bowel syndrome. A prospective study. *Lancet*, **ii**, 753–756.

49 Watson, W. C., Sullivan, S. N., Corke, M. & Rush, D. (1976) Incidence of oesophageal symptoms in patients with irritable bowel syndrome. *Gut*, **17**, 827.

50 Whitehead, W. E., Engel, B. T. & Schuster, M. M. (1980) Irritable bowel syndrome. Physiological and psychological differences between diarrhea-predominant and constipation-predominant patients. *Digestive Diseases and Sciences*, **25**, 404–413.

51 Whitehead, W. E., Winget, C., Fedaravicius, A. S. *et al.* (1982) Learned illness behavior in patients with irritable bowel syndrome and peptic ulcer. *Digestive Diseases and Sciences*, **27**, 202–208.

52 Whorwell, P. J., Clouter, C. & Smith, C. L. (1981) Oesophageal motility in the irritable bowel syndrome. *British Medical Journal*, **282**, 1101–1102.

ENDOMETRIOSIS

Endometriosis is characterized by the identification of extrauterine endometrial tissue. It is a disease of women predominantly in childbearing years with a peak incidence between 30 and 40 years but may occur occasionally in the elderly – the record in the literature stands at 76 years![7] The extrauterine endometrial tissue is under hormonal influence so that the normal cycle occurs with maturation, shedding of the surface endometrial epithelium and bleeding.

Macroscopic appearance in the gastrointestinal tract

The lesions involving the gastrointestinal tract are usually small and multiple and an incidental finding during laparotomy for endometriosis. Larger extramural or intramural lesions of the intestine (endometriomas) may develop occasionally. These lesions if large enough can produce luminal obstruction usually in the sigmoid colon and particularly at the rectosigmoid junction.[2] They occur less frequently in the appendix,[4] caecum[6] or ileum.[2]

Clinical features

Symptoms of the underlying endometriosis include dysmenorrhoea, pelvic pain, sterility, dyspareunia and low backache. Pelvic examination usually reveals tender nodules with areas of irregular induration. The presence of gynaecological and gastrointestinal symptoms in women of childbearing years should raise the possibility of endometriosis. It must be considered particularly in such patients where radiological examination has shown an obstructing lesion at the rectosigmoid junction.

Diagnosis and treatment

Historical perspectives of endometriosis with reviews of the earlier literature have been described by Kratzer and Salvati[3] and Gray.[2] Kratzer and Salvati[3] studied 225 patients with endometriosis diagnosed at laparotomy of whom 77 (34%) had involvement of the sigmoid colon and rectum. The involvement was minor in most cases. In 44 the sigmoid and rectum were adherent to the posterior wall of the uterus, and in 15 to the left tube and ovary. Thirteen had endometrial implants on the surface of the large intestine, but only four had endometriosis in two of whom there were signs of intestinal obstruction from lesions involving the sigmoid colon.

The largest reported series by Gray[2] described 179 cases of endometriosis of the gastrointestinal tract from among 1500 patients undergoing surgical treatment for endometriosis. The majority (142) were lesions on the surface of the large bowel, of which 81 were completely excised. There were only 37 patients aged between 25 and 49 years where the involved bowel required resection. The resection was confined to the anterior wall of the sigmoid or rectosigmoid colon in 27 and only ten patients required resections of segments of the gut with an end-to-end anastomosis; the lower sigmoid was involved in eight and the terminal ileum in two. The intestinal mucosa was not breached in any patient and none presented with rectal bleeding. Meyers and his colleagues[5] recently described seven examples of colonic endometriosis. The lesions were all in the sigmoid or rectosigmoid colon, although one patient also had lesions in the descending colon. They advocated surgical excision of the involved colon since there are no specific radiological signs of endometriosis – the appearances could mimic colorectal cancer or even complicated diverticulitis and also the diagnosis can often only be made on histological grounds.

The current concepts of the management of endometriosis in general have been well reviewed by Dmowski.[1] Four choices of treatment are available: expectant observation, hormone therapy, surgical excision and castration. Only half of the women with rectosigmoid involvement have severe bowel symptoms and it is necessary that the management of endometriosis be flexible and individualized to a particular patient.

Women without significant bowel symptoms or obstruction can be watched without therapeutic intervention. Hormone therapy may be offered to patients with pain, partially obstructing lesions and where the number of endometrial nodules are too extensive for surgical removal. Androgens, progestin agents and the antigonadotrophin agent danazol have all been used; the last mentioned is particularly favoured because it has fewer side-effects and high efficacy.

Surgical intervention may be required for diagnosis where the cause for acute abdominal symptoms is unclear. Surgical removal of constricting lesions is necessary; occasionally it is possible to dissect small implants from the bowel wall without resection of the colon. In women with extensive symptomatic disease who have failed to respond to surgical or hormonal therapy, castration by radiation or surgical excision may be necessary.

Symptoms arising from endometriosis affecting the small bowel, caecum or appendix are uncommon but the principles of treatment are similar to those for colonic endometriosis.

REFERENCES

1 Dmowski, W. P. (1981) Current concepts in the management of endometriosis. *Obstetrics and Gynaecology Annual*, **10**, 279–311.
2 Gray, L. A. (1973) Endometriosis of the bowel: role of bowel resection superficial excision and oophorectomy in treatment. *Annals of Surgery*, **177**, 580–587.
3 Kratzer, G. L. & Salvati, E. P. (1955) Collective review of endometriosis of the colon. *American Journal of Surgery*, **90**, 866–869.
4 Lane, R. E. (1960) Endometriosis of the vermiform appendix. *American Journal of Obstetrics and Gynecology*, **79**, 372.
5 Meyers, W. C., Kelvin, F. M. & Jones, R. S. (1979) Diagnosis and surgical treatment of colonic endometriosis. *Archives of Surgery*, **114**, 169–175.
6 Swann, M. (1962) An endometrioma of the caecum causing an intussusception. *British Journal of Surgery*, **50**, 199.
7 Williams, C. (1963) Endometriosis of the colon in elderly women. *Annals of Surgery*, **157**, 974–979.

PNEUMATOSIS COLI (PNEUMATOSIS CYSTOIDES INTESTINALIS)

Definition and nomenclature

Multiple collections of encysted gas in the submucous and subserous regions of the colon and rectum, which persist for weeks or many years, are referred to as pneumatosis coli or gas cysts of the colon. A similar condition may be seen in the small bowel but in these cases there is always a recognizable associated pathology, usually a peptic ulcer or other ulcerative lesion, which can explain tracking of gas into the bowel wall. A classification of pneumatosis intestinalis is given in Table 11.19. In colonic cases it is most unusual for any other bowel pathology to be demonstrated and thus the condition is often referred to as primary pneumatosis coli.

Differential diagnosis

The frequent diagnostic difficulty in these cases is related to its rarity. Few specialists will see more than one example in a lifetime. When the gas cysts are palpable per rectum the patient is commonly thought to have a rectal neoplasm.

Table 11.19 Classification of pneumatosis cystoides intestinalis.

Catastrophic infective type
Neonatal necrotizing enterocolitis seen in premature and sick newborn infants
Adult: in association with alcoholism, amoebiasis or ischaemia. Necrotizing colitis.

Subacute small bowel type (secondary to mucosal ulceration, disease or other abnormality)
Gastric or duodenal ulcer
Pyloric stenosis
Tuberculosis
Scleroderma
Jejunoileal bypass, etc.

Chronic 'primary' pneumatosis coli (associated with obstructive airways disease in 50% of patients)

The barium enema appearances, although characteristic, are commonly interpreted as being those of polyposis, pseudo-polyposis or the thumb-printing of ischaemic colitis, unless the radiolucency of the filling defects is appreciated. Linear gas shadows in the bowel wall are associated with fulminating clostridial infections as in necrotizing colitis or frank gangrene. Solitary giant gas cysts of the sigmoid colon are probably due to the distension of a diverticulum because of valve formation at its neck. Pathologists unfa-

miliar with pneumatosis coli may interpret biopsies as oleogranulomas because spaces, assumed to have previously contained lipid, in fact contained gas and are associated with granuloma formation.[10]

Pathology

Pneumatosis coli usually affects the left side of the colon, especially the splenic flexure and the sigmoid colon. The right side is rarely affected unless there is concomitant small bowel pneumatosis when secondary pneumatosis intestinalis with an ulcerating intestinal lesion should be suspected. Treatment of the underlying lesion will be followed by resolution of the gas cysts. In the majority of chronic cases the gas cysts extend from the mid-transverse colon to the rectum. Sometimes cysts travel through the wall of the bowel into the omentum and may even occur in the wall of the bladder or vagina.

Macroscopically (Figure 11.72) the gas bubbles are spherical with a typically blue tinge and are situated in the submucosa and subserosa. They produce considerable thickening and stiffening of the bowel wall. The condition can be mimicked by injecting air from a syringe into the submucosa of freshly excised colon.

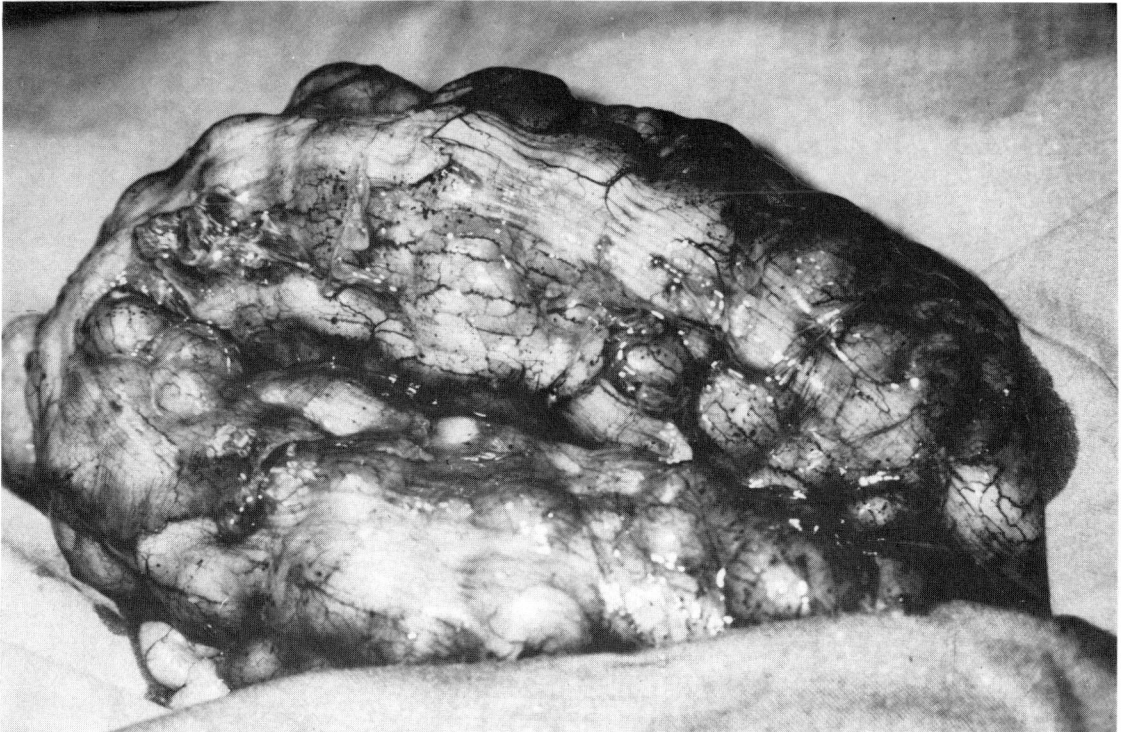

Fig. 11.72 Macroscopic appearance of pneumatosis coli. Sigmoid colon exposed at the time of surgery. Note the large subserosal blebs of gas.

Cysts may vary in diameter from a few millimetres to 2 cm but are never larger. Spontaneous pneumoperitoneum is sometimes seen
with small bowel cysts but not with primary
pneumatosis coli. The mucosal surface of the
colon sometimes appears haemorrhagic in the
region of the cysts but is not otherwise inflamed
and with sigmoidoscopy small submucosal
vessels can be seen coursing over the gas
bubbles.

Microscopically (Figure 11.73) the cystic
spaces are lined with endothelial cells and are
associated with granulomas consisting of collections of endotheloid and foreign body giant
cells. There is no acute inflammatory response.

Patients are usually middle-aged or elderly
and often with multiple pathology. In most large
series half the patients suffer from obstructive
airways disease.[6] Myocardial infarction and
multiple operations are also common and the
condition is reported at the distal end of small
bowel following bypass operations for obesity.[7]

Untreated the condition may persist for many
years. It may recur after apparently successful
medical treatment or surgical excision.[8] On the
other hand spontaneous and prolonged remission may occur without any specific treatment,
but usually only in recently diagnosed cases.

Clinical features

The presenting features are diarrhoea, excessive
flatulence, abdominal pain, bleeding or incontinence. Patients may go to the toilet twenty times
a day but only to pass mucus with flatus and
perhaps some blood. Despite repeated mucous
incontinence the patient will sometimes complain of passing constipated faeces. The symptoms fluctuate considerably and most patients
are unable to relate this fluctuation to diet or
other factors. The pain is usually in the lower
abdomen and colicky but occasionally intestinal
obstruction or volvulus will complicate the condition when severe pain is associated with distension and vomiting.

Clinical examination and investigations

In a slim patient it is often possible to see the
diseased colon through the abdominal wall and
to palpate it as a sausage-shaped mass covered
with knobbly bubbles of gas. Rectal examination will reveal the cysts as rubbery blobs protruding into the lumen in about half the cases. In
almost all cases the cysts can be seen with
sigmoidoscopy as multiple blue-domed swellings (Figure 11.74). Biopsy should be carried out

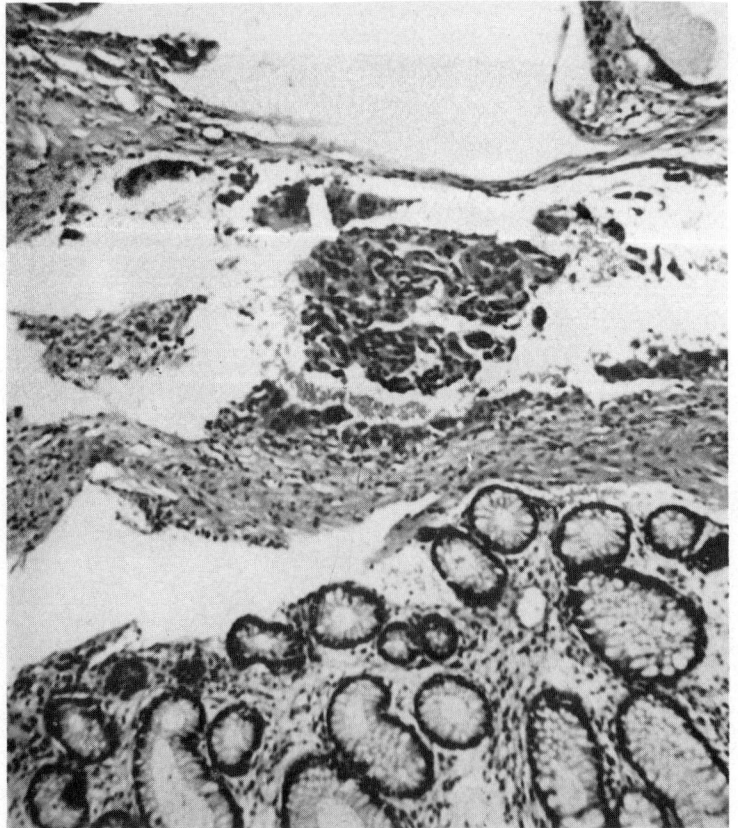

Fig. 11.73 Histological section of
biopsy specimen. Submucosal gas
cyst above, granuloma in centre
and mucous membrane inferiorly (H
& E × 200).

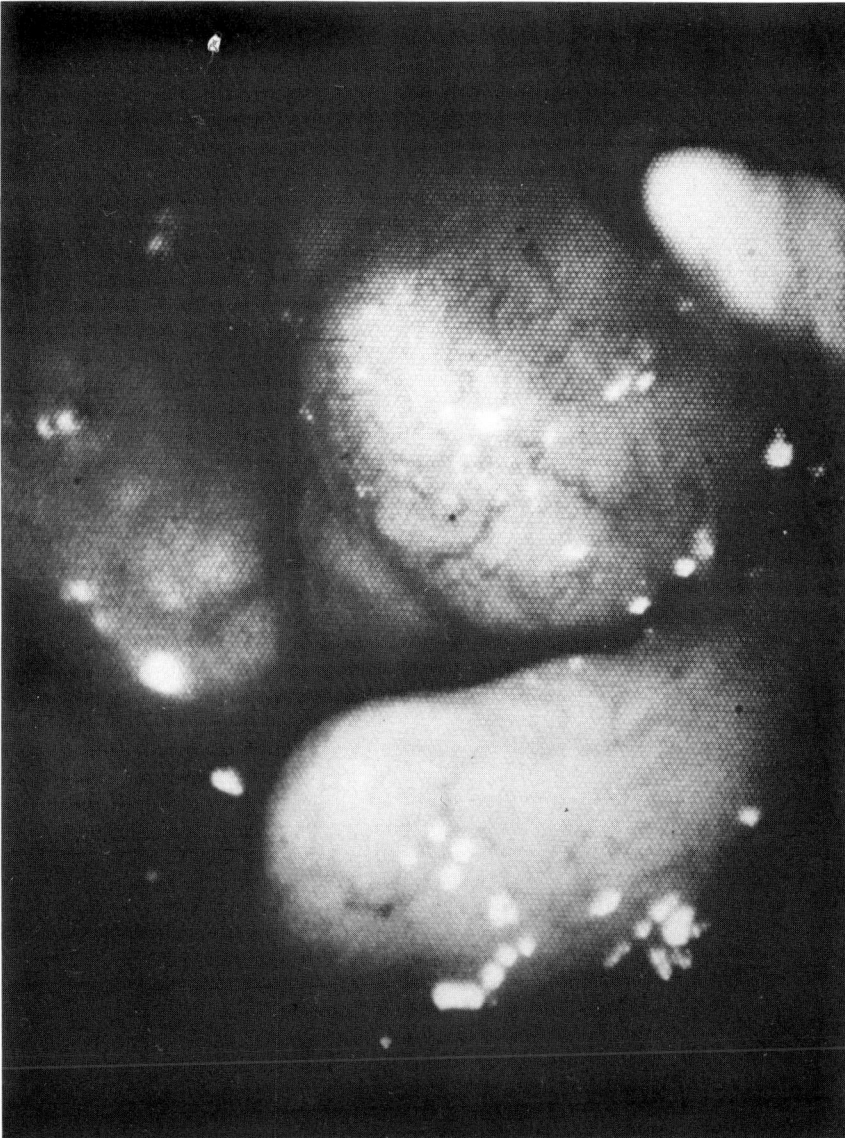

Fig. 11.74   Colonoscopic appearance of multiple gas cysts in sigmoid colon. Note small vessels running over the cysts.

for confirmation when a typical 'pop' will be heard as the cyst ruptures. The biopsy will float in the fixative because of its air content.

A plain X-ray of the abdomen is diagnostic because the multiple radiolucent gas-filled cysts are evident; this proves to be a simple way to document the course of the disease (Figure 11.75). A barium enema examination shows the classical scalloped appearance of cysts protruding into the bowel lumen (Figures 11.76 and 11.77). A chest X-ray should be performed in view of the common association with chest disease. The gas-filled colon may also be seen lying between the right lobe of the liver and the diaphragm (the Chilaiditi's sign) (Figure 11.78).

If cysts are present on the right side of the colon, suggesting the secondary type of pneumatosis, the stomach and small bowel should be investigated by endoscopy and barium studies.

Aetiology

Gas collections in the tissues are normally rapidly absorbed because the total pressure of gases dissolved in venous capillaries is 7.2 kPa (54 mmHg) below atmospheric pressure owing to the removal of O_2. The explanation of persistent gas collections must be either local gas formation in the cysts by bacteria or constant replenishment from the bowel lumen. In the

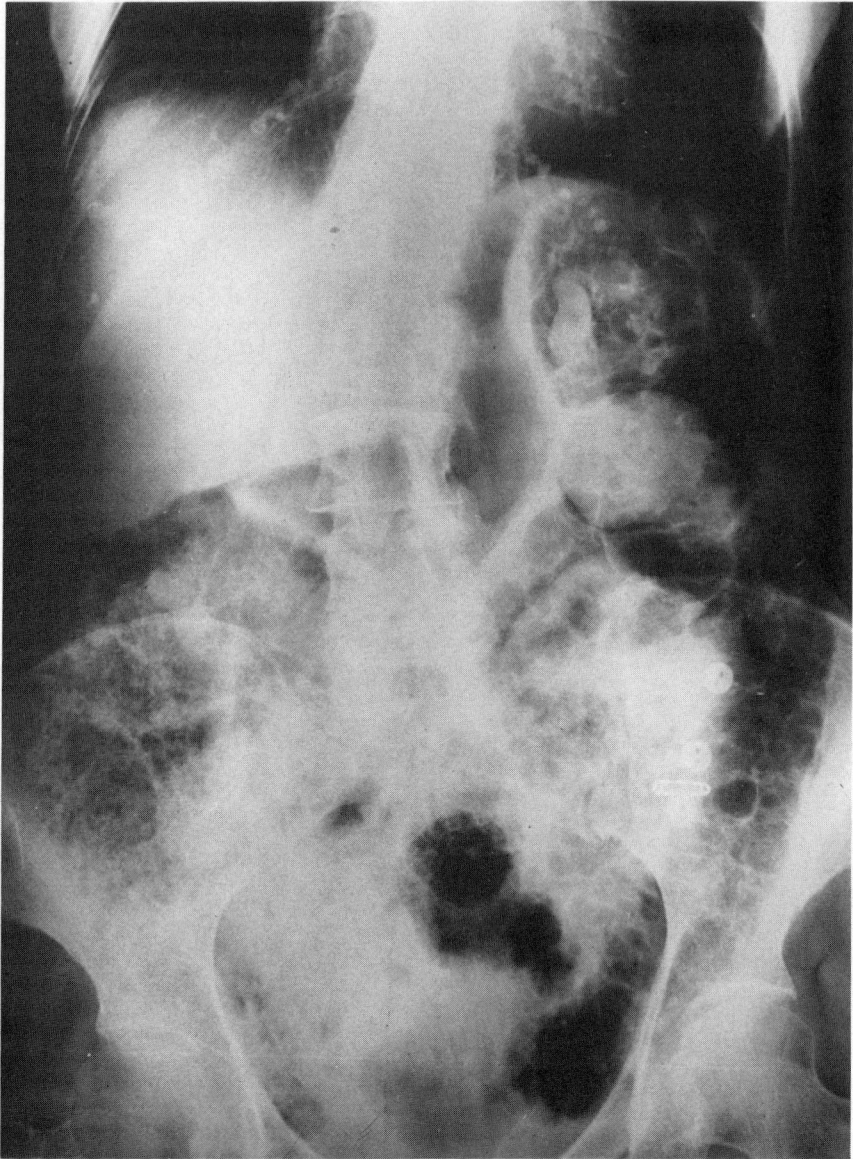

Fig. 11.75   Gas cysts of the colon seen on plain X-ray of the abdomen. Note the cystic collections especially on the left side of the colon.

absence of a mucosal defect in pneumatosis the replenishment is presumably by diffusion from the bowel lumen. There is no convincing evidence in man of bacterial contamination within the cysts. Cyst gas closely resembles bowel gas on analysis, often containing quite large proportions of H_2,[3] and it is conceivable that the cysts grow and multiply because insoluble bowel gas diffuses into the cysts more quickly than it can diffuse from the cysts into the capillaries. The well-known variations in bowel gas with various dietary components[9] probably explains the spontaneous waxing and waning of the size of the cysts and the symptoms they cause. Keyting

et al.[4] proposed that gas originated in the chest as mediastinal emphysema and tracked along the periaortic areolar tissue into the mesentery and then along the mesenteric vessels into the bowel wall. They showed that submucosal colonic cysts could be produced by injection of air into the base of the dogs' mesentery although they failed to persist. We have observed gas in the juxtacolonic mesentery in a patient dying with mediastinal emphysema in association with fibrosing alveolitis. A further piece of evidence has been provided by Gillon *et al.*[2] who showed that many patients with pneumatosis coli during a fast have unusually high levels of breath H_2.

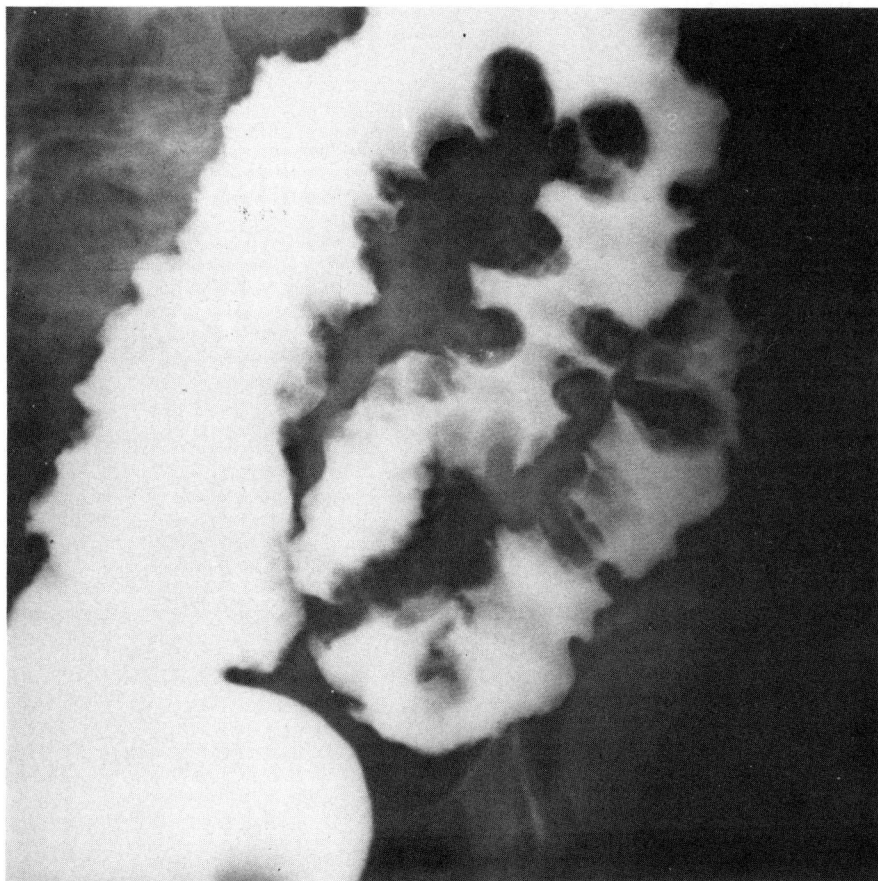

Fig. 11.76 Barium enema in pneumatosis coli. This film shows the characteristic scalloped appearance in the sigmoid colon.

This indicates abnormal bowel gas formation in the presence of unusual bowel organisms, colonic stasis or some form of malabsorption.

Pneumatosis coli probably occurs in patients who form unusually large amounts of H_2 and perhaps other insoluble colonic gases. They then, following the trauma of coughing or some other mechanical insult, develop to surgical emphysema in the colon wall. The emphysema, instead of resolving, extends as the gas bubbles grow, split and migrate round the colon.

There is little evidence to suggest that the gas in these chronic cases originates from gas forming organisms in the bowel wall. It does not involve lymphatic spaces, is not the result of colonic ischaemia and is not a neoplastic process, although all these suggestions have been seriously proposed.

Treatment

Conservative approach
Since this is a benign disease with some spontaneous remissions and a low incidence of serious complications, initially, a conservative approach should be adopted. Antidiarrhoeal drugs help to some extent as well as antibiotics (most recently metronidazole) but these have never been effective in our hands. Dietary advice to reduce the amount of colonic gas production seems sensible and a low residue diet (avoiding husks, bran and beans) can be advocated. Patients placed on an elemental diet rapidly lose their symptoms but will not tolerate the diet for long.

Oxygen
Breathing 70% oxygen at atmospheric pressure for a sufficient period will always result in resolution of colonic gas cysts.[11] First described in 1973,[1] this method of management has now gained wide acceptance and will result in prolonged remission if pursued energetically. There is a high rate of recurrence within two years but the treatment may be repeated. Anxiety about the toxic effects of 70% oxygen have proved unfounded in our experience. Although some authors have used hyperbaric oxygen therapy, theoretically this is unnecessary and practically

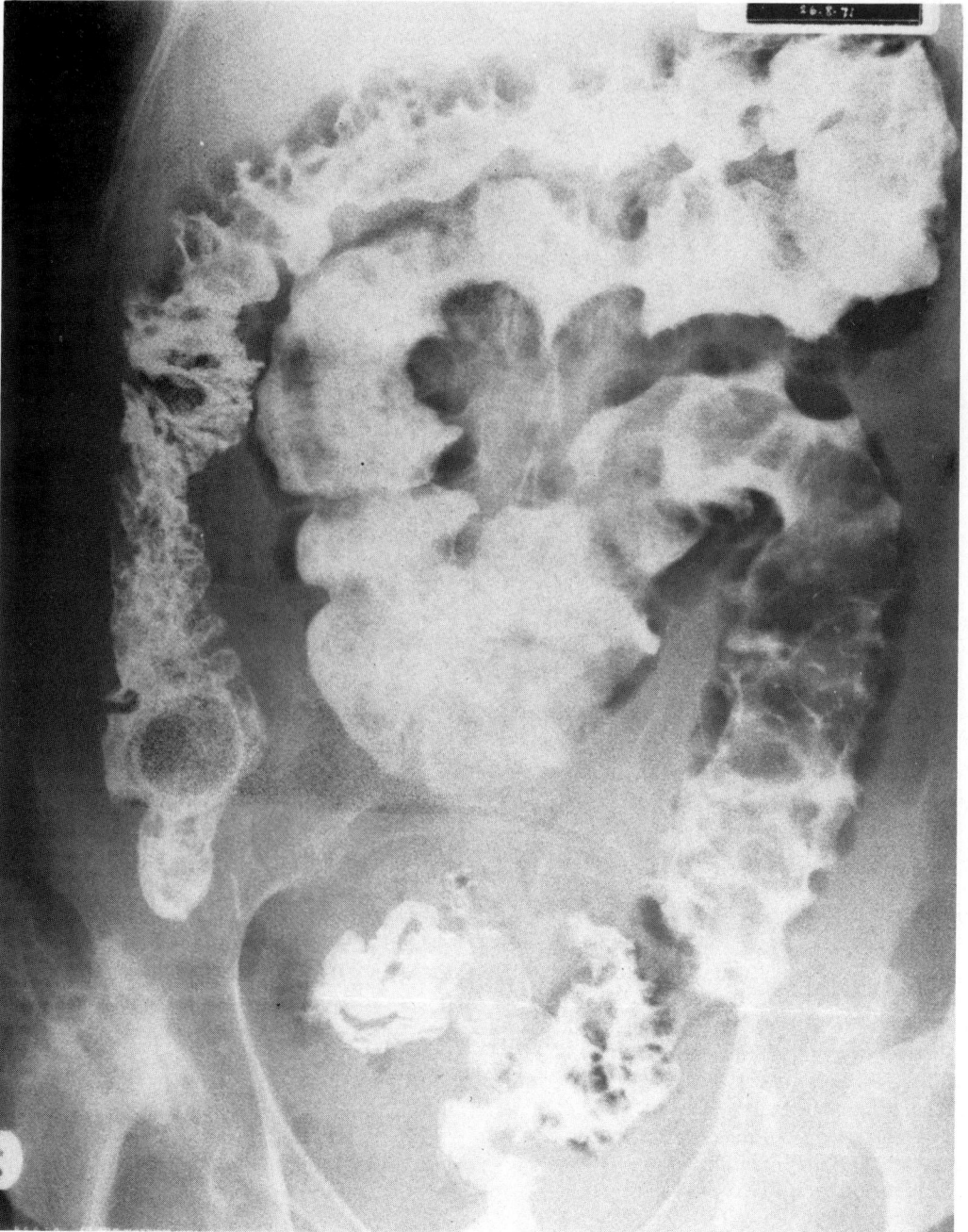

Fig. 11.77 Barium enema in pneumatosis coli. Collections of gas lying in the wall of the colon outside the barium coated mucosa can be easily appreciated.

it is more expensive. The results of treatment are probably inferior in terms of length of remission as it is difficult to give a sufficient number of treatments to induce complete remission. The essential steps in normobaric oxygen treatment are outlined in Table 11.20. It is useless to simply ask the nurse to 'administer oxygen'. Inspired oxygen at 70% is quite difficult to achieve and a close fitting mask (e.g. Ventimask) designed to give high concentrations, together

with high flow rates of humidified oxygen (often 10 l/min), are essential. Adequacy of administration must be monitored by Pa_{O_2} estimations 30 min after commencing treatment. In our experience maintained levels of Pa_{O_2} of 40 kPa (300 mmHg) always result in disappearance of the cysts within five days. Diarrhoea usually ceases immediately treatment is started. Oxygen therapy may be difficult in patients with obstructive airways disease but Klausen et al.[5] have

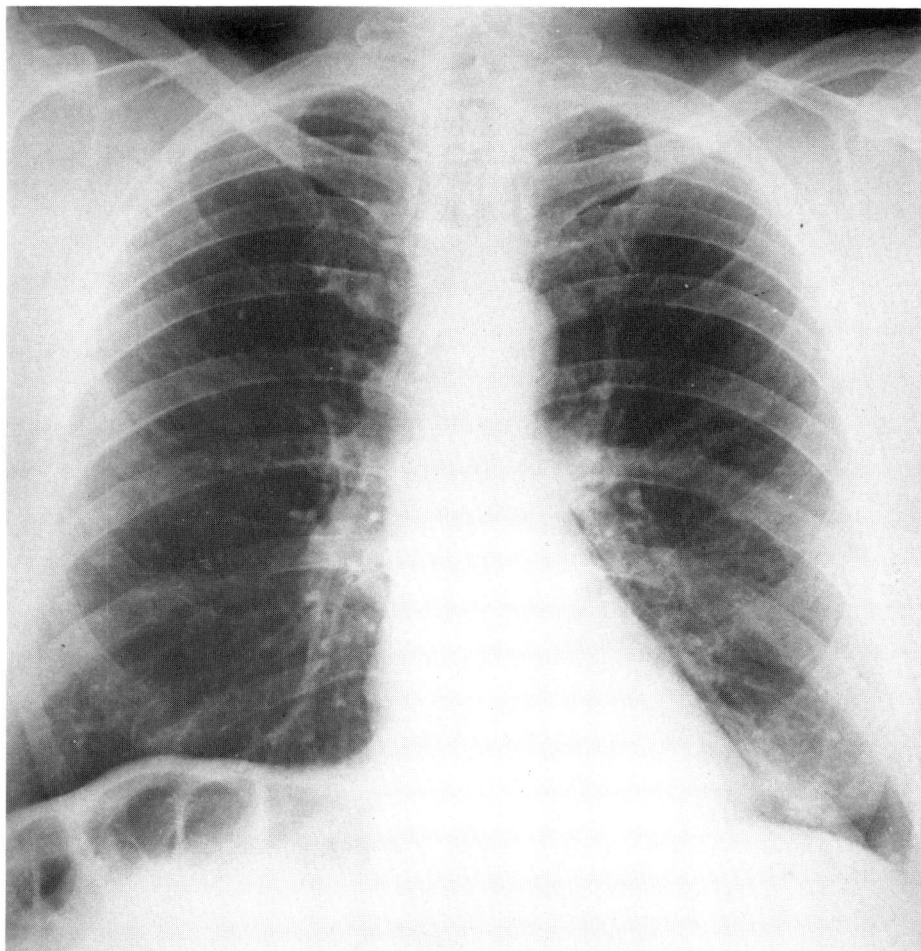

Fig. 11.78   Chilaiditi's sign seen on a chest X-ray. The gas-filled colon lies between the liver and the diaphragm.

Table 11.20   Steps in the treatment of pneumatosis coli with oxygen breathing.

1   Empty the bowel, e.g. Castor oil 30 ml; magnesium sulphate mixture 20 ml two-hourly until diarrhoea

2   Elemental diet or fluid diet only

3   Oxygen by close-fitting mask (humidify or patient will not tolerate) 8–10 l/min or more

4   Estimate PaO_2 after 30 minutes and if below 40 kPa (300 mmHg) increase oxygen flow, replace mask or otherwise adjust until desired PaO_2 is obtained

5   Continue oxygen breathing day and night with only 20-minute breaks for food and toilet – the more the patient wears the mask the quicker the treatment will be completed

6   Monitor progress by plain X-ray of abdomen each day

7   When radiological 'cure' is complete repeat sigmoidoscopy

8   When all cysts have disappeared on the X-ray plate and on sigmoidoscopy continue oxygen therapy for a further 48 hours

9   Arrange a post-treatment barium enema or colonoscopy to exclude other colonic pathology

used doxapram hydrochloride successfully in this situation. Oxygen breathing is continued day and night with only 20 min breaks for refreshment.

Response to therapy is simply monitored by daily abdominal X-rays and the resolution of the cysts can be confirmed with sigmoidoscopy. It has been our practice to continue oxygen treatment for 48 hours after all evidence of the cysts has disappeared because if any cysts remain rapid recurrence of the full syndrome occurs. After therapy a barium enema or colonoscopy should be performed to ensure that there is no underlying colonic pathology.

Surgical treatment

In secondary pneumatosis coli intestinalis surgical management of the primary lesion is frequently necessary and emergency surgery is occasionally required for obstruction or volvulus. Subtotal colectomy may occasionally be required in severely symptomatic patients with recurrent pneumatosis coli despite adequate oxygen therapy.

REFERENCES

1 Forgacs, P., Wright, P. H. & Wyatt, A. P. (1973) Treatment of intestinal gas cysts by oxygen breathing. *Lancet*, **i**, 579–582.

2 Gillon, J., Tadesse, K., Logan, R. F. A. *et al.* (1979) Breath hydrogen in pneumatosis cystoides intestinalis. *Gut*, **20**, 1008–1011.

3 Hughes, D. T. D., Gordon, K. C. D., Swan, J. C. & Bolt, G. L. (1966) Pneumatosis cystoides intestinalis. *Gut*, **7**, 553–557.

4 Keyting, W. S., McCarver, R. R., Kovarik, J. L. & Daywitt, A. L. (1961) Pneumatosis intestinalis: a new concept. *Radiology*, **76**, 733–741.

5 Klausen, N. O., Agner, E., Tougaard, L. & Sorensen, B. (1982) Pneumatosis coli in chronic respiratory failure. *British Medical Journal*, **284**, 1834–1835.

6 Koss, L. G. (1952) Abdominal gas cysts. *American Medical Association Archives of Pathology*, **53**, 523–549.

7 Martyak, S. N. & Curtis, L. E. (1976) Pneumatosis intestinalis; a compilation of jejunoileal bypass. *Journal of the American Medical Association*, **235**, 1038–1039.

8 Sames, C. P. (1964) Pneumatosis cystoides intestinalis (pelvic colon). *Proceedings of the Royal Society of Medicine*, **57**, 400.

9 Sutalf, L. O. & Levitt, M. D. (1979) Follow-up of a flatulent patient. *Digestive Diseases and Sciences (New Series)*, **24**, 652–654.

10 Wyatt, A. P. (1972) Pneumatosis cystoides intestinalis. *Proceedings of the Royal Society of Medicine*, **65**, 780–782.

11 Wyatt, A. P. (1975) Prolonged symptomatic and radiological remission of colonic gas cysts after oxygen therapy. *British Journal of Surgery*, **62**, 837–839.

Chapter 12
Inflammatory Bowel Disease

INCIDENCE, EPIDEMIOLOGY AND GENETICS

DESCRIPTIVE FEATURES

The incidence and prevalence of inflammatory bowel disease in the community can only be measured if all those who have the disease can be identified within a given population. Non-specific inflammatory bowel disease, particularly, poses a number of analytical problems.

DISEASE DEFINITION

The vast majority of cases of non-specific inflammatory bowel disease comprise either ulcerative colitis or Crohn's disease. Although individual features which are discussed elsewhere usually allow clinical distinction to be made between them, there are a minority of individuals in whom the distinction between ulcerative colitis and Crohn's disease cannot be made with certainty. Furthermore, the chance that any disease will be diagnosed depends upon access to sophisticated investigative methods which vary from place to place, especially from tropical underdeveloped areas to others with advanced Western patterns of industrialization. Thirdly, chronic non-specific inflammatory bowel disease is less likely to be recognized in areas where dysenteric illness is endemic. Even in places where infective dysenteric illness is uncommon there will be a pool of cases of unknown and varying size which remain undiagnosed either through failure of presentation or through failure to recognize that the symptoms represent more than a simple disorder of bowel habit.

It is clear therefore that incidence or prevalence data collected in different places or at different times can only be considered together provided these points are taken into account.

INDICES OF FREQUENCY

Death rates

Few people die from Crohn's disease and ulcerative colitis; if they do it is usually from the complications of the disease or the complications of surgery. The chances of dying are also greater in older than in younger people. Fluctuations in death rates can therefore arise from variation in the age pattern of affected individuals, in the efficiency of treatment and in the clinical patterns of disease encountered, as well as from changes in patterns and fashions in death certification.

Hospital admission rates

Although most patients with Crohn's disease are likely to be admitted to hospital at some time or another, this is not true of ulcerative colitis, where the majority of individuals have mild disease limited to the distal large intestine. Outpatient treatment has probably become commoner as medical treatment has improved, and this is likely to be true for both ulcerative colitis and Crohn's disease. It follows that disease frequency could be increasing even though hospital admission rates remain the same or even fall. Admission statistics also seldom allow repeated admissions of a single individual to be distinguished from single admissions of separate people.

Despite these difficulties, hospital admission rates probably form useful indices of Crohn's disease frequency but they are of little value in ulcerative colitis.

Outpatient and other diagnostic referral rates

Few sets of data are available. Even where they do exist the effects of changing diagnostic awareness, increasing diagnostic precision and greater general availability of diagnostic methods must be considered.

INCIDENCE AND PREVALENCE RATES

Tables 12.1 and 12.2 give incidence and prevalence rates recorded predominantly in North

Table 12.1 Average annual incidence and prevalence rates for Crohn's disease per 100 000 population.[a]

		Incidence	Prevalence
England, Oxford[10]	1951–60	0.8	9.0
USA, Baltimore[39]	1960–63	1.8	—
Scotland, Aberdeen[24]	1955–68	2.0	32.5
England, North Tees[8]	1971–77	5.3	35.0
England, Nottingham[36]	1958–72	2.0	26.5
Norway, general survey[41]	1964–69	1.1	—
Switzerland, Basle[11]	1960–69	1.6	—
Denmark, Copenhagen[6]	1970–78	2.7	34.0
Sweden, Malmö[51]	1958–73	4.3	57.0
Sweden, Uppsala and Vastmanland[4]	1968–73	5.0	50.0
Sweden, Stockholm[18]	1970–74	4.5	—
Wales, Cardiff[31]	1966–77	4.0	—
USA, Minnesota[47]	1965–75	6.6	—
New Zealand, Auckland[9]	1969–78	1.8	—

[a] Age-standardized and crude data are not separable in some of these data, and therefore no such distinctions have been attempted in compiling this table.

America. Data are available from these places for a number of reasons which include the high frequency of chronic non-specific inflammatory bowel disease, patterns of organization of medical care which ease the collection of data, and the ready availability of sophisticated diagnostic methods.

Areas of high or likely high incidence or prevalence

Apart from the Scandinavian countries and the United Kingdom, disease frequency is certainly also high throughout North America, though the patterns of health care delivery there militate against the collection of coherent bodies of data.

Table 12.2 Ulcerative colitis: average annual incidence rates (or first hospital admission rates) and prevalence rates per 100 000 population.[a]

		Incidence	Prevalence
Denmark, Copenhagen[6]	1962–78	8.1	117
England, North Tees[8]	1971–77	15.1	99.0
England, Oxford[10]	1951–60	6.5	79.9
Israel, Tel Aviv[13]	1961–70	3.6	37.4
New Zealand, Auckland[9]	1969–78	5.5	41.3
Norway, general survey[41]	1956–60	2.3	—
	1964–69	3.3	—
USA, Baltimore[39]	1960–63	4.6	42.0
USA, Minnesota[47]	1935–44	4.4	—
	1945–54	7.4	—
	1955–64	8.7	88.0 (in 1965)

[a] See footnote to Table 12.1.

Details are available from Australia, New Zealand and white populations in South Africa. Reliable sets of data from elsewhere are sparse, but if the sizes of clinically reported series are reasonable indications, then those living elsewhere seem to be less frequently affected. Few sets of comparative data within countries exist, and even where they do interpretation is difficult given the wide confidence limits around point estimates of prevalence or incidence.[12]

Areas of low or likely low incidence or prevalence

Series of clinical cases tend to be small and are reported infrequently from tropical areas, from Japan and Asia and from eastern and southern Europe and from South America. To decide whether chronic non-specific inflammatory bowel disease is more or less common in these countries depends primarily upon inspired guesswork. The likelihood is that Crohn's disease and ulcerative colitis occur with reasonable if low frequency in southern Europe, but Crohn's disease tends to be under reported in eastern Europe relative to ulcerative colitis, probably because it is relatively rare.

Moderate-sized sets of data have been reported from Czechoslovakia, Spain, Turkey, Japan and some parts of South America, but these probably represent investigator diligence rather than common disease frequency (for a general review see Lee[28]).

Time trends

The frequency with which Crohn's disease has been diagnosed has risen steadily, at least until recently. This rise may in part reflect increasing diagnostic awareness but it undoubtedly arises predominantly from a true rise in disease frequency. Figures covering a reasonable timespan have been reported from Northern Europe, and show a remarkably consistent increase (Figure 12.1) which is approximately an 8% compound rise (Figure 12.2).

The incidence of Crohn's disease may now be falling, or at least have levelled off. Such a plateau effect could arise from a failure to identify cases of recent onset and (more likely) from a pause in the pattern of shortening of the interval between onset and diagnosis (see Figure 12.3); progressive shortening would spuriously increase the frequency of disease because cases identified in a set period would represent those arising in a similar earlier set interval plus an increment representing the element of shortening. Hellers,[18] in recognizing the effects of such changes, concluded that disease frequency had risen in Stockholm county from 1955 to 1969 and had then remained stationary from 1970 to 1974.

Data are too scanty to allow reliable identification of time trends in the frequency of ulcerative colitis, the principal problem being that outpatient diagnoses have seldom been indexed. However, in Norway and in Minnesota,[14, 46] diagnoses of proctitis and colitis have increased in frequency, reflecting a true increase in disease incidence, a better diagnostic awareness, or both.

The apparent increase in the frequency of Crohn's disease could be explained by diagnostic transfer of patients previously considered to have ulcerative colitis. It is uncertain whether

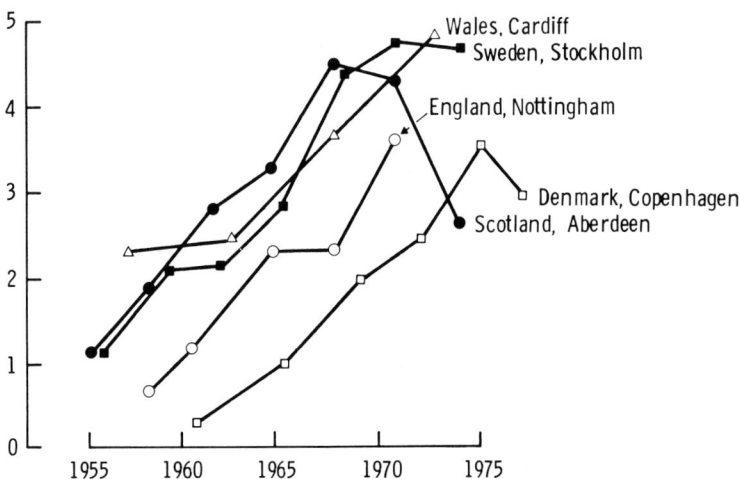

Fig. 12.1 The changing incidence of Crohn's disease. (Figures are average rates per 100 000 population per year.)

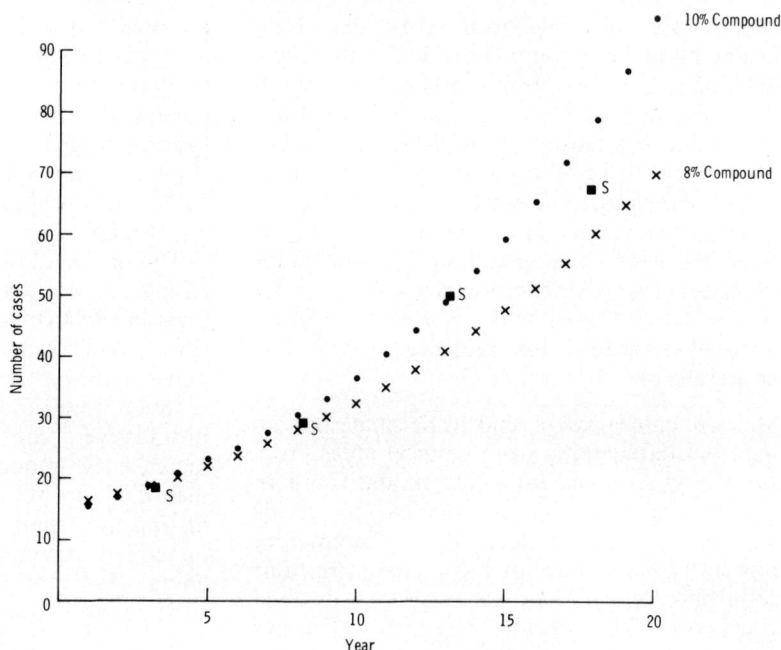

Fig. 12.2 The increased frequency of Crohn's disease: actual numerical growth in Stockholm County ■ S compared with the numbers expected with an 8% or 10% compound rise.

such recategorization has contributed substantially to the recent recorded rise in the frequency of Crohn's disease. However, hospital admission rates for ulcerative colitis have generally changed little, and irregularly, at times when the incidence of Crohn's disease has seemed to be increasing. Several observers have noted a particularly marked increase in the frequency of Crohn's disease of the colon in recent years.

Age and sex incidence

Despite much variation from one set of data to another there is no consistent difference in the sex ratio in Crohn's disease. Ulcerative colitis is slightly commoner in women than in men.

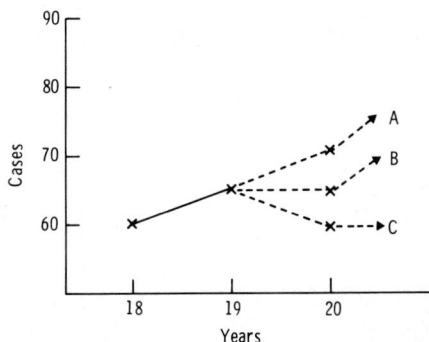

Fig. 12.3 Crohn's disease 'incidence' patterns. A. Incidence continues to increase, time before diagnosis continues to shorten. B. Incidence continues to increase, time before diagnosis does not shorten further. C. Incidence and time before diagnosis both remain the same.

Crohn's disease and ulcerative colitis are more prone to occur in early adult life than at other times. Secondary and even tertiary peaks of frequency have been detected in older people for both ulcerative colitis and Crohn's disease but none of these patterns has been detected consistently. There is general agreement that both diseases are rare in childhood.

Socioeconomic patterns

No particular occupational group seems to be at special risk of developing ulcerative colitis or Crohn's disease, but there may be a general, if slight, tendency for both diseases to occur more often in people of higher socioeconomic grouping.

Urban–rural differences

Differences between urban and rural incidence rates of inflammatory bowel disease have been detected by some,[24, 34] but not others.[18, 42] Overall the disease is rather less common in country dwellers. A reluctance of country dwellers to present with their symptoms could explain such differences as have been found.

Ethnic variation

Available information is limited because most studies of disease frequency have been conducted in places with white populations. In the

United States the incidence of ulcerative colitis and Crohn's disease seems to be much lower in black than in white people.[12] Maoris seem less likely to be affected by inflammatory bowel disease than white New Zealanders, and black (and to a lesser extent Indian) populations in South Africa than white populations.[28, 53]

Jews seem to be more prone to inflammatory bowel disease than non-Jews. Within Israel itself both ulcerative colitis and Crohn's disease seem to be less common than in people living in Northern Europe and North America.[13, 45] Israeli-born and non-Ashkenazi Jews seem to be less susceptible than Jews born in Europe or North America. These differences suggest that environmental influences partly explain the increased susceptibility of Jews to inflammatory bowel disease.

PREDISPOSING FACTORS

Associated disease

An increased frequency of asthma, hay fever, allergic rhinitis and eczema has been detected in patients and their families.[15] As with other associated diseases, there is difficulty in distinguishing between hereditary and environmental effects.

Diet

The tendency for Crohn's disease and ulcerative colitis to occur in populations living in Northern Europe and North America has inevitably suggested a causal association with dietary habits and particularly with a reduced dietary fibre and/or high refined sugar consumption.

Patients with Crohn's disease have been consistently found to consume diets containing an unduly high proportion of refined sugars (Table 12.3). It is difficult to determine whether or not dietary change preceded the onset of disease. Some evidence suggests that the dietary habits may have been long standing. Taste sensitivity

for sugars is not materially altered in Crohn's disease (a reduced sensitivity could explain an increased intake). Parallel changes have not been detected in ulcerative colitis. All these findings are consistent with an association between a high refined-sugar intake and an increased liability to Crohn's disease. This could be either a primary or secondary phenomenon. A secondary effect of reduced dietary fibre intake is unlikely because fibre intake does not seem to be greatly altered in Crohn's disease patients.[3, 44, 50]

Infection

The conflicting and generally disappointing results of experimental studies of the contagion hypothesis are discussed elsewhere. Epidemiological investigations suggest that patients are unable to transmit and to contract infection, but a limiting feature of these studies is that we do not understand what the appropriate timings might be.[36, 37] The detection of lymphocytotoxic antibodies with increased frequency in the sera of family members of patients with inflammatory bowel disease[22] could reflect common exposure to an infectious agent, though such findings are not necessarily specific for infection. If the inverse correlation between the patterns of frequency of endemic dysenteries and of chronic non-specific inflammatory bowel disease is an epidemiological clue, then its nature eludes us.

If Crohn's disease and ulcerative colitis represent abnormal responses to infection from delayed exposure to causal agents which alter the pattern of host response, then the analogies of Hodgkin's disease[14] and paralytic poliomyelitis may be relevant.

Childhood factors

Since both Crohn's disease and ulcerative colitis reach their peak incidence in early adult life, it is natural to consider factors in childhood when seeking epidemiological clues.

Some data suggest that breast feeding exerts a protective influence[2, 19] (Table 12.4), though, if true, it is unclear whether protection is in fact a direct consequence of breast feeding or arises for other associated reasons.

Smoking

It seems that patients with ulcerative colitis are more often non-smokers.[16] The reason for such a difference, which needs confirmation, is unclear.

Table 12.3 Sugar intake (g/day) in Crohn's disease patients and control individuals.

Reference	Average sugar intake in patients	Average sugar intake in controls	No. studied
Martini and Brandes[30]	177	74	63
Miller *et al.*[38]	150	55	34
Thornton *et al.*[50]	122	65	30

Table 12.4 Breast-feeding duration: differences in months, Crohn's disease patients *vs* controls.[19]

	Age			
	10–19	20–29	30–39	40–49
Mean	−1.46	−1.28	−0.67	−0.41
Standard error	0.4	0.4	0.9	1.4
Number	100	137	42	17

GENETIC CONSIDERATIONS

Both ulcerative colitis and Crohn's disease are detected more commonly amongst relatives of patients than in the general population. This increase may be due in part to increased awareness of the significance of symptoms amongst family members, and to common exposure to predisposing environmental factors, but this is very unlikely to be the whole explanation.

Table 12.5 shows the frequency with which ulcerative colitis and Crohn's disease were detected in the relatives of propositi attending the Liverpool colon clinic in England. Similar results have been obtained in Chicago, where 78 first-degree relatives of 646 inflammatory bowel disease patients also had the disease. Commonly recorded relationships are of brothers and sisters being affected, with parent and child being the next most likely. These patterns are summarized by Lewkonia and McConnell.[29] Assessment is complicated, not only by family awareness of symptom patterns, but also by the likelihood that clinics with an established interest in inflammatory bowel disease will inevitably tend to be those to which patients from families with more than one affected member will gravitate.

The tendency for there to be concordance in identical twins argues strongly for inherited factors. If the tendency to develop inflammatory bowel disease is inherited, as seems likely, then this does not follow Mendelian principles.

Table 12.5 Familial relationships in inflammatory bowel disease.[29]

	Crohn's disease	Ulcerative colitis
Number studied	39	103
First-degree relatives affected		
Crohn's disease	7	3
Ulcerative colitis	4	4
Second-degree relatives affected		
Crohn's disease	0	1
Ulcerative colitis	1	—

From Lewkonia and McConnell (1976),[29] with kind permission of the authors and the editor of *Gut*.

Genetic associations

Searches for marker genes have generally been disappointing. No association has been detected for ABO blood group, secretor status and a wide variety of serological markers.[5]

Careful attention has been paid to possible associations with HLA antigens, particularly because of the well-known associations between inflammatory bowel disease and ankylosing spondylitis and between ankylosing spondylitis and HLA-B27. Although possession of HLA-B27 does not of itself increase liability to inflammatory bowel disease, the presence of inflammatory bowel disease does seem to greatly increase the chances that individuals who are B27 will develop ankylosing spondylitis.[29]

Formal searches have yielded no consistent patterns of association between HLA-A or -B status and liability to inflammatory bowel disease. Although various individual series have suggested that associations might exist, the sets of data have been too small to draw reliable conclusions.

There have been few HLA-D antigen studies and no coherent pattern has been detected, although the figures available are enough to indicate that strong associations of the sort detected in systemic lupus erythematosus are unlikely.

Attempts have been made to bring together genetic and epidemiological data in order to account for the observed frequency patterns of ulcerative colitis and Crohn's disease but as yet the data is inadequate to allow any useful conclusions.

REFERENCES

1 Acheson, E. D. (1960) The distribution of ulcerative colitis and regional enteritis in United States veterans with particular reference to the Jewish Religion. *Gut*, **1**, 291–293.
2 Acheson, E. D. & Truelove, S. C. (1961) Early weaning in the aetiology of ulcerative colitis. *British Medical Journal*, **ii**, 929–933.
3 Archer, L. N. J. & Harvey, R. F. (1978) Breakfast and Crohn's disease II. *British Medical Journal*, **ii**, 540.
4 Bergman, L. & Krause, U. (1975) The incidence of Crohn's disease in central Sweden. *Scandinavian Journal of Gastroenterology*, **10**, 725–729.

5 Biemond, I., Weterman, I. T., Rood, J. Jv. *et al.* (1981) Search for genetic markers associated with Crohn's disease in the Netherlands. In *Recent Advances in Crohn's Disease.* (Ed.) Pena, A. S., Weterman, I. T., Booth, C. C. & Strober, W. pp. 197–203. The Hague: Nijhoff.

6 Binder, V., Both, H., Hansen, P. K. *et al.* (1982) Incidence and prevalence of ulcerative colitis and Crohn's disease in the county of Copenhagen 1962–1978. *Gastroenterology*, **83**, 563–568.

7 Bonnevie, O. (1967) A socio-economic study of patients with ulcerative colitis. *Scandinavian Journal of Gastroenterology*, **2**, 129–136.

8 Devlin, H. B., Datta, D. & Dellipiani, A. W. (1980) The incidence and prevalence of inflammatory bowel disease in North Tees Health District. *World Journal of Surgery*, **4**, 183–193.

9 Eason, R. J., Lee, S. P. & Jones, C. T. (1982) Inflammatory bowel disease in Auckland New Zealand. *Australasian and New Zealand Journal of Medicine*, **12**, 128–131.

10 Evans, J. G. & Acheson, E. C. (1965) An epidemiological study of ulcerative colitis and regional enteritis in the Oxford area. *Gut*, **6**, 311–324.

11 Fahrlander, H. & Baerlocher, C. (1970) Epidemiology of Crohn's disease in the Basle area. In *Regional Enteritis: Crohn's Disease* (Ed.) Engel, A. & Larssen, T. pp. 131–141. Fifth Skandia International Symposium. Stockholm: Nordiska Bokhandelus Forlag.

12 Garland, C. F., Lilienfeld, A. M., Mendeloff, A. I. *et al.* (1981) Incidence rates of ulcerative colitis and Crohn's disease in fifteen areas of the United States. *Gastroenterology*, **81**, 1115–1124.

13 Gilat, T., Ribak, J., Benaroya, Y. *et al.* (1974) Ulcerative colitis in the Jewish population of Tel-Aviv-Jafo. *Gastroenterology*, **66**, 335–342.

14 Gutensohn, N. & Cole, P. (1981) Childhood social environment and Hodgkin's disease. *New England Journal of Medicine*, **304**, 135–140.

15 Hammer, B., Ashurst, P. & Naish, J. (1968) Diseases associated with ulcerative colitis and Crohn's disease. *Gut*, **9**, 17–21.

16 Harries, A. D., Baird, A. & Rhodes, J. (1982) Non-smoking. A feature of ulcerative colitis. *British Medical Journal*, **284**, 706.

17 Harries, A. D., Baird, A., Rhodes, J. & Mayberry, J. F. (1982) Has the rising incidence of Crohn's disease reached a plateau? *British Medical Journal*, **284**, 235.

18 Hellers, G. (1979) Crohn's disease in Stockholm County, 1955–1974. A study of epidemiology, results of surgical treatment and long term prognosis. *Acta Chirurgica Scandinavica* (Supplement 490) 1–84.

19 Hellers, G. (1981) Some epidemiological aspects of Crohn's disease in Stockholm County 1955–1979. In *Recent Advances in Crohn's Disease* (Ed.) Pena, A. S., Weterman, I. T., Booth, C. C. & Strober, W. pp. 158–162. The Hague: Nijhoff.

20 Hoj, L., Brix Jensen, P., Bonnevie, O. & Riis, P. (1973) An epidemiological study of regional enteritis and acute ileitis in Copenhagen County. *Scandinavian Journal of Gastroenterology*, **8**, 381–384.

21 Keighley, A., Miller, D. S., Hughes, A. O. & Langman, M. J. S. (1976) The demographic and social characteristics of patients with Crohn's disease in the Nottingham area. *Scandinavian Journal of Gastroenterology*, **11**, 293–296.

22 Korsmeyer, S. J., Williams, R. C., Wilson, I. D. & Strickland, R. G. (1975) Lymphocytotoxic antibody in inflammatory bowel disease: a family study. *New England Journal of Medicine*, **293**, 1117–1120.

23 Kuiper, I., Weterman, I. T., Biemond, I. *et al.* (1981) Lymphocytotoxic antibody in patients with Crohn's disease and family members. In *Recent Advances in Crohn's Disease* (Ed.) Pena, A. G., Weterman, I. T., Booth, C. C. & Strober, W. pp. 341–347. The Hague: Nijhoff.

24 Kyle, J. (1971) An epidemiological study of Crohn's disease in North East Scotland. *Gastroenterology*, **61**, 826–833.

25 Kyle, J. (1972) *Crohn's Disease.* London: Heinemann Medical.

26 Kyle, J. & Stark, J. (1980) Fall in the incidence of Crohn's disease. *Gut*, **21**, 340–343.

27 Langman, M. J. S. (1979) *The Epidemiology of Chronic Intestinal Disease.* London: Arnold.

28 Lee, E. C. G. (1981) *Crohn's Workshop: A Global Assessment of Crohn's Disease.* London: Heyden.

29 Lewkonia, R. M. & McConnell, R. B. (1976) Familial inflammatory bowel disease – heredity or environment? *Gut*, **17**, 235–243.

30 Martini, G. A. & Brandes, J. W. (1976) Increased consumption of refined carbohydrates in patients with Crohn's disease. *Klinische Wochenschrift*, **54**, 357–371.

31 Mayberry, J., Rhodes, J. & Hughes, L. E. (1979) Incidence of Crohn's disease in Cardiff between 1934 & 1977. *Gut*, **20**, 602–608.

32 McDermott, F., Hughes, E. S. R. & Pihl, E. (1980) Mortality and morbidity of Crohn's disease and ulcerative colitis in Australia. *Medical Journal of Australia*, **1**, 534–536.

33 Mendeloff, A. I. & Dunn, J. P. (1971) *Digestive Diseases.* Cambridge, Mass: Harvard University Press.

34 Mendeloff, A. I., Monk, M., Siegal, C. I. & Lilienfeld, A. (1966) Some epidemiological features of ulcerative colitis and regional enteritis – a preliminary report. *Gastroenterology*, **51**, 748–756.

35 Miller, B., Fervers, F., Rohbeck, R. & Strohmeyer, G. (1976) Zuckerkonsum bei patienten mit morbus Crohn. *Verhhandlungen der Deutschen Gesellschaft fur Innere Medizin*, **82**, 922–924.

36 Miller, D. A., Keighley, A. C. & Langman, M. J. S. (1974) Changing patterns in epidemiology of Crohn's disease. *Lancet*, **ii**, 691–693.

37 Miller, D. S., Keighley, A., Smith, P. G. *et al.* (1975) Crohn's disease in Nottingham: a search for time-space clustering. *Gut*, **16**, 454–457.

38 Miller, D. S., Keighley, A., Smith, P. G. *et al.* (1976) A case control method for seeking evidence of contagion in Crohn's disease. *Gastroenterology*, **71**, 385–387.

39 Monk, M., Mendeloff, A. I., Siegel, C. I. & Lilienfeld, A. (1967) An epidemiological study of ulcerative colitis and regional enteritis among adults in Baltimore. I. Hospital incidence and prevalence, 1960–1963. *Gastroenterology*, **53**, 198–210.

40 Monk, M., Mendeloff, A. I., Siegel, C. I. & Lilienfeld, A. (1969) An epidemiological study of ulcerative colitis and regional enteritis among adults in Baltimore. II. Social and demographic factors. *Gastroenterology*, **56**, 847–857.

41 Myren, J., Gjone, E., Hertzberg, J. N. *et al.* (1971) Epidemiology of ulcerative colitis and regional enterocolitis (Crohn's disease) in Norway. *Scandinavian Journal of Gastroenterology*, **6**, 511–514.

42 Norlen, B. J., Krause, U. & Bergman, L. (1970) An epidemiological study of Crohn's disease. *Scandinavian Journal of Gastroenterology*, **5**, 385–390.

43 Paffenbarger, R. S., Wing, A. L. & Hyde, R. T. (1977) Characteristics in youth indicative of adult-onset Hodgkin's disease. *Journal of the National Cancer Institute*, **58**, 1489–1491.

44   Rawcliffe, P. M. & Truelove, S. C. (1978) Breakfast and Crohn's disease I. *British Medical Journal*, **ii**, 539.

45   Rozen, O., Zonia, J., Yekutiel, P. & Gilst, T. (1979) Crohn's disease in the Jewish population of Tel-Aviv-Jafo. *Gastroenterology*, **76**, 25–30.

46   Sedlack, R. E., Nobrega, F. T., Kurland, L. T. & Sauer, W. G. (1972) Inflammatory colon disease in Rochester, Minnesota, 1935–1964. *Gastroenterology*, **62**, 935–941.

47   Sedlack, R. E., Whisnant, J., Elveback, L. R. & Kurland, L. T. (1980) Incidence of Crohn's disease in Olmsted County Minnesota 1935–1975. *American Journal of Epidemiology*, **112**, 759–763.

48   Segal, I., Tim, L. O., Hamilton, D. G. & Mannell, A. (1981) The Baragwanath experience of Crohn's disease and intestinal tuberculosis. In *A Global Assessment of Crohn's Disease* (Ed.) Lee, E. C. G. London: Heyden.

49   Smith, I. S., Young, S., Gillespie, G. *et al.* (1975) Epidemiological aspects of Crohn's disease in Clydesdale 1961–1970. *Gut*, **16**, 62–67.

50   Thornton, J. R., Emmett, P. M. & Heaton, K. W. (1979) Diet and Crohn's disease: characteristics of the pre-illness diet. *British Medical Journal*, **ii**, 762–764.

51   Wenckert, A., Henricksson, A. & Lindstrom, C. (1974) Incidence of Crohn's disease in the city of Malmo. *Scandinavian Journal of Gastroenterology*, **9** (Supplement 27), 42.

52   Whorwell, P. J., Holdstock, G., Whorwell, G. M. & Wright, R. (1979) Bottle feeding, early gastroenteritis and inflammatory bowel disease. *British Medical Journal*, **i**, 382.

53   Wigley, R. D. & MacLaurin, B. P. (1962) A study of ulcerative colitis in New Zealand, showing a low incidence in Maoris. *British Medical Journal*, **ii**, 228–231.

AETIOLOGY AND PATHOGENESIS

At present the term inflammatory bowel disease is used by many to refer solely to ulcerative colitis and Crohn's disease. Yardley and Hamilton[199] have recently suggested that the term inflammatory bowel disease should encompass all forms of inflammatory disease of the intestine, and that ulcerative colitis and Crohn's disease should be categorized within this general heading as idiopathic inflammatory bowel disease. This system has much to commend it, but whether it will be generally adopted, remains to be seen.

Since ulcerative colitis and Crohn's disease are often considered together both clinically and for the purposes of research, it is often assumed that they have the same underlying pathogenesis. The familial incidence of the two disorders and the observation that either can occur within a predisposed family (see earlier) suggests that they are in some way related. However, many of the clinical features tend to favour separate causes. For example, removal of the colon in patients with ulcerative colitis results in cure,

suggesting an organ-specific type of disease. This contrasts with the post-surgical behaviour of Crohn's disease. There is a paucity of reports of the two diseases co-existing in their classic forms, although it should be remembered there are some patients in whom the disease appears to be of an indeterminate nature. Another problem is that the gut can only respond in a limited number of ways to exogenous or endogenous factors and thus disease resulting from different stimuli may be pathologically indistinguishable. For example, rectal biopsies taken from patients with ulcerative colitis and campylobacter colitis are similar.

The resemblance of ulcerative colitis to bacillary dysentery and Crohn's disease to intestinal tuberculosis, together with the available genetic and epidemiological data has lead to a working hypothesis for the aetiology of these conditions (Figure 12.4).

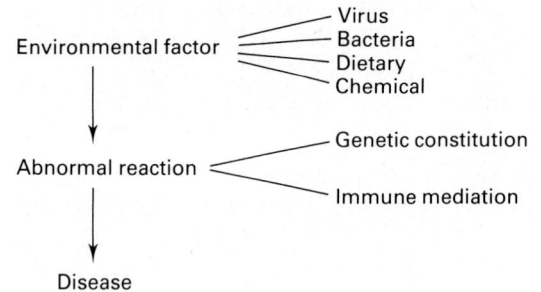

Fig. 12.4   A working hypothesis for the aetiology of inflammatory bowel disease.

Unanswered questions in relation to the pathogenesis of ulcerative colitis and Crohn's disease are:

1   Are they separate entities?
2   Are there single or multiple causes?
3   Do they represent different manifestations of the same cause?
4   Are they mutually exclusive?
5   Do they represent polar ends of a disease spectrum?

TRANSMISSIBLE AGENTS

The concept that inflammatory bowel disease may have an infective aetiology is far from new. However, the report by Mitchell and Rees in 1970[114] on the transmission of granulomas from a patient with Crohn's disease to mice, revived interest in the subject and a surge of research on both transmissible and microbiological aspects has followed. Mitchell's group demonstrated that the transmissible agent was heat labile and passed through a 220-nm filter.[115] Attempts to reproduce this work in other laboratories has produced conflicting results with both negative[3, 16, 17, 27, 67] and positive results.[38, 168, 169] Others have reported atypical changes[46, 158] and the induction of granulomas by non-inflammatory bowel disease tissue.[38, 170] It has also been suggested that antiseptic skin preparations may produce misleading artefacts.[128] An independent review of tissue submitted from the studies which gave positive results has cast serious doubts on some of the results of the transmission work.[199] However, just as the subject seemed to be drawing to a close Das and colleagues have reported further positive data.[43, 44, 194] They demonstrated the induction of lymphomas in nude mice inoculated with Crohn's disease homogenates. In addition, sera from patients appeared to recognize antigenic determinants within the tumours.

With few exceptions,[34, 38] the transmission work has been negative in ulcerative colitis.

Bacteria

MYCOBACTERIA

In 1913 Dalziel,[42] having failed to demonstrate tubercle bacilli in his cases of chronic interstitial enteritis, which were almost certainly Crohn's disease, drew attention to the similarity to Johne's disease of cattle. This disease is caused by *Mycobacterium pseudotuberculosis* but this organism has never been isolated in Crohn's disease. Other attempts to isolate *Mycobacterium tuberculosis* have been negative, and antituberculous therapy is ineffective.[81] In 1974 Watson and Martucci[184] reported sensitivity to mycobacterial antigens in patients with Crohn's disease as determined by a migration-inhibition technique. This was followed by reports of atypical mycobacteria being isolated from Crohn's disease tissue.[32, 33] It was suggested that the organism may be *Mycobacterium kansasii* in the cell wall deficient or L form. However the nature of the organism is still doubtful[161] and it is possible that coryneform bacteria may be producing the acid-fast material.[189]

VARIANT BACTERIA

L-form, or variant, bacteria are those which have lost most if not all of their cell wall components. Their role in the provocation of disease is highly controversial. They can be induced in a variety of ways including exposure to antibiotics and bacteriophages. The resulting organism has atypical properties such as osmotic instability, pleomorphic structure and variable staining characteristics. Pathogenicity and antigenicity are also altered and they have the ability to pass through bacterial filters. Under favourable circumstances they can revert to the normal parent organism. Aluwihare[6] in an electron microscopic study of Crohn's disease tissue found atypical intramural bacteria and speculated that they might be L forms. Orr et al.[128] succeeded in inducing granulomatous change in the terminal ileum of animals by the injection of L forms of *Streptococcus faecalis*. Parent and Mitchell[129, 130] reported the isolation of variants of *Pseudomonas maltophilia* or pseudomonas-like organisms exclusively from patients with Crohn's disease. These organisms did not produce disease when inoculated into animals.[131] To add to the confusion, L forms of a variety of different organisms have recently been reported to be present in both Crohn's disease and ulcerative colitis.[15] The significance of these L forms has yet to be determined, particularly as many patients may have received antimicrobials. Long-term use of sulphasalazine could also induce these variants.

INDIGENOUS BACTERIA

It has been suggested that there may be an imbalance or alteration of the normal flora in inflammatory bowel disease. Wensinck and colleagues[188] have proposed the concept of a Crohn's flora with higher numbers of *Bacteroides*, *Fusobacterium*, *Eubacterium* and *Peptostreptococcus* species and there may be an abnormal antibody response to some of these organisms in such patients.[179] However, Gorbach[58] has shown that changes in microflora can be induced by diarrhoea regardless of the primary cause. Changes in bacterial colonization may also occur with ileal disease and relative stasis. It is unclear whether these changes are of primary or secondary importance, which is critical from an aetiological standpoint.

The observation that diversion of the faecal stream may lead to improvement of disease,[121] taken with recent evidence that metronidazole is useful in the therapy of Crohn's disease,[30, 143, 177] suggests that the gut flora may affect the course of the disease even if they are not of primary aetiological importance. It also suggests that sensitization to bacterial antigens rather than direct infection may be of relevance.

Some strains of *Escherichia coli* have been shown to cross react with antigenic determinants on colonic epithelial cells. This leads to a hypothesis linking sensitization to colonic bacteria with subsequent immunological injury of colonic epithelium (see later in this chapter). *Escherichia coli* can certainly penetrate the mucosa of neonatal pigs[160] and this may lead to sensitization. A similar situation may obtain in man possibly augmented by some other modality such as infant bottle feeding. The enterobacterial common antigen or Kunin antigen is present in nearly all enterobacteriaceae and immunological responsiveness to this has raised considerable interest.

PATHOGENIC BACTERIA

The histological appearances of acute shigella or campylobacter colitis closely resemble ulcerative colitis.[94] These organisms have not been isolated from ulcerative colitis although *Campylobacter* species have been isolated from chronic enteritides in pigs and lambs.[63, 97, 178] Campylobacter colitis may account for some of those patients diagnosed as ulcerative colitis who never experience a relapse.

Clostridium difficile has been identified as the organism responsible for pseudomembranous colitis.[13, 96] Although this disease usually follows the use of antibiotics, it may also undergo person-to-person transmission.[60] There have been conflicting reports on isolation rates from patients with ulcerative colitis and Crohn's disease.[12a, 25, 26, 47, 61, 87, 93, 113, 176] It may sometimes be related to disease relapse. The use of drugs such as sulphasalazine and other specific antimicrobials in inflammatory bowel disease, together with impaired local gut immunity, makes it more likely that these isolations of *Clostridium difficile* represent secondary colonization.

As *Yersinia* can cause an acute terminal ileitis there has been speculation on whether it may lead to chronic disease. No relationship between *Yersinia* infection and Crohn's disease has been identified.[132, 159, 166]

Parasites

Japanese workers have shown that the larvae of the fish nematode *Anisakis* may cause an acute ileitis.[66] This is not directly relevant to disease in the western hemisphere, except to emphasize that a number of different agents may cause terminal ileal disease. Other parasites such as *Giardia lamblia* have been implicated,[11] but

their isolation probably represents a coincidental finding. The disease produced by *Entamoeba histolytica* is usually readily distinguished from ulcerative colitis and there is no evidence that this protozoan is aetiologically related to idiopathic inflammatory bowel disease.

Viruses

Virus exposure early in life is associated with a higher risk of persistent infection. Hepatitis B and subacute sclerosing panencephalitis are good examples.[75, 112] Subacute sclerosing panencephalitis is a chronic measles infection of the brain and thus contacts of patients would not be susceptible to infection unless they lacked previous immunity to measles. In that situation, if the virus were capable of being transmitted, they would be expected to catch measles rather than subacute sclerosing panencephalitis. A similar analogy could be made with inflammatory bowel disease if it were in some way caused by a common viral pathogen. An alternative role for a virus could be by an initiating mechanism such that the organism may have long since been cleared from the body by the time of onset of the chronic disease.

After a series of negative studies,[92, 148, 167] Farmer *et al.*[52] reported the isolation of cytomegalovirus from some patients with inflammatory bowel disease. However, in 1977 Roche and Huang[141] were unable to substantiate a positive role for this virus in idiopathic inflammatory bowel disease. Cytomegalovirus is an opportunistic organism and this probably accounts for its occasional identification in such patients. Evidence that it may modify the course of the disease comes from the detection of a high incidence of cytomegalovirus inclusions in patients developing toxic dilatation.[40]

In 1974, Aronson *et al.*[10] reported evidence of a possible viral agent in patients with Crohn's disease. This lead to a series of studies and the publication of conflicting data. Some workers have shown evidence of RNA viruses of varying sizes,[56, 57, 191] others have had negative results.[118, 133] Other reports have implicated a heat-stable, non-clostridial toxin as the cause for the observed cytopathic effect.[55, 108] Further negative studies include a search for evidence of viruses by immunofluorescence of tissue,[192] lymphocyte reactivity[59] and immune electron microscopy.[190] Examination of tissue by direct electron microscopy has, with a few exceptions,[45, 140] been negative.[6, 39]

In 1970 Hirshaut et al.[71] reported raised titres of antibodies to Epstein–Barr (EB) virus in patients with sarcoidosis. Similar investigations have been negative in idiopathic inflammatory bowel disease.[62, 77, 85]

Frei testing of patients with Crohn's disease has produced both positive[175] and negative results.[142] One serological survey has reported raised antibodies to *Chlamydia*[149] but two others have failed to confirm this finding.[166, 173] Quinn and colleagues[134] have shown that infection of the rectum with *Chlamydia trachomatis* can produce histological changes mimicking Crohn's disease. However, culture of Crohn's disease tissue for *Chlamydia* has been negative.[50]

The case for a viral aetiology for either Crohn's disease or ulcerative colitis, therefore, remains unproven.

DIETARY FACTORS

Andreson[7, 8] and others[144, 146] suggested that ulcerative colitis might be due to milk allergy. In a controlled trial, a milk-free diet has been shown to benefit some patients with ulcerative colitis,[196, 197] but measurement of milk antibodies has produced conflicting results.[48, 78, 107, 152, 172] The presence of eosinophils in the biopsies of some patients[198] and the higher incidence of atopic disease in ulcerative colitis reported by some,[23, 64, 79] suggests an allergic diathesis. However, treatment with mast-cell stabilizers such as sodium cromoglycate has proved disappointing.[4] A much more clear cut relationship with milk-protein intolerance and an ulcerative colitis-like picture has been demonstrated in children.[182] There is little data to suggest that milk allergy is of relevance in Crohn's disease.

In 1961 Acheson and Truelove[2] reported a significant deficit in the incidence of breastfeeding among patients with ulcerative colitis, a finding which has recently been confirmed by others.[193] This implies that either breastfeeding is protective, possibly as a result of antigen exclusion,[163] or that bottle feeding is harmful. This latter effect may be due to sensitization to cow's milk or bacterial antigens as a result of increased intestinal permeability to macromolecules. Bottle feeding certainly promotes the early bacterial colonization of the gut, but although there is undoubtedly increased permeability of the infantile gut in animals, the evidence is not as convincing in man. Breast feeding does not appear to confer protection against Crohn's disease[193] but there has been a suggestion that the duration of breastfeeding may be important.[69]

The recent increase in food processing and the use of additives has prompted considerable speculation on their role in idiopathic inflammatory bowel disease. Carrageenan, which is derived from seaweed, is used extensively in food processing and has therapeutic use as a pepsin inhibitor. Ulcerative disease of the colon has been reported in some animals following the oral administration of this compound.[102, 185, 186] The effect is dependent on the presence of gut bacteria[123, 124, 126] and may be a species-specific phenomenon, particularly as there have been no reports of its deleterious effect in man.[101, 110]

In 1977 James[76] reported a higher consumption of cornflakes in patients with Crohn's disease than controls but this has not been substantiated by others.[9, 105, 136] The higher intake of refined sugar in newly diagnosed patients with Crohn's disease compared with controls seems a more consistent finding.[103, 104, 105, 106, 174] These patients also have a lower intake of fibre, fresh fruit and vegetables. A trial reversing this dietary tendency seemed to have a beneficial effect on patients[68] and is now the subject of a multicentre investigation. The mechanism by which carbohydrate or fibre exert their effects and whether it is a primary or secondary phenomenon remains speculative. It might have some influence on the microbial flora of the gut.

LYMPHATIC OBSTRUCTION

Regional lymphadenopathy, submucosal oedema and evidence of lymphatic obstruction are well described in Crohn's disease.[135, 183] Reichert and Mathes[137] induced mesenteric lymphatic obstruction in dogs by the use of sclerosants and in some instances the additional administration of intravenous *Escherichia coli*. They succeeded in producing thickening and oedema of the bowel but there was little inflammation and no granuloma formation or ulceration. Lymphatic obstruction can produce changes reminiscent of Crohn's disease, particularly if the pig, which has a higher incidence of natural chronic enteritis, is used.[83, 84] Chess et al.[36] suggested that particulate absorption in the terminal ileum might result in lymphatic obstruction and subsequent disease. They administered talcum powder or sand to dogs and were able to induce granulomatous disease. This led Edwards[49] to speculate that toothpaste may be involved in the pathogenesis of Crohn's disease although this has never been substantiated.

Bockus and Lee[24] postulated a rather different role for the lymphatics. They suggested the primary event might be a lymphangitis with impairment of blood supply secondary to inflammation. Attempts to reproduce disease by vascular occlusion have not been successful,[14] although interest in the blood flow and vascular architecture of diseased bowel continues.[29, 73, 90]

RELATIONSHIP TO SARCOIDOSIS

There are striking histological similarities between Crohn's disease and sarcoidosis, except that the granulomata tend to be less well formed in Crohn's disease.

Sarcoidosis is a multi-system disorder where granulomatous involvement may occur in virtually any tissue.[147] It is curious, therefore, how seldom the gastrointestinal tract is involved.[147] It could be that these diseases are mutually exclusive or that they represent separate, perhaps genetically determined, reactions to a similar aetiological event.

A number of clinical features are common to both disorders, such as the development of uveitis, arthritis and erythema nodosum. If, as has been postulated, these symptoms are a reflection of circulating immune complexes, this may be a non-specific finding. Other features such as hypercalcaemia and hyperglobulinaemia are more commonly found in sarcoidosis.

The Kveim test has been assessed in Crohn's disease, but studies have produced conflicting results.[35, 65, 82, 86, 116, 117, 154] Kveim test material can lose its specificity thus inducing false-positive results in many different diseases. This may explain why some workers obtained positive results in Crohn's disease.[95] Sensitivity to Kveim antigen in leucocyte migration inhibition assays has been reported,[31, 139, 195] but a similar finding has also been observed in ulcerative colitis and coeliac disease, suggesting it is a non-specific response. Using thymidine uptake, a low level of lymphocyte reactivity to Kveim antigen has been reported in Crohn's disease,[157] but this study did not use any disease controls. Anergy to tuberculin is a well-recognized feature of sarcoidosis. The situation with respect to Crohn's disease is less clear; most observers consider that anergy, when present, is secondary to the disease process.

Recent investigation of serum angiotensin converting enzyme and T cell subsets has revealed further areas where Crohn's disease and sarcoidosis seem to differ. Elevated levels of angiotensin converting enzyme have been reported in sarcoidosis, particularly when the disease is active.[99, 100] The enzyme is localized in sarcoid granulomas.[155] The levels in Crohn's disease are not raised and, in some instances, may even be depressed, particularly when the patients are taking steroids.[120, 156, 165, 187]

Investigation of T cell subsets in sarcoidosis has suggested that helper T cells are concentrated at the site of disease activity, leaving a relative excess of circulating suppressor cells.[41, 74, 151] The excess of circulating suppressor cells may explain the cutaneous anergy observed in sarcoidosis. The investigation of T cell subsets in Crohn's disease has produced conflicting results.

ANIMAL MODELS

Animal research in the aetiology of inflammatory bowel disease has either examined naturally occurring disease in the animal kingdom or attempted to induce the disease experimentally.

Spontaneous enteritides in animals are well recognized in veterinary practice but unfortunately the nomenclature is confusing, often implying similarities that do not necessarily exist. For instance, granulomatous colitis of Boxer dogs[88, 180] bears a much closer resemblance to Whipple's disease than it does to Crohn's disease. Table 12.6 lists some of the many animal diseases that have been compared with idiopathic inflammatory bowel disease. The spontaneous animal enteritides are of only limited value in aetiological research although they may have a role in testing therapeutic agents. There may be some merit in using a species that has an inherent susceptibility to chronic enteritis in experimental induction of disease.

Kirsner and colleagues described an experimental colitis using the Auer phenomenon.[53, 89, 91] In this model, non-specific colonic inflammation was induced by the instillation of a mild chemical irritant. Circulating antigen/antibody complexes will then localize to the colon, producing a self-limiting colitis. Recent modifications of this system have been reported,[72] and if animals are previously immunized with Kunin antigen, the induced disease becomes more chronic.[109] Clearly an analogous situation could be envisaged in human ulcerative colitis (Figure 12.5).

Table 12.6 Animal enteritides that have been compared with human inflammatory bowel disease.

Animal disease	Reference
Johne's disease of cattle	Dalziel[42]
Regional enteritis of swine	Biester & Schwarte[22] Emsbo[51] Neilson[119]
Regional enterocolitis of Cocker spaniels	Strande *et al.*[162]
Canine colitis	Van Kruiningen[181]
Equine granulomatous colitis	Cimprich[37]
Granulomatous colitis of Boxer dogs	Kennedy & Cello[88] Van Kruiningen[180]
Ulcerative colitis of apes	Scott & Keymer[150]
Ulcerative colitis of Siamang gibbons	Stout & Snyder[164]
Ileitis of hamsters	Boothe & Cheville[28] Johnson & Jacoby[80]
Spontaneous segmental ileitis of rats	Geil *et al.*[54]
Transmissible murine colonic hyperplasia	Barthold *et al.*[12]
Ulcerative colitis-like disease of cotton-top marmosets	Onderdonk[122]
Regional enteritis of lambs	Vanderberghe & Hoorens[178]

Bicks and colleagues have shown that sensitization to 2,4-dinitrochlorobenzene can produce colonic disease.[18, 19, 20, 21] This suggests that the gut can participate in delayed-type hypersensitivity reactions although this particular chemical is unlikely to be of relevance to inflammatory bowel disease.

Following the identification of colonic antibodies in ulcerative colitis, some attempts to induce experimental disease by immunization with gut tissue have been reported. The results have been conflicting.[98, 138, 153] The induced colitis when it has occurred has been self-limiting.

The most promising animal models so far for further investigation of inflammatory bowel disease are the 'Auer colitis' for ulcerative colitis and the inoculation of the nude mouse for Crohn's disease.

OTHER FACTORS

Other factors that have been examined but on which there are, as yet, no firm data include oral contraceptives,[70, 145] detergents,[111] mercury,[1] trauma,[171] psychological aspects[5] and smoking.

REFERENCES

1 Aaronson, R. M. & Spiro, H. M. (1973) Mercury and the gut. *American Journal of Digestive Diseases*, **18**, 583–594.

2 Acheson, E. D. & Truelove, S. C. (1961) Early weaning in aetiology of ulcerative colitis – a study of feeding in infancy in cases and controls. *British Medical Journal*, **ii**, 929–933.

3 Ahlberg, J., Bergstrand, O., Gilstrom, P. *et al.* (1978) Negative findings in search for a transmissible agent in Crohn's disease. *Acta Chirurgica Scandinavica* (Supplementum) **482**, 45–47.

4 Allan, R. N. (1982) Sodium cromoglycate in proctitis and ulcerative colitis. *British Medical Journal*, **284**, 70–71.

5 Alpers, D. H. (1982) Psychiatric illness and inflammatory bowel disease. In *Inflammatory Bowel Diseases* (Ed.) Rachmilewitz, D. pp. 204–212. The Hague: Martinus Nijhoff.

6 Aluwihare, A. P. R. (1971) Electron microscopy in Crohn's disease. *Gut*, **12**, 509–518.

7 Andreson, A. F. R. (1925) Gastrointestinal manifestations of food allergy. *Medical Journal and Record* (Supplement) **122**, 271–275.

8 Andreson, A. F. R. (1953) Allergic manifestations in the gastrointestinal tract. *Gastroenterology*, **23**, 20–35.

9 Archer, L. N. J. & Harvey, R. F. (1978) Breakfast and Crohn's disease II. *British Medical Journal*, **ii**, 540.

10 Aronson, M. D., Phillips, C. A. & Beeken, W. L. (1974) Isolation of a viral agent from intestinal tissue of patients with Crohn's disease and other intestinal disorders. *Gastroenterology*, **66**, 661.

10a Bailas, J. C. (1983) Cigarettes, ulcerative colitis and inferences from uncontrolled data. *New England Journal of Medicine*, **308**, 275–277.

11 Barbour, R. F. & Stokes, A. B. (1936) Chronic cicatrising enteritis. A phase of benign non-specific granuloma of the small intestine. *Lancet*, **i**, 299–303.

12 Barthold, S. W., Coleman, G. L., Bhatt, P. N. *et al.* (1976) The etiology of transmissible murine colonic hyperplasia. *Laboratory Animal Science*, **26**, 889–894.

12a Bartlett, J. G. (1981) *Clostridium difficile* and inflammatory bowel disease. *Gastroenterology*, **80**, 863–865.

13 Bartlett, J. G., Chang, T. W., Gurwith, M. *et al.* (1978) Antibiotic associated pseudomembranous colitis due

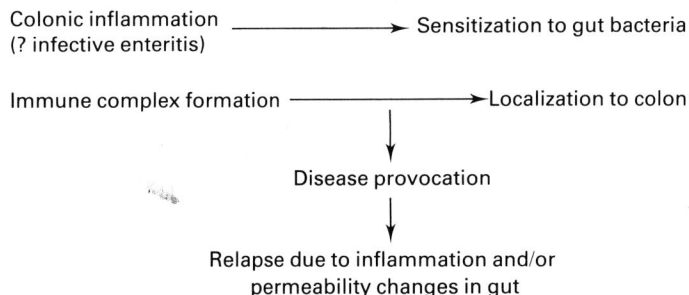

Colonic inflammation ——————→ Sensitization to gut bacteria
(? infective enteritis)

Immune complex formation ——————→ Localization to colon

↓

Disease provocation

↓

Relapse due to inflammation and/or
permeability changes in gut

Fig. 12.5 A proposed aetiology for human ulcerative colitis derived from animal models.

to toxin-producing clostridia. *New England Journal of Medicine*, **298**, 531–534.

14 Bell, H. G. (1934) Chronic cicatrizing enteritis. *California and Western Medicine*, **41**, 239–241.

15 Belsheim, M. R., Darwish, R., Watson, W. L. & Sullivan, S. N. (1980) Bacterial L-forms in inflammatory bowel disease. *Gastroenterology*, **78**, 1139.

16 Bergstrand, O., Holmstrom, B. & Gustafsson, B. E. (1978) Contamination of germ-free animals with intestinal Crohn's tissue. A preliminary report. *Acta Chirurgica Scandinavica* (Supplementum) **482**, 48–50.

17 Bergstrand, O., Gustafsson, B., Holstrom, B. & Norin, K. E. (1981) Ileal Crohn's tissue and concomitant flora inoculated into germ-free rats. *Acta Chirurgica Scandinavica*, **147**, 697–701.

18 Bicks, R. O. & Rosenberg, E. W. (1964) A chronic delayed hypersensitivity reaction in the guinea pig colon. *Gastroenterology*, **46**, 543–549.

19 Bicks, R. O., Brown, G., Hickey, H. D. & Rosenberg, E. W. (1965) Further observations on a delayed hypersensitivity reaction in the guinea pig colon. *Gastroenterology*, **48**, 425–429.

20 Bicks, R. O., Azar, M. M., Rosenberg, E. W. *et al.* (1967) Delayed hypersensitivity reactions in the intestinal tract. 1. Studies of 2,4-dinitrochlorobenzene-caused guinea pig and swine lesions. *Gastroenterology*, **53**, 422–436.

21 Bicks, R. O., Bale, G. F., Goldenberg, J. & Rosenberg, E. W. (1969) Delayed hypersensitivity reactions in the gastrointestinal tract. 4. Effects of chronicity, neostigmine, adjuvant and endotoxin on the pig colon lesion. *American Journal of Digestive Diseases*, **14**, 853–863.

22 Biester, H. E. & Schwarte, L. H. (1931) Intestinal adenoma in swine. *American Journal of Pathology*, **7**, 175–185.

23 Binder, V., Weeke, E., Olsen, J. H. *et al.* (1966) A genetic study of ulcerative colitis. *Scandinavian Journal of Gastroenterology*, **1**, 49–56.

24 Bockus, H. L. & Lee, W. E. (1935) Regional (terminal) ileitis. *Annals of Surgery*, **102**, 416–421.

25 Bolton, R. P. & Read, A. E. (1982) *Clostridium difficile* in toxic megacolon complicating acute inflammatory bowel disease. *British Medical Journal*, **285**, 475–476.

26 Bolton, R. P., Sherriff, R. J. & Read, A. E. (1980) *Clostridium difficile* associated with diarrhoea: a role in inflammatory bowel disease? *Lancet*, **i**, 383–384.

27 Bolton, P. M., Heatley, R. V., Owen, E. *et al.* (1973) Negative findings in laboratory animals for a transmissible agent in Crohn's disease. *Lancet*, **ii**, 1122–1124.

28 Boothe, A. D. & Cheville, N. F. (1967) The pathology of proliferative ileitis of the golden Syrian hamster. *Pathologia Veterinaria (Basel)*, **4**, 31–44.

29 Brahme, F. & Linstrom, C. (1970) A comparative radiographic and pathology study of intestinal vasoarchitecture in Crohn's disease and ulcerative colitis. *Gut*, **11**, 928–940.

30 Brandt, L. J., Benstein, L. H., Boley, S. J. & Frank, M. S. (1982) Metronidazole therapy for perineal Crohn's disease: a follow-up study, *Gastroenterology*, **83**, 383–387.

31 Brostoff, J. & Walker, J. G. (1971) Leucocyte migration inhibition with Kveim antigen in Crohn's disease. *Clinical Experimental Immunology*, **9**, 707–711.

32 Burnham, W. R., Stanford, J. L. & Lennard-Jones, J. E. (1977) Evidence for a mycobacterial aetiology of Crohn's disease. *Gut*, **18**, 965.

33 Burnham, W. R., Lennard-Jones, J. E., Stanford, J. L. & Bird, R. G. (1978) Mycobacteria as a possible cause of inflammatory bowel disease. *Lancet*, **ii**, 693–696.

34 Cave, D. R., Mitchell, D. N. & Brooke, B. N. (1976) Evidence of an agent transmissible from ulcerative colitis tissue. *Lancet*, **i**, 1311–1315.

35 Chapman, J. A., Gleeson, M. H. & Taylor, G. (1971) Kveim tests in Crohn's disease. *Lancet*, **ii**, 1097.

36 Chess, S., O-Lander, G., Puestow, C. B., Benner, W. & Chess, D. (1950) Regional enteritis. Clinical and experimental observations. *Surgery, Gynaecology and Obstetrics*, **91**, 343–350.

37 Cimprich, R. E. (1974) Equine granulomatous enteritis. *Veterinary Pathology*, **11**, 535–547.

38 Cohen, Z., Leving, M. K., Jirsch, D. *et al.* (1981) Transmission of inflammatory bowel disease homogenates in in-bred mice and rabbits. In *Recent Advances in Crohn's Disease* (Ed.) Pena, A. S., Weterman, I. T., Booth, C. C. & Strober, W. pp. 259–265. The Hague: Martinus Nijhoff.

39 Cook, M. G. & Turnbull, G. J. (1975) A hypothesis for the pathogenesis of Crohn's disease based on an ultra structural study. *Virchows Archiv: A. Pathologische Anatomie und Physiologie*, **365**, 327–336.

40 Cooper, H. S., Raffensperger, E. C., Jonas, L. & Fitts, W. T. (1977) Cytomegalovirus inclusions in patients with ulcerative colitis and toxic dilatation requiring colonic resection. *Gastroenterology*, **72**, 1253–1256.

41 Crystal, R. G., Roberts, W. C., Hunninghake, G. W. *et al.* (1981) Pulmonary sarcoidosis: a disease characterised and perpetuated by activated lung T-lymphocytes. *Annals of Internal Medicine*, **94**, 73–94.

42 Dalziel, T. K. (1913) Chronic interstitial enteritis. *British Medical Journal*, **ii**, 1068–1070.

43 Das, K. M., Williams, S. E., Valenzvela, I. & Baum, S. (1981) Induction of lymphoma in athymic (NN/NU) mice by Crohn's disease tissue filtrates: a model for the study of Crohn's disease. In *Recent Advances in Crohn's Disease* (Ed.) Pena, A. S., Weterman, I. T., Booth, C. C. & Strober, W. pp. 266–271. The Hague: Martinus Nijhoff.

44 Das, K. M., Valenzvela, I., Bagchi, S. & Williams, S. E. (1982) Athymic nude mice in studies of Crohn's disease. In *Inflammatory Bowel Diseases* (Ed.) Rachmilewitz, D. pp. 41–55. The Hague: Martinus Nijhoff.

45 Dobbins, W. O. & Siemers, P. T. (1972) A viral etiology for inflammatory bowel disease? *Gastroenterology*, **62**, 742.

46 Donnelly, B. J., Delaney, P. V. & Healy, T. M. (1977) Evidence for a transmissible factor in Crohn's disease. *Gut*, **18**, 360–363.

47 Dorman, S. A., Liggoria, E., Winn, W. C. & Beeken, W. L. (1982) Isolation of *Clostridium difficile* from patients with inactive Crohn's disease. *Gastroenterology*, **82**, 1348–1351.

48 Dudek, B., Spiro, H. M. & Thayer, W. R. (1965) A study of ulcerative colitis and circulating antibodies to milk proteins. *Gastroenterology*, **49**, 544–547.

49 Edwards, H. C. (1958) Crohn's disease and related conditions. In *Modern Trends in Gastroenterology* (Ed.) Avery Jones, F. pp. 262–280. London: Butterworth.

50 Elliot, P. R., Forsey, T., Darougar, S. *et al.* (1981) Chlamydiae and inflammatory bowel disease. *Gut*, **22**, 25–27.

51 Emsbo, P. (1951) Terminal or regional ileitis in swine. *Nordisk Veterinaer Medicin*, **3**, 1–28.

52 Farmer, G. W., Vincent, M. M., Fuccillo, D. A. *et al.* (1973) Viral investigations in ulcerative colitis and regional enteritis. *Gastroenterology*, **65**, 8–18.

53 Ford, H. & Kirsner, J. B. (1964) Auer colitis in rabbits induced by intrarectal antigen. *Proceedings of the*

Society for Experimental Biology and Medicine, **116**, 745–748.

54 Geil, R. G., Davis, C. L. & Thompson, S. W. (1961) Spontaneous ileitis in rats – a report of 64 cases. *American Journal of Veterinary Research*, **22**, 932–936.

55 Gitnick, G. L. (1982) Cytotoxic inducers in Crohn's disease and ulcerative colitis. In *Inflammatory Bowel Diseases* (Ed.) Rachmilewitz, D. pp. 110–125. The Hague: Martinus Nijhoff.

56 Gitnick, G. L. & Rosen, V. J. (1976) Electron microscopic studies of viral agents in Crohn's disease. *Lancet*, **ii**, 217–219.

57 Gitnick, G. L., Rosen, V. J., Arthur, M. H. & Hertweck, S. A. (1979) Evidence for the isolation of a new virus from ulcerative colitis patients: comparison with virus derived from Crohn's disease. *Digestive Diseases and Sciences*, **24**, 609–619.

58 Gorbach, S. L. (1971) Intestinal microflora. *Gastroenterology*, **60**, 1110–1129.

59 Graham, J., Whorwell, P. J., Machen, D. & Wright, R. (1981) Lymphocyte transformation to specific antigens associated with Crohn's disease. *Hepato-Gastroenterology*, **28**, 258–260.

60 Greenfield, C., Szawathowski, M., Noone, P. *et al.* (1981) Is pseudomembranous colitis infectious? *Lancet*, **i**, 371–372.

61 Greenfield, C., Aguilar Ramirez, J. R., Pounder, R. E. *et al.* (1983) *Clostridium difficile* and inflammatory bowel disease. *Gut*, in press.

62 Grotsky, H., Glade, P. R., Hirshaut, Y. *et al.* (1970) Herpes-like virus and granulomatous colitis. *Lancet*, **ii**, 1256–1257.

63 Gunnarsson, A., Hurveil, B., Jonsson, B. *et al.* (1976) Regional ileitis in pigs, isolation of campylobacter from affected ileal mucosa. *Acta Veterinaria Scandinavica*, **17**, 267–269.

64 Hammer, B., Ashurst, P. & Naish, J. (1968) Diseases associated with ulcerative colitis and Crohn's disease. *Gut*, **9**, 17–21.

65 Hannuksela, M., Alkio, H. & Selroos, O. (1971) Kveim reaction in Crohn's disease. *Lancet*, **ii**, 974.

65b Harries, A. D., Baird, A. & Rhodes, J. (1982) Non-smoking: a feature of ulcerative colitis. *British Medical Journal*, **284**, 706.

66 Hayasake, H., Ishikura, H. & Takayama, T. (1971) Acute regional ileitis due to *Anisakis* larvae. *International Surgery*, **55**, 8–14.

67 Heatley, R. V., Bolton, P. M., Owen, E. *et al.* (1975) A search for a transmissible agent in Crohn's disease. *Gut*, **16**, 528–532.

68 Heaton, K. W., Thornton, J. R. & Emmett, P. M. (1979) Treatment of Crohn's disease with an unrefined carbohydrate fibre rich diet. *British Medical Journal*, **ii**, 764–766.

69 Hellers, G. (1981) Some epidemiological aspects of Crohn's disease in Stockholm county 1955–1979. In *Recent Advances In Crohn's Disease* (Ed.) Pena, A. S., Weterman, I. T., Booth, C. C. & Strober, W. pp. 158–162. The Hague: Martinus Nijhoff.

70 Herwitz, R. L., Martin, A. J., Grossman, B. E. & Waddell, W. R. (1970) Oral contraceptives and gastrointestinal disorders. *Annals of Surgery*, **172**, 892–896.

71 Hirshaut, Y., Glade, P., Octavio, L. *et al.* (1970) Sarcoidosis, another disease associated with serologic evidence for herpes-like virus infection. *New England Journal of Medicine*, **283**, 502–506.

72 Hodgson, H. J. F., Potter, B. J., Skinner, J. & Jewell, D. P. (1978) Immune complex mediated colitis in rabbits. An experimental model. *Gut*, **19**, 225–232.

73 Hulton, L., Lindhagen, J., Lundgren, O. *et al.* (1977) Regional intestinal blood flow in ulcerative colitis and Crohn's disease. *Gastroenterology*, **72**, 388–396.

74 Hunninghake, G. W. & Crystal, R. G. (1981) Pulmonary sarcoidosis: a disorder mediated by excess helper T-lymphocyte activity at sites of disease activity. *New England Journal of Medicine*, **305**, 429–434.

75 Jabbour, J. T., Duenas, D. A., Sever, J. L. *et al.* (1972) Epidemiology of sub-acute sclerosing panencephalitis. *Journal of the American Medical Association*, **220**, 959–962.

76 James, A. H. (1977) Breakfast and Crohn's disease. *British Medical Journal*, **i**, 943–945.

77 Jarnerot, G. & Lantrop, K. (1972) Antibodies to EB virus in cases of Crohn's disease. *New England Journal of Medicine*, **286**, 1215–1216.

78 Jewell, D. P. & Truelove, S. C. (1972) Circulating antibodies to cow's milk proteins in ulcerative colitis. *Gut*, **13**, 796–801.

79 Jewell, D. P. & Truelove, S. C. (1972) Reaginic hypersensitivity in ulcerative colitis. *Gut*, **13**, 903–906.

80 Johnson, E. A. & Jacoby, R. O. (1978) Transmissible ileal hyperplasia of hamsters. *American Journal of Pathology*, **91**, 451–459.

81 Jones, J. H., Lennard-Jones, J. C. & Lockhart-Mummery, H. E. (1966) Experience in the treatment of Crohn's disease of the large intestine. *Gut*, **7**, 448–452.

82 Jones-Williams, W. (1971) The Kveim controversy. *Lancet*, **ii**, 926–927.

83 Kalima, T. V. & Collan, Y. (1970) Intestinal villus in experimental lymphatic obstruction: correlation of light and electron microscopic findings with clinical disease. *Scandinavian Journal of Gastroenterology*, **5**, 497–510.

84 Kalima, T. V., Saloniemi, H. & Rahko, T. (1976) Experimental regional enteritis in pigs. *Scandinavian Journal of Gastroenterology*, **11**, 353–362.

85 Kane, S. P. & Nye, F. J. (1971) EB-virus antibody in Crohn's disease. *Lancet*, **i**, 233.

86 Karlish, A. J., Cox, E. V., Hampson, F. & Hemsted, E. H. (1970) Kveim test in Crohn's disease. *Lancet*, **ii**, 977–978.

87 Keighley, M. R. B., Youngs, D., Johnson, M. *et al.* (1982) *Clostridium difficile* toxin in acute diarrhoea complicating inflammatory bowel disease. *Gut*, **23**, 410–414.

88 Kennedy, P. C. & Cello, R. M. (1966) Colitis of boxer dogs. *Gastroenterology*, **51**, 926–929.

89 Kirsner, J. B. (1961) Experimental 'colitis' with particular reference to hypersensitivity reactions in the colon. *Gastroenterology*, **40**, 307–312.

90 Knutson, H., Lunderquist, A. & Lunderquist, A. (1968) Vascular changes in Crohn's disease. *American Journal of Roentenology*, **103**, 380–385.

91 Kraft, S. C., Fitch, F. W. & Kirsner, J. B. (1963) Histologic and immunohistochemical features of the Auer 'colitis' in rabbits. *American Journal of Pathology*, **43**, 913–923.

92 Kyle, J., Bell, T. M., Porteous, I. B. & Blair, D. W. (1963) Factors in the aetiology of regional enteritis. *Bulletin de la Société Internationale de Chirurgie*, **22**, 575–584.

93 La Mont, J. T. & Trnka, Y. M. (1980) Therapeutic implications of *Clostridium difficile* toxin during relapse of chronic inflammatory bowel disease. *Lancet*, **i**, 381–383.

94 Lambert, M. E., Schofield, P. F., Ironside, A. G. & Mandal, B. K. (1979) Campylobacter colitis. *British Medical Journal*, **i**, 857–859.

95 Lancet Editorial (1972) Kveim-Siltzbach test vindicated. *Lancet*, **i**, 188.

96   Larson, H. E., Price, A. B., Honour, P. & Borriello, S. P. (1978) *Clostridium difficile* and the aetiology of pseudomembranous colitis. *Lancet*, **i**, 1063–1066.

97   Lawson, G. J. K., Rowland, A. C. & Wooding, G. (1975) The characterisation of *Campylobacter sputorum* sub-species *mucosalis* isolated from pigs. *Research in Veterinary Science*, **18**, 121–126.

98   Le Veen, H. H., Falk, G. & Schatman, B. (1961) Experimental ulcerative colitis produced by anti-colon sera. *Annals of Surgery*, **154**, 275–280.

99   Lieberman, J. (1975) Elevation of serum angiotensin converting enzyme (ACE) level in sarcoidosis. *American Journal of Medicine*, **59**, 365–372.

100 Lieberman, J., Nosal, A., Schlessner, L. A. & Sastre-Foken, A. (1979) Serum angiotensin converting enzyme for diagnosis and therapeutic evaluation of sarcoidosis. *American Review of Respiratory Disease*, **120**, 329–335.

101 Maillet, M., Bonfils, S. & Lister, R. E. (1970) Carrageenan: effects in animals. *Lancet*, **ii**, 414–415.

102 Marcus, R. & Watt, J. (1974) Ulcerative disease of the colon in laboratory animals induced by pepsin inhibitors. *Gastroenterology*, **67**, 473–483.

103 Martini, G. A. & Brandes, J. W. (1976) Increased consumption of refined carbohydrates in Crohn's disease. *Klinische Wochenschrift*, **54**, 367.

104 Mayberry, J. F. & Rhodes, J. (1981) Studies on the incidence, prevalence, mortality and dietary history of patients with Crohn's disease. In *Recent Advances in Crohn's Disease* (Ed.) Pena, A. S., Weterman, I. T., Booth, C. C. & Strober, W. pp. 163–167. The Hague: Martinus Nijhoff.

105 Mayberry, J. F., Rhodes, J. & Newcombe, R. G. (1978) Breakfast and dietary aspects of Crohn's disease. *British Medical Journal*, **ii**, 1401.

106 Mayberry, J. F., Rhodes, J., Allan, R. *et al.* (1981) Diet in Crohn's disease. *Digestive Diseases and Sciences*, **26**, 444–448.

107 McCaffrey, T. D., Kraft, S. C. & Rothberg, R. M. (1972) The influence of different techniques in characterising human antibodies to cow's milk proteins. *Clinical and Experimental Medicine*, **11**, 225–234.

108 McLaren, L. C. & Gitnick, G. (1982) Ulcerative colitis and Crohn's disease tissue cytotoxins. *Gastroenterology*, **82**, 1381–1388.

109 Mee, A. S., McLaughlin, J. E., Hodgson, H. J. F. & Jewell, D. P. (1978) Chronic immune complex colitis – an experimental model. *Gut*, **19**, 443.

110 Melnyk, C. S. (1975) Experimental colitis. In *Inflammatory Bowel Diseases* (Ed.) Kirsner, J. B. & Shorter, R. G. pp. 23–26. Philadelphia: Lea and Febiger.

111 Mercurius-Taylor, L. A., Jayaraj, A. P. & Clark, C. G. (1982) Are detergents harmful to the gut? *Gut*, **23**, A433.

112 Merril, D. A., Dubois, R. S. & Kohler, D. F. (1972) Neonatal onset of the hepatitis-associated antigen carrier state. *New England Journal of Medicine*, **287**, 1280–1282.

113 Meyers, S., Mayer, L., Buttone, E. *et al.* (1981) Occurrence of *Clostridium difficile* toxin during the course of inflammatory bowel disease. *Gastroenterology*, **80**, 697–700.

114 Mitchell, D. N. & Rees, R. J. W. (1970) Agents transmissible from Crohn's tissue. *Lancet*, **ii**, 168–171.

115 Mitchell, D. N., Rees, R. J. W. & Goswami, K. K. A. (1976) Transmissible agents from human sarcoid in Crohn's disease tissue. *Lancet*, **ii**, 761–765.

116 Mitchell, D. N., Cannon, P., Dyer, N. H. *et al.* (1969) The Kveim test in Crohn's disease. *Lancet*, **ii**, 571–573.

117 Mitchell, D. N., Cannon, P., Dyer, N. H. *et al.* (1970) Further observations on Kveim test in Crohn's disease. *Lancet*, **ii**, 496–498.

118 Morain, C. O., Prestage, H., Harrison, P. *et al.* (1981) Cytopathic effects in cultures inoculated with material from Crohn's disease. *Gut*, **22**, 823–826.

119 Neilson, K. (1971) Regional enteritis in domestic animals. In *Skandia International Symposia Number 5: Regional Enteritis (Crohn's Disease)* (Ed.) Engel, A. & Larsson, T. pp. 266–278. Nordiska Bokhandelns: Forlag.

120 Nunez-Gornes, J. F. & Tewksbury, D. A. (1981) Serum angiotensin converting enzyme in Crohn's disease. *American Journal of Gastroenterology*, **75**, 384–385.

121 Oberhelman, H. A., Kohatsu, S., Taylor, K. B. & Kivel, R. M. (1968) Diverting ileostomy in the surgical management of Crohn's disease of the colon. *American Journal of Surgery*, **115**, 231–240.

122 Onderdonk, A. B. (1982) Ulcerative colitis-like disease of cotton-top marmosets. In *Inflammatory Bowel Diseases* (Ed.) Rachmilewitz, D. pp. 126–134. The Hague: Martinus Nijhoff.

123 Onderdonk, A. B. & Bartlett, J. G. (1979) Bacterial studies of experimental ulcerative colitis. *American Journal of Clinical Nutrition*, **32**, 258–265.

124 Onderdonk, A. B., Franklin, M. L. & Cisneros, R. L. (1981) Production of experimental ulcerative colitis in gnotobiotic guinea pigs with simplified microflora. *Infection and Immunity*, **32**, 225–231.

126 Onderdonk, A. B., Hermos, J. A., Dzink, J. L. & Bartlett, J. G. (1978) Protective effect of metronidazole in experimental ulcerative colitis. *Gastroenterology*, **74**, 521–526.

127 Orr, M. M., Tamarind, D. L., Cook, J. *et al.* (1974) Preliminary studies on the response of rabbit bowel to intramural injection of L-form bacteria. *British Journal of Surgery*, **61**, 921.

128 Orr, M. M., Tamarind, D. L., Cook, J. *et al.* (1975) Chronic lesions of rabbit bowel due to contact with antiseptic skin preparations. *Gut*, **16**, 401.

129 Parent, K. & Mitchell, P. (1976) Bacterial variants: etiologic agent in Crohn's disease. *Gastroenterology*, **71**, 365–368.

130 Parent, K. & Mitchell, P. (1978) Cell wall-defective variants of pseudomonas-like (group Va) bacteria in Crohn's disease. *Gastroenterology*, **75**, 368–372.

131 Parent, K., Mitchell, P. & Beltaos, E. (1980) Pilot animal pathogenicity studies with cell wall-defective pseudomonas-like bacteria isolated from Crohn's disease patients. *Gastroenterology*, **78**, 1233.

132 Persson, S., Danielsson, D., Kjellander, J. & Wallensten, S. (1976) Studies on Crohn's disease. 1. The relationship between *Yersinia enterocolitica* infection and terminal ileitis. *Acta Chirurgica Scandinavica*, **142**, 84–90.

133 Phillpots, R. J., Hermon-Taylor, J. & Brooke, R. N. (1979) Virus isolation studies in Crohn's disease: a negative report. *Gut*, **20**, 1057–1062.

134 Quinn, T. C., Goodell, S. E., Mkrtichian, E. *et al.* (1981) *Chlamydia trachomatis* proctitis. *New England Journal of Medicine*, **305**, 195–200.

135 Rappaport, H., Burgoyne, F. H. & Smetana, H. F. (1951) The pathology of regional enteritis. *The Military Surgeon*, **109**, 463–500.

136 Rawcliffe, P. M. & Truelove, S. C. (1978) Breakfast and Crohn's disease I. *British Medical Journal*, **ii**, 539–540.

137 Reichart, F. L. & Mathes, M. E. (1936) Experimental lymphedema of the intestinal tract and its relation to regional cicatrizing enteritis. *Annals of Surgery*, **104**, 601–616.

138 Richardson, G. S. & Leskowitz, S. (1961) An attempt at production of autoimmunity to tissue of the gastro-intestinal tract. *Proceedings of the Society for Experimental Biology and Medicine*, **106**, 357–359.

139 Richens, E. R., Gough, K. R. & William, M. J. (1973) Leucocyte migration studies with spleen preparations in Crohn's disease. *Gut*, **14**, 376–379.

140 Rieman, J. F. (1977) Further electron microscopic evidence of virus-like particles in Crohn's disease. *Acta Hepato-Gastroenterologica*, **24**, 116–118.

141 Roche, J. K. & Huang, E. S. (1977) Viral DNA in inflammatory bowel disease CMV-bearing cells as a target for immune mediated enterocytolysis. *Gastroenterology*, **72**, 228–233.

142 Rodaniche, E. C., Kirsner, J. B. & Palmer, W. L. (1943) The relationship between lymphogranuloma venereum and regional enteritis. An etiologic study of four cases with negative results. *Gastroenterology*, **1**, 687–689.

143 Rosen, A., Ursing, B., Alm, T. *et al.* (1982) A comparative study of metroinidazole and sulphasalazine for active Crohn's disease I. *Gastroenterology*, **83**, 541–549.

144 Rowe, A. H. (1942) Chronic ulcerative colitis – allergy in its etiology. *Annals of Internal Medicine*, **17**, 83.

145 Royal College of General Practitioners (1974) *Oral Contraceptives and Health.* London: The Whitefriars Press.

146 Sarles, H., Deek, M., Chalvet, K. & Ambrosi, L. (1959) Haemorrhagic rectocolitis and nutritional allergy. *Archives Francaises des Maladies de l'appareil Digestif*, **48**, 907–925.

147 Scadding, J. G. (1967) *Sarcoidosis.* London: Eyre and Spottiswoode.

148 Schneierson, S. S., Garlock, J. H., Shore, B. *et al.* (1962) Studies on the viral aetiology of regional enteritis and colitis: a negative report. *American Journal of Digestive Diseases*, **7**, 839–843.

149 Schuller, J. L., Picket-van-Ulsen, J., Veeken, I. V. D. *et al.* (1979) Antibodies against *Chlamydia* of lymphogranuloma venereum type in Crohn's disease. *Lancet*, **i**, 19–20.

150 Scott, G. B. D. & Keymer, I. F. (1975) Ulcerative colitis in apes: a comparison with the human disease. *Journal of Pathology*, **115**, 241–244.

151 Semenzato, G., Pezzulto, A., Cipriani, A. & Gasparato, G. (1980) Imbalance of Ty and Tu lymphocyte sub-populations in patients with sarcoidosis. *Journal of Clinical and Laboratory Immunology*, **4**, 95–98.

152 Sewell, P., Cooke, W. T., Cox, E. V. & Meynell, M. J. (1963) Milk intolerance in gastrointestinal disorders. *Lancet*, **ii**, 1132–1135.

153 Shean, F. C., Barker, W. F. & Fonkalsrud, E. W. (1964) Studies on active and passive antibody induced colitis in the dog. *American Journal of Surgery*, **107**, 337–339.

154 Siltzbach, L. E., Vieira, L. O. B. D., Topilsky, M. & Janowitz, H. D. (1971) Is there a Kveim responsiveness in Crohn's disease? *Lancet*, **ii**, 634–636.

155 Silverstein, E., Pertschuk, L. P. & Friedland, J. (1979) Immunofluorescent localisation of angiotensin converting enzyme in epithelioid and giant cells of sarcoidosis granulomas. *Proceedings of the National Academy of Sciences USA*, **76**, 6646–6648.

156 Silverstein, E., Fierst, S. M., Simon, M. R. *et al.* (1981) Angiotensin converting enzyme in Crohn's disease and ulcerative colitis. *American Journal of Clinical Pathology*, **75**, 175–178.

157 Simon, M. R., Weinstock, J. V. & Kataria, Y. P. (1980) Kveim-induced lymphocyte reactivity in patients and household contacts of patients with Crohn's disease. *Journal of Clinical and Laboratory Immunology*, **3**, 175–178.

158 Simonowitz, D., Block, G. E., Riddell, R. H. *et al.* (1977) The production of an unusual tissue reaction in rabbit bowel injected with Crohn's disease homogenates. *Surgery*, **82**, 211–218.

159 Sjostrom, B. (1971) Acute terminal ileitis and it's relation to Crohn's disease. In *Skandia International Symposium Number 5: Regional Enteritis (Crohn's Disease)* (Ed.) Engel, A. & Larsson, T. pp. 73–80. Nordiska Bokhandelns: Forlag.

160 Staley, T. E., Corley, L. D. & Jones, E. W. (1970) Early pathogenesis of colitis in neonatal pigs, monocontaminated with *Escherichia coli* – fine structural changes in the colonic epithelium. *American Journal of Digestive Diseases*, **15**, 923–935.

161 Stanford, J. L. (1981) Acid fast organisms in Crohn's disease and ulcerative colitis. In *Inflammatory Bowel Diseases* (Ed.) Rachmilewitz, D. pp. 274–277. The Hague: Martinus Nijhoff.

162 Strande, A., Sommers, S. C. & Petrak, M. (1954) Regional enterocolitis in Cocker Spaniel dogs. *Archives of Pathology*, **57**, 357–362.

163 Stokes, C. R., Soothill, J. F. & Turner, M. W. (1975) Immune exclusion is a function of IgA. *Nature*, **255**, 745–746.

164 Stout, C. & Snyder, R. L. (1969) Ulcerative colitis-like lesion in siamang gibbons. *Gastroenterology*, **57**, 256–261.

165 Studdy, P., Bird, C. & James, D. G. (1978) Serum angiotensin converting enzyme in sarcoidosis and other granulomatous disorders. *Lancet*, **ii**, 1331–1334.

166 Swarbrick, E. T., Price, H. L., Kingham, J. G. C. *et al.* (1979) *Chlamydia*, cytomegalovirus and *Yersinia* in inflammatory bowel disease. *Lancet*, **ii**, 11–12.

167 Syverton, J. T. (1961) Entero viruses. *Gastroenterology*, **40**, 331–337.

168 Taub, R. N. & Siltzbach, L. E. (1974) Induction of granulomas in mice by injection of human sarcoid and ileitis homogenates. In *Proceedings of the 6th International Conference of Sarcoidosis 1972* (Ed.) Iwai, K. & Hosoda, Y. pp. 20–21. University Park Press.

169 Taub, R. N., Sachar, D. B., Siltzbach, L. E. & Janowitz, H. D. (1974) Transmission of ileitis and sarcoid granulomas to mice. *Clinical Research*, **22**, 559.

170 Taub, R. N., Sachar, D. M., Janowitz, H. & Siltzbach, L. E. (1976) Induction of granulomas in mice by inoculation of tissue homogenates from patients with inflammatory bowel disease and sarcoidosis. *Annals of the New York Academy of Sciences*, **278**, 560–564.

171 Taylor, F. W. (1971) Seat injury resulting in regional enteritis and intestinal obstruction. *Journal of American Medical Association*, **215**, 1154–1155.

172 Taylor, K. B. & Truelove, S. C. (1961) Circulating antibodies to milk protein in ulcerative colitis. *British Medical Journal*, **ii**, 924.

173 Taylor-Robinson, D., Morain, C. O., Thomas, B. J. & Levi, A. J. (1979) Low frequency of chlamydial antibodies in patients with Crohn's disease and ulcerative colitis. *Lancet*, **i**, 1162–1163.

174 Thornton, J. R., Emmett, P. M. & Heaton, K. W. (1979) Diet and Crohn's disease: characteristics of the pre-illness diet. *British Medical Journal*, **ii**, 762–764.

175 Tomenius, J., Larre, E., Lindgren, I. *et al.* (1963) Positive Frei tests in the 7 cases of morbus-Crohn's (regional ileitis). *Gastroenterologica*, **99**, 368–373.

176 Trnka, Y. M. & La Mont, J. F. (1981) Associated assessment of *Clostridium difficile* toxin with symp-

tomatic relapse of chronic inflammatory bowel
disease. *Gastroenterology*, **80**, 693–696.

177 Ursing, B., Alm, T., Barany, F. *et al.* (1982) A comparative study of metronidazole and sulphasalazine for
active Crohn's disease 2. *Gastroenterology*, **83**, 550–
561.

178 Vanderberghe, J. & Hoorens, J. (1980) Campylobacter
species and regional enteritis in lambs. *Research and
Veterinary Science*, **29**, 390–391.

179 Van de Merwe, J. P. (1981) A possible role of *Eubac-
terium* and *Peptostreptococcus* species in the aetiology
of Crohn's disease. In *Recent Advances in Crohn's
Disease* (Ed.) Pena, A. S., Weterman, I. T., Booth, C. C.
& Strober, W. pp. 291–296. The Hague: Martinus
Nijhoff.

180 Van Kruiningen, H. J. (1967) Granulomatous colitis of
Boxer dogs: comparative aspects. *Gastroenterology*,
53, 114–122.

181 Van Kruiningen, J. H. (1972) Canine colitis comparable to regional enteritis and mucosal colitis of man.
Gastroenterology, **62**, 1128–1142.

182 Walker-Smith (1980) In press.

183 Warren, S. & Sommers, S. C. (1948) Cicatrizing enteritis (regional ileitis) as a pathologic entity. Analysis of
one hundred and twenty cases. *American Journal of
Pathology*, **24**, 475–501.

184 Watson, D. W. & Martucci, R. (1974) Sensitivity to
microbacterial antigens in patients with Crohn's
disease. *Gastroenterology*, **66**, 794.

185 Watt, J. & Marcus, R. (1971) Carrageenan-induced
ulceration of the large intestine in the guinea pig. *Gut*,
12, 164–171.

186 Watt, J. & Marcus, R. (1973) Experimental ulcerative
disease of the colon in animals. *Gut*, **14**, 506–510.

187 Weaver, L. J., Simonowitz, D., Driscoll, R. & Sololli-
day, N. (1980) Serum angiotensin converting enzyme
in patients with Crohn's disease. *Journal of Surgical
Research*, **29**, 475–478.

188 Wensinck, F. & Schroder, A. M. (1981) Preliminary
study of faecal flora in families of patients with
Crohn's disease. In *Recent Advances in Crohn's
Disease* (Ed.) Pena, A. S., Weterman, I. T., Booth, C. C.
& Strober, W. pp. 286–290. The Hague: Martinus
Nijhoff.

189 White, S. A. (1981) Investigation into the identity of
acid fast organisms isolated from Crohn's disease and
ulcerative colitis. In *Inflammatory Bowel Diseases* (Ed.)
Rachmilewitz, D. pp. 278–282. The Hague: Martinus
Nijhoff.

190 Whorwell, P. J., Baldwin, R. C. & Wright, R. (1976)
Ferritin in Crohn's disease tissue: detection by electron microscopy. *Gut*, **17**, 696–699.

191 Whorwell, P. J., Beeken, W. L., Phillips, C. A. *et al.*
(1977) Isolation of reovirus-like agents from patients
with Crohn's disease. *Lancet*, **i**, 1169–1171.

192 Whorwell, P. J., Beeken, W. L., Davidson, I. W. &
Wright, R. (1978) Search by immunofluorescence for
antigens of rotavirus, *Pseudomonas maltophilia* and
Mycobacterium kansasii in Crohn's disease. *Lancet*, **ii**,
697–698.

193 Whorwell, P. J., Holdstock, G., Whorwell, G. M. &
Wright, R. (1979) Bottle feeding, early gastroenteritis
and inflammatory bowel disease. *British Medical
Journal*, **i**, 382.

194 Williams, S. E., Valenzvela, I., Kadish, A. S. & Das, K.
M. (1982) Glomerular immune complex formation
and induction of lymphoma in athymic nude mice by
tissue filtrates of Crohn's disease patients. *Journal of
Laboratory and Clinical Medicine*, **99**, 827–837.

195 Willoughby, J. M. T. & Mitchell, D. N. (1971) In vitro
inhibition of leucocyte migration in Crohn's disease by
a sarcoid spleen suspension. *British Medical Journal*,
iii, 155–157.

196 Wright, R. & Truelove, S. C. (1965) A controlled therapeutic trial of various diets in ulcerative colitis. *British
Medical Journal*, **ii**, 138–141.

197 Wright, R. & Truelove, S. C. (1966) Serial rectal biopsy
in ulcerative colitis during the course of a controlled
therapeutic trial of various diets. *American Journal of
Digestive Diseases*, **11**, 847–857.

198 Wright, R. & Truelove, S. C. (1966) Circulating and
tissue eosinophils in ulcerative colitis. *American
Journal of Digestive Diseases*, **11**, 831–846.

199 Yardley, J. H. & Hamilton, S. R. (1982) Pathologic
aspects of diagnosis, pathogenesis and etiology of idiopathic inflammatory bowel disease. In *Inflammatory
Bowel Diseases* (Ed.) Rachmilewitz, D. pp. 3–18. The
Hague: Martinus Nijhoff.

IMMUNOLOGICAL ASPECTS

As in many other conditions of unknown aetiology, immunological factors have been extensively investigated in ulcerative colitis and
Crohn's disease. In patients with these conditions, there is an enhanced level of immunological activity, particularly affecting the
gastrointestinal mucosal immune system. Much
evidence suggests that the expression of immune
responses, directed either against the gut itself or
against closely associated antigens such as
enteric bacteria, is responsible for generating
inflammation.[10] It is not clear, however,
whether the development of these immune
responses is the primary event in inflammatory
bowel disease, or whether they merely play a
secondary role in maintaining inflammation. It
also remains a theoretical possibility that there
are powerful immune responses directed against
an as yet unidentified pathogen.

It should also be noted that, almost without
exception, the results of immunological studies
in patients with ulcerative colitis or with
Crohn's disease have yielded similar results.

Evidence suggesting inflammatory bowel disease is of primary immunological origin

There is little direct evidence to support this
hypothesis. An autoimmune mechanism is suggested by the many reported case histories of
individual patients with inflammatory bowel
disease and an autoimmune disease such as thyroiditis,[29] pernicious anaemia[6] or systemic
lupus erythematosus.[4] However, in large surveys
of patients with inflammatory bowel disease,
using serological tests, common autoantibodies
like anti-nuclear factor are found no more often

than normal.[18] The strong familial tendency in inflammatory bowel disease, occurring in up to 30% of patients in some series, might indicate a genetic background of abnormal immune responsiveness. In many autoimmune diseases with a similar familial tendency, this suggestion can be supported by finding linkage of the disease to a particular HLA haplotype, but this is not so in inflammatory bowel disease[8] (unless there is associated ankylosing spondylitis).

Some authors have suggested that the primary abnormality in these diseases may be a deficiency in some part of the system, perhaps at the gut mucosal barrier, which permits increased penetration of antigens through the mucosa. This causes overactivity of other immune mechanisms, resulting in tissue-damaging responses. Although there are a few reported individuals with hypogammaglobulinaemia,[16] or with selective IgA deficiency,[11] who also have inflammatory bowel disease, in the vast majority of individuals the humoral immune system is normal. The evidence for this includes a normal ability to make specific antibodies in response to challenge, and serum immunoglobulins that are normal or raised. The typical pattern is a slight elevation of IgG level, particularly when the colon is involved, a normal or high IgA level, and a normal IgM level which rises in individual patients as they enter remission.[12]

With regard to the cellular (T cell) immune system, there is more evidence to suggest that a degree of immunodeficiency may be present. Cutaneous anergy in Crohn's disease has been recognized for nearly 50 years. Although circulating numbers of T cells are normal, there are differences from normal in T lymphocyte subpopulations and these cells are hyporeactive in in vitro culture.[28] However, the most persuasive evidence suggests that these deficiencies are not present in patients with inflammatory bowel disease of recent onset, but are acquired with time in ill patients.[2]

Thus the basic immunological apparatus in patients with ulcerative colitis and Crohn's disease appears to be normal.

Evidence for tissue-damaging immune responses

Increased numbers of immunologically competent cells – both lymphocytes and plasma cells – are obvious within the lamina propria of the inflamed gut. Recent work has shown marked increases in the numbers of cells producing immunoglobulin of all the main classes – IgG, IgA, IgM and IgE; in particular IgG-producing plasma cells, only sparsely present in normal

gut, are dramatically increased.[3] The predominant lymphocyte type is the T cell, both in diseased bowel and in the sparser cell population of the normal gut mucosa. A recent paper has characterized the subtypes of these cells.[25]

It may be that these increased numbers of lymphocytes and plasma cells are exerting a purely protective function, and indeed similar alterations occur in patients with bacillary dysentery.[24] In the absence of an obvious pathogen, however, and on the basis of a number of observations summarized below, it seems likely that these immune cells mediate tissue damage and inflammation.

ANTIBODY-INDUCED TISSUE DAMAGE

Many patients with inflammatory bowel disease have circulating autoantibodies directed against colonic epithelial cells.[4] Such antibodies theoretically could cause destruction of colonic epithelium, although this has been difficult to demonstrate directly.[5] Studies of these antibodies produced a very striking observation: particular bacterial antigens, notably the lipopolysaccharide of certain *E. coli*, block the reaction of anticolon antibodies with colonic antigen.[23] This suggests that a protective immune response initially developed against colonic bacteria could crossreact with, and potentially damage, colonic epithelium.

Although the concept that autoantibodies against the colon are mediators of inflammation is attractive, similar antibodies have been found in some patients with other colonic diseases in which persistent inflammation does not occur.[19] Therefore other factors are presumably of importance. A number of studies have shown a higher than normal serum titre of antibodies to a variety of colonic bacteria and also to foodstuffs. There is evidence of local production within the mucosa of antibodies to bacteria within the colon.[21] It seems almost inevitable that in the diseased gut mucosa locally produced antibody will meet antigen, leading to immune complex formation. Such local immune complexes would be capable of damaging surrounding tissues, as 'innocent bystanders', as they initiate an inflammatory Arthus-type reaction. This would involve consumption of complement, and attraction of neutrophil leucocytes to the area; both of these occur in active inflammatory bowel disease.[13]

The possibility that antibodies to foodstuffs are relevant to these diseases ties in with longstanding concepts of ulcerative colitis as a food-allergic disorder. As many allergies are mediated by IgE, it is relevant to ask whether IgE-mediated disorders are commonly associated with inflammatory bowel disease. Some authors in fact suggest atopic disorders are more common, whilst others disagree.[9] There is evidence of a greater than normal circulating level of IgE antibodies to a variety of foods, but not in all patients.[20] It might be that in the small group of patients with colitis who appear to respond well to mast-cell stabilizers such as cromoglycate, this mechanism is particularly prominent. Amongst patients as a whole, the evidence for food allergy as a primary cause is notably inadequate.

CELL-MEDIATED TISSUE DAMAGE

In vitro studies have shown that lymphocytes from patients with inflammatory bowel disease are cytotoxic for colonic epithelial cells.[22] This phenomenon, unlike the presence of autoantibodies, is specific for patients with ulcerative colitis or Crohn's disease. The precise form of cytotoxicity is not entirely clear, but involves serum-derived factors, and this may be an example of antibody-dependent cell-mediated cytotoxicity.[27] One reservation for accepting this as the main immunological means of tissue damage in these diseases is that cytotoxicity for ileal epithelium is much less easy to demonstrate, and it seems unlikely that different mechanisms of tissue damage occur in different areas of the gut.[26] However, the in vitro techniques for detecting cellular immunity are considerably less selective than those available for detecting antibodies, so the numerous observations showing some evidence of cell-mediated immunity to the colon, and to enteric bacteria, probably do reflect lymphocyte sensitization to these antigens.

Thus there is evidence of antibody production, of all classes of immunoglobulin, and of cell-mediated immunity, to the gut epithelium and to antigens in the gut lumen closely apposed to the mucosa. The concept that expression of these immune responses causes gut inflammation is further supported by animal models showing both antibody-mediated and cell-mediated inflammation causing colitis.

EXTRAINTESTINAL MANIFESTATIONS

The similarity between certain extraintestinal manifestations of inflammatory bowel disease – peripheral arthropathy, iritis, erythema nodosum – and serum sickness suggests that they have a similar pathogenesis, with deposition of immune complexes from the circulation in these sites. In inflammatory bowel disease these complexes would presumably be formed initially within the gut mucosa. Circulating immune complexes have been detected in ulcerative colitis and Crohn's disease, particularly when the disease is active and extraintestinal manifestations are present.[14] Other theories for these manifestations include the effects of circulating endotoxins from the gut directly activating complement in these sites.[17]

Origin of immunological abnormalities

Why should some individuals develop immune responses against the gut and mucosal antigens and not others? The answer to this must be entirely speculative. In some, it may be that an acute infective episode breaks down the immunological barriers at the mucosal surface and initiates these developments. Others may have defective mucosal immune systems, as in the few patients with hypogammaglobulinaemia. The persistence of damaging immune responses, some authors postulate, may indicate a defective immunoregulatory mechanism; under these circumstances an immune response which was appropriate during an acute infective episode may not be properly controlled, and as a result persists after the infection has passed and continues to cause inflammation. There is evidence for disturbed immunoregulatory function in patients with inflammatory bowel disease, but its relevance is uncertain.[15]

In addition to the immunocompetent cells with the ability to recognize or act against specific antigens, non-specific mediators of inflammation such as macrophages, neutrophil leucocytes and complement, are recruited to the tissues. Whatever the primary cause of these diseases, the presence of tissue-damaging, humoral and cellular, specific and non-specific mediators of inflammation within the mucosa offers a rationale for the use of immunosuppressive and anti-inflammatory drugs in ulcerative colitis and Crohn's disease. Over the next decade, studies on the behaviour of cells isolated from the gut mucosa may bring us nearer to an understanding of these conditions.[7]

REFERENCES

1 Alarcon-Segovia, D., Herskovic, T., Dearing, W. H. *et al.* (1965) Lupus erythematosus cell phenomenon in patients with chronic ulcerative colitis. *Gut,* **6,** 39.
2 Auer, I. O., Wechsler, W., Ziemer, E. *et al.* (1978) Immune status in Crohn's disease. 1. Leucocyte and lymphocyte subpopulations in peripheral blood. *Scandinavian Journal of Gastroenterology,* **13,** 561–571.

3 Brandztaeg, P., Baklien, K., Fausa, O. & Hoel, P. S. (1974) Immunochemical characterisation of local immunoglobulin formation in ulcerative colitis. *Gastroenterology*, **66**, 1123.

4 Broberger, O. & Perlmann, P. (1959) Autoantibodies in human ulcerative colitis. *Journal of Experimental Medicine*, **110**, 657.

5 Broberger, O. & Perlmann, P. (1963) In vitro studies of ulcerative colitis. 1. Reactions of patients' serum with human foetal colon cells in tissue cultures. *Journal of Experimental Medicine*, **117**, 705.

6 Edwards, F. C. & Truelove, S. C. (1964) Course and prognosis of ulcerative colitis. *Gut*, **5**, 1.

7 Fiocchi, C., Youngman, K. R. & Farmer, R. G. (1983) Immunological function of human intestinal lymphoid cells: evidence for enhanced supressor cell activity in inflammatory bowel disease. *Gut*, **24**, 692–701.

8 Gleeson, M. H., Walker, J. S., Wentzel, J. et al. (1972) Human leucocyte antigen in Crohn's disease and ulcerative colitis. *Gut*, **13**, 438.

9 Hammer, B., Ashurst, P. & Naish, J. (1968) Diseases associated with ulcerative colitis and Crohn's disease. *Gut*, **9**, 17.

10 Hodgson, H. J. F. (1980) Immunological aspects of inflammatory bowel disease. In *Inflammatory Disease of the Bowel* (Ed.) Brooke B. V. & Wilkinson, A. pp. 38–52 London: Pitman Medical.

11 Hodgson, H. J. F. & Jewell, D. P. (1977) Selective IgA deficiency and Crohn's disease. *Gut*, **18**, 644–646.

12 Hodgson, H. J. F. & Jewell, D. P. (1978) The humoral immune system in inflammatory bowel disease. *American Journal of Digestive Diseases*, **23**, 123–128.

13 Hodgson, H. J. F., Potter, B. J. & Jewell, D. P. (1977) C_3 metabolism in ulcerative colitis and Crohn's disease. *Clinical and Experimental Immunology*, **28**, 490–495.

14 Hodgson, H. J. F., Potter, B. J. & Jewell, D. P. (1977) Immune complexes in ulcerative colitis and Crohn's disease. *Clinical and Experimental Immunology*, **29**, 187–196.

15 Hodgson, H. J. F., Wands, J. R. & Isselbacher, K. J. (1978) Decreased suppressor cell activity in inflammatory bowel disease. *Clinical and Experimental Immunology*, **32**, 451–458.

16 Kirk, B. W. & Freedman, S. O. (1967) Hypogammaglobulinaemia, thymoma and ulcerative colitis. *Canadian Medical Association Journal*, **96**, 1272.

17 Lake, A. M., Stitzel, A. E., Urmson, R. R. et al. (1979) Complement alterations in inflammatory bowel disease. *Gastroenterology*, **76**, 1374–1379.

18 Lorber, M., Schwartz, L. I. & Wasserman, L. R. (1955) Association of antibody-coated red blood cells with ulcerative colitis. *American Journal of Medicine*, **19**, 889.

19 McGiven, A. R. T., Ghose, T. & Nairn, R. C. (1967a) Autoantibodies in ulcerative colitis. *British Medical Journal*, **ii**, 19.

20 Mee, A. S., Brown, D. & Jewell, D. P. (1979) Atopy in inflammatory bowel disease. *Scandinavian Journal of Gastroenterology*, **14**, 743–746.

21 Monteiro, E., Fossey, J., Shiner, M. et al. (1971) Anti-bacterial antibodies in rectal and colonic mucosa in ulcerative colitis. *Lancet*, **i**, 249.

22 Perlmann, P. & Broberger, O. (1963) Cytotoxic action of white blood cells from patients on human foetal colon cells. Use of isotopes from colon cells as indicator of damage. *Journal of Experimental Medicine*, **117**, 717.

23 Perlmann, P., Hammarstrom, S., Lagercrantz, R. & Gustafsson, B. E. (1965) Antigen from colon of germfree rats and antibodies in human ulcerative colitis. *Annals of New York Academy of Science*, **124**, 377.

24 Scott, B. B., Goodall, A., Stephenson, P. & Jenkins, D. (1983) Rectal mucosal plasma cells in inflammatory bowel disease. *Gut*, **24**, 519–524.

25 Selby, W. S., Janossy, G., Bofill, M. et al. (1982) Mucosal lymphocyte population in inflammatory bowel disease. *Gut*, **23**, 896 (Abstract).

26 Shorter, P. C., Cardoza, M., Spencer, R. J. & Huizenga, K. A. (1969a) Further studies of in vitro cytotoxicity of lymphocytes from patients with ulcerative and granulomatous colitis for allogeneic colonic epithelial cells, including the effects of colectomy. *Gastroenterology*, **56**, 304.

27 Strobo, J. D., Tomasi, T. B., Huizenga, K. A. et al. (1976) In vitro studies of inflammatory bowel disease. Surface receptors of the mononuclear cell required to lyse allogeneic colon epithelial cells. *Gastroenterology*, **70**, 171.

28 Victorino, R. M. M. & Hodgson, H. J. F. (1980) Alteration in T lymphocyte subpopulations in inflammatory bowel disease. *Clinical and Experimental Immunology*, **41**, 156–164.

29 White, R. G., Bass, B. H. & Williams, E. (1961) Lymphadenoid goitre and the syndrome of systemic lupus erythematosus. *Lancet*, **i**, 368.

ULCERATIVE COLITIS

Ulcerative colitis is an inflammatory disease of the colon of unknown aetiology. It virtually always begins in the rectum and extends proximally to affect a variable extent of the colon. Although the first description of the disease is claimed by Wilks and Moxon in 1875, Samuel Wilks gave a very good description of the disease in 1859.[45, 46] He distinguished ulcerative colitis from infective dysenteries, which were extremely common at the time, but it was not until the classical descriptions by Hurst in 1921[15] that the disease entity was fully accepted.

PATHOLOGY

Macroscopic appearances

The disease process starts in the rectum and extends proximally in continuity into the colon. It may be confined to the rectum (usually termed 'haemorrhagic' or 'granular' proctitis) but it is debatable whether this always represents the same disease entity as ulcerative colitis. Certainly only about 10% of patients with a proctitis ultimately develop an extensive colitis.[30] Once the disease extends beyond the rectum, it may be manifest as a proctosigmoiditis, left-sided colitis, subtotal colitis or a universal (total) colitis. In patients with universal disease, there is frequently a mild inflammation of the terminal ileum (backwash ileitis).

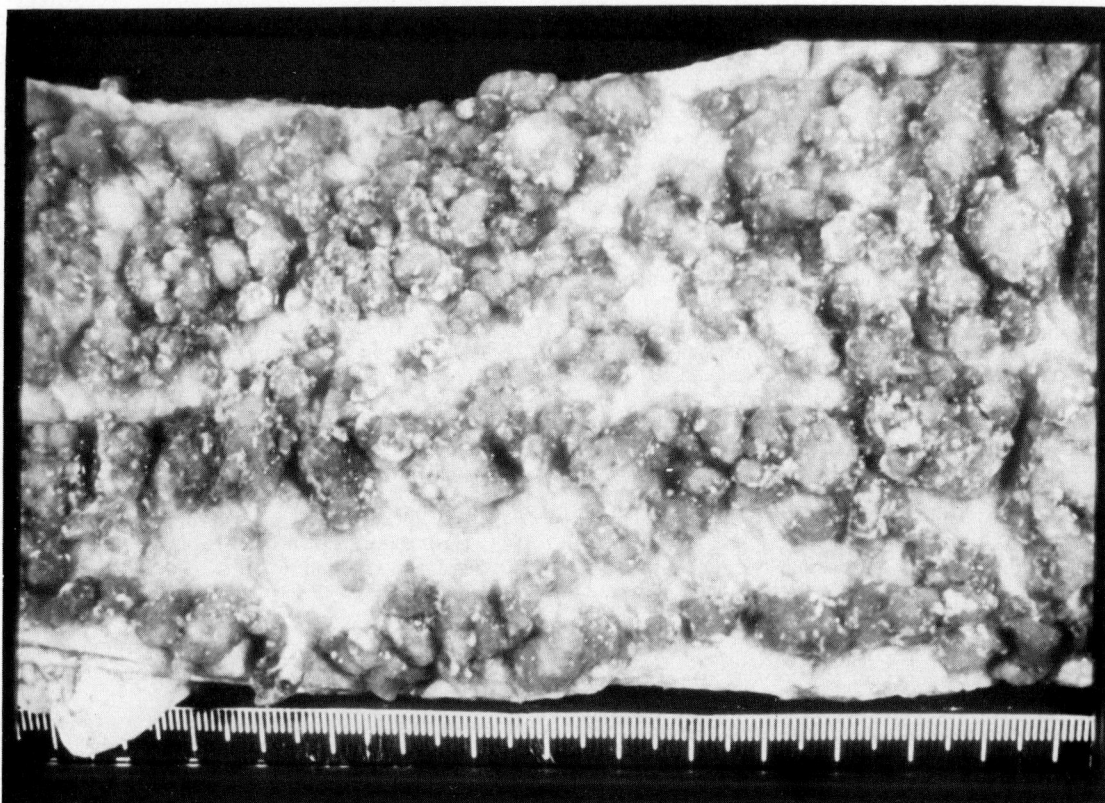

Fig. 12.6   Resected colon from a patient with severe ulcerative colitis. The mucosa is extensively ulcerated.

In active disease, the mucosal surface of the involved colon becomes uniformly haemorrhagic and granular. In severe disease there is ulceration (Figure 12.6), which may be extensive with stripping of large areas of mucous membrane. The ulceration may undermine adjacent mucosa with the formation of inflammatory polyps and mucosal bridges.

As the disease heals, the mucosa may either return to normal or become smooth and atrophic. The inflammatory polyps (pseudopolyps), formed by mucosal undermining and excessive granulation, become epithelialized. Very large numbers of inflammatory polyps may be present. They are mainly found in the colon and are less pronounced in the rectum.

Microscopic appearances

The initial lesion is increasing vascularity and oedema of the mucosa, which becomes infiltrated with acute inflammatory cells – neutrophils, plasma cells and eosinophils – but lymphocytes and macrophages also accumulate. The neutrophils traverse between the epithelial cells into the crypts to form 'crypt abscesses'.

This is characteristically accompanied by discharge of mucus from the goblet cells and this population of cells is therefore reduced in active disease (Figure 12.7). With increasing severity of disease, there is destruction of the glands and the surface epithelium (Figure 12.8). Although the inflammatory and ulcerating process may be severe, it is confined to the mucosa and does not extend appreciably into the deeper layers of the colonic wall except in association with a perforation or an acute dilatation of the colon.

In remission, the histological appearances of the mucosa may return to normal. However, there is usually some degree of mucosal atrophy. The colonic glands may be branched and reduced in number. They are often shorter than normal and do not extend down to the muscularis mucosae. In patients with long-standing disease, there may be hypertrophy of the muscularis and Paneth cell hyperplasia at the base of the crypts.

In patients in whom the risk of developing colorectal cancer is increased, dysplastic lesions may occur which are thought to be precancerous.[28] They may occur anywhere in the colon and, in some cases, can be recognized macroscopically as rather irregular plaque-like lesions

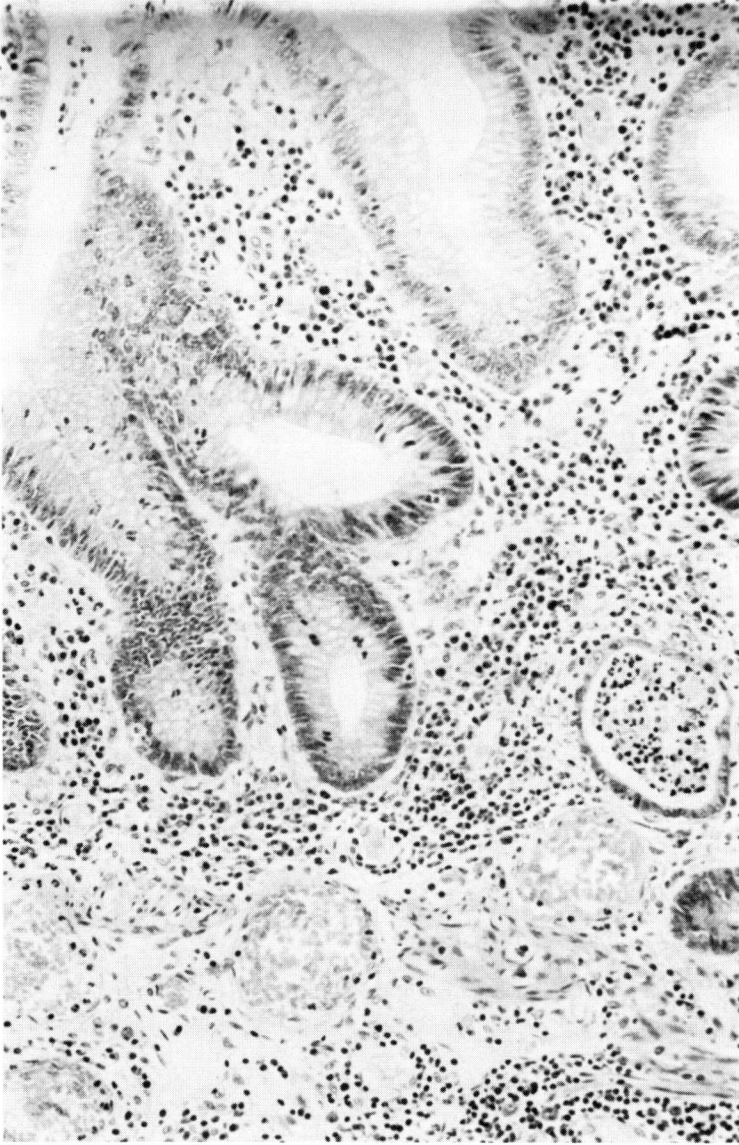

Fig. 12.7 Moderately active ulcerative colitis showing goblet cell depletion, cellular infiltration and increased vascularity. A crypt abscess is present.

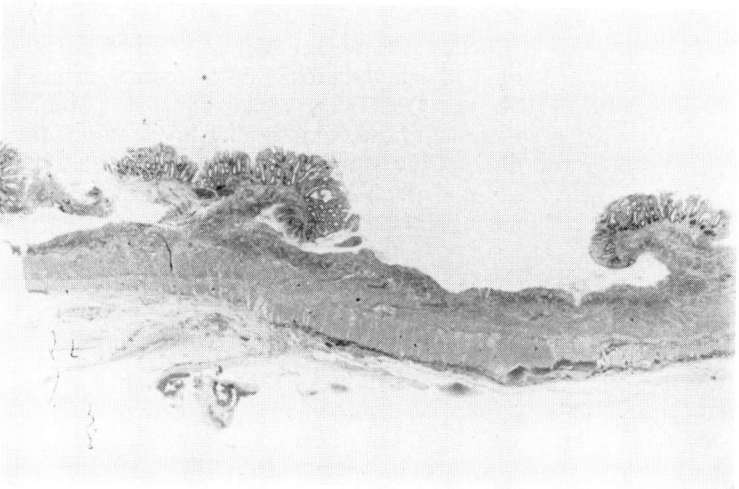

Fig. 12.8 Section from the colon illustrated in Figure 12.6 to show the severe undermining ulceration. The mucosal islands which are shown radiologically in Figure 12.11 are well seen.

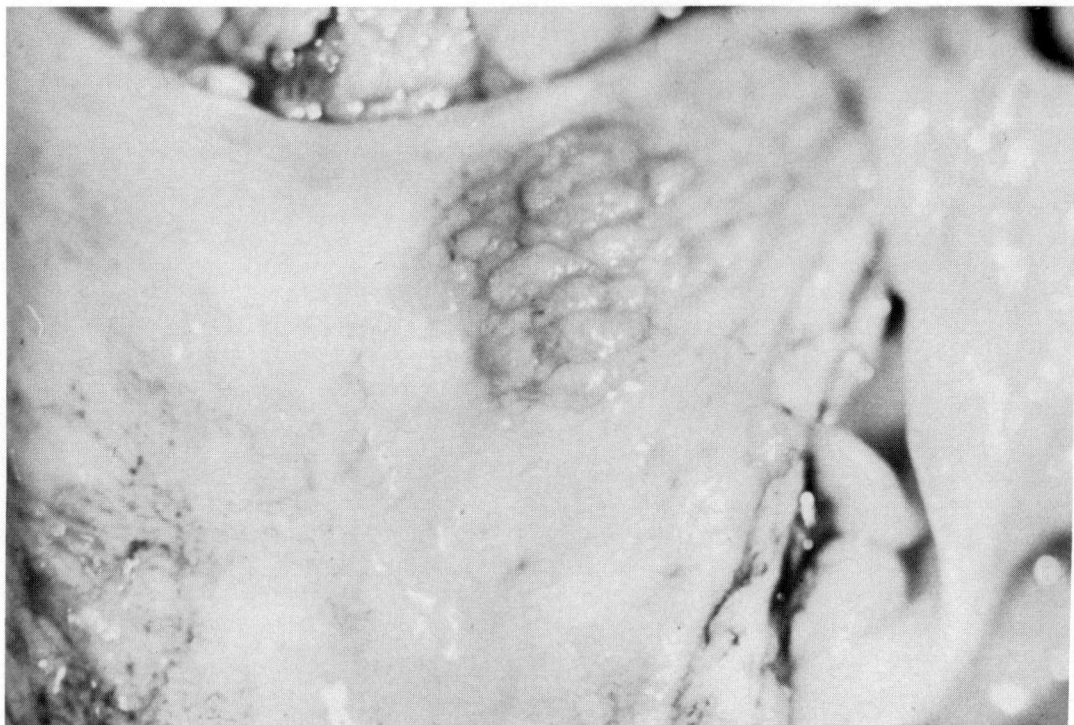

Fig. 12.9   Macroscopic appearances of dysplasia in a patient with long-standing universal colitis.

(Figure 12.9). The larger lesions can be identified radiographically or at colonoscopy. Histologically, there is irregularity of the tubules with crowding of epithelial cells and stratification of the nuclei which are pleomorphic (Figure 12.10). Mucus depletion is commonly present. These changes are present in the absence of acute inflammation and, indeed, this is an important factor since an actively regenerating mucosa may resemble mild dysplasia.

SYMPTOMS AND SIGNS

The cardinal symptoms of ulcerative colitis are rectal bleeding, diarrhoea, the passage of mucus, and abdominal pain, in approximate order of frequency.[7] The severity of the symptoms usually correlates with the severity of the disease. However, it is not uncommon to find active disease on sigmoidoscopy in patients who are asymptomatic. Hence the need for an endoscopic and histological assessment before an asymptomatic patient can be said to be in remission.

Rectal bleeding

Patients with inflammation confined to the rectum (haemorrhagic proctitis) usually notice the passage of fresh blood either streaked on the outside of a normal stool or quite separate from faecal matter. The bleeding is frequently attributed to haemorrhoids by patients and even by their doctors. The passage or leakage of blood-stained mucus is a frequent symptom in these patients and should suggest a proctitis rather than haemorrhoids. With more extensive disease, the blood is mixed with the stool or there is a frank bloody diarrhoea. With severe disease, the stool becomes more like anchovy sauce as the blood is mixed with pus as well as mucus and faecal material.

Diarrhoea

This is variable in degree. Patients with proctitis or proctosigmoiditis often complain of constipation and may never experience diarrhoea, whereas if the whole colon is involved the diarrhoea can be severe and disabling. Most patients

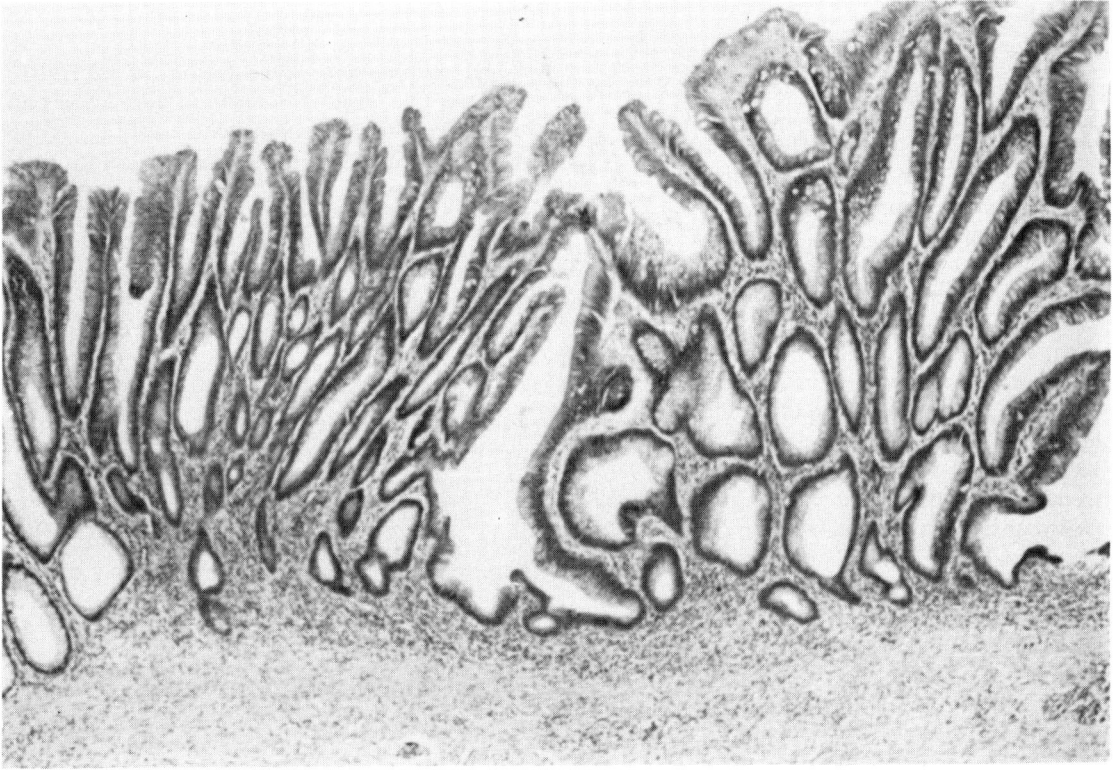

Fig. 12.10 Histological appearance of the lesion shown in Figure 12.9. The hyperplastic epithelium is irregular and the mucosa is becoming polypoid. There is pseudostratification and loss of goblet cells.

with active disease pass several liquid stools daily and may have nocturnal diarrhoea. Urgency and tenesmus are common in association with active disease and patients may be distressed by incontinence. Postprandial diarrhoea is also a common symptom. Mucus or frank pus is commonly mixed with the diarrhoea.

The pathophysiology of the diarrhoea is probably multifactorial. The changes include failure to absorb salt and water, the loss of the rectum's capacity to retain a fluid load and changes in the anorectal distension reflex.[12] Exudation of extracellular fluid, blood loss from the inflamed mucosa, and even an alteration in small intestinal motility,[29] are contributory factors. Motility dysfunction may decrease colonic transit time and explain the chronic diarrhoea in patients with long-standing disease who have a shortened colon.

Abdominal pain

Pain is not a prominent symptom for most patients with ulcerative colitis. Mild colicky pain or lower abdominal discomfort relieved by defecation may be present in some patients. However, severe pain may occur in those with fulminating attacks of the disease.

The cause of the pain is not known with certainty but is probably due to increased tension in the inflamed tissue caused by muscular contraction or distension.

Other symptoms

Patients with severe disease have usually lost weight and complain of malaise and lethargy. Symptoms of anaemia, such as shortness of breath, may also be present and patients may experience ankle swelling secondary to anaemia or hypoproteinaemia.

Weight loss is largely due to diminished food intake as a result of anorexia. Patients with fulminant disease are often nauseated or may even vomit, which further reduces intake. In addition, these patients are hypercatabolic and lose protein through the inflamed colon, both of which contribute to weight loss.

Patients may also present with symptoms referable to the extraintestinal manifestations of ulcerative colitis (see later in this chapter).

Physical signs

Patients with mild disease have few, if any, abnormal physical signs. They are well nourished, are not anaemic, and show no evidence of having a chronic disease. On palpation of the abdomen, the colon may be minimally tender over the affected portion, but this sign is frequently absent.

Patients with more severe disease usually look ill, with evidence of weight loss and salt and water depletion. They are usually febrile and frequently anaemic with signs of iron deficiency. The skin may have the appearances associated with hypoproteinaemia and there may be dependent oedema. Oral candidiasis may be present. Breaking or frank clubbing of the nails often occurs in patients where the disease is chronic. Tachycardia is invariable, and hypotension may be present. Abdominal examination reveals marked tenderness along the length of the colon, and rebound tenderness may be present. The abdomen may be distended and tympanitic but is usually flat. Bowel sounds are often reduced. Minor perianal disease, such as a small fissure, may be present but this is much less common than in patients with Crohn's disease. The signs of associated extraintestinal manifestations may also be present. Mouth ulcers are a common finding in patients with active disease.

Disease severity

It is useful to have a clinical guide to disease severity and the criteria of Truelove and Witts[38] are both simple and practical. *Severe disease* is defined as the passage of more than six stools daily with blood and associated with evidence of systemic disturbance such as fever, tachycardia, anaemia or an ESR elevated to 30 mm/h or more. *Mild disease* consists of four or less stools per day with little or no blood and in the absence of systemic illness or an elevated ESR. *Moderate disease* is intermediate between mild and severe.

For all patients presenting with an acute attack of ulcerative colitis, 15% are severe, 25% moderate and 60% are mild.[10]

Clinical presentation

Patients with a haemorrhagic proctitis usually present either with rectal bleeding associated with a normal bowel habit or they may actually complain of constipation. Since the patient is not systemically ill, several weeks or even months may go by before a patient presents to a doctor. Constipation may also be a feature of any patient with distal disease.

The commonest presentation of ulcerative colitis is the gradual onset of diarrhoea and rectal bleeding. In patients who start by passing blood as their only symptom, small quantities of blood are passed at the time of defecation although they may pass separately some blood and mucus; if this is allowed to persist, diarrhoea usually supervenes within a few weeks. Other patients begin with diarrhoea which, during the course of a few weeks or months, becomes frankly bloody.

Much less commonly, patients may present with an acute onset of bloody diarrhoea and rapidly become ill with anaemia, hypotension, fluid and electrolyte depletion, and may even become septicaemic. The local complications of acute dilatation of the colon, perforation or massive haemorrhage may rarely occur during the initial presenting attack.

COMPLICATIONS

The local complications of ulcerative colitis and their frequency are listed in Table 12.7. The extraintestinal complications, or manifestations, are discussed later in this chapter.

Table 12.7 Local complications of ulcerative colitis and their frequency of occurrence.

Perforation	1–2%
Acute dilatation	2–10%
Massive haemorrhage	3%
Perianal disease	<20%
Strictures	<12%
Carcinoma	3–5%

Perforation

This is the most dangerous of the local complications and is accompanied by faecal peritonitis. It only occurs in patients with severe disease, especially in the first attack. For example, Edwards and Truelove[11] found that 65% of perforations occurred in the first attack. This may be explained by the lack of fibrosis resulting from previous attacks and the absence of adhesions which predisposes to a free perforation. Perforation can complicate an acute dilatation but may occur in the absence of this condition. Most perforations occur on the left side of the colon, especially in the sigmoid. There is no evidence that corticosteroid therapy predisposes to perforation – an assertion that has often been made. Indeed, the incidence of perforation may have diminished as it is now rarely seen, although earlier series quoted a frequency of about 10%.

The diagnosis may be difficult. The classical symptoms and signs of a colonic perforation, such as sudden onset of abdominal pain, distension, rebound tenderness and fever, are frequently absent. The absence of these features is largely due to the occurrence of a faecal peritonitis in a patient who is already severely ill and the signs may be masked by large doses of corticosteroids. The more usual clinical picture is a sudden deterioration in the patient's general condition with a rise in pulse rate. Plain abdominal films with decubitus views should be obtained immediately in order to demonstrate the presence of free air under the diaphragm.

The treatment is surgical with an emergency colectomy but morbidity is high – 75% in the series of Edwards and Truelove.[11]

Acute dilatation

This is another dangerous complication that may be associated with severe attacks of ulcerative colitis. It is often termed a toxic dilatation and mainly affects the transverse colon. Like perforation, the only physical sign may be a sudden deterioration of the patient's general condition, although the abdomen is usually distended and it is often possible to visualize the contour of the colon. Bowel sounds usually disappear and there is a rise in pulse rate. Patients presenting with severe fulminating attacks should have abdominal girth monitored daily during the first few days of treatment and plain X-rays of the abdomen should be obtained at frequent intervals – even daily if there is a suspicion of pending dilatation. The plain films will readily demonstrate the dilated gas-filled colon without haustrations. In addition, 'mucosal islands' may be seen either as polypoid mucosal swellings along the edge of the colon or 'en face'. They represent small, inflamed and oedematous remnants of mucosa surrounded by severely ulcerated areas which have become denuded of most of their mucosa.

Patients in their first attack are particularly liable to this complication,[16] and it is mainly seen in those with a universal colitis. The pathogenesis of the complication is not known. Histologically there is severe inflammation, which usually extends through the muscularis mucosa into the submucosa and muscle layers, together with thinning of the bowel wall.[23] It is possible that the acute inflammatory reaction impairs the myenteric plexus but this is not yet proven.

Various factors have been suggested as possible precipitating events. A metabolic alkalosis or hypokalaemia may be one such factor and rapid correction of these disturbances with intravenous therapy may reverse the dilatation, at least in early cases.[36] Drugs which affect intestinal motility such as opiates, loperamide and anticholinergic agents may also be implicated. As a general rule, these drugs should be avoided in patients with ulcerative colitis and are certainly contraindicated in acute attacks. A barium enema performed in patients with fulminant disease is often assumed to precipitate an acute dilatation but the evidence for this is weak. Finally, patients who have an associated infective diarrhoea (e.g. *Campylobacter*, *Salmonella*, or the toxin of *Clostridium difficile*) may be at particular risk from developing this complication.

Treatment consists of rapid correction of fluid and electrolyte balance and institution of intravenous corticosteroids (see later). Nevertheless, the majority of patients will require urgent colectomy once the initial medical treatment has corrected the major metabolic disturbance.

Massive haemorrhage

This is a rare complication seen in patients with severe disease. The bleeding usually responds to transfusion and treatment of the disease, and is only rarely an indication for an urgent colectomy.

Strictures

Benign fibrous strictures are rare but may occur in patients with long-standing disease. Early series quoted a frequency of 11–12%, but this is almost certainly an exaggerated figure due to the failure to diagnose Crohn's disease. The other major differential diagnosis is that of a carcinoma. Colonoscopy with biopsy is usually helpful in making the correct diagnosis.

Carcinoma

This is considered later in this chapter.

Pseudopolyposis

Pseudopolyps are frequently present in patients who have had recurrent attacks and occur mainly in the descending colon. They may occur singly or in clusters and vary in shape and size from small rounded polypoid lesions to long filiform lesions. They represent excessive granulation tissue (formed in response to the acute inflammation) which has become epithelialized. They may be present for years but can regress with time.[33] They are entirely benign and have no malignant potential.

DIAGNOSIS

The diagnosis of ulcerative colitis is based on the clinical picture, together with a stool examination, sigmoidoscopic and radiological appearances, and the histological assessment of rectal and colonic biopsies.

Stool examination

Stool samples from patients with active ulceration contain large quantities of pus cells and frequently eosinophils. Stools should be cultured to exclude pathogens such as *Salmonella* and *Shigella*, and special cultures should be set up to exclude *Campylobacter* and *Clostridium difficile*. The presence of the toxin of *Clostridium difficile* should also be determined. To exclude amoebiasis, stools should be examined within minutes of obtaining the specimen.

Sigmoidoscopy

This should be performed in all patients with a diarrhoeal illness and is best done in the unprepared patient. This allows minimal changes of early ulcerative colitis to be detected which can otherwise be masked by hyperaemia induced by preparative enemas. The earliest sigmoidoscopic sign of ulcerative colitis is loss of the normal vascular pattern and the mucosa appears hyperaemic and oedematous. The edges of the valves of Houston, which are normally sharp, become blunted. With more severe inflammation, the mucosa becomes granular and eventually friable so that touching or wiping of the mucosa results in small petechial haemorrhages. In patients with severe colitis, the mucosa bleeds spontaneously and becomes ulcerated. In these patients, the lumen usually contains large amounts of liquid reddish-brown stool (a combination of diarrhoea, pus and blood). In patients with long-standing disease, pseudopolyps may be seen on sigmoidoscopy. In remission, the sigmoidoscopic appearances may return to normal, but in patients who have had a long history of repeated attacks, the mucosa becomes pale and atrophic.

There is considerable observer variation in the interpretation of the mild changes, such as hyperaemia, granularity and oedema, but there is much greater uniformity concerning more severe changes such as friability, spontaneous bleeding and ulceration.[3]

Radiology

All patients with a severe attack should have supine and erect films of the abdomen.[5] Normally the interface between the mucosa and air within the colonic lumen is sharp. In the presence of severe disease, this becomes blurred and it is often possible to detect mucosal oedema and ulceration. Thickening of the bowel wall may also be apparent. The plain films are also useful in detecting the presence of faecal material. An inflamed segment of colon does not contain faecal material and, in patients with a severe universal colitis, there are no faeces visible. The presence of faeces in the proximal colon is therefore a good indication that the disease is limited in extent. The films will also demonstrate the width of the colon and an acute dilatation should be suspected if the diameter is greater than 5.5 cm. In severe cases, mucosal islands may be seen (Figure 12.11). The plain films will also help to exclude a perforation.

If the diagnosis is still in doubt, an 'instant' barium enema can be performed. A single-contrast study without preparation is performed, allowing the barium to run in at low pressure without using a balloon catheter. However, barium studies are best avoided in these acutely ill patients and are contraindicated in patients with toxic megacolon.

Even in patients with less severe disease, care has to be taken if a barium enema is performed. Nevertheless, an air contrast procedure is safe providing that adequate preparation is obtained by gentle means, that the radiologist is aware that the disease is active, that the bowel is not over-distended with barium and air, and that the procedure is terminated if pain develops.

In mildly active disease, the mucosa shows fine irregularities or serrations along the edge of the colon and appears granular when seen 'en face' on an air contrast study (Figure 12.12). These abnormalities may be confined to the distal colon but may be present throughout the colon. With increasing severity of the disease, the ulcers become deeper and may appear as 'collar-stud' ulcers penetrating deep into the mucosa (Figure 12.13). As these deep ulcers undermine the epithelium, they may give rise to the radiological appearances of a 'double contour'. Loss of haustral pattern is a common sign and, in patients with long-standing disease, there may be shortening and narrowing of the

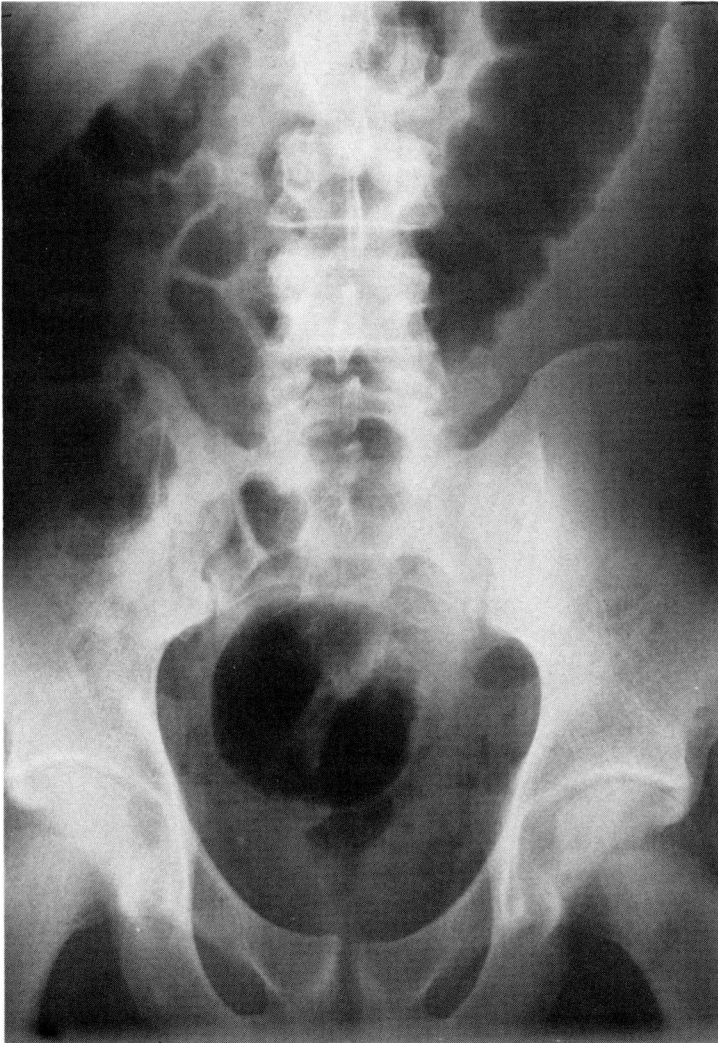

Fig. 12.11 Plain X-ray of a patient with fulminating ulcerative colitis showing mucosal irregularity in the sigmoid and transverse colon. Mucosal islands in the transverse colon are clearly visible.

colon. Pseudopolyps are often present in patients with long-standing disease. Widening of the presacral space seen on a lateral view of the pelvis is also commonly seen. This is probably another sign representing shortening and fibrosis of the rectum and it is not related to active disease and oedema of the pelvic tissues.

If there is doubt about whether the colonic disease is ulcerative colitis or Crohn's disease, a small bowel enema should be obtained to exclude ileal disease. However, for patients with ulcerative colitis, this examination should be normal although the terminal ileum may appear featureless ('backwash ileitis') in those patients with severe universal disease.

Colonoscopy

This procedure is not usually necessary for diagnosis in the majority of patients and is contraindicated in the presence of severe disease as the risk of perforation is high. If there are difficulties in the differential diagnosis, especially with respect to Crohn's disease, it can be useful as it allows multiple biopsies to be obtained. The principal uses of colonoscopy in patients with ulcerative colitis are in cancer surveillance and to determine the nature of a stricture shown radiologically. Colonoscopy is also helpful in defining the extent of disease in those patients whose symptoms are out of proportion to the radiological extent of disease. It is common to find that the disease is much more extensive when assessed using multiple biopsies taken at endoscopy. Indeed, in one series up to 14% of the patients with a universal colitis on colonoscopy had a normal barium enema.[22]

Rectal biopsy

A rectal biopsy should always be performed at the initial sigmoidoscopic examination. Once

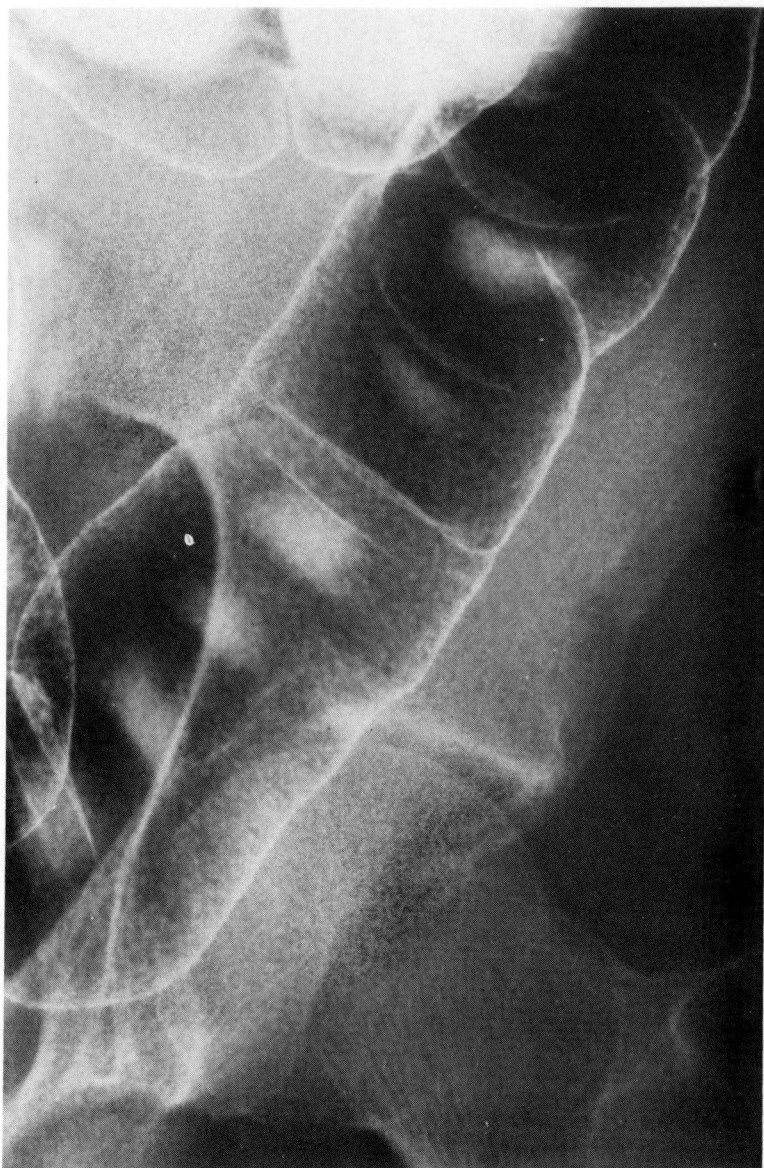

Fig. 12.12 The fine granular
appearances of mild ulcerative
colitis on a double-contrast barium
enema.

the diagnosis is established, some clinicians do not advise that further biopsy specimens be obtained. However, they are frequently useful since there is incomplete agreement between the macroscopic appearances at sigmoidoscopy and the histological appearances.[3, 43] Biopsy specimens should be carefully mounted on card or glass before fixation in order to ensure good orientation. Biopsies should be performed below 10 cm, i.e. below the peritoneal reflection, and preferably on the posterior wall. In this way, the risk of perforation becomes extremely small. The other complication is that of haemorrhage which can be minimized by using small forceps and by ensuring haemostasis before the sigmoidoscope is removed.

Biopsy specimens taken at sigmoidoscopy or at endoscopy can be useful in the differential diagnosis of ulcerative colitis.[44] The characteristic appearances of Crohn's disease or ischaemic colitis may be present. Pseudomembranous colitis can often be diagnosed from biopsy specimens and a skilled histopathologist may distinguish an infective colitis from ulcerative colitis. Search for amoebae in suspected cases of amoebiasis is often rewarding.

Laboratory data

Many patients become iron deficient due to continued blood loss – 0.5 g of elemental iron may be lost during a severe attack.[34] Therefore a

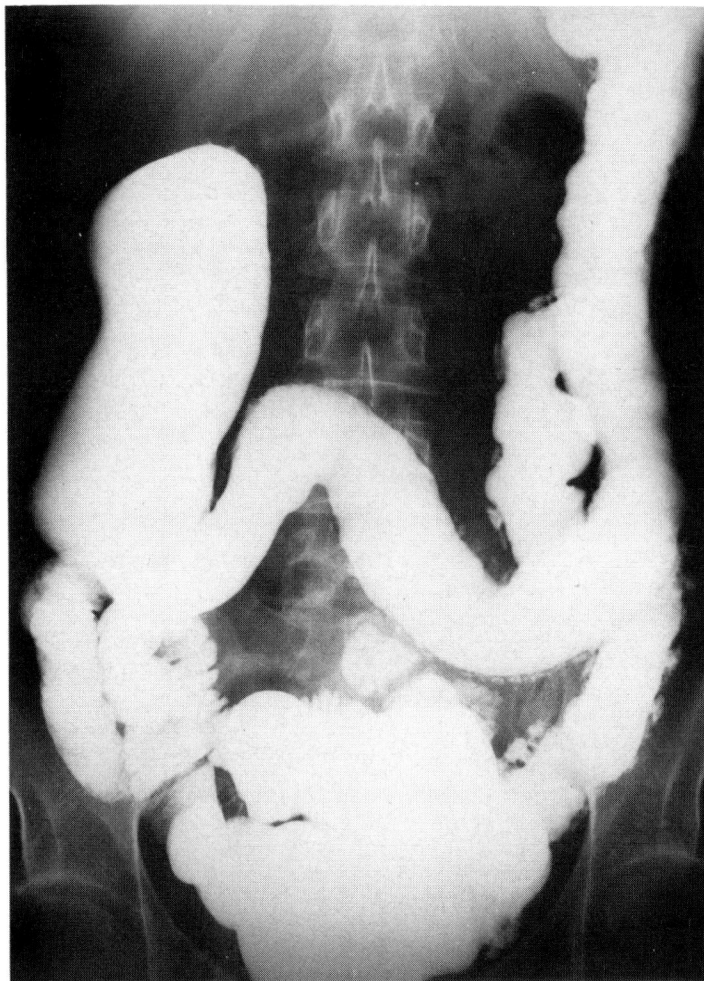

Fig. 12.13 Single-contrast barium enema in a patient with severe ulcerative colitis showing deep ulceration.

hypochromic, microcytic anaemia is commonly associated with active disease, although it is often absent in patients with mild distal disease. Active inflammation is also associated with an eosinophilia, a monocytosis and a thrombocytosis. The ESR is variably raised according to the severity of the disease.

There is rarely any biochemical disturbance in patients with mild or moderate disease but severe attacks are often associated with hypokalaemia, hypoalbuminaemia and a rise in α2-globulins. Serum immunoglobulin concentrations usually increase but remain within the normal range, and fall again as the disease goes into remission. Serum orosomucoid and C-reactive protein concentrations behave as acute phase reactants and are useful in monitoring the inflammatory activity. Liver function tests are commonly abnormal in patients with fulminating attacks and may show elevations of serum aspartate transaminase or alkaline phosphatase. These are transitory changes and prob-

ably reflect a degree of fatty liver or non-specific changes in the liver secondary to toxaemia and undernutrition. About 3% of patients will have persistently abnormal liver enzyme concentrations, even when the disease is in remission, of which the commonest is a rise in serum alkaline phosphatase.[32]

Differential diagnosis

Table 12.8 lists the more common diagnoses that must be considered for patients with suspected ulcerative colitis and provides some practical points in the differential diagnosis. For patients presenting with an acute onset of bloody diarrhoea, an infective cause must be excluded. The introduction of culture techniques for isolating *Campylobacter fetus* subspecies *jejuni*, has highlighted the importance of this organism in causing such symptoms. This is particularly so if pain is a predominant symptom.

Table 12.8 Differential diagnosis of ulcerative colitis.

	Clinical	Radiological	Histological
Ulcerative colitis	Bloody diarrhoea	Extends proximally from rectum; fine mucosal inflammation	Acute inflammatory infiltrate; goblet cell depletion; crypt abscesses
Crohn's disease	Anal lesions common	Segmental disease; rectal sparing; small bowel involvement; strictures and fissure ulcers	Focal inflammation; goblet cell preservation; submucosal involvement; granulomas
Ischaemic colitis	Older age groups; sudden onset; pain often predominant	Splenic flexure; rectal involvement rare; 'thumb-printing'	Mucosal necrosis; ballooning of capillaries; red cell congestion; haemosiderin and fibrosis (long-standing disease)
Infective colitis	Sudden onset usual; identifiable source; other cases known (for example *Salmonella*); pain may predominate (for example *Campylobacter*); pathogens present in stool	Usually normal	Similar to mild ulcerative colitis; neutrophils migrate into epithelium
Amoebic colitis	Travel in endemic area; amoebae in stool	Discrete ulcers; amoeboma or strictures (chronic disease)	Similar to ulcerative colitis; amoebae may be seen within the lamina propria or in the flask-shaped ulcers (readily shown by PAS staining)
Pseudomembranous colitis	May be a history of antibiotics; 'membrane' may be seen on sigmoidoscopy, toxin of *Cl. difficile* detectable in stools	Oedematous; shaggy outline	Similar to acute ischaemic colitis but may show classic summit lesions consisting of a fibropurulent exudate

From Jewell, D. P. Inflammatory bowel disease: diagnosis and medical treatment of ulcerative colitis, *British Journal of Medicine*, May 1982, 456–462, with kind permission of the editor.

Sigmoidoscopic appearances of the infective colitides are similar to ulcerative colitis and it may be difficult for the histopathologist to distinguish between them. Pseudomembranous colitis is also diagnosed more frequently now that the toxin of *Clostridium difficile* can be detected. There is, of course, no reason why patients with ulcerative colitis should not contract an infective colitis. It then becomes arguable whether symptoms are solely due to the infection or whether the infection triggers a relapse. Gonococcal proctitis is easily overlooked in a gastroenterological clinic but, characteristically, it is associated with large quantities of purulent exudate. Chlamydial proctitis is much less common and appears macroscopically similar to ulcerative colitis.

TREATMENT

Medical treatment

All patients with ulcerative colitis must have the nature of the disease explained to them carefully and must appreciate that when symptoms recur they should report to their doctor early so that appropriate treatment can be given. Patients often become psychologically upset by their symptoms, as do their close relatives, so that reassurance and moral support are vital to the overall management.

The major principle of medical therapy is to treat active disease with corticosteroids and, when the acute disease has settled, to maintain the remission with sulphasalazine. The drugs which can be used will be discussed individually and then guidelines for treating attacks of varying severity will be given.

Corticosteroids
The classic trials of Truelove and Witts[38] established the benefit of cortisone in the treatment of acute ulcerative colitis. Oral prednisolone is also effective and this is dose-related, although the higher doses (e.g. 60 mg daily) are associated with appreciable side-effects.[4] When prednisolone is given by mouth, it should be given as a single morning dose since this is as effective as a

divided dose regimen but has fewer side-effects.[26] Intramuscular ACTH may be marginally more effective than cortisone but is seldom needed. Topical corticosteroids, given as a retention enema, are also effective in healing active rectal disease and the combination of oral and topical steroids is more effective than either alone.[37] Absorption of steroid from the rectum is considerable if prednisolone phosphate enemas are used,[27] but this can be minimized either by using betamethasone enemas or, preferably, prednisolone metasulphobenzoate enemas.[19]

Corticosteroids should not be used as maintenance therapy as they are ineffective, at least in doses which are associated with an acceptable incidence of side-effects. Neither cortisone in a dose of 37.5 mg daily,[39] nor prednisolone in a dose of 15 mg daily[20] will maintain a remission. However, an alternate day regime has been advocated as a way of minimizing side-effects.

Sulphasalazine

This drug consists of 5-aminosalicylic acid linked to sulphapyridine by an azo bond. It is poorly absorbed in the small intestine and hence the majority of an orally administered dose is delivered to the colon. The colonic bacteria are able to split the azo bond and thereby release the two individual moieties. Recently it has been shown that the active agent, at least for acute healing, is the 5-aminosalicylic acid.[1, 42] The mode of action of sulphasalazine is unknown. In vitro studies have shown that it has a weak inhibitory effect on prostaglandin synthesis, but it may also reduce prostaglandin catabolism by inhibiting prostaglandin dehydrogenase. It inhibits polymorph and monocyte migration in vitro and this may relate to its ability to inhibit leucotriene synthesis. Sulphasalazine and 5-aminosalicylic acid may also inhibit lymphocyte function and sulphasalazine is known to inhibit folate metabolism.

The dose-related side-effects of sulphasalazine are largely caused by the sulphapyridine and its metabolites, and include nausea, vomiting, diarrhoea, and headache. Many of the non-dose-related side-effects such as erythema nodosum and other hypersensitivity rashes may also be due to the sulphapyridine moiety. Rarely, agranulocytosis and a Heinz body haemolytic anaemia can occur, and recently sulphasalazine has been identified as a cause of male infertility. The drug mainly affects sperm motility but abnormal forms are often present and the total number of spermatozoa may be reduced. These changes are reversible once the drug is stopped.[35] The dose-related side-effects of sulphasalazine can often be overcome by starting at a low dose (e.g., 0.5 g daily) and gradually working up to a full therapeutic dose. For patients with hypersensitivity reactions, desensitization can be achieved by a starting dose of 1 mg daily.[14]

Sulphasalazine is more effective than a placebo in treating active disease although it is not nearly as effective as corticosteroids.[40] Sulphasalazine enemas may be useful for active distal disease,[24] and recently it has been shown that enemas containing a high dose of 5-aminosalicylic acid (4 g) are superior to hydrocortisone enemas (100 mg) in the treatment of active distal disease.[8] However, the major use of sulphasalazine is in long-term maintenance therapy as it reduces the frequency of recurrent attacks, an effect which operates over many years.[9] The optimum dose which gives maximal clinical effect with the least side-effects is 2 g daily.[2]

At the present time, attempts are being made to deliver 5-aminosalicylic acid into the colon either in the form of a slow-release preparation or by linking it to a carrier molecule other than sulphapyridine. One such compound, disodium azodisalicylate, has pharmacodynamics similar to sulphasalazine.[47] It is hoped that such preparations will retain all the beneficial effects of sulphasalazine but without its adverse features.

Azathioprine

There is no evidence that azathioprine is of benefit for active disease. However, it may be of some use as long-term maintenance therapy in a dose of 1.5–2.0 mg/kg, especially for patients with established disease.[17] It should be reserved for those patients who frequently relapse once corticosteroids are tailed off. Azathioprine also has a steroid-sparing effect in those rare patients who appear to benefit from continuous therapy.[18]

Cromoglycate

Despite promising results from early trials, all subsequent studies have shown no benefit, at least in doses up to 800 mg daily.

Antibiotics

Oral antibiotics have no place in the management of ulcerative colitis and may even be responsible for initiating a relapse.

TREATMENT OF ACUTE ATTACKS

Mild attacks

These are defined as the passage of no more than four motions daily, often with blood and mucus, by patients who are not systemically ill. These attacks are best treated with prednisolone in a dose of 20 mg daily in combination with sulphasalazine and a steroid enema. Most patients are able to carry on their normal daily activities. This regimen rapidly renders the overwhelming majority of patients symptom-free. Oral steroids are maintained for at least four weeks before being tailed off. Rectal steroids are usually continued until oral steroids are stopped and they can also be stopped if mucosal healing is apparent on sigmoidoscopy. Patients are maintained on sulphasalazine alone as described above. If a good response is not obtained, the patient should be treated as for a moderate attack or may even require hospital admission.

Moderate attacks

These consist of passing more than four motions daily with blood but in the absence of systemic illness. Prednisolone should be given in a dose of 40 mg daily for at least one week and then reduced over two–three weeks to 20 mg daily. The treatment schedule is otherwise similar to that outlined for mild attacks.

Severe attacks

These are attacks in which there may be severe diarrhoea with bleeding in patients who may show any of the following: tachycardia, obvious salt and water deficiency, fever, anaemia, and hypoalbuminaemia. All such patients must be admitted to hospital. Electrolyte, fluid and blood losses are corrected as quickly as possible and treatment should begin using intravenous fluids, nutrients and prednisolone in a dose of 60 mg daily. Intravenous antibiotics such as tetracycline or metronidazole are often used but whether they have a beneficial role is not clear. Hydrocortisone enemas should also be given using 100 mg twice daily. These enemas are preferable to disposable enemas since they can be dripped into the inflamed colon at a slow rate using a soft catheter and an intravenous infusion set, and are therefore more likely to be retained.

Patients in a severe attack should have careful monitoring of pulse rate, blood pressure and abdominal girth in order to detect the early signs of an acute dilatation or a perforation. Plain X-rays of the abdomen should always be obtained to exclude these complications and are often repeated on a daily basis during the first few days.

About 70% of patients with severe attacks respond rapidly to this form of intravenous therapy in the first five days.[41] Experience has shown that patients not making a satisfactory

response should be considered for urgent colectomy as few do well if medical therapy is continued. The factors which help to identify those patients who are likely to respond poorly and hence come to surgery are a maximum temperature greater than 38°C, a maximum pulse rate of greater than 100/min, or a bowel frequency greater than 12 stools within the first 24 hours of hospital admission. A persistently low serum albumin (< 30 g/l) during the first few days of treatment is another indicator of a poor prognosis.[21]

Patients who respond well to intravenous therapy should then receive oral corticosteroids (e.g. prednisolone 40 mg daily) and sulphasalazine. Hydrocortisone enemas should be continued or changed to a disposable enema (e.g. Predenema). A light diet is given.

There are a few patients who may have severe left-sided disease with proximal constipation. It is common clinical experience that the disease does not settle on intensive corticosteroid therapy unless the constipation is treated, preferably with a gentle osmotic purge.

MANAGEMENT OF PROCTITIS

Patients who have a haemorrhagic proctitis with a normal colon may sometimes be difficult to manage. Initially, topical steroids should be given in the form of a suppository or a foam, together with oral sulphasalazine. However, this regimen frequently fails to heal the inflammation. In these circumstances, oral corticosteroids or a sulphasalazine enema can be tried. If there is still no response, high-dose cromoglycate (1.6 g daily) can be used, although there is little evidence for its value. However, some patients with proctitis may have a type I hypersensitivity reaction within the mucosa[31] and it is conceivable that this might respond to a mast cell stabilizer.

THE ROLE OF DIET

In general, patients should be encouraged to eat a well-balanced high-fibre diet. Milk-free diets have not proved useful for the majority of patients, even though about 20% of patients appeared to benefit under the conditions of a controlled therapeutic trial.[48] Some of these patients probably had hypolactasia which may partly explain the benefit obtained. It should also be noted that patients having severe attacks of ulcerative colitis have a high incidence of hypolactasia.[25]

MAINTENANCE OF REMISSION

Once the patient is in remission, usually defined according to symptoms for the purposes of management, corticosteroids are tailed off as previously described. Sulphasalazine is continued, in a dose of 2 g daily, on a long-term basis since this reduces the risk of a further relapse by about 75% even after many years of treatment. As discussed above, azathioprine may also reduce the rate of relapse, but far less effectively than sulphasalazine, and should only be used in selected patients.

COURSE AND PROGNOSIS

The great majority of patients with ulcerative colitis suffer recurrent attacks of their disease.[10] The number of patients who have only one attack is very small and diminishes even more with increasing length of follow-up. In the few that never relapse, it is conceivable that the initial attack represented a *Campylobacter* or *Clostridium difficile* infection at a time when modern diagnostic techniques were not available. About 8% of patients pursue a chronic continuous course and never have a prolonged remission.

The introduction of corticosteroids greatly reduced the overall mortality of ulcerative colitis but this is mainly in patients with mild or moderate attacks.[10] Severe attacks continue to be dangerous especially when they are of sudden onset and there is delay in making the diagnosis, when the patient is elderly, when universal colitis is present, or when a local complication intervenes. Nevertheless, developments in both medical and surgical treatment have reduced the mortality of severe attacks and, in Oxford, mortality in this situation has fallen from about 33% in the pre-steroid era to about 1% over the past five years.

The long-term prognosis has also probably improved with recent studies showing a survival curve which either does not differ appreciably from the expected survival curve,[6, 30] or is only slightly decreased.[13] This improvement is likely to be due to the reduction in mortality during acute attacks, the reduction in operative mortality, and the use of long-term sulphasalazine which reduces the relapse rate to about one-quarter of that seen in patients who do not receive the drug.[9]

REFERENCES

1 Azad Khan, A. K., Piris, J. & Truelove, S. C. (1977) An experiment to determine the active therapeutic moiety of sulphasalazine. *Lancet*, **ii**, 892–895.

2 Azad Khan, A. K., Howes, D. T., Piris, J. & Truelove, S. C. (1980) Optimum dose of sulphasalazine for maintenance treatment in ulcerative colitis. *Gut*, **21**, 232–240.

3 Baron, J. H., Connell, A. M. & Lennard-Jones, J. E. (1964) Variation between observers in describing mucosal appearances in proctocolitis. *British Medical Journal*, **i**, 89–92.

4 Baron, J. H., Connell, A. M., Kanaghinis, T. G. *et al.* (1962) Outpatient treatment of ulcerative colitis: comparison between three doses of oral prednisolone. *British Medical Journal*, **ii**, 441–443.

5 Bartram, C. I. (1976) Plain abdominal X-ray in acute colitis. *Proceedings of the Royal Society of Medicine*, **67**, 617–618.

6 Bonnevie, O., Binder, V. & Anthonisen, P. (1974) The prognosis of ulcerative colitis. *Scandinavian Journal of Gastroenterology*, **9**, 81–91.

7 Both, H., Torp-Pedersen, K., Kriener, S. *et al.* (1983) Clinical manifestations of ulcerative colitis and Crohn's disease in a regional patient group. *Scandinavian Journal of Gastroenterology*, in press.

8 Campieri, M., Lanfranchi, G. A., Barzzocchi, G. *et al.* (1981) Treatment of ulcerative colitis with high dose 5-aminosalicylic acid enemas. *Lancet*, **ii**, 270–271.

9 Dissanayake, A. S. & Truelove, S. C. (1973) A controlled therapeutic trial of long-term maintenance treatment of ulcerative colitis with sulphasalazine. *Gut*, **14**, 923–926.

10 Edwards, F. C. & Truelove, S. C. (1963) The course and prognosis of ulcerative colitis. *Gut*, **4**, 299–315.

11 Edwards, F. C. & Truelove, S. C. (1964) The course and prognosis of ulcerative colitis. *Gut*, **5**, 1–22.

12 Farthing, M. J. G. & Lennard-Jones, J. E. (1978) Sensibility of the rectum to distension and the anorectal distension reflex in ulcerative colitis. *Gut*, **19**, 64–69.

13 Gyde, S., Prior, P., Dow, M. J. *et al.* (1982) Mortality in ulcerative colitis. *Gastroenterology*, **83**, 36–43.

14 Holdsworth, C. D. (1981) Sulphasalazine desensitisation. *British Medical Journal*, **ii**, 110.

15 Hurst, A. F. (1921) Ulcerative colitis. *Guy's Hospital Report*, **71**, 24–41.

16 Jalan, K. N., Sircus, W., Card, W. I. *et al.* (1969) An experience of ulcerative colitis. 1. Toxic dilatation in 55 cases. *Gastroenterology*, **57**, 68–82.

17 Jewell, D. P. & Truelove, S. C. (1974) Azathioprine in ulcerative colitis: final report on a controlled therapeutic trial. *British Medical Journal*, **ii**, 627–630.

18 Kirk, A. P. & Lennard-Jones, J. E. (1982) Controlled trial of azathioprine in chronic ulcerative colitis. *British Medical Journal*, **ii**, 1291–1292.

19 Lee, D. A. H., Taylor, M., James, V. H. T. & Walker, G. (1980) Rectally administered prenisolone – evidence for a predominantly local action. *Gut*, **21**, 215–218.

20 Lennard-Jones, J. E., Misiewicz, J. J., Connell, A. M. *et al.* (1965) Prednisone as maintenance treatment for ulcerative colitis in remission. *Lancet*, **i**, 188–189.

21 Lennard-Jones, J. E., Ritchie, J. K., Hilder, W. & Spicer, C. C. (1975) Assessment of severity in colitis: a preliminary study. *Gut*, **16**, 579–584.

22 Loose, H. & Williams, C. (1974) Barium enema versus colonoscopy. *Proceedings of the Royal Society of Medicine*, **67**, 1033–1036.

23 Lumb, G., Protheroe, R. H. B. & Ramsay, G. S. (1955) Ulcerative colitis with dilatation of the colon. *British Journal of Surgery*, **43**, 182–188.

24 Palmer, K. R., Goepel, J. R. & Holdsworth, C. D. (1981) Sulphasalazine enemas in ulcerative colitis: a double-blind trial. *British Medical Journal*, **ii**, 1571–1573.

25 Pena, A. S. & Truelove, S. C. (1973) Hypolactasia and ulcerative colitis. *Gastroenterology*, **64**, 400–404.

26 Powell-Tuck, J., Bown, R. L. & Lennard-Jones, J. E. (1978) Comparison of oral prednisolone given as a single or multiple daily dose for active proctocolitis. *Scandinavian Journal of Gastroenterology*, **13**, 833–837.

27 Powell-Tuck, J., Lennard-Jones, J. E., May, C. S. *et al.* (1976) Plasma prednisolone levels after administration of prednisolone-21-phosphate as a retention enema in colitis. *British Medical Journal*, **i**, 193–195.

28 Riddell, R. H. & Morson, B. C. (1979) Value of sigmoidoscopy and biopsy in detection of carcinoma and premalignant change in ulcerative colitis. *Gut*, **20**, 575–580.

29 Ritchie, J. A. & Salem, S. N. (1965) Upper intestinal motility in ulcerative colitis, idiopathic, and the irritable colon syndrome. *Gut*, **6**, 325–337.

30 Ritchie, J. K., Powell-Tuck, J. & Lennard-Jones, J. E. (1978) Clinical outcome of the first ten years of ulcerative colitis and proctitis. *Lancet*, **i**, 1140–1143.

31 Rosekrans, P. C. M., Meijer, C. J. L. M., Wal, A. M. van der & Lindeman, J. (1980) Allergic proctitis, a clinical and immunological entity. *Gut*, **21**, 1017–1023.

32 Shepherd, H. A., Selby, W. S., Chapman, R. W. G. *et al.* (1983) Ulcerative colitis and persistent liver dysfunction. *Quarterly Journal of Medicine*, in press.

33 Sloan, W. P., Bargen, J. A. & Baggenstoss, A. H. (1950) Local complications of chronic ulcerative colitis based on a study of 2000 cases. *Proceedings of Staff Meeting, Mayo Clinic*, **25**, 240–244.

34 Stack, B. H. R., Smith, T., Hywel Jones, J. & Fletcher, J. (1969) Measurement of blood and iron loss in colitis with a whole body counter. *Gut*, **10**, 769–773.

35 Toovey, S., Hudson, E., Hendry, W. F. & Levi, A. J. (1981) Sulphasalazine and male infertility – reversibility and possible mechanism. *Gut*, **22**, 445–451.

36 Torsoli, A. (1981) Toxic megacolon. Part II: prevention. *Clinics in Gastroenterology*, **10**, 117–121.

37 Truelove, S. C. (1960) Systemic and local corticosteroid therapy in ulcerative colitis. *British Medical Journal*, **i**, 464–467.

38 Truelove, S. C. & Witts, L. J. (1955) Cortisone in ulcerative colitis: final report on a therapeutic trial. *British Medical Journal*, **ii**, 1041–1048.

39 Truelove, S. C. & Witts, L. J. (1959) Cortisone and corticotrophin in ulcerative colitis. *British Medical Journal*, **i**, 387–394.

40 Truelove, S. C., Watkinson, G. & Draper, G. (1962) Comparison of corticosteroids and sulphasalazine therapy in ulcerative colitis. *British Medical Journal*, **ii**, 1708–1711.

41 Truelove, S. C., Willoughby, C. P., Lee, E. G. & Kettlewell, M. G. W. (1978) Further experience in the treatment of severe attacks of ulcerative colitis. *Lancet*, **ii**, 1086–1088.

42 Van Hees, P. A. M., Bakker, J. H. & van Tongeren, J. H. M. (1980) Effect of sulphapyridine, 5-aminosalicylic acid, and placebo in patients with idiopathic proctitis: a study to determine the active therapeutic moiety of sulphasalazine. *Gut*, **21**, 632–635.

43 Watts, J. M., Thomson, H. & Goligher, J. C. (1966) Sigmoidoscopy and cytology in the detection of microscopic disease of the rectal mucosa in ulcerative colitis. *Gut*, **7**, 288–294.

44 Whitehead, R. (1973) *Mucosal Biopsy of the Gastrointestinal Tract*. London: W. B. Saunders.

45 Wilks, S. (1859) *Lectures of Pathological Anatomy*, 1st edn. London: Langmans & Roberts.

46 Wilks, S. (1859) Morbid appearances in the intestines of Miss Bankes. *Medical Times and Gazette*, **19**, 264–265.

47 Willoughby, C. P., Aronson, J. K., Agback, H. *et al.* (1982) Distribution and metabolism in healthy volunteers of disodium azodisalicylate, a potential therapeutic agent for ulcerative colitis. *Gut*, **23**, 1081–1087.

48 Wright, R. & Truelove, S. C. (1965) A controlled therapeutic trial of various diets in ulcerative colitis. *British Medical Journal*, **ii**, 138–141.

Surgical treatment

Although the majority of patients with ulcerative colitis can be successfully managed by careful medical treatment, a minority still need surgical treatment either for fulminating disease, or because repeated attacks or continuous symptoms cannot be controlled. During the past decade there has been a marked improvement in the surgical results. This has been achieved by the gradual improvement of existing modes of treatment rather than by dramatic new methods.

When surgery was first attempted for colitis it was used for fulminating disease. Defunctioning operations, such as a diversionary ileostomy or an appendicostomy, were tried but had little effect on the progression of the disease; limited resections of the most severely inflamed segments were gradually extended to a subtotal or total colectomy with ileostomy. Later an increasing proportion of the operations were carried out electively for chronic disease. Since the rectum is always affected, it was often removed, although some surgeons were strong proponents of colectomy with an ileorectal anastomosis. This chapter reviews the changes in established operations made in order to improve the outcome and outlines newer techniques which may enable more patients to avoid having a permanent stoma.

INDICATIONS FOR SURGERY

During an acute attack

A severe exacerbation of ulcerative colitis is a dangerous illness unless treated energetically. In Oxford in the early 1950s the results of medical treatment were reviewed. Between 1938 and 1952, 28% of patients who had been admitted to hospital during a severe attack died during the admission; furthermore, 25% of such patients who were admitted between 1953 and 1962 (the decade following the introduction of corticosteroids) were still dying of the disease.[10, 11] Since then a dramatic fall in mortality has been brought about by changes in the administration of corticosteroid therapy. The regimen introduced by Truelove in Oxford consists of a five-day intensive intravenous administration of prednisolone.[36] Failure to improve during this time is an indication for surgery. Patients who are referred for surgery during an acute attack now come to operation at an earlier stage than used to be the case.

The indications which we still use in Oxford for immediate surgery during an acute attack are:

1 The presence of a major complication such as perforation or acute dilatation on admission to hospital.

2 The development of a severe complication such as a perforation or acute dilatation during the course of the five-day intensive corticosteroids regimen.

3 Re-activation of the colitis after completion of the intravenous corticosteroid regimen.

For chronic disease

About half of the colectomies in Oxford have been carried out as an elective procedure. The most common indications are:

1 Frequent attacks of colitis not adequately controlled by long-term sulphasalazine administration.

2 Continuous symptoms in spite of medical treatment.

3 The development of a major complication. Most local complications are associated with acute attacks of colitis; the majority of remote complications can be dealt with by medical treatment. Rarely we have carried out surgery for a major complication such as a haemorrhage or, in one instance, a septic arthritis. Stricture of the colon has been an indication in a small group of patients, most of whom were thought to have a cancer at the site. Gross perianal fistulas and fissures may be indications for surgery, although most of the patients with serious perianal disease on whom we have carried out a proctocolectomy have subsequently been found to have Crohn's disease.

4 The development of cancer of the colon.

5 To prevent the development of colonic cancer. In the past it was our practice to carry out prophylactic proctocolectomy in patients with extensive ulcerative colitis for ten years or more who, in addition, had presented before puberty and in whom the first attack was severe. Recently fewer patients have been treated surgically for this reason. The introduction of colonoscopy and the detection of dysplastic epithelial changes which can be used as an indicator of potential malignant change[28] has enabled patients with extensive colitis of ten or more years to be included in a surveillance programme. However, there is no general agreement that the epithelial changes are accurate predictors of the development of invasive cancer. Its use alone may mean that a number of patients will unexpectedly develop colorectal cancer.

PREOPERATIVE PREPARATION

For elective surgery sufficient time should be made for careful preoperative preparation of the patient. The use of adequate medication in an acute attack is important because it may delay the need for surgery until the patient is in remission and can be more fully prepared. Anaemia should be corrected and, if the general state of nutrition is poor, periods of intense parenteral feeding may be undertaken. Psychological support is particularly important, especially if the patient is to be left with a permanent ileostomy. The preparation should also consist of a careful explanation to the spouse and an introduction to the stomatherapist who is often best able to explain the technical details of ileostomy life. The patient (and his family) should meet an ileostomist of a similar age, who can provide practical and helpful advice. This type of preparation has been used in Oxford for more than ten years, but it is probably still insufficient. In spite of the most careful attention, a recent study of our patients[21] has shown that the patients still feel that the amount of information they have been given is not adequate. More time should be given to ensure that the patient fully understands the sequelae of the operation. An important aspect of preparation should consist of sexual counselling. Many patients who have been ill with severe colitis suffer from considerable psychosexual disturbance. It is, of course, not possible to undertake such extensive discussions in patients requiring surgery as an emergency, but even a limited preparation of the patient is important in order to achieve a good long-term outcome.

THE CHOICE OF OPERATION

Proctocolectomy

The standard operative procedure which is used by most surgeons when operating as an emergency is a subtotal or total colectomy with a Brooke everted spout ileostomy. This leaves a defunctioned distal sigmoid and rectum, with the proximal end brought out as a mucous fistula. It is often used during elective surgery as a preliminary to ileorectal anastomosis or, if restoration of continuity of the bowel is found to be too dangerous, to proctectomy. In Oxford before 1970 we employed this technique as the standard operation. However, between 1970 and 1982 we have used a single stage proctocolectomy as the operation of choice for the majority of cases even when the colectomy was being undertaken as an emergency.[26]

The policy was changed because we were attracted to proctocolectomy as it was the only procedure which could cure the disease, and a number of surgeons had recorded a fall in mortality using this approach. The disadvantages were a permanent ileostomy, and possible damage to the autonomic nerves in the pelvis during the dissection of the rectum. Recent reports have shown that the long-term outcome with an ileostomy is better than had previously been anticipated.

The long-term results of ileostomy. The first ileostomy operation for ulcerative colitis was carried out before the first World War,[7] it was not until the introduction of the first ileostomy appliance[35] and the improvements in appliances which followed that the operation was used widely. Even then the results were poor. The flush ileostomy often leaked, and the old type of spout ileostomy, which left the peritoneal lining of the ileum exposed to the contents of the stomal bag, became infected and fibrosed. This led to a syndrome of ileostomy diarrhoea due to infection of the ileal contents, with subsequent malnutrition followed by dehydration and renal failure. The poor prognosis which became associated with the old type of stomas can readily be understood. The work of Bryan Brooke in Birmingham changed the outlook dramatically. In 1952 he introduced the everted spout ileostomy which combined the advantage of stomal protrusion into the bag to allow a better water-tight seal of appliance to skin, with a mucosa to skin healing.[6] About the same time ileostomy associations were set up in England and subsequently in the USA. The element of self-help by stoma patients was an important advance.[27] Industry has also played a major role in improving the life of the ileostomy patient, with the introduction of disposable lightweight odour-proof bags, and bag sealants such as Karaya powder, Karaya rings and, more recently, Stomahesive. Finally, the importance of trained stoma nurses must be emphasized. Most countries have stoma clinics run by highly trained specialist nurses who make an important contribution to the life of stoma patients and their families.

A number of surveys have shown that the expectation of life of patients with a permanent ileostomy is very close to that of the normal population, and that the quality of life in the long-term is good.[32] Recently in Oxford Kennedy carried out an extensive study in which he compared the long-term postoperative general health of a group of 39 colitics who had been treated by proctocolectomy and permanent Brooke ileostomy with a control group of healthy volunteers who were matched for age and sex, and with a group of 39 colitics who had not had surgery.[20] He found that the general health of the stoma patients was good or excellent and nearly all were pursuing their normal occupations. The results of standard haematological and biochemical investigations were also normal. Most undertook normal recreations although some had given up swimming. The diets of the stoma patients were virtually normal except that they tended to take more fluid and salt. Despite this there was often evidence of mild dehydration and aldosteronism. Other abnormal findings included increased retention of calcium and mild iron deficiency with a higher than expected incidence of urinary tract stones and gallstones. Psychological abnormalities were minor but not uncommon. There was no impotence in the males and little evidence of sexual dysfunction, though 23% of the male patients reported some psychological difficulty in their sexual relationships. Some of the women with active sex lives complained of dyspareunia in spite of having normal perineal sensation. Most of their trouble lay in feeling less feminine and less attractive than before the operation. Some of these complaints are related to the ileostomy and some to the rectal dissection.

The technique of excision of the rectum. The standard technique of a synchronous abdominoperineal resection of the rectum used for rectal cancer is not appropriate during the operation of proctocolectomy for inflammatory bowel disease. A particularly unpleasant side-effect of the cancer operation is caused by damage to autonomic nerves in the pelvis. Uncommonly this may result in urinary incontinence; more commonly it may lead to male impotence. The incidence of impaired intercourse in males after the standard dissection varies between 11 and 29% in different series, in spite of attempts to preserve the nervi erigentes.[8, 9, 16, 39] To overcome this problem, in the early 1970s we introduced a technique for excising the rectum in a perimuscular plane which seems to have greatly reduced the chance of damaging both the sympathetic and parasympathetic nerves in the pelvis.[25] Figure 12.14 illustrates the importance of using Waldeyer's fascia behind the rectum to direct the dissection into the correct plane. Parks and Lyttle subsequently described a technique of dissection through the intermuscular plane between the intrinsic and external sphincter muscles of the

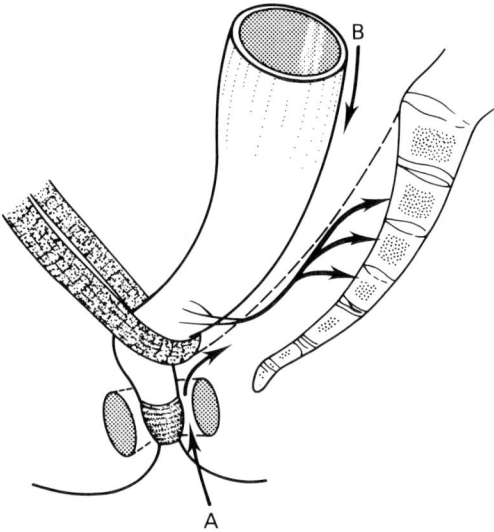

Fig. 12.14 Coronal view of the posterior plane of a perimuscular dissection. Waldeyer's fascia (interrupted line) guides the dissection into the presacral space if it is undertaken from below (A). In this space lie the autonomic nerves. If the dissection is carried out from above (B), the same fascia guides the dissector away from the nerves.

anus.[29] In our initial description of the perimuscular operation we noted that the external sphincter could be removed or left behind. In fact we have almost always retained it, and the term 'perimuscular dissection' relates to the smooth muscle of the upper rectum. A careful reading of the Parks' technique shows that the two operations are virtually identical.

Emergency proctocolectomy. Between 1970 and 1980 we strongly advocated the use of a single stage proctocolectomy in an emergency situation. At the time the results of emergency total colectomy were not good. Ritchie's survey of hospitals in the North-east Metropolitan Region, which comprise two teaching hospitals and 35 non-teaching units, recorded a mortality of 34% for emergency surgery during the period from 1955 to 1966.[32] Our own experience was just as disappointing. A number of authors had begun to record lower mortality figures for proctocolectomy than for total colectomy operations.[18, 34, 37] For example, Koudal and Kristensen from Denmark, during the ten-year period until 1974, recorded a 23% mortality.[24] They found that proctocolectomy carried a lower mortality than the subtotal or total colectomy operation. They suggested that the better results with proctocolectomy may have been an indication only of the severity of the colitis, the subtotal operation having been used on the

more severe cases. However, our own experience before using single stage proctocolectomy was that the inflamed rectum and its proximal mucous colostomy was a cause of some of the major infective complications. In particular, we encountered severe complications as a result of closing the rectal stump and attempting to bury it under the pelvic peritoneum. Severe pelvic infection occurred almost invariably and subsequent anastomosis of the ileum to the retained rectum was extremely difficult.

After adopting the operation as the standard emergency procedure in all cases, except for a few in whom the rectum was left behind for a specific reason, our mortality fell to less than 2% (1 death out of 56 consecutive operations). This compares favourably with other published results. Even St Mark's Hospital reports a mortality in their recent emergency operations of more than 5% when the rectum is retained,[17] and the specialized nature of their institution makes it unlikely that they operate on as many fulminating cases. Nevertheless, during the past few years more patients have the rectum retained in the hope that the new ileoanal operations will have better results than the ileorectal anastomosis.

It is particularly important when mobilizing an acutely dilated colon to avoid perforation and faecal contamination. This is best achieved by leaving the greater omentum attached to the colon and, as soon as a segment has been freed, wrapping the bowel in a crêpe bandage which supports the softened friable wall of the colon and prevents leakage occurring if the tissues tear during the subsequent dissection.

One of the problems associated with an emergency total colectomy lies in siting the distal colostomy. At first the colon was brought out to the lower end of the wound, the incision was closed and the exteriorized gut was then removed. The siting of an end colostomy in the wound was a major cause of infective complications and wound dehiscence. Currently, if the rectum and sigmoid are left in situ it is our practice, after mobilizing the bowel down to the sigmoid colon, to divide the ileum proximal to the ileocaecal bowel and to close both ends of bowel with purse-string sutures using an aseptic technique. Thereafter, after changing gown and gloves, an incision is made in the left iliac fossa (Figure 12.15) and the whole mobilized colon is brought out through the opening. The distal ileum is then exteriorized at the usual site for a Brooke ileostomy, and the abdomen closed. Only when the abdominal wall has been sutured, the skin approximated, and the wound

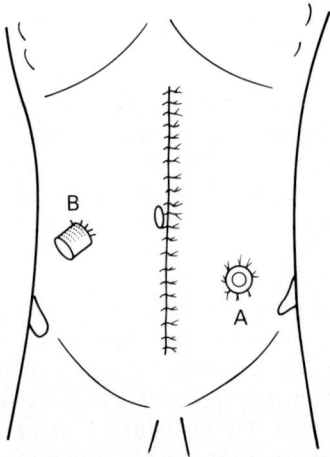

Fig. 12.15 A. The site of the mucous fistula in the left iliac fossa well away from the abdominal incision. B. The site of the Brooke ileostomy. The colon should not be divided until the abdomen has been closed.

sealed are the two stomas fashioned. There has been a much lower incidence of intraperitoneal and wound infection using this technique.

Ileorectal anastomosis

It is desirable to preserve the normal anatomical pathways of excretion if possible. The point of contention is whether this can be safely achieved in patients with ulcerative colitis by total colectomy and ileorectal anastomosis. The disease, although affecting the whole colonic mucosa, is often most severe in the rectum and lower sigmoid although it may spread proximally in time. However, in up to 10% of patients the rectum is spared and it is possible that in such cases the rectum can be retained. Some surgeons advocate the operation in nearly all patients and insist that even when the rectum is the site of severe disease, the majority of patients have an excellent result following colectomy and ileorectal anastomosis.[2] We, on the other hand, have not been able to achieve the same result in our patients. The percentage of patients who fail to do well after the operation has been assessed at between 10 and 50%.[13, 15] In spite of this, Alexander-Williams and Buchmann[1] have suggested that our attitude in advocating procto-colectomy is 'too rigid in the extreme' and that we are 'denying many patients the privilege of normal anal continence'.

The mortality of proctocolectomy is similar to that of the ileorectal operation. It is possible to carry out the latter in one stage and there are some surgeons who do this as a routine, but many units use a two stage technique unless the rectum is spared. A period of defunctioning

gives the inflammation in the rectum time to settle before undertaking ileorectal anastomosis. Aylett[2] has been the prime advocate of the single stage operation whatever the state of inflammation in the rectum. He was able to carry out the operation in 96% of 461 patients treated by colectomy. Most other surgeons have only been able to use the technique in 30–40% of colitics treated surgically. Many patients enjoy improved health after the operation since the majority of the disease has been removed. The advocates of the operation also insist that the majority of patients report normal excretory function, passing a few stools daily. The point of controversy revolves round the proportion of patients who have normal bowel actions. Our experience is that the majority of patients after ileorectal anastomosis have frequent bowel actions, some as many as fifteen stools daily, and many complain of attacks of diarrhoea. In 25% of the patients we have treated in this way, the function has been classified as poor and we have been forced to remove the rectum. Since we have not used the operation extensively the poor results may be the result of inexperience, but there has been a considerable swing away from the operation since the development of ileal pouch operations with ileoanal anastomosis.

In patients where the rectum has been retained, cancer is still a risk. Recent reports on the long-term follow-up of patients who have had an ileorectal operation have shown that the incidence of cancer does increase with time. In Aylett's series only 12 of 461 ileorectal patients developed a tumour,[3] but the long-term follow-up of his cases by Baker *et al.* has shown that the incidence has risen to about 6%.[4] Some patients have died of the tumour and the incidence appears to be rising. Other series have had an even higher incidence.[14] On balance therefore, we still believe that the case against colectomy and ileorectal anastomosis as a standard mode of treatment is strong. In addition, the lifestyle of patients with a permanent ileostomy is not as bad as depicted by the advocates of the ileorectal operation.

The continent ileostomy

In 1967 Professor Kock of Göteborg in Sweden began fashioning the distal ileum into a pouch with a distal valve to form a continent ileostomy.[22] In his operation about 50 cm of terminal ileum are used. The proximal 30 cm are sewn together to form a low-pressure pouch. The distal 15 cm are pushed backwards into the pouch as a retrograde intussusception, which acts as a valve when the pouch is full and prevents leakage onto the surface of the abdomen where the distal end of the ileum is formed into a flush stoma. The stoma is sited much lower on the abdominal wall than the classical Brooke spout ileostomy, because no bag is necessary if continence is complete. The cosmetic result is thus much better than with a spout. The pouch has to be emptied at least three times daily by introducing a plastic tube through the orifice.

Between 1967 and 1979, Kock's unit carried out the operation on 314 patients with inflammatory bowel disease.[23] In 142 patients the ileostomy was fashioned as part of a proctocolectomy operation; in 142 patients it was a secondary operation in which a spout ileostomy was converted to a continent one. A number of other centres have had a similar experience, and some centres such as the Mayo Clinic and the Mount Sinai Hospital of New York have used the operation on a large series of patients.

The operation is not without complications. The mortality in Kock's series is about 2%, although all the deaths occurred before 1975. Until that time the morbidity was substantial, more than 23% of the patients suffering an early postoperative complication. Since then there has been a dramatic fall in the rate of early complications. Between 1975 and 1979 their complication rate fell to 7%. The most important early complication is suture line leakage.

Late complications are also a problem. The most common is related to the formation of the valve. The nipple valve may slide and become incontinent, internal fistulas may form as a result of the sutures or clips which are used to anchor the retrograde intussusception, or eversion of the valve may occur. In the early operations revisional surgery was frequently necessary, but during the last few years a number of modifications have been introduced by different surgeons to prevent valve displacement. These include excision of mesenteric peritoneum and fat to reduce bulk, rotation with respect to each other of the two ileal segments which form the valve, scarification of the peritoneal surfaces of the two segments, multiple stapling of the valve in the pouch and the use of carefully placed sutures on the peritoneal surface of the segments.

Inadequate emptying of the pouch leads to mucosal inflammation similar to that seen with spout ileostomy strictures or with a stagnant loop syndrome. The syndrome of fever and diarrhoea has been called 'pouchitis'. In most cases it can be treated by complete emptying of the pouch more frequently than three times daily. Antibiotics may sometimes be useful. A few cases may need to have the reservoir removed and a spout ileostomy substituted.

The operation is contraindicated in Crohn's disease. Kock found that the rate of early complications was twice as high in 52 Crohn's cases as in those with ulcerative colitis, and that a high proportion of them had the pouch excised. Also a considerable length of ileum may be lost in a group of patients who are very likely to have recurrent disease in the small bowel at a later stage. It is sometimes difficult to make the diagnosis of Crohn's colitis before the whole colon has become available for examination by the histopathologists, so the continent ileostomy should not be used at the primary operation if there is any suspicion that the colitis is due to Crohn's disease.

In spite of these drawbacks, the operation can give excellent results in the right patient. Although the patient wears no ileostomy bags, the continent pouch needs careful handling. Gelernt *et al.*[12] at the Mount Sinai Hospital in New York have stressed that the best results are achieved in well-motivated individuals, and that a negative psychological approach is probably a contraindication to the operation.

Recently surgeons at the Mayo clinic, with considerable experience of the Kock operation, have introduced an indwelling ileostomy device in an attempt to make an ileostomy without a valve continent.[5] The apparatus is very like an inflatable endotracheal tube; the balloon not only obstructs the lumen but helps to maintain the position of the tube. Its simplicity is appealing.

Rectal mucosectomy and ileoanal anastomosis
The problem with a total colectomy and ileorectal anastomosis, as advocated by Aylett, is that the disease is not cured. In 1948, Sabiston and Ravitch[31] tried to overcome this deficiency with an ileoanal anastomosis after carrying out proctocolectomy. The result was severe diarrhoea and the operation was abandoned. Although experimental work by Valiente and Bacon[37] was undertaken to overcome the functional problem by constructing a double-loop pouch which was anastomosed to the anus, this too was associated with a high mortality among the experimental animals. In the late 1970s, Sir Alan Parks *et al.*[30] of St Mark's Hospital took up the idea again, encouraged by Kock's work on ileal pouches. They showed that the rectal mucosa played little part in anal continence. The operation overcomes the two main disadvantages of ileorectal anastomoses: all the mucosa affected by colitis is permanently removed, and

the ileal pouch prevents rapid emptying of the ileum which is the main cause of diarrhoea. Parks' technique consists of the formation of a continent pouch of the lower ileum, and after the rectal mucosa has been dissected off the rectal muscle, the placing of the pouch in the rectal muscle segment with anastomosis of ileal mucosa to the anal verge. Early results are encouraging but the formation of a continent pouch with a valve means that the patient has to catheterize the anus to empty his new rectum.

Other surgeons have tried various modifications of the technique. There is still considerable discussion in the literature about the best method of fashioning the pouch, how much rectal muscle should be retained, and how the operation should be staged. Some advocate a two stage technique with the operation covered by a loop ileostomy; others think that a three stage procedure is safer, with the ileoanal anastomosis being delayed until the patient has got over the primary resection. Goligher stresses that the anastomosis is not infrequently associated with considerable infection, and points out that it may take a considerable time before satisfactory bowel function and continence is achieved.[14] Some surgeons have used a technique in which a pouch is fashioned without a valve. Two types have been described, the 'S' type made by sewing together and opening three segments of ileum,[33] and the more simple 'J' pouch in which two loops are joined together and the distal ileum simply closed. In the latter type, the lowest part of the 'J' is opened and anastomosed to the anal skin from below. Kelly and his colleagues from the Mayo clinic have had the most experience of the operation, and reports are encouraging.[19] As with the Kock ileostomy, the operation is contraindicated in patients with Crohn's colitis.

CONCLUSION

The results of surgery have improved dramatically in the past decade, in the 1960s and early 1970s our main aim was to minimize mortality. The combination of carefully controlled medical treatment, early surgery and the new techniques of dissection dramatically lowered the morbidity and mortality. Most centres can now record a mortality for proctocolectomy of about 2%. Impotence is rarely a problem in the young. Bladder dysfunction should not occur. It is against these results that any new operation must be measured. Life with a permanent ileostomy, although obviously less satisfactory than after an operation in which the anus is retained,

still leaves the patient clear of his disease with an excellent long-term prospect of survival and a tolerable lifestyle. In our opinion total colectomy with an ileorectal anastomosis fails to satisfy the criteria of long-term safety.

The newer operations, such as the Kock's continent pouch and the ileoanal anastomosis, might lead to a further improvement of results, but it must be remembered that here are tens of thousands of patients with Brooke ileostomies living satisfactory lives throughout the world, many having done so for thirty years. There are only a few thousand patients in whom the Brooke stoma has been changed to a Kock's continent ileostomy, and fewer still who have had the operation as a primary procedure. Although up to 50% of the patients have excellent function, the majority have had the operation during the past five years. Complications of the pouch continue to occur and many patients will need a conversion from a Kock pouch to a Brooke spout. Finally, there is the exciting possibility that the new mucosal proctectomy operation with ileoanal anastomosis may eliminate the need for a stoma. However, only a few hundred patients have had the operation in the past few years. The new procedures have still to stand the test of time. The results of proctocolectomy, in spite of its inevitable permanent ileostomy, are the standard against which all new techniques must be measured.

REFERENCES

1   Alexander-Williams, J. & Buchmann, P. (1980) Criteria of assessment for suitability and results of ileorectal anastomosis. *Clinics in Gastroenterology*, **9,** 409.
2   Aylett, S. O. (1966) Three hundred cases of diffuse ulcerative colitis treated by total colectomy and ileorectal anastomosis. *British Medical Journal*, **i,** 1001–1005.
3   Aylett, S. O. (1971) Cancer and ulcerative colitis. *British Medical Journal*, **ii,** 203–205.
4   Baker, W. N. W., Glass, R. E., Ritchie, J. K., *et al.* (1978) Cancer of the rectum following colectomy and ileorectal anastomosis. *British Journal of Surgery*, **65,** 862.
5   Beahrs, O. H., Bess, M. A., Beart, R. W. Jr. *et al.* (1981) Indwelling ileostomy valve device. *American Journal of Surgery*, **141,** 111.
6   Brooke, B. N. (1952) Management of an ileostomy including its complications. *Lancet*, **ii,** 102–104.
7   Brown, J. Y. (1913) The value of complete physiological rest of the large bowel in the treatment of certain ulcerative and obstructive lesions of this organ. *Surgical Gynaecology & Obstetrics*, **16,** 610.
8   Burnham, W. R., Lennard-Jones, J. E. & Brooke, B. N. (1977) Sexual problems amongst married ileostomists. *Gut*, **18,** 673–677.
9   Daly, D. W. (1968) The outcome of surgery for ulcerative colitis. *Annals of the Royal College of Surgeons, England*, **42,** 38.
10   Edwards, F. C. & Truelove, S. C. (1963) The course and prognosis of ulcerative colitis. I–II. *Gut*, **4,** 299–315.

11 Edwards, F. C. & Truelove, S. C. (1964) The course and prognosis of ulcerative colitis. III–IV. *Gut*, **5**, 1–22.

12 Gelernt, I. M. (1983) Personal communication.

13 Goligher, J. C. (1980) *Surgery of the Anus, Rectum, and Colon*, 4th edn. London: Baillière Tindall.

14 Goligher, J. C. (1983) Procedures conserving continence in the surgical management of ulcerative colitis. *Surgical Clinics of North America*, **63**, 49–60.

15 Grundfest, S. F., Fazio, V. W., Weiss, R. A. *et al.* (1981) The risk of cancer following colectomy and ileorectal anastomosis for extensive mucosal ulcerative colitis. *Annals of Surgery*, **193**, 9–14.

16 Gruner, O. P. N., Naas, R., Fretheim, B. & Gjone, E. (1977) Marital status and sexual adjustment after colectomy. Results in 178 patients operated on for ulcerative colitis. *Scandinavian Journal of Gastroenterology*, **12**, 193–197.

17 Hawley, P. (1982) Personal communication during symposium on the treatment of acute colitis, Stockholm.

18 Jones, P. F., Munro, A. & Ewen, S. W. B. (1977) Colectomy and ileorectal anastomosis for colitis: report on a personal series, with critical review. *British Journal of Surgery*, **64**, 615–623.

19 Kelley, K. A. (1983) Personal communication.

20 Kennedy, H. J. (1981) *The Health of Ileostomists*. MD thesis, University of London.

21 Kennedy, H. J., Lee, E. C. G., Claridge, G. & Truelove, S. C. (1982) The health of subjects living with a permanent ileostomy. *Quarterly Journal Medicine*, **51**, 341–357.

22 Kock, N. G. (1969) Intra-abdominal 'reservoir' in patients with permanent ileostomy. *Archives of Surgery*, **99**, 223–231.

23 Kock, N. G. (1982) *Continent Ileostomy in Colo-Rectal Surgery* (Ed.) Heberer, G. & Denecke, H. pp. 57–60. Berlin: Springer-Verlag.

24 Koudahl, G. & Kristensen, M. (1976) Postoperative mortality and complications after colectomy for ulcerative colitis. *Scandinavian Journal of Gastroenterology*, (Supplement) **37**, 117–122.

25 Lee, E. C. G. & Dowling, B. L. (1972) Perimuscular excision of the rectum for Crohn's disease and ulcerative colitis. *British Journal of Surgery*, **59**, 29–32.

26 Lee, E. C. G. & Truelove, S. C. (1980) Proctocolectomy for ulcerative colitis. *World Journal of Surgery*, **4**, 195–201.

27 Lyons, A. S. (1952) An ileostomy club. *Journal of the American Medical Association*, **150**, 812.

28 Morson, B. C. & Pang, L. S. (1967) Rectal biopsy as an aid to cancer control in ulcerative colitis. *Gut*, **8**, 423–424.

29 Parks, A. G. & Lyttle, J. A. (1978) Intersphincteric excision of the rectum. *British Journal of Surgery*, **65**, 862.

30 Parks, A. G., & Nicholls, R. J. (1978) Proctocolectomy without ileostomy for ulcerative colitis. *British Medical Journal*, **ii**, 85–88.

31 Ravitch, M. M., & Sabiston, D. C. Jr (1947) Anal ileostomy with preservation of the sphincter: a proposed operation in patients requiring total colectomy for benign lesions. *Surgery Gynecology & Obstetrics*, **84**, 1095–1099.

32 Ritchie, J. K. (1971) Ileostomy and excisional surgery for chronic inflammatory disease of the colon: a survey of one hospital region. Part II. The health of ileostomists. *Gut*, **12**, 536–540.

33 Rotenberger, D. A., Vermeulen, F. D., Christenson, C. E. *et al.* (1983) Restorative proctocolectomy with ileal reservoir and ileoanal anastomosis. *American Journal of Surgery*, **145**, 82–88.

34 Scott, H. W., Wimbery, J. E., Shull, H. J. & Law, D. H. (1970) IV. Single-stage proctocolectomy for severe ulcerative colitis. *American Journal of Surgery*, **119**, 87–94.

35 Strauss, A. A. & Strauss, S. F. (1944) Surgical treatment of ulcerative colitis. *Surgical Clinics of North America*, **24**, 211.

36 Truelove, S. C. & Jewell, D. P. (1974) Intensive intravenous regimen for severe attacks of ulcerative colitis. *Lancet*, **i**, 1067–1070.

37 Valiente, M. A. & Bacon, H. E. (1955) Construction of pouch using 'pantaloon' technique for pull-through of ileum following total colectomy. *American Journal of Surgery*, **90**, 742–750.

38 Walker, F. C. (1969) *The Surgical Management of Ulcerative Colitis*. New York: Butterworth.

39 Watts, J. McK. de Dombal, F. T. & Goligher, J. C. (1966) Long-term complications and prognosis following major surgery for ulcerative colitis. *British Journal of Surgery*, **53**, 1014–1023.

CANCER IN ULCERATIVE COLITIS

There is conclusive evidence that patients with ulcerative colitis have a higher incidence of colorectal cancer than the general population.[8] The incidence of biliary tract cancer is also increased.[1, 36] The incidence of cancer in all other systems does not differ significantly from the general population.[34]

Colorectal cancer in ulcerative colitis

Although patients with ulcerative colitis have a greater risk of developing colorectal cancer than the general population, the actual numbers of cancers seen in any hospital series under long-term review is small. For example, only 23 colorectal cancers were identified in a series of 676 ulcerative colitis patients from the Queen Elizabeth Hospital and General Hospital, Birmingham over a 32-year review period (1944–1976).[34] These observed cancers, however, constituted an 11-fold risk compared with the relevant general population. Estimates of the apparent cancer risk vary widely from series to series. This probably reflects differing patient selection and methods of analysis in the series under review rather than any real differences in cancer incidence. It is therefore important to first consider the problems involved in the analysis of cancer incidence in hospital series which might help to explain the varying estimates of the cancer risk.

Problems involved in cancer incidence estimation in hospital series

The main problems affecting the apparent cancer risk in a hospital series of ulcerative colitis patients are selection bias at entry into the series, mode of analysis, completeness of follow-up, and status concerning cancer on entry into the series.

SELECTION BIAS AT ENTRY INTO SERIES

Because ulcerative colitis is a rare disorder requiring specialized medical and surgical care, a patient may be initially diagnosed at one hospital and then referred for more specialist attention to a second or even third centre, giving rise to selection, in particular, for severity of disease. These selection biases will affect the apparent incidence of cancer related to severe disease (extensive colitis).[39] One way of minimizing referral bias is to consider only patients diagnosed in a given time period from a defined area or at a defined point in their disease.

Defining the point of entry into the study

Examples of studies establishing entry cohorts. Studies which define how patients enter the series minimize referral bias and enable inter-series comparisons of the cancer incidence to be made. Edwards and Truelove[16] from the Oxford region identified a group of 250 ulcerative colitis patients (from a total series of 624 patients) who were seen at hospital in their first attack ('first attack cohort'). These patients also approximated to a 'regional' cohort in that they were drawn mainly from the Oxford area. This 'first attack' series included some patients who were to die in their first attack, some who would never have another attack and others who developed chronic disease. This eliminated the problem of patients referred late in the course of their disease; these represent a 'survivor' population. Selecting patients in their first attack does, however, select for severity of disease since those patients with milder disease may not be referred to hospital until later in the course of their disease.

Two reports from Scandinavia involve entry cohorts established by collecting all patients with ulcerative colitis diagnosed in a defined region during a defined time period. Bonnevie from Denmark reported all cases of ulcerative colitis diagnosed in Copenhagen County between 1960 and 1971.[4] Kewenter in Sweden reported all cases of extensive colitis diagnosed in the Göteborg region between 1951 and 1974, but gave no information about the total series from which these patients were selected.[24] In Kewenter's series patients were 'near' onset of the disease. In Bonnevie's study 70% of cases were diagnosed within two years of disease onset.

Nefzger and Acheson defined an entry cohort of all cases of ulcerative colitis occurring in males entering the US Army hospitals in 1944.[31] This series probably most nearly reflects the spectrum of disease (in males) occurring in the general population in that even the mildest cases of diarrhoea were admitted, investigated and followed up. However, they were not necessarily near onset of the disease and to some extent would therefore represent a 'survivor' population.

MODE OF ANALYSIS

There are certain problems in estimating the cancer risk in a disease such as ulcerative colitis which is of long duration – patients may be eliminated from the population at risk at any point due to death or surgery (e.g. panproctocolectomy), or lost to follow-up, whereas other patients may enter the series many years after onset of the disease. Early reports expressed the cancer risk as a crude percentage which did not take these factors into account. The recent use of statistical methods of analysis goes some way to correcting these anomalies.

COMPLETENESS OF FOLLOW-UP

It is important that follow-up is as complete as possible since it cannot be assumed that patients lost to follow-up will have a similar cancer incidence to that observed in the group as a whole. The results from series with more than 15% of patients lost to follow-up may be misleading.

STATUS CONCERNING CANCER RISK ON ENTRY TO SERIES

Patients with minimal symptoms may either remain undiagnosed or be treated by their own family practitioner since they are not ill enough to need hospital referral. Some of these patients late in the course of their disease may experience an exacerbation of symptoms initiating hospital referral where on their first visit a diagnosis of colorectal cancer and ulcerative colitis is made. These patients should not be included in the cancer incidence analysis. The cancer risk in these patients belongs to an unknown group of patients with ulcerative colitis in the general population. Patients should have been cancer free for at least one year of follow-up to be eligible for inclusion in any analysis of the cancer risk. Some analyses do not make this stipulation

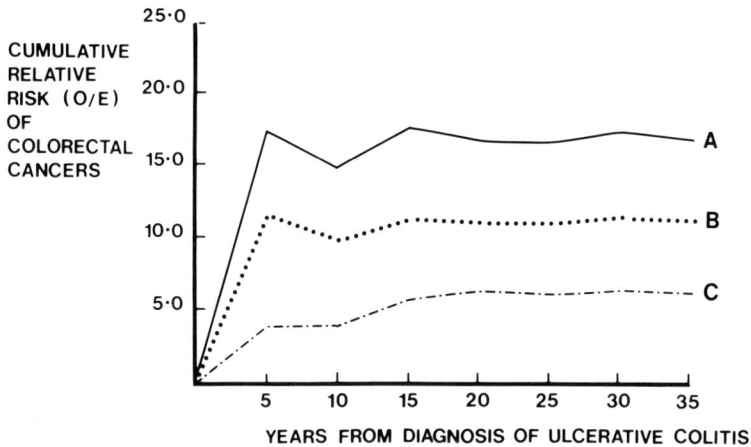

Fig. 12.16 Cumulative relative risk (observed number divided by expected number – O/E) of developing colorectal cancer with time in ulcerative colitis. A. All observed colorectal cancers (n = 35). B. Asymptomatic and interval colorectal cancers (n = 23). C. Interval colorectal cancers (n = 13).

and thus report high cancer incidence rates which do not reflect the real cancer incidence in the series under review.[17]

In a recent analysis from Birmingham, three different groups of cancer patients were defined.[34] Figure 12.16 shows the effect on the apparent cancer incidence in the series by inclusion or exclusion of these groups. Of the 35 colorectal cancers seen over the review period, 12 were referred with cancer on their first hospital visit and classified as 'referred' cancers, 12 were classified as 'asymptomatic' being identified on histopathological examination of the resected specimen following panproctocolectomy for symptomatic disease within the first year of hospital referral, and 13 cancers were diagnosed in the series after a year or more of follow-up. This third group of 'interval' cancers most nearly reflects the cancer incidence occurring in the series under review. The marked effect on the apparent cancer incidence of excluding 'referred' and 'asymptomatic' cancers can be readily appreciated (Figure 12.16).

Cancer incidence in reported series with defined entry cohorts

The results from series in which entry cohorts were defined are summarized in Table 12.9.

Cancer incidence in whole series
Table 12.9 shows a cancer incidence of around 1% at 10 years from onset of disease rising to between 3.5 and 4.5% between 10 and 20 years from onset of disease.[16, 31] Bonnevie did not observe any cancers in his series, presumably due to a surgical policy of elective panproctocolectomy for patients with extensive colitis 10 years from onset of symptoms. This illustrates how the surgical policy in a given hospital can affect the apparent cancer risk in the series.

Cancer incidence in extensive colitis
There are certain difficulties in selecting out a subgroup of patients as having 'extensive colitis' from a total ulcerative colitis series and then subjecting these patients to special analysis as though they were a clearly defined group. Up to a third of ulcerative colitis patients with disease initially confined to the left side of the colon or rectum will at some point in their disease progress to extensive colitis.[16, 45] As patients are not subject to regular barium enema examination or colonoscopy to determine the extent of their disease (these investigations being applied at irregular intervals during follow-up because of exacerbation of symptoms), there must at any one time be a 'hidden' number of patients with extensive colitis classified as having left-sided or distal disease. However, the cancer risk in most series is confined almost exclusively to those patients known to have extensive colitis. This 'hidden' group of extensive colitics classified as having left-sided disease is either not large enough to significantly increase the cancer incidence in left-sided disease or the cancer risk in patients who develop extensive colitis later in the course of their disease is less than in patients developing extensive colitis at or near the onset of their disease.

There is close agreement in the cumulative cancer incidence 20 years from onset of disease in the two series analysing an extensive colitis group separately. Nefzger and Acheson[31] report a cumulative cancer incidence of 13.2% at 17 years and Kewenter et al.[24] of 9.6% at 15 years, and 24.2% at 20 years. The cumulative cancer incidence of 34% at 25 years reported by Kewenter et al.[24] is commonly quoted but this figure has wide confidence limits since it is based on only 73 patient years at risk and two cancers (Table 12.9).

Table 12.9 Colorectal cancer risk in ulcerative colitis – actuarial analysis of series with defined cohorts.

Authors	Composition of series	Review period	Number of patients		Number of cancers			Number of cancers within 10 years of onset of disease		Cumulative cancer incidence		Additional information
			Whole series	Extensive colitis	Whole series	Extensive colitis	Left-sided colitis	Whole series	Extensive colitis	Whole series	Extensive colitis	
Nefzger & Acheson[31]	USA Mortality study, males. All cases of ulcerative colitis entering US Army Hospitals in 1944	1944–1960	525	68	17	NK	NK	4	NK	3.4%, 17 years	13.2%, 17 years	Extent of disease only ascertained in 411 of 525 patients at entry into series. Extensive colitis group drawn from 411 patients
Edwards & Truelove[16]	England Subgroup of whole ulcerative colitis series who were seen in their first attack. Majority of cases drawn from the Oxford region	1938–1962	250	114	4	NK	NK	NK	NK	0.5%, 3–7 years 1.6%, 7–14 years 4.5%, 15–20 years	NK	All four cancers developed in patients with severe or moderately severe first attack. No cancers observed in patients with mild first attack.
Bonnevie et al.[4]	Denmark Mortality study. All cases of ulcerative colitis diagnosed in Copenhagen County, 80% of cases diagnosed within 5 years of onset of disease	1960–1971	332	60	0	0	0	0	0	—	—	Surgical policy of elective panproctocolectomy in extensive colitis patients 10 years from onset of disease
Kewenter et al.[24]	Sweden All cases of extensive colitis diagnosed in Göteborg 'shortly' after diagnosis	1951–1975	NK	234	NK	15	NK	NK	1	NK	3%, 5 years 9.6%, 15 years 24.2%, 20 years	No information given concerning size of whole series from which extensive colitis group were drawn. No information concerning cancer incidence in whole series. Mean observation period short (8.5 years)

NK = Not known.

Actuarial analysis of cancer incidence in hospital series not assembling entry cohorts

The cumulative cancer incidence in series which have varying and unknown levels of referral bias, in particular towards severity of disease, is shown in Table 12.10. These studies, although not necessarily in agreement concerning cancer incidence, do provide useful data on certain aspects of cancer in ulcerative colitis, such as its relation to age at onset, duration and extent of disease. Three factors have a particular bearing on the cancer incidence:

1 Extensive colitis. The cancers occur predominantly in this group of patients.
2 Duration of disease. Very few cancers are observed within the first ten years from onset of disease. The cumulative cancer incidence in the extensive colitis group rises sharply ten years from onset of disease.
3 Age at onset of disease. In an analysis of childhood-onset ulcerative colitis patients, the cumulative cancer risk was 50% at 30 years from the onset of the disease[13] and other series have convincingly shown that early onset of disease increases the cancer risk.[16, 28, 31, 34]

The main determinant of the cancer risk is, however, extensive colitis. Duration of disease and age at onset of disease must be subsidiary factors as they do not appear to increase the cancer risk in patients with left-sided colitis.

Cancer incidence in ileorectal anastomosis

The cancer incidence in two large series of patients with ileorectal anastomosis, carried out predominantly for extensive colitis, is shown in Table 12.11. Baker, Glass and Aylett[2] showed a cumulative cancer incidence of 9% 25 years from onset of disease in close agreement with the results of Grundfest *et al.*[19] who reported a cumulative cancer incidence of 12.9% 25 years from onset of disease. No cancers occurred in either series in the first 10 years from onset of disease. The retained rectum, therefore, in patients with extensive colitis is at increased risk for developing cancer but this risk is less than in patients with extensive colitis and an intact colon where the cumulative cancer risk is between 20 and 30% 20 years from onset of disease (Tables 12.9 and 12.10).

Cancer in left-sided colitis

No series reported has yet shown convincing evidence of an increased cancer incidence in patients with left-sided colitis when compared with the general population. McDougall[28] observed one colorectal cancer in his left-sided colitis group where the expected number of cancers in the general population for this group was 0.95. Greenstein and his colleagues[17] reported a late increase in the cancer risk in patients with left-sided colitis above the general population, but their results are difficult to interpret, since nearly half the patients with colorectal cancer in their analysis were referred on their first visit to the unit with late cancer and therefore do not reflect the real cancer risk in the series.

Distribution of cancer in ulcerative colitis

Langman[25] assembled data on colorectal cancer distribution in colitic and non-colitic patients (Figure 12.17). Colitic cancers are more evenly distributed around the colon than non-colitic, which occur predominantly in the sigmoid colon and rectum. The different distribution of ulcerative colitis cancers might simply be a reflection of a different distribution of cancers occurring in a younger age group. Colorectal cancers in the general population occurring below the age of 40 years, however, seem to have a similar distribution to colorectal cancer occurring later in life,[6] making this explanation unlikely. In clinical practice less colitic cancers will be within the reach of the sigmoidoscope (47.4%) when compared to the general population (76.1%).

Age at diagnosis of cancer in ulcerative colitis

The average age at diagnosis of cancer complicating ulcerative colitis is younger than in the general population. Ritchie, Hawley and Lennard-Jones[35] analysed a large series of 67 colorectal cancers in ulcerative colitis patients from St Mark's Hospital, London. The average age at diagnosis of cancer was 49 years compared with 63 years in 4817 non-colitic colorectal cancers seen over the same review period. This early age at diagnosis of cancer in ulcerative colitis patients has been confirmed by many workers.[21, 26, 41, 44] However, as ulcerative colitis is predominantly a disease of young people (the majority of patients in any hospital series will be below the age of 50 years), it is not surprising that the cancers observed are also in young people. All that can be said is that more cancers are occurring at a younger age than would be expected.

Table 12.10 Colorectal cancer risk in ulcerative colitis: actuarial analyses of series not assembling entry cohorts (unknown referral bias).

Authors	Hospital series	Review period	Number of patients		Number of cancers			Number of cancers within 10 years of onset of disease		Cumulative cancer incidence		Additional information
			Whole series	Extensive colitis	Whole series	Extensive colitis	Left-sided colitis	Whole series	Extensive colitis	Whole series	Extensive colitis	
de Dombal et al.[12]	General Infirmary, Leeds	1952–1963	428	210	8	8	0	1	1	0.1%, 0–10 years 1.4%, 10–19 years 2.9%, >20 years	5%, 10 years 21%, 20 years 41.8%, 25 years	5% yearly increment in cancer risk for patients with ulcerative colitis of more than 20 years standing
McDougall[28]	Gordon Hospital, London	1947–1963	637	196	15	14	1	NK	NK	O = 15 E = 1.47 O/E = 10.2	O = 9 E = 0.31 O/E = 30	Patients entered into the analysis contributed years at risk from date first seen at hospital and not onset of disease. Cancer risk in left-sided colitis: O = 1, E = 0.95
Devroede et al.[13]	Mayo Clinic, USA. Childhood onset series mortality study	1919–1965	396	303	52	NK	NK	NK	NK	3%, 10 years 23%, 20 years 43%, 25 years	3%, 10 years 30%, 20 years 50%, 30 years	20% of patients lost to follow-up. Series selected for severity of disease, 75% of patients had extensive colitis
Lennard-Jones et al.[27]	St Mark's, London. Prospective study of extensive colitic patients	1966–1976	NK	229	NK	5	NK	NK	0	NK	Patients years at risk: 1/200, 12–20 years 1/60, 20–30 years	Severe epithelial dysplasia found in 13 patients. No cancer found in follow-up period without dysplasia
Prior et al.[34]	Queen Elizabeth and General Hospitals, Birmingham	1944–1976	676	462	35	35	0	1	1	8%, 25 years 20%, 30 years	NK	Series selected for severity of disease, 68% of the series had extensive colitis

O = Observed numbers of colorectal cancers; E = Expected numbers of colorectal cancers; NK = Not known.

Table 12.11 Rectal cancer incidence in ileorectal anastomosis.

| Authors | Hospital | Review period | Number of patients | | Number of rectal cancers | | | Number of cancers within 10 years of onset of disease | Cumulative cancer incidence | Duke's classification of cancers at diagnosis | | | Distant metastases |
			Whole series	Extensive colitis	Whole series	Extensive colitis	Left-sided colitis			A	B	C	
Baker et al.[2]	Gordon Hospital, London	1952–1976	374	362	22	21	1	0	0%, 10 years 6%, 20 years 9%, 25 years 15%, 30 years	2	4	12	4
Grundfest et al.[19]	Cleveland Clinic, USA	1957–1977	NK	89	NK	4	NK	0	0%, 10 years 5%, 20 years 12.9%, 25 years	2	0	2	—

NK = Not known.

933

Survival from cancer in ulcerative colitis

Early reports suggested that ulcerative colitis patients developing colorectal cancer had a poor prognosis, considerably worse than the prognosis of patients with colorectal cancer in the general population.[40, 41, 42]

More recently, analyses of survival (some series using the method of matched controls) suggest that the five-year survival of colorectal cancer patients in ulcerative colitis is not significantly different from the general population.[21, 22, 36, 44] Results of these studies are summarized in Table 12.12, the crude five-year survival in both colitic and non-colitic patients ranging from 33 to 55%.

Multiple cancers and differentiation of cancers

All series show a higher incidence of multiple cancers in ulcerative colitis than the control population and cancers in ulcerative colitis tended to be less well differentiated. This higher proportion of less well differentiated cancers did not appear to affect the virulence of the cancers in the colitic group in that the five-year survival of Dukes A classification cancers (i.e. cancers in which survival was long enough for comparisons to be made) was independent of the degree of differentiation, and similar in both groups.

A large proportion of the colitic patients presented with late cancer (Table 12.12). This must

Table 12.12 Survival of patients developing colorectal cancer complicating ulcerative colitis (UC).

Authors	Hospital series	Review period	Control group	Number of cancers	Number of multiple cancers	Number of patients with late cancer on referral	Number of cancers identified on histology of resected specimen for symptomatic colitis
Gyde *et al.*[20]	Queen Elizabeth and General Hospitals, Birmingham. Series of 676 UC patients	1944–1976	Colorectal cancers of the same median age as colitic cancers from West Midlands region	35	4 (11%)	12 (34%)	12
Van Heerden & Beart[44]	Mayo Clinic, USA. Series of 726 patients undergoing surgery for UC	1961–1975	Non-colitic cancers matched for age, sex, Dukes classification and degree of differentiation (Broder's Grade)	70	16 (23%)	17 (24%)	14
Ritchie *et al.*[35]	St Mark's, London. Total series not stated	1947–1980	4817 non-colitic cancers diagnosed at St Mark's over review period	67	15 (26%) (Based on operable cancers, *n* = 57)	19 (28%)	NK
Hughes *et al.*[21]	University of Chicago Hospitals and Clinics, USA. Series of 1142 UC patients diagnosed in review period	1958–1976	Non-colitic cancers matched for age, sex, site and stage	29	4 (14%)	NK	NK
Lavery *et al.*[26]	Cleveland Clinic, USA. Total series not stated	1950–1979	Survival of UC cancers compared with group of non-colitic cancers diagnosed at Cleveland Clinic, 1950–1964	68 (+11 Carcinoma in situ)	3 (4%)	28 (41%)	19 *Duke's classification* A B C 5 6 2 *Carcinoma in situ* 6
Hulten *et al.*[22]	Various Swedish hospitals over 10 year review period	10 years	Non-colitic cancers seen at Sahlgrens Hospital, Göteborg over review period, *n* = 22	25	NK	NK	NK

$^a P < 0.05$. $^b P < 0.01$. NK = Not known.

be due in part to the symptoms of cancer closely mimicking the symptoms of ulcerative colitis which thus do not cause alarm and prompt early investigation. Another factor may be that only 46% of cancers are within reach of the sigmoidoscope as opposed to 76% in the general population, making diagnosis more difficult (Figure 12.17). There are also patients with apparently mild disease not requiring hospital referral until their first visit when they present with late cancer complicating ulcerative colitis. Finally there are some high-risk patients lost to follow-up who only return after developing symptomatic cancer.

Management of patients at high risk of developing cancer

The evidence so far indicates that a small subgroup of patients can be identified who are at high risk for developing cancer, i.e., patients with extensive colitis of more than ten years' duration particularly with early onset of disease. How should these patients be managed? Some clinicians favour elective panproctocolectomy after ten years from onset.[4, 12, 24, 28] This not only removes the cancer risk but restores the patient to good health, free from colitis with minimal follow-up requirements. Certain factors

Mean duration of symptoms to diagnosis of cancer	Mean 5-year survival		Duke's classification at diagnosis of cancer in patients where complete information available	Comparison of Duke's classification and differentiation with controls
	Cases	Controls		
21 years	33.5%	33%	*Duke's classification* A B C Distant metastases 4 5 3 7	NK
17.1 years (operable cases only)	41.7%	47%	*Duke's classification* 6 22 25 17 *Broders Grade* 1 2 3 4 9 27 9 15	NK

10 years in all but two cases	65.1% (in 57 operable cases)	47% rectal cancers, 53% colonic cancers	*Duke's classification*
			A B C
			11 14 17 (n = 42)
			Differentiation
			Well Moderate Poor
			11 17 14
				% incidence of colorectal cancer in patients with simple operable cancers (n = 42) and non-colitic cancers (n = 4472)
				Duke's classification
				        A B C
				With colitis 26^a 33 41
				Without colitis 15 39 46
				Histological grade
				      Low Average High
				With colitis 26 41 33^b
				Without colitis 25 58 17

19.6 years	55.1%	46.9%	NK	NK
17 years	41%	NK	*Duke's classification* A B C Distant metastases 13 15 12 28	% 5-year survival *Duke's classification* A B C With colitis 94 59 57 Without colitis 99 85 67
NK	12%	25%	Surgical specimens not suitable for Duke's staging in UC cancers	*Differentiation* High grade Low grade With colitis 20 5 Without colitis 15 7

mitigate against surgical intervention. Elective surgery carries a small mortality.[37, 38] It leaves often young patients with a permanent stoma and possible further morbidity; the pelvic nerves may on occasion be damaged at operation with ensuing impotence in males. Colectomy and ileorectal anastomosis may be feasible in some patients but the cancer risk persists in the retained rectum (Table 12.11), and the asymptomatic patient with an ileorectal anastomosis may be lost to follow-up, returning only with symptomatic rectal cancer.[2]

CANCER SURVEILLANCE

Although precancerous polypoid lesions were described in ulcerative colitis as early as 1959,[11] the possibility of using precancer (severe epithelial dysplasia) as a marker to define patients at particularly high risk for colorectal cancer was not actively pursued until Morson and Pang[29] produced evidence that dysplasia in rectal biopsies was a good indicator of cancer at some other site in the colon or rectum.

Histopathologists define dysplasia in terms of abnormalities in cell cytology and the architecture of the colorectal mucosa. These dysplastic changes are not uniquely associated with colorectal cancer in ulcerative colitis but are similar to precancerous changes found in other organs, e.g. cervix, bladder and skin.[29] Dysplasia does not consist of one simple change. The pathologist must assess cytological changes in terms of the size, shape and staining properties of the epithelial cell nuclei, changes in proliferation in terms of mitoses (some of which may show abnormal features) in the crypts, and abnormal epithelial cell architecture within the crypts involving adenomatous or villous changes. Even an experienced histopathologist may find dysplastic change difficult to assess in the presence of active inflammation giving rise to reactive hyperplasia. Correct orientation of biopsies is important when interpreting dysplasia.

Assessment of dysplasia is by its nature subjective and even experts may disagree when biopsies are examined 'blind'.[9, 47] Dysplasia has been classified as mild, moderate and severe, with some variation between centres in criteria for defining these groups. International agreement is at present being attempted to clarify and simplify the terminology with a proposal to grade dysplasia more simply as 'high' or 'low' grade.[7, 47]

The clinician needs to know whether dysplasia in rectal biopsies is an effective marker for cancer in the rectum or for cancer elsewhere in the colon, how much additional benefit for cancer diagnosis accrues by including colonoscopy in the surveillance programme and what proportion of cancers may be overlooked even when colonoscopic and rectal biopsies are used routinely.

Dysplasia in the diagnosis of cancer
Retrospective and a few prospective studies have considered the relationship of cancer diagnosis to dysplasia.

Retrospective studies comprise:
1 Colectomy specimens from symptomatic ulcerative colitis patients.
2 Colectomy specimens from patients with colorectal cancer.
3 Rectal biopsy studies and evaluation of the subsequent colectomy specimen undertaken for either colorectal cancer or symptomatic colitis.
4 Rectal biopsies taken to determine the presence of dysplasia in medically treated patients with colitis.

Prospective studies include the incidence of dysplasia in rectal biopsy with the results of subsequent surgery in terms of dysplasia and cancer. The data can be very confusing because there are many reports from different centres where a variety of different types of specimen have been taken from patients with variable duration and extent of disease. There have been several excellent recent reviews.[7, 9, 15, 47]

Retrospective study data. In a summary of eleven recent reports,[15] 108 cancers were analysed from among 453 colectomy specimens. In 95 of the 108 (88%) specimens where cancer was found, dysplastic changes were also present. A combination of colonoscopic and rectal biopsy would therefore have a good chance of making the diagnosis in nearly 90% of the cancers. Dysplasia in the rectum was found in only 33 of the 60 specimens, where enough detail was given to determine rectal dysplasia (66%). This suggests that if rectal biopsy alone were used, 44% of the cancers would have been missed.

Among the 69 reports where enough detail was given, nine cancers occurred less than ten years from the onset of colitis. There may be a need for some form of cancer surveillance, perhaps sigmoidoscopy or rectal biopsy, in patients with disease of less than ten years' duration.

Table 12.13 Incidence of dysplasia in rectal biopsy and subsequent surgery in chronic ulcerative colitis. (Adapted from Butt, Lennard-Jones and Ritchie.[8])

Study	n	High grade dysplasia found in rectum and subsequent surgery	Cancer found in specimen	Cancer found: no high grade rectal dysplasia
Myrvold et al.[30]	47	7	5	0
[a] Yardley & Keren[46]	204	3	5	2
Lennard-Jones et al.[27]	229	12	5	2
Nugent et al.[32]	24	5	2	0
[b] Blackstone et al.[3]	112	0	7	7

[a] Retrospective study.
[b] Colonoscopic biopsy of rectal mucosa only.

Prospective study data. Butt et al.[8] summarized recent data concerning studies of dysplasia in rectal biopsies with subsequent surgery and his results are given in Table 12.13. The data include one retrospective study.[46] In prospective studies the true state of the colon regarding cancer can only be established in patients who subsequently are treated by colectomy. Patients with an intact colon may also be harbouring cancer with no evidence of dysplasia and will not be diagnosed until the cancer becomes symptomatic. The accuracy of the data in prospective studies will improve with time and too much reliance should not be placed on early reports with short follow-up.

Butt, Lennard-Jones and Ritchie[8] estimated that from the available data, 73–87% of the patients with colonic cancer will have dysplasia on rectal biopsy.

Rectal biopsy and colonoscopy – where to biopsy and how often
Most studies show that the extent of dysplasia in association with colon cancer can be very variable – involving most of the colonic mucosa, patchily distributed throughout the colon or even confined to the region of invasive cancer. Occasionally no dysplasia at all is found in association with the cancer. It may be that the latter are examples of colon cancer arising de novo rather than as a complication of ulcerative colitis.

Because of the focal nature of dysplasia, multiple biopsies should be taken preferably from areas where there is no active inflammation. The biopsy sites should be charted so that if dysplasia is found a repeat biopsy can be taken from around the same site. It is well known that dysplasia can occur in flat mucosa with no apparent macroscopic abnormality[29] and random biopsies are therefore necessary. However, Blackstone et al.[3] showed a high cancer incidence in raised lesions which showed dysplasia only on the surface but were subsequently at colectomy found to have frankly invasive carcinoma underlying the dysplasia. Table 12.14 summarizes the data of Butt and Morson,[7] and shows the frequency of the diagnosis of cancer in flat mucosa compared to raised lesions. Cancers diagnosed with dysplasia in flat mucosa as a marker are earlier lesions in terms of the Dukes classification than the cancers diagnosed from dysplasia in raised lesions. Blackstone et al.[3] found that barium enema was helpful in defining raised areas for biopsy on colonoscopy, 7 out of 12 raised lesions found at colonoscopy were also visible on barium enema examinations.

Rectal biopsy and colonoscopy – practical considerations
Rectal biopsy is a simple procedure both for the patient and clinician. Routine regular sigmoidoscopy with multiple biopsies should identify

Table 12.14 Cases detected with macroscopic change associated with dysplasia or cancer (MADC) compared to cases detected with severe dysplasia in flat mucosa in chronic ulcerative colitis. (Adapted from Butt and Morson.[7])

Study	Cases	Cancer cases	MADC	Cancer	Severe dysplasia in flat mucosa	Cancer
Morson and Pang[29]	9	5	2	1	7	4
Yardley et al.[46]	9	7	5	4	3	2
Blackstone et al.[3]	13	8[a]	12	7	1	0

[a] One case without MADC or severe dysplasia in flat mucosa.

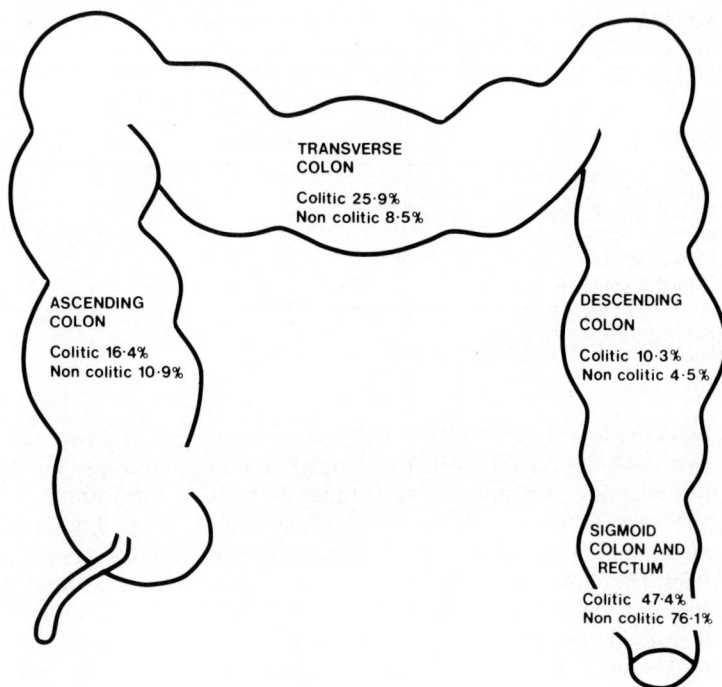

Fig. 12.17 Distribution of colorectal cancers in ulcerative colitis compared to the general population. Colitic cancers, n = 379; non-colitic cancers, n = 6277.

more than a third of the cancers in ulcerative colitis, as at least 40% of colorectal cancers in ulcerative colitis occur within reach of the sigmoidoscope (Figure 12.17).

Colonoscopy may be a time-consuming and unpleasant procedure for the patient and not all centres can offer this service.

Data produced by the histopathologists concerning rectal biopsy and colonoscopy in the diagnosis of cancer is therefore of great clinical interest.

Other methods of cancer surveillance

Carcinoembryonic antigen. Circulating CEA levels have not proved useful in detecting early cancer in ulcerative colitis. Levels are raised in 10% of cases with ulcerative colitis and tend to increase in most patients during active inflammation.[5, 14]

Tissue CEA levels may be of some interest for the future.[18, 23]

Summary

Dysplasia in a rectal biopsy alone should be identified in approximately 60–70% of patients whether the cancer is in the colon or rectum. Addition of colonoscopic biopsies and barium enema will identify approximately 85% of patients with colorectal cancer.

However, some of these cancers particularly in raised lesions will not be diagnosed at an early stage[3, 32] (Table 12.15). Ideally the colon should be removed at the stage of dysplasia, prior to the development of invasive carcinoma. Even with diagnosis of cancer at the Dukes A stage, there will be reccurrence in some patients.

On balance it seems reasonable to discuss the cancer risk with patients putting the case for

Table 12.15 Prospective studies of cancer of the colon in colectomy specimens from patients with chronic ulcerative colitis when either a biopsy exhibiting severe dysplasia in flat mucosa or macroscopic change associated with dysplasia or cancer (MADC) was an important criterion for colectomy. (Adapted from Butt and Morson.[7])

| Study | Total cases | Mode | Cancer cases | Duke's classification | | |
				A	B	C
Lennard-Jones et al.[27]	7	Severe dysplasia	4	4	0	0
Nugent et al.[32]	5	Severe dysplasia	1	0	0	1
Blackstone et al.[3]	12	MADC	7	1	4	2[a]

[a] One case had one Duke's B and two Duke's C cancers in the same patient.

surgery and surveillance. Other considerations such as the patient's age, the severity of colitis symptoms, his reaction to the possibility of a stoma and his marital status will all affect the decision.

However, in patients who have had extensive colitis for 20–25 years particularly those with early onset of disease even in the absence of dysplasia on biopsies, the risk of the patient already having cancer may approach 40%. The clinician's advice should at this point be strongly in favour of panproctocolectomy.

Bile duct cancer in ulcerative colitis

Bile duct cancer is a rare complication of ulcerative colitis.[1, 10, 36] It usually occurs in patients with a long history of extensive colitis. Panproctocolectomy does not prevent this complication which may arise years after surgery and it can occur in patients with previously normal liver function. Ritchie *et al.*[36] reported 15 cases of biliary tract carcinoma complicating ulcerative colitis, only 6 of whom had associated liver disease. Akwari *et al.*[1] reported 13 cases of bile duct carcinoma associated with ulcerative colitis. The presenting symptoms were anorexia, followed by painless jaundice or a sudden deterioration in patients with established liver disease. The mean duration of colitis from onset of symptoms to the diagnosis of bile duct cancer was 19 years, and in 10 patients the carcinoma had spread beyond the bile ducts at the time of diagnosis.[1] They also reviewed the literature and found that in more than 25% of the patients the diagnosis of bile duct cancer was only made at autopsy, and the average survival from onset of symptoms to carcinoma was less than one year. Converse *et al.* (1971), in a report of three cases of bile duct carcinoma complicating ulcerative colitis, reviewed the literature and found that the average age of onset of bile duct carcinoma in ulcerative colitis was 39.8 years (with a range of 20–64 years),[10] compared with the average age at onset of bile duct carcinoma in the general population of 60–70 years.[33, 44] In contrast to the general population, ulcerative colitis patients with bile duct carcinoma seldom have gallstones. This suggests that the cancer in the two groups may have a different aetiology.[1, 10, 36] In a recent report from Birmingham of 676 ulcerative colitis patients under long-term review (1944–1976), 7 liver and biliary tract cancers were observed (1 hepatoma, 6 biliary tract cancers). The expected number was 0.32, giving a 21.9-fold relative risk for liver and bile duct carcinoma above the general population.[34]

REFERENCES

1 Akwari, O., Van Heerden, J., Foulk, W. & Baggenstoss, A. (1975) Cancer of the bile ducts associated with ulcerative colitis. *Annals of Surgery*, 181, 303–309.
2 Baker, W., Glass, R., Ritchie, J. & Aylett, S. (1978) Cancer of the rectum following colectomy and ileorectal anastomosis for ulcerative colitis. *British Journal of Surgery*, 65, 862–868.
3 Blackstone, M., Riddell, R., Rogers, G. & Levin, B. (1981) Dysplasia-associated lesion or mass (DALM) detected by colonoscopy in long-standing ulcerative colitis: an indication for colectomy. *Gastroenterology*, 80, 366–374.
4 Bonnevie, O., Binder, V., Anthonisen, P. & Riis, P. (1974) The prognosis of ulcerative colitis. *Scandinavian Journal of Gastroenterology*, 9, 81–91.
5 Booth, S. N., King, J. P., Lennard-Jones, C. & Dykes, P. W. (1974) The significance of elevation of CEA levels in inflammatory bowel disease of the intestine. *Scandinavian Journal of Gastroenterology*, 9, 651–656.
6 Bulow, S. (1980) Colorectal cancer in patients less than 40 years of age in Denmark 1943–1967. *Diseases of Colon and Rectum*, 23, 327–336.
7 Butt, J. & Morson, B. (1981) Dysplasia and cancer in inflammatory bowel disease (Editorial). *Gastroenterology*, 80, 865–868.
8 Butt, J. H., Lennard-Jones, J. E. & Ritchie, J. K. (1980) A practical approach to the risk of cancer in inflammatory bowel disease. *Medical Clinics of North America*, 64, 1203–1220.
9 Butt, J. H., Price, A. & Williams, C. B. (1983) Dysplasia and cancer in ulcerative colitis. In *Inflammatory Bowel Diseases* (Ed.) Allan, R. N., Keighley, M. R. B., Alexander-Williams, J. & Hawkins, C. F. pp. 140–153. Edinburgh: Churchill Livingstone.
10 Converse, C., Reagan, J. & Decosse, J. (1971) Ulcerative colitis and carcinoma of the bile ducts. *American Journal of Surgery*, 121, 39–45.
11 Dawson, I. M. P. & Pryse Davies, J. (1959) The development of carcinoma of the large intestine in ulcerative colitis. *British Journal of Surgery*, 47, 113–128.
12 de Dombal, F., Watts, J., Watkinson, G. & Goligher, J. (1966) Local complications of ulcerative colitis: stricture, pseudopolyposis and carcinoma of the colon and rectum. *British Medical Journal*, i, 1442–1447.
13 Devroede, G., Taylor, W., Sauer, W. *et al.* (1971) Cancer risk and life expectancy of children with ulcerative colitis. *New England Journal of Medicine*, 285, 17–21.
14 Dilawari, J. B., Lennard-Jones, J. C. & Dykes, P. W. (1974) Serum CEA in clinical disorders. *Gut*, 14, 828.
15 Dobbins, W. O. (1977) Current status of the pre-cancer lesion in ulcerative colitis. *Gastroenterology*, 73, 1431–1433.
16 Edwards, F. C. & Truelove, S. C. (1964) The course and prognosis of ulcerative colitis. Part I, III, IV. Carcinoma of the colon. *Gut*, 4, 299–315.
17 Greenstein, A. J., Sachar, D. B., Smith, H. *et al.* (1979) Cancer risk in universal and left sided ulcerative colitis: factors determining risk. *Gastroenterology*, 77, 290–294.
18 Greenstein, A. J., Panvelliwalla, D. K., Katz, L. B. & Heimann, T. M. (1982) Tissue CEA. Dysplasia and disease duration in colonic inflammatory bowel diseases. *American Journal of Gastroenterology*, 77, 212–215.
19 Grundfest, S. F., Fazio, V., Weiss, R. *et al.* (1981) The cancer risk following colectomy and ileorectal anastomosis for extensive mucosal ulcerative colitis. *Annals of Surgery*, 193, 9–14.

20 Gyde, S. N., Prior, P., Thompson, H. *et al.* (1983) Survival of patients with colorectal cancer complicating ulcerative colitis. *Gut*, in press.

21 Hughes, R., Hall, T., Block, G. *et al.* (1978) The prognosis of carcinoma of the colon and rectum complicating ulcerative colitis. *Surgery, Gynaecology and Obstetrics*, **146**, 46–48.

22 Hulten, L., Kewenter, J., Ahren, C. & Ojewkog, B. (1979) Clinical and morphological characteristics of colitis carcinoma and colorectal carcinoma in young people. *Scandinavian Journal of Gastroenterology*, **14**, 673–678.

23 Isaacson, P. (1976) Tissue demonstration of CEA in ulcerative colitis. *Gut*, **17**, 561–567.

24 Kewenter, J., Ahlman, H. & Hulten. L. (1978) Cancer risk in extensive colitis. *Annals of Surgery*, **188**, 824–827.

25 Langman, M. J. (1966) Epidemiology of cancer of the large intestine. *Proceedings of the Royal Society of Medicine*, **59**, 132–134.

26 Lavery, I., Chiulli, R., Jagelman, D. *et al.* (1982) Survival with carcinoma arising in mucosal ulcerative colitis. *Annals of Surgery*, **195**, 508–512.

27 Lennard-Jones, J., Morson, B., Ritchie, J. *et al.* (1977) Cancer in colitis: assessment of the individual risk by clinical and histological criteria. *Gastroenterology*, **73**, 1280–1289.

28 McDougall, I. (1964) The cancer risk in ulcerative colitis. *Lancet*, **ii**, 655–659.

29 Morson, B. & Pang, L. (1967) Rectal biopsy as an aid to cancer control in ulcerative colitis. *Gut*, **8**, 423–434.

30 Myrvold, H. E., Kock, N. G. & Ahren, C. (1974) Rectal biopsy and pre-cancer in ulcerative colitis. *Gut*, **15**, 301–304.

31 Nefzger, M. & Acheson, E. (1963) Ulcerative colitis in the United States Army in 1944. Follow-up with particular reference to mortality in cases and controls. *Gut*, **4**, 183–192.

32 Nugent, F., Haggitt, R., Colcher, H. & Kutteruf, G. (1979) Malignant potential of chronic ulcerative colitis. *Gastroenterology*, **76**, 1–5.

33 Permen, L. E. & McCollum, E. B. (1963) Primary carcinoma of the extra hepatic biliary ducts. *Henry Ford Hospital Medical Bulletin*, **11**, 167.

34 Prior, P., Gyde, S. N., Macartney, J. C. *et al.* (1982) Cancer morbidity in ulcerative colitis. *Gut*, **23**, 490–497.

35 Ritchie, J., Hawley, P. & Lennard-Jones, J. (1981) Prognosis of carcinoma in ulcerative colitis. *Gut*, **22**, 752–755.

36 Ritchie, J., Allan, R. N., Macartney, J. *et al.* (1974) Biliary tract carcinoma associated with ulcerative colitis. *Quarterly Journal of Medicine*, **170**, 263–279.

37 Ritchie, J. K. (1971) Ileostomy and excisional surgery for chronic inflammatory disease of the colon: a survey of one hospital region. Part I. Results and complications of surgery. Part II. Health of the ileostomists. *Gut*, **12**, 528–540.

38 Ritchie, J. K. (1972) Ileostomy and excisional surgery: 15 years experience at St Mark's Hospital. *British Journal of Surgery*, **59**, 345–351.

39 Sackett, D. & Whelan, G. (1980) Cancer risk in ulcerative colitis. Scientific requirements for the study of prognosis (editorial). *Gastroenterology*, **78**, 1632–1635.

40 Shands, W. C., Dockerty, M. B. & Bargen, J. A. (1952) Adenocarcinoma of the large intestine associated with chronic ulcerative colitis. Clinical and pathological features of 73 cases. *Surgery, Gynaecology and Obstetrics*, **94**, 302–310.

41 Slaney, G. & Brooke, B. N. (1959) Cancer in ulcerative colitis. *Lancet*, **ii**, 694–698.

42 Sloan, W. P. Jr., Bargen, J. A. & Gage, R. P. (1950) Life histories of patients with chronic ulcerative colitis – a review of 2000 cases. *Gastroenterology*, **16**, 25–38.

43 Van Heerden, J. & Beart, R. (1980) Carcinoma of the colon and rectum complicating chronic ulcerative colitis. *Diseases of the Colon and Rectum*, **23**(3), 155–159.

44 Van Heerden, J. A., Judd, E. S. & Dockerty, M. B. (1967) Carcinoma of the extrahepatic bile ducts: a clinicopathologic study. *American Journal of Surgery*, **113**, 49–56.

45 Watts, McK J., de Dombal, F. T., Watkinson, G. & Goligher, J. C. (1966) Early course of ulcerative colitis. *Gut*, **7**, 16–31.

46 Yardley, J. H. & Keren, D. F. (1974) 'Precancer' lesions in ulcerative colitis. *Cancer*, **34**, 835–844.

47 Yardley, J. H., Bayless, T. M. & Diamond, M. P. (1979) Cancer in ulcerative colitis (editorial). *Gastroenterology*, **76**, 221–225.

CROHN'S DISEASE

CLINICAL PRESENTATION

Crohn's disease is a rare disorder with an incidence of the order of 3 per 100 000 population per year and with a prevalence of 40 per 100 000 population.[28] It follows that the number of patients with Crohn's disease seen by any one doctor is usually small. Further, among the many patients referred to hospital, Crohn's disease is a rare explanation for abdominal symptoms. These features explain why the diagnosis is often overlooked.

The modal age at onset of symptoms is 30 years with an equal sex distribution, so that persistent gastrointestinal symptoms in patients of this age group should alert the physician to the possibility of Crohn's disease. However, Crohn's disease may occur at any age and, to compound the difficulty, symptoms may be transient or intermittent or there may be no symptoms whatever at the time of the first consultation. Finally, the term Crohn's disease comprises a spectrum of disorders, the nature of whose presentation will vary according to the site and extent of the macroscopic change and any local complications that have occurred.

History

GENERAL COMMENTS

A careful history should be taken from the symptomatic patient to explore whether there are features suggestive of organic disease which would warrant further investigation. Good quality radiological investigation will usually demonstrate the site of macroscopic disease, but will only do so after the investigation has been requested! Features such as persistent change in bowel habit, urgency, diarrhoea at night, and rectal bleeding, all point to an organic basis for symptoms. Careful assessment should be made of the frequency and severity of abdominal pain, which can often be corroborated by discussion with the family. Clear evidence of a change in appetite or weight loss are also useful pointers. In childhood even severe abdominal symptoms may only be revealed by careful direct questioning. Anorexia is sometimes confused with anorexia nervosa, and the label 'irritable bowel syndrome' should not be applied lightly until organic disease has been carefully considered and excluded. Finally, we have seen a small number of patients with persistent symptoms and initially normal radiological investigations who several years later developed radiological evidence of Crohn's disease. Patients with persistent symptoms should be reviewed at intervals to detect this small group.

Physical examination

Physical examination may reveal clear signs that suggest organic disease and point the way to further investigation. However, since symptoms of Crohn's disease may be intermittent, a completely normal physical examination does not exclude the diagnosis. Extraintestinal manifestations such as finger clubbing, arthritis or erythema nodosum may suggest the diagnosis. There may be clear evidence of recent weight loss. Abdominal examination may reveal palpable masses or fistulas. Since most patients with Crohn's disease have perianal disease, the perianal area should be carefully examined. Skin tags may be a helpful early pointer to the diagnosis.

The history and physical examination will not only suggest whether there are organic features worthy of further investigation, but will also help to determine the site of macroscopic disease and whether local complications are present.

Among a large series of patients with Crohn's disease from our hospital, the distribution of macroscopic disease at presentation was: distal ileum $\pm$ right colon, 66%; extensive colonic involvement, 14%; distal colonic involvement, 5%; diffuse small bowel disease, 5%; others, 7%.[15] The specific presenting features vary according to the macroscopic site of disease. The distal ileum, with or without involvement of the right colon, is the commonest site of macroscopic disease; the symptoms are not dependent on involvement of the right colon. Macroscopic disease of the right colon alone is rare.

Obstructive symptoms

With active mucosal disease
Recurrent bouts of subacute colicky abdominal pain, abdominal distension and rumbling, with systemic features of general malaise, fever, anorexia and weight loss are common.

These symptoms are commonly associated with diarrhoea, probably caused by increased sodium and water secretion from the small intestine proximal to the stenotic segment.

Inactive mucosal fibrous stricture
Distal ileal Crohn's disease has often progressed to fibrous stricture formation by the time of diagnosis. The strictures result in intermittent obstructive symptoms which are usually short-lived and in the ensuing intervals the patient often appears well and symptom-free.

The pain may be vague, intermittent and atypical in site. Persistent or recurrent symptoms should prompt a request for a barium follow-through examination. Some patients elude early diagnosis since the initial investigations usually only include a barium meal and barium enema examination, and the changes in the distal ileum are overlooked, particularly if there is no retrograde filling of distal ileum with contrast during the barium enema examination.

Abscess formation

Abscess formation results from either local perforation proximal to the stricture, perforation through a penetrating ulcer or inflammatory change in locally involved lymph nodes. This complication increases the systemic disturbance and leads to anorexia, weight loss, fever and general malaise. There is usually, but not invariably, a palpable local tender mass in the right iliac fossa.

Local abscess formation, if undetected, can lead to severe malnutrition and is an important example of the hazard of neglected disease. The patient illustrated in Figure 12.18 had undergone a resection of the distal ileum five years previously. When her symptoms recurred she was advised to rest at home. She was first seen three months later: wasted, anaemic, dehydrated and with a palpable mass in the right iliac fossa. At laparotomy a large abscess was drained and recurrent Crohn's disease of the ileum was resected. The stricture which had given rise to such severe complications was only 2 cm in length.

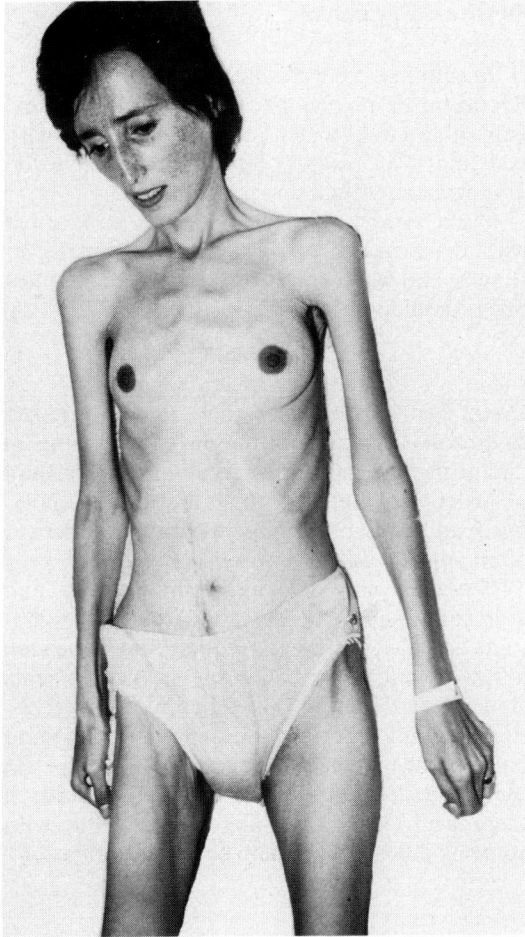

Fig. 12.18 Abscess formation in Crohn's disease. Appearance at presentation after resting at home for three months. Note scar of previous resection of distal ileum for Crohn's disease some five years previously.

Fistula formation

Enterocutaneous fistulas[16]

Enterocutaneous fistulas may follow laparotomy for suspected appendicitis. The fistulas do not arise from the appendix stump but from adjacent loops of ileum damaged at surgery or from the site of a local perforation which has been oversewn. They commonly occur after incision and drainage of a local abscess. Spontaneous enterocutaneous fistulas are rare, but can arise in association with recurrent disease. They must be distinguished from postoperative enterocutaneous fistulas, which are a complication of anastomotic leak where there is no evidence of residual or recurrent Crohn's disease.

Entero-enteric fistulas[12]

These usually occur between adjacent loops of small bowel. They may be demonstrated radio-

logically but are often only identified at laparotomy. They do not usually cause specific symptoms and so do not affect the clinical management, which is determined by the nature and severity of the symptoms from the underlying macroscopic disease. Entero-enteric fistulas (e.g. gastrocolic fistulas) may occasionally give rise to blind loop syndrome or even malabsorption.

Haemorrhage

Massive haemorrhage is a rare but important complication.[34] It may occur from ulcers proximal to a tight stricture or follow infiltration of a major vessel.

'Acute appendix'

Laparotomy may be undertaken to exclude appendicitis when Crohn's disease of the distal ileum is identified. Close questioning will usually reveal symptoms which have been present for some weeks before the acute episode which precipitated the laparotomy.

Colonic involvement[2]

The commonest symptoms of extensive colonic involvement are diarrhoea and general malaise, often associated with anorexia and weight loss. The onset is usually insidious. In a few patients the onset is rapid, leading to a fulminant colitis. Unlike the pattern in small intestinal Crohn's disease, obstructive symptoms are uncommon, though vague persistent abdominal discomfort is often a feature.

Left sided disease

This is commoner in older patients where it may be associated with diverticular disease. The symptoms can mimic the underlying diverticular disease with attacks of pain in the left lower quadrant and intermittent diarrhoea. However, some patients develop fulminating disease with marked general malaise, weight loss, fever and tachycardia. These episodes may be complicated by colonic perforation when the patient presents as an acute abdominal emergency.

Perianal disease[4]

Perianal disease is present in more than two-thirds of patients, though it is usually painless and asymptomatic. Perianal disease is an important pointer to the diagnosis. Perianal disease only becomes painful when there is local abscess formation or active anal fissure. Such episodes alert the clinician to the possibility of Crohn's disease but the diagnosis should have been made in most patients before this stage.

Diffuse small bowel disease[7]

This is a rare site for Crohn's disease though it is commoner in children than adults. Since it may present in a variety of ways, the diagnosis may be elusive, particularly as affected individuals can have a normal bowel habit. Severe symptoms with general malaise, anorexia, weight loss and peripheral oedema, together with a low serum albumin, are common. However, in others, although the radiological examination shows extensive changes, the individual may remain asymptomatic except perhaps for some mild peripheral oedema because of low serum albumin levels.

The pattern at presentation varies according to the interval between the onset of symptoms and diagnosis. With time the diffuse change may revert to normal. During the healing phase strictures may occur which cause symptoms suggestive of subacute intestinal obstruction.

Oesophageal disease

Oesophageal disease is rare. Dyer *et al.*[9] described two cases of Crohn's disease of the oesophagus but could find no other examples in more than 2000 reported cases of Crohn's disease in 12 large series. Huchmerzeyer *et al.*[22] identified 21 cases from the literature including 5 of their own. Thirty-one cases of proven or presumed oesophageal Crohn's disease from the literature have been reviewed by Weterman.[42]

The commonest symptom is progressive dysphagia causing marked weight loss which can become severe within a few weeks. Examination is often unhelpful except to confirm the weight loss. Aphthous ulcers may be present in the mouth.

Confusion can arise with fungal infections such as moniliasis, especially in patients receiving corticosteroids or immunosuppressive therapy.

Gastric and duodenal disease

The first report of duodenal involvement was published by Gottlieb and Aloent in 1937.[14] At least 200 cases have now been reported.[30] The duodenum is more commonly involved than the stomach. Gastroduodenal lesions are usually associated with macroscopic disease in other parts of the gastrointestinal tract.

Epigastric pain is the predominant symptom, which often mimics peptic ulcer, though the poor response to antacids and H_2 blockers may arouse suspicion. The macroscopic lesions may progress to stricture formation which induces anorexia, nausea, vomiting and weight loss. Bleeding is uncommon. Physical examination is usually unhelpful except to confirm weight loss, but occasionally a succussion splash is found. It is surprising how few symptoms may be associated with what appears radiologically to be a tight duodenal stricture.

Extraintestinal manifestations

In some patients extraintestinal manifestations predominate. These features include erythema nodosum, aphthous ulcers of the mouth, acute arthritis, ankylosing spondylitis, ocular lesions or even pyoderma gangrenosum. Growth retardation in children occasionally occurs without abdominal symptoms. However, both these groups usually have gastrointestinal symptoms which can be elicited on careful enquiry.

Summary

The history and physical examination often suggest the presence of organic disease and may suggest the site of macroscopic disease and whether any local complications have developed.

DIAGNOSIS

The diagnosis of the symptomatic patient should follow a clear analytical pathway to determine the site of macroscopic disease, whether it is active or inactive, and to identify or exclude metabolic problems or local complications.

The clinical features that have been described alert the clinician to the possibility that the symptomatic patient has Crohn's disease. Certain uncommon presentations such as ankylosing spondylitis or growth retardation alone may delay the diagnosis. Such examples are the exception to the general pattern. In most patients a good quality barium follow through or barium enema examination will identify the characteristic features and define the site of macroscopic disease. The quality of the films must be considered in interpreting the report since the terminal ileum may not have been displayed well and early lesions in the colon, particularly aphthous ulcers, may have been overlooked. In a few symptomatic patients good quality radiological studies may be entirely normal for several years before unequivocal radiological change develops. The patient who has undergone extensive investigation and acquired a label of functional bowel disorder may be referred later to a colleague. The demonstration of a total colitis on repeat barium enema examination undermines everyone's confidence, except those of the colleague!

Sigmoidoscopy may reveal characteristic perianal disease or patchy mucosal change and rarely the classical aphthous ulcers. Biopsy may be helpful and granulomas may be identified even in apparently normal uninvolved mucosa.

Laboratory tests are helpful, particularly as screening procedures at the first outpatient visit. The symptomatic patient with abdominal pain and diarrhoea can readily be screened by measuring the haemoglobin, packed cell volume, serum iron, total iron binding capacity, serum albumin, serum globulin and acute phase proteins. The ESR is helpful if elevated but normal values do not exclude Crohn's disease, since in some patients the result may be normal in the presence of active macroscopic disease. Normal values for all these indices are common in patients with Crohn's disease where the symptoms are due to an inactive fibrous stricture, or where there are short segments of active disease. In these situations the radiological features are usually characteristic of Crohn's disease.

The symptomatic patient with established Crohn's disease should be subject to a regular critical analysis. The site and extent of macroscopic disease should be reviewed. Contrast radiological examination should be undertaken as often as indicated by the clinical problem. In most patients, particularly those with inactive disease, many years may elapse between examinations. However, patients with severe symptoms may require re-evaluation after only a few weeks. Distal ileal mucosal inflammatory lesions may progress to fibrous strictures which require different management. Patients with aphthous ulceration of the colon who have unexpected or persistent symptoms may require repeat barium enema examinations since the changes can progress to extensive colonic involvement within a few weeks. Patients with diffuse small bowel disease may need reassessment since the changes may either resolve or strictures may develop during the healing phase. The strictures may be amenable to surgical intervention. Diffuse small bowel disease may be followed by the development of extensive colonic involvement.

The possibility of metabolic problems inducing symptoms must be considered, particularly the general malaise associated with fluid and electrolyte depletion (particularly potassium loss). Anaemia is common and may explain the symptoms of general malaise and tiredness. Trace metal deficiency should be considered and corrected especially in patients with persistent diarrhoea. Correction of these metabolic problems will relieve many symptoms previously ascribed to 'the Crohn's disease'.

The local complications which may cause symptoms include stricture, abscess and fistula formation. They should all be considered and identified or excluded.

In patients with abdominal pain the symptoms may be due to an associated disorder such as peptic ulcer, gallstones and renal stones, rather than the underlying disease itself.

Radiology (see also p. 947)

Recent developments have been well reviewed by Goldberg and Jeffrey.[13] The role and value of air contrast studies of the gastrointestinal tract are now well established.

The value of infusion techniques in Crohn's disease of the small intestine have been analysed by Nolan and Gourtsoyiannis.[29] A variety of changes have been identified including discrete, longitudinal and fissure ulcers and sinuses. The double contrast technique may even demonstrate small bowel adhesions. The natural history of the radiographic appearances of discrete mucosal 'aphthous' ulcers has been well documented in serial studies.[24] The radiological findings correlate well with the pathological appearances. Many of the characteristic features are missed using a single contrast technique.[18]

Newer techniques, including gallium scanning,[33] grey scale ultrasound[21] and angiography of the gut[39] may all contribute to diagnosis.

Endoscopy (see also p. 947)

The role of colonoscopy in inflammatory bowel disease has been reviewed recently.[20, 43] While the majority of patients with inflammatory bowel disease do not require colonoscopy, it plays an important role where there are diagnostic doubts or difficulties; it is used to determine the extent or severity of disease, the nature of stricture formation, to take mucosal biopsies to detect dysplasia and for primary diagnosis in children.

The magnifying colonoscope with dye spraying is an interesting technique for demonstrating minute mucosal structure and has been recommended for monitoring response to treatment, the early detection of recurrence and for the prediction of remission.[36]

Histopathology (see also p. 958)

The value of large bowel biopsy in the differential diagnosis of inflammatory bowel disease has been reviewed by Chambers and Morson.[6] Surawicz *et al.*[35] examined 243 rectal biopsies from 90 patients with Crohn's disease and showed that even with multiple serial sectioning epithelioid granulomas were found in only 25%. Granulomas appear to be more common in the rectum and anus than elsewhere in the gastrointestinal tract, although these studies did not correct for variations in mucosal volume.[19] Specific features have been identified by stereomicroscopic examination of rectal biopsies from patients with ulcerative colitis. They include changes in the mucosal pattern, irregular enlarged gland openings filled with exudate, and patchy localization of goblet cells.[31] Scanning electron microscopy studies can readily distinguish between ulcerative colitis and Crohn's disease.

Laboratory indices and diagnosis

Interpretation of laboratory data requires critical analysis. The information that it provides complements the clinical history, physical findings and the results of radiological and sigmoidoscopic examinations.

In most symptomatic patients presenting for the first time the laboratory indices will be abnormal. Unexplained anaemia, elevated ESR or acute phase proteins such as serum orosomucoids, or low serum albumin all point to an organic basis in patients presenting with abdominal symptoms.

Serum albumin levels are useful as indices of activity. They reflect the degree of inflammatory activity in the gut since there is a close relationship between serum albumin levels and gastrointestinal protein loss in inflammatory bowel disease.[23]

Since the half life of serum albumin is of the order of 20 days, serum albumin levels do not alter rapidly but reflect the situation over a period of 1 to 2 weeks.

Acute phase proteins are also useful in determining disease activity. Seromucoids, a group of alpha$_1$ glycoproteins soluble in 0.6 mol/l perchloric acid were first used by Cooke and his colleagues.[8] The predominant protein is orosomucoid (alpha$_1$ acid glycoprotein), for which a specific of assay of alpha$_1$ glycoprotein is now available.[38] The half life of seromucoids is about five days, so the speed of response is much more rapid than serum albumin. A variety of other acute phase proteins have also been utilized.[41]

An elevated ESR is generally a useful index and reflects the increased secretion of alpha-globulin, fibrinogen and gammaglobulin by the liver. However, the ESR is sometimes normal in patients with inflammatory bowel disease, even when the disease is active.

Other useful laboratory indices include C-reactive protein which correlates well with clinical indices of activity.[10] These proteins have a short half life so are a sensitive index for rapid assessment of change in severity.

Problems in diagnosis

The distinction between ulcerative colitis and Crohn's disease is probably still best drawn by Kirsner,[25] while the differential diagnosis of ulcerative colitis and Crohn's disease from other specific inflammatory bowel diseases has been the subject of an excellent review.[37] Tuberculosis of the gastrointestinal tract has to be considered seriously in the differential diagnosis, particularly in the immigrant population.[11] Campylobacter enterocolitis has recently been highlighted in the differential diagnosis.[26] Late-onset Crohn's disease is often found in association with diverticular disease.[3]

The diagnostic errors and reasons for delay in the diagnosis of Crohn's disease have been analysed in a large series of patients.[1] A group of 140 patients with Crohn's disease were grouped according to the site of macroscopic disease – small bowel (61), ileocolic (30), colon alone (40) and anorectal (9). In these patients the mean interval between the onset of symptoms and referral to hospital was only 2.9 months so that the family practitioner is completely exonerated from blame for the delay in establishing the diagnosis.

The correct diagnosis had been established in two-thirds of the patients within two years of the onset of symptoms. The diagnostic problems in 20% were confined to the distinction between ulcerative colitis and Crohn's disease, which had little effect on management.

Mis-diagnosis was most common in small bowel disease. A diagnosis of acute appendicitis which proves to be Crohn's disease may dent the pride of the diagnostician, but has limited impact on management. On careful questioning, most patients with Crohn's disease of the distal ileum mimicking acute appendicitis reveal a history of abdominal symptoms for several months before the acute episode supervened. A label of psychiatric disorder was common. Other patients presenting with abdominal pain had diagnostic labels of peptic ulcer or gallstones attached to them.

The commonest mis-diagnosis in ileocolonic and colonic disease was to attach a psychiatric label to abdominal symptoms which subsequently were shown to have an organic basis. Overall an incorrect diagnosis of psychiatric disorders was made in 19% of the patients.

Simple screening tests for organic disease were helpful but not diagnostic since only half the patients were anaemic and two-thirds had an elevated ESR. The diagnostic confusion commonly arose because of the non-specific nature of the initial symptoms which led the patients to be referred to a number of different specialists.

Diagnostic tests to avoid such pitfalls have always been an attractive proposition. Walker[40] demonstrated that normal buccal mucosa from patients with Crohn's disease incubated with their own serum and then stained with deposited antibody by fluorescent techniques showed a positive reaction not observed in mucosa from normal subjects or patients with ulcerative colitis. Further work suggests that the tests may not be sufficiently specific to be used in differential diagnosis.[27]

REFERENCES

1 Admans, H., Whorwell, P. J. & Wright, R. (1980) Diagnosis of Crohn's disease. *Digestive Diseases and Science*, **25**, 911–915.

2 Allan, R. N., Steinberg, D. M., Alexander-Williams, J. & Cooke, W. T. (1977) Crohn's disease involving the colon: an audit of clinical management. *Gastroenterology*, **73**, 723–732.

3 Berman, I. R., Corman, M. L., Coller, J. A. & Veidenheimer, M.C. (1979) Late onset Crohn's disease in patients with colonic diverticulitis. *Diseases of the Colon and Rectum*, **22**, 524–529.

4 Buchmann, P., Keighley, M. R. B., Alexander-Williams, J. & Allan, R. N. (1980) The natural history of perianal Crohn's disease. *American Journal of Surgery*, **140**, 642–644.

5 Chambers, T. J. & Morson, B. C. (1979) The granuloma in Crohn's disease. *Gut*, **20**, 269–274.

6 Chambers, T. J. & Morson, B. C. (1980) Large bowel biopsy in the differential diagnosis of inflammatory bowel disease. *Investigative Cell Pathology*, **3**, 159–173.

7 Cooke, W. T. & Swan, C. J. H. (1974) Diffuse jejuno ileitis. *Quarterly Journal of Medicine*, **43**, 583.

8 Cooke, W. T., Fowler, D. C. & Cox, E. V. (1958) The clinical significance of seromucoids in regional ileitis and ulcerative colitis. *Gastroenterology*, **34**, 910–919.

9 Dyer, N. K., Cooke, P. I. & Kemp Harper, R. A. (1969) Oesophageal stricture associated with Crohn's disease. *Gut*, **10**, 549–554.

10 Fagan, E. A., Dyck, R. F., Maton, P. N. *et al.* (1982) Serum levels of C-reactive protein in Crohn's disease and ulcerative colitis. *European Journal of Clinical Investigation*, **12**, 351–359.

11 Findlay, J. M. (1979) Tuberculosis of the gastrointestinal tract in Bradford 1967–1977. *Journal of the Royal Society of Medicine*, **72**, 587–590.

12 Givel, J. C., Hawker, P. C., Allan, R. N. & Alexander-Williams, J. (1983) Entero-enteric fistula complicating Crohn's disease. *Journal of Clinical Gastroenterology*, **5**, 321–323.

13 Goldberg, H. I. & Jeffrey, R. B. (1980) Recent advances in the radiographic evaluation of inflammatory bowel disease. *Medical Clinics of North America*, **64**, 1059–1081.

14 Gottlieb, C. H. & Aloent, S. (1937) Regional jejunitis. *American Journal of Roentgenology*, **38**, 881–883.

15 Gyde, S. N., Prior, P., Macartney, J. C. *et al.* (1980) Malignancy in Crohn's disease. *Gut*, **21**, 1024–1029.

16 Hawker, P. C., Givel, J. C., Keighley, M. R. B. *et al.* (1983) Management of enterocutaneous fistulae in Crohn's disease. *Gut*, **24**, 284–287.

17 Higgens, C. S. & Allan, R. N. (1980) Crohn's disease of the distal ileum. *Gut*, **21**, 933–940.

18 Hildell, J., Lindstrom, C. & Wenckert, A. (1979) Radiographic appearances in Crohn's disease. 1. Accuracy of radiographic methods. *Acta Radiologica* (*Diagnostic*), **20**, 609–625.

19 Hill, R. M., Kent, T. H. & Hansen, R. N. (1979) Clinical usefulness of rectal biopsy in Crohn's disease. *Gastroenterology*, **77**, 938–944.

20 Hogan, W. J., Hensley, G. T. & Geenen, J. E. (1980) Endoscopic evaluation of inflammatory bowel disease. *Medical Clinics of North America*, **64**, 1083–1102.

21 Holt, S. & Samuel, E. (1979) Grey scale ultrasound in Crohn's disease. *Gut*, **20**, 590–595.

22 Huchzermyer, G., Paul, F., Seifert, E. *et al.* (1976) Endoscopic results in five patients with Crohn's disease of the oesophagus. *Endoscopy*, **8**, 75–81.

23 Jensen, K. B., Jarnum, S., Koudhal, G. & Kristensen, M. (1976) Serum orosomucoid in ulcerative colitis. Its relation to clinical activity, protein loss and turnover of albumin, IgG. *Scandinavian Journal of Gastroenterology*, **11**, 177–183.

24 Joffe, N. (1980) Radiographic appearances and course of discrete mucosal ulcers in Crohn's disease of the colon. *Gastrointestinal Radiology*, **5**, 371–378.

25 Kirsner, J. B. (1975) Problems in the differentiation of ulcerative colitis and Crohn's disease: the need for repeated diagnostic evaluation. *Gastroenterology*, **68**, 187–191.

26 Loss, R. W., Mangle, J. C. & Pereira, M. (1980) Campylobacter colitis presenting as inflammatory bowel disease with segmental colonic ulceration. *Gastroenterology*, **79**, 138–140.

27 Matthews, N., Tapper-Jones, L., Mayberry, J. F. & Rhodes, J. (1979) Buccal biopsy in diagnosis of Crohn's disease. *Lancet*, **i**, 500–501.

28 Mendeloff, A. I. (1980) The epidemiology of inflammatory bowel disease *Clinics in Gastroenterology*, **9**, 259–270.

29 Nolan, D. J. & Gourtsoyiannis, N. C. (1980) Crohn's disease of the small intestine: a review of the radiological appearances in 100 consecutive patients scanned by a barium infusion technique. *Clinical Radiology*, **31**, 597–603.

30 Nugent, F. W., Richmond, M. & Park, S. K. (1977)

Crohn's disease of the duodenum. *Gut*, **18**, 115–120.

31 Poulsen, S. S., Christensen, K. C., Petri, M. & Jarnum, S. (1980) Stereomicroscopic examination of stained rectal biopsies in ulcerative colitis and Crohn's disease. *Scandinavian Journal of Gastroenterology*, **15**, 535–544.

32 Puntis, J., McNeish, A. S. & Allan, R. N. (1984) Long-term prognosis of childhood onset of Crohn's disease. *Gut*, in press.

33 Rheingold, O. J., Tedesco, F. J., Block, F. E. *et al.* (1979) (^{67}Ga) Citrate scintiscanning in active inflammatory bowel disease. *Digestive Diseases and Science*, **24**, 363–368.

34 Rubin, M., Herrington, J. R. & Schneider, R. (1980) Regional enteritis with major gastrointestinal haemorrhage as the initial manifestation. *Archives of Internal Medicine*, **140**, 217–219.

35 Surawicz, C. M., Meisel, J. L., Ylvisaker, T. *et al.* (1981) Rectal biopsy in the diagnosis of Crohn's disease: value of multiple biopsies and serial sectioning. *Gastroenterology*, **80**, 60–71.

36 Tada, M., Misaki, F., Shimono, M. *et al.* (1978) Endoscopic studies on the muscle structure of colonic mucosa in the follow-up observation of ulcerative colitis. *Gastroenterologica Japonica*, **13**, 72–76.

37 Tedesco, F. H. (1980) Differential diagnosis of ulcerative colitis and Crohn's ileo-colitis and other specific inflammatory disease of the bowel. *Medical Clinics of North America*, **64**, 1173–1183.

38 Thaw, P. A. & Allbutt, E. C. (1980) A critical evaluation of a serum seromucoid assay and its replacement by a serum alpha-1-acid glycoprotein assay. *Annals of Clinical Biochemistry*, **17**, 140–143.

39 Tsuchiya, M., Muira, S., Asakura, H. *et al.* (1980) Angiographic evaluation of vascular changes in ulcerative colitis. *Angiography*, **31**, 147–153.

40 Walker, J. E. (1978) Possible diagnostic test for Crohn's disease by use of buccal mucosa. *Lancet*, **ii**, 759–760.

41 Weeke, B. & Jarnum, S. (1971) Serum concentrations of 19 serum proteins in Crohn's disease and ulcerative colitis. *Gut*, **12**, 297–302.

42 Weterman, I. (1983) Oral, oesophageal and gastroduodenal Crohn's disease. In *Inflammatory Bowel Diseases* (Ed.) Allan, R. N., Keighley, M. R. B., Alexander-Williams, J. & Hawkins, C. F. Edinburgh: Churchill Livingstone.

43 Williams, C. B. & Waye, J. C. (1978) Colonoscopy in inflammatory bowel disease. *Clinics in Gastroenterology*, **7**, 701–717.

RADIOLOGY AND ENDOSCOPY

The roles of endoscopy and radiology in Crohn's disease are complementary. Both are of value in the diagnosis and assessment of upper gastrointestinal and large bowel disease, but radiology is superior for routine use in the small intestine. Endoscopy, in general, allows a more accurate close-up assessment of the gastrointestinal mucosa but good quality double contrast barium radiology also has a high accuracy, approaching, and occasionally superior to, endoscopy. Which of these methods is used depends a great deal upon the experience and availability of the radiologist and endoscopist. Not all patients with known or suspected Crohn's disease warrant endoscopy. A prime indication is to establish the presence and extent of the disease in patients with normal or doubtful radiological studies. The aim of both radiology and endoscopy is to demonstrate the essential pathological features of Crohn's disease – oedema, ulceration, fibrosis and fistulas. The hallmark of Crohn's disease is the asymmetry and discontinuous distribution of the disease process.

The value of radiology

Radiology is widely available and the greater use of double contrast barium examinations using improved barium suspensions and pharmacological techniques has improved the visualization of fine mucosal detail. In general, barium studies are more comfortable for the patient and give a superior overall picture of the extent of the disease. A permanent record of the examination is, of course, an integral part of the procedure.

The value of endoscopy

Medical staff experienced in endoscopy are not so readily available and the examination can be uncomfortable for the patient. Endoscopic procedures require sedation of the patient and are more hazardous than a barium examination. However, in experienced hands, endoscopy gives a better evaluation of the mucosal appearance than radiology. The mucosa is seen in full colour and alteration of mucosal vascularity can be an indication of early disease. Aphthous ulceration is better seen with this method than with radiology. The field of view through an endoscope, however, is small, and the extent of the disease may be difficult to record. Permanent documentation of the mucosal appearance is not a regular feature of endoscopic examinations and the opinion and experience of the examiner is extremely important. A particular and important strength of endoscopy is the ability to obtain tissue for histological examination for an exact diagnosis. Tissue biopsies obtained via an endoscope are small, often involving the surface of the mucosa only. The presence of the diagnostic epithelioid granulomas can usually be found only in a relatively small number of biopsies and the definitive histological diagnosis can be made in less than 25% of patients.[21] It is important, therefore, to take numerous biopsies from several sites.[20] The most reliable site for a successful diagnostic biopsy is from the margin of an early lesion such as an aphthous ulcer.

Oedema

In the early stages, the mucosa becomes swollen. Radiologically this is seen as a coarsening of the fine mucosal detail and can best be shown in the colon on double-contrast barium enema. Endoscopically the vascular pattern may be altered, either becoming more prominent with an overall reddening of the mucosa or the normal vascular pattern may be obscured by thickened oedematous mucosa. In later stages, the mucosal folds become thickened, straightened and distorted and these may be seen both radiologically and at endoscopy. Mucosal nodules may be seen, and these are often discrete. Some nodularity is due to surrounding ulceration, leaving islands of normal mucosa. This is best seen endoscopically. Some nodularity, however, is due to mucosal thickening without associated ulceration (Figure 12.19). Gross oedema may affect the whole thickness of the bowel wall and give rise to 'hosepipe thickening' with swollen loops of intestine. Radiologically this is best seen in the distal ileum where it is shown by separation of the barium-filled bowel (Figure 12.20). Endoscopically areas of hosepipe thickening will be shown as a narrowed lumen with a stiff unpliable wall, often associated with mucosal ulceration.

Ulceration

Shallow aphthous or aphthoid ulceration is probably the earliest stage that can be shown macroscopically.[13] It is intramucosal and cannot be seen radiographically, if viewed in profile, projecting outside the bowel lumen. It is seen 'en face' as a central speck of barium with a surrounding dark translucent halo of mucosal oedema. Endoscopically there is usually an ery-

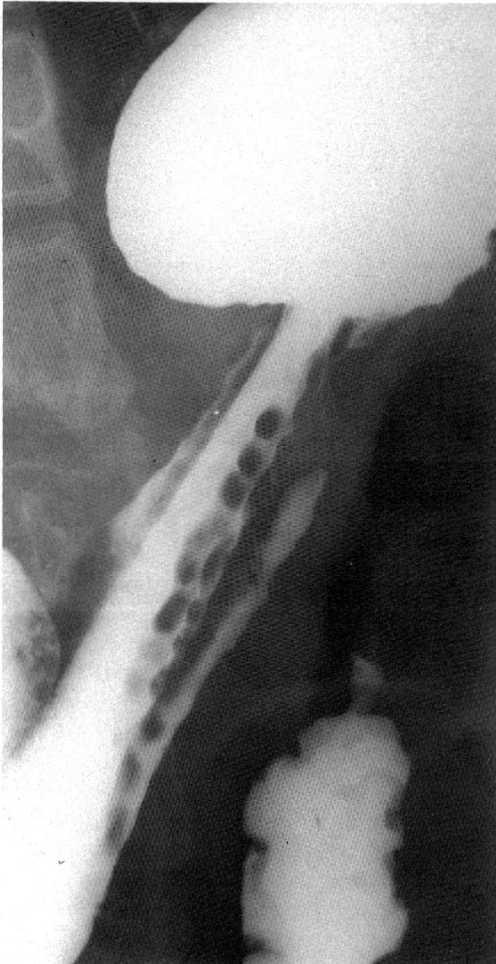

a

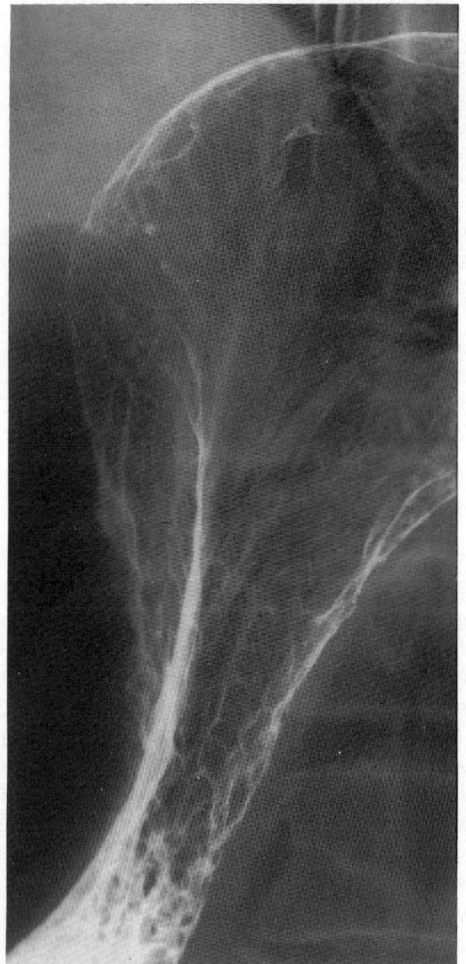

b

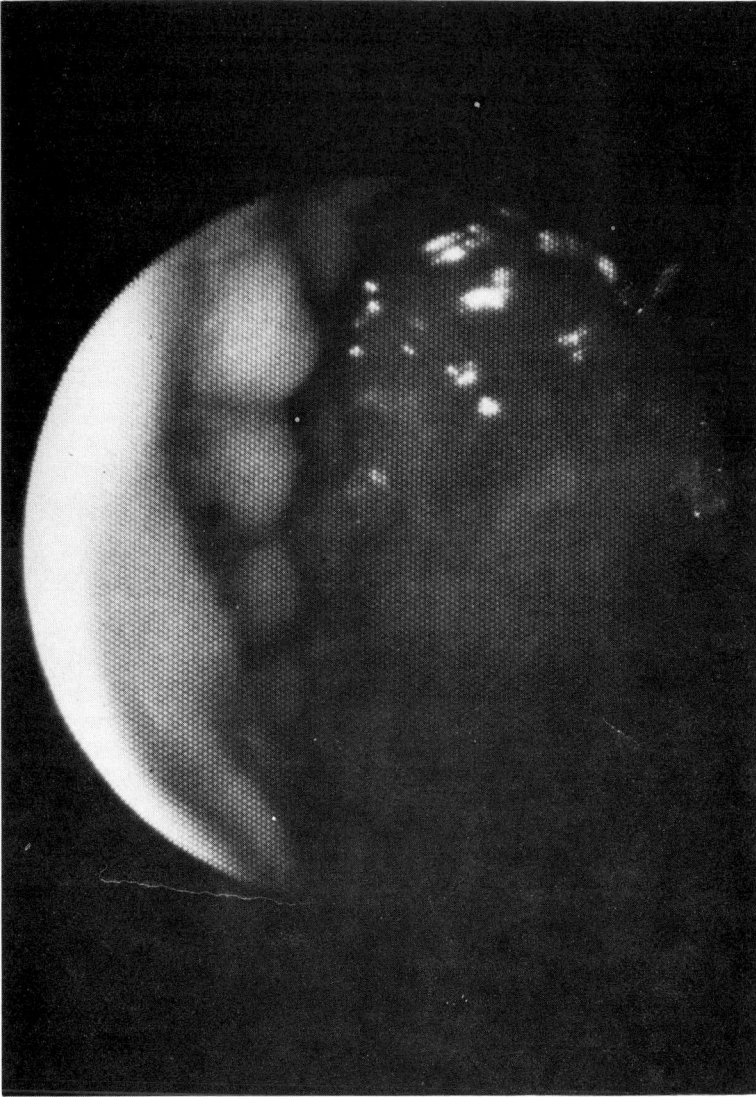

c

Fig. 12.19 (a) Single contrast barium filled phase. Note the marked nodularity along the line of the rugal folds. (b) The same patient in double (air) contrast phase. (c) The endoscopic appearance. Note that there is no ulceration between the nodules.

thematous area with a small central depression and, as the ulcer becomes larger, the central area shows a white slough in the base. Aphthous ulcers may be entirely discrete with large areas of surrounding normal mucosa; both endoscopically and radiographically they are best seen in the colon (Figure 12.21). Progression of the disease leads to more extensive ulceration which may penetrate more deeply into the mucosa and adjacent ulcers may coalesce. This gives rise to a varying pattern of ulceration which is often bizarre. Long linear ulcers may occur, which in the colon lie along the line of the taenia coli (Figure 12.22). Large areas of mucosal ulceration lead to denuded patches.

Linear and transverse ulceration together form a 'cobblestone' pattern (Figure 12.24). Deep penetrating ulcers are said to have a 'rosethorn' appearance radiographically but this is not pathognomonic of Crohn's disease.[17] In the author's experience the use of double-contrast radiography stretches the bowel wall and obliterates some of the deep ulceration, especially in the colon. Intramucosal extension gives rise to a 'collar-stud' lesion[10] which, if multiple, appears radiographically as a continuous track in the submucosa. Varying stages of ulceration may occur at the same time. Severe ulceration is often surrounded at the margin by areas of shallow ulceration.

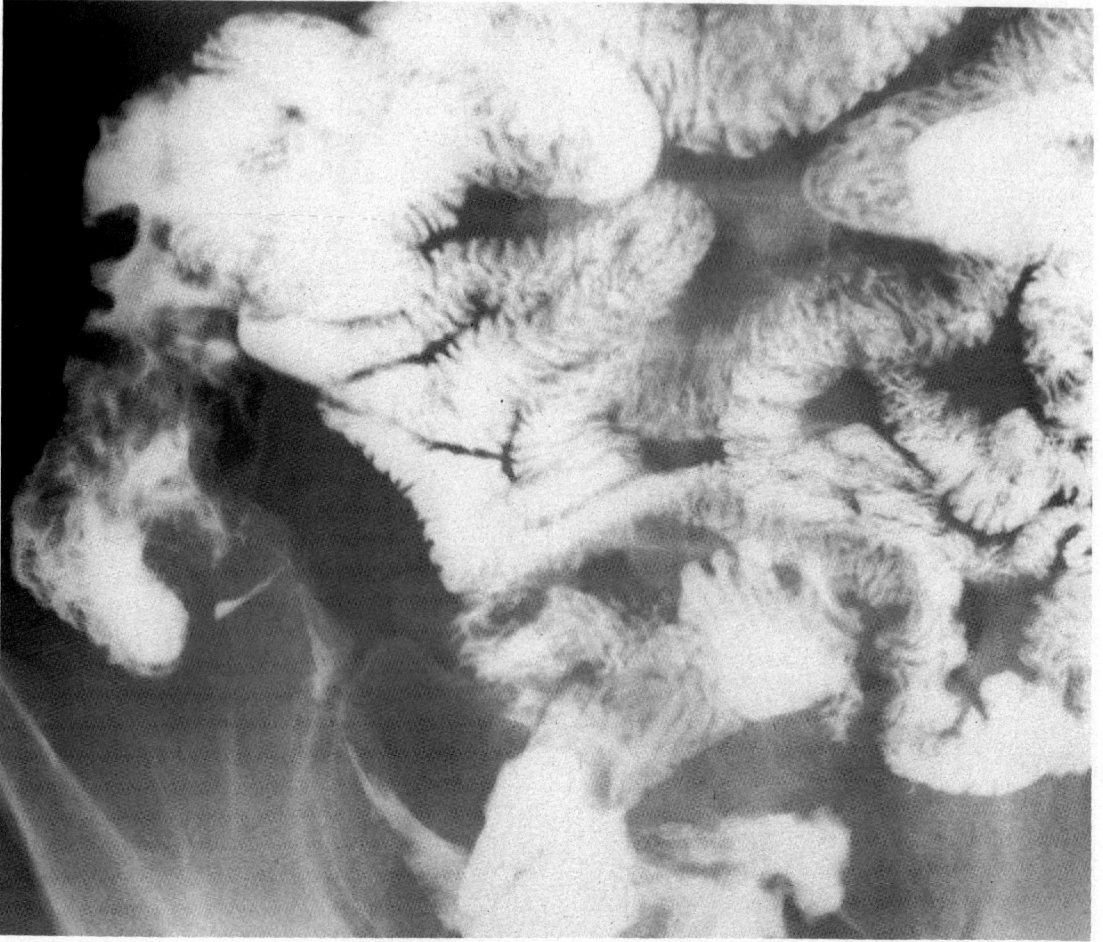

Fig. 12.20 Barium follow through examination showing the narrowed ulcerated terminal ileum showing from adjacent barium-filled bowel by grossly oedematous ileum. There is a deep sinus/fissure 2 cm from the ileocaecal valve.

Fibrosis

Fibrosis develops as the disease heals. If it occurs in a circumferential manner then a stricture will result. Many apparent strictures are, in fact, due to spasm or oedema. Fluoroscopy or endoscopy, aided by an intravenous antispasmodic drug, will normally enable the distinction to be made. Shortening from fibrosis in the long axis of the bowel will often lead to pseudosacculation as the disease process is usually asymmetric; the mesenteric border is frequently more affected.[12] Transmural fibrosis will lead to angulation and adherence of bowel loops, which can cause intestinal obstruction.

Fistulas

Fistulas are probably an extension of deep, transmural ulceration which penetrate into adjacent structures. The most commonly occurring fistulas are entero-enteric; the majority are found within a few centimetres of the ileocaecal valve and are short, giving rise to short bypassed loops. Fistulas between the terminal ileum and sigmoid colon may give rise to symptoms, particularly diarrhoea. Many fistulas are complex, with multiple pathways, and commonly result from abscess formation. Sinuses are the precursor of fistulas, and usually arise from the terminal ileum (Figure 12.20) or the perianal region. Many patients with perianal lesions in Crohn's disease have a normal rectum radiographically.

Features at specific sites

OESOPHAGUS, STOMACH AND DUODENUM

The upper gastrointestinal tract can be examined easily and accurately by endoscopy and

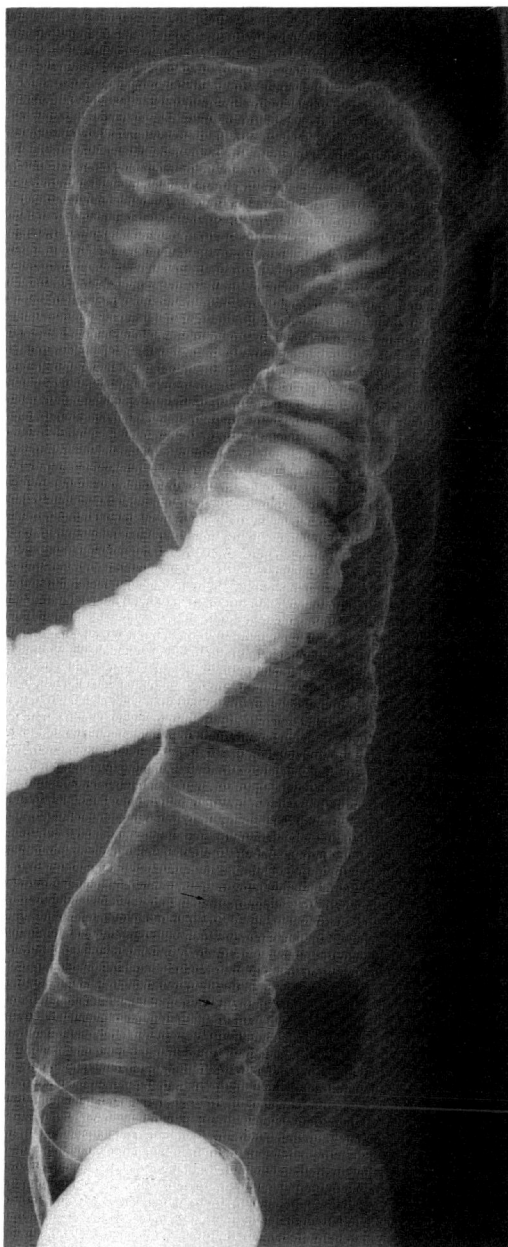

Fig. 12.21 Double contrast barium enema examination in a colon studded with discrete shallow aphthous ulcers of varying size. The white areas represent the shallow ulcer crater and the narrow dark halo represents surrounding oedema. In between the ulcers the colonic mucosa is normal.

double-contrast barium meal examination which has an accuracy approaching that of endoscopy.[5, 9] Crohn's disease of the oesophagus is rare. Its features are mimicked by those of reflux oesophagitis, which is extremely common. Endoscopically they are very similar and Crohn's of the oesophagus is rarely diagnosed radiologically. Oesophageal Crohn's

disease can progress to stricture or fistula formation.[3] The granulomatous process more commonly affects the antrum of the stomach and the first part of the duodenum, usually in continuity. In its severe form it leads to gastric outlet obstruction, which may require surgical bypass to relieve symptoms. Severe disease of the stomach is recorded in 1–4%,[4] and severe duodenal disease in 4–7%, of patients with Crohn's disease elsewhere in the gastrointestinal tract. However, routine demonstration of the surface mucosa by double contrast barium examinations has revealed minor mucosal abnormalities of the stomach and duodenum in up to 40% of patients with Crohn's disease of the ileum or colon;[9] this has also been the author's experience. Mucosal abnormalities are also seen endoscopically in either the oesophagus, stomach or duodenum in approximately 50% of patients with small or large bowel Crohn's disease.[7] The correlation between endoscopy, radiology and histology, is not exact. Minor histological abnormalities, some diagnostic of Crohn's disease, are found in patients who are radiologically and endoscopically normal. The minor changes of oedema and aphthous ulceration are usually indistinguishable, radiologically and endoscopically, from the gastroduodenal erosions seen in peptic ulcer disease. A more unusual appearance which is sometimes seen in the stomach is mucosal irregularity along the line of rugal folds. This appearance seems to be specific to Crohn's disease (Figure 12.19). Radiologically, a mosaic pattern may be seen, either in the stomach or duodenum, which probably represents the end stage of severe ulceration (Figure 12.23).

Differential diagnosis

The main differential diagnosis is peptic ulceration of the oesophagus, stomach and duodenum, in all its manifestations. Both Crohn's disease and peptic ulceration lead to mucosal oedema, shallow aphthous ulceration, deeper ulceration and fibrosis, and peptic perforation may simulate fistulas. Both disease processes may be asymmetrical and discontinuous. A clue to the underlying pathology of Crohn's disease is that the ulceration is more extensive and severe than is normally seen in peptic ulcer disease (Figure 12.24). A further important feature is that, in the author's experience, Crohn's disease of the stomach and duodenum has always occurred with Crohn's disease elsewhere in the gastrointestinal tract. Other differential diagnoses to be considered are neoplasia, lymphoma, sarcoid, and tuberculosis.

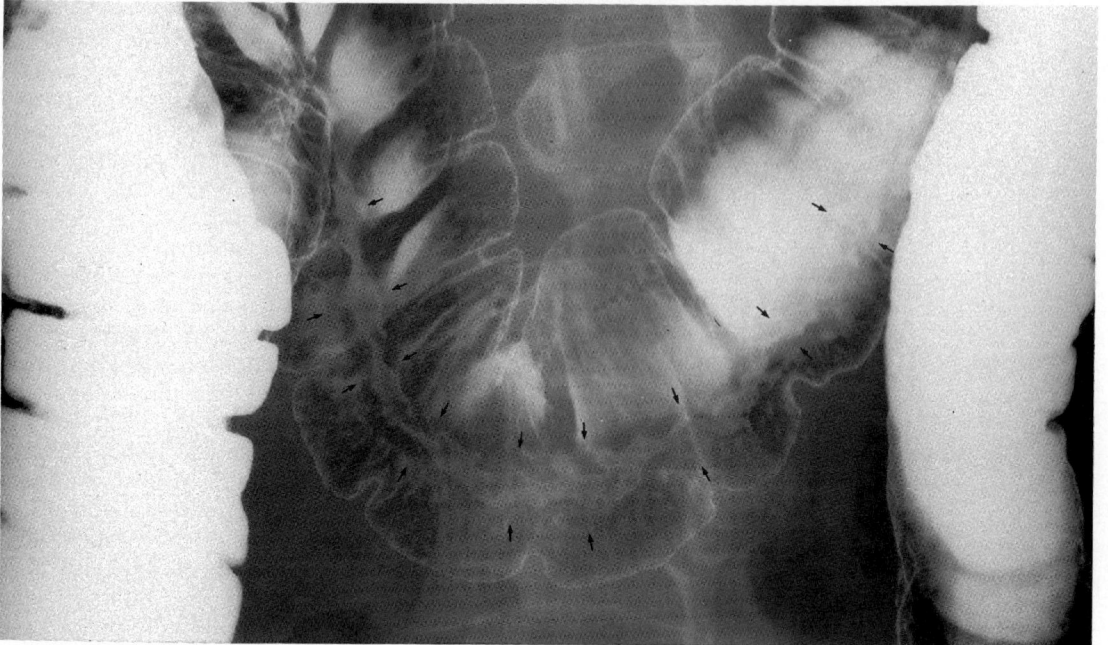

Fig. 12.22 Double contrast barium enema examination showing a long ulcer (arrowed) along the line of a taenia coli in the transverse colon.

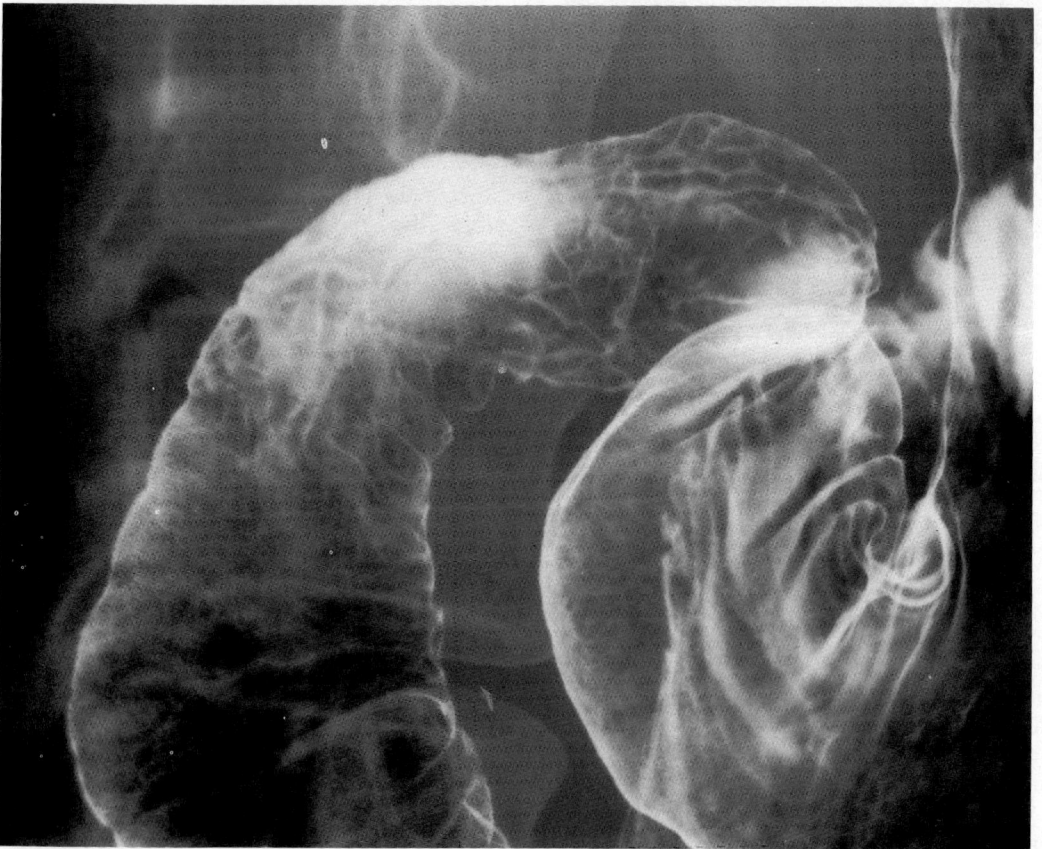

Fig. 12.23 Double contrast barium meal examination showing mosaic appearance of the duodenal cap and proximal part of the descending duodenum. There is an abrupt change to normal mucosa in the remaining parts of the duodenum.

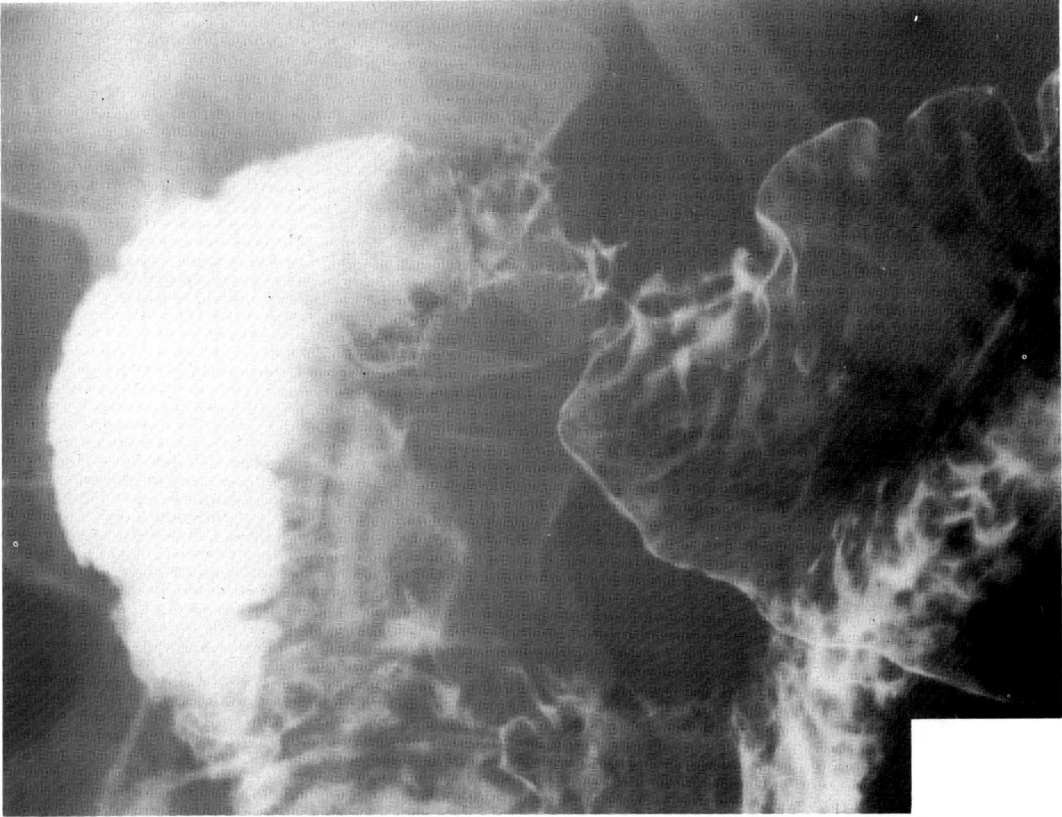

Fig. 12.24 Marked narrowing of the gastric antrum and duodenal cap as shown by a double contrast barium meal examination. The antrum reveals numerous aphthous ulcers.

SMALL INTESTINE

Terminal ileum

This part of the small bowel is the site most commonly affected by Crohn's disease. Unfortunately, it is also the area most difficult to examine by double-contrast radiography and endoscopy unless the patient has an ileostomy. The disease is therefore often well advanced before a diagnosis is established. The early radiographic signs are spasm, irritability and mucosal swelling with nodularity. Shallow ulceration may be seen radiographically and endoscopically. Later, the whole bowel wall becomes thickened (Figure 12.20). In this part of the gastrointestinal tract the disease may present as a long continuous symmetrically affected segment. If severe spasm and oedema are present the classical 'string sign' can be seen on X-ray, but this appearance is rarely due to permanent fibrosis. The thickened terminal ileum may cause indentation of the medial wall of the caecum, and may explain a narrowed caecum identified on barium enema examination.

Jejunoileitis

Diffuse involvement of the proximal small bowel is much less common than disease of the terminal ileum and usually occurs in younger patients. The radiological changes include diffuse thickening and nodularity of the valvulae conniventes, with shallow ulceration at the apices of the mucosal folds. This part of the intestinal tract is rarely examined by an endoscope. More extensive ulceration may lead to large areas of effaced mucosa which may heal later, often with stricture formation (Figure 12.25).

Differential diagnosis

Early disease confined to the terminal ileum may be confused with *Yersinia* enterocolitis. The latter condition, however, is transient and never results in stricture or fistula.[19] Ileocaecal tuberculosis may be identical on radiography, but the presence of longitudinal ulceration helps to distinguish Crohn's disease from tuberculosis.[18] Lymphoma may present a difficult diagnostic problem. The presence of large focal ulceration is in favour of lymphoma. Carcinoid tumours

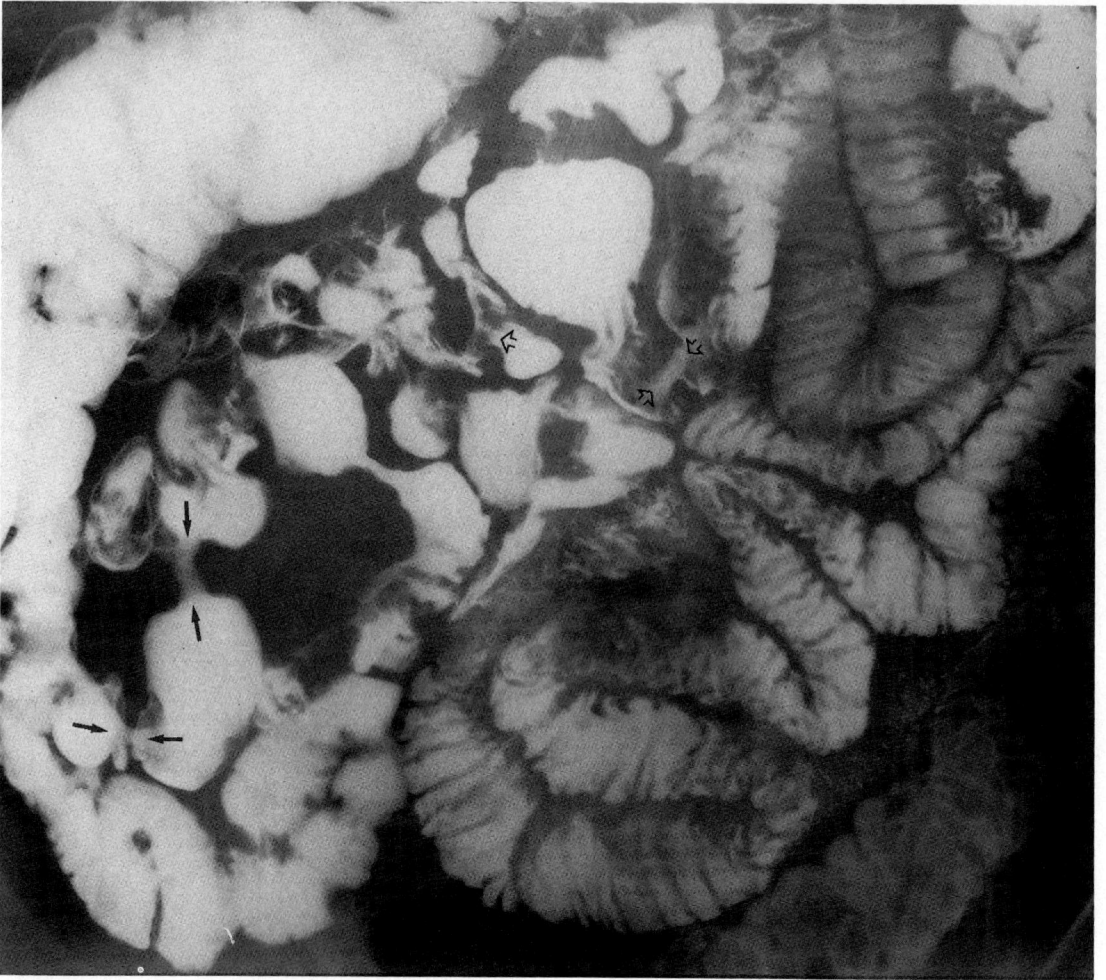

a

with fibrosis occasionally simulate Crohn's disease.[2] Ischaemia rarely causes confusion with Crohn's disease. The sudden onset and rapid resolution or perforation enable the distinction to be readily made.

LARGE INTESTINE

The incidence of colonic Crohn's disease seems to be increasing. This may in part be due to earlier diagnosis by improved radiology and endoscopy which has been aided by more effective large bowel cleansing. It is now recognized that most patients with colitis can safely undergo full bowel preparation without significant systemic disturbance. Only patients with toxic megacolon are exempt from this rule, but this complication is now rarely seen. Crohn's disease classically affects the proximal colon, usually with associated disease in the terminal ileum.[14] The rectum is affected in about 50% of

patients with colonic Crohn's disease[15] unlike ulcerative colitis where the rectum is invariably involved. A few patients with Crohn's disease have continuous total colonic involvement.[6] Shallow aphthous ulceration is seen in the early stages, usually surrounded by normal mucosa (Figure 12.21). Progression of the ulceration leads to a 'cobblestone' or nodular appearance (Figure 12.26), and occasionally large areas of ulceration may be seen. This sometimes occurs in a linear fashion along the line of the taenia coli (Figure 12.22). The ulcerated areas usually show less severe ulceration at the margins, but occasionally the demarcation can be abrupt. Pseudopolyposis, due to inflammatory polyps in areas of quiescent disease, is increasingly seen both endoscopically and on X-ray, the latter due to improvement in barium techniques. The inflammatory polyps in Crohn's disease are asymmetrical and discontinuous (Figure 12.27), unlike those in ulcerative colitis which occur

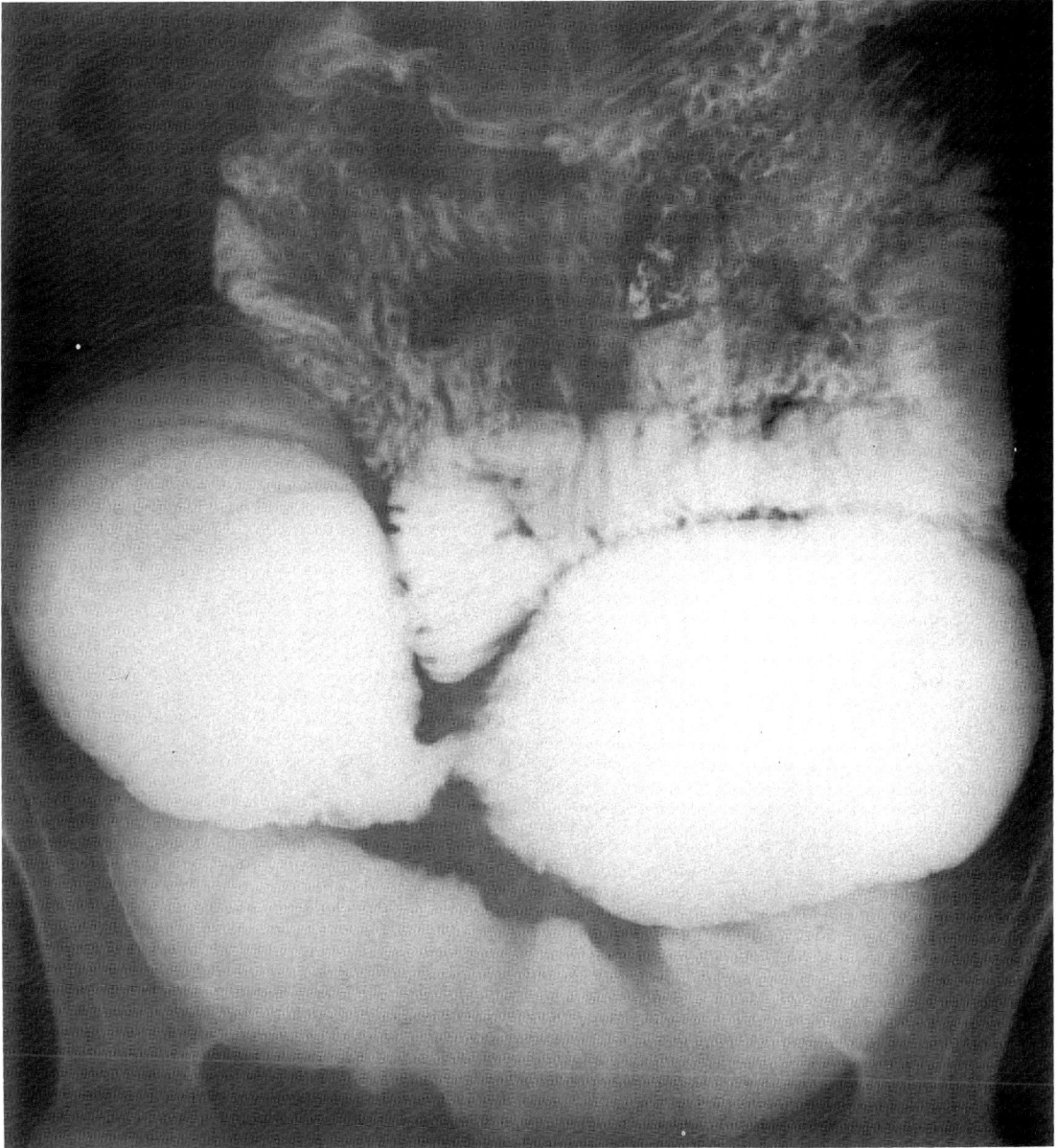

b

Fig. 12.25 (a) Numerous short strictures in the ileum (single arrows). The strictures are typically asymmetric leading to pseudosacculation (open arrows). (b) A single short stricture which has progressed to partial obstruction of the small bowel with gross dilatation.

continuously and distally. Occasionally the polyps may fuse, causing bridges across the intestinal lumen. These are seen well endoscopically but rarely on barium enema examination. Pseudopolyps may be locally grouped and may occlude the bowel lumen, and may be mistaken for a neoplasm.[1] Acute Crohn's colitis may progress to an acute toxic dilatation as in ulcerative colitis. Acute severe colitis is therefore a contraindication for both X-ray examination

and endoscopy. Fibrosis occurring in the circumferential axis will result in strictures which radiologically may be difficult to distinguish from neoplasia. Longitudinal fibrosis on the mesenteric border causes pseudosacculation.

Differential diagnosis

In Western societies the main differential diagnosis is from ulcerative colitis. This disease is continuous proximally from the rectum and

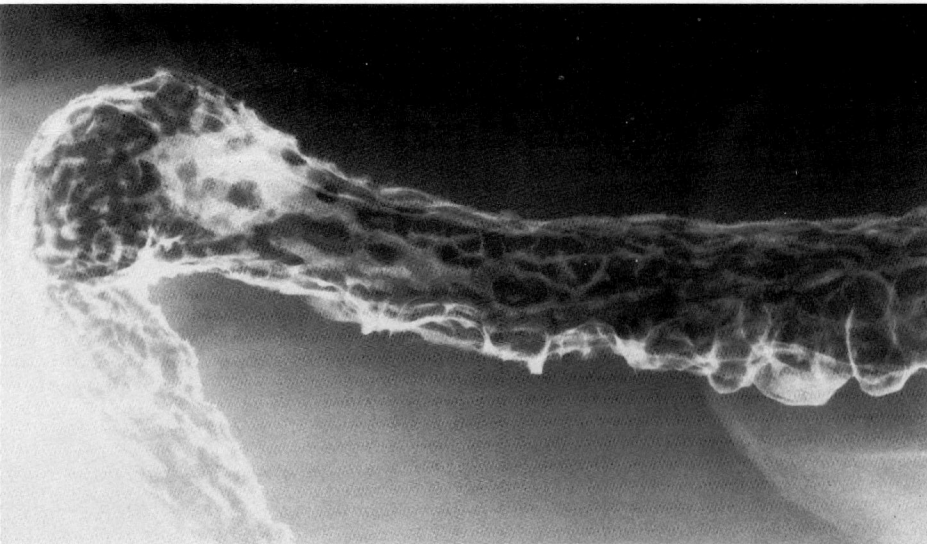

Fig. 12.27 Double contrast barium enema examination showing several features of Crohn's disease. Pseudopolyps are seen in the ascending and transverse colon (filled arrows). Asymmetric involvement of the mesenteric border (open arrows) with normal mucosa on the opposite antimesenteric border. The ileocaecal valve is grossly oedematous (curved arrow).

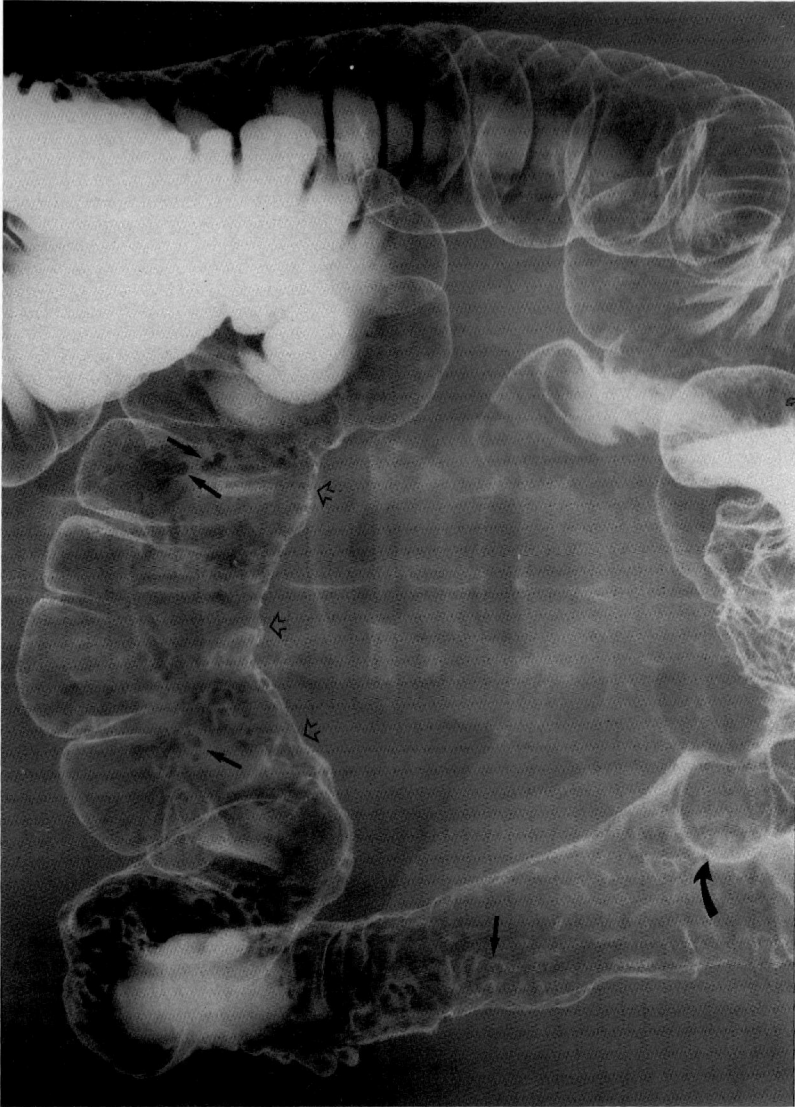

Fig. 12.26 Double contrast barium enema examination showing marked 'cobblestone' formation of the mucosa with longitudinal and transverse ulceration.

956

symmetrical about the colonic circumference. Crohn's disease only rarely manifests both these features. Crohn's disease is more often distributed patchily in the proximal colon with normal intervening mucosa. There is a much higher tendency to form strictures and fistulas in Crohn's disease. Occasionally it may be impossible to distinguish the two conditions radiologically. Endoscopy makes the distinction more readily in the early stages. The diffuse reddened granular mucosa of ulcerative colitis is more easily seen than on X-ray. In severe disease, however, where the ulceration is much more gross and extensive, the distinction on endoscopy may not be made so easily.[21] The underlying pathology may not be apparent for several months or years. It is our experience that when it is difficult to distinguish between the two conditions, Crohn's disease is usually the final diagnosis. Ileocaecal tuberculosis is difficult to distinguish

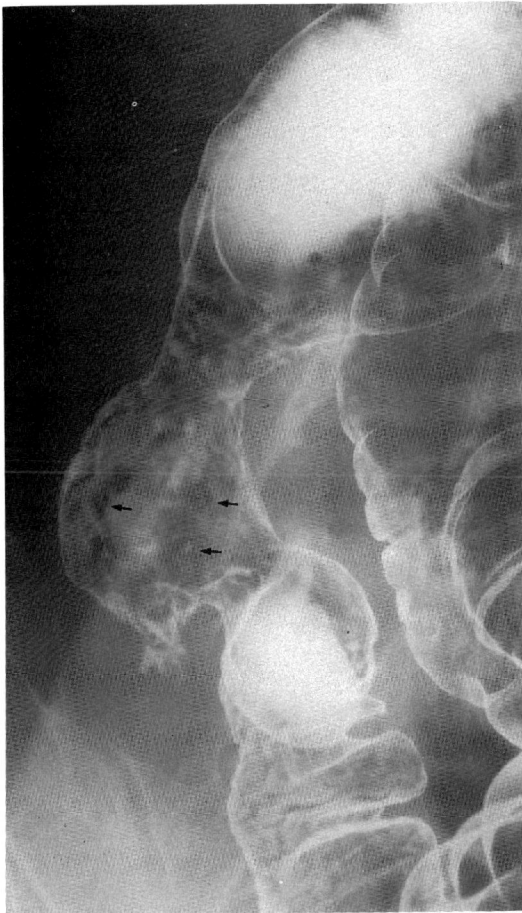

Fig. 12.28 Contracted ulcerated caecum and proximal ascending colon affected by tuberculosis. There are several small aphthous ulcers (arrows). The appearances are indistinguishable from Crohn's disease.

both radiographically and endoscopically (Figure 12.28). Tuberculosis may occasionally affect discontinuous isolated colonic segments and in Western countries the diagnosis may not be made until tissue has been obtained for histological examination. Crohn's strictures in the colon can be confused with neoplasia and occasionally ischaemia. Carcinomatous strictures usually have a shouldered margin with raised edges which are more readily seen at endoscopy. Strictures complicating Crohn's disease tend to be tapered and the margins and transition to normal mucosa less definite. Ischaemia may be extremely difficult to distinguish from Crohn's disease in the elderly. Both conditions in this age group tend to affect the sigmoid colon and are often associated with diverticular disease, giving rise to a confusing appearance both on X-ray and through the endoscope. Ischaemia tends to resolve within a few weeks, so that a repeat examination will usually make the distinction. Both severe diverticular disease and Crohn's disease may give rise to longitudinal submucosal or paracolic sinuses on barium enema examination.[11] In the early stages of the disease, with mucosal oedema and shallow aphthous ulceration, Behçet's disease and amoebic colitis may be considered but in Western countries the demonstration of aphthous ulceration in the colon establishes the diagnosis of Crohn's disease.[16]

Recurrent disease following surgery

The features of recurrent disease are similar to the primary disease and occur in characteristic sites. After ileocaecal resection, for example, recurrent disease almost invariably occurs in the 'new' terminal ileum. The disease often recurs in the jejunum adjacent to the anastomosis after bypass gastrojejunostomy for gastroduodenal disease.

REFERENCES

1 Bernstein, J. R., Ghahremani, G. G., Paige, M. L. & Rosenberg, J. L. (1978) Localized giant pseudo-polyposis of the colon in ulcerative and granulomatous colitis. *Gastrointestinal Radiology*, **3**, 431–435.
2 Chang, S. F., Burrell, M. I., Belleza, N. A. & Spiro, H. M. (1978) Borderlands with diagnosis of regional enteritis: trends in over diagnosis and value of a therapeutic trial. *Gastrointestinal Radiology*, **3**, 67–72.
3 Cynn, W. S., Chon, H., Gureghian, R. A. & Levin, B. L. (1975) Crohn's disease of the oesophagus. *American Journal of Roentgenology*, **125**, 359–364.
4 Fielding, J. F., Toye, D. K. M., Beton, D. C. & Cooke, W. T. (1970) Crohn's disease of the stomach and duodenum. *Gut*, **11**, 1001–1006.

5 Herlinger, H., Glanville, J. N. & Kreel, L. (1977) An evaluation of the double contrast barium meal against endoscopy. *Clinical Radiology*, **28**, 307–314.

6 Joffe, N. (1981) Diffuse mucosal granularity in double contrast studies of Crohn's disease of the colon. *Clinical Radiology*, **32**, 85–90.

7 Korelitz, B. I., Waye, J. S., Kreuning, J. *et al.* (1981) Crohn's disease in endoscopic biopsies of the gastric antrum and duodenum. *American Journal of Gastroenterology*, **76**, 103–109.

8 Laufer, I. (1976) Assessment of the accuracy of double contrast gastroduodenal radiology. *Gastroenterology*, **71**, 874–878.

9 Laufer, I. (1979) *Double Contrast Gastrointestinal Radiology with Endoscopic Correlation.* p. 168 Philadelphia: W. B. Saunders.

10 Lichtenstein, J. E., Madewell, J. E. & Feigin, D. S. (1979) The collar button ulcer. *Gastrointestinal Radiology*, **4**, 79–84.

11 Marshak, R. H. (1975) Granulomatous disease of the intestinal tract (Crohn's disease). *Radiology*, **114**, 3–22.

12 Meyers, M. A. (1976) Clinical involvement of mesenteric and antimesenteric borders of small bowel loops. Radiologic interpretation of pathologic alterations. *Gastrointestinal Radiology*, **1**, 49–58.

13 Morson, B. C. & Dawson, M. P. (Ed.) (1979) *Gastrointestinal Pathology*, 12th edn. pp. 272–336. Oxford: Blackwell Scientific.

14 Nelson, J. A., Margulis, A. R., Goldberg, H. I. & Lawson, T. L. (1973) Granulomatous colitis: significance of involvement of the terminal ileum. *Gastroenterology*, **64**, 1071–1076.

15 Simpkins, K. C. (1976) The barium enema in Crohn's colitis. In *The Management of Crohn's Disease* (Ed.) Weterman, I. T., Pena, A. S. & Booth, C. C. pp. 62–67. Amsterdam, Excerpta Medica.

16 Simpkins, K. C. (1977) Aphthoid ulcers in Crohn's disease. *Clinical Radiology*, **28**, 601–608.

17 Stanley, P., Kelsey Fry, I., Dawson, A. M. & Dyer, N. (1971) Radiological signs of ulcerative colitis and Crohn's disease of the colon. *Clinical Radiology*, **22**, 434–442.

18 Tsukasa, S., Tokjdome, K., Irisa, T. *et al.* (1978) Roentgenographic diagnosis of Crohn's disease of the small intestine. *Stomach and Intestine*, **13**, 335–349.

19 Vantrappen, G., Agg, H. O., Ponette, E. *et al.* (1977) *Yersinia* enteritis and entero-colitis: gastroenterological aspects. *Gastroenterology*, **72**, 220–227.

20 Weterman, I. T. (1981) Colonoscopy in Crohn's disease. In *Crohn's Workshop* (Ed.) Lee E. C. G. pp. 33–38 London: Heyden.

21 Williams, C. B. & Waye, J. D. (1978) Colonoscopy in inflammatory bowel disease. *Clinics in Gastroenterology*, **7**, 701–717.

HISTOPATHOLOGY

The early stages of Crohn's disease are rarely observed and biopsy material may show non-specific inflammatory changes or occasionally granulomas. As the disease develops, ulceration appears in a segment of the gastrointestinal tract or alternatively throughout the colon. Endoscopic examination or double contrast radiology may reveal aphthoid ulcers in the mucosa.

Granulomas can be identified during this stage in biopsies of aphthoid ulcers or in biopsy material from the rectum, colon, perianal area, stomach, jejunum and ileocaecal lymph nodes. As the disease progresses more extensive ulceration associated with fissures develops in the diseased areas accompanied by hosepipe thickening of the bowel wall due to oedema and transmural inflammation. The mesenteric lymph nodes enlarge and show reactive changes with lymphoid hyperplasia, sinus catarrh and scattered granulomas. Jejunal biopsies may show convolutions, oedema and histological evidence of partial villous atrophy.

The gross and histological features of Crohn's disease will be discussed with reference to each anatomical zone.

Involvement of the terminal ileum (regional ileitis)

This is the commonest and most familar lesion in Crohn's disease which leads to ulceration (Figure 12.29) and hosepipe thickening (Figure 12.30) of a variable length of the distal ileum up to the ileocaecal valve. Only a few centimetres may be affected in some patients but more frequently the diseased segment measures 10–12 cm in length; it may extend to 30–40 cm in length with multiple affected segments or skip lesions. Foci of aphthoid ulceration are present in the early stages but in most resected specimens there is extensive ulceration or evidence of linear ulceration along the mesenteric attachment. The mucosa may show a cobblestone pattern or there may be oedema of the circular valvulae conniventes. Pseudopolyps occur in a small proportion of cases and mucosal bridges are occasionally encountered. Stenosis and stricture formation are frequently observed radiologically and on gross examination of the specimen. Fissures, sinuses, fistulas and adhesions with kinking of small intestinal loops are found in patients with longstanding disease. Ulceration at the level of the proximal line of resection indicates that active disease has been left behind in the small intestine. Fruit pulp, tomato skins, fruit stones, a bolus of food debris, and even coins have been discovered in the narrowed segment in patients with intestinal obstruction. Stercoliths resembling gallstones are occasionally found in association with single or multiple strictures. Disease extends into the adjacent caecum in 20% of cases, particularly around the ileocaecal valve. The appendix may be thickened and involved, and Meckel's diverticulum is occasionally affected. Oedema

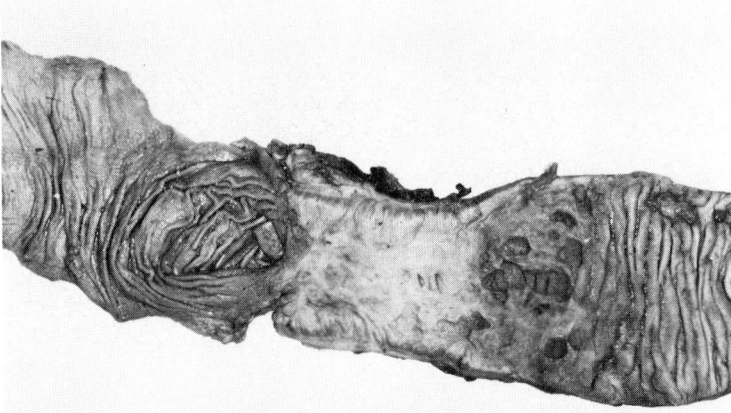

Fig. 12.29 Regional ileitis with ulceration, residual islands of mucosa and hosepipe thickening proximal to ileocaecal valve.

extends into the mesenteric tissues. Abscesses loculate in the ileocaecal region in relation to loops of small bowel and ileocaecal lymph nodes. Recurrent ileal disease following hemicolectomy may be of the simple ulcerative type without hosepipe thickening or strictures.

Histology
There is a wide spectrum of histological features which include ulceration, fissures (Figure 12.31), sinuses, oedema, lymphoid hyperplasia, granulomas, dilatation of lymphatic channels, thickening of the muscularis mucosa, fibrosis, microabscesses, chronic inflammatory cellular infiltration and angiitis. Non-caseating epithelioid cell follicles with Langhan's giant cells (Figure 12.32) are present in the bowel wall in 50–60% of cases and in the lymph nodes in about 25% of cases. Multiple sections must be examined for their detection and foreign body

granulomas, which are frequently present, have to be carefully considered and excluded by polarizing microscopy. Endolymphatic granulomas may be prominent and microgranulomas are present in some cases. More diffuse granulomatous inflammation is found around fissures and sinuses. Eosinophilia is a prominent feature in some cases. Epithelial regenerative changes are usually well developed and may simulate dysplasia. Crypt abscess formation is also seen (Figure 12.33). Pseudopyloric gland metaplasia (Figure 12.34) is present in a high proportion of cases representing a regeneration phenomenon; parietal cells are occasionally identified in the metaplastic tubules. Angiitis is encountered in around 10% of specimens and may be inflammatory, necrotizing or granulomatous (Figure 12.35) in type. Veins may also be involved. Endarteritis obliterans is frequently found and thrombosis is occasionally seen.

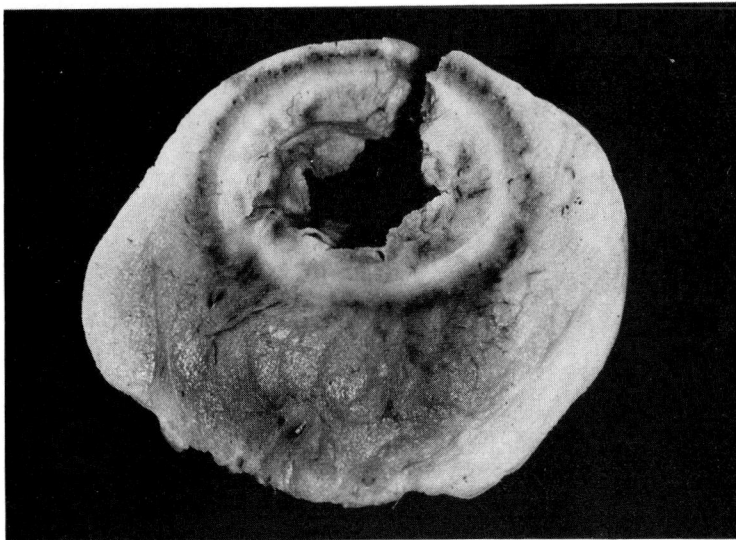

Fig. 12.30 Hosepipe thickening in regional ileitis with oedema extending into mesenteric fat.

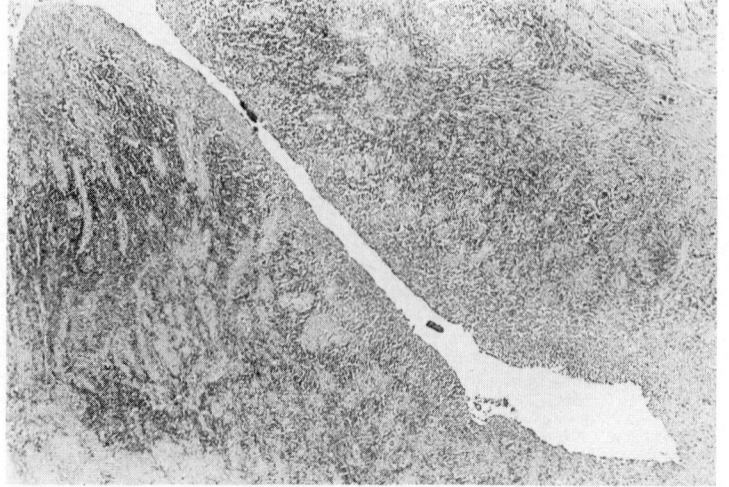

Fig. 12.31 Fissure in ulcerated mucosa in regional ileitis.

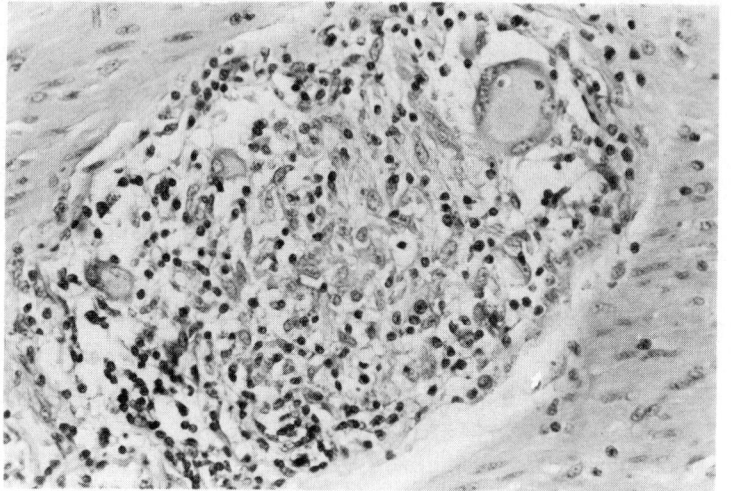

Fig. 12.32 Non-caseating epithelioid cell follicle with Langhan's giant cell.

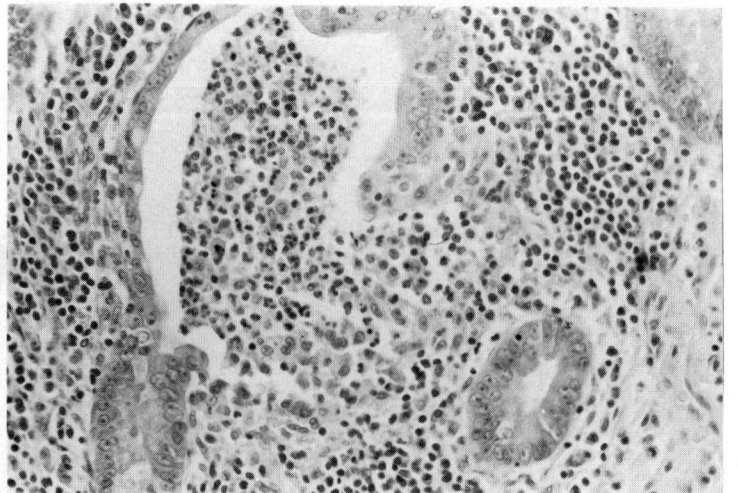

Fig. 12.33 Crypt abscess in Crohn's disease.

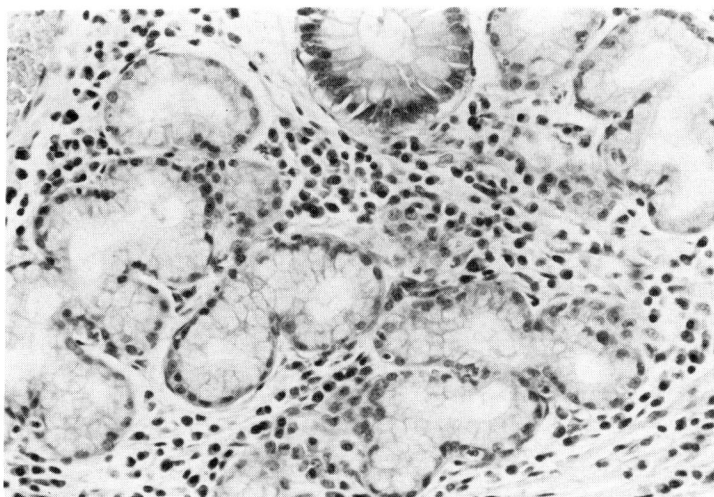

Fig. 12.34 Pseudopyloric gland metaplasia in regional ileitis.

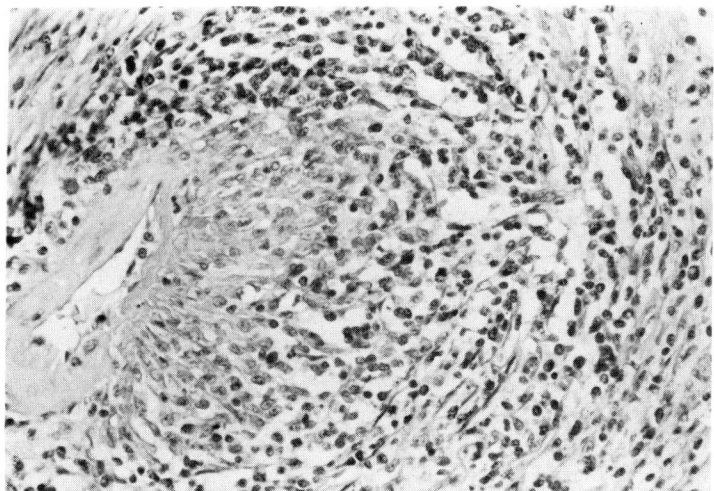

Fig. 12.35 Granulomatous angiitis in Crohn's disease.

Involvement of the colon and rectum

Discrete aphthoid ulcers which can be visualized on endoscopy or double contrast radiography represent the earliest lesions in Crohn's disease. This type of ulceration is not specific since it has been encountered in other infective disorders. Histological examination of aphthoid ulcers reveals focal superficial ulceration, lymphoid hyperplasia, occasional granulomas and even angiitis. As the disease progresses, linear ulceration (Figure 12.36), discrete ulceration, cobblestone mucosa and, frequently, more florid ulceration develop. Fissures appear in the mucosa and may be associated with sinus, fistula or abscess formation particularly in the perianal region. Later in the disease, stenosis occurs either in hosepipe segments (Figure 12.37) or as short strictures. There is usually considerable thickening of the bowel wall as in regional ileitis due to oedema and transmural inflammation. Pseudopolyposis (Figure 12.36) is a further feature of longstanding disease.

Segmental involvement of the colon and rectum is an interesting facet of the disease. Rectal sparing occurs in patients who have the features of segmental or right-sided colitis. The gross appearances are indistinguishable from ulcerative colitis in some cases and the diagnosis can only be established on histological criteria or where there is evidence of small bowel involvement. Local extension into the terminal ileum occurs in approximately 20% of cases of primary Crohn's disease of the colon.

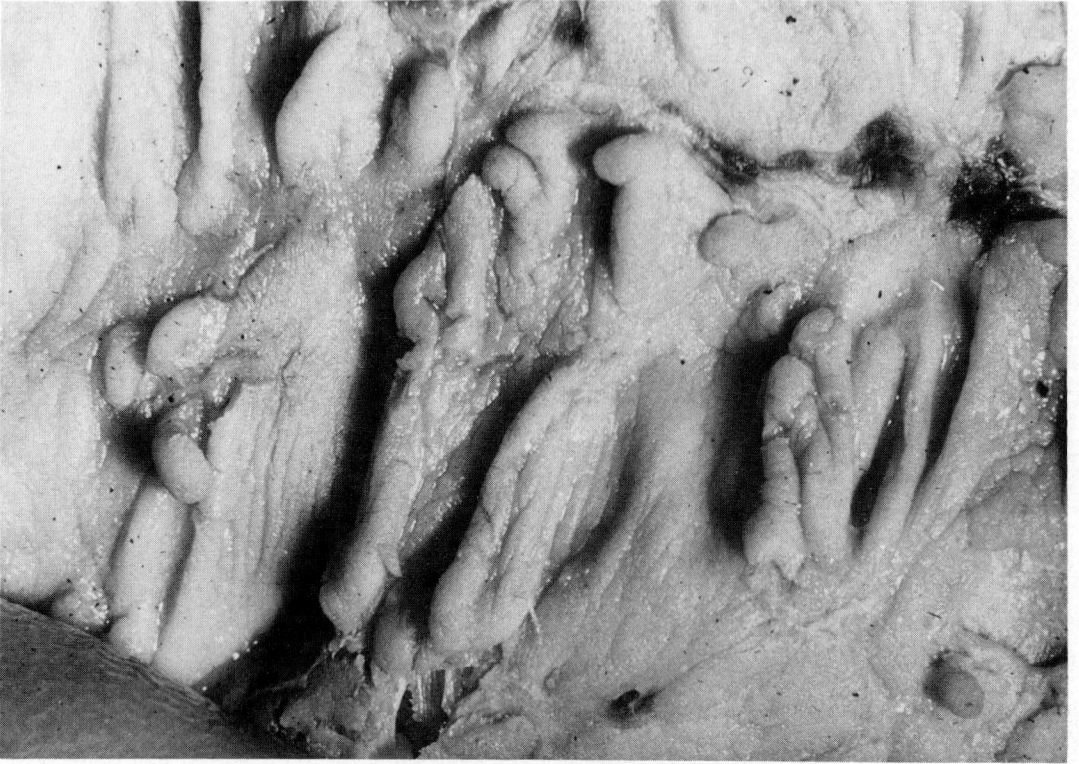

Fig. 12.36   Linear ulceration and pseudopolyposis in Crohn's disease of the colon.

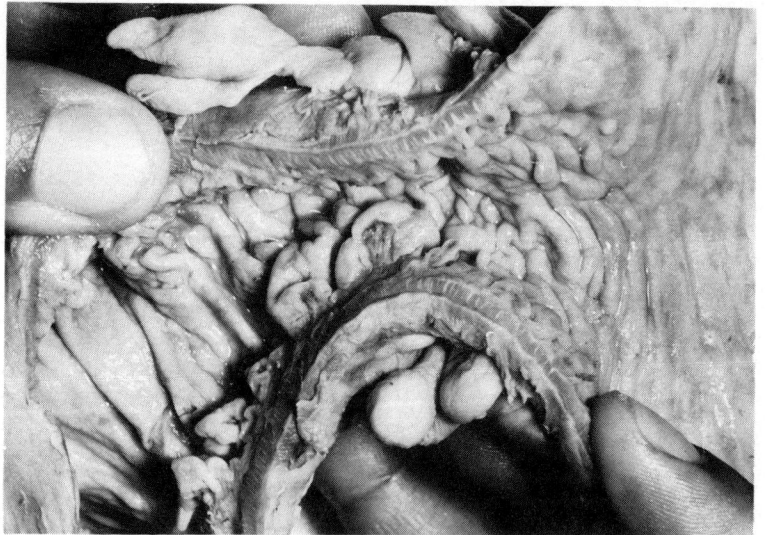

Fig. 12.37   Short hosepipe
segment with pseudopolyposis in
Crohn's disease of the colon.

Histology

The histological appearances are comparable with those found in regional ileitis with ulceration, fissures, lymphoid hyperplasia, oedema, fibrosis, thickening of the muscularis mucosa, and non-caseating granulomas. The incidence of granulomas in Crohn's disease of the colon is around 70% and in rectal biopsy material 27.3% as recorded by Thompson and Bonser,[8] and 25% as recorded by Yardley and Hamilton.[10] Microgranulomas, (Figure 12.38) which represent subtle histological lesions with epithelioid cells and occasional Langhan's giant cells, raise a strong suspicion of Crohn's disease.

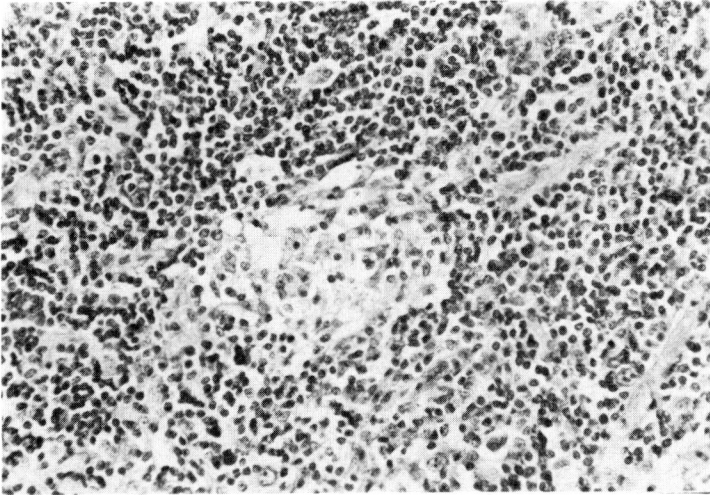

Fig. 12.38 Microgranuloma in Crohn's disease of the colon.

Multiple endoscopic biopsies are more likely to be diagnostic than a single biopsy. Arteritis is a further feature; Thompson and Bonser[8] recorded an incidence of 1.5% in rectal biopsy material. Epithelial regenerative changes occur but tend to be localized to ulcerated areas while the intervening mucosa appears normal. Absence of mucin depletion helps to distinguish Crohn's disease from ulcerative colitis. Focal non-specific inflammation as described by Yardley and Hamilton[10] and disproportionate inflammation are additional features. Granulomatous crypt abscesses are occasionally seen.

Involvement of the jejunum

Primary localization can occur in the jejunum as well as secondary skip lesions complicating regional ileitis. The affected segment shows hosepipe thickening, narrowing and stenosis occasionally amounting to stricture formation. Diaphragms are also occasionally present as an additional congenital anomaly.

Histology
The histological appearances are typical and include ulceration, fissures, lymphoid hyperplasia and granulomas. Ulceration is usually most extensive along the mesenteric attachment. If granulomas are absent then the diagnosis becomes much more difficult since the lesion has to be distinguished from polyarteritis nodosa, simple non-specific ulceration complicating adult coeliac disease, potassium-induced ulceration and ulcerative jejunitis.

Involvement of the duodenum

The incidence of Crohn's disease of the duodenum complicating ileal or colonic disease is 4% in large clinical series. Stenosis is a significant hazard and a bypass operation may be necessary for persistent symptoms. The diagnosis can usually be established by endoscopy, radiology and biopsy. Granulomas are rarely encountered but they may be found in gastric biopsies taken from the same patient. Primary Crohn's disease of the duodenum is exceedingly rare. Duodenal ulcer disease is also a recognized complication of Crohn's disease and may be difficult to distinguish from granulomatous disease. Perforation and haemorrhage represent additional complications of duodenal involvement. Clinical, radiological, endoscopic and pathological observations on Crohn's disease of the duodenum are documented by Fielding *et al.*[3] and by Thompson and Cockel.[9]

Involvement of the stomach

This may be primary or secondary to Crohn's disease elsewhere in the gastrointestinal tract. Random gastric biopsies may show granulomas or an increased population of inflammatory cells. Significant disease is much less common and is associated with ulceration, fissures and thickening of the stomach wall. The pyloric region is most frequently affected but the lesion may be more extensive involving the body mucosa. The gross appearances simulate linitis plastica or 'leather bottle stomach'. Patients with Crohn's disease of the duodenum may also have contiguous gastric disease. Non-caseating granulomas are nearly always present. Primary Crohn's disease of the stomach must be carefully differentiated from sarcoidosis, Wegener's granulomatosis, corrosive poisoning, tuberculosis, histoplasmosis and syphilis.

Involvement of other sites

Crohn's disease of the oesophagus is extremely rare and has to be differentiated from peptic oesophagitis. Crohn's disease of the mouth and lips has been described, supported by histological changes. Crohn's disease of the appendix may be discovered during routine appendicectomy for appendicitis but it should be emphasized that granulomatous disease of the appendix can occur without later development of Crohn's disease. Meckel's diverticulum can be involved by Crohn's disease in association with regional ileitis and it has also been described as a primary lesion. Primary Crohn's disease of the rectum and perianal region are uncommon.

Fistulas and inflammatory changes in Crohn's disease can extend to involve the bladder, urinary tract, ovaries and tubes. More distant granulomatous lesions have also been described in the gallbladder, liver, synovial membranes of joints and the skin surface.

Dysplasia and cancer

There is a fourfold increased incidence of carcinoma of the colon and rectum in patients with longstanding Crohn's disease.[4] We have also encountered carcinoma of the small intestine[5] and cancer in fistulous tracts[1] complicating Crohn's disease. Cancer in the small intestine presents as the occult, diffusely infiltrating variety; colorectal malignant lesions may also be of this type. Dysplasia occurs as a complication of Crohn's disease in the small intestine and also in the colon and rectum. Villous and tubular adenomas are also occasionally encountered.

Involvement of the lymph nodes

Lymph nodes are usually enlarged in association with Crohn's disease. Abscess formation is a problem in the ileocaecal region in association with fissures and sinuses and also between loops of involved small intestine. Sinus catarrh and reactive hyperplasia are prominent. Noncaseating granulomas with epithelioid cells and Langhan's giant cells are found in about 30% of cases. Foreign body giant cells are also occasionally found. Rarely coexistent caseating tuberculosis is discovered in the nodes. Reactive ileocaecal nodes not infrequently show old inactive calcified tuberculosis.

Lymphoid hyperplasia and lymphoma

Rarely lymphoid hyperplasia and lymphocytic plasma cell infiltration are so well developed that they simulate lymphoma. Although malignant lymphoma has been reported in association with both regional ileitis and Crohn's disease of the colon, there is no statistical evidence of an increased incidence.

Hepatic dysfunction

A variety of complications occur in the liver[2] including fatty change, pericholangitis, granulomas, cirrhosis, amyloidosis and stenosing cholangitis. There is also an increased incidence of cholelithiasis and this can be complicated by suppurative cholangitis and multiple liver abscess formation.

Biopsies

The most important clue to the diagnosis of Crohn's disease lies in the identification of noncaseating granulomas or microgranulomas. Sections should be examined from at least three levels in the biopsy. Additional histological features are valuable in the assessment of rectal biopsies such as the presence of focal nonspecific inflammation, disproportionate inflammation, distribution of neutrophils, absence of mucin depletion and relatively normal crypt and surface epithelium. Multiple biopsies are more informative than a single biopsy. Recent attention has focused on the possibility that an increased population of IgM cells in the lamina propria may be a diagnostic feature of Crohn's disease.[6] This claim has been challenged in a more recent study and its specificity has been questioned.[7]

REFERENCES

1 Buchmann, P., Allan, R. N., Thompson, H. & Alexander-Williams, J. (1980) Carcinoma in a rectovaginal fistula in a patient with Crohn's disease. *American Journal of Surgery*, **140**, 462–463.
2 Dew, M. J., Thompson, H. & Allan, R. N. (1979) The spectrum of hepatic dysfunction in inflammatory bowel disease. *Quarterly Journal of Medicine* (*New Series*), **189**, 113–135.
3 Fielding, J. F., Toye, D. K. M., Beton, D. C. & Cooke, W. T. (1970) Crohn's disease of the stomach and duodenum. *Gut*, **11**, 1001–1006.
4 Gyde, S. N., Prior, P., Macartney, J. C. *et al.* (1980) Malignancy in Crohn's disease. *Gut*, **21**, 1024–1029.
5 Hawker, P. C., Gyde, S. N., Thompson, H. & Allan, R. N. (1981) Adenocarcinoma of the small intestine complicating Crohn's disease. *Gut*, **23**, 188–193.
6 Rosekrans, P. C. M., Maijer, C. J. L. M., van der Wal, A. M. *et al.* (1980) Immunoglobulin containing cells in inflammatory bowel disease. *Gut*, **21**, 941–947.
7 Scott, B. B., Goodall, A., Stephenson, P. & Jenkins, R. (1983) Rectal mucosal plasma cells in inflammatory bowel disease. *Gut*, **24**, 519–524.

8 Thompson, H. & Bonser, R. S. (1981) Granuloma, arteritis and inflammatory cell counts in Crohn's disease. In *Recent Advances in Crohn's Disease* (Ed.) Pena, A. S., Weterman, I. T., Booth, C. C. & Stroler, W. pp. 80–83. The Hague: Martinus Nijhoff.

9 Thompson, H. & Cockel, R. (1982) Crohn's disease of the duodenum. *Schweizerische Rundschau fur Medizin (Praxis)*, **71**, 374–377.

10 Yardley, J. H. & Hamilton, S. R. (1981) Focal nonspecific inflammation (FNI) in Crohn's disease. In *Recent Advances in Crohn's Disease* (Ed.) Pena, A. S., Weterman, I. T., Booth, C. C. & Stroler, W. pp. 62–66. The Hague: Martinus Nijhoff.

TREATMENT

Drug treatment

The clinician who seeks in this article anything more than guidance on the treatment of Crohn's disease must look elsewhere. The best way of managing Crohn's disease is to concentrate on a particular current problem rather than to seek long-term ambitious strategies. The results of treatment tend to be unpredictable and a flexible approach is required – trying one measure and, if that fails, trying another. Drug therapy is only one aspect of treatment; dietary manipulation, replacement of nutritional deficits and surgical measures, are all equally important.

Drugs used in the treatment of Crohn's disease may be broadly grouped into anti-inflammatory compounds, drugs that may act by affecting immune responses, antibacterial drugs and symptomatic treatments. The results of controlled trials are summarized and general conclusions are drawn from them about the likely circumstances in which each type of drug may be expected to give benefit. Finally, suggestions are offered about the way in which drugs may be used in different types of Crohn's disease.

ANTI-INFLAMMATORY DRUGS

Sulphasalazine

Pharmacology and metabolism. This drug, salicyl-azo-sulphapyridine, is split at the azo-link by enteric bacteria to yield 5-amino-salicylic acid and sulphapyridine.

Therapeutic experiments in a small number of patients with colonic Crohn's disease, and in a larger number of patients with ulcerative colitis, suggest that sulphasalazine and 5-amino-salicylic acid applied directly to the inflamed colonic mucosa are therapeutically active, but sulphapyridine is not.[14] At present, there is no certainty as to the mode of action of this drug, but it does seem clear that 5-amino-salicylic acid is an important constituent of the molecule and may be the active moiety.

Potential side-effects. The potential side-effects of sulphasalazine are dependent on the blood level of sulphapyridine and on individual hypersensitivity. The blood level of sulphapyridine depends not only on dose but also on the patient's genetic ability to acetylate the drug at a fast or slow rate. High levels of sulphapyridine may be associated with malaise, headache, nausea, dyspepsia and mild haemolysis. The most frequent idiosyncratic reaction is a skin rash; other reactions such as blood dyscrasias are rare. An important side-effect is decreased fertility in men while they are taking sulphasalazine, an adverse effect almost certainly due to the sulphapyridine part of the molecule. There is a decrease in sperm count and motility with an increase in the proportion of abnormal forms. Fertility appears to return within two or three months of stopping the drug.[32]

Evidence for clinical effectiveness. The clinical effectiveness of sulphasalazine will be considered in active disease, in inactive disease, and after resection.

1 Active disease. In the American National Co-operative Crohn's Disease Study (NCCDS), sulphasalazine – 1 g/15 kg body weight (maximum 5 g) daily given over four months – proved no better than placebo in ileal disease, but was effective in ileocolic ($P = 0.027$) and colonic disease ($P = 0.006$).[29] Reanalysis of data in another smaller trial[1] also showed no certain benefit in disease confined to the small bowel but a therapeutic effect in ileocolic and colonic disease ($P < 0.05$). Another controlled trial[35] showed unequivocal benefit of the drug in a dose of 4–6 g daily over a period of 26 weeks; patients with small intestinal disease seemed to do as well as those with disease involving the colon, but the number of patients was small.

2 Inactive disease. In the NCCDS trial, sulphasalazine in a dose of 0.5 g/15 kg body weight (maximum 2.5 g) daily failed to reduce the relapse rate among patients with inactive disease over 1–2 years.

3 After resection. Four trials have failed to show that sulphasalazine given over periods of up to two years reduces the relapse rate after resection.[2, 16, 29, 38] The authors of one trial[38] calculated that between 110 and 130 patients would be needed in each treatment group to ensure a high probability of showing that the

relapse rate is halved by treatment. So far, no trial has achieved this size, and until such a trial is completed the effect of sulphasalazine as a maintenance treatment remains uncertain. However, the results to date are not encouraging.

The role of sulphasalazine in treatment of Crohn's disease. The controlled trials confirm a clinical impression that sulphasalazine is often beneficial in the treatment of active ileocolic or colonic Crohn's disease. Experience suggests that the drug is most effective early in the course of the disease and its effect is often disappointing in patients with a long history. Although there is little evidence from controlled trials to support the use of the drug in extensive small bowel disease, clinical experience suggests that the drug can be effective. There is at present no evidence to support the use of long-term sulphasalazine therapy to reduce the rate of relapse in patients treated medically or the rate of recurrence in patients treated surgically, though individual patients are seen in whom long-term treatment does seem necessary.

Analogues of sulphasalazine and preparations of 5-amino-salicylic acid
One analogue of sulphasalazine has been prepared in which two molecules of 5-amino-salicylic acid are joined by an azo link so that on bacterial cleavage of the diazo bond two molecules of 5-amino-salicylic acid are liberated. Another analogue has been prepared in which 5-amino-salicylic acid is linked to the harmless carrier benzoylalanine. These analogues appear to fulfil their expected function of liberating 5-amino-salicylic acid in the distal part of the intestine. Other analogues have been prepared which are specially potent inhibitors of prostaglandin dehydrogenase. None of these analogues have yet been tested for therapeutic effectiveness in Crohn's disease.

Solutions of 5-amino-salicylic acid tend to become discoloured due to oxidation of this unstable compound. Such solutions have given encouraging results when administered as a retention enema in ulcerative colitis, but no data are yet available on their use in Crohn's disease. If 5-amino-salicylic acid is given by mouth it is likely to be absorbed in the upper small intestine and excreted in the urine. In theory, different delayed release preparations can be prepared which liberate 5-amino-salicylic acid in the small intestine, the proximal or the distal colon. Assessment of the therapeutic effect of such preparations is awaited.

Corticosteroids

Pharmacology and metabolism. The corticosteroids most commonly used in the treatment of Crohn's disease are prednisone or prednisolone. Prednisone is hydroxylated to prednisolone in the body and both are lipid-soluble. For parenteral and topical administration the water-soluble compound prednisolone-21-phosphate may be used. When used as a retention enema, prednisolone metasulphabenzoate is absorbed less than prednisolone-21-phosphate and may be preferable for this reason.

In the blood, cortisol or prednisolone are partially bound to an alphaglobulin, transcortin, and to albumin. Only the unbound steroid is metabolically active and the level of free corticosteroid rises if the serum albumin level falls, with an associated increase in drug side-effects and perhaps therapeutic activity. The biological effects of these drugs on experimentally induced inflammation persist longer than would be predicted from the plasma level. Thus the plasma half life of prednisolone after intravenous administration is around 3–4 hours, but the biological half life is 18–36 hours.

When compared with a normal control group, absorption of prednisolone given by mouth was reduced in seven patients with Crohn's disease.[25] All but one of the patients had ileal disease of mild to moderate severity, but there was no steatorrhoea or excess protein loss from the gut. Other workers have not shown decreased absorption of prednisolone in Crohn's disease, but the results suggest that there may be differences in patients with small or large bowel involvement.[31]

Potential side-effects. The possible side-effects of corticosteroid therapy are well known and limit the therapeutic usefulness of these drugs. Depression of the hypothalamic–pituitary–adrenal axis may be prevented by dosage schedules designed to give intermittent rather than continuous high blood levels, particularly if the high therapeutic level coincides with the physiological peak cortisol level in the morning. It is also likely that intermittent high blood levels, with normal levels for much of the time, cause fewer metabolic side-effects than persistently raised blood levels. Reduced prednisolone absorption in some patients with small intestinal Crohn's disease may lead to fewer side-effects than in patients with normal absorption taking an equivalent dose.

It has been suggested that corticosteroids retard growth in children and that the use of corticotrophin minimizes this side-effect. It is now apparent that growth retardation in Crohn's disease is generally due to poor food intake and the role of corticosteroids in this complication is difficult to assess.[12]

Evidence for therapeutic effectiveness. The clinical effectiveness will be considered in acute disease, active disease and quiescent disease or after resection.

1 Acute disease. The most serious acute form of the disease is severe Crohn's colitis. There has been no controlled trial restricted to Crohn's colitis, but at least one trial[10] has included patients with both Crohn's colitis and ulcerative colitis. This trial showed that corticotrophin, 40 units daily, gave equivalent results to hydrocortisone, 300 mg daily (both drugs given intravenously). Side-effects, especially oedema, tend to be more common with a hydrocortisone infusion than with prednisolone and most clinicians now use the equivalent dose of prednisolone, 60 mg daily, given as a trial of treatment for several days.

2 Active disease. The NCCDS trial showed that prednisone 0.25–0.75 mg/kg body weight (maximum 60 mg) daily given over four months, the dose being adjusted to the activity of the disease, was more effective than placebo ($P < 0.0006$). These results applied to patients with ileal ($P = 0.002$) and ileocolic disease ($P = 0.008$), but the results in patients with colonic disease were not significant, perhaps due to the small size of the group.[29]

3 Quiescent disease or after resection. Three trials have failed to show benefit from low doses of corticosteroids in preventing relapse in patients with inactive disease or after resection. Prednisone, 7.5 mg daily for up to three years, did not reduce the relapse rate not did it affect recurrence or extension of disease among 33 patients when compared with 26 patients who received a control tablet.[28] Prednisone, 0.25 mg/kg body weight (maximum 20 mg) daily, was not apparently superior to placebo over 1–2 years in maintaining remission[29] in the NCCDS trial. A course of prednisolone (with sulphasalazine 3 g daily), beginning with 15 mg and reducing to nil 33 weeks after resection, failed to reduce the recurrence rate over the first three postoperative years.[2]

The role of corticosteroids in Crohn's disease. The main role of corticosteroids in medical treatment is to suppress acute inflammation of the gut. Before starting treatment it is important to ensure, as far as possible, that the symptoms are due to inflammation of the intestine, rather than an abscess or other infective episode. An initial dose of 20–40 mg prednisolone given by mouth, or in severe cases 60 mg prednisolone given intravenously, is advisable with the aim of controlling the symptoms as soon as possible. Thereafter, usually at the end of the first or second week of treatment, the dose can be progressively reduced as long as clinical improvement is maintained and the course of treatment is completed in 4–8 weeks. It is important that neither the patient nor the doctor should regard such treatment as curative; it is best thought of as a measure to control a temporary exacerbation.

Long-term corticosteroid treatment should not be given to a patient who is well in the hope of preventing trouble. However, occasional patients are seen in whom it proves difficult or impossible to withdraw corticosteroid treatment without an immediate recurrence of symptoms. Such patients appear to have 'active chronic' disease which can be suppressed by long-term corticosteroid treatment. In such patients, it may be necessary to continue corticosteroid treatment for a long period provided that the inflammation cannot be controlled by other drugs and that surgical treatment is inappropriate. It is in such patients that the use of azathioprine or 6-mercaptopurine should be considered for its steroid-sparing effect.

Topical corticosteroids are a useful treatment for inflammation of the mouth, distal colon, anal canal or perianal skin.

Combination of a corticosteroid and sulphasalazine

Since both these drugs are effective in the treatment of active Crohn's disease, it is reasonable to ask whether or not the beneficial effects are additive. A controlled trial of prednisone, with or without sulphasalazine, has failed to show that the addition of sulphasalazine increased the rate of remission in active disease or reduced the relapse rate in patients with inactive disease, or that sulphasalazine exerted a steroid-sparing effect.[27] Thus, although this combination of two drugs is often used, it has not been validated by controlled trial. It is probably better to start treatment with sulphasalazine and, if this drug is ineffective, to replace it with prednisolone.

DRUGS WITH A POSSIBLE EFFECT ON IMMUNITY

Azathioprine and 6-mercaptopurine

Pharmacology and metabolism. 6-Mercaptopurine (6-MP) is a purine antagonist which interferes with nucleic acid synthesis. Azathioprine was derived from 6-MP by conjugation of a free SH group with the aim of decreasing toxicity without loss of effectiveness. Azathioprine is largely converted to 6-MP in the body and the similar metabolic pathways suggest that both drugs can be expected to have similar clinical effects.

After oral administration the drugs are absorbed to a variable extent, but there has been no work yet to correlate blood levels with clinical effectiveness in Crohn's disease. Breakdown of these drugs to the urinary metabolite, 6-thiouric acid, requires xanthine oxidase. If the xanthine oxidase inhibitor, allopurinol, is given, the rate of breakdown is reduced and toxic levels may result unless the dose of azathioprine or 6-MP is reduced.

Both drugs have proven immunosuppressant actions and could act in Crohn's disease by altering the immune response in an undefined way. The circulating K cell activity and the plasma cell count in the lamina propria rise in patients with Crohn's disease when the drug is stopped.[7] Patients with Crohn's disease treated with azathioprine have a significantly lower K cell activity than untreated patients.[8] Both drugs have a non-specific anti-inflammatory effect and there is some evidence that azathioprine has antibacterial activity against enteric anaerobes.

Potential side-effects. In high doses, both drugs suppress the bone marrow and this danger sets an upper limit to the doses that can be used for an inflammatory disorder. The dose of azathioprine used in Crohn's disease is usually between 2 and 2.5 mg/kg body weight daily. In the NCCDS trial, two out of 59 patients developed severe and seven moderate leucopenia while taking azathioprine at 2.5 mg/kg body weight daily for up to four months.[26] The only drug-related death among all reported controlled trials occurred from bone marrow failure after treatment with azathioprine in this dose range for 11 years.[20] The starting dose of 6-mercaptopurine used in the one controlled trial was 1.5 mg/kg body weight daily and on this dose most patients developed mild and two developed severe leucopenia.[22] Thus at these doses, regular blood counts, probably monthly, are needed.

About one in ten patients is unable to take these drugs because of some other side-effect. In the two largest controlled trials, one of which included 113 patients given azathioprine, and the other 68 patients given 6-MP, the following

complications caused treatment to be stopped: severe nausea (3), pancreatitis (6), fever (3), and leucopenia (6).[22, 26] All these side-effects resolved without long-term sequelae when the drug was stopped.

There has been concern that an increased frequency of malignant disease might occur among patients treated with immunosuppressive drugs. A prospective survey[11] among patients treated for a variety of disorders, but excluding transplants, included 280 patients with inflammatory bowel disease. Among the total series of 1349 patients, four developed non-Hodgkin's lymphoma (expected number = 0.34, $P < 0.001$), two squamous carcinoma of the skin (expected number = 0.38, $P = 0.06$) and 34 developed other tumours (expected number = 21.74, $P < 0.01$). The increased incidence of malignant disease could be due to other factors, for example some of the diseases treated could be associated with an increased incidence of malignant disease regardless of treatment. However, caution in the use of immunosuppressive drugs is clearly indicated especially as few patients have been followed after treatment for many years.

Evidence of therapeutic effectiveness. The clinical effectiveness will be considered in active disease, chronic active disease and quiescent disease.

1   Active disease. In the NCCDS trial no significant effect of azathioprine in active Crohn's disease was demonstrable, though the published results do show a trend in favour of the drug.[29] Two crossover trials have also failed to show that azathioprine is helpful in active Crohn's disease.[13, 23] These results must be accepted with caution because, in the NCCDS trial, corticosteroids were withdrawn from many patients just before azathioprine was started, and the part played by drug side-effects in limiting numbers of patients who completed the treatment period with azathioprine is difficult to assess. In the other two trials, there was a high proportion of patients with severe structural complications of the disease which would not be expected to respond to drug therapy.

2   Active chronic disease. A trial of 6-mercaptopurine was performed among 83 patients who were chronically ill, with a mean duration of continuous active symptoms of 4.3 years, and had been failures of therapy with sulphasalazine and steroids, but for whom surgery was not imminent.[22] Among 39 patients who received treatment with both 6-mercaptopurine and a control tablet during the two-year cross-

over design, 26 improved with 6-mercaptopurine and only three with placebo ($P < 0.0001$). Of all patients treated during the first year of the trial, 26 out of 36 who received 6-mercaptopurine improved compared with five out of 36 who received a control tablet ($P < 0.001$). In this trial, 60 out of 83 patients were taking prednisone in a mean dose of 20 mg daily and 43 patients were taking sulphasalazine. Among the 44 prednisone-treated patients who received 6-mercaptopurine for at least six months, it was possible to withdraw the steroid in 24 patients and reduce the dose substantially in another nine. By contrast, during placebo treatment, steroids could be discontinued or reduced in only 14 out of 39 patients ($P < 0.001$).

In a trial of azathioprine, prednisolone was given with or without this drug in the treatment of acute disease.[40] It proved possible to withdraw the prednisolone from most of the patients given azathioprine and 10 of these 11 patients remained in remission and completed the trial, whereas eight of 11 receiving placebo were withdrawn early because of relapse ($P < 0.01$). In another trial, 20 patients with Crohn's disease who had received at least 10 mg of prednisone daily over three months were divided equally into two groups and given in addition either azathioprine or a placebo tablet respectively.[24] The mean reduction of 15.5 mg in the daily dose of prednisone among those receiving azathioprine was greater than the mean reduction of 6.1 mg in the placebo group ($P < 0.05$).

3 Quiescent disease. A group of 51 patients who were in good health after treatment of their Crohn's disease with azathioprine, 2 mg/kg body weight daily for at least six months, was divided randomly and in double-blind fashion, either to a group in which azathioprine was continued or to one in which a control tablet was substituted.[20] The trial lasted one year unless relapse occurred earlier. The cumulative probability of relapse was nil at six months and 5% ($\pm$ 5 s.d.) at a year among those on azathioprine, compared with 25% ($\pm$ 9 s.d.) at 6 months and 41% ($\pm$ 11 s.d.) at a year among those in the control group ($P < 0.01$). The relapse rate did not correlate with the duration of pre-trial clinical remission or the duration of azathioprine treatment.

In the NCCDS trial azathioprine, 1 mg/kg body weight daily, was given for one or two years to patients who were well at the start of the trial.[29] Approximately 25% of patients in the trial experienced a relapse by the end of the first year and 40% by the end of the second year.

Patients receiving azathioprine did not rank significantly better than placebo as judged by life table analysis.

The role of azathioprine or 6-mercaptopurine in Crohn's disease. These two drugs act slowly over several months and exert a steroid-sparing and anti-inflammatory effect in patients with chronic active Crohn's disease. In such patients given azathioprine or 6-MP it is often possible to reduce the dose of or withdraw prednisolone. The disease tends to relapse when azathioprine or 6-MP are withdrawn and it is necessary to continue treatment for months or years, provided that the drug is well tolerated. At present, the optimal length of treatment cannot be defined. Since these drugs are potentially dangerous, one of them should be used only if simpler measures have failed, surgical treatment is inappropriate and the disease is causing ill health or disability. Azathioprine is best given in a dose of 2 mg/kg body weight and 6-mercaptopurine in an initial dose of 1.5 mg/kg body weight. Regular blood counts should be performed, probably at monthly intervals, though bone marrow depression is uncommon with these doses.

Other drugs given with the aim of affecting immune responses

Disodium cromoglycate is not absorbed from the gut and it was hoped that it would benefit inflammatory bowel disease by preventing liberation of histamine and other chemical mediators from mast cells, as it appears to do in asthma. Unfortunately, these hopes have not been fulfilled and a controlled trial has failed to show benefit in active or slightly active Crohn's disease.[3] Levamisole,[30, 39] oral BCG,[6] and transfer factor[36] have been tested in controlled trials without demonstrable benefit.

ANTIBACTERIAL DRUGS

Antibacterial drugs may reduce secondary infection or reduce the antigenic stimulus of enteric bacteria to diseased mucosa. An uncontrolled study has suggested that broad-spectrum antibiotics given continuously in various combinations over periods of up to five years can result in considerable benefit.[18] The only antibacterial drugs tested so far by controlled trial have been metronidazole and sulphadoxine/pyrimethamine.

Metronidazole

Metronidazole has a marked antibacterial action against anaerobic organisms such as *Bac-*

teroides species. When given by mouth the proportion of anaerobes in the faecal bacterial flora falls and there is a corresponding increase in aerobes so that the total flora is unchanged.[15]

Clinical experience. In a small double-blind crossover trial,[4] among 20 patients given metronidazole at 1 g daily for two months in addition to other treatments, clinical and haematological improvement ($P < 0.01$) was noted among the six patients with colonic disease but among the group as a whole the only significant effects were a rise in haemoglobin level and fall in sedimentation rate during the metronidazole period.

In a larger randomized double-blind crossover trial over 4 months, metronidazole, 0.4 g twice daily, was compared with sulphasalazine, 1.5 g twice daily, in patients with an elevated clinical activity index and serum orosomucoid level.[34] About one-third of the patients had disease confined to the small bowel and the remainder had colonic disease with or without ileal involvement. The clinical disease activity index improved to the same extent with both drugs during the first four months but the orosomucoid level fell and the haemoglobin level rose further in the metronidazole group. During the second four months after crossover, those patients who had not responded to sulphasalazine responded to metronidazole but there was no response to sulphasalazine after failure of metronidazole. The authors concluded that metronidazole is slightly more effective than sulphasalazine in the treatment of active Crohn's disease.

Uncontrolled observations have suggested that metronidazole, 20 mg/kg body weight, given over months, up to three years, benefited 26 patients with severe perineal Crohn's disease.[5] Deterioration of the perineal lesions occurred in about three-quarters of those in whom withdrawal of metronidazole was attempted.

Side-effects. The major side-effect of metronidazole is a peripheral neuropathy. In the group of patients treated with the drug at a dose of 20 mg/kg body weight daily, one-half developed paraesthesiae, usually of the feet, after a mean of 6.5 months. The neuropathy usually recovered over months when the drug was withdrawn (though it persisted for almost two years in one patient) and it disappeared in some patients when the dose was reduced. Other side-effects can be a metallic taste, nausea, anorexia, headache and a furry tongue. It is said that metronidazole can react with alcohol to give a disulfiram-like effect and moderation in alcohol consumption is usually advised, though few, if any patients complain of this side-effect.

There has been concern that metronidazole might be carcinogenic but no evidence that this is so in man has been forthcoming. Metronidazole did not induce an increased frequency of chromosomal aberrations at a daily dose of 800 mg for four months in a group of patients with Crohn's disease.[34] There is no conclusive evidence at present to suggest that the drug is teratogenic but in the absence of data caution is needed in the use of metronidazole during pregnancy.

Other antibacterial drugs
Sulphadoxine is a long-acting sulphonamide (half life 4–8 days) and pyrimethamine (closely related to trimethoprim, but longer acting) acts in sequential blockade with sulphonamides on folic acid metabolism. Together these drugs are active against a wide range of organisms, including some mycobacteria. In a controlled trial among 51 patients with chronic active Crohn's disease, this drug combination given in one dose weekly was compared with a control tablet; no benefit was apparent from the combined drug.[9]

Dapsone apparently benefited six patients to whom it was given,[37] but no further observations have been published. Antituberculous therapy, before the introduction of rifampicin and other newer drugs, did not appear beneficial.

SYMPTOMATIC DRUG TREATMENT

Anti-diarrhoeal drugs
Double-blind crossover studies have shown that loperamide decreases stool frequency and weight, with a corresponding trend towards solid consistency, in Crohn's disease, after ileocolic resection, or after colectomy and ileorectal anastomosis.[17, 21] In the first of these trials, loperamide in a mean dose of 6.9 mg daily was shown to be superior to diphenoxylate, at a mean dose of 17.7 mg daily, in terms of stool frequency and consistency ($P = 0.01$) and patients' preference ($P = 0.002$). Loperamide[33] and codeine phosphate[19] both reduce ileostomy output by about 20–25%; diphenoxylate appeared less effective.

When the terminal ileum is diseased or after ileal resection, bile salts entering the colon may cause secretion of water and electrolytes, and thus diarrhoea. Cholestyramine, 4 g daily or sometimes smaller doses with meals, can be helpful in this situation, but in practice this treatment is often either ineffective or unacceptable to the patient. In patients with ileal disease and diarrhoea, a trial of cholestyramine in full doses may be made. If there is no response the treatment should be abandoned; if there is a good response, the minimal dose of cholestyramine necessary to maintain improvement should be established by progressive reduction in the total daily use.

Antispasmodic and analgesic drugs
Antispasmodics are of doubtful benefit but are sometimes used in patients with bolus colic when no other treatment is possible. Certain patients with chronic pain, unrelieved by measures already outlined, seem to need regular doses of non-addictive analgesic drugs.

WHICH ASPECTS OF THE DISEASE RESPOND TO DRUG THERAPY?

Drug treatment can reduce inflammation of the gut and to some extent reduce secondary infection. Drugs can affect the function of the intestine to reduce diarrhoea or malabsorption. Lastly, by improving a sense of well-being or reducing local or systemic symptoms, drugs can improve appetite and thus nutrition.

Clinical assessment should define exactly what the patient is complaining of. Since Crohn's disease cannot be cured, treatment should be directed to the disability which it causes. Endoscopic and radiological investigations should be used to assess the detectable extent and structural complications of the disease. Appropriate measurements should be used to define any general or specific nutritional deficits.

Once this assessment is complete, drug therapy may be used, where appropriate, to try and relieve an inflammatory, infective, systemic or symptomatic component of the disorder. A limited goal should be set and simple observations recorded to establish whether or not the goal is achieved within a reasonable time. If no progress is made then a different treatment should be employed until a useful result is obtained. At every stage, all possible drug, nutritional and surgical therapies should be considered in deciding on a treatment policy.

DRUG TREATMENT OF DIFFERENT TYPES OF DISEASE

Crohn's disease of the lips and mouth
Crohn's disease may be associated with ulceration, and sometimes swelling, of the lips, buccal mucosa, gingival sulcus or tongue. Topical corticosteroids often appear helpful. Preparations available are slowly dissolving hydrocortisone lozenges, each containing 2.5 mg of hydrocortisone as the sodium succinate, which should be held between the gum and the cheek near an ulcer four times daily, or triamcinolone dental paste applied to the inflamed area several times daily. In very severe cases, prednisolone-21-phosphate (Prednesol) 5 mg in 30 ml of water can be used as a mouth wash and gargle before being swallowed three or four times daily.

Extensive involvement of the small intestine
Patients with widespread small bowel disease, but without obstructive symptoms due to strictures, often respond well to drug therapy. Some remain well as long as sulphasalazine is continued with a tendency to relapse when it is stopped. Antibacterial drugs may be tried and may be especially helpful if there is bacterial overgrowth in the small bowel. Corticosteroids by mouth generally help but often have to be continued in a maintenance dose equivalent to prednisolone, 10–15 mg daily, over months or years. In such circumstances, azathioprine may be useful for its steroid-sparing and anti-inflammatory effect.

Ileocaecal disease
Disease limited to the ileocaecal region tends to present with obstructive symptoms or local pain and tenderness. Drug therapy can produce temporary relief but rarely leads to satisfactory control of the disease in the long term. Surgical treatment is indicated or often becomes needed for persistent local pain, bolus colic, general ill health or a local complication. Sulphasalazine or metronidazole are worth initial trial if there is no clear indication for operation. Corticosteroid treatment may lead to symptomatic improvement but the drug is difficult to withdraw and local structural complications are liable to develop while treatment is continued.

Ileocolic and colonic disease
Patients with predominantly colonic disease often respond well to drug therapy. Sulphasalazine or metronidazole are usually the first drugs to try and, if successful, can be given over a prolonged period. Severe colitis with fever, anorexia, abdominal pain and tenderness, and diarrhoea often responds to a corticosteroid given intravenously. The usual regimen is to give 20 mg of prednisolone-21-phosphate as a bolus every eight hours. Less severely ill patients often respond to prednisolone 30 or 40 mg daily by

mouth, usually given in one morning dose, and continued for about two weeks before progressive reduction in dose over six to eight weeks once improvement has been obtained; sometimes relapse of symptoms tends to occur when the dose is reduced to 10 mg daily or less. In these circumstances, azathioprine can be given if there is no contraindication and the disease severity warrants its use, to take advantage of its steroid-sparing and anti-inflammatory effect.

Ano-rectal disease
Crohn's disease limited to the rectum and sigmoid colon may respond to topical corticosteroid therapy using suppositories (Predsol), a foam (Colifoam) or retention enemas. Prednisolone as the water-soluble metasulphabenzoate (Predenema) is absorbed less from an enema than prednisolone-21-phosphate (Predsol).

Topical treatment with sulphasalazine or 5-amino-salicylic acid as an enema, or sulphasalazine as a suppository, may also be beneficial.

Anal pain due to a chronic fissure or ulcer may respond to treatment with a steroid cream, such as betamethasone valerate (Betnovate 0.1%), applied by the patient on a rubber finger cot or anal dilator. This cream can also be applied to ulcers on the perineal skin or in the natal cleft or groins.

Perianal fistulas may cause surprisingly little disability, despite their appearance, as long as drainage of pus is free. Such fistulas may close, or become dry and indolent, if the intestinal disease is controlled as already described. Long-term metronidazole has been reported to give good results in a dose of 20 mg/kg body weight daily given over many months, though often results are disappointing. Most clinicians use a rather smaller dose as side-effects are common with this large dose.

Unhealed perineal wounds
In some patients surgical wounds fail to heal after treatment of fistulas or removal of the rectum. Widespread ulceration of the perineum with characteristic ulcers in the natal cleft and groins can develop.

Such patients are very difficult to treat. Surgical toilet and frequent cleansing of the area, with avoidance of maceration of healthy skin, are essential. Topical corticosteroids as a cream or applied as a solution of prednisolone-21-phosphate sometimes appear to help. In severe cases, if there is no response to local measures, systemic corticosteroids in a low dose such as prednisolone 10–20 mg combined with aza-

thioprine 2 mg/kg body weight daily, is a justifiable treatment and often appears to promote healing.

Crohn's disease with associated disorders
Intestinal disease associated with erythema nodosum, pyoderma or arthritis usually responds to systemic (oral or parenteral) corticosteroid therapy. Inflammation of the eye may occur without obvious activity of the intestinal disease and can often be treated by local measures. Sacroiliitis and ankylosing spondylitis tend to follow a course independent of the intestinal disease and require a non-steroidal anti-inflammatory drug for the relief of pain and stiffness.

Internal and external intestinal fistulas
Spontaneous fistulas between neighbouring loops of intestine generally require surgical treatment, though such fistulas can be an incidental finding in a symptomless patient. An enterovesical fistula is generally an indication for operation, but such fistulas can unexpectedly respond to medical treatment, especially if the fistula involves the rectum or distal colon. Some patients have been seen who become symptom-free after treatment with antibacterial drugs or azathioprine.

A spontaneous enterocutaneous fistula is generally the result of chronic intestinal perforation with subsequent rupture or drainage of the resulting abscess through the skin. Such fistulas do not usually close with drug therapy, unlike postoperative fistulas which tend to close spontaneously. Patients have been reported in whom closure of a spontaneous fistula has followed the use of azathioprine or 6-mercaptopurine but this is not the general experience. Antibacterial drugs may reduce the output of pus, but rarely eliminate the abscess cavity.

Intra-abdominal and perianal abscesses
Almost all such abscesses require surgical drainage. Since most are due to a chronic perforation of diseased intestine, the use of antibacterial drugs is unlikely to be successful. Similarly, perianal abscesses rarely respond to antibacterial drugs.

Obstructive episodes
Most obstructive episodes in Crohn's disease are due to structural narrowing of the gut or an adhesion from previous surgery. Occasionally, a corticosteroid given by mouth, perhaps combined with antibacterial drugs, may lead to temporary relief if the obstruction is due to an

exacerbation of Crohn's disease with oedema. Even so, elective surgical treatment is often needed for recurrent episodes. Drug treatment can be useful to obtain a temporary respite during which a patient's nutritional state can be improved before elective, rather than urgent, surgical treatment.

CONCLUSION

Drug treatment in Crohn's disease is only a part of the overall treatment which often includes dietary manipulation, nutritional replacement and surgical measures. Many patients never require any drug therapy, for example those who present with obstructive symptoms due to terminal ileal disease and who are successfully treated by resection of the diseased segment. At present drug treatment of Crohn's disease is non-specific, empirical and often disappointing. The physician looks forward to the day when a specific harmless remedy becomes available which can cure this distressing disorder or at least prevent recurrence after initial medical or surgical treatment.

REFERENCES

1 Anthonisen, P., Bárány, F., Folkenborg, O. et al. (1974) The clinical effect of salazosulphapyridine (Salazopyrin) in Crohn's disease: a controlled double-blind study. *Scandinavian Journal of Gastroenterology*, **9**, 549–554.

2 Bergman, L. & Krause, U. (1976) Postoperative treatment with corticosteroids and salicylazosulphapyridine (Salazopyrin) after radical resection for Crohn's disease. *Scandinavian Journal of Gastroenterology*, **11**, 651–656.

3 Binder, V., Elsborg, L., Greibe, J. et al. (1981) Disodium cromoglycate in the treatment of ulcerative colitis and Crohn's disease. *Gut*, **22**, 55–60.

4 Blichfeldt, P., Blomhoff, J. P., Myhre, E. & Gjone, E. (1978) Metronidazole in Crohn's disease: a double blind cross-over clinical trial. *Scandinavian Journal of Gastroenterology*, **13**, 123–127.

5 Brandt, L. J., Bernstein, L. H., Boley, S. J. & Frank, M. S. (1982) Metronidazole therapy for perineal Crohn's disease: a follow-up study. *Gastroenterology*, **83**, 383–387.

6 Burnham, W. R., Lennard-Jones, J. E., Hecketsweiler, P. et al. (1979) Oral BCG vaccine in Crohn's disease. *Gut*, **20**, 229–233.

7 Campbell, A. C., Skinner, J. M., Hersey, P. et al. (1974) Immunosuppression in the treatment of inflammatory bowel disease. I. Changes in lymphoid sub-populations in the blood and rectal mucosa following cessation of treatment with azathioprine. *Clinical and Experimental Immunology*, **16**, 521–533.

8 Eckhardt, R., Kloos, P., Dierich, M. P. & Meyer zum Büschenfelde, K. H. (1977) K-lymphocytes (Killer cells) in Crohn's disease and acute virus B-hepatitis. *Gut*, **18**, 1010–1016.

9 Elliott, P. R., Burnham, W. R., Berghouse, L. M. et al. (1982) Sulphadoxine–pyrimethamine therapy in Crohn's disease. *Digestion*, **23**, 132–134.

10 Kaplan, H. P., Portnoy, B., Binder, H. J. et al. (1975) A controlled evaluation of intravenous adrenocorticotrophic hormone and hydrocortisone in the treatment of acute colitis. *Gastroenterology*, **69**, 91–95.

11 Kinlen, L. J., Sheil, A. G. R., Peto, J. & Doll, R. (1979) Collaborative United Kingdom–Australasian study of cancer in patients treated with immunosuppressive drugs. *British Medical Journal*, **ii**, 1461–1466.

12 Kirschner, B. S., Voinchet, O. & Rosenberg, I. H. (1978) Growth retardation in inflammatory bowel disease. *Gastroenterology*, **75**, 504–511.

13 Klein, M., Binder, H. J., Mitchell, M. et al. (1974) Treatment of Crohn's disease with azathioprine: a controlled evaluation. *Gastroenterology*, **66**, 916–922.

14 Klotz, U., Maier, K., Fischer, C. & Heinkel, K. (1980) Therapeutic efficacy of sulfasalazine and its metabolites in patients with ulcerative colitis and Crohn's disease. *New England Journal of Medicine*, **303**, 1499–1502.

15 Krook, A., Danielsson, D., Kjellander, J. & Järnerot, G. (1981) The effect of metronidazole and sulfasalazine on the fecal flora in patients with Crohn's disease. *Scandinavian Journal of Gastroenterology*, **16**, 183–192.

16 Lennard-Jones, J. E. (1977) Sulphasalazine in asymptomatic Crohn's disease. *Gut*, **18**, 69–72.

17 Mainguet, P. & Fiasse, R. (1977) Double-blind placebo-controlled study of loperamide (Imodium) in chronic diarrhoea caused by ileocolic disease or resection. *Gut*, **18**, 575–579.

18 Moss, A. A., Carbone, J. V. & Kressel, H. Y. (1978) Radiologic and clinical assessment of broad-spectrum antibiotic therapy in Crohn's disease. *American Journal of Roentgenology*, **131**, 787–790.

19 Newton, C. R. (1978) Effect of codeine phosphate, Lomotil and Isogel on ileostomy function. *Gut*, **19**, 377–383.

20 O'Donoghue, D. P., Dawson, A. M., Powell-Tuck, J. et al. (1978) Double-blind withdrawal trial of azathioprine as maintenance treatment for Crohn's disease. *Lancet*, **ii**, 955–957.

21 Pelemans, W. & Vantrappen, G. (1976) A double-blind crossover comparison of loperamide with diphenoxylate in the symptomatic treatment of chronic diarrhoea. *Gastroenterology*, **70**, 1030–1034.

22 Present, D. H., Korelitz, B. I., Wisch, N. et al. (1980) Treatment of Crohn's disease with 6-mercaptopurine: a long-term randomized double-blind study. *New England Journal of Medicine*, **302**, 981–987.

23 Rhodes, J., Bainton, D., Beck, P. & Campbell, H. (1971) Controlled trial of azathioprine in Crohn's disease. *Lancet*, **ii**, 1273–1276.

24 Rosenberg, J. L., Levin, B., Wall, A. J. & Kirsner, J. B. (1975) A controlled trial of azathioprine in Crohn's disease. *Digestive Diseases*, **20**, 721–726.

25 Shaffer, J. L., Williams, S. E., Turnberg, L. A. et al. (1983) Absorption of prednisolone in patients with Crohn's disease. *Gut*, **24**, 182–186.

26 Singleton, J. W., Law, D. H., Kelley, M. L. jr. et al. (1979) National Co-operative Crohn's Disease Study: adverse reactions to study drugs. *Gastroenterology*, **77**, 870–882.

27 Singleton, J. W., Summers, R. W., Kern, F. jr. et al. (1979) A trial of sulfasalazine as adjunctive therapy in Crohn's disease. *Gastroenterology*, **77**, 887–897.

28 Smith, R. C., Rhodes, J., Heatley, R. V. et al. (1978) Low dose steroids and clinical relapse in Crohn's disease: a controlled trial. *Gut*, **19**, 606–610.

29 Summers, R. W., Switz, D. M., Sessions, J. T. jr. et al. (1979) National Co-operative Crohn's Disease Study: results of drug treatment. *Gastroenterology*, **77**, 847–869.

30 Swarbrick, E. T. & O'Donoghue, D. P. (1979) Levami-sole in Crohn's disease. *Lancet*, **i**, 392.

31 Tanner, A. R., Halliday, J. W. & Powell, L. W. (1981) Serum prednisolone levels in Crohn's disease and coeliac disease following oral prednisolone administration. *Digestion*, **21**, 310–315.

32 Toovey, S., Hudson, E., Hendry, W. F. & Levi, A. J. (1981) Sulphasalazine and male infertility: reversibility and possible mechanism. *Gut*, **22**, 445–451.

33 Tytgat, G. N. & Huibregtse, K. (1975) Loperamide and ileostomy output: placebo-controlled double-blind crossover study. *British Medical Journal*, **ii**, 667.

34 Ursing, B., Alm, T., Bárány, F. *et al.* (1982) A comparative study of metronidazole and sulfasalazine for active Crohn's disease: the Co-operative Crohn's Disease Study in Sweden. *Gastroenterology*, **83**, 550–562.

35 Van Hees, P. A. M., Van Lier, H. J. J., Van Elteren, P. H. *et al.* (1981) Effect of sulphasalazine in patients with active Crohn's disease: a controlled double-blind study. *Gut*, **22**, 404–409.

36 Vicary, F. R., Chambers, J. D. & Dhillon, P. (1979) Double-blind trial of the use of transfer factor in the treatment of Crohn's disease. *Gut*, **20**, 408–413.

37 Ward, M. & McManus, J. P. A. (1975) Dapsone in Crohn's disease. *Lancet*, **i**, 1236–1237.

38 Wenckert, A., Kristensen, M., Eklund, A. E. *et al.* (1978) The long-term prophylactic effect of salazosulphapyridine (Salazopyrin) in primarily resected patients with Crohn's disease. A controlled double-blind trial. *Scandinavian Journal of Gastroenterology*, **13**, 161–167.

39 Wesdorp, E., Schellekens, P. T. A., Weening, R. *et al.* (1977) Levamisole in Crohn's disease: a double-blind controlled trial. *Gut*, **18**, A971–A972.

40 Willoughby, J. M. T., Kumar, P. J., Beckett, J. & Dawson, A. M. (1971) Controlled trial of azathioprine in Crohn's disease. *Lancet*, **ii**, 944–947.

Surgical treatment

More than 80% of patients with Crohn's disease referred to us at the General Hospital, Birmingham, have required at least one operation and some of them have had three or four surgical procedures.[14] The mean number of resections in our patients being followed up with small intestinal disease is between two and four depending on the duration of follow up.[12] Not all operations for Crohn's disease involve major intestinal resection. Surgical management may be required simply to drain an abscess, assess painful disease under anaesthesia, excise a fistulous track, refashion a stoma or even to construct a stoma without resecting the bowel. Surgeons who are extensively involved in the management of patients with Crohn's disease are becoming increasingly conservative in the extent of resection, particularly for small bowel disease, in order to minimize the metabolic sequelae of the short bowel syndrome.

Patients with Crohn's disease face a lifetime disorder which will require metabolic monitoring, and surgical intervention is common (Table 12.16). Some patients will have to face the pro-

Table 12.16 Cumulative recurrence and reoperation rates (The General Hospital, Birmingham).

	5 years	10 years	15 years
Recurrence rates in the ileum			
Small bowel disease and ileal resection	20%	35%	47%
Large bowel disease and ileorectal anastomosis	30%	48%	—
Proctocolectomy and ileostomy	10%	20%	—
Re-operation rates			
Small bowel disease and ileal resection	20%	38%	50%
Large bowel disease and ileorectal anastomosis	50%	68%	—
Proctocolectomy and ileostomy	25%	40%	—

spect of an intestinal stoma, many will be worried about the influence of their disease or its surgical treatment on their sexual, social and family life.[27] Some patients will be receiving drugs which may increase the risk of operation or they may have associated medical disorders which could prove a hazard during anaesthesia. For all these reasons it is crucial that physicians and surgeons should work closely together as a team with specialist nursing staff, stoma therapists, those responsible for managing nutritional support, and dietitians. The group should meet regularly and preferably include a radiologist and histopathologist with a specialist interest in these patients. We have found that a weekly case conference which brings together medical, nursing and laboratory staff is invaluable in the optimum management of patients who have required hospital admission. We also find it helpful to undertake joint follow-up clinics between physician, surgeon and stoma therapists. By these means surgical management includes full discussion with a physician and the nursing staff. Surgical treatment is an important and established method of treatment and, furthermore, there is no evidence that the role of surgery is diminishing despite new therapeutic measures.[1]

GENERAL INDICATIONS FOR OPERATION

Operations for Crohn's disease are usually performed for the complications of the disease (Table 12.17). The most common indication is obstruction, particularly in the small bowel, but sometimes in the duodenum, colon and rectum as well. Abscesses and fistulas are also important indications for operation in Crohn's disease; the problems of management in such patients will

Table 12.17 The main indications for surgical treatment in Crohn's disease.

Obstruction
  Small bowel
  Colon or rectum
  Duodenum
Abscess
  Intra-abdominal
  Pelvic
  Peristomal
Fistulas
  Enterocutaneous
  Enterovaginal
  Enterovesical
  (Entero-enteric are rarely an indication for operation)
Diffuse colitis
  Failure of medical therapy
  Fulminating colitis
Perianal disease
  Gross destruction with incontinence
  Abscess
  (Fistula only in the absence of Crohn's proctitis)
Rare causes
  Haemorrhage
  Perforation
  Growth retardation
  Malignant change
Postoperative complications
  Fistula
  Abscess
  Intestinal obstruction
  Ileal obstruction
  Persistent perineal sinus
Stomal revision
  Recurrence
  Prolapse
  Resiting
  Bleeding
  Retraction

be dealt with separately. Extensive Crohn's colitis which has failed to respond to medical management is the most common indication for colectomy and progressive destructive perianal disease usually eventually requires proctectomy.

Less commonly, operation may be required for acute intestinal haemorrhage, perforation of the small or large bowel, acute fulminating colitis, growth retardation in the adolescent patient and malignant change. It is still sometimes necessary to perform a laparotomy in patients where the diagnosis remains in doubt or when it is impossible to distinguish inflammatory bowel disease from conditions such as a lymphoma, tuberculosis or carcinoma.

Whenever the surgeon is faced with a bowel resection for Crohn's disease he should undertake a very thorough laparotomy and meticulously record his operative findings. He should always perform a thorough pelvic examination and proctosigmoidoscopy preoperatively. The entire intestinal tract should be inspected for skip lesions, ulceration, fistulas and abscess. The

gallbladder should be carefully palpated and it is preferable to perform liver biopsy provided that it is not obscured by adhesions. The length of remaining healthy small bowel should be measured.

It is important that surgeons should appreciate that operations are not designed to cure Crohn's disease but merely to deal with the mechanical complications of fibrosis and sepsis. Hence massive resections, particularly of the small bowel, should be avoided. It must be realized that recurrence occurs and further resection will frequently be necessary. The greatest disservice that surgeons may inflict upon patients is to leave them with insufficient bowel. Care must also be taken to avoid creating a fistula, a blind loop or severe sepsis. Above all, surgeons must avoid postoperative mortality in this young population with non-malignant disease.

GASTRODUODENAL DISEASE

Gastroduodenal Crohn's disease is relatively uncommon,[18] occurring in only 0.4–7% of all patients with Crohn's disease. Fortunately it rarely requires surgical treatment. If the disorder progresses to cause obstructive symptoms an operation may be needed. The obstruction usually occurs in the second part of the duodenum. Alternatively the symptoms of duodenal Crohn's disease may mimic peptic ulcer disease with postprandial pain, vomiting and upper gastrointestinal bleeding. Indeed the Crohn's lesion may have the appearance of a peptic ulcer on barium examination. It is important to make the distinction between peptic ulcer and Crohn's disease and this can sometimes be difficult, particularly as patients after small bowel resection for Crohn's disease have an increased incidence of duodenal ulcer. Duodenal fistula from progressive Crohn's disease is rare and it is likely that most duodenal fistulas occur as a result of damage to the duodenum during excision of the hepatic flexure.

Operation is only advised if there are persistent symptoms and severe stenosis. Resection should be avoided unless the disease is responsible for extensive obstructive disease in the stomach. The treatment of choice is to bypass the stenosis by gastroenterostomy or duodenoenterostomy combined with vagotomy. Because of the risks of exacerbating small bowel diarrhoea, a proximal gastric vagotomy rather than truncal vagotomy is recommended. A Roux Y enteroduodenostomy may be required for the management of a duodenal fistula.

SMALL BOWEL DISEASE

The principal indication for operations on the small bowel is obstruction, particularly if there is no biochemical evidence of active disease.[7] The finding of normal levels of serum albumin, serum orosomucoids and C-reactive protein, haemoglobin and sedimentation rate are all helpful in this respect.

Ileocaecal resection
The majority of patients with small bowel Crohn's disease have a short segment of stenotic terminal ileal disease which stops abruptly at the caecum. The diseased segment may be adherent to other loops of small bowel, the fallopian tubes, the bladder or the sigmoid colon. There may be a small abscess between loops of bowel and the posterior abdominal wall or there may be entero-enteric fistulas. Despite this apparent complexity, it is usually possible to dissect the involved small bowel segment from other structures. Resection should be limited to the diseased segment and the lower pole of the caecum. It is quite unnecessary to perform the classical ileocolectomy to the mid-transverse colon because, after ileal resection, the right colon serves an important role in the absorption of water, electrolytes, vitamins and bile salts.

Small bowel strictures
One of the problems with small bowel Crohn's disease is that there may be multiple strictures. If the bowel between the strictures is grossly dilated or if the segment of healthy bowel between the stricture is less than 10 cm and there is plenty of normal proximal small intestine, then it is probably justified to resect the intervening bowel. If the affected segment is less than 10–20 cm from the ileocaecal valve, then it is probably wise to include the lower pole of the caecum and the appendix in the resection. If longer segments of macroscopically normal intervening bowel are present between these strictures, multiple small bowel resections with end-to-end anastomosis are generally advised. There may be a place for strictureplasty in patients who have had numerous previous small bowel resections with multiple strictures, particularly where there is relatively little healthy residual small bowel.[21] If this operation is being performed it is advisable to biopsy the strictured area, since malignant change cannot always be detected by its macroscopic appearance even when the bowel has been opened. The strictured area is opened by a longitudinal incision which is then closed transversely as in a pyloroplasty.

The principal of this very conservative approach to Crohn's strictures is to minimize the extent of small bowel resection. To date these operations have only been performed in a few specialist centres in patients with little remaining small bowel. These procedures cannot as yet be generally recommended because we do not know the incidence of recurrence or complications when diseased stenotic bowel is deliberately opened and sutured. However, the early results are encouraging.

Bypass procedures
The alternative approach in patients with extensive proximal skip lesions is to bypass the diseased segment by a side-to-side anastomosis. However, this temptation should be resisted unless the surgeon is contemplating total defunction of the segment by raising a proximal stoma. Many of the small intestinal carcinomas reported in the literature have been found in bypassed segments and their prognosis is poor because, as they do not cause obstruction, they present late.[26] Bypass operations also encourage small bowel bacterial overgrowth and may be responsible for malabsorption. There is no justification for performing a bypass in the belief that recurrence is less frequent than after resection. Hence resection should always be advised whenever feasible and safe.

Diffuse or acute disease
Resection should be avoided in diffuse small bowel disease and in acute non-obstructed ileal disease. Acute ileitis may be due to *Yersinia enterocolitica* and, if so, the prognosis without resection is excellent. Acute ileitis due to florid Crohn's disease is best treated by aggressive medical therapy.

Appendicectomy
The question of appendicectomy in Crohn's disease remains controversial. If the patient presents with a short history and physical signs which are indistinguishable from acute appendicitis and the abdomen is explored through a grid iron incision, then removal of a normal or an acutely inflamed appendix is advised even if the small bowel is diseased, since postoperative fistulas are rare and they nearly always arise from the proximal small bowel and not the appendix. If, on the other hand, the history is longer and an exploratory laparotomy is performed, resection is not advised if there is florid ileitis and a normal appendix. Ileocaecal resection may be indicated if, at laparotomy for an acute abdomen, the appendix and terminal

ileum are both chronically diseased and obstructed. However, this last situation should not arise today since all patients with chronic obstructive symptoms should have been thoroughly investigated beforehand.

Recurrence

Recurrence usually occurs at the site of a previous anastomosis and rates vary with duration of follow up. Approximately 20% of patients have developed recurrence at 5 years, 35% at 10 years and 47% at 15 years (Table 12.16). There is no evidence that recurrence is increased in patients who have had repeated operations or in patients presenting at an early age. However, recurrence may be more frequent in patients with a short history of Crohn's disease. At one time there was a vogue amongst surgeons to resect all the macroscopically affected disease and then to undertake an even wider excision if frozen section biopsies from the resection lines showed evidence of granuloma. It is now well established that neither the presence of granuloma at the resection lines nor the extent of resection influence the rate of recurrence. The importance of wide lymphatic clearance remains unanswered. It has been suggested that lymphatic obstruction may increase the risk of recurrence; however, most surgeons take the view that involved lymph nodes should only be resected provided that lymphatic clearance does not jeopardize the blood supply and increase the length of bowel which needs to be resected. Even when the lymph nodes are necrotic and colonized by bacteria, resection of the involved bowel alone is usually associated with complete clinical and radiological resolution of the local disease.

LARGE-BOWEL DISEASE

The indications for elective operation on the large bowel are less precise than for small bowel disease. Many patients with Crohn's colitis are chronically unwell with weight loss, anorexia, disabling diarrhoea or chronic anaemia. Operation in such patients is only indicated if medical treatment with steroids, sulphasalazine, azathioprine or even antimicrobial agents fails. By contrast, the indications for operation in patients with an abscess, an enterocutaneous fistula or a stenotic segment are more clearly defined. Emergency colectomy is sometimes necessary in patients who have not responded to an intensive medical regimen or with acute life-threatening bleeding, toxic dilatation or perforation. Approximately 60% of patients with Crohn's colitis require colectomy.

Emergency operation

It should be remembered that Crohn's colitis may present as acute fulminating colitis which is indistinguishable from acute ulcerative colitis. The prognosis in such patients is extremely poor if surgical treatment is delayed to the stage in which faecal peritonitis occurs.[23] Repeated plain abdominal X-rays should be performed to detect early dilatation. Microscopy of the stool must always be performed to exclude amoebiasis, *Campylobacter*, *Clostridium difficile* colitis and other specific enteropathogens. It is dangerous to try to establish the diagnosis by barium enema but useful information may be obtained by an air contrast examination after sigmoidoscopy. In patients with acute fulminating colitis, failure to respond to medical therapy with steroids, fluid replacement and antibiotics within 72 hours is an absolute indication for colectomy. The most appropriate operation is to excise the colon, establish an end ileostomy and oversew the rectal stump if this is feasible. If the rectum cannot be oversewn, a mucus fistula may be constructed, but they are troublesome to manage and are best avoided if possible. If the rectum is very severely diseased and cannot be oversewn it is usually safe to transect the bowel low in the pelvis and drain the open viscus. It is rarely, if ever, necessary to perform a single stage emergency panproctocolectomy.

Some patients frequently have an initial response to medical therapy but remain ill with fever, profuse diarrhoea, continuing weight loss and progressive hypoalbuminaemia. In such cases, the possibility of surgical treatment and the need for a stoma should be discussed with the patient. If no improvement has been established within three weeks despite steroid therapy then colectomy should be advised, leaving the rectal stump so that subsequent anastomosis is still possible. The place of total parenteral nutrition in patients with acute fulminating colitis remains controversial, but at least one trial has suggested that it did not influence mortality or the colectomy rate.

Elective operation

The type of elective operation appropriate for patients with large bowel Crohn's disease depends to some extent on the wishes of the patient, the location of the disease and the age of presentation.

We and others are increasingly referred elderly patients with Crohn's disease. Many of these patients have coexisting diverticular disease and it is often difficult to distinguish the two disorders. The management of these patients poses special problems. Restoration of intestinal continuity is often not practical because of poor anal tone and rectal involvement. Restorative resection is also hazardous and associated with a high morbidity and mortality. The alternative option of a stoma in the geriatric population with arthritis and poor eyesight is strongly resisted. Hence, every effort is made to avoid surgical intervention in the elderly.

Panproctocolectomy. Radical excision of the entire colon and rectum for Crohn's disease is by panproctocolectomy which involves construction of a permanent ileostomy. A stoma, particularly in younger patients, may be difficult to accept and there may be complications such as skin excoriation, stenosis, retraction, prolapse, bleeding and ileostomy flux, to mention but a few (Table 12.18). However, ileal recurrence rates after proctocolectomy and end ileostomy are lower than after any other operation for Crohn's disease, being approximately 10% at 5 years and 20% at 10 years. The other complications of proctocolectomy include delayed perineal wound healing and sexual dysfunction. Only 60% of perineal wounds are healed six months after operation,[5] and many patients are left with a persistent perineal sinus which intermittently discharges and may be the site of recurrent abscesses. The incidence of sexual problems is difficult to document accurately and must be assessed prospectively.[10] There are

Table 12-18 Late stoma complications.

> *Skin excoriation*
> *Badly sited stoma*
>   Too close to bony prominences
>   Too close to the umbilicus
>   Too close to scars
>   Placed outside the rectus sheath
> *Prolapse of stoma*
> *Interstitial hernia*
> *Parastomal hernia*
> *Intestinal obstruction*
>   Lateral gutter
>   Volvulus
> *Sinuses and parastomal abscess*
> *Parastomal fistulas*
> *Retraction of stoma*
> *Bleeding*
>   Trauma
>   Caput medusae
>   Recurrence
> *Stenosis*
>   Ischaemia
>   Recurrence
> *Ileostomy flux*
>   Intercurrent infection
>   Gastroenteritis
>   Local sepsis
>   Recurrence

some patients with sexual difficulties before operation, some of which are a consequence of their disease. Dyspareunia is the most common difficulty in the female whereas impotence and failure to maintain an erection are the symptoms most frequently reported in men. If there is minimal perianal disease, intersphincteric rectal excision allows excellent primary perineal healing providing there has been no faecal contamination. Furthermore, the incidence of sexual difficulties, particularly in women, is said to be less after this procedure.

Disturbances of the autonomic plexus by the abdominal operator should be avoided at all costs. This is often difficult in Crohn's colitis, particularly if there is extensive perirectal induration as in patients with a rectal stricture or with perirectal fistulas. Nevertheless, a radical vascular clearance as in operations for colorectal cancer are never indicated, and the plane of dissection, though more tedious, must stay close to the bowel distal to the rectosigmoid junction. It is worth reassuring patients that recovery of sexual function may still occur up to 18 months after the resection.

If there is severe perianal disease with established perineal infection or if faecal contamination has occurred, it is wise to leave the perineal and abdominal wounds open. Silastic foam is particularly useful in the management of the open perineal wound.

There is no place for a continent reservoir ileostomy or ileoanal anastomosis with a pelvic pouch in Crohn's disease. Hence, most surgeons rarely advise these procedures as a single stage operation since the true histology of the colon may only become apparent after the bowel has been removed and thoroughly examined by the pathologist.

Abdominoperineal excision. Resection of the rectum with an end colostomy is an operation which is advocated for more elderly patients with severe anal or rectal disease who have an apparently normal colon on barium enema examination or colonoscopy. Unfortunately, the colon in Crohn's disease is never normal and many patients who have had this operation on our unit report dissatisfaction with the flush colostomy which tends to discharge liquid faeces. Although the recurrence rates in these elderly patients is reported to be as low as 6% at 5 years and 11% at 10 years,[24] we have experienced a high incidence of left-sided colonic recurrence in the early postoperative follow-up. For these reasons I find that there are few patients with Crohn's disease suitable for abdominoperineal excision.

Total colectomy and ileorectal anastomosis. Accurate selection of patients who are suitable for restorative resection by ileorectal anastomosis is important, otherwise there is likely to be a high incidence of early rectal recurrence requiring proctectomy and ileostomy. Ileorectal anastomosis is advised only for patients with minimal rectal disease, quiescent anal disease and where an extensive small bowel resection is not needed. Careful evaluation is therefore necessary by rectal examination, proctoscopy, sigmoidoscopy, barium enema and small bowel X-rays. Measurement of rectal capacity with an air-filled balloon is a useful additional assessment, since recurrent rectal disease is uncommon if the rectal capacity is more than 200 cm^3 air.[16]

The operation is particularly useful for younger patients, especially those who are unmarried or who have not had any family. The procedure does not involve a pelvic dissection hence sexual and urinary complications are rare. Furthermore, it is less traumatic physically and psychologically than panproctocolectomy. Recurrence rates vary widely but approximately 40% of patients have had a proctectomy at 5 years and 60% at 10 years. If there are any technical difficulties with the anastomosis or the rectal disease seems more severe than was thought, either a loop ileostomy may be constructed proximal to the anastomosis or the rectal stump oversewn and an end ileostomy fashioned. Although there is a high incidence of recurrence after ileorectal anastomosis, many such recurrences occur in the ileum immediately proximal to the initial anastomosis. Under these circumstances it is possible to resect the ileal recurrence and restore intestinal continuity, provided the rectum remains relatively uninvolved by Crohn's disease.

Faecal diversion alone. There has been recent interest in the place of faecal diversion alone for Crohn's colitis.[20] The protagonists of this approach report that the operative mortality is low and that a prolonged remission may occur in some patients so that the stoma can be closed at a later date. However, the majority of patients require an intestinal resection and the stoma cannot always be safely closed. The procedure has been used for young patients with active acute colonic disease which has not responded to medical treatment and where a major operation might have serious educational, sexual, procreational or financial implications. Faecal diversion has also been advised for some adolescent patients with growth retardation or in young patients with severe perianal disease. The

operation involves a laparotomy, the diversion may be constructed either as a loop ileostomy, in which case laparotomy is not necessary for closure, or as a split ileostomy, in which case another laparotomy is required. However, only 30% of patients after this procedure have been able to have the stoma closed without an intestinal resection, although a further 20% have had a local resection with restoration of intestinal continuity. We prefer the loop ileostomy for faecal diversion since the patients do not have the bother of managing a mucus fistula as well as an ileostomy and closure may be performed without a laparotomy. It has been argued that the loop ileostomy may not completely defunction the distal bowel since ileostomy contents may theoretically enter the distal stoma, but we have never been able to demonstrate this phenomenon radiologically. The loop ileostomy has been a useful means of protecting a difficult anastomosis, avoiding resection of a leaking intestinal suture line and managing certain intestinal fistulas.

PERIANAL DISEASE

Anal disorders such as abscesses, fistulas, fissures, skin tags, ulcers and rectal strictures may precede the clinical manifestations of bowel disease in 7–13% of Crohn's patients. Anal disorders occur in 60–70% of patients at some stage of their disease. Until recently little was known about the natural history of anal Crohn's disease. We have recorded spontaneous healing in 50% of patients with anal fissures and also in a few patients with anal fistulas.[6] Proctectomy is eventually required in only 20% of patients with anal Crohn's disease. It is important to exclude tuberculosis, venereal infections, hydradenitis suppurativa, amoebiasis and malignancy in patients with abnormal anal lesions. Most anal lesions look as though they must be painful but in fact cause patients very little discomfort. Hence surgical treatment should usually be avoided. Incidental lesions such as haemorrhoids or a low-lying fistula should not be treated in the presence of active anorectal inflammatory bowel disease. In quiescent Crohn's disease or where there is no proctitis, haemorrhoids may be treated locally by injection, rubber-band ligation or photocoagulation, but hàemorrhoidectomy is best avoided. Skin tags usually cause very few symptoms and surgical excision should be avoided. Low anorectal fistulas may safely be laid open if there is no rectal disease. Treatment of the specific Crohn's lesion or its complications is straightforward, provided the following principles are adhered to: loculated pus in the perianal region should be drained early, high fistulas are best left alone, a course of metronidazole is often beneficial for patients with diffuse perianal sepsis, and symptomatic strictures can be gently dilated.

SPECIAL SURGICAL CONSIDERATIONS

Abscess

Preoperative abscess. Approximately 10% of patients with Crohn's disease require an operation because of an abscess complicating their intestinal disease. These abscesses may be located in the pelvis, the psoas sheath, between loops of bowel, in the abdominal wall or even under the liver. Such abscesses are often associated with a stenotic segment of bowel and transmural fissures, but they may be due to breakdown of a group of infected lymph nodes. Untreated, many of these lesions progress to form fistulas; entero-enteric fistulas are particularly common when Crohn's disease is associated with an abscess.

Preoperative diagnosis of an abscess may be difficult since fever and leucocytosis are not invariable and also occur as part of the clinical picture of active disease. This distinction is important because steroid therapy is best avoided in patients with an abscess. Most patients with an abscess have marked hypoalbuminaemia with elevated serum alkaline phosphatase levels. Abscess localization may be possible using indium-111-labelled mixed leucocyte scans (Figure 12.39), ultrasonography and CT scanning. These abscesses usually contain mixed organisms principally *Escherichia coli*, a variety of streptococci, and *Bacteroides* sp.[17] Treatment should involve resection of the diseased bowel and drainage of the abscess under antibiotic cover. Recurrence of an intra-abdominal abscess within six months of operation is quite common and has occurred in 30% of our patients; hence, if a patient develops marked anorexia and weight loss after an initial satisfactory postoperative convalescence, a diagnosis of recurrent abscess should be considered. A broad-spectrum penicillin should probably be added to the antibiotic cover in these patients because of a high isolation rate of *Streptococcus milleri*.

Postoperative abscess. Abscesses are an important complication of Crohn's resection and occur in 12–17% of patients. The microbiology of these abscesses do not differ from preoperative lesions but the volume of pus is generally greater and they are frequently multiple. Treatment involves drainage of pus either by a further laparotomy or under X-ray control using percutaneous drainage. The latter technique is particularly useful in seriously ill patients developing an abscess in the early postoperative period. Such procedures demand close cooperation between the surgeon and the radiologist.

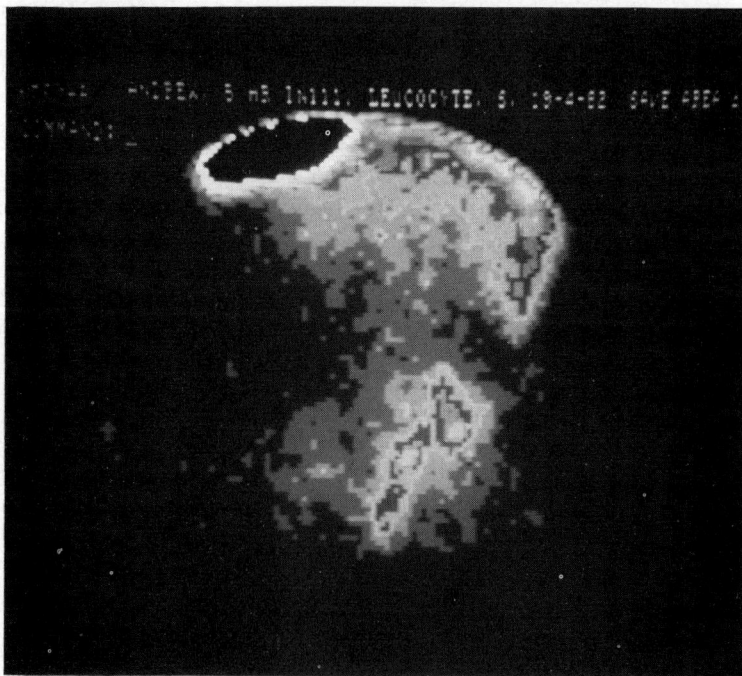

Fig. 12.39 [111]Indium mixed leucocyte scan demonstrating a left psoas abscess.

Abdominal fistulas

Preoperative fistulas. Intestinal fistulas are a common manifestation of Crohn's disease, and are present in 10–15% of patients. Fistulas may be internal, such as ileoileal, ileocolonic, enterovaginal, or enterovesical. External enteroenteric fistulas usually arise from a stenotic segment of disease which has become adherent to a loop of normal intestine as a consequence of deep fissures in the stenotic bowel. They are not in themselves an indication for operation. At operation it is important to identify which is the principal segment of involved intestine since surgical treatment merely involves removing the primary diseased bowel and oversewing the fistulous connection to the macroscopically normal intestine (or bladder or vagina).

Enterocutaneous fistulas require careful preoperative investigation by barium contrast studies of the small and large intestine, contrast studies through the fistula or the stoma if one is present, as well as intravenous pyelography. Many of these fistulas are complex and may enter three or four loops of bowel.[2]

There is no evidence that parenteral or enteral nutrition achieves long-term healing of preoperative enterocutaneous fistulas since there is nearly always distal obstruction, active Crohn's disease or direct mucosal continuity with the skin. The treatment of enterocutaneous fistulas is by surgical resection of the diseased bowel and closure of any fistulous communication to healthy intestine. The skin track should be excised and the skin defect left open to granulate. If the fistula has been complex or if there has been damage to loops of bowel during the dissection, a proximal loop ileostomy is worth considering. An alternative approach is to feed the patient entirely by total parenteral nutrition until the immediate postoperative dangers are past. These operations can be tedious and extremely demanding and require patience. It is often unnecessary to resect a large segment of bowel unless the colon is the site of the fistula.

Postoperative fistulas. Postoperative fistulas are much more difficult to manage and are more demanding on medical resources. These fistulas are usually associated with severe sepsis and malnutrition. There are five phases in the management of postoperative fistulas: resuscitation, drainage of the pus, defining the anatomy of the fistulas, maintaining nutrition, and operation if necessary. Resuscitation by adequate replacement of fluid and electrolytes is mandatory since most patients developing postoperative fistulas

are gravely ill with hypovolaemia, bacteraemic shock, acidosis and prerenal failure. As soon as fluid has been replaced and electrolyte deficiencies corrected (usually this takes 24 hours) the patient should be considered for a laparotomy to drain any areas of localized infection and to exteriorize bowel if necessary. As soon as these measures have been undertaken the patient's general condition improves and nutritional support should be commenced.

It is not always necessary to use parenteral nutrition; enteral nutritional support is safer, cheaper and just as effective provided the fistula arises from the terminal ileum or colon. However, enteral nutrition is rarely feasible at the outset of treatment because the development of a postoperative fistula is usually associated with prolonged paralytic ileus. For these reasons it is usually necessary to provide nutritional support by a central vein using a subcutaneous cannula inserted under strict aseptic conditions. The nutritional fluid is best provided by daily prescription so that all calorie, nitrogen, vitamin and electrolyte replacements are placed in 3 l bags made up under aseptic conditions.

Once the nutritional support has been established, the site of the fistula and the presence of distal obstruction should be carefully assessed by appropriate radiological study. Total parenteral nutrition should be continued for at least six weeks; under these circumstances 60% of postoperative fistulas will heal. If a fistula has not healed by six weeks there is usually an anatomical reason why it has not and surgical treatment will then be necessary.

Urinary complications (Table 12.19)

Urinary infection and stones. Urinary tract disorders are relatively uncommon in patients with Crohn's disease.[19] Cystitis occurs in 5% of patients and does not differ from that occurring in the population at large. Renal or ureteric stones are present in 4% of patients, are usually

Table 12.19 Urinary tract involvement among 429 patients with Crohn's disease.[19]

Complication	No. of patients
Cystitis	70
Pyelonephritis	3
Renal/ureteric calculi	9
Hydronephrosis	9
Ileovesical fistula	9
Retroperitoneal abscess and hydroureter	3
Retention of urine (female)	1
Rectourethral fistula	1

composed of oxalate, and tend to occur after extensive small bowel resection. Calculi are treated by conventional methods but a diet low in oxalate should be advised. Hydronephrosis is present in 2% of patients, is rarely severe, and is often associated with ileocaecal disease, particularly when a psoas abscess is present. The right kidney is more commonly affected than the left. Ureteric obstruction is usually a complication of retroperitoneal fibrosis due to recurrent intestinal disease at the pelvic brim.

Urinary fistulas. Fistulas between the intestinal and urinary tract may be present in 2–4% of patients; they are often complex. The most common communication is between the small bowel and the bladder. Treatment is relatively straightforward since the primary disease is always in the ileum which requires resection, and the bladder lesion can be safely oversewn provided a urethral catheter is left in situ for seven to ten days after the operation. More difficult is the triple fistula between small bowel, sigmoid colon and bladder. Fortunately, most bladder fistulas enter on the dome and not at the trigone. Occasionally, Crohn's disease is associated with recto-urethral, urethroperineal and entero-ureteric fistulas.

Postoperative urinary complications. Postoperative urinary complications are common. There may be voiding difficulties, particularly in female patients, after rectal excision due to loss of the normal urethrovesical angle, or to autonomic damage during proctectomy. Urethroperineal fistulas may occur if the urethra is damaged during proctectomy; they usually take a long time to heal and a urethral stricture is almost inevitable. If there has been damage to the bladder during colectomy resulting in a postoperative enterovesical fistula, healing is often delayed and may be associated with a contracted low-volume bladder, particularly if surgical repair has been necessary.

BOWEL PREPARATION

Mechanical bowel preparation is rarely necessary or indeed desirable for patients requiring intestinal resections for Crohn's disease. Bowel preparation is unnecessary for terminal ileal or ileocaecal resection and for patients requiring a proctocolectomy or abdominoperineal excision with an end ileostomy or colostomy. Mechanical preparation is dangerous in patients with acute colonic disease. It is not really necessary for total colectomy and ileorectal anastomosis since the suture line is well above the sacral promontary and the contents of the colon are liquid. Hence the faecal residue can be milked back into the colon or into the rectum below a soft non-crushing clamp to prevent contamination during suture of the ileorectal anastomosis.

ANTIBIOTIC COVER

Antibiotic cover is advised in all patients requiring an operation for Crohn's disease even though the procedure may seem relatively trivial, as for instance the closure of a colostomy. The organisms which are principally responsible for postoperative infection are *Escherichia coli*, *Proteus* sp., *Klebsiella* sp. and *Bacteroides fragilis*. Certain streptococci may be responsible for persistent intra-abdominal abscess.

I believe that a clear distinction should be made between potentially and frankly contaminated operations. If there has been no gross faecal spillage, in an uncontaminated operative field, short-term perioperative antibiotic prophylaxis is adequate, beginning with a single intravenous bolus dose in the anaesthetic room and continuing for 24 hours after operation. If on the other hand there has been gross contamination at the time of operation or if there is existing sepsis, as for instance in patients with an abscess, fistulas or severe infective perianal disease, the duration of antibiotic cover should be extended to five days.[11]

It is also advisable to leave any grossly contaminated wounds open, closing only the abdominal wall. It is particularly helpful to leave perineal wounds widely open if there has been any operative damage to the rectum or if there has been extensive perianal or perirectal sepsis. Subsequent management of these wounds has been greatly facilitated using silastic foam which forms a sponge dressing to fit the granulating cavity. The foam dressing may be removed whilst taking a bath, soaked in chlorhexidine and easily replaced later.

There is now considerable evidence that systemic perioperative antibiotic cover is as good and certainly safer than giving oral antimicrobials with a mechanical bowel preparation. The dangers of oral antimicrobials are the development of antibiotic resistance, superinfection by staphylococci, and *Clostridium difficile*-associated colitis.[15] Metronidazole has clearly reduced the morbidity of these operations but should be combined with an agent such as an aminoglycoside or a cephalosporin active against the aerobic Gram-negative bacteria. It is also advisable to prescribe a broad-spectrum penicillin if the patient is found at laparotomy to have an intra-abdominal abscess since persistent low-grade streptococcal infection may be responsible for recurrent abscess.

MORTALITY IN CROHN'S SURGERY

The mortality following operations for Crohn's disease is extremely variable, ranging from 1.5 to 18.3%.[1, 17] However, at least 60% of deaths occur after surgical operations. The deaths in all patients with acute colitis requiring operation is still very high and reported as over 40% in non-specialized general hospitals. Mortality is influenced by age, nutritional status, sepsis, whether or not the patient requires an emergency operation, and whether the operation is the first resection or for recurrent disease.[8, 9] It is inappropriate to report on mortality figures following operations performed over 25 years ago when appropriate antibiotics were not available, when anaesthesia was inferior, and when patients received inadequate fluid and electrolyte resuscitation prior to operation. The overall mortality of patients with Crohn's disease in our hospital was reported to be 15%, but the Crohn's disease-related deaths were only 7%. Many of these deaths occurred in the early years of experience and many were from fluid and electrolyte disturbance or from complications of steroid therapy that should now be avoidable. In a personal series over the past six years there were only two deaths following 124 resections for Crohn's disease, one from sepsis and the other from a massive pulmonary embolus. A mortality figure of 2% has been reported from the Cleveland Clinic after initial surgical resection. Goligher[9] also reports operative mortality from initial resections of 4.1%, but the mortality for subsequent operations rose to 8.3%. The units from which low mortality figures emanate nearly always comprise groups of experienced and interested surgeons who work in close collaboration with gastrointestinal physicians.[25] Mortality is frequently associated with delayed operation when patients are grossly malnourished, infected, and have complex fistulas. It is essential, therefore, to consider surgical options at an early stage when medical therapy fails or when patients develop complications of their disease. There is no evidence that total parenteral nutrition has reduced surgical mortality except in the management of serious postoperative complications.

REFERENCES

1 Alexander-Williams, J. (1983) A review of surgical management and directions of future research. In *Inflammatory Bowel Diseases* (Ed.) Allan, R. N., Keighley, M. R. B., Hawkins, C. E. & Alexander-Williams, J. pp. 496–505. Edinburgh: Churchill Livingstone.

2 Alexander-Williams, J. & Irving, M. (1982) *Intestinal Fistula.* Bristol: Wright.

3 Allan, R., Steinberg, D., Alexander-Williams, J. & Cooke, W. T. (1977) Crohn's disease involving the colon: an audit of clinical management. *Gastroenterology*, **73**, 723–732.

4 Ambrose, N. S., Keighley, M. R. B., Alexander-Williams, J. & Allan, R. N. (1983) Clinical impact of colectomy and ileorectal anastomosis in the management of Crohn's disease. *Gut*, in press.

5 Baudot, P., Keighley, M. R. B. & Alexander-Williams, J. (1980) Perineal wound healing after proctectomy for carcinoma and inflammatory disease. *British Journal of Surgery*, **67**, 257–276.

6 Buchmann, P., Keighley, M. R. B., Allan, R. N. *et al.* (1980) Natural history of perianal Crohn's disease. *American Journal of Surgery*, **140**, 642–644.

7 Cooke, W. T., Fowler, D. I., Cox, E. V. *et al.* (1958) The clinical significance of seromucoids in regional ileitis and ulcerative colitis. *Gastroenterology*, **34**, 910–919.

8 Fazio, V. W. (1983) The surgery of Crohn's disease of the small bowel. In *Inflammatory Bowel Diseases* (Ed.) Allan, R. N., Keighley, M. R. B., Hawkins, C. E. & Alexander-Williams, J. pp. 452–461. Edinburgh: Churchill Livingstone.

9 Goligher, J. C. (1980) *Surgery of the Anus, Rectum and Colon*, 4th Edn. London: Baillière Tindall.

10 Gruner, O. P., Naas, R., Frethelm, B. & Gjone, E. (1977) Marital status and sexual adjustment after colectomy. Results in 179 patients operated upon for ulcerative colitis. *Scandinavian Journal of Gastroenterology*, **12**, 1913–1917.

11 Hares, M. M., Bentley, S., Allan, R. N. *et al.* (1982) Clinical trials of the efficacy and duration of anti-bacterial cover for elective resection in inflammatory bowel disease. *British Journal of Surgery*, **69**, 215–217.

12 Higgens, C. S. & Allan, R. N. (1980) Crohn's disease of the distal ileum. *Gut*, **21**, 933–940.

13 Keighley, M. R. B. (1980) Antibiotic associated pseudomembranous colitis: pathogenesis and management. *Drugs*, **20**, 49–56.

14 Keighley, M. R. B. & Ambrose, N. S. (1982) Surgical considerations of Crohn's disease. In *Recent Advances in Surgery* (Ed.) Russell, R. C. G. pp. 197–207. Edinburgh: Churchill Livingstone.

15 Keighley, M. R. B. & Burdon, D. W. (1979) *Antimicrobial Prophylaxis in Surgery.* Tunbridge Wells: Pitman Medical.

16 Keighley, M. R. B., Buchmann, P. & Lee, J. R. (1982) Assessment of anorectal function in selection of patients for ileorectal anastomosis in Crohn's colitis. *Gut*, **23**, 102–107.

17 Keighley, M. R. B., Eastwood, D., Ambrose, N. S. *et al.* (1982) Incidence and microbiology of abdominal and pelvic abscess in Crohn's disease. *Gastroenterology*, **83**, 1271–1275.

18 Kyle, J. (1982) Gastroduodenal involvement of Crohn's disease. *Journal of the Royal College of Surgeons of Edinburgh*, **27**, 327–332.

19 Kyle, J. (1983) Involvement of the urinary tract in Crohn's disease. In *Inflammatory Bowel Diseases* (Ed.) Allan, R. N., Keighley, M. R. B., Hawkins, C. E. & Alexander-Williams, J. pp. 481–486. Edinburgh: Churchill Livingstone.

20 Lee, E. (1975) Split ileostomy in the treatment of Crohn's disease of the colon. *Annals of the Royal College of Surgeons of England*, **56**, 94–102.

21 Lee, E. & Papaioannou, M. D. (1982) Minimal surgery for chronic obstruction in patients with extensive or universal Crohn's disease. *Annals of the Royal College of Surgeons of England*, **64**, 230–233.

22 Pennington, L., Hamilton, S. R., Bayliss, T. M. & Camera, J. L. (1980) Surgical management of Crohn's disease: influence of disease on margin of resections. *Annals of Surgery*, **192**, 311–318.

23 Ritchie, J. K. (1983) Audit of surgery for acute colitis. *Journal of the Royal Society of Medicine*, in press.

24 Ritchie, J. K. & Lennard-Jones, J. E. (1976) Crohn's disease of the distal large bowel. *Scandinavian Journal of Gastroenterology*, **11**, 433–436.

25 Truelove, S. C. & Pena, A. S. (1976) Course and prognosis of Crohn's disease. *Gut*, **17**, 192–201.

26 Weedon, D. D., Shooter, R. G., Ilstrup, D. M. *et al.* (1973) Crohn's disease and cancer. *New England Journal of Medicine*, **289**, 1099–1103.

27 Whelton, M. J. & Findlay, J. M. (1971) Ileostomy and colostomy care. *British Journal of Hospital Medicine*, **24**, 315–322.

CANCER IN CROHN'S DISEASE

Although it seems likely that there is an association between cancer of the gastrointestinal tract and Crohn's disease, it is not as well documented as the association between colorectal cancer and ulcerative colitis. Since Ginzburg[19] first reported a case of cancer of the jejunum complicating Crohn's disease, there have been many case reports of both small and large bowel cancer. Case reports of Crohn's disease and small bowel cancer have been recently reviewed by Hawker *et al.*[25] and large bowel cancer by Zinkin *et al.*[38] In hospital series of Crohn's patients under long-term review, however, very few cancers have been observed in the gastrointestinal tract, in particular in the colon and rectum (Table 12.20).

Two factors will tend to minimize cancers seen in Crohn's disease. First, early surgical resection will prevent macroscopically diseased bowel from remaining in situ long enough to develop cancer. Bypass procedures rather than resection which allow diseased bowel to remain in situ for many years increase the number of observed cancers[21] (Table 12.20). Secondly, misclassification of Crohn's colitis as ulcerative colitis prior to 1960[29] will have tended to reduce the apparent cancer risk in colonic Crohn's disease.

Assessment of the cancer risk in Crohn's disease is more difficult than in ulcerative colitis because macroscopic disease can involve any part of the gastrointestinal tract and, even when there is little evidence of macroscopic disease, patients may have microscopic changes throughout the whole gastrointestinal tract.[3, 13, 15] The three reports which consider the cancer risk in the whole gastrointestinal tract are therefore of particular interest (Table 12.21).[10, 16, 23]

Cancer incidence in Crohn's disease: statistical analyses

Two centres have published statistical analyses of the cancer incidence in Crohn's disease making a comparison with that expected in the general population. Results of these reports are summarized in Tables 12.21 and 12.22. The series from the Mayo Clinic consisted of a retrospective review of 2120 cases of inflammatory bowel disease presenting at the centre between 1919 and 1965 with onset of disease before the age of 21 years. This report confined itself to the colorectal cancer risk and showed an increased risk of 26-fold above the general population in this selected group with early onset disease. The young age at diagnosis of these colorectal cancers was particularly striking, three of them being diagnosed in their second decade.

Three reports from Birmingham concern a consecutive series of 513 patients with Crohn's disease under regular review at one centre. In these reports the cancer risk in the whole gastrointestinal tract was increased between two- and four-fold (Table 12.21). An increased small bowel cancer risk in an early report[16] based on two small bowel cancers was not confirmed in a later report[23] due to re-classification of one of the small bowel cancers. In the later report,[23] a four-fold increase was found in colorectal cancer (Table 12.21) which was not found in the initial report.

Small bowel cancer

Although little statistical proof exists, other evidence supports an association between Crohn's disease and small bowel cancer. Small bowel cancer is extremely rare in the general population with an estimated incidence of 1/100 000 population per year.[2, 24] The 'expected' numbers of small bowel cancers would be less than one in any hospital series of between 200 and 600 patients with Crohn's disease, even under long-term review (Tables 12.20 and 12.22). The four small bowel cancers observed in the Mount Sinai series of 676 patients and the two small bowel cancers observed in the Cleveland Clinic series of 466 patients would therefore constitute a considerably increased risk above the general

Table 12.20 Cancer in Crohn's disease (case reports where series stated).

Authors	Centre	Review period	Number of patients in series	Total number of cancers	Gastrointestinal cancers			Cancers observed less than 10 years from diagnosis	Additional information
					Colorectal	Small bowel	Others		
Van Patter et al.[36]	Mayo Clinic	1912–1949	600	1	1	0	0	NK	
Atwell et al.[4]	Leeds	1934–1962	212	3	3	0	0	NK	
Perrett et al.[30]	Radcliffe Infirmary, Oxford	1938–1968	154	3	3	0	0	3	Three cancers in series diagnosed concurrently with Crohn's disease on first visit to the unit and therefore do not reflect cancer risk in series under review. One more colonic cancer reported at this centre between 1968 and 1970 – series then 221 patients. Diagnosis of cancer made on first visit to the unit but Crohn's disease diagnosed previously – again not reflecting cancer risk in series under review
Farmer et al.[14]	Cleveland Clinic, Ohio	1955–1971	466	3	1	2	0	2	
Darke et al.[12]	The London Hospital	1948–1973	167	3	2	1	0	1	
Brahme et al.[6]	Malmo, Sweden	1958–1973	191	0	0	0	0	0	Epidemiological study of incidence of Crohn's disease with reported mortality of seven in total series but none of these deaths were due to cancer of the gastrointestinal tract
Greenstein et al.[21]	Mount Sinai, New York	1960–1976	579	17	9 (3 in bypassed loops)	4 (All 4 in bypassed loops)	Stomach 1 Duodenum/pancreas 1 Site not known 2	8	Two multiple cancers. Seven cancers in bypassed loops, six out of seven at site of active disease. Four cancers associated with fistulas. One cancer only diagnosed prior to laparotomy. Three five-year survivors

NK = Not known.

Table 12.21 Birmingham series of Crohn's disease patients: incidence of cancer in gastrointestinal tract as a whole.

	Observed	Expected	O/E relative risk
Fielding et al.[16]	7	2.0	3.5[a]
Gyde et al.[23]	18	5.4	3.3[b]
Cooke et al.[10]	7	3.4	2.0

[a] $P < 0.01$.
[b] $P < 0.001$.

population (Table 12.20).[14, 21] Greenstein and Sachar,[20] referring to recent work in their unit, quote an expected number of 0.0466 against an observed number of 4 from small bowel cancers (Table 12.20) giving an increased risk in the small bowel of 85-fold.

A number of series have reported one small bowel cancer which could be a chance occurrence and many series observed no small bowel cancers[4, 6, 30, 36] (Table 12.20).

Clinical data

Many useful clinical features can be derived from individual case reports which have been detailed by Hawker et al.[25] The summary of this clinical data is shown in Table 12.23.

Table 12.23 shows a long latent period between onset of disease and diagnosis of cancer (mean = 18.2 years), most of the small bowel cancers occurring at the site of macroscopic disease.[12, 18, 22, 35] The majority of these cancers occur in the ileum (67%) as opposed to the general population where small bowel cancers are more evenly distributed.[31] Although the cancers appear to occur at a younger age in Crohn's disease than in the general population, this may only be a reflection of the young age of the patients under review. Small bowel cancers have been reported in association with fistulas[8, 17, 22, 34] and in bypassed loops of bowel (Table 12.23).

Macroscopic and histological features

Less than 50% of small bowel cancers are visible to the naked eye,[17] whereas in the general population they are normally apparent as polyps or strictures. This relative 'invisibility' of small bowel cancers in Crohn's disease may be due to the 'endometriosis'-like burrowing nature of many of these cancers.[17] Most of the small bowel cancers in Crohn's disease are adenocarcinomas with few carcinoid tumours or lymphomas reported as distinct from the general population.[1]

Table 12.22 Gastrointestinal cancer in Crohn's disease: actuarial analyses of cancer incidence.

Authors	Review period	Number of patients in series	Follow up	Total number of cancers	Gastrointestinal cancers			Cancers observed less than 10 years from diagnosis
					Colo-rectal	Small bowel	Others	
Weedon et al.,[37] Mayo Clinic	*Diagnosis* 1919–1965 *Follow-up* to Dec. 1972	449	98%	9	8	1	0	1
Fielding et al.,[16] General Hospital, Birmingham	1944–1968	295	99%	7	1	2[a]	Oesophagus 1 Gallbladder 1 Pancreas 2	4
Gyde et al.,[23] General Hospital, Birmingham	1944–1976	513	98%	18	9	1	Pharynx 1 Parotid 1 Oesophagus 1 Stomach 4 Pancreas 1	3
Cooke et al.,[10] General Hospital, Birmingham	1944–1976	174	98%	10	3	1	Pharynx[b] 1 Parotid[b] 1 Oesophagus 2 Stomach 1 Pancreas[b] 1	0

[a] Including one ileocaecal reticulum cell sarcoma.
[b] Not included in statistical analysis.
[c] $P < 0.05$.
[d] $P < 0.01$.
[e] $P < 0.001$.

Colorectal cancer

Tables 12.20 and 12.22 show how few colorectal cancers have been observed in hospital series of Crohn's disease. Because patients with extensive colonic Crohn's disease tend to be symptomatic and require early surgery, few patients remain with intact colons at risk of developing colorectal cancer. Although an increased risk has been shown in the colon,[23, 37] the increased cancer risk in the statistical analyses is based on very few cancers (Table 12.22). Cancers of the large bowel, as in the small bowel, have been described in bypassed loops of bowel and in fistulas.[7, 22, 28, 32, 34] Multiple cancers have been described.[27] The cancers tend to occur in patients with extensive colitis at the site of macroscopic disease and with a more proximal distribution than the general population.[12, 22, 23, 33, 37]

Dysplasia

Dysplasia has been described in association with both small and large bowel cancers in Crohn's disease.[9, 11, 32]

Because of the small numbers of cancers observed in Crohn's disease cancer, surveillance programmes using dysplasia as a marker have not been instituted as in ulcerative colitis.

Cancer incidence at other sites in the gastrointestinal tract

Gyde *et al.*[23] showed a significant increase in cancers of the upper gastrointestinal tract (pharynx to terminal ileum), mainly due to four observed gastric cancers. The site of macroscopic disease in these four patients was distal ileum (2) and distal ileum and right colon (2).

Biliary tract and gallbladder
Although cases of carcinoma of the biliary tree and gallbladder have been reported in association with Crohn's disease,[5, 26] Gyde *et al.*[23] did not confirm an increased incidence of hepatobiliary cancer suggested in an earlier report.[16] No other studies using statistical techniques have been reported on cancer in the biliary tract and gallbladder in Crohn's disease.

Average age at diagnosis of cancer (years)		Cancer incidence			
		Observed (O)	Expected (E)	Relative risk (O/E)	Additional information
33 (Colorectal only)	*Colorectal*	8	0.3	26.6	Retrospective review of 449 patients with Crohn's disease identified by review of hospital records of 2120 patients diagnosed with inflammatory bowel disease between 1919 and 1965 with onset of disease before the age of 21 years
49 (Whole GI tract)	*Whole GI tract*	7	2.02	3.5[d]	
	Small bowel	2	0.02	100[e]	
	Pancreas/gallbladder	3	0.18	17[d]	
57 (Whole GI tract)	*Whole GI tract*	18	5.39	3.3[e]	See Gyde *et al.*[23] for details
57 (Large intestine)	*Colorectal*	9	2.26	4.0[d]	of cancer reclassification from initial reports of
	Upper GI tract	8	2.53	3.2[d]	Fielding *et al.*[16]
57 (Whole GI tract)	*Whole GI tract*	7	3.37	2.1[c]	

Table 12.23 Cancer in Crohn's disease of the small intestine: summary of reported cases.[25]

Total number of cases	61 (45 males, 16 females)
Mean duration of Crohn's disease	18.2 years (1 week – 45 years)
Mean age at diagnosis of cancer	46.9 years (20–80 years)
Site of tumour	
Jejunum	18 (30%)
Ileum	41 (67%)
Other	2 (3%)
Tumours in bypassed loops	
Jejunal	6
Ileal	12
Outcome	
Dead (4 diagnosed at necropsy)	44 (mean survival 7–9 months)
	(1 month – 3 years)
Alive with metastic disease	7
Alive and well without recorded	8 (mean interval 16 months)
metastases at follow-up	(3 months – 3 years)
Not known	2

Cancer in systems other than the gastrointestinal tract

No significant increases or deficits have been observed in any other system.[16, 23]

Summary

There is good statistical and clinical evidence to support an association between Crohn's disease and cancer in the gastrointestinal tract as a whole. The cancers have been reported mainly in the small bowel and colon, usually at the site of macroscopic disease including bypassed loops and fistulas.

The different distribution from the general population of the cancers in both small and large bowel supports an association between the disease and cancer. Because Crohn's disease and cancer is being studied in a relatively young population it is not surprising that the cancers are being found in a younger age range than those found in the general population. However, it is possible to say that more cancer is occurring at a young age than would be expected in the general population.

Cancer complicating Crohn's disease is not a major clinical problem since so few cases are seen in any hospital series, particularly as most patients still undergo resection of macroscopic disease because of persistent symptoms.

REFERENCES

1 Adler, S. N., Lyon, D. T. & Sullivan, P. D. (1982) Adenocarcinoma of the small bowel. *American Journal of Gastroenterology*, 7, 326–330.

2 Ackerman, L. V. & Del Regato, J. A. (1962) *Cancer Diagnosis, Treatment and Prognosis* 3rd edn p. 626. St Louis: Mosby.

3 Allan, R. N., Steinberg, D. N., Dixon, K. & Cooke, W. T. (1975) Changes in bidirectional sodium flux across the intestinal mucosa in Crohn's disease. *Gut*, 15, 201–204.

4 Atwell, J. D., Duthie, H. L. & Goligher, J. C. (1965) The outcome of Crohn's disease. *British Journal of Surgery*, 52, 966–972.

5 Berman, M. D., Falchuk, K. R. & Trey, C. (1980) Carcinoma of the biliary tree complicating Crohn's disease. *Digestive Diseases and Sciences*, 25, 795–797.

6 Brahme, F., Lindstrom, C. & Wenckert, A. (1975) Crohn's disease in a defined population. An epidemiological study of incidence, prevalence, mortality and secular trends in the City of Malmo, Sweden. *Gastroenterology*, 69, 342–351.

7 Buchmann, P., Allan, R. N., Thompson, H. & Alexander-Williams, J. (1980) Carcinoma in a rectovaginal fistula in a patient with Crohn's disease. *American Journal of Surgery*, 140, 462–463.

8 Burbige, E. J., Bedine, M. S. & Handelsman, J. C. (1977) Adenocarcinoma of the small intestine in Crohn's disease involving the small bowel. *Western Journal of Medicine*, 127, 43–45.

9 Butt, J. H. & Morson, B. (1981) Dysplasia and cancer in inflammatory bowel disease. *Gastroenterology*, 80(4), 865–867.

10 Cooke, W. T., Mallas, E., Prior, P. & Allan, R. N. (1980) Crohn's disease: course, treatment and long term prognosis. *Quarterly Journal of Medicine*, 195, 363–384.

11 Craft, C. F., Mendelsohn, G., Cooper, H. S. & Yardley, J. H. (1981) Colonic 'precancer' in Crohn's disease. *Gastroenterology*, 80, 578–584.

12 Darke, S. G., Parks, A. G., Grogono, J. L. & Pollock, D. J. (1973) Adenocarcinoma and Crohn's disease: a report of two cases and analysis of the literature. *British Journal of Surgery*, 60, 169–175.

13 Dunne, W. T., Allan, R. & Cooke, W. T. (1976) Enzymatic and quantitative histological evidence for Crohn's disease as a diffuse lesion of the gastrointestinal tract. *Gut*, 17, 399 (Abstract).

14 Farmer, R. G., Hawk, W. A. & Turnbull, R. B. (1975) Clinical patterns in Crohn's disease. A statistical study of 615 cases. *Gastroenterology*, 68, 627–635.

15 Ferguson, R., Allan, R. N. & Cooke, W. T. (1975) A study of the cellular infiltrate of the proximal jejunal mucosa in ulcerative colitis and Crohn's disease. *Gut*, 16, 205–208.

16 Fielding, J. F., Prior, P., Waterhouse, J. A. & Cooke, W. T. (1972) Malignancy in Crohn's disease. *Scandinavian Journal of Gastroenterology*, **7**, 3–7.

17 Fleming, K. A. & Pollock, A. C. (1975) A case of Crohn's carcinoma. *Gut*, **16**, 533–537.

18 Frank, J. D. & Shorey, B. A. (1973) Adenocarcinoma of the small bowel as a complication of Crohn's disease. *Gut*, **14**, 120–124.

19 Ginzburg, L., Schneider, K. M., Dreisin, D. H. & Levinson, C. (1956) Carcinoma of the jejunum occurring in a case of regional enteritis. *Surgery*, **39**, 347–351.

20 Greenstein, A. J. & Sachar, D. B. (1983) Cancer in Crohn's disease. In *Inflammatory Bowel Diseases* (Ed.) Allan, R. N., Keighley, M. R. B., Alexander-Williams, J. & Hawkins, C. F. pp. 332–337. Edinburgh: Churchill Livingstone.

21 Greenstein, A. J., Sachar, D., Pucillo, A. *et al.* (1978) Cancer in Crohn's disease after diversionary surgery. A report of seven carcinomas occurring in excluded bowel. *American Journal of Surgery*, **135**, 86–90.

22 Greenstein, A. J., Sachar, D. B., Smith, H. *et al.* (1980) Patterns of neoplasia in Crohn's disease and ulcerative colitis. *Cancer*, **46**, 403–407.

23 Gyde, S. N., Prior, P., Macartney, J. C. *et al.* (1980) Malignancy in Crohn's disease. *Gut*, **21**, 1024–1029.

24 Haffner, J. F. W. & Semb, L. S. (1969) Malignant tumours of the small intestine. *Acta Chirurgica Scandinavica*, **135**, 543–548.

25 Hawker, P. C., Gyde, S. N. & Allan, R. N. (1982) Adenocarcinoma of the small intestine complicating Crohn's disease. *Gut*, **23**, 188–193.

26 Joffe, N. & Antonioli, D. A. (1981) Primary carcinoma of the gall bladder associated with chronic inflammatory bowel disease. *Clinical Radiology*, **32**, 319–324.

27 Keighley, M. R. B., Thompson, H. D. & Alexander-Williams, J. (1975) Multifocal colonic carcinoma and Crohn's disease. *Surgery*, **78**(4), 534–537.

28 Lightdale, C. J., Sternberg, S. S., Posner, G. & Sherlock, P. (1975) Carcinoma complicating Crohn's disease. Report of seven cases and review of the literature. *American Journal of Medicine*, **59**, 262–268.

29 Lockhart-Mummery, H. E. & Morson, B. C. (1960) Crohn's disease (regional enteritis) of the large intestine and its distinction from ulcerative colitis. *Gut*, **1**, 87–105.

30 Perrett, A. D., Truelove, S. C. & Massarella, G. R. (1968) Crohn's disease and carcinoma of the colon. *British Medical Journal*, **ii**, 466–468.

31 Rochlin, D. B. & Longmire, W. P. Jr (1961) Primary tumours of the small intestine. *Surgery*, **50**, 586–592.

32 Simpson, S., Traube, J. & Riddell, R. H. (1981) The histologic appearance of dysplasia (precarcinomatous change) in Crohn's disease of the small and large intestine. *Gastroenterology*, **81**, 492–501.

33 Smiddy, F. G. & Goligher, J. C. (1957) Results of surgery in treatment of cancer of the large intestine. *British Medical Journal*, **i**, 793–796.

34 Traube, J., Simpson, S., Riddell, R. H. *et al.* (1980) Crohn's disease and adenocarcinoma of the bowel. *Digestive Diseases and Sciences*, **25**, 939–944.

35 Valdes-Dapena, A., Rudolf, I., Hidayat, A. *et al.* (1976) Adenocarcinoma of the small bowel in association with regional enteritis. Four new cases. *Cancer*, **37**, 2936–2947.

36 Van Patter, W. N., Bargen, J. A., Dockerty, M. B. *et al.* (1954) Regional enteritis. *Gastroenterology*, **26**, 347–450.

37 Weedon, D. D., Shorter, R. G., Ilstrup, D. M. *et al.* (1973) Crohn's disease and cancer. *New England Journal of Medicine*, **289**, 1099–1103.

38 Zinkin, L. D. & Brandwein, C. (1980) Adenocarcinoma in Crohn's colitis. *Diseases of the Colon and Rectum*, **23**, 115–117.

EXTRAINTESTINAL MANIFESTATIONS OF INFLAMMATORY BOWEL DISEASE

The interrelationship between ulcerative colitis and Crohn's disease is not yet clear and their aetiology is unknown. They may share a common aetiology and represent a spectrum of one disease. Extraintestinal manifestations are frequent and common to both forms of inflammatory bowel disease, which may point to a common pathogenesis for both diseases. The complications often influence therapeutic and management decisions. In a minority of patients they are the presenting feature and precede symptoms referable to the gastrointestinal tract. The extraintestinal symptoms may improve with effective medical treatment or surgical resection but this is not always true. Scoring systems devised to assess severity of disease where extraintestinal manifestations are included as indices of disease activity can be criticized on these grounds.

The complications are many and varied. Some may result from drug therapy and electrolyte or nutritional imbalance. The reported incidence rates vary. This may be due to variations in length of follow-up, the criteria for defining complications, or different attitudes to screening for asymptomatic extraintestinal manifestations. Extraintestinal manifestations are commoner in Crohn's colitis than in ileocaecal or small bowel disease.

The extraintestinal manifestations which may occur in inflammatory bowel disease are considered here according to the system involved, though more than one extraintestinal manifestation may occur in any individual.

The liver

Liver disease is one of the most important extracolonic manifestations in terms of morbidity and mortality. The spectrum of liver disease extends from minor abnormalities of the biochemical profile to established cirrhosis, and includes fatty change, pericholangitis, chronic active hepatitis, cirrhosis, granulomas, amyloidosis, hepatic abscess, gallstones, and carcinoma of the biliary tree.

Incidence

In careful microscopic studies of liver biopsies obtained from patients undergoing colectomy for either ulcerative colitis or Crohn's disease, histological abnormalities were found in nearly 90%.[22, 24] In a survey from Birmingham of 1200 patients with inflammatory bowel disease, abnormal liver function tests were present at some time in approximately 8% of patients but in many cases they developed transiently after surgery, associated with abdominal sepsis. One-fifth of patients with abnormal liver function tests had pericholangitis.[19]

Fatty change

The commonest lesion found is fatty infiltration but sepsis and undernutrition may contribute to this finding. In one study, marked liver function abnormalities correlated with extent and severity but not duration of the disease and persisted despite therapy, whereas mildly abnormal liver function tests did not correlate with extent, activity or duration of ulcerative colitis and were usually a self-limiting process.[47]

Pericholangitis

Pericholangitis, also called triaditis, is recognized histologically by cellular infiltration of the portal tracts, portal fibrosis and concentric fibrosis around the intrahepatic and extrahepatic ducts (Figure 12.40).

The aetiology of pericholangitis is unknown, but possible causes include immunological, toxic and infective mechanisms. It is not related to blood transfusions, drug treatment or other systemic manifestations.[22] An infective theory has been proposed as pathogens have been cultured from the portal vein.[23] Experimentally induced chronic portal bacteraemia in calves led to portal inflammation similar but not identical, to pericholangitis.[69] Portal vein bacteraemia could be a consequence of invasion of the bowel flora through a damaged ulcerated bowel wall.

Primary sclerosing cholangitis

Primary sclerosing cholangitis occurs more frequently in association with ulcerative colitis than any other condition, commonly in patients with severe and extensive disease. The extent of the sclerosing cholangitis can be readily identified by endoscopic retrograde cholangiography. Light and electron microscopic studies of biopsies show that the main feature is mesenchymal proliferation involving phagocytic, fibroblastic and immunocytic cells, suggestive of an immunological type of liver injury which may attack bile duct epithelial cells.[51]

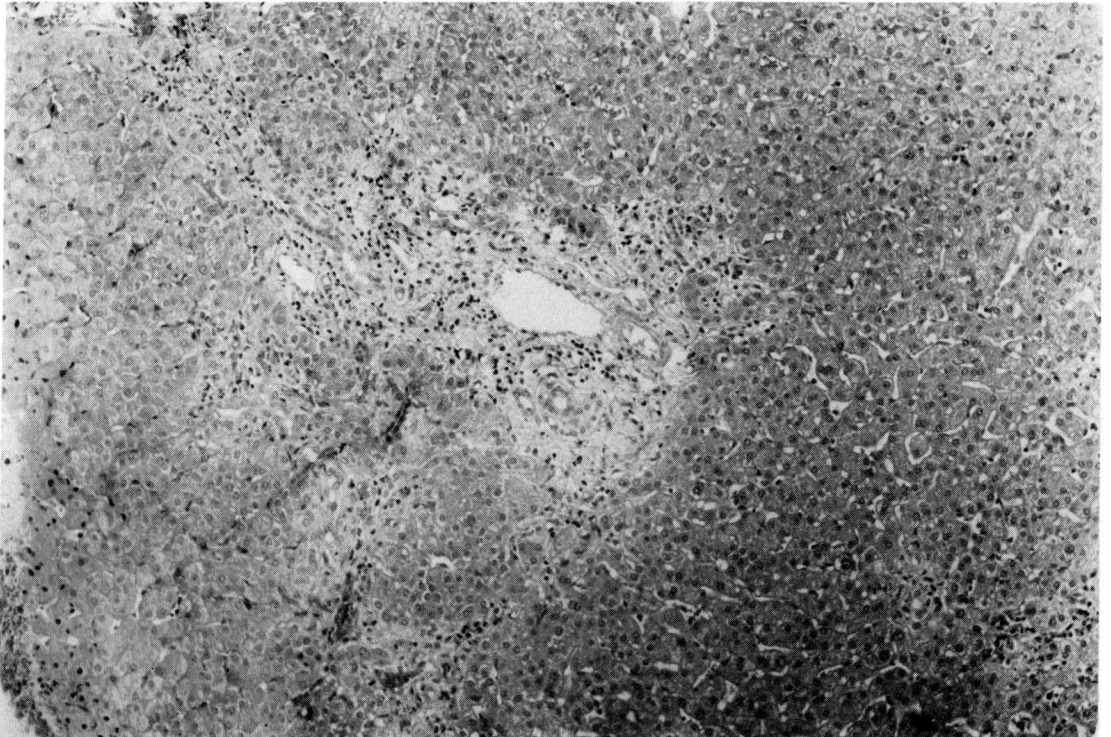

Fig. 12.40 Sclerosing pericholangitis (also called triaditis), showing cellular infiltration of the portal tracts and fibrosis of the portal intra- and extrahepatic ducts. × 140.

A recent study reports the beneficial results of aggressive treatment aimed at promoting biliary drainage and eradication of the biliary infection to prevent progression of the disease.[72] This was achieved by stenting and appropriate antibiotic therapy (cephalosporin or gentamicin $\pm$ metronidazole). The stent was left in place for 12 to 18 months but its care was managed on an outpatient basis.

Cirrhosis of the liver
Cirrhosis of the liver was found in 3 out of 517 patients with Crohn's disease and 11 out of 720 patients with ulcerative colitis.[19] Cirrhosis of the liver associated with ulcerative colitis may sometimes be complicated by hepatoma.

Other conditions
Biliary tract carcinoma is a well recognized complication of ulcerative colitis which in the early stages is often difficult to distinguish from sclerosing cholangitis.

Chronic active hepatitis, amyloidosis, granulomas and hepatic abscess are rare and taken together occurred in only 1–2% of patients in several large series.

Time sequence
Liver abnormalities may precede symptomatic inflammatory bowel disease, so that inflammatory bowel disease must be considered in the differential diagnosis of liver disease. Drug therapy for inflammatory bowel disease, particularly sulphasalazine, and total parenteral nutrition can cause liver function abnormalities.

The skin

Erythema nodosum and pyoderma gangrenosum are important cutaneous manifestations and may be of diagnostic value. The incidence of cutaneous manifestations varies from 2–34%. The latter reports include drug hypersensitivity reactions, perianal and oral lesions. Erythema multiforme has also been documented in association with Crohn's disease, but this may be a chance occurrence.[9] Patients with inflammatory bowel disease also have a higher incidence of atopic skin disease than controls.

Pyoderma gangrenosum
Pyoderma gangrenosum can be recognized as a painful necrotic ulcer with an advancing rolled or undermined border and a pustular centre. Preceding local trauma can be identified in 40% of cases.[5] The lesion most commonly occurs on the pretibial surface but may occur elsewhere.

In one large series, 50% of patients with pyoderma gangrenosum had underlying ulcerative colitis.[58] It may also complicate Crohn's disease. The differential diagnosis of pyoderma gangrenosum includes rheumatoid arthritis, pulmonary infection, diverticulosis, leukaemia, Hodgkin's disease, polycythaemia rubra vera, myeloma, myelofibrosis, Behçet's disease, and chronic active hepatitis. Pyoderma gangrenosum can occur spontaneously without underlying systemic disease, particularly in the elderly.[67]

Decreased neutrophil chemotaxis in vitro has been described in pyoderma gangrenosum due to either an intrinsic neutrophil leucocyte defect or inhibitory serum factors.[37, 62] Neutrophil abnormalities have also been described in Crohn's disease and ulcerative colitis where the number of neutrophils accumulating in response to inflammation is reduced.[54, 70] Defective complement function has also been reported in pyoderma gangrenosum.[17]

Erythema nodosum
The reported incidence of erythema nodosum in inflammatory bowel disease varies from 0.5–9%. Erythema nodosum is a form of panniculitis characterized by red nodules up to several centimetres in diameter, which are painless but tender to touch, on the anterior aspect of the lower limbs. Other sites include the thighs, arms and hands. Women are more commonly affected than men. Unlike pyoderma gangrenosum, the appearance of the nodules usually coincides with an active phase of the disease. Erythema nodosum may precede or coincide with the bowel symptoms. In other patients it only occurs many years after the onset of gastrointestinal disease.[5] Arthralgia or arthropathy commonly coexist. Significant skin involvement may be accompanied by fever and malaise. The lesions may occasionally ulcerate, but usually fade to a bronze discolouration when the underlying bowel disease goes into remission.

Recently a skin lesion has been described in two patients with Crohn's disease that resembles erythema nodosum but runs a different clinical course independent of the activity of Crohn's disease. Steroid therapy proved ineffective.[20] The histological features were also different in that necrobiotic collagen (necrobiosis) was prominent. This variant may have been overlooked since skin biopsy is rarely performed in 'erythema nodosum'. Cutaneous polyarteritis nodosum, which has also been described in Crohn's disease, may be mistaken for erythema nodosum.[41]

Cutaneous polyarteritis nodosum

Cutaneous polyarteritis nodosum is character-ized by a panarteritis of the subcutis and adjac-ent dermis which occasionally involves vessels of the peripheral nerves and skeletal muscle. Clini-cally there may be red subcutaneous nodules of the lower extremities which have a tendency to ulcerate. Peripheral neuropathy, myalgia or arthritis may also be present. In most patients there is a complete spontaneous resolution of the arteritis, while in the remainder cutaneous nodules persist despite resolution of the associ-ated myositis and polyneuritis. Corticosteroids and sulphasalazine seem beneficial. This com-plication is unrelated to the activity of the underlying intestinal disease. Histological examination of biopsies from the lesions shows granulomas with epithelioid cell formation in the vessel wall similar to that observed in Crohn's disease.

Aphthous stomatitis

Aphthous stomatitis is seen in 4% of patients with inflammatory bowel disease.[30] The clinical picture is of ulcers on the floor of the mouth, gums, lower and upper lip, palate and uvula. Their presence usually indicates active disease. Aphthous stomatitis is associated with Behçet's disease, which can involve the gastrointestinal tract. Many cases labelled as Behçet's disease could be Crohn's disease. Aphthous ulceration of the gastrointestinal tract is one of the earliest lesions of Crohn's disease.

Arthritis

Inflammatory bowel disease is often compli-cated by two types of arthritis, an enteropathic arthritis and sacroileitis or ankylosing spondy-litis.[31, 48] The reported incidence varies between 4 and 45%,[30, 74] but this may be explained in part by the selected use of special radiographs of the sacroiliac joints to exclude sacroileitis.[75] Enteropathic arthritis is an inflammatory syn-ovitis limited to a few large joints. The serum from these patients is negative for IgM and rheumatoid factor. Any joint may be affected but most commonly the joints of lower limbs are involved. An acute, sometimes relapsing asym-metric arthritis is characteristic and can precede, coincide with or develop in established bowel disease, but usually accompanies an exacer-bation of the underlying inflammatory bowel disease. The radiological findings of joints involved by enteropathic arthritis are minimal, such as minor joint narrowing, juxta-articular

periostitis, and rarely erosions. Significant per-manent joint disease is rare but may occur and is exacerbated by injury to the inflamed joint. Enteropathic arthritis is more common in Crohn's disease patients with localized colonic disease, but an incidence of 14% has been recorded in patients with small bowel involve-ment.[30]

Arthritis is also observed after intestinal bypass operations for morbid obesity.[71] Cryo-protein complexes can be identified in the serum from these patients including IgG, IgM, IgA, complement components C3, C4, and C5, and IgG antibody against *Escherichia coli* and *Bacil-lus fragilis*. Circulating cryoprotein complexes can activate both the classical and alternative complement pathways which may be important in the pathogenesis of the arthritis. Improve-ment follows treatment with metronidazole or dismantling of the bypass in patients treated for morbid obesity, which suggests that bacterial byproducts originating in the excluded bowel may be important in the aetiology. Endo-toxaemia has been found in patients with active inflammatory bowel disease, which may play a role in the development of extraintestinal mani-festations.[15]

Enteropathic arthritis improves following treatment of the inflammatory bowel disease. Colectomy in a case of fulminant ulcerative colitis led to rapid remission of the concomitant arthritis.[50] Surgical resection of Crohn's disease does not always result in a remission of the arthritis.[28] The enteropathic arthritis is usually self-limiting but symptomatic treatment with non-steroidal anti-inflammatory drugs may be necessary.

Sacroileitis and ankylosing spondylitis

Sacroileitis is thought to be an early manifesta-tion of ankylosing spondylitis. It is frequently asymptomatic, the diagnosis being made on radiological grounds.

Ankylosing spondylitis predominantly affects males (male : female ratio is 4 : 1), but the sex ratio of those with spondylitis complicating inflammatory bowel disease is almost equal. The association between ankylosing spondylitis and HLA-B27 was first noted by Brewerton *et al.*[11] Ninety per cent of patients with sporadic anky-losing spondylitis are HLA-B27 positive, whereas in spondylitis associated with inflam-matory bowel disease only 35% are positive for HLA-B27.[25] HLA-B27 does not predispose to the development of Crohn's disease or ulcerative colitis. The prevalence of inflammatory bowel disease and B27-negative spondylitis in family studies suggests that a non-HLA-linked genetic predisposition to inflammatory bowel disease exists, which also confers susceptibility to spondylitis, even in the absence of expression of bowel disease.

Spondylitis does not correlate with disease activity and is slowly progressive. Effective medical treatment of the inflammatory bowel disease and even colectomy does not alter the clinical course.[28] Treatment regimens include pain relief with analgesic anti-inflammatory drugs such as indomethacin and propionic acid derivatives. Exercise is encouraged and the physiotherapist should recommend back exercises as well as correct posture during work and leisure. Radiotherapy has been used in difficult cases.

Clubbing of the fingers

The association between finger clubbing and inflammatory bowel disease is well recognized. The reported prevalence of finger clubbing in Crohn's disease varies between 31.5 and 58% and 4 and 13% in ulcerative colitis.[42] Hypertrophic osteoarthropathy occurs occasionally. Active disease is significantly associated with finger clubbing in both Crohn's disease and ulcerative colitis. Disease activity, while important in the pathogenesis of the disease, is not the only factor, for finger clubbing may be found in inactive disease. The vagus nerve and possibly other autonomic nerves may act as the afferent pathway of a reflex inducing finger clubbing. The focal stimuli are mucosal inflammatory changes and fibrosis. The efferent pathway of the finger clubbing reflex has not been established. The focal changes include increased blood flow and amount of fibrous connective tissue. Finger clubbing in patients with Crohn's disease tends to regress after resection of macroscopic disease.[42]

Ocular lesions

The reported frequency of eye changes varies widely but was 4% in patients with ulcerative colitis and 13% in patients with granulomatous colitis in a series of 700 cases of inflammatory bowel disease.[30] The commonest eye condition is uveitis, the next commonest being episcleritis. Retrospective studies report a lower incidence, but in these studies the eyes were not checked routinely. Conjunctivitis is uncommon but three patients have been described with inflammatory bowel disease and papillary hypertrophy with fibrovascular membrane formation, pyobleph-

aroconjunctivitis, and eosinophilic microabscess formation.[73] Unilateral corneal lesions have also been described in inactive inflammatory bowel disease.[60] These lesions are small peripheral subepithelial infiltrates of white blood cells associated with mild irritative symptoms. No signs of staphylococcal infection are present. The corneal lesions clear rapidly with topical corticosteroids or systemic indomethacin. They may be due to a leucocyte infiltrate that migrates to a site of antigen–antibody reaction.[14]

Uveitis has been reported as a complication in 4% of patients with inflammatory bowel disease, but a higher incidence is suspected in Crohn's disease localized to the large bowel.[18, 30] There have been associations of uveitis with other systemic disorders. In a review of 100 patients with uveitis, 33 had other systemic disease. More than half the patients with uveitis were positive for HLA-B27 antigen.[10] The patient may be asymptomatic or may complain of blurred vision, eye pain, photophobia and headache. Examination of the eye may show ciliary congestion, extreme turbidity of the aqueous, and iriditic adhesions.

Uveitis can precede the onset of gastrointestinal symptoms and has been reported to occur after colectomy and in inactive inflammatory bowel disease. Uveitis responds to systemic and local steroid therapy.

Haematological disease

A wide range of haematological abnormalities have been described in association with inflammatory bowel disease, ranging from nutritional anaemias to acute myeloid leukaemia. The association of inflammatory bowel disease and malignancy is well described (see earlier in this chapter). In a series of 400 patients with ulcerative colitis recently reported, five patients developed acute myelogenous leukaemia.[27]

Autoimmune haemolytic anaemia
Autoimmune haemolytic anaemia is a rare complication of inflammatory bowel disease, with less than 20 cases recorded in the literature.[1] The diagnosis is based on anaemia, reticulocytosis and a positive Coombs' test. Sulphasalazine can induce these changes and must therefore be excluded. Gastrointestinal haemorrhage and poor nutrition may contribute to the anaemia. Patients with autoimmune haemolytic anaemia associated with ulcerative colitis should be treated in a similar way to idiopathic

autoimmune haemolytic anaemia. Half the patients will respond to corticosteroid therapy. The addition of immunosuppressive therapy to the non-responding corticosteroid-treated patients may induce a remission. Splenectomy produces a remission in the majority of patients.[61] Autoimmune haemolytic anaemia is not an indication for colectomy, as severe haemolysis has been reported many years after colectomy.[1]

Thrombosis

Arterial and venous thrombosis have been described in association with inflammatory bowel disease. The incidence is about 4% with overt clinical signs, but the incidence in post mortem studies is as high at 31%.[4] Extensive thrombosis is a grave complication of both forms of inflammatory bowel disease. Various sites of venous thrombus formation have been recorded, including the cerebral, thoracoepigastric, ileofemoral, portal, and pulmonary veins. Arterial thrombosis is a more serious and poorly understood complication. It has occurred in the carotid, retinal, glans penal, femoral, subclavian, trachial, radial and ulnar arteries. Local vascular factors probably determine the site and whether arterial or venous thrombosis occurs.[7]

Systematic evaluation has revealed a hypercoagulable state in most cases of inflammatory bowel disease.[52] Increased platelet count, accelerated platelet aggregation and platelet retention rate, and increased fibrinogen content, factor VIII and factor IX activity were found. The high platelet count can occur due to the associated anaemia.

In another study, antithrombin III, an important inhibitor of coagulation, was decreased in patients with inflammatory bowel disease compared with hospitalized controls.[45] Decreased levels could predispose to a hypercoaguable state. The levels of clotting factors correlated with the activity of the disease since they are acute phase reactants and decrease with successful medical treatment of the underlying inflammatory bowel disease. However, there is no direct evidence that elevated factors predispose to thrombotic formation.[36] Steroids were considered to play a role, but this theory has now been discredited.[68] Other possible factors include stasis from bed rest, toxaemia, dehydration and immunological mechanisms inducing changes in the vessel wall leading to a vasculitis.

Conversely, thrombocytopenia and purpura have also been reported in ulcerative colitis.[44] Sulphasalazine may be responsible, so platelet counts should be checked at intervals. Malnutrition causing combined iron and B_{12} deficiency may contribute to the thrombocytopenia.

Vasculitis

Isolated cases of vasculitis complicating inflammatory bowel disease have been described. Dermal vasculitis with necrotic skin lesions and pulmonary vasculitis are complications of many systemic diseases, but have also been described in ulcerative colitis.[3, 16] Circulating immune complexes may play a role in initiating the vasculitis.

Takayasu's disease is a rare condition complicating both Crohn's disease and ulcerative colitis and is thought to have an autoimmune basis.[8, 13] Less than ten case reports of this association have been published; all the affected patients were females of child-bearing age and the disease was characterized by a generalized arteritis. Patients with Takayasu's disease without bowel involvement have other manifestations including a peripheral arthritis, skin lesions, erythema nodosum, pyoderma gangrenosum, and uveitis. The arteritis usually responds to high-dose corticosteroid therapy. Some of the histological findings in Crohn's disease, such as granuloma formation, are seen in Takayasu's disease.

Bronchopulmonary disease

Sulphasalazine may cause fibrosing alveolitis. Pulmonary function tests performed on fit patients with underlying inflammatory bowel disease showed a significant decrease in the carbon monoxide transfer factor (TLCO).[21] The observed reduction in TLCO was similar whether or not patients were taking sulphasalazine. The reduction was still observed when TLCO was corrected for the haemoglobin levels.[40] A recent report describes seven patients with advanced lung disease. In three, rapidly progressive bronchiectasis developed within one year of proctocolectomy. In two it developed in association with an exacerbation of colitis and in the other two a milder limited colitis postdated the start of the lung disease. All seven patients had an arthropathy or skin rash and a high incidence of a personal or family history of autoimmune diseases. Antinuclear antibodies were detected in six of the patients and smooth muscle antibodies in five. There was no evidence of hepatic dysfunction. These findings and the clinical response to corticosteroid therapy were highly suggestive of an autoimmune aetiology.

Some patients who were non-smokers had a productive cough and exertional dyspnoea. Bronchial epithelial biopsies from these patients revealed basal cell hyperplastia, basement membrane thickening and submucosal inflammatory changes which are usually only found in cigarette smokers.[32] There are some morphological and developmental similarities between colonic and bronchial epithelium. Both are derived from the primitive gut. Both have columnar epithelial and goblet cells and submucous glands. The nonspecific inflammatory changes beneath the bronchial epithelium are similar to those seen in colonic epithelium in colitis. It is possible that a systemic factor is responsible for the common response at both epithelial sites in patients with colitis. Alternatively, it may be due to contact hypersensitivity to inhaled allergens in the case of bronchial epithelium or ingested allergens in the gut epithelium.

Cardiovascular disease

Only 16 cases of pericarditis complicating inflammatory bowel disease have been described in the literature.[46, 66] It can result in life-threatening cardiac tamponade. It is usually associated with active disease but may predate the onset of bowel symptoms and can occur after colectomy. Pericarditis responds to high-dose corticosteroid therapy but may relapse when the dose is reduced. Pleural effusions have also been noted in these patients.

Renal disease

The incidence of urolithiasis in inflammatory bowel disease is 15%.[43] The pathogenesis of stone formation includes dehydration, corticosteroid treatment, urinary tract infection, and hydronephrosis secondary to ureteric obstruction of the right ureter. The tendency to stone formation is increased following small bowel resection. Bile salt absorption is reduced after ileal resection and their presence in the colon enhances oxalate absorption. However, there is a high incidence of urolithiasis among ileostomy patients, so that other mechanisms must be involved. Steatorrhoea precipitates calcium which normally binds oxalate in the intestine and therefore enhances oxalate absorption. Curiously, a recent study found a similar incidence of urolithiasis in groups of patients with inflammatory bowel disease with hyperoxaluria and normal urinary oxalate excretion.[34]

Dehydration leading to low urinary volume and pH increases uric acid precipitation. The percentage of uric acid stones rises following colectomy, half of the stones contain uric acid compared to an incidence of 10% in the normal population.[49]

Pyelonephritis occurs in 2–4% of patients with ulcerative colitis. The incidence is higher in Crohn's disease due to ureteric obstruction and enterovesical fistulas.[64]

Amyloidosis

Less than 30 cases of amyloidosis complicating Crohn's disease have been reported in the literature. Only a few patients had the diagnosis made during life. The association of amyloid and ulcerative colitis is even rarer. The patients often present in renal failure and may require renal transplantation. It was once thought to occur only with ileal involvement, but a recent report of seven patients, all of whom had had previous resection, makes this untenable.[26] Regression of amyloidosis has followed surgical resection and some think it an indication for surgical resection of the underlying inflammatory bowel disease.

Endocrine disease

There are several reports of coexisting inflammatory bowel disease and hyperthyroidism.[35] Eight per cent had a palpable goitre and 4% had thyrotoxicosis in one large series of patients with ulcerative colitis.[39] Exacerbations of the thyroid disease and ulcerative colitis occurred together and made patient management difficult. Janerot has reported abnormalities of iodine metabolism in patients with inflammatory bowel disease. He noted a decreased 24-hour urine iodine excretion and increased 24-hour ^{131}I uptake, suggesting iodine deficiency.[38] Since thyroxine (T_4) is protein bound and patients with inflammatory bowel disease often have low serum albumin, they also tend to have low levels of thyroxine binding prealbumin and albumin and a higher thyroglobulin compared to controls. This data may erroneously suggest hyperthyroidism so that radioimmunoassay of thyroid hormones should be used in patients with weight loss and diarrhoea if thyroid disease is suspected.

Pathogenesis

The exact mechanism by which the systemic manifestations occur is not known. An immune mechanism has been implicated although this fails to explain all of the manifestations and why only a minority of patients develop them. No linkage with common genetic markers such as blood group or secretor status has been found, and there is no strong association with any of the histocompatibility antigens apart from those who have ankylosing spondylitis and uveitis. The strength of the association between HLA-B27 and inflammatory bowel disease is less strong than in idiopathic spondylitis; this suggests a non-HLA genetic predisposition to inflammatory bowel disease which also confers susceptibility to spondylitis, even in the absence of expression of bowel disease.

In experimental serum sickness, the arthritis, uveitis, glomerulonephritis and skin lesions that occur may be due to circulating immune complexes. Since similar lesions can occur as extra-intestinal manifestations in inflammatory bowel disease, circulating immune complexes formed within the inflamed mucosa may play a role in their initiation. The presence of immune complexes within the intestinal mucosa of patients with inflammatory bowel disease has been inferred from immunofluorescence studies. An increased amount of circulating immune complexes has been described in Crohn's disease using different assay techniques.[33] Some methods of measuring immune complexes may simply be measuring aggregated IgG. When an assay is performed so as to exclude measurement of aggregated IgG, no circulating immune complexes are found in patients with inflammatory bowel disease even among those with extraintestinal manifestation.[63]

It is possible that the perpetuation of inflammatory changes in inflammatory bowel disease is due to complement activation. Immune complexes can activate complement through both the classical and alternative pathways. Evidence for complement activation has come from studies showing the presence of complement breakdown products,[65] antibodies to fixed complement,[57] and increased synthesis and catabolism of C3 and $C1_q$.[59] Complement may be activated by immune complexes and deposited at extravascular sites such as the gastrointestinal tract, skin and joints. Most tests for the presence of immune complexes and antigen–antibody complexes are indirect. They depend upon the biochemistry of complement. This is especially so when the antigen is unknown. The antigen in inflammatory bowel disease could be an infective agent, a dietary component, or altered tissue reaction. Patients who have jejuno-ileal bypass operations for morbid obesity also may develop hepatic and arthritic manifestations. This is

thought to be due to bacteria or bacterial toxins which proliferate in the isolated bowel, get into the circulation and are deposited as antigen–antibody complexes which activate complement and lead to tissue damage. Their symptoms respond to treatment with antibiotics and remit after dismantling of the bypass.

Phagocytic function
The process of localization and elimination of foreign material can be termed an immune effector function and is largely mediated by an immunologically initiated inflammatory response. The local accumulation of immune effector cells such as lymphocytes, macrophages or polymorphonuclear (PMN) leucocytes is instrumental in the localization and destruction of non-self. A defective effector mechanism may explain some of the extraintestinal manifestations of inflammatory bowel disease (Figure 12.41). A neutrophil defect has been described in Crohn's disease, in that they fail to migrate to a site of inflammation.[54] Neutrophil selective enzyme activities are lower and 5'-nucleotidase synthesized by activated macrophages is high in non-involved Crohn's tissue.[56] This indicates that, in the absence of neutrophils, the macrophage has an important role in the pathogenesis of the disease.

The gastrointestinal tract is exposed to multiple antigens in a normal diet. Many of these antigens penetrate the epithelial surface of the gut; most are eliminated by body defence mechanisms. However, patients with Crohn's disease are unable to accumulate sufficient neutrophils to phagocytose foreign material. This may be due to mucosal cells not liberating sufficient amounts of chemotactic factor to attract neutrophils, as the neutrophils have normal migration and phagocytic ability in vitro. This host immune mechanism could be genetically determined, which could account for the increased familial and racial incidence of the disease. It is likely that only some food components, by virtue of their size, configuration or physical state, have this effect. It is possible that the dietary component is a food additive. This could account for the increased incidence of the disease in developed western countries. The dietary component would act as an antigen and cause B cells to secrete antibody, which would escape into the circulation and initiate the extraintestinal manifestation.

An elemental diet is effective treatment in removing the offending dietary antigen, for not only do the patients respond clinically but their extraintestinal manifestations are also resolv-

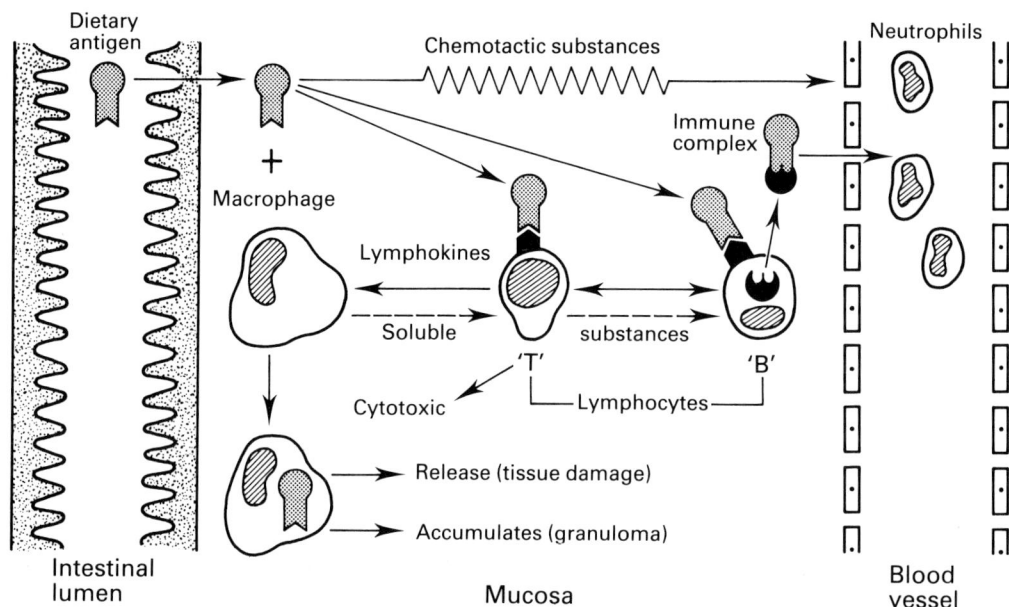

Fig. 12.41 Hypothesis of the pathogenesis of Crohn's disease. A dietary antigen penetrates the mucosa. Chemostactic factors are *not* released in sufficient amounts to attract neutrophils. The dietary antigen persists and interacts with macrophages and lymphocytes. This results in accumulation of macrophages leading to granuloma formation and lymphocyte activation and tissue damage.

ed.[53] A diet rich in fibre may induce remission by binding the offending allergen.

In patients with ulcerative colitis leucocytes are mobilized in normal numbers immediately after eliciting the inflammatory reaction, indicating a normal inflammatory response, but mobilization of neutrophils into skin window chambers subsequently is reduced. This could be due to an intrinsic neutrophil defect or exhaustion of locally produced chemotactic substances. Lysosomal enzyme markers are decreased in rectal biopsies from patients with ulcerative colitis indicating that their release may be important in the pathogenesis of the disease and the extraintestinal manifestations.[29, 55] The failure of neutrophils to continue to accumulate would allow antigens which are normally cleared by innate body defences to persist and set up a secondary immunological reaction.

Summary

The wide variety and similarity of extraintestinal manifestations in both forms of inflammatory bowel disease suggest that a common pathogenesis is involved which is most likely to be immunological. The agent or agents eliciting this response are probably different in both diseases but it may be as a consequence of defective inflammatory response. It is possible that ulcerative colitis and Crohn's disease are generalized diseases in which the major manifestations are in the gastrointestinal tract.

REFERENCES

1 Altman, A. R., Malz, C. & Janowitz, H. D. (1979) Autoimmune haemolytic anaemia in ulcerative colitis. *Digestive Diseases and Sciences*, **24**, 282–285.

2 Balford, J. & Shiner, M. (1974) Evidence of cytotoxicity in ulcerative colitis from immunofluorescent staining of rectal mucosa. *Lancet*, **i**, 1014–1017.

3 Ball, G. V. & Goldman, L. N. (1970) Chronic ulcerative colitis, skin necrosis and cryofibrinogenemia. *Annals of Internal Medicine*, **85**, 464–466.

4 Bargen, I. A. & Barker, N. W. (1936) Extensive arterial and venous thrombosis complicating chronic ulcerative colitis. *Archives of Internal Medicine*, **58**, 17–31.

5 Basler, R. S. W. (1980) Ulcerative colitis and the skin. *Medical Clinics of North America*, **64**, 941–954.

6 Basu, M. K. & Asquith, P. (1980) Oral manifestations of inflammatory bowel disease. *Clinics in Gastroenterology*, **9**, 307–322.

7 Braverman, D. & Bogoch, A. (1978) Arterial thrombosis in ulcerative colitis. *Digestive Diseases*, **23**, 1148–1150.

8 Beau, B., Colasse, W., Le Bihan, G. & Bourreillo, J. (1980) Association d'une maladie de Takayasu et d'une colite inflammatoire. *Semaine des Hospitaux Paris*, **56**, 1841–1845.

9 Brenner, S. M. & Delany, H. M. (1972) Erythema multiforme and Crohn's disease of the large intestine. *Gastroenterology*, **62**, 479–482.

10 Brewerton, D. A., Caffrey, M., Nicholls, A. & Walters, D. (1973) Acute anterior uveitis and HL-AW227. *Lancet*, **ii**, 994–996.

11 Brewerton, D. A., Hart, F. D., Nicholls, A. *et al.* (1973) Ankylosing spondylitis and HLA-B27. *Lancet*, **i**, 904.

12 Butland, R. J. A., Cole, P., Citron, K. M. & Turner-Warwick, M. (1981) Chronic bronchial suppuration and inflammatory bowel disease. *Quarterly Journal of Medicine*, **50**, 63–75.

13 Chapman, R., Dawe, C., Whorwell, P. J. & Wright, R.

(1978) Ulcerative colitis in association with Takayasu's Disease. *Digestive Disease*, **23**, 660–662.

14 Chignall, A. H., Easty, D. L., Chesterton, J. R. & Tomsitt, J. Marginal ulceration of the cornea. *British Journal of Ophthalmology*, **54**, 443–444.

15 Colin, R., Grancher, T., Lemeland, J. F. *et al.* (1979) Recherche d'une endotoxinémie dans les entero-colites inflammatoire cryptogénétiques. *Gastroenterologie Clinique et Biologique*, **3**, 15–19.

16 Collins, W. J., Bendig, D. W. & Taylor, W. F. (1979) Pulmonary vasculitis complicating childhood ulcerative colitis. *Gastroenterology*, **77**, 1091–1093.

17 D'Amelio, R., Rossi, P., Le Moles, S. *et al.* (1981) In vitro studies in cellular and humoral chemotasis in Crohn's disease using the under agarose gel technique. *Gut*, **22**, 566–570.

18 Daum, F., Gould, H. B., Gold, D. *et al.* (1979) Asymptomatic transient uveitis in children with inflammatory bowel disease. *American Journal of Diseases of Children*, **133**, 170–171.

19 Dew, M. J., Thompson, H. & Allan, R. N. (1979) The spectrum of hepatic dysfunction in inflammatory bowel disease. *Quarterly Journal of Medicine*, **48**, 113–135.

20 Du Boulay, C. & Whorwell, P. J. (1982) Nodular necrobiosis: a new cutaneous manifestation of Crohn's disease. *Gut*, **23**, 712–715.

21 Eade, O. E., Smith, C. L., Alexander, J. R. & Whorwell, P. J. (1980) Pulmonary function in patients with inflammatory bowel disease. *American Journal of Gastroenterology*, **73**, 154–156.

22 Eade, M. (1970) Liver disease of ulcerative colitis. *Annals of Internal Medicine*, **72**, 475–487.

23 Eade, M. N. & Brooke, B. N. (1969) Portal bacteremia in cases of ulcerative colitis submitted to colectomy. *Lancet*, **i**, 1008–1009.

24 Eade, M. N., Cooke, W. T., Brooke, B. N. & Thompson, H. (1971) Liver disease in Crohn's colitis. A study of 21 consecutive patients having colectomy. *Annals of Internal Medicine*, **74**, 518.

25 Enlow, R. W., Bias, W. B. & Arnett, F. C. (1980) The spondylitis of inflammatory bowel disease. *Arthritis and Rheumatism*, **23**, 1359–1365.

26 Fausa, O., Nygaard, K. & Elgjo, K. Amyloidosis and Crohn's disease. *Scandinavian Journal of Gastroenterology*, **12**, 657–662.

27 Fabry, T. L., Sachar, D. B. & Janowitz, H. D. (1980) Acute myelogenous leukemia in patients with ulcerative colitis. *Journal of Clinical Gastroenterology*, **2**, 225–227.

28 Ferguson, R. H. (1981) Arthritis associated with inflammatory bowel disease. *Minnesota Medicine*, **64**, 165–166.

29 Gebbers, J. & Otto, H. F. (1978) Immunohisto and ultracytochemical observations on the early lesion in ulcerative colitis. *Gut*, **19**, 989.

30 Greenstein, A. J., Janowitz, H. D. & Sachar, D. B. (1976) The extra-intestinal complications of Crohn's disease and ulcerative colitis. *Medicine*, **55**, 401–412.

31 Haslock, I. (1973) Arthritis and Crohn's disease – a family study. *Annals of the Rheumatic Diseases*, **32**, 479.

32 Higenbottam, T., Cochrane, G. M., Clark, T. J. H. *et al.* (1980) Bronchial disease in ulcerative colitis. *Thorax*, **35**, 581–585.

33 Hodgson, H. J. F., Potter, B. J. & Sewell, D. P. (1977) Immune complexes in ulcerative colitis and Crohn's disease. *Clinical and Experimental Immunology*, **29**, 187–196.

34 Hylander, E., Jarnum, S. & Frandsen, I. (1979) Urolithiasis and hyperoxaluria in chronic inflammatory bowel disease. *Scandinavian Journal of Gastroenterology*, **14**, 475–479.

35 Iyer, S. K. & Karlstadt, R. G. (1980) Hyperthyroidism and ulcerative colitis report of two cases and a review of the literature. *Journal of the National Medical Association*, **72**, 127–131.

36 Iyer, S. K., Handler, L. J. & Johnston, J. S. (1981) Thrombophlebitis migrans in association with ulcerative colitis. *Journal of the National Medical Association*, **73**(10) 987–989.

37 Jacobs, J. C. & Goezl, E. J. (1975) Streaking leucocyte factor, arthritis and pyoderma gangrenosum. *Paediatrics*, **56**, 570–578.

38 Janerot, G. (1975) The thyroid in ulcerative colitis and Crohn's disease. Part 1. Thyroid radioiodide uptake and urinary codine excretion. *Acta Medica Scandinavica*, **197**, 77–81.

39 Järnerot, G., Khan, A. & Truelove, S. (1975) The thyroid in ulcerative colitis and Crohn's disease. Part 2. Thyroid enlargement and hyperthyroidism in ulcerative colitis. *Acta Medica Scandinavica*, **197**, 83–87.

40 Johnson, N., McImee, A. S., Jewell, D. P. & Clarke, S. W. (1978) Pulmonary function in inflammatory bowel disease. *Digestion*, **18**, 416–418.

41 Kahn, E., Daum, F., Aiges, H. W. & Silverberg, M. (1980) Cutaneous polyarteritis nodosa associated with Crohn's disease. *Diseases of the Colon and Rectum*, **23**, 258–262.

42 Kitis, G., Thompson, H. & Allan, R. N. (1979) Finger clubbing in inflammatory bowel disease: its prevalence and pathogenesis. *British Medical Journal*, **ii**, 825–828.

43 Knudsen, L., Marcussen, H., Fleckenstein, P. *et al.* (1978) Urolithiasis in chronic inflammatory bowel disease. *Scandinavian Journal of Gastroenterology*, **13**, 433–436.

44 Kocoshis, S. A., Gartner, J. C., Gaffney, P. C. & Gryboski, J. D. (1979) Thrombocytopenia in ulcerative colitis. *Journal of Pediatrics*, **95**, 83–84.

45 Lam, A. & Borda, I. T. (1975) Coagulation studies in ulcerative colitis and Crohn's disease. *Gastroenterology*, **68**, 245–251.

46 Levin, E. N., Hirschfeld, D. S. & Hersch, R. A. (1979) Pericarditis in association with ulcerative colitis. *Western Journal of Medicine*, **130**, 369–370.

47 Lupmetti, M., Mehigan, D. & Cameron, J. L. (1980) Hepatobiliary complications of ulcerative colitis. *American Journal of Surgery*, **139**, 113–118.

48 Macrae, I. F. & Wright, V. (1973) A family study of ulcerative colitis with particular reference to ankylosing spending and sacro-ileitis. *Annals of the Rheumatic Diseases*, **32**, 10.

49 Maratka, Z. & Nedbal, J. (1964) Urolithiasis as a complication of the surgical treatment of ulcerative colitis. *Gut*, **5**, 214–217.

50 McCullock, D. K., Fraser, D. M. & Turner, A. L. (1980) Arthritis preceding fulminant ulcerative colitis and responding to colectomy. *British Medical Journal*, **i**, 839.

51 Mihas, A. A., Murad, T. M. & Hirschowitz, B. I. (1978) Sclerosing cholangitis associated with ulcerative colitis; light and electron microscopy studies. *American Journal of Gastroenterology*, **70**, 614–619.

52 Mori, K., Watanabe, H., Hiwatashi, N. *et al.* (1980) Studies on blood coagulation in ulcerative colitis and Crohn's disease. *Tohoku Journal Experimental Medicine*, **132**, 93–101.

53 O'Morain, C., Segal, A. W. & Levi, A. J. (1980) Elemental diets in the treatment of acute Crohn's disease. *British Medical Journal*, **i**, 1173–1175.

54 O'Morain, C., Segal, A. W., Walker, D. & Levi, A. J. (1981) Abnormalities of neutrophils function do not cause the migration defect in Crohn's disease. *Gut*, **22**, 817–822.

55 O'Morain, C., Smethurst, P., Levi, A. J. & Peters, T. J. (1983) Organelle pathology in ulcerative colitis with special reference to the lysosomal alterations. *Gut*, in press.

56 O'Morain, C., Smethurst, P., Levi, A. J. & Peters, T. J. (1983) Biochemical analysis of enzymic markers of inflammation in rectal biopsies from patients with ulcerative colitis and Crohn's disease. *Journal of Clinical Pathology*, in press.

57 Pepys, M. B., Druguet, M., Klass, H. J. *et al.* (1977) Immunological studies in inflammatory bowel disease. In *Immunology of the Gut: Ciba Foundation Symposium*. pp. 283–297. Amsterdam: Elsevier.

58 Perry, H. O. (1969) Pyoderma gangrenosum. *Southern Medical Journal*, **62**, 899–908.

59 Potter, B. J., Mee, A. S., Hodgson, H. J. F. & Jewell, D. P. (1978) $C1_q$ metabolism in patients with inflammatory bowel disease. *Gut*, **19**, A443.

60 Schulman, M. F. & Sugar, A. (1981) Peripheral corneal infiltrates in inflammatory bowel disease. *Annals of Ophthalmology (New York)*, **13**, 109–111.

61 Shashaty, G. G., Rath, C. F. & Britt, E. J. (1977) Autoimmune hemolytic anemia associated with ulcerative colitis. *American Journal of Hematology*, **3**, 199–208.

62 Shore, R. N. (1976) Pyoderma gangrenosum, defective neutrophil chemotoxin and leukemia. *Archives of Dermatology*, **112**, 1792–1793.

63 Soltis, R. D. (1981) Circulating immune complexes in Crohn's disease. In *Recent Advances in Crohn's Disease* (Ed.) Pena, A. S., Waterman, I. T., Booth, C. C. & Strober, W. pp. 328–337. The Hague: Martinus Nijhoff.

64 Smith, J. N. & Winship, D. H. (1980) Complications and extraintestinal problems in inflammatory bowel disease. *Medical Clinics of North America*, **64**, 1161–1171.

65 Teisberg, P. & Gjone, E. (1975) Humoral immune system activity in inflammatory bowel disease. *Scandinavian Journal of Gastroenterology*, **10**, 545–550.

66 Thompson, D. G., Lennard Jones, J. E., Swarbrick, E. T. & Bown, R. (1979) Pericarditis and inflammatory bowel disease. *Quarterly Journal of Medicine*, **67**, 93–97.

67 Thornton, J. R., Teague, R. H., Low-Beer, T. S. *et al.* (1980) Pyoderma gangrenosum and ulcerative colitis. *Gut*, **21**, 247–248.

68 Truelove S. C. & Witts, L. J. (1955) Cortisone in ulcerative colitis. Final report on a therapeutic trial. *British Medical Journal*, **ii**, 1041–1048.

69 Vinnick, I. E., Kern, F., Struthers, J. E. *et al.* Experimental chronic portal vein bacteremia. *Proceedings of the Society of Experimental Biology and Medicine*, **115**, 311–314.

70 Wandall, J. H. & Binder, V. (1982) Leucocyte function in ulcerative colitis quantitative leucocyte mobilisation to skin windows and in vitro function of blood leucocytes. *Gut*, **23**, 758–765.

71 Wands, J. R., La Mont, J. T., Mann, E. & Isselbacher, K. J. (1976) Arthritis associated with intestinal bypass procedure for morbid obesity, complement activation and characterization of circulating cryoproteins. *New England Journal of Medicine*, **294**, 121–124.

72 Wood, R. A. B. & Cuschieri, A. (1980) Is sclerosing cholangitis complicating ulcerative colitis a reversible condition? *Lancet*, **ii**, 716–718.

73 Wright, P. (1980) Conjunctival changes associated with inflammatory disease of the bowel. *Transactions of the Ophthalmic Society*, **100**, 96–97.

74 Wright, V. & Watkinson, G. (1965) The arthritis of ulcerative colitis. *British Medical Journal*, **ii**, 670.

75 Wright, R., Lumsden, K., Luntz, M. H. *et al.* (1965) Abnormalities of the sacro-iliac joints and uveitis in ulcerative colitis. *Quarterly Journal of Medicine*, **34**, 229.

INFLAMMATORY BOWEL DISEASE IN CHILDHOOD

Inflammatory bowel disease often becomes evident during childhood and adolescence. Of 844 patients with ulcerative colitis and 489 patients with Crohn's disease diagnosed at the University of Chicago, 40% in each group had the onset of symptoms before age 20 and 20% were under 15 years.[25] The peak ages of onset for both conditions in this retrospective study were 16–20 years. Most children are currently diagnosed between 10 and 18 years of age. Crohn's disease is rarely seen in children less than four years old. At our institution, Crohn's disease is now more common than ulcerative colitis and accounts for approximately two-thirds of the children with inflammatory bowel disease. The prevalence of these disorders varies in different countries. However, a recent survey in Baltimore demonstrated that two-thirds of newly hospitalized children with inflammatory bowel disease had Crohn's disease.[20] Both conditions have become important causes of chronic gastrointestinal disease in children.

Clinical features

The signs and symptoms of childhood inflammatory bowel disease are variable. Indeed, the subtle features of Crohn's disease may delay the correct diagnosis for many months or years.[3] Ulcerative colitis is usually diagnosed more rapidly because of the history of rectal bleeding. Prominent clinical findings are summarized in Table 12.24.

Table 12.24 Children with inflammatory bowel disease: presenting signs and symptoms.

	Crohn's disease ($n = 52$)	Ulcerative colitis ($n = 22$)
Abdominal pain	88%	95%
Altered stool pattern	81%	91%
Rectal bleeding	54%	100%
Weight loss	87%	68%
	($\tilde{x} = 5.7$ kg)	($\tilde{x} = 4.1$ kg)
Fever	44%	41%
Fall in height percentile	36%	14%

Abdominal pain

Abdominal pain is the most common symptom of inflammatory bowel disease in children. In

Crohn's disease, pain is often postprandial. The terminal ileum is affected in at least 80% of children with Crohn's disease, either as ileocolitis or isolated small bowel disease.[10] When disease involves the colon, pain characteristically occurs just prior to defecation. Children attempt to decrease gastrointestinal symptoms by diminishing their dietary intake.[16] Weight loss occurs in 68% of children with ulcerative colitis and the average loss is 9.1 kg. This finding is more frequent in Crohn's disease (87% of patients) and is more marked (12.5 kg).

Stool patterns
A change in stool pattern is the second most common finding (Table 12.24). Diarrhoea is not observed in 20% of children with Crohn's disease, particularly when disease is limited to the terminal ileum. Rectal bleeding occurred in all patients with ulcerative colitis but in only half of those with Crohn's disease.

Systemic signs of inflammatory bowel disease
Recurrent fever (oral temperature > 38°C) was not observed in the majority of our children at the time of diagnosis. However, low-grade temperature elevations may be overlooked.

Arthralgias and arthritis are frequently found. Lindsley and Schaller reported that arthritis occurred in 18 out of 86 (21%) children with ulcerative colitis and 5 out of 50 (10%) with Crohn's disease.[18] Most instances involved peripheral joints (especially knees and ankles) and tended to follow the onset of intestinal symptoms by eight months to eight years. The episodes were usually short-lived (lasting less than four weeks in most patients). No child developed permanent joint damage. These authors were unable to correlate arthritis with the severity of bowel disease, although in most children the intestinal disease was active concurrently with the joint symptoms. Spondylitis occurred in 4% of their patients and did not necessarily occur when the intestinal symptoms were active. This form of arthritis was progressive, resulting in permanent joint damage.

Cutaneous and mucocutaneous lesions have been described, including aphthous ulcers of the oral mucous membranes, erythema nodosum and pyoderma gangrenosum. These complications may be more frequent in ulcerative colitis than Crohn's disease.[1] Resolution usually coincides with satisfactory response of the bowel disease to medical management.

Clubbing of the fingers occurs in up to 25% of children with Crohn's disease.[10] The prevalence is greatest (66%) in children with extensive small

bowel disease. It may improve or disappear following remission of disease activity in the intestine.[1]

Growth failure
Growth failure is a serious complication of childhood inflammatory bowel disease. This finding was observed at the time of diagnosis in 14% of our children with ulcerative colitis and in 36% of those with Crohn's disease. The prevalence varies in reports from different medical centres, occurring in 2.5–21% of children with ulcerative colitis and 13–58% with Crohn's disease.[15] The reasons for these discrepant results include differing definitions of growth failure and utilization of past growth records, referral patterns, and the inclusion of steroid-treated patients.

Genetic short stature
Physicians must recognize that 3% of the normal population will be at the third height percentile for age. These children have genetic short stature and are not growth-impaired. They have normal growth velocity although their height remains at the lower end of normal. Skeletal age is similar to chronological age and there is usually a family history of short stature.

Assessment of impaired growth
In order to document growth retardation, one of two conditions must be present. The child should show an abnormal growth velocity, defined as a subnormal increase in linear growth. Most normal children and teenagers (prior to sexual maturation) increase their height by at least 4 cm/year.[30] If abnormal growth velocity persists for an extended period, a fall in height percentile will follow. Children whose height percentile appears to be normal at the time of diagnosis can be shown to have growth impairment if the height percentile has fallen from previous levels. Skeletal age in these children is usually 18–24 months behind the chronological age when assessed radiologically. Physicians and parents need to recognize that there is unequivocal evidence that inflammatory bowel disease itself causes growth impairment prior to the use of any corticosteroid therapy.[3, 10, 15, 19]

Causes of growth failure
Several explanations of the growth failure have been proposed. These include malabsorption,[2] secondary hypopituitarism with impaired growth hormone secretion,[19] zinc depletion,[27]

and increased protein and energy require-ments.[17] Recent studies from several centres have shown important areas of agreement. First, most children with growth failure do not demonstrate malabsorption based upon mea-surements of D-xylose absorption, Schilling tests, or faecal fat excretion.[12, 16, 17] Plasma zinc levels are not consistently low in children with growth failure[10, 16] and appear to reflect serum albumin concentration.[27] Recent investigations of growth hormone secretion in growth-retarded children, studied prior to receiving steroid medi-cations, have shown consistently normal or even elevated levels of growth hormone.[8, 32] The per-ipheral effects of growth hormone may be blunted in these children. We have recently shown that somatomedin C levels are lower in growth-impaired children with inflammatory bowel disease than normally-growing patients.[13] Furthermore, levels rise after treat-ment and precede improved growth velocity.

Currently there is no evidence to suggest that protein or energy requirements are increased above those needed in healthy children. The basal metabolic rate and nitrogen flux, including protein synthesis and catabolism and nitrogen retention, are not different from normal control children.[12, 22]

Nutritional intervention has resulted in improved growth velocity and allowed some children to reach their pre-illness height percen-tiles. Early studies utilized four to six weeks of total parenteral nutritional support.[17] Sub-sequent reports showed similar results using oral liquid supplements,[16] continuous naso-gastric infusions with elemental formulas,[21] and home total parenteral nutritional support.[29] Growth velocity data in two studies, one using parenteral nutrition and the other using oral supplements, were similar.[12, 16] Growth velocity increased from 1.8–1.9 cm/year prior to treat-ment to 6.2–6.4 cm/year in both centres. Although growth velocity may improve, a return to the pre-illness height percentile may not occur. Three to four years of improved growth velocity may be necessary before the original height percentile is reached.[16] During this inter-val, disease activity must be controlled, particu-larly if adequate energy and protein intake are to be achieved by oral means.

Laboratory tests to assess disease activity

Table 12.25 illustrates the frequency of abnor-mal results in selected tests which are useful in following children with inflammatory bowel disease. The erythrocyte sedimentation rate is a

Table 12.25 Children with inflammatory bowel disease: abnormal laboratory tests at diagnosis.

	Crohn's disease ($n = 52$)	Ulcerative colitis ($n = 22$)
ESR > 20 mm/h	90% ($\bar{x} = 40$ mm/h)	67% ($\bar{x} = 30$ mm/h)
PCV < 33%	38%	50%
< 36%	64%	64%
Iron < 50 μg/dl	68%	55%
Albumin < 3.3 g/dl	46%	45%
Folate < 3.6 ng/dl	34%	44%

more reliable indicator of disease activity in children than adults, and correlates more closely with symptoms in Crohn's disease than in ulcer-ative colitis. Other measures of intestinal absorptive capacity (D-xylose absorption, Schil-ling test and quantitative faecal fat) or nutri-tional status (folate, vitamin B_{12}, vitamin A, vitamin D, zinc) are obtained as indicated. Enteric protein losses are increased in virtually all patients with active disease. There is evidence that protein losses diminish as inflammation decreases.[29]

Lactose intolerance should be evaluated to exclude the possibility that intestinal symptoms are produced by milk products. Dairy products are important sources of energy, protein and calcium and may improve nutrient intake. Children with extensive small bowel disease are likely to have lactose intolerance. Excluding this group, genetic factors become important regard-less of whether disease is localized to the small bowel or colon.[14] Patients belonging to popu-lation groups with a high prevalence of lactase deficiency should be tested for lactose intoler-ance.

Medical treatment

The medical management of children with inflammatory bowel disease is in many ways similar to adults. Sulphasalazine is used as primary therapy and to minimize the cortico-steroid dose. Hypersensitivity reactions are not unusual in children, with 15% developing der-matological lesions and 2.5% manifesting signs of haemolytic anaemia.[10] In these situations, antibiotics such as tetracycline or metronidazole[33] may be tried for Crohn's disease. The risk of complications resulting from long-term continuous metronidizole adminis-tration in children is unknown. Some of the newer experimental salicylate derivatives may be eventually useful in ulcerative colitis, but they are not yet approved for use in children.

Corticosteroids

Corticosteroids are the most effective drug for children with moderately active disease. Once symptoms are controlled with daily administration, the gradual change to an alternate day regimen has definite advantages. Sadeghi-Nejad and Senior[26] reported that growth in children with ulcerative colitis 'approached normal' using an alternate day regimen. Others have described similar findings for children with Crohn's disease.[36] The duration of daily administration varies, depending upon the severity of symptoms. The dose of prednisone is tapered by 2.5–5.0 mg every 1–2 weeks on the alternate day after approximately 6 weeks of daily use. At times this is not possible and the daily regimen continues for a longer period. The dose of prednisone given on the alternate day is usually 20–40 mg or less.

Azathioprine or 6-mercaptopurine

Azathioprine (or 6-mercaptopurine) has been used in adults with Crohn's disease with varying degrees of success.[24] We have used this drug in selected children with reduction in symptoms and lowering of the corticosteroid dose necessary. The problem of long-term safety remains unanswered in the paediatric population. Therefore we tend to restrict its use to patients with extensive small bowel disease, particularly if they have had a previous intestinal resection or severe complications of corticosteroids.

Nutritional intervention

Collection of baseline anthropometric measurements

In order to monitor the extraintestinal effects of inflammatory bowel disease in children, serial height and weight measurements are plotted on standard growth charts. The parents' heights should also be recorded. If there is any question of growth impairment, a bone age determination should be performed to document the delay in skeletal maturation and to estimate growth potential.

Assessment of nutrient intake and goals

Energy and protein intake should be evaluated from food diaries. The energy intake should approach that recommended for normal children of similar age and sex. This is usually 30–45% higher than the mean daily energy intake in untreated symptomatic children.[16] Some authors recommend energy intakes based upon body weight, and suggest 310–335 kJ/kg (75–80 kcal/kg).[12, 17, 21] Concomitant protein intakes of 1.6–3.0 g/kg daily are associated with improved growth. Initially, liquid formula supplements may provide an additional source of nutrients. In addition to energy and protein intake, other nutrients must be provided if tests indicate specific deficiencies. These include iron, folate, vitamin B_{12}, vitamins A and D, and zinc. Because of the wide range of deficiencies reported in these patients, we advise a multivitamin preparation once daily for all children with Crohn's disease. Folate supplementation is given to patients receiving sulphasalazine because of the known interference of sulphasalazine on folate absorption.

Monitoring patient response

The response to treatment is determined by clinical signs and symptoms including weight and height gains and selected laboratory tests (Table 12.25). If clinical improvement does not occur, additional therapeutic manoeuvres may be necessary. A period of bowel rest and parenteral nutritional support or prolonged nasogastric infusion of an elemental diet may initiate a remission, particularly in Crohn's disease.[5, 23] The results of total parenteral support in childhood ulcerative colitis are frequently disappointing, although approximately 30% of children do improve.[34] The availability of home total parenteral nutrition allows children with extensive Crohn's disease the opportunity to resume normal growth and participate in normal social activities without prolonged hospitalization.[29]

Surgical intervention

In ulcerative colitis

Most of the indications for surgery in children with ulcerative colitis are similar to those for adults: haemorrhage, suspected perforation or abscess, toxic megacolon and medical intractibility. In children, impaired growth which does not reverse with medical management is another reason for considering surgery. Recently, there has been renewed interest in mucosal resection and ileoanal anastomosis in children.[6, 31] These procedures may be a promising alternative to the permanent standard or continent ileostomy.

In Crohn's disease

The high risk of recurrence following surgery in children with Crohn's disease has resulted in careful consideration of the indications of surgery in this age group. The frequency of recurrence depends upon the site of involvement and the length of the period of postoperative observation. Fonkalsrud et al.[7] studied recurrence in 50 children with Crohn's disease, an average of $4\frac{1}{2}$ years following surgery. Disease recurred in 7 out of 20 children (35%) with ileocaecal disease after resection of the terminal ileum and ascending colon and re-anastomosis. The results were worse in children with colorectal disease; 64% having recurrence after proctocolectomy. Only two patients had primary small bowel (terminal ileal) resections and one of these had a recurrence. These authors reported that the severity and extent of recurrent disease was greater with colorectal disease than with ileocolitis. These observations differ from those reported in adults and may reflect the greater risk for recurrence in younger patients.[4, 9, 28] High recurrence rates (57%) were also observed in 30 children with Crohn's disease after a follow-up period averaging 6.3 years.[35] Studies in adult patients have suggested a clinical recurrence rate of 94% and a re-operation rate of 89% for the fifteenth year after surgery.[9] For these reasons, medical management, including total parenteral nutritional support, is suggested when absolute indications for surgery (for example, suspected abscess or bowel obstruction) are not present.

When there is growth impairment which does not respond to medical therapy, surgical intervention must be considered. This is particularly true when there is evidence of localized disease amenable to resection. The effect of surgery upon growth has been a controversial matter. This is caused by different definitions of growth and 'catch-up growth' and the substitution of weight gain for linear growth. The degree of skeletal maturation and the period of time available for growth prior to sexual maturation are of critical importance. When puberty advances rapidly, bone maturation may be accelerated and sufficient time may not be available to permit a return to the pre-illness height percentile. Improved linear growth and growth velocity usually occur but the achievement of pre-illness height percentile is variable. Homer and Grand reported that only 2 of 14 prepubertal children with growth retardation reached their pre-illness height percentile following surgery.[11] Wesson showed that two-thirds of children will manifest improved growth velocity, but height percentiles were not reported.[35] Children who are prepubertal or in early stages of sexual development demonstrate greater linear growth than do adolescents who are in the later stages of sexual maturation.

REFERENCES

1   Ament, M. E. (1975) Inflammatory disease of the colon: ulcerative colitis and Crohn's disease. *Journal of Pediatrics*, **86**, 322–334.

2   Beeken, W. (1973) Absorptive defects in young people with regional enteritis. *Pediatrics*, **52**, 69–74.

3   Burbige, E. J., Huang Shi-Shung, & Bayless, T. M. (1975) Clinical manifestations of Crohn's disease in children and adolescents. *Pediatrics*, **55**, 866–871.

4   DeDombal, F. T., Burton, I. & Goligher, J. C. (1971) The early and late results of surgical treatment for Crohn's disease. *British Journal of Surgery*, **58**, 805–816.

5   Elson, C. O., Layden, T. J., Nemchausky, B. A. *et al.* (1980) An evaluation of total parenteral nutrition in the management of inflammatory bowel disease. *Digestive Diseases and Sciences*, **25**, 42–48.

6   Fonkalsrud, E. W., Ament, M. E. & Byrne, W. J. (1979) Clinical experience with total colectomy and endorectal mucosal resection for inflammatory bowel disease. *Gastroenterology*, **77**, 156–160.

7   Fonkalsrud, E. W., Ament, M. E., Fleisher, D. & Byrne, W. (1979) Surgical management of Crohn's disease in children. *American Journal of Surgery*, **138**, 15–20.

8   Gotlin, R. W. & Dubois, R. S. (1973) Nyctohemeral growth hormone levels in children with growth retardation and inflammatory bowel disease. *Gut*, **14**, 191–195.

9   Greenstein, A. J., Sachar, D. B., Pasternack, B. S. & Janowitz, H. D. (1975) Reoperation and recurrence in Crohn's colitis and ileocolitis. *New England Journal of Medicine*, **293**, 685–690.

10 Gryboski, J. D. & Spiro, H. M. (1978) Prognosis in children with Crohn's disease. *Gastroenterology*, **74**, 807–817.

11 Homer, D. R., Grand, R. J. & Colodny, A. H. (1977) Growth, course and prognosis after surgery for Crohn's disease. *Pediatrics*, **59**, 717–725.

12 Kelts, D. G., Grand, R. J., Shen, G. *et al.* (1979) Nutritional basis of growth failure in children and adolescents with Crohn's disease. *Gastroenterology*, **76**, 720–727.

13 Kirschner, B. S. (1981) Somatomedin deficiency: a possible cause of growth failure in children with chronic inflammatory bowel disease. *Abstracts of the Meeting of the American Gastroenterological Association, New York City*, 1192.

14 Kirschner, B. S., deFavaro, M. V. & Jensen, W. (1981) Lactose malabsorption in children and adolescents with inflammatory bowel disease. *Gastroenterology*, **81**, 829–832.

15 Kirschner, B. S., Voinchet, O. & Rosenberg, I. H. (1978) Growth retardation in children with inflammatory bowel disease. *Gastroenterology*, **75**, 504–511.

16 Kirschner, B. S., Klich, J. R., Kalman, S. S. *et al.* (1981) Reversal of growth retardation in Crohn's disease with therapy emphasizing oral nutritional restitution. *Gastroenterology* **80**, 10–15.

17 Layden, T., Rosenberg, T., Nemchansky, B. *et al.* (1976) Reversal of growth arrest in adolescents with Crohn's disease after parenteral alimentation. *Gastroenterology*, **70**, 1017–1026.

18 Lindsley, C. B. & Schaller, J. G. (1974) Arthritis associated with inflammatory bowel disease in children. *Journal of Pediatrics*, **84**, 16–20.

19 McCaffery, T. D., Nasr, K., Lawrence, A. M. & Kirsner, J. B. (1970) Severe growth retardation in children with inflammatory bowel disease. *Journal of Pediatrics*, **45**, 386–393.

20 Mendeloff, A. I. (1982) Personal communication.

21 Morin, C. L., Roulet, M., Roy, C. C. & Weber, A. (1980) Continuous elemental enteral alimentation in children with Crohn's disease and growth failure. *Gastroenterology*, **79**, 1205–1210.

22 Motil, K. J., Grand, R. J. Maletskos, C. J. & Young, V. R. (1982) The effect of disease, drug, and diet on whole body protein metabolism in adolescents with Crohn's disease and growth failure. *Journal of Pediatrics*, **101**, 343–351.

23 Navarro, J., Vargas, J., Cezard, J. P. *et al.* (1982) Prolonged constant rate elemental enteral nutrition in Crohn's disease. *Journal of Pediatric Gastroenterology and Nutrition*, **1**, 541–546.

24 Present, D. H., Korelitz, B. I., Wisch, N. *et al.* (1980) Treatment of Crohn's disease with 6-mercaptopurine. *New England Journal of Medicine*, **302**, 981–987.

25 Rogers, B. H. G., Clark, L. M. & Kirsner, J. B. (1971) The epidemiologic and demographic characteristics of inflammatory bowel disease: an analysis of a computerized file of 1400 patients. *Journal of Chronic Diseases*, **24**, 743–773.

26 Sadeghi-Nejad A. & Senior B. (1968) The treatment of ulcerative colitis in children with alternate-day corticosteroids. *Pediatrics*, **43**, 840–845.

27 Solomons, N. W., Rosenberg, I. H., Sandstead, H. H. & Vo-Khactu, K. P. (1977) Zinc deficiency in Crohn's disease. *Digestion*, **16**, 87–95.

28 Steinberg, D. M., Allan, R. N., Thompson, H. *et al.* (1974) Excisional surgery with ileostomy for Crohn's colitis with particular reference to factors affecting recurrence. *Gut*, **15**, 845–851.

29 Strobel, C. T., Byrne, W. J. & Ament, M. E. (1979) Home parenteral nutrition in children with Crohn's disease: an effective management alternative. *Gastroenterology*, **77**, 272–279.

30 Tanner, J. M., Whitehouse, R. H. & Takaishi, M. (1966) Standards from birth to maturity for height, weight, height velocity, and weight velocity. British children, 1965. Part II. *Archives of Diseases of Childhood*, **41**, 613–635.

31 Telander, R. L. & Perrault, J. (1980) Total colectomy with rectal mucosectomy and ileoanal anastomosis for chronic ulcerative colitis in children and young adults. *Mayo Clinic Proceedings*, **55**, 420–424.

32 Tenore, A., Berman, W. F., Parks, J. S. & Bongiovanni, A. M. (1977) Basal and stimulated serum growth hormone concentrations in inflammatory bowel disease. *Journal of Clinical Endocrinology and Metabolism*, **44**, 622–628.

33 Ursing, B., Alm, T., Barany, F. *et al.* (1982) A comparative study of metronidazole and sulfasalazine for active Crohn's disease: the cooperative Crohn's disease study in Sweden. *Gastroenterology*, **83**, 550–562.

34 Werlin, S. L. & Grand, R. J. (1977) Severe colitis in children and adolescents: diagnosis, course, and treatment. *Gastroenterology*, **73**, 828–832.

35 Wesson, D. E. & Shandling, B. (1981) Results of bowel resection for Crohn's disease in the young. *Journal of Pediatric Surgery*, **16**, 449–452.

36 Whittington, P. F., Barns, H. V. & Bayless, T. M. (1977) Medical management of Crohn's disease in adolescence. *Gastroenterology*, **72**, 1338–1344.

INFLAMMATORY BOWEL DISEASE AND PREGNANCY

In the past patients with inflammatory bowel disease were often advised to avoid pregnancy if at all possible, because conception was likely to result in a marked deterioration in the mother's health, with potential risks for both her life and that of the fetus.[1] Fortunately, more recent experience suggests that childbearing in both ulcerative colitis and Crohn's disease is not particularly hazardous and a favourable outcome to pregnancy is highly probable. This section will summarize current knowledge of the effects of inflammatory bowel disease on pregnancy, and vice versa, and suggest guidelines on management.

Fertility and inflammatory bowel disease

Fertility in women

Ulcerative colitis. There is now general agreement that fertility in women with ulcerative colitis is normal. Early studies were sometimes based on incomplete data, but a recent large survey from Oxford showed that the involuntary infertility rate among 147 married women with the disease was only 6.8%, which is certainly no higher than the infertility rate in the general population.[14]

Crohn's disease. The majority of reports imply that fertility is impaired to some extent in women with Crohn's disease.[7] Subfertility may be particularly common in patients with colonic involvement, but not all authors agree on this point. A number of factors may contribute to reduced fertility, including tubal involvement by the inflammatory reaction, dyspareunia, general ill health interfering with the normal ovulatory cycle, and possibly vitamin B_{12} deficiency.

If a remission of the Crohn's disease can be induced by medical treatment fertility may improve, but sometimes resection of diseased bowel seems to give a better chance of subsequent conception.

Fertility in men

There is no evidence that either ulcerative colitis or Crohn's disease per se impair male fertility. It may be reduced under two particular circumstances.

First, it is now well recognized that maintenance treatment with sulphasalazine interferes with spermatogenesis in a significant proportion of men. Sperm counts and motility are reduced, and there is an increased frequency of abnormal spermatozoal forms.[12] The mechanism of sulphasalazine-induced infertility remains obscure, but the effect seems to be reversible. If the drug can be withdrawn all semen qualities are usually restored after about eight weeks and normal pregnancies have then commonly followed.

Secondly, impaired fertility may occur in men with inflammatory bowel disease treated by proctocolectomy. Wide operative excisions of the rectum may damage the nerves controlling erection and ejaculation, and lead to permanent impotence. However, this problem can almost invariably be avoided if modern surgical techniques involving close dissection of the rectum are used.[10]

The impact of inflammatory bowel disease on pregnancy

Ulcerative colitis

The majority of published studies agree that ulcerative colitis does not reduce the chance of a woman producing a normal healthy baby. The data from the Oxford survey[14] is summarized in Figure 12.42. The outcome of the 209 completed pregnancies was almost identical to that expected for the general population of the United Kingdom. Other studies in North America, Germany and Scandinavia, as well as in the United Kingdom, have given very similar results.[7, 13] Vaginal delivery is the general rule in pregnancies which proceed to term, and the incidence of instrumental or operative deliveries is not increased.

The prognosis for a normal live birth is particularly favourable if the mother's colitis is in established remission when conception occurs. Active disease at the start of pregnancy has, in some studies, been associated with a marginally higher chance of abortion, prematurity or stillbirth. Even if a first attack of ulcerative colitis

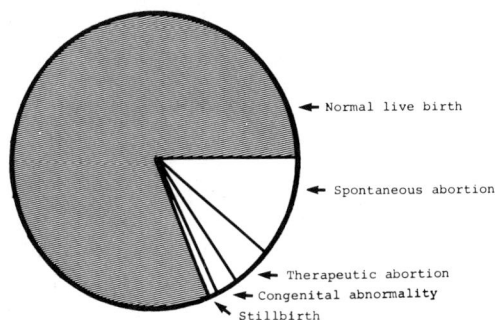

Fig. 12.42 Outcome of 209 completed pregnancies in women with ulcerative colitis.

develops during pregnancy, control of symptoms can almost invariably be achieved with current medical treatment and a normal infant is the usual outcome.

Crohn's disease

Less information is available on the effect of Crohn's disease on the outcome of pregnancy, but the chance of a normal live birth seems good, and in most series has been about 85%.[5] A recent survey on pregnancies in married women with Crohn's disease attending the Oxford inflammatory bowel disease clinic showed a rather lower success rate (70%), but the results were biased by one patient prone to recurrent spontaneous abortions.[9] The incidence of congenital abnormality and stillbirth was not increased.

The state of the Crohn's disease seems to influence the pregnancy outcome, in that active disease at conception may raise the risk of spontaneous abortion,[9] while first attacks of Crohn's disease during pregnancy have often been accompanied by a poor prognosis for a normal live birth.[7]

The effect of pregnancy on inflammatory bowel disease

Ulcerative colitis

Women who conceive when their ulcerative colitis is in stable remission have no excessive risk of a flare-up of their disease during pregnancy or the puerperium than in the general population. Approximately one-third of the patients will develop an exacerbation of their colitis during this period, but this is no higher than the expected recurrence rate for a comparable group of non-pregnant women. Any relapses of ulcerative colitis which do occur are particularly likely during the first trimester of pregnancy, but can easily be controlled by conventional medical treatment in most instances, and nowadays there should be no risk to the mother's life. Exacerbations of colitis were considered likely in the puerperium, but recent studies suggest that this is no longer the case.

The outlook is rather less favourable when the disease is active at the time of conception. Over two-thirds of the patients remain symptomatic or become worse during pregnancy and the puerperium, while the remainder may improve or go into remission. Worsening symptoms are most common early in pregnancy, but severe attacks can usually be prevented by standard medical therapy. At one time, therapeutic abortion was held to be a reliable method of halting relapses of colitis,[1, 3] but there is little clear evidence to support this view and termination of pregnancy cannot be justified purely for this reason.

Sometimes ulcerative colitis starts during pregnancy, and this is especially common during the first trimester. Early studies suggested that this was a grave situation, with a high probability of severe disease and a substantial maternal mortality. More recent studies provide a more optimistic view, in that the colitis usually responds to energetic medical treatment, and maternal deaths have not been observed.

A similar improvement in outlook applies to first attacks of ulcerative colitis in the puerperium. While these also used to carry a poor prognosis and an appreciable maternal risk, nowadays the attacks tend to be mild and readily controlled.

Crohn's disease

Once again, less information is available about the effects of pregnancy on the course of Crohn's disease. In general, however, the patients do well, particularly if the disease is quiescent at conception. Such women have a 60–70% chance overall of remaining symptom-free, and the proportion is probably even higher if the Crohn's disease has been treated surgically before pregnancy.[2, 4] If relapse does occur, the commonest time for recurrence of symptoms seems to be after delivery.

Active disease at conception behaves in a very similar way to active ulcerative colitis in pregnancy, with the majority of patients continuing to have symptoms but a small proportion showing improvement, particularly as the pregnancy progresses.[6]

First attacks of Crohn's disease may coincide with pregnancy, but very few such cases have been reported; the available data imply that the condition often follows a severe course under such circumstances. The same may be true for the onset of Crohn's disease in the puerperium, but again the available information is very limited.

Drug treatment of inflammatory bowel disease in pregnancy

Corticosteroids and sulphasalazine are the most important agents for the treatment of inflammatory bowel disease. Both drugs carry a theoretical risk of teratogenicity (on the basis of animal experiments), but no evidence at all has emerged from recent studies of any increased incidence of congenital abnormality in the babies of mothers treated for inflammatory bowel disease with conventional dosages.[9, 11, 14]

It has been suggested that corticosteroid treatment might lead to impaired placental function and an increased chance of still-birth or prematurity, but again no evidence to support this view has been provided by clinical surveys.

Sulphasalazine and sulphapyridine cross the placenta and could possibly increase the risk of bilirubin displacement from albumin in the neonate, with consequent kernicterus. Neonatal jaundice is not more common in babies of mothers treated with sulphasalazine, and no cases of kernicterus have been reported. Sulphasalazine and its metabolites are secreted into breast milk, and a similar argument might suggest a theoretical risk of kernicterus in breast-fed babies whose mothers took the drug. However, the binding sites for sulphasalazine, sulphapyridine and bilirubin on albumin are different, and the bilirubin-displacing effects of the parent drug and its derivatives are insignificant.[8] There seems no reason, therefore, to advise women who take sulphasalazine to discontinue the drug near to parturition or while they are breastfeeding.

Other drugs such as azathioprine and metronidazole are occasionally used in the treatment of inflammatory bowel disease. Pregnancy is inadvisable in women taking azathioprine because of its potential teratogenic effects. No adverse effects of metronidazole on the fetus have been reported, but as usual it seems sensible to avoid the use of any drug in pregnancy unless there are strong positive reasons for its employment.

Surgical treatment during pregnancy

Surgical intervention during pregnancy is rarely necessary, as even severe attacks can now usually be controlled by medical treatment. Emergency colectomy in cases of severe ulcerative colitis carries a substantial risk to mother and child, but sometimes has to be undertaken because of life-threatening disease. Case reports in recent years imply a more favourable prognosis than was once the case.

Pregnancy in ileostomists

The outlook for a normal pregnancy is very good for women who have a permanent ileostomy. Vaginal delivery is usually possible, although perineal scarring may increase the chance of Caesarean section, particularly in women with Crohn's disease. Minor degrees of ileostomy prolapse are not uncommon as the abdomen enlarges late in pregnancy, but the only other problem which has been reported with any frequency is acute or subacute intestinal obstruction.

Conclusions

Fertility is normal in women with ulcerative colitis, but may be impaired in some women with Crohn's disease. The commonest cause of subfertility in men with inflammatory bowel disease is probably sulphasalazine treatment.

In general, a normal outcome to pregnancy can be expected in women with ulcerative colitis or Crohn's disease. Neither disorder should prevent a woman from embarking on a pregnancy if she so wishes, but ideally she should be symptom-free at the time of conception. If the inflammatory bowel disease is quiescent at the start of pregnancy, there is little or no excess chance of relapse. Any exacerbations which do occur can usually be controlled by medical means, and the commonly used drugs seem to be quite safe. Therapeutic abortion does not help in inducing remission of active disease during pregnancy. Surgical intervention during pregnancy may be hazardous but necessary. Pregnancy in women with a permanent ileostomy usually presents no major problems.

REFERENCES

1 Abramson, D., Jankelson, I. R. & Milner, L. R. (1951) Pregnancy in idiopathic ulcerative colitis. *American Journal of Obstetrics and Gynecology*, **61**, 121–129.

2 Crohn, B. B., Yarnis, H. & Korelitz, B. I. (1956) Regional enteritis complicating pregnancy. *Gastroenterology*, **31**, 615–628.

3 Crohn, B. B., Yarnis, H., Crohn, E. B. *et al.* (1956) Ulcerative colitis and pregnancy. *Gastroenterology*, **30**, 391–403.

4 de Dombal, F. T., Burton, I. L. & Goligher, J. C. (1972) Crohn's disease and pregnancy. *British Medical Journal*, **iii**, 550–553.

5 Fielding, J. F. (1976) Inflammatory bowel disease and pregnancy. *British Journal of Hospital Medicine*, **15**, 345–352.

6 Fielding, J. F. & Cooke, W. T. (1970) Pregnancy and Crohn's disease. *British Medical Journal*, **ii**, 76–77.

7 Järnerot, G. (1982) Fertility, sterility and pregnancy in chronic inflammatory bowel disease. *Scandinavian Journal of Gastroenterology*, **17**, 1–4.

8 Järnerot, G., Andersen, S., Esbjörner, E. *et al.* (1981), Albumin reserve for binding of bilirubin in maternal and cord serum under treatment with sulphasalazine. *Scandinavian Journal of Gastroenterology*, **16**, 1049–1055.

9 Khosla, R., Willoughby, C. P. & Jewell, D. P. (1984) Crohn's disease and pregnancy. *Gut*, **25**, 52–56.

10 Lee, E. C. G. (1980) Proctocolectomy. In *Topics in Gastroenterology, 8* (Ed.) Truelove, S. C. & Kennedy, H. J. pp. 199–205. Oxford: Blackwell Scientific.

11 Mogadam, M., Dobbins, W. O., Korelitz, B. I. & Ahmed, S. W. (1981) Pregnancy in inflammatory bowel disease: effect of sulfasalazine and corticosteroids on fetal outcome. *Gastroenterology*, **80**, 72–76.

12 Toovey, S., Hudson, E., Hendry, W. F. & Levi, A. J. (1981) Sulphasalazine and male infertility: reversibility and possible mechanism. *Gut*, **22**, 445–451.

13 Willoughby, C. P. (1983) Fertility, pregnancy and ulcerative colitis. In *Inflammatory Bowel Diseases* (Ed.). Allan, R. N., Keighley, M. R. B., Hawkins, C. F. & Alexander-Williams, J. pp. 113–120. Edinburgh: Churchill Livingstone.

14 Willoughby, C. P. & Truelove, S. C. (1980) Ulcerative colitis and pregnancy. *Gut*, **21**, 469–474.

Chapter 13
Stomas and Stoma Care

H. B. Devlin

Stomas, either iatrogenic or spontaneous, have been part of the spectrum of intestinal disease since time immemorial.

In the British literature Cheselden[6] described a woman who developed a preternatural colostomy associated with a strangulated umbilical hernia. The first English iatrogenic stoma was described by George Freer of Birmingham,[16] who fashioned a left iliac colostomy for an imperforate anus. The history of stoma surgery has been extensively reviewed by Cromar,[7] Richardson[38] and Devlin.[11]

Stoma surgery is so much a part of gastroenterological practice that the provision of services for the stoma patient is an essential prerequisite of any unit. All surgery brings its train of complications – stoma surgery is no exception to this rule – thus both physicians and surgeons need to know what complications can be expected in stoma patients and how these complications can be managed.

TYPES OF STOMA

Stomas may be constructed to allow *input* to the gut – feeding gastrostomy and jejunostomy; to *divert* the gastro-oesophageal and faecal stream – pharyngostomy, oesophagostomy, ileostomy and colostomy; or as permanent *output* stomas – ileostomy or colostomy. With permanent output stomas the bowel distal to the stoma is usually excised surgically – proctocolectomy and abdominoperineal excision of the rectum. Much surgical invention has been extended recently to develop alternatives to a permanent incontinent stoma, such as the Kock ileostomy pouch,[30] the Parks mucosal proctectomy and pelvic pouch,[35] and stapled or sutured anastomosis for low rectal carcinoma.

The types of stoma employed and their principal indications are summarized in Table 13.1.

INCIDENCE

Upper gastrointestinal tract diverting stomas are used relatively rarely, and, compared with ileostomy or colostomy, feeding stomas are uncommon; no figures for their incidence are available.

Ileostomy and colostomy represent an important aspect of gastroenterology. About 10 000

Table 13.1　Types of gastrointestinal stoma.

Function	Anatomy	Clinical indications
Input stomas (temporary)	Gastrostomy Jejunostomy (fine-tube enterostomy, see text)	Malnutrition, severe catabolic states due to oesophageal obstruction, stricture, corrosive burns, carcinoma, trauma, etc.
		Jejunostomy is a preferred access after gastrectomy or when access to stomach is limited
Diversion stomas (temporary)	Pharyngostomy Oesophagostomy	To divert swallowed saliva and protect the bronchial tree in neonatal oesophageal atresia, tracheo-oesophageal fistula Adult oesophageal obstruction or to divert saliva from the oesophagus
	Ileostomy ('loop' or 'split')	To divert the faecal stream from the colon Anorectal Crohn's disease To 'cover' a distal resection * Non-closed-loop colonic obstruction
	Colostomy ('loop', 'transverse', 'sigmoid') Temporary end colostomy with primary excision of colonic lesion	Anorectal agenesis Trauma Distal inflammatory bowel disease Diverticular disease Colon and rectal carcinoma To 'cover' distal surgical manoeuvres
Output stomas (permanent)	Ileostomy ('terminal')	Ulcerative colitis Colorectal Crohn's disease Familial polyposis coli Ischaemic colitis
	Colostomy ('terminal', 'iliac')	Rectal carcinoma Anal carcinoma Unrepairable anorectal malformations Severe anorectal injuries

ileostomates live in England and Wales and 250–300 new permanent ileostomies are created each year in this population.[23,34] The incidence of inflammatory bowel disease is high in Britain,[12] but the frequency of ileostomy operations has fallen throughout the 1970s.[34]

In the USA it was estimated that 4000 ileostomies were created in 1968 (3480 for ulcerative colitis) and that the average years of life remaining to an ileostomate from the time of operation was 39.3. The cost of ileostomy care was estimated to be $12 400 000 per annum at 1968 prices.[20]

Permanent colostomies are constructed about ten times more frequently than ileostomies. Most permanent colostomies are created for rectal cancer and the life expectation of these elderly patients with malignant disease is less than the younger ileostomy patient with inflammatory bowel disease. In 1980, 5000 permanent colostomy operations for rectal cancer were performed in England and Wales and it was suggested that about 100 000 patients with permanent colostomies were alive in this population. In the Northern Region of England one

colostomy was made per 4000 population at risk per year and two-thirds of all colostomies were permanent.[10,34]

This scene is changing rapidly, particularly since the advent of the stapling gun. Indeed, one report suggests that the number of permanent colostomies performed for rectal cancer may be reduced by 85%.[24] Our own experience is perhaps more cautious, but, undoubtedly, newer techniques have reduced the frequency of new permanent colostomies (Table 13.2). Little is known about the incidence and outcome of temporary stomas, though the experience of appliance manufacturers suggests that British surgeons perform far more of these operations than their European counterparts.

Construction of ileostomies for ulcerative colitis is generally undertaken when patients are in their mid-twenties and rather more frequently in females than males, the ratio of female to male ileostomates being approximately 1.4 : 1. Rectal cancer is a disease of advancing years and the peak incidence of colostomates is in the 65th year; the male/female ratio is 1.2 : 1 or thereabouts.

Table 13.2 Indications for intestinal stomas in a population of 170 000–200 000, North Tees General Hospital 1970–1981.

	Ileostomy		Colostomy		
	Temporary	Permanent	Temporary	Permanent	Total
Colon cancer	}16	2	88	{ 23	}279*
Rectal cancer				{150	
Colon diverticular disease	4	0	51	0	55
Ulcerative colitis	0	39	0	0	39
Crohn's disease	3	16(13)**	6	0	25
Gynaecological cancer	0	1	0	9	10
Sigmoid colon volvulus	0	0	6	0	6
Anorectal trauma	0	0	5	0	5
Miscellaneous	2	1	5	5	13
Total	25	59	161	187	432

* *76 patients with colorectal cancer had 'temporary' stomas performed but no further surgery; i.e., these stomas were permanent because the disease was inoperable.*

** *Only 13 patients had permanent ileostomies for Crohn's disease; however, three patients each had two reoperations requiring new ileostomy construction.*

OPERATIVE TECHNIQUES

Basic principles

Four principles govern the construction of all stomas: the stoma must be *sited* correctly; the bowel must not be *stretched* to the body surface; the mucosa should be immediately *sutured* to the skin margins to prevent *stricture*; and, lastly, no *spaces* should be left in which other viscera could strangulate.

Input enterostomy

The one exception to these principles is the introduction of a fine-bore enteral feeding tube – input gastrostomy or jejunostomy – using the submucosal tunnel technique described by Delaney and Garvey.[8] An input enterostomy can be carried out into the stomach, duodenum or jejunum, though for ease of access the body or fundus of the stomach or an upper loop of jejunum are preferred. If a gastroenteric anastomosis has been performed, the tube can be threaded down into the jejunum well past the anastomosis and then used for immediate post-operative feeding. Narrow catheters should be used; a 16 gauge venous or umbilical catheter is ideal.

Essentially the technique is to introduce the catheter into the gut via a long submucosal tunnel. This is best accomplished by making the tunnel in a mobile loop of intestine. The loop is stretched out and a number 14 needle is placed into the anti-mesenteric border and then along up its hilt in the submucous layer. The bowel is then arranged like a concertina on the needle so

that the needle tip projects into the lumen. The catheter is then threaded in through the needle and the catheter end positioned in the bowel. The needle is withdrawn leaving the catheter in situ. Using the same 14 needle the catheter is threaded through the anterior abdominal wall. To complete the manoeuvre the loop of jejunum is sutured to the parietal peritoneum at the exit site of the catheter. The catheter needs to be fixed to the skin with a silk saxon stocking suture to prevent it accidentally being dislodged. No closure is required when the tube feed is discontinued; the skin suture is cut and the catheter withdrawn. A similar percutaneous technique has been used by introducing a catheter through a needle track placed into the proximal jejunum or the stomach under X-ray control.

Diversion stomas

Pharyngostomy and oesophagostomy are uncommon stomas and details of their construction and management are available in specialist surgical texts. Temporary, 'split' or 'loop', ileostomy and colostomy are common enough; their indications are given in Table 13.1. The relative merits, or demerits, of these stomas should be mentioned; a loop ileostomy discharges faeces at a uniform rate, the faeces are more liquid than solid and it is easy to collect them in an appliance. The stoma is easy to construct and not prone to ischaemia, stenosis or prolapse; it is also easy to close.[1]

If an absorbable rod (Biethium, manufactured by Ethicon Co., Edinburgh) is used to support the stoma, immediate mucocutaneous suturing can be done so that the stoma is functional immediately.[11] Ileal fluid is relatively odourless and wherever possible I would construct a temporary ileostomy rather than a temporary colostomy.

A temporary colostomy is bulky; it needs a support at skin level to ensure that distal defunction is complete and there is not carry over of faeces. The bulk of the stoma and the support make appliance fitting difficult. The stoma discharges semisolid faeces at erratic intervals and colonic contents are very smelly. The loop colostomy is prone to prolapse, making the problem of effluent collection more difficult. The vastness of the stoma greatly upsets many patients and they find the neat small loop ileostomy more acceptable to care for. Many temporary stomas never get closed (Table 13.2); this consideration should also be weighed in the surgical calculus.

Siting

An output stoma should be readily accessible to the patient. Accessibility may be limited by other disabilities; eyesight and arthritis are important considerations. Obesity may pose problems for stoma siting and the use of a mirror for stoma care should be considered.

In general a stoma should be on a flat skin surface to facilitate appliance attachment. The emergent bowel should pass through the rectus muscle to allow fixation to the fascia of the rectus sheath, thereby minimizing the risk of herniation which is common when the bowel is brought through the flank muscles. The stoma should not be too close to the laparotomy incision both to facilitate fitting a leakproof appliance and to prevent wound soiling. Finally, the stoma should not be too close to body creases, flexion lines, the umbilicus, the groin, the waist or the iliac crest.

The stoma site should be tested preoperatively on the patient with an empty appliance. When the best site has been found, the test should be repeated using an appliance full of water. A full stoma appliance should also be tested while the patient sits to eat. Once the ideal site has been identified – it is usually on the cephalad slope of the infraumbilical mound of rectus muscle – it must be marked indelibly preoperatively. This is best done by an intradermal injection of dye, methylene blue or patent blue violet. Turnbull has recommended injecting each layer of the abdominal wall with dye to ensure construction of a direct, straight stoma.[44] Slippage between the abdominal wall layers

after a laparotomy wound has been made can be a problem, and our own preference is to make the stoma track before opening the abdomen in those cases where we have already decided to construct a permanent stoma.

Surgical technique

The bowel must be brought out without any tension, since stretching of the mesentery may make it ischaemic. Tension is most commonly a problem in the fat patient when a loop stoma is being raised. If stretching is a problem the alternative of an end outflow stoma and a distal mucous fistula should be considered. Division of the gut often allows more extensive dissection of the mesentery and better mobilization of the intestine. For defunctioning stomas of the colon, complete transection of the bowel and construction of two stomas prevents carry over of faeces, which can be a troublesome complication of a transverse colostomy.[9]

Immediate mucocutaneous suturing prevents skin level scarring due to healing by granulation and greatly facilitates early postoperative stoma care.[19,36,40] Ileostomies must have a spout to provide a leakproof arrangement with the appliance, as described by Brooke[4] and others.[42,43]

SEQUELAE OF STOMA SURGERY

There are inexorable physical, physiological, psychological, psychosexual and social sequelae of stoma surgery which inevitably interact. Age and sex are important in determining the outcome of stoma surgery. In general, younger patients, particularly ileostomates with ulcerative colitis, adapt more readily than elderly ones with carcinoma of the rectum.

The most immediate physical sequel of stoma surgery is the alteration to the patient's body image. Physiologically there is no control over stoma discharge; apart from stretch sensations there is no awareness of the passage of stool. Flatus emission is identified by smell and copious fluid discharge, diarrhoea by an increase in weight of the bag.

The physiological consequences of a stoma are dictated by its position in the gastrointestinal tract. An ileostomy discharges 400+ ml/day; the effluent has a relatively high sodium content (38–40 mmol daily) compared with the normal daily faecal loss (10 mmol). Magnesium and calcium are lost in excess from an ileostomy; however, potassium losses are small (Table 13.3). As a consequence of this, water and

Table 13.3 Metabolic consequences of ileostomy: average daily losses in faeces and urine.

	Normal subject	Ileostomate
Faeces		
Sodium (mmol)	10	38–40
Potassium (mmol)	12	3–6
Magnesium (mmol)	3–3.5	3.5–4.5
Calcium (mmol)	5.5	7.5–20
Nitrogen (mmol)	up to 107	43–171
Fat (mmol)	11–18	5–13
Bilirubin (mol)	–	118–166
Stercobilinogen (μmol)	35–420	5–52
Volume (ml)	100–150	350–500
Urine		
Volume (ml)	1500	800–1000
Sodium (mmol)	110–240	93
Potassium (mmol)	35–90	114

electrolyte loss, dehydration and hyponatraemia are common in ileostomates. There is an 11% reduction in total body water and a 7% reduction in total body sodium in patients with an ileostomy.[22, 26] Some 30% of ileostomates appear to live on the verge of water and electrolyte depletion despite normal blood electrolyte levels. Such patients may admit to dizziness, muscle cramps and impaired mental concentration. Undoubtedly ileostomates should be advised to take additional salt and water in their diets. Excess water and electrolyte loss from infective diarrhoea, the use of bulking laxatives, excessive alcohol intake and sweating in hot climates are especially dangerous to ileostomates.

The water and electrolyte loss from the ileostomy is matched by a reduction in urine output and an increase in its concentration. Consequently there is an enhanced incidence of urolithiasis variously reported as between 0.7% and 10.8%.[2, 23, 33] If the terminal ileum is diseased or excised, the enterohepatic circulation of bile salts may be interrupted and such patients have a predisposition to gallstones. Long-term studies of British ileostomates have shown cholelithiasis to be more prevalent in them than in a control population but there is, to date, no record of an increased rate of cholecystectomy.[25] Alterations in ileal microbiological flora may also have an adverse effect on vitamin B_{12} absorption.[28]

A colostomy is never associated with the same degree of fluid and electrolyte loss. Colostomies, unmodified by drug therapy or dietary activity, act between one and six times a day and the normal mass action of the colon is apparent. However, in some sigmoid stomas, particularly in patients with Crohn's disease, there may be an almost continuous intermittent discharge of faecal material.[13] A sudden alteration in stoma activity may be indicative of new disease, subacute intestinal obstruction due to an impacted bolus, adhesion bands or volvulus, or intra-abdominal sepsis. Altered colostomy activity, particularly if associated with bleeding, may signify a metachronous colonic tumour.

The psychological consequences of a stoma have attracted much research. There is undoubtedly an alteration in the patient's lifestyle; after all they now have an ectopic anus and are incontinent, so that even with the best stoma care and appliances they can no longer view themselves as normal. This psychological adaptation may vary widely from exhibitionism or obsessionalism to an attempt at concealment. Depression is common, particularly in the elderly, and if unrecognized and untreated may end in suicide. Social isolation and withdrawal from day-to-day contacts may be due to feelings of shame, but the majority stem from a lack of confidence in the appliance and the fear of accidents.

Sexual and psychosexual difficulties receive much attention; their frequency is probably underestimated in the literature and overestimated in some of the paramedical and nursing magazines. Sexual difficulties following nerve damage as a consequence of the pelvic surgery may lead to failure of ejaculation and/or erection in the male and orgasmic disappointment in the female, but this is almost always associated with disorders of micturition. Vaginal scarring and dyspareunia in the female, or mucopurulent discharge from a retained rectal stump, are generally correctable problems. A much greater problem is the management of patients with a loss in libido and embarrassment in normal sexual activity. Estimates of sexual failure in ostomates vary; in general, the younger ostomate with a greater sex drive has fewer problems than the older patient. However, all reports suggest that an ostomy is a sexual deterrent, resulting in reduced sexual experience and a lower incidence of pre- and extramarital activity.[5, 13, 21]

Homosexuals and other sexual aberrants may suffer severely after rectal excision. Hence this aspect of management should be considered before surgery is undertaken.

STOMA CARE

Preoperative

Before undertaking stoma surgery the surgeon must ensure that the patient understands what is being done. If this principle is not followed, the patient may regard the surgeon either as a healer or as a mutilator and violator of their body image. If there has been inadequate preoperative counselling, the ostomate's reaction to the surgeon may be repressed and the patient may not discuss the stoma, its effects on life style and its management with the surgeon. Furthermore, some 30% of patients require stoma surgery as emergencies allowing little time for preoperative preparation and, more importantly, not allowing time to involve their spouse and close family in the decision making. In these circumstances nursing and medical attitudes and support are crucial to long-term success.

Hence the patient should be warned as early as possible in the diagnostic assessment that stoma surgery is a possibility. The spouse, parents, and close friends should be told as well. Soon after the patient has been warned about the possibility of a stoma, an introduction to a stoma care nurse should be made; an ostomate visitor can also be brought in to help. The pre-ostomate will have many fears and questions about recovery, work, home life; these must be heard and evaluated by the surgical team and adequate replies to questions must be provided.

Postoperative

In the immediate postoperative period the patient, despite careful preparation, is usually shocked to see the stoma. The initial response is denial, then gradual adjustment takes place; the patient learns from the stoma nurse how to manage the appliance but all this is within the cocoon of support in hospital. Morale is often much lower than is generally recognized when

the patient is discharged home, and although confidence builds up at home there is a real possibility of anxiety and depression at the time the patient is due to resume work.[14] Depression and denial of rectal loss may be manifest by the development of phantom rectum sensations, a feeling of rectal fullness and a constant desire to defecate, which may persist for months or years after surgery.[15] If depression persists the tricyclic antidepressants are particularly useful, having a powerful mood change potential and an anti-cholinergic action on the gut which becomes more constipated and easier to manage.

Stoma care nurses

Stoma care nurses or enterostomal therapists in the USA are specialist registered nurses who have taken courses in the management of ostomates. Their particular expertise is in pouch management, their knowledge of the range and properties of appliances, skin barriers and odour filters. They have been trained in counselling and psychology so that they can ease the rehabilitation of the patient and his family. They will undertake house calls, advise about housing, toilet and accommodation needs of ostomates. Employers can turn to them for disinterested advice about the employment of ostomates. They are now a vital member of the therapeutic team.

Preoperatively they should be involved in counselling, testing and evaluating appliances, siting the stoma, teaching appliance care postoperatively and in crisis intervention in the longer term.

A stoma nurse will need clinic space with a sluice in the hospital; she needs a telephone, secretarial assistance and records support if she is to provide a worthwhile community-based service. The provision of stoma care is numerically a relatively small commitment. An average family doctor in the UK may have one or two ostomates. He is never going to gain vast knowledge of their needs or of the range of appliances available. Hence the need for specialist nurses and for surgical specialization in this field.

Ostomy clubs

In the British Isles there are three groups providing support for ostomates. The oldest of these is the Ileostomy Association of Great Britain and Ireland; the Colostomy Welfare Group and the Urinary Conduit Association are the others. In the USA all ostomy needs are catered for by the United Ostomy Association. The International Ostomy Association (IOA) provides a liaison between the separate national bodies. The strength of the IOA has been its Professional Advisory Committee which has published excellent pamphlets and acted as a pressure group on behalf of ostomates worldwide.

In the British Isles the voluntary associations have trained 'visitors' who will make hospital and home visits. These visits can often provide a wider dimension of understanding than nurses and surgeons can provide. It could be argued that self-help groups may encourage disability, but to date no evidence for this is available. Our advice is to use the therapeutic skills of these groups in rehabilitation whenever they are available.

APPLIANCES

Modern appliances are generally made of plastic and are disposable. However, there is no doubt that recently lightweight rubber pouches which are reusable have made a comeback on economic grounds.

All appliances consist of a face-plate with an aperture for the stoma, or stoma spout of an ileostomy (Figure 13.1). The face-plate and pouch may be one piece or two pieces. Two pieces have the advantage that once the face-plate is applied and fixed to the skin it can be left in place for days. Each removal involves skin trauma; two piece appliances are consequently more gentle on the skin and more popular. Bags may be disposable and/or drainable. Disposable bags are best for sigmoid end colostomies with hard, formed faeces, drainable bags being preferred for large output stomas. The bags can be emptied of small volumes, obviating the weight problem and the risk of a heavy bag coming adrift and causing an accident.

The choice of an appliance is a personal one, and advice is needed, particularly in the early stages. The variety is now so wide that an expert should be consulted. There are appliances of all shapes, sizes and configurations. The patient needs to make an informed choice with a specialist surgeon or nurse, then the patient needs a check list for reordering. The check list must include the manufacturer's name, the size and the invoice code numbers. This information is a vital part of the patient's armamentarium. On discharge, it is always wise to give the patient at least two weeks' supply of equipment and to include some drainable appliances as a standby in case of a bout of diarrhoea.

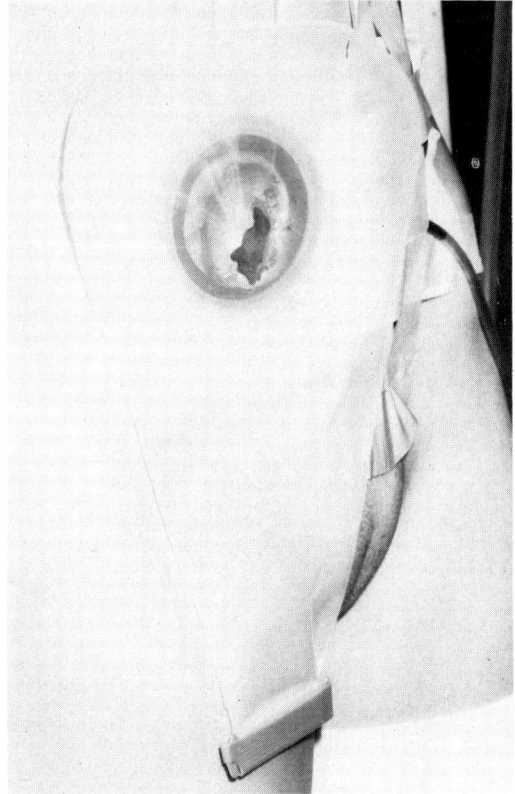

Fig. 13.1 Drainage bag with integral Karaya seal placed over an ileostomy stoma. From Irving[28a] with kind permission of the author and the publisher, W. B. Saunders.

SKIN PROTECTIVES/BARRIERS

The modern era of hypoallergenic skin care dawned in the mid-1960s with Karaya gum.[37, 41] Karaya gum, which can be made into a pliant sheet bonded to a plastic face-plate, is still in use but has been almost superseded by Stomahesive (gelatin, pectin, sodium carboxymethylcellulose and polyisobutylene), Comfeel and Hollihesive. Each of these products is applied directly to the skin, no matter how traumatized it is, and can be moulded to body contours. Each preparation is available in tube paste form which can be used to fill up the skin surface to make it flat enough to take a standard appliance face-plate.

ODOUR

Flatus, which is discharged uncontrolled from a stoma, contains unpleasant smelling compounds – amines, indole, methane and hydrogen sulphide. Hydrogen sulphide molecules are the most obnoxious and are detectable by the human nose at concentrations of 0.01 p.p.m. Flatus is the most threatening breach of cover that the ostomate fears at a cocktail party! So time spent discussing it and dealing with its problems is well spent.

Most intestinal gas is odourless; a normal subject will produce about 500 ml/day (range 300–2000 ml/day). Most of this is odourless nitrogen and carbon dioxide which, although not troublesome to the continent person who can emit it with discretion, is a major problem to the incontinent ostomate, who not only fears odour but also the risk of his bag taking off like a hot air balloon. Most modern appliances incorporate activated odour filters which prevent some of these problems, but the ostomate's apprehension remains.

Some degree of odour prevention can be achieved by avoiding pneumogenic foods; the source of most intestinal gas is swallowed air which is not smelly. However, bacterial degradation of foodstuffs, eggs, beans, onions, cabbage, sprouts, etc., can cause foul-smelling wind and ostomates are best advised to be cautious about ingesting these.

As an alternative to filters, some patients put aspirin or a commercially available instillate into the bag. These include sodium *o*-phenylphenate 0.3% and *p*-chloro-*m*-xylenol 0.2% (Banish), oxychlorodene (Ostobon) and benzalkonium chloride (Zephiran).

Oral preparations, though not well tested, include chlorophyll tablets and bismuth subgallate, which certainly diminish ileostomy odour, probably by reducing the intestinal flora, but do lead to constipation.

Aviation is so much a part of everyday life that mention must be made of the problems that reduced atmospheric pressure causes to the ostomate. As the ambient pressure falls on take-off the appliance may overfill with gas and tear itself adrift, or explode, unless some egress is provided for the excess flatus. Ostomates who contemplate an airborne journey should be warned to use an appliance with a flatus filter and to take all their gear so that they can change the appliance during their journey. They should also avoid taking aerated drinks before and during the flight.

DIET

Ostomates should be encouraged to take a normal unmodified diet; adequate nutritional status will be maintained only if the diet is varied and mixed. The problem of achieving an adequate diet is greatest with the elderly colostomate. Despite all encouragement, many ostomates voluntarily modify their diets to avoid socially embarrassing flatus or liquid motions. Research studies show that just under 50% of ostomates do not vary their diet to achieve stoma outflow modification; the remaining 50% practise dietary modification which may be severe enough to cause malnutrition. The cheapest vegetable foods tend to cause most stomal upset. Beer causes diarrhoea; fizzy drinks should be avoided as they cause wind. Eggs and fish cause odour.

Stoma activity is related to mealtimes; ileostomies are most active about 1 h after the main meal, hence ileostomy activity is greatest in the evening. Colostomies act soon after the first meal of the day; hence colostomy activity is a morning occurrence.[13, 17, 42]

DRUGS

Two aspects of drug therapy concern the ostomate: will the drug be adequately absorbed to achieve its therapeutic effect, and what effect will it have on stoma functions?

Caution should be exercised in prescribing for ostomates. Enteric coated drugs will probably not be adequately absorbed; other tablets may pass into an ileostomy pouch virtually unchanged. For the same reason low-dose contraceptives are not effective in female ileostomates.

Drugs which upset stoma function can disturb fluid and electrolyte balance. Bowel bulking agents attract water and should *never* be given to ileostomates. Oral antibiotics alter the bowel flora causing diarrhoea, fluid loss, debility and candidal superinfections (Table 13.4).

COLOSTOMY IRRIGATION

There is controversy about colostomy care. In the neo-occidental world, irrigation has always been the method of choice while in paleo-occidental Europe a more cautious policy of 'natural' evacuation is more acceptable. These differences have changed with technology in the last few years. All English patients who can irrigate are now taught to do so. Contraindications to irrigation include arthritis, blindness and peristomal hernia.

The new cone-shaped irrigating devices with a plastic outflow conduit have changed the British colostomy scene. The cone is introduced into the colostomy and the colon washed clean with between 1000 ml and 1500 ml of warm water

Table 13.4 Drugs affecting stoma output.

Constipating agents	
Direct action on gut	Opium and its derivatives
	Codeine phosphate, dihydrocodeine
	Loperamide (Imodium)
	Diphenoxylate ⎫
	⎬ Lomotil
	Atropine ⎭
	Tricyclic antidepressants
	Disopyramine (Rythmodan, Norpace)
Indirect action on gut	Quinidine
	Phenothiazine
	Diuretics
*Bulk-forming agents**	Methylcellulose
	Ispagula husk (Isogel)
	Metamucil
Boosters	Oral antibiotics
	Magnesium hydroxide
	Purgatives

* Increased loss from an ileostomy due to bulking agents or laxatives may cause water and electrolyte deficiencies. Bulking agents should never be given to ileostomates.

poured in under gravity from a receptacle placed just above the sitting patient's head. The technique should be taught to the patient by the stoma nurse, and their bathroom at home modified with a hook over the lavatory for the reservoir and cupboards to hold the tackle. The patient rigs up the reservoir, sits on the toilet, leads the outflow conduit between his/her knees into the bowl and runs the irrigation in. The patient may then experience cramping pains as the colon contracts to empty its fluid load; the colon can be helped to contract by massaging the abdomen. Often the effluent does not rush out all at once, and the patient may need to stand up and stretch or crouch to make the last vestiges of effluent flow out.

Irrigation once a day keeps the colon empty, and successfully irrigating patients usually do not require any appliance at all. If properly managed, the modern irrigating cone appliance will last for a considerable time and is a very good alternative to more expensive disposable appliances. Irrigation, to be 100% successful, does, however, need patience and time in the toilet – about an hour each day.

CONTRACEPTION

The options for contraception after stoma surgery require mention. It should be remembered that anatomical dehiscence with sepsis or damage at operation may cause occlusion of the fallopian tubes. In the male, apparent propulsive ejaculation failure does not equate with sterility. If the male can achieve erection and penetration he may cause pregnancy.

The ideal contraceptive for a female ileostomate is a male method; the contraceptive pill may be inadequately absorbed, the disordered vaginal and uterine anatomy make diaphragm occlusive methods insecure, and the distortion of the uterus and the risk of ongoing pelvic sepsis rule out intrauterine devices. Sterilization of the postproctocolectomy female is not recommended; there are often many adhesions and damage to loops of gut with fistula formation is a great hazard.

Hence the male must assume the contraceptive burden with a condom or vasectomy.

PREGNANCY

No obstetrician has reported a large experience with the management of pregnant ostomates. Many female ileostomates successfully complete pregnancy and from the literature some generalizations about their problems can be made.[3, 5, 27, 39]

During the pregnancy, disorders associated with the ileostomy may cause problems. These include dehydration and electrolyte depletion; renal calculi are particularly troublesome in late pregnancy if kidney function becomes impaired. Movements in the anterior abdominal wall and displacement of peritoneal contents by the gravid uterus may cause stoma care problems, such as retraction of the stoma or subacute intestinal obstruction. Previous steroid therapy may affect the pregnancy or the patient particularly immediately post partum when plasma cortisol levels fall.

The management of anaemia in pregnancy requires mention. Oral iron preparations will not be adequately absorbed and if additional small bowel has been resected megaloblastic anaemia due to folate and vitamin B_{12} malabsorption can occur.

Two-thirds of ileostomates who come to full term can be delivered by the normal vaginal route, although instrumental assistance is often required because of a lack of desire to push and disrupt the stoma. A generous episiotomy is usually required because of perineal scarring. If vaginal delivery is impossible a classical caesarean section should be considered because of the difficulties of an approach to the lower abdomen.

Two management problems need to be stressed during pregnancy and the post partum. These are intestinal obstruction and the problems of reconstruction of the perineum after episiotomy, especially in the Crohn's patient. Both are dangerous complications which require skilled surgical intervention which should always be on hand when such a patient is being managed.

COMPLICATIONS OF GASTROENTEROLOGICAL STOMAS

These are summarized in Table 13.5. The aetiology and management of some of these conditions have already been referred to in the text.

Surgical complications

These are all mechanical problems which require active intervention. Two – 'caput medusa' with portal hypertension and traumatic avulsion – are noteworthy. Bleeding from peristomal varices is readily controlled by sclerosant injections or overrunning the varices after mobilization of the mucocutaneous junction and resuture. Avulsion of an ileostomy may be caused by a car seat belt. Patients should be warned of this and advised to adjust the lap strap so that it does not impinge on the stoma. Avulsion, or more correctly ischaemic pressure necrosis, can also be caused by the rim of an ill-fitting ileostomy appliance. Avulsion requires urgent surgical intervention to resite and reconstruct the stoma.

Dermatological complications

Two varieties of peristomal dermatitis can be described but it must be stressed that many patients present with elements of both.

Contact dermatitis is a reaction to the appliance; therefore, the lesion has the same outlines and shape as the offending appliance. Treatment is simply by protecting the skin from the abusing agent. Allergens causing contact dermatitis can be identified by patch testing. Effluent dermatitis is due to digestion of the skin; its outline is geographic with extensions into any skin folds. It is always secondarily infected. The first principle of treatment is to remove the cause and fit an adequate appliance.

Table 13.5 Complications of a stoma.

Surgical		Ischaemia
		Retraction
		Stenosis
		Prolapse
		Herniation
		Obstruction
Dermatological		Effluent dermatitis
		Contact dermatitis
Psychosocial		Odour
		Depression and suicide
		Social deviancy
		Isolation
Sexual	Male	Neurological damage, impotence, etc.
	Female	Neurological and perineal damage
	Both sexes	Psychosexual disorders
Medical		Metabolic disorder
		Dehydration
		Recurrent Crohn's disease
		Recurrent or metachronous cancer
		Liver disease
		Portal hypertension
Trauma		Perforation
		Traumatic avulsion

Damaged skin should be cleansed with warm water without soap; if adhesive is adherent to it a solvent such as trichlorethylene (Zoff) can be used; if soap is required a bland non-scented white soap is best. The skin is dried; cotton wool which may leave wisps adherent to the skin is best avoided and soft paper towels are preferred. Once the skin is cleansed it is best protected with Karaya, or Stomahesive, Comfeel or Hollihesive. With severe skin damage other preparations may be needed in the short term. It should be stressed that corticosteroids cause skin atrophy and topical antibiotics may cause skin sensitivity. The preparations that we advise include: Betnovate Cream (Glaxo; contains 0.1% betamethasone); Betnovate N Cream (Glaxo; 0.1% betamethasone and 0.5% neomycin sulphate); Synalar Cream (ICI; 0.025% fluocinolone acetate, best applied as a 1 : 4 aqueous lotion); Tri Adcortyl Cream (Squibb; 0.1% triamcinolone acetonide, nystatin 100 000 units/g, neomycin 0.25% and gramicidin 0.025%); and Gyno-Daktanin (Janssen; 2% miconazole nitrate).

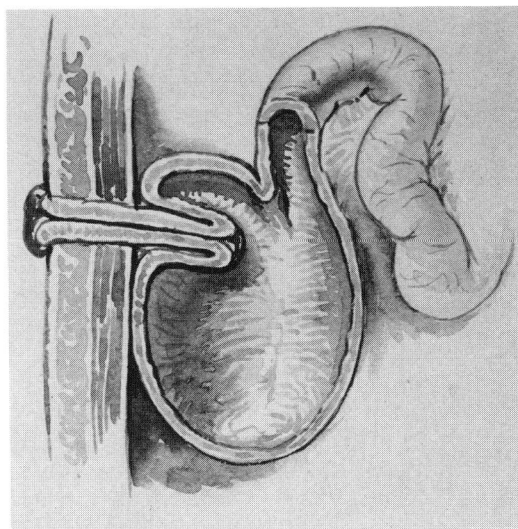

Fig. 13.2 Cut-away view of a continent ileostomy, showing intussusception, or nipple valve. From Palselius[34a] with kind permission of the author and the publisher, W. B. Saunders.

ALTERNATIVES TO PERMANENT STOMAS

No chapter on stoma care would be complete without mention of recent advances in stoma prevention. There are two problems to be overcome in constructing an alternative to the human colon; these are providing a reservoir and ensuring continence. Kock has suggested an intra-abdominal pouch of small gut and an intussuscepted nipple valve to ensure continence. Parks again made a small gut pouch but placed it in the pelvis and used the anal musculature to ensure continence. Although both of these operations are alternatives to a Brooke ileostomy neither of them have overcome the water and electrolyte problems of colectomy.

In the Kock operation a U-loop of distal ileum is opened and sutured side-to-side to make a sac; the distal outflow is then intussuscepted back into it as a nipple valve (Figure 13.2). Evacuation is by regular catheterization. The principal complication is extrusion, and consequent incontinence, of the nipple valve. With the latest techniques valve extrusion rates of 9%[31] and 4.1%[18] are reported. An interesting longer-term complication of the Kock operation has been the development of an enteritis in the pouch. This disorder responds to sulphasalazine therapy. Kock reports that 96% of his patients

($n = 314$) never use appliances, remain in excellent health and have a quality of life superior to conventional ileostomates.[32]

The Parks pelvic ileal pouch and mucosal proctectomy has a shorter history than the Kock operation. In the Parks operation 45 cm of ileum are knuckled up in an 'S' shape; they are then split and joined side-to-side to form a pouch with a capacity of about 400 ml (Figure 13.3). The mucosa is then removed from the rectum down to the dentate line in the anal canal. This manoeuvre is a satisfactory excision in ulcerative colitis (mucosal colitis) and benign polyposis. The pelvirectal muscles are left intact, with their own sensory and reflex circuits; the outflow from the pouch is then threaded through the muscle tube and sutured, mucosa to anal epithelium, at the dentate line. The results of this operation are very encouraging; most patients are fully continent although some do have problems with evacuation and need to intubate their pouches.[29, 35] Our own experience with this operation is very encouraging and we no longer practise rectal excision in ulcerative colitis, preferring retention of the intact sphincters and a pelvic pouch.

The development of intraluminal suturing and stapling techniques has also altered the outlook in rectal cancer. Many more patients are being offered radical excisional surgery with primary anastomosis avoiding a permanent colostomy.

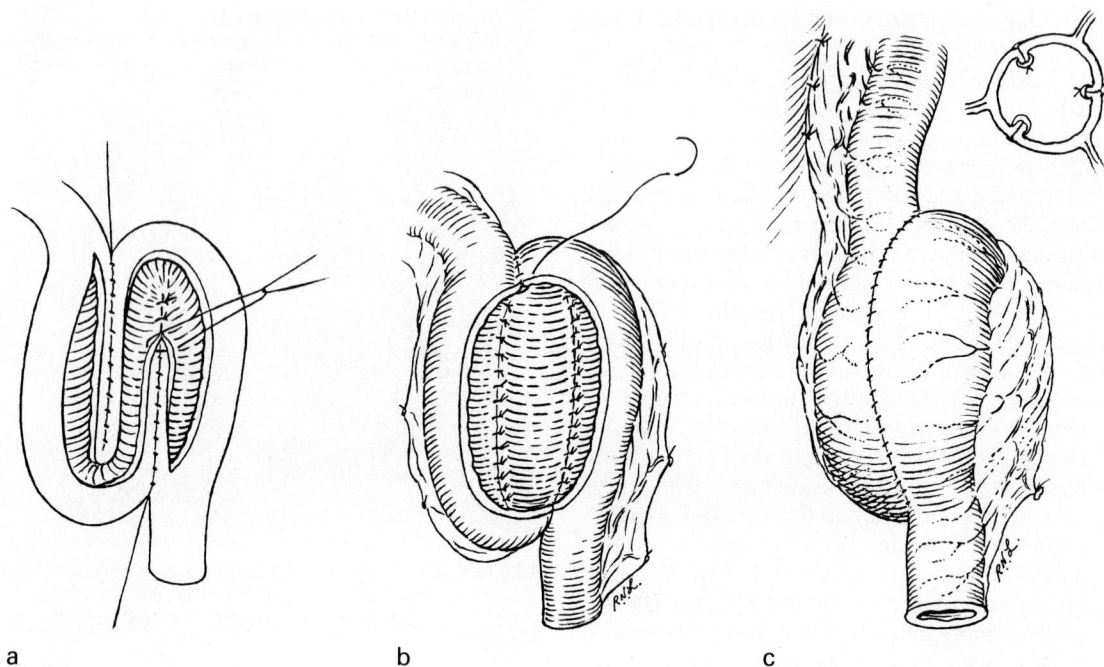

a   b   c

Fig. 13.3 Construction of an ileal pouch. From Nicholls[33a] with kind permission of the author and the publisher, W. B. Saunders.

REFERENCES

1 Alexander-Williams, J. (1974) Loop ileostomy or colostomy for faecal diversion. *Annals of the Royal College of Surgeons of England*, **54**, 141–148.

2 Bennett, R. C. & Hughes, E. S. R. (1972) Urinary calculi and ulcerative colitis. *British Medical Journal*, **i**, 494–496.

3 Boné, J. & Sorensen, F. H. (1974) Life with a conventional ileostomy. *Diseases of the Colon and Rectum*, **17**, 194–199.

4 Brooke, B. N. (1952) The management of an ileostomy including its complications. *Lancet*, **ii**, 102–104.

5 Burnham, W. R., Lennard-Jones, J. E. & Brooke, B. N. (1977) Sexual problems among married ileostomists. *Gut*, **18**, 673–677.

6 Cheselden, W. (1784) Colostomy for strangulated umbilical hernia. *Anatomy*, London.

7 Cromar, C. D. L. (1968) The evolution of colostomy. *Diseases of the Colon and Rectum*, **11**, 256–280, 367–390, 423–446.

8 Delaney, H. M. & Garvey, J. W. (1973) Jejunostomy by needle catheter technique. *Surgery*, **73**, 786–790.

9 Devine, H. (1937) Excision of the rectum. *British Journal of Surgery*, **25**, 351.

10 Devlin, H. B. (1973) Colostomy. *Annals of the Royal College of Surgeons of England*, **52**, 392–408.

11 Devlin, H. B. (1982) Stoma therapy review. *Coloproctology*, **4**, 172–176, 250–259, 298–306, 366–374.

12 Devlin, H. B., Datta, D. & Dellipiani, A. W. (1980) The incidence and prevalence of inflammatory bowel disease in North Tees health district. *World Journal of Surgery*, **4**, 183–193.

13 Devlin, H. B., Plant, J. A. & Griffin, M. (1971) The aftermath of surgery for anorectal cancer. *British Medical Journal*, **iii**, 413–418.

14 Dlin, B. N. & Fischer, H. K. (1976) Psychiatric aspects of colostomy and ileostomy. In *Modern Perspectives in the Psychiatric Aspects of Surgery* (Ed.) Howells, J. G. pp. 321–342. New York: Brunner Mazel.

15 Farley, D. & Smith, I. (1968) Phantom rectum after complete rectal excision. *British Journal of Surgery*, **55**, 40–42.

16 Freer, G. (1821) Reported by Pring, D. 'History of a case of the successful formation of an artificial anus in an adult with an account of an analogous operation in two cases by G. Freer, Esq., of Birmingham.' *Medical and Physical Journal*, **45**, 1–15.

17 Gazzard, B. G., Saunders, B. & Dawson, A. M. (1978) Diets and stoma function. *British Journal of Surgery*, **65**, 642–644.

18 Gerber, A., Apt, M. K. & Craig, P. H. (1983) The Kock continent ileostomy. *Surgery, Gynecology and Obstetrics*, **156**, 345–350.

19 Goligher, J. C. (1958) Extraperitoneal colostomy and ileostomy. *British Journal of Surgery*, **46**, 97.

20 Grogan, J. E. & Smith, M. C. (1973) The economic cost of ulcerative colitis: a national estimate for 1968. *Inquiry*, **10**, 61–68.

21 Gruner, O.-P. N., Nass, R., Fretheim, B. & Gjone, E. (1977) Marital and sexual adjustment after colectomy. *Scandinavian Journal of Gastroenterology*, **12**, 193–197.

22 Haalboom, J. R. E., Poen, H., Struyvenberg, A. & ten Thije, O. J. (1983) Life with an ileostomy. *Lancet*, **i**, 249.

23 Hawley, P. R. & Ritchie, J. K. (1979) Complications of ileostomy and colostomy following excisional surgery. *Clinics in Gastroenterology*, **8**, 403–414.

24 Heald, R. J. (1980) Towards fewer colostomies: the impact of circular stapling devices on the surgery of rectal cancer in a district hospital. *British Journal of Surgery*, **67**, 198–200.

25 Hill, G. L., Mair, W. S. J. & Goligher, J. C. (1975) Gallstones after ileostomy and ileal resection. *Gut*, **16**, 932–936.

26 Hill, G. L., Goligher, J. C., Smith, A. H. & Mair, W. S. J. (1975) Long-term changes in total body water, total exchangeable sodium and total body potassium before and after ileostomy. *British Journal of Surgery*, **62**, 524–527.

27 Hudson, C. N. (1972) Ileostomy in pregnancy. *Proceedings of the Royal Society of Medicine*, **65**, 281–283.

28 Hulten, L., Kewenter, J., Persson, E. & Ahren, C. (1970) Vitamin B12 absorption in ileostomy patients after operation for ulcerative colitis. *Scandinavian Journal of Gastroenterology*, **5**, 113–116.

28a Irving, M. (1982) Ileostomy: surgical procedures, *Clinics in Gastroenterology*, **11**, 2, 237–246.

29 Johnston, D., Williams, N. S., Neal, D. E. & Axon, A. T. R. (1981) The value of preserving the anal sphincter in operations for ulcerative colitis and polyposis: a review of twenty two mucosal proctectomies. *British Journal of Surgery*, **12**, 874–878.

30 Kock, N. G. (1969) Intra-abdominal reservoir in patients with permanent ileostomy. *Archives of Surgery*, **99**, 223–231.

31 Kock, N. G. (1982) The continent ileostomy. In *The Present Management of Ulcerative Colitis and Crohn's Disease* (Ed.) Westbroek, D. L., Tank, K. G. & Bijnen, A. B. Breda, The Netherlands: Medical World Press.

32 Kock, N. G., Myrvold, H. E., Nilsson, L. O. & Philipson, B. M. (1981) Continent ileostomy: an account of 314 patients. *Acta Chirurgica Scandinavica*, **147**, 67–72.

33 Maratka, Z. & Nedbaw, J. (1969) Urolithiasis as a complication of the surgical treatment of ulcerative colitis. *Gut*, **5**, 214–217.

33a Nicholls, R. J. (1982) Ileostomy: surgical procedures. *Clinics in Gastroenterology*, **11**, 2, 247–259.

34 Office of Population Consensus and Surveys (1970–1983) *Report on Hospital Inpatient Enquiry for the Years 1967–1980*. London: HMSO.

34a Palselins, I. (1982) Stoma care in continent ileostomy. *Clinics in Gastroenterology*, **11**, 2, 278–284.

35 Parks, A. G. & Nicholls, J. (1980) Proctocolectomy without ileostomy for ulcerative colitis. *British Medical Journal*, **ii**, 85–88.

36 Patey, D. H. (1957) Primary epithelial apposition in colostomy. *Proceedings of the Royal Society of Medicine*, **44**, 423.

37 Plant, J. A. & Devlin, H. B. (1968) Ileostomy and its management. *Nursing Times*, 711–714.

38 Richardson, R. G. (1973) *The Abominable Stoma, A Historical Survey of the Artificial Anus*. Queensborough, Kent: Abbot Laboratories.

39 Roy, P. H., Sauer, W. G., Beahrs, O. H. & Farrow, G. M. (1970) Experience with ileostomies. *American Journal of Surgery*, **119**, 77–86.

40 Sames, C. P. (1958) Extraperitoneal colostomy. *Lancet*, **i**, 567–568.

41 Sparberg, M., von Prohaska, J. & Kirschner, J. (1966) Solid state Karaya gum ring for use in disposable and permanent ileostomy appliances. *American Journal of Surgery*, **11**, 610–611.

42 Thomson, T. J., Runce, J. & Khan, A. (1970) The effect of diet on ileostomy functions. *Gut*, **11**, 482–485.

43 Todd, I. P. & Fielding, P. (Ed.) (1983) *Operative Surgery: Colorectal Operations*. London: Butterworth.

44 Turnbull, R. B. & Weakley, F. (1967) *An Atlas of Intestinal Stomas*. St. Louis, USA: C. V. Mosby.

Chapter 14
Infections and Infestations of the Gastrointestinal Tract

CHOLERA

Cholera is an infectious disease resulting from colonization of the small intestine by *Vibrio cholerae*, which produces a potent enterotoxin. In its classical form the illness is characterized by severe, watery diarrhoea with resultant life-threatening depletion of body fluids and electrolytes. However, many of those infected are mildly affected or asymptomatic.

The disease occurs in epidemic and endemic forms. It is endemic in many tropical countries in Asia and Africa and is a serious global health problem. Cholera has a short incubation period (usually two to six days), and because of the extent and rapidity of air transport many cases have been imported into Europe and America whilst incubating the disease. Cholera must be considered in the differential diagnosis of acute diarrhoea in people recently arrived from infected areas.

History

Outbreaks of severe diarrhoea that may have been cholera were described by Sanskrit writers and by Hippocrates in 400 BC. There were references to cholera epidemics in India between 1503 and 1817.[28] Since 1817 seven great pandemics have occurred, usually originating in Bengal and spread to Europe and other areas by infected travellers. In the 1840–1849 pandemic one million are said to have died in Russia and 50 000 in England. During this pandemic Snow and Budd proposed their theory of water-borne infection. The disease was often associated with pilgrimages in India and Arabia, when thousands congregated and travelled in insanitary conditions.

During the last 20 years there has been an alarming extension of cholera in Asia and Africa. The latest pandemic began in Sulawesi (Celebes), Indonesia, in 1961. From there it spread to many countries from which it had been absent for decades, including the USSR, Iran and most of Africa.[2] This pandemic was caused by the El-tor variety of cholera vibrio, which differs in some important respects from the classical cholera vibrios responsible for previous epidemics. The El-tor vibrios persist longer in carriers and there is a higher ratio of mildly affected or asymptomatic cases to severely affected patients (probably 10–100 : 1).

Aetiology

The cholera vibrio is a small, motile, gram negative, comma shaped organism 1.5–3 μm by 0.5–0.6 μm, with terminal flagellae. Cholera vibrios are facultative anaerobes preferring alkaline media: optimum growth occurs anaerobically at 37°C at pH 8.0–8.2.[8]

Cholera vibrios have heat-stable somatic O antigens and heat-labile flagellar H antigens. The O antigen is a lipopolysaccharide and the H antigen a protein. Three fractions of the O antigen (A, B and C) determine the three main serotypes of the organism – Ogawa (AB), Inaba (AC), Hikojima (ABC) – and a rare fourth serotype (A). The El-tor biotype, identical serologically with classical cholera vibrios, differs in certain metabolic properties such as resistance to polymyxin B and group IV cholera phages and production of acetoin in culture. Strains of cholera vibrios can be differentiated by bacteriophage sensitivity, but phage typing has proved of limited value in tracing sources of infection. El-tor vibrios may remain viable in well water for over 50 days, in sea water for 6–60 days at 20–30°C and in sweat-stained clothing for about 50 days.

Antibiotic susceptibility

In vitro, *V. cholerae* is usually sensitive to tetracycline (minimal inhibitory concentration (MIC) 2.5 μg/ml), chloramphenicol (MIC 1.5 μg/ml) and sulphafurazole (sulfisoxazole). Recently *V. cholerae* has become resistant to tetracycline in Tanzania.[33] This resistance is plasmid-mediated and related to widespread chemoprophylaxis with tetracycline. The resistant strains disappeared when use of tetracycline was restricted. Cholera vibrios resistant to several antibiotics because of plasmids have been reported from Bangladesh.

Toxin production

The enterotoxin produced by the vibrios is responsible for the pathogenetic effects of cholera; the organisms themselves do not invade the bowel. Before significant toxin production takes place the vibrios must survive the acid barrier of the gastric juice, penetrate the mucous coating of the small intestine and adhere to the brush border of the epithelium. This is believed to occur by specific adhesins on the surface of the vibrios reacting with special receptors on the epithelial cell surface; this complex process has been fully described by Freter.[12] Adhesion of vibrios and its inhibition are probably important factors in bacterial virulence and host resistance.

The cholera enterotoxin causes diarrhoea by stimulating an active secretion of chloride and bicarbonate anions and inhibiting sodium chloride absorption in the small intestine. This follows stimulation of the enzyme adenylate cyclase in the enterocyte by toxin and a consequent increased output of adenosine-3′,5′-cyclic monophosphate (cyclic AMP). The toxin causes a permanent change in the enzyme; recovery follows replacement of the affected cells of the intestinal wall, which can occur within hours. The result is massive secretion of water and electrolytes into the small intestine, exceeding the capacity of colonic resorption.

The cholera toxin has a molecular weight of 84 000 and is a complex of two parts, one molecule of subunit A and an aggregate of five molecules of subunit B.[15,34] The B subunits are not toxic in themselves but are essential for the binding of the complete toxin to specific molecular receptors on the epithelial cell wall and for entry of the active subunit A into the cell to stimulate adenylate cyclase. The receptor is the sialidase-stable ganglioside GGnSLC known as G_{M1}. Discovery of these mechanisms has implications for new approaches to therapy and vaccination in cholera. The heat-labile enterotoxin of enterotoxigenic *E. coli* is similar to the cholera enterotoxin.

Immunity and host susceptibility
There is immunity following an attack of cholera, but its duration is uncertain and second attacks have been recorded. Experiments with volunteers have demonstrated immunity following infection lasting at least three to four years.[18] These subjects did not excrete cholera vibrios after infection, suggesting that immunity is antibacterial rather than antitoxic. These volunteers had IgG antibody to vibrios in their small intestine before reinfection. Protection against clinical cholera has been correlated with the possession of vibriocidal antibodies in the blood. After an attack of cholera there is a rise in serum antibodies – agglutinins (IgM), vibriocidal antibody (IgM), antitoxin (IgG) and coproantibody (IgA). IgG and IgM may lose some of their functions in the gut but it is believed that antibacterial antibody prevents adherence of the vibrios to the gut mucosa and that antitoxic antibodies inhibit combination of the enterotoxin with its receptors.[8] Cell-mediated immunity is not considered important in non-invasive bacterial disease. Local IgA immune bodies in the gut are probably important. The detection of antibodies in the gut is not easy, but anticholera IgA has been demonstrated in the breast milk and saliva of Pakistani women from an endemic cholera area; in most the titre rose after vaccination.[32]

Vaccination with present-day vaccines gives short-term protection of about three to nine months to about 60% of recipients, but this type of protection has a limited impact on public health. Work is proceeding to produce better vaccines, perhaps combining whole cell vaccines with toxin subunit B vaccine, and also oral live vaccines.

There is considerable variation in individual susceptibility to infection with cholera. The dose of cholera vibrios in water to produce infection in 50% of adult volunteers (ID_{50}) was found to be 10^8, 10^{11} being needed to produce cholera-like diarrhoea.[16] If, however, the organisms are administered with $NaHCO_3$ the ID_{50} may be less than 10^3 organisms. Subjects with achlorhydria or after gastrectomy are more easily infected than the average person. Marijuana users are also said to be more susceptible, possibly because the drug may induce achlorhydria.[23] In endemic areas children are the commonest victims, the adults usually having some acquired immunity.

Epidemiology

Cholera is a disease of poor people in developing countries with inadequate sanitation. Sporadic cases may enter developed countries but the disease does not spread there. The sources of infection are mainly human carriers, who outnumber clinical cases by 10–100 : 1. Most carriers do not excrete vibrios for more than two weeks but a few long-term carriers, for example Cholera Dolores,[1] excrete the organisms for longer periods, even up to ten years. In endemic areas about 1% of the population may be carriers in the absence of cases of choleraic diarrhoea.[30] Infection of staff tending cholera patients is uncommon, but carriers among household contacts of patients are frequent. Infection has been spread widely by travellers, refugees, fishermen, pilgrims and smugglers. Cholera vibrios can persist for long periods in water, and in Bangladesh and in many epidemic situations water is the vehicle of transmission. Feachem and his colleagues[11] have reviewed the epidemiology of El-tor cholera and have emphasized the importance of food-borne cholera, particularly in the Sahel region of Africa. This type of transmission is enhanced by burial customs which include expression of the colonic contents of the corpse, washing the body and then sitting down to a funeral feast. Sources of infection include faeces (10^8 vibrios per millilitre), vomitus, sweat and soiled clothing – a faeces, fingers, fomites, flies and food association.

In newly infected areas all ages suffer, but in endemic areas most patients are children under the age of ten. Epidemics fade away as the community gains herd immunity.

There is a seasonal incidence of cholera epidemics. In Bengal cholera increases with rising temperatures in April and decreases when the monsoon comes, in Dacca the maximum prevalence is in November and December and in West Africa the maximum prevalence is in the dry season.[11]

Cholera is not a zoonosis, but recently El-tor cholera has become established as an endemic infection of fish in a salt water atoll in the Gilbert Islands, human infection being acquired by eating the fish.[22] On the Gulf Coast of Lousiana, USA, a few cases have been reported transmitted by shellfish.[4] Cholera has recently been prevalent in most countries of South East Asia and West Africa and in southern Sudan, Uganda, Kenya, Zimbabwe, Angola and Mozambique. It has reached South Africa, Europe and the Pacific islands.

Pathophysiology

The pathophysiological changes in severe cholera are due to profuse isotonic fluid losses through the bowel. These losses are caused by enterotoxin as previously described, and involve vibrios surviving the stomach acid, colonization of the small intestine by a large number of vibrios, and enterotoxin production.

The composition of stools in cholera has been investigated by Watten et al. Their results are summarized in Table 14.1.[6, 24, 36] The stools contain slightly less sodium than plasma but considerably more bicarbonate and potassium. In children the stools have a rather lower electrolyte concentration than in adults. The stools have a low protein content, consistent with a non-invasive process.

The quantity of fluid lost is very variable. Purging may last from a few hours up to eight days. Usually there is a progressive decrease in the rate of fluid lost as the disease continues. In the worst cases initial fluid losses during the first day may exceed one litre per hour, but usually

Table 14.1 Electrolyte contents of the stools in severe cholera.

	Adults	Children
Sodium (mmol/l)	116–135	100
Chloride (mmol/l)	100	75
Potassium (mmol/l)	20–75	25
Bicarbonate (mmol/l)	40–45	32
Osmolarity (mosmol/l)	301	

the loss is less than 500 ml/h. Without antibiotic treatment seriously ill patients may lose twice their body weight in faecal fluid during their illness.[6]

Clearly, the consequences of such fluid losses are hypovolaemic shock, metabolic acidosis and hypokalaemia. Severe metabolic acidosis is associated with a shift of blood volume to the lungs and may result in pulmonary oedema even in hypovolaemic patients. Changes in the blood in severe cholera include a low arterial pH, low plasma bicarbonate, a raised blood urea concentration and a high serum protein concentration.

The serum concentrations of sodium and chloride are usually fairly normal; hypokalaemia becomes marked if patients are rehydrated with potassium-free infusions.

The causes of death in cholera are hypovolaemic shock, acute renal failure due to hypotension and uncompensated metabolic acidosis. Death due to extracellular fluid depletion is usual if there is a loss of 12% of body weight. Patients with 10% weight loss are gravely ill and shocked, while a loss of 5% of body weight is associated with moderate dehydration. Despite the flow of fluid into the bowel the ability to absorb water and electrolytes is retained if glucose is provided and this has important implications for oral rehydration.

MORBID HISTOLOGY

Small intestine histological changes have been studied by intestinal biopsy and at autopsy; they are minimal and non-specific.[13] There is depletion of mucus from mucus-secreting cells, some vasodilation and lymphocytic infiltration of the submucosa. A thick layer of mucus may be present on the bowel wall. The grey, opalescent, 'rice-water' appearance of the stool is caused by excess mucus, clumps of mononuclear cells and ghost epithelial cells. At autopsy the intestines are full of watery stool. Other postmortem changes are the result of fluid and electrolyte losses: the tissues are abnormally dry, the lungs may be dry or sometimes oedematous, and acute tubular necrosis or hypokalaemic nephropathy may be found in the kidneys.

Clinical features

The clinical features of cholera result from gastrointestinal disorder and from fluid losses in the stools.

Incubation period. This ranges from a few hours to six days and may be related to the size of the infecting dose of vibrios reaching the duodenum. Usually it is one to three days.

MILD DISEASE

Many patients have mild or moderate diarrhoea with watery brown stools and sometimes vomiting. The duration of illness ranges from two to five days and if oral fluid intake is maintained marked dehydration does not occur. Fluid losses do not exceed one litre a day and such patients are not seriously incapacitated; however, they are a dangerous and common source of infection. Clinically, the condition is indistinguishable from diarrhoea caused by enterotoxigenic *E. coli*, some enteroviruses and *Salmonella* organisms. The possibility of cholera as a cause of mild diarrhoea should be considered in people coming from infected areas.

SEVERE CHOLERA

The onset is usually sudden, with copious, forceful evacuation of watery stools and vomiting; occasionally, it is more gradual, the severe diarrhoea being preceded by 36–48 hours of mild diarrhoea.

Severe cholera may last for only a few hours, but purging can continue for as long as a week. Diarrhoea tends to diminish progressively after the first 24 hours. Serious dehydration may be present within four hours of the onset but is more usually seen after 12 hours. The stage of collapse is known as the algid stage, and as recovery proceeds it may be succeeded by a febrile stage of reaction.

Gastrointestinal symptoms

'Pints of pale fluid are painlessly poured out'.[9] Initially the stools contain some bile and faecal material but soon light-greyish 'rice-water' stools containing mucus gush forth from the anus. Rarely, some blood is seen in the stools. Evacuation is usually effortless and painless, but muscular cramps occur in the abdomen and limbs later in association with electrolyte depletion. Vomiting occurs in most patients because of reflux of intestinal contents into the stomach. The vomitus is watery, alkaline in reaction and highly infectious.

General symptoms due to isotonic fluid deficit

Isotonic fluid deficit, acidosis and hypokalaemia can develop within hours. The earliest symptom is thirst when the fluid deficit is about 3% of body weight; as dehydration progresses postural

hypotension develops, the pulse races and the blood pressure falls below 90/50 mmHg (12/6.7 kPa). The patient is lethargic, weak and oliguric when about 6% of body weight has been lost. Further unreplaced fluid losses produce a restless, confused and finally comatose, anuric, wizened patient with unrecordable blood pressure. If fluid loss exceeds 12% the patient will die. Recovery is remarkably rapid if rehydration is carried out correctly. Most adults are afebrile, but the temperature may rise with improvement.

Physical signs

These are largely the consequence of extracellular fluid loss and include loss of tissue turgor, sunken eyes, falling-in of the cheeks, wrinkled 'washerwoman's' fingers, peripheral cyanosis, tachycardia and hypotension, depending on the degree of dehydration. The abdomen is flat or sunken and not tender; bowel sounds may be absent. The lungs are usually clear on auscultation but pulmonary oedema due to acidosis may cause auscultatory crackles.

Complications

These are usually due to incorrect and inadequate fluid replacement. They include renal failure associated with hypovolaemic shock. Oliguria or anuria are frequent in cholera, but early and adequate volume replacement causes resumption of urine output in 6–24 hours.[20] Acute pulmonary oedema is associated with metabolic acidosis, particularly if the patient has been given only normal saline while acidotic.

Other recorded complications include abortion, corneal ulcers, pneumonia and hyperpyrexia. Gangrene of the extremities, penis and scrotum was seen formerly.

CHOLERA IN CHILDREN

Cholera is often a paediatric problem and in endemic areas the incidence in children is much higher than in adults. The clinical picture is fairly similar to that in adults but dehydration is more rapidly critical because the ratio of daily water exchange to body weight is considerably higher in children than in adults. The stools of choleraic children contain less sodium and chloride than those of adults.

Certain clinical features are more likely to be seen in children. These include pyrexia, convulsions, paralytic ileus, cardiac arrhythmias, and hypoglycaemia in about 2%.[19] Many children in the tropics are malnourished and cholera may be a particularly serious problem for them.

Cholera is not usually followed by postinfective malabsorption, and early feeding after rehydration is feasible and desirable.

BIOCHEMICAL FINDINGS

These have been summarized by Pierce and Mondal:[25]

1 Base-deficient acidosis is shown by a lowered blood pH of 7.2 or less and a low plasma bicarbonate concentration of about 10 mmol/l, with a lowered arterial P_{CO_2}.

2 Water loss is indicated by a raised plasma osmolarity of 320 mosmol/l or more, a raised haematocrit, an increase in plasma protein levels and an increase in the blood urea concentration. Formerly, determination of the plasma specific gravity was much used in assessing rehydration requirements: it may rise to 1.040 from a normal value of 1.025.

3 Serum sodium and potassium concentrations are often fairly normal, but the latter may fall with rehydration if sufficient potassium is not given.

4 There is a polymorphonuclear leucocytosis.

Diagnosis

Clinical diagnosis is easy in the typical case in the midst of an epidemic, but there is often delay in diagnosing the initial cases seen because of failure of the clinician to consider the possibility of cholera in mildly affected patients, and sometimes because the laboratory is not prepared for cholera diagnosis.

Bacteriological confirmation of cholera is essential. Correct collection of stool specimens is best accomplished by inserting per rectum a sterile, soft rubber catheter lubricated with sterile liquid paraffin and collecting 3 ml of liquid faeces in a sterile container. Glass or cotton wool rectal swabs are less satisfactory. Direct plating on to bile salt agar, thiosulphate–citrate–bile salt agar or gelatin–tellurite–taurocholate medium (GTT) is recommended. If delay in reaching the laboratory is anticipated the specimen can be stored at 4°C, or better put into a transport medium such as alkaline peptone water or Carey–Blair medium. Alkaline peptone water is a cheap, efficient enrichment medium. Rapid preliminary identification of cholera vibrios can be achieved by microscopic observation of the immobilization of comma-shaped vibrios by type-specific antisera using dark-field, phase contrast or immunofluorescent techniques.[35]

Management

The objectives of treatment are:

1 Rapid re-expansion of the extracellular fluid.

2 Replacement of continuing fluid loss.

3 The eradication of *Vibrio cholerae* from the intestines using antibiotics.

4 Prevention of spread to contacts.

5 Possibly diminishing diarrhoea by pharmacological means.

Cholera is often treated by medical auxiliaries in rural areas where medical facilities are basic and intravenous fluids in short supply. Clear, simple guidelines for therapy and patient monitoring are needed in such circumstances. Oral rehydration is used where possible, to conserve intravenous fluids.

REHYDRATION THERAPY IN ADULTS

The route and rate of fluid therapy depend upon the degree of dehydration. Severely dehydrated patients need immediate intravenous therapy using a large-bore needle (18 gauge) in an arm vein or if necessary initially by a hand-held needle in the femoral vein. Fluid should be run in as rapidly as possible so that two litres are delivered in 30 minutes. Then the infusion can be slowed so that 110 ml per kilogram body weight are given within the first four hours of therapy.[3] This should restore lost fluid and improve the patient's condition so that oral rehydration solution (ORS) can then be continued at up to 800 ml/h ($15\ ml \cdot kg^{-1} \cdot h^{-1}$), adjusted as necessary according to continuing losses. Some moderately dehydrated patients can be managed with oral therapy alone but must be carefully watched, and if they fail to improve or if they become hypotensive they must be given intravenous fluids. Mild dehydration can be managed with supervised oral rehydration therapy (ORT). If possible the patient should be weighed on admission. Failing that, the weight is estimated. The degree of dehydration and fluid deficit is assessed according to the features described in the clinical section and in Table 14.2.

Fluids used for rehydration

These should supply the electrolytes lost in the stools (Table 14.1) in more or less the same concentrations. Glucose supplies energy and may prevent the hypoglycaemia which sometimes occurs in children. Rahaman, Majid and Monsur suggest that rehydration solutions should contain at least 44 mmol/l of glucose to

Table 14.2 Assessment of rehydration in cholera.

Degree of dehydration	Signs	Treatment
Severe Fluid deficit 100–110 ml/kg bodyweight	Marked loss of tissue turgor Systolic blood pressure less than 80 mmHg Acidotic breathing Urine output absent	Rapid i.v. infusion 2 litres in 30 min 110 ml/kg bodyweight in 4 hours
Moderate Fluid deficit 60–90 ml/kg bodyweight	Postural hypotension Tachycardia Blood pressure normal or low May be hyperventilation	Some can be managed by oral rehydration If hypotensive give rapid intravenous infusion
Mild Fluid deficit 40–50 ml/kg bodyweight	Thirsty Blood pressure and pulse rate normal Tissue turgor and respiration normal	Oral rehydration

avoid hypoglycaemia.[26] The electrolyte composition of commonly used treatment solutions is shown in Table 14.3. If bicarbonate is used as the base it should be added to the solution shortly before administration. Sodium lactate or acetate are also effective as a diarrhoea treatment solution and have the advantage of long shelf-lives in tropical conditions. Lactate or acetate needs conversion to bicarbonate in the liver but this does not seem to cause problems. Ringer–lactate solution (compound sodium lactate intravenous infusion BP) and 2 : 1 saline–lactate are deficient in potassium, and potassium supplementation is recommended (add 10 mmol KCl to each litre).

Oral rehydration therapy (ORT) is based on the fact that sodium and glucose transport are coupled in the intestine, glucose stimulating salt and water absorption. ORT can be used in mild and moderate dehydration but not in shocked, hypotensive patients. The oral glucose electrolyte solution (Table 14.3) is heated to 40°C and given at a rate of $10\text{--}15 \, \text{ml} \cdot \text{kg}^{-1} \cdot \text{h}^{-1}$. ORT is very important in diminishing mortality in cholera and infantile gastroenteritis.[5]

Monitoring of fluid therapy

Continuous careful observation is essential to steer the patient between under-hydration and over-hydration. Input must be charted clearly and stool output measured hourly. Patients are best nursed on a 'cholera bed' (Figure 14.1). This is a simple bed with a 20 cm hole through the mattress or canvas cover under the buttocks. The patient lies on a plastic sheet with a sleeve going through the hole leading into a calibrated bucket. This allows convenient complete collection of faeces. Replacement therapy is given at a rate of 1–1.5 times the stool output.[7] Urine output may be suppressed for up to 12 hours after therapy begins.

Table 14.3 Composition of commonly used rehydration solutions.

Treatment solution	Electrolyte concentration (mmol/l)				
	Na	K	Cl	Base[a]	Dextrose (D-glucose)
Diarrhoea treatment solution	118	13	83	48	55
Ringer–lactate solution	130	4	109	28	—
Two to one saline–lactate (isotonic saline; $\frac{1}{6}$ molar sodium lactate)	154	—	97	57	—
Oral glucose electrolyte solution[b]	90	20	80	30	111

[a] Base equivalent to mmol/lHCO$_3^-$.
[b] Oral rehydration solution (ORS).

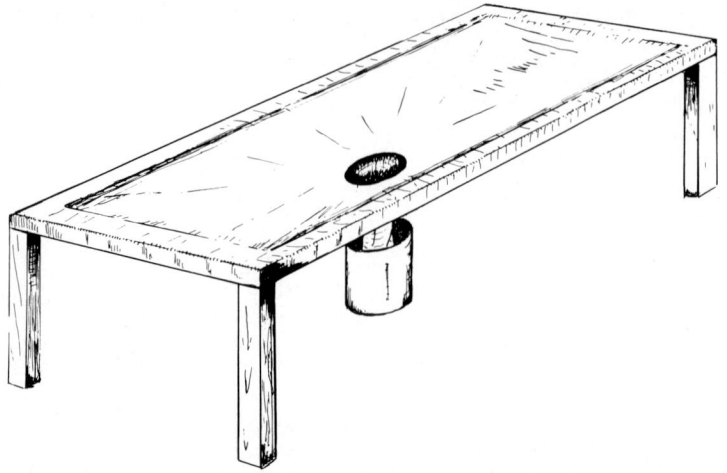

Fig. 14.1 Cholera bed. The plastic sheet is omitted for clarity but its 'sleeve' is shown entering the bucket. (Drawing by J. P. Brady.)

The most important guides to progress are the patient's general condition, the blood pressure and the rate and volume of the radial pulse. Neck veins should be inspected for congestion and lung bases auscultated for crackles as indications of fluid excess. Facial oedema may be found in over-hydrated children. Measurement of central venous pressure is rarely feasible.

Laboratory methods that have been used to measure progress include determination of plasma specific gravity (relative density) using a simple copper sulphate solution method (aiming at a return from a specific gravity of 1.040 to 1.025) and serial estimation of plasma proteins. Blood urea and electrolytes should be determined if possible.

ANTIBIOTICS

Tetracycline is the antibiotic of choice and can eliminate the organism from the small bowel within 24 hours. The duration and amount of diarrhoea is reduced by 50–60%. It will not influence enterotoxin bound to enterocytes, which will continue to cause diarrhoea for about 12 hours. The drug is given orally in doses of 500 mg six-hourly for 48 hours (children: 50 $mg \cdot kg^{-1} \cdot day^{-1}$ in four doses). Resistance of *Vibrio cholerae* to tetracycline has been found in Tanzania and Bangladesh, so the sensitivity to tetracycline should be measured if possible. Alternative, less effective chemotherapy includes furazolidone 100 mg six-hourly (children 5 $mg \cdot kg^{-1} \cdot day^{-1}$), chloramphenicol 500 mg six-hourly (children 75 $mg \cdot kg^{-1} \cdot day^{-1}$) and co-trimoxazole two tablets 12-hourly for adults (children 8 $mg \cdot kg^{-1} \cdot day^{-1}$ of trimethoprim and 40 $mg \cdot kg^{-1} \cdot day^{-1}$ of sulphamethoxazole in two doses). These drugs are given for 72 hours. Parenteral therapy is unnecessary.

PHARMACOLOGICAL METHODS TO REDUCE DIARRHOEA

Chlorpromazine may prove a valuable adjunctive treatment in cholera. It inhibits adenylate cyclase, which is stimulated by cholera enterotoxin. Experimentally, chlorpromazine diminishes intestinal secretion in rats previously given cholera enterotoxin. Rahaman, Greenough, Holmgren and Kirkwood have demonstrated significant reduction in the quantity and duration of diarrhoea in cholera patients treated with the drug in doses of 1 mg/kg given orally or intramuscularly.[27] Mild sedation was induced, vomiting reduced and no serious side-effects found. G_{M1} ganglioside charcoal was found to reduce diarrhoea in one trial.[31] Other supportive measures which have been tried and *not* found useful include plasma volume expanders, steroids, vasopressors, charcoal, kaolin, diphenoxylate and opiates.

PREVENTION OF SPREAD OF CHOLERA IN TREATMENT CENTRES

The patient should be barrier-nursed as far as possible and attendants should wash their hands and then apply a hand lotion containing 0.25% lysol (cresol and soap solution). Clothes and bedpans are soaked in 2% lysol for two hours and then boiled, and utensils should be boiled.[10] Attendants should be vaccinated against cholera.

TEMPORARY TREATMENT CENTRES

Cholera patients will not survive long journeys to hospital. Establishment of local, temporary treatment centres is essential in rural areas in epidemic situations. Ideally they should be organized and stocked with fluids, drugs and equipment as early as possible. Mobile field teams of medical auxiliaries under the supervision of a medical officer staff the centres, often assisted by locally recruited unskilled assistants and patients' relatives.[10] Treatment results at these centres are often as good as in hospitals.[21] Transport to hospital is a problem: home-made stretchers, cycle carriers and boats have all been used. The picture of grieving Ghanaian mothers carrying desperately ill children in their arms or on their backs is a lasting memory.

TREATMENT OF CHILDREN

The same principles apply as in adults. If possible they should be managed in a separate area from the adults. Paediatric scalp vein sets, cholera cots and weighing scales are needed. Whilst intravenous therapy is desirable in seriously dehydrated cases it may be impossible to achieve when management is by medical auxiliaries. Many of these patients can be saved by intraperitoneal infusion. Ringer's lactate can be given in amounts of up to 80 ml/kg through an 18 gauge needle placed in the midline below the umbilicus.[19] The special complications in children should be anticipated and over-rapid infusion must be avoided.

Prognosis

The mortality rate in serious poorly-treated cholera is 50–70%. With correct management at an early stage less than 2% will die, but in many areas the death rate remains much higher.

Principles of prevention

Improvement in hygiene and sanitary conditions and provision of clean water are the most important factors in preventing cholera. Vaccination provides only partial protection for four to six months and has been less cost-effective during cholera epidemics than protecting and chlorinating water supplies. Health education is important as many communities are ignorant about the causation and transmission of cholera. Because only about 4% of cholera patients reach hospital in some areas,[29] hospital treatment will not stop an epidemic. Surveillance, isolation and chemoprophylaxis of household contacts is indicated if possible but mass population chemoprophylaxis is not recommended. Tetracycline 500 mg six-hourly for three days is used for prophylaxis. Surveillance, quarantine and vaccination are important in preventing international spread.

REFERENCES

1 Azurin, J. C., Kobari, K., Barua, D. *et al.* (1967) A long term carrier of cholera, Cholera Dolores. *Bulletin of the World Health Organisation,* **37,** 865–880.

2 Barua, D. & Burrows, W. (1974) *Cholera.* Philadelphia: Saunders.

3 Black, R. E. (1982) The prophylaxis and therapy of secretory diarrhoea. *Medical Clinics of North America,* **66,** 611–619.

4 Blake, P. A., Allegra, D. T., Snyder, D. J. *et al.* (1980) Cholera – a possible endemic focus in the United States. *New England Journal of Medicine,* **302,** 305–309.

5 Carpenter, C. C. J. (1982) Oral rehydration – is it as good as parenteral therapy? *New England Journal of Medicine,* **306,** 1103–1104.

6 Carpenter, C. C. J., Greenough III, W. B. & Gordon, R. S. (1974) Pathogenesis and pathophysiology of cholera. In *Cholera* (Ed.) Barua, D. & Burrows, W. pp. 129–141. Philadelphia: Saunders.

7 Cash, R. A. (1980) Cholera. In *Current Therapy 1980* (Ed.) Conn, H. F. pp. 12–17. Philadelphia: Saunders.

8 Chatterjee, B. D. (1981) Vibrios. In *Medical Microbiology and Infectious Diseases* (Ed.) Braude, A. I. pp. 353–362. Philadelphia: Saunders.

9 Chaudhuri, R. N. (1974a) Cholera. In *Medicine in the Tropics* (Ed.) Woodruff, A. W. pp. 261–268. Edinburgh and London: Churchill Livingstone.

10 Chaudhuri, R. N. (1974b) Management of cholera cases in rural areas. In *Cholera* (Ed.) Barua, D. & Burrows, W. pp. 263–271. Philadelphia: Saunders.

11 Feachem, R., Miller, C. & Bohumie Drasar (1981) Environmental aspects of cholera epidemiology. *Tropical Diseases Bulletin,* **78,** 865–880.

12 Freter, R. (1980) Association of enterotoxigenic bacteria with the mucosa of the small intestine: mechanisms and pathogenic implications. In *Cholera and Related Diarrhoeas* (Ed.) Ouchterlony, O. & Holmgren, J. pp. 155–170. Basel: Karger.

13 Gangarosa, E. J., Beisel, W. R., Benyajati, G. *et al.* (1960) The nature of the gastrointestinal lesion in Asiatic cholera and its relation to pathogenesis: a biopsy study. *American Journal of Tropical Medicine,* **9,** 125–135.

14 Haldar, D., Bal, H. & Chatterjee, A. N. (1961) Screening of some antibiotics on *V. cholerae.* *Annals of Biochemistry and Experimental Medicine,* **21,** 213–214.

15 Holmgren, J. & Lönnroth, I. (1980) Structure and function of enterotoxins and their receptors. In *Cholera and Related Diarrhoeas* (Ed.) Ouchterlony, O. & Holmgren, J. pp. 88–103. Basel: Karger.

16 Hornick, R. B., Music, S. I., Wenzel, R. *et al.* (1971) The Broad Street pump revisited: response of volunteers to ingested cholera vibrios. *Bulletin of the New York Academy of Medicine,* **47,** 1181–1191.

17 Levine, M. M. (1980) Immunity to cholera as evaluated in volunteers. In *Cholera and Related Diarrhoeas* (Ed.) Ouchterlony, O. & Holmgren, J. pp. 195–203. Basel: Karger.

18 Levine, M. M., Nalin, D. R., Craig, J. P. *et al.* (1979) Immunity to cholera in man: relative role of antibacterial versus antitoxic immunity. *Transactions of the Royal Society of Tropical Medicine and Hygiene,* **73,** 3–9.

19 Mahalanabis, D., Watten, R. H. & Wallace, C. K. (1974) Clinical aspects and management of pediatric cholera. In *Cholera* (Ed.) Barua, D., & Burrows, W. pp. 221–233. Philadelphia: Saunders.

20 Mahalanabis, D., Brayton, J. B., Mondal, A. & Pierce, N. F. (1972) The use of Ringer's lactate in treatment of

children with cholera and acute non-cholera diarrhoea. *Bulletin of the World Health Organisation*, **46**, 311–319.

21   Mandara, M. P. & Mhalu, F. S. (1981) Cholera control in an inaccessible district in Tanzania: importance of temporary rural centres. *Medical Journal of Zambia*, **15**, 10–13.

22   McIntyre, R. C., Tira, T., Felood, Y. & Blake, P. A. (1979) Modes of transmission of cholera in a newly infected population on an atoll; implications for control measures. *Lancet*, **i**, 311–314.

23   Nalin, D. R., Levine, M. M., Rhead, J. *et al.* (1978) Cannabis, hypochlorhydria and cholera. *Lancet*, **ii**, 859–861.

24   Pierce, N. F. (1982) Pathophysiology and prophylaxis of infectious diarrhoea. In *New Developments in Tropical Medicine* (Ed.) Strickland, T. pp. 57–62. Washington: National Council for International Health.

25   Pierce, N. F. & Mondal, A. (1974) Clinical aspects and management. In *Cholera* (Ed.) Barua, D. & Burrows, W. pp. 209–218. Philadelphia: Saunders.

26   Rahaman, M. M., Majid, M. A. & Monsur, K. A. (1979) Evaluation of two intravenous solutions in cholera and non-cholera diarrhoea. *Bulletin of the World Health Organisation*, **57**, 977–981.

27   Rahaman, G. H., Greenough III, W. B., Holmgren, J. & Kirkwood, B. (1982) Controlled trial of chlorpromazine as antisecretory agent in patients with cholera hydrated intravenously. *British Medical Journal*, **284**, 1361–1364.

28   Rogers, L. (1950) Cholera. In *British Encyclopaedia of Medical Practice*, 2nd edn, vol. 3 (Ed.) Lord Horder. pp. 443–471. London: Butterworths.

29   Shrivastav, J. B. (1974) Prevention and control of cholera. In *Cholera* (Ed.) Barua, D. & Burrows, W. pp. 405–426. Philadelphia: Saunders.

30   Sinha, R., Deb, B. C., De, S. P., Abou-Gareeb, A. H. & Shrivastav, D. L. (1967) Cholera carriers in Calcutta, 1966–67. *Bulletin of the World Health Organisation*, **37**, 89–100.

31   Stoll, B. J., Holmgren, J., Bardhan, P. K. *et al.* (1980) Binding of intraluminal toxin in cholera: trial of GM1 ganglioside charcoal. *Lancet*, **ii**, 888–891.

32   Svennerholm, L. (1980) Structure and biology of cell membrane gangliosides. In *Cholera and Related Diarrhoeas* (Ed.) Ouchterlony O. & Holmgren, J. pp. 80–87. Basel: Karger.

33   Towner, K. J., Pearson, N. J., Mhalu, F. S. & O'Grady, F. (1980) Resistance to antimicrobial agents of *V. cholerae* El Tor strains isolated during the fourth cholera epidemic in the United Republic of Tanzania. *Bulletin of the World Health Organisation*, **58**, 747–751.

34   van Heynigen, W. E. (1981) Bacterial exotoxins. In *Medical Microbiology and Infectious Diseases* (Ed.) Braude, A. pp. 51–63. Philadelphia: W. B. Saunders.

35   Wallace, C. (1981) Cholera. In *Medical Microbiology and Infectious Diseases* (Ed.) Braude, A. pp. 1058–1062. Philadelphia: Saunders.

36   Watten, R. H., Morgan, F. M., Songkhla, Y. N. *et al.* (1959) Water and electrolyte studies in cholera. *Journal of Clinical Investigation*, **38**, 1879–1889.

SALMONELLA INFECTION

Bacteriology

Salmonella organisms are Gram-negative, aerobic, generally motile bacilli which do not ferment lactose. There are more than 1700 serotypes identified on the basis of their somatic (O) and flagellar (H) antigens. These serotypes can be broadly separated into two categories according to their host-predilection:

1   The organisms responsible for enteric fever, *Salmonella typhi* (*S. typhosa*) and *S. paratyphi A*, *B* and *C*, which are primarily adapted to man.

2   The other serotypes, which are primarily parasites of animals, and generally produce a gastroenteritis type of illness in man, often termed 'food poisoning' because of the predominant source of infection. Although all are potentially pathogenic in humans, a small percentage of the many serotypes account for the vast majority of human infection in the world as a whole. Examples of commonly isolated serotypes are *S. typhimurium*, *S. hadar*, *S. enteritidis*, *S. virchow*, *S. heidelberg*, *S. agona*, *S. saint paul*, *S. montevideo*, *S. derby* and *S. bredeney*. *S. typhimurium* is the most commonly isolated serotype in many parts of the world and regularly accounts for 20% to 30% of all human cases in Britain. *S. typhi*, *S. paratyphi A*, *S. paratyphi B* and some of the other common serotypes can be subdivided by bacteriophage typing which is useful in epidemiological investigations.

TYPHOID AND PARATYPHOID FEVER (SYNONYM: ENTERIC FEVER)

The term enteric fever is frequently used to describe the prolonged febrile state caused by *Salmonella typhi* and *Salmonella paratyphi A*, *B* and *C*. Occasionally, other salmonella serotypes of the food-poisoning variety may produce an invasive illness with prolonged bacteraemia, continued fever, enlargement of spleen, and even the 'rose spots' which are characteristic of enteric fever.

Epidemiology

Typhoid and paratyphoid fevers occur throughout the world, but are most prevalent in the Far East, Central and South America and Africa, reflecting the poor standards of sanitation and water supply in such areas. A significant endemic level also persists in Eastern and Southern Europe, but in the rest of Europe, North America and Australasia enteric fever is now largely an imported disease. The ultimate source of infection is invariably human, and transmission is via the alimentary tract through direct or indirect contact with the faeces or urine of a patient or a carrier. The principal vehicles of spread of typhoid infection are contaminated water and food: paratyphoid infection is less likely to be waterborne because of the necessity for a higher infecting dose, which is unlikely to be found in drinking water unless there is heavy pollution. Raw fruit and vegetables are important vehicles in some tropical countries where use of human faeces for manuring vegetable crops is a common practice. Shellfish harvested in water polluted by sewage have caused outbreaks. Canned meat is generally very safe, but outbreaks have occurred occasionally through faulty canning processes.

Pathogenesis and pathology

Natural infection in enteric fever is by oral ingestion. The size of the infecting dose is important. A dose of 10^9 organisms will induce infection in most, whereas 10^3 organisms will rarely produce symptoms in otherwise healthy individuals.[10] Pathogenicity varies and host factors such as gastric hypoacidity may influence the infecting dose. Strains possessing Vi antigen cause clinical illness more commonly than the non-Vi variants.[10]

After passing the acid barrier of the stomach, the organisms rapidly penetrate the small intestinal mucosa, reach the mesenteric glands via the lymphatics and after a brief period of multiplication spread to the spleen, liver and other reticuloendothelial tissues via the bloodstream. Here they multiply silently for the rest of the incubation period; at the end of this they enter the bloodstream in huge numbers, heralding the onset of the clinical illness. This secondary bacteraemia continues for the greater part of the febrile illness and very few organs of the body escape involvement. However, from a clinical viewpoint the two most important sites affected are the Peyer's patches in the small intestine and the gallbladder. Peyer's patches become hyperplastic, with infiltration of chronic inflammatory cells; later, necrosis of the superficial layer leads to formation of irregular, ovoid ulcers along the long axis of the gut, so stricture formation does not occur. Erosion into the blood vessels may produce severe intestinal haemorrhage or transmural perforation may lead to peritonitis. The lower ileum is the site most severely affected.

The gallbladder is probably affected via the liver; the cholecystitis which results is usually sub-clinical. Pre-existing gallbladder disease predisposes to chronic carrier state, which might explain the rarity of carrier state in children and its frequency in middle-aged women. The organisms may be found incorporated in gallstones.

The pathogenesis of the prolonged fever and toxaemia of enteric fever is far from clear. A major role for endotoxaemia has been discounted after studies in volunteers who were rendered endotoxin-tolerant by repetitive intravenous endotoxin administration but who none the less developed typical typhoid fever when challenged with viable organisms. Furthermore, it is impossible to produce a state of prolonged fever by continuous infusion of endotoxin.[10] It has also not been possible to demonstrate endotoxaemia in natural typhoid fever by the *Limulus* lysate test, a sensitive indicator of endotoxaemia.[4]

Mechanism of immunity

Cell-mediated immunity probably plays an important role in the recovery from infection, while humoral antibody formation has little relevance, because the patient continues to deteriorate even after the appearance of O, H and Vi antibodies. There is no correlation between these antibodies and relapse or reinfection in naturally acquired typhoid fever. Vaccine-induced resistance would seem to be humorally mediated but not related to O, H and Vi antibody formation; antibodies to other, as yet unidentified antigens are probably responsible for protection. Local gut immunity may also play an important role in preventing reinfection.

Natural course

The duration of illness in a case of average severity is approximately four weeks but mild and inapparent cases are common. The incubation period of typhoid fever averages from 10 to 20 days but may be shorter when the infecting dose is large. Paratyphoid fever generally has a shorter incubation period (average 7 to 14 days).

CLINICAL FEATURES

In the *first week* there are few specific features. The onset is insidious, with mounting fever, headache, vague abdominal pain and constipation. There is often relative bradycardia, and the spleen becomes palpable towards the end of the first week. During the *second week* the patient becomes dull and apathetic, with sustained fever and slightly distended abdomen. Crops of 2–4 mm maculopapules (rose spots) appear on the lower chest and upper abdomen between the seventh and tenth day of illness. The rose spots are often more numerous in paratyphoid fever. Cough is commonly present at this stage. During the *third week* the patient gradually lapses into the so-called 'typhoid state', characterized by prolonged apathy and toxaemia with delirium, disorientation or even coma. The abdomen becomes distended, with scanty bowel sounds, and greenish 'pea-soup' diarrhoea is common. Severe intestinal haemorrhage and perforation are prone to occur during this period. During the *fourth week* the temperature gradually returns to normal and the abdominal distension subsides, although the patient remains listless and anorexic for some time afterwards.

There is frequently variation in the clinical picture. Diarrhoea may be present from the onset, particularly in paratyphoid fever, which may behave as simple gastroenteritis. Chronic bacteraemia with fever of many months' duration can occur in association with urinary schistosomiasis and is due to persistence of the organisms within the intestine of the parasites. In children, the onset may be abrupt with vomiting, high fever and often convulsion, and they rarely have a relative bradycardia.

RELAPSE AND REINFECTION

In 10–15% of patients there may be a return of symptoms about ten days after the cessation of antibiotic therapy and the blood culture is again positive, even in the presence of high antibody titre. Such a relapse is usually mild and of short duration. Early antibiotic therapy seems to increase the incidence of relapse by interfering with the development of natural immunity. Relapse occurs less frequently in paratyphoid fever. Natural immunity is generally long-lasting, and reinfection is rare.

CARRIER STATE

During the immediate convalescence stool cultures are frequently positive but their frequency declines rapidly, so that after three months only 4–5% of patients excrete the organism. The 3% of patients who remain positive at the end of one year are regarded as chronic carriers and will remain so for the rest of their lives. Persistent urinary carriage is quite rare beyond the third month in the absence of urinary tract abnormalities, but urinary carriers are common in those countries where urinary tract schistosomiasis is endemic.

Complications

GASTROINTESTINAL TRACT

Haemorrhage
The introduction of chloramphenicol has strikingly reduced the incidence of this dreaded complication, and it is now seen only rarely in the Western world. Frank bleeding is always serious and is most frequent during the third week when the slough in the intestinal ulcers separates. However, trivial bleeding as judged by positive occult blood is not uncommon.

Intestinal perforation
This remains one of the most frequently encountered complications of typhoid fever in countries where it is endemic. The diagnosis may be difficult because the perforation often occurs in a patient who is already severely ill, dehydrated and mentally apathetic with a vaguely tender, distended abdomen, so that the classic signs of perforation may not be present. Rigidity is encountered in less than half of the patients and bowel sounds may not disappear altogether. Free fluid in an already doughy and tender abdomen and gas under the diaphragm may be the only indications of perforation.

Liver and gallbladder
Slight jaundice is not uncommon in typhoid fever and may be due to diffuse hepatitis, cholangitis, cholecystitis or haemolysis. Sub-clinical cholecystitis is a feature of the disease but overt signs of gallbladder inflammation may infrequently appear either during the acute illness or some months later.

CENTRAL NERVOUS SYSTEM

A toxic confusional state characterized by severe disorientation, delirium and restlessness occurs during the second and third weeks of illness, but confusion may dominate the clinical picture from the onset and the patient may be admitted to a psychiatric unit.[11, 18] Paranoid psychosis or catatonia may develop during convalescence and occasionally, the features of acute parkinsonism or encephalomyelitis may complicate the clinical picture.

HAEMATOLOGICAL AND RENAL

Sub-clinical disseminated intravascular coagulation is common in typhoid fever,[4] but there may be frank manifestations of the haemolytic–uraemic syndrome.[2] Immune-complex glomerulitis with deposition of immunoglobulin, C3 complement and salmonella Vi antigen in the glomerular capillary wall has been reported.[25] The nephrotic syndrome develops in some patients with chronic *S. typhi* bacteraemia when there is associated schistosomiasis.[6]

OTHER COMPLICATIONS

Toxic myocarditis is a significant cause of death in countries where enteric fever is endemic. Frank pneumonic consolidation, pancreatitis and abscess formation in such diverse sites as spleen, ovary and bone are other rare complications.

Diagnosis

Definitive diagnosis requires isolation of the organism from blood, bone marrow, faeces or urine. Blood cultures are usually positive in 90% of patients during the first week and in a febrile patient the cultures may remain positive into the second or even third week. The frequency of positive blood culture is much less in patients already given antibiotics, but marrow cultures or clot cultures may remain positive. The organisms can also be cultured from a skin biopsy of the rose-spot lesion. A polymorphonuclear leucopenia is characteristic, particularly during the first week.

With modern techniques, the stool cultures are often positive even during the first week, although the percentage positivity rises steadily as the illness progresses. In some patients the stool culture remains negative throughout the illness, particularly if they have received early antibiotic therapy. Urine culture is positive in 30% of patients during the third week.

SEROLOGICAL DIAGNOSIS

The Widal reaction measures titres of serum agglutinins against somatic (O) and flagellar (H) antigens; these agglutinins begin to appear during the second week. In acute infection, O antibody appears first and becomes negative after several months, whereas H antibody appears a little later but persists for a long time. O antibody generally signifies active infection; H antibody helps to identify the type of enteric infection. Positive O titres of 1/80 in non-immunized people living in non-endemic areas, and titres of 1/160 in people in endemic areas are regarded as significant, but a rising titre has more significance. The Widal test has many limitations: false positives are common because of 'O' and 'H' antigenic similarity among many members of the Enterobacteriaceae and anamnestic reactions are common. Prior immunization makes interpretation of serological tests difficult.

Treatment

Modern treatment has reduced the mortality of enteric fever to negligible levels. Since its introduction in 1948 chloramphenicol has remained the standard therapy because of its efficacy, cheapness, its activity against most isolates and its reliable gastrointestinal absorption. The clinical response to the drug is generally a rapid improvement in the patient's general condition followed by defervescence within two to five days. The drug is generally given orally in a dose of 500 mg every four hours till defervescence, then 500 mg six-hourly, for a total period of 14 days. In anorexic patients and in those having diarrhoea the intravenous route should be used; intramuscular administration gives much lower blood levels and may delay defervescence. Relapses are treated similarly. However, chloramphenicol has certain disadvantages – there is a small risk of marrow toxicity, a high relapse rate of 10–15%, and in recent years plasmid-mediated chloramphenicol-resistant *S. typhi* strains have emerged in many parts of the world. Ampicillin has proved to be distinctly inferior as an alternative drug, but some studies suggest that amoxycillin may be equal or even superior to chloramphenicol in terms of clinical response, subsequent relapse and convalescent carriage rate.[24] Amoxycillin is, however, considerably more expensive than chloramphenicol, and there have been isolated reports of organisms resistant to both chloramphenicol and ampicillin/amoxycillin. Co-trimoxazole is probably the drug of choice in areas where chloramphenicol-resistant typhoid is prevalent, because there is little difference between co-trimoxazole and chloramphenicol in terms of clinical response and relapse rates.[9] It is substantially cheaper than amoxycillin, effective against ampicillin-resistant strains and can also be given parenterally. Among the newer drugs, the semisynthetic beta-lactam amidino-penicillanic acid antibiotic mecillinam has a high in vitro activity against *S. typhi* and *S. paratyphi* and promising results were reported initially,[7] but these could not be confirmed in a later study.[16]

A short course of prednisolone often produces a dramatic response in patients with severe toxaemia.

The management of haemorrhage is non-operative, using sedation and transfusion, unless there is evidence of perforation; then surgery is indicated. Most surgeons prefer simple closure of perforation with drainage of the peritoneum and reserve small bowel resection for patients with multiple perforations.[12] Gentamicin and metronidazole should be added to the treatment regime in these patients.

Treatment of chronic carriers

Attempts to eradicate the chronic carrier state by giving prolonged courses of antibiotics have not been successful. Oral ampicillin, amoxycillin or co-trimoxazole administered for a month will induce a bacteriological cure in 50% of patients provided that the gallbladder is functioning; but as at least three-quarters of chronic carriers have diseased gallbladders success can be expected only in a minority.

Cholecystectomy will eradicate the carrier state in three out of four patients. The likelihood of cure is enhanced by pre- and postoperative treatment with ampicillin. The operation, however, should be reserved for those with symptomatic gallbladder disease and those whose livelihood is threatened, for example food handlers.

Prevention

In areas where the disease is endemic the incidence can only be reduced by government-controlled public health measures to provide pure water supply and safe sanitary disposal of excreta and to encourage high standards in the handling, processing and storage of foodstuffs. Killed typhoid vaccines provide about 70% protection against waterborne infection but a higher infecting dose, as often found in a food-borne infection, will break through this partial immunity. Acetone-inactivated vaccines are slightly more potent than the heat-killed, phenol-preserved vaccine but have a higher incidence of local reaction. The effectiveness of paratyphoid vaccines is doubtful and mono-valent anti-typhoid vaccines are replacing the combined TAB vaccines which tend to cause significant local and general side-effects. For primary immunization, two subcutaneous doses of 0.5 ml each should be given four weeks apart; in case of urgency the interval may be reduced to ten days. Booster doses are necessary every three years – a smaller dose (0.1 ml) of heat-killed phenolized vaccine given intradermally is suitable for this purpose and causes much less reaction.

Trials of oral inactivated vaccines have proved disappointing, but oral live vaccines are being investigated clinically.

OTHER SALMONELLA INFECTIONS

Human salmonellosis has a world-wide distribution and is an increasing public health problem, especially in the economically advanced countries of North America and Western Europe, where much hospital, medical, laboratory and field time and expense are devoted to preventative and control measures, investigation of outbreaks, surveillance and research.[26] Salmonellosis outbreaks account for 10–15% of all adult infective diarrhoea in Britain, and during the decade 1970–79 salmonellosis consistently topped the list of bacterial food poisoning in England and Wales.

Epidemiology

Reservoir of infection

The organisms are widely distributed in the animal kingdom. Domestic species, notably cattle, pigs and poultry, are frequent excretors and the organisms can be found in many wild animals. Household pets such as dogs, cats, birds and turtles are all potential sources of infection. Human cases and convalescent carriers, especially those with mild or unrecognized disease, are other important sources.

Transmission

Transmission is almost always by the oral route following the ingestion of food or drink contaminated either directly or indirectly with animal or human faeces. Chicken and turkey are incriminated most frequently, but other animal meats such as beef, pork and lamb are also important sources. Eggs and egg products have been involved in many outbreaks.

Inadequately cooked meat is a potent hazard because raw meat is frequently contaminated. Salmonellae survive deep freezing and adequate thawing prior to cooking is essential. Adequately cooked meat may later become cross-contaminated in the kitchen from raw meat or by a carrier. Two factors have been primarily responsible for the increasing problem of salmonellosis in the Western world. The spread of infection in animals has been encouraged by large-scale intensive farming methods which confine many animals and fowls in close quarters using bulk-imported, often infected animal feed stuff. Infection in humans has been encouraged by the increasing number of people eating in community catering establishments, which has necessitated more bulk-cooking of food of animal origin and an increased sale of warmed-up pre-cooked foods.

Person-to-person transmission does occur and is particularly relevant in institutional outbreaks. In hospitals and residential institutions most outbreaks are caused by contaminated food, but outbreaks in maternity, children's and geriatric wards may follow admission of patients with undiagnosed salmonella infections.

Unpasteurized milk is a common source of infection in northern Britain. Unusual methods of transmission include the use of inadequately sterilized fibre-optic digestive endoscopes and administration of contaminated commercially produced pancreatic extract to children with cystic fibrosis.[14]

Salmonella infections are commoner during the warmer months when the organisms in the food have a better chance to multiply and reach an optimum infecting dose.

Pathogenesis

The outcome and the severity of illness after an exposure to infection depends on a number of factors.

Host factors
Salmonellosis is generally most severe in the very young and the elderly. The presence of an underlying debilitating or chronic disease increases the susceptibility to bacteraemia. Local factors in the stomach and small intestine appear to play a significant role in the body's resistance to enteric infection. Hypochlorhydria increases susceptibility to clinical salmonellosis[8] and patients who have undergone gastric surgery and those on antacid therapy often develop a severe illness.

Virulence of the organism
There is a marked variability of disease-producing ability among the various serotypes and even among different strains within a given serotype. In general, salmonella infections remain confined to the bowels, but invasion of the bloodstream may occur, presenting either as a typhoidal illness or as septicaemia, with the bacteria being located in various organs. Most serotypes are capable of producing invasive illness, but this occurs more frequently with certain serotypes. Septicaemic illness is common in *S. choleraesuis* infection, which rarely prod-

uces gastroenteritis.[21] Other serotypes may show unusual virulence in certain outbreaks, as reported with *S. virchow*.[17] Multi-resistant clones of *S. typhimurium* with enhanced virulence are currently causing problems in many developing countries in South America, the Middle East and the Far East, giving rise to a higher proportion of cases with septicaemia and meningitis.

Infecting dose
The size of the infecting dose is important in deciding the outcome of a particular infection. The frequency of food-borne outbreaks of salmonellosis and the rarity of water-borne and person-to-person transmission suggest a high infecting dose for salmonella infections. Limited experimental evidence in adult volunteers suggests that an infecting dose of 10^5 or more is necessary to produce clinical illness. Host factors such as gastric hypo-acidity and the virulence of the strain probably influence the size of the infecting dose.

Mechanism of diarrhoea
It was previously believed that the site of disease in salmonellosis was similar to that in enteric fever, with acute inflammatory changes confined to the small intestine (hence the term 'enteritis'). However, recent studies have demonstrated that active proctocolitis occurs commonly in salmonellosis[1, 3, 15] and this correlates well with the observation of blood and pus in the stools of many patients with salmonellosis. Even so, the copious watery diarrhoea seen commonly in salmonella infection indicates a concurrent small bowel dysfunction, and studies in rhesus monkeys have demonstrated a severe defect in jejunal water and electrolyte transport,[19] possibly the effect of an enterotoxin. Several toxins have been found in animal experiments.[13, 20] Thus, it appears that both invasion and production of an enterotoxin may be necessary for the production of diarrhoea in salmonella infection.

Clinical manifestations

Gastroenteritis
After an average incubation period of 12 to 48 hours the illness begins abruptly, with colicky abdominal pain and large quantities of watery diarrhoea, which is often bloody. Vomiting is not a predominant feature. Headache, malaise, fever and shivering are often present, particularly in the initial stages. The abdominal pain may

become intense and more persistent and there may be localized tenderness with some rebound over the sigmoid colon or in the right iliac fossa. Appendicitis may be misdiagnosed in the latter situation: should a laparotomy be undertaken the appendix is generally found to be normal or mildly abnormal, but the terminal ileum is acutely inflamed. Salmonella is an important cause of acute ileitis, along with *Campylobacter* and *Yersinia*.[22]

There is much variation in the severity of the illness. Mild and inapparent infections are common. In extremes of age and in debilitated patients the diarrhoea may be pronounced and protracted, with rapid dehydration leading to renal failure. Those who have undergone gastric surgery previously are particularly prone to develop severe diarrhoea, which is often cholera-like in intensity.

The diarrhoea subsides within a few days in the average patient: persistent diarrhoea for more than three weeks is rare in salmonellosis, although some increased bowel frequency may be observed for a while due to the development of a post-infective irritable bowel state.

Carrier state

After recovery patients usually continue to excrete salmonella in stools for an average period of four to eight weeks; the excretion period is longer in infants and elderly.

Salmonella colitis

A mild degree of colorectal inflammation is not uncommon in salmonellosis, as judged by the frequency of inflammatory exudate in the stools. Colitis may be severe at times with frank bloody stools. Toxic dilatation may complicate the clinical picture.[23] A sigmoidoscopy reveals abnormalities ranging from mucosal oedema and hyperaemia, with or without petechial haemorrhages, to mucosal friability.[15] Gross ulceration and slough formation are rare. The barium enema shows diffuse loss of haustration with fine irregularity of the bowel outline and a disturbance of the mucosal pattern usually confined to the distal colon, but occasionally there may be segmental involvement mimicking Crohn's disease (Figure 14.2).

The rectal biopsy histology is not specific and a similar pattern of inflammation may be seen in other infective colitides, including *Shigella*, *Entamoeba histolytica* and *Clostridium difficile*. The predominant features are those of acute inflammation with oedema and focal collection of polymorphonuclear cells in the mucosa (Figure 14.3).[5] The rectal biopsies may show marked mucus depletion and crypt abscess formation in

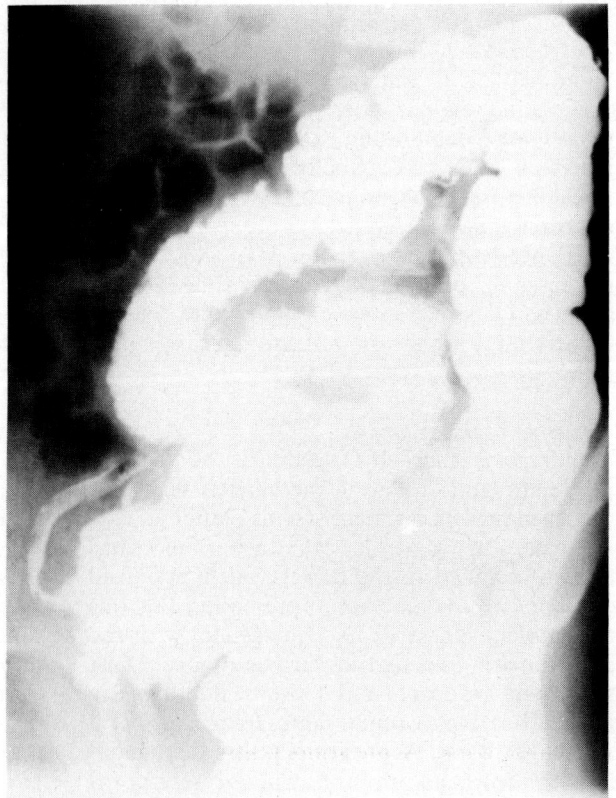

Fig. 14.2 Barium in salmonella colitis, showing a right-sided segmental lesion.

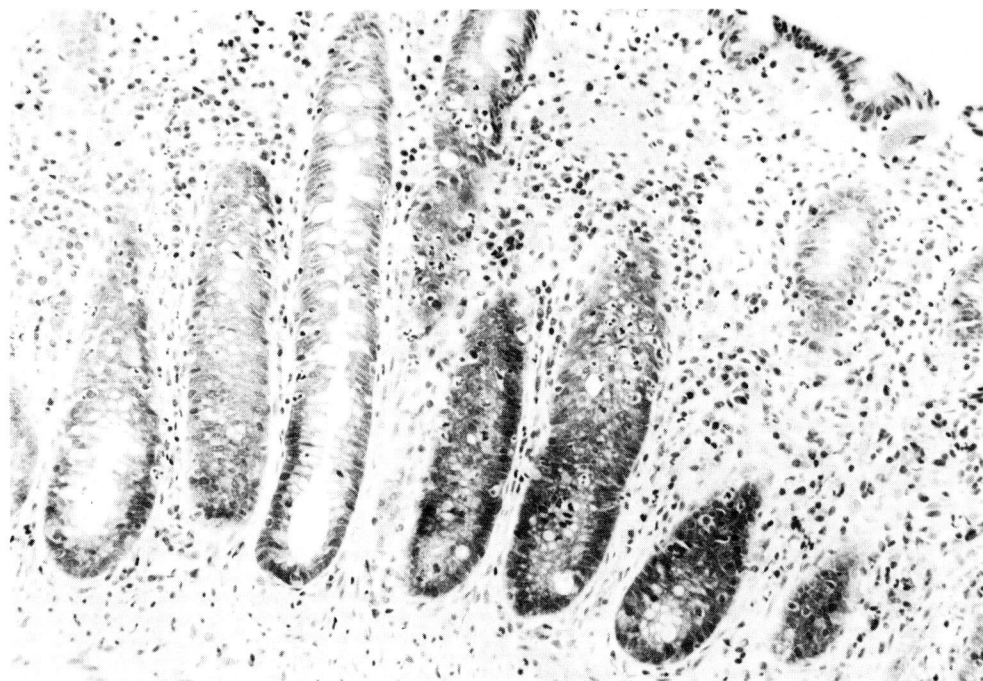

Fig. 14.3 Rectal biopsy appearances in salmonella colitis, showing a polymorphonuclear infiltrate which is invading the crypts, but without any marked increase in chronic inflammatory cell content of the lamina propria. The goblet cell population is relatively well preserved as is the crypt architecture. Haematoxylin and eosin × 500.

severe illness and thus may mimic acute ulcerative colitis of short duration in which abnormalities of crypt architecture have not yet developed.

Invasive salmonellosis
Transient bacteraemia occurs not uncommonly and septicaemic features may dominate in some patients. This may present as a typhoidal illness with sustained fever, splenomegaly and rose spots or with metastatic localization in the meninges, bones and joints, lungs, endocardium, spleen or kidneys. Infants are particularly prone to develop meningitis, and bone involvement is commoner in patients with sickle cell disease.

Reactive arthritis
Sterile synovitis of a reactive nature may follow salmonella infection, particularly in HLA-B27-positive individuals. The symptoms of arthritis usually begin one to two weeks after the infection and any joint may be affected, although the knees and ankles are most frequently involved. Occasionally there is migratory polyarthralgia, resembling acute rheumatic fever, or bilateral proximal interphalangeal joint involvement of rheumatoid type. Acute iridocyclitis may complicate the picture.

PROGNOSIS

The mortality is less than 1%. Most deaths are due to septicaemia or dehydration and renal failure in the elderly or the very young, often in patients who are already suffering from pre-existing disease.

Differential diagnosis

In food-poisoning outbreaks, the longer incubation period, fever and presence of inflammatory exudate in the stools may help to differentiate salmonella infection from 'toxin-type' poisoning caused by *Staphylococcus aureus*, *Clostridium welchii* (*perfringens*) or *Bacillus cereus*. However, definitive diagnosis depends on positive bacteriology because similar clinical features are seen also in *Shigella*, *Campylobacter* and *Yersinia* infections.

The differentiation of severe salmonella colitis from the first episode of inflammatory bowel disease with coincident salmonella infection may pose problems because sigmoidoscopic, radiological and even histological features may be identical. In general, the duration of diarrhoea in salmonella colitis is short, but in more persistent infections steroids together with antibiotics will have to be given to cover both possibilities. In patients who respond promptly to this regimen, the diagnostic dilemma can only be resolved by further rectal biopsies and prolonged follow-up. In primary salmonella colitis, the rectal biopsy histology generally returns to normal after about a month, whereas this is uncommon in inflammatory bowel disease. Those patients who continue to show features of severe colitis for several weeks are usually suffering from underlying inflammatory bowel disease even if the stool cultures remain positive for salmonella.

Treatment

The mainstay of treatment is bed rest with prompt correction of fluid and electrolyte loss. Antibiotics are contraindicated when the infection is confined to the bowel as they do not influence the clinical illness and may prolong the carrier state. Chloramphenicol is the drug of choice in invasive illness, but co-trimoxazole and amoxycillin are satisfactory alternatives. However, multi-resistant strains are encountered and ascertainment of sensitivity is essential. The drugs are given for at least 14 days, but metastatic infections are often slow to respond and require longer courses; relapses are not uncommon.

Prevention

High standards of hygiene are essential in all food premises, including shops, factories, slaughterhouses, kitchens and restaurants. Raw and cooked meat must be handled and stored separately, food should be cooked or thoroughly reheated before use and frozen food should be completely thawed before cooking. Food handlers should be bacteriologically clear before returning to work, but carriers in other occupations may return to work or to school after instruction in personal hygiene.

REFERENCES

1 Appelbaum, P. C., Scragg, J. & Schonland, M. M. (1976) Colonic involvement in salmonellosis. *Lancet*, **ii**, 102.
2 Baker, N. M., Mills, A. E. & Rachman, I. (1974) Haemolytic–uraemic syndrome in typhoid fever. *British Medical Journal*, **ii**, 84–87.
3 Boyd, J. F. (1976) Colonic involvement in salmonellosis. *Lancet*, **i**, 1415.
4 Butler, T., Bell, W. R., Levin, J. *et al.* (1978) Typhoid fever: studies of blood coagulation, bacteraemia and endotoxaemia. *Archives of Internal Medicine*, **138**, 407–410.
5 Day, D. W., Mandal, B. K. & Morson, B. C. (1978) The rectal biopsy appearances in salmonella colitis. *Histopathology*, **2**, 117–131.

6 Farid, Z., Higashi, G. J., Bassily, S., & Miner, W. F. (1975) Immune-complex disease in typhoid and paratyphoid fevers. *Annals of Internal Medicine*, **83**, 432.
7 Geddes, A. M. & Clarke, P. D. (1977) The treatment of enteric fever with mecillinam. *Journal of Antimicrobial Chemotherapy*, **3** (Supplement B), 101–102.
8 Gianella, R. A., Broitman, S. A. & Zamcheck, N. (1973) Influence of gastric acidity on bacterial and parasitic enteric infections. *Annals of Internal Medicine*, **78**, 271–276.
9 Herzog, C. (1976) Chemotherapy of typhoid fever: a review of literature. *Infection*, **4**, 166–173.
10 Hornick, R. B., Greiseman, S. E., Woodward, T. E. *et al.* (1970) Typhoid fever: pathogenesis and immunological control. *New England Journal of Medicine*, **283**, 686–691, 736–746.
11 Khosla, S. M., Srivastava, S. C. & Gupta, S. (1977) Neuro-psychiatric manifestations of typhoid. *Journal of Tropical Medicine and Hygiene*, **80**, 95–98.
12 Kim, J. P., Oh, S. K. & Jarrett, F. (1975) Management of ileal perforation due to typhoid fever. *Annals of Surgery*, **181**, 88–91.
13 Koupal, L. R. & Deibel, R. H. (1975) Assay, characterization, and localization of an enterotoxin produced by salmonella. *Infection and Immunity*, **11**, 14–22.
14 Lipson, A. & Meikle, H. (1977) Porcine pancreatin as a source of salmonella infection in children with cystic fibrosis. *Archives of Diseases in Childhood*, **52**, 569–572.
15 Mandal, B. K. & Mani, V. (1976) Colonic involvement in salmonellosis. *Lancet*, **i**, 887–888.
16 Mandal, B. K., Ironside, A. G. & Brennand, J. (1979) Mecillinam in enteric fever. *British Medical Journal*, **i**, 586–587.
17 Mani, V., Brennand, J. & Mandal, B. K. (1974) Invasive illness with *Salmonella virchow* infection. *British Medical Journal*, **ii**, 143–144.
18 Osuntoken, B. O., Bademosi, O., Ogunremi, K. & Wright, S. G. (1972) Neuropsychiatric manifestations of typhoid fever in 959 patients. *Archives of Neurology*, **27**, 7–13.
19 Rout, W. R., Formal, S. B., Dammin, G. J. & Gianella, R. A. (1974) Pathophysiology of salmonella diarrhoea in the rhesus monkey: intestinal transport, morphological and bacteriological studies. *Gastroenterology*, **67**, 59–70.
20 Sandefur, P. D. & Peterson, J. W. (1976) Isolation of skin permeability factors from culture filtrates of *Salmonella typhimurium*. *Infection and Immunity*, **14**, 671–679.
21 Saphra, J. & Winter, J. W. (1957) Clinical manifestations of salmonellosis in man. An evaluation of 7779 human infections at New York Salmonella Centre. *New England Journal of Medicine*, **256**, 1128–1134.
22 Schofield, P. F. & Mandal, B. K. (1981) Acute ileitis. *British Medical Journal*, **283**, 1545.
23 Schofield, P. F., Mandal, B. K. & Ironside, A. G. (1979) Toxic dilatation of the colon in salmonella colitis and inflammatory bowel disease. *British Journal of Surgery*, **66**, 5–8.
24 Scragg, J. N. (1976) Further experience with amoxycillin in typhoid fever in children. *British Medical Journal*, **ii**, 1031–1033.
25 Sitprija, V., Pipatanagul, V., Boonpucknavig, V. & Boonpucknavig, S. (1974) Glomerulitis in typhoid fever. *Annals of Internal Medicine*, **81**, 210–213.
26 Turnbull, P. C. B. (1979) Food poisoning with special reference to salmonella – its epidemiology, pathogenesis and control. *Clinics in Gastroenterology*, **8**(3), 663–714.

SHIGELLOSIS

Bacillary dysentery due to the genus *Shigella* is an unforgettable illness, for its classical clinical manifestations are remarkably intense and result in considerable distress. Although epidemic dysentery is a disease of antiquity, the causative agent was first adequately described by Kioshi Shiga as late as 1898, thereby permitting the aetiological distinction between amoebic and bacillary dysentery. Since then, the epidemiology of shigellosis has undergone several unexplained shifts that have altered the clinical presentation and severity.[17] In the past decade, epidemic dysentery with high mortality has reappeared in Central America, Asia and Africa. In addition, the infection does occasionally present to the gastroenterologist as an apparently bacteriologically negative chronic inflammatory colitis resembling idiopathic ulcerative colitis.[6]

Microbiology

The organism is a slender, non-motile Gram-negative rod. It is so closely related to *Escherichia coli* that the two are inseparable on the basis of polynucleotide sequence relatedness, and their biochemical characteristics are also, in general, similar. Important distinctions between the two include the inability of shigellae to ferment lactose, their lack of flagella (and hence motility), failure to produce gas from glucose, and inability to decarboxylate lysine (Table 14.4). These characteristics are useful in laboratory identification. The shigellae are highly host-adapted, infecting only humans and a few non-human primates.[17]

SPECIES DEFINITION AND SEROLOGY

Four species have been defined on the basis of biochemical characteristics (Table 14.4) and antigenic differences. They are separable by group-specific polysaccharide antigens, desig-nated A to D, which result in agglutination in the presence of specific antisera. Within these serological groups, however, multiple subtypes are present.

VIRULENCE FACTORS

Epithelial invasion

A virulent shigella is capable of penetrating into epithelial cells in the colon. Cell invasion also occurs in experimental in vivo and in vitro model systems such as the guinea-pig intestine (Figure 14.4) or cornea (Sereny test) and mono-layer cell culture.[9] In the gut, the apical epithe-lial brush border membrane appears to melt away as the organism approaches and pen-etrates into the cytoplasm.[37] The invasive process itself is innocuous and does not kill the cell. With multiplication of the interiorized organism an intracellular microcolony develops and the invaded cell dies. Both chromosomal and plasmid gene products are involved in this complex process.[9, 21] Selection of non-invasive variants results in clinical avirulence in monkeys and human volunteers.[24]

The genetics of invasiveness are complex. Current evidence suggests the involvement of multiple chromosomal loci, although the gene products and their functions are unknown.[32] An exciting recent development has been the finding that large (MW 120 000–140 000) plasmids also carry information essential for invasion by *S. flexneri* and *sonnei* strains.[21, 35] Cure of these plasmids renders the organism non-invasive and avirulent, and their reintroduction restores both properties.

Toxin production

All species produce a protein toxin with diverse biological properties, depending on the model system employed for study.[19] Toxin can display three biological effects:
1 Parenteral injection into sensitive animals causes limb paralysis and death (neurotoxin).

Table 14.4 Usual laboratory characteristics of the genus *Shigella*, compared with those of enterotoxinogenic *Escherichia coli*.

Species	Serological group	Serotypes (subtypes)	Mannitol utilization	Lactose utilization	Gas production	Lysine decarboxylase	Motility
Shigella dysenteriae	A	10	–	–	–	–	–
Shigella flexneri	B	6(12)	+	–	–	–	–
Shigella boydii	C	15	+	–	–	–	–
Shigella sonnei	D	1[a]	+	(late +)	–	–	–
Enterotoxigenic *Escherichia coli*			+	+	+	+	+

[a] Multiple subtypes can be identified by colicin typing.

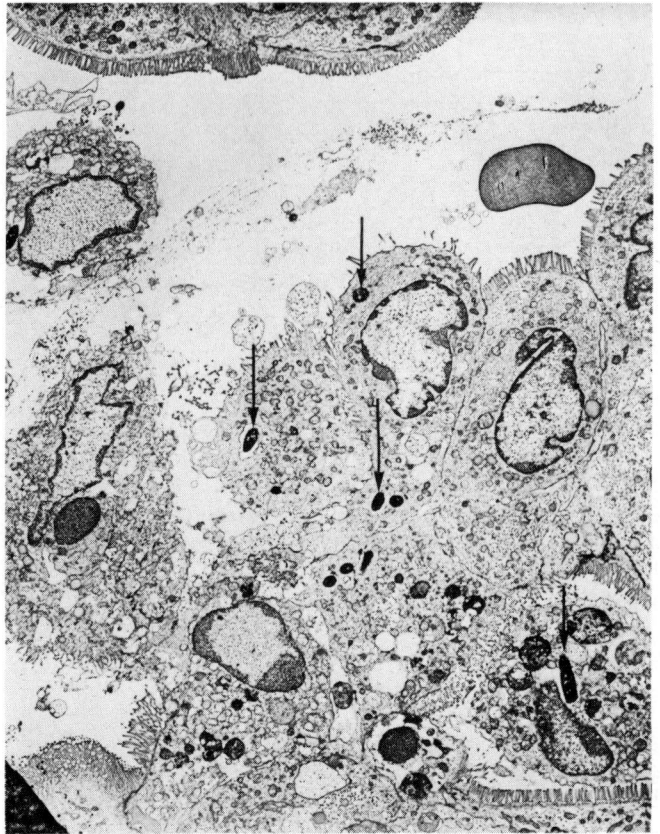

Fig. 14.4 Invasive *Shigella flexneri 2a* in experimental intestinal infection in the guinea pig. The arrows point to the intracellular organisms contained within host cell membrane vesicles. (Courtesy of Drs A. Takeuchi and S. Formal.)

On a weight basis, this is one of the most potent lethal toxins ever described in animal systems, although it is unknown whether it is similarly active in humans.

2 Inoculation into the lumen of rabbit small intestine results in secretion of isotonic fluid (enterotoxin).

3 Addition to sensitive cells in culture leads to cell death (cytotoxin).[18]

The enterotoxin effect in rabbit jejunum is not accompanied by histological changes, whereas in the ileum, epithelial cell death, micro-ulcer formation and haemorrhage, and a marked inflammatory response in the lamina propria occur in addition to fluid secretion.[20]

Pathogenesis

Based on clinical studies, experimental infections in rhesus monkeys, and various other in vivo and in vitro models, a scheme for pathogenesis can be proposed.[19] Relatively few organisms are needed to cause illness, ranging from as few as ten to a few thousand, compared with millions of *Vibrio cholerae* or toxigenic *E. coli*.[17, 24] The organism behaves clinically as if it were indifferent to acid, for buffering of gastric juices does not markedly affect the infectious dose.

Microbial proliferation occurs in the proximal small bowel, without invasion or structural damage of the mucosa, accompanied by net secretion of isotonic fluid similar to that evoked by shigella enterotoxin in rabbit jejunum.[19, 34] It has been proposed that toxin produced in situ is indeed responsible for the net secretion.[19] The ileum is spared in primates and humans, but the colon is heavily involved by an invasive bacterial infection, resulting in dramatic inflammation, epithelial cell sloughing and ulceration, and haemorrhage.[24, 34] As similar histopathology is found in rabbit ileum exposed to toxin, colitis in humans has been thought to be a toxin-related event as well. However, this is dependent upon tissue invasion, multiplication of organisms and delivery of toxin to an intracellular site of action.[20] This scheme is only a working model and should not be considered to be established fact. If true, however, it demonstrates the interaction of multiple virulence factors in disease production, and presents a series of problems as well as opportunities for the development of effective therapeutic or prophylactic measures.

Epidemiology

INCIDENCE AND PREVALENCE

Because of its limited host range, shigellosis is always traceable to a human case or on occasion to a non-human primate infection. Furthermore, because an extremely small infectious inoculum can produce infection, person-to-person contact is highly efficient in transmission. It is unnecessary to involve food or water in which multiplication can take place, although such contaminated common-source vehicles can transmit as well.[17]

Incidence varies considerably according to socioeconomic status and environmental sanitation.[17] The infection is primarily a childhood disease. In children below the age of five years the incidence varies from 100 000–200 000 cases per 100 000 population per year in highly endemic regions in developing countries, to 25/ 100 000 per year in the United States. Even in wealthy nations, when environmental sanitation is poor and uncontrolled faecal contamination occurs, for example in institutions for mentally retarded, the rate rises to as much as 35 000/ 100 000 per year. The ease of person-to-person transmission accounts for the typically high secondary infection rate within families of cases.[17] In Britain and the United States this is reported to be as high as 42% in children under 10 years old, and 15–20% in adults living in the household, although older individuals are less likely to be symptomatic.[13, 38] While the attack rate averages close to 50% in common-source food or water-borne infections, introduction of the organism in closed populations, such as aboard ships, can affect virtually the entire population.[2, 30]

Prolonged convalescent carriage is uncommon in otherwise healthy individuals but may extend beyond eight weeks in 20–30% of poorly-nourished individuals infected with *S. dysenteriae 1* or *S. flexneri* strains.[25] In endemic regions, up to 10% of the population can be bacteriologically positive for the organism at any one time.[17]

EPIDEMIC DYSENTERY

For largely unexplained reasons, epidemic Shiga bacillus (*S. dysenteriae 1*) dysentery decreased in the period between World Wars I and II, with *S. flexneri* becoming the predominant isolate.[17] In the following years, *S. sonnei* emerged as the principal isolate in industrialized nations. It has been suggested that this may relate to the better survival of this species in the cool and moist environment of the water closet (WC).[5] The result of these shifts was a decrease in the severity of clinical disease, with more diarrhoea and less dysentery, and a decrease in the case fatality rate.

Recently, epidemic *S. dysenteriae 1* infection has resurged. Extensive serological surveys in Central America in the 1960s disclosed a highly susceptible population, with only about 1% seropositivity and sporadic isolations of the organism.[26] In 1969, however, a multiply antibiotic-resistant strain appeared and caused an extensive epidemic throughout Mexico and Central America, with high mortality of 10–15% in those untreated.[27] Since then, epidemics have occurred in Bangladesh and most recently in Zaire, due to similarly antibiotic-resistant strains, with high fatality rates as well.[12, 33] The clinical disease is described as intense and severe, as experienced in earlier times, unlike the self-limited watery diarrhoea generally caused by *S. sonnei* with which clinicians in Great Britain and the United States are familiar.

Clinical features

INTESTINAL MANIFESTATIONS

Shigella diarrhoea

Symptoms and signs begin one to five days after ingestion of shigella organisms. The initial clinical presentation is generally with fever, and indeed, experimentally induced *S. flexneri 2a* infection in adult volunteers may cause fever as the sole sign of illness in about 25% of the subjects.[17] In seizure-prone children, the rise in fever is often rapid enough to provoke a febrile convulsion. The speed and extent of the progression of illness is dependent on the virulence of the infecting organism (Table 14.5), and upon clinical epidemiological features of the host. Important host determinants are nutritional status and age, the most susceptible being formula-fed neonates or poorly nourished older infants, and the elderly. Shortly after the fever begins, a mild to moderate, not severely dehydrating watery diarrhoea ensues. Nausea, vomiting and cramps are not usually prominent, and initially the stool is not bloody. When *S. sonnei* is the causal agent, the illness may not worsen and is self-limited in three to seven days. Usually within 24 hours of the onset of diarrhoea numerous pus cells and red cells (but not gross blood) can be readily detected by a wet mount of a drop of liquid stool in one drop of 1% methylene blue

Table 14.5   Clinical features of *Shigella* species.

Species	Convalescent carriage	Frequency of plasmid-mediated antibiotic resistance	Frequency of symptoms		Frequency of haemolytic–uraemic syndrome
			Diarrhoea	Dysentery	
Shigella dysenteriae	< 4 weeks but prolonged in malnourished	+ + +	+	+ + +	+ +
Shigella flexneri	< 4 weeks but prolonged in malnourished	+ +	+ +	+ +	±
Shigella boydii	< 3 weeks	+	+ + +	+	–
Shigella sonnei	< 2 weeks	+ + +	+ + + +	uncommon	–

(Figure 14.5). These findings are indicative of the invasive inflammatory colitis phase of the disease. With a more virulent strain, such as *S. flexneri*, the diarrhoeic stool may become grossly bloody, and with the still more virulent *S. dysenteriae 1* bloody diarrhoea may be present at first examination. While the watery diarrhoea is probably small bowel in origin, the presence of pus and blood is evidence of extension of disease to the colon. It is the extent of colonic invasion that determines whether diarrhoea will become grossly bloody or progress to the dysentery syndrome. None the less, some degree of colonic involvement appears to be a consistent feature of shigellosis.

Bacillary dysentery
With sufficient colonic involvement, a typical triad of signs and symptoms appears. These include intense cramps, tenesmus, and the frequent passage of small volumes of blood, pus and mucus (Figure 14.6). It is the intensity of the discomfort and its repetitive nature over days that makes dysentery such an unforgettable experience. With the most severe infection, such as that due to *S. dysenteriae 1*, the progression to dysentery may be so rapid that the initial presenting symptoms are simply overlooked. When colonic involvement is extensive, fatal necrotizing enterocolitis may occur, with toxic megacolon or overwhelming Gram-negative sepsis as a consequence.[4, 6, 15, 18, 26]

The histopathological features of the colonic disease are reasonably well described. Sigmoidoscopy demonstrates mucosal hyperaemia and/or haemorrhage with mucosal friability, and ulceration with exudate and mucus secretion. Colonic biopsy shows focal epithelial cell damage and sloughing, with intense bleeding and inflammation in the lamina propria (Figure 14.7). Staining with Giemsa or a tissue Gram stain reveals the presence of intraepithelial organisms. Radiological examination of severe cases, usually performed because of suspicion of inflammatory bowel disease, is often consistent with this diagnosis.[8] Segmental involvement of rectum, sigmoid or descending colon is found, with superficial or deep ulcerations, collar-stud

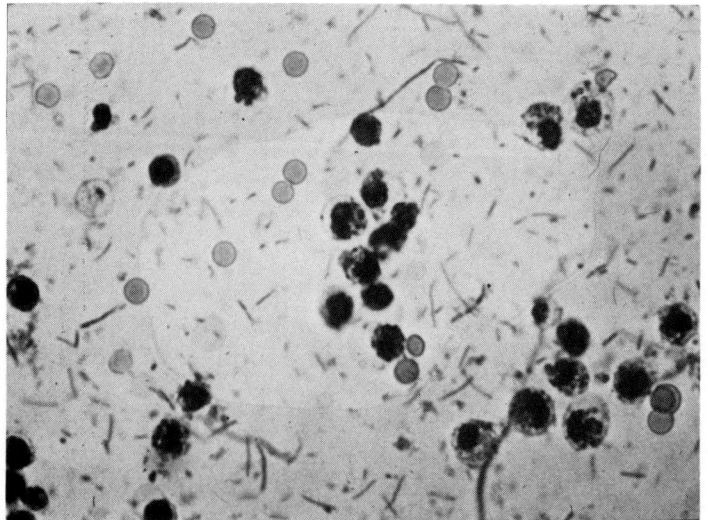

Fig. 14.5   Wet mount of watery diarrhoea stool of patient with *Shigella sonnei* infection. Numerous pus and red cells are present. Courtesy of Dr M. M. Levine.

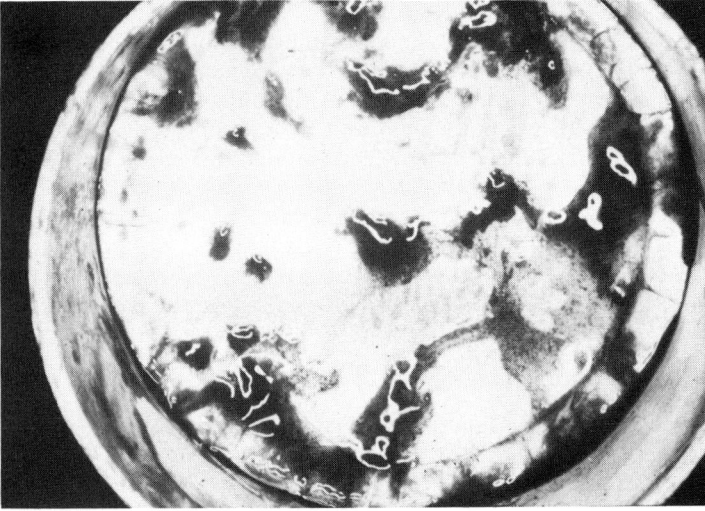

Fig. 14.6 The typical dysentery stool. Patients may pass 30 or more such scanty motions of a bloody muco-purulent nature. Courtesy of Dr M. M. Levine.

ulcers, oedema, spasm and skip areas. The appearance may mimic ulcerative colitis (superficial ulcers) or Crohn's colitis (deep, asymmetric ulcers), or the presence of collar-stud ulcers may suggest ischaemic colitis. Little is known of the small bowel involvement in humans; however, in *S. flexneri 2a* in the rhesus model, the jejunum is histologically normal but actively secreting isotonic fluid.[34] There is no a priori reason to believe that the human responds differently.

Intestinal complications
Necrotizing enterocolitis progressing to toxic megacolon may develop.[4, 15, 26] As with other causes of megacolon, the mortality rate is high, even when surgery is performed prior to perfor-

ation. Extensive mucosal ulceration also predisposes to secondary bacterial invasion and septicaemia, primarily due to *E. coli* or other intestinal coliforms.[18] A second complication of the straining and tenesmus is rectal prolapse (Figure 14.8). Early manual reduction obviates further problems; however, persistent prolapse may compromise blood supply and lead to tissue necrosis.

HAEMOLYTIC–URAEMIC SYNDROME (HUS) AND POST-DYSENTERY REITER'S SYNDROME

Shigella infection, particularly that due to *S. dysenteriae 1*, may initiate fatal HUS. Between the fifth and tenth day of illness, often when the

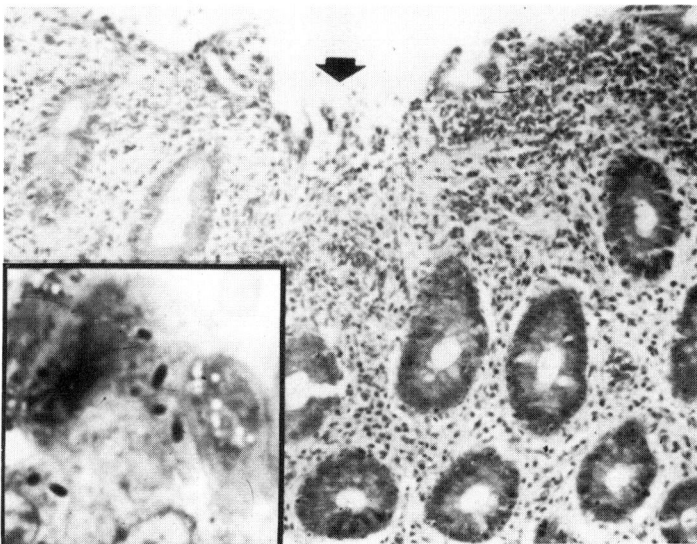

Fig. 14.7 Colonic biopsy in clinical shigellosis. Arrow points to a shallow ulceration. Note marked inflammatory response in the lamina propria. Insert shows an epithelial cell under higher magnification with intracellular micro-organisms stained with Giemsa.

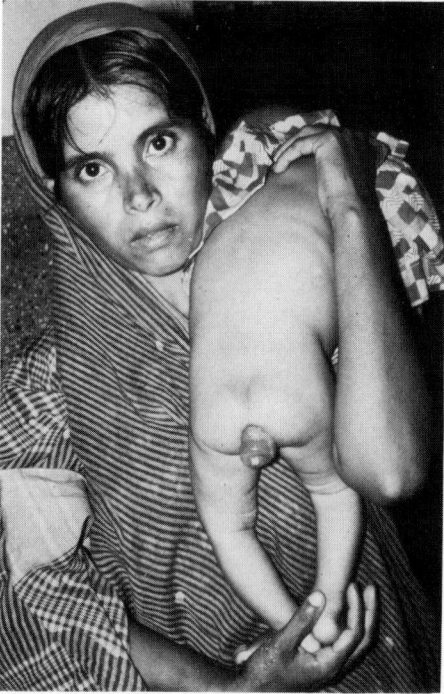

Fig. 14.8 Bangladeshi child with rectal prolapse due to *Shigella flexneri* dysentery. (Courtesy of Dr M. M. Rahaman.)

patient is improving, a marked leukaemoid reaction develops, with peripheral blood counts in excess of $50 \times 10^9/l$.[23] In some of these individuals, microangiopathic haemolytic anaemia develops, with progressive renal failure and death in about 50%.

Reiter's syndrome following shigellosis is similar to that induced by other infectious agents, and it has a predilection for subjects with histocompatibility antigen HLA-B27.[3] In these patients joint manifestations are frequently chronic, destructive and cause a disabling arthritis. The components of the triad (arthritis, iritis and urethritis) may occur in any order, and generally begin within a few weeks or months of the initial episode.

Other rare events
Occasionally, children present with respiratory symptoms and may exhibit rales on auscultation or an infiltrate on radiography.[1] This is a self-limited event which does not require therapy and has been documented to be shigella pneumonia in only one or two instances. The same pertains to the meningismus sometimes observed in young children before intestinal symptoms commence.[1] A lumbar puncture may be performed because of the presence of fever and especially if a seizure has occurred, but this is invariably normal.

Shigella bacteraemia early in infection is probably more common than reported but it is not of clinical consequence and is cleared without therapy.[18] Secondary bacteraemia due to *S. dysenteriae 1* or Enterobacteriaceae entering through the ulcerated mucosa is serious; it can initiate disseminated intravascular coagulation, and may be lethal.[6, 18, 23, 26, 39]

While shigella keratitis is distinctly rare, vaginitis has been reported more frequently in adolescent girls under 15 years of age (Murphy, 1979).

Diagnosis

The clinical presentation may be highly suggestive of shigellosis, and wet mounts of liquid stool to determine the presence of leucocytes and erythrocytes are very helpful.[22] The definitive diagnosis is microbiological. Several simple principles improve the yield of positive cultures.[17] The organism is not hardy in the environment, so specimens should be cultured rapidly, at the bedside if possible, or placed in holding medium if plating is delayed for more than an hour. Stool samples and not swabs should be cultured, selecting bloody or mucoid plugs. If a swab is used, it must pass the sphincter and be streaked directly onto medium. Finally, more than one medium should be used, and never SS agar alone.

Treatment

GENERAL MEASURES

Dehydration can be treated by oral rehydration methods in shigellosis as in cholera or enterotoxigenic *E. coli* infection.[36] Infants can be fed orally if food is tolerated, especially if being breast-fed. In older individuals there is little evidence that antimotility agents are effective and some suggestion that they might worsen the infection by delaying clearance thereby prolonging contact between organism and mucosa.[7]

Febrile convulsions are treated no differently from standard paediatric practice, with temperature reduction and anticonvulsants such as diazepam if indicated.

SPECIFIC THERAPY

Appropriate antimicrobial therapy will shorten the course of shigellosis.[18] Because of spreading transferable antimicrobial resistance in the genus, the problem is to find a drug to which the organism is susceptible. Ampicillin is highly effective but significant resistance is present in some areas, especially in *S. sonnei*. Co-trimoxazole (trimethoprim and sulphameth-oxazole) has been an excellent alternative; unfortunately, transferable resistance to this has appeared recently and may spread. Therefore, it is important that the clinician is aware of the basic principles of antimicrobial therapy of this disease. First, the isolate must be susceptible to the agent in vitro. Second, both tissue and luminal drug must be present; non-absorbable (e.g. neomycin) or highly absorbable agents (e.g. amoxycillin) will fail. Finally, because of the ease of intrafamilial spread, the physician must decide whether or not to treat additional members of the household, especially the young.

Prophylaxis and control

GENERAL MEASURES

Commonsense hygienic practices can reduce person-to-person transmission of shigella infection.[18] Hand-washing with soap has been shown to be effective in reducing the secondary case rate within families, even in a rural setting in Bangladesh. Food preparation and eating should be separated from care for the patient and handling of objects contaminated by faeces.

VACCINES

Parenteral or oral killed vaccines have not been successful.[14] In contrast, live oral vaccines using non-invasive variant organisms or non-proliferating streptomycin-dependent mutants provide significant protection, although such vaccines have not been approved for use.[29] The isolation of plasmids carrying genes essential for invasion which induce protective immunity in experimental animals is most promising. These plasmids have been inserted in the safe and effective type 21a *Salmonella typhi* live oral vaccine strain.[10] Immunization with this engineered vaccine should therefore provide protection against typhoid fever and some forms of shigellosis, and these concepts are currently being tested.[16]

Parenteral immunization of rhesus monkeys with toxoid results in serum neutralizing antibody but no protection against disease following live bacterial challenge.[28] It remains to be determined whether enteral presentation of a toxoid vaccine will be effective.

REFERENCES

1 Barrett-Connor, E. & Connor, J. D. (1970) Extra-intestinal manifestations of shigellosis. *American Journal of Gastroenterology*, **53**, 234–245.

2 Black, R. E., Graun, G. F. & Blake, P. A. (1978) Epidemiology of common-source outbreaks of shigellosis in the United States. *American Journal of Epidemiology*, **108**, 47–52.

3 Calin, A. & Fries, J. F. (1976) An 'experimental' epidemic of Reiter's syndrome revisited. Follow-up evaluation on genetic and environmental factors. *Annals of Internal Medicine*, **85**, 564–566.

4 Chessler, R. K., Rosenthal, W. S. & Pitchumoni, C. S. (1978) Masquerading colitis. Infectious dysentery superimposed on chronic inflammatory bowel disease. *Journal of the Medical Society of New Jersey*, **75**, 161–164.

5 Christie, A. B. (1981) *Infectious Diseases, Epidemiology and Clinical Practice*, 3rd edn, p. 111. Edinburgh: Churchill Livingstone.

6 Counts, G. W., Nitzkin, J. L., Hennekens, C. H. Jr & Ehrenkranz, N. J. (1971) Shiga bacillus dysentery acquired in Nicaragua. *Archives of Internal Medicine*, **128**, 582–584.

7 DuPont, H. L. & Hornick, R. B. (1973) Adverse effect of Lomotil therapy in shigellosis. *Journal of the American Medical Association*, **226**, 1525–1528.

8 Farman, J., Rabinowitz, J. G. Meyers, M. A. (1973) Roentgenology of infectious colitis. *American Journal of Roentgenology*, **119**, 375–381.

9 Formal, S. B., LaBrec, E. H. & Schneider, J. (1965) Pathogenesis of bacillary dysentery in laboratory animals. *Federation Proceedings*, **24**, 29–34.

10 Formal, S. B., LaBrec, E. H., Schneider, E. H. & Falkow, S. (1975) Restoration of virulence to a strain of *S. flexneri* by mating with *Escherichia coli*. *Journal of Bacteriology*, **89**, 835–838.

11 Formal, S. B., Baron, L. S., Kopecko, D. J. *et al*. (1981) Construction of a potential bivalent vaccine strain: introduction of *Shigella sonnei* Form I antigen genes into the *gal E Salmonella typhi* Ty21a typhoid vaccine strain. *Infection and Immunity*, **34**, 387–389.

12 Frost, J. A., Rowe, B., Vandepitte, J. & Threlfall, E. J. (1981) Plasmid characterization in the investigation of an epidemic caused by multiply resistant *Shigella dysenteriae* Type 1 in Central Africa. *Lancet*, **ii**, 1074–1076.

13 Hardy, A. V. & Watt, J. (1948) Studies of the acute diarrhoeal diseases. XVIII. Epidemiology. *Public Health Reports*, **63**, 363–378.

14 Higgins, A. R., Floyd, T. M. & Kader, M. A. (1955) Studies in shigellosis III. A controlled evaluation of a monovalent shigella vaccine in a highly endemic environment. *American Journal of Tropical Medicine Hygiene*, **4**, 281–288.

15 Kelber, M. & Ament, M. E. (1976) *Shigella dysenteriae* 1: a forgotten cause of pseudomembranous colitis. *Journal of Pediatrics*, **89**, 595–596.

16 Keren, D. F., Collins, H. H., Baron, L. S. *et al*. (1982) Intestinal immunoglobulin A response in rabbits to a *Salmonella typhi* strain harboring a *Shigella sonnei* plasmid. *Infection and Immunity*, **37**, 387–389.

17 Keusch, G. T. (1982) Shigellosis. In *Bacterial Infections of Humans*. (Ed.) Evans, A. S. & Feldman, H. pp. 487–509. New York: Plenum.

18 Keusch, G. T. (1982) Shigellosis. In *Critical Reviews in Tropical Medicine*, vol. 1 (Ed.) Chandra, R. K. pp. 77–107. New York: Plenum.

19 Keusch, G. T., Donohue-Rolfe, A. & Jacewicz, M. (1982) Shigella toxin(s): description and role in diarrhea

and dysentery. *Pharmacology Therapeutics*, **15**, 403–438.

20   Keusch, G. T., Grady, G. F., Takeuchi, A. & Sprinz, H. (1972) The pathogenesis of *Shigella* diarrhea. II. Enterotoxin-induced acute enteritis in the rabbit ileum. *Journal of Infectious Diseases*, **126**, 92–95.

21   Kopecko, D. J., Washington, O. & Formal, S. B. (1980) Genetic and physical evidence for plasmid control of *Shigella sonnei* Form I cell surface antigen. *Infection and Immunity*, **29**, 207–214.

22   Korzeniowski, O. M., Varada, F. A., Rouse, J. D. & Guerrant, R. L. (1979) Value of examination for fecal leukocytes in the early diagnosis of shigellosis. *American Journal of Tropical Medicine and Hygiene*, **28**, 1031–1035.

23   Koster, F., Levin, J., Walker, L. *et al.* (1978) Hemolytic–uremic syndrome after shigellosis. Relation to endotoxemia and circulating immune complexes. *New England Journal of Medicine*, **298**, 927–933.

24   Levine, M. M., DuPont, H. L., Formal, S. B. *et al.* (1973) Pathogenesis of *Shigella dysenteriae I* (Shiga) dysentery. *Journal of Infectious Diseases*, **127**, 261–270.

25   Mata, L. J. (1978) *The Children of Santa Maria Cauque: A Prospective Field Study of Health and Growth*, p. 250. Cambridge: MIT Press.

26   Mata, L. J. & Castro, F. (1974) Epidemiology, diagnosis and impact of Shiga dysentery in Central America. In *Industry and Tropical Health VIII. Proceedings of the 8th Conference, Industrial Council for Tropical Health, 1974*. pp. 30–37.

27   Mata, L. J., Gangarosa, E. J., Caceres, A. *et al.* (1970) Epidemic Shiga bacillus dysentery in Central America. I. Etiologic investigations in Guatemala, 1969. *Journal of Infectious Diseases*, **122**, 170–180.

28   McIver, J., Grady, G. F. & Formal, S. B. (1977) Immunization with *Shigella dysenteriae* type 1: evaluation of antitoxic immunity in prevention of experimental disease in rhesus monkeys (*Macaca mulata*). *Journal of Infectious Diseases*, **136**, 416–421.

29   Mel, D. M., Gangarosa, E. J. & Radovanovic, M. L. (1971) Studies on vaccination against bacillary dysentery. 6. Protection of children with oral immunization using streptomycin-dependent shigella strains. *Bulletin of the World Health Organisation*, **45**, 457–464.

30   Merson, M. H., Tenney, J. H., Meyers, J. D. *et al.* (1975) Shigellosis at sea: an outbreak aboard a passenger cruise ship. *American Journal of Epidemiology*, **101**, 165–175.

31   Murphy, T. V. (1979) *Shigella* vaginitis: report of 38 patients and review of the literature. *Pediatrics*, **63**, 511–516.

32   Petrovskaya, V. G. & Licheva, T. A. (1982) A provisional chromosome map of *Shigella* and the regions related to pathogenicity. *Acta Microbiologica Academiae Scientiarum Hungaricae* **29**, 41–53.

33   Rahaman, M. M., Hug, I., Dey, C. R. *et al.* (1974) Ampicillin-resistant Shiga bacillus in Bangladesh. *Lancet*, **i**, 406–407.

34   Rout, W. R., Formal, D. B., Giannella, R. A. & Dammin, G. J. (1975) Pathophysiology of *Shigella* diarrhea in the rhesus monkey: intestinal transport, morphological and bacteriological studies. *Gastroenterology* **68**, 270–278.

35   Sansonetti, P. J., Kopecko, D. J. & Formal, S. B. (1982) Involvement of a plasmid in the invasive ability of *Shigella flexneri*. *Infection and Immunity*, **35**, 852–860.

36   Stoll, B. J., Glass, R. I., Huq, M. I. *et al.* (1982) Epidemiological and clinical features of patients infected with *Shigella* who attended a diarrheal disease hospital in Bangladesh. *Journal of Infectious Diseases*, **146**, 177–183.

37   Takeuchi, A., Sprinz, H., LaBrec, E. H. & Formal, S. B. (1965) Experimental bacillary dysentery: An electron microscopic study of the response of the intestinal mucosa to bacterial invasion. *American Journal of Pathology*, **47**, 1011–1044.

38   Thomas, M. E. M. & Tillett, H. E. (1973) Dysentery in general practice: A study of cases and their contacts in Enfield and an epidemiological comparison with salmonellosis. *Journal of Hygiene*, **71**, 373–389.

39   Ullis, K. C. & Rosenblatt, R. M. (1973) Shiga bacillus dysentery complicated by bacteremia and disseminated intravascular coagulation. *Journal of Pediatrics*, **83**, 90–93.

GIARDIASIS

Intestinal infection due to the protozoan parasite *Giardia lamblia* is common all over the world. It is the most frequent intestinal parasite, detected in 4% of the stool samples examined for parasites at state health laboratories in the USA.[20] Its incidence in the UK has been reported to be 5–16%,[11] in Western Australia 15.2%,[12] in Poland 5.1–10.4%,[21] in Saudi Arabia 14.0%[3] and in India 4–17%.[14] It is evident that *Giardia lamblia* infection is endemic in several countries of the world, but its real prevalence is difficult to deduce from a review of the literature because of variation in survey results influenced by the designs of the studies. Asymptomatic *Giardia lamblia* infection in man is well-known, but its potential pathogenicity, causing outbreaks of diarrhoea amongst travellers and malabsorption syndrome, has attracted the attention of many investigators and physicians.

The parasite

The genus *Giardia* belongs to the phylum Sarcomastigophora, subphylum Mastigophora, class Zoomastigophora, order *Diplomonadorida* and family *Hexamitidae*.[13] About 40 species have been described but Filice's classification of three main species – *Giardia agilis*, *Giardia muris* and *Giardia duodenalis* – is more important;[7] only the last is related to human infection. In Western countries it is called *Giardia lamblia*, a name given by Stiles in honour of Professor A. Giard of Paris and Dr Lambl of Prague.[22] In the Soviet Union and East European countries it is known as *Lamblia intestinalis*.

The parasite has two stages in its life-cycle, the trophozoite and the cyst. The trophozoite is pear-shaped, resembling a tennis racket without a handle. It measures 9–16 μm long, 6–10 μm

wide and 2–4 μm thick, with a broad anterior
and a pointed posterior end. Its dorsal surface is
convex, and the ventral surface is concave with a
sucking disc. It is bilaterally symmetrical. Two
median bodies are seen. It has two ovoid nuclei,
each with a central karyosome. There are two
axonemes and four pairs of flagella (Figure
14.9a). The ultrastructure of the trophozoite has
been studied in detail: the sucking disc has two
lobes, based between the nuclei, and it occupies
the entire cephalic pole on the ventral surface.

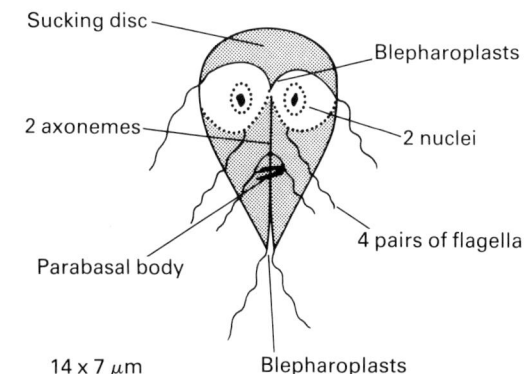

a

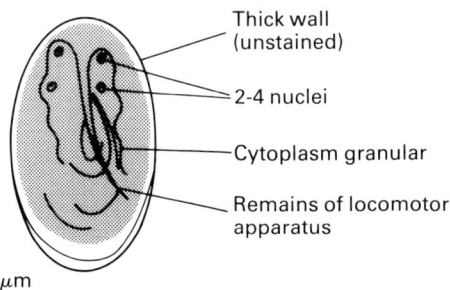

b

Fig. 14.9 *Giardia lamblia*: (a) trophozoite stage; (b) cystic
stage.

There are numerous microtubules in the cytoplasm. Pinocytic vesicles are seen along the
dorsal surface. Abundant ribosomes are
observed, but no Golgi vesicles are present.[8, 15]

The *Giardia* cyst is oval in shape, 8–12 μm in
length and 6–8 μm in width, with a smooth cyst
wall. The fully mature cyst has four nuclei, lying
in a group or with two on either side. A variable
number of fibrillar bodies may be seen in the
cytoplasm (Figure 14.9b). Numerous vacuoles,
possibly phagocytic, have been seen on transmission electronmicroscopy.[14] Endosymbiotic
bacteria, viruses and fungi have been seen within
the cyst.[15]

Infection

Humans are infected by ingesting the viable
mature cysts. Excystation takes place in the
acidic conditions of the stomach,[4] and binu-
cleate trophozoites emerge.[6] Not all *Giardia*
cysts are capable of excystation. Incubation
periods of 1 to 75 days have been reported.
Giardia trophozoites roam the lumen of the
upper two-thirds of the small intestine. They
attach themselves firmly to the epithelial brush
border by means of their ventral sucking discs,
absorb nourishment from the intestinal surface
and reproduce by binary fission. Rarely trophozoites find their way into the bloodstream. Some
detach from the intestinal surface, enter the
faecal stream and encyst during their transit
through the gut. The nuclei in each cyst undergo
a single division to form the quadrinucleate
mature cysts, which are passed out in the faeces.
If environmental conditions are favourable cysts
can survive for up to two months.

Giardia infection spreads through faeces containing the cysts, which contaminate food and
drinking water. Cyst passers who remain asymptomatic themselves are a real hazard to society.
Such people, especially while working as food
handlers, help the spread of infection. Cock-
roaches, flies and other insects can carry the
Giardia cysts from faeces to food. In many
developing countries raw vegetables are often
washed with contaminated, unfiltered water
before sale and this may spread the infection.
There are many communities, particularly in the
developing nations, where the water supply is
chronically infected, and several community-
wide epidemics have been reported as being due
to failure of water purification systems.[5] *Giardia*
cysts settle in water because of their high specific
gravity and are resistant to normal disinfecting
doses of chlorine.

Person-to-person spread of giardiasis has
been strongly suggested among children at day-
care centres and among promiscuous male
homosexuals. *Giardia* infection can even be
acquired through inhalation.[19] The existence of
an animal reservoir for human *Giardia* has been
suspected but not proved.

Clinical features

Most subjects with *Giardia* infection remain
asymptomatic. This has been demonstrated by
human volunteer studies and several epidemiological surveys of the general population of
endemic areas. Indeed, this was the main reason
why *Giardia* was long thought to be a com-

mensal, non-parasitic organism. Clinical manifestations of giardiasis can be classified as (a) acute diarrhoea, (b) chronic malabsorption syndrome or (c) non-specific and extra-intestinal symptoms.

Acute diarrhoea due to giardiasis has been commonly recorded among children in endemic areas and travellers to these areas. The onset is sudden, with the appearance of explosive, foul-smelling, watery diarrhoea. Frequency of stools may be 15 to 20 per day with passage of as much as four litres of liquid stools per day. Abdominal distension, belching, cramping pain and excessive fatigue are present. A small proportion may be febrile. Acute diarrhoea usually stops spontaneously after a few days. Rarely the illness may pass to the subacute or chronic stage and present with the features of malabsorption syndrome.

Patients with malabsorption syndrome present with recurrent or even persistent episodes of loose motions, which may be bulky, frothy, foul-smelling and difficult to flush away. Associated symptoms include flatulence, abdominal pain, anorexia, nausea, weakness and weight loss. Pallor, growth-retardation and other features of undernutrition are recorded among children.

A significant number of patients are recorded in endemic areas who have vague abdominal discomfort, nausea, excessive belching and flatulence and whose stools are positive for *Giardia* cyst. It is tempting to ascribe their symptoms to this parasite though a causal relationship is difficult to establish. Allergic manifestations, such as urticaria, uveitis, arthritis, food intolerance, intermittent fever and infectious lymphocytosis, have been reported in giardiasis. *Giardia* has been suggested as one of the aetiological agents for inflammatory diseases of the biliary tract, pancreas and duodenum.

Diagnosis

Examination of the stool for cysts is a simple test for the diagnosis of giardiasis. The American Society of Parasitologists has recommended examination of at least three consecutive freshly passed stools to detect the maximum proportion of positive cases.[1] Examination of two consecutive stool samples by the formalin–ether concentration method yields almost equally good results. Detection of *Giardia* trophozoites in the duodenal aspirate has been recommended for better results in suspected yet stool-negative patients. Examination of duodenal/jejunal mucosal smears and biopsies has also been

reported, with good results, but these techniques are not recommended as a routine diagnostic approach.

Serodiagnosis of *Giardia* infection is possible by detection of specific antibody by indirect fluorescent antibody methods, indirect haemagglutination test and the microelisa technique.[10, 18, 24] Serodiagnosis is a useful adjunct for diagnosis of giardiasis in situations where stool and duodenal fluid are negative for the parasite.

Patients with giardiasis require other appropriate investigations for malabsorption syndrome, diarrhoea and biliary tract, pancreas and upper gastrointestinal tract symptoms as may be indicated by the clinical presentation.

Immunity, pathogenesis and pathology

Giardiasis is more common and presents with relatively more severe symptoms in young children and particularly in those who have associated malnutrition. However, the exact role of age in the pathogenesis of giardiasis is not known. Clinical observations and experimental studies have demonstrated that protein malnutrition enhances susceptibility to *Giardia* infection. The possibility of genetic factors in the pathogenesis has been suggested by the observation that people with blood group A are more frequently infected with this parasite than those with other blood groups.

Several observations have confirmed a relationship between the host immunity and susceptibility to *Giardia* infection. The infection is higher in hypogammaglobulinaemic subjects, and low levels of IgA and IgG immunoglobulin are associated with more frequent and more severe *Giardia* infection. It has also been demonstrated that infection is more frequent and severe in subjects with lower levels of secretory IgA in the duodenum and reduced gut immunity.[2] Experimental studies have also suggested a role for cell-mediated immunity in enhancing the susceptibility to *Giardia* infection. It has been observed that parasitic resolution in experimental animals is T-cell-dependent. Lymphocytes in the gut also contribute to the protection and help in elimination of parasites from the gut. Further, it has been shown that macrophages help in eliminating *Giardia* infection if they are stimulated by a specific antigen. Two types of phagocytes have been demonstrated: a non-specific variety which persists even in the absence of antibody and complement and a specific type which requires high antibody stimulus.

A parasitic factor has also been incriminated

and strain variations may play an important role in the pathogenesis. Further, the microflora within the parasite may be of significance in making it more virulent.

Diarrhoea is a key manifestation of giardiasis. Recent observations suggest that increased levels of prostaglandins E and F may play an important role in the pathogenesis of the diarrhoea. Elevated prostaglandin levels in giardiasis stimulate the adenylate cyclase system, resulting in an increase in synthesis of cyclic AMP. This inhibits the uptake of sodium chloride and thus leads to diarrhoea.[16]

It is now well established that giardiasis causes malabsorption. However, the exact mechanism of malabsorption is not established. Mechanisms suggested include the following.

1 A large number of parasites adhering to the intestinal villi may act as a mechanical barrier to the absorption of nutrient.

2 Parasites may compete with the host for nutrients.

3 Direct injury to the absorptive epithelial cells by *Giardia* has been demonstrated by light and electron microscopy. Even the penetration of the trophozoites into the epithelium has been shown. This may not only damage the absorptive cells but may also induce hypermotility and thereby reduce the time for absorption of the nutrient by the cells.

4 Damage to the fuzzy coat has been suggested on the basis of electron-microscopic studies of the intestinal biopsies in giardiasis.[23] Depressed brush-border enzymes alter the digestion and absorption of carbohydrate and protein. Recently, experimental studies have shown damage to the brush-border membrane and lowered absorptive capacity for labelled carbohydrate and amino acids, which confirms earlier clinical findings.[9]

5 It has been suggested that giardiasis depresses pancreatic function and thereby leads to exocrine pancreatic insufficiency and malabsorption. However, the significance of pancreatic insufficiency in the aetiology of giardiasis is doubtful, and its role, even if it exists, may be very small.

6 Bacterial overgrowth in the small intestine has been suggested as playing an important role in the pathogenesis of malabsorption. Deconjugation of bile salts and release of toxic bile acids in this situation may result in malabsorption.

It is apparent that several factors may contribute to the pathogenesis of malabsorption in giardiasis. Damage to the fuzzy coat of villi leading to deficiencies of enzyme may be the most important of these.

Pathology

The principal pathological changes in giardiasis are noted in the duodenum and the upper part of the jejunum. Non-specific and mild abnormalities suggestive of reactive hepatitis have been observed in the liver. Chronic inflammatory changes in the gallbladder have also been recorded.

Intestinal villi show atrophy and the crypts are enlarged. The lamina propria is infiltrated with mononuclear, eosinophilic and polymorphonuclear leucocytes. Villous epithelial cells have an increased mitotic index. Invasion of the epithelial cells and mucosa by the parasite is also observed occasionally. All these abnormalities are reversible after treatment with antiparasitic drugs.

Treatment

Until recently, the drug of choice for giardiasis was metronidazole, the usual dose regime being 400 mg thrice daily for seven days. Alternatively, a single dose of two grams per day on three successive days has proved useful, with a parasitological cure rate of 91%. However, it is important to mention that side-effects such as nausea, vomiting, anorexia and a metallic taste are more frequent with the larger doses. A useful compromise therefore is to start with the high-dose schedule and to advise the patient to reduce the dose by half in the event of side-effects.

Recently, a new broad spectrum antiprotozoal drug tinidazole has been introduced. Chemically, it is a nitroimidazole derivative having a close structural similarity to metronidazole, but with certain advantages: it is better tolerated and has fewer gastrointestinal side-effects. The recommended dose schedule is 300 mg daily for seven days or a single dose of 2 g.

An excellent alternative drug is mepacrine (quinacrine, Atabrine) given in a dose of 100 mg three times daily for seven days. The cure rate is of the order of 90–95%. Furazolidone 100 mg four times a day is also quite effective and well tolerated. The efficacy of the drug has ranged from 90% to 100%.

Occasionally, a patient may continue to excrete *Giardia* cysts despite adequate treatment. Reinfection due to poor hygienic conditions or an infected water supply is the main reason, and compromised immune status of the individual is the other possibility. Rarely a true resistance is seen, and in such cases the best treatment is to instil one gram of mepacrine suspended in water directly into the duodenum by intubation.

REFERENCES

1   American Society of Parasitologists (1977) Procedure suggested by the Council for use in examination of clinical specimens for parasitic infections. *Journal of Parasitology*, **63**, 959–960.

2   Andrews, S. J. & Hewlett, E. L. (1981) Proteins against infection with *Giardia muris* by milk littering antibody to giardia. *Journal of Infectious Diseases*, **143**, 242–246.

3   Awadallah, M. A. & Morsy, T. A. (1974) *Ain Shams Medical Journal*, **25**, 835.

4   Bingham, A. K., Jarrol, J. E. Jr. & Meyer, E. A. (1979) Giardia species. Physical factors of excystation in vivo and excystation vs eosin exclusion as determination of viability. *Experimental Parasitology*, **47**, 284–291.

5   Craun, G. D. (1979) Waterborne outbreaks of giardiasis. In *Proceedings of National Symposium on Waterborne Transmission of Giardiasis* (Ed.) Jakubowski, W. & Hoff, J. C. pp. 127–147. Cincinnati: US Environmental Protection Agency.

6   Chatterjee, K. D. (1980) *Parasitology (Protozoology and Helminthology) in Relation to Clinical Medicine*. pp. 37–39. Calcutta: Chaterjee Medical Publishers.

7   Filice, F. P. (1952) Studies on the cytology and life history of a giardia from the laboratory rat. *University of California Publications in Zoology*, **57**, 53–146.

8   Friend, D. S. (1966) The fine structure of *Giardia muris*. *Journal of Cell Biology*, **29**, 317–332.

9   Ganguly, N. K. & Mahajan, R. C. (1983) Personal communication from Department of Parasitology, Postgraduate Institute of Medical Education and Research, Chandigarh.

10 Ganguly, N. K., Mahajan, R. C., Radha Krishna, V. *et al.* (1981) Haemagglutinating antibodies in animal and thymectomised mice infected with *Giardia lamblia*. *Indian Journal of Medical Research*, **75**, 543–547.

11 Hore, C. A. (1949) *Handbook of Medical Protozoology*. pp. 15–334. London: Baillière, Tindall and Cox.

12 Jones, H. I. (1980) Intestinal parasite infections in Western Australian aborigines. *Medical Journal of Australia*, **2**, 375.

13 Levine, N. D., Coliss, J. O., Cox, F. E. G. *et al.* (1980) A newly revised classification of protozoa. *Journal of Protozoology*, **27**, 37–58.

14 Lutchel, D. L., Lawerance, P. W. & DeWald, F. B. (1981) Ultrastructural studies of *Giardia lamblia* cysts. *Applied and Environmental Microbiology*, **40**, 821–831.

15 Nemanic, P., Owen, R. L., Stevens, D. P. & Mueller, J. C. (1979) Ultrastructural observations in giardiasis in a mouse model. II. Endosymbiosis and organelle distribution on *Giardia muris* and comparison with *Giardia lamblia*. *Journal of Infectious Diseases*, **140**, 22–228.

16 Ouchterlony, O. & Holmgren, J. (1978) *Cholera and Related Diarrhoeas. 43rd Nobel Symposium. 1980.* Stockholm: Karger and Basset.

17 Prakash, O. & Tandon, B. N. (1966) Intestinal parasites with special reference to *Entamoeba histolytica* complex as revealed by routine concentration and cultural examination of stool specimens. *Indian Journal of Medical Research*, **54**, 10.

18 Ridley, K. J. & Ridley, D. S. (1976) Serum antibodies and jejunal histology in giardiasis associated with malabsorption. *Journal of Clinical Pathology*, **29**, 30–34.

19 Schuman, H. S., Arnold, T. A. & Rowe, J. R. (1982) Giardiasis by inhalation. *Lancet*, **i**, 53.

20 Smith, J. W. & Wolfe, M. S. (1980) Giardiasis review. *Annual Review of Medicine*, **31**, 373–383.

21 Stelmaszyk, J. L. (1981) *Proceedings of the VIth International Congress of Protozoology, Warsaw*.

22 Stiles (1915) Cited by Craig, C. F. & Faust, C. E. (1970) *Clinical Parasitology* 6th Rev. Edition by Faust, E. C., Russell, P. F. & Jung, C. R. p. 64. Philadelphia: Lea & Febiger.

23 Tandon, B. N., Puri, B. K., Gandhi, P. C. & Tewari, S. G. (1974) Mucosal surface injury of jejunal mucosa in patients with giardiasis: an electron microscopic study. *Indian Journal of Medical Research*, **62**, 1838–1842.

24 Visvesvara, G. S., Smith, P. D., Healy, G. R. & Brown, W. R. (1980) An immunofluorescence test to detect serum antibodies to *Giardia lamblia*. *Annals of Internal Medicine*, **93**, 802–805.

VIRUS INFECTIONS

Acute gastroenteritis is one of the leading causes of morbidity throughout the world. Among healthy adults this infection usually results in only minor inconvenience because recovery generally occurs within a few days. Although it is not a cause of appreciable mortality among children in industrialized countries, it is the leading cause of death among children in many developing countries. Malnutrition and chronic debilitating disease play important contributing roles. Poor sanitation and overcrowding result in repeated exposure to faecal pathogens in infancy, and repeated attacks of severe infectious diarrhoea contribute significantly to the development of protein–energy malnutrition.[39, 104] In such developing countries as India, Indonesia and Guatemala children experience at least one or two episodes of acute gastroenteritis per year during the first three years of life; 1% to 4% of these episodes are fatal. This represents a death rate of 20–55 per 1000 children. Combining this data with recent demographic information, it has been calculated that in Asia, Africa and Latin America 500 million episodes of acute diarrhoeal disease occur among children less than five years old, resulting in the deaths of 5–18 million children.[94]

Improvements in water supplies and sanitation would drastically improve this situation, but limited resources preclude such improvements in many parts of the world. The development of vaccines against major enteric pathogens provides the only alternative approach. However, this approach is dependent on identifying aetiological agents. The accumulated data from a number of studies up to the early 1970s showed that pathogenic bacteria or parasites could be implicated in only 25–40% of episodes of acute gastroenteritis.[97, 104, 113]

These figures were probably an underestimate because techniques to detect enteropathogenicity are recent and have not yet been widely used in most studies conducted in tropical areas. In addition, comparatively few studies have employed tests to detect *Campylobacter* sp., organisms recently recognized as being important causes of gastroenteritis.[108] It has long been assumed by exclusion that viruses caused acute gastroenteritis, but only during the last decade have they been identified. The delay in identifying them is partly because viruses causing gastroenteritis, despite being excreted in very high concentrations, are difficult or impossible to cultivate in vitro, although viruses such as rotaviruses or enteric adenoviruses may be adapted to grow in cell culture by laboratory manipulation.

Those viruses associated with acute gastroenteritis are listed in Table 14.6. The small round viruses associated with acute epidemic gastroenteritis (winter vomiting disease), of which the Norwalk and Ditchling agents are prototypes, although ubiquitous, are not of major significance as the symptoms they induce are generally mild and are of limited duration. However, rotaviruses represent the major pathogens responsible for causing acute diarrhoeal disease among children throughout the world. The enteric or 'fastidious' adenoviruses may be widely distributed and occasionally cause severe infection but they are less frequently associated with acute diarrhoeal disease than rotaviruses. Comparatively little is still known of the role of astroviruses and caliciviruses; they probably represent minor pathogens which tend to be associated with relatively mild disease.

SMALL ROUND VIRUSES AND ACUTE EPIDEMIC GASTROENTERITIS (WINTER VOMITING DISEASE)

Outbreaks of acute gastroenteritis have incubation periods which usually range from 4 to 48 hours. In general, a 4–6-hour incubation period is suggestive of an illness induced by bacterial toxins, while 6–24 hours, but occasionally longer, suggests pathogenic bacteria. However, bacterial causes are much less frequently identified in outbreaks with longer incubation periods (24–48 hours) and it has long been suggested that many of these are caused by viruses. Indeed, it is from the stools of patients involved in such outbreaks that small round viruses have most frequently been identified. The clinical syndrome of acute epidemic non-bacterial gastroenteritis,

also designated winter vomiting disease or perhaps more appropriately epidemic nausea and vomiting, is a self-limiting syndrome in which some or all of the following features occur: fever, nausea, vomiting, vertigo, myalgia, abdominal colic and diarrhoea. Although nausea and vomiting are invariably present, not all patients develop diarrhoea. Symptoms seldom persist for more than a few days. The disease is rarely associated with sufficient prostration to require admission to hospital. Community-wide or family outbreaks with high secondary attack rates are common and all age groups may be affected. Many outbreaks have been described following ingestion of virus-contaminated food and water, particularly raw or improperly cooked shellfish. Person-to-person spread is probably via the faecal–oral route, but since Norwalk virus has been detected in vomitus, this may perhaps also provide a vehicle of transmission, particularly as vomiting is sometimes projectile.[40]

The virus most frequently associated with epidemic gastroenteritis and the one which has been most intensively studied is the Norwalk virus, which was first detected in 1972 by immune electron microscopy (IEM) of a faecal filtrate obtained from a patient during an outbreak in a primary school in Norwalk (Ohio). Numerous small virus-like particles, about 27 nm in diameter, were visualized by IEM.[54] The technique of IEM provides a suitable method for detecting small viruses which cannot be cultivated in vitro and lack a distinct substructure, particularly if they are present in relatively low concentrations. This technique can also detect and quantitate immune responses. Small round virus particles were later implicated as the cause of acute gastroenteritis in two family outbreaks in the USA, one in Montgomery County, Maryland, and one in Hawaii.[131] Virus excretion occurred transiently during the acute phase, was accompanied by an immune response, and when faecal filtrates from such patients were fed to volunteers, they in turn developed immune responses. However, IEM and cross-challenge studies in volunteers showed that whereas the Norwalk and Montgomery County viruses were identical or closely related Hawaii was antigenically distinct.[115, 131] Virus excretion occurs transiently during the acute phase of disease and is accompanied by an immune response. Small round viruses ranging in size from 22 nm to 26 nm were also identified in the UK: the Wollan agent from an outbreak of winter vomiting in a boarding school,[21] the Ditchling agent from a similar outbreak in a primary school[3] and the

Table 14.6 Viruses associated with acute gastroenteritis.

Virus	Size (nm)	Classification	Serotypes	Principal epidemiological features	Usual method of diagnosis Virus	Usual method of diagnosis Serology
Small round structured (Norwalk-like)	30–35	Unclassified (?calicivirus)	At least 3	World-wide distribution. Community and family outbreaks sometimes associated with consumption of contaminated food (shellfish) and water	IEM	IEM, RIA, IAHA
Small round featureless (Ditchling-like)	22–26	Unclassified (?parvovirus)	At least 3		EM	IEM
Rotavirus	70	Rotavirus (family of reoviruses)	2 subgroups 5 serotypes	World-wide; winter disease of infants and children in temperate climates. Approximately 50% of cases of diarrhoea and vomiting in children are rotavirus-induced in UK	EM, ELISA	ELISA, NEUT, CF
'Fastidious' adenovirus	70	Adenovirus	2(Ad40 & 41)	Probably world-wide. Less common cause of diarrhoea and vomiting (5–12%) than rotavirus	EM, ELISA	NEUT
Astrovirus	28–30	'Astrovirus'	2	Mild pathogen of infancy and childhood	EM	IEM, IF
Calicivirus	30–32	Calicivirus	3	Mild pathogen of infancy and childhood. Outbreaks of winter vomiting in schools and geriatric institutions	EM	
Coronavirus-like	80–400	Coronavirus	Unknown	Role in diarrhoeal disease not established. Possible association with neonatal necrotizing enterocolitis	EM	

IEM, immune electron microscopy; EM, electron microscopy; CF, complement fixation; IF, immunofluorescence; ELISA, enzyme-linked immunosorbent assay; NEUT, neutralization; IAHA, immune adherence haemagglutination.

cockle agent in extensive outbreaks of food-poisoning following ingestion of sewage-contaminated cockles in 1976.[2] In contrast to US data, patients in the British outbreaks excreted viruses for a much longer time (4–6 weeks).

The Wollan and Ditchling agents appear closely related antigenically by IEM, but differ from the cockle agent; all the UK strains appear to be unrelated to US viruses. Additional small round viruses, also distinct from Norwalk, have been detected in outbreaks of gastroenteritis. These include the Paramatta agent from Australia,[17] the Marin County agent from California,[91] the Snow Mountain agent, associated with an outbreak in a resort camp,[31] and the Sapporo[63] and Otofuke[112] agents from Japan. The Sapporo and Otofuke agents may represent an additional serotype since they are antigenically related to each other but not to Norwalk agent.

Outbreaks associated with shellfish consumption

Oysters and cockles are filter feeders, and in common with other bivalve molluscs can concentrate viruses from polluted waters, although the number of particles present in the molluscs is likely to be too low to detect by electron microscopy (EM). A marked increase in price of prawns in Britain in the winter of 1976 resulted in restaurants replacing prawn cocktails with seafood cocktails which contained cockles. During December 1976 and January 1977 33 separate episodes of acute gastroenteritis were reported involving 792 people. Numerous 22–26 nm virus particles were detected in faecal filtrates of patients involved in four of the outbreaks studied.[2] No virus was recovered from shellfish. An even more extensive outbreak occurred in Australia in June and July 1978 in which gastroenteritis, often moderate or even severe, occurred in over 2000 people who ingested sewage-contaminated oysters harvested from the Charles River in Sydney (New South Wales). Two viral candidates were identified in patients' stools, the first being 27–30 nm in size and antigenically related to Norwalk virus, and the second somewhat smaller (22–25 nm). The Norwalk-like virus was identified in 39% of faecal specimens examined by EM, but 75% of patients examined had a significant rise in antibody titre to the Norwalk virus. The role of the small virus particles, which closely resembled the cockle agent, is unclear, but since patients did not develop an immune response to it, this virus may not have been of relevance in the outbreak.[87]

Classification of small round viruses associated with epidemic gastroenteritis

These viruses are difficult to characterize, for they cannot be cultivated in vitro and are generally not excreted in high concentrations. Furthermore, their surface structure may be obscured by a coating of gut-derived secretory antibody. Caul and Appleton compared the fine structure and physical properties of a number of small round viruses associated with acute gastroenteritis and proposed that they should be divided into two main groups.[14] The first consists of viruses of which Norwalk is the prototype. They are estimated to be 30–35 nm in diameter and, although amorphous with a feathery or ragged edge, have an obvious surface structure (Figure 14.10). They are, however, quite distinct from such other structural viruses as astroviruses (Figure 14.15) and caliciviruses (Figure 14.16) which also cause acute gastroenteritis. Such viruses as the Norwalk, Hawaii, Sapporo and possibly the Snow Mountain and Marin County agents belong to this group.

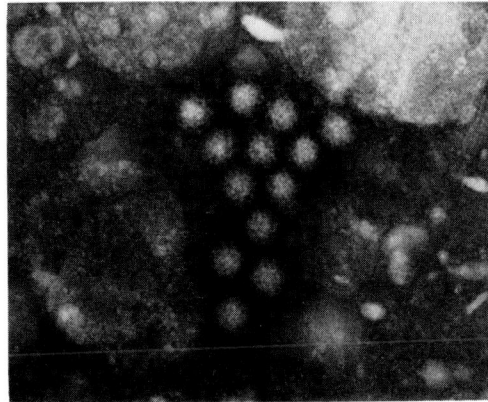

Fig. 14.10 Electron micrograph of negatively stained faecal extract showing Norwalk-like (structured) virus particles (bar = 50 nm).

Viruses in the second group range in size from 22–26 nm and have a smooth entire outer edge but no surface structure (Figure 14.11). Ditchling, Wollan and cockle virus belong to this group. However, the recent finding that Norwalk virus contains a single primary structural protein with a molecular weight of 59 000 suggests that it may be a calicivirus.[44] Although Norwalk virus preparations do not have the cup-like depressions characteristic of the caliciviruses, it is possible that they might be obscured by a coating of secretory antibody.

Table 14.7	Comparison of the properties of two groups of small round viruses associated with acute gastroenteritis.

	Structured virus	Featureless virus
Prototype	Norwalk	Ditchling
Size (nm)	30–35	22–26
Outline	Ragged	Smooth
Buoyant density	1.36–1.41	1.38–1.40
Polypeptide analysis	1 major (55 000)	ND
Provisional classification	Calicivirus	Parvovirus
Main serotypes	Norwalk (USA) } Montgomery County (USA) } 1	Ditchling (UK) } Wollan (UK) } 1
	Hawaii (USA) 2	cockle (UK) 2
	Sapporo (Japan) } Otofuke (Japan) } 3	Paramatta (Australia) 3
Snow Mountain and Marin County agent	Published electron micrographs show virus with addition of antibody. Although both viruses resemble Norwalk, but are antigenically distinct, classification must await further studies.	

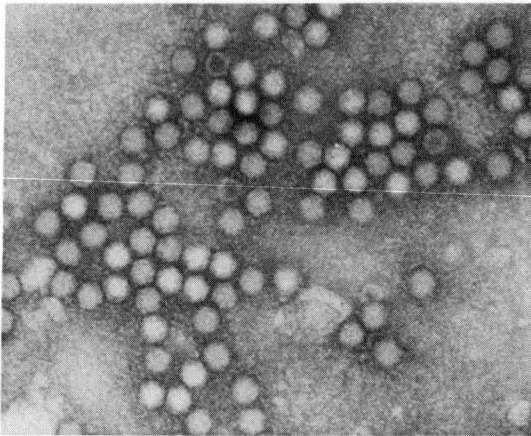

Fig. 14.11 Electron micrograph of negatively stained faecal extract showing Ditchling-like (featureless) virus particles (bar = 50 nm).

The smaller-sized particles may provisionally be classified in the parvoviruses,[14] which induce gastroenteritis in a variety of animal species. Table 14.7 compares and contrasts some of the features of viruses in these two groups.

Pathogenesis

Jejunal biopsies obtained from volunteers infected with Norwalk and Hawaii virus show histological abnormalities within 24–48 hours, which persist for up to two weeks despite clinical recovery within a few days. Such changes also occur in asymptomatic persons.[1, 30, 103] Although jejunal villi are blunted and broadened and contain vacuolated cells, there is no break in the epithelial surface. The lamina propria is infiltrated with mononuclear cells and polymorphonuclear lymphocytes. No histological abnormalities are present in rectal, colonic or gastric biopsies. EM studies of ultra-thin sections of the jejunum fail to reveal virus-like structures. The acute phase of infection is associated with a decrease in brush-border enzymes and a transient impairment of fat and carbohydrate absorption. This also occurs in those who are asymptomatic. There is also a leucopenia involving the lymphocyte subpopulations (T, B and null), which may be the result of a redistribution of cells to the site of virus infection.[30] The mechanism by which diarrhoea is induced has not been established, but since jejunal adenylate cyclase activity is not increased it does not appear to be similar to that induced by enterotoxigenic organisms.[72]

Immunity

Susceptibility to disease correlates poorly with serum antibody levels.[92] Although local intestinal antibody might perhaps be expected to play a more significant role its presence also fails to correlate with resistance to challenge with Norwalk virus. Paradoxically, volunteers developing symptomatic infection had higher local antibody titres in their jejunal fluid than those who were asymptomatic.[10, 45]

Seroepidemiological studies

IEM is an inconvenient method for detecting immune responses and an immune adherence haemagglutination assay and a radioimmunoassay (RIA) have been developed.[58] These methods show that in the USA antibody is acquired gradually and continually, beginning slowly in childhood, until by the fifth decade about 50% have antibody.[41] In contrast, most children, regardless of social class or geographical location, have acquired rotavirus antibody by the age of five.[33] However, in developing countries, antibody to Norwalk virus is acquired at an early age:[42] by the age of five, 80% of children in rural Bangladesh have antibody to Norwalk virus, seroconversion occurring most frequently during cooler, dry periods.[9] Less is known of the role of Norwalk virus as a cause of severe diarrhoeal disease in developing countries, but studies in Bangladesh suggest that Norwalk virus may induce symptoms which are sub-clinical or of much less severity than those due to rotavirus or toxigenic strains of *E. coli*. Nevertheless, repeated episodes of infection by Norwalk or related viruses may induce histological changes which contribute to the malabsorption and chronic diarrhoeal disease which is particularly prevalent in many developing countries.

Although many different small round viruses are associated with epidemic gastroenteritis analyses of serological responses in paired sera obtained from 74 outbreaks of acute gastroenteritis between 1976 and 1980 showed that 42% were associated with Norwalk virus. Outbreaks occurred in families, schools, recreation camps and cruise ships, and were often associated with exposure to contaminated food or drinking or swimming pool water. Norwalk probably represents the major cause of acute non-bacterial epidemic gastroenteritis, with the number of serologically distinct viruses being limited.[54]

ROTAVIRUSES AND THEIR ROLE IN INFANTILE GASTROENTERITIS

Rotaviruses (Figure 14.12) have a wheel-like appearance (Latin *rota* wheel). They have a world-wide distribution and are the commonest cause of acute non-bacterial gastroenteritis in infancy and childhood. They were first identified in ultra-thin sections of jejunal biopsies obtained from young children with acute gastroenteritis in Melbourne, Australia.[6] Virus particles were present only during the acute phase of infection. Thereafter, similar viruses were detected in faecal extracts obtained from children with acute gastroenteritis in many parts of the world.[6, 36, 55] Studies in children from temperate climates show that the highest attack rates occur in those aged between 6 and 24

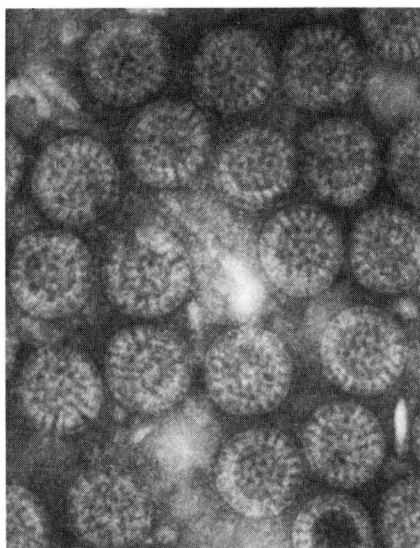

Fig. 14.12 Electron micrograph of negatively stained faecal extract containing rotaviruses (bar = 50 nm).

months and that there is a marked seasonal distribution, infection occurring almost exclusively in winter. Rotaviruses have been detected in faecal extracts of about 25% of acute gastroenteritis patients less than one year old, in 60% of those between one and three years old, and in 20–40% of those between four and six years old (reviewed by Flewett[34]). Apart from neonates, rotaviruses are rarely detected in asymptomatic persons. During the months of peak prevalence as many as 75% of children admitted to hospital with acute gastroenteritis may excrete rotavirus.[27]

After an incubation period of 24–48 hours symptoms begin abruptly, usually with vomiting followed by diarrhoea, this being most profuse on the second to third day of infection, during which time very high concentrations of virus are being excreted (e.g. 10^{11} particles per gram of faeces). Symptoms generally subside within four to five days, following which the amount of virus excreted declines rapidly, but a few patients may excrete virus for 10 to 14 days. Prolonged diarrhoea is uncommon, although protracted diarrhoea associated with rotavirus excretion occurs in patients with immunodeficiency disorders. Such patients may also exhibit uraemia.

Children with immunodeficiency disorders may sometimes also excrete a number of different viruses. Figure 14.13 shows some of the viruses being excreted simultaneously by an infant with severe combined immunodeficiency, failure to thrive, and protracted diarrhoea, who over a period of two months excreted five enteric viruses.[19]

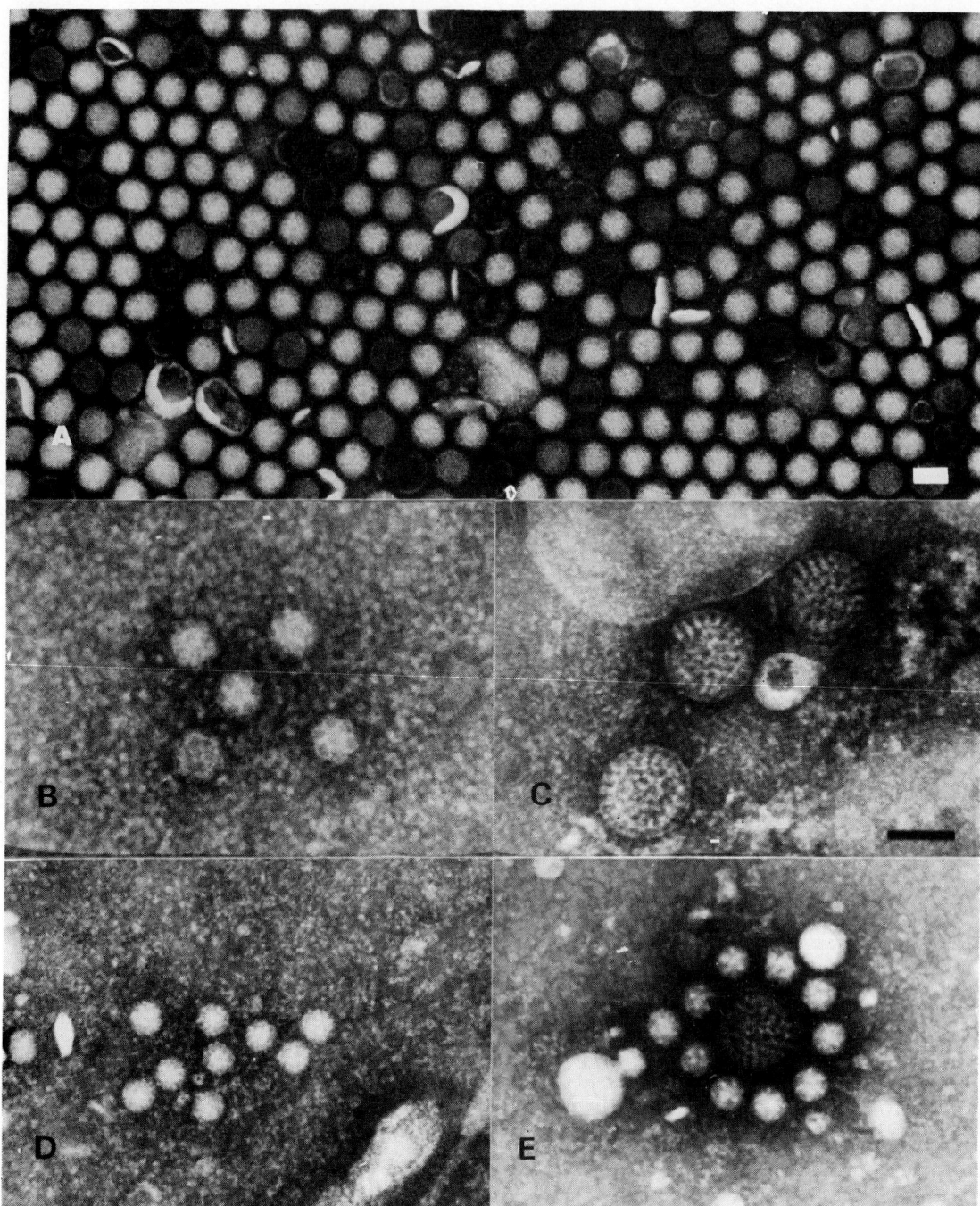

Fig. 14.13 Electron micrographs of negatively stained faecal extracts showing viruses detected in a child with severe combined immunodeficiency. A: adenovirus (bar = 50 nm); B: calicivirus; C: rotavirus; D: small round virus; E: astrovirus + rotavirus (B–E to same scale: bar = 50 nm). From Chrystie *et al.* (1982),[19] with kind permission of the authors and the editor of *Lancet*.

Respiratory symptoms and signs are common in patients with rotavirus-induced diarrhoea. Indeed, the distinct clinical difference between rotavirus-induced diarrhoea and other diarrhoeal infections is a history of preceding cough, nasal discharge and otitis media.[73] Attempts to recover rotavirus from respiratory secretions have been unsuccesful,[38] which suggests that rotavirus infection is spread via the oro-faecal route. Rotaviruses are commonly associated with intussusception in Japan,[64] but not in Australia or France.[85, 88]

Life-threatening rotavirus infection is more common in developing countries, but Carlson and her colleagues reported 21 fatal cases among children in Toronto during a five-year period.[13] Deaths usually resulted from profound dehydration, electrolyte imbalance and cardiac arrest. London children with rotavirus-induced diarrhoea were more likely to be dehydrated than children whose diarrhoea was caused by pathogenic bacteria or other viruses.[73] Dehydration was most severe in infants between the ages of 12 and 18 months. However, it must be pointed out that many of the children in this study were Asian refugees.

It is possible that rotavirus may be implicated in the sudden infant death syndrome.

Rotavirus infection in the tropics

Although results of studies relating to the incidence and seasonal distribution of rotavirus in temperate climates are predominantly in agreement, results of tropical studies show considerable variation. Rotavirus infections are generally more common during the cool season, but in countries with high ambient temperatures throughout the year there may be no marked seasonal variation, unless there is a rainy season. Studies carried out in Asia, Central and South America and Africa show that rotaviruses can be identified in the stools of 14% to 66% of children with acute diarrhoeal disease.[4] In Bangladesh use of techniques to detect rotavirus as well as a wide variety of bacterial pathogens, including enterotoxigenic *Escherichia coli* (ETEC), *Campylobacter jejuni*, *Shigella*, and *Vibrio cholerae*[7, 109] showed that pathogens were present in the stools of 66–70% of patients with acute diarrhoeal disease; mixed infections were common, ETEC (in 20–32% of episodes) and rotaviruses (in 5–24% of episodes) being the pathogens most commonly detected.[7, 109] The major impact of rotavirus infection was on children less than two years old, among whom rotaviruses were the commonest cause of acute diarrhoeal disease (up to 46%), and dehydration was a prominent feature. Infection occurred during the cooler and drier months of December and January. The frequency of rotavirus infection decreased markedly with age. In Bangladesh 77% of episodes of life-threatening dehydration in young children were caused by either rotaviruses or ETEC.

There have been occasional reports of traveller's diarrhoea being associated with viruses. Rotaviruses and Norwalk virus were identified in the diarrhoeal stools of Panamanians touring Mexico[96] (rotavirus in 26%, Norwalk virus in 15%) as well as in 24% of those with diarrhoea in a group of US students attending a Mexican summer school.[121] In addition, serological evidence of rotavirus infection was obtained in 36% of US Peace Corps workers visiting Honduras.[107]

Hospital-acquired infection

The stability of rotaviruses, together with the high concentrations of virus excreted, makes environmental contamination more or less inevitable. In the absence of stringent precautions cross-infection of susceptible contacts is likely. In the Hospital for Sick Children in Toronto about one-third of rotavirus infections during one year were hospital-acquired. Infant surgical wards were the richest source of infection and there was strong evidence that infection was transmitted to patients by attendant staff.[32, 82] A study in London showed that 43% of 51 cases of rotavirus infection diagnosed over a 12-month period were hospital-acquired and resulted in a total of 72 extra days spent in hospital.[89] Although most infections were mild, such complications as delayed healing of surgical wounds and secondary lactose intolerance occurred. The most likely mode of transmission is indirectly from patient-to-patient on the hands of staff. Proper handwashing procedures using such antiseptic preparations as chlorhexidine, although inactivating pathogenic bacteria, have no effect on rotaviruses. A reduction in hospital-acquired rotavirus infection is more likely to be achieved by employing ethanol (with 1% glycerol added as an emollient), since this is virucidal.[111] Alternatively, a preparation of chlorhexidine in 90% ethanol might be used. There is strong circumstantial evidence to suggest that infection is transferred from general paediatric to neonatal units by medical and nursing staff.[117] Once introduced into newborn nurseries, rotavirus infection may persist for many months, the seasonal distribution of infection being less marked than among older children. Most children experiencing neonatal rotavirus infection excrete virus between three and seven days after birth, although excretion has been detected in children less than 24 hours old.[99] Although this suggests that infection may have been acquired in utero, diarrhoeal stools can be produced in newborn calves only 15 hours after rotavirus ingestion.[80] The proportion of infants excreting rotavirus during outbreaks in nurseries for the newborn may be as high as 33–66%.[18, 51, 86] An analysis of data from different parts of the world showed a wide spectrum of infection ranging from subclinical[117] to severe and fatal disease with features compatible with a diagnosis of necrotizing enterocolitis,[11] but studies in nurseries for the newborn suggest that the disease is generally either asymptomatic or relatively mild.

Breastfeeding confers protection, and although this has been shown not to be directly related to the presence of rotavirus antibody[118] orally administered human immunoglobulin may delay excretion of rotavirus and protect low-birth-weight infants from rotavirus-induced diarrhoea.[5] The reason why rotavirus infection causes milder disease among newborns remains to be established; passively transferred maternal antibody does not appear to play a role.[18] It remains to be established whether rotavirus-infected newborn infants are protected from subsequent infection by similar serotypes.

Infection in adults

Sero-epidemiological studies show that most children have acquired rotavirus antibody by the age of five years; after this age rotavirus infections are infrequently reported. However, 30–40% of family contacts of children with rotavirus infection may show booster antibody responses, up to 25% developing mild symptoms.[57, 120] Occasionally, larger outbreaks involving adults who have had little or no recent contact with children are reported.[81, 122] Outbreaks among elderly institutional populations are not uncommon.[22, 47, 126] Decreasing immunity with age and heavy faecal contamination of the environment may be among factors responsible.

Although children may transmit infection to adults, the actual reservoir of infection may well be among adults who excrete low levels of virus from subclinical infections.[62] Veterinary workers have shown that adult cows excrete rotavirus even when asymptomatic, and probably represent the reservoir of infection from which calves are infected.

Animal rotavirus infection

Rotaviruses may induce severe acute diarrhoeal disease in newborn calves and piglets and have also been detected from cases of diarrhoea in lambs, foals, deer, monkeys, rabbits, pronghorn antelopes, kittens and dogs. There is serological evidence of infection in goats, guinea pigs and cats. Rotaviruses have also been detected in turkeys and chickens. Interspecies transmission has been demonstrated experimentally, but whether or not this occurs naturally remains to

be established. Almost all animal and human viruses share common group antigens which are associated with the inner capsid layer of the virus particle. However, the outer capsid layer contains some antigens which are species-specific; as with human viruses it is probable that each species of animal has different rotavirus serotypes. Rotavirus infection in animals has recently been extensively reviewed by Woode.[128]

Classification and antigenicity of rotaviruses

Rotaviruses belong to the family of reoviruses. They are a separate genus within this family, whose viruses contain RNA which is double-stranded and segmented. The inner capsid layer contains *group*-specific antigenic determinants shared by almost all rotaviruses whether human or animal;[130] antigens located on the outer capsid are *type*-specific.[36] Rotaviruses vary antigenically and this appears to be a relatively complex phenomenon. Two main subgroups, determined by differences in the polypeptides associated with the inner capsid layer, have been identified.[43, 137] Five serotypes have so far been detected by neutralization.[100, 116]

Since it is probable that the antigens located on the outer capsid induce protective immune responses, it is important that different serotypes are incorporated in future vaccines. However, the possibility that multiple infection and segment exchange may result in continuous antigen changes could mean that prevention from rotavirus infection by vaccination will be more complex than has hitherto been thought.

Pathogenesis

The histological features of infection are essentially similar in children, calves and piglets.[129] The earliest lesions are present in the proximal end of the small intestine, but in severe cases its entire length may be involved. The essential feature of rotavirus infection is a loss of the absorptive cells lining the small intestine. The villi are blunted, the columnar epithelium being desquamated and replaced by immature cuboidal cells which have migrated rapidly from the crypts. The lamina propria is infiltrated with lymphocytic cells. Vesicles in the villous epithelial cells can be seen by electron microscopy to contain rotaviruses.

The mechanism by which diarrhoea is produced is different to that in cholera and ETEC infections since adenylate cyclase and cyclic AMP levels are not increased. Diarrhoeal symptoms appear to be a result of water malabsorption associated with intestinal hurry. The acute phase of infection is accompanied by a marked defect in D-xylose absorption[79] which improves within a few days as diarrhoea subsides.[90] Although xylose absorption profiles return to normal relatively quickly, lactulose absorption profiles take much longer, which suggests that the gut may be permeable to large molecules for an extended time. The picture is therefore not dissimilar to a short-term coeliac syndrome. Water malabsorption may be largely determined by a temporary failure to absorb solutes. Impairment of intestinal lactose hydrolysis[50] and fat absorption[84] is also a characteristic feature, but this may persist for several weeks (Noone and Menzies, 1983 unpublished observations), which provides a rationale for therapeutic withdrawal of lactose-containing dairy products from the diet.

Laboratory diagnosis

Electron microscopy provides a suitable method for diagnosis when only a few specimens are to be examined and has the advantage that other viruses associated with gastroenteritis may also be detected. Less labour-intensive methods must be used if a large number of specimens are to be tested. Because a high concentration of rotaviruses is usually present in faecal extracts, diagnostic techniques based on immunological identification of rotavirus antigens can be used, and a number of these have been described. The most widely used is enzyme immunoassay,[133] which can be obtained as a kit. This is the most convenient method for detecting immune responses but complement fixation[56] and even neutralization tests[118] may be employed.

Prospects for vaccination

It has recently been shown that human rotaviruses can be adapted to grow in cell culture by prior passage in gnotobiotic piglets.[132] Human strains can also be 'rescued' by co-cultivation with bovine *ts* mutants.[46] In this technique the genes of the fastidious human strains are replaced by corresponding genes of tissue-culture-adapted bovine strains, the resultant hybrid strain having an outer capsid antigen specific for human rotavirus strains. Human strains have also been isolated from faecal preparations by pre-treatment of specimens with trypsin, followed by inoculation into fetal Rhesus monkey kidney cell cultures (MA 104).[101]

Although the development of an attenuated rotavirus vaccine is now technically possible, further information is required relating to the number of serotypes, the degree of protection following infection by antigenically related and unrelated serotypes, and duration of immunity, including local antibody responses. Although it is unlikely that vaccination will prevent reinfection, it may delay it and reduce its severity. This may provide an important contribution to the health of children, particularly in developing countries. Recently an oral live vaccine of bovine origin was shown to induce a serological response in young children. Trials to assess the efficacy of this vaccine are progressing.

'FASTIDIOUS' ADENOVIRUSES

Adenoviruses are double-stranded DNA viruses which are 70–80 nm in diameter and exhibit cubic symmetry (Figure 14.14). They are an

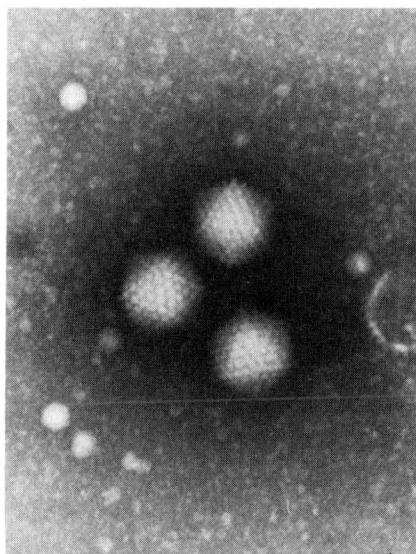

Fig. 14.14 Electron micrograph of negatively stained faecal extract showing adenoviruses (bar = 50 nm).

established cause of respiratory infection including pharyngoconjunctival fever and may also cause follicular conjunctivitis and keratoconjunctivitis. More recently they have been shown to be associated with acute diarrhoeal disease in children. Adenoviruses in the stools of patients with acute diarrhoea, although often present in very high concentrations (Figure 14.13A), resist attempts at propagation in conventional cell cultures. For this reason they are termed 'noncultivable' or 'fastidious' adenoviruses. Recent studies have shown that such adenovirus strains, despite being collected from different parts of the world and over a wide time span, have type-specific antigens which differ from the other 39 'non-fastidious' serotypes.[29] There appear to be only two closely related antigenic variants and these have been provisionally designated Ad40 and 41.[61] Analysis of their DNA profiles following cleavage with restriction enzymes has shown that the genome of these viruses differs from the other serotypes.[28, 124]

Several fastidious strains have recently been cultivated in vitro and as a result seroepidemiological studies have shown that neutralizing antibodies are present in the sera of 15–60% of children under 12 years (living in temperate and tropical countries) without a history of recent diarrhoea; 39% of London children aged less than 7 years were antibody-positive.

Fastidious adenoviruses may be detected in the stools of 5–12% of children with acute diarrhoea,[93] although they are only rarely detected among asymptomatic children. The incubation period may be as long as 8–10 days. Explosive outbreaks in nurseries[37] and community outbreaks involving children[93] have been described. A single fatal case has also been reported.[127] There is often respiratory tract involvement, particularly pneumonia among children admitted to hospital with adenovirus-associated diarrhoea. Although fastidious adenoviruses are generally identified by electron microscopy, enzyme immunoassays capable of detecting type-specific antigens have recently been developed.[52, 136]

THE ROLE OF SMALL ROUND VIRUSES NOT ASSOCIATED WITH WINTER VOMITING

Enterovirus infections and their role in immunocompromised patients

Polio, Coxsackie A and B and echoviruses belong to the genus of enteroviruses, which are included in the family of picornaviruses. Although this group of 27-nm viruses may be isolated from the stools of patients with diarrhoea, particularly children in developing countries, they can be detected equally frequently in matched controls. Coxsackie A virus may be associated with severe gastrointestinal infection in patients who have undergone bone-marrow transplants. Patients on bone-marrow transplant units may experience high mortality rates

associated with gastroenteritis, and a number of organisms including *Clostridium difficile*, adenoviruses and rotaviruses have been implicated; infection with multiple organisms may occur.[135] The mortality rate among bone-marrow transplant patients with diarrhoea associated with enteric pathogens was 55%, whereas only 13% of non-infected patients died.[135] Acute graft-versus-host disease (AGVHD) can also induce severe diarrhoea, but deaths are probably related to infection rather than AGVHD. Because Coxsackie viruses, rotavirus and adenovirus can cause opportunistic infections in severely immunocompromised patients the stools of such patients who had diarrhoea should be examined so that appropriate measures can be taken to prevent transmission to other susceptible contacts.

Astroviruses and caliciviruses

Astroviruses (Figure 14.15) and caliciviruses (Figure 14.16) have been detected in the stools of children with diarrhoea.[76, 77] Morphologically identical viruses have been detected among animals. Both viruses appear to have a worldwide distribution, but are of relatively low pathogenicity and may be excreted by patients with gastroenteritis as well as by people who are asymptomatic; sometimes similtaneous excretion of other enteric pathogens may be observed. Astrovirus and calicivirus infections are more common in infancy than among older persons. Diarrhoea is likely to be the more prominent symptom with astrovirus, but with calicivirus

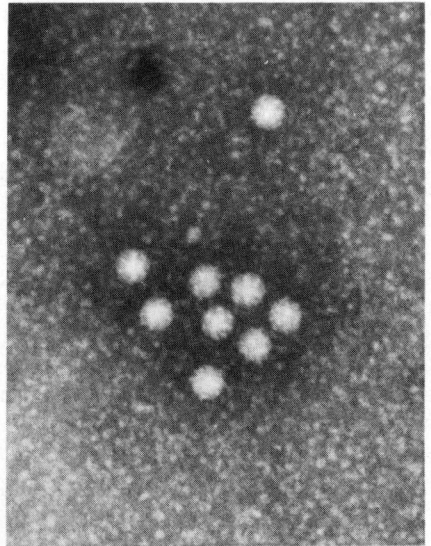

Fig. 14.15 Electron micrograph of negatively stained faecal extract containing astroviruses (bar = 50 nm).

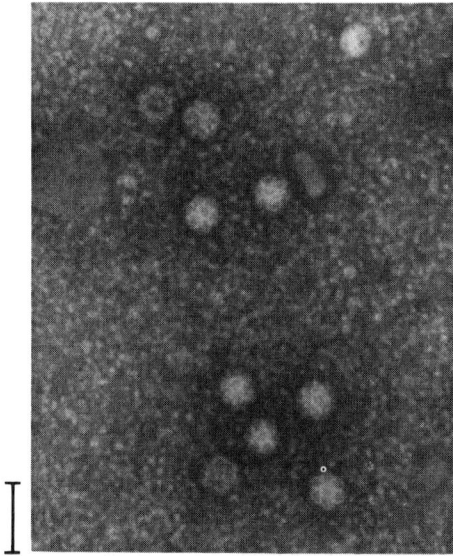

Fig. 14.16 Electron micrograph of negatively stained faecal extract showing caliciviruses (bar = 50 nm).

vomiting may be more marked. Symptoms rarely last for more than 2–3 days and there is no prolonged virus excretion. IEM studies suggest that there are at least two antigenic serotypes of astrovirus[71] and three calicivirus strains.[23] Since acquisition of antibody to astroviruses and caliciviruses has usually occurred by school age, infections in infancy, perhaps often asymptomatic, must be common.[66, 98] Caliciviruses cannot be cultivated in vitro but astroviruses will undergo limited expression but not

serial passage in human embryonic kidney cell cultures.[70] Astroviruses are only mildly pathogenic in adults, causing only occasional mild gastrointestinal symptoms.[68] Some of the morphological features of astrovirus and calicivirus and the infections they induce are compared in Table 14.8.

Coronaviruses

Because coronaviruses are important causes of severe diarrhoeal disease of considerable economic importance in pigs (transmissible gastroenteritis) and calves, and also cause diarrhoea in the young of many other animal species,[20] attempts have been made to identify their human counterpart. However, unlike rotaviruses, evidence that coronaviruses cause gastroenteritis in man is currently somewhat tenuous, although they are an established cause of acute respiratory infection. Coronaviruses are enveloped pleomorphic particles, ranging in diameter from about 80 nm to 400 nm. They are surrounded by a 20-nm fringe-like structure consisting of radiating stalk-like projections which have a tear-drop dilation distally, although with enteric coronavirus-like particles (CVLP), the dilations are more likely to be spherical (Figure 14.17). Although some workers have expressed doubts that these coronavirus-like particles (CVLP) might be bacterial substructures or fragments of gut epithelium,

Table 14.8 Comparison of some of the properties of human astroviruses and caliciviruses and infections induced by them.

	Astroviruses	Caliciviruses
Size (nm)	28–30	30–32
Edge	Unbroken	Feathery
Outline	Circular	Scalloped
Surface hollows	Triangular	Circular
Surface 'stars'	5–6 pointed, with no hollow	6-pointed Star-of-David, with central hollow
Animal virus	Bovine, ovine, feline, canine, deer, turkeys	Porcine, feline, sealions, bovine, mink, chickens, orangeworm
Human serotypes	2	3
Cultivation in vitro	Limited expression in human embryonic kidney cell cultures	No
Age group affected	Infants and young children	Infants, school children and the elderly
Predominant clinical feature	Diarrhoea	Vomiting
Virus excretion	+ + +	+(+)
Immune response	Yes	Yes
Virus-specific IgM	Yes	Yes
Proportion of school children seropositive	~ 70%	~ 70%

Modified from Madeley, C. R. (1979) *Journal of Infectious Diseases*, *139*(5): 519–523, with kind permission of the author and editor.

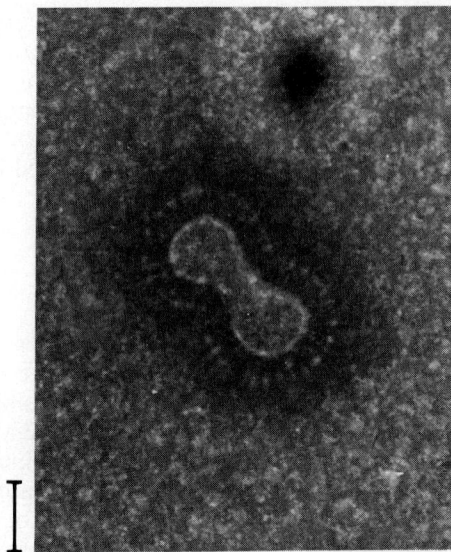

Fig. 14.17 Electron micrograph of negatively stained faecal extract containing coronavirus-like particles (bar = 50 nm).

human CVLPs (HCVLPs) have been propagated in both cell[15] and human intestinal organ cultures.[16]

HCVLPs have been detected in stools of patients with acute and chronic diarrhoea as well as in asymptomatic persons in many parts of the world, including tropical countries (reviewed by MacNaughton and Davies[75]). They are rarely, if ever, seen in the faeces of infants under one year of age, and are rare under the age of five. Virus particles are found in the same proportions in the faeces of normal adults (5.2%) as in adults with gastroenteritis (4.2%).[20] There may be an association of HCVLPs with prolonged diarrhoea. HCVLPs have also been detected in the stools of Australian aboriginal children but are present with equal frequency among children with and without diarrhoea.[105] In rural India, an area in which tropical sprue is endemic, HCVLPs are present in 90% of stools of apparently healthy persons. However, these virus-like particles tend to have T- or Y-shaped structures at the end of the projections attached to the viral envelope, and it remains to be established whether these particles are actually viruses. It has yet to be established whether HCVLPs can induce a low-grade persistent infection that might in turn be involved in producing the enteropathy which is almost universal in parts of southern India.

Most workers have failed to detect viruses, except for the occasional rotavirus, in newborn infants with necrotizing enterocolitis, but a recent report describes an outbreak possibly associated with the excretion of HCVLP.[69]

However, the virus particles closely resembled bovine coronaviruses which were also being studied in the laboratory and cross-contamination remains a possibility.[75] The fact that HCVLP may be associated with some outbreaks of necrotizing enterocolitis among infants is strengthened by a report of an outbreak of necrotizing enterocolitis among newborn infants in Paris.[95] HCVLPs were present in the stools of 77% of babies with the disease but not among asymptomatic infants, and were detected in 9 of 10 specimens of the small gut; the particles were present in necrotic foci in the gut wall. The aetiology of necrotizing enterocolitis may well be complex and the HCVLP may be one of many agents involved in inducing this syndrome.

REFERENCES

1 Agus, S. G., Dolin, R., Wyatt, R. G. *et al.* (1973) Acute infectious nonbacterial gastroenteritis: intestinal histopathology. Histologic and enzymatic alterations during illness produced by the Norwalk agent in man. *Annals of Internal Medicine*, **79**, 18–25.

2 Appleton, H. & Pereira, M. S. (1977) A possible virus aetiology in outbreaks of food poisoning from cockles. *Lancet*, **i**, 780–781.

3 Appleton, H., Buckley, M., Thom, B. T. *et al.* (1977) Virus-like particles in winter vomiting disease. *Lancet*, **i**, 409–411.

4 Banatvala, J. E. (1979) The role of viruses in acute diarrhoeal disease. *Clinics in Gastroenterology*, **8**(3), 569–598.

5 Barnes, G. L., Hewson, P. H., McLellan, J. A. *et al.* (1982) A randomised trial of oral gamma-globulin in low-birth-weight infants infected with rotavirus. *Lancet*, **i**, 1371–1373.

6 Bishop, R. F., Davidson, G. P., Holmes, I. H. & Ruck, B. J. (1973) Virus particles in epithelial cells of duodenal mucosa from children with non-bacterial gastroenteritis. *Lancet*, **ii**, 1281–1283.

7 Black, R. E., Merson, M. H., Rahmann, A. S. M. M. *et al.* (1980) A two-year study of bacterial, viral and parasitic agents associated with diarrhea in rural Bangladesh. *Journal of Infectious Diseases*, **142**, 660–664.

8 Black, R. E., Merson, M. H., Huq, I. *et al.* (1981) Incidence and severity of rotavirus and *Escherichia coli* diarrhoea in rural Bangladesh. *Lancet*, **i**, 141–143.

9 Black, R. E., Greenberg, H. B., Kapikian, A. Z. *et al.* (1982) Acquisition of serum antibody to Norwalk virus and rotavirus and relation to diarrhea in a longitudinal study of young children in rural Bangladesh. *Journal of Infectious Diseases*, **145**, 483–489.

10 Blacklow, N. R., Cukor, G., Bedigian, M. K. *et al.* (1979) Immuno-response and prevalence of antibody to Norwalk enteritis virus as determined by radioimmunoasay. *Journal of Clinical Microbiology*, **10**, 903–909.

11 Brotowasisto (1975) Epidemiology of diarrhoea. In *Diarrhoea*. (in Indonesian) Indonesia: Department of Health.

12 Buffet-Janvresse, C. & Magard, H. (1976) Rotavirus detected in placenta following spontaneous abortion. *La Nouvelle Presse medicale*, **1**, 1249–1251.

disease', which has been attributed to these 27 nm particles generally occurs as outbreaks in schools or isolated communities. Astroviruses (25–28 nm) have been seen in stools of diarrhoeic infants and two hospital outbreaks in children's wards have been documented.[1, 13] Seven per cent of Oxford children between 6 and 12 months old had serum antibodies to astroviruses; the proportion increased to 75% of 5–10-year-olds.[12] Symptoms induced by these viruses include watery stools with occasional vomiting for two to three days.[13] Caliciviruses have been associated with winter vomiting.[5] These are approximately the same size as astroviruses (30 nm) but differ in detailed ultrastructural appearance.[14]

BACTERIAL DIARRHOEA IN CHILDREN

Escherichia coli

Enterotoxigenic E. coli (ETEC). ETEC is an important cause of childhood diarrhoea in tropical countries but occurs rarely in temperate climates,[16] except in areas of poor socio-economic conditions.[23]

Enteroinvasive E. coli (EIEC). With the exception of a Brazilian study[7] EIEC appears to be rare in childhood diarrhoea.

Enteropathogenic E. coli (EPEC). Since the life-threatening outbreaks of EPEC diarrhoea amongst infants in the 1950s and 60s, the importance of this group of diarrhoeagenic E. coli has declined in developed countries; they are, however, frequently found in less developed countries.[22]

Vibrio cholerae

The present pandemic, which began in Sulawesi and has spread eastwards to the West Pacific Islands and westwards to Africa, tends to affect 2–9-year-old children. Disease in the first two years is uncommon; this has been attributed to the protective effect of breastfeeding.[16]

Campylobacter jejuni

C. jejuni has been reported in the stools of approximately 4% of children with acute diarrhoea.[4]

Yersinia enterocolitica

Y. enterocolitica appears to be a common cause of acute diarrhoea in children under five years of age in certain countries of northern Europe and also in Canada, but not elsewhere.[11]

Salmonella

Salmonellae are more frequently isolated from children with diarrhoea in developed countries, possibly because food processing techniques result in greater dissemination. As a group, they probably occur as commonly as C. jejuni.[4]

Shigella

In the USA, the majority of isolates of shigellae are from patients under ten years of age.[20] The incidence of acute diarrhoea in children varies from nil to 12%, the higher incidence being in the Third World.[10]

PARASITIC DIARRHOEA IN CHILDHOOD

Giardia lamblia

G. lamblia is the most ubiquitous protozoal agent causing diarrhoea, and children appear more susceptible than adults.[29] Asymptomatic carriage has also been reported in as many as 10% of children.[9]

Advances in treatment of acute diarrhoea in childhood

Experience in the technique of oral rehydration in developed and underdeveloped countries has challenged the precepts of traditional paediatric teaching on the treatment of acute diarrhoea (see Table 14.9). The emphasis has shifted from intravenous to oral fluid, with resulting economies, improved safety and widespread applicability in areas without sophisticated health care, where the majority of diarrhoea occurs. The regimen recommended by Pizarro et al[19] – administration of twice the estimated fluid deficit over six hours as WHO oral rehydration solution followed by free water (in a ratio of $\frac{2}{3}$ WHO solution to $\frac{1}{3}$ water) followed by a return to breastfeeding or half-strength formula – has proved successful in all age groups including neonates, regardless of the aetiology of the diarrhoea or the underlying biochemical disturbance. Supervision of such a treatment regime is essential, but village health workers should be able to provide such a service in teaching the basis of this regimen to mothers. Controversy still exists about the optimal constituents of oral rehydration solutions, and intravenous fluids will still be required for those in shock, but the widespread application of this therapeutic approach should have a major impact on the appalling mortality and morbidity of acute diarrhoea in childhood.

Table 14.9 Recent changes in the management of acute diarrhoea.

Traditional teaching	Recent concepts
Various fluid and electrolyte disturbances require different treatment	Within broad limits a simple and unified therapeutic approach may be possible
Rehydrate over 24–28 hours with 30 mmol/l Na^+ solution	Rehydrate over 4–6 hours with 75–90 mmol/l Na^+ solution
K^+ given only after urine output established	K^+ in rehydration solution
HCO_3^- only for severe acidosis	HCO_3^- in rehydration solution
Oral intake restricted	Intravenous fluids can be largely eliminated by oral rehydration
Slow reintroduction of diet	Continue breastfeeding if possible. Prompt return to normal diet

Modified from Hirschhorn (1980),[8] with kind permission of the author and the editor of *American Journal of Clinical Nutrition*.

Complications of acute infantile gastroenteritis

Infants under six months of age are the most likely to have complications. Furthermore, pre-existing malnutrition increases susceptibility to all the complications discussed below.

Dehydration develops readily, with accompanying metabolic acidosis and hypokalaemia. Renal failure with renal vein thrombosis or medullary necrosis can ensue. Hypernatraemia may arise in an infant fed unmodified cow's milk or high-solute formulas, with consequent hyperglycaemia, acidosis and convulsions. Hypoglycaemia may also occur, particularly in the malnourished infant.

Acute gastroenteritis is usually a self-limiting illness of a few days duration. On occasion, particularly in young undernourished infants, a syndrome of protracted diarrhoea supervenes.[2] It poses many problems of management and can carry a significant mortality.[24]

The exact mechanisms by which acute gastroenteritis leads to protracted diarrhoea are complex and incompletely understood. Indeed an initial infecting agent is often only inferred, because recognized enteric pathogens are isolated from only a minority of cases of protracted diarrhoea in infants. Acquired intolerance to disaccharides (especially lactose), monosaccharides and food proteins (particularly cow's milk)

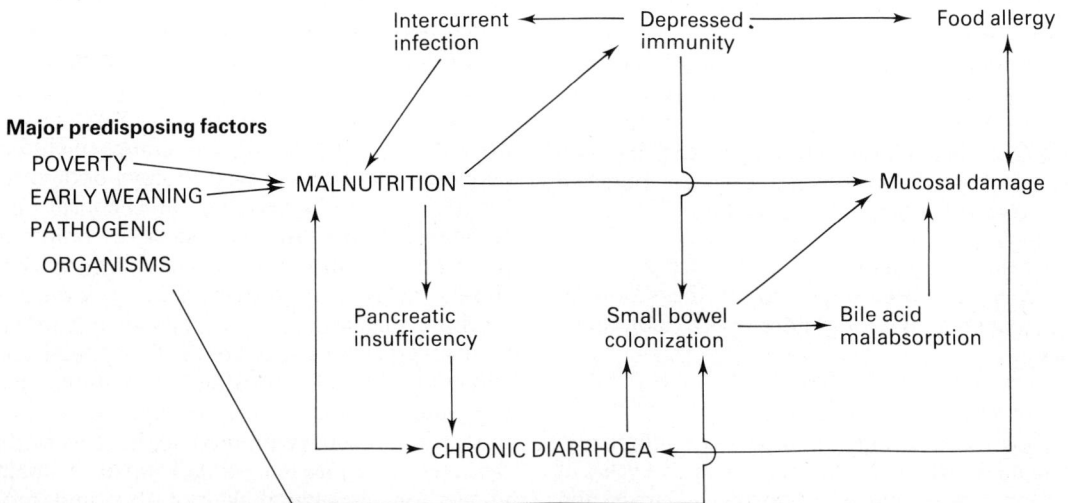

Fig. 14.18 Chronic diarrhoea in infancy – a vicious circle.

may all play a part. Bacterial overgrowth in the small intestine and the altered metabolism of substrates (producing deconjugated bile acids, hydroxy fatty acids and short-chain organic acids) may also be of importance.[21]

Protracted diarrhoea quickly leads to malnutrition and a vicious circle is entered. One possible account of the interrelating factors is shown in Figure 14.18. Interruption of this cycle is seen by many as the outstanding challenge confronting health workers in the developing world.

REFERENCES

1 Ashley, C. R., Caul, E. O. & Paver, W. K. (1978) Astrovirus-associated gastroenteritis in children. *Journal of Clinical Pathology*, **31**, 939–943.
2 Avery, G. B., Villavicencio, D., Lilly, J. R. & Randolph, J. G. (1968) Intractable diarrhea in early infancy. *Pediatrics*, **41**, 712–722.
3 Brown, K. H., Black, R. E., Becker, S. & Hoque, A. (1982) Patterns of physical growth in a longitudinal study of young children in rural Bangladesh. *American Journal of Clinical Nutrition*, **36**, 294–302.
4 Butzler, J. P. & Skirrow, M. B. (1979) Campylobacter enteritis. *Clinics in Gastroenterology*, **8**, 737–765.
5 Cubitt, W. D., McSwiggan, D. A. & Moore, W. (1979) Winter vomiting disease caused by calicivirus. *Journal of Clinical Pathology*, **32**, 786–793.
6 Greenberg, H. B., Valdesuso, J., Yolken, R. H. et al. (1979) Role of Norwalk virus in outbreaks of nonbacterial gastroenteritis. *Journal of Infectious Diseases*, **139**, 564–568.
7 Guerrant, R. L., Moore, R. A., Kirschenfeld, P. M. & Sande, M. A. (1975) Role of toxigenic and invasive bacteria in acute diarrhea of childhood. *New England Journal of Medicine*, **293**, 567–573.
8 Hirschhorn, N. (1980) The treatment of acute diarrhea in children. An historical and physiological perspective. *American Journal of Clinical Nutrition*, **33**, 637–663.
9 Jokipii, L. (1972) Giardiaasia Leningradista. *Duodecim*, **88**, 522–526.
10 Keusch, G. T. (1979) Shigella infections. *Clinics in Gastroenterology*, **8**, 645–662.
11 Kohl, S. (1979) *Yersinia enterocolitica* infections in children. *Pediatric Clinics of North America*, **26**, 433–444.
12 Kurtz, J. & Lee, T. (1978) Astrovirus gastroenteritis. Age distribution of antibody. *Medical Microbiology and Immunology*, **166**, 227–230.
13 Kurtz, J. B., Lee, T. W. & Pickering, D. (1977) Astrovirus associated gastroenteritis in a children's ward. *Journal of Clinical Pathology*, **30**, 948–952.
14 Madeley, C. R. (1979) Comparison of the features of astroviruses and caliciviruses seen in samples of feces by electron microscopy. *Journal of Infectious Diseases*, **139**, 519–523.
15 Merson, M. H. (1982) The global problem of acute diarrhoeal diseases and the WHO Diarrhoeal Disease Control Programme. *Abstract African–Finnish Workshop for Paediatricians and 2nd Regional Congress of UNAPSA, Kaduna, Nigeria, 1982*. Cited by Mäki, M. (1982) *Acute Diarrhoea in Children*. Thesis, University of Tampere.
16 Merson, M. H., Black, R. E., Kahn, M. & Huq, I. (1980) Epidemiology of cholera and enterotoxigenic Escheri-chia coli diarrhoea. *Cholera and Related Diarrheas, 43rd Nobel Symposium, Stockholm, 1978*, pp. 34–45. Basel: Karger.
17 Middleton, P. J., Szymanski, M. T. & Petric, M. (1977) Viruses associated with acute gastroenteritis in young children. *American Journal of Diseases in Children*, **131**, 733–737.
18 Pickering, L. K., Evans, D. J., Munoz, O. et al. (1978) Prospective study of enteropathogens in children with diarrhea in Houston and Mexico. *Journal of Pediatrics*, **93**, 383–388.
19 Pizarro, D., Posada, G., Levine, M. M. & Mohs, E. (1980) Oral rehydration of infants with acute diarrhoeal dehydration: a practical method. *Journal of Tropical Medicine and Hygiene*, **83**, 241–245.
20 Reller, L. B., Gangarosa, E. J. & Brachman, P. S. (1969) Shigellosis in the United States, 1964–1968. *Journal of Infectious Diseases*, **120**, 393–396.
21 Rossi, T. & Lebenthal, E. (1981) Intractable diarrhea of infancy. In *Textbook of Gastroenterology and Nutrition in Infancy* (Ed.) Lebenthal, E. pp. 987–1001. New York: Raven Press.
22 Rowe, B. (1979) The role of *Escherichia coli* in gastroenteritis. *Clinics in Gastroenterology*, **8**, 625–644.
23 Sack, R. B., Hirschhorn, N., Brownlee, I. et al. (1975) Enterotoxigenic *Escherichia coli*-associated diarrheal disease in Apache children. *New England Journal of Medicine*, **292**, 1041–1045.
24 Sunshine, P., Sinatra, F. & Mitchell, C. H. (1977) Intractable diarrhea of infancy. *Clinics in Gastroenterology*, **6**, 445–461.
25 Turnberg, L. A. (1979) The pathophysiology of diarrhoea. *Clinics in Gastroenterology*, **8**, 551–568.
26 Vaughan, V. C. III & McKay, R. J. (1975) The field of paediatrics. In *Textbook of Paediatrics* (10th ed.) (Ed.) Nelson, W. E. p. 4. Philadelphia: Saunders.
27 Vesikari, T., Mäki, M., Sarkkinen, H. K. et al. (1981) Rotavirus, adenovirus and non-viral enteropathogens in diarrhoea. *Archives of Disease in Childhood*, **56**, 264–270.
28 Walker-Smith, J. (1978) Rotavirus gastroenteritis. *Archives of Disease in Childhood*, **53**, 355–362.
29 Wolfe, M. S. (1979) Giardiasis. *Pediatric Clinics of North America*, **26**, 295–303.

CAMPYLOBACTER INFECTIONS

The role of campylobacter infections in human disease has only recently been recognized because their exacting growth requirements delayed identification. Early reports of successful isolations were from blood or other sites which were free from competing organisms. The first stool isolation occurred in 1972,[9] and subsequently these organisms were found to be an important cause of acute diarrhoea in children[7] and adults.[30]

Microbiology

There are three species within the genus *Campylobacter*: *Campylobacter fetus*, *C. sputarum*, and *C. faecalis*. Only *Campylobacter fetus* is of importance in human infection. This species is divided into three subspecies, ssp. *jejuni*, ssp. *intestinalis*, and ssp. *fetus*, which are distinguished by their biochemical characteristics. The last subspecies is not usually responsible for human disease.[31]

These organisms are small Gram-negative microaerophilic curved or spiral rods with a single polar flagellum and a corkscrew motion. The development of selective agar using vancomycin, polymyxin and trimethoprim with incubation at 43°C in a hypoxic environment has proved successful for the isolation of these organisms.[30] Claims of greater sensitivity and selectivity have been made for an alternative method which employs nutrient broth supplemented with saponin-lysed horse blood containing polymyxin, rifampicin, trimethoprim and cycloheximide (Acti-dione).[4]

Epidemiology

Until 1973 there were only 14 reports of campylobacter infections in the literature. The development of improved methodology for the isolation of the organism from faeces lead to the recognition that this infection is a common cause of acute diarrhoea in the community.[7, 30] Campylobacter is an important cause of gastroenteritis in patients who have been admitted to hospital[15] and is worldwide in distribution.[10, 20]

Campylobacter infections are more prevalent in summer months. The organisms are found in the intestine of chickens and may be acquired when meat is inappropriately handled. Infection has been reported following contact with young dogs which had symptoms of diarrhoea and were found to excrete pathogenic campylobacters.[3] Unpasteurized milk or breakdown of the pasteurization process has given rise to several large epidemics,[26] and water contamination has also been implicated in such outbreaks.[20]

Human infectivity appears to be low even though the organism may be excreted for many weeks after an infection because campylobacter organisms survive only briefly outside the body.

Pathogenesis

These organisms are pathogenic because of their invasive activity; the majority of strains are not toxigenic.[6] The jejunum and ileum were considered to be the main sites of involvement, small intestinal biopsies may show broadening and flattening of the villi,[8] haemorrhagic ulcers have been described extending from the jejunum to the proximal ileum[17, 21] and in patients sub-

mitted to laparotomy inflammation of the ileum has been observed.[30] Recently, sigmoidoscopic and histological changes have been found in the rectum in the majority of patients with this infection, and in some the appearances are typical of those found in idiopathic ulcerative colitis.[18]

Clinical features

INTESTINAL DISEASE

Campylobacter gastroenteritis usually presents as a mild self-limiting episode of diarrhoea after an incubation period of three to five days with a range of two to ten days.[6] Many patients are asymptomatic; others develop a more severe illness which is heralded by a febrile prodrome in 50%, characterized by malaise, headache, backache, myalgia and occasional rigors. Abdominal pain is common and may be severe and precede the diarrhoea. The stools are initially green in colour but may subsequently contain blood. The gastrointestinal symptoms usually subside over a few days.

In comparison with salmonella infections vomiting is uncommon, the diarrhoea is less protracted, but abdominal pain is more severe.[30] Severe abdominal pain may result in a laparotomy for a mistaken diagnosis of an acute abdomen. Under these circumstances it is relatively common for a normal appendix to be removed; however, campylobacter infections do sometimes cause appendicitis.[19] Cholecystitis and pancreatitis also occur; the latter is usually mild and recovers spontaneously.[24] Profuse bloody diarrhoea is an occasional feature, and these patients may present the clinical, sigmoidoscopic and histological features of acute idiopathic ulcerative colitis.[18] Alternatively, campylobacter infections may be responsible for a relapse of established inflammatory bowel disease. Under these circumstances treatment of the infection frequently induces a remission of symptoms.[23] Massive lower gastrointestinal haemorrhage due to ulceration of the distal ileum can occur.[21]

EXTRAINTESTINAL MANIFESTATIONS

Extraintestinal manifestations arise as a direct or indirect result of campylobacter infection. Some patients with campylobacter gastroenteritis develop a bacteraemia; this may be more common than is recognized as blood cultures are not routinely obtained from patients with this disease. A septicaemic illness can develop in the absence of gastrointestinal features, and this organism has been responsible for meningitis, pneumonia and endocarditis.[29] Campylobacter meningitis is associated with a pleocytosis of both lymphocytes and polymorphs with a relatively low concentration of glucose in the cerebrospinal fluid.[22] Endocarditis carries a high mortality, possibly due to inappropriate antibiotic therapy.[29]

Reactive arthritis follows campylobacter gastroenteritis in some adult patients with relatively severe infections as with other intestinal bacterial pathogens such as *Clostridium difficile*, *Salmonella*, and *Yersinia*.[13] Reiter's syndrome has also been associated with campylobacter infections.[24, 27] Convulsions have been reported in infected children who are relatively older than those normally prone to febrile convulsions.[14] Patients with campylobacter colitis can develop erythema nodosum.[11]

CAMPYLOBACTER IN PREGNANCY AND IN IMMUNOCOMPROMISED PEOPLE

Fetal death in utero may follow prolonged febrile illnesses due to campylobacter infections at various stages of pregnancy. Necrosis and infarction of the placenta is usually observed. Premature labour with stillbirths or live infants also occurs.[12] Gastrointestinal symptoms are often mild in such patients.

Patients with hypogammaglobulinaemia appear prone to frequent relapses after campylobacter enteritis and may require multiple courses of antibiotic therapy.[1]

Diagnosis

The febrile prodrome and abdominal pain help to distinguish campylobacter gastroenteritis from other forms of infectious gastroenteritis. When abdominal pain is the dominant feature the causes of an acute abdomen such as appendicitis may be diagnosed. Campylobacter colitis may be mistaken for acute idiopathic ulcerative colitis and the use of corticosteroids in these circumstances can be detrimental.

Non-specific findings include a polymorph leucocytosis and an elevated erythrocyte sedimentation rate. Stool microscopy reveals pus cells and red cells, and when a sample has been obtained early in the disease dark-ground microscopy may permit recognition of campylobacter by their characteristic motility.[6] The typical Gram-negative organisms can also be identified by simple Gram staining of stool smears.[28] Confirmation of the diagnosis is usually achieved by stool culture using a selective medium. Serological methods are not widely available. Antibody is detected from the seventh day of illness and declines over two months. Agglutinins are present in 25% of normal sera at low titres ($<1/100$); complement fixation titres of 1/4 or 1/8 are only present in 2% of normal subjects. Although less sensitive the complement fixation test is less strain-specific and more suitable for routine use. Unfortunately studies in patients involved in milk-borne outbreaks have shown a wide variability of antibody response to the same strain.[16] Consequently these techniques are of limited diagnostic value.

Treatment

Most campylobacter infections are mild, self-limiting and require no treatment. When diarrhoea is profuse rehydration is required and can usually be achieved orally. Analgesics or anti-spasmodics such as dicyclomine are sometimes beneficial. If the symptoms are severe, intravenous fluids and specific antimicrobial therapy are required.

The organisms are usually sensitive to a range of antibiotics including gentamicin, clindamycin, erythromycin, chloramphenicol and minocycline, but they are resistant to penicillins and cephalosporins. Erythromycin has been widely used for the treatment of campylobacter infections in the UK because of its narrow spectrum and low toxicity.[6] Whereas most patients respond rapidly to this drug, the routine use of erythromycin confers no advantage in uncomplicated infection.[2]

Antibiotic therapy should be reserved for patients with severe symptoms, suspected bacteraemia, or campylobacter colitis. In the UK erythromycin resistance occurs in only 0.5% of strains, whereas on the continent of Europe 10% of these organisms may be resistant.[5] Because of the possibility of resistance some authorities prefer to use an aminoglycoside to treat suspected or proven bacteraemia, or other forms of systemic infection. Chloramphenicol is the drug of choice for infection of the central nervous system.

Person-to-person spread of this infection is uncommon and isolation of infected individuals is unnecessary.

REFERENCES

1 Ahnen, D. J. & Brown, W. R. (1982) Campylobacter enteritis in immune-deficient patients. *Annals of Internal Medicine*, **96**, 187–188.

2 Anders, B. J., Lauer, B. A., Paisley, J. W. & Reller, L. B. (1982) Double blind placebo controlled trial of erythromicin for treatment of campylobacter enteritis. *Lancet*, **i**, 131–132.

3 Blaser, M. J., Cravens, J., Powers, B. W. & Wang, W. L. (1978) Campylobacter enteritis associated with canine infections. *Lancet*, **ii**, 979–981.

4 Bolton, F. J. & Robertson, L. (1982) A selective medium for isolating *Campylobacter jejuni/coli. Journal of Clinical Pathology*, **35**, 462–467.

5 Brunton, W. A. T., Wilson, A. M. M. & Macrae, R. M. (1978) Erythromicin-resistant campylobacters. *Lancet*, **ii**, 1385.

6 Butzler, J. P. & Skirrow, M. B. (1979) Campylobacter enteritis. *Clinics in Gastroenterology*, **8**, 737–765.

7 Butzler, J. P., DeKeseyer, P., Detrain, M. & Dehain, F. (1973) Related vibrio in stools. *Journal of Paediatrics*, **82**, 493–495.

8 Conrad, S., Roderch, P. & Butzler, J. P. (1973) Enteritis due to 'related vibrio' in children. *American Journal of Diseases of Children*, **126**, 152.

9 Dekeyser, P., Gossiun-Detrain, M., Butzler, J. P. & Steman, J. (1972) Acute enteritis due to related vibrio: first positive stool cultures. *Journal of Infectious Diseases*, **125**, 390–392.

10 De Mol, P. & Bosmans, E. (1978) *Campylobacter* enteritis in Central Africa. *Lancet*, **i**, 604.

11 Ellis, M. E., Pope, J., Mokaski, A. & Dunbar, E. (1982) *Campylobacter* colitis associated with erythema nodosum. *British Medical Journal*, **ii**, 937.

12 Gribble, M. J., Salit, I. E., Isaac-Renton, J. & Chow, A. W. (1981) *Campylobacter* infections in pregnancy: case report and literature review. *Americal Journal of Obstetrics and Gynaecology*, **140**, 423–426.

13 Gumpel, J. M., Martin, C. & Sanderson, P. J. (1981) Reactive arthritis associated with *Campylobacter* enteritis. *Annals of the Rheumatic Diseases*, **40**, 64–65.

14 Havalad, S., Chapple, M. J., Kahakachchi, M. & Hargraves, D. B. (1980) Convulsions associated with *Campylobacter* enteritis. *British Medical Journal*, **280**, 984–985.

15 Jewkes, J., Larson, H. E., Price, A. B. *et al.* (1981) Aetiology of acute diarrhoea in adults. *Gut*, **22**, 388–392.

16 Jones, D. M., Elridge, J. & Dale, B. (1980) Serological response to *Campylobacter jejuni/coli* infection. *Journal of Clinical Pathology*, **33**, 767–769.

17 King, E. O. (1962) The laboratory recognition of *Vibrio Fetus* and a closely related vibrio isolated from cases of human vibriosis. *Annals of New York Academy of Science*, **98**, 700.

18 Lambert, M. E., Schofield, P. F., Ironside, A. G. & Mandal, B. K. (1979) *Campylobacter* colitis. *British Medical Journal*, **i**, 857–859.

19 Megraud, F., Tacharc, C., Latrille, J. & Bondasmy, J. M. (1982) Appendicitis due to *Campylobacter jejuni*. *British Medical Journal*, **ii**, 1165–1166.

20 Mentzing, L. O. (1981) Water-borne outbreak of *Campylobacter* enteritis in central Sweden. *Lancet*, **ii**, 352.

21 Michalak, D. M., Perrault, J., Gilchrist, M. J. *et al.* (1980) *Campylobacter fetus* ss *jejuni*: a cause of massive lower gastrointestinal haemorrhage. *Gastroenterology*, **79**, 742–745.

22 Norrby, R., McCloskey, R. V., Zachrissen, G. & Faken, E. (1980) Meningitis caused by *Campylobacter fetus* ssp *jejuni*. *British Medical Journal*, **280**, 1164.

23 Newman, A. & Lambert, J. R. (1980) *Campylobacter jejuni* causing flare-up in inflammatory bowel disease. *Lancet*, **ii**, 919.

24 Pönkä, A. & Kosunen, T. U. (1981) Pancreas affection in association with enteritis due to *Campylobacter fetus* ssp. *jejuni*. *Acta Medica Scandinavica*, **209**, 239–240.

25 Pontia, A., Martio, J. & Kosunen, T. U. (1981) Reiters syndrome in association with enteritis due to *Campylobacter fetus* ssp. *jejuni*. *Annals of the Rheumatic Diseases*, **40**, 414–415.

26 Robinson, D. A., Edgar, W. M., Gibson, G. L. *et al.* (1979) *Campylobacter* enteritis associated with the consumption of unpasteurised milk. *British Medical Journal*, **i**, 1171–1173.

27 Saari, K. M. & Kauranen, O. (1980) Ocular inflammation in Reiter's syndrome associated with *Campylobacter jejuni* enteritis. *American Journal of Ophthalmology*, **90**, 572–573.

28 Sazie, E. S. M. & Titus, A. E. (1982) Rapid diagnosis of *Campylobacter* enteritis. *Annals of Internal Medicine*, **96**, 62–63.

29 Schmidt, W., Chmel, H., Karunski, Z. & Sen, P. (1980) The clinical spectrum of *Campylobacter fetus* infections: report of five cases and review of the literature. *Quarterly Journal of Medicine*, **49**, 431–442.

30 Skirrow, M. B. (1977) *Campylobacter* enteritis: a new disease. *British Medical Journal*, **ii**, 9–11.

31 Smibert, R. M. (1978) The genus *Campylobacter*. *Annual Review of Microbiology*, **32**, 673–709.

WORM INFECTIONS

Worm infections of the gastrointestinal tract are widely prevalent in the world and pose a major public health problem in many less developed nations. In this section intestinal infection by nematodes (round worms) and cestodes (mostly long, segmented flat worms) is discussed.

Factors in the pathogenicity of worm infections

HOST FACTORS

Host factors that are of importance in the pathogenicity of intestinal worm infections are:

Environmental factors. The most important of these are factors that predispose to infection and reinfection such as water supply, sanitation, defecation habits and conditions of living in communities such as institutions for mentally retarded children.

Innate susceptibility. This feature can be demonstrated to be of importance in animals but is less clearly demonstrable in man. Hormonal influences may be important: strongyloidiasis may become invasive with steroid therapy. Changes in the environment (e.g. pH, short-chain fatty acids) of the intestinal lumen may condition the state of development of worms.

Nutrition. Protein-energy malnutrition depresses cellular immune responses, and this may predispose to infection. Most worm infections may not result in nutritional deficiencies in otherwise well persons with adequate dietary intake but infection may precipitate malnutrition when dietary intake is borderline. The status of a specific nutrient may be important: the available iron stores in patients who are infected with hookworms will condition the rate of development of iron-deficiency anaemia.

Coexistent diseases. It is generally believed that patients with other diseases are predisposed to parasitic infection. For instance, megacolon may favour larval penetration in strongyloidiasis. Systemic diseases such as those that alter immune responses may favour parasitic invasion (for example, the acquired immune deficiency syndrome).

Immune competence. Primary immune deficiency diseases are frequently associated with giardia infections, while secondary immunodeficiency resulting from drug therapy greatly influences the pathogenicity of strongyloidiasis.

PARASITE FACTORS[30]

Parasite factors that influence pathogenicity are considered under the following headings:

Population density. Intestinal parasites require space for living. A population exceeding a threshold will be pathogenic in proportion to its size. For instance, with ascariasis a large worm load will cause greater symptoms than only one or two adult worms in the bowel lumen.

Lifespan of the worm. Since the worms, in general, do not multiply within the definitive host, the duration of infection is regulated by the worms' lifespan and by continued reinfection. However, *Strongyloides stercoralis* and *Capillaria philippinensis* amongst nematodes and *Hymenolepis nana* amongst cestodes can persist by auto-infection and prolonged periods of dormancy have been observed with *Ancylostoma duodenale.*

Pattern of entry. Hookworm disease is usually acquired through the skin; however, if larvae are ingested and enter via the oral cavity, they may cause more severe pulmonary symptoms.

Virulence. Factors that control virulence of specific parasitic strains are not clearly defined in man.

Location. The major site of colonization varies with different worms and leads to varied clinical manifestations.

Response to associated infections. Ascaris may be seen migrating from the mouth and nose during the course of intercurrent infections in children. Combined infections of ascaris with trichuris and hookworm are often encountered.

Response to the modified host. Several parasitic organisms (e.g. strongyloides) will overgrow in debilitated persons.

Prevalence and intensity of infection[11, 40]

The prevalence and intensity of intestinal helminthic infection show considerable variation in distribution and seasonal occurrence. Factors that control the level of endemicity of many infections are poorly understood. The variables influencing the infection pressure are best considered under two headings: environmental factors and socioeconomic factors.

ENVIRONMENTAL FACTORS

The environment has a major role in transmission of many infections. Excretion of large numbers of eggs as by ascaris, hookworm, and trichuris causes extensive contamination in the environment. This contamination is often uneven, occurring close to the house and in areas of defecation. The parasite distribution thus varies over the ground surface. Furthermore, the larvae may enter the soil to different degrees. Aspects of latency and survival under varying climatic conditions are of great importance in the persistence of the parasite: ascaris eggs are resistant and may survive many years in soil and yet remain infective.

SOCIOECONOMIC FACTORS

Socioeconomic factors greatly influence intestinal parasitic infections. Many aspects of human behaviour influence their prevalence and intensity. Some age groups are more exposed than others to infection: young children contract ascaris by playing on contaminated ground around houses and young adult agricultural workers contract hookworm by working in contaminated fields. Occupation may influence exposure: contact with faecal material may be more prevalent among sewage workers. Clustering of cases of parasitic infection may be the result of secondary transmission from an index case or common risk factors (e.g. *Enterobius vermicularis*). Prevalence of soil-transmitted helminthic infections is much higher among the lower socioeconomic classes. Improved general standards of living and sanitation have been shown to reduce the intensity of infection in several populations in Japan, Poland and the USA.

Public health importance[12]

All these intestinal parasitic infections represent large and serious public health problems, particularly in developing countries. This is so especially in tropical regions. Wherever there exists a high prevalence of soil transmitted infections, living conditions are characteristically poor. Thus, the frequency of intestinal parasitic infection has often been considered a general indicator of the level of economic and social development of these communities. Control has been achieved by improved sanitation and alteration in socioeconomic factors with repetitive drug therapy campaigns, but the effects of these interventions have been limited in rural areas of developing countries.

Impact of parasitic infections

Intestinal parasitic infections can influence both social and economic aspects of living. Economic loss due to parasitic infections is impossible to measure with any accuracy; however, the high prevalence of hookworm, ascaris and strongyloides infections indicates major public health importance for these infections. Their importance can be judged by their effects on young populations in causing weight loss, diarrhoea, blood and protein loss from the bowel and the complications that develop. Parasitic infections are often prevalent in areas of the world where other conditions such as impaired nutrition make life-support precarious.

Drug therapy[8]

Important advances have been made in drug therapy recently. The intestinal helminths discussed here are more vulnerable to drug therapy than are some other pathogenic parasitic organisms (e.g. schistosomiasis). In selecting a particular treatment it is important to determine

(a) whether the infection is in an asymptomatic individual, (b) the likelihood of reinfection, (c) the cost of drug therapy to achieve eradication and (d) the consequences of treatment. In developed countries most infections, irrespective of intensity, should be treated unless specific contraindications exist. In contrast, in developing countries, and while planning mass treatment, intensity, economic considerations and the potential for reinfection have to be taken into account. Frequently, a single agent may be used to eradicate several different helminthic infections. Drug therapy for specific parasites will be discussed in relation to each infection.

ASCARIASIS

Ascaris is the largest of the nematodes infecting the human intestinal tract; it is also the worm most frequently infecting man, affecting more than a quarter of the world's population. Prevalence rates for ascariasis of 60–90% are common in many less developed parts of the world.[2, 38]

Most cases of human ascariasis are due to *Ascaris lumbricoides*; a few are due to *A. suis*, the pig roundworm. The larval stages of the dog roundworm, *Toxocara canis*, and of the cat roundworm, *T. cati*, produce the syndrome of visceral larva migrans.

Helminthology[2, 38]

Adult roundworms live in the upper small intestine. A gravid female produces 200 000 eggs per day. The eggs are passed unchanged in the stool. Under suitable environmental conditions the embryo in the egg transforms into an infective larva in 9–12 days. Ascaris eggs can survive six to nine years in the soil. Human infection is usually acquired by the ingestion of infective eggs, although the eggs may be inhaled and then swallowed. Hatching of the egg is believed to occur by the action of the gastric juice on the outer coat and that of the intestinal contents on the inner coat. The hatched larvae penetrate the intestinal mucosa and in 5–15 days are transported to the lungs by way of the portal vein and liver or the lymphatics. In the lung the larvae stay mostly in the capillaries and undergo further development. They then burrow into the alveoli, are coughed up and then swallowed. In the small intestine they develop into adult worms. Their lifespan is about six months to one year.

Pathophysiology

Only minimal tissue reaction occurs when the hatched larvae penetrate the intestine or pass through the liver. Larvae in the lung elicit a predominantly eosinophilic response around the worm and in a perivascular fashion; the associated symptoms are proportional to the larval load. Adult worms rarely produce symptoms in mild infections, but large worm loads may be associated with abdominal symptoms and in patients with borderline nutritional status may be associated with nutritional deficiency states.[42, 45] The in vivo effect, if any, of the trypsin inhibitor associated with the worm is not known.[35] The worms have a tendency to become tangled into a mass, which may produce intestinal obstruction, especially in children. Products of ascaris have been claimed to produce spasm of the host intestinal muscle, which may facilitate intestinal obstruction. Unusual complications result from migration of the worms into sites such as the biliary tract and pancreas; this may occur even in light infections. Such migration is usually associated with the ingestion of a vermifuge, administration of an anaesthetic agent or fever. Perforation of surgical stomas or even intact intestinal wall by worms has been reported.

Clinical features

During larval migration through the lungs patients may present with fever, cough, episodes of asthma and dyspnoea. Physical examination usually shows diffuse crepitations and rhonchi. The sputum is usually mucoid, but may be blood-tinged. Chest radiographs show prominent bronchial markings and, rarely, a diffuse mottled infiltrate. Peripheral blood eosinophilia is common. The sputum usually shows abundant eosinophils but only rarely the nematode larvae. In heavy infections respiratory symptoms may be very severe. Symptoms usually subside in one week to ten days.

Most patients with adult worms in the intestine are asymptomatic. Occasional vague abdominal pain has been attributed to the presence of the worms even in light infection, but is more common in heavy infections. A heavy worm load may lead to nutritional deficiency states in patients with borderline dietary intake. Occasionally patients may present initially after vomiting the worms or passing them in the stool.

The most common intestinal complication of heavy ascaris infection is intestinal obstruction and this is seen mostly in children.[23] In endemic areas ascariasis accounts for 10–15% of the cases of intestinal obstruction and is second only to acute appendicitis as a cause of acute abdomen. The clinical presentation is similar to that of intestinal obstruction from other causes, with abdominal pain, distension, nausea and vomiting. A mass of tangled worms is palpable through the abdominal wall in about half the patients. The most frequent site of obstruction is the terminal ileum. A plain film of the abdomen may demonstrate the mass of worms. Other intestinal complications such as intussusception, volvulus and infarction are rare.

Biliary ascariasis presents usually with biliary colic and is often seen following the use of a vermifuge or anaesthetic or associated with fever from another cause.[37] Jaundice is seen in 20% of patients. The worms return to the intestine with subsidence of symptoms or may stay in the bile duct for a variable period of time. If eggs are laid by a female worm they may move up to the portal tracts and produce a granulomatous reaction and mild chronic liver disease; degeneration of the worm may also have a similar outcome.

Patients may rarely present with pancreatitis or appendicitis caused by an obstructing worm. Perforation of the intestine by the worm, mostly in the distal ileum, is very rare.

Diagnosis

Demonstration of the characteristic eggs in the faeces is the best method for diagnosis of ascaris infection. The fertilized eggs measure 45–75 × 35 μm, are golden brown in colour and mammillated with two distinct envelopes (Figure 14.19a). Unfertilized eggs are usually irregular and longer and have a thin shell (Figure 14.19b). Several concentration techniques for demonstration of eggs are available. The worm burden may be calculated from the egg output in faeces. Occasionally the worm may be detected on an abdominal radiograph,[13] or more often on a barium study (Figure 14.20). Examination of a worm vomited or passed would establish the diagnosis in some. Biliary ascariasis may be suspected from the demonstration of the characteristic shadow in an ultrasonographic or radiographic evaluation of the biliary tract.[9] Serological diagnosis remains unsatisfactory.

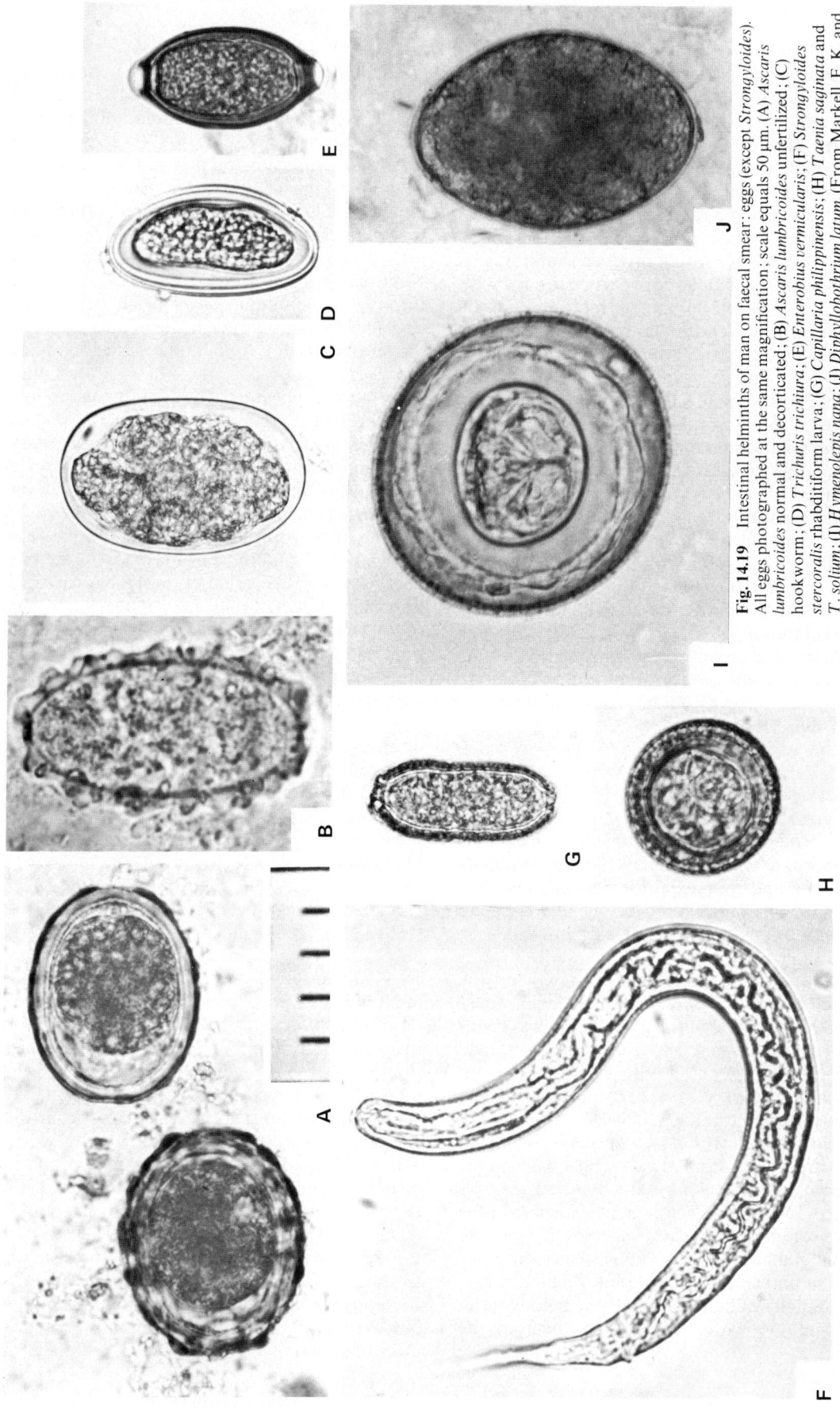

Fig. 14.19 Intestinal helminths of man on faecal smear: eggs (except *Strongyloides*). All eggs photographed at the same magnification; scale equals 50 μm. (A) *Ascaris lumbricoides* normal and decorticated; (B) *Ascaris lumbricoides* unfertilized; (C) hookworm; (D) *Trichuris trichiura*; (E) *Enterobius vermicularis*; (F) *Strongyloides stercoralis* rhabditiform larva; (G) *Capillaria philippinensis*; (H) *Taenia saginata* and *T. solium*; (I) *Hymenolepis nana*; (J) *Diphyllobothrium latum*. (From Markell, E. K. and Voge, M. (1981) *Medical parasitology*, 5th Edition, with kind permission of the authors and the publisher, W. B. Saunders.)

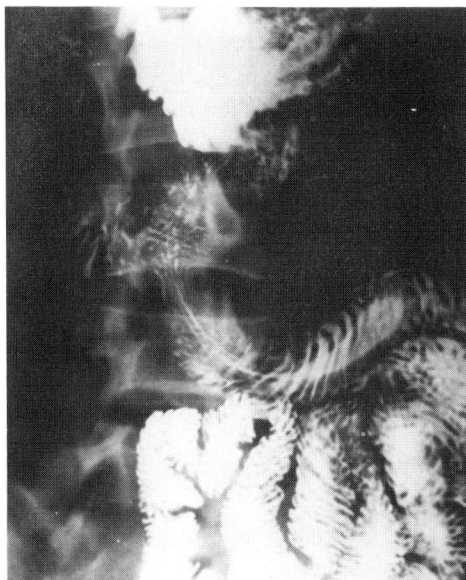

Fig. 14.20 *Ascaris lumbricoides* in the small intestine seen during barium examination as a long filling defect. A portion of the worm's intestine has also been filled with barium. (From Krause, G. R. (1949). In *Radiologic examination of the small intestine*. (Editor: Golden, R.), with kind permission of the author and the publisher, J. B. Lippincott.)

Treatment[8]

There are several effective drugs for the treatment of ascariasis. The choice depends on the clinical presentation and the presence of associated worm infections.

Piperazine salts cause a flaccid paralysis of the ascaris worms and the worms are expelled by host intestinal motility. Several dosage regimes have been found successful. A dose of 75 mg/kg (maximum 3.5 g) given as a single dose daily for two consecutive days is curative in almost 100% of patients. Piperazine is readily absorbed from the intestine. Toxic reactions are rare, and the drug has been safely used during pregnancy. Occasionally, gastrointestinal symptoms, transient neurological or urticarial symptoms have occurred. Piperazine in a longer course is effective against enterobiasis.

Pyrantel is also effective in ascariasis. It produces paralysis of the worm after initial spastic contractions. A single dose of 11 mg/kg (maximum 1.0 g) is curative in over 90% of cases of ascariasis. The drug is poorly absorbed from the intestine and toxicity is infrequent. Occasionally it causes transient gastrointestinal upset, headache and dizziness. Safe use in pregnancy has not been established.

Mebendazole is a broad-spectrum anthelmintic very effective in the treatment of ascariasis. It inhibits glucose uptake by the worm, leading to parasite immobilization and death. It is also ovicidal. Cure rate at a dose of 100 mg twice daily for three consecutive days is almost 100%. It is poorly absorbed from the gut and occasionally produces transient abdominal pain or diarrhoea. It is also effective against hookworm, pinworm, whipworm and strongyloides. It should not be used in pregnancy since embryotoxic and teratogenic effects have been seen in pregnant rats. Safety of its use in children below two years of age has not been established.

Thiabendazole is also a broad-spectrum anthelmintic slightly less effective than mebendazole. Thiabendazole inhibits the helminth-specific enzyme fumarate reductase. It is also ovicidal. At a dose of 25 mg/kg (maximum 3.0 g daily) on two successive days it has a 70–80% cure rate in ascariasis.

Levamisole produces initial stimulation and subsequent paralysis of ascaris worms by ganglionic stimulation. At high concentrations it also inhibits the worm-specific enzyme fumarate reductase. A single dose of 5.0 mg/kg (maximum 150 mg) is over 90% curative. This agent is also an immunostimulant.

When coexisting hookworm infection is treated using tetrachloroethylene pretreatment of ascariasis is essential to avoid migratory complications due to ascaris.

Intestinal obstruction from ascariasis can be managed conservatively in most patients.[23] In addition to supportive therapy piperazine, 75–150 mg/kg, is administered using a nasogastric or intestinal tube. Drug-induced paralysis of the worms relieves the obstruction in most patients. Agents that stimulate worm activity (such as pyrantel, thiabendazole and levamisole) are contraindicated. If the obstruction is not relieved, gentle squeezing of the worms into the colon at surgical exploration may relieve the obstruction. Rarely is enterotomy or intestinal resection needed. During operations care should be taken to prevent migration of the worms into the peritoneal space, which may lead to peritonitis. Biliary ascariasis often responds to conservative management with analgesics.[37] Surgical exploration and worm removal is required if cholangitis ensues.

HOOKWORM INFECTION

Worldwide, hookworm infection is second in prevalence only to ascariasis. Several species of hookworms infect man, but *Ancylostoma duodenale* and *Necator americanus* are the only common species which reach maturity in the human intestine. *A. ceylonicum* is usually a parasite of cats, dogs and other carnivores but may infect man. *A. braziliense* is responsible for creeping eruption (cutaneous larva migrans) but the worm rarely matures in man. *A. caninum*, the common hookworm of dogs and cats, is very rarely a parasite in man.

Helminthology[33]

Adult hookworms are small cylindrical greyish white nematodes. The female worm is larger than the male. The chief morphological differences between species are in the shape of the mouthparts and permit distinction between *Necator* and *Ancylostoma*.

Adult hookworms attach themselves to the mucosa of the small intestine by their buccal capsules; the usual site is the upper intestine but may extend as far down as the lower ileum in heavy infections. Females are prolific egg layers and deposit their ova in the lumen of the intestine. Estimates of fecundity vary, but commonly cited figures are 10 000 eggs per female per day in the case of *N. americanus* and twice that number in the case of *A. duodenale*. Eggs have bluntly rounded ends; they are usually unsegmented but may have divided by the time of examination of fresh faeces.

Eggs leave the host in the faeces. When environmental conditions are favourable, eggs will embryonate and hatch within 24 hours. The larva which emerges from the egg is called a rhabditiform larva. By subsequent growth and moulting, this larva develops into a filariform larva which is infective. Larvae usually penetrate the skin at sites of contact with contaminated material. Infection may also occur via the buccal mucosa: *N. americanus* infects more successfully via the skin than via the mouth, whereas *A. duodenale* is much more efficient in establishing itself via the stomach.[41] Larvae migrate through the circulation to the lungs where they enter the alveoli and move up the respiratory tree to the pharynx. Larvae are then swallowed and complete their development in the intestine. Prolonged dormancy of larvae in man may occur with *A. duodenale*.[40] During these intervals the nematodes are drug-resistant, and their metabolic rate remains low. Transmammary transmission to breastfed babies has been reported with *A. duodenale* but not with *N. americanus*.

Pathophysiology[33, 39, 49]

Hookworms attach to the mucosa of the upper intestine by their buccal capsules; in heavy infections they may be present as low as the ileum.

This distribution has become clear since the observations of Kalkofen in infected dogs.[26] Worms are found to change their site of attachment to the mucosa every four to six hours to seek out new feeding sites. In addition less frequent movements occur for the purpose of mating. The buccal capsule of the worm is apposed to one or two villi or to the upper crypt region of the mucosal surface, and with attachment and suction a plug of the host tissue is drawn into the buccal capsule. Mucosal cells of the tissue plug are pulled free from the lamina propria, villous capillary loops burst and allow blood to flow out. Continuous or intermittent suction by the worm causes tissue and blood to be drawn into the worm's intestinal tract. Within the buccal cavity the mucosal cells show signs of increasing cytolysis as they migrate in a caudal direction; within ten minutes the cells are frequently broken down and digested. Successive plugs of tissue are ingested and the areas of tissue destruction increase in size. The intensity of the inflammatory reaction in the surrounding mucosa is often greater than can be directly attributed to trauma inflicted by the worm. The muscularis mucosae defines the usual maximum depth of penetration of the worm prior to its detachment and fixation at another site. The maximally developed mucosal lesion usually involves about nine villi and an individual worm causes as many as six such lesions or numerous shallow ones each day. Blood loss occurs primarily by passage through the worm's intestinal tract, but bleeding from damaged mucosa external to the worm is also significant. In addition, the major source of nutrient loss to the host is thought to be the plugs of mucosal tissue ingested by the worm. Blood ingestion appears to be of only secondary importance as a food source for the worm since intact erythrocytes are found at all levels in the worm's midgut surrounded by the remains of partially ingested mucosal tissue. After detachment of the worm, changes in the intestinal mucosa are often minimal and consist of general evidence of increased crypt mitotic activity. Repair of the intestinal mucosa is rapid.

It has been clearly shown that blood loss occurs from the mucosal injury. Recorded average blood losses are of the order of 0.03 (ml/day)/worm for *N. americanus*, reaching 0.15 (ml/day)/worm for *A. duodenale* infections.[39] Some of the iron lost as haemoglobin into the intestine is reabsorbed. Patients with hookworm disease retain the ability to absorb orally administered iron. Variations in the rate of development of iron-deficiency anaemia depend on available dietary iron sources and the duration and severity of the hookworm infection. Anaemia responds rapidly to treatment with iron salts. Gastric anacidity and associated vitamin B_{12} and folate deficiency are factors of only limited importance in the pathogenesis of hookworm anaemia.

Studies of infections with the hookworm-like *Nippostrongylus braziliensis* have demonstrated impairment of absorption of salt, water and glucose. A relationship between hookworm infection and impaired absorption in human subjects is, however, complicated by the fact that infection occurs (a) in association with features of malnutrition and hypoproteinaemia, and (b) with other diseases such as tropical sprue. Nevertheless, a variety of studies in Africa and India have demonstrated that no major generalized malabsorptive defect occurs in human hookworm infection.

Hypoproteinaemia with hypoalbuminaemia often accompanies anaemia in patients with hookworm infection.[49] Intestinal protein loss may be severe in association with hookworm infection. Several studies have documented protein-losing enteropathy which responds to treatment of the worm load.[4] Others have suggested that inadequate dietary protein intake is often responsible for the hypoproteinaemia.

Many reports have suggested that infection with hookworms is more severe in the host whose nutritional level is poor, but studies in which nutritional factors have been rigorously controlled have not clearly documented that there is a specific predisposition with malnutrition.[49] Studies with hookworms in dogs support the concept that heavier infections occur in malnourished animals than in those that are well-fed. Recently conducted balance studies in individuals with both hookworm and malnutrition failed to demonstrate that nutritional repletion with high-protein diets altered either quantitative egg counts, intestinal blood loss or the number of spontaneously expelled worms.

Clinical features[41]

When the larvae penetrate the skin maculopapules and localized erythema may occur; this has been termed 'ground itch' or 'dew itch'. Respiratory symptoms are uncommon although cough and wheezing may be associated with worm migration. Chest radiographs taken on these occasions may show fluffy infiltrates representing areas of pneumonitis. Occasionally, severe acute reactions may follow exposure to very large numbers of infective larvae. Such patients may develop allergic reactions associated with skin irritation, pharyngeal itching, cough, dyspnoea, wheezing, vomiting and abdominal pain. Small worm loads may be asymptomatic; however, most patients with significant worm loads will develop chronic symptoms associated with the development of an iron-deficiency anaemia. Gastrointestinal symptoms of epigastric discomfort and tenderness occur with significant infections and may be confused with peptic ulcer disease. Appetite is often increased, but in the later stages of anaemia and congestive heart failure it may be impaired. If serious disease develops during childhood, growth and development may be stunted. Alteration in bowel habit only occurs as a result of change in overall dietary intake. Symptoms of anaemia develop depending on the worm load and dietary intake of iron. Anaemia with haemoglobin values of 80 g/l or less is not uncommon. Cardiac and peripheral vascular manifestations of chronic anaemia are very common.

Diagnosis[24]

Accurate diagnosis is dependent on the identification of hookworm eggs in the faeces. A direct faecal film on a microscope slide mounted in saline or iodine solution is suitable for detection of moderate and severe infections (Figure 14.19c), but light infections (less than 400 eggs per gram of faeces) usually require concentration techniques such as zinc sulphate flotation. Filariform larvae of *N. americanus* and *A. duodenale* can be reared on moist filter paper at 28–30°C. Larvae develop in five to seven days and collect in the reservoir of water at the bottom of the tube. Their distinguishing features can then be defined microscopically.

The worm burden as determined by counting eggs in faecal samples gives only an approximation of the number of adult worms present. A measure of adult worm load can also be obtained after treatment with a vermifuge and the use of a purge, by sieving out the worms from the faecal specimen and directly counting the number of adult worms passed: 85–90% of adult worms can be recovered by this technique.

Antibodies can be detected to third and fourth stage larval antigens; however, they do not have sufficient specificity. Similarly, skin tests have no useful diagnostic purpose.

Treatment[8]

There are several effective drugs for the treatment of hookworm infection and their selection is based on the presence of any associated worm infection and the general and haematological status of the patient.

Mebendazole and pyrantel embonate (pyrantel pamoate) are the drugs of choice in hookworm infection. Mebendazole inhibits glucose uptake by worms, causing depletion of glycogen and ATP and leading to slow death of the worms. The recommended dose in adults and children over two years of age is 100 mg twice daily for three days. Because of its teratogenic effect in rats, mebendazole is not to be used in early pregnancy. Pyrantel embonate produces spastic paralysis of the worms and can be administered as a single dose of 11 mg/kg (maximum 1.0 g); it is less effective against *N. americanus*.

Bephenium hydroxynaphthoate is an alternative drug, but is less effective against *N. americanus*. This drug is a cholinergic agonist and produces spastic paralysis of hookworm and roundworm. Thiabendazole, at a dose of 25 mg/kg (maximum 3.0 g) twice daily for three days is an alternative drug, but is less effective; it is useful against creeping eruption due to *A. braziliense*. Tetrachloroethylene continues to be used in less developed countries; when treating with this agent ascariasis, if present, should be treated first to prevent migratory complications of ascariasis.

Iron-deficiency anaemia accompanying hookworm infection slowly corrects after worm removal but oral iron therapy is beneficial. Careful transfusion of blood or packed cells may be required prior to anthelmintic therapy in patients with severe anaemia. Prevention of reinfection requires wearing of footwear and improvements in sanitation and personal hygiene. Iron supplementation or fortification is useful to prevent hookworm anaemia.

TRICHURIASIS

Infection by *Trichuris trichiura* (whipworm) is worldwide in distribution and is estimated to be the third most prevalent intestinal worm infection.

Helminthology[51]

The adult worms measure 25–50 mm in length and have a whip-like anterior three-fifths; they penetrate into and anchor to the lower bowel mucosa by a spear-like projection. The gravid female worm lays an average of 6000 eggs per day. The eggs are unsegmented on oviposition,

are passed in the stool and become infective with fully developed larvae in approximately three weeks, preferring warm moist soil for their development. Man becomes infected by ingesting infective eggs directly from contaminated soil; no secondary host is required. Young children are much more easily and continuously infected. Infection rates are the greatest in the 5–15-year age group. Larvae are set free in the small intestine, where they penetrate the intestinal villi temporarily. There is no visceral phase in the life cycle. The larvae pass directly downwards into their usual habitat in the caecal lumen, where they mature to adults in 30 to 90 days. Lifespan of adult worms is probably three to five years.[1] The parasite may occur in hogs, which may play a part in transmission.

Pathophysiology[27, 51]

The whip-like portion of the worm attaches to the mucosa of the caecum and ascending colon. Heavy infection may lead to localized superficial inflammation and subepithelial haemorrhages. The infiltration rarely extends deeper than the muscularis mucosae. A diffuse colitis and proctitis with diarrhoea may occur in heavy infections. Rectal prolapse has also been claimed to be a complication of heavy trichuris infection. Large numbers of worms together may occlude the appendiceal orifice and cause appendicitis.

Eosinophilia (range 5% to 15%) may occur. Generalized toxicity is uncommon. Blood loss into the colon occurs and may be significant, reaching 4 ml per day in heavy infections and it may lead to chronic anaemia in susceptible malnourished children.[2] Anaemia is unlikely in adults in whom heavy infections are rare.

Clinical features

Few symptoms accompany light infections. Moderate and heavy infections may cause lower abdominal pain, diarrhoea, which may rarely be bloody, flatulence and distension. Appendicitis may occur and rectal prolapse may be associated with heavy infection and straining.

Diagnosis

The diagnosis is confirmed by the presence of characteristic eggs on examination of a faecal smear or by using concentration techniques (Figure 14.19d). Numerous eggs, barrel-shaped with bipolar translucent plugs, are usually seen. Adult worms may be visualized on proctoscopy or colonoscopy hanging freely from the mucosa.[14]

Treatment[8]

The majority of infections are light: in non-endemic areas these should be treated. In endemic areas symptomatic individuals and those with heavy infections should be treated. Mebendazole is the most useful and effective medication providing egg reduction rates close to 100% and cure rates of about 70%. Patient tolerance to the medication is excellent. Good results have also been obtained with oxantel embonate (oxantel pamoate) but thiabendazole gives poor cure rates.

ENTEROBIASIS

Enterobiasis (oxyuriasis) is a widely prevalent intestinal worm infection, more common in temperate than in tropical climates. It is caused by the small worm *Enterobius vermicularis* (oxyuris, pinworm, seat worm). It is the most prevalent nematode in North America and Europe, where as many as 40 million people may be infected.

Helminthology[34, 51]

E. vermicularis is a small, yellowish spindle-shaped worm living in the caecum and adjacent portions of the large and small intestine. The worms attach to the intestinal mucosa. The male worm is smaller than the female and is rarely seen. The gravid female migrates to the perianal area, usually when the host is asleep, and deposits eggs in the perianal area; the worm most often dies thereafter. Only infrequently are eggs laid in the intestine. The eggs are oval and flattened on one side and have a well developed embryo. The commonest means of infection is by the anus–hand–mouth route, particularly in children and it is aided by the perianal pruritus induced by the migrating female worm. Soiled clothing and sheets are good sources of contamination of the air or dust by ova. Transmission is favoured by overcrowding in institutions and poor hygiene. Rarely, auto-infection by retrograde movement of newly hatched larvae into the colon occurs in adults. Commonly the infection is acquired by ingestion of infective eggs. Eggs hatch into mature larvae in the small intestine – within six hours at body temperature. The larvae moult during their passage into the caecum and develop into adult worms. Egg deposition usually begins 15 to 45 days after ingestion of infective eggs.

Pathophysiology[34, 51]

Worms attached to the mucosal surface of the caecum and proximal colon may cause mild inflammatory reactions associated with minute ulcerations. Eosinophilia (amounting to 6–12% of the total white cell count) can occur in patients with enterobiasis. Migration of the female worms at night with deposition of eggs in the perianal skin may cause severe irritation and lead to eczematous dermatitis and secondary bacterial infection. Obstruction of the lumen of the appendix by worms has been associated with acute appendicitis. Worm migration to other sites is uncommon; rarely, sites such as the vagina, uterus and the fallopian tubes have been involved, leading to vaginitis, endometritis and salpingitis. Granulomas on the peritoneum have been associated with migration of worms via the female genital tract. Occasional hepatic granulomas have been detected in males.[46]

Clinical features[34, 51]

Light infections may be asymptomatic. The most common and significant symptom is perianal pruritus, occurring at night. Scratching may lead to secondary skin changes and associated bacterial infection. Insomnia, restlessness and irritability may occur. Appendicitis and peritonitis may rarely be the presenting problem. Symptoms due to involvement of the genital tract are rare and urinary tract infections are rarely from this cause. Occasionally, thread-like worms may be identified in the perianal area or be seen on the surface of the bowel movements.

Diagnosis[34, 51]

Infection is suggested by symptoms of perianal itching and scratching in children. Diagnosis is dependent on examination of material taken from the perianal region, either at night or early in the morning before bathing. The simplest method to demonstrate the eggs is by applying a length of transparent tape to the perianal region and, after removal, placing the sticky side down in a drop of toluene on a clear microscope slide. Using a low-power objective the typical eggs, flattened on one side and containing an embryonated larva, can be identified (Figure 14.19e). These tape preparations may be stored for several weeks. Swabbing of the perianal area using other techniques is equally valuable. Five examinations are reported to yield a 99% rate of detection. Examination of a faecal smear is not so sensitive. Other family members should be examined when one member is found positive.[3]

Treatment[8]

A variety of drugs are effective in achieving cure rates greater than 90% in enterobiasis. Preferred treatment is with mebendazole. A single 100-mg tablet is usually effective at all ages. Pyrantel embonate is also very effective; dosage should be repeated in two weeks since mature worms seem more vulnerable than young worms to this drug. Viprynium embonate (pyrvinium pamoate) is another useful drug. However, it will cause discoloration of clothing due to excretion of the red dye. Local applications of petroleum jelly or zinc oxide cream to the perianal region may be necessary in addition to antibiotics.[1] Frequent reinfections are likely unless hygienic measures are also carried out and repeated treatments instituted. Handwashing and fingernail scrubbing should be performed frequently. Scrubbing and sterilization of the toilet area are necessary. Underwear should be changed regularly and frequent showers and washing performed. It is important, however, to avoid overzealous decontamination of all clothing in the house since the ova are resistant to ordinary fumigants and disinfectants. It is often more practical to treat reinfections and all likely susceptible subjects with appropriate drugs. An important component of therapy is appropriate reassurance and advice to the family to emphasize the pattern of transmission and the need for retreatment and that inferior hygiene has little role in its persistence.

STRONGYLOIDIASIS

Strongyloides stercoralis is a small nematode parasite infecting humans. It is present worldwide, although it is more prevalent in the tropics. The distribution of strongyloides generally follows that of hookworm. Prevalence rates for infection with *S. stercoralis* of over 80% have been found in low socioeconomic groups in warm humid regions. Because of the ability of the worm to survive by auto-infection, it may persist for long periods; thus 27.5% of Australian ex-prisoners-of-war were found to have the infection more than 30 years after their return from South East Asia.[20] Occasionally, human infection with *S. fullerboni*, which is a common parasite in monkeys, has been noted.

Helminthology[6, 29]

Adult female worms, measuring 2–3 mm × 0.1 mm, live in the crypts of the duodenum and jejunum. They burrow tunnels in the mucosa and lay 30 to 40 eggs each day. The male worm is not usually seen in the intestinal tract. Whether fertilization of the eggs takes place as a result of copulation during migration through the lungs or as a result of parthenogenesis is not clearly established. The eggs are similar in appearance to hookworm eggs, measure 50–60 µm × 30–35 µm and have a thin transparent shell. They soon develop into rhabditiform larvae, which are passed in the stool. Under favourable conditions in the soil the rhabditiform larvae develop into free-living adults and can maintain a free-living cycle. Under unfavourable conditions the rhabditiform larvae transform into infective filariform larvae. The filariform larvae penetrate the skin or the mucosa on contact and are carried to the lungs through the veins. In the lungs they mature into adult worms; after burrowing their way into the respiratory passages, they are swallowed back into the intestine.

Occasionally the rhabditiform larvae, soon after being formed in the host, transform into filariform larvae. This process occurs more frequently when the host immunity is decreased as in malignancy or during glucocorticoid therapy. The infective larvae may invade the colon or perianal area or may disseminate widely in the body to the lung, liver, brain and meninges as a hyperinfection syndrome.

Pathophysiology[6, 22, 29]

When infection is acquired, transient skin and lung symptoms occur as a response to larval migration; the host response is believed to be dependent on larval dose and prior exposure. In the majority of infected people, the adult worms produce no serious consequence to the host. In a few patients infiltration of the small intestine by larvae leads to malabsorption. In hyperinfection infiltration by larvae can produce colitis, pulmonary insufficiency and neurological findings. The larvae are believed to help disseminate enteric bacterial infections, probably due to bacteria adhering to the surface or excreted by the larvae.[22]

Clinical features[6, 20, 29, 32]

The skin manifestations at the time of infection consist of urticarial lesions and petechiae, and are usually termed 'ground itch'. Lung manifestations ranging from mild cough to severe bronchopneumonia were noted in about half of the patients in one series.

The majority of patients with intestinal strongyloidiasis are asymptomatic. However, symptoms of diarrhoea (45%), urticaria (66%), 'indigestion' (73%), pruritus ani (59%) and weight loss (23%) were more common amongst those infected with *S. stercoralis* than amongst controls in a study of Australian ex-prisoners-of-war.[20] Diarrhoea, abdominal pain, nausea, vomiting and weight loss were the common presenting symptoms amongst those with strongyloidiasis seeking medical help.[32] The diarrhoea is often mild, but can be severe. It is usually watery, but in about a fifth of the patients it may be bloody. Abdominal pain is usually epigastric, sometimes cramping, but is often mistaken for peptic ulcer disease. Eosinophilic leucocytosis is common.

Hyperinfection is usually seen in patients immunocompromised by neoplastic disease or glucocorticoid therapy. The commonest neoplastic diseases associated with strongyloides hyperinfection are leukaemias and lymphomas, but a few patients with oat-cell carcinoma of the bronchus have also developed this complication.[22] Symptoms usually depend on the major sites of larval migration. Colonic involvement with bloody diarrhoea is often seen in early hyperinfection. Pulmonary and, less often, neurological manifestations usually predominate the clinical picture. Bacterial sepsis, often with multiple enteric pathogens, is a frequent accompaniment of disseminated strongyloidiasis. Eosinophil counts in peripheral blood are often normal at this stage.

Diagnosis[24]

Careful examination of the stool or duodenal aspirate for larvae is the most important tool for the diagnosis of strongyloidiasis (Figure 14.19f). Routine examination of stools is only 27–37% sensitive and repeated examinations are necessary. Examination of larger stool specimens (1.0 g) detected the infection in 84% of patients in one study.[20] Duodenal samples may be obtained by aspiration or by the use of a string held in a gelatin capsule; these have been claimed to be 90% sensitive in detecting strongyloidiasis, although in one study the string test was only 39% sensitive.[20]

Barium contrast studies are not sensitive; the findings are non-specific and unreliable. Increased or decreased motility, narrowing or dilatation of the lumen and mucosal thickening or ulcerations have been described on barium study. Mucosal biopsies of the affected areas

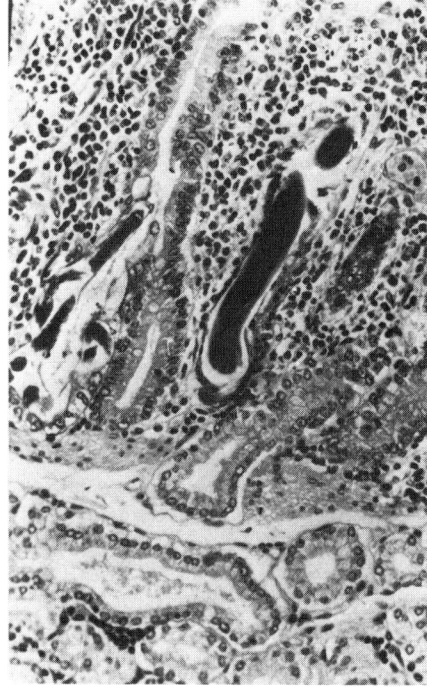

Fig. 14.21 *Strongyloides stercoralis*: section of a mucosal biopsy of small intestine showing larvae invading the mucosa.

may reveal the larvae in cross-section and a mild inflammatory response, often with large numbers of eosinophils, except in cases of hyperinfection (Figure 14.21). With pulmonary involvement the larvae may be detected in the sputum or a lung biopsy specimen (Figure 14.22). When there is meningeal involvement, the larvae are seldom seen in the cerebrospinal fluid specimen obtained by lumbar puncture.

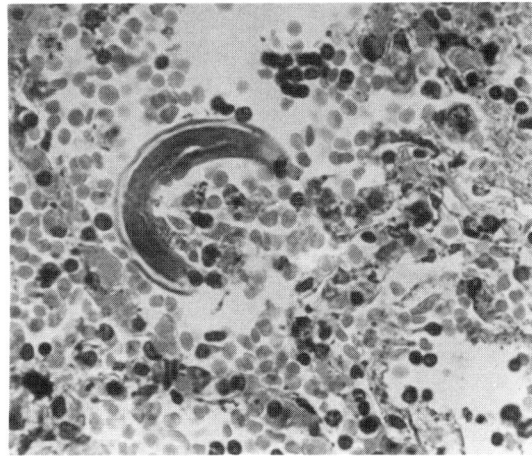

Fig. 14.22 *Strongyloides stercoralis*: a stained touch preparation from cut surface of lung at autopsy showing a larva. Patient with chronic lymphocytic leukaemia who had overwhelming strongyloidiasis.

Serological testing by the ELISA method using an antigen from the related species *Strongyloides ratti* has been found to be 84% sensitive in strongyloidiasis.[36] An indirect immunofluorescent test using the same antigen was reported to be 98% sensitive. These tests are not yet commercially available for routine use. Skin testing has not been found to be a sensitive method for diagnosis.

Treatment[6, 8]

Thiabendazole is considered the drug of choice for the treatment of strongyloidiasis. It is usually administered at a dose of 25 mg/kg for three to eight days. Although reduction or absence of larval excretion in stools is seen in 80% of patients soon after treatment it often recurs later; this is believed to be a result of the major action of the drug being the reduction of fecundity of the female and the drug being not sufficiently larvicidal. Both mebendazole and cambendazole were shown to be superior to thiabendazole against migrating *S. ratti* larvae in mice and *S. stercoralis* larvae in dogs,[21] but there are not sufficient data about their efficacy in treating human infection to recommend their routine use.

INTESTINAL CAPILLARIASIS

Intestinal capillariasis is caused by the small roundworm *Capillaria philippinensis* and has been reported from the northern Philippines and Thailand.[31, 50] Adult worms live in the crypts of the jejunum. The female lays peanut-shaped bi-operculate eggs which are passed in the stools. The embryonated eggs are infective to fish. Human infection is believed to result from the ingestion of raw fish containing infective larvae. Auto-infection with infiltrations of the intestine by newly formed larvae can lead to the development of intestinal malabsorption. Clinical manifestations include watery diarrhoea, often profuse, steatorrhoea and weight loss. Malabsorption of vitamin B_{12} and luminal bile salt deconjugation have also been demonstrated in intestinal capillariasis. Diagnosis is made by the demonstration of the characteristic eggs in stools (Figure 14.19g) but eggs may be difficult to detect and be excreted in cycles. Therapy with mebendazole 300 mg daily for 10 to 30 days has been found to be very effective.[44]

VISCERAL LARVA MIGRANS

Visceral larva migrans (VLM) was originally described as a syndrome consisting of tender hepatomegaly, marked eosinophilia and hyper-gammaglobulinaemia caused by larval nematodes that migrate in the tissues of a non-definitive host.[5] Some authors, however, have described similar manifestations in the definitive host as VLM. Only those under the former definition are discussed here.

Most cases of VLM in humans are caused by the larvae of the dog roundworm, *Toxocara canis*, and the cat roundworm, *T. cati;* rarely, larvae of other nematodes may also cause the same syndrome.[3, 18] VLM is frequently seen even in developed countries, as shown by the high prevalence rates in the south-eastern United States.[17]

Helminthology[3, 17, 18]

Adult toxocara live in the upper intestinal tract of dogs and cats. The eggs laid by the female are passed in the stool. Humans acquire infection by ingestion of eggs, which hatch in the upper intestine. The larvae penetrate the intestine and reach the lung by way of the portal vein and liver or lymphatics. Systemic spread from the lungs may occur but the larvae do not develop into adult worms in humans.

Pathophysiology[17, 18]

Manifestations of VLM are the result of the migration of toxocara larvae in tissues and the host immune response. The symptoms are related to the dose of the inoculum and prior exposure: in general, a large inoculum and prior exposure are associated with more severe features of VLM. Larvae elicit IgM, IgG, and IgE antibody response; the inflammatory cell response to the larvae includes eosinophils, polymorphonuclear leucocytes and macrophages. A marked eosinophilic response often leads to destruction of the larvae but with other types of cellular response the larvae may persist long in tissues and elicit a granulomatous inflammatory response. VLM is mostly a disease of children. Ocular larva migrans (OLM), by contrast, is believed to be associated with a smaller infecting dose, is more frequent in older children and adults and is only infrequently associated with VLM. Titres of antibody against toxocara are much lower in OLM than in VLM.

Clinical features[3, 5, 18]

Young children, 1–5 years of age, in whom pica is common, are the most frequently seen with VLM. The illness manifests as fever (70%), asthmatic symptoms (66%), allergic skin manifestations, nausea, vomiting and abdominal pain (48%), hepatomegaly (70%) and eosinophilia (100%). The illness is generally self-limited. Ocular manifestations are rare in VLM; when present, they consist of diminished visual acuity or a retinal mass which may be mistaken for retinoblastoma.

Diagnosis[18]

Definitive diagnosis of VLM is not possible without the demonstration of the causative larvae in the tissues; this is almost impossible in biopsy specimens. The syndrome has to be suspected on the basis of clinical manifestations and epidemiology. Amongst patients so diagnosed, an ELISA test using an antigen from embryonated eggs of *T. cati* has been shown to be 78% sensitive and 92% specific for the diagnosis of VLM;[10] other serological tests have not been found to be clinically useful.

Treatment[3, 18]

VLM usually runs a benign and self-limited course. Repeated reinfections may cause persistent symptoms. Effective drug therapy regimens have not been established. Diethylcarbamazine has been claimed to be useful while thiabendazole and mebendazole are not thought to be beneficial. The use of glucocorticoids during the acute phase is controversial. Avoiding reinfection by removal or treatment of the pet and controlling the pica are important aspects of therapy.

HELMINTHIC PSEUDOTUMOURS

The larval stages of several roundworms for whom man is not the definitive host, when ingested, may infiltrate or penetrate the intestinal wall and produce inflammatory masses. These pseudotumours may present with signs and symptoms of acute appendicitis or intestinal obstruction. In many of these cases, it is often difficult to demonstrate the causative larvae in the resected tumours.[1, 31]

Anisakiasis

Anisakiasis is caused by larval forms of the genera *Anisakis* and *Phocanema* and has been found mostly in Japan and the Netherlands.[31, 48] Infection is acquired by eating raw, undercooked or pickled fish. Symptoms suggesting acute gastritis may begin soon after ingestion of the larvae, when they reach the stomach. At this stage they have been demonstrated by barium contrast study and upper endoscopy. Removal of the larvae using fibre-optic endoscopes has been claimed to relieve symptoms promptly. The late result of larval ingestion is an eosinophilic phlegmon, most frequently seen in the ileocaecal region and usually presenting with signs and symptoms of appendicitis or intestinal obstruction. Operative treatment may be required for diagnosis and therapy.

Angiostrongyliasis

Abdominal angiostrongyliasis is caused by the larval stages of *Angiostrongylus costaricensis*.[28, 31] The adult worm lives in the mesenteric vessels of a rodent and the eggs passed in the rodent's stools develop into larvae in a slug. Human infection is acquired by the ingestion of the infected slug or its mucus secretions containing the larvae. The larvae penetrate the intestinal wall, most frequently in the ileocaecal region. The illness is common in children, usually begins 20 to 30 days after ingestion and is often confused with appendicitis or intestinal obstruction. Operative treatment is often performed for suspected appendicitis. Untreated, the illness lasts several weeks and may regress. No specific drug therapy regimen has so far been developed.

Gnathostomiasis

Gnathostomiasis is caused by the larval stages of *Gnathostoma spinigerum*, a roundworm of the dog and cat.[31] The eggs develop in fish and human infection results from ingestion of raw or undercooked fish. Commonly, soon after ingestion, a visceral larva migrans syndrome develops, but later inflammatory pseudotumours form in the ileocaecal area. Drug treatment is ineffective and operative intervention is often needed for diagnosis and therapy.

Oesophagostomiasis

Oesophagostomiasis is caused by the larvae of the roundworms of the genus *Oesophagostomum*.[31] Adult worms infect non-human primates in Asia and Africa. The exact mode of human infection is not known. The larvae penetrate the distal ileum or the colon and produce inflammatory masses. Operative treatment is often needed for diagnosis and therapy.

INTESTINAL TAPEWORM INFECTIONS

Intestinal infection by cestodes – long segmented intestinal flatworms or tapeworms – is widely prevalent in the world. The prevalence of the specific tapeworm infection is dependent on the dietary habits and the degree of sanitation. The common cestodes infecting the intestinal tract of man are *Taenia saginata* (beef tapeworm), *T. solium* (pork tapeworm), *Hymenolepis nana* (dwarf tapeworm) and *Diphyllobothrium latum* (fish tapeworm). Occasionally man is infected with *Inermicapsifer madagascariensis*, *Dipylidium caninum*, *Hymenolepis diminuta* and *Echinococcus granulosus*. Infection of humans by the larval stages of tapeworms other than those related to the common intestinal tapeworms is not discussed in this chapter.

Helminthology[7, 24]

Adult tapeworms live in the intestinal tract of the definitive vertebrate host. The anatomical regions of a tapeworm are the head (scolex), the neck and the body, which consists of several segments (proglottides) (Table 14.10). The scolex enables the worm to attach to the intestinal mucosa with the aid of suckers and, in some, with hooklets in an area of the head (the rostellum). Each proglottid has male and female reproductive organs, a primitive nervous system, a muscular system and an excretory system. The surface of the proglottid has microvilli and is capable of absorbing nutrients. The size and branching of the uteri help to differentiate the species. Fertilized eggs accumulate in the gravid uterus and these intact proglottides or the eggs released from them after digestion of the proglottid are passed in the faeces of the definitive host. Larvae released from the eggs (called oncospheres or, in the case of *D. latum*, coracidia) penetrate the intestinal mucosa of the intermediate host and become encysted in the tissues, particularly the skeletal muscles. In the case of *T. solium* and *T. saginata* they develop into fluid-filled sacs called bladder worms (cysticerci), and in the case of *H. nana* they develop into cyst-like 'cysticercoids' that have little or no fluid.

There are two larval stages in the development of *D. latum*: the procercoid in *Cyclops* and the plerocercoid in the fish. Scolices form as an invagination in the wall of the cyst. Human infection is acquired by the ingestion of live encysted larvae. *H. nana* commonly develops also by internal autoinfection.

Pathophysiology[47]

Adult tapeworms do not produce any specific symptoms in the host. Whether in large numbers they produce nutritional deficits in the host is not well established. A trypsin inhibitor has been found on the surface of the rodent tapeworm, *H. diminuta*,[47] but whether such inhibitors are present in the major tapeworms infecting man is not known. Absorption of proteins of the worm has been claimed to lead to eosinophilia, allergic and neurological reactions and 'toxaemia', but these are not well established.

In the case of *T. solium* larval development in humans leads to cysticercosis, which most frequently manifests itself in central nervous system findings.[6] Although eggs may be released from the adult tapeworm and develop in the same host, it is generally believed that human cysticercosis is more likely the result of ingestion of eggs.

D. latum, because of its ability to take up vitamin B_{12} from the intrinsic factor–vitamin B_{12} complex, can lead to deficiency of the vitamin, and thus cause megaloblastic anemia.

Clinical features[7]

Intestinal infection by adult tapeworms is mostly asymptomatic. They may be first discovered during radiological examination (plain X-ray film, barium studies)[19] or stool microscopy. Mild abdominal cramps, 'hunger pains' and dyspepsia have all been described in tapeworm infection, but their relationship to worm infection has not been clearly established. In the presence of marginal nutrition a large worm load may lead to nutritional deficiencies. Occasionally, the finding of a gravid proglottid in the perianal region or stool or the presence of pain and pruritus in the perianal region is the presenting symptom. Intestinal obstruction and appendiceal obstruction with appendicitis have been rarely found with infection by the larger worms. Very rarely worms have been found in the gallbladder or perforating the intestine, leading to peritonitis. As earlier mentioned, *T. solium* infection may present with manifestations

Table 14.10 Intestinal tapeworms of man.

	Taenia solium	*Taenia saginata*	*Hymenolepis nana*	*Diphyllobothrium latum*
Scolex	Four suckers + hooklets	Four suckers	Four suckers + hooklets	Two grooved suckers
Length of worm (metres)	3–10	15–25	0.025–0.040	10–20
Proglottid	Length > Width	Length > Width	Width > Length	Width > Length
Uterus	Central stem with 7–13 lateral projections	Central stem with 15–20 lateral projections	Central sac-like	Central, rosette-shaped
Larval stage/ intermediate host	Cysticercus/pig (man)	Cysticercus/cattle	Cysticercoid/insects (man)	Procercoid in *Cyclops*; plerocercoid in fish
Mode of infection	Pork with live larvae	Beef with live larvae	Ingestion of ova or insects with larvae/eggs	Fish with live larvae

due to the larval stage, with neurological symptoms predominating. *D. latum* infection may present with neurological or haematological manifestations of vitamin B_{12} deficiency.

Diagnosis[7, 24]

The diagnosis of tapeworm infection is usually made by microscopic examination of the stool, when the characteristic eggs are noted (Figure 14.19h–j). Stools may also show the gravid proglottides and this allows identification of the species. Obtaining a sample from the perianal area using adhesive tape, as in the case of pinworm infection, may also be useful to demonstrate eggs or proglottides. Occasionally the tapeworms are seen on a plain X-ray film of the abdomen or a barium meal study.[19] Larval stages of *T. solium* (cysticercosis) may be demonstrated by appropriate scanning studies (e.g. CT scan of head).

Treatment[8, 24]

Niclosamide (Yomesan or Nicloside) is the drug of choice in the treatment of intestinal cestodiasis in man. The drug inhibits glucose uptake by the worm and mitochondrial oxidative phosphorylation and anaerobic metabolism of the worm. It may partially digest the scolex and segments. The usual adult dose is two grams given as a single dose or in two divided doses. The tablets have to be chewed well and taken with plenty of water and may be followed by a purgative. To confirm eradication of the worm the stool should be strained and examined for the scolex (or scolices, depending on number and type of worms), but if this is not possible follow-up stool microscopy a few months later is required. Associated vitamin and nutritional deficiency may also need to be treated.

Praziquantel, an isoquinolene derivative, has been found to be an effective drug in the treatment of intestinal taeniasis and diphyllobothriasis.[15, 43] Early clinical trials indicate that this drug produces 100% cure rates in intestinal taeniasis and diphyllobothriasis with a single dose of 10 mg/kg and 80% cure rate for hymenolepiasis with a single dose of 15–25 mg/kg. It is also one of the most effective agents against cerebral cysticercosis.

Mepacrine (quinacrine) is also an effective drug against intestinal tapeworm infection, but side-effects may be prominent. The usual adult dose of 1.0 g is taken in five equal doses over one hour along with sodium bicarbonate and is followed by a saline purge if spontaneous evacuation does not occur. Mepacrine may also be administered using a duodenal tube. Screening of stool for scolex or scolices and follow-up stool microscopy are needed to confirm worm expulsion.

No drug with ovicidal properties has been identified so far.

REFERENCES

1 Anthony, P. P. & McAdam, W. J. (1972) Helminthic pseudotumours of the bowel. Thirty four cases of helminthoma. *Gut*, **13**, 8–16.

2 Arean, V. M. & Crandall, C. A. (1971) Ascariasis. In *Pathology of Protozoal and Heminthic Diseases with Clinical Correlation* (Ed.) Marcial-Rojas, R. A. pp. 769–807. Baltimore: Williams & Wilkins.

3 Arean, V. M. & Crandall, C. A. (1971) Toxocariasis. In *Pathology of Protozoal and Helminthic Diseases with Clinical Correlation* (Ed.) Marcial-Rojas, R. A. pp. 808–842. Baltimore: Williams & Wilkins.

4 Banwell, J. G., Marsden, P. D., Blackman, V. *et al.* (1976) Hookworm infection and intestinal absorption amongst Africans in Uganda. *American Journal of Tropical Medicine and Hygiene*, **16**, 304–308.

5 Beaver, P. C., Snyder, C. H., Carrera, G. M. *et al.* (1952) Chronic eosinophilia due to visceral larva migrans. Report of three cases. *Pediatrics*, **9**, 7–19.

6 Botero, D. & Castano, S. (1982) Treatment of cerebral cysticercosis with praziquantel in Columbia. *American Journal of Tropical Medicine and Hygiene*, **31**, 810–821.

6 Carvalho-Filho, E. (1978) Strongyloidiasis. *Clinics in Gastroenterology*, **7**, 179–200.

7 Castillo, M. (1971) Intestinal taeniasis. In *Pathology of Protozoal and Helminthic Infections with Clinical Correlation* (Ed.) Marcial-Rojas, R. A. pp. 618–626. Baltimore: Williams & Wilkins.

8 Cline, B. L. (1982) Current drug regimens for the treatment of intestinal helminth infections. *Medical Clinics of North America*, **66**, 721–742.

9 Cremin, B. J. (1982) Ultrasonic diagnosis of biliary ascariasis. *British Journal of Radiology*, **55**, 683–684.

10 Cypress, R. H., Karol, M. H., Zidian, J. L. *et al.* (1977) Larva-specific antibodies in patients with visceral larva migrans. *Journal of Infectious Diseases*, **135**, 633–640.

11 Dorozynski, A. (1976) The altered or tropical disease. *Nature*, **262**, 85–87.

12 Dunn, F. L. (1979) Behavioral aspects of the control of parasitic diseases. *Bulletin of the World Health Organization*, **57**, 499–512.

13 Ellman, B. A., Wynne, J. M. & Freeman, A. (1980) Intestinal ascariasis: new plain film features. *American Journal of Roentgenology*, **135**, 37–42.

14 Fisher, R. M. & Cremin, B. T. (1970) Rectal bleeding due to *Trichuris*. *British Journal of Radiology*, **43**, 214–215.

15 Gemmell, M. A. & Johnstone, P. D. (1981) Cestodes. *Antibiotics and Chemotherapy*, **30**, 54–114.

16 Gill, G. V. & Bell, D. R. (1979) *Strongyloides stercoralis* infection in former Far East prisoners of war. *British Medical Journal*, **iii**, 572–574.

17 Glickman, L. T. & Schantz, P. M. (1981) Epidemiology and pathogenesis of zoonotic toxocariasis. *Epidemiologic Reviews*, **3**, 230–250.

18 Glickman, L. T., Schantz, P. M. & Cypress, R. H. (1979) Canine and human toxocariasis: review of transmission, pathogenesis and clinical disease. *Journal of the*

American Veterinary Medical Association, **175**, 1265–1269.

19 Gold, B. M. & Meyers, M. S. (1977) Radiologic manifestations of *Taenia saginata* infestation. *American Journal of Roentgenology*, **128**, 493–494.

20 Grove, D. I. (1980) Strongyloidiasis in Allied ex-prisoners-of-war in south-east Asia. *British Medical Journal*, **i**, 598–601.

21 Grove, J. I. & Blair, J. (1982) *Strongyloides ratti* and *S. stercoralis*. The effects of thiabendazole, mebendazole and cambendazole in infected mice. *American Journal of Tropical Medicine and Hygiene*, **31**, 469–476.

22 Igra-Siegman, Y., Kapila, R., Sen, P. et al. (1981) Syndrome of hyperinfection with *Strongyloides stercoralis*. *Reviews of Infectious Diseases*, **3**, 397–407.

23 Ihekwaba, F. N. (1980) Intestinal ascariasis and the acute abdomen in the tropics. *Journal of Royal College of Surgeons of Edinburgh*, **25**, 452–456.

24 *Intestinal Protozoan and Heminthic Infections. Report of a WHO Scientific Group (1981)* WHO Technical Report Series 666, Geneva, Switzerland.

25 Jones, T. C. (1978) Cestodes. *Clinics in Gastroenterology*, **7**, 105–128.

26 Kalkofen, U. P. (1974) Intestinal trauma resulting from feeding activities of *Ancylostoma caninum*. *American Journal of Tropical Medicine and Hygiene*, **16**, 613–619.

27 Layrisse, M., Apacedo, C. M. & Roche, M. (1967) Blood loss due to infection with *Trichuris trichiura*. *American Journal of Tropical Medicine and Hygiene*, **17**, 613–619.

28 Loia-Cortis, R. & Lobo-Sanahuja, F. (1980) Clinical abdominal angiostrongylosis. A study of 116 children with intestinal eosinophilic granuloma caused by *Angiostrongylus costaricensis*. *American Journal of Tropical Medicine and Hygiene*, **29**, 538–544.

29 Marcial-Rojas, R. A. (1971) Strongyloidiasis. In *Pathology of Protozoal and Helminthic Disease with Clinical Correlation* (Ed.) Marcial-Rojas, R. A. pp. 711–733. Baltimore: Williams & Wilkins.

30 Marsden, P. D. (Ed.) (1978) Intestinal parasites. *Clinics in Gastroenterology*, **7**(1) 1–243.

31 Marsden, P. D. (1978) Other nematodes. *Clinics in Gastroenterology*, **7**, 219–229.

32 Milder, J. E., Walzer, P. D., Kilgore, G. et al. (1981) Clinical features of *Strongyloides stercoralis* infection in an endemic area of the United States. *Gastroenterology*, **80**, 1481–1488.

33 Miller, T. A. (1979) Hookworm infection in man. *Advances in Parasitology*, **17**, 315–384.

34 Msreno, E. (1971) Enterobiasis. In *Pathology of Protozoal and Helminthic Disease with Clinical Correlation* (Ed.) Marcial-Rojas, R. A. pp. 760–768. Baltimore: Williams & Wilkins.

35 Mukerji, K., Saxena, K. C., Ghatak, S. & Misra, P. K. (1976) Studies on human ascaris: purification of trypsin inhibitor. *Indian Journal of Medical Research*, **64**, 1611–1619.

36 Neva, F. A., Gam, A. A. & Burke, J. (1981) Comparison of larval antigens in an enzyme-linked immunosorbent assay for strongyloidiasis in humans. *Journal of Infectious Diseases*, **144**, 427–432.

37 Ong, G. B. (1979) Helminthic diseases of the liver and biliary tract. In *Liver and Biliary Disease. Pathophysiology, Diagnosis, Management* (Ed.) Wright, R., Alberti, K. G. M. M., Karran, S. & Millward-Sadler, G. H. pp. 1267–1303. London: Saunders.

38 Pawlowski, A. S. (1978) Ascariasis. *Clinics in Gastroenterology*, **7**, 157–178.

39 Roche, M. & Layrisse, M. (1966) The nature and causes of 'hookworm anemia'. *American Journal of Tropical Medicine and Hygiene*, **15**, 1040–1100.

40 Schad, G. A. (1973) Arrested development in human hookworm infection: an adaptation to seasonally unfavorable environment. *Science*, **180**, 502–504.

41 Schad, G. A. & Banwell, J. G. (1978) Hookworm disease. *Clinics in Gastroenterology*, **7**, 129–156.

42 Schultz, M. G. (1982) The effects of *Ascaris lumbricoides* infection on nutritional status. *Reviews of Infectious Disease*, **4**, 815–819.

43 Sharma, S., Dubey, S. K. & Iyer, R. N. (1980) Chemotherapy of cestode infections. *Progress in Drug Research*, **24**, 217–266.

44 Signson, C. N., Banson, T. C. & Cross, J. H. (1975) Mebendazole in the treatment of intestinal capillariasis. *American Journal of Tropical Medicine and Hygiene*, **24**, 932–934.

45 Stephenson, L. S. (1980) The contribution of *Ascaris lumbricoides* to malnutrition in children. *Parasitology*, **81**, 221–233.

46 Symmers, W. C. (1950) Pathology of oxyuriasis. *Archives of Pathology*, **50**, 465–516.

47 Uglem, G. L. & Just, J. J. (1983) Trypsin inhibition by tapeworms: Antienzyme secretion or pH adjustment? *Science*, **220**, 79–81.

48 van Thiel, P. H. (1976) The present state of anisakiasis and its causative worms. *Tropical and Geographic Medicine*, **28**, 75–85.

49 Variyam, E. P. & Banwell, J. G. (1982) Hookworm disease: nutritional implications. *Reviews of Infectious Diseases*, **4**, 830–835.

50 Whalen, G. E., Strickland, G. T., Cross, J. H. et al. (1969) Intestinal capillariasis. A new disease in man. *Lancet*, **i**, 13–16.

51 Wolfe, M. (1978) *Oxyuris, Trichostrongylus* and *Trichuris*. *Clinics in Gastroenterology*, **7**, 201–217.

PSEUDOMEMBRANOUS COLITIS AND ANTIBIOTIC-ASSOCIATED COLITIS

Colitis associated with the use of antimicrobial agents is a relatively frequent and sometimes life-threatening .iatrogenic complication. There has been considerable progress in our understanding of this disease during the past decade. Initial work made extensive use of endoscopy to describe the incidence, pathological features and clinical observations. More recent studies have identified *Clostridium difficile*, a newly detected enteric-toxin-producing bacterium, as the aetiological agent in many or most cases.

Clinical features

Antibiotic-associated colitis is described as inflammation of the colon which occurs in association with the use of antimicrobial agents and is otherwise unexplained. Nearly all agents with a spectrum of activity against bacteria have been implicated, whereas drugs with activity restricted to mycobacteria, parasites or fungi do not appear to cause this complication. The most frequent offending agents are the lincomycins, ampicillin and the cephalosporins.[2] With these drugs, the incidence and severity of symptoms do not appear to correlate with the route of administration, dose or duration of treatment.

Most patients with antibiotic-associated colitis have diarrhoea as the initial and most prominent complaint. The stool in these cases is usually watery or mucoid; gross blood is relatively uncommon except in the haemorrhagic colitis which has been noted most frequently with ampicillin. The onset of diarrhoea is usually noted during the first four to ten days of antibiotic administration. However, at least one-third of patients note the initial change in bowel habits at any time up to four to six weeks after the implicated agent has been discontinued.[39] Common additional findings include abdominal cramps, abdominal tenderness, fever and leucocytosis. The spectrum of clinical findings ranges from 'simple' self-limited diarrhoea with no systemic complaints to severe colitis which may simulate an acute abdominal catastrophe. Late and serious complications include severe dehydration, electrolyte imbalance, hypotension, hypoalbuminaemia with anasarca, toxic megacolon or colonic perforation. Extraintestinal symptoms are rare, although occasional patients have polyarthritis. The natural course of the disease in different studies shows mortality rates which vary from nil[39] to 20%.[29]

Diagnosis

The most characteristic lesion is pseudomembranous colitis (PMC), with multiple elevated yellowish-white plaques which vary in size from a few millimetres to 15–20 mm in diameter.[36] The intervening mucosa may appear normal or show hyperaemia and oedema. Occasionally, the pseudomembranes coalesce to involve large segments of the colonic mucosa; these may slough to leave large denuded areas of mucosa. Histological studies show that pseudomembranes arise from a point of superficial ulceration on the intact mucosa. Lesions have been classified in three categories, which appear to be rather uniform in an individual patient.[32] The earliest or most mild form consists of focal necrosis with polymorphonuclear cells and an eosinophilic exudate in the lamina propria. Splaying out from the necrotic focus is a collection of fibrin and acute inflammatory cells which form the characteristic 'summit lesion'. The second category shows disrupted glands containing mucin and polymorphonuclear cells sur-

mounted by typical pseudomembranes. Both types of lesion show areas of intervening normal mucosa, and the inflammatory changes are limited to the superficial portion of the lamina propria, predominantly subepithelial in location. The third and most advanced form of the disease shows complete structural necrosis with extensive involvement of the lamina propria, which is overlaid by a thick confluent pseudomembrane. Pseudomembranous colitis is the most severe form of colitis noted with antibiotic-associated diarrhoea. Patients without demonstrable pseudomembranes may also have granularity and friability of the intestinal mucosa visible on gross inspection, and histological changes may resemble those noted with idiopathic ulcerative colitis.

The preferred method to establish the diagnosis is by endoscopy. The distal colon is involved in the majority of patients, so that sigmoidoscopy is generally adequate. However, about 20% have typical lesions restricted to the right colon, necessitating the use of colonoscopy. Care must be exercised in endoscopic technique in order to detect and biopsy appropriate lesions.[36] Copious amounts of mucus must often be removed with caution in order to avoid separation of pseudomembranes from the typical stalk attachment which is necessary for histological confirmation of PMC. Radiological studies, especially air-contrast examinations, may show typical lesions of PMC.[34] However, this procedure must be performed with caution because of the potential complication of colonic perforation; it is not considered to be as sensitive or specific as endoscopy.

Microbiology

Studies from the 1950s suggested that *Staphylococcus aureus* was responsible for most cases of antibiotic-associated colitis.[3] The diagnosis at that time was usually based on the detection of this organism with direct stains and culture of stool specimens. Many now regard this work as rather inconclusive because of the frequency with which staphylococci may be found in the stools of healthy persons, especially those who have received antibiotics. It is not possible in retrospect to know if 'staphylococcal enterocolitis' was a valid diagnosis or simply a reflection of the keen concern devoted to the organism at that time.[3] At any rate, this organism does not appear to be an important cause of antibiotic-associated colitis according to more recent reviews.[22]

The only currently recognized agent of antibiotic-associated colitis is *Clostridium difficile*. This organism was originally described in 1935 as a component of the normal faecal flora of newborn infants.[19] Studies at that time showed that the isolates produced a toxin which proved lethal to a variety of experimental animals. Nevertheless, the role of *C. difficile* as a clinically significant pathogen was not recognized until 1977, when Koch's postulates were satisfied for this as the agent of antibiotic-associated colitis.[4, 5]

The preferred method to implicate *C. difficile* as a cause of colitis is a tissue culture assay on stool to detect a cytopathic toxin which is neutralized by *C. sordellii* or *C. difficile* antitoxin.[5, 21, 25] This is recognized as a highly sensitive and specific test which is preferred to stool cultures because of its relative simplicity and improved specificity according to clinical correlations.[42] The cytopathic toxin produced by this organism shows highly characteristic actinomorphic changes in cell lines containing fibroblast cells; the quantity necessary to elicit these changes is only 0.2–5 pg.[35] The cytotoxin is thermolabile, showing decreases in titre which correlate directly with time and temperature.[18] Thus, specimens which must be referred to laboratories at distant locations should be sent utilizing a transport system that will ensure delivery within 24 hours, or the specimens should be maintained in a frozen state prior to processing. Results of the assay are available in 24 hours. Titres may be determined using serial dilutions, but these do not correlate with the severity of clinical symptoms.[8] Thus, the most important feature of the test is to demonstrate the toxin: concentrations are of little value in judging severity.

The clinical experience with *C. difficile* toxin assays indicates that nearly all patients with antibiotic-associated pseudomembranous colitis have positive tests (Table 14.11). The incidence among patients with other forms of colitis associated with antibiotic usage is 50–75%. Approximately 10–20% of patients with 'simple' diarrhoea complicating a course of antibiotic exposure will have this toxin. These data indicate that *C. difficile* has been implicated in the entire spectrum of clinical and pathological changes noted in patients with antibiotic-associated diarrhoea and colitis. However, the incidence of the toxin seems to increase with the severity of the disease process. Nevertheless, it is necessary to emphasize that some patients with antibiotic exposure will have positive assays with no change in bowel habits and many have very trivial bouts of self-limited diarrhoeal disease. The only other patient population in which this toxin has been detected with any frequency is infants.[23, 27, 33, 42] The incidence in this population is between 14% and 43% and it is not associated with overt symptoms in the vast majority. Carriage rates for the organism and the toxin decrease during the first year of life so that virtually all children over two years old have negative toxin assays unless there is antibiotic exposure. Pseudomembranous colitis was reported long before antibiotics were available and, although most cases occur in this setting, there are other identifiable risk factors. Limited experience in patients with PMC which occurs independently of antibiotic exposure shows that *C. difficile* is usually implicated. Some investigators have noted high rates of positive assays in patients with inflammatory bowel disease and severe relapse,[41] but this has not been a consistent observation.[28]

Table 14.11 Incidence of *Clostridium difficile* toxin assay in various patient populations.

Patient category	Author's experience[a]	Literature experience[b]
Antibiotic-associated pseudomembranous colitis (PMC)	136/141 (96%)	83–100%
Antibiotic-associated diarrhoea or colitis without PMC	193/710 (27%)	17–34%
Gastrointestinal diseases unrelated to antibiotic usage	9/562 (2%)	2%
Antibiotic exposure without diarrhoea	2/110 (2%)	2–8%
Healthy adults	0/60	0–0.5%
Healthy neonates	12/45 (27%)	14–43%

[a] Number positive/number of patients examined.
[b] Incidence range based on reported experience.[1, 15, 18, 21, 23, 25, 26, 27, 29, 33]

Pathogenesis

The pathogenesis of antibiotic-associated colitis involving *C. difficile* appears to require antibiotic exposure, a source of the organism and toxin production.

The organism appears to be a component of the normal flora of approximately 3% of healthy adults who are presumed to be at risk when given an appropriate inducing agent. However, outbreaks of this complication have been reported in hospitals, suggesting exogenous sources of the organism as well.[29] Environmental cultures show excessive recovery rates in case-associated areas compared to control sites, the most common sources being toilets, bedpans and floors, as well as the hands and stools of asymptomatic hospital personnel caring for these patients.[16] Another potential source is endoscopy equipment, which appears to have been implicated in at least one major outbreak.[29] These data suggest that *C. difficile*-induced disease occurs sporadically among previously asymptomatic carriers and may also reflect acquisition of the organism from contaminated sources by patients who are rendered susceptible by administration of antimicrobial agents.

An impressive feature of *C. difficile*-induced enteric disease is that it occurs almost exclusively in the presence of antibiotic exposure. An attractive thesis is that this represents a superinfection involving the selection of resistant strains which are allowed to flourish when the competing flora is inhibited. In vitro susceptibility tests do not support this concept in either experimental animals or patients, since the organisms recovered are often susceptible to the agent implicated in causing the disease.[43] For example, ampicillin represents one of the most frequent offending agents despite the fact that this antibiotic is almost uniformly active against *C. difficile*. Similarly, approximately half of the strains recovered in patients with clindamycin-induced colitis are highly susceptible to this antibiotic. The implication is that sensitivity profiles of *C. difficile* isolates are not particularly useful in determining drugs which are likely to cause the complication, although they may prove useful in determining potential therapeutic agents. The role of antimicrobial agents in altering the normal colonic flora with the elimination of colonization resistance appears to be a critical factor in pathogenesis. Studies in experimental animals have shown three models of *C. difficile*-induced colonic disease: lethal diarrhoea in newborn hares,[14] mono-contaminated germ-free mice[31] and guinea pigs or hamsters given a variety of antimicrobial agents.[4] The common denominator in all three examples is an alteration of the normal flora found in healthy adult animals.

C. difficile-induced colitis is a toxin-mediated enteric disease in which typical pathological changes are noted after intraluminal challenge using the cell-free supernatant of *C. difficile* or its partially purified toxins.[4, 38] Mucosal invasion by the organism has not been observed. Studies of the toxin per se are somewhat complicated since this work indicates that the organism produces at least two toxins, designated toxin A and toxin B.[35, 38] These are large-molecular-weight proteins with somewhat different biological activities. Toxin B is a potent cytotoxin which presumably accounts for the changes noted in tissue-cultured cells. Toxin A is more active in animal models of enteric disease such as the rabbit ileal loop assay; this toxin may be more important in clinical expression and pathological changes associated with *C. difficile*-induced disease. The organism produces both toxins at the termination of log-phase growth, suggesting release with lysis of replicating strains. Most strains of *C. difficile* are toxigenic, although there is considerable variation in the amount of toxin produced in vitro.[42] This work suggests that the central role of antibiotics is a reflection of their impact on the normal flora, resulting in deregulated growth of *C. difficile* which is present either as a component of the normal flora or acquired from an environmental source. Toxin levels measured in the cytotoxicity assay and differences in clinical expression may reflect, in part, variations in toxigenic potential as well as growth rates.

An additional factor to emphasize in pathogenesis concerns the apparent age-related risk. As previously noted, infants often harbour *C. difficile* and its toxins with no deleterious consequences. *C. difficile* has been clearly implicated in antibiotic-associated diarrhoea and colitis in older children, but the incidence appears to be substantially less than in older individuals, considering the frequency with which ampicillin and other antibiotics are used in this population. Prospective studies of antibiotic-associated diarrhoea show an age-related risk for this complication. Studies in the pre-antibiotic era indicated that the patients most vulnerable to PMC were those with intestinal neoplasms, ischaemia or surgery.[21] The implication is that age and physiological disturbances of the colon may enhance susceptibility to *C. difficile* toxin.

Treatment

Colitis should be suspected in any patient who develops diarrhoea which is otherwise unexplained and occurs during or up to six weeks following antibiotic exposure. As previously noted, this complication has been most frequently seen in patients given ampicillin, lincomycins or cephalosporins, although almost any drug with antibacterial activity may be responsible. These include some cancer-chemotherapeutic agents as well.[13] Stool examination may show leucocytes, especially with pancolitis, but this is a relatively non-specific observation and not consistently seen. The preferred method to establish the diagnosis of colitis or PMC is endoscopy. The preferred method to detect *C. difficile*, the major recognized putative agent, is the tissue-culture assay to detect *C. difficile* toxin. It is emphasized that this organism has been implicated in the entire spectrum of anatomical changes found in the colon of patients with antibiotic-associated diarrhoea ranging from an entirely normal mucosa to the most serious and characteristic form of colitis, PMC. Thus, a distinction is made between studies done to establish the anatomical diagnosis and those used for an aetiological diagnosis. Utilization of either endoscopy or the toxin assay is considered cost-effective only for patients with severe or persistent symptoms. The major indications are for patients with systemic complaints, those with severe or debilitating diarrhoea, patients undergoing diagnostic evaluation for other causes of gastrointestinal complaints and patients with prolonged diarrhoea following discontinuation of the implicated agent. Previous studies indicate that most patients with antibiotic-associated diarrhoea have resolution of their bowel complaints within one to two weeks without specific therapy other than discontinuation of the implicated agent.

Patients with severe disease should be treated with appropriate supportive measures including intravenous fluids to correct fluid and electrolyte disturbances. Antiperistaltic drugs should be avoided.[30] The use of corticosteroids is controversial, although some recommend these drugs for severely ill individuals. Patients with *C. difficile*-induced disease pose an epidemiological hazard to susceptible hosts within the hospital setting, especially if they are incontinent. Specific guidelines to eliminate spread are limited, although many authorities recommend enteric precautions at least until diarrhoea resolves or the organism is eliminated.[16]

Specific forms of therapy are available only for *C. difficile*, utilizing antibiotics directed against the putative agent or anion-exchange resins to bind *C. difficile* toxin (Table 14.12). Vancomycin is the most frequently advocated antibiotic for several reasons. This drug is active against virtually all strains of *C. difficile*, and it is not absorbed when given orally so that levels within the colonic lumen are extremely high while systemic absorption is nil.[21, 40] The clinical experience with this drug indicates that most patients have a prompt eradication of fever and other systemic complaints within 24–48 hours and a gradual resolution of diarrhoea over two to fourteen days. Nearly all patients respond. The major problems are the high cost of the drug, its unpalatable taste and a relatively high incidence of relapses. The incidence of relapses in our experience is 24% among 189 patients with *C. difficile*-induced disease, and some of these individuals suffered repeated relapses with sequential courses. Other investigators have noted the incidence of relapse to vary from nil[21] to 35%.[17] Relapses are characterized by the recurrence of diarrhoeal symptoms with positive toxin assays for *C. difficile* at 2–30 days following discontinuation of oral vancomycin treatment.[6] Cultures at this time indicate that the

Table 14.12   Treatment of *Clostridoum difficile*-induced colitis

1   Seriously ill patients
   a   Oral regimen (preferred): vancomycin 125–500 mg orally, 4 times daily, 7–14 days
   b   Parenteral regimen: metronidazole 500 mg intravenously every 6 hours until patient will tolerate oral medications

2   Moderately ill patients
   a   Vancomycin, 125–500 mg orally, 4 times daily, 7–14 days
   b   Bacitracin, 500 mg (25 000 units) orally, 4 times daily, 7–14 days
   c   Metronidazole, 250 mg orally, 3 times daily, 7–14 days
   d   Cholestyramine, 4 g packet orally, 4 times daily, 7–14 days

3   Relapses following treatment
   a   Repeat any of above regimens
   b   Vancomycin, 125–500 mg orally, 4 times daily, 7–14 days; followed by cholestyramine, 4 g orally, 4 times daily, 2–3 weeks

implicated strains are susceptible to vancomycin. Two postulated mechanisms for relapse are (a) that the organism is never eliminated from the intestinal tract because of sporulation or (b) that a new strain is acquired from environmental sources in a host who is susceptible owing to reduced colonization resistance following vancomycin treatment.

Alternative antibiotics which may be used include bacitracin and metronidazole. Bacitracin has the same potential advantages as vancomycin in that it is active against most strains of *C. difficile* and it is poorly absorbed when given by the oral route so that levels in the colonic lumen are exceptionally high.[11] Metronidazole is extremely active against *C. difficile* in vitro. However, this drug is well absorbed when given orally, levels in the colonic lumen are modest and this drug has been implicated in causing *C. difficile* disease in occasional patients. Despite these disadvantages, the initial experience is favourable, the drug is considerably cheaper than vancomycin and it may be preferred for parenteral therapy among patients who are too seriously ill to receive oral medications.[12, 27]

The anion-exchange resin most frequently used is cholestyramine but the clinical experience with these resins is highly variable, ranging from universal success[24] to almost no detectable response.[20] In view of this erratic track record, cholestyramine is generally reserved for patients who are less seriously ill or have contraindications to vancomycin. This drug should not be given concurrently with vancomycin since it binds the antibiotic to produce a marked reduction in stool levels of biologically active drug.[37]

The loss of colonization resistance is a fundamental factor in the pathophysiology of *C. difficile*-induced enteric disease, so attempts to re-establish the normal flora are a theoretically attractive approach to treatment. Recolonization with lactobacilli has not been extensively studied, although previous experience with this approach shows that repopulation may be difficult to achieve, possibly reflecting the fact that these organisms are not prevalent components of the normal flora. A more physiological approach is use of faecal enemas; this has proved modestly successful in animal models as well as in patients with antibiotic-associated colitis.[7] Despite theoretical advantages, this approach is unlikely to gain wide acceptance owing to its lack of aesthetic appeal as well as the possibility of transmitting an enteric pathogen.

REFERENCES

1 Aronsson, B., Mollby, R. & Nord, C. E. (1981) Occurrence of toxin-producing *Clostridium difficile* in antibiotic-associated diarrhea in Sweden. *Medical Microbiology and Immunology*, **170**, 27–35.

2 Bartlett, J. G. (1981) Antimicrobial agents implicated in *Clostridium difficile* toxin-associated diarrhea or colitis. *Johns Hopkins Medical Journal*, **149**, 6–9.

3 Bartlett, J. G. & Gorbach, S. L. (1977) Pseudomembranous colitis. In *Advances in Internal Medicine* (Ed.) Stollerman, G. H. pp. 455–476. Chicago: Yearbook Medical Publishers.

4 Bartlett, J. G., Onderdonk, A. B., Cisneros, A. B. & Kasper, D. L. (1977) Clindamycin-associated colitis due to toxin-producing species of clostridium in hamsters. *Journal of Infectious Disease*, **136**, 701–705.

5 Bartlett, J. G., Chang, T. W., Gurwith, M. *et al.* (1978) Antibiotic associated pseudomembranous colitis due to toxin-producing clostridia. *New England Journal of Medicine*, **198**, 531–534.

6 Bartlett, J. G., Tedesco, F. J., Shull, S. & Lowe, B. (1979) Relapse following oral vancomycin therapy of antibiotic-associated pseudomembranous colitis. *Gastroenterology*, **78**, 431–434.

7 Bowden, T. A. Jr., Mansberger, A. R. Jr. & Lykins, L. E. (1981) Pseudomembranous enterocolitis: mechanism for restoring floral homeostasis. *American Surgery*, **47**, 178–183.

8 Burdon, D. W., George, R. H. & Mogg, G. (1981) Faecal toxin and severity of antibiotic-associated pseudomembranous colitis. *Journal of Clinical Pathology*, **34**, 548–551.

9 Chang, T. W., Lauermann, M. & Bartlett, J. G. (1979) Cytotoxicity assay in antibiotic-associated colitis. *Journal of Infectious Disease*, **140**, 765–770.

10 Chang, T. W., Lin, P. S., Gorbach, S. L. & Bartlett, J. G. (1979) Ultrastructural changes of cultured human amnion cells by *Clostridium difficile* toxin. *Infection and Immunology*, **23**, 795–798.

11 Chang, T. W., Gorbach, S. L., Bartlett, J. G. & Saginur, R. (1980) Bacitracin treatment of antibiotic-associated colitis and diarrhea caused by *Clostridium difficile*. *Gastroenterology*, **78**, 1584–1586.

12 Cherry, R. D., Portnoy, D., Jabbari, M. *et al.* (1982) Metronidazole: an alternate therapy for antibiotic-associated colitis. *Gastroenterology*, **82**, 849–851.

13 Cudmore, M. A., Silva, J. Jr., Fekety, R. *et al.* (1982) *Clostridium difficile* colitis associated with cancer chemotherapy. *Archives of Internal Medicine*, **142**, 333–335.

14 Dabard, J., Dubos, F., Martinet, L. & Ducluzeau, R. (1979) Experimental reproduction of neonatal diarrhea in young gnotobiotic hares simultaneously associated with *Clostridium difficile* and other clostridial species. *Infection and Immunology*, **24**, 7–11.

15 Delmee, M. & Wauters, G. (1981) Rôle de *Clostridium difficile* dans les diarrhées survenant après antibiothérapie: étude de 87 cas. *Acta Clinica Belgica*, **36**, 178–184.

16 Fekety, R., Kim, K-H., Brown, D. *et al.* (1981) Epidemiology of antibiotic-associated colitis. *American Journal of Medicine*, **70**, 906–908.

17 George, W. L., Rolfe, R. D., Harding, G. K. M. *et al.* (1982) *Clostridium difficile* and cytotoxin in feces of patients with antimicrobial agent-associated pseudomembranous colitis. *Infection*, **10**, 205–207.

18 Gilligan, P. H., McCarthy, L. R. & Genta, V. M. (1981) Relative frequency of *Clostridium difficile* in patients with diarrheal disease. *Journal of Clinical Microbiology*, **14**, 26–31.

19 Hall, I. C. & O'Toole, E. (1935) Intestinal flora in newborn infants with description of a new pathogenic anaerobe, *Bacillus difficilis. American Journal of Diseases of Children*, **49**, 390–402.

20 Keighley, M. R. B. (1980) Antibiotic-associated pseudomembranous colitis. Pathogenesis and management. *Drugs*, **20**, 49–56.

21 Keighley, M. R. B., Burdon, D. W., Arabi, Y. *et al.* (1978) Randomized controlled trial of vancomycin for pseudomembranous colitis and postoperative diarrhoea. *British Medical Journal*, **ii**, 1667–1669.

22 Keusch, G. T. & Present, D. H. (1976) Summary of workshop on clindamycin colitis. *Journal of Infectious Disease*, **133**, 578–587.

23 Kim, K-H., Fekety, R., Botts, D. H. *et al.* (1981) Isolation of *Clostridium difficile* from the environment and contacts of patients with antibiotic-associated colitis. *Journal of Infectious Disease*, **143**, 42–50.

24 Kreutzer, E. W. & Milligan, F. D. (1978) Treatment of antibiotic-associated pseudomembranous colitis with cholestyramine resin. *Johns Hopkins Medical Journal*, **143**, 67–72.

25 Larson, H. E., Price, A. B., Honour, P. & Borriello, S. P. (1978) *Clostridium difficile* and the aetiology of pseudomembranous colitis. *Lancet*, **i**, 1062–1066.

26 Lishman, A. H., Al-Jumaili, I. J. & Record, C. O. (1981) Spectrum of antibiotic-associated diarrhea. *Gut*, **22**, 34–37.

27 Meuwissen, S. G. M. & Rietra, P. J. G. M. (1980) Antibiotic-associated pseudomembranous colitis. *Acta Gastro-enterologica Belgica*, **43**, 377–385.

28 Meyers, S., Mayer, L., Bottone, E. *et al.* (1981) Occurrence of *Clostridium difficile* toxin during the course of inflammatory bowel disease. *Gastroenterology*, **80**, 697–700.

29 Mogg, G. M., Keighley, M., Burdon D. *et al.* (1979) Antibiotic-associated colitis – a review of 66 cases. *British Journal of Surgery*, **66**, 738.

30 Novak, E., Lee, J. G., Seckman, C. E. *et al.* (1976) Unfavorable effect of atropinediphenoxylate (Lomotil) therapy in clindamycin-caused diarrhea. *Journal of the American Medical Association*, **235**, 1451–1454.

31 Onderdonk, A. B., Cisneros, R. L., & Bartlett, J. G. (1980) Study of *Clostridium difficile* in gnotobiotic mice. *Infection and Immunity*, **28**, 227–282.

32 Price, A. B. & Davies, D. R. (1977) Pseudomembranous colitis. *Journal of Clinical Pathology*, **30**, 1–12.

33 Sheretz, R. J. & Sarubbi, F. A. (1982) The prevalence of *Clostridium difficile* and toxin in a nursery population: a comparison between patients with necrotizing enterocolitis and an asymptomatic group. *Journal of Pediatrics*, **100**, 435–439.

34 Stanley, R. J., Melson, G. L. & Tedesco, F. J. (1974) The spectrum of radiographic findings in antibiotic-related pseudomembranous colitis. *Radiology*, **111**, 519–524.

35 Sullivan, N. M., Pellett, S. & Wilkins, T. D. (1982) Purification and characterization of toxins A and B of *Clostridium difficile. Infection and Immunology*, **35**, 1032–1040.

36 Sumner, H. W. & Tedesco, F. J. (1975) Rectal biopsy in clindamycin-associated colitis. *Archives of Pathology*, **9**, 237.

37 Taylor, N. S. & Bartlett, J. G. (1980) Binding of *Clostridium difficile* cytotoxin and vancomycin by anion exchange resins. *Journal of Infectious Disease*, **141**, 92–97.

38 Taylor, N. S., Thorne, G. M. & Bartlett, J. G. (1981) Comparison of two toxins produced by *Clostridium difficile. Infection and Immunology*, **34**, 1036–1043.

39 Tedesco, F. J., Barton, R. W. & Alpers, H. D. (1974) Clindamycin-associated colitis. *Annals of Internal Medicine*, **81**, 429–433.

40 Tedesco, F. J., Markam, R., Gurwith, M. *et al.* (1978) Oral vancomycin therapy of antibiotic-associated pseudomembranous colitis. *Lancet*, **ii**, 226–228.

41 Trnka, Y. M. & LaMont, J. T. (1981) Association of *Clostridium difficile* toxin with symptomatic relapse of chronic inflammatory bowel disease. *Gastroenterology*, **80**, 693–696.

42 Viscidi, R., Willey, S. & Bartlett, J. G. (1981) Isolation rates and toxigenic potential of *Clostridium difficile* isolates from various patient populations. *Gastroenterology*, **81**, 5–9.

43 Willey, S. H. & Bartlett, J. G. (1979) Cultures for *Clostridium difficile* in stools containing a cytotoxin neutralized by *Clostridium sordellii* antitoxin. *Journal of Clinical Microbiology*, **10**, 880–884.

TRAVELLER'S DIARRHOEA

With the considerable increase in international travel during the last decade there has been an explosive increase in the number of acute attacks of diarrhoea among visitors (on holiday or on business) and temporary residents (volunteers or contract workers) in areas where sanitation and hygiene are poor.[14] The attacks are most frequent in tropical areas and instructive eponyms such as Delhi Belly, the Aztec Two-Step and Basrah Belly are used to describe the illness. However in southern Europe (particularly the Mediterranean), some areas of Russia and parts of the USA there have also been epidemics of acute diarrhoea among travellers.

Microbiology

Traveller's diarrhoea may be caused by a variety of bacteria, viruses and parasites. Although certain enteropathogens such as *Shigella* spp.,[2] *Salmonella* spp. and *Campylobacter* spp.[1] can be identified by the use of appropriate culture media and incubation conditions, the commonest bacterial enteropathogens, such as *Escherichia coli* which produce enterotoxins (ETEC), have only been recognized during the last decade because of the development of appropriate methods for toxin detection.[7] ETEC may produce two main types of enterotoxin: heat-labile (LT) and heat-stable (ST). LT used to be detected by measurements of the quantity of fluid secretion when bacterial filtrates were inoculated into a loop of rabbit ileum, but recently characteristic effects on tissue culture cell lines (especially Y-1 adrenal and CHO) have been demonstrated. LT has a large molecular weight (about 100 000) and immunological methods such as the enzyme-linked immunosorbent assay (ELISA) and the gel precipitation (BIKEN) test may be used for its detection. ST is rather small (molecular weight around 4000) for satisfactory immunological tests and has no effect on tissue culture cells. It is usually detected by observing the fluid secretion in the intestine of weanling mice.

Both ST and LT produce fluid secretion without damaging the intestinal mucosa. The toxins bind to the enterocytes, enter the cells and increase the intracellular concentrations of adenylate cyclase. This in turn increases the concentrations of the cyclic nucleotides (cGMP or cAMP), which stimulate secretion of fluid and electrolytes from the enterocytes into the intestinal lumen. There is also a third group of toxins called CT toxins characterized by their cytopathic effects on tissue-culture cell lines; these effects are distinguishable from those of LT.

ETEC should be differentiated from two other types of *E. coli*, which cause diarrhoea by other mechanisms: firstly, enteroinvasive *E. coli* (EIEC) damage the mucosal epithelium (especially in the colon) to produce a typical dysentery syndrome of blood and mucus, and secondly, enteropathogenic *E. coli* (EPEC). The latter have traditionally been identified by serotyping because of the characteristic presence of these organisms in epidemics of diarrhoea in infants and children and, less commonly, in adults. Their mechanism of action is not well defined and conventional tests for enterotoxin are negative. However, EPEC can cause diarrhoea in volunteers and when filtrates are perfused into the intestines of experimental animals they induce secretion of fluid and electrolytes.

Rotavirus and Norwalk agent are recognized as important causes of traveller's diarrhoea.[13] Both cause tissue destruction of the jejunal mucosa and there is acute watery diarrhoea without blood or mucus. Although the viruses are most reliably detected by electron microscopy, recent ELISA techniques applied to whole faecal homogenates have been successful. A rising titre of serum antibodies may be used to confirm a diagnosis retrospectively.

Parasitic infections are diagnosed microscopically on appropriately prepared samples. It is important to recognize that cysts and trophozoites of *Giardia lamblia* are intermittently excreted and a single microscopic examination may miss the diagnosis.[15] Trophozoites of *Entamoeba histolytica* may be identified microscopically if fresh specimens are examined.

Clinical features

Diarrhoea often occurs within a few days of arriving in a contaminated area. The attack may be brief, lasting less than 24 hours, but often lasts for three to five days.[6] There are several forms of clinical presentation, which vary according to the nature of the infecting organism:

1 Watery diarrhoea with normally coloured stools. This is the most frequent presentation, commonly due to ETEC, rotavirus, Norwalk agent or *Campylobacter*.
2 Initial watery diarrhoea progressing to malabsorption. This suggests the presence of *Giardia lamblia*.
3 Dysentery (blood and mucus). This suggests the presence of EIEC, *Shigella* spp., *Salmonella* spp. or *Entamoeba histolytica*.

Nausea and abdominal pain may be common and vomiting (especially with Norwalk agent) also occurs. Pyrexia, headache and rigors are often experienced in the first few days. A few patients have severe fluid and electrolyte loss, with hypokalaemia in severe illness. The combination of nausea, anorexia and vomiting causes some weight loss in most patients but this is usually regained quickly.

Prognosis

Most sufferers from traveller's diarrhoea, particularly those with acute watery diarrhoea syndrome, recover within the first week. In others, for example those with *Giardia lamblia* or *Entamoeba histolytica*, symptoms can persist for many weeks. A further group recovers from the initial watery diarrhoea, but protracted diarrhoea with symptoms of malabsorption occurs. This postinfective malabsorption syndrome appears to be related to bacterial colonization of the upper intestine which develops at the time of, or soon after, the acute diarrhoea.

Investigations

These should be considered in relation to treatment, because the bacteriological findings do not influence management in the majority of patients who have a brief, self-limiting disease. When there is acute watery diarrhoea the diagnosis of ETEC, rotavirus and Norwalk agent can be made on single faecal specimens by a combination of ELISA tests and bioassay. Most laboratories can offer routine diagnosis of rotavirus and Norwalk agent by ELISA but documentation of ETEC requires referral to a specialist laboratory. In dysenteric diarrhoea it is essential to culture on specific media for *Salmonella* spp. and *Shigella* spp. and to use specific culture media and incubation conditions for *Campylobacter*, which are microaerophilic. EPEC may be identified by serotyping. It is important to subject the stools to light microscopy for the detection of trophozoites and cysts of *Entamoeba histolytica* and *Giardia lamblia* in traveller's diarrhoea that persists for more than one week.

Differential diagnosis

There are several groups of diseases which should be considered: firstly, other diarrhoeal diseases that are endemic in a particular area (e.g. *Vibrio cholerae, Aeromonas* spp., *Yersinia enterocolitica, Vibrio parahaemolyticus*); secondly, diarrhoea which presents as part of a food-poisoning syndrome, in which nausea and vomiting are classically the dominant symptoms (e.g. *Staphylococcus aureus, Bacillus cereus, Clostridium perfringens*); thirdly, diarrhoea which is the presenting symptom in the first attack of inflammatory bowel disease.

Treatment

The majority of patients require an explanation of the expected natural history and cause of the disease together with symptomatic therapy and reassurance. Antibiotics are rarely indicated.

SYMPTOMATIC TREATMENT

Complete rest and a liquid diet for 48 hours will often improve the diarrhoea. It is best to replace fluid and electrolyte losses at an early stage. This may be achieved using the WHO formula oral rehydration solution glucose–electrolyte packets, which are made up in water to give a fluid concentration of glucose 110 mmol/l, sodium 90 mmol/l and potassium 20 mmol/l.[11] These concentrations ensure that the glucose stimulates the absorption of sodium and water, even in the presence of a damaged mucosa. If the packets are not available travellers can make a sugar and salt solution themselves, using a small soft-drink bottle (300 ml) and its cap as a measure (one level capful of salt plus eight level capfuls of sugar in three bottles of water gives a sodium concentration of about 90 mmol/l). Lucozade (a soft drink containing glucose) is a good source of sugar and water but it requires the addition of salt. A cup of Marmite yeast extract (constituted using one level teaspoon of Marmite in 150 ml of water) is another useful source of sodium – this recipe provides 60 mmol/l of sodium. However, it requires glucose or sugar to stimulate the sodium absorption.

ANTIDIARRHOEAL AGENTS

In the majority of patients symptomatic therapy alone is sufficient, but if abdominal discomfort is severe it is advisable to use drugs which reduce intestinal motility, such as loperamide, diphenoxylate or codeine phosphate. Their use should be restricted to adults because in young children they tend to permit some enteropathogens to proliferate to dangerous levels in the intestine. Drugs which make the stool more formed by increasing its bulk, such as kaolin, have a good reputation for reducing the explosive watery stools. They are generally safe but they do nothing to reduce the electrolyte or water loss. A recently introduced drug, bismuth salicylate (subsalicylate), does reduce the fluid loss and abdominal pain. So far, unfortunately, it has been proven to be effective only in traveller's diarrhoea due to ETEC; it does not improve the diarrhoea caused by EIEC or *Shigella* spp. *Lactobacillus* has been prescribed for diarrhoea, usually in the form of yoghurt or in dried bacterial form. The rationale is sound in that lactobacilli may produce an intestinal milieu which is inhibitory to several enteropathogens, but unfortunately several trials have failed to show any significant benefit in traveller's diarrhoea.

ANTIBIOTICS

There are only a few indications for antibiotic administration and it is essential to consider the local pattern of drug resistance. This may be a severe problem and recently there has been a striking increase in the numbers of strains of *Shigella* spp. and *Salmonella* spp. with multiple antibiotic resistance patterns among travellers returning to the UK from abroad, especially the subcontinent of India. The most appropriate antibiotic will be indicated by the drug sensitivity pattern but ampicillin, tetracycline and co-trimoxazole (trimethoprim plus sulphamethoxazole) may be useful. Antibiotics should be reserved for patients with moderate or severe dysentery; those in whom diarrhoea is improving spontaneously and those who are asymptomatic carriers should not receive antibiotics.

Similar indications apply in those with *Salmonella* spp. infections. Mild dysentery or watery diarrhoea is best left untreated. Indeed, antibiotic therapy may actually prolong excretion in asymptomatic carriers. Ampicillin, chloramphenicol and co-trimoxazole are the most useful for those with severe dysentery.

Giardia lamblia is treated with metronidazole or tinidazole.

Entamoeba histolytica is treated with a combination of metronidazole, which is active against trophozoites, and diloxanide furoate, which is active against cysts.

Prophylaxis

The best way to avoid diarrhoea is by avoiding those foods or drinks which are faecally contaminated.[5] The traveller should be made aware of the high-risk areas. Among British travellers most cases of diarrhoea occur in those who visit the Mediterranean, North Africa, the Middle East, the Far East, the Indian subcontinent or Central America. Any food, however well presented, can be bacteriologically contaminated, but salads, fresh fruits and fruit juices, especially those bought from street vendors, are all hazardous. It is often valuable to use local knowledge about which restaurants and cafés have reliable reputations. If the visitor is self-catering then salads, vegetables and fruit can be soaked in solutions of potassium permanganate or sodium hypochlorite. Although most enteropathogens are contracted from food rather than water it is important to caution against drinking any tapwater. Bottled drinks and boiled beverages are usually safe. If it is essential to drink local water, purifying tablets can be used, and lightweight portable water filters suitable for packing in a small suitcase are available.

Chemoprophylaxis is becoming more popular but not all drugs are effective. Of the antimicrobials there is some evidence that sulphathiazole, clioquinol,[10] Streptotriad (sulphadiazine, sulphadimidine, sulphathiazole and streptomycin), neomycin, trimethoprim,[4] co-trimoxazole[4] and doxycycline[12] protect against diarrhoea. However, side-effects are important: these include optic nerve damage (clioquinol), mucosal damage (neomycin), skin rashes (co-trimoxazole) and increased excretion rates of *Salmonella* spp.[8] Many authorities believe that clioquinol (Entero-Vioform) should not be used, because of its capacity to cause serious toxic reactions. Furthermore, there is evidence that drug resistance is increased by the indiscriminate use of antimicrobials.[9] Recent studies show that bismuth subsalicylate can be used to prevent traveller's diarrhoea and is also effective in controlling the disease once it is established.[3] In general it is best to limit the use of chemoprophylaxis to certain groups of patients: firstly, those whose mission is very important (travellers on business, politicians, athletes and others who are on a brief visit); secondly, individuals whose resistance to infection is low (for example those with achlorhydria, whether idiopathic or due to cimetidine, those with previous gastric surgery and the elderly); thirdly, those who seem to experience diarrhoea particularly frequently when they go abroad.

REFERENCES

1   Butzler, J. P. & Skirrow, M. B. (1979) *Campylobacter enteritis. Clinics in Gastroenterology*, **8**, 737–765.
2   DuPont H. L., Olarte, J., Evans D. G. et al. (1976) Comparative susceptibility of Latin American and United States students to enteric pathogens. *New England Journal of Medicine*, **295**, 1520–1521.
3   DuPont, H. L., Sullivan, P., Evans, D. G. et al. (1980) Prevention of travellers' diarrhoea (emporiatric enteritis): prophylactic administration of subsalicylate bismuth. *Journal of the American Medical Association*, **243**, 237–241.
4   DuPont, H. L., Galindo, E., Evans, D. G. et al. (1983) Prevention of travellers' diarrhoea with trimethoprim-sulfamethoxazole and trimethoprim alone. *Gastroenterology*, **84**, 75–80.
5   Ericsson, C. D., Pickering, L. K., Sullivan, P. & DuPont, H. L. (1980) The role of location of food consumption in the prevention of travelers' diarrhoea in Mexico. *Gastroenterology*, **79**, 812–816.
6   Farmer, R. G., Gulya, A. J. & Whelan, G. (1981) Traveller's diarrhoea: clinical observations. *Journal of Clinical Gastroenterology*, **3**(1) 27–29.
7   Gorbach, S. L., Kean B. H., Evans, D. G. et al. (1975) Travellers' diarrhoea and toxigenic *Escherichia coli*. *New England Journal of Medicine*, **292**, 933–936.
8   Mentzing, L. O. & Ringertz, O. (1968) Salmonella infection in tourists. 2. Prophylaxis against salmonellosis. *Acta Patholologica Microbiologia Scandinavica*, **74**, 405–413.
9   Murray, B. E., Rensimer, E. R. & DuPont, H. L. (1982) Emergence of high-level trimethoprim resistance in fecal *Escherichia coli* during oral administration of trimethoprim or trimethoprim-sulfamethoxazole. *New England Journal of Medicine*, **306**, 130–135.
10 Richards, D. A. (1970) A controlled trial in travellers' diarrhoea. *Practitioner*, **204**, 822–824.
11 Sack, R. B., Pierce, N. F. & Hirschhorn, N. (1978) The current status of oral therapy in the treatment of acute diarrhoeal illness. *American Journal of Clinical Nutrition*, **31**, 2251–2257.
12 Santosham, M., Sack, R. B., Froehlich, J. et al. (1981) Biweekly prophylactic doxycycline for travellers' diarrhoea. *Journal of Infectious Disease*, **143**, 598–608.
13 Sheridan, J. F., Aurelian, L., Barbour, G. et al. (1981) Traveller's diarrhoea associated with rotavirus infection: analysis of virus-specific immunoglobulin classes. An enzyme-linked immunosorbent assay for the detection of rotavirus-specific immunoglobulin G (IgG). *Infection and Immunity*, **31**(1), 419–429.
14 Turner, A. C. (1967) Travellers' diarrhoea: a survey of symptoms, occurrence and possible prophylaxis. *British Medical Journal*, **iv**, 653–654.
15 Wright, S. G., Tomkins, A. M. & Ridley, D. S. (1977) Giardiasis: clinical and therapeutic aspects. *Gut*, **18**, 343–350.

YERSINIA INFECTIONS

The genus *Yersinia* currently includes four species. These are *Y. pestis*, the plague organism, *Y. ruckeri*, a fish pathogen, *Y. enterocolitica* and *Y. pseudotuberculosis*. The latter two species may cause illness with major gastrointestinal manifestations in humans.

Pathogenesis

YERSINIA ENTEROCOLITICA

The pathogenesis of *Yersinia enterocolitica* infection usually involves ingestion of the organism. The only successful human infection experiment recorded involved ingestion of 3.5×10^9 organisms.[4] Similar large numbers of organisms via the oral route have been required to produce infection in animal models. Infection is usually via the faecal–oral route or by contaminated food. The incubation period appears to range from four to ten days. The organisms invade the epithelial lining of the ileum and colon, creating small focal ulcerations associated with neutrophils and a pyroninophilic response with numerous mitotic figures in regional lymph nodes. At the same time a systemic inflammatory response is manifested by an elevated erythrocyte sedimentation rate, a leucocytosis and an increase in immature polymorphonuclear leucocytes in peripheral blood. When invasion proceeds beyond the gastrointestinal tract the involved systems (liver, joints and, rarely, the central nervous system) also manifest a polymorphonuclear leucocyte invasion with micro- or gross abscess formation. During the gastrointestinal illness blood and pus can often be found in the stool, as befitting an invasive pathogen.[1, 2, 8]

Much recent work has centred about differences in the virulence properties characterizing the environmental strains which rarely cause human disease and the 0:3, 0:5, 27, 0:8 and 0:9 serotypes, which are most often pathogenic in man. It now appears that the ability of strains to invade HeLa cells, resist the lethal effect of fresh serum, and possibly replicate within macrophages correlates well with their in vivo virulence as judged by presence in fresh human isolates and isolates which are virulent in animal models. Recent demonstration of the V and W antigens, which are dependent on the presence of calcium for their expression at 37°C, and the property of auto-agglutination have been linked to the presence of one or more 42–48 000 MW plasmids and an 82 000 MW plasmid.[6, 10] These factors for virulence in *Y. enterocolitica* are similar to those seen in *Y. pestis* and *Y. pseudotuberculosis*.

Most strains of *Y. enterocolitica* produce a 10 000 MW heat-stable enterotoxin antigenically similar to that produced by some enterotoxigenic *E. coli*. The presence of this toxin in nearly all strains of *Y. enterocolitica*, including environmental strains, the report of toxin-negative isolates causing illness in animals and man, the inability to detect the toxin in the stools of infected animals, and the ability of the bacteria to produce the toxin at 25°C but not at 37°C, have cast doubt on its role in the pathogenesis of enteric disease.[6, 10]

Recovery from illness in humans and animals has been associated with antibody production. Protection from an intravenous challenge with *Y. enterocolitica* in mice is mediated by antibody but not by immune cells. Immunodeficient animals (cytotoxin-treated, nude or irradiated mice) and humans (neonates, patients with haemoglobinopathy, haemochromatosis or malignancy and those receiving immunosuppressive therapy) have increased susceptibility to unusually severe and life-threatening yersiniosis, often complicated by sepsis. This suggests an important role for lymphocyte or macrophage function as well as antibody in recovery from this infection.[1, 2]

YERSINIA PSEUDOTUBERCULOSIS

The pathogenesis of *Y. pseudotuberculosis* is much like that of *Y. enterocolitica* except that it appears to be more invasive in animals and man, usually causing impressive purulent mesenteric adenitis and, less commonly, pyogenic extension to other organs. The pathological hallmark is the epithelial granuloma with microabscesses in the affected mesenteric nodes, appendix and terminal ileum.[7]

Epidemiology

YERSINIA ENTEROCOLITICA

There has been an increasing number of cases of *Y. enterocolitica* reported in the past two decades. Whether this is due to improved recognition or a change in incidence is difficult to ascertain, although a serological study performed in Finland demonstrated a tenfold increase in the prevalence of high levels of anti-*Y. enterocolitica* antibody in donors in 1973 as compared with 1969.

By 1979, over 8000 isolates of *Y. enterocolitica* had been reported worldwide. *Y. enterocolitica* has been reported from every continent except

Antarctica, with the majority of cases from Western Europe and Canada. In general, serotypes 0:3 (80%) and 0:9 (10–15%) account for most European cases, 0:3 for most Japanese and Canadian cases, and 0:8, 0:5, 27 and more recently 0:3 for most United States cases. Worldwide, 0:3 and 0:9 account for the majority of isolates.[1, 2, 4]

The actual incidence of this infection has wide geographic variation, with an apparent predilection for colder temperate-climate regions, including Scandinavia, Canada and the northern United States. In most series, except for that from Montreal, Canada, there is an increased incidence of illness in the late autumn and winter months. In prospective studies, 2.8% of ill Canadian children and 5% of Swedish, 1.5% of German and 1.3% of Belgium patients with apparent appendicitis had yersiniosis. In the United States, 0.7% to 2% of stool cultures from northern states and almost none from southern states have contained yersinia in large prospective studies employing techniques of cold enrichment. In most series, asymptomatic carriage is unusual except in family outbreaks. There does not appear to be a sex predilection for the gastrointestinal syndromes of *Y. enterocolitica*.[1, 2, 4]

While many non-human serotypes of *Y. enterocolitica* have been isolated from such environmental sources as water, wild and domestic animals and animal products (milk and cheese), there is convincing evidence to implicate contaminated water, milk, pork and family dogs in the spread of *Y. enterocolitica* to man. Family studies have revealed a considerable risk of intrafamily spread. Nearly 30% of families in one large study had multiple cases.[9] More extensive family outbreaks, hospital outbreaks in Finland and Canada, and very large outbreaks in Japan and the United States, including two in the United States linked to contaminated milk, have occurred. There are several reports implicating drinking water as a source of this organism for human infection in single cases and outbreaks.

YERSINIA PSEUDOTUBERCULOSIS

The reservoir of *Y. pseudotuberculosis* appears to be similar to that for *Y. enterocolitica*. It is commonly found in domestic and wild animals, and small family outbreaks have been linked to disease in dogs, cats, chickens and canaries. The cold weather predominance for human disease mirrors that seen in animals. Males are much more frequently infected than females, and the peak age is 5–15 years.

Clinical syndromes

YERSINIA ENTEROCOLITICA

The major clinical syndromes associated with *Y. enterocolitica* include acute febrile gastroenteritis, terminal ileitis and mesenteric adenitis. Less common syndromes include a typhoidal-like septicaemic syndrome, extraintestinal pyogenic localized syndromes such as arthritis, meningitis, cellulitis, liver abscess and a host of reactive syndromes such as erythema nodosum, reactive arthritis and possibly autoimmune thyroiditis.[1, 2, 4, 8]

The most common syndrome (75–80% of cases) is a self-limiting acute febrile gastroenteritis. This resembles that seen with other invasive bacterial pathogens such as shigella, campylobacter, salmonella, enteroinvasive *E. coli* and *Entamoeba histolytica*. The clinical features include fever of a few days' duration (in 50–90%), vomiting (in 20–40%), abdominal pain (in 20–65%) and diarrhoea (five to ten stools per day) of two to three weeks' duration. There are case reports of more chronic illness lasting several months which simulates chronic inflammatory bowel disease. Radiographs reveal regional colitis, swollen mucosa, ulcerations and 'cobblestoning' of the mucosa, nodular filling defects and occasionally polyp-like structures. Lesions are usually confined to 10–20 cm of the distal ileum or less commonly the ascending colon. Fistulas and strictures are not seen. Sigmoidoscopy reveals ulcerations or swollen friable mucosa.[5, 11] In a quarter of patients the stool contains blood, and 80% of the time it contains polymorphonuclear leucocytes. Rarely, cases of intestinal ulceration, massive bleeding, perforation and peritonitis have been reported. In most patients blood cultures are negative and diagnosis is established by recovery of the organism from the stool. This is usually an illness of children under five years of age.[8]

In older children or adults, or possibly in association with more invasive organisms, a pseudoappendicitis syndrome is encountered in addition to gastroenteritis. This accounts for 10–15% of *Y. enterocolitica* cases and is clinically identical to classical appendicitis, with right lower quadrant tenderness and fever. Radiological examination reveals coarse, irregular nodularity of the intestinal mucosa and ulcerations which resolve over several months. Endoscopy has revealed colitis, aphthoid ulcers and rarely pseudomembranes.[5, 11] The findings at surgery are usually terminal ileitis or mesenteric lymphadenitis. Diagnosis can be established by culture of the stool and also the involved mesenteric nodes or peritoneal fluid. All cases of mesenteric adenitis should have the involved nodes cultured for *Yersinia*; as well, all cases of acute febrile enteritis and chronic inflammatory bowel disease should have stool cultures performed to exclude yersiniosis.

Cutaneous manifestations including erythematous maculopapular rashes, ulcerative skin lesions, wound infections and erysipelas-like rashes have been reported either in association with the gastrointestinal manifestations or alone. Erythema nodosum, especially in older European women, is not an uncommon finding with or following yersiniosis. Arthritis, most commonly of the culture-negative reactive variety, involving multiple joints in individuals with HLA-B27 has also been reported. This manifestation is much more common in Europe (one-third of cases) than the United States, giving rise to the hypothesis that certain strains, such as 0:3, are more arthritogenic than others. Carditis, haemolytic anaemia, thyroiditis and Reiter's syndrome are less commonly reported non-suppurative sequelae of infection.[1, 2, 4, 8]

Septicaemia is unusual and most often reported in children or adults compromised by aplastic anaemia, malnutrition, haemoglobinopathy (especially thalassaemia), malignant disease, liver disease, haemochromatosis or immunosuppressive therapy. Septicaemia in apparently otherwise healthy children and adults has also been reported. Typical manifestations include fever, headache, malaise and depressed sensorium. Hepatic involvement, with hepatomegaly and abscess, may also occur. The most serious manifestation of *Yersinia* infection, septicaemia, is associated with a case-fatality ratio of approximately 50% despite antibiotic treatment.

Focal pyogenic infections, which are probably secondary to sepsis and which usually occur in similarly immunocompromised individuals, have been reported infrequently. These manifestations, more common in adults than in children, include intra-abdominal abscess, suppurative arthritis, hepatitis, urethritis, meningitis, cholangitis, ophthalmitis, osteomyelitis, endocarditis and lung abscess.

YERSINIA PSEUDOTUBERCULOSIS

The clinical manifestations of *Y. pseudotuberculosis*, a much rarer disease then *Y. enterocolitica*, are nearly identical to those of the latter agent except for the relative rarity of the typical febrile gastroenteritis syndrome. Instead, the mesenteric adenitis–pseudoappendicitis syndrome is the most common clinical manifestation of infection with *Y. pseudotuberculosis*, followed by the reactive syndromes (arthritis, erythema nodosum) and sepsis in the categories of patients also susceptible to *Y. enterocolitica* sepsis.[7] Diagnosis is by appropriate cultures of blood and tissue, especially mesenteric lymph nodes and peritoneal fluid at the time of appendicectomy. Laparoscopy has been utilized to obtain culture material.

Microbiology and diagnosis

Yersinia belongs to the family Enterobacteriaceae and is a Gram-negative coccobacillary rod. *Y. enterocolitica*, originally isolated from humans and first described in the 1930s, has been previously referred to as *Bacterium enterocoliticum*, 'Germe X', *Pasteurella X*, *Pasteurella pseudotuberculosis B* and *Pasteurella pseudotuberculosis rodentium*. *Yersinia pseudotuberculosis* was first described as an animal pathogen in 1883, with the first human case reported 75 years later.

YERSINIA ENTEROCOLITICA

Y. enterocolitica is motile at 25°C but not at 37°C. It does not generally ferment lactose, but ferments glucose, sucrose, xylose, mannitol, maltose, arabinose, galactose, fructose, mannose, trehalose, sorbitol and cellobiose. It is negative for oxidase, gelatine hydrolysis, lysine decarboxylase, phenylalanine deaminase and arginine dihydrolase. It produces catalase and is positive for ornithine decarboxylase and urease. The triple-sugar/iron/agar slant is acid/acid. The lysine/iron/agar reaction produces an alkaline slant and acid butt.[1]

Recent DNA homology and biochemical studies have demonstrated four major subgroups of *Y. enterocolitica*, which have been proposed to represent separate species. The newly proposed species are *Y. enterocolitica*, which includes the serotypes most frequently associated with human disease, and *Y. fredrikenii*, *Y. intermedia* and *Y. kristensenii*.[3]

The major diagnostic test for yersiniosis is a positive culture. *Y. enterocolitica* is relatively easy to isolate from otherwise uncontaminated specimens. It grows well on blood agar as well as on eosin–methylene blue and other Enterobacteriaceae differential plating media such as MacConkey, deoxycholate, and in most cases shigella–salmonella agar. Since *Y. enterocolitica* grows slower at 37°C than most enteric pathogens it may be somewhat difficult to isolate from heavily contaminated specimens such as stool. During the acute enteric phase of illness, especially in children infected with the 0:3 serotype, shedding is so heavy that the organism is relatively easily isolated on the above media in laboratories familiar with the morphology of the 0.5–1.0-mm colonies. For optimal isolation of the organism from heavily contaminated clinical specimens (such as stool or other enteric contents) or environmental sources, cold enrichment utilizing the ability of yersinia to grow at a temperature as low as 4°C has proven valuable. Phosphate-buffered saline (volume 5 ml, pH 7.6, 0.067 mol/l) or Rappaport broth is generally inoculated with 0.5 g of faeces and incubated at 4°C for three to four weeks with weekly or biweekly subculturing of three separate specimens. Because these techniques are not routine, they require specific communication between the clinician and the microbiology laboratory. A recently described technique of rapid isolation of yersinia from stool by mixture with 0.5% KOH for two minutes prior to plating on Mac-Conkey, salmonella–shigella and cellobiose–arginine–lysine media may markedly shorten the time for isolation.[12]

Subsequent identification by biochemical reactions, motility and serotyping (over 500 serotypes) is performed by standard methods. Antibiotic susceptibility tests by disc and agar-diffusion methods have demonstrated susceptibility to co-trimoxazole (trimethoprim–sulphamethoxazole), aminoglycosides (gentamicin, kanamycin, amikacin), chloramphenicol and the newer cephalosporins, for example cefamandole and cefotaxime. *Y. enterocolitica* is usually resistant to ampicillin, carbenicillin, erythromycin and the older cephalosporins, and has been shown to contain beta-lactamases, which probably mediate some of these resistance patterns. It is of interest that clavulanic acid, a beta-lactamase blocker, can increase the organism's sensitivity to ampicillin.

Antibodies in animals and humans to various serotypes of *Y. enterocolitica* have been measured by agglutination of organisms and more recently by enzyme-linked immunosorbent assays (ELISA) and radioimmune assays which have demonstrated IgM and IgG rises. These techniques have been primarily utilized for epidemiological studies or diagnosis of the extra-intestinal manifestations of yersinia. There have been reports of cross-reactions with the genera *Brucella*, *Vibrio* and *Salmonella*, resulting in false positive serological results, and false negative results can also occur, especially in young children. Where certain serotypes predominate, for example 0:3 and 0:9 in Europe or 0:3 in Canada, serodiagnosis is feasible.

YERSINIA PSEUDOTUBERCULOSIS

Yersinia pseudotuberculosis shares many of the biochemical and motility characteristics of *Y. enterocolitica* but is sucrose-, ornithine-decarboxylase-, cellobiose- and sorbitol-negative. There are five serotypes, with strain I causing 60–80% of human disease. Isolation techniques for its growth are similar to those for *Y. enterocolitica*.

DIFFERENTIAL DIAGNOSIS

The differential diagnosis of yersinia gastroenteritis and mesenteric adenitis includes infection by shigella, salmonella, campylobacter, *Entamoeba histolytica*, enteroinvasive *E. coli*, antibiotic-associated colitis, chronic inflammatory bowel disease and rarely tuberculosis, tularaemia, brucellosis, sarcoid and Epstein–Barr virus infection. The typhoidal-sepsis syndrome can be simulated by any organism causing septicaemia, but especially salmonella.

Therapy

Therapy for the milder yersinia syndromes such as gastroenteritis and mesenteric adenitis and for the reactive syndromes such as erythema nodosum and arthritis remains controversial. There is no evidence that antimicrobial treatment either modifies the clinical syndrome or the duration of shedding of the organism. Supportive therapy with fluids and electrolytes as well as anti-inflammatory agents in the reactive syndromes are indicated.[2, 4, 8]

Specific antimicrobial therapy is indicated in the *Yersinia enterocolitica*-caused typhoidal-sepsis syndrome and the rare pyogenic complications (wound infections, hepatic abscess, meningitis and septic arthritis). In these settings chloramphenicol ($50–75$ $mg \cdot kg^{-1} \cdot day^{-1}$), aminoglycosides (gentamicin, $5–7.5$ $mg \cdot kg^{-1} \cdot day^{-1}$) and tetracycline ($20–30$ $mg \cdot kg^{-1} \cdot day^{-1}$) have had apparently beneficial effects. It would be anticipated from in vitro susceptibility testing and experiences with shigellosis and salmonellosis that trimethoprim–sulphamethoxazole (10–20 milligrams trimethoprim per kilogram per day orally or intravenously) would be efficacious. In gastroenteritis in a highly susceptible host, such as a neonate or a patient with malnutrition, cancer, haemochromatosis or haemoglobinopathy or receiving immunosuppressive therapy specific antimicrobial therapy is probably indicated to treat 'incipient' sepsis.[2, 8]

Similar principles probably hold true for therapy of *Y. pseudotuberculosis*, with therapy including ampicillin ($100–200\,\text{mg}\cdot\text{kg}^{-1}\cdot\text{day}^{-1}$), tetracycline ($20–30\,\text{mg}\cdot\text{kg}^{-1}\cdot\text{day}^{-1}$ orally) or streptomycin ($20–30\,\text{mg}\cdot\text{kg}^{-1}\cdot\text{day}^{-1}$ intramuscularly).

Control, prevention and prognosis

Basic control measures rely on appropriate personal and food hygiene to prevent spread from animals to man and from man to man. This is especially important in families with an index case and in hospitals. Patients with yersiniosis must be cared for with enteric isolation strictly enforced. The normal period of shedding of *Y. enterocolitica* in stools of convalescing humans varies from two weeks to as long as four months, with a mean of 42 days in one large prospective series. There is no vaccine for this illness or any data regarding the value of prophylactic antimicrobial therapy. In a common-source outbreak, rapid identification of the source will help to curtail the spread of illness as well as possibly prevent unnecessary operations for the pseudoappendicitis syndrome. Unfortunately, it may be necessary to perform an appendicectomy to exclude true appendicitis.

Nearly all the syndromes caused by *Y. enterocolitica* and *Y. pseudotuberculosis* are self-limiting with full recovery. The exceptions are those cases of sepsis with a 50% to 75% mortality rate, and septic complications, which may require prolonged antimicrobial therapy as well as drainage of areas of purulence.[1, 2, 4, 8, 9]

It is hoped that further understanding of the virulence factors and basic immunity will allow the development of an efficacious vaccine for use in high-risk settings. At present, a high index of suspicion in the appropriate setting and communication between the clinician and the microbiology laboratory will facilitate diagnosis and our further understanding of these fascinating organisms.

REFERENCES

1 Bottone, E. J. (1977) *Yersinia enterocolitica:* a panoramic view of a charismatic microorganism. *CRC Critical Reviews in Microbiology,* **5,** 211–241.

2 Bottone, E. J. (1981) *Yersinia Enterocolitica.* Boca Raton, Florida: CRC Press.

3 Brenner, D. J., Ursing, J., Benovier, H. *et al.* (1980) Deoxyribonucleic acid relatedness in *Yersinia enterocolitica* and *Yersinia enterocolitica*-like organisms. *Current Microbiology,* **4,** 195–200.

4 Carter, P. B., LaFleur, L. & Toma, S. (1979) *Yersinia enterolitica.* Biology, epidemiology and pathology. In *Microbiology and Immunology,* vol. 5. Basel: Karger.

5 El-Maraghi, N. R. H. & Main, N. S. (1979) The histopathology of enteric infection with *Yersinia pseudotuberculosis. American Journal of Clinical Pathology,* **71,** 631–639.

6 Gemski, P., Lazere, J. R. & Casey, T. (1980) Plasmid associated with pathogenicity and calcium dependency of *Yersinia enterocolitica. Infection and Immunity,* **27,** 682–685.

7 Knapp, W. (1958) Mesenteric adenitis due to *Pasteurella pseudotuberculosis* in young people. *New England Journal of Medicine,* **259,** 776–778.

8 Kohl, S. (1979) *Yersinia enterocolitica* infections. *Pediatric Clinics of North America,* **26,** 433–444.

9 Marks, M. I., Pai, C. H., LaFleur, L. *et al.* (1980) *Yersinia enterocolitica* gastroenteritis. A prospective study of clinical, bacteriologic, and epidemiologic features. *Journal of Pediatrics,* **96,** 26–31.

10 Portney, D. A., Moseley, S. L. & Falkow, S. (1981) Characterization of plasmids and plasmid-associated determinants of *Yersinia enterocolitis* pathogenesis. *Infection and Immunity,* **31,** 775–782.

11 Vantrappen, G., Agg, H. O., Ponette, E. *et al.* (1977) Yersinia enteritis and enterocolitis: gastroenterological aspects. *Gastroenterology,* **72,** 220–227.

12 Weissfeld, A. S. & Sonnenwirth, A. C. (1982) Rapid isolation of *Yersinia* spp. from feces. *Journal of Clinical Microbiology,* **15,** 508–510.

SCHISTOSOMIASIS (BILHARZIASIS)

Some 200 million people are probably infected with schistosomiasis and 500–600 millions exposed to the risk of infection.[45] Three main species of schistosomes or 'blood flukes' cause human infections, *Schistosoma haematobium, S. mansoni* and *S. japonicum* (see Table 14.13).

Cercariae of other mammalian schistosomes, such as *S. margrebowiei* (Le Roux, 1933) and *S. rodhaini* (Brumpt, 1931) also penetrate man, as do schistosomes of birds, and may cause cercarial dermatitis ('swimmer's itch').[46]

LIFE-CYCLE AND BIOLOGY

The species of human schistosomes are similar in their basic life-cycles, but they exhibit pronounced differences in their infectivity to the particular groups of snails which they utilize as intermediate hosts and in their infectivity to other mammalian hosts.

The adult schistosomes are approximately 10–20 mm in length and superficially resemble roundworms, this being an adaptation to their habitat inside blood vessels. The filiform female worm is held within the 'schist' or gynaecophoric canal of the shorter male worm. The integument of the schistosome is a living tissue

Table 14.13. Important species of *Schistosoma*, their geographical distribution and some characteristics

	S. haematobium (Bilharz, 1852)	*S. mansoni* (Sambon, 1907)	*S. japonicum* (Katsurada, 1904)
Distribution	Most African, some middle-eastern countries	Most African countries, parts of Arabia, northern and eastern parts of South America, some Caribbean islands	Mainland China, Philippines, Japan (very small extent), Celebes, Malaysia
Molluscs	Genus *Bulinus* (aquatic)	Genus *Biomphalaria* (aquatic)[7,29]	Genus *Oncomelania* (amphibious)[14]
Location of adult worms	Veins of vesical plexus	Inferior mesenteric vein and tributaries	Superior and inferior mesenteric veins and tributaries
Eggs	Terminal spine, passed in urine and sometimes faeces 20–300 per worm pair per day	Lateral spine, passed in faeces and sometimes urine 100–300 per worm pair per day	Vestigial spine, passed in faeces. >3000 per worm pair per day
Infection	Urinary or vesical schistosomiasis	Intestinal schistosomiasis	Intestinal schistosomiasis

	S. mekongi (Voge et al., 1978)	*S. intercalatum* (Fisher, 1934)	*S. mattheei* (Veglia and LeRoux, 1929)
Distribution	Laos, Cambodia, Thailand	Zaire, Cameroon, Gabon, Central African Republic	Southern Africa, where it replaces *S. bovis*
Molluscs	Genus *Tricula*[14]	Genus *Bulinus*	Genus *Bulinus* Parasite of cattle, infections in man together with *S. haematobium* or *S. mansoni*
Location of adult worms	Superior and inferior mesenteric veins and tributaries	Inferior mesenteric vein and tributaries	Probably veins of vesical plexus and inferior mesenteric vein and tributaries
Eggs	Vestigial spine; smaller than *S. japonicum*	Large terminal spine, passed in faeces	Terminal spine, passed in urine and faeces
Infection	Intestinal schistosomiasis[39]	Intestinal schistosomiasis[51]	Urinary and intestinal symptoms[32]

rather than a chitinous protective sheath and it is an important site for host–antigen attachment. The worms ingest red blood cells and possess a protease that breaks down globin and haemoglobin, releasing tyrosine. The black haematin-like pigment which is regurgitated by the adult worms is taken up by reticuloendothelial cells in the liver and spleen. The adult worms may live for 20–30 years, but the mean lifespan is probably much shorter (three to eight years). Each worm pair, according to the species of schistosome, produces 300–3000 or more eggs per day. The schistosomes do not multiply in the definitive host, and the infection process produces, or tends to produce, an over-dispersed distribution of parasites within the host population, in which most individuals carry few parasites and a small proportion are heavily infected. Thus, in schistosomiasis, although the proportion of those with infections of high intensity is relatively low, morbidity may be appreciable.

The complex life-cycle involves alternating parasitic and free-living stages: egg, miracidium, first-stage (mother) sporocyst, second-stage (daughter) sporocyst, cercaria, schistosomulum, and adult schistosome. The sexual generation of adult schistosomes is present in the definitive vertebrate host and the multiplicative asexual phase in a molluscan host (see Figures 14.23 and 14.24).

The non-operculate yellowish eggs contain the embryo (miracidium), which develops inside over a period of six days. If the egg remains in the tissues, it lives for a further fifteen days, secreting histiolytic antigenic material. The egg dies some 21 days after oviposition, releasing products of autolysis. The eggshell is destroyed over a period of weeks or months depending on whether or not calcification has taken place. The ova which pass through the bladder or intestinal wall (probably less than 50% of total egg production) contain embryos which are usually visibly motile and ready to hatch when the eggs are passed. When urine or faeces are diluted by fresh water, and usually under the influence of warmth (10–30°C) and light, the miracidia become active and emerge from the eggshells.

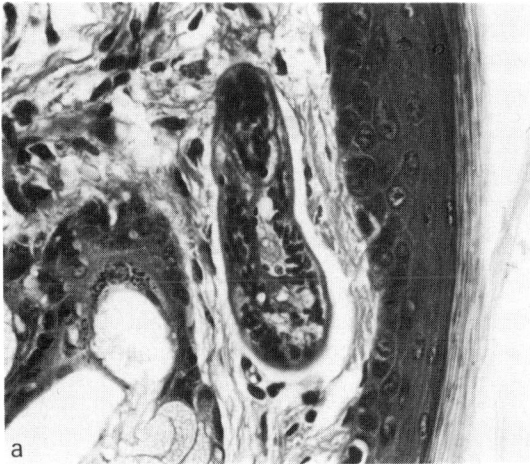

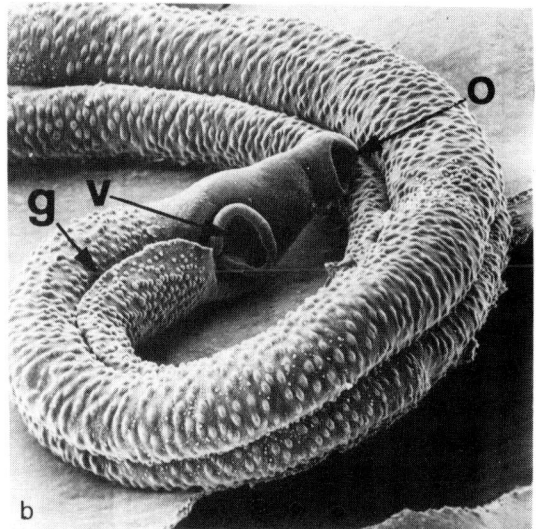

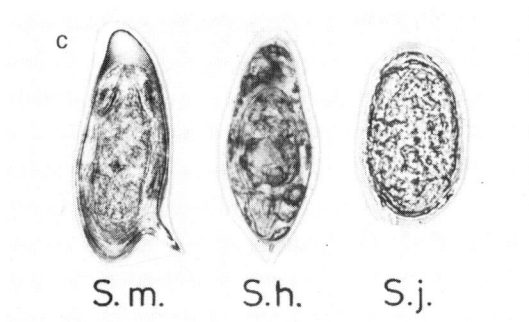

S.m.   S.h.   S.j.

Fig. 14.23 (a) Schistosomulum (*Schistosoma haematobium*, 6 μm long, stained with haematoxylin + eosin) in the dermis of a mouse two days post-infection. (Photomicrograph courtesy of Dr M. Nilsson.) (b) Adult male *Schistosoma haematobium*, showing oral (o) and ventral (v) suckers, integument with tubercles and gynaecophoric canal (g). (Scanning electron micrograph, × 30, courtesy of Professor M. Hicks.) (c) Eggs of *S. mansoni* (S.m.), *S. haematobium* (S.h.) and *S. japonicum* (S.j.) × 200.

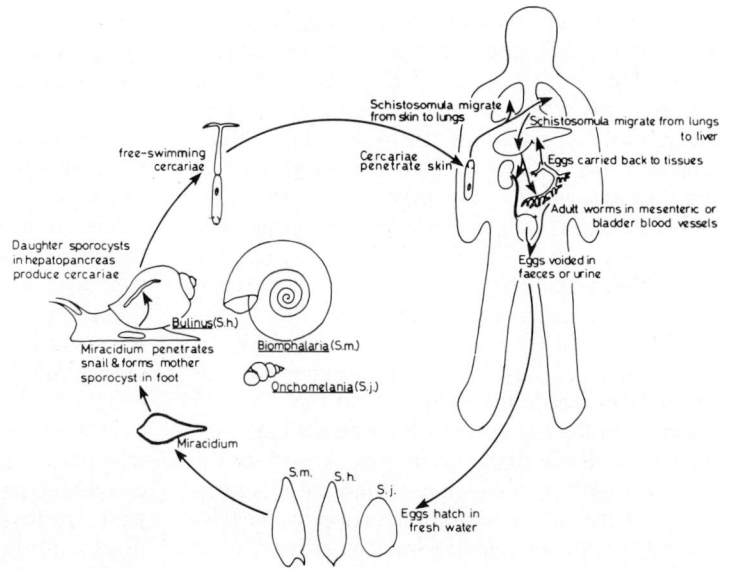

Fig. 14.24 Schistosome life cycle (*S. mansoni*, S.m.; *S. haematobium*, S.h.; *S. japonicum*, S.j.). (Diagram courtesy of Dr E. James.)

The miracidia of the schistosomes that infect man differ in size but are similar in their behaviour and morphology. Penetration of the miracidium occurs when the larva becomes attached to the body surface of the snail by a secretion from the apical gland cells. The cycle within the snail intermediate host (sporocysts) between the penetration of the miracidium larva and the production of mature cercariae lasts approximately four to five weeks for *S. mansoni*, five to six weeks for *S. haematobium* and seven or more weeks for *S. japonicum*.

Daily output of infective cercariae from the snail may vary from one or two to several thousand. The penetration process of the cercaria is quite rapid, and many penetrate the stratum corneum within a few minutes, and at the same time the larva changes in appearance to become a worm-like schistosomulum. Within a few hours of penetration the trilaminate membrane of the cercaria is replaced by the multilaminate integument of the schistosomulum and adult. The passage through the subcutaneous tissue may be effected within 48 hours. Peripheral lymphatic and venous vessels are penetrated and from them transportation to the right heart and the lungs is achieved. Available evidence suggests that worms leave the lungs via the pulmonary veins and pass through the heart to the systemic circulation, and that an individual worm may make several circuits of the pulmonary/systemic circulation before entering a blood vessel which leads to the hepatic portal system. Most sexually mature worms leave the liver when they have mated and, depending on the species, migrate to the different egg-laying

sites. A period of some 30–40 days may elapse between successful cercarial penetration and the appearance of eggs in the urine or stools of the definitive host, but it may be much longer.[47]

PATHOLOGY AND CLINICAL FEATURES

Three disease syndromes are associated with schistosome infection: dermatitis, which results from cercarial penetration of the skin, acute schistosomiasis, or Katayama fever, which occurs in intense initial infection and usually coincides with the onset of egg-laying by the worms, and chronic schistosomiasis, in which lesions in different organs are dependent on the main egg-laying sites of the adult worms. Approximately 4–12% of patients in endemic areas show advanced disease, but the large majority of patients are asymptomatic carriers of the parasite, or show a mild non-specific symptomatology, the pathology of the schistosome infection being represented by a few scattered granulomas around eggs in different organs (see Table 14.14).

The major parasite factor responsible for the occurrence of chronic disease is the egg. The host-granulomatous response to the egg plays an essential part in the pathogenesis of the various disease syndromes (see Table 14.15).[42]

An exaggerated fibroblastic reaction to focally accumulated eggs may give rise to a pseudoneoplastic lesion and patients with such lesions may even be falsely diagnosed as malignancy, especially if they have obstructive intestinal masses.

Table 14.14 Pathology and clinical features of *Schistosoma* infection.[43, 48]

Stage	Parasitological	Clinical	Pathological
1 Invasive	Penetration – cercariae	Hypersensitivity reaction – immediate and delayed types	Papular dermatitis
	Migration – schistosomula	Fever and cough	Inflammatory reactions in lungs and liver
2 Maturation	Maturation – adult worms, migration to egg-laying sites, early oviposition	Acute febrile illness, Katayama fever – form of serum sickness or immune complex disease	Intense reactions, general and local to products of eggs and/or young chistosomes
3 Established infection	Intense oviposition: high levels of egg excretion. Severity of disease related to worm burden and intensity of host response Initial massive infection produces –	Early chronic disease, digestive symptoms, haematuria	Reaction around viable eggs is destructive. Peri-ovular area of necrosis with or without deposition of hyaline eosinophilic band (Hoeppli phenomenon), surrounded by exudative cellular reaction with many eosinophils. New eggs produced as infection progresses, but reaction around them becomes smaller (modulates), more discrete and purely proliferative. Granuloma formation with little fibrosis in early stages
		more severe clinical symptoms	
4 Chronic	Prolonged duration, often with reduced egg excretion	Chronic diseases, portal hypertension, pulmonary hypertension, cor pulmonale, obstruction of gastrointestinal tract, obstructive uropathy	Development of fibrous tissue in different sites according to species of schistosome with lesions in different organs

Table 14.15 The schistosome egg granuloma or pseudotubercle

	Mechanisms of formation	Cellular constituents
S. mansoni *S. haematobium*	A cell-mediated immune reaction dependent on thymus-derived lymphocytes and formed independently of humoral antibody	Ovum engulfed by multinucleated giant cells surrounded by macrophages, eosinophils, polymorphonuclear and mono-nuclear leucocytes, round cells and plasma cells – in contrast to tubercle granulomas which consist almost entirely of macrophages. Fibroblasts replace some cells as healing takes place.
S. japonicum	Possibly an immediate hypersensitivity (antibody-mediated) response or 'foreign-body' type of reaction.	In *S. japonicum* infection, granulomas contain more neutrophils and plasma cells; necrosis and exudation occur with Hoeppli phenomenon frequently present – also less frequently seen in *S. mansoni* and *S. haematobium* infections. Hoeppli phenomenon is an eosinophilic corona around usually viable *S. japonicum* ova within about 10% of granulomas in heavy infections. Precipitate is an antigen–antibody complex with gradient to antibody excess at periphery.

The cause of such a pseudoneoplastic lesion is apparently local, since host reaction to the schistosome eggs in other areas may be focal and limited.[2] In tissue sections, live schistosome worms usually appear inside blood vessels unaccompanied by any local reaction (Figure 14.25b). When the worm dies and disintegrates it may, however, produce vascular thrombosis and inflammation.

Infection with *S. mansoni*

The worm burden in the human population increases with age, and usually reaches a maximum between ten and twenty years old, after which it declines. Some people have high levels of egg excretion but do not appear to show or develop severe disease. Other factors in addition to the parasite load may influence the development of severe manifestations.

ACUTE SCHISTOSOMIASIS

The incubation period may be as short as two to three weeks or as long as eight weeks, and severity is usually related to intensity of infection. In most infections, reaction to cercarial penetration is unnoticed, but a few allergic manifestations with eosinophilia, diarrhoea, hepatosplenomegaly and lymphadenopathy may occur.[33]

Pathology

The liver may show evidence of hepatitis on needle biopsy, and the spleen may show signs of acute infectious splenitis, with intense eosinophilic infiltrates. The intestinal mucosa, including the jejunum and ileum, may show superficial necrotic and haemorrhagic ulcers. The acute phase is characterized by large granulomas, which are found mainly in the liver and intestine and less frequently in other organs. Intralobular foci of necrosis and destruction of hepatocytes occur in the enlarged liver, with portal infiltration of histiocytes, eosinophils, lymphocytes, and hyperplasia and hypertrophy of the Kupffer cells.[6] The spleen enlarges, with intensive eosinophilia and congestion of the sinuses. In severe cases a necrotizing arteritis may occur in the lungs, with miliary dissemination of eggs, and granulomas with exudate and necrosis in the liver, intestines, peritoneum, abdominal and pulmonary lymphatic glands, pleura, lungs and pancreas. Severe oedema, erythema, haemorrhages, petechiae, small ulcerations and punctate elevations are found in the rectum and sigmoid.

Clinical features

In *S. mansoni* infections the clinical picture only rarely presents as an acute febrile illness, and usually this phase is asymptomatic or a mild febrile episode. An irritating maculo-papular rash may occur and persist for some days, the symptoms of the acute phase being due to hypersensitivity. Constitutional symptoms presenting in many other infections may occur with an abrupt onset. Prolonged diarrhoea or dysentery is reported with epigastric discomfort, abdominal pain and distension. Urticaria, facial oedema and erythematous or purpuric lesions may occur.

There is weight loss with tender hepatomegaly, but liver enlargement also occurs in the absence of symptoms. The spleen is usually palpable but soft and not as enlarged as in chronic cases. Generalized enlargement of lymph nodes occurs, but the hepatosplenomegaly regresses in a few months.

There may be evidence of hypochromic anaemia and the sedimentation rate is raised. Eosinophilia may reach 70%. Serum globulin is increased, particularly the gamma globulin fraction, and changes may occur in the cephalin flocculation test, thymol turbidity and bromsulphathalein retention. Liver biopsy shows periportal infiltration with a predominantly eosinophilic reaction. Deaths during the acute phase are rare and the severe forms of the disease seldom develop early, but coma or an acute abdomen may develop and spinal cord complications have been reported.[33]

CHRONIC SCHISTOSOMIASIS

The established infection may not give rise to symptoms, and the majority of infections are described as the 'intestinal' form of the disease, with vague poorly defined complaints or no symptoms. This depends, however, on the intensity of infection. An increasing number of eggs are carried to the liver in the portal vein and liver enlargement occurs in either the left or right lobes, with or without splenomegaly, both in the intestinal and later hepatointestinal forms of the disease.

Pathology

Variable degrees of fibrosis are seen in the portal tracts of the liver, with eggs, granulomas and cellular infiltrates (Figure 14.25c, d). These are also found in the intestines (Figure 14.25a) and, less often, in the lungs and other organs. Eggs

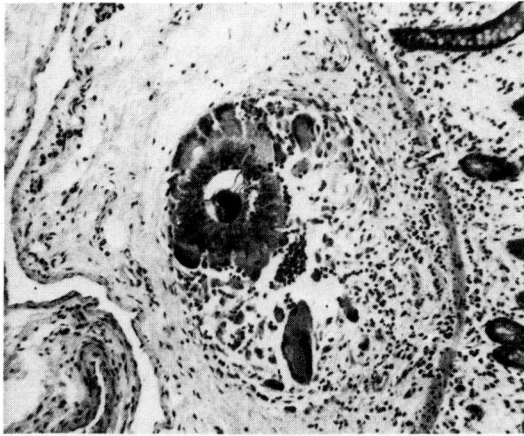

a

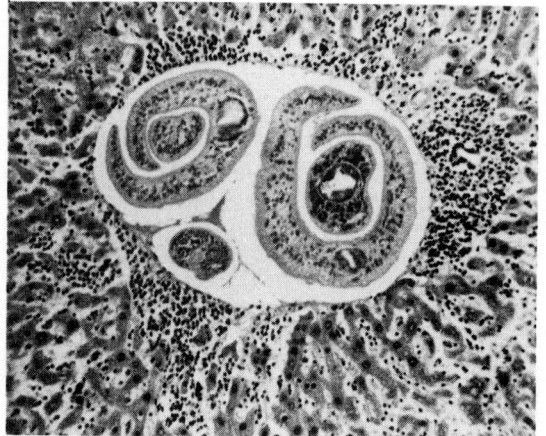

b

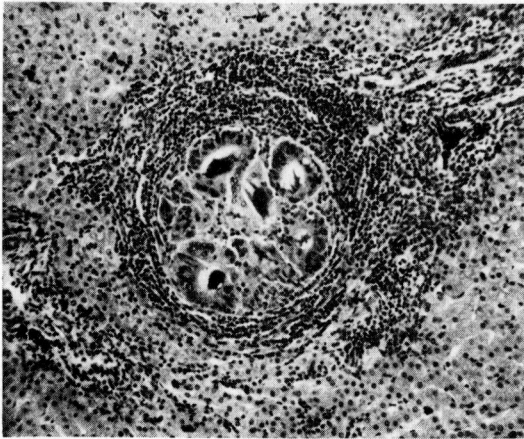

c

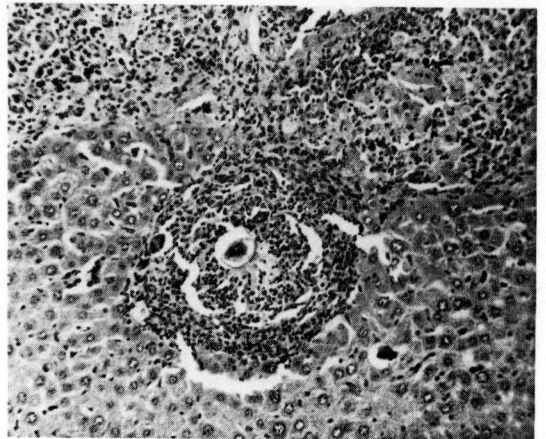

d

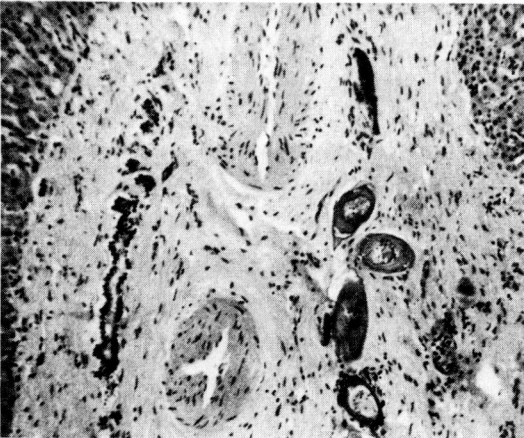

e

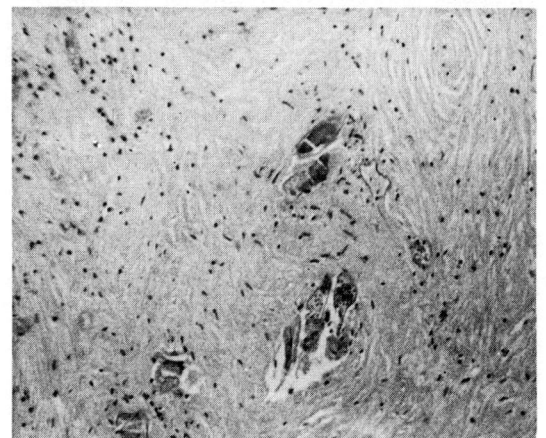

f

Fig. 14.25 (a) Section of large intestine showing Hoeppli reaction around a *Schistosoma mansoni* egg; the surrounding cellular infiltrate contains giant cells. (b) Transverse section of a vessel showing two pairs of adult schistosomes, the females lying in the gynaecophoric canals of the male worms. (c) Schistosome granuloma in liver; a clump of eggs and surrounding giant cells with an intense cellular infiltrate. (d) Granuloma around a *Schistosoma japonicum* egg in liver section. (e) Symmers' fibrosis: increased periportal connective tissue and bundles of fibrous tissue surrounding a large clump of eggs. (f) *Schistosoma haematobium* eggs surrounded by concentric rings of loose fibrous tissue in a peritoneal mass. Five-micrometre sections, stained with haematoxylin + eosin, kindly provided by Mr H. Furse.

are trapped in the mucosa and submucosa of the large intestines, where they produce granulomatous reactions and are eventually destroyed. Bilharziomas are localized masses of fibrous and inflammatory tissue which usually contain many eggs. They develop most frequently in the intestinal serosa or in the mesentery. *S. mansoni* eggs become calcified much less frequently than do those of *S. japonicum*, however, and severe changes are rarely seen. Increased vascularity of the mucosa of the large intestine is common and small papillomatous growths may occur.[15] Extreme fibrosis and oedema of the intestinal wall and of the retroperitoneal tissues has been reported. Granulomatous tumours on the anti-mesenteric surface of the small intestine with intestinal obstruction have also been reported from Africa.[52] Schistosomal stenosis has been recorded in Brazil.[9]

Despite the almost universal involvement of the intestine in *S. mansoni* infection, there are virtually no reports of malabsorption.[42] Another manifestation of intestinal pathology, protein-losing enteropathy, does not occur in most cases of schistosomiasis, but has been recorded in patients in Egypt with intestinal polyposis.[23] Schistosomal colitis is reported to be very rare in Brazil, and while sessile and pedunculated polyps are frequently reported from Egypt, these lesions are not seen in Brazil.[9]

With the development of hepatosplenomegaly the disease is considered chronic and more severe. The fibrotic changes in the liver lead to portal hypertension with enlargement of the spleen.

Symmer's 'clay-pipe-stem' fibrosis occurs in the 6–20-year-old age-group some five to fifteen years after the onset of infection (Figure 14.25e). The liver and spleen are palpable, the liver eventually becoming hard and nodular.[5] Symmer's fibrosis is an irreversible but not necessarily inevitable lesion of chronic *S. mansoni* and *S. japonicum* infection. Portal tracts become surrounded by broad bands of fibrotic (collagen-rich) tissue, with a macroscopic appearance similar to clay pipe stems (Figure 14.26e).[8] It is always found with evidence of portal hypertension and all cases of portal hypertension attributed to schistosomiasis have Symmer's fibrosis.[9] Diffuse bilharzial fibrosis also occurs when ova are deposited in small numbers over a period of time.[18]

The left lobe of the liver is often affected more than the right and the basic lesion is fibrosis in the portal tracts accompanied by phlebitis and periphlebitis. Unlike that of cirrhosis, when fibrosis follows degeneration of the liver cells, fibrosis is interstitial and invasive being unique to schistosomiasis.[18] Granulomas around ova are numerous in the portal spaces and smaller than in the early stages of infection, and may disappear completely. The liver parenchyma remains intact except in focal areas of necrosis.[9] The portal hypertension produces oesophageal varices, a common site of haematemesis.

In many cases of Symmer's fibrosis, the spleen increases in size due to congestion caused by portal hypertension, and hyperplasia of the reticuloendothelial elements results. In some patients with hepatosplenic schistosomiasis in Brazil, progressive glomerulosclerotic changes have been noted leading to glomerulonephritis. IgG and IgM complexes have been found in kidney biopsy specimens of patients with *S. mansoni* infections with or without nephrosis.[3, 34]

Hepatosplenic involvement occurs in two forms. In the first, compensated liver disease, liver function is only slightly affected and a collateral circulation is established; eggs bypassing the liver through collaterals become embolized and induce granulomas in the lungs, with possible subsequent development of obstructing and destructive arteritis and cor pulmonale. The other form, decompensated liver disease, may occur with evidence of reduced liver function, jaundice, cirrhosis, oedema and ascites. It is not clear why or at what stage decompensation occurs. Splenectomy with spleno-renal anastomosis has been used in the treatment of portal hypertension in Brazil, but portacaval anastomosis has lead to encephalopathy in 35–40% of patients. Although many patients with well developed hepatosplenomegaly may have massive oesophageal varices which can rupture, most of them are functioning members of society with a better prognosis than patients with non-schistosomal cirrhosis.[40] Haematemesis, although difficult to treat, is rarely fatal and relatively few patients develop hepatic coma. As portal hypertension increases, so does the chance of developing pulmonary hypertension. A cyanotic syndrome with clubbing of the fingers is rarely reported in patients with portal hypertension and hepatosplenomegaly.[1]

Liver changes in *S. mansoni*, *S. japonicum* and *S. haematobium* infections are similar but differ in degree. In addition to granuloma formation, portal inflammation is seen, with possible invasion of the parenchymal border by lymphocytes and histiocyctes. Portal inflammation is thought to be due to toxins from ova, possibly being a delayed hypersensitivity reaction due to schistosome antigen.

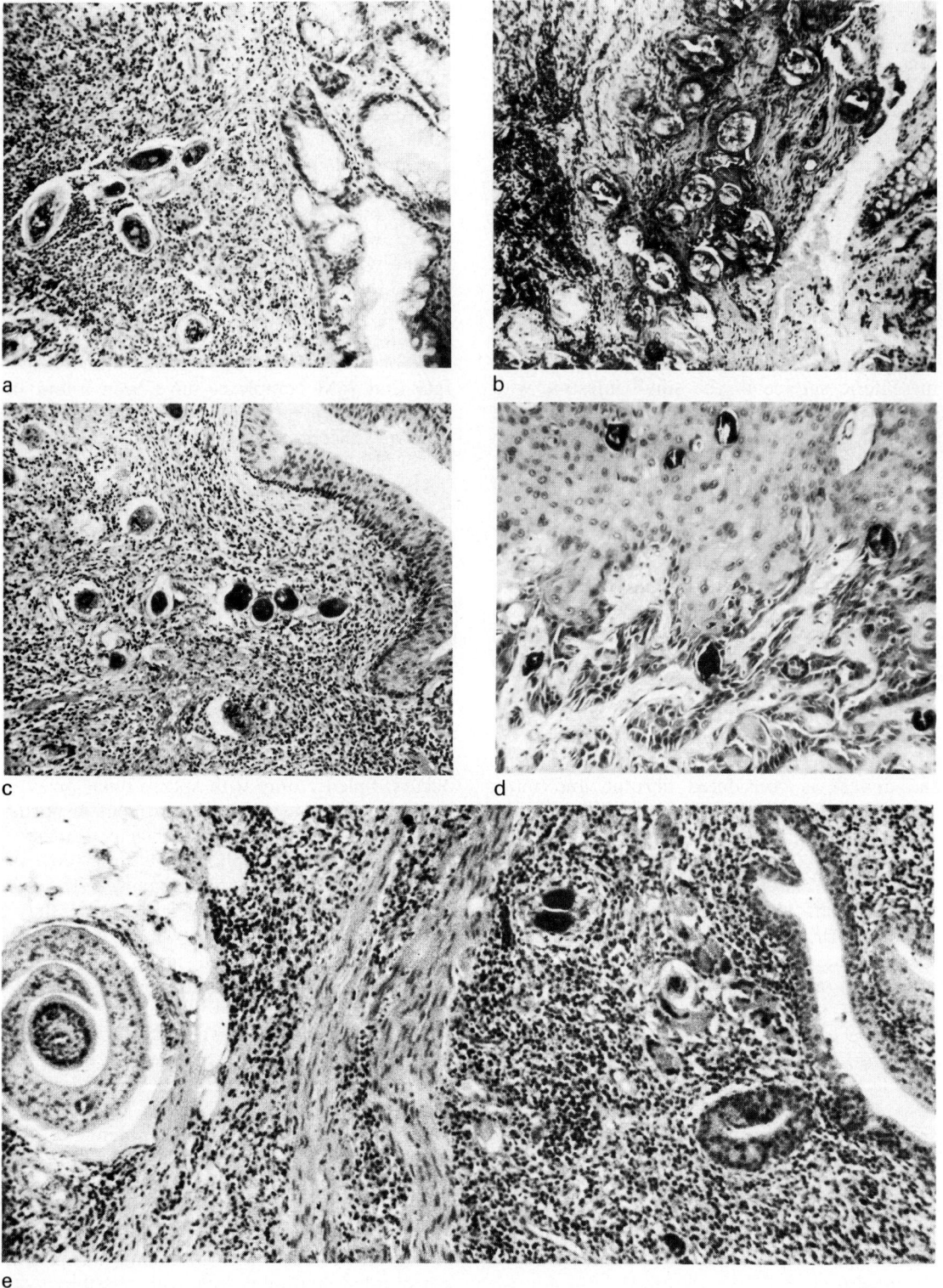

Fig. 14.26 (a) Numerous eggs of *Schistosoma mansoni* in the submucosa of a rectal polyp with surrounding haemorrhage and intense cellular infiltrate. (b) Nests of *Schistosoma mansoni* eggs in the mucosa of a rectal polyp. (c) Nest of *Schistosoma haematobium* eggs in the bladder wall; acute stage with cellular reaction around the eggs. (d) Section of bladder wall showing squamous cell carcinoma with *Schistosoma haematobium* ova. (e) Section across ureter showing adult worms in a vessel and eggs surrounded by intense cellular reaction in the ureteric wall, Five-micrometre sections, stained with haematoxylin + eosin, kindly provided by Mr H. Furse.

Infection with *S. japonicum*

Peak prevalence and intensity of infection are generally observed in the 15–20-year-old age groups, but older persons have also been found to have high prevalence and intensity of infection.[49] The course of the infection is similar to *S. mansoni* infection. While *S. japonicum* is generally thought to cause greater disease, the available evidence does not support this.[28]

PATHOLOGY

Changes in the liver are similar to those in *S. mansoni* infections. As well as the pipe-stem portal fibrosis, extensive intralobular fibrosis may be present. The gastrointestinal tract lesions tend to be focal, isolated and more proliferate than with *S. mansoni* infection.[37, 38]

The pathogenesis of the brain lesions seen is not clearly understood. An intense granulomatous reaction is caused in the central vessels and in the surrounding brain or there may be diffuse involvement with scattered lesions.[22]

CLINICAL FEATURES

Acute infection
Little evidence exists that *S. japonicum* cercariae produce swimmer's itch. The 'Kabure' syndrome of Japan is generally thought to be due to non-human cercariae.[41] There may be early skin manifestations following cercarial penetration, which, with the accompanying pruritus, has been ascribed to anaphylaxis. The acute stage or 'Katayama fever' most commonly found in *S. japonicum* infections is characterized by fever, eosinophilia (30–80%), splenomegaly, lymphadenopathy, urticaria and frequently diarrhoea or dysentery. It is usually seen in heavy primary infections and may result in death.[41] The incubation period usually lasts some 40 days with a range of 14 to 84 days.[10, 36]

Chronic infection
The early chronic stages of the disease are usually asymptomatic as in *S. mansoni*, but diarrhoea and abdominal pain related to intensity of infection are common. Hepatic coma is frequently observed as a terminal event in China, but in the Philippines the main terminal episode is massive bleeding in the upper gastrointestinal tract.[35] *S. japonicum* infection has been implicated as a co-carcinogen in carcinoma of the rectum and carcinoma of the liver. Granulomatous disease of the rectum and sigmoid colon with mucosal hyperplasia, pseudopolyposis,

ulceration, thickening of the bowel wall and stenosis may occur. These pathological changes may be the substrate for malignant transformation, although the prevalence in endemic areas is unknown. In a large autopsy series in Japan, the rate of carcinoma of the colon in infected persons was 25 times greater than that of non-infected persons. The associated carcinoma of the colon has been histologically described as a well differentiated adenocarcinoma with pseudopolyps, calcified eggs being identified in the tissues.[28]

The frequency of severe portal hypertension, associated with shunting of eggs to the pulmonary circulation and cor pulmonale, depends upon the intensity of infection. The brain is principally involved in *S. japonicum* infection, in contrast to the spinal cord which is involved in *S. mansoni* and *S. haematobium* infections. Clinically the latter infections are manifested by the occurrence of transverse myelitis. The first clinical manifestations of cerebral schistosomiasis are Jacksonian-type paroxysmal seizures, usually in people over 20 years of age, followed by grand-mal seizures in many fatal cases.[4, 22]

Schistosomal dwarfism is reported from China and Brazil. It is accompanied by impairment of gonad formation and sexual immaturity, and is thought to be due to depressed activity of the anterior lobe of the pituitary gland.[19]

Infection with *S. haematobium*

Cercarial dermatitis may occur some 24 hours after infection and lasts approximately 48 hours. The acute or toxaemic stage usually begins eight weeks after infection (range 5–12 weeks). Haematuria is seen in 50% of cases. Although there is evidence of urinary tract disease with kidney involvement, no hypertension occurs, and in East Africa low blood pressures are recorded. Pulmonary changes due to *S. haematobium* may lead to cor pulmonale. Cutaneous manifestations are reported, with lesions in the genital and perigenital areas, and severe urinary schistosomiasis may be associated with osteoporosis.[17, 22]

Kidneys, ureters, urinary bladder, urethra and genital tissues may be involved, but eggs are most numerous in the bladder, ureters and seminal vesicles. Lung, colon, and appendix also contain *S. haematobium* ova in almost all infections. The worms tend to remain in one location for prolonged periods laying large numbers of eggs which accumulate at one site, thus causing focal lesions.[26] The eggs calcify and produce granulomata which are generally smaller than those of *S. mansoni* but have the same cellular composition.[44, 50]

In the bladder polypoid, fibrous and sandy patches, ulceration, stricture, leucoplakia and cystitis glandularis, fibrosis and calcification of the bladder wall and bladder neck may occur.[15] Secondary bacterial infection sometimes occurs, but is not usually related to the infection, with consequent pyelonephritis. In Egypt *S. haematobium* infection is associated with a high prevalence of cancer of the bladder and, in particular, squamous cell carcinomas (Figure 14.26d).[25] Obstructive uropathy is clearly demonstrated by intravenous pyelography,[16] and the development of hydronephrosis and hydroureter is commonly seen in children and adolescents. Associated bacteriuria and hydronephrosis may impair urine concentrating ability.[24]

Involvement of the rectum occurs in 70% of *S. haematobium* infections, and the remainder of the large intestine and appendix may also be involved. While gross lesions are rare, granular areas in the mucosa resembling sandy patches are common. Granulomas may cause acute obstruction in the large intestine.[15]

SYNERGISTIC AND ANTAGONISTIC EFFECTS

Synergistic and antagonistic interrelations between schistosomiasis and salmonellosis are suggested to explain the recorded associations of these infections in China, Brazil and Egypt. Experimental evidence also exists for such interrelations with hepatitis, malaria and *Entamoeba histolytica*.[42] Further investigations are required into the importance of other infections and of malnutrition in relation to the course of human schistosomiasis.

DIAGNOSIS

The definitive diagnosis of an active infection is only made by detecting schistosome ova in concentrated urine, faeces or biopsy material. Eggs may be found in excreta as early as five to six weeks after infection with *S. mansoni* or *S. japonicum*, and some ten to twelve weeks with *S. haematobium*. Longer delays between exposure and patency are common, and in the case of *S. japonicum* repeated stool examinations may be necessary since in light infections ova are laid in clusters in the faeces and tend to be aggregated.[28] Qualitative techniques for detection of

ova are used in clinical practice, but quantitative techniques are mainly used for research in the fields of epidemiology, control, clinicopathology and drug trials.[20]

Quantitative techniques to examine stools now include modifications of the Kato method – that is, the quick Kato method and the Kato/Katz method – and nucleopore filtration of urine specimens has been developed.[31]

Special stains are sometimes useful. The eggshells of *S. mansoni* are acid-fast, while those of *S. haematobium* are not. The shells of *S. intercalatum*, which are very similar to *S. haematobium*, are acid-fast after Bouin's fixation. In patients with light or inactive infections, rectal biopsy is particularly effective in detecting eggs. They are best seen by crushing the biopsy between glass slides. Eggs may also be recovered by hydrolysis of tissues in 4% KOH for 18 hours, incubating at 37°C for fresh tissues and 56°C for fixed tissues.[26]

Promising immunodiagnostic tests are now also available including radioimmunoassay and enzyme-linked immunosorbent assay (ELISA).[27, 30]

TREATMENT

A number of highly effective drugs are available for the treatment of schistosomiasis and these have now largely displaced the tri- and pentavalent antimonials and the later generation of non-antimonial compounds such as lucanthone, hycanthone and niridazole.[11] The drugs currently in use are metriphonate, oxamniquine and praziquantel.

Metriphonate (Bilarcil), although only effective against *S. haematobium*, is very cheap and of low toxicity. A widely used schedule of 7.5 mg/kg, given in three oral doses at intervals of 14 days, is the standard treatment regimen.[12] Cholinergic symptoms may be expected during treatment, but tolerance is extremely good, and such symptoms, if they occur, are mild and disappear spontaneously in a few hours. High cure rates and substantial reductions in egg output are reported in selective population chemotherapy programmes. The drug is extensively used in Egypt and elsewhere.

Oxamniquine (Mansil, Vansil), which is highly effective against *S. mansoni* only, being administered as a single oral dose with few side-effects, is used clinically in the treatment of acute, subacute, chronic, and complicated cases of *S. mansoni* infection with excellent results. In the Western hemisphere, a single oral dose of

15 mg/kg bodyweight in adults produces high cure rates, but in children under 30 kg in weight the optimum regimen is a total dose of 20 mg/kg given in two divided doses of 10 mg/kg four to six hours apart. In Africa total doses of 40 and 60 mg/kg administered over two or three days are found necessary to obtain good therapeutic response; even if parasitological cure is not achieved, egg output is reduced by 80–90%. The drug is very suitable for population-based chemotherapy and is being widely used in South America.[11]

Praziquantel (Biltricide), which is highly effective against all human schistosome species, is unquestionably a major advance in the chemotherapy of the disease. It is highly effective when given in a single oral dose of 40 mg/kg bodyweight for *S. haematobium*. For *S. mansoni* in a single dose of 40 mg/kg or 2 × 20 mg/kg at an interval of four hours in one day is recommended. For *S. japonicum* the present recommended regimen is two doses of 30 mg/kg at an interval of four hours in one day or three of 20 mg/kg in one day. The available evidence shows that patients with advanced disease from infection with *S. japonicum* or *S. mansoni*, with ascites or portal hypertension, tolerate the drug very well, which offers an optimistic outlook for the future treatment of advanced cases.[13]

PROGNOSIS

It is now considered that the prognosis of uncomplicated cases of the schistosome infections is generally very good, provided that specific treatment is given. Improvement in the function and structure of damaged organ systems can be expected.[11]

ACKNOWLEDGEMENTS

I am indebted to members of my staff, including Dr E. R. James and Mr H. Furse, for their assistance in the preparation of photomicrographs, to Professor Marian Hicks and Dr Margaretha Nilsson, who kindly provided illustrative material, and to Mrs Diana Mulholland for preparation of the manuscript.

REFERENCES

1 Andrade, Z. A. & Andrade, S. G. (1970) Pathogenesis of schistosoma pulmonary arteritis. *American Journal of Tropical Medicine and Hygiene*, **19**(2), 305–310.

2 Andrade, Z. A. & Rodrigues, G. (1954) Pseudoneoplastic manifestations of intestinal schistosomiasis. *Archives of Brazilian Medicine*, **44**, 437–444.

3 Andrade, Z. A., Andrade, S. G. & Sadigursky, M. (1971) Renal changes in patients with hepatosplenic schistosomiasis. *American Journal of Tropical Medicine and Hygiene*, **20**(1), 77–83.

4 Ariizumi, M. (1963) Cerebral Schistosomiasis japonica: report of one operated case and fifty clinical cases. *American Journal of Tropical Medicine and Hygiene*, **12**, 40–45.

5 Bogliolo, L. (1957) Anatomical picture of the liver in hepato-splenic *Schistosomiasis mansoni*. *Annals of Tropical Medicine and Parasitology*, **51**, 1–14.

6 Bogliolo, L. (1967) The pathogenesis of Schistosomiasismansoni. In *Bilharziasis* (Ed.) Mostofi, F. K. pp. 184–196. Berlin, Heidelberg & New York: Springer-Verlag.

7 Brown, D. S. (1980) *Freshwater Snails of Africa and their Medical Importance*. London: Taylor Francis.

8 Cheever, A. W. (1972) Pipe-stem fibrosis of the liver. (Correspondence) *Transactions of the Royal Society of Tropical Medicine and Hygiene*, **66**, 946–948.

9 Cheever, A. W. & Andrade, Z. A. (1967) Clinical and pathological aspects of schistosomiasis in Brazil. In *Bilharziasis* (Ed.) Mostofi, F. K. pp. 157–166. Berlin, Heidelberg & New York: Springer-Verlag.

10 Chen, W. C., Lui, H., Hu, S. Y. *et al.* (1964) Clinical analysis of 580 cases of acute schistosomiasis (Chinese). *Chinese Journal of Internal Medicine*, **12**, 259–262.

11 Davis, A. (1982) Management of the patient. In *Schistosomiasis: Treatment, Epidemiology and Control* (Ed.) Jordan, P. & Webbe, G. pp. 184–226. London: Heinemann Medical Books.

12 Davis, A. & Bailey, D. R. (1969) Metrifonate in urinary schistosomiasis. *Bulletin of the World Health Organization*, **41**, 209–224.

13 Davis, A. & Wegner, D. H. G. (1979) Multicentre trials of praziquantel in human schistosomiasis: design and techniques. *Bulletin of the World Health Organization*, **57**, 761–771.

14 Davis, G. M. (1979) The origin and evolution of the gastropod family Pomatiopsidae, with emphasis on the Mekong River Triculinae. *Monograph of the Academy of Natural Sciences of Philadelphia*, **20**, 1–120.

15 Edington, G. M. & Gilles, H. M. (1969) *Pathology in the Tropics*. Baltimore: Williams & Wilkins.

16 Forsyth, D. M. & Bradley, D. J. (1964) Irreversible damage by *Schistosoma haematobium* in schoolchildren. *Lancet*, **ii**, 169–171.

17 Gilles, H. M. (1982) Infection with *S. haematobium*. In *Schistosomiasis: Treatment, Epidemiology and Control* (Ed.) Jordan, P. & Webbe, G. pp. 79–104. London: Heinemann Medical Books.

18 Hashem, M. (1947) The etiology and pathogenesis of the endemic form of splenomegaly: Egyptian splenomegaly. *Journal of the Egyptian Medical Association*, **30**, 48–79.

19 Hsueh, C. H. & Wu, Y. H. (1963) Endocrine disturbances in late schistosomiasis: a clinical study of 17 cases. *Chinese Medical Journal*, **82**, 519–527.

20 Jordan, P. (1982) Diagnostic and laboratory techniques. In *Schistosomiasis: Treatment, Epidemiology and Control* (Ed.) Jordan, P. & Webbe, G. pp. 165–183. London: Heinemann Medical Books.

21 Jordan, P. & Webbe, G. (1969) *Human Schistosomiasis*. London: Heinemann Medical Books.

22 Kane, C. A. & Most, H. (1948) Schistosomiasis of the central nervous system. Experiences in World War II and a review of the literature. *Archives of Neurological Psychiatry* (Chicago), **59**(2), 141–183.

23 Lehman, J. S., Farid, Z., Bassily, S. *et al.* (1970) Intestinal protein loss in schistosomal polyposis of the colon. *Gastroenterology*, **59**(3), 433–436.

24 Lehman, J. S., Farid, Z., Bassily, S. & Kent, D. C. (1971) Hydronephrosis, bacteriuria and maximal urine concentration in urinary bilharziasis. *Annals of Internal Medicine*, **75**(1), 49–55.

25 Makar, M. (1967) Some clinopathological aspects of urinary bilharziasis. In *Bilharziasis* (Ed.) Mostofi, F. K. pp. 45–47. Berlin: Springer-Verlag.

26 McCully, R. M., Barron, C. H. & Cheever, A. W. (1976) Schistosomiasis: diseases caused by trematodes. In *Pathology of Tropical and Extraordinary Diseases*, vol. 2 (Ed.) Bindford, C. H. & Connor, D. H. pp. 482–508. Washington D.C.: Armed Forces Institute of Pathology.

27 McLaren, M. L., Lilleywhite, J. E., Dunne, D. W. & Doenhoff, M. J. (1981) Serodiagnosis of human *Schistosoma mansoni* infections: enhanced sensitivity and specificity in ELISA using a fraction containing *S. mansoni* egg antigens ω_1 and α_1. *Transactions of the Royal Society of Tropical Medicine and Hygiene*, **75**, 72–79.

28 Mott, K. S. (1982) *S. japonicum* and *S. japonicum*-like infections. In *Schistosomiasis: Treatment, Epidemiology and Control* (Ed.) Jordan, P. & Webbe, G. pp. 128–149. London: Heinemann Medical Books.

29 PAHO/WHO (1968) *An Introductory Guide for Intermediate Hosts of Schistosomiasis in the Americas*. Washington D.C.: World Health Organization.

30 Pelley, R. P., Warren, K. S. & Jordan, P. (1977) Purified antigen radioimmunoassay in serological diagnosis of *Schistosoma mansoni*. *Lancet*, **ii**, 781–786.

31 Peters, P. A., Warren, K. S. & Mahmoud, A. A. F. (1976) Rapid, accurate quantification of schistosome eggs in nucleopore filters. *Journal of Parasitology*, **62**, 145–155.

32 Pitchford, R. J. (1959) Cattle schistosomiasis in man in the eastern Transvaal. *Transactions of the Royal Society of Tropical Medicine and Hygiene*, **54**(3), 285–290.

33 Prata, A. (1982) Infection with *S. mansoni*. In *Schistosomiasis: Treatment, Epidemiology and Control* (Ed.) Jordan, P. & Webbe, G. pp. 105–127. London: Heinemann Medical Books.

34 Silva, L. C. da, Brito, T. de, Camargo, M. E. *et al.* (1970) Kidney biopsy in the hepatosplenic form of infection with *Schistosoma mansoni* in man. *Bulletin of the World Health Organization*, **42**(6), 907–910.

35 Sulit, Y. S. M., Domingo, E. O., Dalmucio-Cruz, A. E. *et al.* (1964) Parasitic cirrhosis among Filipinos. *Journal of the Philippine Medicine Association*, **40** (12, 11), 1021–1038.

36 Tsai, C. Y. & Yu, W. (1966) Investigation in incubation period of acute schistosomiasis. *Chinese Medical Journal*, **85**, 183–185.

37 Tsutsumi, H. & Hasada, A. (1964) Studies in liver fibrosis (cirrhosis) due to *Schistosomiasis japonica*. III. The state of intervention of ova in the digestive tract. *Kurume Medical Journal*, **11**, 80–87.

38 Tsutsumi, H., Watanabe, A. & Nakashima, T. (1963) Studies on fibrosis (cirrhosis) due to *Schistosomiasis japonica*. Morphology of liver: Parts 1 & 2. *Kurume Medical Journal*, **10**, 51–59, 269–274.

39 Voge, M., Bruckner, D. & Bruce, J. I. (1978) *Schistosoma mekongi* sp. n. from man and animals, compared with four geographic strains of *Schistosoma japonicum*. *Journal of Parasitology*, **64**, 577–584.

40 Warren, K. S. (1968) Pathophysiology and pathogenesis of hepatosplenic schistosomiasis mansoni. *Bulletin of the New York Academy of Medicine*, **44**(3), 280–294.

41 Warren, K. S. (1971) Worms. In *Cecil-Loeb Textbook of Medicine*, 13th edn (Ed.) Beeson, P. B. & McDermott, W. pp. 745–752. Philadelphia: Saunders.

42 Warren, K. S. (1973) The pathology of schistosome infections. *Helminthological Abstracts, Series A, Animal and Human Helminthology*, **42**, 592–633.

43 Warren, K. S. (1977) Modulation of immunopathology and disease in schistosomiasis. *American Journal of Tropical Medicine and Hygiene*, **26**, 113–119.

44 Warren, K. S. & Domingo, E. O. (1970) Granuloma formation around *Schistosoma mansoni*, *S. haematobium* and *S. japonicum* eggs. Size and rate of development, cellular composition, cross-sensitivity and rate of egg destruction. *American Journal of Tropical Medicine and Hygiene*, **29**(2), 292–304.

45 Webbe, G. (1981) Schistosomiasis: some advances. *British Medical Journal*, **283**, 1104–1106.

46 Webbe, G. (1982) The parasites. In *Schistosomiasis: Treatment, Epidemiology and Control* (Ed.) Jordan, P. & Webbe, G. pp. 1–15. London: Heinemann Medical Books.

47 Webbe, G. (1982) The life-cycle of the parasites. In *Schistosomiasis: Treatment, Epidemiology and Control* (Ed.) Jordan, P. & Webbe, G. pp. 50–77. London: Heinemann Medical Books.

48 WHO Memorandum (1974) Immunology of schistosomiasis. *Bulletin of the World Health Organization*, **51**, 553–595.

49 WHO Workshop (1980) Quantitative aspects of the epidemiology of *Schistosoma japonicum* infection in a rural community in Luzon, Philippines. *Bulletin of the World Health Organization*, **58**, 629–638.

50 Winslow, D. J. (1967) Histopathology of schistosomiasis. In *Bilharziasis* (Ed.) Mostofi, F. K. pp. 230–241. Berlin, Heidelberg & New York: Springer-Verlag.

51 Wright, C. A., Southgate, V. R. & Knowles, R. J. (1972) What is *Schistosoma intercalatum* Fisher 1934? *Transactions of the Royal Society of Tropical Medicine and Hygiene*, **66**, 28–64.

52 Wydell, S. H. (1958) Some abdominal complications of *S. mansoni* as seen on Ukerewe Island. *East African Medical Journal*, **35**(8), 413–426.

INTESTINAL AMOEBIASIS

Fedor Losch first gave a detailed description of amoebic dysentery in 1875,[13] and since then much progress has been made in the understanding of this disease. Amoebiasis may be acute or chronic, symptomatic or asymptomatic infestation of the bowel. Extraintestinal disease, particularly amoebic liver abscess, is also quite common, and pulmonary, skin and neurological disease may occur.

Previously, the infection was thought of as a tropical disease, peculiar to underdeveloped countries, but the parasite can subsist in temperate climates, and a high incidence has been observed in developed countries, particularly in recent years.

Incidence and epidemiology

Until recently, amoebiasis was considered to be a disease transmitted through the ingestion of contaminated food and water and occurring in underdeveloped countries, where poor sanitary conditions prevail.[24] While this is basically true, and the highest incidence is found in tropical countries of South America and southern Asia, a drastic change in the incidence of amoebic infestation has occurred in the past ten years, with an alarming spread of the disease in the developed world. This is due to a new factor, namely that in the United States and Britain amoebiasis has become a venereal disease transmitted through widespread homosexual practices.

Numerous epidemiological studies have been undertaken using serological diagnosis. One such survey showed a 12% positivity for indirect haemagglutination in the general population of San José, Costa Rica, 30% in Medellín, Colombia, 58% in Bangkok, Thailand, and 76% in Calcutta. This high incidence of seropositivity coincides with the degree of invasive amoebiasis observed.[15]

In Mexico City 4–6% positivity is reported and amoebic liver abscess has been found in 2% of patients hospitalized in the National Medical Centre of Mexico City and in 3.2–4% of postmortems.[12] In Maracaibo, Venezuela, seropositivity ranged from 4.4% to 6.5%, depending on the population studied,[3] and amoebic liver abscess is found in 0.3–0.8% of hospitalized patients.[31]

The homosexual communities in New York and San Francisco have a high incidence of amoebiasis. In a VD clinic in Manhattan, Phillips, Mildram and William found *Entamoeba histolytica* in 25.5% of homosexual men, 6.2% of bisexual men and 0% of heterosexual men and women.[23]

Pomerantz, Marr and Goldman report a sharp increase in the number of cases of amoebiasis reported in recent years, and state that 'the incidence of amebiasis in New York City exceeded totals for most other major infectious diseases of public health importance such as tuberculosis and hepatitis, and was almost as prevalent as syphilis'.[24] Between 1958 and 1970, 47.8% of the cases were reported in males, and this figure increased to 65% of all cases between 1977 and 1978. Similar data have been reported from other cities in the United States and Britain.[7, 16, 20]

Pathology and pathogenesis

Classically, amoebiasis is contracted through the ingestion of contaminated food and water containing cysts of *Entamoeba histolytica*. These cysts have a considerable capacity for survival under most conditions. The route is faecal–oral. Ingested trophozoites are destroyed by gastric juices. In the small intestine, the cysts develop into trophozoites which invade the tissues, mainly in the colon, involving the caecum and rectosigmoid area, although all portions of the bowel may be involved.

The increased frequency of amoebiasis in homosexuals is thought to be due to the transmission of parasitic and other infections through frequent oral–anal sexual contact, and it is probable that promiscuity will result in severe disease because of frequent reinfection. There are other questions yet to be solved concerning the transmission of amoebiasis in non-tropical areas and in the developed world, such as contamination of public facilities, the role of food handlers, the importance of immigration and the eventual development of the disease in asymptomatic carriers.[8]

When *E. histolytica* comes in contact with intestinal cells, the first lesion produced is necrosis of the microvilli, followed by degeneration of the cells and infiltration of the surrounding tissues by polymorphonuclear leucocytes. *E. histolytica* separates the intercellular junctions, penetrates the lamina propria and invades all the layers of the intestinal wall. There is further necrosis, followed by the formation of an amoebic ulcer surrounded by a dense inflammatory infiltrate. Occasionally, a desmoplastic inflammatory reaction occurs, leading to the development of a pseudotumour known as an amoeboma.

E. histolytica is only capable of killing and phagocytizing cells on direct contact: neighbouring cells not in contact with amoebae remain intact.[25] Cell damage is not mediated by a cell-free cytotoxin, and there is no evidence that *E. histolytica* produces a cyto-lethal substance. Although microfilaments are apparently required for a contact-dependent extracellular cytopathic effect, the exact mechanism involved has yet to be identified. Phagocytosis is important, but apparently not essential.

Host factors are also important, including intestinal bacterial flora, nutritional condition and general immunological status. It has been speculated that the extreme rarity of small bowel involvement can be attributed to the sterility of that part of the gut.

A puzzling problem is the failure of some infected individuals to develop invasive disease. They remain asymptomatic carriers for long periods of time. Brumpt believed that the virulence of amoebae varies, and he actually described two varieties of morphologically indistinguishable amoebae, one pathogenic and one inoffensive.[2] The amoebae present in asymptomatic carriers may be less virulent than those present in acute clinical cases, and it is also possible that virulence follows a changing pattern which is related to the parasite itself or to immune factors present in the host.[35]

Lysates from different strains of amoebae have been studied by thin-layer starch electrophoresis for isoenzyme patterns, and it has been possible to identify and differentiate the special and unique patterns associated with 11 different types of amoebae.[27, 28] Those taken from asymptomatic carriers are clearly different from those from individuals with clinical disease. It is not known whether these differences are the cause or effect of some associated factor, or whether the isoenzyme pattern changes from pathogenic to non-pathogenic. If these findings prove to be valid and are confirmed, they have important implications.[11]

Immune response to *E. histolytica*

Amoebae are recognized by the immune system and antibodies form to amoebic antigens.[29] Their effectiveness as a mechanism of host resistance is uncertain. Cellular immune mechanisms may be an important factor in the control of amoebiasis.[18] There is evidence that patients cured of amoebic liver abscess will not be reinfected.[5] Amoebic antigen can produce antibodies in experimental animals and in turn protect such animals when they are challenged with large doses of pathogenic parasites.[4] The antibodies can also produce passive immunization in suckling hamsters.[32]

Clinical features

The manifestations of amoebiasis encompass a broad spectrum of disease, ranging from the asymptomatic carrier state to acute dysentery or chronic bowel disease.

ACUTE AMOEBIC DYSENTERY

At the onset the disease usually takes the form of a non-specific diarrhoea and subsequently develops into a more severe illness, with abdominal pain, cramps and severe tenesmus. The stools are liquid with an abundance of mucus and bright red blood. There is seldom fever, but as the disease develops the patient may become seriously ill. In some patients the initial diarrhoea may stop spontaneously, or

with non-specific treatment, and then recur within weeks or months.

A prolonged dysenteric disease may be encountered in young or older patients, with bloody diarrhoea and rather severe deterioration of general health. This condition is clinically indistinguishable from chronic ulcerative colitis, and some of the patients have actually been treated with steroids and sulphasalazine (Azulfidine) on the basis of a diagnosis of ulcerative colitis made endoscopically and radiologically. Such treatment in amoebiasis only makes the condition worse. It is extremely difficult to differentiate between the two diseases in endemic areas because they not infrequently coexist. In ulcerative colitis the diseased mucosa might be more susceptible to invasive amoebiasis and consequently amoebic infection should be carefully excluded in every new patient with ulcerative colitis. Likewise, patients with ulcerative colitis should undergo periodic surveillance to detect possible amoebic infestation.

Three main clinical settings are seen in non-tropical countries.[9]

1 Amoebiasis in groups of middle-aged people who contracted the disease while abroad. Frequently this is initially interpreted as being traveller's diarrhoea. The illness may remain as a diarrhoea or develop into full-blown dysenteric amoebiasis.

2 Amoebiasis in immigrants from tropical countries, who have brought the disease with them.

3 Male homosexuals who develop intestinal disease due to amoebae alone or in combination with a number of bacterial and parasitic infections. Association with giardia is common in this clinical setting.

Occasionally the disease may be severe, with dehydration, toxic shock and peritonitis, and toxic megacolon may develop because of transmural ulceration. The colon may perforate freely, and a tender mass can be felt in the abdomen when a perforation has been sealed with omentum. Abdominal rigidity is often absent. Leucocytosis is present and disassociated fever has been observed as in typhoid fever.[17] A liver abscess is a frequent accompanying lesion and this extremely severe clinical picture is invariably lethal if left untreated.

Amoebomas are pseudotumoral lesions which may follow an acute or a chronic course. They are usually located in the caecum or rectosigmoid portion of the colon. The main differential diagnosis is carcinoma of the bowel; this is most important because amoebomas are usually cured by medical treatment but are associated with a high mortality rate if they are submitted to surgery. A positive diagnosis can only be established by biopsy to exclude the possibility of a carcinoma and to demonstrate the amoebae in the histology sections. Positive serology is also of much diagnostic value.

CHRONIC AMOEBIASIS

Non-dysenteric colitis is a highly debatable entity. The clinical picture is one of irritable bowel, with or without pain, constipation or diarrhoea, and with cysts present in the stools. It is difficult to determine whether the cysts are responsible for the symptoms or whether there is an underlying irritable bowel syndrome. In any event caution is required before attributing the symptoms to the amoebae because the complaints frequently persist after successful treatment of the cysts. The persistence of an irritable bowel syndrome following successful treatment of acute dysenteric disease has been attributed to residual damage to the bowel wall but there is no evidence in support of this assumption. It is wise to refrain from attaching excessive importance to the diagnosis of chronic amoebic colitis, but cyst shedders, even when asymptomatic, should be treated because of their potential infectivity.

AMOEBIC LIVER ABSCESS

Amoebic liver abscess is a frequent complication in the more severe forms of amoebic colitis, or it may present as a primary disease without previous intestinal symptoms. These abscesses are usually located posteriorly in the right lobe of the liver but may occur in the left and may follow an acute or chronic course. The presentation may be with fever, sweating and weight-loss in the absence of localizing signs. In other patients there is hepatic tenderness, hepatomegaly and a pleural reaction above the affected diaphragm. Isotopic liver scans or ultrasonography are of diagnostic help. The extension of a right lobe abscess to the pleura and lung, and that of a left lobe abscess to the pericardium, or perforation into the peritoneal cavity are life-threatening complications.

Rare manifestations of amoebiasis are skin infections, either perianal, genital or at the opening of a sinus tract from a draining abscess. They may imitate squamous cell carcinoma and present as an ulcer or fungating mass.

Diagnosis

MICROSCOPIC DIAGNOSIS

Amoebiasis is best diagnosed on stool examination by an able and experienced technician. Stools must be examined within the hour of passing, because trophozoites lyse and become unrecognizable on storage at room temperature. The stool specimen must be free of contaminants such as barium, castor oil, mineral oil or magnesium hydroxide, since these substances interfere with parasite identification. Pretreatment with tetracyclines, sulphonamides, bismuth and kaolin compounds will prevent an adequate diagnosis.

Trophozoites may be confused with polymorphonuclear leucocytes and macrophages, and the innocuous trophozoites of *Entamoeba coli* can be mistaken for *E. histolytica*. Likewise, the cysts of *Entamoeba hartmani* should be differentiated from the cysts of *E. histolytica*.

If fresh stools are not available for examination for technical or geographical reasons, fixed or preserved specimens must be used. Ten-per-cent formalin should be used for cysts and polyvinyl alcohol (PVA) for trophozoites.[6] The formalin–ether method should be used for concentration of the fixed specimen. The specimen preserved in PVA should be smeared on cover slips and stained with iron haematoxylin or Gomori's trichrome stain.

The examination of three to six samples, if carried out adequately, allows the diagnosis of 80–90% of patients.

ENDOSCOPIC DIAGNOSIS

The most important evidence of acute amoebic colitis is provided by proctoscopic examination, which should be undertaken routinely. Normal mucosa, generalized erythema and, most frequently, amoebic ulcers can be observed using the rigid sigmoidoscope. These ulcers are usually 1–5 mm in diameter, randomly distributed in the mucosa and located over relatively normal mucosa (Plate 14.1). In the more severely affected patients there is diffuse inflammation of the mucosa with large ulcers which are extremely difficult to differentiate from those of ulcerative colitis (Plate 14.2). In the majority of patients colonoscopic examination shows that the lesions stop at the descending colon, but in some the whole colon is involved. Colonoscopic examination is vital for the diagnosis of amoeboma of the caecum. A large ulcerated mass is seen, often fungating, with freely bleeding ulcers which make it difficult to distinguish from adenocarcinoma. Biopsy is essential and the presence of parasites in the fibrous tissue indicates a diagnosis of amoeboma.

Scrapings of any ulcers should always be taken and examined while fresh. Amoebae can be identified with the aid of ferric haematoxylin or PAS staining of biopsy material (Plate 14.3).

RADIOLOGY

A barium enema is not usually performed in acute amoebic dysentery. In the more chronic infections or in the event of any diagnostic doubt, the enema shows ulcerations along the margin of the gut, either in the form of fine serrations or as larger ulcers which, when present, extend throughout the whole length of the colon, but are more marked in the sigmoid and descending colon. The 'thumb-prints' appearance is occasionally seen and the mucosa has a cobblestone appearance. Radiological differential diagnosis of these atypical pictures is not easy and it is often very difficult to exclude ulcerative colitis. However, once the disease has responded to treatment the lesions heal completely and the colon returns to normal (Figures 14.27 and 14.28).

In amoebic toxic dilatation of the colon, plain films of the abdomen are similar to those seen in ulcerative colitis.[36] All segments of the colon are dilated and the haustral pattern is absent. An amoeboma appears as an irregular filling defect with ulceration located in the caecum or in the left colon. The diagnosis of amoeboma may be suspected from the clinical picture and epidemiologic situation, but endoscopic and histological confirmation is always necessary.

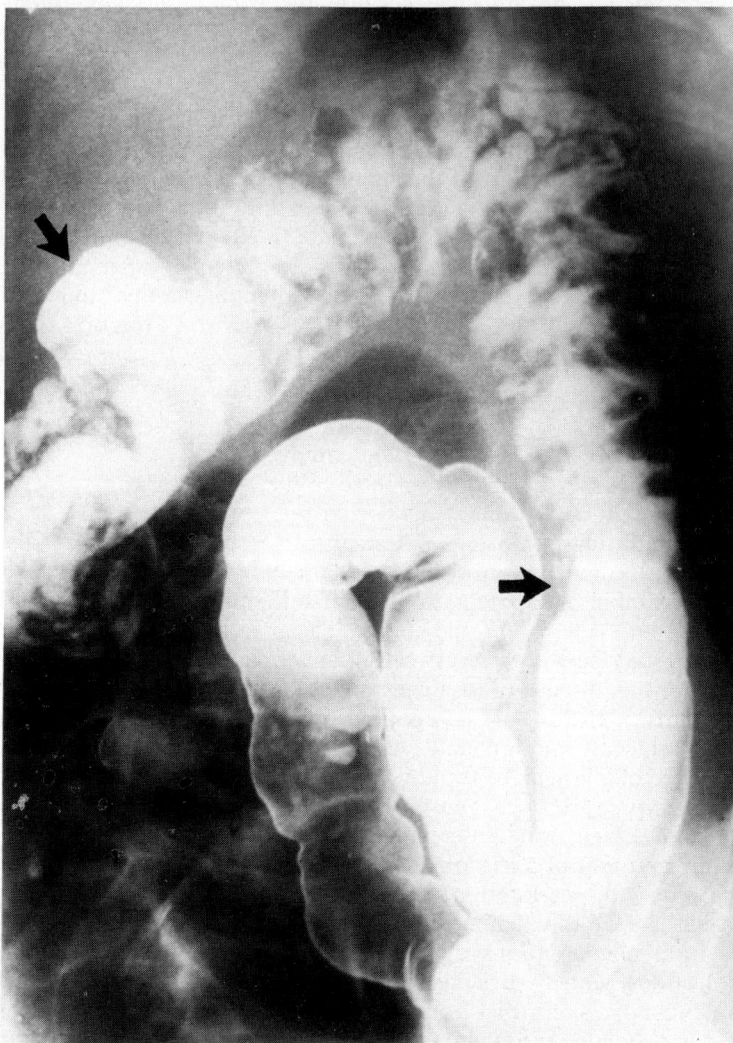

Fig. 14.27 A 65-year-old woman with very severe and protracted bloody diarrhoea resembling ulcerative colitis. There are large ulcers in the left colon (arrowed), which appear to stop beyond the splenic flexure. There is a very large ulcer in the transverse colon, near the splenic flexure. Endoscopy shows lesions in the more distal bowel. *E. histolytica* was found in the stools and in the mucosal biopsy.

a

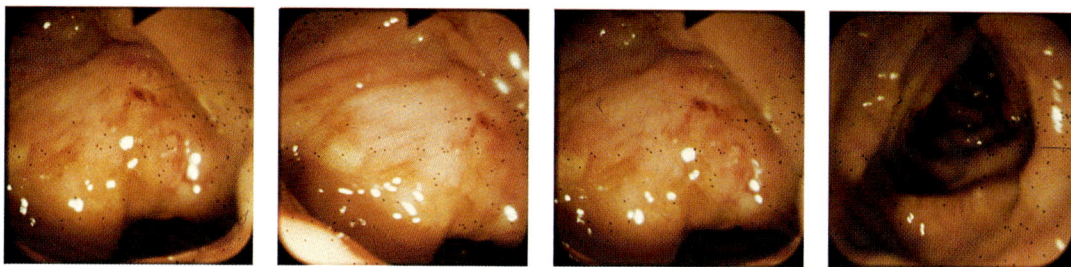

Plate 14.1 The rectal mucosa appears to be oedematous and there is a scattering of shallow, bleeding ulcers in the mucosa in the typical case of amoebic dysentery. Usually the sigmoid and the more proximal colon are normal, or there is only slight oedema.

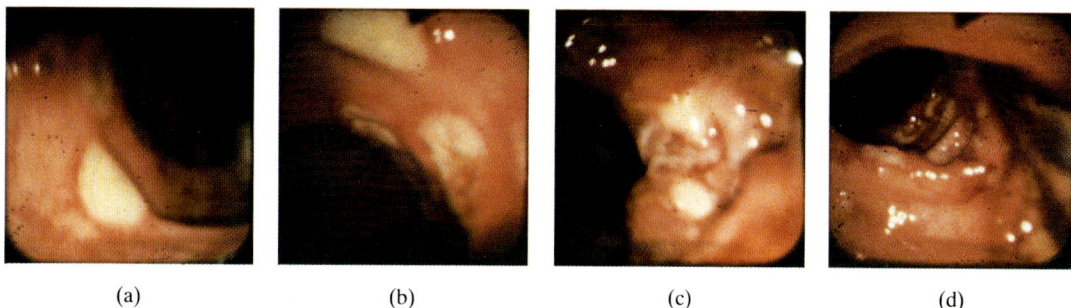

(a)   (b)   (c)   (d)

Plate 14.2 In very severe infections the ulcers become very deep and large (a,b), but the mucosa between has a fairly normal appearance. Some ulcers (c) have an irregular base and swollen border. There are deep, bleeding ulcers in the sigmoid and descending colon. *Entamoeba histolytica* was found in the stools and in the mucosal biopsy of this patient.

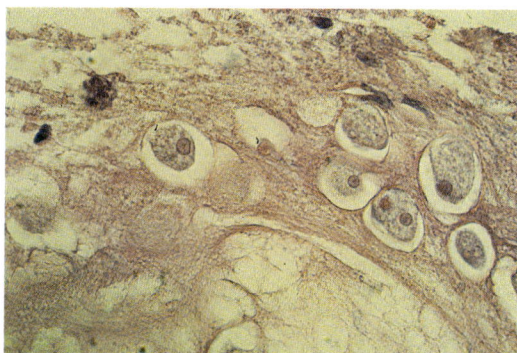

Plate 14.3 Multiple trophozoites are present in the exudate and necrotic material on the surface of the ulcer. Haematoxylin and eosin, ×900.

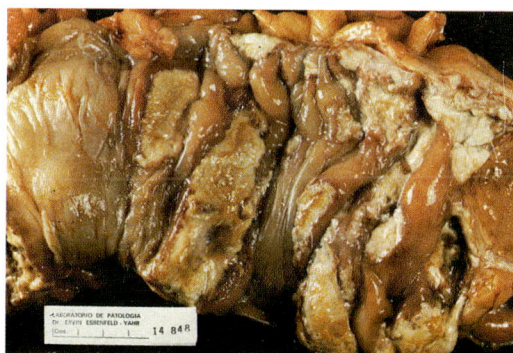

Plate 14.4 Resected colon from patient with amoebiasis.

Colour by courtesy of the President of the Venezuelan Cancer Society.

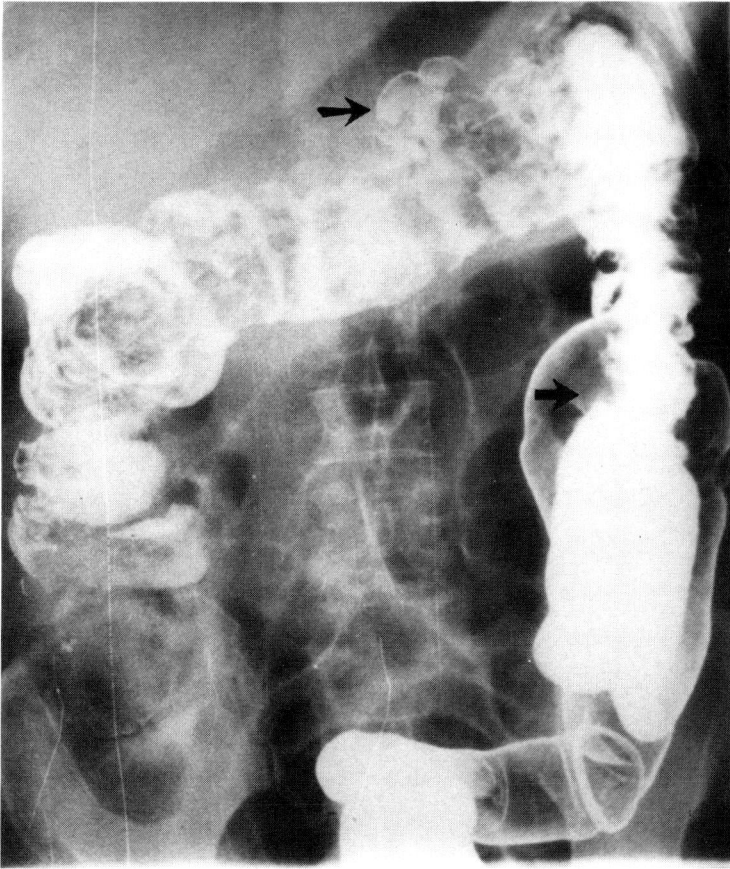

b

Fig. 14.27(b)

SEROLOGIC DIAGNOSIS

E. histolytica is antigenic and produces an immune response in the host. The antibodies usually persist for a long time, making it difficult to differentiate between a previous infection and existing disease. Positive reactions always indicate invasive amoebiasis and are most useful in the diagnosis of extraintestinal disease. Nevertheless, epidemiological studies can best be done by serological methods, even though they will not distinguish between active disease, postinfection and asymptomatic carriers.

Indirect haemagglutination,[19, 22] latex agglutination,[19] cellulose acetate precipitation,[19, 22] counter immunoelectrophoresis,[30, 34] complement fixation,[10] gel diffusion precipitin test[22] and fluorescent immunoassay[33] have all been used with varying degrees of sensitivity and specificity. In general, they will give a 90–98% positive response in extraintestinal disease and 80–90% in intestinal infection.[10, 22, 30, 34]

The enzyme-linked immunosorbent assay (ELISA) method for detection of amoebic antigen in stools is a very simple and highly sensitive method,[21, 26] but it has not yet been completely evaluated. However, should future experience show a good clinical and parasitological correlation, this could become a most useful diagnostic test.

Treatment

Ipecacuana has been used in the treatment of dysentery since the 19th century, and its alkaloid, emetine, which was isolated in 1912, has been effective in intestinal and invasive amoebiasis, but because of its side-effects other drugs have been introduced in the management of amoebiasis.

Oxyquinolines, arsenicals and antibiotics including paromomycin and erythromycin and tetracyclines have been used. Chloroquine also possesses amoebicidal properties, but only in extraintestinal disease. Dehydroemetine has the same properties as emetine, but without the neuromuscular and cardiac side-effects.

In 1966, Powel and Elsdon Dew demonstrated that metronidazole was highly effective

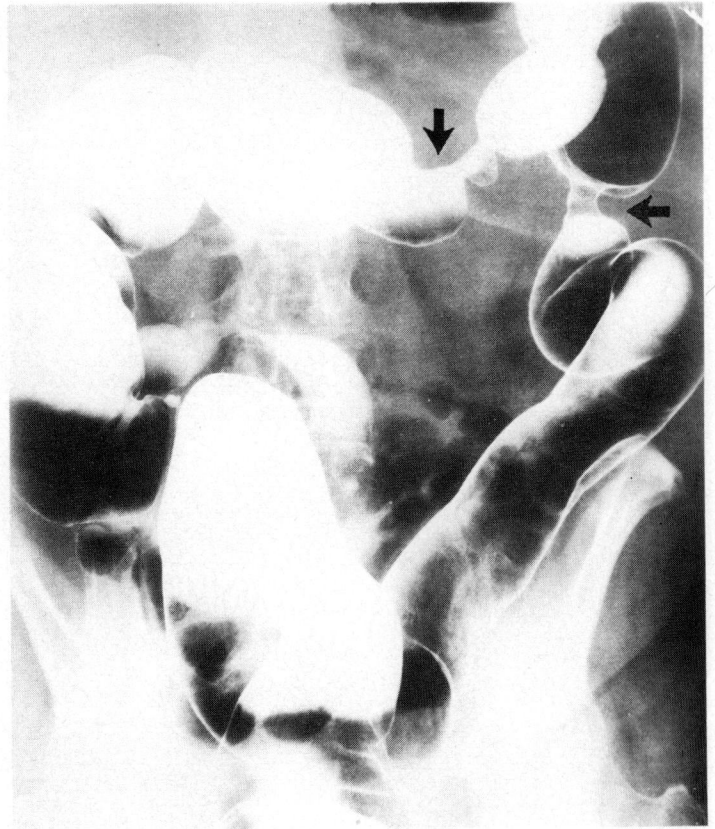

Fig. 14.28 Same patient as Figure 14.27: X-ray taken six months after healing. The colon is normal except for two strictures: one in the distal transverse colon probably where the large ulcer was, and one in the descending colon at the junction of the diseased and apparently healthy mucosa.

and well tolerated in intestinal disease as well as tissue invasion. Although some resistance has been reported occasionally, most of the infections respond well, with prompt resolution of symptoms. A number of metronidazole derivatives, including ornidazole and tinidazole, are in common use. Parenteral metronidazole and ornidazole are also available, for severe intestinal amoebiasis and liver abscess, or when the drug cannot be administered orally.

The effect of metronidazole and its derivative compounds on anaerobic intestinal flora is thought to be beneficial and despite the observation of its carcinogenicity in rats and mutagenic action in bacteria, it is currently the drug of choice in the treatment of intestinal amoebiasis. Patients with acute amoebic colitis who do not respond to metronidazole, should receive parenteral dehydroemetine.

The treatment of the asymptomatic cyst shedder is problematic. Clioquinol (iodochlorhydroxyquin) is a highly effective drug, but it is no longer used following reports that it can cause a subacute myelo-optic neuropathy. At present the choice of drug lies between metronidazole, di-iodohydroxyquinoline (iodoquinol), diloxanide furoate and the antibiotic paro-

momycin; they can be administered in subsequent series if necessary. Table 14.16 summarizes the most useful drugs and their dosage for the management of intestinal and extraintestinal infections.

In cases of toxic megacolon, or when perforation occurs, treatment should be initiated as soon as possible once the diagnosis has been established, together with general supportive measures. Surgery may be necessary on an emergency basis and must then be radical, that is, partial or total colonic resection (Plate 14.4 shows a section of resected colon). Primary anastomosis must be avoided.[1, 17] The mortality is extremely high if this form of amoebic colitis is left untreated but with vigorous medical and surgical treatment it has been reduced to 45–55%.

The treatment for amoeboma is parenteral dehydroemetine and metronidazole. The patients usually heal on medical therapy alone but they will perforate occasionally and emergency surgery will be required. Amoebomas and acute fulminant colitis often coexist with liver abscesses and the latter should be sought out and treated using oral or parenteral metronidazole or its derivatives.

Table 14.16 Drugs used in intestinal and extraintestinal amoebic infections.

Form of infection	Dosage	Route
Intestinal		
Trophozoites in stool		
Metronidazole ⎫		
Ornidazole ⎬	500–750 mg t.i.d. for 5–10 days	Oral
Tinidazole ⎭		
Dehydroemetine	$1 \text{ mg} \cdot \text{kg}^{-1} \cdot \text{day}^{-1}$ for 10 days	Subcutaneous
Cysts		
Metronidazole ⎫		
Ornidazole ⎬	500–750 mg t.i.d. for 5–10 days	Oral
Tinidazole ⎭		
Diloxanide furoate	500 mg t.i.d. for 10 days	Oral
Paromomycin sulphate	500 mg t.i.d. for 5–10 days	Oral
Di-iodohydroxyquinoline (iodoquinol)	650 mg t.i.d. for 20 days	Oral
Extraintestinal		
Metronidazole ⎫		
Ornidazole ⎬	500–750 mg t.i.d. for 5–10 days	Oral
Tinidazole ⎭		
Dehydroemetine	$1 \text{ mg} \cdot \text{kg}^{-1} \cdot \text{day}^{-1}$ for 10 days	Subcutaneous
Dehydroemetine +	$1 \text{ mg} \cdot \text{kg}^{-1} \cdot \text{day}^{-1}$ for 10 days +	Subcutaneous
metronidazole	500 mg t.i.d. for 5–10 days	Oral
Tetracycline	500 mg every 6 hours for 10 days	Oral
Metronidazole ⎫		
Ornidazole ⎭	500 mg every 6–8 hours for 5 days	Intravenous

t.i.d. = three times a day.

It is sometimes necessary to resect an amoeboma, particularly if there has been no response to medical therapy or where there is doubt about the underlying diagnosis. Although amoebic abscess should resolve on medical therapy, surgical drainage may be necessary if the abscess is very large.

REFERENCES

1 Bautista, J. (1978) Tratamiento quirúrgico de las complicaciones de la amibiasis invasora. *Archivos de Investigacion Medica (Mexico)*, **9**, 411–415.
2 Brumpt, E. (1925) *Entamoeba dispar* n. sp.; ameba with quadrinuclear cysts, parasite in man. *Bulletin de l'Académie de Médicine* (Paris), **94**, 943. Cited in *Lancet*, **i**, 303 (1979).
3 Chacin-Bonilla, L. & Bonpart, D. (1981) A seroepidemiological study of amebiasis in adults in Maracaibo, Venezuela. *American Journal of Tropical Medicine and Hygiene*, **30**, 1201–1205.
4 De La Torre, M., Ortiz-Ortiz, L., De La Hoz, R. & Sepulveda, B. (1973) Acción del suero humano inmune de la gammaglobulina antiamibiana sobre los cultivos de *E. histolytica*. *Archivos de Investigacion Medica (Mexico)*, **4**, 155.
5 De Leon, A. (1970) Pronóstico tardío en el absceso hepático amibiano. *Archivos de Investigacion Medica (Mexico)*, **1**, 205.
6 Despommier, D. D. (1981) The laboratory diagnosis of *Entamoeba histolytica*. *Bulletin of the New York Academy of Medicine*, **57**, 212–216.
7 Dritz, S. K., Ainsworth, T. E., Back, A. *et al.* (1977) Patterns of sexually transmitted enteric diseases in a city. *Lancet*, **ii**, 3–4.

8 Fodor, T. (1981) Unanswered questions about the transmission of amebiasis. *Bulletin of the New York Academy of Medicine*, **57**, 224–226.
9 Kean, B. H. (1981) Clinical amebiasis in New York City: symptoms, signs and treatment. *Bulletin of the New York Academy of Medicine*, **57**, 207–211.
10 Kim, H. & Finkelstein, S. (1978) Serologic responses in amebiasis. *Archivos de Investigacion Medica (Mexico)*, **9**, 357–361.
11 Lancet (1979) Pathogenic *Entamoeba histolytica*. (Editorial.) *Lancet*, **i**, 303.
12 Landa, L., Aubanel, M., Segovid, E. & Sepulveda, B. (1972) Seroepidemiología de la amibiasis en adultos. *Archivos Investigacion Medica (Mexico)*, **3**, 377–380.
13 Losch, F. (1875) Massenhafte Entwickelung von Amoeben in Dickdarm. *Archiv für Pathologische Anatomie*, **211**(65), 196.
14 Marr, J. S. (1981) Amebiasis in New York City: a changing pattern of transmission. *Bulletin of the New York Academy of Medicine*, **57**, 188–200.
15 Meerovitch, E., Healy, G. R. & Ambroise-Thomas, P. (1978) Amoebiasis survey in Calcutta (India), Bangkok (Thailand), Medellin (Colombia) and San José (Costa Rica). *Canadian Journal of Public Health*, **69**, 286–288.
16 Monillan, A. & Robertson, D. H. (1977) Sexually transmitted diseases in homosexual males in Edinburgh. *Health Bulletin (Edinburgh)*, **35**, 266–271.
17 Nicholls, J. C. (1981) Amoebiasis: a surgeon's view. *Annals of the Royal College of Surgery of England*, **63**, 25–27.
18 Ortiz-Ortiz, L., Garmilla, C., Tanimoto-Weki, M. & Zamacona-Ravelo, G. (1973) Hipersensibilidad celular en amibiasis. I. Reacciones en hamsters inoculados con *E. histolytica*. *Archivos de Investigacion Medica (Mexico)*, **4**, 141.
19 Ortiz-Ortiz, L., Capin, N. R., Capin, R. & Zamacona, G. (1978) Un nuevo método de hemaglutinación para

determinar anticuerpos contra entamoeba histolytica. *Archivos de Investigacion Medica (Mexico)*, **9**, 351–356.

20 Ostrow, D. G. & Shaskey, G. M. (1977) The experience of the Howard Brown Memorial Clinic of Chicago with sexually transmitted diseases. *Sexually Transmitted Diseases*, **4**, 53–55.

21 Palacios, O., De La Hoz, R. & Sosa, H. (1978) Determinación del antígeno amibiano en heces por el método ELISA. *Archivos de Investigacion Medica (Mexico)*, **9**, 339–348.

22 Patterson, M., Healy, G. R. & Shabot, J. M. (1980) Serologic testing for amoebiasis. *Gastroenterology*, **78**, 136–141.

23 Phillips, S. C., Mildram, D. & William, D. C. (1981) Sexual transmission of enteric protozoa and helminths in a venereal disease clinic population. *New England Journal of Medicine*, **305**, 603–606.

24 Pomerantz, B. M., Marr, J. S. & Goldman, W. D. (1980) Amebiasis in New York City 1958–1978: identification of the male homosexual high-risk population. *Bulletin of the New York Academy of Medicine*, **56**, 232–244.

25 Ravdin, J. I., Croft, B. Y. & Guerrant, R. L. (1980) Cytopathogenic mechanisms of *Entamoeba histolytica*. *Journal of Experimental Medicine*, **152**, 377–390.

26 Root, D. M., Cole, F. X. & Williamson, J. A. (1978) The development and standardization of an ELISA method for the detection of *Entamoeba histolytica* antigens in stool samples. *Archivos de Investigacion Medica (Mexico)*, **9**, 203–210.

27 Sargeaunt, P. G. & Williams, J. E. (1978) The differentiation of invasive and non-invasive *Entamoeba histolytica* by isoenzyme electrophoresis. *Transactions of the Royal Society of Tropical Medicine and Hygiene*, **72**, 519–521.

28 Sargeaunt, P. G., Williams, J. E., Kumate, S. & Jimenez, E. (1980) The epidemiology of *Entamoeba histolytica* in Mexico City. *Transactions of the Royal Society of Tropical Medicine and Hygiene*, **74**, 653–656.

29 Sepulveda, B., Tanimoto, M., Vazquez-Saavedra, J. A. & Landa, L. (1971) Inducción de inmunidad antiamibiana en el hamster, con antígeno obtenido de cultivos axénicos de *Entamoeba histolytica*. *Archivos de Investigacion Medica (Mexico)*, **2**, 289.

30 Sharma, P., Das, P. & Dutta, G. P. (1981) Rapid diagnosis amoebic liver abscess using *Entamoeba histolytica* antigen. *Archivos de Investigacion Medica (Mexico)*, **12**, 558.

31 Sociedad Venezolana de Gastroenterologia (1972) Amibiasis en Venezuela. *Revista Venezolana de Sanidad y Asistencia Social*, **37**, 716–763.

32 Tanimoto-Weki, M., Vazquez-Saavedra, J. A., Calderon-Lara, P. & Aguirre-Garcia, J. (1973) Inmunidad consecutiva a la inyección de antígeno amibiano axénico en el hamster. *Archivos de Investigacion Medica (Mexico)*, **4**, 147.

33 Taylor, R. G. & Perez, T. R. (1978) Serology of amebiasis using the Fiax TM System. *Archivos de Investigacion Medica (Mexico)*, **9**, 363–366.

34 Tosswill, J. H. C., Ridley, D. S. & Warhurst, D. C. (1980) Counter inmunoelectrophoresis as a rapid screening test for amoebic liver abscess. *Journal of Clinical Pathology*, **33**, 33–35.

35 Vinayak, V. K., Naik, S. R., Sawhney, S. *et al.* (1977) Pathogenicity of *Entamoeba histolytica* – virulence of strains of amoeba from symptomatic and asymptomatic cases of amoebiasis. *Indian Journal of Medical Research*, **66**, 935–941.

36 Wig, J. D., Talwar, B. L. & Bushnurmath, S. R. (1981) Toxic dilatation complicating amoebic colitis. *British Journal of Surgery*, **68**, 135–136.

37 Wolfe, M. S. (1973) Non-dysenteric intestinal amebiasis: treatment with diloxamide furoate. *Journal of the American Medical Association*, **224**, 1601–1604.

38 Is Flagyl dangerous? (1975) *Medical Letter on Drugs and Therapeutics*, **17**, 53–54.

GASTROINTESTINAL TUBERCULOSIS

Most people would consider that the virtual elimination of tuberculosis in dairy cattle and the pasteurization of milk would have effectively eliminated the disease, particularly in the United Kingdom, but in fact the disease is still present, although it is almost never due to *Mycobacterium bovis*, and is now almost exclusively caused by *Mycobacterium tuberculosis*. In the Third World the disease is far more common: in Delhi it accounts for 0.8% of hospital admissions[13] and nearly 11% of patients with intestinal obstruction and 5.7% of patients with intestinal perforation.[8, 9, 10]

In the last decade there has been a series of reports from authors working in a number of British cities with large immigrant populations[16, 29, 30, 37, 46] coming predominantly from the Indian subcontinent. There is, however, a very definite prevalence of the disease in the indigenous population. The clinician is advised always to bear gastrointestinal tuberculosis in mind as the differential diagnosis of both Crohn's disease and ulcerative colitis.

Clinical presentation

In the United Kingdom the disease is predominantly seen in immigrants, principally those from the Indian subcontinent, though it is seen in the West Indian community. In the Bradford series the disease was present in Ukrainian, Polish and Irish immigrants as well as those from the Third World. Reports from North America also draw attention to the occurrence of the disease in the Caucasian immigrant community rather than in the indigenous community.[24, 35]

In the United Kingdom the disease is seen more frequently in men than women, mainly because there are more men than women in the immigrant community. The housing conditions of these men are frequently poor, they often work shifts and the almost hostel-like conditions, with the absence of women, leads to poor nutritional standards.

Patients are mainly affected in the fourth decade, when they present with two groups of symptoms: those of a chronic inflammatory illness, and symptoms more directly related to the part of the gastrointestinal tract that has been affected. The chronic inflammatory illness symptoms are vague and non-specific and include anorexia, fatigue, weight loss, asthenia, depression and fever.

It is not clear why gastrointestinal tuberculosis should occur at such varying times after the patient's immigration, following initial primary infection.[35] The interval varied from six months to 16 years with a mean of some 6 years in the Bradford series.[16] Studies in patients with pulmonary disease have shown that phage typing of the organism was identical to that found in the patient's country of origin.[22] There is some evidence that the stress of immigration itself may modify immune mechanisms, but there is still no clear explanation of why the time interval is so variable.

Pathology

Gastrointestinal tuberculosis may be classified as primary or secondary. Primary tuberculosis nearly always occurs following ingestion of *Mycobacterium bovis*, and the very strict monitoring of dairy herds and pasteurization of milk have reduced the incidence of the disease in the UK. Maintenance of this strict monitoring continues, as does elimination of other vectors of the disease, such as the infected badger population. Only 1.3% of the patients with gastrointestinal tuberculosis in Bradford have *Mycobacterium bovis*.

Secondary gastrointestinal tuberculosis represents recrudescence of previous disease, frequently pulmonary, though women may acquire the infection initially via the genital tract. The disease assumes two types: first, peritoneal disease, which may be acute or chronic, and, secondly, direct involvement of the gastrointestinal tract. The omentum may become thickened and form plaque-like masses.

Histology

The classical tuberculous granuloma is not always found and caseation may be present in only 32.7% of patients.[26, 27] The absence of caseation may be due to an abnormality of host reaction, modification of the immune response, attenuation of disease or the partial effects of treatment. The demonstration of acid-fast bacilli is relatively uncommon despite the fact that the lesion may be typical of tuberculosis. This observation remains true despite the use of auromine–rhodamine and Ziehl–Neelsen staining techniques.

Investigations

The diagnosis of any chronic inflammatory disease depends on the results of a variety of fairly non-specific investigations and some specific investigations. In gastrointestinal tuberculosis there might be evidence of a mild normocytic normochromic anaemia, although a fairly typical iron-deficiency-pattern anaemia can be found. The erythrocyte sedimentation rate (ESR) may be elevated, but the Bradford series and others have indicated that it may be raised in as few as 56%. A low serum iron with a normal iron binding capacity may be found as in any chronic inflammatory disorder. There may be disturbance of proteins with a low serum albumin. The more specific investigations are of variable usefulness; for example, Heaf and Mantoux testing was positive in only 31% of patients in the Bradford series,[16] 60% of the Manchester series[30] and 100% of the small Southampton series.[44]

The critical investigation is to demonstrate the presence of tubercle bacilli, in tissue obtained by biopsy or laparotomy, by culture of stools, peritoneal fluids, sputum, high vaginal swabs or gastric aspiration or by culture of liver tissue, endometrial biopsy material, liver biopsy or tissue from the gastrointestinal tract itself. Good contact between physician and bacteriologist or pathologist is desirable, because demonstration of the bacteria on culture or histologically requires persistence and meticulous care. At least six stool specimens should be sent for culture. The recovery of *Mycobacterium tuberculosis* from the stools does not always indicate active gastrointestinal disease because the bacilli from infected sputum can survive passage through the gastrointestinal tract. Investigations such as faecal fat, Schilling test, xylose absorption and glucose tolerance tests can be normal even in the presence of very extensive disease. A fall in alpha-2-globulins was considered by Pimparker to indicate a deterioration in gastrointestinal tuberculosis.[33] Plain X-rays of the abdomen are essential, because they may reveal abscess cavities, calcification, small bowel fluid levels and evidence of peritoneal fluid. Barium studies are valuable and may frequently demonstrate the site and extent of disease, but do not define the cause with certainty.

SPECIFIC INVESTIGATIONS

Udwadia[42] and Wolfe, Behn and Jackson[46] have drawn attention to the very considerable value of laparoscopy and target biopsy. The procedure is straightforward in those with established ascites but there may be problems where there is fibro-caseous disease. Udwadia[42] reported 29 lesions in a series of 34 laparoscopies in patients whose symptoms and abdominal signs raised the possibility of gastrointestinal tuberculosis. When abdominal pain, a mass, ascites and a history of pyrexia and weight loss were present the appropriate investigation was laparoscopy and biopsy. Lymphangiography is of considerable value,[6] but, unfortunately, similar abnormalities can arise owing to non-specific reactive hyperplasia, lymphoma and metastatic malignant disease. Beetlestone *et al.*[6] and Witte, Horowitz and Dumont[45] have reviewed the role of thoracic duct cannulation with subsequent staining and culture of the aspirate.

Isotopic techniques have been tried. Techniques such as ^{67}Ga-citrate scanning[5, 40] and ^{111}In-labelled leucocyte scanning[34] may be helpful, but they too are non-specific and other forms of intra-abdominal sepsis such as pyogenic abscesses and those associated with Crohn's disease may give similar appearances. CT scanning has been described by Gleason *et al.*,[17] as being of value in the diagnosis of duodenal disease, but there are no extensive series considering its role in gastrointestinal tuberculosis. The problem with these techniques is that they are expensive, high-technology procedures and are not likely to be available in the countries where gastrointestinal tuberculosis is most likely to occur. ^{67}Ga-citrate scanning is helpful when tuberculosis affects the liver: multiple small abscess cavities can be demonstrated.

Clinical features

OROPHARYNGEAL TUBERCULOSIS

Oropharyngeal tuberculosis is extremely uncommon. Cowan and Jones have described a single case and given an extensive review of the topic.[15] Tuberculous laryngitis was common in the days prior to antituberculous therapy and was frequently present in those with extensive pulmonary tuberculosis. In the United Kingdom pulmonary tuberculosis very rarely proceeds to the extensive fulminating disease associated with laryngeal involvement.

OESOPHAGEAL DISEASE

Oesophageal disease is exceedingly rare and the majority of patients with oesophageal symptoms have them as a result of extrinsic compression of the oesophagus by lymphatic gland masses (Figure 14.29), although these may eventually erode the oesophagus, causing a broncho-oesophageal fistula. Fortunately, when these fistulas do occur they heal very rapidly with effective antituberculous therapy and surgical intervention is rarely indicated.

GASTRIC TUBERCULOSIS

Gastric tuberculosis is very unusual and in my experience has only accounted for 1.5% of the patients with abdominal tuberculosis, but figures of up to 2.8 per cent in a larger series of 500 patients have been reported by Mukerjee and Singal.[31] The patient may present with gastric ulcers or with a narrowing of the pyloric antrum (Figure 14.30a) which might be mistaken for a malignant lesion. The lesion responds well to antituberculous therapy (Figure 14.30b).

DUODENAL DISEASE

Duodenal disease, like the other forms of upper gastrointestinal tract tuberculosis, is unusual; it may be associated with symptoms due simply to extrinsic pressure on the duodenal loop. Direct involvement of the duodenal mucosa can occur (Figure 14.31); indeed, tuberculous duodenal ulceration was recognized as a clinical entity long before peptic ulceration. Treatment may lead to healing with stricture formation which can cause high small bowel obstruction. Complications of the duodenal disease may include fistula formation (Figure 14.32); these fistulas, like the oesophageal fistulas heal rapidly on antituberculous treatment.

TUBERCULOUS PERITONITIS

The view is widely held, incorrectly, that tuberculous peritonitis is due to extension from contiguous disease; in fact, it occurs following reactivation of latent tuberculosis in the peritoneum that was a result of haematogenous spread from a primary focus.[32] Only 6% of patients have concurrent parenchymal pulmonary disease.[38] The clinical presentation is that of anorexia, debility, weight loss and fever coupled with the development of ascites. 65% of patients have abdominal tenderness.[38] A 'doughy abdomen' is a very rare finding.[7] Often, the

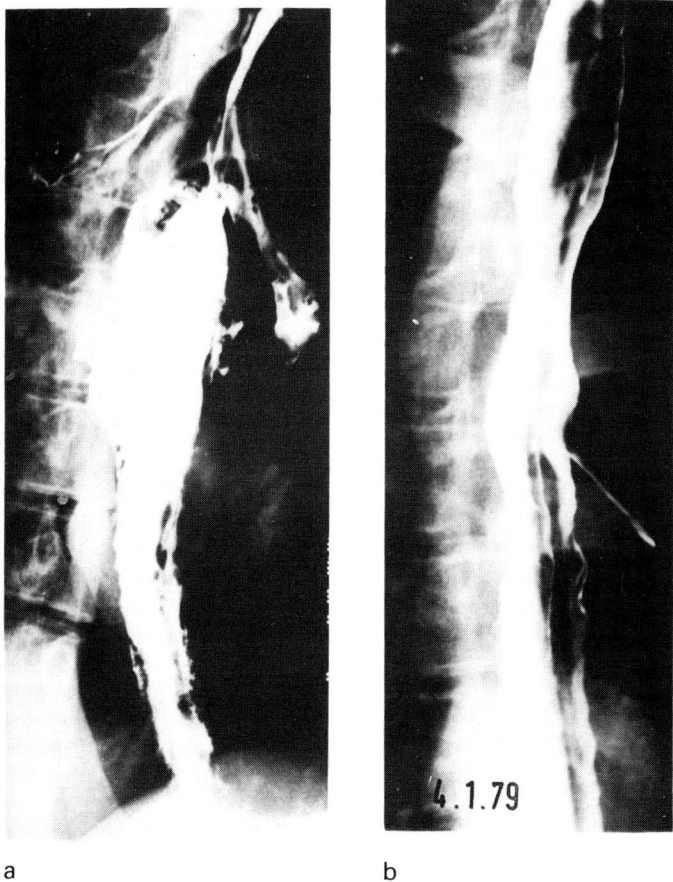

Fig. 14.29 (a) Compression of the oesophagus by mediastinal glands presenting with dysphagia in a 23-year-old Indian woman. (b) The radiological appearances when the patient was free of symptoms, three weeks after commencing treatment.

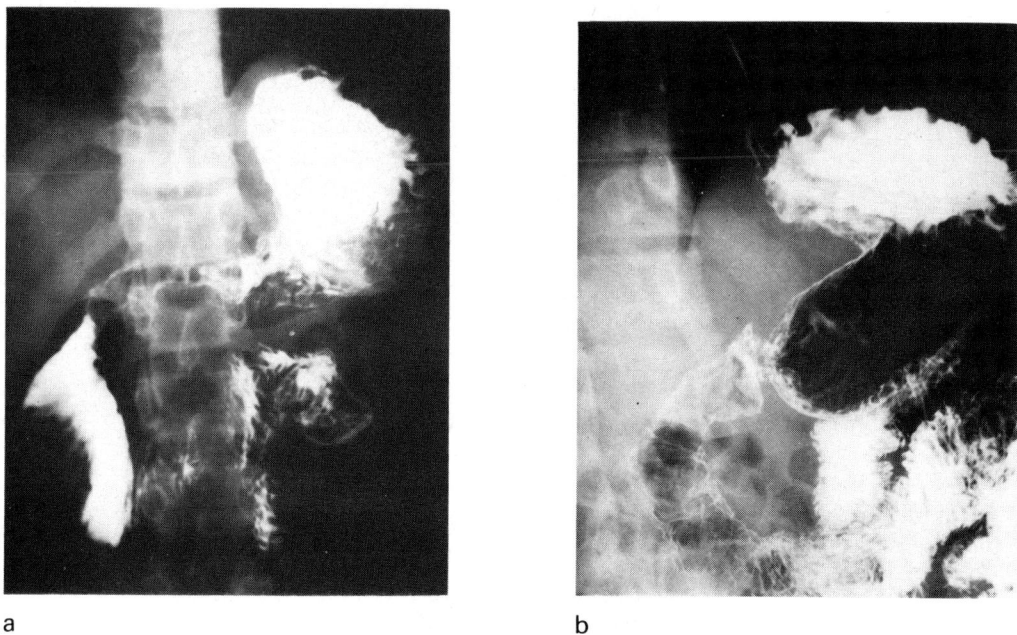

Fig. 14.30 (a) Barium swallow X-ray of a young Asian man presenting with anorexia and weight loss, showing narrowing of the antrum. (b) Barium meal examination after nine months treatment, showing normal appearances.

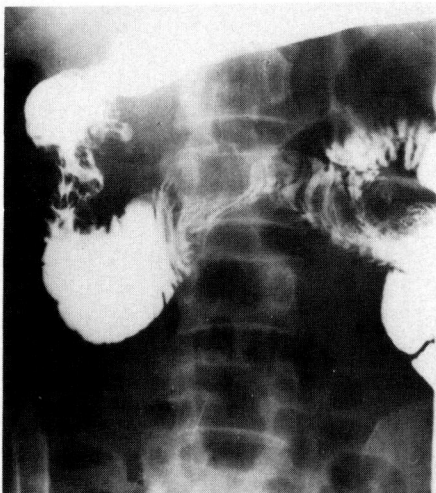

Fig. 14.31 Barium meal showing mural involvement of the second part of the duodenum by tuberculosis and compression of the distal duodenum by an extrinsic gland mass. From Findlay *et al.* (1979),[16] with kind permission of the authors and the editor of *Journal of the Royal Society of Medicine.*

other serous membranes are involved; for example a pleural effusion occurred in 32% of one series.[38] A pericardial effusion may occur coincidentally with peritonitis,[39] and there may be ECG evidence of myocardial involvement in association with peritonitis. ST depression and widespread T wave inversion were noted in 13% of patients.[38] Constrictive pericarditis may rarely develop as a complication of treatment of gastrointestinal tuberculosis with conventional anti-tuberculous therapy.

DISEASE OF THE JEJUNUM AND ILEUM

The jejunum and ileum are areas more frequently affected by ..berculosis. Twenty-eight patients out of 102 had ileal disease independant of associated caecal involvement.[43] Pimparker[33] reviewed the topic and claimed that ileal disease could occur in 31–89% of patients. The characteristic presentation is with pain, a change in bowel habit, malabsorption and ultimately symptoms of obstruction (Figure 14.33).

Ileo-caecal disease is by far the most common type infection, probably because of the considerable lymphatic gland mass present in this area. Pimparker reported an incidence of 21–87% for various authors,[33] while Homan, Grafe and Dineen reported an incidence of some 52%[25] and in the Bradford series the incidence was 62%.[16]

Radiologically, the principal characteristics are a string-like narrowing of the ileum and a high-riding contracted caecum (Figure 14.34). The lesion often presents to the clinician as a mass in the right iliac fossa.

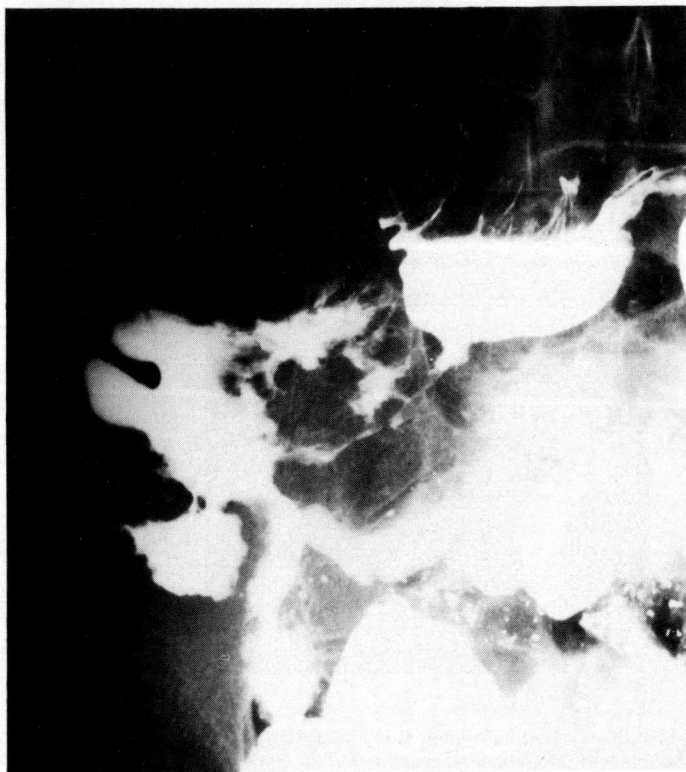

Fig. 14.32 (a) Barium meal examination showing a duodeno-colic fistula and extensive disease of the ascending colon and caecum. (b) Barium meal examination taken six months later showing closure of the duodeno-colic fistula.

a

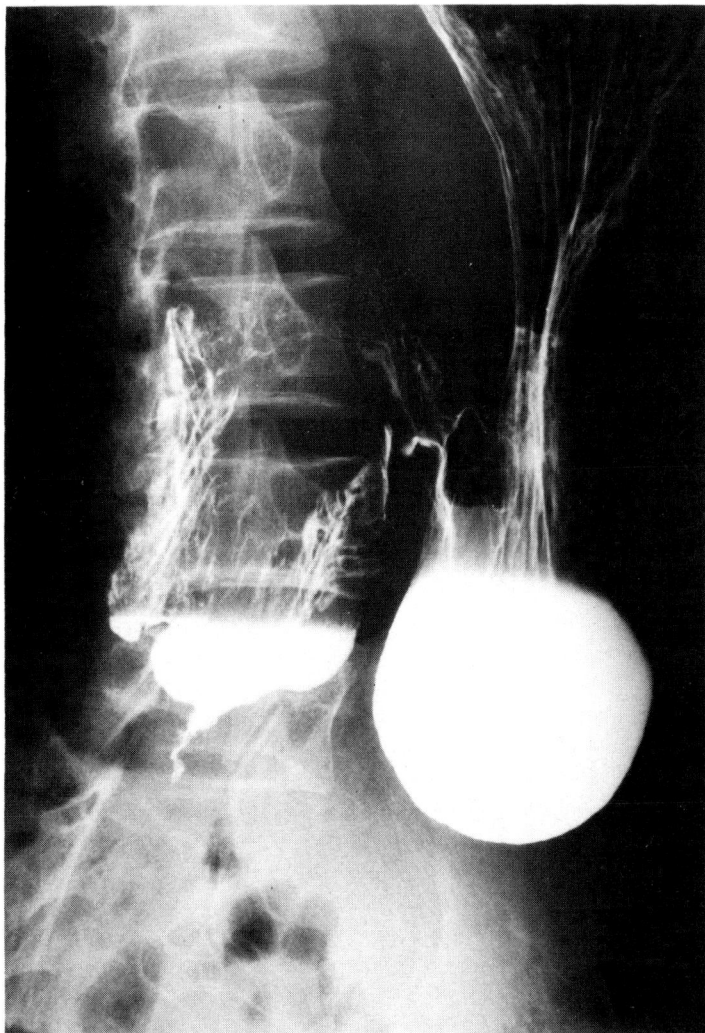

Fig. 14.32(b)

TUBERCULOSIS OF THE APPENDIX

This is uncommon and is most frequently found in association with ileo-caecal tuberculosis. Shah, Mehta and Jalundhwala[36] studied 20 patients and Anand[3] 50 with ileo-caecal tuberculosis and not one had appendicular involvement. There are three presentations.[11] The first is a form of chronic disease with low-grade intermittent pain, occasional vomiting and diarrhoea; examination reveals tenderness, guarding and an occasional mass. This presentation is almost indistinguishable from ileo-caecal disease. The second is an acute illness similar to acute appendicitis. The third is the so-called 'latent type', where the appendix looks normal at the time of removal but is found to be heavily involved by tuberculous disease. The last is the rarest of the three presentations.

TUBERCULOUS COLITIS

Tuberculous colitis is, like Crohn's disease, a granulomatous disease that is essentially a transmural process and may, therefore, progress to fistula or stricture formation. Ahuja, Gaiha and Sachdev characterized two forms; the hyperplastic and the ulcerative.[2] Tuberculous colitis occurring without associated ileo-caecal disease is very rare.[1, 12, 18] The differential diagnosis of the condition in temperate climates is large: carcinoma, non-specific ulcerative colitis, Crohn's disease, amoebiasis, pseudomembranous colitis and ischaemic colitis may all mimic the condition. In the tropics amoebiasis, bacterial dysentery and granuloma have to be considered. Granet[21] described a patient with tuberculous salpingitis that spread to involve the colon. Goldfischer and Janis provide a fasci-

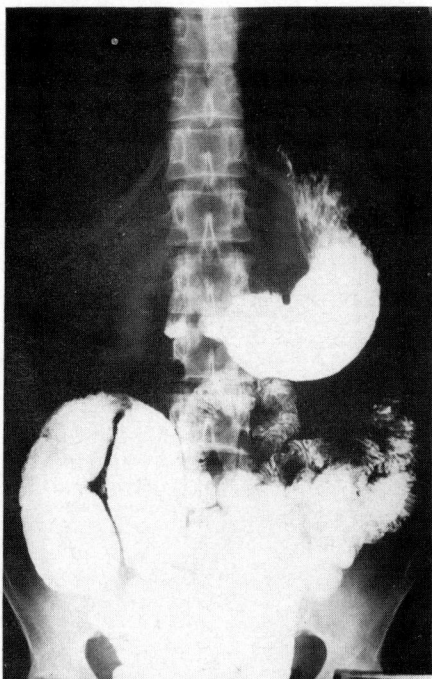

Fig. 14.33 Barium meal and follow-through examination showing gross distension of the ileum. This patient developed intestinal perforation 48 hours after this examination and a tight fibrous band associated with the tuberculous process was found to be obstructing the loops.

nating account of the postmortem on Louis XIII, King of France, with excellent descriptions of the autopsy findings and an interesting discussion of the problems of distinguishing between ulcerative colitis and tuberculous colitis.[19] Like Crohn's disease tuberculous colitis can be segmental and associated with skin lesions. Ulcerating lesions may occur and can go on to produce single or multiple strictures. Figure 14.35 illustrates the change shown on a barium enema in a patient with tuberculous colitis. Rectal biopsy is still of immense value. Details and extensive descriptions of the condition are provided by Ahuja, Gaiha and Sachdev[2] and Balikian, Uthman and Kabakian.[4]

ANORECTAL DISEASE

Anorectal tuberculosis is extremely unusual and only occurred in 3 out of 66 patients reported by Goyal *et al.*[20] and in 5 out of 75 patients described by Gupta, Sharma and Rathi.[23] The commonest variety is the ulcerative type, which is associated with blue and pink rectal lesions that may resemble amoebic ulcers because both have undermined edges. A thick mucopurulent discharge may frequently be produced. The

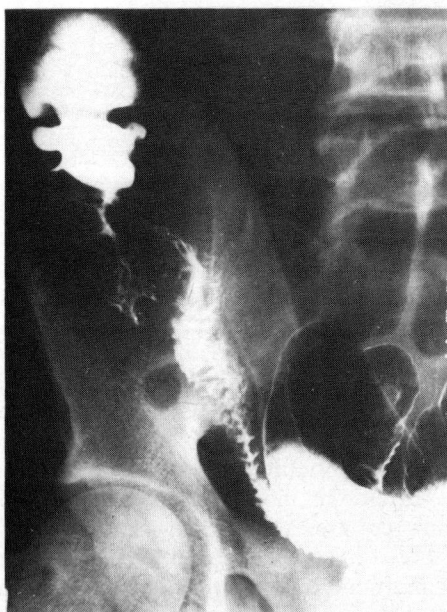

a

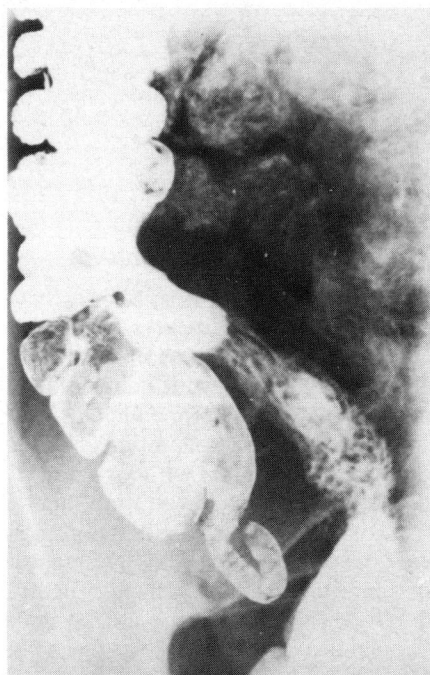

b

Fig. 14.34 (a) Barium meal showing a contracted string-like terminal ileum with a high-riding contracted caecum, (b) Radiological appearances of the same patient after 18 months of treatment.

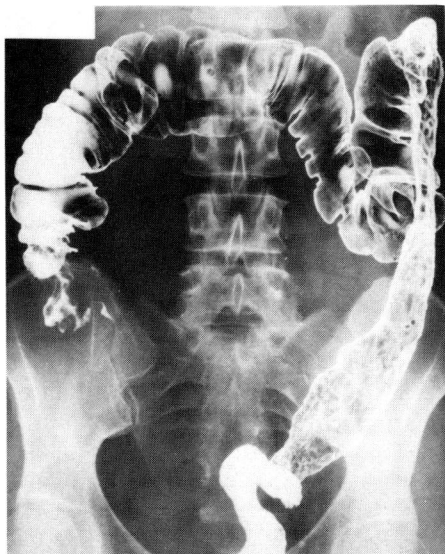

Fig. 14.35 Barium enema X-ray of an Asian patient showing extensive colitic changes shown to be due to tuberculosis.

other forms are a varicose type which is associated with warty excrescences and may resemble condylomata acuminata and a lupoid type which is uncommon and may be nodular and ulcerated. Fistulas may occur. The differential diagnosis is considerable and includes Crohn's disease, cancer of the rectum, amoebiasis, sarcoidosis, granuloma venereum and actinomycosis. The ulcers of Crohn's disease are greater in number and smaller in size.

HEPATIC TUBERCULOSIS

Hepatic tuberculosis occurs most frequently in patients with evidence of a disseminated tuberculous illness but Cleve, Gibson and Webb[14] also describe 'atypical tuberculosis of the liver' where the disease is apparently entirely confined to the liver. A liver biopsy is of considerable diagnostic value. These patients can be difficult to manage because of the hepatotoxicity of antituberculous therapy.

CROHN'S DISEASE AND GASTROINTESTINAL TUBERCULOSIS

The distinction between these two conditions is the most important decision the clinician has to make. In the United Kingdom if a white person presents with fever, anorexia, weight loss, diarrhoea, abdominal pain and a mass in the right iliac fossa, the condition is probably Crohn's disease. Exactly the same group of symptoms occurring in a patient from the Indian subcontinent would strongly suggest tuberculous gastrointestinal disease. Crohn's disease is associated with the satellite complications of skin involvement, uveitis, clubbing, spondylitis, sacro-iliitis, ascending cholangitis and sclerosing cholangitis. The skin may be involved directly, with the typical magenta-colour perineal involvement which frequently involves the gluteal region, and the disease can affect the mouth and sub-mammary skin tissue. Episcleritis is common to both conditions, whereas phlyctenular conjunctivitis is indicative of tuberculosis. Lupus vulgaris is characteristic of tuberculous infection of the skin but is caused by *Mycobacterium bovis* rather than *Mycobacterium tuberculosis*. Tuberculosis affects the joints, particularly the larger synovial joints such as the ankle, knee and spine and produces a different picture to that normally seen in the bony involvement of patients with Crohn's disease. Ascites is very unusual in Crohn's disease and is more commonly a feature of tuberculosis. The aphthous ulcers which are so common in patients with Crohn's disease are not characteristic of tuberculous disease. Taylor observed in 1945 that 'Crohn's disease has received a too enthusiastic and uncritical reception, while ileocaecal tuberculosis has been too lightly discarded.'[41] Nearly forty years later this statement is still true and the clinician would do well to remember that corticosteroids (or even azathioprine) administered to a patient with tuberculosis in the mistaken belief that the illness is Crohn's disease may rapidly prove to be very hazardous, if not fatal.

Treatment

SURGERY—THE ACUTE SITUATION

The principal roles of surgery are diagnosis at laparotomy when the diagnosis is obscure and assisting in the management of chronic complications.

Intestinal obstruction is the most frequent presentation requiring surgical intervention; far less frequently, perforation and bleeding may need surgical management. Obstruction occurs most commonly as a result of ileocaecal lesions, for which a limited right hemicolectomy remains the most widely used treatment. Bypass ileo-transverse-colostomy should be avoided as should division of terminal ileum and implantation of the proximal loop into the transverse colon. These latter two procedures may be associated with blind-loop syndrome and fistula and abscess formation. It may, however, be necessary to bypass lesions when the obstruction is very proximal, as may occur when there is duodenal disease. An ileoplasty has been suggested when there are small well-defined strictures in the small bowel, and Katariya *et al.* have reported a series of patients in whom multiple strictures were dealt with by this procedure with good results.[28] Medical treatment is obligatory.

The other situation requiring emergency operation is where a patient presents with symptoms suggesting acute appendicitis. If on opening the abdomen the surgeon can see that the probable diagnosis is that of tuberculosis gland or omental biopsies or both should be taken and the material examined both histologically and bacteriologically.

MEDICAL MANAGEMENT

The principal aim of medical treatment is the elimination of the tubercle bacilli using antituberculous treatment, but it is also important to treat the patient's general condition by dealing with anaemia, hypoproteinaemia and vitamin deficiencies and to manage complications such as subacute intestinal obstruction. Blood transfusions, oral courses of iron and vitamins, and parenteral vitamin B_{12} may all be necessary. Ideally the patient should receive a high-protein diet, but some patients are so ill that they are unable to tolerate such a diet; such patients should be managed by hyperalimentation with low-residue diets, and in the case of high small bowel disease it may be necessary to resort to intravenous feeding regimes.

When using antituberculous therapy the ideal is to give a drug that is indicated by culture and sensitivity. However, this is a long process and management should start before the results of any sensitivity testing are available. Modern triple treatment is rifampicin (rifampin), isoniazid and ethambutol. Isoniazid, aminosalicylic acid and streptomycin has been shown to be less satisfactory than the combination of rifampicin, isoniazid and ethambutol. Rifampicin is prescribed in a daily dose of 450 mg for those whose body weight is below 50 kg and 600 mg for those whose body weight is greater. Isoniazid is normally given in a single dose of 300 mg a day and ethambutol is given in a single dose of 15–25 mg per kilogram bodyweight for the first two months.

Rifampicin (Rifampin)
One of the problems in the use of rifampicin in patients with gastrointestinal tuberculosis is that the drug may cause disturbance of liver function,

and this can be masked in the initial phase because the patient may frequently have abnormal liver function as an inherent part of the tuberculous disease process. Where rifampicin therapy does cause disturbance of liver function it will normally settle within the first few weeks of treatment; occasionally, however, there may be a very severe hepatic reaction.

The drug will induce liver enzymes, thereby compromising the efficacy of certain drugs, including corticosteroids, some narcotics, oral contraceptives, oral hypoglycaemics and digoxin.

Intermittent therapy has been introduced for patients with pulmonary tuberculosis, but this is unwise for patients with gastrointestinal tract disease because of the uncertainty about absorption. Any failure of absorption would be exacerbated if the drug is given on an intermittent basis. A flu-like illness, the so called 'flu syndrome' may develop on intermittent rifampicin treatment. Patients on rifampicin may produce pink urine.

Ethambutol
Ethambutol may rarely cause liver disturbance, but the most widely recognized complication of the drug is retrobulbar neuritis, which occurs in 3% of patients.

Isoniazid
Isoniazid produces the most dangerous form of hepatitis of all the drugs used for antituberculous therapy. Although rare this complication may be fatal.

The peripheral neuropathy that is associated with isoniazid therapy occurs in slow acetylators far more frequently than it occurs in fast acetylators and can be prevented by the administration of pyridoxine in a dose of 10 mg thrice daily. Patients with gastrointestinal tract disease are more prone to the development of the peripheral neuropathy because they are more likely to suffer from malnutrition and vitamin depletion.

Corticosteroids
There is little information from controlled trials about the value of corticosteroids in the management of gastrointestinal tract disease. The rationale for their use is that the combination of corticosteroids with antituberculous treatment will prevent healing occurring with fibrosis that will eventually cause obstruction. Prednisolone in a daily dose of 20–30 mg together with antituberculous therapy may well produce healing without the lesion proceeding to fibrosis. Other situations where corticosteroids should be

administered are cases of associated tuberculous meningitis and Addison's disease and in patients on treatment with corticosteroids for other conditions such as rheumatoid arthritis at the time when they develop their gastrointestinal problems.

Second-line drugs
Where sensitivity testing shows that the above regimens are unsatisfactory, the second-line drugs, cycloserine, ethionamide and pyrazinamide, should be used.

FOLLOW-UP AND OUTCOME OF
TREATMENT

It is essential that the families of patients should be contacted, and appropriate follow-up involving contact and family tracing undertaken.

The successful outcome of treatment depends on the return of haematological, biochemical and frequently even radiological changes to normal. It is usually necessary to continue treatment for about 18 months. The mortality rate in our experience is about 4% and is due to problems such as failure to take treatment, deliberate avoidance of follow-up and, most commonly, presentation with an advanced stage of the disease.

The increasing armamentarium of diagnostic techniques has allowed clinicians to make an early and precise diagnosis of gastrointestinal tuberculosis. Modern treatment has led to a most satisfactory outcome and the majority of patients can expect to make a complete recovery.

ACKNOWLEDGEMENTS

The following are reproduced with kind permission of the authors, editors and publishers: Figs. 14.29, 14.30, 14.34a, from Findlay, J. M. (1980) in *Recent Advances in Surgery* (Ed.) Taylor, S. (Churchill Livingstone); Figs. 14.33, 14.35 from Findlay, J. M. (1984) in *Inflammatory Bowel Disease* (Ed.) Allan, R. N., Keighley, M. R. B., Hawkins, C. & Alexander-Williams, J. (Churchill Livingstone); Fig. 14.34b from Addison, N. V. & Findlay, J. M. (1981) in *Current Surgical Practice III* (Ed.) Hadfield, J. & Hobsley, M. (Edward Arnold).

REFERENCES

1 Abrams, J. S. & Holden, W. D. (1964) Tuberculosis of the gastrointestinal tract. *Archives of Surgery*, **89,** 282–293.
2 Ahuja, S. K., Gaiha, M. & Sachdev, S. (1976) Tubercular colitis simulating ulcerative colitis. *Journal of the Association of Physicians of India*, **24,** 617–619.
3 Anand, S. S. (1956) Hypertrophic ileo-caecal tuberculosis in India with a record of 50 hemicolectomies: Hunterian lecture. *Annals of the Royal College of Surgeons of England*, **19,** 205–222.

4 Balikian, J. P., Uthman, S. M. & Kabakian, H. A. (1977) Tuberculous colitis. *American Journal of Proctology*, **28,** 75–79.
5 Baran, R. J. & Fratkin, M. J. (1976) Gallium scanning of tuberculous peritonitis. (Letter.) *Journal of Nuclear Medicine*, **17,** 1020–1021.
6 Beetlestone, C. A., Wieland, W., Lewis, E. A. & Itayemi, S. O. (1977) Lymphogram in abdominal tuberculosis. *Clinical Radiology*, **28,** 653–658.
7 Bender, M. D. & Ockner, R. K. (1973) Diseases of the peritoneum, mesentery and diaphragm. In *Gastrointestinal Disease: Pathophysiology, Diagnosis, Management.* (Ed.) Sleisenger, M. H. & Fordtran, J. S. pp. 1578–1600. Philadelphia: W. B. Saunders.
8 Bhansali, S. K. (1967) Gastrointestinal perforations: a clinical study of 96 cases. *Journal of Postgraduate Medicine*, **13,** 1–12.
9 Bhansali, S. K. & Desai, A. N. (1968) Abdominal tuberculosis: clinical analysis of 135 cases. *Indian Journal of Surgery*, **30,** 218–232.
10 Bhansali, S. K., Desai, A. N. & Dhaboowala, C. B. (1968) Tuberculous perforation of the small intestine: a clinical analysis of 19 cases. *Journal of the Association of Physicians of India*, **16,** 351–355.
11 Bobrow, M. L. & Friedman, S. (1956) Tuberculous appendicitis. *American Journal of Surgery*, **91,** 389–393.
12 Camiel, M. R. (1945) Ileocaecal tuberculosis. *Radiology*, **44,** 344–351.
13 Chuttani, H. K. (1970) Intestinal tuberculosis. In *Modern Trends in Gastroenterology* (Ed.) Card, W. I. & Creamer, B. pp. 309–327. London: Butterworths.
14 Cleve, E. A., Gibson, J. R. & Webb, W. M. (1954) A typical tuberculosis of liver with jaundice. *Annals of Internal Medicine*, **41,** 251–260.
15 Cowan, D. L. & Jones, G. R. (1972) Tuberculosis of the tonsil: case report and review. *Tubercle*, **53,** 255–258.
16 Findlay, J. M., Addison, N. V., Stevenson, B. K. & Mirza Z. A. (1979) Tuberculosis of the gastrointestinal tract in Bradford 1967–1977. *Journal of the Royal Society of Medicine* **72,** 587–590.
17 Gleason, T., Prinz, R. A., Kirsh, E. P. *et al.* (1979) Tuberculosis of the duodenum. *American Journal of Surgery*, **72,** 36–40.
18 Goldberg, H. I. & Reeder, M. M. (1973) Infections and infestations of the gastrointestinal tract. In *Alimentary Tract Roentgenology*, 2nd edn (Ed.) Margulis, A. R. & Burhenne, H. J. pp. 1575–1607. St Louis: Mosby.
19 Goldfischer, S. & Janis, M. (1981) A 42-year-old King with a cavitary pulmonary lesion and intestinal perforation. *Bulletin of the New York Academy of Medicine*, **57,** 139–143.
20 Goyal, S. C., Singh, K. P., Sabharwal, B. D. & Bhandari, Y. P. (1977) Granulomatous lesions of rectum. *Journal of the Indian Medical Association*, **69,** 16–17.
21 Granet, E. (1935) Intestinal tuberculosis: a clinical roentgenological and pathological study of 2086 patients affected with pulmonary tuberculosis. *American Journal of Digestive Diseases*, **2,** 209–214.
22 Grange, J. M., Aber, V. R., Allen, B. W. *et al.* (1977) Comparison of strains of mycobacterium tuberculosis from British, Ugandan and Asian immigrant patients: a study in bacteriophage typing, susceptibility to hydrogen peroxide and sensitivity to ghiopen-a-carbonic acid hydrazide. *Tubercle*, **58,** 207–215.
23 Gupta, A. S., Sharma, V. P. & Rathi, G. L. (1976) Anorectal tuberculosis simulating carcinoma. *American Journal of Proctology*, **27,** 33–38.
24 Hill, G. S. Jr., Tabrisky, J. & Peter, M. E. (1976) Tuberculous enteritis. *Western Journal of Medicine*, **124,** 440–445.

25   Homan, W. P., Graffe, W. R. & Dineen, P. (1977) A 44-year experience with tuberculous enterocolitis. *World Journal of Surgery*, **2**, 245–250.

26   Hoon, J. R., Dockerty, M. B. & Pemberton, J. de J. (1950) Collective review: ileocecal tuberculosis including a comparison of this disease with non-specific regional enterocolitis and non-caseous tuberculated enterocolitis, *International Abstracts of Surgery*, **60**, 417–440: In *Surgery, Gynecology and Obstetrics*, **91**.

27   Horsfield, G. I. (1978) personal communication.

28   Katariya, R. N., Sood, S., Rao, P. G. & Rao, P. L. (1977) Stricture-plasty for tubercular strictures of the gastrointestinal tract. *British Journal of Surgery*, **64**, 496–498.

29   Kaufman, H. D. & Donovan, I. (1974) Tuberculous disease of the abdomen. *Journal of the Royal College of Surgeons of Edinburgh*, **19**, 377–380.

30   Mandal, B. K. & Schofield, P. F. (1976) Abdominal tuberculosis in Britain. *Practitioner*, **216**, 683–689.

31   Mukerjee, P. & Singal, A. K. (1979) Intestinal tuberculosis: 500 operated cases. *Proceedings of the Association of Surgeons of East Africa*, **2**, 70–75.

32   Nice, C. M. Jr (1950) Pathogenesis of tuberculosis. *Diseases of the Chest*, **17**, 550–560.

33   Pimparker, B. D. (1977) Abdominal tuberculosis. *Journal of the Association of Physicians of India*, **25**, 801–811.

34   Saverymuttu, S. H., Peters, A. M., Hodgson, H. J. *et al.* (1982) Indium-111 autologous leucocyte scanning: a comparison with radiology for imaging the colon in inflammatory bowel disease. *British Medical Journal*, **285**, 255–257.

35   Schulze, K., Warner, H. A. & Murray, D. (1977) Intestinal tuberculosis: experience at a Canadian teaching institution. *American Journal of Medicine*, **63**, 735–745.

36   Shah, R. C., Mehta, K. N. & Jalundhwala, J. M. (1967) Tuberculosis of the appendix. *Journal of the Indian Medical Association*, **49**, 138–140.

37   Shukla, H. S. & Hughes, L. E. (1978) Abdominal tuberculosis in the 1970s: a continuing problem. *British Journal of Surgery*, **65**, 403–405.

38   Singh, M. M., Bhargava, A. N. & Jain, K. P. (1969) Tuberculous peritonitis; an evaluation of pathogenic mechanisms, diagnostic procedures and therapeutic measures. *New England Journal of Medicine*, **281**, 1091–1094.

39   Sochocky, S. (1967) Tuberculous peritonitis: a review of 100 cases. *American Review of Respiratory Diseases*, **95**, 398–401.

40   Steinbach, J. J. (1976) Abnormal ^{67}Ga-citrate scan of the abdomen in tuberculous peritonitis: case report. *Journal of Nuclear Medicine*, **17**, 272–273.

41   Taylor, A. W. (1945) Chronic hypertrophic ileocaecal tuberculosis, and its relation to regional ileitis (Crohn's disease). *British Journal of Surgery*, **33**, 178–181.

42   Udwadia, T. E. (1978) Peritoneoscopy in the diagnosis of abdominal tuberculosis. *Indian Journal of Surgery*, **40**, 91–95.

43   Vaidya, M. G. & Sodhi, J. S. (1978) Gastrointestinal tract tuberculosis: a study of 102 cases including 55 hemicolectomies. *Clinical Radiology*, **29**, 189–195.

44   Wales, J. M., Mumtaz, H. & MacLeod, W. M. (1976) Gastrointestinal tuberculosis. *British Journal of Diseases of the Chest*, **70**, 39–57.

45   Witte, M. H., Horowitz, L. & Dumont, A. E. (1963) Use of thoracic-duct cannulation in the diagnosis of tuberculous enteritis. *New England Journal of Medicine*, **268**, 1125–1126.

46   Wolfe, J. H. N., Behn, A. R. & Jackson, B. T. (1979) Tuberculous peritonitis and role of diagnostic laparoscopy. *Lancet*, **i**, 852–853.

CHAGAS' DISEASE

Chagas' disease is endemic in extensive areas of Latin America. In the rural areas of Central Brazil alone there are around eight million who are affected by *Trypanosoma cruzi*, and in 10% one or more of the clinical forms of the disease is present, especially involvement of the digestive tract or heart. Cardiac damage is the most frequent cause of death in these patients.

The number of organs involved varies between different geographical areas. Pathological alterations without corresponding clinical manifestations can be detected in various organs. In 800 postmortem examinations performed in patients with Chagas' disease, Köberle found megacolon in 188, megaoesophagus in 188 and megaduodenum in 20.[13] The occurrence of damage to several organs in the same patient is not rare.[7] The correlation between involvement of the digestive system and Chagas' disease has been established on the basis of the following observations: (a) a similar geographical distribution between patients with Chagas' disease and those with gut abnormality, (b) follow-up observations from the acute phase of Chagas' disease to the chronic phase, with the development of megaoesophagus, (c) the presence of nests of leishmanias in the smooth muscle of patients with Chagas' disease[12] and (d) the occurrence of megacolon and megaoesophagus in 20% of rats inoculated with *T. cruzi*.[19]

Pathogenesis

Chagas' disease is caused by the flagellate protozoan *T. cruzi* and is transmitted by the infected reduviid bug Triatoma which first bites the host and then defecates over the wound. After the inoculation, a marked parasitaemia develops, lasting only a few days. Some patients present the features of myocarditis or meningoencephalitis at this stage, while in others only fever occurs. Even in this phase the parasite can be localized in different organs, where it reproduces to form a leishmania in the interior of the different tissues, particularly the smooth muscle of the gut and the myocardium. The proliferating leishmanias give rise to a pseudocyst which eventually bursts to release different forms of the parasite.

The parasites are either destroyed by the local cellular mechanisms or penetrate into the cells, including the nerve plexuses; some reach the bloodstream or lymphatic channels and infect tissues at a distance. The affected cell remains intact until the rupture of the pseudocyst when various morphological changes appear, including vacuolization, karyorrhexis, karyolysis, nuclear pyknosis and neurophagia. In most patients the acute phase subsides spontaneously.

The patient then remains asymptomatic for a long period; at this stage the diagnosis of Chagas' disease can only be established by xeno-diagnosis or by demonstrating a positive Guerreiro-Machado's serum immunoreaction. Many patients remain asymptomatic all their lives – the indeterminate form of the disease – while others will present symptoms depending on the organs involved, especially the myocardium and the gut.

In the chronic phase the following histological findings can be observed: absence or scarcity of parasites in the tissues, an inflammatory reaction in the tissues, and lesions of either the nerve plexuses or smooth muscle.

Until recently it was thought that the destruction of the muscle fibres was a direct action of *T. cruzi*, while the lesion of the neural plexuses depended on the liberation by the parasite of a conjectural neurotoxin.[12, 13] However, several observations suggest the participation of an immunological mechanism, humoral and cellular, in the development of chronic Chagas' disease. Thus the *T. cruzi* determines the formation of specific humoral antibodies, IgM in the acute phase, and IgG and IgA in the chronic phases.[29] More recently, Ribeiro dos Santos, Ramos de Oliveira and Koberle[26] demonstrated the presence of antineurone antibodies in the serum of chronic chagasic patients. In 83% the antibody was of the IgG type, and 7% presented concomitantly antibody of the IgM type. The presence of IgM indicates that in chronic chagasic patients continuous destruction of neurones occurs, because this immunoglobulin appears exclusively in the active phase of the immune response.

The basic element of the cellular-type response is the thymus-dependent (T) lymphocyte, which is sensitized during the infection by appropriate antigens.[27] The lymphocyte sensitized by the *T. cruzi*, in the presence of an antigen of crossed reactivity in the surface of the myocardial cells, is the basis for the tissue lesion in the chronic phase of the disease.

These immunological humoral and cellular mechanisms probably function together to cause the tissue damage. There is progressive destruction of the myenteric plexuses, the muscle fibres along the gut and the myocardium. Other organs can also be involved: the bladder, ureters, bronchi, salivary glands and central nervous system; primary involvement of the liver, pancreas or kidney has not been demonstrated.

Pathology

In the gut the basic lesion of Chagas' disease is the destruction of the cells of the myenteric plexuses; this begins in the early phases of the disease and progresses with time. This destruction is not limited to the narrowed segments in the megaoesophagus and in the megacolon but extends diffusely and extensively along the oesophagus and colon.[13, 14]

The destruction of neurones increases as the organ dilates.[13] The number of neurones destroyed is smaller in the non-dilated organs, suggesting that a critical number of myenteric cells must be destroyed before the development of the dyskinetic alterations and mega-bowel. Destruction of 50% of the cells of the plexuses of Meissner and Auerbach is necessary before alterations in motor function of the oesophagus occur, and destruction of 90% is required for the development of megaoesophagus. Fifty-five per cent destruction of myenteric plexuses is necessary for the appearance of megacolon.

Although this correlation has not been established in relation to other organs of the digestive system, a reduction or total absence of myenteric cells is observed in the presence of mega-duodenum and the same occurs in the stomach at the level of the pylorus and in the small bowel. Total absence of these plexuses occurs in the gallbladder of chagasic patients with mega-oesophagus.

The decrease or destruction of myenteric cells along the digestive tube leads to motor alterations which, in turn, cause modifications of the smooth muscle fibres of the affected segment. Thus, in the initial phase of the megaoesophagus the circular muscle layer is hypertrophied to a greater degree than the longitudinal layer.[17] The intense motor activity of the oesophagus in this phase would be the factor responsible for this hypertrophy. There is food stasis in association with the dyskinesia of the oesophagus and there is progressive dilatation which causes thinning of the muscle wall. A similar sequence occurs in the chagasic colon as a result of the stasis of the faecal bolus at the level of the rectosigmoid.

Megajejunum or megaileum are rare because the content of the lumen of the small bowel is liquid and the motor dysfunction is rarely accompanied by stasis. The muscle mass of the pylorus may become hypertrophied in the late stages of the disease. However, megagastria is very rare, probably because the content of the stomach is liquid or semi-liquid. Mega-gallbladder and megacholedochus are rare.

Abnormal function

The disordered function of the digestive system in Chagas' disease depends basically on the variable denervation of the parasympathetic nervous system, which causes motor and secretory alterations, and possibly affects the liberation and action of hormones. The number of cells of the plexuses of Meissner and Auerbach that must be destroyed for motor alterations to be detected will depend on the degree of physiological control performed by the myenteric plexus in relation to each organ.

MOTOR ALTERATIONS

Although motor alterations of the oesophagus in the megaoesophagus can be observed radiologically, they are better detected by an electro-manometric examination. The principal

observations are as follows:[1]
a there is aperistalsis during swallowing, with waves of smaller amplitude than in controls;
b there are spontaneous waves independent of swallowing, or iterative waves after swallowing;
c there is a lack of response to swallowing;
d the amplitude of the pressure of the upper sphincter of the oesophagus is similar to that of the controls;
e in patients with a more dilated oesophagus the amplitude of pressure of the lower sphincter of the oesophagus is similar to that of the controls or elevated. The 'pull through' technique shows values which are higher than those of the controls (Figures 14.36 and 14.37).

During the swallowing there is achalasia, delay or incomplete opening of the sphincter.[23] The sphincter dysfunction is more accentuated in the more advanced cases of megaoesophagus. Achalasia was observed in 100% of patients with dysphagia and oesophageal dilatation.[23]

Gastro-oesophageal reflux is not observed in patients with chagasic megaoesophagus as the pressure of the lower sphincter of the oesoph-

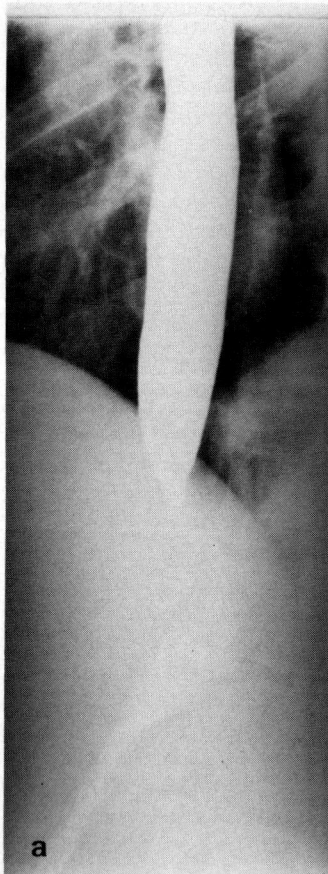

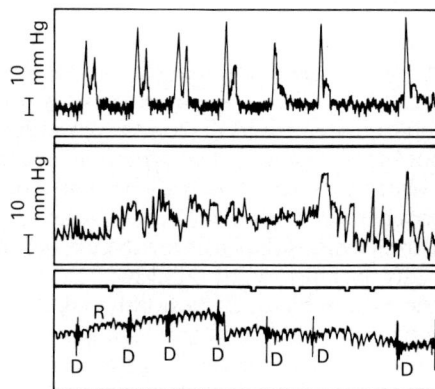

Fig. 14.36 X-ray (a) and electromanometric (b) study of early-stage megaoesophagus.

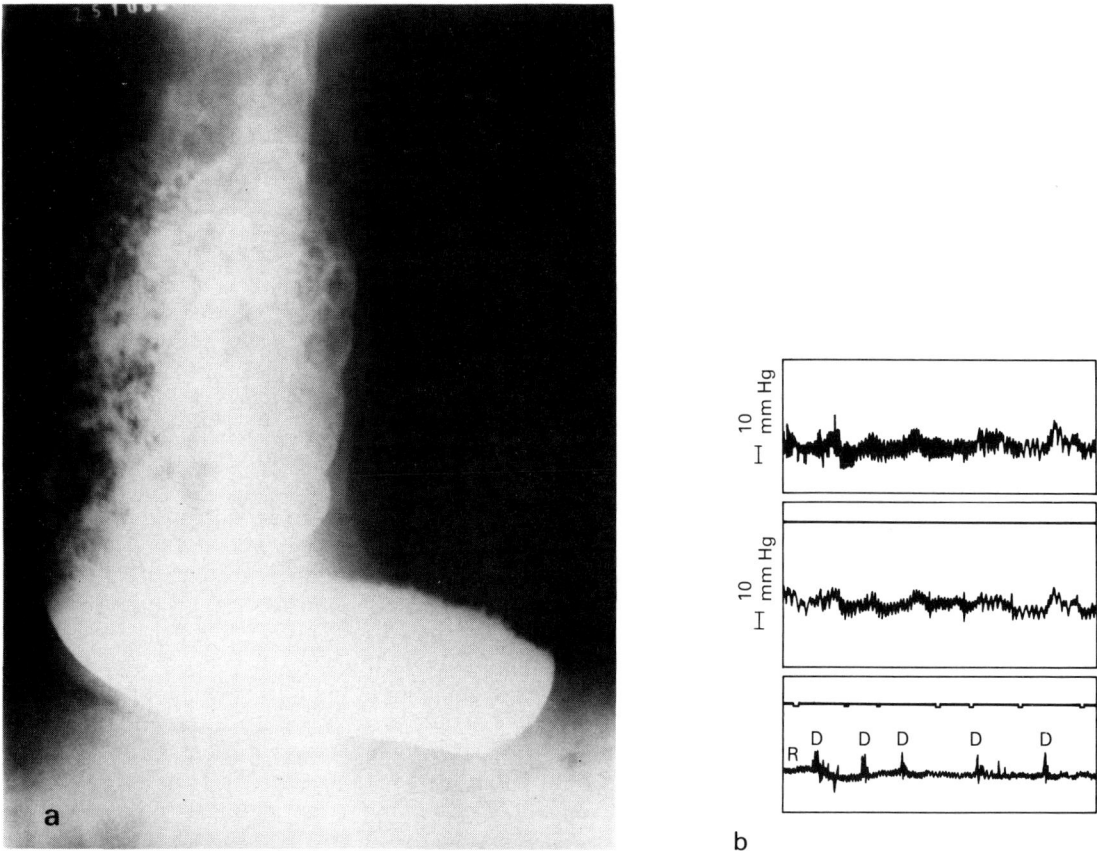

Fig. 14.37 X-ray (a) and electromanometric (b) study of advanced-stage megaoesophagus.

agus is normal or elevated. The oesophagitis observed is secondary to food stasis.

Gastric emptying is accelerated in the initial phases of Chagas' disease and related to elevated intragastric pressures. This suggests that in chagasic patients the lesions in the intramural nerve plexuses decrease the vagal action in the phenomenon of gastric accommodation to distension.[20] Alterations of gastric motility may appear in the more advanced phases and lead to delay in emptying of the stomach and gastric stasis. Such stasis is rarely accompanied by gastric dilatation. Studies of gastric emptying of solid meals labelled with technetium-99m and tracked with a gamma camera showed a delay compared with controls in 65.5% of chagasic patients without megaoesophagus[16].

Fluoroscopic examination reveals dyskinetic segments characterized by hypertony or dyskinesia in the small bowel. These alterations may accelerate or delay the time of transit in the bowel.

The studies of the motor activity in patients with chagasic megacolon had varying results. In some patients with chagasic megacolon there is

motor hyperactivity characterized by an increase in the number of waves, which have greater amplitude and duration than waves in controls,[10] while in others colonic motor activity is reduced.[8] The waves recorded in the sigmoid and rectum are synchronous,[10] which may contribute to the disordered propulsive activity of the colon.

Under basal conditions the motor activity of the internal sphincter of the anus in chagasic patients with megacolon is similar to that of controls. However, the response of chagasic patients to distension of the rectum is different from that of controls: an insufflation above 150 ml (sometimes up to 300 or 500 ml) is required to produce the desire to evacuate. This suggests that in the chagasic megacolon there is a decrease in sensitivity of the walls of the rectum because of the intrinsic denervation. There is no drop in the pressure of the internal sphincter of the anus; indeed, it may be elevated.[19]

The emptying of the gallbladder in chagasic patients with megaoesophagus may be affected in different ways. When cerulein is used as a stimulant, both hyperkinesia and hypokinesia may occur. In comparison with normal controls both the basal pressure and the phasic contraction of the sphincter of Oddi are elevated. These alterations, however, remain to be correlated with clinical features.[8]

Whether or not the digestive tract is dilated in Chagas' disease, it is sensitive to cholinergic drugs because of denervation of the parasympathetic plexuses. In patients with Chagas' disease the response of the lower sphincter of the oesophagus to gastrin is smaller than in controls,[21] and the sigmoid colon shows no response to gastrin.[17] An absence or decrease of the myenteric plexuses, with a consequent diminution in acetylcholine could explain these observations.

SECRETORY ALTERATIONS

The volume of saliva is increased and the concentrations of amylase, total protein and phosphorus are elevated. The salivary glands in chagasic patients are hypersensitive to mechanical stimuli and to pilocarpine.[30] Both the basal and the pentagastrin-stimulated acid output is significantly lower in patients with Chagas' disease.[3]

INTESTINAL ABSORPTION

A glucose-tolerance test shows hyperglycaemia at 30 minutes and normal values after 120–180 minutes.[17] The absorption of D-xylose is also elevated at 30 minutes. Long *et al.* have reported low levels of blood insulin after oral glucose in chagasic patients which might explain the hyperglycaemia.[15] Partial denervation of the pancreas could explain the low insulin levels.

Clinical findings

The clinical picture of Chagas' disease varies from patient to patient. In the digestive system the complaints are mainly related to involvement of the oesophagus and colon; gastric and salivary complaints are infrequent. There is a long delay between the acute phase of the disease and the beginning of the chronic phase, usually 15 to 20 years. Complaints start between the third and fourth decades of life. For unknown reasons, megaoesophagus is three times as common in men as in women.

Progressive dysphagia, at first intermittent and later continuous, is the most common complaint in patients with oesophageal involvement and may develop even in the absence of dilatation of the oesophagus. Eventually the patient can swallow only fluids. Retrosternal pain is rare, except in the early phase of the disease when the oesophageal muscle has good tone but incoordinate function.

The incidence of cancer of the oesophagus in patients with megaoesophagus is around 3%. The diagnosis of the tumours is often delayed because the symptoms are confused with those of the underlying Chagas' disease.

Sialorrhoea and hypertrophy of salivary glands (especially the parotids) can be present in the early phases of megaoesophagus. Regurgitation of saliva or food into the respiratory tract occurs in the late phases of the disease, particularly during sleep. Under these circumstances the patient is awakened with coughing. Aspiration pneumonia is commonly observed in this phase of megaoesophagus.

Dyspeptic complaints, with or without delay in gastric emptying, are frequent and when there is pyloric dysfunction or dyskinesia of the duodenal loop the patient has profuse vomiting. Epigastric pain occurs if a peptic ulcer develops. This complication may be more frequent in chagasic patients than in the normal population.[4]

Chronic progressive constipation is the most common complaint of patients with chagasic colonopathy; it develops before the appearance of megacolon. Large amounts of laxatives are used. As the disease worsens the laxatives cease to be effective, leading the patients to use enemas. When the patient manages to have a bowel movement the calibre and volume of the faecal bolus are great, causing anal pain and requiring great effort for its evacuation. Faecal impaction occurs. Volvulus of the sigmoid is a well-recognized complication.

Gallstones are reported in 12% of patients with advanced forms of megaoesophagus but the stones are usually asymptomatic. This could be explained by the small meals usually eaten by patients, which are a weak stimulus for gallbladder contraction. Patients usually lose weight and in more advanced disease become cachectic.

Hypertrophy of the parotid glands is frequent in patients with megaoesophagus.[1, 30] In advanced megacolon the abdomen becomes distended, particularly in the left lower quadrant which corresponds to the dilated faeces-filled sigmoid colon. Other symptoms may follow involvement of other viscera, particularly the myocardium.

Diagnosis

The information that the patient lives or has lived in an endemic area for Chagas' disease is an important clue for the diagnosis of the disease. It can be confirmed by Guerreiro-

Machado's complement fixation test or by immunofluorescence and haemagglutination. Sensitivity and specificity of these methods are 95–100%.[2]

In the acute phase, *T. cruzi* can be identified by examination of fresh peripheral blood samples or using Romanovsky's stain. In the chronic phase when the parasitaemia is smaller, the parasite can be detected by xenodiagnosis (a laboratory-reared *Triatoma* vector, known to be parasite-free, is allowed to sting the patient and the parasite is recognized in the enteric tube or the stools of the bug).

Once the diagnosis of Chagas' disease is established it is necessary to identify which organ (or organs) are involved. Investigations will depend on the patient's symptoms. In the early phases the oesophagus is not dilated, but barium examination will show motor alterations with a degree of stasis. These alterations can be identified more easily by manometry, particularly when the oesophagus is not dilated. In the more advanced stages, varying degrees of dilatation can be observed radiologically and it is not uncommon to find the oesophageal diameter to be greater than 10 cm.[1]

Dyskinesia of the sigmoid has been observed radiologically in the early phases of chagasic colonopathy, but colonic involvement is usually only established when the rectum or sigmoid dilates (Figure 14.38). Manometric examination of the rectum and sigmoid has little place in the diagnosis of chagasic colonopathy.

If the stomach and duodenum are involved, the radiological examination shows a delay in the gastric emptying and food stasis, as well as dyskinetic alterations and dilatation of the duodenal arch. A delay in gastric emptying was observed radiologically in 23.6% of our patients with megaoesophagus. The administration of cholinergic drugs (methacholine) will demonstrate motor hyperactivity of the involved organ if there are doubts about the diagnosis after X-ray or electromanometric examinations. However, when the oesophagus is heavily dilated the response is poor because of the severe muscle weakness. There is no practical method for establishing the diagnosis of involvement of the extrahepatic biliary ducts apart from demonstrating megagallbladder or megacholedochus radiologically.

It must be stressed that a chagasic cardiopathy is present in 50% of patients with chagasic megaoesophagus. In these patients the ECG reveals involvement of the conduction system, particularly right bundle branch block, and this is of diagnostic value.

Treatment

In the last few years two trypanosomicide drugs have been used in the treatment of Chagas' disease: nifurtimox and benznidazole which are administered orally in the dosage of 5–10 mg/kg daily for 30 to 120 days. These drugs are effective in the treatment of the acute phase when *T. cruzi* is detected in the peripheral blood; they are more effective at eliminating the acute symptoms than at clearing the parasites from the blood. In the chronic phase when definite tissue alterations are present the use of these drugs is controversial. Peripheral neuropathy is a common side-effect.

TREATMENT OF MEGAOESOPHAGUS

A liquid or semi-fluid diet, which is not irritating to the mucous membrane of the oesophagus is recommended. Extreme temperature should also be avoided. The patient must not eat before going to bed or there will be regurgitation into the airways.

Dilatation treatment

The forced dilatation of the gastro-oesophageal junction can be undertaken with Hurst bougies, but this only has a temporary effect and is used as a preliminary measure for other forms of treatment; balloons may be used.[22] Dilatation is reserved for the following situations:

a serious cardiac involvement caused by the chagasic carditis, when there is a major surgical

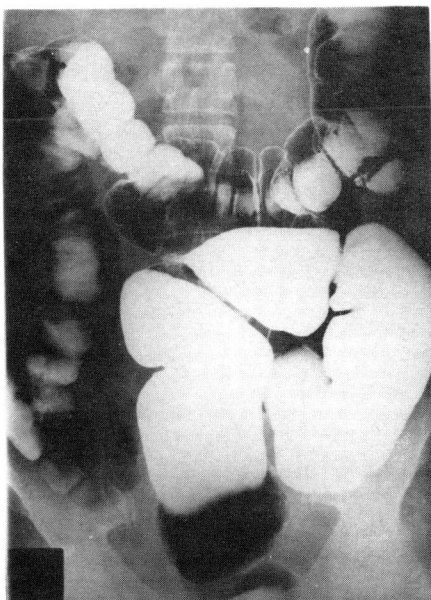

Fig. 14.38 Barium enema showing dilatation of the descending colon, sigmoid and rectum.

risk, or when surgery is contraindicated for example by serious neurological, vascular or renal disease.

b the presence of complications secondary to the involvement of the oesophagus itself, such as marked undernourishment, aspiration pneumonia, bronchiectasis and severe bronchitis. In these situations the dilatation ensures improved emptying of the oesophagus, enabling the patient to be fed and improving the clinical conditions to make surgery possible.

c disease in the earliest phase with motor disturbances but no oesophageal dilatation.

Apart from these situations, all patients must be operated on, even the elderly: old age is not a contraindication to surgery.

Surgical treatment
The oldest and most widely used procedure is Heller's operation or one of its variants. These operations may be followed by regurgitation in 10–15% of patients because the gastro-oesophageal sphincter mechanism is destroyed. Several operations using anti-reflux manoeuvres have been suggested to avoid this complication. The type of surgery to be performed will depend on the degree of the megaoesophagus. In the non-advanced form a long cardiomyotomy involving 6 cm of the distal oesophagus and 3 cm of the proximal stomach is performed. This is accompanied by a fundoplication to prevent reflux: two-thirds of the circumference of the distal oesophagus is fixed to the gastric fundus (Figure 14.39). In 410 patients operated on by this technique, good results were obtained in 95.52%.[24]

In advanced megaoesophagus in which the oesophagus is over 10 cm in diameter, the organ becomes inert, with no power of contraction and conduction of food. Here subtotal resection of the organ is indicated. Considering that these patients are frequently undernourished and have pulmonary disease secondary to the bronchial aspiration, procedures which require a thoracotomy represent a major risk. In these patients a cervicoabdominal oesophagectomy via the transmediastinal route and without thoracotomy has been performed, with the stomach mobilized into the chest and sutured to the cervical oesophagus. Some authors regard coloplasty as the procedure of choice whenever these patients require an oesophagectomy.

TREATMENT OF ANTROPYLORIC DYSFUNCTION

An antropyloromyotomy is performed by resecting a band of the seromuscular layer (0.5 cm wide × 5 cm long) of the anterior part of the antrum and pylorus. This operation is usually performed on patients who have megaoesophagus and antropyloric dysfunction.

TREATMENT OF MEGACOLON

Medical treatment of the megacolon is indicated in patients with mild or no dilatation of the colon or whenever there is a contraindication to surgical treatment. A high-fibre diet is encouraged and laxatives and enemas are used liberally.

Surgical treatment
Based on the observation that the functional alterations and alterations of the myenteric plexuses are most marked in the distal segment of the colon, rectosigmoidectomy in its different variations has been the operation for chagasic megacolon most widely performed in Brazil. The modifications introduced to this technique aim to decrease morbidity, particularly wound

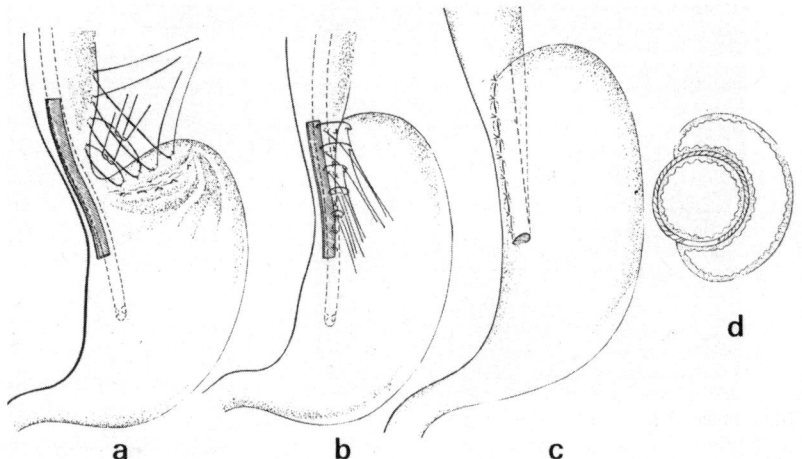

Fig. 14.39 Surgical treatment of the non-advanced megaoesophagus: (a) cardiomyotomy; (b) suture of the posterior aspect of the stomach to the posterior wall of the oesophagus; (c) suture of the anterior surface of the stomach to the left and right lateral margins of the myotomy; (d) transverse section of the stomach and oesophagus at the level of the surgical intervention.

dehiscence, stenosis of the anastomosis, pelvic abscesses, anal incontinence and sexual impotence. Among the modifications that have been introduced are those of Cutait[6] (abdomino-perineal rectosigmoidectomy with delayed anastomosis), Simonsen, Babr and Gazal[28] (abdomino-endoanal rectosigmoidectomy), and Duhamel modified by Haddad.[11] The morbidity rate has been progressively reduced by these techniques.[9]

Prognosis

The prognosis of Chagas' disease with gut involvement depends on the presence of complications: carcinoma of the oesophagus, bronchopneumonia, cachexia, rectal abscesses and sepsis. However, chronic myocarditis is the most frequent cause of death in patients, either by cardiac failure or by arrhythmias such as ventricular fibrillation or Stokes–Adams syndrome.

REFERENCES

1 Bettarello, A. & Pinotti, H. W. (1976) Oesophageal involvement in Chagas' disease. *Clinics in Gastroenterology*, **5**, 103–105.
2 Camargo, M. F. (1971) Hemagglutination test for Chagas' disease with chromium chloride, formalin-treated erythrocytes, sensitized with *Trypanosoma cruzi* extracts. *Revisto do Instituto de medicina tropical de São Paulo*, **13**, 45–50.
3 Carneiro-Leão, G. J., Zaterka, S., Neves, D. P. & Bettarello, A. (1981) Acid secretion in patients with Chagas' disease. *Acta Gastroenterologico Latoamericana*, **11**, 273–278.
4 Ceneviva, R., Modena, G. L. P. & Castelfranchi, P. L. (1971) Doença de Chagas e úlcera gástrica. *Arquivos de Gastroenterologia*, **8**, 85–88.
5 Conte, V. P., Pinotti, H. W. & Bettarello, A. (1983) Normal neuronal clustering in the neck region of the human gallbladder wall and corresponding neuronal denudement in Chagas' disease. *Ohio Journal of Science*, **83**, 28–30.
6 Cutait, D. (1965) Technique of recosigmoidectomy for megacolon. Report of 425 resections. *Diseases of the Colon Rectum*, **8**, 107–114.
7 Ferreira-Santos, R. (1961) Aperistalsis of the esophagus and colon (megaesophagus and megacolon) etiologically related to Chagas' disease. *American Journal of Digestive Diseases*, **6**, 700–726.
8 Gelrud, M., Bettarello, A., Pinotti, H. W. *et al.* (1982) Sphincter of Oddi (30). Pressure in chagasic patients with megaesophagus. Presented to the *World Congress of Gastroenterology, Stockholm, Sweden, 1982.*
9 Habr-Gama, A. (1983) Tratamento cirúrgico do megacolon chagásico. In *Conduta em cirurgia do aparelho digestivo* (Ed.) Pinotti, H. W.
10 Habr-Gama, A., Haberkorn, S., Gama-Rodrigues, J. J. *et al.* (1974) Manometria ano-reto-cólica. Comportamento motor normal e patológico. *Arquivos de Gastroenterologia São Paulo*, **11**, 201–216.
11 Haddad, J. (1968) Tratamento do megacolo adquirido pelo abaixamento retroretal do colo com colostomia perineal. Operação de Duhamel modificada. *Revista do Hospital das clínicas de Faculdade de medicina da Universidade de São Paulo*, **23**, 235–253.
12 Koberle, F. (1968) Chagas' disease and Chagas' syndrome: the pathology of American trypanosomiasis. *Advances in Parasitology*, **6**, 63–116.
13 Koberle, F. (1968) Patogenia da moléstia de Chagas. In *Doença de Chagas* (Ed.) Cançado, J. R. pp. 238–260. Belo Horizonte: Imp. Oficial do Estado Minas Gerais.
14 Koberle, F. & Nador, F. (1955) Etiologia e patogenia do megaesôfago no Brasil. *Revista paulista de medicina*, **47**, 643–661.
15 Long, R. G., Albuquerque, R. H., Prata, A. *et al.* (1980) Response of plasma pancreatic and gastrointestinal hormone and growth hormone to oral and intravenous glucose and insulin hypoglycaemia in Chagas' disease. *Gut*, **21**, 772–777.
16 Lopasso, F. P., Pinto, R. E., Meneghetti, J. C. *et al.* (1979) Estudo do esvaziamento gástrico com ^{99m}Tc. *Revista paulista de medicina*, **93**, 127–128.
17 Meneghelli, U. G. (1969) Estudos sobre a absorção intestinal de glicose, xilose e ácido oléico I^{131} na forma crônica em moléstia de Chagas. *Thesis, Faculdade de Medicina de Ribeirão Preto.*
18 Meneghelli, U. G. (1977) Motilidade do sigmoide e do reto de portadores de moléstia de Chagas em condições basais e sob ação da pentagastrina. Ribeirão Preto, *Thesis, Faculdade de Medicina de Ribeirão Preto.*
19 Okumura, M. & Corrêa-Neto, A. (1961) Produção experimental de 'megas' em animais inoculados com *Trypanosoma cruzi. Revista do Hospital das clínicas da Faculdade de medicina da Universidade de São Paulo*, **16**, 338–341.
20 Oliveira, R. B., Troncon, L. E. A., Meneghelli, U. G. *et al.* (1980) Impaired gastric accommodation to distention and rapid gastric emptying in patients with Chagas' disease. *Digestive Diseases and Sciences* **25**, 790–794.
21 Padovan, W. (1977) Ação da pentagastrina sobre a pressão do EIE avaliada pela relação dose/resposta em indivíduos controles e chagásicos crônicos. Ribeirão Preto, *Thesis, Faculdade de Medicina de Ribeirão Preto.*
22 Pinotti, H. W. (1969) Instrumento dilatador da cárdia para tratamento do megaesôfago. *Revista da Associação, médica brasiliera*, **15**, 271–274.
23 Pinotti, H. W., Raia, A., Corrêa-Neto, A. & Bettarello, A. (1968) The sphincter of the lower esophagus in various stages of megaesophagus provoked by Chagas' disease. *Arquivos de Gastroentologia*, **5**, 51–58.
24 Pinotti, H. W., Ellenbogen, G., Gama-Rodrigues, J. J. & Raia, A. (1977) Surgical treatment of the megaesophagus. *Chirurgia Gastroenterologica*, **11**, 7–13.
25 Pinotti, H. W., Zilberstein, B., Pollara, W. M. & Raia, A. (1981) Esophagectomy without thoracotomy. *Surgery, Gynecology and Obstetrics*, **153**, 344–346.
26 Ribeiro Dos Santos, R., Ramos de Oliveira, J. C. & Köberle, F. (1976) Aspectos imunopatológicos da destruição neuronal na moléstia de Chagas. *Revista goiana de medicina*, **22**, 235–243.
27 Santos-Bush, C. A. & Teixeira, A. R. L. (1974) The immunology of experimental Chagas' disease. III Rejection of allogenic heart cells in vitro. *Journal of Experimental Medicine*, **140**, 38–53.
28 Simonsen, O., Babr, A. K. & Gazal, P. (1960) Retosigmoidectomia endoanal com ressecção da mucosa retal. *Revista paulista de medicina*, **57**, 116–118.
29 Teixeira, A. R. L. & Santos-Bush, C. A. (1974) The immunology of experimental Chagas' disease. I. Preparation of *Trypanosoma cruzi* antigens and humoral antibody response to these antigens. *Journal of Immunology*, **113**, 859–869.
30 Vieira, C. B. (1961) Hyperamilasemia and hyperactivity of salivary glands associated with megaesophagus. *American Journal of Digestive Diseases*, **6**, 727–740.

SEXUALLY TRANSMITTED DISEASES

In British law, the venereal diseases are defined as syphilis, gonorrhoea and chancroid, but a considerably larger number of conditions are now recognized as being sexually transmitted.

The majority of patients at risk for sexually transmitted infections who present with gastro-enterological problems are likely to be male homosexuals. Fortunately, they will normally have taken the precaution of having themselves checked beforehand to exclude syphilis, gonorrhoea and chancroid and most venereal disease or genitourinary medicine clinics will now wish to exclude the presence of gastrointestinal pathogens, at least in symptomatic patients. Nevertheless, there are large geographical variations in the numbers of practising homosexuals, in the incidence of health risks and in referral patterns, so local knowledge and evaluation are important to both specialties.

The hazards of homosexuality

INFECTIONS

The risks of infection relate to the numbers of partners, anonymity of contacts, prevalence of infection within the sexual circle and types of sexual practice. For example, mutual masturbation is relatively free of health risk and exclusively homosexual females very rarely contract sexually transmitted disease, while oroanal contact and anogenital contact followed by fellatio predispose to certain gastrointestinal infections and infestations.

Homosexual men who present to the sexually transmitted disease surveillance services tend to be highly promiscuous, to have internationally mobile links and to be subject to multiple and repeated infections.

ASSOCIATED RISKS

Those homosexuals who are selected by their attendance at sexually transmitted disease clinics give high scores for neuroticism, but it is unclear how much of this is constitutionally determined and how much is related to the stress of a particular lifestyle.

In some circles, there are fashions for the use of 'recreational' and addictive drugs, for the wearing of varied genital ornaments whose use involves actual or potential trauma and for the insertion of foreign bodies (including the much publicized practice of 'fist fornication', which can lead to perforation of the bowel and peritonitis). Homosexuals are prone to anal fissures and fistulas, anorectal abscesses, unexplained (but probably traumatic) proctitis and ulcers, pruritus ani with or without fungal infection, sphincter damage and possible haemorrhoids and cloacogenic or squamous carcinoma. They also form the bulk of reported cases of the acquired immune deficiency syndrome (AIDS).

It is not possible to differentiate between homosexuals and heterosexuals by rectal examination; moreover, many homosexuals are married and relatively few conform to recognizable stereotypes.

Syphilis

Venereal syphilis is a relatively uncommon condition in the Western world but homosexual males form a high-risk group, some of them contracting the infection several times.

Primary syphilis may present as an ulcer or mass involving the anorectum, with or without inguinal lymphadenopathy (Figure 14.40). It

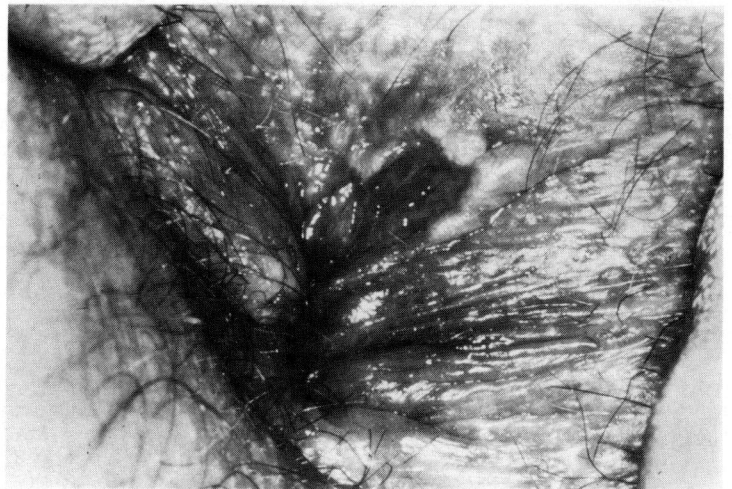

Fig. 14.40 Primary syphilis around the anal canal.

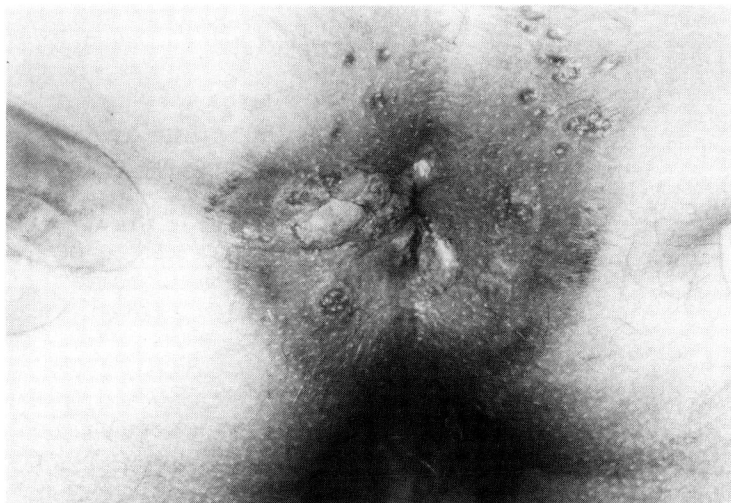

Fig. 14.41 Secondary syphilis around the anus.

may be a source of diagnostic confusion, particularly since the serological tests for syphilis may take up to three months to become positive. Dark-ground examination of material from lesions is definitely a task for the expert, especially in differentiating between *Treponema pallidum* and various saprophytic spirochaetes.

Condylomata lata or mucous patches may be the only manifestation of secondary syphilis and their siting cannot be assumed to indicate the type of sexual practice (Figure 14.41). In most cases the infecting contact will have taken place in the previous six months, but relapses can occur up to the end of the second year. The serological tests for syphilis are almost invariably strongly positive and usually spirochaetes are demonstrable in large numbers in the local lesions.

In the West, gummata are currently rare in all parts of the body, and strongly positive serology is the rule. Treatment, follow-up and contact tracing should be in specialist hands.

Gonorrhoea

Infection with *Neisseria gonorrhoeae* is even more common among homosexuals and bisexual males than among heterosexuals. In men urethral infections are usually symptomatic, anorectal infections usually silent and oropharyngeal infections almost invariably so. Only half of women with genital gonorrhoea have any symptoms, and anorectal infections are less likely to be noticed than in men. There is a high risk of anorectal contamination – of the order of 40% – in women with urogenital infection even in the absence of anal intercourse. Such anorectal symptoms that are present are generally mild and consist of slight discharge,

soreness, irritation and a feeling of fullness leading to increased frequency of defaecation. Asymptomatic infections in either sex predispose to gonococcal septicaemia.

Diagnosis requires repeated sampling of the sites at risk: urethra, anorectum, pharynx and cervical os (not high vagina). The finding by an experienced microscopist of Gram-negative intracellular diplococci in material from a man with urethritis is a highly specific and sensitive indicator of gonococcal infection, but the same cannot be said of other sites. Ideally, samples should be inoculated directly onto a selective medium (such as Modified New York City medium) and chocolate agar to minimize loss of organisms either through overgrowth by other bacteria or through suppression of vancomycin-sensitive gonococci. Plates should be incubated immediately at 37°C in an appropriate CO_2-enriched moist atmosphere. Amies transport medium with plain swabs or Stuarts medium with charcoal-impregnated swabs must be used if direct inoculation is impossible; transport to the laboratory within six hours should give near perfect results.[10] The laboratory needs to exercise a high degree of quality control to ensure the growth of this delicate organism, and additional procedures are required to exclude the presence of other organisms, particularly meningococci, and to identify penicillinase-producing gonococci.

Treatment will depend on local antibiotic resistance patterns,[2] sites of infection and presence or absence of complications or other infections. If the condition is to be treated by the non-expert, advice should be sought about therapy, other conditions to be excluded, follow-up, and, most important of all, contact tracing.

Non-specific infections

There are considerable problems in the definition of non-specific urogenital and anorectal infection and in unravelling the relative roles of various putative and proven pathogens at different sites.

Chlamydia trachomatis is an obligate human intracellular energy parasite which causes, among other conditions, urogenital and anorectal infections. It is an extremely common infection and accounts for 50% of cases of non-specific urethritis (a condition to which homosexuals are relatively less prone than heterosexuals), but available information on rectal carriage rates is scanty and conflicting. Certainly, *Chlamydia trachomatis* will cause various degrees of clinical and subclinical proctitis, the most severe granulomatous forms usually being related to the lymphogranuloma venereum (LGV) serotypes.

The proctitis of LGV is not generally preceded by the multilocular buboes typical of the infection (Figure 14.42) and the evanescent painless primary vesicle, papule or ulcer will tend to go unnoticed at a site not visible to the patient. It is mainly a condition of tropical and subtropical climates. In females it tends to involve the rectum late in the course of the disease by spreading via the lymphatics in the rectovaginal septum. In most men proctitis arises from the practice of anal intercourse, it may present early and a history of travel to an endemic area may well be absent. Annular strictures occur 3–10 cm from the anal verge and may exceptionally produce severe obstructive symptoms necessitating colostomy. Other complications include perirectal abscess, fistula-in-ano, rectovaginal fistula, lymphoedema, secondary ulceration and, later, malignant change.

Diagnosis of chlamydial infections of the anorectum is by tissue culture, and in the case of LGV by serological tests with additional information from biopsy. Treatment is with tetracyclines or, as second choice, erythromycin. In the case of LGV or complicated infections, therapy may need to be taken for several weeks and sometimes in repeated courses. Buboes should be aspirated rather than incised as incision predisposes to chronic fistula formation and scarring. As would be expected, surgical procedures in the presence of active infection or scarring lead to poor results, so strictures, for example, are managed with antibiotic therapy and progressive dilatation wherever possible.

A variety of articular and extra-articular 'reactive' manifestations are encountered in association with inflammatory bowel disease and with certain gastrointestinal and genital tract infections. These joint complications usually run their course irrespective of treatment and the underlying condition.

Chancroid

One can no longer assume that chancroid in the West has been acquired in the classical endemic areas; furthermore, with reasonable standards of hygiene the clinical picture may be less dramatic than expected. The full-blown condition consists of multiple, painful, ragged-edged, destructive-looking ulcers which bleed easily, followed in many cases by unilocular abscess formation in the draining lymph nodes.

The typical 'school-of-fish' morphology of *Haemophilus ducreyi* is best preserved by gently rolling the swab once across the slide, and defined media have made the organism easier to isolate. However, in practice, the diagnosis is usually made on clinical grounds, combined with the response to chemotherapy. The drug of choice is co-trimoxazole, which will not obscure the diagnosis of syphilis, but local antibiotic susceptibilities of *Haemophilus ducreyi* vary.[1] The sometimes very destructive nature of the condition is related to superadded anaerobic infection, which will normally respond to the use of metronidazole, so that surgical removal of dead tissue is rarely necessary.

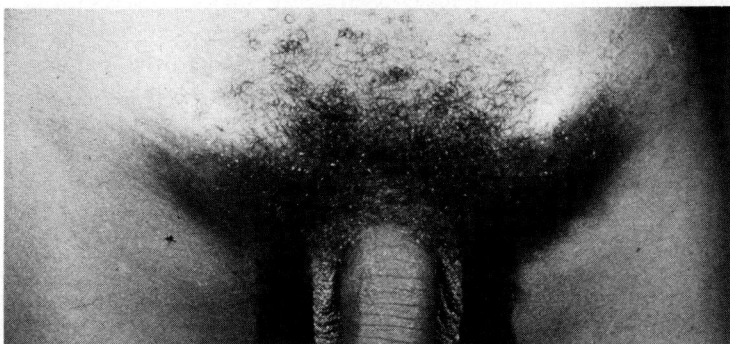

Fig. 14.42 Typical inguinal buboes of lymphogranuloma venereum.

Warts

Viral warts of the anal and perianal region are commonly associated with genital warts, particularly in females. Warts are often found in homosexual males, and are more frequent in the perianal than in the genital region. This is mainly a result of the moister environment, which favours growth, but is possibly partly explained by concealment of sexual orientation in those with genital lesions alone. Anyone who treats large numbers of patients with perianal warts will be aware that they can occur in exclusively heterosexual men.

The typical filiform or cauliflower morphology makes the diagnosis clear (Figure 14.43), but condylomata lata should be excluded and

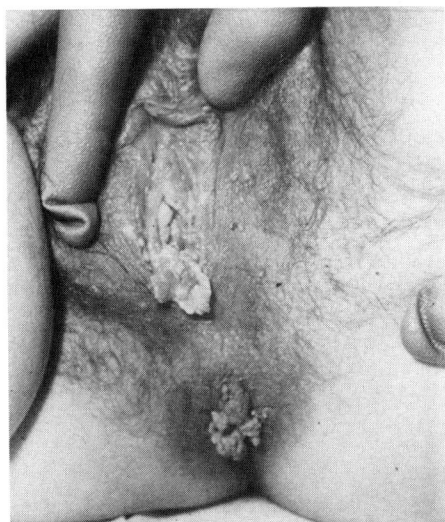

Fig. 14.43 Anal and vulval warts.

biopsy made if there is any suspicion of a malignant lesion. Previous warts of the vulva are a predictor for malignancy at that site and the same may be true of the cervix and anus. Other sexually transmitted agents or factors may be involved in oncogenesis but we are far from proving causes. Treatment of warts is by local destruction with, for example, podophyllin paint or cryocautery. There is a tendency to short-term recurrences and eventual spontaneous resolution. Large or persistent lesions may require diathermy or heat cautery under general anaesthesia, but if normal tissue is damaged the result may be extensive and disabling scarring. One useful alternative is the use of saline/adrenaline (epinephrine) solution to distend

tissue followed by cropping with scissors, under general anaesthesia or caudal block. Gigantic recurrent forms may respond to immunotherapy with autogenous vaccine, while the Buschke–Loewenstein tumour, which behaves in a locally malignant fashion, requires complete surgical removal.

Herpes

Herpes simplex of the anogenital region is a relatively uncommon condition, but in the United Kingdom the incidence is increasing more rapidly than that of any other sexually transmitted condition. Most facial herpes is caused by type I herpes simplex virus (HSV) while anogenital herpes tends to be associated with type II. Anorectal infection occurs predominantly in homosexual men but may coexist with genital infections in women or occur in isolation. The primary attack is usually accompanied by fever and malaise, and local pain is usually moderate to severe, commonly leading to inhibition of defecation and sometimes of micturition. Recurrences cause minimal to moderately severe local symptoms. Open lesions at all stages are infectious and viral particles have occasionally been recovered from apparently intact skin and normal rectal mucosa.

Visualization of typical vesicles is virtually diagnostic (Figure 14.44), but tissue culture is essential when ulcers alone are seen and should be considered in diffuse non-ulcerative proctitis. Cultures are more likely to be positive if obtained early in the illness but delay may be necessary for the patient to tolerate examination.

Acyclovir, preferably given by mouth, appears to be the only antiviral agent with useful activity in the primary attack. It is too early to say if treatment in the primary attack will influence the chance of recurrence or whether long-term suppressive therapy is feasible. Saline baths reduce swelling and pain and help to clear secondary infection. Unless the lesions appear destructive, antibiotics are best avoided since they predispose to yeast infection. Moreover, syphilis may mimic or coexist with herpes, and most commonly used antibiotics, with the exception of co-trimoxazole, tend to mask the diagnosis. Simple analgesics have little impact on the pain in severe cases and it is worth remembering that lignocaine (lidocaine) does not share the sensitizing properties of older local anaesthetics and may be applied by the patient in the form of a gel.

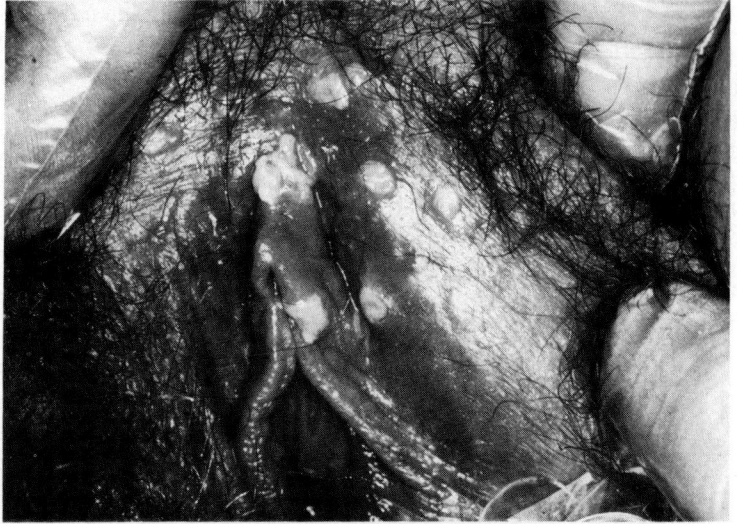

Fig. 14.44   Genital herpes.

Gastrointestinal infections and infestations

Homosexuals have been incriminated in the increased incidence of amoebiasis in New York, and this observation should serve as an object lesson to anyone who feels that a homosexual contribution to any individual gastroenterological practice may be dismissed without proper evaluation.[6] The surgeon, in particular, will wish to have information about the hepatitis B antigen status of patients in order to minimize the risk of transmission to staff.

The gastrointestinal pathogens and non-pathogenic contaminants so far detected in homosexuals are listed in Table 14.17. No doubt reports will follow of other organisms capable of transmission by the direct faecal–oral route.[7]

Table 14.17   Gastrointestinal organisms associated with homosexuality.

Hepatitis A	*Dientamoeba fragilis*
shigellae	*Entamoeba hartmanni*
Giardia lamblia	*Entamoeba coli*
Enterobius vermicularis	*Entamoeba histolytica*
? salmonellae	*Iodamoeba buetschlii*
? *Campylobacter fetus*	*Endolimax nana*

Appropriate control groups are essential since homosexuals in one area may be less at risk of some conditions than the general population in an entirely different area.

It has long been known that the clinical picture and histology of inflammatory bowel disease and LGV can be indistinguishable, and more recently the possibility of similar confusion between inflammatory bowel disease and campylobacter infection has been recognized. In this connection it is worth noting that certain media used for isolating *Neisseria gonorrhoeae* are ideal for isolating *Campylobacter fetus* under different cultural conditions – a happy coincidence which should stimulate gastroenterologists and venereologists alike to assess the area of overlap.[11] Both disciplines should make the maximum use of direct microscopy within the clinic to examine warm stools for the presence of ova, cysts and parasites.

Acquired immune deficiency syndrome (AIDS)

Most reports of this condition have come from the Center for Disease Control in the USA, where, since 1979, rates have approximately doubled every six months (see Table 14.18). Reports of rare malignancies, particularly diffuse undifferentiated non-Hodgkins lymphoma, are also being sought by the same agency, but are not as yet included in the definition of AIDS. Suggested factors contributing to the development of AIDS include a new strain of cytomegalovirus, multiple viral infections and drug abuse.[11]

The type of Kaposi sarcoma seen occurs in a younger age group than is usual in temperate zones and runs a more aggressive course, with visceral involvement. Gastrointestinal invasion occurs late in the disease and only rarely has it been reported as the sole and presenting feature. However, patients may present because of other gastrointestinal sexually associated conditions.[9]

Table 14.18 Conditions seen in cases of acquired immune deficiency syndrome between 1 June 1981 and 15 September 1982 studied by the US Center for Disease Control.

Condition	Proportion of cases
Pneumocystis carinii pneumonia ± other opportunistic infections	51%
Kaposi sarcoma ± other opportunistic infections	30%
Kaposi sarcoma + *Pneumocystis carinii* pneumonia ± other opportunistic infections	7%
Other opportunistic infections only	12%

The other opportunistic infections include:

a *pneumonia, meningitis* or *encephalitis* due to aspergillosis, candidiasis, cryptococcosis, cytomegalovirus, nocardiasis, strongyloidosis, toxoplasmosis, zygomycosis or atypical mycobacteriosis,

b *oesophagitis* due to candidiasis, cytomegalovirus or herpes simplex virus,

c *progressive multifocal leucoencephalopathy,*

d *chronic enterocolitis* (more than four weeks' duration) due to cryptosporidiosis, or

e unusually extensive *mucocutaneous herpes simplex* of more than five weeks' duration.

Other sexually transmitted conditions

Scabies and molluscum contagiosum in adults and pediculosis pubis are all sexually associated and easily diagnosed clinically. Donovanosis (granuloma inguinale) is extremely rare outside endemic areas and is diagnosed by microscopy of smears prepared from deep biopsy material.

Patients with one sexually transmitted condition often have one or several others simultaneously and some patients continue in a lifestyle which predisposes to serial infections. The single most profitable means of assessment is a well-taken history; with practice, embarrassment on both sides will disappear and more accurate answers will be obtained.

REFERENCES

1 Bilgeri, Y. R., Ballard, R. C., Duncan, M. O. *et al.* (1982) Antimicrobial susceptibility of 103 strains of *Haemophilus ducreyi* isolated in Johannesburg. *Antimicrobial Agents and Chemotherapy*, **22**, 686–688.

2 Brown, S., Warnissorn, T., Biddle, J. *et al.* (1982) Antimicrobial resistance of *Neisseria gonorrhoeae* in Bangkok: is single drug treatment passé? *Lancet*, **ii**, 1366–1368.

3 Center for Disease Control (1982) Sexually transmitted disease treatment guidelines 1982. *Morbidity and Mortality Weekly Report (supplement)*, **31**, 355–605.

4 Center for Disease Control (1982) Update on acquired immune deficiency syndrome (AIDS) – United States. *Morbidity and Mortality Weekly Report*, **37**, 507–508, 513–514.

5 King, A., Nicol, C. & Rodin, P. (1980) *Venereal Diseases*, 4th edn. London: Baillière Tindall.

6 Marr, J. S. (1981) Amebiosis in New York City: a changing pattern of transmission. *Bulletin of the New York Academy of Medicine*, **57**, 188–200.

7 Quinn, T. C., Corey, L., Chaffee, R. G. *et al.* (1981) The etiology of anorectal infections in homosexual men. *American Journal of Medicine*, **71**, 395–406.

8 Robertson, D. H. H., McMillan, A. & Young, M. (1980) *Clinical Practice in Sexually Transmissible Diseases*. Tunbridge Wells: Pitman Medical.

9 Rose, H. S., Balthazar, E. J., Megibow, A. J. *et al.* (1982) Alimentary tract involvement in Kaposi sarcoma: radiographic and endoscopic findings in 25 homosexual men. *American Journal of Roentgenology*, **139**, 661–666.

10 Taylor, E. & Phillips, I. (1980) Assessment of transport and isolation methods for gonococci. *British Journal of Venereal Disease*, **56**, 390–393.

11 Wright, E. P., Balsden, M. J. & Okubadejo, O. A. (1982) Isolation of *Campylobacter jejuni* from cervix. (Letter.) *Lancet*, **ii**, 380.

Chapter 15
Anal and Perirectal Problems

CONDITIONS OF THE PELVIC FLOOR

RECTAL PROLAPSE

Rectal prolapse can occur at any age. Prolapse of the mucosa alone commonly occurs in childhood, particularly within the first two years of life; thereafter it becomes increasingly rare.[8] In adults mucosal prolapse may be due to haemorrhoids or may be associated with the descending perineum syndrome (see below). The term rectal prolapse implies a full thickness prolapse where both the mucosa and the rectal wall are extruded beyond the anus (Figure 15.1). Full thickness prolapse occurs most commonly in women of advanced age, the maximum incidence being in the fifth, sixth and seventh decades.[14] It is rarely a condition of childhood, although it is occasionally a complication of cystic fibrosis.

Aetiology

MUCOSAL PROLAPSE

In children mucosal prolapse appears to be the result of an abnormal pattern of defecation whereby abnormally raised intra-abdominal pressures sustained during straining lead to simple extrusion of the anal mucosa. When not due to haemorrhoids, mucosal prolapse in the adult may be a complicating feature of the descending perineum syndrome (see below).

FULL THICKNESS PROLAPSE

A variety of theories have been advanced based upon the following observations:
1 An abnormally deep pouch between the rectum and the vagina (or bladder in men) is usually found in these patients. Moschcowitz[21]

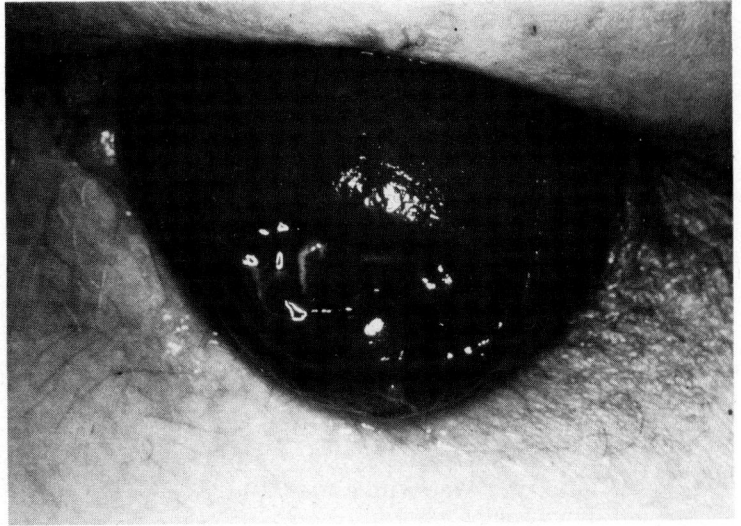

Fig. 15.1 Full thickness rectal prolapse.

claimed that this was a true hernia of the pouch of Douglas through a defect in the endopelvic fascia onto the rectal wall and subsequently into the rectal lumen. It seems possible that these are secondary events since there is no evidence of primary weakness in the supporting connective tissue of the pelvis which might permit herniation to occur.

2 Cineradiography of the rectum during defecation in patients with rectal prolapse has demonstrated that prolapse is nearly always initiated by an intussusception of the rectum 6–8 cm from the anal verge.[4] This would appear to be a clear account of the dynamics involved, but does not explain what pathological processes permit the intussusception to develop.

3 The internal anal sphincter tone is usually greatly diminished in patients with a prolapse as a result of being stretched by the four layers of the prolapse as it advances through the anal canal. Of even greater interest is the observation that the external anal sphincter and puborectalis muscles are also deficient. Using specialized histochemical staining techniques, structural changes consistent with denervation have been seen in biopsies from these muscles in patients with full thickness rectal prolapse.[1, 29] These histological changes may result from localized damage to the neuronal supply, as indicated by a delay in the initiation of the anal reflex[12] and by the changes observed during single fibre electromyography.[23] Further clinical evidence in favour of a neurological 'element' to the development of rectal prolapse is supported by the observation that prolapse is extremely common in patients with cauda equina lesions.[42]

In some patients, denervation of the pelvic floor muscles causes an increased obliquity of the anorectal angle. The straightened anorectal funnel then permits prolapse of the anterior rectal wall, thereby initiating a circumferential intussusception of the rectal wall into, and subsequently through, the anal canal.

Clinical features

MUCOSAL PROLAPSE

The symptoms of mucosal prolapse may be indistinguishable from patients with haemorrhoids, unless there is abnormal perineal descent (see below). In children, the symptoms are minor and are usually accompanied by an abnormal pattern of defecation.

FULL THICKNESS PROLAPSE

Symptoms
The prolapse may appear only during defecation with spontaneous reduction; alternatively the prolapse may be permanently down and require manual replacement. Although the physical presence of prolapsing bowel can be the origin of some distress, particularly if associated with incontinence, it is rarely a source of discomfort, although mucous discharge is common. In some patients the prolapse itself is asymptomatic.

The most serious and disabling sequel is faecal incontinence. Penfold and Hawley[30] reported that 62% of patients were incontinent of liquid stool[3] and 42% were incontinent of formed stool. Apart from weakness of the sphincters and pelvic floor some patients cannot distinguish impending prolapse from a faecal bolus.

Irregular bowel function, particularly constipation, often precedes the onset of prolapse.

Examination

The diagnosis is not always readily realized either because patients are not observed during straining or because of the understandable reluctance of some patients to reproduce a defecatory effort on an examination couch. Examination with the patient in the squatting position may help to obviate this problem.

Inspection of the perineum may reveal signs of soiling, an absent anal reflex, abnormal perineal descent and a patulous anus. Digital examination of the anal canal may reveal poor resting tone, a deficient anorectal angle and a poor squeeze during voluntary contraction of the external anal sphincter. Sigmoidoscopic examination of the rectum and lower sigmoid colon may be normal but the macroscopic appearances of a mild proctitis due to trauma is quite common. Such patients have on occasions been mis-diagnosed as having inflammatory bowel disease.

Treatment

MUCOSAL PROLAPSE

Treatment is rarely indicated in children since spontaneous resolution usually occurs.[38] Bowel habit should be improved by dietary measures and bulking agents. Local measures can be applied to the prolapsing mucosa but are rarely necessary. In the adult, mucosal prolapse may be treated by excision, rubber band ligation or injection, but there is usually a primary abnormality of defecation which should be attended to first (see descending perineum syndrome).

FULL THICKNESS PROLAPSE

Once a complete prolapse has developed, resolution of the problem cannot be achieved by medical treatment. The only effective means of controlling prolapse and improving faecal continence is by an operation which should always be offered even though many of the patients are elderly.

The Thiersch operation

The most minor procedure for treating prolapse is by the insertion of silver wire or Teflon subcutaneously around the lax anal canal; these materials may be placed under local anaesthesia, which is an advantage for the elderly patient. However, there is a 68% recurrence rate[32] and complications such as secondary infection, faecal impaction and wire fractures are common. The procedure should probably be abandoned, although more promising results have been reported using silastic slings around the anus. The chief criticism is that the technique is not curative but merely contains the prolapse within the anal canal.

Rectosigmoidectomy

Excision of the upper rectum and sigmoid colon was initially advocated by Miles[18] and more recently by Muir.[22] However, this is a major procedure with all the attendant risks of anastomotic leakage. The chief criticism is the high recurrence rate which Porter[32] found to be of the order of 58% in the first three years.

Rectopexy implantation techniques

Ripstein[33] devised a technique whereby a rectangular implant is sutured onto the anterior aspect of the rectum leaving two lateral flaps which are sutured onto the anterior surface of the sacrum. A sling is thus created which is in contact with the anterior two-thirds of the circumference of the rectum and which fixes it to the sacrum. The implanted material was initially fascia lata and later changed to a Teflon mesh.

A similar technique was later devised by Wells[44] who tethered the rectum to the hollow of the sacrum by means of a strip of polyvinyl alcohol (Ivalon) sponge. The technique differs from the Ripstein approach in that the midpoint of a rectangle of sponge is first sutured to the anterior surface of the sacrum thereby creating two flaps which are sutured to the anterior aspect of the rectum in such a way as to leave the anterior third uncovered by the material. Similar techniques are also described using the more inert polypropylene (Marlex) mesh with excellent functional results.[17]

Both operations appear to be safe, and relatively free of complications (Figure 15.2). Recurrence rates are more common after the Ripstein operation (2–6%) than the posterior rectopexy (0–3%). The Ripstein operation may be associated with subsequent stricture at the site of rectopexy sufficient to cause intestinal obstruction or faecal impaction.[9] Ripstein and Lanter[34]

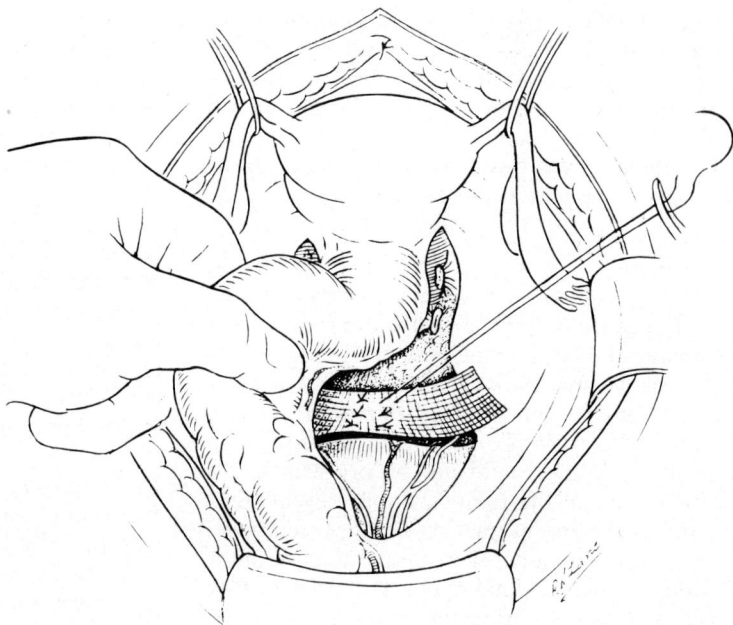

Fig. 15.2 Abdominal rectopexy. From Keighley, Fielding and Alexander-Williams (1983)[17] with kind permission of the authors and the editor of *British Journal of Surgery.*

recorded one recurrence out of 45 operations although at the Lahey Clinic the recurrence rate was 7.5%.[15] In a series of 150 patients treated by the Wells' operation, Morgan and his colleagues[20] found a recurrence rate of 3.2%. There were no recurrences in the Marlex mesh posterior rectopexy procedures performed in Birmingham.[17]

Delorme's operation
There has been renewed interest in the procedure devised by Delorme[6] whereby the rectal mucosa is peeled off the muscle wall and then plicated. The operation has been advocated in high risk patients since the approach is transanal thereby reducing the potential risks of an abdominal procedure. Christianssen and Kirkegaard[5] reported satisfactory results in 12 patients (median age 73 years) but recurrence rates as high as 31% have been reported following Delorme's operation.[40]

Successful correction of the rectal prolapse leads to return of continence in 70% of patients who were incontinent before their operation. For patients with persistent incontinence, which is extremely uncommon, subsequent postanal repair provides excellent functional results.

FAECAL INCONTINENCE

Individuals affected by faecal incontinence have a feeling of social alienation; there is also an economic factor related to district nursing time and laundry costs.[3, 25]

Mechanisms of continence

Anal continence is dependent on several factors:
1 The angle between the lower rectum and anus (anorectal angle) created by contraction of the pubo-rectalis muscle is probably the single most important factor.
Extensive division of the internal and external sphincter can be performed with little functional disability provided that the pubo-rectalis muscle is not damaged.[19] Continence is largely achieved by a flap valve mechanism.[25] Elevation of intra-abdominal pressure causes the anterior rectal wall to close over the upper anal canal. Continuous electrical activity occurs in the pubo-rectalis muscle[7] which maintains the anorectal angle even during sleep. This function is facilitated by means of a spinal reflex arc.[28]
2 The internal sphincter is probably implicated in providing fine control (i.e. continence to flatus and to liquid stool).[2]
3 The external sphincter assists in maintaining continence over short periods. When the sphincter mechanism becomes threatened by liquid stool, vigorous contraction, which can be maintained for approximately one minute, may provide sufficient time to prevent accidental soiling.
4 The sensation of rectal filling and appreciation of the nature of rectal contents are important for faecal continence. The former probably depends on sensory receptors in the levator muscles and the latter depends on a locally mediated visceral reflex (the rectosphincteric reflex). When the rectum is distended by a

bolus of air or faeces, the internal sphincter reflexly relaxes. This allows a sample of rectal contents to enter the anal canal and provide an afferent stimulus to the sensory fibres in the lower anal canal. In this way sensory discrimination is permitted.

Incontinence (Table 15.1)

Table 15.1 Causes of faecal incontinence.

Spinal cord lesion
Diabetic neuropathy
Trauma to the perineum
Inflammatory bowel disease
Tumours: villous adenoma, carcinoma
Rectal prolapse
Descending perineum syndrome
Congenital: imperforate anus
Postoperative: anal dilatation, sphincterotomy,
  laying open fistulas
Obstetric trauma

AETIOLOGY

Diarrhoea

Copious liquid stools from whatever cause may overwhelm the normal anal sphincter mechanisms and lead to incontinence. Diarrhoea may be secondary to infestation or infection of the gut, to inflammatory bowel disease or to intestinal resection.

Faecal impaction

In the elderly, and in some patients with upper motor neurone lesions, incontinence may be the result of faecal impaction. Faecal impaction causes chronic rectal distension and stimulation of the rectosphincteric reflex so that internal sphincter tone is persistently reduced. In this way, semi-solid stool leaks through the sphincters and soiling occurs. Major incontinence of formed stool rarely occurs in these patients.

Internal anal sphincter deficiency

Rectal prolapse, and certain surgical procedures such as anal sphincterotomy and manual dilatation of the anus, may render the internal anal sphincter deficient. The degree of disability is slight and usually confined to loss of control to liquid stool and flatus. Examination may reveal scarring from previous surgery or the presence of a mucosal or full thickness prolapse.

External sphincter deficiency

The skeletal muscle component of the anal canal can be affected alone or in combination with deficiency of the internal sphincter. Such damage may occur in full thickness rectal prolapse as well as following operations for anal fistulas, perineal trauma and obstetric injuries. Rarely, some infections such as lymphogranuloma, Crohn's disease and occasionally malignant tumours cause local destruction of the sphincter apparatus.

Traumatic disruption of the external sphincter ring may lead to incontinence, particularly if the pubo-rectalis muscle is damaged. This may arise following an impalement injury or road traffic accident, or be iatrogenic following inexpert fistula surgery or obstetric injuries.

Neurological

Spinal cord lesions such as tumours involving the anterior horn cells supplying the pelvic floor muscles (i.e. probably segments S2–S4) may lead to a lower motor neurone lesion and incontinence. The history is often brief and attended by perineal pain. There are usually other neurological features with disturbances of bladder function. Diabetes mellitus can also cause a peripheral neuropathy affecting the motor innervation of the pelvic floor and sphincters.

Congenital

Congenital anorectal atresia is associated with incontinence particularly if the levator plate fails to develop normally.

Idiopathic

In the majority of patients with faecal incontinence none of these aetiological factors applies. Histochemical staining of biopsies from the pelvic floor muscles in patients with idiopathic incontinence show the same denervation changes as observed in patients with rectal prolapse.[29] Supportive evidence for a neuropathy has also been provided by electrophysiological investigation.[12, 23] The cause of the neuronal damage remains speculative. Many women give a history of preceding difficult and prolonged labour. Neuronal damage may be caused by undue compression by the fetal head of the nerves supplying the pelvic floor; these nerves lie in side walls of the pelvic outlet. Perineal descent may be another factor. In some patients the nerves become damaged by entrapment either in Alcock's canal or beneath the sacrospinal ligaments. The pudendal nerve supplying the levator ani and the sphincter are often tightly bound in connective tissue as they leave the pelvis and are occasionally transmitted through the sacrospinal ligaments to gain access to the perineum.

CLINICAL FEATURES

Because of embarrassment felt by the patient there is often a considerable delay between the onset of symptoms and presentation to the doctor. Usually symptoms are sufficiently distressing to make it necessary for patients to wear a pad requiring frequent changes throughout the day. Such individuals often become isolated and housebound.

Digital examination will reveal reduced resting tone. The bar of muscle in the upper posterior part of the anal canal caused by tonic contraction of the pubo-rectalis will be less obvious or absent. Contraction in the external sphincter, induced either voluntarily or reflexly by coughing, will also be reduced or absent.

TREATMENT

Partial incontinence
Where the problem is one of soiling due to faecal impaction, treatment with aperients supported where necessary by infrequent irritant suppositories and enemas is successful in restoring continence. Those patients with an internal anal deficiency and diarrhoea can be adequately managed by constipating agents.

Severe incontinence
Simple measures can rarely be applied with success to this group of patients, particularly if there is a rectal prolapse or gross sphincter deficiency and most patients require operative repair.

OPERATIVE MEASURES

Congenital atresia
In the surgical treatment of congenital anorectal disorders it is most important that the neoanus and rectum should be sited accurately in relationship to the pelvic floor muscles and the external sphincter if continence is to be restored (Figure 15.3).[24] Where incontinence develops secondary to the disruption of the external sphincter ring, sphincter reconstruction (Figure 15.4), accompanied by a temporary defunctioning colostomy, will restore continence to 70% of patients.[26]

A variety of operations have been devised to treat idiopathic incontinence. The gracilis sling procedure is advocated, particularly in the United States of America.[31] Both gracilis tendons are transplanted so as to encircle the anus and act as a sphincter substitute. The results of the operation are variable probably because the gracilis is electrically silent at rest and hence there is no muscle tone at rest or during sleep. The benefits from such a technique are probably the result of fibrosis around the anal canal.

Since the anorectal angle seems to be a major factor in continence, procedures attempting to restore this angle should prove satisfactory. Hakelius and his colleagues[10] described an operation to transplant the palmaris longus or sartorius muscle inserted as a U-shaped sling around the rectum. The transplanted muscle was shown to be capable of function, possibly due to reinnervation from collateral sprouting of nearby axons supplying healthy muscle.

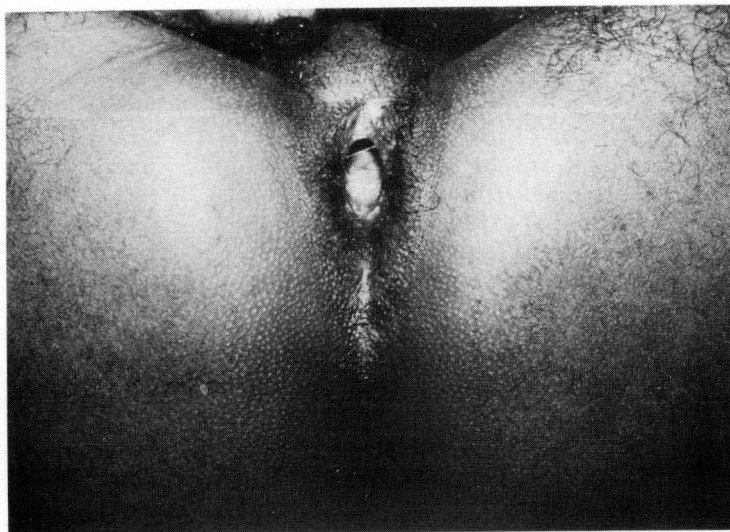

Fig. 15.3 Imperforate anus, treated at birth but anal canal open outside the sphincter. Continence was restored after re-routing the anal canal.

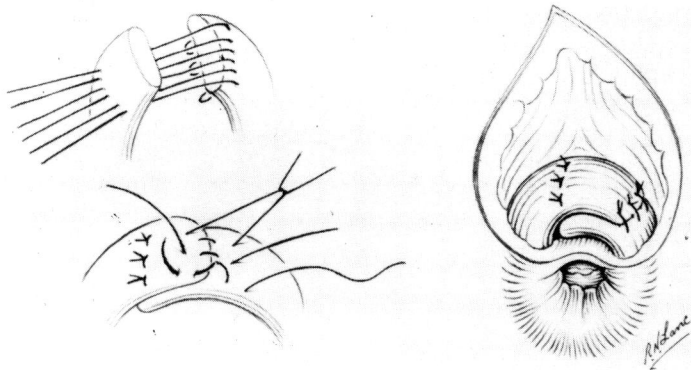

Fig. 15.4 Sphincter reconstruction. From Keighley and Fielding (1983)[16] with kind permission of the authors and the editors of *British Journal of Surgery*.

Parks[29] and others[16] have achieved the same purpose using a simpler technique. The anorectal angle is restored by insertion of a lattice of sutures into the pubo-coccygeus and pubo-rectalis muscle behind the rectum through an intersphinteric approach (Figure 15.5).

THE DESCENDING PERINEUM SYNDROME

A syndrome associated with abnormal descent of the pelvic floor was initially described by Parks and his colleagues.[27] Since that time little interest has been shown in the problem despite the problems of associated incontinence. The incidence is unknown but it is a frequent finding in patients attending rectal clinics. Perineal descent is common in women over the age of 30 years.

Definition

Hardcastle and Parks[11] defined the syndrome by measurement of the anorectal angle in relation to the bony pelvis by radiographic techniques. Descent can be assessed clinically by observing the relationship between the ischial tuberosities and the plane of the perineum at rest and during straining. In normal controls at rest the perineum lies at a level of 2.5 cm above the ischial tuberosities. During straining the perineum descends by 1.6 cm. In patients with the descending perineum syndrome the perineum descends 3.7 cm from its resting position to 1.2 cm *below* the ischial tuberosities.[13]

Aetiology

Most patients with this syndrome admit to long-standing difficulties with having a bowel action

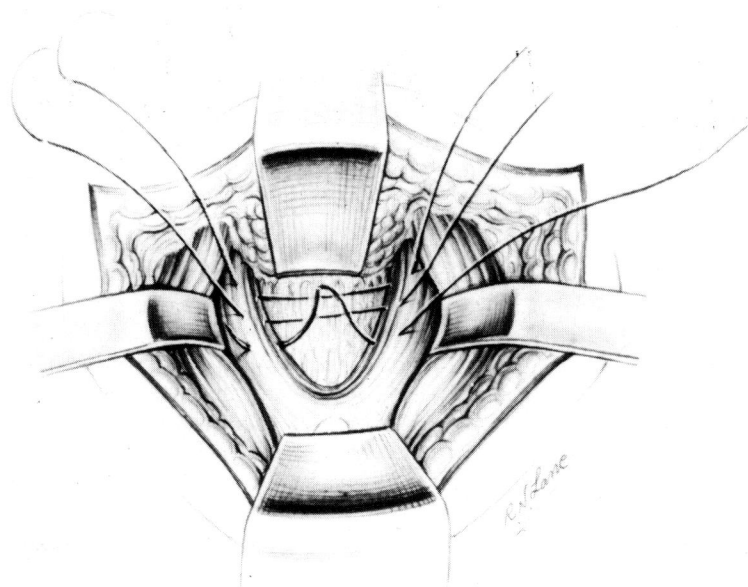

Fig. 15.5 Post anal repair. From Keighley and Fielding (1983)[16] with kind permission of the authors and the editor of *British Journal of Surgery*.

necessitating prolonged straining. It has been suggested that constant straining leads to weakness of the pelvic floor because of denervation.[13] It is not clear if denervation is a cause or a consequence of perineal descent. As the perineum descends there is a considerable stretching force applied to the perineal course of the pudendal nerves causing elongation of at least 20% of its normal length.[13] Since irreversible damage occurs when nerves are stretched by as little as 12%[39] it is possible that perineal descent may lead to, rather than be the consequence of, nerve damage.

Clinical features

Symptoms
Patients give a history of straining and there is often chronic constipation followed by incontinence. There is usually an obvious anterior mucosal prolapse which causes a localized obstruction to the passage of faecal contents such that these patients can only defecate by inserting a finger into the anal canal to push the prolapse aside. The problem may be compounded by tenesmus.

There are often episodes of rectal bleeding, mucous discharge, pruritus ani or overt prolapse. Occasionally patients describe severe pain or a dull ache often precipitated by prolonged standing and relieved by lying flat.

Clinical findings
There is obvious and abnormal perineal descent during straining. The anal reflex may be reduced or absent and the anorectal angle is deficient. At proctoscopy the anterior rectal wall may occupy the lumen of the instrument either with the patient in the resting state or during a period of straining. Sigmoidoscopy may reveal a solitary ulcer (see below).

Treatment

Management is by attempting to improve bowel function by bulking agents and irritant suppositories to avoid straining. The prolapsing mucosa may be treated by injection sclerotherapy, banding, cryotherapy or surgical excision. Postanal repair is rewarding in patients with perineal descent who become incontinent.

Treatment of the abnormal defecation pattern is often unrewarding since the disorder has usually been established since birth and proves refractory to cure. Hence, no matter how enthusiastic local treatment to the prolapsing mucosa may be, early recurrence is inevitable.

SOLITARY ULCER SYNDROME OF THE RECTUM

This syndrome is closely related to the descending perineum syndrome. The term was introduced by Lloyd-Davies in the 1930s to describe a symptom complex associated with a shallow ulcer situated usually in the low anterior rectal wall.

Aetiology

In company with the descending perineum syndrome, many of these patients strain excessively at defecation and anterior rectal mucosal prolapse is common. The histological features are non-specific with smooth muscle hypertrophy.[36] Ulceration may arise either from ischaemia when the tip of the prolapse becomes impacted in the anal canal or alternatively from trauma due to the pubo-rectalis muscle which fails to relax during defecation.[35] This theory does not explain the small proportion of posterior ulcers, but here the ulceration may be due to digital trauma.[41]

Clinical features

The condition is most common in women in their third decade. Rutter and Riddell found that 68% of ulcers were situated either anteriorly or anterolaterally,[36] fourteen per cent were situated in the lateral position, while only 18% were posterior. Almost all the ulcers were situated 4 to 10 cm from the anal verge.

Symptoms
In addition to disordered defecation, patients commonly have intermittent rectal bleeding, which is occasionally severe causing chronic anaemia. Mucous discharge and soiling is common and a high proportion of patients complain of perineal pain, probably due to inflammation and stimulation of the sensory receptors in the pelvic floor.

Examination
There may be perineal descent, occasionally a complete prolapse is seen but more commonly an anterior mucosal prolapse is observed during straining. On digital examination both sphincters may be deficient and the ulcer with a surrounding area of induration may be palpable on the anterior rectal wall. With sigmoidoscopy, the ulcer is seen usually as a shallow well-demarcated lesion with a grey coloured slough over its base. The outline may be irregular and the edge may be polypoidal.

Treatment

Treatment is identical to that described for patients with the descending perineum syndrome. Excision of the ulcer may be performed either locally using an intra-anal approach or by anterior resection. However, both operations are associated with a high recurrence rate. In the belief that rectal prolapse is a major aetiological factor Schweiger and Alexander-Williams[37] treated patients by rectopexy and reported success in 10 out of 12 patients with solitary rectal ulcers, but long-term results were poor in patients who did not have a rectal prolapse.

Clinicians must be aware of this syndrome. Sometimes the macroscopic appearances closely resemble a carcinoma and patients have in the past been treated by rectal excision. It is therefore mandatory that all ulcers in the rectum should be biopsied before considering excisional surgery.

REFERENCES

1 Beersiek, F., Parks, A. G. & Swash, M. (1979) Pathogenesis of ano-rectal incontinence: a histometric study of the anal sphincter musculature. *Journal of the Neurological Sciences*, **42**, 111–127.

2 Bennett, R. C. & Duthie, H. L. (1964) The functional importance of the internal anal sphincter. *British Journal of Surgery*, **51**, 355–357.

3 Brocklehurst, J. C. (1975) Management of anal incontinence. *Clinics in Gastroenterology*, **4**, 479–487.

4 Broden, B. & Snellman, B. (1968) Procidentia of the rectum studied with cineradiography: a contribution to the discussion of causative mechanism. *Diseases of the Colon and Rectum*, **11**, 330–347.

5 Christianssen, J. & Kirkegaard, P. (1981) Delorme's operation for complete rectal prolapse. *British Journal of Surgery*, **68**, 537–538.

6 Delorme, R. (1900) Sur le traitement des prolapsus du rectum totaux pour l'excision de la muquese rectable au rectocolique. *Bulletin Membres Societe Chirurgical Paris*, **26**, 498–499.

7 Floyd, W. F. & Walls, E. W. (1953) Electromyography of the sphincter ani externus in man. *Journal of Physiology*, **122**, 599–609.

8 Goligher, J. C. (1980) *Surgery of the Anus, Rectum and Colon*. 4th Edition. London: Baillière Tindall.

9 Gordon, P. H. & Hoexter, B. (1978) Complications of the Ripstein procedure. *Diseases of Colon and Rectum*, **21**, 277–280.

10 Hakelius, L., Gierup, J., Grotte, G. & Jorulf, H. (1978) A new treatment of anal incontinence in children: free autogenous muscle transplantation. *Journal of Paediatric Surgery*, **13**, 77–82.

11 Hardcastle, J. D. & Parks, A. G. (1970) A study of anal incontinence and some principles of surgical treatment. *Proceedings of the Royal Society of Medicine*, **63** (Supplement), 116–118.

12 Henry, M. M., Parks, A. G. & Swash, M. (1980) The anal reflex in idiopathic faecal incontinence; an electrophysiological study. *British Journal of Surgery*, **67**, 781–783.

13 Henry, M. M., Parks, A. G. & Swash, M. (1982) The pelvic floor musculature in the descending perineum syndrome. *British Journal of Surgery*, **69**, 470–472.

14 Hughes, E. S. R. & Gleadell, L. W. (1966) Complete prolapse of the rectum. *British Journal of Surgery*, **53**, 760–765.

15 Jurgeleit, H. C., Corman, M. L., Coller, J. A. & Veidenheimer, M. C. (1975) Procidentia of the rectum: Teflon sling repair of rectal prolapse, Lahey Clinic experience. *Diseases of the Colon and Rectum*, **18**, 464–467.

16 Keighley, M. R. B. & Fielding, J. L. (1983) Surgical management of forced incontinence. *British Journal of Surgery*, **70**, in press.

17 Keighley, M. R. B., Fielding, J. L. & Alexander-Williams, J. (1983) Results of abdominal rectopexy using polypropylene (Marlex) mesh in 100 consecutive patients. *British Journal of Surgery*, **70**, in press.

18 Miles, W. E. (1933) Recto-sigmoidectomy as a method of treatment for procidentia recti. *Proceedings of the Royal Society of Medicine*, **26**, 1445–1452.

19 Milligan, E. T. C. & Morgan, C. N. (1934) Surgical anatomy of the anal canal with special reference to anorectal fistulae. *Lancet*, **ii**, 1150.

20 Morgan, C. N., Porter, N. H. & Klugman, D. J. (1972) Ivalon (polyvinyl alcohol) sponge in the repair of complete rectal prolapse. *British Journal of Surgery*, **59**, 841–846.

21 Moschcowitz, A. V. (1912) The pathogenesis, anatomy and cure of prolapse of the rectum. *Surgery, Gynecology and Obstetrics*, **15**, 7–21.

22 Muir, E. G. (1954) Rectal prolapse. *Proceedings of the Royal Society of Medicine*, **48**, 33–44.

23 Neill, M. E. & Swash, M. (1980) Increased motor unit fibre density in the external anal sphincter muscle in ano-rectal incontinence: a single fibre EMG study. *Journal of Neurology, Neurosurgery and Psychiatry*, **43**, 343–347.

24 Nixon, H. H. (1980) Congenital deformities of the anorectal region. In *Surgery of the Anus, Rectum and Colon* (Ed.) Goligher, J. C., 4th Edition, pp. 259–278. London: Baillière Tindall.

25 Parks, A. G. (1975) Anorectal incontinence. *Proceedings of the Royal Society of Medicine*, **68**, 681–690.

26 Parks, A. G. & McPartlin, J. F. (1971) Late repair of injuries of the anal sphincter. *Proceedings of the Royal Society of Medicine*, **64**, 1187–1189.

27 Parks, A. G., Porter, N. H. & Hardcastle, J. D. (1966) The syndrome of the descending perineum syndrome. *Proceedings of the Royal Society of Medicine*, **59**, 477–482.

28 Parks, A. G., Porter, N. H. & Melzak, J. (1962) Experimental study of the reflex mechanism controlling the muscles of the pelvic floor. *Diseases of the Colon and Rectum*, **5**, 407–414.

29 Parks, A. G., Swash, M. & Urich, H. (1977) Sphincter denervation in anorectal incontinence and rectal prolapse. *Gut*, **18**, 656–665.

30 Penfold, J. C. B. & Hawley, P. R. (1972) Experiences of ivalon-sponge implant for complete rectal prolapse at St. Mark's Hospital, 1960–1970. *British Journal of Surgery*, **59**, 846–848.

31 Pickrell, K. L., Broadbent, T. R., Masters, F. W. & Metzger, J. T. (1952) Construction of a rectal sphincter and restoration of anal continence by transplanting the gracilis muscle. *Annals of Surgery*, **135**, 853–862.

32 Porter, N. H. (1962) Collective results of operations for rectal prolapse. *Proceedings of the Royal Society of Medicine*, **55**, 1087–1091.

33 Ripstein, C. B. (1952) Treatment of massive rectal prolapse. *American Journal of Surgery*, **83**, 68–71.

34 Ripstein, C. B. & Lanter, B. (1963) Etiology and surgical therapy of massive prolapse of the rectum. *Annals of Surgery*, **157**, 259–264.

35 Rutter, K. R. P. (1974) Electromyographic changes in certain pelvic floor abnormalities. *Proceedings of the Royal Society of Medicine*, **67**, 53–56.

36 Rutter, K. R. P. & Riddell, R. H. (1975) The solitary ulcer syndrome of the rectum. *Clinics in Gastroenterology*, **4**, 505–530.

37 Schweiger, M. & Alexander-Williams, J. (1977) Solitary ulcer syndrome of the rectum: its association with occult rectal prolapse. *Lancet*, **i**, 170.

38 Stephens, F. D. (1958) Minor surgical conditions of the anus and perineum. *Medical Journal of Australia*, **1**, 244–246.

39 Sunderland, S. (1978) *Nerve and Nerve Injuries*, pp. 62–66. Edinburgh: Churchill Livingstone.

40 Swinton, N. W. & Palmer, T. E. (1960) The management of rectal prolapse and procidentia. *American Journal of Surgery*, **99**, 144–151.

41 Thomson, H. & Hill, D. (1980) Solitary rectal ulcer: always a self-induced condition? *British Journal of Surgery*, **67**, 784–785.

42 Todd, I. P. (1959) Etiological factors in the production of complete rectal prolapse. *Postgraduate Medical Journal*, **35**, 97–100.

43 Todd, I. P. & Porter, N. H. (1977) In *Operative Surgery: Colon, Rectum and Anus*, p. 255. London: Butterworths.

44 Wells, C. H. (1959) New operation for rectal prolapse. *Proceedings of the Royal Society of Medicine*, **52**, 602–603.

HAEMORRHOIDS

Over 50% of patients attending a rectal clinic have haemorrhoids. The condition is thus common, it is only recently that surgeons have begun to undertake serious research into the subject. Consequently it has become a controversial subject, especially when treatment is considered.

The nature of haemorrhoids

In his interesting essay 'De Haemorrhois' Parks[13] outlined the surgical history of haemorrhoids over four millenia. More recently W. H. F. Thomson[16] conducted an elegant anatomical study of the nature of haemorrhoids and reviewed some of the theories concerning this. He undertook injection studies to demonstrate the arterial and the venous system as well as any arteriovenous communications. He also studied the smooth muscle in the anal submucosa, first described by Treitz in 1853, and gave an account of the anal cushions.

The injection studies showed that the anal canal receives a rich blood supply from the superior, middle and inferior rectal arteries, whose branches reach the anal submucosa in a variety of ways. The previous finding of dilated veins forming the haemorrhoidal plexus was confirmed. This observation was also present in eight out of ten neonates that were studied. Using serial section and radiological techniques, the presence of arteriovenous communications was also substantiated.

Treitz described the venous plexus being surrounded by smooth muscle in the submucosa and Thomson[16] verified this finding, believing that this muscle acts as a support to the anal lining during defecation. The anal cushions were demonstrated proctoscopically even in the neonate. The anal lumen was shown to be a triradiate slit with the stem of the 'Y' directed posteriorly. These anatomical studies demonstrated that the cushions consisted of an area of venous dilatation covered by smooth muscle with intervening elastic and fibrous tissue. These cushions are found in infants and asymptomatic people and must be regarded as normal structures.

There are a number of theories concerning the aetiology of haemorrhoids; one theory is that they are merely varicose veins, another is that they represent an area of vascular hyperplasia. A small proportion may also represent a true porto-systemic communication in the anal submucosa. Thomson considered the nature of haemorrhoids to be due primarily to a lax anal mucosa which slides downward causing distal displacement of the anal cushions. This is specially liable to occur where there is a history of constipation or prolonged straining at stool leading to stretching or disruption of Treitz's muscle and venous engorgement. Once displaced, a tight internal sphincter is liable to perpetuate the venous engorgement.

Haemorrhoids occur at the site of the primary venous cushions and so are found at three sites around the circumference of the anal canal – left lateral, right posterior and right anterior. When the primary haemorrhoids are large, secondary haemorrhoids often develop in between.

Large haemorrhoids usually consist of an internal and external component, the external component having an epithelial lining and lying below the line of the anal valves (dentate line). The portion of the haemorrhoid above the dentate line is covered with columnar epithelium but there are sometimes areas of squamous change in patients with a long history of prolapse. Below the dentate line the haemorrhoid is covered with stratified squamous epithelium and skin (Figure 15.6). The external component is frequently overlooked by the clinician but is often responsible for the symptoms. Skin tags also occur which may be troublesome and can impair cleaning of the perineum after defecation.

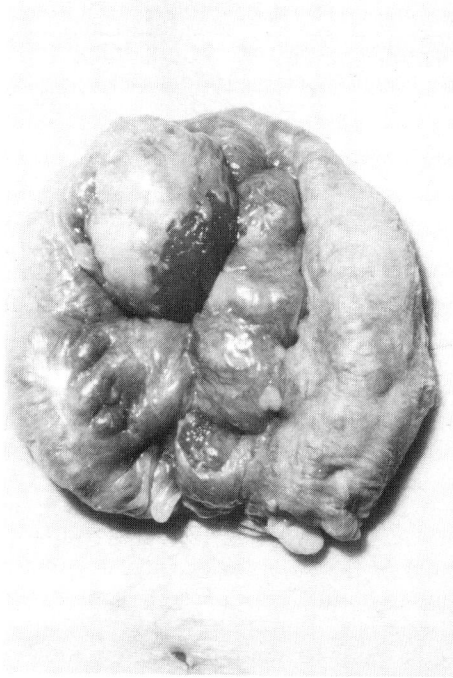

Fig. 15.6 Prolapsed haemorrhoids. Note the squamous epithelial change on the right anterior haemorrhoid.

Predisposing factors

Reference has already been made to the role of constipation and straining at defecation in the pathogenesis of haemorrhoids. However, a recent study of consecutive new patients attending a rectal clinic found a history of straining in only 1 out of 8 patients.[9] A family predisposition to haemorrhoids (50%) seemed to be more important.

Pregnancy is often accompanied by the onset of haemorrhoidal symptoms (see below) which are aggravated during labour. This often contributes to marked discomfort in the early puerperium. A few patients with pelvic disease, such as large ovarian or uterine masses, present with haemorrhoids but all the symptoms disappear after removal of the pelvic mass. Recent work has suggested that certain hormones, such as FSH, prolactin and glucocorticoids, may be responsible for initiating some of the symptoms in female patients.[15]

The relationship between carcinoma of the rectum and haemorrhoids is probably coincidental rather than causal. Haemorrhoids do not occur more commonly in patients with portal hypertension and when varices about the anus do occur in such patients they are quite different in appearance from true haemorrhoids.

Haemorrhoids are very unusual below the age of 20, and if they do occur the diagnosis of an haemangioma of the rectum should be considered. It must be recognized, that in the majority of patients no explanation for the onset of symptoms due to haemorrhoids can be found.

Complications

A fissure may complicate prolapsing haemorrhoids. Other complications include a prolapsing anal polyp or a hypertrophied anal papilla.

Thrombosis is a frequent, painful occurrence in patients with haemorrhoids and may occur in the external venous plexus or in the internal and external venous plexus of a prolapsed haemorrhoid (Figure 15.7). This condition is somewhat confusingly referred to as a strangulated haemorrhoid. This process may involve one or more

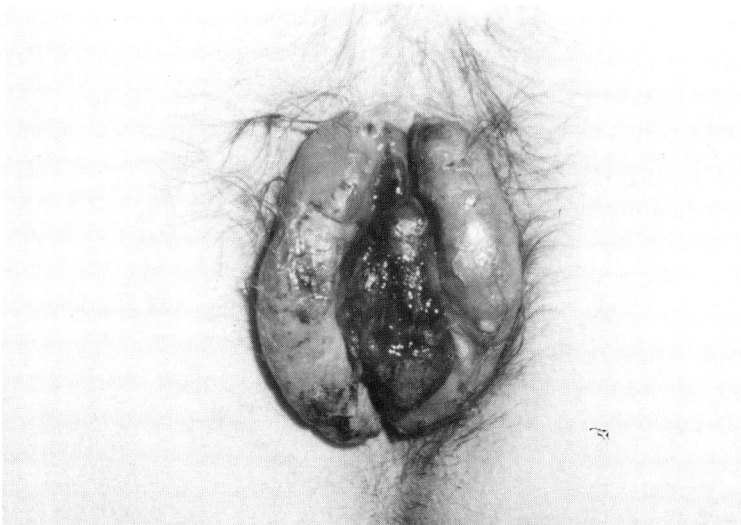

Fig. 15.7 Circumferential thrombosed, prolapsed haemorrhoids. Note the groove between the internal and external components.

of the primary sites of haemorrhoids, and in its most severe form the whole circumference of the anal canal. A very localized form of thrombosis is now called a clotted venous saccule[17] or thrombosed perianal varix having previously been incorrectly called perianal haematoma (Figure 15.8) see p. 1191.

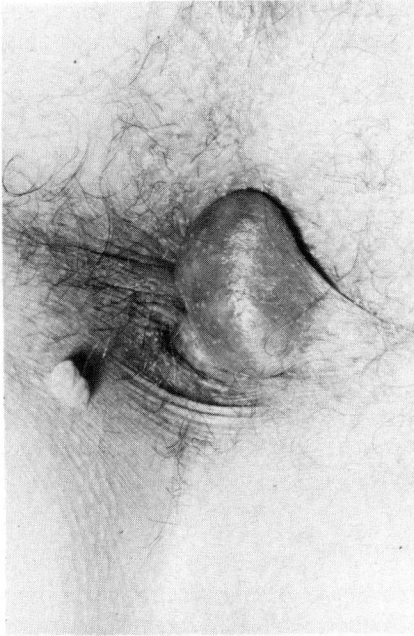

Fig. 15.8   Clotted venous saccule (perianal haematoma).

Clinical features

Haemorrhoids occur in either sex and usually present in patients over 20 years of age. Often there is a long history of symptoms before the patient seeks advice. The symptoms of haemorrhoids may be similar to those of serious disease, namely, neoplastic and inflammatory bowel disease. The widespread custom by some physicians to prescribe treatment for symptoms with one of the many proprietary brands of suppository without a full proctological assessment will achieve very little and is to be condemned since other more sinister diseases may be missed. The patient must be fully assessed to establish the exact diagnosis and, if the haemorrhoids warrant it, appropriate treatment instituted. In many instances the patient merely wishes for some reassurance that the symptoms do not indicate that there is underlying colitis or cancer.

SYMPTOMS

The traditional classification of haemorrhoids (Table 15.2) is based on two symptoms only:

Table 15.2   Traditional classification of haemorrhoids.

First degree	Bleeding
Second degree	Prolapse (with or without bleeding)
Third degree	Prolapse (with or without bleeding) requiring replacement

bleeding and prolapse. Although it is clear that these are important, there are others which if present may trouble the patient more. These symptoms, together with the frequency of their occurrence and their incidence as the first symptom, are shown in Table 15.3.

Anorectal bleeding is a most important feature, particularly as it may be the only presenting symptom of adenomas, adenocarcinomas and inflammatory bowel disease. It always requires full assessment. Bleeding from haemorrhoids is at the time of defecation, often after passage of the stool, when there is a spurt of bright red blood. The bleeding may drip into the pan especially during straining at stool. The bleeding may be episodic or continuous, but iron deficiency anaemia only occurs in about 1% of patients. Sometimes haemorrhoidal bleeding occurs into the rectum, rather than externally after defecation. This may result in dark blood being passed at the next time of defecation or dark blood being noted on the rectal mucosa at sigmoidoscopy at levels up to 15 cm from the anus. Although bleeding from haemorrhoids may present in this way, it is rare and a tumour in the colon must always be excluded by barium enema, flexible sigmoidoscopy or colonoscopy.

Discomfort and pain are different degrees of the same symptom and contrary to what is often taught are relatively common in patients with haemorrhoids.[12] In most patients this is due to engorgement of the external haemorrhoidal component with stretching of the sensitive overlying epithelium or due to excessive internal sphincter overactivity. Pain may also be due to an associated fissure, thrombosis of the external plexus or a clotted venous saccule.

Table 15.3   The symptoms of haemorrhoids.

Symptoms	Occurrence (%)	Incidence as first symptom (%)
Bleeding	81	39
Discomfort	64	13
Pruritus ani	62	8
Prolapse	50	20
Swelling	49	11
Pain	35	9
Discharge	29	Nil

Pruritus ani commonly occurs in association with haemorrhoids and is mainly due to the swelling of the external component or to skin tags leading to inability to achieve perfect cleansing after defecation. The patient will often give a history that there is faecal staining of his underwear. Faeces contain bacteria which produce endopeptidases and these chemicals are some of the most powerful itch producing substances known. Mucous discharge may also be responsible Other possible causes of pruritus must be excluded.

Prolapse of haemorrhoids occurs usually at the time of defecation, although patients with large haemorrhoids may experience prolapse at other times of exertion such as when lifting heavy objects or playing certain sports. As prolapse is often associated with external haemorrhoidal venous engorgement, discomfort or pain may also be present.

A swelling at the anal margin may be the way a patient describes prolapse, but more usually it is due to the external component of a haemorrhoid. Such a swelling can reach a considerable size, particularly if there has been straining at stool and there is a tight sphincter. Thrombosis of the external plexus will result in a painful swelling.

Discharge is from excessive mucus production as a consequence of a reddened mucosa (traumatic proctitis) or from the prolapsed internal pile.

PHYSICAL SIGNS

In all patients a full rectal examination, consisting of inspection, palpation, sigmoidoscopy and proctoscopy, is essential.

With inspection, skin tags, a thrombosed external haemorrhoidal plexus or permanent prolapse will be detected. Gentle parting of the anal margin should indicate whether or not a fissure is present. An essential step in this part of the examination is to ask the patient to strain as on defecation (Valsalva manoeuvre). A good indication of the degree of prolapse and engorgement of the external plexus can be obtained in this way. Also any descent of the perineum will be detected. This finding may suggest a long history of straining at defecation with consequent weakening of the pelvic floor.

Palpation will detect areas of thrombosis, or an hypertrophied anal papilla or fibrous anal polyp (Figure 15.9). Uncomplicated haemorrhoids are impalpable.

Sigmoidoscopy is always the next part of the examination which is aimed not at assessing the

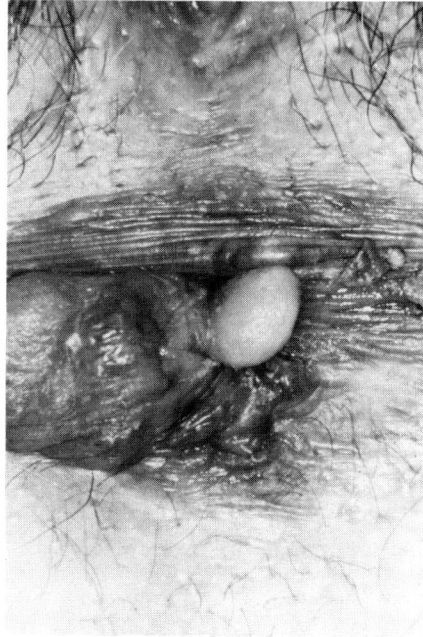

Fig. 15.9 Prolapsed fibrous anal polyp.

haemorrhoids, but excluding other more serious diseases. It must be remembered that more of the rectum can be felt with the finger than seen with the proctoscope, so it is logical to pass the sigmoidoscope after the digital examination. The presence of inflammatory bowel disease will modify the approach to any haemorrhoids that may require treatment and tumours must be excluded. Haemangioma of the rectum may be detected.

Proctoscopy is only of value to examine the lowermost rectum and the anal canal and is essential for outpatient treatment. Proctoscopy will allow examination of the anal cushions for enlargement and prolapse and squamous epithelial change may be detected, as may reddening of the mucosa. Hypertrophied anal papillae and anal polyps occur in approximately 20% of patients and bleeding may be produced by the examination in about 5%.

Special investigations

Barium enema, flexible sigmoidoscopy and colonoscopy may be required to complete the assessment, particularly in patients with bleeding, or in whom blood is found on sigmoidoscopy. Anal canal manometry has been recommended to define treatment groups, but more work is required to determine if this has any useful routine clinical application.

Treatment

Some patients with haemorrhoidal symptoms do not require any specific treatment – it is an explanation for their symptoms that is required and reassurance that they do not have a serious problem. If the patients have constipation and difficulty with defecation, they require advice about fluid intake and diet or the use of laxatives and suppositories to ensure a regular, easy bowel movement without excessive straining.

Many patients, will require treatment of the actual haemorrhoids. Proprietary suppositories are widely used but of dubious value, although critical assessment is wanting.[2] There is, however, a wide range of different techniques (Table 15.4) available and these will be discussed

Table 15.4 The methods for treating haemorrhoids.

Fixation of the mucosa	Injection sclerotherapy; infrared coagulation
Fixation of the mucosa and removal of redundant internal component	Elastic band ligation; cryotherapy
Relaxation of internal sphincter	Maximal anal dilatation; partial internal sphincterotomy
Radical excision of internal and external component	Haemorrhoidectomy

but there is some difficulty in evaluating the effectiveness of the various treatment methods since there is no acceptable method of classifying patients. The traditional classification of 1st, 2nd and 3rd degree haemorrhoids only takes into account two of the symptoms, and does not indicate the state of the external component. There is no way at present to assess treatment other than taking each symptom in turn. Furthermore, most available studies only report short-term results. It should also be stressed that treatment should be directed towards control of symptoms and not anatomical perfection. A patient whose symptoms have disappeared requires no more treatment even if there are still abnormal signs on proctoscopy. It must be remembered that anal cushions are normal.

Injection sclerotherapy

A submucosal injection of 5% phenol in arachis oil is given at the anorectal junction, usually at the three primary sites. This induces submucosal inflammation and fixation of the mucosa and perhaps occlusion of some of the haemorrhoidal vessels. This technique may cause some discomfort and can be complicated by mucosal ulceration if the injection is too superficial. Other complications include oleogranuloma formation and prostatitis if the injection is too deep. Injection is a simple outpatient procedure and can be repeated. The only administrative burden is in preparing the syringes with the sclerosant. Injection sclerotherapy has been used for over 100 years and is effective in controlling bleeding, but of little value in patients with prolapse.

Infrared coagulation

Infrared coagulation is a recent innovation. A small controlled area of coagulation to tissue is created at the anorectal junction by a light beam. The area becomes fibrosed and leads to mucosal fixation. This treatment is as effective as injection sclerotherapy and elastic band ligation and has the advantage of being less invasive and causing fewer side effects. The risk of secondary haemorrhage is small and postoperative pain is rare, but the equipment required is more expensive.[3, 9]

Elastic band ligation

The principle of elastic band ligation is to apply a tight elastic band above the internal (insensitive) haemorrhoid and the mucosa above it (Figure 15.10). Not only does this remove some of the redundant mucosa, but also fixes it at the site of banding to the underlying muscle by scar tissue, thereby preventing the haemorrhoid from sliding down the anal canal.

This procedure can be done in the office or on an outpatient basis, but it is usual to band above only two haemorrhoids at any one time. Further bands may be applied after four weeks. Elastic band ligation reduces many of the symptoms of haemorrhoids, including prolapse, for several years. A complication of treatment is pain, which occurs about one week after therapy and may be severe even when the band is correctly placed. If the band is placed too low in the anal canal, onto the sensitive epithelium, it causes immediate pain and a general anaesthetic may be necessary to remove it. Secondary haemorrhage may also be a problem and is reported in 10% of patients, occurring any time up to three weeks after application.

Cryotherapy

Cryotherapy freezes living tissue. The application of a closed probe in which liquid nitrogen ($-180°C$) is allowed to boil off, or in which pressurized nitrous oxide is allowed to expand rapidly ($-75°C$), may be employed to achieve

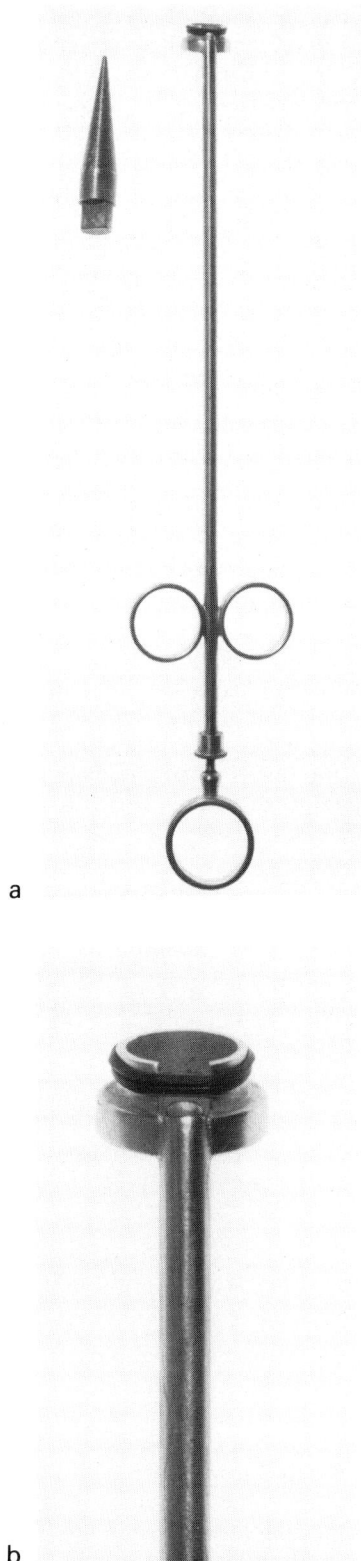

a

b

Fig. 15.10 The banding of haemorrhoids. (a) One design of band applicator. The loading cone is to the left. (b) Enlargement showing the bands stretched around the ring of the applicator.

this. As the tissues freeze they become solid and white. When rewarming occurs, the tissues look normal. Six hours later swelling occurs, followed in 24 hours by thrombosis and infarction. The area then becomes black and over a 10–14 day period separates from the surrounding healthy tissue. Although this technique is probably suitable for internal haemorrhoids, the external component often does not respond well. Internal haemorrhoids can be treated on an outpatient basis, but external piles usually require general or local anaesthesia.[18]

Freezing of haemorrhoids has its advocates who are pleased with the results, but it is not widely used. Cryotherapy is associated with considerable discomfort and a troublesome discharge while the frozen area sloughs. Cryosurgery is often incapable of eradicating the external component and has the further disadvantage of needing special apparatus.

Maximal anal dilatation
It has been argued that the displaced anal cushions become engorged not only during defecation but also as the result of a tight unyielding internal sphincter. Maximal anal dilatation is used to disrupt this tight band and reduce the activity of the internal anal sphincter. A short-acting general anaesthetic is required and the anal canal is gently dilated until it accommodates six to eight fingers. A sponge is then inserted to exert gentle pressure on the wall of the anal canal and reduce the risk of haematoma, and left for one hour. A postoperative regimen of a regular bulk laxative and the passage of an anal dilator is recommended by some for six months.[10]

There is no doubt that this procedure reduces many of the symptoms of haemorrhoids, particularly in young male patients. It should be used with extreme caution in the elderly and never in those with a pelvic floor neuropathy (descending perineum syndrome). It is contraindicated if there is a history of obstetric trauma as there is a 2–4% incidence of incontinence (of not only flatus but also solid faeces) which may be permanent.

Partial internal sphincterotomy
Surgical division of the tight unyielding distal internal sphincter only is an alternative to maximal anal dilatation. This avoids dilatation of the proximal internal sphincter, the external sphincter and also muscles of the pelvic floor. The operation is best performed in the lateral rather than the midline position, under general anaesthesia. This simple and safe procedure has

been widely adopted in the treatment of fissure, but its use in the management of haemorrhoids is inferior to anal dilatation.[7]

Haemorrhoidectomy

There is no doubt that a correctly performed haemorrhoidectomy is the best treatment for curing a patient of haemorrhoids. Often, though, it is not done well and symptoms persist or return early. In most series only 5–10% of all patients with haemorrhoids need this operation. The following criteria are used in the selection of patients for haemorrhoidectomy: those who have large prolapsing haemorrhoids with areas of squamous epithelial change and a large external component (see Figure 15.6); those whose symptoms have not responded to other treatments; and those who have recurrent episodes of thrombosis in the external component.

The principle of the operation is the removal of the three primary haemorrhoids, taking care not to damage either of the underlying sphincters and to preserve a bridge of mucosa and skin between each wound to ensure healing without stenosis. However, the mucocutaneous bridges often cover secondary haemorrhoidal tissue and are often redundant themselves. This secondary haemorrhoidal tissue can be dissected from under the bridges, which are then sewn into the anal canal so that there is no external redundancy. The operation is based on that described by Milligan and Morgan in 1934[11] and is widely used.

The first bowel movement and dressings on the first few postoperative days are painful and although this can be dealt with quite simply with analgesics, surgeons have developed other operations aimed at reducing this problem, such as the Parks' submucous haemorrhoidectomy[14] and Ferguson's closed haemorrhoidectomy.[4] However, because they are more complicated they have not been widely adopted.

Apart from pain, other complications of haemorrhoidectomy include retention of urine, which may occur in 2% of patients, faecal impaction, secondary haemorrhage, occurring also in 2%, and impaired healing of the anal wounds which is often due to excessive granulation tissue that can be cauterized readily with silver nitrate. Once the anal canal has healed, the majority of patients are delighted with the result.

CRITIQUE OF AVAILABLE THERAPY

Which of these various treatments are generally used? Injection sclerotherapy is still the most popular first treatment for internal haemorrhoids and elastic band ligation is becoming widely used for other patients, often avoiding the need for operation. The place of infrared coagulation, cryotherapy, maximal and dilatation and internal sphincterotomy still requires evaluation. Although less radical methods of treatment for haemorrhoids should be tried first, haemorrhoidectomy has a definite place in the treatment of persistent or complicated piles, provided the patient requests it.

Treatment of complications

A fissure sometimes accompanies large prolapsing haemorrhoids. It is usual to treat these patients with a haemorrhoidectomy and a partial internal sphincterotomy.

Thrombosed external and thrombosed prolapsed haemorrhoids may be treated by bedrest, the application of an evaporating and therefore cooling lotion (lead and spirit lotion) or ice packs, and the administration of non-constipating analgesics and a lubricant laxative (liquid paraffin). It may take as long as ten days for the acute symptoms to resolve. Definitive treatment for the haemorrhoids will subsequently be required in most patients. Some surgeons therefore advocate an emergency haemorrhoidectomy, although this may be technically difficult when dealing with thrombosis which involves the whole circumference of the anal canal. Maximal dilatation of the anus or partial internal sphincterotomy may reduce the patient's pain, but the cosmetic results are bad and most patients require a haemorrhoidectomy later.

Clotted venous saccule may be treated in the first 24 hours by evacuation of the clot under local anaesthesia. However, most cases are allowed to resolve spontaneously.

Haemorrhoids in patients with inflammatory bowel disease

All patients with haemorrhoids should be assessed to determine whether or not there is evidence of underlying inflammatory bowel disease. Patients with Crohn's disease often have oedematous skin tags (Figure 15.11) which are not seen in any other condition and must be distinguished from ordinary skin tags or thrombosed external haemorrhoids.

There is a low incidence of complications in patients with idiopathic proctocolitis (ulcerative colitis) who require outpatient or operative

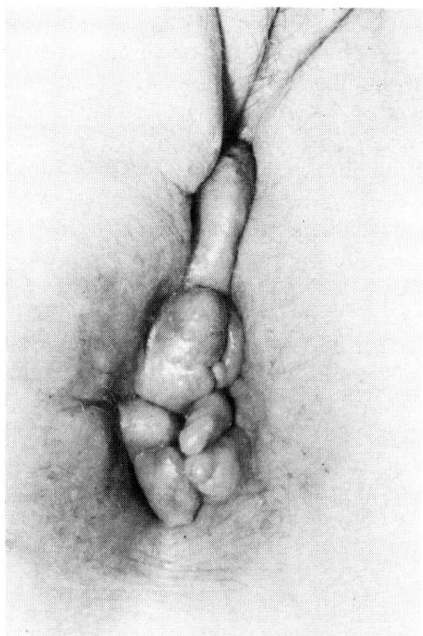

Fig. 15.11 Crohn's disease. Oedematous skin tags should *not* be operated upon.

treatment of haemorrhoids.[6] This is not the case with Crohn's disease where such treatments may lead to severe ulceration and sepsis. Local treatment of haemorrhoids is rarely necessary and is never advised in Crohn's disease.

REFERENCES

1 Alexander-Williams, J. (1981) Haemorrhoids. In *Colorectal Disease* (Ed.) Thomson, J. P. S., Nicholls, R. J. & Williams, C. B. pp. 331–344. London: Heinemann.
2 Alexander-Williams, J. (1982) The management of piles. *British Medical Journal*, **285**, 1137–1139.
3 Ambrose, N. S., Hares, M. M., Alexander-Williams, J. & Keighley, M. R. B. (1983) Prospective randomised comparison of photocoagulation and rubber band ligation in treatment of haemorrhoids. *British Medical Journal*, **286**, 1389–1391.
4 Goldberg, S. M. (1983) Closed haemorrhoidectomy. In *Rob and Smith's Operative Surgery* (Ed.) Todd, I. P. & Fielding, L. P. 4th Edition. Alimentary Tract and Abdominal Wall. 3. Colon, Rectum and Anus pp. 489–494. London: Butterworths.
5 Goligher, J. C. (1980) *Surgery of the Anus, Rectum and Colon.* pp. 93–135. 4th Edition. London: Baillière Tindall.
6 Jeffrey, P. J., Ritchie, J. K. & Parks, A. G. (1977) Treatment of haemorrhoids in patients with inflammatory bowel disease. *Lancet*, **i**, 1084–1085.
7 Keighley, M. R. B., Alexander-Williams, J., Buchmann, P. *et al.* (1979) Prospective trials of minor surgical procedures and high fibre diet for haemorrhoids. *British Medical Journal*, **ii**, 967–969.
8 Leicester, R. J., Nicholls, R. J. & Mann, C. V. (1981) Infrared coagulation – a new treatment for haemorrhoids. *Diseases of the Colon and Rectum*, **23**, 602–605.
9 Leicester, R. J., Nicholls, R. J. & Thomson, J. P. S. (1983) Unpublished data.
10 Lord, P. H. (1983) Maximal anal dilatation. In *Rob and Smith's Operative Surgery* (Ed.) Todd, I. P. & Fielding, L. P. 4th Edition. Alimentary Tract and Abdominal Wall. 3. Colon, Rectum and Anus pp. 474–479. London: Butterworths.
11 Mann, C. V. (1983) Open haemorrhoidectomy (St. Mark's ligation/excision method). In *Rob and Smith's Operative Surgery* (Ed.) Todd, I. P. & Fielding, L. P. 4th Edition. Alimentary Tract and Abdominal Wall. 3. Colon, Rectum and Anus pp. 495–502. London: Butterworths.
12 Murie, J. A., Sim, A. J. W. & Mackenzie, I. (1981) The importance of pain, pruritus and soiling as symptoms of haemorrhoids and their response to haemorrhoidectomy or rubber band ligation. *British Journal of Surgery*, **68**, 247–249.
13 Parks, A. G. (1956) De Haemorrhois – a study in surgical history. *Guy's Hospital Reports*, **104**, 135–156.
14 Parks, A. G. (1983) Haemorrhoidectomy. In *Rob and Smith's Operative Surgery* (Ed.) Todd, I. P. & Fielding, L. P. 4th Edition. Alimentary Tract and Abdominal Wall. 3. Colon, Rectum and Anus. pp. 480–488. London: Butterworths.
15 Saint-Pierre, A., Treffot, M. J. & Martin, P. M. (1982) Hormone receptors and haemorrhoidal disease. *Coloproctology*, **4**, 116–120.
16 Thomson, W. H. F. (1975) The nature of haemorrhoids. *British Journal of Surgery*, **62**, 542–552.
17 Thomson, W. H. F. (1982) The real nature of 'perianal haematoma'. *Lancet*, **ii**, 467–468.
18 Williams, K. L. (1983) Cryosurgery of haemorrhoids. In *Rob and Smith's Operative Surgery* (Ed.) Todd, I. P. & Fielding, L. P. 4th Edition. Alimentary Tract and Abdominal Wall. 3. Colon, Rectum and Anus pp. 503–508. London: Butterworths.

ANAL FISSURE

An anal fissure (fissure-in-ano) is a disruption in the lining of the anal canal usually beginning at or distal to the pectinate line and extending to or beyond the anal verge.

Classification

Fissures may be classified as either acute or chronic and further subdivided as either primary or secondary.[8] A primary fissure is 'idiopathic' since there is no satisfactory explanation for its occurrence. A secondary fissure is either linked to a known disorder, such as Crohn's disease or leukaemia, or to a cause and effect relationship, such as following damage from a foreign body, childbirth or previous anal surgery.

An acute fissure is superficial and amounts to a crack in the anoderm without any surrounding fibrosis. The floor of the acute fissure is formed by the brick-red longitudinal fibres of the muscularis mucosa. It resolves spontaneously or after conservative treatment. On the other hand, the chronic fissure represents true ulceration of the anoderm with surrounding fibrosis, exposure of the underlying transverse fibres of the internal sphincter muscle and/or the triad of ulcer, hypertrophied papilla, and a sentinel pile. Chronic fissures do not usually heal with conservative treatment.

Aetiology

In spite of the common occurrence and 'apparent simplicity' of anal fissure, its aetiology remains an enigma. The concept that all fissures result from the passage of a constipated stool is an oversimplification. In one report only 20% of patients gave a history of constipation.[18] Other possible causes include cryptitis, venous stasis and diarrhoea.

Primary fissure

There has been much discussion about spasm or hypertonicity of the internal sphincter and its relationship to anal fissures. Recent studies show an increase in the resting internal sphincter pressures in patients with anal fissure.[2, 11]

Nothmann and Schuster[22] have recognized an 'overshoot' contraction occurring in the internal sphincter after receptive relaxation of the rectum in patients with anal fissure (Figure 15.12). This phenomenon is almost certainly related to spasm of the internal sphincter in patients with anal fissure. These changes disappear after successful treatment. It is impossible at present to know whether these findings represent cause or effect. However, the concept of

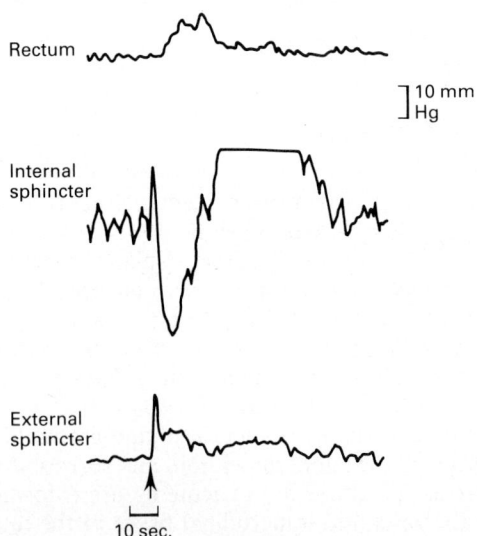

Fig. 15.12 Contraction of internal sphincter in a patient with anal fissure. After Nothmann and Schuster.[22]

internal sphincter spasm provides a rationale for the present day medical and surgical treatments.

Eisenhammer[7] postulated a number of reasons for the common posterior occurrence of anal fissure. He put forward the idea that the posterior midline was the most unsupported point of the anal skin because of the V-shaped divergence of the subcutaneous external sphincter and undermining of the anoderm in the posterior quadrant by deep crypts. However, he felt that the most important factor was the bilateral pull by the corrugator cutis ani in the posterior midline superimposed on a loss of elasticity and mobility of the anoderm by acute or chronic irritation. Oh[23] believes that acute primary fissures occur in the posterior or anterior midline because of greater expansibility in this direction and the elliptical shape of the anus.

Secondary fissure

Crohn's fissures are probably much more common than is generally recognized. Fielding reported a 51% incidence of fissures in Crohn's disease[5] and found them to be asymptomatic in over 90%. Other causes of secondary fissures include syphilis, tuberculosis, leukaemia, anorectal surgery, anal carcinoma, childbirth and prolonged diarrhoea secondary to laxative abuse.

Clinical presentation

OCCURRENCE

Although the peak incidence is in the second and third decades, all age groups are affected. Both sexes are equally affected. Approximately 10% of fissures in females are anterior compared with only 1% in males.[10]

SYMPTOMS

The principal symptom is painful defecation. The pain is described as sharp or burning and may persist for hours after defecation. Pain can lead to constipation and symptoms are aggravated by the eventual passage of a constipated stool thus creating a vicious circle.

Bleeding is also a common symptom. It is usually scanty and is always bright red in colour. Frequently it is noticed only on the toilet paper. A chronic discharge may lead to soiling of the underclothes and pruritus ani. Urinary tract symptoms, such as frequency, dysuria and even urinary retention, may occur. Dyspareunia has also been reported.

EXAMINATION

Anal fissures can almost always be detected by inspection alone. A few words of reassurance followed by slow, gentle separation of the buttocks will usually reveal the fissure and the associated 'sentinel pile'. If an acute fissure is seen, no further examination is necessary, conservative treatment should be instituted if appropriate and the patient brought back a few weeks later for completion of the examination. Occasionally there is such severe spasm that the fissure cannot be visualized and in such cases intersphincteric abscess must be considered in the differential diagnosis. If in doubt, a gentle digital examination aided by a topical, local or even a general anaesthetic may be necessary.

For chronic fissures, a complete anorectal examination can usually be performed at the initial visit. Occasionally, a topical or local anaesthetic may be necessary. Any chronic fissure in which Crohn's disease or carcinoma is suspected should be biopsied. Beware of the laterally placed fissure since this usually is a secondary fissure. Broad-based or multiple fissures, regardless of location, should arouse suspicion. Tuberculous fissures are rare and may be difficult to distinguish from Crohn's. Leukaemic fissures are usually a sign of advanced disease and can be extremely painful. No treatment is indicated except occasionally to drain an abscess.[9]

Treatment

Conservative therapy is the treatment of choice for acute primary fissure, whereas operative intervention is indicated for chronic primary fissure. The treatment of a secondary fissure is directed to the underlying problem.

Acute fissure
Conservative treatment consists of avoiding constipation by the use of bulk laxatives (psyllium seed or bran) and symptomatic measures such as a warm sitz-bath. An additional advantage of increased dietary fibre is the resulting dilatation of the anal sphincter as a consequence of increased stool weight. Anaesthetic ointments, suppositories, anal dilators and injection of long-acting local anaesthetics are of unproven effectiveness but nevertheless play a role in conservative therapy.

Chronic fissure
Although there are no satisfactory explanations for why some acute fissures become chronic, once chronicity occurs, further conservative treatment is usually unsuccessful. The basis for

present day surgical treatment of chronic anal fissure is 'pectenotomy'.[19] Eisenhammer[6] later recognized that 'pectenotomy' is actually an internal sphincterotomy.

Excision of anal fissure was popularized by Gabriel.[10] He excised a triangle of skin with the ulcer, removed a small triangle of internal sphincter muscle and stretched the anal sphincter. However, a 'keyhole' deformity sometimes develops, resulting in soiling, and the popularity of the procedure has waned.

In many centres, sphincterotomy gave way to anal stretching.[17] However, following reports of high failure rates and occasional incontinence, the value of sphincter stretching likewise came under question.

Lateral internal sphincterotomy subsequently became popular. This sphincterotomy ignored the fissure site and thus the 'keyhole' deformity was avoided. Variations in the basic technique have been described by Parks (Figure 15.13)[24] and Notaras (Figure 15.14).[21] These techniques avoid an anal incision, thus theoretically reducing postoperative discomfort. Many reports have shown that lateral internal sphincterotomy achieves the best results with the least morbidity (Table 15.5).[1, 4, 10, 12] A major advantage is that it can be performed under local anaesthesia. Minor degrees of incontinence, such as mucous drainage and staining of the underclothes, appear to be rare and recurrence rates are low (see Table 15.5).

More recently, Theuerkauf[26] introduced

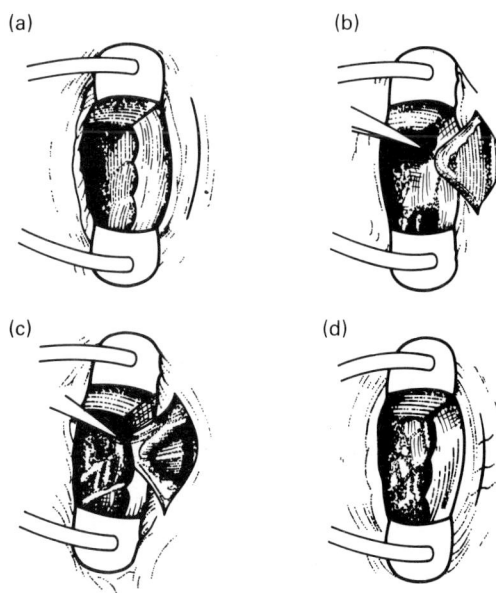

Fig. 15.13 Lateral internal sphincterotomy, perianal incision (after Parks[24]): (a) lateral skin incision; (b) division of the lower border of the internal sphincter; (c) division of the internal sphincter to dentate line; (d) closure of wound.

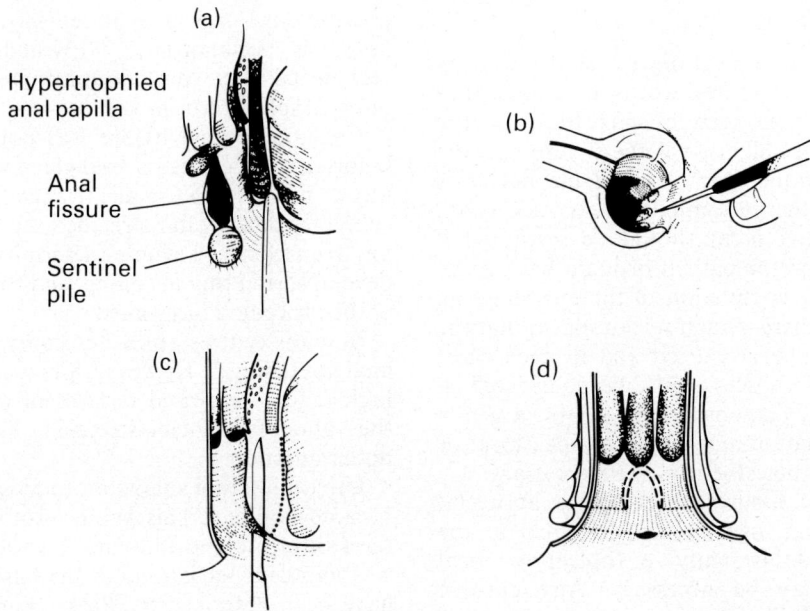

Fig. 15.14 Lateral internal sphincterotomy, stab-wound technique (after Notaras[21]): (a) anal fissure; (b, c) insertion of blade between the epithelium of the anal canal and the internal sphincter as far as the dentate line; (d) after the subcutaneous sphincterotomy the divided sphincter separates under a bridge of skin.

bilateral superficial distal internal sphincterotomy. In this procedure, the internal sphincter muscle is superficially incised in two quadrants through half of its thickness rather than a full thickness one-quadrant division as in the conventional lateral internal sphincterotomy. Results in his first 100 patients have been excellent with a recurrence rate of 1% and a 1% incidence of incontinence.

At the present time, we favour one-quadrant

lateral internal sphincterotomy. Keighley, Greca and Nevah[15] achieved better results when lateral internal sphincterotomy was performed under general anaesthesia compared with local anaesthesia. However, we believe that with proper patient selection the use of local anaesthesia is satisfactory. The technique recently described by Nivatvongs[20] allows the local anaesthesia to be performed with minimal or no discomfort (Figure 15.15).

Table 15.5 Comparisons of procedures for anal fissure.

	No. of patients	Impaired control for: Flatus (%)	Faeces (%)	Faecal soiling (%)	Unhealed or recurrence (%)
Lateral internal sphincterotomy					
Hoffman and Goligher[14]	99	6	1	7	3
Hawley[12]	24	?	0	0	0
Abcarian[1]	150	30[a] 0[b]	0	0	1.3
Collopy and Ryan[3]	86	17	12	19	15
Sphincter stretch					
Watts, Bennett and Goligher[27]	95	12	2	20	16
Hawley[12]	18	?	0	0	28
Abcarian[1]	—	—	—	—	—
Collopy and Ryan[3]	74	30	16	34	30
Posterior internal sphincterotomy					
Bennett and Goligher[3]	127	24	11	28	7
Hawley[12]	32	?	0	8	8
Abcarian[1]	150	40[a] 5[b]	5	5	1.3
Collopy and Ryan[3]	—	—	—	—	—

[a] Temporary; [b] permanent.

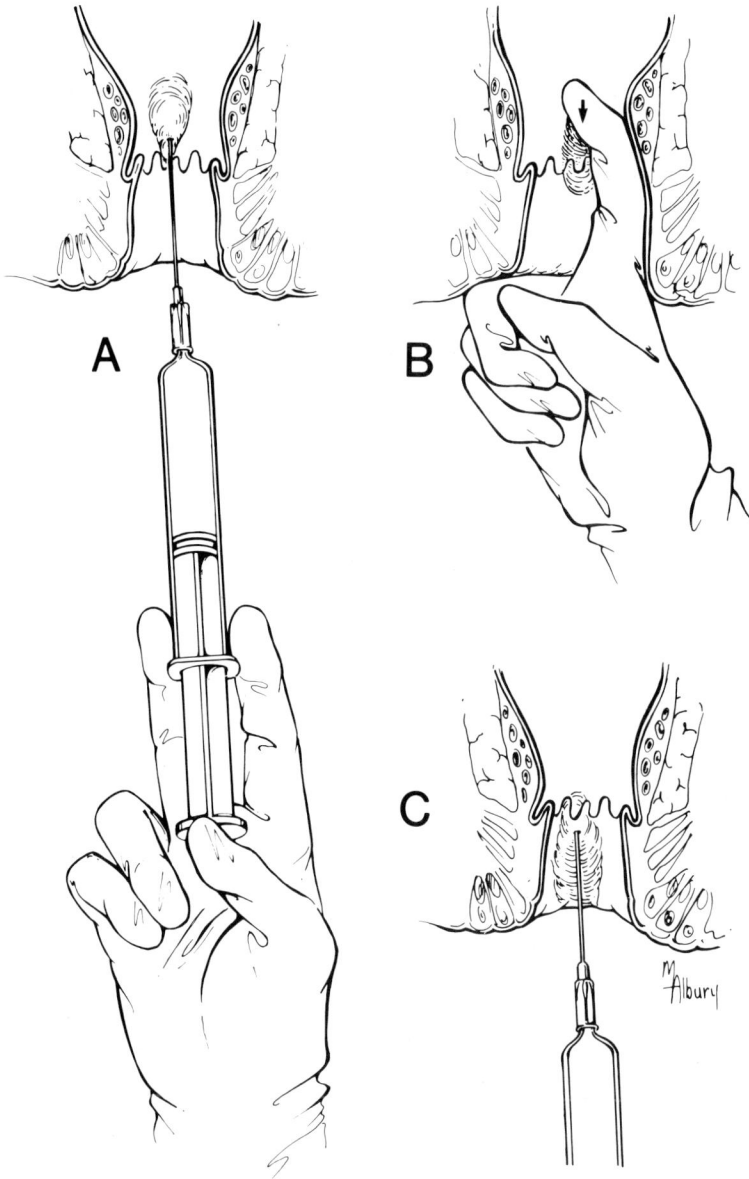

Fig. 15.15 Technique of local anaesthesia. A. Injection of the anaesthetic solution 2 mm proximal to the pectinate line. B. The anaesthetic solution is squeezed into the anoderm. C. Injection of the anaesthetic solution 2 mm distal to the pectinate line. From Nivatvongs (1982)[20] with kind permission of the editor of *Diseases of the Colon and Rectum.*

Anal fissure in children

Anal fissure is the most common cause of rectal bleeding in infants[13] but the bleeding is rarely profuse. Anal fissure is extremely rare in breast fed infants.[25] The fissures in children are almost always acute and therefore superficial. Unlike adults, acute primary fissures in children are often multiple and commonly located laterally.[16] In older children, the presence of a fissure-in-ano should signal the possibility of leukaemia.[25]

As a rule, the diagnosis can easily be confirmed by inspection. Sometimes the fissure will have healed by the time the parents seek medical attention for the child. However, the characteristic history and lack of symptoms at the time of examination usually make the diagnosis obvious.

Medical therapy consists mainly of bulk laxatives, stool softeners, mineral oil, or simple dietary regulation. Only approximately 1% of acute fissures in children become chronic.[25] These are treated quite successfully under general anaesthesia by dilatation of the anus with excision of any chronic scar tissue or papilla if necessary.[16, 25] Dilatation alone is usually the only form of treatment required in children who develop a chronic fissure.

REFERENCES

1 Abcarian, H. (1980) Surgical correction of chronic anal fissure: results of lateral internal sphincterotomy vs. fissurectomy-midline sphincterotomy. *Diseases of the Colon and Rectum*, **23**, 31–36.

2 Arabi, Y., Alexander-Williams, J. & Keighley, M. R. B. (1977) Anal pressures in hemorrhoids and anal fissure. *American Journal of Surgery*, **134**, 608–610.

3 Bennett, R. C. & Goligher, J. C. (1962) Results of internal sphincterotomy for anal fissure. *British Medical Journal*, **2**, 1500–1503.

4 Collopy, B. & Ryan, P. (1979) Comparison of lateral subcutaneous sphincterotomy with anal dilatation in the treatment of fissure-in-ano. *Medical Journal of Australia*, **2**, 461–462 and 495.

5 Crapp, A. R. & Alexander-Williams, J. (1975) Fissure-in-ano and anal stenosis. Part I: Conservative management. *Clinics in Gastroenterology*, **4**, 619–628.

6 Eisenhammer, S. (1953) The internal anal sphincter: its surgical importance. *South African Medical Journal*, **27**, 266–270.

7 Eisenhammer, S. (1959) The evaluation of the internal anal sphincterotomy operation with special reference to anal fissure. *Surgery, Gynecology and Obstetrics*, **109**, 583–590.

8 Eisenhammer, S. (1974) Internal anal sphincterotomy plus free dilatation versus anal stretch with special criticism of the anal stretch procedure for hemorrhoids: the recommended modern approach to hemorrhoid treatment. *Diseases of the Colon and Rectum*, **17**, 493–522.

9 Goldberg, S. M., Gordon, P. H. & Nivatvongs, S. (1980) Fissure-in-ano. In *Essentials of Anorectal Surgery*. 1st edition, pp. 86–99. Philadelphia: J. B. Lippincott.

10 Goligher, J. C. (1980) Anal fissure. In *Surgery of the Anus, Rectum and Colon*. 4th edition, pp. 136–153. London: Baillière Tindall.

11 Hancock, B. D. (1977) The internal sphincter and anal fissure. *British Journal of Surgery*, **64**, 92–95.

12 Hawley, P. R. (1969) The treatment of chronic fissure-in-ano: a trial of methods. *British Journal of Surgery*, **56**, 915–918.

13 Holder, T. M. & Ashcraft, K. W. (1980) Acquired anorectal lesions–fissure-in-ano. In *Pediatric Surgery*. 1st edition, p. 429. Philadelphia: W. B. Saunders.

14 Hoffman, D. C. & Goligher, J. C. (1970) Lateral subcutaneous internal sphincterotomy in treatment of anal fissure. *British Medical Journal*, **3**, 673–675.

15 Keighley, M. R. B., Greca, F. & Nevah, E. *et al.* (1981) Treatment of anal fissure by lateral subcutaneous sphincterotomy should be under general anaesthesia. *British Journal of Surgery*, **68**, 400–401.

16 Kleinhaus, S. (1979) Miscellaneous anal disorders. In *Pediatric Surgery* (Ed.) Ravitch, M. M. 3rd edition, p. 1078. Chicago: Year Book Medical Publishers.

17 Lord, P. H. (1969) A day-case procedure for the cure of third-degree haemorrhoids. *British Journal of Surgery*, **56**, 747–749.

18 Mazier, W. P., De Moraes, R. T. & Dignan, R. D. (1978) Anal fissure and anal ulcers. *Surgical Clinics of North America*, **58**, 479–485.

19 Miles, E. W. (1939) Anal fissure. In *Rectal Surgery: A Practical Guide to the Modern Surgical Treatment of Rectal Diseases*. 1st edition, pp. 147–157. London: Cassell.

20 Nivatvongs, S. (1982) An improved technique of local anesthesia for anorectal surgery. *Diseases of the Colon and Rectum*, **25**, 259–260.

21 Notaras, M. J. (1971) The treatment of anal fissure by lateral subcutaneous internal sphincterotomy – a technique and results. *British Journal of Surgery*, **58**, 96–100.

22 Nothmann, B. J. & Schuster, M. M. (1974) Internal anal sphincter derangement with anal fissures. *Gastroenterology*, **67**, 216–220.

23 Oh, C. (1975) Lateral subcutaneous internal sphincterotomy for anal fissure. *Mount Sinai Journal of Medicine*, **42**, 596–601.

24 Parks, A. G. (1967) The management of fissure-in-ano. *Hospital Medicine*, **1**, 737.

25 Raffensperger, J. G. (1980) Gastrointestinal hemorrhage. In *Swenson's Pediatric Surgery*. 4th edition, pp. 425–458. New York: Appleton-Century-Crofts.

26 Theuerkauf, F. J. (1981) Bilateral superficial distal internal sphincterotomy. *Presentation at American Society of Colon and Rectal Surgeons Meeting*, Colorado Springs, Colorado, 1981.

27 Watts, J. M., Bennett, R. C. & Goligher, J. C. (1964) Stretching of anal sphincters in treatment of fissure-in-ano. *British Medical Journal*, **2**, 342–343.

ANORECTAL SEPSIS

Anorectal sepsis is a common surgical emergency. The latest available figures show that 6970 patients were admitted to hospital in 1978 in England and Wales with anorectal sepsis.[12] There is also a population which is treated outside hospital practice and which is not referred until the patient presents with a fistula or further episodes of sepsis. Sepsis is commoner in men than women and while occurring in the young and the old, it is commonest in the third and fourth decades.[12] Two to three per cent of all admissions with anorectal sepsis are associated with underlying inflammatory bowel disease; the primary diagnosis is more likely to be Crohn's disease than ulcerative colitis. Perianal abscess is about three times more common than ischiorectal abscess. Supralevator abscess is rare in spite of Prasad's recent claim that supralevator sepsis accounted for 9.1% of their series.[20]

Anorectal sepsis usually begins with an infection of the anal glands to form an intermuscular abscess;[4, 5, 6, 18] this abscess then tracks through or around the sphincter to present at one of the standard sites (Figure 15.16). Although there is strong evidence for this aetiology, Goligher[9] was able to identify only eight intermuscular abscesses in 28 patients carefully explored. In addition, recent microbiological studies have suggested that an intermuscular abscess or fistula is only likely to be present when culture of the pus has demonstrated a bowel-derived organism.[11] Staphylococcal abscesses orginate from skin and not from anal glands. We do not know why these abscesses should be commoner in men than in women and why the anal glands

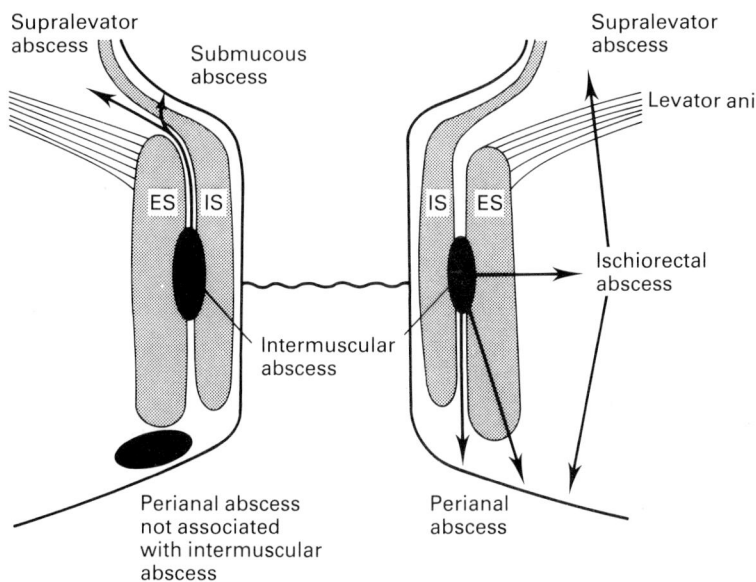

Fig. 15.16 Anatomy of anorectal abscess, IS = internal sphincter; ES = external sphincter.

should be more susceptible to sepsis in the third and fourth decades.

Although this is a common problem, management may be poor and the recurrence rate is high. Correct management depends upon:

1 An understanding of the anatomy of the anal canal with particular reference to the anatomy of abscesses and fistulas.
2 The correct diagnosis.
3 Microbiology.
4 An understanding of the objectives of surgical management.

Anatomy

ABSCESS

An understanding of the anatomy of the anal canal is essential when considering the management of all abscesses, but especially those which originate in the intermuscular plane. The potential space between the internal and external sphincters contains the anal glands whose ducts open into the anal canal at the dentate line. The type of abscess depends upon the direction that the pus tracks from the intermuscular space.
The pus may track along three planes (Figure 15.16):
1 Between the internal and external components of the sphincter, or sometimes through the lowermost fibres of the external sphincter, to present as a perianal abscess.
2 Laterally through the external sphincter to present as an ischiorectal abscess. Occasionally an ischiorectal abscess may also track through the levator ani to present with a supralevator component.

3 Proximally between the sphincters to present as a submucous abscess or very rarely in the supralevator space as a supralevator abscess.

Any abscess which does not originate in the intermuscular space will lie subcutaneously and will be perianal rather than ischiorectal.

FISTULA

It has been suggested that fistulas are either low, common and easy to manage or high, rare and difficult to manage. This generalization is true. Over 90% of fistulas are low and they are easy to manage while the rare high fistulas may be very difficult. The terms low and high have been applied rather loosely but generally refer to the anatomical relationship that the fistula track bears to the external sphincter. A high fistula, however, may not be difficult to manage if it is merely called high because the track extends proximally in the intersphincteric space to open into the rectum. In this situation, little of the sphincter has to be divided. The relative incidence of these anatomical variations is difficult to establish, but Parks'[19] series which is commonly quoted contained a large number of referals to a specialist centre (Table 15.6) with a

Table 15.6 Incidence of anal fistula.[a]

Intersphincteric	183 (46.1%)
low	137
high (to rectum)	46
Trans-sphincteric	116 (29.3%)
Suprasphincteric	78 (19.6%)
Extrasphincteric	20 (5.0%)

[a] Parks[18] 397 patients.

much higher incidence of high fistula than is commonly seen by most surgeons whose experience is that 90% are of the low intersphincteric variety. Most anal fistulas originate as an intermuscular abscess with the internal opening at the dentate line. The direction that the fistula track takes before opening at skin level determines the type of fistula. Fistulas secondary to pelvic sepsis are not true anal fistulas but because of their anatomical relationship to the anal canal tend to be classified in the same group.

Anal fistulas secondary to anal sepsis (Figure 15.17)

There are three principal anatomical varieties of fistula:

1 Intersphincteric. The track runs between the internal and external components of the sphincter. The normal direction (low intersphincteric) is distal, to open onto the skin close to the anal canal but occasionally the track runs proximally to open into the rectum (high intersphincteric) above the internal sphincter.

2 Trans-sphincteric. The track runs through the external sphincter and through the ischiorectal fossa to perianal skin. The amount of external sphincter below the track defines the height of the fistula and thereby the difficulty in surgical management.

3 Suprasphincteric. The track passes upwards in the intersphincteric space, above the external sphincter and then back through levator ani, into the ischiorectal fossa and thence to the perianal skin.

'Anal' fistula secondary to pelvic sepsis

An extrasphincteric fistula is nearly always secondary to pelvic sepsis which discharges through the levator ani into the ischiorectal fossa and then to perianal skin.

The correct diagnosis

ABSCESS

The diagnosis of sepsis is usually easy with the patient complaining of a painful lump in the region of the anal canal. On examination there is erythema overlying an obviously tender swelling. A large area of erythema, however, does not necessarily mean that the abscess is ischiorectal; those abscesses which are close to the anal canal are likely to be perianal. Occasionally a patient may complain of acute anal pain but, in spite of tenderness, there is nothing abnormal to see. An examination under anaesthetic is required to make the diagnosis, and usually pus may be identified either under the submucosa of the anal canal or in the intermuscular plane, which is more difficult to detect. An intersphincteric abscess may defy diagnosis and must always be considered in a patient with anal pain and no evidence of an anal fissure.

FISTULA

The external opening of a fistula is obvious with inspection of the perianal skin. It is thought by many that the further away the opening is from the anal canal, the more likely the fistula is to be

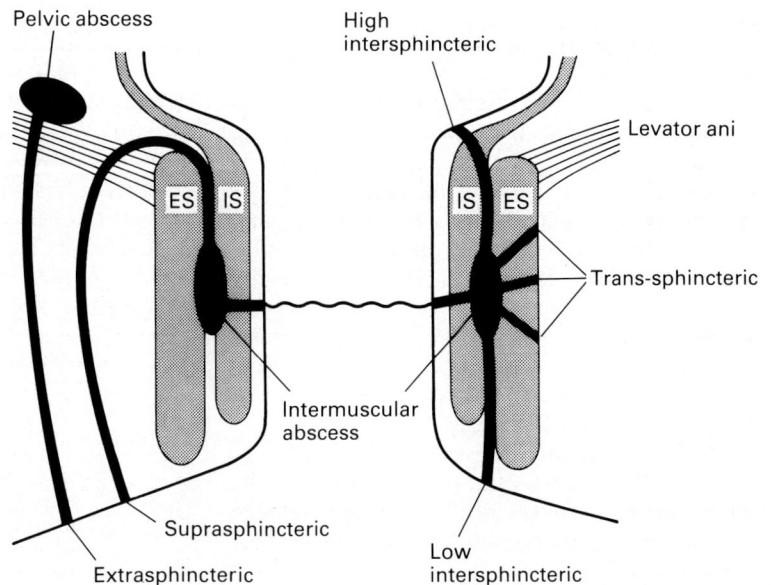

Fig. 15.17 Anatomy of anal fistulas. IS = internal sphincter; ES = external sphincter.

high but this is not necessarily true. Goodsall's law is useful but not absolute; anterior fistulas open directly into the anal canal, whereas fistulas between 3 and 9 o'clock open posteriorly in the midline. The track of a low fistula can usually be easily palpated; it feels like a firm piece of string running towards the anal canal from the external opening. The fistula is probably high if no track can be palpated.

Microbiology

Until recently very little interest has been taken in the microbiology of anorectal sepsis. Coliforms have been the most commonly isolated organism but recent surgical interest in the obligate anaerobes has demonstrated *Bacteroides fragilis* in a high proportion of anorectal abscess. The incidence of isolating *B. fragilis* varies, Abcarian[1] found occasional colonies, but Meislin[16] suggested that the incidence was as high as 47%. However, his study was small with only 21 patients. Whitehead[24] reported that 32/74 patients had 'gut-specific' *Bacteroides*. Other authors have emphasized the frequency with which skin organisms such as *Staphylococcus aureus* are identified; they are responsible for 15–25% of the organisms cultured.[2, 8, 17, 25] A recent study confirmed this incidence and then suggested that associated fistulas are only found when a bowel-derived organism is grown in culture.[11] This view was supported by Wilson[25] who related recurrent sepsis to the original organism cultured; there were seven recurrent fistulas and in each case the original was bowel-derived. In contrast, however, Whitehead[24] claimed that fistulas were found when skin organisms were cultured but his study does not say whether or not the *Staphylococci* were found in pure culture and the operations in this study were performed by surgeons of varying experience.

The objectives of surgical treatment

PRINCIPLES OF MANAGEMENT

The aims of surgical management are threefold:
1 To relieve symptoms;
2 To achieve rapid healing, thereby ensuring early return of the patient to work;
3 To avoid recurrent sepsis.

There are two distinct schools of thought concerning immediate surgical management. One argues that the relief of symptoms with an early return to work is of prime importance, while suggesting that even if the recurrence rate is high the remaining patients have no further trouble. It is further claimed that definitive surgery in the acute phase to an associated fistula may cause damage to the sphincter and thereby incontinence. It is suggested that this approach is associated with an unacceptable risk of incontinence particularly as the surgery for anorectal sepsis is often performed by surgeons in training. This concept of management prevails in the United States and may reflect the very large number of surgeons operating on small numbers of patients. This view, however, also has support in the United Kingdom.

The second and more positive school argues that, whatever the surgical diagnosis, a high recurrence rate is unacceptable as a principle of correct surgical management. Surgery should therefore aim to prevent recurrence as well as alleviate symptoms and ensure an early return to work.

The relief of symptoms. The pain of anorectal sepsis is caused by the pressure of pus within the abscess cavity; any surgical manoeuvre that removes the pus will relieve the symptoms.

Rapid healing. The smaller the wound, the more rapid will be the healing providing that the pus does not re-collect; healing may be aided by antibiotics.

The prevention of recurrent sepsis. An anorectal abscess will recur or the patient will be left with an anal fistula if the presenting abscess is secondary to an intermuscular abscess and if a fistula is not laid open during the acute episode. Most of these recurrences will present within two years but the time interval may be much longer.

There are few good studies of recurrence since the length of follow-up is either inadequate or the number of patients successfully followed is too small.[7, 14, 15] The incidence of recurrent sepsis reported in Cardiff was 25%[2] which was comparable to that of Wilson.[25] In 1982 we showed that 68/165 (41.2%) of the patients presenting with anorectal sepsis had had a previous abscess;[11] 30 of these patients had a fistula demonstrated at operation. Chrabot, Prasad and Abcarian[3] demonstrated fistulas in 53 out of 68 patients presenting with recurrent anorectal sepsis.

SURGICAL TECHNIQUES

Aspiration of the pus. This will relieve the acute symptoms but the pus will almost certainly re-collect unless aspiration is followed by a more definitive surgical procedure. Successful aspiration may be associated with an immediate return to work but does nothing to prevent recurrent sepsis.

Drainage of the abscess. Simple drainage will relieve the acute symptoms, and is associated with rapid healing and an early return to work, but does nothing to prevent recurrence.

Incision and primary suture (under antibiotic cover). This will relieve the symptoms and is associated with rapid healing and an early return to work but it does nothing to prevent recurrence. Originally described by Ellis,[8] Wilson[25] demonstrated a recurrence rate of 22% within the relatively short mean follow-up period of just over two years while a later study from the same unit[14] showed a recurrence rate of 8/66 patients successfully followed over one year; 44 patients, however, were lost to follow-up. These studies emphasize the problems associated with inadequate follow-up. It has recently been suggested that suture of the wound after drainage of soft tissue abscesses holds no advantage over simple drainage provided that each procedure is covered by systemic antibiotic therapy.[21] This study and that of Leaper[14] used Clindamycin as the antibiotic of choice.

Saucerization. This previously popular management was based on the misconception that the large wound would 'heal from the bottom' and would be associated with a low incidence of recurrence. This concept, however, ignored the presence of the intermuscular cavity and the internal opening. The technique is associated with a large wound, slow healing and a long period of time off work. That it does nothing to prevent recurrence was demonstrated by Leaper[14] with 23 (21.1%) recurrences in 109 patients within one year.

Incision and drainage/laying open the fistula. Drainage relieves the symptoms; laying open of the fistula prevents recurrent sepsis but the patient has to accept slower healing of the wound and a longer period lost from work.
It is suggested that the correct management of anorectal abscess is as follows:
1 Examination under anaesthesia (EUA) drainage of abscess (laying open of fistula).

The patient is examined under anaesthetic and the abscess is drained. A search is made for a fistula remembering that this should be done with great care as the tissues are friable and false tracks can easily be produced. Pressure on the abscess from outside prior to drainage may define the internal opening by demonstrating pus at the dentate line.
2 Microbiology of the pus. The pus should be sent for both aerobic and anaerobic culture. No further surgical procedure will be required if culture grows a skin-derived organism.[11]
3 Second EUA (laying open of fistula). A second EUA is performed after 7–10 days and any fistula track demonstrated is laid open.

These techniques have recently been described in *Rob and Smith's Operative Surgery.*[10]

SURGICAL MANAGEMENT OF THE ANAL FISTULA

It is emphasized that the laying open of any fistula in a patient with acute anorectal sepsis should be approached with caution and is the province of experienced surgeons rather than surgeons in training. The management of fistulas not associated with acute sepsis should also be approached with care but low (intersphincteric) fistulas are generally easy to treat and associated with minimal morbidity. The management of high fistulas, however, is difficult and faecal incontinence as a result of surgical damage to the sphincter is a disaster. Fistula tracks are best identified initially by palpation if it is low, and then by using the Lockhart–Mummery fistula probe. The probe should be passed carefully into the track which is laid open along the groove of the probe. An injection of dye is never required as the granulation tissue along the track is itself the perfect marker and even vigorous curettage of the granulation tissue will always leave some granulation tissue indicating the next part of the track to be laid open.

The low intersphincteric fistula is usually easily identified running from the external opening into the anal canal opening at the dentate line. The high intersphincteric fistula merely requires the laying open of the upper part of the internal sphincter.

The trans-sphincteric fistula may run to the apex of the ischiorectal fossa before turning and passing through the sphincter much lower than might be thought from where the track runs to the apex of the fossa. The surgeon may also be deceived when a secondary track passes up to the apex of the ischiorectal fossa, while the primary track runs posteriorly, passing through the sphincter in the mid line. On occasion the track may run in the intersphincteric plane such that its passage through the two components of the sphincter may not be adjacent. Extreme care is needed if there is an extension into the supra-levator space because surgical damage to the rectum will convert a trans-sphincteric fistula into a suprasphincteric fistula.

The suprasphincteric fistula may be best treated by division of the sphincter, excision of the track, and primary suture under cover of a left iliac fossa loop colostomy.

High trans-sphincteric, and sometimes supra-sphincteric fistulas, may be treated using the seton suture. The lower part of the track is laid open with division of the sphincter as necessary. The seton suture is then tied without tension around the remaining sphincter; healing with fibrosis takes place as the seton migrates through the remaining part of the sphincter and continence is maintained. This process may be rather slow.

The extrasphincteric track requires treatment to the primary pelvic pathology with simple curettage of the fistula track. Successful treatment of the pelvic sepsis will result in spontaneous closure of the fistula without any further surgical procedure.[23]

Inflammatory bowel disease

Anorectal sepsis is commoner in Crohn's disease than ulcerative colitis and commoner in Crohn's colitis than small bowel disease.

Crohn's disease
Management of anorectal sepsis in Crohn's disease is never easy. The basic principle is that surgical intervention should be the minimal required to relieve symptoms while remembering that anal Crohn's disease is merely a manifestation of total gut disease which may require systemic therapy as well as local treatment. Abscesses should be drained and very low fistulas may be laid open; however, the wounds do not heal well and laying open of high fistulas should be avoided if possible. Partial internal anal fistulotomy with curettage of the track has recently been advocated with some success.[22] The presence of multiple fistulas and recurrent sepsis may be an indication for excision of the rectum. There may be a place for azathioprine and recently it has been suggested that a combination of metronidazole and Septrin will help to control the problem but no data are yet available.

Ulcerative colitis
Abscesses should be drained and low fistulas may be laid open with reasonable confidence that the wound will heal. High fistulas are uncommon in ulcerative colitis and should be approached with caution.

Tuberculosis
Tuberculous perianal disease is usually associated with systemic disease and in the UK this is usually only seen in the immigrant population. Surgical drainage, combined with anti-tuberculous therapy, will control the problem.

Hidradenitis suppurativa
Hidradenitis is a curious problem which may cause debilitating disease; the pus can be very offensive. Sepsis arises in abnormal apocrine sweat glands and anal manifestations are often associated with axillary, cervical, groin and scrotal disease. The infecting organism is usually *Staphylococcus aureus* but *Bacteroides* has recently been implicated.[13] Surgical management varies from wide excision of the affected areas to simple laying open of the tracks with careful postoperative nursing care.

Fulminating gangrene
This is not a common condition but the extent of the sepsis is generally so severe that diagnosis is easy; management, however, is more difficult. There is a high incidence of associated disease, particularly diabetes mellitus. This problem is variously described as acute dermal gangrene, invasive necrotizing infection, or loosely associated with scrotal gangrene (Fournier's disease). Surgical excision should be vigorous, with excision of the involved tissue leaving healthy, bleeding wound edges. The infecting organism is not necessarily clostridial but there may be a place for hyperbaric oxygen.

REFERENCES

1 Abcarian, H. (1976) Acute suppurations of the anorectum. *Surgery Annual*, **8**, 305–333.
2 Buchan, R. & Grace, R. H. (1973) Anorectal suppuration: the results of treatment and the factors influencing the recurrence rate. *British Journal of Surgery*, **60**, 537–540.
3 Chrabot, C. M., Prasad, M. L. & Abcarian, H. (1983) Recurrent anorectal abscesses. *Diseases of the Colon and Rectum*, **26**, 105–108.
4 Eisenhammer, S. (1956) The internal anal sphincter and the anorectal abscess. *Surgery, Gynecology and Obstetrics*, **103**, 501–506.
5 Eisenhammer, S. (1958) A new approach to the anorectal fistulous abscess based on the high inter-muscular

lesion. *Surgery, Gynecology and Obstetrics*, **106**, 595–599.

6 Eisenhammer, S. (1961) The anorectal and anovulval fistulous abscess. *Surgery, Gynecology and Obstetrics*, **113**, 519–520.

7 Eisenhammer, S. (1978) The final evaluation and classification of the surgical treatment of the primary anorectal cryptoglandular intermuscular (intersphincteric) fistulous abscess and fistula. *Diseases of the Colon and Rectum*, **21** (3), 237–254.

8 Ellis, M. (1960) Incision and primary suture of abscesses of the anal region. *Proceedings of the Royal Society of Medicine*, **53**, 652–653.

9 Goligher, J. C., Ellis, M. & Pissidis, A. G. (1967) A critique of anal glandular infection in the aetiology and treatment of idiopathic anorectal abscesses and fistulas. *Diseases of the Colon and Rectum*, **17**, 357–359.

10 Grace, R. H. (1983) Ano-rectal sepsis. In *Rob and Smith's Operative Surgery* (Ed.) Todd, I. P. & Fielding, L. P. 4th Edition, Section 3 – Colon, Rectum and Anus. pp. 516–523. London: Butterworth.

11 Grace, R. H., Harper, I. A. & Thompson, R. G. (1982) Ano-rectal sepsis: microbiology in relation to fistula-in-ano. *British Journal of Surgery*, **69**, 401–403.

12 HIPE (1978) Hospital in-patient enquiry.

13 Leach, R. D., Eykyn, S. J., Phillips, A. *et al.* (1979) Anaerobic axillary abscess. *British Medical Journal*, **ii**, 5–7.

14 Leaper, D. J., Page, R. E., Rosenberg, I. L. *et al.* (1976) A controlled study comparing the conventional treatment of idiopathic anorectal abscess with that of incision, curettage and primary suture under antibiotic cover. *Diseases of the Colon and Rectum*, **19**, 46–50.

15 McElwain, J. W., Alexander, R. M. & MacLean, M. D. (1966) Primary fistulectomy for anorectal abscess: a clinical study of 500 cases. *Diseases of the Colon and Rectum*, **9**, 181–185.

16 Meislin, H. W., Lerner, S. A., Graves, M. H. *et al.* (1977) Anaerobic and aerobic bacteriology and outpatient management. *Annals of Internal Medicine*, **87**, 145–149.

17 Page, R. E. & Freeman, R. (1977) Superficial sepsis: the antibiotic of choice for blind treatment. *British Journal of Surgery*, **64**, 281–284.

18 Parks, A. G. (1961) Pathogenesis and treatment of fistula-in-ano. *British Medical Journal*, **i**, 463–469.

19 Parks, A. G., Gordon, P. H. & Hardcastle, J. D. (1976) A classification of fistula-in-ano. *British Journal of Surgery*, **63**, 1–12.

20 Prasad, A. L., Read, D. R. & Abcarian, H. (1981) Supralevator abscesses: diagnosis and treatment. *Diseases of the Colon and Rectum*, **24**, 456–461.

21 Simms, M. H., Curran, F., Johnson, R. A. *et al.* (1982) Treatment of acute abscesses in the casualty department. *British Medical Journal*, **284**, 1827–1829.

22 Sohn, N., Korelitz, B. I. & Weinstein, M. A. (1980) Anorectal Crohn's disease: definitive surgery for fistulas and recurrent abscesses. *American Journal of Surgery*, **139**, 394–397.

23 Todd, I. P. & Lockhart–Mummery, Sir H. E. (1983) Fistula-in-ano. In *Rob and Smith's Operative Surgery* (Ed.) Todd, I. P. & Fielding, L. P. 4th Edition, Section 3 – Colon, Rectum and Anus. pp. 524–537. London: Butterworth.

24 Whitehead, S. M., Leach, R. D., Eykyn, S. J. & Phillips, I. (1982) The aetiology of perirectal sepsis. *British Journal of Surgery*, **69**, 166–168.

25 Wilson, D. H. (1964) The late results of anorectal abscess treated by incision, curettage, and primary suture under antibiotic cover. *British Journal of Surgery*, **51**, 828–831.

PRURITUS ANI AND PROCTALGIA FUGAX

PRURITUS ANI

Pruritus ani is a symptom of itching and irritation in the perianal region but does not designate a specific aetiology. The symptom complex is exceedingly common since the skin is covered, often moist, and soiled by faeces. Often the patient enters a cycle of irritation which leads to scratching of the area and continued irritation. Treatment must be directed at breaking this cycle.

Aetiology

The majority of cases are idiopathic and a specific cause cannot be determined.[1] The known causes are:

1 Proctological disorders. Skin tags, mucus-producing prolapsing internal haemorrhoids or polyps, draining fistulas or sinuses, fissures, condyloma acuminatum and hidradenitis suppurativa.

2 Dermatological conditions. Psoriasis, seborrhoeic dermatitis and atopic eczema.

3 Contact dermatitis. Soaps with irritating chemicals and alkaline pH, local analgesic compounds and other topical ointments.

4 Fungal. Candidiasis and dermatophytosis.

5 Bacterial. Secondary to scratching and infection.

6 Parasitic. Pinworms (*Enterobius vermicularis*), pediculosis and scabies.

7 After oral antibiotic therapy. Frequently related to diarrhoea and altered intestinal microflora.

8 Systemic diseases. Diabetes mellitus.

9 Neoplasms. Intraepithelial carcinoma (Bowen's disease) and extramammary Paget's disease.

10 Hygiene. Poor hygiene as well as overmeticulous hygiene using excessive soap.

11 Warmth and hyperhidrosis. Related to underclothing, obesity, moisture and climate.

12 Dietary. Excessive consumption of coffee, alcohol, milk and fruit juices.

13 Psychogenic. Perpetuation of the cycle of anxiety–itch–anxiety cycle may be present in certain patients.

14 Idiopathic. Represents around 50% of cases but there is some evidence that these patients have faecal soiling and imperfect anal function.

Clinical features

The symptoms of pruritus ani may range from mild to severe, for periods of from days to years.

Careful history must be obtained regarding the onset of the problem and associated factors, such as diet, drugs, stool consistency and skin eruptions.[5] A careful dietary history should be taken, paying particular attention to excessive coffee consumption. Other dermatological problems should be sought as well as the use of drugs or chemicals applied to the perianal area. A history of anorectal surgery is important.

Examination of the perianal area may reveal, on the one hand, normal appearing skin and, at the other extreme, severe inflammation with thickening and lichenification.[2] Specific dermatological conditions may be recognized (such as psoriasis) by its gross appearance or on biopsy.

Specific anorectal diseases should be identified and corrected, particularly disorders which allow moisture to escape from the rectum. These include chronic abscesses and fistulas which drain pus as well as prolapse of mucosa from the rectum which allows mucus to continually seep onto the perianal skin. Evaluation of the sphincter is important since seepage may occur following laying open a fistula where a portion of the sphincteric ring is divided. A sulcus may result which allows for continuous seepage from the rectum with concomitant moisture to the perianal skin.

Laboratory tests are rarely helpful but should be performed in refractory cases. Specifically, scrapings may reveal yeast and a tape test may disclose pinworm infestation. Biopsy of the involved skin may be useful to exclude a malignancy or other specific dermatological conditions.

Treatment

Since most cases are idiopathic, patients should be made to understand that a specific cause does not exist. Frequently, there is concern about cancer or other serious conditions. When a specific aetiology is determined, treatment is directed appropriately. This includes medical treatment of fungal, yeast and parasitic involvement, as well as surgical treatment of anorectal disease which permits moisture accumulation. Band ligation or sclerotherapy of prolapsing internal haemorrhoids may control mucus production by decreasing redundant tissue without resorting to haemorrhoidectomy. Drainage of abscesses, laying open of fistulas, removal of condylomas, and treatment of fissure with lateral internal sphincterotomy should be advised. These surgical problems account for 5–10% of all patients.

Where a specific aetiology has not been determined, a more general approach must be used.

Dietary restrictions may be indicated and specifically directed towards coffee and alcohol. Faulty hygiene is also a precipitating cause of pruritus ani since many patients, when they begin to have irritation, shower and bathe the area more vigorously which may perpetuate the cycle. Refraining from the use of soap in the perianal region is important since soap is slightly alkaline in pH and often remains in contact with the skin after bathing. Soap should not be used during the active treatment phase in the perianal region. All other topical medications in use should be stopped to avoid contact dermatitis. Following bathing, the area must be thoroughly blotted and dried to prevent maceration. Dry cotton is often useful during the day to prevent moisture accumulation. Bathing should be performed after bowel movements, if possible, or the area cleansed thoroughly with moistened tissue paper. Nylon underwear must not be worn.

Suppositories and analgesic agents should be avoided. A water soluble 0.25% or 1% steroidal cream with an acid pH may be helpful if used sparingly, twice a day, in the involved area.[4]

Tension and stress, in certain individuals, may promote this condition as may an irritable bowel with irritating loose, frequent bowel movements. These patients will benefit from counselling, dietary restrictions to avoid loose bowel movements, and the use of hydrophilic bulk agents.

In difficult and refractory cases, dermatological consultation may be of value. There is no role for wide surgical excision of the involved skin or radiation as used in the past. However, surgical reconstruction of sphincter deficiency may be helpful and postanal repair is worth considering in patients with gross faecal soiling.

PROCTALGIA FUGAX

Aetiology

Proctalgia fugax (fleeting rectal pain) commonly occurs in young adults, yet is rarely complained about.[6] The pain is sudden, sharp and electrical in nature, and lasts from seconds to 45 minutes. It may awaken patients at night, is more common in men than in women and may be incapacitating in its severity.

The cause of proctalgia fugax is unknown but may be related to stress, fatigue or functional gastrointestinal disorders. A number of reports support the association with proctalgia fugax[3] of functional disorders with loose frequent bowel movements, passage of mucus and abdominal bloating and pain. Other causes of pain in the rectum should be excluded such as coccygeal (coccygodynia), infections of the rectum and perianal area, thrombosed haemorrhoids, anal fissure, solitary rectal ulcer and tumour. Consideration should also be given to radicular pain originating in the spine.

Tenderness may be elicited in the pubococcygeous muscle on performing digital rectal examination which may mimic the pain of proctalgia fugax. Proctoscopic evaluation reveals normal rectal and colonic mucosa.

Treatment

Treatment is non-specific and is begun only after excluding other possible causes for the pain. Patients must be reassured and instructed as to the harmless nature of the attacks. Because the cause is unknown, treatment is non-specific and may include warm baths, muscle relaxants or periodic massage of painful spastic muscle of the levator mechanism. Individual patients may express relief by defecation.

REFERENCES

1 Friend, W. G. (1977) The cause and treatment of idiopathic pruritus ani. *Diseases of the Colon and Rectum*, **20**, 40–42.
2 Gallagher, D. M. (1971) Pruritus ani. *Modern Treatment*, **8**, 963–970.
3 Pilling, L. F., Swenson, W. M. & Hill, J. R. (1972) The psychologic aspects of proctalgia fugax. *Diseases of the Colon and Rectum*, **8**, 372–376.
4 Smith, L. E., Henrichs, D. & McCullah, R. D. (1982) Prospective studies on etiology and treatment of pruritus ani. *Diseases of the Colon and Rectum*, **25**, 358–363.
5 Sullivan, E. S. & Garnjobst (1978) Pruritus ani: a practical approach. *Surgical Clinics of North America*, **58**, 505–512.
6 Thompson, W. G. (1981) Proctalgia fugax. *Digestive Diseases and Sciences*, **26**, 1121–1124.

ANAL TUMOURS

BENIGN POLYPS

Benign polyps of the anal canal are relatively rare and may consist of hyperplastic polyps, adenomatous polyps, or villous adenomas which are found with more regularity in the rectum and colon. Inflammatory polyps accompanying fissures or pseudopolyps as a manifestation of inflammatory bowel disease are seen more frequently. Also very common is the hypertrophied anal papilla. The most common benign polyp of the anal canal and perianal area is the papilloma of the anus, or condyloma acuminatum.

Symptoms, if present at all, usually appear as bleeding or mucous discharge. Treatment of adenomatous polyps and villous adenoma should consist of complete local excision or fulguration. Hyperplastic polyps, inflammatory polyps or condylomas may be treated likewise with fulguration or excision.

ANAL MALIGNANCY

Malignant anal tumours comprise only about 1–4% of colon and anorectal malignant growths.[7, 39] However, if only the distal 2 cm of the rectum, anal canal and anus are considered, anal canal carcinoma represents one-third[35] of malignant tumours found in the rectum.

In the most recent review from the Mayo Clinic,[3] the following distribution of malignant lesions was noted: squamous cell carcinoma (55%), basaloid carcinoma (31%), Paget's disease (4%), melanoma (3.5%), basal cell carcinoma (3.5%) and adenocarcinoma (3.5%). Additional tumours include lymphosarcoma, leiomyosarcoma, rhabdomyosarcoma, haemangiopericytoma, plasmacytoma and endothelioma.

The complexity and multiplicity of cellular elements involved in the formation of the anal canal is responsible for this diversity of tumour types. Although first described in detail by the French anatomists Hermann and Desfosses,[21] Grinvalsky and Helwig[18] were responsible for the clear anatomical and histological areas illustrated in Figure 15.18. The basaloid squamous

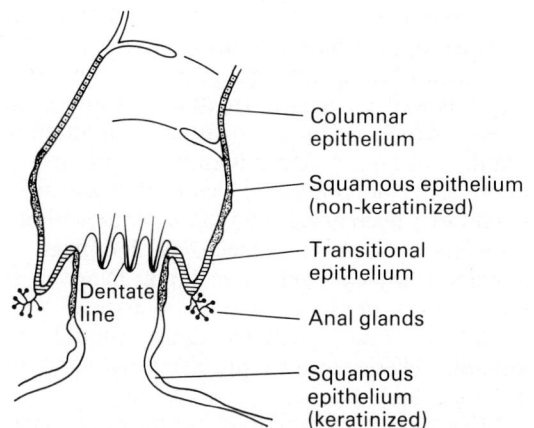

Fig. 15.18   Anatomy of anal canal.

type of cloacogenic carcinoma and its glandular variants (adenocystic or mucoepidermoid) originate from the 'transitional zone' between the non-keratinized squamous portion of the anal canal and the keratinized epithelium (anoderm) of the anus. This 'transitional zone' results from remnants of the embryonal cloacal membrane, formed as a horizontal plate consisting of cloacal and surface ectoderm.[23] This membrane later disappears, giving the anal canal continuity. Also arising from or just above the transitional zone are small cell carcinomas which are of neuroendocrine origin.[41] The rare adenocarcinoma of the anal canal arises from the anal glands located in the crypts of Morgagni.

The unique anatomy of the anal canal gives rise to several patterns of metastatic spread. This may be by direct extension through the anal wall, regionally to pelvic or inguinal lymph nodes, or via systemic or portal venous routes of drainage. The rarity of these tumours, the diverse nature of histological types, their nomenclature and the anatomical variance from other areas have made standard regimens of treatment for these carcinomas difficult to develop and assess.

Traditionally, surgery alone, either by local excision for low grade squamous lesions or abdomino-perineal excision for other types, has been the primary mode of treatment. Radiation has been generally reserved for salvage therapy. Staging has followed closely the Dukes' classification or that described by Richards *et al.*[34] (Table 15.7).

Table 15.7 Classification of anal malignancy.

ABC classification
  A. Growth limited to anal epithelium
  B. Local extension, no nodal involvement
  C. Regional node metastasis

Roswell Park classification[33]
  0. Carcinoma in situ
  I. Sphincter muscle not involved (100% five-year survival)
  II. Sphincter muscle involved (50% five-year survival)
  III. Regional metastasis
    (a) Perirectal nodes
    (b) Inguinal nodes
  IV. Distant metastasis

Mayo Clinic classification[5]
  A. Growth limited to mucosa and submucosa
  B. Muscular penetration
    B_1 – Internal sphincter
    B_2 – External sphincter
    B_3 – Ischiorectal fat or adjacent tissues
  C. Regional nodes
  D. Distant metastasis or unresectable local tumour

Squamous cell carcinoma/basaloid carcinoma

Squamous cell carcinoma and basaloid carcinoma occur predominantly in women (2 : 1) during the fifth and sixth decades. Typically squamous carcinoma of the anal margin and perianal region is well differentiated and of low metastatic potential making wide local resection eminently satisfactory. By contrast, squamous carcinoma of the anal canal is poorly differentiated and more malignant, necessitating abdomino-perineal excision. Morson[26] considers 'transitional cell carcinoma', basaloid carcinoma and cloacogenic carcinoma to be non-keratinizing squamous carcinomas, resembling an adenocarcinoma of the rectum in behaviour.[14] The major presenting symptoms are bleeding, pain or an anal mass.[27, 29, 35] Unlike basaloid carcinoma, squamous cell carcinoma is frequently associated (50%) with pruritus ani.[4]

Early lesions may manifest themselves as a localized ulcer or warty growth with raised, irregular and ulcerated borders. Later the lesion is often hard and projecting, with or without ulceration. The smaller tumours may be confused with condylomas, a papilloma, a primary chancre, an anal fissure or a prolapsed and thrombosed internal haemorrhoid. Goligher[14] stresses that suspicion of a carcinoma should be aroused if there is induration. Any such lesion should undergo biopsy.

Squamous carcinomas of the anus and perianal region, if superficial and of low grade (and if they are less than 2 cm in diameter) are generally best treated with wide local excision.[7, 12, 14, 24, 29] Recently, there has been much interest in the use of supervoltage radiation for treatment of perianal carcinoma.[17] If the carcinoma is invasive, radiation may be used with mitomycin C.[17, 31, 37]

Papillon,[32] using primary radiation therapy alone, in 98 highly selected cases, has recently reported a 68% five-year survival rate with no evidence of recurrent disease and with a very low incidence of complications. He believes that faulty technique was responsible for the poor results in earlier radiation series. Owen and associates[31] indicate that a regimen of mitomycin C, 5-fluorouracil and radiation with subsequent surgical excision has been very effective in ten patients. Nigro and colleagues[28] have used mitomycin C, 5-fluorouracil and radiation therapy in 27 patients, who underwent abdominoperineal resection afterwards. Tumour size was considerably reduced in all patients and survival seems to be improved so far.[35]

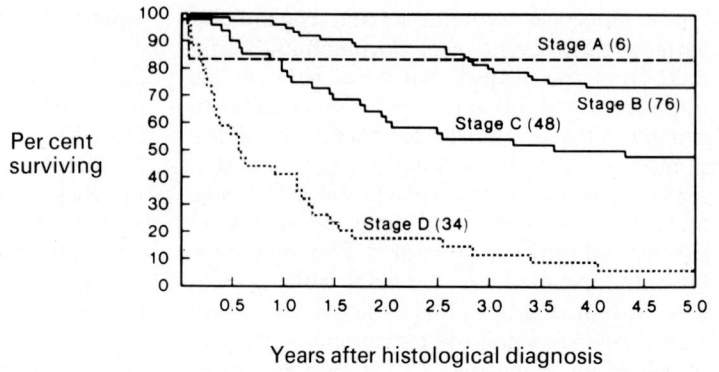

Years after histological diagnosis

Fig. 15.19 Survival in anal carcinoma by stage of patients without local excisions or elective radiation.

The best proven treatment for invasive squamous cell or basaloid carcinoma is abdomino-perineal excision. Survival statistics are similar for squamous cell and basaloid carcinoma except when lymph nodes are involved, in which case, survival is better for basaloid carcinoma.[3, 28] Survival does not appear to be influenced by therapeutic or prophylactic inguinal lymph node dissections. In 1958, Stearns[38] demonstrated that the morbidity of prophylactic groin dissection was high and advocated unilateral therapeutic dissection of the groin when nodes became involved clinically.

In a recent review of anal canal carcinoma, Schneider and Schulte[35] found that patients who had tumours confined to the anal sphincters had a 60% five-year survival rate. Penetration through the sphincters decreased five-year survival rate to 25%. Furthermore, patients with nodal or venous involvement carried a prognosis of only a 14% five-year survival rate.

Radiation therapy of relatively advanced lesions has given a 10–35% five-year survival rate.[22] However, colostomy was required in 20–25% of the cases and necrosis of the irradiated area was noted in 14% of the cases. Lesser complications were seen in up to 50% of the cases. Local recurrence after radiation therapy was 40%; Dalby and associates in an earlier series[9] reported a more optimistic five-year corrected survival of 51.2%. However, there were 23 instances of necrosis, of which ten were serious. A recently reported study by Cummings and associates from the Princess Margaret Hospital in Toronto noted a five-year uncorrected survival of 59%, and a corrected five-year survival of 71% in patients with primary anal carcinoma treated with external beam and interstitial radiation.[8] When used as a preoperative or postoperative adjuvant therapy, radiation with 4000 to 5000 rad eliminated local or pelvic recurrence.[35, 40]

In a Mayo Clinic series of 194 patients treated between 1950 and 1976, a classification was described[5] in which the depth of penetration into the anal musculature (see Figure 15.19) was used in an attempt to determine the limits of efficacy of surgical treatment and to determine in which patients adjuvant radiotherapy or chemotherapy should be used. Nineteen patients in this series underwent wide local excision for tumours equal to or less than 2 cm in diameter. Twelve patients had stage A disease, and although one had a recurrence requiring a subsequent abdomino-perineal excision, all survived five years. Of seven stage B patients who had a local excision, five also had local radium application and four of the seven survived five years (Table 15.8).

Table 15.8 Local excision of anal carcinoma.[a]

Stage	Number of patients	Number of recurrences	5-year survival
A	12	1 (8%)	12 (100%)
B	7	4	4

[a] All lesions ≤2 cm in diameter.

Radiation therapy in this series was selected as primary treatment in 11 patients, who presented with clinically unresectable disease (surgical refusal, poor condition). Survival was poor, although four out of the 11 lived longer than five years free of their disease. Survival was also poor (one out of 13) in a group of patients with very extensive disease who were treated with a variety of radiation techniques (Table 15.9). No judgement should be made as to efficacy of radiation treatment from this small early series.

One hundred and thirty patients underwent abdomino-perineal excision for potential cure.

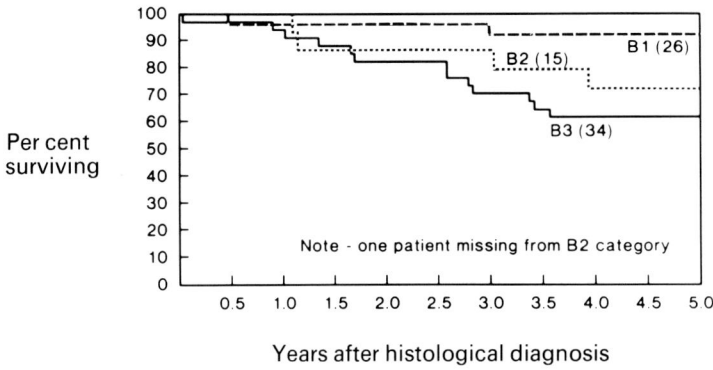

Fig. 15.20 Survival in anal carcinoma of surgical stage B patients (after abdomino-perineal excision) surgically staged and all tumour removed.

Table 15.9 Primary radiation therapy of anal carcinoma.

Reason no surgery	Number of patients	5-year survival
Elective decision	11	4 (36%)
Extensive disease	13	1 (8%)

There were six stage A patients, 76 stage B patients, and 48 stage C patients. Fifty-one developed recurrent disease. Survival for stage A was 83%, for stage B 74% and for stage C 48%. Only 6% of stage D patients survived five years (Figure 15.19). Figure 15.20 depicts the survival for the B group. There was a 92% five-year survival for B_1 patients as opposed to 63% survival for B_3 patients. Subclassification of C patients by inguinal or pelvic nodal involvement, number of nodes involved, or depth of penetration did not affect prognosis in this group.

In addition to stage, tumour size was a significant factor in survival. Four centimetres was found to distinguish patients with a good or poor survival. Tumour histology was a further significant factor in survival. Low grade squamous cell carcinoma had the best prognosis (approximately 90% five-year survival) followed by high grade squamous and basaloid lesions (approximately 63% five-year survival), and

small cell carcinoma had a poor survival (approximately 13% five-year survival) (Figure 15.21). It is interesting to note that the majority of recurrences were local rather than distant (Figure 15.22) which is somewhat different from the pattern seen in adenocarcinoma of the rectum. Patients with small cell carcinoma tend to develop local and distant metastases.

Adjuvant radiation has been established as effective therapy following surgical resection of adenocarcinoma of the rectum.[19] From our experience all stage C and B_3 patients, plus B_2 patients with lesions greater than 4 cm benefit from adjuvant radiation. The authors suggest that since the small cell tumour is of neuroendocrine origin and frequently recurs as disseminated disease, it may be responsive to chemotherapy. The glandular variants of basaloid carcinoma, which are highly malignant,[30] may also benefit from this combined approach.

In order to generate adequate numbers for a controlled prospective trial of combined therapy, a multi-institutional study will have to be inaugurated.

Melanoma

Melanoma of the anorectum was first described in 1812, and first diagnosed in 1857. There are only about 250 cases described in the literature.[6]

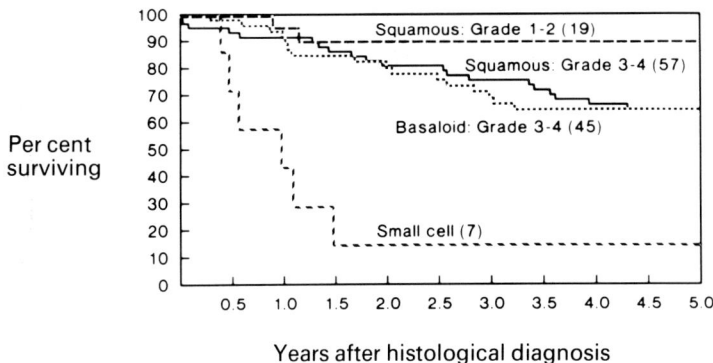

Fig. 15.21 Survival in anal carcinoma by histology (after abdomino-perineal excision) surgically staged and all tumour removed.

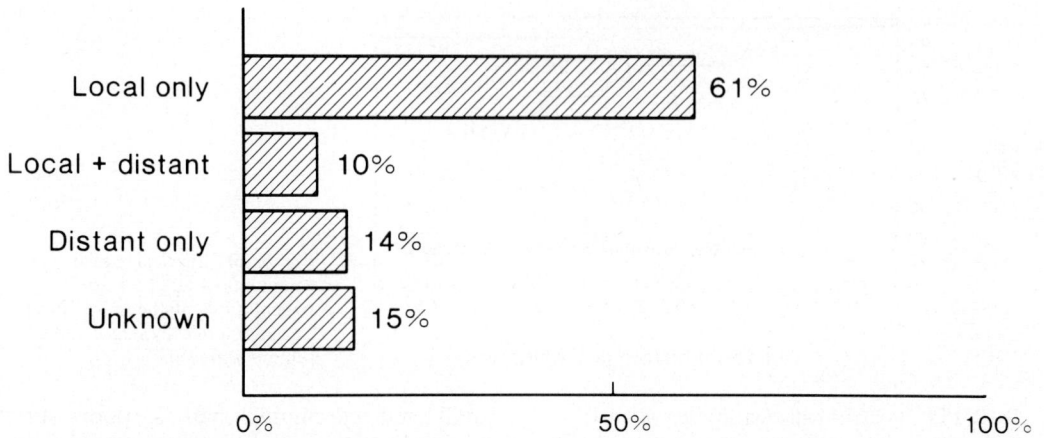

Fig. 15.22   Surgically treated anal carcinoma. Sites of initial recurrence (51 patients).

After the skin and eye, the anal canal is the next most common site for primary melanoma, although less than 1% of all melanomas arise here.[25] In a recent review from the Mayo Clinic, a total of 37 cases were carefully documented, analysed, and followed for at least five years. Twenty-four were females and 13 were males. The ages of patients ranged from 22 to 79 years with an average of 62 years. Symptoms included bleeding (25), pain (15), mass (14), constipation (10), diarrhoea (4) and tenesmus (1). Melanoma of the anal canal may present as a polypoid bluish-black lesion which may be mistaken for a thrombosed haemorrhoid, or there may be ulceration and marked induration. The majority (19/37) of tumours were larger than 2 cm. Twelve were ulcerating, 11 were verrucous and four were flat. Twenty-four of 37 were amelanotic.

Six patients had distant disease at presentation. Of the 31 patients treated surgically (wide local excision: 12, abdomino-perineal excision: 19) only four are alive, and only three survived for more than five years. There is a recent report[2] in which a 50% five-year survival was achieved in six patients treated with a posterior pelvic exenteration with incontinuity bilateral groin and pelvic nodal dissections.

Basal cell carcinoma

Basal cell carcinoma are typically firm lesions with an irregular raised edge and central ulceration. They comprise less than 1% of anorectal neoplasms[13, 30] and occur three times more commonly in men than women. These tumours must not be confused with basaloid carcinoma, and are similar to basal cell carcinoma located elsewhere. They are slow-growing and of very low malignant potential. Metastasis is very rare. Local excision is the treatment of choice.[10]

Bowen's disease

Bowen's disease, described by the pathologist of that name in 1912, is a low grade in situ intraepidermal squamous carcinoma. It most often appears as discrete, scaly, erythematous plaques. Itching or burning are common clinical features. Histologically there are multinucleate giant cells with vacuolation. This lesion may be a harbinger of other cutaneous, respiratory, gastrointestinal, genitourinary or other malignancies which occur within ten years of the diagnosis of Bowen's disease in 40% of patients.[16] Ten per cent of patients with Bowen's disease will develop invasive squamous cell carcinoma and 35% of those will later metastasize unless treated. There is also a high (20%) incidence of local recurrence following excision.[16] Local excision with careful follow-up is the treatment of choice. Split-thickness skin grafting may be necessary after excising larger lesions.

Perianal Paget's disease

Paget's disease presents as a pruritic, scaling, plaque-like area similar in appearance to Bowen's disease. A distinction may be made between the two based on the content of acid mucosubstance,[1] and other histological grounds. The lesion may be indistinguishable from a carcinoma of a local apocrine gland (50% of cases),[16] or may be associated with de facto or future visceral carcinoma (85% of patients).[20] For localized lesions, a wide local excision with supervital staining,[11] to obtain adequate margins of excision, is recommended. For Paget's disease with an underlying carcinoma, abdomino-perineal excision with or without inguinal node dissection is the treatment of choice.

Buschke–Lowenstein tumour

The Buschke–Lowenstein tumour is a variant of the squamous cell carcinoma and is frequently mistaken for condyloma acuminata. Radiation and chemotherapy have been conspicuously ineffective and radical excision is the only hope for cure.

REFERENCES

1　Ackerman, L. V. & Rosai, J. (1981) Gastrointestinal/anus. In *Surgical Pathology*, p. 568. St. Louis: C. V. Mosby.

2　Baskies, A. M., Sugerbaker, E. V., Chretien, P. B. & Deckers, P. J. (1982) Anorectal melanoma: the role of posterior pelvic exenteration. *Diseases of the Colon and Rectum*, **25**, 772–777.

3　Beahrs, O. H. Wilson, S. H. (1976) Carcinoma of the anus. *Annals of Surgery*, **184**, 422–428.

4　Beart, R. W., Jr (1980) Rare anal tumors (unpublished review).

5　Boman, B. M., O'Connell, M. J., Moertel, C. G. *et al.* Cancer of the anal canal. The Mayo Clinic experience, 1950–1976. Submitted for publication.

6　Chiu, Y. S., Unni, K. K. & Beart, R. W., Jr (1980) Malignant melanoma of the anorectum. *Diseases of the Colon and Rectum*, **23** (2), 122–124.

7　Corman, M. L. & Heggilt, R. C. (1977) Carcinoma of the anal canal. *Surgery, Gynecology and Obstetrics*, **145**, 674–676.

8　Cummings, B. J., Thomas, G. M., Keane, T. J. *et al.* (1982) Primary radiation therapy in the treatment of anal canal carcinoma. *Diseases of the Colon and Rectum*, **25**, 778–782.

9　Dalby, J. E., Chir, B. & Pointer, R. S. (1961) The treatment of anal cancer by interstitial irradiation. *American Journal of Roentgenology*, **85**, 515–520.

10　Goldberg, S. M., Gordon, P. H. & Nivatvongs, S. (1980) Neoplasms of the anal canal. In *Essentials of Anorectal Surgery*. p. 162 Philadelphia: Lippincott.

11　Goldberg, S. M., Gordon, P. H. & Nivatvongs, S. (1980) Neoplasms of the anal canal. In *Essentials of Anorectal Surgery*. Chapter 14, p. 164 Philadelphia: Lippincott.

12　Golden, G. T. & Horsly, J. G. (1976) Surgical management of epidermoid carcinoma of the anus. *American Journal of Surgery*, **131**, 275–280.

13　Goligher, J. C. (1980) *Surgery of the Anus, Rectum and Colon*. Fourth Edition, p. 675. London: Baillière Tindall.

14　Goligher, J. C. (1980) *Surgery of the Anus, Rectum and Colon*, fourth edition. pp. 667–677. London: Baillière Tindall.

15　Gradsky, L. (1965) Uncommon nonkeratinizing cancers of the anal canal and perianal region. *New York State Journal of Medicine*, **65**, 894.

16　Graham, J. H. & Helwig, E. B. (1961) Bowen's disease and its relationship to systemic cancer. *Archives of Dermatology*, **83**, 738.

17　Green, J. P. & Schaupp, W. C. (1980) Anal carcinoma; current therapeutic concepts. *American Journal of Surgery*, **140**, 151–155.

18　Grinvalsky, H. T. & Helwig, E. B. (1956) Carcinoma of the anorectal junction: histologic considerations. *Cancer*, **9**, 480–488.

19　Gunderson, L. L. & Sosin, H. (1974) Areas of failure found at reoperation (second or symptomatic look) following curative surgery for adenocarcinoma of the rectum. *Cancer*, **34**, 1278–1992.

20　Helwig, E. G. & Graham, J. H. (1963) Anogenital and extramammary Paget's disease. A clinicopathological study. *Cancer*, **16**, 387.

21　Hermann, G. & Desfosses, L. (1880) Sur la muquese de la region cloacle de rectum. *Comptes Rendus Academie des Sciences*, **90**, 1201–1203.

22　Hintz, B. L., Cheryielu, K. K. N. & Surdarsanam, A. (1978) Anal carcinoma: basic concepts and management. *Journal of Surgical Oncology*, **10**, 141–150.

23　Houser, S. & Johnston, W. (1977) Anal carcinoma. *Review of Surgery*, **34**, 439–441.

24　Kuehn, P. G., Beckett, R., Eisenberg, H. *et al.* (1964) Epidermoid carcinoma of the perianal skin and anal cervix. *New England Journal of Medicine*, **270**, 614.

25　Mason, J. K. & Helwig, E. B. (1966) Anorectal melanoma. *Cancer*, **19**, 39–50.

26　Morson, B. C. (1959) The pathology and results of treatment of cancer of the anal region. *Proceedings of the Royal Society of Medicine* (Supplement), **52**, 117.

27　Morson, B. C. (1960) Pathology and results of treatment of squamous cell carcinoma of anal region in neoplastic disease at various sites. *Cancer of the Rectum* (Ed.) Dukes, C. E. Baltimore: Williams and Wilkins.

28　Nigro, N. D., Vaithevicius, U. K. & Considen, B. (1974) Combined therapy for cancer of the anal canal: a preliminary report. *Diseases of the Colon and Rectum*, **17**, 354–356.

29　O'Brien, P. H., Jennette, J. M., Wallace, K. M. & Metcalf, J. S. (1982) Epidermoid carcinoma of the anus. *Surgery, Gynecology and Obstetrics*, **155**, 745–751.

30　Owen, S. H. Q. (1978) Anal and para-anal tumors. *Surgical Clinics of North America*, **58**, 591.

31　Owen, S. H. Q., Magill, G. B., Learing, R. H. *et al.* (1978) Multidisciplinary preoperative approach to the management of epidermoid carcinoma of the anus and anorectum. *Diseases of the Colon and Rectum*, **21**, 89.

32　Papillon, J. (1981) Radiation therapy in the management of epidermoid carcinoma of the anorectum. *Cancer*, **47**, 2817–2826.

33　Paradis, P., Douglass, H. O., Jr & Holyoke, E. D. (1975) The clinical implications of a staging system for carcinoma of the anus. *Surgery, Gynecology and Obstetrics*, **141**, 411–416.

34　Richards, J. C., Beahrs, O. H. & Woolner, L. B. (1962) Squamous cell carcinoma of the anus, anal canal and rectum in 109 patients. *Surgery, Gynecology and Obstetrics*, **114**, 475–482.

35　Schneider, T. C. & Schulte, W. J. (1981) Management of carcinoma of anal canal. *Surgery*, **90** (4), 729–732.

36　Serota, A. I., Weil, M., Williams, R. A. *et al.* (1981) Anal cloacogenic carcinoma: classification and clinical behavior. *Archives of Surgery*, **116**, 456–459.

37　Sescky, B. & Remmington, J. H. (1980) Treatment of carcinoma of the rectum and squamous carcinoma of the anus by combination chemotherapy, radiotherapy, and operation. *Surgery, Gynecology and Obstetrics*, **151**, 369–371.

38　Stearns, M. W. (1958) Epidermoid carcinoma of the anal region. *Surgery, Gynecology and Obstetrics*, **106**, 92–96.

39　Stearns, M. W. & Quam, S. H. Q. (1970) Epidermoid carcinoma of the anorectum. *Surgery, Gynecology and Obstetrics*, **131**, 953–957.

40　Stearns, M. W., Urmacker, C., Steinberg, S. S. *et al.* (1980) Cancer of the anal canal. *Current Problems in Cancer*, **4**, 12.

41　Weatherly, P. R., Wick, M. R., Kosten, W. R. & Weiland, L. H. (1983) Small cell undifferentiated (neuroendocrine) carcinomas of the colon, rectum and anus. (In preparation).

PERIANAL CROHN'S DISEASE

Perianal Crohn's disease attracted little attention until Morson and Lockhart-Mummery[12] described the classical sarcoid-like features seen on histological examination of biopsy material from anal fistulas. They subsequently showed that anal lesions could predate the onset of overt intestinal disease by many years. Since then an extensive literature on the subject has developed but there is little agreement over the frequency of anal involvement, the natural history and the best methods of management.

Much of the uncertainty stems from a failure to define the specific condition in question since a number of different anal lesions may be seen; some are specific to Crohn's disease, others are incidental, some are frequently associated with severe complications and others are trivial. It is crucial therefore to define the lesions present in clinico-pathological terms[9] if one is to assess the probable outcome in an individual patient, and to plan logical and effective treatment.

Classification of anal lesions (Table 15.10)

PRIMARY LESIONS

These are important for three reasons: they are helpful in diagnosing Crohn's disease, they tend to reflect general disease activity, and one lesion – the cavitating ulcer – is responsible for most of the severe morbidity associated with anal Crohn's disease.

Table 15.10 Classification of anal lesions.

Primary lesions
Crohn's fissures
Oedematous skin tags
Cavitating ulcers
Secondary lesions
Abscesses/fistulas
Skin tags
Strictures
Incidental lesions
Haemorrhoids
Skin tags
Abscesses
Fistulas

Crohn's fissure (Figure 15.23)

The highly characteristic appearance of this lesion strongly suggests the diagnosis of Crohn's disease. An ulcer 5–10 mm wide extends from the dentate line to the anal verge, where the distal rolled edge, sometimes with a small perforation in it, is seen. The ulcer is shallow, the transverse fibres of the internal sphincter can be seen in its base, but it appears much deeper because of the oedema of its rolled undermined edges. The oedema also gives the edge a translucent, watery pink appearance – sometimes with a blueish tinge. The ulcer usually lies in the midline posteriorly, sometimes anteriorly as well, and is surprisingly painless. The appearance contrasts sharply with the classical anal fissure which is painful and tightly closed by anal spasm, and with margins of normal opaque skin.

The pale oedematous appearance is seen when the disease process is 'active' and this activity is usually obvious in intestinal as well as

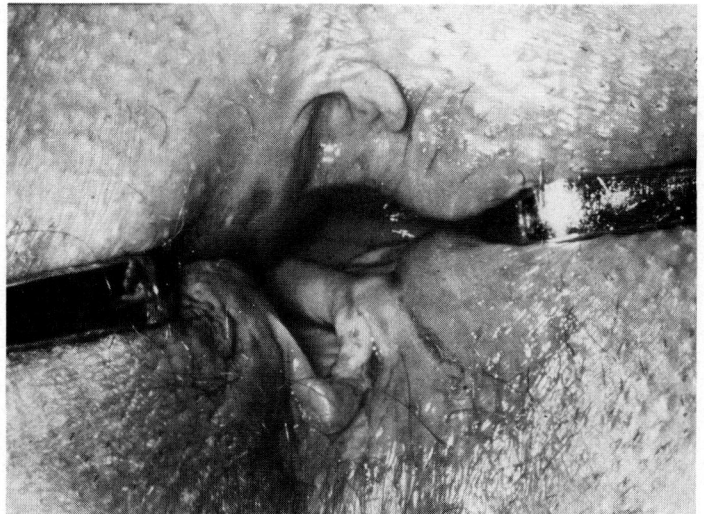

Fig. 15.23 Primary Crohn's anal fissure. Large posterior and small (healed) anterior.

anal lesions. When the disease is quiescent, whether as a result of medical treatment, surgical resection of proximal disease or spontaneous resolution, the oedema resolves, the edge flattens and the base scars over covered by a fragile epithelial layer which is an easily recognized relic of the earlier active fissure.

Oedematous skin tags (Figure 15.24)
The presence of very large oedematous skin tags – much larger than those seen with haemorrhoids or anal irritation – is also very characteristic of Crohn's disease. There is often a shallow, linear ulcer on the inner aspect of each tag.

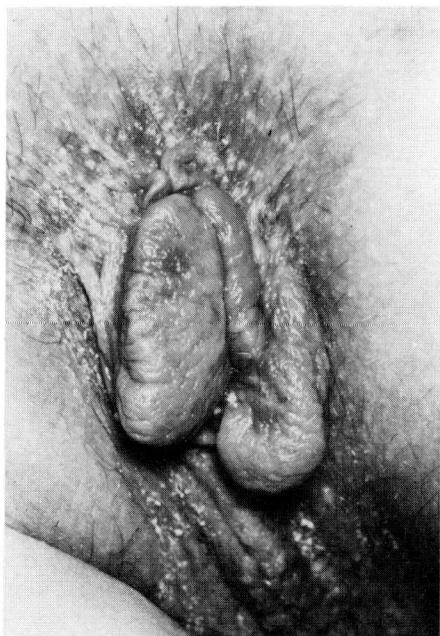

Fig. 15.25   A cavitating ulcer at the anorectal junction.

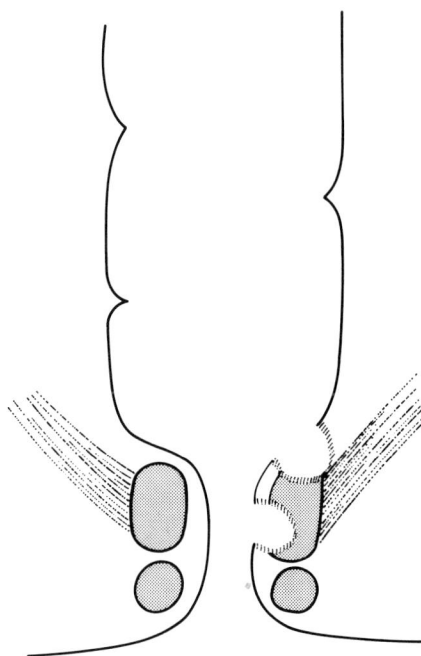

Fig. 15.24   Oedematous skin tags.

The cavitating ulcer (Figure 15.25)
This is felt as a deep craggy ulcer within the anal canal or lower rectum (Figure 15.26). It erodes through the sphincter mechanism without respect for the usual anatomical barriers, allows egress of faecal material and becomes infected, leading to the complicated and unpredictable fistulas so characteristic of severe Crohn's disease. A cavitating ulcer is usually intensely painful. An anterior suprasphincteric ulcer in the female will readily traverse the rectovaginal septum to produce a short direct fistula. A cavitating ulcer indicates the presence or likely future development of severe perianal complications.

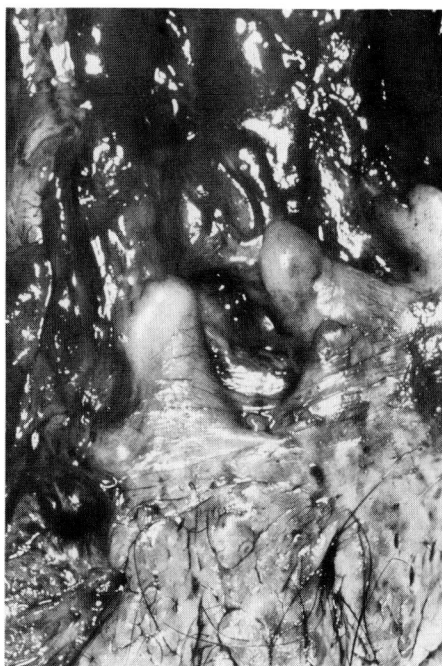

Fig. 15.26   The common sites of cavitating ulcer.

SECONDARY LESIONS

As disease activity wanes the Crohn's fissure usually heals and oedematous skin tags resolve, leaving large but less obtrusive tags. By contrast cavitating ulcers tend to produce serious secondary complications. Even if the primary ulcer resolves and attempts to heal by epithelialization, faecal material continues to enter the track which is kept open by mechanical pressure. Consequently, deep fistulas arising from cavitating ulcers may show some improvement in keeping with the patient's general condition, but they rarely heal completely, and probably never do so when the cavitating ulcer is suprasphincteric.

Healing of fissures or ulcers may lead to anal stenosis, but narrowing of the anal canal in Crohn's disease is mostly due to a combination of sphincter spasm and perianal fibrosis, both of which are due to deep perianal sepsis as a consequence of cavitating ulceration.

INCIDENTAL LESIONS

The incidental lesions (haemorrhoids, abscess and low lying fistulas) may occur as isolated findings in patients known to have Crohn's disease or in conjunction with unrelated primary lesions (active or healed) while something which looks similar may have arisen from a primary lesion. Hence an abscess or fistula may be either incidental or secondary to a cavitating ulcer and it is important to make this distinction by careful examination.

The presence of any of the three primary lesions makes a diagnosis of Crohn's disease very likely, even when there is no history of intestinal disease. However, we have occasionally seen a classical Crohn's fissure, sometimes with granulomas, in association with other conditions such as ulcerative colitis, diverticulitis, pseudomembranous colitis, and occasionally with no disease at all. At present, most of these patients have not developed overt Crohn's disease.

Biopsy under local anaesthetic of the distal margin of an active anal fissure is a useful procedure since it yields a higher incidence of granulomas than rectal mucosa biopsy from the same patient.

Incidence

The frequency with which anal lesions have been reported in Crohn's disease varies from 25 to 80%.[5, 10] Lower figures usually emanate from retrospective surveys, and it is likely that the higher figure of 80% is closer to the truth. The incidence of anal lesions is greater with colonic Crohn's disease than in small bowel disease.

Aetiology

There has been much speculation as to why Crohn's disease should show a special tendency to affect the anal region. No convincing reason has been proposed and one can only note the general tendency for Crohn's disease to affect either narrowed areas of the bowel, such as the pylorus, ileocaecal region or proximal to an anastomosis, or areas with abundant lymphoid tissue.

Natural history

Of several studies of the natural history of anal Crohn's disease, the most detailed is that of Buchmann et al.[4] who reassessed the patients studied by Fielding[5] ten years earlier. They were able to follow up about half the original series and showed that many lesions had healed or remained quiescent, though sometimes leaving induration or stenosis. In general the degree of disability was limited, but ten patients from the series had required abdomino-perineal excision, half of them primarily for perianal disease. Other authors have reported a much more serious outcome, particularly in those who also have rectal involvement.[2, 7]

It is likely that the differing viewpoints reflect the patients studied. Simple fissures and skin tags are common in population surveys but trivial in significance, while cavitating ulcers are seen more commonly in referral centres and have a marked tendency to progress to serious perianal fistulas and sepsis. Long-term studies have shown that patients with extensive perianal fistulas may remain quiescent for years without radical treatment. However, some patients with fistulas have serious limitations to the quality of life they lead and this is not always apparent from casual outpatient attendances.

Differential diagnosis

The commonest diagnostic problem is to determine whether multiple or slightly atypical anal fistulas occurring in the absence of overt intestinal disease are due to Crohn's disease. The presence of a classical primary lesion, or granulomas with a biopsy, makes Crohn's disease very likely. In their absence one can only await the outcome of events.

A number of conditions are sometimes misdiagnosed as anal Crohn's disease. Perianal hidradenitis suppurativa can closely simulate multiple fistulas of Crohn's disease. Careful examination of the anal canal will allow differentiation since the skin of the anal canal is spared in hidradenitis, whereas evidence of a primary lesion is usually present in the anal canal of patients with Crohn's disease.

The craggy edge of a cavitating ulcer may sometimes be mistaken for anal carcinoma; conversely, a carcinoma developing in a chronic anal or rectal stricture of Crohn's disease may go undiagnosed. A variety of less common conditions needs to be considered in the differential diagnosis, including perianal pilonidal sinus, infection in immunosuppressed patients (for example, in leukaemia or those on chemotherapy), venereal disease and a variety of dermatological conditions.

Treatment

GENERAL PRINCIPLES

1 The patient should be treated according to symptoms rather than objective findings because patients with gross disease may continue for many years with relatively little trouble. On the other hand, Crohn's disease is a very chronic process and patients may come to accept severe morbidity as part of their way of life. Such patients may greatly appreciate being steered towards radical treatment if careful assessment of their anal lesion shows that the prognosis is poor.
2 The exact nature of the anal lesion (primary, secondary or incidental) should be determined and disease 'activity' assessed, both in relation to the intestine and to the anal lesions. Both elements of assessment are important in determining treatment.
3 Significance of disease activity. Signs of disease activity in primary anal lesions tend to reflect activity of proximal disease. They are usually associated with the presence of granulomas in the perianal tissues and with slow healing of perianal wounds. When the proximal disease comes under control, as a result of specific medical or surgical therapy or by spontaneous remission, the signs of local activity wane and normal healing may occur. Improvement in primary lesions with decreasing disease activity does not necessarily lead to relief of symptoms since incidental lesions will be unaffected and the behaviour of secondary complications is also dependent on mechanical factors.

TREATMENT OF MINOR LESIONS

Uncomplicated primary lesions usually require no treatment. Steroid cream may give temporary relief but the natural history of the disease is probably unaltered.

Incidental lesions should be treated conservatively as far as possible. However, where primary lesions are absent or quiescent, incidental lesions causing troublesome symptoms in the absence of anorectal Crohn's disease may be treated as they would in normal subjects but preferably by the most conservative method. Haemorrhoids are usually treated by band ligation, low lying fistulas by laying open the track and abscesses by drainage.

Secondary complications are treated with the same regard to disease activity as incidental lesions but cause problems more frequently. When pus is diagnosed it is best drained immediately by simple incision and light curettage. This should be done even when the abscess is painless because pus is destructive to tissue and, if left undrained, will often spread widely leading to complicated fistulas which might be avoided by early drainage.

Most anal strictures cause little problem in the absence of an associated abscess or fistula. If the stricture is troublesome, regular use of an anal dilator or gentle dilatation under general anaesthetic can be tried, although the long-term benefit is uncertain. Anal stricture with a cavitating ulcer and recurrent fistulas is a combination which is usually best treated by rectal excision.

RECURRENT ABSCESS AND FISTULAS

This group of conditions constitutes the principal management problem of anal Crohn's disease. There is a wide spectrum of disorders, from an occasional abscess to almost continuous disability with multiple fistulas extending far into the buttocks, sacral region and scrotum. The first step in management must be a careful assessment of the pathology underlying the clinical picture. A cavitating ulcer, especially suprasphincteric or high in the anal canal and associated with severe rectal involvement, carries a poor prognosis and radical surgery must be considered. With less severe cases a number of approaches may be used for general management.

DRUG THERAPY

Metronidazole has been the drug most widely recommended for anal Crohn's disease and many reports have been favourable.[1, 3] Intermittent treatment is useful for acute symptoms, but it is doubtful whether it has a major effect on the long-term outcome of the disease. While metronidazole is the most effective drug, improved results are often obtained when combined with an antibiotic effective against aerobic organisms such as a cephalosporin or co-trimoxazole. Pain is reduced and discharge decreases, but symptoms rapidly recur when the drug is stopped. Many patients find that side-effects make long-term administration of metronidazole unpleasant.

LOCAL SURGERY

Any abscess should be drained at an early stage by local incision. Many fistulas are low in relation to the sphincters and can be laid open in the same way as would be done in the absence of Crohn's disease.[11] However, surgery should always tend towards a conservative rather than radical approach, particularly when there are signs of disease activity.

Where a cavitating ulcer is present, operation should be limited to laying open superficial tracks only as far as the sphincter. The use of a silicone seton has been recommended when a number of fistulous tracks lead from a cavitating ulcer which is situated in the deep portion of the sphincter. The seton is passed from the anal canal through the cavitating ulcer outside the sphincter to the perianal skin, ensuring a direct track from the outer aspect of the cavitating ulcer to the skin. Peripheral fistulous tracks are then opened as far as the seton and often heal by granulation since the seton ensures that faecal matter and infection have a good drainage track to the surface. In our hands this technique has been moderately successful.

PROXIMAL DIVERSION

Proximal loop ileostomy or split ileostomy is recommended by some authors[6] as a definitive treatment in the belief that the anal lesions will heal and allow later closure of the diversion. This often leads to local improvement, but from the results so far reported it is questionable whether the combined disability of stoma and anal disease gives better results than selective conservative therapy and radical surgery. Proximal diversion has a place in women with a persisting short direct rectovaginal fistula which may be amenable to repair. Younger patients who find it difficult to accept a permanent stoma may adapt to a temporary stoma, and then are often willing to accept a definitive stoma and rectal excision.

The place of proximal diversion with reparative fistula surgery is not well defined at present, but is more attractive where the intestinal disease appears to have become inactive.

Resection of proximal disease with restoration of intestinal continuity results in improvement in perianal lesions in some patients,[8] but the perianal disease is rarely the sole indication for intestinal resection.

RECTAL EXCISION

To recommend rectal excision is perhaps the most difficult decision to be made for perianal disease. The decision is made on the severity of symptoms, especially poorly controlled abscesses and extensive fistulas, and the presence of severe rectal disease or a high cavitating ulcer. With this combination, the outcome is poor and rectal excision can be recommended. These patients constitute only 5% of those with perianal disease and most welcome life with a stoma when compared to their previous disease.

In the past, healing of the perineal wound has been a major problem after rectal excision for Crohn's disease. Conservative excision of perianal tissue which has now gained favour gives fewer problems with perineal healing, and in resistant cases a gracilis muscle flap will bring new tissue with a good blood supply into the cavity leading to satisfactory healing.

REFERENCES

1 Allan, R. N. & Cooke, W. T. (1977) Evaluation of metronidazole in the management of Crohn's disease. *Gut*, **18**, 422–425.
2 Baker, W. N. W. & Milton-Thompson, G. J. (1974) Management of anal fistulae in Crohn's disease. *Proceedings of the Royal Society of Medicine*, **67**, 58.
3 Brandt, L. J., Bernstein, L. H., Boley, S. J. & Frank, M. S. (1982) Metronidazole therapy for perineal Crohn's disease: a follow up study. *Gastroenterology*, **83**, 383–387.
4 Buchmann, P., Keighley, M. R. B., Allan, R. N. *et al.* (1980) Natural history of perianal Crohn's disease. *American Journal of Surgery*, **140**, 642–644.
5 Fielding, J. F. (1972) Perianal lesions in Crohn's disease. *Journal of The Royal College of Surgeons* (*Edinburgh*), **17**, 32–37.
6 Harper, P. H., Kettlewell, M. G. W. & Lee, E. C. G. (1982) The effect of split ileostomy on perianal Crohn's disease. *British Journal of Surgery*, **69**, 608–610.
7 Hellers, T., Bergstrand, O., Ewerth, S. & Holmstrom, B. (1980) Occurrence and outcome after primary treatment of anal fistulae in Crohn's disease. *Gut*, **21**, 525–527.
8 Heuman, R., Bolin, T., Sjodahl, R. & Tagesson, C. (1981) The incidence and course of perianal complications and arthralgia after intestinal resection with restoration of continuity for Crohn's disease. *British Journal of Surgery*, **68**, 528–530.
9 Hughes, L. E. (1978) Surgical pathology and management of anorectal Crohn's disease. *Journal of the Royal Society of Medicine*, **71**, 644–651.
10 Lockhart-Mummery, H. E. & Morson, B. C. (1964) Crohn's disease of the large intestine. *Gut*, **5**, 493–509.

11 Marks, C. G., Ritchie, J. K. & Lockhart-Mummery, H. E. (1981) Anal fistulae in Crohn's disease. *British Journal of Surgery*, **68**, 525–527.
12 Morson, B. C. & Lockhart-Mummery, H. E. (1959) Anal lesions in Crohn's disease. *Lancet*, **ii**, 1122–1123.
13 Sachar, D. B. (1980) Metronidazole for Crohn's disease – breakthrough or ballyhoo? *Gastroenterology*, **79**, 393–395.

OTHER PROBLEMS

SKIN TAGS

Skin tags are very common and are usually of no pathological significance. Redundancy of the perianal skin may occur in association with internal haemorrhoids where there is a tendency for the lining of the anal canal to slide downwards. A tag may accompany an anal fissure and its presence is one indication of chronicity of the lesion. It may be a manifestation of anal Crohn's disease especially if oedematous.

Skin tags are usually asymptomatic but sometimes the patient finds their presence uncomfortable. Patients with pruritus ani are often found to have tags which in some cases may contribute to the condition owing to difficulty in cleaning the anus of faeces after defecation.

The diagnosis is made on inspection. Tags can be confused with other perianal lesions (e.g. condylomas or even carcinoma) and with any prolapsing swelling. However, with the observation that they are formed by normal skin the diagnosis should not be in doubt.

Asymptomatic tags do not need treatment. When associated with a fissure, excision should be accompanied with a sphincterotomy or anal dilatation. A haemorrhoidectomy may be the only effective means in dealing with large tags occurring with internal haemorrhoids. It is unwise to remove tags in Crohn's disease since a chronic unhealing wound may be produced.

THROMBOSED PERIANAL VARIX (CLOTTED VENOUS SACCULE, EXTERNAL PLEXUS HAEMATOMA)

This is a common self-limiting condition caused by acute thrombosis in the perianal subcutaneous venous plexus.[10] It is an intravascular lesion and thus does not spread diffusely in the perianal region but remains localized. It may occur in isolation or in association with thrombosed prolapsed internal haemorrhoids. In all likelihood, raised venous pressure causing congestion of the veins and stasis of blood leads to its formation. Frequently the patient gives a history of straining, for example during defecation or rigorous exercise, and shortly afterwards notices pain at the anal verge. Over the next few hours a painful swelling develops which becomes worse over the next 24–48 hours. The pain is often severe and throbbing and is exacerbated by defecation which is often avoided. These symptoms continue for several days and gradually subside. A few weeks later a small firm painless nodule may be all that remains.

In the acute stage, the lesion appears as a localized swelling just outside the anal orifice. The overlying skin is usually oedematous and sometimes a dark blue colour due to the underlying clot is discernible. It may be confused with a prolapsing swelling but inspection and gentle palpation will reveal it to be a perianal lesion. Rectal examination and sigmoidoscopy should be deferred until after resolution but should not be omitted.

The only other common anal conditions causing severe acute pain are an anal fissure (fissure-in-ano) and an anorectal abscess. It is usually possible to diagnose the former on inspection but an abscess may produce a perianal swelling which may be hard to distinguish from a thrombosed perianal varix. Under these circumstances examination under anaesthesia may be helpful.

If the patient presents within the first 48 hours, surgical evacuation of the clot or complete excision of the lesion, if small, usually produces immediate relief and rapid resolution. Either procedure can be done under local anaesthetic (lignocaine 0.5%) in the outpatient department with the patient in the left lateral position.

More often, however, the patient presents at a later stage when the symptoms have begun to resolve, at which time reassurance and symptomatic treatment are all that are required. Non-constipating analgesics and aperients are prescribed, with the local application of hypertonic solutions to reduce oedema if necessary.

HYPERTROPHIED PAPILLA (FIBROUS ANAL POLYP)

This lesion arises from one of the papillary processes of the dentate line, i.e. between the cusps of an anal valve. It is often pedunculated and the stalk may be long and attenuated. The lesion is composed of fibrous tissue covered by squamous epithelium in keeping with its origin from the cutaneous lining of the anal canal.

The aetiology is unknown, but a hypertrophied papilla may be associated with a chronic anal fissure with or without an accompanying skin tag or with haemorrhoids. It may, however, occur in the absence of any other lesion.

The condition is often asymptomatic, being found on routine anorectal examination. In other cases the patient complains of a prolapsing swelling often requiring digital replacement, which is frequently described as haemorrhoids. Treatment is by excision which can easily be performed under local anaesthesia.

CONDYLOMATA ACUMINATA

These lesions are very common. They are caused by an antigenic variant of the papilloma virus responsible for cutaneous warts. Condylomata acuminata are transmitted by direct contact and over 50% of patients are homosexual males. It is essential to exclude other sexually transmitted diseases, particularly syphilis and gonorrhoea (see Chapter 14). Serology should be routinely carried out and a sigmoidoscopy, taking a rectal swab if there is any suspicion of gonococcal proctitis. A follow-up of sexual partners should be carried out wherever possible.

The warts usually measure a few millimetres across but they may vary from minute pinhead lesions to one or two centimetres in diameter. Small lesions are sessile and hemispherical but as they enlarge they become pedunculated and develop a finely serrated surface. They are usually multiple and sometimes cover the anal orifice and perianal region in a carpet-like manner. Extension onto the labia or scrotum and groin may occur and the penis is often involved. In about 50% of patients anal warts encroach into the anal canal and in about 10% the lower rectum is affected. There is a tendency for spontaneous involution, and lesions in this phase have a smooth surface often surmounted by a dark punctum. Occasionally condylomata acuminata may invade the surrounding tissues and in about 1–2% of cases a frank squamous cell carcinoma is found.[7]

The patient may notice the swelling but often only complains of irritation and discharge, sometimes observing blood on the toilet paper after wiping. Difficulty in maintaining anal hygiene is responsible for an unpleasant smell due partly to faecal soiling and partly to malodorous discharge.

Condylomata acuminata must be distinguished from skin tags, condylomata lata and squamous cell carcinoma. If in doubt, examination of exudate under dark ground illumination and histological examination of biopsy material is necessary.

The disease can be treated by the local application of podophyllin (20%) in spirit, injection of cytotoxic agents, e.g. bleomycin directly into the lesions, or by surgical destruction or excision. Podophyllin is suitable if few warts are present. It is a skin irritant and should therefore be carefully applied to the lesions alone and must never be used where open wounds or fissuring are present. Two applications per week by a nurse using a pledget of gauze mounted on an orange stick are continued until the warts have disappeared. This treatment is unsuitable where the anal canal and rectum are involved. It has the further disadvantage that regular and frequent outpatient visits are required. Injection of bleomycin into the lesions has been claimed to be successful in about 70% of cases.[2]

Surgical treatment is necessary if the warts are extensive, particularly when the anal canal is involved. Destruction can be affected by diathermy fulguration or by cryotherapy, but both methods cause damage to the surrounding normal skin causing pain, discharge and delayed healing. Scissor excision[11] avoids these drawbacks, removing the wart while leaving a clean wound without damaged edges. The excision is facilitated by the subcutaneous injection of 1 : 200 000 adrenaline in saline. This tends to separate the lesions as the skin is stretched by the injection, making accurate excision easier while the adrenaline acts as a haemostatic agent. Surgical treatment also permits removal of lesions in the anal canal and rectum.

About 60% of patients are cured by scissor excision in one treatment and a further 30% by two. Three or more treatments are required in the remaining 10%.

ANAL STENOSIS

Narrowing of the anal canal is due to a variety of causes. It may be congenital or acquired.

Congenital

Anal stenosis may occur as the sole defect or in association with ectopic anus or incomplete covered anus.[9] Agenesis of the anal canal presents with neonatal obstruction but anal stenosis may not be recognized for some months or longer if the degree of stenosis is mild. It will cause constipation and may result in megarectum. Faecal retention leads to soiling which is often only recognized as abnormal some years later. Abdominal distension may be present.

The condition may be recognized at birth where an ectopic or covered anus is apparent. A simple stenosis is diagnosed on digital examination. Treatment is by careful dilatation repeated as necessary over several months. This may need to be combined with a cut-back operation where there is a covered anus.

Acquired

Anal stenosis may be caused by trauma, irradiation or local anorectal disease (e.g. carcinoma and inflammations such as Crohn's disease) or rarely tuberculosis or lymphogranuloma venereum. The patient complains of difficulty in evacuation and often notices thin ribbon-like stools. There may be tenesmus with faecal retention and overflow incontinence. A full anorectal examination, and if necessary examination under anaesthetic with biopsies where indicated, is essential.

Perineal injuries involving the anus may heal by scarring causing stenosis and any damage to the anal sphincter mechanism may cause incontinence. Stenosis may follow anal operations where there has been excessive removal or destruction of the anoderm, e.g. haemorrhoidectomy or diathermy fulguration of warts. It may occur at the site of an ileo- or colo-anal anastomosis especially after local sepsis or dehiscence. High-dose irradiation (e.g. in treating anal carcinoma) causes stenosis in about 20% of cases. Crohn's disease is probably the commonest cause of anal stenosis.

Treatment depends on the cause and the degree of narrowing. Mild traumatic or post-operative stenosis will respond to dilatation, repeated as necessary. If this fails some form of operation, either division of the stenosis, advancing a plastic perianal skin flap into the anal canal or a sphincter reconstruction depending on the circumstances, may be needed. A colostomy may be necessary in post-irradiation stricture unresponsive to dilatation. Most patients with strictures in Crohn's disease can be managed satisfactorily by repeated dilatation and only rarely is the severity of anal disease a reason for total rectal excision.

HIDRADENITIS SUPPURATIVA

Hidradenitis suppurativa is caused by infection of apocrine glands which are found in the axilla, groin, external genitalia, the nape of the neck, areola of the nipples, as well as in the perianal region. The disease predominantly affects young adults and does not appear until after puberty when the glands begin to function. The sex ratio is approximately equal, although perianal involvement may be more common in males. There is an association with acne vulgaris. The cause is unknown, but it is likely that there is an abnormality in the material secreted by the glands. Retention of secretion results in stasis and infection leading to abscess formation. The glands are deeply placed in the dermis and suppuration may extend into the subcutaneous tissues forming tracks or large areas of undermining lined by granulation tissue. Subcutaneous extension may break through to the surface as sinuses some distance from the original lesion. This infective process is accompanied by attempts at repair with fibrosis in the skin and subcutaneous tissue.

An acute lesion begins as a localized tender nodule around an apocrine gland which gradually resolves over a few days with or without a small discharge of pus. There may then be recurrent exacerbations at the same site, while other lesions may form. Discharge from sinuses is intermittent producing relief of pain when it occurs.

Anal lesions occur in about one-third of patients with hidradenitis.[3] On inspecting the perianal region localized nodules and sinuses will be seen. In severe cases, obvious thickening and oedema of the surrounding skin and induration along subcutaneous tracts will be evident. The disease may be confused with furunculosis, an infected sebaceous cyst, acute perianal abscess or with the external opening of an anal fistula, but the typical appearance of the lesions and their presence in other sites will confirm the diagnosis.

A full anorectal examination is important since there appears to be an association between hidradenitis and anal fistula and possibly also with squamous cell carcinoma of the perianal skin.[12]

Treatment is surgical. A localized abscess should be incised and the granulations in the cavity curetted. Subcutaneous tracks should be laid open and curetted, the wounds being left open to heal by secondary intention. Occasionally where there is extensive involvement a wider excision is necessary. These large open wounds almost always heal satisfactorily. Incision and laying open can be repeated as new lesions develop.

PILONIDAL SINUS

Pilonidal sinus is a common condition which affects young adults with males outnumbering females by a ratio of 3 : 1. It is rare in individuals over the age of 40 and in children and adolescents. While not a disease of the gastrointestinal tract, it may be confused with anorectal sepsis owing to its proximity to the anal region.

Pathology

Pilonidal sinus is a chronic inflammatory lesion occurring between the buttocks consisting of one or more primary openings communicating with a subcutaneous cavity. The primary track is situated in the natal cleft and is lined at its origin by cutaneous epithelium. This soon gives way to chronic inflammatory granulation tissue within the cavity, often containing foreign body giant cells. Frequently the cavity ramifies in various directions to open onto the surface via one or more secondary tracks. The primary tracks usually extend in a cephalad direction and the secondary openings are usually situated on either side of the midline, sometimes a considerable distance away.

Hairs are almost always found in the primary track. Some are detached but others may be rooted in hair follicles in the surrounding skin. Hair follicles are not present in the primary track.

Pathogenesis

There has been controversy as to whether the disease is congenital or acquired. For many years a congenital origin was accepted and numerous theories were proposed. These all had one feature in common, namely the presence of an abnormal epithelially lined structure in the natal cleft, be it a pit or a subcutaneous cyst. Remnants of the medullary canal and dermoid inclusion cysts were postulated and it was also suggested that cutaneous pits could occur as a result of retraction of the tail bud during embryological development. The failure to find any epithelium within excised pilonidal sinuses when examined histologically and the observation that recurrence may occur after excision were the two most important pieces of evidence against the congenital theory.

It is now generally accepted that an acquired cause is more likely.[6] The presence of hairs in the primary track and the occurrence of pilonidal sinuses containing hairs elsewhere in the body (e.g. in the finger webs of barbers, at the umbilicus and in the axillae) strongly suggest that the lesion starts by penetration of the skin by hairs. Most patients (but not all) are hirsute with considerable hair growth in the region of the sinus. How the penetration starts is not clear. It may be that the point of a hair still rooted in the surrounding area punctures the skin and is propelled deeper by the movement of the buttocks. However, more commonly the hairs found in the sinus are detached and are lying in the opposite direction, namely with their tips projecting from the opening. Some are too long to have originated from the immediate vicinity. It may be, therefore, that the penetration is made by loose hairs, for example, from the head. This agrees with the observation that a detached hair when gently rolled between a finger and the palm of the hand will tend to move in the direction of its root. This appears to be due to the orientation of the scales on the hair which project outwards from the shaft at an acute angle toward the tip. It may also be that there is some susceptibility of the skin to penetration by hairs.

Whatever the precise means of penetration, infection occurs leading to abscess formation in the subcutaneous tissue which may drain spontaneously via the primary site of entry or point elsewhere to form a secondary opening. The latter will also be created by surgical drainage.

Clinical presentation

There are two forms of clinical presentation, namely as an acute abscess and as a chronic discharging sinus. The patient with a pilonidal abscess complains of a tender swelling in the natal cleft or buttock developing over a few days. The lesion can be distinguished from an anorectal abscess both by its position and by the absence of tenderness, swelling and induration in the immediate perianal region. Untreated it may settle spontaneously, but usually it bursts and discharges to form a chronic pilonidal sinus. This requires surgical drainage because complete resolution is rare.

The natural history of pilonidal sinus is characterized by relapses and remissions. The discharge may vary considerably and there is often recurrent abscess formation. Pilonidal sinus may be confused with an anal fistula particularly if there is a posterior opening, hidradenitis suppurativa or a simple furuncle.

Treatment

A pilonidal abscess should be drained to permit the acute inflammation to settle. Cure is very unlikely and it is usually necessary to deal at a later date with the resulting pilonidal sinus.

The treatment of a pilonidal sinus depends on the size of the lesion and the severity of symptoms. A small sinus which gives rise to only an occasional discharge of a small amount of material can be managed by conservative means, which include attention to hygiene, the removal of hairs from the track, and shaving the area or the application of depilatory creams. This treatment sometimes results in complete healing but in most cases some form of operation is necessary. The procedures described can be divided into two types: first, those in which the whole lesion is widely excised, and second, those in which the tracks are laid open and abscess cavities deroofed.

Wide excision

The patient is anaesthetized and placed in the jack-knife or the left lateral position and the buttocks are strapped apart. An elliptical incision to include all primary and secondary openings is made and continued through the subcutaneous fat to the fascia over the sacrum and coccyx. The fat is separated from the fascia by sharp dissection and the specimen is removed. It may help to have previously injected dilute methylene blue into the sinus so that any track that has been opened by the dissection can be more easily identified.

The resulting wound may be left open to heal by secondary intention or closed by primary suture. With the former method healing takes a few weeks depending on the size of the wound but the patient can be ambulant for most of this time. A silicone foam stent (Dow Corning) moulded to the shape of the cavity is a convenient dressing, new moulds being made as the wound contracts. During this time the wound edges should be kept shaved since hairs can grow into it and impede healing. The majority of cases heal satisfactorily by this method but recurrences occur in up to 10%.[5, 8] Simple primary suture may be suitable for small wounds but plastic techniques to close large defects without tension are not popular. The recurrence rate is at least 20% after primary suture.[5, 8]

Laying open

A probe is inserted into the primary opening and an incision is made along its direction to open the track and any main abscess cavity. Secondary tracks are laid open in a similar manner. After removal of hairs and curettage of granulation tissue, the wound edges are trimmed to obtain as flat a contour as possible to facilitate healing by secondary intention. With this method the resulting wound is smaller than with wide excision and the results are similar.[5] In a more conservative variant of laying open, the primary and secondary openings are enlarged by circumcision and the cavity is cleaned by brushing or curettage leaving the overlying skin intact.[4] This operation can be carried out under local anaesthetic as an outpatient procedure. Provided the wound is correctly dressed cure rates of 90% can be obtained.[1]

Injection of the track with pure liquid phenol has been reported to produce satisfactory results in a similar proportion of patients.[8]

REFERENCES

1 Edwards, M. H. (1977) Pilonidal sinus: a 5-year appraisal of the Millar–Lord operation. *British Journal of Surgery*, **64**, 867–868.
2 Figueroa, S. & Gennaro, A. R. (1980) Intralesion bleomycin injection in treatment of condylomata acuminata. *Diseases of the Colon and Rectum*, **23**, 550–551.
3 Jackman, R. J. & McQuarrie, H. B. (1949) Hidradenitis suppurativa: its confusion with pilonidal disease and anal fistula. *American Journal of Surgery*, **77**, 349.
4 Lord, P. H. & Miller, D. M. (1965) Pilonidal sinus: a simple treatment. *British Journal of Surgery*, **52**, 298–300.
5 Notaras, M. J. (1970) A review of three popular methods of treatment of post natal (pilonidal) sinus disease. *British Journal of Surgery*, **57**, 886–890.
6 Patey, D. H. (1969) A reappraisal of the acquired theory of sacrococcygeal pilonidal sinus and an assessment of its influence on surgical practice. *British Journal of Surgery*, **56**, 463–466.
7 Prasad, M. L. & Abcarian, H. (1980) Malignant potential of perianal condyloma acuminata. *Diseases of the Colon and Rectum*, **23**, 191–197.
8 Shorey, B. A. (1975) Pilonidal sinus treated by phenol injection. *British Journal of Surgery*, **62**, 407–408.
9 Stephens, F. D. & Smith, E. D. (1971) *Anorectal Malformations in Children*. Chicago: Year Book Medical Publishers.
10 Thomson, H. (1982) The real nature of perianal haematoma. *Lancet*, **ii**, 467–468.
11 Thomson, J. P. S. & Grace, R. (1978) Peri-anal and anal condylomata acuminata – a new operative technique. *Journal of the Royal Society of Medicine*, **71**, 180–185.
12 Thornton, J. P. & Abcarian, H. (1978) Surgical treatment of perianal and perineal hidradenitis suppurativa. *Diseases of the Colon and Rectum*, **21**, 573–577.

Chapter 16
The Functional Gut

APPETITE AND SATIETY

Anorexia is common in many gastrointestinal diseases. Many reasons for this have been suggested, such as pain and gastric distension in obstructive lesions, pyrexia in inflammatory conditions and some enigmatic anorectic factor released by cancerous tissue.[6] However, it is only recently that some progress has been made in the understanding of appetite control, especially in the linkage of psychological factors with physiological and metabolic events and the influence of peptide and monoamine neurotransmitters on the control of food intake.

PSYCHOLOGICAL FACTORS

Four factors influence eating in animals and man.[16]

1 Incentive properties of food. This refers to a preference for one food rather than another.

2 Level of arousal. It is possible to induce eating in satiated animals by a mild stress such as tail pinching. Stress can also result in overeating in satiated people, as can be shown by the excess consumption of food by students during examinations and by some women suffering loneliness or depression.

3 Environmental stimuli. This is best illustrated by the classic experiment of making food especially noticeable by directing light on it: obese subjects will then eat more than if the food is poorly lit.[17]

4 Learning. This is intertwined with all the other factors.

PHYSIOLOGICAL DEVELOPMENTS

Traditionally, the hypothalamus has been considered to contain both the 'satiety' and 'feeding' centres. As bilateral lesions in the ventromedial hypothalamus (VMH) result in hyperphagia and electrical stimulation induces satiety, this area has been known as the 'satiety' centre. The lateral hypothalamus (LH) has been known as the 'feeding' centre because lesions in this area stop eating and electrical stimulation induces feeding.[5] However, problems have arisen with this 'dual centre' hypothesis.

Lateral hypothalamus – feeding centre

It has been shown that the LH lesions which were particularly effective in producing aphagia were situated far lateral and were actually damaging pallidofugal fibre pathways, including a dopaminergic nigrostriatal bundle; if the latter was damaged outside the hypothalamus, aphagia was also produced.[9] This dopaminergic pathway appears important in tail-pinch arousal: such arousal does not produce eating in the presence of dopaminergic blockade.[15]

Recent neurophysiological studies in rat, cat and monkey have shown that the firing rate of LH neurones can alter both before and during feeding, and this has indicated a physiological basis for the psychological factors.[14]. The LH neurones involved appear to extend out lateral to the LH into the substantia innominata. Some of the neurones are associated with just the sight of food, these neurones firing only when the monkey actually sees food and responding most to the animal's preferred food. These sight-responsive neurones only fire if the animal has learnt that the object visualized is actually food. Other neurones respond to the taste of food, again with greater firing in response to preferred tastes already learnt. Such neurones only respond to the sight or taste of food if the animal is hungry, and the response diminishes as the intensity of satiety increases. Interestingly, a specific neurone which has ceased to respond to the sight of food on which the monkey has been fed to satiety, can still respond to the sight of a different food. This is the physiological explanation of 'sensory-specific satiety', where the desire for the particular food being eaten decreases more than for foods that have not been eaten.

The importance of the hypothalamus in feeding is its close relation to the forebrain, through which it receives learning-related visualized olfactory inputs, and its ability to then modulate autonomic, endocrine and feeding responses in the hungry animal when food is sighted or scented.

Ventromedial hypothalamus – satiety centre

It is now thought that the real effects of neuro-surgical destruction of the VMH are slight and that hyperphagia may only be induced if the adjacent ventral noradrenergic bundle which courses in the region of the VMH is damaged.[4] This bundle, after arising from the lateral tegmental cell groups (A1–A5), ascends to join the medial forebrain bundle in the mesencephalon and courses through the periventricular region of the diencephalon, providing a few fibres to the VMH nucleus. These fibres may exert a dual effect depending on whether alpha- or beta-adrenergic receptors are involved; an alpha stimulus produces feeding, whereas eating is

inhibited by a beta stimulus.[7] Lesions of this bundle produce behavioural changes similar to those described in VMH-lesioned animals, suggesting that they may result from depletion of hypothalamic noradrenaline. These behavioural changes involve an exaggeration of those psychological factors (incentive properties, arousal, cue stimulus) which are important in the control of feeding, and result in the animal overreacting to environmental stimuli. It is now thought that this overreaction is a primary effect of the lesion and not secondary to metabolic changes such as the hyperinsulinaemia seen in such lesioned animals. This can be demonstrated by a unilateral VMH lesion, which produces hyperactivity and excessive eating only in response to those environmental stimuli on the side opposite to the lesion despite the general presence of mild hyperinsulinaemia and gastric acid hypersecretion.[8] Consequently Powley has proposed that in the VMH-lesioned animal the exaggerated sensory reaction to stimuli results in exaggerated food-related reflexes (cephalic reflexes) such as insulin and gastric acid secretion, which then make the animal 'feel' more hungry than it really is, resulting in the consumption of more food.[12]

Nevertheless, even when pair-fed, the VMH-lesioned animal gains more weight than the sham-lesioned control, indicating enhanced metabolic efficiency, which may be a consequence of a decrease in brown fat activity.[22] Recently, a close link has been shown to exist between the VMH area and brown fat; electrical stimulation of this area enhances specifically lipogenesis and heat production in brown fat but not in liver or white fat.[11,18] This has led to the view that satiety may be associated with a stimulation of brown fat thermogenesis to burn off excess energy consumed.

How is this related to man? Quaade has electrically stimulated the LH in (obese) humans and reported 'convincing hunger responses' whereas damage to the VMH area in man can result in hyperphagia, obesity and hyper-insulinaemia.[13] Obese man has also been shown to have a significantly greater rise of insulin in response to food presentation than non-obese controls, and there may be a relationship between the degree of obesity and the size of cephalic insulin secretion.[19] Thus, it might be that heightened cephalic responses are one cause of overeating and might predict hyperphagia in those obese subjects who are secret, compulsive or 'craving' eaters. Also, reduced cephalic responses may be implicated in the loss of appetite in disease states.

NEUROTRANSMITTER DEVELOPMENTS

In 1972 Smith and his colleagues clearly demonstrated that a decrease in glucose utilization was not the dominant mechanism for the initiation of eating an ordinary meal (the 'glucostatic control theory').[21] In the same year Yaksh and Myers showed that when a monkey was fed, the VMH released a substance which, on cross-perfusion into the VMH area of a hungry monkey, inhibited feeding.[23] These reports stimulated further research into the role that monoamines, hormones and peptides play in the modulation of food intake. Serotonin agonists have been found to produce satiety, whereas opiates stimulate feeding.[10] Opiates also modulate the dopaminergic stimulus to feeding induced by arousal, such as occurs with tail pinching, for naloxone will significantly decrease food ingestion in this model in a dose-related fashion. This has led to the suggestion that the endogenous opiates may be the neurotransmitter stimulant of food intake in the lateral hypothalamus.

As injected cholecystokinin (CCK) reduces feeding in rats and monkeys[26] its role as a satiety factor has been extensively investigated. The major objection to the experiments using parenteral administration is that the dosages were such as to produce gastrointestinal colic and nausea which themselves could have produced satiety.[2] The finding that L-phenylalanine, a potent releaser of CCK, can reduce food intake, whereas D-phenylalanine (which does not release CCK) does not, suggests that endogenous CCK may act as a satiety signal.[3] However, the evidence is more in favour of a central than a peripheral role for CCK on satiety, for not only is CCK present in the hypothalamus but also intraventricular infusion of CCK produces satiety.[1] Likewise, when injected intraventricularly, thyrotrophin-releasing hormone, somatostatin and bombesin also produce satiety, whereas gamma-aminobutyric acid and diazepam stimulate appetite, and thus these peptides have also been suggested as possible neurotransmitters involved in appetite control.[10]

REFERENCES

1 Della-Fera, M. A. & Baile, C. A. (1979) Cholecystokinin octapeptide: continuous picomole injections into the cerebral ventricles of sheep suppress feeding. *Science*, **206**, 471–473.

2 Deutsch, J. A. & Hardy, W. T. (1977) Cholecystokinin produces bait shyness in rats. *Nature*, **266**, 196.

3 Gibbs, J., Falasco, J. D. & McHugh, P. R. (1976) Cholecystokinin-decreased food intake in rhesus monkeys. *American Journal of Physiology*, **230**, 15–18.

4 Gold, R. M. (1973) Hypothalamic obesity: the myth of the ventromedial nucleus. *Science*, **182**, 488–490.

5 Grossman, S. P. (1976) Neuroanatomy of food and water intake. In *Hunger: Basic Mechanisms and Clinical Implications*. (Ed.) Novin, D., Wyrwicka, W. & Bray, G. pp. 51–59. New York: Raven Press.

6 Hall, R. J. (1975) Progress report; normal and abnormal food intake. *Gut*, **16**, 744–752.

7 Liebowitz, S. F. (1976) Brain catecholaminergic mechanisms for control of hunger. In *Hunger: Basic Mechanisms and Clinical Implications*. (Ed.) Novin D., Wyrwicka, W. & Bray, G. pp. 1–18. New York: Raven Press.

8 Marshall, J. F. (1975) Increased orientation to sensory stimuli following medial hypothalamic damage in rats. *Brain Research*, **86**, 373–387.

9 Marshall, J. F., Richardson, J. S. & Teitelbaum, P. (1974) Nigro-striatal bundle damage and the lateral hypothalamic syndrome. *Journal of Comparative Physiology and Psychology*, **87**, 808–830.

10 Morley, J. E. (1980) The neuroendocrine control of appetite: the role of the endogenous opiates, cholecystokinin, TRH, gamma-amino-butyric acid and the diazepam receptor. *Life Sciences*, **27**, 355–368.

11 Perkins, M. N., Rothwell, N. J., Stock, M. J. & Stone, T. W. (1981) Activation of brown adipose tissue thermogenesis by the ventromedial hypothalamus, *Nature*, **289**, 401–402.

12 Powley, T. L. (1977) The ventromedial hypothalamic syndrome, satiety and a cephalic phase hypothesis. *Psychological Review*, **84**, 89–126.

13 Quaade, F. (1974) Stereotaxy for obesity. *Lancet*, **i**, 267.

14 Rolls, E. T. (1981) Central nervous mechanisms related to feeding and appetite. *British Medical Bulletin*, **37**, 131–134.

15 Rowland, N. E. & Antelman, S. M. (1976) Stress-induced hyperphagia and obesity in rats: a possible model for understanding human obesity. *Science*, **191**, 310–311.

16 Sahakian, B. J. (1982) The interaction of psychological and metabolic factors in the control of eating and obesity. *Scandinavian Journal of Psychology* (in press).

17 Schacter, S. & Rodin, J. (1974) *Obese Humans and Rats*. Potomac, Maryland: Lawrence Erlbaum Associates.

18 Shimazu, T. & Takahashi, A. (1980) Stimulation of hypothalamic nuclei has differential effects on lipid synthesis in brown and white adipose tissue. *Nature*, **284**, 62–63.

19 Sjöström, L., Garellick, G., Krotkiewski, M. & Luyskx, A. (1980) Peripheral insulin in response to the sight and smell of food. *Metabolism*, **29**, 901–909.

20 Smith, G. P. & Gibbs, J. (1976) Cholecystokinin and satiety: theoretic and therapeutic implications. In *Hunger: Basic Mechanisms and Clinical Implications*. (Ed.) Novin, D., Wyrwicka, W. & Bray, G., pp. 349–355. New York: Raven Press.

21 Smith, G. P., Gibbs, J., Strohmayer, A. J. & Stokes, P. E. (1972) Threshold doses of 2-deoxy-D-glucose for hyperglycaemia and feeding in rats and monkeys. *American Journal of Physiology*, **222**, 77–81.

22 Trayhurn, P. & James, W. P. (1981) Thermogenesis: dietary and non-shivering aspects. In *The Body Weight Regulatory System: Normal and Disturbed Mechanisms* (Ed.) Cioffi, L. A., James, W. P. T. & Van Itallie, T. B. New York: Raven Press.

23 Yaksh, T. L. & Myers, R. D. (1972) Neurohumoral substances released from the hypothalamus of the monkey during hunger and satiety. *American Journal of Physiology*, **222**, 503–515.

AN APPROACH TO THE PATIENT WITH CHRONIC ABDOMINAL PAIN

Chronic abdominal pain commonly provides a perplexing problem for doctors, because physical signs of disease are usually absent and investigations negative apart from incidental findings which confuse the issue. Furthermore, pain is subjective and no one except the patient knows its intensity; nor is there any method of measuring it. Chronic pain can be defined as pain continuing longer than three months, but often patients appear after years of uncertainty, the victims of numerous erroneous diagnoses. The longer the duration, the less likely is organic disease; yet even when time has excluded any reasonable possibility of malignant disease, fear of this – in the minds of both the patient and the doctor – may linger, and the longer the duration of the trouble the more difficult it is to cure.

Every gastrointestinal clinic contains many who suffer from pain which is not of organic origin; the incidence varies from 31%[5] to 50% or more.[11] Hospital beds are also occupied: in Britain, in the Oxford region, Rang, Fairbairn and Acheson[16] reported that this was the tenth commonest cause of admission to hospital in males and sixth in females. There were no fewer than 682 discharges in 1966 where the final diagnosis was unexplained abdominal pain. Many were young women who underwent appendicectomy for removal of a normal appendix. Follow-up showed that 24% of males and 38% of females were re-admitted to hospital once or more often either because of the pain itself or for other abdominal symptoms, or for psychiatric reasons.

No age is exempt. Ten per cent of children suffer from it and Apley could detect organic disease in only 7% of 200 children with recurrent abdominal pain.[1] That children may not 'grow out' of these pains was shown by his follow-up of 30 who were reviewed eight to twenty years after attending a children's hospital; 9 were completely well, but 12 continued to have abdominal pain, frequently accompanied by headaches or other symptoms, and 9, though free from abdominal pains, had continued with symptoms like migraine or dysmenorrhoea. The proportion of children with bodily or nervous complaints was several times higher than in a control group who had attended the same children's hospital for minor physical disorders.

Adults may present with symptoms that can mimic peptic ulcer, disease of the gallbladder, or carcinoma. Some are even admitted as an acute abdominal emergency.[4] Three questions must be answered when a patient presents with pain of undetermined origin:

1 Does the pain resemble any known disorder?
2 Have appropriate investigations been carried out satisfactorily and relevant diseases been excluded?
3 Do the description of the pain and any associated symptoms point towards an organic or psychosomatic disorder?

METHODS OF DIAGNOSIS

The mental process of diagnosis depends upon pattern-matching and here lies a source of error: the stereotypes of disease used for teaching can be wrong and so-called classic descriptions are seldom seen. Furthermore, though chronic abdominal pain is so common in practice, the subject is often missing from textbooks, even from those on gastroenterology.

Importance of the history

Most diagnoses are made from the history, and this is even more so with abdominal pain. Yet it is only too easy for the family doctor, instead of listening, to write a prescription for tablets in order to keep the queue of patients moving, or for the hospital doctor to fill up a form for yet another X-ray to save spending time in extracting the whole story. Careful analysis of symptoms or data-collecting can so easily be overlooked. Also, much depends upon the patient's lucidity and the doctor's ability to interpret lay words. Indigestion, acidity, bile and heartburn may mean almost anything and wind often implies epigastric discomfort or pain. Some symptoms have greater discriminating value than others. For example, the rating for postural heartburn in diagnosing reflux oesophagitis would be high, and night pain points towards organic disease like duodenal ulcer.[12] A low value would be awarded to nausea, aerophagy or even loss of weight, which can occur in those with nervous dyspepsia.[8] A detailed analysis of the pain is essential:

1 Character. Organic pain is often described as aching, boring or gripping and not, for example, as pricking or stabbing.

2 Severity. Exaggerated descriptions such as 'like a two-edged sword being plunged into various parts of my belly' are unlikely to be used by those with organic disease and indeed have seldom been experienced.

3 Situation. Organic disease is likely to be localized to one area, and the more diffuse the pain, especially if in the upper and lower abdomen, the less likely is disease.

4 Frequency. Organic disease fluctuates in severity and is usually intermittent, whereas *continuous* pain, perhaps present day and night for weeks or years, is probably psychosomatic.

5 Any special times of occurrence. Is the pain related to the periods? Does it follow stress?

6 Factors that aggravate or relieve the pain. Important clues can be obtained by enquiry as to the effect of food, drink, alkali, defecation and so on.

Sometimes the sole complaint is of pain, though often associated symptoms may guide towards a diagnosis. Abdominal symptoms which seldom have an organic basis include feelings of fullness and bloating, continuous nausea, belching and prolonged burning sensations. Complaints which are usually psychogenic are listed in Table 16.1. The previous or family history may

Table 16.1 Complaints that are more likely to originate from the psyche than the soma – especially if several are present.

Tiredness
Headache
Dizziness
Depression
Dyspareunia
Sexual difficulties
Insomnia

be important. Operations for removal of normal viscera like the appendix or gallbladder may have been performed or a nervous breakdown or other psychiatric illness may have occurred. Occasionally, abdominal pain is familial and a reaction to stress which is part of the family pattern.

Clinical examination

The object of examining the patient should be:

To detect signs of disease.

To achieve rapport. Important details may be obtained only when the patient is relaxed and lying on the couch. For example, the standard answer to the standard question 'is your marriage satisfactory?' is often yes. When rephrased

more sympathetically – 'tell me about problems at home' – facts may pour out.

To reassure. Most patients are anxious, especially if their chronic pain has been neither diagnosed nor alleviated. Also, some may have been subjected to numerous tests without being properly examined even at the start. A painstaking examination can be therapeutic, especially when the doctor talks reassuringly at the same time.

A complete examination is always necessary, just as the patient must be considered as a whole person, but in this section the focus will be only on the abdomen. The manner of the patient should be observed. Some prod themselves to find areas of tenderness and others lie on the couch with the eyes closed – as if brave sufferers of pain; both are unlikely with organic disease.

Abdominal tenderness is often misleading. True tenderness is an index of inflammation as in acute appendicitis; it is seldom a sign of peptic ulcer unless this is penetrating the peritoneum, nor is it a sign of malignant disease. Tenderness from organic disease is usually localized, constant in its position and may be associated with an increase in pulse rate, whereas tenderness due to anxiety is diffuse and may change during the course of examination, or disappear when the patient is diverted by asking a question or suchlike. Exquisite pain occurring even with light touch is of no organic significance, and pain or tenderness in one spot, often superficial, virtually excludes intra-abdominal disease; for example, a doctor when trying to prove disease in the gallbladder by Murphy's sign may cause a tender area on a rib or induce an anxiety pain at that spot. Rebound tenderness, even when examining an 'acute abdomen', often has little significance;[15] in chronic cases, it is of no value and guarding is more often due to apprehension or failure to relax.

The inexperienced must beware of mistaking structures that can be felt in a normal abdomen for disease; these include the liver edge, lower pole of right kidney, pulsating aorta, colon when loaded with faeces or felt in the left iliac fossa, cervix at rectal examination in women, and congenital abnormalities like Riedel's lobe or horseshoe kidney. The patient should be told whether anything relevant is found or be reassured completely.

How far to investigate

There are many reasons for requesting investigations, but in these patients the motives are usually the fear of missing organic disease (often unnecessary if a careful history is taken), the desire to reassure with a normal result, or the urge to do something – the 'desperation test'. Many will have been investigated already, so radiographs and other results should be studied and not repeated unless necessary. For example, endoscopy must be done during a painful phase and not in a remission when any ulcer may be healed. Routine tests will have included blood counts and serum biochemistry.

Blood count

Anaemia, unless due to some other cause (e.g. menorrhagia), implies disease of the alimentary tract. A raised erythrocyte sedimentation rate (ESR) or increased orosomucoids suggests inflammatory bowel disease or connective tissue disorder, perhaps causing vasculitis affecting the gut. A normal ESR makes organic disease unlikely though it does not exclude it.

Tests to be done in special cases are a reticulocyte count for spherocytosis and to exclude sickle cell disease.

Serum biochemistry

A biochemical profile is often available, providing results of 10 or 12 routine tests. The serum calcium occasionally suggests the diagnosis missed by the clinician: hypocalcaemia points to adult coeliac disease, which can be painful, whereas hypercalcaemia, perhaps due to hyperparathyroidism or sarcoidosis, causes vague abdominal symptoms. The serum amylase level is likely to be normal in chronic pancreatitis unless measured during an episode of pain.

Rarely, hyperlipaemia may be associated with pain like pancreatitis; inspection of serum stored overnight in the refrigerator may show it to be milky, and the level of fasting triglycerides may be high. Porphyria, though also rare, can cause psychiatric symptoms and result in unnecessary laparotomies because of abdominal pain; it can easily be excluded at the bedside by testing the urine with Ehrlich's aldehyde reagent.

Complicated and expensive tests such as ultrasound or CT scanning should not be ordered without good reason; for example to exclude cancer of the body of the pancreas. Laparoscopy is seldom indicated. The final investigation – direct inspection by laparotomy – is sometimes advised but it carries the risk of the surgeon blaming the pain upon some irrelevant finding like an adhesion, and motility defects like irritable bowel cannot be seen.

A healthy person has been defined as 'someone not fully investigated', meaning that abnormal but symptomless conditions are not uncommon. Unfortunately, a mania for investigating often seems to permeate hospital practice, and the more the investigations, the greater the anxiety created, especially when the patient is not told the result.

Admission of the patient to hospital

Admission is often a better policy than trying to solve a long-standing case by visits to the outpatient clinic, and watching and talking to the patient in the ward is usually more rewarding than an extensive 'work-up' of tests, and a psychiatric assessment may more easily be done.

Observation during an attack of pain is invaluable. Sometimes hysterical features are prominent, and those with organic disease are likely to have an increase in pulse or other concomitant of pain like sweating. Examination may, though rarely, reveal a lump due to intermittent intussusception and the stethoscope may reveal loud peristaltic sounds when colic is suspected, perhaps due to subacute obstruction.

A sample of blood is taken for the serum bilirubin and amylase measurements to exclude possible biliary or pancreatic disease, and urine is examined for evidence of renal disease and to exclude porphyria. The temperature is taken, and sometimes a plain radiograph of the abdomen may show a dilated loop of gut due to obstruction by volvulus or internal hernia. When psychogenic pain is suspected, an injection of saline sometimes stops it instantaneously, though up to 20% of those with organic disease could be placebo reactors.

DISORDERS CAUSING CHRONIC PAIN OF FUNCTIONAL ORIGIN

In the past, various labels (Table 16.2) have been given to abdominal pain of undetermined origin, but these are now obsolete. Today the term functional is often used but this can have two

Table 16.2 Diagnoses formerly used to explain abdominal pain but now obsolete.

Adhesions
Chronic appendicitis
Chronic cholecystitis
Displaced uterus
Visceroptosis

meanings: (a) psychogenic or (b) a disturbance of physiological function. Both of these may, in fact, be appropriate for patients with irritable bowel. Most cases can be fitted into one of the following conditions though there is much overlap.

Worry pain

Transient aches and pains are common in the healthy but may continue in someone with an emotional problem or who unduly fears cancer.

Worry pain perpetuated by non-disease

This happens when a normal or irrelevant finding is wrongly regarded by the doctor as significant. Meador in his article 'The Art and Science of Non-disease' classified the various types.[13] Findings which are often symptomless can too easily be accepted as causing the pain instead of being coincidental (Table 16.3). The

Table 16.3 Findings that are often incidental and symptomless – a cause of non-disease.

Chronic gastritis
Duodenitis
Hiatus hernia
Gallstones
Diverticulosis
Cyst on the ovary

same applies to blood tests; laboratory errors or normal variations can mislead; for example, a slightly raised serum bilirubin as in Gilbert's syndrome.

Abdominal neurosis

The abdomen frequently acts as a sounding board for the emotions, so symptoms may be part of a psychoneurosis. This is easily overlooked, for it is a common assumption that pain is a prima facie sign of physical illness. Surgeons sometimes seem unaware that neurosis exists and surgical books – including monographs about abdominal pain – even fail to mention it. Similarly, medical books provide lists of differential diagnoses unrelated to the reality of practice. Yet psychiatric factors are a common cause of abdominal pain; this was shown in a study of 96 patients complaining of recurrent or persistent abdominal pain investigated by Gomez and Dally, for only 15 had organic disease that could have explained their symptoms.[6]

Support for a psychogenic disorder may be provided by the personality of the patient. An exaggerated description of symptoms is common; for example, one woman smilingly and even laughingly said that the pain was so ghastly that life had become unbearable. Weeping during a consultation indicates depression and seldom occurs even with severe organic disease. Patients vary strikingly in their complaint threshold, some first visiting the doctor when their disease is advanced. Others may have a low pain and complaint threshold and notice sensations which would pass unobserved by the average person. Then symptoms pour out in profusion; the greater the number the less likely is organic disease. Sometimes examination becomes impossible because of continuous talking; then the clinical thermometer comes in useful as it compels silence when placed under the tongue.

The complaint of other bodily feelings likely to be psychosomatic (Table 16.1) provides a positive factor in diagnosing neurosis, and details from the previous history may be important. Psychological factors superimposed upon organic disease provide a snare for the unwary. Also, neurotic patients are not immortal and may develop organic disease. Caution is necessary in those over 50 years old who have never suffered from nervous illness or such symptoms before as an organic cause is more likely. However, although a mistaken label of neurosis may be bad for the doctor's reputation, an unwarranted organic diagnosis may be disastrous for the patient as it can cause invalidism, unnecessary operations and deprivation of much of the enjoyment of eating. Treatment is most effective when carried out before patients have been confused by doing the round of various hospitals and different specialists.

An occasional patient makes a career of suffering and as Szasz wrote, 'In the game of painsmanship, the patient's aim is to produce undiagnosable pain and unrelievable suffering. This creates meaning for his life and power to control his human environment.... Such persons crave medical and surgical (and *not* psychiatric) intervention to make their role as sick patients legitimate'.[17]

Irritable bowel

This explains much abdominal pain. It is due to a disturbance of motility and can affect any part of the alimentary tract from oesophagus to anus. Morarty and Dawson performed balloon distension of the distal oesophagus, second part of the duodenum, proximal jejunum and distal ileum.[14] Pain was noticed in sites throughout the abdomen and was sometimes referred elsewhere. The same pain of which the patients complained could be reproduced in 14 of the 21 patients, and in three of these it was also reproduced by distension through the colonoscope. Yet, though it is due to a disturbance of function of the bowel, there is often a psychological factor.

The term irritable bowel is used to indicate that sometimes the whole gut may be involved and be a basis for nervous dyspepsia, but here the term will refer to the colon and will only be dealt with briefly as a full account is given in Chapter 11. Its incidence in the general population is not known but many people probably have symptoms and do not attend hospitals. Labels given to it resemble a veritable Tower of Babel and vary from spastic colon, through dyskinesia of the colon to mucous colitis. The last must be avoided; otherwise an intelligent patient may become worried about the need for colectomy and ileostomy.

Pain is most likely in the left iliac fossa or lower abdomen though may occur elsewhere. Diarrhoea may alternate with the passage of rabbit-like stools. There may be scars of unnecessary operations. Indeed, Chaudhary and Truelove found that one-third of the men in their series had had an appendicectomy and one-third of the women had had either this or a gynaecological operation.[3] Now that irritable colon is diagnosed earlier, this happens less frequently.

Diagnosis must be made from the presence of definite and positive symptoms as well as by the exclusion of relevant organic disease by routine blood tests, sigmoidoscopy and barium enema X-ray. The X-ray may be omitted in young women at the first visit; it can be arranged if symptoms persist or if the ESR is raised.

Two problems commonly arise and may add to the patient's anxiety: first, a label of diverticulitis may be given merely because a few diverticula of the colon are seen on X-ray – a normal finding in older people; secondly, the fear of organic disease may lead to fruitless and unnecessary investigations. Reassurance is essential as many fear cancer or are frightened by mucus. Other treatments, such as high-fibre diets, are dealt with in Chapter 11.

Nervous dyspepsia

Dyspepsia often arises from problems in the psyche. Pain or discomfort may be localized to the epigastrium, though they more often occur elsewhere as well. It starts immediately after eating, in contrast to ulcer pain, which is not aggravated but is relieved by food.[8] Alkalis may have little effect and victims are not awakened from sleep because of pain as in peptic ulcer; more often they are unable to sleep because of a disturbed mind.

Other symptoms (Table 16.4) distinguish these patients. Appetite may be good, yet a feeling of satiety develops after a few mouthfuls

Table 16.4 Differential diagnosis between dyspepsia due to peptic ulcer and nervous dyspepsia.

	Ulcer	Nervous dyspepsia
Complaint	Pain	Various symptoms: wind, discomfort, burning, acidity, dislike of clothes touching abdomen or tight garments around waist
Reaction to foods	Eats anything (except perhaps fat)	'Sensitivity' to various foods
Effect of alkali	Immediate relief	Variable
Pointing test	+ (pain confined to epigastrium)	– (pain also elsewhere in abdomen)
Health otherwise	Fit	Tiredness, headaches insomnia, etc.

so that the meal has to be discontinued. Sensitivity to food occurs and patients become introspective about eating, finding that various and in some cases every type of food and drink causes symptoms. Even the smell of food may start trouble. One patient stated that she knew by telepathy whether food was about even if she could not see or smell it. Another was able to enjoy New Zealand lamb but English lamb made her ill for several days afterwards. No one's stomach has this remarkable power of discrimination and any 'allergy' usually lies in the psyche and not in the gastric mucosa. Vomiting may be prominent and even continue for years without loss of weight; indeed, the patient may appear remarkably robust in spite of it.

Other symptoms which support the diagnosis are nausea, burning feelings, dislike of anything tight around the waist and so on. 'Heartburn' may be a complaint, but this is not true heartburn, which lasts for two or three minutes; it may continue for 24 hours and is a typical nervous symptom. In contrast to the peptic ulcer patient, who is usually fit apart from the dyspepsia, these patients are often unwell in other ways, with symptoms of nervous origin (Table 16.1).

Reassurance after thorough examination and investigation often cures. Unfortunately, this may not happen: instead of immediate reassurance when the barium meal is normal, the patient may be told that this does not exclude an ulcer and put on the list for endoscopy; this puts doubt in the mind, particularly if the examination is delayed for two or three months. If endoscopy is normal, reassurance may be ineffective because of amnesia from diazepam. Next the patient may fail to contact the general practitioner or communication from the hospital may be defective. Worst of all is the doubt cast by reporting a mucosal variation such as gastritis, for neither the doctor nor colleagues in other specialities may know its significance. It is always more rewarding to 'find something' especially for junior staff whose clinical acumen may lag behind their technical competence. However, both gastritis and duodenitis are often incidental. If given an organic label, neurosis may be perpetuated and patients condemned to dieting or tablets instead of being cured by reassurance. Correct diagnosis must be made before treatment. Prescribing an H_2-receptor antagonist may cure by a placebo effect but can do harm; instead of instant reassurance, it fixes the idea of the trouble being organic and due to acid.

Fear of cancer, so often present, must be dispelled. Faulty ideas concerning digestion must be corrected. The idea that some foods cannot be digested is imaginary, as could be proved by sampling through a stomach tube. Similarly, worry is caused by so-called wind, which is sometimes thought to be a form of marsh gas due to unnatural fermentation; most is swallowed air (aerophagy) and explaining this will relieve anxiety. A normal diet should be prescribed with confidence as some will have developed food fads. A careful search for an emotional cause should be made.

'Chronic appendicitis'

Pain in the right iliac fossa is a common manifestation of anxiety in young women and may have replaced the swooning of the Victorian era. A nagging pain, often *continuous* with occasional stabs, develops, often after worry such as an upset love affair. Fear of appendicitis may have been made worse by the suggestion of a 'grumbling appendix'. It is unaffected by eating, defaecation, micturition, menses or

movement, but is worse when the patient is worried or fatigued. Many thousands of normal appendices are removed each year because of this. Sometimes the appendix is described as abnormally long or kinked – perhaps as a face-saving manoeuvre by the surgeon – or the pathologist reports minor inflammatory changes which are really variations of normal.[2] The pain may disappear after operation, probably from suggestion. If it continues, a diagnosis of adhesions is often made; adhesions, however, cause no symptoms except by mechanical obstruction and occur in the healthy. Ingram and Evans found that more than half of such patients were dissatisfied after appendicectomy; their pain recurred or they developed other psychosomatic symptoms.[10] The poor result of removing a normal appendix was confirmed by Howie and he suggested 'that the place of planned appendicectomy for mild or recurrent iliac fossa pain was a very restricted one'.[9]

'Chronic cholecystitis'

Gallstones cause acute cholecystitis, obstructive jaundice and attacks of subacute pain in the epigastrium and right hypochondrium. Complaints of vague discomfort together with belching and dyspepsia after eating fats or other food are not due to gallbladder disease and were found to be more common in those with normal cholecystograms by Hinkel and Moller.[7] These workers also questioned patients with gallstones and found that most enjoyed eating fat and that intolerance usually developed only after medical advice to avoid eating it. Cholecystectomy for these symptoms, especially when the gallbladder is normal, is ineffective: so often the same trouble continues.

Deliberate disability

The clandestine taking of purgatives can mimic colonic disease and is easily overlooked. It is detected by testing the faeces or urine for cascara and phenolphthalein.

Munchausen's syndrome

Patients travel from hospital to hospital seeking medical attention and operations by inventing symptoms.

Pain of undetermined origin

Occasionally, pain is the only symptom and cannot be fitted into any category. New methods of investigation may, in the future, provide some physiological explanation.

GUIDELINES FOR HANDLING THE PATIENTS

Many patients are easily cured by reassurance; the doctor may arrange a follow-up visit so as to be certain that symptoms have improved or gone. Some, especially those with long-standing pain, provide a challenge. Handling the patient is made difficult by lack of confidence in doctors, anxiety created by fruitless investigations and operations, and bitterness that no one is able to produce a cure. Aggression may be marked; this may conceal anxiety or a desire to escape the detection of the real emotional problem. They ascribe their pains to some disease or dysfunction of their bodies and never to an emotional cause, in contrast to those with organic disease, who may even suggest that the trouble is nervous. Self-opinionated theories abound and the patient may try to 'out-talk' his doctor. Doctor–patient relationships can be strained to the utmost from mutual frustration and antagonism, so that only a sense of detachment by the doctor will save the situation.

A sympathetic and confident approach is essential. These patients are not imposters and the pain, whether organic or psychogenic, to the patient is the same. The idea that it is imaginary is naturally resented. Unfortunately, when no organic trouble is found, all that may happen is the frustrating statement, 'There is nothing wrong with you', which is bound to create hostility whereas the alternative, 'There is nothing *seriously* wrong with you', can have a very beneficial effect, especially if the mechanism of pain is discussed.

Correction of faulty physiological ideas

This may take time, and providing a suitable booklet written for the lay person can be helpful. Many have wrong ideas about digestion: they blame acid and fear bile if they see it in vomit, not realizing that this is an essential physiological substance. The same applies to mucus which may be detected by studying stools.

Providing an explanation

It is hardly surprising that this is so necessary; it satisfies the ego and provides an alibi for the reality of the pain. The term 'spasm' is easily accepted without causing anxiety; then antispasmodic tablets can be prescribed to 'relax the bowel', though often any drug will help if dispensed by a sympathetic doctor. Discussion about nerves must be approached cautiously as many wrongly associate this suggestion with lack of courage and take offence, not realizing that the bravest person is sometimes neurotic. The problem of nervous tension and its effect upon the body can be explained. Headache can be given as an example of pain caused by worry, as this idea is so easily accepted by lay people.

Counteracting any iatrogenic component

Doctors feel compelled to tell the patient something and to proclaim a diagnosis. It is a pity if this is dogmatic and frightening; for example, one surgeon proudly stated that 'the abdomen was in a mess', meaning that he found many adhesions, though these were in fact symptomless. Even a gastroenterologist may remark that he is sure that the pain is organic or a psychiatrist may state that the patient is as normal a person as he is. Diplomacy is needed to counteract these statements without letting a colleague down.

Conflicting information commonly confuses. Different explanations and diagnoses may be given, even by doctors working in the same department. What the patient is told should be written in the case notes for all to see and, most important, reported to the general practitioner.

Searching for an emotional cause

This may be simple, as in a child developing stomach ache to avoid going to school. In adults it is usually more complicated and difficult to extract. Time and privacy are needed for talking and listening to the patient. Problems may involve domestic upsets, business strains or difficulties with sex, or the patient may be attempting to attract sympathy and attention. The help of a psychiatrist may be needed, but patients whose complaints are almost entirely somatic are often dealt with better by a sympathetic physician who can speak authoritatively. However, the psychiatrist can be of great help for certain patients, especially those who may have delusions about their bodily functions or suffer from serious depression. Treatment of depression may cure abdominal pain.

Drugs and other treatment of pain

The effect of drugs is difficult to assess as any new one may be effective, at any rate temporarily. Analgesics and antispasmodics may be tried but addiction-forming drugs like pethidine (meperidine) must be avoided. Cure may be effected by any form of suggestion, whether by hypnotism (though no controlled trials are available) or by the magic of fringe medicine like acupuncture. One patient underwent laparotomy: nothing abnormal was found but the explanation that one coil of bowel was longer than another produced a cure.

Importance of a combined approach

Needless to say, the spouse must be kept fully in the picture, with emphasis that the symptoms are genuine. All those who come into contact with the patient – other doctors, nurses and relatives – must also know what has been said so as to take the same hopeful approach. For example, the endoscopist and radiologist can be told of the presumptive diagnosis and act as psychotherapists in reassuring the patient at the time of investigation. Once the decision has been taken that organic disease is absent, the same supportive and reassuring attitude is taken by all.

REFERENCES

1 Apley, J. (1959) *The Child with Abdominal Pains.* Oxford: Blackwell Scientific.
2 Campbell, J. S., Fourier, P. & Da Silva, T. (1961) When is the appendix normal? *Canadian Medical Association Journal,* **85,** 1155–1157.
3 Chaudhary, N. A. & Truelove, S. C. (1962) The irritable colon syndrome: a study of the classical features, predisposing causes and prognosis in 130 cases. *Quarterly Journal of Medicine,* **31,** 307–322.
4 De Dombal, F. T., Leaper, D. J., Jane, C. et al (1974) Human and computer-aided diagnosis of abdominal pain. *British Medical Journal,* **1,** 376–380.
5 Ferguson A., Sircus, W. & Eastwood, M. A. (1977) Frequency of functional gastrointestinal disorders (Letter). *Lancet,* **ii,** 613–614.
6 Gomez, J. & Dally, P. (1977) Psychologically mediated abdominal pain in surgical and medical outpatient clinics. *British Medical Journal,* **i,** 1451–1453.
7 Hinkel, C. L. & Moller, G. A. (1957) Correlation of symptoms, age, sex and habits with cholecystographic findings in 1000 consecutive examinations. *Gastroenterology,* **32,** 807–815.
8 Horrocks, J. C. & De Dombal, F. T. (1978) Clinical presentation of patients with dyspepsia. Symptomatic study of 360 patients. *Gut,* **19,** 19–26.
9 Howie, J. G. R. (1968) The place of appendicectomy in the treatment of young adults with possible appendicitis. *Lancet,* **1,** 1365–1367.
10 Ingram, P. W. & Evans, G. (1965) Right iliac-fossa pain in young women. *British Medical Journal,* **ii,** 149–151.
11 Kirsner, J. B. & Palmer, W. L. (1958) The irritable colon. *Gastroenterology,* **34,** 490–501.
12 Lawson, M. J., Grant, A. K., Paull, A. & Read, T. R. (1980) Significance of nocturnal abdominal pain: a prospective study. *British Medical Journal,* **i,** 1302.
13 Meador, C. K. (1965) The art and science of nondisease. *New England Journal of Medicine,* **i,** 92–95.
14 Moriarty, K. J. & Dawson, A. M. (1982) Functional abdominal pain: further evidence that the whole gut is affected. *British Medical Journal,* **i,** 1670–1672.
15 Prout, W. G. (1970) The significance of rebound tenderness in the acute abdomen. *British Journal of Surgery,* **57,** 508–511.
16 Rang, E. H., Fairbairn, A. S. & Acheson, E. D. (1970) An enquiry into the incidence and prognosis of undiagnosed abdominal pain treated in hospital. *British Journal of Preventive and Social Medicine,* **24,** 47–51.
17 Szasz, T. S. (1968) The psychology of persistent pain. In *Pain. Proceedings of the International Symposium on Pain Organised by the Laboratory of Psychophysiology. Faculty of Science, Paris April 11–13, 1967* (Ed.) Soulairac, A., Cahn, J. & Charpentier, J. London and New York: Academic Press.

ANOREXIA NERVOSA AND RELATED DISTURBANCES

There is a spectrum of eating disorders and disturbed attitudes to weight which converge in anorexia nervosa. Bulimia and self-induced or spontaneous vomiting and purgative addiction are frequently found in anorexia nervosa but may also exist independently in patients who maintain a normal weight.

ANOREXIA NERVOSA

Anorexia nervosa can be defined as a state of voluntary undernutrition, due to morbid attitudes to food and weight, that results in an impairment of physiological function. Attempts have been made to define the illness in a more comprehensive fashion. The 'medical' approach is exemplified by Feighner et al. who assembled the following criteria for the diagnosis.[10]

1 Onset before 25 years of age.
2 Anorexia with accompanying weight loss of at least 25% of original body weight.
3 A distorted, implacable attitude toward eating, food, or weight that overrides hunger, admonitions, reassurance and threats, for example:
 denial of illness, with a failure to recognize nutritional needs;
 apparent enjoyment in losing weight, with the overt manifestation that food refusal is pleasurable indulgence.
4 A desired body image of extreme thinness, with overt evidence that it is rewarding to the patient to achieve and maintain this state.
5 Unusual hoarding or handling of food.
6 No known medical illness that could account for the anorexia and weight loss.
7 No other known psychiatric disorder, with particular reference to primary affective disorders, schizophrenia, obsessive–compulsive and phobic neurosis.

8   At least two of the following manifestations:
amenorrhoea;
lanugo;
bradycardia (persistent resting pulse of
   60 or less);
periods of overactivity;
episodes of bulimia;
vomiting (may be self-induced).

The drawback of this approach is that it defines only the very severe case and dilutes the emphasis on attitudes to eating and weight that many consider to be more at the heart of the disturbance. Bruch has described the typical anorexic position as 'a struggle for control, for a sense of identity and effectiveness, with relentless pursuit of thinness as a final step in this effort'.[2] Crisp has used the term 'weight phobia' as a more apt description than the misleading term anorexia nervosa.[3] These patients are usually not anorexic but are fighting their hunger in order to attain a desired shape. 50% of the patients in the series of Halmi *et al.* experienced a strong appetite; characteristically, 80% of the series indulged in excessive cooking for their families.[15]

A typical history would be of a plump girl in her teens teased about her weight at school, kept rather immature by an over-protective mother, the mother and the girl both frightened by her burgeoning sexuality. The girl then decides to diet, finds it very easy and experiences a psychological 'high' at her success, and as a result of multiple secondary gains maintains the behaviour until she is seriously underweight. Although this would be a typical presentation, anorexia nervosa may occur in a wider age range, both before the menarche and after the menopause, and can also affect males.

Incidence

Until the early 1960s anorexia nervosa was considered to be a rare disease, but in more recent times it has become commonplace. It is not easy to arrive at the true incidence of anorexia nervosa in the general population, as it is only a highly selected segment of the sick population that presents itself for medical attention. The patient with anorexia nervosa is commonly very reluctant to recognize that there is anything wrong with her and to seek medical help. It is often the incontrovertible abnormality of amenorrhoea rather than low weight that convinces the patient that she should seek help and even then help is sought more because of parental insistence than on the patient's own initiative. In

males, unpropelled by amenorrhoea in the direction of medical help, the unidentified population is likely to be even larger than in females. There is also a bimodal distribution of age at onset among the males, with a peak at 12 and in the early 20s,[18] as against 17–18 among the women.[15] Although increasing knowledge about anorexia nervosa amongst the lay public and doctors must result in the more frequent identification of cases it seems likely that there has been a real increase in the prevalence of anorexia nervosa; we can only speculate about the reasons for this. A cult of thinness has developed. Huenemann *et al.* studied attitudes to food and weight in American teenagers.[20] Of the girls who considered themselves to be overweight only half were actually overweight according to standard tables. The males had far more realistic attitudes to their weight.

One of the major problems of most anorexics is coping with their developing sexuality. Anorexia nervosa is the perfect device for such individuals in that it turns the clock back and they regain the prepubertal state. Increasing pressures for earlier sexual activity may be increasing the difficulties of the vulnerable portion of the population. Strains in the parental marriage may contribute to the development of anorexia nervosa, and the patient with anorexia nervosa may also consciously or unconsciously seek through her illness to keep her parents together. There is a very low incidence of divorce amongst the parents of anorexics, for example 3 out of 44 in the series of Halmi *et al.*,[15] a possible proof of the effectiveness with which the anorexia serves to keep parents together. The pressure from the general increase in broken marriages may be contributing to the increase in anorexia nervosa.

Population studies

There have been no random population studies but special populations such as female university students and girls' sixth forms (16–18-year-olds) have been investigated. Due to the increased frequency of the illness in social classes I.II these surveys are likely to overestimate the incidence.

Russell studied school girls aged 16 to 18, female nurses and medical students.[31] He enquired after amenorrhoea and a weight loss of at least seven pounds (≈ 3 kg). He found that 4% of the population had at some time experienced a combination of these two factors. The number of these individuals that suffered an unequivocal anorexia nervosa was not ascertained, but if we accept that anorexia nervosa may exist in a less severe form, it seems likely that many of these individuals with weight loss and amenorrhoea were actual cases or on the fringe of anorexia nervosa.

The true incidence of anorexia nervosa in males is even less sure than that in females as male cases are more difficult to identify. The ratio of male to female of 1 : 15 reported by Crisp and Toms[5] accords with general experience.

Familial factors

Crisp and Toms[5] found that in their series of 13 males, 3 had affected siblings. In females, Theander observed a 6% risk for the development of anorexia nervosa in the sisters of anorexic probands.[33] It is not possible to conclude from these studies whether the increased risk to a sibling is by a genetic mechanism or in the sharing of a common experience.

Physiological changes associated with anorexia nervosa[18]

Hormones

Gonadotrophin levels are reduced. Luteinizing hormone (LH) and follicle stimulating hormone (FSH) levels are low. When the system is stimulated by the injection of gonadotrophin-releasing hormone the LH response is reduced until the patient has almost regained ideal body weight; then the response becomes normal. The FSH response is greater at all weights than in the normal individual.[14] The response is similar to that of the prepubertal girl. Growth hormone and plasma cortisol levels are raised,[12] the raised growth hormone level being associated with a low serum somatomedin level.[28]

Reports on thyroid status have varied. The consensus is that thyroid-stimulating-hormone is normal or a little raised, thyroxine (T_4) is low normal and triiodothyronine (T_3) is reduced, probably because of a peripheral failure in the conversion of T_4 to T_3.[27] Testosterone metabolism is affected in the female but this is thought to be secondary to the reduced T_3.[1] In the male serum testosterone is substantially reduced[11] and when the anorexia occurs before puberty is completed this may lead to an arrest of development, with a resumption after refeeding and normalization of testosterone levels.

Prolactin levels are usually normal.[24]

Insulin

The blood sugar and insulin response to intravenous dextrose are both raised in the anorexic, and this is one of the few functional abnormalities that persist when weight is regained.[6]

Water regulation

Anorexics show a deficient response to water deprivation[24] and a delayed excretion of a water load.[30]

Temperature regulation

Anorexics maintain a lower than normal basal temperature and have an impaired response both to heating and cooling.[24] This abnormality persists even when normal body weight is regained. There are also abnormal thermogenic responses to food.[23]

Body image

Anorexics tend to overestimate their body size when underweight and often show more accurate judgement when refed but there are many exceptions.[18]

Conclusion

Most of the physiological changes of anorexia nervosa are a non-specific response to starvation, apart from the disturbances of insulin and temperature regulation. If anorexics are constitutionally different, it is more likely to be in the way that their metabolism allows them to sustain such low body weights without collapse rather than in any primary interference with appetite and eating. In primitive conditions, with cycles of glut and famine, bulimia and the ability to cope with starvation must have had a valuable adaptive advantage.

Clinical presentation

The patient may often not complain of weight loss, and even though the loss may be extreme, will only admit to being 'a little thin'. Other patients may accept that they are underweight but assert that they are perplexed as to the cause as they are eating huge meals. On further investigation they may prove to secretly vomit their food or the 'huge' meals may prove to be in reality very small ones. They may complain of a lack of appetite or admit the appetite but avoid food because it induces abdominal pain (previous appendicectomy is a common finding among anorexics). Diarrhoea is commonly present and is usually due to purgation. Many patients use exercise as a means of keeping their weight low, and one of the intriguing aspects of anorexia nervosa lies in the patients' ability to remain active when grossly undernourished. Amenorrhoea is a necessary feature in the female and may be a very early feature, sometimes coming before there has been any significant loss of weight.

The patient has commonly been obese.[4] They often look and behave younger than their chronological age. They work hard at school to the exclusion of all other interests. There is often a hostile dependent relationship with the mother.

In males the presentation is either in a younger age group, in which it is often part of a school-refusal type of problem, or in older males, in whom problems of coping with homosexual feelings are prominent.

Treatment and progress

Treatment must be initially directed at regaining an ideal weight with subsequent sorting out of the problems that led to the illness. This sequence may seem illogical, but in practice it is extremely difficult to get the anorexic to look at her problems realistically while she is underweight. As she gets near to her ideal weight there is often a surprisingly rapid transformation from infantile to mature attitudes.

Patients vary in the degree of cooperation that they will offer to a refeeding programme. In the most difficult cases the patient will have to remain on strict bedrest, with the plumbing arrangements such that she cannot secretly dispose of food or vomit. The patient should be given regular meals and snacks with an adequate carbohydrate content such that she will gain up to 2 kg per week. If she gains quicker than this she is likely to feel out of control and in terror of a relentless progress to obesity. The patient also requires time to become accustomed to her new body shape and to acquire new eating habits. The patient should be forbidden food other than at set meals, thus avoiding the risk of a bulimic episode and subsequent panic. The patient should be sat with during meal times and for an hour thereafter. The time can be used to ensure that she finishes her meal and does not subsequently dispose of it. This time also provides an opportunity for getting to know the patient and dealing with problems as they arise. Chlorpromazine may be a helpful adjunct to treatment and may be required in a dosage of up to 600 mg/day in order to help the patient cope with the anxieties of eating and the tedium of her regime. It is important that the patient regains her target weight and spends further time in hospital maintaining that weight

in conditions of increasing independence. The ideal weight can be assessed from standard tables, but it is also important to take into account the patient's premorbid healthy weight, the weight at which ovulation ceased and familial factors. Thus, in a lean family a lower weight than in the tables might be acceptable, but where the patient ceased menstruation at a weight above the ideal it may be necessary to accept that her physiology is set to function normally at that higher weight, which should then be the target weight.

Other family members must be seen as part of the assessment, and it will usually be necessary to work with the mother to help her cope with the problems of her relationship and to help in rendering the patient more independent and self-confident. As the patient becomes more realistic about the problems she should have the opportunity of regular psychotherapeutic sessions for sorting out the underlying problems. Minuchin, Rosman and Baker have advocated a family therapy approach which as practised by them has given good results in the younger, less severely ill patients, treated outside hospital.[25]

Prognosis

The prognosis for anorexia nervosa will vary with the severity of the underlying personal and social disturbance and the adequacy of treatment. Generally speaking, in most large series some 40% to 60% of all patients make excellent and lasting recoveries. Some 5% die prematurely from the metabolic effects of starvation or suicide.[26, 32]

BULIMIA NERVOSA

Otherwise known as 'binge eating' or 'dietary chaos syndrome', bulimia nervosa has been defined by Russell.[29] It is a condition in which the subject eats and then vomits considerable quantities of food. The behaviour induces feelings of guilt and self-disgust. This behaviour is well-known in anorexia nervosa, but in recent years it has been found in association with normal weight. It may present diagnostic difficulties because even more than in anorexia nervosa these patients are very secretive and misleading about the true state of affairs and may complain of distension, abdominal pain, vomiting and so on, without revealing the cause. The habit can lead to hypokalaemia, metabolic alkalosis and acute dilatation of the stomach.

A less obvious complication of the syndrome is parotid enlargement,[22] which may be due to a hypersecretory response to the excessive quantities of food that are eaten, particularly following on a period of abstinence. Dental enamel may be destroyed by the acid contents of the stomach (perimolysis) and this may lead to the detection of a surreptitious vomiter.[19]

Fairburn and Cooper have demonstrated that the syndrome is exceedingly common in the community.[9] They advertised in a woman's magazine for individuals who used vomiting as a means of controlling weight and asked them to complete a questionnaire. They received 620 completed questionnaires; 83% of the respondents clearly had bulimia nervosa. Half of these felt that they needed medical help but only 2.5% were receiving any treatment, emphasizing the discrepancy between medically identified cases and the prevalence of the problem in the community.

In view of the frequency of anorexic/bulimic behaviour in the community it could be of value to screen routinely those attending a gastroenterological clinic, either while taking the history or by the use of a questionnaire. A suitable questionnaire could be the Eating Attitudes Test,[13] although there are some reservations about its interpretation for population studies.[34]

Clinical features

This is a predominantly female syndrome, and about half the patients have had an episode of anorexia nervosa. The peak age of onset of bulimia nervosa is 17–20; for those patients who come to medical attention the syndrome has been in existence for an average of four years. Patients are very secretive about their habit and when they are unable to pursue the habit undetected they avoid bulimic episodes.

Their psychological problems are similar to those found in anorexia nervosa, but they tend to be more outgoing and more sexually experienced. A minority abuse alcohol and drugs and are promiscuous.

Johnson and Larson found that bulimics suffered more episodes of dysphoria and social withdrawal than a control population.[21] They conceptualized the bulimia thus: initially food is used in an attempt to relieve unpleasant feelings, with the development of addiction and the use of vomiting to avoid obesity; this complex of behaviour produces a vicious circle. As with any morbid habit, it may so dominate the patient's awareness that it obscures the underlying problems that produce the behaviour, and this may

contribute to the powerful hold that the habit gains on the patient and act as a barrier to coming to grips with the underlying problems.

The condition may be physically and psychologically disabling. The metabolic complications are potentially life-threatening and the patients' lives are dominated by their habit. The syndrome may also reflect underlying handicaps of personality, which could constitute a problem even apart from the bulimia.

Treatment

There is no well-developed scheme of treatment like that for anorexia nervosa. The two main lines of approach, which can also be pursued simultaneously, are psychotherapeutic help with the underlying conflicts and a behavioural approach aimed at giving the patient better control over the habit. Such measures as keeping a diary of food consumed, a chart of binges and strategies that can be used for distracting the mind when working up to a binge may all be helpful.[8] Lacey has evolved a programme of treatment in which the patient keeps a diary of food eaten and of vomiting.[21a] She contracts to maintain her weight constant and to eat three meals a day at set times even when she has binged. She has individual sessions with a therapist, largely devoted to planning and monitoring behaviour, and group sessions devoted to sorting out interpersonal problems. Excellent results have been obtained in ten sessions at weekly intervals.

As yet there is little knowledge about the natural history and the long-term response to treatment of this condition.

PURGATIVE ADDICTION

Purgative abuse is common in bulimia nervosa and anorexia nervosa (40% in the series of Halmi *et al.*[15]), but severe abuse amounting to addiction can exist independently. The patients are nearly always women. They feel dirty inside and have a horror of inadequate evacuation of faeces, which with older patients may be iatrogenic. Purgation has played a major role in therapeutics for many centuries and concepts of colonic stasis and toxins have been widely held by the medical profession in the earlier part of the twentieth century.

Unfortunately, once the habit is established patients will not have a bowel action without purgation, and should they become oedematous and bloated owing to an associated electrolyte disturbance may purge themselves even more in an attempt to get rid of excessive fluid. They are usually secretive about their habit and will go to great lengths in order to acquire purgatives while in hospital for investigation, presenting considerable diagnostic difficulty. The physical aspects of this condition are further discussed in Chapter 11.

Treatment

Treatment is difficult. Even when confronted about the habit some patients will continue to deny that they take purgatives. There is usually a serious underlying disorder of personality, which may sometimes be amenable to psychotherapeutic help. At a simpler level it may be possible to wean patients on to safer methods of purgation. A mixture of psychological support and monitoring of electrolytes may prevent serious crises.

PSYCHOGENIC VOMITING

Psychogenic vomiting is an involuntary response to psychological strain and must be distinguished from self-induced vomiting such as is found in anorexia nervosa, bulimia nervosa and sometimes in peptic ulcer,[7] where it is used to relieve ulcer pain.

In a group of psychogenic vomiters studied by Hill, two-thirds of the patients were women.[17] The average age of the group was 38 and the current episode of vomiting had lasted from six months to seven years.

Although there had sometimes been earlier episodes of vomiting the older age at onset distinguishes the condition from anorexia and bulimia nervosa. Contrary to the popular misconception that such patients are unaffected by their vomiting, half of the group had lost 6 kg or more in weight and a number had developed metabolic complications.[16] There is always a danger that, because these patients are labelled as neurotic, physical reactions to hypokalaemia and hyperventilation will be misdiagnosed as hysterical phenomena.

These patients were often living with spouses or elderly parents whom they found difficult to tolerate: their relatives were literally 'making them sick'. Their histories often revealed that they had been vomiters in childhood. They had experienced an excessive amount of parental loss by death and separation and some could remember that they responded with vomiting at the time of their loss. There were also strong family histories of vomiting. It may be that these patients, in response to an early loss, maintained unrewarding relationships as adults that more secure individuals might have abandoned, and this has activated their tendency to vomit.

Treatment

These patients respond very well to the opportunity of 'bringing up' their difficulties verbally: it may give considerable relief. They are often rather dependent individuals and are also helped by consistent medical support. Symptomatic treatment with one of the phenothiazine tranquillizers may also be helpful.

REFERENCES

1   Boyar, R. M. & Bradlow, H. L. (1977) Studies of testosterone metabolism in anorexia nervosa. In *Anorexia Nervosa* (Ed.) Vigersky, R. A. pp. 271–276. New York: Raven Press.
2   Bruch, H. (1966) Anorexia nervosa and its differential diagnosis. *Journal of Nervous and Mental Disorders,* **141,** 555–566.
3   Crisp, A. H. (1970) Psychological aspects of some disorders of weight. In *Modern Trends in Psychosomatic Medicine,* Vol. 2 (Ed.) Hill, O. W. pp. 124–146. London: Butterworths.
4   Crisp, A. H. & Stonehill, E. (1971) Relation between aspects of nutritional disturbance and menstrual activity in primary anorexia nervosa. *British Medical Journal,* **iii,** 149–151.
5   Crisp, A. H. & Toms, D. A. (1972) Primary anorexia nervosa or weight phobia in the male: report on 13 cases. *British Medical Journal,* **i,** 334–338.
6   Crisp, A. H., Ellis, J. & Lowry, C. (1967) Insulin response to a rapid intravenous injection of dextrose in patients with anorexia nervosa and obesity. *Postgraduate Medical Journal,* **43,** 97–102.
7   Edwards, F. C. & Coghill, N. F. (1968) Clinical manifestations in patients with chronic atrophic gastritis, gastric ulcer and duodenal ulcer. *Quarterly Journal of Medicine,* **37,** 337–360.
8   Fairburn, C. G. (1982) Binge eating and its management. *British Journal of Psychiatry,* **141,** 631–633.
9   Fairburn, C. G. & Cooper, P. J. (1982) Self-induced vomiting and bulimia nervosa: an undetected problem. *British Medical Journal,* **284,** 1153–1155.
10 Feighner, J. P., Robins, E., Guze, S. B. *et al.* (1972) Diagnostic criteria for use in psychiatric research. *Archives of General Psychiatry,* **26,** 57–63.
11 Frankel, R. J. & Jenkins, J. S. (1975) Hypothalamic–pituitary function in anorexia nervosa. *Acta Endocrinologica,* **78,** 209–221.
12 Garfinkel, P. E., Brown, G. M., Stancer, H. C. & Moldofsky, H. (1965) Hypothalamic–pituitary function in anorexia nervosa. *Archives of General Psychiatry,* **32,** 739–744.
13 Garner, D. M., Olmsted, M. P., Bohr, Y. & Garfinkel, P. E. (1982) The Eating Attitudes Test: Psychometric features and clinical correlates. *Psychological Medicine,* **12,** 871–878.
14 Halmi, K. A., Sherman, B. M. & Zamudio, R. (1975) Impaired LH response to gonadotrophin-releasing

hormone (GnRH) in women with anorexia nervosa. *Psychosomatic Medicine*, **37**, 82–83.

15 Halmi, K. A., Goldberg, S. C., Eckert, E. *et al.* (1977) Pretreatment evaluation in anorexia nervosa. In *Anorexia* Nervosa (Ed.) Vigersky, R. A. pp. 43–54. New York: Raven Press.

16 Hill, O. W. (1967) Psychogenic vomiting and hypokalaemia. *Gut*, **8**, 98–101.

17 Hill, O. W. (1968) Psychogenic vomiting. *Gut*, **9**, 348–352.

18 Hill, O. W. (1976) Anorexia nervosa. In *Modern Trends in Psychosomatic Medicine*, Vol. 3 (Ed.) Hill, O. W. pp. 793–403. London: Butterworth.

19 House, R. C., Grisius, R., Bliziotes, M. M. & Licht, J. H. (1981) Perimolysis: Unveiling the surreptitious vomiter. *Oral Surgery*, **51**, 152–155.

20 Huenemann, R. L., Shapiro, L. R., Hampton, M. C. & Mitchell B. W. (1966) A longitudinal study of gross body composition and body conformation and their association with food and activity in a teenage population. *American Journal of Clinical Nutrition*, **18**, 325–338.

21 Johnson, C. & Larson, R. (1982) Bulimia: An analysis of moods and behaviour. *Psychosomatic Medicine*, **44**, 341–351.

21a Lacey, J. H. (1983) Bulimia nervosa, binge eating, and psychogenic vomiting: a controlled treatment study and long term outcome. *British Medical Journal*, **286**, 1609–1613.

22 Levin, P. A., Falko, J. M., Dixon, K. *et al.* (1980) Benign parotid enlargement in bulimia. *Annals of Internal Medicine*, **93**, 827–829.

23 Luck, P. & Wakeling, A. (1980) Altered thresholds for thermoregulatory sweating and vasodilatation in anorexia nervosa. *British Medical Journal*, **28**, 906–908.

24 Mecklenburg, T. S., Loriaux, D. C., Thompson, R. H. *et al.* (1974) Hypothalamic dysfunction in patients with anorexia nervosa. *Medicine*, **53**, 147–159.

25 Minuchin, S., Rosman B. L. & Baker, L. (1978) *Psychosomatic Families – Anorexia Nervosa in Context*. Cambridge, Massachusetts: Harvard University Press.

26 Morgan, H. G. & Russell, G. F. M. (1975) Value of family background and clinical features as predictors of long-term outcome in anorexia nervosa: four-year follow-up study of 41 patients. *Psychological Medicine*, **5**, 355–371.

27 Moshang, T., Jr, Parks, J. S., Baker, L. *et al.* (1975) Low serum triiodothyronine in patients with anorexia nervosa. *Journal of Clinical Endocrinology and Metabolism*, **40**, 470–473.

28 Rappoport, R., Prevot, C. & Czernichow, P. (1978) Growth hormone and somatomedin activity in children with anorexia nervosa in relation to weight changes. *Annales d'endocrinologie (Paris)*, **39**, 259–260.

29 Russell, G. F. M. (1979) Bulimia nervosa: an ominous variant of anorexia nervosa. *Psychological Medicine*, **9**, 429–448.

30 Russell G. F. M. & Bruce J. T. (1966) Impaired water diuresis in patients with anorexia nervosa. *American Journal of Medicine*, **40**, 38–48.

31 Russell, J. A. O. (1972) Psycho-social aspects of weight loss and amenorrhoea in adolescent girls. In *Psychosomatic Medicine in Obstetrics and Gynaecology* (Ed.) Morris, N. pp. 593–595. Basel: Karger.

32 Stonehill, E. & Crisp A. H. (1977) Psychoneurotic characteristics of patients with anorexia nervosa before and after treatment and at follow-up 4–7 years later. *Journal of Psychosomatic Research*, **21**, 187–193.

33 Theander, S. (1970) Anorexia nervosa. *Acta Psychiatrica Scandinavica* (Supplement 214).

34 Williams, P., Hand, O. & Tarnopolsky, A. (1982) The problem of screening for uncommon disorders – a comment on the Eating Attitudes Test. *Psychological Medicine*, **12**, 431–434.

Chapter 17
Nutrition

DEFICIENCY DISEASES

Normal body function requires adequate intake of nutrients. Malfunction can result from lack of macronutrients – energy or protein – or micronutrients such as vitamins or minerals which are needed in small amounts for specific biochemical roles.

MACRONUTRIENT DEFICIENCIES

Starvation

When dietary intake ceases totally, rapid adaptation occurs.[6] Liver glycogen is consumed and fat breakdown increases, supplying ketones as alternatives to glucose for brain metabolism. Insulin levels fall, and cortisol, glucagon and growth hormone levels rise. The inhibitory effect of insulin on lipolysis decreases, and fat is broken down into fatty acids and glycerol. Gluconeogenesis from protein increases and muscle wasting occurs through the alanine–gluconeogenesis cycle. There are rapid decreases in basal metabolic rate and body temperature, mediated through a fall in triiodothyronine (T_3) and an increase in reverse T_3 (rT_3), while thyroxine (T_4) levels are unchanged. The increased energy supply from fat conserves glucose and prevents hypoglycaemia. Protein catabolism is slowed and serum albumin levels are maintained, at least initially.

The absence of nutrients in the gut results in a very rapid loss of cellular mass, even when nutrition is maintained by parenteral feeding. The rate of DNA synthesis falls, cellularity declines and disaccharidase levels fall. The pancreas loses cell mass and exocrine secretions decrease.[12]

Protein–energy malnutrition

In contrast to starvation, which is acute, protein–energy malnutrition (PEM) is a chronic state resulting from the interaction of dietary deficiencies and infection (Figure 17.1). *Marasmus* resembles starvation: there is severe wasting of fat and muscle, but physiological adaption is good. When provided with energy, the children recover quickly. In *kwashiorkor* there is maladaption: fat stores are increased even when energy deficiency is acute and low levels of important proteins such as albumin lead to clinical problems such as oedema.[2]

FACTORS DETERMINING THE DEVELOPMENT OF KWASHIORKOR OR MARASMUS

The factors which determine the type of PEM a given child develops are not clear. Originally, it was thought that children who developed

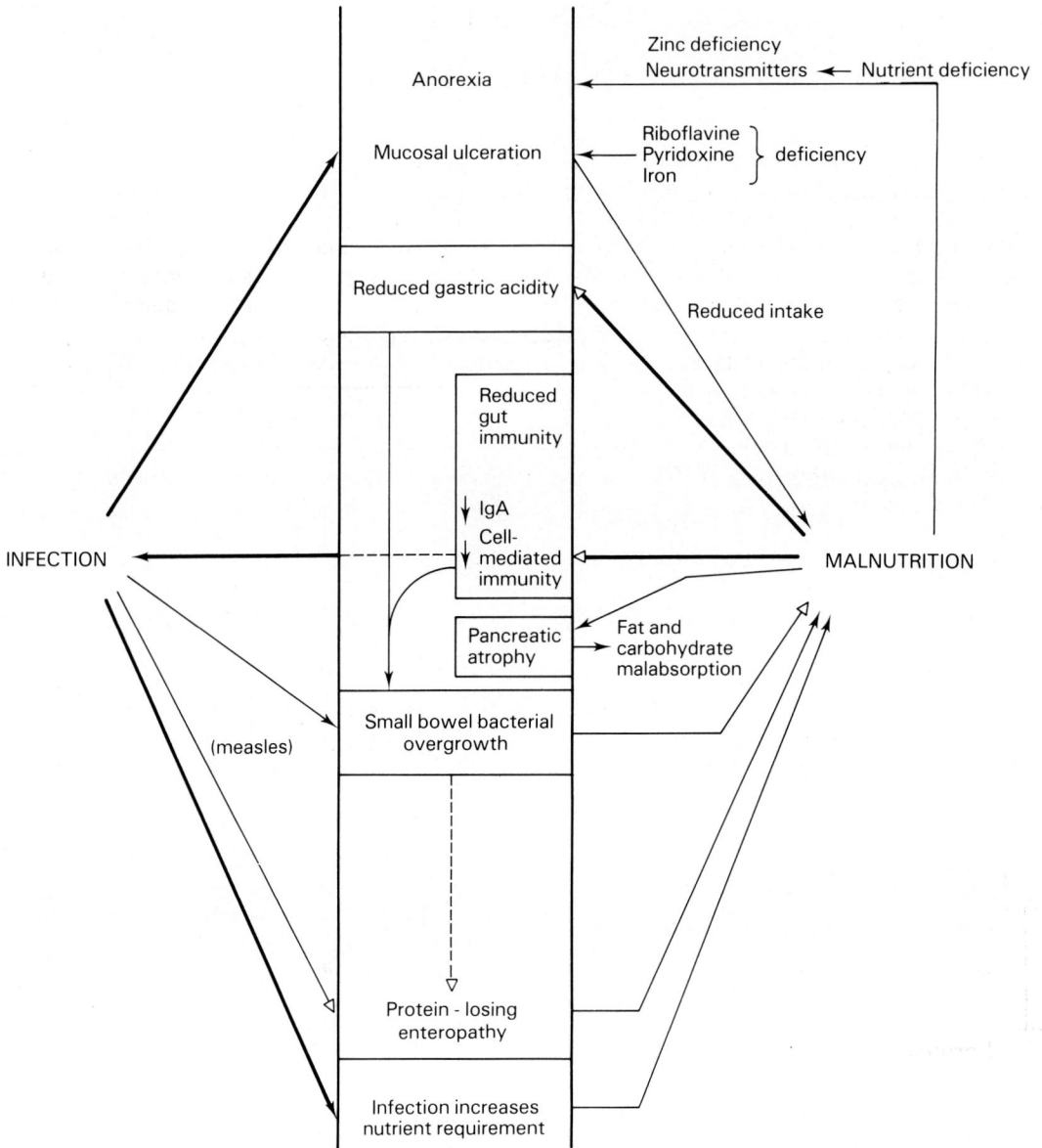

Fig. 17.1 The interaction of malnutrition and infection in the aetiology of protein–energy malnutrition.

kwashiorkor suffered from protein deficiency in the face of excess carbohydrate, while marasmus resulted from lack of energy. However, dietary analysis shows that protein deficiency when measured as the proportion of energy intake derived from protein rarely falls below calculated requirements even in places where kwashiorkor is common. In Nigeria, children with kwashiorkor were found to have consumed 7% of their diet as protein, but had only taken 25% of their energy requirement.[26] Unless energy requirements are satisfied, protein is broken down to supply the energy deficit and thus is not available for protein synthesis. Efforts to prevent

kwashiorkor solely by increasing the protein in the diet are doomed to failure unless energy requirements are satisfied. The protein content of most Third World diets is adequate, but energy requirements are not.[25]

PEM is usually precipitated by infection. In the Gambia, marasmus is more common than in Uganda, which may be because of the higher prevalence of infection in the former. Cortisol levels were found to be higher as a result of the infection, and this might favour the wasting of muscle and preservation of serum albumin, leading to a marasmic type of PEM.[40a] Infection can lead to malnutrition through repeated episodes of diarrhoea or pneumonia associated with respiratory infections. The weight loss is not fully recovered because of the high bulk and low energy density of the diet.[24, 34]

The importance of imbalance in nutrient deficiency as a factor is suggested by the epidemiological data: kwashiorkor is less common where a wide variety of foods is consumed, for example among the Sandawe of Tanzania.[28] Recent evidence implicates zinc deficiency as the critical factor responsible for immune deficiency and the skin lesions which are characteristic of the disease.[16] Children with kwashiorkor may lose their oedema on a low-protein or even a no-protein diet, highlighting the role of sodium pump abnormalities, perhaps mediated through deficiencies of vanadium or other trace elements.[14] Other proposed explanations include variations in individual protein or energy needs and, more recently, release of serum proteinase inhibitors.

THE ECOLOGY OF DEFICIENCY DISEASES

Man's ancestors were probably hunter–gatherers whose way of life was similar to the Bushmen of Africa. The type of diet consumed would have been one of great variety – traditional diets of the !Kung Bushmen include 40 different plants, besides insects and animals. Such a diet is also rich in 'fibre', lacks refined carbohydrate and is low in fat. Leafy vegetables and berries would have a high content of folic acid, ascorbic acid and trace elements, and the animal protein would be rich in essential amino acids and fats. Because of frequent droughts, however, such populations would often be subject to famine.

With the development of agriculture, the dietary patterns changed. Storage carbohydrates of manioc (cassava or yucca) became the chief energy sources. Such diets contain less protein and trace elements and the amino acid and vitamin pattern is often imbalanced.

With the coming of industrialization, food consumption changed yet again, with the introduction of 'junk foods', further refinement of staples, removing fibre and vitamins, and the introduction of chemicals to prevent decay in storage, and to enhance flavour and appearance.

These changes are reflected in the type of deficiency diseases seen in these communities. In hunter–gatherer or pastoral societies, gross starvation is frequent; however, specific syndromes such as kwashiorkor and vitamin deficiencies

are uncommon. With colonization, the East African staple food changed from millet to maize and pellagra appeared. The habit of polishing rice appeared in Malaysia and caused beri beri.

In societies with a long stable history methods have evolved to maximize the utilization of diets. For example, in Central America cooking maize with ash increases the availability of tryptophan and niacin, thus preventing pellagra. In the Indian subcontinent an adequate protein intake is provided, with little or no animal protein, by mixing foods of complementary amino acid composition.

In the Third World, the process of industrialization changes the patterns of deficiency disease. Urbanization is associated with more marasmus and infection owing to crowding and lack of sanitation. As infection and malnutrition nearly always go together it is often difficult to distinguish their individual effects.

In fully industrialized societies, overnutrition is the problem and deficiency diseases tend to be confined to high-risk groups such as the elderly and 'alternative culture' groups eating fad diets such as macrobiotic diets.

Isolated deficiency diseases

Specific isolated deficiencies are seldom seen. A diet high in protein, for example, tends also to be high in trace elements such as zinc. The diet of the urban poor tends to be based on one or two foods such as flour or rice and hence lacks micronutrients as well as being energy-deficient. When the general level of nutrition is suboptimal, the syndrome of marasmus or general wasting is seen, but as the intake level falls, deficiencies of other micronutrients are exposed.

Energy deficiency may result from failure to eat sufficient amounts of local food. Typical diets in Africa consist of banana, yam, and cassava, which have a low energy density. Having a small stomach volume, the child cannot obtain sufficient energy before becoming satiated.[34] Also, social customs often allocate pure staple to the mother and child and the 'sauce' to the father and most of the energy content is derived from the staple carbohydrate, while the sauce often contains beans, fat, meat, peanuts and other appetizing and energy-rich ingredients. The low energy density of the common staples also prevents children who have suffered from infections such as gastroenteritis from catching up by increasing their food intake during convalescence, although in New Guinea, for example, high-energy pork is reserved for feasts and convalescence.

1218   *Nutrition*

The availability of nutrients in these diets is also reduced because of the high content of fibre and phytates. The fibre not only satiates appetite because of its bulk and water content, but also impairs digestion of nutrients such as zinc, iron and calcium which may be bound by the high phytate content.

CLINICAL SYNDROMES OF
PROTEIN–ENERGY MALNUTRITION

The classical syndromes of marasmus and kwashiorkor are the tip of the iceberg. The prevalence is only 1% to 2%, although 10% to 50% of children in the non-industrial world suffer from growth failure. This is measured by comparing their weight and height against standards from adequately nourished communities.

PEM can be classified by comparing the child's weight with the 50th centile of weight for his age according to WHO or Stuart standards. By using the 'Wellcome criteria'[13] children can be classified according to severity as undernourished, marasmus, marasmic kwashiorkor or kwashiorkor (Table 17.1).

Table 17.1   A classification of protein–energy malnutrition.[13]

| | Percentage of expected weight for age | |
	<60%	60–80%
Oedema	Marasmic kwashiorkor	Kwashiorkor
No oedema	Marasmus	Underweight

The Wellcome classification does not take failure to grow into account. Children with chronic malnutrition may be stunted (below 90% height for age). If their body weight loss is in proportion to their height deficit they are perfectly proportioned dwarfs.

Waterlow has proposed a classification in which weight-for-height is used as an indication of current nutritional status and height-for-age as an indication of past nutritional history.[40] In a population children can be divided into broad categories: normal, wasted but not stunted (acute malnutrition), wasted and stunted (acute on chronic), and stunted but not wasted (chronic).

Infant and child mortality rates in developing countries range from 170 to 20 per 1000 live births. A high proportion of those who survive fail to attain their full genetic potential for either intelligence or growth. The main reason for this is subclinical protein–energy malnutrition. The

Table 17.2   Clinical differences between kwashiorkor and marasmus.

	Kwashiorkor	Marasmus
Oedema	Yes	No
Hair	Pale/easily pluckable	Normal
Skin	Flaky-paint rash	Normal
Muscle wasting	Moderate	Severe
Appetite	Poor	Good
Mental state	Apathy/irritability	Alert
Hypothermia	Moderate	Severe
Liver	Enlarged	Normal
Tonsils/spleen	Reduced	Reduced
Face	Moon-shaped	Wasted

functional value of these criteria in terms of the quality of adult performance is poorly understood. The final adult height in developing countries is reduced, but the delay in skeletal maturation allows some catch-up in height, providing that the nutritional insult was not too early in development.

Table 17.2 summarizes the clinical differences between kwashiorkor and marasmus, while Table 17.3, 17.4 and 17.5 summarize the effects of PEM on biochemical values, blood constituents and hormones respectively.

Marasmus
The marasmic child has the classical appearance of starvation. There is gross wasting of muscle and fat, but skin and hair are usually normal.

Table 17.3   Biochemical changes in protein–energy malnutrition.

Electrolytes	Plasma	Intracellular
Na^+	Normal	↑
K^+	Normal	↓
Mg^{2+}	Normal or ↓	↓
Ca^{2+} (serum)	Normal	?
Zn^{2+}	Normal or ↓	↓
Water	—	↑
Serum protein		
Albumin	Reduced	
Immunoglobulin	Increased	
Transferrin	Reduced	
Transcortin (cortisol-binding protein)	Reduced	
Retinol-binding protein	Reduced	
Lipids		
Lipoprotein	Reduced	
Cholesterol	Reduced	
Glucose	Often reduced	

↑ = increased; ↓ = reduced.

Table 17.4 Blood constituents in protein–energy malnutrition.

	Marasmus	Kwashiorkor
Total protein	Normal	↑↓
Albumin	Normal	↓
Transferrin	?	↓
Transcortin (cortisol-binding protein	Normal	↓
Immunoglobulins	↑	↑
Lipoprotein	Normal	↓
Complement C3	?	↓

There is no oedema and the child is alert and hungry if fed. The patient usually sits immobile, the limbs are flexed and permanent flexion deformities of the hips may result. The temperature may be reduced, even in tropical countries. The intercostal muscles are wasted and coughing is weak. Clinical signs are often absent even in the presence of infection. The pulse is normal, the heart may be small and cardiac sounds muffled. The abdomen is usually distended, but in contrast to kwashiorkor the liver is not enlarged. The rectum is sometimes prolapsed. The stools are usually soft, and chronic diarrhoea may occur. Careful palpation may reveal enlarged abdominal nodes suggestive of tuberculosis. The tonsils are small because of wasting of the lymphoreticular system. Splenic enlargement is usually the consequence of malaria or sickle cell anaemia.

This condition arises during famines when there is a general reduction in energy intake, in children of six months or less whose mothers fail to breastfeed, and in children with chronic infection (such as tuberculosis), severe mental retardation or congenital heart disease.

Kwashiorkor

The characteristic features of kwashiorkor have been summarized by Trowell *et al.*[38] The early changes in the skin are hyperkeratotic; it then flakes, leaving a weeping dermatosis characteristically distributed in the flexures. In mild cases, hypopigmentation of the face and flexor surfaces is seen. The hair shows dyspigmentation, especially at the hair line. The hairs themselves are atrophic and brittle and are easily plucked without pain. Curiously, the eyelashes are often luxuriant and thick. The face is 'moon-shaped' and body fat is normal or increased. Muscle wasting is concealed and the appearance of the body suggests Cushing's disease.

Hypothermia occurs, but is less marked than in marasmus. The blood pressure may be reduced, and the heart sounds are soft. In severe cases, the extremities are cold and peripheral perfusion is reduced. During refeeding, cardiac failure with gallop rhythm may develop if excessive energy is given too early.

Many cases are precipitated by diarrhoea, which leads to dehydration. This may be masked by oedema, and it is not uncommon to find both oedema and dehydration in the same patient. The abdomen is distended and the liver markedly enlarged, with a soft smooth edge. The mucous membranes usually show chronic ulceration, especially at the corner of the mouth. Candidiasis is usual, especially after measles, and may also be seen at the anus.

The patient's behaviour is characterized by lethargy and lack of interest in the surroundings. On stimulation, the child is intensely irritable and peevish. There is muscular weakness and hypotonia, the reflexes often showing markedly prolonged relaxation. Severe anorexia occurs and tube feeding is often necessary.

INFECTION IN THE AETIOLOGY
OF PEM

The environment of children in developing countries is highly contaminated with pathogens. The climate favours the transmission of malaria, poor sanitation results in contamination of water with faecal organisms, the humidity and constant warmth encourages bacteria and flies, and lack of water discourages hygiene. Consequently, children and adults are infected most of the time.

In Uganda the incidence of PEM increased after the rains with the rise in malaria and respiratory infections rather than at times of drought or food shortage.[32] Children attending a 'well child clinic' were almost always colonized by entero and respiratory viruses.[11] Guatemalan children are infected almost constantly, and longitudinal studies have demonstrated that recurrent infections result in anorexia, loss of weight, and eventually in frank PEM.[24] These frequent bouts of gastroenteritis are thought to result from infection with specific enteroviruses such as rotavirus or from infection with enterotoxigenic bacteria.

Bacteriological studies of staple foods such as tortillas in Guatemala and porridges in the Gambia and artificial milks show very heavy bacterial contamination. Ingestion of these diets may contribute to small bowel overgrowth.

BREASTFEEDING AND
PROTEIN–ENERGY MALNUTRITION

The traditional pattern of breastfeeding in developing countries is rapidly being eroded.

Breastfeeding protects infants from PEM by providing immunological factors such as virus- and bacteria-specific sIgA and cell-mediated immunity, as well as non-specific antiviral and antibacterial factors. Artificial feeds are usually contaminated and prepared wrongly and contribute to malnutrition.

MALNUTRITION AND THE GUT

Diarrhoea is a common complication of PEM. Between the ages of seven and thirteen months, children in the Gambia have diarrhoea on six days in each month on average. The main aetiological factor is very heavy bacterial colonization of the upper bowel and reduced concentration of bile salts.[33] Rotavirus infection is the commonest aetiological factor in Guatemala, while in the crowded cities enterotoxinogenic *E. coli*, *Salmonella* and *Shigella* are prevalent. Acute secretory diarrhoea causes death by electrolyte depletion. It may also be followed by prolonged chronic diarrhoea in the survivors.

In children with PEM, measles presents with severe diarrhoea caused by 'Koplik's' lesions throughout the intestine. Measles is often followed by *Candida* infection of the mouth and gastrointestinal tract.

Enteric bacterial infections are frequent because faeces contaminate the drinking water, personal hygiene is poor owing to lack of water, and flies and the warm weather encourage bacterial growth and dispersion. In addition, indigenous methods of preparing food often involve leaving warm foods overnight, thus encouraging bacterial growth.[24]

The effect of diarrhoea is often worsened by incorrect attempts at treatment: very often the children are starved or put on clear fluids for long periods. During recovery prolonged hypokalaemia results in anorexia, intestinal ileus and weakness. The introduction of WHO Oral Rehydration Fluid as the first line of treatment has greatly reduced these complications and the decline in the practice of 'resting' the bowel and the early reintroduction of food reduces the risk of malnutrition and promotes mucosal healing.

Clinical effects of diarrhoea

The anorexia associated with gastroenteritis significantly decreases intake. Repeated attacks of gastroenteritis produce significant weight loss, especially in children already malnourished. Viral infections complicated by vitamin deficiencies lead to a painful mouth, which inhibits eating. The associated fever, mobilization of immune mechanisms, increased basal metabolic rate and the losses due to diarrhoea, sweating and vomiting increase nutrient requirements.[5] Changes in function of the gut interfere with absorption. Reduced D-xylose absorption accompanies systemic infection.[9]

After the episode of infection, failure to replace potassium leads to prolonged weakness, atonia of the gut and anorexia. In 10% of cases, chronic diarrhoea may follow an acute episode. This may be due to damage to the intestinal mucosa, reduction in brush border lactase or contamination of the small bowel. The child's ability to catch up when he regains his appetite is hampered by the very low energy density and high bulk of many tropical staple foods. The small child cannot eat enough to satisfy his needs, unless provided with a high-energy rehabilitation food.

GASTROINTESTINAL ABNORMALITIES

The mouth

The mucosa of the mouth and tongue is atrophic in PEM, the sign of 'sordes' resulting from chronic infection with bacteria, virus such as herpes, or thrush; such infection commonly occurs as a result of depression of local immunity and the resulting sore mouth is an important cause of anorexia. In severe malnutrition, infection with *Leptotrichea buccalis* (*Fusiformis fusiformis*) can lead to cancrum oris, a necrotic lesion which exposes underlying bone.

The tongue is smooth, with papillary atrophy and fissuring, which is also typical of associated dietary deficiencies such as iron deficiency and vitamin B_{12} deficiency.

The small intestine

Intestinal biopsy shows that in early PEM the villus and crypt cellularity is equally affected, but in more severe cases villous atrophy occurs. The normal finger villi are replaced by ridges and convolutions, and the surface area is markedly reduced.[36] As villous cells predominantly subserve absorption and crypt cells secretion, this may contribute to the frequency with which diarrhoea occurs. The bowel wall is permeable to dietary peptides, giving rise to elevated levels of food antibodies.[7, 8]

Brush-border lactase levels are diminished and xylose tolerance is impaired. Reduced absorption of sucrose and glucose can be detected when these sugars are given in hypertonic solutions. When administered isotonically in small boluses, absorption is satisfactory.[20]

Reduced absorption of fat and vitamin A has also been demonstrated, but amino acid absorption is only affected in severe cases.[1]

Follow-up studies after treatment of PEM show that these changes persist for years. Similar changes occur in adults in the tropics. It seems likely that chronic infection may be responsible for these changes, perhaps through immune damage caused by T cell cytolysis.

The significance of malabsorption is controversial: the bowel reserve capacity is such that treatment of PEM with high-fat, lactose-containing diets can be initiated within a few days of commencing therapy.[3]

The contaminated bowel syndrome in PEM. Bacterial counts in the small intestine show an increase in *E. coli* and anaerobes such as *Bacteroides* spp., anaerobic lactobacilli and clostridia which are able to deconjugate bile salts to form free bile salts. When the level of conjugated biles salts falls below the level necessary for micelle formation, fat malabsorption occurs.[17] In addition, a high proportion of people living in these contaminated environments have elevated levels of breath hydrogen. As a result of bacterial contamination, a spectrum of absorptive defects occurs – in absorption of fat, carbohydrate, vitamin B_{12}, water and electrolytes. It has been suggested that this causes the chronic diarrhoea seen so frequently in PEM. Why this contamination occurs is unknown; decreased gastric acidity, high levels of environmental contamination and reduced gut immunity are all possible causes.

The large intestine
The large intestine is usually dilated, giving rise to the pot belly of PEM. Intestinal transit times are accelerated, but fluid absorption is probably unaffected. Prolapse of the rectum is often found, especially in children with heavy *Trichuris* infection.

The exocrine pancreas
In malnourished animals, the weight of the pancreas decreases proportionately more than body weight; this is due to loss of DNA content and cell number. In PEM the pancreas is atrophic, with loss of cellularity, reduced levels of lipase, trypsin and amylase and an impaired response to pancreozymin stimulation. There is no evidence that chronic pancreatitis follows PEM.

The liver in PEM
Fatty infiltration of the liver is a cardinal feature of kwashiorkor. Liver failure, with jaundice, clotting defects and raised transaminase levels, has been described in very severe cases in Jamaica, but not in Africa. Jamaican cases of kwashiorkor also tend to have more fat infiltration than those in Africa. In a baboon model of kwashiorkor, the addition of sucrose to the protein-deficient diet increased fat deposition.[10] This observation may be relevant, since Jamaican children have a very high sucrose intake. The fat deposition starts in the portal tracts and spreads towards the centre. It results from impaired hepatic synthesis of very-low-density lipoproteins,[2] which prevent fat from being transported or utilized. The protein matrix is wasted, cell atrophy occurs and the endoplasmic reticulum disappears. Children with marasmus do not have fatty livers. Liver glycogen stores are increased; the release by glucagon is not significantly reduced. Bile production is also diminished.

Albumin levels are reduced in kwashiorkor, especially in African children, but not in marasmus. The rate of synthesis is depressed and despite a slower catabolic rate serum levels are low (10–20 g/l). This may play a role in the aetiology of the characteristic oedema. It results from a reduction in the pool of amino acids available for synthesis.[39]

The endocrine pancreas
The effects of the endocrine adaptations (Table 17.5) in PEM are to maintain blood glucose. Insulin levels are low and the response to intravenous glucose is blunted. When children are supplemented with potassium, the insulin response improves.[22] An additional factor may be chromium deficiency. Persistence of low insulin levels after treatment has been reported; its significance is uncertain.

The blood glucose level is low in PEM. The adrenergic response is defective. Blood glucagon levels are reduced in fasting, hypoglycaemic children. Hypoglycaemia contributes to hypothermia, and increased death rates occur in children allowed to get cold or fed at infrequent intervals. The normal shivering and sweating effect of adrenal secretion does not occur.[19]

IMPAIRED IMMUNE RESPONSE IN PEM

Deficiency of the immune response is an important complication of PEM.

Delayed hypersensitivity. Skin reactions to both *Candida* and tuberculin are impaired. This is associated with reduced T cell populations

Table 17.5 Endocrine changes in protein–energy malnutrition.

		Kwashiorkor	Marasmus
Adrenocortical	Cortisol total	↑	↑
axis	free	↑	?
	Diurnal rhythm	Abolished	Normal
	ACTH response	↓	↑
	Dexamethazone suppression	Normal	?
Thyroid function	Protein-bound iodine	↓	Normal
	Thyroxine (T₄)	↑ or normal	↓ or normal
	Thyroid-stimulating hormone	↓ or normal or ↑	↓ or normal or ↑
	^{131}I uptake	Normal	↓ or normal
Glucose metabolism	Insulin	↓ or normal	↓
	Glucose	↓ or normal	↓ or normal
	Glucose tolerance	↓	Normal
	Glucagon response	↓ or normal	?
	Growth hormone	↑	?
Growth	Somatomedin	↓	?

↑ = increased; ↓ = reduced. Data from Pimstone (1976).[31a]

and diminished mitogen-stimulated transformation.[7, 8] In the gut, the evidence for depressed T cell function is that protein-deficient young animals have reduction of absolute and relative numbers of intraepithelial lymphocytes. It has been postulated that the villous atrophy in PEM could be the result of T-cell-induced damage from the immunostimulation caused by chronic infection.

Humoral immunity. In general, serum immunoglobulin levels are increased in PEM. The response to antibody stimulation is also normal. However, IgA levels are reduced: young rats have reduced IgA in colostrum, and the response of secretory IgA to immunization with measles is reduced.[7, 8]

Structural changes in the cysternae of B lymphocytes have been reported.[23]

The immune response to polio immunization is diminished in children in developing countries, but this does not appear to be related to their nutritional state, but rather to the frequency of competing enterovirus infection and by the presence in saliva of an inhibitor which can be neutralized with horse antihuman globulin.

Macrophage function. Clearance of PVP and antibody affinity are diminished in children with PEM and in protein-deficient rats. However, the numbers and appearance of macrophages in the gut and liver are normal.

Iron deficiency. This almost invariably accompanies PEM and contributes to the immunodepression.

The role of iron is complex: on the one hand, it is a component of the cytochrome system and necessary for the integrity of cell function; on the other, excess free iron is required for the multiplication of bacteria. When the binding capacity of transferrin is exceeded, free iron enhances bacterial multiplication, and exacerbation of bacterial infection and malaria has been suggested. Lack of iron impairs the delayed hypersensitivity response and, more specifically, reduces the capacity of neutrophils to kill bacteria.

Zinc deficiency. Zinc seems to play a crucial role in the immune depression associated with PEM. The atrophy of the thymus is reversed by zinc supplementation. Zinc also influences T cell function since local application of zinc sulphate can repair the depressed cutaneous delayed hypersensitivity response to *Candida* antigen.[16] Zinc is also necessary for in vitro lymphocyte transformation. The presence of zinc–transferrin is a critical factor.

Vitamin deficiency. The most important vitamin concerned with gut function is pyridoxine, because of its central role in nucleic acid synthesis. It is associated with reduced numbers of lymphocytes and thymus involution.

TREATMENT OF DIARRHOEA WITH
ORAL REHYDRATION IN PEM

The development of a balanced oral electrolyte solution – WHO oral rehydration fluid[27] – has revolutionized treatment of diarrhoea in the developing world. Treatment can be given to moderately dehydrated children orally at a rate of 100 ml/kg over four hours. Because of low glucose concentration (110 mmol/l), it is adequately absorbed despite the suboptimal function of the small gut and facilitates the absorption of sodium and potassium. Rehydration occurs rapidly and breast or weaning feed is commenced after four hours. Rapid provision of nutrients in the gut encourages early healing of the gut mucosa. The rapid replacement of potassium leads to resolution of hypotonia, improved appetite and recovery of weight loss. Field trials in the Philippines and elsewhere have confirmed the value and practicality of this method of treatment. The early refeeding does not lead to prolongation of diarrhoea, provided that small boluses of isosmotic feeds are given frequently.

Children examined repeatedly show impaired growth associated with each bout of infection, with very poor catch-up between bouts. The impaired immune response to infection increases the clinical severity of many diseases.

THE EFFECT OF MEASLES ON THE GUT IN PEM

In measles, the 'Koplik's' lesions are extensively distributed through the gut, giving rise to a bloody diarrhoea. The desquamation of skin, fever and anorexia further erode the nutritional state of the child. A protein-losing enteropathy can develop. After the acute phase, staphylococcal pneumonia often develops. Severe *Candida* infection with extensive involvement of the alimentary tract may then follow. Not surprisingly, measles epidemics are often followed by kwashiorkor: the mortality in the Congo, for example, can be as high as 30%. The stress of measles in the malnourished child can expose other deficiency disease, especially vitamin A deficiency, which produces rapid onset of xerophthalmia and blindness.

TREATMENT OF PEM

Mortality rates in the 1960s were between 5% and 10%, but in the 1970s the rate fell to less than 1% in many units. The principles of treatment are:

1 Initiation of cure by giving only basal energy requirements as frequent small boluses of a diet containing 0.7 $g \cdot kg^{-1} \cdot day^{-1}$ protein and 380 $kJ \cdot kg^{-1} \cdot day^{-1}$ (90 $kcal \cdot kg^{-1} \cdot day^{-1}$).

2 Correction of electrolyte disturbances using oral rehydration fluid.

3 Prevention of hypoglycaemia by frequent feeding and by giving a porridge feed at night to cover the long night and cold dawn.

4 Enteral feeding if the patient is anorexic.

5 Gradual increase of energy from basal (**1** above) to 630–840 $kJ \cdot kg^{-1} \cdot day^{-1}$ (150–200 $kcal \cdot kg^{-1} \cdot day^{-1}$) and protein to 2.5 $g \cdot kg^{-1} \cdot day^{-1}$ using a milk- and vegetable-oil-reinforced diet.

6 Replacement of potassium and magnesium deficits.

7 Replacement of trace elements and vitamins during the period of rapid weight gain.

Despite the impaired absorption of lactose and fat, providing small boluses of isotonic feed are offered, absorption and then weight gain are usually very fast and should exceed 10 $g \cdot kg^{-1} \cdot day^{-1}$. In cases with prolonged diarrhoea metronidazole has been found useful, but its value is not yet proven.

During recovery, feeding with excess energy can lead to cardiac failure and massive fluid secretion into the gut due to excessive sodium pump action.[29]

During refeeding, the voluntary appetite is enormous. When feeds containing energy reinforcement in the form of added fat to bring the energy content up to 6.3 MJ/l (1500 kcal/l) are offered, weight increases rapidly, then falls as the child attains his expected weight-for-height.[3] During this phase of rapid growth, balanced vitamin and trace element supplementation is vital.

MICRONUTRIENT DEFICIENCY DISEASES

Man is omnivorous, eats a wide range of foods and seems to have a relatively high requirement for vitamins and trace elements. When a high-protein diet is consumed, trace elements are present as fellow travellers. While energy foods such as carbohydrates and fats are difficult to destroy, the quantity of trace elements and vitamins may be influenced by a number of factors.

The geology of the environment. Zinc deficiency occurs in areas of the Middle East with low soil zinc levels. In China and Southern Africa, geological mineral deficiencies are responsible for trace element imbalance in the diet.[41]

Phytate and fibre in the diet. These reduce the availability of calcium in wheat flour and in millet-based diets. The absorption of zinc from such diets is also impaired.

Preparation. Ascorbic acid (vitamin C) is destroyed by prolonged boiling in traditional British cooking. In Tanzania, soaking of maize and removal of the supernatant reduces riboflavine (vitamin B_2) and nicotinic acid by 50%. Removal of the husks from rice eliminates most of the thiamine (vitamin B_1) and causes beri beri in South East Asia. In contrast, the preparation of soya bean curd (tofu) by fermentation increases the vitamin concentration and allows increased absorption of amino acids. Native beers made from fermented millet, yams or bananas yield significant amounts of B vitamins.

Nutrient imbalance. When growth and cell multiplication are suppressed by PEM, underlying deficiency can be exposed if treatment is started with energy and protein, but without minerals and vitamins. Blindness from vitamin A deficiency can occur during the treatment of kwashiorkor. Pellagra can be produced by excess lysine in the diet, and excess zinc supplementation can precipitate copper deficiency.

Selection of diets. Many people have dietary restrictions which deprive them of essential nutrients. In East Africa eggs are forbidden to pregnant women because they are thought to result in deafness of the baby. In times of famine, when only storage foods are available, deficiency diseases occur. Many deficiency diseases are seasonal. Low levels of vitamin D occur in some Middle Eastern countries due to lack of exposure to sunlight. Lack of fruit and green vegetables causes scurvy, which is now seen increasingly in the elderly poor. With economic hardship, city dwellers living on maize flour, bread and refined foods are prone to vitamin deficiency. Alcoholism is the most common cause of vitamin deficiencies in the industrialized nations, but an increasingly important cause of deficiency diseases is the dietary restrictions of some religious cults and other groups: vegan diets are deficient in vitamin B_{12} and zen macrobiotic diets may produce frank PEM.

Trace elements

The importance of minute amounts of trace elements in the diet reflects their indispensable role in the structure of specific enzymes. These metalloenzymes are essential in many metabolic functions.

ZINC DEFICIENCY

Zinc deficiency occurs as a primary deficiency disease. In the Middle East it has been described in adolescent boys with growth failure and delayed sexual development. It has also been described in poorer socioeconomic groups in the USA and Australia. The clinical symptoms include anorexia and loss of taste acuity. The appetite is reduced and there are mucocutaneous lesions around the mouth and anus. The skin lesions are both hyperkeratotic and bullous in appearance. In Jamaica, low levels of zinc are associated with reduced taste acuity in pregnancy.

In PEM, serum zinc levels are normal in marasmus but low in kwashiorkor. Unless supplementation is given during treatment, levels fall.[15] The skin lesions of kwashiorkor respond to local applications of zinc and the impaired cutaneous delayed hypersensitivity is also reversed. Supplementation with zinc also hastens thymus regeneration during refeeding.

Zinc is an important cofactor in enzymes concerned with DNA synthesis and lymphocyte transformation. It is also associated with insulin release. Severe zinc deficiency occurs in acrodermatitis enteropathica, because of a congenital defect in zinc absorption from the intestinal mucosa. In breast milk zinc is transported with a ligand which facilitates delivery to and absorption from the mucosa. In foods high in phytates such as soya-based 'milks', it is chelated and deficiency can result.

Vitamins

VITAMIN A DEFICIENCY

Vitamin A deficiency damages the ability of epithelial cells to differentiate and causes keratinizing metaplasia of mucous epithelium and ciliated epithelium. The vitamin inhibits the conversion of cysteine to cystine and oxidation of sulphydryl groups, thereby preventing keratinization. When vitamin A is deficient local infection is inadequately contained and wound healing is delayed. Vitamin A has a protective effect from carcinogenesis and deficiency is implicated in carcinoma of the stomach and nasopharynx.[35] Adequate amounts of vitamin A occur in tissue fluids and are present in milk, liver, eggs and meat. Carotenes, precursors of the vitamin, are present in leafy vegetables and fruits and are the chief sources in developing countries. Deficiency is prevalent in Central America and Africa. It may be seasonal; on the other hand, the mango season in Central America and the Caribbean may supply sufficient stores for the rest of the year.

Release of vitamin A from liver stores is defective in PEM due to the failure of the liver to synthesize retinol binding protein. In vitamin-A-deficient children blood levels may rise when the PEM is treated. Absorption of the vitamin is impaired in ascariasis. Treatment of vitamin A deficiency is urgent in PEM, because treatment with energy and protein alone may precipitate xerophthalmia and blindness. The vitamin should be given intramuscularly, or in a water-soluble form because of impaired fat absorption in PEM.

NICOTINIC ACID DEFICIENCY

Nicotinic acid (niacin) occupies a central place in energy metabolism. It is an essential component of coenzyme I (nicotinamide adenine dinucleotide) and coenzyme II (nicotinamide adenine dinucleotide phosphate). These enzymes mediate energy transport, amino acid metabolism and pentose synthesis. Pellagra is caused by a deficiency of nicotinic acid or nicotinamide, or of their precursor tryptophan. It is prevalent where maize provides more than 50% of the energy intake. In Central America, preparation of maize using traditional methods involves soaking it in lime. This alkaline digestion makes tryptophan more available. In Africa, the custom of soaking the maize and discarding the supernatant results in a 50% loss of the vitamin. Requirements are proportional to the energy intake: 1.05 mg/MJ (4.4 mg/1000 kcal) or 9 mg per day.

Pellagra manifests itself in tissues with rapid cell turnover – the classic skin changes characteristically occur in areas exposed to sunlight, producing 'Casal's necklace'. In the mouth it produces a bright red mucosa and ulceration. There is desquamation of the tongue and hypertrophy of fungiform papillae. In the stomach mucosal atrophy and hypochlorhydria ensue, while in the small intestine atrophy and non-specific inflammation cause the characteristic diarrhoea.

VITAMIN C DEFICIENCY

Ascorbic acid (vitamin C) deficiency causes scurvy due to defective formation of collagen. In addition, bone formation is abnormal and increased vascular permeability results in bleeding gums and brittle loose teeth. The gum changes start as small haemorrhages in the tips of the interdental papillae and progress to generalized spongyness. Deficiency does not have any specific action on the gut. In animals, ascorbic

acid deficiency produces hypercholesterol-aemia. Eventually, the incidence of gallstones increases.[18] Lack of ascorbic acid appears to decrease the liver synthesis of bile salts, while cholesterol production is increased. Consumption of ascorbic acid also inhibits the conversion of nitrites to nitrosamine. The traditional Yorkshire custom of eating lettuce with Yorkshire pudding before the meat course may thus protect against gastric tumours.

VITAMIN D DEFICIENCY

Vitamin D deficiency retards tooth development and produces abnormal dentine. It is essential for absorption of calcium from the gut. The active form, 1,25-dihydroxycholecalciferol ($1,25(OH)_2D_3$), increases brush border permeability to calcium. In steatorrhoea, vitamin D enterohepatic circulation is blocked. Vitamin D deficiency causes rickets because of low calcium and phosphate. It is especially common in strict Moslem women who are not exposed to sunlight. The low breast milk levels of vitamin in these women increases the risk of infantile rickets. Their diet of unleavened wheat, which contains phytates, may also contribute by chelating dietary calcium. Vitamin D absorption is impaired in liver disease and tropical sprue.

NUTRITIONAL DEFICIENCY IN GUT DISEASES

Nutrition and gut function are intimately related, as malnutrition rapidly impairs gut function. The resulting reduction in absorption of nutrients essential for gut function then compounds the malnutrition.

Congenital disaccharidase deficiency causes chronic diarrhoea in children. Other rare congenital defects include congenital malabsorption of zinc in acrodermatitis enteropathica, B_{12} transport deficiency, and Hartnup's disease, which causes tryptophan malabsorption.

In chronic bowel disease such as Crohn's disease and ulcerative colitis, secondary malnutrition occurs, because of lack of appetite and increased protein losses. Appropriate enteral or parenteral feeding with attention to vitamin and trace element needs can improve the patient's well-being and resistance to infection and can promote growth in children.

In blind loop syndromes, bacterial overgrowth produces secondary nutritional deficiency of folate and B_{12}. Folate deficiency may produce malabsorption by itself, but it is so often accompanied by bacterial overgrowth and systemic infection that its role as a primary cause of malabsorption is in doubt.

Iron deficiency and nutritional immuno-paresis significantly impairs resistance to parasitic infection. Heavy infestation with *Ascaris* may compete with the host for nutrients, but deworming does not seem to improve nutrition. *Strongyloides stercoralis* superinfection, however, produces significant malabsorption and is seen in patients with depressed immunity. While the presence of *Giardia* in the gut is associated with malabsorption, it may not be directly causative since bacterial overgrowth may also be present. In animal experiments, iron and protein deficiency is associated with impairment of the immune clearance of *Nippostrongylus* infection.

All the above conditions can lead to a vicious circle, where nutritional deficiency damages gut absorption, thereby worsening the nutritional status. Parenteral nutrition may be necessary to break the circle, but balanced mineral and high-energy feeds can accomplish the same objective in skilled hands.

NUTRITIONAL DEFICIENCY IN CANCER OF THE GUT

Nutritional deficiencies and imbalances appear to be important in the aetiology of several forms of malignant disease, especially in cancer of the gut.

There are great epidemiological variations in the incidence of oesophageal cancer. The incidence is low where staples such as millet, cassava or yams are common, but high where maize or wheat is the staple. In Kazakhstan, north-eastern Iran and Transkei the rate exceeds 100/100 000 p.a.[41] The risks are higher in populations deriving a high proportion of their energy from one staple. In such groups, there is a good inverse correlation between the cancer rate and the amount of magnesium, zinc and nicotinic acid in the diet.[41]

Vitamin A has been linked to carcinogenesis. When it is deficient, epithelial surfaces develop into keratinizing squamous cells, a premalignant change. High doses of vitamin A can reverse these changes. Experimentally, retinoids have been shown to suppress the malignant behaviour of cultured cells previously transformed by viruses or radiation. The mechanism is unknown.

Epidemiological studies have indicated that people with above-average betacarotene intake and those with above-average retinol levels are at below-average risk of cancer. Several large prospective studies are in progress to assess whether higher carotenoid intakes can protect against cancer.[31] On the other hand, low levels of vitamin A appear to protect against the carcinogenic effects of aflatoxin.

When meat is cooked at high temperatures for long periods, nitrites are converted to nitrosamines, which are carcinogenic. The consumption of ascorbic acid with the meal may reduce this effect by detoxicating these substances.

Cancer of the large bowel may be induced by carcinogens resulting from bacterial metabolites or foods. The lower incidence of cancer of the colon in populations living on a high fibre intake is striking. This may be because such people have rapid intestinal transit times which reduce the exposure of the bowel to carcinogens.

Liver tumours in animals can be induced by selenium deficiency, but this has not been shown in man.

REFERENCES

1 Abidi, S. A. & Mercer, D. W. (1973) Protein digestion in human intestine as reflected in luminal mucosal and plasma amino acids concentrations after meals. *Journal of Clinical Investigation*, **52**, 1586–1594.
2 Alleyne, G. A. O., Hay, R. W., Picou, D. I. *et al.* (1977) *Protein Energy Malnutrition.* London: Edward Arnold.
3 Ashworth, A. (1979) Progress in the treatment of protein energy malnutrition. *Proceedings of the Nutrition Society*, **38**, 89–97.
4 Ball, P. C. (1975) The effect on oral tissues of dietary deficiencies and hormonal imbalance. In *Applied Physiology of the Mouth* (Ed.) Lavalle, C. L. B. Bristol: John Wright.
5 Beisel, W. R. (1982) Single nutrients and immunity. *American Journal of Clinical Nutrition*, **35** (supplement), 417–468.
6 Cahill, G. F. (1966) Starvation in man. *New England Journal of Medicine*, **282**, 668–675.
7 Chandra, R. K. (1980) Food antibodies in malnutrition. *Archives of Disease in Childhood*, **50**, 532.
8 Chandra, R. K. (1980) *Immunology of Nutritional Disorders.* London: Edward Arnold.
9 Cook. G. (1972) Impairment of D-xylose absorption in Zambian patients with systemic infection. *American Journal of Clinical Nutrition*, **25**, 490.
10 Coward, W. A. & Lunn, P. G. (1981) The biochemistry and physiology of kwashiorkor and marasmus. *British Medical Bulletin*, **37**(1), 19–24.
11 Domok, I., Fayinka, D. A., Skritic, N. *et al.* (1974) Factors affecting the efficacy of live polio vaccine in warm climates. *Bulletin of the World Health Organisation*, **51**, 347.
12 Duthie, H. L. & Wormsley, K. G. (1979) *Scientific Basis of Gastroenterology.* Edinburgh: Churchill Livingstone.
13 Editorial (1970) Classification of infantile malnutrition. *Lancet*, **ii**, 302–303.
14 Golden, M. H. N., (1982) Protein deficiency, energy deficiency and the oedema of malnutrition *Lancet*, **i**, 1261–1265.
15 Golden, M. H. N. & Golden, B. E. (1981) *American Journal of Clinical Nutrition*, **34**, 892–899.

16 Golden, M. H. N., Harland, P. S. E. G., Golden, B. E. & Jackson, A. A. (1978) Zinc and immunocompetence in protein energy malnutrition. *Lancet*, **i**, 1226–1228.

17 Gracey, M. (1979) The contaminated small bowel syndrome: pathogenesis, diagnosis and treatment. *American Journal of Clinical Nutrition*, **32**, 234–243.

18 Harris, W. S., Kottke, B. A. & Subbiah, M. T. R. (1979) Bile acid metabolism in ascorbic-acid-deficient guinea pigs. *American Journal of Clinical Nutrition*, **32**, 837–841.

19 Heard, C. R. C. (1978) The effects of protein energy malnutrition on blood glucose homeostasis. *World Review of Nutrition and Dietetics*, **30**, 107–147.

20 James, W. P. T. (1970) Sugar absorption and intestinal motility in children when malnourished and after treatment. *Clinical Science*, **38**, 305–318.

21 Lunn, P. G., Whitehead, R. G., Cole, T. J. & Austin, S. (1979) The relationship between hormonal balance and growth in malnourished children and rats. *British Journal of Nutrition*, **41**(1), 73–84.

22 Mann, M. D., Becker, B. L., Pimstone, B. L. & Hanson, J. D. L. (1975) Total body potassium, serum immunoreactive insulin concentration and glucose tolerance in protein energy malnutrition. *British Journal of Nutrition*, **33**, 55–61.

23 Martins Campos, J. V., Fagundes Neto, U., Patricio, F. R. S. *et al.* Jejunal mucosa in marasmic children. *American Journal of Clinical Nutrition*, **32**, 1575–1591.

24 Mata, L. Kromal, R. A., Urrutia, J. J. & Garcia, B. (1977) Effect of infection on food intake and the nutritional state: perspectives as viewed from the village. *American Journal of Clinical Nutrition*, **30**, 1215–1227.

25 McLaren, D. S. (1974) The great protein fiasco. *Lancet*, **ii**, 93.

26 Naismith, D. J. (1973) Kwashiorkor in western Nigeria: a study of traditional weaning foods with particular reference to energy and linoleic acid. *British Journal of Nutrition*, **30**, 567.

27 Nalin, D. R., Cash, R. A., Islam, R. *et al.* (1968) Oral maintenance therapy for cholera in adults. *Lancet*, **ii**, 370–373.

28 Newman, J. L. (1970) Dimensions of the Sandawe diet. *Ecology of Food and Nutrition*, **4**, 33–39.

29 Patrick, J. (1977) Death during recovery from severe malnutrition and its possible relationship to sodium pump activity in the leucocyte. *British Medical Journal*, **i**, 1051–1054.

30 Patrick, R. S., Mackays, A. M., Coward, D. G. & Whitehead, R. G. (1979) Experimental protein energy malnutrition in baby baboons. 2. Liver pathology. *British Journal of Nutrition*, **30**, 171.

31 Peto, R., Doll, R., Buckley, J. D. & Sporn, M. B. (1981) Can dietary beta-carotene materially reduce human cancer rates? *Nature*, **290**, 201–208.

31a Pimstone, B. (1976) Endocrine function in protein–calorie malnutrition. *Clinical Endocrinology*, **5**, 79–95.

32 Poskitt, E. M. E. (1971) Seasonal variation in infection and malnutrition at a rural paediatric clinic in Uganda. *Lancet*, **ii**, 517.

33 Rowland, M. G. H. & McCollum, J. P. K. (1977) Malnutrition and gastroenteritis in the Gambia. *Transactions of the Royal Society of Tropical Medicine and Hygiene*, **71**(3), 199–203.

34 Rustihauser, I. H. E. & Frood, J. D. L. (1973) The effect of a traditional low fat diet. *British Journal of Nutrition*, **29**, 261.

35 Sporn, M. M., Dunlop, N. M., Newton, D. L. & Smith, J. M. (1976) Prevention of chemical carcinogenesis by vitamin A and its chemical analogs. *Federation Proceedings*, **35**, 1332–1338.

36 Stanfield, J. P., Hutt, M. S. R. & Tunnicliffe, R. (1965) Intestinal biopsy in kwashiorkor. *Lancet*, **ii**, 519–523.

37 Stuart, H. C. & Stevenson, S. S. (1954) In *Textbook of Pediatrics* (Ed.) Nelson, W. E. Philadelphia: Saunders.

38 Trowell, H. C., Davies, J. N. P. & Dean, R. F. A. (1954) *Kwashiorkor*. London: Edward Arnold.

39 Waterlow, J. C. & Jackson, A. A. (1981) Nutrition and protein turnover in a man. *British Medical Bulletin*, **37**(1), 5–10.

40 Waterlow, J. V. (1976) Classification and definition of protein energy malnutrition. In *Nutrition in Preventive Medicine* (Ed.) Beeton, G. H. & Bengoa, J. M. p. 52 *World Health Organisation Monograph Series No. 62*.

40a Whitehead, R. G. & Lunn, P. G. (1979) Endocrines in protein–energy malnutrition. *Proceedings of the Nutrition Society*, **38**, 69.

41 Van Rensburg, S. J. (1981) Epidemiologic and dietary evidence for a specific nutritional predisposition to esophageal cancer. *Journal of the National Cancer Institute*, **67**, 243–250.

THERAPEUTIC NUTRITION

Since the introduction of total parenteral nutrition as a safe form of therapy for the restoration and maintenance of protein and energy stores of patients with gastroenterological disease, the relevance and importance of nutrition has become increasingly recognized. Nutritional disorders resulting from severe gastrointestinal pathology can now be effectively treated and there is growing awareness of the prevalence and prognostic implications of malnutrition in hospital patients.

NORMAL DIETARY REQUIREMENTS

Energy

A basic requirement of living organisms is for energy to maintain cellular function and structure. Energy is stored as chemical energy inherent in the covalent bonding structure of the terminal phosphate group of the adenosine triphosphate (ATP) molecule. The ATP is free to diffuse to sites where energy is required in the cell. Although some ATP is formed from glycolytic pathways outside the mitochondria, most is formed within the mitochondria in the tricarboxylic cycle. The major body store of energy is fat, with a limited amount of carbohydrate stored as glycogen. Protein is not an energy store as such, but structural proteins are used as an energy source through gluconeogenesis in some situations.

Energy requirements
A patient's total daily requirement for energy is the sum of his basal energy expenditure, his dietary induced energy expenditure, and his activity energy expenditure.

Basal energy expenditure is closely related to body size and represents the energy necessary for the work of the heart and lungs, work for the synthesis of new chemical bondings and work to maintain electricochemical gradients in cells. Approximately 97 $kJ \cdot kg^{-1} \cdot day^{-1}$ (23 $kcal \cdot kg^{-1} \cdot day^{-1}$) are usually required by normal adults for basal energy expenditure.[42]

Activity energy expenditure depends on the amount of physical work performed, and varies in active people from 2 MJ (500 kcal) per day in sedentary individuals to 13 MJ (3000 kcal) per day for manual labourers. In hospital patients spending much of the day lying in bed it is less than 2 MJ per day, although this will be increased if the patients are restless or hypoxic. In addition, there is energy expended in the assimilation of nutrients, whether given by mouth or vein. This is called *dietary induced thermogenesis* and it varies with the type of food ingested and the metabolic state of the patient. For example, protein sufficient to provide 1 MJ increases the basal metabolic rate by 300 kJ, whereas 1 MJ of glucose increases it by 60 kJ and 1 MJ of fat increases it by 40 kJ. In very septic patients, high glucose intake may induce a significant rise in dietary induced thermogenesis, an effect which is not seen with similar intakes of fat. Sick gastroenterological patients may have additional energy requirements due to fever, major surgery, sepsis and disseminated carcinoma.[44]

Generally speaking, gastroenterological patients having intravenous feeding require about 170 $kJ \cdot kg^{-1} \cdot day^{-1}$ (40 $kcal \cdot kg^{-1} \cdot day^{-1}$) to reach energy balance.[60] Depleted patients have a smaller requirement for energy but if there is extensive sepsis or widespread inflammatory bowel disease, energy requirements will be higher.[20] For example, in patients with peritonitis, intra-abdominal abscesses or extensive pancreatic necrosis, energy requirements can reach 250 $kJ \cdot kg^{-1} \cdot day^{-1}$ (60 $kcal \cdot kg^{-1} \cdot day^{-1}$). It is important to remember that it can be quite difficult to administer high energy intakes to very sick patients. In particular, glucose is not oxidized at high rates of energy intake and fat may be needed as a substitute if energy balance is to be attained.[45]

Energy sources

Carbohydrate. Carbohydrate is an essential energy source for the brain, erythrocytes, neural tissue, renal medulla and cells involved in inflammation and repair. Sixty per cent of ingested glucose is phosphorylated in the liver to glucose-6-phosphate and is then converted to glycogen, fatty acids or blood glucose. Carbohydrate is stored as glycogen in the liver (1.3 MJ/300 kcal) and in muscle (2.5 MJ/600 kcal) but these stores are rapidly depleted in fasting (in 18 hours) and exercise (in minutes). Carbohydrate sources provided in commercially available enteral diets include sucrose, liquid glucose (corn syrup), lactose, maltodextrins and starch. For intravenous use glucose is the safest and most widely used energy source in therapeutic nutrition, but alternative carbohydrate energy sources are fructose, maltose and the polyols sorbitol, xylitol and glycerol.

Fat. Fat is the main energy store of the body, accounting for over 400 MJ (100 000 kcal). Besides insulating and protective functions, its main reason for existence is as an energy store. Some fat is stored as triglyceride in adipose tissue and transported in various forms (lipoprotein complexes) to sites where energy is required. In fasting states, fat is metabolized by the liver to ketone bodies, and this decreases the glucose requirements of neural tissue.[4]

There is a group of fats with unsaturated bonds in their carbon chains which are precursors of prostaglandins and are considered essential fatty acids. About 4% of the total energy intake should consist of such polyunsaturated fats from vegetable sources, according to recommended dietary allowances. Normal ratios of fatty acids in the blood are maintained if 1% to 2% of energy is supplied as linoleic acid.[20] For clinical use, fat is supplied in commercially available enteral preparations as whole milk fat, vegetable oil, coconut oil or hydrogenated soya oil. Medium-chain triglycerides are indicated for some malabsorption states and when long-chain fatty acids are contraindicated. For intravenous use fat is supplied as soya oil and egg yolk phospholipid emulsions which have the same properties as chylomicrons.

Protein

Protein forms 16% of the body mass and forms its major structural component, being an integral part of cell walls, cytoplasm, nuclei and intracellular matrix. Any breakdown of protein as an energy source, therefore, will have an effect on structure and compromise body function. Collagen is the main extracellular protein of the body, while actin and myosin form a large part of intracellular total body protein. Plasma proteins play an important part in immunological and transport functions and have effects in processes of inflammation and repair.

Protein requirements

Because body protein is constantly being broken down and remodelled, a certain amount of nitrogen from the pool of amino acids is excreted as urea and needs to be replaced. About 50 grams a day (100 mg $N \cdot kg^{-1} \cdot day^{-1}$) of good quality protein is required to balance this loss.[12] Quality of protein, however, is important and while a Western diet may contain more than twice the amount of protein required, the biological value of that protein may only be 50%.

There are eight essential amino acids (isoleucine, leucine, lysine, methionine, phenylalanine, threonine, tryptophan and valine), which cannot be synthesized from other amino acids in the body. Amino acids absorbed from the intestine are used by the liver for manufacture of export proteins and to maintain constant turnover in peripheral tissues. The process of gluconeogenesis occurs to supply essential glucose requirements in starvation. It also occurs in catabolic states such as trauma and sepsis.[4] With excess protein, the liver can eliminate amino acids, form urea, and feed the remaining carbon chains into the Krebs cycle for energy production. When the liver is damaged urea synthesis may stop and free ammonia ions are formed.

The protein requirements of gastroenterological patients on parenteral feeding regimens vary according to their nutritional and metabolic state.[20] Gastroenterological patients who present for intravenous feeding require about 300 mg $N \cdot kg^{-1} \cdot day^{-1}$ (i.e. nearly 2 grams of protein per kilogram) with an adequate energy intake to maintain nitrogen balance.[60] This greatly exceeds the recommended dietary allowances for normal subjects.[12] When patients are very septic, however, positive nitrogen balance may not be possible. Patients recovering from sepsis need an increased amount of nitrogen (400 mg $\cdot kg^{-1} \cdot day^{-1}$) to replace the protein lost.[34]

Protein sources

From a therapeutic point of view, protein can be given either enterally or by the intravenous route. Studies of nitrogen balance comparing the oral and intravenous routes of administration of casein hydrolysates suggest that both routes are comparable and that there is no significant advantage in enteral feeding.[50] Intravenous protein requirements can be supplied either as protein hydrolysates or as synthetic crystalline amino acid solutions. Although protein hydrolysates may produce positive nitrogen balance, they are less effective than crystalline amino acids and have more often been associated with adverse effects.[43] Special amino acid mixtures may be required in renal failure[27] and hepatic failure,[28] although indications for their use have not yet been clearly defined.

Inter-relationships of protein and energy

Within certain limits of energy and protein intake there is a region where increases in either will result in protein retention.[20] Normally-nourished patients lay down protein only when energy requirements are met but depleted patients retain protein at lesser energy intakes. In this respect depleted patients behave as growing children. Nevertheless, authorities agree that high rates of restoration of lean body mass require high protein intake and that by proper manipulation of energy and protein intake it is possible to increase lean body mass or body fat in proportions appropriate to the individual.[20, 34]

Vitamins and trace elements

Vitamins

Vitamins are organic substances required to maintain normal cellular activity. Deficiency states do not usually single out a particular vitamin and the clinical syndromes observed often combine deficiencies of protein, energy and multiple vitamins. Table 17.6 shows the major vitamins, their normal action, the effects of deficiency, and the recommended daily allowances. Recommended intravenous allowances are based on dietary allowances in healthy individuals and patients with deficiencies will need more.[48]

Trace elements

Trace elements are found in micromolar amounts in the tissues and are essential for normal cellular function. The place of iron in haem, cobalt in vitamin B_{12} and iodine in thyroid metabolism has been known for some time. Deficiencies of zinc, copper, selenium and chromium have also been described and these are listed along with other elements considered essential in Table 17.7.[49]

Zinc is one important element which often needs to be given in increased amounts in gastroenterological patients.[65] About 2 mg/day of elemental zinc is lost in the urine and this increases with sepsis or injury. Patients with diarrhoea or ileostomies lose about 17 milligrams per litre, but with a high small bowel

Table 17.6 Recommended daily allowances of vitamins.

	Action	Effect of deficiency	Dietary[a]	Intravenous[b]
Water-soluble				
Thiamine (B$_1$)	Glucose metabolism	Beriberi	1.4 mg	3 mg
Riboflavine (B$_2$)	Energy transfer	Glossitis, chelosis	1.6 mg	3.6 mg
Nicotinic acid (niacin) (B$_3$)	Energy transfer	Pellagra	18 mg	40 mg
Pyridoxine (B$_6$)	Decarboxylation and transamination	Convulsions	2.2 mg	4 mg
Pantothenic acid	Part of CoA	Dermatitis, enteritis	NR	15 mg
Folate	Coenzyme with B$_{12}$	Anaemia	400 μg	400 μg
B$_{12}$	Coenzyme in nucleic acid synthesis	Pernicious anaemia	3 μg	5 mg
C	Collagen synthesis	Scurvy	60 mg	100 mg
Fat-soluble				
A	Visual pigments	Night blindness	1000 μg RE[c]	1135 μg RE[c]
D	Calcium and phosphate utilization	Rickets	5 μg	5 μg
E	Energy transfer	?	10 mg[d]	210 mg[d]
K	Prothrombin synthesis	Bleeding disorder	NR	500 μg

[a] Committee on Dietary Allowances (1980) (males 23–50 years old)[12]
[b] Nutrition Advisory Group (1979a)[48]
[c] Retinol equivalents. 1 μg retinol equivalent corresponds to 1 μg retinol or 6 μg betacarotene
[d] Alpha-tocopherol equivalents. 1 mg alpha-tocopherol equivalent has the same activity as 1 mg *d*-alpha-tocopherol.
   NR = no recommendation

fistula the losses are less (12 mg/l). The suggested replacement of elemental zinc in milligrams per day for patients with abnormal losses is:

$$2 + 17.1 \times \text{stool mass (kg)} + 12.2$$

$$\times \text{fistula output mass (kg)}$$

If given as zinc sulphate this needs to be multiplied by 2.5. As only 20% of orally administered zinc is absorbed, a further multiplication by 5 is required if given orally. Zinc levels in the blood reflect zinc ingestion rather than balance. While 4 mg elemental zinc is sufficient for parenteral regimens to maintain most patients in zinc balance, many gastroenterological patients will require more than this and 10 mg as a basic requirement is suggested.

Copper requirements are not increased in gastroenterological patients above 300–500 μg/day.[59]

Other elements listed in Table 17.7 have not been specifically studied in gastroenterological patients.

ASSESSMENT OF NUTRITIONAL STATUS

Surveys of hospital patients in Western countries have revealed a high incidence of protein–energy malnutrition.[35] Nutritional assessment should make it possible to select patients whose nutritional status adversely affects the outcome of their illness. Clinically significant malnutrition has not yet been simply defined in spite of the multitude of nutritional markers available. For this reason, broadly based nutritional syndromes are suggested here to aid assessment and give guidance in the management of patients with nutritional disorders.[34]

Table 17.7 Recommended daily allowances of trace elements.

Element	Effect of deficiency	Dietary[a]	Intravenous
Zinc	Impaired wound healing and growth, dermatitis, alopecia	15 mg	2.5–4 mg[b] 4–14 mg[c]
Copper	Anaemia, neutropenia, bone demineralization	2–3 mg	0.5–1.5 mg[b]
Chromium	Impaired glucose handling	0.05–0.2 mg	10–15 μg[b]
Iodine	Goitre, hypothyroidism	150 μg	150 μg[c]
Iron	Anaemia	10–20 mg	1–4 mg[c]
Fluorine	Dental susceptibility to caries	1.5–4 mg	0.4 mg[c]
Manganese	Vit K deficiency	2.5–5.0 mg	0.15–0.8 mg[b]
Molybdenum	?	0.15–0.5 μg	20 μg[c]
Selenium	Muscle weakness and pain	0.05–0.2 mg	30 μg[c]

[a] Committee on Dietary Allowances (1980)[12]
[b] Nutrition Advisory Group (1979b)[49]
[c] Shenkin & Wretlind (1977)[57]

NUTRITIONAL SYNDROMES

Gastroenterological patients can be affected by two metabolic and nutritional processes. Semi-starvation in patients with anorexia, vomiting or a partial obstruction results in gradual wasting of muscle and fat stores, with lowered metabolic rate. Compensatory mechanisms are designed to conserve energy and body protein. Sepsis or other severe types of stress result in rapid breakdown of protein for gluconeogenesis with raised metabolic rate. Compensatory mechanisms are designed to provide essential protein and energy components for healing and repair. From the combination of these two processes, semi-starvation and stress, four nutritional syndromes can be identified.

The normal state
The majority of gastroenterological patients do not have a clinically relevant nutritional problem. Food intake has been normal, they are not septic and clinically they have normal stores of subcutaneous fat and muscle. Such patients can be maintained on an adequate oral diet unless the pathology of their disorder requires a specific therapeutic measure (such as a gluten-free diet in coeliac disease). After surgery there is a loss of body weight (about 6%) and a temporary fall in plasma protein levels. These return to normal when normal oral intake resumes, usually during the second postoperative week.

Nutritional depletion
Patients with this syndrome have an overall deficit in their intake or utilization of food or both. Weight loss is marked, with clinical evidence of subcutaneous fat loss and wasting of muscles. Metabolic rate is low and urinary nitrogen loss is small. Plasma proteins remain normal. Examples of this syndrome include cachexia seen in patients with strictures of the oesophagus or cancer of the stomach. The patient, if the condition is severe, looks like a 'walking skeleton'.

Normal with sepsis
These patients are usually quite easily picked out, for they either are septic or have recently been so. In gastroenterological patients the classic causes of this syndrome are acute attacks of inflammatory bowel disease and pancreatic abscess. Clinically, such patients may have normal stores of muscle and fat, but there are clear signs of sepsis and plasma albumin levels are low. If this situation persists muscle wasting follows, although fat stores are preserved (see below). Nutritional therapy will be required in these patients if the increased metabolic rate is prolonged and cannot be reduced by draining abscesses, controlling sepsis or treatment of the underlying problem.

Nutritional depletion and sepsis
This occurs in two situations: (a) in depleted patients who have a metabolic insult such as sepsis, or a major operation or (b) in normally nourished patients who have a severe metabolic stress and rapidly become depleted of their nutritional reserves. Examples of the first situation are depleted patients with carcinoma of the oesophagus or stomach who develop septic complications after oesophagectomy or gastrectomy. Examples of the second situation are normally nourished patients with prolonged severe pancreatitis with sepsis, or prolonged exacerbations of colitis. These patients are obviously unwell, with tachycardia, fever and low intravascular volume. However, the degree of depletion may not be apparent from the history and may be masked on physical examination by preservation of body fat stores or oedema. However, muscle wasting is a constant feature of all these patients, along with a low plasma albumin. While treatment must be aimed at identifying the septic source and controlling the hypermetabolic stimulus, these patients need early nutritional support.

PRIMARY ASSESSMENT

The identification of these nutritional syndromes relies on a good history and a physical examination supported by a few basic measurements.

History
The history should determine the energy balance of the patient, and consider his energy intake and energy output to arrive at an estimate of nutritional depletion and the time scale over which this has occurred. Particular attention should be paid to a clinical history of anorexia, vomiting, nausea, diarrhoea and abnormal losses from diarrhoea or fistulas. A detailed dietary history may be helpful in identifying the patient's food fads, proportions of fat, carbohydrate and proteins in the diet, use of dietary supplements and vitamins, and additional calories from alcohol which may be associated with other nutritional deficiencies. Dietary recall beyond 24 hours, however, is not very accurate, and dietetic assessment has been shown to be of little help in the classification of patients.

Weight loss is of major importance in the clinical history. Changes in weight over very short periods of time reflect fluid balance, but changes over a period of weeks or months indicate loss of body tissue. Excluding fluid balance problems, rapid changes in weight are associated with hypermetabolism and sepsis while long-term changes in weight are associated with depletion syndromes. With severe sepsis up to 1 kg of wet lean tissue may be lost each day, whereas in total starvation only half this amount is lost. Assessment of weight loss relies on an accurate recall of well weight, but this may be difficult in very sick or elderly patients. However, using recalled well weight is more accurate than using standard tables of predicted weight for height.[47]

Physical examination

Physical examination should aim to estimate the nutritional reserves of the patient, look for signs of hypermetabolism and assess the state of hydration. Fat stores are estimated by gently pinching the skinfolds on the arms, back and abdomen to feel the amount of subcutaneous fat present. Muscle wasting is best observed in muscles around the scapulae and in the temporalis fossae, the interossei and the muscle bellies on the upper arm. Hydration needs to be assessed by looking for oedema in the lower legs and sacral area. If oedema is present, weight loss may be greater than that estimated from the history. Unlike childhood kwashiorkor, oedema is seldom observed in malnourished adult patients unless other factors such as cardiac, renal or hepatic dysfunction are present. Subtle skin and hair changes are described in association with different vitamin and trace metal deficiencies, but these are not usually specific in gastroenterological patients in whom protein–energy malnutrition has complex manifestations.

Basic measurements

A nutritional assessment is incomplete without a few basic measurements. The patient's weight should be recorded, and weight loss estimated by subtracting this from the recalled well weight. Apart from clinical evidence of sepsis the most useful measurement associated with the hypermetabolic and stress syndromes is a low level of plasma albumin. Low plasma albumin reflects protein losses into inflamed tissues, alterations in protein turnover and changes in intravascular/extravascular distribution of albumin and water.[30] From this primary assessment the nutritional syndromes categorized above are identified.

In the clinical setting it will be found that there is considerable overlap in the clinical picture of these syndromes; they form a spectrum of nutritional disorders rather than defined categories.

SECONDARY ASSESSMENT TECHNIQUES

Further information may be gained by more detailed measurements using anthropometry, immunology, calorimetry, body composition and biochemistry.

Anthropometry

This includes the measurement of weight, height, skinfold thickness (by calipers) and upper arm circumference.[6] Various ratios of weight to height have been suggested to indicate obesity and depleted states (weight/height, weight/height^2, weight/height^3). Recent population-based studies have made anthropometric measurements more meaningful, especially if age-, sex- and race-specific standards are based on large studies. Probably, where good local standards are available weight/height^2 is the best of these estimates.

Skinfold thickness measurements are usually taken at the midpoint of the upper arm over the biceps and triceps. Other skinfolds that may be measured include the subscapular skinfold and the suprailiac skinfold. From the triceps skinfold and arm circumference measurements, mid-arm muscle circumference can be derived as an index of muscle wasting. There are large random errors in the measurement of skin folds and they have little meaning in the individual patient. They are useful, however, in evaluating groups of patients.[11]

Immunological assessment

Protein–energy malnutrition is associated with impaired immunological responses.[13] Defects in B and T cell function as well as impaired inflammatory responses have been described. In clinical practice, total lymphocyte count and delayed hypersensitivity skin tests have been routinely used. While a total lymphocyte count below 10^9 per litre has been observed in groups of patients with severe nutritional depletion, the association is tenuous and does not help to distinguish nutritional syndromes.

Cell-mediated immunity as tested by the delayed hypersensitivity skin test is impaired in depleted states.[13] A battery of recall antigens (purified protein derivative, mumps, candida, trichophyton, streptokinase/streptodornase) are injected intradermally on the forearm and read at 24 and 48 hours. Reactions are scored according to the diameter of induration produced at the injection sites. Problems are recognized in standardizing the administration, recording and interpretation of the results.[2] There are many conditions apart from disorders of nutritional state associated with absent skin test reactions (anergy): these include sepsis, advanced cancer, trauma, old age, diabetes mellitus, steroid administration and immunosuppressive disorders. It is questionable whether skin testing, although widely practised, is of any use in the clinical evaluation of nutritional status and it probably does not justify the discomfort to patients and the expense of the tests.[64]

CALORIMETRY

Energy requirements should be tailored to the energy needs of individual patients. Of the methods available for measurement of metabolic expenditure at rest, the only practical method for clinical practice is indirect calorimetry. Expired gases are collected and analysed to determine oxygen consumption and carbon dioxide output of fasting patients at rest. This is referred to as resting metabolic expenditure. Variations occur with body build, age, sex and physical activity. Estimates of total energy expenditure can be made from equations which have been derived for males and females, using weight, height and age with additional factors added for activity and injury. Table 17.8 shows the components of energy expenditure and total energy requirements of gastroenterological patients according to the nutritional syndromes detailed above.

Body composition analysis
Most body composition analysis methods use the dilution of administered radioisotopes to measure various body spaces or compartments. Assessment of total body water is made using deuterated or tritiated water. Total exchangeable sodium and potassium are estimated from the rapid dilution in the body of the appropriate isotope. Total body potassium can also be mea-

sured in a whole body counter and this can be used as an estimate of body cell mass. In vivo neutron activation analysis is a new method of measuring total body nitrogen that can be used in sick patients.[33] Two techniques of measuring total body nitrogen have been developed. With the delayed technique, the patient is irradiated with fast neutrons, then moved to a whole body counter and the resulting radiation decay measured. With the prompt gamma technique the patient is irradiated with neutrons and the resulting radiation is counted at the same time. In combination with total body water measurements, the total body content of protein, water, fat and minerals can be determined. These methods are currently research tools and have been used to detect changes in body nitrogen in groups of patients undergoing specific nutritional regimens.

Plasma proteins
There are four plasma proteins synthesized in the liver which are currently used in the assessment of nutritional status.

Albumin. Within 24 hours of protein being eliminated from the diet, albumin synthesis is halved. However, this dramatic fall in synthesis is not reflected in the plasma albumin level for many weeks. Studies in primates indicate that unless the protein content of the diet is less than 3%, plasma albumin levels do not fall even after several months.[30] The reasons why plasma albumin levels are maintained are related to the shifts of extravascular albumin (comprising 50% of total albumin) into the intravascular compartment, contraction of the albumin pool and a lowered albumin breakdown rate. Furthermore, albumin has a long half-life of about 21 days. Changes in plasma albumin, therefore, do not reflect a patient's total protein status.[30] Low plasma albumin seen in gastroenterological patients is most often associated with leakage of albumin in inflammatory conditions of the gastrointestinal tract and increased capillary permeability, which occurs in trauma (including operations) and sepsis.[16, 62]

Table 17.8 Energy expenditure in gastroenterological patients.

Nutritional syndromes	Resting energy expenditure $kJ \cdot kg^{-1} \cdot day^{-1}$ ($kcal \cdot kg^{-1} \cdot day^{-1}$)	Activity energy expenditure $kJ \cdot kg^{-1} \cdot day^{-1}$ ($kcal \cdot kg^{-1} \cdot day^{-1}$)	Total energy expenditure $kJ \cdot kg^{-1} \cdot day^{-1}$ ($kcal \cdot kg^{-1} \cdot day^{-1}$)
Normal: operative	109(26)	42(10)	151(36)
Normal: postoperative	122(29)	29(7)	151(36)
Nutritional depletion	92(22)	42(10)	134(32)
Nutritional depletion and sepsis	147(35)	29(7)	176(42)
Septic (not depleted)	189(45)	29(7)	218(52)

Transferrin. Transferrin has a short half-life of seven days and responds more rapidly than albumin to nutritional changes. Although transferrin is less affected by fluid changes than albumin, its plasma level is greatly influenced by iron deficiency, which can be associated with malnutrition. While a low level of plasma transferrin present before surgery is an adverse prognostic factor,[8] its association with total body protein status is uncertain.[30]

Prealbumin and retinol binding protein. Prealbumin is the transport protein for thyroxine and is linked in a constant molar ratio with retinol binding protein, which transports retinol (vitamin A). Retinol binding protein is metabolized by the kidney and may be markedly elevated in chronic renal failure.[30] Because the half-lives of these proteins are much shorter than those of albumin and transferrin (two days for prealbumin, 12 hours for retinol binding protein) they more accurately reflect acute changes in nutritional status.[58] There is some confusion, however, about whether these proteins are markers of energy status or protein status.[30]

DYNAMIC NUTRITIONAL ASSESSMENT

The problem with the nutritional measurements outlined so far is that as single static measurements they cannot give information on the dynamics of the nutritional state. Most markers change so slowly that it can be many weeks before repeated measurements will show a clear indication of change in nutritional stores. Nitrogen balance studies can determine whether positive nitrogen balance is being achieved but need repetitive and time-consuming nitrogen analyses of urine and faeces and other secretions. In ordinary clinical care nitrogen balance studies are often inaccurate and misleading. Recently, the short half-life plasma proteins transferrin and prealbumin have been suggested as indicating dynamic nutritional state.[10] Prealbumin responds rapidly to nutritional improvement over a few days whereas transferrin responds more slowly. A normal level of transferrin with a low prealbumin level indicates recent deterioration in nutritional status, whereas recent improvement would be indicated by a rising prealbumin level with a low transferrin level.

PREOPERATIVE ASSESSMENT
OF SURGICAL RISK

It has been suggested that gastroenterological patients who are nutritionally depleted have a higher risk of major complications after surgery than patients who are not depleted. Various formulae, all of which reflect low levels of plasma proteins, are available for use in individual patients to assess risk from a surgical operation.[8] It is now realized that most of these risk factors are associated with manifest or occult sepsis rather than nutritional depletion alone, and that a careful clinical appraisal along the lines set out above may be just as effective in identifying patients at risk from major surgery.[1]

The question of which patients will benefit from specific nutritional therapy before their operation has not been answered. It appears that marginally depleted patients do not need preoperative therapy unless major postoperative complications are anticipated. This is probably because fewer problems are encountered in the surgery of lean individuals. Very depleted patients, especially those who are hypoalbuminaemic, undergoing major surgery should receive perioperative nutritional support.

NUTRITION AND INFECTION

The metabolic and nutritional consequences of sepsis have important implications in the planning of nutritional therapy. In many gastroenterological patients, metabolism may change from the low protein turnover, low energy requirement of nutritional depletion, to the high protein turnover, high energy requirement of sepsis. The extent of these changes will depend on the source of infection, the virulence of the organism and the host response. It is the host response (particularly immunological defence mechanisms) that is affected by nutritional status.

EVIDENCE FOR INCREASED
SUSCEPTIBILITY IN MALNUTRITION

Nutritional depletion is known to affect the structure and function of the immune system.[9] There are marked histomorphological changes in the thymus, with depletion of lymphocytes, reduction in size and loss of corticomedullary differentiation. Similar changes occur in the spleen and lymph nodes. More important, however, are the functional changes. T cell function, assessed by delayed hypersensitivity skin testing, blast transformation of lymphocytes to mitogens and lymphokinin production, is reduced, while B cell function is not affected to the same extent. Polymorphonuclear leucocytes ingest bacteria normally, but their intracellular killing is reduced in depleted patients. Lower liver synthesis of some complement components has been noted, and lysozyme production is reduced in plasma, tears, saliva and other secretions.

These impaired responses, which can be observed in nutritionally depleted patients, are complex.[13] Iron deficiency has been shown to affect lymphocyte distribution by complex mechanisms, while zinc deficiency is known to alter the delayed hypersensitivity skin test results and impair thymic development and in vitro lymphocyte activation. Deficiencies of the vitamins pyridoxine, folate and vitamins A, C and E affect lymphocyte function. Certain fatty acids have been shown to inhibit phytohaemagglutinin and purified protein derivative immune responses. Among these factors, the place of protein and energy depletion is difficult to ascertain. There is evidence that children with kwashiorkor are more susceptible to infection than those with marasmus.[56] Rats fed a protein-depleted diet succumb to infections more readily than rats fed a normal diet.[38] The clinical impression is that malnourished patients are more susceptible to septic complications, but a clear association between protein–energy malnutrition and susceptibility to infection has been difficult to show.

THE PATIENT'S RESPONSE TO SEPSIS

The challenge of sepsis sets in motion a series of cellular, metabolic and hormonal effects leading to a catabolic state which, if left unchecked, rapidly exhausts the nutritional reserves of the patient, particularly those of protein.

Cellular responses
The initial recognition and defence against sepsis rests with the leucocytes. In their mediation of the inflammatory response they synthesize small proteins known as leucocyte endogenous mediator (LEM), which acts on a large number of organ systems.[51] In the hypothalamus LEM produces fever, while in the bone marrow it induces neutrophil release and increased granulopoiesis. In the liver, acute phase protein synthesis is stimulated and redistributions of zinc, copper and iron occur because of alterations in the serum proteins. LEM induces muscle release of amino acids for protein synthesis in the liver and wound and stimulates other granulocytes to release lysozyme. The effect of these cellular changes is to enhance the inflammatory response, stimulate immunity and make available nutrients for eventual wound healing.

The effect of malnutrition on these cellular responses is still being determined. It appears that wasted individuals are still able to manufacture LEM to initiate these changes effectively, whereas stressed patients cannot mount such an effective response.[37] The clinical consequences of stress to patients may be in impaired ability to heal wounds, poor inflammatory responses and decreased immunity to infection.

Endocrine responses
The metabolic response to infection is mediated by hormones released by the changes in circulating blood volume and the metabolites released from damaged tissues which affect the neuro-endocrine system. The catecholamines adrenaline (epinephrine) and noradrenaline (norepinephrine), released from the adrenal medulla, are essential for survival during stress. Their effects on cardiac function and respiration are well known, but they also affect glucose metabolism in liver and muscle and mobilize free fatty acids. Adrenocorticotrophic hormone (ACTH) acts on the adrenal cortex to release glucocorticoids which may increase tenfold in sepsis, stimulating gluconeogenesis in conjunction with peripheral breakdown of protein in muscle and augmenting lipolysis.[4] The increased insulin observed in septic states is counteracted by a greater increase in glucagon with a resultant fall in the insulin/glucagon ratio. This interaction between the catecholamines and pancreatic endocrine hormones is fundamental to the regulation of substrates during infection. Growth hormone also increases in sepsis.

Metabolic responses
The main metabolic changes in severe sepsis are an increase in protein breakdown, a smaller increase in protein synthesis and an alteration in glucose metabolism.[4] The increased requirement for energy of cellular metabolism (ATP) is seen as a rise in whole body oxygen consumption and resting metabolic expenditure. The magnitude of increase in energy expenditure and acceleration of the flux of substrates through organ systems is small in mild infections, but up to 50% above resting expenditure in septicaemic patients. In sick patients, the extra energy requirement cannot be met by increasing energy intake. Clinically, the results are early weight loss from loss of muscle and fat and hypoproteinaemia. The major change in energy metabolism in septic patients is an acceleration of gluconeogenesis.[4] Both glucagon and the catecholamines stimulate the accelerated hepatic production of glucose. In many of the rapidly healing tissues of

the inflammatory process the metabolism of glucose to lactate provides the main energy source. However, for other energy needs in the body fat is still the principal energy source. The protein for gluconeogenesis comes from muscle catabolism. Alanine, the main amino acid released from muscle, is the principal gluconeogenic precursor. The branched-chain amino acids released by muscle catabolism can become a fuel source for the remaining muscle. The nitrogen residues are processed to urea in the liver and excreted in the urine. The amount of nitrogen lost in the urine can be up to 40 grams per day in severe sepsis. Most of this nitrogen loss is from muscle, which also contributes to an increased urinary loss of potassium, phosphate, magnesium and zinc.

The metabolic events change with time following infection. The earliest response to sepsis may be a transient depression of physiological responses (ebb phase) followed by the increase in metabolic reactions just described (flow phase). This phase depends on the severity of the sepsis and the host's ability to deal with it successfully. It is followed by a convalescent phase in which muscle protein and fat are resynthesized over a period of months.

IMPLICATIONS FOR THE MANAGEMENT OF THE SEPTIC PATIENT

The different hormonal and metabolic environment of the septic patient compared with that of the non-septic patient means that nutritional requirements are different. The aim should be to remove the source of the sepsis, with nutritional therapy providing a supportive role as other therapeutic measures take effect. Because positive nitrogen balance is very difficult, if not impossible, to achieve in the hormonal and metabolic environment of uncontrolled sepsis, the nutritional goals in the septic patient are to prevent or minimize tissue losses. However, as the patient recovers, there is not only a need to maintain the patient's nutritional state, but to replenish the deficits that have occurred during the septic insult.

Currently there is no consensus as to the optimal energy source for septic patients. Because of the impaired glucose metabolism in septic patients, infusions of glucose are handled poorly, often requiring large amounts of insulin to prevent glycosuria.[5] Such glucose may be deposited as excess glycogen and constitute a metabolic stress rather than effective nutrient support.[20] Most energy sources containing fat are carnitine-dependent, and in septic conditions carnitine may be reduced in the mitochondria. However, combinations of fat and glucose are recommended in septic patients as a compromise, though not optimal regimen.[45]

Many gastroenterological patients have septic foci but the intensity of the sepsis is not sufficient to require initiation of nutritional support. In septicaemic patients, or those with undrained or undrainable collections, the administration of large amounts of nitrogen is wasteful and may be harmful.[20]

In septic patients, vitamins and trace metals may need to be given in increasing amounts. Hypermetabolic patients receiving maintenance amounts of zinc[65] and folate[3] have been shown to become deficient in these nutrients, particularly when moving into an anabolic phase.

NUTRITIONAL SUPPORT

Oral intake

There is no doubt that the natural route for the ingestion and assimilation of nutrients is the cheapest, most efficient, and preferred route. For an adequate oral intake, an intact gastrointestinal tract, an ability to absorb nutrients, a favourable metabolic environment and a motivated patient are required. There are many gastroenterological disorders where modification of the diet is an essential part of therapy. Removal of gluten from the diet in coeliac disease, and of lactose in disaccharidase deficiency are such situations. However, the benefits of other dietary modifications are not so easily demonstrated. The use of bland diets in peptic ulcer disease has shown no advantage over normal diets in clinical trials.[7] Symptomatic relief of diverticular disease has been demonstrated to follow the addition of fibre to the diet. Chronic hepatic encephalopathy, usually treated with protein restriction, has shown improvement with diets containing high proportions of branched-chain amino acids.[28] Low-protein diets enriched with essential amino acids have been given orally in chronic renal failure patients with benefit.[29] Patients with steatorrhoea may benefit from the use of medium-chain triglycerides, available as an oil for cooking, or baking, or as a drink. Medium-chain triglycerides do not require bile acids or pancreatic lipase for absorption and pass into the portal circulation for oxidation in the liver. Dietary modification for patients with dumping after gastric surgery is often successful with low-carbohydrate and high-fat diets[52] or by adding pectin to the diet.[40]

There are other gastroenterological disorders where modification of the diet cannot overcome problems of ingestion and absorption of nutrients. Anorexia, nausea and vomiting affect the ability of the patient to take an adequate oral diet.

Despite good dietetic services and ingenious manipulation of the presentation of food, many patients fail to increase energy intake sufficiently to maintain body weight. The causes are many. Alterations in taste and sensation of satiety have been shown in cancer patients:[15] 30% have an elevation in the recognition threshold for sweetness, and in patients with upper gastrointestinal carcinoma meat aversion has been correlated with altered sensations of bitterness. Catecholamine release in response to stress depresses eating by neuroendocrine changes in hypothalamic centres. In advanced carcinoma, patients also complain of fullness, further decreasing their motivation to eat. The ability of dietary manipulation to meet the requirements of patients with these gastrointestinal disorders is therefore limited and other therapeutic measures are often required.

Postoperative patients do not usually require specific nutritional therapy. Usually, oral fluids can be commenced within a few days of surgery and the patient progresses to a light diet. The loss of body weight (about 6% after the average major operation) and the deficit of nitrogen and energy occurring during this time are replenished over the next few months. It must be remembered, however, that it takes at least 10 to 14 days after commencing oral intake for a patient to reach normal energy requirements, even with careful dietary manipulation and supplemental feeding.[31] While this deficit can be tolerated reasonably well in properly nourished patients, those malnourished prior to surgery may not be able to cope with this degree of weight loss. Furthermore, postoperative complications, especially sepsis, magnify the deficit and may further extend the convalescence of the patient. In such circumstances the early use of an alternative nutritional therapy must be considered.

Enteral therapy

Enteral feeding can be used to supplement oral intake or as a method of using the gastrointestinal tract where disorders of the mouth, oesophagus or stomach prevent natural delivery of food to the absorptive areas. The recent development of fine-bore nasogastric tubes has enabled commercially available liquid diets to be delivered with minimal patient discomfort.

INDICATIONS

There are three conditions which need to be fulfilled before nutritional therapy via the enteral route should be considered.

1 Spontaneous oral intake must be inadequate for nutritional requirements. A careful dietary assessment is needed to determine if energy and protein intake meet estimated requirements.

2 The proximal small intestine needs to be functional. Often fine-bore tubes can be fed past obstructions in the oesophagus or stomach to the functional area of the digestive tract.

3 The gastrointestinal tract needs to be an appropriate route for administration of nutrients for the patient's condition. This particularly applies in conditions where gut rest is considered part of management despite a functional gastrointestinal tract. Such conditions as pancreatitis or high small bowel fistulas are not appropriately treated by enteral therapy.

Conditions which particularly fulfil these criteria include non-gastrointestinal problems such as severe head injury, central nervous system disorders, burns and major trauma. Among the gastroenterological disorders which may be treated with enteral diets are ileal or colonic fistulas, non-obstructive problems in the large bowel, and obstructive lesions in the upper gastroenterological tract.

METHODS

Nasogastric tube

There is no indication for the use of wide-bore nasogastric tubes in enteral feeding. They are uncomfortable for the patient and increase the incidence of aspiration and ulceration. There are many fine-bore tubes on the market, with variations of weighted ends, side and end holes, and adaptations to aid placement. As these tubes do not permit aspiration, the position needs to be checked by X-ray before feeding commences. Feeding tubes, which may become blocked when the consistency of the nutrient is too thick for the size of the tube, can be irrigated with water to overcome the obstruction. Regurgitation may still occur with fine-bore tubes, particularly at night, and patients should be encouraged to sleep semi-recumbent to avoid this potentially serious problem.

Tube enterostomy

This technique, which has been widely practised in the past, is not frequently used today.[63] Feeding enterostomies, created surgically, usually into the stomach or jejunum, use large-bore tubes. The feeding fistula usually closes spontaneously once the tube is removed. It may be a useful alternative to total parenteral nutrition in neonates with tracheo-oesophageal fistulas.

Fine-needle catheter jejunostomy
Recently, the technique of fine-needle catheter jejunostomy has been re-evaluated as a method of infusing nutrients directly into the jejunum postoperatively. The catheter is inserted by a needle tunnelled sub-mucosally along a 10 cm length of the jejunum at the time of operation, and the bowel segment is secured to the anterior abdominal wall. This catheter can then be used for early postoperative feeding.[67] The catheters may leak into the abdominal cavity. However, for those who do not have access to safe parenteral nutrition, the technique, if used properly, can be a valuable aid.

ADMINISTRATION

With fine-bore nasogastric tubes, continuous infusion of nutrients is preferable because nursing care is easier, and there is less diarrhoea and fewer problems with nausea and vomiting. Although three litres of nutrient solution can quite easily be administered by gravity feeding over a 24-hour period, the use of a pump enables a more constant infusion to be maintained.

Enteral feeding should be commenced gradually, usually with quarter-strength or half-strength solutions, progressing to a full nutrient load over the next two days as the patient's condition and tolerance allows. As with all forms of nutritional therapy, there is need for careful monitoring of the patient with regard to fluid and electrolytes, watching for fluid retention,

hyperglycaemia and electrolyte imbalances. Diarrhoea, which is a common complication, is usually corrected by slowing the rate of delivery or reducing the osmotic load.

TYPES OF ENTERAL DIETS

There are many types of liquid feeding formulas available and to the uninitiated the choice seems overwhelming. The ideal complete formula should have about 4 MJ (1000 kcal) per litre, with a nitrogen : energy ratio (g : kJ) of about 1 : 840 (a g : kcal ratio of about 1 : 200).

Formulas can be classified into four groups, each with particular indications as shown in Table 17.9.

ELEMENTAL DIETS

Elemental diets were developed in the 1960s for astronauts, to eliminate problems of storage, ingestion and waste disposal. They are composed of amino acids or small peptides as the nitrogen source, with up to 30% of the energy supplied as fat. They have no lactose or digestive residues and have added to them recommended daily allowances of trace metals and vitamins. They have been demonstrated to maintain nitrogen and energy balance in normal subjects for up to six months. However, they are unpalatable, expensive, and their indications for use in gastroenterological patients have been seriously questioned.[41]

The clinical application of elemental diets has been based on the premise that they are more easily absorbed, do not stimulate gastrointestinal secretions and have low residue. While the last premise is unquestioned, the first two have not found support in experimental or clinical situations. Particular situations where these

Table 17.9 Enteral nutrition formulae.

Classification	Constituents	Use	Examples
Meal replacements	Balanced proportions of protein, carbohydrate and fat with electrolytes	Provide complete and balanced meals	Ensure, Isocal, Osmolite, Clinifeed
Supplements	Proportions of protein, carbohydrate and fat with particular emphasis on either protein or carbohydrate	Added to regular meals to provide the extra calories or protein	Sustacal (extra calories) Sustagen (extra protein)
Feeding components	Only one or two components	Used to make up specific diets for specific purposes	Caloreen (carbohydrate) Polycose (carbohydrate) MCT oil (fat) Casec (protein)
Elemental diets	No-residue balanced diets with protein components reduced to basic elements (amino acids, simple sugars)	Suggested for malabsorption, pancreatic insufficiency (see text)	Flexical Vivonex Aminaid (essential amino acids) Hepaticaid (branched-chain-enriched amino acids)

diets may be indicated include the short bowel syndrome, gastrointestinal fistulas, inflammatory bowel disease, pancreatic disease, chronic intestinal obstruction, diverticulitis and various diarrhoeas. While most trials of elemental diets have a satisfactory outcome, it cannot be certain that other less expensive and more palatable diets may have been just as effective. One study comparing the effectiveness of elemental diets with total parenteral nutrition in gastroenterological patients showed that nitrogen retention was equivalent.[66]

A number of side-effects have been reported with these diets, including gastric retention, altered bowel habits, fluid balance problems, hyperglycaemia and deficiencies of vitamins or fatty acids. Most can be corrected by careful attention to the composition of the diet or by slowing delivery to the gut.

After initial enthusiasm, elemental diets have only a limited role in gastroenterological patients.[41] Patients with malabsorption problems such as exocrine pancreatic insufficiency or the short gut syndrome, who have failed on conventional dietary manipulation, should be tried on an elemental diet.

Parenteral therapy

In the early decades of this century, the feasibility of using nutritional therapy by intravenous routes was established. In 1937 Elman showed that a protein hydrolysate of casein could be given intravenously to humans.

Isotonic dextrose solutions were used in the 1920s, but fat solutions initially produced in the 1930s were found to be unstable. The major problem in developing effective nutritional therapy, however, was related to administration of the hypertonic nutrient solutions. The successful development in the late 1960s of central venous catheterization techniques enabled hypertonic solutions to be infused safely, which led to the successful management of patients who previously would have died of the nutritional consequences of their disease.

INDICATIONS

The indications for using the parenteral route for feeding patients are related to the inability of the intestine to adequately absorb sufficient nutrients for the patient's needs. Thus, intravenous nutrition is indicated when the intestinal tract is blocked, too short, inflamed or simply cannot cope.

When the gastrointestinal tract is blocked
Although acute obstruction of the intestine is usually treated as a surgical emergency regardless of the nutritional state of the patient, conditions which gradually produce obstruction of the pharynx, oesophagus, stomach or duodenum may first require intravenous nutrition to treat the insidious and often far advanced protein–energy malnutrition that has occurred. Available evidence suggests that weight loss must be large (probably more than 20%) and plasma proteins very low (albumin less than 30 g/l) before it can be said that the patient has a 'dangerous' level of malnutrition. Nevertheless, it must be remembered that if an already malnourished patient should sustain a postoperative complication, his nutritional reserves may be unable to withstand the consequent nutritional assault. Thus, although patients with weight loss of more than 20% and those with very low concentrations of plasma proteins should be fed intravenously for two weeks before a major operation, others, who on physical examination have depleted reserves of protein and fat yet do not fulfil these criteria, should be considered carefully for intravenous nutrition. This is particularly so if it is considered that the postoperative course may be complicated.

When the gastrointestinal tract is too short
This category includes not only those patients who have had massive small bowel resections but also those with fistulas where the effective length of the gut is reduced. Intravenous nutrition is particularly effective in high-output small-intestinal fistulas, where oral feeding produces an increase in fistula output and greater morbidity and mortality.[32] In patients with a short gut syndrome, parenteral therapy is necessary to maintain nutrition until it is possible to gradually introduce enteral feeding.[25]

When the gastrointestinal tract is inflamed
Nutritional depletion is a common feature of inflammatory bowel disease. More than 50% of patients requiring urgent surgery for acute colitis suffer from protein–energy malnutrition.[35] There is some evidence that postoperative parenteral nutritional may be beneficial in such patients.[68]

Although some patients with intractable Crohn's enteritis go into remission when the gut is rested and vigorous nutritional therapy is instituted,[18] there does not appear to be any primary effect of total bowel rest and intravenous nutrition on acute colitis.[17]

In summary, intravenous nutrition is indicated in severely malnourished patients about to undergo major surgery for inflammatory bowel disease. It should also be used in some patients with Crohn's disease of the small intestine, particularly where there is evidence of obstruction. Here, nutritional integrity can be preserved while the gut is rested and time is gained which may allow spontaneous remission. Other patients with intestinal inflammation may also receive benefit from gut rest and parenteral nutrition. There is some evidence that fluorouracil toxicity is less when the gut is rested, and patients with radiation enteritis and protein–energy malnutrition may also be helped by a period of such treatment.

When the gastrointestinal tract cannot cope

Whenever there is an intra-abdominal abscess or septic focus, it is difficult to administer nutrients via the enteral route. Patients with complications of pancreatitis, in particular, come into this category. Prolonged attacks of acute pancreatitis can be associated with rapid deterioration in nutritional state and treatment with total gut rest and intravenous nutrition appears to be effective.

Pancreatic pseudocysts often resolve spontaneously but those in which this does not occur need drainage. A period of gut rest and parenteral nutrition buys time, allows the cyst wall to mature and thicken and enables subsequent drainage to be more straightforward. Pancreatic abscesses, too, need surgical drainage but this may need to be repeated on a number of occasions; without nutritional therapy the associated hypermetabolism and starvation can lead to advanced protein–energy malnutrition. Prolonged postoperative ileus, pseudo-obstruction of the colon and idiopathic pseudo-obstruction of the intestine may all require intravenous nutrition for varying periods while awaiting spontaneous remission. In idiopathic pseudo-obstruction of the intestine[55] very prolonged periods of feeding may be required and some patients may need to be fed intravenously permanently.

METHODS

There are three forms of parenteral nutritional support currently used. While each has a place in the nutritional support of patients, central venous administration of adequate energy and nitrogen remains the standard method for providing total balanced nutritional support.

Protein-sparing therapy

Dextrose-free amino acid solutions have been shown to have a nitrogen-sparing effect. The concept is to promote low glucose and low insulin concentrations in plasma, allow mobilization of endogenous fat stores and satisfy the energy deficit by ketogenesis. Some workers believe that if additional glucose is given nitrogen-sparing is less and that elevation of insulin impairs visceral protein synthesis. After many studies it is now clear that amino acids alone are protein-sparing, can be given via peripheral veins and are associated with fewer side-effects than when dextrose is given. Nevertheless, the provision of an energy supply with the amino acids has marked clinical and metabolic advantages[68] and there are very few indications for isotonic dextrose-free amino acid solutions in gastroenterological patients.

Peripheral total parenteral nutrition

The early attempts to give glucose in sufficient quantity for energy needs were limited by the inability of the peripheral veins to accept hypertonic solutions. With the development of isotonic fat solutions, energy needs can be met more easily when the sole access is by the peripheral route. By combining amino acids and fat with a small quantity of isotonic glucose for essential cellular metabolism, the nutritional needs of an average patient can be met. There are, however, disadvantages in this approach. Peripheral lines are more cumbersome for the patient than central lines, and despite meticulous care, they do need changing frequently as phlebitis and venous occlusion occurs with these solutions. The place of peripheral total parenteral nutrition is therefore limited to those occasional patients in whom a central line is contraindicated or is impossible to insert.

Central total parenteral nutrition

The development of central venous catheterization has enabled the delivery of hypertonic glucose solutions to be given safely. The glucose and amino acids are given simultaneously through a central venous line with its tip in the superior vena cava. On such therapy, patients gain weight and may be put into positive nitrogen balance. Fat can be administered through this line or peripherally and a balanced nutritional regimen tailored to the patient's needs administered.

There are a number of techniques for placement of central venous catheters, with the infraclavicular puncture being recommended. The use of long catheters from the antecubital fossa is not recommended because they are associated with a high rate of catheter tip misplacement and the patient's movements may be restricted. Complications of insertion include arterial puncture, air embolism, pneumothorax and misplaced tip. Air embolism is reduced if the catheter is inserted with the patient tilted head-down. A chest X-ray after the procedure is important to check for pneumothorax and the position of the catheter tip. The incidence of venous thrombosis increases if the tip is in any other vessel than the superior vena cava.

The most important complication of central parenteral nutrition is catheter tip sepsis. The main source of organisms contaminating central venous catheters is the skin puncture site. However, with meticulous nursing care a central line may be maintained for many months without adverse effects. Catheter sepsis has an incidence of 3% to 10%, much higher rates occurring in units dealing with major complicated gastrointestinal patients.[46] It is clear, however, that the colonization of central catheters is very much more common than the reported clinical sepsis rate. The potential for septic problems is therefore great. When a patient with a central venous line develops clinical signs of sepsis, the catheter must be suspected. If no other source of infection is found, the catheter is removed. About 75% of catheters removed for suspected catheter sepsis, however, are eventually exonerated as the source of sepsis.[54]

ADMINISTRATION AND MONITORING

Ideally, administration of the nutrient solution should be managed by a team of clinicians, nursing staff, pharmacists and technicians. The incidence of complications and catheter sepsis increases in situations where only an occasional patient is treated. Solutions need to be prepared under aseptic conditions, preferably in the pharmacy under a laminar flow hood. The attending physician each day evaluates the patient's clinical situation, and appropriate amounts of glucose, amino acids and electrolytes are prescribed. Vitamins and trace metals are added and the solution is infused over a 24-hour period. Fat is not added to the nutrient solution but is given by a peripheral line or a Y connection at the central venous catheter. Delivery of the nutrient solution is best carried out by a modern intravenous pump with microprocessor control which will administer solutions at specified volume rates very accurately. This not only reduces the problems of nursing care in adjusting drip flow rates but ensures that solutions are administered evenly over 24-hour periods, minimizing problems of hyperglycaemia and glycosuria.

When starting glucose-based parenteral nutrition, it is important to commence with less than half the glucose load intended and gradually increase the glucose over the first 24 to 48 hours, to prevent hyperglycaemia and glycosuria. Similarly, when stopping parenteral nutrition, a solution of 10% dextrose should be given for 12 to 24 hours after finishing to prevent rebound hypoglycaemia.

Patients receiving parenteral nutrition need to be monitored daily with clinical and biochemical assessments. Daily weighing is important to indicate hydration and is more accurate than fluid balance records. Urine testing for glycosuria is required to check that prescribed glucose is not being lost, and the regular recording of body temperature is an essential part of monitoring for catheter sepsis. Daily biochemistry monitoring should include electrolytes, urea, chloride and phosphate, and two to three times a week liver function tests need to be checked. Other ions such as zinc, copper and magnesium should be monitored weekly. If fat is being used, the blood should be centrifuged and the plasma assessed for opalescence.

PRESCRIBING

The basis for prescribing parenteral nutritional therapy when the patient is not oedematous is the weight of the patient. Weight is used to calculate energy requirements for maintenance of body protein and further increments allowed for depleted patients and hypermetabolic patients.

Energy

Glucose remains the most commonly used source of energy for most parenteral nutrition regimens. For most gastroenterological patients 170 $kJ \cdot kg^{-1} \cdot day^{-1}$ (40 $kcal \cdot kg^{-1} \cdot day^{-1}$) is sufficient. Infusion rates of glucose above 170 $kJ \cdot kg^{-1} \cdot day^{-1}$ result in fat synthesis and occasionally may be harmful.[60] Very septic patients need up to 250 $kJ \cdot kg^{-1} \cdot day^{-1}$. This additional requirement should probably be given as fat. However, there are problems in the utilization of fat in hypermetabolic patients as well, and the optimal solution for these patients awaits definition.[34]

Other energy sources such as fructose, sorbitol, xylitol and ethanol have been used but advantages over the cheaper and more readily available dextrose solutions have not been demonstrated.

Besides giving fat solutions when energy requirements are high, the two other occasions where fat should be given are where peripheral veins are being used and to prevent or treat fatty acid deficiency. One litre of 10% fat solution per week is sufficient to prevent this problem.[20]

Protein

Hydrolysates of casein have been superseded by crystalline amino acids in balanced proportions.[43] There are many commercial preparations, some with electrolytes and energy added. Protein should be given in proportion to the energy: the nitrogen : energy ratio (grams : kilojoules) should be between 1 : 420 and 1 : 630 (a gram : kilocalorie ratio between 1 : 100 and 1 : 150).[60]

The requirement for protein varies according to the state of depletion. Generally, most gastroenterological patients will go into positive balance when $300\ mg \cdot kg^{-1} \cdot day^{-1}$ of nitrogen are given. Depleted patients will readily utilize protein even when less than optimal energy is supplied.[20] Hypermetabolic patients have an increased nitrogen and energy requirement as most of the losses are from the protein compartment. Table 17.10, which outlines the energy and protein requirements of patients with the nutritional syndromes, is a fair guide suitable for use in gastroenterological patients.[34]

Fluid and electrolytes

In patients receiving total parenteral nutrition, deficiencies of sodium, phosphate, or potassium will cause a fall in nitrogen retention while fat accumulation still occurs.[53] Adequate replacement of electrolyte losses and continued maintenance are therefore critical to successful nutritional therapy.

The protein and energy are supplied in a fluid load which is appropriate to the patient's needs. Usually two to three litres are required, but losses from fistulas, diarrhoea and nasogastric tubes and extra renal losses all need to be accounted for. Elderly patients in particular are easy to overload with total parenteral nutrition and some restriction of the sodium is usually necessary. Large increases in weight due to water in any patient may be countered by sodium restriction.

Malnourished patients starting parenteral nutritional therapy have a marked avidity for potassium. As cells are turned from catabolism to anabolism, extra potassium is required for glycogen storage and increased cell growth. Phosphate is another ion which may fall precipitously in malnourished patients starting intravenous nutrition. About 15 millimoles per litre per day is required and blood levels should be carefully monitored.

Magnesium is given at 4 millimoles per litre per day. Most of the anion is given as chloride, but if hyperchloraemic metabolic acidosis becomes a problem some should be substituted by acetate in the formula, acetate being metabolized to bicarbonate. Gastroenterological patients with acid loss from fistulas, nasogastric tubes or vomiting usually do not require acetate.

Table 17.10 Guidelines for intravenous administration of energy and nitrogen in different categories of gastroenterological patients.

Nutritional syndrome	Energy $kJ \cdot kg^{-1} \cdot day^{-1}$ (kcal $\cdot kg^{-1} \cdot day^{-1}$)	Nitrogen $mg \cdot kg^{-1} \cdot day^{-1}$	Remarks
Normal: preoperative	170(40)	250	Glucose intake above this level is not oxidized
Normal: postoperative	170(40)	300	Energy requirements do not increase significantly but increased nitrogen loss occurs owing to decrease in protein synthesis
Nutritional depletion	170(40)	300	The aim is to replenish body fat stores and lean body mass. Energy needs are low with nutritional depletion and moderate gains in fat and protein will occur.
Nutritional depletion and sepsis	190(45)	350	Energy stores and protein compartment are depleted, but energy requirements and protein loss are high. There is a need to match losses and provide extra nitrogen for repletion. Part of the energy load should be given as fat ($42\ kJ \cdot kg^{-1} \cdot day^{-1}$)
Septic	210(50)	400	This group has the highest requirements for energy and nitrogen, although the aim is to prevent loss, not to replete. At least $42\ kJ \cdot kg^{-1} \cdot day^{-1}$ should be given as fat

Vitamins and trace elements

A suitable preparation of fat- and water-soluble vitamins should be added daily to the nutrient solution. Of the many preparations available, none supply all vitamins, and vitamins B_{12} and K need to be given intramuscularly as injections usually once a week. Folic acid should be given also at 1 mg/day to the intravenous solution. This should be increased to 5 mg/day in trauma or septic patients as megaloblastic anaemias have been demonstrated in these circumstances on smaller doses of folate.[3]

Ideally, trace elements should be given daily, especially in children and debilitated patients. With fistulas and in inflammatory conditions increased losses of zinc occur in the bowel as well as in the urine. The daily requirement of about 10 mg of zinc may need to be increased in these situations. Other elements given daily are copper (1.5 mg/day), manganese (0.5 mg/day), chromium (20 μg/day), iodine (100 μg/day) and selenium (50 μg/day). Such solutions need to be made up for intravenous administration. A weekly infusion of fresh plasma, suggested by some to supply trace elements, will not compensate for increased losses or make up deficits that have occurred.

Other additives

In general, the central venous line used for parenteral nutrients should not be used for any other additives. However, insulin may be added by the pharmacy if required. Cimetidine has also been given in nutrient solutions, but other drugs such as antibiotics should be given through separate intravenous lines as compatibility with nutrients is not known.

COMPLICATIONS

Complications of parenteral nutrition are either metabolic or related to the catheter. The most important catheter complication is sepsis, and meticulous nursing care is essential to minimize this. Other catheter complications occur at insertion (pneumothorax, arterial puncture, etc.), from disconnection of the line (air embolus) or from thrombosis of a large vein, almost always because the nutrients were infused into a vein other than the superior vena cava.

Metabolic complications are uncommon if the patient is monitored carefully each day. Hyperosmolar crises usually occur with too rapid infusion of glucose. Hypoglycaemia may occur if the infusion is stopped suddenly. Other metabolic complications occur with deficiencies of vitamins, trace metals or electrolytes.

SPECIAL CONDITIONS

Hepatic failure

In patients with fulminant hepatic failure, administration of conventional amino acid solutions may worsen encephalopathy. Hepatic encephalopathy has been related to the high levels of aromatic amino acids (phenylalanine, tyrosine and tryptophan) in the plasma acting as precursors of false neurotransmitter amines in the central and peripheral nervous systems.[23] Administration of branched-chain amino acid solutions (enriched with leucine, isoleucine and valine) will normalize the plasma aminogram and possibly reverse the coma in patients with chronic hepatic encephalopathy.[24] Glucose should be used as the energy source in hepatic failure, but it needs careful monitoring. Blood levels may fluctuate widely because carbohydrate tolerance is impaired as a result of peripheral insulin resistance. Intravenous lipid infusions are contraindicated as they have a synergistic effect in producing coma, particularly with ammonia and they may exacerbate coma by displacing tryptophan from plasma protein binding sites.[14] Patients with chronic hepatic failure should also receive increased amounts of vitamins.

Renal failure

Patients with acute renal failure are usually hypercatabolic and have increased requirements for energy and nitrogen.[61] Because of limited fluid volumes and the increased blood urea from protein administration, modified nutritional regimens have been suggested in such patients. However, with the early use of dialysis, many of these problems can be overcome and a full nutritional regimen prescribed. It has been suggested that the use of essential amino acids only may improve survival as well as improving blood urea levels.[27] Others have shown that the administration of adequate amounts of protein and energy with haemodialysis is more important in improving survival than the use of essential or non-essential amino acids.[22] Careful monitoring of potassium, phosphate, hydrogen, magnesium and calcium ions in patients with renal failure on parenteral nutrition is essential.

Respiratory failure

Administration of high doses of glucose to patients with borderline respiratory function may increase their carbon dioxide production to the point of compromising respiratory function.[20] Such patients in intensive care may benefit from the replacement of some glucose energy intake with fat. High rates of infusion of amino acids may increase respiratory drive in some patients; this may be important therapeutically.[21]

Home parenteral nutrition

There are a small number of gastroenterological patients who are unable to survive without prolonged intravenous nutrition. Most of these patients have had massive small bowel resections for vascular problems or Crohn's disease, and are left with insufficient absorptive surface to maintain protein and energy balance. The development of regimens and equipment suitable for long-term intravenous administration outside the hospital setting has vastly improved the lifestyle of these patients and some have been maintained on such therapy for up to ten years.[26]

Solutions are prepared in the pharmacy and given intermittently, usually overnight so the patient is free of the infusion apparatus during the day.[39] A vest with a small pump has been devised to enable continuous infusion of nutrients throughout the day if required.[19]

REFERENCES

1   Baker, J. P., Detsky, A. S., Whitwell, J. *et al.* (1982) A comparison of the predictive value of nutritional assessment techniques. *Human Nutrition: Clinical Nutrition,* **36,** 233–241.
2   Bates, S. E., Suen, J. Y. & Tranum, B. L. (1979) Immunological skin testing and interpretation – a plea for uniformity. *Cancer,* **43,** 2306–2314.
3   Beard, M. E. J., Hatipov, C. S. & Hamer, J. W. (1980) Acute onset of folate deficiency in patients under intensive care. *Critical Care Medicine,* **8,** 500–503.
4   Beisel, W. R. & Wannemacher, R. W. (1980) Gluconeogenesis, ureagenesis and ketogenesis during sepsis. *Journal of Parenteral and Enteral Nutrition* **4,** 277–285.
5   Black, P. R., Brooks, D. C., Bessey, P. Q. *et al.* (1982) Mechanisms of insulin resistance following injury. *Annals of Surgery,* **196,** 420–435.
6   Blackburn, G. L., Bistrian, B. R., Maini, B. S. *et al.* (1977) Nutritional and metabolic assessment of the hospitalised patient. *Journal of Parenteral and Enteral Nutrition,* **1,** 11–22.
7   Buchman, E., Kaung, D. T., Dolan K. & Knapp, R. N. (1969) Unrestricted diet in the treatment of duodenal ulcer. *Gastroenterology,* **56,** 1016–1020.
8   Buzby, G. P., Mullen, J. L., Matthews, D. C. *et al.* (1980) Prognostic nutritional index in gastrointestinal surgery. *American Journal of Surgery,* **139,** 159–167.
9   Chandra, R. K. (1981) Immunocompetence as a functional index of nutritional status. *British Medical Bulletin,* **37,** 89–94.
10 Church, J. C. & Hill, G. L. (1983) Personal communication.
11 Collins, J. P., McCarthy, I. D. & Hill, G. L. (1979) Assessment of protein nutrition in surgical patients – the value of anthropometrics. *American Journal of Clinical Nutrition,* **32,** 1527–1530.
12 Committee on Dietary Allowances (1980) *Recommend-ed Dietary Allowances* 9th edition. Washington DC: National Academy of Sciences.
13 Cunningham-Rundles, S. (1982) Effects of nutritional status on immunological function. *American Journal of Clinical Nutrition,* **35,** 1202–1210.
14 Davis, M. & Williams, R. (1977) Nutritional problems in fulminant hepatic failure. In *Nutritional Aspects of Care of the Critically Ill* (Ed.) Richards, J. R. & Kinney, J. M., pp. 487–498. Edinburgh: Churchill Livingstone.
15 DeWys, W. D. (1978) Changes in taste sensation and feeding behavior in cancer patients: a review. *Journal of Human Nutrition,* **32,** 447–453.
16 Deysine, M. & Stein, S. (1980) Albumin shifts across the extracellular space secondary to experimental infections. *Surgery, Gynecology and Obstetrics,* **151,** 617–620.
17 Dickinson, R. J., Ashton, M. G., Axon, A. T. R. *et al.* (1980) Controlled trial of intravenous hyperalimentation and total bowel rest as an adjunct to the routine therapy of acute colitis. *Gastroenterology,* **79,** 1199–1204.
18 Driscoll, R. H. & Rosenberg, I. H. (1978) Total parenteral nutrition in inflammatory bowel disease. *Medical Clinics of North America,* **62,** 185–201.
19 Dudrick, S. J., Englert, D. M., Van Buren, C. T. *et al.* (1979) New concepts of ambulatory home hyperalimentation. *Journal of Parenteral and Enteral Nutrition,* **3,** 72–76.
20 Elwyn, D. H. (1980) Nutritional requirements of adult surgical patients. *Critical Care Medicine,* **8,** 9–20.
21 Elwyn, D. H., Askanazi, J., Kinney, J. M. & Gump, F. E. (1980) Kinetics of energy substrates. *Acta Chirurgica Scandinavica* (supplement) **507,** 209–219.
22 Feinstein, E. I., Blumenkrantz, M. J., Healy, M. *et al.* (1981) Clinical and metabolic responses to parenteral nutrition in acute renal failure – a controlled double-blind study. *Medicine,* **60,** 124–137.
23 Fischer, J. E. & Baldessarini, R. J. (1971) False neuro-transmitters and hepatic failure. *Lancet,* **ii,** 75.
24 Fischer, J. E., Rosen, H. M., Ebeid, A. M. *et al.* (1976) The effect of normalization of plasma aminoacids on hepatic encephalopathy in man. *Surgery,* **80,** 77–91.
25 Fleming, C. R. & Remington, M. (1981) Intestinal failure. In *Nutrition and the Surgical Patient* (Ed.) Hill, G. L., pp. 219–235. Edinburgh: Churchill Livingstone.
26 Fleming, C. R., Beart, R. W., Berkner, S. *et al.* (1980) Home parenteral nutrition for management of the severely malnourished adult patient. *Gastroenterology,* **79,** 11–18.
27 Freund, H. & Fischer, J. (1980) Comparative study of parenteral nutrition in renal failure using essential and non essential aminoacid containing solutions. *Surgery, Gynecology and Obstetrics,* **151,** 652–656.
28 Freund, H., Yoshimura, N. & Fischer, J. E. (1979) Chronic hepatic encephalopathy – long term therapy with a branched-chain aminoacid enriched elemental diet. *Journal of American Medical Association,* **242,** 347–349.
29 Giovannetti, S. & Maggiore, Q. (1964) A low-nitrogen diet with proteins of high biological value for severe chronic uraemia. *Lancet,* **i,** 1000–1003.
30 Golden, M. H. N. (1982) Transport proteins as indices of protein status. *American Journal of Clinical Nutrition,* **35,** 1159–1165.
31 Hackett, A. F., Yeung, C. K. & Hill, G. L. (1979) Eating patterns in patients recovering from major surgery – a study of voluntary food intake and energy balance. *British Journal of Surgery,* **66,** 415–418.
32 Hill, G. L. (1983) Operative strategy in the treatment of enterocutaneous fistulas. *World Journal of Surgery,* **1,** 495–501.

33 Hill, G. L. & Beddoe, A. H. (1982) In vivo neutron activation in metabolic and nutritional studies. (i) Introduction. *Journal of Clinical Surgery*, **1**, 270–279. (ii) Clinical applications. *Journal of Clinical Surgery*, **1**, 333–345.

34 Hill, G. L. & Church, J. M. (1983) Energy and protein requirements of general surgical patients requiring intravenous nutrition. *British Journal of Surgery* (in press).

35 Hill, G. L., Blackett, R. L., Pickford, I. R. & Bradley, J. A. (1977) A survey of protein nutrition in patients with inflammatory bowel disease. A rational basis for nutritional therapy. *British Journal of Surgery*, **64**, 894–896.

36 Hill, G. L., Blackett, R. L., Pickford, I. *et al.* (1977) Malnutrition in surgical patients: an unrecognised problem. *Lancet*, **i**, 689–692.

37 Hoffman-Goetz, L., McFarlane, D., Bistrian, B. R. & Blackburn, G. L. (1981) Febrile and plasma iron responses of rabbits injected with endogenous pyrogen from malnourished patients. *American Journal of Clinical Nutrition*, **34**, 1109–1116.

38 Ing, A. F. M., Meakins, J. L., McLean, A. P. H. & Christou, N. V. (1982) Determinants of susceptibility to sepsis and mortality: malnutrition *vs* anergy. *Journal of Surgical Research*, **32**, 249–255.

39 Jeejeebhoy, K. N., Langer, B., Tsalla, G. *et al.* (1976) Total parenteral nutrition at home: studies in patients surviving 4 months to 5 years. *Gastroenterology*, **71**, 943–953.

40 Jenkins, D. J. A., Gassull, M. A., Leeds, A. R. *et al.* (1977) Effect of dietary fibre on complications of gastric surgery: prevention of post-prandial hypoglycaemia by pectin. *Gastroenterology*, **73**, 215–217.

41 Koretz, R. L. & Meyer, J. H. (1980) Elemental diets – facts and fantasies. *Gastroenterology*, **78**, 393–410.

42 Long, C. L. & Blakemore, W. S. (1979) Energy and protein requirements in the hospitalized patient. *Journal of Parenteral and Enteral Nutrition*, **3**, 69–71.

43 Long, C. L., Zikria, B. A., Kinney, J. M. & Geiger, J. W. (1974) Comparison of fibrin hydrolysates and crystalline amino acid solutions in parenteral nutrition. *American Journal of Clinical Nutrition*, **27**, 163–174.

44 Long, C. L., Schaffel, N., Geiger, J. W. *et al.* (1979) Metabolic response to injury and illness: estimation of energy and protein needs from indirect calorimetry and nitrogen balance. *Journal of Parenteral and Enteral Nutrition*, **3**, 452–456.

45 MacFie, J., Smith, R. C. & Hill, G. L. (1981) Glucose or fat as a nonprotein energy source? *Gastroenterology*, **80**, 103–107.

46 Maki, D. G. (1982) Infections associated with intravascular lines. In *Current Clinical Topics in Infectious Diseases* (Ed.) Remington, J. S. and Swartz, M. N. pp. 309–363. New York: McGraw Hill.

47 Morgan, D. B., Hill, G. L. & Burkinshaw, L. (1980) The assessment of weight loss from a single measurement of body weight: the problems and limitations. *American Journal of Clinical Nutrition*, **33**, 2101–2105.

48 Nutrition Advisory Group (1979a) Multivitamin preparations for parenteral use – a statement by the Nutrition Advisory Group (AMA). *Journal of Parenteral and Enteral Nutrition*, **3**, 258–262.

49 Nutrition Advisory Group (1979b) Guidelines for essential trace element preparations for parenteral use. *Journal of the American Medical Association*, **241**, 2051–2054.

50 Patel, D., Anderson, G. H. & Jeejeebhoy, K. N. (1973) Amino acid adequacy of parenteral casein hydrolysate and oral cottage cheese in patients with gastrointestinal disease as measured by nitrogen balance and blood aminogram. *Gastroenterology*, **65**, 427–437.

51 Powanda, M. C. (1977) Changes in body balances of nitrogen and other key nutrients: description and underlying mechanisms. *American Journal of Clinical Nutrition*, **30**, 1254–1268.

52 Robinson, F. W. & Pittman, A. C. (1957) Dietary management of postgastrectomy dumping syndrome. *Surgery, Gynecology and Obstetrics*, **104**, 529–534.

53 Rudman, D., Millikan, W. J., Richardson, J. *et al.* (1975) Elemental balances during intravenous hyperalimentation of underweight adult subjects. *Journal of Clinical Investigation*, **55**, 94–101.

54 Ryan, J. A., Abel, R. M., Abbott, W. M. *et al.* (1974) Catheter complications in total parenteral nutrition – a prospective study of 200 consecutive patients. *New England Journal of Medicine*, **290**, 757–761.

55 Schufflers, M. D., Lowe, M. C. & Bill, A. H. (1977) Studies of idiopathic intestinal pseudoobstruction. Hereditary hollow visceral myopathy: clinical pathological studies. *Gastroenterology*, **73**, 327–338.

56 Scrimshaw, N. S., Taylor, C. E. & Gordon, J. E. (1968) *Interactions of Nutrition and Infection*. World Health Organisation Monograph Series, No. 57.

57 Shenkin, A. & Wretlind, A. (1977) Complete intravenous nutrition including amino acids, glucose and lipids. In *Nutritional Aspects of Care in the Critically Ill* (Ed.) Richards, J. R. & Kinney, J. M. pp. 345–365. Edinburgh: Churchill Livingstone.

58 Shetty, P. S., Watrasiewicz, K. E., Jung, R. T. & James, W. P. T. (1979) Rapid-turnover transport proteins: an index of subclinical protein energy malnutrition. *Lancet*, **ii**, 230–232.

59 Shike, M., Roulet, M., Kurian, R. *et al.* (1981) Copper metabolism and requirements in total parenteral nutrition. *Gastroenterology*, **81**, 290–297.

60 Smith, R. C., Burkinshaw, L. & Hill, G. L. (1982) Optimal energy and nitrogen intake for gastroenterological patients requiring intravenous nutrition. *Gastroenterology*, **82**, 445–452.

61 Spreiter, S. C., Myers, B. D. & Swenson, R. S. (1980) Protein–energy requirements in subjects with acute renal failure receiving intermittent haemodialysis. *American Journal of Clinical Nutrition*, **33**, 1433–1437.

62 Starker, P. M., Gump, F. E., Askanazi, J. *et al.* (1982) Serum albumin levels as an index of nutritional support. *Surgery*, **91**, 194–199.

63 Torosian, M. H. & Rombeau, J. L. (1980) Feeding by tube enterostomy. *Surgery, Gynecology and Obstetrics*, **150**, 918–927.

64 Twomey, P., Ziegler, D. & Rombeau, J. (1982) Utility of skin testing in nutritional assessment: a critical review. *Journal of Parenteral and Enteral Nutrition*, **6**, 50–58.

65 Wolman, S. L., Anderson, H., Marliss, E. B. & Jeejeebhoy, K. N. (1979) Zinc in total parenteral nutrition: requirements and metabolic effects. *Gastroenterology*, **76**, 458–467.

66 Yeung, C. K., Smith, R. C. & Hill, G. L. (1979) Effect of an elemental diet on body composition: a comparison with intravenous nutrition. *Gastroenterology*, **77**, 652–657.

67 Yeung, C. K., Young, G. A., Hackett, A. F. & Hill, G. L. (1979) Fine needle catheter jejunostomy – an assessment of a new method of nutritional support after major gastrointestinal surgery. *British Journal of Surgery*, **66**, 727–732.

68 Young, G. A. & Hill, G. L. (1980) A controlled study of protein sparing therapy after excision of the rectum. Effects of intravenous aminoacids and hyperalimentation on body composition and plasma amino acids. *Annals of Surgery*, **192**, 183–191.

OBESITY

Definition

Obesity is an excessive accumulation of adipose tissue. The term 'overweight' is now used to describe a body weight of 110 to 119% above an ideal reference weight (equivalent to 100%) for height and sex, and the term 'obesity' is used when the body weight is 120% or more above this reference. Until recently there was no precise formula for calculating the ideal reference weight and thus no precise definition of 'obesity'. In 1960 the Metropolitan Life Insurance Company of New York issued tables of actuarial optimal weights for three frame sizes (small, medium, large) according to height and sex.[10] The optimal weights referred to individuals wearing shoes and indoor clothing and no firm guidance was given regarding the definition of frame size. This has led to several definitions of the ideal reference weight, including the average value for the whole range of frame sizes, the upper limit of the large frame size or even the upper limit of an approximation of frame size for each individual. The difference can be as much as 9 kg. In 1979, the American Build Study considered this problem and reaffirmed earlier recommendations that the ideal reference weight should refer to the upper limit of the 'large' frame size and that the use of frame size should henceforth be abandoned.[14]

This has resulted in generous allowances for those individuals of small build. However, recent insurance studies of mortality risk tend to confirm that this definition of ideal reference weight is appropriate (see Table 17.11).

Aetiology

Obesity is only rarely associated with a clear genetic defect. The Laurence–Moon–Biedl syndrome is inherited as a recessive trait and is characterized by obesity, mental retardation, retinitis pigmentosa and hypogonadism. In the Prader–Willi syndrome the obesity is associated with diabetes mellitus, hypotonia, mental retardation and hypogonadism. The Morgagni–Stewart–Morel syndrome appears mainly in women and is inherited as a dominant trait. It is characterized by obesity, hypertension, hirsutism, hyperostosis of the frontal bones, hypogonadism and mental abnormalities. In all three syndromes the obesity is associated with hyperphagia, although a temperature-regulating defect has been discovered in some individuals with the Prader–Willi syndrome.

Table 17.11 Appropriate body weight and the lower limits for defining overweight and obesity.

Height (cm)	Men Average (kg)	Men Acceptable range (kg)	Men Overweight (kg)	Men Obese (kg)	Women Average (kg)	Women Acceptable range (kg)	Women Overweight (kg)	Women Obese (kg)
145					46.0	37–53	58	64
148					46.5	37–54	59	65
150					47.0	38–55	61	66
152					48.5	39–57	63	68
156					49.5	39–58	64	70
158	55.8	44–64	70	77	50.4	40–58	64	70
160	57.6	45–65	72	78	51.3	41–59	65	71
162	58.6	46–66	73	79	52.6	42–61	67	73
164	59.6	47–67	74	80	54.0	43–62	68	74
166	60.6	48–69	76	83	55.4	44–64	70	77
168	61.7	49–71	78	85	56.8	45–65	72	78
170	63.5	51–73	80	88	58.1	45–66	73	79
172	65.0	52–74	81	89	60.0	46–67	74	80
174	66.5	53–75	83	90	61.3	48–69	76	83
176	68.0	54–77	85	92	62.6	49–70	77	84
178	69.4	55–79	87	95	64.0	51–72	79	86
180	71.0	58–80	88	96	65.3	52–74	81	89
182	72.6	59–82	90	98				
184	74.2	60–84	92	101				
186	75.8	62–86	95	103				
188	77.6	64–88	97	106				
190	79.3	66–90	99	108				
192	81.0	68–93	102	112				

Figures adjusted to take account of extended lower range suggested by the Society of Actuaries 1979 Build Study. Limits of overweight taken to be 110–119% of upper limit, with obesity present when weight is 120% or more.

Hypothalamic damage due to trauma, inflammation or neoplasm are also rare causes of obesity in man. An endocrine basis for obesity has long been sought but in only a few cases can a hormonal defect such as occurs in Cushing's syndrome, myxoedema, insulinoma and steroid medication be identified. In the vast majority the aetiology of the obesity has eluded investigators. Recent interest has centred on studies of genetically obese mice, especially the *ob/ob* mouse, where the obesity appears to be mainly related to a defect in non-shivering thermogenesis due to an abnormality in the thermogenic activity of brown fat.[5]

Whether a similar mechanism could account for obesity in man is now under investigation and a defect in noradrenergic-stimulated thermogenesis has been reported in obese human subjects.[6] Dietary-induced thermogenesis is reduced in those with a propensity for obesity both after a single meal[12] and following six days over-feeding of an extra 4.2 MJ (1000 kcal) of fat.[15] Although anatomical studies have indicated the presence of brown fat in adult man[3] its involvement in thermogenesis in man is, as yet, unproven.

Mortality and morbidity from digestive diseases

In a recent analysis of mortality by weight in 750 000 men and women in the USA, the mortality rates for weights (relative to the ideal reference weights) of 120%–129%, 130%–139%, and 140% or more were respectively 28%, 46% and 88% higher than for the optimal-weight group.[8] While coronary heart disease was the major factor in the higher mortality of obese individuals, the highest relative mortality for both sexes was from diabetes mellitus and the next highest from digestive diseases. In those with a weight of 140% or more, the mortality from digestive diseases for males was four times as great, and that for females 2.25 times as great, as in those of optimal weight. The Build and Blood Pressure Study of 1959, covering 4 500 000 people, also showed high mortality rates from digestive diseases in obese individuals.[13] Cancer mortality was elevated only among those weighing 140% or more, being 1.33 and 1.55 times as great in males and females respectively. Colorectal cancer was the principal site of excess cancer mortality in males (relative rates: 1.73 in males; 1.22 in females), whereas in females the highest incidence was from cancer of the gallbladder and biliary passages (relative mortality 3.6). The relative mortality rates for cancer of the stomach

and pancreas were higher in males (1.88 and 1.62 respectively) than in females, where the relative mortality rate for stomach cancer (1.03) was similar to that in the optimal weight group and that for pancreatic cancer (0.61) was significantly lower.

Obese women also have a high incidence of gallbladder disease. Rimm *et al.* in a study of over 70 000 obese women reported a 2.7-fold increased incidence of gallbladder disease.[11] There was an increased incidence of diabetes mellitus (4.5-fold), hypertension (3.3-fold), gout (2.6-fold) and jaundice of all types (1.4-fold). Gallbladder disease in obese women has been subject to particular scrutiny recently. As obesity develops there is an increase in the endogenous synthesis of cholesterol by the liver and other tissues. The body pool of cholesterol expands with an increase in the rate at which cholesterol is excreted into the bile.[9] The catabolism of cholesterol to bile salts, the other major route for cholesterol excretion, does not seem to compensate, so biliary cholesterol increases disproportionately, exceeding the capacity of bile salts to solubilize cholesterol. The bile, therefore, becomes supersaturated with respect to cholesterol, which precipitates out. The high incidence of gallstones in young obese females may also be associated with other factors. The contraceptive pill both increases biliary cholesterol saturation and by eliminating ovulation reduces the usual surge in metabolism which occurs at this time. The latter effect could result in as much as a 5% reduction in the monthly energy expenditure, which if unaccompanied by a reduction in food intake, or compensatory thermogenesis, could result in weight gain. Many women attempt to slim by specifically limiting those foods containing carbohydrates such as potatoes and bread. This lowers their intake of fibre, so reducing the bile salt pool,[4] decreasing the solubilization of excreted cholesterol and thus increasing the tendency to gallstone formation. It may be that the low intake of cereal fibre in most slimming diets could increase the incidence of diverticular disease.

Treatment

DIET

The treatment of obesity consists of a suitable reduction in energy intake with the maintenance of an adequate intake of protein, fibre and electrolytes. Diets which only involve reducing carbohydrate intake are not to be recommended as they foster an excess intake of fat-enriched foods. Such regimens can also produce postural hypotension, which may be a consequence of a reduction in sympathetic outflow; starch will relieve or prevent this postural hypotension. Protein-only diets should also be avoided since they have been associated with an increased incidence of arrhythmias and sudden death, possibly due to an associated low potassium intake.[7] Similarly, total starvation is never justified since it can cause large losses in electrolytes, especially potassium, and result in sudden death.

In designing a diet, consideration must be given to individual energy needs, personal idiosyncrasies and home circumstances. Also, the individual must be provided with more than just an outline of the diet: in practice, such cursory dietary advice can result in the individual ingesting up to 70% more calories than expected.

Restriction of energy intake results in a fall in the basal metabolic rate by as much as 15% early in the dieting period. With substantial weight loss there is also less metabolically active lean tissue, which further reduces the basal metabolic rate. Hence, weight loss can be arrested despite strict adherence to the diet because the energy intake of the diet is balanced by the reduction in the basal metabolic rate. One should aim at achieving a 4.2 MJ (1000 kcal) energy deficit each day, but in short individuals with limited mobility (e.g. the elderly) this may not be possible without developing a special low-energy regimen with additional vitamins and electrolytes. All dietary regimens should be supported by patient-monitoring, which seems to be most effectively carried out by group therapy with the incorporation of behaviour modification into the diet schedule.

Special care is required for those who achieve the desired weight loss. It can be estimated that with every 10 kg loss in weight the individual loses about 420 kJ (100 kcal) of basal metabolic activity per day because of a decline in lean tissue. The individual who loses 30 kg and reaches the ideal weight may consider dieting as over and neglect the fact that there is a permanent loss of about 1.05 MJ (300 kcal) of metabolizing lean tissue and hence dietary intake must be restricted accordingly. Long-term dietary changes are, therefore, essential if the individual is not to regain the lost weight.

DRUGS

Anorectic drugs should not be used as the sole method for treating obesity and are best used as an adjunct to appropriate dietary therapy if hunger is a problem after a fortnight of strict dietary perseverance. Intermittent therapy is not recommended, especially if fenfluramine is prescribed since depression may occur if the drug is suddenly stopped. The value of thermogenic drugs such as ephedrine is limited because of cardiovascular side-effects. Thyroid hormones have been used widely but their role is limited since they cause a marked loss in lean body mass.

SURGERY

Jaw wiring is sometimes used as a temporary measure to limit food intake. It should only be used in selected patients, for example those needing rapid weight loss prior to surgery. Careful dental hygiene is required. The patient relies on liquid nutrients such as milk with vitamin supplements. The patients can still gain weight if they so wish by ingesting large volumes of energy-rich fluid and they often rapidly gain weight once the wires are removed despite a suitable dietary regimen. The use of a welded nylon cord around the waist, which reminds the subject of minor degrees of weight gain, has also been suggested.[2]

Jejuno-ileal bypass in which the first 14 inches of jejunum are anastomosed to the last 4 inches of the ileum has been used with success. The operation is very successful in achieving rapid early weight loss by a permanent reduction in appetite. Although malabsorption is responsible for much of the early loss of weight, absorption improves after 6 to 12 months as the intestine adapts.[1] The operative mortality (5%) and high morbidity (up to 70%) after this operation has greatly reduced its role in management. The operation is associated with serious metabolic sequelae: hypoproteinaemia, hypocalcaemia, alkalosis and deficiency of certain trace elements. There is also a high incidence of hepatocellular change; ultimately this may progress to cirrhosis which is not always reversible by restoring intestinal continuity. (see also Chapter 8, p. 527.)

Gastric plication has the advantage that it has a much lower morbidity than jejuno-ileal bypass. Staples are used to fashion an upper pouch with a volume of 50–60 ml. The aperture from the upper pouch is limited to a 12 mm ring, which should be reinforced to prevent later dilatation. Further evaluation of this approach is required.

REFERENCES

1 Faloon, W. W. (1977) Symposium on jejunoileostomy for obesity. *American Journal of Clinical Nutrition*, **30**, 1–128.
2 Garrow, J. S. & Gardiner, G. T. (1981) Maintenance of weight loss in obese patients after jaw wiring. *British Medical Journal*, **282**, 858–860.
3 Heaton, J. M. (1972) The distribution of brown adipose tissue in the human. *Journal of Anatomy*, **112**, 35–39.
4 Heaton, K. W. (1975) Bile salts and fibre. In *Fiber Deficiency and Colonic Disorders* (Ed.) Reilly, R. W. & Kirsner, J. B. New York & London: Plenum Medical Books.
5 James, W. P. T. & Trayhurn, P. (1981) Thermogenesis and obesity. *British Medical Bulletin*, **37**, 43–46.
6 Jung, R. T., Shetty, P. S., James, W. P. T. *et al.* (1979) Reduced thermogenesis in obesity. *Nature*, **279**, 322–323.
7 Lantigua, R. A., Amatruda, J. M., Biddle, T. L. *et al.* (1980) Cardiac arrhythmias associated with a liquid protein diet for the treatment of obesity. *New England Journal of Medicine*, **303**, 735–738.
8 Lew, E. A. & Garfinkel, L. (1979) Variations in mortality by weight among 750 000 men and women. *Journal of Chronic Diseases*, **32**, 563–576.
9 Mabee, T. M., Meyer, P., Den Besten, L. & Mason, E. E. (1976) The mechanism of increased gallstone formation in obese human subjects. *Surgery*, **79**, 460–468.
10 Metropolitan Life Insurance Company, New York (1960) *Statistical Bulletin*, **41**, Feb. p. 6, March p. 7.
11 Rimm, A. A., Werner, L. H., Yserloo, B. van. & Bernstein, R. A. (1975) Relationship of obesity and disease in 73 532 weight-conscious women. *Public Health Reports*, **90**, 44–51.
12 Shetty, P. S., Jung, R. T., James, W. P. T. *et al.* (1981) Postprandial thermogenesis in obesity. *Clinical Science*, **60**, 519–525.
13 Society of Actuaries (1959) *Build and Blood Pressure Study 1959*, Vol. 1. Chicago: The Society of Actuaries.
14 Society of Actuaries (1979) *Build Study 1979*. Association of Life Insurance Medical Directors of America.
15 Zed, C. A. & James, W. P. T. (1982) Thermic response to fat feeding in lean and obese subjects. *Proceedings of Nutrition Society*, **41**, 32A.

THE AGED GUT

It is often difficult to separate the changes in gut function which occur with increasing age from the effects of diseases which become more frequent with longevity. It is also difficult to decide whether malnutrition in an elderly individual is due to impaired absorption caused by disease or merely to poor diet alone.

Nutritional measurements in old age

It has been suggested on the basis of anthropometric, haematological and biochemical measurements that about 3% of persons over age 65 living at home in Britain are malnourished. In half malnutrition was ascribed to underlying disease, in half to poor diet alone.[9] The proportion of malnourished patients entering acute geriatric wards in Britain is of the order of 10%.

Advancing years are accompanied by loss of height and weight. There is an increased proportion of body fat and a decrease in lean body mass as indicated by measurements of total body potassium and total body water, or by densitometry or anthropometry; there may also be a shift of fat to non-subcutaneous sites with ageing. Anthropometric data have only recently been provided for normal, healthy people over 65 years old so that useful comparisons of nutritional status can be made in this age group.[15] Measurements of triceps skinfold thickness (TSF) and mid-arm circumference (MAC) with the derived arm muscle circumference in healthy normal subjects in England, Wales, Sweden, the United States and Canada show that there is no marked change in these indicators of nutrition until about 75 years of age, although Burr, Milbank and Gibbs suggest that TSF and MAC decline steadily from age 65, indicating progressive loss of subcutaneous tissue.[7] There is no age-related fall in plasma haemoglobin or plasma protein concentration in healthy individuals.

Gut function

STOMACH

Gastric acid output
Both basal and peak gastric acid output decrease with increasing age[3] and there is a correlation between decreased numbers of gastric parietal cells, associated gastric atrophy, and the degree of achlorhydria.[2] Perhaps more important, some individuals appear to retain near-normal gastric acid secretion in response to pentagastrin stimulation despite a diminished parietal cell mass, while an increasingly higher proportion of individuals become virtually achlorhydric with advancing age.

Histology
Most studies suggest that a large proportion of 'normal' asymptomatic individuals over 60 years old have atrophic gastritis. Andrews *et al.* found that 23 out of 24 biopsies in this group showed some degree of atrophic gastritis.[2] Bird, Hall and Schade found only 50 histologically normal gastric biopsies in 201 asymptomatic subjects aged 65 to 90 years, but there was no relation between age and the degree of gastric atrophy in this range.[5]

Gastric emptying

Few studies using acceptable methodology have been carried out to examine the effect of age on gastric emptying. However, two groups using isotopic markers have shown considerable prolongation of gastric emptying for liquids in healthy elderly subjects compared with younger controls[10,19]. In one study there was no significant difference in the rate of gastric emptying of solid foods between young and aged men[19]. Since delayed gastric emptying could impair digestion and lead to delayed bioavailability or decreased serum concentration of drugs these findings must be confirmed.

SMALL INTESTINE

Histology

There is an age-related reduction in the villus height of small intestinal mucosa and a slight increase in the breadth of villi. The enterocyte height and intraepithelial lymphocyte counts are unchanged.[21] Together these changes reduce the estimated mucosal surface area.

Absorption

Passive. D-xylose has been used as a model for passive absorption. The measurement of urinary xylose excretion after an oral load does not accurately reflect small bowel absorptive function in the elderly because of decreased urinary clearance, but Haeney et al. used a one-hour serum sample of xylose following a five-gram oral load to demonstrate that there is no decline in xylose absorption with increasing age up to 92 years.[11]

Most drugs are absorbed passively via the small intestine. No significant impairment of drug absorption has been demonstrated in the few instances where it has been examined (paracetamol (acetaminophen), digoxin, practolol and aspirin).[12]

Minerals and vitamins. The subject of vitamin B_{12} absorption, in common with other aspects of normal ageing, is beset with problems of methodology, particularly as the Schilling test assumes both normal renal function and complete urinary collection. Previous gastric surgery is probably the commonest cause of malabsorption of vitamin B_{12} and iron in the elderly. Pernicious anaemia and severe atrophic gastritis are also increasingly frequent. Vitamin B_{12} and iron absorption is normal in healthy elderly individuals.[16] Marx, using ^{59}Fe with ^{51}Cr as an inert marker, found no difference between the young and the elderly in respect of either mucosal uptake or transfer of iron.[13] Iron up-take and transfer increased to a similar extent in young and elderly patients with iron deficiency.

Fats and calcium. There are no definitive studies on the effect of age on fat absorption in normal man. Webster, Wilkinson and Gowland, using serum micronephelometry, found that the maximum value of fat in serum after a standard fatty meal was lower in the elderly than in young subjects,[22] and Citi and Salvini found reduced absorption of ^{131}I-labelled olein and triolein in 60-to-80-year-olds,[8] but these methods have been challenged: using [^{14}C] triolein, McEvoy found no age-related decline in fat absorption.[14]

Calcium absorption probably does decline over 60 years of age,[6] but it has not been established whether this is because of vitamin D deficiency in a number of elderly individuals or whether calcium absorption declines with age independent of vitamin D status.

PANCREAS

Structure

There is a steady increase in the calibre of the main pancreatic duct with age, and the other branches show areas of focal dilatation or stenosis not associated with any other abnormality.[20] This suggests that pancreatograms obtained in elderly patients should be interpreted with caution.

Secretion

Secretion rate and bicarbonate output probably decrease with increased age, at least after secretin stimulation. Moesner et al. also found decreased output of lipase, amylase and trypsin after pancreozymin stimulation.[17]

SPLANCHNIC BLOOD FLOW

Splanchnic blood flow declines with increasing age both absolutely and as a fraction of cardiac output.[4] The splanchnic circulation is also susceptible to hypoxia associated with cardiac or respiratory insufficiency and to hypovolaemia or systemic hypotension.[1] Very few cases of painless occult malabsorption due to vascular insufficiency have been described in geriatric patients. The classical syndromes associated with vascular insufficiency of both small and large intestine (almost always painful) are usually seen in older individuals.

Summary

Few gastrointestinal functions decline to an important extent as a result of old age alone. There is little clinical evidence that significant malnutrition occurs in any normal elderly individual as a result of the ageing process itself. Nevertheless, such factors as achlorhydria, delayed gastric emptying, decreased pancreatic function and subclinical vitamin D deficiency may contribute to maldigestion or malabsorption which could be important in any individual faced with the stress of a marginally inadequate diet or intercurrent illness.

REFERENCES

1 Almy, T. P. (1981) Factors leading to digestive disorders in the elderly. *Proceedings of the New York Academy of Science*, **57**, 709–717.
2 Andrews, G. R., Haneman, B., Arnold, B. J. *et al.* (1967) Atrophic gastritis in the aged. *Australian Annals of Medicine*, **16**, 230–235.
3 Baron, J. H. (1963) Studies of basal and peak acid output with an augmented histamine meal. *Gut*, **4**, 136–144.
4 Bender, A. D. (1965) The effect of increasing age on the distribution of peripheral blood flow in man. *Journal of American Geriatric Society*, **13**, 192–201.
5 Bird, T., Hall, M. R. P. & Schade, R. O. K. (1977) Gastric histology and its relation to anaemia in the elderly. *Gerontologia*, **23**, 309–321.
6 Bullamore, J. R., Wilkinson, R., Gallacher, J. C. *et al.* (1970) Effect of age on calcium absorption. *Lancet*, **ii**, 535–537.
7 Burr, M. L., Milbank, J. E. & Gibbs, D. (1982) The nutritional status of the elderly. *Age and Ageing*, **11**, 89–96.
8 Citi, S. & Salvini, L. (1961) The intestinal absorption of ^{131}I-labelled olein and triolein, of ^{58}Co-vitamin B and ^{59}Fe in aged subjects. *Journal of Gerontology*, **12**, 123–126.
9 DHSS (Department of Health and Social Security) (1979) *Nutrition and Health in Old Age. Report on Health and Social Subjects, No. 16.* London: HMSO.
10 Evans, M. A., Triggs, E. J. & Cheung, M. (1981) Gastric emptying rate in the elderly. Implications for drug therapy. *Journal of the American Geriatric Society*, **29**, 201–205.
11 Haeney, M. R., Culank, L. S., Montgomery, R. D. & Sammons, H. G. (1978) Evaluation of xylose absorption as measured in blood and urine: a one-hour blood xylose screening test in malabsorption. *Gastroenterology*, **75**, 393–400.
12 James O. F. W. (1981) Absorption and distribution of drugs in the elderly. In *Advanced Geriatric Medicine* (Ed) Caird, F. & Evans, J. G., pp. 1–14. London: Pitman.
13 Marx, J. J. M. (1979) Normal iron absorption and decreased red cell iron uptake in the aged. *Blood*, **53**, 204–211.
14 McEvoy, A. (1982) Investigation of intestinal malabsorption in the elderly. In *Advanced Geriatric Medicine 2* (Ed) Evans, J. G. & Caird, F. I. pp. 100–110. London: Pitman.
15 McEvoy, A. W. & James, O. F. W. (1982) Anthropometric indices in normal elderly subjects. *Age and Ageing*, **11**, 97–100.
16 McEvoy, A. W., Fenwick, J. D., Boddy, K. & James, O. F. W. (1982) Vitamin B_{12} absorption from the gut does not decline with age in normal elderly humans. *Age and Ageing*, **11**, 180–183.
17 Moessner, J., Pusch, H. J. & Koch, W. (1982) Die excretorische Pankreas Funktion Altersveränderungen: Ja oder Nein? *Aktuel Gerontologie*, **12**, 40–43.
18 Montgomery, R. D., Haeney, M. R., Ross, I. N. *et al.* (1978) The ageing gut: a study of intestinal absorption in relation to nutrition in the elderly. *Quarterly Journal of Medicine*, **47**, 197–211.
19 Moore, J. G., Tweedy, C., Christian, P. E. & Datz, F. L. (1983) Effect of age on gastric emptying of liquids/solid meals in man. *Digestive Diseases and Sciences*, **28**, 340–344.
20 Sahel, J., Cros, R. C., Lombard, C. & Sarles, H. (1979) Morphometrique de la pancreatographie endoscopique normale du sujet agé. *Gastroenterologie Hepatologie*, **15**, 574–577.
21 Warren, P. M., Pepperman, M. A. & Montgomery, R. D. (1978) Age changes in small-intestinal mucosa. *Lancet*, **ii**, 849–850.
22 Webster, S. G., Wilkinson, E. M. & Gowland, E. (1977) A comparison of fat absorption in young and old subjects. *Age and Ageing*, **6**, 113–117.

Chapter 18
The Pancreas

CLINICAL ANATOMY AND CONGENITAL ABNORMALITIES

With increasing use of endoscopic retrograde pancreatography (ERCP), knowledge of the anatomy of the pancreas, and particularly of the duct system, has rapidly expanded in recent years, and radiological anatomy (including ultrasonography and computed tomography) must be included with any topographical account of the gland. The variations in normal anatomy are now better known, and with use of electron micrography, consideration must also be taken of the constituent cells.

DEVELOPMENT

Developmental anomalies occur mainly because the pancreas derives from two separate buds, ventral (or anterior) and dorsal (or posterior), arising from the primitive duodenum. With unequal growth of the duodenal circumference, so-called 'migration', the buds come to lie close together with fusion of their parenchymal masses and, normally, anastomosis of their ducts. There is also a rotation of the duodenum such that its original ventral surface faces to the right. In the adult, the ventral pancreas is represented by the lower part of the head and the uncinate process, and its duct forms the proximal, or right, end of the main pancreatic duct (of Wirsung) which usually opens with the common bile duct, by way of the ampulla of Vater, into the duodenum. The remainder of the pancreas with the distal main duct is derived from the dorsal pancreas. The proximal part of the original dorsal pancreatic duct may persist as an accessory duct (of Santorini) which opens into the duodenum at a more cranial level than the ampulla of Vater.

ANATOMY

The adult pancreas is traditionally divided into the head with uncinate process, neck, body and tail, but for clinical purposes it is probably more satisfactory to define only two parts, the head to the right of the superior mesenteric vein, and the body to the left of the vein.

ANTERIOR ASPECT

The head of the pancreas is largely encircled by the 'C' of the duodenum, and the uncinate process extends behind the superior mesenteric vessels and lies to the right of the ascending, or fourth, part of the duodenum. The gastric antrum and pylorus lie with the duodenal bulb on the anterior surface of the upper part of the head, so that tumours may invade the antrum and bulb and mimic peptic ulceration. The gastroduodenal artery passes behind the first part of the duodenum and in front of the head parallel with the second part. The root of the transverse mesocolon lies along the anterior surface of the pancreas, and the posterior aspect of the body of the stomach lies on the pancreas to the left of the superior mesenteric vessels.

POSTERIOR ASPECT

Behind the head of the pancreas are the right kidney, inferior vena cava and aorta, with the body in front of the splenic and portal veins and just below the trifurcation of the coeliac trunk. Vascular changes in pancreatic carcinoma are frequent, being detectable on angiography in some 70–80% of cases.[6] Pseudocyst formation may show displacement of the right kidney and ureter on urography. The splenic artery and vein are intimately related to the posterior and superior surfaces of the pancreas, and narrowing and irregularity of the splenic and gastroduodenal arteries occur frequently with a carcinoma of the pancreas. The common bile duct grooves the head of the pancreas close to the medial margin of the second part of the duodenum, so that it is frequently obstructed by a carcinoma of the head; a smooth, long stricture may occur in chronic pancreatitis. The neck of the pancreas overlies the cysterna chyli and abdominal thoracic duct, and a pancreatic carcinoma may occasionally produce chylous ascites. The tail of the pancreas reaches to the angle between the spleen and the left kidney and lies in front of the left suprarenal gland.

BLOOD SUPPLY AND VENOUS DRAINAGE

The pancreas has an arterial supply, above, from the common hepatic, splenic and gastroduodenal arteries, below, from the superior mesenteric artery, and anastomotic arcades form between them. There is a free arterial plexus around the gland and an interlobular plexus from which vessels pass to the gland parenchyma. A single artery reaches each lobule, and this then divides to form a sinusoidal vascular bed for the islet cells which, in turn, is connected to an interacinar capillary plexus serving the exocrine cells and forming an insuloacinar portal system.[3] The venous drainage of the pancreas is to the splenic, superior mesenteric and portal veins. These may be used for venous sampling, for example, in the investigation of endocrine tumours.

LYMPHATICS

Lymphatic capillaries accompany the terminal vascular plexuses of the acini and islets, and drain into three regional groups of lymph nodes: the pancreatico-duodenal, the superior mesenteric and the pancreaticosplenic nodes, which lie along the upper border of the pancreas. From these nodes, efferent lymphatics pass mainly to the preaortic nodes, but some may pass in the lesser omentum to the hepatic nodes. The multiple lymph nodes on the posterior and anterior margin of the head of the pancreas adjacent to the duodenum may when enlarged indent the duodenal margin on radiography.

INNERVATION

The paravascular nerve plexuses which enter the pancreas have both motor and sensory components.[7] The sympathetic motor contribution to these plexuses is derived from postganglionic fibres from neurones in the coeliac plexus and the plexus round the origin of the superior mesenteric artery. Secretory stimulation of the exocrine cells occurs via preganglionic parasympathetic fibres which synapse with cholinergic neurones situated in tissue spaces in the gland; they are vagal in origin and derived from the posterior gastric nerve via the coeliac and superior mesenteric plexuses. Pacinian corpuscles are present in the pancreas, and the sensory fibres from them pass through the paravascular plexuses and sympathetic chains to reach the posterior root ganglion cells from T5 to T9.

THE DUCT SYSTEM

In 90% of individuals the main pancreatic duct joins the common bile duct to enter the duodenum as a single duct on the summit of the papilla. The ampulla of Vater lies in the second part of the duodenum in 75% of the population, in 15% at the angle between the second and third parts, and in 9% in the horizontal third part of the duodenum.[14] The accessory duct reaches the duodenum in about 60%, but only opens onto the duodenum in 20%.[6] It usually communicates with the main duct as it passes upwards and in front of it from the lower part of the head of the pancreas, and its ampulla, when present, lies about 2 cm above the ampulla of Vater. A normal main pancreatic duct is about 3.5 mm wide at the head, 3 mm in the body and 2.5 mm at the tail, but can be up to 10 mm wide at the head and still be within normal limits.[6] The direction taken by the main pancreatic duct varies considerably (Figure 18.1); it often makes a sharp bend in its course and even turns back on itself. It does not show any gross irregularity and tends to taper from head to tail. There are side branches at regular intervals, and sometimes the main duct bifurcates in the body of the pancreas.[1]

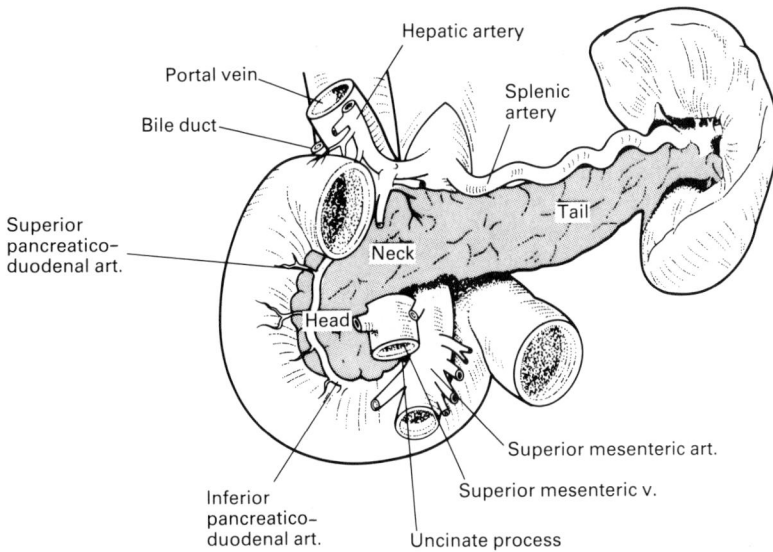

a

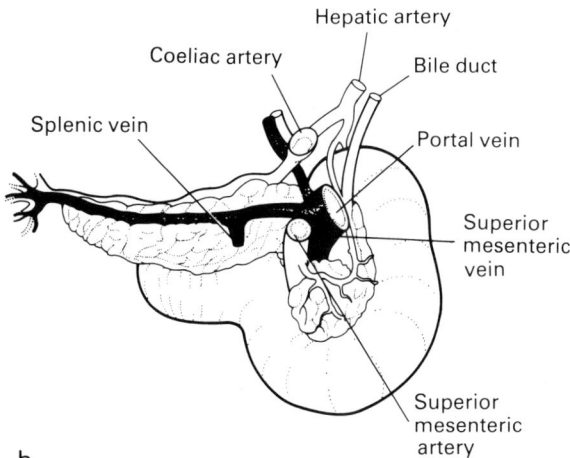

b

Fig. 18.1 The pancreas: (a) anterior view; (b) posterior view.

Radiological anatomy ultrasound and computed tomography

The outline of the pancreas is not definable on plain films as its soft tissue density is similar to that of its surroundings. With the development of grey-scale ultrasound and computed axial tomography, it has been possible to visualize the pancreas, and it has become necessary to know the variations of normal anatomy, not only of the pancreas, but also of the duodenum, the arteries and veins, and the duct system. The variations include those of age and posture, and during ERCP there are frequently marked changes in the position of the duct system with manipulation of the endoscope.

The proximal half of the duodenum is narrower than the distal half, with a sudden transition at the level of the ampulla of Vater. This is well shown on double-contrast tube duodenography in which the ampulla shows a filling defect on the medial wall in 25% of examinations.[6] The posterior gastric wall may be displaced or indented by a pancreatic mass.

The pancreas appears on pancreatograms as straight, L-shaped, oblique or horizontal, sigmoid or inverted V- or U-shaped.[6] The head usually lies just to the right of the T12/L1 vertebra, but may be as high as T11, or as low as L5/S1 in the elderly, visceroptotic patient. It may lie completely to the right of the spine, over the spine or even to its left. With pneumatography and computed tomography (CT), the maximum anteroposterior diameters of the gland are 3 cm, 2.5 cm and 2 cm for head, body and tail, respectively and the margins are smooth and regular; in 20% the tail may appear lobulated.[6]

The pancreas can be displayed on CT by 4–8 sections at 1-cm intervals in the region of L1 and L2, depending where the gland lies. Its body curves over the superior mesenteric artery, and the head lies in front of the inferior vena cava where it is joined by the left renal vein. Frequently, the portal and splenic veins, and the splenic artery, can be distinguished from the pancreas. Ultrasound gives similar, if less well-defined, appearances, but when the retroperitoneal fat planes are not well-defined, or absent, the pancreas may be better defined than when shown by CT. Ultrasound is also better for distinguishing the splenic and portal veins, and can also be used for longitudinal scans at 5-mm intervals near the midline to identify the aorta and inferior vena cava. In these scans, the body of the pancreas may be defined, as well as the superior mesenteric artery; and the

formation of the portal vein by the junction of splenic and superior mesenteric veins may be distinguished behind the head of the pancreas. Bowel gas interferes with ultrasound examination (but not CT), and in 10–20% of cases the head and body of the pancreas cannot be shown by this technique.[6]

HISTOLOGY

The exocrine cells

The name 'pancreas' implies that the gland contains relatively little connective tissue, and of 100 g of human pancreas, 98 g are composed of exocrine cells. Interlobular ducts are lined with cuboidal cells and enter the substance of the lobules to join the lumen formed by the acinar cells which are wrapped around it in mulberry fashion.[15]

The pancreatic acinar cell is a model of protein synthesis in its ultrastructure. The cells are derived from a primitive duct system and their basal lamina is continuous with that of the duct system into which it leads. Closely associated with the lamina and just outside it is the neurovascular stroma. The acinar cell shows an endoplasmic reticulum with ribosomes attached to it and mitochondria sandwiched between its layers. The synthesis of the pancreatic enzymes occurs on the ribosomal granules, from where they are transported to the Golgi complex. Here the polypeptides are condensed into a granule that is eventually coated by a membrane which it is thought might protect the cytoplasm from their action until their discharge into the acinar lumen.[15] It has been suggested that a network of intercellular canaliculi might allow enzymes to enter the stromal tissue in pancreatitis, but their presence has not been confirmed.[12]

The mechanism of the production of non-enzyme bicarbonate-rich pancreatic juice is discussed on p. 1261, but the ultrastructure of the ductal cells is against their active secretion of water and electrolytes. Some ductal cells may produce mucus, and goblet cells are present in the larger ducts.

Sympathetic vasoconstriction inhibits exocrine secretion, and the space between the acinar cells and the nerve fibres occupied by cholinergic synaptic vesicles suggests a diffusion of parasympathetic mediators across the space before enzymes can be secreted.[15]

The endocrine cells

The endocrine cells of the pancreas are arranged in nests, or islets, which are spherical in outline and diffusely distributed in the parenchyma. The islets vary greatly in number (from 170 000 to 2 000 000) and occupy about 1% of the volume of the pancreas. They are surrounded by connective tissue fibres continuous with those of the exocrine interstitial septa, and have a rich vascular supply. Peripheral nerve fibres are closely associated with the endocrine cells, and both cholinergic and adrenergic neural elements have been identified. The innervation has not been fully elucidated, but it is known that sympathetic stimulation causes inhibition of insulin release, and parasympathetic stimulation causes insulin secretion, whereas the opposite is true of glucagon release.[2]

The endocrine cells are derived from the ductal system, but no new formation of these cells occurs after birth. The mitotic activity of islet cells in the adult is low but may be increased under some conditions. In spontaneous diabetes mellitus there may be decreased B cell volume, especially if it is of the juvenile type. Diet and hormones play a part in the regulatory mechanism of the growth of the endocrine pancreas – cortisone and growth hormone stimulate islet growth, as does food intake. Hyperplasia of the B cells may occur in obesity and maturity-onset diabetes mellitus.[2]

There are different islet cell types, of which four have been particularly identified by their secretory granules. These granules are membrane-bound cytoplasmic particles containing stored hormones: B cells produce insulin; A cells, glucagon; D cells, somatostatin; and PP cells, pancreatic polypeptide. Usually the B cells predominate in number. The hormones are synthesized in the endoplasmic reticulum and stored in the cytoplasmic granules from which they are released by the appropriate stimulus. Hyperplasia and tumour formation may not necessarily produce hyperfunction, and the primary tumours may be composed of more than one endocrine cell type.[2]

CONGENITAL ABNORMALITIES

The most important congenital abnormality affecting the pancreas is cystic fibrosis, which is inherited as an autosomal recessive trait. This is described on p. 1286. Heterotopic pancreatic tissue is common and usually has little clinical significance.

The heterotopic pancreas

The heterotopic pancreas, which has also been called 'accessory pancreas' or 'aberrant pancreas', may be defined as the presence of pancreatic tissue that lacks anatomical and vascular continuity with the main body of the pancreas. The frequency at autopsy has varied from 0.55% to 13.7%, the lower figure being the more likely. It occurs about once in every 500 operations in the upper abdomen.[13] There are several theories for its origin but none is convincing. Most islands of aberrant pancreatic tissue lie within the wall of the intestine and stomach; others are associated with the spleen and omentum. They form firm, yellow intramural nodules varying in size from 2 mm to 4 mm which are often described as being submucosal or subserosal. On histology, there may be pancreatic lobules with ducts, acini and islets, or only a few widely separated ducts. There may be characteristic central umbilication gastroscopically and on radiography, with a submucosal filling defect and appearances difficult to distinguish from that of a leiomyoma. If the umbilication is large there may be confusion with a peptic ulcer.

There may be an association with a diverticulum of the intestine, and this must be distinguished from the presence of pancreatic tissue in a Meckel's diverticulum. Heterotopic pancreatic tissue may be subject to pancreatitis or superficial ulceration with intestinal bleeding, as well as carcinoma, cyst formation, intussusception and intestinal obstruction. Symptoms are often vague and of uncertain mechanism, and any diagnosis is made retrospectively, with the possible exception of Meckel's diverticulum. Haemorrhage from the intestine is the easiest to associate with such tissue. Ectopically located pancreatic tissue should be sought at operation for insulinoma if the tumour cannot be located in the pancreas. The most common location for a tumour not in the pancreas will be beneath the mucosa of the duodenum and a duodenotomy with palpation of its lumen should be undertaken in these circumstances.[4]

Anomalies of the pancreatic duct

The commonest duct anomaly is lack of anastomosis between the ducts of the developing ventral and dorsal pancreatic buds.[1] The definitive main pancreatic duct is derived in fetal life by fusion of the dorsal duct, which provides the drainage for the tail and body of the pancreas, with the ventral duct which drains the head of the gland. Should there be failure of the two ducts to fuse, the dorsal pancreatic duct will empty into the duodenum through the accessory ampulla, while the ventral duct drains the pancreatic head with the lower end of the common

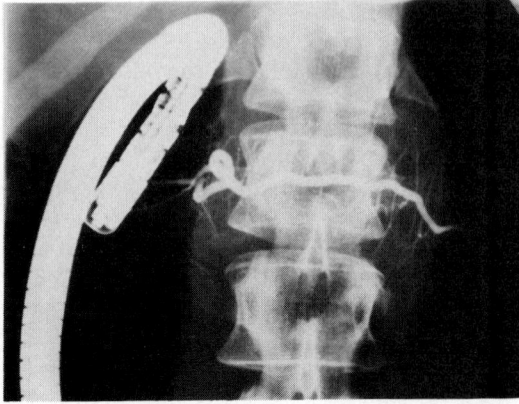

a

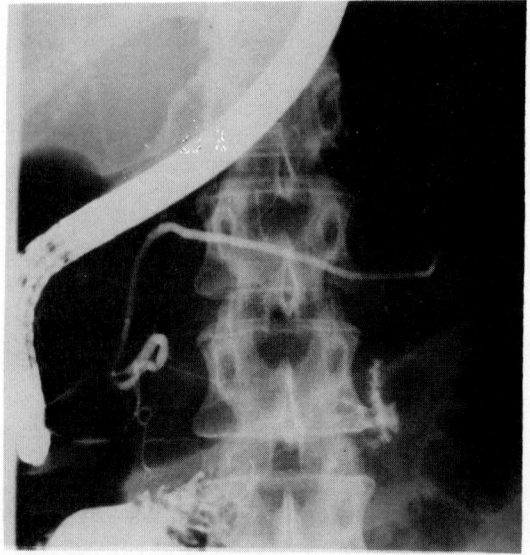

b

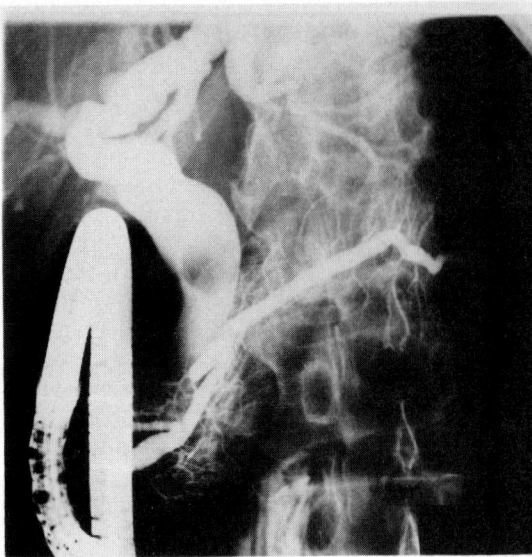

c

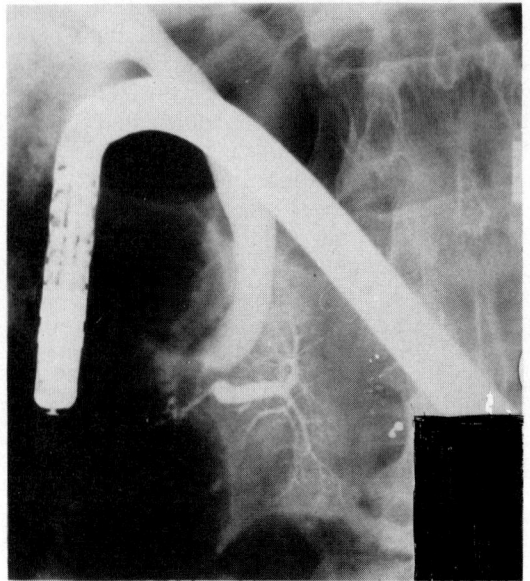

d

Fig. 18.2   Three normal pancreatograms (a), (b) and (c) obtained on ERCP. (c) also shows a dilated common bile duct with a stone in it and some acinar filling. (d) Unfused ventral pancreas shown on ERCP with filling of the common bile duct. Courtesy of Dr A. T. R. Axon.

bile duct at the ampulla of Vater (see Figure 18.2). An unfused ventral duct is found in up to 5% of normal individuals[1] with completely independent ducts of Santorini and Wirsung. The main pancreatic duct opens into the duodenum separately from the common bile duct in 10% of the population, and in 2% the dorsal pancreatic duct becomes the main duct with drainage of the ventral duct into it.[6] Occasionally there may be absence of the part of

the pancreas derived from the dorsal bud, as well as failure of union between the dorsal and ventral components.

Annular pancreas

The congenital anomaly of annular pancreas, first described in 1862, has an incidence of 6 in 100 000 in adults, although personal experience of six patients with this condition in eight years

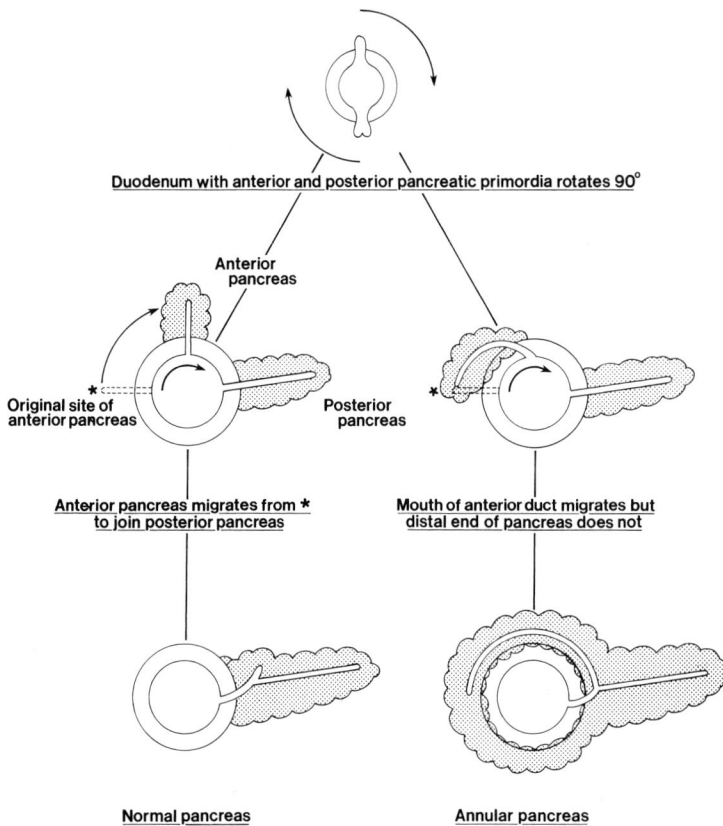

Fig. 18.3 Development of normal and annular pancreas. From Morrell, M. T. & Keynes, W. M. (1981),[11] with kind permission of the authors and the publisher, Heinemann Medical Books.

suggests that the incidence is likely to be greater. The disorder may become symptomatic in neonates, in adult life or not at all. It consists of a ring of pancreatic tissue totally or partially encircling the second part of the duodenum. On pancreatography there is usually a normal main duct, but not necessarily a branch encircling the duodenum.[1] The diagnosis is simple in the neonate, but difficult in the adult in whom the usual dyspeptic symptoms may be explained away by associated disorders or the cause remain unrecognized. There is a particular association with peptic ulceration, pancreatitis and jaundice.[11] The cause of the condition is a matter for speculation (Figure 18.3).

ANNULAR PANCREAS IN NEONATES

In the neonate, multiple associated abnormalities are usual, such as duodenal atresia, stenosis or obstruction, and an immediate operation may be required. The condition may be suggested on plain X-ray of the abdomen by two adjacent fluid levels, one in the stomach and one in the dilated proximal duodenum, with absence of air in the rest of the abdomen. The treatment is with a duodenojejunostomy or duodeno-duodenostomy. Jaundice is rare.

ADULT ANNULAR PANCREAS

Annular pancreas rarely presents after the neonatal period until adulthood. The symptoms most often begin in the fifth decade. There is usually an insidious history of intermittent epigastric pain, bloating and vomiting, with a long history of mild indigestion, or abdominal discomfort unrelated to meals. Vomiting may be at night with partly digested food. A peptic ulcer is found in a third of patients, and pancreatitis in a fifth, as well as gallstones, hiatal hernia, gastritis and duodenitis. The symptoms may be due to the concomitant lesion, or mimic a duodenal ulcer.[10] Persistent symptoms are due to duodenal obstruction (Figure 18.4). Presentation may be from bleeding from the upper intestinal tract.

Barium meal examination may show an eccentric stricture of the second part of the duodenum over 1–3 cm long with proximal dilatation of the duodenum (Figure 18.4). The commonest misinterpretation is stenosis due to duodenal ulceration even though the narrowing is unusually more distal; a concomitant duodenal ulcer may disguise these findings. Endoscopy is helpful in the diagnosis, but the condition is easily missed at laparotomy. There

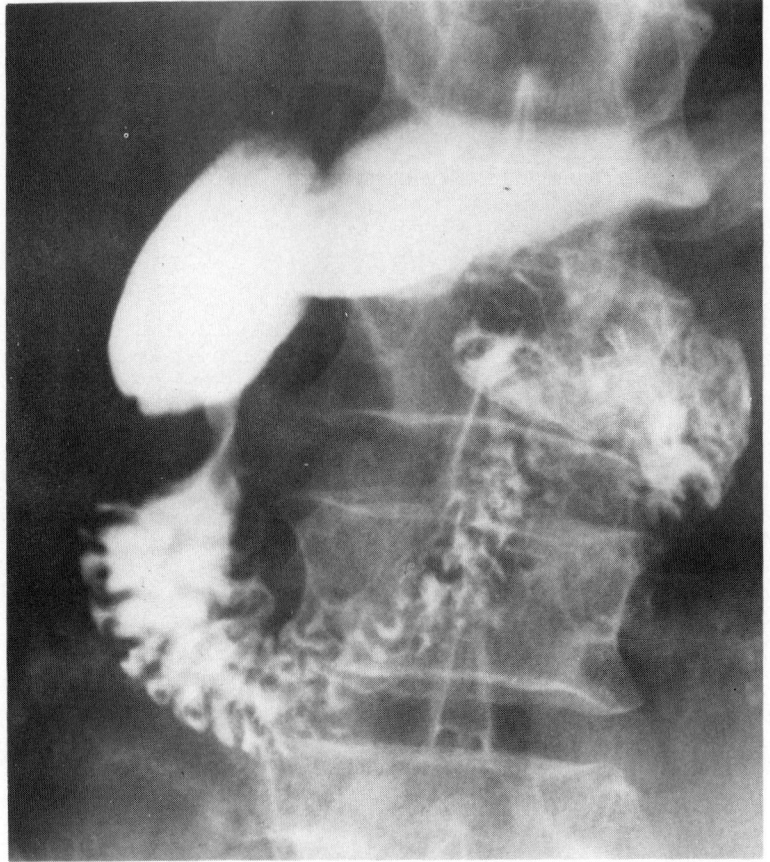

Fig. 18.4 Barium filling the duodenum with constriction in the second part produced by an annular pancreas. From Morrell, M. T. & Keynes, W. M. (1981),[11] with kind permission of the authors and the publisher, Heinemann Medical Books.

may be non-specific relief from symptoms and the only cure is by operation; gastrojejunostomy with vagotomy has given the best results.[11] Division (or resection) of the annulus has been followed by complications or persistence of the symptoms and should be avoided.

Gastric acid output may be high when there is an annular pancreas and this might induce more proximal peptic ulceration with obstruction to the outflow of food and secretions. Acute pancreatitis may be the presenting complaint[5] and there has been histological evidence of pancreatitis on resection of the annulus and at autopsy. The pancreatitis is usually confined to the annulus and adjoining part of the head, and it occurs more frequently than the suggested 21%.[8, 9]

The diagnosis is easiest to make when there are recurrent attacks of moderately severe upper abdominal pain accompanied by obstructive jaundice. Already narrowed by the annular pancreas, the common bile duct is presumably further obstructed by inflammatory oedema or possibly by a gallstone. Of fourteen recorded patients, four had common bile duct stones, two of which had impacted. In ten patients, the jaun-

dice was due to pancreatitis. The duct was dilated in seven patients in whom it was visualized[11] and dilatation of the duct has also been reported with no history of jaundice. The removal of a fixed, impacted ampullary stone can present a technical problem to the surgeon because a transduodenal approach may be impossible when there is an annular pancreas. The stone may be removed through the common bile duct after duodenotomy below the annulus, but the annulus should not be incised.

REFERENCES

1 Axon, A. T. R. (1981) Endoscopic retrograde pancreatography. In *The Pancreas* (Ed.) Keynes, W. M. & Keith, R. G. pp. 117–141. London: Heinemann Medical Books.

2 Boquist, L. (1981) The endocrine cells. In *The Pancreas* (Ed.) Keynes, W. M. & Keith, R. G. pp. 31–40. London: Heinemann Medical Books.

3 Fujita, T., Yanatori, Y. & Murakami, T. (1976) Insulo-acinar axis, its vascular basis and its functional and morphological changes caused by CCK-PZ and caerulein. In *Endocrine Gut and Pancreas* (Ed.) Fujita, T. Chapter 30. Amsterdam: Elsevier.

4 Harrison, T. S. (1978) The hypoglycemic syndrome: endogenous hyperinsulinism. In *Surgical Endocrinology*

(Ed.) Friesen, S. R. pp. 150–167. Philadelphia: Lippincott.

5 Jackson, J. M. (1963) Annular pancreas and duodenal obstruction in the neonate. *Archives of Surgery*, **87**, 379–383.

6 Kreel, L. (1981) Applied and radiological anatomy. In *The Pancreas* (Ed.) Keynes, W. M. & Keith, R. G. pp. 8–22. London: Heinemann Medical Books.

7 Lever, J. D. (1981) General anatomy of the human pancreas. In *The Pancreas* (Ed.) Keynes, W. M. & Keith, R. G. pp. 3–7. London: Heinemann Medical Books.

8 Lloyd-Jones, W., Mountain, J. C. & Warren, K. W. (1972) Annular pancreas in the adult. *Annals of Surgery*, **176**, 163–170.

9 McGregor, A. M. C., Green, B. J. & Stein, M. A. (1969) Symptomatic annular pancreas in the adult. *British Journal of Surgery*, **56**, 713–715.

10 Morrell, M. T. & Keynes, W. M. (1970) Annular pancreas and jaundice. *British Journal of Surgery*, **57**, 814–816.

11 Morrell, M. T. & Keynes, W. M. (1981) Annular pancreas. In *The Pancreas* (Ed.) Keynes, W. M. & Keith, R. G. pp. 159–168. London: Heinemann Medical Books.

12 Munger, B. L. (1973) The ultrastructure of the exocrine pancreas. In *The Pancreas* (Ed.) Carey, L. p. 17. St Louis: Mosby.

13 ReMine, W. H. & van Heerden, J. A. (1978) Rare endocrine tumors and syndromes. In *Surgical Endocrinology* (Ed.) Friesen, S. R. pp. 393–403. Philadelphia: Lippincott.

14 Schwartz, A. & Birnbaum, D. (1962) Roentgenologic study of the topography of the choledocho-duodenal junction. *American Journal of Roentgenology*, **87**, 772–776.

15 Tompkins, R. K. & Traverso, L. W. (1981) The exocrine cells. In *The Pancreas* (Ed.) Keynes, W. M. & Keith, R. G. pp. 23–30. London: Heinemann Medical Books.

PHYSIOLOGY

The pancreas contains exocrine and endocrine components, and although the emphasis in this section is on the exocrine tissue, there are important endocrine–exocrine functional relationships that have to be considered. In terms of volume percentages, the pancreas comprises 82% acinar cells, 4% duct cells, 4% blood vessels, 2% endocrine cells and 8% extracellular matrix.[1] The acinar cell is thus by far the dominant cell type as well as being the most important for the exocrine function. The acinar cell itself is not, however, the functional unit in this tissue since acinar cells are organized in a network comprising up to several hundred intercommunicating cells (functional syncytium) surrounding complexly shaped lumina.[9] The exocrine pancreas, apart from being an extremely important organ in its own right, has also served as the most useful model system for the study of protein secretion and its control.

The pancreatic juice

COMPOSITION AND SECRETORY RATE

The exocrine pancreas secretes a fluid containing electrolytes as well as a large number of functionally important digestive enzymes. Pancreatic juice collected in a physiological situation (after a meal) will have been produced as a result of a complex mixture of physiochemical processes evoked by a combination of chemical signals. Pancreatic secretion is evoked by both nervous and hormonal mechanisms, and the most important signalling molecules are cholecystokinin (CCK), acetylcholine (ACh), secretin and vasoactive intestinal polypeptide (VIP). Although the precise electrolyte composition will vary with the type of stimulation some general features are always observed. The juice is isosmolal with plasma and the sodium and potassium concentrations are virtually constant and approximately plasma-like. The sum of the chloride and bicarbonate concentrations is constant in spite of wide variations in the individual concentrations (Figure 18.5). Although it is possible to obtain pure human pancreatic juice, the most detailed studies have been undertaken in the dog, cat, rat and pig.[4] There seem to be species differences, particularly in regard to the ability of CCK to evoke fluid secretion, but most work has been in vivo where many interactions between nervous and hormonal mechanisms may occur and will complicate the analysis.

In contrast to the view presented in many textbooks, pure CCK alone evokes marked fluid secretion at least in the isolated perfused rat and pig pancreas.[11, 16] In both the intact rat and the isolated perfused rat pancreas pure CCK can evoke higher rates of fluid secretion than can be obtained with secretin stimulation.[16, 22] VIP evokes marked fluid secretion at least in the pig.[6] ACh activates exactly the same type of secretory process as CCK. ACh interacts with muscarinic receptors and its effect on fluid secretion is blocked by atropine. This antagonist does not interfere with the action of CCK and related peptides (e.g. gastrin). CCK interacts with specific CCK receptors and its effects on fluid secretion can be blocked by the specific and competitive CCK antagonist dibutyryl cyclic guanosine monophosphate which does not interfere with the action of ACh.[15] Another peptide, totally unrelated to the CCK–gastrin family, bombesin (or gastrin-releasing peptide, GRP), and other members of the bombesin family can also stimulate the same fluid secretion mechanism as CCK and ACh. Bombesin

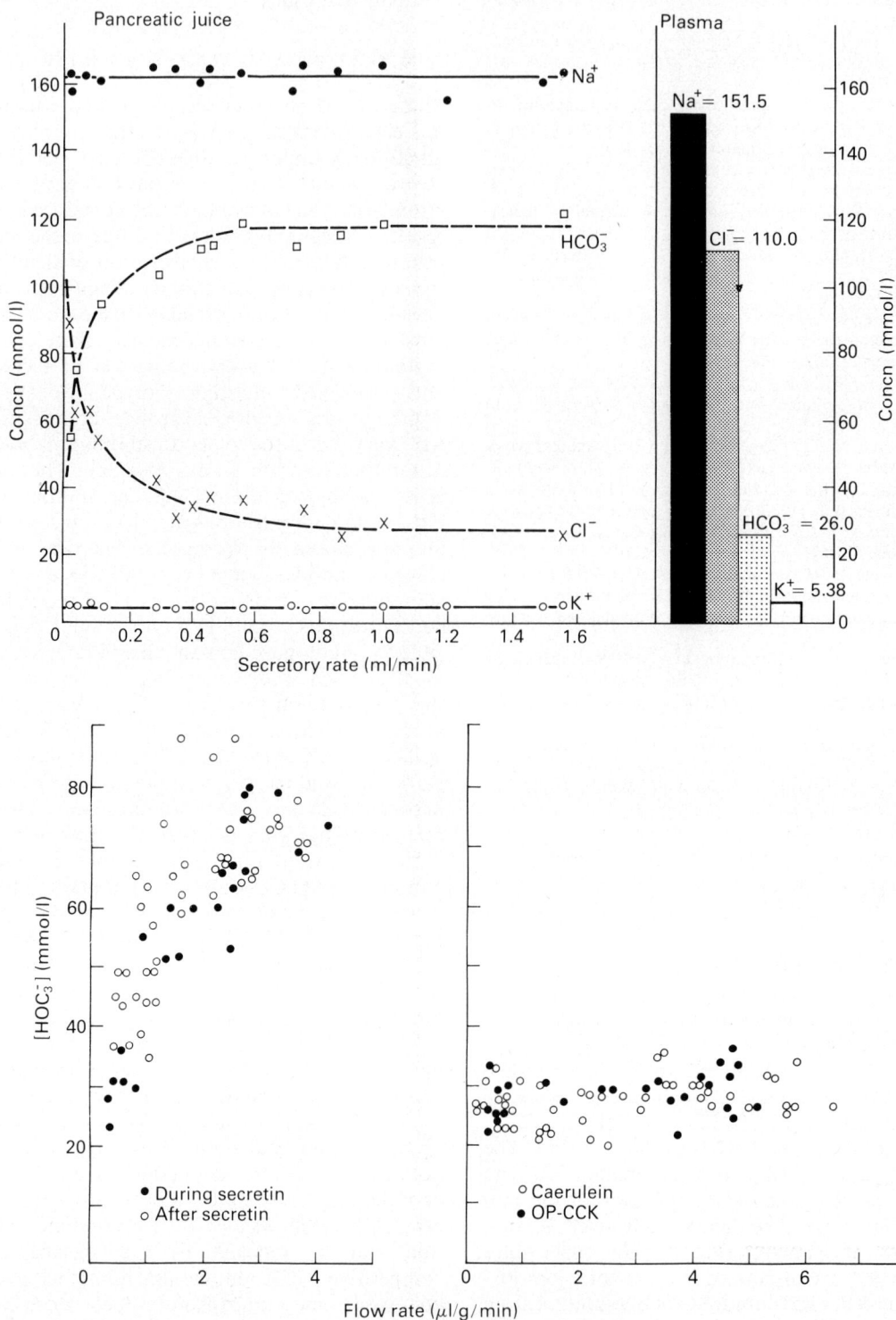

Fig. 18.5 Relationship between pancreatic juice flow and electrolyte concentration in juice. Upper part shows results from dog pancreas stimulated with secretin. From Bro-Rasmussen, F. *et al.* (1956),[2] with kind permission of the authors and the editor of *Acta Physiologica Scandinavica.* Lower part shows results from the rat pancreas stimulated with secretin, CCK or the CCK analogue caerulein. From Sewell, W. A. & Young, J. A. (1975),[22] with kind permission of the authors and the editor of *Journal of Physiology.*

also acts in the presence of complete blockage of ACh and CCK receptors. VIP evokes formation of fluid with the same composition as that evoked by secretin.

Figure 18.5 illustrates the relationship between electrolyte concentration and secretory rate in the cat and the rat during stimulation with secretin or CCK. CCK evokes the formation of a juice with a plasma-like composition in both the rat and the pig and there is no tendency for the bicarbonate concentration to rise with increasing flow rate. In the case of secretin stimulation, however, there is a clear pattern of increase in bicarbonate and decrease in chloride concentration as the flow rate goes up.

THE COMPONENTS OF FLUID SECRETION

CCK clearly evokes the formation of a fluid with a composition that is quite different from that evoked by secretin. CCK receptors have been localized to acinar cells, whereas there is no evidence available to suggest the existence of such receptors on duct cells. On the other hand, duct cells have secretin receptors although they are not the only site for specific secretin binding, since acinar cells have also been shown to possess such receptors.[20] There is otherwise substantial, but still indirect, evidence showing that the CCK-evoked secretion originates from the acinar cells whereas the secretin-evoked juice comes from duct cells.[17]

The mechanisms underlying the two types of fluid secretion are also different. In experiments on the isolated perfused rat pancreas, it has been shown that the acinar fluid secretion evoked by activation of CCK receptors is acutely dependent on the presence of calcium in the extracellular fluid whereas this is not the case with respect to the secretin-evoked fluid secretion. On the other hand, secretin-evoked fluid secretion is markedly dependent on the presence of CO_2/HCO_3 in the perfusion fluid whereas this is not the case for CCK-evoked secretion.[17]

PROTEIN SECRETION

The pancreatic acinar cells secrete a large number of proteins, electrolytes and water. Amongst the secreted proteins are many important digestive enzymes such as lipase, α-amylase, four (pro)carboxypeptidases, three trypsin-(ogen)s, chymotrypsin(ogen), two (pro)elastases, two colipases and (pro)phospholipase A_2. It is generally accepted that these proteins are synthesized at the rough endoplasmic reticulum, processed through the Golgi complex

and stored in the zymogen granules. Stimulation of the acinar cells results in the fusion of zymogen granule membrane with luminal plasma membrane, with an opening developing at the point of fusion establishing continuity between the interior of the zymogen granule and the acinar lumen through which the stored proteins can escape. This mode of secretion has been termed exocytosis. The granule membrane inserted into the luminal plasma membrane during exocytosis is subsequently recaptured and can be reutilized (membrane recycling).[8] In many species, certainly in the rat and the pig, acinar enzyme secretion is accompanied by acinar fluid secretion. The fluid secretion is not merely a passive process secondary to enzyme secretion, since it is possible to reduce CCK-evoked fluid secretion markedly by the specific sodium–potassium pump inhibitor ouabain without reducing amylase output.[16]

HORMONAL AND NERVOUS CONTROL OF EXOCRINE SECRETION

The most important control of acinar enzyme and fluid secretion is exerted by the hormone cholecystokinin (CCK) and by the parasympathetic nerves with acetylcholine (ACh) as the transmitter, but several other control mechanisms have also been identified (Figure 18.6).

Cholecystokinin (CCK)

CCK exists in different molecular forms with CCK_{39}, CCK_{33} and CCK_8 being the most important. The C-terminal CCK octapeptide (CCK_8) appears to dominate in the gut. Recent studies, using much improved radioimmunoassay procedures and comparison with effects on pancreatic secretion after exogenous CCK application in man, indicate that the responses to fat can be accounted for in terms of CCK release whereas pancreatic responses to a normal light meal cannot be explained solely as due to CCK release.[5]

Acetylcholine

The acinar cells have a good functional innervation because electrophysiological studies on mouse and rat show that every single acinar cell investigated with an intracellular microelectrode responded with depolarization when the nerves were stimulated.[14] There is now also good evidence from studies in vivo indicating the importance of nervous control. In dogs with a transplanted pancreas the response to intraduodenal stimuli is reduced to about 50% of control

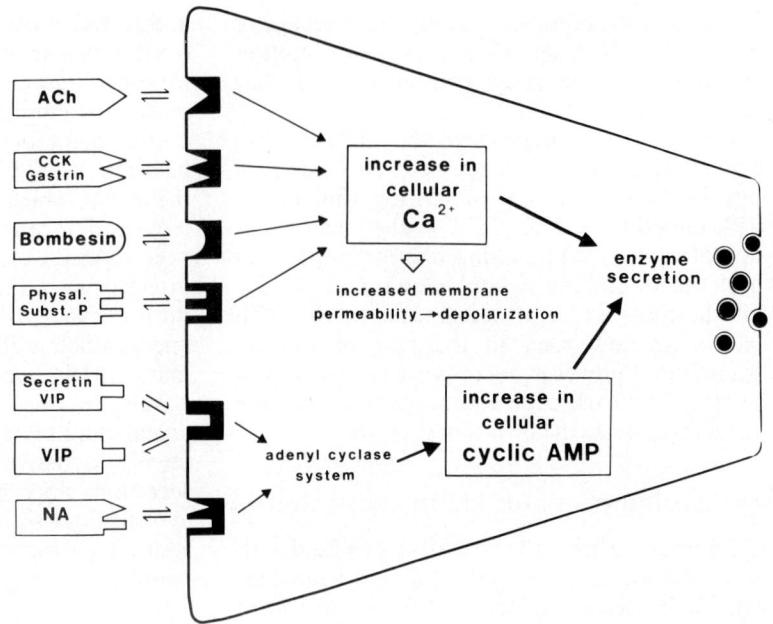

Fig. 18.6 Schematic diagram showing different specific receptors controlling acinar enzyme secretion. All the receptors shown here are not necessarily found on the pancreatic acinar cells in all species. Receptors for ACh and CCK seem always to be present. Bombesin and secretin/VIP receptors are present in several species. Substance P receptors have so far only been demonstrated in the guinea pig pancreas, and catecholamine receptors (NA = noradrenaline) have so far only been demonstrated in the rat pancreas.

indicating a substantial nervous component in the normal response. Furthermore, it has been shown that the pancreatic response to intraduodenal tryptophan or oleate instillation occurs much quicker than can be accounted for by CCK release. Atropine or vagotomy markedly delays the response, again indicating the functional importance of the vagal cholinergic pathway.[13]

Other transmitters

A number of putative hormones and transmitters can stimulate the acinar cells, but in most circumstances there is still uncertainty about their physiological role in the normal intact organism. The list of substances that can directly activate the acinar cells to secrete includes peptides belonging to the bombesin group, VIP, substance P, noradrenaline and adrenaline. Specific acinar receptor sites for many different agonists seem to coexist in the same acinar units (Figure 18.6). A detailed mapping of the control mechanisms has unfortunately only been undertaken in very few species and not in man. The bombesin peptides are perhaps of special interest. Bombesin was originally isolated from amphibian skin but mammalian bombesin (also called gastrin-releasing peptide) has also been isolated. Although bombesin undoubtedly releases gastrin (GRP) there is little doubt that it also directly activates acinar cells via the same intracellular mechanism employed by CCK and ACh.[10]

Cellular secretion processes

Polypeptide hormones in general activate cellular processes by increasing or decreasing the cytoplasmic level of a messenger. The roles of cyclic nucleotides (cyclic adenosine $3',5'$-monophosphate and cyclic guanosine $3',5'$-monophosphate) and ionized calcium as intracellular mediators of contraction, secretion and changes in metabolism are widely recognized. The most direct evidence for intracellular messenger effects mediating the action of hormones or neurotransmitters on the acinar cells comes from two different types of electrophysiological studies. In microelectrode investigations (Figure 18.7) it has been possible to apply substances inside or immediately outside the plasma membrane. It transpires that the peptide secretagogues as well as ACh evoke membrane depolarization when applied to the outside of the plasma membrane, after a minimum delay of about 0.5 s, whereas application inside has no effect. Intracellular injection of the calcium chelator EDTA inhibits the depolarizing effect of extracellular secretagogue application whereas intracellular calcium injection mimics the depolarizing action following extracellular ACh or peptide hormone application.[14, 15] In recent patch-clamp single-channel current recording investigations (Figure 18.7) it has been shown that ACh or CCK when applied extracellularly, outside a small area of plasma membrane to which there is no access, evokes opening of single ionic channels in that same area. When

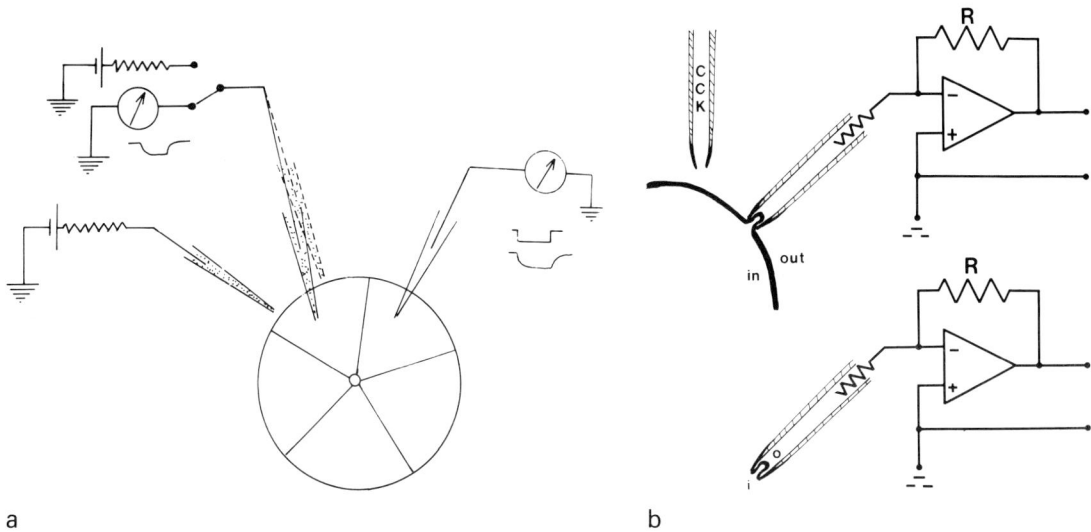

a   b

Fig. 18.7 Micropipette techniques for investigating messenger functions. (a) Microelectrode set-up to probe the effects of intra- and extracellular applications of secretagogues, calcium and calcium chelators on membrane potential and resistance. (This is the arrangement used in ref. 18.) (b) Patch-clamp set up to study picoampere currents through single ionic channels. A small area of plasma membrane (about 10 μm^2) is electrically isolated by sealing a fire-polished glass micropipette against the cleaned outer membrane surface (treated with collagenase). The acinar cell unit is stimulated by CCK release from another extracellular pipette. In the study of Maruyama and Petersen[12] this procedure was shown to open channels in the isolated membrane patch. The electrically isolated membrane patch area can also be excised from the cell (lower part of diagram) and thus the effect of possible internal messengers (e.g. calcium) on ion channel opening can be directly investigated under well-controlled conditions. From Maruyama, Y. & Petersen, O. H. (1982),[12] by kind permission of the authors and the editor of *Nature*.

the isolated membrane patch is excised from the cell it can be shown that the same channels can be activated by calcium from the internal side.[12] Many other less direct approaches confirm that ACh, CCK and bombesin actions on acinar cells are mediated by a rise in internal ionized calcium concentration.[15, 21] The precise mechanism by which internal calcium activates enzyme secretion by exocytosis is still unknown. It seems likely that the calcium-mediated opening of membrane ion channels allows salt loading of the acinar cells during stimulation and therefore is important for the formation of the acinar neutral fluid secretion.[12]

The mechanism of action of VIP and secretin on both the acinar cells and the duct cells is perhaps less clear. There are strong arguments in favour of cyclic AMP as an intracellular messenger.[17, 20] The specific ion transports activated by cyclic AMP have not, however, been identified.

For the bicarbonate-secreting duct cell the only transport pathway to have been definitively localized is the sodium–potassium pump at the basal plasma membrane.[3] There are plenty of (different) schematic models for the cellular transports involved in the formation of the sodium bicarbonate rich fluid, but at this stage it

is not possible to choose between them as real knowledge is lacking.

In the acinar cells certain transport pathways have been precisely localized and fragments of a picture are available (Figure 18.8).

There are marked potentiating interactions between the secretagogues acting via changes in internal ionized calcium concentration (CCK, ACh and bombesin) and those acting via changes in intracellular cyclic AMP concentration (secretin and VIP).[7, 16] The mechanism underlying this phenomenon is unknown.

Endocrine–exocrine interaction

It is now clear that a significant proportion of blood draining the islets enters capillaries in the exocrine tissue. Islet hormones can therefore be present in relatively high concentrations in the extracellular fluid surrounding the acinar cells. It has been shown that both exogenous and endogenous insulin markedly augments CCK-evoked fluid and amylase secretion in the isolated perfused rat pancreas, while having no effect on secretion alone.[19] Glucagon can act as a secretagogue at very high concentrations,[23] but the physiological significance of this finding is still unclear.

BASAL

CCK

Bom

ACh

Ca^{2+}

LUMEN

Na^+

K^+

Na^+

amino
acid

Na^+

K^+

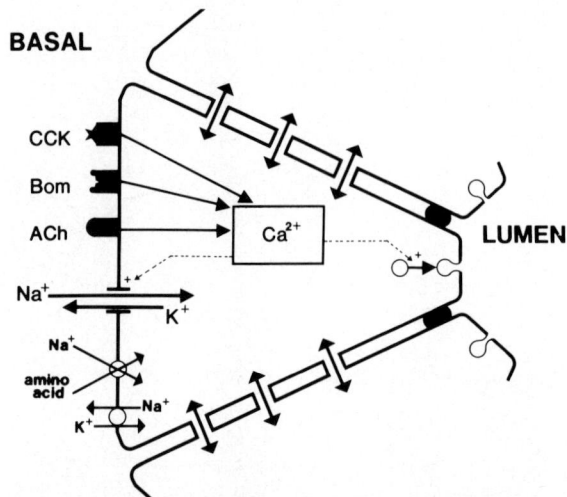

Fig. 18.8 Schematic diagram showing specific transport pathways *that have been identified* in pancreatic acinar cells. There are without any doubt many other transport pathways, but direct evidence for their localization is lacking. Interaction with three specific receptor sites (for CCK, ACh and bombesin) evokes an increase in cytoplasmic ionized calcium concentration.[15] The precise mechanism by which this is achieved is not clear. Internal calcium acts to evoke exocytosis at the luminal membrane (but the molecular mechanism of the control is unknown) and to open up channels mainly permeable to monovalent cations in the basolateral plasma membrane.[12] The sodium influx is probably an important element of the transacinar electrolyte and fluid secretion process. Specific luminal ion translocations must also be involved, but nothing is known about this aspect. Sodium–amino acid cotransport proteins are present in the plasma membrane. They allow 'uphill' transport of a variety of amino acids by exploiting the sodium concentration gradient across the plasma membrane. The sodium gradient (low intracellular sodium concentration in relation to the extracellular sodium concentration) is maintained by the sodium–potassium pump. This pump extrudes sodium and accumulates potassium using ATP as energy [$(Na^+ + K^+)$-activated ATPase]. The acinar cells within individual units are linked together by junctional channels allowing passage of ions as well as organic molecules (at least up to a molecular weight of about 800). The tight junctions close the intercellular space close to the acinar lumen. These junctions act as a barrier to transport between the interstitial fluid and the lumen. They also act as a barrier to lateral diffusion of integral membrane proteins in the plasma membrane thus maintaining the different composition and therefore function of the basolateral and luminal plasma membrane. All receptors, channels and pumps shown localized to the basal plasma membrane are probably distributed all over the basolateral plasma membrane.[15]

Conclusion

The exocrine pancreas secretes fluid containing a large number of important digestive enzymes. The mechanism of secretion appears to be exocytosis in the acinar cells. Fluid is secreted in both acinar and duct cells in response to a variety of hormonal and nervous stimuli. In the acinar cells a number of specific transport pathways have been identified and localized. Insulin markedly potentiates the action of the major pancreatic secretagogue cholecystokinin.

REFERENCES

1 Bolender, R. P. (1974) Stereological analysis of the guinea pig pancreas. *Journal of Cell Biology*, **61**, 269–287.

2 Bro-Rasmussen, F., Killmann, S. A. & Thaysen, J. H. (1956) The composition of pancreatic juice as compared to sweat, parotid saliva and tears. *Acta Physiologica Scandinavica*, **37**, 97–113.

3 Bundgaard, M., Moller, M. & Poulsen, J. H. (1981) Localization of sodium pump sites in cat pancreas. *Journal of Physiology*, **313**, 405–414.

4 Denyer, M. E. & Cotton, P. B. (1979) Pure pancreatic juice studies in normal subjects and patients with chronic pancreatitis. *Gut*, **20**, 89–97.

5 Dockray, G. J. (1982) The physiology of cholecystokinin in brain and gut. *British Medical Bulletin*, **38**, 253–258.

6 Fahrenkrug, J., Schaffalitzky De Muckadell, O. B., Holst, J. J. & Lindkaer Jensen, S. (1979) Vasoactive intestinal polypeptide in vagally mediated pancreatic secretion of fluid and HCO_3^-. *American Journal of Physiology*, **237**, E535-E540.

7 Gardner, J. D. & Jensen, R. T. (1981) Regulation of pancreatic enzyme secretion in vitro. In *Physiology of the Gastrointestinal Tract* (Ed.) Johnson, L. R. pp. 831–871, New York: Raven Press.

8 Gorelick, F. S. & Jamieson, J. D. (1981) Structure–function relationships of the pancreas. In *Physiology of the Gastrointestinal Tract* (Ed.) Johnson, L. R. pp. 773–794, New York: Raven Press.

9 Iwatsuki, N. & Petersen, O. H. (1978) Electrical coupling and uncoupling of exocrine acinar cells. *Journal of Cell Biology*, **79**, 533–545.

10 Iwatsuki, N. & Petersen, O. H. (1978) In vitro action of bombesin on amylase secretion, membrane potential and membrane resistance in rat and mouse pancreatic acinar cells. A comparison with other secretagogues. *Journal of Clinical Investigation*, **61**, 41–46.

11 Lindkaer Jensen, S., Rehfeld, J. F., Holst, J. J. et al. (1981) Secretory effects of cholecystokinins on the isolated perfused porcine pancreas. *Acta Physiologica Scandinavica*, **111**, 225–231.

12 Maruyama, Y. & Petersen, O. H. (1982) Cholecystokinin activation of single-channel currents is mediated by internal messenger in pancreatic acinar cells. *Nature,* **300,** 61–63.

13 Meyer, J. H. (1981) Control of exocrine secretion. In *Physiology of the Gastrointestinal Tract* (Ed.) Johnson, L. R. pp. 821–829. New York: Raven Press.

14 Petersen, O. H. (1981) Electrophysiology of exocrine gland cells. In *Physiology of the Gastrointestinal Tract* (Ed.) Johnson, L. R. pp. 749–772. New York: Raven Press.

15 Petersen, O. H. (1982) Stimulus–excitation coupling in plasma membranes of pancreatic acinar cells. *Biochimica et Biophysica Acta,* **694,** 163–184.

16 Petersen, O. H. & Ueda, N. (1977) Secretion of fluid and amylase in the perfused rat pancreas. *Journal of Physiology,* **264,** 819–835.

17 Petersen, O. H., Maruyama, Y., Graf, J. *et al.* (1981) Ionic currents across pancreatic acinar cell membranes and their role in fluid secretion. *Philosophical Transactions of the Royal Society of London Series B,* **296,** 151–166.

18 Philpott, H. G. & Petersen, O. H. (1979) Extracellular but not intracellular application of peptide hormones activate pancreatic acinar cells. *Nature,* **281,** 684–686.

19 Saito, A., Williams, J. A. & Kanno, T. (1980) Potentiation of cholecystokinin-induced exocrine secretion by both exogenous and endogenous insulin in isolated and perfused rat pancreas. *Journal of Clinical Investigation,* **65,** 777–782.

20 Schulz, I. (1981) Electrolyte and fluid secretion in the exocrine pancreas. In *Physiology of the Gastrointestinal Tract* (Ed.) Johnson, L. R. pp. 795–819 New York: Raven Press.

21 Schulz, I. & Stolze, H. H. (1980) The exocrine pancreas: the role of secretagogues, cyclic nucleotides and calcium in enzyme secretion. *Annual Review of Physiology,* **42,** 127–156.

22 Sewell, W. A. & Young, J. A. (1975) Secretion of electrolytes by the pancreas of the anaesthetized rat. *Journal of Physiology,* **252,** 379–396.

23 Singh, M. (1980) Effect of glucagon and digestive enzyme synthesis, transport and secretion in mouse pancreatic acinar cells. *Journal of Physiology,* **306,** 307–322.

EVALUATION OF PANCREATIC DISEASE

The investigation and evaluation of pancreatic disease remains one of the more difficult problems in gastroenterology. The diseases considered here are chronic pancreatitis and pancreatic adenocarcinoma. The diagnosis of acute pancreatitis, endocrine pancreatic neoplasms, fibrocystic disease, and childhood pancreatic disorders are discussed later in this chapter.

The plethora of available pancreatic investigations is a poor testament to their individual usefulness, and highlights the lack of a reliable standard investigation. Many are expensive,

others invasive, and some poorly tolerated by ill patients. Before requesting pancreatic investigations the clinician should ask himself what question needs to be answered and whether it will affect management. Sometimes the clinical history, examination, and a plain abdominal X-ray are all that is required to make a diagnosis and institute treatment, but usually a number of fairly sophisticated procedures are needed since one test will often complement another. In this chapter we describe the different pancreatic investigations available and discuss their use in specific situations.

It is convenient to divide pancreatic investigations into three groups, namely *morphological* or *imaging* tests which detect changes in the shape and size of the pancreas and abnormalities of its duct systems, tests which aim to detect pancreatic disease by alteration in *function*, and other investigations designed to detect abnormal patterns or constituents in blood, urine, faeces or pancreatic juice to provide *markers* of pancreatic disease.

MARKERS OF PANCREATIC DISEASE

Serum markers

Amylase and isoamylase
The measurement of serum and urinary amylase levels and the amylase : creatinine clearance ratio is largely of relevance to the diagnosis of acute pancreatitis. Total serum amylase levels are so variable in chronic pancreatitis and carcinoma as to be of little diagnostic value.

The pancreatic isoenzyme of amylase can now be separated using chromatography, electrophoresis or isoelectric focusing and has been claimed to be useful diagnostically.[95] These techniques are unsuitable for large-scale or rapid analysis, but the development of a rapid assay now available commercially which selectively inhibits salivary amylase has renewed the interest in isoamylase determination. The initial reports were encouraging[79] with low pancreatic isoamylase levels occurring in chronic pancreatitis, but further experience has been disappointing; only a minority of patients with chronic pancreatitis studied by O'Donnell, Fitzgerald and McGeeney[79] had a low pancreatic isoamylase. We also found that the wide range of normal values severely restricted the usefulness of the test even when severe exocrine insufficiency was present.[60]

Immunoreactive trypsin

A radioimmunoassay for the measurement of serum immunoreactive trypsin (IRT) is commercially available. Initial reports by Temler and Felber[98] and Elias, Redshaw and Wood[33] showed high serum IRT levels in acute pancreatitis and low levels in chronic pancreatitis, especially when steatorrhoea was present;[2] variable levels occurred with carcinoma of the pancreas. A more recent study by Koop *et al.*[61] reporting variable serum IRT values (even with pancreatic exocrine insufficiency) accords with our experience that normal IRT levels occurred in half the chronic pancreatitis patients studied and that a significant proportion of those without pancreatic disease had abnormal IRT levels.[87] Serum IRT is therefore of little diagnostic value but trypsin assay in pancreatic juice may be more valuable (vide infra).

Gastrointestinal hormones

Radioimmunoassay techniques are available for measurement of serum levels of gut hormones but most assays are complicated and not widely available. Pancreatic polypeptide (PP) release following a test meal or secretin stimulation is impaired in patients with steatorrhoea due to chronic pancreatitis compared to coeliac disease or controls.[13] High levels of motilin and enteroglucagon occur in pancreatitis, but insulin, glucagon, gastrin and gastric inhibitory peptide are not affected.[11] These findings – particularly for PP assay, which is commercially available – are of interest but more rigorous clinical evaluation is still needed.

Other serum markers

These tests aim to provide early diagnostic tests for pancreatic cancer. Serum carcinoembryonic antigen (CEA) levels are non-specific for pancreatic carcinoma[105] and raised levels also occur in pancreatitis and liver disease.[27] Alphafetoprotein (AFP) levels in serum are elevated in 25% of those with pancreatic cancer[2] but are too nonspecific for diagnostic purposes. Pancreatic oncofetal antigen (POA), initially reported to be highly specific for pancreatic carcinoma,[10] has now also been shown by Wood and Moosa[102] to be non-specific although false-negative results were rare. This study also found no use for AFP or CEA determinations.

Pancreatic juice markers

The development of endoscopic retrograde cholangiopancreatography (ERCP) provides the opportunity to collect secretions from the can-

nulated pancreatic duct. Attempts to use the technique for pancreatic function testing have been disappointing and collections are probably incomplete. Significant differences in volume, bicarbonate and protein output occur between normals and pancreatic disease, but there is considerable overlap.[26] The more promising line of investigation now appears to be the qualitative measurement of pancreatic juice constituents from a single sample at ERCP. Cytology of pancreatic juice increases diagnostic accuracy.[34, 49] Albumin, IgA and IgG levels in pancreatic juice are all raised in the presence of carcinoma, the former also rising in other types of pancreatic disease.[43, 77] Pancreatic juice lactoferrin levels are increased in chronic pancreatitis, but not in pancreatic carcinoma – in which immunoreactive trypsin levels are low – so that measurement of these two analytes enables distinction of pancreatitis from carcinoma and both groups from controls.[36] More detailed analysis of pancreatic juice proteins, such as isoelectric focusing,[5] shows abnormal profiles in the presence of pancreatic disease, especially carcinoma. All these analyses should prove of increasing value in combination with ERCP, especially when radiology is equivocal, and, it is hoped, in patients with early pancreatic disease not detectable by other methods.

Faecal analyses

A spectacular degree of steatorrhoea may be observed in patients with pancreatic insufficiency which is most unusual in other malabsorptive states. Faecal fat estimation is useful in identifying patients requiring enzyme replacement therapy and the response to treatment, but not for differential diagnosis; furthermore, accurate and reproducible results require a sevenday constant fat diet with markers.[94] Faecal triglyceride measurement is non-specific and sample collection and storage problems have led to this test not being widely favoured.

Low outputs of pancreatic enzymes in faeces should occur in pancreatic insufficiency although significant destruction occurs during intestinal transit making trypsin assay too unreliable for diagnostic purposes. However, faecal chymotrypsin assay has been extensively studied and is stable on storage. Clinical experience shows widely divergent results, probably due to the variations in technique. In a recent review Kelleher[59] concluded that faecal chymotrypsin estimation is a useful test if steatorrhoea is present, especially in cystic fibrosis; in less florid pancreatic disease, where screening tests are really needed, false-negative results are frequent (16–100%) as they are in pancreatic carcinoma (45%).[6, 97] The test has been shown to be more reliable if a 24-h faecal collection is made with hormonal stimulation and purgation,[89] but this makes for a less attractive screening test.

Urinary estimations

Urinary amylase and the amylase : creatinine ratio is discussed on p. 1298. Urinary trypsin radioimmunoassay has not proved a useful test. An underestimated and simple test is the measurement of urinary indican, whose levels are extremely low in pancreatic insufficiency and rise with replacement therapy.[69]

Fat absorption tests

In pancreatic disease the failure to assimilate fat is caused by impaired enzymatic triglyceride digestion rather than failure to absorb the fatty acids produced. This has resulted in the development of fat absorption tests, mainly using radio-labelled triglycerides and fatty acids, since the latter should be preferentially absorbed in the presence of pancreatic disease. These tests are unreliable[74, 81] and have now been largely abandoned. Breath tests measuring $^{14}CO_2$ after oral [^{14}C]tripalmitin[19] or [^{14}C]triolein[42] have also been employed, but will probably not stand up to more rigorous evaluation.

PANCREATIC FUNCTION TESTING

Tests involving duodenal intubation

These tests measure exocrine function by analysing duodenal aspirate after either direct stimulation of pancreatic secretion using secretin, cholecystokinin (CCK) or caerulein[18, 32] or indirect stimulation by the use of a standard test meal, usually that of Lundh.[66]

For direct stimulation tests, the intubation system must be reliable, because incomplete collection or gastric juice contamination of the duodenal aspirates invalidates the results. A multi-lumen tube is positioned fluoroscopically to enable duodenal and gastric contents to be collected separately. Basal and sequential 10-min collections are collected on ice over 30–80 min.

The types, dosage and methods of giving stimulation vary widely, as do the preparations of secretin and CCK used. High doses of secretin

(4 CU/kg) administered by infusion are claimed to provide the most reliable index of function from measuring maximal bicarbonate output rather than concentration, but this hormone is unreliable to stimulate enzyme output for which CCK must be used. Reported studies have employed secretin stimulation alone,[32] secretin followed by CCK,[18] or secretin and CCK infusion combined.[103] Aspirates are analysed for secretion rate, bicarbonate concentration and output; enzyme output is also measured if CCK stimulation is used, in which case each centre must establish a normal range because of inter-laboratory variation. It is thus clear that meticulous adherence to technique is required to produce meaningful results with direct stimulation tests, and their performance is not justified in centres performing only a few tests annually. The characteristic finding in severe exocrine insufficiency or large pancreatic neoplasms is a depression of volume secreted and bicarbonate and enzyme concentrations. When duct obstruction (usually neoplastic) is present a diminished volume with normal bicarbonate and enzyme concentration occurs;[32] this will not be detected by indirect tests nor will impaired bicarbonate secretion which precedes loss of enzyme output in the progression of pancreatitis.

The indirect test of Lundh[66] is easier to perform and has a more standard protocol. A single lumen tube is positioned fluoroscopically in the duodenum. A test meal of glucose, corn oil, and casilan is given orally and four 30-min aspirates are collected on ice to measure tryptic activity. This test is dependent upon extra-pancreatic factors, such as gastric and vagal function or endogenous secretin and CCK release; abnormal results should be interpreted with caution, especially in the presence of small bowel disease. Both direct and indirect tests will not distinguish pancreatitis from carcinoma but provide an opportunity to collect duodenal aspirates for cytological examination.

The diagnostic accuracy of both types of tests is now well documented, although largely in retrospective series. For the largest series of secretin tests, misleading results occurred in only 5.1% of controls and 5.2% of patients with pancreatic disease.[31] For the secretin–CCK test an accuracy of 88% in detection of pancreatic disease with a 7% false-positive rate is representative.[16] For the Lundh test most studies report overall accuracies of 80–90% in detecting chronic pancreatitis and around 75% for carcinoma of the pancreas.[57, 76] Test failures occur with appreciable frequency and are more common with direct (10%) than indirect (7%) tests; inexperienced investigators can expect a higher failure rate. In spite of the theoretical advantages of direct stimulation tests, comparisons with the Lundh test have not shown an increased sensitivity for the former in the detection of pancreatic disease.[15, 46, 101] The Lundh test will probably meet the needs of most clinicians outside specialized centres.

Oral (tubeless) pancreatic function tests

There are obvious practical disadvantages to duodenal intubation tests, which are time-consuming, unpleasant, and have to be carefully performed. All of the new oral pancreatic function tests (PFTs) are based on similar principles. A pancreatic enzyme substrate is given by mouth and is hydrolysed by the enzyme to produce a metabolite that is absorbed and subsequently excreted in the urine. Urinary recovery of the metabolite provides an indirect index of pancreatic exocrine function. Whilst this avoids duodenal intubation, it is evident that urinary recovery of the metabolite depends upon its absorption, intermediary metabolism and urinary excretion in addition to pancreatic function.

The most widely studied test uses a synthetic tripeptide *N*-benzoyl-1-tyrosyl-*p*-aminobenzoic acid (BTP) which is hydrolysed by chymotrypsin to release *p*-aminobenzoic acid (PABA).[55] After absorption, most PABA is conjugated in the liver before urinary excretion. Laboratory estimation of PABA uses a relatively simple colorimetric method, but some drugs, notably paracetamol and sulphonamides, interfere with the estimation. Oral doses of BTP used range from 150 to 2000 mg with or without a Lundh meal, and urine is collected for 6 or 8 h, the latter period conferring no demonstrable advantage. No toxic effects have been described to date. The result of the test is expressed as the percentage of the oral dose of BTP in the PABA recovered from the urine during the collection time. Clinical experience of the BTP test now amounts to about 2000 patient studies. Recent reviews by Lang, Gyr, Stalder and Gillessen[62] and Mitchell[70] indicate accuracies of 86% and 76% in the diagnosis of chronic pancreatitis and pancreatic carcinoma, respectively. Although only 10% of patients with other gastrointestinal disease have a falsely abnormal test, this rises to over 50% in patients with non-pancreatic steatorrhoea or cirrhosis. We modified the BTP test to overcome this problem using a two-day test, since which the incorporation of a tracer dose of

$[^{14}C]$-PABA with the BTP allows a more accurate assessment from a single 6-h urine.[73, 99] The ratio of urinary recovery of PABA (dependent upon pancreatic function, absorption and conjugation) to ^{14}C (independent of pancreatic function) eliminated the falsely abnormal results due to intestinal or liver disease which occur with the unmodified BTP test. The initial encouraging results still require more extensive and rigorous prospective evaluation.

The fluorescein dilaurate (FDL) test[67] uses this substrate for pancreatic esterases that hydrolyse FDL to release fluorescein which is absorbed and excreted in the urine; on a second occasion fluorescein alone is administered. From the two 10-h urine recoveries of fluorescein, a ratio is derived in a similar way to the modified BTP test. Clinical studies[63, 68] are less extensive than for the BTP test. Over 90% of patients with documented exocrine insufficiency have an abnormal test with about a 7% false-positive rate for controls, but more studies are needed. Esterases are bile-dependent and the need for two 10-h urine collections is a practical disadvantage. Comparisons of the BTP and FDL tests demonstrate similar accuracies and both correlate well with standard duodenal intubation tests.[63]

The most recent test is the dual-labelled Schilling (DLS) test,[17] based on the observation that cobalamin can only be transferred to intrinsic factor (by which it is carried in the small intestine) from its complex with R protein if this protein has been degraded by pancreatic proteases. The DLS test distinguished normals from patients with pancreatic steatorrhoea and with small bowel disease (except, worryingly, for those with steatorrhoea). A 24-h urine collection is needed because of low isotope recoveries.

These new tests still require fuller evaluation, and duodenal intubation tests remain the standard function tests.[28] Theoretically the oral PFTs are less sensitive because they should not become abnormal until much of the pancreas is destroyed,[29] yet clinical studies have now shown normal results in pancreatitis with no greater frequency than with duodenal intubation tests,[17, 63, 73] and the overall sensitivity in reports to date is similar to duodenal intubation tests.

IMAGING

Until recently the pancreas was inaccessible and an anatomical assessment could be made only by laparotomy. Recent advances in imaging

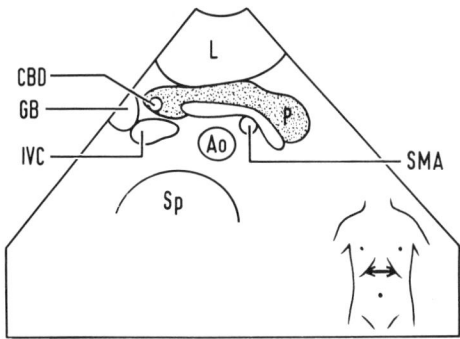

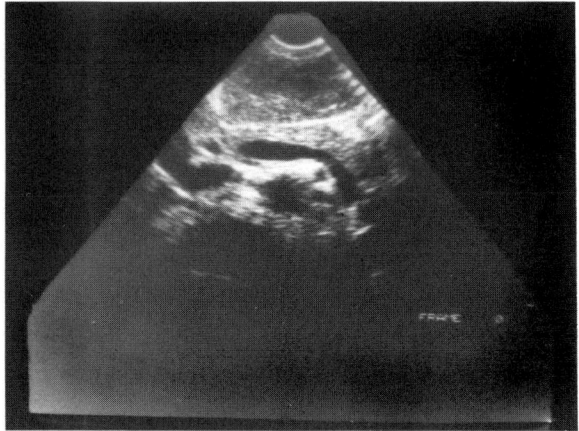

Figure 18.9 Transverse US scan showing the normal pancreas. P = pancreas, L = liver, Ao = aorta, IVC = inferior vena cava, SMA = superior mesenteric artery, CBD = common bile duct, GB = gallbladder, Sp = spine. Courtesy of Dr J. Watters.

have not only improved diagnostic ability, but are providing valuable information about the natural history of pancreatic disease.[78] Information about both the parenchyma and ductular system of the pancreas is required. Although a percutaneous method has been used,[20] endoscopic retrograde pancreatography (ERCP) is the most practicable non-operative method of imaging the ductular system, whilst computed tomography (CT) and ultrasound (US) demonstrate the parenchyma.

Ultrasound and computerized tomography

ULTRASOUND

Ultrasound is widely available as a quick and cheap form of imaging, but it does depend on considerable operator skill. High frequency ultrasound in the 3.5–5 MHz range is usually employed for pancreatic techniques, a pulse echo technique being used. A transducer trans-mits the ultrasound which is reflected at the interface between tissues and receives the incoming echo which is converted electronically into an image for display. The image produced is a section through the patient (Figure 18.9) which may be in any axis chosen by the operator. Different echo amplitudes are represented by different shades of grey, hence the term 'greyscale'. Either of two types of equipment in common use ('real-time' and 'static') may be used for pancreatic imaging, but recent advances with real-time apparatus have improved resolution substantially and this will probably become the examination of choice in the future. Different tissues give different appearances. For example fluid filled cysts appear black with no 'echoes' (Figure 18.10). Solid tumours, on the other hand, may be either echo-poor or echogenic depending on the amount of vascular tissue, collagen and their structure (Figure 18.11). Ultrasound is almost totally reflected at gas interfaces and is attenuated by bone so that structures behind both are

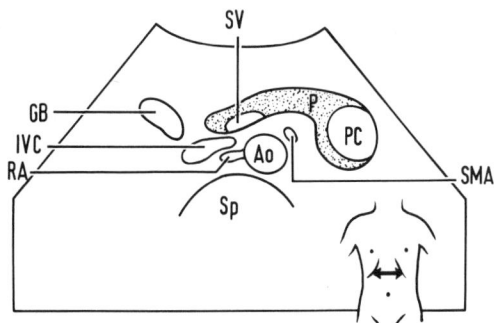

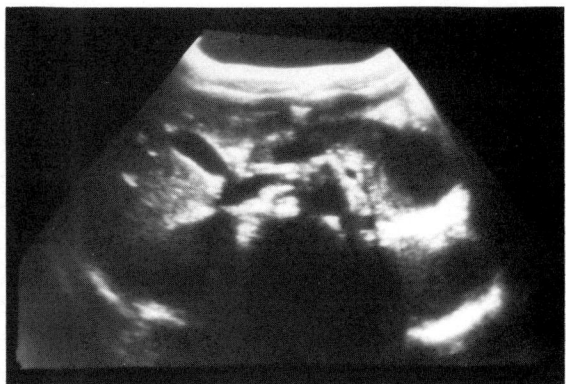

Fig. 18.10 Transverse US scan showing pseudocyst developing in a patient with acute pancreatitis. PC = pseudocyst, RA = right renal artery. Courtesy of Dr J. Watters.

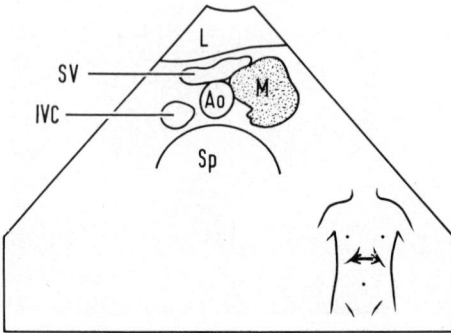

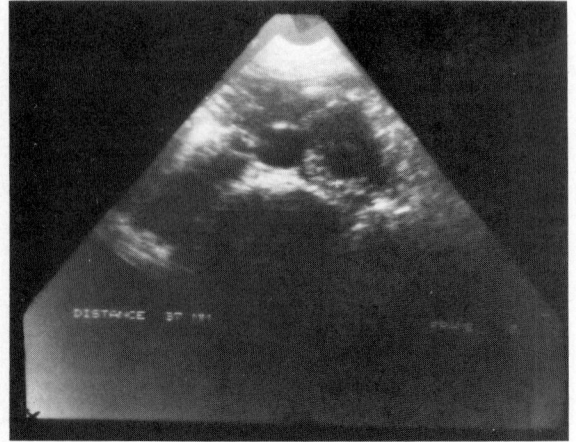

Fig. 18.11 Transverse US scan of the pancreas showing solid echo-poor tumour in the body of the pancreas. M = tumour mass. Courtesy of Dr J. Watters.

difficult to see. Scanning may be difficult in patients who are either very fat or very muscular.

Ultrasound has the advantage over CT scanning of being quick and cheap and, although resolution is usually not as good as with CT, the echogenicity of tissues differs more than their X-ray attenuation. This may enable an ultrasonographer to detect a tumour in the pancreas even though the overall contour of the gland remains unaltered. Its disadvantage is that it is less objective than a CT scan, and is therefore very much more dependent upon the skill of the operator. Sensitivities and specificities for ultrasound of over 90% have been reported from specialized centres,[64] but others have been less convincing and CT is generally considered to be a more accurate and sensitive investigation.

COMPUTED TOMOGRAPHY (CT)

X-Rays are directed sequentially through a thin section of the body, detected by a scintillation or ionization counter and a computer then calculates their attenuation and constructs a two-dimensional image (Figure 18.12). Considerable technical progress has been made with CT since its inception in 1972.[52] The time taken to scan a segment has been reduced to 1–5 s and the thickness of a transverse section can be as little as 1.5 mm. These developments have improved resolution and discrimination.[83] Organs are distinguished by differences in X-ray attenuation, but unfortunately most soft intra-abdominal organs are similar in this respect and the radiologist has to use his knowledge of tissue planes and landmarks in order to interpret the scan. Interpretation is helped by the use of oral and intravenous radiopaque contrast media, but it may still be impossible to distinguish a pancreatic cancer from normal pancreatic tissue unless there is overall enlargement, distortion of outline or infiltration across tissue planes. Up to eight sections may be needed to see the whole pancreas. Its advantages over US are its objectivity, that it is unaffected by intestinal gas or by

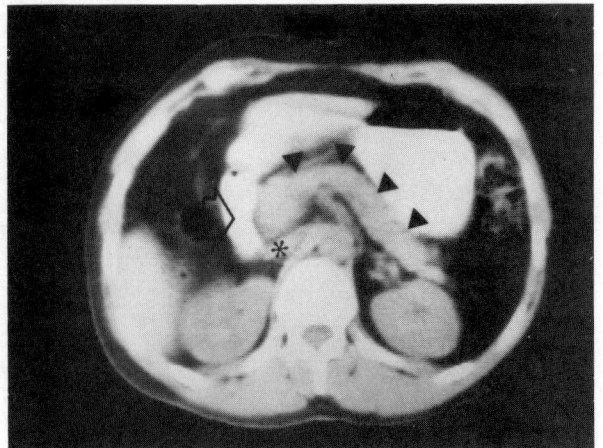

Fig. 18.12 CT scan of normal pancreas (arrowheads) showing relation of the pancreatic head to the inferior vena cava (*) and second part of duodenum which contains contrast medium (open arrow). Courtesy of Dr. P. J. Robinson.

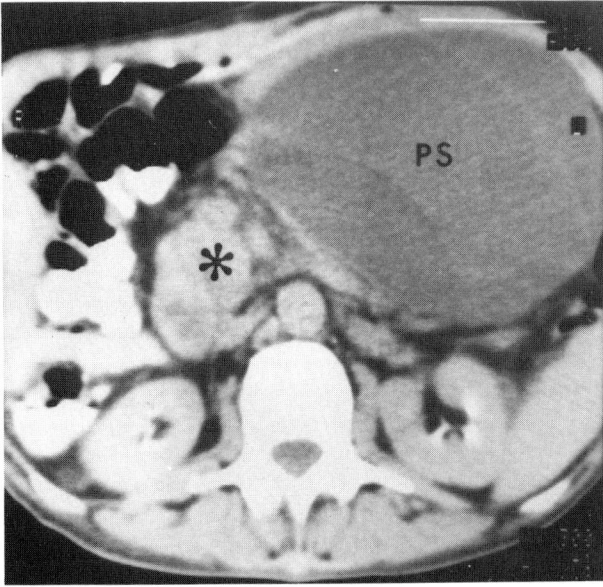

Fig. 18.13 Large pseudocyst (PS) replacing most of the body and tail of the pancreas in association with an inflammatory enlargement of the pancreatic head (*). Courtesy of Dr P. J. Robinson.

fat, and that resolution is the same throughout the image. However, it is more expensive, time consuming, and carries a small radiation hazard. Recent series[39, 51] have shown CT to be a more sensitive and specific examination than ultrasound.

CT AND ULTRASOUND IN CHRONIC PANCREATITIS

Parenchymal changes are not always demonstrable in chronic pancreatitis. The size of the pancreas may be increased or decreased, but is often within normal limits.[38] The main diagnostic feature using ultrasound is increased echogenicity caused by areas of fibrosis and calcification[93] which may be generalized or patchy in distribution; dilated pancreatic ducts may be visualized.[65] Cysts and pseudocysts are well demonstrated by ultrasound (Figure 18.10) appearing as well circumscribed echo-free areas. Similar changes are found using CT (Figure 18.13).[35] Calcification (Figure 18.14) may be detected when invisible on a plain abdominal film.[38] Inflammatory masses, duct calculi, dilatation of the main pancreatic duct, cysts and abscesses (Figure 18.15) may be seen.

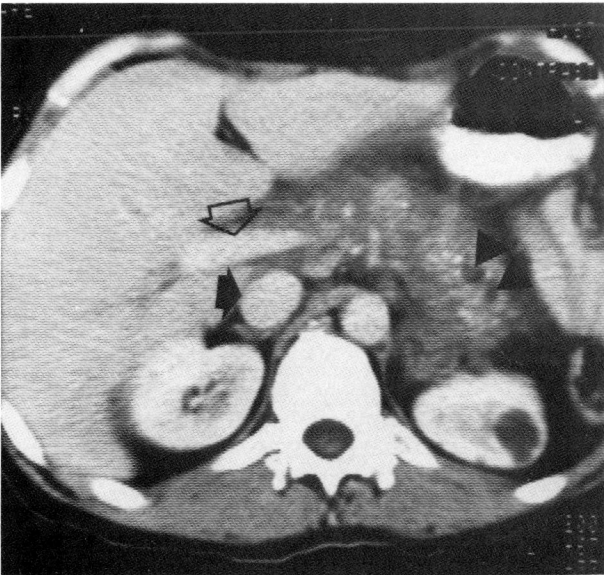

Fig. 18.14 CT scan showing chronic pancreatitis with irregular outline, effects of calcification in body and areas of duct dilatation (arrowheads). Open arrow: portal vein; closed arrow: inferior vena cava. Courtesy of Dr P. J. Robinson.

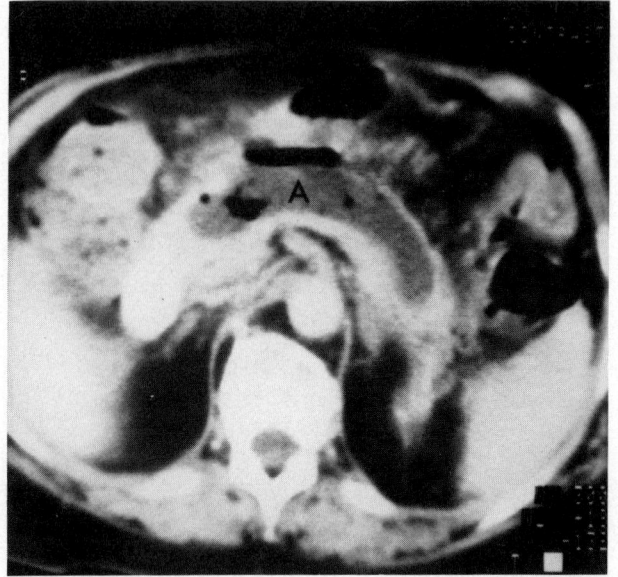

Fig. 18.15 CT scan showing pancreatic abscess; the pancreas is almost entirely replaced by low density material (A) containing pockets of gas and a larger air fluid level. Courtesy of Dr P. J. Robinson.

CT AND ULTRASOUND IN PANCREATIC CANCER

Both ultrasound and CT may show mass lesions down to a diameter of 2–3 cm depending on the site.[83] Diffuse enlargement of the pancreas can be seen in some cases as a result of oedema and obstruction distal to the tumour (Figure 18.16). Similarly, a dilated pancreatic duct, dilated bile ducts, and occasional pseudocysts may be seen as well. Ultrasound will, on occasions, show varying echogenicity within a pancreatic mass suggesting a neoplastic aetiology. These imaging techniques may demonstrate invasion across tissue planes, involved lymph nodes, and metastases in the liver which may help in assessing operability.

Nuclear magnetic resonance (NMR)

Nuclear magnetic resonance (NMR) imaging is the newest of the imaging techniques and only research prototypes are available at present. Preliminary reports suggest that in the future it may be a valuable diagnostic tool.

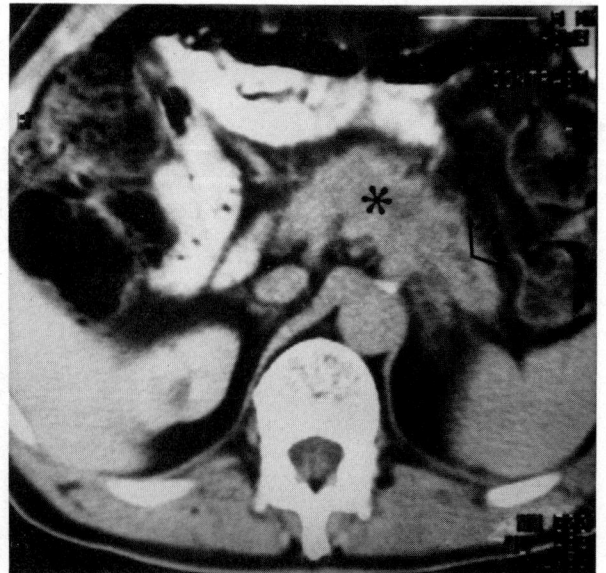

Fig. 18.16 CT scan showing carcinoma of the body of the pancreas (*) causing localized enlargement with loss of the normal outline and proximal duct dilatation (open arrow). Courtesy of Dr P. J. Robinson.

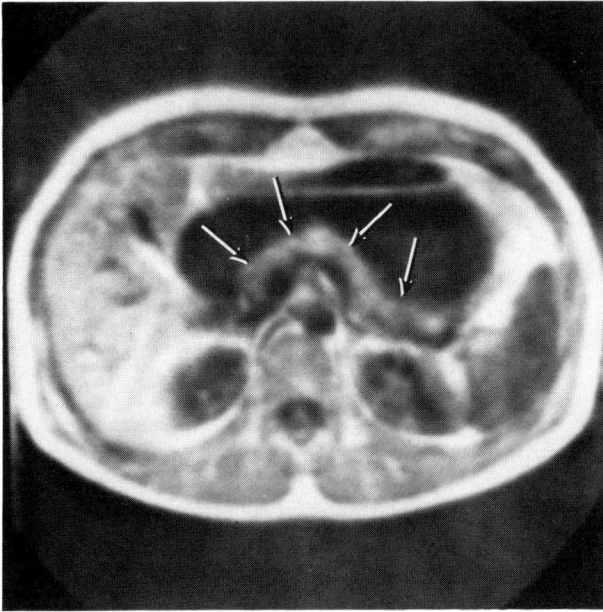

Fig. 18.17 NMR image showing normal pancreas (arrowed). Courtesy of Dr G. Bydder.

NMR depends upon the fact that certain nuclei (such as protons) behave like tiny spinning magnets: in the presence of a large static magnetic field these nuclei are selectively aligned in the direction of the field. Additional pulsed magnetic fields are applied to change the direction of this magnetization, following which it returns to or recovers its original position. The rate at which it does this depends on the exchange of energy between nuclei and other surrounding atoms and molecules ('spin-lattice relaxation'). During the relaxation phase an electrical voltage is detected in a coil surrounding the patient and this signal is used to reconstruct a tomographic image (Figure 18.17).

NMR differs from CT in several important respects. Scanning of one section takes 2–4 min (as opposed to 5–10 s for CT), although multiple slice options permitting simultaneous scanning of up to 15 slices have recently become available. The resolution of NMR images is less than CT, but frequently there is greater contrast between normal and abnormal tissue with NMR than with CT. Very little work has yet been done on the pancreas, but abnormalities have been seen in pancreatitis[104] and carcinoma.[96] Nuclei other than protons such as ^{23}Na and ^{31}P are other possibilities for imaging studies.

Pancreatic angiography

The need for this technique has been reduced greatly by the development of less invasive imaging methods requiring less expertise. Only careful studies using selective techniques by expert personnel are justified and they need suitably sophisticated (and expensive) equipment which can demonstrate small intrapancreatic carcinomas (1.0–1.5 cm in diameter). Overall sensitivities and specificities of up to 90% have been achieved, but angiography is less reliable in diagnosing periampullary tumours, particularly of bile duct origin.[50] Islet cell tumours still provide a major indication for angiography because they usually present clinically when undetectable by other techniques; transhepatic pancreatic venous cannulation also enables sampling for hormone assays.[56] There is no place for angiography in the diagnosis of pancreatitis, and the distinction from carcinoma is unreliable. Angiography can provide useful preoperative information concerning vascular anatomy, particularly when the resectability of a carcinoma remains in doubt. Nowadays the most frequent indication for angiography is when other investigations have yielded conflicting or unsatisfactory results.[41]

Radioisotope scanning

The most suitable isotope, [^{75}Se]selenomethionine, has a long half-life (120 days) and only 7% of the dose reaches the pancreas. Significant hepatic and intestinal uptake necessitates long scanning times and liver image subtraction. A normal scan is a reliable indicator of a normal pancreas with a false-negative rate of 5% for carcinoma or chronic pancreatitis,[4] but there is an unacceptably high false-positive rate of up to 30% and the scan does not distinguish carcinoma from pancreatitis.[3] Much previous enthusiasm for isotope scanning[16, 71] was engendered because alternatives such as ERCP, CT scanning or ultrasound (all of which still show a higher false-negative rate) were not available or were still being developed. Most centres now prefer to accept the slightly higher-false-negative rates in exchange for the differentiation between carcinoma and pancreatitis provided by ultrasound or CT.

Endoscopic retrograde cholangiopancreatography (ERCP)

ERCP has been widely used as a diagnostic tool since 1972. It is a combined endoscopic and radiological procedure performed in the X-ray department on a high-quality fluoroscopy table with facilities for radiography. A side-viewing duodenoscope is used, except after Polya partial gastrectomy, when an end-viewing or fore-oblique endoscope may be easier.

Initial preparation is as for routine oesophagogastroduodenoscopy. The patient is sedated usually with diazepam and peristalsis is arrested with hyoscine butylbromide (Buscopan).

The duodenoscope is passed blindly to 40–50 cm and gastric landmarks are sought; full gastroscopy is not usually attempted. The pylorus is identified, and with it virtually filling the field of view, the tip and instrument are angulated up so that with gentle pressure the duodenum is entered after a temporary 'red-out'. The cap is examined and the superior duodenal angle identified. The 'scope is rotated approximately 90° clockwise with upward angulation to enter the second part of the duodenum. After next rotating it about 180° anti-clockwise, the instrument is advanced well down into the second part of the duodenum. The papilla is identified at the cephalad end of a longitudinal fold on the medial wall. An accessory papilla is commonly present anteriorly and proximally. The patient is turned prone and a full-faced view of the papilla obtained. This is the most critical phase because with poor positioning subsequent cannulation may be impossible.

The cannula, completely filled with contrast medium, is directed at the apex of the papilla. An orifice is often visible but, if not, probing of the tip usually results in cannulation. Approaching at right-angles favours the pancreatic duct whilst upwards angulation favours the bile duct. Deep cannulation selectively opacifies one duct whilst insertion of a few millimetres may result in both ducts filling. Contrast medium is injected under fluoroscopic control; and radiographs are taken of the pancreatic duct with the cannula in place, and demonstrate the main pancreatic duct and the first and second generation of side branches (Figure 18.18). Films of the biliary system may be obtained after withdrawing the endoscope completely. Although ERCP has been used to demonstrate pancreatic parenchyma by acinar opacification, this cannot be recommended as it is associated with an unacceptably high incidence of post-pancreatography pancreatitis even when non-ionic contrast media are used.[100] The procedure is expensive both in time and labour, it requires some expertise, and there is a 3% risk of complications following the procedure.[12] These include acute pancreatitis and, rarely, cholangitis, but they are fewer when ERCP is performed by an experienced endoscopist.

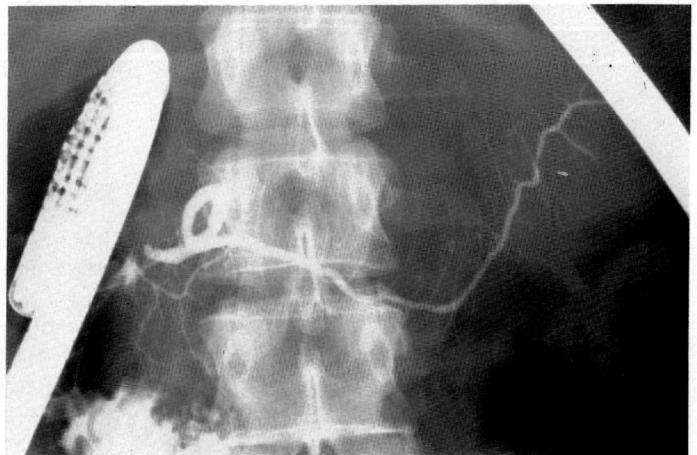

Fig. 18.18 Retrograde pancreatogram showing a normal pancreas.

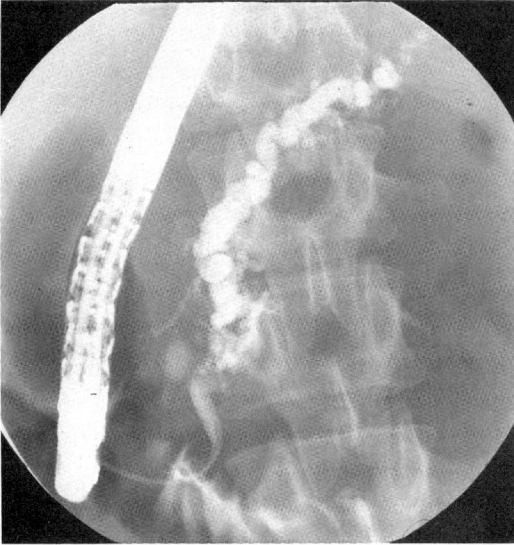

Fig. 18.19 Pancreatogram of a patient with alcoholic pancreatitis showing dilatation and tortuosity of the main pancreatic duct, dilatation, shortening, and nipping of side branches. A cyst can be seen in the head of the pancreas.

ERCP IN CHRONIC PANCREATITIS

Retrograde pancreatography is probably the most sensitive of the imaging methods in the diagnosis of chronic pancreatitis.[23] Changes are found in the main pancreatic duct and side branches.[58, 90] The main duct may be dilated or narrowed. Dilatation is generalized (Figure 18.19) or localized to one part of the gland (Figure 18.20); narrowing too may be generalized, giving a shrunken appearance (Figure 18.21). Obstruction of the main duct may be demonstrated but it is seen more often in the presence of pseudocysts which on other occasions may communicate with a duct (Figure 18.22). Other abnormalities include intraduct calculi, and small cysts in continuity with the main duct. Side branch changes are similar to those seen in the main duct and include narrowing, dilatation, and irregularity (Figure 18.23). Branches may be tortuous or leave the main duct at irregular intervals; often they are nipped at their origins and dilated peripherally: sometimes they are shortened and do not branch normally to a second generation. Occasionally coarse parenchymal opacification is seen.

The diagnosis of gross chronic pancreatitis is simple as usually the main duct and side branches are all abnormal. However, sometimes side branches alone are affected and problems arise in interpretation. 'Minimal change' disease[58] is usually defined as a pancreatogram with a normal main pancreatic duct and some normal but at least three affected side branches. It is the concept of 'minimal change' disease that is controversial[8] as it may be difficult to distinguish from the normal. A number of studies have shown that pancreatic function is depressed in these patients, but may not be outside the normal range,[7, 84, 91] implying that in some cases pancreatography is more sensitive than function tests in detecting chronic pancreatitis. ERCP compares favourably with ultrasound and CT in the diagnosis of pancreatic cancer with an accuracy of 88–100%, but CT detects some cases of chronic pancreatitis missed by ERCP.[39, 75]

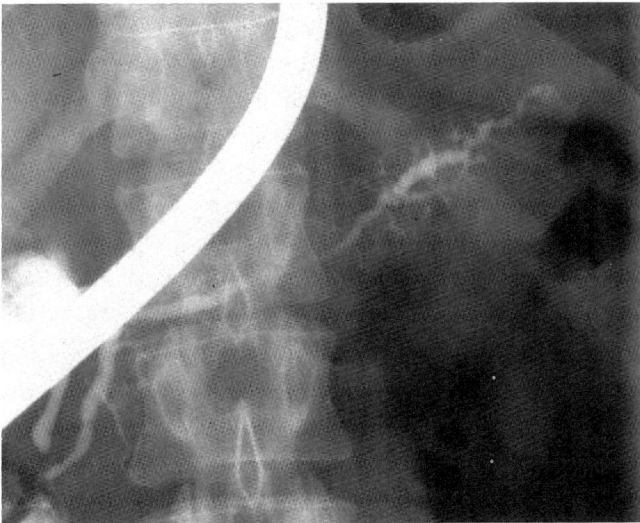

Fig. 18.20 Pancreatogram of a patient with alcoholic pancreatitis showing a stricture in the body of the pancreas with upstream dilatation and side branch changes.

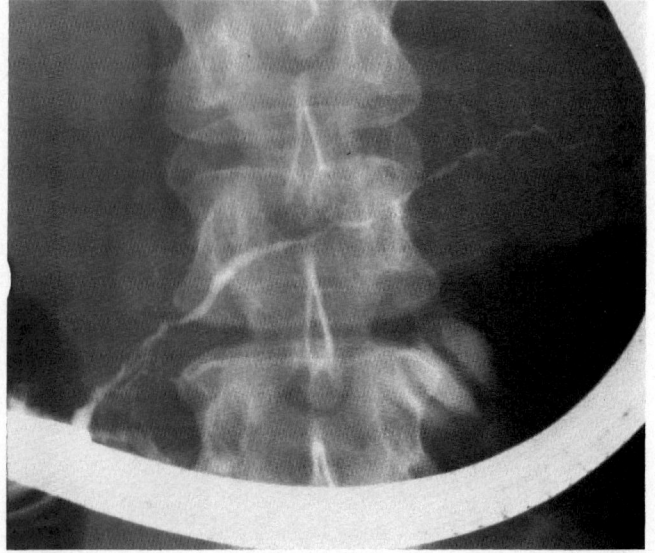

Fig. 18.21 Pancreatogram of a patient with idiopathic chronic pancreatitis showing diffuse narrowing of the main pancreatic duct and side branches.

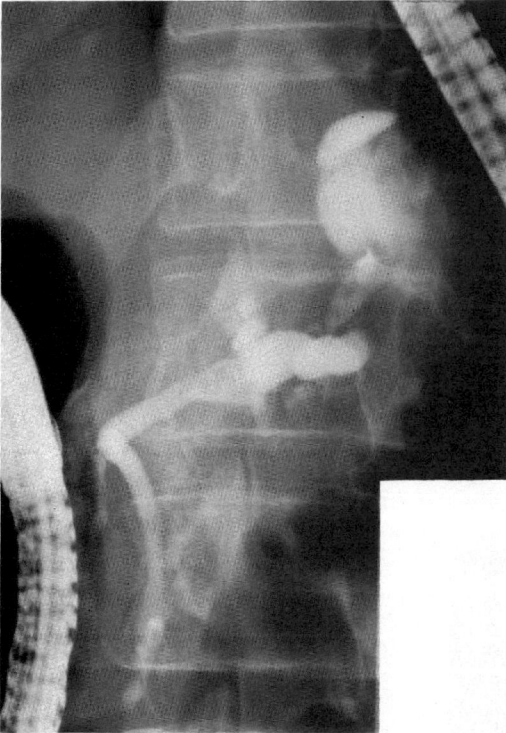

Fig. 18.22 Pancreatogram showing pseudocyst.

ERCP IN PANCREATIC CANCER

The typical ERCP changes of pancreatic cancer are those of a stenosed or obstructed pancreatic duct (Figure 18.24).[82] If the lesion is in the head of the pancreas the bile duct may be obstructed as well. Contrast medium passing upstream from the obstruction will enter a dilated duct system (Figure 18.25). Downstream, the pancre-

atic ducts should be within normal limits, but parenchymal abnormalities may be found in the region of the obstruction due to the seepage of X-ray contrast medium into necrotic areas of tumour. Occasionally a long stricture of the main pancreatic duct is seen, presumably the result of encasement by extensive cancer. Cytology obtained from pure juice or brushings may be helpful.

INVESTIGATION OF SUSPECTED PANCREATIC DISEASE

In the following section pancreatic cancer and chronic pancreatitis are considered separately, but the diagnostic approach in patients presenting with syndromes suggestive of underlying pancreatic disease is also discussed. These include pancreatic insufficiency, relapsing pancreatitis, the abdominal mass, chronic abdominal pain, and jaundice.

Chronic pancreatitis

Since the Marseilles classification[92] new pancreatic investigations have cast doubt on previous assumptions, and the diagnosis and assessment of chronic pancreatitis is both difficult and controversial. There are no agreed definitions or generally accepted criteria for a diagnosis of chronic pancreatitis; thus certain patients with severe symptomatic disease may have normal or equivocal tests and in other asymptomatic patients anatomical tests carried out for other

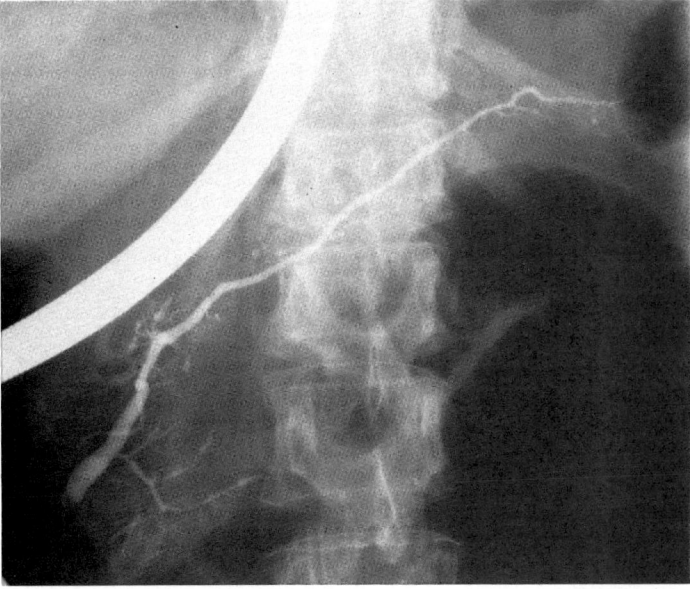

Fig. 18.23 Pancreatogram of a patient with chronic pancreatitis secondary to gallstones, showing normal main pancreatic duct but nipping irregularity, narrowing, and dilatation of the side branches typical of generalized pancreatitis.

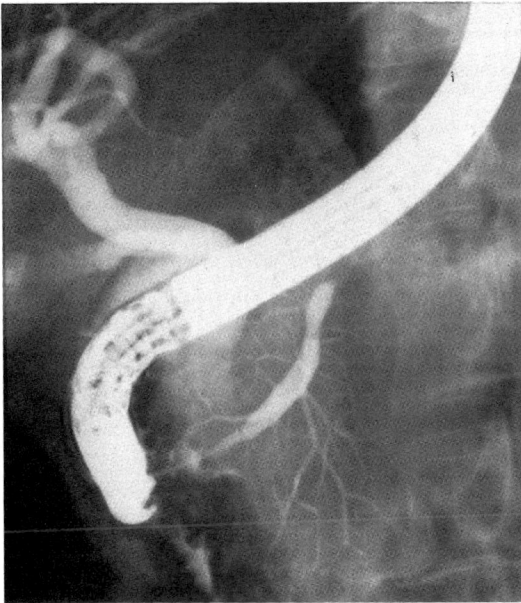

Fig. 18.24 Pancreatogram showing total obstruction of the pancreatic duct in the neck of the gland due to pancreatic cancer.

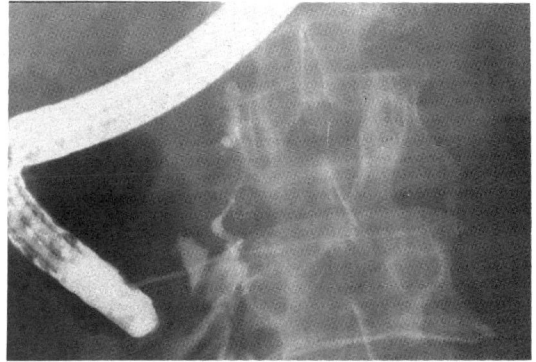

Fig. 18.25 Pancreatogram showing stenosis in the neck of the pancreas with upstream dilatation due to carcinoma of the pancreas.

reasons incidentally show quite severe abnormalities.[9] Experts disagree over the significance of certain radiological changes[24, 45] and the normal ranges for pancreatic function tests. There are geographical differences in referral patterns and in the natural history of pancreatitis; expertise, techniques, and equipment are not uniform. Nevertheless most agree that some permanent anatomical or functional abnormality should be demonstrable to diagnose chronic pancreatitis in the form of functional, parenchymal or ductular abnormality. All three of these parameters are abnormal in many patients, but in others tests are equivocal or normal and assessment is difficult because no one investigation is ideal. If pancreatic calcification is seen on plain abdominal X-ray other diagnostic tests are unnecessary.

Pancreatic cancer

With the exception of ampullary neoplasms and tumours of islet cell origin, the prognosis of pancreatic cancer is appalling, but a positive diagnosis should be sought to exclude treatable conditions and help management. A diagnosis can be made with varying degrees of confidence by ultrasound, CT, or ERCP, but an abnormal function test does not distinguish between an inflammatory and a neoplastic process and may be normal in the absence of duct obstruction.

Material for cytological examination may be obtained by duodenal aspiration during oral pancreatic function tests, from pure juice or brushings taken at ERCP, or at percutaneous thin-needle aspiration guided by CT or ultrasound. There is no diagnostic advantage in obtaining pure juice samples rather than duodenal aspiration (both give accuracies of between 50 and 90%),[80] but pure juice contains more cells and the results are easier to interpret.

Fine-needle percutaneous aspiration biopsy of the pancreas is a safe and simple technique giving a positive result in about 80% of patients.[48, 53]

Relapsing pancreatitis

Relapsing pancreatitis is subclassified into acute relapsing and chronic relapsing pancreatitis, the latter being associated with permanent anatomical or functional damage. Modern imaging techniques show that cases previously thought to be acute relapsing pancreatitis often have anatomical changes.[47] The diagnosis of relapsing pancreatitis is usually made on clinical grounds and elevated plasma amylase, but some require pancreatic function tests or imaging. After diagnosis the main purpose of investigation is to discover some remediable cause for the disease[22] or to exclude cancer-related pancreatitis and for this imaging is required. The surgeon is looking for distal disease, localized main duct strictures, pancreatic cysts and pseudocysts, congenital abnormalities of the pancreas, mass lesions, and evidence of biliary disease.

ERCP is the investigation of choice in patients with relapsing pancreatitis because in experienced hands it will provide an outline of the entire duct system in over 90% of patients demonstrating localized pancreatitis, duct strictures, pancreas divisum[21, 72] or widespread total disease. Cysts and pseudocysts may be filled but this should be avoided if possible because of the danger of infection.[25] In over 80% of patients a cholangiogram will be obtained. Direct cholangiography, either by ERCP or a percutaneous technique, is the best method of delineating the bile ducts and demonstrating calculi within them[44] (Figure 18.26), but is of less value in demonstrating stones in the gallbladder where oral cholecystography or ultrasound are superior. Common duct stones can be removed by endoscopic sphincterotomy if indicated.[88] For

these reasons ERCP is particularly valuable in those with symptoms following cholecystectomy[86] in whom both retained stones and chronic pancreatitis are common and may coexist.

Pancreatic insufficiency

If a pancreatic cause for steatorrhoea seems likely, most of the available tests should be reliable since gross disease must be present. Initially function tests may be carried out to confirm that the pancreas is the seat of the problem, but, if positive, an imaging investigation will probably be needed in order to distinguish pancreatitis from carcinoma. A similar sequence applies in patients presenting with diabetes mellitus.

Abdominal mass

Pancreatic disease may present as a palpable abdominal mass with or without pain or other symptoms to suggest pancreatic disease. The investigation of choice here is either ultrasound or CT. These techniques reliably demonstrate whether or not the mass is arising from the pancreas, and will, in addition, provide other valuable information about the tumour. If the lesion is cystic, aspiration can be carried out using a thin needle or, if solid, a sample can be taken for cytology during the examination. Ultrasound and CT indicate whether the tumour has invaded across tissue planes and whether liver metastases are present. If a pancreatic mass is large enough to be palpable it is most unusual for these techniques not to provide an accurate diagnosis. ERCP and pancreatic function tests are rarely necessary.

Chronic abdominal pain

Many patients are referred with suspected pancreatic disease because of undiagnosed abdominal pain and most do not have chronic pancreatitis. Before embarking on a pancreatic assessment it is essential that an abdominal X-ray, upper digestive endoscopy, and cholecystogram or ultrasound are performed. Other common causes of abdominal pain should also be considered, and only then should the patient be subjected to pancreatic investigation. It is in these patients that a simple, reliable non-invasive test is most needed. US can perhaps provide this in the most skilled hands,[65] but not all major centres can produce such reliable results[30, 45] and this investigation alone is

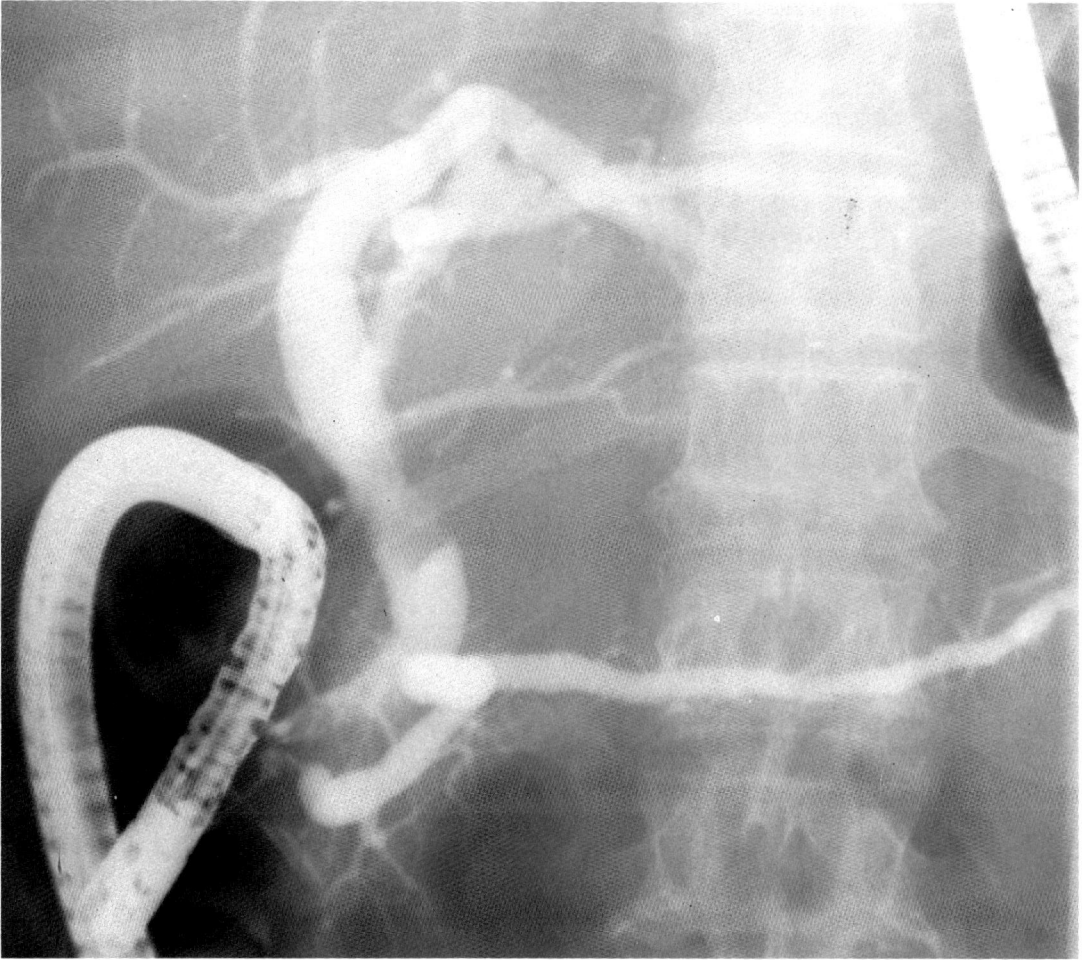

Fig. 18.26 Pancreatogram showing irregularity of the main pancreatic duct and side branch changes typical of chronic pancreatitis. A large faceted lucent stone can be seen in the common bile duct.

unlikely to be enough in a district hospital. For similar reasons, CT is also unsuitable. Our experience of serum isoamylase and trypsin determination for screening purposes has been disappointing and we doubt that any of the oral PFTs will prove accurate enough as a single screening test. ERCP alone will provide a positive diagnosis in about 24% of patients,[85] but this figure includes gallstones and peptic ulcers missed by other techniques. The high specificities and sensitivities reported for any of the above tests originate from specialized centres with a particular expertise in their performance, and many studies are retrospective and/or contain an unrealistically high proportion of patients who do have pancreatic disease. These are not the conditions under which most clinicians operate. A recently completed study in Leeds[40] supports this view; a prospective study of ultrasonography, CT scanning, and the modified BTP test in 85 patients suspected to have pancreatic disease (of whom 10% were subsequently proved to have it) showed lower sensitivities and specificities for each investigation than previously reported by ourselves or others.

For these reasons the combination of a function test and a morphological test is probably the best approach. A duodenal intubation test and ERCP provide the most accurate combination at present. Each test detects some patients missed by the other: function tests diagnose more pancreatitis and ERCP more carcinoma.[1, 30, 84] When either test is performed, there is an opportunity to take samples for cytology or biochemical analysis. This combination, however, is time consuming, unpleasant for the patient, and may not be available. An alternative less invasive approach is to use ultrasound or CT and an oral PFT to select those requiring a more detailed study. Once pancreatic disease has been found, doubts about its nature are best resolved by imaging and cytology.

Jaundice

Pancreatic cancer usually presents as progressive, cholestatic jaundice. Investigations are needed to exclude benign and operable lesions and to assess the best form of palliation. It is essential to obtain good radiographs of the common bile duct and as ultrasound may not detect intraduct calculi a contrast examination is desirable. This is most easily done by percutaneous cholangiography. The differential diagnosis for lesions at the lower end of the bile duct lies between carcinoma, benign ampullary papilloma, and chronic pancreatitis. Until recently laparotomy was the usual next step, but malignant obstruction of the bile duct can sometimes be relieved by the insertion of a percutaneous[37] or endoscopic prosthetic tube,[54] and if either of these procedures are to be carried out further investigations are needed to exclude chronic pancreatitis or an operable ampullary lesion amenable to surgery.

ACKNOWLEDGEMENTS

We would like to thank our radiological colleagues Dr D. J. Lintott, Dr J. Watters, and Dr P. J. Robinson from St James's University Hospital and the General Infirmary at Leeds for providing radiographs and for helpful criticism during the preparation of this section. We also thank Dr G. Bydder, Senior Research Fellow, Hammersmith Hospital, for his contribution on NMR imaging.

Line drawings were provided by the University of Leeds Medical Illustration Department.

REFERENCES

1   Adler, M., Waye, J. D. & Dreiling, D. (1976) A correlation of function structure and histopathology. *Acta Gastro-Enterologica Belgica*, **29**, 502–508.

2   Adrian, T. E., Besterman, H. S., Mallinson, C. N. *et al.* (1978) Plasma trypsin in patients with steatorrhoea due to chronic pancreatitis. *Clinical Science and Molecular Medicine*, **54**, 24.

3   Agnew, J. E., Maze, M. & Mitchell, C. J. (1976) Review article: pancreatic scanning. *British Journal of Radiology*, **49**, 979–995.

4   Agnew, J. E., Youngs, G. R. & Bouchier, I. A. D. (1973) Conventional and subtraction scanning of the pancreas on assessment based on blind reporting. *British Journal of Radiology*, **46**, 83–98.

5   Allan, B. J. & White, T. T. (1979) Pancreatic juice proteins in pancreatic carcinoma. *New England Journal of Medicine*, **300**, 94–95.

6   Amman, R. W., Tagwercher, E., Kashiwagi, H. & Rosenmund, H. (1968) Diagnostic value of fecal chymotrypsin and trypsin assessment for detection of pancreatic disease: a comparative study. *American Journal of Digestive Diseases*, **13**, 123–146.

7   Ashton, M. G., Axon, A. T. R. & Lintott, D. J. (1978) Lundh test and ERCP in pancreatic disease. *Gut*, **19**, 910–915.

8   Axon, A. T. R. (1981) Minimal change pancreatitis. In *Pancreatic Disease in Clinical Practice* (Ed.) Mitchell, C. J. & Kelleher, J. pp. 399–403. London: Pitman Medical.

9   Axon, A. T. R., Ashton, M. G. & Lintott, D. J. (1979) Pancreatogram changes in patients with calculous biliary disease. *British Journal of Surgery*, **66**, 466–470.

10 Banwo, O., Versey, J. & Hobbs, J. R. (1974) New oncofetal antigen for human pancreas. *Lancet*, **i**, 643–645.

11 Besterman, H. S., Adrian, T. E., Bloom, S. R. *et al.* (1982) Pancreatic and gastrointestinal hormone in chronic pancreatitis. *Digestion*, **24**, 195–208.

12 Bilbao, M. K., Dotter, C. T., Lee, T. G. & Katon, R. M. (1976) Complications of endoscopic retrograde cholangiopancreatography (ERCP) a study of 10,000 cases. *Gastroenterology*, **70**, 314–320.

13 Bloom, S. R., Besterman, H. S., Adrian, T. E. & Mallinson, C. N. (1977) Pancreatic polypeptide in the diagnosis of pancreatic insufficiency. *Irish Journal of Medical Science*, **iv** (1), 37 (abstract).

14 Braganza, J., Critchley, M., Howat, H. T. *et al.* (1973) An evaluation of ^{75}Se-selenomethionine scanning as a test of pancreatic function compared with the secretin–pancreozymin test. *Gut*, **14**, 383–389.

15 Braganza, J. M. & Rao, J. J. (1978) Disproportionate reduction in tryptic response to endogenous compared to exogenous stimulation in chronic pancreatitis. *British Medical Journal*, **ii**, 392–394.

16 Braganza, J. M., Fawcitt, R. A., Forbes, W. St. C. *et al.* (1978) A clinical evaluation of isotope scanning, ultrasonography and computed tomography in pancreatic disease. *Clinical Radiology*, **29**, 639–646.

17 Brugge, W. R., Goffe, J. S., Allen, N. C. *et al.* (1980) Development of a dual label Schilling test for pancreatic exocrine function based on the differential absorption of cobalamin bound to intrinsic factor and R protein. *Gastroenterology*, **78**, 937–949.

18 Burton, P., Evans, D. G., Harper, A. A. *et al.* (1960) A test of pancreatic function based on the analysis of duodenal contents after administration of secretin and pancreozymin. *Gut*, **1**, 111–124.

19 Chen, I. W., Azmundeth, K., Connell, A. M. & Saenger, E. L. (1974) ^{14}C-tripalmitin breath test as a diagnostic aid for fat malabsorption due to pancreatic insufficiency. *Journal of Nuclear Medicine*, **15**, 1125–1129.

20 Cooperberg, P. L., Cohen, M. M. & Graham, M. (1979) Ultrasonographically guided percutaneous pancreatography: report of two cases. *American Journal of Roentgenology*, **132**, 662–663.

21 Cotton, P. B. (1980) Congenital anomaly of pancreas divisum as cause of obstructive pain and pancreatitis. *Gut*, **21**, 105–114.

22 Cotton, P. B. & Beales, J. S. M. (1974) Endoscopic pancreatography in the management of relapsing pancreatitis. *British Medical Journal*, **i**, 608–611.

23 Cotton, P. B., Denyer, M. E., Kreel, L. *et al.* (1978) Comparative clinical impact of endoscopic pancreatography, grey-scale ultrasonography, and computed tomography (EMI scanning) in pancreatic disease: preliminary report. *Gut*, **19**, 679–684.

24 Cotton, P. B., Lees, W. R., Vallon, A. G. *et al.* (1980) Grey scale ultrasonography and endoscopic pancreatography in pancreatic diagnosis. *Radiology*, **134**, 453–459.

25 Davis, J. L., Milligan, F. D. & Cameron, J. L. (1975) Septic complications following endoscopic retrograde cholangiopancreatography. *Surgery, Gynecology and Obstetrics*, **140**, 365–367.

26 Denyer, M. E. & Cotton, P. B. (1979) Pure pancreatic juice studies in normal subjects and patients with chronic pancreatitis. *Gut*, **20**, 89–97.

27 Dilawari, J. B., Blendis, L. M., Waller, S. L. *et al.* (1973) Can carcinoembryonic antigen (CEA) differentiate carcinoma pancreas from chronic pancreatitis? *Gut*, **14**, 827–828.

28 Di Magno, E. P. (1982) Editorial: Diagnosis of chronic pancreatitis: are non-invasive tests of exocrine pancreatic function sensitive and specific? *Gastroenterology*, **83**, 143–146.

29 Di Magno, E. P., Go, V. L. W. & Summerskill, W. H. J. (1973) Relations between pancreatic enzyme outputs and malabsorption in severe pancreatic insufficiency. *New England Journal of Medicine*, **288**, 813–815.

30 Di Magno, E. P., Magelada, J. R., Taylor, W. P. & Go, V. L. W. (1977) A prospective comparison of current diagnostic tests in pancreatic cancer. *New England Journal of Medicine*, **297**, 737–742.

31 Dreiling, D. A. (1975) Pancreatic secretory testing in 1974. *Gut*, **16**, 653–656.

32 Dreiling, D. A. & Janowitz, H. D. (1962) The measurement of pancreatic secretory function. In *The Exocrine Pancreas. CIBA Foundation Symposium* (Ed.) de Reuck, A. V. S. & Cameron, M. P. London: Churchill.

33 Elias, E., Redshaw, M. & Wood, T. (1977) Diagnostic importance of changes in circulating concentration of immunoreactive trypsin. *Lancet*, **ii**, 66–68.

34 Endo, Y., Morii, T., Tamura, H. & Okuda, S. (1974) Cytodiagnosis of pancreatic tumours by aspiration under direct vision using a duodenal fibrescope. *Gastroenterology*, **67**, 944–951.

35 Fawcitt, R. A., Forbes, W. St. C., Isherwood, I. *et al.* (1978) Computed tomography in pancreatic disease. *British Journal of Radiology*, **51**, 1–4.

36 Fedail, S. S., Harvey, R. F., Salmon, P. R. *et al.* (1979) Trypsin and lactoferrin levels in pure pancreatic juice in patients with pancreatic disease. *Gut*, **20**, 983–986.

37 Ferucci, J. T. & Mueller, P. R. (1982) Interventional radiology of the biliary tract. *Gastroenterology*, **84**, 974–985.

38 Ferucci, J. T., Wittenberg, J., Black, E. B. *et al.* (1979) Computed body tomography in chronic pancreatitis. *Radiology*, **130**, 175–182.

39 Foley, W. D., Stewart, E. T., Lawson, T. L. *et al.* (1980) Computed tomography, ultrasonography and endoscopic retrograde cholangiopancreatography in diagnosis of pancreatic disease: A comparative study. *Gastrointestinal Radiology*, **5**, 29–35.

40 Foster, P. N., Mitchell, C. J., Robertson, D. R. C. *et al.* (1982) Screening tests for pancreatic disease. *Presented to European Pancreatic Club, Essen.*

41 Freeny, P. C., Bull, J. T. & Ryan, J. (1979) Impact of new diagnostic imaging methods on pancreatic angiography. *American Journal of Roentgenology*, **133**, 619–624.

42 Goff, J. S. (1982) A two stage triolein breath test differentiates pancreatic insufficiency from other causes of malabsorption. *Gastroenterology*, **83**, 44–46.

43 Goodale, R. L., Condie, R. M., Dressel, R. D. *et al.* (1979) A study of secretory protein, cytology and tumour site in pancreatic cancer. *Annals of Surgery*, **189**, 340–344.

44 Goodman, M. W., Ansel, H. J., Vennes, J. A. *et al.* (1980) Is intravenous cholangiography still useful? *Gastroenterology*, **79**, 642–645.

45 Gowland, M., Warwick, F., Kalantzis, N. & Braganza, J. (1981) Relative efficiency and predictive value of ultrasonography and endoscopic retrograde pancreatography in diagnosis of pancreatic disease. *Lancet*, **ii**, 190–193.

46 Gyr, K., Agrawal, N. N., Felsenfeld, D. & Font, R. G. (1975) Comparative study of secretin and Lundh tests. *American Journal of Digestive Diseases*, **20**, 506–512.

47 Hamilton, I., Bradley, P., Lintott, D. J. *et al.* (1982) Endoscopic retrograde cholangiopancreatography in the investigation and management of patients after acute pancreatitis. *British Journal of Surgery*, **69**, 504–506.

48 Hancke, S., Holm, H. H. & Koch, F. (1975) Ultrasonically guided percutaneous fine needle biopsy of the pancreas. *Surgery, Gynecology and Obstetrics*, **140**, 361–364.

49 Hatfield, A. R. W., Smythies, A., Wilkins, R. & Levi, A. J. (1976) Assessment of endoscopic retrograde cholangiopancreatography (ERCP) and pure pancreatic juice cytology in patients with pancreatic disease. *Gut*, **17**, 14–21.

50 Herlinger, H. & Finlay, D. B. L. (1978) Evaluation and follow up of pancreatic arteriograms. A new role for angiography in the diagnosis of carcinoma of the pancreas. *Clinical Radiology*, **29**, 277–284.

51 Hessel, S. J., Siegelman, S. O. S., McNeil, B. J. *et al.* (1982) A prospective evaluation of computed tomography and ultrasound of the pancreas. *Radiology*, **143**, 129–133.

52 Hounsfield, G. N. (1973) Computerised transverse axial scanning (tomography) part 1: description of system. *British Journal of Radiology*, **46**, 1016–1022.

53 Hudson, E. A. & Price, A. B. (1981) In *Pancreatic Disease in Clinical Practice* (Ed.) Mitchell, C. J. & Kelleher, J. London: Pitman Medical.

54 Huibregtse, K. & Tytgat, G. N. (1982) Palliative treatment of obstructive jaundice by transpapillary introduction of a large bore bile duct prosthesis. *Gut*, **23**, 371–375.

55 Imondi, A. R., Stradley, R. P. & Wolgemuth, R. (1972) Synthetic peptides in the diagnosis of exocrine pancreatic insufficiency in animals. *Gut*, **13**, 726–731.

56 Ingermasson, S., Kulal, C., Larsson, L. I. *et al.* (1977) Islet cell hyperplasia localised by pancreatic vein catheterisation and insulin radioimmunoassay. *American Journal of Surgery*, **133**, 643–645.

57 James, O. (1973) The Lundh test. *Gut*, **14**, 582–591.

58 Kasugai, T., Kuno, N. & Kizu, M. (1974) Manometric endoscopic retrograde pancreatocholangiography: technique, significance and evaluation. *American Journal of Digestive Diseases*, **19**, 485–502.

59 Kelleher, J. (1981) Other biochemical screening tests. In *Pancreatic Disease in Clinical Practice* (Ed.) Mitchell, C. J. & Kelleher, J. pp. 212–215. London: Pitman Medical.

60 Kelleher, J., Mitchell, C. J., Ruddell, W. S. J. *et al.* (1983) Assessment of a rapid pancreatic isoamylase method. *Scandinavian Journal of Gastroenterology* (in press).

61 Koop, H., Lankisch, P. G., Stockmann, F. & Arnold, R. (1980) Trypsin radioimmunoassay in the diagnosis of chronic pancreatitis. *Digestion*, **20**, 151–156.

62 Lang, D., Gyr, K., Stalder, G. A. & Gillessen, D. (1981) Assessment of exocrine pancreatic function by oral administration of *N*-benzoyl-L-tyrosyl-*p*-aminobenzoic acid; 5 years' clinical experience. *British Journal of Surgery*, **68**, 771–775.

63 Lankisch, P. G. (1981) Comparison of oral and duodenal intubation tests. In *Pancreatic Disease in Clinical Practice* (Ed.) Mitchell, C. J. & Kelleher, J. pp. 166–170. London: Pitman Medical.

64 Lees, W. R. (1981) In *Pancreatic Disease in Clinical Practice* (Ed.) Mitchell, C. J. & Kelleher, J. pp. 18–35. London: Pitman Medical.

65 Lees, W. R., Vallon, A. G., Denyer, M. E. *et al.* (1979)

Prospective study of ultrasonography in chronic pancreatitis. *British Medical Journal*, **i**, 162–164.

66 Lundh, G. (1962) Pancreatic exocrine function in neoplastic and inflammatory disease: a simple and reliable new test. *Gastroenterology*, **42**, 275–280.

67 Meyer-Bertenrath, J. G. & Kaffarnik, H. (1968) Egenschafter neuer Substrate zur Bestimmung von Pankreas Enzymen. *Zeitschrift für Klinische Chemie und Klinische Biochemie*, **6**, 484–488.

68 Meyer-Bertenrath, J. G., Heckmann, G. & Kaffarnik, H. (1978) Zur Biochemie und klinischen Bedeutung des oralen Pankreasfunctiontests mit Fluorescein-diläurinaureester. *Klinische Wochenschrift*, **56**, 917–920.

69 Miloszewski, K., Kelleher, J., Walker, B. E. *et al.* (1975) Increase in urinary indican excretion in pancreatic steatorrhoea. *Scandinavian Journal of Gastroenterology*, **10**, 481–485.

70 Mitchell, C. J. (1981) Assessment of pancreatic function. In *Topics in Gastroenterology* (Ed.) Jewell, D. P. & Lee, E. Oxford: Blackwell Scientific.

71 Mitchell, C. J., Elias, E., Agnew, J. E. *et al.* (1976) Rational sequence of tests for the assessment of pancreatic function. *British Medical Journal*, **ii**, 1307–1309.

72 Mitchell, C. J., Lintott, D. J., Ruddell, W. S. J. *et al.* (1979) Clinical relevance of an unfused pancreatic duct system. *Gut*, **20**, 1066–1071.

73 Mitchell, C. J., Field, H. P., Simpson, F. G. *et al.* (1981) Preliminary evaluation of a single-day tubeless test of pancreatic function. *British Medical Journal*, **282**, 1751–1753.

74 Moore, J. G., Englert, R., Bigler, A. H. & Clark, R. W. (1971) Simple faecal tests of absorption. A prospective study and critique. *American Journal of Digestive Diseases*, **16**, 97–105.

75 Moss, A. A., Federle, M., Shapiro, H. A. *et al.* (1980) The combined use of computed tomography and endoscopic retrograde cholangiopancreatography in the assessment of suspected pancreatic neoplasm: A blind clinical evaluation. *Radiology*, **134**, 159–163.

76 Mottaleb, A., Kapp, F., Noguera, E. C. A. *et al.* (1973) The Lundh test in the diagnosis of pancreatic disease: a review of five years experience. *Gut*, **14**, 835–841.

77 Multigner, L., Figarella, C., Sahel, J. & Sarles, H. (1980) Lactoferrin and albumin in human pancreatic juice: a valuable test for diagnosis of pancreatic disease. *Digestive Diseases and Science*, **25**, 173–178.

78 Nagata, A., Homma, T., Tamai, K. *et al.* (1981) A study of chronic pancreatitis by serial endoscopic pancreatography. *Gastroenterology*, **81**, 884–891.

79 O'Donnell, M. D., Fitzgerald, O. & McGeeney, K. F. (1977) Differential serum amylase determination by use of an inhibitor, and design of a routine procedure. *Clinical Chemistry*, **23**, 560–566.

80 Osnes, M., Serck-Hanssen, A., Kristensen, A. *et al.* (1979) Endoscopic retrograde brush cytology in patients with primary and secondary malignancies of the pancreas. *Gut*, **20**, 279–284.

81 Pimparkar, B. D., Tulsky, E. G., Kalser, M. H. & Bockus, H. L. (1961) Correlation of radioactive and chemical fecal fat determinations in various malabsorption syndromes. *American Journal of Medicine*, **30**, 927–939.

82 Reuben, A. & Cotton, P. B., (1979) Endoscopic retrograde cholangiopancreatography in cancer of the pancreas. *Surgery, Gynecology and Obstetrics*, **148**, 179–184.

83 Robinson, P. J. A. (1981) In *Pancreatic Disease in Clinical Practice* (Ed.) Mitchell, C. J. & Kelleher, J. pp. 35–55. London: Pitman Medical.

84 Rolny, P., Lukes, P. J., Gamklou, R. *et al.* (1978) A comparative evaluation of endoscopic retrograde pancreatography and secretin–CCK test in the diagnosis of pancreatic disease. *Scandinavian Journal of Gastroenterology*, **13**, 777–781.

85 Ruddell, W. S. J., Lintott, D. J. & Axon, A. T. R. (1983) The diagnostic yield of ERCP in the investigation of unexplained abdominal pain. *British Journal of Surgery*, **70**, 74–75.

86 Ruddell, W. S. J., Lintott, D. J., Ashton, M. G. & Axon, A. T. R. (1980) Endoscopic retrograde cholangiography and pancreatography in the investigation of post cholecystectomy patients. *Lancet*, **i**, 444–447.

87 Ruddell, W. S. J., Mitchell, C. J., Hamilton, I. *et al.* (1981) Clinical value of serum immunoreactive trypsin concentration. *British Medical Journal*, **ii**, 1429–1432.

88 Safrany, L. (1977) Duodenoscopic sphincterotomy and gallstone removal. *Gastroenterology*, **72**, 338–343.

89 Sale, J. K., Goldberg, D. M., Thjodleifsson, B. & Wormsley, K. G. (1974) Trypsin and chymotrypsin in duodenal aspirate and faeces in response to secretin and cholecystokinin – pancreozymin. *Gut*, **15**, 132–138.

90 Salmon, P. R. (1975) Endoscopic retrograde choledochopancreatography in the diagnosis of pancreatic disease. *Gut*, **16**, 658–663.

91 Salmon, P. R., Baddeley, H., Machado, G. *et al.* (1975) Endoscopic pancreatography, scintigraphy and exocrine function in pancreatitis. A comparative study. *Gut*, **16**, 830–831.

92 Sarles, H. (1963) *Pancreatitis. Symposium, Marseilles 1963.* Basel: Karger.

93 Sarti, D. A. & King, W. (1980) The ultrasonic findings in inflammatory pancreatic disease. *Seminars in Ultrasound*, **1**, 178–191.

94 Simpson, F. G., Hall, G. P., Kelleher, J. & Losowsky, M. S. (1979) Radio-opaque pellets as faecal markers for faecal fat estimation in malabsorption. *Gut*, **20**, 581–584.

95 Skude, G. & Eriksson, S. (1976) Serum isoamylases in chronic pancreatitis. *Scandinavian Journal of Gastroenterology*, **11**, 525–527.

96 Smith, F. W., Hutchison, J. M. S. & Mallard, J. R. (1982) Nuclear magnetic resonance imaging of the pancreas. *Radiology*, **146**, 677–680.

97 Smith, J. S., Ediss, I., Mullinger, M. A. & Boguch, A. (1971) Faecal chymotrypsin and trypsin determination. *Canadian Medical Association Journal*, **104**, 691–694.

98 Temler, R. S. & Felber, J. P. (1976) Radioimmunoassay of human plasma trypsin. *Biochimica et Biophysica Acta*, **445**, 720–728.

99 Tetlow, V. A., Lobley, R. W., Herman, K. & Braganza, J. (1980) A one-day oral pancreatic function test using a chymotrypsin-labile peptide and a radioactive marker. *Clinical Trials Journal*, **17**, 121–128.

100 Twomey, B., Wilkins, R. A. & Levi, A. J. (1982) Pancreatic parenchymography using metrizamide. *Gut*, **5**, A432.

101 Waller, S. L. (1975) The Lundh test in the diagnosis of pancreatic disease. *Gut*, **16**, 657–658.

102 Wood, R. W. & Moosa, R. (1977) The prospective evaluation of tumour associated antigen for the early diagnosis of pancreatic cancer. *British Journal of Surgery*, **64**, 718–720.

103 Wormsley, K. G. (1972) Pancreatic function tests. *Clinics in Gastroenterology*, **1**, 27–42.

104 Young, I. R., Bailes, D. R., Burl, M. *et al.* (1982) Initial clinical evaluation of a whole body tomograph. *Journal of Computer Assisted Tomography*, **6**, 1–18.

105 Zamcheck, N. (1974) Carcinoembryonic antigen in benign and malignant digestive tract disease. *Advances in Internal Medicine*, **19**, 413–433.

MACROAMYLASAEMIA

Macroamylasaemia is a term coined by Berk, Kizu and Wilding[3] to describe the presence in serum of an amylase with an unusually high molecular weight. The phenomenon is clinically significant because the resulting hyper-amylasaemia may be incorrectly construed as indicative of pancreatic disease.

Composition of macroamylase

Macroamylase dissociates at acid pH[10, 16] to yield normal salivary and pancreatic amylase, and a protein capable of combining with serum amylase of normal subjects to form macro-amylase. Thus, macroamylasaemia results from the presence of an abnormal serum protein capable of binding normal amylase.

The most striking feature of these amylase binding proteins is their heterogeneity. Binding proteins identified to date include immuno-globulins G[7] and A,[10] as well as non-immunologic glycoproteins.[14] The immuno-globulins usually have a single type of light chain, suggesting development from a single clone.[15] The molecular weights of the binding proteins range from 200 000 to several million.

The affinity of the binding proteins for amylase ranges from the tight binding character-istic of an antigen–antibody reaction to a weak interaction which dissociates during gentle iso-lation procedures.[6] The serum concentration of macroamylase (a reflection of the quantity and affinity of the binding protein) ranges from a small fraction of the normal serum amylase level of 300 iu/l to several thousand iu/l. The binding protein usually persists indefinitely but can dis-appear spontaneously.[8]

Physiology of macroamylase

Bound and unbound amylase have roughly similar enzymatic activity,[11] and the elevated serum amylase level in macroamylasaemia pre-sumably results from a decreased serum clear-ance of the bound enzyme. The kidney plays a major role in the turnover of low molecular weight proteins (such as normal amylase) which are filtered at the glomerulus and then cata-bolized by the renal tubule. Macroamylase is too large to be filtered at the glomerulus and never appears in the urine. Thus, failure of the kidney (and perhaps other organs) to clear macroamylase results in an excessive accumula-tion of serum amylase activity.

Clinical aspects of macroamylasaemia

Prevalence

Macroamylasaemia is not a rare phenomenon; well over 100 cases have been reported in the literature since 1967 with a roughly equal male : female distribution.[6] A prevalence of 1.3% was found during routine screening of 622 sera of hospitalized subjects.[9] Macro-amylasaemia was found in 1.6% of all elevated serum amylase levels[5] and in 20% of all patients with asymptomatic chronic hyper-amylasaemia.[12]

Health implications

While there is no evidence to suggest that the amylase complex is deleterious to health, several clinical conditions are associated with macro-amylasaemia. Serum amylase measurements are obtained almost solely to evaluate abdominal pain, and nearly all macroamylasaemic patients have a past history of abdominal discomfort. A high prevalence of alcoholism has been reported in macroamylasaemic subjects,[1] but this associ-ation may merely reflect the frequency with which serum amylase levels are obtained to evaluate the possibility of alcoholic pancreatitis. A small minority of macroamylase patients have a syndrome consisting of villus atrophy, malab-sorption and serum immunoglobulin abnormali-ties.[4, 10] A small fraction of the serum paraprotein binds amylase.

Diagnosis

Failure to identify macroamylasaemia as the cause of hyperamylasaemia usually leads to a costly evaluation of the pancreas. Although occasionally transient, macroamylasaemia is usually chronic and should be considered in any patient with raised serum amylase levels that persist for more than one week. In particular, this condition should be suspected when a patient with normal renal function has hyper-amylasaemia associated with a normal or low urinary amylase excretion rate. More specific is the finding of a renal clearance of amylase : cre-atinine of less than 1%,[13] although marked sali-vary hyperamylasaemia can also yield low clearance ratios.[2]

A number of techniques specifically identify macroamylase, including gel filtration, thin-layer chromatography, electrophoresis and thermal lability.[6] Unfortunately these techniques are time-consuming and are seldom provided by the routine clinical chemistry laboratory.

Although non-specific, the lipase assay is a simple means of evaluating unexplained chronic hyperamylasaemia. Serum lipase is elevated if pancreatic isoamylase is the cause of hyperamylasaemia, whereas lipase is normal in macroamylasaemia or salivary hyperamylasaemia. Because the latter two conditions have no pathological implications, a normal lipase indicates that hyperamylasaemia is clinically unimportant, while an elevated lipase indicates a need to evaluate the pancreas.

Treatment

The only 'treatment' required for macroamylasaemia is to inform the patient of the benign nature of the hyperamylasaemia. In particular, he should be told that the amylase elevation is likely to persist indefinitely and that any subsequent medical attendants must be apprised of the macroamylasaemic origin of the amylase elevation.

REFERENCES

1 Ammon, R. K. (1969) A case of macroamylasemia. *Medical Journal of Australia*, **2**, 31–33.
2 Berk, J. E., Fridhandler, L. & Montgomery, K. (1973) Simulation of macroamylasemia by salivary-type 'S-type' hyperamylasemia. *Gut*, **14**, 726–729.
3 Berk, J. C., Kizu, H. & Wilding, P. (1967) A newly recognized cause for elevated serum amylase activity. *New England Journal of Medicine*, **277**, 941–946.
4 Bosseckert, H., Winnefeld, K. & Seidel, K. (1969) *Macro-amylasaemia with Paraproteinaemia and the Malabsorption Syndrome*, Vol. 14. pp. 133–135. Germany: GMM.
5 Durr, H. K., Bindrich, D. & Bode, J. C. (1977) The frequency of macroamylasemia and the diagnostic value of the amylase to creatinine clearance ratio in patients with elevated serum amylase activity. *Scandinavian Journal of Gastroenterology*, **12**, 701–705.
6 Fridhandler, L. & Berk, J. E. (1978) Macroamylasemia. *Advances in Clinical Chemistry*, **20**, 267–286.
7 Harada, K., Nakayama, T., Kitamura, M. & Sugimoto, T. (1975) Immunological and electrophoretical approaches to macroamylase analysis. *Clinica Chimica Acta*, **59**, 291–299.
8 Hedger, R. W. & Hardison, G. M. (1971) Transient macroamylasemia during an exacerbation of acute intermittent porphyria. *Gastroenterology*, **60**, 963–968.
9 Helfat, A., Berk, J. E. & Fridhandler, L. (1974) The prevalence of macroamylasemia. *American Journal of Gastroenterology*, **62**, 54–58.
10 Levitt, M. D. & Cooperband, S. R. (1978) Hyperamylasemia from the binding of serum amylase by an 11S IgA globulin. *New England Journal of Medicine*, **278**, 474–478.
11 Levitt, M. D., Duane, W. C. & Cooperband, S. R. (1972) Study of macroamylase complexes. *Journal of Laboratory and Clinical Medicine*, **80**, 414–422.
12 Levitt, M. D., Ellis, C. J. & Meier, P. B. (1980) Extrapancreatic origin of chronic unexplained hyperamylasemia. *New England Journal of Medicine*, **302**, 670–671.
13 Levitt, M. D., Rapoport, M. & Cooperband, S. R. (1969) The renal clearance of amylase in renal insufficiency, acute pancreatitis and macroamylasemia. *Annals of Internal Medicine*, **71**, 919–925.
14 Kitamura, T., Yoshioka, K., Ehara, M. & Akedo, H. (1977) A study on the nature of macroamylase complex: Dissociation of macroamylase by substrates. *Gastroenterology*, **73**, 46–51.
15 Kobayashi, T., Nakayama, T. & Kitamura, M. (1978) Electrophoretic identification of serum immunoglobulins linked to amylase : macroamylase. *Clinica Chimica Acta*, **86**, 261–265.
16 Ueda, M., Berk, J. E. & Fridhandler, L. (1971) Macroamylasemia: Variation in the response of the macroamylase complex to acidification. *Proceedings of the Society of Experimental Biology and Medicine*, **137**, 1152–1156.

CYSTIC FIBROSIS

GENERAL FEATURES

Cystic fibrosis is an inherited disease which primarily affects the pancreas and lungs, but is characterized by abnormal secretion from many exocrine glands. It was first separated from other 'coeliac' syndromes and the relationship between the pancreatic and lung lesions clarified by Fanconi, Uehlinger and Knauer[15] in Germany and Dorothy Andersen[1] in the United States. The demonstration of pancreatic insufficiency was the key to the clinical diagnosis until di Sant'Agnese et al.[10] showed that patients uniformly secreted sweat containing high concentrations of sodium chloride. The one absolute essential for diagnosis continues to be the finding of a high sweat sodium or chloride. Gibbs, Bostick and Smith[21] showed that steatorrhea was not seen in all patients. Since then it has gradually become apparent that the clinical expression of the disease may be quite variable.

AETIOLOGY AND PATHOGENESIS

The electrolyte abnormalities in sweat reflect a secretory lesion which is probably expressed in all epithelial cells. At maximal flow rates the concentration of sodium and chloride is much greater in sweat from cystic fibrosis patients than in sweat from normal individuals, and the sweat bicarbonate concentration is lower.[37] The

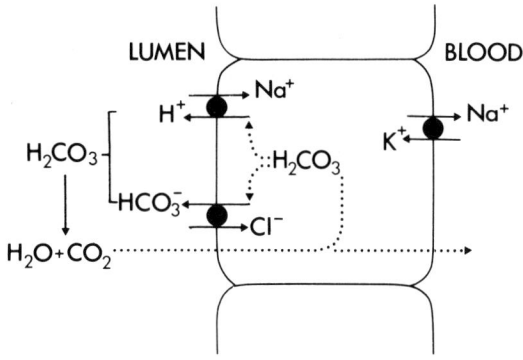

Fig. 18.27 The transport systems of the sweat duct cell (modified from Quinton).[37] The reabsorption of NaCl from the duct lumen depends upon Na^+/H^+ and HCO_3^-/Cl^- exchange systems. Low HCO_3^- concentrations in the sweat duct lumen can only be explained by malfunction of the HCO_3^-/Cl^- system.

reabsorption of sodium and chloride from the lumen of the sweat duct is a product of at least three transport systems (Figure 18.27), the Na^+/K^+ exchange pump driven by a $(Na^+ + K^+)$-ATPase, the Na^+/H^+ exchange system and the Cl^-/HCO_3^- exchange systems. The Na^+/K^+ pump is ubiquitous and not affected by cystic fibrosis. If the Na^+/H^+ exchange system were involved, the inward transport of sodium would be reduced, but so would the luminal appearance of proton and the net result would be a decrease in the consumption of bicarbonate by conversion to H_2CO_3. As a consequence the ductal bicarbonate concentration would be increased in cystic fibrosis, whereas it is decreased. The transport abnor-

malities are therefore most consistent with defective bicarbonate generation via Cl^-/HCO_3^- exchange. The possibility that defective bicarbonate generation may underlie other lesions in cystic fibrosis is supported by recent evidence[19] which shows that pancreatic HCO_3^- secretion is reduced, not only in patients with severe pancreatic disease, but even in patients with normal levels of acinar function where the defect could not possibly be secondary to destructive pathology.

Electrolyte abnormalities are associated with increased viscosity of secretions and a tendency to develop highly proteinaceous or mucoid plugging. Mucus glycoproteins appear to be chemically altered with a high ratio of fucose : sialic acid, and the carbohydrate chains are elongated.[46] Mucus is particularly thick, tenacious and copious. The result, as shown in Figure 18.28, is an obstructive tubulopathy which affects multiple organs, including the pancreas, gut, liver, lungs and testes. Interestingly, the urinary tract is functionally spared, perhaps because high passive fluid flow and low protein concentration prevent the accumulation of organic plugs.

INHERITANCE

Cystic fibrosis is inherited as an autosomal recessive trait, with a very high incidence in Caucasians compared to other races. Approximately one individual for every 20 in the population is a heterozygote or gene carrier, and homozygotes occur with a frequency of one in

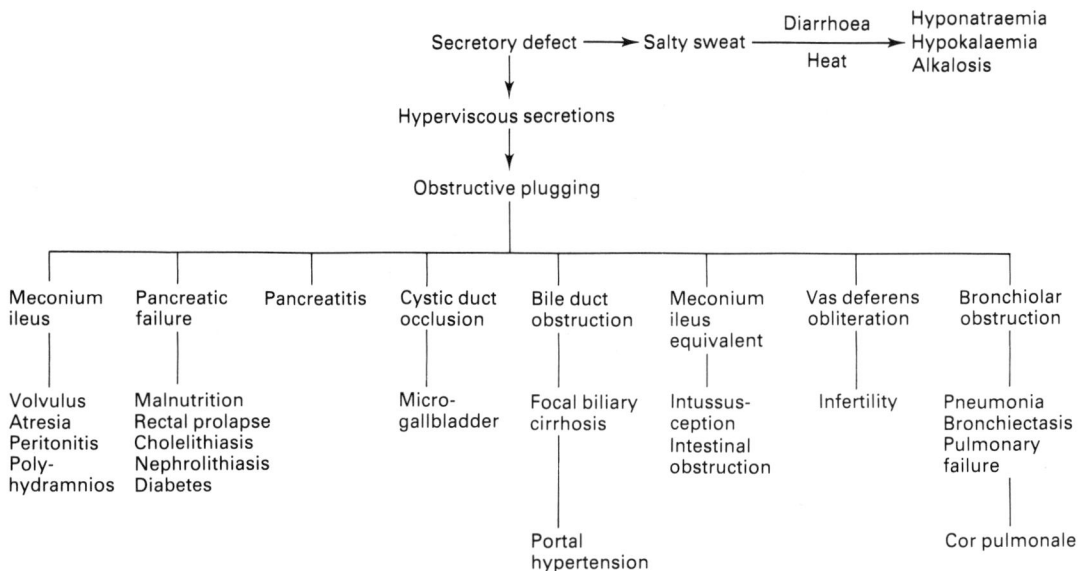

Fig. 18.28 Consequences of the secretory defect in cystic fibrosis.

every 2000 live births. The carrier state cannot be identified with certainty in spite of a continuous flow of claims to the contrary.

PROGNOSIS

In most patients the outcome of the disease depends almost entirely on the pulmonary complications. These begin, often insidiously, as a chronic pulmonary infection caused by the plugging of small airways by thick, viscid secretions and lead eventually to widespread destruction of terminal bronchioles, bronchiectasis, atelectasis and emphysema with associated respiratory failure, haemoptyses and cor pulmonale. Death results from respiratory failure or overwhelming pulmonary infection. The median survival for patients in Canada is 28 years for males and 19 years for females. There is no explanation for the great discrepancy between the sexes. Girls appear to do as well as boys until the early teens, but worsen subsequently at a much faster rate.

Gastrointestinal factors may play an important role in deciding overall prognosis, because both male and female patients who lack sufficient pancreatic disease to produce steatorrhoea have been shown to have remarkably well preserved pulmonary function, at least into the third decade.[17]

PANCREATIC DISEASE

The classification of pancreatic disease in cystic fibrosis can be quite confusing. Patients who have steatorrhoea are generally considered to have pancreatic insufficiency, while those who absorb fat normally are said to have retained pancreatic function. Neither term is satisfactory, as many patients in the latter category lack pancreatic function, and many of the former have some pancreatic function. Nevertheless, a classification based on the presence or absence of fat malabsorption has merit because the clinical course of the disease is quite different in patients from each category. Pancreatic disease will be discussed, therefore, under two headings, pancreatic insufficiency and pancreatic sufficiency, arbitrarily defined by the presence or absence of steatorrhoea.

Pancreatic insufficiency (patients with steatorrhoea)

PATHOLOGY

Pancreatic damage begins in utero and first appears as an arrest of acinar development.[27, 36]

At birth intralobular ductules are filled with mucus and many are dilated. Acini are still relatively intact, although there is evidence of early atrophy and there are variable degrees of interstitial fibrosis. By the end of the first year of life, advanced acinar destruction is always present and exocrine elements are progressively replaced by fibrous tissue and fat.[28] With time, ductules and acini disappear. Endocrine elements are relatively preserved but as patients grow older there is islet cell loss and the gland becomes completely replaced by a fibroadipose stroma.

CLINICAL FEATURES

In our clinic approximately 60% of patients are diagnosed before the age of one year, 85% before the age of five years. Although pancreatic acini appear to be relatively preserved in infancy, most patients have steatorrhoea at diagnosis. Stools are bulky, greasy, malodorous, loose and often more frequent than normal, although diarrhoea is rarely reported. In the absence of chest complications the appetite is often well maintained and growth may be unimpaired. If chest problems are severe the appetite falls and there is rapid and profound weight loss. On physical examination infants are often thin with wasted limbs and buttocks and a protuberant abdomen. Rectal prolapse occurs in 20% of patients and should suggest the diagnosis. Finger clubbing is an early and impressive sign. Deficiencies of fat soluble vitamins are common biochemically but rare clinically. At birth, bruising and intracranial and gastrointestinal bleeding due to vitamin K deficiency have been reported.[43] In older children it is common to find evidence of vitamin E deficiency but clinical sequelae are unusual. Ophthalmoplegia, absent deep tendon reflexes, hand tremors and positive Rombergism have been described, however,[14] and raise the possibility of vitamin E deficiency (see also p. 677). Overt rickets does not occur in cystic fibrosis but in older children bony demineralization is not uncommon, and in some patients 25-hydroxy-vitamin D levels may be low. Although vitamin B_{12} may be malabsorbed in untreated patients, megaloblastic anaemia has not been reported. Most patients with pancreatic insufficiency have low plasma and tissue levels of linoleic acid, while other fatty acids such as palmitoleic, oleic and eicosotrienoic may be elevated, suggesting a mild essential fatty acid deficiency.[25] Urinary oxalate excretion may be increased as with other causes of steatorrhoea.

DIAGNOSIS

The diagnosis of pancreatic insufficiency can usually be made by looking at the stool smear which is loaded with neutral fat droplets. Deficient secretion of pancreatic enzymes may be suspected from low random or 24-h stool chymotrypsin activity.[5] Serum levels of pancreatic amylase or trypsinogen may be reduced. Most patients with steatorrhoea will have abnormal excretion of *p*-aminobenzoic acid (PABA) following the administration of *N*-benzoyl-L-tyrosyl-PABA.[34] Quantitative determination of a three- or five-day faecal fat excretion with a known fat intake will establish the presence of steatorrhoea. Faecal fat excretion is surprisingly variable, amounting to as much as 80% of intake in some patients, with a mean of 38% (Figure 18.29).

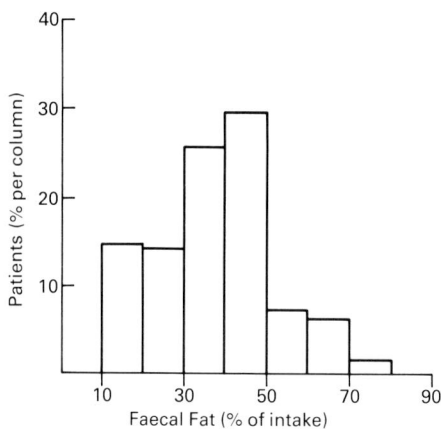

Fig. 18.29 Range of steatorrhoea in 190 patients, untreated, with cystic fibrosis, registered with the Cystic Fibrosis Clinic in Toronto, Canada. Note that most of the cases are concentrated in the 10–50% range. From Forstner *et al.* (1980),[16] with kind permission of the authors and the publisher, Imperial Press.

The only truly definitive test for pancreatic insufficiency continues to be the documentation of very low enzyme output from the pancreas following stimulation by secretin and cholecystokinin. Our studies on patients with steatorrhoea show that all had a lipase output which was less than 1.5% of the average for controls.[20]

Paradoxically, pancreatic insufficiency in very early infancy is associated with elevated levels of serum trypsinogen; high serum trypsinogen values at this age appear to be a very satisfactory screening technique for the 80% of the cystic fibrosis population with pancreatic insufficiency.[7] The high serum trypsinogen levels must be due to reflux from obstructed acini since most patients have evidence of pancreatic insufficiency at this time. Serum trypsinogen levels fall as patients become older, but low activities do not appear until six years of age, and therefore a normal value in a young patient does not exclude pancreatic insufficiency.

TREATMENT

All patients should receive regular supplementation with pancreatic enzymes. Enteric-coated, acid-resistant microspheres which release their pancreatic enzymes at a pH of 5.5–6.0 have largely replaced capsules containing pancreatic extract powders, because in this way the number of capsules required for symptomatic relief is greatly reduced. The recommended dose is 3–4 capsules per meal, and one with each snack, with each capsule containing approximately 30 000 NF (USP) units of protease. It seems reasonable to take the capsules at regular intervals throughout the meal, but this has not been tested systematically. A very few patients appear to be made worse by the acid-resistant preparations and these may have unusually high gastric acid output preventing neutralization of duodenal and upper jejunal secretions to the degree required for pancreatic enzyme release.

It is uncommon to correct the steatorrhoea completely. Our patients with cystic fibrosis excreted 18 times as much fat per gram of fat intake as the normal average when no pancreatic supplement was given, and only improved to twelve times the normal with pancreatic extract powders.[16] When cimetidine and bicarbonate were added to inhibit and neutralize gastric acid secretion, absorption improved significantly but stool fat excretion fell to less than 7% of intake in only three of 45 tests. The enteric-coated microspheres have not improved this performance. The response to pancreatic supplementation depends on the amount of fat in the diet.[12] Patients taking more than 100 g of fat daily may require one or two additional capsules with meals and snacks. The diet should be calorically adequate. Since fat is the most economical and appetizing energy source, it should not be restricted, but encouraged. When patients are given adequate diets they exhibit normal growth velocity for both height and weight until they develop advanced respiratory failure in their teens.[6]

Vitamins should be given in large daily doses in water-soluble form. Recommended amounts are: vitamin A, 8000 iu; vitamin D, 800 iu; water-soluble vitamin K (menadiol sodium phosphate), 5.0 mg; and water-soluble vitamin E (DL-α-tocopherol acetate), 300 iu. B vitamins should be administered in twice the daily minimum requirements.

Amino acid hydrolysate, medium-chain triglycerides (MCT) and polysaccharide supplements are rarely indicated. In infants under six months' old with severe pulmonary problems it is useful to begin feeding with MCT and hydrolysate formulae because it may be difficult to ensure delivery of pancreatic enzymes with liquid formulae. The MCT mixes should be supplemented with essential fatty acids.[22] An attempt should be made to give pancreatic supplements along with the MCT formula because the absorption of fat will be improved.[13]

There is no solution for the anorexia and profound malnutrition which overcomes the steatorrhoeic patient as pulmonary function enters the stage of terminal deterioration. These patients are usually adolescents or young adults and girls fail earlier than boys. Oral supplementation with elemental and high caloric diets are of no value. Nocturnal caloric supplementation by intubation has had little long-term effect, and a tube is poorly tolerated by patients with a chronic cough. Intravenous alimentation or supplements with intralipid succeed only in younger patients with relatively good pulmonary function who appear to have been underweight on other grounds.

SPECIFIC SYNDROMES ASSOCIATED WITH PANCREATIC INSUFFICIENCY

Hypoalbuminaemia, oedema and anaemia
These problems coalesce in infants under the age of six months, with a peak incidence at 3–4 months. Affected patients are almost always untreated and often undiagnosed. The cause appears to be profound maldigestion and malnutrition, often aggravated by an inadequate caloric intake due to a poor supply of breast milk or intercurrent illness. Vitamin E levels are low, but the cause of the anaemia is not known. Soy protein has been incriminated because of its low digestibility, but the syndrome occurs on all formulae. Patients improve rapidly with pancreatic supplementation and adequate caloric intake. The diagnosis of cystic fibrosis may be difficult to confirm if the initial presentation is with fluid retention, because oedema may produce spurious low sweat chloride estimations.[30] A negative sweat test should always be repeated in a suspicious case when the oedema subsides.

Rectal prolapse
Rectal prolapse is a useful sign of pancreatic insufficiency because in almost half of those patients who have cystic fibrosis the episodes of prolapse precede the diagnosis.[41] Prolapse usually develops between one and 2.5 years and has a tendency to spontaneous resolution even without treatment. Patients who have not received pancreatic supplements are often improved dramatically when these are given; but if episodes of rectal prolapse develop while on pancreatic supplements, dietary and supplement manipulation rarely improve the situation.[41] With time, children learn to reduce the prolapsed mucosa themselves and the problem seems to fade in significance. Approximately 10% of patients require surgical correction, usually for repeated episodes which are either painful or a nuisance.

Diabetes mellitus
Pancreatic islets are almost the last element to disappear as pancreatic fibrosis develops, but biochemical evidence of insulin deficiency becomes more frequent with increasing age and can be detected in one-third of patients.[38, 47] Clinically significant diabetes mellitus is rare and easily controlled with small doses of insulin. The immunoreactive insulin response to glucose is delayed and diminished, even before glucose intolerance can be demonstrated.[48]

Gallstones
Gallstones develop in 11% of patients with cystic fibrosis,[29] the incidence rising with advancing age. Steatorrhoea is associated with an excessive loss of faecal bile acids, a decreased bile acid pool, a shortage of taurine conjugates and increased cholesterol saturation.[22] Excessive leakage of bile acid is the primary problem. It occurs only in patients with steatorrhoea and responds well to pancreatic supplementation.[45] One suspects that cholelithiasis would cease to be a significant complication of cystic fibrosis if it were possible to correct pancreatic insufficiency completely.

Renal stones
Patients with pancreatic insufficiency are at risk to develop both oxalate and uric acid stones but this is a rare complication. The interest in uricolithiasis is in its relationship to pancreatic supplementation. Pancreatic extracts are rich in purine. Patients who take more than 20 capsules of pancreatic powder daily ingest in excess of 150 mg purine, doubling or tripling their normal intake. Both hyperuricosuria and hyper-

uricosaemia occur. Enteric microspheres virtually eliminate this risk since the total dose of pancreatic extract is reduced by 60–80%.

Pancreatic sufficiency (patients without steatorrhoea)

PATHOLOGY

In perhaps one-fifth of all patients with cystic fibrosis, the relentless progression of pancreatic disease either does not occur or seems to be retarded for one or two decades. Pancreatic morphology has been studied in relatively few instances, but there is ample evidence that there can be considerable pancreatic damage in many of these patients. Large portions of the pancreas are often atrophic and in areas of relative preservation there is irregular plugging of the large and small ducts and variable amounts of fibrous tissue.[9, 40] In some patients, however, pancreatic function is within the normal range, presumably a sign that the pancreas is spared pathologically.

CLINICAL FEATURES

The outstanding feature of these patients is their relative freedom from pulmonary disease.[18] Figure 18.30 summarizes the difference in the rates of deterioration of the 1-s forced expiratory volume, in pancreatic sufficient and insufficient patients and shows progressive deterioration in the patients with pancreatic insufficiency, with minimal change in the pancreatic sufficient group. Similar results were obtained with a variety of other pulmonary function tests. There is no doubt that pancreatic sufficient patients have cystic fibrosis. In our series the mean sweat chloride estimation was 105 mequiv./l compared with 120 mequiv./l in the patients with steatorrhoea, well above the normal range. The mean age at presentation was five years, considerably later than that of the patients with pancreatic insufficiency, but the range was one month to 22 years. Approximately one-quarter of our patients presented with respiratory symptoms, 75% exhibited some evidence of clinical chest disease, 39% had clubbing, 30% nasal polyps; and 4% had a rectal prolapse, which suggests that this complication may not be restricted to patients with pancreatic insufficiency.

Eight per cent of the group had had pancreatitis. This is the only complication of cystic fibrosis that appears to be exclusively restricted to patients with pancreatic sufficiency, almost certainly because they are the only patients with sufficient surviving pancreatic tissue after the first few years of life to generate an active inflammatory response.

DIAGNOSIS

Patients with pancreatic sufficiency are diagnosed most commonly as a result of a routine sweat chloride test performed for respiratory symptoms or because of a family history of cystic fibrosis. Occasionally metabolic alkalosis, rectal prolapse, loose stools or an unexplained attack of pancreatitis may prompt investigation.

The range of pancreatic function in these patients stretches from 1–2% to 100% of normal. In contrast to patients with Shwachman's syndrome in whom the level of pancreatic insufficiency is often in a borderline zone of 1–10%,[23] 64% of 33 patients that we have examined by quantitative pancreatic function testing have had greater than 20% pancreatic function.

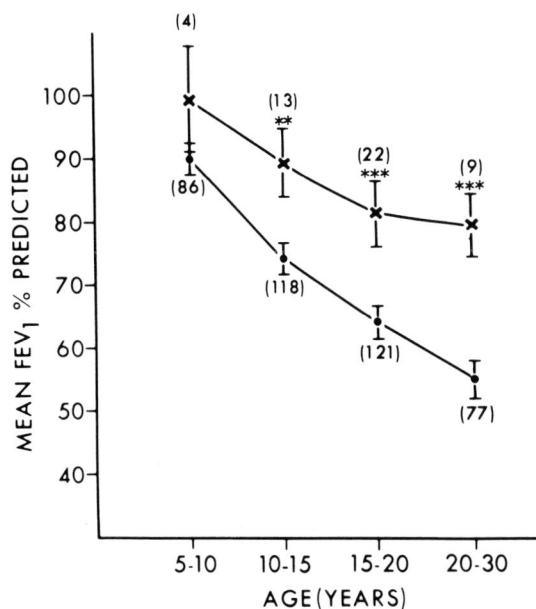

Fig. 18.30 Mean FEV_1 (forced expiratory volume in 1 s) as a percentage of the predicted value versus age in cystic fibrosis patients without (X) and with (O) steatorrhoea. The values are mean ±s.e. (mean), **$P < 0.05$, ***$P < 0.02$. From Forstner *et al.* (1980),[16] with kind permission of the authors and the publisher, Imperial Press.

INTESTINAL TRACT DISEASE

Pathology

The intestinal mucosa is unaffected by cystic fibrosis. Villus structure and absorptive cells are normal. Disaccharidase activities may even be

1292 *The Pancreas*

increased.[2] Surface and crypt mucus is often increased. Some crypts may be greatly distended and even cyst-like, as if obstructed. At birth and throughout life the lumen contains masses of rubbery, green-black meconium which adhere very strongly to the intestinal surface. Undegraded proteins, particularly albumin, are the major constituents. The meconium protein content at birth is approximately 6–8 times that of normal meconium.[39]

MECONIUM ILEUS

Approximately 10–15% of patients with cystic fibrosis present at birth or shortly thereafter with signs and symptoms of small bowel obstruction. The cause is a plug of meconium in the terminal ileum which is acquired in utero as perhaps the first overt manifestation of pancreatic insufficiency. Typically no meconium is passed and there is progressive abdominal distension. Rubbery, firm loops of bowel may be visible or palpable and the rectal examination is unproductive. A history of polyhydramnios may be obtained.

The radiologic findings are quite characteristic (Figure 18.31). In addition to air fluid levels and distended loops of small bowel, small bubbles of gas can be seen trapped in the meconium of the distal small bowel, giving a ground glass appearance. A barium enema will demonstrate a small collapsed microcolon.

Half of the cases of meconium ileus are complicated by volvulus, atresia and/or meconium peritonitis. Atresia and meconium peritonitis usually result from intrauterine events associated with volvulus or extravasation of meconium through a perforation. Intraperitoneal calcification may be apparent on plain radiographs. Meconium pseudocysts may appear in the inflammatory reaction, ascites may develop and an infective peritonitis may occur if the perforation does not close.

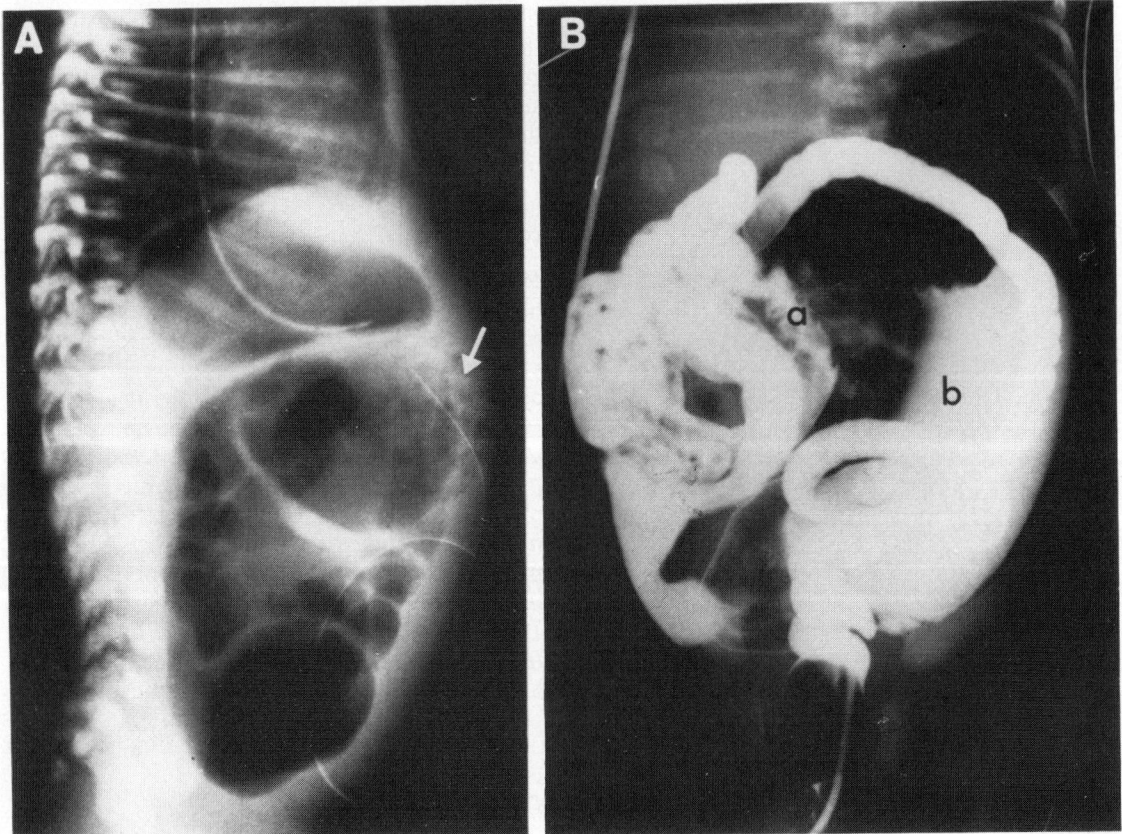

Fig. 18.31 Radiological abnormalities in meconium ileus. A: The plain roentgenogram shows greatly distended loops of bowel filled with air. The arrow points to a bubbly mass which is typical of meconium. B: A Gastrografin enema was performed which outlined the small, unexpanded colon. At 'a' the Gastrografin has entered the meconium mass in the distal ileum. At 'b' the Gastrografin has refluxed proximally through an area of incomplete obstruction to fill a huge loop of bowel which proved to be part of a volvulus.

Meconium ileus is almost always associated with cystic fibrosis, but rare reports of the condition have appeared in association with stenosis of the pancreatic duct,[26] with partial pancreatic aplasia,[3] and with a normal gastrointestinal tract.[11] Approximately one-third of patients with meconium peritonitis and one-fifth of patients with atresia of the small bowel[33] will have cystic fibrosis.

Treatment

Most patients can be relieved of their intestinal obstruction with diatrizoate (Gastrografin or Hypaque) enemas. The major hazard is that these hypertonic solutions may cause a dangerous loss of fluid and electrolytes into the bowel. Infants ought to be supported with continuous intravenous fluids during the procedure. Colonic perforation has been reported[44] but is rare. Gastrografin enemas are not indicated for complicated meconium ileus. The surgical approach to meconium ileus usually involves removal of the plug with irrigation at the time of surgery and, if there is atresia or peritonitis, a limited resection. The survival of these patients has continued to improve from decade to decade.

MECONIUM ILEUS EQUIVALENT

Later in life, about 10% of patients with cystic fibrosis[31] suffer from recurrent complaints attributable to partial or complete bowel obstruction. Although inspissated masses of meconium play an aetiological role, the resemblance to meconium ileus is somewhat tenuous. Large faecal masses can be palpated in the abdomen, particularly in the caecal area. These masses may persist for many months in spite of the daily passage of several stools. Intermittent abdominal distension and cramping may also occur without further disturbance. Rarely the putty-like obstructive masses in the right colon and terminal ileum precipitate acute obstructive episodes with ileus and vomiting. Holsclaw, Rocmans and Shwachman[24] found that 1% of patients with cystic fibrosis presented with intussusception, presumably using an adherent faecal mass as the lead point. In 22 episodes in 19 patients, only two required intestinal resection. The common site for the intussusception was ileocolic.

Treatment

Meconium ileus equivalent is usually responsive to medical management. The most urgent task is to ensure that the presence of faecal masses and

X-ray evidence of bubbly faecal material in the distal small bowel and colon are not regarded as a surgical emergency. In chronic cases it is important to ensure adequate pancreatic replacement therapy because the failure to digest intraluminal protein is a major cause of constipation and obstruction. A diet which is high in roughage and a mild laxative, such as mineral oil, may be all that is required to relieve the patient. In acute obstructive episodes, characterized by clear evidence of small bowel obstruction, such as vomiting or air fluid levels throughout the small intestine, a nasogastric tube should be introduced and the impaction should be cleared with enemas. Most centres use 10% *N*-acetylcysteine as a mucus clearing agent. Even though the masses are not particularly mucoid, this agent seems to be sufficiently irritating to dislodge the faecal plugs. *N*-Acetylcysteine may be introduced by mouth, by D-tube or Miller-Abbott tube, depending upon the indication. Gastrografin enemas may be used as a last resort.

Surgery is reserved for those rare patients with intussusception that cannot be relieved by enema, or for the even more unusual patient with clear evidence of an obstructive mass which cannot be removed by the persistent application of conservative measures.

GASTRO-OESOPHAGEAL REFLUX (SEE CHAPTER 2)

Oesophagitis and oesophageal stricture occur secondary to oesophageal reflux and usually in the absence of any evidence of hiatal hernia.[4] Chronic pulmonary disease and multiple medications are probable predisposing factors. The incidence is approximately the same as that of overt diabetes mellitus and patients are usually of the same age. Oesophageal reflux should always be considered as a cause of anorexia and weight loss in an adolescent.

RADIOLOGY

The pancreas

Plain roentgenograms, barium studies, ultrasonography, computerized tomography and cholangiopancreatography may all provide useful information with regard to the pancreas. Calcification and macroscopic cyst formation are both relatively rare, but their demonstration may provide the explanation for an extrinsic mass compressing the duodenum.[8] Recurrent episodes of obstructive jaundice have occurred as a result of intrapancreatic compression of the common duct by fibrous tissue, and a similar narrowing and distortion of pancreatic ducts may be seen in patients with pancreatic sufficiency and recurrent pancreatitis.

The intestinal tract

Barium examinations frequently reveal thickened and coarse mucosal folds or nodular indentations which may lead to mistaken diagnoses of duodenal ulcer, neoplasia or inflammatory bowel disease. Adherent faecal masses compound the interpretive difficulties if the primary diagnosis is unclear. Taussig, Saldino and di Sant'Agnese[42] found radiological abnormalities in one-third of colonic and small intestinal studies, and in 80% of duodenal studies. If an ulcer or a neoplasm is suspected, the diagnosis should be confirmed independently by endoscopy.

REFERENCES

1 Andersen, D. (1938) Cystic fibrosis of the pancreas and its relation to celiac disease. *American Journal of Diseases of Children*, **56**, 344–399.

2 Antonowicz, I., Lebenthal, E. & Shwachman, H. (1978) Disaccharidase activities in small intestinal mucosa in patients with cystic fibrosis. *Journal of Pediatrics*, **92**, 214–219.

3 Auburn, R., Feldman, S., Gadacz, T. & Rowe, M. (1969) Meconium ileus secondary to partial aplasia of the pancreas: report of a case. *Surgery*, **65**, 689–693.

4 Bendig, D. W., Seilheimer, D. K., Wagner, M. L. et al. (1982) Complications of gastroesophageal reflux in patients with cystic fibrosis. *Journal of Pediatrics*, **100**, 536–540.

5 Bonin, A., Roy, C., LaSalle, R. et al. (1973) Fecal chymotrypsin, a reliable index of exocrine pancreatic function in children. *Journal of Pediatrics*, **83**, 594–600.

6 Corey, M. L. (1980) Longitudinal studies in cystic fibrosis. In *Perspectives in Cystic Fibrosis, Proceedings of the 8th International Congress on Cystic Fibrosis* (Ed.) Sturgess, J. pp. 246–255. Mississauga: Imperial Press.

7 Crossley, J. R., Smith, P. A., Edgar, B. W. et al. (1981) Neonatal screening for cystic fibrosis, using immunoreactive trypsin assay in dried blood spots. *Clinica Chimica Acta*, **113**, 111–121.

8 Cunningham, D. G., Henkin, R. E. & Reynes, C. J. (1981) Macroscopic cysts of the pancreas in cystic fibrosis demonstrated by multiple radiological modalities. *Journal of the American Medical Association*, **245**, 72–74.

9 di Sant'Agnese, P. (1955) Fibrocystic disease of the pancreas with normal or partial pancreatic function. *Pediatrics*, **15**, 683–695.

10 di Sant'Agnese, P., Darling, R., Perera, G. & Shea, E. (1953) Abnormal electrolyte composition of sweat in cystic fibrosis of the pancreas. *Pediatrics*, **12**, 549–563.

11 Dolan, T. & Touloukian, R. (1974) Familial meconium ileus not associated with cystic fibrosis. *Journal of Pediatric Surgery*, **9**, 821–824.

12 Durie, P. R., Bell, L., Linton, W. et al. (1980) Effect of cimetidine and sodium bicarbonate on pancreatic replacement therapy in cystic fibrosis. *Gut*, **21**, 778–786.

13 Durie, P. R., Newth, C. J., Forstner, G. G. & Gall, D. G. (1980) Malabsorption of medium-chain triglycerides in infants with cystic fibrosis: correction with pancreatic enzyme supplements. *Journal of Pediatrics*, **96**, 862–864.

14 Elias, E., Muller, D. P. & Scott, J. (1981) Association of spinocerebellar disorders with cystic fibrosis or chronic childhood cholestasis and very low vitamin E. *Lancet*, **ii**, 1319–1321.

15 Fanconi, G., Uehlinger, E. & Knauer, C. (1936) Das Coelioksyndrom bei angeborener zystisher Pankreas Fibromatose und Bronchiektasis. *Wiener Medizinische Wochenschrift*, **86**, 753–756.

16 Forstner, G., Gall, G., Corey, M. et al. (1980) Digestion and absorption of nutrients in cystic fibrosis. In *Perspectives in Cystic Fibrosis. Proceedings of the 8th International Congress on Cystic Fibrosis* (Ed.) Sturgess, J. pp. 137–148. Mississauga: Imperial Press.

17 Gaskin, K., Gurwitz, D., Corey, M. et al. (1980) Improved pulmonary function in cystic fibrosis patients without pancreatic insufficiency. In *Perspectives in Cystic Fibrosis, Proceedings of the 8th International Congress on Cystic Fibrosis* (Ed.) Sturgess, J. pp. 226–228. Mississauga: Imperial Press.

18 Gaskin, K., Gurwitz, D., Durie, P. R. et al. (1982) Improved respiratory prognosis in patients with cystic fibrosis with normal fat absorption. *Journal of Pediatrics*, **100**, 857–862.

19 Gaskin, K. J., Durie, P. R., Corey, M. et al. (1982) Evidence for a primary defect of pancreatic HCO_3^- secretion in cystic fibrosis. *Pediatric Research*, **16**, 554–557.

20 Gaskin, K. J., Durie, P. R., Lee, L. et al. (1984) Colipase and lipase secretion in childhood onset pancreatic insufficiency. Delineation of patients with steatorrhea secondary to relative colipase deficiency. *Gastroenterology*, **86**, 1–7.

21 Gibbs, G. E., Bostick, W. L. & Smith, P. M. (1950) Incomplete pancreatic deficiency in cystic fibrosis of the pancreas. *Journal of Pediatrics*, **37**, 320–325.

22 Harries, T. J., Muller, D. P. R., McCollum, J. P. K. et al. (1979) Intestinal bile salts in CF. Studies in the patient and experimental animal. *Archives of Disease in Childhood*, **54**, 19–24.

23 Hill, R. E., Durie, P. R., Gaskin, K. J. et al. (1982) Steatorrhea and pancreatic insufficiency in Shwachman syndrome. *Gastroenterology*, **83**, 22–27.

24 Holsclaw, D., Rocmans, C. & Shwachman, H. (1971) Intussusception in patients with cystic fibrosis. *Pediatrics*, **48**, 51–58.

25 Hubbard, V. S., Dunn, G. D. & di Sant'Agnese, P. A. (1977) Abnormal fatty acid composition of plasma lipids in cystic fibrosis. *Lancet*, **ii**, 1302–1304.

26 Hurwitt, E. & Arnheim, E. (1942) Meconium ileus associated with stenosis of the pancreatic ducts. *American Journal of Diseases of Children*, **64**, 443–454.

27 Imrie, J., Fagan, D. & Sturgess, J. (1979) Quantitative evaluation of the development of the exocrine pancreas in CF and control infants. *American Journal of Pathology*, **95**, 697–707.

28 Kopito, L., Shwachman, H., Vawter, G. & Edlow, J. (1976) The pancreas in cystic fibrosis: chemical composition and comparative morphology. *Pediatric Research*, **10**, 742–749.

29 L'Heureux, P., Isenberg, J., Sharp, H. & Warwick, W. (1977) Gallbladder disease in cystic fibrosis. *American Journal of Roentgenology*, **128**, 953–956.

30 Maclean, W. & Tripp, R. (1973) Cystic fibrosis with edema and falsely negative sweat test. *Journal of Pediatrics*, **83**, 85–90.

31 Matseshe, J., Go, V. & DiMagno, E. (1977) Meconium ileus equivalent complicating cystic fibrosis in post neonatal children and young adults. *Gastroenterology*, **72**, 732–736.

32 McPartlin, J., Dickson, J. & Swain, V. (1972) Meconium ileus, immediate and long term survival. *Archives of Diseases in Childhood*, **47**, 207–210.

33 Noblett, H. (1979) Meconium ileus. In *Pediatric Surgery* (Ed.) Ravitch, M., Welch, K., Benson, C. *et al.* pp. 943–952. Chicago and London: Year Book Medical Publishers.

34 Nousia-Arvanitakis, S., Arvanitakis, C. & Greenberger, N. J. (1978) Diagnosis of exocrine pancreatic insufficiency in cystic fibrosis by the synthetic peptide *N*-benzoyl-L-tyrosyl-*p*-aminobenzoic acid. *Journal of Pediatrics*, **92**, 734–737.

35 Nousia-Arvanitakis, S., Stapleton, F., Linshaw, M. & Kennedy, J. (1977) Therapeutic approach to pancreatic extract-induced hyperuricosuria in cystic fibrosis. *Journal of Pediatrics*, **90**, 302–305.

36 Oppenheimer, E. & Esterly, J. (1973) Cystic fibrosis of the pancreas. *Archives of Pathology*, **96**, 149–154.

37 Quinton, P. A. (1982) Suggestion of an abnormal anion exchange mechanism in sweat glands of cystic fibrosis patients. *Pediatric Research*, **16**, 533–537.

38 Rosan, R., Shwachman, H. & Kulczycki, L. (1962) Diabetes mellitus and cystic fibrosis of pancreas. *American Journal of Diseases of Children*, **104**, 625–634.

39 Schutt, W. & Isles, T. (1968) Protein in meconium ileus. *Archives of Disease in Childhood*, **43**, 178–181.

40 Shwachman, H., Lebenthal, E. & Khaw, K. (1975) Recurrent acute pancreatitis in patients with cystic fibrosis with normal pancreatic enzymes. *Pediatrics*, **55**, 86–94.

41 Stern, R., Izant, R. J., Boat, T. F. *et al.* (1982) Treatment and prognosis of rectal prolapse in cystic fibrosis. *Gastroenterology*, **82**, 707–710.

42 Taussig, L. M., Saldino, R. M. & di Sant'Agnese, P. A. (1973) Radiographic abnormalities of the duodenum and small bowel in cystic fibrosis of the pancreas. *Radiology*, **106**, 369–376.

43 Torstenson, O., Humphrey, G., Edson, J. & Warwick, W. (1970) Cystic fibrosis presenting with severe hemorrhage due to vitamin K malabsorption. A report of 3 cases. *Pediatrics*, **45**, 857–860.

44 Wagget, H., Bishop, H. & Koop, E. (1970) Experience with Gastrografin enema in the treatment of meconium ileus. *Journal of Pediatric Surgery*, **5**, 649–654.

45 Weber, A., Roy, C., Morin, C. & LaSalle, R. (1973) Malabsorption of bile acids in children with cystic fibrosis. *New England Journal of Medicine*, **289**, 1001–1005.

46 Wesley, A., Forstner, J., Qureshi, R. *et al.* (1983) Human intestinal mucin in cystic fibrosis. *Pediatric Research*, **17**, 65–69.

47 Wilmshurst, E., Soeldner, J., Holsclaw, D. *et al.* (1975) Endogenous and exogenous insulin responses in patients with cystic fibrosis. *Pediatrics*, **55**, 75–82.

48 Yeates, D., Sturgess, J., Kahn, S. *et al.* (1970) Mucociliary transport in trachea of patients with cystic fibrosis. *Archives of Disease in Childhood*, **51**, 28–33.

ACUTE PANCREATITIS

Acute pancreatitis is a condition resulting from an acute inflammatory process in the pancreas usually characterized by upper abdominal pain and raised concentrations of pancreatic enzymes in blood, urine and peritoneal fluid.

AETIOLOGY

The two most common aetiological factors identified from prospective series of patients are biliary disease and alcohol abuse,[28, 37, 48] and together account for approximately 80% of patients. Any patient who has suffered an attack of acute pancreatitis may suffer a further attack after recovery from their acute illness when the precipitating factor, for example gallstones, persists. It is therefore mandatory that an immediate search for a possible cause is undertaken and appropriate therapeutic measures instituted. It is customary to describe a patient suffering a series of attacks of acute pancreatitis with full clinical recovery between each attack as having *recurrent acute pancreatitis*. Occasionally subsequent attacks may occur prior to complete recovery and this may be related to the rapid reintroduction of a normal diet, re-exposure to alcohol or the passage of small stones from the gallbladder down the lower common bile duct in the recovery phase of the disease.

Although sporadic reports of acute pancreatitis and its complications extend back four centuries, it has been well established for approximately a century[19, 41, 44] that both gallstones and alcohol abuse are aetiological factors. In the United Kingdom it is usual to find that approximately half the patients have gallstones[28, 37] which characteristically are smaller than the gallstones in patients presenting with predominantly biliary symptoms. An incidence varying from 9% to almost 40% for alcohol abuse has been reported in the UK[28, 48] with the maximal incidence being found in Scotland. In these patients there is usually a characteristic time interval of 12–36 h following a bout of heavy alcohol abuse prior to the onset of the signs and symptoms of acute pancreatitis. In any individual patient this period can be remarkably constant where recurrent attacks of acute pancreatitis occur.

There are in addition a considerable number of *minor aetiological factors*, most of which are listed in Table 18.1. As with the major factors the relative incidence of these minor factors varies from area to area within one country and also from country to country. No single factor in this group would be expected to account for more than 5% of all patients with 'de novo' or primary acute pancreatitis.

One prospective study indicated that *viral infections* accounted for approximately 4% of the total patients with primary acute pancreatitis and that the most commonly implicated viruses were the Coxsackie B group and also the

Table 18.1   Acute pancreatitis: aetiology.

'De novo' acute pancreatitis
   Major factors
      Biliary disease (gallstones)
      Alcohol abuse

   Minor factors
      Viral infections (Coxsackie B and mumps)
      Tumours (pancreatic and ampullary)
      Ischaemia
      Metastatic tumours
      Hyperparathyroidism
      Hyperlipoproteinaemia
      Drugs
      Previous 'blind loop' surgery

Iatrogenic acute pancreatitis
   Postoperative (especially lower common bile duct
      exploration and sphincteroplasty)
   After endoscopic retrograde
      cholangiopancreatography (ERCP)
   After translumbar arteriography

---

mumps virus.[25] These viruses probably attack the pancreatic tissue directly in a preferential fashion and the real incidence of this problem has not yet been studied adequately. It should be also noted that both the hepatitis and Marburg viruses which tend to affect the liver primarily may, coincidentally with the severe hepatitis, cause focal areas of pancreatic necrosis and clinical signs of acute pancreatitis.

Both *primary*[21] and *secondary*[34, 40] *pancreatic tumours* may present initially as an attack of acute pancreatitis, and histologically it is not unusual to find a considerable degree of surrounding inflammation in the tissue immediately adjacent to a carcinoma. Carcinoma of the ampulla of Vater is not infrequently associated with the presence of gallstones and may present clinically with acute pancreatitis. Ischaemic pancreatitis occurs in relation to dissecting aortic aneurysm, mesenteric vascular thrombosis and hypothermia.[20]

The association between *hypercalcaemia, hyperparathyroidism* and acute pancreatitis is ill understood but this is a much less frequent association than is suggested by many textbooks. Two series each containing over 500 patients identified no more than four with hyperparathyroidism[22, 23, 28, 55] and some of these patients had one of the two major aetiological factors present in addition.[7] Recent suggestions from Australia[50] that the association between recent parathyroidectomy and acute pancreatitis occurred in 9% of patients have been discounted by other authors who found no cases in 334 parathyroidectomies.[57] *Hyperlipaemia* has been claimed to be a causal factor in the pathogenesis of acute pancreatitis[11] but it

may well be that while this metabolic abnormality can induce inflammation in a minority of patients it is more customary to find hyperlipoproteinemia as an incidental factor associated with alcohol abuse.[16] In the majority of patients it is type IV or type V hyperlipoproteinaemia,[13] but the occasional patient with the rare type I has been described. (See also Chapter 9.)

Many drugs have been implicated in the precipitation of attacks of acute pancreatitis. It is both dangerous and irresponsible to attribute commonly used drugs as possible causative factors in acute pancreatitis without full exploration of the possibilities of the major and minor factors already listed being the cause in an individual patient. Nevertheless, numerous anecdotal reports have appeared over the last 20 or 30 years suggesting that frusemide, cimetidine and oral contraceptives may be involved. Considering the frequency of prescription of these drugs the association with acute pancreatitis may be no more than spurious (Table 18.2), but a stronger case can be made for thiazide diuretics. Another group of drugs which have been recorded as precipitants of acute pancreatitis are steroids.[39] It is recognized that the relatively high incidence of acute pancreatitis in recipients of renal transplants may partly be due to the use of steroids. The incidence in renal transplant patients varies from 2% to 5.6%. The mortality tends to be high and many of the patients are on both steroids and azathioprine, another drug which is thought to precipitate acute pancreatitis. All of the many drugs listed in Table 18.2 have been implicated occasionally as major causative factors of acute pancreatitis. There is no evidence to implicate cimetidine in the pathogenesis of acute pancreatitis. The overall incidence of drug-induced pancreatitis may be much higher than has been appreciated because so few studies have been carried out prospectively with an adequate comparison group such as that reported from Nottingham in

Table 18.2   Drugs believed to precipitate acute pancreatitis.

	Reports	Patients
Steroids	Several	50
Oral contraceptives	Several	50
Thiazide diuretics	Several	Few
Azathioprine	Several	Very few
Frusemide (very high dosage)	Several	Very few
Valproic acid	3	Few
L-Asparaginase	3	Few
Phenformin	2	Few
Paracetamol	1	Very few
Warfarin	1	Very few

1978.[8] In that particular study a diuretic (cyclopenthiazide) together with potassium chloride was found to have been used regularly in 11 of the pancreatitis patients and in only one of the controls. There was no significant difference between the two groups in the use of antihypertensive agents including beta-blockers.

Patients who have previously undergone a Billroth II or Polya type gastrectomy creating a blind duodenal loop are significantly more at risk than those who have undergone a Billroth I type gastrectomy,[52, 58] and the mechanism of acute pancreatitis in these patients may be related to partial obstruction of the blind loop creating a situation similar to the experimental Pfeffer preparation for induction of acute pancreatitis.

Iatrogenic acute pancreatitis

This includes pancreatitis that occurs soon after a surgical operation, diagnostic or therapeutic retrograde pancreatography (ERCP) and immediately following translumbar aortography (Table 18.1).

It has been known for a long time that patients subject to surgical procedures involving instrumentation of the lower end of the common bile duct and sphincteroplasty procedures at the ampulla of Vater are particularly prone to postoperative acute pancreatitis which can be difficult to diagnose.[30] Associated with this delay in diagnosis is an increased mortality which is at least partly attributable to the delay in recognition of hypovolaemia with consequent increased risk of acute renal failure. Partial gastrectomy which may involve direct damage to the pancreas is known to precipitate immediate postoperative acute pancreatitis, but in addition to those procedures which are performed in the immediate locality of the pancreas, there are a considerable number of isolated reports of pancreatitis occurring after orthopaedic, urological, and cardiac[18] operations. In such situations it is believed that pancreatic ischaemia has occurred either during or after surgery.

Although diagnostic ERCP is believed to be innocuous there are a number of reports of major attacks of acute pancreatitis following cannulation of the ampulla, some of which have been fatal.[4, 51] Therapeutic ERCP, where stones are removed from the lower common bile duct with sphincteroplasty carried out using a diathermy apparatus, is associated with a somewhat higher incidence of post-instrumentation pancreatitis which can be particularly severe.

Percutaneous translumbar aortography may be associated with direct damage to the pancreas along the course of the needle and a number of patients have been reported with this complication occurring immediately after the investigation.[27] It is necessary to aim the needle at the aorta away from the level of the pancreas to avoid this complication.

Acute pancreatitis may be induced by penetrating injuries to the pancreas but is more frequently associated with blunt abdominal injuries, e.g. that inflicted by a seat-belt or steering wheel. In contrast to other forms of acute pancreatitis, where initial conservative management is generally acceptable, direct surgical intervention is warranted as completion of the partial transection of the pancreas against the vertebral column is often the best therapy. Particular difficulty is encountered when the right side of the pancreas is injured by blunt trauma. In such situations the duodenum and the lower end of the common bile duct, as well as the head of the pancreas, are damaged, and resection with reconstruction is exceedingly difficult. Roux loop drainage and external tube drainage can be fraught with complications but represent possible therapies.

PATHOGENESIS

In clinical acute pancreatitis, material for histology is rarely obtained in vivo. Major changes of autolysis readily occur post mortem and it is only those specimens obtained for histological purposes within a few hours of death or at operation which are entirely satisfactory. In acute pancreatitis from biliary disease and alcohol abuse *periductal necrosis* is the common histological finding at autopsy, while ischaemic forms of pancreatitis are typified by a *perilobular necrosis*.[20] A combination of these elements may be seen in some of the most severe forms of pancreatitis. The details of events in pancreatitis associated with alcohol abuse and gallstones are poorly understood.

In biliary associated pancreatitis it is typical to find small stones in considerable numbers in the gallbladder and common bile duct. Several studies have shown that it is usually the transient passage of stones through the common bile duct which is associated with acute pancreatitis,[1, 31] and it is believed that such a stone or stones are held up at the ampulla of Vater for a varying time only; complete impaction in this area is unusual. The events during the period of impaction are not agreed but the possibilities include duodenal reflux and/or biliary reflux along the pancreatic duct which acts as the trigger to initiate acute pancreatitis. In therapeutic terms the eradication of gallstones from the biliary tract invariably prevents further episodes of acute pancreatitis while the presence of even a single stone may allow recurrent attacks to take place.

The traditional explanation for alcohol induced acute pancreatitis has been that an increase of pancreatic secretion associated with spasm at the sphincter of Oddi are important factors. More recently several groups have shown in laboratory studies that both increased vascular levels of ethanol and reflux of ethanol, with or without bile salts being present, increase the permeability of the pancreatitic duct epithelium. In addition, in a clinical study from Baltimore of a selected group of patients with previous alcohol induced acute pancreatitis with induced hyperlipaemia, pain developed. In a proportion of these patients there was elevation of serum amylase, but the small numbers and the lack of a control group of patients causes scepticism that this is the major mechanism in alcohol induced pancreatitis.[12]

Acute pancreatitis associated with viral infection has been shown in both animals and man to be due to direct attack on the acinar cells by the virus.

CLINICAL FEATURES

The most important feature of acute pancreatitis is abdominal pain. This is usually sudden in onset and increases rapidly to reach maximal intensity within a few hours. Indeed such is the rapidity and severity of the pain that it resembles closely that experienced in a perforated viscus. The pain is usually felt in the epigastrium but other common sites for pain are the right and left upper quadrants. Less frequently pain is periumbilical or hypogastric. Characteristically, but only in 50% of patients, the pain radiates centrally through to the back, being felt in the lower thoracic, upper lumbar region.

In the average patient pain lasts for about 48 h. Occasionally pain persists for up to a week; rarely an episode of acute pancreatitis is completely painless. Vomiting may be the most clamant symptom and exceed pain as a problem.

Physical examination will reveal varying degrees of shock depending upon the severity of the attack. A modest fever is often encountered and there will be tachycardia and hypotension, although a transitory rise in blood pressure is found in 10% of patients. Half the patients show guarding or rigidity and it is a frequent observa-

tion that the severity of the pain appears to be out of proportion to the abdominal signs. An epigastric mass is felt in 10–20% of patients. Most patients have a paralytic ileus for 24 to 96 h. Other features which occur less commonly and which are discussed below include tachypnoea, hypoxia, ascites and pleural effusions.

Severe hyperglycaemia and diabetic ketoacidosis may be a presenting feature. A fall in serum calcium may be sufficient to cause tetany. Mental confusion may be prominent, particularly in the alcoholic and where hypoxia is profound. Cardiac failure, pulmonary insufficiency and acute respiratory distress are encountered. Uncommonly, fat necrosis in the subcutaneous tissues manifests as painful areas, particularly in the legs, and there may be associated arthralgia and a mild eosinophilia.

Table 18.3   Complications in severe acute pancreatitis.

Cardiac insufficiency
Renal insufficiency
Respiratory insufficiency
Haematological abnormalities
Anaemia
Disseminated intravascular coagulation
Thrombosis of portal and/or splenic veins
Biochemical abnormalities (see text)

The complications encountered with acute pancreatitis are listed in Table 18.3 and the late complications are shown in Table 18.4. The biochemical changes in themselves are not specific, but taken together with the clinical setting they often provide a characteristic diagnostic picture and, furthermore, they can be used to grade the severity of the illness. Mild anaemia, a leucocytosis, hyperglycaemia and glycosuria are found fairly frequently. Other changes include elevated serum bilirubin, alkaline phosphatase and transaminase levels and methaemalbuminaemia.

Table 18.4   Late complications of acute pancreatitis.

Pseudocyst
Abscess
Fistula
Stricture of pancreatic duct
Pancreatic ascites
Diabetes mellitus

DIAGNOSIS

Acute pancreatitis should be considered in the differential diagnosis of upper abdominal disease and shock syndromes (Table 18.5).

Table 18.5 Differential diagnosis of acute pancreatitis.

Mild pancreatitis
  Acute cholecystitis
  Peptic ulceration
  Intestinal obstruction with ileus
  Acute intermittent porphyria
  Diaphragmatic pleurisy

Severe pancreatitis
  Perforated peptic ulcer
  Gangrenous cholecystitis
  Intestinal strangulation
  Mesenteric artery occlusion
  Ruptured abdominal aneurysm
  Myocardial infarction

The most widely used test is serum amylase which may be elevated in acute pancreatitis. Values four times greater than normal favour the diagnosis. However, acute inflammation can occasionally occur in the absence of raised amylase values, and there are a number of situations in which serum amylase values are increased apart from pancreatitis; these are listed in Table 18.6. They usually follow a different clinical course to acute pancreatitis.

Table 18.6 Other causes of an elevated serum amylase.

Perforated peptic ulcer	Intestinal obstruction
Ruptured ectopic pregnancy	Mesenteric infarction
Burns	Renal failure
Drugs including morphine	Diabetic ketoacidosis

The amylase may be of salivary origin or macroamylasaemia (p. 1285) and the estimation of isoenzymes can be helpful. If there is hypertriglyceridaemia in association with pancreatitis there is a tendency for the serum, but not the urinary, amylase concentrations to be normal. The rise in amylase level has little prognostic value. Serum amylase levels usually return to normal within one week.

Amylase appears in excess in the urine before the serum and some authorities believe that the estimation of urinary amylase is of more help than its serum concentration; but hyperamylasuria has similar problems of interpretation to the serum concentration. Increased amylase levels may also be found in pleural effusions or ascites should these occur.

Early suggestions that a raised amylase : creatinine clearance ratio is of precise diagnostic value have not been substantiated and this ratio is no longer regarded as being informative. Serum lipase values are increased in the acute episode and are more specific than amylase as an indication that pancreatitis is present, but not pathognomic because serum concentrations may be raised in perforated peptic ulcer, mesenteric vein thrombosis and following the administration of morphine.

Although the plain film of the abdomen may show a localized ileus of small bowel ('sentinel loop') or colon (colon cut-off sign), the information is of limited diagnostic value. Gallstones may be seen. Ultrasonography and computerized tomography have had no immediate role in the diagnosis of acute pancreatitis but are of great help in identifying pancreatic pseudocysts and abscesses. In the future, CT scanning may have an important practical role in confirming the diagnosis and the severity of acute pancreatitis.

ASSESSMENT OF SEVERITY

Attempts before 1974 to grade the severity of acute pancreatitis objectively depended on single or multiple clinical signs, and findings at laparotomy.

Clinical assessment

A major drawback of most of the many clinical features is that they take a number of hours or days to develop. Only *hypotension* (systolic blood pressure less than 90 mmHg) is a prognostic sign occurring sufficiently early in the course of the disease to be of much value. It is true that it is usually associated with fairly severe acute pancreatitis but it may simply reflect a delay in hospitalization in the milder case with associated hypovolaemia, rather than intrinsically severe pancreatitis. The use of hypotension as an objective factor in one recent prospective study from Bristol proved a little disappointing.[14]

Renal failure rarely occurs as a single system failure in hospitals where care is taken in monitoring both urine output and central venous pressure. This regulates the often considerable intravenous volumes required in the initial stages of disease to achieve a minimum 30 ml of urine per hour. At the present time, provided prophylactic steps are taken, renal failure only occurs as a preterminal event associated with other major system failures.[28]

The *duration of paralytic ileus* and the presence or absence of abdominal distension are signs that must be monitored for several days and they are therefore of limited value.

Small *pleural effusions*, especially on the left side, occur with great frequency when daily radiological examinations are performed. They do not correlate well with severity but the larger effusions are associated with those patients with the worst prognosis.

Body wall ecchymosis, either at the umbilicus (Cullen's sign) or in the flank, usually on the left side (Grey Turner's sign), occurs in 3% of patients and takes over 24 h to develop.[17] The signs are undoubtedly associated with a most severe form of acute pancreatitis but cannot be applied universally as an objective grading system. Very recently it has been shown that 65% of patients developing these clinical signs survive the pancreatitis, provided active conservative supportive measures are taken.[17]

The development of a *pancreatic abscess or pseudocyst*, while serious for the individual patient, is not necessarily related to an initially severe form of disease. They take a considerable time to develop and cannot be used in a prospective study of any new therapy confined to patients with severe acute pancreatitis where an early separation of severe and mild cases is necessary.

Assessment at operation

The presence or absence of fat necrosis, and the volume and colour of free fluid at operation have not been clearly related to outcome. The presence of blood-stained fluid may well be associated with a poorer outcome but less than 10% of patients today undergo early laparotomy. Only a minority of surgeons carefully dissect the anterior surface of the whole pancreas and of these only a few remove any possible peripancreatic necrotic tissue to assess the gland directly. This may explain the findings in one French study of over 50 patients where the surgeon considered necrotic pancreatitis to be present and in exactly 50% the pathologist disagreed because the necrotic process was confined to the surrounding tissue rather than the pancreas itself.[33]

Multiple factor objective assessment

The drawbacks associated with clinical approaches to grading of severity of pancreatitis prompted Ranson to examine retrospectively a large number of patients admitted to the New York University Hospital with a diagnosis of acute pancreatitis. Of 40 biochemical, haematological and clinical factors which were assessed only 11 were found to be significantly related to the outcome[49] (Table 18.7). These 11 factors were then employed prospectively to delineate patients with severe disease from those with a

Table 18.7 The eleven early objective signs used to classify the severity of pancreatitis.[48]

At admission
Age > 55 years
White blood cell count > 16 000 per mm^3
Blood glucose > 200 mg/100 ml
Serum lactate dehydrogenase > 350 iu/l
Serum glutamic-oxaloacetic transaminase (aspartate transaminase) > 250 Sigma-Frankel units/100 ml
During initial 48 h
Haematocrit fall > 10 percentage points
Blood urea nitrogen rise > 5 mg/100 ml
Serum calcium level below 8 mg/100 ml
Pa_{O_2} below 60 mmHg
Base deficit > 4 mEq/l
Estimated fluid sequestration > 6000 ml

milder form of acute pancreatitis. A minimum of three prognostic factors had to be present for the patient to be considered in the severe category.[48, 49] The greater the number of prognostic factors the more severe the disease and the more likely death the outcome. A statistical analysis of this approach validated its use,[46] and in the following year a report from the UK showed that a similar grading system had proved useful in the assessment of 161 patients admitted to one Glasgow hospital.[28] In this modified system only nine factors were employed, but again a minimum of three were taken to indicate severe disease (Table 18.8). Comparison of individual factors occurring in the total patients in New York and Glasgow graded as having severe acute pancreatitis indicated that nearly all were more abnormal in the patients with alcohol abuse as the aetiology of the pancreatitis compared to biliary disease (Table 18.9).

The major problem of the multiple factor grading scheme was that too many patients with a gallstone aetiology met the criteria for severe disease without running a clinical course of comparable severity to those with the alcohol aetiology. This was because of the higher mean age of patients with biliary disease and the greater frequency of gross elevations in transaminase (transferase) levels. By omitting age

Table 18.8 Prognostic factors in patients with acute pancreatitis used by Imrie *et al.* (1978).[30]

White blood cell count (WBC) > 15 × 10^9/l
Glucose > 10 mmol/l (no diabetic history)
Urea > 16 mmol/l (no response to i.v. fluids)
Pa_{O_2} < 60 mmHg (8.0 kPa)
Calcium < 2.0 mmol/l
Albumin < 32 g/l
LDH > 600 units/l
SGOT/SGPT > 100 units/l
Age > 55 years

Table 18.9 Mean levels of different prognostic factors in severe acute pancreatitis of biliary or alcohol abuse aetiology (grading as in Table 18.8).

	Alcohol	Biliary
WBC	18 900	15 240
Glucose	36.1	13.2
Urea	11.7	7.9
Pao_2	52.7	57.7
Calcium	1.87	1.99
Albumin	35.9	34.4
LDH	1429	712
SGOT	303	231
SGPT	151	239
Age	47.7	62.6

as a criterion and increasing the 'cut-off' of the SGOT (serum glutamic-oxaloacetic transaminase) level to 200 units per litre, a more precise system of analysis was produced in which almost half the previously included biliary patients were excluded from the severe category[42] (Table 18.10). Although Ranson did not have such a large number of gallstone patients to assess he has reached a similar conclusion.[45, 47]

Table 18.10 Prognostic factors in patients with acute pancreatitis used by Osborne, Imrie and Carter (1981).[42]

WBC $>15 \times 10^9/l$
Glucose >10 mmol/l (no diabetic history)
Urea >16 mmol/l (no response to i.v. fluids)
Pao_2 <60 mmHg (8.0 kPa)
Calcium <2.0 mmol/l
Albumin <32 g/l
LDH >600 units/l
SGOT >200 units/l

If three or more adverse prognostic factors are present within 48 h of hospitalization, severe acute pancreatitis is confirmed.

Analysis of peritoneal aspirate or lavage fluid

An alternative to the assessment of multiple biochemical factors is the analysis of the free peritoneal fluid withdrawn by a catheter introduced below the umbilicus. The presence of a minimum of 10 ml, or preferably 20 ml, of free fluid, especially if dark in colour, can be considered a good index of the severity of disease.[36] If no free fluid is obtained after the insertion of the peritoneal catheter, 1 l of isotonic dialysis fluid or saline is run into the peritoneal cavity for 10–15 min. The patient is moved from side to side to allow an even distribution of the fluid and aspiration of this lavage fluid is performed.

The presence of a dark-coloured fluid with a very high amylase content (with no bacteria present) is indicative of severe acute pancreatitis. The presence of organisms on an immediate Gram film makes the diagnosis of acute pancreatitis very unlikely.[10] Immediate laparotomy is recommended in this situation because bowel ischaemia or perforation is the most likely cause. This is an alternative to the multiple factor grading system and it has the additional advantage of speed and ready availability. The other systems depend on the prompt return of biochemical and haematological assessments which are not necessarily available 24 h a day.

Single factor assessment

Attempts have been made to grade patients into severe disease categories on the basis of only one prognostic factor being present.[54] While this type of system is easier to apply it is inferior to the multiple factor grading systems.

Of the single factors employed hypocalcaemia and a high level of lactate dehydrogenase (LDH) are less generally applicable than a single arterial oxygen sample. The oxygen results can be obtained rapidly night or day, while the others are much more dependent on daytime facilities and can be restricted to certain days of the week. A Pao_2 level of less than 60 mmHg will delineate a group of patients with a mortality around 20%;[14, 54] and hypoxia of a more severe degree, Pao_2 less than 52.5 mmHg (7 kPa), will identify a group of patients with a mortality rate over 30%. Thus a single arterial blood gas sample may be the nearest to an ideal quick single factor assessment for severity of disease (Table 18.11).

Table 18.11 Arterial hypoxia in the initial 48 h of acute pancreatitis and its related mortality ($n = 255$ patients).

Lowest Pao_2	n	Died
Less than 8 kPa (60 mmHg)	96	17 (17.7%)
Less than 7 kPa (52.5 mmHg)	43	13 (30.2%)

While many patients may be accurately graded on clinical grounds, a significant proportion are particularly difficult to assess at an early stage of their illness and this is one of the strengths of an objective system of grading severity. Such a system permits a comparison of results from centre to centre and limits trials of new therapy to those patients with severe disease because the mortality rate of the milder forms of the disease is less than 2%. The ideal method of assessing severity is not yet available but it may be best to employ a combination of peritoneal aspiration or lavage with one of the multiple criteria grading systems. It is possible that a combination of laboratory tests and a CT scan may provide an alternative method of grading severity of disease.

TREATMENT

The two main aims in the treatment of acute pancreatitis are to restore fluid and electrolyte balance and to provide adequate analgesia. In all but the mildest of cases it is preferable to monitor the central venous pressure and rehydrate rapidly with isotonic saline. It is advisable to administer plasma and occasionally blood as well should the haematocrit fall. The volume replacement is monitored according to the central venous pressure and urinary output.

Patients may require up to 8 l in the first 24 h. Intravenous therapy is maintained until the circulatory state is stable, and this usually occurs within four days. Attempts are made to reduce pancreatic secretory activity by avoiding oral feeding during the initial few days of hospitalization, and adequate intravenous calorie supplementation is necessary. Most patients require nasogastric suction for the first 24–48 h and this is maintained if a paralytic ileus occurs. Oral feeding is commenced on around the 3rd–4th day in moderately severe pancreatitis, but delayed longer in severe episodes particularly if a paralytic ileus is present. Anticholinergic drugs are best avoided because they have no proven value.

Morphine and its derivatives are contraindicated because they cause spasm of the sphincter of Oddi and may worsen the inflammation. Pethidine is usually recommended in doses of 50–150 mg 4–8 hourly either i.m. or i.v. depending on the condition of the patient. Good results are also obtained using buprenorphine hydrochloride (Temgesic) 300–600 μg 4–8 hourly by i.m. or slow i.v. injection. Most patients require pain relief for 48–72 h. When the pain is very severe and persists for a prolonged period, the addition of diazepam is advisable and this also helps those patients who find the nasogastric tube unpleasant.

Broad-spectrum antibiotic therapy is not indicated for it does not prevent abscess formation. Antibiotics are indicated only when there is clear evidence of an identified infecting organism, preferably with sensitivity data. This is unusual. Steroids have not been assessed in the therapy of acute pancreatitis.

Specific drugs utilized in acute pancreatitis such as glucagon[37] and aprotinin (Trasylol)[28, 37] have been shown to be ineffective. Likewise, cimetidine and calcitonin are of no value, while a degree of uncertainty still remains as to the potential benefit of a combination of low molecular weight dextran and heparin. Claims have been advanced that the proteinase inhibitor gabexate mesylate (Foy) and leupeptin might represent a significant therapeutic advance but these have not been fully assessed.

The position regarding *peritoneal lavage* as a therapeutic adjunct in the management of severe acute pancreatitis remains unresolved. This is perhaps the single most important area of debate in current therapy. There are those who strongly advocate the use of peritoneal lavage, usually based on uncontrolled or poorly controlled studies and with differing proportions of patients having alcohol abuse pancreatitis and gallstone associated pancreatitis in the respective studies.[5, 47, 54] A uniform claim that respiratory problems are lessened by peritoneal lavage has been advanced by most groups studying the problem but this is counterbalanced with the late problem of peripancreatic sepsis which may negate any benefit derived from peritoneal lavage.[47] There is debate whether antiseptics or antibiotics should be added to the peritoneal lavage fluid and, if so, which drug. Ampicillin,[47] cephalosporins,[54] doxycycline (Vibramycin)[5] and taurolidine (a new antiendotoxin agent) have all been used. It is possible that peritoneal lavage may be most beneficial to the patients with alcohol abuse pancreatitis.[54] At the present time the advice to any clinician managing a patient with severe acute pancreatitis is to utilize peritoneal lavage but to be aware that large amounts of protein may be lost during the procedure, and that a considerable increase in the exogenous albumin administered may be necessary.

As well as the investigation and the identification of gallstones there is a considerable debate as to the *optimum time for biliary intervention* whether it be by surgical means or by endoscopic sphincterotomy. There are three schools of thought: The first supports immediate surgery within 48 h of admission; the second supports surgical intervention about a week after the onset of pancreatitis in the patients with mild disease; and finally there is a view that the attack should be allowed to settle completely, investigations be carried out as an outpatient and readmission be planned for definitive biliary surgery at a later date. These approaches have variously been described as immediate surgery[2] (within 48 h of hospitalization), early surgery[45] (3–8 days after admission) and late or delayed surgery (usually performed at subsequent admission after out-patient investigation of biliary tract disease). No study has been mounted to compare these three options. The major drawback to the immediate surgical policy is the difficulty of accurately identifying at an early stage that gallstones are the aetiology. The majority view is that early surgery performed within 3–8 days of admission with a mild form of acute pancreatitis is a per-fectly sensible form of treatment[42, 45] somewhat similar to the surgical approach to acute chole-cystitis favoured by many at this time. The ques-tion as to the optimum timing of surgery in severe acute pancreatitis must be treated on an individual basis as many other factors need to be taken into account, including the cardiorespira-tory and renal status of the patient.

COMPLICATIONS

Complications of severe acute pancreatitis

One of the major purposes in early grading of a patient in the category of severe pancreatitis is to alert the clinician to the danger and likeli-hood of certain system failures and to the com-plications which may develop. A minimum of 50% of patients with severe acute pancreatitis will be candidates for the most intensive conser-vative, non-surgical therapy, as first-line man-agement.

CARDIAC INSUFFICIENCY OR FAILURE

It has been known for many years that ECG changes occur in patients with acute pancreatitis but their significance is unknown.[43] This problem is further complicated by the fact that occasional patients present with a clinical condi-tion simulating myocardial infarct, especially when left upper quadrant abdominal pain is the predominant feature. The suggestion that cardiac muscle may be particularly vulnerable in acute pancreatitis is supported by the finding that six out of 14 patients who died in one pro-spective study showed unequivocal evidence of myocardial infarction.[28]

The mechanism of the problem is incom-pletely understood and has been the subject of remarkably little study. It may be necessary to digitalize all older patients with acute pancrea-titis and many patients do benefit from low dose dopamine. Until there is a more rational under-standing of the pathogenesis of this problem therapy will remain empirical.

RENAL INSUFFICIENCY OR FAILURE

This was formerly a major problem because of the failure to recognize the degree of hypo-volaemia present in many patients, but it is now an uncommon complication in centres where active supportive measures are the routine form of treatment. A minimum urine output of 30 ml/h can usually be ensured by an appropri-ate rate of i.v. infusion; many of the severely ill patients require a minimum of 4 l and often as many as 8 or 9 l of fluid in the first 24 h of therapy. It is particularly important to appre-ciate the need for early reversal of hypovolaemia within the first few hours of hospitalization and for the employment of plasma or albumin-rich fluids as well as electrolyte solutions. In all the severely ill patients a central venous pressure line is mandatory. Failure to achieve a minimum urine output of 30 ml/h is an indication for a 20 g bolus of mannitol once hypovolaemia has been reversed. If this is unsuccessful a repeat of the 20 g bolus is advised and consideration should be given to peritoneal dialysis. Custom-ary thresholds of blood urea or creatinine should not be used as indicators for the intro-duction of peritoneal dialysis; the main index is the failure to produce an adequate urinary output. The response to peritoneal dialysis when incipient renal failure is present is usually most gratifying, provided there are no other com-plications.

RESPIRATORY INSUFFICIENCY OR FAILURE

This is the complication which is most feared and which occurs with greatest fre-quency.[26, 28, 38, 48] The clinical presentation is insidious with only tachypnoea as an indication of the degree of respiratory insufficiency.[15] Cyanosis is unusual and respiratory distress dif-ficult to detect on clinical grounds alone. It is mandatory that arterial blood gas measure-ments be performed regularly, especially during the initial period. The levels of arterial gases should be measured at least twice daily, and when the PaO_2 is less than 60 mmHg (8 kPa) supplementary humidified oxygen should be provided. A check of the PaO_2 levels after the provision of oxygen is required to assess whether sufficient reversal of the hypoxaemia has occurred. Restoration of PaO_2 levels to above 70 mmHg is usual, provided a flow rate in the region of 10 l/min of 70% oxygen can be achieved.[26] If hypoxaemia cannot be reversed and particularly when the PaO_2 is less than 52.5 mmHg (7 kPa), assisted ventilation therapy is indicated. The exact mechanism of the hypoxaemia is ill understood but there is right to left shunting of around 25–30% of cardiac output[38] although this is not the sole factor. The possible causes of the right to left shunting include atelectasis and pulmonary capillary blockage either due to platelet thrombi or leucocyte clumping or to combinations of these factors. In addition, hyaline membrane disease has been documented in fatal acute pancreatitis with respiratory failure.[32]

Another factor causing the adult respiratory distress syndrome associated with acute pancreatitis is varying pressure in the pulmonary artery which has been recorded in severe acute pancreatitis. Airways closure is not an important feature.[32] The presence of pleural effusions, atelectasis and pulmonary oedema may be observed but some patients who are severely hypoxic have remarkably few radiologic abnormalities.[25] This respiratory complication is a variant of the adult respiratory distress syndrome with pleural effusions being a particular feature; these require aspiration should they persist. The effusion fluid characteristically has not only a high amylase content but also a high albumin and calcium concentration.[24] In a study involving young patients with no previous history of respiratory disease who suffered from acute pancreatitis, it was shown that a period of 6–12 weeks was required for the hypoxaemia to resolve.[38] This correlates with the length of time a patient may require to remain on assisted ventilator therapy, since patients kept on this type of life support system for periods of around 6–8 weeks may recover sufficiently at this stage to be weaned off the ventilator therapy. Such patients may also develop *peripancreatic sepsis* and require some form of intra-abdominal drainage procedure prior to withdrawal of the respiratory support. An outline of the steps involved in the management of the respiratory insufficiency of these patients is indicated in Table 18.12.

Table 18.12 Management of respiratory insufficiency in acute pancreatitis.

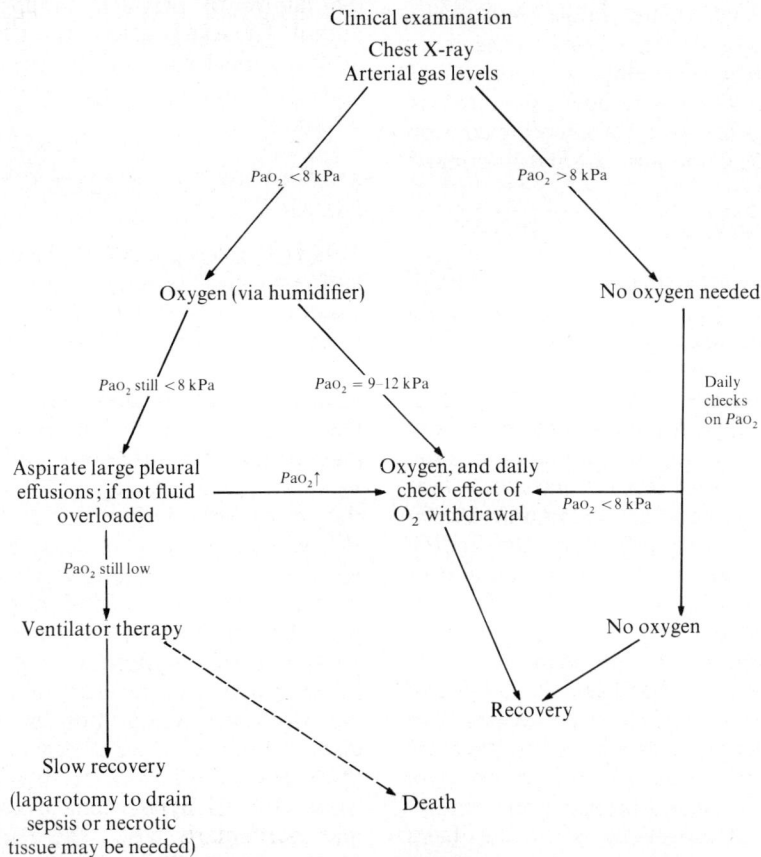

Clinical examination
Chest X-ray
Arterial gas levels

$Pao_2 < 8\,kPa$ $Pao_2 > 8\,kPa$

Oxygen (via humidifier)   No oxygen needed

Pao_2 still $< 8\,kPa$ $Pao_2 = 9\text{–}12\,kPa$ Daily checks on Pao_2

Aspirate large pleural effusions; if not fluid overloaded $Pao_2\uparrow$ Oxygen, and daily check effect of O_2 withdrawal $Pao_2 < 8\,kPa$

Pao_2 still low

Ventilator therapy   No oxygen

Recovery

Slow recovery
(laparotomy to drain sepsis or necrotic tissue may be needed)   Death

HAEMATOLOGICAL ABNORMALITIES

The most frequent haematological abnormality is an *apparent drop in haemoglobin* associated with restoration of circulating blood volume. Most patients initially are admitted with a considerable degree of dehydration and have elevated levels of haemoglobin and haematocrit. After restoration of circulating fluid the haemoglobin may fall markedly and this can be accentuated by any bleeding in or around the pancreas. Only occasionally is blood transfusion required but this aspect requires careful monitoring in every patient. Elevated fibrinogen levels have been documented early in the disease[6] and rise progressively to around 300% of normal levels at 5–6 days after admission. Factor V and factor VIII also rise and probably behave as acute phase reactants rather than from any specific coagulopathy. Levels of fibrin degradation products often show a small rise. About one third of patients with acute pancreatitis have a significant shortening of their clotting time as measured by the kaolin–cephalin clotting time. Although disseminated intravascular coagulation has been described in acute pancreatitis it is unusual, and a consecutive study of 161 patients revealed no evidence of this phenomenon.[28] Deep vein thrombosis and major pulmonary emboli are not common complicating factors.

An activation of the complement system occurs in acute pancreatitis; but it is unclear whether this is simply another manifestation of the response to trauma or whether a more specific explanation must be found.

BIOCHEMICAL ABNORMALITIES

For many years much attention has been focused on the problem of hypocalcaemia, which is mainly due to the loss of circulating albumin from the intravascular space[24] into the retroperitoneum, peritoneal cavity and pleural cavity. This *albumin loss* is an important biochemical phenomenon and requires correction. However, the restoration of normal serum albumin levels is often impossible in the severely ill patient because of the 'porosity' of the endothelial layer lining capillaries.[3]

There is also a tendency for the ionized fragment of circulating serum calcium to fall and this is associated with elevated parathyroid hormone levels which indicate a satisfactorily functioning calcium homeostatic mechanism.[29] The restoration of circulating ionized calcium

by means of infusions of calcium gluconate is rarely necessary, but if it is required it is essential that sufficient calcium gluconate be given and 50–60 ml of isotonic calcium gluconate are administered slowly intravenously.

Occasionally, in the most severely ill patients, profound falls in extracellular sodium and elevations of potassium may occur, indicative of the so-called 'sick cell syndrome'. We have documented one such patient who responded well to hourly pulses of 50% dextrose and insulin via a central line.[3] Using this approach not only did the ionized calcium level rise but the sodium and potassium levels returned to normal.

Later complications of acute pancreatitis

These are summarized in Table 18.4, and of the list shown pancreatic pseudocyst and abscess are the most common problems.

PANCREATIC PSEUDOCYST

This invariably follows moderate or severe attacks of acute pancreatitis, usually within 2–4 weeks. The pseudocyst arises from blockage of the foramen of Winslow by fibrinous material with consequent collection of pancreatic juice in the lesser sac. ERCP evidence indicates that most major pancreatic pseudocysts are directly linked to the main duct system. Approximately 50% resolve spontaneously and the remainder require some form of drainage procedure. Traditionally this has been a surgical approach usually by draining the pseudocyst directly into the posterior aspect of the stomach, i.e., cystogastrostomy. In this operation it is usual to suture the posterior wall of the stomach to the anterior wall of the pseudocyst, with the size of the incision in the posterior wall of the stomach being 8–10 cm. If the pseudocyst does not lie in direct relationship to the posterior wall of the stomach, drainage by alternative means is necessary; this can be by an anastomosis to a loop of jejunum, or a Roux loop, or less frequently to the duodenum. It is possible to simply aspirate small cysts of the head of the pancreas which can be responsible for considerable symptoms of pain and vomiting.[53] Recently percutaneous aspiration of pseudocysts guided either by ultrasound or CT scanning has been used. This method is particularly attractive in older patients with cardiorespiratory or other complications. However, a major drawback is the reaccumulation of fluid in the pseudocyst which occurs particularly in larger cysts communicating directly with the main pancreatic duct. Repeated aspirations may be carried out but they increase the risk of introducing sepsis and converting a sterile collection into a pancreatic abscess. A further problem is that many larger pseudocysts following attacks of severe acute pancreatitis contain peripancreatic necrotic debris and slough. It is not possible to aspirate this type of material through a percutaneous needle and for these reasons it is likely that surgical treatment will remain the major definitive approach to established pseudocysts.

Conservative management beyond six weeks after diagnosis of pseudocyst is associated with unpredictable complications both in timing and severity. Even with hindsight the problems of pseudocyst rupture or haemorrhage cannot be anticipated. These complications are of sufficient severity to warrant active surgical intervention for pseudocysts at around six weeks because patients treated by surgery at six weeks after the diagnosis was established have a better outcome than if surgery is delayed.[9] Occasionally it is necessary to perform a drainage procedure at an earlier stage if pain cannot be relieved, if jaundice occurs due to external pressure on the common bile duct or if haemorrhage occurs from the pseudocyst.

Most of the deaths associated with pancreatic pseudocyst can be accounted for by the development of *haemorrhage* or *sepsis*. Mortality rates associated with the treatment of pancreatic pseudocyst are 8–15%. Pancreatic pseudocyst is much more commonly associated with alcohol abuse, occurring 5–6 times more frequently than with biliary tract disease.

The complication of haemorrhage from the pseudocyst is frequently due to incorporation of either splenic artery or vein into the posterior wall of the pseudocyst but may also be due to leakage from aneurysmal new vessel formation in the wall. An additional source of bleeding can be rupture of an attenuated vessel across the central area of an enlarging pseudocyst, but this is the least common of the causes of haemorrhage, all of which are associated with a poor prognosis. Unsuspected and less vigorous bleeding into a pancreatic pseudocyst can be detected at operation by needle aspiration prior to decompression of the pseudocyst. Controlled decompression of the pseudocyst is desirable, if bleeding is encountered with early ligation of the splenic vessels. This may be very difficult, especially with adjacent necrotic tissue. *Upper gastrointestinal bleeding* may be a presentation of

haemorrhage from a pancreatic pseudocyst. Bleeding from a duodenal ulcer, gastric ulcer or gastric erosion may occur during the acute phase of pancreatitis or in the recovery period.

Pancreatic pseudocysts in chronic pancreatitis are discussed on p. 1316 and in pancreatic injury on p. 1330.

PANCREATIC ABSCESS

This is a serious complication of acute pancreatitis, occurring in 1–5% of patients. It occurs more commonly in pancreatitis due to gallstones than in association with alcohol abuse. The complication usually manifests in the third week, but may be as late as 3–4 months after the initial illnesses. The patient may have persistent abdominal pain and there is anorexia, weight loss, fever and leucocytosis. The usual organism involved is *Escherichia coli* and this may be detected in blood cultures. Pancreatic abscesses seem to be a particular complication of patients who are hypoxic and require assisted ventilation.

The diagnosis is confirmed by an ultrasonic scan or computerized tomography. This is easy if the abscess is well circumscribed but more difficult if there is diffuse retroperitoneal sepsis.

The treatment of a pancreatic abscess is always surgical under appropriate antibiotic cover. A circumscribed abscess is localized and drained externally either surgically or by the insertion of percutaneous drains under ultrasonic scan guidance. While the use of a percutaneous approach has clear attractions, there is as yet insufficient experience with this form of drainage to predict if it will replace conventional surgery.

Diffuse retroperitoneal sepsis presents a particular problem. Even with open drainage the mortality rate varies between 30–80%. This complication is not amenable to conventional surgery and it may be necessary to re-enter the abdomen frequently to drain abscesses which occur in the peripancreatic, retropancreatic, paracolic gutters and subhepatic and subphrenic spaces. Secondary complications of haemorrhage, ileus and fistula all occur. Prolonged periods of parenteral nutrition are needed and it is essential that great care is afforded to the overall nutritional support of the patient.

Pancreatic abscess following pancreatic injury is discussed on p. 1330.

DIABETES MELLITUS

The incidence of diabetes mellitus observed in the recovery phase of acute pancreatitis is between 2% and 4%. This is a remarkably low figure but does indicate the relative sparing of the endocrine tissue. In the most severe necrotizing forms of acute pancreatitis the islet tissue is also destroyed. The urine is monitored for sugar and ketones, and patients will require soluble insulin initially and subsequently appropriate long-acting insulin. The diabetic state is usually not permanent.

RECURRENT ACUTE PANCREATITIS

The diagnosis of recurrent acute pancreatitis is given to those patients who suffer from more than one attack of pancreatitis but who show no morphological or functional evidence of pancreatic disease between episodes of pain. The episodes do not differ in any way from those of acute pancreatitis and it is not possible to predict whether a patient will have further episodes of inflammation during and immediately after an isolated attack of pancreatitis. Most frequently such patients have fine biliary sand or very small stones and benefit from cholecystectomy. Persistent secret alcohol abuse must be excluded. Rarely hereditary pancreatitis or an ampullary cancer may be found. A proportion may be identified as having 'pancreas divisum' at ERCP and Santorini sphincterotomy may help.

Where the label of idiopathic or hereditary pancreatitis is applicable, then the diagnostic procedures and immediate management are similar to those for acute pancreatitis, and the main problem is to find a satisfactory regimen to avoid further episodes. Regular light meals, total abstinence from alcohol and smoking and avoidance of morphine derivatives are advised. Regular oral anti-cholinergic therapy is occasionally helpful. Surgical intervention is seldom advisable.

REFERENCES

1 Acosta, J. M. & Ledesma, C. L. (1974) Gallstone migration as a cause for acute pancreatitis. *New England Journal of Medicine*, **290**, 484–487.
2 Acosta, J. M., Rossi, R., Galli, O. M. R. *et al.* (1978) Early surgery for acute gallstone pancreatitis: Evaluation of a systemic approach. *Surgery*, **83**, 367–370.
3 Allam, B. F. & Imrie, C. W. (1977) Serum ionized calcium in acute pancreatitis. *British Journal of Surgery*, **64**, 665–668.
4 Ammann, R. W., Deyhle, P. & Butikofer, E. (1973) Fatal necrotizing pancreatitis after peroral cholangiopancreatography. *Gastroenterology*, **64**, 320–323.
5 Balldin, G. & Ohlsson, K. (1979) Demonstration of pancreatic protease–antiprotease complexes in the peritoneal fluid of patients with acute pancreatitis. *Surgery*,

85, 451–456.
6 Berry, A. R., Taylor, T. V. & Davies, G. C. (1982) Diagnostic tests and prognostic indicators in acute pancreatitis. *Journal of the Royal College of Surgeons Edinburgh*, **27**, 345–352.
7 Bess, M. A., Edis, A. J. & Van Heerden, J. A. (1980) Hyperparathyroidism and pancreatitis. *Journal of the American Medical Association*, **234**, 246–247.
8 Bourke, J. B., Mead, G. M., McIllmurray, M. B. & Longman, M. J. S. (1978) Drug-associated primary acute pancreatitis. *Lancet*, **i**, 706–708.
9 Bradley, E. L., Clements, J. L. & Gonzalez, A. C. (1979) The natural history of pancreatic pseudocysts. A verified concept of management. *American Journal of Surgery*, **137**, 135–141.
10 Bradley, J. S., Bradley, P., Cameron, J. L. & McMahon, M. J. (1981) Diagnostic peritoneal lavage in acute pancreatitis, the value of microscopy of the fluid. *British Journal of Surgery*, **68**, 245–246.
11 Buch, A., Buch, J., Carlsen, A. & Schmidt, A. (1980) Hyperlipoidemia and pancreatitis. *World Journal of Surgery*, **4**, 307–314.
12 Cameron, J. L., Zuidema, G. D. & Margolis, S. (1975) A pathogenesis for alcoholic pancreatitis. *Surgery*, **77**, 754–763.
13 Cameron, J. L., Capuzzi, D. M., Zinderman, G. D. & Margolis, S. (1975) Acute pancreatitis with hyperlipaemia. *Annals of Surgery*, **177**, 483–499.
14 Cooper, M. J., Williamson, R. C. N. & Pollock, A. V. (1982) The role of peritoneal lavage in the prediction and treatment of severe acute pancreatitis. *Annals of the Royal College of Surgery*, **64**, 422–27.
15 Croton, R. S., Warren, R. A., Scott, A. & Roberts, N. B. (1981) Ionized calcium in acute pancreatitis. *British Journal of Surgery*, **68**, 241–243.
16 Dickson, A. P. & Imrie, C. W. (1984) Hyperlipidaemia, alcohol abuse and acute pancreatitis, a prospective study. *British Journal of Surgery* (in press).
17 Dickson, A. P. & Imrie, C. W. (1984) Body wall ecchymosis in patients with acute pancreatitis. *Surgery, Gynecology and Obstetrics* (in press).
18 Feiner, H. (1976) Pancreatitis after cardiac surgery. *American Journal of Surgery*, **131**, 684–688.
19 Fitz, R. H. (1889) Acute pancreatitis. *Boston Medical and Surgical Journal*, **120**, 181, 205, 229.
20 Foulis, A. K. (1982) Morphological study of the relation between accidental hypothermia and acute pancreatitis. *Journal of Clinical Pathology*, **35**, 1244–1248.
21 Gambill, E. E. (1971) Pancreatitis associated with pancreatic carcinoma. *Mayo Clinic Proceedings*, **46**, 174–177.
22 Imrie, C. W. (1974) Observations on acute pancreatitis. *British Journal of Surgery*, **61**, 539–544.
23 Imrie, C. W. & Blumgart, L. H. (1975) Acute pancreatitis; a prospective study of some factors in mortality. *Bulletin Société Internationale de Chirurgie*, **34**, 601–603.
24 Imrie, C. W., Allam, B. F. & Ferguson, J. C. (1976) Hypocalcaemia of acute pancreatitis: the effect of hypoalbuminaemia. *Current Medical Research Opinion*, **4**, 101–116.
25 Imrie, C. W., Ferguson, J. C. & Sommerville, R. G. (1977) Coxsackie and mumps virus infection in a prospective study of acute pancreatitis. *Gut*, **18**, 53–56.
26 Imrie, C. W., Ferguson, J. C., Murphy, D. & Blumgart, L. H. (1977) Arterial hypoxia in acute pancreatitis. *British Journal of Surgery*, **64**, 185–188.
27 Imrie, C. W., Goldring, J., Pollock, J. G. & Watt, J. K. (1977) Acute pancreatitis after translumbar aortography. *British Medical Journal*, **ii**, 681.

28 Imrie, C. W., Benjamin, I. S., Ferguson, J. C. *et al.* (1978) A single centre double blind trial of trasylol therapy in primary acute pancreatitis. *British Journal of Surgery*, **65**, 337–341.

29 Imrie, C. W., Beastall, G. H., Allam, B. F. *et al.* (1978) Parathyroid hormone and calcium homeostasis in acute pancreatitis. *British Journal of Surgery*, **65**, 717–720.

30 Imrie, C. W., McKay, A. J., Benjamin, I. S. & Blumgart, L. H. (1978) Secondary acute pancreatitis: aetiology, prevention, diagnosis and management. *British Journal of Surgery*, **65**, 399–402.

31 Kelly, T. R. (1976) Gallstone pancreatitis: pathophysiology. *Surgery*, **80**, 488–492.

32 Lankisch, P. G., Rahlf, G. & Koop, H. (1983) Pulmonary complications in fatal acute haemorrhagic pancreatitis. *Digestive Diseases and Sciences*, **28**, 111–116.

33 Leger, L., Lenriot, J. P. & Lemaigre, G. (1974) Five to twenty year follow-up after surgery for chronic pancreatitis in 148 patients. *Annals of Surgery*, **180**, 185–191.

34 McLatchie, G. R. & Imrie, C. W. (1981) Acute pancreatitis associated with tumour metastases in the pancreas. *Digestion*, **21**, 13–17.

35 McMahon, M. J., Playforth, M. J. & Booth, E. W. (1981) Identification of risk factors for acute pancreatitis from routine radiological investigation of the biliary tract. *British Journal of Surgery*, **68**, 465–467.

36 McMahon, M. J., Playforth, M. J. & Pickford, I. R. (1980) A comparative study of methods for the prediction of severity of attacks of acute pancreatitis. *British Journal of Surgery*, **67**, 22–25.

37 MRC Multicentre Trial Study Group (1977) Death from acute pancreatitis. MRC multicentre trial of glucagon and aprotinin. *Lancet*, **ii**, 632–635.

38 Murphy, D., Pack, A. I. & Imrie, C. W. (1980) The mechanism of arterial hypoxia occurring in acute pancreatitis. *Quarterly Journal of Medicine*, **49**, 151–160.

39 Nakashima, Y. & Howard, J. M. (1977) Drug induced acute pancreatitis. *Surgery, Gynecology and Obstetrics*, **145**, 105–109.

40 Niccolini, D. G., Graham, J. H. & Banks, P. A. (1976) Tumour-induced pancreatitis. *Gastroenterology*, **71**, 141–145.

41 Opie, E. L. (1901) The relation of cholelithiasis to disease of the pancreas and to fat necrosis. *Johns Hopkins Hospital Bulletin*, **12**, 19.

42 Osborne, D. H., Imrie, C. W. & Carter, D. C. (1981) Biliary surgery at the same admission for gallstone associated pancreatitis. *British Journal of Surgery*, **68**, 758–761.

43 Pollock, A. V. (1959) Acute pancreatitis. *British Medical Journal*, **i**, 6–14.

44 Prince, M. (1882) Pancreatic apoplexy with a report of two cases. *Boston Medical and Surgical Journal*, **107**, 28, 55.

45 Ranson, J. H. C. (1979) The timing of biliary surgery in acute pancreatitis. *Annals of Surgery*, **189**, 654–663.

46 Ranson, J. H. C. & Pasternack, B. S. (1977) Statistical methods for quantifying the severity of clinical acute pancreatitis. *Journal of Surgical Research*, **22**, 79–91.

47 Ranson, J. H. C. & Spencer, F. C. (1978) The role of peritoneal lavage in severe acute pancreatitis. *Annals of Surgery*, **187**, 565–574.

48 Ranson, J. H. C., Rifkind, K. M. & Turner, J. W. (1976) Prognostic signs and nonoperative peritoneal lavage in acute pancreatitis. *Surgery, Gynecology and Obstetrics*, **143**, 209–219.

49 Ranson, J. H. C., Rifkind, K. M., Roses, D. F. *et al.* (1974) Prognostic signs and the role of operative management in acute pancreatitis. *Surgery, Gynecology and Obstetrics*, **139**, 69–81.

50 Reeve, T. S. & Delbridge, L. W. (1982) Pancreatitis following parathyroid surgery. *Annals of Surgery*, **195**, 158–162.

51 Ruppin, H., Amon, R. & Ettl, W. (1974) Acute pancreatitis after endoscopic radiological pancreatography. *Endoscopy*, **6**, 94–98.

52 Saidi, F. & Donaldson, G. A. (1963) Acute pancreatitis following distal gastrectomy for benign ulcer. *American Journal of Surgery*, **105**, 87–92.

53 Sankaran, S. & Walt, A. J. (1975) The natural and unnatural history of pancreatic pseudocysts. *British Journal of Surgery*, **62**, 37–44.

54 Stone, H. H. & Fabian, T. C. (1980) Peritoneal dialysis in the treatment of acute alcoholic pancreatitis. *Surgery, Gynecology and Obstetrics*, **150**, 878–882.

55 Trapnell, J. E. & Duncan, E. H. L. (1975) Patterns of incidence in acute pancreatitis. *British Medical Journal*, **ii**, 179–183.

56 Trapnell, J. E., Rigby, C. C., Talbot, C. H. & Duncan, E. H. L. (1974) A controlled trial of Trasylol in the treatment of acute pancreatitis. *British Journal of Surgery*, **61**, 177–182.

57 van Lanschott, J. J. B. & Bruining, H. A. (1982) Parathyroidectomy as a cause of pancreatitis. *Langenbecks Archiv für Chirurgie*, **357**, 186–187.

58 Wallensten, S. (1958) Acute pancreatitis and hyperdiasturia after partial gastrectomy. *Acta Chirurgica Scandinavica*, **115**, 182–188.

CHRONIC PANCREATITIS

A classification of pancreatitis into four types was proposed (at a symposium on the aetiology and pathology of pancreatitis held at Marseilles in 1963). Type I is acute pancreatitis and type II is recurrent acute pancreatitis. In these conditions the pancreas returns to normal clinically and histologically after each attack. When aetiologic factors are removed, there is no recurrence of the pancreatitis and no residual disease in the gland. Type III and type IV are recurrent chronic pancreatitis and chronic pancreatitis. In these forms there is permanent histological damage to the gland. Type III and type IV are distinguished by clinical manifestations such as pain, which are episodic in type III, even though the gland is permanently damaged. In type IV pain is either always present or nearly so, or there is permanent exocrine or endocrine insufficiency. This classification, the best available, is inadequate because the distinctions between the acute and chronic subdivisions are dependent upon knowing whether or not there is irreversible fibrosis or destruction of glandular tissue, facts which cannot always be ascertained. In addition, many management decisions are based on specific aetiology, clinical manifestations and complications which are not part of the classification. It is exceptional that acute pancreatitis (type I or II) progresses to chronic pancreatitis (type III or IV). Chronic pancreatitis is a different disease or group of diseases from acute pancreatitis, arising from different causes and by different mechanisms. Although chronic pancreatitis may manifest itself initially as recurrent acute attacks, there is good reason to believe that chronic injury to the pancreas has long become established in these glands.[44]

AETIOLOGY

By far the most common cause of chronic pancreatitis in Western cultures is alcohol abuse.[44, 51] There is marked individual variation in the exact amount of alcohol necessary to induce chronic pancreatitis, but it has been estimated that the average consumption approaches 150 ml daily for 20 years. There is no relationship between the type of alcohol (such as wine, beer, or whisky), or the pattern of consumption (daily versus intermittent binge-drinking) in the induction of alcoholic pancreatitis. In spite of the common toxic insult a surprisingly small number of alcoholic patients with chronic pancreatitis also develop cirrhosis of the liver.

Alcohol ingestion stimulates pancreatic secretion, increases the protein concentration and lowers bicarbonate concentration.[44] This pancreatic juice contains more protein precipitates than that from normal people, especially immediately after a period of alcohol abuse.[26] The changes in the composition of the pancreatic secretion cannot be explained by modifications of gastrointestinal hormones and appear to be due to a direct toxic effect of alcohol on the pancreatic parenchyma. At least one of the proteins in the pancreatic secretion has a high affinity for calcium and may form a stable precipitate which remains within the smaller ducts. It has been hypothesized that these intraductal precipitates occlude the lumen causing atrophy of the epithelium followed by inflammation and scarring of the parenchyma.[44] Although the 'protein plug' theory for the pathogenesis of alcoholic pancreatitis is widely accepted, there is no evidence that the precipitates do act as plugs or cause injury to the pancreas; the precipitates may be harmless products of the disease, rather than its cause.

While gallstones frequently cause acute pancreatitis, they rarely cause chronic pancreatitis, and any chronic pancreatic lesions due to gallstone pancreatitis are residual scars from pancreatic necrosis, abscess, or pseudocyst following the acute inflammatory episode. Unlike alcohol-induced pancreatitis, removal of the precipitating factor (by cholecystectomy) results in resolution or arrest of the progression of the disease. There are no proven cases of gallstone-induced ampullary stenosis leading to chronic pancreatitis.

Metabolic factors are more likely to produce acute rather than chronic pancreatitis. Hypercalcaemia, predominantly due to hyperparathyroidism, can cause either acute or chronic pancreatitis,[12] but it probably accounts for less than 1% of all cases of clinically recognized chronic pancreatitis. Hyperlipidaemia is always in the form of elevated triglycerides, usually as chylomicrons in type I or type V hyperlipoproteinaemia, but also as very low density lipoproteins in type IV.

Trauma is a common cause of acute pancreatitis and may result in chronic pancreatitis if there is sufficient disruption of the major pancreatic ductal system.

Several kindreds of hereditary chronic pancreatitis have been reported.[65] The onset is typically in adolescence, and males are affected slightly more frequently than females. An aminoaciduria has been associated with the disease but is inconsistently found. Pancreatitis seems to be passed in an autosomal dominant fashion with incomplete penetrance. Cystic fibrosis is an important cause of pancreatic insufficiency during childhood and is discussed in detail elsewhere in this chapter.

Chronic severe protein malnutrition may result in pancreatic insufficiency, especially in childhood.[7] Clinical evidence of pain, inflammation, and endocrine insufficiency is absent. Pancreatic ducts are normal and fibrosis is uncommon. Pancreatic function returns when nutrition is improved if fibrosis is not extensive. Another form of pancreatitis which may be associated with malnutrition occurs in some tropical regions and is almost endemic on the Indian subcontinent, particularly in the state of Kerala where a limited vegetarian diet is common. Most patients have recurrent abdominal pain beginning in childhood. Pancreatic insufficiency, calcification, and diabetes mellitus are frequent and are not reversed by improved nutrition.

Recent studies have demonstrated that pancreatitis occurs more frequently in persons with the congenital anomaly *pancreas divisum*.[41] In this condition there is failure of fusion of the dorsal and ventral buds of the pancreas. The majority of the gland is drained through the duct of Santorini and the accessory ampulla.

Although most individuals with this condition have no clinical pancreatic disease, there is a four-fold increased risk of the development of acute, otherwise inexplicable pancreatitis. There is a strong tendency for pancreatitis to occur in young women, though it may occur in both sexes and at all ages. The initial clinical pattern is of recurrent acute pancreatitis, but chronic pancreatitis may develop later. The disease seems to be caused by relative obstruction to the flow of pancreatic juice through an inadequate orifice at the accessory ampulla, and, at least until there is irreversible fibrosis of the gland, may be treated by a surgical sphincteroplasty.[61]

Other uncommon but identifiable causes of chronic pancreatitis include haemochromatosis, sclerosing cholangitis,[54] and primary biliary cirrhosis.[18] Chronic pancreatitis is associated with choledochal cysts, at least in adults, probably because of a congenital malformation of the proximal pancreatic duct.[39] No aetiology can be identified in a substantial number of cases; these are unsatisfactorily grouped and described as idiopathic.[56]

PATHOLOGY

The gross appearance of the pancreas may remain normal both to inspection and palpation at the onset of clinical disease. During exacerbations the gland is swollen and inflamed, but later the gland becomes indurated and may be distorted and irregular. Atrophy and extensive scarring develop last, leaving the shrunken pancreas with a firm hard texture and a relatively tubular, rather than flattened, configuration.

The pancreatic ducts remain normal in early stages of the disease, but later become progressively distorted. Most characteristically there is dilation of the duct, sometimes interrupted by strictures (Figure 18.32). However, the duct may instead be shrunken and pruned of its branches (Figure 18.33). It is not known if the duct changes are primary, associated directly with the pathogenesis of the disease, or if they are secondary to scarring from chronic parenchymal inflammation or duct disruption during acute pancreatitis. Intraductal calculi (Fig. 18.34) are present in about half the patients with advanced pancreatitis and may be large enough to occlude the lumen of the duct at the ampulla or at a stricture.

Histologically, chronic pancreatitis involves all parts of the exocrine pancreas, although adjacent lobules may be affected to different degrees. Frequently an entire segment of the pancreas, such as the head or the tail, may be comparatively much more diseased than other

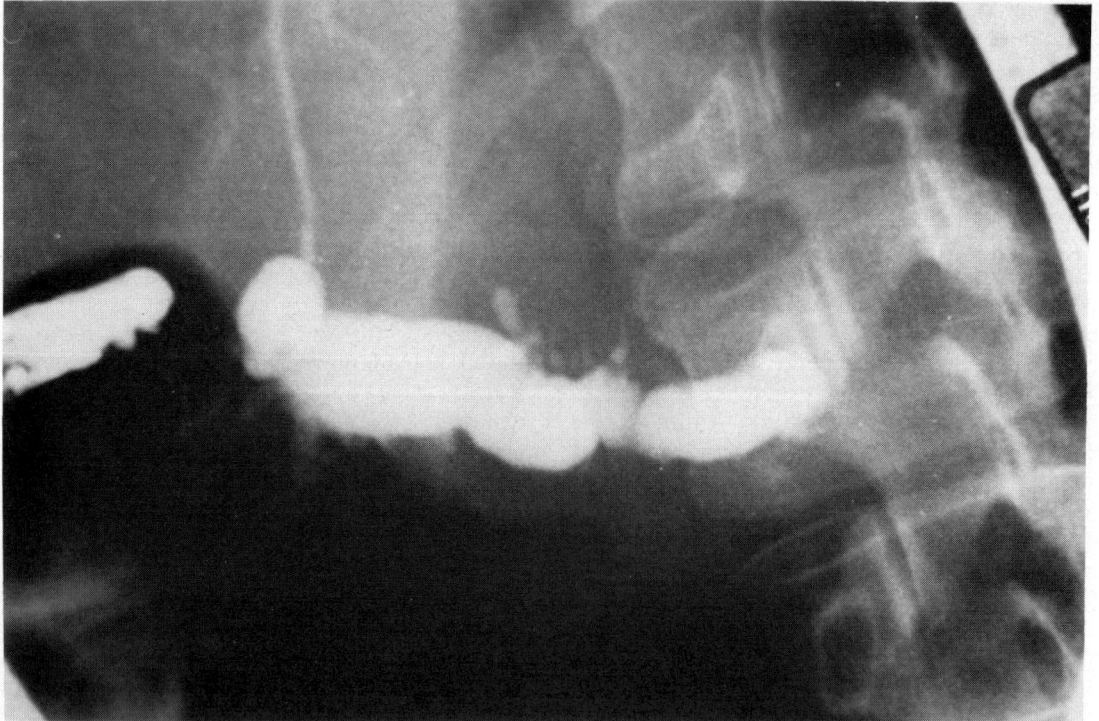

Fig. 18.32   An endoscopic retrograde pancreatogram showing a dilated, intermittently narrowed pancreatic duct.

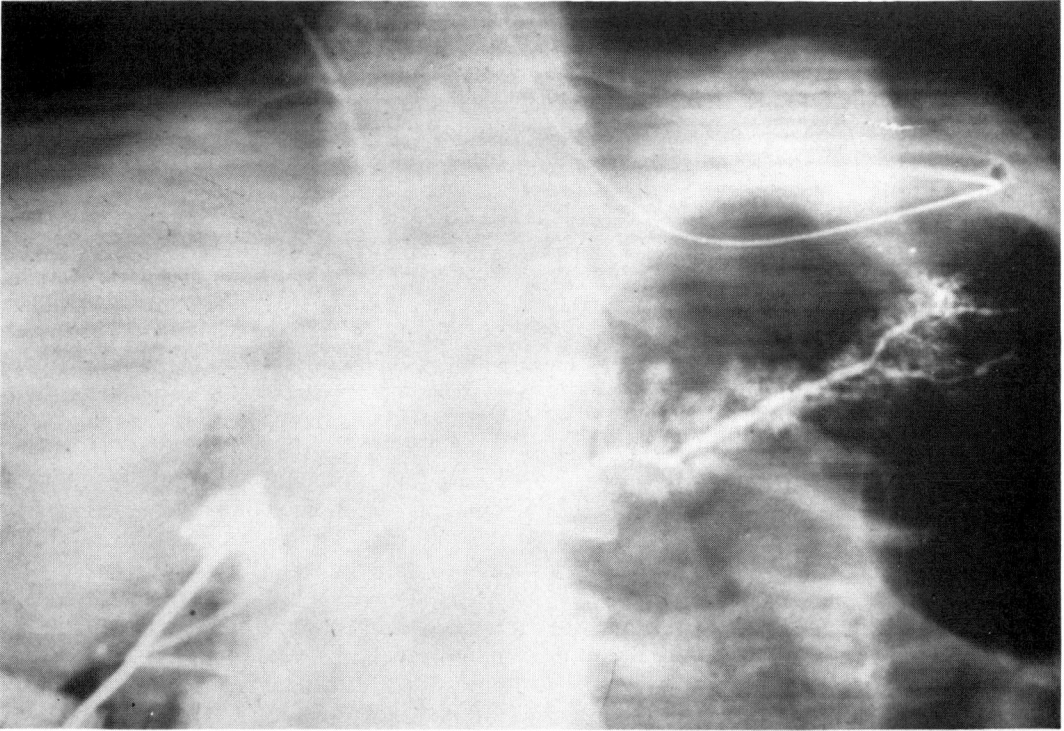

Fig. 18.33 An operative pancreatogram demonstrating a diffusely small pancreatic duct.

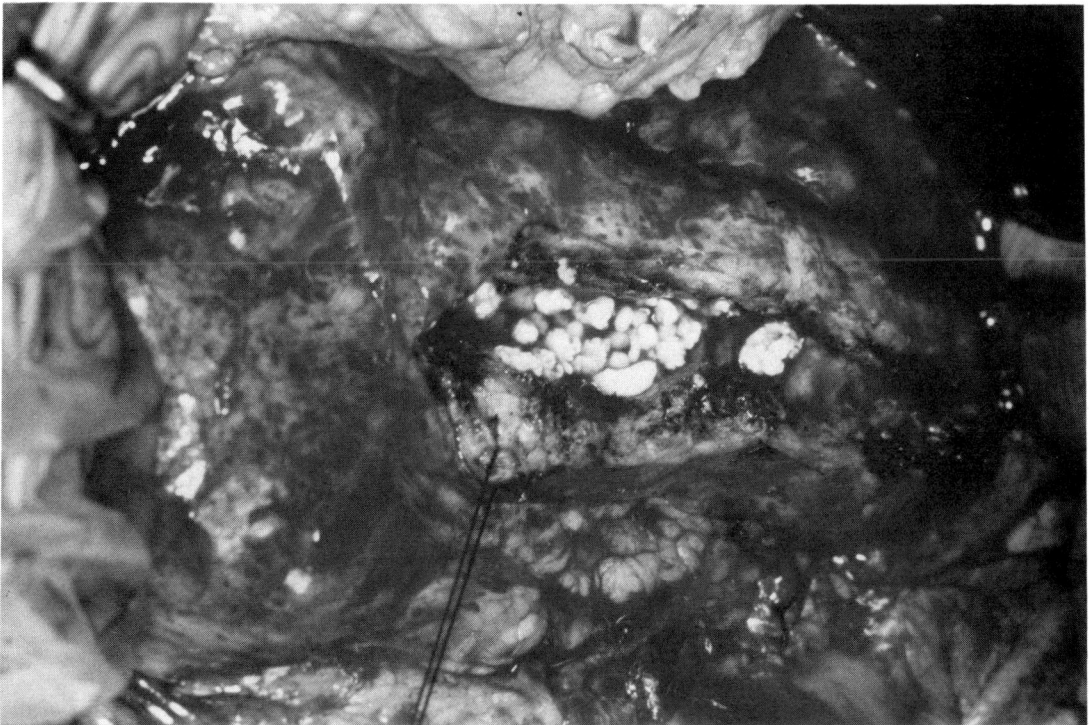

Fig. 18.34 An operative photograph showing multiple calculi in a dilated pancreatic duct.

parts. There is acinar destruction and the functioning exocrine tissue is replaced by dense scar tissue. The islets of Langerhans become encased in fibrous tissue but retain adequate function until late in the disease.

CLINICAL FEATURES

Abdominal pain is the cardinal symptom of chronic pancreatitis. It generally first appears as an attack indistinguishable from type I acute pancreatitis, although the inflammatory destruction and fibrotic replacement of the gland may have occurred unnoticed for years.[44, 51, 56] The pain, characteristically severe, constant, and penetrating, may occasionally be described as heaviness but rarely as burning. It is almost always located in the upper half of the abdomen, from which it can radiate directly through to the back or laterally around to the left or right flank. Less frequently pain is referred to the inferior abdomen or anterior chest. Initially the duration of pain is quite variable, lasting several hours to several days, but as the disease progresses the attacks become more frequent and pain-free intervals shrink and vanish. Painless chronic pancreatitis presenting as pancreatic insufficiency is much less common.

Precipitating factors are difficult to identify. In individuals who drink alcohol sporadically, the pain tends to occur 12–24 h after episodes of alcohol intake. The influence of meals is not usually significant. Once pain has begun, eating frequently exacerbates the discomfort regardless of the composition of the meal while prolonged fasting may relieve it. Pain is not relieved by antacids, though some patients feel improved by vomiting. Others feel better when sitting up and leaning slightly forward. The pain seems to grow worse with fatigue.

The mechanism of pain in chronic pancreatitis is not well understood. The inflammatory reaction involving the pancreas and nearby parietal peritoneum is important in the early episodic form of the pain; later when chronic continuous pain becomes established there is entrapment of nerve fibres in scar tissue. It is possible that obstruction of the pancreatic ducts by strictures and intraluminal precipitates contribute to the pain.

Episodes of anorexia, nausea, and vomiting are associated with abdominal pain due to acute exacerbation of inflammation. In these instances loss of weight is due to decreased caloric intake, even in the absence of pancreatic insufficiency.

Pain is the commonest early feature of chronic pancreatitis, but it is not a *sine qua non.* Some patients will be found to have asymptomatic chronic pancreatitis, perhaps by the incidental finding of pancreatic calcifications seen on an X-ray examination or as an unexpected finding at laparotomy for other reasons. Others will present without pain but with advanced disease producing pancreatic insufficiency. When inflammation, atrophy and fibrosis have reduced pancreatic secretion of enzymes and bicarbonate to 10% of normal, significant maldigestion of fat and protein occurs with consequent malabsorption of these nutrients and steatorrhoea.[15] There is also malabsorption of fat-soluble vitamins, especially vitamin D.[10] At this stage, the steatorrhoea causes frequent loose, foul, floating greasy stools, along with bloating, cramping and flatulence. Initially patients may compensate for their malabsorption by hyperphagia, but as the disease advances weight loss becomes the rule. Some patients will also develop deficiencies of water-soluble vitamins, especially vitamin B_{12}. This defective absorption is reversed by replacement of pancreatic enzymes and seems to be due to a binding of vitamin B_{12} to non-intrinsic factor polypeptides.[55]

Approximately one-third of patients with chronic pancreatitis will have overt diabetes mellitus and another third will have abnormal glucose tolerance at some time during the course of their disease. The first manifestation will be transient hyperglycaemia associated with an episode of acute pancreatitis or an exacerbation of pain. Diabetes mellitus usually develops about one decade after the onset of symptoms, but can be the first sign of painless chronic pancreatitis. Because the islets of Langerhans tend to resist injury by inflammation and fibrosis longer than the exocrine tissues, most patients who develop diabetes will also have pancreatic exocrine insufficiency and steatorrhoea.

The symptoms associated with a pseudocyst are similar to those of chronic pancreatitis and may provide its first manifestations. Obstructive jaundice,[50, 62] gastric outlet obstruction,[8] pancreatic ascites,[11, 22] and upper gastrointestinal bleeding from oesophageal varices[32] are uncommon *presenting* features of chronic pancreatitis, usually appearing later in the course of the disease.

PHYSICAL EXAMINATION

There are few pertinent physical findings, the most common being weight loss, of a degree generally proportional to the severity of anorexia, and steatorrhoea. Tenderness in the upper abdomen is common, especially during times of acute inflammation. An enlarged pancreas is occasionally palpable, especially in a thin person, but the finding of a mass usually indicates a pseudocyst. Rare findings include: jaundice when there is a stricture of the common bile duct; an enlarged spleen when there is thrombosis of the splenic vein; ascites when there is a pancreatic–peritoneal fistula; or a succussion splash when there is duodenal obstruction.

INVESTIGATIONS

Laboratory investigations (see also p. 1267)

There is no good test for chronic pancreatitis, particularly in the earlier stages or milder forms. Serum amylase and lipase are helpful for the diagnosis of acute pancreatitis but are of much less use to evaluate chronic pancreatitis.[3] Serum levels of these enzymes rise with acute exacerbations of inflammation or pancreatic duct obstruction, but are usually normal for much of the time in otherwise uncomplicated chronic pancreatitis. If the amylase isoenzymes in serum or urine are analysed, pancreatic isoamylase can be shown to decrease in chronic pancreatitis. However, the decline of circulating pancreatic isoamylase is an insensitive index for the disease because it probably occurs only in moderately advanced stages when there has been considerable loss of functioning tissue. Abnormal 'aged' pancreatic isoamylases, altered during stagnant incubation, are found in pseudocysts and in the serum of patients with pseudocysts.[58]

The loss of pancreatic function has been used as a test to indicate chronic pancreatitis. The stool is examined for fat using Sudan stain as a crude qualitative screening test, the presence of neutral fat suggesting pancreatic insufficiency. It is more accurate to measure the faecal fat excretion over 72 h on a diet of defined fat intake. If steatorrhoea is found, maldigestion due to pancreatic insufficiency, rather than malabsorption due to intestinal disease, can be demonstrated by normal D-xylose absorption or partial reversal of the steatorrhoea with oral pancreatic enzyme replacement. Severe pancreatic exocrine insufficiency may also be documented by measurement of reduced faecal chymotrypsin. The concentration of the protein lactoferrin is increased in pancreatic secretions in chronic pancreatitis and measurement of pancreatic juice lactoferrin levels can be used to diagnose chronic pancreatitis.[35] However, it has not been shown that the abnormality occurs in early stages of the disease, and the usefulness of this phenomenon is therefore unknown.

Direct measurement of pancreatic secretory capacity provides a more sensitive index of pancreatic function.[17] The secretin test measures pancreatic output of fluid, bicarbonate and enzymes into the duodenum, from which they are collected via a duodenal tube, in response to a standard dose of secretin. Low values indicate pancreatic glandular insufficiency or duct obstruction. Pancreatic exocrine function may also be quantitated using the Lundh test.[4] In this test a standard meal is given to the patient to stimulate endogenous secretin and cholecystokinin, and the output of trypsin into the duodenum is measured.

Function of the endocrine pancreas can be estimated by determining the fasting and 2-h postprandial blood glucose levels, or more formally with a glucose tolerance test.

Biochemical tests of liver function may demonstrate cholestasis in proportion to the degree of stricture of the common bile duct by surrounding fibrosis. The serum alkaline phosphatase is the most sensitive index and has been reported to be increased in up to one-third of patients.[59, 62] The serum bilirubin rises later, as the bile duct obstruction worsens or secondary biliary cirrhosis develops. Fluctuation and transient rises in serum bilirubin also occur with superimposed bouts of pancreatic inflammation or with recurrent cholangitis.[62]

Radiography

Plain films of the abdomen remain valuable for the detection of patients with suspected chronic pancreatitis.[49] Pancreatic calcifications are found in 50–60% of patients with advanced disease and 30% of patients at earlier stages (Figure 18.35). Barium contrast studies of the digestive tract are not helpful except when duodenal stenosis is suspected or to define coincident alimentary pathology. Ultrasonography has proved to be invaluable for the diagnosis of certain aspects of chronic pancreatitis,[28, 29, 43] particularly the demonstration of pseudocysts. The gland itself is usually normal in size and configuration but may show swelling or even a mass when there is active inflammation. Dilatation of the pancreatic duct may be detected using real-time instruments. The major limitation of ultrasound is the inability to image the entire gland in at least 30% of patients because of overlying bowel gas. Ultrasonography has largely replaced selenomethionine radionuclide scanning of the pancreas as a non-invasive test.[5]

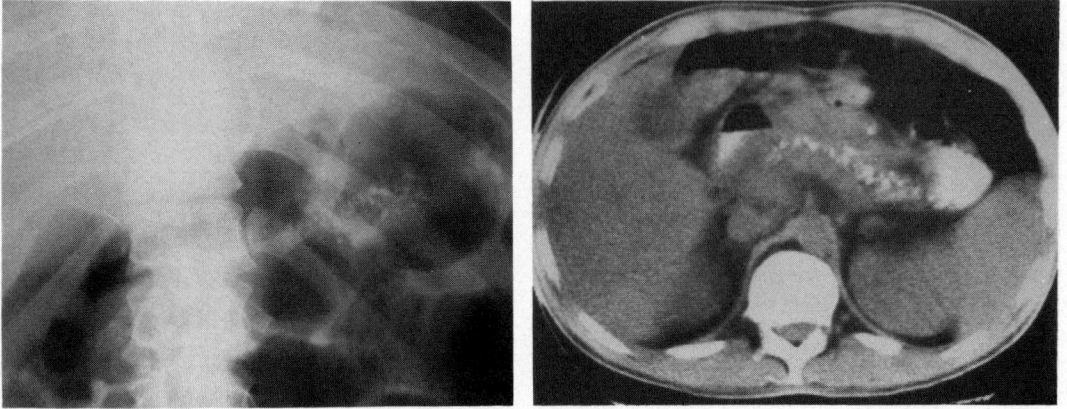

Fig. 18.35 A plain radiograph of the abdomen demonstrating calcification of the pancreas (left). A computerized tomogram of the same patient showing enhancement of the calcifications (right).

The radioisotope scan suffers from a high frequency of false-positive results, but because of its low false-negative rate of about 10%, some still use it as a screen to rule out pancreatic disease.

Computerized tomography has better resolution than ultrasonography and does not suffer from the inability to image through bowel gas.[19, 27] However, computerized tomography relies on contrast of tissue density, particularly fat, and good imaging may therefore be difficult in emaciated patients. Both ultrasonography and CT scanning may have difficulty in differen-

tiating chronic pancreatitis from pancreatic carcinoma. Percutaneous 'skinny needle' aspiration may be indicated to obtain cytological aspirates if cancer is in question. Cytological proof of malignancy can be obtained in nearly 90% of pancreatic cancers and false-positive findings are very rare.[68] However, scanning techniques rarely provide sufficiently detailed information about the anatomy of the pancreatic ducts to plan surgical therapy.

Delineation of the pancreatic ducts requires direct opacification with contrast material, which can be accomplished by endoscopic retro-

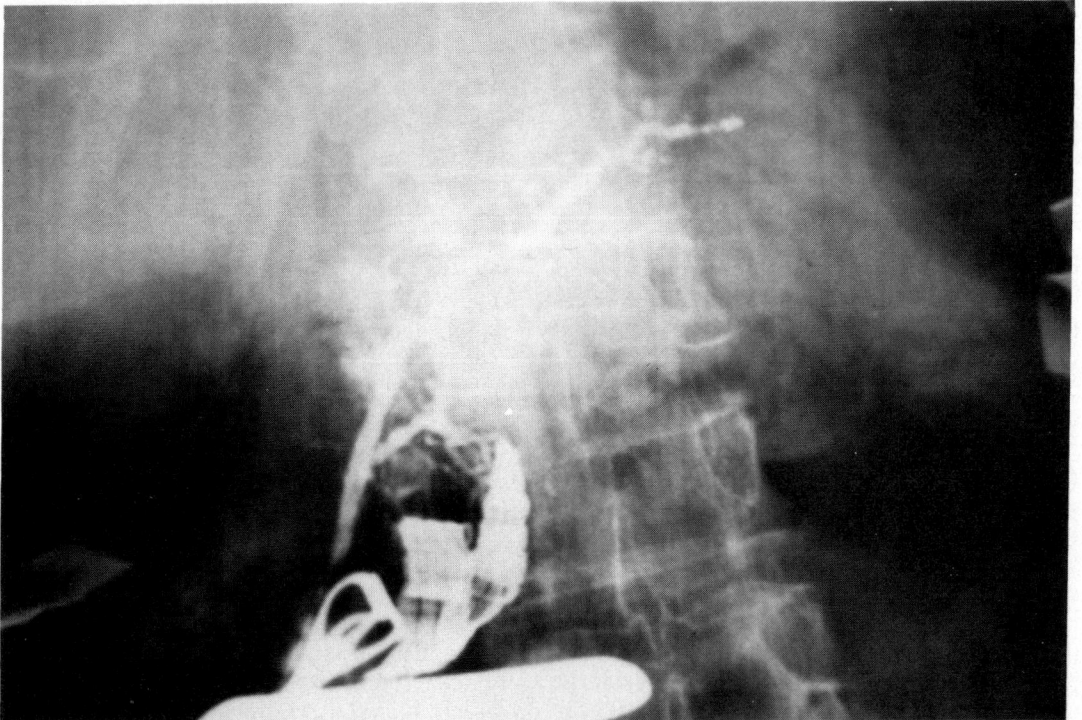

Fig. 18.36 Pancreatogram showing mild dilatation, tortuosity and irregularity of the pancreatic duct.

grade pancreatography[4, 20] (ERCP). Although the duct appears normal in early stages, abnormalities are regularly observed in moderate or advanced disease.[36] The principal earlier changes are irregular dilatation of the main pancreatic duct with occasional narrowing or diffuse constriction and pruning of the ductal system (Figure 18.36). Later, the main pancreatic duct either dilates several-fold (Figure 18.32), or may have segmental constrictions ('chain of lakes') or even complete obstruction, sometimes by an intraluminal stone. The presence of pancreatic stones on plain abdominal radiographs tends to correlate with pancreatic duct dilatation. About 30% of patients will have dilated major ducts but well over 50% of those with pancreatic stones have such dilatation. Because the stenotic segments may empty poorly, there is a risk of introducing infection during pancreatography; prophylactic antibiotics substantially decrease the incidence of clinical infection.

Extrinsic compression of the common bile duct within the substance of the pancreas occurs in up to one-third of patients with moderate or advanced chronic pancreatitis.[59, 62] The typical long, tapered, smooth stricture of the intrapancreatic portion of the bile duct can be shown by endoscopic retrograde cholangiography or by percutaneous transhepatic cholangiography (Figure 18.37). One of these investigations is indicated in any patient with chronic pancreatitis who is jaundiced or who has a persistently raised serum alkaline phosphatase.

Selective coeliac angiography is used mainly when splenic or portal venous occlusion is suspected, or to detect vascular anomalies in advance of major surgical resections.[32]

An integrated diagnostic approach to the patient with suspected chronic pancreatitis

The diagnosis of chronic pancreatitis is generally considered in patients who present with chronic epigastric pain, steatorrhoea, or weight loss. Diagnostic evaluation of a patient presenting with pain generally begins with radiographic and then endoscopic studies of the upper digestive tracts if there are aspects of the history that suggest gastric or duodenal pathology. A plain film of the abdomen demonstrating characteristic pancreatic calcification virtually establishes the diagnosis. If needed, the diagnostic evaluation then proceeds with an ultrasonographic examination of the biliary tree and pancreas. When the diagnosis is still in doubt, the evaluation may proceed with computerized tomography (CT) in order to image the gland

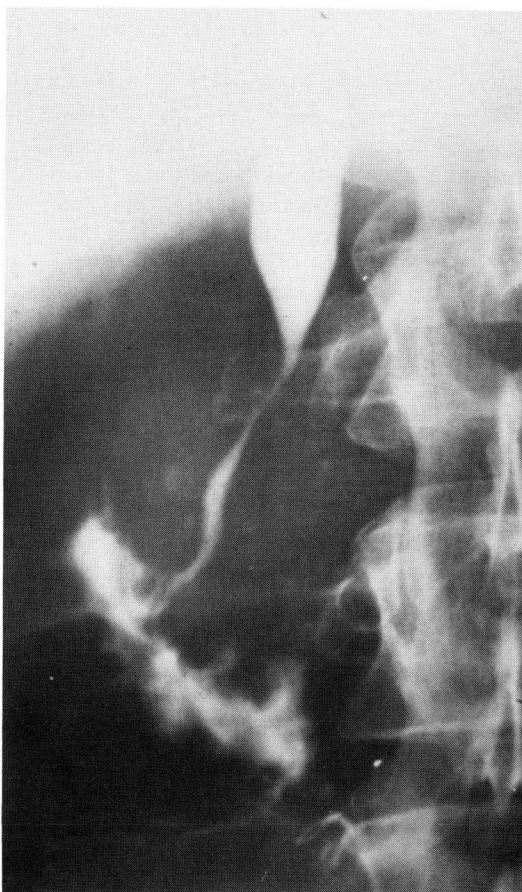

Fig. 18.37 A cholangiogram demonstrating a stenotic distal common bile duct due to chronic pancreatitis.

more fully. Calcifications undetected on plain film may be observed, and solitary solid masses may be identified. Diffuse disease of the pancreas supports the diagnosis of chronic pancreatitis, but localized solid lesions must be distinguished from pancreatic cancer. This may be most easily accomplished by a percutaneous needle aspiration of the mass under ultrasonographic or CT guidance.[68] Occasionally endoscopic pancreatography, arteriography, or even laparotomy may be necessary to distinguish the two diseases.[20] The diagnosis of chronic pancreatitis may be confirmed by the demonstration of decreased pancreatic exocrine function using the secretin stimulation test or the Lundh meal test. Often when the clinical history is particularly compelling, a clinical diagnosis of chronic pancreatitis may be made without a complete radiological or secretory evaluation.

Patients with painless chronic pancreatitis presenting as steatorrhoea and weight loss require a different diagnostic evaluation. The first step is to document fat malabsorption either with a qualitative stool examination or with a 72-h stool collection on a defined diet. A faecal chymotrypsin test may be helpful in identifying pancreatic disease, though a D-xylose test or intestinal biopsy may be needed to exclude intestinal causes in malabsorption. A plain film of the abdomen demonstrating characteristic calcification is once again quite helpful in establishing a diagnosis of chronic pancreatitis. In ambiguous cases direct measurement of pancreatic exocrine function is helpful. In the absence of the availability of these tests an empiric trial of therapy with oral pancreatic enzymes may suffice. When the diagnosis of pancreatic cancer is also being entertained, evaluation should proceed with ultrasonography and the other studies as discussed above.

NATURAL HISTORY

The natural history of chronic pancreatitis varies substantially with the underlying aetiology. Since the most common cause of pancreatitis in Western countries is alcohol, most is known about the course of this form of the disease.

Chronic alcoholic pancreatitis tends to become symptomatic in early adulthood after 10–20 years of heavy alcohol abuse. At least 95% of patients with alcoholic pancreatitis will present with acute abdominal pain and the clinical features of acute pancreatitis. Physiological or histological studies, however, will demonstrate established chronic pancreatitis even at presentation.[44] The first attack of pain generally resolves completely, but if alcohol abuse continues there will be a relapse of pain or acute pancreatitis. With the passage of time attacks of pain seems to depend less upon alcohol ingestion and resolve more slowly. Initially the serum amylase is significantly elevated with acute attacks, while later the amylase remains at normal concentrations even during symptomatic exacerbations. After a mean of ten years the discomfort tends to subside in a number of patients. Some authorities believe that this improvement correlates with the development of pancreatic exocrine and endocrine insufficiency, indicative of 'burning out' of the pancreas.[2, 23] Although it is also claimed that the appearance of calcifications on abdominal radiography similarly heralds the abatement of pain, our experience demonstrates many exceptions and we do not find it a clinically useful observation. The role of abstinence in the treatment of chronic pancreatitis is unproven, but common

wisdom emphasizes its importance in limiting the recurrence of acute pancreatitis early in the disease. Later pancreatic insufficiency progresses relentlessly even with faithful abstinence from alcohol.

Although many of these patients develop diabetes mellitus, the long-term vascular degenerative complications of diabetes, such as retinopathy, nephropathy, and peripheral arterial atherosclerosis, occur less frequently in the secondary diabetes of chronic pancreatitis than in spontaneous diabetes.[31] It is not known whether this difference is due to the later onset and shorter duration of diabetes mellitus in patients with chronic pancreatitis, who also as a group have decreased longevity, or whether the vascular complications of spontaneous diabetes are promoted by associated genetic or environmental factors which are not necessarily present in patients with pancreatitis.

Most patients survive at least two decades following initial symptoms of chronic pancreatitis. Death directly related to pancreatitis or its complications occurs in only a minority of patients and is usually due to cardiovascular, malignant, or hepatic disease. The incidence of cancer of the pancreas itself is probably not significantly increased in patients with chronic pancreatitis, with a probable exception in the rare kindreds of hereditary pancreatitis.

COMPLICATIONS

Pseudocyst (see also p. 1306)

Pancreatic pseudocysts complicate both acute and chronic pancreatitis.[8, 12, 66] At least 10% of patients with pancreatitis develop clinically apparent pseudocysts. A pseudocyst is a collection of escaped pancreatic fluid and liquefied tissue which forms in pancreatic or peripancreatic tissues. The walls of the pseudocyst are composed of granulation and fibrous tissue but are not lined by epithelium. There are probably two kinds of pseudocysts: those that form as a result of injury to the pancreas during an acute episode of pancreatitis and those that appear in chronic pancreatitis without an identifiable antecedent acute attack of inflammation, perhaps related to duct obstruction by a stricture or pancreatic calculus.[13] Pseudocysts vary in size from 1 to 20 cm in diameter and may be found in any portion of the gland or outside it from the neck to the pelvis. The propensity of pseudocysts to track widely throughout the retroperitoneum and out into the mesenteries, up into the thorax, and to fistulize into viscera is thought to be caused by tissue erosion by the activated proteolytic enzymes in the cyst contents.

Pseudocysts most commonly present with abdominal pain, usually in the epigastrium and are frequently aggravated by eating. Some signal their presence by their impingement upon the stomach or duodenum, causing vomiting, or upon the bile duct, causing jaundice. Some patients with pseudocysts will develop fever, perhaps but not necessarily because of infection of the pseudocyst. Other pseudocysts do not cause symptoms but are discovered because a mass is palpated, the serum amylase is found to be increased, or are even an unanticipated finding from ultrasound or CT scanning (Figure 18.38) or ERCP.

The concept of the natural history of pseudocysts is changing now that the new diagnostic techniques, particularly ultrasound and CT, have shown that many pseudocysts remain silent and some resolve spontaneously. It has been estimated that approximately 30% of pseudocysts following an attack of acute pancreatitis will resolve spontaneously within six weeks of the attack.[9] After that time the chances of resolution diminish markedly, except for the smallest cysts. The rate of spontaneous resolution of pseudocyst developing in chronic pancreatitis in the absence of an identifiable superimposed acute attack is much less.

Other than pain, the acute life-threatening complications of pancreatic pseudocysts are rupture into the free peritoneal cavity, rupture into a viscus (usually with fatal haemorrhage into the gastrointestinal tract), evolution into a pancreatic abscess, and erosion of a major blood vessel with massive bleeding into the pseudocyst cavity. It is partly the fear of those consequences that motivates the surgical treatment of symptomatic, persistent pseudocysts, especially those greater than 5 cm in diameter. In one series of 93 patients with pseudocysts the incidence of complications in medically treated patients was 41%, compared with a 20% incidence of complications in surgically treated patients.[9] It should be recognized that most of the pseudocysts in that series were the product of acute pancreatitis; pseudocysts arising in chronic pancreatitis are much less prone to spontaneous complications, and their surgical treatment should be attended by a morbidity rate of less than 5%.

Common bile duct stricture

The pancreatic fibrosis of chronic pancreatitis surrounds and encases the distal several centimetres of the common bile duct, which is normally intrapancreatic. In as many as one-third of patients with known chronic pancreatitis this process causes a long stricture of the duct

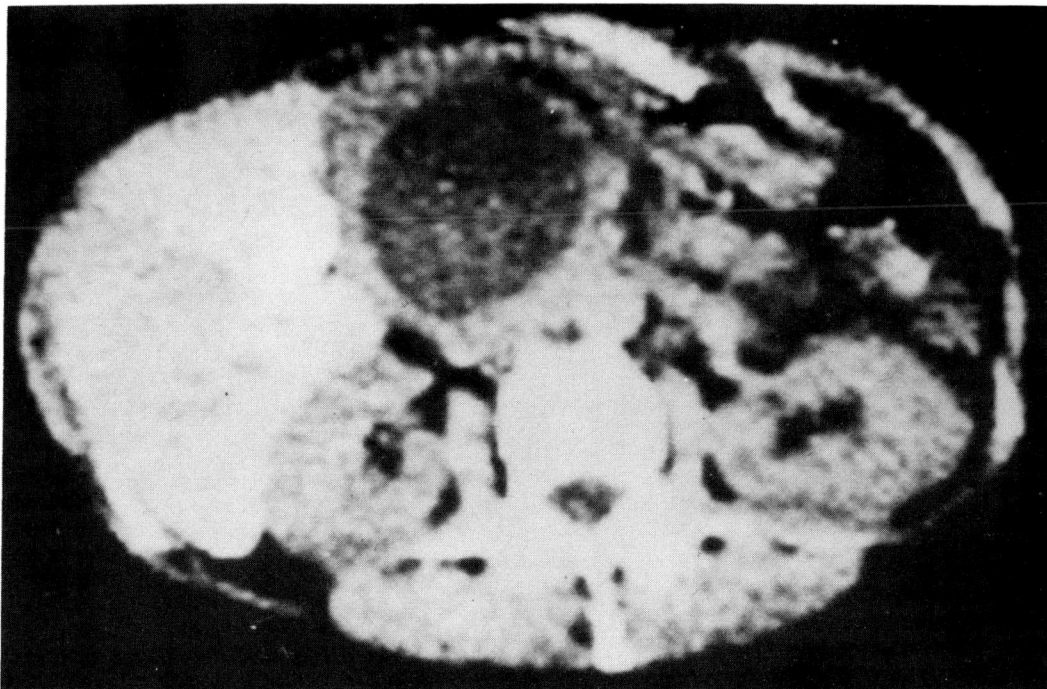

Fig. 18.38   A computerized tomogram showing a large mature pancreatic pseudocyst.

(Figure 18.37).[45, 50] The earliest functional consequence is cholestasis, first indicated by a persistent increase of serum alkaline phosphatase and later by hyperbilirubinaemia. The levels of bilirubin and indeed clinical jaundice can fluctuate during periods of active pancreatic inflammation or low-grade cholangitis.[62] Some patients without previously symptomatic chronic pancreatitis may first present with obstructive jaundice, and it is easy to misinterpret this as cancer, especially in the absence of accompanying pain. Untreated, the chronic cholestasis can lead to secondary biliary cirrhosis.[62] A pseudocyst adjacent to the bile duct can also compress the duct and cause jaundice, but irreversible fibrosis of the duct is usually present.[59]

Intestinal obstruction

Obstruction of the upper gastrointestinal tract is much less common than biliary obstruction, but fibrotic strictures of the second portion of duodenum do occur.[8] Pseudocysts in the head of the pancreas occasionally will compress the duodenum or pyloric antrum. Transient obstruction of the duodenum due to swelling or ileus may occur during periods of acute inflammation.

Ascites (see also Chapter 20)

Ascites in an alcoholic patient is usually due to hepatic cirrhosis. However, ascites may form in chronic pancreatitis when a direct communication develops between the pancreatic duct system and the peritoneal cavity, usually the consequence of a ruptured pseudocyst, but sometimes from rupture and necrosis of a duct near the surface of the gland.[11, 22] These patients present with ascites, with or without chronic discomfort, but not with an acute abdominal catastrophe. The diagnosis of chronic pancreatic ascites is established by paracentesis with the finding of high concentrations of amylase in the ascitic fluid, as well as the raised protein content of an exudate. The pancreatico-peritoneal fistula can often be shown by pancreatography.[30]

Pleural effusion

Chronic pleural effusions may develop in a manner similar to that of pancreatic ascites.[11] The pancreatic secretions from a ruptured pseudocyst or pancreatic duct leak into the retroperitoneum and dissect cephalad through the oesophageal foramen or behind the attachments of the diaphragm into the chest and break through into the pleural space. There may also be a fistula into the pericardium. Patients present with dyspnoea and cough due to the large effusion which is usually unilateral and more often left-sided. In contrast to the pleural effusions which may follow an attack of acute pancreatitis, there is usually no recent acute episode antecedent to the development of pancreatic pleural effusions. They do not resolve spontaneously and recur rapidly after thoracentesis. The diagnosis is indicated by the

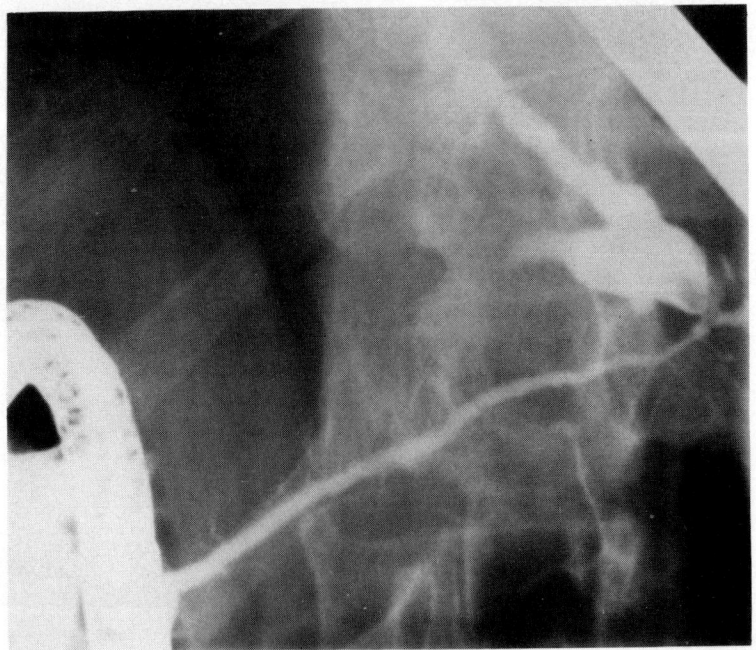

Fig. 18.39 An endoscopic retrograde pancreatogram showing a fistula tracking superiorly toward the oesophageal hiatus from a ruptured pseudocyst.

finding of a very high amylase concentration in the effusion and can be established by demonstrating the pancreatico-pleural fistula with ERCP (Figure 18.39).

Splenic vein thrombosis

Obstruction of the splenic vein, which lies partly within the pancreatic substance, may happen as a consequence of constriction by fibrosis or thrombosis caused by narrowing and continuous inflammation. The spleen enlarges, but usually the event comes about slowly and remains asymptomatic due to the adequate collateral venous drainage through the gastric veins. In some cases, the splenic vein obstruction can cause hypersplenism or acute rupture of the spleen. Localized portal hypertension in the gastric wall may lead to gastric varices, but these rarely rupture or bleed. Much more uncommonly the portal vein itself becomes obstructed either by propagation of thrombus from the splenic vein or by constriction of the portal and superior mesenteric veins as they course through the pancreas (Figure 18.40). This circumstance produces more generalized portal hypertension and is more likely to lead to bleeding oesophageal varices.[32, 34]

Aneurysm

False aneurysms of the arteries in and around the pancreas can be produced by erosion and weakening of the arterial walls by inflammation and enzymatic digestion of an affected vessel in the wall of the pseudocyst. The splenic, gastroduodenal, and pancreaticoduodenal arteries are most likely to be injured. If the aneurysm wall gives way and ruptures, the haemorrhage into the cyst cavity is massive although it can be intermittent. Blood may reach the intestinal tract via the pancreatic duct and present as apparent gastrointestinal bleeding.[33] The bleeding vessel can be identified and haemorrhage controlled by angiographic embolization. Definitive treatment must be directed at the time of surgery for the pseudocyst with ligation of the communicating artery.

TREATMENT

Medical treatment

The treatment of chronic pancreatitis begins by the identification of aetiologic factors and their correction when possible.[42] Alcoholic pancreatitis is often particularly resistant to therapy,

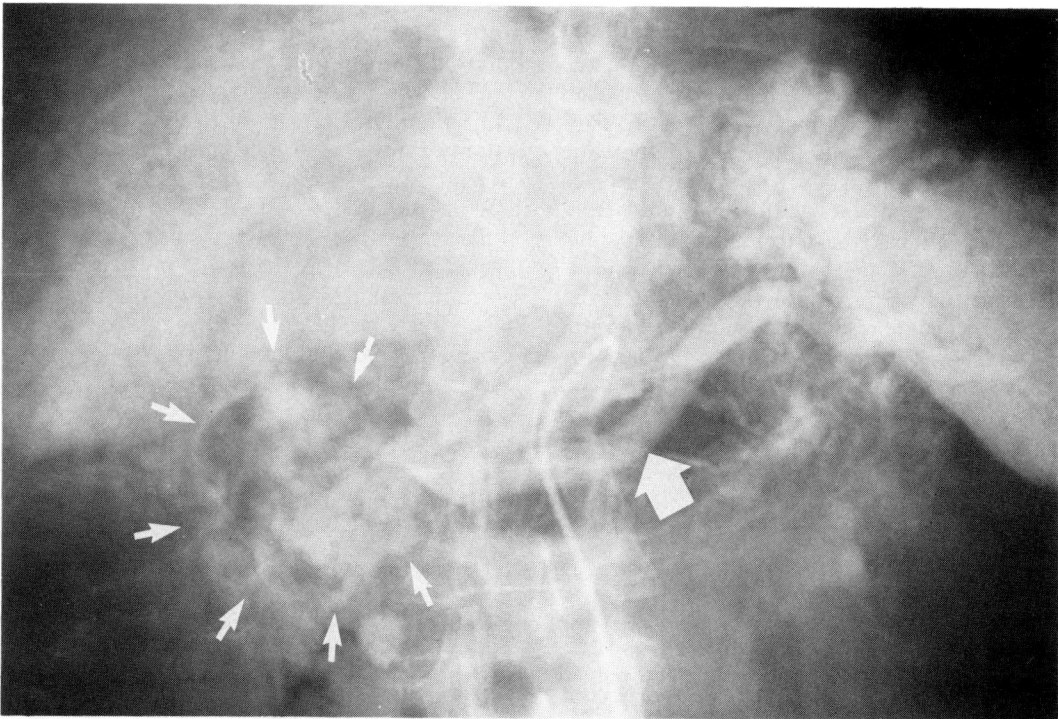

Fig. 18.40 Angiogram showing obstruction of the superior mesenteric and portal veins. The splenic vein (large arrow) terminates in a nest of vericeal collateral veins (small arrows).

both because of the difficulties in ending the alcohol abuse and because cessation of excessive drinking may come too late to be of substantial benefit. If the symptoms are intermittent (Marseilles type III), abstinence may be rewarded, but as the periods of pain become more frequent and even to merge into continuous discomfort, the likelihood of abatement diminishes. At this point, the pain seems to become established and often progresses unremittingly without further exposure to alcohol; none the less, any patient with chronic pancreatitis should severely restrict his alcohol consumption.

Beyond the further limitation of toxic factors, only the manifestations and complications of chronic pancreatitis can be treated. There is no present remedy to relieve or even to halt the inflammation and scarring of the gland. In any stage of chronic pancreatitis pain control is likely to be the biggest problem. Episodes of acute pancreatitis should be treated as discussed earlier in this chapter. Aspirin or other non-steroidal anti-inflammatory drugs are worth trying, but narcotics are usually needed. Codeine or pethidine (meperidine) are suitable for intermittent use, but methadone is better for long-term maintenance analgesia. Habituation or addiction to narcotics becomes inextricably entwined with the pain of the disease, and it is virtually impossible to differentiate the demands of the two contributing elements. Low-fat diets and anticholinergic medications theoretically decrease stimulation of the pancreas but do not reliably lessen the pain. It has been proposed that oral pancreatic enzymes may reduce pancreatic pain by feedback inhibition of pancreatic secretion, but there is no proof that they are effective. Some patients with persistent severe abdominal pain have been treated by splanchnic nerve block with alcohol.[28] This technique is effective in only 15–20% of patients and even then the pain tends to return after several months. It is therefore much less valued for chronic pancreatitis than for pancreatic cancer, wherein the objectives are short-term. The possibility must be kept in mind that the pain may be due to a treatable complication of pancreatitis, such as a pseudocyst, or the development of a coincident treatable disease, for example peptic ulcer.

Maintenance of good nutrition is critical to the management of patients with chronic pancreatitis. Even before the development of pancreatic exocrine insufficiency and steatorrhoea many patients with chronic pancreatitis have periods of anorexia, nausea, and vomiting which significantly limit their ability to take a satisfactory diet, and the problem is magnified in alcoholic patients with irregular eating habits. Diets that are rich in carbohydrates and somewhat restricted in fat and protein are better tolerated.[52] Care should be taken to anticipate and treat vitamin deficiencies (such as B_2, B_{12}, and D).

When pancreatic exocrine capacity falls below 10% of normal, steatorrhoea develops and malnutrition becomes significant.[15] At first, patients may compensate by increasing their total caloric intake, but most patients will benefit from oral replacement of pancreatic enzymes. Enzyme preparations that are rich in pancreatic lipase are most effective in limiting steatorrhoea. Treatment usually begins with two tablets of pancreatin with each meal and one tablet with each snack,[14, 24] the dose increasing until symptoms of diarrhoea and flatulence are controlled. Although malabsorption should be abolished by the replacement of 10–20% of normal enzyme activity in the duodenum, this is seldom accomplished. These less-than-perfect results seem to be due to inactivation of enzymes by gastric acid and failure of sufficient mixing of food and pancreatic enzymes.[16] The efficacy of enzymes are improved by the coincident administration of antacids, especially aluminium hydroxide or sodium bicarbonate,[24] or H_2-receptor antagonist drugs such as cimetidine 300 mg three times daily.[40] Microencapsulated enteric coated preparations of pancreatic enzymes are an expensive alternative to adjuvant antacids.

Diabetes mellitus complicating pancreatitis may initially be treated with a diet and careful attention to overall good nutrition.[6] Later oral hypoglycaemic agents or insulin therapy are frequently required. Control of the diabetes is often difficult because of the propensity to hypoglycaemic attacks,[31] perhaps due in part to irregular food intake during attacks of abdominal pain or anorexia, and perhaps to impaired release of glucagon. Diabetic ketoacidosis is not seen often except after major pancreatic resections.

Surgical treatment

The most common indication for surgery is abdominal pain uncontrolled by medical therapy.[64] Surgery is also required for the treatment of complications of chronic pancreatitis, such as obstruction of the common bile duct or duodenum or the persistence of a pancreatic pseudocyst.

The two major surgical alternatives for reducing pancreatic pain are operations to improve the drainage of the pancreatic duct or to resect pancreatic tissue.[1, 37] When possible, drainage (decompressive) procedures are preferable because they conserve pancreatic tissue and any residual exocrine and endocrine function. Drainage procedures require that there be a dilated pancreatic duct, usually greater than 7 mm. For this reason, ERCP has become invaluable for demonstrating the size and configuration of the pancreatic ducts and thereby for planning the best surgical approach.[67]

Of the patients failing medical therapy for pancreatic pain 30–40% will be found to have a dilated main pancreatic duct. In most patients there is no evidence of obstruction, even though the duct may be 3–4 times its normal diameter; contrast medium injected into the duct flows in easily and drains without delay. True strictures and obstructed segments occur in the minority of patients. If the main duct is over 7 mm in diameter, the pancreatic duct is opened along its length for 8–10 cm and a Roux-en-Y loop of jejunum sutured to it (modified Puestow procedure, Figure 18.41).[60, 63] Long-term follow-up has demonstrated continued patency of the anastomosis in up to 100% of patients,[60] and effective pain relief in greater than 70%.[63] Although no pancreatic tissue is sacrificed and the gland is adequately decompressed, pancreatic insufficiency develops eventually in at least 35% of patients.[60] Caudal pancreaticojejunostomy (Duval procedure), in which the

transected tail of the pancreas is anastomosed to a Roux-en-Y loop of jejunum for retrograde drainage, is less successful than lateral anastomosis because the connection is too small to decompress the entire length of gland effectively and is more likely to occlude in time. Transduodenal sphincteroplasty is generally ineffective for chronic pancreatitis because the treated segment is too short to accomplish decompression of the greater portion of the pancreatic duct.

Patients whose main pancreatic duct is not dilated are not candidates for pancreaticojejunostomy. Resection of the distal 50–60% of the pancreas has been used with little success. The principal indication for this operation is treatment of patients with obstructing lesions of the midpancreatic duct and the rare situation of chronic pancreatitis localized to the distal portion of the gland. Distal subtotal (95%) pancreatectomy (the Child procedure) has had better success in relieving severe chronic pain.[21] In this operation all of the pancreas is resected except for a small amount of tissue along the sweep of the duodenum. It is effective for the relief of pain in just over half the patients, though virtually all patients so treated will develop pancreatic insufficiency and diabetes. If the pancreatitis appears to be disproportionately localized to the head of the pancreas, perhaps with a mass, resection of the head (pancreaticoduodenectomy, the Whipple

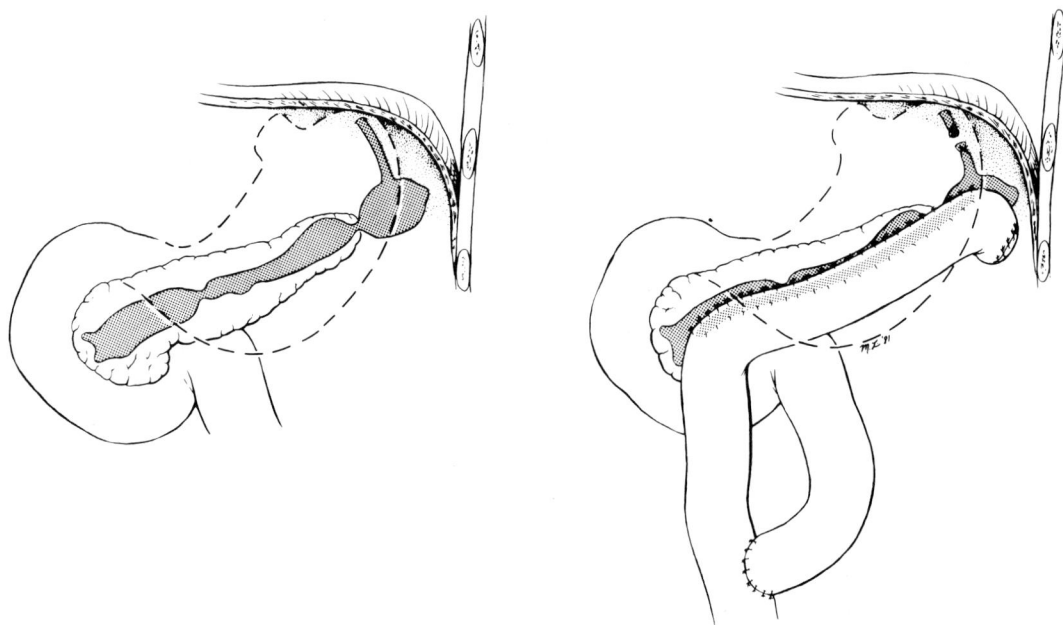

Fig. 18.41 A schematic diagram showing (left) a dilated pancreatic duct, with a distal pseudocyst and pancreatico-pleural fistula. It is treated surgically (right) by lateral pancreaticojejunostomy (modified Puestow procedure) and ligation of the fistula tract.

procedure) may be the best alternative. This is a major operation, requiring special skills, but in appropriately selected patients the incidence of satisfactory pain relief exceeds 70% and enough pancreas is preserved to avoid the development of diabetes mellitus.

Total pancreatectomy is the procedure of last resort. Although it is usually effective for the relief of pain, all patients are left with pancreatic insufficiency and diabetes mellitus that must be managed carefully. Without endogenous glucagon, insulin reaction and profound hypoglycaemia are greater threats than hyperglycaemia and ketoacidosis. Because diet and insulin must be carefully and regularly controlled, patients who continue to drink after total pancreatectomy are at high risk of dying from the acute complications of diabetes. Total pancreatectomy should not be offered to unreformed alcoholics. If autologous islet cell transplantation, currently under investigation, proves to be practical, it may considerably reduce the morbidity of total exocrine pancreatectomy.[56]

Vagotomy and antrectomy with a Billroth II gastrojejunostomy has been used in some patients,[37] the rationale being to reduce the normal stimulation of pancreatic secretion by duodenal hormones, gastrin, and vagal innervation. This approach has had occasional success, particularly in those patients whose pain is aggravated by eating, and should be tried before resorting to a total pancreatectomy.

Patients with the congenital anomaly pancreas divisum are at increased risk for developing acute recurrent pancreatitis because of a stenosis at the orifice of the duct of Santorini, the main pancreatic duct in these individuals.[41] In time there may be permanent damage to the gland, causing chronic pancreatitis.[61] When patients are discovered sufficiently early in the course of their disease, recurrent pancreatitis is prevented by transduodenal sphincteroplasty of the accessory ampulla.[61] If chronic pancreatitis has become established, treatment is more complex and follows the principle outlined previously for other forms of chronic pancreatitis.

Chronic pancreatitis may cause stenosis of the distal common bile duct by extrinsic compression and by fibrosis (Figure 18.37).[50, 62] If the fibrosis has functional significance, the serum alkaline phosphatase will always be increased. Later the patient may become jaundiced and in time develop secondary biliary cirrhosis. Surgical decompression of the bile duct is indicated when a significantly elevated alkaline phosphatase persists. Choledochoduodenostomy and choledochojejunostomy have been the preferred

surgical tactics.

Obstruction of the duodenum in chronic pancreatitis is due to fibrosis rather than to transient oedema as in acute pancreatitis. The narrowing is progressive and unremitting and is corrected by bypass with a gastrojejunostomy.

Pancreatic pseudocysts associated with chronic pancreatitis or with resolving acute pancreatitis should be treated surgically if symptomatic, or larger than 4 cm, or persistent for more than six weeks.[9, 48] Internal drainage to the stomach, duodenum, or a Roux-en-Y loop of jejunum is preferred.[48, 66] Recurrence after cyst enterostomy is about 5%. External drainage may be used when the cyst wall is too flimsy to hold sutures, but has a high recurrence rate of 25%. Percutaneous catheter drainage of pseudocysts is being studied as a definitive treatment; preliminary results show an unacceptably high frequency of infection and recurrence of the cyst.

Chronic pancreatic ascites and pleural effusions, caused by an internal fistula from the pancreas to the peritoneum or pleural space, occasionally respond to repeated withdrawal of the fluid and pharmacological reduction of pancreatic secretion with acetazolamide and anticholinergic drugs. In most patients surgical treatment is necessary.[11] The location of the leak from the pancreatic duct, usually due to a ruptured pseudocyst, can be demonstrated by ERCP (Figure 18.39) in more than 80% of patients.[30] The most common surgical procedure used is to bring a Roux-en-Y loop of jejunum up to the site of the leak, thereby channelling the pancreatic secretions into the intestinal tract. When the disruption is in the tail of the pancreas, distal pancreatectomy may provide a simple and effective solution. In patients with pancreatic pleural effusions, the retroperitoneal fistula into the chest can be interrupted below the diaphragm (Figure 18.41). Once the origin of the fistula has been dealt with, nothing need be done to the pleural end of the tract other than emptying the fluid from the pleural cavity. The interrupted fistula tract will heal and the pleural effusion will not reaccumulate.

Frequently more than one of the indications for surgery will coexist. Pseudocysts are present in about one quarter of all patients requiring surgery for chronic pancreatitis, and bile duct stenoses occur in about 30%. Duodenal obstruction is apparent in about 5%. The surgical plan must deal with as many of these problems as necessary. Combined drainage of multiple organs – pancreatic duct, bile duct, stomach – into the jejunum is effective and not difficult.

REFERENCES

1 Adson, M. A. (1979) Surgical treatment of pancreatitis, review of a series. *Mayo Clinic Proceedings*, **54**, 443–448.

2 Amman, R. W., Largiader, F. & Akoubrantz, A. (1979) Pain relief by surgery in chronic pancreatitis? Relationship between pain relief, pancreatic dysfunction, and alcohol withdrawal. *Scandinavian Journal of Gastroenterology*, **14**, 209–215.

3 Anonymous (1982) Diagnosis of chronic pancreatitis. *Lancet*, **i**, 719–720.

4 Ashton, M. G., Axon, A. T. R. & Lintott, D. J. (1978) Lundh test and ERCP in pancreatic disease. *Gut*, **19**, 910–915.

5 Bachrach, W. H., Birsner, J. W., Izenstark, J. L. & Smith, U. L. (1972) Pancreatic scanning: A review. *Gastroenterology*, **63**, 890–910.

6 Bank, S., Marks, I. N. & Vinik, A. L. (1975) Clinical and hormonal aspects of pancreatic diabetes. *American Journal of Gastroenterology*, **64**, 13–22.

7 Banwell, J. G., Hutt, M. R. S., Leonard, P. J. et al. (1967) Exocrine pancreatic disease and the malabsorption syndrome in tropical Africa. *Gut*, **8**, 388–401.

8 Bradley, E. L. & Clements, J. L., Jr. (1981) Idiopathic duodenal obstruction, an unappreciated complication of pancreatitis. *Annals of Surgery*, **193**, 638–648.

9 Bradley, E. L., Clements, J. L. & Gonzales, A. C. (1979) The natural history of pancreatic pseudocysts: a unified concept of management. *American Journal of Surgery*, **137**, 135–141.

10 Braunstein, H. (1961) Tocopherol deficiency in adults with chronic pancreatitis. *Gastroenterology*, **40**, 224–231.

11 Cameron, J. L. (1979) Chronic pancreatic ascites and pleural effusions. *Gastroenterology*, **74**, 134–140.

12 Carey, M. C. & Fitzgerald, O. (1969) Hyperparathyroidism associated with chronic pancreatitis in a family. *Gut*, **9**, 700–703.

13 Crass, R. A. & Way, L. W. (1981) Acute and chronic pseudocysts are different. *American Journal of Surgery*, **142**, 660–663.

14 DiMagno, E. P. (1979) Medical treatment of pancreatic insufficiency. *Mayo Clinic Proceedings*, **54**, 435–442.

15 DiMagno, E. P., Go, V. L. W. & Summerskill, W. H. J. (1973) Relations between pancreatic enzyme outputs and malabsorption in severe pancreatic insufficiency. *New England Journal of Medicine*, **288**, 813–815.

16 DiMagno, E. P., Malagelada, J. R., Go, V. L. W. & Moertel, C. G. (1977) Fate of orally ingested enzymes in pancreatic insufficiency. *New England Journal of Medicine*, **296**, 1318–1322.

17 Dreiling, D. A. (1975) Pancreatic-secretory testing in 1974. *Gut*, **16**, 653–657.

18 Epstein, O., Chapman, R. W. G., Lake-Bakaar, G. et al. (1982) The pancreas in primary biliary cirrhosis and primary sclerosing cholangitis. *Gastroenterology*, **83**, 1177–1182.

19 Ferrucci, J. T., Jr., Wittenberg, J., Black, E. B. et al. (1979) Computed body tomography in chronic pancreatitis. *Radiology*, **130**, 175–182.

20 Freeny, P. C., Bilbao, M. K. & Katon, R. M. (1976) 'Blind' evaluation of endoscopic retrograde cholangiopancreatography (ERCP) in the diagnosis of pancreatic carcinoma: The 'double duct' and other signs. *Radiology*, **119**, 271–274.

21 Frey, C. F., Child, C. G., III. & Fry, W. (1976) Pancreatectomy for chronic pancreatitis. *Annals of Surgery*, **184**, 403–412.

22 Gambill, E. E., Walters, W. & Scanlon, D. W. (1960) Chronic relapsing pancreatitis with extensive subacute peritonitis and chronic, recurrent massive 'chylous' ascites. *American Journal of Medicine*, **28**, 668–670.

23 Girdwood, A. H., Marks, I. N., Bornman, P. C. et al. (1981) Does progressive pancreatic insufficiency limit pain in calcific pancreatitis with duct stricture or continued alcohol insult? *Journal of Clinical Gastroenterology*, **3**, 241–245.

24 Graham, D. Y. (1977) Enzyme replacement therapy of exocrine pancreatic insufficiency in man. *New England Journal of Medicine*, **296**, 1314–1317.

25 Graham, D. Y. (1982) Pancreatic enzyme replacement; The effect of antacids or cimetidine. *Digestive Diseases and Sciences*, **27**, 485–490.

26 Guy, O., Robles-Diaz, G., Adrich, Z. et al. (1983) Protein content of precipitates present in pancreatic juice of alcoholic subjects and patients with chronic calcifying pancreatitis. *Gastroenterology*, **84**, 102–107.

27 Hasga, J. R., Alfidi, R. J., Harrilla, T. R. et al. (1977) Definitive role of CT scanning of the pancreas. *Radiology*, **124**, 723–730.

28 Hegedus, V. (1979) Relief of pancreatic pain by radiology-guided block. *American Journal of Roentgenology*, **133**, 1101–1103.

29 Lees, W. R., Vallon, A. G., Denyer, M. E. et al. (1977) Prospective study of ultrasonography in chronic pancreatitis. *British Medical Journal*, **i**, 162–164.

30 Levine, J. B., Warshaw, A. L., Falchuk, K. R. & Schaprio, R. H. (1977) The value of endoscopic retrograde pancreatography in the management of pancreatic ascites. *Surgery*, **81**, 300–302.

31 Linde, J., Nilsson, L. & Barany, F. R. (1977) Diabetes and hypoglycemia in chronic pancreatitis. *Scandinavian Journal of Gastroenterology*, **12**, 369–373.

32 Little, A. G. & Moossa, A. R. (1981) Gastrointestinal hemorrhage from left-sided portal hypertension, an unappreciated complication of pancreatitis. *American Journal of Surgery*, **141**, 153–158.

33 Longmire, W. P., Jr. & Rose, A. S. III. (1973) Hemoductal pancreatitis. *Surgery, Gynecology and Obstetrics*, **136**, 246–250.

34 McDermott, W. V., Jr. (1960) Portal hypertension secondary to pancreatic disease. *Annals of Surgery*, **132**, 147–150.

35 Multigner, L., Figarella, C. & Sarles, H. (1981) Diagnosis of chronic pancreatitis by measurement of lactoferrin in duodenal juice. *Gut*, **22**, 350–354.

36 Nagata, A., Homma, T., Tamai, K. et al. (1981) A study of chronic pancreatitis by serial endoscopic pancreatography. *Gastroenterology*, **81**, 884–891.

37 Potts, J. R. & Moody, F. G. (1981) Surgical therapy for chronic pancreatitis: Selecting the appropriate approach. *American Journal of Surgery*, **142**, 654–659.

38 Pradham, D. J., Leveque, H., Juanteguy, J. M. & Seligman, A. M. (1972) Pancreatitis. The role of vagotomy, antrectomy, and Billroth II gastroenterostomy in the treatment of alcoholic pancreatitis. *American Journal of Surgery*, **124**, 21–27.

39 Rattner, D. W., Schapiro, R. H. & Warshaw, A. L. (1983) Abnormalities of the pancreatic and biliary ducts in adult patients with choledochal cysts. *Archives of Surgery* (in press).

40 Regan, P. T., Malagelada, J. R., Dimagno, E. P. et al. (1977) Comparative effects of antacids, cimetidine, and enteric coating on the therapeutic response to oral enzymes in severe pancreatic insufficiency. *New England Journal of Medicine*, **297**, 854–858.

41 Richter, J. M., Schapiro, R. H., Mulley, A. G. & Warshaw, A. L. (1981) Association of pancreas divisum and pancreatitis and its treatment by sphincteroplasty

of the accessory ampulla. *Gastroenterology*, **81**, 1104–1110.

42 Roller, R. J., Mallory, A., Caruthers, S. B., Jr. & Schaefer, J. W. (1977) Oral cholecystography after alcoholic pancreatitis. *Gastroenterology*, **73**, 218–220.

43 Russell, J. G. B., Vallon, A. G., Braganza, J. M. & Howat, H. T. (1978) Ultrasonic scanning in pancreatic disease. *Gut*, **19**, 1027–1033.

44 Sarles, H. & Laugier, R. (1981) Alcoholic pancreatitis. *Clinics in Gastroenterology*, **10**, 401–415.

45 Sarles, H. & Sahel, J. (1978) Cholestasis and lesions of the biliary tract in chronic pancreatitis. *Gut*, **19**, 851–857.

46 Sato, T., Noto, N., Matsuno, S. & Miyakawa, K. (1981) Follow-up results of surgical treatment for chronic pancreatitis, present status in Japan. *American Journal of Surgery*, **142**, 317–323.

47 Schindler, S. C., Schaeffer, J. W., Hall, D. & Griffin, W. O. (1970) Chronic pancreatic ascites. *Gastroenterology*, **59**, 453–459.

48 Shatney, C. H. & Lillehei, R. C. (1979) Surgical treatment of pancreatic pseudocysts. Analysis of 119 cases. *Annals of Surgery*, **189**, 386–901.

49 Simeone, J. F., Wittenberg, J. & Ferrucci, J. T., Jr. (1980) Modern concepts of imaging the pancreas. *Investigative Radiology*, **1**, 6–18.

50 Snape, W. J., Long, W. B., Trotman, B. W. *et al.* (1976) Marked alkaline phosphatase elevation with partial common bile duct obstruction due to calcific pancreatitis. *Gastroenterology*, **70**, 70–73.

51 Strum, W. B. & Spiro, H. M. (1971) Chronic pancreatitis. *Annals of Internal Medicine*, **74**, 264–277.

52 Taubin, H. C. & Spiro, H. M. (1973) Nutritional aspects of chronic pancreatitis. *American Journal of Clinical Nutrition*, **26**, 367–373.

53 Taylor, R. H., Bagley, F. H., Braasch, J. W. & Warren, K. W. (1981) Ductal drainage or resection for chronic pancreatitis. *American Journal of Surgery*, **141**, 28–33.

54 Thompson, H. H., Pitt, H. A., Tompkins, R. K. & Longmire, W. P., Jr. (1982) Primary sclerosing cholangitis, a heterogeneous disease. *Annals of Surgery*, **196**, 127–136.

55 Toskes, P. P., Hansell, J., Cerda, J. & Deren, J. J. (1971) Vitamin B_{12} malabsorption in chronic pancreatic insufficiency; studies suggesting the presence of a pancreatic 'Intrinsic Factor'. *New England Journal of Medicine*, **284**, 627–631.

56 Trapnell, J. E. (1979) Chronic relapsing pancreatitis: a review of 64 cases. *British Journal of Surgery*, **66**, 471–475.

57 Traverso, L. W., Abou-Zamzam, A. M. & Longmire, W. P., Jr. (1981) Human pancreatic cell autotransplantation following total pancreatectomy. *Annals of Surgery*, **193**, 191–195.

58 Warshaw, A. L. & Lee, K.-H. (1980) Aging changes of pancreatic isoamylases and the appearance of 'old amylase' in the serum of patients with pancreatic pseudocysts. *Gastroenterology*, **79**, 1246–1251.

59 Warshaw, A. L. & Rattner, D. W. (1980) Facts and fallacies of common bile duct obstruction by pancreatic pseudocysts. *Annals of Surgery*, **192**, 33–37.

60 Warshaw, A. L., Popp, J. W., Jr. & Schapiro, R. H. (1980) Long-term patency, pancreatic function, and pain relief after lateral pancreaticojejunostomy for chronic pancreatitis. *Gastroenterology*, **79**, 289–293.

61 Warshaw, A. L., Richter, J. M. & Schapiro, R. H. (1983) The cause and treatment of pancreatitis associated with pancreas divisum. *Annals of Surgery*, **198**, 443–452.

62 Warshaw, A. L., Schapiro, R. H., Ferrucci, J. T., Jr. & Galdabini, J. J. (1976) Persistent obstructive jaundice, cholangitis, and biliary cirrhosis due to common bile duct stenosis in chronic pancreatitis. *Gastroenterology*, **70**, 562–567.

63 White, T. T. & Keith, R. G. (1973) Long-term follow-up study of fifty patients with pancreaticojejunostomy. *Surgery, Gynecology and Obstetrics*, **136**, 353–358.

64 White, T. T. & Savotinek, A. H. (1979) Results of surgical treatment of chronic pancreatitis. Report of 142 cases. *Annals of Surgery*, **189**, 217–224.

65 Williams, R. A., Caldwell, B. F. & Wilson, S. E. (1982) Idiopathic hereditary pancreatitis. Experience with surgical treatment. *Archives of Surgery*, **117**, 408–412.

66 Winship, D., Butt, J., Henstorf, H. *et al.* (1977) Pancreatitis: pancreatic pseudocysts and their complications. *Gastroenterology*, **73**, 593–603.

67 Wong, D. H., Schuman, B. M. & Grodsinsky, C. (1980) The value of endoscopic retrograde cholangiopancreatography in the surgical management of chronic pancreatitis. *American Journal of Gastroenterology*, **73**, 353–356.

68 Yamanaka, T. & Kimara, K. (1979) Differential diagnosis of pancreatic mass lesion with percutaneous fine-needle aspiration biopsy under ultrasonic guidance. *Digestive Diseases and Sciences*, **24**, 694–699.

INJURIES TO THE PANCREAS

The incidence of pancreatic trauma is increasing in all parts of the world and numerous comprehensive reports on pancreatic trauma are available.[1, 3, 9, 11] The morbidity and mortality of these injuries varies widely between 10 and 25% depending on the nature of the injuring agent, the time that elapses before definitive treatment and the preinjury physiological reserves of the patient.

ANATOMICAL CONSIDERATIONS

In the treatment of pancreatic injury, careful adherence to a series of fundamental principles is vital, particularly with regard to operative decisions. The pancreas is a retroperitoneal organ overlying the rigid spinal column centrally and the firm posterior muscles on each side. In front, the pancreas is protected by the anterior abdominal wall and overlying intestinal loops. On the right side, the horseshoe of the duodenum may cushion the local effects of trauma. In close proximity to the pancreas are major vascular structures. The liver and common bile duct are above and to the right and the spleen is immediately adjacent to the tail of the pancreas on the left. All these viscera and structures are easily damaged, especially by blows to a relaxed abdominal wall.

FACTORS INFLUENCING MORTALITY AND MORBIDITY

In view of these anatomical relations, it is not surprising that injuries to the pancreas are localized in only 2% of patients with penetrating trauma and about 33% with blunt trauma. If an isolated injury is diagnosed promptly and dealt with without delay, prognosis is excellent. The dominant factor influencing outcome, however, is the concomitant visceral injury occurring in 98% of penetrating injuries and about 66% of blunt injuries. The high mortality is largely due to the close relationship between the pancreas and nearby arteries, veins and the pancreatic duct, which is highly susceptible to trauma. If neglected, damage to the pancreatic duct results in extravasation of pancreatic enzymes into the parenchyma of the gland and surrounding tissues. These enzymes when activated by intestinal contents cause local digestion, inflammation and necrosis of tissue with severe loss of fluid and blood into the area. The resultant hypovolaemia may be so extensive as to cause shock. In addition, vasoactive substances such as bradykinin are released causing vasodilatation, which accounts for some of the severe systemic haemodynamic changes that may occur. Although these physiological changes are potentially important, it is the blood loss and concomitant damage to the duodenum, spleen, kidneys, liver and overlying intestine that usually determine survival.

Mortality rates rise with the number of structures injured: 5% with a single organ and 43% with four organs.[11] In blunt trauma, the liver, duodenum and spleen are the most likely organs to be injured. In penetrating wounds, the stomach, adjacent vessels, the liver and spleen are most often affected. The extent, degree, and multiplicity of injury vary but the two most lethal factors are bleeding from a peripancreatic vessel (such as the portal vein or superior mesenteric vessels) and sepsis consequent on bowel disruption (most often of the transverse colon). Other obvious factors that influence morbidity, include (1) the injuring agent, for example a gunshot as opposed to a stab wound, (2) the extent of pancreatic injury, (3) the presence of extra-abdominal injury, such as head injury or thoracic trauma, (4) the degree of blood loss, (5) the degree of contamination by intestinal organisms, (6) the age of the patient, (7) the presence and degree of hypovolaemic shock, and (8) the time lapse between injury and treatment.

Although fewer than 2% of all intra-abdominal injuries involve the pancreas, the overall mortality rate for pancreatic injuries in the USA remains between 10% and 20%.[4, 7, 14] Shotgun wounds produce a mortality rate in excess of 50%, gunshot wounds about 15%, blunt injuries 10–15%, and stab wounds about 5%.

In 98% of penetrating wounds, viscera other than the pancreas will also be damaged. Death is seldom due to the pancreatic injury itself but usually results from the associated injuries. Apart from the effects of haemorrhage from adjacent vessels, colonic injury is the most threatening complication. The transverse colon is injured in about 25% of penetrating wounds but in only about 2% of blunt injuries. The deleterious effects of colonic damage occur through contamination of the peritoneal cavity and subsequent infection rather than any intrinsic colonic damage which can easily be dealt with at operation by primary repair, excision with colostomy or by exteriorization. Concomitant shock increases the morbidity and mortality rate to about 40% and reflects the volume of blood loss, which usually originates from peripancreatic vessels rather than from parenchymal pancreatic damage. Haemorrhage is the primary cause of death in about two-thirds of fatalities and sepsis in about a quarter. Other lesions such as head injury or thoracic trauma are responsible for the remainder of the deaths.

Any part of the pancreas may be injured, depending on the track of the missile or, in blunt trauma, the site of impact. In blunt trauma the basic injury is identical whether due to steering wheel, handlebar, boot or stake although the degree and extent may vary widely. The head of the pancreas bears the brunt of the injury in about 40% of patients, the body in about 15% and the tail in about 30%. In 15% of patients, multiple separated injuries of the pancreas that involve more than one segment are present. Loss of integrity of the adjacent duodenum plays an important role in determining the final outcome. Concomitant duodenal injury may range from contusion or haematoma to severe disruption of duct structures with spillage of bile, pancreatic juice and chyme. Approximately 20% of all pancreatic injuries will be associated with damage to the duodenum but this figure rises to 50% when injuries are confined to the head of the pancreas.[5]

A retroperitoneal haematoma is present in about 50% of pancreatic injuries and may obscure the degree of underlying damage. The consequences of knife wounds and gunshot wounds differ greatly, ranging from small clean holes with little surrounding necrotic tissue and minor bleeding caused by knives to widespread disruption of the pancreatic parenchyma from gunshot trauma. Debridement of the pancreas requires great discretion and should veer towards being conservative. It is important, however, that all peripancreatic haematomas be opened and fully explored. Unless this is done, serious pancreatic injury may be missed. The size of a peripancreatic haematoma does not necessarily reflect the severity of the underlying injury; large haematomas may have little or no associated pancreatic injury and conversely a small haematoma may mask a ductal disruption. It is also important to realize that an apparently intact anterior pancreatic wall may nevertheless be associated with posterior parenchymal damage of a degree to cause disruption of the main pancreatic duct.

ASSESSMENT

Although the immediate causes of death in patients with pancreatic injury are intra-abdominal haemorrhage, head injury or thoracic trauma, the main threat generated by the pancreas itself is the leakage of pancreatic juice from a damaged main pancreatic duct. Failure to recognize and seal a damaged main duct or to control the production and diversion of pancreatic juice is the greatest local cause of morbidity and mortality. Leakage from minor ducts creates a pancreatic fistula which will close spontaneously within 4–6 weeks. Rupture of a main duct, however, may predispose to the development of hypovolaemia, sepsis, erosive lesions of the abdominal cavity and soft tissues, and a more permanent fistula.

Consequently, the main objective at the time of the initial operative exploration is accurate determination of the integrity of the main pancreatic duct.[6] In most cases, this can be made by simple inspection and palpation. In some patients the field is grossly obscured by oedema and fragmentation of the pancreatic surface making determination of ductal integrity extremely difficult. A number of approaches to this important decision have been proposed. Some surgeons have advocated endoscopic retrograde pancreatography (ERCP) to delineate the state of the pancreatic duct. This is seldom feasible in severely injured patients as it presupposes that the patient is stable, that there is a substantial chance of the duct being injured and that operation may be delayed for a few hours without harm to the patient. In practice, ERCP is very rarely performed in the acute situation. Other proposals are the use of intraoperative pancreatography through a duodenotomy, or through the cut tail of the pancreas deliberately transected for the purpose of identifying the distal pancreatic duct. Most surgeons agree that these iatrogenic invasions of the duodenum or the pancreas are time consuming, potentially hazardous and usually impractical. The intraoperative administration of secretin may be helpful in identifying a leaking duct by increasing the amount of secretion so that the site of leakage is visible. Generally, however, when the main damage is to the body or the tail, the decision to resect is made on clinical observation and judgment. As resection of the body and tail may be done with relative ease and safety, this approach is justifiable where substantial doubt about the integrity of the duct remains.

In contrast, when the traumatic lesion is situated in the head of the pancreas, the risk–benefit ratio of resection is usually unacceptable. Greater surgical caution is therefore advisable when debriding this area so as not to damage a duct which is intact or only contused. In such patients, careful placement of sump drains around the area and tacit acceptance of an unavoidable fistula if the duct is injured is necessary.

DIAGNOSIS

Penetrating wounds of the abdomen which involve the pancreas may enter from the neck through the chest into the peritoneal cavity, or through the thoracic cage and diaphragm into the pancreas, or, most often, entry is through the anterior or posterior abdominal wall. In deep penetrating wounds, the clinical indications for laparotomy are nearly always present and the track of the knife or missile should be followed to its termination.

In recent years, patients in whom the anterior peritoneum is penetrated but who show no overt abnormal clinical signs are investigated with peritoneal lavage to determine whether blood, bile or amylase is present, indicating a potential need for laparotomy. The measurement of amylase in the lavage fluid has been recently challenged and has largely been abandoned in many centres. The presence of blood (RBC $> 50\,000/cm^3$), bile or intestinal content in the lavage would automatically indicate the need for laparotomy and direct inspection of the pancreas. Because of the posterior situation of the pancreas, amylase elevation alone, without evidence of blood or intestinal content in the lavage return, is very rare.

By contrast, blunt trauma of the pancreas is associated with concomitant visceral injury in only two-thirds of cases and the signs and symptoms of pancreatic injury may be very slow to evolve. The retroperitoneal location of the pancreas and an intact posterior peritoneum tends to contain any leaking pancreatic fluid or slowly evolving haematoma. In these circumstances, the patient may deny all abdominal pain and tenderness for 12–24 h, thereafter abdominal distension develops due to an increasing ileus. This sequence is particularly likely to occur in those patients in whom the blow has been transmitted through the rib cage rather than directly through the softer anterior abdominal wall. The combination of fractured ribs on the left and abdominal pain always raises questions about associated splenic injury but the possibility of pancreatic damage should also be kept in mind. Peritoneal lavage is often negative in these circumstances even though subsequent operation may reveal a badly damaged pancreas to the point of complete transection.

SPECIAL INVESTIGATIONS

Amylase levels

In 1929, Elman *et al.*[2] suggested that hyperamylasaemia may be a valuable method of diagnosing pancreatic disease, and in 1943 Naffziger and McCorkle[10] used this observation to draw attention to an association between hyperamylasaemia and pancreatic trauma. Unfortunately, the relationship between the levels of serum amylase and the presence and degree of pancreatic injury in abdominal trauma is complex and often perplexing.[12] Many observations have been made on this subject, some of which have been contradictory. Current views on hyperamylasaemia, abdominal trauma and pancreatic injury may be briefly summarized by the following statements. (1) The presence of hyperamylasaemia may be deceptive since an elevated serum amylase may be a reflection of the salivary rather than the pancreatic isoenzyme. In an unpublished series from our institution, hyperamylasaemia in blunt trauma was due to non-pancreatic amylase in 18% of cases. (2) The serum amylase level may rise slowly following pancreatic injury and about one-half of patients with a subsequently proven transected pancreas will have normal serum levels at the time of operation. (3) Only about 8% of patients with hyperamylasaemia have *pancreatic* injuries requiring operation. Other causes for the elevated serum amylase include the presence of a ruptured bowel, thoracic injuries (the lung produces non-pancreatic amylase), head injury which is known to stimulate hyperamylasaemia, and administration of narcotics causing spasm of the sphincter of Oddi. In patients who have been taking alcohol, the hyperamylasaemia may be due to acute erosive gastritis or alcohol rather than traumatic pancreatitis.

With the availability of rapid isoamylase studies in the emergency department, it is now possible to distinguish pancreatic amylase from non-pancreatic amylase. Even in these circumstances, the presence of an elevated pancreatic isoenzyme component does not make a case for immediate laparotomy, for although many of these patients will have had some pancreatic damage, presumably against the lumbar spine, the injury is sometimes self-limiting.

It is necessary to be cautious about the use of serum amylase levels as a determinant of whether or not to operate. Clinical observation remains paramount and the main value of the serum amylase levels is in those patients in whom the level is raised and continues to rise. In these circumstances, the possibility of a leak from the pancreatic duct or the development of a pseudocyst of the pancreas is sufficiently high to warrant operative intervention.

Radiographic assessment

Traditionally, radiographic studies of the abdomen have formed part of the diagnostic investigations. Reliance is placed on extrapancreatic changes which might reflect parenchymal damage. These include (a) obliteration of the psoas shadow, (b) the presence of ileus and so-called sentinel loops, often with fluid levels, and (c) the presence of any fracture of a lumbar spine or pedicle. It was hoped that with the advent of ultrasonography, a clearer picture of the damaged pancreas might be obtained. By and large, ultrasonography has not been helpful, partly because of the frequently associated ileus and the presence of concomitant injuries. The value of computerized tomography (CT) is currently being evaluated. It has been postulated that a CT scan may become an integral and very early part of the examination of patients known to have sustained severe blunt trauma. Many examples of damage to the pancreas, sometimes clinically unsuspected at the time, have been encountered. CT scanning, when available, may be extremely helpful in determining the need for operation in those patients with minimal symptoms and signs.

SURGICAL TREATMENT

Initial assessment

Operations for pancreatic injury are more often performed because of the knowledge that multiple organs are injured rather than for specific evidence of pancreatic damage. In either event, a long midline incision is the most versatile approach. When the abdomen is opened, priority is given to control of bleeding which may well come from multiple sources such as the liver, the mesenteric and splenic vessels surrounding the pancreas, the portal vein and its tributaries, or the inferior vena cava. Alarming bleeding from intrapancreatic vessels is seldom encountered. When major bleeding has been controlled, a thorough abdominal exploration should be performed with particular attention to examination of the small and large intestine. Any leaking areas are approximated with tissue forceps to preclude further contamination of the peritoneal cavity. Individual lesions may or may not be repaired definitively at this time or may be left until the pancreas has been explored and dealt with if necessary.

Whenever pancreatic injury is suspected, the lesser sac is opened by detaching the greater omentum from the transverse colon to give a clear view of the organ. With an injury on the right side, full mobilization of the duodenum must be performed so that the head of the pancreas can be palpated both anteriorly and posteriorly. Similarly, on the left side, the tail of the pancreas should be mobilized so as to give access to the posterior aspect of the body of the pancreas. This mobilization may be done with or without reflection of the spleen medially. Any haematoma overlying the pancreas must be opened. Unless this is done, a serious lesion of the pancreas and of its main duct may be missed. At worst, such an omission will result in peritonitis and possibly death; at best, fluid may collect in the lesser sac leading to the formation of a pancreatic pseudocyst.

Lacerations without pancreatic duct damage

Simple lacerations of the parenchyma which do not extend to the main pancreatic duct are closed with a series of interrupted non-absorbable sutures. If sufficient pancreatic tissue has been debrided so as to make this difficult, there is no need to approximate the pancreas for the purpose of producing cosmetic normality. Such attempts may in fact be harmful if these result in the accumulation of fluid intraparenchymally. As the area must always be accurately drained with sump drains, a track will be provided for any pancreatic juice that may be secreted postoperatively from the open surface of any unapproximated parenchyma.

Damage to the pancreatic duct

If the main pancreatic duct is transected or ischaemic, the pancreas should be transected just beyond that point. In the past, attempts have been made to repair the duct and to preserve the pancreas. Most of these technical efforts have resulted in failure, which may cause serious morbidity and possibly the death of the patient. While no surgeon wishes to sacrifice pancreatic tissue unnecessarily, the organ is known to have a substantial reserve capacity and diabetes mellitus does not occur until more than 80% of the pancreas is resected unless a predisposition towards diabetes already exists.

If the pancreas is to be resected, an attempt should be made to identify the main pancreatic duct and to close it very carefully with interrupted non-absorbable sutures. This transection is preceded by suture-ligation of the splenic vessels approximately 1 cm behind the upper border of the pancreas. The cut end of the pancreas is closed by approximating the anterior and posterior borders with a series of interrupted non-absorbable sutures in an attempt to produce a fluid-tight closure. Some surgeons have advocated closure by a double layer of staples when the pancreas is soft and not the site of chronic pancreatitis. Sump drains are placed in the bed of the resected pancreas and brought out laterally in such a way as not to overlie the colon where erosion may cause a subsequent colonic fistula.

Preservation of the spleen

The desirability of preserving the spleen is now well accepted. In the past, the spleen was automatically sacrificed in all resections of the body and tail of the pancreas. Recently it has been demonstrated in selected cases of pancreatectomy that the spleen may be preserved by careful techniques.[13]

Damage to the head of the pancreas

A far more complex problem is present when the pancreas is transected close to the head or when the head of the pancreas is partially shattered. In the former case, when it is obvious that about

80% of the pancreas lies to the left of the rupture, an attempt may be made to save the distal half of the pancreas and to anastomose the pancreatic duct to a Roux Y jejunal loop, primarily to preserve the islet cell population of this large segment. The proximal line of resection may be closed as previously described. When the duct is stenotic between the transected end and the ampulla of Vater due to previous alcoholic pancreatitis, a Roux Y loop may be brought over the proximal end to contain a pancreatic fistula if this should develop.

THE DIFFICULT DECISIONS

Massive damage to the head of the pancreas with parenchymal disruption

In this situation, the alternatives lie between simple drainage and a pancreatectomy which carries a high mortality rate (about 40%) due partly to the concomitant injuries which are so frequent in this type of lesion, whether it is caused by blunt trauma or a gunshot wound. The more conservative approach consists of wide local drainage by a series of sump tubes and Penrose drains with the surgeon accepting the overwhelming probability of a pancreatic fistula. In accepting this, however, one is also ensuring with relative certainty that the fistula will be controlled.

Pancreatoduodenal injury

Not infrequently, severe damage to the pancreatic head occurs in conjunction with damage to the duodenal wall. Graham *et al.*[5] reported a 25.5% mortality rate in 68 patients with combined duodenopancreatic injuries. In these circumstances, two problems must be resolved – repair of the duodenum and physiological rest of the pancreas. To achieve the latter, a so-called 'diverticulization of the duodenum' is performed in which an incision is made through the antrum of the stomach that permits the pylorus to be closed from within the stomach by a continuous suture of polyglycolic acid which will dissolve spontaneously in about three weeks, and the establishment of a gastroenterostomy at the point of gastrotomy to provide for gastric emptying. Vagotomy is not necessary for this brief period of pyloric occlusion.[17] If desired, an H_2-receptor antagonist may be administered to produce hypochlorhydria during this period. A T-tube may be inserted into the common bile duct to divert the bile. In addition, intravenous

parenteral hyperalimentation is instituted to improve nutrition and to reduce the volume of pancreatic secretion. With this approach, both the pancreas and the duodenal repair are rested.

The method of duodenal closure will be dictated by the extent of the injury. If possible, the edges of the defect are excised and closed by a double layer of sutures after a good blood supply is assured. This repair may be horizontal or vertical provided an adequate duodenal lumen is preserved. If the defect is so large as to preclude this possibility, two alternatives other than pancreatoduodenectomy remain. Either a loop of jejunum may be attached around the edges of the defect as an onlay graft, or the terminal end of a Roux Y jejunal loop may be anastomosed as a duodenojejunostomy. Resection of the duodenum and primary anastomosis is rarely feasible. Insufficient cases are available to assess the relative efficacy of these procedures, but if the condition of the patient permits prolongation of the operation, Roux Y duodenojejunostomy is much preferred to an onlay graft.

Damage to the retropancreatic common bile duct

This dilemma may be posed by a through-and-through wound to the head of the pancreas which has damaged the common bile duct in its juxtapancreatic course and probably the main pancreatic duct too. This combination of injury may be identified by an intraoperative cholangiogram. If possible, the approach to the injured common bile duct should be divorced from that of the pancreatic duct. If injury to the common bile duct is relatively minor, a T-tube may be inserted in the hope that spontaneous healing will occur. More often, however, the nature of the lesion is such that it is imperative to bypass the bile to prevent local leakage. In such cases, the bile duct is mobilized as far distally as possible and transected just above the area of injury. The distal cut end is oversewn and the proximal end placed into a Roux Y jejunal loop with an end-to-side anastomosis. The peripancreatic tissues are then drained and the possibility of a controlled fistula is accepted.

The available alternatives are limited by the patient's condition, the surgeon's experience and the general lack of reliable data on this injury. Pancreatoduodenectomy may be unavoidable if destruction is extensive, but where the missile tract is small, conservative treatment is favoured by many. This conservative approach includes diverticulization of the duodenum, diversion of bile by the insertion of a T-tube into the common bile duct, drainage of the pancreas anteriorly and posteriorly, or the placement of a Roux Y jejunal loop over the pancreatic head with drainage of the posterior aspect of the pancreas.

Unsalvageable duodenopancreatic injury

A small number of cases of pancreatic injury are so extensive as to preclude any approach other than pancreatoduodenectomy.[8, 18] In the case of blunt trauma, in which a shearing force has torn the common bile duct and caused a large retroperitoneal haemorrhage, a substantial portion of the operation may have been performed by the injury itself. In these circumstances, the surgeon needs to complete the transection at the junction of the head and the body of the pancreas and perform the various necessary anastomoses. In the absence of other serious injury, these patients frequently survive. There is an extremely high mortality rate when patients requiring pancreatoduodenectomy also have damage to the colon, deep fractures of the liver and other associated visceral injuries. About 50% of these patients will also have a major vascular injury. Experience of pancreatoduodenectomy for trauma is described by Yellin and Rossoff,[18] who showed that the mortality in carefully selected patients is in the order of 40%. In the hands of less experienced surgeons the mortality approaches 100%. The technique advocated by Traverso and Longmire[15] may be used, thereby preserving the antrum of the stomach if the anatomical distribution of the injuries does not preclude this technique.

COMPLICATIONS

Major complications of pancreatic injury are (1) pancreatic fistulas occurring in approximately 20%, (2) pseudocysts in about 10%, (3) pancreatic abscesses in about 5%, and (4) occasionally delayed pancreatic ductal stenosis.

Fistula

While fistula is listed as a complication, its presence is often accepted as an inevitable result of initial conservative management. The fistula may result from leakage of an inadequately ligated main pancreatic duct, which could not be identified at the time of pancreatic transection, or from one of a myriad of smaller pancreatic ducts in the resected parenchyma. Until about ten years ago, a pancreatic fistula was greatly

feared. Today, it is recognized that most pancreatic fistulas will close spontaneously in about six weeks in patients whose nutrition is maintained by parenteral hyperalimentation. After this time, if the fistula has not closed spontaneously, a second operation should be undertaken provided the patient is in positive nitrogen balance. At this operation, a Roux-en-Y anastomosis may be successfully placed over the area of drainage or an elective resection of the area may be carried out in selected cases.

Pseudocyst

Pancreatic pseudocysts are most likely to develop when peripancreatic haematomas are not explored and leakage of pancreatic juice is confined within the lesser sac. As long as infection does not occur, the patient may only develop symptoms 3–6 months after the injury. These symptoms are characterized by increasing epigastric discomfort, loss of appetite, nausea, vomiting, and a palpable intra-abdominal mass. The evolution of such a mass may easily be delineated by sequential ultrasonography, and the site of pancreatic ductal leakage may be demonstrated by ERCP. As these pseudocysts connect with a major pancreatic duct, percutaneous needle aspiration is likely to be unsuccessful as definitive treatment. Analysis of serum amylase will show a zymogram characteristic of deaminated pancreatic isoenzymes (so-called 'old' amylase). The treatment of these pseudocysts in most cases is resection of the pancreas just proximal to the leaking duct. In selected cases, it is feasible to anastomose the pancreatic pseudocyst to adjacent stomach or to the jejunum using a Roux Y reconstruction. In our experience, posttraumatic pseudocysts of the pancreas rarely regress spontaneously.

Pseudocysts occurring in acute and chronic pancreatitis are on p. 1306 and p. 1316, respectively.

Pancreatic abscess

Infection of a pancreatic pseudocyst or a frank pancreatic abscess due to infection of damaged pancreatic tissue is always serious. The development of sepsis is identified by increasing fever, leucocytosis, abdominal pain, and later by signs of generalized sepsis. If these signs are neglected, the patient often develops septicaemia and septic shock. A pancreatic abscess has a high mortality and should be identified early by clinical suspicion confirmed on CT scan or ultrasonography. Treatment of infected pancreatic tissue is by surgical removal and thorough debridement. Such debridement may need to be repeated on a number of occasions as delineation of the necrotic pancreas is not always easy and the surgeon is hesitant to excise more tissue than is necessary in a difficult area where haemorrhage is an ever present danger. The recurrence of fever should be regarded as evidence of undrained infected tissue and should always indicate the need for urgent re-exploration. Unless this is done, the patient is likely to develop continuing signs of sepsis and the adult respiratory distress syndrome, which is frequently fatal.

Pancreatic abscess in acute pancreatitis is discussed on p. 1306.

Chronic pancreatic duct stenosis

The development of abdominal pain suggestive of chronic pancreatitis in a patient who has had blunt upper abdominal trauma treated either conservatively or by operation should raise the question of ductal stenosis or a small undetected pseudocyst, especially in the presence of a hyperamylasaemia. The diagnosis of chronic duct stenosis is only achieved by ERCP.[16]

REFERENCES

1 Balasegaram, M. (1979) Surgical management of pancreatic trauma. *Current Problems in Surgery*, **16**, 1–59.
2 Elman, R., Arnesan, N. & Graham, E. A. (1929) Value of blood amylase estimations in the diagnosis of pancreatic disease. *Archives of Surgery*, **19**, 943.
3 Frey, C. (1982) Trauma to the pancreas and duodenum. In *Abdominal Trauma* (Ed.) Blaisdell, W. F. pp. 87–122. New York: Thieme-Stratton.
4 Graham, J. M., Mattox, K. L. & Jordan, G. L. (1978) Traumatic injuries of the pancreas. *American Journal of Surgery*, **136**, 744–748.
5 Graham, J. M., Mattox, K. L., Vaughan, G. D. III & Jordan, G. L. (1979) Combined pancreatoduodenal injuries. *Journal of Trauma*, **19**, 340–346.
6 Heitsch, R. C., Knutson, C. O., Fulton, R. L. & Jones, C. E. (1976) Delineation of critical factors in the treatment of pancreatic trauma. *Surgery*, **80**, 523–529.
7 Jones, R. C. (1978) Management of pancreatic trauma. *Annals of Surgery*, **187**, 555–564.
8 Lowe, R. J., Saletta, J. D. & Moss, G. S. (1977) Pancreaticoduodenectomy for penetrating pancreatic trauma. *Journal of Trauma*, **17**, 732–747.
9 Lucas, C. E. (1977) Diagnosis and treatment of pancreatic and duodenal injury. *Surgical Clinics of North America*, **57**, 49–65.
10 Naffziger, H. C., McCorkle, H. J. (1943) The recognition and management of acute trauma of the pancreas, with particular reference to the use of the serum amylase test. *Annals of Surgery*, **118**, 594–602.
11 Northrup, W. & Simmons, R. L. (1972) Pancreatic trauma: a review. *Surgery*, **71**, 27–43.
12 Olsen, W. R. (1973) The serum amylase in blunt abdominal trauma. *Journal of Trauma*, **13**, 201–204.
13 Robey, E., Mullen, J. T. & Schwab, C. W. (1982) Blunt transection of the pancreas treated by distal pancreatectomy, splenic salvage and hyperalimentation: four cases and review of the literature. *Annals of Surgery*, **196**, 695–699.
14 Stone, H. H., Fabian, T. C., Satiani, B. & Turkleson, M. L. (1981) Experiences in the management of pancreatic trauma. *Journal of Trauma*, **21**, 257–262.
15 Traverso, W. L. & Longmire, W. (1978) Preservation of the pylorus during pancreaticoduodenectomy. *Surgery, Gynecology and Obstetrics*, **146**, 959.
16 Vallon, A. G., Lees, W. R. & Cotton, P. B. (1979) Grey-scale ultrasonography and endoscopic pancreatography after pancreatic trauma. *British Journal of Surgery*, **66**, 169–172.
17 Vaughan, G. D., Frazier, O. H., Graham, D. Y. *et al.* (1975) The use of pyloric exclusion in the management of severe duodenal injuries. *American Journal of Surgery*, **134**, 785–790.
18 Yellin, N. E. & Rosoff, I. (1975) Pancreaticoduodenectomy for combined pancreaticoduodenal injuries. *Archives of Surgery*, **110**, 1177–1182.

CANCER OF THE EXOCRINE PANCREAS

The most important tumours of the pancreas clinically are cancer and endocrine tumours. The former is common but presents late and with few specific features; the latter are rare but often have striking and characteristic presentations.

Exocrine pancreatic cancer is responsible for 5.5% of all cancer deaths. It is the second most frequent cause of death from gastrointestinal cancer and the fourth in overall cancer related mortality following lung, colorectal and breast cancer. The incidence has doubled in Western Europe, tripled in the USA and quadrupled in Japan over the past 40 years. The rising incidence of pancreatic cancer is generally attributed to enhanced exposure to environmental carcinogens, but the influence of the increased frequency of diseases associated with pancreatic cancer cannot be ignored.[26]

The overall prognosis is poor with five-year survival rates of only 1–2%, 85% of the victims being dead within one year of presentation. The topographical anatomy of the pancreas is such that the presence of symptoms usually indicates that the disease has progressed beyond our current ability to effect a cure. The situation is further compounded by delay in diagnosis. Thus only 15% of symptomatic patients consult a physician within one month of the development of symptoms and 10% of patients have undergone cholecystectomy within two years before diagnosis of pancreatic cancer.

Epidemiology

AGE AND SEX

Incidence of pancreatic cancer increases with age and 75% of patients are more than 60 years old at diagnosis. Overall incidence is 8–10 per 100 000 for the USA and Western Europe, increasing to 100 per 100 000 for those aged 75 or older. Males are usually more frequently afflicted than females, as evidenced by a median ratio of 1.6 : 1 around the world. This varies from 1.1 : 1 in Israel to 1.9 : 1 in South Africa.[1]

RACIAL, GEOGRAPHIC AND ETHNIC DIFFERENCES

American blacks have incidence rates 43% higher for men and 48% higher for women than their white counterparts. By contrast African blacks do not have such a correspondingly high incidence. Especially high rates of pancreatic cancer have been reported in Hawaiian men and New Zealand Maori men with incidence rates twice those of their Anglo-Saxon male counterparts.[1]

Japan has one of the lowest rates of pancreatic cancer, but Japanese migrating to the USA have rates higher than both native Japanese and US residents. The incidence rate for second generation US Japanese is significantly below that of US residents – more akin to the native Japanese. This has been interpreted as evidence for exposure of the first generation migrants to carcinogens associated with lower socioeconomic groups in which incidence of pancreatic carcinoma is increased. Pancreatic cancer occurs least frequently in Africa, Asia and Latin America.

SPECIFIC RISK FACTORS

The available information can only be interpreted as indicating a multi-factorial aetiology.

Among environmental factors which have been implicated are occupation, diet and smoking.

Occupation

High rates have been reported in metal workers, coke and gas plant workers and chemists (Table 18.13). Non-oven coke workers have a 4.5-fold increased risk of pancreatic cancer. Specific potential carcinogens include benzidine, beta-naphthylamine and alkylating chemotherapeutic drugs.[19, 20]

Diet

An association between per capita animal fat consumption and disease incidence has been noted. Japanese data link the 4-fold increased incidence of pancreatic cancer to rising consumption of fat and animal protein. Japanese immigrants to the US have been shown to Westernize their diet relatively quickly and have a higher incidence of pancreatic cancer than native Japanese.[13] A relationship between coffee consumption and pancreatic cancer has been reported, with the risk of pancreatic cancer being increased by a factor of 2.7 as coffee consumption increases to three or more cups per day. Although these data were adjusted for smoking the evidence must still be regarded as inconclusive.

Smoking

Cigarette smokers have been shown to have an increased incidence of pancreatic carcinoma which is dose related. This increased incidence tapers off at high doses of tobacco exposure, which may be due to mortality from other tobacco related disease processes. Postulated mechanisms include: secretion and concentration of the carcinogen in bile (including modified bile acids) with subsequent reflux into the pancreatic duct; blood-borne transport of carcinogen to the pancreas; and cigarette-stimulated increase in serum lipid concentration.

Table 18.13 British occupations with highest incidence of cancer of the pancreas.[19, 20]

1968–1970		1959–1963	
Textile workers	117	Furnace, forge, foundry	131
Paper and printing workers	134	Clothing	185
Administrators and managers	124	Service, sport, recreation	117
Professional, technical workers and artists	117	Armed forces	238

(Reported in age-standardized registration ratio for occupied and retired males; 100 = expected incidence.) From the Registrar General (1971, 1975),[19, 20] with kind permission of the authors and the publisher, Her Majesty's Stationery Office.

DISEASES ASSOCIATED WITH PANCREATIC CANCER

Diabetes mellitus
In a study of over 20 000 diabetics, the mortality rate from pancreatic cancer was increased by a factor of 1.82, and the average time interval between diagnosis of diabetes and death from pancreatic carcinoma was 11.4 years. The effect appears to be more pronounced in female diabetics.

Gallstones
A positive association between gallstones and pancreatic cancer has been noted. Autopsy study of pancreatic cancer patients reveals 13.9% of males and 37.9% of females to have gallstones. In a retrospective series, 15% of women with pancreatic cancer had previous cholecystectomy.

Alcoholism and chronic pancreatitis
Epidemiological studies have not demonstrated an association between chronic alcoholism and pancreatic cancer. Acute pancreatitis is not associated with pancreatic carcinoma and data regarding chronic pancreatitis are inconclusive. The pathological changes of chronic pancreatitis, including pancreatic calcification, may occur concurrently with development of pancreatic carcinoma. There is, however, an increased incidence of pancreatic cancer in patients with hereditary pancreatitis.

Pathology

Pancreatic cancer can be of ductal or acinar cell origin. Connective tissue tumours are rare, as are those of uncertain histogenesis. The most common type is duct cell adenocarcinoma; Table 18.14 lists the various subclassifications as delineated in the Memorial Hospital series.

Ductular cell origin
Pancreatic duct cancer arises from duct epithelium and is a mucinous adenocarcinoma. *Giant cell carcinoma* is characterized by bizarre giant cells and sarcomatous elements. A more differentiated variant, the *epulis–osteoid* type, may have a less aggressive course. Prognosis in these tumours is poor.
Adenoacanthoma (*adenosquamous cancer*) is an uncommon tumour containing the elements of an adenocarcinoma and a squamous cell cancer. There is argument over the pathogenesis but these tumours are probably adenocarcinomas with squamous metaplasia. The clinical presen-

Table 18.14 Classification of primary non-endocrine cancers of the pancreas.

Duct (ductular) cell origin		572 (89%)
Duct cell adenocarcinoma	494	
Giant cell carcinoma	27	
Giant cell carcinoma (epulis–osteoid)	1	
Adenosquamous carcinoma	20	
Microadenocarcinoma	16	
Mucinous ('colloid') carcinoma	9	
Cystadenocarcinoma	5	
Acinar cell origin		8 (1%)
Acinar cell carcinoma	7	
Acinar cell cystadenocarcinoma	1	
Uncertain histogenesis		61 (9%)
Pancreaticoblastoma	1	
Papillary and cystic tumour	1	
Mixed type: duct and islet cells	1	
Unclassified	58	
Connective tissue origin		4 (1%)
Osteogenic sarcoma	1	
Leiomyosarcoma	1	
Haemangiopericytoma	1	
Malignant fibrous histiocytoma	1	
Total		645 (100%)

From Cubilla, A. C. & Fitzgerald, P. J. (1980),[3] with kind permission of the authors and the publisher, Williams & Wilkins.

tation is similar to adenocancers and they share a similar degree of malignancy.

Microadenocarcinoma is composed of smaller acini than duct cell adenocarcinoma and is characterized by less fibrosis. *Mucinous adenocarcinoma* produces excessive amounts of mucin; mucinous obstruction of the biliary tract has been reported and renal tubular obstruction due to mucoprotein can occasionally occur with the tumour. Histologically it is characterized by large cystic mucin-filled spaces with clumps of carcinoma cells. *Cystadenoma/carcinoma* is also a mucin-producing tumour and consists of multi-loculated cysts filled with haemorrhagic/ necrotic material. Histologically there is a wide range of cells present ranging from benign to obvious adenocarcinoma. Prognosis in these last two subtypes is better than for duct cell adenocarcinoma.

Acinal cell origin
These rare tumours may comprise purely acinar cells or have a mixture of acinar and ductal elements. The tumours are easily overlooked histologically and labelled as an undifferentiated cancer. They may bear a superficial resemblance to islet cell cancers or oat cell cancers. The tumours occur in younger patients with a clinical presentation similar to that of duct cell adenocarcinoma, but it is possible that widespread

fat necrosis (panniculitis) is a particular association of disseminated acinar cell cancers which contain much lipase activity. Survival is poor.

Connective tissue origin

Rare cancers of uncertain histogenesis and of connective tissue origin have been described and all have a poor prognosis. Of interest in this group is *pancreatoblastoma* which can be mistakenly identified as a neuroblastoma. *Papillary cystic carcinoma* is a relatively rare tumour consisting of sheets of cells arranged in a characteristic periangiomatous manner, and carries a good prognosis. *Mixed islet and duct cell carcinoma* is reported. *Anaplastic carcinoma* which cannot be specifically classified accounts for 5–8% of pancreatic tumours. *Primary sarcoma* of the pancreas is reported although the diagnosis is difficult and can be questioned in the older literature. Several appear to be well documented, however, including osteogenic sarcoma, leiomyosarcoma, haemangiopericytoma and malignant fibrous histocytoma. These comprise less than 0.1% of most series.[3]

Pancreatic lymphoma

These are very rare tumours but are clinically important because they may respond to radiotherapy or chemotherapy. The pathologist may have considerable difficulty in distinguishing a pancreatic lymphoma, particularly reticulum cell sarcoma, from undifferentiated anaplastic cancers.

Benign tumours

Benign tumours are exceptionally uncommon. Adenomas are reported as having arisen from ductular or acinar elements and they have a tendency to become cystic.

Clinical features

The most common presenting symptoms of pancreatic cancer are weight loss, jaundice and pain (Table 18.15). Weight loss is probably the earliest feature and is present initially in 70% of patients. Abdominal pain occurs in 54% of patients at presentation and jaundice in about 20–30%. Cholestasis due to common bile duct obstruction does affect all but a few patients late in the disease; only 20% of jaundiced patients will have an entirely pain free course.

The frequency of an abnormal glucose tolerance test in patients with pancreatic cancer may be as high as 70%. Thus the development of diabetes mellitus in the absence of a positive family history should raise suspicion of a pancreatic tumour. Other symptoms are non-

Table 18.15 Presenting symptoms and physical signs of pancreatic cancer.

	Percentage of patients
Symptoms	
Loss of weight	70–90
Jaundice	20–30
Pain	50–60
Vomiting	15–25
Change in bowel habits	5–20
Pruritus	20
Signs	
Hepatomegaly	60–70
Jaundice (noted by physician)	54
Abdominal mass	33
Palpable gallbladder	15–20
Thrombophlebitis	10
Ascites	5

specific and include nausea, vomiting, pruritus, flatulence, change in bowel habits and generalized weakness.

Physical examination frequently reveals jaundice, hepatomegaly, abdominal mass with or without tenderness, a palpable gallbladder or ascites. Only one third of patients with clinical hepatomegaly have an enlarged liver at laparotomy; the remainder have a pancreatic mass erroneously perceived as the liver. Venous thrombosis develops in about 10% of patients. The polyarthritis–panniculitis–eosinophilia syndrome is rare and is associated with an extensive metastasizing pancreatic carcinoma which secretes excessive amounts of lipase, causing widespread fat necrosis predominantly of the subcutaneous fat and fatty bone marrow.[24]

Diagnostic investigations

Pancreatic cancer is frequently diagnosed after the tumour has advanced beyond cure because of the infrequent recognition of early non-specific symptoms, a late presentation, the lack of reliable screening tests and poor definition of the population at risk. A high index of suspicion and a thorough understanding of available diagnostic techniques are essential for early diagnosis and effective treatment. The advantages and limitations of each diagnostic investigation must be considered in approaching the symptomatic patient.

Biochemistry

Serum alkaline phosphatase is raised in more than 80% of patients. Hyperamylasaemia occurs in 15%. Up to 80% of patients will have glucose intolerance when challenged with a 5-h glucose tolerance test.[7]

Radiology

The abdominal plain film should be examined for pancreatic calcification, a mass, fat necrosis, pancreatic abscess and changes in bowel gas pattern. The pancreatic mass effect is more frequently due to benign pseudocysts than to carcinoma. Fat necrosis and changes in bowel gas pattern are usually secondary to pancreatitis. Up to 4% of patients with pancreatic calcification will have a coexisting pancreatic carcinoma. If the calcification is the result of hereditary pancreatitis, however, the incidence is significantly higher; 20% of these patients eventually die of pancreatic malignancy.

Patients presenting with upper abdominal complaints are frequently first studied with a barium meal, but this will miss 50% of cancers of the head of the pancreas and all but the most extensive tumours of the body and tail. With the addition of hypotonic duodenography and double contrast technique, accuracy is increased to 80% for head of pancreas lesions but this still leaves most distal disease unrecognized.[9]

Ultrasound

Sensitivity in prospective studies ranges from 80 to 95% and specificity from 85 to 99%. Ultrasound can routinely identify tumours down to 2 cm in size. Small defects in the parenchyma can be detected prior to changes in size and contour of the gland as a whole. In pancreatic cancer true diagnostic advance is measured by ability to discriminate resectable tumours; ultrasound appears to have this capacity, detecting up to 88% of resectable cancers prospectively.[22]

Ultrasound is the initial procedure of choice in patients with a suspected pancreatic cancer; it fulfils many criteria for a screening test, being safe, non-invasive, repeatable, available to outpatients, and relatively inexpensive. When used by skilled personnel, highly reliable results are obtained. Ultrasound, however, is observer dependent and its main limitations include significant variation in technical capability and high frequency of failed or inconclusive examination. Failed or technically inadequate studies occur in 20–30% of cases and are usually not included in the calculation of sensitivity of the test.

Computerized tomography (CT)

Pancreatic carcinoma is detected by CT as a focal or diffuse mass altering the contour of the pancreas. Small lesions may be missed because the attenuation of the tumour tissue is similar to that of the surrounding normal parenchyma. An abnormal pancreas can be identified by CT scan in 80% of patients. The differentiation between neoplastic and inflammatory disease of the pancreas, however, is quite difficult with CT. The advantages include a very low incidence of failed examination, the ability to outline reliably the whole of the gland, and the detection of deposits in regional lymph nodes and liver.[23]

At present CT scan is best utilized in conjunction with other available radiological techniques when assessing patients with early, potentially resectable pancreatic cancer.[16] Lack of specificity and sensitivity along with expense and radiation exposure make CT a poor candidate for pancreatic cancer screening. In more advanced disease it is useful to define extent of local tumour and metastasis. Its ability to image the pancreas successfully when other sensitive techniques have failed make it particularly useful in the overall approach to diagnosing pancreatic cancer. The performance of CT scanning in diagnosing early pancreatic cancer may well improve as new-generation scanners with better resolution emerge.[11]

Nuclear magnetic resonance (NMR) computerized scanners may also prove to have the discriminatory capability required to detect early lesions.

Endoscopic retrograde cholangio-pancreatography (ERCP)

ERCP has proved very sensitive in the diagnosis of pancreatic carcinoma. Delineation of ductal anatomy enables early diagnosis of resectable tumours, and cannulation of the ampulla can produce adequate specimens for reliable cytological diagnosis of pancreatic cancer.

The technique has a sensitivity of 85–95% and a specificity of 90%. A positive test is predictive in 85% of cases and a negative test reliably excludes pancreatic cancer in greater than 90%. ERCP is the most accurate test to discriminate between pancreatitis and pancreatic cancer. In combination with cytology and stimulated pancreatic secretion assay as a single procedure, it is the single most useful investigation overall in the diagnosis of pancreatic cancer.[15]

The ability of ERCP to detect duodenal and ampullary tumours, both frequently resectable lesions and often missed using other diagnostic techniques, provides further reason to include this investigation as part of the evaluation of a patient suspected of having pancreatic cancer. Limitations include a cannulation failure of 15–20% in experienced hands and sepsis or pancreatitis following injection of contrast into pancreatic ducts.

Angiography, venography

Pancreatic arteriography with visualization of small, intrapancreatic arteries can detect and differentiate small, resectable pancreatic neoplasms. It is also useful in staging and in determining the resectability of neoplasms. The accuracy of diagnosis with arteriography varies from 40 to 96%. The degree of visualization of the pancreatic vasculature relates directly to the diagnostic sensitivity of the technique with coeliac and superior mesenteric artery injections being only 60–70% accurate. With the use of vasoconstrictors, magnification, and side-hole catheters, more selective arteriography is possible. Superselective angiography is possible in 85–95% of patients, and diagnostic accuracy improves to 90% with detection of tumours as small as 2 cm.

Several prospective studies using selective (coeliac and superior mesenteric artery) injections for 80% of patients and superselective (splenic, gastroduodenal, and dorsal pancreatic artery) injections in 20% of patients show diagnostic sensitivity of 70–75% and specificity of 71–91%. Thus the diagnostic yield for angiography is low, but its main value lies in the identification of the anatomy of the arterial supply of the foregut before surgery. It may also provide evidence of non-resectability, i.e. large vessel encasement or major venous obstruction. Identification of resectable tumours of the pancreas using combined arteriography and ERCP may be as high as 94%.[21]

Duodenal drainage studies

Decreased volume, bicarbonate and enzyme content are the most frequent abnormalities. Abnormalities in secretion occur in 90% of patients with either pancreatitis or pancreatic cancer, and duodenal drainage studies are not very useful in differentiating the two diseases. Cytological findings when positive are discriminative. The limitations of duodenal drainage are lack of specificity and the necessary expertise to make an accurate cytological diagnosis.[18]

Pancreatic cytology

Preoperative cytological diagnosis is possible using either a percutaneous fine needle aspiration technique or at ERCP. The sensitivity rate is 80–95% using fine needle aspiration techniques with very low morbidity. CT and ultrasound guidance for fine needle placement affords an opportunity to confirm the nature of suspect lesions. The technique may be used intraoperatively.

The collection of cytological specimens during ERCP is more accurate than collection by duodenal drainage. Methods include collection of pancreatic juice, brushings of pancreatic duct and ERCP-fine needle aspiration. A diagnostic sensitivity of 50–85% can be expected, although evidence for good correlation with resectable tumours is lacking at present. Preoperative cytology when positive is quite useful. In patients without biliary or duodenal obstruction, positive cytology will obviate laparotomy. The limitations include the need for an experienced cytologist, potential needle tract dissemination of tumour and the specialized technique for the collection of specimens.[12]

Tumour markers

At present no single tumour marker has been identified to be useful in identifying patients with early, resectable carcinoma of the pancreas. An oncofetal antigen complex present in human fetal pancreas has been evaluated for its prognostic value and has proved to be the most valuable of the markers identified so far with a sensitivity of 91%; the false-positive rate, however, is 30%. The true negative accuracy determined prospectively is 94%, making the test clinically useful in excluding disease. Because many of the false-positives are patients with pancreaticobiliary disease, the test may have value in screening. Other pancreatic cancer associated antigens have been identified but have similar specificity problems.

Carcinoembryonic antigen (CEA) has not proved useful in the early diagnosis of pancreatic cancer; the false-positive rate among patients with other cancers and gastric diseases is excessively high. High or rising CEA levels are indicative of extensive and metastatic tumours. Alpha-fetoprotein is of no value in the diagnosis of pancreatic cancer.

Specific isoenzymes of ribonuclease, deoxyribonuclease, amylase and galactosyl transferase are elevated in pancreatic cancer. Hormones including gastrin, parathyroid hormone, glucagon, insulin, C-peptide and human chorionic gonadotropin have been screened prospectively. Complement fragments related to the presence of tumour and immunological monitoring for pancreatic cancer have been identified. However, none of these tests has been sufficiently sensitive or specific for clinical use.[25]

Radionuclide scanning and thermography

Selenomethionine scanning of the pancreas is non-specific and overall accuracy is about 50%.

Thermography is also insensitive. At present neither test has a role in routine diagnosis of pancreatic cancer.

Laparoscopy
Laparoscopy is an under-utilized but effective diagnostic tool. Its value lies in the ability to visualize the pancreas and liver directly, and to biopsy suspicious nodules. Visualization of the pancreas with target cytological specimens is possible in 70% of patients. Its limitations include the need for technical proficiency, and the difficulties when there is obesity or adhesions from previous surgery. Laparoscopy often obviates the necessity for laparotomy in advanced intra-abdominal disease whilst enabling a histological diagnosis to be made.[5]

Laparotomy with pancreatic biopsy
Histological confirmation of pancreatic cancer should be sought during the time that the patient is being evaluated. If metastatic disease is identified, malignant tissue is usually available from the liver by percutaneous needle biopsy, laparoscopy or minilaparotomy with liver biopsy. If there is no evidence of metastatic tumour and cytological methods fail to identify malignant cells, operative confirmation of the diagnosis should be sought with simultaneous biopsy and assessment of resectability. Pancreatic resection is probably not indicated in the absence of histological confirmation of malignant disease.[4]

The techniques for pancreatic biopsy include needle biopsy which may be direct or trans-duodenal, fine needle aspiration for cytology, and wedge biopsy. Complications include haemorrhage, pancreatitis, pancreatic fistula and duodenotomy leaks, all of which are potentially fatal. The morbidity for the procedure is 5%, death occurs in 1.7%, and the false-negative rate is 10–15%. A wedge biopsy is associated with fewer complications and false-negative results than needle biopsy. The technique of intraoperative fine needle aspiration and cytological examination may reduce complications and has comparable diagnostic accuracy.

Laparotomy is often used in evaluating a patient for pancreatic cancer because it allows immediate histological confirmation of cancer, adequate staging, palliative bypass procedures and definitive evaluation of resectability.

Clinical staging (Table 18.16) is a useful prognostic tool, and also enables comparisons to be made of treatment results in various cancer patient groups.[17]

Table 18.16 Staging of pancreatic cancer.

Stage I
T_1, T_2, N_0, M_0 – No direct extension (or unknown) or limited direct extension of tumour to adjacent viscera, with no (or unknown) regional metastases. Limited direct extension is defined as involvement of organs adjacent to the pancreas (duodenum, common bile duct or stomach) that could be removed en bloc with the pancreas if a curative resection was attempted

Stage II
T_3, N_0, M_0 – Further direct extension of tumour into adjacent viscera, with no (or unknown) lymph node involvement and no distant metastases

Stage III
T_{1-3}, N_1, M_0 – Regional node metastases without clinical evidence of distant metastases

Stage IV
T_{1-3}, N_{0_1}, M_1 – Distant metastatic disease in liver and other sites present

Treatment

SURGICAL

Surgical cure of pancreatic carcinoma is possible in a small number of patients who present at an early stage. For many others meaningful palliation can be achieved surgically through biliary and enteric diversion procedures. With an average operative mortality of 20% and an overall five-year survival of less than 5%, some authorities recommend bypass rather than pancreatoduodenectomy for all pancreatic cancer patients.[14]

The average survival following a bypass procedure is 4.3 months (3–8.1 months) compared to 16.5 months (10.3–22.3 months) following resection of all types. If the surgeon is able to resect with histologically tumour-free margins, average survival is 30.3 months. The operative mortality from bypass procedures is 6%, but in specialized centres it may be 10% or less for pancreatoduodenectomy. It is important to appreciate that periampullary tumours other than pancreatic cancer have five-year survival rates of 25% or greater; these tumours are often impossible to distinguish from pancreatic cancer at laparotomy, thus improving overall rate of cure in resection procedures.

The use of resection as a palliative procedure in pancreatic cancer cannot be justified. If lymph node metastases are demonstrated at laparotomy, a bypass is just as effective as resection. The best palliation is an end-to-side choledochojejunostomy using a Roux-en-Y jejunal limb. Cholecystojejunostomy is acceptable if the gallbladder is distended and the cystic duct is widely patent, and then an enteroenterostomy some 40 cm distal to the anastomosis is required to divert the stream of enteric contents. It is advisable to employ gastric drainage routinely because 13% of patients having a biliary bypass alone are reported to require a second laparotomy for duodenal obstruction. A definitive biopsy is essential even if resection is not contemplated.

Resective procedures include radical pancreatoduodenectomy (Whipple procedure), total pancreatectomy and regional pancreatectomy. In considering the choice between the Whipple procedure and a total pancreatectomy for cancer of the head of the pancreas, the multifocal potential of the tumour must be appreciated. Pathological examination of total pancreatectomy specimens reveals tumour multi-centricity in 15–40% of cases, and 20% of partial pancreatectomy specimens from Whipple procedures reveal tumour at the line of resection. Total pancreatectomy avoids the need for the potentially dangerous pancreatic–jejunal anastomosis and allows for an en-bloc tumour resection with larger numbers of harvested nodes;[2, 8] but diabetes mellitus is difficult to control.

On the other hand, the theoretical increase in morbidity from partial pancreatectomy (Whipple procedure) is not apparent and the five-year survival does not seem to be affected by choice of operative procedure. Partial pancreatectomy leads to salvage of exocrine and endocrine pancreatic function in some patients, although less frequently than one might hope. Thus the controversy between partial and total pancreatectomy for cancer of the head persists. Our practice is the selective use of total pancreatectomy for patients who are insulin-dependent diabetics and when tumour is found on frozen section at the margins of the resected head.

Gastrointestinal bleeding is a late complication in 6% of patients with a pancreaticoduodenectomy. Anastomotic ulcers occur frequently following total pancreatectomy, and a vagotomy or antral resection following subtotal or total pancreatectomy has been recommended. Relief from pain is best obtained by a percutaneous coeliac plexus block.

RADIATION AND CHEMOTHERAPY

Preoperative radiation has improved resectability in patients considered unresectable at a first laparotomy. Prospective randomized studies, however, have shown that radiation therapy alone is not effective in treating unresectable pancreatic carcinoma. Intraoperative implantation of iodine-125 combined with external beam irradiation may be useful in patients with localized but unresectable tumours.[6]

5-Fluorouracil (5-FU) is the most extensively studied chemotherapeutic agent for pancreatic cancer; generally less than 20% of patients show any response. Mitomycin C has activity similar to that of 5-FU. Streptozotocin and doxorubicin (Adriamycin) have also been used. Combination chemotherapy using these agents has been reported to improve response rate to 30–43%, but this is probably an optimistic figure.[27]

The combination of radiation therapy with chemotherapy holds some promise. Patients receiving 5-FU plus either 4000 or 6000 rads via external beam showed statistically improved survival over radiation alone.

REFERENCES

1 Berg, J. W. & Connelly, R. R. (1979) Updating the epidemiologic data on pancreatic cancer. *Seminars in Oncology*, **6**, 275–283.
2 Cooperman, A. M., Herter, F. P., Marboe, C. A. *et al.* (1981) Pancreatoduodenal resection and total pancreatectomy – an institutional review. *Surgery*, **90**, 707–712.
3 Cubilla, A. L. & Fitzgerald, P. J. (1980) Surgical pathology of tumours of the exocrine pancreas. In *Tumours of the Pancreas* (Ed.) Moossa, A. R., pp. 159–193. London: Williams & Wilkins.
4 Cuschieri, A. & Wormsley, K. G. (1980) The pancreas. *Recent Advances in Gastroenterology*, No. 4 (Ed.) Bouchier, I. A. D., p. 223. London: Churchill Livingstone.
5 Cuschieri, A., Hall, A. W. & Clark, J. (1978) Value of laparoscopy in the diagnosis and management of pancreatic carcinoma. *Gut*, **19**, 672–678.
6 Dobelbower, R. R. (1981) Current radiotherapeutic approaches to pancreatic cancer. *Cancer*, **47**, 1729–1733.
7 Fitzgerald, P. J., Fortner, J. G., Watson, R. C. *et al.* (1978) The value of diagnostic aids in detecting pancreatic cancer. *Cancer*, **41**, 868–879.
8 Fortner, J. G. (1981) Surgical principles for pancreatic cancer: Regional total and sub-total pancreatectomy. *Cancer*, **47**, 1712–1718.
9 Frank, P. H. & Moossa, A. R. (1980) The value of standard radiological investigations in the diagnosis of pancreatic neoplasms. In *Tumours of the Pancreas* (Ed.) Moossa, A. R. London: Williams & Wilkins.
10 Go, V. L. W., Taylor, W. F. & DiMagno, E. P. (1981) Efforts at early diagnosis of pancreatic cancer: The Mayo Clinic experience. *Cancer*, **47**, 1698–1703.
11 Kolmannskog, F., Schrumpf, E., Bergan, A. & Larsen, S. (1982) Diagnostic value of computed tomography in pancreatic carcinoma: a comparison with other radiologic methods. *Acta Radiologica, Diagnosis*, **23**, 131–141.
12 Kolins, M. D., Bernacki, E. G. & Schwab, R. (1981) Diagnosis of pancreatic lesions by percutaneous aspiration biopsy. *Acta Cytologica*, **25**, 675–677.
13 Lin, R. S. & Kessler, I. I. (1981) A multifactorial model for pancreatic cancer in man. *Journal of the American Medical Association*, **245**, 147–152.
14 Moossa, A. R. (1980) Surgical treatment of pancreatic cancer. In *Tumours of the Pancreas* (Ed.) Moossa, A. R., pp. 443–467. London: Williams & Wilkins.

15 Moossa, A. R. & Levin, B. (1979) Collaborative studies in the diagnosis of pancreatic cancer. *Seminars in Oncology*, **6**, 298–308.

16 Moss, A. A., Federle, M. F., Shapiro, H. A. *et al.* (1980) The combined uses of computed tomography and endoscopic retrograde cholangiopancreatography in the assessment of suspected pancreatic neoplasm: A blind clinical evaluation. *Radiology*, **134**, 159–163.

17 Pollard, H. M. (1981) Cancer of the pancreas task force: staging of cancer of the pancreas. *Cancer*, **47**, 1631–1637.

18 Reber, H. A., Tweedie, J. H. & Austin, J. L. (1981) Pancreatic secretions as a clue to the presence of pancreatic cancer. *Cancer*, **47**, 1646–1651.

19 Registrar General (1971) *Decennial Supplement – England and Wales 1961, Occupational Mortality Table.* London: HMSO.

20 Registrar General (1975) *Statistical Review of England and Wales for Three Years 1968–1970, Supplement on Cancer.* London: HMSO.

21 Rosch, J. & Keller, F. S. (1981) Pancreatic arteriography, transhepatic pancreatic venography and pancreatic venous sampling in diagnosis of pancreatic cancer. *Cancer*, **47**, 1679–1684.

22 Taylor, K. J. W., Buchin, P. J., Viscomi, G. N. & Rosenfield, A. T. (1981) Ultrasonic scanning of the pancreas. *Radiology*, **138**, 211–213.

23 Weyman, P. J., Stanley, R. J. & Levitt, R. G. (1981) Computed tomography in evaluation of the pancreas. *Seminars in Roentgenology*, **16**, 301–311.

24 Wood, R. A. B. (1981) The diagnosis of pancreatic cancer. In *Surgical Review 2* (Ed.) Lumley, J. S. P. & Craven, J. L. pp. 107–117. London: Pitman Medical.

25 Wood, R. A. B. & Moossa, A. R. (1977) The prospective evaluation of tumour–associated antigens for the early diagnosis of pancreatic cancer. *British Journal of Surgery*, **64**, 718–720.

26 Young, J. L., Jr., Asine, A. J. & Pollock, E. S. (1978) *SEER Program. Cancer Incidence and Mortality in the United States 1973–1976.* Bethesda: US Department of Health Education and Welfare.

27 Zimmerman, S. E., Smith, F. P. & Schein, P. S. (1981) Chemotherapy of pancreatic carcinoma. *Cancer*, **47**, 1724–1728.

TUMOURS OF THE ENDOCRINE PANCREAS

ZOLLINGER–ELLISON SYNDROME (GASTRINOMA)

Zollinger and Ellison in 1955 described a syndrome with a diagnostic triad of (1) fulminating ulcer diathesis, (2) recurrent ulceration unresponsive to standard medical and surgical approaches, and (3) the presence of non-beta-cell islet tumours of the pancreas.[8] That this was an endocrine syndrome was proved when Gregory *et al.* extracted gastrin from these tumours in 1960.[3] It has since become appreciated that many of these tumours can be malignant. In addition, the impact of a precise diagnostic tool

in gastrin radioimmunoassay (RIA) and the discovery of potent H_2-receptor antagonist drugs have changed the natural history and therapy of the disorder.

Epidemiology

In Northern Ireland the incidence is in the order of 1 per 1.5 million of the population, which is somewhat less than half that of insulinoma. It can be calculated from the incidence of peptic ulcer in the population that in 0.7 per 1000 patients with peptic ulceration, the disease will be due to a gastrinoma.[1] However, the incidence of gastrinoma is likely to be higher among peptic ulcer sufferers referred to hospital for diagnostic purposes and in particular in those with a disease either severe enough or with complications to require surgery. Many patients will present to surgeons, who must therefore be on the alert for the syndrome.

Approximately one third of patients have the autosomal dominant syndrome of multiple endocrine adenomatosis, type I (MEA I), where tumours can also be found most commonly in the parathyroids but also in adrenals, pituitary, ovaries and thyroid (see Chapter 9).

Aetiology

In the majority, a tumour is sited in the pancreas. However, tumours can also be located in the duodenum or stomach, in structures adjacent to the pancreas, for example regional lymph nodes or the omentum mesentery, and rarely in the ovary or parathyroid. Most of the pancreatic tumours are islet cell adenomas or adenocarcinomas, but tumours of ductal origin, microadenomas, islet cell nests and focal or generalized nesidioblastosis have been recorded. The quantitation of hyperplasia of islets is difficult, and the islets should be clearly shown to contain gastrin before they can be considered as contributing to the syndrome.

Patients with the sporadic disease tend to exhibit metastases most frequently to liver and regional lymph nodes. Patients with the MEA syndrome usually have benign tumours but they may have these in multiple primary sites.

Gastrin is invariably produced from the tumour although it is conceivable that other peptide hormones which stimulate acid secretion may cause the syndrome, but this has so far not been described. Other peptides might also be secreted from the tumour, particularly pancreatic polypeptide.[7] The presence of multiple hormones being secreted from the tumour may give rise to other associated syndromes such as insulinoma, glucagonoma, the watery diarrhoea, hypokalaemic and achlorhydric syndrome, etc. In the MEA subjects separate discrete tumours may secrete different peptides whereas in the sporadic cases the different peptides are produced within the same tumour.

Pathogenesis

Nearly all the features of the disease can be explained by the excessive production of gastrin from tumour cells, causing hypersecretion of acid which leads to peptic ulceration. The syndrome can be controlled by inhibiting gastric acid secretion either surgically or pharmacologically.

Clinical features

The history is usually short (less than two years). The peptic ulcers are often multiple and atypical in site including oesophagus, distal duodenum and upper jejunum. Complications are frequent including perforation, pyloric stenosis, haemorrhage and gastro-jejuno-colic fistulas. The syndrome inevitably recurs after standard surgical procedures. Hepatomegaly may be present indicating metastases and one third of patients have evidence of the MEA syndrome, particularly hyperparathyroidism. Diarrhoea is quoted as a feature but is relatively uncommon in the Northern Irish series and may suggest secretion of peptides in addition to gastrin.

The impact of the diagnostic procedure of gastrin RIA and the therapeutic intervention of the H_2-receptor antagonist drugs is only now being assessed, but they undoubtedly have an impact on the classical features of the Zollinger–Ellison syndrome. The early use of the gastrin RIA should lead to early diagnosis and an avoidance of catastrophic complications. Although H_2-receptor antagonist drugs can be life saving in this syndrome, they can nevertheless delay the diagnosis, for if they are introduced prior to establishing an accurate diagnosis, the patient will improve, and the clinician will be lulled into a situation of false security. There are patients with gastrinoma who cannot be differentiated on clinical grounds from the many patients with peptic ulcer who do not have the syndrome.

Diagnosis

The clinician is confronted with the problem of attempting to differentiate the uncommon gastrinoma patient from the mass of peptic ulcer sufferers who do not have a gastrinoma. Clinical features alone are not helpful although any of the following observations will increase the probability of a gastrinoma: multiple ulcers in unusual sites, diarrhoea, complications of peptic ulcer, recurrence after gastric surgery, a family history of peptic ulcer, hepatomegaly, other endocrine disorders particularly hyperparathyroidism. However, the absence of any of these features does not exclude the diagnosis.

The main, specific, diagnostic tool is the RIA of gastrin. Some authorities hold that a gastrin assay should be performed on every peptic ulcer patient whose symptoms are severe enough to be referred to a hospital for management. Such an approach may not be feasible in some centres, but if such a policy is not undertaken, gastrinoma patients will not be diagnosed, or they will be diagnosed later in their disease when management becomes more difficult.

Gastrin RIA

The gastrin assay used should be one which identifies the two major gastrin species G17 and G34. In the authors' laboratory 95% of normal subjects have levels <100 ng/l in the fasting state, and <300 ng/l after a meal. The diagnostic value of a fasting sample is greater than a random sample, although if a random sample falls within the normal fasting range, a sample in the fasting state is not required. All gastrinoma patients in the Northern Irish series have had elevated fasting gastrin levels,[2] although other centres have occasionally reported gastrinoma patients with normal levels. If the condition is strongly suspected then fasting samples on three separate days would eliminate the possibility that the diagnosis may be missed.

Gastric hypersecretion

Patients with a gastrinoma will exhibit gastric hypersecretion. This should be greater than 1 l containing more than 100 mmol/l acid on a 12-h overnight secretion. However, a 1-h basal acid output (BAO) usually suffices, and should exceed 15 mmol/l. Patients who have been subjected to previous gastric surgical procedures will meet the same criteria, but in such patients the diagnosis should be considered when the BAO exceeds 5 mmol/l. Patients with gastrinoma have a poor response to maximal stimulation with pentagastrin (maximum acid output, MAO) and therefore have reduced MAO/BAO ratios.

The combination of an elevated fasting gastrin and an elevated BAO makes the diagnosis of a gastrinoma almost certain.

Tumour localization

Ultrasound (US), isotope scanning, and computerized axial tomography (CT) have revolutionized the location of tumours. The liver should be scanned for metastases. As the primary tumour is most likely to be present in the pancreas this organ should receive the closest scrutiny. US and CT scanning of the pancreas should be the first approach and coeliac axis angiography only undertaken if these procedures are negative or indeterminate. Should pancreatic radiology prove negative then the clinician should be aware of the possibility of a tumour in unusual sites (see above). It is conceivable that some tumours may be too small to identify, or that hyperplasia of islets may be the underlying abnormality, although this is exceedingly rare. If a tumour cannot be identified then the condition of antral G cell hyperplasia should be excluded (see below).

Other hormone assays

Plasma secretin is elevated in patients with a gastrinoma[6] because of the acid hypersecretion. Circulating pancreatic polypeptide is frequently elevated in these patients and in those with other islet cell tumours. Increased secretion of pancreatic polypeptide gives rise to no specific clinical syndrome, and although a normal level does not exclude an islet cell tumour, the finding of an elevated level is strongly in support of the diagnosis. The relevance of pancreatic polypeptide in the syndrome is still being assessed, but elevated levels are encountered in subjects with and without liver metastases.

Assessment of the parathyroids, adrenals and pituitary should be undertaken to exclude the MEA syndrome. A number of other pancreatic and gut hormones should be assayed to exclude multiple hormone involvement; e.g., insulin, glucagon, somatostatin, vasoactive intestinal polypeptide, substance P, neurotensin, calcitonin, etc.

Provocative tests for gastrin release have been advocated, e.g. intravenous secretin, calcium and glucagon,[5] when gastrin levels have been in the borderline range. Patients with a gastrinoma are reported to have a significant release of gastrin after these tests but in the authors' experience there are so many false-positives and false-negatives with the secretin test, that it has proved unhelpful.

Patients with a gastrinoma show a poor gastrin response to eating, suggesting autonomous secretion from the tumour or a feedback effect of the tumour on normal gastrin cells.

Differential diagnosis

This involves an assessment of the causes of hypergastrinaemia once the raised hormone level is identified in a patient with peptic ulceration.

Antral G-cell hyperplasia

Antral G cells become hyperplastic in hypo- or achlorhydric states, although rarely this is associated with hypersecretion of acid when the diagnosis of a gastrinoma is mimicked.[4] Such patients will have fasting hypergastrinaemia and hypersecretion of acid within the range of the Zollinger–Ellison syndrome, but they do not harbour a tumour. The gastrin response to a standard meal is helpful in that patients with antral G-cell hyperplasia have excessive gastrin release whereas patients with a gastrinoma have impaired release. Endoscopic biopsy of the antrum with estimation of gastrin content by RIA and immunohistochemistry may be helpful, gastrinoma patients having reduced gastrin, and patients with antral G-cell hyperplasia having increased gastrin levels and increased numbers of gastrin cells. However, such data should be interpreted with caution because of the variable scatter and distribution of G cells in the antrum, making a small biopsy sample potentially unrepresentative.

Hypo- or achlorhydric states

Patients with achlorhydria and hypochlorhydria exhibit circulating hypergastrinaemia due to the loss of the normal feedback mechanism on gastrin release. Patients with achlorhydria, especially those with pernicious anaemia, can have massive elevations of circulating gastrin. Hypochlorhydric states associated with gastric cancer or gastric ulcer show more modest elevations of circulating gastrin. Estimation of gastric secretion and, where relevant, of circulating parietal cell and intrinsic factor antibodies, and a gastric biopsy indicating atrophic gastritis will clearly differentiate such patients from those with a gastrinoma.

Postvagotomy state

Mild elevations (100–200 ng/l, fasting) of gastrin are encountered after a vagotomy, presumably related to hypochlorhydria.

Renal failure

Patients with renal failure exhibit elevated gastrin levels probably because of failure of renal clearance of the peptide. Frequently such patients have atrophic gastritis but some may exhibit the features of a pseudogastrinoma when recognition and prompt management is required.

H_2-Receptor antagonist therapy

This therapy causes elevation of postprandial gastrin levels but has only a slight effect on fasting levels. However, since, by definition, the drugs inhibit acid secretion, the measurement of acid secretion must only be undertaken when the patient has discontinued therapy for at least 48 h. Therapy during this period can be replaced by adequate antacids. As newer and more potent H_2-receptor antagonist drugs become available, the effects on circulating gastrin may become more marked.

Miscellaneous

A number of miscellaneous causes of hypergastrinaemia are rarely encountered: short gut syndrome, and retained and isolated antrum.

Treatment

Management should be directed along two fronts: (1) the control of the hormone (gastrin) and its action, and (2) the control of the tumour, which, if effectively dealt with, will also eradicate the hormonal effects. The ultimate aim should be to extinguish or eradicate the tumour and thus the syndrome. However, this is only sometimes possible. A number of different approaches are open to the clinician depending upon the circumstances.

1 Surgical excision of the tumour with resultant cure of the syndrome without resort to control of the target organ (stomach). This is indicated in the rare circumstances when a single, simple tumour is clearly identified and amenable to surgical resection. Cure would be indicated by a return of circulating gastrin and acid secretion to normal levels. Failure to remove the tumour might either necessitate further excision or control of the target organ by gastrectomy or H_2-receptor antagonist therapy, although many would advocate this approach initially.

2 Where a surgical cure appears less likely (e.g., multiple tumours, local metastases, etc.) then the surgeon when possible should still attempt surgical excision but must combine this with either total gastrectomy or H_2-receptor antagonist therapy.

3 When the tumour cannot be resected, usually due to liver metastases, then manage-

ment is by total gastrectomy or H_2-receptor antagonist therapy. The tumour can then be treated with cytotoxic therapy, usually streptozotocin or by embolization procedures.

Control of the target organ

Prior to the availability of H_2-receptor antagonist therapy, the target organ could only be controlled by total gastrectomy. H_2-receptor antagonist therapy is clearly indicated during the control of the syndrome prior to surgery when the patient may be severely ill and requiring considerable rehabilitation. Most authors, post tumour surgery, would now advocate the use of H_2-receptor antagonist therapy rather than total gastrectomy. Patients who have undergone total gastrectomy face nutritional disturbances and dumping symptoms, although these can usually be controlled. Clinicians advocating total gastrectomy point to its lasting control of the syndrome.

H_2-receptor antagonist drugs should be given in a dose and frequency necessary to render the patients hypochlorhydric. Either cimetidine (200 mg t.d.s. and 400 mg nocte) or ranitidine (150 mg b.d.) may be used, and doses larger than conventional may be needed. Should one drug be ineffective then another may be effective. Occasionally acid secretion cannot be controlled and total gastrectomy should then be undertaken. Advocates of H_2-receptor antagonist therapy point to its effectiveness, and the avoidance of a mutilating total gastrectomy. However, adequate control may not be achieved and the patients must comply fully.

Metastatic disease

Metastatic disease, usually hepatic, presents a problem in management. Before undertaking major therapeutic intervention a decision must be made whether the metastatic disease is significantly impairing the patient's quality of life, given that the clinical features are adequately controlled (vide supra). Many patients with a gastrinoma with metastases can lead lives of excellent quality, and it should be clearly decided whether intervention will lead to further clinical improvement.

Further intervention is justifiable in the following circumstances: if eradication of the tumour and a cure is a possibility; if the metastatic tumour is exerting effects on organs by pressure or replacement; or if the general health of the patient is deteriorating due to the large tumour mass. The following options may be considered: further surgical excision of tumour mass; cytotoxic therapy (streptozotocin); or embolization of tumour masses.

Streptozotocin (500 mg/m² body surface) has been found to be effective in the management of islet cell tumours including gastrinomas. The drug is given into a peripheral vein by bolus, the dose being repeated daily for five consecutive days. The regimen is repeated at signs of recurrence of tumour. Gastrointestinal effects, mainly anorexia, nausea and vomiting are frequent and occasional renal side-effects are a more serious problem. Most tumours will regress with such therapy. Should the response be poor, an increased dose, direct administration into the arterial supply of the tumour, or combination with 5-fluorouracil can sometimes succeed. Experience with other cytotoxic drugs in gastrinoma is negligible and anecdotal, but clearly if the patient's condition is deteriorating then resort to other drugs effective in the management of other solid tumours should be undertaken.

Patients with the MEA I syndrome often have multiple adenomas and are usually not cured by surgery. They may require management of other endocrine syndromes, for example hyperparathyroidism, and first-degree relatives of the patients should be screened particularly for parathyroid and islet cell abnormalities.

Prognosis

It is important to realize that gastrinomas, despite widespread metastases, are relatively indolent and slow growing, and years of good quality life can be enjoyed despite large masses of tumour. Mortality usually occurs because the syndrome is not adequately controlled, tragically in circumstances where the true nature of the disease has not been realized. Very difficult management problems arise where the syndrome is unsuspected and the patient has multiple complications worsened by inadequate surgical operations. It is strongly emphasized that such patients should be under the care of a skilled team experienced in the management of islet tumours and with access to necessary radiological and biochemical diagnostic tools.

Should the syndrome be controlled and the tumour excised, then the prognosis is excellent, even if small metastatic deposits in regional lymph nodes are not resected. The prognosis is more guarded when there are metastases to the liver but even in the absence of effective management, patients may live for several years.

Conclusion

Despite new approaches to therapy of patients with a gastrinoma, it is strongly emphasized that all patients should undergo a laparotomy even if the initial impression is that surgical cure is impossible or that management by other means might be more effective. This approach is justified because a laparotomy provides the opportunity to examine the extent of the tumour directly, and to obtain biopsy material for a specific diagnosis. Unless this is performed the certain diagnosis and defined nature of the tumour will never be ascertained and management may be irrational. The biopsy tissue if correctly stored may provide the unique means to approach future therapy with the developing disciplines of tissue culture, monoclonal antibodies and genetic engineering.

Appendix

Circulating gastrin assay
Blood (a minimum of 2 ml) should be taken into a heparinized tube, after an overnight fast. Gastrin is relatively stable in blood but if transfer to the laboratory is not assured within six hours, the plasma should be separated and stored frozen ($-20°C$) pending transport.

Tissue samples for gastrin analysis
At laparotomy, if the tumour cannot be excised, multiple sites including metastases should be biopsied as there is significant regional variation of hormone(s) content from site to site.

Tissue should be processed for: routine histopathology; electron microscopy; and specific immunohistochemistry for hormones (special fixatives are required so the specialized laboratory should be contacted). Tissue should be frozen ($-20°C$ and $-80°C$) for RIA of hormone content, characterization of molecular species, possible preparation of monoclonal antibodies to surface antigens, and possible isolation of genetic material for genetic engineering of human peptides.

REFERENCES

1 Buchanan, K. D. (1980) Gut hormones and gut endocrine tumour syndromes. *British Journal of Hospital Medicine*, **24**, 190–197.
2 Buchanan, K. D. & Ardill, J. E. S. (1978) Pathophysiology of gastrin and secretin. *Journal of Clinical Pathology*, **33** (Supplement 8), 17–25.
3 Gregory, R. A., Tracy, H. J., French, J. & Sircus, M. (1960) Extraction of a gastrin-like substance from a pancreatic tumor in a case of Zollinger–Ellison syndrome. *Lancet*, **i**, 1045–1048.

4   Lamers, C. B. H., Ruland, C. M., Joosten, H. J. M. *et al.* (1978) Hypergastrinemia of antral origin in duodenal ulcer. *Digestive Diseases,* **23,** 998–1002.

5   McGuigan, J. E. & Wolfe, M. M. (1980) Secretin injection test in the diagnosis of gastrinoma. *Gastroenterology,* **79,** 1324–1331.

6   Strauss, E., Greenstein, R. J. & Yalow, R. S. (1978) Plasma-secretin in the management of cimetidine therapy for Zollinger–Ellison syndrome. *Lancet,* **ii,** 73–75.

7   Taylor, I. L., Walsh, J. H., Rotter, J. & Passaro, E. (1978) Is pancreatic polypeptide a marker for Zollinger–Ellison syndrome? *Lancet,* **i,** 845–848.

8   Zollinger, R. M. & Ellison, E. H. (1955) Primary peptic ulcerations of the jejunum associated with islet cell tumors of the pancreas. *Annals of Surgery,* **142,** 709–728.

INSULINOMA INCLUDING NESIDIOBLASTOSIS

Insulinomas are tumours of pancreatic B-cells which secrete inappropriate amounts of insulin into the circulation and cause hypoglycaemia; i.e., a blood glucose level of below 2.2 mmol/l. They are the longest recognized and commonest functioning pancreatic islet-cell tumours and have been well reviewed.[3, 5, 6] Approximately 70% are small single benign tumours, 10% are multiple (usually microadenomata), 10% are part of multiple endocrine adenomatosis type I (see Chapter 9), and 10% are malignant with metastases. Occasional cases of hyperplasia and nesidioblastosis are recorded. Identification is made by histological methods, immunocytochemistry and the presence of insulin in tumour extracts.

Clinical features

Symptoms are due to the effect of hypoglycaemia on the nervous system – neuroglycopenia. The excessive insulin secretion is offset by eating and symptoms are therefore commonest in the early morning and late afternoon and are increased by alcohol and attempts to diet and exercise. Sympathetic stimulation is rare since the blood glucose falls slowly, thus the characteristic features of iatrogenic insulin overdosage are not seen. Weight gain is not common except in those who treat their symptoms by overeating.

Psychological disturbances
These are often subtle and are noticed either because they become more severe or are cumulatively striking. Episodes occur during fasting and are stopped by eating: alterations of mood, attitude, behaviour and personality are each or all seen. The subtlety of the changes commonly leads to a delay in diagnosis, the mean interval between the onset of symptoms and diagnosis being four years and periods of 10–20 years being common. The differential diagnosis is usually of psychological disorder, temporal lobe epilepsy or abuse of pharmaceuticals.

Neurological disturbances
The most common are circumoral paraesthesiae and numbness, headaches which may be severe, and mental dysfunction which may progress to coma. Many organic neurological syndromes have been described. The differential diagnosis is of cerebrovascular disease, cerebral tumour or infiltrative or metabolic syndromes.

Once the diagnosis of hypoglycaemia has been made the differential diagnosis is between factitious insulin abuse and reactive hypoglycaemia. The hypoglycaemia complicating endocrine and hepatic disease rarely causes diagnostic problems.

Diagnosis

Symptoms occur in the fasting state; they are accompanied by hypoglycaemia and inappropriately raised plasma insulin levels, and are relieved by the ingestion of carbohydrate (Whipple's triad updated).

Blood is taken after several 12-h overnight fasts. If the blood glucose is below 2.2 mmol/l plasma, insulin is measured as well. If hypoglycaemia is not detected the patient is admitted for a 24–72-h fast in which free fluids are given, exercise is encouraged and blood is drawn at 4-h intervals until the patient experiences symptoms. At this point two more samples are taken rapidly and glucose is given. Blood glucose in healthy males rarely falls below 2.8 mmol/l after 72 h; in females it may fall to 1.7 mmol/l,[3] but no symptoms occur and insulin levels are extremely low or undetectable. If the candidate shows no symptoms or hypoglycaemia after 72 h the diagnosis can usually be excluded. If doubt remains, sophisticated tests of induced hypoglycaemia can be performed using fish insulin or measuring C-peptide levels.[3]

Localization

Most insulinomas are 4 cm or less in diameter, are highly vascular and are found in all parts of the pancreas and, occasionally, in the duodenal wall or the hilum of the spleen. The radiological technique of choice is selective coeliac and superior mesenteric angiography.[4] This is variably reliable; an accuracy of 55–75% is quoted.[2, 4] If doubt remains, portal and splenic venous blood samples are obtained for insulin assay by percutaneous transhepatic puncture of a portal vein branch.[8] This gives the best chance of locating microadenomata albeit with occasional serious morbidity.

In many centres laparotomy is still preferred to angiographic techniques and 80% accuracy of localization has been achieved.[2]

Treatment

The majority of patients with single benign tumours are usually cured by resection, but tumours must be accurately localized; random left hemipancreatectomy only cures 25% of patients. During the operation blood sugar levels fall and afterwards hyperglycaemia is seen and must be monitored for at least 24 h. When benign tumours remain the patient is treated by appropriately spaced carbohydrate feeds and diazoxide 5–15 mg/kg body weight, with a diuretic if fluid retention occurs on this dose. Hirsuties is common but nausea and hypotension are rare at these doses. Long-acting glucagon, glucocorticoids and phenylhydantoin have also been used in occasional patients.

In malignant disease the primary growth is reduced surgically in bulk as much as possible to reduce secreting mass, and the residual tumour is treated by cytotoxic chemotherapy while the secretory capacity of hepatic metastases may be reduced by hepatic arterial embolization.

Chemotherapy
This has been improved by the combined use of streptozotocin and 5-fluorouracil.[7] Six out of seven malignant insulinomas showed reduction in size and insulin secretion on this regimen compared with three out of eight with streptozotocin alone. The treatment is toxic with severe vomiting, renal impairment and marrow suppression. Chlorozotocin is a less toxic analogue of streptozotocin and may be as effective. Adriamycin is under study.

Hepatic arterial embolization
This is indicated where cytotoxic drugs fail or are intolerable. It is only appropriate to the treatment of hepatic metastases and may have to be repeated depending on insulin secretion and tumour pain.

Prognosis

Benign tumours are notoriously prolonged in course and 20 or 30 years may elapse before the diagnosis is made. The median survival of malignant tumours is approximately 40 months but extreme variation is encountered.

Nesidioblastosis

In this rare condition nesidioblasts differentiate from pancreatic duct epithelium and form A, B, D and PP cells, which are separate from the true islets and increase the endocrine content of the pancreas five-fold.[1] The picture is of a baby with somnolence, ataxia, fits and coma, frequently with permanent brain damage, all due to hypoglycaemia and hyperinsulinism, which does not improve with time in contrast to other forms of neonatal hypoglycaemia. Diagnosis is by fasting hypoglycaemia and hyperinsulinism, true insulinomas being very rare in infancy. Treatment is by frequent feeds and diazoxide, usually in an attempt to gain time and weight before partial or total pancreatectomy. The incidence of nesidioblastosis as a cause of unexpected 'cot' death is unknown.

REFERENCES

1 Aynsley-Green, A., Polak, J. M., Keeling, J. *et al.* (1978) Averted sudden neo-natal death due to pancreatic nesidioblastosis. *Lancet*, **i**, 550.
2 Case Records of the Massachusetts General Hospital (1983) *New England Journal of Medicine*, **308**, 30–37.
3 Fajans, S. S. (1979) Diagnosis and medical treatment of insulinomas. *Annual Review of Medicine*, **30**, 313–329.
4 Gray, R. K., Rosch, J. & Grollman, J. H. (1970) Arteriography in the diagnosis of islet-cell tumours. *Radiology*, **97**, 39–44.
5 Hall, R., Anderson, J., Smart, G. A. & Breese, M. (1978) Hypoglycaemia. *Fundamentals of Clinical Endocrinology* 3rd ed, pp. 583–599. Tunbridge Wells: Atman.
6 Marks, V. & Samols, E. (1974) Insulinoma: Natural history and diagnosis. *Clinics in Gastroenterology*, **3**, 559–573.
7 Moertel, C. G., Hanley, J. A. & Johnson, L. A. (1980) Streptozotocin alone compared with streptozotocin plus fluorouracil in the treatment of advanced islet-cell carcinoma. *New England Journal of Medicine*, **303**, 1189–1194.
8 Turner, R. C., Morris, P. J., Lee, E. C. G. & Harris, E. A. (1978) Localisation of insulinomas. *Lancet*, **i**, 515–518.

VIPOMAS AND OTHER TUMOURS

Over the last two decades a considerable number of regulatory peptides have been isolated. These are now known to be important neurotransmitters in the central and peripheral nervous system and a number of them also have a role as circulating hormones. Surprisingly, they are often produced by endocrine tumours

Table 18.17   Regulatory peptides and their associated clinical syndromes.

Peptide	Action	Syndrome
Insulin	Hypoglycaemia	Neuroglycopenia
Gastrin	Acid secretion	Peptic ulcer
	Mucosal growth	Diarrhoea
VIP (and PHI)	Intestinal secretion	Watery diarrhoea
	Smooth muscle relaxation	Low blood pressure
	Acid inhibition	Low acid
Glucagon	Stimulates hepatic gluconeogenesis	Rash
		Hyperglycaemia
		Weight loss
Pancreatic polypeptide	Weakly inhibits pancreatic enzyme secretion and gallbladder contraction	Nil
Somatostatin	Inhibits all digestive functions	Diabetes mellitus
		Gallstones
		Steatorrhoea
Neurotensin	Inhibits acid	?Diarrhoea
	Stimulates intestinal secretion and motor activity	
Growth hormone releasing factor	Stimulates growth hormone	Acromegaly
Corticotrophin releasing factor	Stimulates ACTH	Cushing's syndrome
Neuropeptide Y	Hypertension	Unknown
	Inhibits pancreatic secretion	

of the pancreas, but the reason why this tissue bed should be such a fertile source of tumour production of these regulatory peptides is not known. The tumours usually produce more than one, and frequently many, of the peptides simultaneously. However, the clinical picture is dominated by the peptide which is produced in greatest quantity and, although the clinical picture can switch from one tumour syndrome to another, this is the exception (Table 18.17). The tumours are slow growing, and often the history can be traced back many years prior to the time of diagnosis. With this relatively long cell doubling time, extrapolation backwards to the moment when the first abnormal cell appeared sometimes suggests a fetal origin. Although the patient's eventual demise may be the result of increasing tumour mass, the course is slow and, at least initially, clinical symptoms result from excess production of the respective regulatory peptide. Amongst the different types of pancreatic endocrine tumour, insulinomas stand out as usually being benign (and therefore curable by resection). Of the other tumour types, low grade malignancy is the commonest pattern and late recurrence is frequent after apparently successful resection of a tumour.

Clinical features

VASOACTIVE INTESTINAL PEPTIDE

Vasoactive intestinal peptide (VIP) is composed of 28 amino acids and its structure puts it in the glucagon–secretin family of peptides. VIP relaxes smooth muscle, lowers blood pressure and stimulates watery juice secretion from the intestine and pancreas.[23] VIP is widely distributed throughout the body in both the central and peripheral nervous system. It is thought to act physiologically as a neurotransmitter or neuromodulator rather than as a circulating hormone. A new peptide has recently been isolated with a histidine at one end and an isoleucine at the other; it has therefore been given the name PHI (peptide histidine isoleucine).[27] Subsequently this peptide was found to have an identical distribution to VIP in all species examined and also to be always coproduced with VIP from tumours.[11] VIP infusion can cause watery diarrhoea in animals,[19] and has dramatic effects on water and ion transport in the human small and large bowel.[15] PHI, which has considerable sequence similarities to VIP, also stimulates intestinal juice production in animals[13] and in man.[4] The potency and effects of PHI are thus similar to those of VIP with the exception of PHI on blood vessels, where it is markedly less potent than VIP.[18]

In 1958 Verner and Morrison[29] described two cases of severe watery diarrhoea associated with non-insulin-secreting islet cell adenomas of the pancreas. The syndrome became known as the Verner–Morrison syndrome, alternatively the watery diarrhoea syndrome, the watery diarrhoea, hypokalaemia and achlorhydria syndrome (WDHA), or pancreatic cholera syndrome. None of these terms gives a precise indication of aetiology. Bloom, Polak and Pearse[8] were able to show that these tumours were associated with VIP production and, in a larger series, Long *et al.*[17] found that all pancreatic tumours associated with severe watery diarrhoea were producing VIP. In this series of 62 patients, ten of them were shown to have ganglioneuroblastomas, which are the main extrapancreatic VIP-producing tumours. It is therefore appropriate now to use the term VIPoma for those tumours producing VIP; this term is useful because it is aetiologically informative. These tumours have now all been shown to also produce PHI-like peptide;[9] this peptide is obligatorily cosynthesized as it is coded for in the same messenger RNA as VIP. Other tumours producing watery diarrhoea, including medullary carcinoma of the thyroid, carcinoma of the bronchus, carcinoid syndrome and gastrinoma, do so by mechanisms other than production of VIP, which is not raised in plasma from these patients. Similarly, other non-tumour causes of diarrhoea, including purgative abuse, active Crohn's disease, active ulcerative colitis, acute infection, pancreatic insufficiency, short gut syndrome and diabetic diarrhoea, are not associated with excess VIP production.[17]

The most important clinical feature of the VIPoma syndrome is the very severe watery diarrhoea which almost inevitably leads to hypokalaemia, and this is associated with acidosis, an unusual feature to be present with hypokalaemia. This diarrhoea may be initially intermittent but when severe the hypotensive action of VIP may precipitate vascular collapse and even death. Weight loss is not an early feature but it can become extreme in advanced cases. Mild diabetes mellitus and mild hypercalcaemia occur in a sizable minority of cases, and the cause of both is multi-factorial, though VIP has been shown to have a direct glucagon-like effect in causing increased hepatic gluconeogenesis. The possible reasons for the effect of VIP on calcium metabolism are uncertain. Although a low gastric acid secretion distinguishes the VIPoma syndrome from the Zollinger–Ellison (gastrinoma) syndrome, also associated with diarrhoea, about a third of the VIPoma patients have normal gastric acid secretion.[17]

NEUROTENSINOMAS

Neurotensin is a peptide of 13 amino acids which inhibits gastric acid and stimulates small intestinal juice production and small intestine motor activity.[22] Neurotensin is particularly· potent in stimulating contractions of the large bowel.[10] VIPomas have been found also to secrete neurotensin in about 10% of cases,[6] and occasionally neurotensin is produced by other types of tumour.[14] However, no particular clinical syndrome has been associated with neurotensin production by pancreatic tumours.[22]

PANCREATIC POLYPEPTIDE (PP)

PP is a peptide of 36 amino acids which was accidentally discovered to contaminate insulin preparations. It has been demonstrated to have a weak action in man, inhibiting gallbladder contraction and pancreatic enzyme secretion.[1] Unlike VIP (including PHI-like materials) and neurotensin, whose origins in the pancreas are unclear, PP is produced by PP cells, which comprise approximately 10% of the population of the islet of Langerhans. It is perhaps not surprising, therefore, that pancreatic endocrine tumours frequently secrete PP;[21] indeed, approximately a third of gastrinomas, three-quarters of VIPomas, half the glucagonomas and one-quarter of the insulinomas are also found to release very large amounts of PP into the circulation,[3] and nearly 100% of pancreatic endocrine tumours contain significant amounts of extractable PP. Although measurement of PP in the blood is a good indication of the presence of a pancreatic endocrine tumour, no clinical features have yet been recognized in association with elevation of plasma PP. Recently, marginal elevations of PP in association with possible tumours have been distinguished from physiological PP elevation by means of the atropine suppression test (atropine suppresses physiological elevation).[3]

SOMATOSTATIN

Somatostatin is a peptide produced by the D cell of the islets of Langerhans (like the PP cell, the D cell forms about 10% of the cells of the normal islet). Somatostatin is remarkable for its wide inhibitory actions on the release of gastrointestinal hormones and also a direct inhibitory action on the target tissue of these same hormones.[12, 24] Somatostatinomas were found to be associated with steatorrhoea, diabetes mellitus and gallstones, as well as a reduced gastric acid secretion.[16] These tumours are often extremely slow growing and are not always associated with the full, or indeed any part of, the syndrome.[25] It seems likely that escape occurs from the powerful effects of somatostatin when secretion is long continued, the mechanism of which is unknown.

ENTEROGLUCAGONOMA

Only one patient has been reported with entero-glucagonoma, a renal tumour associated with gross slowing of gastrointestinal transit and a striking elongation of small intestinal mucosal villi.[2]

OTHER PEPTIDES

Recently pancreatic endocrine tumours have been described which secrete growth hormone releasing factor,[28] and other peptides including corticotrophin-releasing factor, neuropeptide tyrosine, etc.[2]

Diagnosis

The diagnosis of VIPomas and other endocrine tumours is based mainly on clinical awareness of the particular syndrome. Once the possibility has been raised, a fresh fasting plasma sample containing the enzyme inhibitor aprotinin (Trasylol) is taken and sent to the nearest major radioimmunoassay laboratory (in the United Kingdom via the Supra Regional Assay Service). Plasma levels of the respective peptide are usually extremely elevated and provide no diagnostic problem. In the case of VIP, for example, levels above 60 pmol/l can be considered diagnostic of a tumour, while levels above 30 pmol/l require to be repeated, with re-examination of the clinical situation. Healthy subjects normally have VIP concentrations of approximately 2 pmol/l. The presence of more than one tumour-related peptide obviously helps confirm the diagnosis and in the author's laboratory gastrin, glucagon, VIP, somatostatin and neurotensin are routinely assayed together. Additional help can be obtained from chromatography of the plasma sample to demonstrate that the majority of the elevated peptide-like immunoreactivity is associated with a peptide molecule of approximately the correct size. Tumours frequently have abnormal post-translational enzymic processing of the prohormone and thus secrete large forms of the peptide in addition to the normal moiety.

Localization

While the diagnosis is usually straightforward, localization of the tumour and/or any secondaries is more difficult. Non-invasive procedures such as computerized tomography (CT scan), ultrasound or liver scintigraphy are followed by arteriography, preferably highly selective and with background subtraction. Nuclear magnetic resonance scanning can be helpful, particularly for secondaries in liver. In future, high-speed CT scanning combined with arteriography (perhaps digital radiography) may also prove helpful. Isotopic means for localizing the tumour, for example using ions such as zinc which are specifically concentrated in the tumour or monoclonal antibodies which react with tumour surface components, are still in the early stages of testing. The use of selective venous sampling using a transhepatic portal venous catheter can be helpful but is associated with significant risk. It is necessary to cannulate all the tributaries of the pancreatic vein and take simultaneous hepatic venous samplings (to control for spontaneous fluctuations in tumour peptide output) and such a procedure may take many hours. Aberrant tumour drainage can still cause false localization, but the most significant problem is that much of the elevated hormone levels in the plasma is the result of large molecular weight forms with very slow plasma clearance. Thus a relatively small percentage of new hormone is added per single passage and it is difficult to distinguish a small increase from assay noise. Selective venous sampling is a procedure to be undertaken only in highly experienced centres and the authors' laboratory does not now recommend it because of the improvements in other localization procedures.

Once tissue is obtained by hepatic biopsy or surgically, it can be examined histologically. The appearance of the tissue gives little indication as to a tumour's metastatic potential and cannot usually be used to indicate prognosis. Immunocytochemical staining with antibodies to neurone-specific enolase, an enzyme present only in neuroendocrine tissue, is an excellent marker to confirm the endocrine nature of a tumour.[26] Since some endocrine tumours are clinically silent yet have the same biological behaviour as other endocrine tumours (i.e., grow very slowly), this can be very helpful. Further, it is possible to identify the specific hormone produced by each of the component cell types by means of immunocytochemical staining with antibodies to each of the known peptides. It is often found that tumours have more than one cell type, even though secretion of a single hormone is responsible for the clinical picture.

Radioimmunoassay of tumour extracts can provide further confirmation of the multiple hormone production. Electron microscopy enables identification of the secretory granules and it is often found that there is a mixture of typical and atypical granule forms. This may be important as the different cell populations may respond differently to cytotoxic therapy.

Treatment

SURGICAL

Surgical removal of a lone tumour is optimal, but, even when achieved, late recurrences are common to all pancreatic endocrine tumours other than insulinoma. Since the tumours are slow growing and produce their clinical symptoms by elevated circulating hormone concentrations, excellent palliation can be achieved by tumour bulk reduction if total excision is impossible. By far the commonest site of initial metastases is the liver, but surgical removal of hepatic metastases is now less commonly performed than previously following the introduction of hepatic arterial embolization.[5] Removal of the arterial blood supply to the liver produces little symptomatic (or biochemical) effect and may therefore be performed in elderly or preterminal patients under local anaesthesia. The most significant complication is infection in necrotic tumour mass and the risk of this is reduced by heavy antibiotic cover.

DRUG THERAPY

The cytotoxic antibiotic streptozotocin (500 mg/ m^2/day)[30] is dramatically effective on the VIPoma (Figure 18.42). Remissions are obtained in nearly 100% of patients and may last many years. This agent is associated with acute fever and nausea and is best administered intermittently in hospital with aspirin and antiemetics. It is toxic to the kidney; thus patients with impaired renal function are at considerable risk and the dose should be greatly reduced if this drug is to be used.[30] Unfortunately the number of individual tumour syndromes is too small for a clinical trial to be mounted comparing various cytotoxic agents. The exception is 5-fluorouracil but combination with streptozotocin does not produce any marked benefit.[20] Temporary remission can be obtained by administration of high-dose steroids and thus these agents will not distinguish this condition from inflammatory bowel disease as remission will occur in both situations. A number of other drugs, including trifluoperazine, lithium and metoclopramide have been helpful in individual patients but improvement has not been reproducible. Long-acting somatostatin analogues administered by subcutaneous injection will suppress the diarrhoea in VIPomas. Whether any reduction of tumour mass will result or, alternatively whether escape will rapidly occur, awaits further clinical trial.

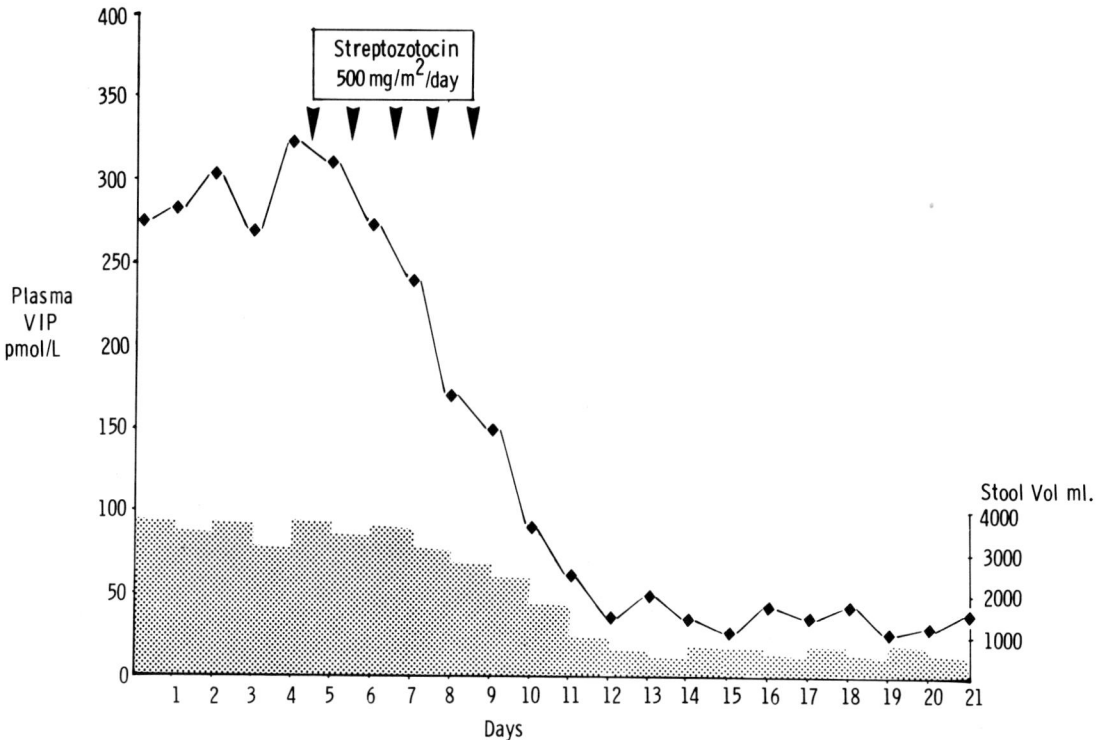

Fig. 18.42 Plasma VIP level and stool volume in a VIPoma patient undergoing therapy with streptozotocin on five days. All clinical symptoms remitted in parallel with the fall of plasma VIP.

Conclusions

The prognosis of endocrine pancreatic tumours is surprisingly good. Indeed the patient may first present as a cachetic, with apparent carcinoma of the pancreas but who still attends the clinic a year later. Palliation is very worthwhile. Whether earlier diagnosis (greater clinical awareness of the syndromes) will result in a higher cure rate is at present unknown. From the authors' experience there are about 200 new endocrine tumour cases in the United Kingdom per year that are diagnosed and approximately an equal number that are missed. These tumours are of great interest and illustrate the mechanism of the regulatory peptide system, but they are rare in any one physician's clinical practice.

REFERENCES

1   Adrian, T. E., Greenberg, G. R. & Bloom, S. R. (1981) Actions of pancreatic polypeptide in man. In *Gut Hormones* (Ed.) Bloom, S. R. & Polak, J. M. pp. 206–212. Edinburgh: Churchill Livingstone.
2   Adrian, T. E., Allen, J. M., Terenghi, G. *et al.* (1983) Neuropeptide Y in pheochromocytomas and ganglioneuroblastomas. *Lancet*, **ii**, 540–542.
3   Adrian, T. E., Yeats, J., Wood, S. M. *et al.* (1983) Pancreatic polypeptide secretion by pancreatic apudomas and its lack of suppression by cholinergic blockade. *Gut*, **24**, A596.
4   Agnostides, A. A., Christofides, N. D., Chadwick, V. S. & Bloom, S. R. (1983) Peptide histidine isoleucine (PHI): a secretagogue in human intestine. *Gut* (in press).
5   Alison, D. J. (1978) Therapeutic embolisation. *British Journal of Hospital Medicine*, **20**, 705–715.
6   Blackburn, A. M., Bryant, M. G., Adrian, T. E. & Bloom, S. R. (1981) Pancreatic tumours produce neurotensin. *Journal of Clinical Endocrinology and Metabolism*, **52**, 820–822.
7   Bloom, S. R. (1972) An enteroglucagon tumour. *Gut*, **13**, 520–523.
8   Bloom, S. R., Polak, J. M. & Pearse, A. G. E. (1973) Vasoactive intestinal peptide and watery diarrhoea syndrome. *Lancet*, **ii**, 14–16.
9   Bloom, S. R., Christofides, N. D., Yiangou, Y. *et al.* (1983) Peptide histidine isoleucine (PHI) and the Verner–Morrison syndrome. *Gut*, **24**, A473.
10 Calam, J., Unwin, R. & Peart, W. S. (1983) Neurotensin stimulates defaecation in man. *Lancet*, **i**, 737–738.
11 Christofides, N. D., Yiangou, Y., Blank, M. A. *et al.* (1982) Are peptide histidine isoleucine and vasoactive intestinal peptide cosynthesized in the same prohormone? *Lancet*, **ii**, 1398.
12 Gerich, J. (1982) Regulation of somatostatin secretion and its biologic actions. In *Hormones in Normal and Abnormal Human Tissues* Vol. 2 (Ed.) Fotherby, K. & Pal, S. B. pp. 475–518. Berlin, New York: Walter de Gruyter.
13 Ghiglione, M., Christofides, N. D., Yiangou, Y. *et al.* (1982) PHI stimulates intestinal fluid secretion. *Neuropeptides*, **3**, 79–82.
14 Gutniak, M., Rosenquist, U., Grimelius, L. *et al.* (1980) Report on a patient with watery diarrhoea syndrome caused by a pancreatic tumour containing neurotensin, enkephalin and calcitonin. *Acta Medica Scandinavica*, **208**, 95–100.
15 Krejs, G. J. (1980) Effect of VIP infusion on water and ion transport in the human large intestine. *Gastroenterology*, **78**, 1200–1204.
16 Krejs, G. J., Orci, L., Conlon, J. M. *et al.* (1979) Somatostatinoma syndrome, biochemical, morphological and clinical features. *New England Journal of Medicine*, **301**, 285–292.
17 Long, R. G., Bryant, M. G., Mitchell, S. J. *et al.* (1981) Clinicopathological study of pancreatic and ganglioneuroblastoma tumours secreting vasoactive intestinal polypeptide (VIPomas). *British Medical Journal*, **282**, 1767–1771.
18 Lundberg, J. M. & Tatemoto, K. (1982) Vascular effects of the peptides PYY and PHI: comparison with APP and VIP. *European Journal of Pharmacology*, **143**, 143–146.
19 Modlin, I. M., Bloom, S. R. & Mitchell, S. J. (1978) Experimental evidence for vasoactive intestinal peptide as the cause of the watery diarrhoea syndrome. *Gastroenterology*, **75**, 1051–1054.
20 Mortal, C., Hanley, J. A. & Johnson, L. A. (1980) Streptozotocin alone compared with streptozotocin plus fluoro-uracil in the treatment of advanced islet cell carcinoma. *New England Journal of Medicine*, **303**, 1189–1192.
21 Polak, J. M., Bloom, S. R., Adrian, T. E. *et al.* (1976) Pancreatic polypeptide in insulinomas, gastrinomas, VIPomas and glucagonomas. *Lancet*, **i**, 328–330.
22 Rosell, S., Rokaeus, A. & Theodorsson-Norheim, E. (1983) The role of neurotensin in disease. *Scandinavian Journal of Gastroenterology*, **18** (Supplement 82), 59–67.
23 Said, S. I. (Ed.) 1982 *Vasoactive Intestinal Peptide*. New York: Raven Press.
24 Schuszdiarra, V. (1983) Somatostatin – physiological and pathophysiological aspects. *Scandinavian Journal of Gastroenterology*, **18** (Supplement 82), 69–84.
25 Stacpoole, P. W., Kassleberg, A. G., Berelewitz, M. & Chey, W. Y. (1983) Somatostatinoma syndrome: does a clinical entity exist? *Acta Endocrinologica*, **102**, 80–87.
26 Tapia, F. J., Polak, J. M., Barbarosa, A. J. A. *et al.* (1981) Neuron-specific enolase is produced by neuroendocrine tumours. *Lancet*, **i**, 808–811.
27 Tatemoto, K. & Mutt, V. (1981) Isolation and characterization of the intestinal peptide porcine PHI (PHI-27), a new member of the glucagon–secretin family. *Proceedings of the National Academy of Sciences USA*, **78**, 6603–6607.
28 Thorner, M. O., Perriman, R. L., Cronin, M. J. *et al.* (1982) Somatotrophin hyperplasia. Successful treatment of acromegaly by removal of a pancreatic islet tumor secreting a growth hormone-releasing factor. *Journal of Clinical Investigation*, **70**, 965–977.
29 Verner, J. V. & Morrison, A. B. (1958) Islet cell tumour and a syndrome of refractory watery diarrhoea and hypokalaemia. *American Journal of Medicine*, **25**, 374–380.
30 Weiss, R. B. (1982) Streptozotocin: A review of its pharmacology, efficacy, and toxicity. *Cancer Treatment Reports*, **66**, 427–438.

GLUCAGONOMA

Glucagonomas are pancreatic islet cell tumours containing or secreting pancreatic glucagon and are commonly malignant. They produce a characteristic, largely unexplained, clinical syndrome which has, since its recognition, led to the diagnosis of approximately 200 tumours.[1]

Clinical features

Skin rash.[3] The rash is a characteristic erythema with a distinct margin which migrates and shows histological changes of necrolysis confined to the superficial epidermis. It is termed necrolytic migratory erythema[3] and is histologically and clinically similar to the rash of acrodermatitis enteropathica of children and iatrogenic zinc deficiency; all three respond to oral zinc treatment.

Diabetes mellitus. All patients have impaired glucose tolerance tests but usually only mild diabetes. Pancreatic glucagon stimulates endogenous insulin secretion, and in all patients plasma insulin or C-peptide levels are high. Ketoacidosis has only been described once and the combined secretion of insulin and glucagon causes a unique depression of all plasma amino acid levels.

Blood disorders. Patients usually have moderate normochromic anaemia but a marked tendency to severe, life-threatening venous thrombosis. This is unexplained and resistant to conventional treatment. Weight loss, intermittent diarrhoea and severe depression are less reliable features of the syndrome.

These clinical features develop in random order and may have been present for many years before diagnosis, even with malignant tumours. Recently a patient without a rash has been diagnosed prospectively who had diabetes with aggressive venous thrombosis. Before 1974 glucagonomas were seldom diagnosed specifically or other than retrospectively.[2] Occasionally patients with the glucagonoma syndrome show evidence of clinically significant secretion of other peptides, particularly gastrin or insulin.

Diagnosis

Plasma glucagon levels are usually elevated 10–20-fold, much higher than in stress, burns or ketoacidosis. Plasma pancreatic polypeptide levels are also increased in 50% of cases. Plasma amino acids, where available, are also diagnostic.

Localization of tumour is again by abdominal angiography but routine scanning techniques are often capable of detecting metastases in the liver and upper abdomen. Portal sampling is seldom required.

Treatment

Surgery is curative in a minority of patients but debulking of the primary tumour is often all that can be achieved. Treatment with streptozotocin alone or in combination with 5-fluorouracil and, latterly, doxorubicin, has variable and occasionally very dramatic results. Otherwise hepatic arterial embolization can reduce secretion and improve the patient's general condition.

The skin rash is probably best treated with oral zinc sulphate 200 mg daily, while intravenous amino acids, antibiotics and corticosteroids have all been advocated.

Prognosis

Again this is highly variable and depends entirely on the response to treatment. The majority of patients have had symptoms for many years before diagnosis, even with widespread metastases.

REFERENCES

1 Mallinson, C. N., Bloom, S. R., Warin, A. P. *et al.* (1974) A glucagonoma syndrome. *Lancet,* **ii,** 1–3.
2 McGavran, M., Unger, R. H., Recant, L. *et al.* (1966) A glucagon secreting alpha-cell carcinoma of the pancreas. *New England Journal of Medicine,* **274,** 1408.
3 Wilkinson, D. S. (1973) Necrolytic migratory erythema with carcinoma of the pancreas. *Transactions of the St. John's Hospital Dermatological Society,* **59,** 244.

FAMILIAL PANCREATITIS

The differential diagnosis of familial causes of pancreatitis is shown in Table 18.18. The severity and frequency of the attacks of pancreatitis may vary widely between individual patients as well as between disease entities. Whatever the cause of the pancreatitis, progressive destruction of the pancreas may ensue, resulting in calcification, exocrine pancreatic insufficiency and diabetes mellitus.

'Familial pancreatitis' implies a causal relationship between an individual genotype and a predisposition to develop pancreatitis.

Table 18.18 Differential diagnosis of familial pancreatitis.

Cystic fibrosis
Hereditary pancreatitis
Metabolic pancreatitis
    Hyperlipidaemia
    Hyperparathyroidism
    α_1-Antitrypsin deficiency
Miscellaneous disorders
    Annular pancreas
    Pancreatic tumours
    Gallstones

Whilst this may be the case in a number of the conditions discussed, it should be stressed that this has not been established from the available published studies, and careful prospective studies are required to clarify this important issue.

Cystic fibrosis (see also p. 1286)

This is by far the most common genetically determined disorder of the pancreas, occurring in approximately 1 in 2000 live Caucasian births, being inherited in an autosomal recessive fashion. Fifteen to twenty per cent of patients with cystic fibrosis do not have any clinical evidence of exocrine pancreatic insufficiency, and interestingly, it is this group of patients who tend to develop attacks of acute pancreatitis accounting for about 0.5% of all patients with cystic fibrosis.[36] In this particular series of patients, the majority presented with abdominal pain and only later was the diagnosis of cystic fibrosis firmly established. The youngest patient presenting with abdominal pain and pancreatitis was seven years' old. Thus, a diagnosis of cystic fibrosis should be considered in any patient with pancreatitis, and conversely pancreatitis must be considered in the older child with cystic fibrosis who develops acute abdominal pain.

Hereditary pancreatitis

This is the second commonest genetically determined disorder of the pancreas, and is inherited in an autosomal dominant fashion; penetrance varies from 40 to 80%.[17, 30, 37] Although the pathogenesis has not been defined, the presence of a structurally abnormal protein has been suggested;[8] anatomical defects such as abnormalities of the pancreatic ducts[2, 4, 7, 11, 12, 19, 29, 30, 34, 40] and of the sphincter of Oddi[13, 31] could also play a role in pathogenesis.

CLINICAL MANIFESTATIONS, COMPLICATIONS AND PATHOLOGY

Both sexes are equally affected with respect to severity and frequency of attacks, and the average age at onset of symptoms is 10–12 years, with a range from infancy to old age;[17, 30, 37] 80% of patients, however, present before the age of 20 years. The attacks of pancreatitis may become progressively less severe with age in some patients,[23, 37] whereas in others this is by no means the case and major surgery may be required to relieve pain.[2, 4, 11, 34, 40] Malabsorption leading to failure to thrive is uncommon unless the disease is particularly severe or extensive surgery has been necessary.

In marked contrast to cystic fibrosis, calcification of the pancreas is common, occurring in about 50% of patients, and exocrine pancreatic insufficiency and diabetes mellitus may develop in severely affected patients;[13, 23, 37] haemorrhagic pancreatitis has been reported.[29] There appears to be an association between carcinoma of the pancreas and other intra-abdominal tumours, and hereditary pancreatitis,[7, 17] but the nature of the association is speculative and not clear. The tumours usually develop after the disease has been present for several years, suggesting that the inflammatory process may predispose to the development of carcinoma. This possibility, however, is not supported by the fact that family members who do not have pancreatitis may develop carcinoma, and many affected families without carcinoma have been described.[37]

As in other forms of pancreatitis pseudocysts may be a complication,[13, 37] and portal and splenic vein thrombosis have been reported.[23] Aminoaciduria occurs in some patients, which may reflect non-specific renal tubular dysfunction secondary to acute pancreatitis irrespective of the cause, or alternatively the presence of two separate disease entities.[18, 20, 30]

Reports on the pathological changes are derived largely from patients with long-standing severe disease. Macroscopically the gland is shrunken with calculi frequently present in the pancreatic ducts. Microscopically, the appearances are similar to those seen in cystic fibrosis with widespread interstitial fibrosis and loss of acinar tissue, but relative preservation of islet cells.[17]

DIAGNOSIS AND TREATMENT

The diagnosis of hereditary pancreatitis must always be suspected if more than one member of a family develops pancreatitis at an early age, particularly if other causes of pancreatitis, such as gallstones and alcoholism, have been excluded;[14] radiological visualization of large rounded areas of calcification support the diagnosis. Although endoscopic retrograde cholangiopancreatography (ERCP) is not diagnostic, the procedure is useful in establishing abnormalities such as stones, pseudocysts, and areas of narrowing or dilatation in the ducts. ERCP should probably be performed in all patients at the time of diagnosis and surgery considered if duct disease is present. No specific therapy is available and the management of acute or chronic disease is similar to that in any other form of acute/chronic pancreatitis. Theoretically, early surgical intervention for duct disease should be beneficial but no systematic prospective studies have been performed. The traditionally accepted indications for surgery in this disorder are intractable severe pain and/or duct obstruction.

Metabolic pancreatitis

FAMILIAL HYPERLIPIDAEMIC STATES

Acute and recurrent episodes of pancreatitis may occur in patients with familial hyperlipidaemic states particularly in types I, IV, and V, incidence rates being about 30, 15 and 40%, respectively.[6] The presence of a raised serum triglyceride in a patient with pancreatitis should alert one to this association and the appropriate investigations instituted. Although there is some experimental evidence for a causal relationship between hypertriglyceridaemia and pancreatitis, the mechanisms involved in the genesis of the pancreatitis occurring in patients with familial hyperlipidaemic states have not been defined. Sarharia *et al.*[33] speculated that toxic free fatty acids may be liberated from the excessive triglycerides in the pancreas. Of interest is a case report of a patient with glycogen storage disease, and hyperlipidaemia, who died from an episode of haemorrhagic pancreatitis following several years of recurrent abdominal pain.[25]

HYPERPARATHYROIDISM

Early reports indicated that approximately 7% of patients with hyperparathyroidism developed pancreatitis,[26, 35] but more recent reports suggest a much lower incidence of 1–2%.[5, 32, 39] Despite the fact that acute pancreatitis secondary to iatrogenic hypercalcaemia has been described,[5, 22] any causal relationship between hyperparathyroidism and pancreatitis remains to be established.

α_1-ANTITRYPSIN DEFICIENCY

α_1-Antitrypsin is a glycoprotein serum protease inhibitor (Pi) which is synthesized by the liver; deficient individuals have only 10–20% of the normal serum concentration. A number of genetically determined alleles of α_1-antitrypsin can be distinguished, and have been labelled according to their electrophoretic mobility. Normal individuals have clear M bands with a Pi phenotype M, whilst deficient subjects have

fainter, slower moving Z bands and a Pi phenotype Z. Less marked reductions of α_1-antitrypsin levels are found in subjects with Pi genotype MZ, SZ, with very low concentrations in Pi nil individuals.

Novis *et al.*[28] have screened a large group of patients with alcoholic pancreatitis for Pi type and serum α_1-antitrypsin. These workers found Pi phenotype MZ to be commoner and MM to be less common than in controls; α_1-antitrypsin levels were also lower in the patients. In contrast, Mero and Sandholm[24] found elevated α_1-antitrypsin concentrations in a group of patients with acute pancreatitis. Whether there is a causal relationship between this protease inhibitor and pancreatitis is unclear, but it seems unlikely.

Miscellaneous disorders

Pancreatic tumours,[9, 10, 21, 38] gallstones[1, 3] and annular pancreas[16, 27] can be familial and associated with pancreatitis.

REFERENCES

1 Acosta, J. M. & Ledesma, C. L. (1974) Gallstone migration as a cause of acute pancreatitis. *New England Journal of Medicine*, **290**, 484–487.
2 Appel, M. F. (1974) Hereditary pancreatitis. *Archives of Surgery*, **108**, 63–65.
3 Auidist, A. W. (1972) Pancreatitis and choledocholithiasis in childhood. *Journal of Pediatric Surgery*, **7**, 78.
4 Bergstrom, K., Hellstrom, K., Kallner, M. & Lundh, G. (1973) Familial pancreatitis associated with hyperglycinuria. *Scandinavian Journal of Gastroenterology*, **8**, 217–223.
5 Bess, M. A., Edis, A. J. & van Heerden, J. A. (1980) Hyperparathyroidism and pancreatitis. *Journal of the American Medical Association*, **243**, 246–247.
6 Buch, A., Buch, J., Carlsen, A. & Schmidt, A. (1980) Hyperlipidaemia and pancreatitis. *World Journal of Surgery*, **4**, 307–314.
7 Castleman, B., Scully, R. E. & McNeely, B. U. (1972) Case records of the Massachusetts General Hospital (Case 25-1972). *New England Journal of Medicine*, **286**, 1353–1356.
8 Erbe, R. W. (1976) Current concepts in genetics. *New England Journal of Medicine*, **294**, 480–482.
9 Fishman, R. S. & Bartholomew, L. G. (1979) Severe pancreatic involvement in three generations in von Hippel–Lindau disease. *Mayo Clinic Proceedings*, **54**, 329–331.
10 Friedman, Z., Shochat, S. J., Maisels, M. J. et al. (1976) Correction of essential fatty acid deficiency in newborn infants by cutaneous application of sun-flower-seed oil. *Pediatrics*, **58**, 650–654.
11 Gerber, B. C. & Aberdeen, S. D. (1963) Hereditary pancreatitis. *Archives of Surgery*, **87**, 86–96.
12 Girard, R. M. & Archambault, A. (1980) Hereditary chronic pancreatitis (CPC 25-1972). *New England Journal of Medicine*, **303**, 286–287.
13 Gross, J. B. & Comfort, M. W. (1957) Hereditary pancreatitis: report on two additional families. *Gastroenterology*, **32**, 829–854.

14 Gross, J. B., Gambill, E. E. & Ulrich, J. A. (1962) Hereditary pancreatitis. *American Journal of Medicine*, **33**, 358–364.

15 Hochgelerent, E. L. & David, D. S. (1974) Acute pancreatitis secondary to calcium infusion in a dialysis patient. *Archives of Surgery*, **108**, 218–219.

16 Jackson, L. G. & Apostolides, P. (1978) Autosomal dominant inheritance of annular pancreas. *American Journal of Medical Genetics*, **1**, 319–321.

17 Kattwinkel, J., Lapey, A., di Sant'Agnese, P. A. *et al.* (1973) Hereditary pancreatitis: three new kindreds and a critical review of the literature. *Pediatrics*, **51**, 55–59.

18 Lapey, A., Kattwinkel, J., di Sant'Agnese, P. & Laster, L. (1971) Hereditary pancreatitis without aminoaciduria: two new kindreds. *Pediatric Research*, **5**, 389 (Abst.).

19 Lilja, P., Evander, A. & Ihse, I. (1978) Hereditary pancreatitis – a report on two kindreds. *Acta Chirurgica Scandinavica*, **144**, 35–37.

20 Logan, A., Jr., Schlicke, P. & Manning, G. B. (1968) Familial pancreatitis. *American Journal of Surgery*, **115**, 112–117.

21 MacDermott, R. F. & Kramer, P. (1973) Adenocarcinoma of the pancreas in four siblings. *Gastroenterology*, **65**, 137–139.

22 Manson, R. R. (1974) Acute pancreatitis secondary to iatrogenic hypercalcemia. *Archives of Surgery*, **108**, 213–215.

23 McElroy, R. & Christiansen, P. A. (1972) Hereditary pancreatitis in a kinship associated with portal vein thrombosis. *American Journal of Medicine*, **52**, 228–241.

24 Mero, M. & Sandholm, M. (1979) Alpha$_1$-antitrypsin and total trypsin-inhibitor capacity in acute pancreatitis. *Annales Chirurgiae et Gynaecologiae Fenniae*, **68**, 39–40.

25 Michels, V. V. & Beaudet, A. L. (1980) Hemorrhagic pancreatitis in a patient with glycogen storage disease type 1. *Clinical Genetics*, **17**, 220–222.

26 Mixter, C. G., Jr., Keynes, W. M. & Cope, O. (1962) Further experience with pancreatitis as a diagnostic clue to hyperparathyroidism. *New England Journal of Medicine*, **266**, 265–272.

27 Montgomery, R. C., Poindexter, M. H., Hall, G. H. & Leigh, J. E. (1971) Report of a case of annular pancreas of the newborn in two consecutive siblings. *Pediatrics*, **48**, 148–149.

28 Novis, B. H., Bank, S., Young, G. O. & Marks, I. N. (1975) Chronic pancreatitis and alpha-1-antitrypsin. *Lancet*, **ii**, 748–749.

29 Perrault, J., Gross, J. B. & King, J. E. (1976) Endoscopic retrograde cholangiopancreatography in familial pancreatitis. *Gastroenterology*, **71**, 138–144.

30 Riccardi, V. M., Shih, V. E., Holmes, L. B. & Nardi, G. L. (1975) Hereditary pancreatitis. *Archives of Internal Medicine*, **135**, 822–825.

31 Robechek, P. J. (1967) Hereditary chronic relapsing pancreatitis. *American Journal of Surgery*, **113**, 819–824.

32 Romanus, R., Heimann, P., Nilsson, O. & Hansson, G. (1973) Surgical treatment of hyperparathyroidism. *Progress in Surgery*, **12**, 22–76.

33 Saharia, P., Margolis, S., Zuidema, G. D. & Cameron, J. L. (1977) Acute pancreatitis with hyperlipemia: studies with an isolated perfused canine pancreas. *Surgery*, **82**, 60–67.

34 Sato, T. & Saitoh, Y. (1974) Familial chronic pancreatitis associated with pancreatic lithiasis. *American Journal of Surgery*, **127**, 511–517.

35 Schmidt, H. & Creutzfeldt, W. (1970) Calciphylactic pancreatitis and pancreatitis in hyperparathyroidism.

Clinical Orthopaedics and Related Research, **69**, 135–145.

36 Shwachman, H., Lebenthal, E. & Khaw, K. T. (1975) Recurrent acute pancreatitis in patients with cystic fibrosis with normal pancreatic enzymes. *Pediatrics*, **55**, 86–95.

37 Sibert, J. R. (1978) Hereditary pancreatitis in England and Wales. *Journal of Medical Genetics*, **15**, 189–201.

38 Swift, M., Sholman, L., Perry, M. & Chase, C. (1976) Malignant neoplasms in the families of patients with ataxia-telangiectasia. *Cancer Research*, **36**, 209–215.

39 Werner, S., Hjern, B. & Sjoberg, H. E. (1974) Primary hyperparathyroidism: Analysis of findings in a series of 129 patients. *Acta Chirurgica Scandinavica*, **140**, 618–625.

40 Whitten, D. M. & Feingold, M. (1968) Hereditary pancreatitis. *American Journal of Diseases of Children*, **116**, 426–428.

CALCIFIC PANCREATITIS

Pancreatic lithiasis has a world-wide distribution, the incidence varying from 9.4% to 74.4% of patients with chronic pancreatitis.[12] Calcification seems to follow the process of pancreatitis although evidence for this is often lacking.

Aetiology

Alcoholism and malnutrition are the major aetiological factors. While alcoholism plays the dominant role in calcific pancreatitis in the developed nations of the West, malnutrition is the common association in developing Asian and African countries.[8] Rarer causes include hereditary pancreatitis with aminoaciduria, hypercalcaemia, hyperlipoproteinaemia, abdominal trauma and mumps. Gallstone pancreatitis rarely develops calcification. Some cases of 'idiopathic pancreatitis' may be due to stenosis of the sphincter of Oddi or a congenital malformation of the duct system.

Pathogenesis

Ductular reduplication following injury with increased secretion and accumulation of proteinaceous material has been clearly documented in alcoholic calcific pancreatitis. The proteinaceous material encourages concretions which later cause destruction of the ductular epithelium followed by dilatation and strictures. Whether the primary changes occur at the ductular level[9] or at the acinar level[3] is disputed.

A close association with protein malnutrition has been recorded in calcific pancreatitis reported from Asian and African countries.[10, 13] Functional and structural alterations in the pancreas in protein malnutrition are well documented.[2, 11] The pancreas, an organ with a very high protein turnover, is vulnerable to protein deprivation, particularly the essential amino acids methionine, leucine, isoleucine and valine. Although the early changes are reversible, prolonged protein deficiency in childhood may initiate irreversible structural changes in the gland. Parotid enlargement, fatty liver and occasionally cirrhosis are also found and reflect protein malnutrition. Genetic factors or other precipitating events like viral infections or ingestion of dietetic toxins might well contribute to the pancreatic injury. Identical twins and siblings may share the disease but vertical transmission does not occur. The role of viral infections is currently under study. Cassava (tapioca or manihot), by virtue of its cyanogenic content, is postulated to have a role in pathogenesis;[6] it may also deplete marginal methionine stores in the conversion of hydrocyanic acid to thiocyanate before excretion. There is a strong geographical correlation between tapioca consumption and incidence of calcific pancreatitis in the state of Kerala in India. Immunological changes may have a role in perpetuating the injury. Depressed T lymphocytes, elevation in serum IgG and IgM levels, and the presence of antipancreatic antibodies have been demonstrated, although other markers of autoimmunity were absent.[7]

Pathology

The alcoholic variety of calcific pancreatitis shows pathological changes very similar to that found in non-calcific disease.

When malnutrition predominates, the gland is small, atrophic, fibrosed and, later, calcified.[4] Calcification is almost always intraductal and the calculi vary from a few millimetres to a few centimetres in size. There is extensive atrophy of the acini with replacement by broad sheets of fibrous tissue. The ductular epithelium is destroyed with dilatation of the ductular spaces. These contain inspissated mucoid material, organic debris, desquamated cells and calcareous material. The islets of Langerhans may be normal, hypertrophic or atrophic.

Analysis of the calculi reveals a predominance of carbonates of calcium with traces of phosphates, oxalates and magnesium and proteins.

The liver shows focal fatty changes, deposition of glycogen in the nuclei and, occasionally, cirrhosis.

Clinical presentation

The cardinal symptom of calcific pancreatitis is severe, recurrent upper abdominal pain, which is refractory to analgesics, but a 'painless' variety of pancreatitis with calcification has been reported from the USA. The calcific pancreatitis occurring in tropical countries of Asia and Africa presents features distinct from the alcoholic variety. The patients commonly present in the second decade of life with abdominal pain, diabetes mellitus, or incidentally detected pancreatic calculi on radiology. They are non-alcoholic and show no evidence of biliary tract disease. There is a characteristic appearance with cyanosed lips, enlarged parotids, pot belly, poor nutrition and defective growth. Diabetes mellitus is a presenting feature in more than 90% of patients. Ketosis is common, but coma is unusual. Diarrhoea is rare although steatorrhoea may develop on a high fat diet.

Unusual complications include obstructive jaundice, pancreatic malignancy, pseudocyst formation and ascites. Complications secondary to diabetes such as recurrent infections, angiopathy, nephropathy, and neuropathy develop by the third decade causing death within a few years. Females with calcific pancreatitis can conceive, go to full term and deliver healthy babies.

Investigations

Demonstration of pancreatic calculi on radiology is diagnostic of chronic pancreatitis. The calculi may be solitary or multiple (Figure 18.43). Hyperglycaemia and ketonuria are common. There is reduction in insulin secretion in response to oral glucose and intravenous tolbutamide.[5] Biochemical steatorrhoea occurs in 60% of patients; serum amylase and lipase values are normal, but the Lundh and secretin–pancreozymin tests are abnormal with tryptic activity being maximally depressed in the calcific cases.

Ultrasonography rarely adds to the information obtained from routine radiography. ERCP findings (Figure 18.44) of ductal dilatation, cyst formation and strictures are similar to those seen in advanced pancreatitis secondary to alcoholism.[1]

Treatment

The aims of treatment are relief of pain, correction of exocrine and endocrine deficiency, and management of complications. Pain responds poorly to analgesics. Diabetes mellitus is

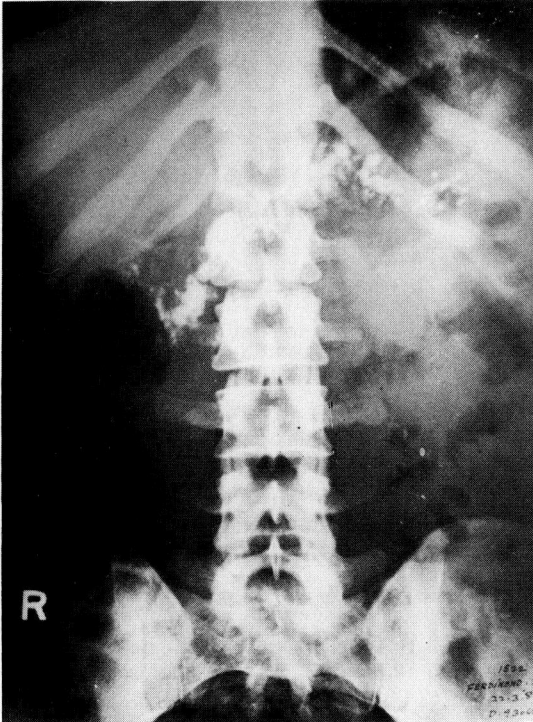

Fig. 18.43   Plain film of abdomen showing diffuse pancreatic calcification.

insulin-dependent, requiring large doses (100–200 units) of soluble insulin. Steatorrhoea is controlled with large doses of pancreatic extracts.

The main indication for surgery is pain and the operative procedures which have been used include sphincteroplasty, opening the main pancreatic duct with removal of stones, partial pancreatectomy, retrograde pancreaticojejunostomy, Puestow's procedure and sympathectomy. Pain relief follows most of the operations,

but relapse is common within 3–5 years. These operations have no effect on insulin requirements.

REFERENCES

1 Balakrishnan, V., Rao, V. R. K., Meenu Hariharan & Anand, B. S. (1982) ERCP findings in tropical pancreatitis syndrome. Presented at the Annual Conference of the Indian Society of Gastroenterology, Srinagar.
2 Barbezat, G. O. & Hansen, J. D. L. (1968) The exocrine pancreas and protein-calorie malnutrition. *Pediatrics*, **42**, 77–92.
3 Dreiling, D. A. (1975) Alcohol, alcoholic pancreatitis, and pancreatic secretion. *Annals of the New York Academy of Sciences*, **252**, 187–199.
4 Geevarghese, P. J. (1968) *Pancreatic Diabetes*. Bombay: Popular Prakashan.
5 Kannan, V. (1981) Insulin secretion in pancreatic diabetes mellitus. *Journal of the Association of Physicians of India*, **29**, 321–331.
6 Pitchumoni, C. S. (1973) Pancreas in primary malnutrition disorders. *American Journal of Clinical Nutrition*, **26**, 374–379.
7 Raji, E. K., Balakrishnan, V., Prabha, B. *et al.* (1982) Immunological aspects of chronic calcific pancreatitis of Kerala (tropical pancreatitis). *Abstracts of the 7th World Congress of Gastroenterology*, Stockholm, Sweden.
8 Sarles, H. (1973) An international survey on nutrition and pancreatitis. *Digestion*, **9**, 389–403.
9 Sarles, H. (1974) Chronic calcifying pancreatitis: chronic alcoholic pancreatitis. *Gastroenterology*, **66**, 604–616.
10 Shaper, A. G. (1960) Chronic pancreatic disease and protein malnutrition. *Lancet*, **i**, 1223–1224.
11 Thompson, M. D. & Trowell, H. C. (1952) Pancreatic enzyme activity in duodenal contents of children with a type of kwashiorkor. *Lancet*, **i**, 1031–1035.
12 Wellmann, K. F. & Volk, B. W. (1977) Pancreatitis, pancreatic lithiasis, and diabetes mellitus. In *The Diabetic Pancreas* (Ed.) Volk, B. W. & Wellmann, K. F. pp. 291–309. New York and London: Plenum Press.
13 Zuidema, P. J. (1959) Cirrhosis and disseminated calcification of the pancreas in patients with malnutrition. *Tropical and Geographical Medicine*, **11**, 70–74.

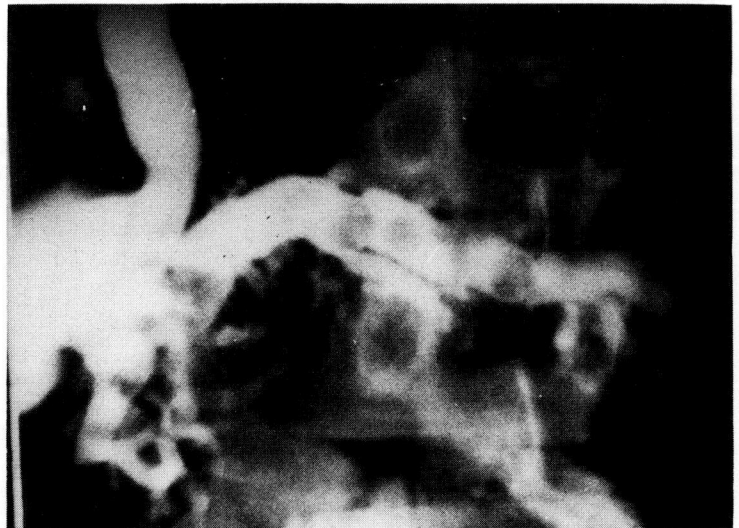

Fig. 18.44   ERCP in chronic calcific pancreatitis of the tropics. The pancreatic duct is markedly dilated with intraductal calculi. The secondary branches are also dilated and distorted.

SHWACHMAN SYNDROME

The clinical association of pancreatic insufficiency with neutropenia and other haematological abnormalities was first described by Shwachman *et al.*[4] and Bodian, Sheldon and Lightwood.[1] Schmerling, *et al.*[3] have given a detailed description of the disorder.

The syndrome is a major cause of pancreatic insufficiency of childhood. It can be distinguished from cystic fibrosis by the absence of pulmonary lesions and normal sweat chloride values. Affected children present with diarrhoea, failure to thrive, exocrine pancreatic insufficiency, and growth retardation. Neutropenia is a prominent feature, and there may be anaemia, thrombocytopenia and bone marrow hypoplasia. Metaphyseal dysostosis and short stature are frequent. The syndrome is inherited probably as an autosomal recessive and siblings may be affected. Improvement in bowel habits is well known in spite of persistence of pancreatic insufficiency, but symptomatic improvement may also reflect reversion of fat absorption to normal. Recently, sensitive techniques have demonstrated a correlation between the correction of steatorrhoea and improved pancreatic function.[2] This points to a functional reserve of pancreatic tissue in these patients.

The prognosis is generally good. Early detection of the syndrome by screening for pancreatic function is required, particularly in the adult patient, to provide nutritional support and to prevent infections. Steatorrhoea calls for substitution therapy with pancreatic extracts.

REFERENCES

1 Bodian, M., Sheldon, W. & Lightwood, R. (1964) Congenital hypoplasia of the exocrine pancreas. *Acta Paediatrica*, **53**, 282–293.
2 Hill, R. E., Durie, P. R., Gaskin, K. J. *et al.* (1982) Steatorrhoea and pancreatic insufficiency in Shwachman syndrome. *Gastroenterology*, **83**, 22–27.
3 Schmerling, D. H., Prader, A., Hitzig, W. H. *et al.* (1969) The syndrome of exocrine pancreatic insufficiency, neutropenia, metaphyseal dysostosis and dwarfism. *Helvetica Paediatrica Acta*, **24**, 547–575.
4 Shwachman, H., Diamond, L. K., Oski, F. A. & Khaw kon, T. (1964) The syndrome of pancreatic insufficiency and bone marrow dysfunction. *Journal of Pediatrics*, **65**, 645–663.

Chapter 19
The Gallbladder and Biliary Tract

ANATOMY AND EMBRYOLOGY

The liver primordium appears in the third week of growth of the conceptus. The hepatic diverticulum is an outgrowth from the foregut which penetrates the septum transversum to form both the liver and bile ducts. A small outgrowth is formed from the developing bile duct and develops into the gallbladder and cystic duct (Figure 19.1).

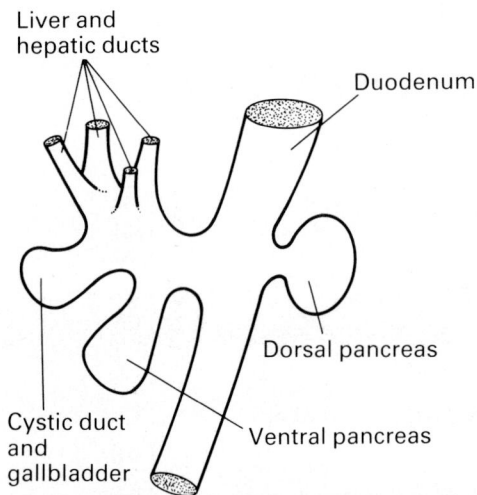

Fig. 19.1 Embryology of the biliary system: the four primordia of the hepaticopancreatic complex in the fifth week. From S. E. Gray & J. E. Skandalakis, (1972) *Embryology for Surgeons*, p. 252, with kind permission of the authors and the publisher, W. B. Saunders.

Grossly, the gallbladder is pear shaped, some 6–8 cm long and 2–3 cm in diameter, partly embedded in the underside of the right lobe of the liver covered by peritoneum, holding some 50 ml of bile with the fundus anteriorly. The body gives rise to the neck from which a small pouch, probably pathological in origin (Hartmann's) may project. From here the cystic duct (3–4 cm) runs to join the common hepatic duct which together then form the common bile duct (Figure 19.2). The cystic duct lumen contains a series of crescentic folds derived from its mucosa, which form the spiral valve of Heister. This may help to hold the lumen open. There is considerable variation from this general description in the relations of the various components of the biliary system, both with themselves and with the vascular supply of this area which itself shows considerable variation.[3]

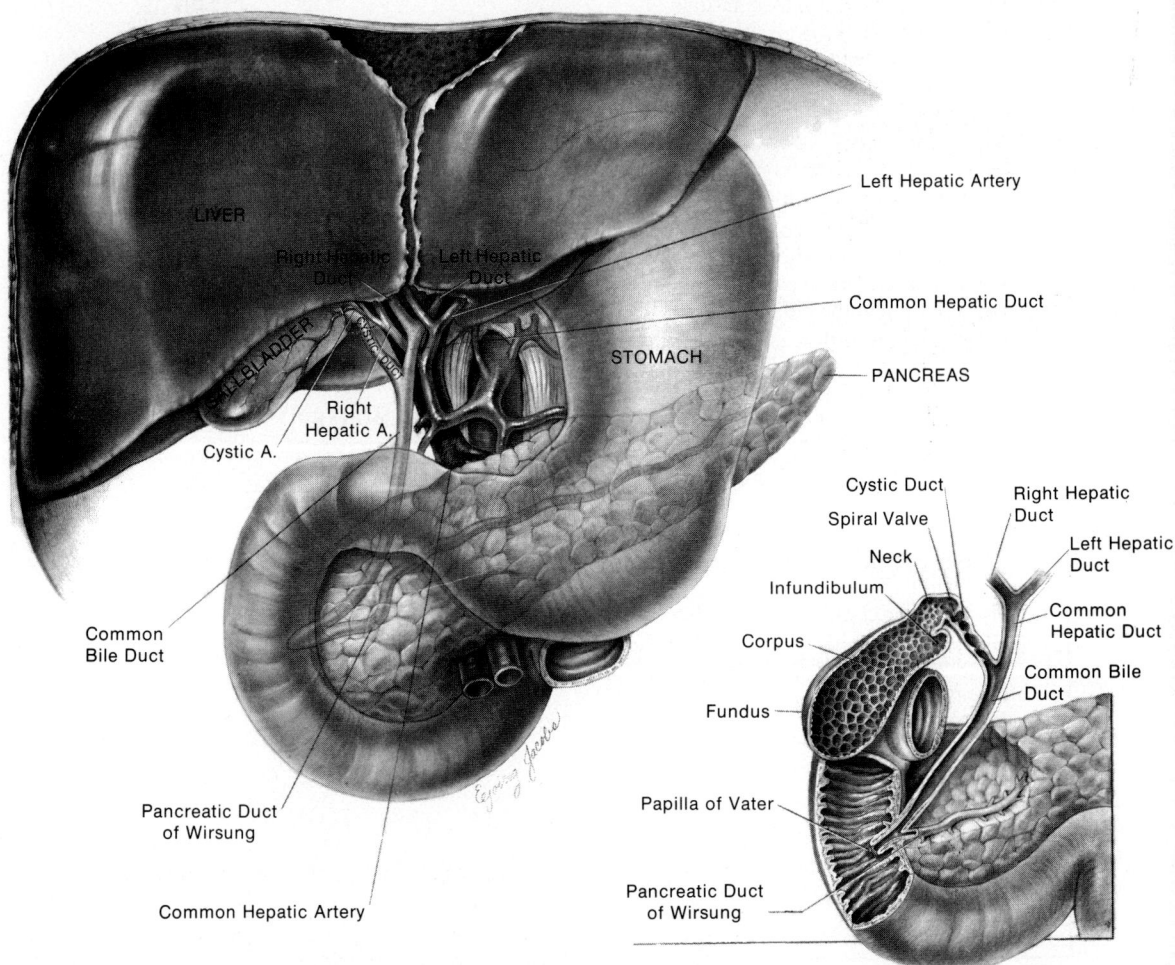

Fig. 19.2 Anatomy of the biliary system. From M. J. Orloff, (1981) The biliary system. In *Davis-Christopher Textbook of Surgery* (Ed.) Sabiston, D. C. p. 1230, with kind permission of the author, the editor and the publisher, W. B. Saunders.

The biliary tract receives both sympathetic (from the coeliac plexus) and parasympathetic (vagal) innervation. Afferent fibres are also present. The sympathetic fibres supply the muscle coat which also receives a small cholinergic innervation. A myenteric plexus is present in the submucosa and subserosa. Receptors for VIP have been described on gallbladder nerve fibres and pharmacological techniques have revealed a variety of receptors on the smooth muscle.

HISTOCHEMISTRY

Enzymes

Acid phosphatase activity has been demonstrated in human gallbladder epithelium at the ultrastructural level[19] chiefly in the lysosomes, although some is seen in the Golgi apparatus. Thiamine pyrophosphatase is present in the Golgi apparatus too, and small amounts are also seen in mucous droplets. This may represent a route for various lysosomal enzymes to be secreted into the bile along with mucus.[29] Mucosal β-glucuronidase activity measured biochemically is higher in acalculous patients which is compatible with the concept that this enzyme may play a role in the formation of the nidus for lithogenesis.

Alkaline phosphatase has been demonstrated in gallbladder capillary endothelium[37] and in the brush border of the epithelium[20] (Figure 19.3). Three patterns are found: complete, patchy and absent which can be related to the biliary lipid composition suggesting that the biliary epithelium may be able to modify biliary lipid composition. Alkaline phosphatase is found on the embryologically related small intestinal brush border, a known site of lipid absorption. Human gallbladder epithelial esterase activity is chiefly lysosomal (Figure 19.4). Using inhibitors and activators, it appears that at least two enzyme complexes are involved, one of which has cholesterol esterase activity. Bile acids are able to modulate the mucosal enzyme activity.

Mucosubstances

Wallraff *et al.*[37] provided one of the earliest comprehensive surveys of gallbladder histochemistry, documenting the presence of glycoproteins, neutral and acid mucosubstances in the apical epithelium. This was confirmed by Esterly and Spicer[9] who showed that the amount of mucus present increased with inflammation and this has also been described in experimental lithogenesis in animals.[14, 23] The neck cells secrete both neutral and carboxymucins. In carcinoma, carboxymucins predominate. Immunological techniques[13] have demonstrated a sulphoglycoprotein specific for the human gallbladder, and three others which are common to the stomach and intestine. These biochemical similarities reflect metaplastic potential. There are a few reports of the localization of mucosubstances at the ultrastructural level.[18, 24]

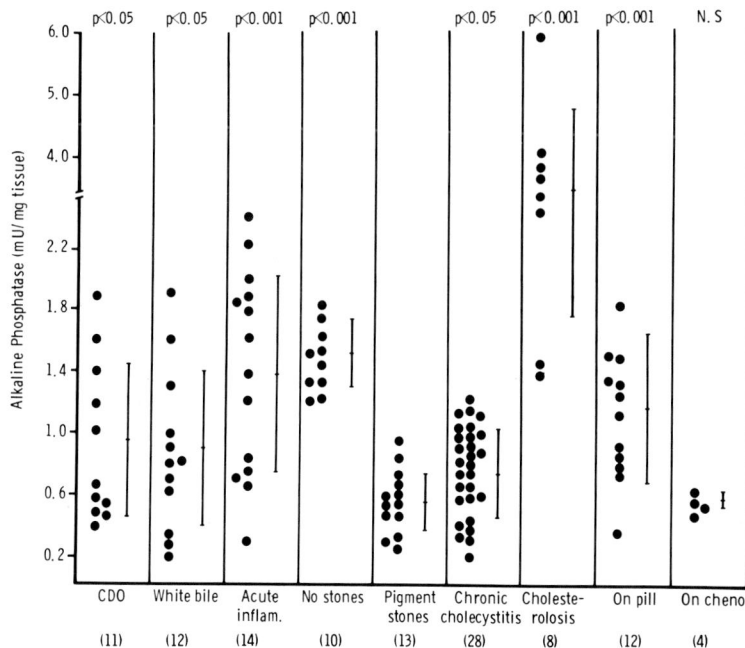

Fig. 19.3 Alkaline phosphatase (mU/(mg tissue)) activity in gallbladder mucosa of various groups of patients (numbers are given in parentheses). The pigment stone group are taken as an arbitrary control for comparison and statistical differences between the groups are shown at the tops of the columns. CDO: common duct obstruction.

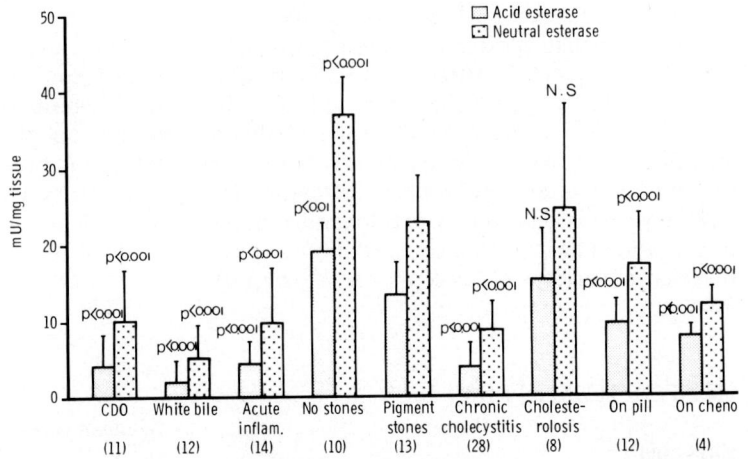

Fig. 19.4 Acid and neutral esterase activity (mU/(mg tissue)) in gallbladder mucosa from various groups of patients (numbers are shown in parentheses). The pigment stone group are taken as an arbitrary control for comparison and statistical differences between the groups are shown at the tops of the columns. DCO: common duct obstruction.

Lipids

Lipid droplets were first described in the gallbladder epithelium by Virchow.[35] More recently cholesterol and its esters, fatty acids and some unsaturated lipids have been documented.[4, 17] There is evidence of lipid uptake from the lumen by the epithelial cells in guinea pig using labelled oleic acid, cholesterol lecithin and lysolecithin.[27] Extremes of this phenomenon may lead to cholesterolosis while it is possible that one of the lipid components may act as an irritating agent to initiate and maintain cholecystitis.

HISTOLOGY

Electron microscopy

There are a number of reports of transmission electron microscopy on human gallbladder, most of them perforce on diseased tissue.[16] Three epithelial cell types have been described in the fundus. The principal ordinary cells have regular microvilli on their apical cell membrane with some intervening pits. Anions may play a role in the stability of the apical cell membrane.[31] The lateral cell border has irregular microvilli and the space between the cells varies with their functional state.[2] The cells are joined at their apices by tight junctions but these are not the site for net fluid transport.[11] Coated and non-coated pits may be found on the basolateral membrane. The epithelium rests on a basement membrane. There is a normal complement of organelles. At the apex, there are secretory droplets derived from a well-developed Golgi apparatus. The residual bodies have many forms and some with lipid inclusions. A fibrillary system is well developed by the lateral cell membrane and as a terminal web. Lipid droplets may be found especially in the basal part of the cells.

Pencil cells may be seen in over 60% of gallbladders with compact cytosol but their exact state is uncertain. Basal cells represent intraepithelial lymphocytes, probably T, and mast cells. Macrophages, some containing lipid are also found between the epithelial cells and in the lamina propria.

Various cell types have been described in the neck glands.[21, 22] The glands have tall antral cells with numerous pale secretory droplets and tall microvilli, whereas the cells in the neck are cuboid with short irregular microvilli and few or no secretory granules. Endocrine-like cells are also present.

There are several scanning electron microscopy reports on normal and pathological material.[25] Mucosal folds are seen and at higher magnifications the hexagonal boundaries of the cells and the apical microvilli are identified. Cholesterolosis produces broadened folds. Chronic cholecystitis effaces the folds to give irregular undulating areas.

Tracers

The principal function of the gallbladder is to concentrate bile 4–10-fold by the absorption of water and electrolytes. Horseradish peroxidase (MW 40 000) and cationized ferritin (MW 480 000) are absorbed in vivo.[5, 15] Horseradish peroxidase, following fluid phase endocytosis, appears in the lateral intercellular space within 5 minutes of an intraluminal injection. Cationized ferritin is internalized by adsorption endocytosis, is stripped from the membrane, and after 2 hours exocytosed in clumps into the lateral intercellular space (Figures 19.5 and 19.6). These observations represent both rapid and somewhat slower pathways for the transport of large molecules from the bile to the lamina propria.

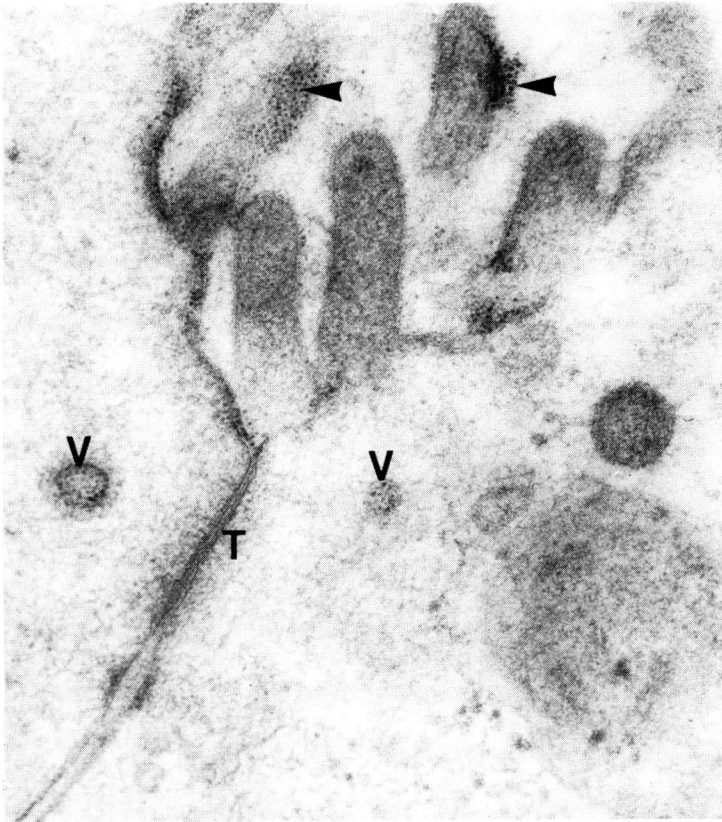

Fig. 19.5 Apex of guinea-pig gallbladder epithelial cell showing binding within five minutes' exposure of cationized ferritin by microvilli (arrowheads) and internalization in vesicles (V). There is no marker in the tight junction (T). Uncounterstained electron micrograph, × 70 000.

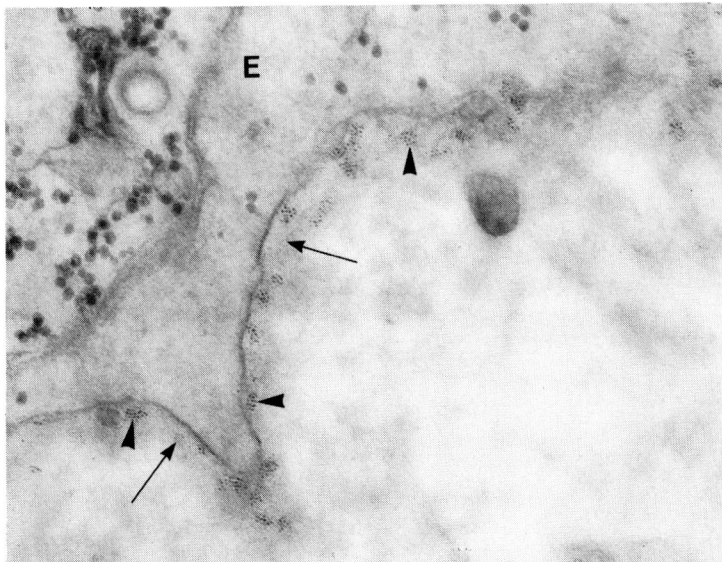

Fig. 19.6 Base of guinea-pig gallbladder epithelial cell (E) showing clumps of cationized ferritin against the basement membrane (arrow). At this stage (2 h after labelling) no marker has passed into the underlying connective tissue. Uncounterstained electron micrograph, × 60 000.

Cell proliferation

The labelling index is very low in 'normal' gall-bladder, some 10 times lower than the 1–1.5% reported for laboratory animals.[30] There is a significantly higher labelling index in distended gallbladders, for example carcinomatous obstruction of the gallbladder. There was no preferential site for cell labelling on the crests or valleys of the mucosal folds.

Tissue culture

It is possible to culture guinea-pig gallbladder epithelium in a number of media.[8] Growth of epithelial cells is established by 1–2 days into culture extending over the explant and into colonies. The fine structure and biochemical activity is maintained for at least 7 days, as is the ability to take up cationized ferritin in vitro, as an index of integrated behaviour.

Secretion of mucus

The secretion of mucus is one of the chief functions of gallbladder epithelium. This is a spontaneously occurring phenomenon but it may be induced by various means. Wahlin and his colleagues[36] have shown that intragastric olive oil and injections of cholecystokinin will cause the discharge of mucous droplets. Vagal stimulation produces the same effect as does pilocarpine.[1] The secretion of mucus by exocytosis will place more packages of membrane into the apical cell membrane and this will induce membrane retrieval.

Immunocytes

Lymphocytes and plasma cells predominantly IgA are found in the lamina propria of the gallbladder and their numbers increase with the severity of cholecystitis. IgA and IgM cells also increase in severe cholecystitis.[12] IgM cells are the most numerous in the muscle layers. These cells also increase in chronic inflammation. Using electron immunoperoxidase techniques, Nagura et al.[26] have shown the basolateral distribution of IgA over bile duct epithelium which suggests a secretory component-mediated transfer of IgA. There are coated pits on the basolateral surface of gallbladder epithelium.

Eosinophils may be noted in increased numbers infiltrating the gallbladder in 2.5% of specimens, often simply a prominent component of a mixed inflammatory cell infiltrate. Rarely, there may be a purely eosinophilic cholecystitis.[10]

Mast cells

Mast cells are found in relatively small numbers in the gallbladder.[28] Their ratios are 40 : 20 : 10 in serosa, muscle and mucosa per high power field. Mast cells are also present between the epithelial cells where they stain relatively little, possibly due to low quantities of heparin in the granules and the presence of lower sulphated glycosaminoglycans.[34]

Metaplasia-ectopia

Chronic inflammation and the presence of stones may induce metaplasia, usually in the form of cells resembling pyloric antrum or goblet cells but occasionally as squamous cells. Argentaffin cells occur chiefly in relation to neck glands.[7] Enterochromaffin cells are common in the gallbladders of some species e.g. ox, pig, guinea pig. Endocrine cell types and Paneth cells are seen on electron microscopy of metaplastic gallbladders removed for stones.[21] Inappropriate mucin secretion with the production of CEA and intestinal mucin has been noted in metaplasia.[6] Ectopic gastric mucosa occurs rarely and contains gastric mucous cells and parietal cells. Such patients may present with cholecystitis.[32]

REFERENCES

1 Axelsson, H., Danielsson, A., Henriksson, R. & Wahlin, R. (1979) Secretory behaviour and ultrastructural changes in mouse gallbladder principal cells after stimulation with cholinergic and adrenergic nerves. *Gastroenterology*, **76**, 335–340.
2 Blom, H. & Helander, H. F. (1977) Quantitative electron microscopical studies on in vitro incubated rabbit gallbladder epithelium. *Journal of Membrane Biology*, **37**, 45–61.
3 Blumgart, L. H. (Ed.) (1982) *The Biliary Tract*. Edinburgh: Churchill Livingstone.
4 Boyd, W. (1922) Studies in gallbladder pathology. *British Journal of Surgery*, **10**, 337–356.
5 Coghill, S. B., Hopwood, D. & Milne, G. (1983) The uptake of horseradish peroxidase and its subsequent redistribution by guinea pig gallbladder in vivo. *Journal of Pathology* **139**, 89–95.
6 De Boer, W. G. R. M., Ma, J., Rees, J. W. & Nayman, J. (1981) Inappropriate mucin producer in gallbladder metaplasia and neoplasia: an immunological study. *Histopathology*, **5**, 295–303.
7 Delaquerriere, L., Tremblay, G. & Riopelle, J. L. (1962) Argentaffine cell in chronic cholecystitis. *Archives of Pathology*, **74**, 142–151.
8 Elhamady, M. S., Hopwood, D., Milne, G. et al. (1983) Tissue culture of guinea pig gallbladder. *Journal of Pathology*, **140**, 221–235.
9 Esterly, J. R. & Spicer, S. S. (1968) Mucin histochemistry of human gallbladder and changes in adenocarcinoma, gastric fibrosis and cholecystitis. *Journal of National Cancer Institute*, **40**, 1–11.

10 Fox, H. & Mainwaring, A. R. (1972) Eosinophilic infiltration of the gallbladder. *Gastroenterology*, **63**, 1049–1052.

11 Frederiksen, D., Møllgaard, K. & Rostgaard, J. (1979) Lack of correlation between transepithelial transport capacity and paracellular pathway ultrastructure in Alcian Blue treated rabbit gallbladder. *Journal of Cell Biology*, **83**, 383–393.

12 Green, F. H. Y. & Fox, H. (1972) An immunofluorescent study of the distribution of immunoglobulin containing cells in the normal and inflamed human gallbladder. *Gut*, **13**, 379–384.

13 Häkkinen, I. & Laito, M. (1970) Epithelial glycoproteins of human gallbladder. *Archives of Pathology*, **90**, 137–142.

14 Hayward, A. F., Freston, J. W. & Bouchier, I. A. D. (1968) Changes in the ultrastructure of gallbladder epithelium in rabbits with experimental gallstones. *Gut*, **9**, 550–556.

15 Hopwood, D., Milne, G. & Wood, R. A. B. (1982) The uptake of cationized ferritin and its subsequent redistribution by gallbladder epithelium in vivo. *Journal of Pathology*, **136**, 95–109.

16 Hopwood, D., Kouroumalis, E., Milne, G. & Bouchier, I. A. D. (1980) Cholecystitis: a fine structural analysis. *Journal of Pathology*, **130**, 1–14.

17 Illingworth, C. F. W. (1929) Cholesterolosis of the gallbladder. *British Journal of Surgery*, **17**, 203–229.

18 Koga, A. (1973) Electron microscopic observations on the mucous secretory activity of the human gallbladder epithelium. *Zeitschrift für Zellforschung*, **139**, 463–471.

19 Kouroumalis, E., Hopwood, D., Ross, P. E. et al. (1983) Gallbladder epithelial acid hydrolases in human cholecystitis. *Journal of Pathology*, **139**, 179–191.

20 Kouroumalis, E., Hopwood, D., Ross, P. E. & Bouchier, I. A. D. (1983) Mucosal alkaline phosphatase and bile lipids in gallbladders in cholecystitis. *Journal of Pathology*, **141**, 169–179.

21 Laitio, M. & Nevalainen, T. (1975) Ultrastructure of endocrine cells in metaplastic epithelium of human gallbladder. *Journal of Anatomy*, **120**, 219–225.

22 Laitio, M. & Nevalainen, T. (1975) Gland ultrastructure in human gallbladder. *Journal of Anatomy*, **120**, 105–112.

23 Lee, S. P. (1981) Hypersecretion of mucous glycoprotein by the gallbladder epithelium in experimental cholecystitis. *Journal of Pathology*, **134**, 199–207.

24 Luciano, L., Reale, E. & Wolpers, C. (1974) Die Feinstruktur der Gallenblase und Gallengänge V. Histochemische Lokalisierung von Mukosubstanzen in menschlichen Gallenblasenepithel. *Histochemistry*, **38**, 57–70.

25 Myllärniemi, H. & Nickels, J. I. (1972) Observations by scanning electron microscopy of normal and pathological human gallbladder epithelium. *Acta Pathologica et Microbiologica Scandinavica*, A**85**, 42–48.

26 Nagura, H., Smith, P. D., Nakane, P. K. & Brown, W. R. (1981) IgA in human bile and liver. *Journal of Immunology*, **126**, 587–595.

27 Neiderhiser, D. H., Harmon, C. K. & Roth, H. P. (1976) Absorption of cholesterol by the gallbladder. *Journal of Lipid Research*, **17**, 117–124.

28 Norris, H. T., Zamcheck, N. & Gottlieb, L. S. (1963) The presence and distribution of mast cells in the human gastrointestinal tract at autopsy. *Gastroenterology*, **44**, 448–455.

29 Palade, G. (1975) Ultracellular aspects of the process of protein secretion. *Science*, **189**, 347–358.

30 Putz, P. & Willems, G. (1979) Cell proliferation in the human gallbladder epithelium: effect of distension. *Gut*, **20**, 246–248.

31 Quinton, P. M. & Philpott, C. W. (1973) A role for anionic sites in epithelial architecture. *Journal of Cell Biology*, **56**, 787–796.

32 Runge, P. M., Schwartz, J. N., Seigler, H. F. et al. (1978) Gallbladder with ectopic gastric mucosa. *Archives of Pathology*, **102**, 209–211.

33 Smith, R. & Sherlock, S. (1981) *Surgery of the Gallbladder and Bile Ducts*. 2nd edition. London: Butterworth.

34 Tas, J. & Berndsen, R. G. (1977) Does heparin occur in mucosal mast cells of the rat small intestine. *Journal of Histochemistry and Cytochemistry* **35**, 1058–1062.

35 Virchow, R. (1857) Uber das Epithel der Gallenblase und über einen intermediaren Stoffwechsel das Fettes. *Virchows Archiv*, **11**, 574–578.

36 Wahlin, T., Bloom, G. D. & Danielsson, Å. (1976) Effect of cholecystokinin-pancriozymin (CCK-PZ) on glycoprotein secretia from mouse gallbladder epithelium. *Cell Tissue Research*, **171**, 425–435.

37 Wallraff, J. & Dietrich, K. F. (1957) Die Morphologie und Histochemie der Steingallenblase des Menschen. *Zeitschrift für Zellforschung*, **46**, 155–231.

CONGENITAL ABNORMALITIES

Most apparent congenital anomalies of the gallbladder and biliary tract are really variants of the normal anatomy. The rare anomalies that do occur are related to alterations and variations in embryological budding from the foregut. These abnormalities are usually asymptomatic and of no clinical significance but may occasionally predispose to stasis, inflammation and stone formation. They are, however, important to the radiologist in interpreting radiographic investigations and to the surgeon when operating on the biliary system.

ANOMALIES OF THE BILE DUCTS

Hepatic ducts (Figure 19.7)

The intrahepatic ducts are remarkably constant and drain named segments of the liver. The confluence of the right and left hepatic ducts is always extrahepatic. In 75% of individuals there is a single right hepatic duct but in 25% the right anterior and posterior segmental ducts enter the left hepatic duct separately, which has led to the erroneous concept of an 'accessory' hepatic duct. This is a variant of normal and not a congenital anomaly.[11] Occasionally the hepatic ducts enter the duodenum separately, with the cystic duct joining the right hepatic duct. This has been termed duplication of the common bile duct. Bile ducts passing directly from the liver to the gallbladder are rare, and probably secondary to disease rather than congenital.[12]

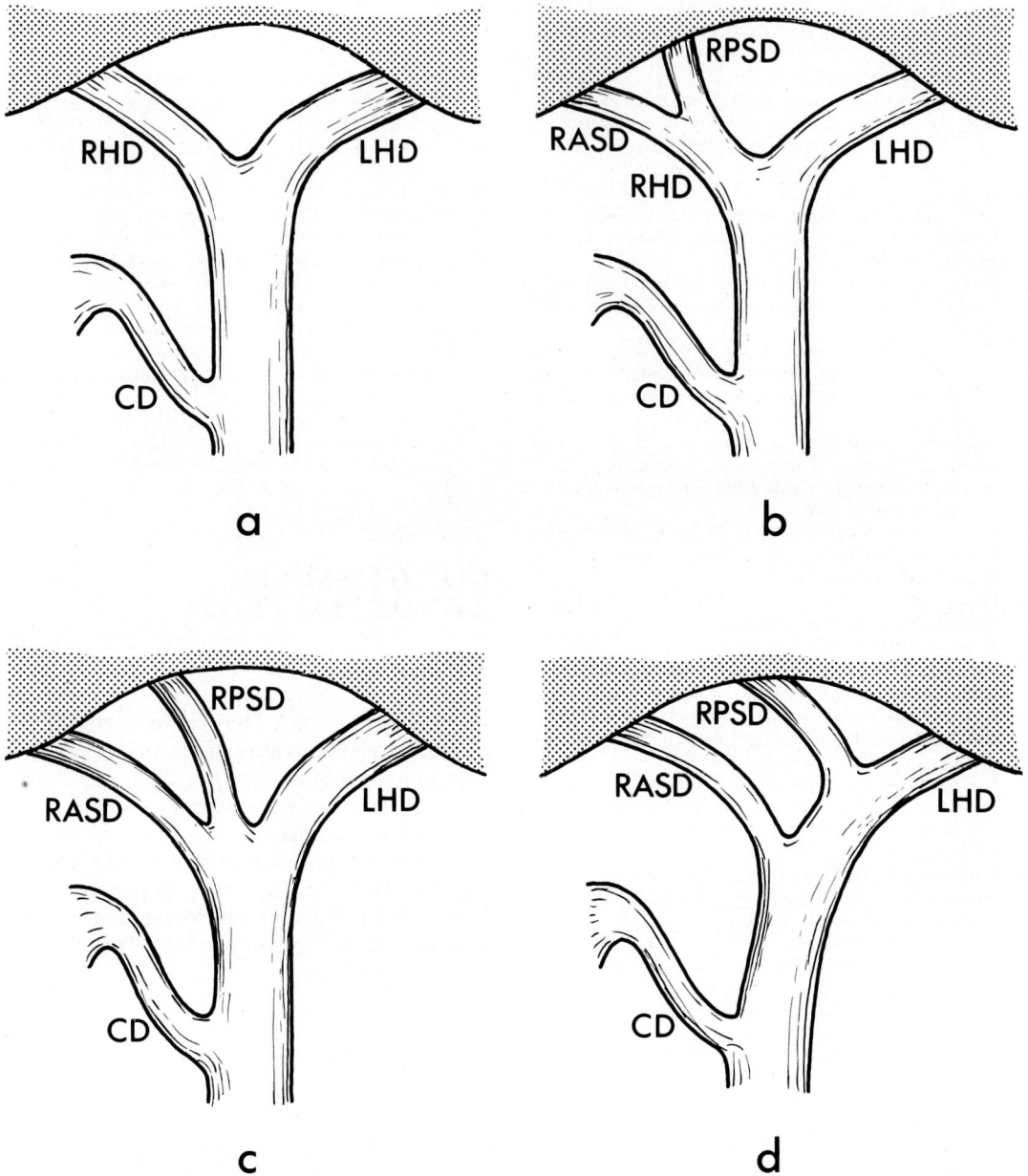

Fig. 19.7 Variations of the hepatic ducts. (a) A single right hepatic duct (RHD) is usually formed within the liver and is present in 75% of individuals; (b) sometimes it is formed outside the liver; (c) in 25% the segmental ducts form a triple confluence with the left hepatic duct (LHD); or (d) join it separately. (RASD = right anterior segmental duct; RPSD = right posterior segmental duct; CD = cystic duct).

Common hepatic and common bile duct

Most anomalies are variants of normal anatomy. Variations of the intrapancreatic portion depend on the extent to which the common duct is covered by the pancreas. Although of no functional significance they are important to the surgeon. Very rarely the retroduodenal portion may be atretic and bypassed by an accessory duct.

The relationship of the bile duct to the pancreatic duct at the ampulla and the site of opening of the bile duct into the duodenum are also variants of normal anatomy. With duplications of the bile duct, two separate openings may be present. Duplications may be associated with duodenal atresia with separate openings proximal and distal to the atresia.

Congenital cystic dilatation of the common bile duct – choledochal cysts

The currently accepted classification (Figure 19.8) is a modification of the original of Alonso-Lej *et al.*[1] by the addition of intrahepatic cystic or fusiform dilatation.[15] (a) Concentric dilatation: this is the classical choledochal cyst (over 90%) which is usually cystic but may be fusiform; (b) Diverticulum or eccentric dilatation of

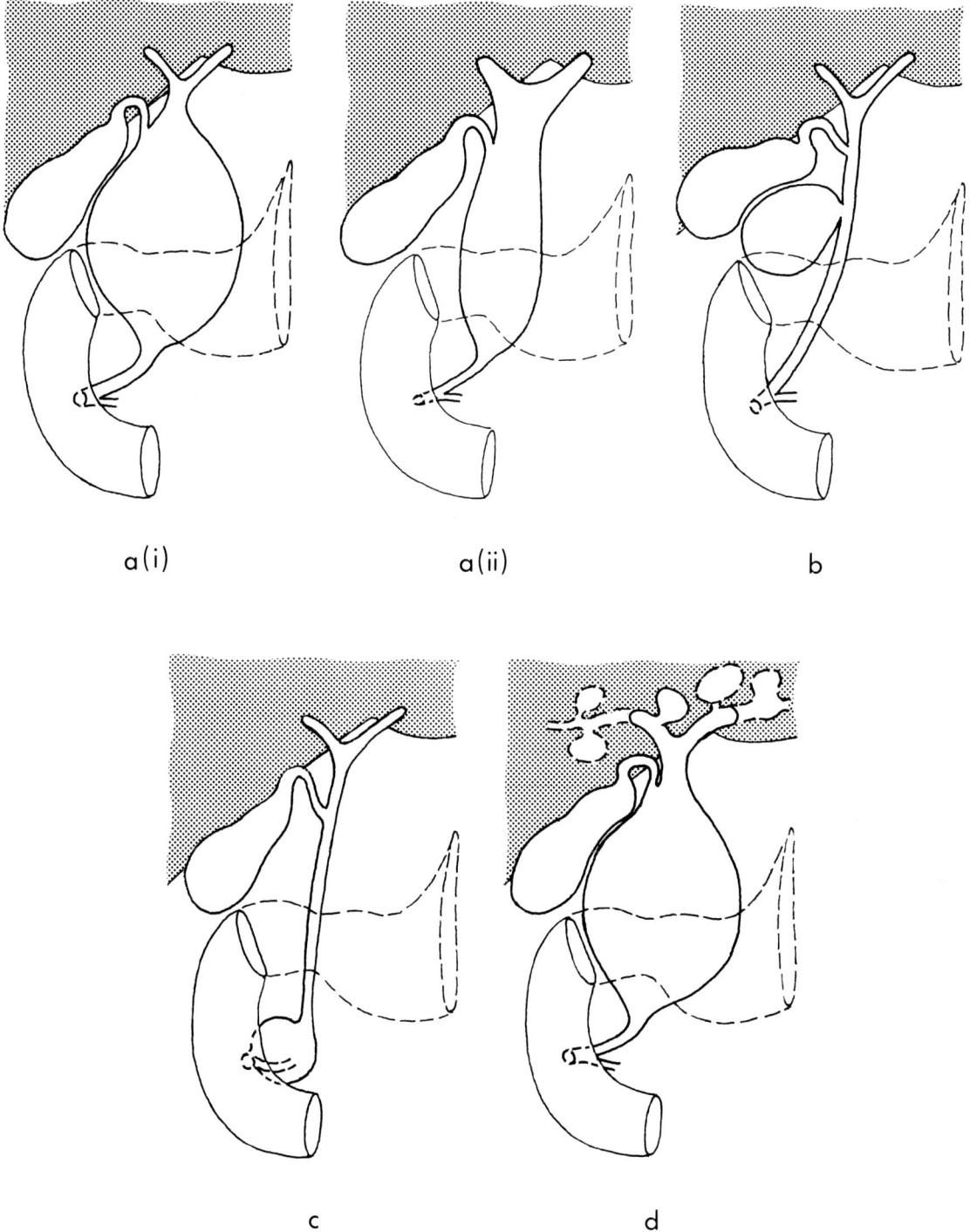

Fig. 19.8 Varieties of choledochal cyst. (*ai*) Concentric dilatation of the common bile duct; (*aii*) fusiform dilatation; (b) diverticulum or eccentric dilatation; (c) choledochocoele, which may be extra- or intramural; (d) intrahepatic cystic dilatation – Caroli's disease.

the common bile duct; (c) Choledochocoele: this may be extra- or intramural; (d) Intrahepatic cystic dilatation – Caroli's disease.[2]

All forms are uncommon in Western countries, where choledochal cyst is usually unassociated with intrahepatic cystic dilatation. Choledochal cysts are commoner in Oriental countries and are four times more common in the Japanese than in other races. About half of the patients have associated intrahepatic cystic dilatation.[19, 24] Increasing use of endoscopic retrograde cholangiopancreatography (ERCP) has indicated that choledochocoeles may be more common than previously suspected. The relationship between Caroli's disease and congenital hepatic fibrosis, of which it may be a variant, is recognized.

One quarter of choledochal cysts present during the first year of life, some 60% between one and 10 years of age and the remaining 10–20% during the second decade. Patients rarely present later in life. Although many patients are diagnosed after the age of one year, very few are symptom-free during the first year of life. Choledochal cysts are commoner in females (3 to 1).

PATHOLOGY

Choledochal cysts vary greatly in size and may contain from a few millilitres to several litres of fluid. The content is usually inspissated bile but rarely frankly purulent. Associated gallstones are rarely found in children (two out of 28 patients in Cape Town), but may be more frequent in adults. The gallbladder is usually normal. The cyst wall varies in thickness from 1 mm to about 1 cm and microscopically it consists of fibrous tissue. Muscle is conspicuously absent although smooth muscle fibres may occasionally be identified. There is no epithelial lining although islets of cuboidal or columnar mucosa may remain. The incidence of carcinoma is approximately 20 times greater than in the normal population.[16]

AETIOLOGY

The aetiology is unknown but suggested aetiological mechanisms range from distal common bile duct obstruction to congenital weakness of the wall. Distal obstruction alone is an insufficient mechanism and requires concomitant damage to epithelium and duct wall to produce a choledochal cyst.[9] Reflux of pancreatic juice, in situations where a common channel of pancreatic and bile duct above the ampulla have

been shown, could cause the damage, and this theory is supported by the finding of elevated amylase concentrations in the cyst.[10] Although not previously suggested, we consider that an intrauterine vascular accident affecting the recently recognized tenuous blood supply to the supraduodenal bile duct could be an alternative mechanism.[18]

CLINICAL FEATURES

The classical triad is intermittent obstructive jaundice, abdominal pain and an abdominal mass. Jaundice is the most constant feature, occurring in about 75% of reported cases. Pain is usually a feature in about two-thirds but occurred in only half of our patients. A smooth mass continuous with the liver is palpable in the right upper quadrant in about half the patients. The full triad was only present in 20% of Cape Town patients.[17] In infancy the most common symptom is persistent jaundice often associated with abdominal distension, fever and vomiting while in older children there is frequently a history of recurrent mild episodes of jaundice with pale stools and dark urine. Important late complications include cholangitis and cirrhosis.

LABORATORY AND RADIOLOGICAL STUDIES

Liver function tests will merely confirm obstructive jaundice, when present. The most important definitive diagnostic tests today are ultrasound (Figure 19.9) or computerized tomographic (CT) scanning to demonstrate the cyst and the status of the intrahepatic ducts. In older children and adults ERCP will confirm the diagnosis. This technique has replaced operative cholangiography, except in the case of small children (Figure 19.10). Modern radionuclide scanning can be helpful. These methods have superseded previously used radiological investigations.

TREATMENT

The only acceptable treatment today for the classical choledochal cyst is surgical excision of the cyst with reconstruction of the bile duct by hepatico-jejunostomy using a Roux-en-Y loop. An alternative, which is seldom used, is interposition of an isolated segment of jejunum between the proximal bile duct and the duodenum. To protect the adjacent vascular structures, which are adherent to the cyst, the anterior wall is excised. Posteriorly the cyst lining is stripped leaving the outer wall intact

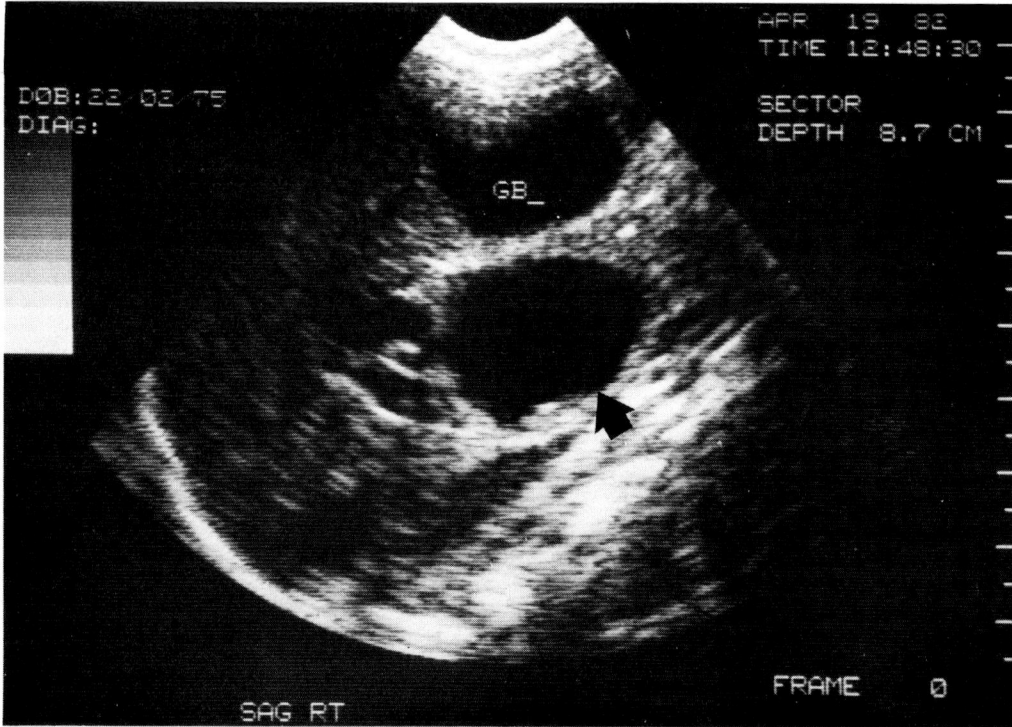

Fig. 19.9 Ultrasonogram of choledochal cyst. The echolucent choledochal cyst is indicated by the arrow.

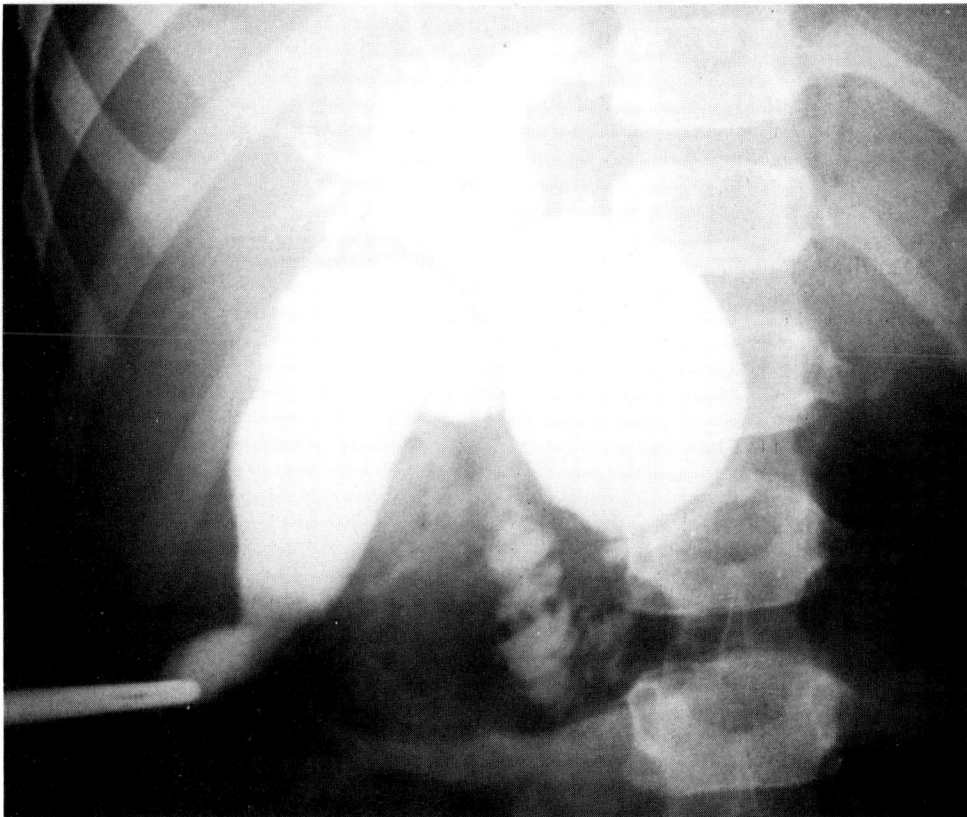

a

Fig. 19.10 Operative cholangiograms. (a) The concentric dilatation of the common bile duct is outlined on cholangiography; (b & c: overleaf).

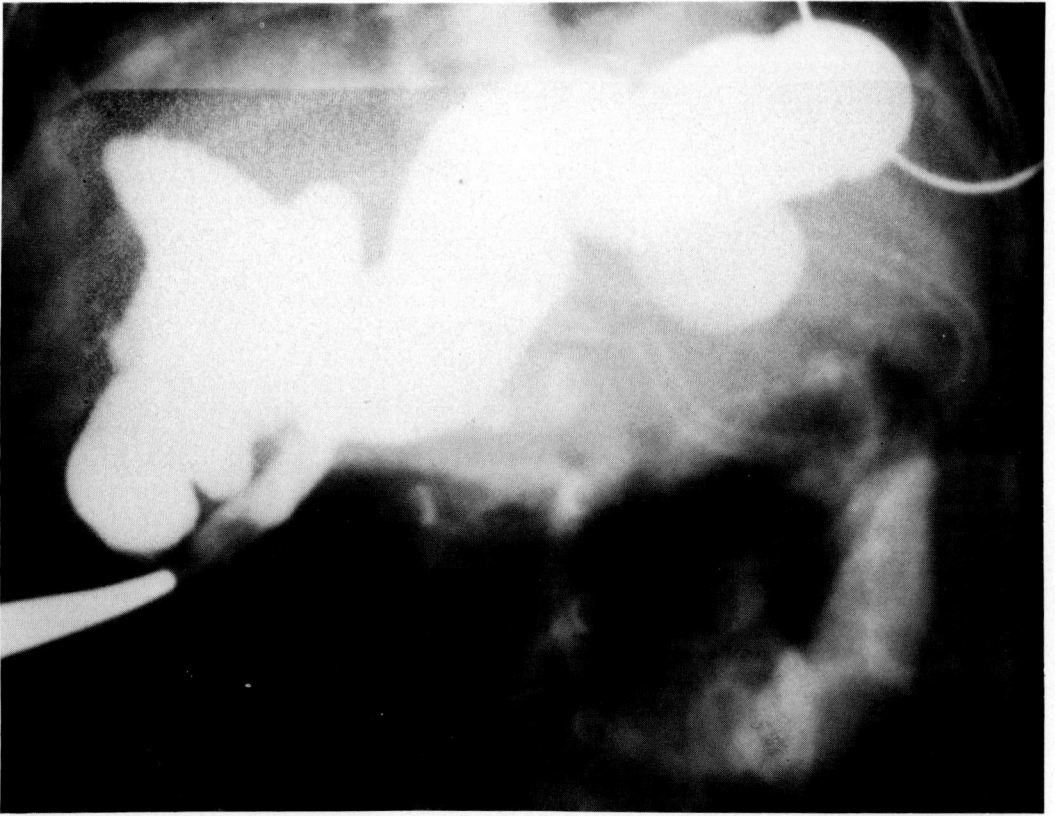

b

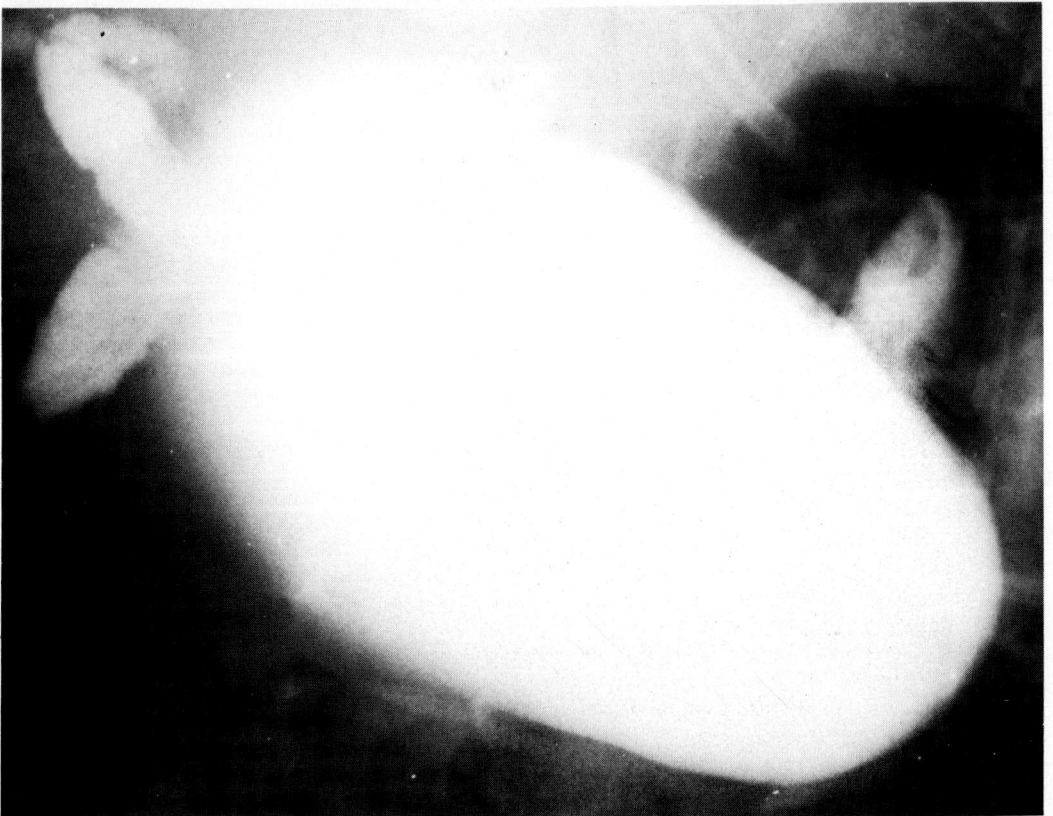

c

Fig. 19.10(continued) Operative cholangiograms. (b & c). A large choledochal cyst with gross dilatation of the intrahepatic ducts in a three-week-old baby.

where it abuts on the portal vein and hepatic artery.[14] The upper anastomosis should be performed to normal duct above the cyst or to the confluence of the ducts in the porta hepatis to prevent subsequent stricture.[22] The distal portion of the cyst is left and the opening of the bile duct oversewn taking care not to damage the pancreatic duct.

External drainage is unjustified. Internal drainage to the duodenum or a Roux loop of jejunum was practised in the past, but is unacceptable because drainage is inadequate, anastomotic strictures form and recurrent cholangitis leads to secondary biliary cirrhosis and portal hypertension. In addition the increased hazard of carcinoma persists unless the cyst is excised.

The treatment of other varieties of choledochal cyst depends upon the symptoms and the type of anomaly. Eccentric diverticula should be excised. Treatment for Caroli's disease remains unsatisfactory. Choledochocoeles should only be treated if symptomatic, as the pancreatic duct is in danger at operation. Vaterian cysts can be treated by sphincteroplasty or endoscopic sphincterotomy. Symptomatic peri-vaterian cysts pose a very difficult management problem but partial excision was successful in one of our patients.

ANOMALIES OF THE GALLBLADDER AND CYSTIC DUCT

Gallbladder anomalies

This is the least variable part of the biliary tree. The only common anomaly (18%) is the Phrygian cap deformity, in which the distal fundus of the gallbladder is folded upon itself. Very rarely the gallbladder may be absent, vestigial, duplicated, bilobed, or may be misplaced. A mobile gallbladder, attached by a mesentery, may undergo torsion and strangulation. If the gallbladder is absent so is the cystic duct. Duplications are rare. Only two abnormalities of position are of importance to the surgeon: very rarely the gallbladder may lie on the left side of the liver without situs inversus, but more important is an intrahepatic gallbladder which is completely submerged in the liver substance. It may be missed and mistaken for absence of the gallbladder. When associated with symptomatic gallstones, treatment is difficult. The alternatives are cholecystostomy and removal of the gallstones or preferably a partial cholecystectomy and ligation of the cystic duct if possible.

Cystic duct anomalies

The cystic duct may be absent with the gallbladder draining directly into the common duct. This is almost certainly not a congenital defect, but due to erosion of a large gallstone, which is invariably present, into the duct.[12] Most cystic duct anomalies are variants of the normal anatomy, in which the duct runs a longer course parallel with or spiralling around the common hepatic duct (Figure 19.11). Double cystic ducts may drain a single normal gallbladder and enter the bile duct or right hepatic duct.

BILIARY ATRESIA

Although considered here, biliary atresia should be regarded as an acquired and not a congenital or developmental anomaly. In the past it was regarded as congenital and classified into 'correctable' and 'non-correctable' types. In the 'correctable' type (10%) the proximal bile ducts are patent but end blindly before the duodenum. In 'non-correctable' types the proximal extrahepatic bile ducts are obliterated and may extend throughout the entire liver. The modern concept is based on the work of Kasai *et al.*,[8] who demonstrated convincingly that biliary atresia was a treatable, and in some instances a curable condition. The common anatomical types encountered at operation are depicted in Figure 19.12.

AETIOLOGY AND PATHOLOGY

Biliary atresia arises as a result of an inflammatory process, best described as a progressive sclerosing cholangitis, which usually affects both the extrahepatic and intrahepatic biliary tree but may occasionally be segmental and localized. No specific agents have consistently been identified although an infective viral agent seems most likely. Rubella and hepatitis A and B viruses and more recently the REO virus have been implicated. There appears to be a progression from hepatitis to ductal hypoplasia or obliteration. Liver damage is present in all patients but the extent of the damage varies. The rarity of the disease in the immediate neonatal period or in stillborns, suggests that complete obliteration of the bile ducts occurs some time after birth. It is thought to occur in about 1 in 10 000 infants.

CLINICAL FEATURES AND DIAGNOSIS

The clinical features are persistent jaundice, clay-coloured faeces and hepatomegaly. The

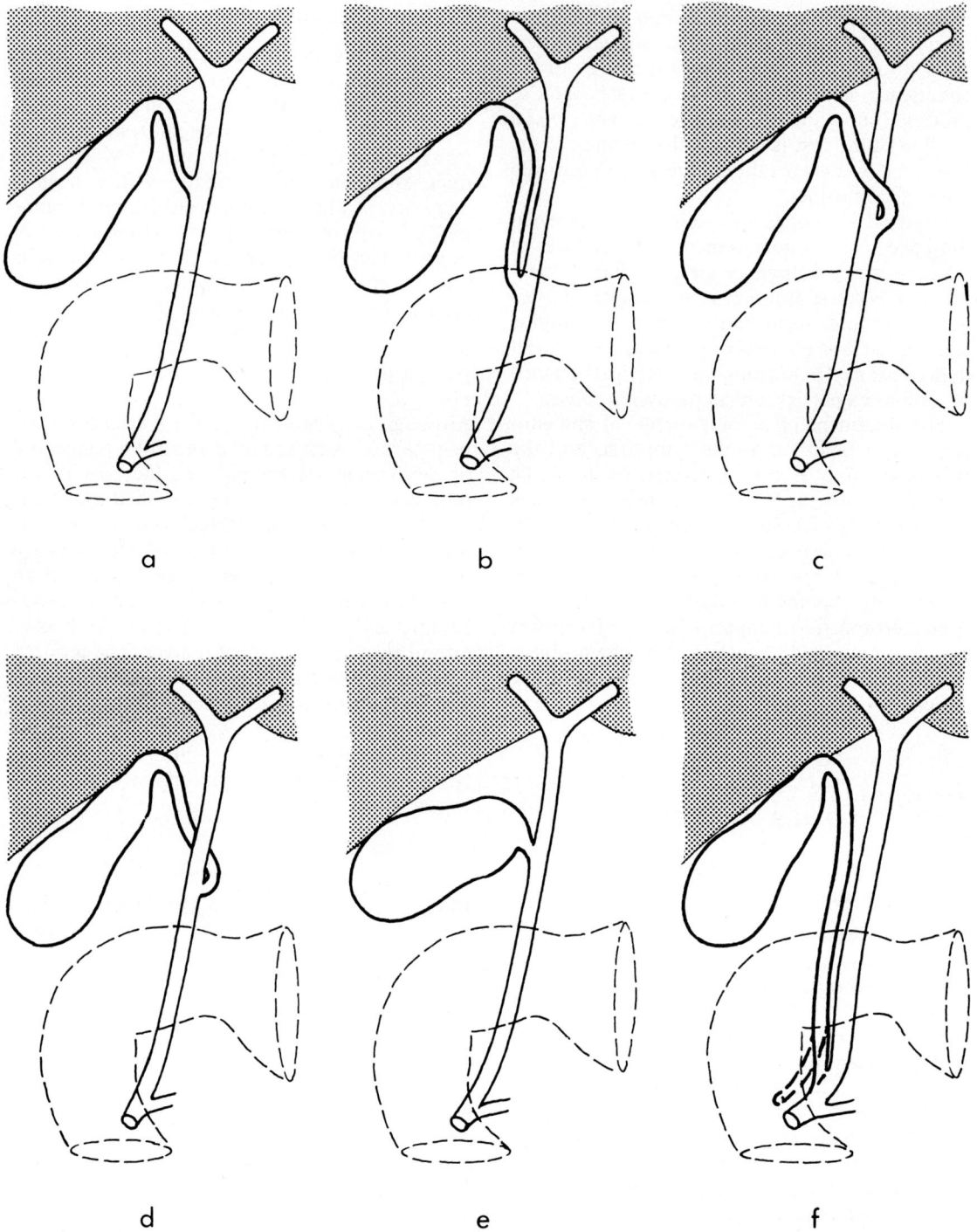

Fig. 19.11 Variations of the cystic duct. (a) The cystic duct joins the common hepatic duct at an angle entering its right side in about two-thirds of individuals. In the remaining one-third (b) it either runs parallel with the duct, often incorporated in its wall or (c) and (d) spirals around it, entering on the left side. The cystic duct may be (e) short or (f) long, entering separately into the duodenum or joining the common hepatic duct low down giving a short common duct. In these situations, the common duct or its blood supply may be damaged when removing the whole cystic duct.

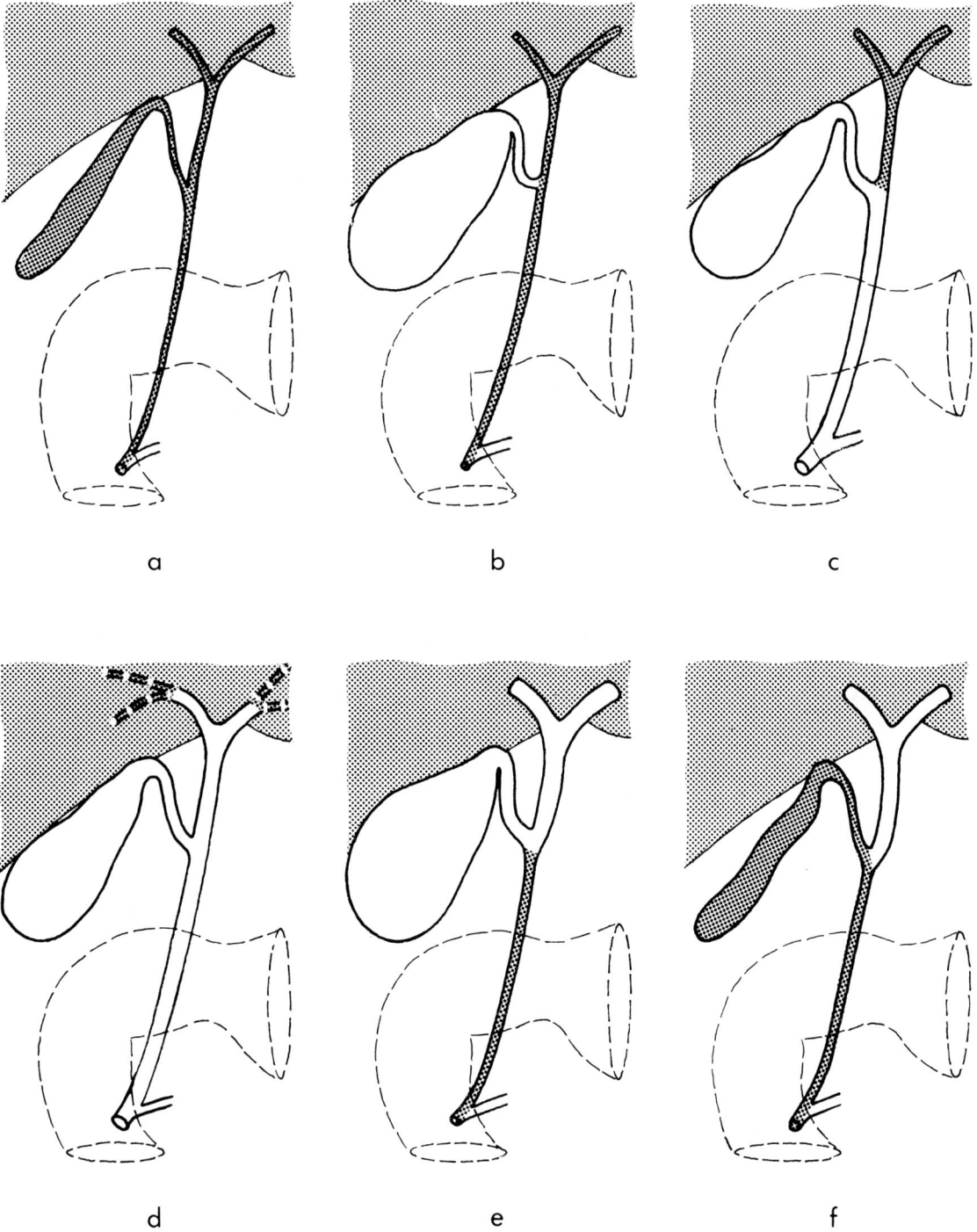

Fig. 19.12 Common anatomical types of biliary atresia. Obliteration of (a) the gallbladder and extrahepatic bile duct, (b) the extrahepatic bile duct, (c) the common hepatic bile duct, (d) the intrahepatic bile ducts, (e) the common bile duct and (f) the gallbladder and common bile duct. Types (a) to (d) were formerly considered 'non-correctable' and (e) and (f) 'correctable' biliary atresia.

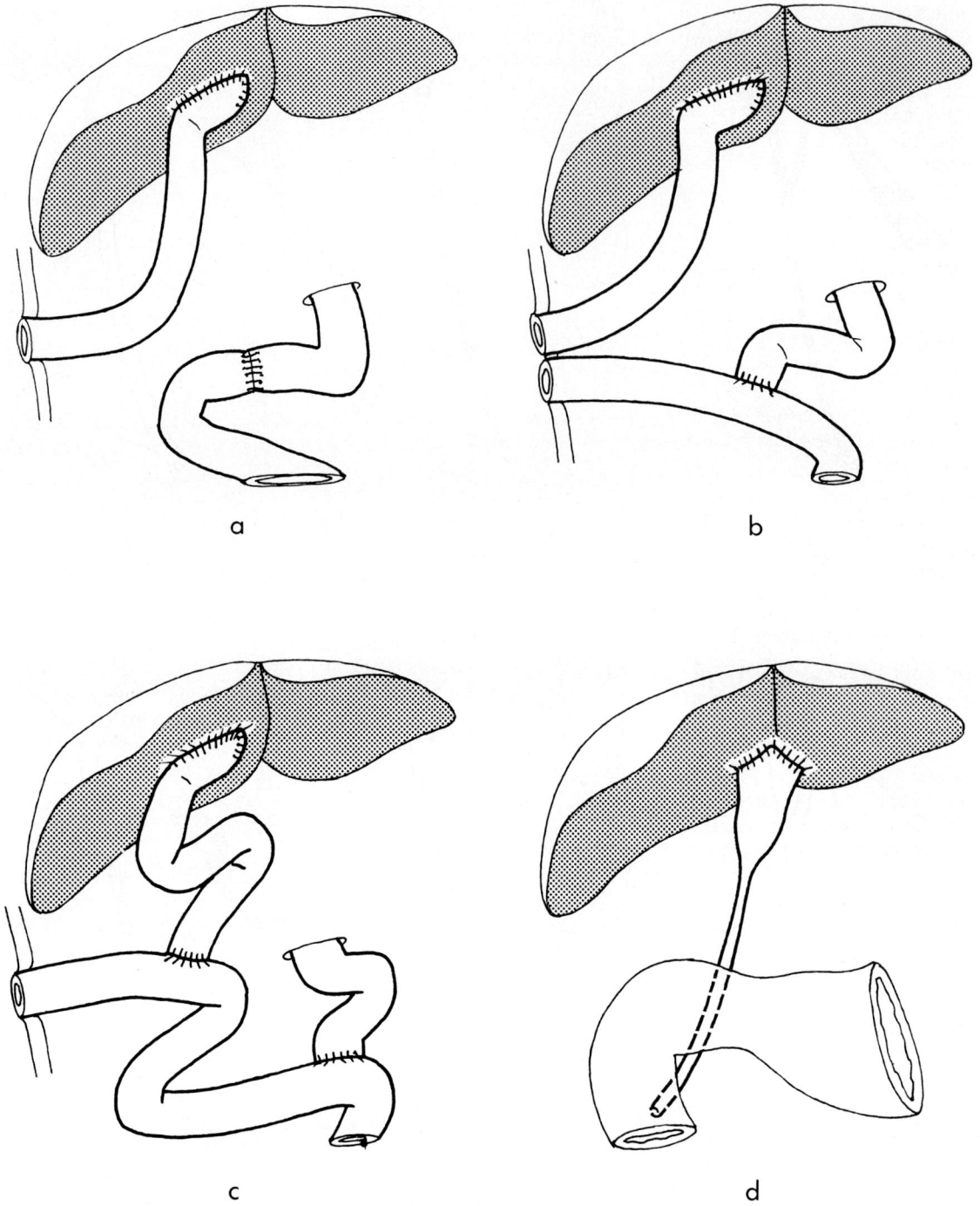

Fig. 19.13 Various modifications of portoenterostomy to prevent ascending cholangitis. (a) The Sawaguchi procedure completely diverts biliary flow to an abdominal wall stoma. (b) In the Suruga procedure a double-barrelled stoma is devised. (c) The Kasai II procedure provides a biliary conduit system that is not completely diverting but allows decompression of the conduit via a stoma. (d) The Kasai gallbladder operation or hepatic portocholecystostomy, is performed where the gall-bladder, cystic duct, and common bile duct are patent.

jaundice is usually noticed within the first few weeks after birth. An infant with persistent jaundice requires urgent investigation to determine the cause. Full investigations must be undertaken to exclude other causes of jaundice and to determine ductal patency. There are no absolutely reliable tests available to confirm a diagnosis of biliary atresia and percutaneous liver biopsy can be misleading. Furthermore, extensive tests are time-consuming and time is crucial for successful surgical management. Ultrasound is being used more often to identify the ductal system and gallbladder. Once biliary atresia is strongly suspected or cannot be ruled out, surgical exploration for definitive diagnosis is essential. The diagnosis depends on surgical biopsy of the liver, which is submitted to an expert pathologist for frozen section, and operative cholangiography. Surgical treatment depends on the findings. The earlier laparotomy policy improves the results of treatment for biliary atresia at the expense of a more accurate preoperative diagnosis.

SURGICAL TREATMENT

In approximately 10% of patients a large enough extrahepatic bile duct is found to permit an anastomosis to a Roux loop of jejunum. In the remainder, a hepatic portoenterostomy (Kasai operation) is performed. The basis of hepatic portoenterostomy is that the intrahepatic bile ducts are patent in early infancy and extend 1–2 mm from the porta hepatis into the fibrous tissue which replaces the extrahepatic biliary ducts. When this portal fibrous tissue is transected deep in the porta hepatis, minute bile ducts communicating with intrahepatic ducts are opened and bile drainage can be established in many patients younger than three months of age. With time the intrahepatic ductules are progressively destroyed and by the age of two months there is a rapid decrease in the rate of cure by surgery. Thus an operation should be performed within 60 days of birth.

The Kasai operation (hepatic portoenterostomy) has been fully described in standard texts,[7] and various modifications devised to prevent post-operative cholangitis are demonstrated in Figure 19.13.

RESULTS

The results largely depend upon (a) the age at the time of operation; (b) the degree of cirrhosis and liver damage; (c) the presence (or absence) of microscopically demonstrable ducts in the

fibrous mass at the porta hepatis; (d) the technique of the surgical procedure; and (e) the incidence of post-operative portal hypertension.

A 'cure rate' of 40–50% in infants operated on at less than 90 days of age has been quoted from various centres. However this 'cure' means bile drainage and loss of jaundice with survival for more than one year. Even when good bile drainage has been achieved and the serum bilirubin returns to normal, progression of fibrosis may occur after portoenterostomy. This fibrosis is often aggravated by recurrent attacks of cholangitis. Persisting long-term problems are those of cirrhosis and portal hypertension.

Where bile drainage stops and jaundice returns some time after an early successful result, re-exploration and removal of the fibrous plaque in the porta hepatis with a revision of the portoenterostomy may re-establish bile flow.

LIVER TRANSPLANTATION

Liver transplantation remains controversial in children with liver failure due to biliary atresia.[23] Starzl and his associates have performed transplants in 48 children for biliary atresia between 1963 and 1977 with a one year survival rate of 33%.[21] However, long-term survival is rare and we do not believe the procedure is acceptable for biliary atresia at the present stage of the development of liver transplantation.

REFERENCES

1 Alonso-Lej, F., Rever, W. G. Jr. & Pessagno, D. J. (1959) Congenital choledochal cyst, with report of 2, and an analysis of 94 cases. *International Abstracts of Surgery*, **108**, 1–30.
2 Caroli, J., Soupalt, R., Kossakowski, J. *et al.* (1958) 'La dilatation polycystique congénitale des voies biliares intrahépatiques. Essai de classification. *Semaine des Hôpitaux De Paris*, **34**, 488–495.
3. Donahue, P. K. & Hendren, W. H. (1976) Bile duct perforation in a newborn with stenosis of the ampulla of Vater. *Journal of Pediatric Surgery*, **11**, 823–825.
4 Gray, S. W. & Skandalakis, J. E. (1972) *Embryology for Surgeons*. Philadelphia: Saunders.
5 Hays, D. M. & Kimura, K. (1980) *Biliary Atresia: The Japanese Experience*. Cambridge, Mass.: Harvard University Press.
6 Hays, D. M. & Kimura, K. (1981) Biliary atresia: new concepts of management. *Current Problems in Surgery*, **18**, 541–608.
7 Kasai, M. (1974) Treatment of biliary atresia with special reference to hepatic porto-enterostomy and its modifications. *Progress in Pediatric Surgery*, **6**, 5–52.
8 Kasai, M., Kimura, S., Asakura, Y. *et al.* (1968) Surgical treatment of biliary atresia. *Journal of Pediatric Surgery*, **3**, 665–675.
9 Kato, T., Asakura, Y. & Kasai, M. (1974) An attempt to produce choledochal cyst in puppies. *Journal of Pediatric Surgery*, **4**, 509–513.

10 Kimura, K., Tsugawa, C., Ogawa, K. *et al.* (1978) Choledochal cyst. *Archives of Surgery*, **113**, 159–163.

11 Kune, G. A. (1970) The influence of structure and function in the surgery of the biliary tract. *Annals of the Royal College of Surgeons of England*, **47**, 78–91.

12 Kune, G. A. & Sali, A. (1980) *The Practice of Biliary Surgery* 2nd edn. Oxford: Blackwell Scientific Publication.

13 Lilly, J. R. (1977) Surgical jaundice in infancy. *Annals of Surgery*, **186**, 549–558.

14 Lilly, J. R. (1978) Total excision of choledochal cyst. *Surgery, Gynecology and Obstetrics*, **146**, 254–256.

15 Longmire, W. P., Mandiola, S. A. & Gordon, H. E. (1971) Congenital cystic disease of the liver and biliary system. *Annals of Surgery*, **174**, 711–726.

16 Lorenzo, G. A., Seed, R. W. & Beal, J. M. (1971) Congenital dilatation of the biliary tract. *American Journal of Surgery*, **121**, 510–517.

17 Louw, J. H. (1975) Choledochal cysts. *South African Journal of Surgery*, **13**, 199–205.

18 Northover, J. M. A. & Terblanche, J. (1979) A new look at the arterial supply of the bile duct in man and its surgical implications. *British Journal of Surgery*, **66**, 379–384.

19 Saito, S. & Ishida, M. (1974) Congenital choledochal cyst (cystic dilatation of the common bile duct). *Progress in Pediatric Surgery*, **6**, 63–90.

20 Shim, W. K. T., Kasai, M. & Spence, M. A. (1974) Racial influence on the incidence of biliary atresia. *Progress in Pediatric Surgery*, **6**, 53–62.

21 Starzl, T. E., Koep, L. J., Schröter, G. P. J. *et al.* (1979) Liver replacement for pediatric patients. *Pediatrics*, **63**, 825–829.

22 Terblanche, J., Allison, H. F. & Northover, J. M. A. (1983) An ischaemic basis for biliary strictures. *Surgery*, in press.

23 Terblanche, J., Koep, L. J. & Starzl, T. E. (1979) Liver transplantation. *Medical Clinics of North America*, **63**, 507–521.

24 Tsuchida, Y. & Ishida, M. (1971) Dilatation of the intrahepatic bile ducts in congenital cystic dilatation of the common bile duct. *Surgery*, **69**, 776–781.

PHYSIOLOGY OF EXTRAHEPATIC BILE TRANSPORT

The flow of bile is determined by the pressure difference between the hepatocytes and the intestinal lumen. The origin of this gradient is the 'secretory pressure' of the hepatocytes themselves, which in man is about 29–39 mmHg. However, control of the gradient, and thus of bile flow, is achieved mainly by regulating the resistance of the gallbladder and biliary duct system.

GALLBLADDER FILLING

During the interdigestive period, bile flows into the gallbladder because for much of the time the sphincter of Oddi remains closed. Closure of the common bile duct, however, depends not only on the activity of the sphincter muscle but also on the state of tone of surrounding duodenal muscle. The gallbladder tone at this stage is low, as is the resistance of the cystic duct, thus favouring flow into the gallbladder. This is generally regarded as being due simply to the intrinsic properties of the gallbladder and cystic duct muscle in the absence of the excitatory hormonal and neural stimuli which operate during feeding. However, recent evidence suggests that there may be active inhibition of muscle tone by vagal, non-adrenergic non-cholinergic inhibitory nerves during this period.[2] Thus the gallbladder may demonstrate receptive relaxation

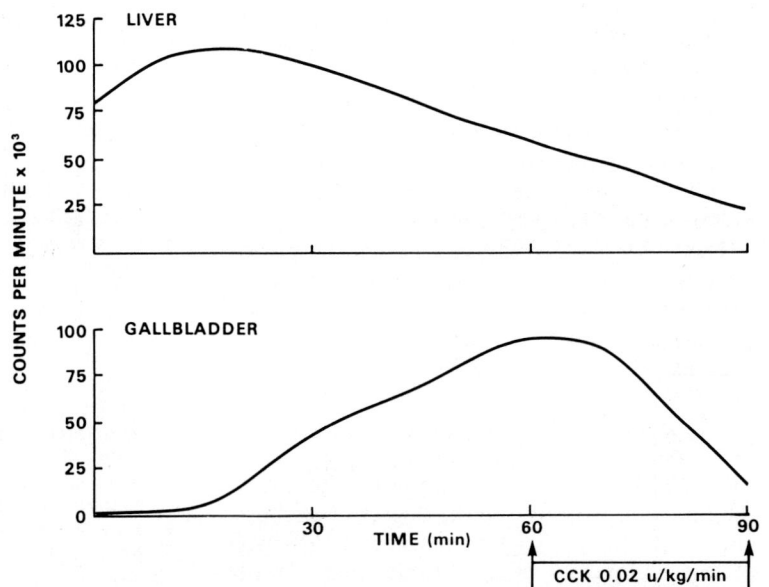

Fig. 19.14 Dynamic curves from a $^{99}Tc^m$-HIDA scan in a normal subject showing the time course of gallbladder filling in relation to hepatic secretion and gallbladder emptying in response to intravenous CCK infusion.[7]

analogous to that of other storage organs such as the gastric corpus.[1] Gallbladder filling in man can be observed by HIDA scanning[7] and typically has a time course as shown in Figure 19.14.

GALLBLADDER EPITHELIAL TRANSPORT

During this phase of filling and storage there is rapid absorption of fluid by the gallbladder epithelium. This is significant, not so much as a device for water conservation by the body, but as a means of preventing the build-up of an excessive volume because the capacity of the gallbladder in man is limited to 50–60 ml. As a consequence of the absorption of water and electrolytes there is a five- to ten-fold increase in concentration in the gallbladder bile of organic constituents such as bile salts, bile pigments, cholesterol and other biliary lipids (Table 19.1).

Table 19.1 Composition of normal bile.

	Hepatic bile (mmol/l)	Gallbladder bile (mmol/l)
Bile salts[a]	0.8–38.1	47.9–275.4
Bilirubin	6.8	51.0
Cholesterol[a]	0.3–3.0	0.1–87.1
Fatty acids[a]	0.1–2.9	0.1–55.4
Lecithin[a]	4.1–6.6	11.2–39.0
Na^+	145	130
K^+	5	12
Ca^{2+}	10	46
Cl^-	100	25
HCO_3^-	28	10

[a] Data provided by Dr P. E. Ross.

Fluxes of water occur in both directions across gallbladder epithelium but the net flux is from gallbladder to blood. The absorptive capacity of the gallbladder epithelium is greater than that of the ileum or the urinary bladder and for that reason the gallbladder has become a widely used model for electrolyte and water transport across epithelia.

As in other transport systems, the movement of water is passive and secondary to the active uptake of other substances, principally sodium. The fluid absorbed from the gallbladder is iso-osmotic with respect to plasma but the passive permeability of the epithelium to water is too low to permit simple iso-osmotic fluid absorption. Hence a mechanism exists which restricts the diffusion into the blood, of the actively transported solutes until sufficient water has followed. The lateral intercellular spaces play an important part in this process.[3]

Until recently, the most widely accepted explanation was the standing gradient hypothesis (Figure 19.15a). Solute, actively pumped into the long lateral intercellular space, diffuses along its concentration gradient to emerge at the serosal end of the space. Water can then diffuse from the epithelial cells along their entire length. Hence in the steady state of fluid absorption there will be an osmotic gradient along the length of the intercellular space. Recent evidence, however, has shown that the so-called 'tight' junctions between gallbladder epithelial cells are leaky to water and small solute molecules and that most of the fluid transported by the gallbladder epithelium follows a paracellular route (i.e. via the junctions and spaces) rather than a transcellular route through the epithelial cells. Moreover, micropuncture studies of intercellular space fluid have not confirmed the existence of an osmotic gradient. Hence, the older, and until recently less accepted, serial membrane model (Figure 19.15b) might provide a better explanation. In this model, the solute is pumped into the intercellular space but does not readily diffuse out of this region because of a non-specific barrier provided by the basal clefts and lamina propria. Water can then diffuse into the intercellular space, producing an osmotic equilibrium and, of course, increasing the hydrostatic pressure. This predicted rise in pressure would account for the observed swelling on the intercellular spaces during fluid absorption and is consistent with micropuncture studies showing an iso-osmotic intercellular fluid.

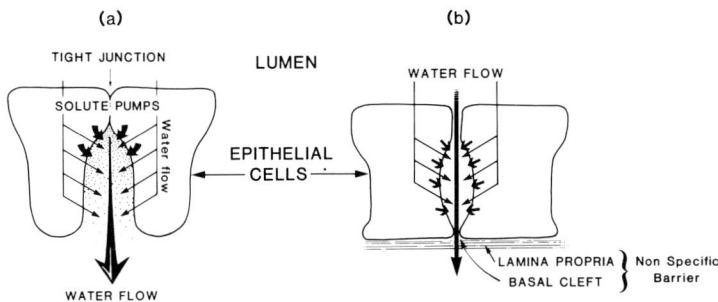

Fig. 19.15 Two hypotheses for iso-osmotic fluid absorption by the gallbladder epithelium. (a) The standing gradient hypothesis and (b) the serial membrane hypothesis. In (a) the osmotic gradient is indicated by the density of stippling (for explanation see text). In (b) the paracellular route for water movement is shown in addition to the originally proposed transcellular route.

Moreover, although the original hypothesis envisaged a transcellular route for water movements, a paracellular route would still be consistent with the model.

GALLBLADDER EMPTYING

Throughout the interdigestive period there is periodic emptying of the gallbladder.[4] These bouts of emptying are associated with phase 2 of the migrating myoelectrical complexes (MMCs), recurring bursts of electrical activity, and associated mechanical activity, which sweep down the gut during periods of fasting. While some of the mechanisms controlling the MMCs have been identified, nothing is known about what links gallbladder and biliary tract motility to this intestinal activity.

The physiological significance of this periodic emptying, however, is readily evident. It prevents stasis of bile in the gallbladder and, hence, reduces the risk of gallstone formation. Stasis is now recognized as an important contributing factor in the genesis of cholesterol gallstones. In part, this is simply because of an increased probability of crystal formation during prolonged storage of lithogenic bile. However, stasis may itself contribute to the production of lithogenic bile – not because of the concentrating effect of epithelial absorption of water which also increases bile salt concentration in proportion to the increase in biliary lipid concentration – but because of the effect of stasis on the enterohepatic circulation of bile salts. It is established that a reduction in the enterohepatic circulation of bile salts results in the production of a more lithogenic bile. So by maintaining the enterohepatic circulation, the periodic emptying of the gallbladder, linked to the propulsive activity of the ileum during the final phase (3) of the MMC, should reduce the likelihood of lithogenic bile being formed and, hence, of cholesterol stone formation. The 'housekeeper' role of the MMC may apply also to the biliary tract in that periodic emptying may prevent the build-up of bacterial flora and cell debris in the biliary tree.

In normal subjects the gallbladder empties rapidly after ingestion of a meal. The gallbladder contracts, increasing the intravesicular pressure. Since, at the same time, the resistance to bile flow through the sphincter decreases, bile enters the duodenum. The cystic duct resistance increases in response to the same mechanisms which elevate gallbladder pressure. This probably has less effect in restricting the expulsion of bile from the gallbladder than in preventing the

diversion of hepatic bile into the gallbladder. Hepatic secretion increases as a result of the increase in the rate of the enterohepatic circulation of the bile salt pool, and perhaps as a consequence of neural and hormonal signals.

The mechanisms controlling gallbladder emptying are summarized in Figure 19.16. The principal mechanism for the stimulation of gallbladder emptying has long been considered to be the release of the hormone cholecystokinin (CCK) from the duodenal mucosa, stimulated by the presence of food. The establishment of this hormonal mechanism by classical physiological methods involving transplanted intestinal loops or cross circulation experiments, was eventually followed by the isolation and purification of CCK. It is a linear polypeptide containing 33 amino acids of which the *C*-terminal octapeptide is considered to be the biologically active fragment although the *C*-terminal tetrapeptide retains much of the activity.

CCK is released from the endocrine cells of the small intestine in response to stimulation by a variety of digestion products including amino acids such as phenylalanine and tryptophan, fatty acids and hydrogen ions.

CCK acts directly on gallbladder smooth muscle and appears to mediate its effects through changes in intracellular cyclic nucleotide concentrations.[6] Contraction of the gallbladder induced by CCK is preceded by an increase in phosphodiesterase activity leading to a fall in intracellular cyclic AMP levels. There is also a significant rise in cyclic GMP levels and there is dispute over which of these two nucleotides is actually responsible for the contraction. In contrast CCK causes relaxation of the sphincter of Oddi.

Other hormones and peptides will also stimulate or inhibit gallbladder contraction.[6] Gastrin and the amphibian peptide caerulein are structurally similar to CCK and can both activate the CCK receptors, leading to gallbladder contraction. Gastrin, although less potent than CCK, may play a physiological role in the regulation of gallbladder contraction during the gastric phase of digestion. Caerulein is not a physiological regulator of gallbladder contractility but is a potentially useful alternative to CCK in clinical or scientific studies because of its high potency. Secretin is without effect on the gallbladder when administered alone but augments responses to CCK. Vasoactive Intestinal Peptide (VIP) inhibits responses to CCK but the physiological significance of this remains obscure particularly since VIP-like immunoreactivity is localized in neurones and the exis-

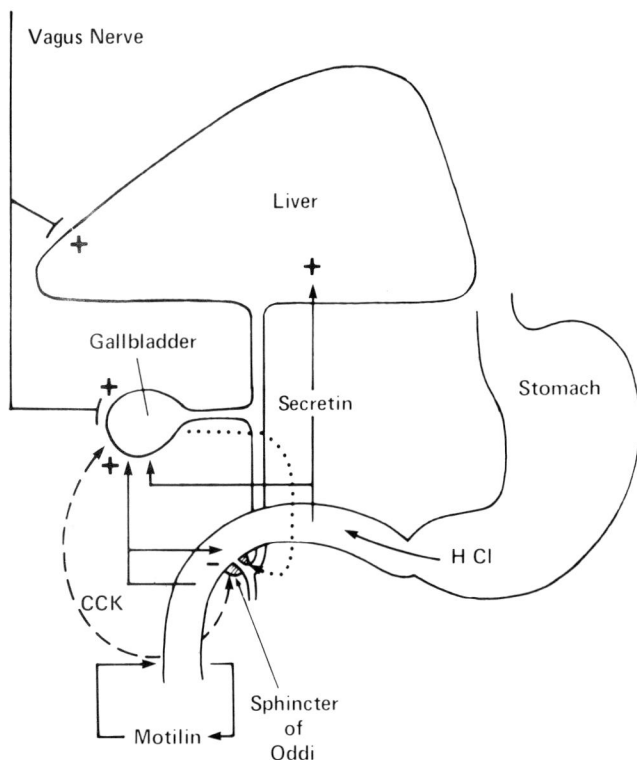

Fig. 19.16 Control of gallbladder emptying. During a meal CCK released from the duodenal mucosa contracts the gallbladder and relaxes the sphincter of Oddi. Secretin, released by gastric acid passing into the duodenum, can enhance the cholecystokinin action on the gallbladder contraction. The vagus nerve also stimulates gallbladder contraction. Bile flow into the duodenum is also enhanced by the actions of the vagus and secretin on hepatic bile secretion. A pathway between the gallbladder and sphincter of Oddi has been postulated (dotted line). Pathways also exist which link gallbladder emptying to fasting duodenal motility (dashed lines) and these probably account for the action of motilin.

tence of non-adrenergic non-cholinergic inhibitory nerves to the gallbladder is still not widely accepted.

Motilin and pancreatic polypeptide also appear to influence gallbladder contractility, the former causing gallbladder contraction and the latter relaxation. In both cases, isolated gallbladder strips from several species, including man, fail to respond to these peptides indicating that their site of action is probably remote from the gallbladder muscle. In the case of motilin, activation of gallbladder contraction may be secondary to initiation of MMCs by this peptide. The mode of action of pancreatic polypeptide on the gallbladder muscle is obscure.

Neural control of gallbladder emptying generally has been relegated to a fairly unimportant role. Although the vagus appears to have little importance in regulating the sphincter of Oddi, it is well established that stimulation of cholinergic, parasympathetic nerves, or exogenous administration of acetylcholine or cholinomimetic drugs will stimulate vigorous gallbladder contractions, though less powerfully than CCK. Perhaps more significantly, concomitant cholinergic nerve and CCK (or gastrin) stimulation will produce synergistic responses (i.e. greater than the sum of the responses to each individual stimulus)[5] and this is largely ignored in most text-book accounts of the control of gallbladder emptying.

The time course of gallbladder emptying also suggests that the control mechanism involves much more than merely the release of CCK consequent upon entry of chyme into the duodenum. The gallbladder emptying response to a liquid meal in man is very rapid and cannot be accounted for by release of CCK alone. The gallbladder can empty by over 50% in the first 15 minutes before any appreciable gastric emptying has occurred and long before there is any real elevation of serum CCK levels. It seems probable that there are significant cephalic and gastric phases of gallbladder emptying involving vagal cholinergic nerves and perhaps gastrin and an early intestinal phase which may involve complex neurohormonal and hormonal–hormonal interactions. While individual mechanisms have been identified (see Figure 19.16) we need much more information about the integration of these processes before we can evaluate their physiological importance in the regulation of the motility of the gallbladder and biliary tree.

REFERENCES

1 Davison, J. S. & Al-Hassani, M. (1980) The role of non-cholinergic, nonadrenergic nerves in regulating distensibility of the guinea-pig gallbladder. In *Gastrointestinal*

Motility. (Ed.) Christensen, J. pp. 89–95. New York: Raven.

2 Davison, J. S., Al-Hassani, M., Crowe, R. & Burnstock, G. (1978) The non-adrenergic inhibitory innervation of the guinea-pig gallbladder. *Pflugers Archivs*, **337**, 43–49.

3 Diamond, J. M. (1979) Osmotic water flow in leaky epithelia. *Journal of Membrane Biology*, **51**, 195–216.

4 Itoh, Z., Takahashi, I., Nakaya, M. *et al.* (1982) Inter-digestive gallbladder bile concentration in relation to periodic contraction of gallbladder in the dog. *Gastroenterology*, **83**, 645–651.

5 Pallin, B. & Skoglund, S. (1964) Neural and humoral control of the gallbladder-emptying mechanism in the cat. *Acta Physiologica Scandinavica*, **60**, 358–362.

6 Ryan, J. P. (1981) Motility of the gallbladder and biliary tree. In *Physiology of the Gastrointestinal Tract* (Ed.) Johnson, L. R. pp. 473–494. New York: Raven.

7 Shaffer, E. A., McOrmond, P. & Duggan, H. (1980) Quantitative cholescintigraphy: assessment of gallbladder filling and emptying and duodenogastric reflux. *Gastroenterology*, **79**, 899–906.

PHYSIOLOGY OF BILE SECRETION

Bile secretion is one of the major functions of the liver. Bile is an aqueous solution of organic and inorganic compounds. Bile acids, bile pigments, cholesterol and phospholipids are the chief organic compounds. Bile also contains small amounts of proteins. Because of the peculiar aggregation properties of the bile acids, which readily form micelles at physiological concentrations, bile is more complex than most other secretions, especially in regard to the osmotic properties of its constituents. Bile formed by the hepatocytes is secreted into the bile canaliculi. It is then modified during its passage in the bile ductules and ducts, and in the gallbladder, where water and inorganic electrolytes are reabsorbed, with, as a result, concentration of the organic constituents. Most conclusions regarding canalicular bile formation are derived from indirect evidence and are hypothetical. Here the available experimental data are summarized and

the current theories of hepatic bile formation discussed. More detailed references may be found in several recent reviews.[7, 9, 17, 18, 23]

BILE COMPOSITION

In general, *inorganic electrolytes* are present in common duct bile at concentrations closely reflecting those in plasma (Table 19.2). Bile concentrations of sodium, potassium, calcium and bicarbonate may, however, be appreciably higher than in plasma, while chloride level may be lower.

In spite of these variations bile *osmolality*, as measured by freezing point depression, is usually approximately 300 mosmol/kg and it varies in parallel to plasma osmolality. The total osmotic activity is accounted for only by the inorganic electrolytes because it is generally assumed that bile acids, which are. in micellar form, have little or no osmotic activity.

The concentration of bicarbonate in bile is often higher than that in plasma. This may be due to bicarbonate transport mechanisms, which have been postulated in the hepatocytes[14] and in the bile ductules and ducts, in response to secretin (see below).

The major *organic constituents* of bile are the conjugated bile acids, the bile pigments, cholesterol and phospholipids. The concentration and physicochemical properties of these compounds, which are important for the understanding of cholesterol and pigment gallstone formation, will be discussed on page 1389.

STRUCTURE–FUNCTION RELATIONSHIPS IN THE BILIARY SYSTEM

Bile is secreted primarily by the hepatocytes into bile canaliculi which are formed by a groove of

Table 19.2 Flow and electrolyte concentrations of hepatic bile.

Species	Flow ($\mu l \cdot min^{-1} \cdot kg^{-1}$)	Concentration (mmol/l)						
		Na^+	K^+	Ca^{2+}	Mg^{2+}	Cl^-	HCO_3^-	Bile acids
Man	1.5–15.4	132–165	4.2–5.6	0.6–2.4	0.7–1.5	96–126	17–55	3–45
Dog	10	141–230	4.5–11.9	1.5–6.9	1.1–2.7	31–107	14–61	16–187
Sheep	9.4	159.6	5.3	–	—	95	21.2	42.5
Rabbit	90	148–156	3.6–6.7	1.3–3.3	0.15–0.35	77–99	40–63	6–24
Rat	30–150	157–166	5.8–6.4	—	—	94–98	22–26	8–25
Guinea pig	115.9	175	6.3	—	—	69	49–65	—

Numbers indicate range or means of published values.

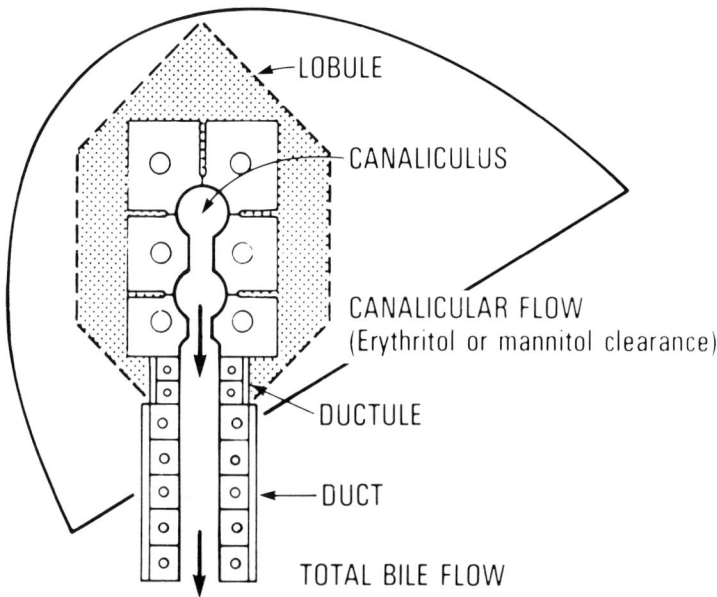

Fig. 19.17 Schematic diagram of the biliary system. From Erlinger (1982)[18] with kind permission of the publisher, J. B. Lippincott.

the lateral plasma membrane between two hepatocytes[33] and are about 1 μm in diameter. The membrane forms numerous microvilli which increase the surface area. The bile canalicular membrane represents about 13% of the hepatocyte plasma membrane. The bile canaliculi connect to bile ducts, lined by biliary epithelial cells. The smallest bile duct, the ductule, connects the canaliculus with the portal (interlobular) bile ducts. The interlobular bile ducts drain into larger bile ducts which form the intra- and extrahepatic biliary tree (Figure 19.17). With respect to bile secretion, the liver may be regarded as an epithelium transporting a variety of substrates from blood to bile. This vectorial transport is made possible by the high degree of polarization of the hepatocyte plasma membrane. As in other transporting epithelia, the canalicular lumen is sealed by intercellular junctions.

The polarization of the hepatocyte plasma membrane

Three domains of the hepatocyte plasma membrane may be recognized: sinusoidal (facing the blood sinusoids), lateral (or intercellular) and canalicular. They demonstrate important morphological, biochemical and enzymatic differences. Especially important for transepithelial transport is the localization of the Na^+,K^+-activated adenosine triphosphatase (Na^+,K^+-ATPase) which is mainly in the sinusoidal and intercellular membrane, with little or no activity in the canalicular membrane.[6, 29] A wide range

of epithelia, including iso-osmotic and hyperosmotic absorbers and secretors have (with the exception of the choroid plexus) the Na^+ pump (the Na^+,K^+-ATPase) preferentially on the basolateral surface of the epithelial cells.[11] In the hepatocyte, the sinusoidal and intercellular membrane is the equivalent of the basolateral membrane of other epithelial cells: the liver is therefore no exception among transporting epithelia regarding the localization of the enzyme.

Alkaline phosphatase, whose role in transport and in bile secretion is unknown, is, in contrast, preferentially located on the canalicular membrane.[6]

The tight junction and the paracellular pathway

A substrate in plasma can enter canalicular bile in one of two ways (Figure 19.18): the transcellular pathway (entering the hepatocyte through the sinusoidal membrane, crossing the hepatocyte and entering the canaliculus through the canalicular membrane) or the paracellular pathway. In the latter case, the solute crosses the intercellular junction. The junction includes the tight junction, which is a sealing structure between the lumen of the bile canaliculus and the intercellular space and, hence, the sinusoidal blood. Tight junctions differ among epithelia. In impermeable epithelia (such as the toad bladder), the tight junction provides a high transepithelial resistance to the movement of water and ions (and, hence, to electrical current) whereas in relatively permeable epithelia (such

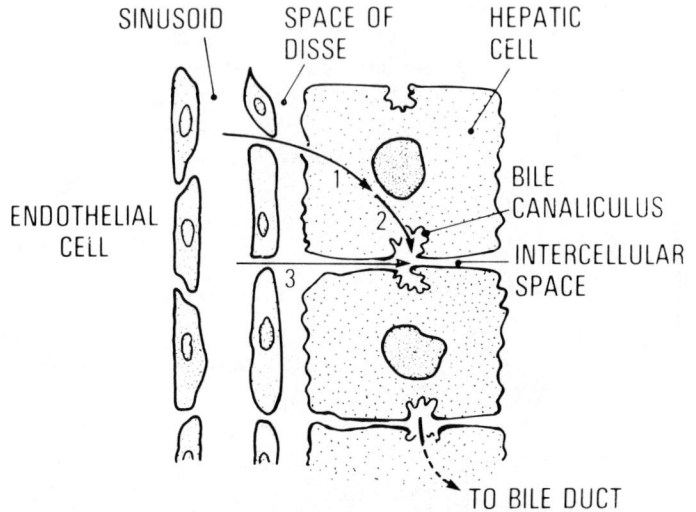

Fig. 19.18 Possible anatomic pathways of bile formation. A substrate can enter bile either after being taken up by the sinusoidal membrane (1) and transported into the cell (2) (transcellular pathway) or directly from the intercellular space through the tight junction (paracellular pathway.) From Erlinger (1982),[18] with kind permission of the publisher, J. B. Lippincott.

as the gallbladder, intestine or proximal kidney tubule), the tight junction is 'leaky' permitting some passage of water and ions (with, as a result, a low electrical resistance). The liver is of an intermediate type and there is evidence for a paracellular ion and fluid flux into bile which could play an important role in choleresis and possibly cholestasis. The existence of a negative charge barrier in the tight junction has also been postulated.[10]

The hepatocyte cytoskeleton

The canaliculus is surrounded by a narrow zone of organelle-poor cytoplasm, known as peri-canalicular ectoplasm, where actin micro-filaments (7 nm in diameter) are present particularly. They form a pericanalicular network, insert in the intercellular junction and extend into the microvilli where they appear to insert on the inner part of the membrane. They may have a key role in maintaining the shape of the cell, particularly its microvilli. Agents that interfere with the structure and function of microfilaments affect bile flow which suggests a role for these organelles in secretion.

Microtubules, which are 24 nm in diameter, are more randomly distributed within the liver cell cytoplasm than are microfilaments. They play a role in the intracellular transport and secretion by the liver cell of proteins and lipo-proteins. Antimicrotubular agents may also affect bile formation (see below).

CANALICULAR BILE FLOW

The maximal bile secretory pressure (about 25–30 cm H_2O) exceeds the sinusoidal perfusion pressure (about 5–10 cm H_2O) which excludes hydrostatic filtration as an important mechanism of canalicular bile secretion. Canalicular bile flow is regarded mainly as an osmotic water flow in response to active solute transport. *Bile acids*, which are potent choleretics, are most probably one of these solutes but the active transport of *inorganic ions* also plays a role.

Estimation of canalicular bile flow

Canalicular bile flow may be estimated by measuring the biliary clearance of non-metabolized solutes that enter canalicular bile by passive processes and are neither secreted nor reabsorbed by the biliary epithelium.[20, 45] The most widely used of such solutes are erythritol and mannitol (labelled with ^{14}C). In brief, when injected into the systemic circulation, the biliary secretion rate of such a solute during a steady state should depend on the permeability of the canaliculus and on canalicular bile flow. The biliary clearance (C) is calculated as $C = F \times [B]/[P]$ where F is bile flow, [B] and [P] the biliary and plasma concentrations respectively. The technique implies that the selected solute: (i) is unable to cross the biliary epithelium; (ii) has a permeability in the canaliculi high enough to achieve diffusion equilibrium at the highest rates of canalicular flow. Neither of these assumptions is presently accessible to direct experimental testing. However, an operational test of adequate canalicular permeability is the finding that increments in bile flow induced by bile acids are accompanied by parallel increases in solute clearance. Depending on the species, erythritol (MW 122) and mannitol (MW 182) meet these requirements.

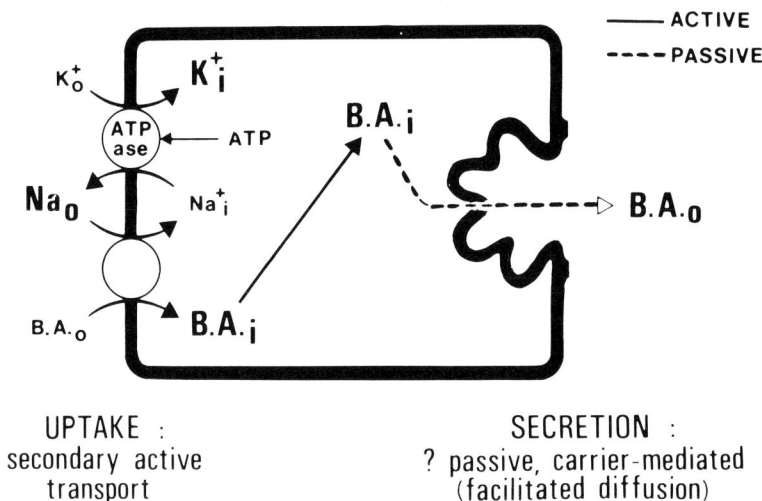

Fig. 19.19 Mechanisms of transport of bile acids by the liver cell. The uptake is thought to be a secondary active transport energized by the Na^+ gradient. The biliary secretion is probably a facilitated diffusion process. (K_o^+ = extracellular K^+ concentration; K_i^+ = intracellular K^+ concentration; Na_o^+ = extracellular Na^+ concentration; Na_i^+ = intracellular Na^+ concentration; $B.A._o$ = extracellular bile acid concentration; $B.A._i$ = intracellular bile acid concentration). From Erlinger (1981),[16] with kind permission of the editor of *Hepatology*.

The original assumption that erythritol and mannitol do not cross the biliary epithelium was based on the observation that their clearance was not modified by secretin[20, 45] which acts presumably on the ductules or ducts. However, small increases in erythritol and mannitol biliary clearance in response to secretin have been observed in dogs[3, 32, 34] because either canalicular bile flow is stimulated by this hormone, or there is some permeability of the bile ductules or ducts to erythritol and mannitol.

The observation that the biliary clearance of polyethylene glycol 900 (a solute much larger than erythritol and mannitol) is greater than that of erythritol and mannitol[27] suggests that reabsorption of water may occur, either in the canaliculus itself or distally. If reabsorption occurs in the canaliculus itself, erythritol and mannitol clearance may reflect *net* canalicular flow, while polyethylene glycol clearance may estimate *total* canalicular flow. If reabsorption of water and erythritol occurs distally, erythritol clearance may underestimate canalicular flow.

Bile acids and bile flow

BILE ACID TRANSPORT BY THE LIVER (FIGURE 19.19)

The liver has an extraction efficiency for bile acids of approximately 90%. The *uptake* of bile acids by the hepatocyte is a saturable, carrier-mediated process[24, 37] (Figure 19.20) exhibiting

(especially for conjugated bile acids) a strong sodium dependence.[39] Such Na^+ dependence is highly suggestive of a sodium-coupled transport (or symport) process which is energized by the Na^+ gradient maintained by the Na^+ pump (or Na^+,K^+-ATPase). It allows accumulation of bile acids within the hepatocyte against their electrochemical gradient: it is therefore referred to as *active* (because it is not directly linked to the energy source – ATP – but rather to an ion gradient, it is called secondary active).

Once concentrated into the cell, the bile acid anion will tend to move out of the cell into the canalicular lumen along its electrochemical gradient, a movement favoured by the negative membrane potential which will drive anions out of the cell. Because canalicular secretion is limited by a maximal secretory capacity it is assumed that the process is carrier-mediated. It is not known whether the putative carrier, possibly the bile acid binding protein identified by Accatino and Simon,[1] uses an additional source of energy or is a passive mediated transport, for example facilitated diffusion. The very high biliary bile acid concentration (up to the 100 mmol/l range) is probably related to the formation of micelles.

EFFECT OF BILE ACID SECRETION ON CANALICULAR FLOW

An apparently linear relationship between bile acid secretion rate and bile flow has been

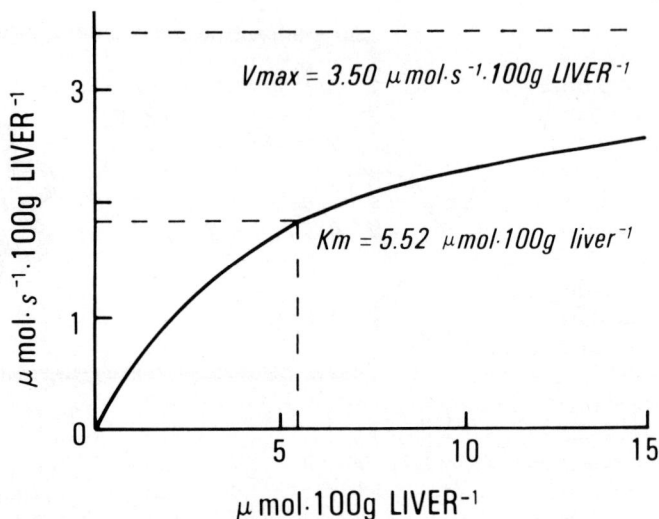

Fig. 19.20 Relationship between [^{14}C]taurocholate uptake velocity (ordinate) and taurocholate dose (abscissa). The technique used was the multiple indicator dilution method in the anaesthetized dog. Note that the non-linear increase in uptake velocity with the dose of taurocholate. After Glasinović, Dumont, Duval & Erlinger (1975)[24] and Erlinger (1982).[17]

demonstrated in many animal species, including dog[36] and man[35] (Figure 19.21). Bile acid-induced choleresis is presumably of canalicular origin; it is accompanied by a parallel increase in erythritol clearance and a linear relationship is also found between erythritol clearance and bile acid secretion (Figure 19.21).

The hypothesis that bile acids increase bile flow by providing an osmotic driving force for water and electrolytes was proposed by Sperber,[42] but because bile acids are in the micellar form most of the osmotic activity must be accounted for by their counter-ions (cations accompanying the bile acid anions to maintain electroneutrality).

Alternatively their choleretic effect could be due, at least in part, to their regulating the activity of other solute pumps. Experimental studies of selective biliary obstruction demonstrated an increased bile acid flux through the non-obstructed liver and a disproportionate increase in bile flow, together with an increase in Na$^+$, K$^+$-ATPase activity of liver cell plasma membranes.[44] In other experiments ursodeoxycholic acid (and 7-ketolithocholic acid) was 'hypercholeretic' (more choleretic than physiological bile acids) and, simultaneously, stimulated biliary bicarbonate secretion,[14] an apparently important flow-generating system[26] (see below).

PATHWAY OF FLUID MOVEMENT

Because bile acids are transported through the canalicular membrane of the hepatocyte, it is often thought that the associated osmotic water flow also occurs through the canalicular membrane. However, the ionic composition of bile closely resembles that of the extracellular fluid

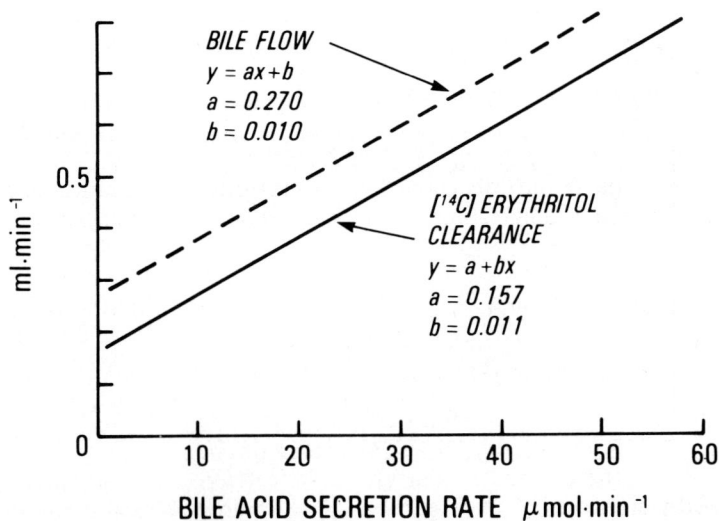

Fig. 19.21 Relationship between the bile flow (dotted line), [^{14}C]erythritol clearance (full line) and bile acid secretion in cholecystectomized patients with T-tubes in the common bile duct. After Prandi, Erlinger, Glasinović & Dumont (1975)[35] and Erlinger (1982).[17]

so it is necessary to postulate either an equilibration downstream along the biliary channels, or a paracellular water and ionic pathway from the intercellular space into the bile canaliculi. The first possibility seems unlikely but as discussed earlier, the tight junction between liver cells is probably relatively 'leaky'. The bile-to-plasma concentration ratio of large solutes stabilizes well before the liver-to-plasma ratio,[22] suggesting either a restricted (for example vesicular) pathway within the hepatocytes, or, alternatively, a direct passage through the paracellular pathway. Polyethylene glycol 4000 appears very rapidly in bile even though its size precludes a rapid entry into the hepatocytes. Experiments with the potent choleretics dehydrocholate and taurodehydrocholate have demonstrated a progressive increase in the bile-to-plasma concentration ratio of sucrose, penetration of ionic lanthanum into the tight junctions and increase in the number of intercellular 'blisters'. These observations suggest that the paracellular pathway may be an important site for bile acid-induced water and ion movement into bile.[31]

Other mechanisms in canalicular bile flow (canalicular bile acid-independent flow)

Although there is a good correlation between bile flow and bile acid secretion under physiological circumstances, studies at low bile acid secretion rates have shown an increase in slope of the bile flow–bile acid secretion relationship,[2] possibly due to a fall in the concentration of bile acids below the critical micellar concentration and, hence, an increase in their osmotic activity. Because of endogenous bile acid synthesis, it is practically impossible to obtain bile without bile acids. Therefore, one can postulate either a fall of bile flow to zero, or a positive extrapolation of the bile flow–bile acid secretion relationship for a zero bile acid secretion.[8, 19]

In the former case, bile acids would be the only active flow-generating solute ('one component theory'). In the latter case, flow could be generated without bile acids by one (or even several) other mechanisms ('two component theory'). The best piece of evidence in favour of the second view is the possibility of an increase in canalicular bile flow without any increase in bile acid secretion, for example with phenobarbital[5, 28] (Figure 19.22) and a variety of other agents. The term canalicular bile acid-independent flow is generally used to describe this fraction of bile flow but this may not be adequate because interrelationships between the two fractions have been observed. Better terms must await the identification of the cellular mechanisms involved.

Role of Na$^+$, K$^+$-ATPase

The question of the role of Na$^+$,K$^+$-ATPase in canalicular transport processes other than bile acid transport remains controversial. Evidence

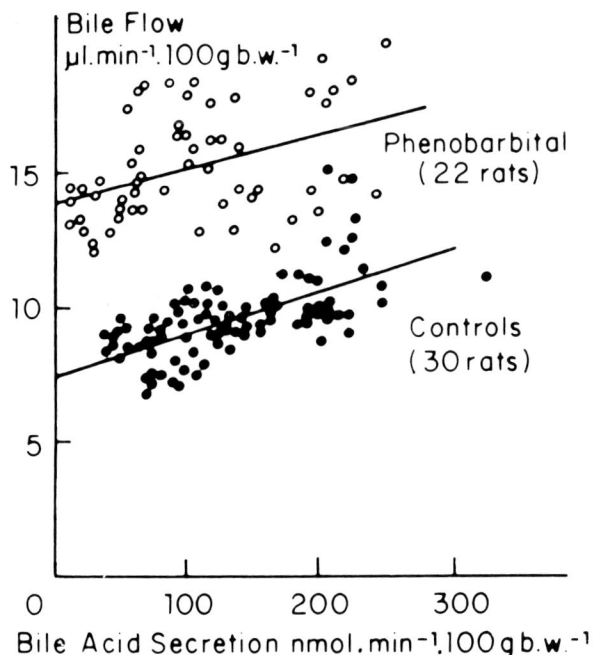

Fig. 19.22 Effect of phenobarbital on bile flow and bile acid secretion in the rat. After Berthelot, Erlinger, Dhumeaux and Préaux (1970).[5]

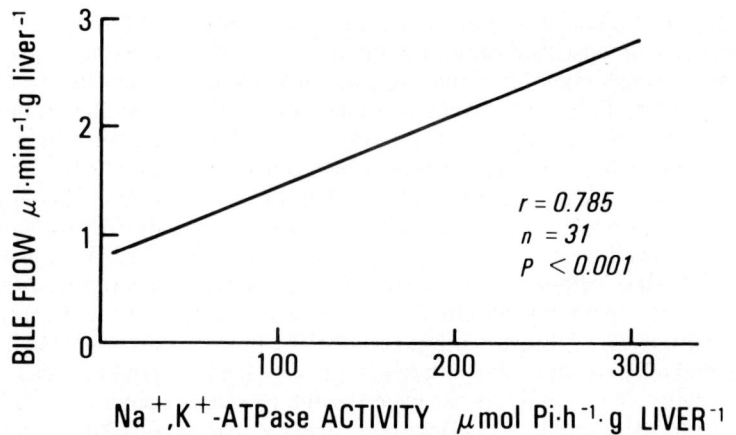

Fig. 19.23 Relationship between bile flow and Na$^+$, K$^+$-ATPase activity in liver plasma membrane preparations in the rat. After Reichen and Paumgartner (1977)[38] and Erlinger (1982).[17]

for a role for this enzyme was originally derived from studies of the effect of inhibitors of Na$^+$ transport on bile flow.[19] However, interpretation of the effect of drugs such as ouabain, ethacrynic acid or amiloride in vivo is complex, the overall effect being the result of both a choleretic and an inhibitory effect.

More direct evidence for a role of Na$^+$,K$^+$-ATPase has been sought by studying the relationship between bile flow and Na$^+$,K$^+$-ATPase in liver cell plasma membranes and a good correlation has been found between bile flow and Na$^+$,K$^+$-ATPase activity[31, 38, 41] (Figure 19.23). It is difficult to understand the mode of coupling between enzyme activity and secretion because the bulk of Na$^+$,K$^+$-ATPase activity is located not on the canalicular membrane, but on the sinusoidal and intercellular membrane opposite to the net direction of Na$^+$ transport. Two ways of coupling between enzyme activity and transport are proposed:[16] firstly active transport of Na$^+$ into the intercellular space followed by passive movement into the canalicular lumen, secondly the transport of an anion, such as Cl$^-$ or HCO$_3^-$ (or some other) using the Na$^+$ gradient. Sodium-driven Cl$^-$ transport is widespread among epithelia. However studies on cultured hepatocytes do not support the latter mechanism.[40] Bicarbonate transport is also conceivable.

Role of bicarbonate transport

A bicarbonate transport mechanism may have a role in the elaboration of canalicular bile.[3, 14, 26, 43] The cellular mechanism is not known. Attempts to demonstrate a bicarbonate-sensitive ATPase in liver cell plasma membranes have failed but other mechanisms (such as the Na$^+$/H$^+$ antiport of the kidney tubule) are possible.

ROLE OF DUCTULES AND DUCTS

Secretion (ductular/ductal bile acid-independent flow)

Secretion occurs in the ductules and ducts in many species including man, mostly in response to secretin administration.[36] Secretin choleresis is generally accompanied by changes in bile composition, chiefly a rise in bicarbonate and pH, and a fall in bile acids.[25] The intraduodenal infusion of HCl in dogs induces the same response as endogenous secretin.

The evidence for a ductular/ductal site of action of secretin is: (1) secretin choleresis does not enhance the maximal biliary secretory capacity of BSP whereas bile acids, which act on the bile canaliculi do; (2) the biliary 'wash-out' volume during constant rate BSP infusions is less with secretin choleresis than bile acid choleresis suggesting that secretin acts distal to the canaliculi; (3) biliary clearances of erythritol and mannitol are increased during bile acid choleresis and not during secretin choleresis.

The secretory activity of the bile ductules and ducts explains the choleresis that occurs in certain diseases. Elevated bile flows have been recorded in patients with cirrhosis, other chronic liver diseases associated with ductular proliferation, and in congenital dilatation of the intrahepatic biliary tree. An augmented surface of the biliary epithelium is common to these conditions.

Reabsorption

The bile ductules or ducts may also have a reabsorptive function. Thus in cholecystectomized dogs, the composition of bile stored in the common bile duct was similar to typical gallbladder bile. Bile-to-plasma concentration ratios above unity in the steady state have been found for mannitol and erythritol in various species which suggest there is water reabsorption distal to the canaliculi because neither solute is thought to be transported by concentrative processes. No studies in man are available.

MECHANISMS OF CHOLESTASIS

Cholestasis is defined as a diminution (or cessation) of bile flow and is subdivided as extrahepatic and intrahepatic. *Extrahepatic cholestasis* is the result of mechanical obstruction of the extrahepatic bile ducts usually by a gallstone or a tumour. *Intrahepatic cholestasis* may be the result of two different mechanisms: (i) mechanical obstruction of intrahepatic bile ducts, for example by a primary or secondary liver tumour, granulomas, infiltration by lymphoma or any other space-occupying lesion; (ii) disturbance of canalicular bile flow, for example during viral or drug-induced hepatitis, or drug-induced cholestasis. Cholestasis must be distinguished from necrosis during liver parenchymal disease: both can occur separately or together. For instance, during viral hepatitis, necrosis can occur alone (anicteric hepatitis), or in association with cholestasis (common acute hepatitis with jaundice), while cholestasis can occur alone or predominantly (cholestatic hepatitis).

The cellular mechanisms of intrahepatic cholestasis due to disturbance of canalicular bile flow are not well understood[15] and it is possible that there are several. Experimentally, three main mechanisms have been implicated.

(a) *A decrease in* Na^+,K^+*-ATPase.* In this case, cholestasis could result from decreased bile acid secretion due to a decreased Na^+ gradient, or from decreased Na^+,K^+-ATPase mediated transport. Drugs which affect the Na^+,K^+-ATPase activity to produce cholestasis include oestrogens, chlorpromazine, and 17α-alkylated steroids. Interference with hepatocyte membrane transport processes is a common mechanism of cholestasis.

(b) *An alteration of the cytoskeleton.* Interference with *microfilament* structure and function by cytochalasin B or phalloidin[12] causes a decrease or even a complete cessation of bile flow, and provides circumstantial evidence that microfilament dysfunction leads to cholestasis and that microfilaments may have a role in secretion. This could be by (i) altering the structural organ-

ization necessary for normal secretion, particularly microvilli; (ii) interfering with a *contractile* function; (iii) modifying the *permeability* of the *paracellular* pathway that may be regulated by microfilaments.

The role of *microtubules* has been studied with colchicine and vinblastine. No effect on basal (spontaneous) bile flow was observed but colchicine markedly decreased bile flow and bile acid secretion induced by a bile acid load.[13]

(c) *An increase in the permeability of the paracellular pathway.* This was first postulated to explain oestrogen-induced cholestasis.[21] Any increased permeability may allow regurgitation of bile constituents (such as bile acids or bilirubin, and water) from the canalicular lumen into the circulation. Structural evidence that absorption (regurgitation) can take place in human bile ductules has been obtained in cholestasis from various causes.

CHOLERETICS: MECHANISMS OF ACTION

A choleretic drug might act by one of several possible mechanisms: (i) concentrative (usually active) secretion into bile canaliculi followed by osmotic filtration of water and electrolytes. This process may be conveniently called 'bile acid-like choleresis' and operates for most commercial choleretics. However, this type of choleresis is not accompanied by an increase in biliary lipid secretion, in contrast to the choleresis induced by physiological bile acids. (ii) Stimulation of 'bile acid-independent mechanisms' as with phenobarbital and other drugs (spironolactone or clofibrate in the rat) that are microsomal enzyme inducers. (iii) Stimulation of secretion by the ductules or ducts for example with secretin.

There is no evidence that any of these choleretics are of therapeutic value in patients with cholestasis, with the possible exception of phenobarbitone (phenobarbital) in children with intrahepatic cholestasis.

BILIARY SECRETION IN MAN

Although the existence of most of the processes described previously has been inferred from animal studies, similar processes may well operate in man (Figure 19.24). Patients with T-tubes in the common bile duct show a linear relationship between bile flow (and erythritol or

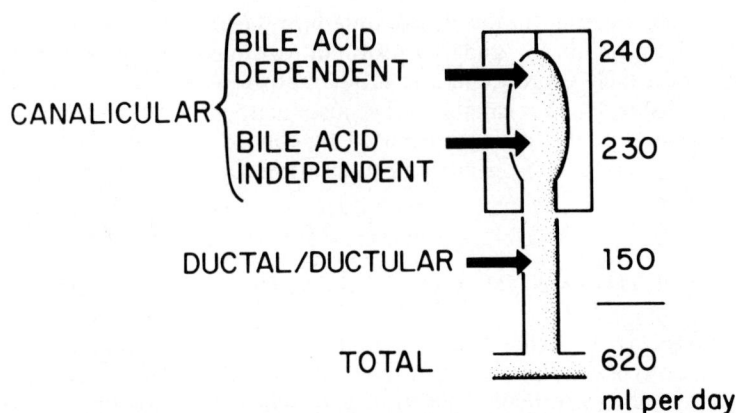

Fig. 19.24 Bile secretion in man. From data collected in cholecystectomized patients with T-tubes in the common bile duct.

mannitol clearance) and bile acid secretion rate, with a mean of 11 µl of *canalicular* bile secreted per µmol of bile acids. When the enterohepatic circulation is intact, a mean of approximately 15 µmol of bile acids is secreted per min, which gives a mean flow associated with bile acids of 0.15–0.16 ml/min. The estimated canalicular bile acid-independent flow is 0.16–0.17 ml/min, and the estimated ductular/ductal secretion is about 0.11 ml/min. The daily hepatic bile production under these circumstances (i.e. after cholecystectomy) is therefore approximately 600 ml.

REFERENCES

1 Accatino, L. & Simon, F. R. (1976) Identification and characterization of a bile acid receptor in isolated liver surface membranes. *Journal of Clinical Investigation*, **56**, 496–508.

2 Balabaud, C., Kron, K. A. & Gumucio, J. J. (1977) The assessment of the bile salt-non-dependent fraction of canalicular bile water in the rat. *Journal of Laboratory and Clinical Medicine*, **89**, 393–399.

3 Barnhart, J. L. & Combes, B. (1978) Erythritol and mannitol clearances with taurocholate and secretin-induced cholereses. *American Journal of Physiology*, **234**, E146–E156.

4 Barnhart, J. L. & Combes, B. (1978) Characterization of SC 2644-induced choleresis in the dog. Evidence for canalicular bicarbonate secretion. *Journal of Pharmacology and Experimental Therapeutics*, **206**, 190–197.

5 Berthelot, P., Erlinger, S., Dhumeaux, D. & Préaux, A. M. (1970) Mechanism of phenobarbital-induced hypercholeresis in the rat. *American Journal of Physiology*, **219**, 809–813.

6 Blitzer, B. L. & Boyer, J. L. (1978) Cytochemical localization of Na^+,K^+-ATPase in the rat hepatocyte. *Journal of Clinical Investigation*, **62**, 1104–1108.

7 Blitzer, B. L. & Boyer, J. L. (1982) Cellular mechanisms of bile formation. *Gastroenterology*, **82**, 346–347.

8 Boyer, J. L. (1971) Bile formation in the isolated perfused rat liver. *American Journal of Physiology*, **221**, 1156–1163.

9 Boyer, J. L. (1980) New concepts of mechanisms of hepatocytic bile formation. *Physiological Reviews*, **60**, 303–326.

10 Bradley, S. E. & Herz, R. (1978) Permselectivity of biliary canalicular membrane in rats: clearance probe analysis. *American Journal of Physiology*, **235**, E570–E576.

11 Di Bona, D. R. & Mills, J. W. (1979) Distribution of Na^+-pump sites in transporting epithelia. *Federation Proceedings*, **38**, 134–143.

12 Dubin, M., Maurice, M., Feldmann, G. & Erlinger, S. (1978) Phalloidin-induced cholestasis in the rat: Relation to changes of microfilaments. *Gastroenterology*, **75**, 450–455.

13 Dubin, M. Maurice, M., Feldmann, G. & Erlinger, S. (1981) Influence of colchicine and phalloidin on bile secretion and hepatic ultrastructure in the rat. Possible interaction between microtubules and microfilaments. *Gastroenterology*, **79**, 646–654.

14 Dumont, M., Uchman, S. & Erlinger, S. (1981) Hypercholeresis induced by ursodeoxycholic acid and 7-ketolithocholic acid in the rat. Possible role of bicarbonate transport. *Gastroenterology*, **79**, 82–89.

15 Erlinger, S. (1978) Cholestasis: pump failure, microvilli defect or both? *Lancet*, **i**, 533–534.

16 Erlinger, S. (1981) Hepatocyte bile secretion: current views and controversies. *Hepatology*, **1**, 352–359.

17 Erlinger, S. (1982) Bile flow. In *The Liver: Biology and Pathobiology* (Ed.) Arias, I., Popper, H., Schachter, D. & Schafritz, D. A. pp. 407–427. New York: Raven Press.

18 Erlinger, S. (1982) Secretion of bile. In *Diseases of the Liver*. 5th Edition. (Ed.) Schiff, L. & Schiff, E. pp. 93–119. Philadelphia: J. B. Lippincott.

19 Erlinger, S., Dhumeaux, D., Berthelot, P. & Dumont, M. (1970) Effect of inhibitors of sodium transport on bile formation in the rabbit. *American Journal of Physiology*, **219**, 416–422.

20 Forker, E. L. (1967) Two sites of bile formation as determined by mannitol and erythritol clearance in the guinea pig. *Journal of Clinical Investigation*, **46**, 1189–1195.

21 Forker, E. L. (1969) The effect of estrogen on bile formation in the rat. *Journal of Clinical Investigation*, **48**, 654–663.

22 Forker, E. L. (1970) Hepatocellular uptake of inulin, sucrose and mannitol in rats. *American Journal of Physiology*, **219**, 1568–1573.

23 Forker, E. L. (1977) Mechanisms of hepatic bile formation. *Annual Review of Physiology*, **39**, 323–347.

24 Glasinović, J. C., Dumont, M., Duval, M. & Erlinger, S. (1975) Hepatocellular uptake of taurocholate in the dog. *Journal of Clinical Investigation*, **55**, 419–426.

25 Hardison, W. G. M. & Norman, J. C. (1968) Electrolyte composition of the secretin fraction of bile from the perfused pig liver. *American Journal of Physiology*, **214**, 758–763.

26 Hardison, W. G. M. & Wood, C. A. (1978) Importance of bicarbonate in bile salt independent fraction of bile flow. *American Journal of Physiology*, **235**, E158–E164.

27 Javitt, N. B. & Wachtel, N. (1981) Hepatic bile formation: quantitative estimates of canalicular water flow. *Abstracts of the Fourth International Gstaad Symposium: The Liver: Dynamics of Structure and Function; Gstaad, 1981.* p. 23.

28 Klaassen, C. D. (1971) Studies on the increased biliary flow produced by phenobarbital in rats. *Journal of Pharmacology and Experimental Therapeutics*, **176**, 743–751.

29 Latham, P. S. & Kashgarian, M. (1979) The ultrastructural localization of transport ATPase in the rat liver at non-bile canalicular plasma membranes. *Gastroenterology*, **76**, 988–996.

30 Layden, T. J. & Boyer, J. L. (1976) The effect of thyroid hormone on bile salt-independent bile flow and Na^+, K^+-ATPase activity in liver plasma membranes enriched in bile canaliculi. *Journal of Clinical Investigation*, **57**, 1009–1018.

31 Layden, T. J., Elias, E. & Boyer, J. L. (1978) Bile formation in the rat. The role of the paracellular shunt pathway. *Journal of Clinical Investigation*, **62**, 1375–1385.

32 Lewis, M. H., Baker, A. L., Dhorajiwala, J. & Moosa, A. R. (1982) Secretin enhances [^{14}C]erythritol clearance in unanesthetized dogs. *Digestive Diseases and Sciences*, **27**, 57–64.

33 Millward-Sadler, G. H. & Jezequel, A. M. (1979) Normal histology and ultrastructure. In *Liver and Biliary Disease*. (Ed.) Wright, R., Alberti, K. G. M. M., Karran, S. & Millward-Sadler, G. H. pp. 13–43. London: Saunders.

34 Nicholls, R. J. (1979) Biliary mannitol clearance and bile salt output before and during secretin choleresis in the dog. *Gastroenterology*, **76**, 983–987.

35 Prandi, D., Erlinger, S., Glasinović, J. C. & Dumont, M. (1975) Canalicular bile production in man. *European Journal of Clinical Investigation*, **5**, 1–6.

36 Preisig, R., Cooper, H. L. & Wheeler, H. O. (1962) The relationship between taurocholate secretion rate and bile production in the unanesthetized dog during cholinergic blockade and during secretin administration. *Journal of Clinical Investigation*, **41**, 1152–1162.

37 Reichen, J. & Paumgartner, G. (1975) Kinetics of taurocholate uptake by the perfused rat liver. *Gastroenterology*, **68**, 132–136.

38 Reichen, J. & Paumgartner, G. (1977) Relationship between bile flow and Na^+,K^+-adenosinetriphosphatase in liver plasma membranes enriched in bile canaliculi. *Journal of Clinical Investigation*, **60**, 429–434.

39 Ruifrok, P. G. & Meijer, D. K. (1982) Sodium ion-coupled uptake of taurocholate by rat-liver plasma membrane vesicles. *Liver*, **2**, 28–34.

40 Scharschmidt, B. F., Van Kyde, R. W. & Stephens, J. E. (1982) Chloride transport by intact rat liver and cultured rat hepatocytes. *American Journal of Physiology*, **242**, G628–G633.

41 Simon, F. R., Sutherland, E. & Accatino, L. (1977) Stimulation of hepatic sodium and potassium-activated adenosine triphosphatase activity by phenobarbital. Its possible role in regulation of bile flow. *Journal of Clinical Investigation*, **59**, 849–861.

42 Sperber, I. (1959) Secretion of organic anions in the formation of urine and bile. *Pharmacological Reviews*, **11**, 109–134.

43 Van Dyke, R. W., Stephens, J. E. & Scharschmidt, B. F. (1982) Effect of ion substitution on bile acid-dependent and -independent bile formation by rat liver. *Journal of Clinical Investigation*, **70**, 505–517.

44 Wannagat, F. J., Adler, R. D. & Ockner, R. K. (1978) Bile acid-induced increase in bile acid-independent flow and plasma membrane Na,K-ATPase activity in rat liver. *Journal of Clinical Investigation*, **61**, 297–307.

45 Wheeler, H. O., Ross, E. D. & Bradley, S. E. (1968) Canalicular bile production in dogs. *American Journal of Physiology*, **214**, 866–874.

FORMATION OF CHOLESTEROL GALLSTONES

Cholesterol gallstone formation consists of six sequential steps: (i) a metabolic defect involving altered synthesis, metabolism or hepatic processing of biliary lipids; (ii) augmented hepatic secretion of cholesterol and/or decreased hepatic secretion of bile salts together with a change in the chemistry of biliary lecithin; (iii) altered relative lipid composition of hepatic and gallbladder bile resulting in excessive cholesterol supersaturation; (iv) a change in gallbladder function characterized by decreased contractility and mucin hypersecretion; (v) nucleation and precipitation of cholesterol supersaturated bile in the gallbladder with the eventual formation of cholesterol monohydrate crystals; and (vi) retention of cholesterol monohydrate crystals in the gallbladder, followed by their agglomeration and progressive growth into macroscopic stones. This section will outline the physicochemical and metabolic abnormalities responsible for each of these steps, classify the pathophysiological basis of abnormal bile in terms of specific kinetic defects in the enterohepatic circulation of bile salts and/or hepatic cholesterol secretion and suggest how extrahepatic factors may be responsible for lithogenic bile in many gallstone patients.

Biliary bile salts, phospholipids and cholesterol

Bile salts are the major solutes of human bile (Figure 19.25). The primary bile salts (cholates and chenodeoxycholates are formed in the liver which are the major catabolic products of cholesterol). The secondary bile salts (deoxycholates and lithocholates) are bacterial products of the primary bile salts via selective removal of a single hydroxyl function. Tertiary bile salts (ursodeoxycholates and lithocholate

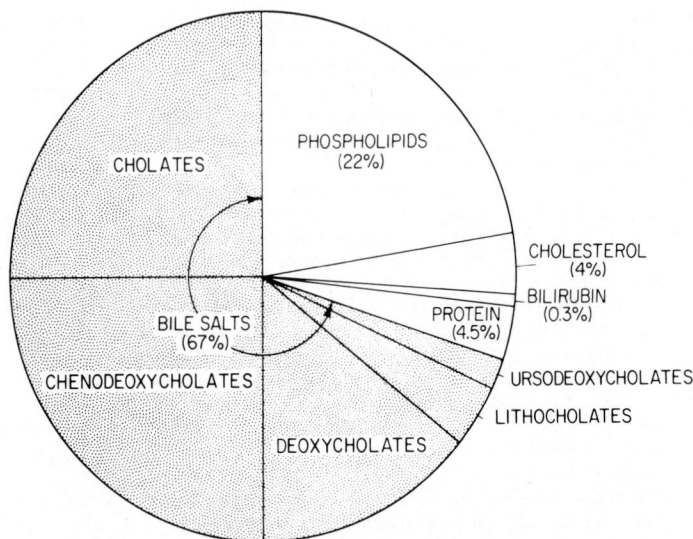

Fig. 19.25 Typical solute composition (weight %) of gallbladder and hepatic bile in healthy man.

sulphates) are bacterial and hepatic metabolites, respectively, of secondary bile salts. Each bile salt is conjugated in amide linkage with an amino acid, glycine or taurine. These bile salt conjugates constitute a family of molecules that share many detergent-like functions in bile and upper small intestine. However, individual bile salts exhibit specific pathophysiological effects within the organs of the enterohepatic circulation.[3]

Bile phospholipids are principally (>95%) lecithins (phosphatidylcholines). More than 80% of bile lecithin has palmitic acid (C16) esterified at the sn-1 position and an unsaturated fatty acid, oleic (C18 : 1), linoleic (C18 : 2) or arachidonic acid (C20 : 4) esterified at the sn-2 position. The di- and tetraenoic fatty acids are precursors of prostaglandin synthesis by the gallbladder mucosa; the chemistry of biliary lecithins appears to change considerably in lithogenic bile.[2] The predominant sterol of bile is cholesterol monohydrate (>98%); in addition, small amounts of cholesterol precursors, cholesterol derivatives and dietary phytosterols can be detected. Bilirubin conjugates and a large variety of proteins are minor components of bile (Figure 19.25).

The conventional and space-filling structures and physicochemical behaviour of the major biliary lipids are displayed in Figure 19.26. Each molecule is partly hydrophobic (literally, water fearing) and partly hydrophilic (literally, water loving); for this reason they are called amphiphiles. The molecules align at an oil–water interface with their hydrophobic portions directed towards the oil and their hydrophilic portions directed towards the water.

The hydrophobic portion of cholesterol (A) (Figure 19.26) is the steroid nucleus (cross hatched) and branched hydrocarbon side chain and the hydrophilic portion is the single hydroxyl function (closed oval). Cholesterol is insoluble in bulk water and crystallizes out as cholesterol monohydrate crystals. The hydrophobic portions of lecithin (B) consist of two long fatty acid chains (R, R′) with glycerol (closed oval) and phosphorylcholine (positive and negative charged groups) constituting the hydrophilic portions. Lecithin is an insoluble swelling amphiphile, and in water forms hydrated crystals called liquid-crystals. The cholestane steroid nucleus (cross hatched) constitutes the hydrophobic portion of bile salts (C) and the hydrophilic portions consist of polyhydroxyl functions and an ionic side chain. Bile salts are soluble amphiphiles with appreciable solubility as monomers (0.6–5 mmol/l); however, once they exceed this concentration the monomers self-associate to form small molecular aggregates called micelles. By forming mixed molecular aggregates in bile, i.e. mixed micellar and liquid crystalline vesicles, bile salts act as solvents for lecithin and cholesterol.

The physical–chemical state of normal bile[8]

Depending principally on bile salt concentration the biliary lipids interact to form a variety of macromolecular structures which can occur singly or as mixtures in the enterohepatic organs. Bile salt concentrations vary between 0.1–0.3 mmol/l in the hepatocyte, 20–50 mmol/l in the hepatic ducts, 100–400 mmol/l in the gallbladder, 2–8 mmol/l in the upper small intestine,

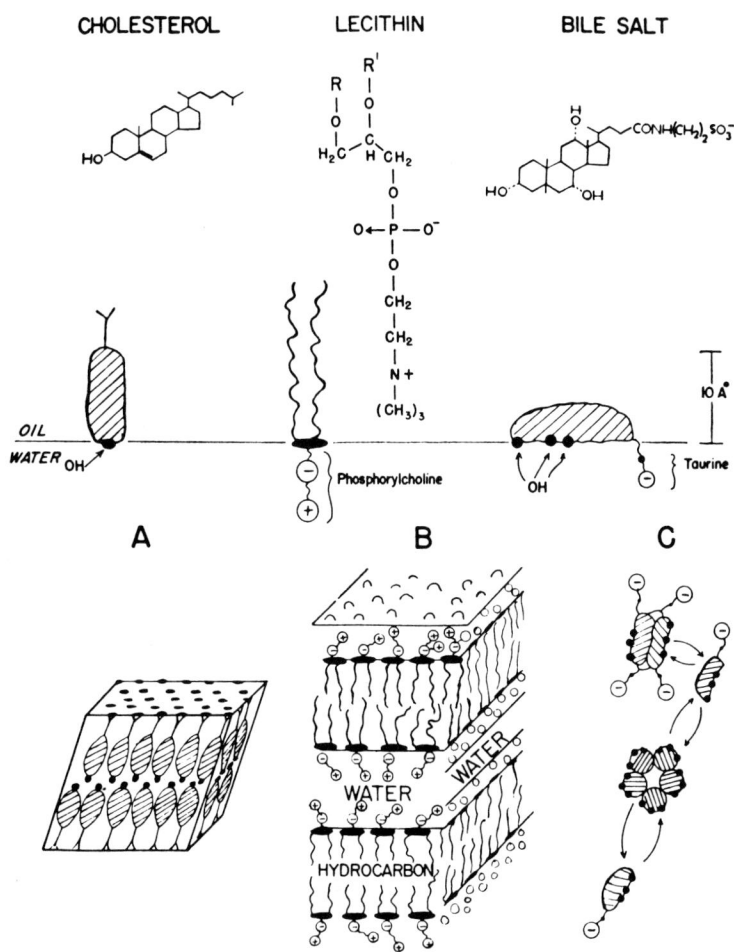

Fig. 19.26 Conventional and short-hand space-filling structures, amphiphilic orientation at an oil–water interface and physicochemical characteristics in bulk water of the major biliary lipids (for details see text).

and 0.5–2 mmol/l in the ileum. In the hepatocyte the diluted bile salt–lecithin–cholesterol complexes form liquid crystalline vesicles, which are probably unilamellar and about 100 nm in diameter (Figure 19.27). After exocytosis into the canalicular lumen these are transformed, probably incompletely, into bilayered disc-shaped structures called mixed micelles. With progressive removal of water along the ductular system the large mixed micelles subdivide into small globular simple micelles, i.e. bile salt–cholesterol micelles, and small disc-shaped mixed micelles, i.e. bile salt–lecithin–cholesterol micelles. In the gallbladder, the rapid removal of water and electrolytes induces more subtle changes: the size of the mixed micelles decreases slightly and the size of coexisting simple micelles increases. The mean diameter of particles in the gallbladder is about 5 nm. Dilution of bile in the upper small intestine during fat digestion and the solubilization of hydrolytic products (monoglycerides and 'fatty acid soaps') lead to a reversal in physical state; the simple and mixed

micelles of bile become transformed into large disc-shaped mixed micelles which now coexist with unilamellar vesicles or liposomes composed of the same lipids (Figure 19.27). Intestinal absorption of the dispersed digestion products reduces the sizes and alters the structures of the particles and when the ileum is reached only small simple bile salt micelles remain (Figure 19.27). Bile salts are transferred as monomers into ileal enterocytes by an active sodium-coupled transport system. From the absorptive cells, they enter portal blood where they are bound to albumin and high-density lipoprotein and return to the liver for reextraction and secretion into bile. This continuous recycling of bile salts is called the enterohepatic circulation.

The physical–chemical state of abnormal bile[4, 8]

Abnormal bile, that is, bile relatively enriched in cholesterol, differs physicochemically from normal bile in several ways (Figure 19.28). The

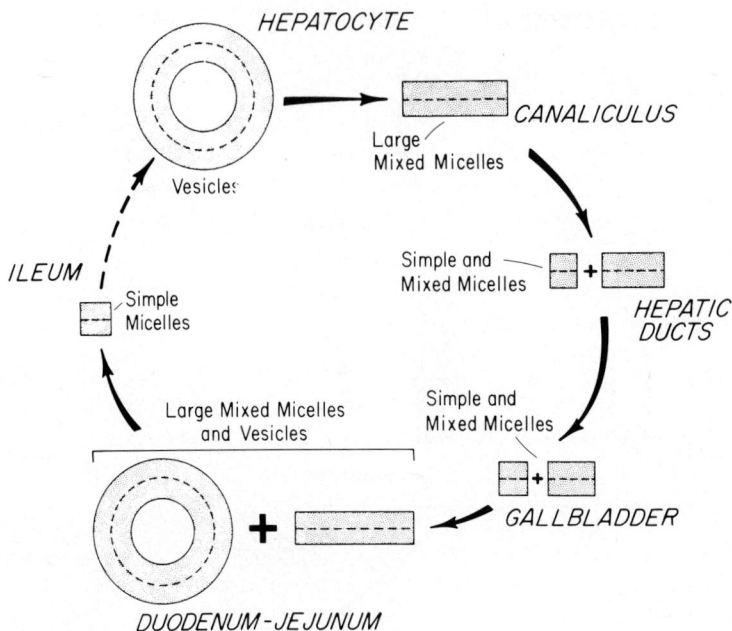

Fig. 19.27 Physicochemical state of normal bile in various organs of the enterohepatic circulation. For details see text.

biliary lipid vesicles produced by the liver are either deficient in bile salts (and lecithin) or enriched in cholesterol or both. It appears that only a portion of these are transformed into large mixed micelles within the canaliculus; the others persist in dilute hepatic bile as stable cholesterol-rich liquid crystalline vesicles. The mixed micelles have the same fate as the normal micelles depicted in Figure 19.27. In model hepatic bile the cholesterol-rich vesicles have been shown to form spontaneously and remain stable, without precipitating or fusing, for intervals of several days to weeks. Within the gallbladder the vesicles may also remain stable but in gallstone-prone individuals they precipitate to form microscopic or macroscopic cholesterol-rich liquid crystals. If the precipitated liquid crystals are retained in the gallbladder, they are progressively transformed into cholesterol monohydrate crystals and the remaining lecithin is redissolved by bile salts to form mixed micelles (Figure 19.28).

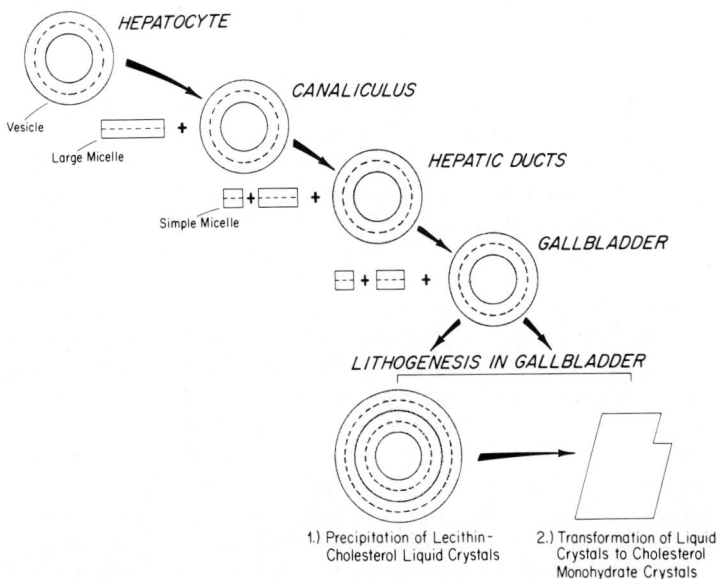

Fig. 19.28 Physicochemical state of abnormal bile: a cholesterol-enriched unilamellar vesicle (liposome) is synthesized and secreted by the liver. For details see text.

The identification of abnormal bile

Abnormal bile can be distinguished from normal bile by plotting relative biliary lipid compositions on phase diagrams, as shown in Figure 19.29. In hepatic bile, of average total lipid concentration of 3 g/100 ml, there is a small micellar zone and two metastable zones. When bile compositions fall within the micellar zone, they are unsaturated with cholesterol; those falling on the phase boundary are just saturated with cholesterol. Relative compositions falling within the one-phase metastable zone contain micelles that are supersaturated with cholesterol. Within the two-phase metastable zone, cholesterol-rich liquid crystalline vesicles in addition to supersaturated micelles solubilize excess cholesterol. The compositions of normal hepatic biles fall on the boundary between these two zones, i.e. they are supersaturated with cholesterol and their physical state may be micellar or micellar plus liquid crystalline. The compositions of hepatic biles from gallstone patients uniformly fall in the two-phase metastable zone, where the physical state consists of supersaturated micelles and cholesterol-rich liquid-crystalline vesicles (Figure 19.28).

Being more concentrated, the phase diagram of gallbladder bile contains a larger micellar zone (Figure 19.29). However, gallbladder bile has only a single one-phase metastable zone containing cholesterol supersaturated micelles. The relative lipid composition of most normal gallbladder biles falls within the micellar zone, on the micellar-metastable limit, or within the metastable zone where the cholesterol is solubilized in unsaturated, saturated or supersaturated micelles, respectively. In contrast, the relative lipid compositions of biles from gallstone patients fall outside these regions and lie in a labile zone from which rapid precipitation is possible. As in hepatic bile, it is probable that the excess cholesterol in such biles is solubilized in cholesterol-rich liquid crystals; however, 'abnormal' bile in gallstone-immune individuals probably contains vesicles which are stabilized by other biliary factors.

Pathophysiological basis of abnormal bile

The development of cholesterol enriched (supersaturated or lithogenic) bile has many causes and may be subdivided into six pathophysiological types (Table 19.3). In general, lithogenic bile and cholesterol gallstones can arise as part of any syndrome which results in a deficiency in hepatic bile salt secretion, an excessive cholesterol secretion, or a combination of both. In rare cases, abnormal bile is produced extrahepatically, a result of an alteration in bile composition in the gallbladder. The kinetics of an abnormal enterohepatic circulation and cholesterol secretion rates in each pathophysiological type are shown in Table 19.4. Two pathophysiological principles which control the formation of lithogenic bile are displayed in Figure 19.30.

The normal individual has an approximate bile salt synthetic rate, pool size, enterohepatic circulatory dynamics and cholesterol secretion rate as shown in Table 19.4. Pathophysiological principle A (Figure 19.30) demonstrates the complex inverse relationship between hepatic bile salt synthesis and bile salt return to the liver. In normal subjects the bile salt return rate is ~ 30 g/100 ml and de novo synthesis is repressed to a low level, approximately 0.5 g/100 ml. Pathophysiological principle B relates the physicochemical state of bile, as expressed by the saturation index, to the bile salt secretion rate. In normals, a high bile salt secretion rate engenders a saturation index less than 1, i.e. bile is unsaturated with cholesterol.

In Type 1 gallstone disease there is defective bile salt synthesis (Table 19.3). The size of the bile salt pool contracts to a new steady state,

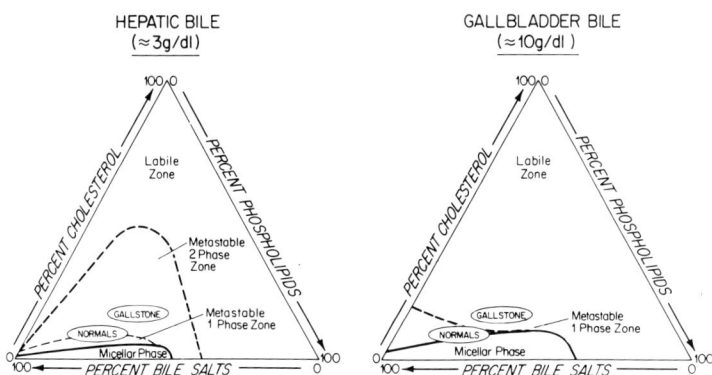

Fig. 19.29 Phase diagrams of hepatic and gallbladder biles with plots of the relative lipid (bile salt–lecithin–cholesterol) compositions for normal individuals and cholesterol gallstone patients. Precipitation is slow when relative lipid compositions fall within metastable zones but fast when relative lipid compositions fall within labile zones (see text for other details).

Table 19.3 Aetiological classification of cholesterol gallstones.

Type	Abnormality	Causes
1	Defective bile salt synthesis	Congenital 12α-hydroxylase deficiency, cerebrotendinous xanthomatosis, oestrogens, possibly Type IIb hyperlipo-proteinaemia, chronic cholestatic liver disease and primary biliary cirrhosis
2	Excessive bile salt loss	Ileectomy, ileal bypass, regional ileitis, cystic fibrosis with pancreatic insufficiency, primary bile salt malabsorption, possibly bile salt sequestering agents
3	Oversensitive bile salt feedback	Reduced bile salt secretion in some Caucasians with gallstones
4	Excessive cholesterol secretion	Obesity, Type IV hyperlipo-proteinaemia, clofibrate therapy, high caloric intake, massive cholesterol intake, oestrogens
5	Mixed defect (types 3 and 4)	Reduced bile salt secretion and excessive cholesterol secretion in American Indians and perhaps many Caucasians with gallstones
6	Primary extrahepatic gallstone disease	Cholecystitis (acalculous and bacterial), salmonellosis, somatostatinoma syndrome, post-truncal vagotomy, phaeochromocytoma, other stasis syndromes, total parenteral nutrition

there is low hepatic return of bile salts, low synthesis rates and low hepatic secretion rates (Table 19.4). Pathophysiological principle A is abnormal (Figure 19.30) and pathophysiological principle B shows that because of the curvilinear relationship between the supersaturation index and the low secretion rate of bile salts, there is a very high saturation index (Figure 19.30). These individuals have, in general, a 50–70% chance of developing cholesterol gallstones.

In Type 2 gallstone disease there is excessive bile salt loss from the alimentary tract (Table 19.3). The bile salt pool contracts to a new steady state with a low hepatic bile salt return

Table 19.4 Kinetics of the enterohepatic circulation and biliary cholesterol secretion in normals, types 1–6 gallstone disease and after medical or surgical therapy.

	Bile salts					Cholesterol Secretion rate
	Return rate	Synthetic rate	Pool size	Circulations of pool	Secretion rate	
Normal	30 g	0.5 g	3 g	10	30.5 g	0.7 g
Gallstone disease						
type 1	L	L	L	N	L	L
2	L	H	L	L	L	L
3	L	N(L)	L	N(L)	L	N
4	N(H)	N(H)	N(H)	N	N(H)	H
5	L	N(L)	L	N(L)	L	H
6	N(L)	N(H)	N	N(L)	N(L)	N
CDCA/UDCA therapy	N(H)	L	N(H)	N(H)	N(H)	L
Cholecystectomy	H	N(L)	L	H	H	N
Gallstone-induced gallbladder dysfunction	H	N(L)	L	H	H	N

L, low; N, normal; H, high.

Pathophysiological Principle A

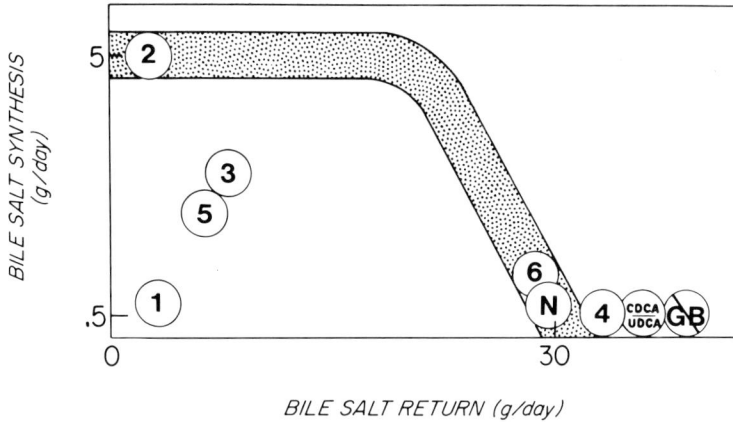

Pathophysiological Principle B

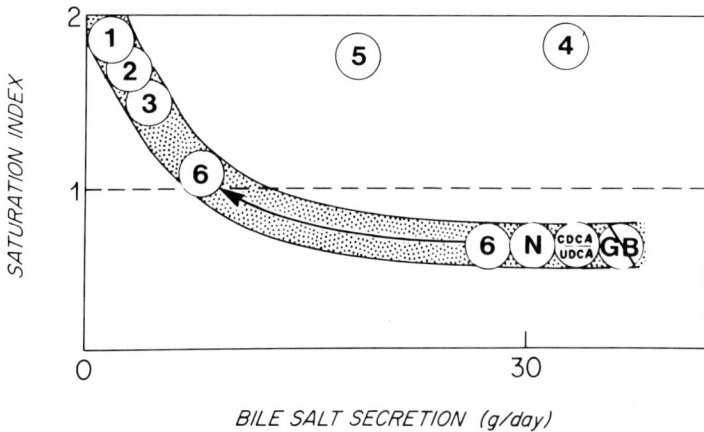

Fig. 19.30 The pathophysiological principles underlying gallstone disease. Principle A is control of bile salt synthesis by the bile salt return to the liver and Principle B is control of saturation index of bile by the bile salt secretion rate. N = normal; numbers 1 → 6 correspond to six pathophysiological types of gallstone diseases. The aetiology of each is given in Table 19.3, and the kinetics of the enterohepatic circulation of bile salts and cholesterol secretion are shown in Table 19.4. CDCA/UDCA = bile salt therapy with chenodeoxycholic

acid or ursodeoxycholic acid; (GB) = cholecystectomy or disease-induced malfunction of the gallbladder (see text for description).

and low hepatic secretion rates. This occurs because de novo bile salt synthesis, while maximal, cannot keep pace with intestinal loss (Table 19.4). Pathophysiological principle A is obeyed (Figure 19.30) but because maximum de novo synthesis cannot compensate for the intestinal loss of bile salt there is a very low secretion rate. Hence pathophysiological principle B is abnormal and the saturation index is extremely high. These individuals have a 30–40% chance of developing cholesterol gallstones.

In Type 3 gallstone disease, there is oversensitive bile salt feedback on de novo bile salt synthesis (Table 19.3). The precise aetiology is not known but there may be a constitutional or acquired synthesis defect, coupled with a low return of bile salts to the liver. This results in a contraction of the bile salt pool with low hepatic bile salt return and low secretion rates (Table 19.4). The combined defect leads to an abnormal pathophysiological principle A, i.e. de novo synthesis does not keep pace with a low return and

because the bile salt secretion rates are also low (pathophysiological principle B) the saturation index is high (Figure 19.30). Such individuals have a 20–50% chance of developing gallstones.

In Type 4 gallstone disease, the sole abnormality is excessive hepatic cholesterol secretion which can have many causes (Table 19.3). The kinetics of the enterohepatic circulation may be completely normal or supranormal in such patients (Table 19.4), hence pathophysiological principle A is normal (Figure 19.30). Because of the massive increase in biliary cholesterol secretion, pathophysiological principle B is disobeyed, i.e. the saturation index is very high, even though bile salt secretion rates may also be high (Figure 19.30). Such patients have about a 50% chance of developing cholesterol gallstones.

In Type 5 gallstone disease there is a mixed defect (Table 19.3), characterized by hyposecretion of bile salts from a contracted bile salt pool and hypersecretion of cholesterol (Table

19.4). The aetiology is uncertain, but a constitutional defect in the synthesis of bile salts and an increased hepatic synthesis of cholesterol have been suggested. Figure 19.30 shows that both pathophysiological principles A and B are abnormal in that there is defective bile salt synthesis in the face of a diminished bile salt return, and a very high saturation index even at moderate bile salt secretion rates. This syndrome is seen in members of certain American Indian tribes who have a 70–80% prevalence of cholesterol gallstones. However, a less severe degree of this mixed defect may constitute the major pathophysiological basis of gallstone formation in many individuals.

In Type 6 gallstone disease, the primary pathogenesis lies in the gallbladder (Table 19.3) and the kinetics of the enterohepatic circulation and biliary cholesterol secretion rates are completely normal (Table 19.4), hence the two pathophysiological principles are initially normal (Figure 19.30). Owing to absorption of bile salts and phospholipids in the gallbladder and possibly cholesterol secretion by the gallbladder mucosa, pathophysiological principle B becomes progressively abnormal as bile is stored in the gallbladder. Both the mechanisms involved and the aetiological entities are, as yet, poorly defined (Table 19.3).

The pathophysiological consequences of the two interventions for treating gallstone disease are also displayed in Table 19.4 and Figure 19.30. Bile acid therapy, i.e. chronic ingestion of chenodeoxycholic acid (CDCA) or ursodeoxycholic acid (UDCA), alters the enterohepatic circulation (Table 19.4) by suppressing endogenous bile salt synthesis and usually by expanding the bile salt pool. The expanded bile salt pool may or may not give rise to an increase in bile salt secretion. The major salutary hepato-biliary effect of these bile salts is to induce a profound decrease in the rate of hepatic cholesterol secretion (Table 19.4). Cholecystectomy removes both the gallstones and the gallbladder. As a result of the loss of the gallbladder which normally sequesters most of the bile salt pool during fasting, bile salt secretion rates become high postoperatively[10, 11] (Table 19.4). With either mode of therapy, the pre-existing Type 1–6 abnormalities (see pathophysiological principles A and B, Figure 19.30) become normal – in the former due to bile salt-induced hyposecretion of cholesterol, and in the latter due to hypersecretion of endogenous bile salts.

Pathophysiological basis of gallstone disease in the average patient

The average patient with cholesterol gallstones is usually of normal weight or slightly obese and has neither gastrointestinal disease leading to bile salt malabsorption, nor hepatic disease causing impaired bile salt synthesis. These patients appear to have a mixed defect (pathophysiological type 5), similar to that of the American Indian but of milder degree. By combining secretory data from many investigations this double defect is displayed in Figure 19.31. The dependence of saturation index on the bile salt secretion rate is slightly but distinctly different in these gallstone patients compared with controls. Thus for any bile salt secretion rate greater than ~ 8 $\mu mol \cdot kg^{-1} \cdot h^{-1}$, the gallstone patients secrete

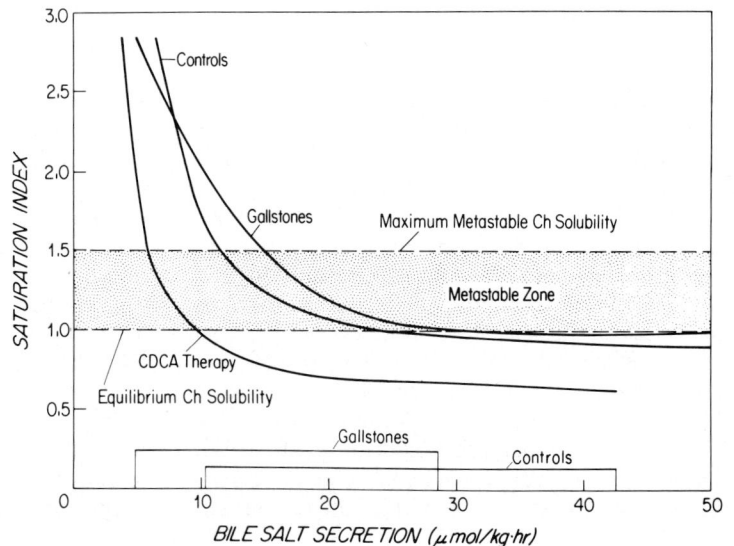

Fig. 19.31 Curves of saturation index versus bile salt secretion rate for controls, average 'non-obese' whites with gallstones and gallstone patients during chenodeoxycholic acid (CDCA) therapy; Ch = cholesterol. The ranges of bile salt secretion rates for controls and gallstone patients are displayed on the abscissa (discussed in text).

slightly more cholesterol than normals. The curves show that the threshold bile salt secretion rate required to exceed the maximum metastable cholesterol solubility is ~ 14 $\mu mol \cdot kg^{-1} \cdot h^{-1}$ in gallstone patients compared with ~ 11 $\mu mol \cdot kg^{-1} \cdot h^{-1}$ in controls. The second and, perhaps, more detrimental defect is shown along the abscissa. The range of bile salt secretion rates in gallstone patients, while overlapping with controls, can fall as low as 4 $\mu mol \cdot kg^{-1} \cdot h^{-1}$ compared with 11 $\mu mol \cdot kg^{-1} \cdot h^{-1}$ in controls. In the latter group bile salt secretion rates can rise to 43 $\mu mol \cdot kg^{-1} \cdot h^{-1}$ in contrast to an upper limit of 28 $\mu mol \cdot kg^{-1} \cdot h^{-1}$ in the gallstone patients. Thus hyposecretion of bile salts particularly during fasting coupled to hypersecretion of cholesterol places such patients at greater risk of developing supersaturated bile and gallstones. In all pathophysiological types of gallstone disease, CDCA/UDCA therapy profoundly depresses the saturation index so that over all physiological bile salt secretion rates bile becomes unsaturated with cholesterol (Figure 19.31).

The evolution of lithogenic bile in the average gallstone patient

Although the immediate source of lithogenic bile is the liver, the ultimate determinants may involve colonic, intestinal, plasma and hepatic factors (Figure 19.32).

COLONIC FACTORS

The activity of colonic bacteria coupled with alterations in bowel motility and diet may be involved in increasing the formation and colonic absorption of secondary bile salts. This increases the hepatic return of deoxycholate and decreases the hepatic return of chenodeoxycholate (and cholate). In fact there is an increased proportion of secondary bile salts in most gallstone patients, deoxycholate levels correlate positively with the saturation index of bile and interventions that decrease the production/absorption of deoxycholate can deplete bile with cholesterol.

LIVER FACTORS

Increased levels of returning deoxycholate suppress endogenous chenodeoxycholate synthesis; this, coupled with a decrease in chenodeoxycholate returning from the colon, leads to a contraction of the chenodeoxycholate pool. A contracted chenodeoxycholate pool is observed in many patients with lithogenic bile and its size correlates inversely with the saturation index. The small chenodeoxycholate pool plus increased recycling of deoxycholate could have several consequences. (a) Hepatic cholesterol secretion will increase as a result of less chenodeoxycholate, normally a suppressor of cholesterol secretion, coupled with more deoxycholate which has a strong detergent effect on liver cell membranes. (b) Deoxycholate conjugates, being the most hydrophobic molecules in the bile salt pool, complete a very short enterohepatic cycle by being absorbed principally from the jejunum – hence, while their absolute concentration in bile may be only slightly increased, their effective flux through the liver cells may be dramatically increased and thereby become potent suppressors of de novo bile salt synthesis. (c) Low levels of chenodeoxycholate in bile also appear to increase the percentage of biliary lecithin composed of arachidonic acid in the sn-2

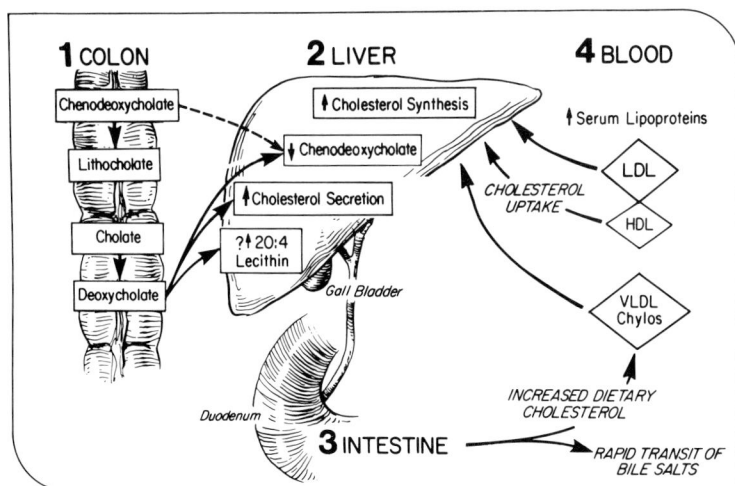

Fig. 19.32 Scenarios for the evolution of supersaturated lithogenic bile in man. The ultimate predisposing abnormalities may involve colonic, hepatic, small intestine and blood factors (see text for discussion).

position – a substrate for prostaglandin synthesis by the gallbladder mucosa. This may also be induced directly by the greater return and recycling of deoxycholate. There is evidence that hepatic cholesterol synthesis is increased in some patients with gallstones and that the fraction of cholesterol diverted to de novo bile salts is decreased.

INTESTINAL FACTORS

The small intestine may play two roles. (a) Rapid intestinal transit times are known to induce faster recycling of the bile salt pool by accelerating the delivery of bile salt to active ileal transport sites. Rapid transit also allows for a greater spill-over of bile salts into the colon. The more rapid return of bile salts to the liver suppresses de novo bile salt synthesis and the increased conversion of primary into secondary bile salts will secondarily have adverse effects on cholesterol secretion by the liver. (b) Cholesterol of both dietary and biliary origin is absorbed with about 40% efficacy from the small intestine. Increased dietary cholesterol intake increases absorption, and is taken up by the liver in very-low-density lipoprotein (VLDL) and chylomicron remnants. It has been shown in man that increased intake of dietary cholesterol can increase hepatic cholesterol secretion and thereby increase the cholesterol content of bile.

PLASMA FACTORS

Both plasma low-density and high-density lipoproteins (LDL and HDL) are recognized by high-affinity receptors on sinusoidal membranes; in man the liver is the major catabolic organ for the cholesterol of these lipoproteins. The free cholesterol derived from both lipoprotein particles is used in part for de novo bile salt synthesis and also for biliary cholesterol secretion. Any factor that increases the hepatic uptake of these lipoproteins (higher blood levels, increased activity, number or affinity of sinusoidal receptors, etc.) could contribute to hypersecretion of biliary cholesterol and the formation of lithogenic bile. In non-obese individuals there is epidemiological evidence of a positive correlation between LDL plus VLDL cholesterol and cholesterol saturation index of bile; in the same subjects there is a negative correlation between HDL cholesterol and saturation index.

The role of the gallbladder

The gallbladder is the organ in which most gallstones form and plays several roles in their formation. First, it responds to lithogenic bile in a distinct way and provides an environment favourable to nucleation, precipitation and crystal growth. Second, the absorption function of the gallbladder mucosa alters the composition of bile and changes the phase equilibria of biliary lipids. Third, through its influence on the enterohepatic circulation of bile salts, the gallbladder affects the relative composition of bile and may augment and perpetuate lithogenic potential and the growth of stones through altered contractility, concentrating capacity and filling efficiency.

MUCIN HYPERSECRETION AND STASIS

In animal models and in man, lithogenic bile has two important effects on gallbladder function: there is a depression of gallbladder contractility, and stimulation of mucin hypersecretion with the formation of mucin gels in bile.[7] Both appear to be related to increased prostaglandin production in the gallbladder mucosa (Figure 19.33).

Recent human and animal studies suggest that the trigger for increased prostaglandin synthesis may be a subtle imbalance in the fatty acid precursors that are esterified to the sn-2 position of biliary lecithin. For example, there is an increase of sn-2 arachidonyl lecithin (C20 : 4) and a decrease in sn-2 linoleyl lecithin in bile of experimental animals and in man with gallstones. Further, in gallstone patients the levels of arachidonyl lecithin correlate inversely with the percentage of endogenous chenodeoxycholate in bile.[2] The chemistry of biliary lecithin is rendered normal by feeding chenodeoxycholate and cholate.[1] During early lithogenesis in the prairie dog there is increased activity of mucosal phospholipase A_2, as inferred from increased production of palmitoyl lysolecithin in sterile bile. Non-steroidal anti-inflammatory drugs (aspirin and indomethacin) which inhibit cyclooxygenase are capable of inhibiting mucin hypersecretion and gel formation.[6, 12] Lithogenesis in this animal model is inhibited by these agents despite the persistence of cholesterol supersaturated bile. Gallbladder compliance in the lithogenic baboon is also normalized by both aspirin and indomethacin.

NUCLEATION AND PRECIPITATION

Despite similar degrees of cholesterol supersaturation, human lithogenic biles nucleate about five times faster than non-lithogenic supersaturated biles, suggesting the presence of nucleators

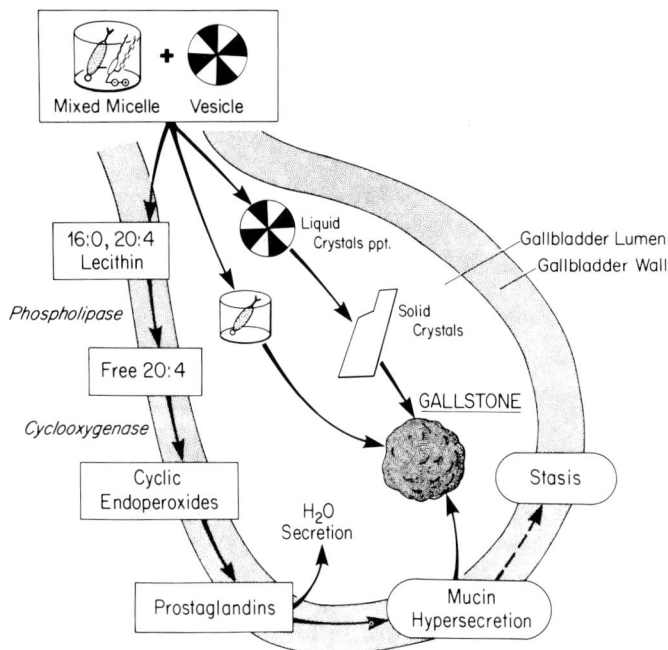

Fig. 19.33 Postulated gallbladder mucosal and luminal events during cholesterol lithogenesis in man (For details see text).

or reduction in anti-nucleating agents in abnormal bile.[5] A possible nucleating agent is excess mucin glycoproteins in the lithogenic gallbladder. Mucin gels may act as epitactic surfaces to lower the energy of nucleation and enhance nucleation and initial growth of gallstones by the slowing of molecular movement due to their viscoelasticity. Extensive model and animal studies suggest that the initial biliary precipitates are liquid crystals of lecithin and cholesterol (homogeneous nucleation) and *not* cholesterol monohydrate crystals (Figure 19.33). Once the liquid crystals have precipitated a transition to cholesterol monohydrate crystals may take place. Thereafter liquid crystals are no longer evident in bile and further precipitation onto coexisting crystals occurs in the form of molecular cholesterol from mixed micelles or liquid-crystalline vesicles (heterogeneous nucleation).

CRYSTALLIZATION AND STONE GROWTH

The transformation of the initial liquid crystalline precipitate into solid cholesterol crystals may take many days or weeks. The gallbladder factors that may accelerate or retard the conversion are not known but it is possible that mucin gels may act as a 'three dimensional crucible' for supporting liquid crystals during these transitional steps. Liquid crystals are now known to be an important component of biliary sludge and may be an early event in sludge formation. It is also possible that mucin gels and stasis are responsible for the trapping of precipitates and

preventing their discharge during gallbladder contraction. The potential importance of other nucleating and/or anti-nucleating factors in native bile, including those that could retard the liquid → solid crystal formation, have yet to be rigorously explored.

Cholesterol gallstones are formed by myriads of small cholesterol monohydrate crystals. Human gallstones are either single or, if numerous, are usually equal in size, an indication of multiple nucleation at one point in time. From studies in vitro[13] and studies in squirrel monkeys,[9] there appear to be three mechanisms of crystal growth: two-dimensional layer growth, crystal aggregation and amorphous assembly of fragmented crystals. In prairie dogs and squirrel monkeys homogeneous nucleation appears to predominate since the central zone of the crystal aggregate does not contain bilirubin precipitates, calcium salts or glycoprotein and concentric layer or ring formation in gallstones is not observed. In contrast, the centre of human gallstones is likely to have an amorphous substrate (pigment, glycoprotein, etc.) containing randomly arranged cholesterol crystal plates. The outer crystals are oriented perpendicularly to the surface and pigmented or calcium-containing concentric rings in the stones are common. These rings separate two layers of cholesterol crystals which have different axial orientations and may represent points of temporary cessation in stone growth. Liesegang's phenomenon, a mineralogical term describing the periodic precipitation of crystals in gels, has also been invoked to explain the ring phenomenon. Nevertheless it is likely that 'rings' are related to changes in the degree of cholesterol saturation of bile with periodic interruption of gallstone growth or even dissolution, followed by reorientation of crystal direction when growth is resumed. The striking differences in gallstone petrology in man versus experimental animals could be related to numerous factors which include the great differences in the time required for stone growth, the fluctuating variations in bile composition and the doping effects of mineral, drug and bilirubin precipitates.

REFERENCES

1 Ahlberg, J., Curstedt, T., Einarsson, K. & Sjövall, J. (1981) Molecular species of biliary phosphatidylcholines in gallstone patients: the influence of treatment with cholic acid and chenodeoxycholic acid. *Journal of Lipid Research*, **22**, 404–409.
2 Cantafora, A., Angelico, M., Di Base, A. *et al.* (1981) Structure of biliary phosphatidylcholine in cholesterol gallstone patients. *Lipids*, **16**, 589–592.
3 Carey, M. C. (1982) The enterohepatic circulation. In *The Liver: Biology and Pathobiology* (Ed.) Arias, I. M., Popper, H., Schacter, D. & Shafritz, D. pp. 429–465. New York: Raven.
4 Carey, M. C. & Small, D. M. (1978) Physical-chemistry of cholesterol solubility in bile. Relationship to gallstone formation and dissolution in man. *Journal of Clinical Investigation*, **61**, 998–1026.
5 Holan, K. R., Holzbach, R. T., Hermann, R. E. *et al.* (1979) Nucleation time: a key factor in the pathogenesis of cholesterol gallstone disease. *Gastroenterology*, **77**, 611–617.
6 Lee, S. P., Carey, M. C. & Lamont, J. T. (1981) Aspirin prevention of cholesterol gallstone formation in prairie dogs. *Science (Washington, D.C.)*, **211**, 1429–1431.
7 Lee, S. P., Lamont, J. T. & Carey, M. C. (1981) Role of mucus hypersecretion in the evolution of cholesterol gallstones: studies in the prairie dog. *Journal of Clinical Investigation*, **67**, 1712–1723.
8 Mazer, N. A. & Carey, M. C. (1983) Quasielastic light scattering studies of aqueous biliary lipid systems. Cholesterol solubilization and precipitation in model bile solutions. *Biochemistry (USA)*, **22**, 426–442.
9 Portman, O. W., Osuga, T. & Tanaka, N. (1975) Biliary lipids and cholesterol gallstone formation. *Advances in Lipid Research*, **13**, 135–194.
10 Shaffer, E. A. & Small, D. M. (1976) Gallstone disease: pathogenesis and management. *Current Problems in Surgery*, **13**, 1–72.
11 Shaffer, E. A. & Small, D. M. (1977) Biliary lipid secretion in cholesterol gallstone disease. The effect of cholecystectomy and obesity. *Journal of Clinical Investigation*, **59**, 828–840.
12 Thornell, E. (1982) Mechanisms in the development of acute cholecystitis and biliary pain: a study on the role of prostaglandins and effects of indomethacin. *Scandinavian Journal of Gastroenterology*, **17** (Supplement 76) 1–31.
13 Toor, E. W., Evans, D. F. & Cussler, E. R. (1978) Cholesterol monohydrate growth in model bile solution. *Proceedings of the National Academy of Sciences (USA)*, **75**, 6230–6234.

FORMATION OF PIGMENT GALLSTONES

Classification

Pigment gallstone disease is a relatively neglected, but important cause of biliary tract pathology in Occidental and Oriental subjects.[10, 14]

All pigment gallstones contain calcium bilirubinate and related derivatives as a major or minor component, but as shown in Table 19.5, there are two major types of pigment gallstones descriptively known as brown or black stones. The brown pigment gallstone, also called bilirubin or bile pigment calcium stone, commonly occurs in Oriental subjects. The black or pure pigment gallstone occurs in Occidental patients. These two types of calcium bilirubinate pigment gallstones are morphologically, chemically and clinically distinct (Table 19.5). Despite geographic differences, some recurrent common bile duct stones in Occidental patients are qualitatively similar to brown pigment stones in Orientals. Likewise, the black pigment stones in the general population are similar to those found in patients with cirrhosis or haemolysis.

The remaining types of pigment stones usually consist of a calcium salt, e.g. calcium carbonate, phosphate or calcium palmitate with calcium bilirubinate as a minor component.[11]

Epidemiology

The prevalence of pigment gallstone disease varies throughout the world. In the United States, black pigment gallstones accounted for 20–30% of cholecystectomies performed at a major urban medical centre.[13] In Japan the incidence of brown pigment stone disease is decreasing, whereas that of black and cholesterol stones is increasing.[7]

Gallstones occur rarely before the age of 10. From puberty through to the sixth decade, cholesterol stone disease predominates. However, from the seventh decade pigment stones occur more frequently than cholesterol stones in the general American population undergoing cholecystectomy.[13] In patients with haemolysis or cirrhosis, the incidence of black pigment stones increases with age.[10] In Japan, the incidence of brown pigment stone increases with age.[7]

Pigment gallstones occur as frequently in black as in white subjects[13] but are rare in certain ethnic groups, such as native Americans, Scandinavians, or Bolivians.

Table 19.5 Features of black and brown pigment gallstones[14]

	Black	Brown
Clinical associations		
Incidence increases with age	Yes	Yes
Female predominance	Yes	Yes
Haemolysis and/or cirrhosis	Yes	No
Low protein diet	No	Yes
Bacterial infection in bile	Uncommon	Nearly 100%
Recurrent stones	Uncommon	Quite frequent
Location in biliary tree	Usually limited to gallbladder	Intra- and extra-hepatic ducts and gallbladder
Morphology	Black to brown, 50% amorphous, remainder crystalline	Brown, laminated
Radiodensity	50% opaque	Lucent
Major stone components (% *dry weight*)		
Calcium bilirubinate	40	60
Calcium palmitate	Rare	15
Calcium phosphate	9	Absent
Calcium carbonate	6	Rare
Cholesterol	2	15
Bile salts	2	2
Unmeasured	30	10

Females are at relatively less risk of pigment stone disease than cholesterol stones.

Black or brown pigment stone disease may develop in both Oriental and Occidental patients without a predisposing clinical disorder such as malaria, haemolysis or cirrhosis. In the US, black pigment stones are limited to the gallbladder; whereas in the Orient, brown pigment stones occur both in the gallbladder and in the extra- and intrahepatic ducts.

Stone and bile composition

Profiles of brown and black stones have been determined by American, European and Japanese investigators using a variety of chemical, chromatographic and analytical techniques.[8, 15, 20] A typical brown pigment stone is composed of calcium salts of bilirubin, fatty acids (mostly palmitate), and cholesterol in a glycoprotein matrix. It is laminated, easily fragmented, and usually radiolucent on an abdominal flat film. A black stone also contains calcium bilirubinate and varying proportions of calcium phosphate and carbonate; minimal amounts of cholesterol and rarely calcium palmitate are present. The outer surface is black, but the interior is brown. Half of these black stones is amorphous, radiopaque, and brittle when crushed. A major qualitative difference between brown and black pigment gallstones is that the calcium bilirubinate may be polymerized to a greater degree in black than in brown stones.[2, 3, 21]

The gallbladder bile surrounding either brown or black pigment gallstones is usually not saturated with cholesterol and may contain an increased proportion of mono- and unconjugated bilirubin IXα.[6, 12] Bacterial infection with enteric bacteria approaches 100% in brown pigment stone disease whereas in black pigment stone disease the bile is sterile. Ionized calcium in bile determined by several different methods is approximately 0.75–1.0 mmol/l in human hepatic and gallbladder bile.[9] Whether ionized calcium concentrations vary in pigment compared with cholesterol stone disease remains to be determined. At present it seems likely that the ionized calcium concentration in bile is influenced by bile salt binding[19] and pH.

Pathogenesis

The usual steps in gallstone formation include supersaturation, nidation, sequestration and aggregation. This sequence may vary from a matter of days or many years. Brown and black pigment stones show different features and because both stone types contain calcium bilirubinate the conditions leading to precipitation of calcium bilirubinate may differ. Maki[5] suggested that brown pigment stones resulted from the hydrolysis of conjugated bilirubin to its unconjugated form and that this was mediated by β-glucuronidase of bacterial origin. This attractive hypothesis remains unproven because bacterial infection has not been documented as an initial event. Another possibility is that stasis of the biliary tree, perhaps due to a motility disturbance, enables hydrolytic enzymes that originate from the liver, pancreatic juice, ductal mucosa or bacteria to hydrolyse not only conjugated bilirubin but also biliary lecithins which would result in increased concentrations of bilirubin IXα and perhaps monoconjugated bilirubin. In addition, hydrolysis of biliary lecithins would decrease the capacity of the remaining mixed micelles of bile salts and lecithin to solubilize cholesterol; consequently, precipitation of cholesterol as well as calcium bilirubinate and fatty acids would occur and this may be on a glycoprotein skeleton.

Black pigment stone disease develops in the gallbladder in the absence of bacterial infection and the postulation is that local gallbladder conditions contribute. These stones occur in the elderly and contain calcium bilirubinate as well as calcium salts of phosphate and carbonate[15] with minimal cholesterol. Because anions like carbonate and phosphate are present only in miniscule concentrations at the normal pH of bile, it may be that the microenvironment near the gallbladder epithelium may contribute to stone formation. The secretion of glycoprotein may also be important because mucin can bind calcium and bilirubinate and provide a framework upon which calcium salts like carbonate and phosphate may grow. It remains unproven whether spontaneous hydrolysis of conjugated bilirubin is a mechanism.[1]

A tenfold increase in bilirubin and its conjugates occurs in the T-tube bile of patients with chronic haemolytic anaemia which results in a higher incidence of stones at a younger age in subjects with haemolysis than in the general population. Factors promoting solubilization of bilirubin IXα relate primarily to bile acid and hydrogen ion concentrations. As the pH of human bile decreases within the gallbladder, the limits of solubility of bilirubin in bile may be exceeded and influence the precipitation of calcium bilirubinate. In patients with cirrhosis, a decrease in bile acid concentration in bile may predispose to the formation of black pigment stones.

Mouse model of human pigment gallstones

Over the past several years the laboratory mouse (genotype *nb/nb*) with hereditary haemolytic anaemia has been used as a model of human pigment gallstone disease.[16] Because *nb/nb* mice are genetically homogeneous, they provide an excellent animal model that avoids the genetic heterogeneity of the human disease and the effects of treatment. As a result of increased bilirubin production, *nb/nb* mice *spontaneously* develop calcium bilirubinate (black) gallstones which are nearly identical to those from patients with sickle cell disease. The higher levels of plasma bilirubin and reticulocytosis in *nb/nb* mice than in control mice indicate that haemolysis is a prerequisite and significant risk factor for gallstone formation.[16] The development of gallstones in mice with haemolysis depends upon hepatic bile composition, gallbladder modification of hepatic bile, local events within the gallbladder, and characteristics of a specific genotype. The secretion of increased concentrations of bilirubin IXα and its conjugates is the primary abnormality in the hepatic bile of *nb/nb* mice. Hepatic bile of *nb/nb* mice contains high concentrations of bilirubinate that in the presence of ionized calcium exceed the solubility product of calcium bilirubinate to form calcium bilirubinate stones. Infection and inflammation do not play a role.

The contribution of the gallbladder to haemolysis-induced pigment gallstone disease in mice is important. Bile pigment precipitates occur within the glands located in the gallbladder neck *before* luminal stones develop.[18] Mucin glycoprotein secretion by the glands in the gallbladder neck is enhanced in *nb/nb* mice with luminal stones suggesting a local response to microscopic stone disease.[4]

REFERENCES

1 Boonyapisit, S. T., Trotman, B. W. & Ostrow, J. D. (1978) Unconjugated bilirubin and the hydrolysis of conjugated bilirubin, in gallbladder bile of patients with cholelithiasis. *Gastroenterology*, **74**, 70–74.

2 Burnett, W., Dwyer, K. R. & Kennard, C. H. (1981) Black pigment or polybilirubinate gallstones: composition and formation. *Annals of Surgery*, **193**, 331–333.

3 Carr, S. H. & Ostrow, J. D. (1981) Equilibrium swelling of pigment gallstones: evidence for network polymer

structure. *Hepatology Rapid Literature Review*, **11**, 1657–1658 (abstract).

4 LaMont, J. T., Turner, B. S., Bernstein, S. E. & Trotman, B. W. (1983) Gallbladder glycoprotein secretion in mice with hemolytic anemia and pigment gallstones. *Hepatology* (in press).

5 Maki, T. (1966) Pathogenesis of calcium bilirubinate gallstone. *Annals of Surgery*, **164**, 90–100.

6 Masuda, H. & Nakayama, F. (1979) Composition of bile pigment in gallstones and bile and their etiological significance. *Journal of Laboratory and Clinical Medicine*, **93**, 353–360.

7 Nagase, M., Tanimura, H., Setoyama, M. & Hikasa, Y. (1978) Present features of gallstones in Japan. A collective review of 2144 cases. *American Journal of Surgery*, **135**, 788–790.

8 Nakayama, F. (1969) Quantitative microanalysis of gallstones. *Journal of Laboratory and Clinical Medicine*, **72**, 602–611.

9 Robertson, W. G. & Marshall, R. W. (1981) Ionized calcium in body fluids. *CRC Critical Reviews in Clinical and Laboratory Sciences*, **15**, 85–125.

10 Soloway, R. D., Trotman, B. W. & Ostrow, J. D. (1977) Pigment gallstones. *Gastroenterology*, **72**, 167–182.

11 Sutor, D. J. & Wooley, S. E. (1973) The nature and incidence of gallstones containing calcium. *Gut*, **14**, 215–220.

12 Tritapepe, R., DiPadova, C. & Rovagnati, P. (1980) Are pigmented gallstones caused by a 'metabolic' liver defect? *British Medical Journal*, **i** 832.

13 Trotman, B. W. & Soloway, R. D. (1975) Pigment vs cholesterol cholelithiasis. Clinical and epidemiological aspects. *American Journal of Digestive Diseases*, **20**, 735–740.

14 Trotman, B. W. & Soloway, R. D. (1982) Pigment gallstone disease: summary of the National Institutes of Health – International Workshop. *Hepatology*, **2**, 879–884.

15 Trotman, B. W., Ostrow, J. D. & Soloway, R. D. (1974) Pigment vs cholesterol cholelithiasis: comparison of stone and bile composition. *American Journal of Digestive Diseases*, **19**, 585–590.

16 Trotman, B. W., Bernstein, S. E., Bove, K. E. & Wirt, G. D. (1980) Studies on the pathogenesis of pigment gallstones in hemolytic anemia. Description and characteristics of a mouse model. *Journal of Clinical Investigation*, **65**, 1301–1308.

17 Trotman, B. W., Bernstein, S. E., Balistreri, W. F. *et al.* (1981) Hemolysis-induced gallstones in mice: increased unconjugated bilirubin in hepatic bile predisposes to gallstone formation. *Gastroenterology*, **81**, 232–236.

18 Trotman, B. W., Bongiovanni, M. D., Kahn, M. J. & Bernstein, S. E. (1982) A morphological study of the liver and gallbladder in hemolysis induced gallstone in mice. *Hepatology*, **2**, 863–869.

19 Williamson, B. W. A. & Percy-Robb, I. W. (1980) Contribution of biliary lipids to calcium binding in bile. *Gastroenterology*, **78**, 696–702.

20 Wosiewitz, W. (1981) Common duct pigment stones (CDPS) and gallbladder pigment stones (GBPS): a comparative morphological and analytical investigation. *Hepatology Rapid Literature Review*, **11**, 1650–1652 (abstract).

21 Zilm, K. W., Grant, D. M., Englert, E., Jr. & Straight, R. C. (1980) The use of solid ^{13}C nuclear magnetic resonance for the characterization of cholesterol and bilirubin pigment composition of human gallstones. *Biochemical Biophysical Research Communications*, **93**, 857–866.

CLINICAL FEATURES AND MEDICAL TREATMENT OF GALLSTONES

INCIDENCE AND CLINICAL ASSOCIATIONS

Gallstones tend to occur more frequently in premenopausal women than males (female-to-male ratio approximately 2 : 1). Obesity and parity are almost certainly contributory factors and a positive family history is not infrequent. After the menopause the male-to-female ratio becomes closer to one. The prevalence of gallstones in the adult population in the United Kingdom is about 15%. This figure however hides the fact that the incidence increases with age so that by the time a patient reaches the age of 80 years or above, the chance of gallstones being present is of the order of 40–50%. There are probably about 5 million people with gallstones in Great Britain. Pigment stones in this country form a relatively small percentage of all gallstones but should be remembered in any patient with a chronic haemolytic disorder (e.g. congenital spherocytosis, sickle cell anaemia, thalassaemia) – where the incidence is approximately 33% – or with cirrhosis of the liver. Most gallstones formed by patients in the Western Hemisphere consist predominantly of crystalline cholesterol monohydrate. Drugs such as clofibrate and exogenous oestrogens undoubtedly increase the cholesterol saturation of the patient's bile and predispose to gallstone formation. In the case of exogenous oestrogens (as used in oral contraceptive preparations or for postmenopausal symptoms) the degree of risk of developing cholelithiasis associated with long-term ingestion has been overstated. Recent evidence suggests that only a small susceptible subpopulation of all 'pill takers' will develop gallstones – and those that do so usually present within one to four years of oral contraceptive use.[10]

There is an increased incidence of cholesterol gallstones in patients who have a broken enterohepatic circulation of bile salts, for example patients with Crohn's disease of the terminal ileum, ileal resection and short-circuit operations for morbid obesity. Male patients with type IV hyperlipidaemia (isolated elevation of serum triglycerides carried in the prebeta-lipoprotein fraction) also have an increased incidence of cholesterol gallstones. It is relevant that there is an inverse relationship between serum triglyceride levels and serum high density lipoprotein cholesterol (HDL-C) concentrations as well as evidence to suggest that the lower the serum HDL-C level the more saturated the patient's bile.[15] There is no obvious relationship between serum total cholesterol (most of which is carried in the low density lipoprotein (LDL) fraction) and either biliary cholesterol saturation or the incidence of gallstones. Thus, patients with type II hyperlipidaemia (familial hypercholesterolaemia) do not form more gallstones than the general population as a whole. The frequently quoted association between diabetes mellitus and gallstones on the one hand and hyperparathyroidism and gallstones on the other does not stand up to careful scrutiny.[9]

CLINICAL FEATURES

It is important to appreciate that more than 50% of patients with gallstones never have symptoms and never present with the clinical syndromes of cholelithiasis – 'silent gallstones'. Their stones are usually discovered as an incidental finding at post-mortem examination. No pain will be experienced and complications will not occur provided the stones remain free in the lumen of the gallbladder and do not migrate into the cystic duct or bile duct.

A further 5% of gallstones are discovered incidentally as a result of laparotomy or radiological investigation performed for some other reason. Until recently, only those gallstones which contained enough calcium to render them radiopaque tended to be identified, for instance at the time of a barium meal or intravenous pyelogram. With the increasingly wide use of abdominal ultrasound and whole body CT and NMR scanners many more radiolucent gallstones are likely to be discovered.

Biliary colic, obstructive jaundice and acute cholecystitis are all specific symptoms or complications that can be ascribed to gallstones. In contrast, symptoms such as fatty food intolerance, 'dyspepsia', eructation, flatulence, pyrosis, bad breath and vague epigastric discomfort occur with equal frequency in patients with and without gallstones. Such non-specific symptomatology should not be taken as an indication that gallstones are causing symptoms. It is probable that about 15% of all patients with cholelithiasis are identified not because they have specific symptoms but rather because they have complained to their medical practitioner of a variety of these non-specific symptoms that have

served as an indication for an oral cholecystogram which subsequently demonstrates gallstones. If the 50% of all patients whose stones are discovered at autopsy are excluded together with the 5% discovered incidentally and the 15% whose stones are not giving rise to true symptoms, a hard core of 35% of patients remains who have genuine signs and symptoms or complications which develop as a result of cholelithiasis.

Pain

If a gallstone becomes acutely impacted in the cystic duct the patient will experience pain as the gallbladder responds by contracting down in an attempt to expel the stone. The term gallbladder or biliary 'colic' is a misnomer, because the pain does not increase and decrease in intensity (as occurs in intestinal colic). Instead, the pain is of sudden onset, is severe and constant for up to three hours and does not have the characteristic waxing and waning element of colic. The pain lasts less than an hour in 40% of patients. Should the pain continue for more than six hours it is probable that some other complication such as cholecystitis or pancreatitis has developed.[12]

The pain of biliary origin is usually located in the epigastrium or upper right quadrant and classically radiates to the intrascapular region or tip of the right scapula. The patient frequently describes the pain as band-like extending round the upper abdomen, through into the back. Less commonly discomfort is experienced in the lower chest, when it may be confused with intrathoracic diseases such as oesophagitis, myocardial infarction or a dissecting aneurysm. Conversely, the pain associated with myocardial infarction or ischaemia may be upper abdominal and band-like and may mimic gallbladder disease. It is less well recognized that biliary colic pain may occasionally be felt predominantly or exclusively in the left upper quadrant, which may suggest a high posterior gastric ulcer, pancreatitis or even renal disease especially when the pain radiates into the back.

One of the commonest conditions to be confused with biliary disease is a variant of the irritable bowel syndrome which is sometimes referred to as the 'hepatic flexure syndrome'. In this disorder the symptoms of fatty intolerance and right hypochondrial pain radiating into the back appears indistinguishable from those of gallbladder disease but the association with other symptoms such as abdominal bloating, alternating diarrhoea and constipation and the fact that the pain is relieved by defecation should suggest a diagnosis of functional colonic disorder rather than gallstones. Typical biliary pain associated with an elevation of serum conjugated bilirubin, alkaline phosphatase or transaminase is virtually diagnostic of biliary tract disease; bilirubin and alkaline phosphatase levels are higher in common duct obstruction than in cystic duct obstruction.

Acute cholecystitis

The pain associated with the acute impaction of a stone in the cystic duct is relieved if the stone disimpacts or passes. If, on the other hand, the stone stays impacted an attack of acute cholecystitis may be initiated and the longer the stone is impacted, the greater the risk of the bile becoming secondarily infected. In 80% of patients the attack subsides as the stone is passed or falls back into the gallbladder lumen. The complications of acute cholecystitis include localized avascular necrosis and gangrene of the gallbladder wall with perforation which may become walled off or, less frequently, free perforation with biliary peritonitis. Chronic cholecystitis – a condition where the gallbladder becomes thickened, fibrosed and shrunken – occurs as a consequence of either recurrent attacks of acute cholecystitis or failure of the stone of the cystic duct to disimpact.

Hydrops of the gallbladder

Another consequence of persistent occlusion of the cystic duct is the development of hydrops of the gallbladder. This is a relatively painless condition, possibly because there is slow distension of the gallbladder from the continuous secretion of mucus. If the material in the obstructed gallbladder becomes infected and purulent, an *empyema* of the gallbladder develops. Calcium may be secreted into the lumen of the hydropic gallbladder, causing 'limey' bile; if calcium salts accumulate in the wall of the gallbladder it is known as a porcelain gallbladder.

Choledocholithiasis

About 10–20% of patients with gallstones in the gallbladder also have choledocholithiasis (see p. 1412). Usually the passage of a stone into the common bile duct is associated with biliary colic because the duct is suddenly obstructed and distends acutely. However, if duct occlusion by the calculus is only partial and there is gradual distension no pain may be experienced; this occurs in 25% of patients with common bile duct stones. The stone(s) may remain free in the common bile duct, impact, disimpact, re-impact or pass and the degree of obstruction will be variable.

If the obstruction to the bile duct is complete, extrahepatic obstructive jaundice or cholestasis develops. How rapidly the jaundice becomes clinically manifest will depend on whether or not the cystic duct is patent. If it is, the gallbladder can store the bile secreted by the liver in the early stages. In these circumstances the jaundice may not appear obvious for 48 hours. Conversely patients with choledocholithiasis who develop complete bile obstruction and have either a non-functioning gallbladder or a previous cholecystectomy may become jaundiced in less than 24 hours, and this is particularly so if the obstruction is complicated by cholangitis. Cholangitis is readily diagnosed in the presence of fever, rigors, right-sided abdominal pains and obstructive jaundice with pale stools and dark urine. What is less widely appreciated is that in some patients with a very dilated bile duct and only partial bile duct obstruction, cholangitis may be a subacute illness with the symptoms of malaise, weakness, shivering, anorexia, general lack of energy and a complete absence of jaundice, pruritus or abdominal pain. Frequently, such patients have a very high serum alkaline phosphatase level in the absence of raised bilirubin. The complications of cholangitis especially the more serious suppurative form include septic shock and hepatic abscess. There are two further complications of choledocholithiasis: acute pancreatitis, which is relatively common, and secondary biliary cirrhosis, which is rare.

Fistulas

Recurrent bouts of acute cholecystitis usually lead to adhesions between the gallbladder and the duodenum, colon, or stomach and provide the basis for the location of a subsequent biliary fistula. These fistulous tracts tend to heal after the gallstones have passed – in 85% of patients this is per rectum. If, however, the stone is over 2.5 cm in diameter it usually impacts in the terminal ileum or very occasionally in the duodenum or sigmoid colon, particularly if there is gross diverticular disease, causing intestinal obstruction – 'gallstone ileus'. The types of biliary fistula which may occur secondary to cholelithiasis are shown in Figure 19.34.

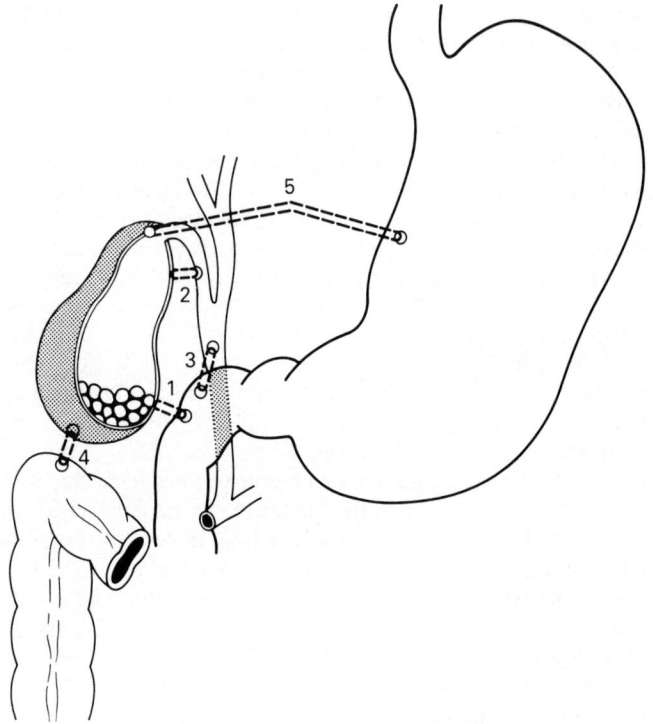

Fig. 19.34 Types of biliary fistulas secondary to cholelithiasis. 1: cholecystoduodenal (70%); 2: cholecystocholedochal (rare); 3: choledochoduodenal (rare); 4: cholecystocolic (14%); 5: cholecystogastric (6%); 6: biliary cutaneous fistula (rare). Fistulas may also occur from the gallbladder to the bronchial tree, pericardium, hepatic artery, portal vein, ovary, renal pelvis, vagina, bladder or uterus. These are uncommon, however. From G. D. Bell (1978) *Medicine*, 3rd series, p. 896, with kind permission of the editor.

Cancer

Carcinoma of the bladder is an infrequent complication of cholelithiasis occurring in less than 0.5% of patients but over 95% of all cases of this tumour occur in patients with gallstones. The patients affected are usually those whose gallstones have been associated with long-standing chronic cholecystitis.

MEDICAL TREATMENT

The two main drugs currently available with proven efficacy for dissolving gallstones are the bile acids chenodeoxycholic acid (CDCA – 3α, 7α-dihydroxycholanoic acid) and its 7β epimer ursodeoxycholic acid (UDCA). It is essential that patients are selected correctly for medical dissolution. Patients whose gallstones are radiopaque or who have stones in a gallbladder which is non-functioning following cystic duct obstruction should not be managed medically. Furthermore even if the gallbladder shows radiological function and the gallstones are radiotranslucent there is still a one in five chance that the stones will be of the non-cholesterol variety and consequently fail to respond to bile acid therapy. Both CDCA and UDCA desaturate the bile of cholesterol gallstone patients but the exact mechanism of action (if indeed it is the same for the two

drugs) is controversial. Although both drugs lower the hepatic levels of β-hydroxy-β-methylglutaryl CoA reductase (HMGCoA reductase), the rate-limiting enzyme for cholesterogenesis, this mechanism may well not be the major mode of action. Other mechanisms include a reduction in the cholesterol absorption from the gut, and an acute effect to limit the amount of cholesterol leaving the hepatocyte. The fact that in man both CDCA and UDCA but not cholic acid reduce the output of cholesterol into bile relative to bile salts and phospholipids, and therefore desaturate bile, possibly reflects the varying ability of the bile acids to solubilize lipid from the canalicular membrane of the hepatocyte.

Small gallstones, especially those which float, often dissolve in less than six months, but larger stones (up to 1.5 cm) frequently take one to two years to disappear. Stones in excess of 1.5 cm take so long to dissolve that many authorities believe that such patients should not be offered dissolution therapy. Because of the time taken to dissolve gallstones medically, only those patients with relatively mild or infrequent symptoms should normally be offered medical treatment. Obese patients tend to have high pretreatment hepatic HMGCoA reductase levels; they also secrete excessive amounts of cholesterol into their bile and consequently it is difficult to desaturate the bile of such patients with either CDCA or UDCA. The success rate of gallstone dissolution in obesity is poor.

After excluding (a) obese patients, (b) patients with stones in excess of 1.5 cm diameter, (c) those unable to tolerate optimum doses, (d) those whose bile fails to desaturate and (e) those who fail to complete one year of treatment, a success rate defined as complete gallstone dissolution with either CDCA or UDCA is reported to be about 65%. Such figures however do not reflect the overall experience with treating unselected patients where the results indicate that the success rate for CDCA is about 20–30% complete dissolution at two years.[13] Double-blind studies comparing the efficacy of CDCA with the newer drug UDCA suggest that the dissolution rates are similar. The optimum dose of CDCA is about 10–15 mg·kg body weight^{-1}·day^{-1}, whereas that of UDCA is about 8–10 mg·kg body weight^{-1}·day^{-1}.

CDCA and UDCA are equally, or possibly more, effective if the whole or majority of the dose is given at night before going to bed. The combination of a night time dose of CDCA with a low-cholesterol diet gives better results than if the drug is taken in three equally divided doses combined with a normal diet. Curiously the efficacy of UDCA does not seem to be increased by giving it with a low cholesterol diet.

Diarrhoea and hypertransaminasaemia occur as a dose-related side effect in approximately 30% of patients treated with CDCA.[13] The diarrhoea can often be prevented by gradually building up the dose of CDCA over 2–3 weeks and frequently improves when the patient has remained on the drug for more than a month. Diarrhoea does not occur with UDCA so patients who develop troublesome symptoms on CDCA should be switched to the alternative drug. Until recently it was believed that the reason why patients taking CDCA, but not UDCA, developed raised serum transaminase levels was because of bacterial conversion in the gut of CDCA into lithocholic acid, a known hepatotoxin in many animal species. This idea is unlikely to be the complete answer because it has been shown that lithocholate can be formed equally rapidly from UDCA and CDCA.[2] Man has the capacity to sulphate lithocholic acid thereby rendering it less toxic and more readily excretable in the stool. Prolonged ingestion of CDCA does not cause any serious histological damage in the liver or gut.[5] Many gastroenterologists use CDCA in preference to UDCA for most patients because it has been used more extensively and more is known about the drug, but it is probable that UDCA will become widely prescribed. Comprehensive reviews of both CDCA[7] and UDCA[1] discuss these and other topics in detail.

A side effect which occurs in about 10% of patients taking UDCA is the formation of a calcified rim around previously radiotranslucent stones. It is generally held that the formation of a calcified coating around a cholesterol gallstone effectively precludes its subsequent dissolution, but there are also isolated reports of stones continuing to reduce in size with UDCA therapy despite the presence of calcification.

The other agent available in Great Britain for dissolving gallstones is the plant monoterpene mixture, Rowachol. The major constituent, menthol, is known to inhibit the synthesis of hepatic HMGCoA reductase.[3] Our own experience in Nottingham[4] suggests Rowachol is best used in combination with CDCA in a dose of two to three capsules daily, which is equivalent to 10–15 drops of the liquid Rowachol formulation.

There are no sound data to support any specific diet in the treatment of gallstones or cholecystitis. None the less, it is traditional practice to recommend a low-fat, low-energy diet with, in recent years, an emphasis on a high fibre content.

Common bile duct stones can be dissolved, fragmented or flushed from the bile duct by a variety of substances. Most experience has been with mono-octanoin[8] and heparinized saline which are instilled directly into the duct via either a T-tube or an endoscopically placed naso-biliary catheter or via a catheter inserted at the time of percutaneous transhepatic cholangiography. Mono-octanoin is currently the agent of choice.

The success rate for dissolving common bile duct stones with orally administered drugs such as chenodeoxycholic acid and ursodeoxycholic acid has varied from 10% to 65%. Many clinicians will not use oral agents to dissolve common bile duct stones because of the high incidence of complications arising from the retention of the stones; other authorities do treat selected patients, generally the elderly, with oral cholelitholytics. The patients, their relatives, and general practitioners are made aware of the risks of dissolution therapy, and are given instructions to contact their medical attendant so that prompt hospital admission can be given should complications develop. The success rate for complete stone dissolution in a series of 30 patients which we have treated is 53%; 17% have required surgery while 20% have undergone endoscopic papillotomy.

Gallstone recurrence after stopping bile acid treatment

Usually a patient embarking on a course of CDCA or UDCA will have a pretreatment oral cholecystogram (OCG) and a repeat OCG at 6–9 month intervals until the gallstones are no longer visible. The policy in most centres is to maintain the patient on full dose therapy for a further three months and then repeat the OCG. Only if the second OCG is negative as well is the treatment stopped. Our policy is to confirm by ultrasonography with a real time sector scanner attachment that complete dissolution really has taken place.[14]

The bile of patients with cholesterol gallstones is supersaturated with cholesterol before treatment, but during therapy with CDCA and UDCA the bile becomes unsaturated; on withdrawing treatment the bile reverts to its supersaturated state in one to three weeks. Ruppin and Dowling[11] reported 46 patients whose gallstones had been dissolved with one course of treatment and who underwent follow-up X-rays. The overall recurrence rate was 54% and a similar figure was obtained when the results of patients with recurrent stones dissolved by a second course of medical treatment were included: 30 recurrences from the 60 occasions when complete gallstone dissolution was recorded. Post-dissolution maintenance trials are in progress to determine whether low dose night time UDCA or bran supplements will reduce the incidence of gallstone recurrence.

REFERENCES

1   Bachrach, W. R. & Hofmann, A. F. (1982) Ursodeoxycholic acid in the treatment of cholesterol cholelithiasis. *Digestive Diseases and Sciences*, **27**, 737–761 (Part I), 833–856 (Part II).
2   Bazzoli, F., Fromm, H., Sarua, R. P. *et al.* (1982) Comparative formation of lithocholic acid from chenodeoxycholic acid and ursodeoxycholic acids in the colon. *Gastroenterology*, **83**, 753–760.
3   Clegg, R. J., Middleton, B., Bell, G. D. & White, D. A. (1982) The mechanism of cyclic monoterpene inhibition of hepatic-3-hydroxy-3-methylglutaryl Coenzyme A Reductase in vivo in the rat. *Journal of Biological Chemistry*, **257**, 2294–2299.
4   Ellis, W. R., Bell, G. D., Middleton, B. & White, D. A. (1981) Adjunct to bile acid treatment for gallstone dissolution: low dose chenodeoxycholic acid combined with a terpene preparation. *British Medical Journal*, **282**, 611.
5   Fisher, R. L., Anderson, D. W., Boyer, J. L. *et al.* (1982) A prospective morphologic evaluation of hepatic toxicity of Chenodeoxycholic acid in patients with cholelithiasis: the National Co-operative Gallstone Study. *Hepatology*, **2**, 187–201.
6   Gracie, W. A. & Ransohoff, D. F. (1982) The natural history of silent gallstones: the innocent gallstone is not a myth. *New England Journal of Medicine*, **307**, 798–800.
7   Iser, J. H. & Sali, A. (1981) Chenodeoxycholic acid. A review of its pharmacological properties and therapeutic use. *Drugs*, **21**, 90–119.
8   Jarrett, L. N., Balfour, T. W., Bell, G. D., Knapp, D. R. & Rose D. H. (1981) Intraductal infusion of monooctanoin. Experience in 24 patients with retained common duct stones. *Lancet*, **i**, 68–70.
9   Langman, M. J. S. (1979) Gallstones. In *The Epidemiology of Chronic Digestive Disease*, pp. 114–128. London: Edward Arnold.
10 Royal College of General Practitioners' Oral Contraceptive Study (1982) Oral contraceptives and gallbladder disease. *Lancet*, **ii**, 957–959.
11 Ruppin, D. C. & Dowling, R. H. (1982) Is recurrence inevitable after gallstone dissolution by bile acid treatment? *Lancet*, **i**, 181–195.
12 Schoenfield, L. J. (1977) *Diseases of the Gallbladder and Biliary System*. New York: John Wiley.
13 Schoenfield, L. J. & Lachin, J. M. (1981) Chenodiol (Chenodeoxycholic acid) for dissolution of gallstones: the National Co-operative Gallstone Study. *Annals of Internal Medicine*, **95**, 257–281.
14 Somerville, K. W., Rose, D. H., Bell, G. D., Ellis, W. R. & Knapp, D. R. (1982) Gallstone dissolution and recurrence: are we being misled? *British Medical Journal*, **284**, 1295–1297.
15 Thornton, J. R., Heaton, K. W. & Macfarlane, D. G. (1981) A relation between high density lipoprotein cholesterol and bile cholesterol saturation. *British Medical Journal*, **283**, 1352–1354.

CHOLECYSTITIS AND CHOLEDOCHOLITHIASIS

The presence of gallstones usually leads to inflammation of the wall of the gallbladder or bile ducts. Less frequently, the stones enter the cystic duct or common bile duct and may partially or completely obstruct the flow of bile. These events are usually expressed clinically as recurrent biliary pain, acute cholecystitis or obstructive (cholestatic) jaundice.

ACUTE CHOLECYSTITIS

Acute cholecystitis is a common admission diagnosis in patients admitted to the surgical wards of developed countries. It usually occurs in the presence of gallstones but may also occur rarely in the absence of any pre-existing gallbladder disease.

Acute calculous cholecystitis

AETIOLOGY

Acute cholecystitis almost always occurs as a result of obstruction of the cystic duct or Hartmann's pouch by a gallstone. The inflammation often develops in the absence of bacteria because cultures from the gallbladder lumen or wall are sterile in up to 50% of patients. Non-bacterial sources of inflammation may be prostaglandins released from cells in the gallbladder wall or lysolecithin which is produced from biliary lecithin by the action of lysosomal enzymes derived from either damaged epithelial cells or bacteria.

PATHOLOGY

The gallbladder wall is tense, oedematous and inflamed, the process often extending to surrounding structures such as the free edge of the lesser omentum, the duodenum, the hepatic flexure of the colon and the greater omentum. This acute inflammatory process may be superimposed on a chronically thickened and fibrotic gallbladder wall, a legacy of previous inflammatory attacks.

In 90–95% of patients, the inflammation subsides spontaneously but in a few it progresses to empyema of the gallbladder, gangrene of the wall or free perforation of the gallbladder. A local abscess (pericholecystic or subphrenic) may occur, the natural history of which is to discharge into the gut, the pleural cavity or a bronchus, or rarely to present on the anterior abdominal wall.

CLINICAL FEATURES

The patient has severe upper abdominal pain, which is usually felt in the epigastrium or in the right upper quadrant. The pain often radiates to the back, particularly to the right scapular area. Nausea, anorexia and occasional vomiting also occur. The physical findings include low-grade fever, tachycardia and a variable degree of tenderness and guarding or rigidity over the site of the inflamed gallbladder. Careful palpation may reveal a tender mass under the right costal margin.

The physical signs may resolve over a period of days, or less commonly may progress with increasing tenderness and enlargement of the gallbladder mass. Mild jaundice may develop but rarely progresses unless there is an associated calculous obstruction of the common bile duct.

INVESTIGATIONS

There are many acute abdominal conditions which may mimic acute cholecystitis – for example, hepatitis, peptic ulcer, pancreatitis and pyelonephritis. It is therefore mandatory to confirm the diagnosis, particularly if an early operation is contemplated. All patients require a full blood examination, liver function tests, serum amylase estimation and microscopy of the urine. Demonstration of cystic duct obstruction will confirm the diagnosis; currently, the best investigation to confirm this is biliary scintigraphy. In a modern hospital, oral cholecystography or intravenous cholangiography have no place in investigating acute cholecystitis as the sensitivity of these examinations is much less than radionuclide scanning. Ultrasound examination will demonstrate gallstones but cannot demonstrate whether the gallbladder is obstructed. Enlargement of the gallbladder or thickening of the wall on ultrasound are unreliable signs of acute cholecystitis. However, it has been claimed that the finding of gallstones by ultrasound and confirmation that the site of maximum tenderness is over the gallbladder is a reliable method of reaching the diagnosis.

TREATMENT

Antibiotics (a cephalosporin or an aminoglycoside) are usually prescribed although they are unnecessary if the disease is mild. The patient's fluid requirements are given intravenously.

Following confirmation of the diagnosis by cholescintigraphy or other means, the following plan of management is recommended:

1 Immediate cholecystectomy if a tender, enlarging gallbladder mass is present or the patient fails to improve on conservative treatment.

2 Planned early cholecystectomy within two to three days even if the clinical signs of inflammation have subsided.

As an alternative, for those patients whose disease settles on conservative treatment, the operation can be delayed for several weeks or months. This is probably a safe option but requires a further hospital admission and an increased total hospital stay. There is also a risk that a further attack will occur before the patient is readmitted for cholecystectomy.

Acute acalculous cholecystitis

This condition is uncommon because more than 95% of patients with acute cholecystitis have stones in the gallbladder.

AETIOLOGY

Acute acalculous cholecystitis may occur in a wide variety of clinical circumstances. It may be precipitated by abdominal and extra-abdominal operations, bacteraemia, trauma, fractures, pancreatitis, burns and other serious illnesses. The disease also has an association with diabetes mellitus and may develop in children with congenital biliary anomalies or following infectious diseases. A particular form of the disease occurs in fasting patients undergoing parenteral nutrition, usually in the setting of an intensive care ward.

PATHOLOGY

There is a spectrum of pathological changes in the gallbladder ranging from mild acute inflammation and oedema to gangrene and perforation. The cause of acalculous cholecystitis is unknown but is almost certainly multifactorial. Stasis of the gallbladder may occur in the fasting patient from lack of cholecystokinin release. Chemical changes in bile constituents such as lecithin or bile salts may initiate inflammation and oedema leading to blockage of the cystic duct; bacterial infection may then occur. Hypoxia and hypovolaemia following a serious illness may cause further damage to the gallbladder, leading to gangrene and perforation.

CLINICAL FEATURES

The symptoms and signs are similar to those of acute calculous cholecystitis, but the setting of the illness, particularly in very ill patients, may make early diagnosis very difficult. The diagnosis should be suspected in any sick patient who develops pain, tenderness or a mass in the right upper quadrant. There are no specific investigations which are useful and decisions about diagnosis and treatment must be determined on clinical grounds alone, bearing in mind that early gangrene and perforation may occur.

TREATMENT

The frequency of gangrene and perforation make surgical treatment mandatory. Cholecystectomy is the treatment of choice but, rarely, the local conditions or the general state of the patient may justify cholecystostomy.

CHRONIC CHOLECYSTITIS

Chronic inflammation of the gallbladder is almost exclusively associated with the presence of gallstones. Other less common forms of chronic cholecystitis are described later in this chapter (p. 1473).

Chronic calculous cholecystitis

This is the commonest form of gallbladder disease although there is little correlation between the severity of the pathological changes in the gallbladder and the form of clinical presentation.

AETIOLOGY

It is not at all clear whether gallstones have to be present before chronic inflammation occurs in the gallbladder wall. Indeed, minor degrees of obstruction at the cystic duct or at the sphincter of Oddi or the presence of bile supersaturated with cholesterol in the gallbladder lumen may induce changes in mucus production and nucleation of cholesterol microliths before inflammatory changes occur in the gallbladder wall. The presence of gallstones may then induce cholecystitis, obstruction of the cystic duct and/or secondary bacterial invasion of the gallbladder.

PATHOLOGY

The earliest changes of chronic cholecystitis are seen in the mucosa where epithelial cells show excessive secretory activity. As the disease progresses, outpouching of the mucosa between muscle bundles is seen. These intramural pouches, termed Rokitansky Aschoff sinuses, may sometimes contain tiny flecks of black pigment.

The characteristic changes in the gallbladder wall are a chronic inflammatory cellular infiltrate and fibrosis. Generally, these changes are of greater severity with increasing size and number of gallbladder stones.

Acute complications of chronic calculous cholecystitis may follow obstruction of the cystic duct by a stone. This event may lead to accumulation of mucus in the gallbladder lumen (a mucocoele) or pus may accumulate in the gallbladder lumen if secondary bacterial infection ensues (an empyema). The gallbladder wall may also become acutely inflamed (acute on chronic cholecystitis) or gangrenous (gangrenous cholecystitis).

In the presence of large gallstones and cystic duct obstruction, an intramural abscess may penetrate into an adjacent viscus leading to a fistula (cholecysto-duodenal or cholecystocolic fistula). Rarely, the abscess may point through the anterior abdominal wall (cholecysto-cutaneous fistula). A large gallstone may pass via a cholecysto-duodenal fistula into the gut and lodge in the terminal ileum producing intestinal obstruction (gallstone ileus). There is also an association between gallstones, chronic cholecystitis and cancer of the gallbladder (see p. 1459).

CLINICAL FEATURES

Many patients with chronic calculous cholecystitis have no symptoms for many years; indeed, it is not rare to find a fibrotic gallbladder containing stones at autopsy in a patient who has had few if any symptoms of biliary disease. The events leading to clinical symptoms are not known and, except in acute or complicated disease, there is little correlation between the severity of clinical symptoms and the pathological changes in the biliary tract.

Recurrent attacks of upper abdominal pain are the typical and common clinical presentation of chronic calculous cholecystitis. A typical attack occurs at night, sometimes after a heavy meal. The onset is rapid rather than sudden, being severe and usually constant rather than colicky (the term biliary colic is usually a misnomer). The site is epigastric or under the right costal margin and the pain commonly radiates to the right scapular area. Biliary pain may also be felt substernally or, uncommonly, under the left costal margin.

Untreated, the pain lasts for 1–6 h, relief occurring gradually. Nausea and vomiting may accompany the pain but vomiting provides no relief. The patient moves around the bed frequently because of the severity of the pain. Fever and jaundice are not usually present.

Examination of the abdomen usually reveals mild tenderness in the upper abdomen which is as common in the epigastrium as over the gallbladder. The gallbladder is rarely palpable unless the cystic duct is obstructed and a mucocoele has developed.

Murphy's sign was originally described to indicate the presence of chronic calculous cholecystitis. This sign is present when pressure by the examining hand under the right costal margin produces discomfort at the height of inspiration when the patient is asked to take a deep breath. Often, the finding of tenderness under the right costal margin before deep inspiration is interpreted mistakenly as a positive Murphy's sign by clinicians when examining a patient with suspected gallstone disease. Murphy's sign has no place in any description of physical findings. Its interpretation is confusing and it is certainly not specific for gallbladder disease, often being positive in patients in whom the disease is absent.

TREATMENT

Pain relief
The patient is treated with a parenteral analgesic such as pethidine, one or two injections usually being sufficient. An anti-emetic agent such as prochlorperazine maleate or metoclopramide may be given to control nausea. Reports have also indicated that the inhibitor of prostaglandin synthesis, indomethacin, is effective in relieving biliary pain. Intravenous fluids are not usually necessary as fluids can be taken as soon as the attack subsides.

Confirmation of the diagnosis
There are many causes of acute upper abdominal pain so a clinical diagnosis of chronic calculous cholecystitis must be confirmed by investigation. The investigations commonly used to demonstrate gallstones are ultrasound and oral cholecystography. These investigations are not mutually exclusive and both should be performed if one is negative when there is a strong clinical suspicion of gallstones. Rarely, ERCP or microscopic examination of gallbladder bile obtained by duodenal intubation may be used if other investigations fail to show stones and the patient continues to have troublesome biliary type symptoms.

Treatment
The treatment options in a patient with gallstones are either surgical (cholecystectomy) or conservative (no further treatment or dissolution of stones by orally administered bile salts). Cholecystectomy should be advised for all patients with severe symptoms, especially if attacks occur at regular intervals. Surgery is also strongly advised if the gallbladder fails to opacify on cholecystography or cholescintigraphy because complications such as acute cholecystitis or empyema are very common when the cystic duct is obstructed.

It would be an advantage to know the natural history of gallstones in making decisions about patients with few or no symptoms, but this has not been clearly defined. However, the following observations are relevant to this decision:

1   Gallstones have a low clinical 'penetrance' as indicated by X-ray studies on asymptomatic people and the frequency of apparently 'silent' gallstones in patients at autopsy.

2   No more than 50% of patients known to have gallstones and presenting with biliary pain are likely to suffer a further attack of pain or biliary complication within the ensuing 10 years. Patients with an obstructed neck of the gallbladder (non-opacification on oral cholecystogram or cholescintigraphy) are at higher risk from acute disease, particularly acute cholecystitis.

3   Gallbladder cancer usually occurs in the presence of gallstones. The annual risk of cancer of the gallbladder in white females (the group with the highest prevalence of gallstones) has been estimated at 2.1 per 100 000 persons. The mortality of elective cholecystectomy in patients aged less than 50 years is 0.1–0.2% in good circumstances. The morbidity is also extremely low and in countries with a good standard of surgical training damage to bile ducts is extremely uncommon. The mortality and morbidity of surgery increases with age-related diseases and particularly in the presence of biliary complications, such as obstructive jaundice and cholangitis.

It is reasonable therefore to advise cholecystectomy to all patients with symptoms, except those with severe cardiac or respiratory disease or other conditions rendering surgery unsafe.

Asymptomatic patients, 'silent gallstones', with a long life expectancy may be wise to have surgery when young and fit because the morbidity and mortality of biliary disease and biliary surgery increases with age, the stones become larger and the pathological changes in the gallbladder become more severe. One argument used for advising cholecystectomy in asymptomatic patients is the risk of gallbladder cancer, but the low prevalence of this disease does not justify either population screening or a prophylactic cholecystectomy. Several series of patients with 'silent' gallstones have been studied and the number of patients who eventually require a cholecystectomy or who develop serious complications as a result of an expectant policy is small. The management of the 'silent' gallstone is controversial. Perhaps all 'silent' stones should be left alone. On the one hand there is the view that they should be removed in younger patients while older patients should be managed by medical dissolution if possible; on the other hand arguments have been put forward to treat younger patients conservatively and older patients by cholecystectomy.

Dissolution of stones by oral chenodeoxycholic acid or ursodeoxycholic acid has a limited place in treatment because less than one in ten patients presenting to hospital has conditions and stones suitable for this form of treatment (see p. 1406).

COMPLICATIONS OF CHRONIC CALCULOUS CHOLECYSTITIS

The following complications may occur as a result of gallbladder stones: acute cholecystitis, choledocholithiasis, acute pancreatitis, biliary enteric fistula and gallstone ileus.

Chronic acalculous cholecystitis (syn hyperplastic cholecystoses)

The commonest pathological forms of these conditions are adenomyosis of the gallbladder, cholesterolosis of the gallbladder and calcified (porcelain) gallbladder. These conditions are commonly associated with gallstones but may occur in their absence (see pages 1429 and 1472).

CHOLEDOCHOLITHIASIS

Stones are found in the common bile duct in 10–15% of patients with gallbladder stones. More than 80% of common duct stones are similar in appearance and chemical composition to those in the gallbladder, presumably due to migration of gallbladder stones along the cystic duct. These are termed *secondary bile duct stones* and are composed principally of cholesterol (80%) or black pigment (20%). *Primary bile duct stones* are red–brown in colour, soft in consistency and composed principally of calcium bilirubinate. This material may also be found in the bile duct as biliary mud. These primary duct stones may occur in the bile duct when either cholesterol stones or pigment stones are present in the gallbladder. Characteristically, however, they are found in the bile duct months or years after cholecystectomy and are believed to occur as a result of sphincter of Oddi dysfunction, usually associated with secondary bacterial infection in the bile duct.

Primary bile duct stones may also occur as a result of the following: biliary strictures; parasitic infestation – *Clonorchis sinensis, Ascaris lumbricoides* or *Fasciola hepatica*; foreign bodies

– non-absorbable suture material or metallic clips placed on the cystic duct or used to close the common bile duct during previous biliary surgery may migrate into the common duct lumen and form the nidus of a gallstone.

CLINICAL MANIFESTATIONS OF CHOLEDOCHOLITHIASIS

The natural history of stones in the common bile duct is unknown. What is clear is that their presence is commonly associated with partial or complete bile duct obstruction which may be complicated by secondary bacterial infection (cholangitis) or infection in the blood stream (septicaemia). Prolonged partial obstruction and cholangitis may ultimately lead to biliary cirrhosis of the liver with manifestations of chronic liver failure and portal hypertension.

Stones in the common bile duct therefore present clinically in one of the following ways: recurrent upper abdominal pain with or without jaundice; obstructive (cholestatic) jaundice; cholangitis ± septicaemia and liver abscesses; symptoms and signs of chronic liver failure; recurrent pyrexia.

The upper abdominal pain associated with common duct stones is indistinguishable from that of stones in the gallbladder. Obstructive jaundice is associated with pruritus, dark urine and clay-coloured stools. Within 48 hours of the beginning of obstruction, the lack of bile in the gut leads to a prolongation of the prothrombin time due to diminished absorption of vitamin K from the small intestine.

Physical examination usually provides no clue to the diagnosis. The gallbladder is not usually palpable in patients with extrahepatic obstructive jaundice due to gallstones, because it is unable to distend following fibrosis in the wall secondary to chronic inflammation. The gallbladder is usually palpable if a mucocoele is present, but this is uncommon.

MANAGEMENT OF CHOLEDOCHOLITHIASIS

Diagnosis

The most common method for diagnosing common bile duct stones is by operative cholangiography at the time of biliary surgery. In patients with gallbladder stones and biochemical signs suggestive of a stone in the common bile duct, it is often unnecessary to confirm the latter diagnosis prior to surgery as the intraoperative investigations will do this. It is generally accepted that either an operative cholangiogram via the cystic duct or choledochoscopy should be performed in all patients with gallstones in the gallbladder or bile ducts. However, in patients who have had a previous cholecystectomy, preoperative confirmation of choledocholithiasis is essential. It is recommended that an ultrasound be performed first in order to assess the calibre of the bile ducts. However, ultrasonography has a very low sensitivity for diagnosing stones in the common bile duct, and a contrast study is preferable either by ERCP or percutaneous transhepatic cholangiography.

Treatment

There is little or no place for conservative treatment in this disease and the stones must be removed surgically, either by an abdominal operation or via endoscopic sphincterotomy.

Complications of choledocholithiasis

CHOLANGITIS

The clinical manifestations of cholangitis are jaundice, high swinging fever and extreme toxicity, probably due to septicaemia and endotoxaemia. The bile ducts may become distended with pus (suppurative cholangitis). This condition is highly dangerous and without appropriate intervention the patient may die of septic shock, liver abscess, or liver and renal failure.

The treatment of cholangitis must include the following:

Antibiotics. Broad spectrum antibiotic treatment against aerobic and anaerobic organisms is used. Intravenous ampicillin, gentamicin and metronidazole is an appropriate combination of drugs. Blood cultures are taken before antibiotics are administered.

Intravenous fluids. These are necessary while repeated measurements of blood pressure, pulse, central venous pressure and urinary output are obtained.

Biliary drainage. The method by which the drainage of the bile ducts is achieved is controversial, but either endoscopic sphincterotomy or percutaneous transhepatic drainage of the common duct should be attempted. These techniques, especially endoscopic sphincterotomy, have now replaced surgical drainage at laparotomy as the best immediate form of biliary decompression. Endoscopic drainage can be performed immediately after the diagnosis has been confirmed by ERCP.

Surgery. Ultimately, duct stones must be removed and this may have been achieved by endoscopic sphincterotomy. In patients who have had a previous cholecystectomy this may be the only treatment necessary. Furthermore, if the patient is elderly or unfit, clearing of the common bile duct may be sufficient treatment, even if gallbladder stones are present. Elective cholecystectomy together with exploration of the common bile duct is performed in all other patients when the patient has fully recovered from the cholangitis.

OBSTRUCTIVE JAUNDICE

The clinical features of cholestatic jaundice due to stones often include biliary type pain associated with increasing jaundice on a background of recurrent episodes of biliary pain over a number of years. Occasionally, and especially in elderly patients, the jaundice may be painless and a clinical diagnosis of extrahepatic obstructive jaundice due to neoplasm will be made.

The management of obstructive jaundice requires that the diagnosis be established by either ERCP or percutaneous transhepatic cholangiography. Treatment may take the form of an endoscopic sphincterotomy or transperitoneal exploration of the bile duct.

BILIARY ENTERIC FISTULAS CAUSED BY GALLSTONES

Fistulas from the biliary tract (usually the gallbladder) develop only in patients with advanced biliary disease, usually in the presence of large stones. Enteric fistulas usually occur between the gallbladder and the duodenum or common bile duct; less commonly, they involve the colon and the stomach. Fistulas to the renal tract and bronchial tree have been described. The clinical features of biliary intestinal fistulas are similar to those of chronic cholecystitis although recurrent jaundice and fever may occur if stones are present in the common bile duct. A plain radiograph of the biliary tract often demonstrates gas in the biliary tree, which is diagnostic of a biliary-enteric communication. A barium meal with the addition of effervescent tablets can delineate the fistula and the biliary tract with barium and gas.

Treatment
Symptoms usually demand that cholecystectomy be undertaken together with common duct exploration if stones are present in the bile duct. The fistulous communication to the gut is closed.

A biliary enteric fistula may be left untreated in aged or unfit patients if the stones have been discharged into the gut and there is free biliary drainage because the risks of a complicated biliary exploration may exceed those of the untreated biliary disease.

Gallstone ileus

A large gallstone which passes into the gut through a cholecyst-enteric fistula may impact in the narrowest part of the small intestine, the terminal ileum, 25–50 cm from the ileocaecal valve. Acute mechanical small intestinal obstruction occurs with characteristic clinical and radiological signs. The main radiological signs of gallstone ileus are the finding of gas in the biliary tree (indicating the biliary-enteric fistula) and a large radiopaque stone in the right lower abdomen in association with the multiple distended small bowel loops and fluid levels of low small bowel obstruction.

The patient with gallstone ileus is usually elderly and may have had recurrent attacks of upper abdominal pain; usually there have been no biliary symptoms. The diagnosis of gallstone ileus should always be entertained in aged patients presenting with small bowel obstruction, particularly if there are no external hernias or scars indicating a previous laparotomy.

The treatment is by surgery. The gallstone is removed through a small enterotomy, taking care to avoid contamination by intestinal contents. Peroperative antibiotic prophylaxis is employed. Although the source of the mischief is the gallbladder, it is inadvisable to deal with the biliary tract at this time. This should be attempted at a later operation in patients who are fit, (see under biliary-enteric fistula) whereas in the aged and infirm, it is unnecessary to deal with the biliary tract unless obstruction or cholangitis is present or occurs subsequently.

Very rarely, gallstones may impact at other sites in the intestine, particularly at sites of narrowing due to disease (e.g. sigmoid diverticulitis). Management of these patients follows similar principles to that outlined above.

RECURRENT PYOGENIC CHOLANGITIS (ASIATIC CHOLANGIOHEPATITIS)

This disease occurs in the Chinese population of Hong Kong, Korea and South East Asia. The primary lesion is believed to be the formation of calcium bilirubinate mud and stones in intrahepatic bile ducts, followed by secondary enteric bacterial infection. It is held that these patients have a protein-deficient diet and excrete less than normal amounts of the β-glucuronidase inhibitor glucuro-1,4-lactone. Beta-glucuronidase hydrolyses bilirubin glucuronide in bile, allowing bilirubin to combine with calcium to form insoluble calcium bilirubinate which precipitates in the bile. The accumulation of calcium bilirubinate promotes bile stasis, secondary infection, and recurrent cholangitis.

Patients present with recurrent attacks of upper abdominal pain and fever accompanied by varying degrees of extra- and intrahepatic obstructive jaundice. Radiological examination of the bile ducts demonstrates dilated intrahepatic ducts containing stones and biliary mud, the left hepatic ducts often being affected to a greater degree than the right. Intrahepatic and extrahepatic bile duct strictures occur in advanced disease with proximal duct dilatation and stone formation. The liver becomes scarred and atrophic and liver abscesses may develop. Unlike chronic cholecystitis, the primary pathology is in the bile ducts and the gallbladder is often free of disease although it may contain

stones and become distended and infected in association with bile duct obstruction. There may also be the complications of choledocho-enteric fistulas, pancreatitis and Gram-negative septicaemia.

The management of this condition is difficult but in principle is no different from other forms of bile duct disease associated with stones and obstruction. It consists of: treatment of cholangitis (see p. 1425); drainage of the biliary tract and extraction of stones, the site of drainage depending on the level of obstruction; and in badly affected patients partial hepatic resection of severely affected areas.

BACTERIA IN THE BILE IN GALLSTONE DISEASE

The normal biliary tract is sterile but is invaded and colonized by intestinal bacteria in the presence of stones or obstruction. In a study of 267 consecutive patients undergoing biliary surgery for gallstone disease in Adelaide, bacteria were cultured from the bile in 38% (Table 19.6).

Table 19.6 Bacteria recovered from bile[a] in 267 patients with gallstones.

Group	Gallbladder bile	Common duct bile
Gram-positive facultative bacteria		
Staphylococcus		
coagulase negative	22 (25%)	34 (40%)
S. aureus	2 (2%)	
Streptococcus		
S. viridans		
Enterococcus	10 (11%)	4 (5%)
Diphtheroids	3 (4%)	1 (1%)
Total	37 (42%)	40 (47%)
Gram-negative aerobic or facultative bacteria		
Aeromonas	2 (2%)	1 (1%)
Enterobacteriaceae		
E. coli	17 (19%)	18 (21%)
Enterobacter spp.	9 (10%)	4 (5%)
Klebsiella spp.	6 (7%)	6 (7%)
Proteus spp.	1 (1%)	3 (4%)
Salmonella spp.	1 (1%)	1 (1%)
Total	36 (40%)	33 (39%)
Anaerobic organisms		
Bacteroides		
B. fragilis	5 (6%)	4 (5%)
Other	4 (4%)	3 (4%)
Clostridium		
C. perfringens	2 (2%)	2 (3%)
Other	3 (4%)	2 (3%)
Anaerobic cocci	2 (2%)	1 (1%)
Total	16 (18%)	12 (14%)
Total isolates	89 (100%)	85 (100%)

[a] Percentages are of all species isolated; some patients had more than one species isolated.

Enterobacteriaceae were the most common of the enteric organisms and anaerobes were cultured in only 19% of positive bile cultures (7% of all patients). Staphylococci were rarely grown from bile.

Bacterbilia is found most frequently in patients with stones in the common bile duct, particularly if the duct is obstructed. There is also a high risk of bacterbilia in patients aged over 60 years (Table 19.7). Bacteraemia or septicaemia may occur during investigative manipulations or operations on patients whose biliary

Table 19.7 Conditions associated with an increased risk of bacterbilia in patients with gallstones.

Previous biliary surgery
Common duct obstruction due to stone
Stones in the common bile duct
Age greater than 60 years
Acute cholecystitis

disease is often associated with bacterbilia. Under these circumstances, it is prudent to administer a short course of a prophylactic antibiotic directed against the Enterobacteriaceae.

INVESTIGATION OF THE BILIARY TRACT

Abdominal X-ray

A plain abdominal X-ray should be obtained in all patients with suspected gallbladder disease.

Between 10% and 30% of all gallstones are radiopaque because of their calcium content, and over 80% of radiolucent stones contain more than 70% cholesterol. Occasionally, a hydrops or empyema of the gallbladder may be seen as a right upper quadrant mass, while limey bile and porcelain gallbladder are readily seen as calcified shadows in the right upper quadrant. Acute emphysematous cholecystitis which occurs more often in diabetics also has a classic radiological appearance of air limited to the gallbladder wall or lumen. Air in the biliary tree may be seen after choledochoduodenostomy or may occur spontaneously if a fistula has developed. A combination of air in the biliary tree and intestinal obstruction seen on a plain radiograph is virtually diagnostic of gallstone ileus.

Ultrasound

Ultrasonography has evolved to be one of the most useful methods of investigation of the biliary tract (Figure 19.35). Ultrasound examination requires skin contact with a sound transducer 1–2 cm in diameter with a mineral oil or water-soluble gel between the transducer and the skin to facilitate contact. Emitted sound waves are differentially absorbed and echoed by the intra-abdominal organs, which form characteristic images. Grey-scale ultrasonography produces sharp images, and the use of real time allows for accurate localization of the region to be examined. For optimal imaging, the part of

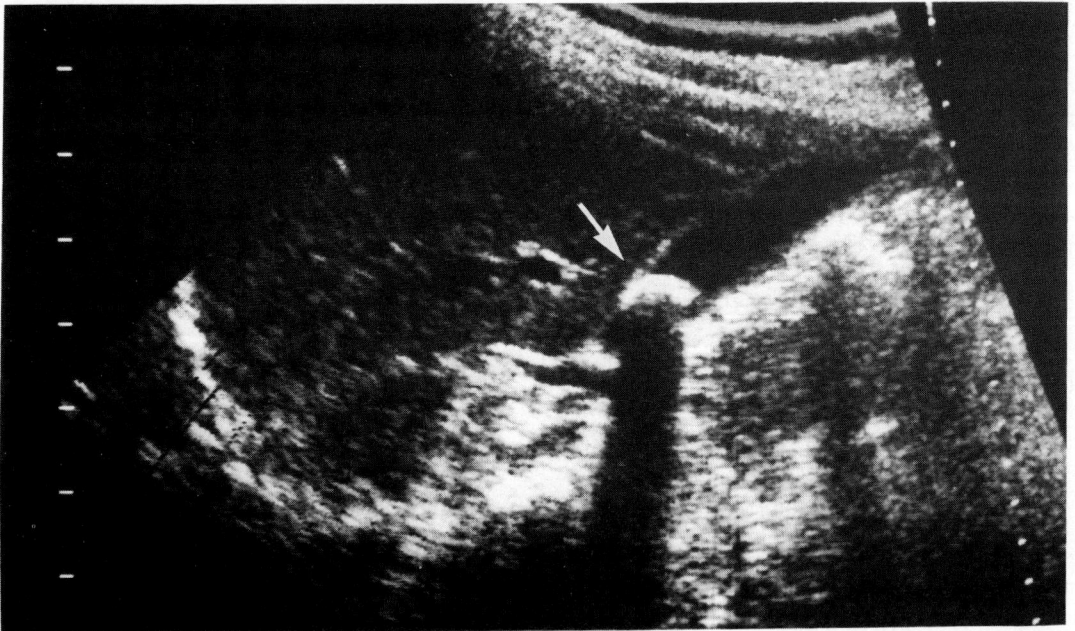

Fig. 19.35 Ultrasound of the gallbladder, showing a large calculus (arrow) in the fundus of the gallbladder casting a prominent acoustic shadow.

the anatomy to be studied must be investigated by the shortest and most direct route to the transducer. Therefore, factors such as bowel distended with gas, or thick adipose tissue interposed between the transducer and the structure, will interfere with good imaging. The obvious advantage of ultrasound over other imaging techniques is its safety. It is now the optimum first investigation in the diagnosis of gallstones, and its accuracy for stones in the gallbladder is at least equal to that of oral cholecystography. In addition, ultrasound examination will provide information about the liver parenchyma, the calibre of the intrahepatic ducts and common bile duct and the state of the pancreas.

Gallstones may still be seen when the gallbladder is radiologically non-functioning and an idea of gallbladder wall thickening and contractility can also be obtained. Stones which have been missed at oral cholecystography may be discovered by this technique and, unlike oral or intravenous cholangiography it provides information in patients with jaundice. If dilated intrahepatic ducts are demonstrated a percutaneous transhepatic cholangiography may be helpful in outlining the site and nature of the obstruction. However, jaundice produced by gallstones in the common bile duct is often intermittent because of a 'ball valve' effect, and the ultrasound may show the intrahepatic ducts to be of normal calibre. Another difficulty in the diagnosis of stones in the common bile duct is that the image is often obscured by gas in the colon or duodenum.

Biliary scintigraphy

The introduction of radionuclide techniques for imaging of the biliary tree has allowed investigation of the dynamics of the biliary tract. The first agent used in hepatobiliary scanning was ^{131}I-labelled rose bengal. However, this radionuclide did not gain wide acceptance because of its long half-life, its relatively high radiation dose to bowel mucosa, and its low counting statistics which provided a poor image of the biliary tree. Recently, a new series of [99]Tc^m-labelled radiopharmaceuticals has been developed which rapidly concentrate in the biliary tree and these agents provide a high counting rate, a short half-life, a relatively low dose of radiation to the patient and satisfactory imaging of the biliary tree and the gallbladder.

The radionuclide is injected intravenously as a sterile solution. It is rapidly cleared from the blood stream by the liver and excreted in bile while a small proportion of the radionuclide is excreted by the kidneys, although recently developed radiopharmaceuticals show only minimal renal excretion. The radionuclide in bile emits gamma radiation that is readily recorded by standard gamma cameras, and the image may be stored on magnetic tape for later playback to highlight areas of interest. In clinical application, the radionuclide is injected in fasting patients and views of the biliary tree are taken one hour after injection (Figure 19.36). If the gallbladder is not seen, further views are obtained at 2 hours and at 4 hours. Non-visualization of the gallbladder in the presence of a clinical picture consistent with acute cholecystitis is diagnostic of obstruction of the cystic duct provided hypertransaminasaemia is absent (Figure 19.37). The investigation is very accurate in the diagnosis of cystic duct obstruction even in the presence of mild jaundice (with a serum bilirubin up to 75 μmol/l).

These investigations may also give functional information about gallbladder emptying and the rate of bile clearance into the intestine.

Oral cholecystogram

Oral cholecystography was introduced by Graham and Cole in 1924.[12] Improved contrast agents have done much to increase the accuracy of the investigation. The currently used contrast medium is iopanoic acid, a lipid-soluble weak acid which is absorbed in the small intestine and colon, transported in the blood bound to albumin, and selectively taken up by the liver, conjugated and excreted into the bile as the glucuronide. The contrast material then enters the gallbladder where it is concentrated by the reabsorption of water from the bile. X-ray images of the gallbladder containing contrast are obtained 12–15 hours after oral ingestion of the contrast medium (Figure 19.38).

With visualization of the gallbladder, radiolucent stones may be diagnosed and the sensitivity approaches 95%. Non-visualization of the gallbladder has numerous causes including failure to ingest the agent, intestinal obstruction preventing passage through the small bowel, malabsorption of the contrast, liver dysfunction and biliary tract abnormalities preventing flow of contrast into the gallbladder. Oral cholecystography is most useful in the diagnosis of gallstones in patients presenting with recurrent biliary-type pain. It is of less use in the assessment of the acutely ill patient, where techniques such as biliary scintigraphy and ultrasonography have greater utility. It has no place in the assessment of the jaundiced patient.

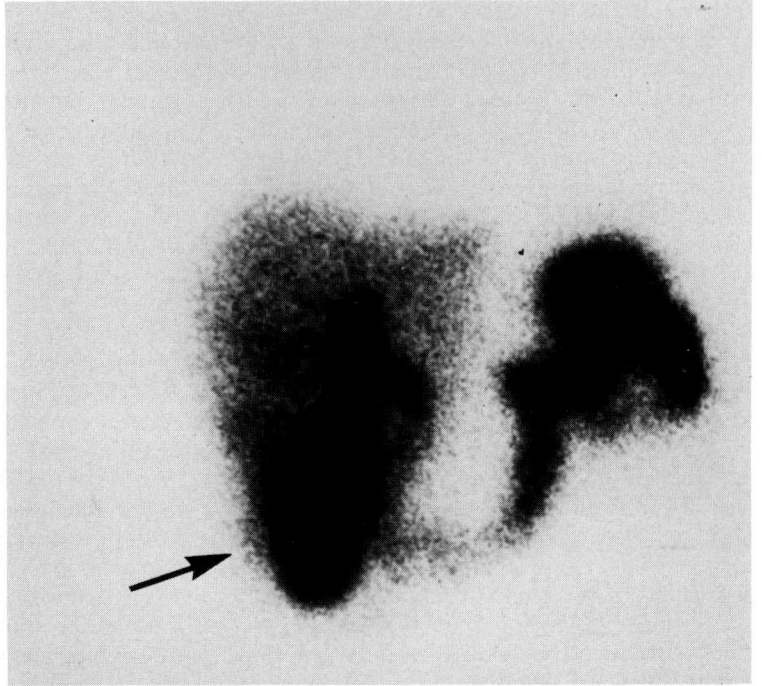

Fig. 19.36 DIDA scintigram in left anterior oblique position at one hour after injection of radionuclide, showing take-up of the radionuclide in a normal gallbladder (arrow).

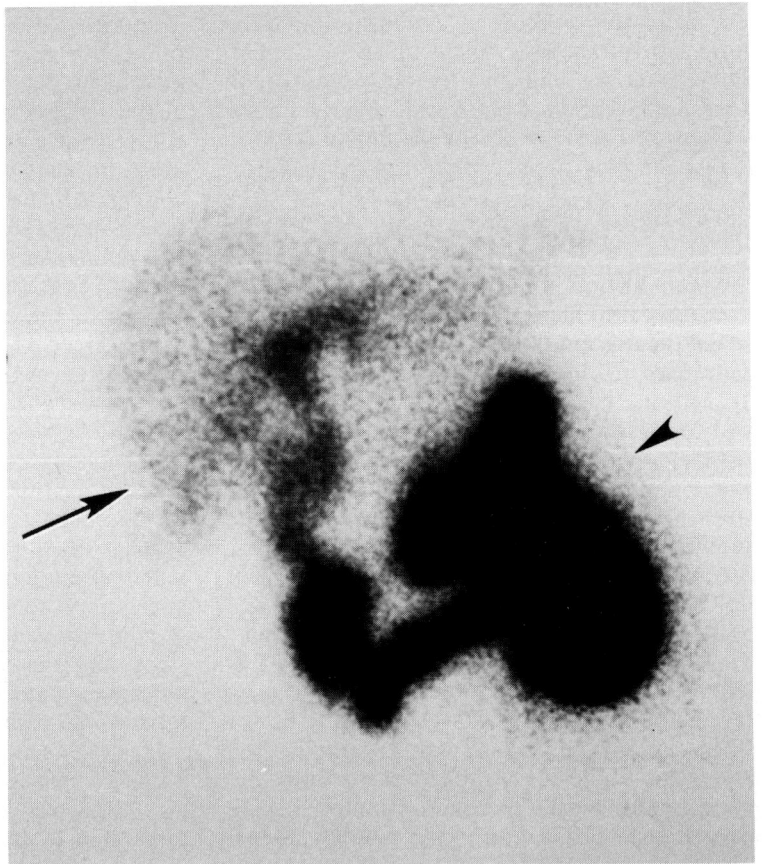

Fig. 19.37 DIDA scintigram in left anterior oblique position at one hour after injection of the radionuclide, showing no uptake in the gallbladder (arrow). Most of the radionuclide is in the small intestine (arrowhead). This appearance is consistent with an obstructed cystic duct and a diseased gallbladder.

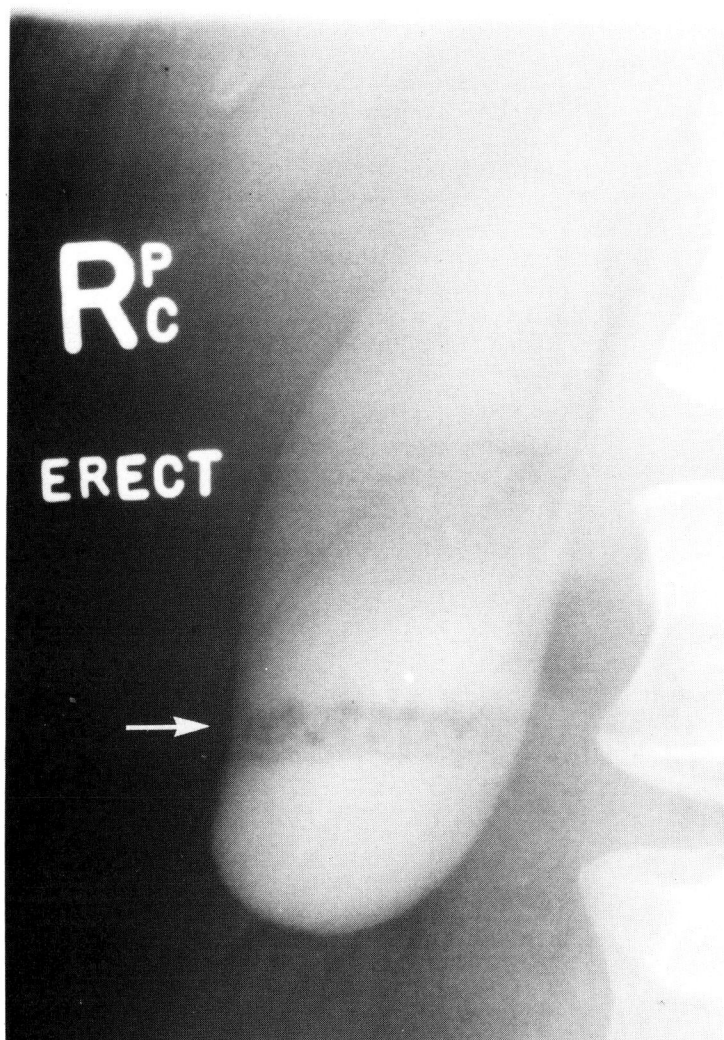

Fig. 19.38 Oral cholecystogram taken with the patient in the erect position demonstrating multiple small stones floating in the gallbladder (arrow). This appearance is typical of cholesterol calculi.

About 10% of patients with nonvisualization and 60% of those with poor visualization have a normal cholecystogram at a second examination, and for this reason should the gallbladder be non-functioning on the first examination a second cholecystogram is necessary, or alternatively an intravenous cholangiogram (IVC) or ultrasound scan. If the oral cholecystogram is normal but the clinical history and biochemical tests are very suggestive of gallstone disease an IVC or ultrasound or endoscopic retrograde cholangiopancreatography (ERCP) should be considered.

Intravenous cholangiogram

Enthusiasm for the use of intravenous cholangiography in the diagnosis of biliary disease has fluctuated since its introduction in 1953. The test is performed by intravenous infusion of sodium or meglumine iodipamide which is cleared from the bloodstream by the liver and excreted into bile. Non-visualization of the gallbladder in patients with suspected acute cholecystitis suggests an obstructed cystic duct, so long as the common bile duct is seen. The intravenous cholangiogram is also used to outline the common bile duct in patients after cholecystectomy. Evaluation of the usefulness of intravenous cholangiography shows that only 50% of studies produce optimum images and of those studies judged to be diagnostic, the error rate for diagnosis of stones in the common bile duct is approximately 40%. The major problem with the procedure is insufficient visualization of the biliary tree and of poor excretion in the jaundiced patient. Further, fatal anaphylactic reactions to the contrast medium may occur. The first generation of intravenous cholangiographic agents such as iodipamide and ioglycamate should be discarded in favour of either iotroxamide or iodoxamide which are safer and give higher biliary iodine concentrations and as a consequence better bile duct visualization. Optimum results are obtained by infusing intravenous iotroxamide (Biliscopin) of about $4 \, mg \cdot kg$ body $wt^{-1} \cdot min^{-1}$ for one hour. Better and safer biliary imaging techniques are now available so intravenous cholangiograms should rarely be used for the investigation of patients with biliary tract problems.

Percutaneous transhepatic cholangiogram (PTC)

Visualization of the obstructed biliary tree is obtained by percutaneous transhepatic injection of contrast medium into the dilated bile ducts (Figure 19.39). Before the introduction of fine needles, the procedure had a low diagnostic success rate and was associated with a high incidence of bile leakage or haemorrhage. Since 23 gauge Chiba needles have been used the incidence of complications has fallen and a recent large study reported a complication rate of only 3.4%. In this study, the success rate for visualization of dilated bile ducts was 99% whilst visualization of non-dilated ducts was achieved in 70% of patients. Percutaneous transhepatic cholangiography is used in jaundiced patients in whom a preceding ultrasound examination reveals dilated intrahepatic ducts. It is contraindicated in patients with bleeding diathesis and is unlikely to be successful in patients with liver cirrhosis.

Transhepatic tubes placed in the bile duct by this technique may be used for preoperative drainage of an obstructed biliary tract and for long-term drainage of an obstructed duct in patients unsuitable for surgical treatment.

Endoscopic retrograde cholangiopancreatography (ERCP)

Direct cannulation of the pancreatic duct and common bile duct through the papilla of Vater allows filling of these ducts with radiopaque contrast material and delineation of the biliary and pancreatic ducts (Figure 19.40). ERCP is the optimal investigation for patients suspected to have stones in the bile duct after a previous cholecystectomy. In such patients the intrahepatic ducts are often of normal calibre and PTC has

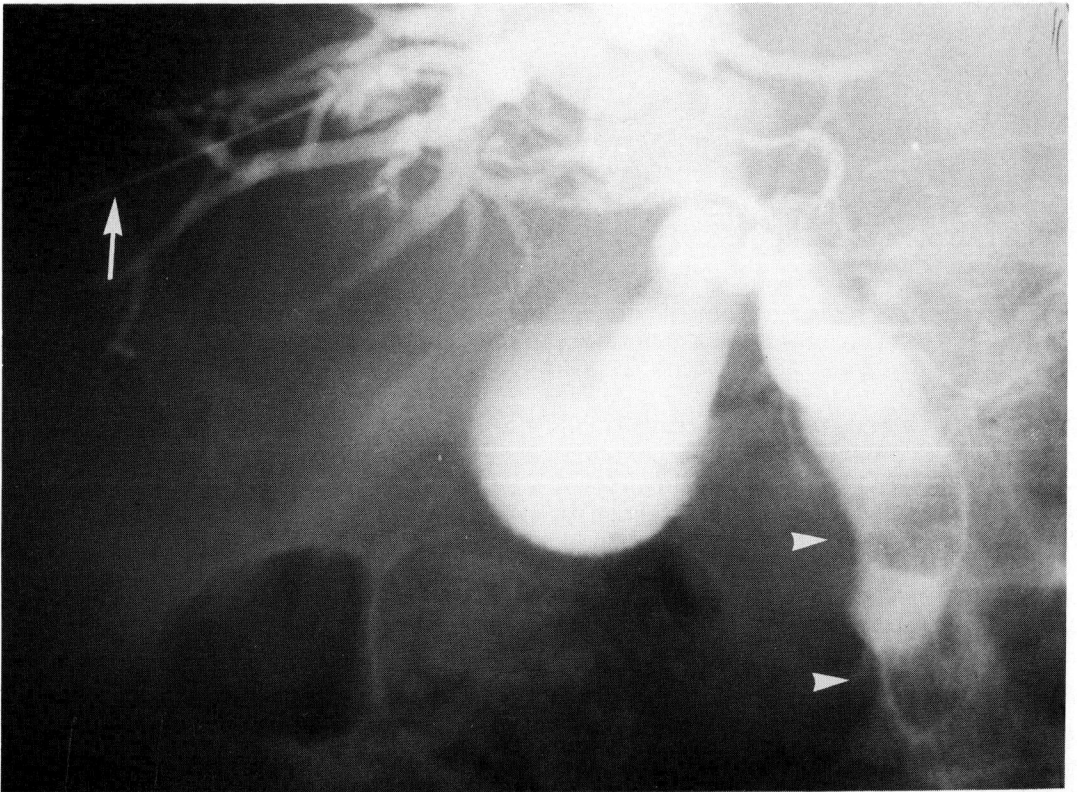

Fig. 19.39 Percutaneous transhepatic cholangiogram performed with a 23 gauge needle (arrow). Contrast introduced into the dilated intrahepatic ducts has opacified the gallbladder and common bile duct. Two large stones are shown in the common bile duct (arrowheads).

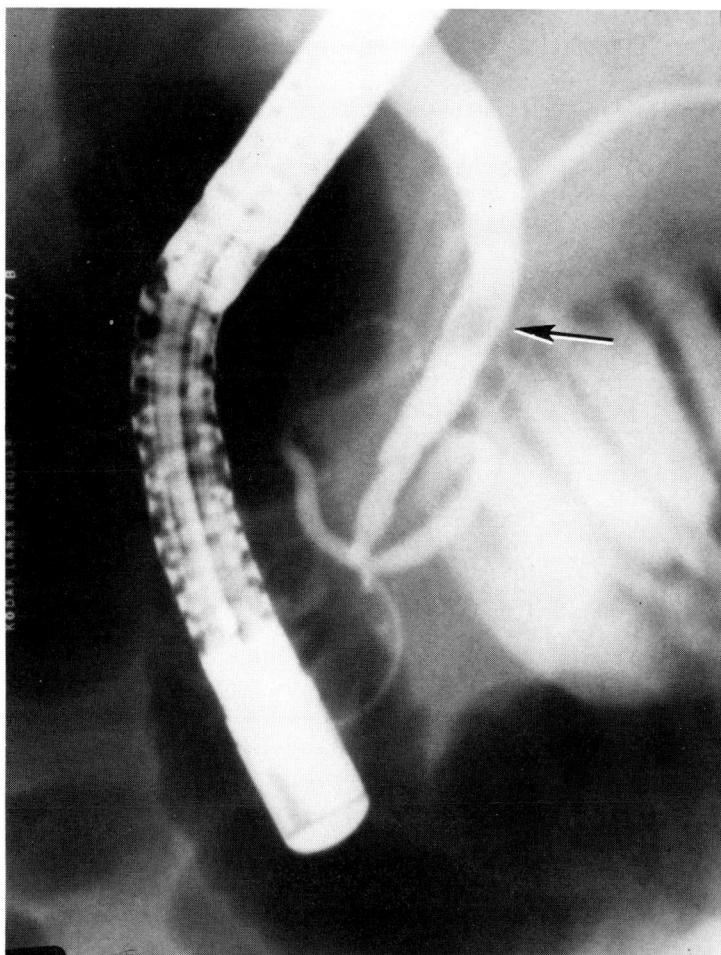

Fig. 19.40 ERCP showing contrast in the common bile duct and pancreatic duct. A radiolucent stone is demonstrated in the common bile duct (arrow).

only a 70% success rate and a higher morbidity than ERCP, which has a success rate exceeding 90%. Further, if a stone is diagnosed by ERCP, the endoscopist may proceed to sphincterotomy for its removal, thereby avoiding the need for abdominal surgery.

In the presence of a dilated extrahepatic biliary tree, as assessed by ultrasonography, there is little to choose between PTC and ERCP. In many institutions, local expertise will determine which of the two investigations is used. However, ERCP allows additional information to be obtained, such as endoscopic examination of the stomach and duodenum, and cannulation of the pancreatic duct.

T-Tube cholangiography

A T-tube is usually inserted in the common bile duct following exploration of the common bile duct for stones. The T-tube drains the duct and allows radiological examination of the biliary tree to be performed 5–7 days after the oper-

ation. T-tube cholangiography is performed by injecting a small volume of Hypaque 30% contrast medium into the biliary tree via the tube under fluoroscopic control. The biliary tree is examined for retained stones and for free passage of contrast medium from the common bile duct into the duodenum.

Computerized axial tomography (CT)

CT scanning of the biliary tree can demonstrate the gallbladder and extrahepatic bile ducts but does not offer any advantages over ultrasonography. In view of the relatively high radiation exposure of CT, there is little, if any, indication for this investigation in the diagnosis of biliary tract disease.

Bile microscopy

A diagnosis of stones can be made with confidence in at least 95% of patients with gallstones by using radiological and ultrasonic investigations of the biliary tract. In the remaining patients, small stones in the gallbladder may remain undetected. There is a high correlation between the presence of cholesterol crystals and/or pigment granules in bile and gallstones in the gallbladder.

After an overnight fast, a mercury tip weighted catheter is swallowed and its tip positioned in the third part of the duodenum. The fasting gallbladder is stimulated to contract by an intravenous bolus of cholecystokinin-octapeptide and dark gallbladder bile is aspirated through the catheter. The bile is centrifuged and examined for cholesterol crystals and pigment granules, the presence of which is invariably associated with gallbladder disease and stones.

SURGERY FOR GALLSTONES

Surgery for gallstones is principally by laparotomy although access may also be obtained to the common bile duct either endoscopically after sphincterotomy or by instruments passed percutaneously through an established T-tube tract.

Cholecystectomy

This operation involves removal of the gallbladder and stones through an upper abdominal incision. The cystic artery is identified and ligated before it is divided. The cystic duct is identified and the common bile duct and common hepatic duct are also exposed in order to prevent damage to these structures. The cystic duct is then ligated with absorbable suture material. The cystic duct commonly enters the common hepatic duct after running posteriorly and even then may join to the left of this structure. Attempts to remove all the cystic duct under these circumstances are hazardous and should be avoided. However, it is important that stones are not left within it. An operative cholangiogram is performed if possible in all patients, but this examination is mandatory if either the clinical history or the operative findings indicate any possibility of stones in the common bile duct (see Table 19.8).

The timing of surgery depends on the speed with which the appropriate investigations can be carried out. There is debate about the timing of a cholecystectomy in a patient with acute cholecystitis but accumulating evidence favours early cholecystectomy because it reduces the time in hospital and decreases the risk of serious com-

Table 19.8 Clinical, investigative and operative indicators of stones in the common bile duct.

Clinical
   Obstructive jaundice
   Acute pancreatitis

Investigative
   Raised alkaline phosphatase
   Common duct dilated on ultrasound

Operative
   Palpable stone in duct
   Dilated common bile duct
   Multiple small stones in gallbladder with wide cystic duct

---

plications. It must be emphasized that early cholecystectomy does not mean emergency cholecystectomy, which is often performed at night by inexperienced junior staff in an ill-prepared patient who has been inadequately investigated. Unless there is evidence to suggest free perforation or the patient's condition is rapidly deteriorating, time should be allowed for radiological confirmation of cholelithiasis. Opportunity is given for resuscitation and assessment of the patient as well as consultation with an experienced anaesthetist.

OPERATIVE CHOLANGIOGRAPHY

During cholecystectomy, the cholangiogram is performed through a small cannula introduced into the common bile duct via the cystic duct. Meticulous attention to the technical aspects of performing the examination is essential for high quality radiographs and this can be achieved only by cooperation between the surgeon, radiographer and anaesthetist. The position of the patient on the operating table is checked so that the right upper quadrant is central over the X-ray plate. Either the X-ray tube or the operating table is tilted 15° to the right so that the vertebral column does not overlie the region of the common bile duct. A preliminary X-ray is taken to check the exposure and alterations are made to the settings if the exposure is incorrect. Once the cannula has been inserted into the cystic duct, bile is allowed to drain from the common bile duct to enable it to fill the cannula.

The syringe containing the contrast medium is then connected to the cannula ensuring that no air bubbles are introduced. Hypaque 30% is used as the contrast medium and three X-rays are taken. For the first, 1–1.5 ml of contrast is injected into the biliary tree. The anaesthetist stops the ventilator and the X-ray is taken. The second X-ray is taken after injection of a further 1–2 ml of contrast medium and the third obtained after an injection of a further 5 ml. In a normal operating cholangiogram, the entire biliary tree is seen, there is unrestricted flow of contrast medium into the duodenum and no evidence of radiolucent defects within the ducts. Occasionally, flow of contrast into the duodenum may be restricted by a contracted sphincter of Oddi, giving the appearance of a stricture or a small stone impacted at the lower end of the bile duct. This contraction of the sphincter may be caused by opiate administration during anaesthesia. Administration of the opiate antagonist nalorphine usually will relax the sphincter and allow the contrast to flow into the duodenum as demonstrated on a further radiograph.

It is usually unhelpful to perform postexploratory operative cholangiography after exploration of the common bile duct and the removal of stones because it is almost impossible to remove the air bubbles from the biliary tree. Our current practice is to examine the biliary tree with a rigid choledochoscope at the completion of the common bile duct exploration. However, if completion cholangiography is essential, this is best undertaken by using a small balloon catheter, the distended balloon preventing leakage of the contrast through the choledochotomy incision. The advantages of routine operative cholangiography have been demonstrated in numerous studies over the last decade, although there is still controversy about whether it should be used selectively or routinely. Its use has reduced both the incidence of stones retained in the common bile duct after cholecystectomy and the incidence of negative common bile duct explorations. An added bonus of operative cholangiography is the delineation of the duct anatomy in a difficult operative procedure.

CHOLEDOCHOSCOPY

The reported incidence of stones retained in the common bile duct after operative stone removal is between 2% and 7%. One of the major reasons for retention of stones is the inadequacy of post-exploratory cholangiography. Operative choledochoscopy serves to examine the bile ducts following surgical exploration. Two types of endoscope are available, the rigid right-angled choledochoscope (using a Hopkins lens system) and the fibre-optic flexible choledochoscope. The rigid choledochoscope is preferred as it provides excellent views of the bile ducts and the ampulla of Vater and is easier to handle. Additional stones are visualized in approximately 10% of patients by using the choledo-

choscope at the end of the duct exploration for stones. Choledochoscopy adds only about 10 minutes to operating time and has few complications. Its use after duct exploration for stones is recommended as a routine procedure.

Cholecystostomy

Cholecystostomy involves drainage of the gallbladder contents and extraction of any contained stones if this is technically feasible. A drainage tube is inserted into the fundus of the gallbladder, fixed with a purse-string suture and brought to the skin surface through a stab incision separate from the laparotomy wound. This operation is rarely performed unless the general condition of the patient is extremely poor, and an obstructed inflamed gallbladder must be drained. It may also be performed if local conditions or the skill of the surgeon make cholecystectomy hazardous.

Extraction of stones from the common bile duct

AT LAPAROTOMY

Supraduodenal exploration. The duct is exposed and a longitudinal incision made in its supraduodenal segment. Stones are extracted by employing a variety of techniques which include the use of forceps, irrigation and passage of balloon catheters. All stones identified on the operative cholangiogram should be found and their removal finally confirmed by inspecting the duct with a rigid choledochoscope. A T-tube is inserted into the common bile duct which is closed with a continuous absorbable suture. The T-tube should have a large external limb and be exteriorized through as short a distance as possible through a stab incision separate from the laparotomy wound. Bile should flow freely to a drainage bag through this tube.

Transduodenal exploration. This is indicated only if a stone is impacted in the ampulla of Vater and cannot be extracted by supraduodenal manipulation. Extraction of the stone may be achieved either by a formal sphincteroplasty or by a simple sphincterotomy. The duodenum is mobilized and opened on the opposite wall to the papilla of Vater. In most patients, a sphincteroplasty is required and the terminal 2 cm of the duct are opened into the duodenum, the incision being continued through the sphincter until the bile duct is widely open. Fine catgut sutures are used to oppose the duodenal and bile duct mucosa.

Stones in the ampulla or lower bile duct are then easily extracted through the sphincteroplasty. Occasionally, a single stone may be impacted at the terminal end of the ampulla and it suffices to make a slit over the stone, in other words a sphincterotomy, so that it may be extracted. The duodenum is then closed. T-tube drainage is only required if the common duct has been opened above the duodenum.

AT ENDOSCOPY

The treatment of stones in the common bile duct in individuals with a prior cholecystectomy has been revolutionized in recent years by the ability to divide the sphincter of Oddi by instruments introduced through an endoscope. The patient is mildly sedated usually with diazepam, and the endoscope inserted in the usual manner for an ERCP (see Chapter 18). The common bile duct is selectively cannulated and contrast medium injected to demonstrate the stone. A wire papillotome is then inserted into the common bile duct making sure that it is freely positioned in the duct and orientated away from the pancreatic duct. The wire is positioned within the sphincter of Oddi and the papillotome is bowed to place the sphincter on a stretch. A combination of cutting and coagulation diathermy current is then applied, making a cut of sufficient length through the sphincter muscle to allow the passage of the stone. The orifice is usually between 1 and 2 cm in length. The stone may be extracted by inserting either a balloon catheter or a flexible wire basket into the common bile duct and pulling the stone through the sphincterotomy opening. With increasing experience the rate for successful removal of stones from the bile duct is in excess of 90% and the mortality and morbidity possibly lower than surgical exploration by laparotomy.

THROUGH A T-TUBE TRACT

Stones retained in the bile duct following duct exploration may be extracted by manipulation of a steerable catheter and a stone basket through an established T-tube tract. To facilitate such a procedure, the external limb of any T-tube inserted into the common duct after exploration should be large (at least 14F gauge) and its route to the surface should be almost direct.

Stone extraction by this route is highly successful but should not be attempted until at least 4 weeks after operation when enough fibrosis has occurred around the tube to prevent rupture of the tract during these manipulations.

CHEMICAL DISSOLUTION OF RETAINED COMMON DUCT STONES

Some common duct stones may be dissolved by infusion of agents directly into the duct via a T-tube or through tubes inserted at ERCP (see above). Agents which effectively dissolve cholesterol stones are mono-octanoin and cholic acid. It is also claimed that the addition of EDTA may dissolve stones composed of calcium bilirubinate. These measures are useful but require careful control and admission of the patient to hospital. Cholic acid infusion (and less so mono-octanoin) may cause severe diarrhoea which can be prevented by simultaneous oral administration of the bile-salt-absorbing resin, cholestyramine. Infusions of these substances through a T-tube have been generally replaced by manipulative removal of stones through the T-tube tract, because this procedure may be performed on an outpatient basis and is far more cost-effective when compared to dissolution treatment.

RECURRENT COMMON BILE DUCT STONES

Problems associated with retained or recurrent common bile duct stones are discussed in more detail on page 1455.

REFERENCES

1 Berci, G. & Hamlin, J. A. (1981) *Operative Biliary Radiology.* Baltimore: Williams and Wilkins.
2 Blumgart, L. H. (1982) *The Biliary Tract.* Edinburgh: Churchill Livingstone.
3 Burhenne, H. J. (1980) Percutaneous extraction of retained biliary stones: 661 patients. *American Journal of Radiology,* **134,** 888.
4 Cooperberg, P. L. & Burhenne, H. J. (1980) Real-time ultrasonography: diagnostic technique of choice in calculous gallbladder disease. *New England Journal of Medicine,* **302,** 1277–1279.
5 Cotton, P. B. (1972) Cannulation of the papilla of Vater by endoscopy and retrograde cholangiopancreatography (ERCP). *Gut,* **13,** 1014–1025.
6 Cotton, P. B. (1980) Non-operative removal of bile duct stones by duodenoscopic sphincterotomy. *British Journal of Surgery,* **67,** 1–5.
7 Down, R. H. L., Arnold, J., Goldin, A. et al. (1979) Comparison of accuracy of ^{99}Tc-pyridoxylidene glutamate scanning with oral cholecystography and ultrasonography in the diagnosis of acute cholecystitis. *Lancet,* **ii,** 1094–1096.
8 Elias, E., Hamblyn, A. N., Jain, S. et al. (1976) A randomized trial of percutaneous transhepatic cholangiography with the Chiba needle versus endoscopic retrograde cholangiography for bile duct visualization in jaundice. *Gastroenterology,* **71,** 439–443.
9 Goodman, M. W., Ansel, H. J., Vennes, J. A. et al. (1980) Is intravenous cholangiography still useful? *Gastroenterology,* **79,** 642–645.

10 Gottfries, A. (1969) Lysolecithin: a factor in the pathogenesis of acute cholecystitis. *Acta Chirurgica Scandinavica*, **135**, 213–217.

11 Gracie, W. A. & Ransohoff, D. F. (1982) The natural history of silent gallstones: the innocent gallstone is not a myth. *New England Journal of Medicine*, **307**, 798–800.

12 Graham, E. A., Cole, W. H. & Copher, G. H. (1924) Visualisation of the gallbladder by the sodium salt of tetrabromophthalein. *Journal of the American Medical Association*, **82**, 1777–1778.

13 Jolly, P. C., Baker, J. W., Schmidt, H. M. *et al.* (1968) Operative cholangiography: a case for its routine use. *Annals of Surgery*, **168**, 551–565.

14 Kune, G. A. & Sali, A. (1981) *The Practice of Biliary Surgery* 2nd edn. Oxford: Blackwell.

15 Long, T. N., Beimback, D. M. & Camio, C. J. (1978) Acalculous cholecystitis in critically ill patients. *American Journal of Surgery*, **136**, 31–36.

16 McArthur, P., Cushieri, A., Sells, R. A. & Shields, R. (1975) Controlled clinical trial comparing early with interval cholecystectomy of acute cholecystitis. *British Journal of Surgery*, **62**, 850–852.

17 Nora, P. F., Berci, G., Dorazio, R. *et al.* (1977) Operative choledochoscopy. *American Journal of Surgery*, **133**, 105–110.

18 Rosenthall, L., Shaffer, E. A. & Lisbona, R. (1978) Diagnosis of hepatobiliary disease by ^{99m}Tc HIDA cholescintigraphy. *Radiology*, **126**, 467–474.

19 Safrany, L. (1977) Duodenoscopic sphincterotomy and gallstone removal. *Gastroenterology*, **72**, 338–343.

20 Schoenfield, L. J. (1977) *Diseases of the Gallbladder and Biliary System*. New York: John Wiley.

21 Thistle, J. L., Carlson, G. L., Hofmann, A. F. *et al.* (1980) Mono-octanoin, a dissolution agent for retained cholesterol bile duct stones. Physical properties and clinical application. *Gastroenterology*, **78**, 1016–1022.

22 Toouli, J., Jablonski, P. & Watts, J. McK. (1974) Dissolution of stones in the common bile duct with bile salt solutions. *Australian and New Zealand Journal of Surgery*, **44**, 335–340.

23 Toouli, J., Geenen, J. E., Hogan, W. J. *et al.* (1982) Sphincter of Oddi motor activity: a comparison between patients with common duct stones and controls. *Gastroenterology*, **82**, 111–117.

24 Way, L., Admirand, W. H. & Dunphy, J. E. (1972) Management of choledocholithiasis. *Annals of Surgery*, **176**, 347–359.

SCLEROSING CHOLANGITIS

This is a rare disease of unknown cause. The accepted criteria for the primary disease[2] excludes many patients who have the disorder but in addition have concomitant gallstones within the biliary tree. Differentiation from other conditions such as cholangiocarcinoma is difficult. Several aetiological theories have been proposed and some consider sclerosing cholangitis as a reaction of the biliary tree, perhaps immunologically based, to a group of heterogeneous agents or stimuli.[4]

Incidence

About 0.06% of patients undergoing biliary surgery[3] have primary sclerosing cholangitis which occurs slightly more frequently in males. When sclerosing cholangitis is associated with other diseases such as ulcerative colitis the sex incidence is equal and the frequency is 0.8%.[7] In this setting the term secondary sclerosing cholangitis is best avoided because the aetiology of ulcerative colitis and other associated diseases is also unknown.

Pathology

The condition affects both extra- and intrahepatic bile ducts. The ducts are indurated and irregularly thickened with a reduced lumen and many adhesions between the extrahepatic biliary tree and adjacent organs even before surgical exploration. The fibrosis extends from the submucosal to the subserous layers and is characterized by a cellular infiltrate of lymphocytes, plasma cells, polymorphs and eosinophils.[5] The condition usually spares the mucosa of the biliary tree but the gallbladder may be involved in the same process. Areas of proliferation of ductular epithelial cells with distortion of the periductal glands and fibrous tissue often makes histological differentiation from cholangiocarcinoma of the bile duct difficult. This difficulty may become less common because the advent of operative biliary endoscopy permits a good specimen of bile duct to be obtained. However, it is often difficult to introduce the choledochoscope into the narrowed bile duct in these patients. Even so there remains the possibility of a cholangiocarcinoma in another part of the biliary tree which has not been biopsied.[1] This problem is more common in patients with associated ulcerative colitis in whom cholangiocarcinoma may appear many years after the cholangitis has been diagnosed.[6] The initial intrahepatic disorder may be a peri-cholangitis and this may be found in conjunction with the typical concentric fibrosis which occurs around hepatic bile ducts and characterizes chronic pericholangitis. This may progress to secondary biliary cirrhosis.[1]

Clinical features

The condition often has a vague onset, usually between the ages of 30 and 60 years, with right hypochondrial pain and intermittent obstructive jaundice and pruritus. The jaundice usually becomes a constant feature and eventually the patient progresses to liver failure in 5–15 years.

Anorexia, weight loss, nausea, vomiting and episodes of cholangitis can occur, but bleeding from oesophageal varices is uncommon. On occasions the associated ulcerative colitis may be symptomatically mild but colonoscopy will demonstrate the colitis which may be total.[8]

Laboratory investigations

These reveal an obstructive (cholestatic) jaundice with a marked elevation of serum alkaline phosphatase concentration. Initially the serum bilirubin concentration may be disproportionately slight. A raised erythrocyte sedimentation rate often precedes elevation of serum aspartate and alanine transaminases. The prothrombin time may be prolonged. The hepatitis antigens are not present.

Radiological investigations

Ultrasound demonstrates an absence of dilated intra- and extrahepatic ducts, but may show coincidental gallstones. Endoscopic retrograde cholangiography and percutaneous transhepatic cholangiograms may both be necessary to demonstrate the full extent of the disease (Figure 19.41). Many patients still provide a taxing problem for the surgeon who at operation has difficulty in performing operative cholangiography and in this way overlooks the diagnosis.

The diagnosis may be made by liver biopsy if the typical whorled fibrotic appearance of the bile ducts is seen. Biopsy of a thin sliver of bile duct wall from a choledochotomy incision may be helpful but must be carefully performed. The diagnosis may be obtained by a biopsy of the narrow bile duct mucosa using the rigid choledochoscope. Unfortunately these methods of biopsy will not exclude a cholangiocarcinoma in another area of the liver. Patients with ulcerative colitis who are seen early in the disease may have either pericholangitis or a normal liver biopsy.[8]

Treatment

The natural history of the disease is one of fluctuation. Corticosteroids have no proven value.

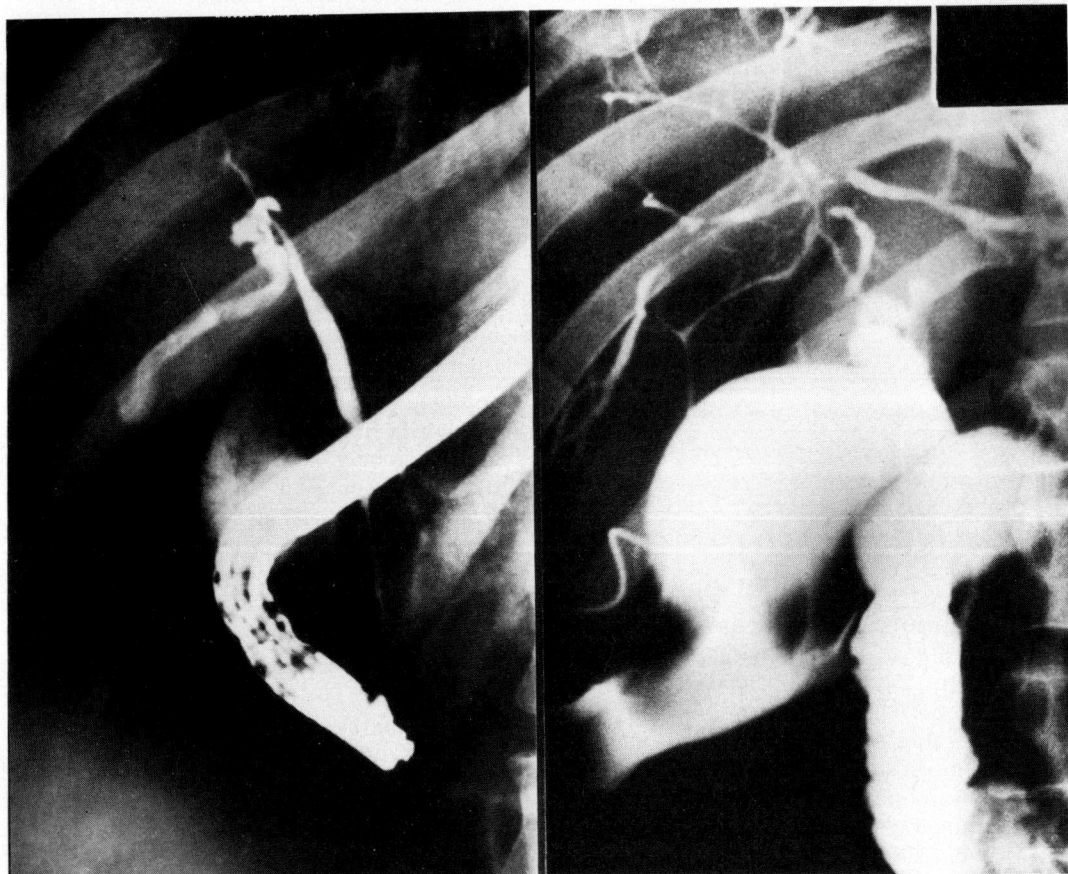

Fig. 19.41 A patient with sclerosing cholangitis. Left: endoscopic retrograde cholangiography has outlined the stricture at the lower end of the common bile duct. Right: it was necessary to do a laparoscopy and direct puncture of the gallbladder through the liver to outline the intrahepatic biliary tree and show the strictures and beading.

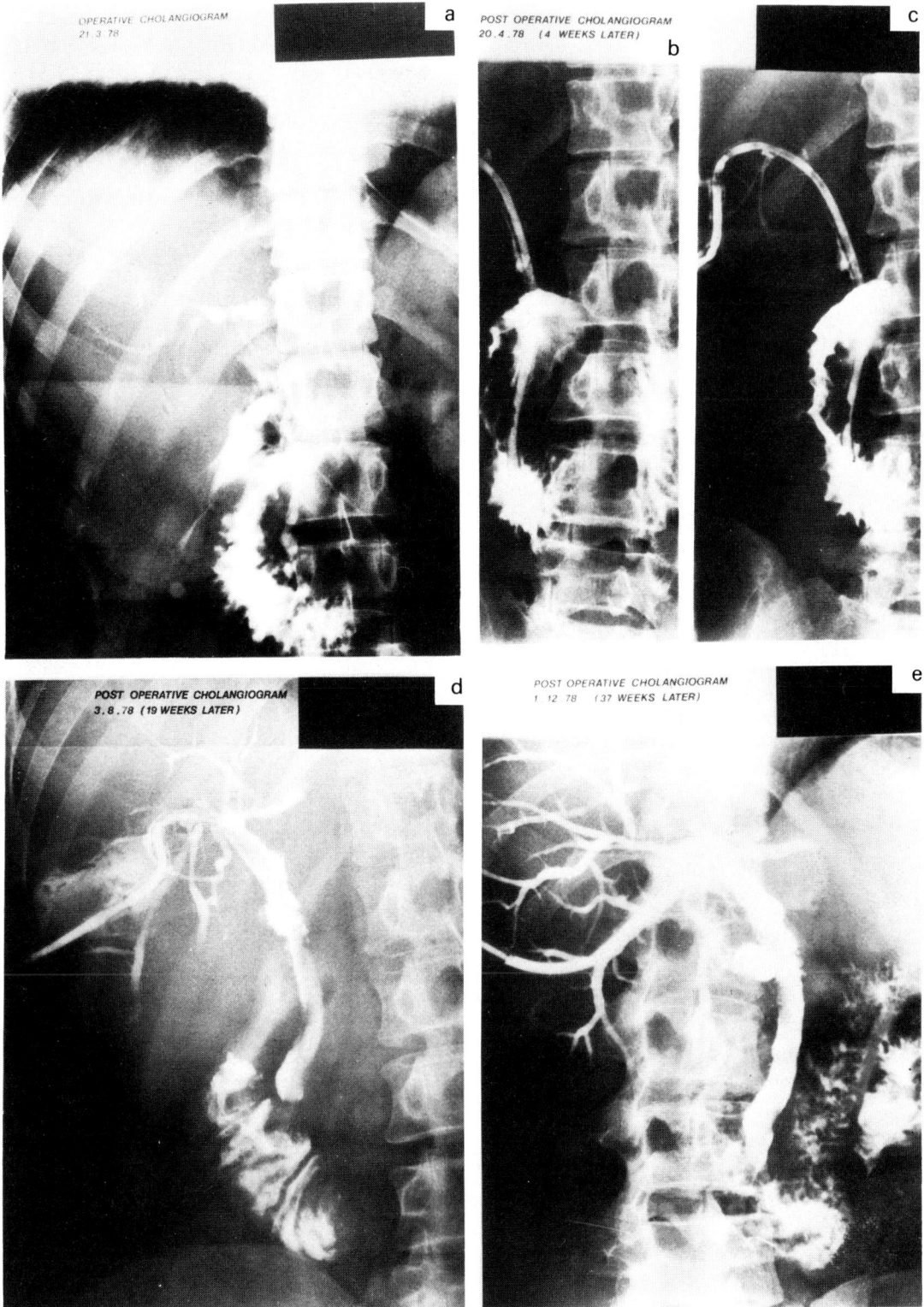

Fig. 19.42 A patient treated for one year with a silicone tube biliary stent. (a) 21/3/78, shows direct puncture of the common bile duct at operation and the multiple strictures in the biliary tree. (b, c) 20/4/78, shows the silicone tube in place with a tube cholangiogram. (d) 3/8/78, shows dilatation of the extra- and intrahepatic biliary tree with the tube still in place. (e) 1/12/78, shows that dilatation of the biliary tree has been maintained; following removal of the silicone tube the patient has continued to have a normal bilirubin level. From Wood and Cuschieri (1980),[8] with kind permission of the authors and the editor of *Lancet*.

Antibiotics should be used for an attack of cholangitis but their long-term use encourages resistant organisms. The administration of fat-soluble vitamins will improve the prothrombin time in patients who do not have established cirrhosis. Coexistent gallstone disease should be dealt with by cholecystectomy and choledochotomy if the stones are in the biliary tree. If there is evidence of biliary obstruction in the extrahepatic ducts, the ducts should be dilated up by introduction at the choledochotomy incision of fine Lister bougies which are then passed into the intrahepatic biliary tree. A transhepatic silicone stent with multiple spirally disposed holes along the transhepatic portion can be pulled through the right lobe of the liver, and via the extrahepatic biliary tree into the duodenum.[8] This procedure may not be successful if cirrhosis is present. A daily wash-out of the hepatostomy tube with saline is essential to assure continued patency and occasionally it is necessary to insert a second tube using a guide wire technique should the first tube become blocked. The material is usually a deposit of calcium bilirubinate. This technique has resulted in marked radiological, clinical and biochemical improvement (Figure 19.42). Colectomy should be recommended if an associated ulcerative colitis is shown to involve the whole colon even if this is relatively symptomless. If there is established cirrhosis the prognosis is poor even if the ducts are stented.

REFERENCES

1   Mistilis, S. P. (1975) Liver disease in bowel disorders. In *Diseases of the Liver* (Ed.) Schiff, J. D., pp. 1373–1383. Philadelphia: J. B. Lippencott.
2   Myers, R. N., Cooper, J. H. & Padis, N. (1970) Primary sclerosing cholangitis. Complete gross and histologic reversal after long term steroid therapy. *American Journal of Gastroenterology*, **53**, 527–538.
3   Oviedo, M. A., Volkomer, D. & Scanlon, E. F. (1974) Primary sclerosing cholangitis. *Archives of Surgery*, **109**, 747–749.
4   Peck, J. J., Kern, W. H. & Mikkelsen, W. P. (1974) Sclerosis of the extrahepatic bile ducts. *Archives of Surgery*, **108**, 798–800.
5   Roberts, J. M. (1955) Stenosing cholangitis. *Western Journal of Surgery, Obstetrics and Gynecology*, **63**, 253–259.
6   Thorpe, M. E. C., Scheuer, P. J. & Sherlock, S. (1967) Primary sclerosing cholangitis, the biliary tree and ulcerative colitis. *Gut*, **8**, 435–448.
7   Warren, K. W., Athanassiades, S. & Monge, J. I. (1966) Primary sclerosing cholangitis – a study of forty-two cases. *American Journal of Surgery*, **III**, 22–38.
8   Wood, R. A. B. & Cuschieri, A. (1980) Is sclerosing cholangitis complicating ulcerative colitis a reversible condition? *Lancet*, **ii**, 716–718.

BILIARY DYSKINESIA: GALLBLADDER DYSKINESIA AND PAPILLARY STENOSIS

The only universally accepted cause of typical recurrent biliary pain in the absence of previous surgery or trauma is gallstones. Patients with abdominal pain of biliary type with 'normal' investigations are generally considered to have psychosomatic disease. It seems unreasonable, however, when we accept that chest pain results from diffuse oesophageal spasm, and bowel disturbance from irritable bowel syndrome that we should not countenance the possibility of biliary symptoms from a motility disorder of the biliary tract or biliary dyskinesia.

A plethora of papers over the last 40 years about right upper quadrant abdominal pain without gallstones and the liberal use of various terms purporting to define particular disorders of biliary tract motility has given no understanding of the possible disease entities involved.

Table 19.9   Classification of biliary dysmotility syndromes.

Acalculous gallbladder disease
Cystic duct syndrome
Gallbladder hypercontraction
Gallbladder hypocontraction or hypotonia
Sphincter of Oddi disease (papillary stenosis)
Hypertonia, spasm, hypermotility or hypertrophy
Fibrous stenosis

Table 19.9 presents a simplified view to include all previously described forms of biliary dyskinesia. The two principal areas of putative dysmotility in the biliary tract are the two structures containing significant muscle layers known to undergo regular contraction and relaxation, namely, the gallbladder and the sphincter of Oddi. It should be emphasized, however, that consideration of the bile duct sphincter without reference to the pancreatic duct sphincter is artificial as these two muscular mechanisms are closely linked. This interrelationship may have important clinical implications because some patients with papillary stenosis (see below) undoubtedly suffer from pancreatic rather than biliary pain.

HISTORICAL BACKGROUND AND CURRENT VIEW

Sphincter of Oddi dysfunction and stenosis

Oddi[27] first put forward the concept that 'dysfunction of the choledochal sphincter' might explain certain 'morbid affections of the biliary tract' particularly after removal of the gallbladder. Ivy[22] again propounded the idea that a motor dysfunction of the biliary tract or biliary dyskinesia could cause symptoms. Mirizzi[25] and Best and Hicken[4] redescribed this as biliary dyssynergia, implicating spasm of the lower end of the common bile duct. Numerous reports, predominantly surgical, have subsequently described the recognition and treatment of sphincter of Oddi fibrosis[26] in patients with recurrent biliary and/or pancreatic symptoms especially after cholecystectomy.

It is suggested that in the postcholecystectomy situation, the terms biliary dyskinesia, biliary dystonia, biliary dysmotility, biliary dyssynergia, sphincter of Oddi fibrosis, sphincter of Oddi dyskinesia, papillary and ampullary stenosis all relate to a single pathophysiological entity, namely, that of common bile duct and/or pancreatic duct obstruction by an abnormal pancreaticobiliary sphincter mechanism. Papillary stenosis is recommended as the appropriate term as this also allows for pancreatic involvement which would otherwise be excluded by the term biliary dyskinesia. In parallel with other sphincter stenoses such as pyloric stenosis, two varieties of this condition are proposed although the symptomatology and standard investigative findings may be indistinguishable (Table 19.9).

Gallbladder dysmotility

The concept of gallbladder dyskinesia, acalculous gallbladder disease or acalculous cholecystitis is a more recent one.[7] There has been a proliferation of descriptive terms, often based on cholecystographic appearances, which have implied pathophysiological processes without any hard evidence and a better approach is to describe three possible variants under the collective term acalculous gallbladder disease (Table 19.9). Acalculous cholecystitis may be a misnomer as pathological examination of cholecystectomy specimens demonstrate inflammation in less than 50%. It has been suggested that inappropriate early and sustained contraction of the cystic duct prevents gallbladder evacuation following the stimulus of a meal and thereby gives rise to the gallbladder pain of cystic duct syndrome. Gallbladder hypercontraction is meant to denote accelerated gallbladder emptying in response to a normal stimulus giving rise to pain and gallbladder hypocontraction or hypotonia indicates sluggish or absent response to normal stimuli with the result that pain ensues from gallbladder distension.

WORKING DEFINITIONS

The following working definitions are suggested for dysmotility syndromes.

Papillary stenosis is a benign condition affecting one or more of the two main muscular components of the pancreaticobiliary sphincter mechanism[5] in which obstruction to the normal flow of bile and/or pancreatic juice occurs. The obstruction may be functional owing to increased sphincter activity or mechanical owing to fibrosis and may occur intermittently or continuously. This definition excludes calculous and neoplastic obstruction at the level of the papilla and benign ductal obstructions more proximal to the papilla. Papillary stenosis may give rise to biliary symptoms indistinguishable from common bile duct obstruction due to other causes.

Gallbladder dyskinesia or acalculous gallbladder disease is a benign condition affecting the muscular wall of the gallbladder and cystic duct in which abnormal speed (dyskinesia), tone (dystonia) or coordination (dyssynergia) of contraction may be present alone or in combination in response to normal stimuli of gallbladder contraction. These abnormalities of motility may give rise to biliary symptoms indistinguishable from those of gallstone disease.

RECOGNITION AND SYMPTOMATOLOGY

Recognition of biliary dyskinesia and appropriate investigations are summarized in Table 19.10. The overall incidence of these conditions is unknown. Estimates of gallbladder dysmotility range up to 10% of all gallbladder disease, papillary stenosis in 0–40% of all patients with postcholecystectomy pain and 5% of all cholecystectomies.[34]

The patient with acalculous gallbladder disease or papillary stenosis is predominantly female and presents with right upper quadrant abdominal pain of variable severity, episodic in nature, occasionally continuous, and varying from minutes to hours. It often follows food and is associated with fatty food intolerance, heartburn, flatulence, epigastric fullness, sweating, nausea and faintness. The pain may radiate to the epigastrium, right costal margin, back at the same level or to the right scapula and is usually labelled as biliary colic.

The patient with papillary stenosis presents between a few weeks and several years after cholecystectomy and usually no definitive diagnosis is made. Symptoms of obstructive jaundice

Table 19.10 Recognition of biliary dyskinesia.

Patient status	Presentation	Investigations	Diagnosis to consider
Gallbladder in situ	Recurrent biliary colic	Apparently normal gallbladder	Acalculous gallbladder disease ± papillary stenosis
Gallbladder in situ	Recurrent pancreatic pain or acute relapsing pancreatitis of unknown cause	Normal biliary tract and pancreatic duct	Papillary stenosis
Common bile duct stones ± gallbladder in situ ± gallbladder stones	Biliary pain, jaundice, cholangitis	Unsuspected papillary abnormality as well as common bile duct stones	Papillary stenosis
Postcholecystectomy	Biliary or pancreatic pain, jaundice, cholangitis	No stones	Papillary stenosis

occur in under 10% of patients with papillary stenosis and rigors or pyrexia occur in less than 5%. Characteristically attacks of pain are precipitated by fat ingestion and opiate-like drugs but not all the attacks are meal-related and many are spontaneous and have no obvious precipitating factor. This pattern of postcholecystectomy pain is often reported by the patient to be indistinguishable from that present prior to the operation. The patients are quite well between attacks. Approximately 20% of patients will experience increasing numbers of attacks with time and in some the pain may become continuous which may erroneously suggest chronic pancreatic disease.

INVESTIGATIONS AND DIAGNOSTIC CRITERIA

The patient with biliary dysmotility usually has undergone many biliary investigations, over a long period of time, with apparently negative findings. Such patients are often labelled as neurotic, menopausal, 'functional' or hysterical. Table 19.11 outlines the diagnostic approach to biliary dyskinesia.

Suspected gallbladder dysmotility (acalculous gallbladder disease)

ORAL CHOLECYSTOGRAPHY AND FATTY MEAL

Fatty meal stimulation of gallbladder contraction as an adjunct to standard oral cholecystography has been largely ignored by the clinician and the cholecystokinetic effects of a fatty meal are so variable that its diagnostic value has been questioned. Attempts to remove subjective judg-

Table 19.11 Diagnostic approach in biliary dyskinesia.

Suspected gallbladder dysmotility
    Oral cholecystography
    Cholecystokinin cholecystography
    Biliary drainage

Papillary stenosis
    Suspected papillary stenosis with gallbladder in situ
        Oral cholecystography and intravenous cholangiography
        Biliary drainage
        Evocative biochemistry tests
        Endoscopic retrograde cholangiopancreatography
        Endoscopic manometry
    Suspected papillary stenosis at surgery
        Intra-operative cholangiography
        Intra-operative manometry and radiomanometry
        Intra-operative flow measurement during bile duct perfusion
        Surgical examination of the papilla
    Suspected papillary stenosis following cholecystectomy
        T-tube cholangiography, radiomanometry and flow measurements
        Evocative biochemical tests
        Intravenous cholangiography
        Endoscopic retrograde cholangiopancreatography
        Endoscopic manometry

ments of gallbladder contraction from radiographs have been made by various mapping techniques[14] but these have not been widely accepted.

CHOLECYSTOKININ CHOLECYSTOGRAPHY

A recent refinement has been the use of cholecystokinin (CCK) or its octapeptide in which one Ivy Dog Unit/kg CCK or 75 Ivy Dog Units CCK or 20 ng/kg CCK-octapeptide is injected intravenously over 2–3 min after gallbladder opacification by standard cholecystography. Serial gallbladder radiographs are then taken at 5, 10, 15, 20 and 30 min and clinical observations are made for symptoms. Different investigators have used different criteria for diagnosing an abnormal response and include reproduction of the patient's symptoms, incomplete gallbladder emptying of less than 20–50% of the starting volume and spasm of various parts of the gallbladder and cystic duct[3] to distinguish cystic duct syndrome, gallbladder hypercontraction and gallbladder hypocontraction (Figure 19.43). However false negative rates are unknown, duration of follow-up is too short in most reports and improvement may represent the placebo effect of surgery.

BILIARY DRAINAGE

Duodenal intubation and aspiration of its contents during gallbladder contraction after a fatty stimulus, duodenal instillation of 50% magnesium sulphate or CCK have been used alone (Meltzer-Lyon Test) or in combination with oral cholecystography. This cumbersome technique has not been widely used.

Suspected papillary stenosis

BIOCHEMICAL TESTS

Measurement of serum liver enzymes, bilirubin and pancreatic enzyme concentrations in patients with papillary stenosis is of limited value as less than 25% of patients demonstrate significant abnormalities unless seen during a prolonged acute attack. Attempts to reproduce an acute attack pharmacologically and so produce an evocative biochemical test have employed morphine alone or in combination with secretin, carbachol, neostigmine (Prostigmin) or a meal to cause variable elevations of amylase, lipase and trypsin. The morphine–Prostigmin test[26] has not gained wide acceptance.[24] Normal limits for this test have been difficult to establish and different workers have used different diagnostic criteria to regard a test as abnormal. Carr-Locke and Gregg[9] studied 24 healthy subjects, 13 patients with chronic relapsing pancreatitis, 20 patients with papillary stenosis and 13 patients with a combination of stenosis and chronic pancreatitis. The serum amylase and lipase responses to intramuscular injection of 10 mg morphine sulphate and 1 mg neostigmine were assessed. Significant abdominal pain occurred in all patients with papillary stenosis, 62% of those with stenosis and pancreatitis and 8% with only pancreatitis. Normal responses are shown in Figure 19.44 and patients shared the same pattern although maximum enzyme concentrations were significantly higher in papillary stenosis and controls. Setting a limit of three times normal allowed a correct diagnosis of 65% of patients with papillary stenosis. Although the test has some use in separating patients for further investigation it is unpleasant, distressing when pain is reproduced and chronic pancreatitis needs to be excluded in order to validate the results.

ORAL CHOLECYSTOGRAPHY AND INTRAVENOUS CHOLANGIOGRAPHY

Advocates of CCK cholecystography for gallbladder dyskinesia also suggest its use for diagnosing papillary stenosis. Characteristically the gallbladder fails to empty normally, the common bile duct is 'overfilled', hepatic ducts become visible, little or no contrast enters the duodenum and pain accompanies the examination.

In symptomatic post-cholecystectomy patients intravenous cholangiography is often the first radiological investigation employed to exclude common duct stones but its value in papillary stenosis is limited. Common duct dilatation and delayed contrast evacuation beyond three hours may be present[23] but often radiographic definition is insufficient to permit accurate quantification (Figure 19.45).

SURGICAL EXAMINATION OF THE DUODENAL PAPILLA

Although Del Valle and Donovan[13] described the surgical treatment of fibrotic papillary stenosis in 1926 it is only since 1950 that reports of this condition have appeared, principally in patients undergoing a second or subsequent exploration of the common bile duct for post-cholecystectomy symptoms. Papillary stenosis can be defined as the inability to pass a Bakes No. 3 dilator or 3 mm probe across the papilla from the bile duct, or a lacrimal probe into the pancreatic duct although this will detect only the most severe stenosis. Palpation by probing through the duodenal wall has many pitfalls and an erroneous diagnosis may be made; if there is any doubt the surgeon should inspect the papilla through a duodenotomy. If stenosis is present a transduodenal sphincterotomy or sphincteroplasty is performed and a papillary biopsy taken. The place of choledochoscopy in this condition has yet to be determined.

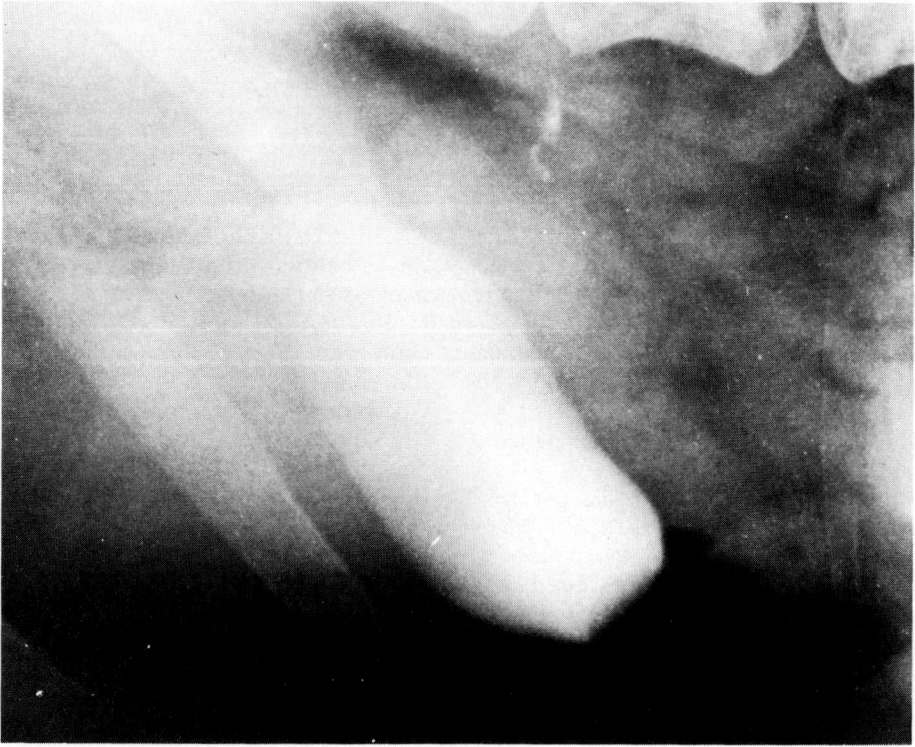

Fig. 19.43 Oral cholecystographs showing (a) normal resting appearance 10 hours after contrast ingestion, (b) same patient 20 min after fat stimulus with faint common bile duct opacification and about 50% gallbladder contraction (normal); (c) appearance of cystic duct syndrome with globular configuration of gallbladder 20 min after fat stimulus accompanied by right upper quadrant pain and no gallbladder emptying, relieved by glyceryl trinitrate; (d) appearance of gallbladder hypercontraction 10 min after fat stimulus with 80% emptying and filling of common bile duct with accompanying discomfort.

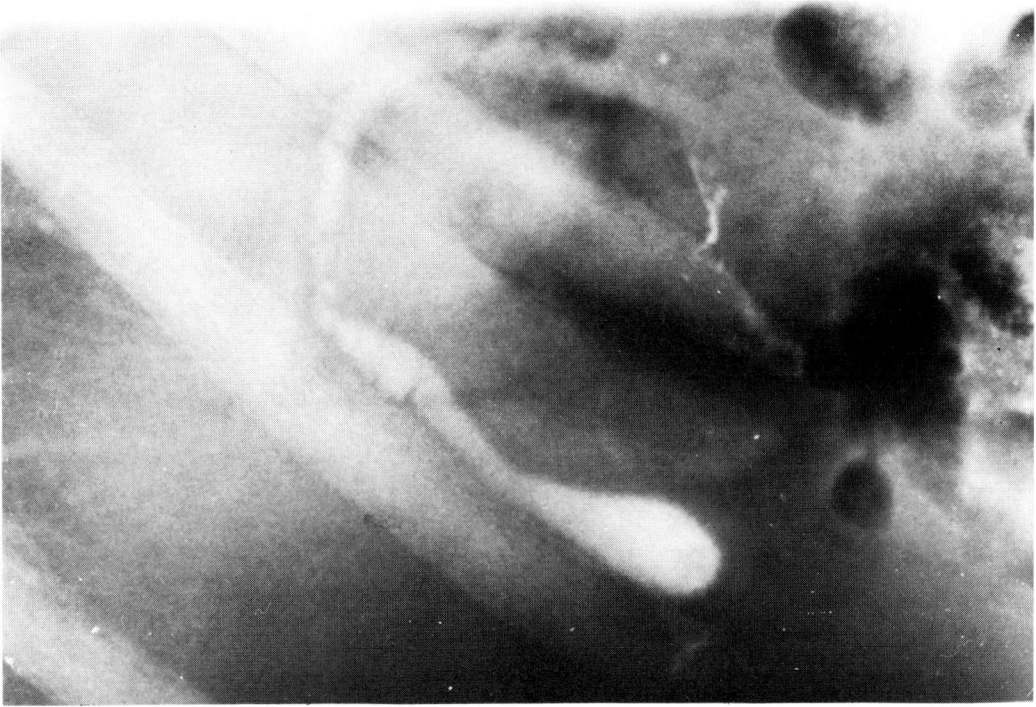

d

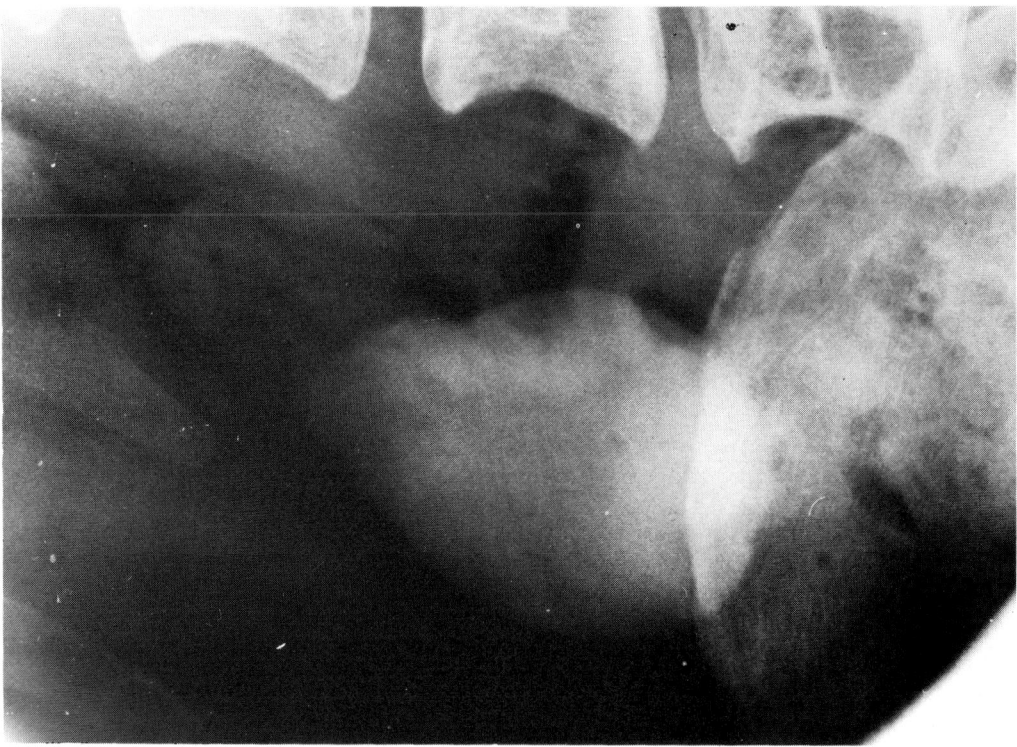

c

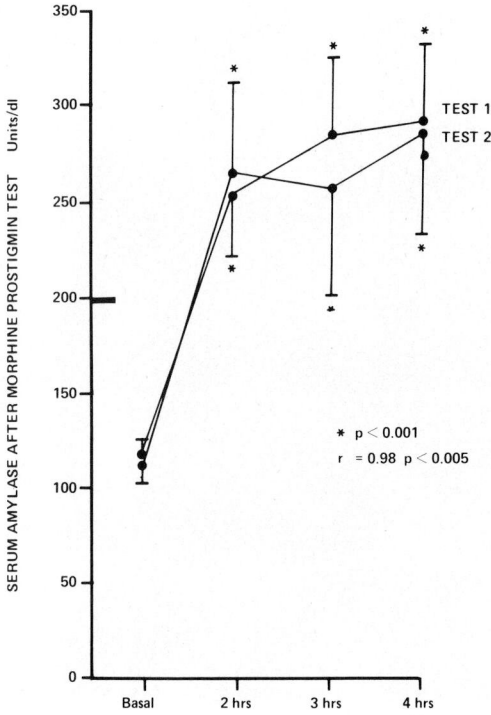

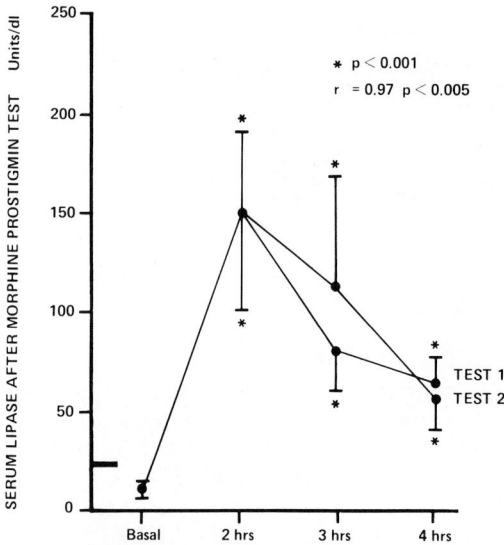

Fig. 19.45 Tomographic radiograph of intravenous cholangiogram in postcholecystectomy patient with papillary stenosis. Common bile duct is dated at 12 mm and no drainage of contrast has occurred after 3 hours.

Fig. 19.44 (a) Serum amylase concentrations before (basal) and 2, 3, and 4 h after morphine-neostigmine(Prostigmin) injection in 24 normal subjects (Test 1) and in 14 of these who underwent a second test (Test 2). Values are mean ± SE. Correlation between Tests 1 and 2 and statistical difference from basal values are shown. Horizontal bar is upper limit of normal. (b) As for (a) showing serum lipase response.

OPERATIVE INVESTIGATION

Three basic techniques have been employed to assist diagnosis of papillary disease during biliary surgery: cholangiography, biliary manometry and measurement of flow rates during common bile duct perfusion (Table 19.11). These have been described as single procedures or as combinations, e.g. radiomanometry (cholangiography combined with manometry)[6] and flowmetry (manometry plus flow rate measurements).[21] Cholangiography may be supplemented by the use of cineradiography,[8] television fluoroscopy[21] or the use of small (dental) intra-abdominal retroduodenal films.[36]

Intra-operative cholangiography
Standard intra-operative cholangiography by hand injection of contrast from a syringe is the mainstay of gallstone detection in the common

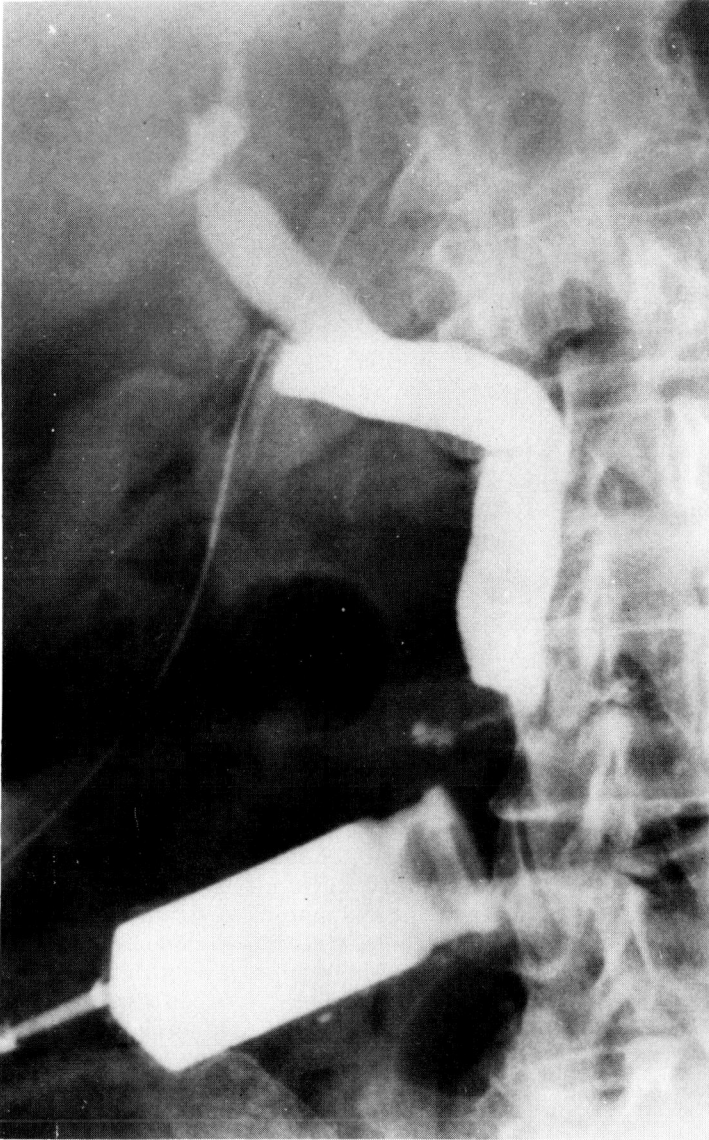

Fig. 19.46 Papillary stenosis: intra-operative cholangiogram showing complete filling of the biliary tract but no contrast draining into the duodenum.

bile duct during biliary surgery but no universally accepted appearances for sphincter stenosis have been described. A peroperative cholangiogram with no calculi, a maximum bile duct diameter of 10 mm or greater, and in which little or no contrast enters the duodenum with or without a fixed minute channel in the sphincter of Oddi area (malignant papillary disease having been excluded) provides reasonable evidence to proceed further with investigation of the papilla with a view to surgical treatment (Figure 19.46).

Intra-operative manometry
There are several methods for combining pressure and flow measurements with cholangiography.[35] The simplest technique employs a vertical and movable reservoir containing dilute radiographic contrast connected via a tube manometer to a biliary cannula. As the reservoir is raised, flow of contrast commences as the resistance of the sphincter of Oddi is overcome and biliary compliance fully accommodated and this is the opening or 'passage pressure'. With the reservoir disconnected fluid flows until the sphincter closes and a 'closing', 'resting', or 'residual' pressure is recorded. Simultaneous cholangiography may be taken as these events occur. Yvergneaux *et al.*[36] have provided diagnostic criteria for papillary stenosis using this method (Table 19.12). Some authors have stressed a need to differentiate between sphincter spasm and stenosis and have used various

Table 19.12 Diagnostic criteria for papillary stenosis on intra-operative radiomanometry.[36]

1   Elevated passage and residual pressures (>15 cmH$_2$O)
2   Radiographs at normal passage pressures (15 cmH$_2$O) delineate constant obstruction in sphincter channel
3   Radiographs at high pressures (up to 45 cmH$_2$O) overcome obstruction and reveal absent rhythmic sphincter activity
4   Radiographic signs of chronic biliary stasis
5   Infrequent pancreatic reflux of contrast (22% compared with 74% normally)

antispasmodics to accomplish this.[28] White *et al.*[35] reported a 92% correct diagnosis of abnormalities from cholangiography alone and increased this to 98.8% when cholangiography was combined with manometry.

Flow measurement
Some consider flow rate to be a more accurate index of papillary obstruction and Hess[21] has investigated the relationship between perfusion pressure and flow rate in controls and patients with papillary stenosis. Although there was overlap at low perfusion pressures the groups were distinct at 30 cm of water: controls had flow rates of over 15 ml/minute whereas in stenosis rates were 10 ml/minute or less. White *et al.*[35] obtained 91.5% accuracy for operative cholangiography alone, 92% for pressures alone (16 cm of water taken as the normal limit) and 95.5% for flow measurement alone (10 ml/minute at 30 cm perfusion pressure taken as normal limit). Combining cholangiography and manometry gave correct diagnoses in 94.5% of cases, cholangiography and flow measurements in 99.1% and manometry and flow measurements in 99.1%. This study included patients with common duct calculi and sphincter spasm relieved by amylnitrite.

T-TUBE STUDIES

Although theoretically all the intra-operative techniques already mentioned can be applied via the T-tube for diagnosis of papillary disease, this does not seem to have been a useful mode of investigation from the lack of reports in the literature.

ENDOSCOPIC RETROGRADE
CHOLANGIOPANCREATOGRAPHY (ERCP)

The development, uses and techniques of ERCP have been well described[12] but its application to diagnosis of papillary stenosis has been discussed much less. The papilla in papillary stenosis usually appears normal endoscopically although peripapillary distortion, hypertrophy of the papilla and hyperaemia are occasionally seen. Cannulation of the papillary orifice with a standard 1.7 mm diameter (5 French gauge) ERCP catheter may prove difficult or impossible in moderate or severe fibrotic stenosis[19, 37] and retrograde cholangiopancreatography may only be achieved by impaction of the catheter during contrast injection. With less severe stenosis the catheter may be deeply inserted into the common bile duct or pancreatic duct but the papilla moves with the cannula on withdrawal. Recently developed tapered tip catheters for ERCP are of considerable help in this situation. In the dyskinetic form of stenosis cannulation is usually normal. Common bile duct or pancreatic duct dilatation is present in the majority of patients with papillary stenosis[17, 19, 32, 37] with upper normal limits of 10–12 mm for the common bile duct and 5–7 mm for the pancreatic duct. Of more value is the demonstration of progressive bile duct dilatation on serial examinations for comparison with previous operative or intravenous cholangiograms (Figure 19.47).

The most significant radiological sign of papillary disease is delayed drainage of contrast after removal of the endoscope in the absence of any drug which might influence normal sphincter and duodenal motility. A common bile duct retaining contrast beyond 45 minutes is always abnormal and in the absence of other pathology this is due to sphincter of Oddi disease.[2] There is a characteristic absence of normal sphincter phasic activity on fluoroscopy with either the complete loss of sphincter channel opening, or partial opening movements of the sphincter without obvious drainage of contrast into the duodenum. The normal pancreatic duct empties contrast within about five minutes so that persistence of a pancreatogram when no main ductal stricture has been shown is indicative of papillary disease. Pancreatic duct sphincter phasic activity is also absent in these cases but is more difficult to visualize on fluoroscopy (Figure 19.48).

Reproduction of the symptoms by filling of the common bile duct with contrast during ERCP is common in papillary stenosis and occurs with much smaller volumes injected than in patients with normal findings or other hepato-biliary diseases, although it is probable that pain can be produced in almost anyone by continued filling of the biliary tree after full opacification in the postcholecystectomy state.

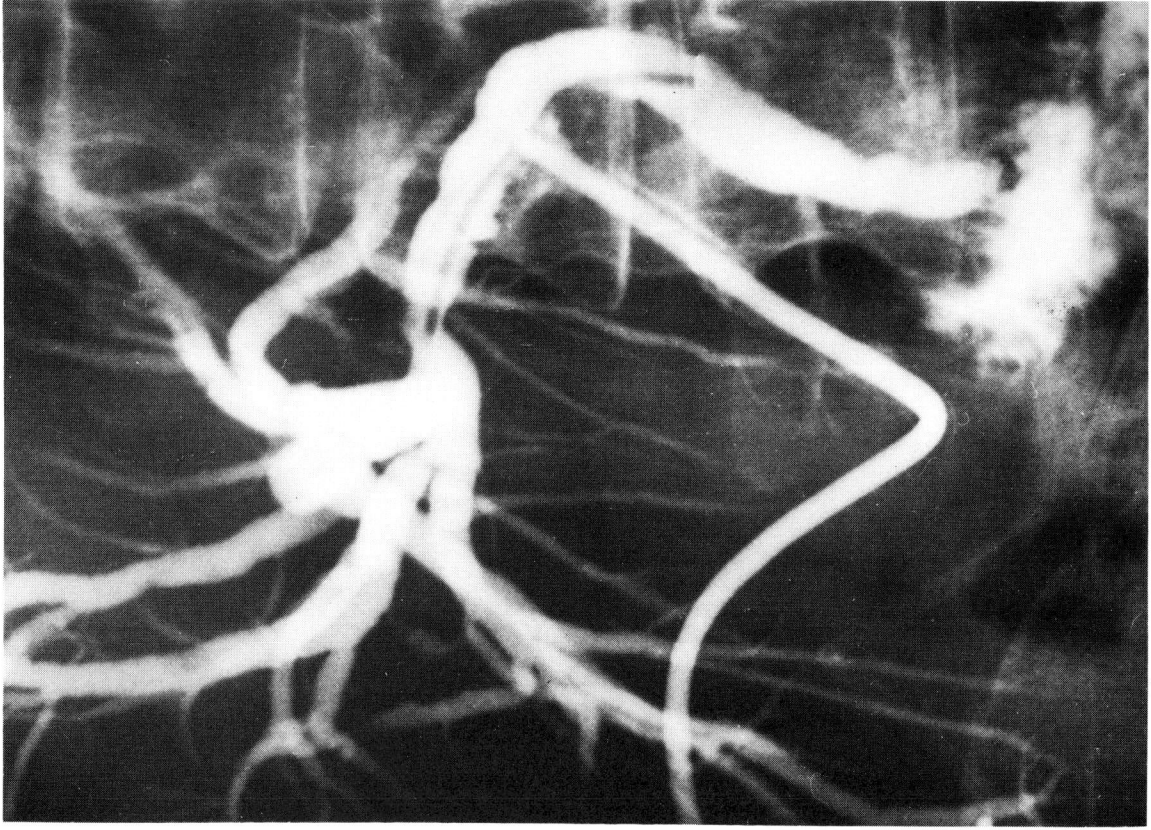

b

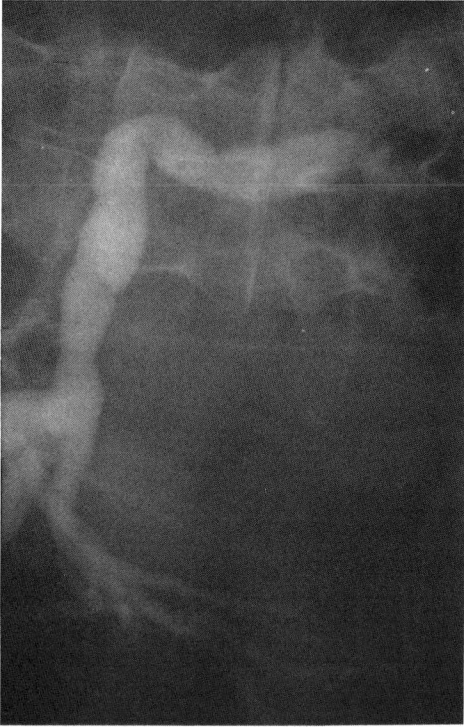

a

Fig. 19.47 Sequence of radiological studies in same patient with previous Billroth 1 partial gastrectomy and recurrent papillary stenosis over 6.5 years. (a) Intra-operative cholangiogram after cholecystectomy showing dilated common bile duct (12 mm) without duodenal drainage, no specific treatment (2.4.76). (b) Post-operative T-tube cholangiogram showing diminution in common bile duct diameter (10 mm) during T-tube drainage (12.4.76). (c)–(h): overleaf.

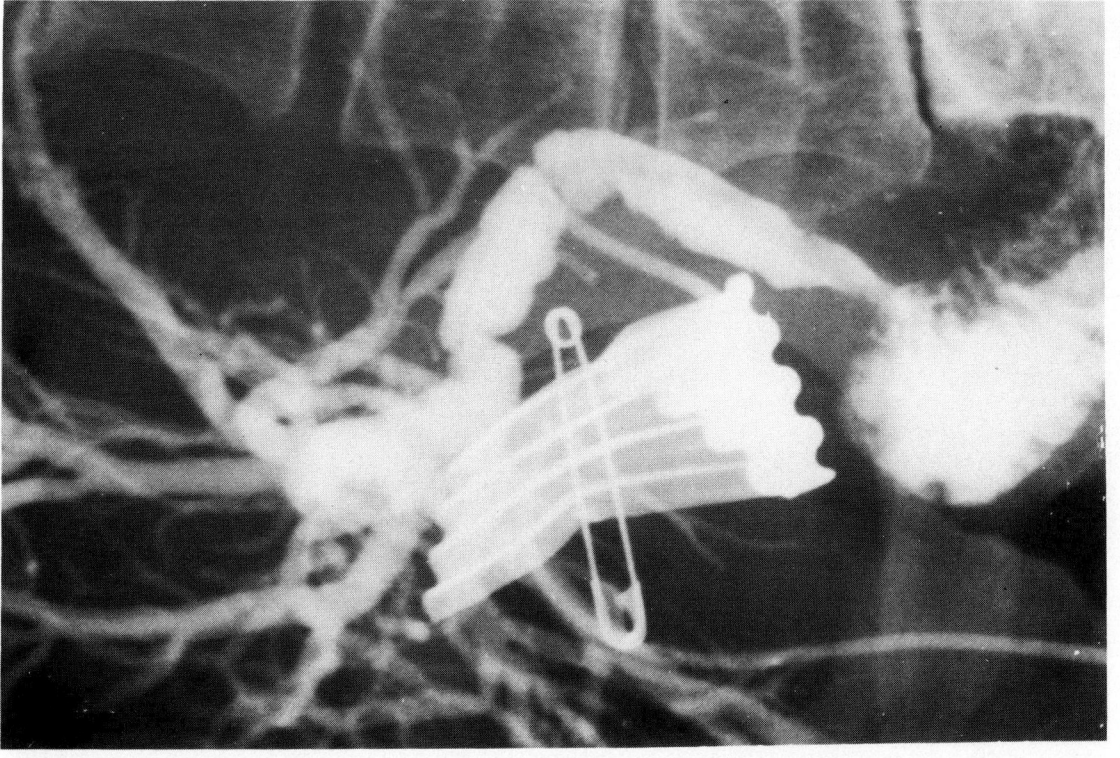

c

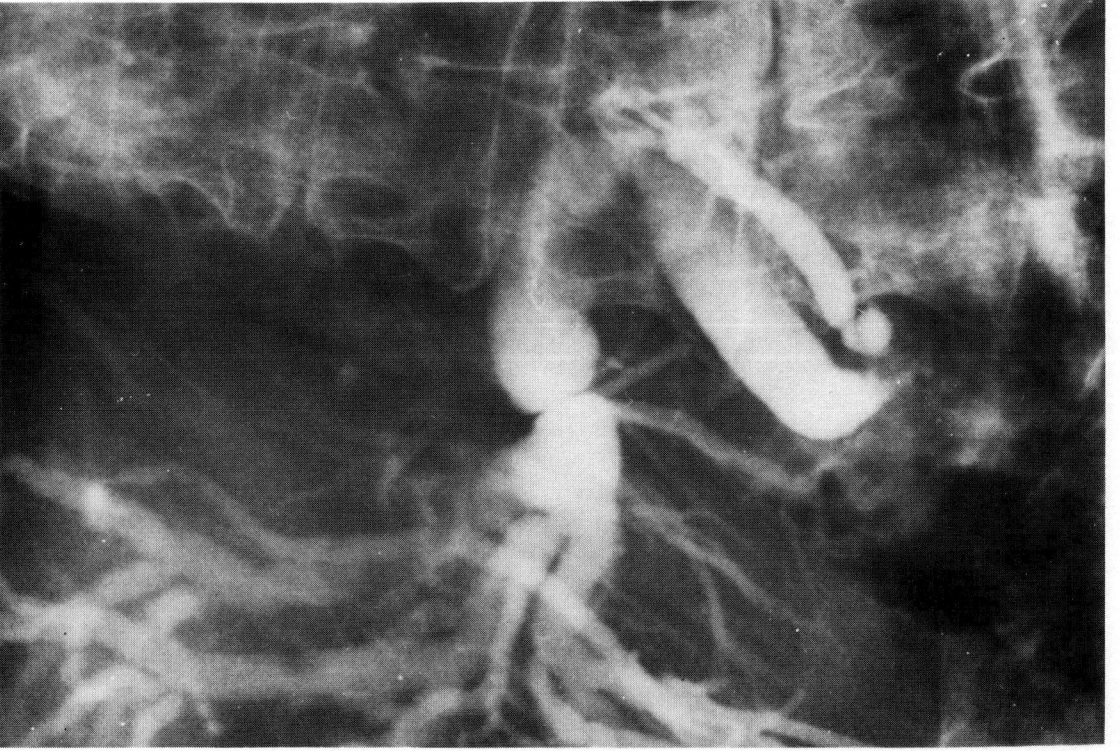

d

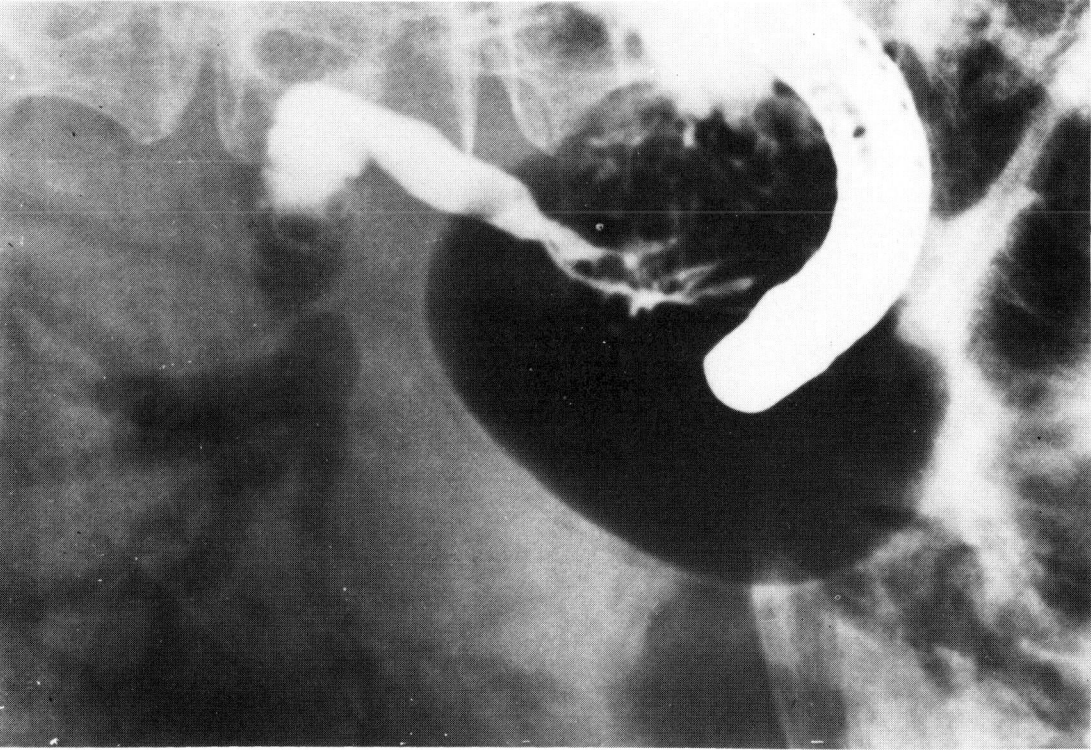

f

Fig. 19.47 (continued) (c) ERCP showing dilated common bile duct (12 mm), pancreas divisum with chronic pancreatitis and no drainage 30 min after ERCP (14.6.80). (d) Post-operative T-tube cholangiogram following surgical sphincteroplasty for confirmed papillary stenosis with common bile duct 11 mm diameter (18.8.80). (e) Follow up ERCP 5 months later showing 8 mm common bile duct containing air, wide sphincteroplasty and air in upper biliary tract. Patient asymptomatic (26.1.81). (f) ERCP (3.3.82) showing 17 mm common bile duct and no drainage at 30 min. Endoscopic sphincter performed. (g), (h): overleaf.

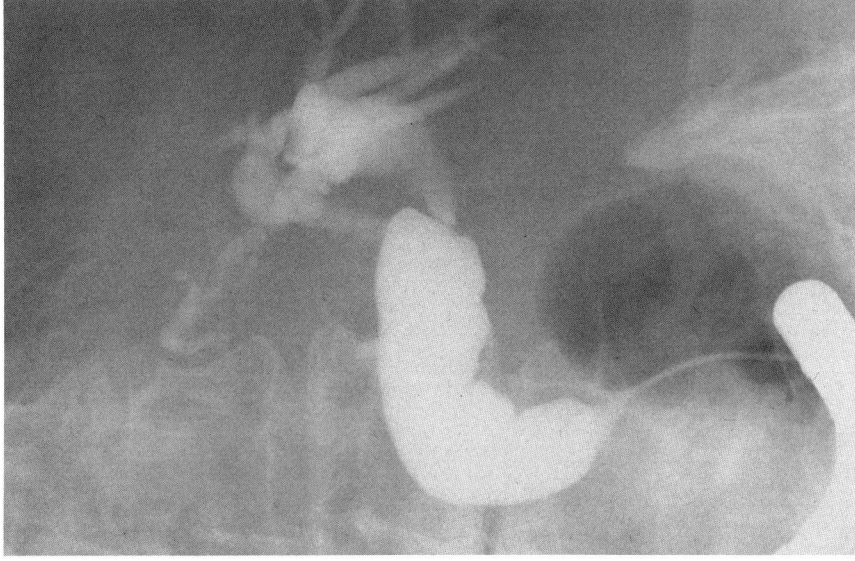

e

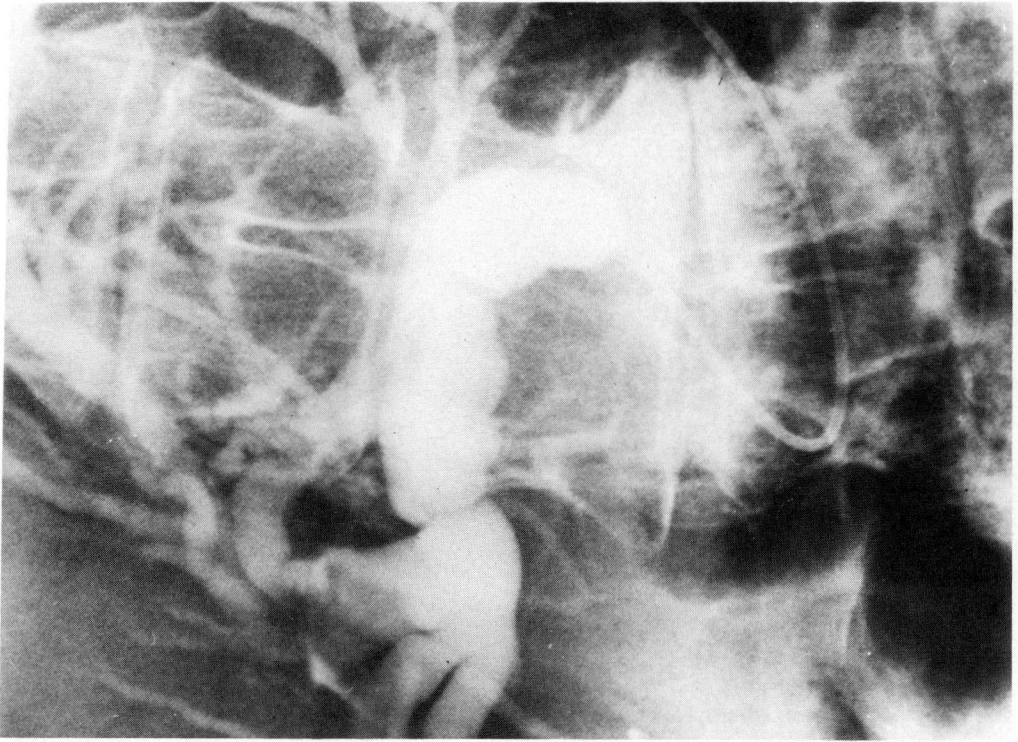

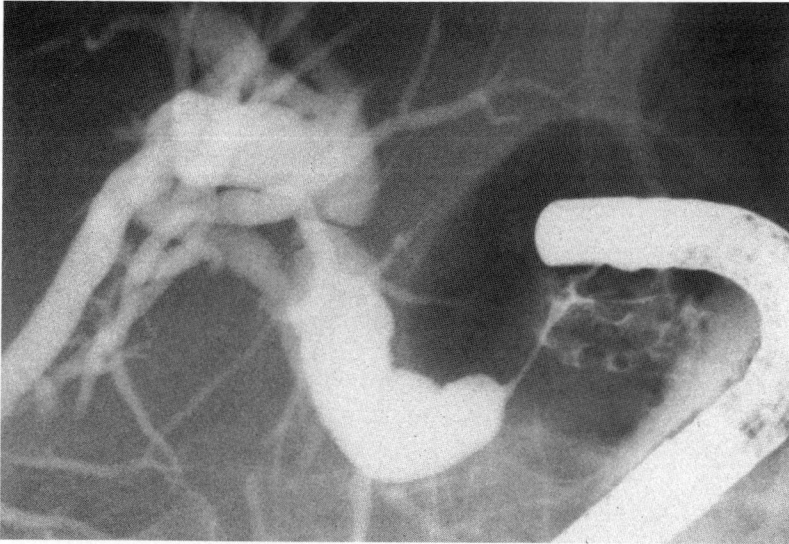

Fig. 19.47 (continued) (g) ERCP for further pain showing common bile duct with long papillary stricture and closed sphincterotomy (8.9.82). (h) Same ERCP with nasobiliary catheter inserted. Treated by choledochoduodenostomy (9.9.82).

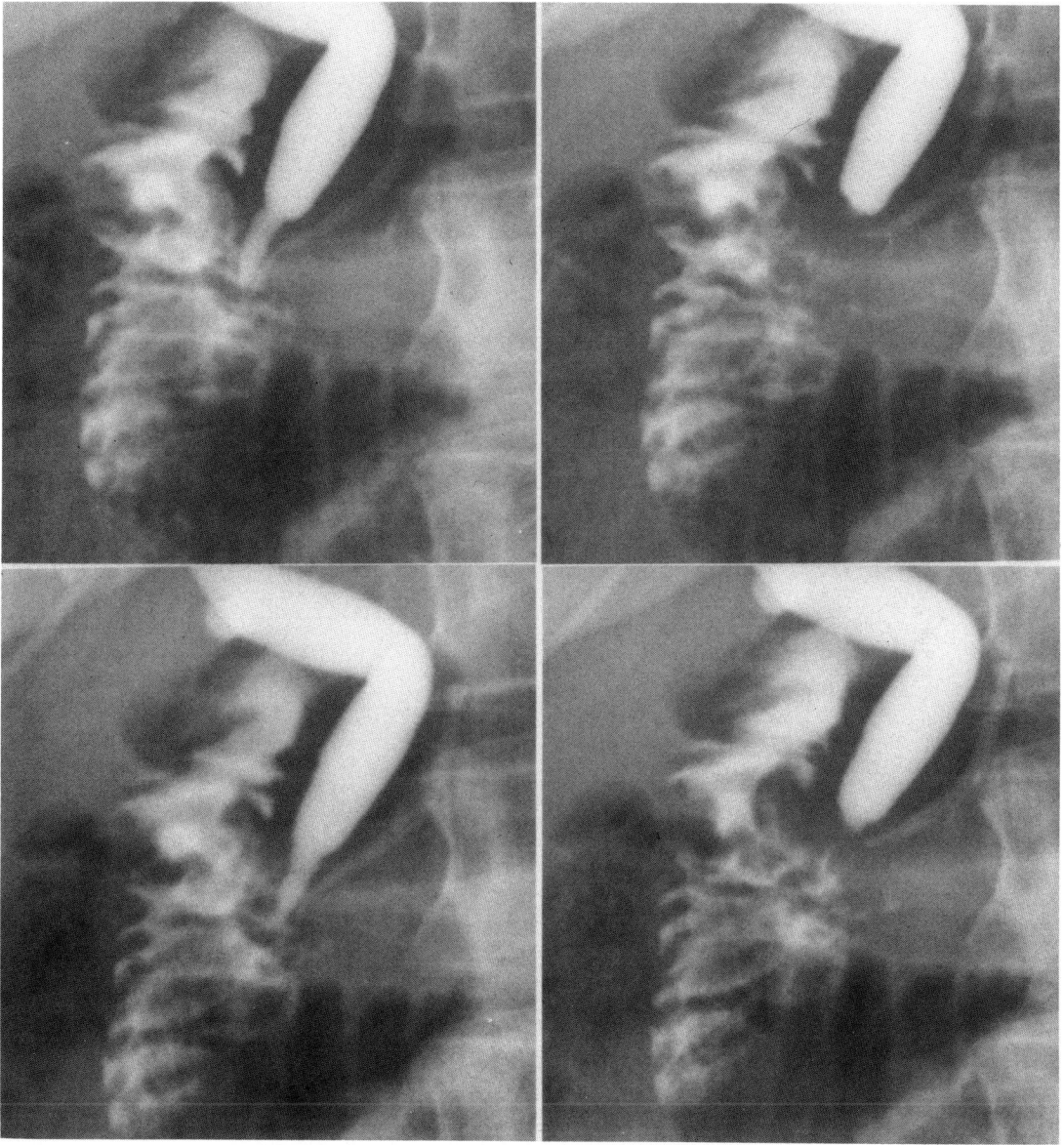

a

Fig. 19.48 (a) Post-ERCP sequence to demonstrate normal bile duct sphincter activity through two cycles of opening and closing. (b)–(f): continued overleaf.

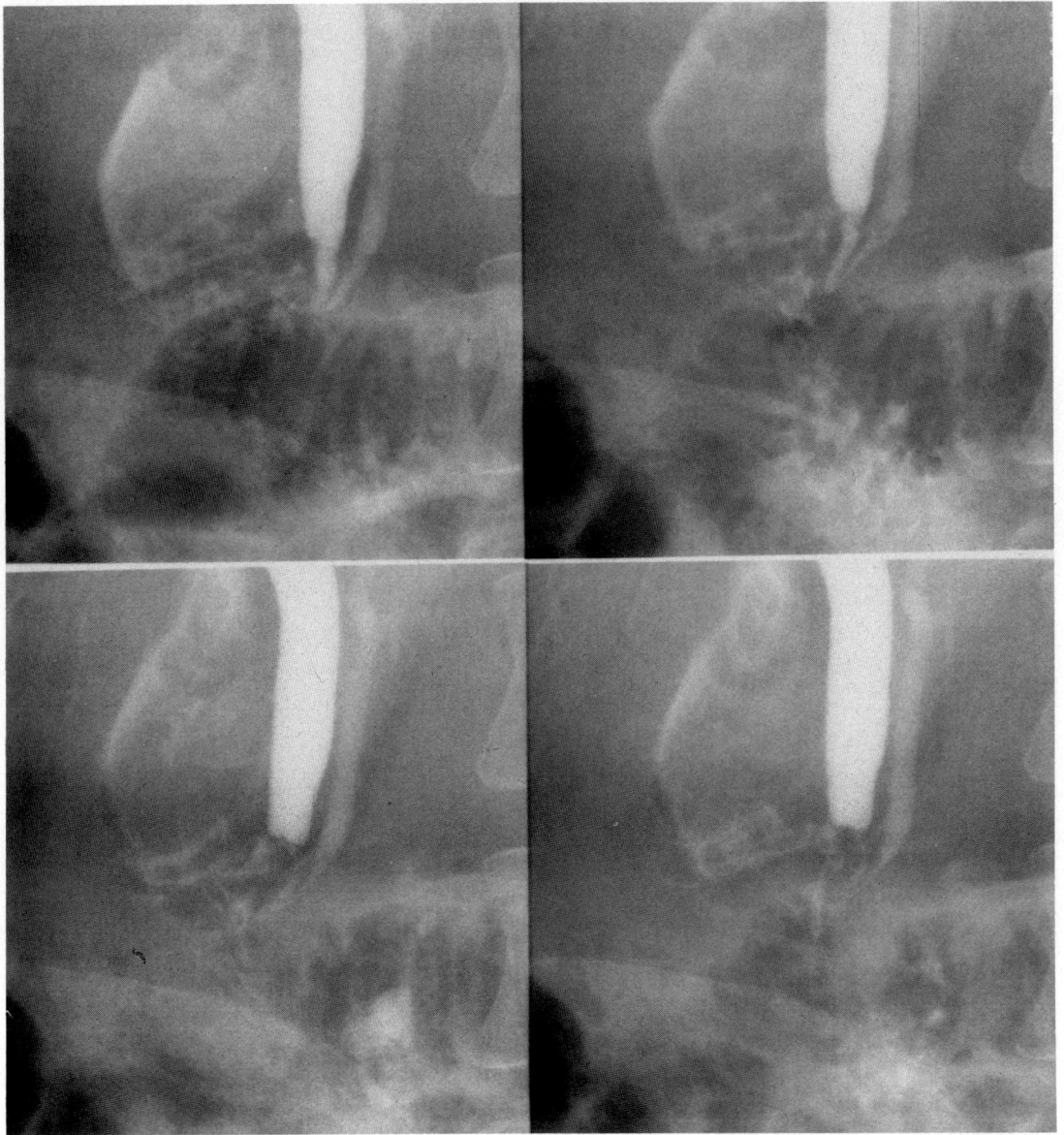

b

Fig. 19.48(continued)   (b) Bile duct and pancreatic duct sphincters through one cycle from open to closed.

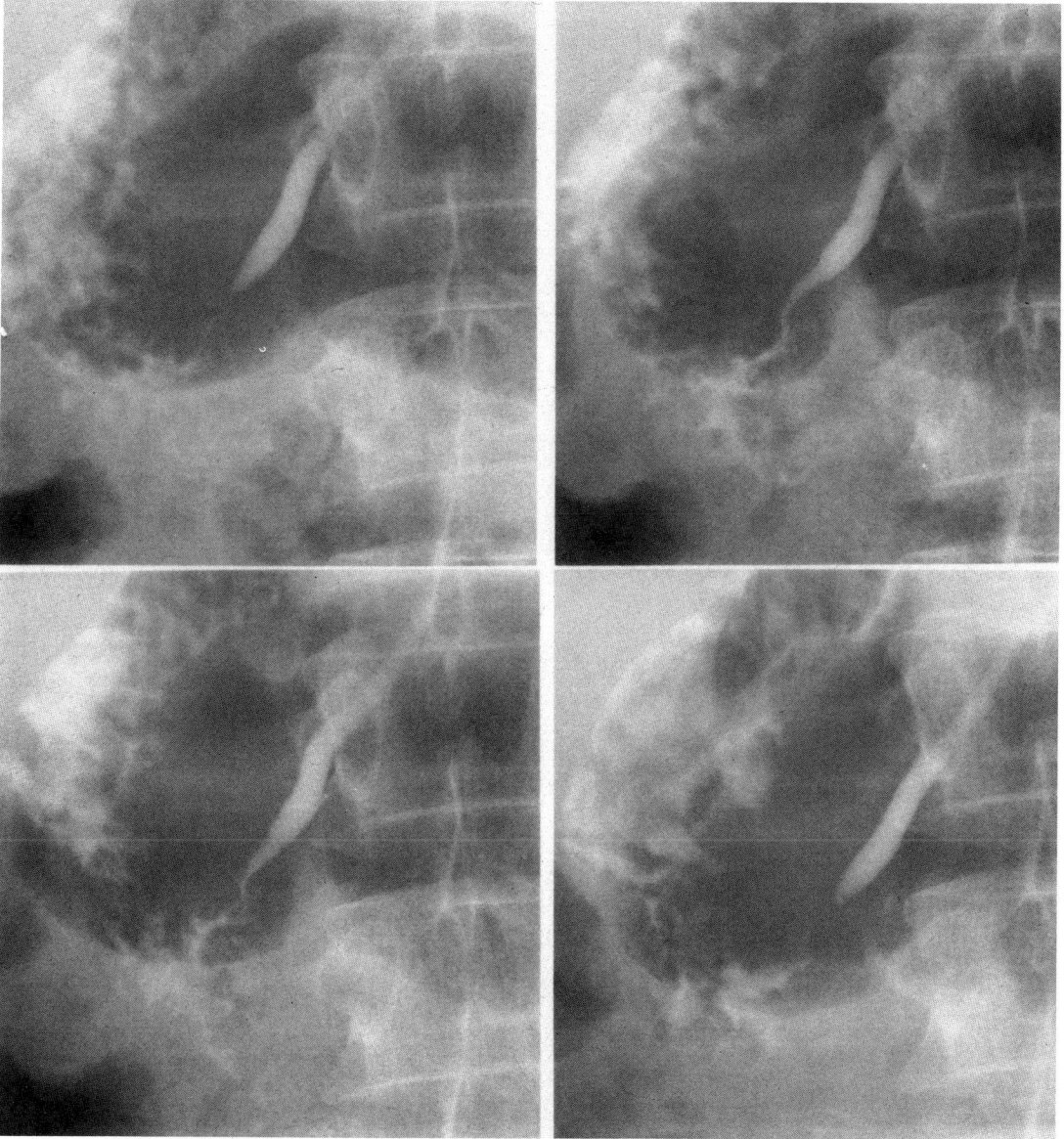

c

Fig. 19.48(continued) (c) Pancreatic duct sphincter through two cycles of opening and closing. (d)–(f): continued overleaf.

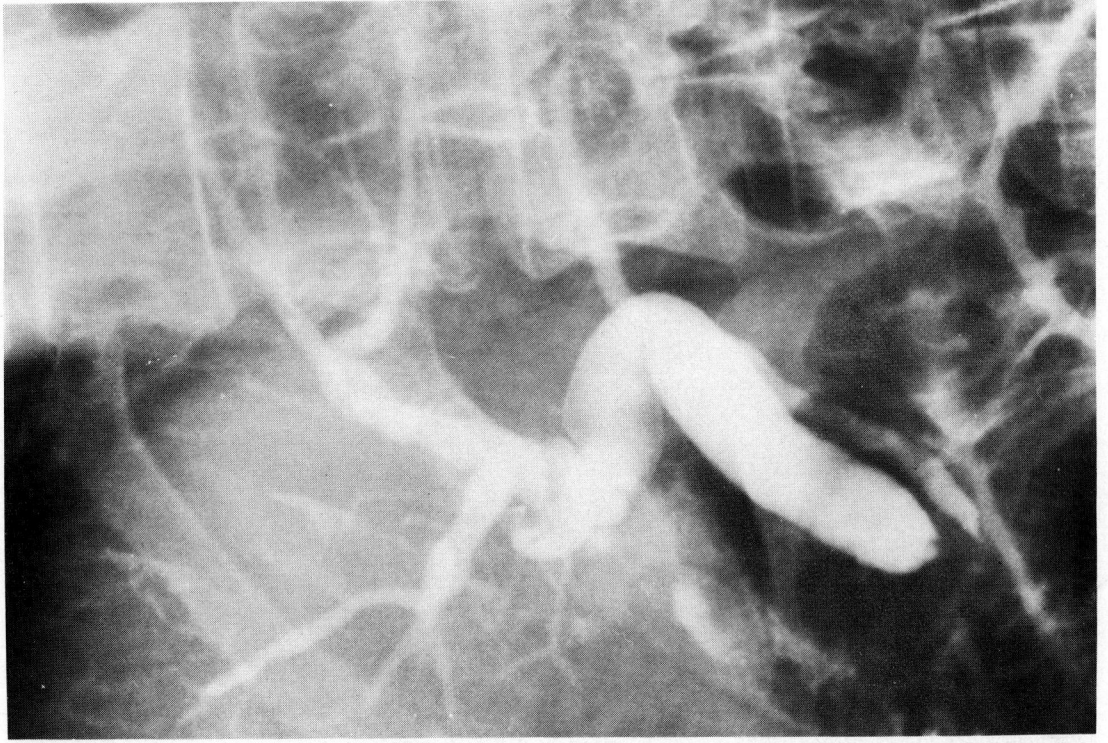

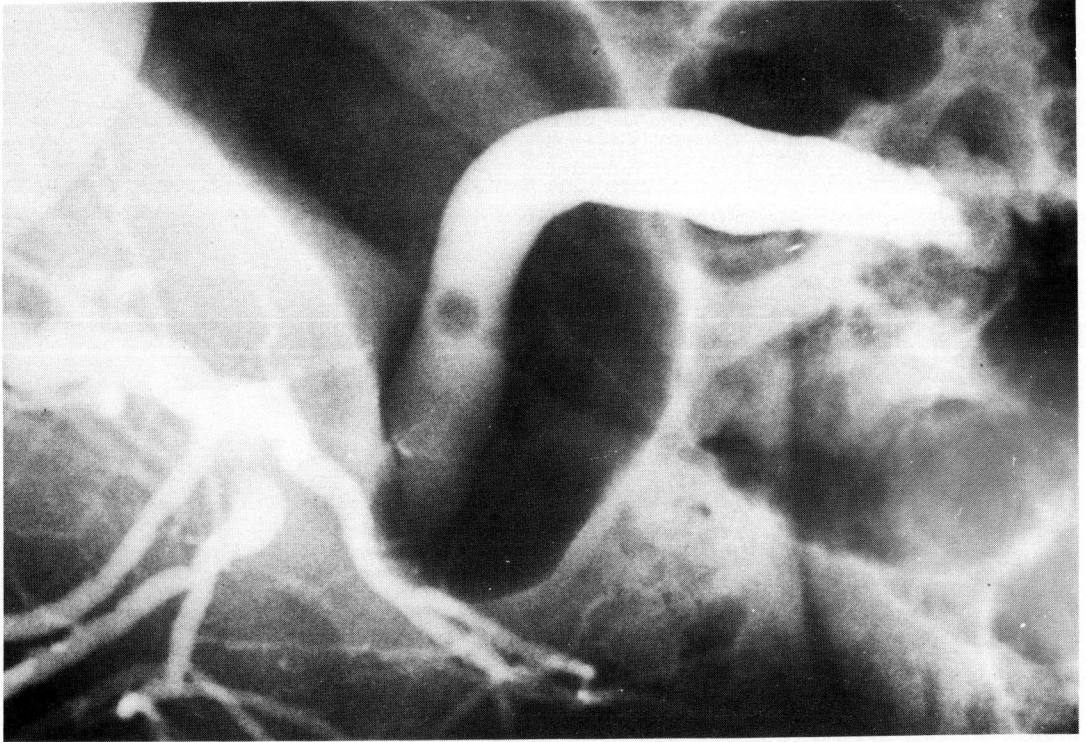

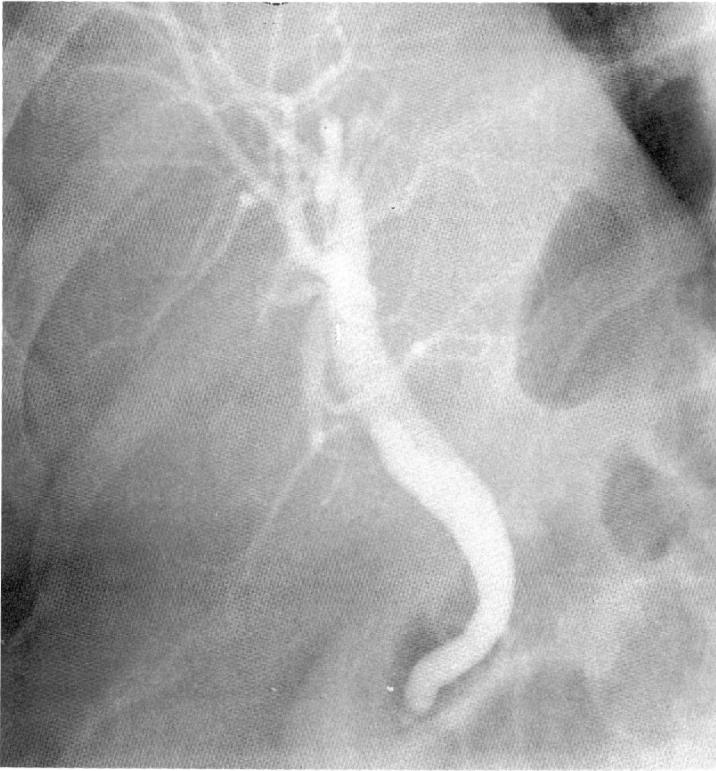

Fig. 19.48 (continued) (d) 30 min after ERCP in papillary stenosis showing dilated common bile duct (13 mm) containing a stone and no drainage or sphincter activity. (e) Papillary stenosis showing dilated common bile duct (11 mm) and normal pancreatic duct but no drainage or sphincter activity. (f) Papillary stenosis showing dilated common hepatic duct (12 mm) and no drainage or sphincter activity.

f

The ERCP criteria suggested for the diagnosis of papillary stenosis are shown in Table 19.13; at least three should be present.

Table 19.13   ERCP diagnosis of papillary stenosis

1 Difficulty in papillary cannulation with 1.7 mm ERCP catheter
2 Dilatation of common bile duct to 10 mm or greater and pancreatic duct to 5 mm or greater
3 Delayed drainage of contrast medium to 30 minutes or more following ERCP
4 Absence of normal phasic activity of sphincteric mechanism in absence of drug effects
5 Reproduction of patient's symptoms on common bile duct contrast injection

ENDOSCOPIC MANOMETRY

The technique of endoscopic manometry using perfused catheters has been described from many centres[11] and pressure gradients have been demonstrated between common bile duct, pancreatic duct and duodenum. On pull-through recordings through the papilla a phasic wave-form has been seen consistently and is thought to represent sphincteric activity.

In papillary stenosis common bile duct–duodenal gradients are elevated compared with controls (Table 19.14).[1, 10, 20, 29] Only Carr-Locke and Gregg[10] reported an increased pancreatic duct–duodenal gradient. Hagenmuller et al.[20] suggest that papillary stenosis is present if common bile duct pressure exceeds 15 cm of water and Rosch et al.[29] 15 mmHg. Bar-Meir et al.[1] found too much overlap with normal controls and Carr-Locke and Gregg[10] found 75% of 44 patients with papillary stenosis had common bile duct pressures above 9.6 mmHg (mean $\pm$ 2 SD for asymptomatic postcholecystectomy controls) but only 40% had pancreatic duct pressures greater than 18.5 mmHg (mean + 2 SD for normal controls). A normal limit of 45 mmHg for basal sphincter of Oddi pressures has been suggested.[1] Carr-Locke and Gregg[10] found elevated peak and trough (basal) phasic pancreatic duct sphincter and bile duct sphincter pressures compared with normal controls (Table 19.14) and they, and Bar-Meir et al.,[1] have used these criteria to identify patients with stenosis who might benefit from sphincterotomy.

In addition Carr-Locke and Gregg[10] noticed two types of endoscopic manometry recordings

Table 19.14   Endoscopic manometry findings in papillary stenosis.

Authors	Common bile duct-duodenal gradient (mm Hg)[a]	Pancreatic duct-duodenal gradient (mm Hg)	Sphincter pressures (mmHg)	
Hagenmuller *et al.*[20]	18.1 ± 8.0 (PS) 4.6 ± 2.8 (N)	—	—	—
Rosch *et al.*[29]	17.8 (PS) 8.8 ± 2.1 (N)	—	—	—
Bar-Meir *et al.*[1]	19 ± 2 (PS) 12 ± 1 (N)	12 ± 1 (PS) 15 ± 1 (N)	*Basal* 62 ± 9 (PS) 34 ± 1 (N) ($P < 0.01$)	*Amplitude* 213 ± 21 (PS) 134 ± 10 (N) ($P < 0.01$)
Carr-Locke and Gregg[10]	9.9 ± 4 (PS) 2.0 ± 1.7 (N) ($P < 0.001$) 6.0 ± 1.8 (APC) ($P < 0.05$)	18.9 ± 6.8 (PS) 10.7 ± 3.9 (N) ($P < 0.001$)	*Trough* (PDS) 23.5 ± 11.1 (PS) 15.9 ± 6.6 (N) ($P < 0.001$)	*Peak* (PDS) 72.5 ± 21.1 (PS) 47.2 ± 8.4 (N) ($P < 0.001$)
			Trough (BDS) 26.4 ± 14.2 (PS) 13.4 ± 6.2 (N) ($P < 0.001$)	*Peak* (BDS) 67.2 ± 11.9 (PS) 51.2 ± 6.7 (N) ($P < 0.001$)

PS = papillary stenosis; N = normal; APC = asymptomatic postcholecystectomy; PDS = pancreatic duct sphincter; BDS = bile duct sphincter.
[a] 1 mmHg = 133 Pa.

in patients with stenosis (Figure 19.49) one characterized by high amplitude waves with elevated trough pressures and the other by a high pressure zone with little or no phasic activity. These may represent the dyskinetic and fibrotic forms of papillary stenosis.

PATHOGENESIS AND PATHOPHYSIOLOGY

The aetiology of the conditions collectively known as biliary dyskinesia is completely unknown. Examination of cholecystectomy specimens is commonly normal but a variety of chronic inflammatory changes has been seen.[16] Fibrosis and inflammation in and around the cystic duct occur in 60% of patients operated on for cystic duct stenosis[18] and there is a link between the pathology of the hypercontractile type of dyskinesia and the hyperplastic cholecystoses. These changes are variable and do not correlate with the type of dysmotility which suggests that dyskinesia is not secondary to cholecystitis but perhaps induces changes in the gallbladder when relative bile stasis is present.

There are predominantly chronic inflammation and fibrosis in benign papillary stenosis[26] giving rise to a variety of descriptive terms: papillitis, oddis, chronic papillo-odditis, sclerosing

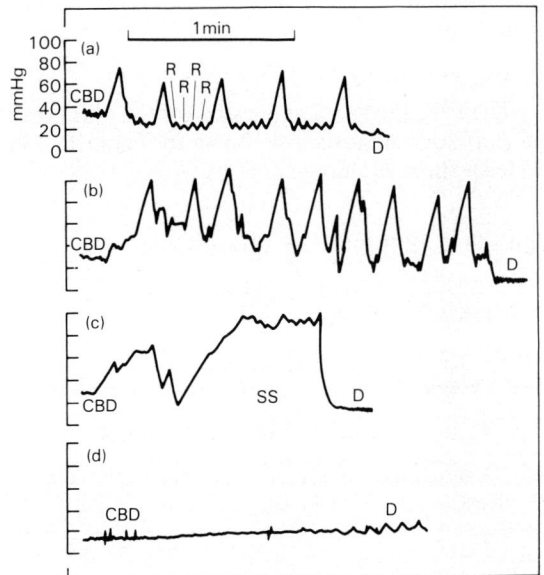

Fig. 19.49 Endoscopic manometry recording from (a) normal subject showing duodenal pressure (D) and bile duct pull-through phasic activity (bile duct sphincter), (b) patient with papillary stenosis showing elevated common bile duct and phasic pressures, (c) papillary stenosis with high non-phasic pressure in presumed stenotic segment (SS), and (d) same patient as (c) after endoscopic sphincterotomy with loss of all phasic activity and common bile duct–duodenal gradient.

choledocho-odditis, papillite icterigeni primitive and enfermedod del coledocho terminal.[30] Stolte *et al.*[33] proposed a sequence of acute papillitis progressing to granulation tissue and chronic papillitis with eventual stenosis as a primary phenomenon or, more commonly, secondary to damage from pancreatic, duodenal or bile duct disease. Papillary fibrosis is associated in almost 90% of patients with present or previous gallbladder or common duct stones.[19, 34] The passage of a stone through the papilla and papillary trauma during surgery may initiate papillitis and lead to stenosis; rarely stenosis occurs primarily without stone disease[28] (Figure 19.50).

TREATMENT

Gallbladder dyskinesia

Patients with gallbladder dyskinesia who are at the most severe end of the symptomatic spectrum should undergo cholecystectomy. Fat restriction and antispasmodic drugs (glyceryl trinitrate, hyoscine, propantheline and mebeverine) are unhelpful. Favourable results are reported in suitably selected patients who have undergone surgery[16] but no controlled trials exist.

Papillary stenosis

Patients with severe symptoms rarely respond to medical therapy (dietary approaches, choleretics, progesterones and antispasmodics) or reassurance and are repeatedly referred for investigation and treatment. Once the diagnosis has been confirmed, operative treatment is indicated and this may be surgical or endoscopic. Surgical sphincterotomy or sphincteroplasty with or without pancreatic sphincteroplasty is the surgical treatment of choice and long-term experience in appropriately selected patients has been good with an operative mortality of 4.5% and good clinical results in 93.3%.[15, 26, 34]

Endoscopic sphincterotomy is the logical treatment in patients diagnosed by ERCP. The technique involved is identical to that used for common duct stones except that a pre-cut papillotomy may be necessary for full insertion of the sphincterotome. The complications of haemorrhage, pancreatitis and perforation are more common in papillary stenosis (8.9%) than for common duct stones (7.5%) and the mortality is 2.2% (18 of 813) compared with 1% (77 of 7583) for stones.[32] Papillary re-stenosis was found in 11.5% of patients; nonetheless 87.4% of these were free of symptoms at the time of follow-up. From a personal experience of 37 endoscopic

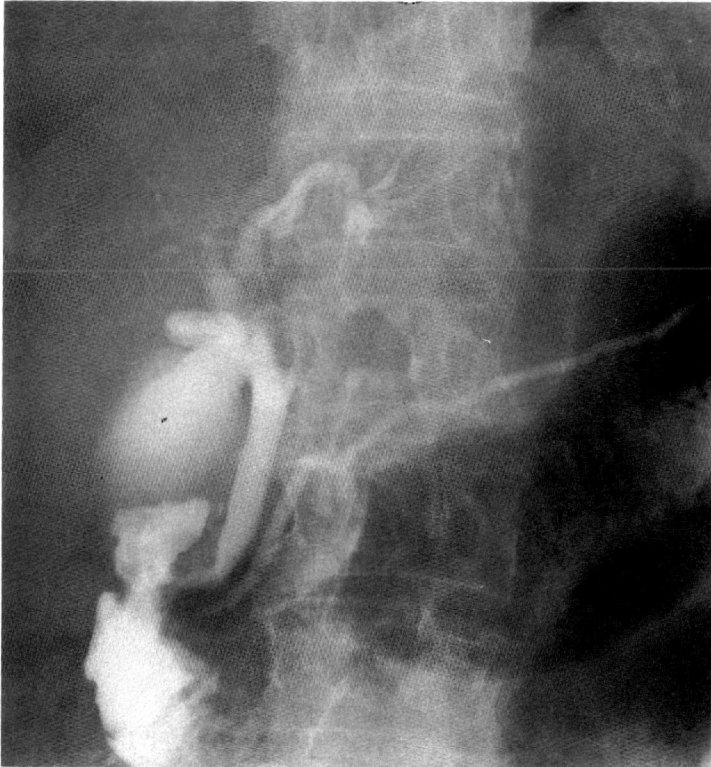

Fig. 19.50 ERCP sequence in a patient with primary papillary stenosis showing: (a) dilated common bile duct (17 mm), normal gallbladder (partly filled), and normal pancreatic duct; (b) & (c) overleaf.

a

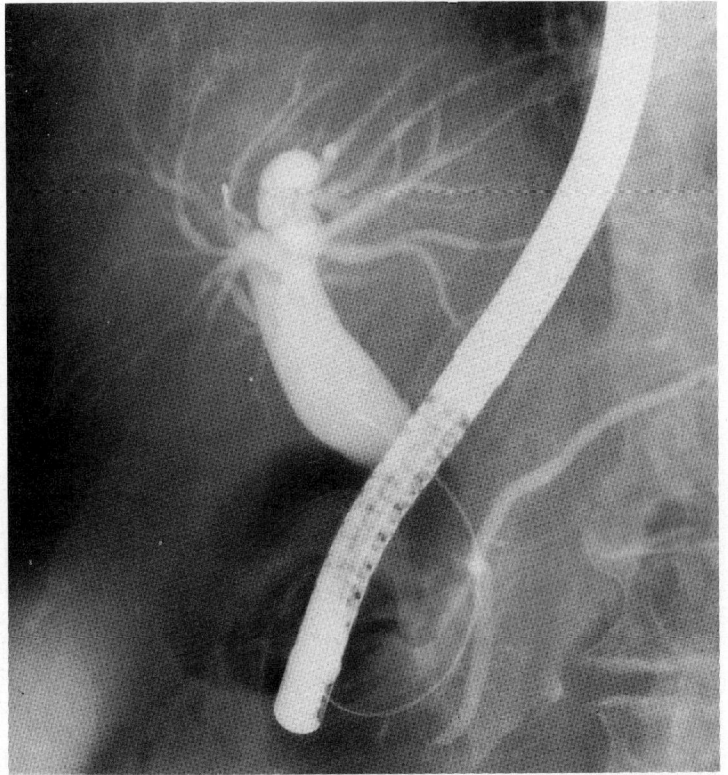

b

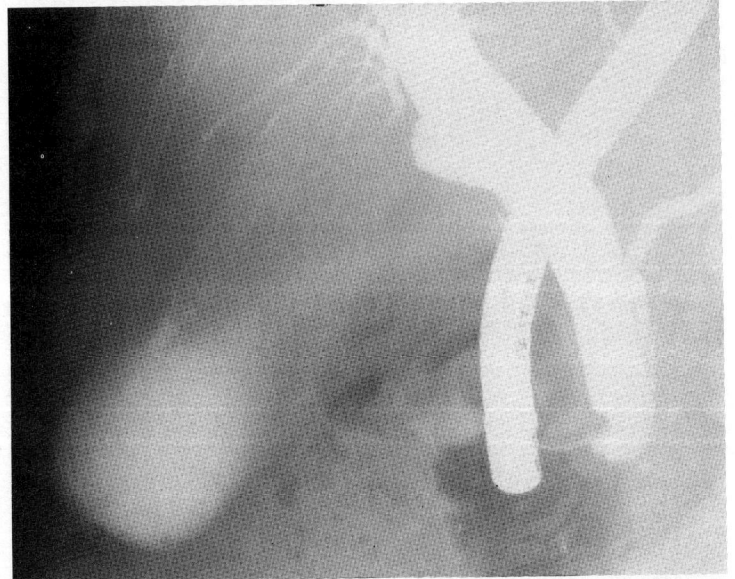

Fig. 19.50(continued) ERCP
sequence in a patient with primary
papillary stenosis showing: (b)
basket passed after endoscopic
sphincterotomy to exclude stones;
(c) immediate postsphincterotomy
diminution in common bile duct
diameter (10 mm) with rapid
drainage of contrast.

c

sphincterotomies for papillary stenosis there
were complications in six (16.2%) compared
with 10% in 319 patients with common duct
stones. These were acute pancreatitis in two
patients, haemorrhage in three, all treated conservatively, and combined haemorrhage and
pancreatitis in another requiring emergency
surgery. There were no deaths and one patient
required surgery six months later for re-stenosis
of the papilla. Six months to five years after the
procedure 33 patients have been rendered free of
pain and one is improved (Figure 19.51).

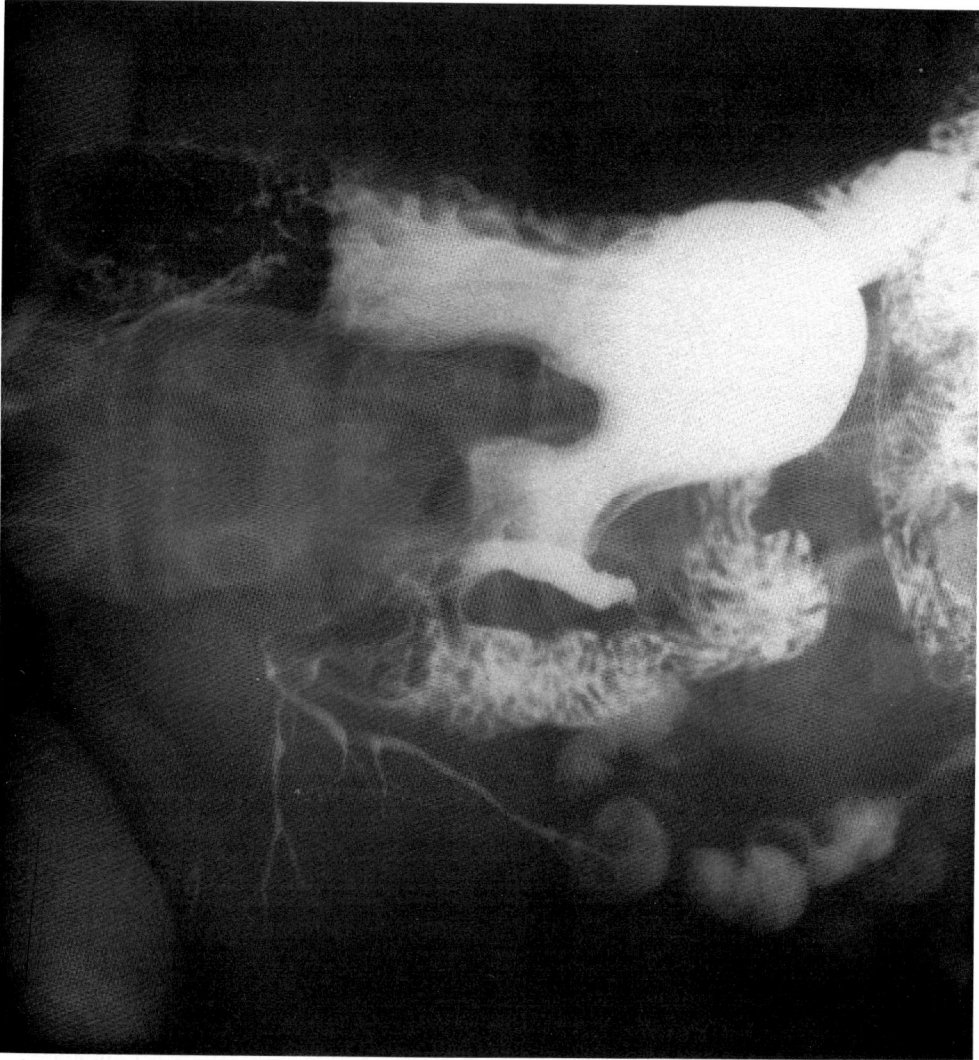

b

a

Fig. 19.51 (a) 30 min post-ERCP in papillary stenosis showing dilated common bile duct (12 mm) and no drainage of contrast. (b) Barium meal in same patient one year later with reflux into common bile duct through patent sphincterotomy.

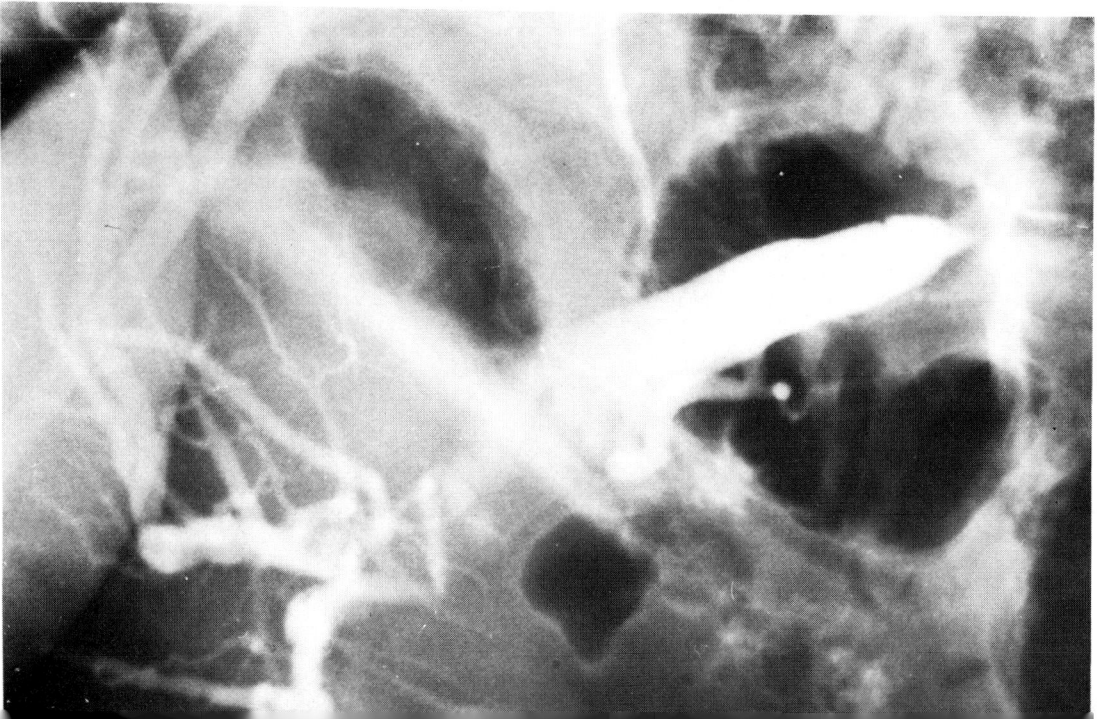

REFERENCES

1 Bar-Meir, S., Geenen, J. E., Hogan, W. J. *et al.* (1979) Biliary and pancreatic duct pressures measured by ERCP manometry in patients with suspected papillary stenosis. *Digestive Diseases and Sciences*, **24**, 209–213.

2 Belsito, A. A., Marta, J. B., Cramer, G. G. & Dickinson, P. D. (1977) Measurement of biliary tract size and drainage time. *Radiology*, **122**, 65–69.

3 Berk, R. N. (1977) Cholecystokinin cholecystography in the diagnosis of chronic acalculous cholecystitis and biliary dyskinesia. *Gastrointestinal Radiology*, **1**, 325–330.

4 Best, R. R. & Hicken, N. F. (1936) Cholangiographic demonstration of biliary dyssynergia. *Journal of the American Medical Association*, **107**, 1615–1620.

5 Boyden, E. A. (1957) The anatomy of the choledochoduodenal junction in man. *Surgery, Gynecology and Obstetrics*, **104**, 641–652.

6 Caroli, J. (1946) La Radiomanometrie biliare. *Semaine Hopital Paris*, **21**, 1278–1282.

7 Caroli, J. & Hepp, J. (1948) La coudure douloureuse intermitente du col de la vesicule – variete frequente des dyskinesies biliaires pures – demonstration radiomanometrique. *Semaine Hopital Paris*, **24**, 526–532.

8 Caroli, J., Porcher, P., Pequignot, G. & Delattre, M. (1960) Contribution of cineradiography to study the function of human biliary tract. *American Journal of Digestive Diseases*, **5**, 677–696.

9 Carr-Locke, D. L. & Gregg, J. A. (1984) Does the morphine prostigmine test predict the presence of papillary stenosis (in preparation).

10 Carr-Locke, D. L. & Gregg, J. A. (1979) Endoscopic manometry of biliary and pancreatic sphincters. Findings in biliary and pancreatic disease and after sphincter surgery. *American Journal of Gastroenterology*, **72**, 333.

11 Carr-Locke, D. L. & Gregg, J. A. (1981) Endoscopic manometry of pancreatic and biliary sphincter zones in man. Basal results in healthy volunteers. *Digestive Diseases and Sciences*, **26**, 7–15.

12 Cotton, P. B. (1977) Progress report ERCP. *Gut*, **18**, 316–341.

13 Del Valle, D. & Donovan, R. D. (1926) Odditis, esclero-retractil. *Archivos Argentinos de Engermedades del Aparato Digestivo y de la Nutricion*, **1**, 605–615.

14 Dudfield Rose, J. (1959) Serial cholecystography – a means of pre-operative diagnosis of biliary dyskinesia. *Archives of Surgery*, **78**, 56–66.

15 Farthmann, E. H., Soehendra, M. & Schreiber, H. W. (1978) Results of surgical papillotomy. In *Endoscopic Sphincterotomy of the Papilla of Vater* (Ed.) Demling, L. & Classen, M. pp. 31–35. Stuttgart: Georg Thieme.

16 Freeman, J. B., Cohen, W. N. & DenBesten, L. (1975) Cholecystokinin cholangiography and analysis of duodenal bile in the investigation of pain in the right upper quadrant of the abdomen without gallstones. *Surgery, Gynecology and Obstetrics*, **141**, 371–376.

17 Geenen, J. E. (1982) New diagnostic and treatment modalities involving endoscopic retrograde cholangiopancreatography and esophagogastroduodenoscopy. *Scandinavian Journal of Gastroenterology*, **17** (supplement 77), 93–106.

18 Goldstein, F., Grunt, R. & Margulies, M. (1974) Cholecystokinin cholecystography in the differential diagnosis of acalculous gallbladder disease. *Digestive Diseases*, **19**, 835–849.

19 Gregg, J. A., Clark, G., Barr, C. *et al.* (1980) Post-cholecystectomy syndrome and its association with ampullary stenosis. *American Journal of Surgery*, **139**, 374–378.

20 Hagenmuller, F., Ossenberg, F. W. & Classen, M. (1977) Duodenoscopic manometry of the common bile duct. In *The Sphincter of Oddi. Proceedings of Third Gastroenterological Symposium, Nice, 1976.* pp. 72–76. Basel: Karger.

21 Hess, W. (1978) Manometry and radiography in the biliary system during surgery. In *Endoscopic Sphincterotomy of the Papilla of Vater*. (Ed.) Demling, L. and Classen, M. pp. 19–23. Stuttgart: Georg Thieme.

22 Ivy, A. C. (1934) Biliary dyskinesia. *Annals of Internal Medicine*, **8**, 115–122.

23 Leonard, P. & Massion, J. (1965) L'Apport pre-operatoire du medecin de l'indication de la sphincterotomie. *Reviews of International Hepatology*, **15**, 967–983.

24 Logiudice, J. A., Geenen, J. E., Hogan, W. J. & Dodds, W. J. (1979) Efficacy of the morphine-prostigmine test for evaluating patients with suspected papillary stenosis. *Digestive Diseases and Sciences*, **24**, 455–458.

25 Mirizzi, P. L. (1932) La colangiografia durante las operaciones de la vias biliares. *Boletin Sociedad de Cirugia la Plata*, **16**, 1325.

26 Nardi, G. L. & Acosta, J. M. (1966) Papillitis as a cause of pancreatitis and abdominal pain. Role of evocative test, operative pancreatography and histologic evaluation. *Annals of Surgery*, **164**, 611–621.

27 Oddi, R. (1887) D'une disposition sphincter speciale de l'ouverture du canal choledoque. *Archives Italiennes de Biologie*, **8**, 317–322.

28 Peel, A. L. G. & Thompson, H. H. (1981) The biliary sphincter. In *Alimentary Sphincters and their Disorders* (Ed.) Thomas, P. A. & Mann, C. V. p. 153. London: Macmillan.

29 Rosch, W., Coch, H. & Demling, L. (1976) Manometric studies during ERCP and endoscopic papillotomy. *Endoscopy*, **8**, 30–33.

30 Schein, C. J. (1978) Choledochoduodenal junctional stenosis. In *Post Cholecystectomy Syndromes. A Clinical Approach to Etiology, Diagnosis and Management.* pp. 119–127. New York: Harper & Row.

31 Seifert, E., Gail, K. & Weismuller, J. (1982) Langzeitresultate nach endoskopischer Sphinkterotomie. *Deutsche medizinische Wochenschrift*, **107**, 610–614.

32 Siegel, J. H. (1979) Endoscopic management of choledocholithiasis and papillary stenosis. *Surgery, Gynecology and Obstetrics*, **148**, 747–752.

33 Stolte, M., Becker, V., Assmus, K. D. & Trommsdorff, L. (1978) Pathological anatomy of the papilla of Vater. In *Endoscopic Sphincterotomy of the Papilla of Vater* (Ed.) Demling, L. & Classon, M. Stuttgart: Georg Thieme.

34 Tondelli, P., Gyr, K., Stalder, G. A. & Allgower, M. (1979) The post-cholecystectomy syndrome. *Clinics in Gastroenterology*, **8**, 487–505.

35 White, T. T., Waisman, H., Hopton, D. & Kavlie, H. (1972) Radiomanometry, flow rates and cholangiography in the evaluation of common bile disease. A study of 220 cases. *American Journal of Surgery*, **123**, 73–79.

36 Yvergneaux, J. P., Bauwens, E., Van Outryve, L. & Yvergneaux, E. (1977) Benign stenosis of the papilla of Vater. Diagnosis of 119 cases with conventional and selective low radiomanometry. *Acta Chirurgica Belgique*, **6**, 523–532.

37 Zimmon, D. S., Ferrara, T. P. & Clemetts, A. R. (1978) Radiology of papilla of Vater stenosis. *Gastrointestinal Radiology*, **3**, 343–348.

LATE PROBLEMS AFTER CHOLECYSTECTOMY

Although cholecystectomy is regarded as a highly successful operation, symptoms persist or recur in many patients. Hunt[10] found only three out of four patients symptom free after cholecystectomy and others report a figure as low as 50%. Problems are usually mild, although a minority are disabling or even potentially fatal. The term postcholecystectomy syndrome is best avoided as there is no evidence that this is an entity.[2] Immediate postoperative complications are not discussed in this section.

Clinical features

The predominant clinical feature is pain, sometimes accompanied by jaundice, with fever on occasion. Symptoms are similar to or identical with those preceding surgery.

Pain is usually situated in the epigastrium or right hypochondrium, and sometimes radiates to the back or shoulders, especially on the right. It may be related to meals or occur at night. There are often associated nausea, heartburn and flatulence. Vomiting may occur and the onset can be marked with diarrhoea. There may be transient jaundice but, if due to obstruction of the extrahepatic bile ducts, it can become deep, with pruritus, pale stools and dark urine and is sometimes complicated by fever and rigors. When jaundice occurs, the cause can be assigned to the hepato-biliary system with confidence.

Abdominal examination is usually normal. Epigastric and right subcostal tenderness is present in the acute situation, but does not help to define the exact cause. Abnormal liver function tests are sometimes discovered incidentally and may be attributed to a previous cholecystectomy.

Aetiology

Although postcholecystectomy symptoms often show a similar pattern, they can result from a wide variety of causes many of which are extrabiliary. Occasionally no organic disease is present as the patient's original symptoms were due to non-organic disease.

INITIAL DIAGNOSIS INCORRECT

Cholecystectomy may have been performed inappropriately for extrabiliary problems. 'Silent' gallstones often co-exist with reflux oesophagitis, peptic ulceration, the irritable bowel syndrome and diverticular disease of the colon which may have been the true cause of the symptoms. Angina pectoris can cause similar pain related to meals as well as exercise. Pain from the right kidney in the 'anterior renal area' is identical to that referred from the gallbladder to the right hypochondrium. Other causes of referred pain include spinal disease and conditions of the lower part of the chest on the right. The discovery of gallstones, unless clinically typical in every way, should prompt an effort to exclude other diagnoses before ascribing the symptoms to the gallstones.

EXTRAHEPATIC BILIARY TRACT DISEASE

Disease of the bile ducts may be (a) *residual* – missed, not corrected during, or resulting from the original cholecystectomy, or (b) *recurrent* – appearing sometimes years later, following an immediately satisfactory postoperative course.

These conditions include calculi, stricture, fistula and carcinoma. The incidence of *stones* occurring in the common duct after cholecystectomy varies from 0.26[4] to 22%[5] (Figure 19.52). An average figure is probably 5%, and the incidence is higher where the common duct has been explored than in simple cholecystectomy.[9] Stones can form in a dilated common duct after cholecystectomy, but this is uncommon and probably does not happen in ducts of normal calibre. Retained stones remain asymptomatic in a minority of patients; in most patients they are a serious cause of trouble with the acute hazard of cholangitis or the chronic complication of biliary cirrhosis.[9] Postcholecystectomy *biliary strictures* are either traumatic or inflammatory. The former group is commoner, resulting from an operative error (Figure 19.53). This may be due to a congenital anomaly at the junction of the cystic and common ducts, or clamping the common bile duct when pulling on a short cystic duct (Figure 19.54), or ligating the common hepatic duct in mistake for the cystic duct, or due to an inflamed Hartmann's pouch adherent to the main duct. Although complete biliary obstruction may take years to develop, jaundice and liver damage inevitably ensue, and the result is a disaster which is technically difficult to resolve surgically. Inflammatory strictures occur at the lower end of the common bile duct, and are the sequelae of stones and infection. A stone impacted here will often cause mucosal ulceration with ensuing contracture of

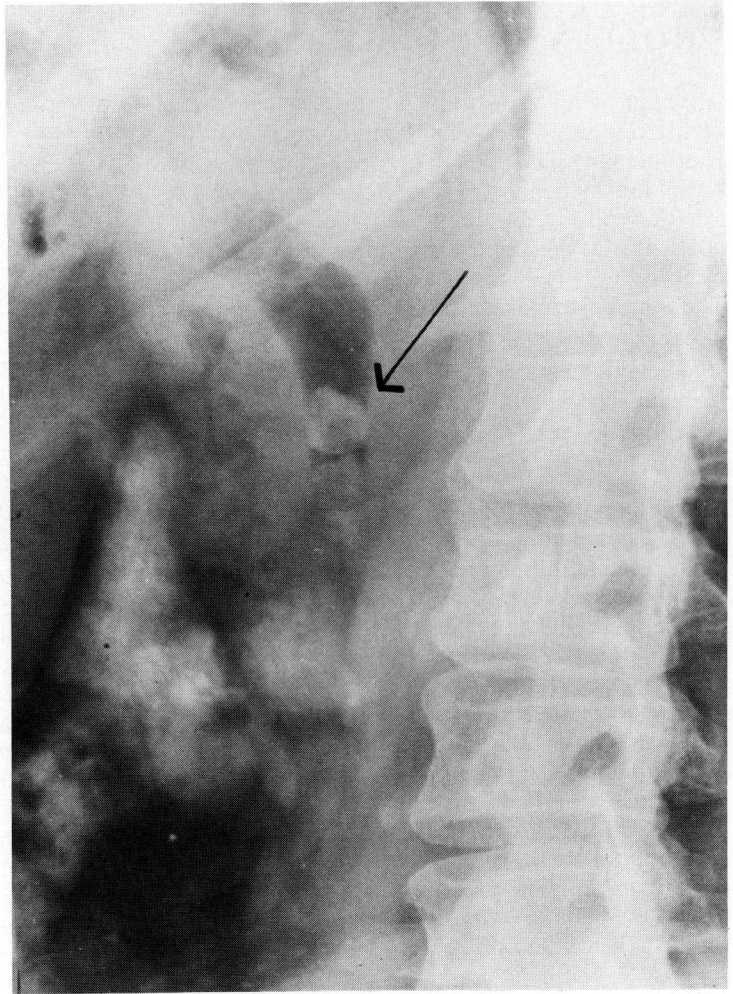

Fig. 19.52 Radiograph showing stones in air-filled common bile duct ten years after cholecystectomy, with a choledochoduodenal fistula (arrowed).

the common duct sphincter. This type of stricture is commonly 1 cm in length and quite distinct from papillary stenosis of the ampulla. A less common complication is the development of a *fistula* between the lower third of the common bile duct and the wall of the duodenum due to pressure necrosis from a large retained stone. Spontaneous resolution of an attack of jaundice and cholangitis may result; further treatment may not be needed. *Carcinoma* of the head of pancreas or lower end of the bile duct appearing after cholecystectomy must be considered as a possible cause of symptoms. A mass of doubtful aetiology in the head of pancreas at the initial procedure usually in the presence of jaundice should not be dismissed as inflammatory, but exact diagnosis ascertained by transduodenal thin needle aspiration cytology, or 'Trucut' needle biopsy.

STUMP AND SUMP SYNDROMES

Most surgeons leave a cystic duct remnant of about 2 cm length. This is because the cystic duct often enters the common duct at a level lower than that suggested from the external appearance, and common bile and cystic ducts share a wall at this point (Figure 19.55). The stump has been blamed for postcholecystectomy symptoms, but this is unlikely, unless it contains a stone. Millbourn[14] described 21 operations performed for a stump remnant and causes for the symptoms other than the stump were found in every case. The existence of a cystic stump syndrome has not been established.

Sump syndrome
Following side-to-side choledochoduodenostomy the lower end of the common bile duct occasionally becomes a poorly draining sump.

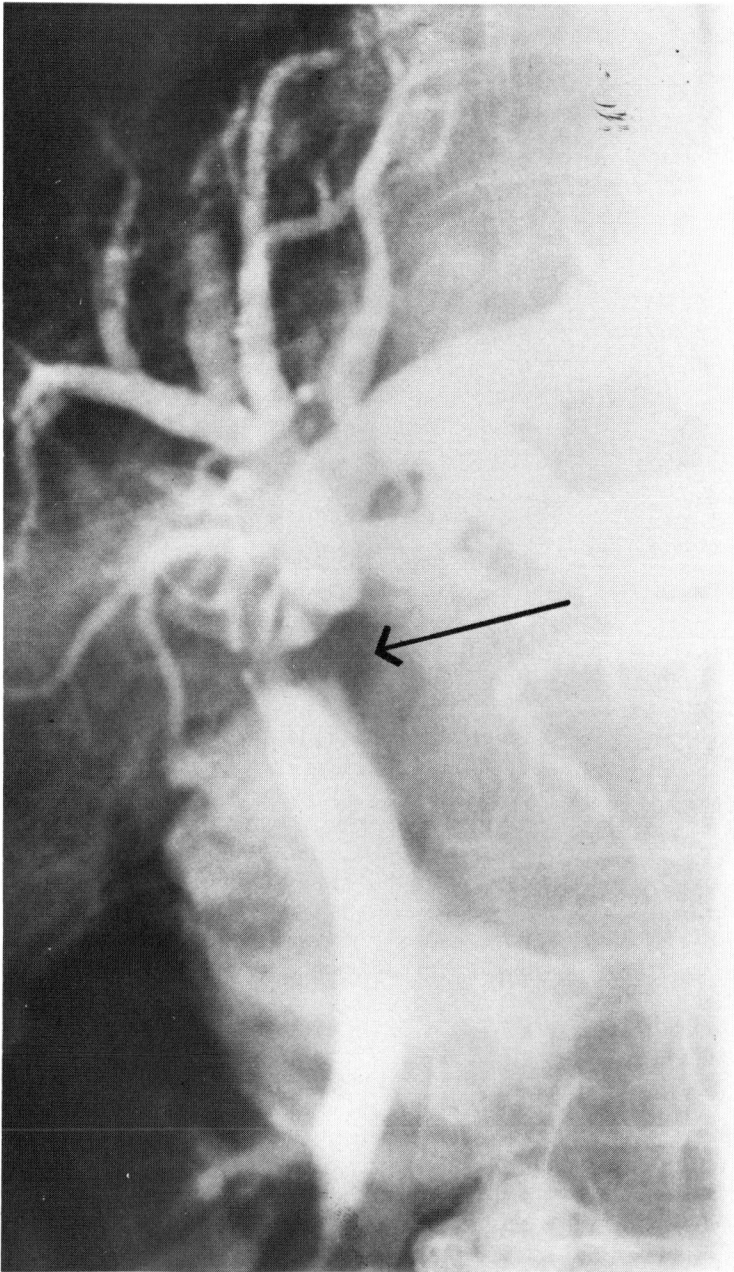

Fig. 19.53 Percutaneous transhepatic cholangiogram showing high hepatic duct stricture (arrowed).

Residual gall stones may be present and food debris is liable to collect. Pancreatitis or cholangitis can result, especially if the anastomosis is smaller than the usually recommended 2 cm. Treatment is either by duodenoscopic sphincterotomy to allow free drainage of the lower end of the duct or alternatively by surgical reconstruction.

BILIARY DYSKINESIA

This produces symptoms by disordered neuromuscular motility interfering with the passage of bile from the common duct into the duodenum, and is described elsewhere in this chapter (pp. 1428–1450).

PANCREATITIS

Cholelithiasis is the commonest cause of acute pancreatitis in Britain. Most surgeons perform a cholecystectomy as soon as active inflammation in the pancreas has settled, to prevent further attacks. The first attack of pancreatitis, when stones are present in the common duct, is often associated with inflammatory papillitis or stricture which may lead to acute relapsing pancrea-

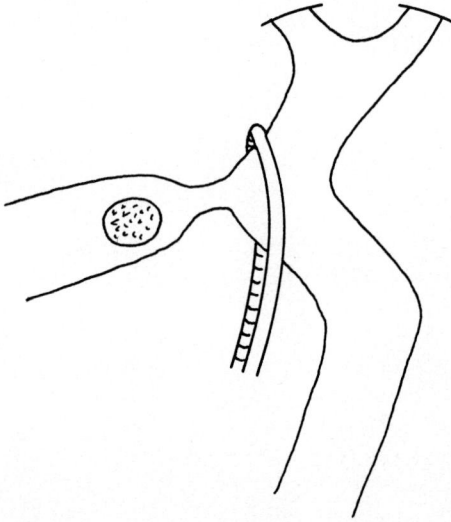

Fig. 19.54 Common cause of hepatic duct stricture at cholecystectomy.

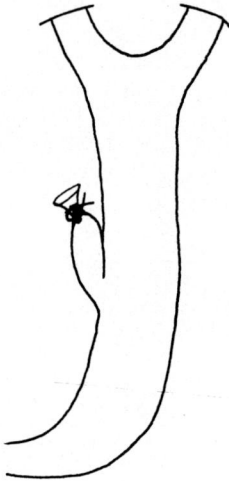

Fig. 19.55 Cystic duct stump, with common and cystic ducts sharing a common wall.

titis, and require secondary correction by either endoscopic sphincterotomy or operative sphincteroplasty. Occasionally undiagnosed pancreatitis may be the cause of initial symptoms, erroneously attributed to the gallbladder, for which cholecystectomy was performed. In this situation attacks of pain will continue postoperatively.

LIVER DISEASE

Chronic liver disease does not result if the primary operation has been completely effective in eliminating gallstones and restoring the extrahepatic biliary tract to normal. However, abnormal liver function tests are sometimes discovered postoperatively when pre-operative assessment has been inadequate. Nonopacification of the gallbladder at cholecystography may be due to failure of excretion of the contrast medium by an abnormal liver rather than from malfunction of the gallbladder. Some patients are thus submitted to cholecystectomy because of misinterpretation of tests and this error is avoided by employing pre-operative liver function tests routinely and the addition of an ultrasound in dubious cases. Nevertheless gallstones and liver disease may co-exist, and this may necessitate an evaluation both in the pre-operative and postcholecystectomy situations by immunological tests, ERCP, and liver biopsy.

FLATULENT DYSPEPSIA

About half the patients with gallstones who present with flatulent dyspepsia lose their symptoms after cholecystectomy. Rains[15] suggested that this type of dyspepsia is of gastric rather than biliary origin. Johnson[12] showed that after cholecystectomy some patients develop a disorder of gastroduodenal motility whereby the duodenum contracts but the pylorus does not, in response to a swallowed meal. The result is reflux of bile from the duodenum through the open pylorus into the stomach and sometimes even into the oesophagus. This sequence of events is more liable to occur in patients who have had a functioning gallbladder removed. Treatment can only be symptomatic.

OTHER DISEASES

Attention has been drawn to the increased risk of carcinoma of the colon developing in cholecystectomized patients, especially carcinoma of the right side of the colon in women.[13, 18] It is possible that altered bile acid metabolism after cholecystectomy results in the formation of carcinogens.

ABDOMINAL WALL

Occasionally symptoms may be due to causes in the incision, such as hernia or neuroma. Intraperitoneal adhesions involving the parietes may cause similar problems. Painful conditions in the ribs and costal cartilages must not be forgotten.

Investigations

Biochemical liver function tests
Elevation of serum alkaline phosphatase (and 5'-nucleotidase) with or without elevation of the

serum bilirubin suggests obstruction of the biliary system or residual calculi. Any elevation of aspartate transaminase implies hepatocellular damage possibly from cholangitis. Disturbances of serum proteins are unusual with structural biliary disease and normally indicate chronic hepatocellular disease which may antedate the cholecystectomy. Immunological tests, anti-mitochondrial antibodies, anti-smooth muscle antibodies and anti-nuclear factor are negative in primary biliary disease.

Ultrasound scan
Dilated intra- and extrahepatic bile ducts are easily shown as are larger stones in the common bile duct (Figure 19.56). Small stones, which may impact at the lower end of the common bile duct causing proximal duct dilatation are frequently overlooked. Ultrasound is especially useful in the jaundiced patient to decide whether percutaneous or retrograde cholangiography is the more appropriate next diagnostic step.

Intravenous cholangiography (IVC)
The intravenous infusion of modern contrast agents allows good demonstration of the biliary system in the presence of normal liver function and may show residual calculi and strictures. Tomography is a useful addition especially when contrast density is low. Iodine sensitivity is a contraindication to IVC and even if this is not previously known in a particular patient, 'allergic' reactions are quite frequent.

Percutaneous transhepatic cholangiography (PTC)
This technique is quick and reliable using the narrow diameter Chiba needle. It almost always demonstrates dilated ducts and in expert hands a large proportion of normal-sized ducts.

Uncorrected bleeding disorders and untreated biliary sepsis are contraindications. PTC is particularly indicated when ultrasound examination has demonstrated dilated intrahepatic ducts.

Endoscopic retrograde cholangiopancreatography (ERCP)[1, 16]
Retrograde cannulation of the papilla of Vater using a side-viewing duodenoscope allows instillation of contrast material directly into the biliary system and pancreatic duct. The technique is fully described by Cotton.[6] ERCP is particularly appropriate when ultrasound has shown normal-sized bile ducts and intravenous cholangiography is unsuccessful for example in the presence of jaundice. Residual or recurrent stones and structural abnormalities of the biliary system may be demonstrated. Furthermore when definition is poor by IVC the greater contrast density of ERCP may resolve diagnostic doubts. It is simple to proceed to corrective duodenoscopic sphincterotomy if stones are shown in the bile ducts or if there is papillary stenosis. Manometric studies help to elucidate biliary dyskinesia and papillary stenosis. Another advantage of ERCP in investigation of postcholecystectomy symptoms is that it allows simultaneous examination of the pancreatic ducts and may reveal features of chronic pancreatitis.

Treatment

Retained or recurrent common duct stones are so likely to cause obstructive jaundice and cholangitis with possibly fatal consequences that they should always be removed if possible (see p. 1423. In older patients or in those with co-existent serious disease duodenoscopic sphinc-

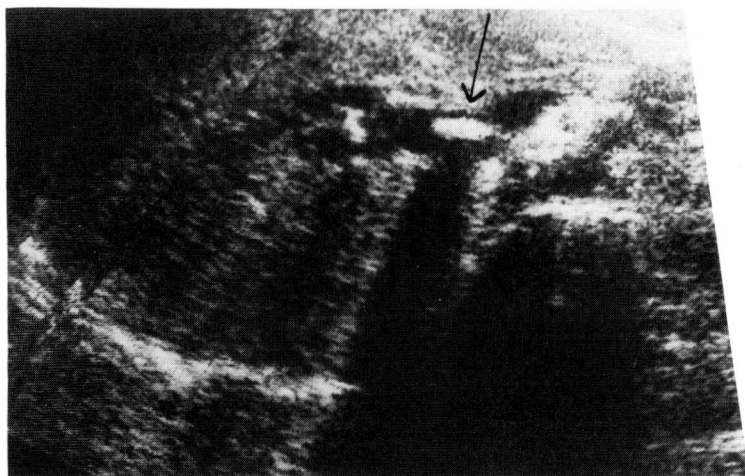

Fig. 19.56 Ultrasound scan showing a stone in a dilated common bile duct (longitudinal section).

terotomy is the method of choice as surgical mortality for re-exploration of the bile duct is 5–12.3%.[7] Younger patients who are fit are probably best treated surgically at least until the long-term safety of diathermy sphincterotomy has been established. Follow up studies so far have revealed no serious consequences within 5 years. Dissolution of retained common duct stones has been reported by some authors. Orally administered bile salts are probably less effective than a terpene preparation ('Rowachol') which dissolves approximately 50% of stones.[8] Perfusion of the bile duct with mono-octanoin via a naso-biliary tube placed endoscopically has occasionally been successful.[19] Similarly strictures of the bile duct, serious enough to cause abnormal liver function tests, are likely to be complicated by cholangitis or secondary biliary cirrhosis. They are treated best by surgery although there is increasing interest in endoscopic and transhepatic dilatation.

Papillary stenosis with biliary dilatation, especially if complicated by recurrent cholangitis, is suitable for treatment by duodenoscopic sphincterotomy. The management of patients in whom pain is dominant but without dilatation of the bile duct is more controversial. If pressure studies show a gradient across the papilla then satisfactory results may be expected from sphincterotomy but when there is no such gradient results are disappointing. Drug treatment with anticholinergics or nitrites may provide relief in acute attacks of biliary spasm but in many cases an alternative cause for pain may be found.

Cholangitis following cholecystectomy is likely to be due to retained stones or poor drainage in association with stenosis of the duct. Urgent treatment with antibiotics is essential to control the infection, and emergency or early elective treatment of the underlying cause.

DUODENOSCOPIC SPHINCTEROTOMY (ENDOSCOPIC PAPILLOTOMY)[6]

The lower end of the common bile duct can be opened into the duodenum by a diathermy incision through the papilla of Vater employing a side-viewing duodenoscope. This procedure permits removal of stones from the bile ducts and allows free drainage of bile in cases of papillary stenosis.

Technique

Before considering sphincterotomy the patient's coagulation status should be checked and deficiencies corrected. It is a wise precaution to have available 2 units of compatible blood in case of severe primary haemorrhage.

Routine retrograde cholangiography demonstrates the ductal anatomy and excludes a stricture of the bile duct above the papilla. The papillotome is then inserted selectively into the bile duct and the position checked by fluoroscopy. After satisfactory placement the diathermy wire is tightened, bowing the papillotome. A blended or cutting current is applied and a controlled incision is made in a cephalad direction, between '11 and 1 o'clock'. The length of the incision is 'tailored' to the size of the stone – a minimum incision passing just through the papillary muscle and appropriately larger for stones up to about 2 cm diameter. Stones may either be extracted immediately using a balloon catheter or Dormia basket, or allowed to pass spontaneously.

In the latter event a check retrograde cholangiogram after 2–4 weeks is required to ensure satisfactory duct clearance or in the case of failure to permit delayed basket-extraction or even extension of the sphincterotomy.

Complications occur in about 10% of patients, haemorrhage being the most common, pancreatitis, stone impaction with cholangitis, and perforation are less frequent. About 2% of patients may require urgent surgery for treatment of these complications. The overall mortality rate of the procedure is about 1%.

Results

Successful sphincterotomy is achieved in over 95% of patients and in 90% the ducts are cleared of stones.

RETAINED GALL STONES WITH T-TUBE IN PLACE

Early after cholecystectomy stones may be found in the bile ducts by T-tube cholangiography. The frequency of this complication is reduced by routine intra-operative cholangiography and/or choledochoscopy. Such stones inevitably increase in size if left and eventually cause symptoms; removal is therefore mandatory.

Formerly surgical re-exploration was required for residual calculi, but recently several non-operative techniques have been developed. In the early days after operation saline irrigation and periodic clamping of the T-tube may permit spontaneous passage. If the ducts are not clear in about one week, dissolution of stones can be attempted by T-tube perfusion with mono-octanoin. When solubility of a sister stone in organic solvents (e.g. acetone) has been shown to be successful, dissolution can be expected in over 50% of cases after infusion of mono-octanoin for 10 days.[11]

Insoluble stones and those not responding to the above treatments can usually be removed either by instrumentation via the T-tube track or endoscopic sphincterotomy. The relative roles of these two approaches are currently under discussion and preference depends to some extent upon available skills. Before safe instrumentation of the T-tube track is possible it is necessary to wait about 6 weeks after operation to allow a secure track to form. A large T-tube (greater than 12F) inserted laterally is required. If these conditions are met a steerable catheter can be inserted under fluoroscopy into the bile duct and the stones grasped with a wire basket and either delivered intact or after fragmentation. In skilled hands complications are infrequent and the success rate is over 90%.[3] An alternative percutaneous technique avoiding radiology employs a narrow diameter fibre-endoscope inserted through the T-tube track allowing the stones to be grasped in a basket under direct vision.

It is now rare for surgery to be required for stones when there is a T-tube in situ. Indications are failure of the non-operative techniques, complications arising, or rarely for very large stones.

SURGERY

If the above methods fail, surgical re-exploration is usually necessary. The common bile duct is exposed through the original incision, opened and the stone(s) removed. It is important to look for a stricture at the lower end of the duct.

Sphincteroplasty

This procedure is indicated for a stricture of the lower end of the choledochus, as distinct from ampullary stenosis. The second part of the duodenum is opened with a vertical anterior incision, the ampulla identified and a small probe passed. The duodenal wall is incised for 2 cm upward, and the incision deepened to divide the common bile duct wall until a wide opening is obtained. Sutures are placed on each side between the duodenal and choledochal edges, to prevent later stenosis (Figure 19.57). If relapsing pancreatitis has occurred, sphincteroplasty of the first centimetre of the pancreatic duct is also performed.

Choledochoduodenostomy

This operation is easier to perform than sphincteroplasty and is indicated when the common bile duct is widely dilated and obstructed at its lower end. A vertical incision is made in the duct at the upper border of the first part of the duodenum and another incision in the corresponding part of the duodenum longitudinally. The two openings are then anastomosed with interrupted sutures, and the opening should be at least 2 cm across. The disadvantage of this procedure is the liability to attacks of acute pancreatitis due to stones, debris and sepsis collecting in the lower end of the common bile duct, particularly if there is obstruction (Figure 19.58).

Stricture repair

A stricture at the upper end of the duct, if only partial, can sometimes be repaired by choledochoplasty, dividing the stricture longitudinally

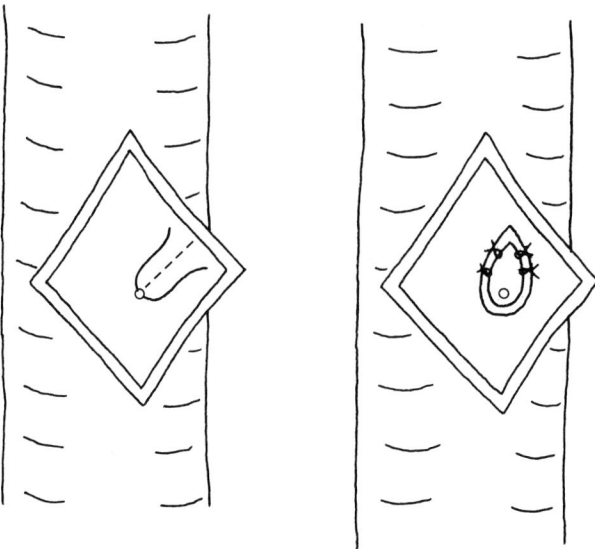

Fig. 19.57 Transduodenal operative sphincteroplasty.

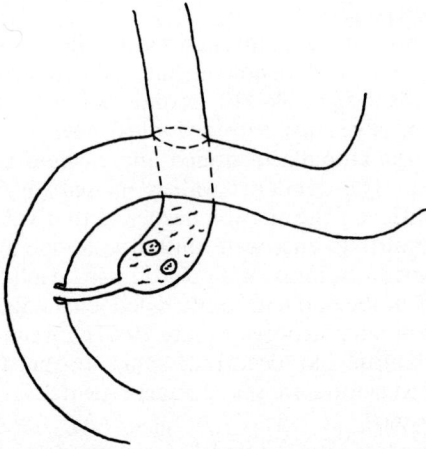

Fig. 19.58 Choledochoduodenostomy, with biliary debris and stones collecting in the lower end of the common bile duct, and distal stenosis.

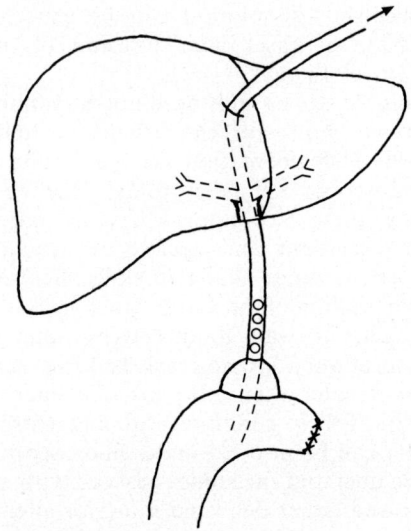

Fig. 19.60 Smith's mucosal graft reconstruction for very high common hepatic duct stricture.

and suturing it transversely, as in a Mickulicz pyloroplasty (Figure 19.59). Failing this, and if there is no loss of length of the common bile duct, resection of the stricture may be possible, and end-to-end anastomosis carried out over a tube.

With strictures high in the common hepatic duct, direct repair is usually impossible. A Roux loop of upper jejunum is fashioned, 45 cm in length, and sutured to the edges of the hole after opening the bile duct above the stricture. The recurrent stricture rate is high, and the last resort is the technique of mucosal graft described by Smith,[17] employing a transhepatic multi-hole catheter, with a mucosal patch of the Roux loop sutured over the lower end of the catheter and drawn up into contact with the edge of the hepatic duct opening (Figure 19.60).

REFERENCES

1 Blumgart, L. H., Carachi, R., Imrie, C. W. *et al.* (1977) Diagnosis and management of post-cholecystectomy symptoms: the place of endoscopy and retrograde choledochopancreatography. *British Journal of Surgery*, **64**, 809–816.

2 Bolton, J. P. & LeQuesne, L. P. (1981) Postcholecystectomy symptoms. In *Surgery of the Gall Bladder and Bile Ducts*. (Ed.) Lord Smith & Sherlock S. 2nd edn. pp. 337–359. London: Butterworth.

3 Burhenne, H. J. (1981) Radiological retrieval of bile duct stones. In *Therapeutic Endoscopy and Radiology of the Gut* (Ed.) Bennett, J. R. pp. 185–204. London: Chapman & Hall.

4 Cassie, G. F. & Kapadia, C. R. (1981) Operative cholangiography or extraductal palpation: an analysis of 418 cholecystectomies. *British Journal of Surgery*, **68**, 516–517.

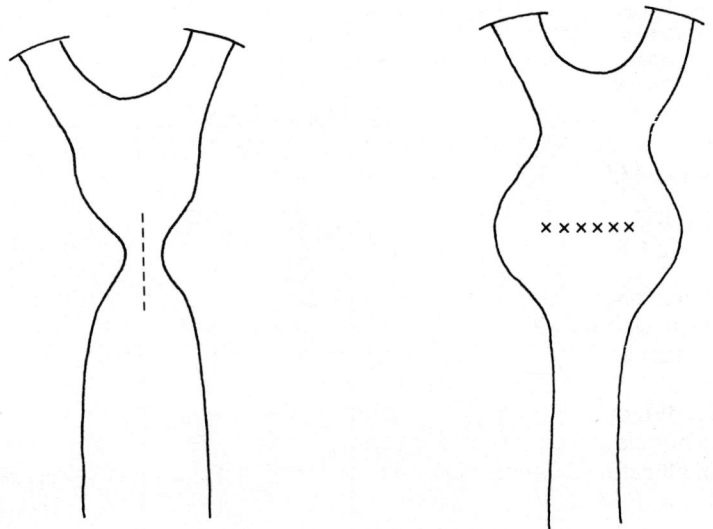

Fig. 19.59 Choledochoplasty for partial stricture of common duct.

5 Corlette, M. B. & Schatzki, S. (1978) Operative cholangiography and overlooked stones. *Archives of Surgery*, **113**, 729–734.

6 Cotton, P. B. (1980) Endoscopic retrograde cholangiopancreatography (ERCP). In *Practical Gastrointestinal Endoscopy*, Cotton, P. B. & Williams, C. B. pp. 55–76. Oxford: Blackwell.

7 Cotton, P. B. (1981) Duodenoscopic sphincterotomy and bile duct stone removal. In *Therapeutic Endoscopy and Radiology of the Gut* (Ed.) Bennett, J. R. pp. 169–184. London: Chapman & Hall.

8 Ellis, W. R. & Bell, G. D. (1981) Treatment of biliary duct stones with a terpene preparation. *British Medical Journal*, **282**, 611.

9 Havard, C. (1960) Non-malignant bile duct obstruction. *Annals of the Royal College of Surgeons of England*, **26**, 88–114.

10 Hunt, D. (1982) Investigation of postcholecystectomy problems. *Medical Journal of Australia*, **1**, 214–216.

11 Jarrett, L. N., Balfour, T. W., Bell, G. D. *et al.* (1981) Intraductal infusion of mono-octanoin: experience of 24 patients with retained common duct stones. *Lancet*, **i**, 68–70.

12 Johnson, A. G. (1975) Cholecystectomy and gallstone dyspepsia. *Annals of the Royal College of Surgeons of England*, **56**, 69–80.

13 Linos, D. A., O'Fallen, W. M., Beart, R. W. Jr *et al.* (1981) Cholecystectomy and carcinoma of the colon. *Lancet*, **ii**, 379–381.

14 Millbourn, E. (1950) On the importance of the remnant cystic duct in the development of post-operative biliary distress following cholecystectomy. A study partly based on a cholangiography series. *Acta Chirurgica Scandinavica*, **100**, 448–465.

15 Rains, A. J. H. (1964) The effects and clinical features of gallstones. In *Gallstones, Causes and Treatment*. p. 101. London: Heinemann.

16 Ruddell, W. S. J., Lintott, D. J., Ashton, M. G. & Axon, A. T. R. (1980) Endoscopic retrograde cholangiography and pancreatography in investigation of postcholecystectomy patients. *Lancet*, **i**, 444–447.

17 Smith, R. (1964) Hepaticojejunostomy with transhepatic intubation. A technique for very high strictures of the hepatic ducts. *British Journal of Surgery*, **51**, 186–194.

18 Vernick, L. J. & Kuller, L. H. (1981) Cholecystectomy and right-sided colon cancer: an epidemiological study. *Lancet*, **ii**, 381–383.

19 Witzel, L., Wiederholt, J. & Wolbergs, E. (1981) Dissolution of retained duct stones by perfusion with monooctanoin via a Teflon catheter introduced endoscopically. *Gastrointestinal Endoscopy*, **27**, 63–65.

TUMOURS

CARCINOMA OF THE GALLBLADDER

While often thought of as a rare condition it has been claimed that gallbladder carcinoma represents almost 20% of all gastrointestinal carcinomas.[16] Others have stressed the frequency of the tumour.[4, 18, 31, 32, 37, 71] While the incidence is not clear the tumour has been found in 0.2% of all gallbladder operations in Sweden[90] and at the M.D. Anderson Hospital and Tumour Institute over a 36 year period 0.08% of all patients admitted had gallbladder cancer.[62]

There are racial and ethnic differences in the incidence of gallbladder cancer. Caucasians in the United States have an incidence 50% higher than that of Negroid peoples and the rate in the south-west of America is particularly high in American Indians compared to Caucasians.[20]

The tumour is more common in women and has a peak incidence in the 70–75 year old group and a female to male ratio of approximately 3.1.[21, 29, 75, 77] There is a close association with cholelithiasis and less than 10% of patients with gallbladder cancer have no gallstones. It has been suggested that the presence of the stone and associated inflammation and infection may be causal or contributory aetiological factors. However, the great majority of patients with gallstones never develop a cancer. Since 1968 the total deaths and total crude mortality for gallbladder cancer have fallen in the United States, but the number of cholecystectomies has risen.[20] While this may indicate that an increased removal of the gallbladder lowers the risk of dying from gallbladder cancer, it may be but a coincidental observation.[82] No human carcinogen has been identified which might be responsible for gallbladder cancer.

Histologically 75–90% of tumours are well-differentiated mucin-secreting adenocarcinomas, while 5% are squamous cell and approximately 10% anaplastic. The mode of spread of gallbladder carcinoma is mainly by the lymphatics along the cystic duct and thence to the common bile duct, or by direct extension into the adjacent liver. The common hepatic duct is frequently involved by direct extension and presentation is then with painless progressive jaundice, which must be distinguished from cholangiocarcinoma at the confluence of the bile ducts. This mode of spread through Calot's triangle to the common hepatic duct is frequent with tumours which commence in the region of the neck of the gallbladder or Hartmann's pouch, but less so with tumours commencing close to the fundus of the gallbladder which tend to involve at an early stage the duct to the antero-inferior segment of the liver. The demonstration of selective involvement of ducts and vessels in the anterior-inferior part of the right lobe of the liver on cholangiography or angiography, particularly in the presence of obstructive jaundice, should arouse suspicion of gallbladder cancer and CT-scanning may suggest the diagnosis. A calcified gallbladder (porcelain gallbladder) seen on X-ray may indicate carcinoma.[64] Occasionally, endoscopic retrograde cholangiopancreatography reveals an irregular filling defect within the gallbladder or obstruction of the common hepatic duct close to the hilus and a failure of the gallbladder to fill.

None the less preoperative diagnosis is uncommon and while many patients may have a history of biliary disease extending over one year in duration 50% will not.[21] The majority of patients are diagnosed either as an incidental finding at elective biliary surgery or during laparotomy for suspected cholangiocarcinoma at the confluence of the ducts. In a recent experience of 95 cases of carcinoma affecting the confluence of the bile ducts seen over a period of 4.5 years, we have encountered 16 cases of gallbladder cancer. Although some patients gave a history of biliary symptoms the majority presented with obstructive jaundice. A correct preoperative diagnosis was considered in 5 of the 16 patients, this being significantly higher than the 8.6% preoperative diagnostic rate recorded by Piehler and Crichlow.[63] This high yield of preoperative diagnosis has been dependent upon a high index of clinical suspicion and critical appraisal of percutaneous cholangiograms, particularly involvement of the antero-inferior biliary radicles in patients with obstructive jaundice.

Some patients who undergo cholecystectomy for cholelithiasis will be found to have either frank gallbladder carcinoma at the time of operation or the tumour will be discovered microscopically after removal of the gallbladder. These patients are presenting at an earlier stage of the disease. Cancer of the gallbladder tends to be locally invasive until late in the course of the disease when the presentation is with a widely spreading growth.[26]

Treatment

Unfortunately most gallbladder cancers are diagnosed late and there is extensive involvement of the liver and structures in the porta hepatis by the time operation is performed so that only biopsy or palliative bypass are possible.

The results of excisional treatment are usually poor, but where cholecystectomy has been carried out for cancer which has only involved the gallbladder microscopically the results are better. Bergdahl[6] observed that patients with mucosal and submucosal cancers had a five year survival of 63.6% and a ten year survival of 45.5% whereas patients with full thickness involvement of the gallbladder wall were all dead within 2.5 years. He recommends that if microscopic carcinoma is discovered after removal of the gallbladder for presumed benign disease patients should be re-operated and a wedge resection of approximately 5 cm of normal liver tissue and dissection of the regional lymph nodes performed. A similar suggestion for improvement of results was made by Nevin *et al.*[58] who suggested that simple cholecystectomy be employed for lesions involving the mucosa or the muscularis mucosae and a radical cholecystectomy be undertaken for more advanced cases. Moosa *et al.*[55] reported a five year survival of only 4.9% but if the patients who underwent cholecystectomy were considered the five year survival was 14.3%. Others have not been able to demonstrate improved results by the use of radical procedures for cancer of the gallbladder.[24, 45] Nevertheless, it does seem that the only possibility of cure lies in identifying patients with early growths or in a more radical operation for selected cases.

Tompkins[82] recommends radical cholecystectomy (removal of the gallbladder with adjacent wedge of liver tissue and regional lymphatics) in patients with a small tumour localized to the gallbladder and believes that in more advanced lesions palliative decompression is indicated. Radiotherapy and chemotherapy may also be considered but response is generally poor.

Excellent palliation can be obtained by a biliary enteric bypass utilizing the left hepatic duct system approached via the umbilical fissure[8, 36, 76] and this can usually be carried out to a dilated ductal system at a good distance from the primary lesion. The anastomosis tends to be involved by tumour extension only late in the disease. The surgical approach includes dissection above the ligamentum teres exposing the left hepatic ducts at the point of their confluence of drainage from the anterior and posterior elements of the left lateral segment. Biliary enteric anastomosis carried out at this point allows a wide stoma with excellent drainage (Figure 19.61) and often excellent quality of survival.

Early diagnosis is usually made at operation and early cholecystectomy for cholelithiasis may account for increased salvage in some more recent series.[61] As pointed out by Tompkins[82] it is hard to justify cholecystectomy for the prevention of cancer because the risk of dying after cholecystectomy is probably very similar to that of developing a cancer of the gallbladder but more support can be found for the recommendation of early cholecystectomy for the prevention of possible gallstone complications, such as jaundice, pancreatitis, acute cholecystitis and perforation, which have a higher incidence and a greater associated mortality.

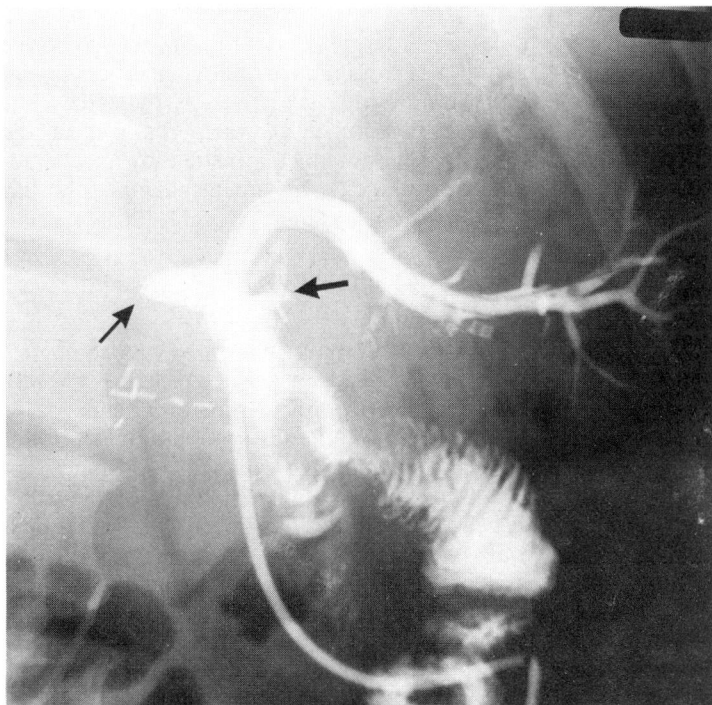

Fig. 19.61 Tubogram obtained by injection of contrast through a transanastomotic–transjejunal tube. The patient presented with obstructive jaundice due to malignant involvement of the bile ducts at the confluence by extension of a large gallbladder carcinoma. There was wide involvement of the right hepatic and intrahepatic ducts. An anastomosis to the left hepatic ductal system, at the base of the ligamentum teres, has been undertaken by side-to-side anastomosis using a Roux-en-Y loop of jejunum (large arrow). Note the transanastomotic tube running well into the left hepatic ductal system. The main left hepatic duct is patent and runs towards the obstruction at the confluence (small arrow). Excellent relief of the symptoms was obtained with complete relief of jaundice and pruritus, and the patient is free of symptoms four months after operation.

At cholecystectomy the surgeon should open the gallbladder and inspect the lining. Frozen section examination of suspicious areas should be performed. If an early cancer is identified immediate consideration should be given to a more radical excision, including lymph node clearance. It is much more difficult to recommend re-operation several days later in a patient recovering from cholecystectomy.

Right hepatic lobectomy is seldom applicable for gallbladder cancer because the gallbladder lies in the anatomical plane between the right and left lobe of the liver and an extended right hepatic lobectomy is usually all that is possible or reasonable if a lobectomy is considered essential. This is the minimum procedure necessary to remove all potential local invasive tumour.

There is little evidence that adjunctive chemotherapy or radiotherapy produces any marked improvements in outcome although some have reported a modest prolongation of survival after treatment.[62, 85]

CARCINOMA OF THE CYSTIC DUCT

This is an extremely rare lesion and usually only found incidentally at operation for obstruction of the gallbladder or in the specimen removed at cholecystectomy.

In the advanced stages the disease is indistinguishable from cancer arising in the mid-portion of the bile ducts or the gallbladder. Nishimura *et al.*[59] recommend operative removal of the gallbladder, entire cystic duct and peri-ductal lymphatics for localized lesions. If the adjacent common bile duct is involved radical resection of the duct from the hilus to the pancreas is indicated with reconstruction by Roux-en-Y hepaticojejunostomy.

TUMOURS OF THE BILE DUCTS

Benign tumours

Non-malignant tumours of the bile ducts are uncommon, but the exact incidence of the lesions is not known since many are probably asymptomatic. Epithelial benign tumours of the bile duct are of two varieties.

A *papilloma* is the commonest and is usually situated in the region of the papilla of Vater. The tumours, polypoid in character, are rarely bigger than 2 cm in diameter and are covered by columnar cells with a minimum of associated subepithelial inflammatory change. Histological distinction from hyperplasia may be difficult, but in cases of hyperplasia the subepithelial chronic inflammatory reaction is greater. These tumours may have a malignant potential.[15]

Multiple papillomatosis presenting as diffuse intrahepatic and extrahepatic biliary papillomata is extremely rare.[35, 60] Most patients manifest as obstructive jaundice, frequently intermittent and often complicated by cholangitis. This complication is a result of partial and intermittent obstruction of the bile duct by fragments from the villous tumour.[14] In some patients the only symptom is abdominal pain.[23] The history may extend for more than 20 years and be associated with anaemia as a result of bleeding from the growth. In only two reports has there been associated cholelithiasis.

Preoperative diagnosis is made radiologically. Filling defects seen have in the past been attributed to air bubbles or intrabiliary blood clots.[40] Diagnosis has become more precise since the widespread availability of percutaneous, retrograde, and operative cholangiography. It is best to regard these tumours as having low-grade malignant potential (Figure 19.62).[1, 15, 30, 35, 57]

Treatment of this uncommon tumour is difficult. Most patients have been treated by palliative surgical techniques, usually cholecystectomy, curettage and an internal surgical drainage procedure or even T-tube drainage. However, the majority of patients have had recurrence associated with jaundice and cholangitis.

Attempted radical curative surgery by means of hepatic lobectomy has been reported in only five patients[14, 30, 35, 41, 52] but major resectional surgery for this lesion has a high recurrence rate, and in 12 patients for whom adequate follow up figures were available (mean age 54 years) the mean survival was 28 months.[30] It should be noted, however, that although no patient survived more than six years the only five year survivals were in three patients submitted to radical surgery.

A reasonable approach to this rare condition includes preoperative and operative cholangiographic diagnosis, early choledochotomy and assessment of the intrahepatic biliary tree by choledochoscopy. If the tumour is bulky then curettage may be necessary in order to identify the sites of origin within the bile duct. Care must be taken to perform choledochoscopy of all accessible intrahepatic ducts. When the papillomatosis appears to be confined to one lobe a radical resection consisting of partial hepatectomy with excision of the involved ducts should be performed for although this does not guarantee freedom from recurrence it carries the best possibility of long-term cure in a young patient. In cases of papillomatosis involving both the right and left ducts radical surgery is not applicable. Long-term external drainage should be avoided as a primary palliative manoeuvre and curettage or internal bypass is indicated. The outlook is poor if complete removal of the tumour is impossible.[30] Instillation of chemotherapeutic agents by an intraductal tube has been reported in a single patient.[7]

Carcinoma of the bile duct

Adenocarcinoma of the bile duct (cholangiocarcinoma) has three morphological variants; the *papillary* lesion which grows within the lumen of the duct and has a tendency to produce a field change with multiple tumour sites; the *nodular* type which forms a small well-localized mass involving a portion of the ductal system; and the *diffuse* variety where the duct wall is thickened over an extensive area, the lumen narrowed and the surrounding tissues of the hepatoduodenal ligament often inflamed. This last type of lesion is very difficult to differentiate from sclerosing cholangitis.

Incidence and natural history
The incidence of bile duct tumours at autopsy varies from 0.01% to 0.2% and may constitute about 2% of all cancers found at autopsy.[43, 46, 47] While still a relatively rare form of cancer, 4500 new cases per annum may be expected in the United States, an incidence similar to that of carcinoma of the tongue.[49] The incidence of the disease may be increasing,[13, 17, 83] although the advent of the new diagnostic methods may have enabled many more of these lesions, almost certainly misdiagnosed in the past, to be diagnosed. Thus, in a specialist referral centre in the UK 37 cases were seen in one 17 month period.[86] Most tumours occur in the age group 50–70 years, although very young patients may be affected. Males are more frequently affected than females.

The majority of patients with bile duct cancer die within 6–12 months of diagnosis from biliary obstruction, cholangitis and liver failure.[47] The prognosis is worst for lesions affecting the confluence of the bile ducts, and best for lesions close to the papilla.

Aetiology
The cause is unknown and although there is no convincing link with the presence of gallstones they were present in 33 of 84 patients.[12] There may be a relationship between ulcerative colitis and cholangiocarcinoma. The disease may present either some years after proctocolectomy or as the presenting feature, with ulcerative colitis only being discovered subsequently.

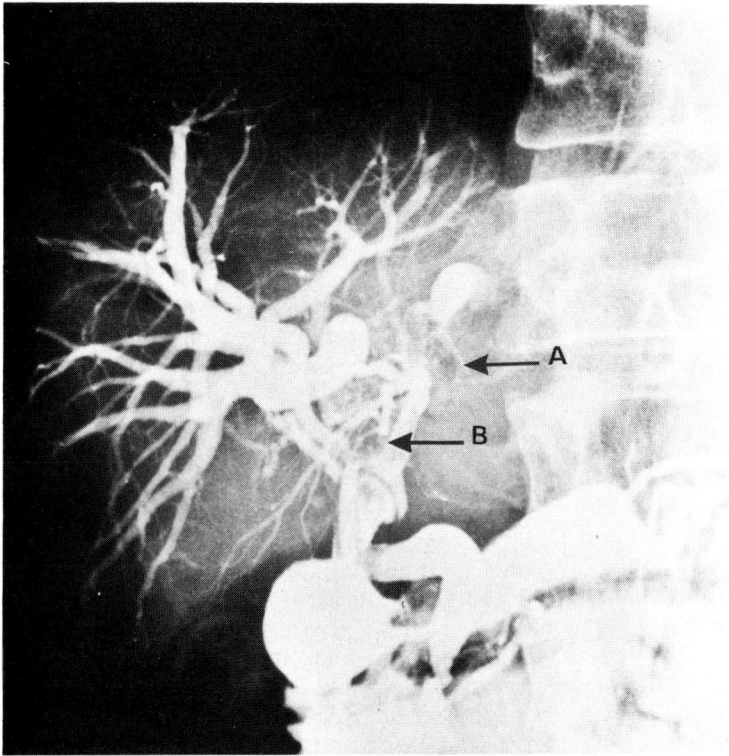

a

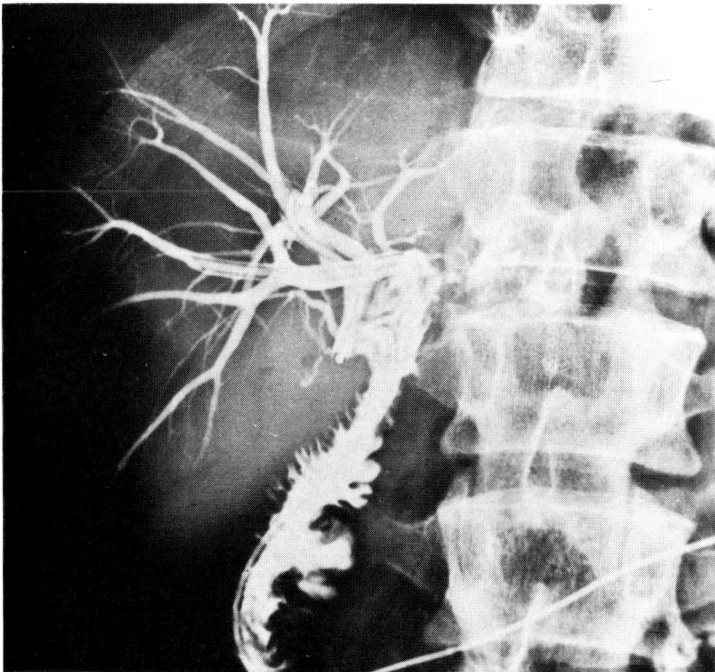

b

Fig. 19.62 T-tube cholangiography obtained in a 44-year-old man referred from management of an intrahepatic biliary papilloma occupying the confluence of the bile ducts but arising in the left hepatic ductal system. Note the filling defect (arrowed) in the left hepatic duct and at the confluence.
(b) Postoperative tube cholangiogram of this patient after a left hepatic lobectomy and reconstruction by means of hepaticojejunostomy Roux-en-Y over a transanastomotic-transjejunal tube. The patient remains well and free of symptoms nine months after surgery.

Roberts-Thomson et al.[69] considered there is a clear relationship between the two diseases. It is possible that infection and bile stasis may be important and a relationship has been demonstrated between congenital hepatic fibrosis or polycystic disease and the presence of these tumours.[9, 44] Long-standing poorly drained choledochal cysts may also undergo neoplastic change.

Welton et al.[90] report that chronic typhoid carriers in New York died of hepatobiliary cancer six times more often than matched controls and suggest that bacterial degradation of bile salts might be implicated.

Location

Cancer of the extrahepatic biliary system may be classified into three anatomical areas: the upper third, comprising the common hepatic duct and the confluence of the hepatic ducts; the middle third, comprising the common bile duct between the cystic duct and the upper border of the duodenum; and the lower third, between the upper border of the duodenum and the papilla of Vater. Diagnosis, prognosis and treatment of these tumours vary. Growths in the upper third present the greatest challenge in pre-operative diagnosis and in acquisition of histological material for confirmation of diagnosis. They have the worst prognosis and are the most difficult group to treat.

BILE DUCT CANCER AT THE HILUS OF THE LIVER

Altemeier et al.[3] and subsequently Klatskin[44] first described the features of adenocarcinoma at the bifurcation of the bile ducts and ever since there has been pessimism about these tumours. A number of concepts have been generally accepted: (1) pre-operative diagnosis is frequently not possible; (2) histological confirmation is difficult to obtain; (3) excisional therapy for cure is rarely possible; and (4) biliary-enteric anastomosis is very difficult for palliation with intubation being preferred.

The recent experience in our unit in which a policy of detailed pre-operative investigation to define the extent of the lesion, an aggressive surgical approach directed at excision whenever possible and an appraisal of tubal drainage compared with cholangio-enteric anastomoses suggests that these assumptions can be challenged. The study indicates that: (1) preoperative diagnosis is nearly always possible; (2) histological or cytological material is usually obtainable; (3) preoperative cholangiography combined with angiography gives an excellent guide to the extent of tumour and to resectability; (4) resection can be accomplished in 20% of patients with an acceptable post-operative mortality; and (5) biliary-enteric anastomosis is often possible and is preferable to intubational methods.[11, 86]

Diagnosis

An ordered use of ultrasonography, fine needle percutaneous transhepatic cholangiography (PTC) and endoscopic retrograde cholangio-pancreatography (ERCP) should be successful in imaging the obstructive lesion in most patients. In particular, fine needle PTC is successful in nearly all who have dilated ducts[5, 10] and is the most useful and accurate technique in hilar cholangiocarcinoma (Figure 19.63). A simple cholangiographic diagnosis should not be accepted and the examination must be pursued until the entire intrahepatic biliary tree on both left and right sides has been outlined, because this gives a valuable guide to resectability and to later operative approaches.[86]

Fine needle aspiration cytology of masses at the hilus carried out under radiological control at the time of PTC is useful. The method relies on expert cytological opinion. Cytological examination of bile samples has also yielded reliable positive results, although a negative report is of no value. Cytological specimens and intra-operative biopsy provide a diagnosis in the majority of patients.

A major diagnostic problem is the differential diagnosis between the diffuse form of cholangiocarcinoma and sclerosing cholangitis.[50] On the other hand the appearances at the hilus of the liver may be those of malignant obstruction, with a stricture localized to the confluence of the ducts without diffuse involvement, either of the common bile duct or intrahepatic ducts. The newer diagnostic means permit the detection of early sclerosing cholangitis localized to a small area of the biliary tree which closely resembles the focal type of cholangiocarcinoma. Similarly a localized benign stricture may occur in association with cholelithiasis and may present diagnostic difficulties.

Patients who are found on routine investigation to have an isolated rise in serum alkaline phosphatase require immediate and full investigation. In this situation where the bile ducts are not completely occluded or where there may be obstruction to isolated segments of the liver an ERCP should be performed particularly if preliminary ultrasound reveals no dilatation of the intrahepatic biliary tree.

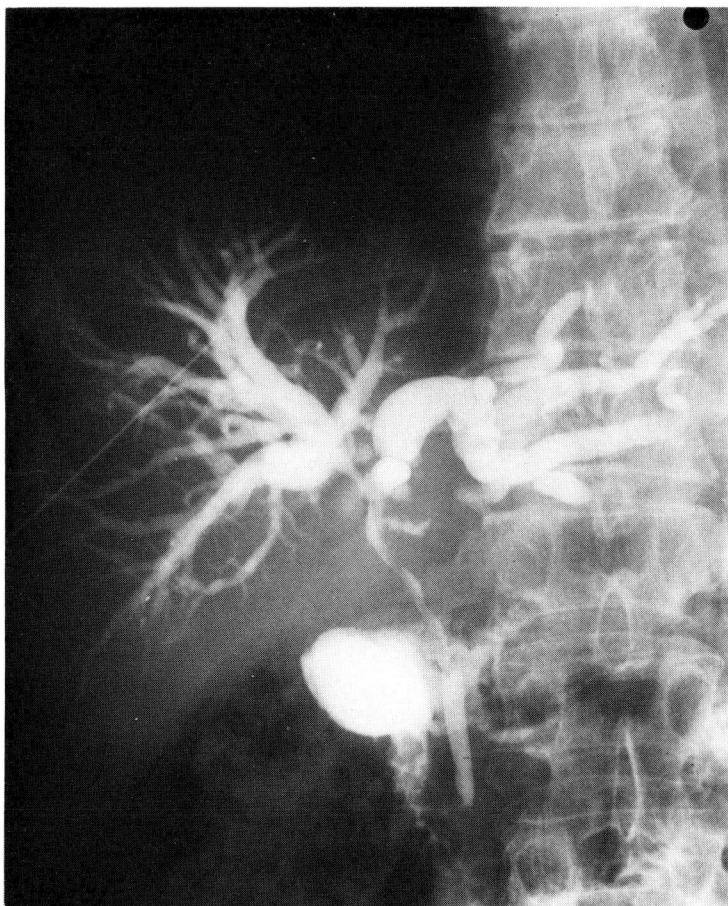

Fig. 19.63 Percutaneous transhepatic cholangiogram in a patient presenting with relentlessly progressive obstructive jaundice. Note the long stricture occupying the common bile duct and common hepatic duct and extending into the right ductal system. The origin of the left duct is also occluded. The gallbladder is not outlined. Late-phase portography revealed involvement of the portal vein.

Assessment of the extent of tumour

Involvement of adjacent blood vessels and the extent of spread along the ducts into the liver may compromise complete excision of the tumour without concomitant extensive resection of the liver and its blood supply. Because it is very difficult to be sure at operation of the extent of the involvement of vessels an approach aimed at full radiological diagnosis must be made. Involvement of the main stem portal vein *or* contralateral involvement of the hepatic artery to one side of the liver and the portal vein to the other were always associated with irresectability.[92] Unilateral involvement of the artery or the vein or both was compatible with resection. The length of the biliary stricture is not a sufficient guide to resectability.

On the basis of studies by Voyles *et al.*[86] a judgement of *irresectability* at pre-operative investigation can be made according to the following criteria: (a) bilateral intrahepatic bile duct spread of the disease so extensive as to preclude resection (or multifocal disease) on cholangiography; (b) involvement of the main trunk of the portal vein; (c) involvement of both branches of the portal vein or bilateral involvement of hepatic artery and portal vein; (d) a combination of vascular involvement to one side of the liver with extensive cholangiographic involvement contralaterally, so that it is impossible to preserve a vascularized segment of the liver with complete excision of tumour. Inaccuracies in this approach include the fact that it is not possible to detect lymph node metastases, the caudate lobe of the liver is not well visualized, and inferior vena cavography is difficult to assess. CT scanning may improve assessment in the future.

Cholangiography on its own has one further important advantage in allowing assessment of the possibilities for palliative treatment, being extremely valuable in demonstrating preoperatively the likely ducts available for biliary-enteric anastomosis (vide infra). Dilated ducts should not be accepted as a sole criterion of suitability for decompression because they may be present in atrophic segments of the liver which function poorly. Such segmental atrophy is not uncommon in hilar cholangiocarcinoma if there is long-standing unilateral ductal or portal venous obstruction.

Treatment

Experience with resection of hilar cholangiocarcinoma is small and the place of resection debated. The resectability rate varies from 5%[8] to 58%.[48] Thus, Longmire was only able to resect six out of 33 lesions and[50] and Smith,[74] who treated 33 cases in 33 years, excised only five. Tompkins and his colleagues[84] have reported 47 cases in whom resection was possible in 22, hepatic resection being part of the procedure in five. Mortality rates for resection vary from 0%[2] to 50%[28] but it should be appreciated that the mortality for simple drainage in biliary tract obstruction is high and that mortality rates will differ according to whether a particular series contains a high proportion of patients with simple excision of the tumor or with excision combined with hepatic resection.

Patients have been approached in the Hepatobiliary Unit at the Royal Postgraduate Medical School, London, with the objective of full preoperative investigation and resection whenever possible, as indicated by the preoperative studies and the general status of the patient. In our experience of 94 patients with hilar cholangiocarcinoma, resection for attempted cure was carried out in 18, with hepatic resection necessary in 12 of these. Three patients, all subjected to hepatic resection, died in hospital, all of infective complications. In two of these the patient had been subjected to long-term preliminary percutaneous transhepatic biliary catheter drainage. A further 15 left the hospital, the mean survival for the entire group being 17 months. Eight patients died at 6–28 months, with a mean survival of 13 months; two of these patients died at seven and nine months of causes unrelated to cholangiocarcinoma, but the remainder died of the effects of recurrent tumours. Seven patients are alive, with a mean survival of 22.2 months (range 9–58). The longest survivor in this group had a tumour affecting the right branch of the portal vein, and treatment consisted of excision of the tumour together with extended right hepatic lobectomy and reconstruction by hepaticojejunostomy to the liver. The postoperative quality of life was studied and the patients submitted to resection were found to have a combined total of 248 months of evaluable survival time, 218 (88%) of which were spent in good health. Patients who were submitted to palliative surgery had a total of 300 months of evaluable time, of which 18 months (6%) were spent symptom free.[12]

Few others have pursued a policy of radical excision of hilar cholangiocarcinoma but some, and in particular workers in Sweden and France, agree with the concept and make a case for tumour excision, either for potential cure or for palliation. Thus, Launois[48] reports 11 patients in whom tumour resection was carried out followed by reconstruction of the biliary tree. Of these, four had simple hepatic duct resection but in the others some form of hepatic lobectomy was necessary. The mean survival time of nine patients was 1.5 years, but five were alive at intervals up to 3.25 years. Similarly, Bengmark's group in Lund[25] recorded 16 of 34 hilar tumours resected, the results in terms of quality of life and survival being better for patients submitted to resection than for bypass. Clearly it is very difficult to compare patients submitted to resection with those submitted to palliation only since the extent of tumour is almost certainly less in the former group, and the general status of the patients almost certainly better. However, it is important not to deny a patient who can tolerate operation the possibility of cure or the best possible palliation, and not simply to resort to intubational methods or bypass as a panacea.[78]

Other forms of treatment

The majority of patients with hilar cholangiocarcinoma will not be suitable for resection and many will be old or have coincident disease. The options open in the management of this group of patients are either some form of biliary decompression by means of biliary-enteric anastomosis or the passage of a trans-tumour tube allowing relief of biliary obstruction. Bypass or intubation may be combined with radiotherapeutic approaches.

Assessment of the results of such palliative methods is no less difficult than for resection. A major problem is that many series of patients submitted to surgical decompression contain some patients who might have been suitable for resection, and therefore constitute a better risk group, and others possibly too ill to tolerate any form of treatment at all. In some reports, histological confirmation of the nature of the stricture has not been available. More recently, percutaneous transhepatic intubational techniques (Figure 19.64) have allowed biliary decompression without laparotomy, and the method is being used for definitive treatment in some cases without due consideration as to the possiblity of resection, or indeed as to whether biliary-enteric bypass might provide a better form of palliation.

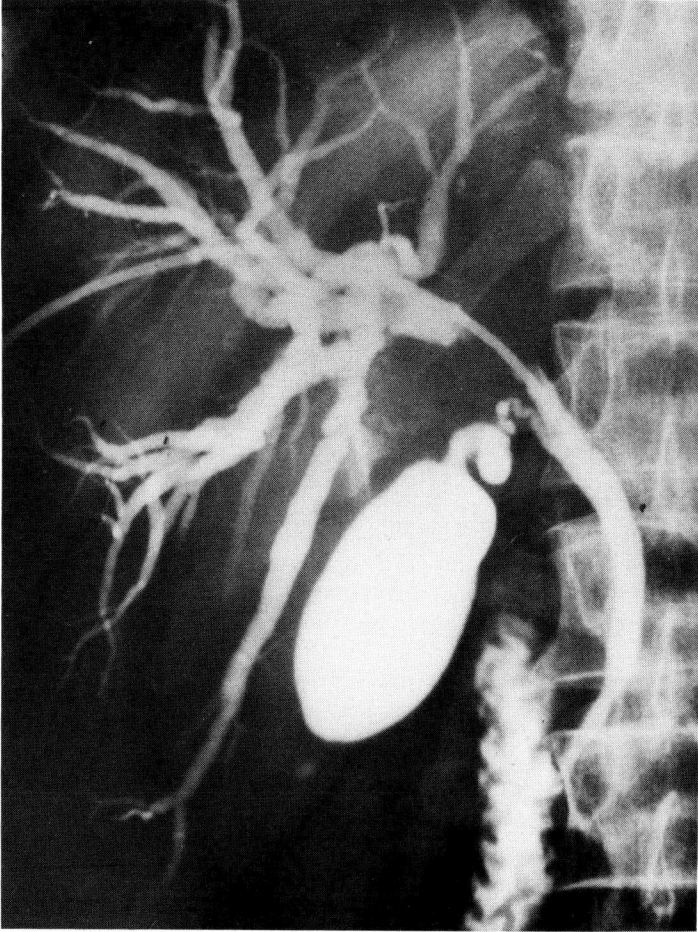

Fig. 19.64 Cholangiocarcinoma at the confluence of the bile ducts traversed by the introduction of a percutaneous transhepatic tube. The left ductal system is not outlined. The tube traverses the tumour and is lying within the distal bile duct. Such tubes may be replaced by means of an indwelling endoprosthesis.

The 'U'-tube technique initially described by Praderi[65, 66, 67] and popularized by Terblanche[79, 80, 81] has been utilized by many. There is no doubt that the method does give palliation, sometimes for several years, in a proportion of patients. Thus Longmire[50] reports relief of jaundice in 15 patients, partial relief in nine but no relief at all in six. One patient lived 4.5 years after operation but it is not stated that histological confirmation was obtained. The series studied in London, at the Royal Postgraduate Medical School, has also yielded a few such successful cases but the period of symptom-free survival is short. Of 32 cases treated by intubation and/or bypass, nine died in hospital (28%) and of the 23 who survived only five are alive at periods from one to 15 months, the mean period of survival being only 8.5 months. Terblanche[78] has stated that he does not believe that resection should be done for lesions in the area of the confluence of the bile duct. He recommends intubation of these tumours and treatment with radiotherapy. In a recent update[79] it is reported that two out of 15

patients treated by this method survived eight and ten years and of the 13 who died the longest survivor was five years. However, there is some doubt that these were biopsy proven carcinomas of the bile ducts and it is important that care is taken to prove the diagnosis before claims of long survival after intubation can be accepted.[82] Indeed, as pointed out earlier in this chapter, benign localized strictures do occur.[72]

Finally, and importantly, despite efforts to maintain sterility, these tubes invariably become infected, and recurrent low grade cholangitis and progressive liver damage is the fate of nearly all the patients. Alternative methods of tubal drainage, such as the placement of a transhepatic endoprosthesis introduced perioperatively or the more recently introduced percutaneous transhepatic drainage, have similar disadvantages and carry with them the potential for serious infection.[54] Launois[48] surveyed the collected results of 12 reports of palliative biliary-jejunal anastomoses, including his own work, and found that the postoperative death rate was 40% and the mean survival only seven months. Biliary fistulation and cholangitis were the most frequent complications and cholangitis the most lethal. It is important to note that included within this survey were satisfactory results from three centres.[8, 68, 70]

Recently, and disappointed with our results of palliative tubal drianage, we have, using detailed PTC studies to select the site of anastomosis, made more use of internal biliary-enteric bypass as described by Bismuth and Corlette.[8] These authors report 80 patients with hilar carcinoma of whom four were resected, ten were deemed inoperable and in six no palliative bypass was possible. Forty-five mucosa-to-mucosa bypass procedures were performed with only two postoperative deaths and three biliary fistulas, the average survival being 13 months. The techniques used by Bismuth's group rely heavily on anastomosis to the left duct, approached through the umbilical fissure by the technique of Soupault and Couinaud[76] (see Figure 19.61). We have recently employed this technique in a series of 18 patients with malignant strictures affecting the confluence of the bile ducts and found it to be highly satisfactory, allowing anastomosis in a high proportion of patients in whom we have previously thought good biliary-enteric drainage was impossible. Drainage of only the left side gives perfectly satisfactory results in terms of relief of jaundice in the majority of cases.

A number of authors have used external irradiation in conjunction with tubal placement,[50, 80] and some long-term survivors have been reported. However, we have encountered severe complications following internal irradiation, including duodenal stenosis and severe irradiation duodenitis with intractable gastrointestinal bleeding in three patients, and have now temporarily suspended its use. More recently Japanese workers have published preliminary results of intraoperative radiotherapy for lesions of this type and the initial findings are encouraging.[42] A small group of patients treated at King's College Hospital, London, have been managed by means of internal radiotherapy by means of an iridium-192 wire passed down a U-tube.[27] This gives the advantage of high dose local irradiation without the side-effects mentioned above. Six out of eight patients so managed were alive up to 23 months after treatment, but as with all tubal drainage systems maintenance of drainage was a problem and tubes required changing in several patients. In two, bile drainage was not achieved, both patients dying at six and 22 months from a combination of cholangitis and tumour extension. Tumour recurrence causing further biliary obstruction occurred in one patient. The authors point out that cholangitis is likely to remain a problem in patients so treated.

The use of percutaneously placed endoprostheses appears an attractive option, but in these high-risk patients even this procedure may carry a mortality of 25–31%.[22, 23] Endoscopically placed prostheses may have a place but are more successful with tumours lower in the biliary tree (see below).[19] Possibly no treatment at all would be the best approach for some elderly and infirm patients.

In conclusion, hilar cholangiocarcinoma continues to pose major problems, but recent advances in imaging methods should allow preoperative diagnosis in most cases. An ordered use of cholangiography combined with angiographic techniques will give an excellent index of irresectability and of the anatomical possibilities for biliary-enteric anastomosis which is probably superior to any form of tubal drainage. Transhepatic intubational techniques may allow preparation of some patients for resectional surgery, but the true benefits of such preoperative decompression await the results of controlled studies. Local irradiation may have a place in the management of these tumours.

Perhaps the most important points to emphasize are first that three studies, including our own, have indicated that resection may be carried out in approximately 20% of patients with an acceptable operative mortality,[25, 48, 86] and one group has a resectability rate of 47%.[82, 84] Operative/hospital mortality must be compared to the high mortality for palliative treatment alone. Adequate investigation also allows a reasonable selection of patients, not only for resection but for biliary-enteric anastomosis, the approach of the French school being particularly valuable.[8, 36] Patients should not be denied a chance for cure, and be submitted to intubational methods for decompression which, whether operative or percutaneous, have a considerable mortality and morbidity, without careful studies to define their selection. Surgical approaches to these lesions require specialist expertise and patients should be referred if possible to centres where adequately trained teams are available.

TUMOURS IN THE MID- AND LOW COMMON BILE DUCT

These tumours are best managed by surgical excision and this is possible in most patients with lesions arising in the middle or lower third of the bile duct. Occasionally, if a tumour involves the mid-portion of the bile duct, local resection with anastomosis or reconstruction by means of a Roux-en-Y loop is sufficient, but most such lesions, if resectable, require wide excision including the head of the pancreas.

It is not clearly understood that the presentation of these lesions may be with intermittent or indeed sometimes with only one attack of jaundice. Here also, as for the high lesions, there remains a belief that the mortality for surgical resection is prohibitive and that the outcome is uniformly poor. However, a nihilistic attitude is not warrented provided precise diagnosis is used and the operation is performed by an experienced surgeon.

Pancreaticoduodenectomy, originally introduced as a two-staged procedure,[91] is now frequently performed in centres specializing in this type of surgery with a mortality of less than 6%.[38, 51, 73, 87] Even in large series, when the patients are drawn from multiple hospitals and not treated by specialist surgeons, the overall hospital mortality for all types of tumour in the peripapillary area is no higher than 21%.[56] Resectability rates vary, with the origin of the tumour being over 70% for ampullary carcinoma and probably about 50% for carcinoma of the bile ducts.[56, 88, 89] The mortality rate also varies with the origin of the tumour, ampullary carcinoma having the lowest mortality within one month of surgery.

The majority of low bile duct cancers are well differentiated but local extension to the pancreas, duodenum and lymph nodes is present in almost half.[88] The lesion may be very difficult and sometimes impossible to differentiate from small carcinomas of the head of the pancreas, although involvement of both the pancreatic and biliary ductal system at ERCP is highly suggestive of pancreatic tumour rather than a lesion of bile duct origin, and occasionally ERCP clearly shows the biliary origin of the lesion (Figure 19.65). The hospital mortality for pancreaticoduodenectomy carried out for bile duct cancer ranges from 8 to 22%. The five-year survival figures of 25% are less good than those for duodenal and ampullary cancer.[89] Curative surgery should usually be attempted, however, provided it can be carried out with an acceptable mortality rate. The results for excision of bile duct cancers in the lower portion of the duct are much better than for the high duct, and long-term survival is recorded.[82, 84] The passage of a

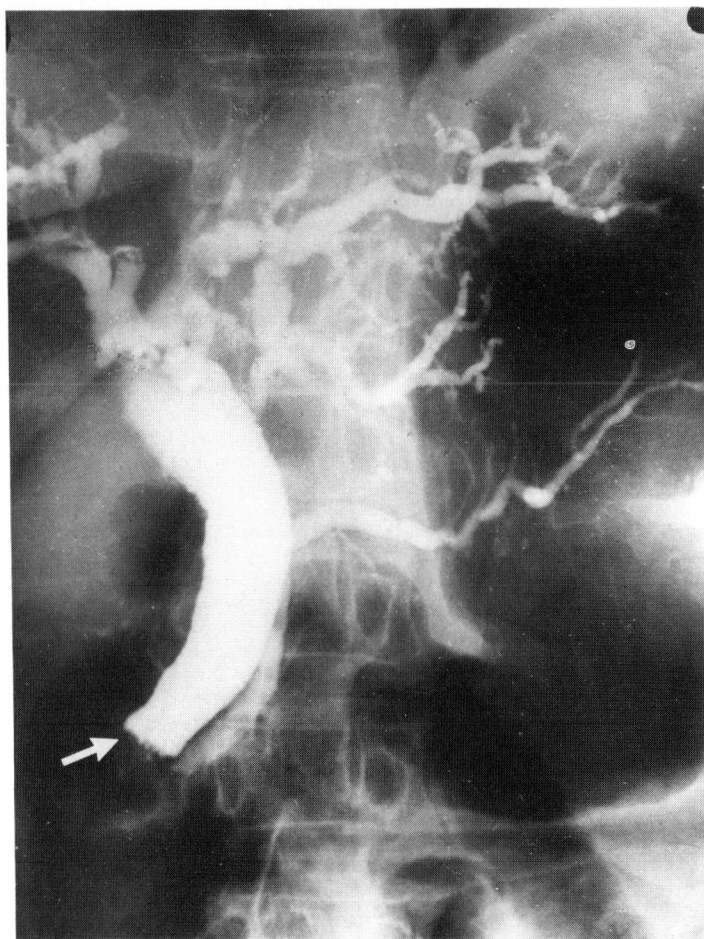

Fig. 19.65 ERCP in a patient who presented with obstructive jaundice. There is a carcinoma involving the lower end of the common bile duct (arrowed), the biliary system being dilated proximally. The lesion is clearly separate from the pancreatic duct and at endoscopy was shown to be not of papillary origin. The diagnosis of a cholangiocarcinoma affecting the lower bile-duct was confirmed at subsequent pancreaticoduodenectomy.

percutaneous drainage catheter as a preliminary to resective surgery may have a place but to date available data suggest this is of limited value.[22, 34, 53, 54] Percutaneous or endoscopic placement of biliary endoprostheses[19, 39] may provide effective palliation, but published results are preliminary and reflect a significant incidence of infection and a high hospital mortality. The place of these techniques, their relationship to surgery and indications for their employment in preference to operative bypass or resection awaits full evaluation.

REFERENCES

1 Adolphs, H. D., Schlachetzki, J., Breining, H. & Karhoff, B. (1974) Maligne Papillomatose der extrahepatischen Gallenwege. *Medizinische Klinik*, 69, 1899–1902.

2 Akwari, O. E. & Kelly, K. A. (1979) Surgical treatment of adenocarcinoma location: junction of the right, left and common hepatic biliary ducts. *Archives of Surgery*, 114, 22–25.

3 Altemeier, W. A., Gall, E. A., Zinninger, M. M. & Hoxworth, P. I. (1957) Sclerosing carcinoma of the major intrahepatic bile ducts. *Archives of Surgery*, 75, 450–460.

4 Arminski, T. C. (1949) Primary carcinoma of the gall bladder. *Cancer*, 2, 397–398.

5 Benjamin, I. S. & Blumgart, L. H. (1979) Biliary bypass and reconstructive surgery. In *Liver and Biliary Disease: Pathophysiology, Diagnosis, Management* (Ed.) Wright, R., Alberti, K. G. M. M., Karran, S. & Millward-Sadler, G. H. pp. 1219–1246. London: W. B. Saunders.

6 Bergdahl, L. (1980) Gallbladder carcinoma first diagnosed at microscopic examination of gallbladders removed for presumed benign disease. *Annals of Surgery*, 191, 19–22.

7 Bernauer, B. & Deucher, F. (1967) Die aszendierende Choledochuspapillomatose. *Schweizerische medizinische Wochenschrift*, 97, 652–654.

8 Bismuth, H. & Corlett, M. B. (1975) Intrahepatic cholangioenteric anastomosis in carcinoma of the hilus of the liver. *Surgery, Gynecology and Obstetrics*, 140, 170–178.

9 Bloustein, P. A. (1977) Association of carcinoma with congenital cystic conditions of the liver and bile ducts. *American Journal of Gastroenterology*, 67, 40–46.

10 Blumgart, L. H. (1978) Biliary tract obstruction – New approaches to old problems. *American Journal of Surgery*, 135, 19–31.

11 Blumgart, L. H., & Kelley, C. J. (1984) Hepaticojejunostomy in benign and malignant high bile duct stricture: approaches to the left hepatic ducts. *British Journal of Surgery* (in press).

12 Blumgart, L. H., Hadjis, N. S., Benjamin, I. S. & Beazley, R. (1984) Surgical approaches to cholangicocarcinoma at confluence of hepatic ducts. *Lancet*, i, 66–70.

13 Broden, G., Ahliberg, J., Bengtsson, L. & Hellers, G. (1978) The incidence of carcinoma of the gallbladder and bile ducts in Sweden, 1958 to 1972. *Acta Chirurgica Scandinavica* (Supplement) 482, 24–25.

14 Caroli, J. (1973) Disease of the intrahepatic biliary tree. *Clinical Gastroenterology*, 2, 147–161.

15 Cattell, R. B., Braasch, J. W. & Kahn, F. (1962) Polypoid epithelial tumors of the bile ducts. *New England Journal of Medicine*, 266, 57–61.

16 Chandler, J. G. & Fletcher, W. S. (1963) A clinical study of primary carcinoma of the gall bladder. *Surgery, Gynecology and Obstetrics*, 117, 297–300.

17 Cohn, I. Jr (1978) Gastrointestinal cancer. Surgical survey of abdominal tragedy. *American Journal of Surgery*, 135, 3–11.

18 Cooke, L., Avery-Jones, F. & Keich, M. K. (1953) Carcinoma of the gallbladder. A statistical study. *Lancet*, ii, 585–587.

19 Cotton, P. B. (1982) Duodenoscopic placement of biliary prostheses to relieve malignant obstructive jaundice. *British Journal of Surgery*, 69, 501–503.

20 Diehl, A. K. (1980) Epidemiology of gallbladder cancer: a synthesis of recent data. *Journal of the National Cancer Institute*, 65, 1209–1214.

21 Donaldson, L. A. & Busutill, A. (1975) A clinicopathological review of 68 carcinomas of the gallbladder. *British Journal of Surgery*, 62, 26–32.

22 Dooley, S., Dick, R., Irving, D. *et al.* (1981) Relief of bileduct obstruction by the percutaneous transhepatic insertion of an endoprosthesis. *Clinical Radiology*, 32, 163–172.

23 Eiss, S., Di Maio, D. & Caedo, J. P. (1960) Multiple papillomas of the entire biliary tract. *Annals of Surgery*, 152, 320–324.

24 Evander, A. & Ihse, I. (1981) Evaluation of intended radical surgery in carcinoma of the gallbladder. *British Journal of Surgery*, 68, 158–160.

25 Evander, A., Fredlund, P., Hoevels, J. *et al.* (1980) Evaluation of aggressive surgery for carcinoma of the extrahepatic bile ducts. *Annals of Surgery*, 191, 23–29.

26 Fahim, R. B., McDonald, J. R., Richards, J. C. & Ferris, D. O. (1962) Carcinoma of the gallbladder; a study of its modes of spread. *Annals of Surgery*, 156, 114–122.

27 Fletcher, M. S., Dawson, J. L., Wheeler, P. G. *et al.* (1981) Treatment of high bile duct carcinoma by internal radiotherapy with Iridium 192 wire. *Lancet*, ii, 172–174.

28 Fortner, J. G., Kallum, B. O. & Kim, D. K. (1976) Surgical management of carcinoma of the junction of the main hepatic ducts. *Annals of Surgery*, 184, 68–73.

29 Gerst, P. H. (1961) Primary carcinoma of the gallbladder. A thirty year summary. *Annals of Surgery*, 153, 369–372.

30 Gouma, D. J., Mutum, S. S., Benjamin, I. S. & Blumgart, L. H. (1984) Intrahepatic biliary papillomatosis. *British Journal of Surgery*, accepted for publication.

31 Graham, E. A. (1931) Prevention of carcinoma of the gallbladder. *Annals of Surgery*, 93, 317–322.

32 Hamrick, R. E. Jr, Liner F. J., Hastings, P. R. & Cohn, I. Jr (1982) Primary carcinoma of the gallbladder. *Annals of Surgery*, 195, 270–273.

33 Harbin, W. P., Mueller, P. R. & Ferrucci, J. T. Jr (1980) Transhepatic cholangiography: complications and use patterns of the fine needle technique. *Radiology*, 135, 15.

34 Hatfield, A. R. W., Terblanche, J., Fataar, S. *et al.* (1982) Preoperative external biliary drainage in obstructive biliary jaundice. *Lancet*, ii, 896–899.

35 Helpap, B. (1977) Malignant papillomatosis of the intrahepatic bile ducts. *Acta Hepato-Gastroenterologica*, 24, 419–425.

36 Hepp, J. & Couinaud, C. (1956) L'abord et l'utilisation du canal hepatique gauch dans les reparations de la voie biliaire principale. *Presse Medicale*, 64, 947–948.

37 Horwitz, A. & Rosenweig, J. (1960) Carcinoma of the gallbladder – a real hazard. A summary of twenty cases. *Journal of the American Medical Association*, 173, 234–236.

38 Howard, J. M. (1968) Pancreatico-duodenectomy. 41 consecutive Whipple resections without an operative mortality. *Annals of Surgery*, **168**, 629–640.

39 Huibregtse, K., Haverkamp, H. J. & Tytgat, G. N. (1981) Transpapillary positioning of a large 3.2 mm biliary endoprosthesis. *Endoscopy*, **13**, 217–219.

40 Hulten, O. (1960) On precancerous bile duct tumours. *Archives Chirurgica Scandinavica*, **119**, 122–125.

41 Huguet, C., Gasne, G. & Caroli, J. (1971) Papillomatose des voies biliaires intrahepatiques. *Revue Medico-chirurgicale des Maladies du Foie, de la Rate et du Pancreas*, **46**, 189–193.

42 Iwasaki, Y., Ohto, M., Todoroki, T. *et al.* (1977) Treatment of carcinoma of the biliary system. *Surgery, Gynecology and Obstetrics*, **144**, 219–224.

43 Kirschbaum, J. D. & Kozoll, D. C. (1941) Carcinoma of the gallbladder and extrahepatic bile ducts. *Surgery, Gynecology and Obstetrics*, **73**, 740–754.

44 Klatskin, G. (1965) Adenocarcinoma of the hepatic duct at its bifurcation within the porta hepatis. *American Journal of Medicine*, **38**, 241–256.

45 Koo, J., Wong, J., Cheng, F. C. Y. & Ong, G. B. (1981) Carcinoma of the gallbladder. *British Journal of Surgery*, **68**, 161–165.

46 Krain, L. S. (1972) Gallbladder and extrahepatic bile duct carcinoma. Analysis of 1808 cases. *Geriatrics*, **27**, 111–117.

47 Kuwayti, K., Baggenstoss, A. H., Stauffer, M. H. & Priestly, J. I. (1957) Carcinoma of the major intrahepatic and the extrahepatic bile ducts exclusive of the papilla of Vater. *Surgery, Gynecology and Obstetrics*, **104**, 357–366.

48 Launois, B., Campion, J.-P., Brissot, P. & Gosselin, M. (1979) Carcinoma of the hepatic hilus. Surgical management and the case for resection. *Annals of Surgery*, **190**, 151–157.

49 Longmire, W. P. Jr (1976) Tumours of the extrahepatic biliary radicals. In *Current Problems in Cancer* (Ed.) Hickey, R. C. pp. 1–45. Chicago: Year Book Medical Publishers.

50 Longmire, W. P. Jr (1977) The diverse causes of biliary obstruction and their remedies. In *Current Problems in Surgery*, **XIV**, 7. p. 29. Chicago: Yearbook Medical Publishers.

51 Longmire, W. P. Jr & Shaffy, O. A. (1966) Certain factors influencing survival after pancreatico-duodenal resection for carcinoma. *American Journal of Surgery*, **111**, 8–12.

52 Madden, J. J. Jr & Smith, G. W. (1974) Multiple biliary papillomatosis. *Cancer*, **34**, 1316–1320.

53 McPherson, G. A. D., Benjamin, I. S. & Blumgart, L. H. (1982) Percutaneous drainage in biliary obstruction. *Lancet*, **ii**, 1155–1156.

54 McPherson, G. A. D., Blenkharn, J. I. & Blumgart, L. H. (1982) The significance of bacteria in external biliary drainage systems. A possible role for antisepsis. *Journal of Clinical Surgery*, **1**, 22–26.

55 Moosa, A. R., Anagnost, M., Hall, A. W. *et al.* (1975) The continuing challenge of gallbladder cancer. Survey of thirty years experience at the University of Chicago. *American Journal of Surgery*, **130**, 57–62.

56 Nakase, A., Mautsumoto, Y., Uchida, K. & Honjo, I. (1977) Surgical treatment of cancer of the pancreas and periampullary region. *Annals of Surgery*, **185**, 52–57.

57 Neumann, R. D., Li Volsi, V. A., Rosenthal, N. S. *et al.* (1976) Adenocarcinoma in biliary papillomatosis. *Gastroenterology*, **70**, 779–782.

58 Nevin, J. E., Moran, T. J., Kay, S. & King, R. (1976) Carcinoma of the gallbladder. *Cancer*, **37**, 141–148.

59 Nishimura, A., Mayama, S., Nakano, K. *et al.* (1975) Carcinoma of the cystic duct: case report. *Japanese*

Journal of Surgery, **5**, 109–117.

60 Okulski, E. G., Dolin, B. J. & Kandawalla, N. M. (1979) Intrahepatic biliary papillomatosis. *Archives of Pathology and Laboratory Medicine*, **103**, 647–649.

61 Pemberton, L. B., Diffenbaugh, W. F. & Strohl, E. L. (1971) The surgical significance of carcinoma of the gallbladder. *American Journal of Surgery*, **122**, 381–383.

62 Perpetuo, M. D. C. M. O., Valdivieso, M., Heilbrun, L. K. *et al.* (1978) Natural history study of gallbladder cancer. *Cancer*, **42**, 330–335.

63 Piehler, J. M. & Crichlow, R. W. (1978) Primary carcinoma of the gallbladder. *Surgery, Gynecology and Obstetrics*, **147**, 929–942.

64 Polk, H. C. (1966) Carcinoma and the calcified gallbladder. *Gastroenterology*, **50**, 582–585.

65 Praderi, R. (1963) El drenaje biliar externo o interno por el hepatico izquierdo. *Revista da Associačao Medica Brasileira*, **9**, 401–403.

66 Praderi, R. (1971) Obstruccion neoplasia de los hepaticos. *Revista Argentina Cirurgica*, **20**, 115.

67 Praderi, R., Parodi, H. & Delgado, B. (1964) Tratamiento de las obstrucciones neoplasicas de la via biliar suprapancreatica. *Anais da Faculdade de Medicina Montevideo*, **49**, 221–241.

68 Ragins, H., Diamond, A. & Meng, C. H. (1973) Intrahepatic cholangiojejunostomy in the management of malignant biliary obstruction. *Surgery, Gynecology and Obstetrics*, **136**, 27–32.

69 Roberts-Thompson, I. C., Strickland, R. J. & Mackay, I. R. (1973) Bile duct carcinoma in chronic ulcerative 0colitis. *Australian and New Zealand Journal of Medicine*, **3**, 264–267.

70 Ross, A. P., Braasch, J. W. & Warren, K. W. (1973) Carcinoma of the proximal bile ducts. *Surgery, Gynecology and Obstetrics*, **136**, 923–928.

71 Ross, F. P. & Hickok, D. F. (1960) Hernia and gallbladder surgery in patients over seventy. *New England Journal of Medicine*, **262**, 501–505.

72 Smadja, C., Bowley, N. & Blumgart, L. H. (1983) Idiopathic localised bile duct strictures. Relationship to primary sclerosing cholangitis (in press).

73 Smith, R. (1973) Progress in the surgical treatment of pancreatic disease. *American Journal of Surgery*, **125**, 143–153.

74 Smith, R. (1981) Injuries of the bile ducts. In *Surgery of the Gallbladder and Bile Ducts*, 2nd edn (Ed.) Lord Smith of Marlow & Sherlock, S. ch. 16, p. 361. London: Butterworths.

75 Solan, M. J. & Jackson, B. T. (1971) Carcinoma of the gallbladder – a clinical appraisal and review of 57 cases. *British Journal of Surgery*, **58**, 593–597.

76 Soupault, R. & Couinaud, C. L. (1957) Sur un procede nouveau de derivation biliaire intra-hepatique. Les cholangio-jejunostomies gauches sans sacrifice hepatique. *La Presse Medicale*, **65**, 1157–1159.

77 Strauch, G. O. (1960) Primary carcinoma of the gallbladder. *Surgery*, **47**, 368–383.

78 Terblanche, J. (1979) Carcinoma of the proximal extrahepatic biliary tree – definitive and palliative treatment. *Surgery Annual*, **11**, 249–265.

79 Terblanche, J. (1981) Discussion of a paper. *Annals of Surgery*, **194**, 455–456.

80 Terblanche, J. & Louw, J. W. (1973) 'U' tube drainage in the palliative therapy of carcinoma of the main hepatic duct system. *Surgical Clinics of North America*, **53**, 1245–1256.

81 Terblanche, J., Saunders, S. G. & Louw, J. W. (1972) Prolonged palliation in carcinoma of the main hepatic duct junction. *Surgery*, **71**, 720–731.

82 Tompkins, R. K. (1982) Carcinoma of the gallbladder and biliary ducts. In *The Biliary Tract. Clinical Surgery*

International Vol. 5 (Ed.) Blumgart, L. H. pp. 183–196. Edinburgh: Churchill Livingstone.

83   Tompkins, R. K. & Berci, G. (1981) Operative cholangioscopy. *Surgical Rounds,* **4,** 20–28.

84   Tompkins, R. K., Thomas, D., While, A. & Longmire, W. P. Jr (1981) Prognostic factors in bile duct cancer. *Annals of Surgery,* **194,** 447–457.

85   Treadwell, T. A. & Hardin, W. J. (1976) Primary carcinoma of the gallbladder: the role of adjunctive therapy in its treatment. *American Journal of Surgery,* **132,** 703–706.

86   Voyles, C. R., Bowley, N. B., Allison, D. J. *et al.* (1983) Carcinoma of the proximal extrahepatic biliary tree. Radiological assessment and therapeutic alternatives. *Annals of Surgery,* **197,** 188–194.

87   Warren, K. W. & Jefferson, M. F. (1973) Carcinoma of the exocrine pancreas. In *The Pancreas* (Ed.) Carey, L. C. p. 243. St Louis: Mosby.

88   Warren, K. W., Veidenheimer, M. C. & Pratt, H. S. (1967) Pancreato-duodenectomy for periampullary cancer. *Surgical Clinics of North America,* **47,** 639–645.

89   Warren, K. W., Choe, D. S., Plaza, J. & Relihan, M. (1975) Results of radical resection for periampullary cancer. *Annals of Surgery,* **181,** 534–540.

90   Welton, J. C., Marr, J. S. & Friedman, S. M. (1979) Association between hepatobiliary cancer and typhoid carrier state. *Lancet,* **i,** 791–794.

91   Whipple, A. O., Parsons, W. B. & Mullins, C. R. (1935) Treatment of carcinoma of ampulla of Vater. *Annals of Surgery,* **102,** 763–799.

92   Williamson, B. W., Blumgart, L. H. & McKellar, N. J. (1980) Management of tumours of the liver. Combined use of arteriography and venography in the assessment of resectability especially in hilar tumours. *American Journal of Surgery,* **139,** 210–215.

OTHER DISORDERS OF THE GALLBLADDER AND BILIARY TRACT

Gallbladder disease in children

Cholelithiasis and cholecystitis are rare in children and neonates[5] but present clinically in a manner similar to adults: right upper quadrant pain, nausea, vomiting and jaundice. The diagnosis can be made by a plain abdominal radiograph for there is a greater possibility of the gallstones being calcified in children than adults, cholecystography, ultrasonography and radionuclide scanning.

A variety of causes has been implicated in the genesis of gallbladder disease in children including congenital abnormalities in the case of neonates, systemic infections in young children, and cholelithiasis in older children. It is claimed that acalculous cholelithiasis is commoner in children than adults. Haemolytic disease is uncommonly responsible for gallstones in children. There is a prominent association between cholelithiasis and early pregnancy in adolescents.

Many of the children are obese and, in contrast to adults, gallstones in children occur with almost equal frequency in males and females.[3]

The management of children follows the same principles as for adults and a cholecystectomy is recommended.

Hyperplastic cholecystoses

This term has been used to describe a variety of degenerative and non-inflammatory hyperplastic disorders involving the gallbladder mucosa and muscle. The unitary concept remains controversial and includes such conditions as adenomyomatosis, cholesterolosis, neuromatosis, lipomatosis, fibromatosis and calcified gallbladder.[1] The lesions may be generalized, localized or segmental.

Adenomyomatosis

In this disorder there is hyperplasia of the muscle and mucosa of the gallbladder. The projection of pouches of mucous membrane through weak points in the muscle coat, possibly due to raised intracystic pressure, produces the so-called Rokitansky–Aschoff sinuses or crypts. These are probably identical with intramural diverticula.[6] The diverticula (or sinuses or crypts) are usually intramural and are not recognized with the naked eye. The diverticula may opacify on cholecystography and are best seen after gallbladder contraction when they appear as a 'halo' or ring of opacified beads around the gallbladder. Other appearances include deformity of the body of the gallbladder or marked irregularity of outline. Localized adenomyomatosis is responsible for the appearance of a phrygian cap at the gallbladder fundus.

Cholesterolosis

In this condition there is deposition of cholesterol esters and other lipids in the mucosa in the absence of inflammation. If diffuse it appears as a 'strawberry gallbladder' but the lesion may be patchy. Radiological features are those of small fixed filling defects on cholecystography.

CLINICAL FEATURES

There is much disagreement over the clinical significance of the hyperplastic cholecystoses and whether or not they produce symptoms. Some authors attribute right upper quadrant pain and other digestive disorders to the condition[4] whereas others are more cautious in ascribing a clinical syndrome to the pathology. Hyperplastic cholecystoses are probably common, one or other of the features being recognized histologically in up to 50% of resected gallbladders. Cholecystitis and cholelithiasis may be superimposed on a gallbladder with hyperplastic cholecystosis.

Management is controversial and depends on whether or not there is a belief that the disorder is a cause of symptoms in which event cholecystectomy is recommended. The indication for surgery is more certain when there is in addition cholecystitis or cholelithiasis.

Vasculitis

Cholecystitis may occur as a rare complication in polyarteritis nodosa, systemic lupus erythematosis and giant cell arteritis. The gallbladder disease takes the form of an acute acalculous cholecystitis and is managed by a cholecystectomy.

Emphysematous cholecystitis

In this disorder there is acute cholecystitis with the formation of gas in the wall or lumen of the gallbladder and in the biliary tract. The organisms are similar to those found in the more commonly encountered variety of cholecystitis. The condition is rare and found particularly in aged patients and those with diabetes mellitus.

The presentation is that of an acute severe cholecystitis and plain radiographs reveal gas in the biliary system. The patient requires an urgent cholecystectomy with adequate antibiotic cover particularly with penicillin and an aminoglycoside since the most common gas-forming bacteria in bile are *Clostridia* and *Escherichia coli*.

Haemobilia

Bleeding from the gallbladder is rare and the term 'haemocholecyst' has been suggested to distinguish gallbladder bleeding from bleeding into the extra- and intrahepatic ducts.[2] The causes of gallbladder bleeding include erosion of the cystic artery by a gallstone, haemorrhagic cholecystitis, cancer of the gallbladder and aberrant pancreatic tissue in the gallbladder wall. Rarely the bleeding may produce sufficient pressure to rupture the viscus thereby inducing a haemoperitoneum.

Intrahepatic lithiasis

Three varieties of intrahepatic gallstones have been described:[7] (1) primary intrahepatic gallstones when stones are present only in the intrahepatic biliary radicles; (2) intrahepatic gallstones secondary to infection or biliary stasis; (3) mixed intrahepatic and extrahepatic bile duct gallstones.

Primary intrahepatic gallstones are usually found in the Far East and are related particularly to the parasitic infections ascariasis and clonorchiasis. These parasites, together with the liver flukes *Opisthorchis sinens* (Chinese liver fluke) and *Fasciola hepatica* (sheep liver fluke), may be a cause for acalculous cholecystitis or gallstones.

Mixed intrahepatic and extrahepatic bile duct stones are a complication in 1–2.5% of patients with gallstones in the West. The presentation is with right-sided abdominal pain, fever and jaundice, and the diagnosis is established either by percutaneous transhepatic cholangiography or endoscopic retrograde cholangiography. The management is by surgical removal of the gallstones, flushing of the biliary tree and the establishment of permanent, adequate biliary drainage. Usually a papillostomy or choledochotomy is sufficient, but occasionally it is necessary to perform a segmental hepatic resection. A Roux-en-Y hepaticojejunostomy is advised if the calibre of the biliary tree is greater than 2 cm.

Surgical drainage is not always successful and about 10% of patients suffer from recurrent bile stasis and cholangitis and eventually develop liver failure.

REFERENCES

1 Aguirre, J. R., Boher, R. O. & Guraeib, S. (1969) Hyperplastic cholecystoses: a new contribution to the unitarian theory. *American Journal of Roentgenology*, **107**, 1–13.
2 Bismuth, H. (1973) Hemobilia. *New England Journal of Medicine*, **288**, 617–619.
3 Crichlow, R. W., Seltzer, M. H. & Jannetta, P. J. (1972) Cholecystitis in adolescents. *American Journal of Digestive Diseases*, **17**, 68–72.
4 Elfving, G., Lehtonen, T. & Teir, H. (1967) Clinical significance of primary hyperplasia of gallbladder mucosa. *Annals of Surgery*, **165**, 61–69.
5 Harned, R. K. & Babbitt, D. P. (1975) Cholelithiasis in children. *Radiology*, **117**, 391–393.
6 Ochsner, S. F. (1971) Intramural lesions of the gallbladder. *American Journal of Roentgenology*, **113**, 1–9.
7 Simi, M., Loriga, P., Basoli, A. *et al.* (1979) Intrahepatic lithiasis. *American Journal of Surgery*, **137**, 317–322.

Chapter 20
The Peritoneum

CONGENITAL ABNORMALITIES OF THE ANTERIOR ABDOMINAL WALL, PERITONEUM AND MESENTERY

THE ANTERIOR ABDOMINAL WALL

The anterior abdominal wall contains and protects the abdominal viscera. During early intra-uterine life the wall is severely deficient, permitting herniation of the midgut loop into the extra-embryonic coelom. In this way a 'physiological' umbilical hernia is produced. By the tenth week of intrauterine life the midgut returns to the abdominal cavity and simultaneously the abdominal wall develops to completely enclose the abdominal viscera. The umbilical cord is attached to the abdominal wall at the umbilical ring. Within about ten days of birth the cord shrivels, dries and separates at its junction with the skin, and the umbilical ring closes.

Congenital abnormalities of the abdominal wall and umbilicus are common although the majority are of a minor nature.

Umbilical hernia

This is due to failure of the umbilical ring to completely close. A small sac of peritoneum is forced through the gap in the linea alba and becomes adherent to the overlying skin. During crying or straining, bowel or omentum bulges through the gap into the peritoneal sac. The hernia is almost always easily reducible and incarceration is rare. In the majority of children the gap closes spontaneously and the hernia disappears. However, if the hernia persists after the age of three years, it is unlikely to close spontaneously and surgical repair should be carried out.

Paraumbilical hernia

In this condition the umbilical ring closes normally after birth, but there is a small defect usually just above, or less commonly just below, the umbilicus, giving rise to a paraumbilical hernia. This will not close spontaneously and requires to be closed surgically.

Epigastric hernia

This is due to a defect in the linea alba, usually located midway between the xiphoid process and the umbilicus. A small piece of extra-peritoneal fat protrudes through the defect, causing a swelling. This will often cause pain and tenderness. The fat should be removed and the defect repaired surgically.

Exomphalos (omphalocoele)

This is a rare but serious major hernia through the anterior abdominal wall at the umbilicus. The intestine is covered by a glistening, transparent membrane consisting of amniotic sac lined by peritoneum. As the membrane is avascular, it disintegrates rapidly, becoming opaque in 12 hours and rupturing by 36 hours, thus exposing the abdominal viscera. Prompt surgical intervention is essential if the life of the baby is to be saved.

Two main types are described: hernia into the umbilical cord (exomphalos minor) and exomphalos major.

HERNIA INTO THE UMBILICAL CORD (EXOMPHALOS MINOR)

In this condition the midgut loop has failed to return normally into the abdominal cavity. The neck of the sac is an abnormally wide umbilical ring but is usually less than 5 cm in diameter. The herniated loops of gut occupy the base of the cord. It is often possible to reduce the hernia by simply twisting the cord. Because the umbilical defect is usually small, it is possible to excise the avascular sac and repair the abdominal wall in layers.

EXOMPHALOS MAJOR

In exomphalos major the defect in the abdominal wall is much larger. The avascular sac contains multiple loops of small intestine and often also liver. Because the physiological umbilical hernia of intrauterine life fails to return to the abdominal cavity, it is common to have associated malrotation of the midgut loop. There is also a high incidence of other congenital defects, especially cardiac and renal tract abnormalities.

Immediate treatment consists of covering the sac with a sterile plastic bag. Definitive treatment should be carried out within a few hours of delivery. However, the abdominal cavity is often too small to allow reduction of the hernia to be carried out. The aim of the operation is, therefore, to remove the avascular sac, to mobilize skin flaps from the remainder of the abdominal wall and to suture the skin over the defect. No attempt is made to repair the muscle layers. In this way skin cover is produced but with a ventral hernia. A formal repair of the abdominal musculature is performed at about two years of age.[1]

If skin cover is not possible, as is often the case, two alternative methods of management are available. The sac may be painted regularly with 2% aqueous mercurochrome; within a few days a dry eschar is formed which allows granulation tissue to form beneath it. Epithelialization then occurs slowly from the periphery as the eschar separates. The alternative is to carry out a staged repair of the defect using silastic sheeting.[2] This method has proved to be extremely useful in dealing with very large defects. The sac is excised and the skin is undercut from the margins of the defect. Silastic sheets are then sutured to each other over the exposed viscera

like the ridge of a tent. The skin is sutured to the silastic sheets as far up the side of the sheeting as possible. Every two to three days the abdominal contents are squeezed further into the abdominal cavity and a fresh row of sutures is placed between the silastic sheets. Thus the length of the sheets covering the defect is gradually shortened and the skin and rectus muscle of each side are brought closer together. After two weeks it is usually possible to remove the silastic sheets and to approximate the rectus muscles and skin.

Gastroschisis

In gastroschisis there is also a defect in the anterior abdominal wall in the region of the umbilicus allowing loops of bowel to protrude. There are, however, several important differences between this condition and exomphalos. In gastroschisis, the umbilical cord is normally situated and the defect is usually just to the right of the cord. There is no sac and the herniated viscera are completely exposed. Unlike exomphalos, associated congenital abnormalities are rare, which improves the prognosis. Treatment is, however, similar, the aim being to return the bowel to the abdominal cavity and to obtain skin cover in a similar fashion to that described for exomphalos (see above).

Persistence of the vitellointestinal duct

In early intrauterine life the vitellointestinal duct connects the apex of the midgut loop with the vitelline sac. It normally becomes obliterated and disappears completely. However, the whole or part of the vitellointestinal duct may occasionally persist, giving rise to several characteristic congenital abnormalities. If the entire duct remains, there is a patent communication between the ileum and the umbilicus which may discharge faeces or flatus; if only the proximal end persists, a Meckel's diverticulum is formed. Persistence of the distal part of the duct leads to an umbilical sinus which is lined by intestinal mucosa and secretes mucus. Rarely, the proximal and distal ends of the vitellointestinal duct are closed but the middle part remains patent. Mucus is secreted into the open part causing cystic dilatation.

THE PERITONEUM AND MESENTERY

Major abnormalities of fixation of the mesentery to the posterior abdominal wall are rare and are associated with either nonrotation, incomplete rotation or malrotation of the midgut loop. Incomplete fixation of the small intestinal mesentery, which is then free to twist, may give rise to neonatal volvulus of the small intestine.

Minor abnormalities of peritoneal fixation are common, especially at the duodenojejunal junction and in the ileocaecal region. The peritoneum may be folded beneath the bowel and reflected on to the posterior abdominal wall forming a pouch. Such pouches are of clinical importance since loops of small intestine may be trapped within them, causing internal herniation and intestinal obstruction.

Occasionally abnormal peritoneal bands are present, passing between the intestine and the posterior abdominal wall. These may cause compression of the small intestine and mechanical obstruction.

Congenital cysts of the mesentery

Congenital cysts are occasionally found within the peritoneal cavity. They may be small and asymptomatic, being only an incidental finding at laparotomy or they may become very large and present either as a painless abdominal swelling or as recurrent attacks of abdominal pain and vomiting. Acute abdominal symptoms may be precipitated by infection, torsion or rupture. The most common congenital cysts of the mesentery are the chylolymphatic cyst and the enterogenous cyst.

The *chylolymphatic cyst* arises in congenitally abnormal lymphatic tissue. There is no efferent communication with the rest of the lymphatic system and cystic dilatation occurs. The commonest site is in the small bowel mesentery. The cyst may be multilocular or unilocular and contains either clear lymph or chyle. Treatment is by surgical excision.

An *enterogenous cyst* arises as a result of duplication of the intestine and is usually situated on the mesenteric side of the small intestine. Its wall is similar to that of the small intestine, being lined by mucous membrane. There is no communication with the adjacent intestine but the cyst shares the same blood supply; hence enucleation is impossible and resection of the affected part of the intestine is necessary.

REFERENCES

1 Gross, R. E. (1948) A new method for surgical treatment of large omphalocoeles. *Surgery*, **24**, 277.
2 Schuster, S. R. (1967) A new method for the staged repair of large omphalocoeles. *Surgery, Gynecology and Obstetrics*, **125**, 837.

ASCITES

The peritoneum

The peritoneum is a complex serous membrane which lines the abdominal wall and is reflected over the viscera within the abdomen. The parietal and visceral layers are developed, respectively, from the somatopleural and splanchnopleural layers of the lateral plate mesoderm. The peritoneal cavity is closed in the male but communicates with the open ends of the uterine tubes in females. There are many ligaments, two omenta, a greater and a lesser mesentery, and many peritoneal recesses and folds between the organs. The total area of peritoneal surface in the adult is between 1.5 and 2.0 m^2, approximately equal to the total body surface area. The blood flow to the peritoneum is from 50 to 70 ml/min.

The normal peritoneum consists of a single layer of flattened mesothelial cells with round or oval nuclei and a submesothelial layer of collagen and reticular fibres. Microvilli protrude from the free mesothelial surface, which is lubricated by a small volume of serous fluid.[13] In women of reproductive age the amount of fluid varies, being greatest (20 ± 6 ml) during the early luteal phase. If the ovaries are inactive the volume is 4 ± 2 ml.[24] It seems that peritoneal fluid in females may be derived in part from ovarian exudation.

The peritoneum participates in solute exchange and is permeable to molecules of small and intermediate molecular weight (500–5 000 daltons). Transfer of substances occurs probably by both simple intercellular and transcellular movement. Diffusion of ions is quantitatively greater across the mesentery than by transfer across the parietal peritoneum. Particulate material is taken up by phagocytic cells.

There is still controversy over the mechanism of peritoneal repair. The most favoured concept is that healing occurs by the development of new mesothelial cells from metaplasia of subperitoneal fibroblasts. It is unlikely that the mechanism is by transformation of peritoneal macrophages or by the seeding of mesothelial cells from adjacent normal peritoneal surfaces.[13] Three phases are discernible in the development of adhesions: firstly, from 0 to 7 hours after injury, degeneration and desquamation of mesothelial cells occurs; secondly, from 7 hours to 10 days, fibrin is deposited on the exposed basement membrane and fibrinous adhesions are formed; thirdly, from 10 to 30 days, the transformation of fibrinous to fibrous adhesions occurs.[30]

The Peritoneum

Ascites is the accumulation of excessive fluid in the peritoneal cavity. The causes are listed in Table 20.1, the commonest in the United Kingdom being malignant disease and cirrhosis of the liver. Fluid accumulates when it enters the peritoneal cavity from the mesenteries, the peritoneum and the hepatic surface at a rate greater than can be returned to the circulation via the capillaries and lymphatics.

Clinical features

The patient may be unaware of the presence of ascites, but sudden and marked accumulation of peritoneal fluid is accompanied by abdominal discomfort, which may be severe, and dyspnoea. Pain is often a feature of malignant ascites.

The classic physical sign of free fluid is shifting dullness; less satisfactory is the demonstration of a fluid thrill. However, the clinical detection of ascites is unreliable. At least one litre of fluid is necessary to detect shifting dullness and the sign can be mimicked by a loaded colon with a mesentery. It is claimed that as little as 120 ml of fluid can be detected when the abdomen is percussed with the patient in the knee-chest position – the 'puddle' sign, but this is an inelegant and uncomfortable examination. With greater accumulation of fluid there is bulging of the flanks, elevation of the diaphragm, eversion of the umbilicus, and scrotal and lower limb oedema, probably from pressure upon the inferior vena cava. Renal function may be compromised by compression of the renal veins and proteinuria ensues. In gross ascites, slightly elevated jugular venous pressure may be observed. A pleural effusion develops in about 10% of patients and is believed to result from the passage of ascitic fluid through small tears in the peritoneum overlying defects in the diaphragm. The effusion is usually found in the right pleural cavity.

Ascites must be differentiated from gaseous distention of the bowel (the abdomen is resonant and the umbilicus never becomes everted), obesity, pregnancy, large intra-abdominal tumours, and ovarian cysts. Characteristically ovarian cysts demonstrate dullness in the centre of the abdomen and resonance in the flanks – the very opposite of the findings in ascites.

Investigations

The clinical diagnosis of gross ascites is generally easy, but if there is any doubt the fluid may be demonstrated by radiological means, or by diagnostic paracentesis. Paracentesis with

Table 20.1 Causes of ascites

Liver disease (see Table 20.2)	cirrhosis
	Budd–Chiari syndrome
	subacute hepatic necrosis
	fulminant viral hepatitis
	malignant infiltration
	veno-occlusive disease
	hepatocellular cancer
	cholangiocarcinoma
Cardiac	congestive cardiac failure
	constrictive pericarditis
	tricuspid insufficiency
Renal	nephrotic syndrome
	acute glomerulonephritis
	chronic peritoneal dialysis
	long-term haemodialysis
	renal transplant
Pancreatic	malignant disease
	chronic pancreatitis
	acute pancreatitis
	pseudocyst
Infection/Inflammation	intestinal perforation
	tuberculosis
	syphilis
	pyogenic infections
	filariasis
	candidiasis
Malignant disease	ovary
	uterus
	stomach
	prostate
	mesothelioma
	leukaemia
	sarcoma
	colon
	testes
	breast
	neuroblastoma
	lymphoma
	myeloma
Venous thrombosis	portal vein obstruction
	inferior vena caval obstruction
Malnutrition/Protein-energy malnutrition	protein-losing enteropathy
Miscellaneous	trauma
	bile leak
	endometriosis
	myxoedema
	recurrent polyserositis (familial Mediterranean fever)
	Whipple's disease
	congenital dysplasia of the lymphatic system
	vasculitis
	systemic lupus erythematosus
	Henoch–Schonlein purpura
	Crohn's disease
	sarcoidosis
	eosinophilic ascites
	urinary ascites of newborn (see Table 20.4)

chemical, microbiological and cytological examination of the fluid is mandatory in all patients presenting for the first time with ascites, unless there are specific contraindications.

PLAIN RADIOGRAPH OF THE ABDOMEN

In the presence of ascites there is a generalized loss of density and detail, particularly at the hepatic angle. Supine and lateral views show the gut to be floating on fluid.

ULTRASONIC SCAN

Scanning can be performed with a gray-scale B-scanner or a real-time B-scanner. Longitudinal and transverse abdominal scans are performed on patients who are supine, but occasionally other positions are used to demonstrate a fluid shift. The technique is more sensitive than radiology and can detect as little as 300 ml of fluid. Early features on the scan are free fluid in the superior right paracolic gutter, lateral to the liver, or in the pelvis. As fluid accumulates it is detected around and beneath the liver and in the lesser sac, the transverse colon floats on the surface of the fluid and loops of small intestine are arranged around the mesentery (Figure 20.1). The bowel has a characteristic polycystic or arcuate appearance; it usually floats but sinks when empty. Ultrasonography can differentiate between free and loculated fluid, and between fluid in the gallbladder, urinary bladder or an ovarian cyst.[16] The features of a *transudate* are homogeneous echo-free areas surrounding and interposed between the loops of bowel and the viscera in a uniform manner; the features of an *exudate* are small amorphous echos, septa and matted loops of bowel.

COMPUTERIZED TOMOGRAPHY

This technique accurately detects small volumes of fluid, particularly when in the pelvic, perihepatic or perisplenic regions. It is of especial help in the diagnosis of intra-abdominal masses associated with ascites.

PARACENTESIS

This simple and safe procedure can be undertaken for diagnostic purposes, but also may be used to relieve the discomfort of massive ascites. The patient should first empty the bladder. Aspiration is made under local anaesthesia via a 21 gauge needle. The usual site is in either of the iliac fossae, midway between the anterior superior iliac spine and the umbilicus. For diagnostic purposes about 50 ml of fluid is aspirated and examined macroscopically, microbiologically, chemically and cytologically.[3]

Macroscopic appearances

The fluid in cirrhosis is generally translucent and yellow to light green in appearance, deriving some of its colour from bilirubin. Blood-stained ascites is a feature of trauma, neoplastic involvement of the peritoneum or tuberculosis. The fluid may be bile-stained or chylous which can be recognized by the white, turbid appearance. A cloudy fluid suggests infection, but this appearance also occurs in one third of patients with uninfected ascites, and in the absence of raised white blood cell concentrations.[2]

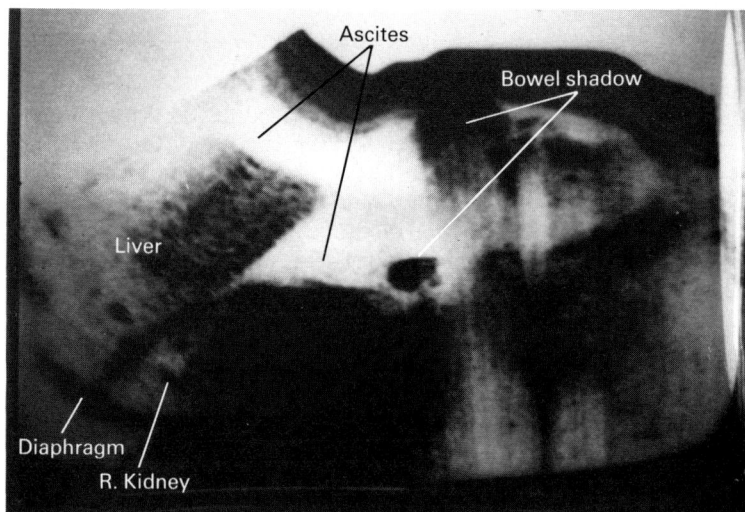

Fig. 20.1 Ultrasonic scan of a patient with ascites: longitudinal scan through right lobe of liver.

Biochemistry

Protein. The protein content is used to distinguish a transudate, which has a total protein less than 25 g/l, from an exudate, which has a greater protein concentration. A transudate is typical in cirrhosis of the liver, cardiac failure and those diseases with a low serum albumin. However, protein levels as high as 50 g/l have been reported in chronic liver disease, congestive cardiac failure and constrictive pericarditis, when the protein is believed to originate from the lymphatics. Seventeen per cent of patients with liver disease have an ascitic fluid protein greater than 30 g/l and 12% have concentrations greater than 40 g/l. An exudate suggests that the fluid is inflammatory, malignant or traumatic in origin, but rarely malignant ascites has a protein level less than 20 g/l.

Glucose. Ascitic glucose concentration is generally low in bacterial infections, tuberculosis and malignant ascites, but the results are variable and the measurement does not have diagnostic value.

Enzymes. Amylase concentrations greater than 2 000 U and elevated lipase levels occur in ascites of pancreatic origin. Lactic dehydrogenase levels greater than 500 Sigma units occur in malignant disease, but this enzyme does not distinguish clearly between a transudate and an exudate.

pH. The ascitic fluid in patients with bacterial peritonitis has been shown to have a low pH, being from 7.12 to 7.31 in contrast to the normal range of 7.39 to 7.58.[20]

Cytology

White cell count. A white cell count greater than 500/mm^3 with more than 50% polymorphonuclear cells suggests bacterial peritonitis. Only 10% of cirrhotic patients with uninfected ascites have a cell count greater than 500 cells/mm^3, and 90% of the cells in such effusions are mononuclear. If mononuclear cells predominate in a raised ascitic white cell count, tuberculosis, neoplasm, and pancreatic ascites should be considered.[8] The presence of candida in the absence of peritoneal dialysis suggests intestinal perforation.

Cytodiagnosis. Cells are exfoliated from the peritoneum in the presence of ascites, but they are often so grossly deformed and coated with mucus and fibrin that conventional light and electron microscopy are unhelpful. These techniques lack both specificity and sensitivity. Scanning electron microscopy holds more promise because it provides a three-dimensional view and it is possible to distinguish lymphocytes (with short microvilli), mesothelial cells (with denser microvilli), histocytes (with laminar-shaped microvilli) and adenocarcinoma (with very dense microvilli).

DIAGNOSTIC PARACENTESIS IN THE ACUTE ABDOMEN

A variety of methods has been described. A four-quadrant tap is regarded as unnecessary. Either needle aspiration under local anaesthesia is performed at the point of maximum abdominal tenderness, or a dialysis catheter is introduced in the midline below the umbilicus and manipulated into the pelvis. Aspiration of more than 1 ml of fluid is regarded as a positive indication of intraperitoneal disease. This technique is useful in assessing abdominal trauma, acute pancreatitis and in the assessment of postoperative complications.[21]

OTHER INVESTIGATIONS

Other investigations which may provide diagnostic help include peritoneal biopsy (of particular value in tuberculous peritonitis rather than malignant disease), laparoscopy and serum thyroxine levels.

Ascites in cirrhosis of the liver

The process of fluid accumulation in cirrhotic patients has been studied intensively and a number of mechanisms are recognized which operate to varying degrees in individual patients.

PORTAL HYPERTENSION

The causes of an increased portal venous pressure, that is a pressure greater than 14 mmHg, are shown in Table 20.2. Under normal resting conditions only one fifth of the sinusoids are perfused by portal blood; there is no increase in the portal blood pressure until the portal blood flow has increased five fold.[10] Conversely, small increases in portal blood flow (which occur after meals and with splenic enlargement) readily increase the portal pressure in patients with cirrhosis. Increased vascular resistance to hepatic outflow develops in cirrhotic patients for several reasons. Vascular channels in the liver may be compressed by fibrosis and regenerating

Table 20.2 Classification of portal hypertension

Suprahepatic	veno-occlusive disease
	hepatic vein occlusion
	(Budd–Chiari syndrome)
	constrictive pericarditis
	right-sided heart failure
Intrahepatic	cirrhosis – from any cause
	hepatitis
	congenital hepatic fibrosis
	partial nodular transformation
	idiopathic non-cirrhotic portal
	hypertension
	sarcoidosis
	schistosomiasis
	reticulo-endothelial system
	diseases
	veno-occlusive disease
Extra(pre)hepatic	portal vein thrombosis due to
	pancreatic disease, sepsis,
	thrombotic states, trauma,
	malignant disease
Increased hepatic blood flow	tropical splenomegaly syndrome
	blood dyscrasias
	cirrhosis with congestive
	splenomegaly

nodules, and there is a decrease in hepatic outflow tracts because of a reduction in the number of central and hepatic veins in association with an increase in hepatic arterial channels.[27] Arteriovenous shunts may develop and contribute to portal hypertension.

Portal vein occlusion is rarely accompanied by ascites, whereas the accumulation of fluid in the peritoneum is a common association of obstruction to the hepatic veins.

HYPOALBUMINAEMIA

Hypoalbuminaemia accompanies chronic or subacute liver disease, renal disease and protein-losing enteropathies. In cirrhosis of the liver there is reduced hepatic albumin synthesis, and the combination of a low serum albumin concentration and raised portal pressure causes increased exudation of fluid from the arteriolar end of the capillary and reduced reabsorption of fluid at the venous end. However, the presence of a reduced plasma colloid oncotic pressure and an increase in the splanchnic venous hydrostatic pressure does not always predict accurately the development of ascites in the cirrhotic patient.

INCREASED LYMPH FLOW

Cirrhosis of the liver is characterized by the production of large volumes of splanchnic lymph consequent upon the high hydrostatic pressure that accompanies portal hypertension. The narrow plasma/tissue oncotic gradient associated with hypoalbuminaemia and the discontinuous endothelial lining of the hepatic sinusoids allow plasma proteins to pass into the interstitial tissue, thereby further reducing the colloid osmotic gradient. Normally filtration occurs at a very low sinusoidal pressure, and a small increase in hydrostatic pressure will encourage the outpouring of protein-rich hepatic lymph.[34] Thoracic lymph flow rises to 10–12 ml/min from a normal of 1 ml/min, and ascites develops when the capacity of the intra-abdominal lymphatics to remove the fluid is exceeded. Hepatic lymph drainage may be impaired not only by lymphatic obstruction from fibrous tissue and regenerating nodules, but also by obstruction at the junction of the thoracic duct and the subclavian vein.[14]

In hepatic venous obstruction there is a leak of high-protein lymph from the liver itself; in portal vein obstruction the fluid tends to originate from the extensive surface of the peritoneum and is low in protein. The combination of fluid originating from these two separate sites, with differing protein content, explains the variation that is encountered in the protein content of the ascitic fluid in cirrhosis of the liver.

DISORDERED SODIUM AND WATER METABOLISM

A feature of hepatic cirrhosis is loss of the normal diurnal rhythm of urinary sodium excretion and an inability to excrete a large sodium load. Patients with hepatic decompensation and ascites excrete little sodium and ultimately develop oliguria and renal failure. It is possible that this avid conservation of sodium is secondary to a reduced effective circulatory volume following the sequestration of fluid in the splanchnic and hepatic tissues, and ultimately in the peritoneal cavity. Furthermore, a decrease in effective central blood volume might activate baroreceptors which inhibit vagal afferent impulses to the midbrain and hypothalamus, increase the sympathetic efferent discharge, and activate the renin–angiotensin–aldosterone axis with enhancement of distal tubular sodium reabsorption.[5] Alternatively the primary defect may be an abnormality of renal sodium concentration, which then causes an increased extracellular volume and overflow of fluid into the peritoneal cavity in association with altered portal vascular system haemodynamics. The immersion studies of Epstein[17] support the concept that a reduced effective intravascular volume is the major factor in sodium retention.

The traditional view that hyperaldosteronism is the mechanism involved in producing renal sodium conservation following a reduction in effective circulatory volume has been questioned. Two thirds of patients with cirrhosis of the liver who also have fluid retention do not have increased renin or aldosterone activity.[33] An excess antidiuretic hormone (ADH) activity may contribute to fluid retention. Higher than normal levels of circulating ADH have been observed in cirrhosis[6] and water retention has been reversed by alcohol[31] and demeclocycline[12] which are known to impair ADH secretion. An elevation of vasoactive inhibitory peptide or a deficiency of humoral naturetic factor have also been suggested to have a role in the genesis of ascites.

TREATMENT

Ascites complicating chronic liver disease is treated with a combination of a low sodium diet and diuretics. The daily intake of sodium should not exceed 25–50 mmol, but there are advantages in permitting the patient to have a combination of effective diuretics and an unrestricted sodium intake – food is more palatable and there is a reduced tendency to hyponatraemia.[29] The initial diuretic agents to be used are aldosterone antagonists such as spironolactone at a starting dose of 200 mg daily; this can be increased to 400 mg daily in order to achieve a urinary sodium : potassium ratio greater than one. The addition of a loop diuretic such as frusemide, ethacrynic acid or bumetamide may be necessary to achieve a satisfactory diuresis. The initial dose of frusemide is 40 mg daily with a maximum daily dose of 250 mg. All loop diuretics must be used with caution, particularly in patients without peripheral oedema when the rate of diuresis must be restricted to produce a weight loss of around 0.6 kg daily; there is a limit to the rate at which fluid can be mobilized from the peritoneal cavity and more vigorous diuresis will contract the circulatory volume, particularly in the presence of hypoalbuminaemia.[15, 19] Used judiciously, diuretic therapy is safe and is not associated with serious complications. It is seldom necessary to remove all the ascitic fluid; indeed there are advantages if the amount of peritoneal fluid is reduced only as far as is necessary to ensure the comfort of the patient. Potassium depletion must be avoided and, although drugs like spironolactone, amiloride and triamterene have a potassium-sparing action, potassium (in the form of potassium chloride and at a daily dose of 100 mmol) is frequently required.

The majority of patients respond to a regimen of initial bed rest, salt restriction and diuretics, but in a few the additional step of water restriction to one litre daily is required. The rapid removal of fluid by abdominal paracentesis must be avoided because of the danger of precipitating hepatic encephalopathy; however, between three and four litres may be removed slowly through a narrow-bore cannula when the ascites is painfully tense or if there is respiratory embarrassment. Ultrafiltration of ascites through a plate dialyser followed by intravenous infusion of the concentrated peritoneal fluid will remove excess water and induce a diuresis in those patients in whom a rapid reduction in ascitic fluid is required, for example in patients who require urgent abdominal surgery. The technique is not without difficulties and fluid tends to reaccumulate, but in 50% of these patients the ascites is eventually controlled by diuretics.[26, 28]

In the small group of patients who are resistant to all combinations of diuretic therapy the ascites can be controlled by insertion of a peritoneovenous shunt under local anaesthetic. The LeVeen shunt[25] comprises a pressure-sensitive valve placed in the extraperitoneal tissues deep to the abdominal muscles, a perforated tube inserted into the abdominal cavity, and a subcutaneous tube draining into the jugular vein. Newer modifications of the valve create turbulence and reduce the tendency to occlusion.[18]

Insertion of a peritoneovenous shunt is associated with a marked natriuresis and diuresis but some patients require additional diuretic therapy to control the ascites. The use of the shunt in cirrhosis of the liver is not without hazard for there is an operative mortality of up to 20%, and morbid events, including fever, disseminated intravascular coagulation, sepsis, ascites leak, pulmonary oedema, small bowel obstruction and shunt occlusion, occur in two thirds of the recipients.[7, 18]

Malignant ascites

Those tumours responsible for malignant ascites are shown in Table 20.1. Ultrasonography demonstrates that the fluid is irregularly distributed into pockets. The carcinoembryonic antigen (CEA) titre may be helpful since in malignant ascites the titre ranges from 1.6 to 26 500 ng/ml and is usually greater than 10 ng/ml, whereas in only 2% of those with non-malignant ascites is the titre greater than 5 ng/ml. If the ascitic fluid titre is between 5.0 and 9.9 ng/ml, and is twice that in the plasma, a diagnosis of malignant ascites is suggested. Gastrointestinal and breast cancers often have high ascitic CEA titres. As it can be very difficult to distinguish between mesothelial cells which are found in chronic congestive cardiac failure, the nephrotic syndrome and cirrhosis, and the cells in malignant ascites, cytological diagnosis is accurate in only 55–75% of patients, whereas CEA titres are only 34–74% sensitive but 100% specific. The addition of an estimation of human chorionic gonadotrophin in the fluid has been claimed to increase sensitivity to greater than 70% in ovarian, breast and lung cancers.[11] A new and very useful marker of human cancer cells is the CaI antibody, which reacts with a determinant which is present on two glycoproteins on the cell membrane. This test is very specific and is particularly helpful in distinguishing benign (reactive) mesothelial cells from a mesothelioma.[35]

PSEUDOMYXOMA PERITONEI

Pseudomyxoma peritonei is an uncommon disorder in which the peritoneum is filled with large quantities of yellow-green mucus. It arises from either a mucus-secreting ovarian cancer or, rarely, a mucus-secreting cancer of the appendix.

TREATMENT

The treatment of malignant ascites is unsatisfactory. The usual management is to perform recurrent abdominal paracentesis via a trochar, with the attendant problem of fluid, electrolyte and protein depletion. The rapid loss of fluid can precipitate shock and so drainage should be undertaken using 16 gauge catheters inserted via a 14 gauge needle. Radioactive isotopes, radiation therapy, sclerosing agents and alkylating drugs have all been used with limited success. Bleomycin has been recommended because it has low systemic toxicity and can be injected directly into the peritoneal cavity at a dose of 60–120 mg in 100 ml normal saline. 5-Fluorouracil (2.5 mg) has also been used but, like other cytotoxic agents, it is less effective when large intra-abdominal tumour masses are present in association with the ascites. The injection of *Corynebacterium parvum* intraperitoneally and oral spironolactone have also been tried. The LeVeen peritoneovenous shunt[25] can be used in exceptional circumstances as it may make a ter-

minal illness more comfortable, although life is not necessarily prolonged and there is the danger not only of disseminating the tumour but also of early occlusion of the shunt.

Meig's syndrome

This syndrome originally associated ascites with benign ovarian fibromas, but the term has been widened to include ascites and hydrothorax in the presence of other ovarian tumours including thecomas, granulosa cell tumours, Brenner tumours and mucinous cystadenomas. Meig's syndrome, therefore, can be applied to ascites and all ovarian tumours, not only fibromas, as long as there is no evidence that the ascites results from malignant extension of the tumour. The cause is uncertain and has been ascribed to pressure on the lymphatics (the ascites may be chylous), recurrent torsion of the tumour, and secretion of fluid by the tumour.

Tuberculous ascites

Tuberculous peritonitis is frequently unsuspected and is easily missed, particularly when the infection complicates cirrhosis of the liver. The chest X-ray is normal in 35% of patients. The usual presentation is with abdominal swelling and discomfort; a 'doughy' feel to the abdomen is a rare physical finding. The fluid is usually a yellow, turgid exudate, and contains more than 250 white cells/mm^3, the majority of which are mononuclear. Rarely the ascites is haemorrhagic. The identification of organisms may be difficult, but the disease is readily diagnosed by peritoneal biopsy. The treatment is along conventional lines for pulmonary tuberculosis (see Chapter 14).

Chylous ascites

In chylous ascites there is an accumulation of lymph or lymph-like fluid which has a milky appearance. The triglyceride content is high (often greater than 5 g/l) and on centrifugation a clear subnatant fluid separates from a floating layer of chylomicrons. Chylous ascites is rare but may be caused by many intra-abdominal situations (Table 20.3) in which there is either a direct leak of lymph from traumatized or obstructed lymphatics, or transudation of lymph from the surface of the intestine, liver, or porta hepatis.[32] The commoner causes are inflammatory disease (35%), neoplasms (30%); no cause is identified in 20% of patients.

Table 20.3   Causes of chylous ascites

Infections	tuberculosis
	filariasis
	dysentery
	syphilis
Neoplastic	lymphoma
	leukaemia
	cancer of the stomach,
	pancreas, ovary
Trauma	
Congenital	dysplasia of the lymphatic
	system
Cirrhosis of the liver	
Protein-losing enteropathy	

Haemorrhagic ascites

Ascites is considered haemorrhagic if there are more than 50 000 red cells/mm^3. It may follow damage to large vessels, invasion of Glisson's capsule, rupture of mesenteric varices or lymphomatous involvement of the spleen. Other causes include tuberculous peritonitis, malignant involvement of the peritoneum (usually hepatocellular cancer or peritoneal carcinomatosis), trauma, mesothelioma, mesenteric cysts, hepatic vein thrombosis, multiple myeloma, perforated viscus, lymphoma, and endometriosis. Ultrasonography or computerized tomography are valuable techniques in the evaluation of haemorrhagic ascites since if a solid peritoneal mass is identified a guided needle biopsy can be used to establish the diagnosis.[23]

Pancreatic ascites

Ascites develops in 10–20% of patients with cancer of the pancreas who have widespread peritoneal metastases. On the other hand ascites and pleural effusions are unusual in chronic pancreatitis; about 60% of such patients have an accompanying pseudocyst of the pancreas. Ascites may also complicate acute pancreatitis.

Pancreatic ascites usually develops when there has been a rupture of the pancreatic duct and pancreatic secretions leak into the peritoneal cavity; this mechanism operates in both chronic and acute pancreatitis. The internal fistula may communicate directly with the peritoneal cavity, the pleura or the mediastinum. Fluid accumulation is often insidious and relatively painless, but the ascites is usually described as 'massive'.

The diagnosis is established by demonstrating a markedly elevated ascitic amylase concentration (greater than 2 000 U) or lipase content in a fluid which has a protein concentration in the range typical of exudates. The serum amylase may also be elevated. Endoscopic retrograde pancreatography is helpful in defining the anatomy prior to surgery.

The management of patients with pancreatic ascites is initially by nasogastric suction, atropine, acetazolamide (Diamox) 500 mg twice daily and repeated abdominal paracentesis to encourage spontaneous closure of the leak. If the patient is in poor nutritional condition, as is frequently the case in the alcohol abuser, parenteral hyperalimentation is recommended. If medical management is unsuccessful after 3 weeks, surgical intervention is advisable. Small pseudocysts are resected; if large, drainage is required. A direct leak into the peritoneum is managed by appropriate drainage or resection. Radiotherapy in the form of a single dose of 500 rads has been used in patients who have a high operative risk.[9]

Bile ascites

The free escape of bile into the peritoneal cavity is usually an acute, serious event with a mortality rate from 10 to 80%. Bile evokes a brisk chemical peritonitis and there is severe pain, shock, dehydration, and eventually sepsis and renal failure. Bile ascites has been reported after trauma, percutaneous transhepatic cholangiography and liver biopsy, particularly when extrahepatic bile duct obstruction is present. Other causes are following cholecystectomy, in acute or chronic cholecystitis, typhoid fever, steroid therapy, and acute pancreatitis. Spontaneous rupture of the biliary tree is a rare event which has been recorded in infants and children. The treatment of bile peritonitis requires initial resuscitation with fluid replacement, analgesics and antibiotics, and thereafter a prompt laparotomy to repair the bile leak.

Ascites in renal disease

Ascites occurs in the nephrotic syndrome as a consequence of severe hypoalbuminaemia. The fluid may become infected; however, pneumococcal peritonitis is now very rare. Acute glomerulonephritis may be complicated by ascites. Uraemic patients frequently accumulate peritoneal fluid which can be improved by haemodialysis or peritoneal dialysis.

Ascites develops in some patients who are receiving maintenance dialysis, and the nephrotic syndrome, circulatory overload, infection or inferior vena caval compression have all been implicated. Candidal infection may be present.[4] The mechanism is uncertain in 2–3% of patients. The protein content varies from 12 to 63 g/l in these patients and they respond poorly to a low sodium intake and diuretics.[1] In a few patients the ascites responds dramatically to renal transplantation. Rarely and inexplicably, ascites may develop for the first time following renal transplantation.

Ascites in the newborn

Neonates who develop ascites present with abdominal distension and the diagnosis of fluid can be made on plain abdominal radiograph or by ultrasound, and confirmed by an ascitic tap. The presence of calcium on a plain radiograph suggests meconium peritonitis.[22] The causes of ascites in the newborn are listed in Table 20.4. About 25% of neonatal ascites is urinary in nature and the common predisposing factor is posterior urethral valves with resultant leak of urine from the kidney. Urine enters the peritoneal space by diffusion, or rarely by rupture of

Table 20.4 Causes of neonatal ascites

Urinary	urethral stricture/atresia
	renal vein thrombosis
	congenital nephrosis
	perforated bladder
	posterior urethral valve
	pelvic neuroblastoma
	uterocoele
Gastrointestinal	perforated appendix
	perforated Meckel's diverticulum
	perforated ileum
	meconium peritonitis
	imperforate anus
Cardiac	all causes of congestive cardiac failure
Hepatobiliary	polycystic disease of the liver
	Meckel–Gruber syndrome
	biliary atresia
	perforation of the biliary tract
	cirrhosis of the liver
	portal vein hypoplasia/ obstruction
Infection	sepsis
	syphilis
	toxoplasmosis
	cytomegalovirus infection
Chylous	constricting peritoneal band
	thoracic duct occlusion/stenosis
Erythroblastosis fetalis	
Hydrometrocolpos	
Unknown	

the overlying peritoneum. Urinary ascites is seven times more common in male than female children and carries a mortality rate greater than 70%. It is treated by prompt decompression of the urinary tract using a temporary diversion procedure followed by relief of the obstruction.

Eosinophilic ascites

A raised concentration of eosinophilic cells in ascitic fluid is encountered in the hypereosinophilic syndrome, eosinophilic gastroenteritis, chronic peritoneal dialysis, metastatic malignant disease, abdominal lymphoma, ruptured hydatid cyst, and vasculitis. The hypereosinophilic syndrome is more frequent in males and is characterized by mitral valve disease, congestive cardiac failure, segmental small bowel deformities, hepatomegaly, malabsorption and peripheral eosinophilia.

Myxoedema ascites

Ascites is rarely encountered in myxoedema; pleural and pericardial effusions occur much more frequently. The mechanism is not known but the fluid usually has a protein content of 40–60 g/l and responds readily to thyroid replacement.

Spontaneous bacterial peritonitis

This complication occurs in 8–10% of patients with alcoholic cirrhosis. The presentation is very varied and may be asymptomatic or with fever, pain, reduced bowel sounds and liver failure. The patient frequently develops renal failure and the mortality varies from 14 to 80%. Little help is given by the gross appearance of the fluid or by chemical analysis, and the diagnosis is made on the basis of an ascitic white count greater than 1 000 cells/mm^3 or a polymorphonuclear ascitic count greater than 500 cells/mm^3, organisms seen on the Gram stain (which may be negative in 25% of patients with a positive culture), a positive bacterial culture, and a lactic acid content greater than 32 mg/100 ml. These tests are all time-consuming and the observation that the pH of the ascitic fluid is significantly lower (7.12–7.31) than normal (7.39–7.58) has important diagnostic advantages over them. Five millilitres of ascitic fluid is aspirated and maintained anaerobically in a sealed non-heparinized plastic syringe, and analysed for pH on a blood gas analyser.[20]

REFERENCES

1 Arismendi, G. S., Izard, M. W., Hampton, W. R. & Maher, J. F. (1976) The clinical spectrum of ascites associated with maintenance dialysis. *American Journal of Medicine*, **60,** 46–51.

2 Bar-Meir, S., Lerner, E. & Conn, H. O. (1979) Analysis of ascitic fluid in cirrhosis. *Digestive Diseases and Sciences*, **24,** 136–144.

3 Bateson, M. C. & Bouchier, I. A. D. (1981) *Clinical Investigation of Gastrointestinal Function*, 2nd edn. Oxford: Blackwell Scientific Publications.

4 Bayer, A. S., Blumenkrantz, M. J., Montgomerie, J. Z. *et al.* (1976) Candida peritonitis. Report of 22 cases and review of the English literature. *American Journal of Medicine*, **61,** 832–840.

5 Bichet, D. G., Van Putten, V. J. & Schrier, R. W. (1982) Potential role of increased sympathetic activity in impaired sodium and water excretion in cirrhosis. *New England Journal of Medicine*, **307,** 1552–1557.

6 Bichet, D. G., Szatalowicz, V., Chaimowitz, C. & Schrier, R. W. (1982) Role of vasopressin in abnormal water excretion in cirrhotic patients. *Annals of Internal Medicine*, **96,** 413–417.

7 Blendis, L. M., Greig, P. D., Langer, B. *et al.* (1979) The renal and hemodynamic effects of the peritoneovenous shunt for intractable hepatic ascites. *Gastroenterology*, **77,** 250–257.

8 Boyer, T. D., Kahn, A. M. & Reynolds, T. B. (1978) Diagnostic value of ascitic fluid lactic dehydrogenase, protein and WBC levels. *Archives of Internal Medicine*, **138,** 1103–1105.

9 Cameron, J. L. (1978) Chronic pancreatic ascites and pancreatic pleural effusions. *Gastroenterology*, **74,** 134–140.

10 Conn, H. O. (1979) Portal hypertension and its consequences. In *Current Gastroenterology and Hepatology* (Ed.) Gitnick, G. L. pp. 338–402. Boston: Houghton Mifflin.

11 Couch, W. D. (1981) Combined effusion fluid tumour marker assay, carcinoembryonic antigen (CEA) and human chorionic gonadotropin (hCG) in the detection of malignant tumours. *Cancer*, **48,** 2475–2479.

12 De Troyer, A., Pilloy, W., Broechaert, I. & Demanet, J-C. (1976) Demeclocycline treatment of water retention in cirrhosis. *Annals of Internal Medicine*, **85,** 336–337.

13 Dobbie, J. W., Zaki, M. & Wilson, L. (1981) Ultrastructural studies on the peritoneum with special reference to chronic ambulatory peritoneal dialysis. *Scottish Medical Journal*, **26,** 213–223.

14 Dumont, A. E. & Mulholland J. H. (1960) Flow rate and composition of thoracic-duct lymph in patients with cirrhosis. *New England Journal of Medicine*, **263,** 471–474.

15 Earley, L. E. (1970) Pathogenesis of oliguric acute renal failure. *New England Journal of Medicine*, **282,** 1370–1371.

16 Edell, S. L. & Gefter, W. B. (1979) Ultrasonic differentiation of types of ascitic fluid. *American Journal of Roentgenology*, **133,** 111–114.

17 Epstein, M. (1979) Deranged sodium homeostasis in cirrhosis. *Gastroenterology*, **76,** 622–635.

18 Epstein, M. (1982) Peritoneovenous shunt in the management of ascites and the hepatorenal syndrome. *Gastroenterology*, **82,** 790–799.

19 Gabuzda, G. J. (1970) Cirrhosis, ascites and edema. Clinical course related to management. *Gastroenterology*, **58,** 546–553.

20 Gitlin, N., Stauffer, J. L. & Silvestri, P. C. (1982) The pH of ascitic fluid in the diagnosis of spontaneous bacterial peritonitis in alcoholic cirrhosis. *Hepatology*, **2,** 408–411.

21 Gjessing, J., Oskarsson, B. M., Tomlin, P. J. & Brock-Utne, J. (1972) Diagnostic abdominal paracentesis. *British Medical Journal*, **i,** 617–619.

22 Griscom, N. T., Colodny, A. H., Rosenberg, H. K. *et al.* (1977) Diagnostic aspects of neonatal ascites: report of 27 cases. *American Journal of Roentology*, **128,** 961–970.

23 Hackner, J. F. III, Richter, J. E., Pyatt, R. S. & Fink, M. P. (1982) Haemorrhagic ascites: an unusual presentation of splenic lymphoma. *Gastroenterology*, **83,** 470–473.

24 Koninckx, P. R., Renaer, M. & Brosens, I. A. (1980) Origin of peritoneal fluid in women: an ovarian exudation product. *British Journal of Obstetrics and Gynaecology*, **87,** 177–183.

25 LeVeen, H. H., Christoudias, G., Moon, I. P. *et al.* (1974) Peritoneovenous shunting for ascites. *Annals of Surgery*, **180,** 580–591.

26 Levy, V. G., Opolon, P., Pauleau, N. & Caroli, J. (1975) Treatment of ascites by reinfusion of concentrated peritoneal fluid – review of 318 procedures in 210 patients. *Postgraduate Medical Journal*, **51,** 564–566.

27 Madden, J. L., Lore, J. M. Jr, Gerold, F. P. & Ravid, J. M. (1954) The pathogenesis of ascites and a consideration of its treatment. *Surgery, Gynaecology and Obstetrics*, **99,** 385–391.

28 Parbhoo, S. P., Azdukiewicz, A. & Sherlock, S. (1974) Treatment of ascites by continuous ultrafiltration and reinfusion of protein concentrate. *Lancet*, **i,** 949–952.

29 Reynolds, T. B., Lieberman, F. L. & Goodman, A. R. (1978) Advantages of treatment of ascites without sodium restriction and without complete removal of excess fluid. *Gut*, **19,** 549–553.

30 Schade, D. S. & Williamson, J. R. (1968) The pathogenesis of peritoneal adhesions: an ultrastructural study. *Annals of Surgery*, **167,** 500–510.

31 Strauss, M. P., Birchard, W. H. & Saxon, L. (1956) Correction of impaired water excretion in cirrhosis of the liver by alcohol ingestion or expansion of extracellular fluid volume: the role of antidiuretic hormone. *Transactions of the Association of American Physicians*, **69,** 222–228.

32 Tsuchiya, M., Okazaki, I., Maruyama, K. *et al.* (1973) Chylous ascites formation and a review of 84 cases. *Angiology*, **24,** 576–584.

33 Wilkinson, S. P. & Williams, R. (1980) Renin-angiotensin-aldosterone system in cirrhosis. *Gut*, **21,** 545–554.

34 Witte, C. L., Witte, M. H. & Dumont, A. E. (1980) Lymph imbalance in the genesis and perpetuation of the ascites syndrome in hepatic cirrhosis. *Gastroenterology*, **78,** 1059–1068.

35 Woods, J. C., Harris, H., Spriggs, A. I. & McGee J. O'D. (1982) A new marker for human cancer cells. Immunocytochemical detections of malignant cells in serous fluids with the CaI antibody. *Lancet*, **ii,** 512–515.

FAMILIAL MEDITERRANEAN FEVER (RECURRENT POLYSEROSITIS)

Familial Mediterranean fever (FMF) is a rare, inherited disorder characterized by spontaneous, irregularly occurring attacks of fever and serosal inflammation involving the peritoneum, pleura and synovia. Amyloidosis occurs frequently in some ethnic groups, but not in others.

FMF is most often found in persons of Mediterranean ancestry. Although Sephardic Jews and Armenians are regarded as the major populations at risk, substantial numbers of cases have been reported from Egypt, Turkey, Lebanon, Italy and other Mediterranean countries. Jews in the United States who develop FMF are more frequently Ashkenazi than Sephardic. In addition, irrefutable instances of FMF in other ethnic groups (such as Anglo-Saxon, Japanese, American Indian) suggest that no person exhibiting typical symptoms should be excluded from diagnostic consideration on the basis of ancestry. This, together with the absence of a positive family history in many patients, has raised appropriate concern about the aptness of the term FMF to designate this disease. One suggested alternative – recurrent polyserositis – is more accurate than FMF, but has not achieved wide acceptance as yet.

Aetiology and pathogenesis

The most careful genetic studies of FMF, performed in Israel, suggest that the disorder is inherited as an autosomal recessive trait. However, the underlying mechanisms that tend to trigger attacks remain a complete mystery. There is no body of evidence to support any infectious agent, or an autoimmune or hypersensitivity basis for the disease, nor is there any consistent biochemical deviation that would suggest an inborn error of metabolism.[8]

Clinical features

Most patients with FMF report the onset of disease during childhood or adolescence, but initial attacks have been reported in infancy as well as during the sixth decade of life. Attacks vary in frequency, occurring once every three to four weeks in many patients, but happening as often as once a week or as seldom as once a year in others. There is no temporal regularity to their onset, and interval periods are generally characterized by robust health with complete freedom from symptoms. A typical peritoneal or pleural attack will last from 24 to 72 hours. The onset is usually abrupt with a peak in fever and pain intensity occurring within the first 12 hours. Occasionally, mild prodromal symptoms, such as fatigue or minor abdominal discomfort, may signal a full-blown attack.

FEVER

Fever either precedes or accompanies serosal manifestations of the disease. The temperature rise is usually brisk and may be accompanied by a rigor. Typical temperature elevations range between 38.5 and 40°C. At times, fever may be the sole manifestation of an attack, and patients have been reported whose serosal symptoms began only after years of recurrent episodes of unexplained fever. On occasions, serosal symptoms occur without fever.

PERITONEAL SYMPTOMS

The peritoneum is by far the most frequently involved serosal surface. Nearly all FMF patients have been stricken with peritonitis which is, for most, the principal manifestation of each attack. Pain and tenderness is usually initially localized to one sector of the abdomen; this progresses to more generalized pain and distension. Classical signs of peritonitis (guarding, rebound tenderness, board-like rigidity, absent bowel sounds) parallel the severity of the attack.

These findings, together with fever and leucocytosis, often lead to early surgical exploration if a diagnosis of FMF has not been made. Conversely, the concern that any single peritoneal attack could represent an unrelated abdominal emergency has prompted some physicians to recommend prophylactic appendectomy for the patient with FMF.

PLEURAL SYMPTOMS

Many patients experience referred chest and shoulder pain from diaphragmatic irritation during bouts of peritonitis. In addition, typical unilateral pleuritic chest pain with an accompanying pleural effusion may occur with or without peritonitis. Isolated pleuritic episodes were reported in 40% of a large group of patients seen at the Tel Hashomer Hospital in Tel Aviv.

SYNOVIAL SYMPTOMS

Approximately 75% of FMF patients seen in Israel have experienced at least one episode of acute arthritis. This contrasts sharply with the rarity of inflammatory joint disease among Armenian and Jewish FMF patients reported from the United States. The reason for this discrepancy is not known. The arthritis of FMF is usually restricted to a single joint at any one time, and has a predilection for the large joints, in particular the knee, ankle, hip and elbow, in order of frequency. Synovitis can occur independently of other manifestations of FMF, and tends to last longer than peritoneal or pleuritic attacks. Effusions are common. Radiographs and joint fluid analyses show only non-specific changes. Short attacks of arthritis, which last only one to two weeks, undergo complete resolution. However, protracted forms, which may last as long as a year, may result in serious consequences, including osteoporosis with peri-articular fractures and aseptic necrosis of the femoral head.

SKIN MANIFESTATIONS

An erysipeloid erythema is commonly observed in FMF patients in Israel, but is rare elsewhere. Typical lesions occupy between 15 and 50 cm^2 of skin surface, are fairly sharply defined, and almost always occur below the knee.

AMYLOIDOSIS

The complication of amyloidosis is commonly seen in the Mediterranean region, but is extremely rare in the United States. Approximately 25% of FMF patients in Israel develop amyloidosis and the incidence in Turkey may approach 60%. In Israel the development of amyloidosis bears no relationship to the frequency or severity of serosal attacks, and in some instances may precede any episodes of inflammation. The characteristic pathological features of FMF-associated amyloidosis is the deposition of serum amyloid A (SAA) protein in the intima and media of arterioles. The two organs most heavily involved are the kidneys and spleen; the liver is spared. The clinical hallmark of FMF-associated amyloidosis is nephropathy, which presents as the nephrotic syndrome before proceeding to progressive renal failure. Death due to FMF is almost always a consequence of renal amyloidosis.

OTHER MANIFESTATIONS

Rarely episodes of non-infectious, self-limited pericarditis and meningitis occur. Intestinal obstruction due to bowel adhesions has also been observed. The most disturbing complications of FMF observed in the United States – depression and drug addiction – have diminished considerably since the advent of effective treatment to prevent attacks.

Laboratory findings

Although typical attacks of serositis are accompanied by elevated markers of inflammation (leucocytosis, and elevated sedimentation rate, C-reactive protein, fibrinogen and haptoglobin), there are no laboratory findings specific for, or even particularly suggestive of, FMF. Biochemical assessment of renal and hepatic function is normal, as are lipid studies and a variety of serological tests. Patients with associated amyloidosis show proteinuria and the biochemical abnormalities consistent with the stage of renal failure. Examination of serosal effusions typically show sterile exudates with a predominance of neutrophils and fibrin strands. Radiological studies may show the expected small pleural effusions (for pleural attacks) and non-obstructive ileus (for peritoneal attacks).[2, 9]

Treatment

A variety of treatments have been used in the past to ameliorate or prevent FMF attacks including dietary regimens, immunotherapy, antibiotics, hormones (oestrogens and adrenal corticosteroids), antipyretics, anti-inflammatory drugs, and psychotherapy; none has been shown to be effective. However, during the past 10 years there has been ample confirmation of the value of prophylactic colchicine therapy, first reported to be effective in 1972.[3] While intravenous colchicine has no value in treating full-blown attacks of FMF, when taken orally at a dose of 0.6 mg (one tablet) twice daily, approximately 85% of FMF patients experience complete cessation of their attacks or marked reduction in frequency and severity. A few patients require a third colchicine tablet, while others manage on just one a day. Many describe the value of an extra tablet to abort the progression of prodromal symptoms, which may still appear during maintenance colchicine treatment.[1, 3, 4, 8, 11] Children with FMF have a lower response rate, even when adult dosage is employed; the reason for this is unclear. Long-term studies have shown that prophylactic colchicine treatment is safe; in particular, adverse effects upon bone marrow, liver or renal function have not been detected.[5, 6] Additional medication for control of loose stools may be required by some patients. Because of colchicine's potential to produce chromosomal damage, patients contemplating childbearing are advised to discontinue treatment three months before planned conception, and for the duration of pregnancy. There has been no report of excess fetal damage when such precautions are taken. Wright *et al.*[10] have introduced, as an alternative to daily maintenance colchicine, a protocol for more intensive colchicine therapy to be initiated at the first premonition of an attack. This benefits the majority of patients and is the treatment of choice for infrequent attacks. The value of prodrome-initiated therapy in patients with frequent attacks will depend on the pace of an attack following its first signal, the amount of amelioration afforded by colchicine, and the degree of bowel upset caused by the higher dose of colchicine.

REFERENCES

1　Dinarello, C. A., Wolff, S. M., Goldfinger, S. E. *et al.* (1974) Colchicine therapy for familial Mediterranean fever. A double-blind trial. *New England Journal of Medicine*, **291**, 934–937.
2　Ehrenfeld, E. N., Eliakim, M. & Rachmilewitz, M. (1961) Recurrent polyserositis (familial Mediterranean fever, periodic disease). A report of fifty-five cases. *American Journal of Medicine*, **31**, 107–123.
3　Goldfinger, S. E. (1972) Colchicine for familial Mediterranean fever. *New England Journal of Medicine*, **287**, 1302.
4　Goldfinger, S. E. (1975) Colchicine suppression of attacks of familial Mediterranean fever. *Frontiers of Internal Medicine: 12th International Congress of Internal Medicine*. Tel Aviv 1974. pp. 334–338. Basel: Karger.
5　Goldstein, R. C. & Schwabe, A. D. (1974) Prophylactic colchicine therapy in familial Mediterranean fever. A controlled double-blind study. *Annals of Internal Medicine*, **81**, 792–794.
6　Ravid, M., Robson, M. & Kedar (Keizman), I. (1977) Prolonged colchicine treatment in four patients with amyloidosis. *Annals of Internal Medicine*, **87**, 568–570.
7　Schwabe, A. D. & Peters, R. S. (1974) Familial Mediterranean fever in Armenians. Analysis of 100 cases. *Medicine (Baltimore)*, **53**, 453–462.
8　Schwabe, A. D., Terasaki, P. I., Barnett, E. V. *et al.* (1977) Familial Mediterranean fever: recent advances in pathogenesis and management. *Western Journal of Medicine*, **127**, 15–23.
9　Sohar, E., Gafni, J., Pras, M. & Heller, H. (1967) Familial Mediterranean fever. A survey of 470 cases and review of the literature. *American Journal of Medicine*, **43**, 227–253.
10　Wright, D. G., Wolff, S. M., Fauci, A. S. & Alling, D. W. (1977) Efficacy of intermittent colchicine therapy in familial Mediterranean fever. *Annals of Internal Medicine*, **86**, 162–165.
11　Zemer, D., Revach, M., Pras, M. *et al.* (1974) A controlled trial of colchicine in preventing attacks of familial Mediterranean fever. *New England Journal of Medicine*, **291**, 932–934.

RETROPERITONEAL FIBROSIS (ORMOND'S DISEASE)

Retroperitoneal fibrosis is a rare disease of uncertain aetiology. It is characterized by the deposition of fibrous tissue in the retroperitoneal space extending from the aortic bifurcation upwards to approximately the level of the renal arteries. The clinical picture is usually the result of compression of important retroperitoneal structures, in particular the ureters.

Pathology

The fibrous tissue deposited forms a thick rubbery plaque lying mainly over the bodies of the third and fourth lumbar vertebrae. It is in close apposition to the aorta below the renal arteries, and spreads laterally over the psoas muscles. There is no involvement of the peritoneum itself, and the mesentery is usually also free of fibrosis. Extension may occur along the course of the common iliac arteries, but usually stops at the brim of the pelvis. Upward extension may occasionally lead to involvement of the mediastinum. The ureters, major veins, aorta and lumbar nerves may all be involved in the fibrotic process. Histologically dense collagen tissue is seen. In the early stages, this is cellular with a prominent lymphocytic and polymorph infiltration, and with a vascular stroma; later the fibrous tissue becomes avascular and acellular. The abdominal aorta is often the site of severe atherosclerosis, though whether this is more than an incidental finding is uncertain.[16]

Aetiology

In up to 10% of patients the fibrotic process develops in relation to a malignant tumour.[10, 11] It may be associated with carcinoid, which has a particular propensity to cause widespread fibrosis, but neoplasms of the breast[1] and stomach, lymphoma[4] and lymphosarcoma are also rare causes.

Some of the patients develop evidence of an abnormal tendency to fibrosis in other organs, and the following disorders are recorded as occurring with retroperitoneal fibrosis: scleroderma, mediastinal fibrosis, Riedel's thyroiditis, pseudotumour of the orbit,[18] retractile mesenteritis, and sclerosing cholangitis. Generally these disorders are thought to represent the effects of an abnormal immunological and fibrotic response to some unknown antigen and may pre- or post-date the retroperitoneal fibrosis.

Interest has centred recently around the possibility that beta-blocking drugs could be a factor in the production of retroperitoneal fibrosis.[2, 14, 19] Up until July 1981 there had been 17 such reports in the United Kingdom on the

Adverse Reaction Register of the Committee on Safety of Medicines. Seven different beta-blockers were involved and were either given alone or in combination with a diuretic. These reports are of interest in view of the abnormal fibrous reaction to the beta-blocker practolol seen in the visceral peritoneum.[13] The other important drug association of retroperitoneal fibrosis is with the serotonin antagonist, methysergide. About 12% of cases of retroperitoneal fibrosis have been associated with this drug which is used in the treatment of migraine. The association is of practical importance since the process commonly remits on withdrawal of the methysergide. The disorder has occasionally been associated with therapy with dihydroergotamine, hydralazine, methyldopa, and some analgesics.

A variety of autoimmune disorders, and disorders of uncertain aetiology apart from those associated with fibrosis, may occur with retroperitoneal fibrosis. Thus Raynaud's phenomenon, arteritis, polyarthritis, sarcoidosis,[7] Crohn's disease, interstitial nephritis,[9] and scleroderma[12] are all recorded accompaniments.

The precise cause of the disease remains uncertain. The close relationship of the fibrosis to the abdominal aorta and the presence of severe aortic atheroma[6] has led to the suggestion that the process develops in relation to a slow leakage of blood, or some specific component of the blood, from this vessel. A similar type of reaction occurs rarely in relation to an abdominal aortic aneurysm. Similarly the possibility that chronic leakage of urine from an obstructed kidney could cause a fibrous reaction has been entertained, because a granulomatous and fibrotic reaction around the renal pelvis is sometimes recorded with obstructed kidneys. Most observers, however, feel that this disease represents the effects of some immunological stimulation of collagen formation.

Clinical features

This is a rare disorder. Up to 1977 only approximately 500 cases were recorded in the world literature. The incidence is uncertain as it is probable that some examples are not associated with clinical consequences. Very rarely the disorder is familial.

Characteristically, except in the cases following methysergide, males are more commonly affected than females. Most patients are between 50 and 70 years of age. The symptoms are often non-specific and insidious, and are usually related primarily to obstruction of the ureters.

Loin pain, lower abdominal pain or backache are early symptoms. The pain is often poorly localized, and dull and aching in character; there may also be abdominal tenderness and distension on palpation. When the ureters are completely or partially occluded the patient develops attacks of renal colic and the features of oliguric renal failure. Partial ureteric obstruction causes abdominal pain, frequency and lassitude. Obstruction of the ureters also leads to the onset of hypertension with retinopathy, dyspnoea and headaches. Occasionally generalized oedema occurs due to associated nephrotic syndrome following involvement of the renal veins.

Compression of the inferior vena cava, and the iliac veins and lymphatics results in swelling of one or both legs due to oedema and occasionally a varicocoele or hydrocoele develops in males. Involvement of the lumbar nerve roots may give rise to backache with radiation of pain into the thigh and leg, and pain on movement of the hip. Accompanying these symptoms there is often systemic upset, including lassitude, weight loss and occasionally fever.[3]

Physical signs are remarkably few and no doubt this causes the recognized delay in diagnosis. A palpable mass due to the fibrotic process is unlikely, presumably because of its deep, mid-line position. Nevertheless, about 30% of patients have an abdominal mass or a mass felt rectally or vaginally. Involvement of the ureters may result in one or more enlarged, palpable kidneys.

Additional features in patients with other types of fibrotic disease include a hard woody goitre with stridor (Reidel's thyroiditis), venous obstruction due to superior vena caval obstruction (mediastinal fibrosis) and proptosis (pseudotumour of the orbit).

Differential diagnosis

This is extremely wide because of the comparative lack of physical signs and the vagueness of the symptoms. Because swelling of the ankles may occur, a diagnosis of venous insufficiency or heart failure may be made. Back and hip pain may simulate a primary orthopaedic disorder of the back or hip, whilst reference of the pain to the abdomen without physical signs may lead to a diagnosis of renal tract disease or irritable bowel syndrome. The presence of hypertension, proteinuria and elevated blood urea may suggest a diagnosis of chronic renal failure of uncertain cause with secondary hypertension. There is a considerable risk, however, that patients with this disorder will be labelled as 'functional' or 'neurotic'.

The following are rare but recognized complications of the disease which can lead to unusual abdominal manifestations:

1 A mass is sometimes felt on rectal examination due to the fibrotic process involving the pelvis; this may simulate a rectal or pararectal tumour.

2 Portal hypertension with bleeding oesophageal varices can follow secondary involvement of the porta hepatis and the portal vein.

3 Obstructive jaundice due to common bile duct constriction may rarely be seen.

4 Nausea, vomiting and weight loss may occur and may closely simulate gastric ulceration or neoplasia.

5 Toxic megacolon, proctitis and rectal stenosis are all rarely recorded.

Investigation

BLOOD AND URINE TESTS

Three blood tests provide helpful but nonspecific evidence of the presence of this disease: the haemoglobin, which is unexplainedly reduced so that a mild and usually normochromic anaemia results; the ESR, which is elevated in over 50% of patients; and the serum albumin, which is reduced.

Where there is secondary involvement of the kidneys and ureteric obstruction, proteinuria or frank evidence of renal tract infection (pyuria, proteinuria casts and organisms) can be seen on microscopy or are revealed by culture or simple clinical tests. Once renal function is deranged there is evidence of impaired creatinine clearance and later elevation of the blood urea.

THE INTRAVENOUS PYELOGRAM

Until recently this was the main investigation by which a definite diagnosis could be made and it still has an important part to play in diagnosis, although its specificity has been questioned. Obstruction of the ureters may cause dilatation of the upper third, medial deviation, particularly of the middle third, due to involvement of the ureters in the fibrotic process, which contract to produce ureteric tethering, and hydronephrosis affecting one or both kidneys. Of these radiological signs, dilatation and medial deviation are non-specific; it is well recognized that some medial deviation of the ureters may be seen in normal pyelograms. Nevertheless, these findings, particularly in the face of a compatible history

and physical examination and with suggestive results from simple blood tests, makes the diagnosis probable. The value of the intravenous pyelogram diminishes with increasing evidence of secondary renal failure.

ULTRASONIC AND CT SCANNING

Both of these techniques have a useful part to play in diagnosis, although experience with them in this rare disease is small. Fagan, Larrieu and Amparo[5] studied three patients with retroperitoneal fibrosis in whom ultrasound showed the presence of an anechogenic mass with clear margins and irregular contours enveloping but not displacing structures such as the aorta, vena cava and ureters. The kidney may be pushed anteriorly by the mass. There was a clear margin between the mass and the posterior peritoneum anteriorly. Similar features are shown on CT scanning. The density of the fibrous tissue is similar to that of the muscles which it covers, and the infiltration of tissue planes between muscles is clearly shown. CT scanning is particularly good at defining the extent of the fibrotic process and monitoring its progress.

BIOPSY

A biopsy for histological examination is taken at laparotomy (see below).

Treatment

An accurate diagnosis must always be made where this is feasible,[8, 15] which usually requires surgery and biopsy with careful histology. This is to ensure that cases due to malignant disease are diagnosed, as the prognosis is much worse than in idiopathic cases. However, even with careful scrutiny of the tissue obtained malignant fibrosis may be missed and the diagnosis becomes apparent by the subsequent clinical course. A laparotomy is necessary to expose both ureters and retroperitoneal spaces, to mobilize the ascending and descending colon and to dissect the retroperitoneal tissues.

If the ureters are involved in the fibrous tissue they are first mobilized in their upper and lower portions. The part encased in fibrous tissue is freed by blunt dissection following incision through the fibrous plaque along the course of the ureter (ureterolysis). This procedure is worthwhile even if it is known that the diagnosis is one of malignant retroperitoneal fibrosis. Once freed the ureters are placed laterally and retained by stitching the peritoneum onto the psoas muscles.

Most patients in whom this operation is performed improve, and long-term survival for 10–20 years is possible. There is argument as to whether patients in whom the diagnosis has been confirmed histologically and in whom bilateral ureterolysis has been performed should also be given steroid drugs. Reports of successful corticosteroid therapy are found in the literature, and relapse is recorded following cessation of this treatment. Nevertheless, biopsy and ureterolysis should invariably be the first procedure – this would be mandatory to make a diagnosis and preserve renal function – whereas corticosteroids might be considered when there is continuing evidence of progression as judged by repeated CT scanning. In a group of patients who are usually over 50 and with possible complicating hypertension and renal impairment, the point at which to introduce corticosteroids (usually prednisolone 40 mg daily, reducing to 5 mg three times a day) may be difficult to decide. Haematological and CT monitoring may help in making such a decision.

Prognosis

Any potentially causative drug treatment must be stopped. Patients who present with acute oliguric renal failure or renal failure which does not respond to ureterolysis alone or coupled with corticosteroids have a poor prognosis; about 10% of all patients die from these causes. The others are usually cured, and apart from the complications of hypertension, survive normally. The prognosis may be altered by the presence of another fibrosing disease.

REFERENCES

1 Blairon, J., Paulet, P., Rutsaert, J. & Limbosch, J. M. (1979) Oesophageal stenosis and retroperitoneal fibrosis appearing as a late consequence of a breast carcinoma. *Acta Gastroenterologica Belgica*, **42**, 285–293.

2 Bullimore, D. W. (1980) Retroperitoneal fibrosis associated with atenolol. *British Medical Journal*, **281**, 59–60.

3 Byrd, W. E., Hunt, R. E. & Burgess, R. (1981) Retroperitoneal fibrosis as a cause of fever of undetermined origin. *Western Journal of Medicine*, **134**, 357–361.

4 Dlabel, P. W., Mullins, J. D. & Coltman, C. A. Jr. (1980) An unusual manifestation of non-Hodgkins lymphoma fibrosis masquerading as Ormond's disease. *Journal of the American Medical Association*, **243**, 1161–1162.

5 Fagan C. J., Larnieu, A. J. & Amparo, E. G. (1979) Retroperitoneal fibrosis: ultrasound and CT features. *American Journal of Roentgenology*, **133**, 239–243.

6 Gabrielli, L. & Lorenzi, G. (1979) Arteriosclerotic obliteration of the infrarenal aorta and retroperitoneal fibrosis. *Angiologia*, **31**, 105–111.

7 Godin, M., Fillastre, J. P., Ducastelle, T. *et al.* (1980) Sarcoidosis. Retroperitoneal fibrosis, renal arterial involvement and unilateral focal glomerulosclerosis. *Archives of Internal Medicine*, **140**, 1240–1242.

8 Kinder, C. H. (1979) Retroperitoneal fibrosis (editorial). *Journal of the Royal Society of Medicine*, **22**, 63–67.

9 Kirschbaum, B. B., Koontz, W. W. & Olichney, M. J. (1981) Association of retroperitoneal fibrosis and interstitial nephritis. *Archives of Internal Medicine*, **141**, 1361–1363.

10 Koep, L. & Zuidema, G. D. (1977) The clinical significance of retroperitoneal fibrosis. *Surgery*, **81**, 250–257.

11 Larrieu, A. J., Weiner, I., Abston, S. & Warren, M. M. (1980) Retroperitoneal fibrosis. *Surgery, Gynaecology and Obstetrics*, **150**, 699–702.

12 Mansell, M. A. & Watts, R. W. (1980) Retroperitoneal fibrosis and scleroderma. *Postgraduate Medical Journal*, **56**, 730–733.

13 Marshall, A. J., Baddeley, H., Barritt, D. W. *et al.* (1977) Practolol peritonitis. *Quarterly Journal of Medicine*, **46**, 135–149.

14 McClusky, D. R., Donaldson, R. A. & McGeown M. G. (1980) Oxprenolol and retroperitoneal fibrosis. *British Medical Journal*, **281**, 1459–1460.

15 McComb, J. E. & Gall, E. P. (1979) Retroperitoneal fibrosis. *Arizona Medicine*, **36**, 41–44.

16 Mitchinson, M. J. (1970) The pathology of idiopathic retroperitoneal fibrosis. *Journal of Clinical Pathology*, **23**, 681–689.

17 Mosimann, F. & Mange, B. (1980) Portal hypertension as a complication of idiopathic retroperitoneal fibrosis. *British Journal of Surgery*, **67**, 804.

18 Richards, A. B., Shalka, H. W., Roberts, F. J. & Flint, A. (1980) Pseudotumour of the orbit and retroperitoneal fibrosis. A form of multifocal fibrosclerosis. *Archives of Ophthalmology*, **98**, 1617–1620.

19 Thompson, J. & Julian, D. G. (1982) Retroperitoneal fibrosis associated with metoprolol. *British Medical Journal*, **284**, 83–84.

Chapter 21
Reference Ranges in Theory and Practice

D. N. Baron

THE IDEA OF A REFERENCE RANGE

What used to be called 'normal values' or 'normal range' is now preferably called 'reference range' or 'reference interval'. The former term is more common and more euphonious; the latter is preferred by metrologists. 'Reference values' are the results obtained from the sample of the 'reference population'; from the reference values the reference range can be calculated. Why should we abandon 'normal values', and what do we mean by 'reference range' – and are they necessary? In this chapter I shall be mainly referring to the interpretation of the numerical result of a single chemical pathology investigation, but the same arguments apply to patients' height, blood pressure, lymphocyte count or any other numerically measurable value.

Disease and abnormality

Clinicians request investigations as extensions of their clinical skills. A common use is to obtain an analytical result that gives help with diagnosis. However, probably the most important and productive use of tests in chemical pathology (not discussed further here) is as part of a series to help in monitoring progress: patients act as their own references, with 'subject-specific reference ranges', and population reference ranges are less important. To oversimplify, a clinician would like to interpret a particular laboratory result as 'abnormal', the fact that this result is outside the normal range identifying the patient as having the disease under consideration. It is not nearly so simple. 'Disease' is a convenient reification for the use of authors of chapters in textbooks, and for vital statisticians. There are interactions of pathological processes with people, converting people into patients, that often give end-results so similar that they can be conveniently grouped into diseases.

'Normal', 'healthy', and 'non-diseased' are not the same. Because of the impossibility of defining normal in this respect, which could lead to the false view that there is a strict boundary between normal and abnormal, and also because of other meanings of normal such as the normal or Gaussian distribution, 'reference range' is used without commitment, to define a set of results to which one compares and refers the patient's result. The simultaneous comparison of a group of results in a profile with a group of reference ranges, for example by multivariate analysis, will not be considered further here. In such a group of results each individual result may be within its reference range, but the pattern of combination be abnormal.

CHOICE OF REFERENCE RANGES

Reference ranges and population subgroups

For any given analyte (a new and useful word meaning any substance whose concentration, activity and so on can be established by analysis of plasma, urine etc.) there can be a number of reference ranges. That for fasting recumbent patients in hospital not having the disease in question may be different from that for ambulant healthy subjects out of hospital. Depending on the analyte, we might need to have separate reference ranges for different ages, for men and women – on and off the Pill and at different stages of the menstrual cycle – for omnivores, vegetarians and vegans, for different ethnic groups and perhaps for different blood groups, for different climates and environments, for various times of the day and for different seasons of the year, and for differing body build and degrees of physical fitness. Then there is the question of drugs: can one say what proportion of the population needs to be regularly on a drug, such as alcohol, nicotine or aspirin, for this group to be a 'normal' and to need its own set of reference ranges? In practice, when reporting reference ranges from 'healthy' 'normal' subjects, the criteria that have been adopted must be recognized, and defined or implied.

Because most individual results are method-dependent, and to some extent collection-procedure-dependent and even laboratory-dependent, reference ranges are equally method-dependent. For this discussion we will assume initially that the analytical results are accurate and precise, and we need take account only of biological variation within our defined reference population.

Calculation of reference ranges

A reference range, of reference values bounded by reference limits, is needed because of the impossibility of comparing a patient's result with all the results from the reference population. By convention, unless otherwise stated, the 0.025 and 0.975 fractiles (2.5th and 97.5th percentiles) of the sample of the reference population are used as the lower and upper reference limits, thus excluding the lower 2.5% and the upper 2.5%. Because there is usually only a small sample, any such reference range should be accompanied by its confidence limits (as should the other derived values mentioned below), though this information is rarely provided. There are a variety of mathematical procedures to calculate these reference limits. If the distribution of the reference values is approximately Gaussian, or can be so transformed by a simple procedure such as taking logarithms (many actual distributions are positively skewed and are log-normal), then a parametric method can be applied: mean ± 1.960 standard deviations (s.d.) – usually taken as mean ± 2 s.d. –

yields the fractile limits defined above. For other distributions a non-parametric method is used.

The conventional reference range leads to the apparent paradox that if, for example, a dozen independent tests are done simultaneously, then there is a probability of 50% per specimen of finding at least one 'abnormal' result. If these tests are repeated, different results outside the reference ranges may be found. It has been suggested that for such multiple testing mean ± 3 s.d. should be used for reference ranges.

A healthy person is one who has been insufficiently investigated.

Effects of different settings of the reference limits

Figure 21.1 shows a model with the reference distribution of, say, a plasma analyte concentration being Gaussian, and the overlapping distribution of raised values in disease being skewed. It may be assumed that there is a similar pattern of lowered values in a different disease.

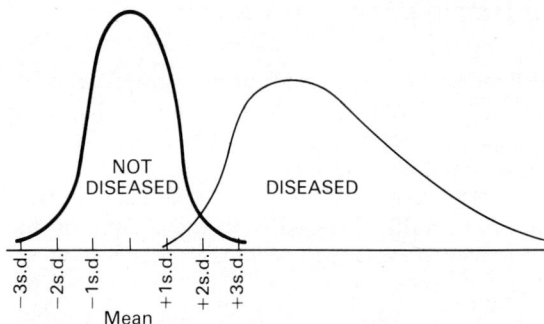

Fig. 21.1 Theoretical Gaussian curve for the distribution of a component (e.g. measurements of plasma concentration) in a non-diseased population, showing the range at different multiples of one standard deviation (s.d.) from the mean. This is compared with a positively skewed curve for the same component in a theoretical diseased population, showing overlap between the values found with and without disease.

Figure 21.2 imposes the reference range of the central 95% of the population as defined above. False positives are results above the reference range in healthy subjects, and false negatives are results within the reference range in diseased patients. The conventional reference range yields an obligatory 2.5% false positive rate at the upper end, and 2.5% at the lower end. From this overlap, and the position of the reference limits, can be derived the sensitivity (percentage of all patients with the disease that the test classifies as positive for the disease) and the specificity (percentage of normal results in subjects without the disease). False decisions (posi-

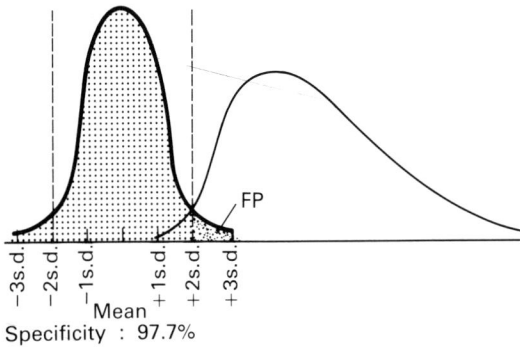

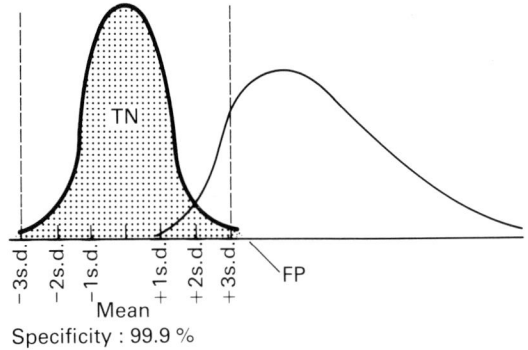

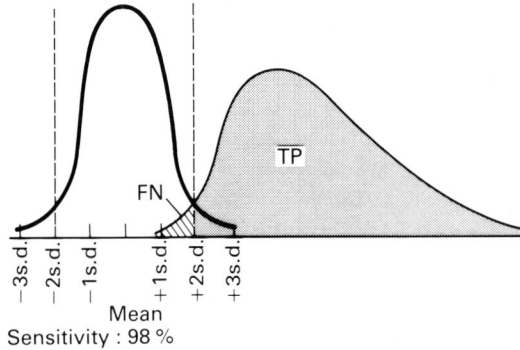

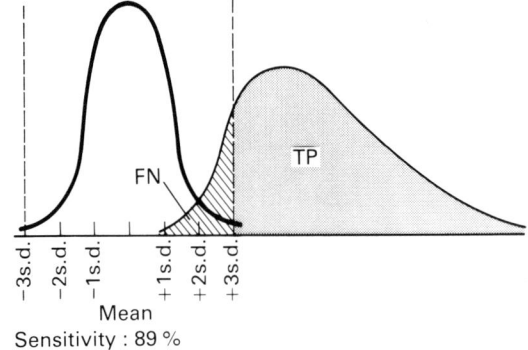

Fig. 21.2 The use of mean ±2 s.d. (≃ 95% of population) as reference range, and its effect on the distribution of true and false positives (TP and FP) and of true and false negatives (TN and FN), and on specificity and sensitivity. The specificity is 97.7% and not 97.5% because mean ±2 s.d. has been used and not ±1.96 s.d. (see text). The distributions are the same as in Figure 21.1.

Fig. 21.3 The use of mean ±3 s.d. (≃ 99.7% of population) as reference range.

tive + negative) are at a minimum and efficiency is highest when the reference limit is at the point of intersection of the 'non-diseased' and the 'diseased' distribution, as shown here.

However, for different clinical circumstances different settings of the reference limits, leading to different reference ranges, may be necessary. If, for example, treatment is hazardous and must be avoided for the non-diseased, whereas failure to recognize and treat a diseased person is not so crucial, then by setting the reference range to include more than 99% of the population, such as mean ±3 s.d. (Figure 21.3), the false positives are reduced and the false negatives necessarily increased. If there is great clinical risk in missing positive cases, and treating the non-diseased is not hazardous, then by setting the reference ranges to include a lower proportion of the population, such as mean ±1 s.d. (Figure 21.4), the false negatives are reduced and the false positives thereby increased. These changes alter the sensitivity and specificity.

Imprecision of results, due to poor methodology or to laboratory or collection error, will

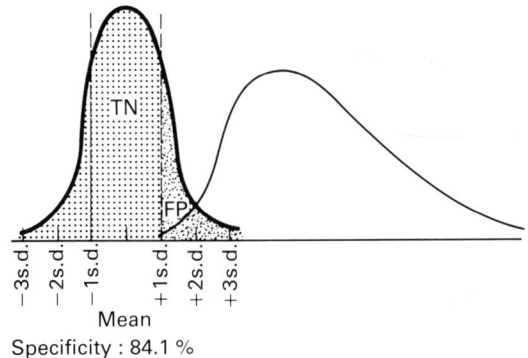

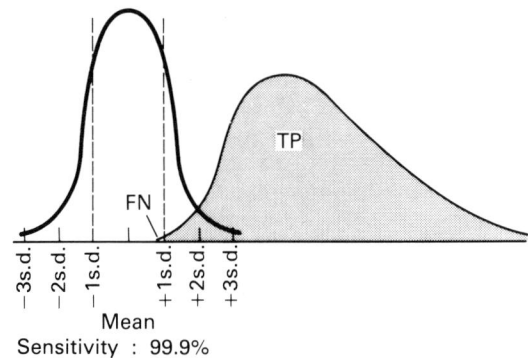

Fig. 21.4 The use of mean ±1 s.d. (≃ 67% of population) as reference range.

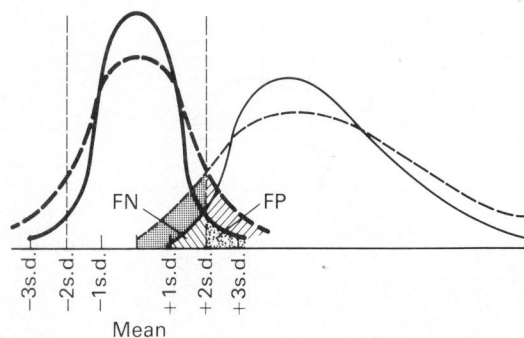

Fig. 21.5 Effect of imprecision of laboratory results (curves with broken lines) on the distribution of values in the diseased and non-diseased subjects shown in Figure 21.2.

make a test at the same time less specific and less sensitive by increasing the proportion both of false positives and of false negatives (Figure 21.5).

OTHER USEFUL DERIVED VALUES

A further concept, derived from the Bayesian approach, is that of predictive values; this takes account of the prevalence of the disease in the specific population to which the patient under study belongs, for example the general population for screening, outpatients with suggestive clinical picture, or ward patients with relatively certain diagnosis. The predictive value of a positive test is the percentage in that population, with and without the disease under consideration, of positive results that are true positives – and vice versa for a negative test result. Ideally, no test would be in general clinical diagnostic use unless its predictive values had been found to be satisfactory.

Improvements have been suggested, rather than the laboratory just quoting the result with its appropriate reference range. One is to ignore reference ranges, and to use decision levels which have been established by experience and agreement between clinician and chemical pathologist as markers for suitable action. For example, in the upper levels plasma potassium concentration has a conventional reference limit of 5.0 mmol/l. A decision level for the laboratory could be 6.0 mmol/l, at which the clinician must be telephoned; a decision level for the clinician could be 7.5 mmol/l, at which urgent therapy must be begun.

Another suggested improvement is to use one of the mathematical procedures that adjust the result, or observed value (o.v.), in relation to the reference distribution. Perhaps the most studied has been the s.d. unit, calculated as (o.v. − mean)/s.d. for a Gaussian distribution; for example, with this system any test result with a value at its upper reference limit would be reported as +2 s.d. units. It may also be possible, using a Bayesian procedure, to calculate the probability that the observed patient belongs to the reference population. Laboratories that have computer-assisted reporting systems can program the computer to flag the result when reference limits or decision levels are passed, or to report the results in adjusted units. One can use a graphic presentation of results and also indicate the reference ranges: such presentation, especially when in multiple radial form, may help in interpreting a group of related results. Delta checks, for significant differences between present and previous results, can also be flagged.

REFERENCE RANGES IN PRACTICE

Provided that the reservations above are understood, reference ranges are a valuable guide to the initial interpretation of a laboratory result. The tables list reference ranges for the results of the most commonly requested static laboratory investigations in chemical pathology on plasma (Table 21.1), urine (Table 21.2) and faeces (Table 21.3). A separate table (21.4) lists certain reference ranges for children of different ages. Changes for age, sex and so on in adults can be found in textbooks of chemical pathology, as can reference ranges for results of dynamic tests: many of these in gastroenterology are described elsewhere in this book.

The ranges are derived from UK populations, and the methods are those commonly used in British laboratories. Most large laboratories throughout the world issue their own sets of reference ranges, and these may differ in detail from those presented here because of different populations and different methods.

In the tables for adults the results are given both in SI units (with emphasis on moles) and in traditional units, with rounded-off conversions. The principles of SI units, and their application to medicine, are discussed in the final part of this Chapter.

Table 21.1   Reference ranges – plasma/serum.

Constituent	SI or other international units	Traditional units	Notes
Aldosterone	100–500 pmol/l	3.5–18 ng/100 ml	
Amino acid nitrogen	2.5–4.0 mmol/l	3.5–5.5 mg/100 ml	Fasting
Aminotransferases – see transaminases			
Ammonia (whole blood)	12–60 μmol/l	20–100 μg/100 ml	
Amylase	70–300 U/l	40–160 Somogyi units/100 ml	
Anion gap	6–16 mmol/l	6–16 mEq/l	As $[Na^+] - ([Cl^-] + [HCO_3^-])$
Bicarbonate	24–30 mmol/l	24–30 mEq/l	As CO_2 content
Bilirubin			
total	5.0–17 μmol/l	0.3–1.0 mg/100 ml	
conjugated	<3.0 μmol/l	<0.2 mg/100 ml	
Caeruloplasmin	0.3–0.6 g/l	30–60 mg/100 ml	
Calcium	2.1–2.6 mmol/l	8.5–10.5 mg/100 ml	1.0–1.2 mmol/l is ionized
Carbon dioxide (whole blood)	4.5–6.0 kPa	35–46 mmHg	As PCO_2
Carbonic acid	1.1–1.4 mmol/l	1.1–1.4 mEq/l	
Carotenoids	1.0–5.5 μmol/l	50–300 μg/100 ml	
Chloride	95–105 mmol/l	95–105 mEq/l	
Cholesterol – total	4.0–6.5 mmol/l	160–260 mg/100 ml	
Cholinesterase	2–5 kU/l	2000–5000 iu/l	at 37°C: Dibucaine Number > 80
Copper	13–24 μmol/l	80–150 μg/100 ml	
Cortisol	200–700 nmol/l	8–35 μg/100 ml	Marked circadian rhythm; at 09:00
Creatine	15–60 μmol/l	0.2–0.8 mg/100 ml	
Creatinine	60–120 μmol/l	0.7–1.4 mg/100 ml	
Creatine kinase	3–150 U/l	3–150 iu/l	At 37°C
Enzymes – see individual enzymes			
Fatty acids – free	0.3–0.6 mmol/l	0.3–0.6 mEq/l	Fasting
Ferritin	15–250 μg/l	1.5–25 μg/100 ml	
Folate	5.0–20 μg/l	5.0–20 ng/ml	
Gastrin	5–50 pmol/l	10–100 pg/ml	
Glucose (whole blood)			
venous	3.0–5.0 mmol/l	55–90 mg/100 ml	Fasting values; plasma concentrations
capillary	3.2–5.2 mmol/l	60–95 mg/100 ml	are 10–15 per cent higher
γ-Glutamyltransferase	5–45 U/l	5–45 iu/l	At 37°C
Haptoglobins	5–30 μmol/l	30–180 mg/100 ml	
Hydrogen ion activity exponent (pH)	7.36–7.42	7.36–7.42	(Whole blood)
Insulin	10–30 mU/l	10–30 μu/ml	Fasting
Iron	11–34 μmol/l	60–190 μg/100 ml	Marked circadian rhythm; at 08:00
Iron-binding capacity – total	45–75 μmol/l	250–400 μg/100 ml	
Ketones	0.06–0.2 mmol/l	0.06–0.2 mEq/l	As acetoacetate
Lactate	0.75–2.0 mmol/l	0.75–2.0 mEq/l	Fasting
Lactate dehydrogenase			
total	130–500 U/l	130–500 iu/l	At 37°C
'heart specific'	120–260 U/l	120–260 iu/l	As 'hydroxybutyrate dehydrogenase'
Lead (whole blood)	0.5–1.7 μmol/l	10–35 μg/100 ml	
Lipase	18–280 U/l	0–1.5 Cherry-Crandall units	
Lipids – total	4.5–10 g/l	450–1000 mg/100 ml	Fasting
Magnesium	0.7–1.0 mmol/l	1.8–2.4 mg/100 ml	
5'-Nucleotidase	2–15 U/l	2–15 iu/l	At 37°C
Osmolality	275–295 mmol/kg	275–295 mosmol/kg	
Oxygen (whole blood)	11–15 kPa	85–105 mmHg	As PO_2
Phosphatases			
acid – total	0.5–5.5 U/l	0.3–3.0 KAu/100 ml	1–10 U/l with a 4-NPP method
—'prostatic'	0–1 U/l	0–0.5 KAu/100 ml	0–4 U/l (NPP)
alkaline – total	20–95 U/l	3–13 KAu/100 ml	30–110 U/l (NPP)
Phosphate – inorganic	0.8–1.4 mmol/l	2.5–4.5 mg/100 ml	As phosphorus
Phospholipids	1.8–3.0 mmol/l	150–250 mg/100 ml	As lecithin
Potassium	3.5–5.0 mmol/l	3.5–5.0 mEq/l	

continued

Table 21.1 (*Cont.*)

Constituent	SI or other international units	Traditional units	Notes
Protein			
Total	60–80 g/l	6.0–8.0 g/100 ml	
Albumin	35–50 g/l	3.5–5.0 g/100 ml	50–70 µmol/l
Globulin—total	18–32 g/l	1.8–3.2 g/100 ml	
γ-Globulin—total	7–15 g/l	0.7–1.5 g/100 ml	
IgA	1.0–4.0 g/l	100–400 mg/100 ml	
IgG	8.0–16.0 g/l	800–1600 mg/100 ml	
IgM	0.5–2.5 g/l	50–250 mg/100 ml	
Fibrinogen	2–4 g/l	0.2–0.4 g/100 ml	
Pyruvate	50–80 µmol/l	0.4–0.7 mg/100 ml	Fasting
Sodium	135–145 mmol/l	135–145 mEq/l	
Thyrotrophic hormone	0–5 mU/l	0–5 mU/l	
Thyroxine	60–130 nmol/l	4.5–10 µg/100 ml	
Transaminases			
alanine	5–25 U/l	5–25 iu/l	At 37°C
aspartate	5–35 U/l	5–35 iu/l	At 37°C
Transferrin	1.2–2.0 g/l	120–200 mg/100 ml	
Triglyceride	0.3–1.8 mmol/l	25–150 mg/100 ml	Fasting, as glycerol
Trypsin	140–400 µg/l	140–400 ng/ml	Immunoreactive
Urea	3.0–6.5 mmol/l	18–40 mg/100 ml	
Urate	0.1–0.4 mmol/l	1.5–7.0 mg/100 ml	
Vitamin A	1.0–3.0 µmol/l	30–90 µg/100 ml	
Vitamin B_{12}	160–900 ng/l	160–900 pg/ml	Microbiological assay
Vitamin D	8–60 nmol/l	3–24 ng/ml	As 25-hydroxycholecalciferol
Zinc	12–17 µmol/l	80–110 µg/100 ml	

Table 21.2   Reference ranges – urine: values per 24-hour excretion.

Constituent	SI or other international units	Traditional units	Notes
Aldosterone	15–50 nmol	5–18 µg	
Amino acid nitrogen – free	4–20 mmol	50–300 mg	
Amylase	200–1500 U	10–7000 Henry–Chiamori units	
Ascorbic acid	0–45 µmol/8 h	0–8 mg/8 h	Overnight sample
Calcium	2.5–7.5 mmol	100–300 mg	
Chloride	170–250 mmol	170–250 mEq	
Copper	0.2–1.5 µmol	10–100 µg	
Creatine	0–0.4 mmol	0–50 mg	
Creatinine	9–18 mmol	1.0–2.0 g	
Glucose	0.1–1.0 mmol	20–200 mg	
Hydrogen ion activity exponent (pH)	5.5–8.0	5.5–8.0	Range over 24 h
5-Hydroxyindoleacetic acid	10–45 µmol	2–8 mg	
Hydroxyproline	80–250 µmol	10–35 mg	
Indicans	0.1–0.4 mmol	20–80 mg	
Lead	0–0.3 µmol	0–60 µg	
Nitrogen – total	0.7–1.5 mol	10–20 g	
Osmolality	700–1500 mmol	700–1500 mosmol	Total solute excretion
Phosphate	15–50 mmol	0.5–1.5 g	As phosphorus
Porphyrins			
δ-Aminolaevulinic acid	1–40 µmol	0.1–5.0 mg	
Porphobilinogen	1–12 µmol	0.2–2.0 mg	
Coproporphyrin	0.15–0.3 µmol	100–200 µg	
Uroporphyrin	6–40 nmol	5–30 µg	
Potassium	40–120 mmol	40–120 mEq	
Protein—total	40–120 mg	40–120 mg	
Sodium	100–250 mmol	100–250 mEq	

continued

Table 21.2 (*Cont.*)

Constituent	SI or other international units	Traditional units	Notes
Steroid hormones			Varies with time of menstrual period or pregnancy
Oestriol		µg × 0.0035 = µmol ⎫	
Pregnanediol		mg × 3.1 = µmol ⎭	
17-Oxosteroids: *men*	25–80 µmol	7–24 mg	
women	15–60 µmol	4–17 mg	
17-Oxogenic steroids: *men*	20–75 µmol	6–22 mg	
women	15–60 µmol	4–17 mg	
Urea	250–600 mmol	15–35 g	
Uric acid	1.5–4.5 mmol	250–750 mg	
Urobilinogen	0.5–5.0 µmol	0.3–3.0 mg	
Vanilmandelic acid	10–35 µmol	2–7 mg	Or HMMA
Volume	750–2000 ml	750–2000 ml	

Table 21.3 Reference ranges – faeces: values per 24-hour excretion.

Constituent	SI or other international units	Traditional units	Notes
Total wet weight	60–250 g	60–250 g	
Total dry weight	20–60 g	20–60 g	
Coproporphyrin	0.15–0.5 mmol	0.1–0.3 mg	
Fat – total	10–18 mmol	3–5 g	As stearic acid
Nitrogen – total	70–110 mmol	1–1.5 g	
Urobilinogen	100–500 µmol	60–300 mg	

Table 21.4 Reference ranges – infants and children.

Constituent		Birth (full term)	1 Week	1 Month	3 Years	6 Years	15 Years	Adult
Blood								
Glucose – fasting	(mmol/l)	1.2–4.5	2.5–4.7					3.0–5.0
Serum/Plasma								
Urea	(mmol/l)			1.5–4.0		2.5–6.0		3.0–6.5
Bicarbonate	(mmol/l)			18–24				24–30
Chloride	(mmol/l)			98–106				95–105
Potassium	(mmol/l)	3.5–6.5		4.0–5.8				3.5–5.0
Sodium	(mmol/l)			134–142				135–145
Calcium	(mmol/l)	1.8–3.0		2.2–2.8				2.1–2.6
Phosphate	(mmol/l)	1.2–2.8		1.5–2.3		1.0–1.8		0.8–1.4
Alkaline phosphatase	(U/l – KA)	35–105		70–230		70–175	70–210	20–95
Aspartate transaminase	(U/l)			4–80		5–40		5–35
Bilirubin – total	(mmol/l)	10–110	20–140	5–17				5–17
Protein – total	(g/l)	50–70		55–70	58–75			60–80
Albumin	(g/l)	25–40		33–45	35–48			36–50
Cholesterol	(mmol/l)		2.2–5.2		3.0–6.2			4.0–6.5
Urine								
Creatinine	(µmol/kg · 24 h)		45–120			90–160		130–220
17-Oxogenic steroids	(µmol/24 h)					3–20	10–45	15–75
17-Oxosteroids	(µmol/24 h)					0–7	10–30	15–80
Volume	(ml)		50–300		500–700	600–1000		750–2000

SI IN RELATION TO MEDICAL AND LABORATORY PRACTICE

DEVELOPMENT OF THE SYSTÈME INTERNATIONAL D'UNITÉS (SI)

The international organization responsible since 1875 for weights and measures is the Conférence générale des Poids et Mesures (CGPM), whose recommendations are accepted for medicine as a whole by the World Health Organization.

In 1960 CGPM codified the current revisions and extensions of the metric system as 'Système International d'Unités' (abbreviated as SI in all languages), to include agreed later modifications. Since then a few additions and minor changes have been made to SI, and this is now the internationally accepted 'language' for measurement throughout science and technology, which includes medicine.

In the early 1970s the relevant international organizations in pathology and laboratory medicine reviewed SI and recommended its adoption. They drew up guidelines for the use of SI in laboratory reporting, and in particular made recommendations on the introduction of *amount of substance* (unit: the mole), and the preferred use of molar concentration for measurement of components of known relative molecular mass ('molecular weight') in body fluids.

THE UNITS AND THEIR PRESENTATION

The current SI base units are listed in Table 21.5.

The primary units of SI are called *base* units and not *basic* units because, for example, length is not more basic in the fundamental behaviour of the universe than is velocity: it is merely, in the present stage of science, generally more convenient to use as a base.

Derived units, for more complex physical quantities, are formed from the base units by simple multiplication and division.

SI, as well as being *decimal* and *metric* (and using approved prefixes for multiples and submultiples), is *coherent*. This means that the unit for any such complex quantity can be derived from the units for other quantities without the use of numerical factors. In contrast, for example, a few metric and Imperial units of

Table 21.5 The independent base units of SI.

Physical quantity	Name of SI unit	Symbol for SI unit
Length	metre	m
Mass	kilogram	kg
Time	second	s
Electric current	ampere	A
Thermodynamic temperature	kelvin	K
Luminous intensity	candela	cd
Amount of substance	mole	mol

There are also the supplementary units of radian (plane angle) and steradian (solid angle)

force involve the use of a numerical constant representing gravitational acceleration. Very many derived units have special names and symbols, an example being the unit of force, the newton (symbol: N), derived as $kg \cdot m \cdot s^{-2}$. When one unit is divided by another (e.g. grams per litre), this may be expressed either by using a solidus (g/l), or by a negative exponent ($g \cdot l^{-1}$). The use of negative exponents is desirable, to avoid ambiguity, for all complex symbols containing more than two units. To include raised multiplying points within complex symbols is not essential, but makes for clarity. There are many other derived units that do not have special names and symbols, an example being the unit of velocity, derived as m/s.

Decimal multiples and submultiples of the units are formed by prefixes (Table 21.6).

Compound prefixes must never be used: for example, 10^{-9} g is a nanogram (ng) and not a millimicrogram (mμg). The use by pharmacists and some others of mcg (?millicentigram!) as an abbreviation for microgram causes great confusion.

Length

The SI unit is the metre (m).

The ångström (Å) should not be used, and the measurement should be converted to nanometres (1 Å = 10^{-1} nm).

Table 21.6 Prefixes for multiples and submultiples.

Multiple	Prefix	Symbol	Sub-multiple	Prefix	Symbol
10^1	deca	da	10^{-1}	deci	d
10^2	hecto	h	10^{-2}	centi	c
10^3	kilo	k	10^{-3}	milli	m
10^6	mega	M	10^{-6}	micro	μ
10^9	giga	G	10^{-9}	nano	n
10^{12}	tera	T	10^{-12}	pico	p
10^{15}	peta	P	10^{-15}	femto	f
10^{18}	exa	E	10^{-18}	atto	a

The micron (μ) as a name for a unit of length is obsolete: the correct name for this unit is the micrometre (μm).

Volume

The SI unit is the cubic metre (m^3). Because this is inconvenient and unfamiliar the working unit that is accepted for medicine and related sciences is the litre (l), which is an alternative special name for the cubic decimetre (dm^3: $1000\ cm^3$) – with its submultiples. The widely used '100 ml' is a decilitre (dl).

In American laboratories and clinical journals there is a tendency to use L as the symbol for litre, to avoid possible lack of distinction between l and 1: this alternative is now internationally accepted.

The lambda (λ) as a name for a unit of volume (10^{-6} l) is obsolete: the correct name for this unit is the microlitre (μl).

Per cent (%) means 'per hundred parts of the same'. Thus 'mg%' means 'milligrams per hundred milligrams' and must *never* be used to mean 'milligrams per hundred millilitres', which differs by a factor of the order of one thousand, depending on the density of the solvent. If in doubt, use % only for countable numbers, such as 'X% of the population'.

Mass

The SI unit is the kilogram (kg); the working unit is the gram (g). Multiples and submultiples are expressed in terms of the original metric unit, the gram, and not in terms of the SI base unit.

The gamma (γ) as a name for a unit of mass (10^{-6} g) is obsolete: the correct name for this unit is the microgram (μg).

The dalton (Da) – and its multiples e.g. kDa – is widely used as an alternative name for atomic mass unit.

Amount of substance

The SI unit is the mole (mol). This is the amount of substance that contains a standard number of specific particles (referred to the mole of ^{12}C atoms which has a mass of exactly 12 g), whether atoms, ion, radicals or molecules. This new unit was sometimes found confusing by non-chemists on its first introduction. 1 mole of H^+ (hydrogen ions) has a mass equal to 1.008 grams (usually taken in medicine as 1 g), 1 mole of H_2 (molecular hydrogen) has a mass of about 2 g, 1 mole of H_2O (water) has a mass of about 18 g and 1 mole of glucose has a mass of about 180 g.

Concentration

SI includes several types of concentration: particularly relevant to medicine and laboratory analyses are mass concentration (derived unit kg/m^3, working unit g/l) and amount of substance concentration (derived unit mol/m^3, working unit mol/l).

All concentrations of components are to be expressed per litre. Mole (substance) concentrations are to be used to express the results of all components of known molecular/ionic/atomic mass that are measured in blood plasma and other body fluids, and mole contents will be used for timed excretions and similar measurements. Results of protein analyses continue to be expressed in mass/volume units when they are measured in mixtures (e.g. total IgG) or when their exact molecular mass is unknown. However, the quoting of protein results as mole concentrations is beginning as specific protein analyses become more common, and is already in use by some laboratories for albumin. Mass concentrations are used for some other mixtures, such as plasma total lipids; for many mixtures, however, results are given as moles of a predominant constituent, such as stearic acid for faecal fat.

The change from mass to substance amounts and concentrations requires more than just a change in numerical values (as, for example, from °F to °C), because it involves a conceptual change in dimensions: there is a parallel situation in the change from weight to mass. As the chemical, physiological and pharmacological activity of a component is generally proportional to the concentration of molecules or ions present and not to the mass concentration, the use of the mole expresses amounts or concentrations in biologically relevant terms.

The mole avoids certain ambiguities in the use of the equivalent, and brings in non-ionized components whose concentration could not be expressed on the equivalent scale. For monovalent ions, for example Na^+, one mole is numerically the same as one equivalent, so for sodium 140 milliequivalents per litre becomes 140 mmol/l; 1 mole of NaCl contains 1 mole of Na^+ and 1 mole of Cl^-. As the molar mass of glucose is 180 g, a plasma glucose concentration of 90 mg/dl becomes 5.0 mmol/l; as the molar mass of thyroxine is 777 g, a plasma thyroxine concentration of 10 µg/dl becomes 130 nmol/l; and as the molar mass of phenobarbitone is 232 g, a plasma phenobarbitone concentration of 4.6 mg/dl becomes 0.2 mmol/l.

Introduction of the molar system for expressing drug concentration in plasma is under discussion. Moles are always used for prescription of electrolytes, often for intravenous nutrients, but not yet for other therapy.

Particle counts

These are expressed per litre. For example, a blood erythrocyte count of $4.5 \times 10^6/mm^3$ becomes $4.5 \times 10^{12}/l$: leucocyte and platelet counts are to be expressed as $\times 10^9/l$.

Time

The SI unit is the second (s).

Working units are minute (min), hour (h), day (d) and year (a) – yr is conventional, but it is better not to abbreviate. Note that '24 h' may be necessary to avoid ambiguity when 'day' is contrasted to 'night', as for urine volume collection periods.

Frequency

The SI unit is the hertz (Hz).

This replaces cycles per second for frequency of periodic phenomena. It should not be used for discontinuous events such as dispensing of doses of medicine, or urinating.

Temperature

The SI unit, both for thermodynamic temperature and for temperature interval, is the kelvin (K). The working unit (for customary temperature) is the degree Celsius (°C). It should be noted that C here is the symbol for Celsius, not for centigrade.

The kelvin thermodynamic temperature scale starts at absolute zero (-273.16°C). This is inconvenient so the familiar Celsius scale, starting at the freezing point of water (0°C), will be retained in medicine for all clinical purposes. The kelvin temperature *interval* is identical with the degree Celsius temperature *interval*.

Pressure

The SI unit is the pascal (Pa).

In medicine pressure is very often measured as the height of a liquid column, either as millimetres of mercury (mmHg) or as centimetres or millimetres of water (mmH_2O); 1 mmHg = 1 Torr. These measures are not SI so cannot be used without conversion in calculations involving pressure (such as flow rate), are artificial when applied to instruments such as transducers that do not involve a column, and vary very slightly with column temperature and with gravity (height above sea level). However, as there are so many existing clinical sphygmomanometers, column measurements will remain in clinical use for a very considerable time, until new ideas are accepted and new instruments available. It would be a great convenience if the manufacturers would provide stick-on scales graduated in kilopascals for their current instruments.

Although the pascal has been readily accepted, because of its advantages, by laboratory workers and by medical research scientists, it has been accepted for bedside measurement of blood pressure by few clinicians. In Britain a group of physicians set up a Society for the Preservation of the Millimetre of Mercury!

Energy

The SI unit is the joule (J).

This is to be used for all forms of energy, including heat energy. To be abandoned is the traditional unit for heat energy, the calorie (cal: strictly the gram-calorie); this was used in nutrition as the kilocalorie (kcal), often called the Medical Calorie (Cal) or to everyone's confusion, just Calorie. For general use we should refer, for example, to a low-energy instead of a low-calorie diet.

Enzyme activity

Originally, units for measurement of enzyme activity, particularly in body fluids, were arbitrary. They were usually named after the originators of the analytical method, such as the King–Armstrong unit for alkaline phosphatase. International agreement led to a unit applicable to any enzyme, which is the amount that will catalyse the transformation of one micromole of substrate per minute – under defined conditions. This is used in. laboratories now for most enzymes and has the symbol U; plasma enzyme activities are generally quoted as U/l.

There is a recommendation for a unit of enzyme catalytic activity related to SI, being that which produces an observed catalysed reaction rate of substrate transformation of one mole per second – under defined conditions. The unit is called the katal (kat), and its introduction to clinical measurement is under discussion. Conversion factor: 1 U $\simeq$ 16.7 nkat.

Other physical quantities

For current usage in radiation physics, physicians are referred to their local department of nuclear medicine, medical physics, etc. Similar specialist consultation is advised for problems of units and symbols arising in relation to bioengineering and to electronics.

ACKNOWLEDGEMENTS

I am grateful to Dr R. E. Pounder for critical comments on the manuscript. I wish to thank Mrs Ksenia Wilding for the graphic work, and Miss Jane Lytle for skilled secretarial help.

Hodder and Stoughton Educational kindly gave permission for the reproduction, in modified form, of Tables 21.1, 21.2, 21.3, and 21.4; and of Figures 21.1, 21.2, 21.3, and 21.4, from Baron (1982), *A Short Textbook of Chemical Pathology.*

FURTHER READING

Baron, D. N. (1982) *A Short Textbook of Chemical Pathology*, 4th edn. London: Hodder and Stoughton Educational.
Galen, R. S. & Gambino, S. R. (1975) *Beyond Normality: The Predictive Value and Efficiency of Medical Diagnoses.* New York: Wiley.
Gräsbeck, R. & Alström, T. (1981) eds. *Reference Values in Laboratory Medicine: The Current State of the Art.* Chichester: Wiley.
World Health Organization (1977) *The SI for the Health Professions.* Geneva: World Health Organization.

Index